Textbook of
Pathology
VOLUME I

Textbook of Pathology
VOLUME I

Chief Editor
Vinay Kamal
Director Professor of Pathology
Maulana Azad Medical College
Bahadur Shah Zafar Marg
New Delhi (India)

Editors
Anubhav MD
Vigyat MD

Illustrations by
Ram Murti Senior Graphic Artist

Volume I contains: General Pathology, Hematology including Recent Diagnostic Techniques
Volume II contains: Systemic Pathology

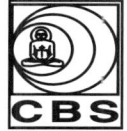

CBS Publishers & Distributors Pvt Ltd

New Delhi • Bengaluru • Chennai • Kochi • Kolkata • Mumbai
Hyderabad • Jharkhand • Nagpur • Patna • Pune • Uttarakhand

Disclaimer

Science and technology are constantly changing fields. New research and experience broaden the scope of information and knowledge. The editors have tried their best in giving information available to them while preparing the material for this book. Although, all efforts have been made to ensure optimum accuracy of the material, yet it is quite possible some errors might have been left uncorrected. The publisher, the printer and the editors will not be held responsible for any inadvertent errors, omissions or inaccuracies.

Textbook of
Pathology
Volume I

ISBN: 978-93-86478-39-9

Copyright © Author and Publisher

First Edition: 2017

All rights reserved. No part of this book may be reproduced or transmitted in any form or by any means, electronic or mechanical, including photocopying, recording, or any information storage and retrieval system without permission, in writing, from the editors and the publisher.

Published by Satish Kumar Jain and produced by Varun Jain for

CBS Publishers & Distributors Pvt Ltd
4819/XI Prahlad Street, 24 Ansari Road, Daryaganj, New Delhi 110 002, India.
Ph: 23289259, 23266861, 23266867 Website: www.cbspd.com
Fax: 011-23243014   e-mail: delhi@cbspd.com; cbspubs@airtelmail.in

Corporate Office: 204 FIE, Industrial Area, Patparganj, Delhi 110 092
Ph: 4934 4934 Fax: 4934 4935 e-mail: publishing@cbspd.com; publicity@cbspd.com

Branches

- **Bengaluru:** Seema House 2975, 17th Cross, K.R. Road, Banasankari 2nd Stage, Bengaluru 560 070, Karnataka
  Ph: +91-80-26771678/79 Fax: +91-80-26771680 e-mail: bangalore@cbspd.com
- **Chennai:** 7, Subbaraya Street, Shenoy Nagar, Chennai 600 030, Tamil Nadu
  Ph: +91-44-26680620/26681266 Fax: +91-44-42032115 e-mail: chennai@cbspd.com
- **Kochi:** Ashana House, No. 39/1904, AM Thomas Road, Valanjambalam, Ernakulam 682 016, Kochi, Kerala
  Ph: +91-484-4059061–65 Fax: +91-484-4059065 e-mail: kochi@cbspd.com
- **Kolkata:** 6/B, Ground Floor, Rameswar Shaw Road, Kolkata-700 014, West Bengal
  Ph: +91-33-22891126, 22891127, 22891128 e-mail: kolkata@cbspd.com
- **Mumbai:** 83-C, Dr E Moses Road, Worli, Mumbai-400018, Maharashtra
  Ph: +91-22-24902340/41 Fax: +91-22-24902342 e-mail: mumbai@cbspd.com

Representatives

• **Hyderabad**	0-9885175004	• **Jharkhand**	0-9811541605	• **Nagpur**	0-9021734563
• **Patna**	0-9334159340	• **Pune**	0-9623451994	• **Uttarakhand**	0-9716462459

Printed at: Thomson Press India Ltd., Faridabad, Haryana, India

Eminent worthy teachers, our promising students and
esteemed faculty members for enduring inspiration
and
My loving soulmate Dr (Mrs) Manita Kamal,
dear Dr Spriha Arun, Dr Mansi Dhende, Dr Anubhav and
Dr Vigyat for always being there with me. This book could be
completed due to their outstanding support and
encouragement at every step.

Contents

Preface — xi
Foreword by Dr Meera Sikka — xiii
Foreword by Dr Rajeev Sen — xiv
Foreword by Dr Ezhil Arasi N — xv
Foreword by Dr Nita Khurana — xvi
Foreword by Dr Sunita Sharma — xvi
Foreword by Dr Kuldeep Kumar Kaul — xvii
Foreword by Dr Syed Besina Yasin — xix
Foreword by Dr Sujata Kanetkar — xx
Foreword by Dr Hansa Goswami — xxi

Section I: General Pathology

1. Cellular Adaptations, Cell Injury, Apoptosis, Pigments Calcification, Cellular Accumulations and Aging — 3
   Cellular Adaptations 4
   Cell Injury 14
   Apoptosis 32
   Subcellular Response to Injury 37
   Pigments 38
   Calcification 42
   Intracellular Accumulations 44
   Extracellular Accumulations 47
   Cellular Aging 48

2. Inflammation, Tissue Healing and Repair — 51
   Acute Inflammation 53
   Chronic Inflammation 96
   Tissue Healing and Repair 110

3. Disorders of Hemostasis — 134
   Hyperemia and Congestion 134
   Hemorrhage 137
   Hemostasis 139
   Thrombosis 147
   Embolism 156
   Infarction 160
   Edema 165
   Shock 170

4. Immunopathology including Amyloidosis — 177
   Immune System 178
   Nonspecific (Innate or Inborn) Immune Response 182
   Specific Immune Response 187
   Immunization and Vaccines 211
   Immunodeficiency Disorders 215
   Hypersensitivity Reactions 230
   Immunologic Tolerance 250
   Autoimmune Diseases 254
   HLA System 264
   Transplantation Immunology 266
   Amyloidosis 273

5. **Genetic Disorders** — 282
   Human Genome 282
   Chromosomal Disorders 292
   Single Gene Mutation (Mendelian Disorders) 301
   Disorders of Sexual Differentiation 312
   Work up of Genetic Disorders 313

6. **Neoplasia: Molecular Basis, Metastasis, Clinical Oncology and Laboratory Diagnosis** — 316
   Neoplasia 317
   Nomenclature and Classification 321
   Characteristic Features of Tumors 332
   Epidemiology of Tumors 335
   Cell Cycle and Cancer 337
   Genetic Preposition of Cancer 341
   Acquired Preneoplastic Lesions 343
   Molecular Basis of Cancer: Role of Genetic and Epigenetic Alterations 345
   Multistep Carcinogenesis 380
   Invasion and Metastasis 392
   Routes of Metastasis of Tumors 395
   Clinical Oncology 400
   Laboratory Diagnosis 412

7. **Nutritional and Infectious Diseases** — 417
   Nutritional Diseases 417
   Bacterial Infections 430
   Viral Infections 446
   Fungal Infections 450
   Parasitic Diseases 452

Section II: Hematology

8. **Red Blood Cells** — 459
   Hematopoiesis 459
   Red Blood Cell, Hemoglobin and Classification of Anemias 474
   Iron Deficiency Anemia 481
   Megaloblastic Anemia: Vitamin B_{12} and Folic Acid Deficiency 487
   Red Blood Cells Destruction and Classification of Hemolytic Anemia 495
   Hereditary Spherocytosis, Ovalocytosis and Stomatocytosis 499
   Thalassemias 502
   Sickle Cell Disorders and Other Hemoglobinopathies 509
   Glucose-6-Phosphate Dehydrogenase Deficiency and Pyruvate Kinase Deficiency 514
   Immune Hemolytic Anemia 516
   Paroxysmal Nocturnal Hemoglobinuria 521
   RBCs Fragmentation Syndromes 522
   Diagnostic Approach of Hemolytic Anemia 523
   Bone Marrow Failure Syndromes 528

9. **White Blood Cells** — 533
   Leukocytes and their Quantitative and Qualitative Disorders 533
   Acute Leukemias 539
   Myelodysplastic Syndromes/Myeloproliferative Neoplasms 559
   Myeloproliferative Neoplasms 562
   Chronic Lymphoproliferative Disorders 574
   Multiple Myeloma and Waldenström Macroglobulinemia 580
   Disorders of Mononuclear Phagocytic System 588
   Hematopoietic Stem Cell Transplantation 592

10. **Bleeding Disorders** — 596
    Normal and Disorders of Hemostasis 596
    Platelet Disorders 600
    Thrombocytopenias 602
    Platelet Function Disorders 605
    Vascular Purpura 607

11. **Coagulation Disorders** — 609
    Inherited and Acquired Coagulation Disorders 609
    Thrombophilia (Hypercoagulable State) 618
    Clinical Aspects of Bleeding Diathesis 620

12. **Blood Groups and Blood Transfusion** — 626
    Blood Group Systems 626
    Blood Collection, Processing and Storage 631
    Blood Grouping 632
    Blood Cross-matching (Compatibility Test) 634
    Blood Components Therapy 634
    Autologous Blood Transfusion and Plasma Exchange 637
    Adverse Blood Transfusion Reactions 639

13. **Lymph Nodes, Spleen and Thymus** — 641
    Disorders of Lymph Node 641
    Hodgkin's Disease 648
    Non-Hodgkin's Lymphoma 658
    Spleen 677
    Thymus Gland 682

14. **Advanced Diagnostic Techniques** — 687
    Frozen Section Technique 687
    Electron Microscopy and Polarizing Light Microscopy 688
    Histology and Histochemical Stains 691
    Immunohistochemistry 698

Immunofluorescence Microscopy 703
Chemiluminescence vs Chemifluorescence 705
Flow Cytometry 706
Cytogenetic Analysis 709
Fluorescence in situ Hybridization 716
Enzyme-linked Immunosorbent Assay (ELISA) 721

Methods for DNA Sequences 724
Tissue Microarray 731
High Performance Liquid Chromatography (HPLC) 733
Electrophoresis 734

Index I–XXV

Section III: Systemic Pathology

15. Blood Vessels 741
Arteriosclerosis 742
Atherosclerosis 744
Aneurysms 755
Vasculitis 760
Veins 767
Lymphatic System 769
Tumors of Blood Vessels 769
Hypertension 772

16. Heart 781
Ischemic Heart Disease 783
Rheumatic Fever and RHD 798
Myocardium 806
Endocardium 811
Cardiac Valves 818
Pericardium 821
Congestive Heart Failure 826
Cardiac Hypertrophy 829
Cardiac Tumors 830
Congenital Heart Diseases 831

17. Nasal Cavity, Nasopharynx, Paranasal Sinuses, Ear, Larynx and Neck 836
Inflammation and Infections 836
Neoplastic Disorders 838
Miscellaneous Disorders 845
Ear 845
Larynx 849
Neck 851

18. Lung 856
Pneumonias 860
Lung Abscess 869
Tuberculosis 870
Chronic Obstructive Pulmonary Disease 876
Restrictive Pulmonary Diseases 886
Pneumothorax and Atelectasis Lung 898
Pulmonary Vascular Disorders 900
Lung Tumors 906
Pleural Diseases 927

19. Oral Cavity and Salivary Glands 932
Oral Cavity 932
Salivary Glands 938
Jaw 950

20. Gastrointestinal Tract 957
Esophagus 959
Stomach 967
Small Intestine 986
Large Intestine 1002
Appendix 1029
Anus and Perianal Region 1031
Peritoneum 1034
Investigations of Gastrointestinal Disorders 1036

21. Liver, Gallbladder and Exocrine Pancreas 1040
Liver 1041
Jaundice and Cholestasis 1050
Hepatitis 1058
Bacterial and Parasitic Infections of Liver 1077
Cirrhosis 1082
Metabolic Liver Diseases 1094
Bile Duct Disorders 1107
Vascular Disorders 1110
Liver Tumors 1113
Gallbladder 1126
Common Neoplasms and Precursor Lesions of Gallbladder 1137
Pancreas 1139
Pancreatitis 1140
Pancreatic Tumors 1145

22. Kidney and Ureter 1150
Anatomy 1150
Physiology 1153
Glomeruli 1157
Glomerulonephritis 1161
Nephrotic Syndrome 1171
Acute Nephritic Syndrome 1187
Chronic Glomerulonephritis 1197
Evaluation of Renal Biopsy 1201
Diseases of the Tubules 1205

Tubulointerstitial Disorders 1209
Obstructive Uropathy and Hydronephrosis 1217
Renal Stones (Nephrolithiasis and Urolithiasis) 1218
Vascular Disorders 1221
Cystic Diseases of Kidney 1226
Congenital Anomalies of the Urinary Tract 1229
Neoplasms of the Kidney 1230
Laboratory Diagnosis 1242

23. Urinary Bladder and Male Reproductive System — 1245
Urinary Bladder 1245
Testes 1255
Prostate Gland 1276
Penis 1282

24. Female Reproductive System — 1284
Vulva 1287
Vagina 1291
Cervix 1297
Fallopian Tubes 1306
Endometrium 1308
Ovary 1321
Gestational Trophoblastic Tumors 1349
Pregnancy Associated Diseases 1353

25. Breast — 1358
Female Breasts 1358
Inflammatory Disorders 1364
Fibrocystic Disease 1366
WHO Classification: Breast Tumors 1370
Breast Carcinoma 1376
Male Breasts 1407

26. Endocrine System: Pancreas, Thyroid, Parathyroid, Adrenal and Pituitary Glands — 1409
Endocrine Pancreas 1409
Diabetes Mellitus 1412
Thyroid Gland 1425
Parathyroid Glands 1452
Adrenal Glands 1457
Pituitary Gland 1467

27. Bones and Joints — 1475
Bones 1475
Osteomyelitis 1477
Metabolic Bone Diseases 1479
Bone Tumors 1484
Joints 1517

28. Soft Tissue Tumors and Skeletal Myopathies — 1524
Soft Tissue Tumors 1524
Skeletal Muscles 1542

29. Skin — 1549
Normal Skin 1550
Inflammatory Disorders 1555
Cutaneous Infections 1558
Autoimmune Disorders 1562
Nonmelanocytic Lesions and Tumors 1565
Pigmentation Disorders and Melanocytic Tumors 1569
Fibrous and Fibrohistiocytic Tumors 1573
Neural and Neuroendocrine Tumors 1574
Vascular Tumors 1575
Tumors of Cutaneous Appendages 1576
Cutaneous Metastases 1577
Miscellaneous Disorders 1577

30. Nervous System — 1580
CNS Infections 1584
CNS Tumors 1590
Reaction of CNS to Injury 1611
Cerebrovascular Diseases 1611
Head Injuries 1615
Demyelinating Disorders 1616
Congenital Disorders 1617

Index — 1621

Preface

The study of pathology is essential for safe clinical practice. In modern era, tremendous growth is in progress in diagnostic pathology with recent advances in molecular methods, cytogenetics and immunohistochemistry. Rapidly changing hematology needs integration of recent guidelines and diagnostic criteria of hematological disorders.

I joined India's premier institution in Department of Pathology, Maulana Azad Medical College, New Delhi. I puzzled over the fact that the students admitted of very high caliber still had problems in grasping the teaching material. I interacted with students and eminent faculty members across country. I discussed problems faced by the students in reproducing text. I analyzed their inputs and then started working on Textbook of Pathology in 2007. Primary aim of this book is to discuss complex topics in a straightforward, clear and organized manner.

All the chapters have been shared with the eminent teachers and young budding residents across country. Their valuable opinion on various aspects has been taken positively during drafting of the chapters to meet the need of the young generation of pathologists. Each chapter focuses on the essentials necessary to build a broad fundamentals backed up with numerous colored figures, gross morphology, light microscopy, photographs, tables and flow diagrams.

I trust you will enjoy reading this book. I have spent a great deal of time and energy ensuring easy grasp and retaining the topics. I am inviting your comments, valuable suggestions and criticism.

Chief Editor
Vinay Kamal
Email: vinaykamal@hotmail.com
Mobile: 09818001202

Foreword

The *Textbook of Pathology* by Dr Vinay Kamal, Director Professor, Department of Pathology, Maulana Azad Medical College, New Delhi, covers various aspects of pathology in a systematic manner. The book includes several strong points such as a reader-friendly font size of text and the simple language used in the text making it easy to understand.

The text is very well illustrated in the form of gross and microscopic pictures. An attempt has been made to include the recent advances specially the current WHO classifications wherever applicable. Key points have been placed separately in a box to facilitate quick revision by the students. The clinical features of disease along with their pathologic basis have also been included which will greatly help the students. The flow diagrams provided along with the text will aid in understanding. The text is accompanied by several tables particularly useful for the professional examination. All these features reflect the author's vast experience as a teacher. I am sure the students will find the book easy to read and comprehend.

Dr Meera Sikka
Director Professor and Head
Department of Pathology
University College of Medical Sciences
and
GTB Hospital, New Delhi

Foreword

I have known Dr Vinay Kamal, ever since I joined the then Govt Medical College, Rohtak, on December 31st, 1983, with deepening bond of friendship between us. I have been witness to his commitment to the undergraduate and postgraduate students and his evolution as a teacher. He would deliver a lecture in a lucid fashion, yet will ensure that it is conceptually comprehensible.

I have seen glimpses of the *Textbook of Pathology* comprising of high resolution figures, numerous tables and recent WHO classifications with clinicopathological correlation. It holds a wealth of information for undergraduate students, postgraduate scholars and practicing pathologists.

It connects from basic understanding learnt by a medical student in preclinical courses to genesis of diseases, its manifestations and contemporary practice of the science of clinical pathology using bridge of contemporary knowledge.

Without prejudice of our friendship, I am sure that this textbook is going to provide answers to most of the questions, a medical student is seeking in pathology.

Dr Rajeev Sen
Senior Professor and Head
Department of Pathology
Post Graduate Institute of Medical Sciences
Rohtak (Haryana)

Foreword

It gives me immense pleasure and privilege for having given me the opportunity to contribute to the publication of *Textbook of Pathology* by Dr Vinay Kamal, Director Professor, Department of Pathology, Maulana Azad Medical College, New Delhi. He has covered recent concepts of pathology in a systemic manner in easy language. Book contains recent WHO classification whereever applicable, clinicopathological correlation, diagnostic approach, numerous colored figures, gross morphology, light microscopy and flow diagrams.

The book will be of a great source of enlightenment to the students reflecting the zeal and enthusiasm of the author. I wish him all the success in his endeavor and sincerely pray that the book will be of much help to the budding doctors all over the nation and abroad.

Dr Ezhil Arasi N
Vice Principal (Administration)
Professor and Head
Department of Pathology
Osmania Medical College
Hyderabad (Telangana)

Foreword

I feel pleased and honored to be given an opportunity to write the foreword for the first edition of the *Text book of Pathology* written by Dr Vinay Kamal, Director Professor, Department of Pathology at India's premier medical institute, Maulana Azad Medical College, New Delhi. I have known him since 1990 when I joined MAMC as a postgraduate student. He connects with the students and takes keen interest in their learning and tries to help them out in all their personal and academic problems. A similar helpful attitude towards staff with all help extended to them has been his nature at all times.

I have reviewed all the chapters of this *Textbook of Pathology*. From its inception the book was intended to fulfill the needs of the medical students to understand the basic principles of pathology in a simple language and concise format. I convey my heartfelt appreciation for the hard work done by Dr Vinay Kamal for conceptualizing and executing this body of work.

The author with his more than three decades of teaching experience has put the essential elements of the subject in a student-friendly format complete with high resolution of 1533 figures and 1097 tables, inclusion of up-to-date recent advances and recent diagnostic techniques. Emphasis has been kept on the section on hematology and hematolymphoid disorders so that the students use this book as a complete package.

The enormous time and effort put into creating tables and key points so as to clarify the subject and help in distinguishing closely related terms and disorders particularly useful to undergraduate student and ready resource for the postgraduate students. The chapters of this textbook have been shared with the eminent teachers and young budding residents across country. Their valuable opinion on various aspects has been taken positively during the drafting of the chapters to meet the need of the young generation of pathologists. This positive attitude towards suggestions for betterment was greatly appreciated by the colleagues and students alike. This Herculean task is the result of many months of sleepless nights and hard work.

The experience and enthusiasm of the author to help the learning of the student is evident in the simple format and comprehensive information provided in a context necessary to translate knowledge of pathology into clinical practice.

I hope the students and pathologists will enjoy the book and it will be a ready tool for updating knowledge for the postgraduates and teachers alike. The balance of detail and brevity and integrated coverage of clinical information and pathology will serve its intended purpose of building a solid foundation in pathology for the future doctors to better serve their patients.

Dr Nita Khurana
Director Professor
Department of Pathology
Maulana Azad Medical College
New Delhi

Foreword

It is a proud moment for me to write a brief review of the first edition of the *Text book of Pathology* written by Dr Vinay Kamal. It provides a comprehensive coverage to all the diseases. Each chapter starts with learning objectives. This textbook contains 1533 illustrations and 1097 tables, recent WHO classification, recent concepts in pathology, recent diagnostic techniques, gross morphology, light microscopy and flow diagrams. These have simplified the subject in making the concepts easily understandable. I convey my heartfelt appreciation for the hard work done by Dr Vinay Kamal for conceptualizing and executing this body of work. I hope that the students will enjoy reading this book and will find pathology a much easier and interesting subject.

Dr Sunita Sharma
Director Professor and Head
Department of Pathology
Lady Hardinge Medical College
New Delhi

Foreword

I have been associated with Dr Vinay Kamal, Director Professor, Department of Pathology, Maulana Azad Medical College, New Delhi, for the last two decades. We have been together as examiners on various occasions. His positive attitude towards students, clear and honest thoughts impressed me. We had long discussions on many academic topics and the problems faced by the students in their examinations.

Our department had an opportunity to review many of the chapters of the forthcoming *Textbook of Pathology*. He shared these chapters with senior faculty and postgraduates across country to seek their opinion. He used to analyze their suggestions and incorporated relevant matter in the book.

Highlights of this *Textbook of Pathology* include recent WHO classification, 1533 figures, 1097 tables, recent concepts in pathology, immunohistochemistry, molecular biology, recent diagnostic techniques and clinicopathological correlation. For a quick revision, the tables, pictures and diagrams are given in such a nice way, which reflects that the author has taken due care of all these areas that makes the book a unique.

Hence, it is an ideal comprehensive *Textbook of Pathology* for undergraduates, postgraduates, consultants and clinicians. I am confident that his contribution in pathology shall be remembered forever.

Dr Kuldeep Kumar Kaul
Professor and Head
Department of Pathology
Govt Medical College, Jammu
Jammu and Kashmir

Foreword

Good teachers are the reason why ordinary students dream to do extraordinary things. Dr Vinay Kamal, Director Professor, Department of Pathology, besides being a pathologist par excellence is a dedicated teacher for whom the welfare of students is of prime importance.

I have known him for the last 15 years. What has impressed me most is his sincerity, honesty and desire to help others. He has played a pivotal role in getting the MD pathology degrees recognized both at Govt Medical College, Srinagar as well as Sher-I-Kashmir Institute of Medical Sciences, Srinagar. Credit goes to him in enhancement of postgraduates intake in these institutions. His contributions in the specialty of pathology as a teacher, educator and consultant is praiseworthy.

Now as an author he has this prestigious *Textbook of Pathology* to his credit. Our department has reviewed his chapters. He has worked hard to complete the project in 11 years. *Textbook of Pathology* is well written with 1533 high resolution figures and 1097 tables. Latest WHO classifications and recent advances have been incorporated appropriately. It holds a wealth of information for undergraduate students, postgraduate scholars and practicing pathologists. I congratulate him for this phenomenal effort. I am sure reading this book will enrich all the readers.

Dr Syed Besina Yasin
Additional Professor and Head
Department of Pathology
Sher-I-Kashmir Institute of Medical Sciences
Srinagar, Jammu and Kashmir

Foreword

Dr Vinay Kamal, Director Professor, Department of Pathology, has illustrious teaching career of 35 years. His *Textbook of Pathology* is a fruit of his tireless, meticulous efforts for quality, simplicity and standardization. The author shared some topics and illustrations with me.

The topics have been covered in such a way to make things easy to understand as well as assure success in various competitive examinations. This textbook is rich with high resolution 1533 illustrations as well as 1097 tables, which provide key points for better understanding. It covers all the recent updates in the medical field. I am confident that it will be appreciated and will be useful for both undergraduates and postgraduates in pathology.

Dr Sujata Kanetkar
Professor and Head
Department of Pathology
Krishna Institute of Medical Sciences
Satara, Karad, Maharashtra

Foreword

I have been interacting with Dr Vinay Kamal on various occasions on the subject of pathology for the last 15 years. The undaunted association with teaching undergraduates and postgraduates at premier institution as Director Professor, Department of Pathology, Maulana Azad Medical College, New Delhi since many years, distinguishes him from many other academicians by way of his integrated innovative approach, to make the subject of pathology simple and easy. He has vast teaching experience of more than three decades.

I have reviewed some of the chapters of forthcoming *Textbook of Pathology* by Dr Vinay Kamal. Salient features of textbook include comprehensive knowledge of pathology with recent WHO classification, recent concepts in pathology, 1533 figures and 1097 tabulated data analysis, molecular pathology, immunohistochemistry, recent advanced techniques, clinicopathological correlation, gross morphology, light microscopy and flow diagrams. This book will go long away in making students understand pathology and its relevance, significance and importance in medicine. This book is the eventual result of his immense passion of teaching students, without compromising quality. I wish great success to his new endeavor.

Dr Hansa Goswami
Professor and Head
Department of Pathology
BJ Medical College
Ahmedabad, Gujarat

Acknowledgments

Foremost acknowledgement is gratefulness to Almighty for guiding me all time during preparation of first edition of *Textbook of Pathology*. I express my gratitude to Mr Satish Kumar Jain CHAIRMAN and Mr Varun Jain MANAGING DIRECTOR of CBS Publishers & Distributors Pvt. Ltd. for extending their whole hearted support at every step in completion of book.

I am grateful to Mr YN Arjuna VICE PRESIDENT—PUBLISHING, EDITORIAL AND PRODUCTION, Mrs Ritu Chawla AGM and Dr Krishna Garg. I express my gratitude to Mr Sunil Dutt PROMOTION MANAGER, who has been main guiding force behind in completion of the book.

Credit goes to the outstanding team comprising of Mr Ram Murti SENIOR GRAPHIC ARTIST, Mrs Sunita Rautela SENIOR DTP OPERATOR and Mr Ananda Mohanty SENIOR PROOF READER for their devotion and excellent work in the book. Mr Ram Murti and Mrs Sunita Rautela deserve special mention in preparation of layout of the book. Mr Ram Murti put sincere efforts in finalizing 1533 figures.

The magnitude of the work pertaining to first edition of *Textbook of Pathology* has been possible for outstanding support and cooperation from friends, well-wishers, my departmental colleagues and especially residents, the backbone of department across the country.

The chapters of this textbook have been shared with the eminent teachers and young budding residents across country. Their valuable opinion on various aspects has been taken positively during the drafting of the chapters to meet the need of the young generation of pathologists. This positive attitude towards suggestions for betterment was greatly appreciated by the colleagues and students alike.

I express my gratitude especially to Dr Meera Sikka, Dr Rajeev Sen, Dr Ezhil Arasi N, Dr Nita Khurana, Dr Sunita Sharma, Dr Kuldeep Kumar Kaul, Dr Hansa Goswami, Dr Syed Besina Yasin, Dr Sandeep Mathur, Dr Narender Kumar Mogra, Dr SS Surana, Dr Surender Pal, Dr Archna Buch, Dr Seema Rao, Dr Uday, Dr Abhijit Das, Mr GD Manoj and Mr Rajiv Aggarwal for extending whole hearted support and advice.

Andhra Pradesh

Sidhartha Medical College, Vijayawada
Professor of Pathology
Dr Venkata Rama Reddy Bollareddy

Bihar

Govt Medical College, Patna
Assistant Professor of Pathology
Dr Pallavi Agrawal

All India Institute of Medical Sciences, Patna
Senior Resident/Tutor of Pathology
Dr Iffat Jamal

Chandigarh (Union Territory)

Post Graduate Institute, Chandigarh
Assistant Professor of Hematology
Dr Prashant Sharma

Senior Resident of Pathology
Dr Chandni Garg

Post Graduate Residents of Pathology
Dr Archana Sundram, Dr Shilpi Thakur, Dr Debajyoti Chatterji

Govt Medical College, Chandigarh
Professor of Pathology
Dr RPS Punia

Senior Resident of Pathology
Dr Garima Rakheja

Former Senior Resident of Pathology
Dr Vidhu Jaswal Wadhwa

Post Graduate Resident of Pathology
Dr Nayan Koul

Delhi

Maulana Azad Medical College, New Delhi
Former Director Professor and Head of Pathology
Dr Tejinder Singh

Former Professors
Dr Nita Kumar, Dr DK Shome, Dr Sonu Nigam

Director Professor of Pathology
Dr Nita Khurana

Director Professor of Community Medicine
Dr GK Ingle

Director Professor of Microbiology
Dr Surinder Kumar

Professor of Pathology
Dr Sarika Singh

Associate Professors of Pathology
Dr Richa Gupta, Dr Sharmana Mandal

Assistant Professors of Pathology
Dr Prerna Arora, Dr Reena Tomar, Dr Meeta Singh, Dr Nidhi Verma, Dr Varuna Mallya Ashwin, Dr Priyanka Saxena, Dr Ritika Walia

Senior Residents of Pathology
Dr Surekha Yadav, Dr Latika Gupta, Dr Barkha Maheswari, Dr Nishant Sagar, Dr Sushil Kumar Sharma, Dr Ashutosh Rath, Dr Dimple Chaudhary, Dr Radhika Agarwal, Dr Vishal Singh

Post Graduate Residents of Pathology
Dr Usha Rani, Dr Neelam Singh, Dr Gunjan Nain, Dr Jyotsna Ranjan, Dr Lalnunsangi Saila, Dr Pritika Kushwaha, Dr Sneha Goswami, Dr Kirti Balhara, Dr Neelakashi Goyal, Dr Rabish Kumar

Alumni Post Graduate Residents of Pathology since 1990
Dr Neelam Sood, Dr Rajeev Bajaj, Dr Promila Gautam, Dr Rajiv Sharma, Dr Pooja Sakhuja, Dr Sangita Sarkar Basu, Dr Sandhya Bajaj, Dr Anand Verma, Dr Debadutt Basu, Dr Sangita Lamba, Dr Sangita Saigal, Dr Sunanda, Dr Meenakshi Gupta, Dr Sangita Sonkar, Dr Nita Khurana, Dr Anju Goyal, Dr Rupa Sarma, Dr Jyotika, Dr Rekha Aggarwal, Dr Ira Gulati, Dr Neerja Vajpayee, Dr Meena Sidhu, Dr Nakhat, Dr Anju Jain, Dr Ramona Chopra, Dr Renu Das, Dr Dinesh Rakheja, Dr Nilanjana, Dr Sonu Nigam, Dr Deepali Gupta, Dr Shobini Rajan, Dr Shikha Gupta, Dr Sameer Gupta, Dr Haimanti Sarin, Dr Meenashi Sidar, Dr Pragati Narula Kumar, Dr Naveen Sharma, Dr Payal Kapur, Dr Pradeep Suri, Dr Som Pal Singh, Dr Archana, Dr Ruma Pahwa, Dr Deepali Verma, Dr Deepika Sharma, Dr Kirti Sharma, Dr Niti Singhal, Dr Sandeep Singhal, Dr Ritesh Sachdeva, Dr Divya Chhabra, Dr Abha Goel, Dr Prashant Sharma, Dr Sanjeev Gupta, Dr Samhita Bhattacharya, Dr Shyam Sunder, Dr Ruchika Aggarwal, Dr Parul Jain, Dr Reema Gulati, Dr Shubhita Bhatnagar, Dr Kajal Puneet Phull, Dr Deepti Mahajan, Dr Deepak Kumar Singh, Dr Nidhi Goyal, Dr Sukriti Singhal, Dr Prerna Arora, Dr Kavita Kohli, Dr Namarta Setia, Dr Somak Roy, Dr Vijay Saroha, Dr Debpriya Ghosh, Dr Doris Zaultei, Dr Meeta Singh, Dr Ankur Garg, Dr Akhila Lakshmikantha, Dr Vibha Chhabra, Dr Nidhi Mahajan, Dr Nivedita Ghosh, Dr Pallavi Aggarwal, Dr Ashumi Gupta, Dr Swapnil Agarwal, Dr Jyotsna Nigam, Dr Rachna Khera, Dr Sangita Tripathi, Dr Parul Sobti, Dr Alphy Sara Verghese, Dr Ruchi Jha, Dr Reema Dahiya, Dr Poonam Rani, Dr Divya Sharma, Dr Jenna Bhattacharya, Dr Devi Subarayan, Dr Amita Jain, Dr Bembem Khuraijam, Dr Barkha Maheshwari, Dr Parul Gautam, Dr Annapurna Saxena, Dr Chandni Garg, Dr Vasudha Goyal, Dr Parth Desai, Dr Prasad S Dange, Dr Roopali Rathi, Dr Garima Rakheja, Dr Suniti Pahwa Sikund, Dr Vikram Raj Gopinathan, Dr Ashna Mittal, Dr Ashu Singh, Dr Sushil Kumar Sharma, Dr Nishant Sagar, Dr Uday, Dr Darilin, Dr Vijaya Vaishnav, Dr Radhika Aggarwal, Dr Dimple Chaudhary, Dr Kamal Wadhwa, Dr Vishal Chauhan, Dr Anusha S Bhat, Dr Chetna Mehrol, Dr Shubhra Narayan, Dr Pomilla Singh, Dr Saumya Pandey, Dr Tushar Kalonia, Dr Babita Khangar

Former Senior Residents of Pathology
Dr Rashmi Jain, Dr Sabita Basu, Dr Kachnar Verma, Dr Neha Singh, Dr Garima Goyal, Dr Rekha Boyal, Dr Sharmana Mandal, Dr Sangita Sonkar, Dr Arun Kumar Thakran, Dr Ankita Jaswal

Technical Staff of Pathology
Mr Ashok Aggarwal, Mr Vinod Sharma, Mr Ramesh Kumar, Mr Rajan, Mr Narender Singh, Mr Rakesh Kumar, Mrs Sudha Roy, Mrs Promila, Mrs Ranjana, Mrs Bindu, Mrs Aji, Mrs Soffie, Mrs Neelam, Mrs Geeta Verma

Photography Section of Pathology
Mr Subhankar Ghosh

Office of Pathology
Mrs Bimla Devi

Avni Book Depot, MAMC, New Delhi
Mr Varis Sharma

Photocopy Center
Mr Narender Kumar

University College of Medical Sciences, New Delhi
Director Professor and Head of Pathology
Dr Meera Sikka

Director Professors/Professors
Dr Satinder Sharma, Dr VK Arora, Dr Sonal Sharma, Dr Mrinalini Kotru

Lady Hardinge Medical College, New Delhi
Director Professor and Head of Pathology
Dr Sunita Sharma

Director Professors/Professors of Pathology
Dr Manjula Jain, Dr Monisha Chaudhary, Dr Kiran Aggarwal, Dr Shilpi Aggarwal, Dr Selja Shukla

Assistant Professors of Pathology
Dr Vandana Puri Tiwari, Dr Lalita Jyotsna Prakhya, Dr Shivali Sehgal

All India Institute of Medical Sciences, New Delhi
Professor of Pathology
Dr Sandeep Mathur

Acknowledgments

Assistant Professor of Internal Medicine
Dr Arvind Kumar

Assistant Professor of Hematoncology
Dr Sanjiv Gupta

Assistant Professors of Pathology
Dr Shipra Goel, Dr Seema Kaushal

DM Residents Hematology
Dr Uday, Dr Prasad S Dange

Senior Resident of Pathology
Dr Vikram Raj Gopinathan

Vardhman Medical College, New Delhi
Director Professor/Professor of Pathology
Dr Ashish Kumar Mandal, Dr Rashmi Arora

Senior Resident of Pathology
Dr Tanvi Aggarwal

Intern Trainee
Dr Sugandha Bansal

Ambedkar Medical College, Rohini
Assistant Professors of Pathology
Dr Bembem Khuraijam, Dr Divya Sharma

PGIMER, Ram Manohar Lohia Hospital, New Delhi
Director Professor of Orthopedics
Dr Anil Mehtani

Professor of Dermatology
Dr Kabir Sardana

Senior Resident Anesthesiology
Dr Monika Chandra

North DMC Hindu Rao Medical College, New Delhi
Professor of Pathology
Dr Raj Bala Yadav

Consultant Pathologist
Dr Som Pal Singh

Chacha Nehru Bal Chikitsalaya, Geeta Colony
Assistant Professor of Pathology
Dr Nidhi Mahajan

Sir Ganga Ram Hospital, Rajinder Nagar
Consultant Pathologist
Dr Seema Rao

Central Govt Health Scheme, New Delhi
Consultant Pathologist
Dr Ila Tyagi

Janakpuri Super Speciality Hospital, New Delhi
Director
Dr MM Mehandiratta

Assistant Professor of Pathology
Dr Abhijit Das

Institute of Human Behaviour and Allied Sciences, New Delhi
Professor of Pathology
Dr Sujata Chaturvedi

Gujarat
BJ Medical College, Ahmedabad
Professor and Head of Pathology
Dr Hansa Goswami

Professors of Pathology
Dr HA Oza, Dr Smita Shah, Dr Nandita Mehta, Dr Mahesh Patel, Dr Sanjay Dhotre, Dr Ina Shah

Associate Professor of Pathology
Dr Hemina Desai, Dr Ami Shah, Dr Monika Kohli

Assistant Professor of Pathology
Dr Meena Patel, Dr Purvi Patel, Dr Sakera Baji, Dr Hetal Jani, Dr Ami Shah, Dr Uvri Parikh, Dr Vashali Anand, Dr Hitender Barot

Tutors of Pathology
Dr Prabha Rathod, Dr Bharat Pateliya, Dr Shivani Dixit, Dr Bhavesh Faldu, Dr Pooja Dave, Dr Garshma Jobanputra, Dr Neelam Mehta, Dr Amit Satasiya, Dr Kajal Parikh, Dr Priyanka Gohel, Dr Mital Chokshi, Dr Binal Vagh, Dr Taruna Hadiya

Post Graduate Residents of Pathology
Dr Hiralben Patel, Dr Ruchira Wadhwa, Dr Devanshi Gosai, Dr Nishith Thakor, Dr Pratibha Vyas, Dr Mehul Kumar Patel, Dr Varsha Dhuliya, Dr Shalibhadra Shah, Dr Hiren Mandiya, Dr Tripuli Sonawan, Dr Ritesh Gohail, Dr Komalben Joshi, Dr Jaymalakumari Solanki, Dr Aritra Aash, Dr Juhi Khanna, Dr Ronnak Jain, Dr Neeraja Barve, Dr Vivek Kumar, Dr Ruchi Patel, Dr Sneha Patel, Dr Dhruti Patel, Dr Neetal Desai, Dr Mital Yadav, Dr Yamini Rana, Dr Kajal Parikh, Dr Taruna Hidiya, Dr Binal Vaghani, Dr Bharat Pateliya, Dr Prabha Rathod, Dr Garishma Jobanputra, Dr Sonali Timaniya, Dr Siddhartha Ghelani, Dr Payal Malviya, Dr Jaimin Manek, Dr Vaibhavi Dhimmar, Dr Avani Oza, Dr Dhaval Vaghela, Dr Niraj Maiyad, Dr Khushali Parikh, Dr Shreya Solanki, Dr Nikita Patel, Dr Hemangi Mehta, Dr Alisha Mody, Dr Ajay Devraniya, Dr Akash Thakkar

NHL Medical College, Ahmedabad
Associate Professor of Pathology
Dr Anjali Goyal

GCS Medical College, Ahmedabad
Professor and Head of Pathology
Dr Deepak Joshi

PDU Medical College, Rajkot
Associate Professor of Pathology
Dr Amit Agravat

Post Graduate Resident of Pathology
Dr Rashi Garg

GMERS Medical College, Himmat Nagar
Associate Professor of Pathology
Dr Atul Shrivastav

Haryana
Post Graduate Institute of Medical Sciences, Rohtak
Former Senior Professors of Pathology
Dr Uma Singh, Dr SK Mathur

Senior Professor and Head of Pathology
Dr Rajeev Sen

Senior Professor of Pathology
Dr Sunita Singh

Professors of Pathology
Dr Nisha Marwah, Dr Rajnish Kalra, Dr Sanjay Kumar, Dr Veena Gupta, Dr Meenu Gill, Dr Sant Parkash, Dr Sumiti Gupta, Dr Sonia Chhabra

Associate Professor of Pathology
Dr Gajender Singh

Assistant Professors of Pathology
Dr Monika Gupta, Dr Promil Gupta, Dr Shivani Dua Batra, Dr Renuka Verma

Senior Residents of Pathology
Dr Hemant, Dr Padam, Dr Deepika, Dr Neha Singh, Dr Richa, Dr Sonu, Dr Pansi, Dr Sucheta, Dr Gauri, Dr Dimple, Dr Shivani, Dr Mansi, Dr Shilpi, Dr Divya, Dr Nitika

Post Graduate Residents of Pathology
Dr Mega, Dr Suma, Dr Tapsya, Dr Vasundhra, Dr Komal, Dr Saurav, Dr Ajay, Dr Neha, Dr Namita, Dr Yashika, Dr Sweta, Dr Shruti, Dr Vikas, Dr Sakshi, Dr Manpreet, Dr Gurupriya, Dr Nitish, Dr Roomi, Dr Madhulika, Dr Deepshika, Dr Meena, Dr Ritesh, Dr Gurjeet, Dr Nidhi, Dr Bharti, Dr Vipul, Dr Lalit, Dr Aayushi, Dr Reeti, Dr Himadri, Dr Aardhna, Dr Sandeep, Dr Manish, Dr Raman Kapil

SHKM Govt Medical College, Nalhar
Principal
Dr Sansar Sharma

Professor and Head of Pathology
Dr Shivani Kalhan

Associate Professor of Pathology
Dr Pawan Singh Bodwal

BPS Govt Medical College, Khanpur, Sonepat
Associate Professor of Pathology
Dr Kulwant Singh

Post Graduate Resident of Pathology
Dr Kanika Makkar

ESIC Medical College, Faridabad
Assistant Professor of Pathology
Dr Nimisha Sharma

Maharishi Markandeshwar University, Mullana, Ambala
Professors of Pathology
Dr Sanjay Bedi, Dr Prem Singh Madhan

Shanti Diagnostic Center, Faridabad
Managing Director
Dr Satya Pal Jayant

Maharishi Dayanand University, Rohtak
Professor and Head of Music Department
Dr (Mrs) Vimal Dinesh

Himachal Pradesh
Indira Gandhi Medical College, Simla
Professor and Head of Pathology
Dr Vijay Kaushal

Professor of Pathology
Dr Kavita Mardi

Maharishi Markandeshwar University, Solan
Professor and Head of Pathology
Dr Manohar Lal Gupta

Jammu & Kashmir
Govt Medical College, Jammu
Former Professor and Head of Pathology
Dr Yudhvir Gupta

Professor and Head of Pathology
Dr Kuldeep Kumar Kaul

Professors of Pathology
Dr Kuldeep Singh, Dr Subhash Bhardwaj, Dr Jyotsna Suri

Associate Professors of Pathology
Dr Surender Atri, Dr Ruchi Khajuria, Dr Deepti Mahajan, Dr Sindhu Sharma, Dr Rupali Bargotra

Lecturers of Pathology
Dr Deepa Hans, Dr Ameet Kaur, Dr Teepulsher, Dr Navneet Naaz

Senior Residents of Pathology
Dr Vidhu Mahajan, Dr Anu Gupta, Dr Mansi Sharma, Dr Deepti Gupta, Dr Akhtar Salaria, Dr Sunil Raina, Dr Sailja Kotwal, Dr Gousia Rather, Dr Poonam Sharma, Dr Virender Rana, Dr Ritu Bhagat, Dr Megha Sharma, Dr Sharoly Singh, Dr Bahrti Thaker, Dr Jagriti, Dr Suby Singh

Post Graduate Residents of Pathology
Dr Neha Bharti, Dr Chiterlekha Bhasin, Dr Anu Mangoch, Dr Sonia Nagyal, Dr Bhavneet Kour, Dr Priyanka, Dr Navkiran Kaur, Dr Anjali Saini, Dr Shelly Singh, Dr Isha Sharma, Dr Sunali Gupta, Dr Shweta Bhagat, Dr Usha Kiran, Dr Monika Pangotra, Dr Shabnam Sarfaraz, Dr Sovia Anand, Dr Madhubala, Dr Aashna Gupta, Dr Sonika Rukhwal, Dr Chhavi Gupta, Dr Himanshu Rana, Dr Abhishek Dogra, Dr Faiza Hafiz, Dr Wasim-Ul-Shafi, Dr Shazia Khatana, Dr Saba Mustaq, Dr Faisal Bashir, Dr Rashmi Aithmia

Govt Medical College, Srinagar
Professor and Head of Pathology
Dr Ruby Reshi

Professor of Pathology
Dr Riyaz Ahmad Tasleem

Associate Professors of Pathology
Dr Bilal Sheikh, Dr Lateef A Wani, Dr Mehnaaz Sultan

Assistant Professors of Pathology
Dr Salma Bhat, Dr Sheema Sheikh, Dr Shazia Handoo

Lecturers of Pathology
Dr Adil Sidique, Dr Nusrat Baseer

Assistant Surgeons of Pathology
Dr Ruksana, Dr Nazia Quyoom, Dr Bilal Banday

Demonstrators of Pathology
Dr Summiya, Dr Baba Iqbal Khaliq, Dr S Imtiyaz, Dr Jibrna, Dr Suhail, Dr Nusart Ali, Dr Manzoor, Dr Shaheen, Dr Irfan

Post Graduate Residents of Pathology
Dr Farooq, Dr Aijaz Amin, Dr Farzana, Dr Arshi, Dr Saymah

Sher-I-Kashmir Institute of Medical Sciences, Srinagar
Former Professors and Heads of Pathology
Dr KM Baba, Dr Parveen Shah

Acknowledgments

Former Professors of Pathology
Dr Nassima Chanda, Dr GN Sofi

Additional Professor and Head of Pathology
Dr Syed Besina Yasin

Additional Professors of Pathology
Dr Rumana Makhdooni, Dr Mohd Iqbal Lone

Associate Professor of Pathology
Dr Zubaida Rasool

Senior Residents of Pathology
Dr Danish Khan, Dr Tazeen Jeelani, Dr Suhail Mushtaq, Dr Nuzhat Samoon, Dr Sumat Khursheed, Dr Imza Feroz, Dr Ozma Masoodi, Dr Duri Mateen, Dr Huzaifa Tak, Dr Nazia Bhat, Dr Naheena Bashir, Dr Mir Wajahat

Post Graduate Residents of Pathology
Dr Shaziya Ashraf, Dr Farhat Abbas, Dr Sagir Akhtar, Dr Zarka Nabi, Dr Faizan Mir, Dr Salma Gull, Dr Prabhleen Kaur, Dr Nazia Tabassum, Dr Majid Khan, Dr Salma Yaseen, Dr Ishrat Younis, Dr Muneera Gul, Dr Asima Aijaz, Dr Mehak Shafat, Dr Subuh Parvez Khan, Dr Fiza Parvez khan, Dr Barqul Afaq, Dr Showkat Ahmed, Dr Shazieya Akhtar, Dr Noor Jahan

Former Post Graduate Residents of Pathology
Dr Sumaira Qadri, Dr Iram Naaz

SKIMS Medical College, Srinagar
Professor and Head of Pathology
Dr Rasheed Khan

Associate Professors of Pathology
Dr Afiya Shafi, Dr JB Singh

Acharya Shri Chander College of Medical Sciences, Jammu
Professor and Head of Pathology
Dr Arvind Khajuria

Professor of Pathology
Dr KC Gosain

Associate Professor of Pathology
Dr Mahima Sharma

Assistant Professor of Pathology
Dr Nitin Gupta

Karnataka
Sri Devraj Urs Medical College, Kolar
Professor of Pathology
Dr CSBR Prasad

VIMS, Bellary
Post Graduate Resident of Pathology
Dr Prachi Singhal

Sapthagiri Institute of Medical Sciences, Bangalore
Executive Director
Mr GD Manoj

Professor and Head of Pathology
Dr Vijaya C

Associate Professors of Pathology
Dr Aparana Narasimha, Dr AH Nagarajappa, Dr Amoolya Bhat, Dr Arachana C Shetty

Assistant Professors of Pathology
Dr Smita S Massarnatti, Dr Padma Priya Kasukurti, Dr Suraksha Rao B

Madhya Pradesh
Mahatma Gandhi Memorial Medical College, Indore
Professor and Head of Pathology
Dr CV Kulkarni

Bundelkhand Medical College, Sagar
Professor and Head of Pathology
Dr Bharat Jain

Index Medical College, Indore
Professor and Head of Pathology
Dr Shri Kant Nema

Professors of Pathology
Dr Sanjeev Narang, Dr Anil Kapoor, Dr Arjun Singh

Assistant Professors of Pathology
Dr Anjali Singh, Dr Parul Dargar, Dr Priyanka Sachdeva

Post Graduate Residents of Pathology
Dr Akanchha, Dr Harmeet Choudhary, Dr Radhika Rathi, Dr Randeep Kaur Bal, Dr Saniya Sharma, Dr Snehil Agrawal, Dr Somendra Dhariwal, Dr Surekha Sharma, Dr Aditya Tignath, Dr Apurrva Malhotra, Dr Awani Jain, Dr Himani, Dr Jai Singh, Dr Neelambara Bidwai, Dr Rahul Krode, Dr Shahar Bano Khan, Dr Vikas Mishra, Dr Atul Partap Singh, Dr Prachi Mehla, Dr Priya Roy, Dr Pulkit, Dr Rajesh, Dr Ranu Yadav, Dr Rohit Sangtani, Dr Shipra Yadav, Dr Vinitha Jose

All India Institute of Medical Sciences, Bhopal
Professor and Head of Pathology
Dr Neelkamal Kapur

Assistant Professor of Pathology
Dr Garima Goyal

Netaji Subhash Chandra Bose Medical College, Jabalpur
Post Graduate Resident of Pathology
Dr Amita Gupta

Sri Aurobindo Institute of Medical Sciences, Indore
Post Graduate Resident of Pathology
Dr Priyanka Kiyawat Jain

Maharashtra
Seth GS Medical College and KEM Hospital, Mumbai
Associate Professor of Pathology
Dr Rachna Chaturvedi

Post Graduate Resident of Pathology
Dr Pranav Patwardhan

Grant Medical College and Sir JJ Group of Hospitals, Mumbai
Associate Professor of Pathology
Dr Kalpana Anand Deshpande

Tata Memorial Hospital, Mumbai
Associate Professor of Pathology
Dr Asawari Patil

DR DY Patil Medical College, Navi Mumbai
Medical Director and Trustee
Dr Priya Darshini

Mahatma Gandhi Mission Medical College, Navi Mumbai
Dean
Dr GS Narshetty

Professor and Head of Pathology
Dr Rita Dhar

Professors of Pathology
Dr Ujwala Maheshwari, Dr BD Bolker

Alumni of the Institution
Dr Akshun Kalia, Dr Anubhav, Dr Harman Preet Chinna, Dr Manan Dave, Dr Amit Sharma, Dr Anurag Tiwary, Dr Saurabh Kumar

Mahatma Gandhi Mission Medical College, Aurangabad
Professor and Head of Pathology
Dr Bhale

Professor of Pathology
Dr Smita Mulay

Dr DY Patil Medical College, Pune
Former Vice Chancellor
Dr Amarjit Singh

Dean
Dr Jitender Bhowalkar

Professor and Head of Pathology
Dr Harsh Kumar

Professors of Pathology
Dr SS Chandanwale, Dr Charusheela Gore, Dr Archna Buch, Dr Pagaro Pradhan

Associate Professors of Pathology
Dr Rupali Bavikar, Dr Shruti Vimal, Dr Arpana Dharwadkar, Dr Tushar Kamble, Dr Iqbal Banymme

Lecturers of Pathology
Dr Vidya Vishvanathan, Dr Sushama Kulkarni, Dr Yamini Ingale, Dr Shubhangi Tayade, Dr Yogesh Tayade, Dr Dadaso Baravkar

Demonstrators of Pathology
Dr Anjali Deshpande, Dr WC Raut, Dr AJ Nagarkar, Dr Monali Kadam, Dr Kamini Masul, Dr Sharad Pole

Post Graduate Resident of Surgery
Dr Mansi Dhende

Post Graduate Resident of Pediatrics
Dr Udit Sihag

Alumnus of Ophthalmology
Dr Spriha Arun

Bhartiya Vidyapeeth Medical College, Pune
Principal
Dr Vivek Saoji

Professor and Head of Pathology
Dr NS Mani

Professors of Pathology
Dr Manjiri Karandikar, Dr Ravinder C Nimbargi

Krishna Institute of Medical Sciences, Krar
Former Professor and Head of Pathology
Dr Sushma Desai

Medical Superintendent of Krishna Hospital
Dr Ashok Yadavrao Kshirsagar

Professor and Head of Pathology
Dr Sujata Kanetkar

Professor of Pathology
Dr Jyotsna Wadar

Assistant Professor of Pathology
Dr Dhiraj Shukla

MPV Vasantrao Medical College, Nasik
Professor and Head of Pathology
Dr Preeti Bajaj

ESI Post Graduate Institute of Medical Sciences, Mumbai
Professor and Head of Pathology
Dr Madhuri Kate

Odisha

Kalinga Institute of Medical Sciences, Bhubaneshwar
Professor and Head of Pathology
Dr Urmila Senapati

Professors of Pathology
Dr Jayasree Rath, Dr Kanakalata Dash, Dr Amit Kumar Adhya

Associate Professors of Pathology
Dr Ranjita Panigrahi, Dr Ranjana Giri

Assistant Professors of Pathology
Dr Sarojini Raman, Dr Nageshwar Sahu, Dr Pranati Misra, Dr Prajna Das, Dr Madhusmita Mohanty, Dr Rajni Sharma, Dr Prita Pradhan

Post Graduate Residents of Pathology
Dr Soma Pradhan, Dr Malvika Mgadhi, Dr Monideepa Chattopadhyay, Dr Rituparna Ghosh, Dr Sandhya Biswal, Dr Chinmayee Panigrahi, Dr Pallavi Mishra

MKCG Medical College and Hospital, Berhampur
Post Graduate Residents of Pathology
Dr Chandan Bajad, Dr Kamal Kant

Pondicherry

JIPMER, Pondicherry
Professors of Pathology
Dr Bhawana Ashok Badhe, Dr Debdatta Basu, Dr N Siddaraju, Dr Surendra Kumar Verma, Dr Rakhee Kar

Aarpaddai Veedu Medical College, Kirumampakkam
Assistant Professor of Pathology
Dr Ashu Singh

Punjab

Govt Medical College, Amritsar
Former Professor and Head of Pathology
Dr SK Kahlon

Professor and Head of Pathology
Dr Surender Pal

Professors of Pathology
Dr Amarjit Singh, Dr Kuldeep Singh Chahal

Associate Professors of Pathology
Dr Vijay Mehra, Dr Permeet Kaur Bagga

Assistant Professors of Pathology
Dr Jagdeep, Dr Ram Krishan Sharma, Dr Navjot Kaur, Dr Mandeep Randhawa, Dr Jaspreet Singh

Senior Residents of Pathology
Dr Poonam Katru, Dr Harkirat Kaur, Dr Sofia, Dr Neeraj Bisht, Dr Rekha, Dr Sanjeev Kohli, Dr Vinay Sharma, Dr Hardeep Sethi, Dr Jagpal Kaur

Post Graduate Residents of Pathology
Dr Sonal Aggarwal, Dr Swati Sharma, Dr Navpreet Kaur, Dr Vrinda Aggarwal, Dr Moninder Kaur, Dr Krishma Goyal, Dr Gaurav, Dr Supreet Kaur, Dr Babita Rani, Dr Shweta Mahajan, Dr Utkarshni, Dr Gurpal Kaur, Dr Anamika Sharma, Dr Nidhima Aggarwal, Dr Megha Bansal, Dr Dikshi Aneja, Dr Neha Saini, Dr Kanika Wadhwa, Dr Saloni Saini, Dr Gurinderpal Kaur

Dayanand Medical College, Ludhiana
Former Professor and Head of Pathology
Dr Vinita Malhotra

Former Professor of Pathology
Dr BS Shah

Professor and Head of Pathology
Dr Neena Sood

Professor
Dr Harpreet Kaur

Christian Medical College, Ludhiana
Professors of Pathology
Dr Roma Issac, Dr Rupinder Kaur

Govt Medical College, Patiala
Professor and Head of Pathology
Dr Ramesh Kundal

Assistant Professor of Pathology
Dr Chetan Dass

Adesh Medical College, Bhatinda
Professor and Head of Pathology
Dr Vijay Suri

Senior Resident of Pathology
Dr Saumya Bhagat

Sri Guru Ramdas Medical College, Amritsar
Professor and Head of Pathology
Dr Mridu Manjiri

Associate Professor of Pathology
Dr Manisha Sharma

Assistant Professor of Pathology
Dr Neha Sharma

Punjab Institute of Medical Sciences, Jalandhar
Professor and Head of Pathology
Dr Usha Bandish

Port Blair Union Territory
Andaman and Nicobar Islands Institute of Medical Sciences, Port Blair
Assistant Professors of Pathology
Dr Jyotsna Nigam, Dr Jitender Nigam

Rajasthan
Geetanjali Medical College, Udaipur
Professor and Head of Pathology
Dr Narender Kumar Mogra

Assistant Professor of Pathology
Dr Tarang Patel

Pacific Medical College, Udaipur
Professor of Pathology
Dr SS Surana

Pacific Institute of Medical Sciences, Udaipur
Professor of Pathology and Medical Superintendent
Dr DR Mathur

RNT Medical College, Udaipur
Professor and Head of Pathology
Dr Sunita Bhargav

Post Graduate Resident of Pathology
Dr Pupul Bose

SMS Medical College, Jaipur
Professor and Head of Pathology
Dr Ajay Yadav

Associate Professor of Pathology
Dr Ranjana Solanki

Assistant Professor of Pathology
Dr Subhash Sharma, Dr Vidhi Sharma

Jawahar Lal Nehru Medical College, Ajmer
Professor and Head of Pathology
Dr Geeta Pachauri

Sardar Patel Medical College, Bikaner
Professor and Head of Pathology
Dr Neelu Gupta

Associate Professor of Biochemistry
Dr Anita Verma

SN Medical College, Jodhpur, Rajasthan
Professor of Pathology
Dr Ajay Malviya

Senior Resident of Pathology
Dr Praveen Verma

Medical College, Kota
Professor of Pathology
Dr Rajeev Saxena

National Institute of Medical Sciences, Jaipur
Professor of Pathology
Dr Vineet Choudhary

Mahatma Gandhi Medical College, Jaipur
Post Graduate Resident of Pathology
Dr Shubhi Saxena

All India Institute of Medical Sciences, Jodhpur
Senior Resident of Pathology
Dr Parul Gautam

Tamil Nadu

SRM Medical College, Kuttankuathur, Chennai
Professor and Head of Pathology
Dr John Jaison

Chettinad Medical College, Chennai
Assistant Professor of Pathology
Dr Devi Subbarayan

Telangana

Osmania Medical College, Hyderabad
Vice Principal-cum-Professor and Head of Pathology
Dr Ezhil Arasi N

Associate Professor of Pathology
Dr BS Nithyanand

Gandhi Medical College, Secunderabad
Professor and Head of Pathology
Dr O Sharvan Kumar

Bhaskar Medical College, Moinabad, Hyderabad
Principal-cum-Professor of Pathology
Dr Narsing Rao

Professor of Pathology
Dr Vijay Sreedhar

Govt Medical College, Mehboob Nagar
Associate Professor and Head of Pathology
Dr Devojee Nayak

Rajiv Gandhi Institute of Medical Sciences, Adilabad
Professor and Head of Pathology
Dr Chandra Shekhar

Mallareddy Women Institute of Medical Sciences, Surram, Hyderabad
Professor and Head of Pathology
Dr Jijiya Bai

Mallareddy Institute of Medical Sciences, Surram, Hyderabad
Professor and Head of Medicine
Dr EA Ashok Kumar

MNR Medical College, Fasalwadi
Professor and Head of Pathology
Dr Asoka RS Kumar

Shadan Institute of Medical Sciences, Perranchuru
Professor of Pathology
Dr Salma Mahajbeen

Kamineni Institute of Medical Sciences, Narkatpally
Professor and Head of Pathology
Dr V Sathyanarayana

Uttar Pradesh

SN Medical College, Agra
Professor and Head of Pathology
Dr Atul Gupta

King George Medical University, Lucknow
Professors of Pathology
Dr Suresh Babu, Dr Uma Shankar Singh

Assistant Professor of Pathology
Dr Chanchal Rana

MLN Medical College, Allahabad
Professor of Pathology
Dr Kachnar Varma

Post Graduate Resident of Pathology
Dr Faheema Hasan Younus

Rohilkhand Medical College, Bareilly
Professor and Head of Pathology
Dr Parbodh Kumar Kakkar

Professor
Dr Ranjan Aggarwal

Hind Institute of Medical Sciences, Safedabad
Assistant Professor of Pathology
Dr Sangita Tripathi

Sharda Medical College, Noida
Professor and Head of Pathology
Dr Geeta Desmukh

Muzaffarnagar Medical College, Muzaffarnagar
Professor
Dr Anupam Varshney

Uttarakhand

All India Institute of Medical Sciences, Rishikesh
Director
Padma Shree Dr Ravi Kant

Jolly Grant Medical College, Dehradun
Assistant Professor of Pathology
Dr Ankita Katara Pandey

All India Institute of Medical Sciences, Dehradun
Assistant Professor of Pathology
Dr Neha Singh

West Bengal

Vivekanand Institute of Medical Sciences, Kolkata
Professor and Head of Pathology
Dr Debashish Bandopadhyaya

Section I

General Pathology

1. Cellular Adaptations, Cell Injury, Apoptosis, Pigments, Calcification, Cellular Accumulations and Aging
2. Inflammation, Tissue Healing and Repair
3. Disorders of Hemostasis
4. Immunopathology including Amyloidosis
5. Genetic Disorders
6. Neoplasia: Molecular Basis, Metastasis, Clinical Oncology and Laboratory Diagnosis
7. Nutritional and Infectious Diseases

CHAPTER 1

Cellular Adaptations, Cell Injury, Apoptosis, Pigments, Calcification, Cellular Accumulations and Aging

Learning Objectives

CELLULAR ADAPTATIONS
- Atrophy
- Hypertrophy
- Hyperplasia
- Metaplasia
- Dysplasia
- Reduction in Size of Organs

CELL INJURY
- Overview
  - Causes of Cell Injury
  - Main Targets of Cell Injury
  - Types of Cell Injury
  - Vulnerability of Cells to Ischemic Injury
- Reversible Cell Injury
  - Hydropic Change
  - Fatty Change
  - Hyaline Change
- Irreversible Cell Injury
- Morphological Patterns of Necrosis
  - Coagulative Necrosis
  - Liquefactive Necrosis
  - Caseous Necrosis
  - Fat Necrosis
  - Gangrenous Necrosis
  - Fibrinoid Necrosis
  - Gummatous Necrosis
  - Postmortem Autolysis
  - Zenker's Necrosis
- Outcome of Necrosis
  - Complete Resolution
  - Repair by Fibrosis
  - Dystrophic Calcification
  - Resorption of Necrotic Tissue

APOPTOSIS
- Extrinsic (Death Receptor) Pathway
- Intrinsic Mitochondrial Pathway

SUBCELLULAR RESPONSE TO INJURY
- Lysosomal Dysfunction
- Induction (Hypertrophy) of Endoplasmic Reticulum
- Mitochondrial Dysfunction
- Cytoskeleton Abnormalities

PIGMENTS
- Endogenous Pigments
  - Melanin
  - Bilirubin
  - Hemosiderin
  - Lipofuscin
  - Homogentisic Acid
  - Hamazaki-Weissenberg Bodies
- Exogenous Pigments
  - Coal Dust
  - Tattooing

CALCIFICATION
- Dystrophic Calcification and Metastatic Calcification

INTRACELLULAR ACCUMULATIONS
- Lipids
- Cholesterol and Cholesterol Esters
- Proteins and Glycogen

EXTRACELLULAR ACCUMULATIONS
- Amyloidosis
- Hyaline Change

CELLULAR AGING
- Theories of Aging
- Genetic Disorders
- Mammalian Sirtuin System

Section I: General Pathology

CELLULAR ADAPTATIONS

Cells are the structural and functional units of tissues. These are capable of adjusting their structure and functions in response to various physiological and pathological stimuli. This capability is called cellular adaptation depending on the ability of cells to divide.

Cellular adaptations include *atrophy (shrinkage of cells), hypertrophy (increase in the size of cells which results in enlargement of the organs), hyperplasia (increased number of cells in an organ or tissue) and metaplasia (transformation or replacement of one adult cell type with another).*

Cells based on proliferative activity in the context of the cell cycle are shown in Table 1.1. Cellular adaptations showing type and duration of injurious stimuli are shown in Fig. 1.1.

Physiological State

Normal cellular adaptation occurs in response to an appropriate stimulus and ceases once the need for adaptation has ceased. Under physiological state, cells are adaptable within physiological limits. Hormones synthesized during pregnancy induce changes in breast and uterus.

Table 1.1: Cells based on proliferative activity in the context of the cell cycle

Type of cells	Organs
Labile cells	Bone marrow
	Epidermis
	Epithelium lining (gastrointestinal tract, bronchi and vagina)
	Epithelium lining excretory ducts (salivary glands, pancreas, and biliary tract)
Stable cells	Liver
	Kidney
	Smooth muscle
	Striated muscle
	Fibroblasts
	Vascular endothelium
	Cartilage
	Bone
Permanent cells	Central nervous system
	Sensory organs
	Cardiac muscle
	Skeletal muscle
	Renal glomeruli

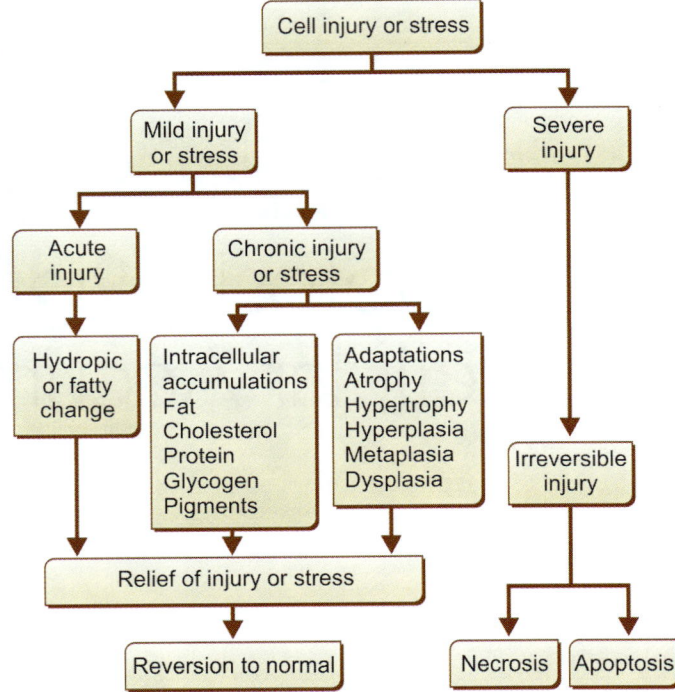

Fig. 1.1: Cellular adaptations showing type and duration of injurious stimuli.

Pathological State

Under pathological state, cells can respond to injury by producing cell stress proteins, which protect from damage and help in recovery.

Pathological adaptations include *atrophy, hypertrophy, hyperplasia and metaplasia*. Cell loss from tissues can be achieved by programmed cell death (apoptosis). Cellular adaptations showing atrophy, hypertrophy, hyperplasia, and metaplasia are shown in Fig. 1.2.

Atrophy: Atrophy is a reversible reduction in the size of the cell. The number of cells is the same as before the atrophy occurred, but the size of some fibers is reduced. This is a response to injury by *downsizing* to conserve the cell. Atrophy occurs as a result of insufficient blood flow, disuse of organs, denervation, or reduced endocrine stimulation (Fig. 1.3).

Hypertrophy: Hypertrophy is an enlargement of a cell without cell division due to an increased workload. It can result from normal physiological and pathological conditions (Fig. 1.4).

Hyperplasia: Hyperplasia is an increase in the number of cells of a tissue due to increased rate caused by increased workload, hormonal stimulation, or decreased tissue cells (Fig. 1.5).

Cellular Adaptations, Cell Injury, Apoptosis, Pigments, Calcification, Cellular Accumulations and Aging

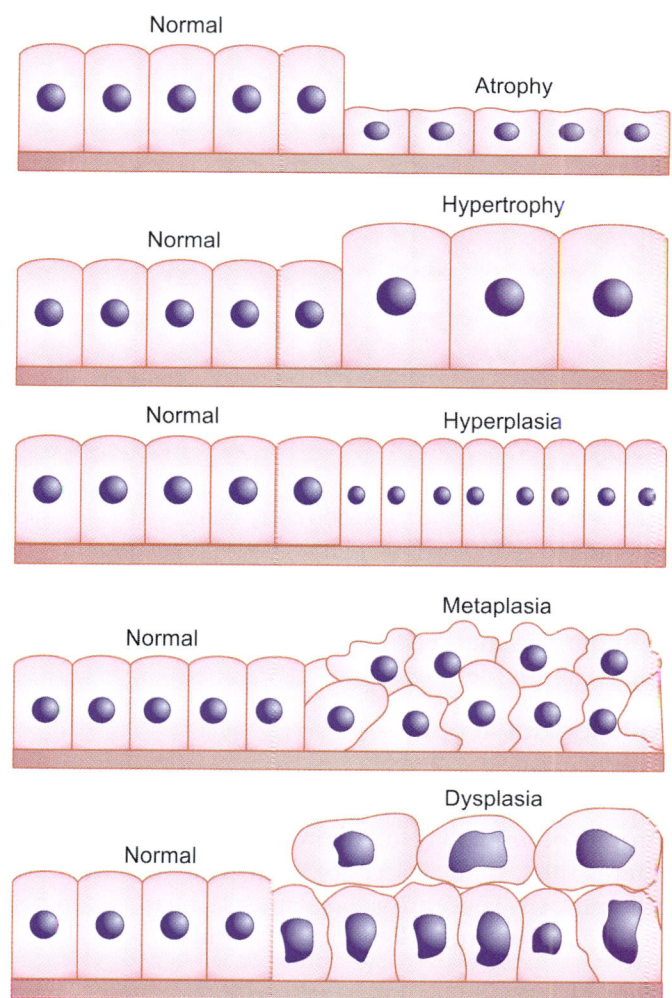

Fig. 1.2: Cellular adaptations showing atrophy, hypertrophy, hyperplasia, metaplasia and dysplasia.

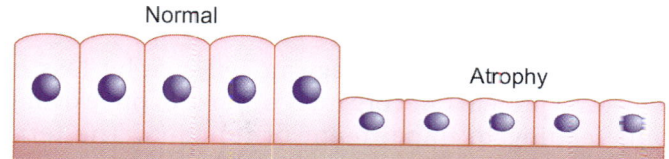

Fig. 1.3: Atrophy showing reversible reduction in the size of the cells.

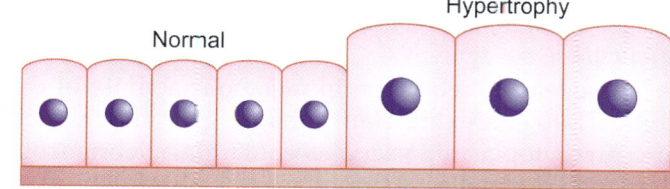

Fig. 1.4: Hypertrophy showing enlargement of a cells without cell division.

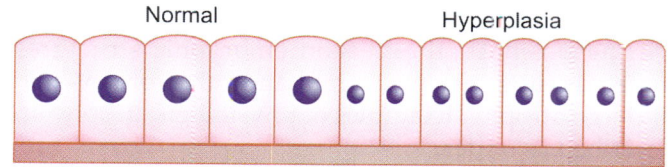

Fig. 1.5: Hyperplasia showing an increase in the number of cells of a tissue.

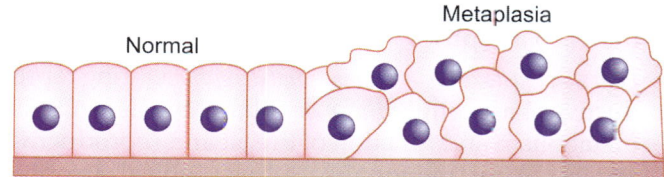

Fig. 1.6: Metaplasia showing replacement of an adult cell with another adult cell as a response to chronic inflammation or irritation.

Metaplasia: Metaplasia is transformation or replacement of one adult cell type to another adult cell type. It is thought to arise from reprogramming of stem or undifferentiated cells present in adult tissue.

Metaplastic changes most often occur due to chronic irritation. Metaplastic cells can better endure the change of stress. It usually occurs as a response to persistent injury (chronic inflammation or irritation). It is thought to be an adaptive mechanism (Figs 1.6 and 1.7).

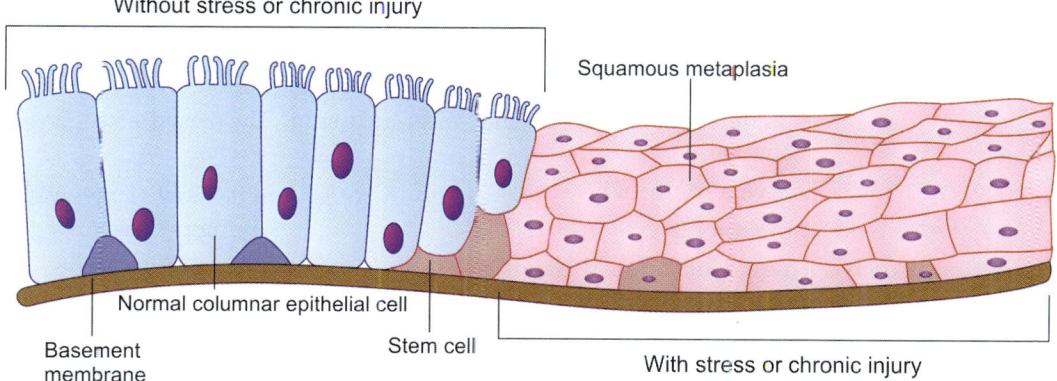

Fig. 1.7: Squamous metaplasia. Columnar epithelium is replaced by squamous epithelium as a response to chronic irritation in tobacco smokers.

ATROPHY

Atrophy refers to shrinkage in cell size by loss of structural proteins and organelles in size of pre-existing cells leading to impairment of function. The term atrophy is most often used to describe reduced organ size that may be related to cell loss rather than shrinkage. Causes of atrophy are *reduced workload, loss of innervation, reduced blood supply, inadequate nutrition, loss of endocrine stimulation and aging.*

These lead to reduction in metabolic activity of the cells. The cells exhibit autophagic granules, which are intracytoplasmic vacuoles containing debris from degraded organelles. Atrophy may be physiological or pathological (generalized or localized) (Table 1.2).

Physiological Atrophy

During postnatal life, certain embryonic structures, female breasts, uterus, vagina and other organs may undergo atrophy. Examples of physiologic atrophy are described as under:

- *Embryonic structures atrophy:* During fetal development, some embryonic structures, such as notochord, thyroglossal duct and patent ductus arteriosus undergo atrophy.
- *Female breasts, uterus and vaginal atrophy:* During reproductive phase, *estrogen hormone* plays key role in normal metabolism and function of breast and reproductive organs. After menopause, physiological atrophic changes occur in breast, endometrium, and vaginal epithelium due to decreased levels of estrogens in body.
- *Brown atrophy of organs:* Lipofuscin is a finely granular yellow brown *wear and tear* pigment due to aging process. This pigment contains lipid formed as residue of lysosomal digestion. It is accumulated in **liver, heart muscle, adrenal glands** and **ganglion cells**, producing condition brown atrophy (Fig. 1.8).

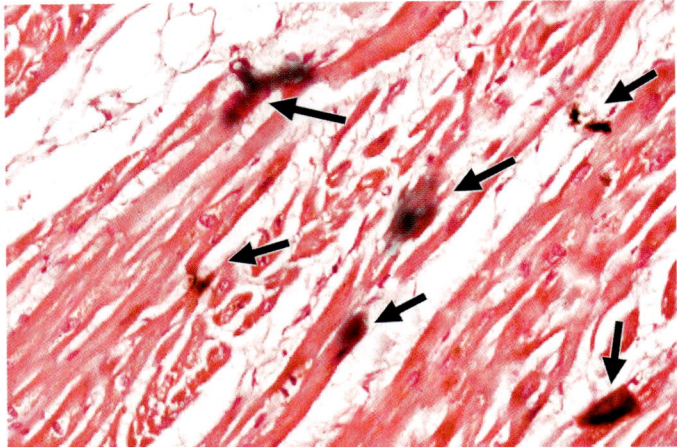

Fig. 1.8: Accumulation of intracellular lipofuscin pigment. Liver of 80 years old man shows golden cytoplasmic granules, which represent lysosomal storage of lipofuscin (arrows) (400X).

- *Brain atrophy due to aging:* In old age, frontal cortex undergoes marked atrophy revealing thinning of the gyri and widening of the sulci.

Pathological Atrophy

Pathological atrophy depends on the underlying cause and can be generalized or localized. Generalized atrophy occurs as a result of protein calorie malnutrition (marasmus), senile (old age), endocrine disorders and osteoporosis. These are skeletal muscle, heart, secondary sex organs, brain, and endocrine glands.

Pathological Generalized Atrophy

- *Endocrine glands atrophy:* Decreased endocrine stimulation due to hypopituitarism leads to atrophy of thyroid and adrenal glands.
- *Cachexia:* Increased synthesis of cytokines and TNF-α in cancer and chronic inflammatory diseases cause marked muscle wasting (cachexia), anorexia and lipid depletion.

Table 1.2: Physiological atrophy and pathological atrophy

Type of atrophy	Atrophy of organs	Etiology
Physiological atrophy	Embryonic structures (notochord, thyroglossal duct and patent ductus arteriosus)	Physiological phenomenon
	Female breasts, uterus and vagina during menopause	Decreased estrogens in menopausal women
	Brown atrophy of heart	Lipofuscin (wear and tear pigment)
	Brain atrophy	Aging process
Pathological generalized atrophy	Thyroid and adrenal glands	Hypopituitarism
Pathological local atrophy	Skeletal muscles	Denervation
	Renal cortex (due to stones)	Renal stones
	Exocrine gland (due to cystic fibrosis)	Cystic fibrosis
	Brain atrophy	Alzheimer disease

Cellular Adaptations, Cell Injury, Apoptosis, Pigments, Calcification, Cellular Accumulations and Aging

Pathological Localized Atrophy

- *Skeletal muscle atrophy:* Skeletal muscles undergo atrophy with reduced muscular strength in patients, when a fractured bone is immobilized in a plaster cast for prolonged period.

  Denervation causes skeletal muscle atrophy due to loss of lower motor neurons which adversely affect their normal metabolism.

- *Renal atrophy:* Renal stones obstructing urine outflow produce hydronephrosis resulting in atrophy of renal cortex and medulla.

- *Exocrine glands atrophy:* In cystic fibrosis of pancreas, thick secretion increases pressure in duct resulting in atrophy of exocrine gland. It is autosomal recessive disorder with fatal outcome among white population.

  Normally, transmembrane conductance regulator (CFTr) gene located on long arm of chromosome 7 codes for a membrane protein that participates in the movement of chloride and other ions across membranes.

  Mutation of CFTr gene causes malfunction of exocrine glands results in *increased viscosity of mucus and chloride* concentration in sweat and tears. Patient develops *recurrent respiratory infections, meconium ileus* and *sterility* in males. *Sweat chloride test* is an important diagnostic tool.

- *Brain atrophy:* Alzheimer disease is secondary to extensive cell death resulting in marked atrophy of the frontal lobe, thinning of gyri and widening of sulci.

HYPERTROPHY

Hypertrophy refers to increase in cell size, and resultant increase in organ size. It is a response to increased functional demand or trophic signals such as hormones and growth factors.

It occurs in permanent cells due to synthesis of more cellular structural components. Hypertrophy occurs due to physiological or pathological causes.

Molecular Basis

The molecular basis of hypertrophy reflects increased expression of growth-promoting genes (proto-oncogenes) such as *c-jun, c-fos, c-myc* and RAS (*nuclear transcription factors*).

It leads to increase synthesis of cellular proteins and number of intracellular organelles (e.g. mitochondria, Golgi apparatus). Only labile and stable cells are able to undergo hypertrophy as well as hyperplasia. Hypertrophy may be physiological, pathological, subcellular and compensatory (Table 1.3).

Physiological Hypertrophy

Physiological hypertrophy is an adaptive response to normal changes in various organs. Examples of physiological hypertrophy are as follows:

- *Skeletal muscle hypertrophy:* Skeletal muscle undergo hypertrophy due to hard physical labor or weight training. Phosphoinositide-3 kinase pathway is postulated to play role in exercise induced hypertrophy. Skeletal muscle shows increased number of myofilaments and mitochondria; abundant endoplasmic reticulum, mild nuclear enlargement. It leads to synthesis of more membranes, enzymes, ATP and higher levels of aerobic respiration.

- *Uterine hypertrophy during pregnancy:* During pregnancy, increased estrogen levels stimulate smooth muscle cells to synthesize more proteins and lead to smooth muscle hyperplasia and hypertrophy of uterus.

Pathological Hypertrophy

Cardiac hypertrophy: Cardiac hypertrophy occurs due to increased functional demand in patients with hypertension and valvular heart disease. Since the heart muscle is composed of terminally differentiated myocytes that cannot divide. Increased demand for action can be met only by increased size of the muscle cells. Pathogenesis of cardiac hypertrophy is described as under.

Table 1.3: Physiological and pathological hypertrophy

Type of hypertrophy	Organs involved	Mechanism
Physiological hypertrophy	Skeletal muscle hypertrophy	Physical labor
		Weight training
	Uterus in pregnancy (hyperplasia and hypertrophy)	Hormones
Pathological hypertrophy	Cardiac hypertrophy	Hypertension
		Valvular heart disease
	Subcellular hypertrophy of liver organelles	Barbiturates
		Alcoholism
Compensatory hypertrophy	Renal hypertrophy	Following nephrectomy of opposite side

- *Mechanical stretch* induces production of growth factors such as *TGF-β, FGF, insulin-like growth factor-1* and *vasoactive agents (angiotensin II* and *endothelin).* These *bind to G-protein coupled receptors,* induce signal to synthesize *increased synthesis of contractile proteins, embryonic genes (e.g. cardiac α-actin and ANF)* and *growth factors.*
- *Hypertrophy resulting* from transcriptional regulation leads to *increased synthesis of mRNA, rRNA, and protein.* These increase the strength and work capacity of heart. Cardiac muscles show increased cytosol, number of organelles and DNA content (Fig. 1.9).

Subcellular Hypertrophy of Liver Organelles

- *Barbiturates therapy:* It induces endoplasmic reticulum hypertrophy in liver, which increases the synthesis of cytochrome P450 oxidase available to detoxify the drugs.
- *Alcohol intake:* It may also cause endoplasmic reticulum hypertrophy in liver.

Compensatory hypertrophy: Compensatory renal hypertrophy occurs following nephrectomy or congenital absence of one kidney or nonfunctional kidney. Differences between atrophy and hypertrophy are shown in Table 1.4.

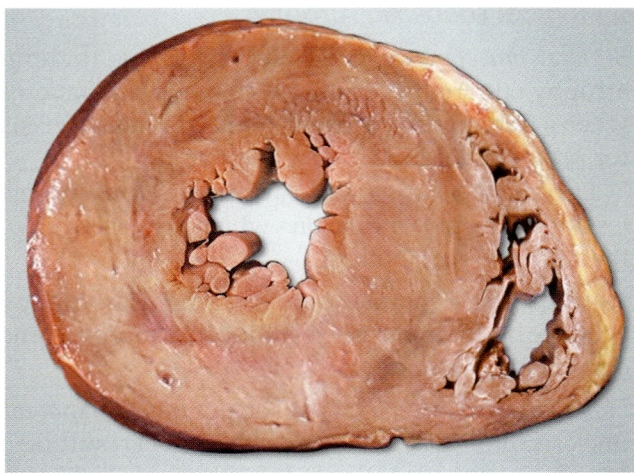

Fig. 1.9: Left ventricular hypertrophy. The left ventricle is markedly thickened in this patient with severe hypertension that was untreated for many years. The myocardial fibers have undergone hypertrophy. Normal thickness of wall of left ventricle is 1.2–1.5 cm.

Table 1.4: Differences between atrophy and hypertrophy

Parameters	Atrophy	Hypertrophy
Definition	A decrease in the size of cells by loss of cell substance with subsequent decrease in the size of affected part	Increased in size of organs due to an increased size of constituents without cell division
Physiological state	Embryonic structures (notochord, thyroglossal duct and patent ductus arteriosus)	Skeletal muscle undergo hypertrophy due to hard physical labor or weight training
	Breast, uterus and vaginal atrophy after menopause due to decreased levels of estrogens in body	Uterine hypertrophy due to increased synthesis of estrogens in pregnant women
	Brown atrophy of organs due to deposition of lipofuscin pigment (liver, heart muscle, adrenal gland and ganglion cells)	
	Brain atrophy in old age	
Pathological state	Protein calorie malnutrition (generalized atrophy of skeletal muscle, heart, secondary sex organs, brain, and endocrine glands)	Cardiac hypertrophy either due to hypertension or damaged cardiac valves
	Hypopituitarism induced atrophy of thyroid and adrenal glands	Barbiturates therapy (hypertrophy of endoplasmic reticulum liver)
	Cancer and chronic inflammation in marked muscle wasting (cachexia) due to synthesis of cytokines and TNF-α	Alcohol intake (hypertrophy of endoplasmic reticulum in liver)
	Skeletal muscle atrophy due to denervation and immobilized in a plaster cast in case of fracture	
	Renal cortex and medulla atrophy due to hydronephrosis induced by renal stone.	
	Atrophy of exocrine gland due to thick secretion in duct in case of cystic fibrosis	
	Brain atrophy (thinning of gyri and widening of sulci in frontal due to Alzheimer disease)	

HYPERPLASIA

Hyperplasia refers to increase in the number of cells in an organ or tissue, which may then have an increased size. It can only occur in tissues containing labile or stable cells. Physiological, pathological and compensatory hyperplasias are shown in Table 1.5.

Differences between hypertrophy and hyperplasia are shown in Table 1.6.

Physiological Hyperplasia

Physiological hyperplasia is an adaptive response to normal changes in various organs.

Table 1.5: Physiological, pathological and compensatory hyperplasias

Types of hyperplasia	Organs	Mechanism
Physiological hyperplasia	Uterine endometrial hyperplasia	Estrogen induced
	Uterine muscle hypertrophy	Pregnancy
	Breast glandular epithelium	Pregnancy
	Bone marrow hyperplasia	Higher altitude
	Islet β-cells hyperplasia of fetus	Diabetic mother
Pathological hyperplasia	Ductal hyperplasia of breast	Hormonal imbalance induced fibrocystic disease
	Cystoglandular or adenomatous or atypical hyperplasia of endometrium	Hormonal imbalance
	Thyroid follicular hyperplasia	Increased TSH level
	Hyperplasia of surface epithelium of skin	Wound-healing by primary intention
	Skin epidermal cell hyperplasia	Psoriasis
Compensatory hyperplasia	Hyperplasia of hepatocytes (TGF-α, TGF-β, HGF)	Following partial hepatectomy

Table 1.6: Differences between hypertrophy and hyperplasia

Features	Hypertrophy	Hyperplasia
Definition	Increased in size of organs due to an increased size of constituents without cell division	Increase in the number of cells in an organ or tissue in response to increased functional demand, where the cells are capable of mitotic division
Process	Physical/hormonal stimuli such as trophic hormones, vasoactive agents, hemodynamic factors; there is synthesis of cellular constituents resulting in increased size	Physical/hormonal stimuli; there is increase in number of cells due to cell division resulting in increased size of organ
Cell features	Cell size and cytoplasm is increased	Cell size usually remains normal, cytoplasm may be reduced
Mitosis	Absent	Present
Conversion to tumor	Never	May transform to neoplasia
Physiological	A demand for additional work met by skeletal muscle hypertrophy	Hormone induced hyperplasia in female breast
		Uterus during pregnancy
		Erythroid bone marrow hyperplasia at altitude
		Compensatory hyperplasia after partial hepatectomy and nephrectomy
Pathological	Cardiac hypertrophy (hypertension, valvular disease)	Cystoglandular and adenomatous hyperplasia of endometrium
	Uterus hypertrophy during pregnancy	Atypical hyperplasia of the endometrium
	Urinary bladder hyperplasia during obstruction to urine outflow due to prostate enlargement	Prostatic hyperplasia (prostatic glands and stromal smooth muscle cells)
		Thyroid gland hyperplasia (toxic or nontoxic goiter)
		Hyperplasia of epidermis in wound healing

Examples of physiological hyperplasia are as follows:

- *Uterine endometrial hyperplasia:* During menstrual cycle, there is increase in number of endometrial cells in response to estrogen stimulation after ovulation.
- *Uterus muscle hyperplasia during pregnancy:* During pregnancy, smooth muscle cells of uterus undergo physiological hyperplasia and hypertrophy.
- *Breasts during pregnancy:* During pregnancy, hormones stimulate breast glandular epithelium cells leading to physiological hyperplasia.
- *Thyroid gland hyperplasia:* During puberty and pregnancy, there is increased demand of thyroid hormones. Increased TSH stimulate thyroid follicular cells to undergo physiological hyperplasia leading to thyroid enlargement.
- *Bone marrow hyperplasia:* Erythroid bone marrow hyperplasia is typically seen in people living at high altitude. Low oxygen tension stimulates production of erythropoietin, which promotes the survival and proliferation of erythroid precursors in the bone marrow.
- *Islet β cells hyperplasia of the pancreas:* During intrauterine life in diabetic mothers, fetus develops islet β cells hyperplasia in response to hyperglycemia and increased demand of insulin during early gestation. Pancreatic β cells, which may secrete insulin autonomously and cause hypoglycemia at birth in newborn.

Pathological Hyperplasia

Pathological hyperplasia is a response to either excessive hormonal stimulation or abnormal production of hormonal growth factors. Proto-oncogenes code for growth factors, growth factor receptors, signal transducers (e.g. mitogen-induced protein kinases), and DNA transcription factors to initiate cell mitosis. It may be associated with increased risk for cancer.

Examples of pathological hyperplasia are described as under:

- *Endometrial hyperplasia:* Hormonal imbalance may lead to cystoglandular, adenomatous and atypical hyperplasia of endometrium.
- *Prostatic hyperplasia:* Dihydrotestosterone stimulates prostate glandular acini leading to prostatic hyperplasia (Fig. 1.10).
- *Thyroid gland hyperplasia:* It occurs as a consequence of increased serum levels of thyroid stimulating hormone.
- *Primary intention of wound healing:* Hyperplasia of surface epithelium of skin occurs in wound healing.
- *Psoriasis:* It is disease of the epidermis and dermis characterized by persistent epithelial hyperplasia. It may be caused by defective epidermal cell surface receptors and altered intracellular signaling. Patient develops erythematous, scaly plaques, commonly on the dorsal extensor cutaneous surfaces (Fig. 1.11).

Compensatory Hyperplasia

Partial surgical removal of diseased liver is frequently a stimulus for regeneration of hepatocytes by *TGF-α, TGF-β* and *HGF*.

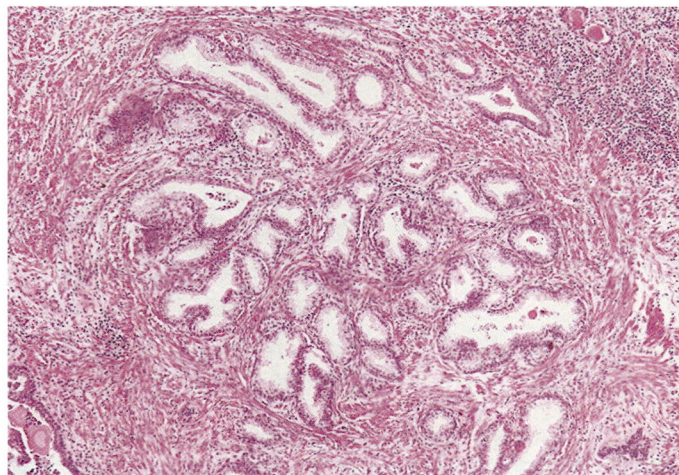

Fig. 1.10: Nodular hyperplasia prostate. The acini are relatively uniform and evenly spaced. The acini are lined by columnar secretory cells. The basal cell layers may be inconspicuous, but may be highlighted by high molecular weight cytokeratin immunostain (400X).

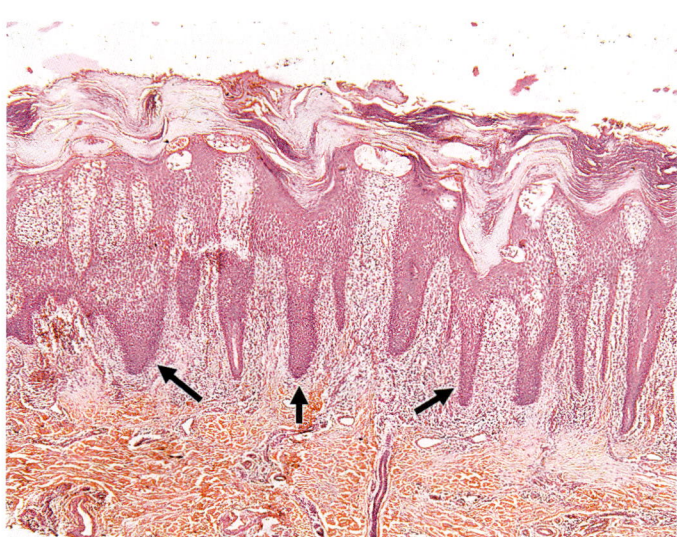

Fig. 1.11: Psoriasis showing downward elongation of the rete ridges (arrows) with thinning of overlying stratum granulosum, with parakeratosis above this. Small aggregates of neutrophils with surrounding spongiform change are seen in the superficial epidermis. Capillaries within dermal papillae are brought close to the surface (400X).

METAPLASIA

Metaplasia is the reversible replacement of one differentiated mature tissue by another. It is an adaptive response to various stimuli. New metaplastic cells are better adapted to exposure to the stimulus. Metaplasia in mesenchymal tissues is often less clearly adaptive. Differences between physiological metaplasia and pathological metaplasia are shown in Table 1.7.

Physiological Metaplasia

Physiological metaplasia is generally a normal transient response to changing conditions. For example, in the body's normal response to inflammation, monocytes migrate to inflamed tissues and transform into macrophages.

Pathological Metaplasia

Pathological metaplasia is usually a response to chronic irritation (e.g. smoking) or chronic inflammation. This process is usually reversible. Examples of pathological hyperplasia are described as under.

Squamous Metaplasia

- *Tobacco smoking:* Though metaplasia is considered to be a protective mechanism, yet it may be harmful. Prolonged exposure of the bronchi to tobacco smoke leads to squamous metaplasia of the bronchial epithelium. It also impairs the production of mucus and ciliary clearance of debris (Fig. 1.12).

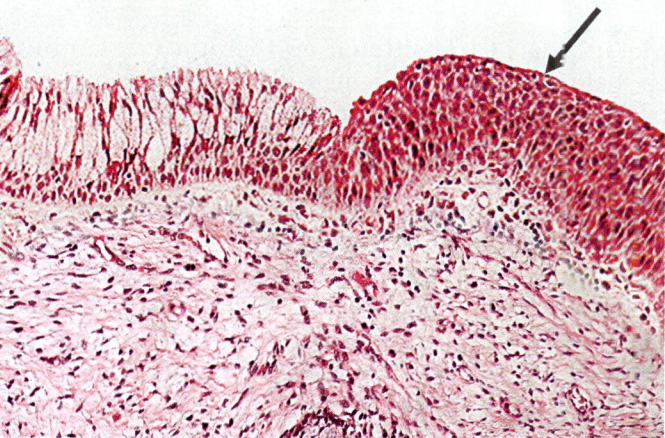

Fig. 1.12: Squamous metaplasia of bronchi in tobacco smoker showing replacement of columnar epithelium of bronchi by squamous epithelium (arrow) (100X).

- *Vitamin A deficiency:* Squamous metaplasia occurs in pancreatic duct due to vitamin A deficiency.
- *Stone in urinary tract:* Chronic irritation due to stone in urinary bladder may transform normal transitional epithelium to squamous epithelium.

Columnar Metaplasia in Barrett's Esophagus

In Barrett's esophagus, esophageal squamous epithelium is replaced by intestinal-like columnar epithelium as a result of chronic irritation by gastric acid in gastroesophageal reflux disease. There is increased risk of development of gastric carcinoma in Barrett's esophagus.

Table 1.7: Physiological metaplasia and pathological metaplasia

Parameter	Original tissue	Stimulus	Metaplastic tissue
Physiological metaplasia	Monocytes in blood circulation	Under physiological state	Tissue macrophages
Pathological metaplasia	Ciliated columnar in bronchial tree	Tobacco smoking	Squamous metaplasia
	Columnar glandular epithelium lining ducts pancreas	Vitamin A deficiency	Squamous metaplasia
	Transitional epithelium in urinary bladder	Renal stones	Squamous metaplasia
	Squamous epithelium in Barrett's esophagus	Gastric acid (gastroesophageal reflux disease)	Columnar metaplasia
	Transitional epithelium in urinary bladder	Chronic inflammation prostatitis	Glandular epithelium (cystitis glandularis)
	Fibrocollagenous tissue	Trauma	Osseous metaplasia (myositis ossificans)
	Myeloid metaplasia in liver and spleen	Agnogenic myeloid metaplasia, myelofibrosis, polycythemia vera	Hematopoiesis outside bone marrow
	Metaplasia in benign neoplasm	Benign neoplastic process	Cartilaginous and bony tissue in pleomorphic adenoma
	Squamous or osseous metaplasia in malignant neoplasm	Malignant neoplastic process	Breast carcinoma

Transitional to Glandular Epithelial Metaplasia

Metaplasia of transitional epithelium to glandular epithelium is seen in patients with chronic inflammation of the bladder (cystitis glandularis).

Osseous Metaplasia in Myositis Ossificans

Osseous metaplasia is the formation of bony trabeculae within striated muscle at the site of tissue injury. Fibrocollagenous tissue transforming to osseous tissue is known as *myositis ossificans*. It is worth mentioning that dystrophic calcification occurring at injury site does not lead to the formation of bone trabeculae.

Myeloid Metaplasia

Myeloid metaplasia occurs due to proliferation of hematopoietic cells at the site other than bone marrow, such as liver and spleen. It is known as *extramedullary hemopoiesis*. Various causes of myeloid metaplasia are *agnogenic myeloid metaplasia, myelofibrosis and polycythemia vera*.

Metaplasia in Neoplasm

Metaplasia is seen in pleomorphic adenoma of salivary gland. Tumor shows areas of cartilage and bone. Breast carcinoma may show squamous or osseous metaplasia in some cases. Prognosis of metaplastic breast carcinoma is poor.

DYSPLASIA

Dysplasia means loss of regular appearance of cells in epithelium. It is characterized by variations in size and shape of dividing cells with mitotic activity arranged in disordered fashion with loss of cell maturation as cells progress to the surface, as a result of chronic irritation or inflammation. It may revert to normal, if stimulus is removed. If stimulus persists, it can precede malignant change. Differences between metaplasia and dysplasia are shown in Table 1.8.

- *Cervical intraepithelial dysplasia:* Human papillomavirus 16 causes cervical intraepithelial dysplasia. The

Table 1.8: Differences between metaplasia and dysplasia

Features	Metaplasia	Dysplasia
Definition	The transformation of one type of cell (epithelial or mesenchymal) into another adult cell type known as *metaplasia*	Disordered cell growth may or may not progress to cancer
Pleomorphism	Absent	Present
Nuclei	Normal	Hyperchromatic and large
Mitotic figures	Very less	More mitotic figures
Architecture of cells in tissues	Architecture is not lost	Loss of ordered maturation
Reversible/irreversible	Reversible, if stimuli are removed	Irreversible change, if whole thickness involved
Role	Adaptive change	Not adaptive change
Examples	Ciliated columnar to squamous metaplasia in trachea and bronchi (smoking)	Cervical dysplasia due to human papillomavirus 16
	Columnar to squamous metaplasia due to stones in the ducts of salivary gland, pancreas and biliary system; and vitamin A deficiency	Dysplasia of the bronchus due to cigarette smoking causing squamous metaplasia progressing to squamous dysplasia
	Squamous to columnar metaplasia in Barrett's esophagus caused by chronic irritation by gastric juices in gastroesophageal reflux	Skin dysplasia due to exposure to sun ultraviolet light causing skin dysplasia
	Transitional to squamous metaplasia of urinary bladder due to trauma	On light microscopy, showing increased nuclear size and chromatin showing mitotic activity, with normal spindles. The cells arranged in disordered fashion with loss of cell maturation as cells progress to the surface
	Fibrocollagenous tissue to osseous metaplasia in myositis ossifcans	
	Tumor metaplasia (adenosquamous cell carcinoma, stromal mucinous metaplasia in pleomorphic adenoma, and squamous or osseous metaplasia in breast carcinoma)	

Cellular Adaptations, Cell Injury, Apoptosis, Pigments, Calcification, Cellular Accumulations and Aging

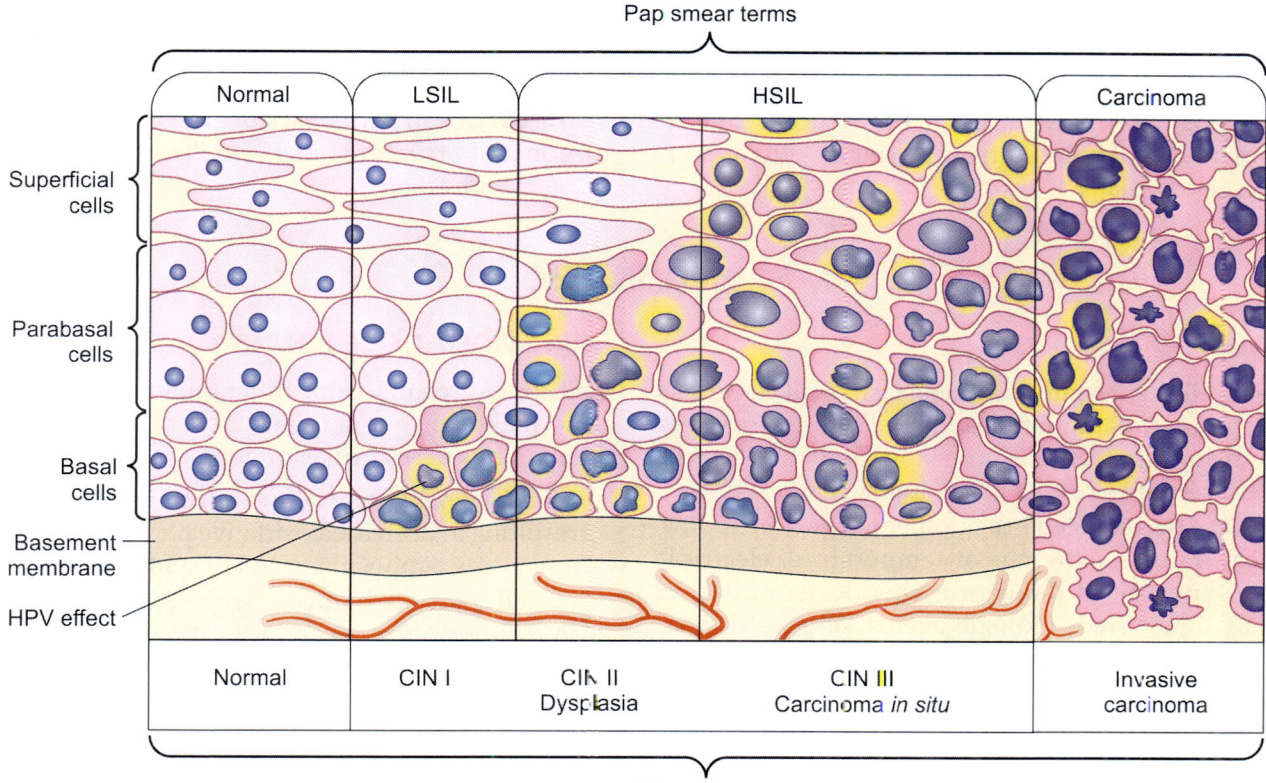

Fig. 1.13: Development of cervical intraepithelial neoplasia (CIN I, CIN II, CIN III) and invasive cervical carcinoma.

distinction between severe dysplasia and early cancer of the cervix is a common diagnostic problem for the pathologist (Figs 1.13 and 1.14).

- *Dysplasia in bronchial epithelium:* Tobacco smoking produces dysplasia in respiratory epithelium. It is potentially reversible if the patient stops smoking. It may progress to bronchogenic carcinoma in heavy tobacco smokers.
- *Skin dysplasia:* Exposure to sun ultraviolet light causes skin dysplasia.
- *Actinic keratosis:* It is a form of dysplasia in *sun-exposed skin*. Histologic examination reveals atypical cells, varying in size and shape. These cells show no signs of regular maturation as the cells move from the basal layer of the epidermis to the surface.

REDUCTION IN SIZE OF ORGANS IN OTHER PATHOLOGICAL PROCESSES

Pathological processes other than atrophy associated with reduced organ size include agenesis, aplasia and hypoplasia.

Agenesis

Agenesis refers to absence of organ resulting from failure to develop during embryonic development (e.g. renal agenesis). Renal agenesis differs from atrophy, in which a decrease in the size of an organ results from a decrease in pre-existing cells. Bilateral renal agenesis is incompatible with life. Unilateral renal agenesis causes compensatory hypertrophy of opposite kidney.

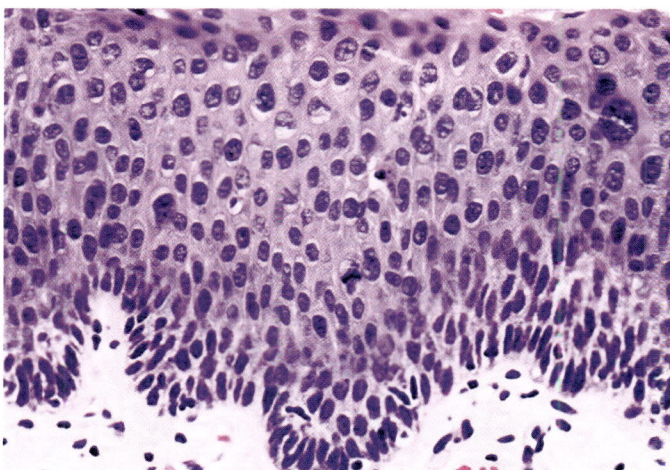

Fig. 1.14: CIN III (cervical intraepithelial neoplasia). This is cervical squamous dysplasia at high magnification extending from the center to the right. The epithelium is normal at the left. Note how the dysplastic cell nuclei are larger and darker, and the dysplastic cells have a disorderly arrangement (400X).

Aplasia

Aplasia refers to failure of cell production. During fetal development, there is no development of adrenal cortex. During postnatal period, aplasia may occur due to permanent loss of bone marrow precursor cells as seen in aplastic anemia.

Hypoplasia

Hypoplasia refers to incomplete development of an organ due to decrease in cell production. It may also occur due to partial lack of growth and maturation of gonadal structures in *Klinefelter's* syndrome and *Turner* syndrome.

CELL INJURY

OVERVIEW

Normal cell is in a state of homeostasis. Cell continues to function by adaptation despite mild to severe stress through its life. Cellular stress beyond the level of adaptive response results in cell injury.

Cells can be damaged in a number of ways, including physical trauma, extremes of temperature, electrical injury, exposure to damaging chemicals, radiation damage, injury from biologic agents, and nutritional factors.

Most injurious agents exert their damaging effects through uncontrolled free radical production, impaired oxygen delivery or utilization, or the destructive effects of uncontrolled intracellular calcium release.

CAUSES OF CELL INJURY

Cell injury depends on cellular response to (a) injurious stimuli, i.e. (type, duration and severity of injury), (b) ability of the tissues to regenerate, e.g. (labile or dividing cells/stable cells/permanent cells), (c) metabolic needs of cell, (d) adaptability of cell, and (e) genetic constitution. Following mechanisms are responsible for cell injury. Cell injury may result from several intrinsic or extrinsic causes shown in Table 1.9.

MAIN TARGETS OF CELL INJURY

Cell injury results from functional and biochemical abnormalities in one or more of several essential cellular components described as under:

- *Mitochondria:* Hypoxia first affects the mitochondria resulting in decreased oxidative phosphorylation and adenosine triphosphate (ATP) synthesis.

  Cell injury is induced, when ATP production in mitochondria reduces to 5–10% of normal levels. Anaerobic glycolysis occurs with loss of glycogen, accumulation of lactic acid, acid pH which interferes with enzymes.

- *Cell membranes:* Injury adversely affects cell membranes such as plasma membranes, mitochondrial, lysosomal and other organelle membranes. Ionic and osmotic homeostasis of the cell and its organelles depend on cell membranes.

  There is reduced sodium pump function leading to influx of sodium and water; and efflux of potassium. Failure of the calcium pump leads to influx of Ca^{++} into the cell, activate various enzymes causing damage to the cell. Myelin fibers are derived from damaged membranes of mitochondria, or rough endoplasmic reticulum and plasma membrane.

Table 1.9: Causes of cell injury

Parameters	Causes
Infectious agents	Bacteria, viruses, parasites and fungi
Hypoxia	Myocardial infarction due to atherosclerosis of coronary arteries
	Gangrene intestine
Ischemia	Cardiopulmonary failure (hypotension, shock)
Physical injury	Burn, trauma, severe cold, radiation
Chemical injury	Mercury, cyanide, arsenic, carbon monoxide poisoning; acid or alkali induced burns
Drug induced injury	Drugs toxicity
Immunologic injury	Anaphylactic reaction, autoimmune diseases
Nutritional injury	Protein energy malnutrition (marasmus, Kwashiorkor)
	Vitamin A deficiency

- *Rough endoplasmic reticulum:* Injury to rough endoplasmic reticulum leads to decreased synthesis of protein due to detachment of ribosomes. Increased intracellular calcium and reactive oxygen species adversely affect endoplasmic reticulum leading to decreased protein synthesis. Misfolded proteins lead to the unfolded protein response which may further injure the cell.
- *Cytoskeleton:* Injury may cause damage to cytoskeleton. Blebs are observed on cell surface, most likely caused by disorderly function of the cellular cytoskeleton.
- *Genetic apparatus:* Injury may cause damage to DNA. Increased intracellular calcium and reactive oxygen species cause DNA damage.

TYPES OF CELL INJURY

Depending on severity of cell injury, various cellular changes occur. Differences between reversible and irreversible cell injury are shown in Table 1.10.

Subcellular and Cellular Alterations

These are characterized by intracellular accumulation of biomolecules and calcium.

Reversible Cell Injury

Reversible cell injury is acute sub-lethal injury to cytoplasmic organelles sparing nucleus. It affects metabolically active cells of *liver, heart and kidneys.* Swelling of mitochondria, organelles, glycogen depletion, cell blebs and myelin figures is signs of reversible injury.

Blebs are observed on cell surface, most likely caused by disorderly function of the cellular cytoskeleton. Myelin figures are derived from damaged membranes of mitochondria, or rough endoplasmic reticulum and the plasma membrane; demonstrated in cytoplasm on electron microscopy. Examples of reversible cell injury are hydropic change and fatty change in organs.

Irreversible Cell Injury

Irreversible cell injury is characterized by necrosis/cell death. Lipid peroxidation is often a feature of irreversible cell injury.

- *Nuclear changes*: Pyknosis, karyorrhexis, and karyolysis are signs of cell death.
- *Blebs:* These are observed on cell surface, most likely caused by disorderly function of the cellular cytoskeleton.
- *Myelin figures:* These are derived from damaged membranes of mitochondria, or rough endoplasmic reticulum and the plasma membrane; demonstrated in cytoplasm on electron microscopy.

These myelin figures first appear during the reversible stage and become more pronounced in irreversibly damaged cells. Pathophysiology of reversible and irreversible cell injury is shown in Fig. 1.15.

Ischemic/Reperfusion Injury

Ischemic/reperfusion injury is a common clinical problem that arises in occlusive cardiovascular disease, infection, transplantation, shock, and many other circumstances.

If cells are reversibly injured due to ischemia, complete recovery occurs following restoration of blood flow. However, reperfusion can result in more damage including cell death.

During ischemia, cellular damage generates oxygen derived free radicals. On reestablishment of blood flow (reperfusion), abundant molecular oxygen (O_2) is available, which combines with free radicals to form reactive oxygen species. Oxygen derived free radicals are formed inside cells through the xanthine oxidase pathway and released from activated neutrophils.

Table 1.10: Differences between reversible cell injury and irreversible cell injury

Features	Reversible cell injury	Irreversible cell injury
Cell swelling	Moderate	Marked
Cell membrane changes	Aggregation of intramembraneous particles	Defects in cell membrane
Myelin fibers (laminated structures)	Derived from damaged plasma membrane and organelles (less pronounced)	Derived from damaged plasma membrane and organelles (more pronounced)
Endoplasmic reticulum (ER)	Swelling of ER	Lysis of ER and detachment of ribosomes
Mitochondrial changes	Moderate	Marked
Mitochondrial densities	Small size densities (amorphous) derived from proteins and calcium deposition	Large size densities derived from proteins and calcium deposition
Lysosomal changes	Autophagy by lysosomes	Autolysis by rupture of lysosomes
Nuclear changes	Clumping of nuclear chromatin	Pyknosis, karyorrhexis and karyolysis
Examples	Hydropic change, fatty change in liver	Necrosis (myocardial infarction)

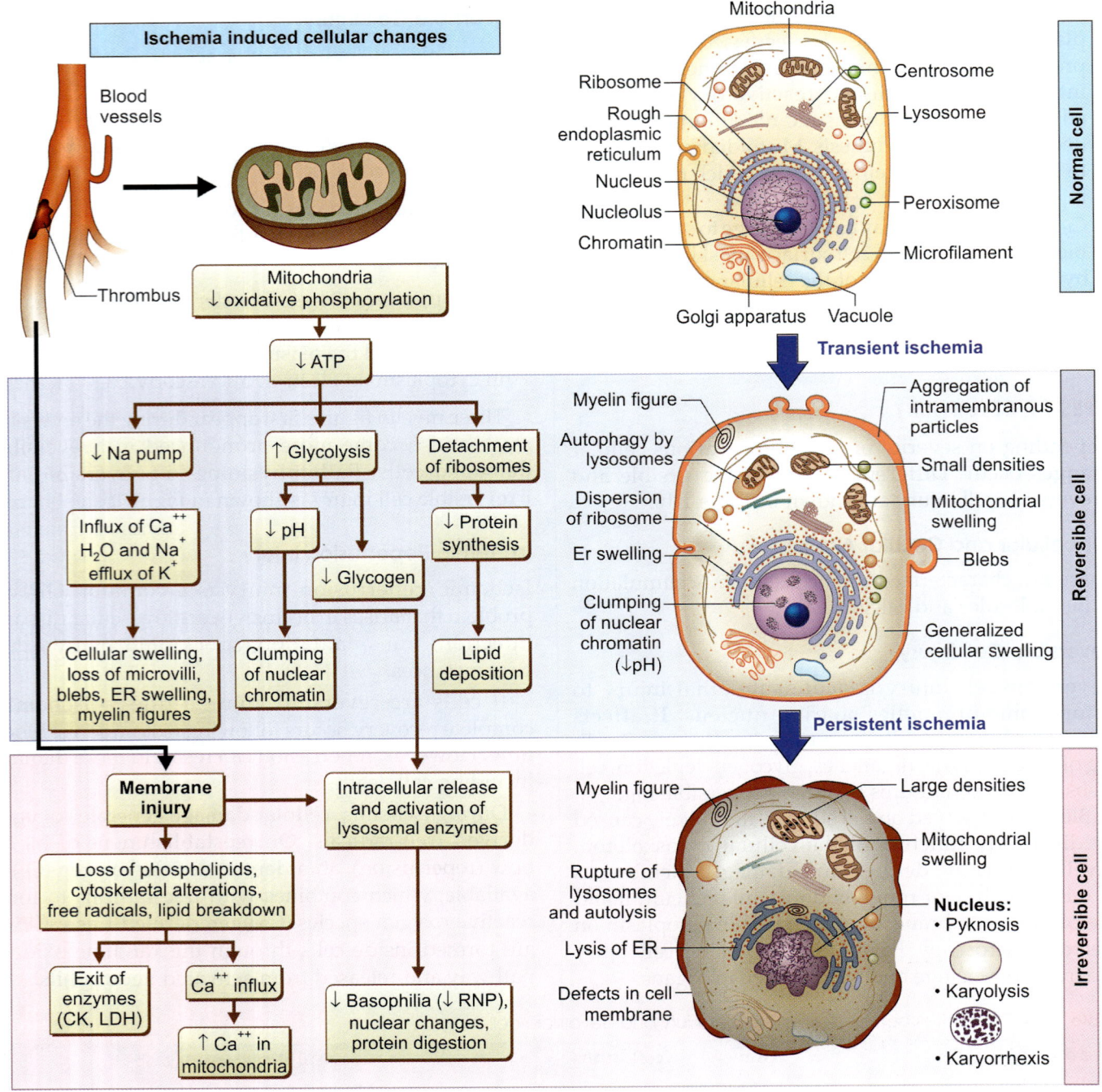

Fig. 1.15: Pathophysiology of reversible and irreversible cell injury.

Apoptosis

Apoptosis is genetically programmed pathway of programmed cell death. Increased intracellular calcium triggers the release of intracellular apoptotic signals by injured cell.

Apoptosis occurs by two mechanisms, e.g. signals initiating apoptosis by acting caspases and gene regulating proteins.

Necroptosis

Necroptosis is hybrid of necrosis and apoptosis. It is a *programmed cell death without activation of caspases*. It shows cell swelling, cell membrane damage, increased lysosomal permeability and signs of inflammation.

- *TNFR1 is activated by tumor necrosis-α.* It leads to recruitment of RIP1, RIP3 and other proteins to form complex comprising of RIP, RIP3 and caspase 8.

- *Caspase 8 is not activated* in this process. Necroptosis plays important role in *ischemic brain injury* and *neurodegenerative disorders*.

Pyroptosis

Pyroptosis is form of programmed cell death associated with antimicrobial response during inflammation (innate immune response).

VULNERABILITY OF CELLS TO ISCHEMIC INJURY

Ischemic injury depends on the type of cells or tissues undergoing ischemic necrosis (Table 1.11).

Nervous System

Complete interruption of blood supply to brain causes irreversible damage to neurons within 3–5 minutes. Cerebellum's Purkinje cells and hippocampus area are more susceptible to ischemic injury.

Myocardium and Liver

Ischemic necrosis of myocardial cells and hepatocytes cause irreversible cell death within 1–2 hours.

Skeletal Muscles

Ischemic necrosis of skeletal muscle cells causes irreversible cell death within many hours.

REVERSIBLE CELL INJURY

Reversible cell injury is acute sub-lethal injury to cytoplasmic organelles sparing nucleus. It affects metabolically active cells of liver, heart and kidneys. Swelling of mitochondria, organelles, glycogen depletion, cell blebs and myelin figures are signs of reversible injury.

DECREASED ATP PRODUCTION

ATP depletion occurs due to reduced supply of oxygen and nutrients to the cells. It also occurs due to mitochondrial damage and chemical toxins (cyanide). Hypoxia first affects the mitochondria resulting in decreased oxidative phosphorylation and adenosine triphosphate (ATP) synthesis. Cell injury is induced, when ATP production in mitochondria reduces to 5–10% of normal levels.

FAILURE OF Na^+/K^+ ATPASE PUMP

Under physiological state, membrane Na^+/K^+ pumps (Oubain-sensitive sodium and potassium ATPase) that are responsible for maintaining relatively high potassium and low levels of sodium concentration within cells are dependent on an adequate supply of ATP. Cell membrane permeability is increased due to depletion of ATP.

Swelling of Cell

Decreased availability of ATP results in failure of the $Na^+ K^+$ ATPase pump. It causes *influx of sodium ions* along with water into cell. *Potassium diffuses out of cell*. These changes cause *swelling of endoplasmic reticulum* as well as hydropic change in cytoplasm of cells.

Exchange of H^+ and Na^+

When intracellular acidosis threatens cell due to anaerobic glycolysis, it pumps out H^+ of the cell in exchange of Na^+ to maintain proper intracellular pH.

FAILURE OF ATP-DEPENDENT CALCIUM PUMP

Influx of calcium: Under physiologic state, excess intracellular Ca^{++} is extruded by a calcium pump that is ATP-dependent. Increased sodium inhibits efflux of calcium due to activation of sodium/calcium exchanger. It leads to excessive accumulation of calcium in the cell resulting in mitochondrial dysfunction.

CELL BLEBS FORMATION

Blebs are observed on cell surface, most likely caused by disorderly function of the cellular cytoskeleton.

MYELIN FIGURES

Myelin figures are derived from damaged membranes of mitochondria, rough endoplasmic reticulum and the plasma membrane; demonstrated in cytoplasm on electron microscopy.

Examples of reversible cell injury are *hydropic change*, *fatty change* and *hyaline change* in organs discussed as under.

Table 1.11: Vulnerability of cells (organs) to ischemic irreversible cell injury

Organs	Cells/Tissues	Duration of irreversible injury
Nervous system	Neurons (cerebellum's Purkinje cells and hippocampus area most susceptible to injury)	3–5 minutes
Heart	Myocardium	20–30 minutes
Liver	Hepatocytes	1–2 hours
Skeletal muscle	Skeletal muscle fibers	Many hours
Fibrous tissue	Fibroblasts	Resistant to ischemic changes

Hydropic Change

Hydropic change is acute sublethal reversible cell injury characterized by accumulation of fluid in cytoplasm resulting in pale and swollen cytoplasm.

- *Etiology:* Hydropic change is caused by *hypoxia, chemical poisoning, biologic toxins and chemical agents*.
- *Mechanism:* These injurious agents cause hydropic swelling by (i) *increasing the permeability of the plasma membrane to sodium*, (ii) *damaging the membrane sodium-potassium ATPase (pump)*, and (iii) *interfering with the synthesis of ATP*, thereby depriving the pump of its fuel.

  Accumulation of sodium in the cell leads to an increase in water content to maintain isosmotic conditions, and the cell then swells.

Fatty Change

Fatty change is also known as *fatty metamorphosis* or *steatosis*. It is acute sublethal reversible cell injury characterized by accumulation of lipid droplets as a result of disturbance of ribosomal function and uncoupling of lipid from protein metabolism. Moderate degree of fatty change is reversible, but severe fatty change may not be reversible. Fatty change is observed most frequently in the *liver, heart,* and *kidney*.

Etiology

Fatty change may be secondary to *alcoholism, diabetes mellitus, malnutrition, obesity, or carbon tetrachloride poisoning*. It results from an imbalance *between the uptake, utilization, and mobilization of fat from liver cells*. Alcoholic fatty liver may be reversible with complete abstinence from alcohol.

Mechanism

Fatty change in liver can result from any of the mechanisms: (i) increased transport of triglycerides in hepatocytes, (ii) decreased mobilization of fat from liver due to decreased synthesis of transporting apolipoproteins, (iii) decreased utilization of fat by the cells, and (iv) increased concentration of lipoproteins in cells.

Fatty change is thus linked to the disaggregation of ribosomes and consequent decreased protein synthesis caused by failure of ATP production in CCl_4 induced injured cells. Mechanism of fatty change liver is shown in Fig. 1.16.

Hyaline Change

This term *hyaline change* denotes a characteristic *homogeneous, glassy,* and *eosinophilic appearance* in hematoxylin and eosin sections. It is caused most often by nonspecific accumulations of proteinaceous material.

Alcohol
- Mobilization of fatty acids from peripheral tissue
- Altering mitochondrial and smooth endoplasmic reticulum leading to inhibit fatty acids oxidation
- Decreasing synthesis of lipoprotein synthesis

Diabetes mellitus
- Increased lipoprotein lipase
- Mobilization of FFA

Increased intake of fats (obesity)

Decreased uptake of fats (genetically inherited hyperlipidemias)

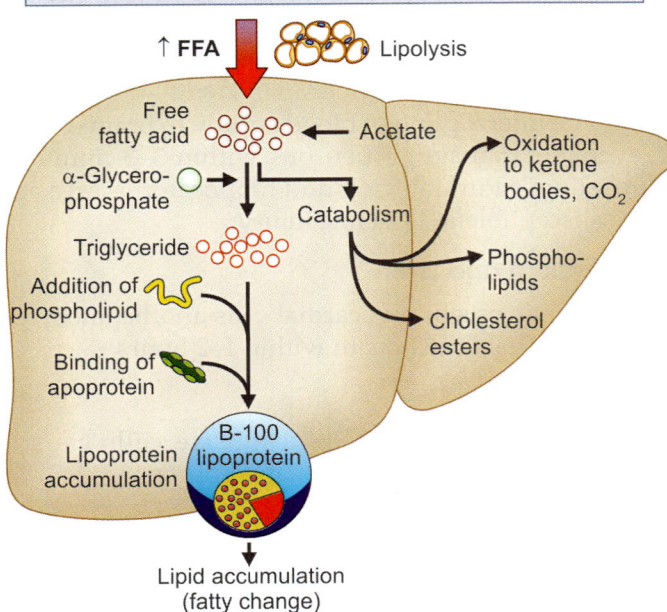

Fig. 1.16: Mechanism of fatty change liver. It occurs due to increased transport of triglycerides in hepatocytes, decreased mobilization of fat from liver due to decreased synthesis of transporting apolipoproteins, decreased utilization of fat by the cells and increased concentration of lipoproteins in cells.

IRREVERSIBLE CELL INJURY

Persistent severe cell injury transforms reversible into irreversible cell injury. It is characterized by necrosis/cell death. Lipid peroxidation and nuclear changes such as pyknosis, karyorrhexis, and karyolysis are signs of irreversible cell injury (cell death).

Light Microscopy

On light microscopy, cellular outlines in irreversible cell injury are maintained with loss of structural details.

Hematoxylin and eosin stained section shows intense cytoplasmic eosinophilia of dead cell due to loss of cytoplasmic RNA and denaturation (coagulation) of proteins. Loss of basophilia is a sign of cell injury, indicating a cessation of protein synthesis.

Mechanism

- *Plasma membrane damage:* It occurs due to prolonged ischemia, mechanical disruption, chemical agents, infectious agents, complement components and phospholipase activation and free radical injury.
- *Defects in cell membranes:* Defects in plasma membrane and membranes of cell organelles (mitochondria and lysosomes) leads to decreased phospholipid synthesis, increased breakdown of phospholipids and cytoskeleton abnormality.
- *Mitochondrial damage:* It leads to depletion of ATP and influx of calcium. Oxidative stress leads to accumulation of oxygen-derived free radicals. DNA damage caused by ionizing radiation, chemotherapy and free radicals adversely affects endoplasmic reticulum to synthesize proteins (Table 1.12).

Cellular Proteins in Blood

In irreversible cell injury, intracellular enzymes and proteins released from the dead cells into the blood circulation are used as diagnostic parameters.

- *Myocardial infarction:* Creatine kinase-MB fraction enzyme and cardiac troponins are estimated in patients with myocardial infarction.
- *Liver cell necrosis:* Liver cell necrosis releases enzymes (*transaminases, alkaline phosphatase and glutamyltransferase*) and enter blood circulation, which are estimated.
- *Skeletal muscle injury:* Creatine kinase levels are increased in cardiac and skeletal muscle injury.

Sequence of Events

Sequence of events in irreversible cell injury are described as under.

DEPLETION OF ATP PRODUCTION

Physiological state: Under physiological state, adenosine triphosphate (ATP) synthesized by mitochondria-oxidative phosphorylation is required for synthetic and degradation processes.

Pathological state: Persistent ischemia or chemical cyanide cause mitochondrial damage affecting adversely ATP production due to failure of oxidative phosphorylation. Cell injury is induced, when ATP production in mitochondria reduces to 5–10% of normal levels. Decreased ATP production due to persistent hypoxia produces following cellular changes as described under:

- *Failure of oxidative phosphorylation in mitochondria:* Interruption in blood supply due to atherosclerosis and blood loss decreases the delivery of O_2 and glucose to the cells. Ischemia impairs mitochondrial

Table 1.12: Mechanism of irreversible injury

Mechanism	Effects on cell membranes	Cellular changes
Loss of selective membrane permeability due to depletion of ATP and activation of phospholipases	Plasma membrane	Influx of fluid and ions
	Mitochondrial membrane	Influx of fluid and ions
	Lysosomal membrane	Lysosomes releasing enzymes
	Mitochondrial damage leading formation of pores in its membrane	Causing leakage of mitochondrial cytochrome 'c' from mitochondrial pore, which may trigger apoptotic pathway resulting in cell death
		Increased intracellular calcium level triggering activation of cellular enzymes resulting in irreversible injury
	ATP depletion produce multiple cellular effects	Failure of sodium pump causing influx of sodium ions along with water into cell. Potassium diffusing out of cell
		Failure of calcium pump causing damage to cellular components
		Disruption of protein synthesis due to detachment of ribosomes from rough endoplasmic reticulum
		Increased rate of anaerobic glycolysis leading to accumulation of lactic acid and decrease in intracellular pH resulting in inactivation of enzymes
		Membrane misfolding leading to cell injury and death
Accumulation of free radicals	Cellular reduction of oxygen leads to accumulation of oxygen derived free radicals	Oxygen derived free radicals causing lipid peroxidation of cell membranes, protein fragmentation as a result of oxidation of amino acids residue side chain, and DNA breaks

electron transport, thereby decreasing ATP synthesis due to failure of oxidative phosphorylation. It leads to increase in adenosine monophosphate and adenosine diphosphate (ADP).

- *Failure of Na$^+$/K$^+$ pump:* Depletion of ATP leads to influx of sodium, water and calcium, efflux of potassium ions, swelling of endoplasmic reticulum and loss of microvilli resulting in blebs formation.
- *Failure of calcium pump:* ATP depletion causes failure of calcium pump across the plasma membrane. Increased sodium inhibits efflux of calcium due to activation of sodium/calcium exchanger. It leads to excessive accumulation of calcium in the cell resulting in *mitochondrial dysfunction*.
- *Increased anaerobic glycolysis:* ATP depletion leads to overproduction of lactic acid due to increased activities of phosphofructokinase and phosphorylase.

    Mitochondria fail to oxidize lactic acid to pyruvate. Instead pyruvate is reduced to lactate in cytosol, and its accumulation in the cytosol lowers the intracellular pH resulting in clumping of nuclear chromatin.
- *Detachment of ribosomes:* Decreased ATP production cause detachment of ribosomes leading to decreased protein synthesis.
- *Lipid deposition:* Decreased ATP production leads to increased lipid deposition.

FAILURE OF NA$^+$ AND K$^+$ ATPASE

Physiological state: Adequate supply of ATP is essential to maintain high potassium and low sodium levels in cell with membrane Na$^+$/K$^+$ pumps (Oubain-sensitive sodium and potassium ATPase).

Pathological state: Due to decreased ATP production, cellular swelling and increased cytosolic calcium occurs.

- *Swelling of cell:* Cell membrane permeability is increased due to depletion of ATP generation. Decreased availability of ATP results in failure of the Na$^+$ K$^+$ ATPase pump.

    It causes influx of sodium ions along with water into cell. Potassium diffuses out of cell. These changes cause swelling of endoplasmic reticulum as well as hydropic change in cytoplasm of cells.
- *Exchange of H$^+$ and Na$^+$:* When intracellular acidosis threatens cell due to anaerobic glycolysis, it pumps out cellular hydrogen ions in exchange of sodium to maintain proper intracellular pH. Increased intracellular sodium level activates the sodium/calcium exchanger, thereby enhancing calcium accumulation inside cell and mitochondrial dysfunction.

FAILURE OF CALCIUM PUMP

Under physiological state, cytosolic calcium is maintained at extremely low levels by energy dependent transport in a normal cell. Excess intracellular Ca^{++} is extruded by a calcium pump that is ATP dependent.

Pathological State

Under pathological state, ATP depletion causes failure of calcium pump across the plasma membrane. Increased sodium inhibits efflux of calcium due to activation of sodium/calcium exchanger.

It leads to excessive accumulation of calcium in the cell resulting in mitochondrial dysfunction. Influx of calcium to the cytosol comes from the extracellular fluid and stores in mitochondria and endoplasmic reticulum.

Significance of Calcium Influx in Cytoplasm

Increased level of free calcium in the cytosol causes extensive calcification of mitochondria and activates intracellular enzymes resulting in damage to cellular components and finally cell death. Following cellular enzymes are activated by increased cytosolic calcium level (Fig. 1.17).

- *Activation of phospholipases:* High cytosolic calcium activates phospholipases, which degrades the membrane phospholipids releasing free fatty acids as well as lysophospholipids.

    These are *potent mediators of inflammation*. These also act as detergent that *solubilize cell membrane*. It results in decreased synthesis of phospholipids of all cellular membranes of including mitochondria.
- *Activation of proteases:* High cytosolic calcium also activates a series of proteases that *attack the cytoskeleton* and its attachments to the cell membrane. As the interactions between cytoskeleton proteins and the plasma membrane are disrupted, it leads to formation of membrane blebs, and alteration of shape of the cell.
- *Activation of ATPase:* High cytosolic calcium activates of ATPase, resulting in ATP depletion.
- *Activation of endonuclease:* Activation of endonuclease causes fragmentation of DNA.

Cellular Adaptations, Cell Injury, Apoptosis, Pigments, Calcification, Cellular Accumulations and Aging

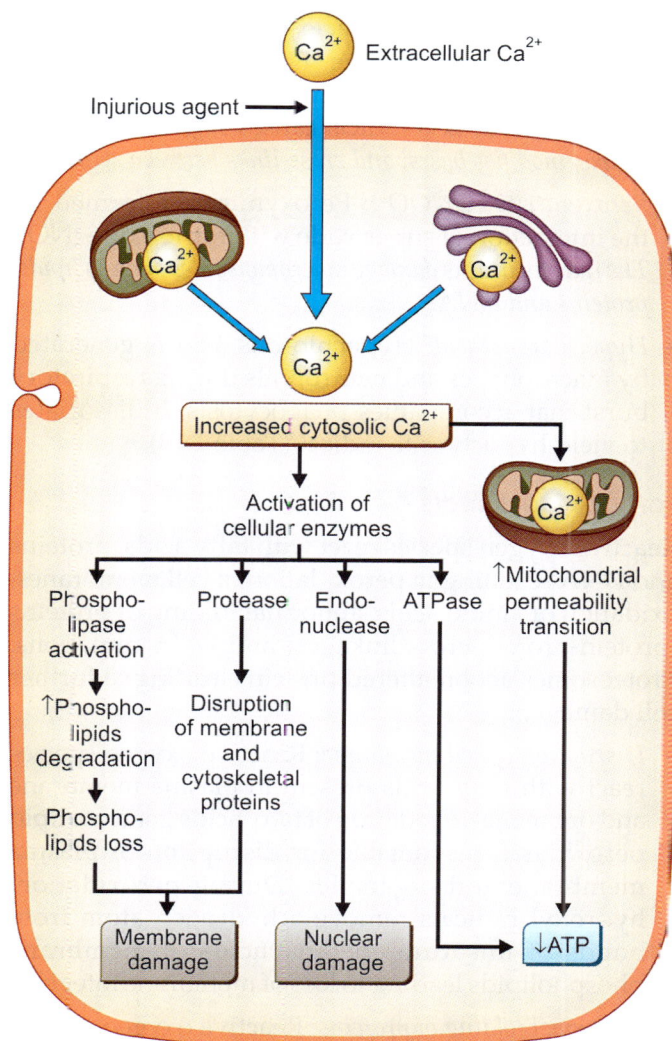

Fig. 1.17: Role of increased cytosolic calcium in pathogenesis of cell injury. Increased cytosolic calcium activating cellular enzymes resulting to membrane and nuclear damage.

MITOCHONDRIAL DYSFUNCTION

In normal cells the *mitochondrial permeability transition pore (MPTP)* opens and closes sporadically.

Pathological state: Prolonged mitochondrial injury leads to sustained opening of MPTP and release of *mitochondrial cytochrome-c* from electron transport chain in cytosol.

This process further diminishes ATP synthesis. Under certain circumstances, it may also trigger apoptotic pathway resulting in cell death.

DISRUPTION OF PROTEIN SYNTHESIS

Mitochondrial and lysosomal damage leads to detachment of ribosomes from rough endoplasmic reticulum. Rough endoplasmic reticulum is the first ultrastructural changes seen in irreversible cell injury. Intense eosinophilia of dead cell occurs due to loss of RNA and coagulation of proteins. Cellular outlines are well preserved.

INCREASED RATE OF ANAEROBIC GLYCOLYSIS

Anaerobic glycolysis leads to accumulation of lactic acid and decrease in intracellular pH resulting in inactivation of enzymes.

ROLE OF REACTIVE OXYGEN SPECIES

Physiological state: Free radicals have a single unpaired electron in the outer orbit. During normal cellular respiration, about 3% of the oxygen entering the mitochondrial electron transport chain is reduced to generate oxygen derived free radicals.

- *Oxygen derived* free radicals produce highly reactive oxygen species, *superoxide, hydroxyl radicals, H_2O_2*. In addition to oxygen-derived free radicals, nitric oxide (NO) can act as a free radical and be converted to an even more reactive anion.
- *Copper and iron catalyze* to form free radical leading to generation of reactive oxygen species.
- *Protective molecules* include *superoxide dismutase, glutathione peroxidase, vitamin E, vitamin C and catalase*.

Pathological state: When reactive oxygen species are produced in excess, they react with, and damage proteins, lipids, carbohydrates, nucleic acids. These damaged molecules may themselves be reactive species with a chain reaction being set up with widespread damage. During pathological state, oxidative stress to cell leads to generation of reactive oxygen species by following mechanisms:

- *Injurious stimulus:* Inflammation, ionization radiation, chemical agents and reperfusion injury generate reactive oxygen species such as *superoxide anionic radical, H_2O_2 and hydroxyl radical* in the target cells.
- *Generation of reactive oxygen species:* O_2 is converted to reactive oxygen species by oxidative enzymes present in the mitochondria (respiratory enzymes), peroxisome (peroxisome oxidase) and endoplasmic reticulum (cytochrome P450). During ischemia, reactive oxygen species generation is increased due to damage to electron transport chain and reduced activity of superoxide dismutase (SOD). Induction of free radicals cause additional free radicals formation in an autocatalytic chain reaction (called *propagation*).
- *Accumulation of reactive oxygen species:* Oxidative stress leads to accumulation of reactive oxygen species in the cells.

Reactive Oxygen Species

- *Superoxide anion:* Superoxide anion is generated by leaks in the electron transport chain, which is then converted to H_2O_2, eventually to other ROS. It does not readily diffuse far from its origin.

- *Hydrogen peroxide:* Under physiological state, superoxide dismutase derived from cytoplasm and mitochondria participates in generation of hydrogen peroxide in small concentration. Hydrogen peroxide is converted to water by catalase within peroxisomes and glutathione peroxidase in both the cytosol and the mitochondria.

    Under pathological state, hydrogen peroxide forms oxygen derived free radicals via Fe^{++} catalyzed *Fenton reaction*. When hydrogen peroxide is produced in excess, it is converted to *highly reactive hydroxyl radicals*. In neutrophils, myeloperoxidase transforms hydrogen peroxide to the potent radical hypochlorite, which is lethal for microorganisms and cells.

- *Hydroxyl radicals:* During physiological state, hydroxyl radicals are formed by the hydrolysis of water, the reaction of H_2O_2 with ferrous ions (the Fenton reaction), and the reaction of O_2^- with H_2O_2 (Haber-Weiss reaction).

    Under pathological state hydroxyl radical is the most reactive intracellular molecule of reactive oxygen species (ROS) responsible for attack on macromolecules. During peroxidation, hydroxyl radicals remove a hydrogen atom from bonds of unsaturated fatty acids of membrane phospholipids leading to loss of membrane integrity.

    Hydroxyl radicals cause *lipid peroxidation, oxidative damage to proteins* by cross-linking of amino acids, (sulfur containing amino acids—cysteine and methionine, as well as arginine, histidine, and proline), fragmentation of polypeptide chains and DNA damage. Hydroxyl radical causes *single DNA strand breaks, modifies bases, and cross-links between strands*.

- *Peroxynitrite ($ONOO^-$):* Peroxynitrite is formed by the interaction of superoxide with nitric oxide (NO). *The radical attacks damage macromolecules such as lipids, proteins and DNA.*

- *Hypochlorous acid:* Hypochlorous acid is generated by macrophages and neutrophils during respiratory burst that accompanies phagocytosis. It dissociates to yield hypochlorite radical (Table 1.13).

Pathological Effects

Reactive oxygen species react with fatty acids, proteins and DNA resulting in peroxidation of cell membranes, oxidation of amino acids, abnormal folding of proteins (protein-protein cross linkages) and DNA mutations. Proteosomes act on altered proteins leading to further cell damage.

- *Disruption of cell membrane:* Reactive oxygen species react with fatty acids present in plasma membrane and organelles. Oxidation of fatty acids generate lipid peroxidases responsible for disruption of plasma membrane and organelles. During peroxidation, hydroxyl radicals remove a hydrogen atom from bonds of unsaturated fatty acids of membrane phospholipids leading to loss of membrane integrity.

- *Abnormal folding of proteins:* Reactive oxygen species adversely affects rough endoplasmic reticulum leading to decreased synthesis of proteins. Protein fragmentation occurs as a result of oxidation of amino

Table 1.13: Reactions involving reactive oxygen metabolites produced by phagocytic cells

Reactive oxygen metabolites	Generation by reactions	Actions
Hydroxyl radical (OH)	Fenton reaction $Fe^{2+} + H_2O_2 \rightarrow Fe^{3+} + OH^- + OH$ Haber-Weiss reaction $O_2^- + H^+ + H_2O_2 \rightarrow O_2 + H_2O_2 + OH$	Hydroxyl radical attacking cellular macromolecules
Hydrogen peroxide	Superoxide dismutase by Fenton reaction	Diffusing within cells
Superoxide anion	Reduction of molecular oxygen by leaks in the electron transport chain	Not diffusing far from its origin
Peroxynitrite (ONOO)	$NO + O_2^- \rightarrow (ONOO.)$	Damaging macromolecules
Lipid peroxide radical (RCOO.)	Generated during lipid peroxidation	Initiating chain breakage, destroying unsaturated fatty acids resulting in a loss of membrane integrity
Hypochlorous acid (HOCl)	Generated by neutrophils (myeloperoxidase) and macrophages during respiratory burst that accompanying phagocytosis	Dissociating to yield hypochlorite radical

acids residue side chain by reactive oxygen species. Oxidation of proteins lead to loss of enzymatic activity and abnormal folding of proteins.

- *DNA damage:* Reactive oxygen species react and cause oxidation of DNA leading to mutations and DNA breaks. Role of cellular enzymes in generation and removal of reactive oxygen species are shown in Table 1.14.

Conditions Generating Activated Oxygen Species

Conditions generating activated oxygen species (O_2^-, H_2O_2 and $-OH$) are shown in Table 1.15.

- *Ionizing radiation (X-rays):* These can hydrolyze H_2O into hydroxyl (OH^-) and hydrogen (H^+) free radicals.
- *Enzymatic metabolism of chemicals (CCl_4)/drugs (barbiturates):* These toxic products (CCl_4 as well as barbiturates) cause proliferation of smooth endoplasmic reticulum. These also induce P450 oxidase system of smooth endoplasmic reticulum of hepatocytes.
- *Reperfusion cell injury:* Free radicals generated as a result of reperfusion can cause damage to normal cells by generation of free radicals.
- *Nitric oxide (NO):* Nitric oxide can act directly as a free radical or be converted to other highly reactive forms (Fig. 1.18).

Degradation of O_2 Derived Free Radicals

Fortunately free radicals are inherently unstable and generally decay spontaneously. Antioxidants either block the initiation of free radical formation or scavenge free radicals. In addition, several systems, i.e. detoxifying enzymes, antioxidants and transporting proteins contribute to free radical inactivation. Mechanism of inactivation of reactive oxygen species is shown in Table 1.16.

CYTOSKELETON ABNORMALITIES

Cytoskeleton filaments serve as anchors connecting the plasma membrane to the cell interior.

- *Activation of proteases* by increased cytosolic Ca^{++} may cause damage to elements of the cytoskeleton.
- *Increased cytosolic* Ca^{++} activates proteases, which cause damage to the elements of cytoskeleton, e.g. thin actin filaments, thick myosin filaments, microtubules and intermediate filaments. Intermediate filaments include *keratin filaments, neurofilaments, desmin filaments, vimentin filaments and glial filaments*.

LIPID BREAKDOWN PRODUCTS

During lipid peroxidation, hydroxyl radicals remove a hydrogen atom from the unsaturated fatty acids of membrane phospholipids.

Table 1.14: Role of cellular enzymes in generation and removal of reactive oxygen species

Cell organelle	Oxidative enzymes participating in generation reactive oxygen species	Removal of reactive oxygen species (antioxidant mechanism)
Mitochondria	Respiratory enzymes	Superoxide dismutase (SOD) in mitochondria converting oxygen to hydrogen peroxide
		Glutathione converting hydroxyl ion to hydrogen peroxide
Cytosolic peroxisome	Peroxisome oxidase	Catalase in peroxisome converting hydrogen peroxide to water and oxygen
Endoplasmic reticulum	Cytochrome P450	–

Table 1.15: Conditions generating activated oxygen species (O_2^-, H_2O_2 and $-OH$)

Condition	Mechanism
Oxygen therapy	Excessive O_2
X-rays	Ionization radiation hydrolyze H_2O into hydroxyl (OH^-) and hydrogen (H^+) free radicals
Radiotherapy	Ionization radiation hydrolyze H_2O into hydroxyl (OH^-) and hydrogen (H^+) free radicals
PMN cells and macrophages	Inflammation
PMN cells xanthine oxidase	Reperfusion injury after ischemia
CCl_4 and barbiturates toxicity	Inducing P450 oxidase system of smooth endoplasmic reticulum of hepatocytes
Mutagens	Chemical carcinogenesis
Mitochondrial metabolism	Biological aging

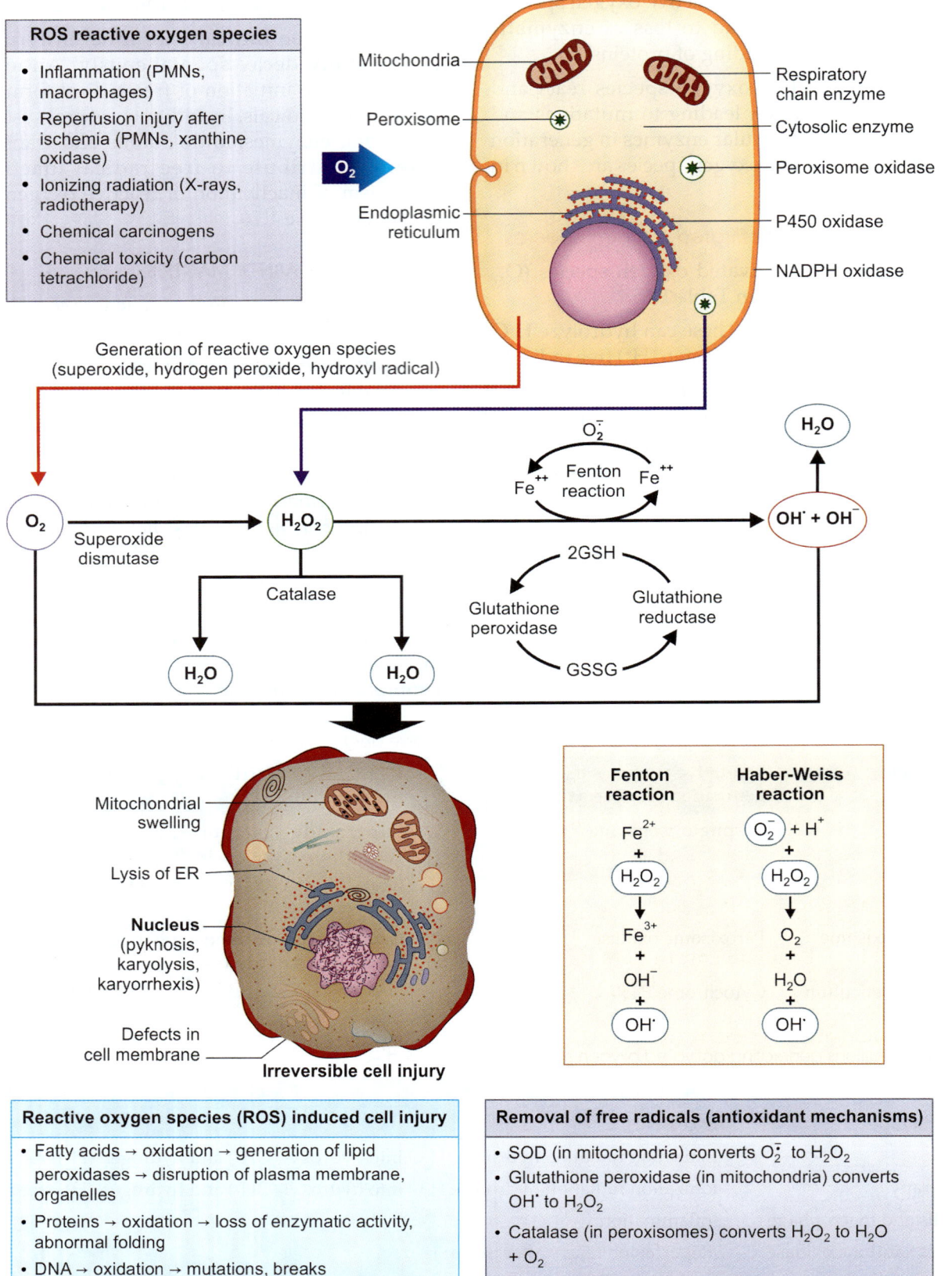

Fig. 1.18: Role of reactive oxygen species (ROS) in cell injury. Oxidative enzymes generating reactive oxygen species are located in mitochondria, peroxisome and endoplasmic reticulum. Reactive oxygen species (hydroxyl ions, hydrogen peroxide and superoxide) react with cellular fatty acids, proteins and DNA leading to irreversible cell injury.

Table 1.16: Mechanism of inactivation of free radicals

Parameters	Categories	Mechanism of action
Intracellular oxidative enzymes	Superoxide dismutase (SOD)	First-line of defense against O_2^-, converting it to H_2O_2 and O_2 in cytosol and mitochondria
		Cytosol also containing P450 oxidase in endoplasmic reticulum
	Catalase	Catalase located in peroxisomes
		Catalase eliminating H_2O_2 to O_2
		Completing the dissolution of O_2^- by eliminating H_2O_2 and, therefore, its potential conversion to OH
	Glutathione peroxidase (GPX)	Catalyzing the reduction of H_2O_2 and lipid peroxides in mitochondria and the cytosol
Exogenous antioxidants (either inhibit synthesis or scavenge free radicals)	Vitamin E (α-tocopherol)	Fat-soluble vitamin protecting cell membranes against peroxidation by blocking free radical chain reaction
	Retinoids	Precursor of fat-soluble vitamin A. These function as chain breaking antioxidants
	Vitamin C (ascorbate)	Water-soluble and reacting directly with O_2, hydroxyl and some products of lipid peroxidation
		Serving to regenerate the reduced form of vitamin E
Transport proteins	Transferrin, ferritin, lactoferritin, ceruloplasmin	Endogenous antioxidants minimizing the generation of reactive forms by transition metals

- The *lipid radicals* so formed react with molecular oxygen and form a lipid peroxide radical. A chain reaction is initiated.
- *Lipid peroxides* are unstable and break down into smaller molecules. The destruction of the unsaturated fatty acids of phospholipids results in a loss of membrane integrity.
- *Unesterified* free fatty acids, acyl carnitine, and lysophospholipids, catabolic products accumulate in the injured cells as a result of phospholipid degradation. They have a detergent effect on membranes. They also either insert into the lipid bilayer of the membrane or exchange with membrane phospholipids, potentially causing changes in permeability and electrophysiological alterations. The important sites of membrane damage are as mentioned below.

Lipid Peroxidation Induced Cellular Membranes Damage

- *Mitochondrial membrane damage:* Damage to mitochondrial membrane results in decreased ATP production, culminating in necrosis, and release of proteins that trigger apoptotic death.
- *Plasma membrane damage:* Plasma membrane damage leads to loss of osmotic balance and influx of fluids and ions, as well as loss of cellular contents. The cells may also leak metabolites that are vital for the reconstitution of ATP, thus further depleting energy stores.
- *Lysosomal membrane damage:* Injury to lysosomal membrane results in leakage of their enzymes into the cytoplasm and activation of the acid hydrolases in the acidic intracellular pH the injured (e.g. ischemic) cell. Lysosomes contain RNases, DNases, proteases, glucosidases, and other enzymes. Activation of these enzymes leads to enzymatic digestion of cell components, and the cells die by necrosis.

DAMAGE TO DNA PROTEINS

Cells have manifestations that repair damage to DNA. Ionizing radiation and oxidative stress cause necrosis or apoptosis. A similar reaction is triggered by improperly folded proteins, which may be the result of inherited mutations or external triggers such as free radicals.

CELL DEATH

When the cell can no longer maintain itself as a metabolic unit, necrotic cell death occurs. Disruption of electron transport system and sustained opening of mitochondrial permeability transition pore (MPTP) indicate irreparable cell injury.

- *Nuclear changes:* Nuclear changes include condensation of chromatin (*pyknosis*), fragmentation of the chromatin (*karyorrhexis*) and lysis of chromatin due to the action of endonuclease (*karyolysis*) leaving a shrunken cell devoid of nucleus.

- *Cytoplasmic changes:* Hematoxylin and eosin stained section shows intense cytoplasmic eosinophilia of dead cell due to loss of cytoplasmic RNA and denaturation (*coagulation*) of proteins. Loss of basophilia is a sign of cell injury, indicating a cessation of protein synthesis.

MORPHOLOGICAL PATTERNS OF NECROSIS

Irreversible cell injury leads to necrosis (cell death). Types of necrosis, mechanism and pathological changes are shown in Table 1.17. Differences between autolysis and necrosis are shown in Table 1.18.

Various morphological patterns of necrosis are described as under.

COAGULATIVE NECROSIS

Coagulative necrosis refers to light microscopic changes in the dying cells as a result of ischemia. Cellular outlines are maintained but structural details are lost. Widespread tissue necrosis, is called as an *infarction*.

Etiology

- *Ischemia:* Coagulative necrosis results most often from sudden interruption of blood supply to an organ with normal protein content supplied by end arteries with limited collateral circulation (*heart, kidney, spleen, adrenal gland except brain*).

Table 1.17: Types of necrosis, mechanism and pathological changes

Type	Mechanism	Pathological changes
Coagulative necrosis	Most often resulting from interruption of blood supply, resulting in denaturation of proteins	Architecture of cells well preserved, but structural details (nuclear changes) lost
	Best seen in organs supplied by end arteries with limited collateral circulation, such as the heart and kidney	Increased cytoplasmic binding of acidophilic dyes
Liquefactive necrosis	Enzymatic liquefaction of necrotic tissue in brain due to ischemia and areas of bacterial infection	Necrotic tissue soft and liquefied
Caseous necrosis	Sharing features of both coagulation and liquefaction necrosis	Architecture not preserved but tissue not liquefied; gross appearance is soft and cheese-like
	Most commonly seen in tuberculous granuloma	Histological appearance is amorphous, with increased affinity for acidophilic dyes
Fat necrosis	Liberation of pancreatic enzymes with auto-digestion of pancreatic parenchyma and trauma to breast parenchyma	Necrotical fat cells, acute inflammation, hemorrhage, calcium soap formation, clustering of lipid-laden macrophages (in the pancreas)
Gangrenous necrosis	Most often resulting from interruption of blood supply to a lower extremity or the bowel	Changes depending on tissue involved and whether gangrene is dry or wet
Fibrinoid necrosis	Characterized by deposition of fibrin-like proteinaceous material in walls of arteries; often observed as part of immune-mediated vasculitis	Smudgy pink appearance in vascular walls; actual necrosis may or may not be present

Table 1.18: Differences between autolysis and necrosis

Features	Autolysis	Necrosis
Definition	Self-digestion or disintegration of cells by its own enzymes liberated from lysosomes	Spectrum of morphologic changes that follow cell death in living tissue, largely resulting from the progressive action of enzymes on lethally injured cells
Occurrence	After death autolysis occurring not showing inflammatory infiltrate	Occurs only in living tissue, infiltrated by inflammatory cells
Calcification	Absent	Dystrophic calcification may be present

Brain does not contain protein content hence shows liquefactive necrosis due to ischemia.

- *Exposure to heavy metals:* Exposure of cells to heavy metals (e.g. lead and mercury) and ionization radiation also results in intracellular accumulation of lactate anions (intracellular acidosis); which cause denaturation of lysosomal hydrolytic enzymes and structural proteins. Renal cortical coagulative necrosis is seen in *mercurial poisoning.*

Pathogenesis

Under physiological state, calcium concentration in interstitial fluids is 10,000 times higher than that inside the cell. Under pathological state, pathogenesis of coagulative necrosis is described as under:

- *Depletion of ATP:* Lack of O_2 impairs mitochondrial electron transport results in depletion of ATP. It facilitates the synthesis of oxygen derived free radicals.
- *Influx of calcium:* Following damage to plasma membrane, massive influx of calcium into the dead cell.
- *Inhibition of lysosomal enzymes:* Ischemia inhibits activity of lysosomal hydrolytic enzymes in the cells, so there is no dissolution of dead cells.
- *Release of mitochondrial cytochrome-c:* Mitochondrial damage promotes the release of cytochrome-c to the cytosol, and the cell dies.
- *Dissolution of cell:* Cell death releases intracellular enzymes, which start to dissolve cellular components, and triggers an acute inflammatory reaction in which white blood cells migrate to the necrotic area and begin to digest the dead cells.

Cellular Changes

- *Cytoplasmic changes:* Hematoxylin and eosin stained section shows intense cytoplasmic eosinophilia with dead cell is due to loss of cytoplasmic RNA and denaturation (coagulation) of proteins. Loss of basophilia is a sign of cell injury, indicating a cessation of protein synthesis.
- *Nuclear changes:* Nuclear fragmentation (karyorrhexis and karyolysis) is a *hallmark of coagulative necrosis*. Nuclei undergo phases of condensation of chromatin along the nuclear membrane (pyknosis), fragmentation of the chromatin (karyorrhexis) and lysis of chromatin due to the action of endonuclease (karyolysis) leaving a shrunken cell devoid of nucleus.

Gross Morphology

Infarction is gross manifestation of coagulative necrosis. Infarcts are of two types, i.e. pale infarct and hemorrhagic infarct depending on the consistency of the tissue.

Pale (ischemic) infarct: Pale infarct is secondary to the sudden occlusion of a vessel. It is commonly seen in solid organs such as *heart, kidney,* and *spleen.*

- Increased density of solid tissue prevents RBCs from diffusing through necrotic tissue. It produces *wedge shaped infarct with apex pointing to the source of obstruction, and the base of infarct at the periphery of the organ* (Fig. 1.19).
- Myocardial infarct is most often caused by ischemia related to coronary artery occlusion by atheromatous plaque.

Hemorrhagic (red) infarct: Hemorrhagic infarct is present in *loose-textured tissue* such as that found in the organs (e.g. *lung and small intestine, ovaries, testis*) allowing RBCs to diffuse through necrotic tissue.

- Hemorrhagic infarct is *wedge shaped* area of hemorrhage extending to the pleural surface due to embolus in one of the pulmonary artery tributaries.
- Venous occlusion also causes hemorrhagic infarcts (e.g. splenic *vein thrombosis*).

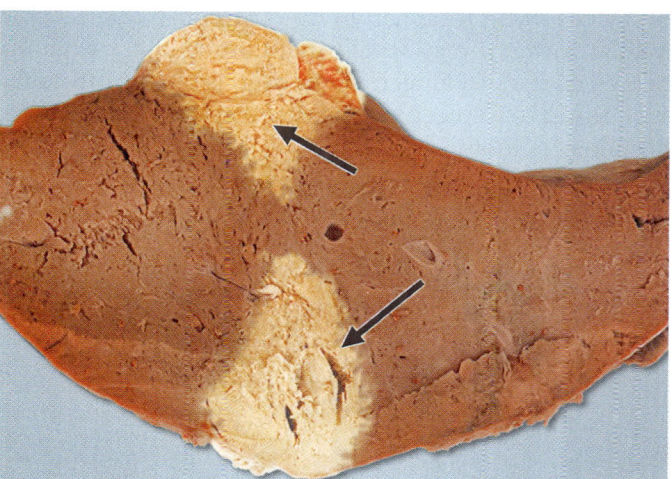

Fig. 1.19: Multiple pale infarcts in spleen (arrows).

LIQUEFACTIVE NECROSIS

Liquefactive necrosis (colliquative necrosis) transforms the tissues into liquid viscous mass.

- Liquefactive necrosis most often occurs as a result of ischemic necrosis of brain and suppurative infections bacterial or fungal (lung abscess) in lungs.

Table 1.19: Differences between coagulative necrosis and liquefactive necrosis

Features	Coagulative necrosis	Liquefactive necrosis
Cause	Hypoxic injury except in brain	Hypoxic injury in CNS. Bacterial and fungal infections (abscess)
Organs involves	Heart, kidney, spleen	Brain, small intestine and appendix
Cellular outline	The cellular outlines are maintained but structural details, e.g. nucleus are completely lost	Both cell outlines as well as structural details are completely lost
Mechanism	Due to intracellular acidosis (due to hypoxia) structural as well as enzymatic denaturation of proteins occurs. Dead cells are removed by fragmentation and phagocytosis	Bacteria and fungi stimulate accumulation of inflammatory cells. Hydrolytic enzymes (autolysis and heterolysis) result in complete digestion of dead cells
Gross morphology	Firm in texture	Formation of liquid viscous mass
Light microscopy	Conversion of cells into acidophilic coagulated, devoid of nuclear details	Cellular architecture not recognized rather than liquid viscous mass is seen. It is creamy in acute inflammation

- Liquefactive necrosis is seen in brain and lung. Hydrolytic enzymes liberated by neutrophils and macrophages digest the tissue resulting in transformation of the tissue into soft, circumscribed creamy liquid viscous. Differences between coagulative necrosis and liquefactive necrosis are shown in Table 1.19.

Liquefactive Necrosis in Brain

Brain does not contain proteins, hence ischemia produces liquefactive necrosis. Hydrolytic enzymes liberated by phagocytes cause necrosis of affected brain tissue resulting in creamy liquid viscous. Later a cyst wall is formed. It is worth mentioning that ischemia causes coagulative necrosis in organs rich in proteins such as kidney, spleen and heart; except brain, that lacks proteins contents.

- *Gross morphology:* Brain tissue is creamy liquid viscous. It may show cyst formation (Fig. 1.20).
- *Light microscopy:* It reveals cystic space contains necrotic cell debris. The cyst wall is formed by proliferating capillaries, neutrophils, macrophages and gliosis (proliferating glial cells).

Liquefactive Necrosis in Lungs

Suppurative infections such as bacterial or fungal cause liquefactive necrosis in lungs (lung abscess).

- *Gross morphology:* Hydrolytic enzymes by phagocytes convert affected lung parenchyma in creamy liquid viscous.
- *Light microscopy:* The cyst wall is formed by proliferating capillaries, neutrophils, macrophages and proliferating fibroblasts in lung abscess.

CASEOUS NECROSIS

Caseous necrosis is a combination of coagulative and liquefactive necrosis seen in tuberculosis, in which cellular outlines as well as structural details are lost. *Caseous necrosis is hallmark of tuberculosis.*

Caseous material appears as amorphous, coarsely granular, eosinophilic debris. It is derived from the lipid-rich cell walls of the pathogens (e.g. *Mycobacterium tuberculosis*) destroyed by activated macrophages by the interaction of T-lymphocytes and probably cytokines such as interferon-γ (IFN-γ) derived from these cells.

It is a delayed-type hypersensitivity reaction (type IV cellular immunity). Differences between coagulative and caseous necroses are shown in Table 1.20.

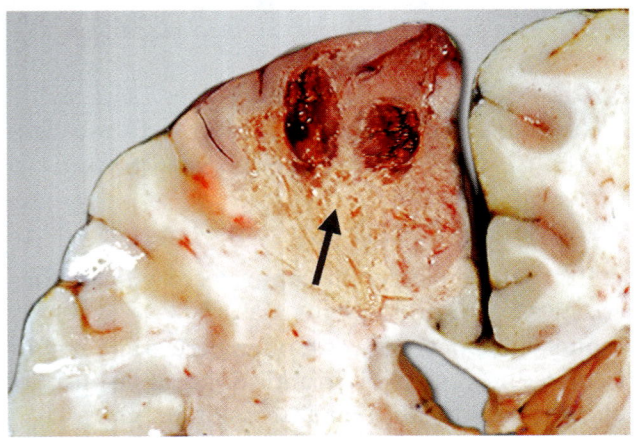

Fig. 1.20: Liquefactive necrosis in the frontal lobe of brain with formation of cystic spaces (arrow).

> **Gross Morphology**
>
> Caseous material resembles clumpy cheese-like consistency, hence the name caseous necrosis. It is formed by the release of lipid from the cell walls of Mycobacterium tubercle bacilli after destruction by macrophages. This type of appearance also occurs in systemic fungal infection by *Histoplasma capsulatum*.

Cellular Adaptations, Cell Injury, Apoptosis, Pigments, Calcification, Cellular Accumulations and Aging

Table 1.20: Differences between coagulative and caseous necroses

Features	Coagulative necrosis	Caseous necrosis
Causes	Hypoxia, e.g. heart, kidney and spleen	Mycobacterium tubercle bacillus
Mechanism	Due to intracellular acidosis (due to hypoxia) structural as well as enzymatic denaturation of proteins occurs. Dead cells are removed by fragmentation and phagocytosis. Cellular outlines are preserved, but structural details are lost	It is reaction between Mycobacterium tubercle bacillus antigens and inflammatory cells. Cellular outlines are completely obscured
Gross examination	Firm texture of organs	Cheesy white appearance
Microscopic examination	Cellular outlines are maintained and structural details are lost. Cells are acidophilic, coagulated with loss of nuclear details due to blockage of cytoplasmic hydrolytic enzymes. There is no dissolution of tissue	Cellular outline as well as structural details is lost. It is amorphous granular debris (fragmented, coagulated cells and granular debris) surrounded by chronic inflammatory cells. Epithelioid granulomas and giant cells are present

Light Microscopy

- The tubercular lesion is composed of epithelioid granulomas (activated macrophages, CD4+ T cells), caseous necrosis and Langhans' type giant cells.
- Caseous necrotic tissue lack cellular outlines as well as cellular details, which appears amorphous finely granular, eosinophilic appearance with increased affinity for acidophilic dye (Figs 1.21 and 1.22).

FAT NECROSIS

Fat necrosis occurs in two forms, i.e. enzymatic and traumatic. Fat necrosis in omentum occurs following acute pancreatitis. Traumatic fat necrosis, unlike enzymatic fat necrosis, is not enzyme mediated but is secondary to direct severe trauma to organs rich in fat, i.e. female breast, surgical trauma in abdominal wall and omentum.

Pancreatic Enzymatic Fat Necrosis

Pancreatic enzymatic fat necrosis represents auto-digestion by pancreatic enzymes such as *lipases and proteases released from pancreatic cells*. These enzymes damage peripancreatic fat cells laden with triglycerides leading to liberation of free fatty acids. These fatty acids combine calcium ions, sodium, or magnesium to form *calcium soaps (saponification)*. Hemorrhage occurs as a result of vessel erosion.

- *Predisposing factors:* Predisposing factors of acute pancreatitis include alcoholism, hypercalcemia, hyperlidemia and autoimmune etiology.
- *Radiological findings:* The precipitated calcium in the soaps can be visualized by radiological imaging.
- *Serum calcium:* Serum calcium level is decreased in patients who had a recent bout of acute pancreatitis.
- *Gross morphology:* Macroscopically, fat necrosis looks like opaque *chalky-white* nodules composed of calcium soaps in the fat surrounding the pancreas or in the abdominal cavity.

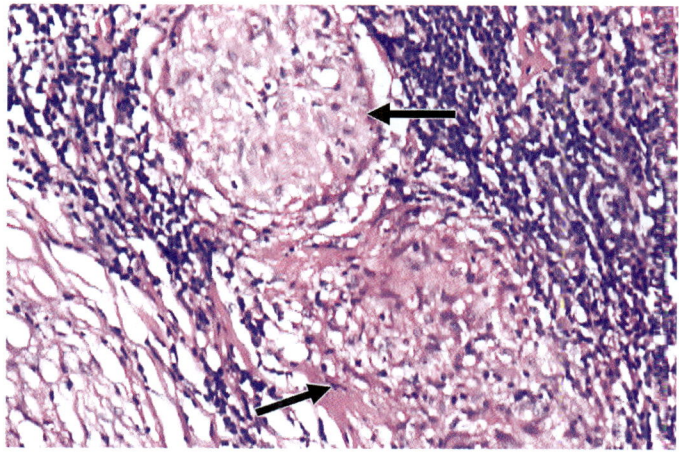

Fig. 1.21: Tuberculosis of lymph node showing epithelioid granulomas (arrows) caseous necrosis and Langhans' giant cells (400X).

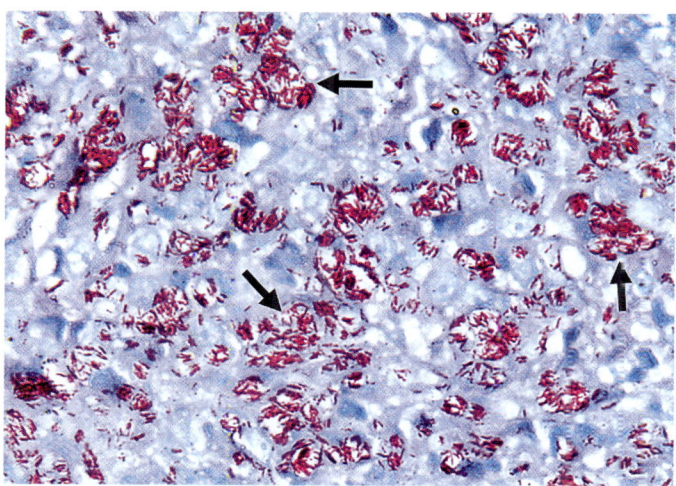

Fig. 1.22: AFB demonstrated by ZN stain (arrows) (400X).

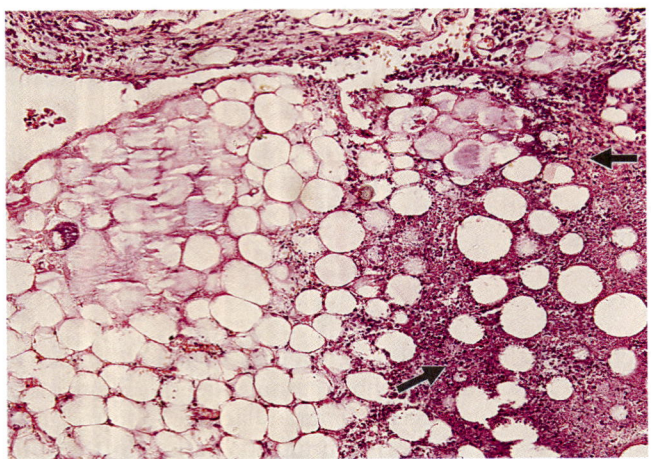

Fig. 1.23: Fat necrosis of pancareas showing irregular islands of necrotic fat cells, which have lost their outlines. There is presence of chronic inflammatory cells. Macrophages are filled with fat and calcium (arrows) (100X).

- *Light microscopy:* Microscopic examination reveals irregular islands of necrotic fat cells, which lose their outlines and become indistinct. There is presence of inflammatory cells, macrophages filled with fat and calcium deposits. Deposition of calcium around the periphery of necrotic fat cells gives a basophilic tinge. Giant cell reaction around these foam cells may occur (Fig. 1.23).
- *Clinical features:* Patients with acute pancreatitis experience sudden-onset abdominal pain, distention, and vomiting.

Fat Necrosis in Female Breast

Trauma to the breast is most common cause of fat necrosis in women >55 years. It may occur in women, who had *prior surgical intervention* or *radiation therapy*.

Lipase enzyme liberated from traumatized adipose tissue breaks down intracellular triglycerides into free fatty acids. These free fatty acids combine with sodium, magnesium or calcium ions to form soaps. The tissue becomes opaque and chalky white demonstrated as calcified lesion on radiograph.

- *Clinical features:* Patient presents with unilateral painful localized superficial irregular breast mass in acute stage. On clinical examination, affected breast is firm, erythema of the overlying skin, dimpling and nipple retraction mimicking breast cancer.
- *Gross morphology:* It shows chalky white areas of *fat saponification*. Variegated color and areas of hemorrhage are demonstrated on the cut surface of this lump. It is gritty to cut because of the presence of spotty calcification.
- *Light microscopy:* Initially, acute inflammatory reaction consists of necrosis of adipocytes and hemorrhage. *Chronic inflammatory lesion* is composed of plasma cells, macrophages, multinucleated giant cells, foam cells termed as lipophages.

There is presence of foreign body giant cells and dystrophic calcification demonstrated by imaging techniques. Fibroblastic proliferation leads to fibrosis. As a result, an irregular, fixed, hard mass may ensue and clinically *resemble breast cancer. Thus, the lesions often require biopsy to establish their benign character.*

GANGRENOUS NECROSIS

Gangrenous necrosis occurs most often from interruption of blood supply to *intestine* and *lower extremities*. Morphological changes depend on tissues affected, which may be dry or wet gangrene discussed as under. Differences between dry gangrene and wet gangrene are shown in Table 1.21.

Differences between caseous and necrosis gangrenous necrosis are shown in Table 1.22.

Table 1.21: Differences between dry gangrene and wet gangrene

Parameters	Dry gangrene	Wet gangrene
Mechanism	Slow occlusion of arteries	Sudden interruption of blood flow in both artery and vein
Underlying disorders	Atheromatous plaques	Emboli, ligation, crush injuries
Organ involved	Limbs (small area involved due to presence of collaterals)	Bowel (large area involved due to absence of collaterals)
Gross morphology	Dry, decreased in size with black discoloration	Wet, swollen, edematous and soft in consistency
Odor	Absent	Present
Line of demarcation	Present at the junction of healthy and gangrenous part	Clear line demarcation absent
Infection	Absent	Most often present
Prognosis	Most often better due to little septicemia	Most often poor due to profound toxemia
Treatment	Conservative amputation	Major surgical resection essential

Cellular Adaptations, Cell Injury, Apoptosis, Pigments, Calcification, Cellular Accumulations and Aging

Table 1.22: Differences between caseous necrosis and gangrenous necrosis

Features	Caseous necrosis	Gangrenous necrosis
Definition	Reaction between Mycobacterium tubercle bacillus antigens and inflammatory cells	Form of coagulative necrosis, which may be followed by liquefactive necrosis, when an organ loses its blood supply and followed by infection Types of gangrene, e.g. dry gangrene, wet gangrene and gas gangrene
Gross examination	Cheesy white appearance	Organs appearance varies
Histology	Showing amorphous granular debris (fragmented, coagulated cells and granular debris) surrounded by chronic inflammatory cells. Epithelioid granulomas and giant cells present	Cellular outlines maintained and structural details lost
Granulomatous reaction	Present	Absent

Types of Gangrene

- *Dry gangrene:* It is a variant of coagulative necrosis due to ischemia with minimal bacterial invasion. It commonly affects foot in diabetic patients as a result of formation of atheromatous plaques in tibial and popliteal arteries of lower extremities. The affected tissues appear black because of the deposition of iron sulphide from degraded hemoglobin.
- *Wet gangrene:* It refers to superimposed infection with liquefactive necrosis of organ. Liquefactive necrosis occurs due to extensive lytic activity from bacteria and white blood cells that produce a liquid center in the affected area. It is commonly seen in lower extremities and intestine as a complication of acute appendicitis (Fig. 1.24).
- *Gas gangrene:* It is not caused by ischemia. *Clostridium perfringens*, anaerobe bacterial toxin causes muscle injury releasing gas bubbles, which spread in the tissues. It is more likely to follow severe trauma and may be fatal.

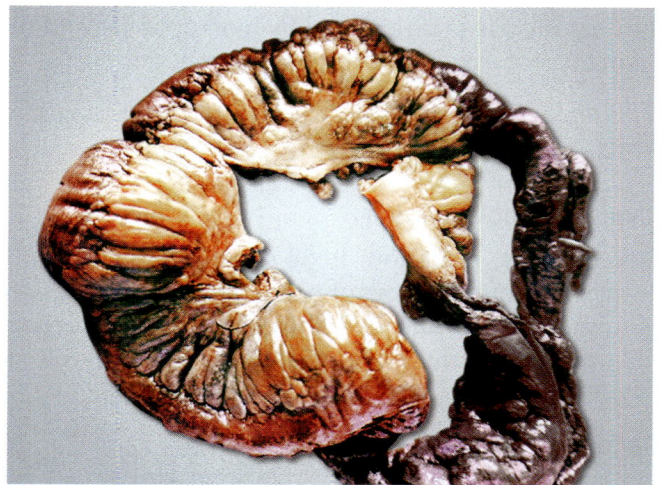

Fig. 1.24: Ischemic bowel disease (gangrene intestine) showing dusky blackish discoloration.

FIBRINOID NECROSIS

Fibrinoid necrosis is observed in areas of necrotizing vasculitis due to insudation and accumulation of plasma proteins in the wall of injured small blood vessels such as arterioles and small muscular arteries.

Fibrinoid necrosis appears as eosinophilic material in hematoxylin and eosin stained sections. It has no distinct gross features. It is most commonly seen in malignant hypertension, immune-mediated vasculitis (Henoch-Schönlein purpura, lupus erythematosus and polyarteritis nodosa).

GUMMATOUS NECROSIS

Gummatous necrosis is a granulomatous destructive rubbery lesion seen in tertiary syphilis. It most often occurs in the liver (*gumma hepatitis*). It may also be demonstrated in *brain, heart, testes* and *bone*. Patient may have neurological and cardiac valve disorders.

- *Gross morphology:* Gumma has firm necrotic amorphous proteinaceous mass that may be partly hyalinized.
- *Light microscopy:* Central area of gumma shows necrosis with partly retaining structural details of previously normal tissue.

There is presence of epithelioid cell granulomas, multinucleated giant cells in the central region of gumma. Peripheral zone of gumma shows fibroblasts, capillaries, lymphocytes and plasma cells.

POSTMORTEM AUTOLYSIS

Postmortem autolysis occurs secondary to the release of endogenously derived intracellular enzymes moments after death.

There is no inflammatory infiltrate, since an inflammatory response occurs only in living tissue.

SUBCUTANEOUS NECROSIS OF NEWBORN

Subcutaneous necrosis of newborn is self-limited disease affecting term neonates and young infants. It is characterized by circumscribed, indurated, nodular areas of fat necrosis. It is related to *trauma on bony prominences during delivery or maternal diabetes mellitus*. It resolves spontaneously by 2 to 4 weeks without fibrosis. It is also called adiponecrosis neonatorum.

ZENKER'S NECROSIS

Zenker's necrosis refers to glassy waxy necrosis of the striated muscle such as *rectus abdominis* and *diaphragm* in acute severe infectious diseases like typhoid fever and burns. It has been named by *Friedrich Albert von Zenker*.

- *Gross examination:* Affected skeletal muscle appears pale and friable.
- *Light microscopy:* Muscle fibers undergoing swelling and loss of striations show hyaline appearance. Small areas of hemorrhage may be seen.

OUTCOME OF NECROSIS

Necrosis may have following outcome described as under.

COMPLETE RESOLUTION

Complete resolution occurs by regeneration of cells by mitoses in organs such as the kidney or liver. Liver comprises stable cells and possess limited proliferative activity. Liver regeneration occurs by two mechanisms: Proliferation of remaining hepatocytes and repopulation from progenitor cells.

REPAIR BY FIBROSIS

In the heart, the dead myocardial cells are removed by inflammatory cells and replaced by a fibrous scar.
- *Healing starts* with granulation tissue formation by first week.

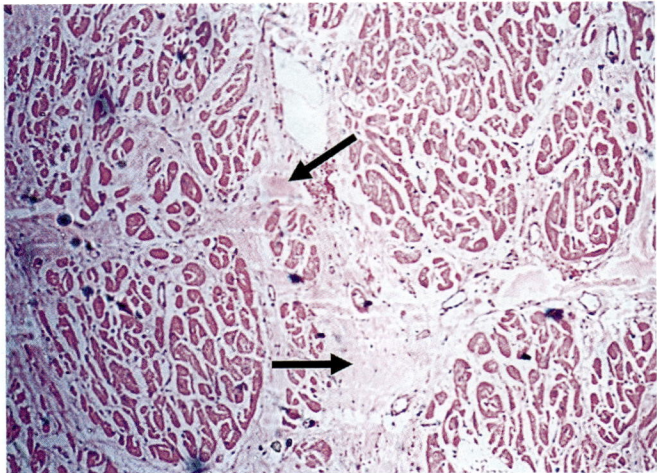

Fig. 1.25: Healed myocardium after infarction showing fibrosis (arrows) (100X).

- By *second week* granulation tissue is replaced by yellow necrotic myocardium.
- By *third week*, yellow necrotic myocardium is replaced by fibrous scar. Phagocytosis of necrotic debris by macrophages is complete.
- By *sixth week*, infarct tissue is replaced by white, patchy and non-contractile scar tissue (Fig. 1.25).

DYSTROPHIC CALCIFICATION

Dystrophic calcification has its origin in direct cell injury. Calcium is deposited in dead or dying tissues. Serum calcium concentration is within normal limits. The necrotic tissue is impregnated with deposition of calcium salts. It occurs by two processes: Initiation and propagation.

RESORPTION OF NECROTIC TISSUE

In the ischemic brain and suppurative infections of lung, the necrotic tissue is removed by macrophages and the infarct transforms into a fluid-filled pseudocyst.

APOPTOSIS

OVERVIEW

Apoptosis is a process of genetically programmed cell death that occurs in multicellular organisms. It is characterized by individual cell death without inflammatory reaction. On the other hand, tissue necrosis is associated with inflammatory reaction.

Biochemical changes in apoptosis include blebbing cell shrinkage, nuclear fragmentation, chromatin condensation, DNA fragmentation and mRNA decay.

Diverse Injurious Stimuli

Free radicals, radiation, toxic substances, and withdrawal of growth factors or hormones trigger a variety of stimuli, including cell surface receptors such as FAS, mitochondrial response to stress, and cytotoxic T lymphocytes.

Cellular Changes

During apoptosis, cell plasma membrane shows irregular buds known as *blebs*. There is loss of cell surface microvilli. Caspases degrade cytoskeleton resulting in shrinkage of the cytoplasm.

- *Cell organelles* are tightly packed and preserved. Nuclear chromatin undergoes condensation known as *pyknosis*, a hallmark of apoptosis. It is followed by DNA fragmentation known as *karyorrhexis*.
- *Cell fragments* formed as a result of apoptosis are known as *apoptotic bodies*. These are phagocytosed and rapidly degraded by phagocytic cells, before cellular lysosomal enzymes may spill over surrounding cells and cause tissue damage. Differences between necrosis and apoptosis are shown in Table 1.23.

Mechanism of Apoptosis

Apoptosis is triggered by a variety of extracellular and intracellular signals in response to a stress. Increased intracellular calcium triggers the release of intracellular apoptotic signals by damaged cell. It is often a self-defense mechanism, destroying cells that have been infected with pathogens or those in which genomic alterations have occurred.

- *Cellular components* such as poly ADPase polymerase may also participate in regulation of apoptosis.
- *Activation of cellular enzymes* degrades the cells own nuclear DNA as well nuclear and cytoplasmic proteins. It is second morphologic pattern of cell death. Before the actual process of cell death is precipitated by cellular enzymes, apoptotic signal must cause regulatory proteins to initiate the apoptosis pathway.
- *Apoptosis* detects and destroys cells that harbor dangerous mutations, thereby maintaining genetic consistency and *preventing the development of cancer*.

Apoptosis during Embryogenesis

- *Involution of structures:* During development of human embryo, apoptosis plays important role in involution of Müllerian and Wolffian structures.
- *Development of lumen in hollow organs:* Apoptosis participates in development of lumens in hollow organs such as the heart and bowels.
- *Formation of digits:* Apoptosis participates in the formation of digits during embryogenesis, because cells between the digits undergo apoptosis.

Apoptosis during Adult Life

- *Elimination of self-reacting lymphocytes:* Apoptosis eliminates potentially harmful self-reactive lymphocytes. Cell death is induced by cytotoxic T cells.
- *Menstrual cycle:* Apoptosis participates in normal endometrial cell breakdown after withdrawal of estrogen and progesterone in the menstrual cycle.

Table 1.23: Differences between necrosis and apoptosis

Features	Necrosis	Apoptosis
Definition	It is caused by injurious agents, e.g. hypoxia, toxins	Programmed cell death
Induction	Pathological role—hypoxia, toxins mainly	Often physiological and may be pathologic especially DNA damage
Mechanism	Cell death by ATP depletion due to hypoxia or hydrolytic enzymes digestion	Programmed cell death
Extent	Death of many contiguous cells	Death of single cells
Inflammatory response in adjacent cells	Present	Absent
Cell size	Enlarged	Cell shrinkage
Cell membrane integrity	Plasma membrane disruption	Plasma membrane lost Cytoplasmic blebbing
Morphology	Cell swelling	Cell shrinkage and fragmentation to form apoptotic bodies
Nuclear changes	Nuclear changes (pyknosis, karyorrhexis and karyolysis)	Nucleus fragmentation into nucleosome-size fragments
Lysosomes	Lysosomal breakdown liberating enzymes	Intact lysosomes and other organelles
Fate of dead cells	Phagocytosis by inflammatory cells, e.g. polymorphonuclear cells and macrophages	Phagocytosed by adjacent cells

- *Councilman bodies in viral hepatitis:* Apoptosis removes viral infected hepatocytes. Apoptotic cells represent membrane-bound cellular chromatin remnants that are extruded into the hepatic sinusoids in cases of viral hepatitis.

  These appear as eosinophilic stained structures in hematoxylin and eosin stained sections seen under light microscope.

- *Skin's keratin layer turnover:* It accounts for constant cell turnover in the skin's outer keratin layer.

- *Tumor cells destruction:* Apoptosis is often a self-defense mechanism for destruction of cells infected with viruses or irreparable DNA damaged cells by cytotoxic T cells, thus protecting against neoplastic transformation. Radiation and cytotoxic anticancer drugs induce apoptosis of cancer cells.

- *Red neurons in brain:* Red neurons represent dead neuron in the brain in hypoxic injury.

- *Apoptosis in parenchymal organs:* Apoptosis occurs in parenchymal organs after obstruction of ducts.

MECHANISM OF APOPTOSIS

Apoptosis is mainly initiated by extrinsic (death receptor) and intrinsic (mitochondrial) pathways. Both pathways converge to activate caspases and participate in execution.

Third mechanism is mediated by influx of calcium within cell due to binding of a drug to calcium binding protease *caplin*. Mechanisms of apoptosis is shown in Fig. 1.26.

There are two phases of apoptosis: initiation and execution. Initiation phase comprises extrinsic (death

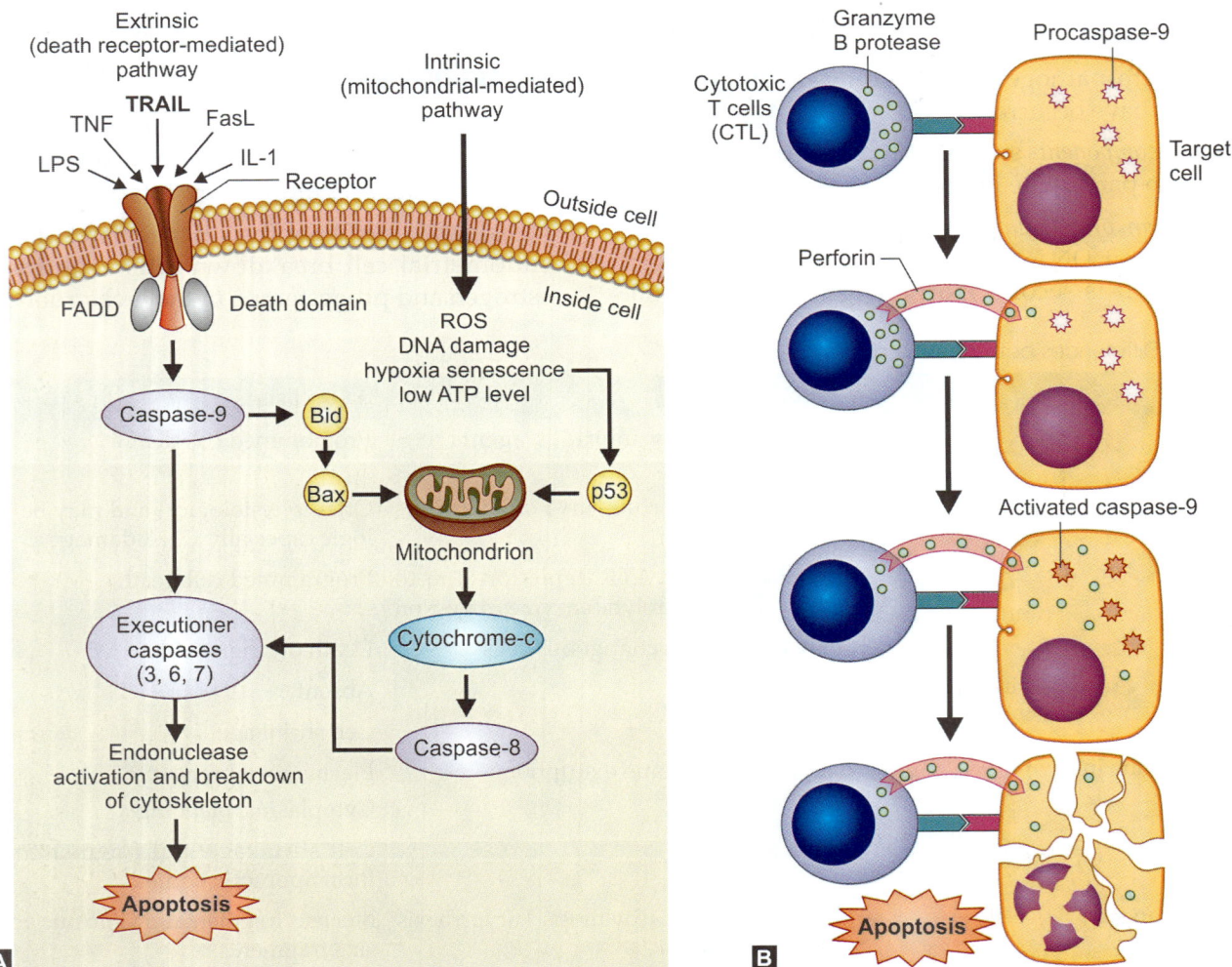

Fig. 1.26: (A) Mechanisms of apoptosis occurring by extrinsic (death receptor) pathway, intrinsic (mitochondrial) pathway. The extrinsic pathway is activated by signal such as Fas ligand (FasL), that on binding to the Fas receptor, forming a death-inducing complex by joining the Fas-associated death domain (FADD) to the death domain of the Fas receptor. Instrinsic pathway is activated by injurious stimuli such as reactive oxygen species and DNA damage that induce the release of mitochondrial cytochrome-c into the cytoplasm. Both pathways of apoptosis differ in their induction and regulation. Both pathways culminate in the activation of 'executioner' caspases and (B) showing activation of caspases by cytotoxic T cells.

receptor) and intrinsic mitochondrial pathways described as under.

INITIATION PHASE

Extrinsic (Death Receptor) Pathway

Extrinsic pathway is also known as cell surface death receptor pathway. Tumor necrosis factor (TNF), synthesized by activated macrophages mediates apoptosis by extrinsic pathway.
- Most of the human cells possess two receptors for TNF-R1 and TNF-R2.
- TNF-R1 binds and activates caspases via intermediate death domain proteins such as TNF receptor-associated death domain and Fas-associated death domain.

Mechanism

Fas receptor: Fas receptor is first apoptosis signal also known as Apo-1 or CD95. It is a member of TNF family. Fas receptor contains a cytoplasmic domain (i.e. death domain) involved in protein-protein interactions, which is essential for delivering apoptotic signals.

Binding of Fas to FasL: Fas bind Fas ligand (FasL), a transmembrane protein part of TNF family. The interaction of Fas and FasL leads to formation of death inducing signal complex (DISC). It forms a binding site for an adapter protein FADD (Fas-associated death domain).

Generation of caspases: FADD binds to pro-caspases-8 via (inactive form) a death domain. Multiple pro-caspase-8 molecules come into proximately, and cleave one another to generate caspase-8 (active form).
- The initial activating caspases are caspase-8 and caspase-9, and the terminal caspases (executioners) include caspase-3 and caspase-6.
- Caspases are aspartate-specific cysteine proteases, which mediate the execution phase of apoptosis or 'molecular guillotines'.
- This pathway of apoptosis can be inhibited by a protein called FLIP (caspases-8 inhibitor).
- In some cells, caspases-8 directly activates other members of the caspases, and triggers the execution of apoptosis of the cell. In other cells, the Fas-DISC starts a feedback loop that spirals into increasing release of pro-apoptotic factors from mitochondria and the amplified activation of caspases-8.

Intrinsic Mitochondrial Pathway

Mitochondria are essential for aerobic respiration to human life. Without them, a cell ceases to respire aerobically and rapidly dies. This forms the basis of apoptosis by mitochondrial pathway.
- The mitochondrial membrane is a key regulator of apoptosis. There is no role of death receptors in this pathway.
- The essence of this intrinsic pathway is a balance between pro-apoptotic and protective molecules that regulate mitochondrial permeability and the release of death inducers that are normally sequestered within the mitochondria. Mitochondria contain cysteine derived caspases, which induces apoptosis.

Physiological state: Normally mitochondrial IAPs (inhibitor of apoptosis proteins) suppress the activity of cysteine proteases called caspases.

Pathological state: Caspases participate in inducing apoptosis. Increased permeability of mitochondria leads to release of SMACs (small mitochondria-derived activator of caspases). Caspases inhibit the activity of IAPs, thus allowing apoptosis to proceed.

Caspases and Apoptosis

- *Release of mitochondrial c:* Apoptotic proteins (e.g. caspases and apoptotic proteins Bax, Bak and Bim) target mitochondria and create mitochondrial apoptosis-induced channel (MAC) in the outer mitochondrial membrane resulting in leakage of apoptotic effectors such as cytochrome-c and apoptosis inducing factor (AIF). Nitric oxide is inducer of apoptosis by making mitochondria more permeable.

- *Activation of caspases by mitochondrial cytochrome-c:* Cytochrome-c binds with apoptosis protease activating factor-1 (Apaf-1) and ATP, which then binds to procaspase-9 to create a protein complex known as an *apoptosome*. The apoptosome cleaves pro-caspase to its active form of caspases-9, which in turn activates the effector caspases-3.

- *Apoptosis inducing factor:* Other mitochondrial protein such as apoptosis inducing factor (AIF), enter the cytoplasm, where they bind to and neutralize various inhibitors of apoptosis. Function of inhibitors of apoptosis is to block caspase activation. The net result is the initiation of a caspase cascade.

- *Action of caspases:* These effector caspases cleave target proteins, including endonucleases nuclear proteins, and cytoskeletal proteins to mediate the varied morphological and biochemical changes that accompany apoptosis.

Regulation of Apoptosis by Gene Products

Apoptosis is regulated by caspases and gene regulating proteins such as antiapoptotic proteins, apoptotic proteins and p53 tumor suppressor proteins.

- *Antiapoptotic proteins (BCL-2 and BCL-x):* These inhibit apoptosis. These anti-apoptotic proteins normally reside in mitochondrial membranes and the cytoplasm. Growth factors and other survival signals stimulate the production of anti-apoptotic members of the BCL-2 family of protein.
- *Apoptotic proteins (Bax, Bak, Bim):* These facilitate apoptosis. When cells are deprived of survival signals or subjected to stress, BCL-2 and/or BCL-x are lost from the mitochondrial membrane and replaced by pro-apoptotic members of the family, such as Bax, Bak, and Bim.
- *Role of p53 tumor suppressor protein:* DNA is protected by p53 tumor suppressor gene. The p53 gene induces apoptosis by several mechanisms:
    - It downregulates transcription of the antiapoptotic protein: BCL-2.
    - It upregulates transcription of the pro-apoptotic genes: Bax, Bak and Bim.
    - It activates proteins that arrest the cell in G1 phase of cell cycle, permitting time for DNA repair to go ahead.

    If the DNA damage is irreparable, p53 tumor suppressor gene activates mechanisms that terminate in apoptosis.

Degradation of Nucleus

Degradation of DNA by endonucleases into nucleosomal chromatin fragments. These are multiples of 180 to 200 base pairs. These are demonstrated by *laddering* appearance of DNA on electrophoresis. This phenomenon is characteristic but not specific for apoptosis.

Role of Transaminases

These cross-link apoptotic cytoplasmic proteins.

Activation of Caspases by Cytotoxic T Cells

Granzyme B protease synthesized by cytotoxic T cells, activates caspase cascade. The entry of granzyme B into target cells is mediated by *perforin*, a cytotoxic T cell protein. *Granzyme B* protease synthesized by cytotoxic T cells, activates caspase cascade.

The entry of granzyme B into target cells is mediated by **perforin**, *a cytotoxic T cell protein.*

EXECUTION PHASE

The caspases consist of a group of aspartic acid-specific cysteine proteases that which mediate the execution phase of apoptosis. Caspase possesses two properties: The *'c' refers to a cysteine protease* (i.e. an enzyme with cysteine in its active site), and *caspase* refers to the unique ability of these enzymes to cleave after aspartic acid residues. The caspase family has more than 10 members. These are divided into two major groups: Initiator and executioner depending on the order, in which they are activated during apoptosis.

Initiator Caspases

These include caspases 2, 8, 9, 10, 11, 12. Initiator caspases are cleaved to generate its active form; the enzymatic death program is set in motion by rapid and sequential activation of other caspases.

Executioner Caspases

Executioner caspases include caspase-3, caspase-6 and caspase 7. Executioner caspases act on many cellular components such as cytoskeleton and nucleus.

- These caspases disrupt cytoskeleton and degradation of nucleus. These also target various proteins involved in transcription, DNA replication, and DNA repair.
- Caspase-3 converts a cytoplasmic DNase into an active form, which induces the characteristic internucleosomal cleavage of DNA. Dead cells are removed by following mechanisms.

Mechanism of Removal of Cells

- *Efferocytosis:* At early stages of apoptosis, dying cells secrete soluble factors that recruit phagocytes. This process facilitating prompt clearance of apoptotic cells is called efferocytosis.
- *Phosphatidylserine role:* Phosphatidylserine is normally present on the cytosolic surface of the plasma membrane. During apoptosis, scramblase causes redistribution of phosphatidylserine to the extracellular surface. These molecules mark the cell for phagocytosis by phagocytic cells possessing appropriate receptors.
- *Engulfment of cell:* Upon recognition, the phagocyte recognizes its cytoskeleton for engulfment of the cell. The removal of dying cells by phagocytes occurs in an orderly manner *without eliciting an inflammatory response.*

SUBCELLULAR RESPONSE TO INJURY

Certain conditions are associated with alterations in cell organelles (lysosomes, smooth endoplasmic reticulum, and mitochondria) or the cytoskeleton (microtubules). Certain substances are not metabolized by cells resulting in accumulation and impairment of functions.

Deficiency of enzyme results in accumulation of endogenous substances (lysosomal storage diseases). Insoluble endogenous pigments such as lipofuscin and melanin accumulate in cells. Exogenous particulates accumulate such as silica, carbon and asbestos in the lungs.

LYSOSOMAL DYSFUNCTION

Lysosomes contain many hydrolytic enzymes, including acid phosphatase, glucuronidase, sulfatase, ribonuclease, and collagenase. These participate in the *degradation of endogenous substances*. Lysosomal enzymes degrade most of proteins and carbohydrates, but some lipids remain undigested.

Mechanism

Lysosomes participate in the breakdown of phagocytosed material in one of two ways: Autophagy or heterophagy described as under:

- *Autophagy:* Autophagy refers to lysosomal digestion of the cell's own components. It participates in removal of damaged organelles during cell injury and the cellular remodeling of differentiation, and atrophic cells due to nutrient deprivation.
- *Chloroquine antimalarial drug raises the intracellular pH of the lysosomes, thus inactivating its enzymes reduces tissue damage in inflammatory reactions.* The same inhibition of enzymes, however, can result in abnormal accumulation of glycogen and phospholipids in lysosomes, causing *myopathy*.
- *Heterophagy:* Heterophagy is process of lysosomal digestion of materials ingested from extracellular compartment by phagocytosis and pinocytosis. It occurs in neutrophils to degrade bacteria and macrophages to remove apoptotic cells.

Examples of Lysosomal Disorders

Hurler's syndrome: Hurler syndrome is an example of lysosomal disorder. It refers to increased deposition of glycosaminoglycans due to deficiency of lysosomal enzyme.

Glycogen storage disease: Glycogen storage is an example of lysosomal disorder. Due to deficiency of lysosomal enzymes, accumulation of metabolites occurs due to incomplete degradation.

- *Glycogen storage disease or von Gierke's disease:* It occurs due to glucose-6-phosphatase deficiency.
- *McArdle syndrome type V:* It occurs due to deficiency of phosphorylase enzymes in skeletal muscles.
- *Pompe disease type II:* It occurs due to deficiency of glucosidase.

HYPERTROPHY OF ENDOPLASMIC RETICULUM

Smooth endoplasmic reticulum participates in the metabolism of chemicals. When cells exposed to chemicals, the endoplasmic reticulum shows hypertrophy as an adaptive response.

MITOCHONDRIAL DYSFUNCTION

The mitochondrial dysfunction plays an important role in cell injury and apoptosis. Mitochondrial number is increased in hypertrophy and decreased in atrophy. Abnormal mitochondria (megamitochondria) may be seen in *alcohol liver disease*, mitochondrial *myopathies*, certain nutritional diseases and benign tumors arising from oncocytes of salivary glands, thyroid, parathyroid and kidneys (known as *oncocytes*).

CYTOSKELETON ABNORMALITIES

Cytoskeleton represents network of protein filaments in the cytosol that maintains cell structure (shape), and in some cases, assists in the motility of the cell. It allows coordinated intracellular transport of organelles and molecules.

- The membrane skeleton composed of spectrin, actin, and protein provides structural integrity to the cell membrane of red blood cells.
- Hereditary spherocytosis, an autosomal dominant disease, is an example of a defect in spectrin resulting in a hemolytic anemia. Components of cytoskeleton, their arrangement, functions and disorders are shown in Table 1.24.

Composition

Cytoskeleton is composed of actin filaments (6–8 nm), thick myosin filaments (15 nm), microtubules (20–25 nm); and intermediate filaments. Functions of actin filaments, microtubules and intermediate filaments.

- *Actin filaments:* Normally, actin filaments in leukocytes participate in leukocytic movement and phagocytosis. These are also involved in the contractile process of muscle cells. *Phalloidin toxin (Amanita phalloides)*

Table 1.24: Components of cytoskeleton, their arrangement, functions and disorders

Components of cytoskeleton	Size	Arrangement	Functions	Disorders
Actin filaments	8 nm	Microfilaments thin, twisted strands of protein molecules. Scattered or organized actin like protein	Movements of pigment granules, amoeboid movement and protoplasmic streaming	Impairment of leukocytic movement and phagocytosis
Microtubules	25 nm	Microtubules hollow fibers made of a spiral arrangement of protein subunits, tough durable fibers	Maintaining shape of cell and participate in intracellular transport, movement of organelles and chromosomes (colchicine drug disrupting microtubules hence impairing movement of chromosomes)	Male sterility, Kartagener's syndrome, dysfunctional leukocytes and Chèdiak-Higashi syndrome
Intermediate filaments	8–10 nm	Intermediate filaments thicker hollow tubes, twisted protein strands, examples (*keratin, microfilaments, glial filaments, desmin and vimentin*)	In most of the cells, forming a basket around the nucleus and present in cell to cell junction	Mallory's hyaline, α_1-antitrypsin deficiency and Parkinson disease

inhibit actin filaments resulting in disruption of phagocytic activity of the cells.

- *Microtubules:* Microtubules are polymers composed of the protein tubulin capable of undergoing rapid assembly and disassembly in the cytosol. These are essential for leukocytic migration and phagocytosis. *Cytochalasin B drug prevents the assembly of microtubules also resulting in disruption of phagocytic activity of the cells.*
- *Intermediate filaments:* Intermediate filaments, such as *keratin, microfilaments, glial filaments, desmin and vimentin*, are important in the integration of cell organelles. Immunochemical stains utilizing monoclonal antibodies against individual intermediate filaments (e.g. desmin to identify muscle) are useful in identifying the origin of neoplasms.

Disorders of Microtubules

- *Male sterility:* Defects in microtubules inhibit sperm motility and results in sterility.
- *Kartagener's syndrome or immotile cilia syndrome:* It refers to immobilization of cilia of respiratory epithelium causes *interference of clearance of pathogens resulting in bronchiectasis.*
- *Dysfunctional leukocytes:* Colchicine drug used in acute attacks of gout binds to tubulin and prevents the assembly of microtubules, thus *prevents migration and phagocytosis of leukocytes in response to urate crystals.*
- *Chèdiak-Higashi syndrome:* It is autosomal recessive disorder. Main *defect is in the assembly (polymerization) of microtubules* in the cytoplasm. It is characterized by defective degranulation of neutrophils, impaired microbial killing, and recurrent *Staphylococcus aureus* bacterial infections forming soft tissue abscess.

  This disorder results from a mutation in the 'LYST gene' on chromosome 1q42 that encodes a protein for microtubules involved in intracellular trafficking of proteins.

Disorders of Intermediate Filaments

- *Mallory hyaline:* In chronic alcoholic persons, Mallory hyaline demonstrated in hepatocytes. It is an example of intermediate filaments (cytokeratins) abnormality.
- *α_1-antitrypsin deficiency:* Structurally abnormal α_1-antitrypsin molecules accumulate in the liver.
- *Parkinson disease:* α-Synuclein accumulates in neurons in the substantia nigra of patients with Parkinson disease.

PIGMENTS

Pigments are colored substances which absorb visible light. These are either present in normal cells or introduced from exogenous source. Examples of endogenous pigments synthesized within the body are melanin, bilirubin, hemosiderin, lipofuscin, homogentisic acid. Exogenous pigments introduced from exogenous source include carbon (anthracotic) pigment, tattooing, β-carotene and arsenic (Table 1.25).

Table 1.25: Type of pigments

Source of pigment	Pigments
Endogenous pigments	Melanin
	Bilirubin
	Hemosiderin
	Hematin
	Lipofuscin
	Homogentisic acid
	Hamazaki-Weissenberg bodies
Exogenous pigments	Carbon (anthracotic) pigment
	Tattooing
	β-carotene
	Arsenic

ENDOGENOUS PIGMENTS

Endogenous pigments deposited in the body are melanin, bilirubin, hemosiderin, lipofuscin, homogentisic acid and Hamazaki-Weissenberg bodies.

MELANIN PIGMENT

Melanin pigment is the only endogenous black-brown pigment derived from tyrosine. Melanin is distributed in *skin, hair, adrenal gland, nerve cells and substantia nigra*. Disorders of melanin pigment are shown in Table 1.26.

Synthesis

Melanin is formed in melanocyte or its precursor derived from neural crest. Tyrosinase in melanocytes present in the epidermis oxidizes tyrosine to dihydroxy phenyl alanine (DOPA). The product is transferred to adjacent clusters of keratinocytes and macrophages (melanophores) in the dermis. Melanin combines with proteins to form melanoprotein.

Hyperpigmentation

Increased melanin pigmentation is associated with sun tanning and with a wide variety of disorders due to over activity of ACTH, estrogens, Peutz-Jeghers syndrome and freckles.

Hypopigmentation

Decreased melanin pigmentation is observed in albinism and vitiligo.

BILIRUBIN PIGMENT

Bilirubin is the normal pigment present in bile. It is derived from hemoglobin but contains no iron. RBCs are normally destroyed by reticuloendothelial system (spleen and bone marrow) and liberate hemoglobin, which dissociates to form haem moiety porphyrin and iron and globin.

Bilirubin derived from porphyrin is an unconjugated (lipid soluble) form, which is conjugated into water-soluble form in the liver by glucuronyl transferase

Table 1.26: Disorders of melanin pigment

Mechanism	Underlying causes and clinical features
Hyperpigmentation	
ACTH overactivity	Cushing's syndrome
ACTH producing tumors	Small cell carcinoma lung, pancreatic carcinoma and medullary carcinoma thyroid
Addison's disease	Pigmentation of breast areola, gums, elbow and skin
Estrogen overactivity	Pregnancy, oral contraceptive pills, chronic liver disease and estrogen therapy in prostate carcinoma
Focal hyperpigmentation	*Peutz-Jeghers syndrome* (familial syndrome characterized by multiple polyps in stomach and bowel associated with brownish pigmentation around mouth and lips)
	Freckles: Skin shows focal areas of pigmentation throughout the skin
Hypopigmentation	
Albinism	It occurs due to defective tyrosine activity. Patient develops generalized hypo-pigmentation
Vitiligo (leukoderma)	It is most common type of focal hypopigmentation. Patient suffers from inborn total absence of melanocytes. Patient presents with lack of pigmentation on the face, hands and genital organs
Leprosy, poikiloderma or following burns	These are common examples of acquired hypopigmentation

enzyme and excreted into bile. Its normal synthesis and excretion are vital to health.

Jaundice (*yellow discoloration*) is a clinical disorder caused by excess of this pigment in the body, which gets deposited in *sclerae*, mucosae, and internal organs.

Bilirubin level is increased due to hemolytic anemia (spherocytosis), liver etiology (uptake and conjugation defect of unconjugated bilirubin) and posthepatic obstruction.

Hemolytic jaundice, which is associated with the destruction of red cells in hemolytic anemia. In hemolytic disease of newborns, an increase in unbound conjugated bilirubin may result in 'kernicterus' when it enters the central nervous system and dissolves in brain tissue.

Conjugated bilirubin is primarily increased in viral hepatitis (hepatocellular) and obstructive jaundice (intrahepatic or extrahepatic obstruction of the biliary tract). Bilirubin may accumulate in liver cells.

HEMOSIDERIN PIGMENT

Hemosiderin pigment is a hemoglobin-derived golden brown granular or crystalline pigment. It is also known as *iron pigment*. It consists of partially degraded apoprotein, lipid and iron. Hemosiderin is a partially denatured form of ferritin present in the form of aggregates in tissues.

Iron Metabolism

Apoferritin takes up excess of iron and oxidizes ferrous form to ferric form. This iron deposited in the core and surrounded by apoprotein is known as *ferritin*. Then ferritin is broken down to hemosiderin. Unlike ferritin, iron in the hemosiderin goes back to metabolic pool of the body in a slow fashion.

Storage

Normally, hemosiderin and ferritin exists normally in small amounts as physiologic iron stores within tissue macrophages of the *bone marrow, liver, and spleen*, all actively engaged in red cell breakdown.

> ### Light Microscopy
> Hemosiderin appears as globular and golden brown granules. This pigment becomes refractile, when condenser of the microscope is lowered down (Fig. 1.27).

Perl's Stain

Perl's stain is also known as *iron stain*. Perl's stain turns hemosiderin to blue by Prussian blue reaction (Fig. 1.28).

Distribution of iron in adults is shown in Table 1.27 and difference between ferritin and hemosiderin is shown in Table 1.28.

Hemosiderin is absent in bone marrow macrophages in iron deficiency. It accumulates pathologically in tissues in excess amounts.

Table 1.27: Distribution of iron in adults

Total body iron (3.0–5.0 gm)		
Functional iron	Hemoglobin	1.5–3.0 gm
	Essential nonavailable iron	0.3 gm
	Myoglobin and enzymes of cellular respiration	0.05 gm
Storage/available tissue iron	Ferritin and hemosiderin	1.2–2.0 gm
Plasma	Transferrin transport iron	3–4 mg

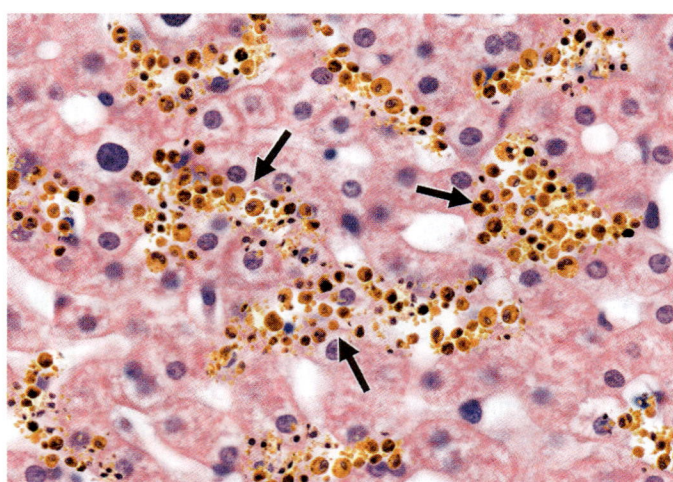

Fig. 1.27: Hemosiderin granules in liver seen as golden brown finely granular pigment (arrows).

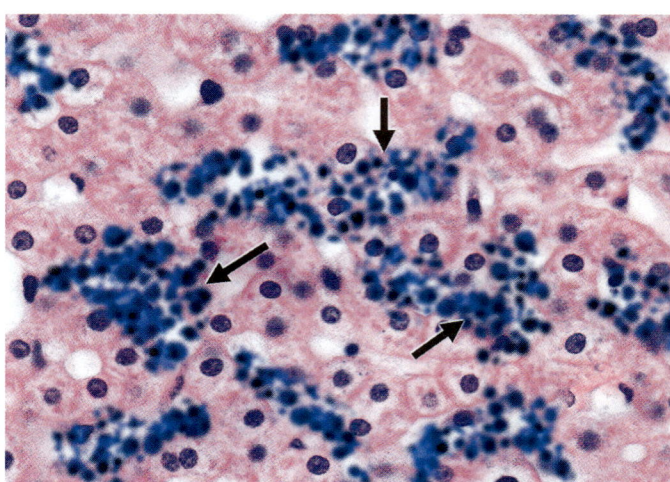

Fig. 1.28: Hemosiderin granules in liver demonstrated by Prussian blue stain specific for iron (arrows).

Table 1.28: Differences between ferritin and hemosiderin

Ferritin	Hemosiderin
Colorless (unstained smear)	Golden yellow (unstained smear)
Water soluble	Water insoluble
Contains less iron	Contains more iron
Storage: Bone marrow, liver and spleen	Storage: Bone marrow, liver and spleen

Hemosiderosis

Hemosiderosis represents intracellular storage of hemosiderin located in the fixed macrophages of the bone marrow without associated tissue or organ damage. In congestive heart failure, small hemorrhages occur in the lungs. Red blood cells are phagocytozed by alveolar macrophages. These alveolar macrophages laden with hemosiderin are known as *heart failure cells*. Pulmonary hemosiderosis along with fibrosis is known as *brown induration of lung*. Examples of localized hemosiderosis are *organized hematoma, hemorrhagic infarcts* and *bone fractures*.

Hemochromatosis

Hemochromatosis refers to extensive accumulation of hemosiderin primarily within parenchymal cells with accompanying tissue damage, scarring, and organ dysfunction. Excessive iron deposition occurs in primary or secondary hemochromatosis.

Primary Hemochromatosis

- *Basic defect:* It is autosomal dominant inborn disorder of iron metabolism resulting in dysregulation of iron metabolism. It most often occurs due to mutation of HFE gene on chromosome 6. Other gene mutations seen include C282Y, followed by the H63D.
- *Organs damage:* It increases iron absorption in the small intestine, excess iron is stored mostly in the form of hemosiderin, primarily in the liver, pancreas, myocardium, and multiple endocrine glands. Prussian blue staining marks the intraparenchymal deposition of hemosiderin.
- *Bronze diabetes:* Primary hemochromatosis results in 'bronze diabetes' characterized by micronodular cirrhosis, diabetes mellitus, and skin pigmentation (melanin).

Secondary Hemochromatosis

Secondary hemochromatosis is most often caused by multiple blood transfusions especially in β-thalassemia major. Iron is deposited in parenchyma of various organs.

HEMATIN PIGMENT

Hematin is derived from the breakdown of hemoglobin by macrophages in the spleen and bone marrow that have phagocytozed red blood cells (RBCs).

It is a Prussian blue-negative, black, crystalline product originating from the oxidation of heme from the ferrous to the ferric state in conditions associated with macrophage removal of RBCs in the spleen (e.g. malaria, methemoglobinemia and schistosomiasis).

LIPOFUSCIN PIGMENT

The term is derived from the Latin (fuscus-brown), thus brown lipid. It is an insoluble pigment, also known as *lipochrome* or *wear and tear* or aging pigment. It is composed of polymers of lipids and phospholipids complexed with proteins.

- *Organs involved:* Lipofuscin pigment accumulates in liver, heart muscle, adrenal gland and ganglion cells, producing *brown atrophy*.
- *Synthesis:* Lipofuscin is derived from continuing lipid peroxidation of lipids present in cellular membranes as a result of inadequate defenses against activated oxygen-derived free radicals. Lipid peroxides are unstable and breaking down into smaller molecules Lipofuscin does not injure cells or impair their functions.
- *Light microscopy:* Lipofuscin appears as a yellow brown finely granular pigment in cytoplasm often in perinuclear region in *liver, heart muscle, adrenal glands* and *ganglion cells* especially of aging persons or patients with cancer cachexia or severe malnutrition.
- *Histochemistry:* Lipofuscin is acid-fast and demonstrated by Sudan black and basic fuscin stains.
- *Electron microscopy:* Lipofuscin pigment deposition appear as electron dense granules located in a perinuclear region.

HOMOGENTISIC ACID

Homogentisic acid is a black pigment that occurs in patients with alkaptonuria. It is a rare inborn error of metabolism due to homogentisic oxidase deficiency. The term alkaptonuria refers to urinary excretion of metabolized homogentisic acid imparting a *dark color to urine on standing*.

The term *ochronosis* refers to deposition of this pigment prominently in *cartilage* and *connective tissue*. Other affected structures include the *eyes, larynx* and *bronchi, heart* and *vessels, prostate*, and *sweat glands*. Most symptoms result from joint involvement, which can lead to *disabling arthritis* as patient ages.

HAMAZAKI-WEISSENBERG BODIES

Hamazaki-Weissenberg bodies appear as small, yellow brown spindle-shaped structures in the sinuses of lymph nodes either lying free or as cytoplasmic inclusions. Their significance is not known.

EXOGENOUS PIGMENTS

COAL DUST

Deposition of coal dust (anthracotic pigment) derived from coal mines and tobacco smoke in the interstitial tissue of lungs, peribronchial lymphatics and hilar lymph nodes is known as *coal worker pneumoconiosis*. Alveolar macrophages laden with anthracotic pigment are called as *dust cells*. Pathological lesions depend upon duration of exposure and magnitude of coal dust.

TATTOOING

Tattooing is a form of localized exogenous pigment inoculated into the skin. It is phagocytozed by dermal macrophages. It resides in dermal macrophages forever. This pigment does not evoke inflammatory response.

CALCIFICATION

Physiological calcification: Normally, calcium salts comprised of calcium phosphate, calcium carbonates are deposited in bone and teeth. In hematoxylin and eosin stained sections, calcium appears as basophilic amorphous, granular and clumped in intracellular as well as extracellular sites.

Pathological calcification: Pathological calcification occurs by two processes: Dystrophic calcification and metastatic calcification. Dystrophic calcification reflects underlying cell injury. Metastatic calcification reflects an underlying disorder in calcium metabolism.

DYSTROPHIC CALCIFICATION

Dystrophic calcification has its origin in direct cell injury. Calcium is deposited in dead or dying tissues. Serum calcium concentration is within normal limits. It occurs by two processes: Initiation and propagation. These are described as under.

PROCESS OF CALCIFICATION

Initiation

Calcium is deposited inside cells or in extracellular compartment. Calcium inside cell is present in the form of membrane bound vesicles containing acidic phospholipids.
- Calcium has strong affinity for phospholipids. Phosphatase participates in deposition of phosphates.
- Now tiny crystals of calcium are released from membrane bound vesicles into the extracellular compartment.

Propagation

Further deposition of calcium is known as *propagation*. It depends on level of calcium and phosphate in the extracellular compartment, presence of collagen fibers and other proteins. Propagation enhances deposition of calcium. Calcium now binds with osteopontin. Under physiological state, osteopontin participates in mineralization of bone.

EXAMPLES OF DYSTROPHIC CALCIFICATION

- *Necrosis:* Calcium is deposited in dead and dying tissues, i.e. coagulative necrosis, liquefactive necrosis, fat necrosis and caseous necrosis.
- *Neoplastic conditions:* Psammoma bodies are calcific spherules seen in papillary carcinoma of thyroid, meningioma, uterine leiomyomas and serous cystadenoma, serous cyst borderline tumor and serous cyst adenocarcinoma.
- *Parasitic diseases:* Calcium is deposited in sites of dead parasites, i.e. cysticercosis, filariasis and hydatid cyst.
- *Trauma:* Calcium deposition in muscles after trauma is called as 'myositis ossificans'.
- *Tissue repair:* Calcium deposition takes place in hyalinized scar.
- *Lithopodion:* Calcium deposition in dead fetus after ruptured tubal pregnancy is called lithopodion.
- *Cardiovascular system:* Calcium is deposited in arteriosclerosis, atheromatous plaques, venous thrombi and scarred heart valves.
- *Thyroid gland:* Calcium deposition occurs in multinodular goiter.
- *Calcinosis:* It is type of dystrophic calcification seen under skin.
- *Intrauterine toxoplasma infection:* It affects approximately 0.1% of all pregnancies. Acute encephalitis in the fetus afflicted with TORCH syndrome may be associated with foci of necrosis that become calcified.

METASTATIC CALCIFICATION

Metastatic calcification reflects an underlying disorder in calcium metabolism. Calcium is deposited in normal tissues. Serum calcium and phosphate concentration is increased.

Etiology

Metastatic calcification occurs in primary hyperparathyroidism and tumor metastases to the bone with increased osteolytic activity leading to mobilization of calcium and phosphate, resulting in hypercalcemia.

Disturbance of calcium metabolism occurs in milk alkali syndrome, hypervitaminosis D, destructive bone disease (multiple myeloma and metastatic bone tumors), prolonged immobilization and advanced renal disease with phosphate retention in secondary hyperparathyroidism.

Due to excess calcium intake in the form of milk and self-antacid therapy causes milk-alkali syndrome, and the patient develops nephrocalcinosis and renal stones. Etiology of metastatic calcification is shown in Table 1.29 and differences between dystrophic calcification and metastatic calcification are shown in Table 1.30.

Table 1.29: Etiology of metastatic calcification

Disorders
Primary hyperparathyroidism
Secondary hyperparathyroidism due to advanced renal disease with phosphate retention
Milk alkali syndrome (milk ingestion and self-antacid therapy)
Hypervitaminosis D
Destructive bone disease (multiple myeloma and metastatic bone tumors)
Prolonged immobilization

Examples

Calcium is deposited in the alveolar septa of the lung (*pulmonary alveolar microlithiasis*), renal tubular basement membrane (nephrolithiasis), cornea, blood vessels and fundal glands of stomach because relative alkalinity left after their acid secretions favors it (Fig. 1.29A and B).

Table 1.30: Differences between dystrophic calcification and metastatic calcification

Features	Dystrophic calcification	Metastatic calcification
Definition	Calcium is deposited in previously damaged tissues	Calcium deposited in normal tissues
Calcium metabolism	No systemic disturbance of calcium metabolism	Systemic disturbance of calcium metabolism
Serum calcium concentration	Normal range	Increased levels
Organs involved	Organs affected due to necrosis, e.g. parasitic infections as mentioned and some tumors as mentioned below	Renal tubular basement membrane, lungs, cornea, blood vessels, fundal glands of stomach due to relative alkalinity left after their acid secretions favors it
Etiology	*Necrosis:* Coagulative, liquefactive, fat and caseous necrosis	Hyperparathyroidism
	Parasites: Cysticercosis (dead parasite) and filariasis	Milk alkali syndrome
	Venous thrombi (phleboliths)	Hypervitaminosis D
	Tumors: Psamomma bodies in papillary carcinoma thyroid, meningiomas, serous cystadenoma, serous borderline tumor, serous cystadenocarcinoma of ovary and leiomyoma	*Destructive bone disease due to multiple myeloma*, carcinomas of thyroid, gastrointestinal tract, breast, kidney (renal cell carcinoma), neuroblastoma, and malignant melanoma
	Blood vessels: Complicated atheromatous plaque, venous thrombi and Monkeberg's calcific sclerosis	
	Others: Dead fetus (lithopodion), traumatic myositis ossificans, hyalinized scar tissue goiter undergoing degeneration and acute encephalitis in fetus afflicted, with TORCH syndrome are examples of dystrophic calcification	Prolonged immobilization and pulmonary alveolar microliths
		Secondary hyperparathyroidism due to chronic renal disease with phosphate retention

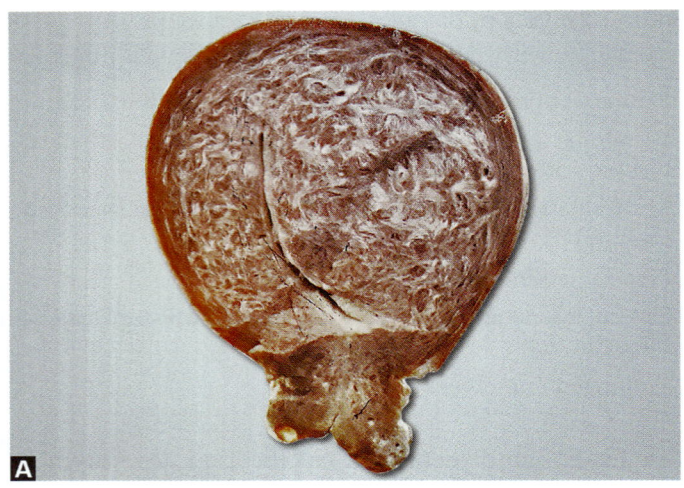
Fig. 1.29A: Showing calcified Leiomyoma.

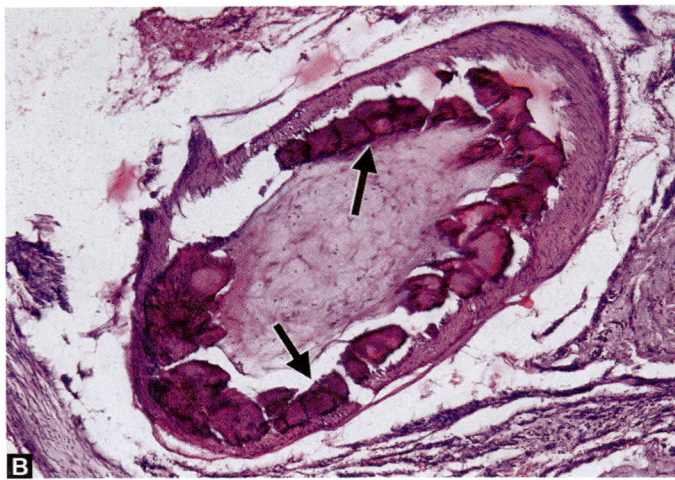
Fig. 1.29B: Medial calcification of artery (arrows) (400X).

INTRACELLULAR ACCUMULATIONS

LIPIDS

Fatty change refers to any abnormal accumulation of triglycerides, cholesterol/cholesterol esters and phospholipids within parenchymal cells of liver, heart, skeletal muscle and kidneys. Defects in any of the steps of uptake, catabolism or secretion may result in lipid accumulation in cells. Skeletal muscle may show mild fatty change as a result of ischemia and severe fatty change due to diphtheria.

FATTY CHANGE LIVER (STEATOSIS)

Liver is the major organ involved in fat metabolism. Therefore, fatty change most often occurs in liver due to accumulation of triglycerides.

Etiology

The lipid accumulates when lipoprotein transport is disrupted and/or when fatty acids accumulate.

- Alcohol abuse and diabetes mellitus associated with obesity are the most common causes of fatty change in liver. Alcohol interferes with mitochondrial and microsomal function in hepatocytes, leading to an accumulation of lipid.
- Other causes of fatty change include toxins, protein malnutrition (kwashiorkor), anoxia and severe gastrointestinal malabsorption. Tetracycline can cause microvesicular fatty change in liver.

Pathogenesis

Physiological state: Free fatty acids from adipose tissue or ingested FFA are normally transported into hepatocytes, where they are esterified to triglycerides, converted into cholesterol or phospholipids, or oxidized to ketone bodies. Some of the fatty acids are synthesized from acetate within hepatocytes as well. Egress of the triglyceride requires the formation of complexes with apoproteins to form lipoproteins, which are able to enter the circulation.

Pathological state: Defects in any of the steps of uptake, catabolism, or secretion can lead to accumulation of triglycerides in fatty liver. Hepatotoxins (e.g. alcohol) alter mitochondrial and smooth endoplasmic reticulum function and thus inhibit fatty acid oxidation. Carbon tetrachloride and protein malnutrition decrease the synthesis of apoproteins. Anoxia inhibits fatty acid oxidation, and starvation increase fatty acid mobilization from peripheral stores.

Clinical Significance

Mild fatty change has no effect on cellular functions. Severe fatty change may transiently impair cellular functions. But in carbon tetrachloride poisoning, fatty change is irreversible.

Gross Morphology

Mild fatty change in liver may not affect the gross appearance. Severe fatty change results in enlargement of liver. It becomes progressively yellow on cut surface until it may weigh 3 to 6 kg. This uniform change is consistent with fatty metamorphosis (fatty change).

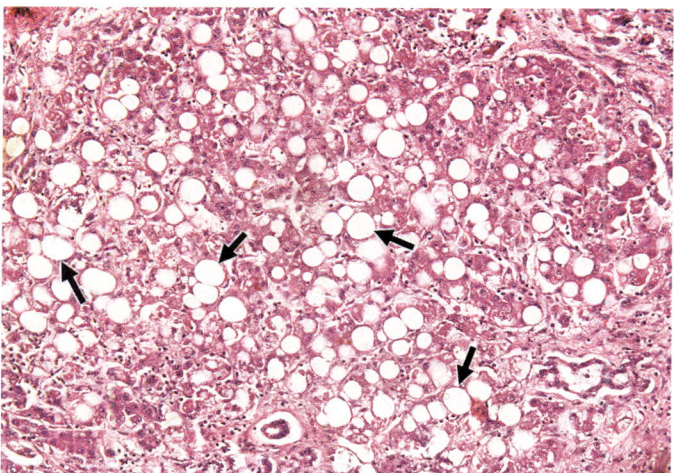

Fig. 1.30: Fatty change liver showing preservation of cells with nuclei displaced towards periphery with abundant clear looking cytoplasm (arrows) (400X).

Light Microscopy

Initially, hepatocytes show small fat vacuoles around nucleus (mild fatty change or microvesicular) in hematoxylin and eosin stained sections.

- Progressive accumulation of fat vacuoles in the cytoplasm coalesce to create spaces that displace the nucleus toward periphery (severe fatty change). Occasionally contiguous cells rupture, and the enclosed fat globules unite to produce so-called fatty cysts.
- Distribution of lipid vacuoles may be diffuse, focal or zonal, midzonal or peripheral depending on severity and etiology (Fig. 1.30).

Frozen Section Technique

In paraffin embedded sections, fat is dissolved during processing of tissue in tissue processor. Fat can be demonstrated by frozen section technique with the fat stains such as *Sudan III, Sudan IV, Sudan black, Oil red O and osmic acid*.

CHOLESTEROL AND CHOLESTEROL ESTERS

Most cells utilize cholesterol for the synthesis of cell membranes without intracellular accumulation. Accumulation of cholesterol and its esters is demonstrated in various pathological states: *Atherosclerosis, xanthomas, cholesterolosis (gallbladder) and Niemann-Pick disease* described as under.

Atherosclerosis

Atherosclerosis means hardening (sclerosis) or loss of elasticity of large elastic arteries and medium-sized arteries due to atheromatous plaque formation. It is composed of smooth muscle cells, foam cells, fibrin, and extracellular matrix material, such as collagen, elastin, glycosaminoglycans, and proteoglycans. Endothelium over the surface of the fibrous cap frequently appears intact.

Xanthomas

Patient with familial or acquired hyperlipidemia presents with masses known as *xanthomas* in skin and tendon. These are formed due to accumulation of cholesterol or cholesterol esters within macrophages in these areas.

Cholesterolosis of Gallbladder

Presence of cholesterol laden macrophages in the lamina propria of the gallbladder gives mucosa, a yellow-speckled appearance known as *strawberry gallbladder*. There is no association with inflammatory changes and cholelithiasis. Cholesterolosis of gallbladder is shown in Fig. 1.31.

Niemann-Pick Disease

Niemann-Pick disease is a hereditary lysosomal storage disease caused by deficiency of sphingomyelinase results in accumulation of sphingomyelin in phagocytes (types A and B Niemann-Pick disease).

- Type C Niemann-Pick disease is caused by defect in a gene involved in cholesterol transport with cholesterol accumulation within phagocytes.
- Diagnostic hallmark is presence of *foamy histiocytes* containing sphingomyelin in liver, spleen, lymph nodes, and skin.

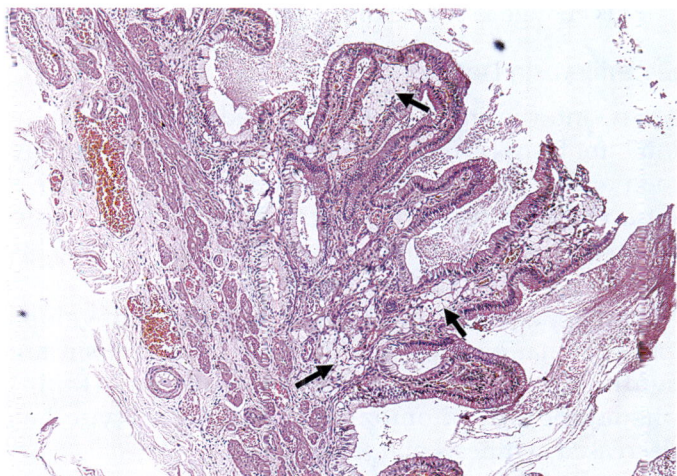

Fig. 1.31: Cholesterolosis of gallbladder. Cholesterol laden macrophages are seen in gallbladder (arrows) (100X).

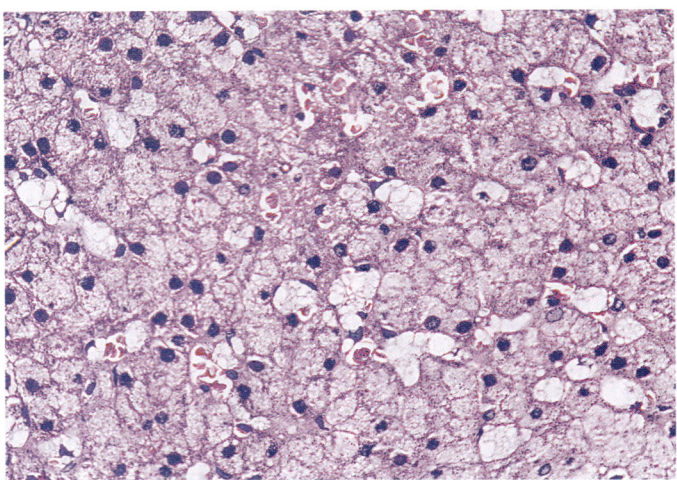

Fig. 1.32: Niemann-Pick disease showing foamy histiocytes' containing sphingomyelin (400X).

- Child presents with hepatosplenomegaly, anemia, fever, and in some variants, neurologic manifestations.
- Approximately 50% of the patients develop cherry red spot in the macula similar to that of Tay-Sachs disease. Death occurs by 3 years of age (Fig. 1.32).

PROTEINS

Intracellular accumulation of proteins occurs in renal diseases associated with proteinuria, *a_1-antitrypsin deficiency*, accumulation of cytoskeletal proteins and *amyloidosis*.

Renal Disease with Proteinuria

Proximal tubules reabsorb droplets of protein in patient with nephritic or nephrotic syndrome. These proteins in cells appear as rounded eosinophilic droplets, vacuoles or aggregates.

This change is reversible, if proteinuria diminishes.

α_1-antitrypsin Deficiency

The α_1-antitrypsin is a protein encoded on the proteinase inhibitor locus (Pi) on chromosome 14. It affects equally men and women. Gene mutation leads to defective intracellular transport and secretion of proteins due to accumulation in endoplasmic reticulum in liver. This protein is not secreted by liver.

Patient with α_1-antitrypsin deficiency develops emphysema. Normal amounts of α_1-antitrypsin are synthesized in normal genotype persons (PiMM phenotype). But homozygous PiZZ genotype has decreased synthesis of α_1-antitrypsin.

Serum electrophoresis reveals absence of α_1-globulin peak.

GLYCOGEN

In diabetes mellitus, glycogen is demonstrated in renal tubular cells, β-cells of islet of Langerhans, liver and myocardium. Glycogen is demonstrated by best carmine or PAS. Glycogen is also accumulated in cells in genetic disorders, known as *glycogen storage diseases*.

Glycogen Storage Disease

Due to deficiency of lysosomal enzymes, accumulation of metabolites occurs due to incomplete degradation. Examples are glycogen storage disease or von Gierke's disease due to glucose-6-phosphatase deficiency. These are described as under:

- *Hepatorenal or von Gierke disease type I:* It occurs due to deficiency of glucose-6-phosphatase. Glycogen is accumulated in *hepatocytes* and *cortical tubular cells*. Failure of glucose mobilization results in hypoglycemia and convulsions.

  Deranged glucose metabolism may result in hyperlipidemia and xanthomas. Patient presents with failure to thrive, *hepatomegaly* or enlargement of kidneys. Glycogen storage disease of liver is shown in Fig. 1.33.

- *McArdle syndrome type V:* It occurs due to deficiency of phosphorylase enzymes in *skeletal muscles*. Glycogen is deposited in subsarcolemal region. Creatine kinase enzyme is raised. Patient presents with exercise induced *painful cramp*. Myoglobinuria occurs in 50% of patients. Patient lives a compatible life.

- *Pompe disease type II:* It is generalized glycogen storage disorder due to deficiency of glucosidase. Patient presents with *massive cardiomegaly*, and *muscle hypotonia*. Children under 2 years may develop cardiorespiratory failure. But adults present with myopathy.

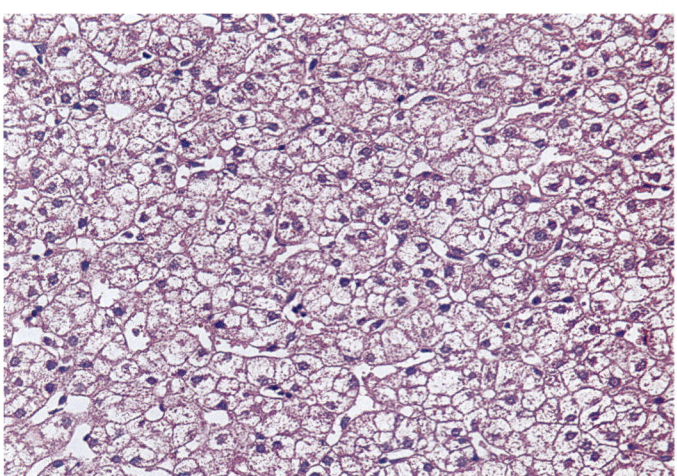

Fig. 1.33: Glycogen storage disease of liver (400X).

Cellular Adaptations, Cell Injury, Apoptosis, Pigments, Calcification, Cellular Accumulations and Aging

EXTRACELLULAR ACCUMULATIONS

AMYLOIDOSIS

Amyloidosis is fundamentally a disorder of protein misfolding. More than 20 different proteins result in aggregation to form insoluble fibrils. These insoluble fibrils are deposited in extracellular tissue in one organ or many organs resulting in tissue damage. Amyloidosis may be localized or systemic. It is not a single disease entity but rather a diverse group of inherited or acquired disorders. Most important organs involved are *kidney, spleen and liver*. Morphology of these organs is described as under.

RENAL AMYLOIDOSIS

Kidney amyloidosis is the most common serious complication in the disease.

Gross Morphology
Kidney is enlarged, pale, and waxy with smooth surface with firm consistency. In advanced cases, the kidneys are contracted and shrunken due to vascular narrowing induced by deposition of amyloid.

Light Microscopy
- Kidney biopsy shows amyloid deposits primarily affecting glomeruli and renal blood vessels, often causing marked vascular narrowing.
- Peritubular tissue is also involved.

Electron Microscopy
Electron microscopy reveals deposition of amyloid fibrils in subendothelial region of glomerular basement membrane.

Clinical Correlation
Patient presents with proteinuria in nephritic/nephrotic range and ultimately go into renal failure.

SPLEEN AMYLOIDOSIS

Amyloidosis of the spleen often causes moderate or even marked enlargement (200–800 gm). Amyloidosis of the spleen has two different anatomical patterns such as *sago spleen* or *lardaceous spleen*. In both the patterns, amyloid spleen is firm in consistency, and cut surfaces reveal pale gray, waxy deposits (Fig. 1.34).

Sago Spleen
Most commonly, the amyloid deposition is limited to the splenic follicles, resulting in the gross appearance of a moderately enlarged spleen dotted with *tapioca-like gray nodules* (so-called *sago* spleen).

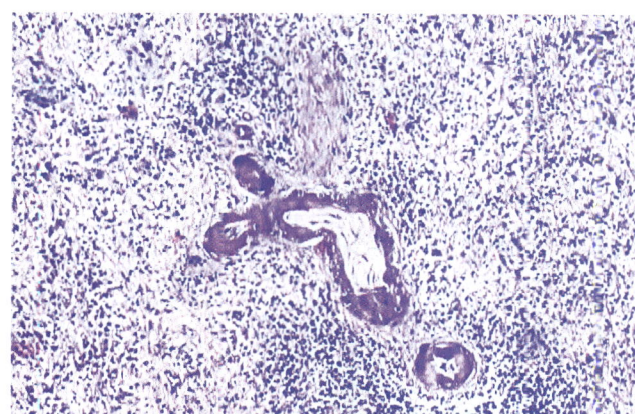

Fig. 1.34: Amyloid deposition in spleen (100X).

Lardaceous Spleen
Alternatively, the amyloid deposits may spare the follicles and mainly infiltrate the red pulp sinuses, producing a large, firm spleen mottled with waxy discolorations (*lardaceous* spleen).

LIVER AMYLOIDOSIS

Secondary amyloidosis most often involves liver leading to hepatomegaly.

Gross Morphology
The amyloid liver is usually grossly enlarged (as much as 900 gm), pale, and smooth surface, firm consistency. When sectioned, it has sharp rigid edges.

Light Microscopy
- Amyloid material is initially deposited in the spaces of Disse between the hepatocytes and vascular sinusoids. As more amyloid accumulates, it compresses the hepatic cords and sinusoids
- The hepatic cords undergo nutritional and pressure atrophy and become displaced or replaced by bands and nodules of amyloid.

HYALINE CHANGE

Hyaline change refers to an alteration within cells or extracellular space. Intracellular hyaline material is demonstrated as Russel bodies in plasma cells and alcoholic hyaline in liver.

Hyaline arteriosclerosis is characterized by hyaline thickening of arteriolar walls. It accompanies *benign hypertension* and *diabetes mellitus*.

Light Microscopy
It reveals eosinophilic glassy appearance in hematoxylin and eosin sections.

CELLULAR AGING

It has been proposed that cells have a programmed capacity for a limited number of cell divisions, after which cells are not replaced and atrophy ensues, with loss of function.

THEORIES OF AGING

Alternative theories suggest that essential neuroendocrine biological stimuli from brain or endocrine glands are programmed to stop at a certain biological age, resulting in lack of essential trophic factors to maintain cell growth.

Other proposals suggest inefficient DNA repair, free radical damage, or failure of protein catabolism as the root cause of aging. Cumulative injury theories propose that aging is the result of all cellular impairments sustained throughout life, whether through DNA damage, protein modification, free radical damage, or disease.

DNA DEFECTS

It has been suggested that aging is merely the result of the known inefficiencies in repair of DNA, which occurs at a low level in normal people. With time the proportion of cells carrying abnormal DNA increases and tissue function is impaired. This applies not only to nuclear DNA but also to mitochondrial DNA, which has much less effective systems for repairing damage.

DEGENERATION IN EXTRACELLULAR MATERIAL

Through protein cross-linking, modification such as glycosylation, and oxidation, has been proposed as a mechanism that impairs function of the specialized parenchymal cells, leading to cell dysfunction with age.

FREE RADICAL INJURY

Decrease in the availability of free radical scavenging systems has been proposed as the mechanism whereby free radical-mediated damage becomes more significant with age and begins to cause cellular dysfunction and death. This would also cause damage to DNA, as well as to proteins (Fig. 1.35).

GENETIC DISORDERS

Patient with genetic disorders like Hutchinson-Gilford progeria or Werner syndrome develop premature aging process.

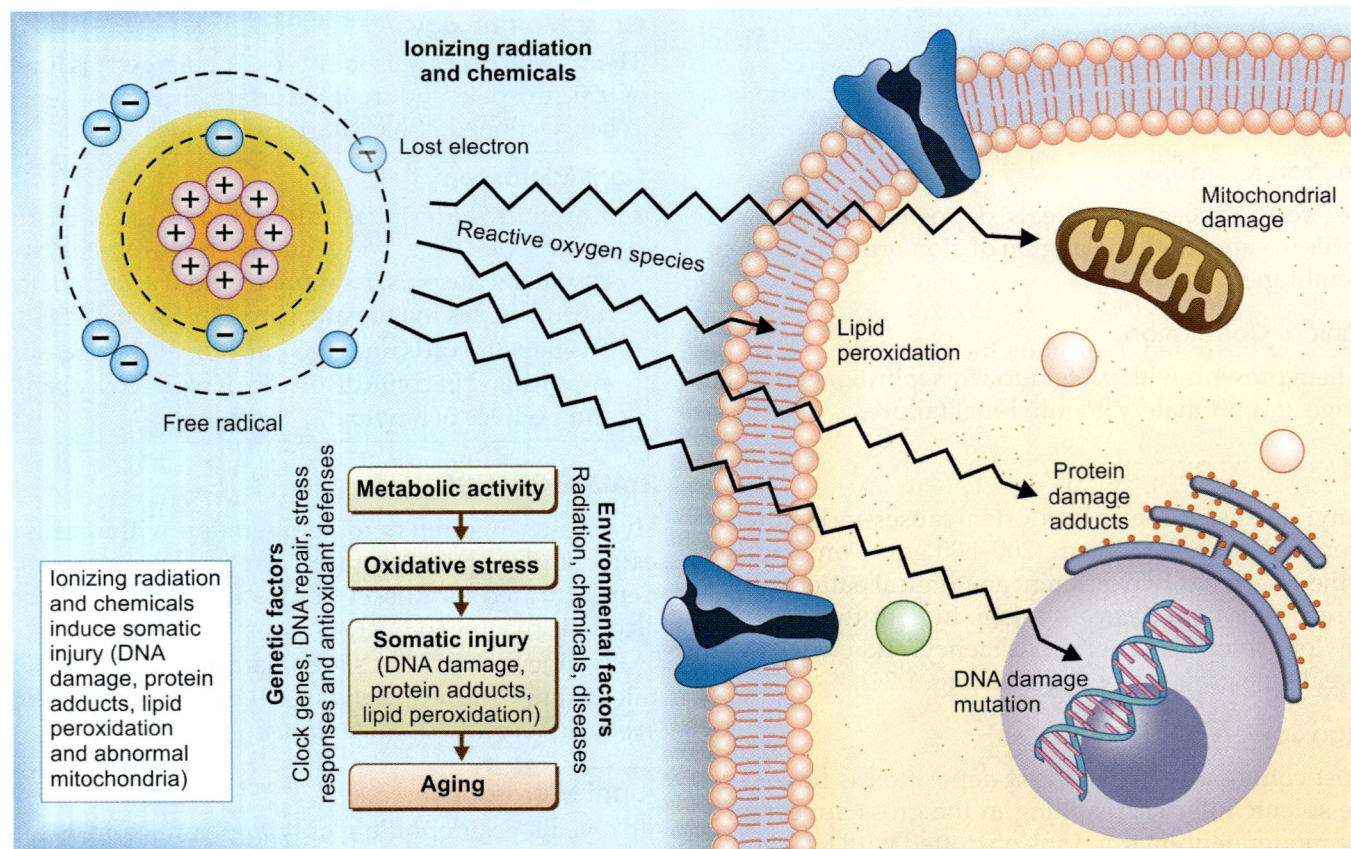

Fig. 1.35: The free radical theory of human aging.

Cellular Adaptations, Cell Injury, Apoptosis, Pigments, Calcification, Cellular Accumulations and Aging

These disorders are described as under.

Hutchinson-Gilford Progeria

- *Basic defect:* Lamins are intermediate filament proteins that form a fibrous meshwork beneath the nuclear envelope. Lamin A (LMNA) gene mutation is thought to make the nucleus unstable, leading to cell injury and death.
- *Clinical features:* It is a rare genetic disease causing premature aging in children. Patient presents with early cataracts, hairloss, skin atrophy, osteoporosis, and atherosclerosis.

Werner Syndrome

- *Basic defect:* This is a autosomal recessive disorder which occurs due to mutation in the WRN gene, which effects multiple DNA-dependent enzymatic functions, including proteins with ATPase, helicase, and exonuclease activity.
- *Clinical features:* Patient presents with early cataracts, hairloss, skin atrophy, osteoporosis, and accelerated atherosclerosis. Patient with Werner syndrome die in the fifth decade from either cancer or cardiovascular disease.

MAMMALIAN SIRTUIN SYSTEM

The salient information regulator (SIR) genes (sirtuins) comprise highly conserved family of proteins present in all species. Seven sirtuin genes (SIRT1 to SIRT7) have been identified in mammals. These seven sirtuin genes code for seven distinct sirtuin enzymes dependent on oxidized nicotinamide adenine dinucleotide. *Sirtuin system controls other genes thus influence other regulatory molecules.* Sirtuin system is influenced by environmental and nutritional factors. Expression and activity of sirtuins are strongly influenced by *dietary, lifestyle or environmental factors.* Increased expression of SIRT1 has been demonstrated to prolong the lifespan.

Subcellular Location

Nucleus contains SIRT1, SIRT2, SIRT6 and SIRT7. SIRT1 and SIRT2 are also located in the cytoplasm. Mitochondria contain SIRT3, SIRT4 and SIRT5. SIRT1 has been widely studied.

SIRT1 hydrolyzes NAD^+ into ADP-ribose moiety and nicotinamide. It removes an acetyl group from a protein acetyllysine. It transfers acetyl group to the ADP-ribose moiety leading to formation of 2'-O-acetyl-ADP-ribose. Sirtuin enzyme activities and subcellular locations are shown in Fig. 1.36 and Table 1.31.

Calorie restriction and tissue levels of specific sirtuins: Calorie restriction (or complete fasting) affect the level of specific sirtuins. The sirtuin system is involved in mediating the increase in lifespan by calorie restriction. There is *increased gluconeogenesis, cholesterol metabolism, fatty acid oxidation, fatty acid mobilization and increased insulin activity.*

There is decreased glycolysis and adipogenesis. Calorie restriction and its effect on the level of sirtuins in various tissues is shown in Table 1.32.

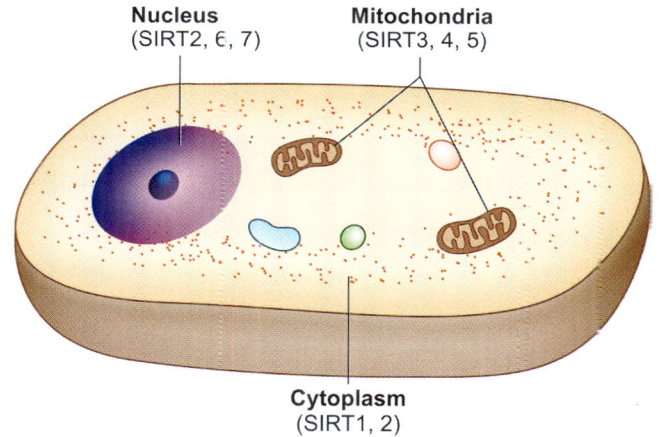

Fig. 1.36: Location of sirtuins in mammalian cellular compartments.

Table 1.31: Mammalian sirtuin enzyme activities and subcellular locations

Subcellular location	Sirtuin	Location in organs	Type of enzyme
Nucleus and cytoplasm	SIRT1	Brain, hypothalamus, heart, kidney, liver, pancreas, spleen, skeletal muscle and white adipose tissue	Deacetylase
	SIRT2	Adipose tissue	Deacetylase
Mitochondria	SIRT3	Skeletal muscle, brown adipose tissue, white adipose tissue, heart, kidney, liver	Deacetylase and ADP-ribosyltransferase
	SIRT4	Islets of Langerhans in the pancreas	ADP-ribosyltransferase
	SIRT5	Liver	Deacetylase
Nucleus	SIRT6	Adipose tissue, skeletal muscle, brain, and heart	Deacetylase and ADP-ribosyltransferase
	SIRT7	Adipose tissue and cardiac muscle	Deacetylase

Table 1.32: Calorie restriction and its effect on the level of sirtuins in various tissues

Sirtuin	Tissue upregulation	Tissue downregulation
SIRT1	Increased level of SIRT1 in liver, kidney, intestine, skeletal muscle and white adipose tissue	Decreased level of SIRT1 in hypothalamus
SIRT2	Increased level of SIRT2 in adipose tissue	No downregulation in any other tissue
SIRT3	Increased level of SIRT3 in liver, skeletal muscle, white adipose tissue and brown adipose tissue	No downregulation in any other tissue
SIRT5	Increased level of SIRT5 in liver	No downregulation in any other tissue

- *Tissue upregulation of SIT1:* There is upregulation of SIRT1 in the *liver, kidney, intestine, skeletal muscle and white adipose tissue*, but its downregulation in the hypothalamus. SIRT1 is involved in regulating expression of adipokines such as adiponectin and tumor necrosis factor.

    SIRT1 expression has negative association with fatty change in human beings. SIRT1 stimulates nitric oxide synthase leading to increased production of nitric oxide responsible for vasodilation. SIRT2 level is increased in adipose tissue.

- *Tissue upregulation of SIRT3:* There is upregulation of SIRT3 in the liver, skeletal muscle, white adipose tissue and brown adipose tissue.

- *Tissue upregulation of SIRT5:* SIRT5 level is *increased the liver.*

Tobacco smoking and its effect on tissue SIRT1 activity: Tobacco smoke extract adversely affect tissue SIRT1 levels. SIRT1 activity is decreased in tobacco smokers in the pulmonary monocyte-macrophage cells and epithelial cells. Their level is also decreased in human umbilical vein and endothelial cells in smokers.

Resveratrol and its effect on tissue SIRT1 activity: Resveratrol increases SIRT1 activity in adipose tissue, skeletal muscle, liver, β cells of islets of Langerhans in pancreas, heart and endothelial cells.

Sirtuin system and its role in cancer: SIRT1 level is increased in some cancers. Research work suggested that SIRT1 acts as tumor promotor by deactivating proteins like p53, p300 and foxhead transcriptional factor involved in DNA repair.

CHAPTER 2

Inflammation, Tissue Healing and Repair

Learning Objectives

ACUTE INFLAMMATION
- Cellular Events
- Outcome of Acute Inflammation
- Morphologic Patterns of Acute Inflammation
- Chemical Mediators
- Defects in Leukocytes and Complement
- Anti-inflammatory Therapeutic Agents
- Systemic Effects of Inflammation

CHRONIC INFLAMMATION
- Nonspecific Chronic Inflammation
- Granulomatous Inflammation

TISSUE HEALING AND REPAIR
- Control of Normal Cell Proliferation and Tissue Growth
- Cell Cycle and its Regulation
- Regeneration of Tissue and Organ
- Extracellular Matrix (ECM)
- Mechanism of Tissue Repair
- Factors Affecting Wound Healing

OVERVIEW OF INFLAMMATION

Inflammation is a tissue response at microcirculation level to nonself injurious agents. Inflammatory response is expressed through vascular (arterioles, capillaries and venules) and cellular functions that are coordinated by chemical mediators. Increased vascular permeability due to widened intercellular junctions and contraction of endothelial cells by chemical mediators such as histamine, VEGF, and bradykinin leads to extravasation of proteins, inflammatory cells and red blood cells resulting in exudate formation.

Transudate is poor in protein. Macrophages and lymphocytes participate in repair either by complete resolution and return of tissue to normal state or by formation of scar tissue.

Classification

- *According to duration:* Inflammation may be acute (seconds, minutes or <48 hours), subacute or chronic (>48 hours, days, weeks, months or years).
- *According to predominant component:* Inflammation may cause necrosis, fibrinous inflammation of coelomic cavities and thickening of wall, e.g gallbladder in chronic cholecystitis.
- *According to histological features:* Inflammation is nonspecific in majority of cases. There is specific cause of inflammation in tuberculosis, leprosy and syphilis.
- *According to causative agent:* Aseptic inflammation due to sterile chemical agents, radiation has a reparative character. Septic inflammation caused by pathogens has a protective character.

Stages of Inflammation

The process of inflammation is a dynamic sequence of events: Acute or chronic depending on the persistence of the injury, clinical symptoms, and the nature of the inflammatory response. Acute and chronic inflammatory responses are shown in Fig. 2.1 and differences between acute and chronic inflammation are shown in Table 2.1.

Section I: General Pathology

Acute Inflammatory Response

- Acute inflammatory response is transient, rapid onset early response of short duration og injury lasting from a few minutes to <48 hours. It dilutes, neutralizes and eliminates the injurious agents by exudation of plasma proteins, fluid along with neutrophils.
- Neutrophils are the dominant players of acute inflammation. These clear debris and begin the process of wound healing. During mild tissue injury, inflammatory exudate is removed resulting in restoration of normal tissue architecture (resolution). Transition to chronic inflammation occurs in cases of persistent injury.

Chronic Inflammatory Response

Chronic inflammatory response has the potential to cause *tissue destruction, fibrosis and disease*. It lasts for days, weeks or years.

It is associated with *influx of macrophages, lymphocytes and plasma cells*, proliferation of blood vessels (*angiogenesis*), *fibrosis* (role of fibroblasts, macrophages); and *tissue necrosis* (organ damage).

- *Pathogenesis:* Chronic inflammation is mediated by *reactive oxygen species, hydrolytic enzymes, IFN-γ, other cytokines and growth factors. Macrophages and fibroblasts regulate scar tissue formation.*
- *Examples of chronic inflammation:* These include *tuberculosis, chronic sinusitis, chronic hepatitis, autoimmune diseases (i.e. ulcerative colitis, Crohn's disease).*

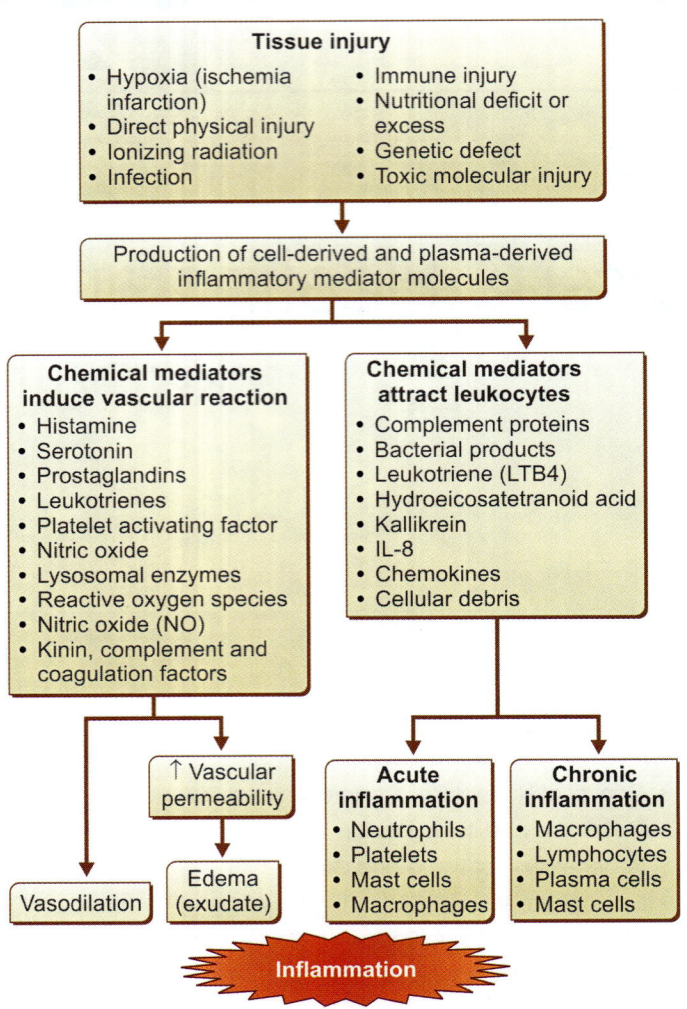

Fig. 2.1: Acute and chronic inflammatory responses.

Table 2.1: Differences between acute and chronic inflammation

Parameters	Acute inflammation	Chronic inflammation
Pathogenesis	Pathogens, trauma, burns	Progression of persistent acute inflammation, foreign bodies, tuberculosis, autoimmune diseases
Onset	Immediate (rapid onset within seconds)	Delayed (slow onset)
Cells involved	PMNs cells	Lymphocytes and macrophages
Chemical mediators	Histamine (key mediator), prostaglandins, TxA_2, prostacyclin, leukotrienes, lipoxins	Cytokines (IL-1), growth factors
Immunoglobulin	IgM	IgG
Duration	Shorter (lasting for a few hours to days)	Longer duration (lasting for weeks, months, or years)
Exudation	Present	Absent
Tissue necrosis	Present	Less prominent
Tissue fibrosis	Absent	Present
Angiogenesis	Absent	Present
Outcome	Complete resolution, tissue destruction (abscess), progression to chronic inflammation	Scar tissue formation, secondary amyloidosis
Peripheral blood leukocytic response	Neutrophilic leukocytosis	Lymphocytosis or monocytosis

ACUTE INFLAMMATION

Acute inflammation is transient, rapid response to tissue injury. It participates in delivery of leukocytes (PMNs cells) and plasma proteins to the site of injury. Macrophages and mast cells play an important role in inflammation. Acute inflammation is mediated by chemical mediators, which act on nearby blood vessels. Resident tissue macrophages recognize inflammatory inducers such as bacterial products, immune complexes, toxins, physical injury, or dead cells and attempt to eliminate them. Macrophages synthesize master cytokines such as IL-1 and TNF-α.

Chemical Mediators

Chemical mediators are derived from plasma proteins, tissue macrophages, mast cells, platelets and endothelial cells, local injured tissue, and bacterial products. These increase the vascular permeability, with exudation of water, salts and plasma proteins including fibrinogen along with numerous PMNs cells to eliminate injurious agent.

Macrophage Functions

Inflammatory inducers such as bacterial products, immune complexes, toxins, physical injury activate tissue macrophages participate in synthesis of cytokines (IL-1 and TNF-α), which activate neutrophils and venular endothelium.

Local Effects

- *Activation of leukocytes:* Cytokines (IL-1 and TNF-α) activate neutrophils, which synthesize arachidonic acid metabolites (leukotrienes and prostaglandins), interleukins (IL-1 and IL-6). Neutrophils express adhesion molecule, i.e. Sialyl-Lewis X-modified glycoprotein, integrin (low affinity state) and L-selectin. Neutrophils participate in bacterial killing by degranulation and formation of oxidative burst.
- *Activation of endothelium:* Cytokines (IL-1 and TNF-α) activate endothelium, which leads to expression of adhesion molecules, i.e. selectins (E selectin, P selectin), ICAM and VCAM. Activated endothelium synthesizes prostaglandin (PGI), interleukins (IL-1, IL-6, and IL-8) and PDGF. There is increased procoagulant activity of endothelium.
- *Fibroblasts:* These enhance the proliferation of fibroblasts, collagen synthesis. These synthesize collagenase and protease and prostaglandin E.

Systemic Effects

Cytokines (IL-1 and TNF-α) synthesized by macrophages increase the synthesis of acute phase reactants. These also cause fever, loss of appetite, sleep, neutrophilia and hemodynamic effects (shock). Il-6 increases erythrocyte sedimentation rate.

Anti-inflammatory Agents

Glucocorticoids are broad spectrum powerful anti-inflammatory agents, which participate in downregulating expression of genes encoding proinflammatory cytokines (IL-1 and TNF-α) and nitric oxide synthase.

Causes of Tissue Injury

Each of the stimuli may induce reactions with some distinctive characteristics, but all inflammatory reactions have the same features. When a deficit of water, oxygen, or nutrients occurs or if constant temperature and adequate waste disposal are not maintained, cellular synthesis does not take place. A lack of just one of these basic requirements can cause cell disruption or death.

- *Infectious agents:* Bacteria, viruses, fungi, and parasites can cause cell injury or death. Mammal's cells possess family of *toll-like receptors* and several cytoplasmic receptors, which can detect pathogens resulting in synthesis of chemical mediators of inflammation. These organisms affect cell integrity, usually by interfering with cell synthesis, producing mutant cells. Human immunodeficiency virus alters the cell, when virus is replicated in the cells.
- *Physical agents:* Mechanical injury (trauma or surgery) includes blunt or penetrating injuries (cutaneous laceration, osseous fracture). Physical injury disrupts cell's organelles (such as mitochondria, nuclei, lysosomes, and ribosomes). Thermal injury includes burns, or frostbite and irradiation.
- *Toxic agents:* Endogenous and exogenous toxic agents cause cell injury.
- *Endogenous agents:* These include genetically determined metabolic errors, gross malformations, and hypersensitivity reactions.
- *Exogenous agents:* These include alcohol, lead, carbon monoxide (toxic gas), acids, alkali, and drugs that alter cellular function such as chemotherapeutic agents or immunosuppressive drugs.
- *Foreign bodies:* Foreign bodies (sutures, splinters, dirt) elicit inflammation, because these cause tissue injury.
- *Immunological reactions: Immunological reactions include:* (i) hypersensitivity reactions due to environmental antigens including bee sting or self-antigens, and (ii) autoimmune disorders. Since these stimuli for the inflammatory response cannot be eliminated, such reactions tend to be persistent, and often have

features of chronic inflammation. These are important causes of morbidity and mortality.

- *Endogenous causes:* Circulation disorders include thrombosis, acute myocardial infarction, and hemorrhage. Activation of pancreatic enzymes results in acute pancreatitis. Metabolic products such as uric acid may cause inflammatory response.

Beneficial effects: During acute inflammation, neutrophils are recruited at injured site. These inflammatory cells eliminate injurious agent, removes cellular debris from injured area.

Inflammatory exudates dilute or neutralize the injurious agent. Inflammation prevents the spread of infection followed by resolution. Without inflammation, infections would go unchecked and wound would never heal.

Harmful effects: Tissue damage occurs due to liberation of lysosomal enzymes into the extracellular tissue, especially due to prolonged unregulated inflammatory response in chronic inflammation and hypersensitivity reactions. Tissue damage may also occur in space occupying lesions in brain compressing vital structures.

Major Components

Acute inflammation has two major components: Vascular and cellular responses (Fig. 2.2).

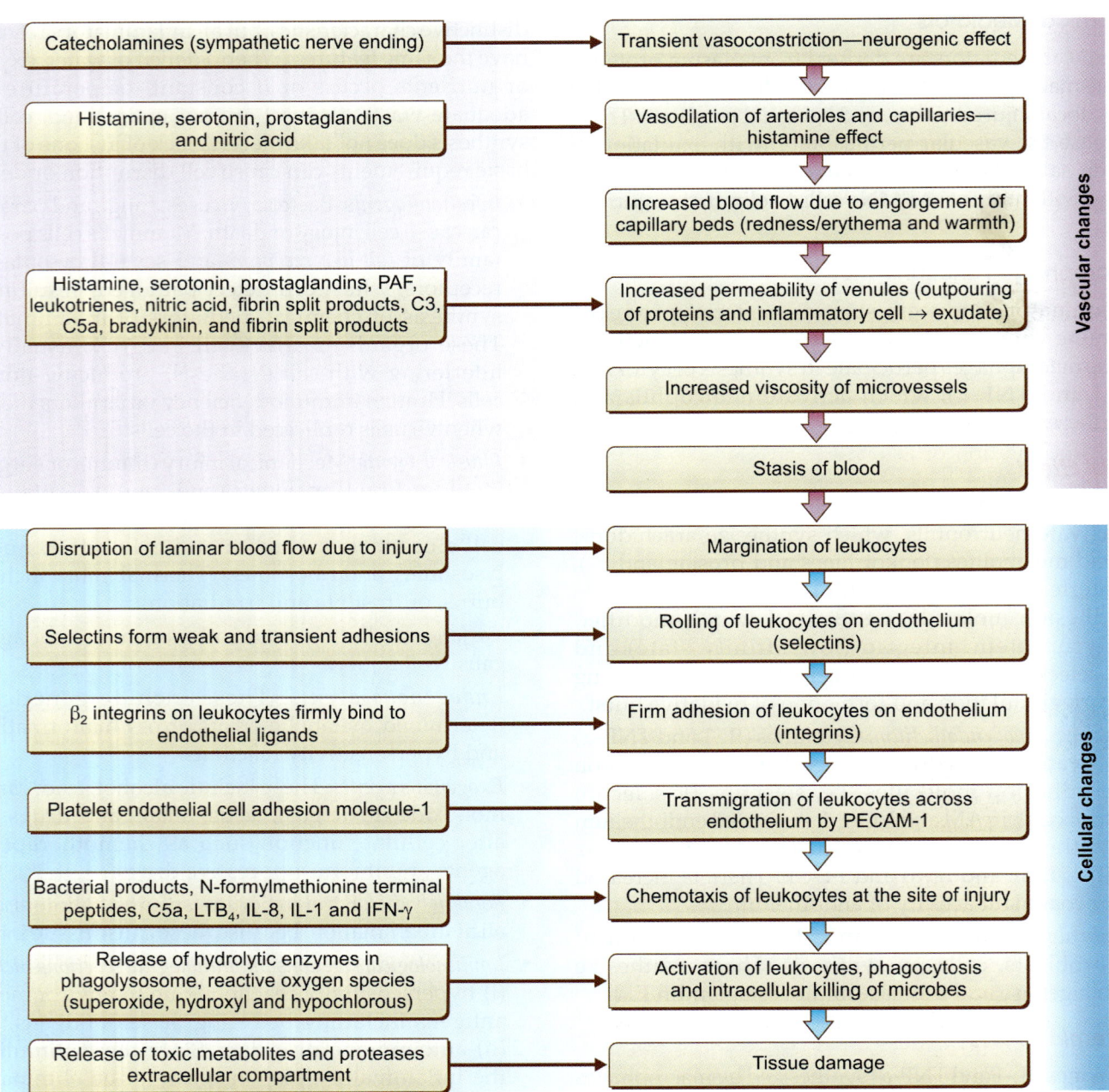

Fig. 2.2: Vascular and cellular events in acute inflammation.

Vascular Response

Vascular response depends on nature and severity of inflammatory stimulus. These include alterations in vascular blood flow and structural changes in the microvasculature (vasodilatation and increased vascular permeability). These changes result in extravasation of plasma fluid and proteins (edema) along with leukocytes to the site of injury.

Cellular Response

Inflammatory cells are recruited from circulation, which migrates to the injurious tissue by margination, rolling, adhesion, transmigration to initiate inflammation and eliminate injurious stimulus. Chemotaxis occurs due to endogenous signaling molecules such as lymphokines and exogenous toxins.

Neutrophils are dominant cells in acute inflammation during 1–2 days. These phagocytose and degrade injurious agent by lysosomal enzymes, free radicals, oxidative burst. Macrophages and mast cells play an important role in inflammation.

Vascular Events

Normally, most of the capillary bed is closed down by precapillary sphincters. In acute inflammation, the sphincters open, causing blood to flow through all capillaries. During acute inflammation, vascular changes start with a transient neurogenic-mediated vasoconstriction of arterioles. It is shortly followed by vasodilatation of arterioles, capillaries, and postcapillary venules. It leads to increased blood flow to the injured area, which becomes red and warm.

Cardinal Signs

Under optimal conditions, the inflammatory response remains confined to a localized area (i.e. redness, swelling, heat, pain and loss of function).

The four cardinal signs of acute inflammation were described nearly 2000 years ago by Celcius, which include rubor (redness), calor (heat), dolor (pain), and tumor (swelling). Virchow added functio laesa (loss of function) sign. Rubor, calor, and tumor are mediated by histamine. These cardinal signs result from vascular changes, neutrophilic recruitment to the site of injury, synthesis of chemical mediators, and leukocytes induced tissue injury. Acute inflammation subsides after elimination of injurious agents.

- *Rubor (redness):* Increased blood flow due to vascular dilatation gives redness and heat. Histamine causes vasodilatation of arterioles resulting in increased blood flow through all capillaries to the inflamed area. The inflamed area becomes red and hot in acute inflammation.
- *Calor (heat):* It occurs due to increased blood flow in the injured area, mediated by chemical mediators such as histamine, serotonin, C3a, C5a, prostaglandins (PGI_2, PGD_2, PGE_2, and $PGF_{2\alpha}$).
- *Dolor (pain):* Certain chemical mediators stimulate sensory nerve endings giving pain. Nerves also stimulated by stretching from edema. The inflamed area becomes painful, when touched. Pain occurs due to pressure on nerve endings from swelling; and direct effect of *prostaglandin E_2 (PGE_2)* and *bradykinin* on nerve endings.
- *Tumor (swelling):* Increased vascular permeability gives edema causing tissue swelling. Chemical mediators such as *histamine, bradykinin* and *prostaglandins* increase vascular permeability leading to extravasation of inflammatory exudate into the interstitial tissue (edema).
- *Functio laesa (loss of function):* Pain and swelling result in loss of *function*. When swelling and pain are marked, there is loss of function (partial or complete) of the inflamed structure. This clinical sign was added by Virchow in 1800s.

VASCULAR RESPONSE

Vascular component in acute inflammation comes into play when tissue is damaged by infectious agents, trauma, toxic agents, endogenous product (uric acid), immunological reactions and foreign bodies (sutures, splinters, dirt). Vascular response in acute inflammation includes immediate (e.g. immediate transient and sustained) and late response. Vascular response in acute inflammation is shown in Table 2.2.

Vasoconstriction of Arterioles

Initially, rapid transient vasoconstriction of arterioles occurs after minor tissue injury. It is mediated by neurologic and liberation of catecholamines from sympathetic nerve endings. This process lasts for 30 seconds. It is followed by vasodilatation of microvasculature.

Vasodilation of Arterioles and Capillaries

Vasodilation of arterioles and capillaries increases blood flow to injured site referred to as active hyperemia responsible for redness (rubor), increased local temperature (heat = calor) and removal of toxins. It is immediate sustained response after tissue injury. It starts 2–3 hours after injury and lasts for about 8 hours. It is mediated by chemical mediators synthesized by damaged tissue and mast cells such as *histamine, serotonin,* and sustained by prostaglandins (PGI_2, PGD_2, PGE_2, $PGF_{2\alpha}$) and nitric oxide.

Table 2.2: Vascular response in acute inflammation

Vascular response	Blood vessels	Mediated by neurologic/chemical mediators	Net effect
Transient vasoconstriction	Microvasculature	Neurologic mechanism by liberation of catecholamines from sympathetic nerve endings	Blood flow decreased
Vasodilatation	Arterioles and capillaries	Histamine Serotonin Sustained by prostaglandins (PGI_2, PGD_2, PGE_2, $PGF_{2\alpha}$) and nitric oxide	Blood flow increased (redness/erythema and warmth)
Increased vascular permeability	Venules	Histamine, serotonin, bradykinin, C3a, C5a, fibrin split products, prostaglandins, leukotrienes, platelet activating factor, nitric oxide	Inflammatory exudate and increased viscosity of blood

Increased Vascular Permeability

Increased vascular permeability is the hallmark of acute inflammation affecting postcapillary venules.

Physiological state: Normally, the wall of the normal venules is sealed by tight junctions between adjacent endothelial cells. Fluid leaving and entering blood vessels is in equilibrium.

Pathological state: Increased vascular permeability occurs due to various plasma derived (*fibrin split products, bradykinin, C3a, C5a*) and cells derived (*histamine, serotonin, prostaglandins, leukotrienes, platelet activating factor, nitric oxide*) chemical mediators.

Due to widening of inter-endothelial junctions, there will be outside movement of the fluid rich in plasma proteins and inflammatory cells (exudate) from the blood vessels to the site of injury.

MECHANISM OF INCREASED VASCULAR PERMEABILITY

Increased vascular permeability is caused by chemical mediators, bacterial toxins, chemical agents, physical agents, severe burns, thermal injuries, X-rays, ultraviolet rays, leukocyte induced endothelial injury, widening of venular inter-endothelial cells and leakage from newly formed vessels described as under. Chemical mediators responsible for increased vascular permeability are shown in Table 2.3.

Chemical Mediators

Histamine (mast cells, platelets, basophils), serotonin, prostaglandins, C3a and C5a increase permeability of postcapillary venules, which last for 15–20 minutes. Histamine binds and induces intracellular signaling pathway by phosphorylation of contractile myosin cytoskeleton proteins leading to increased vascular permeability.

Table 2.3: Chemical mediators responsible for increased vascular permeability

Characteristics	Examples	Chemical mediators
Plasma derived	Coagulation/fibrinolytic systems	Fibrin split products
	Kallikrein-kinin system	Kinins (bradykinin)
	Complement system	C3a, C5a
Cell derived	Mast cells, platelets	Histamine
	Platelets	Serotonin
	Inflammatory cells	Prostaglandins
		Leukotrienes
		Platelet activating factor
	Endothelium	Prostaglandins
		Nitric oxide
		Platelet activating factor

Bacterial Toxins, Chemicals, Physical Agents, and Severe Burns

These injurious agents cause necrosis of endothelium of microvasculature. It leads to prolonged vascular leakage of fluid elements into interstitial tissue persisting for several hours to days until the damaged endothelium is thrombosed or repaired.

Thermal Injury, X-rays and Ultraviolet Rays

Delayed prolonged vascular leakage starts 2–12 hours after injury and lasts for several hours or days due to mild to moderate thermal injury, X-rays, and ultraviolet rays.

Leukocyte-dependent Endothelial Injury

In acute inflammation, leukocytes liberate oxygen derived free radicals and proteolytic enzymes. These cause detachment of venular endothelial cells leading to increased permeability. It is a delayed response, which persists for hours. Glomeruli and pulmonary capillaries are also affected by this mechanism.

Vascular Endothelial Growth Factor

Vascular endothelial growth factor acts on vesiculovacuolar organelles located close to intercellular junction of venules increase the size and number of these channels leading to increased vascular permeability.

Leakage from Newly Formed Vessels

New vessels formed are responsible for persistent leakage of fluid. Increased expression of receptors for histamine and VEGF further increases vascular permeability.

TRANSUDATE FORMATION

A transudate is ultrafiltrate of plasma. Permeability of vascular endothelium is usually normal. It has a low protein content mostly albumin. It is usually caused by alterations in hydrostatic pressure or oncotic pressure. It implies a problem due to increased hydrostatic pressure. Transudate is formed when fluid escapes from the normal endothelium of microvasculature. It occurs in non-inflammatory conditions.

Causes

Transudate occurs either due to increased *hydrostatic pressure (congestive heart failure)* or decreased *osmotic pressure (decreased protein synthesis in liver diseases, malnutrition, protein loss in kidney diseases such as nephritic or nephrotic syndrome)*, and lymphatic obstruction. Lymphatic flow obstruction due to *filariasis* leads to edema. Woman with *breast cancer develops edema arm*, which has undergone *mastectomy along with removal of lymph nodes and lymphatic channels.*

Composition

Transudate is straw-colored ultrafiltrate of blood plasma with low protein content with specific gravity <1.012. It is composed of mainly water, dissolved electrolytes, and low protein.

INFLAMMATORY EXUDATE

An exudate has a high protein content caused by increased vascular permeability of postcapillary venules during acute inflammatory process. Contraction of endothelial cells of postcapillary venules results in widening of inter-endothelial space and extravasation of plasma proteins and neutrophils known as *exudate*. Severe injury to microvasculature causes extravasation of excessive inflammatory exudate into interstitial space. *Because the metabolically active leukocytes consume glucose, the glucose content in blood is often greatly reduced*

Composition

Exudate is rich in fibrinogen/fibrin, immunoglobulins, salts, water and neutrophils. It has specific gravity >1020.

Clinical Correlation

Acute inflammation brings chemical mediators of inflammation into injured site, which act on nearby blood vessels. It is responsible for swelling (edema), pain, and impaired function. *Exudates formed in severe burns are life-threatening. Fibrin formation in the injured area aids in localizing the spread of infectious microorganisms.* Exudates dilute bacterial toxins and provide opsonins (IgG, C3b) to *assist in phagocytosis.* Formation of transudate and exudate is shown in Figs 2.3 and 2.4. Differences between exudate and transudate are shown in Table 2.4.

STASIS OF BLOOD DUE TO REDUCED BLOOD FLOW

Escape of fluid from microvasculature into the interstitial tissue increases the concentration of the red blood cells and blood viscosity leading to slowing of blood flow (stasis). These small vessels are dilated and congested. Leukocytes principally neutrophils now begin to accumulate along the endothelial surface, a process called *margination*.

RESPONSE OF LYMPHATIC CHANNELS

Normal hydrostatic pressure in capillaries at arterial end is 32 mm Hg and 12 mm Hg at venous end. Osmotic

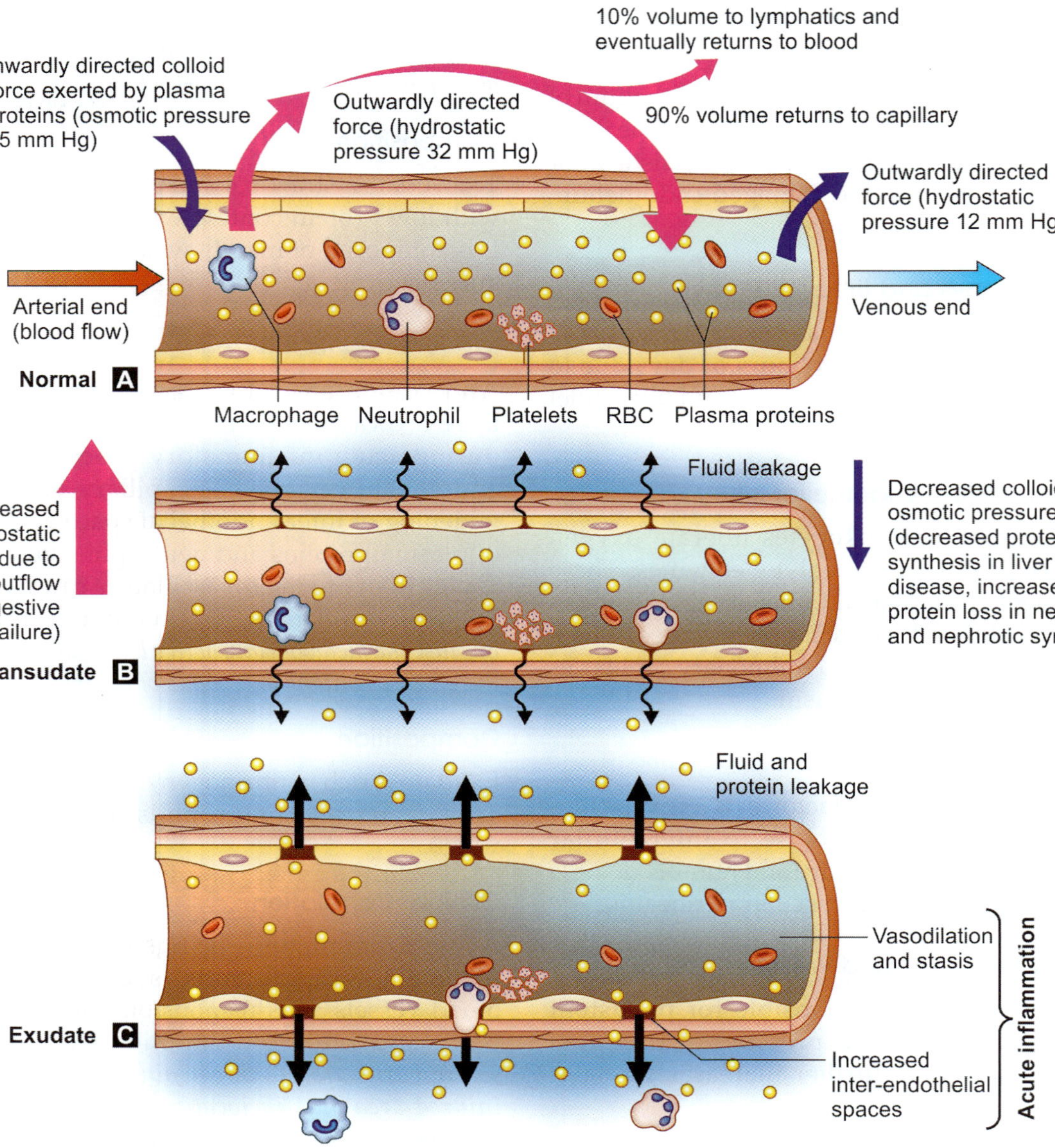

Fig. 2.3: Formation of transudate and exudate. (A) Normal hydrostatic pressure at arterial end of capillary is 32 mm Hg and 12 mm at venous end. Oncotic pressure exerted by plasma proteins is 25 mm Hg. Approximately 90% of fluid is drained back to capillary, while 10% of interstitial fluid drained by lymphatic channels to venous circulation; (B) Transudate is formed as a result of increased hydrostatic pressure or decreased oncotic pressure; (C) An exudate is formed due to increased vascular permeability.

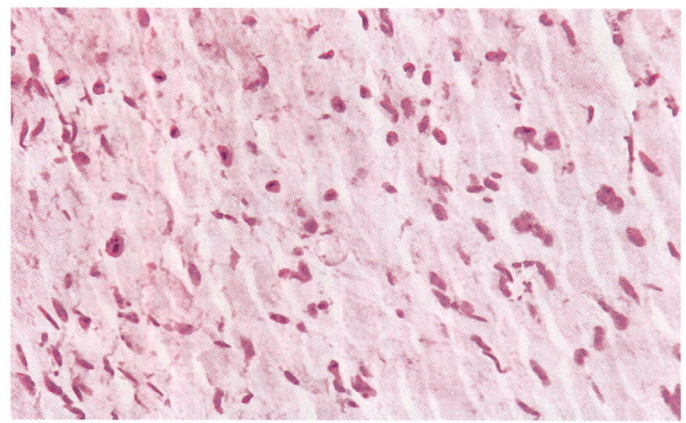

Fig. 2.4: Acute inflammatory exudate (400X).

pressure exerted by plasma proteins is 25 mm Hg in capillaries.

Physiological state

- Due to pressure gradient, hydrostatic blood pressure forces water out of capillaries at the arterial end. At the venous end, 90% of extravasated fluid is drained back in capillaries at venous end due to oncotic pressure exerted by plasma albumin.
- Remaining 10% fluid in interstitial tissue is drained via lymphatic channels into circulation. When the balance of these forces is altered, the net result is accumulation of fluid in the interstitial spaces (i.e. edema).

Inflammation, Tissue Healing and Repair

Table 2.4: Differences between exudate and transudate

Characteristics	Exudate	Transudate
Cause	Increased permeability of postcapillary venules in inflammation	Increased hydrostatic pressure or decreased oncotic pressure
Pathological state	Acute inflammation	Congestive heart failure
		Hypoproteinemia (malnutrition)
		Nephrotic syndrome (protein loss)
Endothelial permeability	Altered endothelial permeability	Normal endothelial permeability
Fluid nature	Inflammatory extravascular fluid	Ultrafiltrate of blood plasma
Composition	Mainly protein and cellular debris	Mainly water and dissolved electrolytes
Color	Yellowish-white opaque appearance	Transparent/light straw colored
pH	Less alkaline (<7.3)	More alkaline (>7.3)
Specific gravity	>1.020 due to raised proteins content in exudate	<1.012
Proteins content	High protein content, which raises specific gravity	Low protein fluid (<5 gm/dl)
Glucose concentration	Low in case of association with infections and cancer	Same as that of blood
Ratio of LDH levels in fluids and serum	High (>0.6)	Low (<0.6)
Light microscopy	PMN cells in acute inflammation	Inflammatory cells absent
	Macrophages and lymphocytes in chronic inflammation	

Pathological state
- During acute inflammation, lymph flow is increased. It helps to remove edema fluid from extravascular fluid along with cell debris. Severe cases result in inflammation of lymphatic channels and lymph nodes.
- There is presence of red streaks near a skin wound due to lymphangitis.

CELLULAR EVENTS

The cellular response in acute inflammation is a multi-step process, marked by recruitment of phagocytic cells (e.g. neutrophils and monocytes) into extravascular tissue to the site of injury.

Neutrophils are the primary leukocytes in acute inflammation, i.e. *Staphylococcus aureus* infection. Macrophages and mast cells play an important role in acute inflammation. On the other hand, macrophages, lymphocytes and plasma cells participate in chronic inflammation.

Mechanism

The leukocytes first roll, then become activated and adhere to endothelium, then transmigrate across the endothelium, pierce the basement membrane, and migrate to site of injury by chemotaxis.

- PECAM-1 (platelet endothelial cell adhesion molecule-1) synthesized by inter-endothelial junctions and platelets participate in transmigration of leukocytes.
- Chemoattractants, i.e. bacterial products (peptides with N-formylmethionine termini), plasma proteins (C5a), cells (IL-8, LTB_4), and cellular debris attract neutrophils to the site of injury.

Role of Selectins

These participate in rolling of leukocytes on endothelium by forming loose transient adhesions.
- Selectin family is comprised of *E selectins* (endothelial cells), *P selectins* (platelets and endothelial cells) and *L selectins* (leukocytes).
- Leukocytes with the help of their Sialyl-Lewis X (oligosaccharides) bind to E and P selectins expressed on vascular endothelial cells. These mediate the initial adhesion of leukocytes (primarily neutrophils) to endothelial cells at sites of inflammation.
- P selectin is a cell adhesion molecule that mediates the *margination of neutrophils* during acute inflammation.

Role of Integrins

Integrins are a family of cell surface receptors that mediate interactions with extracellular matrix components and with other cells.

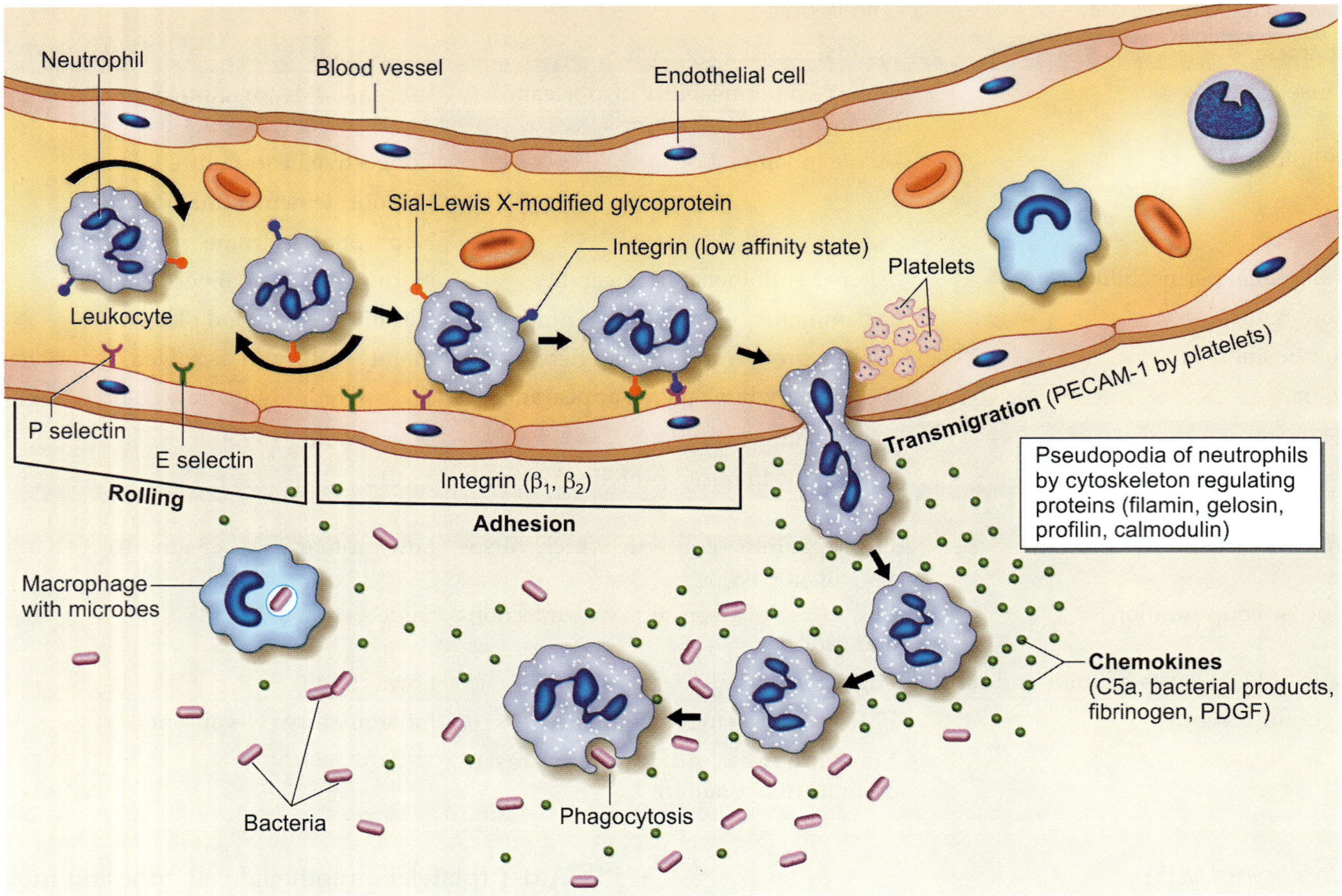

Fig. 2.5: Mechanism of leukocyte emigration involving rolling, adhesion, transmigration, chemotaxis and phagocytosis of injurious agent. Rolling is mediated by selectins, firm adhesion by β integrin, and transmigration by platelet endothelial cell adhesion molecule-1.

- During inflammation, β_2 integrins form firm adhesion of leukocytes to Ig family adhesion proteins expressed on vascular endothelium. These are involved in leukocyte recruitment to the injury site in acute inflammation.
- Integrins expressed on various inflammatory cells include lymphocyte function—associated antigen-1 (*LFA-1*), macrophage antigen-1 (*MAC-1*), and very late antigen-4 (*VLA-4*). These bind to Ig family adhesion proteins expressed on endothelium.

Emigration

Emigration is escape of inflammatory leukocytes between endothelial cells into surrounding interstitial tissue. It occurs by *margination, rolling, firm adhesion, and transmigration processes.*

Mechanism of leukocyte emigration is shown in Fig. 2.5. Cellular changes in acute inflammation are shown in Table 2.5.

MARGINATION

Margination occurs due to localization of leukocytes from central axial column along the vascular endothelium. Margination of leukocytes in microvessel is shown in Fig. 2.6.

Physiological State

Normally, 50% of neutrophils travel in laminar flow, while 50% are circulating along venular endothelial cells (marginating zone). *Red blood cells being smaller*: In size move faster than large-sized white blood cells.

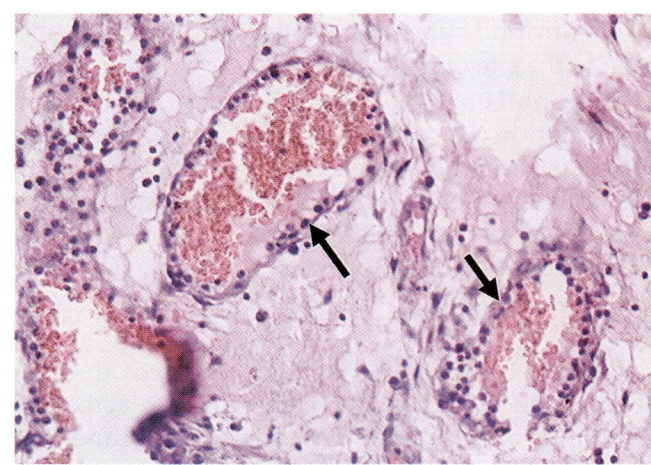

Fig. 2.6: Margination of leukocytes in microvessel (arrows)(100X).

Table 2.5: Cellular changes in acute inflammation

Process	Definition	Role
Margination	Localization of leukocytes from central axial column along the vascular endothelium	Disruption of laminar blood flow due to injury
Rolling	Rolling (or tumbling) along the vascular endothelium	Selectins form weak and transient adhesions.
Firm adhesion	Leukocytes bind firmly to endothelium	β_2 integrin on leukocytes firmly bind to endothelial ligands
Transmigration (diapedesis)	Movement of leukocytes across venular endothelium	PECAM-1—*platelet endothelial cell adhesion molecule-1*
Chemotaxis	Recruitment of leukocytes at the site of tissue injury site known as chemotaxis	C5a, bacterial products, N-formylmethionine terminal peptides, leukotrienes ($LT3_4$) hydro-eicosatetraenoic acid, kallikrein and IL-8, IL-1 and IFN-γ); and cellular debris
Phagocytosis	Phagocytes (neutrophils and macrophages) eliminate microbes and cellular debris by process of phagocytosis	Opsonization, binding, engulfment, phagolyso some formation, release of hydrolytic enzymes in phagolysosome
Intracellular killing of microbes	Killing and degradation of microbes in neutrophils	• Oxygen dependent (superoxide, highly reactive hydroxyl molecule, hypochlorous (HOCl) free radical • Oxygen independent system (lactoferrin, defensins, bactericidal permeability increasing protein, lysosomal enzyme and major basic proteins)

Pathological State

During acute inflammation, release of chemical mediators (i.e. histamine, leukotrienes and kinins) and cytokines act on endothelial cells of capillaries and leukocytes leading to *increased expression of adhesion molecules* and slowing down of leukocytes.

Margination (pavementing) occurs as all leukocytes line the endothelial surface, *due to activating and deactivating neutrophilic adhesive molecules*. RBCs also aggregate into rouleaux *(stacks of coins)* in venules.

ROLLING

After margination, the leukocytes start rolling (or tumbling) along the vascular endothelium by forming weak and transient adhesions mediated by 'selectins' family of adhesive molecules.

Selectins Family

Selectin family consists of three types of structurally related selectins. E selectin is found on endothelial cells. P selectin is expressed on platelets and endothelial cells. L selectin is present on leukocytes except T cells.

- E and P selectins expressed on endothelial cells bind to oligosaccharides such as Sialyl-Lewis X on the surface of leukocytes.
- These mediate the *initial adhesion of leukocytes (primarily neutrophils)* to endothelial cells in acute inflammation.

Regulation of Selectins

Selectin family is regulated by the following mechanisms:
- *E selectins (CD62E):* These are stored in *Weibel-Palade bodies of resting endothelial cells. Upon activation, E-selectins are redistributed along the luminal surface of the endothelial cells*, where they mediate the initial adhesion and rolling of leukocytes.
- *P selectins (CD62P):* These are stored in *endothelial Weibel-Palade bodies and platelet α-granules; relocate to the plasma membrane after stimulation by mediators* such as histamine and thrombin.
- *L selectins (CD62L):* These are *expressed on all leukocytes except T cells* and bind to endothelial mucin-like molecules such as GlyCam-1.

FIRM ADHESION

During inflammation, β_2 integrins expressed over leukocytes firmly bind to ligands expressed on venular endothelium.

Leukocyte and endothelial adhesion molecules are shown in Fig. 2.7 and Table 2.6.

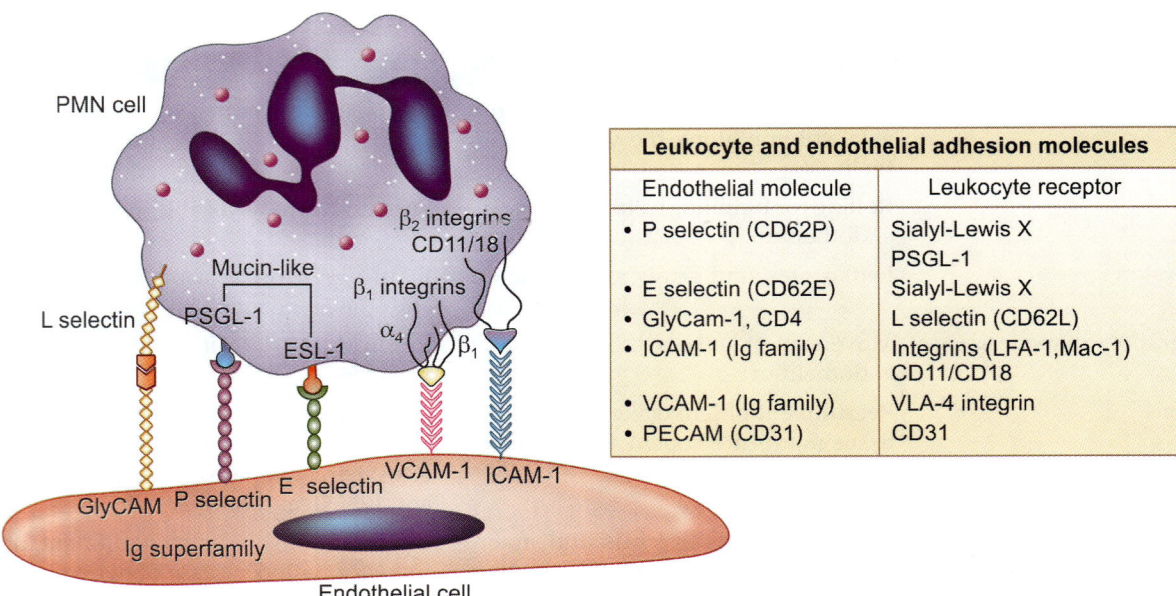

Fig. 2.7: Leukocyte and endothelial adhesion molecules.

Table 2.6: Endothelial/leukocyte adhesion molecules

Endothelial adhesion molecule	Leukocyte adhesion receptor	Major role
P selectin (CD62P)	Sialyl-Lewis X PSGL-1	Rolling of PMNs cells
		Rolling of monocytes
		Rolling of lymphocytes
E selectin (CD62E)	Sialyl-Lewis X	Rolling of leukocytes
		Adhesion of leukocytes
GlyCam-1, CD4	L selectin (CD62L)	Rolling of PMNs cells
		Rolling of monocytes
ICAM-1 (Ig family)	Integrins (LFA-1, Mac-1) CD11/CD18	Adhesion, arrest and transmigration of PMNs, monocytes and lymphocytes
VCAM-1 (Ig family)	VLA-4 integrin	Adhesion of PMNs, monocytes and lymphocytes
PECAM (CD31)	CD31	Transmigration of all leukocytes through endothelium

Integrins on Leukocytes

Physiological state: Normally, β_2 integrins (LFA-1, MAC-1, and VLA-4) are expressed in low concentration on leukocytes. Hence, leukocytes do not adhere firmly to their appropriate ligands endothelial surface, unless activated by chemokines (C5a, LTB_4 and bacterial endotoxins) during acute inflammation.

Pathological state: Leukocytic activation leads to increased concentration and conformational changes of β_2 integrins on their surface. Corticosteroids, lithium and catecholamines inhibit activation of adhesion molecules.

Ligands on Venular Endothelium

Chemical mediators (chemokines, IL-1 and TNF-α) increase the expression of ligands ICAM (intercellular adhesion molecule) and VCAM (vascular cell adhesion molecule) over vascular endothelium. *VCAM-1 also participates in adhesion of eosinophils, monocytes, lymphocytes to venular endothelium.*

Mechanism of Firm Adhesion

Leukocytic β_2 integrin binds to ligands expressed over venular endothelium. During acute inflammation, binding of integrin to heparin sulphate glycosaminoglycans causes *stoppage of rolling of leukocytes*. Net result is formation of firm adhesion of leukocytes to endothelial surface.

Defects of Adhesion of Leukocytes and Clinical Correlation

Leukocytic adhesion is impaired in diabetes mellitus and patient on steroid therapy and hemodialysis.

LAD-1 mutation: Gene mutation of leukocyte adhesion molecules (LAD-1) causes deficiency of β_2 integrins (LFA-1 and Mac-1) expressed on leukocytes. It impairs adhesion of leukocytes to venular endothelium. *Patients suffer from recurrent bacterial infections, delayed wound healing and delayed separation of umbilical cord in newborns.*

LAD-2 mutation: Gene mutation of LAD-2 causes mild disorder.

TRANSMIGRATION

Transmigration is the movement of leukocytes across venular endothelium. It is also known as diapedesis. Transmigration of leukocytes occurs in venules in all tissues except lung where it occurs via capillaries.

Mechanism

- *Synthesis of PECAM-1:* Inter-endothelial junctions of postcapillary venules and platelets synthesize a chemokine known as *Platelet endothelial cell adhesion molecule-1* (PECAM-1).
- *Action of PECAM-1:* It stimulates adherent neutrophils to produce *collagenase, elastase, and metalloproteinases* leading to *focal digestion* of venular basement membrane.
- *Transmigration of neutrophils:* Neutrophils start inserting pseudopodia; migrate into the interstitial tissue spaces towards chemotatic stimulus. Red blood cells also transmigrate along with neutrophils towards site of injury.

CHEMOTAXIS

Recruitment of leukocytes at the site of tissue injury site is known as *chemotaxis*.

Chemotactic Factors

Chemotaxis occurs under the influence of chemotactic mediators derived from (i) complement proteins (C5a), (ii) bacteria and mitochondrial products, particularly low molecular weight N-formylmethionine terminal peptides, (iii) cell-derived arachidonic acid metabolites (LTB$_4$, hydroeicosatetranoic acid, kallikrein and IL-8), (iv) chemokines (e.g. IL-1 and IFN-γ); and (v) cellular debris.

Chemotactic factors for various cells in inflammation are shown in Table 2.7.

Table 2.7: Chemotactic factors for various cells in inflammation

Factor	Source	Chemotaxis
Formylated peptides	Bacterial products of *Escherichia coli*	Neutrophils
C5a	Activated complement component	Neutrophils
Kallikrein	Product of factor XIIa-mediated conversion of prekallikrein	Neutrophils
Fibrinogen	Plasma protein	Neutrophils
PAF (AGEPC)	Basophils	Eosinophils
	Mast cells	
PDGF	Platelets	Neutrophils and macrophages
	Monocytes	
	Macrophages	
	Smooth muscle cells	
	Endothelial cells	
TGF-β	Platelets	Macrophages and fibroblasts
	Neutrophils	
	Macrophages	
	Lymphocytes	
	Fibroblasts	
Fibronectin	Extracellular matrix protein	Fibroblasts and endothelial cells

Steps of Chemotaxis

Binding of chemokines on leukocytes: Chemotactic mediators bind to seven transmembrane G-protein coupled receptors (GPCRs) family on leukocytes. G-protein mediated signal transduction leads to generation of lipid second messengers and increased cytosolic calcium.

Enhancement of neutrophilic motility: Calcium causes contraction of *cytoskeleton actin regulating proteins* (filamin, gelosin, profilin and calmodulin), which are necessary for pseudopodia that anchor to the ECM. These pull the leukocytes in the direction toward injury site.

Recruitment of leukocytes

- *Neutrophils predominance:* Neutrophils predominate in the acute inflammatory infiltrate during the first 6–24 hours, which are short lived. Cellular infiltrate is dominated by continuously recruited neutrophils for several days in Pseudomonas infection.

- *Macrophages predominance:* Neutrophils undergo apoptosis and disappear after 24 to 48 hours. Then neutrophils are replaced by monocytes in 24–48 hours, which survive longer. *Inflammation lasting more than a few days attracts macrophages and lymphocytes.* Macrophages participate in clearance of pus, cellular debris, damaged tissue and dead neutrophils.

- *Lymphocytes predominance:* In acute viral infections, lymphocytes may be the first cells to arrive.

- *Eosinophils predominance:* In hypersensitivity reactions, eosinophils may be the main cell type.

Defects of chemotaxis and clinical correlation: Chemotaxis is impaired in *diabetes mellitus, cancer, sepsis, immunodeficiency disorders and thermal injuries.*

ACTIVATION OF LEUKOCYTES

Leukocytes express on their surface different kinds of receptors that recognize different stimuli. After recruitment of leukocytes to the injured site, *microbes, products of necrotic cells and chemical mediators activate the leukocytes.*

These activated leukocytes participate in *phagocytosis and degradation of injurious agents.* Synthesis of chemical mediators amplifies the inflammatory reaction. *Various receptors expressed on leukocytes are discussed below.*

Toll-like Receptors (TLRs) on Leukocytes

- *Cells expressing Toll-like receptors:* Macrophages, neutrophils, dendritic cells, microglial cells, eosinophils, mast cells, endothelial cells, mucosal cells and lymphocytes express toll-like receptors (TLRs). TLRs provide defense against invasion by microorganisms. Each TLR recognizes and binds distinct microbial molecules called pathogen-associated molecular proteins (PAMPs).

- *Pathogen-associated molecular proteins:* PAMPs present in pathogens include such as gram-positive cocci (lipoprotein, lipotectoic acid), gram-negative cell wall lipopolysaccharides (LPS), bacteria with flagella (flagellin) viruses (single-stranded or double-stranded RNA molecules) and fungi (zymosan).

- *Mechanism:* TLR binds and relays a signal to the nucleus resulting in activation of nuclear synthesis of transcription factors (chemical mediators) such as (i) arachidonic acid metabolites and cytokines amplifying the inflammatory reactions, and (ii) production of microbiocidal reactive oxygen species and lysosomal enzymes killing the microbes. Toll-like receptors and their actions are shown in Fig. 2.8 and pathogen-associated molecular proteins (PAMPs) are shown in Table 2.8.

Seven α-Helical Transmembrane G-protein Coupled Receptors

- *Binding of products:* Certain bacterial N-formyl-methionyl peptides, lipid mediators, chemokines, C5a, platelet activating factor, prostaglandin E and leukotrienes bind to seven α-helical transmembrane G-protein coupled receptors on leukocytes.

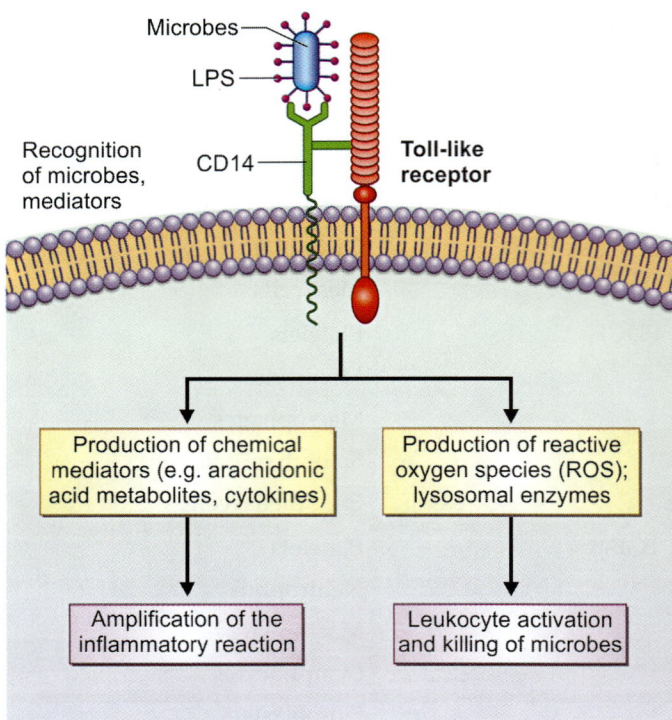

Fig. 2.8: Toll-like receptors and their actions.

Inflammation, Tissue Healing and Repair

Table 2.8: Pathogen-associated molecular proteins (PAMPs)

Pathogens	Pathogen-associated molecular proteins (PAMPs)
Gram-negative bacterial cell wall	Lipopolysaccharides (LPS): Endotoxin
Gram-positive bacteria cocci	Peptidoglycan such as lipoprotein, lipotectoic acid
Bacteria with flagella	Flagellin
Viruses	Single-stranded or double-stranded RNA molecules
Fungi	Zymosan

- *Cellular changes in leukocytes:* It leads to (i) cytoskeleton changes by signal transduction, (ii) increased expression of integrin adhesion molecules leading to adhesion of leukocytes to endothelium, and (iii) transmigration and chemotaxis of leukocytes into site of tissue injury by activation of the respiratory burst.

  Seven α-helical transmembrane G-protein coupled receptors and their actions are shown in Fig. 2.9.

Phagocytic Receptors

Microbes bind to phagocytic receptors leading to killing of bacteria by production of microbiocidal reactive oxygen species, release of lysosomal enzymes, leukocytic activation and killing the microbes. Phagocytic receptors and their actions are shown in Fig. 2.10

Opsonin Receptors on Leukocytes

Macrophages express opsonin receptors (FcR1, CR1 and C1q), scavenger receptors, macrophage integrin receptors MAC1 (CD11 and CD18). FcR1, CR1, C1q receptors recognize microbes coated by IgG, C3 (classical and alternate pathways) and plasma proteins derived mannose binding lectin (MBL). Scavenger receptors bind microbes and modified LDL. Opsonin receptors on leukocytes are shown in Fig. 2.11.

Cytokine Receptors

- *Activation of leukocytes:* Cytokine IFN-γ synthesized by natural killer cells and T cells bind to cytokine receptor superfamily on leukocytes. It leads to activation of leukocytes results in production of reactive oxygen species, release of lysosomal enzymes and ultimately killing of microbes.

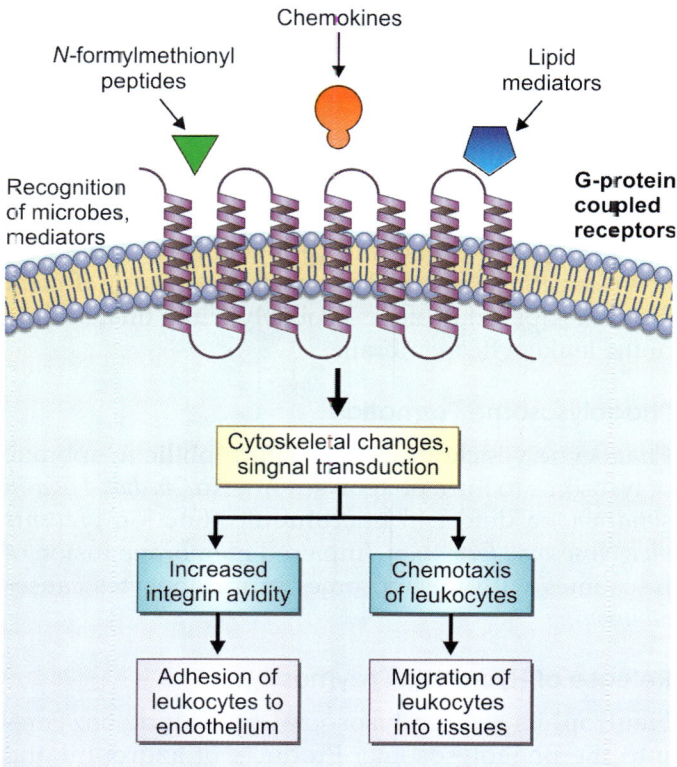

Fig. 2.9: Seven α-helical transmembrane G-protein–coupled receptors and their actions.

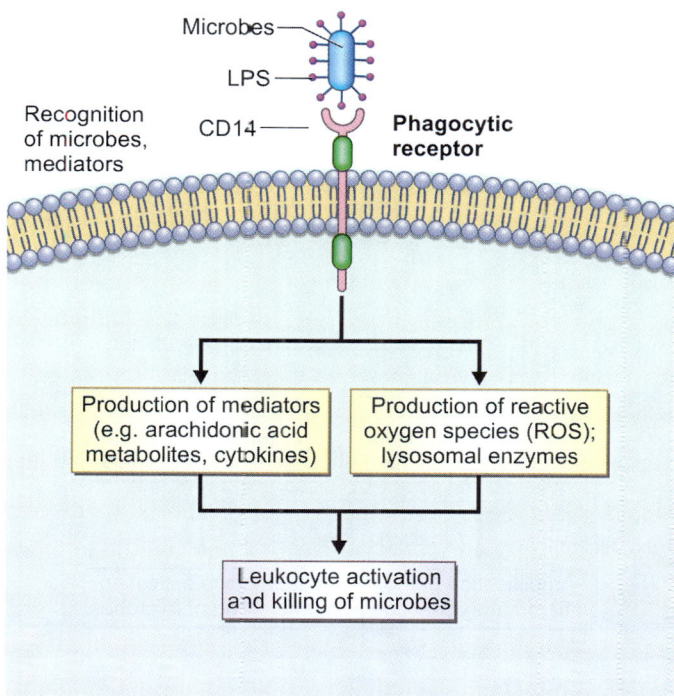

Fig. 2.10: Phagocytic receptors and their actions.

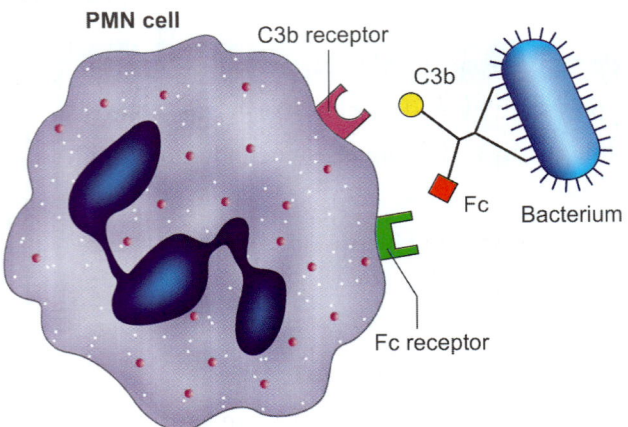

Fig. 2.11: Opsonin receptors on leukocytes.

- *Signaling by cytokine receptors:* It depends upon their association with the Janus kinases (JAKs), which couple ligand binding to tyrosine phosphorylation of signaling proteins recruited to cytokine receptor complex.
- *Signaling proteins:* Among these signaling proteins are unique family of transcription factors named the signal transducers and activators of transcription (STAT).

The receptors and their corresponding cytokines have been divided into several families based on their structure and activities. Cytokine receptors and their actions are shown in Fig. 2.12.

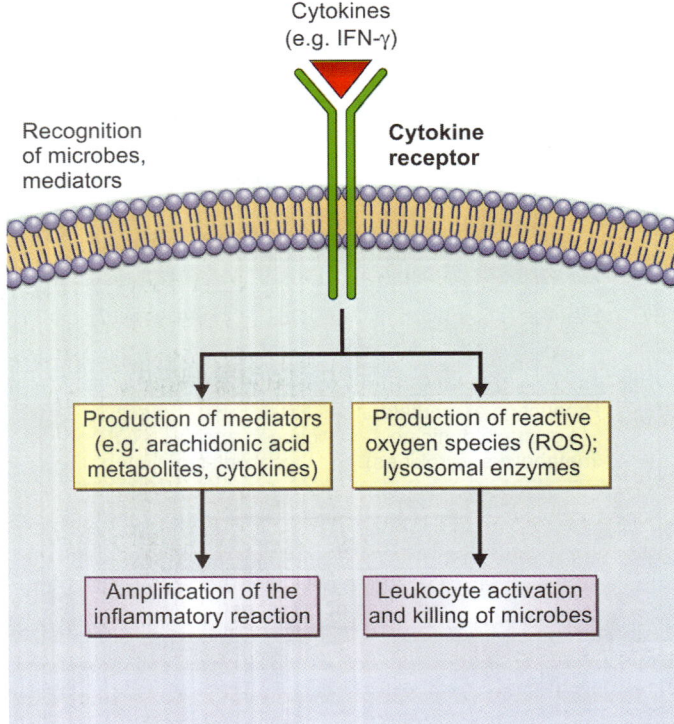

Fig. 2.12: Cytokine receptors and their actions.

PHAGOCYTOSIS

Phagocytes (neutrophils and macrophages) eliminate microbes and cellular debris by process of phagocytosis. Activated phagocytes recognize, internalize, and *degrade the injurious agent and dead cells by releasing oxygen derived free radicals, nitrogen species (ROS, NO) and lysosomal enzymes in phagolysosomes*. Phagocytosis involves distinct steps, i.e. *recognition, opsonization, binding, engulfment, phagolysosome formation, intracellular killing and degradation.* Sequential steps in phagocytosis are shown in Fig. 2.13 and phagocytosis of injurious agent is shown in Fig. 2.14.

Opsonization of Injurious Agents

Opsonization is a process by which injurious stimulus coated by opsonins, i.e. IgG, C3b and complement mannose binding lectin (MBL). Opsonization enhances binding of injurious agent to membrane receptors (e.g. FcR1, CR1 and MBL) expressed on activated neutrophils. Defects in opsonization results in *Bruton's agammaglobulinemia*.

Binding Opsonized Fragment to Cellular Receptors

Microbes are coated (opsonized) by *immunoglobulin* (IgG), *complement* (C3b) and *mannose binding lectin* (MBL). Opsonized microbes bind to cell surface receptors of leukocytes. Fc portion of the IgG binds to FcR1 and C3b to FcR1 of leukocytes. Bacterial polysaccharide binds to mannose binding lectin (MBL) receptors on leukocytes.

Engulfment of Injurious Agent

Neutrophils push out pseudopodia to surround the injurious particle completely, forming an endocytic phagocytic vacuole (phagosome), driven by *polymerization* (assembly and disassembly) *of actin filaments*. Special proteins probably allow final sealing of the leukocytic membrane.

Phagolysosome Formation

Phagocytic vesicle fuses with neutrophilic membrane of lysosome to form phagolysosome. In *Chédiak-Higashi syndrome*, a defect in microtubule function *prevents phagolysosome formation*. Impaired membrane fusion of lysosomes with melanosomes in melanocytes causes *albinism*.

Release of Hydrolytic Enzymes

Neutrophils release lysosomal hydrolytic enzymes into the phagolysosome. Products of azurophil and specific granules of neutrophils participate in *vascular permeability, chemotaxis and tissue damage*.

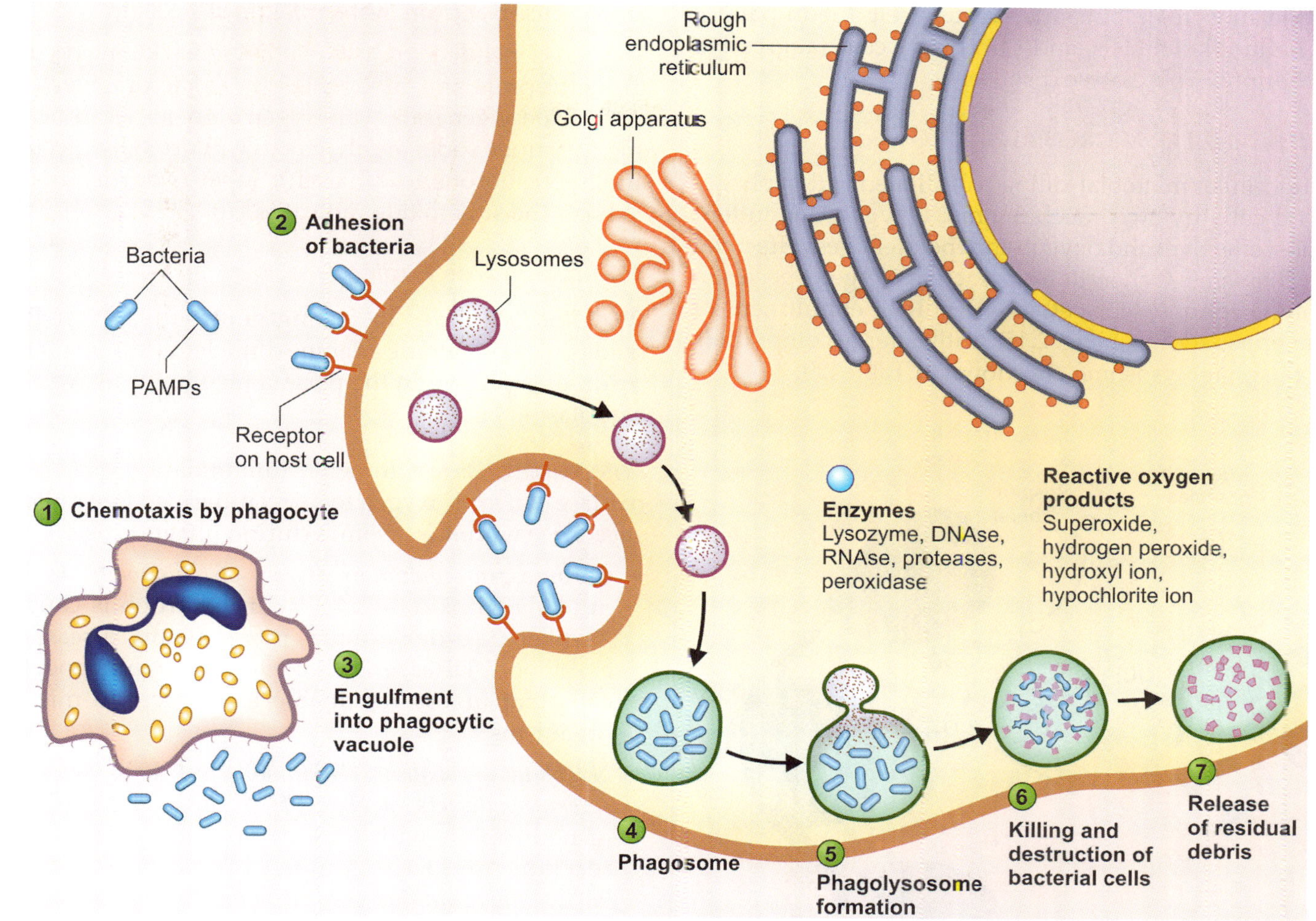

Inflammation, Tissue Healing and Repair

Fig. 2.13: Sequential steps in phagocytosis showing chemotaxis of phagocyte towards injurious agent, recognition of injurious agent, adhesion, engulfment, formation of phagolysosome, killing of pathogens by lysosomal enzyme, reactive oxygen species, and release of apoptotic body.

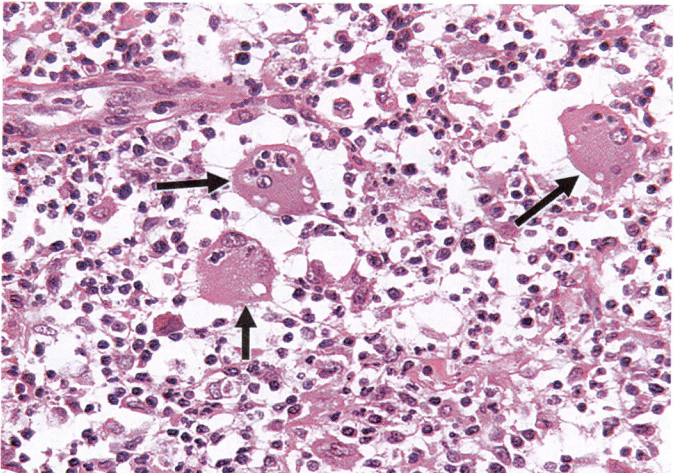

Fig. 2.14: Phagocytosis. Phagocytes showing ingested injurious agent (arrows) 400X).

Phagocytosis and Clinical Correlation

Defects in opsonization: Defects in opsonization causes Bruton's agammaglobulinemia.

Defective phagocytosis: Phagocytosis is impaired leukemias, diabetes mellitus, malnutrition and neonates.

Defective phagolysosome formation: In *Chédiak-Higashi syndrome*, a defect in microtubule function prevents phagolysosome formation. Impaired membrane fusion of lysosomes with melanosomes in melanocytes causes *albinism*.

Defective degranulation of neutrophils: Chédiak-Higashi syndrome is an example of defective degranulation of neutrophils.
- *Physiological state.* LYST gene located on chromosome 1q42 encodes a protein essential for assembly of microtubules in the cytoplasm.
- *Pathological state:* Mutation of LYST gene occurs in *Chédiak-Higashi syndrome*. It is characterized by *defective degranulation of neutrophils, impaired microbial killing, and recurrent bacterial infections* (*Staphylococcus aureus*) forming soft tissue abscess. Neutrophils contain giant granules due to aberrant organelles. This order affects other cells such as platelets (bleeding).

melanocytes (albinism), Schwann cells (neuropathy), natural killer cells, and cytotoxic T cells (aggressive lymphoproliferative disorder).

INTRACELLULAR MICROBIAL KILLING

Intracellular microbial killing is facilitated within phagocytic cells by two mechanisms: Oxygen-dependent (most effective) and oxygen-independent (less effective) mechanisms. Generation of reactive oxygen species in polymorphonuclear cell as a result of engulfment of bacteria is shown in Fig. 2.15. Antibacterial compounds of the phagolysosome are shown in Table 2.9.

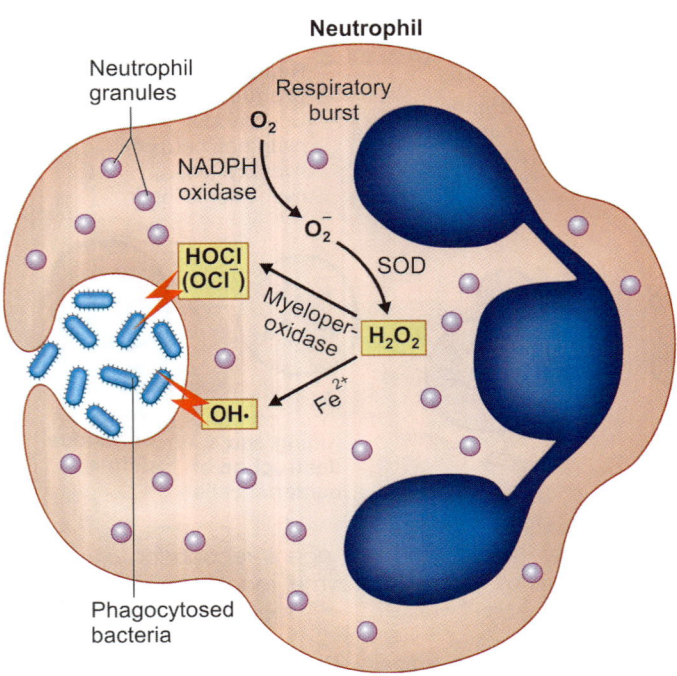

Fig. 2.15: Generation of reactive oxygen species in polymorphonuclear cell as a result of engulfment of bacteria.

Oxygen-dependent System Microbial Killing

Oxygen-dependent intracellular microbial killing occurs in neutrophils and monocytes (not macrophages). It occurs due to generation of oxygen derived free radicals such as superoxide, highly reactive hydroxyl molecule and hypochlorous acid (bleach). Superoxide dismutase reduces the superoxide radical to H_2O_2.

Superoxide Free Radical

Physiological state: In resting neutrophils, NADPH oxidase (nicotinamide adenine dinucleotide phosphate oxidase) is present in the plasma membrane as well as cytoplasm.

Pathological state: In acute inflammation, NADPH oxidase converts oxygen to oxygen-derived free radical *superoxide* within lysosomes during phagocytosis.

- *Chronic granulomatous disease of childhood:* Defect in NADPH oxidase activity in neutrophils causes X-linked disorder chronic granulomatous disease of childhood. Disease is characterized by phagocytic cells that ingest but unable to kill certain microorganisms.
- *Nitroblue tetrazolium (NBT) slide test:* It is used for *screening defects in NADPH oxidase*. The number of neutrophils with dark cytoplasmic granules of reaction product is counted. *Normally, more than 95% of the granulocytes containing NADPH oxidase are positive for nitroblue tetrazolium (NBT).* In chronic granulomatous disease, less than 5% of neutrophils are stained by NBT slide test.
- *Highly reactive hydroxyl molecule:* During phagocytosis, superoxide dismutase converts superoxide radical to hydrogen peroxide (H_2O_2). This reaction is

Table 2.9: Antibacterial compounds of the phagolysosome

System	Compound	Actions
Oxygen-dependent system	*Superoxide:* Deficiency develops chronic granulomatous disease of childhood	These are oxygen derived free radicals. These participate in intracellular killing of microbes in neutrophils and (not macrophages)
	Hydroxyl molecule	Microbiocidal action
	Hypochlorous	Microbiocidal action
Oxygen-independent system	Lactoferrin	Lactoferrin binds iron in neutrophils leading to inhibition of bacterial reproduction
	Defensins	Cytotoxic to microbes
	Bactericidal permeability increasing protein	It activates phospholipase, which degrades phospholipids of bacterial cell wall resulting in killing of microbes
	Lysosomal enzyme	It hydrolyzes the muramic acid N-acetylglucosamine bond of bacterial glycopeptides resulting killing of microbes
	Major basic proteins	Major basic protein is a cationic protein in eosinophilic granules, is cytotoxic to helminths

neutralized by glutathione peroxidase. Hydrogen peroxide dissociates to highly reactive hydroxyl molecule.

- *Hypochlorous (HOCl⁻) free radical (bleach):* MPO (myeloperoxidase) enzyme in phagocytic vacuole H_2O_2 combines with chloride ions (Cl^-) to form hypochlorous ($HOCl^-$) free radicals, which kills bacteria by halogenization, in which halide is bound covalently to cellular constituents or by oxidation of proteins and lipids (lipid peroxidation).

  Patients deficient in myeloperoxidase cannot produce hypochlorous ($HOCl^-$) acid. It leads to increased susceptibility to Candida infections. It is rarely associated with recurrent bacterial infections.

Oxygen-independent Microbial Killing

This process is much less effective than oxygen-dependent microbial killing.

- *Lactoferrin:* Normally, bacteria require iron for reproduction. Binding of lactoferrin present in neutrophilic granules to iron leads to *inhibition of bacterial reproduction.*
- *Defensins:* Defensins are cationic arginine-rich granule peptides in neutrophils. These are *cytotoxic to microbes.*
- *Bactericidal permeability increasing protein:* Bactericidal permeability increasing protein activates phospholipase, which degrades phospholipids of bacterial cell wall leading to *killing of microbes.*
- *Lysosomal enzyme:* Lysosomal enzyme present in azurophilic granules hydrolyzes the muramic acid N-acetylglucosamine bond of bacterial glycopeptides leading to *killing of microbes.*
- *Major basic proteins:* Major basic proteins, a cationic protein in eosinophilic granules is *cytotoxic to helminthes.*

LEUKOCYTES INDUCED INJURY

Inflammation plays an important role to eliminate the initial cause of cell injury as well as the necrotic cells and tissues, but it is itself capable of causing tissue damage by liberation of products by neutrophils and macrophages.

During phagocytosis, leukocytes release microbiocidal and other products (e.g. lysosomal enzymes, reactive oxygen species, arachidonic acid products, prostaglandins and leukotrienes) within phagolysosomes, but also into extracellular space causing tissue damage and may amplify the effects of injurious stimulus.

Mechanism of Tissue Damage

- *Digestion of basement membranes:* During transmigration, leukocytes release *elastase* and *metalloproteinases*, which digest the basement membrane.
- *Regurgitation during feeding:* It may occur if the phagocytic vacuole remains transiently open to outside before complete closure of the phagolysosomes.
- *Frustrated (regurgitated) phagocytosis:* Deposition of immune complex on the flat surface of glomerular basement membrane activates complement system and recruitment of leukocytes.

  Leukocytes fail to engulf these immune complexes. These release lysosomal hydrolytic enzymes and Oxygen-derived free radicals leading to *glomerular basement membrane injury.* It leads to increased permeability and protein loss in urine.

  After phagocytosis, potentially cytotoxic substances such as urate crystals are released, which damage the membrane of phagolysosomes. This leukocytes induced injury mechanism is known as *frustrated (regurgitated) phagocytosis.*

  In addition, there is some evidence that substances in secondary granules of neutrophils may be directly secreted by exocytosis. After phagocytosis, neutrophils rapidly undergo apoptotic cell death and are digested by macrophages.

- *Chemical mediators:* Inflammatory chemical mediators produced by phagocytes such as *prostaglandins* and *leukotrienes* play key role in tissue damage.
- *Necrosis by phagocytes in situ:* Prolonged severe injury causes necrosis of tissue.
- *Leukocyte-induced disorders:* Leukocyte-induced injury may cause acute injury (e.g. *glomerulonephritis, acute transplant rejection, bronchial asthma, acute adult respiratory syndrome, septic shock, vasculitis; and chronic injury* (e.g. chronic graft rejection, atherosclerosis, arthritis and chronic lung disease). Leukocyte-induced injury is shown in Table 2.10.

OUTCOME OF ACUTE INFLAMMATION

Acute inflammation may have one of the following outcomes (complete resolution, pus formation, fibrosis, and progression to chronic inflammation). Outcome of acute inflammation is shown in Fig. 2.16.

COMPLETE RESOLUTION

Resolution of normal structure and function of tissue occurs without scarring, if the injurious agent is eliminated. Lymphatics and macrophages play central role in complete resolution of acute inflammation

Table 2.10: Leukocyte-induced injury

Disorder	Cells and molecules involved
Acute respiratory distress syndrome	Neutrophils
Bronchial asthma	Eosinophils, IgE
Glomerulonephritis	Neutrophils, macrophages, antigen, antibody
Vasculitis	Neutrophils, antibody, complement
Acute organ transplant rejection	Lymphocytes, complement, antibody
Chronic organ transplant rejection	Lymphocytes, cytokines
Atherosclerosis	Macrophages
Pulmonary fibrosis	Macrophages

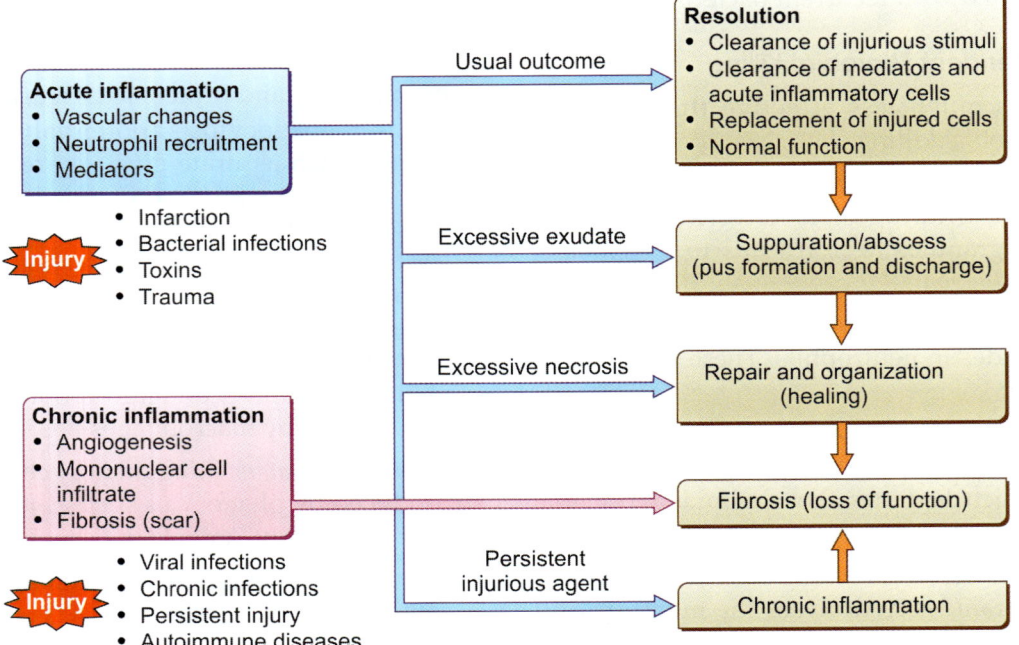

Fig. 2.16: Outcome of acute inflammation—resolution, suppuration, healing by fibrosis, loss of function and chronic inflammation. The components of the various reactions and outcome are depicted here.

(e.g. restoration of structure and function of tissue without scarring).

Role of Cells Entering in Cell Cycle

Complete resolution occurs with mild injury (bee sting or first degree burns) to those cells, which are capable to enter the cell cycle (e.g. labile and stable cells).

Mechanism

- *Apoptosis of neutrophils:* Neutrophils start disappearing as a result of apoptosis from injury site.
- *Chemical mediators:* Leukotrienes undergo decay after neutralizing the injurious agent.
- *Vascular permeability:* Normalization of vascular permeability occurs.
- *Macrophages:* These phagocytose necrotic cellular debris and apoptotic neutrophils leading to removal from injured site.
- *Drainage of edema fluid:* Edema fluid and proteins are finally drained into the lymphatics.
- *Restoration of normal structure:* Injured cells with intact supporting stroma undergo regeneration (e.g. labile and stable cells) with restoration of normal structure and function.

TISSUE DESTRUCTION

Oxygen-derived free radicals released by mononuclear cells are injurious to the own tissues as well as invading agents.

Pus Formation (Abscess)

Production of large amounts of thick yellow pus or purulent exudate (PMN cells) by pyogenic bacteria such as *Staphylococcus aureus* is accompanied by significant liquefactive necrosis. The destroyed tissue is restored and eventually replaced by fibrosis.

Skin Ulcer

Loss of surface epithelium or skin results in ulcer formation. It can be caused by acute inflammation of epithelial surfaces (e.g. ulcer of the skin and peptic ulcer).

Ulcers in Stomach and Duodenum

These heal by regeneration of mucosa close to its edge, perforation in ulcer involving full thickness of the wall, or chronic ulcer persisting for years. *Gastric ulcer is deep, with its floor covered by debris and neutrophils. Beneath this is granulation tissue and dense fibrosis replacing muscle coat.*

Suppurative Fistula

Suppurative fistula is an abnormal communication between two organs or between an organ and a surface due to suppurative infection.

PROGRESSION TO CHRONIC INFLAMMATION

Persistent or recurrent acute infection >48 hours progress to chronic inflammation. It occurs when host response fails to degrade the injurious agent (e.g. pathogen, tissue debris and foreign bodies) that incites gradual onset inflammatory reaction. It usually occurs as *de novo*, without a preceding acute inflammation.

- This process is characterized by disappearance of neutrophils from the injury site; followed by influx of mononuclear cells (e.g. *macrophages, lymphocytes and plasma cells*), *angiogenesis* and *fibrosis* in the injured tissue. Plasma cells produce *immunoglobulins*. Some of the macrophages may become multinucleate giant cells.
- Fibroblasts migrate into the injured area and lay down collagen fibers. Consequently, chronic inflammation is *almost always accompanied by tissue destruction*.

HEALING BY CONNECTIVE TISSUE REPLACEMENT

Healing by fibrosis is the final result of tissue destruction, with resultant distortion of structure and, in some cases, altered function. *Growth factors synthesized by macrophages* initiate the subsequent process of repair forming scar composed primarily of collagen fibers. The scar does not contain parenchymal cells, hence functional impairment may occur.

Third Degree Burns

These occur with extensive injury or damage to permanent cells, which are incapable of regeneration. Fibrous scarring occurs in these areas of damage, forming a scar composed primarily of collagen. It leads to functional impairment of tissue.

Fibrinous Exudate Organization

Organization occurs in fibrinous inflammation seen in coelomic cavities (*pericardium, pleura and peritoneum*), in which excessive fibrinous exudates cannot be cleared. These cavities are organized by growing of capillary loops into the exudates accompanied by fibroblasts and capillaries forming adhesions. Mass of fibrous tissue is called *organization*.

MORPHOLOGIC PATTERNS OF ACUTE INFLAMMATION

Vascular and cellular responses in acute inflammation produce distinctive morphological patterns in various tissues. Location, cause, and duration of inflammation determine the morphology of an inflammatory reaction. Reactive gliosis is a normal response of the brain to injury and infection but is not visible on the cut surface of the brain at autopsy. These are described below.

SEROUS INFLAMMATION

Serous inflammation of coelomic cavities: Serous inflammation occurs in coelomic cavities (e.g. *pleural, pericardial and peritoneal cavities*) and *skin*. Serous fluid is yellow and straw-colored with scant cells. It is either derived from plasma proteins or secretion of mesothelial cells of serous cavities. Tissue looks dull engorged with blood vessels.

Skin blisters: These are caused by burns and viral infection. Serous fluid is accumulated either within or immediately beneath the epidermis of the skin.

FIBRINOUS INFLAMMATION

Deposition of fibrin-rich exudates in meninges and coelomic surfaces (pleura, pericardium and peritoneum) is known as *fibrinous inflammation*. It occurs as a result of increased vascular permeability due to acute inflammation and malignancy leading to extravasation of fibrinogen over coelomic surfaces. Surface of the heart is covered by shaggy fibrinous exudates giving *bread and butter* appearance.

- Fibrinous exudate may be removed by fibrinolysis. Cellular debris is cleared by macrophages.
- When fibrin is not removed, it may stimulate the growth of fibroblasts and capillaries and thus leading to organization (fibrous strands) and obliteration of the pericardial sac.

PURULENT (SUPPURATIVE) INFLAMMATION

Pyogenic bacteria such as *staphylococci* cause liquefactive necrosis of tissue leading to formation of opaque pus due to excessive inflammatory exudates. Pus contains cellular debris derived from damaged tissue and polymorphonuclear cells. The destroyed tissue is restored and eventually replaced by fibrosis.

Clinical Features

Patient presents with pain induced by bradykinin and edema fluid.

Examples of Purulent Infection

- *Abscess in organs:* These include *skin abscess, brain abscess, pyogenic meningitis, lung abscess, lobar pneumonia, bronchopneumonia, splenic abscess, breast abscess, empyema gallbladder and acute appendicitis.*

    There is danger of perforation of *suppurative acute appendicitis;* hence early appendectomy is the treatment of choice. Multiple splenic abscesses are shown in Fig. 2.17. Histopathology of acute inflammation in appendix, lymph node, bone and lung is shown in Figs 2.18 to 2.21.

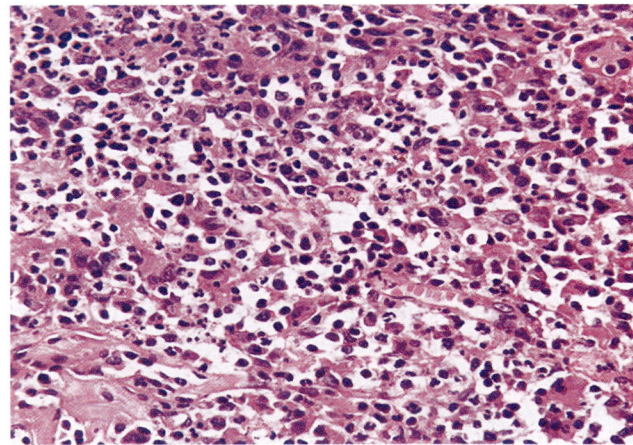

Fig. 2.19: Acute lymphadenitis showing infiltration by polymorphonuclear cells (400X).

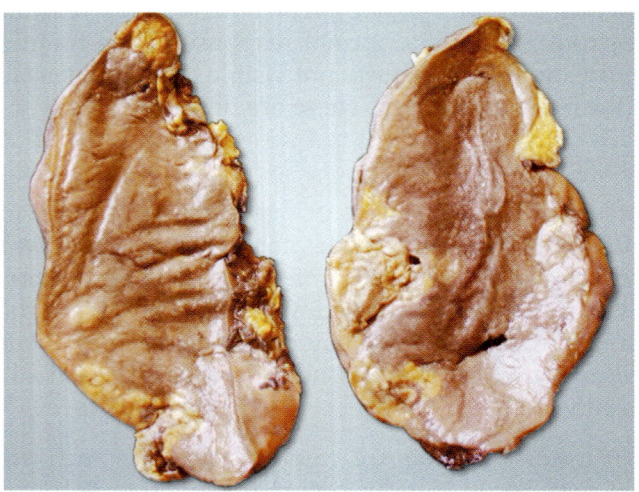

Fig. 2.17: Multiple abscesses in spleen.

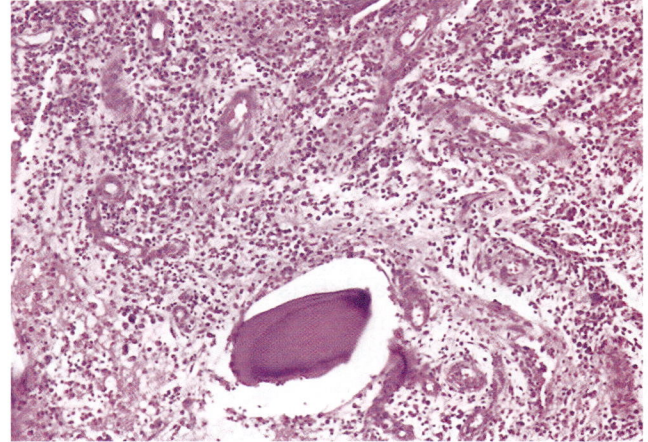

Fig. 2.20: Acute osteomyelitis. It shows infiltration by polymorphonuclear cells (400X).

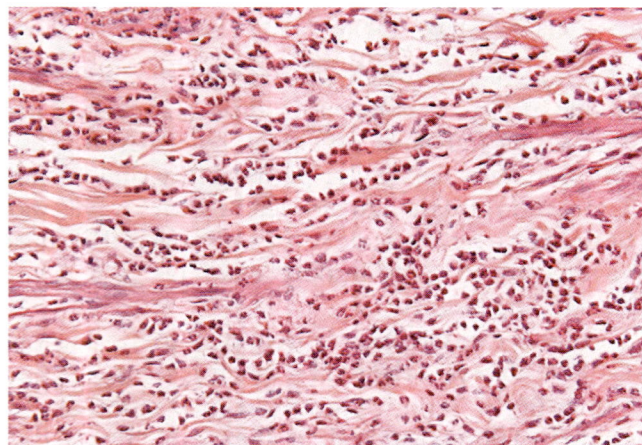

Fig. 2.18: Acute appendicitis showing infiltration of muscular coat by neutrophils (400X).

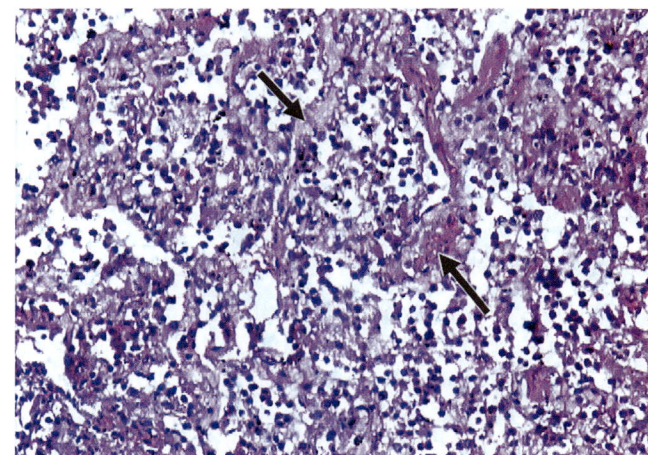

Fig. 2.21: Lobar pneumonia showing alveoli packed with polymorphonuclear cells (arrows) (400X).

- *Carbuncle:* It is an extensive form of abscess in the *back of the neck and scalp due to collection of pus in multiple loci.* Patient presents with multiple discharging sinuses at the surface.
- *Furuncle or boil:* It is small abscess related to hair follicles or sebaceous glands.
- *Cellulitis:* It refers to acute diffuse suppurative inflammation caused by streptococci. These bacteria synthesize *hyaluronidase* and *streptokinase enzymes* that *dissolve the ground substances* and facilitate the spread of infection in areolar tissue of orbit, pelvis, and subcutaneous tissue.

Complications

Complications include thrombophlebitis, massive bacteremia, and septic shock, embolization to various solid organs producing septic infarcts, lymphangitis and lymphadenitis.

PSEUDOMEMBRANOUS INFLAMMATION

Deposition of yellow-colored exudate over mucosal surfaces produces a shaggy membrane composed of necrotic tissue. *Corynebacterium diphtheria* liberates toxin, which forms pseudomembrane in the pharynx and trachea of children leading to severe respiratory distress.

Clostridium difficile's toxin in adults produces *pseudomembranous colitis.*

HEMORRHAGIC INFLAMMATION

Hemorrhagic inflammation is seen in pancreatitis.

GANGRENOUS INFLAMMATION

Gangrenous inflammation is seen in gangrenous appendicitis and gangrene gut.

CATARRHAL INFLAMMATION

Catarrhal inflammation involves mucosal surfaces (e.g. catarrhal rhinitis, catarrhal conjunctivitis) containing mixture of serous and mucous secretions.

CHEMICAL MEDIATORS

Chemical mediators mediate specific response by acting on the blood vessels, inflammatory cells or other cells in tissues. These regulate inflammation and immunity. These are synthesized either at injury site (local synthesis by cells) or plasma derived (distant synthesis).

- *Synthesis:* Chemical mediators are derived from (i) *plasma proteins* (complement system, kinins, and clotting factors), (ii) *cells* (leukocytes, tissue macrophages, endothelial cells of blood vessels, mast cells and platelets), (iii) *bacterial products,* and (iv) *fibroblasts of damaged tissues* in response to tissue injurious stimulus.
- *Properties:* Chemical mediators have short lifespan (e.g. seconds to minutes). These possess enzymatic or toxic activity. These have potential to cause harmful effects.
- *Mechanism:* These bind to specific receptors on single or multiple target cells, and stimulate them to release secondary molecules, which may direct enzymatic effects and/or systemic toxic effects.
- *Categories:* Chemical mediators are derived from plasma proteins or inflammatory cells. Plasma and cell derived chemical mediators and their functions are shown in Fig. 2.22.
- *Functional categories:* Chemical mediators produce vascular and cellular changes in inflammation. Based on functions, these are classified into following categories: *Vasoactive, chemotactic* and *combined chemotactic as well as vasoactive* and *chemical mediators.*

Functional Categories

Chemical mediators are categorized according to their actions described as under. Functional categories of chemical mediators and their inflammatory response are shown in Fig. 2.23 and Table 2.11.

Chemical Mediators with Vasoactive Actions

- *Vasodilation of arterioles and capillaries:* Chemical mediators such as histamine, serotonin, nitric oxide, bradykinin, platelet activating factor cause vasodilation of microvasculature and sustained by prostaglandins (PGI_2, PGD_2, PGE_2, $PGF_{2\alpha}$) resulting in increased blood flow to injury site. It is responsible for *redness (rubor) and increased local temperature (heat = calor).*
- *Increased permeability of venules:* Chemical mediators such as histamine, serotonin, bradykinin, anaphylatoxins (C3a, C5a), prostaglandins (PGD_2, PGE_2, $PGF_{2\alpha}$), leukotrienes (LTC_4, LTD_4, LTE_4), platelet activating factor (PAF) and neuropeptide (substance P) increase the permeability of venules and result in *inflammatory exudates.*

Chemical Mediators with Chemotactic Actions

Chemotactic agents include such as C5a, chemokines, leukotrienes (LTB_4, LTC_4), collagen, fibrin and bacterial peptides (pathogen-associated molecular patterns—PAMPs).

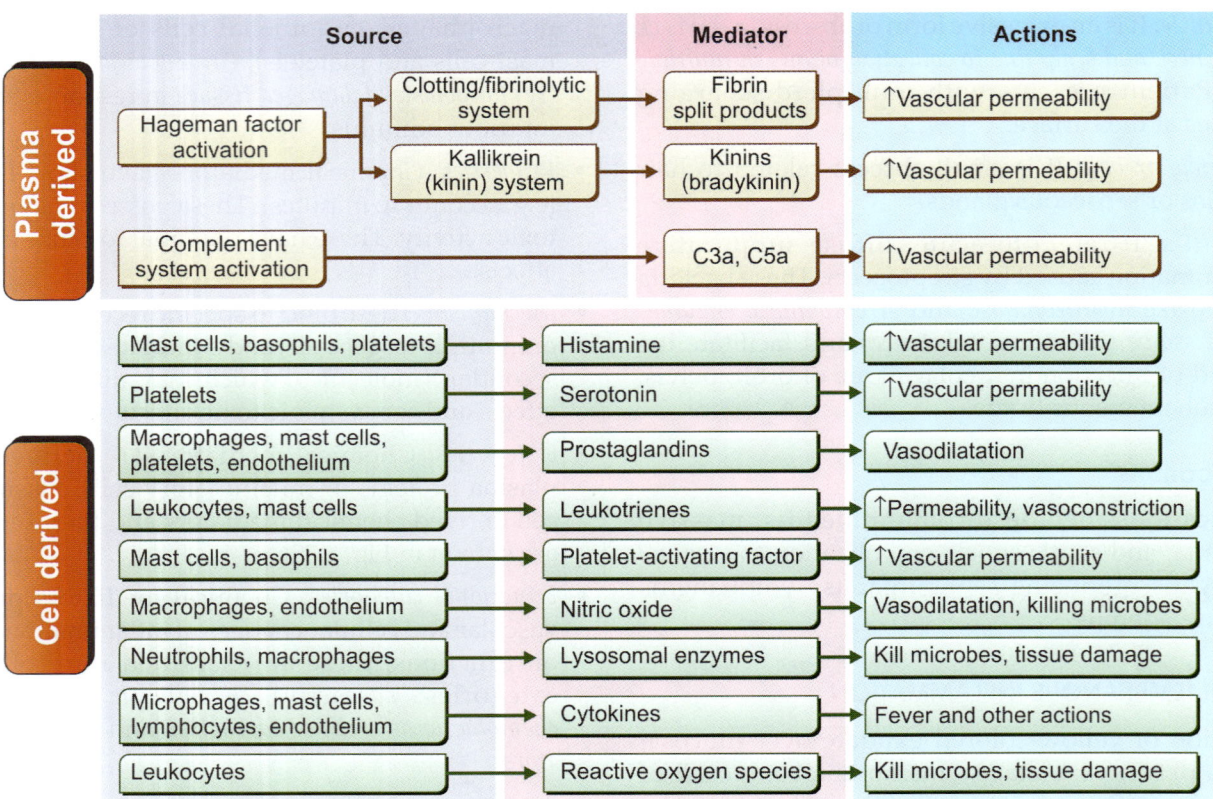

Fig. 2.22: Plasma and cell derived chemical mediators and their functions.

Chemical Mediators with Vasoactive and Chemotactic Actions

Complement components, cytokines (interferon and interleukins), products of arachidonic acid metabolism, and platelet activating factor produce vasoactive and chemotactic effects.

Source of Chemical Mediators

Plasma Derived Chemical Mediators

These include kinin system, fibrinolytic system, coagulation system, and complement system. These are synthesized by liver.

Cell Derived Chemical Mediators

These are synthesized by monocytes, macrophages, lymphocytes, fibroblasts, mast cells, platelets, and endothelial cells of blood vessels. Chemical mediators may be preformed or newly synthesized.

PLASMA DERIVED CHEMICAL MEDIATORS

Plasma proteins derived chemical mediators mediate inflammatory response. Hageman factor (XII) synthesized by liver is the key source of vasoactive chemical mediators.

It is activated by negatively charged surfaces (collagen, basement membrane), activated platelets and high molecular weight kininogen). Hageman factor activates kinin system resulting in activation of fibrinolytic system, coagulation system (intrinsic pathway) and complement system at the site of injury.

Plasma proteins derived chemical mediators in inflammation are shown in Fig. 2.24.

Kallikrein (Kinin) System

Kallikrein (kinin) system is activated by Hageman factor, plasmin and leukocyte protease. It is degraded by kininase and angiotensin converting enzyme (ACE) in the lungs.

Mechanism of Actions

Kinin system activates *coagulation system* (intrinsic pathway) and *fibrinolytic system*. It also activates *complement system* to generate C3, C5a, C5–9, which participate in *chemotaxis of leukocytes, opsonization* and *phagocytosis of microbes*. It converts kininogen to *bradykinin*, which mediates *vascular permeability, arteriolar dilation,* and *pain*.

Fibrinolytic System

Plasminogen activator synthesized by *endothelium* and *leukocytes* activates fibrinolytic system. Fibrinolytic system converts plasminogen to *plasmin*, which degrades

Inflammation, Tissue Healing and Repair

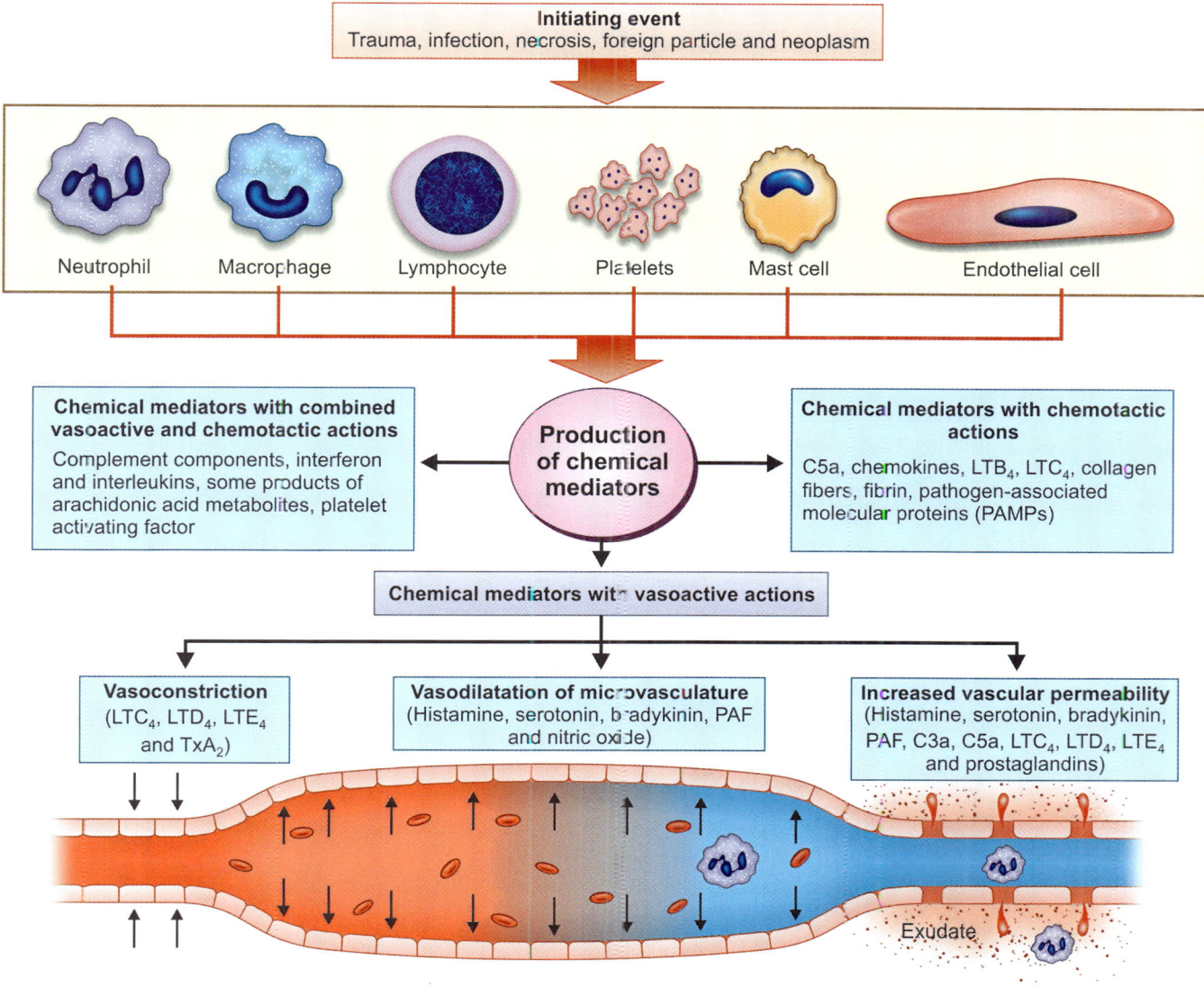

Fig. 2.23: Functional categories of chemical mediators and their inflammatory response.

fibrin into *fibrin peptides*. Fibrinolytic system participates in *vascular phase of inflammation* as mentioned below.

Mechanism of Actions

- Plasmin activates Hageman factor XII to synthesize plasma proteins related bradykinin (kinin). Bradykinin mediates *vascular permeability*, arteriolar dilation, and *pain*.
- Fibrinolytic system cleaves C3 to C3a. Plasmin, fibrin peptides, C3a and bradykinin *increase vascular permeability*.

Coagulation System

Coagulation system and inflammation are tightly linked. During final stage of coagulation, thrombin and insoluble fibrin are formed. These bind to seven-transmembrane G-protein coupled receptors expressed on platelets, endothelial cells, smooth muscle cells and other cells.

Thrombin and insoluble fibrin participate in vascular phase of inflammation. Coagulation system products and their actions are shown in Table 2.12.

Mechanism of Actions

- Thrombin and insoluble fibrin increase expression of *adhesion molecule* by mobilization (P selectin) on vascular endothelium. These also induce integrin synthesis, resulting in *leukocytic adhesion to vascular endothelium*.
- Factor Xa and fibrin peptides *increase vascular permeability*.

Table 2.11: Functional categories of chemical mediators

Functional categories	Inflammatory response	Chemical mediators	Source
Chemical mediators with vasoactive actions	Vasodilation of arterioles and capillaries	Histamine	Mast cells, basophils, platelets
		Serotonin	Platelets
		Bradykinin	Liver (plasma derived)
		Platelet activating factor	Mast cells, basophils
		Nitric oxide	Macrophages, endothelium
	Vasoconstriction	Leukotrienes (LTC_4, LTD_4, LTE_4)	Leukocytes, mast cells
		Thromboxane A_2	Macrophages, mast cells, platelets, endothelium
	Increased vascular permeability of venules	Histamine	Mast cells, basophils, platelets
		Serotonin	Platelets
		Bradykinin	Liver (plasma derived)
		Platelet activating factor (PAF)	Mast cells, basophils
		Anaphylatoxins (C3a, C5a)	Liver (plasma derived)
		Prostaglandins (PGD_2, PGE_2, $PGF_{2\alpha}$)	Macrophages, mast cells, platelets, endothelium
		Leukotrienes (LTC_4, LTD_4, LTE_4)	Leukocytes, mast cells
		Neuropeptide (substance P)	
Chemical mediators with chemotactic actions	Chemotaxis of leukocytes	C5a	Liver (plasma derived)
		Chemokines	Leukocytes, endothelial cells
		Leukotrienes (LTB_4, LTC_4)	Leukocytes, mast cells
		Collagen fibers	Tissue
		Fibrin (plasma derived)	Liver (plasma derived)
		Pathogen-associated molecular proteins (PAMPs)	Bacterial peptides
Chemical mediators with combined vasoactive and chemotactic actions	Vasoactive and chemotaxis of leukocytes	Complement components (C3a, C5a)	Liver (plasma derived)
		Interleukins	Macrophages, dendritic cells, fibroblasts, hepatocytes
		Chemokines	Leukocytes, endothelial cells
		LTC_4, LTD_4, LTE_4	Macrophages, mast cells, endothelial cells
		Platelet activating factor	Mast cells, basophils

- Factor Xa participates in *emigration of leukocytes*. Thrombin and fibrin peptides participate in *recruitment of leukocytes* to the site of injury.

    These also *enhance the synthesis of chemical mediators such as chemokines, prostaglandins, platelet activating factor, nitric oxide.*

Complement System

Complement system consists of a group of soluble plasma proteins synthesized by liver present in its inactive form that interact with one another in three distinct enzymatic-activation cascades. These are numbered C1 to C9 (C3 most abundant).

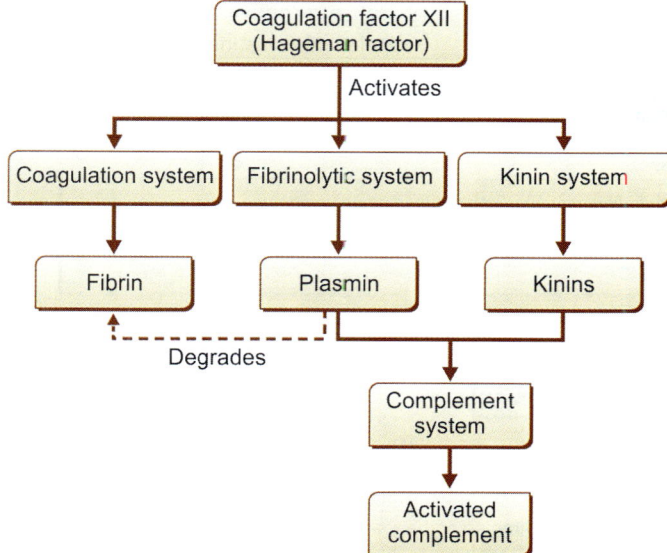

Fig. 2.24: Plasma proteins derived chemical mediators in inflammation.

Mechanism of Action

Complement proteins participate in innate and adaptive immunity during inflammation. These cause immune lysis of cells. Many regulatory proteins expressed by mammals prevent inappropriate activation of complement.

Complement Pathways

Three pathways of complement have different triggers at starting points, but all converge at the same place, C3 convertase. This enzyme begins the formation of tiny openings in the cell membrane and the destruction of target pathogen. Three pathways of complement are described as under.

- *Classical pathway:* It is also known as *immunologic pathway*. This pathway involves *fixation of antibodies* (IgG and IgM) and complement (C1). It is rapid and nonspecific. C1q, C1, C1s are converted to form C4, C2, C3.
- *Alternate pathway:* It is *antibody independent pathway*. It is activated by *bacteria, fungi, viruses and parasites and venom*. Factor B and factor D are converted to C3. *Deficiency of C3 affects alternate pathway of complement activation resulting to recurrent infections with fatal outcome, until treated.*
- *MB-lectin pathway:* It is also *antibody independent pathway*. It binds mannose (carbohydrate) on pathogen surfaces. It is *nonspecific for bacteria and viruses*. MBL, MASP-1, MASP-2 are converted to form C4, C2, C3.

Complement System Activation

All these three pathways converge to form C3. C3 convertase enzyme converts C3 molecule into an activator—C3b. C3 convertase enzyme and C3b are the central features of complement system activation. Activation of complement produces C3a, C5a and C5–9. Mechanism of action of complement is described as under.

- *C3 convertase enzyme:* It activates complement system and splits C3 into two functionally distinct C3a and C3b. C3a is released, while C3b binds to C5 convertase.
- *Binding of C3b to C5 convertase:* C3b–C5 convertase complex cleaves C5 to C5a and C5b. C5a is released, while remaining C5b binds to C5–C9. Other molecules given of C3a, C5a, which are peptide mediators of inflammation. These participate in chemotaxis of leukocytes and phagocytosis of bacteria.
- *Binding of C3b to C5–C9:* C5b is a reactive site for the final assembly of an attack complex. C5b fragment polymerizes with complement proteins C6–C9, resulting in the formation of membrane attack complex (MAC). Insertion of MACs produces hundreds of tiny holes in the lipid bilayer cell membrane results in cell lysis.

Complement Actions

Complement system cascade and its actions is shown in Fig. 2.25 and Table 2.13. Breakdown products of complement system mediates acute inflammation by following mechanisms:

Table 2.12: Coagulation system products and their actions

Coagulation system	Actions
Thrombin and insoluble fibrin	Mobilization of adhesion molecule (*P selectin*) and its expression on vascular endothelium.
	Induction of *integrin synthesis*, resulting to *leukocytic adhesion* to vascular endothelium
Factor Xa and fibrin peptides	Increased vascular permeability
Factor Xa	Emigration of leukocytes
Thrombin and fibrin peptides	Recruitment of leukocytes to the site of injury
	Enhancing synthesis of *chemical mediators* such as chemokines, prostaglandins, platelet activating factor, nitric oxide

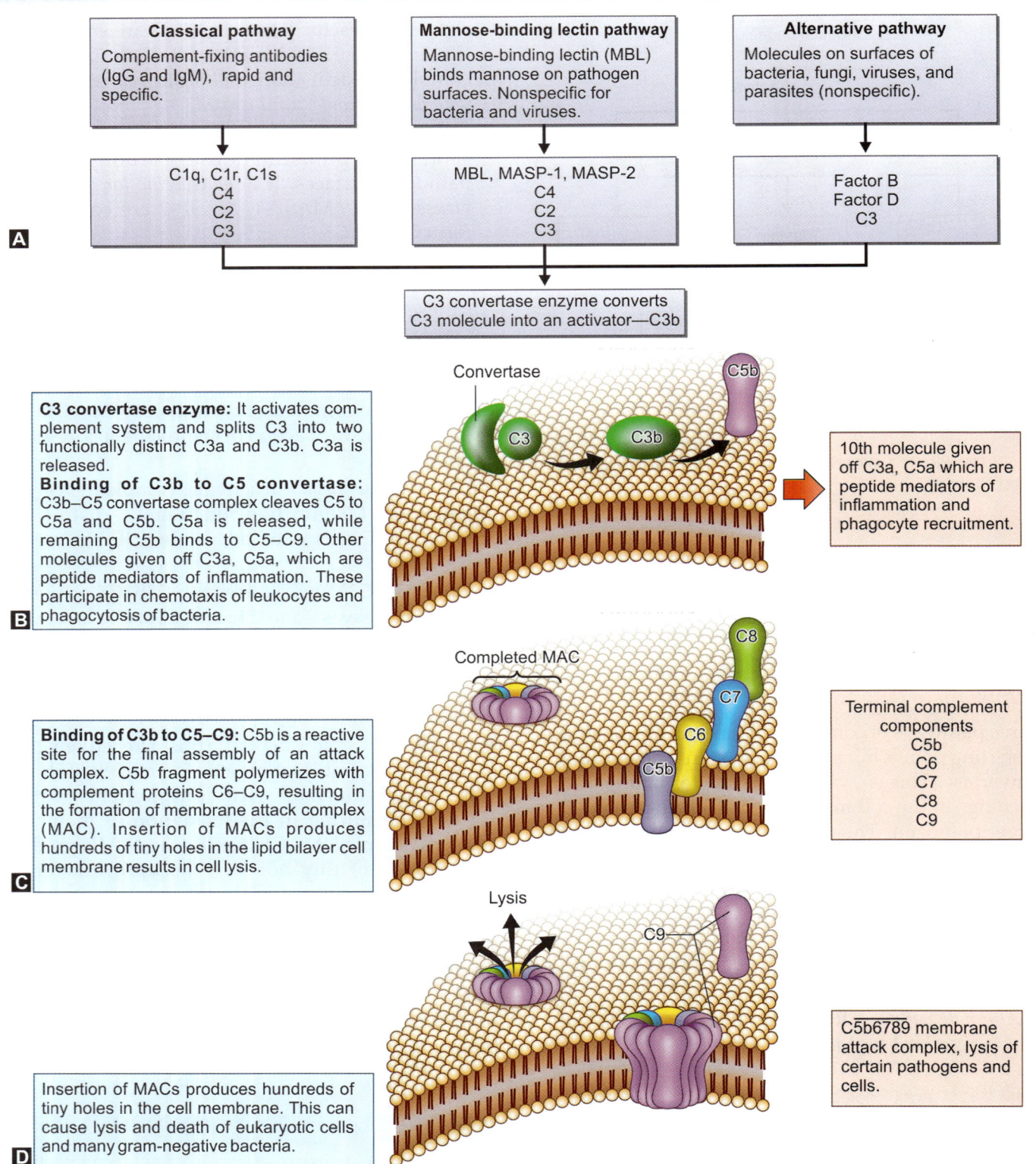

Fig. 2.25: Complement system cascade and its actions.

- *Opsonization and phagocytosis:* C3b acts as opsonins, which *coat the bacteria leading to phagocytosis by neutrophils and macrophages.*
- *Increased vascular permeability:* C3a and C5a cause increased vascular permeability.
- *Leukocytic adhesion, transmigration and chemotaxis:* C5a fragment is a *chemotactic agent,* which mediates the release of histamine from platelet-dense granules. *It induces the expression of leukocyte adhesion molecules.* It participates in *transmigration and chemotaxis of leukocytes.*

Table 2.13: Complement system cascade and its actions

Complement system cascade	Actions
C3b	Opsonization of microbes
	Phagocytosis of microbes
C3a and C5a	Increased vascular permeability
C5a	Adhesion of leukocytes
	Transmigration of leukocytes
	Chemotaxis of leukocytes
C3a, C5a and C4	Anaphylactic shock (due to excessive release of histamine)
C5a	Synthesis of arachidonic acid metabolites (lipooxygenase pathway)
C5b–C9 membrane attack complex (MAC)	Degradation of microbes and enhancing arachidonic acid metabolism and producing reactive oxygen metabolites
Defective formation of membrane attack complex (MAC) leads to increased susceptibility to Neisseria organisms.	

- *Anaphylactic shock:* C3a, C5a and C4 are called *anaphylatoxins*. These stimulate degranulation of mast cells and basophils liberating histamine. Histamine causes *increased vascular permeability, vasodilatation and smooth muscle contraction.* Patient develops anaphylactic shock.
- *Synthesis of arachidonic acid metabolites:* C5a fragment activates lipooxygenase enzyme, which acts on membrane of neutrophils and monocytes resulting to synthesis of arachidonic metabolites (lipooxygenase pathway).
- *Membrane attack complex (MAC):* C5b–C9 is a lytic agent for bacteria and target cells. It stimulates arachidonic acid metabolism and produces reactive oxygen metabolites. *Defective formation of membrane attack complex (MAC) leads to increased susceptibility to infections by Neisseria organisms.*

Disorders of Complement System

Disorders of complement system cascade are shown in Table 2.14. Patients develop increased susceptibility to infections due to defects in complement proteins, pathological activation and deficiency of regulatory proteins.

Recurrent Infections

Patient presents with increased susceptibility to infection due to deficiency of complement components such as C2, C3, and C5. Defective formation of membrane attack complex (MAC) leads to increased susceptibility to infections by Neisseria organisms.

Hereditary Angioneurotic Edema

Physiological state: Normally, classical pathway involves fixation antibodies (IgG and IgM) and complement (C1). C1 is inhibited by plasma protein C1 inhibitor (C1 INH).

Pathological state: Hereditary deficiency of C1 inhibitor (C1 INH) causes improper activation of C1 by immune complex resulting to excessive breakdown of C2 and C4.

Complement C2 molecule generates vasoactive peptide (bradykinin), which produces painless non-pitting edema of soft tissues especially *laryngeal edema, which may be life-threatening.*

Table 2.14: Disorders of complement system cascade

Disorder	Complement system cascade defects
Recurrent infections	C2, C3, and C5 deficiency
Neisseria infections	C5b–C9 defective formation of membrane attack complex (MAC)
Laryngeal edema	Hereditary deficiency of C1 inhibitor (C1 INH)
Systemic lupus erythematosus	C2 and C4 deficiency leading to improper clearance of immune complex
Paroxysmal nocturnal hemoglobinuria	PIG-A gene mutation encoding phosphatidylinositol linked membrane proteins leading to uncontrolled activation of complement resulting from recurrent bouts of intravascular complement mediated hemolysis
	Flow cytometry demonstrating *diminished CD55 and CD59 expression on red blood cells, leukocytes and platelets*

Systemic Lupus Erythematosus

Patient with C2 and C4 deficiencies may develop autoimmune disease SLE due to failure to clear immune complexes.

Paroxysmal Nocturnal Hemoglobinuria

- *Physiological state:* Under physiological state, glycosylphosphatidylinositol (GPI) anchor regulatory proteins such as CD55, CD59 and C8, which are required for the protection of *red blood cells, granulocytes,* and *platelets* from complement-mediated lysis. CD55 known as *DAF* (decay accelerating factor) cleaves C3b. CD59 known as *MIRL* (membrane inhibitor reactive lysis) participates in cleaving C5–C9.
- *Gene mutation:* PIG-A gene mutation encoding phosphatidylinositol linked membrane proteins leads to *uncontrolled activation of complement* resulting to *recurrent bouts of intravascular complement mediated hemolysis.*
- *Clinical manifestations:* The condition is often marked by the *passage of hemoglobin-containing urine on awakening.*

During hemolytic episodes, patients develop normocytic or macrocytic anemia, accompanied by an appropriate *reticulocyte response.* PNH may develop as a primary disorder or evolve from preexisting case of aplastic anemia.

- *Laboratory diagnosis:* Flow cytometry demonstrates *diminished CD55 and CD59 expression on red blood cells, leukocytes and platelets.* Traditional diagnostic test was based on hemolysis in sucrose (*sucrose hemolysis test*) or *acidified serum* (*Ham test*) *in vitro.*

CELL DERIVED CHEMICAL MEDIATORS

Cell derived chemical mediators may be preformed or newly synthesized are shown in Table 2.15. These are synthesized by *monocytes, macrophages, lymphocytes, fibroblasts, mast cells, platelets, and endothelial cells* of blood vessels. These participate in acute inflammation by *increasing vascular permeability* resulting in extravasation of plasma protein rich fluid along with inflammatory cells in interstitial tissue *exudate.*

Vasoactive Amines

Vasoactive amines include histamine, serotonin and bradykinin. Vasoactive amines chemical mediators are shown in Table 2.16.

Histamine

Histamine is stored in the secretory granules of *mast cells, basophils and platelets.* It release is triggered by *immune complexes, C3a, C5a, IL-1, IL-8, neuropeptide* into the extracellular tissues. It also increases *secretion of salivary, lacrimal, respiratory and gastric glands.* Histamine action

Table 2.15: Cells derived preformed and newly synthesized chemical mediators

Subcategories	Source	Chemical mediators
Preformed cell derived chemical mediators	Stored in the secretory granules of mast cells, basophils and platelets	Histamine
	Stored in dense bodies of platelets	Serotonin
	Neutrophils and macrophages	Lysosomal enzymes
Newly synthesized cell derived chemical mediators	Arachidonic acid metabolites (cyclooxygenase pathway)	Prostaglandins
		Prostacyclin (PGI_2)
		Thromboxane A_2 (TXA_2)
	Arachidonic acid metabolites (lipooxygenase pathway)	Leukotrienes
		Lipoxins
	Cytokines	Interleukins
		Tumor necrosis factor-α (TNF-α)
		Interferons (IFN-α, IFN-β, IFN-γ)
		Chemokines
		Growth factors
	Other chemical mediators	O_2 derived free radicals
		Nitric oxide
		Platelet activating factor
		Neuropeptides (substance P)
		Hypoxia induced factor-α (HIF-α)

Table 2.16: Vasoactive amines chemical mediators

Chemical mediators	Source	Actions
Histamine	Mast cells, basophils, platelets, enterochromaffin cells	Increased vascular permeability (exudate)
		Bronchoconstriction (bronchial asthma)
		Anaphylactic shock (circulatory collapse)
Serotonin	Platelets	Increased permeability of venules (exudate)
		Vasodilation
		Increased collagen synthesis
Bradykinin	Plasma proteins (kinin)	Increased vascular permeability (exudate)
		Vasodilation
		Induction of pain

on smooth muscle varies with location. It increases *intestinal motility*. It is responsible for the *wheal* and *flare* reaction in skin, pruritus and headache. It mediates *acute inflammation, bronchial asthma and anaphylactic shock*. Histamine is *inactivated by histaminase*.

- *Acute inflammation:* Histamine binds to specific H1 receptors in the vascular wall, inducing endothelial cell contraction gap formation, *increasing vascular permeability and edema formation* (exudate) in acute inflammation. It occurs due to phosphorylation of contractile myosin and cytoskeleton proteins. It causes smooth muscle relaxation of arterioles resulting in *vasodilation*.

- *Bronchial asthma:* Histamine is *potent fast acting chemical mediator in allergic disorders*. It causes *smooth muscle contraction of bronchioles*. It increases *mucus secretion in bronchioles*. It increases synthesis of *eotaxin*, which attract eosinophils.

- *Anaphylactic shock:* Massive release of histamine may cause *circulatory collapse* (anaphylactic shock). Patient develops *hypotension, tachycardia, circulatory failure*, and *shock*.

Serotonin

Serotonin is stored in dense bodies of *platelets*. Its release is triggered by immune complexes, C3a, C5a, IL-1, IL-8, neuropeptide into the extracellular tissues. It increases *permeability of microvasculature* and *vasodilatation*. It causes *smooth muscle contraction* and inhibits gastric secretion.

Bradykinin

Bradykinin is related to plasma proteins known as *kinins*. Kinin system converts kininogen to bradykinin. It causes *vasodilation of peripheral arterioles*, increased capillary permeability and induction of *pain*. In allergy, it causes *prolonged smooth muscle contraction of bronchioles*

and *increased mucus secretion*. It activates complement system to generate C3, C5a, C5–9, which participate in *chemotaxis of leukocytes, opsonization* and *phagocytosis of microbes*.

Lysosomal Enzymes of Phagocytes

Macrophages and neutrophils contain lysosomal enzymes in their granules. During inflammation, lysosomal enzymes (preformed chemical mediators) are released at the site of tissue injury resulting in degradation of injurious agents. Liberation of lysosomal enzymes in the interstitial tissue may cause tissue damage.

Neutrophils

Neutrophils contain azurophilic and specific granules. Specific granules are released more easily in extracellular compartment even in low concentration, in comparison to azurophilic granules. Their actions are described as under:

- *Degradation of pathogens:* Myeloperoxidase, lactoferrin, lysozyme, major basic proteins degrade bacteria, and debris within phagolysosomes. Neutral elastases degrade virulence factors of bacteria and thus *combat bacterial infection*.

- *Degradation of extracellular matrix:* During acute inflammation, *neutrophilic collagenase, hydrolase, protease* and *elastase* degrade extracellular matrix composed of collagen fibers, basement membrane, elastin and cartilage.

- *Synthesis of anaphylatoxins:* These also cleave C3 and C5 directly releasing anaphylatoxins (C3a, C5a) and release a kinin-like peptide from kininogen.

Macrophages

Macrophages contain acid hydrolases; collagenases, elastases, phospholipases and plasminogen activator participate in chronic inflammation.

Arachidonic Acid Metabolites

Arachidonic Acid

Arachidonic acid (AA) is 20-carbon polyunsaturated fatty acid (4 double bonds) obtained from *dietary linoleic acid* (essential fatty acid). It is present in its esterified form as a component of *cell membrane phospholipids of tissue macrophages, mast cells, endothelial cells and recruited leukocytes*.

Arachidonic Acid Metabolite Pathways

Tissue injury leads to influx of cytosolic calcium in *tissue macrophages, mast cells, endothelial cells and recruited leukocytes*. Increased cytosolic calcium activates membrane phospholipase A_2 enzyme resulting in synthesis of arachidonic acid known as *eicosanoids*. PGH_2 serves as a substrate for *cyclooxygenase and lipooxygenase enzymatic pathways*. These enzymatic pathways synthesize various arachidonic acid metabolites.

Generation of arachidonic acid metabolites and their roles in inflammation is shown in Fig. 2.26. The spectrum inflammatory cytokines are released by mast cell. These cytokines elicit overlapping extensive effects in target cells are shown in Fig. 2.27. Arachidonic acid metabolites, their source and actions are shown in Table 2.17.

- *Cyclooxygenase pathway:* This pathway produces *prostaglandins, prostacyclin* and *thromboxane A_2*. This

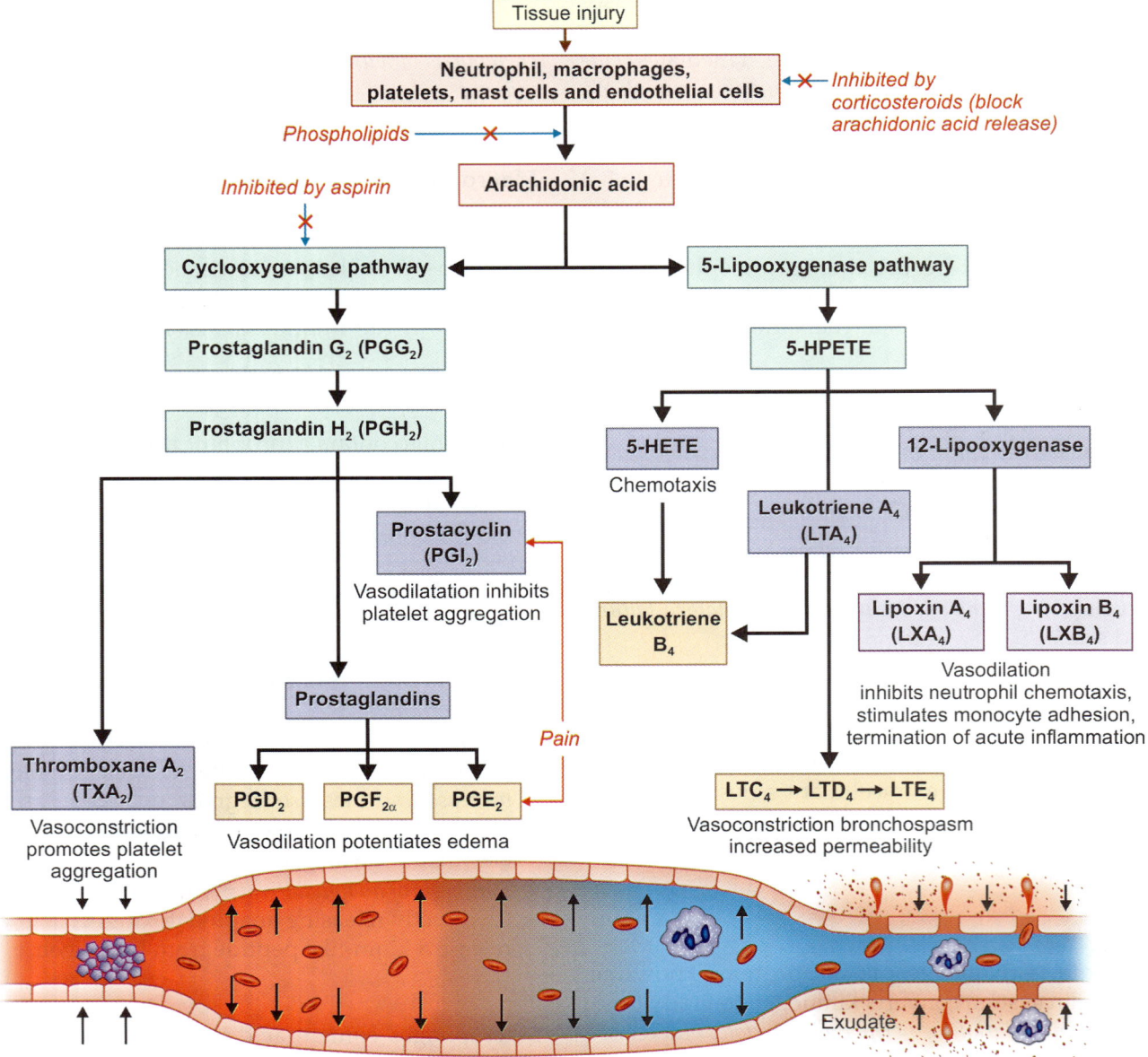

Fig. 2.26: Generation of arachidonic acid metabolites and their roles in inflammation.

Inflammation, Tissue Healing and Repair

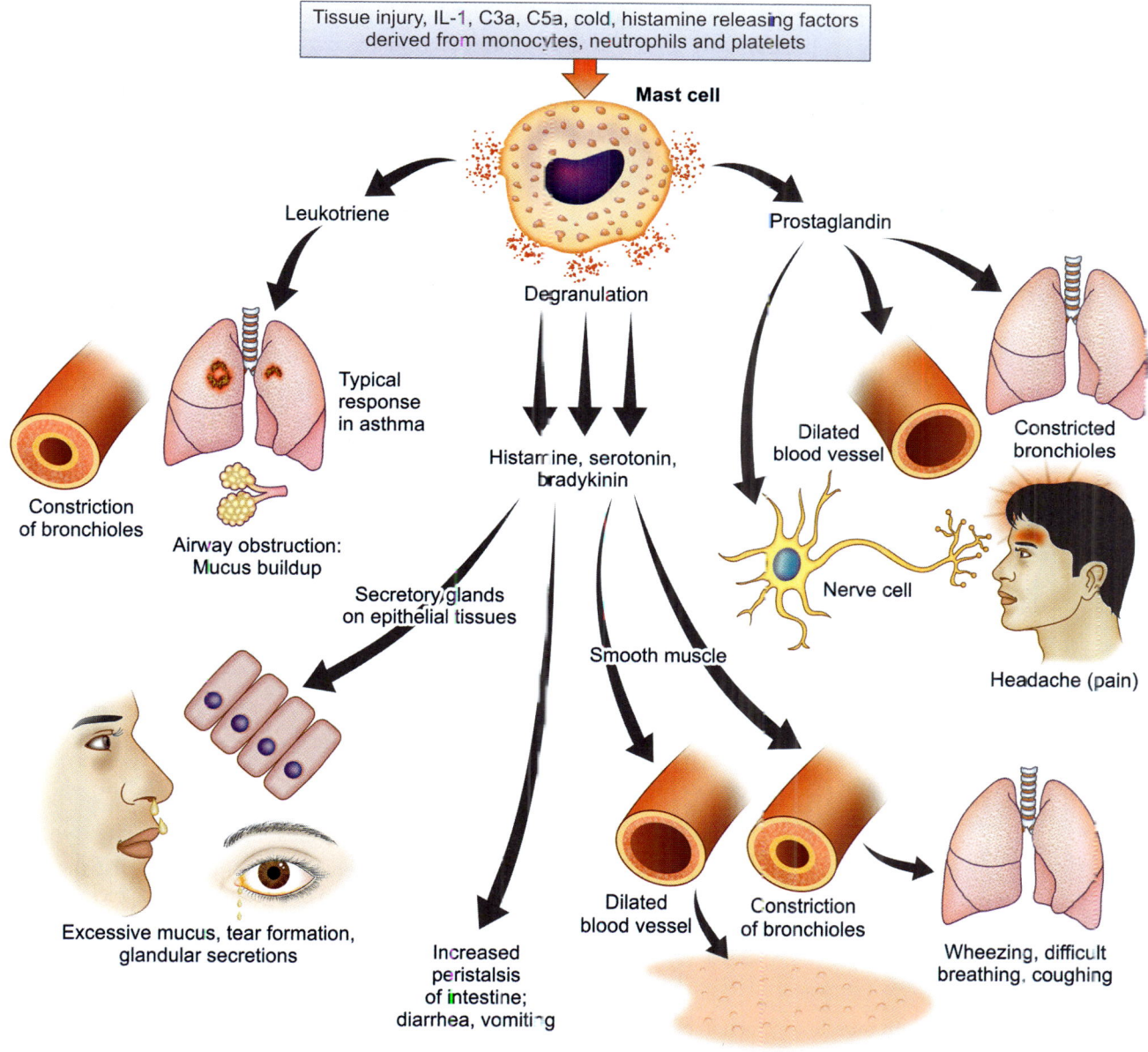

Fig. 2.27: The spectrum of reactions to inflammatory cytokines released by mast cell. These cytokines elicit overlapping extensive effects in target cells.

pathway is affected by anti-inflammatory drugs (NSAIDs and corticosteroids). COX-2 inhibitor drugs produce less toxicity than COX-1.

- *Lipooxygenase pathway:* This pathway synthesizes leukotrienes (LTB_4, LTC_4, LTD_4, and LTE_4) and lipoxins (LXA_4, LXB_4). Arachidonic acid metabolites such as leukotrienes and lipoxins are synthesized by cell-cell interactions (neutrophils-platelets).

Arachidonic acid metabolites and their actions
- *Prostaglandins (PGI_2, PGE_2 and PGD_2):* These promote *platelet aggregation*. These cause *vasodilatation and increased vascular permeability* with exudation (edema).

These modulate *phagocytic activity* of leukocytes. These are responsible for *pain* and *fever*.

- *Leukotrienes (LTC_4, LTD_4 and LTE_4):* These are potent chemical mediators of inflammation. Leukotrienes have histamine like actions. These cause *vasodilation and increased vascular permeability*.

  These activate PMNs leukocytes leading to adhesion on venular endothelium, *chemotaxis*, and generation of oxygen derived free radicals and release of lysosomal enzymes.

- *Prostacyclin:* It causes *vasodilatation* and *inhibits platelets aggregation*. It enhances the action of other

Table 2.17: Arachidonic acid metabolites, their source and actions

Pathways	Category of chemical mediators	Source	Chemical mediators	Actions
Cyclo-oxygenase pathway	Prostaglandins*	Macrophages, endothelial cells, mast cells, platelets	PGD_2	Promotes platelets aggregation
				Vasodilation
				Increased vascular permeability
			PGE_2	Pain, fever, edema
			PGD_2, PGE_2	Modulation of phagocytic activity of leukocytes
	Prostacyclin (PGI_2)	Vascular endothelium (prostacyclin synthase enzyme)	PGI_2	Activating adenylyl cyclase and increases intra-cellular levels of cAMP
				Inhibiting platelets aggregation
	Thromboxane A_2 (TxA_2)	PGI_2 is converted to TxA_2 by thromboxane synthase in platelets	TxA_2	Platelet aggregation (due to activation of guanylyl cyclase increasing intracellular levels of cGMP)
				Increased vascular permeability (serotonin released due to interaction of platelets, thrombin and collagen fibers)
				Vasoconstriction
				Smooth muscle contraction
Lipooxygenase pathway (5) in neutrophils	Leukotrienes**	Leukocytes and mast cells	LTB_4	Adhesion, chemotaxis and activation of neutrophils
			LTC_4, LTD_4, LTE_4	Vasoconstriction
				Increased permeability of venules
				Bronchoconstriction (monteleukast therapeutic agent used to block leukotrienes receptors)
Lipooxygenase pathway (12) in platelets	Lipoxins (LXA_4, LXB_4)	Platelets	LXA_4, LXB_4	Termination of acute inflammation by inhibiting adhesion, chemotaxis of leukocytes
				Vasodilatation

*Prostaglandins regulate smooth muscle contraction of uterus during delivery.
**Leukotrienes: LTA_4 is converted to LTB_4, LTC_4, LTD_4 and LTE_4), LTC_4 synthase enzyme in platelets converts (LTA_4) to LTC_4. Simultaneously, this pathway cnoverts 5-HPETE (5-hydroperoxyeicosatetraenoic acid) to 5-HETE (chemotactic action).

chemical mediators leading to increased vascular permeability and chemotaxis.

- *Thromboxane A_2:* It is synthesized by *platelets* with its thromboxane synthase enzyme. It *promotes platelets aggregation*. It causes *vasoconstriction*.
- *Lipoxins (LXA_4, LXB_4):* These terminate acute inflammation in the first few hours of injurious stimulus. *Lipoxins inhibit adhesion of leukocytes to endothelium as well as chemotaxis. These also cause vasodilatation.*

Cyclooxygenase Pathway

This pathway leads to formation of *prostaglandins, prostacyclin* and *thromboxane A_2*. Anti-inflammatory therapeutic agents such as NSAIDs and corticosteroids inhibit the synthesis of prostaglandins. *Prolonged administration of non-steroidal anti-inflammatory drugs may increase risk of arterial thrombosis* in people possibly due to reduced prostacyclin in endothelial cells. COX-2 inhibitor drugs produce less toxicity than COX-1. Anti-inflammatory agents inhibiting cyclo-oxygenase pathway are shown in Table 2.18.

Prostaglandins

- *Synthesis:* Prostaglandins are synthesized by *macrophages, endothelial cells, mast cells and platelets.*
- *Actions:* PGD_2 causes *vasodilation, increased vascular permeability* and *aggregation of platelets*. PGE_2 is

Table 2.18: Anti-inflammatory agents inhibiting cyclooxygenase pathway

Therapeutic agents	Actions
Aspirin (NSAIDs)	Inhibits the action of both COX-1 and COX-2
Meloxicam and carprofen (NSAIDs)	Inhibit the action of COX-2 without toxic effects
Glucocorticoids	Downregulate expression of gene encoding COX-2 without toxic effects
Omega-3 fatty acid consumption	Serves as poor substrates for synthesizing prostaglandins

Prolonged administration of non-steroidal anti-inflammatory drugs may increase risk of arterial thrombosis in people possibly due to reduced prostacyclin in endothelial cells.

responsible for pain, fever and edema. PGD_2 and PGE_2 modulate phagocytic activity of leukocytes.

Prostacyclin (PGI_2)

- *Synthesis:* Prostacyclin synthase enzyme in *vascular endothelium* synthesizes prostacyclin. Prostacyclin activates adenylyl cyclase and increases *intracellular levels of cAMP*.
- *Actions:* Prostacyclin inhibits *platelets aggregation*. It participates in *vasodilatation, increased vascular permeability and chemotaxis*.

Thromboxane A_2 (TxA_2)

- *Synthesis:* Thromboxane synthase enzyme in platelets synthesizes TXA_2. Thromboxane A_2 activates guanylyl cyclase and increases intracellular levels of cGMP.
- *Actions:* TXA_2 promotes *platelets aggregation*. It causes *vasoconstriction*. It mediates smooth muscle contraction. Platelets come in contact with thrombin and fibrillar collagen fibers liberate serotonin resulting in *increased vascular permeability*.

Lipoxygenase Pathway Products

Arachidonic acid metabolites such as leukotrienes and lipoxins are synthesized by cell-cell interactions (neutrophils-platelets) by following mechanisms:

5-Lipooxygenase pathway in neutrophils: Arachidonic acid metabolites of this pathway include leukotrienes and 5-HETE. Leukotrienes are synthesized by leukocytes and mast cells. Mechanism of actions of leukotrienes and therapeutic correlation is shown in Table 2.19

- *Synthesis:* Injurious stimulus activates 5-lipooxygenase enzymatic pathway in neutrophils resulting in synthesis of LTA_4. Simultaneously LTA_4 is converted to leukotrienes, e.g. LTB_4 (chemotactic), LTC_4, LTD_4, and LTE_4.
- *Actions:* Leukotrienes and histamine have similar functions. Histamine is less potent with rapid action. While *leukotrienes are more potent chemical mediator of inflammation*, but *slow reacting substance of anaphylaxis (SRS-A)*.

12-Lipooxygenase pathway in platelets: This pathway converts arachidonic acid to lipoxins (LXA_4 and LXB_4) in platelets. After an inflammatory response, neutrophils promote the *switch in* arachidonic acid derived prostaglandins and leukotrienes to anti-inflammatory lipoxins.

- *Termination of acute inflammation:* Lipoxins terminate acute inflammation in the first few hours of injurious stimulus by *inhibiting adhesion of leukocytes to endothelium* as well as chemotaxis in the first few hours. These also cause vasodilatation.
- *Apoptosis of neutrophils:* Lipoxins transmit signal to macrophages, which phagocytose apoptotic bodies of *neutrophils (programmed death)*.

Table 2.19: Mechanism of actions of leukotrienes and therapeutic correlation

Leukotrienes	Actions	Therapeutic correlation
LTC_4, LTD_4 and LTE_4	Binding to cyst LT1 and cyst LT2 receptors on bronchial smooth muscles leading to prolonged bronchospasm, increased vascular permeability, and mucus secretion of the asthmatic persons	Therapeutic agent (monteleukast) administered for treatment of bronchial asthma blocking cysteinyl leukotrienes receptors (cyst LT1 and cyst LT2) expressed in bronchi
		Zileutin inhibits 5-lipooxygenase and thus decreases synthesis of LTC_4, LTD_4 and LTE_4
		Consumption of fish-rich in omega-3 fatty acid serves as poor substrates for synthesizing leukotrienes (lipooxygenase pathway)
		Non-steroidal anti-inflammatory drugs are not effective in inhibiting the synthesis of metabolites by lipooxygenase pathway
LTB_4	Increasing PMNs adhesion to endothelium and recruitment to site of tissue injury	Not applicable

Leukotrienes also participate in generation of oxygen derived free radicals and release of lysosomal enzymes

- *Anti-inflammatory action:* Lipoxins are *potent anti-inflammatory chemical mediators* that may have therapeutic significance.

Cytokines

Cytokines are proteins synthesized by activated macrophages, mast cells and endothelial cells. These usually act at short range. In inflammation, these have multiple effects such as activation of inflammatory cells which result in degradation of injurious agents.

Cytokines include interleukins, tumor necrosis factor-α, interferons (IFN-α, IFN-β, and IFN-γ), chemokines and growth factors (Table 2.20).

Interleukins

Interleukins, source and their actions are shown in Table 2.21.

- *Synthesis:* These cytokines are soluble proteins synthesized by *lymphocytes, monocytes/macrophages, NK cells, fibroblasts, hepatocytes and epithelial cells.* Macrophages

Table 2.20: Cytokines chemical mediators and their actions

Chemical mediators	Source	Specific cytokine	Actions
Interleukins: IL-1, IL-6, IL-8, IL-10, IL-13	Monocytes/macrophages, lymphocytes, dendritic cells, fibroblasts, hepatocytes and epithelial cells	IL-1	Adhesion, chemotaxis of leukocytes and phagocytosis
			Synthesis of acute phase reactants
		IL-6	It increases liver synthesis of acute phase reactants
		IL-8	Chemotaxis of leukocytes
Tumor necrosis factors	TNF-α synthesis by macrophages, T cells, and NK cells	TNF-α	Adhesion of leukocytes
			Synthesis of acute phase reactants
	TNF-β synthesis by T cells	TNF-β	T cell proliferation
			Cytotoxic to some tumor cells
Interferons	IFN-α synthesis by macrophages, T cells, and NK cells	IFN-α	Antiviral activity
	IFN-β synthesis by fibroblasts	IFN-β	Antiviral activity
	IFN-γ synthesis of T cells and NK cells	IFN-γ	Antiviral activity
			Activation of macrophages and T cells during chronic inflammation
			Increase cytotoxicity of natural killer cells
Chemokines: C-X-C(α), C-C(β) XC(γ) and CX3C	Leukocytes, endothelial cells	C-X-C (α)	Chemotaxis of neutrophils
		C-C (β-Chemokine)	Chemotaxis of monocytes
		XC (γ-Chemokine)	Chemotaxis of lymphocytes
		CX3C	Chemotaxis of monocytes and T cells
Growth factors: G-CSF, GM-CSF, IL-7, and IL-13	G-CSF synthesis by macrophages, neutrophils and T cells, fibroblasts and vascular endothelium	G-CSF	Activation and differentiation of neutrophils
	GM-CSF synthesis by fibroblasts and vascular endothelium	G-CSF	Hematopoiesis
		GM-CSF	Promote the growth and development of macrophages from undifferentiated precursor stem cells
			Activation of natural killer cells and dendritic cells
	IL-7 synthesis by stromal cells in bone marrow, dendritic cells, hepatocytes, keratinocytes, neurons and epithelial cells except normal lymphocytes	IL-7	Act as a growth factor for bone marrow stem cells
	IL-13 synthesis by T cells	IL-13	Act as a growth factor for bone marrow stem cells

Table 2.21: Interleukins, source and their actions

Characteristics	Interleukin	Source	Actions
Chemotactic activity	IL-I	Macrophages/monocytes	Master cytokine stimulating T cells proliferation and IL-2 synthesis
			Adhesion of neutrophils
			Chemotaxis of neutrophils
			Phagocytosis of injurious agent by neutrophils
			Inducing fever
	IL-8	Macrophages/monocytes	Chemotaxis of neutrophils
	IL-9	CD4+ T cells	Chemotaxis of neutrophils and fever
	IL-16	T-suppressor cells and eosinophils	Chemotaxis of T-helper cells
Synthesis of acute phase reactants	IL-6	T cells, B cells, macrophages and fibroblasts	Stimulate liver to synthesize acute phase reactants
	IL-11	Bone marrow stromal cells	Stimulate liver to synthesize acute phase reactants
Synthesis of other cytokines	IL-17	T-helper cells	Synthesis of IL-6, IL-8, G-CSF and PGE2
Regulation of lymphocytes	IL-2	T cells, NK cells and macrophages	Stimulate proliferation of T cells, B cells (immunoglobulin synthesis), and NK cells; activates monocytes
			Activated natural killer cells kill of cancer cells, fungi and virally infected cells by antibody-dependent cell-mediated cytotoxicity (ADCC)
	IL-4, IL-13 (both have similar functions)	T cells	IL-4 and IL-13 promote growth of B and T cells
			IL-4 and IL-13 switching B cells to synthesize IgE antibody in type I hypersensitivity reactions
			IL-4 also enhance expression of HLA class II antigens
Specific immune response	IL-5	T cells	IL-5 promotes end-stage maturation of B cells into plasma cells
			Priming of basophils to release histamine and leukotrienes and chemotaxis of eosinophils in type I hypersensitivity reaction
	IL-6	T cells, B cells, macrophages and fibroblasts	Promote maturation of B and T cells
			Inhibit growth of fibroblasts
			Induce synthesis of acute phase reactants by liver
			Promote mucus secretion
	IL-9	T cells	Proliferation of T cells
	IL-12	T cells	Activate T cells and natural killer cells
	IL-15	Monocytes	Proliferation of T cells and B cells
	IL-10	T cells	Inhibiting macrophages, B cells and synthesis of interferons
Growth factors activity	IL-3	T cells	Act as a growth factor for tissue mast cells and hematopoietic stem cells
	IL-4	T cells	Promote growth of B and T cells; enhances expression of HLA class II antigens
	IL-7	Stromal cells in bone marrow, dendritic cells, hepatocytes, keratinocytes, neurons and epithelial cells	Act as a growth factor for bone marrow stem cells

synthesize IL-1, IL-8, and IL-12. T cells synthesize IL-2 to IL-5, IL-9, IL-10, IL-13, and IL-16. Stromal cells synthesize IL-7.

- *Actions:* These mediate communications between leukocytes such as B cells, T cells, NK cells, monocytes, macrophages, hematopoietic cells and many other cell types. IL-2 and IL-4 favor lymphocytes growth. IL-10 and TGF-β disfavor lymphocytes growth.

Tumor Necrosis Factor-α or β

- *Tumor necrosis factor-α (TNF-α, cachectin):* It is synthesized by macrophages, T cells, and NK cells. It stimulates T cell proliferation and IL-2 production; *cytotoxic to some tumor cells.*
- *Tumor necrosis factor-β (TNF-β):* It is synthesized by T cells. It stimulates T cell proliferation and IL-2 production. *It is cytotoxic to some tumor cells.*

Interferons (IFN-α, IFN-β, and IFN-γ)

These are antiviral and activate leukocytes. The antiviral activity of interferon is shown in Fig. 2.28. Interferons, source and their actions are shown in Table 2.22.

- *Interferon-α (IFN-α):* It is synthesized by macrophages and T cells. It has *antiviral activity.*
- *Interferon-β (IFN-β):* It is synthesized by fibroblasts. It has *antiviral activity.*
- *Interferon-γ (IFN-γ):* It is synthesized by activated T cells and NK cells. It has *antiviral activity.* It activates macrophages and T cells during chronic inflammation. It enhances expression of HLA class II antigens.

  It participates in *differentiation of T and B cells.* It increases the *cytotoxicity of natural killer cells.* It activates neutrophils and stimulates diapedesis.

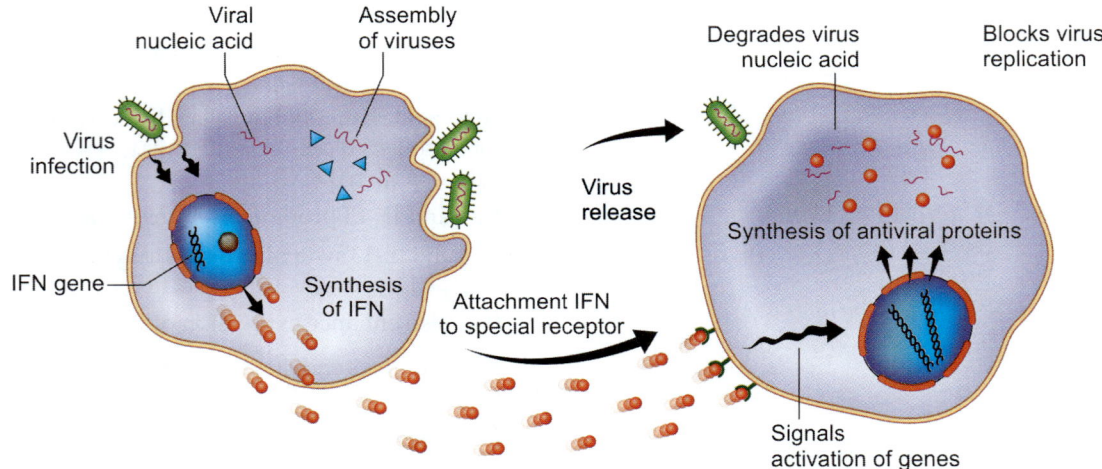

Fig. 2.28: The antiviral activity of interferon. When a cell is infected by a virus, its nucleus is triggered to transcribe interferon (IFN) gene. Interferon diffuses out of the cell and then binds to IFN receptors on nearby uninfected cells, where it induces production of proteins that eliminate viral genes and block viral replication. Note that the original cell is not protected by IFN and that does not prevent viruses from invading the protected cells.

Table 2.22: Interferons, source and their actions

Chemical mediator	Source	Specific cytokine	Actions
Tumor necrosis factors	TNF-α synthesis by macrophages, T cells, and NK cells	TNF-α	Adhesion of leukocytes
			Synthesis of acute phase reactants
	TNF-β synthesis by T cells	TNF-β	T cell proliferation
			Cytotoxic to some tumor cells
Interferons	IFN-α synthesis by macrophages, T cells, and NK cells	IFN-α	Antiviral activity
	IFN-β synthesis by fibroblasts	IFN-β	Antiviral activity
	IFN-γ synthesis of T cells and NK cells	IFN-γ	Antiviral activity
			Activation of macrophages and T cells during chronic inflammation
			Increase cytotoxicity of natural killer cells

Chemokines

- *Synthesis:* These are synthesized by macrophages and endothelial cells.
- *Classification:* Chemokines are classified into four groups according to the arrangement of the conserved cysteine (CC) residues in the mature proteins—(i) C-X-C chemokine (α-chemokine), (ii) C-C chemokine (β-chemokine), (iii) C-chemokine (γ-chemokine) and (iv) CX3C chemokine.
- *Actions:* These participate in recruitment of inflammatory cells (neutrophils, monocytes, T cells) to the injured site. These also increase enhance the adhesion integrin affinity of leukocytes to ligand on vascular endothelium. Chemokines bind to G-protein coupled receptors and exert biological effects. *HIV enters in to lymphocytes via G-protein coupled receptors (CXCR4, CCR5).* Other chemokines include C5a, IL-8 and platelet activating factor. Chemokines and their actions are shown in Table 2.23.

Growth factors: Growth factors, source and their actions are shown in Table 2.24.

- *Interleukin-4 (IL-4):* It is synthesized by T cells. It promotes growth of B and T cells and enhances expression of HLA class II antigens.
- *Interleukin-7 (IL-7):* It is synthesized by *stromal cells in bone marrow, dendritic cells, hepatocytes, keratinocytes, neurons and epithelial cells except normal lymphocytes.* It is a hematopoietic growth factor for bone marrow stem cells.
- *Interleukin-13 (IL-13):* It is synthesized by *T cells.* It acts as a growth factor for bone marrow stem cells.
- *Granulocyte colony stimulating factor (G-CSF):* It participates in activation and differentiation of neutrophils. It is synthesized by *macrophages, neutrophils and T cells.*
- *Macrophage stimulating factor (GM-CSF):* It is synthesized by fibroblasts and vascular endothelium. It participates in *hematopoiesis.* It promotes the growth and development of macrophages from undifferentiated precursor stem cells. It also *activates natural killer cells and dendritic cells.*

Oxygen Derived Free Radicals (Reactive Oxygen Species)

Oxygen derived free radicals (reactive oxygen species) play key role in microbial killing and tissue injury.

- *Synthesis:* Injurious stimulus activates neutrophils and macrophages, which synthesize oxygen derived free radicals via NADPH oxidase pathway, i.e. superoxide anion (O_2^-), hydrogen peroxide (H_2O_2) and hydroxyl ions (OH). These metabolites combine with nitric oxide to form nitrogen intermediates.
- *Actions:* Oxygen derived free radicals play an important role in *microbial killing in phagolysosome and tissue injury.* These cause damage to vascular endothelium resulting in increase *vascular permeability.* These also increase synthesis of cytokines and adhesive molecules, thus amplify the cascade of inflammatory mediators.
- *Antioxidants:* Serum, tissue fluids and host cells possess antioxidant mechanisms that protect against these potentially harmful oxygen derived radicals. These include: (i) ceruloplasmin-copper binding serum protein, (ii) transferrin-iron free fraction of serum, (iii) superoxide dismutase enzyme, (iv) catalase-H_2O_2 detoxifier, and (v) glutathione peroxidase, another powerful H_2O_2 detoxifier.

Nitric Oxide

Nitric oxide is synthesized by macrophages and endothelium. Free radical gas released during conversion of arginine to citrulline by NO synthase. Actions

Table 2.23: Chemokines and their actions

Chemokines category	Specific chemokine	Actions
C–X–C chemokine (α-chemokine)	α-Chemokine	Activation and chemotaxis of neutrophils
*C–C chemokine (β-chemokine) examples	MCP-1 (monocyte chemotactic protein-1)	Chemotaxis of monocytes
	RANTES (regulated and named T cell expressed and secreted)	Chemotaxis of lymphocytes
	Eotaxin	Chemotaxis of eosinophils or basophils
C-chemokine (γ-chemokine)	Lymphotaxin	Chemotaxis of lymphocytes
CX3C chemokine	Fractalkine	Chemotaxis of monocytes and T cells
		Promote strong adhesion of monocytes and T cells

*C–C chemokine (β-chemokine) molecule does not attract neutrophils.

Table 2.24: Growth factors, source and their actions

Category	Interleukin	Source	Actions
Growth factors activity	IL-3	T cells	Act as a growth factor for tissue mast cells and hematopoietic stem cells
	IL-4	T cells	IL-4 promoting growth of B and T cells; enhances expression of HLA class II antigens.
	IL-7	Stromal cells in bone marrow, dendritic cells, hepatocytes, keratinocytes, neurons and epithelial cells	IL-7 acting as a growth factor for bone marrow stem cells
	G-CSF synthesis by macrophages, neutrophils, T cells, fibroblasts and vascular endothelium	G-CSF	Activation and differentiation of neutrophils
	GM-CSF synthesis by fibroblasts and vascular endothelium	G-CSF	Hematopoiesis
		GM-CSF	Promote the growth and development of macrophages from undifferentiated precursor stem cells.
			Activation of natural killer cells and dendritic cells
	IL-7 synthesis by stromal cells in bone marrow, dendritic cells, hepatocytes, keratinocytes, neurons and epithelial cells except normal lymphocytes	IL-7	Act as a growth factor for bone marrow stem cells
	IL-13 synthesis by T cells	IL-13	Act as a growth factor for bone marrow stem cells

of nitric oxide (NO) are shown in Fig. 2.29. Mechanism of actions of nitric oxide on target cells is shown in Table 2.25.

Physiological state: Nitric oxide (NO), which was previously known as *endothelium derived relaxing factor*. It is a free radical soluble gas synthesized in low concentration. It has half-life in seconds (short lived) *in vivo*. Nitric oxide synthase enzyme converts L-arginine to citrulline resulting in release of nitric oxide in *vascular endothelium (endothelial inducible eNO)*, *macrophages (macrophage-inducible iNO)* and *neurons (nNO)*.

Pathological state: During inflammation, *inflammatory cytokines* (IL-1, TNF-α and interferon-γ) and *bacterial endotoxin* participate in synthesis of nitric oxide. *Calcium influx in vascular endothelium and neurons stimulates synthase enzyme* resulting in synthesis of nitric oxide. TNF-α and interferon-γ stimulate macrophage inducible synthase enzyme to synthesize nitric oxide (iNO).

Mechanism of action: Nitric oxide acts in paracrine manner on target cells through induction of cyclic guanosine monophosphate (GMP), which initiates intracellular events. *Nitric oxide and platelet acting factor (PAF) have opposite action.*

Table 2.25: Mechanism of actions of nitric oxide on target cells

Target organs	Actions
Blood vessels	Vasodilatation by relaxation of smooth muscle cells
	Hypotensive shock in septic patients
Leukocytes	Decrease adhesion of leukocytes to vascular endothelium
Platelets	Inhibit platelets aggregation and degranulation
	Prevent thrombus formation
Brain	Regulation of neurotransmitter by increasing blood flow to brain
Microbes	Killing of microbes (nitric oxide derived reactive oxygen metabolites toxic to microbes)
Tumor cells	Killing of tumor cells by macrophages

Inflammation, Tissue Healing and Repair

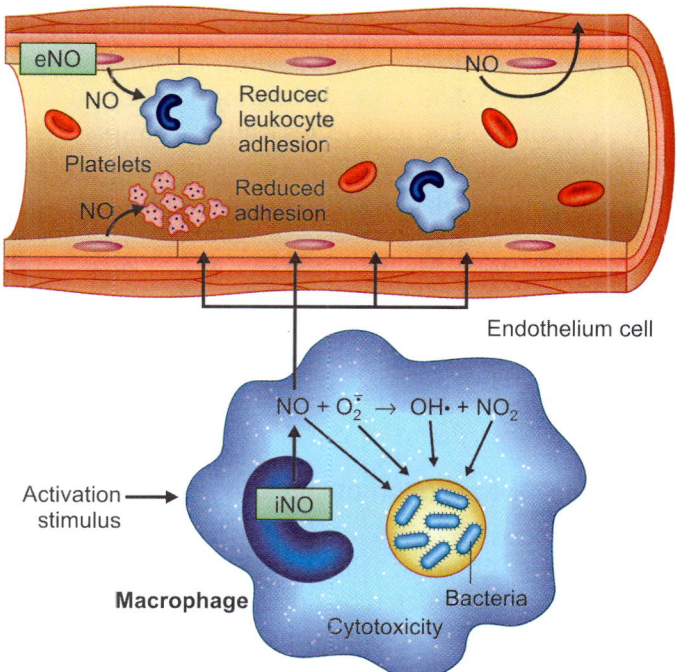

Fig. 2.29: Actions of nitric oxide (NO). It is produced by vascular endothelium and macrophages. It causes vasodilatation. Sustained synthesis of nitric oxide in patient with septicemia develops hypotensive shock. It inhibits platelets aggregation and thus prevents thrombus formation. Nitric oxide derived free radicals cause degradation of microbes.

Platelet Activating Factor

Platelet activating factor is cell membrane phospholipid synthesized by platelets, mast cells/basophils, neutrophils, macrophages, monocytes, endothelial cells, and vascular endothelium. Physiological actions of platelet activating factor and histamine are similar.

Platelet activating factors and their actions are shown in Table 2.26. Differences between nitric oxide and platelet activating factor are shown in Table 2.27.

- *Mechanism of action:* Platelet activating factor acts via G-protein coupled receptor and can elicit most of the cardinal features of inflammation. Platelet activating factor and nitric oxide have opposite action.
- *Target organs:* Platelet activating factor increases *vascular permeability, smooth muscle contraction of bronchioles, pulmonary edema, hypotension, and wheal and flare in the skin*. It kills bacteria and tumor cells.

Neuropeptides (Substance P)

Neuropeptides (substance P) are small proteins synthesized by nerve fibers mainly in *lungs* and *gastrointestinal tract*. It is related to kinin family. Substance P and bradykinin have similar functions. Its synthesis is activated by capsaicin (chiles).

Table 2.26: Platelet activating factors and their actions

Platelet activating factor	Actions
Mast cells/basophils derived PAF	Increases vascular permeability leading to edema
	Vasoconstriction
Endothelial derived PAF	Priming and chemotaxis of leukocytes
Neutrophils derived PAF	Increase leukocyte adhesion to endothelium by integrin mediated mechanism
	Chemotaxis, degranulation and oxidative burst of leukocytes
	Enhances synthesis of eicosanoids by leukocytes
Monocytes/macrophages derived PAF	Adhesion of leukocytes of vascular endothelium
Platelets derived PAF	Platelets aggregation
	Thrombus formation

Platelet activating factor is more potent mediator than histamine.

Table 2.27: Differences between nitric oxide and platelet activating factor

Characteristics	Nitric oxide	Platelet activating factor
Blood vessels	Vasodilatation	Vasoconstriction and increased vascular permeability
Leukocytes	Inhibits leukocyte recruitment	Enhance chemotaxis, degranulation and oxidative burst
Platelets	Inhibits platelet aggregation	Enhances platelet aggregation
Killing of microbes/tumor cells	Absent	Present
Respiratory bronchi/bronchioles	No effect	Bronchospasm

Neuropeptides (substance P) and its actions are shown in Table 2.28.

Actions

Substance P transmits pain signals, regulates blood pressure, modulates vascular permeability; and stimulates secretion of endocrine cells. It also synthesizes other pro-inflammatory molecules, which are thought to link the sensing of dangerous stimuli to development of protective host responses.

Hypoxia Inducible Factor (HIF)

Hypoxia inducible factor-α, a protein released from injured cells mediates cell injury and inflammatory response. It activates many genes involved in inflammation, including VEGF, which increases vascular permeability. Local and systemic effects of chemical mediators are shown in Table 2.29.

DEFECTS IN LEUKOCYTES AND COMPLEMENT

Defects in leukocytes and complement lead to recurrent infections and other fatal disorders.

Defects of Adhesion of Leukocytes

Leukocytic adhesion is impaired in *diabetes mellitus* and patient on *steroid therapy* and *hemodialysis*. Gene mutation of *LAD-1* causes deficiency of β_2 integrins (LFA-1 and MAC-1) expressed on leukocytes leading to impairment of adhesion of leukocytes to venular endothelium.

Patients suffer from *recurrent bacterial infections, delayed wound healing and delayed separation of umbilical cord in newborns*. Gene mutation of LAD-2 causes mild disorder.

Defects in Chemotaxis of Leukocytes

Chemotaxis is impaired in *diabetes mellitus, cancer, sepsis, immunodeficiency disorders* and *thermal injuries*.

Defects in Opsonization of Injurious Agents

Defects in opsonization results in *Bruton's agammaglobulinemia*. Opsonization is a process by which injurious stimulus coated by opsonins, i.e. *IgG, C3b and complement mannose binding lectin (MBL)*.

Opsonization enhances binding of injurious agent to membrane receptors (e.g. FcR1, CR1 and MBL) expressed on activated neutrophils.

Table 2.28: Neuropeptides (substance P) and its actions

Synthesis	Actions
Nerve fibers mainly in lungs and gastrointestinal tract	Transmission of pain signals
	Regulation of blood pressure
	Modulation of vascular permeability
	Stimulation of secretion of endocrine cells
	Synthesis of other pro-inflammatory molecules, which are thought to link the sensing of dangerous stimuli to that development of protective host responses

Table 2.29: Local and systemic effects of chemical mediators

Local and systemic effects	Chemical mediators
Increased vascular permeability and edema	Histamine, anaphylatoxins (C3a, C5a), bradykinin, leukotrienes (LTC_4, LTD_4, and LTE_4), nitric oxide, platelet activating factor and neuropeptide (substance P)
Vasodilatation	Histamine, serotonin, bradykinin, platelet activating factor, nitric oxide
Vasoconstriction	LTC_4, LTD_4, LTE_4, TxA_2
Adhesion of neutrophils to endothelium	C5a, LTB_4, IL-1, TNF-α, chemokines and platelet activating factor
Chemotaxis of leukocytes and their activation	C5a, LTB_4, IL-1, TNF-α, chemokines and bacterial products
Pain	Prostaglandins, bradykinin, and neuropeptides (substance P)
Fever	Prostaglandins, IL-1 acting on hypothalamic thermoregulatory centers
Bronchoconstriction	Histamine and leukotrienes
Tissue damage	Lysosomal enzymes, oxygen derived free radicals, hypochlorous acid, prostaglandins, leukotrienes, and nitric oxide

Defects in Phagolysosme Formation

Chédiak-Higashi syndrome and *albinism* are examples of defects in phagolysosome formation. Phagocytic vesicle fuses with neutrophilic membrane of lysosome to form phagolysosome. In *Chédiak-Higashi syndrome a defect in microtubule function prevents phagolysosome formation.* Impaired membrane fusion of lysosomes with melanosomes in melanocytes causes *albinism*.

Defects in Phagocytosis

Defects in Opsonization

Defects in opsonization causes *Bruton's agammaglobulinemia*.

Defective Phagocytosis

Phagocytosis is impaired in leukemias, diabetes mellitus, malnutrition and neonates.

Defective Phagolysosome Formation

In *Chédiak-Higashi syndrome, a defect in microtubule function prevents phagolysosome formation.* Impaired membrane fusion of lysosomes with melanosomes in melanocytes causes *albinism*.

Defective Degranulation of Neutrophils

Chédiak-Higashi syndrome is an example of defective degranulation of neutrophils.

LYST gene located on chromosome 1q42 encodes a protein essential for assembly of microtubules in the cytoplasm. Mutation of LYST gene occurs in Chédiak-Higashi syndrome. It is characterized by *defective degranulation of neutrophils, impaired microbial killing, and recurrent bacterial infections (Staphylococcus aureus)* forming soft tissue abscess. *Neutrophils contain giant granules due to aberrant organelles.*

Defects in Complement System

Disorders of complement system cascade are shown in Table 2.30. Patients develop increased susceptibility to infections due to defects in complement proteins, pathological activation and deficiency of regulatory proteins.

ANTI-INFLAMMATORY THERAPEUTIC AGENTS

The acute inflammatory response can be treated with anti-inflammatory drugs, which can prevent production of key mediators of inflammation. Phospholipase A_2 activity is inhibited by corticosteroids, limiting the production of arachidonic acid and, therefore, the formation of arachidonic acid metabolites.

Anti-inflammatory therapeutic agents can be directed at many targets along the eicosanoid biosynthetic cyclooxygenase and lipooxygenase pathways. Anti-inflammatory agents inhibiting lipooxygenase pathway are shown in Table 2.31.

Cyclooxygenase Pathway

Various anti-inflammatory therapeutic agents are used to inhibit the action of COX-1 and COX-2 (cyclooxygenase pathway). COX-2 inhibitor drugs produce less toxicity than COX-1.

- *Non-selective therapeutic agent:* NSAID such as aspirin inhibits the action of both COX-1 and COX-2, preventing synthesis of prostaglandins.

Table 2.30: Disorders of complement system cascade

Disorder	Complement system cascade defects
Recurrent pyogenic infections and membranous glomerulonephritis	C2, C3b, and C5 deficiency
Neisseria and pneumococcal infections	C5b–C9 defective formation of membrane attack complex (MAC)
Hereditary angioneurotic edema (laryngeal edema)	Hereditary deficiency of C1 inhibitor (C1 INH)
Systemic lupus erythematosus	C1q, C1r and C1s, C2, C4 deficiency leading to improper clearance of immune complex
Hemolytic-uremic syndrome and membranoproliferative glomerulonephritis	Factor H and factor 1
Paroxysmal nocturnal hemoglobinuria	CD55 (DAF deficiency) and CD59 (MIRL) deficiency
	PIG-A gene mutation encoding phosphatidylinositol linked membrane proteins leading to uncontrolled activation of complement resulting in recurrent bouts of intravascular complement mediated hemolysis
	Flow cytometry demonstrates diminished CD55 and CD59 expression on red blood cells, leukocytes and platelets

Table 2.31: Anti-inflammatory agents inhibiting lipooxygenase pathway

Therapeutic agents	Actions
Montelukast	Inhibits leukotrienes synthesis or block leukotrienes receeptors (e.g. cyst LT1 and cyst LT2)
Zileutin	Inhibits 5-lipooxygenase and thus decreasing synthesis of LTC_4, LTD_4 and LTE_4
Glucocorticoids	Downregulate expression of gene encoding COX-2 without toxic effects
Omega-3 fatty acid consumption	Serves as poor substrates for synthesizing prostaglandins

Prolonged administration of non-steroidal anti-inflammatory drugs may increase risk of arterial thrombosis in people possibly due to reduced prostacyclin in endothelial cells.

- *Selective anti-inflammatory therapeutic agents:* Meloxicam and *carprofen* inhibit the action of COX-2 without toxic effects. Prolonged administration may *increase risk of arterial thrombosis* in people possibly due to reduced prostacyclin in endothelial cells, while sparing of COX-1 mediated production of TxA_2 in platelets.

Lipooxygenase Pathway

5-Lipooxygenase pathway is *not affected by non-steroidal anti-inflammatory drugs (NSAIDs).* Pharmacological agent such as *montelukast* is used to inhibit leukotrienes synthesis or *block leukotrienes receptors* (e.g. cyst LT1 and cyst LT2). It is useful in the treatment of *bronchial asthma.*

Zileutin inhibits 5-lipooxygenase and thus decreasing synthesis of LTC_4, LTD_4 and LTE_4.

Fish oil is a source of omega-3 fatty acid. Consumption of fish oil (omega-3 fatty acid) may modify inflammatory response. Omega-3 fatty acid serves as poor substrates for synthesizing prostaglandins (cyclooxygenase pathway) and leukotrienes (lipooxygenase pathway). In contrast, omega 3 fatty acid serves as excellent substrate for the synthesis of anti-inflammatory products (e.g. *resolvins* and *protectins*).

Glucocorticoids are *broad spectrum powerful anti-inflammatory agents,* which downregulate expression of genes encoding phospholipase, COX-2, pro-inflammatory cytokines (IL-1 and TNF-α) and nitric oxide synthase. *Glucocorticoids also upregulate genes that encode potent anti-inflammatory protein such as lipocortin-1.*

SYSTEMIC EFFECTS OF INFLAMMATION

In some cases, local tissue injury can result in prominent systemic inflammatory manifestations as a result of release of chemical mediators into the circulation.

SYNTHESIS OF ACUTE PHASE PROTEINS BY LIVER

Within hours on onset of inflammation, leukocytes release cytokines (IL-1, IL-6, and TNF-α), which stimulate liver to synthesize acute phase proteins such as *C-reactive proteins, serum amyloid A, haptoglobin and fibrinogen.* These reach to the site of inflammation to kill the pathogens by opsonization (CRP and SAA), clearing necrotic cells and activating complement pathways.

Serum Levels of Acute Phase Proteins

C-Reactive Proteins (CRP) Level

C-reactive protein (IL-6) is a sensitive marker of cell necrosis associated with acute inflammation and disease activity. Its concentration is increased in *disrupted atheromatous plaques in coronary artery disease,* which may predispose to thrombosis and myocardial infarction. On this basis; anti-inflammatory agents are being tested in patients to reduce the risk of myocardial infarction. It is *excellent monitor* of the disease activity in patient suffering from *rheumatoid arthritis.*

Serum Amyloid Associated (SAA) Level

SAA (IL-1 and TNF-α) also replaces apolipoprotein A (component of HDLs). HDLs are used by macrophages as a source of energy producing lipids. Prolonged synthesis of SAA results in *secondary amyloidosis.*

Serum Fibrinogen Level

Erythrocyte sedimentation rate (ESR) is increased in inflammation. Increased synthesis of fibrinogen promotes RBCs rouleaux formation, which is the basis of increased ESR in inflammation.

Clinical Correlation

Fever

Patient has above normal temperature (>1 to 4°C) due to bacterial products and cytokines, which act as pyrogen. Fever plays an important role in providing a *hostile environment for bacterial and viral reproduction. More oxygen is available for the oxygen dependent MPO system.* Mechanism of fever and therapeutic agent is described as follows:

- *Exogenous pyrogens released by bacteria or injured cells* stimulate macrophages to synthesize IL-1 and TNF-α (endogenous pyrogens). IL-1 stimulates prostaglandin (PGE_2) synthesis in the *hypothalamic thermoregulatory centers,* thereby resets the body temperature set point at higher level (fever).

Inflammation, Tissue Healing and Repair

- Profound chills with *shivering, sweating* and *piloerection* are associated with *fever*. Inhibitors of cyclooxygenase (e.g. aspirin) block the fever response by inhibiting PGE_2 synthesis in the hypothalamus.
- *Non-steroidal anti-inflammatory drugs* (NSAIDs) including aspirin *reduce fever by inhibiting cyclooxygenase* and thus *blocking prostaglandins synthesis*.

Lethargy

Lethargy, a common feature of the acute phase response, results from the effects of IL-1 and TNF-α on the *central nervous system*.

Other Manifestations

Patient presents with *increased pulse rate, hypotension, rigors (shivering), chills (search for warmth), anorexia, somnolence, and malaise* (probably because of the actions of cytokines on brain cells). Patient has decreased sweating due to redirection of blood flow from cutaneous to deep vascular beds leads to minimize heat loss.

HEMATOLOGICAL FINDINGS

Leukocytosis

Leukocytosis is defined as an absolute increase in the circulating WBC count. In acute inflammation (bacterial infection), cytokine (IL-1, TNF-α) released by leukocytes stimulates bone marrow leading to leukocytosis (TLC 15,000–20,000/cumm). In prolonged infection, colony stimulating factors (CSFs) induce proliferation of precursors in the bone marrow. There is shift to the left, which is defined as greater than 10% band form neutrophils or the presence of metamyelocytes. Neutrophils contain *toxic granules* (e.g. prominence of azurophil granules in lysosomes).

Leukemoid Reaction

In some cases, bone marrow produces more immature leukocytes in increased number to the circulation (i.e. shift to the left) showing leukocytosis as high as 40,000–100,000/cumm (leukemoid reactions). It is sometimes difficult to differentiate from leukemia.

Leukopenia

Leukopenia is defined as an absolute decrease in the circulating WBC count. It is occasionally encountered under conditions of chronic inflammation, especially in patients who are malnourished or who suffer from a chronic debilitating disease.

Monocytosis

In chronic inflammation, peripheral blood shows absolute monocytosis (e.g. *tuberculosis, rheumatoid arthritis*). There is increase in serum IgG.

Leukopenia Conditions

Leukopenia conditions are seen in typhoid fever, viruses, rickettsiae, certain protozoa, disseminated cancer and rampant tuberculosis.

Lymphopenia

Lymphopenia occurs due to sequestration of B- and T-lymphocytes in lymph nodes. *It indicates apoptosis of lymphocytes.*

Lymphocytosis

Lymphocytosis is defined as an increase in the absolute peripheral blood lymphocyte count above the normal range (<4,000/μl in children and 9,000/μl in infants). Lymphocytosis is seen in acute viral infections (*infectious mononucleosis, mumps and German measles*), *whooping cough, tuberculosis, brucellosis* and *lymphoproliferative diseases*.

Eosinophilia

Eosinophilia is demonstrated in bronchial asthma, hay fever and parasitic infections.

Erythrocyte Sedimentation Rate (ESR)

Increased plasma levels of acute phase reactants accelerate erythrocyte sedimentation rate. ESR index estimated by *Wintrobe's tube or Westergren's pipette* expressed as mm/hour is important to monitor the activity of many inflammatory diseases such as tuberculosis and rheumatoid arthritis.

SEPTIC SHOCK

Septicemia denotes the clinical condition in which bacteria are found in the circulation. Final diagnosis is made by culturing the organisms from the blood. In these patients, lipopolysaccharide (LPS) released by gram-negative bacteria activates monocytes/macrophages to synthesize large quantity of cytokines (IL-1 and TNF-α). These cytokines cause direct systemic cytotoxic damage to capillary endothelial cells resulting in *generalized vasodilatation, platelet aggregation and widespread organ dysfunction, particularly in the lungs, kidneys, liver, and heart.*

SYTEMIC INFLAMMATORY RESPONSE

Systemic inflammatory response is a clinical triad characterized by (i) disseminated intravascular coagulation, and (ii) cardiovascular failure and hypoglycemia.

Disseminated Intravascular Coagulation (DIC)

Patient develops disseminated intravascular coagulation by the action of bacterial products (lipopolysaccharide) and TNF-α. These bacterial products and

TNF-α stimulate endothelial cells to express tissue factor and promote platelets aggregation.

These also inhibit anticoagulant mechanism by (i) *decreasing synthesis of thrombomodulin by endothelial cells*, and (ii) *decreasing the expression of tissue factor pathway inhibitor* (TFPI). This condition is always fatal.

Cardiovascular Failure

Cytokines (IL-1 and TNF-α) activate cardiac myocytes and vascular smooth muscle cells to synthesize NO, which causes heart failure and hemodynamic shock due to loss of perfusion pressure.

Patient may develop *acute respiratory distress syndrome (ARDS)* is neutrophil-mediated endothelial injury characterized by escape of fluid from blood in the lung air spaces.

METABOLIC CHANGES

Inflammation produces various metabolic effects described as under.

Negative Nitrogen Balance

Negative nitrogen balance occurs due to protein catabolism. Metabolic products increase the osmotic pressure in interstitial space which attracts water and thus contribute to edema (swelling tumor).

Skeletal Muscle Catabolism

Skeletal muscle catabolism provides amino acids that can be used in the immune response and for tissue repair.

Glucose Metabolism

Cytokines (IL-1 and TNF-α) cause liver injury and impair liver function, resulting in a failure to maintain normal blood glucose levels due to lack glycolysis from stored glycogen. Anaerobe utilization of glucose is increased because of hypoxia with increased formation of lactic and pyruvic acids.

Lipid Metabolism

Lipid metabolism leads to increased formation of ketone bodies and fatty acids.

Mineral Metabolism

There is increased extracellular K^+ concentration.

Acid–base Balance

Metabolic acidosis occurs as a result of formation of ketone bodies and lactic acid.

RELEASE OF VARIOUS HORMONES

TNF-α and IL-1 synthesized by macrophages play key role in release of norepinephrine, vasopressin and activation of the renin-angiotensin-aldosterone system.

CHRONIC INFLAMMATION

Chronic inflammation is an immune reaction to persistent and recurrent injury greater than 48 hours to weeks or months or years. It occurs when host response fails to degrade the injurious agent (e.g. pathogen, tissue debris and foreign bodies) that incites gradual onset inflammatory reaction. It usually occurs as *de novo*, without a preceding acute inflammation.

Histologic Features

Injured tissue shows infiltration by macrophages, lymphocytes (T cells and B cells) and plasma cells. Tissue destruction is induced by persistent agent or inflammatory cells. Healing occurs by replacement of damaged tissue with formation of granulation tissue (proliferation of fibroblasts and capillaries) and fibrosis.

Etiopathogenesis

Chronic inflammation occurs due to persistent infectious agents, prolonged exposure to potentially toxic agents and autoimmune disorders. It occurs by following mechanisms:

- *Progression of acute inflammation:* In acute inflammation, if the injurious agent persists for longer period, it will progress to chronic inflammation accompanied by tissue destruction. *Pneumonic focus results in extensive destruction and formation of a cavity in extensive fibrosis. Peptic ulcer is manifested by acute and chronic inflammatory phases.*

- *Persistent infections:* Chronic inflammation due to microorganisms with low virulence resisting elimination results in delayed hypersensitivity reaction. These organisms include *Mycobacterium tubercle bacilli, Mycobacterium leprae bacilli, Treponema pallidum*, cat-scratch disease, fungi, brucellosis, and viruses. All these conditions except brucellosis and viral infections cause granulomatous inflammation. Later two organisms resist phagocytosis and intracellular killing, but granulomas are absent.

- *Prolonged exposure to potentially toxic agents:* Prolonged exposure to exogenous and endogenous substances may cause chronic inflammation.

- *Autoimmunity:* Autoimmunity is altered long-standing immune response to self antigens. It initiates chronic inflammation affecting various organs.

Major Histological Patterns

Chronic inflammation occurs in two patterns: chronic nonspecific inflammation and granulomatous inflammation.

NONSPECIFIC CHRONIC INFLAMMATION

Tissue injury and healing proceed simultaneously in chronic inflammation. Neutrophils have disappeared from the site. There is influx of macrophages, lymphocytes, plasma cells, associated with granulation tissue formation (proliferation of fibroblasts and capillaries) resulting in tissue scarring and architecture distortion.

Chronic nonspecific inflammation is mediated by the interaction of monocytes/macrophages with lymphocytes. Cytokines synthesized by macrophages and lymphocytes activate each other. Macrophages display antigens to T cells resulting in synthesis of antibody-producing plasma cells.

Components of nonspecific chronic inflammation: These include inflammatory cells (macrophages, lymphocytes and their cytokines), tissue destruction, formation of granulation tissue and tissue fibrosis. Other inflammatory cells such as eosinophils, mast cells, platelets and neutrophils also participate in chronic inflammation.

ROLE OF INFLAMMATORY CELLS

Macrophages

Macrophages are the dominant player of chronic inflammation. Monocytes begin to emigrate into extravascular tissues quite early in acute inflammation. In chronic inflammation, macrophage accumulation persists as a result of continuous recruitment from the circulation and local proliferation at the site of inflammation. Macrophages regulate lymphocyte responses to antigens and secrete a variety of mediators that modulate the proliferation and function of fibroblasts and endothelial cells.

Origin and Distribution

Mononuclear phagocytes are derived from a common precursor in the bone marrow, which give rise to monocytes. Blood monocytes migrate and differentiate into tissue macrophages known as *reticuloendothelial cells* diffusely distributed in the connective tissues in various organs (Fig. 2.30 and Table 2.32).

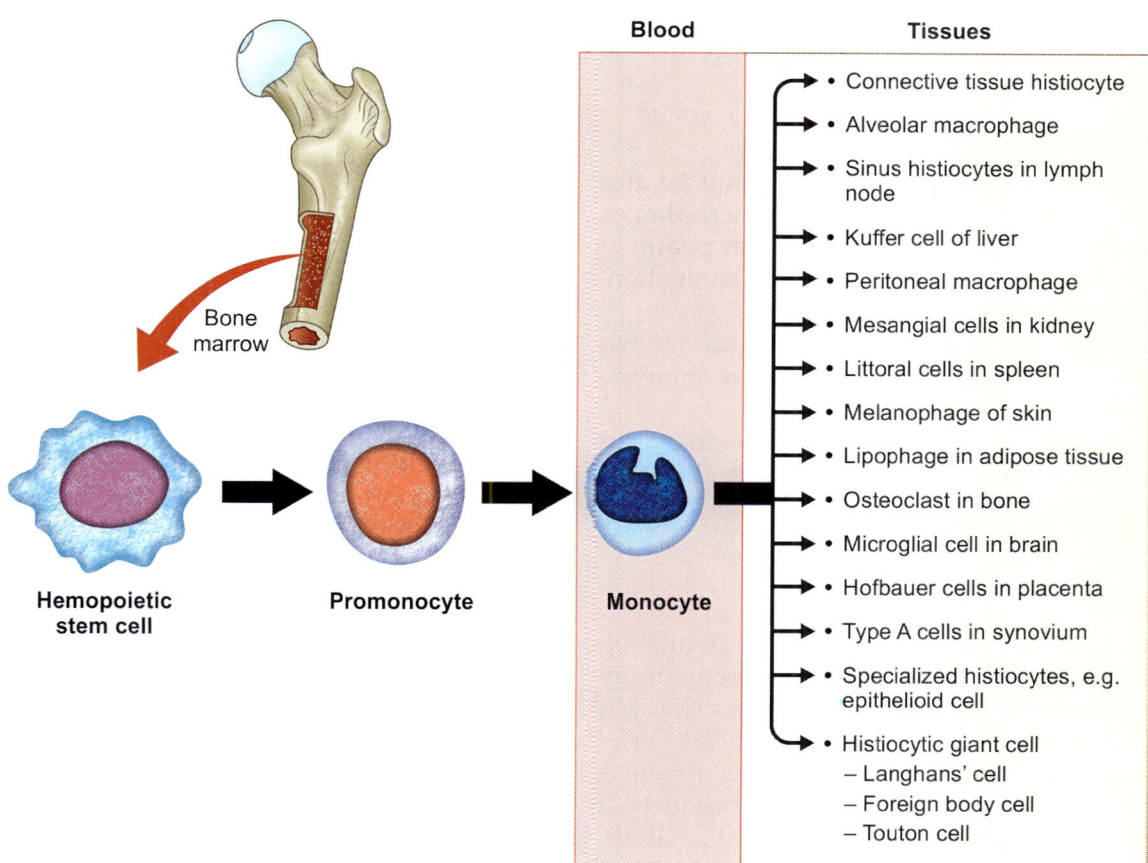

Fig. 2.30: Reticuloendothelial cells distribution in various tissues.

Table 2.32: Reticuloendothelial cells distribution in various tissues

Tissue	Reticuloendothelial cells
Blood	Monocytes
Connective tissue	Macrophages
Lung	Alveolar macrophages
Peritoneum	Peritoneal macrophages
Kidney	Mesangial cells
Liver	Kupffer's cells
Lymph nodes	Sinus histiocytes
Spleen	Littoral cells
Placenta	Hofbauer cells
Skin	Melanophages
Brain	Microglial cells
Synovium	Type I (type A cells)
Bone	Osteoclasts
Adipose tissue	Lipophage
Specialized histiocytes	Epithelioid cells, histiocytic giant cells, Langhan's giant cells, foreign body giant cells, Touton giant cells

Lifespan

Half-life of blood monocytes is *one day*, while lifespan of *tissue macrophage* is *several months* or years. If the injurious agent is eliminated, macrophages eventually disappear either dying off or making their way into the lymphatic channels and lymph nodes.

Activation of Macrophages

Activation of macrophages occurs by immune and non-immune mechanisms. Activated macrophages synthesize TNF-α, IL-1, chemokines that promote leukocyte recruitment and participate in inflammation, tissue injury and repair.

- *Immune mechanism:* T cells synthesize interferon-γ (IFN-γ), which activate macrophages by immune mechanism.
- *Non-immune mechanism:* Bacterial endotoxins, dead cells, fibronectin-matrix proteins and chemical mediators activate macrophages by non-immune mechanism.

Recruitment

Chemotaxis plays key role in migration of circulating monocytes similar to PMNs cells to injured site by chemokines, where these are called *tissue macrophages*. Chemokines are derived from *mononuclear cells* (macrophages, T cells), *bacterial products, products derived from injured tissue* (e.g. breakdown products of collagen, fibronectin), growth factors (PDGF, TGF-α), *fibrinopeptides,* and complement cascade product (C5a) (Table 2.33).

Table 2.33: Sources of chemokines and their role in chemotaxis of macrophages

Source of chemokines	Examples of chemokines
Blood cells	Macrophage chemotactic protein I (MCP-1)
Bacteria	Bacterial products
Injured tissue	Breakdown products of collagen fibers and fibronectin
Growth factors	PDGF, TGF-α
Fibrinopeptides	Fibrin degradation products
Complement	C5a

Proliferation of Tissue Macrophages

Growth factors derived from T cells and tissue play an important role in proliferation of macrophages leading to increased number of macrophages at persistent injury site.

- Macrophages engulf particulate, process and present to T cells.
- Activated T cells synthesize IFN-γ, which activates macrophages and transform into epithelioid cells and multinucleated giant cells.

Macrophage Immobilization

Certain cytokines and oxidized lipids can cause such immobilization.

Macrophage Products

Macrophages possess receptors for *IgG* and *C3b*, which process antigen, enhance immune response, and participate in phagocytosis of injurious agent. *Activated macrophages synthesize many products, which participate in elimination of injurious agent and initiation of tissue repair by fibrosis and tissue destruction in chronic inflammation.* This ongoing tissue destruction can activate the inflammatory cascade by diverse mechanisms, so that features of both acute and chronic inflammation may coexist in certain circumstances (Table 2.34). Lifespan of blood cells in tissues is shown in Table 2.35.

- *Cytokines:* Macrophages synthesize IL-1, TNF-α, IL-6, IL-8 and MCP-1. These *attract inflammatory cells* at the site of tissue injury.
- *Reactive oxygen and nitrogen species:* These are toxic to microbes as well as host cells.
- *Neutral proteases:* These may cause degradation of extracellular matrix.
- *Metalloproteinases (MMPs):* Metalloproteinases are synthesized by *polymorphonuclear cells, macrophages, fibroblasts, synovial cells* and *some epithelial cells.* These cause breakdown of type III collagen fibers. Deposition of type I collagen fibers increases tensile strength by 80%.

Table 2.34: Macrophage products and their actions

Category	Inflammatory mediators	Actions
Cytokines	IL-1, TNF-α	Chemotaxis of inflammatory cells
	IL-6	Synthesis of acute phase reactant by liver
	IL-2	Autocrine action
Chemokines	IL-8	Chemotaxis of inflammatory cells and paracrine action
	MCP-1	
Lysosomal enzymes	Neutral hydrolases	Toxic to extracellular matrix
	Acid hydrolase	Hydrolyzing the muramic acid N-acetylglucosamine bond of bacterial glycopeptides leading to killing of microbes
	Serine protease	
	Metalloproteinases* (MMPs)	Degradation of type III collagen fibers
		Deposition of type I collagen fibers leading to increased tensile strength
Cell derived arachidonic metabolites	Prostaglandins	Platelet aggregation
		Vasodilatation
		Increase vascular permeability with formation of inflammatory exudate
		Modulation of phagocytic activity of leukocytes
		Pain
		Fever
	Leukotrienes	Vasoconstriction
		Increase vascular permeability
		Bronchospasm
Plasminogen activator	–	Cleave plasminogen to form plasmin, that degrades fibrin strands resulting in dissolution of blood clot
Procoagulant activator	–	Activation of coagulation system
Reactive oxygen and nitrogen species	Superoxide, highly reactive hydroxyl molecule and hypochlorous acid (bleach)	Toxic to microbes and host cells
Growth factors, fibrogenic and angiogenic factors	PDGF, FGF, and TGF-β	Fibroblast proliferation
		Collagen deposition
		Angiogenesis

*Metalloproteinases (MMPs) also known as *collagenases synthesized by* macrophages, neutrophils, fibroblasts, synovial cells and some epithelial cells.

Table 2.35: Lifespan of blood cells in tissues

Blood cells	Lifespan
Neutrophils	6 hours in peripheral blood
	4 days in tissues during acute inflammation
Lymphocytes	2 weeks to 2 years
Monocytes	1–3 days in peripheral blood
	Months to years in tissues (tissue macrophages)
Platelets	7–10 days

- *Growth factors (PDGF, FGF, and TGF-β):* These growth factors participate in *proliferation of fibroblasts, deposition of collagen fibers* and *angiogenesis*.
- *Macrophage membrane products:* Arachidonic acid metabolites such as prostaglandins and leukotrienes participate in inflammatory process (Fig. 2.31).

Lymphocytes

Multiple subtypes of lymphocytes are shown in Table 2.36.

- *T cells* participate in cell mediated immunity. Activated macrophages display antigens to T cells. Macrophages synthesize IL-12 that stimulates T cell responses. Activated T cells recruit monocytes from the circulation with IFN-γ, a powerful activator of macrophages.
- *B cells,* when stimulated with antigen, become plasma cells and secrete immunoglobulins (e.g. IgG, IgA, IgM, IgD and IgE). Plasma cells participate in humoral immunity.
- *Natural killer cells:* These kill tumor cells and virus infected cells by lysing or damaging plasma membranes.

Macrophages and Lymphocytes Interaction

Poorly digested antigen is presented by macrophages to CD4+ T cells. Interaction between macrophages and T cells triggers the release of cytokines (especially interferon-γ by CD4+ T cells), mediate the transformation of monocytes/macrophages to epithelioid cells and giant cells (Fig. 2.32).

Eosinophils

Eosinophils are abundant in immune reactions mediated by IgE and in parasitic infections, recruited by chemokine (*eotaxin*). Eosinophilic granules contain major basic protein, a highly cationic protein that is toxic

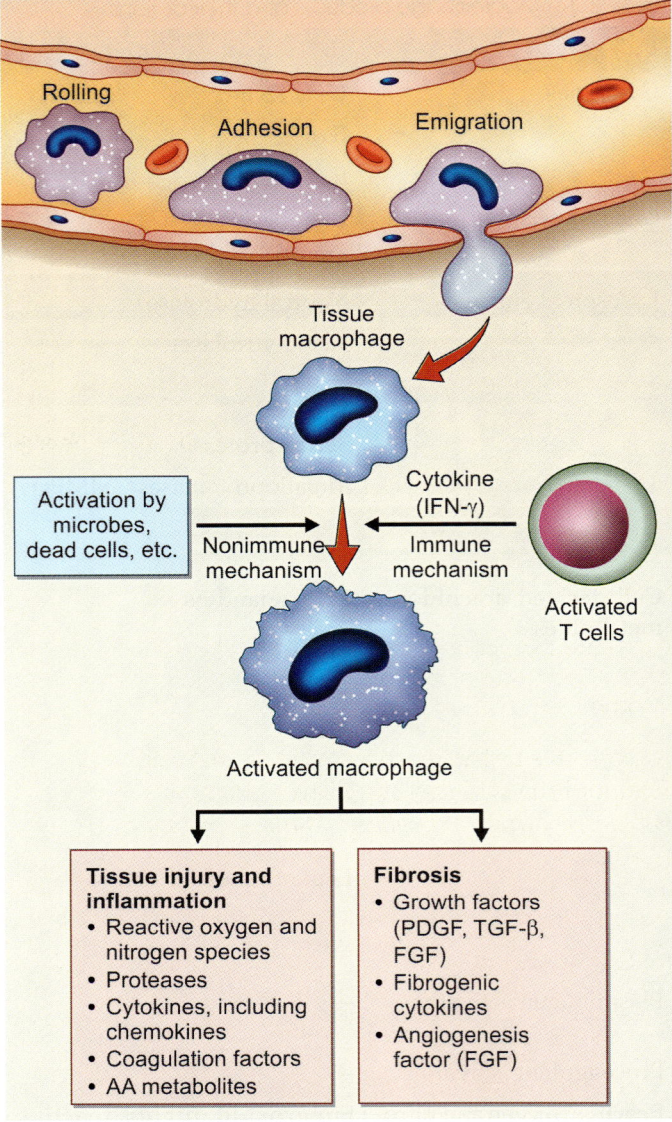

Fig. 2.31: Role of activated macrophages in chronic inflammation. Macrophages are activated by immunological or nonimmunological mechanisms. Various products synthesized by activated macrophages participate in tissue injury and fibrosis.

Table 2.36: Multiple subtypes of lymphocytes

Lymphocytes	Subtype	Actions
B cell	Plasma cell	Synthesis of antibodies either against persistent antigen to injury site or against altered tissue components in chronic inflammation
T cell	Effector T cells	Delayed hypersensitivity
		Showing mixed lymphocytic reactivity
		Cytotoxic killer cells (K cells)
	Regulatory T cells	Helper T cells
		Suppressor T cells
Natural killer cells (NK cells)	Cytotoxic cells	Kill tumor cells
		Virus infected cells by lysing or damaging plasma membranes

Inflammation, Tissue Healing and Repair

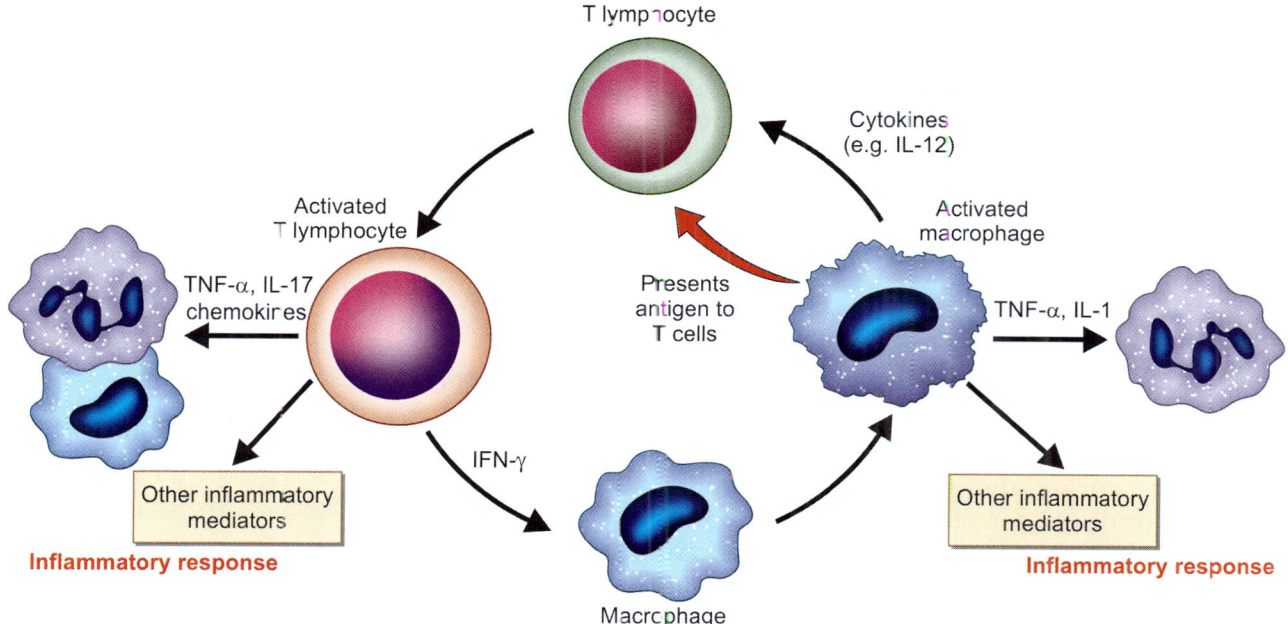

Fig. 2.32: Macrophage–lymphocyte interactions in chronic inflammation. Activated T cells synthesize cytokines (TNF, IL-17 and chemokines) cause chemotaxis of neutrophils and macrophages. Macrophages synthesize (TNF, IL-1 and chemokines) also recruit inflammatory cells.

to parasites but also causes lysis of host epithelial cells. Eosinophilia is highly suggestive of response to *invasive helminthes, arthropods, allergic rhinitis and bronchial asthma* (Table 2.37).

- Eosinophilic specific granules contain preformed chemical mediator, i.e. major basic protein (MBP), which *kills only invasive helminthes by type II hypersensitivity reaction.* It has *no effect on pinworms*

Table 2.37: Primary inflammatory mediators of eosinophils

Inflammatory mediators	Specific mediators	Actions
Reactive oxygen metabolites	Superoxide, highly reactive hydroxyl molecule and hypochlorous acid	These participate in inflammatory reactions
Lysosomal granules enzymes (also known primary crystalloid granules)	Major basic proteins (highly cationic protein)	Modulation of hypersensitivity reactions
		Killing only invasive helminthes by type II hypersensitivity reaction
		No effect on noninvasive parasites such as pinworms and *Ascaris lumbricoides*
		Lysis of host epithelial cells
	Histaminase	Modulation of hypersensitivity reactions
		Neutralization of histamine
	Aryl sulphatase B	Neutralization of leukotrienes
	Eosinophil cationic protein	Damaging schistosomula of *Schistosoma mansoni*
	Eosinophil peroxidase	Functions unknown
	Acid hydrolase	Functions unknown
	β-glucuronidase	Functions unknown
Phospholipase D	–	Specific functions unknown
Prostaglandins of E series	–	Specific functions unknown
Cytokines	–	Specific functions unknown

and round worms (*Ascaris lumbricoides*), which are not invasive.
- Eosinophils *modulate hypersensitivity reactions* with the help of histaminase and arylsulfatase. *Histaminase neutralizes histamine, whereas arylsulfatase neutralizes leukotrienes*. Eosinophilic red granules contain crystalline material in cytoplasm, which become Charcoat-Leydon crystals in the sputum of asthmatics patients.

Mast Cells

Mast cells express on their surface the *receptor* (FcERI) *that binds the Fc portion of IgE antibody*. Mast cell granules release *histamine, leukotrienes, prostaglandins, and platelet activating factor* during allergic reactions to foods, insect venom, or drugs, sometimes with catastrophic results (e.g. *anaphylactic shock*). Mast cells may produce cytokines (TNF-α and IL-4), that contribute fibrosis in chronic inflammation (Fig. 2.33).

Platelets

Platelets regulate *vascular permeability* and *proliferation of mesenchymal cells* in chronic inflammation. These also participate in *thrombosis* and *clot formation*. Platelets contain primary inflammatory mediators in dense granules and α-granules. Dense granules contain serotonin, calcium and ADP. Platelets' α-granules contain cationic proteins, fibrinogen and coagulation proteins, platelet derived growth factors, acid hydrolases and thromboxane A_2.

Neutrophils

Neutrophilic exudate can persist for many months in osteomyelitis because of persistent infection and mediators produced by activated macrophages and T cells.

TISSUE DESTRUCTION

Tissue destruction leads to loss of organ function, and healing occurs by fibrosis. Inappropriate activation of macrophages causes tissue destruction in chronic inflammation.

- *Multinucleated giant cells formation:* Some of the macrophages may become multinucleate giant cells. Fibroblasts migrate into the area and lay down collagen.
- *Synthesis of chemical mediators:* Necrotic tissue also stimulates leukocytes to release *cell derived chemical mediators*. It also activates *plasma derived chemical mediators (kinin system, coagulation system, complement system and fibrinolytic system)*. Necrosed cells liberate uric acid at persisting injurious agent.

  In cellular immune reactions, *T cells may directly kill cells. This ongoing tissue destruction can activate the inflammatory cascade by diverse mechanisms, so that features of both acute and chronic inflammation may coexist in certain circumstances.*

FORMATION OF GRANULATION TISSUE

Granulation tissue is *highly vascular tissue composed of newly formed blood vessels and activated fibroblasts*. Fibronectin is required for granulation tissue formation. It is a cell adhesion glycoprotein which binds collagen, fibrin, and cell surface receptors (e.g. integrins).

- *Angiogenesis:* It is a process of new blood vessels development from existing blood vessels. It is essential in *tissue development, reproduction, and wound healing*. It occurs by mobilization of endothelial precursor cells (EPSc) from bone marrow and *pre-existing vessels* at the site of injury chemotactic factors (VEGF, FGF) recruit endothelial cells from pre-existing blood vessels to form new blood vessels (angiogenesis).
- *Synthesis of collagen fibers:* Collagen fibers are the most abundant protein in the body. They form the major structural component of many organs. These provide tensile strength of healing wounds. *Chemotactic factors recruit fibroblasts*. PDGF, EGF, TGF-α, FGF-β,

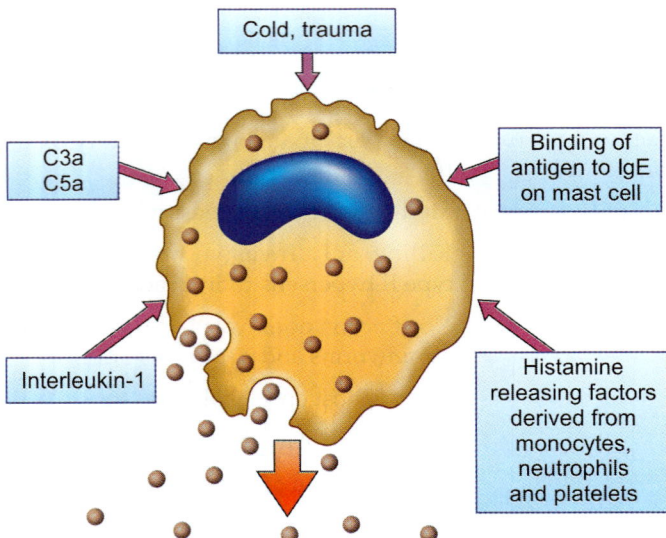

Fig. 2.33: Mast cells degranulation and their actions.

IGF-1, IL-1 and TGF-β participate in proliferation of fibroblasts resulting in synthesis of collagen fibers in early wound healing (3 to 5 days).

TISSUE FIBROSIS

Growth factors (PDGF, FGF, and TGF-β) synthesized by macrophages participate in migration of fibroblasts, their proliferation, and synthesis of collagen into the area.

- Angiogenic factors (VEGF, FGF) also participate in new vessels formation (angiogenesis).
- Fibrogenic cytokines synthesized by macrophages serve to eliminate injurious agents, process of repair in chronic inflammation.

GRANULOMATOUS INFLAMMATION

Granulomatous inflammation is a distinctive form of chronic inflammation. It is characterized by the presence of granulomas admixed with mononuclear infiltration (macrophages, lymphocytes and plasma cells). Differences between granuloma and granulation tissue are shown in Table 2.38 and some examples of chronic granulomatous inflammation are shown in Table 2.39.

Table 2.38: Differences between granuloma and granulation tissue

Characteristics	Granuloma	Granulation tissue
Features	Well circumscribed collection of modified macrophages (epithelioid cells) surrounded by lymphocytes and fibroblasts	Hallmark of healing process composed of proliferation of fibroblasts and new blood vessels formation embedded in loose edematous matrix along with inflammatory cells such as neutrophils, lymphocytes and plasma cells
Examples	Tuberculosis, tuberculoid leprosy, sarcoidosis, rheumatoid arthritis	Normal physiological response after an injury
Vascularization	Granuloma not vascularized	Highly vascularized due to angiogenesis
Proliferation of fibroblasts	Proliferation of fibroblasts is minimal	Proliferation of fibroblasts marked
Consequence	Damage to host tissues	Physiological process

Table 2.39: Some examples of chronic granulomatous inflammation

Disorder	Characteristics
Persistence of infectious agents due to failure of phagocytosis	
Tuberculosis	Mycobacterium tubercle bacilli induced caseous necrosis, epithelioid granulomas and Langhans' giant cells. AFB may be demonstrated by ZN staining
Leprosy	*Mycobacterium leprae* bacilli induced noncaseating granulomas
Syphilis	*Treponema pallidum* induced with gumma (microscopic to grossly visible lesion), with central necrotic cells, surrounded by macrophages and plasma cell infiltrate
Cat-scratch disease	Gram-negative bacteria forms rounded or stellate granuloma containing central granular debris
Prolonged exposure to exogenous and endogenous substances	
Endogenous materials	Necrotic adipose tissue and bone
	Uric acid crystals (gouty tophus)
Exogenous materials	Suture materials, implanted prosthesis, asbestos fibers, silicosis, berylliosis
Autoimmune diseases	
Organ specific diseases	Hashimoto's thyroiditis
	Pernicious anemia
	Rheumatoid arthritis
Contact hypersensitivity reactions	Self-antigens altered by exposure to nickel
Diseases of unknown etiology	Ulcerative colitis
	Crohn's disease
	Sarcoidosis

COMPOSITION OF GRANULOMA

Granuloma consists of three components: (i) *Epithelioid cells (activated macrophages) contain eosinophilic cytoplasm and oval or elongate nuclei, which may show folding of nuclear membrane,* (ii) *collar of lymphocytes plasma cells and reactive fibroblasts*, and (iii) *multinucleated giant cells formed by fusion of epithelioid cells.*

Epithelioid cells show increased endoplasmic reticulum and a few phagolysosomes on electron microscopy. Demonstration of granulomas in biopsy specimen has diagnostic significance associated with the lesions.

ETIOPATHOGENESIS OF GRANULOMA

Granulomas are formed in various pathological conditions due to bacteria, fungi, parasites, inorganic compounds (silicosis, berylliosis), foreign bodies (sutures, implants, accidents) and sarcoidosis (unknown etiology). Brucellosis and viral infections resist phagocytosis and intracellular killing, but granulomas are absent. Granulomas are seen in primary or secondary granulomatous conditions.

Persistence of Infectious Agents

Persistence of infectious agents occurs due to failure of phagocytosis.
- *Tuberculosis:* Mycobacterium tubercle bacilli cause caseous necrosis, epithelioid granulomas and Langhans' giant cells. AFB is seen in macrophages.
- *Leprosy:* Macrophages are laden with *Mycobacterium leprae* bacilli. Noncaseating granulomas are present.
- *Syphilis:* It is caused by *Treponema pallidum* with formation of gumma (microscopic to grossly visible lesion), with central necrotic cells, surrounded by macrophages and plasma cell infiltrate.
- *Fungal granuloma:* Granulomas may be seen in fungal infections (e.g. histoplasmosis, blastomycosis, cryptococcosis, coccidioidomycosis).
- *Parasitic infections:* Granulomas are seen in schistosomiasis.
- *Cat-scratch disease:* Gram-negative bacteria form rounded or stellate granuloma containing central granular debris.

Prolonged Exposure to Substances

Prolonged exposure to exogenous and endogenous substances cause chronic inflammation.
- *Exogenous substance:* Granulomas are seen in vicinity of necrotic adipose tissue, necrotic and bone and gouty tophus (uric acid crystals).
- *Endogenous substance:* Foreign body granulomas are seen around surgical suture materials, implanted prosthesis, asbestos fibers, silica and beryllium. Silica is a man-made non-degradable substance, which causes silicosis of lung.

Autoimmune Disorders

Organ Specific Disorders

- *Hashimoto's thyroiditis:* It is an autoimmune disease characterized by *destruction of thyroid follicles by autoantibodies* such as *antithyroid peroxidase antibody, antithyroglobulin antibody and anti-TSH antibody.* Patient presents with diffuse painless thyroid enlargement, transient hyperthyroidism from excessive release of thyroid hormones from damaged follicles, but later hypothyroidism in 40–50% of cases.
- *Pernicious anemia:* Parietal cells in stomach synthesizes *intrinsic factor* required for absorption of vitamin B_{12}. *Autoantibodies* formed against parietal cells in stomach cause pernicious anemia.
- *Rheumatoid arthritis:* In long-standing cases, rheumatoid nodules are formed in synovium. Rheumatoid nodule is composed of macrophages, lymphocytes and plasma cells.

Contact Hypersensitivity Reactions

Self-antigens are altered by exposure to nickel. Patient develops contact hypersensitivity reactions.

Disorders of Unknown Etiology

- *Ulcerative colitis:* It is characterized by ulcerations of mucosa and submucosa with formation of pseudopolyps in colon. *Disease begins in the rectum as friable red mucosa and extends in continuity to involve part or the entire colon. It does not form fistulous tract.* Light microscopy shows crypt abscesses due to PMNs infiltration. Patient may develop adenocarcinoma in these pateints. Patient presents with abdominal cramping, diarrhea with blood and mucus, rectal bleeding, and tenesmus (ineffective and painful straining of stool).
- *Crohn's disease:* It is autoimmune disorder characterized by *discontinuous/skipped lesions involving all layers of small or large intestine*. On light microscopy, intestinal wall shows non-caseating granulomas along with dense chronic inflammatory infiltrate. Patient presents with colicky pain in right lower quadrant due to intestinal obstruction, diarrhea and anal bleeding. It is located in the terminal ileum (30%), colon and small bowel (50%), colon alone (20%).
- *Sarcoidosis:* Sarcoidosis is an idiopathic disorder in which abnormal immune system leads to formation of noncaseating granulomas and collection of activated macrophages. These trigger an inflammatory response leading to extensive tissue damage and scarring. *It is essential to exclude tuberculosis, fungal infection*

and *berylliosis*. Relative frequency of organs involved in sarcoidosis is shown in Table 2.40 and differences between sarcoidosis and tuberculosis are shown in Table 2.41.

GRANULOMA FORMATION

Exposure to antigen activates macrophages resulting in synthesis IFN-γ. Then IFN-γ activates T-helper cells (CD4+ T cell) leads to synthesis of IFN-γ. IFN-γ synthesized by activated macrophages and T-helper cells (CD4+ T cell) plays key role in formation of granuloma. IFN-γ activates macrophages to become epithelioid cells. IFN-γ also participates in proliferation and differentiation of T cells.

MAINTENANCE OF GRANULOMA

Cytokines TNF-α and IFN-γ participate in recruitment of chronic inflammatory cells, formation and maintenance of tuberculous and systemic fungal granulomas.

BREAKDOWN OF GRANULOMA

Inhibitors of TNF-α cause the *breakdown of granulomas resulting in dissemination of disease.*

TYPE OF GRANULOMAS

There are two type of granulomas: *immunological* (caseating and non-caseating granulomas) and *non-immunological* (foreign body granulomas). Immunological granulomas are mediated by lymphocytes.

Examples of *immunological mediated granulomas are tuberculosis, leprosy, cat-scratch fever, sarcoidosis, histoplasmosis* and *Hodgkin's disease*. Foreign body granulomas are formed by poorly digestible particles seen in *silicosis, surgical sutures, implanted prosthesis, asbestosis*, and beryllium exposure. Mechanism of granuloma formation is shown in Figs 2.34, 2.35 and Table 2.42.

Table 2.40: Relative frequency of organs involved in sarcoidosis

Organs	Frequency	
Lymph nodes	80%	Hilar, mediastinal. Cervical, epitrochlear, preauricular and post-auricular lymph nodes
Lungs	80%	Diffuse consolidation without cavities
Liver	70%	Noncaseating granulomas in portal tracts
Skin	30%	Small erythematous nodules on back
Eyes	20%	Lacrimal gland involvement
Heart	20%	Light microscopy showing noncaseating granulomas in heart
Brain	15%	Noncaseating granulomas are present in brain
Spleen	15%	Nodules visible in 15% cases on gross examination. Light microscopy showing noncaseating granulomas in 75% cases
Bone	15%	Destruction of terminal phalanges
Nasal and pharyngeal mucosa and tonsils	10%	Light microscopy showing noncaseating granulomas in these regions
Salivary gland	1%	Bilateral parotid gland enlargement but may involve all salivary glands

Table 2.41: Differences between sarcoidosis and tuberculosis

Characteristics	Sarcoidosis	Tuberculosis
Etiology	Unknown etiology	Mycobacterium tubercle bacilli
Granuloma	Noncaseating granulomas	Caseating granuloma
Cytoplasmic inclusions in giant cells	Presence of Schaumann bodies, asteroid bodies and birefringent crystals	Absence of Schaumann bodies, asteroid bodies and birefringent crystals
Steroid therapy	Improvement	Worsens the disease
Diagnosis	Done by excluding causes of granulomatous lesions	Acid-fast bacilli demonstration

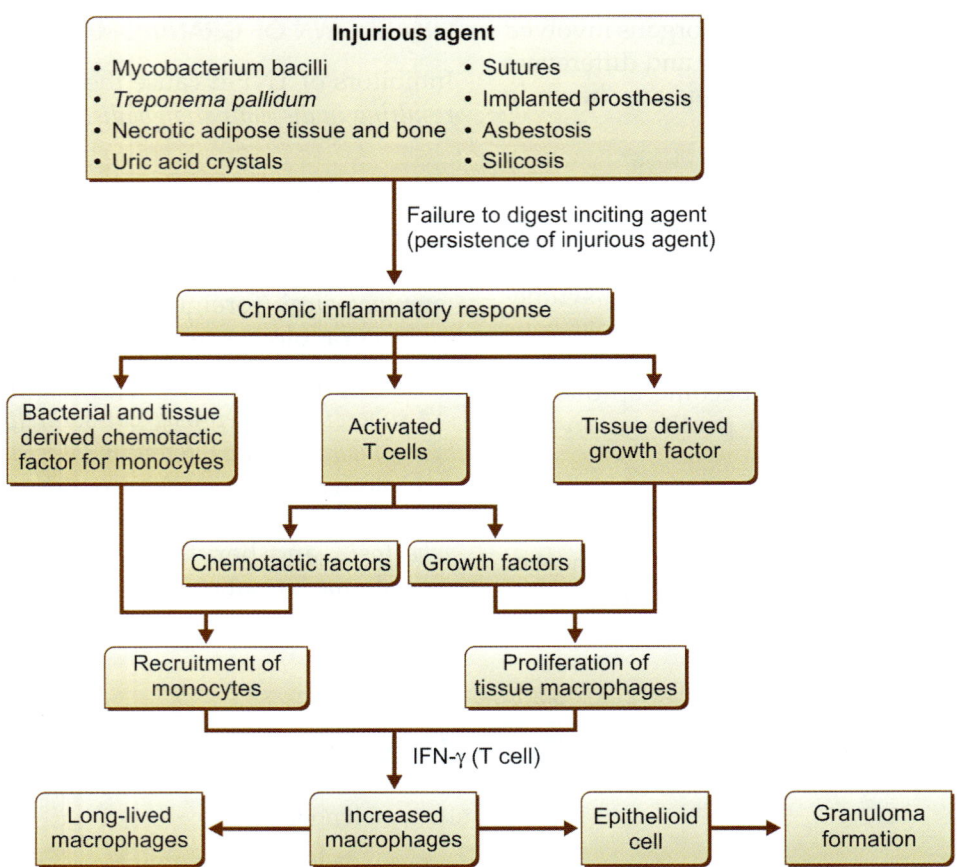

Fig. 2.34: Mechanism of granuloma formation. Persistence of injurious agent leads to chronic inflammatory response resulting in formation of granulomas.

Table 2.42: Mechanism of formation and causes of granulomatous inflammation

Mechanism	Examples
Immunological mechanism	Tuberculosis
	Leprosy
	Cat-scratch fever
	Sarcoidosis
	Histoplasmosis
	Blastomycosis
	Cryptococcosis
	Coccidioidomycosis
	Hodgkin's disease (mixed cellularity variant)
Non-immunological mechanism	Silicosis
	Berylliosis
	Asbestosis
	Surgical sutures
	Implanted prosthesis
	Foreign body induced pneumonia

Immunological Mediated Granulomas

- *Caseating granulomas:* These are demonstrated in *tuberculosis* (Fig. 2.36). In tuberculosis, caseating granulomas are formed when tubercle bacilli are poorly degradable by macrophages. These are characterized by the *presence of central caseous necrosis and Langhans' giant cells with nuclei arranged peripherally (in horseshoe/ring form or clustered at two poles)* in tuberculosis (Fig. 2.37).

  Diagnostic techniques for tuberculosis include by demonstration of *AFB* (Ziehl-Neelsen stain), *culture on LJ medium, serological PCR technique* (Fig. 2.38). Differences of tumor and Langhans' giant cells are shown in Table 2.43.

- *Non-caseating granulomas:* These are composed of multinucleated giant cells without necrosis. These are caused by *fungi, cat-scratch fever, syphilis, sarcoidosis, schistosomiasis and Hodgkin's disease* (Fig. 2.39).

Nonimmunological Mediated Granulomas

Foreign Body Granuloma

Foreign body giant cells are associated with inert foreign body with or without necrosis.

Inflammation, Tissue Healing and Repair

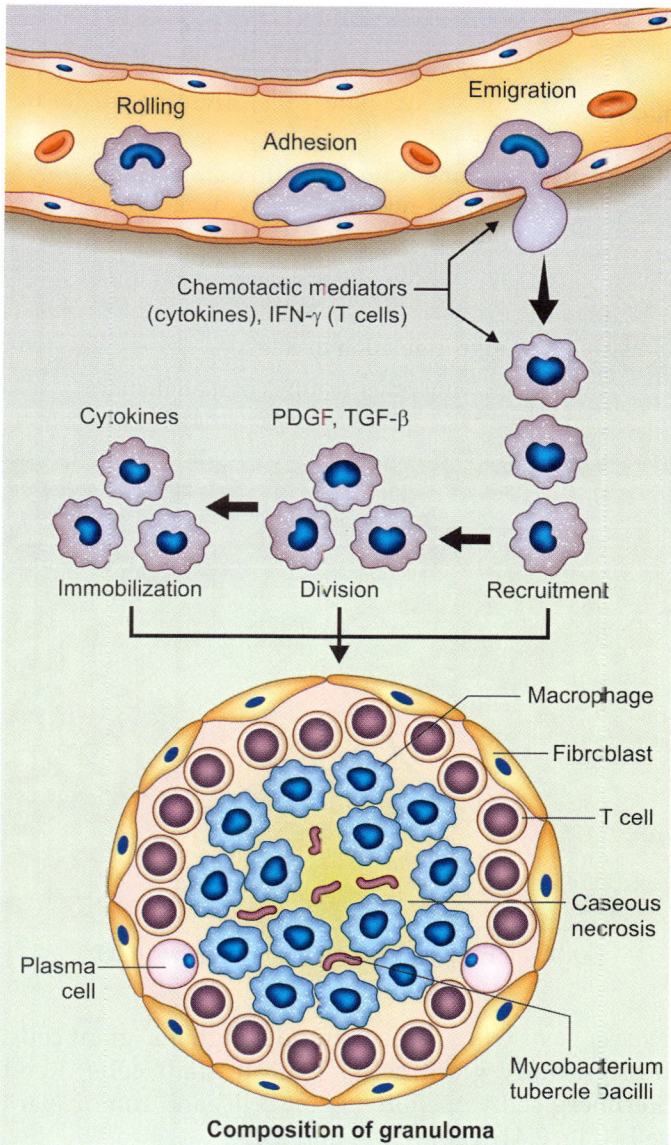

Fig. 2.35: Mechanism of granuloma formation.

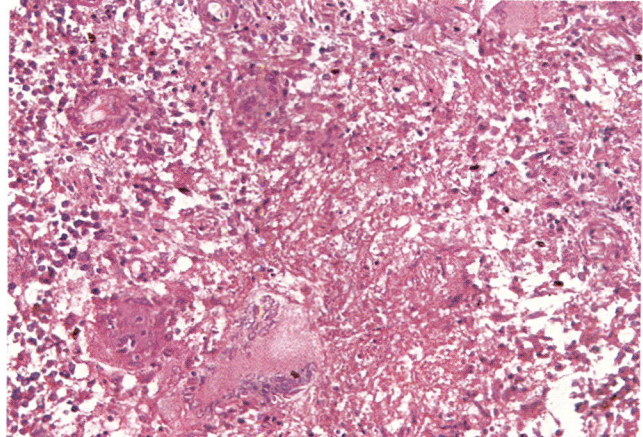

Fig. 2.36: Tubercular lymphadenitis showing epithelioid granulomas, caseous necrosis and Langhans' cells (100X).

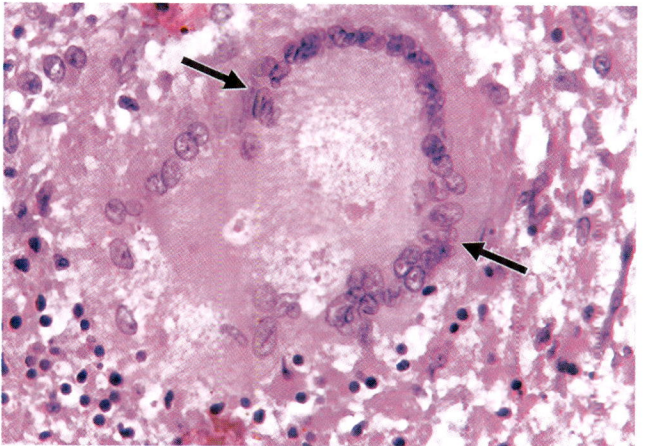

Fig. 2.37: Langhans' giant cell showing many small nuclei around the periphery in horseshoe/ring form (arrows) (400X).

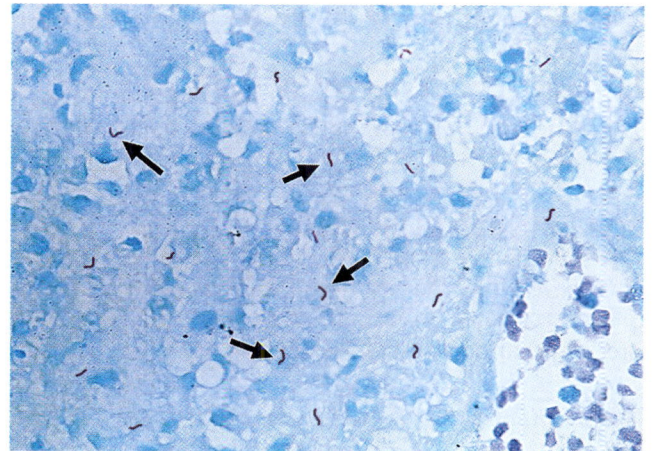

Fig. 2.38: Tubercular lymphadenitis showing acid-fast bacilli demonstrated by ZN stain (arrows) (400X).

- Inert foreign body incites granuloma formation such as talc associated with intravenous drug abuse, sutures and other fibers.
- Foreign bodies can usually be identified in the center of the granulomas, particularly if viewed with polarized light, in which it appears refractile. Foreign body granuloma is shown in Fig. 2.40.

Special Form of Granuloma

These are satellate granuloma and Durck's granuloma.
- *Satellite granulomas:* These are demonstrated in cat-scratch fever and lymphogranuloma venereum.

Table 2.43: Differences between Langhans' giant cells and anaplastic tumor giant cells

Features	Langhans' giant cells	Anaplastic tumor giant cells
Origin	Fusion of epithelioid cells in response to chronic inflammation	Anaplastic giant cells, dividing nuclei of neoplastic cells
Number of nucleus/nuclei	Containing 20 or more small nuclei around the periphery in horseshoe/ring form or clustered at two poles	Prominent nuclei, either single huge polymorphic nucleus or may have two or more nuclei
Nucleus morphology	Normal appearing nucleus, same as macrophage and epithelioid cells	Hyperchromatic nuclei
Size of nucleus	Normal	Large in relation to cells
Associated features	Absent	Showing other features of malignancy

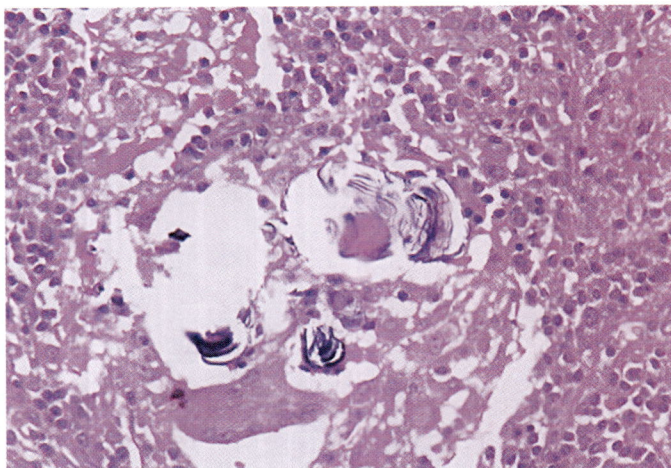

Fig. 2.39: Noncaseating granuloma in sarcoidosis showing laminated concretions composed of calcium and proteins measuring up to 50 micrometer in diameter known as *Schaumann bodies*. It is worth mentioning that Schaumann bodies are also seen in berylliosis (400X).

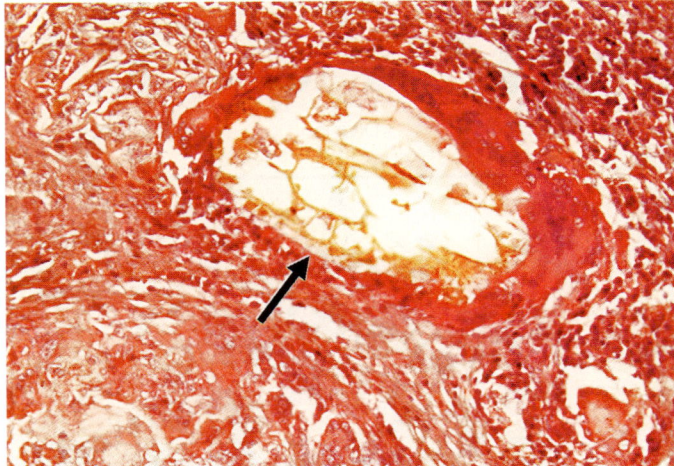

Fig. 2.40: Foreign body granuloma (arrow) (400X).

Satellite granulomas show central neutrophilic infiltrate.

- *Durck's granuloma:* It is demonstrated in brain as a result of cerebral malaria caused by *Plasmodium falciparum*.

MULTINUCLEATED GIANT CELLS

Physiological state: Multinucleated giant cells are present in bone marrow (megakaryocytes), bone (osteoclast) and placenta (syncytiotrophoblasts).

Pathological state: Multinucleated giant cells are formed by fusion of activated macrophages (epithelioid cells) showing multiple nuclei.

Epithelioid cells are recruited by IL-4 and IFN-γ. These measure 40–50 micron in diameter. Cytoplasm of giant cells is abundant and contains 15 or more small nuclei.

Type of giant cells: These include Langhans' giant cells, foreign body giant cells, Touton giant cells, Reed Sternberg cells, Aschoff's giant cells, and tumor giant cells (Fig. 2.41, Tables 2.44 and 2.45).

Table 2.44: Giant cells seen in bone tumors and tumor-like conditions

Benign tumors or tumor-like conditions
Osteoclastoma
Benign fibrous histiocytoma
Chondroblastoma
Chondromyxoid fibroma
Fibrous dysplasia
Metaphyseal fibrous defects (non-ossifying fibroma)
Aneurysmal bone cyst
Malignant tumors
Malignant fibrous histiocytoma
Fibrosarcoma
Giant cell variant of osteosarcoma

Inflammation, Tissue Healing and Repair

Table 2.45: Giant cells in various pathological conditions

Giant cells	Pathological disorders	Morphology and condition
Langhans' giant cells	Tuberculosis	Contain peripherally arranged nuclei in a horseshoe-shaped pattern
Foreign body giant cells	Prolonged exposure to exogenous or endogenous substances	Foreign body granulomas showing haphazardly scattered nuclei around foreign material
	Surgical suture materials, implanted prosthesis, asbestos fibers, silica, beryllium, necrotic adipose tissue, necrotic and bone and gouty tophus (uric acid crystals)	
Touton giant cells	Juvenile xanthogranuloma, xanthoma disseminatum and dermatofibroma	Touton giant cells show ring of nuclei separating outer foamy cytoplasm
Aschoff's giant cell	Rheumatic heart disease	Aschoff's nodule composed of swollen eosinophilic collagen fibers, central fibrinoid necrosis surrounded by macrophages lymphocytes, plasma cells and occasional multinucleated giant cells
Reed-Sternberg cells	Hodgkin's disease	Popcorn cells (lymphohistiocytic cells) in lymphocytic rich variant
		Lacunar cells in nodular sclerosis variant Classic RS cells in mixed cellularity variant
Warthin-Finkeldey giant cells	Measles	Giant cells
Tumor giant cells	Tumors	Benign and malignant bone lesions
Giant cell	Physiological state	Morphology
Under physiological giant cells present in various sites	Bone	Osteoclasts
	Bone marrow	Megakaryocytes
	Placenta	Syncytiotrophoblastic giant cells

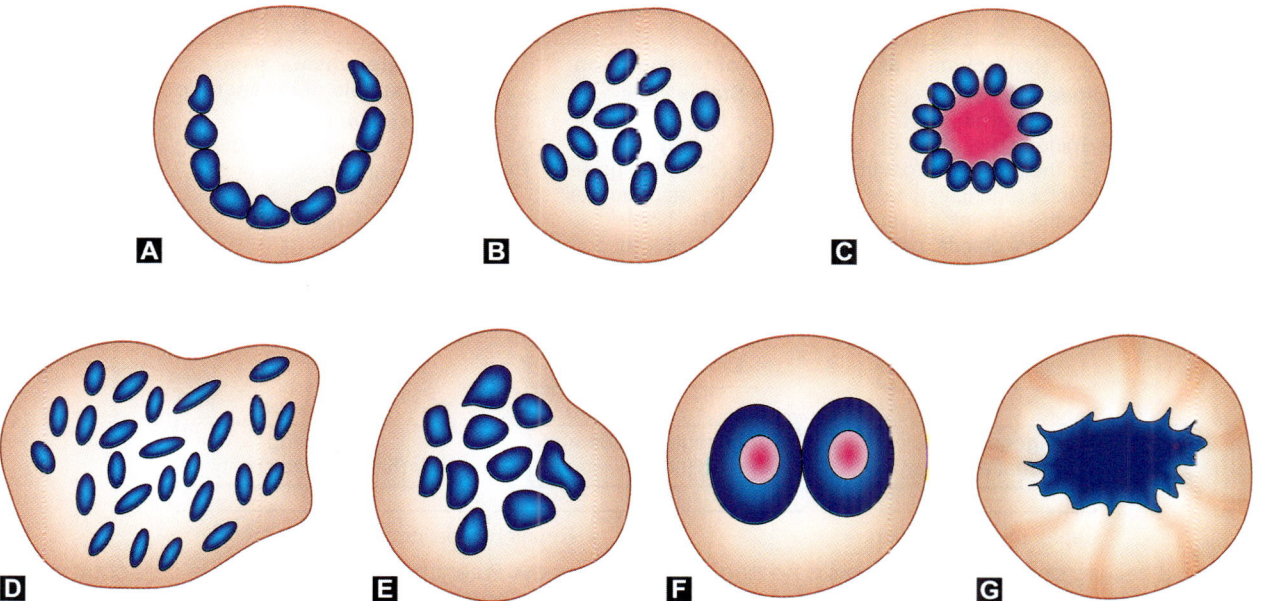

Fig. 2.41: Types of giant cells. (A) Langhans' giant cell; (B) Foreign body giant cell; (C) Touton giant cell; (D) Osteoclastic giant cell (E) Tumor giant cell; (F) Reed-Sternberg giant cell; (G) Aschoff giant cell.

TISSUE HEALING AND REPAIR

Tissue destruction occurs due to loss of blood supply (ischemic necrosis), inflammatory agents, trauma and radiotherapy. Healing is the replacement of destroyed or lost tissue by viable tissue.

Wound healing is the *final stage of the response of tissue to the injury*. It fills the vacant gap created by tissue destruction by migration of survival cells. It requires the *highly coordinated interaction of vascular component, cellular component and chemical mediators* (Fig. 2.42).

CONTROL OF NORMAL CELL PROLIFERATION AND TISSUE GROWTH

Size of cell populations in adult tissue is determined by *rate of cell proliferation, differentiation and apoptosis*. Increased cell numbers may result from either increased proliferation or decreased cell death by apoptosis.

- *Apoptosis:* Apoptosis is a *physiological process* required for tissue homeostasis, but it can also be *induced by a variety of pathologic stimuli* (*refer* to Chapter 1).
- *Hyperplasia:* Hyperplasia is *an increase in the number of cells of a tissue due* to increased rate of cell division due to increased functional demand, hormonal stimulation. It may be *physiological, compensatory* or *pathological conditions* (*refer* to Chapter 1).

Mechanism of Healing

- Healing occurs *by removal of the damaged tissue by phagocytosis, lymphatic drainage of exudates, angiogenesis, and regeneration of residual stem cells*. It restores the continuity of the injured tissue.
- *Damage to residual stem cells leads to fibrosis resulting in malfunction of organs.* Both platelet derived growth factor (*PDGF*) and fibroblast growth factor (*FGF*) participate in *migration, proliferation of fibroblasts leading to synthesis and deposition of extracellular matrix leading to wound healing*. Most of the organs heal by regeneration and fibrosis.

TISSUE PROLIFERATIVE ACTIVITY

Tissue proliferative activity is a process of *replacement of damaged components and returning to normal state*. It requires *preservation of the basement membrane, residual*

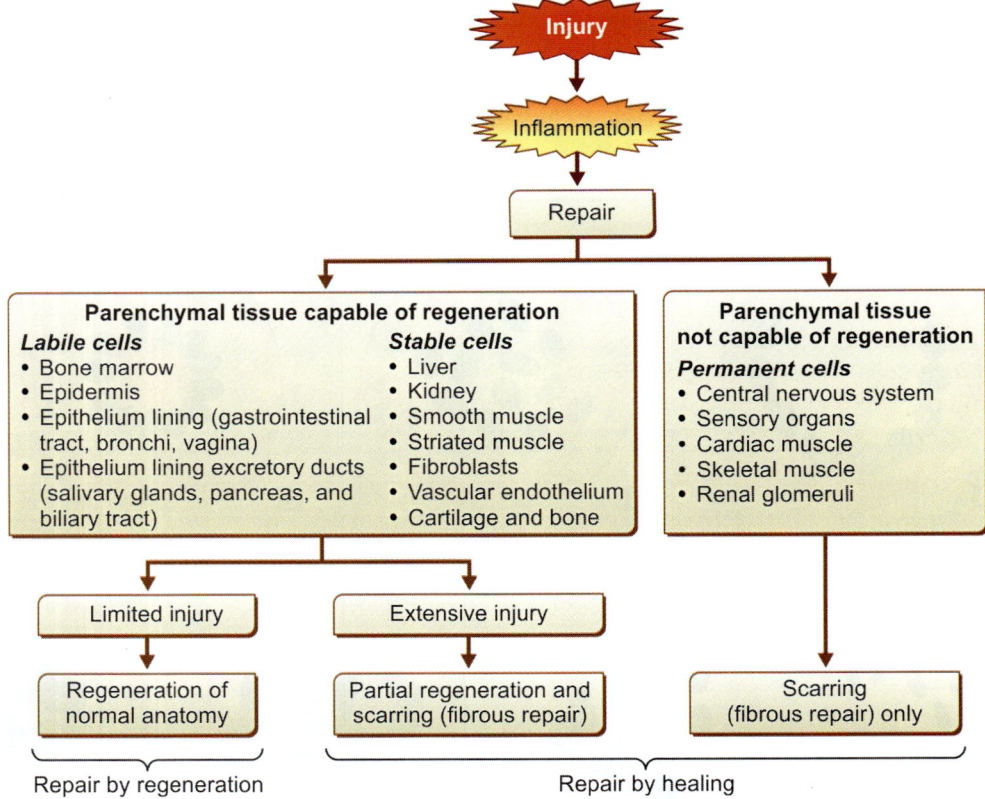

Fig. 2.42: Tissue healing and repair. Labile cells in healing and repair process. Parenchymal tissue with labile cells contain stem cells that continuously regenerate new stem cells. Tissue with labile cells repairs by regeneration. Parenchymal tissue with stable cells contain stem cells that reproduce rapidly as a result of injury. Tissues with stable cells repair by regeneration. Tissues with permanent cells do not contain stem cells. Hence, injury to tissues with permanent cells repair by fibrosis only.

stem cells and *intact extracellular matrix (collagen fibers type III and fibronectin)*. Regeneration is *not possible if the stem cells are destroyed*.

Prerequisite of Regeneration

Healing involves two processes, e.g. *proliferation of surviving cells to replace lost tissue; and migration of surviving cells into the vacant space*. Regeneration of cells *depends on the ability of cells to replicate* (e.g. labile cells, stable cells and permanent cells) and *growth factors such as VEGF, FGF-β, and EGF*. These growth factors stimulate cell division resulting in restoration of tissue to normal.

Broad Group of Cells

The tissues of the body are divided into three groups based on proliferative activity of their cells in the context of the cell cycle. These are labile cells, stable cells and permanent cells described as under, also shown in Table 2.46.

Labile cells: Labile cells enter cell cycle *continuously and proliferate throughout life*. Regeneration of cells is excellent, if stem cells are not destroyed. Examples are *bone marrow cells and epithelium lining epidermis, oral cavity, gastrointestinal tract, genitourinary tract, uterus, and cervix, and vagina, excretory ducts of salivary glands, pancreas, and biliary tract*. Organs with labile cells heal by *regeneration with a little or without fibrosis*.

Stable cells: These cells normally have *a little proliferative activity* but remain capable of more rapid cell division following injury, e.g. *liver, renal tubular epithelium smooth muscle, fibroblasts, vascular endothelium, cartilage and bone*. That is the reason that these cells *regenerate from G_0 cells (quiescent)* when needed.

Permanent cells: These are *irreversibly post-mitotic terminally differentiated cells*. These cells are incapable of division and regeneration in postnatal life. *Healing occurs by fibrosis*. Examples are *neurons of central nervous system, sensory organs, renal glomeruli, myocardial muscle, and striated muscle*. Injury to adult neurons is replaced by glial cells (gliosis in CNS), cardiac muscle in acute myocardial infarction by fibrosis, and skeletal muscle through the differentiation of the satellite cells located beneath myocytes basal lamina.

STEM CELLS

Stem cells possess self-renewal properties to generate differentiated cell lineages. Stem cells are essential to give rise to these lineages during life. *Embryonic and adult stem cells can be used to repopulate damaged cells* (Fig. 2.43). Stem cells therapy in clinical practice are shown in Table 2.47.

Table 2.46: Cells based on proliferative activity in the context of cell cycle

Type of cells	Organs
Labile cells	Bone marrow
	Epidermis
	Epithelium lining gastrointestinal tract, bronchi and vagina
	Epithelium lining excretory ducts of salivary glands, pancreas, and biliary tract
Stable cells	Liver
	kidney
	Smooth muscle
	Striated muscle
	Fibroblasts
	Vascular endothelium
	Cartilage
	Bone
Permanent cells	Brain
	Cardiac muscle
	Skeletal muscle

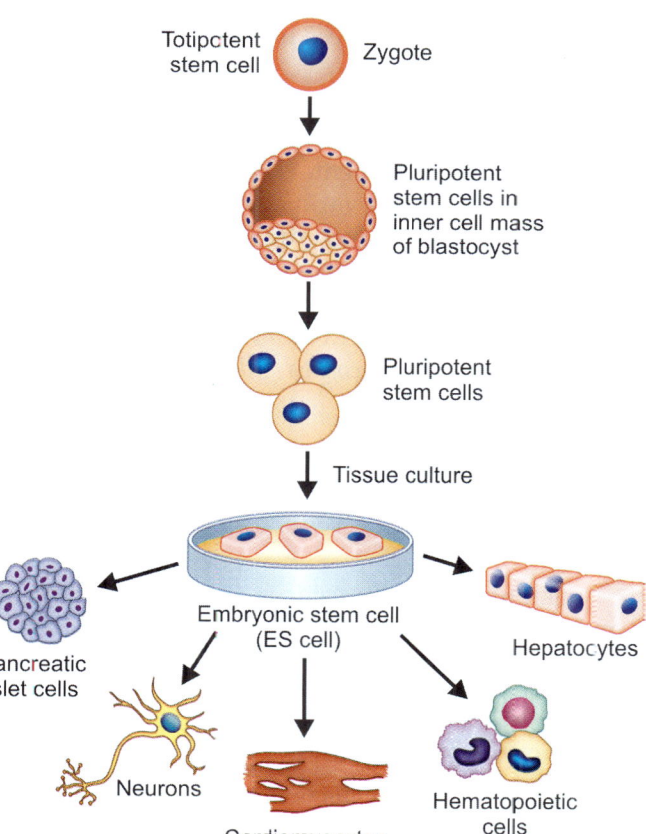

Fig. 2.43: Generation and differentiation of stem cells. Embryonic pluripotent stem cells obtained from inner cell mass of blastocyst are cultured and induced to obtain differentiated cells such as hepatocytes, pancreatic islets of Langerhans' cardiomyocyte and neurons.

Table 2.47: Stem cells therapy in clinical practice

Stem cell type	Disease	Stem cell therapy
Embryonic stem cells	Diabetes mellitus	β cells embryonic stem cells
	Myocardial infarction	Myocardial embryonic stem cells
	Liver damage	Hepatocytic embryonic stem cells
Adult stem cells	Restricted use skin, lining epithelia of gut, cornea and hematopoietic tissue	Reprogramming of adult stem cells into pluripotent cells, similar to embryonic cells, by the transduction of genes encoding embryonic stem cell transcription

Embryonic Stem Cells

- *Blastocyst formation:* Zygote is formed by union of ovum and sperm. Two-cell stage zygote divides by mitosis to form morula and then 32 cells blastocyst. This blastocyst gets implanted into uterine endometrium. Cells of the inner mass of blastocyst are known as *pluripotent embryonic stem (ES) cells. Inner cell mass of the blastocyst generates embryo.*

- *Clinical aspect:* These embryonic stem cells are cultured and used to *repopulate damaged cells* in various organs such as β *cells of Langerhans' in diabetes mellitus, myocardial cells in acute myocardial infarction* and *hepatocytes in liver cell injury.*

Adult Stem Cells

- *Differentiation of embryonic pluripotent stem cells:* During embryonic development, *embryonic pluripotent stem cells develop* through various stage into multipotent stem cells, lineage committed stem cells and differentiated cells. These differentiated cells form *endoderm, mesoderm and ectoderm.* These *possess restricted capacity* to form different cell types (e.g. *skin, lining epithelia of gut, cornea and hematopoietic tissue*).

- *Clinical aspect:* These cells can be *reprogrammed into pluripotent cells,* similar to embryonic cells, by the *transduction of genes encoding embryonic stem cell transcription.* ES cells may be used to *repopulate damaged organs.*

  Somatic stem cells reside in special microenvironments called *niches.* These niche cells *generate or transmit stimuli that regulate stem cell self-renewal and the generation of progeny cells.*

Maintenance of Stem Cells

Maintenance of stem cells is achieved by two mechanisms described as under:

- *Obligatory asymmetric replication:* Each stem cell division *produces two daughter cells.* One of the daughter cells retains self-renewal property, while other enters a differentiation pathway.

- *Stochastic differentiation:* Stem cells division *generates either two self-renewing stem cells or two cells* that will differentiate.

Stem Cell Therapy

Both embryonic stem (ES) and induced pluripotent stem (iPS) cells are capable of differentiating into various cell types. Stem cells, their location and clinical aspect are shown in Table 2.48.

Embryonic Stem Cells Therapy

Therapeutic cloning using embryonic stem cells is done by *introducing diploid nucleus of an adult cell in to an anucleate oocyte.* The oocyte is activated, and the zygote divides to become a blastocyst that contains the donor DNA. The blastocyst is dissociated to obtain embryonic stem cells.

Differentiated cells of adult tissues can be reprogrammed to become pluripotent by transferring their nucleus to an enucleated oocyte.

Induced Pluripotent Stem Cells (iPS Cells) Therapy

- The cells of a patient are placed in *culture and transduced with genes encoding transcription factors,* to generate iPS cells.

- The goal of stem cell therapy is to *repopulate damaged organs* of a patient or *to correct a genetic defect,* using the cells of the same patient to avoid immunological rejection.

Stem Cells in Tissue Homeostasis

Bone Marrow Stem Cells

Bone marrow consists of hematopoietic and marrow stromal stem cells.

- *Hematopoietic stem cells (HSCs):* Hematopoietic stem cells are *pluripotent labile cells participating in the hematopoiesis.* Labile cells enter cell cycle continuously and proliferate throughout life. *Regeneration of cells is excellent, if stem cells are not destroyed.* Hematopoietic stem cells are *used in various hematological disorders.* These cells are obtained from *bone marrow, umbilical*

Inflammation, Tissue Healing and Repair

Table 2.43: Stem cells, their location and clinical aspect

Organ	Location of stem cells	Clinical aspect
Bone marrow stem cells	Hematopoietic stem cells	Various hematological disorders
	Marrow stem cells	Generation of osteoblasts, chondroblasts, endothelial cells, myoblasts and adipocytes
Liver stem cells	Canals of Hering	Oval cells prominent in recovery phase of fulminant hepatic failure, liver tumors, chronic hepatitis and cirrhosis
Neural stem cells	Subventricular zone (SVZ) and dentate nuclei	Generate neurons, astrocytes, oligodendrocytes in Parkinson's disease, Alzheimer disease and spinal cord injury
Epidermis stem cells	Hair follicle bulge, interfollicular areas of epidermis and sebaceous glands	Wound healing
Skeletal muscle stem cells	Satellite cells located beneath the myocyte basal lamina	Regeneration of injured skeletal muscle
Cardiac muscle stem cells	Under debate	May be used in injured myocardium
Intestinal stem cells	Located immediately above Paneth cells in the small intestine, or at the base of the crypts in the colon	Regeneration of crypts of small intestine
Limbal stem cells in cornea	Located at the junction between the epithelium of the cornea and the conjunctiva	Corneal opacity and correction of photoreceptors

cord and blood. Granulocyte macrophage colony stimulating factors are administered to obtain hematopoietic stem cells.

- *Marrow stromal cells (MSCs):* Marrow stromal cells are multipotent. These do not participate in normal hemostasis. These are important for *therapeutic applications to generate osteoblasts, chondroblasts, endothelial cells, myoblasts and adipocytes*. Marrow stromal cells are obtained and administered to generate cells depending on the tissues.

Liver Stem Cells

- *Locations:* Liver stem cells are present in *canals of Hering* at the junction between parenchymal hepatocytes and biliary ductal system.
- *Stem cells role:* Liver stem cells located *in this niche* may undergo transformation to bipotential progenitor *oval cells*. These oval cells are capable of *differentiating into parenchymal hepatocytes and biliary ductular system*.
- *Clinical correlation:* Oval cells are prominent in the patients with *liver diseases* such as recovery phase of *fulminant hepatic failure, liver tumors, chronic hepatitis* (some cases) and *advanced liver cirrhosis*.

Neural Stem Cells in Brain

- *Locations:* Brain contains neural stem cells (NSCs) also known as *neural precursor cells*. These cells are capable to *generate neurons, astrocytes and oligodendrocytes*. Neural stem cells have been demonstrated in two areas of brain such as *subventricular zone (SVZ)* and *dentate nuclei*.

- *Clinical aspect:* Research is in progress for neural stem transplantation in patients suffering from *Parkinson's disease, Alzheimer's disease* and *spinal cord injury*.

Epidermis Stem Cells

- *Locations:* Skin consists of stem cells in the epidermis regions: *The hair follicle bulge, interfollicular areas of epidermis and sebaceous glands* (Fig. 2.44).

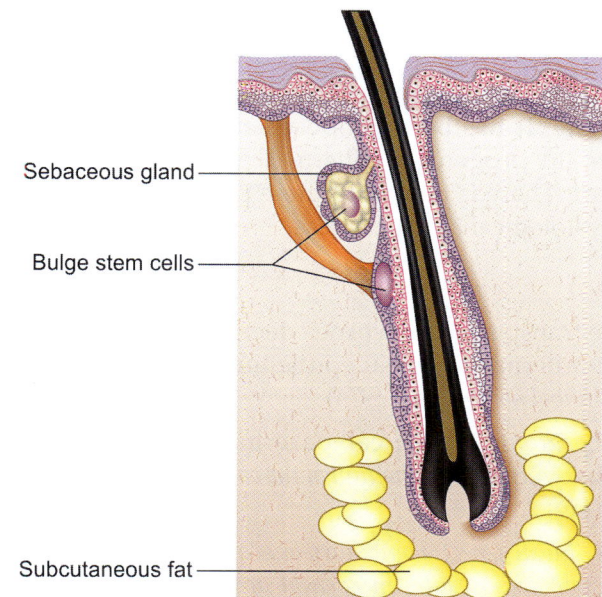

Fig. 2.44: Stem cells in skin. These are located in the bulge area of the hair follicle, sebaceous glands and lower layer of the epidermis. These cells replenish surface epithelial cells after skin wounding.

- *Regulation:* These stem cells are regulated by two mechanisms: *Wnt pathway stimulates these stem cells. Bone morphogenic protein (BMP) inhibits these stem cells.*
- *Clinical aspect:* Bulge area of hair follicle is niche for stem cells. These cells are able to generate all the cell lineages of the hair follicle. Human skin consists of labile cells capable of high turnover rate of about 4 weeks. These cells replenish surface epithelial cells after skin wounding. These cells do not participate in normal hemostasis.

Intestinal Epithelium Stem Cells

- *Locations:* Intestinal stem cells are located immediately above *Paneth cells in the small intestine, or at the base of the crypts in the colon.*
- *Regulation:* These are regulated by *Wnt pathway* and bone morphogenic protein (BMP) similar to that seen in skin epidermis.
- *Clinical aspect:* Stem cell participates in formation of crypts in the villous structures of intestine. Stem cells in crypts of small intestine *regenerate crypts in about 3–5 days.*

Skeletal Muscle Stem Cells

- *Locations:* Skeletal muscle consists of *satellite cells located beneath the myocyte basal lamina.*
- *Clinical aspect:* These cells participate in regeneration of injured skeletal muscle. Notch signaling regulate satellite stem cells by upregulation of delta-like ligands and angiogenesis.

Cardiac Muscle Stem Cells

Presence of progenitor cells in myocardium is under debate. It has been proposed that myocardium may contain progenitor cells, which may repair injured heart. There is no role of these progenitor cells during physiological aging process.

Stem Cells in Cornea

The transparency of cornea depends on the integrity of the outermost corneal epithelium, which is *maintained by limbal stem cells* (LSCs).

- *Locations:* These cells are located at the junction between the *epithelium of the cornea and the conjunctiva* (Fig. 2.45).
- *Clinical aspect: Hereditary or acquired deficiency of limbal stem cells results in corneal opacity.* It can be treated by *transplantation of limbal stem cells* (LSCs). Retinal stem cells transplantation may correct the loss of photoreceptors that occurs in degenerative diseases of the retina.

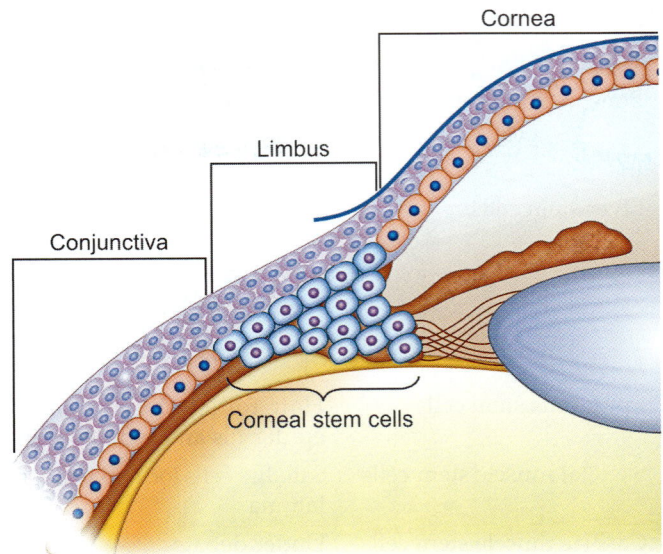

Fig. 2.45: Stem cells in cornea. These are located in the limbus region between the cornea and conjunctiva.

CELL CYCLE AND ITS REGULATION

CELL CYCLE

Phases of cell cycle comprises G_0, G_1, G_2 and M phases (Fig. 2.46).

- *M (mitotic phase):* This phase describes the interval between the onset of prophase and conclusion of telophase. Two daughter cells are produced in this phase. Division of nucleus is followed by division of cytoplasm resulting in formation of two new cells.
- G_1 *(pre-synthetic phase):* Following mitosis, the cell enters this phase. Synthesis of RNA, protein, organelles and cyclin D occurs in this phase. The main difference between slowly and rapidly dividing cells is the length of the G_1 phase of cell cycle.
- *S (synthetic phase):* Synthesis of DNA, RNA, and protein occurs in this phase. *Labile cells undergo mitosis throughout life.* Doubling of DNA occurs in this phase.
- G_2 *(pre-mitotic phase):* After completion of nuclear DNA duplication, cell enters this phase. Synthesis of tubulin is necessary for formation of mitotic spindle.
- G_0 *phase:* It is the resting phase of stable parenchymal cells. Quiescent cells that have not entered the cell cycle are in the G_0 state. This phase consists of stable and permanent cells. Stable cells may enter cell cycle. Permanent cells do not enter cell cycle.

Regulation of Cell Cycle

Regulation of the G_1, checkpoint (G_1 to S) phase is the most critical phase of the cycle. It is controlled by cyclin D and cyclin-dependent kinase-4 (Cdk-4).

Inflammation, Tissue Healing and Repair

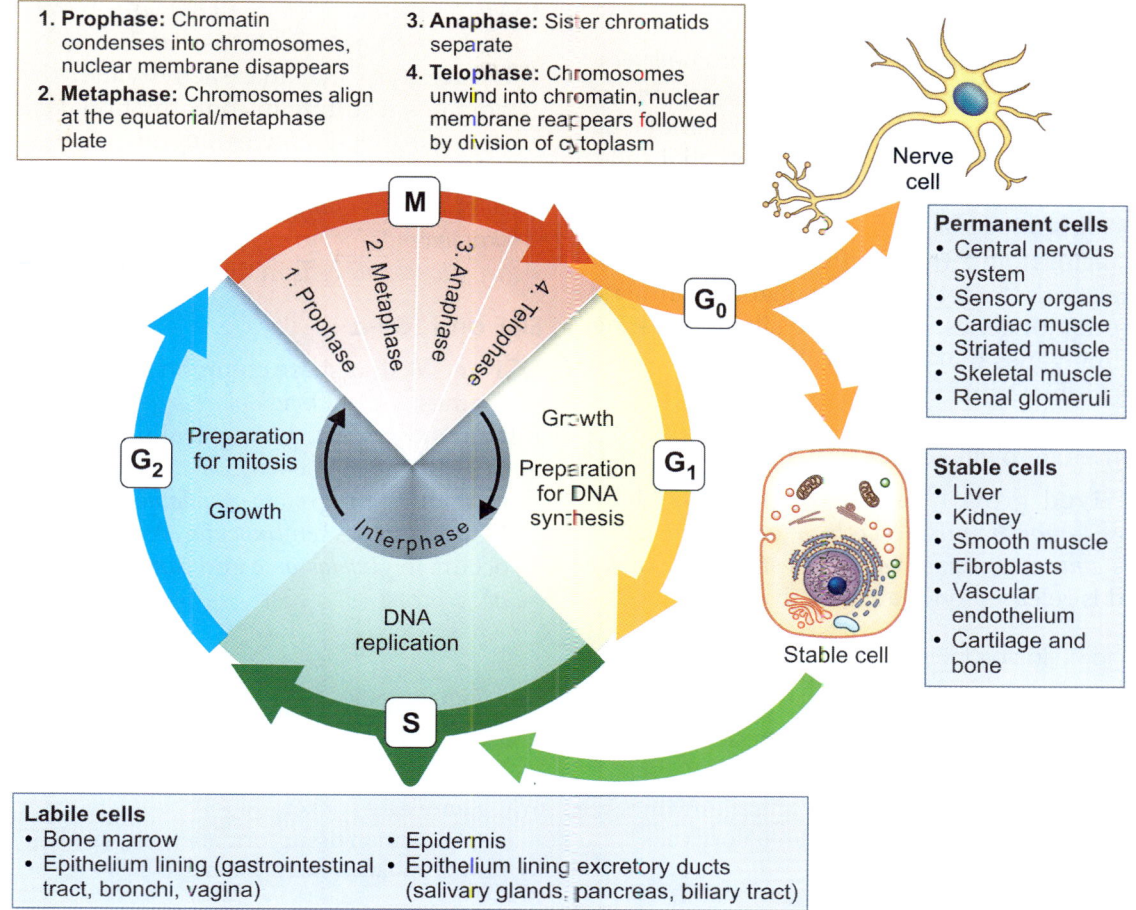

Fig. 2.46: Cell cycle shows G_0, G_1, G_2, G_3, S and M phases. Location of the G_1 is the restriction point. G_1/S and G_2/M are checkpoints of cell cycle. Cells from labile tissues such as bone marrow, epidermis, epithelial lining gastrointestinal tract, bronchi and vagina may cycle continuously.

Cyclin D and Cdk-4 Synthesis

Growth factors activate nuclear transcribing proto-oncogenes to produce cyclin D and Cdk-4.

Mechanism

- *Binding of cyclin D to Cdk-4:* Cyclin D binds to Cdk-4 to form a complex; that causes the cell to enter the S phase by phosphorylation of RB proteins. *RB proteins normally arrest the cell in the G_1 phase.* Cdk-4 phosphorylates the RB protein causing the cell to enter the S phase.

- *TP53 suppressor gene:* It arrests the cell in G phase by inhibiting Cdk-4. It prevents *RB protein phosphorylation.* It may *provide time for repair of DNA in the cell.*

- *BAX gene:* When there is excessive DNA damage, *BAX gene* is activated. BAX gene inhibits BCL2 antiapoptotic gene causing release of cytochrome-c from the mitochondria and apoptosis of the cell.

CONTROL OF REGENERATION

Regeneration is controlled by stimulatory and inhibitory factors. Stimulation is a three-stage process described as under:

- *Initiation:* Cells in growth arrested phase (G_0) are primed for progression to cell division. Initiation is brought about by tissue specific growth factors such as *epidermal growth factor (EGF) and platelet derived growth factor* (PDGF). It is worth mentioning that growth factors play an important role in cancers.

- *Potentiation:* Non-specific growth factors such as *insulin, hydrocortisone, growth hormone and ACTH* stimulate cells which have already been primed by the appropriate initiator to enter S phase.

- *Signaling through integrin:* It participates in *enhancing contact with basement membranes and adjacent cells.*

GROWTH FACTORS

Growth factors (polypeptides) synthesized by macrophages, damaged cells and platelets play an important role in the healing process by cell regeneration. These are chemotactic for white blood cells, fibroblasts and endothelial cells. These also act as mitogens, which increase proliferation of cells in healing process.

Growth factors bind to specific receptors, which deliver signals to the target cells. These signals stimulate the transcription of genes that may be silent in resting cells, including genes that control cell cycle entry and progression (Table 2.49).

Platelet Derived Growth Factor (PDGF)

Platelet derived growth factor is synthesized by *macrophages, smooth muscle cells, endothelial cells, keratinocytes and many tumor cells.* It is *stored in platelet granules* and is released on platelet activation.

- *Mechanism of action:* PDGF binds to specific cell surface receptors (transmembrane proteins) and induces tyrosine kinase activity in their intracellular domains resulting in conformational changes.
- *Actions:* PDGF causes *migration (chemotaxis)* and *proliferation of fibroblasts, smooth muscle cells* and *monocytes to areas of inflammation.* It participates in *healing skin wounds by process of wound contraction.* It *activates hepatic stellate cells* in the initial steps of liver fibrosis.

EGF and TGF-α

EGF and TGF-α share common biologic activities. EGF is synthesized by *macrophages, keratinocytes*, and other inflammatory cells during healing of skin wounds.

- *EGF:* It participates in *formation of granulation tissue* by promoting the *growth of endothelial cells* and *fibroblasts*. EGF *stimulates keratinocytes*. Amplification of EGFR-1 occurs in *glioblastoma* and *cancers of the lung, head and neck, breast*.

Table 2.49: Growth factors involved in tissue healing and repair

Growth factor	Source/Synthesis	Functions
PDGF (stored in platelets)	Macrophages, smooth muscle cells, endothelial cells, keratinocytes	Migration and proliferation of smooth muscle cells, fibroblasts, endothelial cells and monocytes
EGF and TGF-α Both have similar actions	Macrophages, keratinocytes and other inflammatory cells	Stimulation of keratinocytes. Granulation tissue formation as a result of proliferation of fibroblasts and endothelial cells
FGF-β	Macrophages, T cells, endothelial cells, platelets, many other cells	Angiogenesis. Synthesis of extracellular matrix proteins
TGF-β	Macrophages, T cells, endothelial cells, platelets	Chemotaxis of fibroblasts, macrophages, and lymphocytes. Stimulation of fibroblasts to synthesize collagen fibers. Modulation of repair process by inhibiting collagen degradation. Decreases the synthesis of metalloproteinase enzymes and enhances protease inhibitor activities
IL-1 and TNF-α	Macrophages	Proliferation of fibroblasts, smooth muscle cells, and endothelial cells in wound healing. Chemotaxis of neutrophils. Regeneration of hepatocytes. Synthesis of metalloproteinases and acute phase reactants
Fibronectin	Blood plasma	Chemotaxis of fibroblasts and endothelial cells. Angiogenesis and extracellular matrix deposition
VEGF	Endothelial cells and many other cells	Angiogenesis in chronic inflammation and tumors. Healing of wounds
Hepatocyte growth factor (HGF)	Fibroblasts, endothelial cells, and mesenchymal cells of liver	Proliferation of hepatocytes, epithelia of biliary tract, lungs, kidney, mammary gland and skin
Keratinocyte growth factor (FGF-7)	Fibroblasts	Migration, proliferation and differentiation of keratinocytes
Insulin growth factor-1 (IGF-1)	Liver	Synthesis of collagen fibers. Migration of keratinocyte

- *TGF-α:* It is involved in *epithelial cell proliferation in embryos* and *adults.* It also participates in *transformation of normal cells to cancer cells.*

Fibroblastic Growth Factor-β

FGF-β is synthesized by *macrophages, T cells, endothelial cells, and many other cells.*

Actions

- *Synthesis:* It stimulates *fibroblasts to synthesize extracellular matrix proteins* (including fibronectin) and epithelialization of skin.
- *Angiogenesis:* It simulates *endothelial cells to synthesize new vessels* (angiogenesis).
- *Maturation of organs:* It participates in *development of skeletal and cardiac muscles, and lung maturation.*
- *Lineage:* It differentiates specific lineages of *hematopoietic cells.*

Transforming Growth Factor-β

TGF-β is synthesized by *macrophages, T cells, endothelial cells, platelets, and many other cells.*

Actions

- *Chemotaxis:* It is chemotactic for *fibroblasts, macrophages and lymphocytes.*
- *Synthesis:* It stimulates *fibroblasts and enhances synthesis of collagen fibers, fibronectin and proteoglycans.*
- *Modulation of repair:* It modulates the repair process by *inhibiting collagen degradation by downregulating metalloproteinase enzymes and upregulating protease inhibitor activities.* It causes *fibrosis of the lung, kidney, and liver during chronic inflammation.*

IL-1 and TNF-α

IL-1 and TNF-α synthesized by macrophages promote the proliferation of fibroblasts, smooth muscle cells, and endothelial cells.

Actions

- *Chemotaxis:* These are chemotactic for neutrophils at the site of injury.
- *Liver regeneration:* These are involved in the initiation of liver regeneration.
- *Synthesis of MMPs:* IL-1 stimulates metalloproteinases synthesis.
- *Synthesis of acute phase reactants:* It participates in synthesis of acute phase reactants.

Fibronectin

Fibronectin (glycoprotein) links other extracellular matrix components (e.g. collagen and proteoglycans) and macromolecules (e.g. fibrin and heparin) to cell surface integrins.

Actions

- *Chemotaxis:* It participates in chemotaxis of *fibroblasts and endothelial cells.*
- *Angiogenesis:* It promotes *angiogenesis* (new vessel formation).

Vascular Endothelial Growth Factor

VEGFR-2 is located in endothelial cells and many other cells. VEGF family comprises VEGF-C and VEGF-D. These bind to VEGFR-3 and signal through three tyrosine kinase receptors. VEGF is potent *inducer of blood vessel formation during intrauterine life.*

- *Physiological state:* It plays central role in *angiogenesis (capillaries and lymphatic channels)* in adults.
- *Pathological state:* It promotes *angiogenesis in chronic inflammation,* healing of *wounds, and in tumors.*

Insulin-like Growth Factor-1

Insulin like growth factor-1 (IGF-1) is synthesized by liver. It participates in *proliferation of collagen fibers.* It participates in *migration of keratinocytes.*

Hepatocyte Growth Factor (HGF)

Hepatocyte growth factor (HGF) is synthesized by *fibroblasts, endothelial cells and liver mesenchymal cells.*

Actions

- *Proliferation of cells:* Hepatocyte growth factor participates in *proliferation of hepatocytes, epithelia of biliary tract, lungs, kidney, mammary gland, and skin.*
- *Embryo development:* HGF acts as a morphogen in embryonic development. It promotes cell scattering and migration, and enhances survival of hepatocytes.

SIGNALLING MECHANISM IN CELL GROWTH

The process of *receptor mediated signal transduction* is activated by the binding of ligands such as growth factors, and cytokines to specific receptors. It leads to expression of specific genes. Biochemical pathways and transcriptional regulation mediates growth factor activity.

According to the source of the ligand and the location of its receptors, there are four modes of signaling mechanisms, i.e. autocrine (in the same cell), paracrine (adjacent cells), endocrine (distant cells), and juxtacrine (cell to cell or cell to extracellular matrix) based on source of the ligand and the location of receptors (Fig. 2.47 and Table 2.50).

Autocrine Signaling

Cells respond to signaling molecules and synthesize growth factors, which act on the same cells, thus establishing an autocrine loop. Autocrine signaling participates in liver regeneration and proliferation of antigen-stimulated lymphocytes.

Tumors frequently overproduce growth factors and their receptors, thus stimulating their own proliferation through an autocrine loop.

Paracrine Signaling

One cell type synthesizes the ligand, which acts on adjacent target cells that express the appropriate receptor. The responding cells are in close proximity to the ligand-producing cells and are generally of a different type.

Paracrine stimulation is common in connective tissue repair of healing wounds, in which a factor produced by one cell (e.g. macrophage) has growth effect on adjacent cells (e.g. a fibroblast). It is also necessary for hepatocyte replication during liver regeneration, and notch effects in embryonic development, wound healing, and renewing tissues.

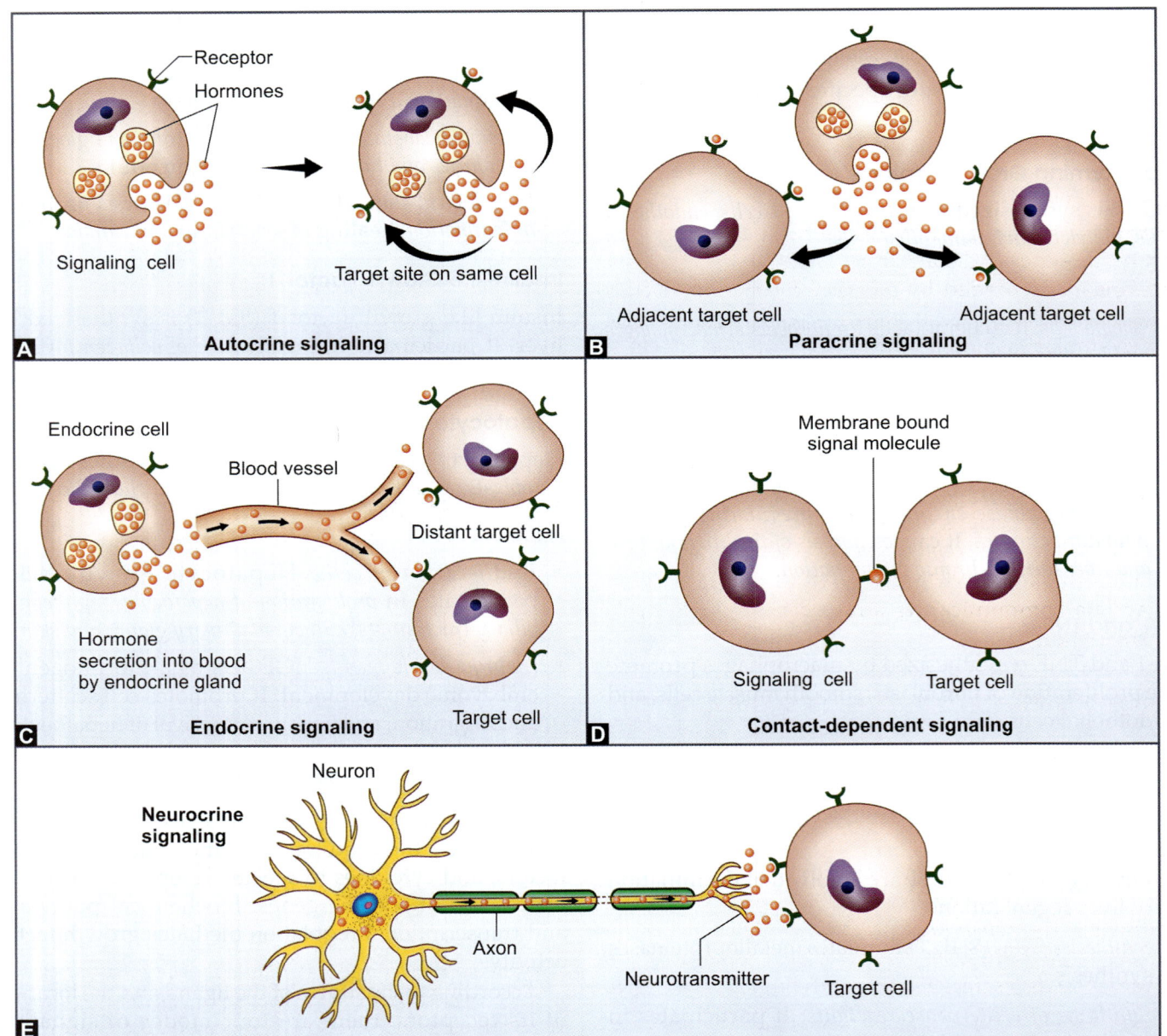

Fig. 2.47: General patterns of intercellular signaling demonstrating autocrine, paracrine, endocrine, contact-dependent and neurocrine signaling.

Inflammation, Tissue Healing and Repair

Table 2.50: Modes of cell signaling

Signaling mechanism	Mechanism	Regulation cell growth in organs
Autocrine signaling	Cells synthesize molecules, which act on same cells forming autocrine loop	Liver regeneration Proliferation of antigen stimulated lymphocytes
Paracrine signaling	Cells synthesize molecules, which act on adjacent cells	Connective tissue repair of wound healing Hepatocyte replication during regeneration Notch effects in embryonic development, wound healing and renewing tissues
Endocrine signaling	Cells synthesize hormones, which act on distant target cells from their site of synthesis	Endocrine glands synthesize hormones, which act on distant target cells Hepatocyte growth factor acting at distant target cells Several cytokines produce systemic effects in inflammation
Juxtacrine signaling	Known as *contact-dependent signaling* (cell to cell or cell to extracellular matrix signaling)	Two adjacent cells interacting with the help of membrane ligand membrane protein Intracellular compartment of two adjacent cells interacting via communicating junction permit relatively small molecules Two adjacent cells interacting via extracellular matrix glycoprotein and membrane protein

Endocrine Signaling

Hormone synthesized by cells of endocrine organs act on target cells distant from their site of synthesis, being usually carried by blood. Growth factors may also circulate and act at distant sites. Cytokines also act in similar fashion and produce systemic effects of inflammation.

Juxtacrine Signaling

Juxtacrine signaling requires close contact in multicellular organisms. There are three types of juxtacrine signaling described as under: *Two adjacent cells interact with the help of membrane ligand protein.*

- Intracellular compartment of two adjacent cells interact via communicating junction permit relatively small molecules.
- Two adjacent cells interact via extracellular matrix glycoprotein and membrane protein.

Cell Surface Receptors and Signal Transduction Pathways

Binding of a ligand to its receptor induces a series of events by which extracellular signals lead to expression of genes. Behavior of cells in healing process are initiated by three receptor systems that share integrated signaling pathways: (i) *Protein tyrosine kinase receptors for peptide growth receptors*, (ii) *seven transmembrane G-protein coupled receptors for chemokines and other factors*, and (iii) *integrin receptors for extracellular matrix* (Fig. 2.48).

Protein tyrosine kinase (growth factor) receptors: When protein kinase receptors bound to growth factors such as *EGF, TGF-α, HGF, PDGF, VEFG, FGH, c-kit ligand and insulin*. These receptors *activate GTPase cascade and Pl3 kinase pathway.* Both these pathways initiate a cascade of events leading to *several signaling pathways.*

Signaling Transduction Pathways

MAP kinase pathway: Adaptor protein GRB2 binds a guanosine triphosphate-guanosine diphosphate (GTP-GDP) exchanger factor called SOS. It acts on the GTP binding protein RAS and catalyzes the formation of RAS-GTP. This product activates MAP kinase pathway and stimulates phosphorylation and synthesis of transcriptional factors such as FOS and JUN.

IP3 pathway: PLC-γ catalyzes the breakdown of membrane inositol phospholipids into inositol 1, 4, 5-triphosphate (IP3). IP3 increases concentration of calcium and results in activation of serine threonine kinase protein C. Net result is *activation of transcription factors.*

Phosphatidylinositol-3 kinase (PI3 kinase) pathway: PI3 phosphorylates a membrane phospholipid results in generation of product that activates kinase Akt (also known as *protein kinase B*). Net result is *cell proliferation* and *survival through inhibiting apoptosis.*

Cell Surface Receptors

Seven transmembrane G-protein coupled receptors: These receptors bind to *chemokines, vasopressin, serotonin, histamine, epinephrine, norepinephrine, calcitonin, glucagon, parathormone, corticotropin and rhodopsin.* Binding of these receptors to ligands (chemokines) trigger cyclic AMP leading to multiple effects.

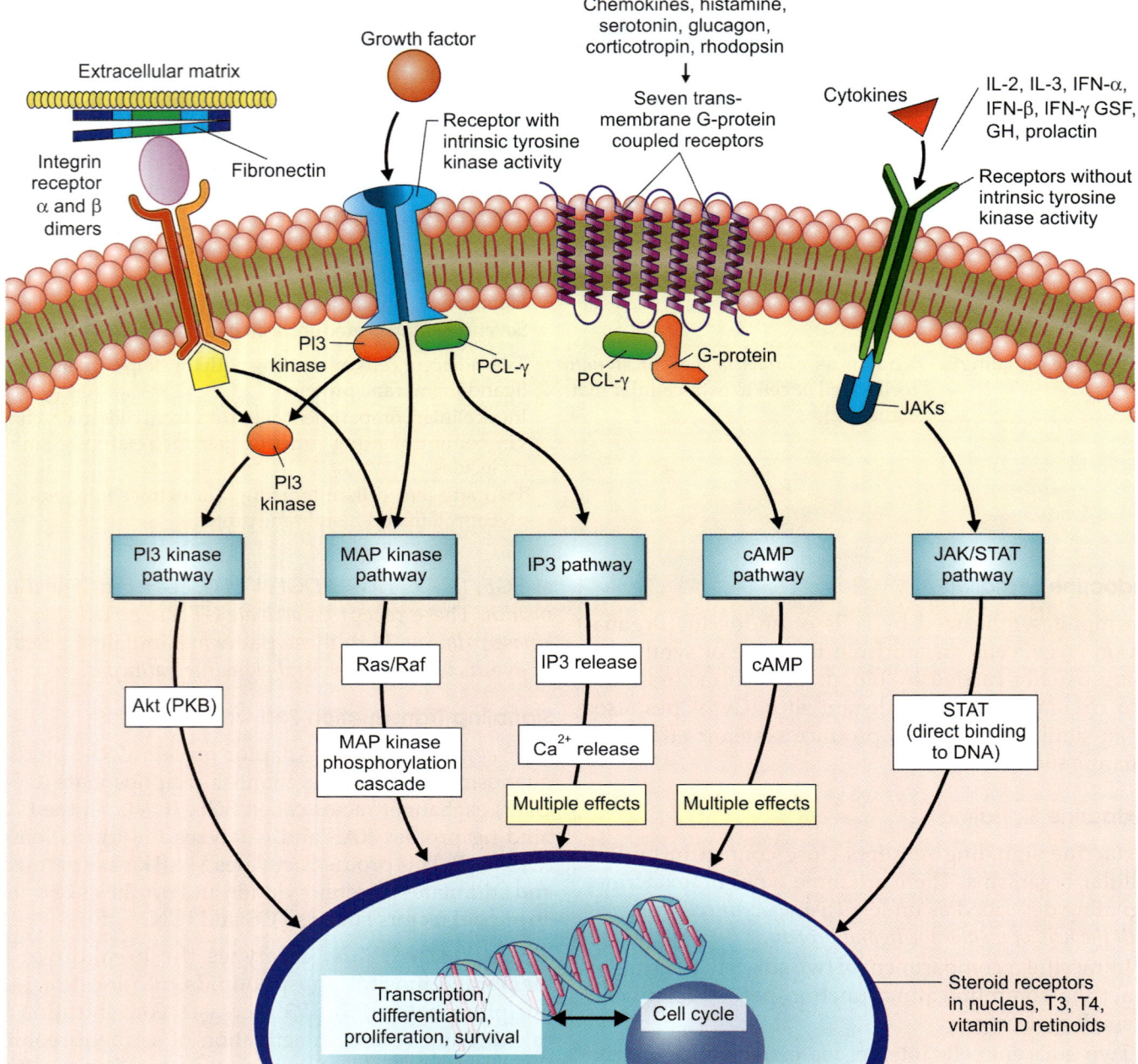

Fig. 2.48: Cell surface receptors and their principal signal transduction pathways. It shows receptors with intrinsic tyrosine kinase activity, seven transmembrane G proteins, and receptors without tyrosine kinase activity. Cyclic adenosine monophosphate (cAMP): Inositol triphosphate (IP3); Janus kinase (JAK); Mitogen activated protein (MAP) kinase; Signal transducers and activators of transcription (STATs).

Receptors without tyrosine kinase activity: These receptors bind to IF-α, IF-β, IF-γ, erythropoietin, granulocyte stimulating factor, growth hormone transmit extracellular signals to the nucleus by activating JAK-STAT (Janus kinase) pathway. JAKs link the receptors and activates cytoplasmic transcription factors known as STAT (signal transducers and activation of transcription). Cytokines may also activate MAP kinase pathways.

Integrin receptors for extracellular matrix: These receptors transmit chemical and physical information in the extracellular matrix. These create attachment sites for *the actin filaments of cytoskeleton*. These receptors activate PI3 kinase and MAP kinase pathways leading to *proliferation and differentiation of cells*.

Steroid receptors: These receptors are most often located in the nucleus. These function as ligand dependent transcription factors. These bind to *steroid hormones, thyroid hormone, vitamin D and retinoids*. Activated receptors then bind to specific DNA sequences known as *hormone response elements*. These are involved in inflammation, atherosclerosis and adipogenesis.

Mechanism: Transducing signals transmit the information to the nucleus and *modulate gene transcription* through the activity of transcriptional factors. Transcriptional factors *regulating cell proliferation* include products of *growth promoting genes such as c-JUN and c-MYC, and cell cycle-suppressing p53*.

REGENERATION OF TISSUE AND ORGAN

LIVER REGENERATION

Liver comprises stable cells and possess limited proliferative activity. Liver regeneration occurs by two mechanisms: Proliferation of remaining hepatocytes and repopulation from progenitor cells.

Proliferation of Remaining Hepatocytes

- *Priming phase:* IL-6 synthesized by Kupffer cells acts on the uninjured hepatocytes. It makes the hepatocytes to receive and respond to growth factor.
- *Growth factor action:* Hepatocyte growth factor (HGF) and TGF-α act on primed hepatocytes. Hepatocyte replication is followed by replication of non-parenchymal cells.
- *Termination phase:* The hepatocytes turn to quiescence. The nature of the stop signal is poorly understood. It may be due to synthesis of TGF-β that inhibits further proliferation of liver parenchyma.

Repopulation From Progenitor Cells

Fulminant hepatic necrosis, if the patient survives, usually regenerates. Progenitor cells in the liver contribute to repopulation. Patient suffering from chronic viral hepatitis develops cirrhosis.

There is development of broad collagenous scars within the hepatic parenchyma. Hepatocytes form regenerative nodules that lack central veins and expand to obstruct blood vessels and bile flow.

HEALING OF CENTRAL NERVOUS SYSTEM

Central nervous system comprises permanent cells. In spinal cord injuries, axonal regeneration can be seen up to 2 weeks after injury.

- *Damage to the brain or spinal cord* results in proliferation of capillaries and gliosis (permanent scar formation). Gliosis occurs due to proliferation of astrocytes and microglia.
- *After two weeks, axonal regeneration occurs* only in the hypothalamohypophysial region, because *capillary and glial barriers do not interfere with axonal regeneration.* Axonal regeneration seems to require contact with extracellular fluid containing plasma proteins.

HEALING OF PERIPHERAL NERVOUS SYSTEM

Neurons in the peripheral nervous system can regenerate their axons. Patient develops a bulbous lesion known as *traumatic neuroma*, if cut ends are not in perfect alignment. Light microscopy shows *disorganized axons and proliferating Schwann cells and fibroblasts.* The nerve is surrounded by dense collagenous tissue, which appears dark blue in trichrome stain.

BONE FRACTURE HEALING

Bone fracture is usually accompanied by trauma to adjacent soft tissues with hemorrhage. Healing occurs by the process of organization, while the bone is repaired by regeneration. Pathological fractures may occur due to *osteoporosis, especially steroid induced, metastatic tumors, primary tumors (benign and malignant), Paget's disease, and bone lesions of hyperparathyroidism and osteogenesis imperfecta* (Fig. 2.49).

Phases of Healing of Bone Fractures due to Trauma

- *Inflammatory phase:* It starts 4–5 days after bone fracture. Inflammatory cells degrade the debris. It is followed by early organization by proliferation of fibroblasts and new capillaries formation.
- *Repair phase:* Procallous formation: It consists of fibrocartilaginous callus. Early bone regeneration by osteoblasts occurs after one week of fracture. Provisional callus bridges the gap-first, osteoid tissue (may include cartilage), then woven bone.
- *Mature callous formation:* It occurs from 3 weeks onwards. Cortical gap is healed by ossification. Osteoclastic and osteoblastic activity is proceeding.
- *Remodeling of callus:* Definite weeks to months. Osteoblasts and osteoclasts are active. Lamellar bone is laid down.
- *Final reconstruction:* It occurs months later. Fracture site may be almost invisible.

Complications of Bone Fracture

- *Fat embolism:* It may occur in fracture of the long bones due to entry of fat from the marrow cavity into the torn ends of veins.
- *Infection:* If the overlying skin is breached in any way, the fracture is compound, the risk of infection is greatly increased; this is an important adverse factor in the healing process.
- *Other complications:* These include *excess callus formation, delayed union of fracture, malunion (angulation and shortening) of fracture.* Non-union of fracture and *pseudoarthrosis.* Non-union occurs if soft tissues such as muscle or fat are interposed between the severed ends. Fibrous union results from excessive movement, infection and ischemia.

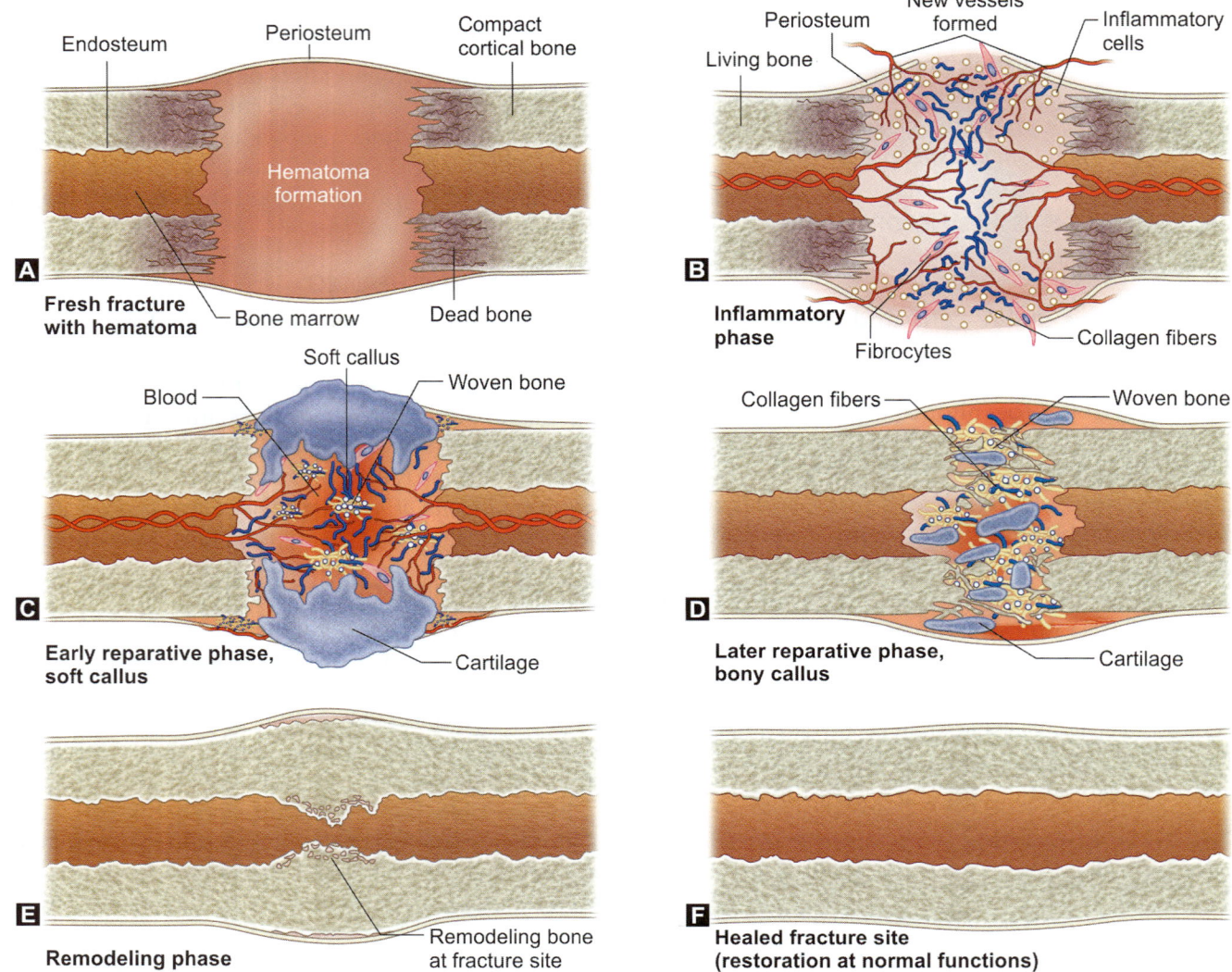

Fig. 2.49: Healing of bone fracture. (A) Hematoma is formed in recent fracture; (B) During inflammatory phase (2–7 days), neovascularization, early fibrosis and woven bone occur; (C) during reparative phase (2–6 weeks), there is gradual decrease in inflammation and granulation tissue. Soft callus is formed. Abundant woven bone is formed. Cartilage appears at the periphery; (D) During later reparative phase, bony callus is formed; (E) During remodeling phase in later months, linear stress causes alignment of new bone and formation of compact bone joining new bone to original bone; (F) Healed bone is formed.

Factors Influencing Fracture Healing

- *Local causes:* These include infection (open fractures), inadequate blood supply, and avascular necrosis of head of femur and scaphoid, interposition of soft tissues, type of fracture, type of bone, large hematoma and imperfect immobilization.
- *General causes:* These include age, malnutrition, diabetes mellitus, decreased calcium and phosphate levels and systemic infections.

EXTRACELLULAR MATRIX (ECM)

Spaces between cells are filled with extracellular matrix (ECM). Epithelial cells rest on a dense sheet of ECM called the basement membrane. Mesenchymal cells are surrounded by a diffuse ECM. Extracellular matrix plays an important role in tissue repair (Figs 2.50 and 2.51).

Extracellular matrix is *essential for wound healing*, which provides *framework for cell migration, cell shape, gene expression* and *differentiation*. It also participates in *angiogenesis* and *maintenance* of correct polarity for the *re-assembly of multicellular structures*. Actions of extracellular matrix are shown in Table 2.51.

Composition of ECM: ECM consists of structural fibrous glycoproteins and amorphous ground substance. Structural fibrous glycoproteins are composed of collagen fibers, fibronectin, laminin, and elastin. These reinforce the ground substance. Amorphous ground substance is a gel-like material that absorbs water.

Inflammation, Tissue Healing and Repair

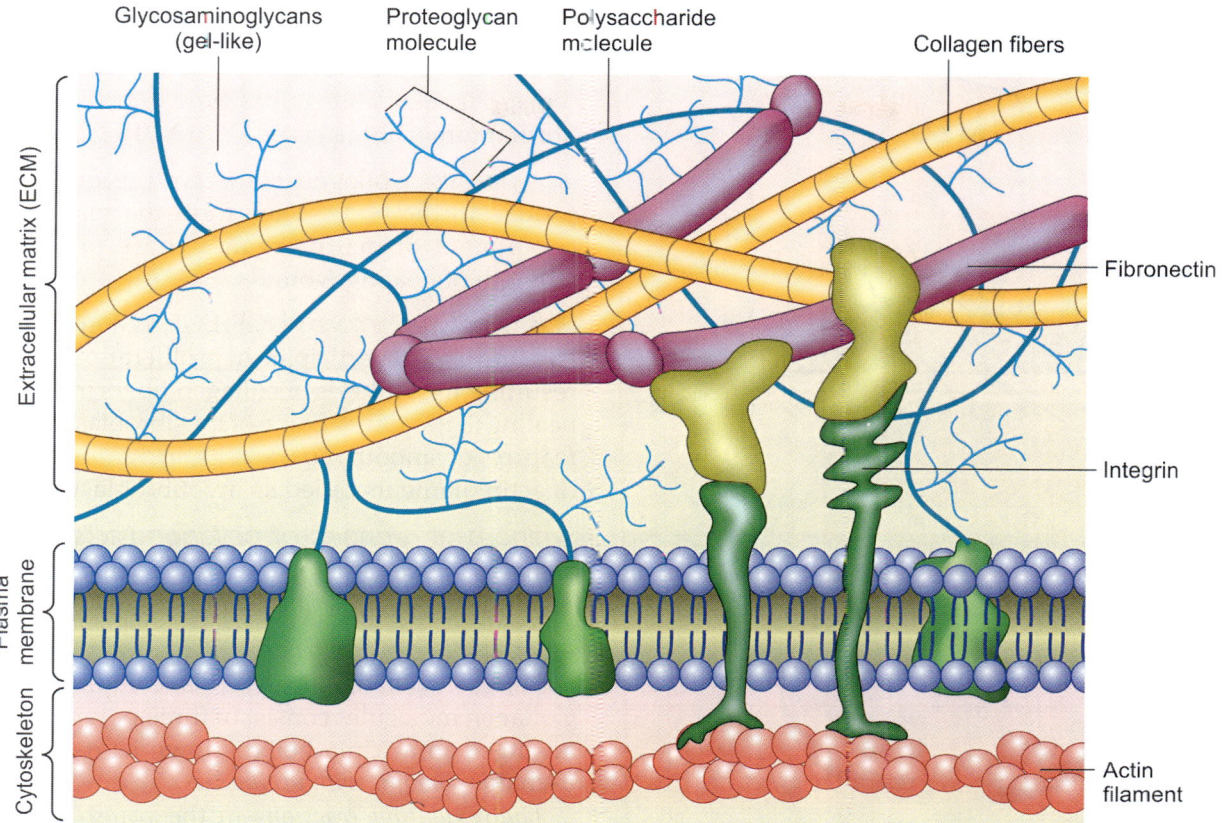

Fig. 2.50: Composition of extracellular matrix (ECM). ECM consists of *structural fibrous glycoproteins* and amorphous ground substance. *Structural fibrous glycoproteins* are composed of collagen fibers, fibronectin, laminin, and elastin. These reinforce the ground substance. *Amorphous ground substance* is a gel-like material composed of glycosaminoglycans (*hyaluronic acid, chondroitin sulfate, heparin, and heparin sulfate*) and proteoglycans (carbohydrate and proteins). Both epithelial and mesenchymal cells interact with extracellular matrix via integrins.

Table 2.51: Actions of extracellular matrix

Parameters	Actions of extracellular matrix
Mechanical support	Cell anchorage Cell migration Maintenance of cell integrity
Control of growth	Regulation of cell proliferation by signaling mechanism via cellular receptors of the integrin family
Maintenance of differentiation	Regulation of differentiation of the cells in tissues via acting cell surface integrin
Scaffoldings for tissue renewal	Regeneration of labile and stable cells if intact ECM Scar formation due to disruption of ECM
Establishment of tissue microenvironment	Forming boundary between epithelial cells and underlying connective tissue
Storage of regulatory molecules	Storage of growth factors in ECM during regeneration of cells at injured site

Structural Fibrous Glycoproteins

Structural fibrous glycoproteins consist of 3 major fibrous glycoproteins: *Collagen fibers, fibronectin and laminin.*

- *Collagen fibers:* Collagen fibers are the *most abundant glycoprotein in humans* (>25% total protein). There are numerous genes that encode different collagen molecules. Mnemonic, collagen fibers go from hard to soft types. These are distributed in various organs.

- *Fibronectin:* It is a fibrous protein participating in motility. It has binding sites for cells and other ECM proteins. *It links cells to the ECM. Sequence of fibronectin such as arginine, glycine, and aspartate binds to cells avidly.*

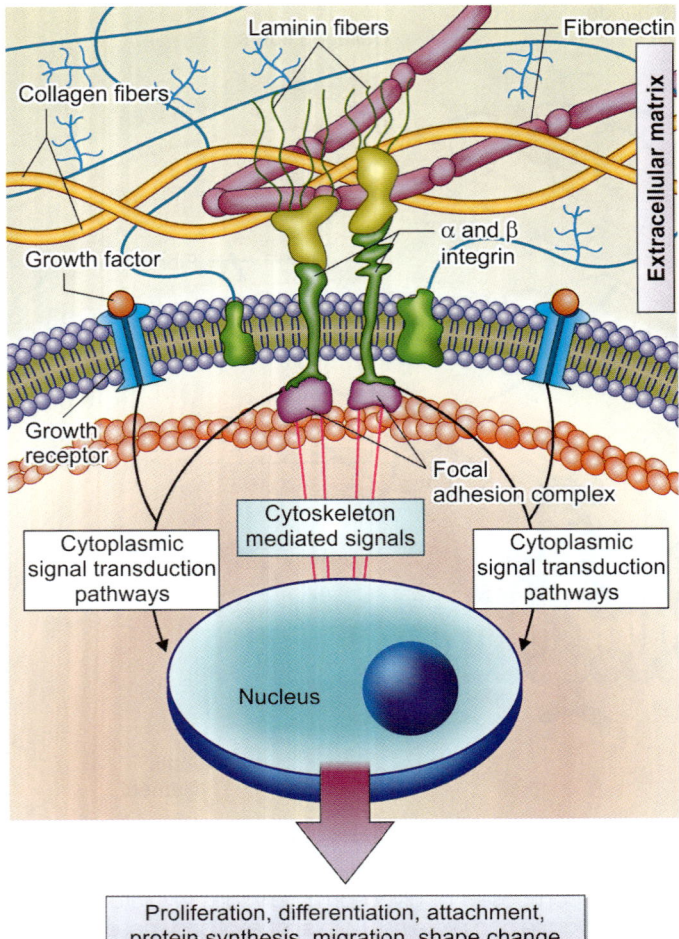

Fig. 2.51: Mechanisms by which ECM components and growth factors interact and activate signaling pathways. Integrins bind to cytoskeleton proteins and mediate nuclear signaling. Growth factors bind to cell receptors and activate signal transduction pathways. These signaling from ECM components and growth factors produce various responses such as proliferation, locomotion and differentiation.

- *Laminin:* It is abundant in *basement membranes* where they *promote adhesion* of many types of cells. Laminin present participates in attachment of endothelial and visceral cells to glomerular basement membrane.

Amorphous Ground Substance

Amorphous ground substance is a gel-like material comprising glycosaminoglycans and proteoglycans that absorbs water and sodium. They also bind and selectively release growth factors.

- *Glycosaminoglycans:* The most abundant glycosaminoglycans are *hyaluronic acid, chondroitin sulfate, heparin, and heparin sulfate.*
- *Proteoglycans:* Proteoglycans are *ground substance* of connective tissues consisting of carbohydrate (>50% carbohydrate) with some proteins.

COLLAGEN FIBERS

Collagen may be fibrillar or non-fibrillar (amorphous) types. Fibrillar collagen is type I, II, III; while non-fibrillar (amorphous) type IV to XVIII (Table 2.52).

Biosynthesis: Collagen fibers are the most abundant protein in the body. They form the major structural component of many organs. These provide tensile strength of healing wounds.

Role of growth factors: PDGF, EGF, TGF-α, FGF-β, IGF-1, IL-1 and TGF-β participate in proliferation of fibroblasts resulting in synthesis of collagen fibers in early wound healing (3 to 5 days). Some of the fibroblasts also acquire features of smooth muscle cells, including the presence of actin filaments called as myofibroblasts.

Synthesis of α-chains of collagen fibrils: DNA sends signal to messenger RNA, where splicing occurs, where α-chains of collagen fibrils are formed.

Assembly of collagen fibrils: Structural unit of collagen is tropocollagen (collagen fibrils) comprising α-chains. Collagen molecules consist of three polypeptide chains arranged in a triple helix, known as α-chains. These α-chains *combine with proline.*

Hydroxylation reactions in the rough endoplasmic reticulum *convert proline to hydroxyproline;* and *lysine to hydrolysine.* Ascorbic acid is required in these hydroxylation reactions. It leads to assembly of triple helix of α-chains.

Stabilization of triple helix of α-chains: Hydroxyproline residues produce bonds that stabilize the triple helix in the tropocollagen molecule.

Cross linkage of triple helix α-chains: Transportation of triple helix α-chains through Golgi apparatus results in formation of true fibrils in extracellular space.

- *Oxidation:* Oxidation of hydroxylysine by lysyl oxidase (MMP enzyme) results in cross linkage of α-chains occurs. *Lysyl oxidase is a metalloproteinase enzyme containing copper.* Fibrils are arranged in *quarter stagger* mode to form insoluble fibers. *Inhibition of lysine oxidation* results in malformation of skeleton, blood vessels seen in *Marfan's syndrome.*
- *Cross-linking:* Cross-linkage of collagen fibrils gives *structural stability to tropocollagen.* These are relatively *resistant to general proteases; slow remodeling by specific collagenases.* Decreased cross-linking (e.g. *vitamin C deficiency*) reduces the tensile strength of collagen. In vitamin C deficiency, the structurally weakened collagen is responsible for a bleeding diathesis (e.g. *bleeding into skin and joints*) and poor wound healing. Decreased cross-linking with *advancing age* leads to *decreased elasticity of skin, joints, and blood vessels.*

Table 2.52: Collagen fibrils and their distribution

Collagen fibrils	Property	Distribution	Genetic disorders
Fibrillar collagen			
Type I	Greatest tensile strength	Bones, tendons and skin (90%)	Osteogenesis imperfecta; Ehlers-Danlos syndrome; Arthrocalasis I
Type II	Thin collagen fibrils	Cartilage (50%) and vitreous humor	Achondrogenesis type II
Type III	Thin collagen fibrils	Blood vessels, uterus, skin (10%) and granulation tissue	Vascular Ehlers-Danlos syndrome
Type V	Amorphous fibrils	Cell surfaces, hair and placenta	Classical Ehlers-Danlos syndrome
Type IX	Amorphous fibrils	Soft tissue, blood vessels, cartilage, intervertebral discs	Stickler syndrome; Multiple epiphyseal dysplasias
Collagen fibrils in glomerular basement membrane			
Type IV	Amorphous fibrils	Basement membranes (glomerular basement membrane) and basal lamina	Alport's syndrome
Distribution of collagen fibrils in other tissues			
Type VI	Amorphous microfibrils	Various organs	Bethlem myopathy
Type VII	Anchoring fibrils at dermal-epidermal junctions	Skin	Dystrophic epidermolysis bullosae
Type IX	Amorphous microfibrils	Cartilage and intervertebral disc	Multiple epiphyseal dysplasias
Type XVII	Transmembrane collagen	Skin	Benign atrophic generalized epidermolysis bullosae
Type XV, XVIII	Endostatin-forming collagen	Endothelial cells	Knobloch syndrome Type XVIII collagen

Ehlers-Danlos syndrome (EDS) is characterized by defects of type I and type III collagen synthesis and structure. Clinical findings include *hypermobile joints, aortic dissection* (most common cause of death), bleeding into the skin (*ecchymosis*), rupture of the bowel, and poor wound healing.

ELASTIN, FIBRILLIN AND ELASTIC FIBERS

Blood vessels, lungs, skin and *uterus* require elasticity to perform functions. Collagen fibers provide tensile strength to the tissues. On the other hand elastic fibers can stretch up to 1.5 times their length and snap back to their original length when relaxed.

Composition

Elastic fibers consist of a central core made of elastin, surrounded by network of fibrils. Elastic fibers are synthesized by fibroblasts and smooth muscle cells in arteries. *Substantial quantity of elastin is found in aorta, skin, ligaments and uterus.*

Synthesis

Elastic fibers are derived from elastic microfibril. *The microfibril consists of numerous proteins such as microfibrillar associated glycoproteins, fibrillin and fibrullin.* Elastic fibers are also derived from amorphous elastin. Microfibrils scaffold and organize the deposition of amorphous elastin. These also influence the availability of active TGF-β in the ECM. *Genetic defect in synthesis of fibrillin causes Marfan's syndrome.* Inhibition of lysine oxidation results in malformation of skeleton, blood vessels seen in Marfan's syndrome.

CELL ADHESION PROTEINS

Adhesion molecules enable cells to contact and specifically interact with each other in multicellular organisms. Specialized *cell-cell and cell-matrix interactions permit communication between cells* and their surrounding environment necessary for development and functional activity. Several different families of receptors mediate these interactions. These are three categories of adhesion molecules described as follows.

- *Cell junctions:* These are formed slowly but generate very stable and durable connections such as tight junctions, desmosomes, and gap junctions.
- *Cell surface adhesion molecules:* These include *selectins, immunoglobulin-like cell adhesive molecules, and integrins*. Their function is adhesion of cells to extracellular matrix or to neighboring cells, rather than cell activation. These play an important role in *acute inflammation*. These ensure *arrival of cells to the required locations*. These are selective and quickly formed. Adhesions are relatively weak in comparison to cell junctions.
- *Substrate adhesion molecules:* These consist of *extracellular matrix molecules* and *matched receptors*. These are expressed on the cell surface.

FAMILIES OF ADHESION MOLECULES

Several different families of receptors mediate these interactions. The families of cell adhesion molecules include *selectins, integrins, immunoglobulin (Ig) super family members and cadherins*.

Members of these adhesion receptor families are critical in embryonic development, differentiation, migration, inflammation, and wound healing and cancer metastases.

Selectin Family

Selectins are cell adhesion molecules mediating initial adhesion of leukocytes (primarily neutrophils) to endothelial cells at sites of inflammation.

- *E selectins (CD62E):* These are stored in *Weibel-Palade bodies* of resting endothelial cells. Upon activation, E selectins are redistributed along the luminal surface of the endothelial cells, where they *mediate the initial adhesion and rolling of leukocytes*.
- *P selectins (CD62P):* These are stored in *Weibel-Palade bodies* of endothelium and platelet α-granules, relocate to the plasma membrane after stimulation by mediators such as *histamine and thrombin*.
- *L selectins (CD62L):* These are expressed on neutrophils. These bind to *endothelial mucin-like molecules such as GlyCam-1*.

Lectins

Lectins are expressed on cells and endothelial cells. Glycosyl transferases are lectin-related cell adhesive molecules (CAMs). These transfer monosaccharides to an oligosaccharide chain on an adjacent cell.

Immunoglobulin Family Adhesion Proteins

Intercellular adhesion molecules such as ICAM-1 and ICAM-2 are expressed on the endothelial cells. These bind to integrin expressed on leukocytes.

Integrins

Integrins contain 2-α and 2-β chains. These belong to immunoglobulin supergene family. α-chain has ligand binding sites for Ca^{++} and Mg^{++} which are needed for integrin to adhere. *During inflammation, integrin participates in adhesion of leukocytes to vascular endothelium leading to chemotaxis of leukocytes to the injury site.* Integrin family is shown in Table 2.53.

Cadherins

Cadherin participate in forming stable adhesion. These are expressed on all cells forming solid organs.

- *Cadherin family:* It includes cadherin E, P, N and L members. E-cadherin is present in desmosomes of *epithelial cells*. P-cadherin is expressed in *placenta*. N-cadherin is present in *neural tissue*. L-cadherin is demonstrated in *liver*.
- *Actions:* In adults, cadherins are responsible for *tight cell-to cell associations within tissues*. These are *intimately associated with the cytoskeleton*, interacting via other proteins with both *microfilaments* and *intermediate filaments*. These *mediate homotype interactions* in *zonula adherens, tight junctions, gap junctions,* and *desmosomes*.
- *Degradation:* Cadherins are rapidly degraded by proteases in the absence of Ca^{++}.

Cadherin-catenin Linkage

Catenin family includes α-catenin, β-catenin and γ-catenin. The β-catenin is a membrane protein associated with cell adhesion molecules. These link cadherin to the cytoskeleton. If this cadherin-catenin

Table 2.53: Integrin family

Integrins	Mechanism of actions
$β_1$ integrin	Binding of cells to extracellular matrix
	β-chain using CD29
$β_2$ integrin (LeuCAMs)	Leukocyte adhesion to endothelium during inflammation
	β-chain using CD18
$β_3$ integrin (cytoadhesions)	Interactions of platelets and neutrophils at inflammatory sites or sites of vascular damage

linkage is disturbed, cadherin does not work. It leads to disruption of embryonic development especially of brain neural tissue.

GLYCOSAMINOGLYCANS AND PROTEOGLYCANS

Amorphous ground substance is a *gel-like material comprising glycosaminoglycans and proteoglycans that absorbs water*. These are covalently *linked to core proteins*. The core proteins have many side chains of glycosaminoglycans. *They attract Na^+ and water* and expand to form gels that occupy space between cells. They also bind and selectively release growth factors.

Glycosaminoglycans

These are long unbranched polysaccharide chains composed of repeating units of disaccharides. One sugar is an amino sugar (N-acetyl glucosamine) and the other is glucuronic acid. The most abundant glycosaminoglycans are hyaluronic acid, chondroitin sulfate, heparin, and heparin sulfate.

Proteoglycans

Proteoglycans consist of carbohydrate (>50% carbohydrate) with some protein. These are *ground substance* of connective tissues. These possess an extracellular and intracellular domain. These interact with collagen, fibronectin, and other ECM molecules. These are categorized into *sulfated* and *non-sulfated*. Sulfated proteoglycans include heparin sulfate, keratin sulfate and chondroitin sulfate (A, B, and C). Hyaluronic acid is example of non-sulfated proteoglycans.

MECHANISM OF TISSUE REPAIR

Tissue repair involves five mechanisms: Removal of injured tissue by inflammation, angiogenesis, migration and proliferation of fibroblasts, scar formation and remodeling of connective tissue. Organization refers to replacement of dead tissue or hematoma by granulation tissue. It is seen in *hematoma (wound and bone fracture), thrombi, infarcts and fibrinous exudates*.

Removal of Injured Tissue

In early stage of injury, *polymorphonuclear cells are recruited to the site of injury*. Chemical mediators released by injured cells, plasma proteins, tissue macrophages, mast cells, platelets and endothelial cells increase vascular permeability resulting in inflammatory exudates. Polymorphonuclear cells liquefy the injured tissue and remove dead cellular debris.

Stages of Wound Healing

There are two stages in wound healing: Proliferative stage and progressive fibrosis. Proliferative stage comprises formation of granulation tissue. Angiogenesis is regulated by various angiogenic cytokines (e.g. *VEGF, FGF*). Fibrosis occurs by various pro-fibrotic cytokines (e.g. *TGF-β, PDGF*).

PROLIFERATIVE PHASE

In proliferative stage, specific cells migrate, proliferate and fill the gap created by tissue destruction. It occurs by formation of granulation tissue and angiogenesis.

Formation of Granulation Tissue

Granulation tissue is soft, pink and highly vascular young immature tissue seen in chronic inflammation. It fills defects created by liquefaction of cellular debris. It serves as the foundation for scar tissue development. Due to presence of numerous, newly developed capillaries, granulation tissue is fragile. These capillaries bleed easily and permit leakage of plasma proteins and white blood cells into the tissues.

Pathogenesis

- *Formation of granulation tissue:* Granulation tissue is formed by proliferation of fibroblasts, myofibroblasts delicate collagen fibrils, macrophages and vascular endothelial cells. Capillaries arise from adjacent blood vessels by division of endothelial cells in a process termed angiogenesis. Newly formed blood vessels supply blood to the granulation tissue. Granulation tissue supplies antibacterial antibodies and growth factors.

- *Role of macrophages:* Macrophages synthesize growth factors and remove cellular debris.

- *Scar formation:* If the damage affects deeper layers of tissue, fibroblasts proliferate resulting in synthesis of collagen fibers. Granulation tissue can mature into fibrous tissue (scar formation).

Angiogenesis

Angiogenesis is a process of new blood vessels development from existing blood vessels. It is essential in tissue development, reproduction, and wound healing. Angiogenesis occurs as a result of mobilization of endothelial precursor cells (EPCS) from bone marrow and pre-existing vessels at the site of injury (Fig. 2.52).

Mechanism

Bone marrow *endothelial precursor cells (EPCS) migrate to a site of injury* and proliferate to form a mature network by linking with pre-existing vessels. *Endothelial cells from pre-existing blood vessels become motile and proliferate to form capillary sprouts*. Regardless of the mechanism of

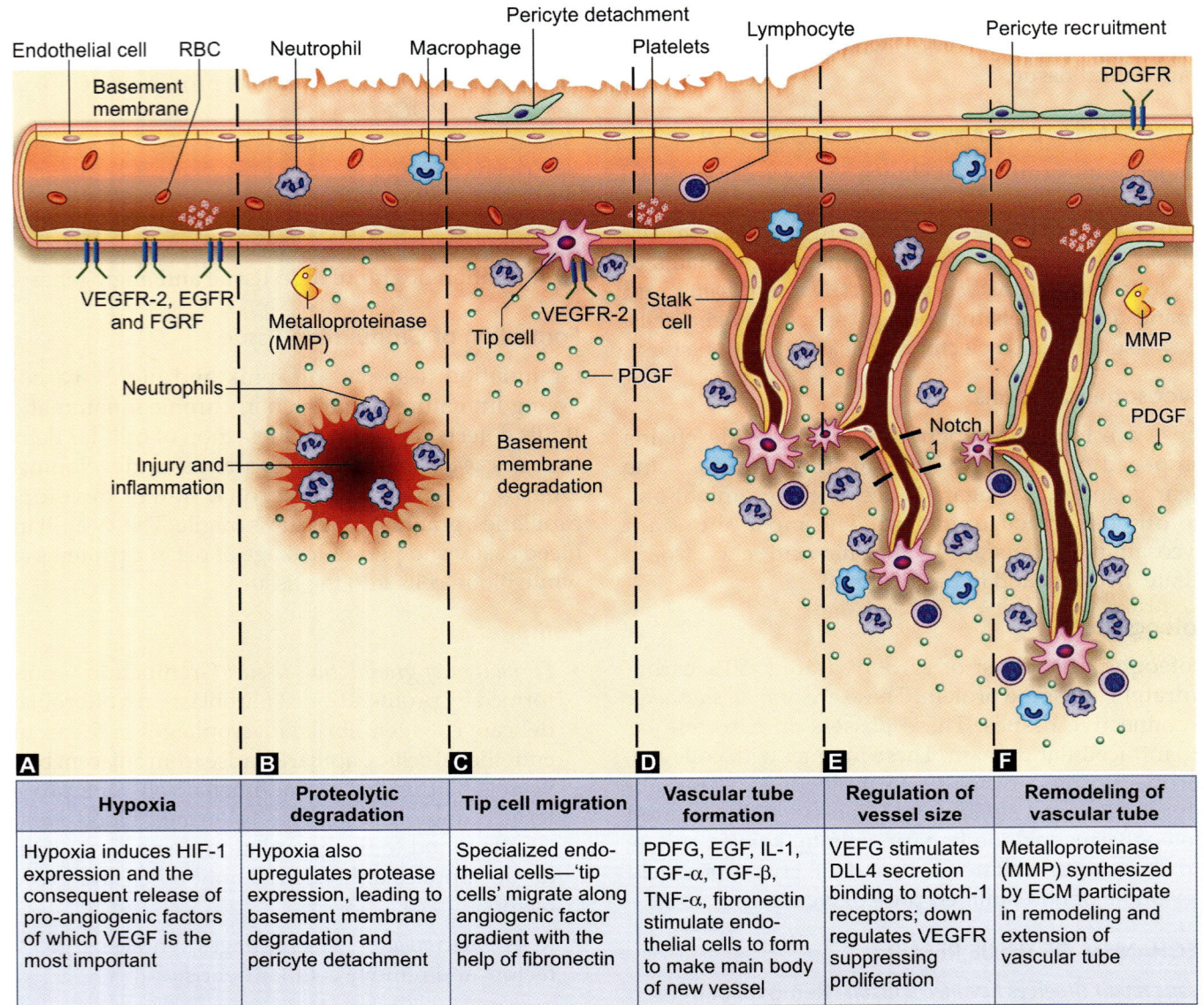

Fig. 2.52: Angiogenesis. Endothelial precursor cells are mobilized from bone marrow and pre-existing capillaries. Endothelial cells become motile, proliferate to form capillary sprouts. It is followed by maturation (stabilization) by recruitment of pericytes and smooth muscle to form periendothelial layer. Blockage of DLL4 leads to sprouting, proliferation of endothelial cells, decrease in vascular lumen size and organization. Blockage of VEGF leads to decrease in sprouting, proliferation of endothelial cells, decrease in vascular lumen size and organization.

angiogenesis, *vessel maturation requires the recruitment of pericytes and smooth muscle cells to form the periendothelial layer*. Mechanism of angiogenesis by following steps is described below:

- *Sprouting of vessel:* It occurs by *separation of pericytes. Notch signaling pathway regulates sprouting and branching of new vessels.* Growth factors synthesized by extracellular proteins participate in this process.
- *Chemotaxis of endothelial cells:* Fibronectin participates in *recruitment (migration) of these endothelial cells* toward the site of tissue injury.
- *Proliferation of endothelial cells:* Endothelial cells proliferate just behind the leading front (tip) of the migrating cells. This function is mediated by growth factors such as *PDGF, EGF, TG-α, FGF-β, fibronectin, IL-1 and TNF-α*.

These growth factors act on VEGF-1, VEFG-2 and VEGF-3 receptors. *Targeted mutations in these receptors result in lack of angiogenesis.*

- *Remodeling and extension of the vascular tube:* Metalloproteinases synthesized by extracellular matrix degrade ECM to permit remodeling and extension of the vascular tube.
- *Formation of mature vessels: Recruitment of periendothelial cells to form the mature blood vessels.* This function is mediated by proteins such as *fibronectin, VEGF-A,*

VEGF-B, VEGF-C, VEGF-D, angiopoietin-1 and angiopoietin-2. VEGF-C especially induces *hyperplasia of lymphatic vasculature*. Targeted mutations in these VEGFs result in lack of angiogenesis.

- *Modulation:* TGF-β modulates the repair process by inhibiting proliferation of endothelial cells and migration. It also suppresses deposition of basement membrane.

Regulation of Angiogenesis by ECM Proteins

Angiogenesis is regulated by extracellular matrix proteins by following mechanisms:

- *Formation and maintenance:* Integrin α and β play key role in formation and maintenance of angiogenesis.
- *Destabilization of cell matrix interactions:* ECM protein ssuch as *thrombospondin-1, SPARC and tenacin* destabilize cell-matrix interactions promote angiogenesis.
- *Tissue modeling during endothelial invasion:* ECM proteins such as *metalloproteinases and plasminogen activators* are essential in tissue remodeling during endothelial invasion. These ECM proteins cleave ECM proteins and release VEGF and FGF-2 leading to induction of angiogenesis. On the other hand, ECM protein such as endostatin inhibits proliferation of endothelial cells and angiogenesis.

Interactions between Notch and VEGF

VEGF induces delta 4 (DLL4) notch that inhibits VEGFR signaling.

- *Blockage of DLL4:* It leads to sprouting, proliferation of endothelial cells, decrease in vascular lumen size and organization.
- *Blockage of VEGF:* It leads to decrease in sprouting, proliferation of endothelial cells, decrease in vascular lumen size and organization.

PROGRESSIVE FIBROSIS

Steps in scar formation involve angiogenesis, deposition of connective tissue and remodeling.

Collagen type III fibers synthesis reaches a peak within 5 to 7 days and continues for several weeks, depending on wound size.

- *Decreased cellularity:* As the amount of collagen in granulation tissue progressively increases, the tissue becomes gradually *less vascular* and *less cellular*. Cellularity and edema is diminished with formation of *an avascular, hypocellular scar*.
- *Increased deposition of ECM:* The fibroblasts assume a more synthetic property. Therefore, there is *increased deposition of extracellular matrix*. It leads to *formation of scar*.

Remodeling of Wound

After deposition of extracellular matrix, the connective tissue in the scar continues to be modified and remodeled. Collagen fibers become denser and align according to force as seen in muscle, tendon or ligament. It is known as *remodeling*. Remodeling increases the tensile strength of scar tissue.

Metalloproteinases (MMPs)

- *Synthesis:* Metalloproteinases (collagenases) are synthesized by polymorphonuclear cells, macrophages, fibroblasts, synovial cells and some epithelial cells.
- *Actions:* These degrade collagen fibers III and replace with type I collagen fibers, increasing tensile strength to approximately 80% of the original. Metalloproteinases cut triple helix collagen into two unequal fragments, which are susceptible to digestion by other macrophages.

Wound Contraction

Proliferation of myofibroblasts causes progressive wound contraction and deformity. These cells are bound together by tight junctions *forming syncytia*. These cells express *smooth muscle actin, desmin,* and *vimentin*. By contrast, fibroblasts tend to be solitary cells, surrounded by collagen fibers. A mature scar is composed of *type I collagen fibers*. Further changes in scars occur such as *cicatrization*—a late diminution in size resulting in *deformity, calcification* and *ossification*.

Cell-matrix Interactions

- *Fibronectin:* It attaches fibroblasts to collagen fibers.
- *Chondronectin:* It *binds chondrocytes to type II collagen*, the matrix of cartilage.
- *Laminin:* It binds epithelial cells to type IV collagen of basement membranes.
- *Osteonectin:* It binds hydroxyapatite and calcium ions to type I collagen (bone matrix) and initiates mineralization.

CUTANEOUS WOUND HEALING

Wound healing occurs by primary or secondary intention. Surgical clean incised wound with closely apposed margins heals by primary intention. An open or excised wound (healing by secondary intention).

There are no fundamental differences between these two types, they merely differ in the degree to which the various stages apply (Fig. 2.53). Growth factors, enzymes and other factors regulating tissue healing and repair are shown in Table 2.54.

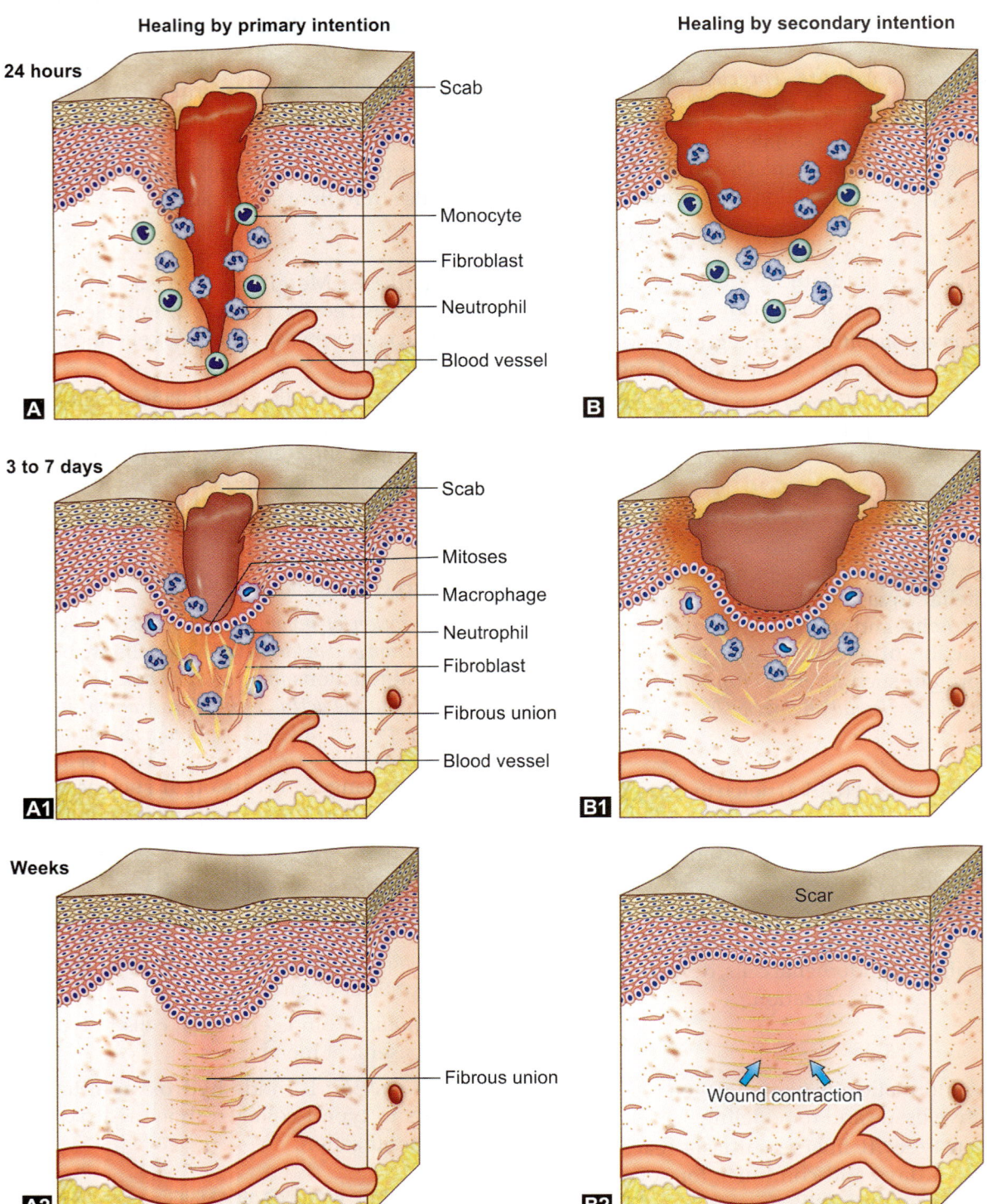

Fig. 2.53: Wound healing. (A) Healing of skin wound by primary intention—it occurs in surgical wound with closely opposed edges with minimum tissue loss. Healing requires only minimal proliferation of cells and neovascularization with formation of small scar; (B) Healing of wound by secondary intention—it occurs in wound with far apart edges with substantial tissue loss. This wound requires contraction, extensive proliferation of cells and neovascularization. Re-epithelization of wound starts from the margins with deposition of collagen fibers and granulation tissue leading to resorption of granulation tissue and formation of large scar.

Stages of wound healing: Acute inflammatory response begins at the margins of wound. Hardening of the surface occurs by formation of scab. Macrophages participate in removal of necrotic debris. It is followed by epidermal proliferation, contraction of the wound, progressive increase in collagen fibers, loss of vascularity, and shrinkage of the scar. The primary function of the skin is to serve as a protective barrier against the environment.

Table 2.54: Growth factors, enzymes and other factors regulating tissue healing and repair

Growth factors and cytokines	Functions
EGF, TNF-α, HGF	Proliferation of epithelial cells
PDGF, FGF-β, TGF-β	Chemotaxis of monocytes
	Migration of fibroblasts
PDGF, FGF-β, TGF-β, EGF	Fibroblasts proliferation
PDGF	Collagen synthesis
Lysyl oxidase	Collagen cross-linking and maturation
TGF-β	Inhibition of collagen secretion
ECM proteins such as *thrombospondin-1, SPARC and tenacin destabilizing* cell-matrix interactions	Promotion of angiogenesis
Integrin α and β	Formation and maintenance of angiogenesis
VEGF-A, VEGF-B, VEGF-C, VEGF-D, angiopoietin-1 and angiopoietin-2, fibronectin, TGF-β	Maturation of blood vessels during angiogenesis
ECM protein such as endostatin	Inhibiting proliferation of endothelial cells and angiogenesis
PDGF, FGF, EGF, EGF, TNF-β, TGF-β	Synthesis of collagenases
ECM proteins such as metalloproteinases (MMP-1, MMP-2, MMP-3, MMP-13)	Tissue remodeling by movement of surface and stromal cells

Healing by Primary Intention

Healing by primary intention occurs in *clean surgical superficial skin wounds* with *closely apposed edges and minimal tissue loss*. Normally, maturation of the epidermis requires an intact layer of basal cells that are in direct contact with one and another. Disruption of this contact *activates basal cells* which results in *migration, proliferation* and *epithelialization of skin wound*.

Contact Inhibition of Growth and Motility

When epithelial continuity is re-established, migration and cell division cease, and the epidermis resumes its normal cycle of maturation and shedding. This process of epithelial growth regulation is referred to as *contact inhibition of growth and motility*. Such a wound requires only minimal cell proliferation and neovascularization to heal, and the result is a small scar.

Healing in Surgical Wound

Suturing of apposed edges by sutures used for clean surgical wounds. Surgical clean wound with opposed margins heals by *primary intention*. Epithelial regeneration predominates over fibrosis. *Healing is fast with minimal scarring/infection.*

There is *regeneration of epidermis*. Dermis undergoes fibrous repair. *Sutures are taken out on 5–10 days after surgery.* This scar provides 10% normal strength. *Minimal scarring gives good strength.* Maturation of scar continues up to 2 years. Risk of trapping infection under skin produces abscess.

Healing by Secondary Intention

Healing by secondary intention *occurs in open gaping or infected wounds*, in which the edges are far apart and in which there is substantial tissue loss. Healing of such wound requires extensive cell proliferation and granulation tissue formation. Resorption of granulation tissue is replaced by deposition of collagen-rich scar tissue.

Examples of open gaping or infected wounds are large *third degree burns, ulcers, extraction, sockets, and external bevel gingivectomies.* Tissues in the third stage burn do not restore to normal owing to *loss of skin, basement membrane and connective tissue infrastructure.*

Mechanism

Extensive proliferation of epithelial cells and formation of granulation tissue are essential for healing of such wound.

- Healing *is slower in open gaping or infected wounds. Fibrosis predominates over epithelial regeneration.* Resorption of granulation tissue is replaced by deposition of collagen-rich scar tissue. There is more inflammatory exudate to *remove necrotic tissue.* Wound contraction is necessary. Initially contraction occurs, then clot dries to form a *scab*.

- There is increased liability to infection in the presence of granulation tissue. Healing takes longer time. It produces a larger scar; not necessarily weaker resulting in fibrosis.

FACTORS AFFECTING WOUND HEALING

FACTORS ADVERSELY AFFECTING WOUND HEALING

- *Type of injurious agent:* Blunt, crushing or tearing of tissues adversely affect wound healing.
- *Retention of debris:* These include foreign bodies, dirt, sutures, hematoma, necrotic tissue and denervation.
- *Poor apposition of wound margins:* Due to poor opposition of wound margins leads to large hematoma formation. It retards wound healing.
- *Impaired circulation:* Molecular oxygen is required for collagen synthesis. It has been shown that even a temporary lack of oxygen due to cardiovascular pathology can result in the formation of less stable collagen fibers.

  Failure of proper collagen synthesis leads to delayed healing and weak scars.
- *Persistent infection:* Wounds in ischemic tissue become infected more frequently. Polymorphonuclear cells and macrophages require oxygen for destruction of microorganisms.

  Staphylococcus aureus is the most common cause of impaired wound healing. Gangrene, suppuration and secondary hemorrhage delay wound healing.
- *Metabolic disorders:* Diabetes mellitus is associated with susceptibility to infection, impaired circulation and increasing tissue levels of glucose.
- *Glucocorticoids excess:* These interfere with collagen formation and thus decrease tensile strength. Glucocorticoids along with antibiotic are occasionally used to prevent scar formation (e.g. bacterial meningitis).
- *Proteins deficiency:* Proteins rich in sulfur amino acids are essential for wound healing. Protein deficiency leads to delayed wound healing.
- *Vitamin C (ascorbic acid):* It is a powerful, biologic reducing agent. It is necessary for the *hydroxylation of proline residues in collagen*.

  Deficiency of vitamin forms an abnormal collagen that lacks tensile strength. Patients with vitamin C deficiency exhibit poor wound healing.
- *Vitamin A:* It stimulates epithelialization, capillary formation, and collagen synthesis. Deficiency of vitamin A retards wound healing.
- *Vitamin K:* It plays an indirect role in wound healing by preventing bleeding disorders. Deficiency of vitamin K retards wound healing.
- *Vitamin B complex:* These are important cofactors in enzymatic reactions that contribute to the wound-healing process. Deficiency of vitamin B-complex retards wound healing.
- *Zinc:* During wound healing, zinc maintains the structural integrity of dermal tissue and mucosal membranes. It also aids in division of cells responsible for creating new tissue.

FACTORS ACCELERATING WOUND HEALING

These include ultraviolet light, administration of anabolic steroids, deoxycorticosterone acetate, and growth hormone, rise in temperature and hyperbaric oxygen.

COMPLICATIONS OF WOUND HEALING

- *Wound rupture:* It occurs due to infections and hematoma formation.
- *Deficient scar formation:* These include wound dehiscence and ulceration.
- *Excessive fibrosis:* It leads to cosmotic scarring, hypertrophic scar and keloid formation. Keloid is formed due to excessive scar formation (hypertrophic scars).

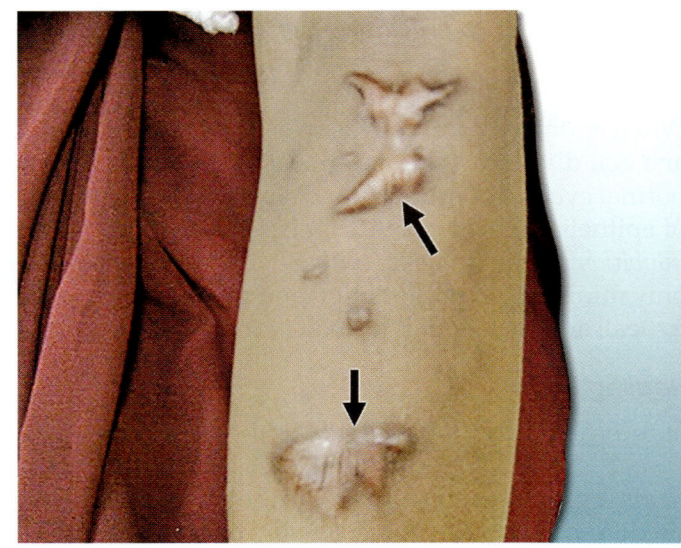

Fig. 2.54: Keloid is an exaggerated response to injury that produces abundant collagenous soft tissue, forming a large nodular scar. It often follows trauma to the skin, such as ear-piercing or surgical wounds. It most often occurs in dark-skinned persons especially of African lineage. It tends to recur after resection (arrows).

Table 2.55: Differences between primary intention and secondary intention

Parameters	Primary intention	Secondary intention
Site	Clean, uninfected surgical incision approximated by surgical sutures	In all natural, open wounds like abscess, surface wounds in road accidents. Infection may be present
Tissue injury	Limited to superficial layer of epithelium and connective tissues	Extensive, causing cells death and necrosis in larger area; larger defect
Inflammatory reaction	Less intense	More intense for clearing large amount of fibrin, necrotic debris and exudate
Granulomatous tissue	Small amount of granulation tissue is formed	Larger amount of granulation tissue is formed to fill large defect
Wound contraction	Absent	Present due to presence of fibroblasts
Scarring	Less scarring	More scarring
Keloid	Absent	May be formed later transforming into squamous cell carcinoma
		Skin appendages destroyed do not regenerate in either type of wound healing

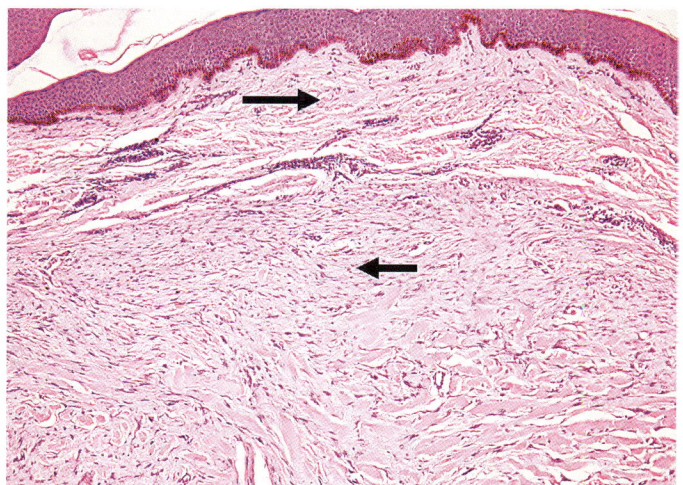

Fig. 2.55: Keloid is composed of dense bundles of collagen in the dermis (arrows) (100X).

It is caused by *excessive synthesis of type III collagen as a result of third degree burns.*

Light microcopy reveals irregular, thick collagen bundles that extend beyond the confines of the original injury (Figs 2.54 and 2.55).

- *Excessive contraction:* Limitation of movements occur due to contractures. Excessive contraction may cause strictures formation of tubular structures.
- *Epidermoid cyst:* Implantation of epidermal cells giving rise to keratin-filled epidermoid cyst.
- *Proud flesh:* The swollen flesh surrounding a healing wound is caused by excessive granulation tissue.
- *Malignant change:* Healed lesion may undergo malignant transformation. Differences between healing by primary and secondary intention are shown in Table 2.55.

CHAPTER 3

Disorders of Hemostasis

Learning Objectives

HYPEREMIA AND CONGESTION
- Overview
- Chronic Venous Congestion

HEMORRHAGE
- Overview
- Examples of Hemorrhage

HEMOSTASIS
- Components of Hemostasis
- Mechanism of Hemostasis
- Control of Hemostasis

THROMBOSIS
- Overview
- Pathogenesis of Thrombosis
- Thrombotic Disorders
- Arterial and Venous Thrombi

EMBOLISM
- Overview
- Thromboembolism
- Etiology of Embolism

INFARCTION
- Overview
- Factors Influencing Infarction
- Type of Infarcts

EDEMA
- Type of Edema Fluid
- Clinical Types of Edema
- Pathophysiology of Edema

SHOCK
- Stages of Shock
- Hypovolemic Shock
- Cardiogenic Shock
- Septic Shock
- Neurogenic Shock
- Anaphylactic Shock

HYPEREMIA AND CONGESTION

OVERVIEW

ACTIVE HYPEREMIA

Hyperemia refers to increased blood supply via capillaries and small vessels in a tissue or organ. Active hyperemia is usually a physiological response to an increased functional demand associated with inflammation.

PASSIVE VENOUS CONGESTION

Passive congestion refers to the engorgement of an organ with venous blood. *Acute passive congestion occurs in shock or sudden right-sided heart failure.* It occurs due to obstruction to venous return or increased back flow from congestive heart failure.

Deep venous thrombosis of the leg veins causes edema of the lower extremity. *Thrombosis of the hepatic*

Disorders of Hemostasis

Table 3.1: Differences between hyperemia and congestion

Parameters	Hyperemia	Congestion
Process	*Active process*	*Passive process*
Blood flow	Increased blood flow due to arteriolar dilatation in inflammation or skeletal muscles during exercise	Blood pooling due to impaired venous blood flow in congestive heart failure or isolated venous obstruction
Edema	*Absent*	*Present*
Gross morphology	Organs with reddish discoloration due to engorgement with oxygenated blood	Organs with blue–red color (cyanosis) due to accumulation of deoxygenated hemoglobin
Light microscopy	Acute pulmonary congestion with engorged capillaries, septal edema and minute intra-alveolar hemorrhage	Chronic pulmonary congestion with alveolar spaces containing numerous hemosiderin laden macrophages, 'heart failure cells' and thickened septa
	Acute liver congestion with distended sinusoids and fatty change	Chronic liver congestion with dilated central vein, distended sinusoids, fatty change progressing to cardiac cirrhosis

veins (Budd-Chiari syndrome) causes chronic passive congestion of the liver. Differences between hyperemia and congestion are shown in Table 3.1.

CHRONIC VENOUS CONGESTION

CHRONIC VENOUS CONGESTION OF LIVER

Long-standing chronic right-sided heart failure increases venous pressure resulting in chronic venous congestion of liver, because hepatic veins drain into inferior vena cava. Pitting edema is seen in lower extremities.

Gross Morphology

Cut surface of the liver can assume an appearance referred to as *nutmeg liver*, with dark red congested centrilobular areas alternating with pale unaffected peripheral portions of the lobules (Fig. 3.1).

Light Microscopy

- The central veins and sinusoids are dilated and congested. Surrounding hepatocytes show brownish-yellow discoloration and fatty change.
- The increased venous pressure leads to dilation of the sinusoids and pressure atrophy of the centrilobular hepatocytes.
- Long-standing chronic passive congestion of liver leads to bridging fibrosis in extreme cases resulting in cardiac cirrhosis (Fig. 3.2).

BUDD-CHIARI SYNDROME

The cause is thrombotic occlusion of the major hepatic veins, resulting in hepatomegaly. It is most often associated with *hepatocellular carcinoma, polycythemia vera or other abdominal tumors.* It may also occur as a complication of pregnancy. Less common causes

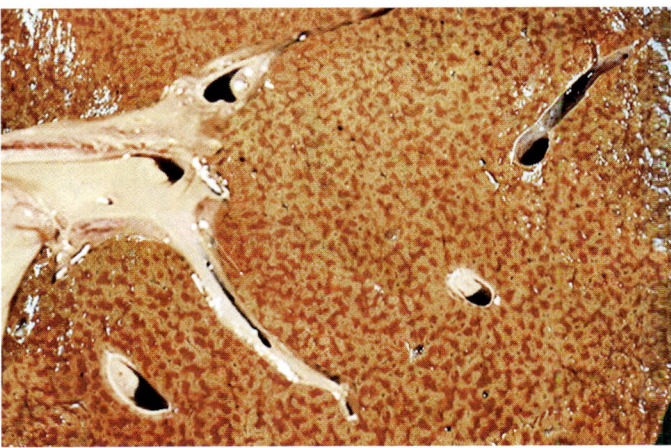

Fig. 3.1: Central venous congestion. Here is an example of a *nutmeg* liver seen with chronic passive congestion of the liver. Note the dark red congested regions that represent accumulation of RBCs in centrilobular regions.

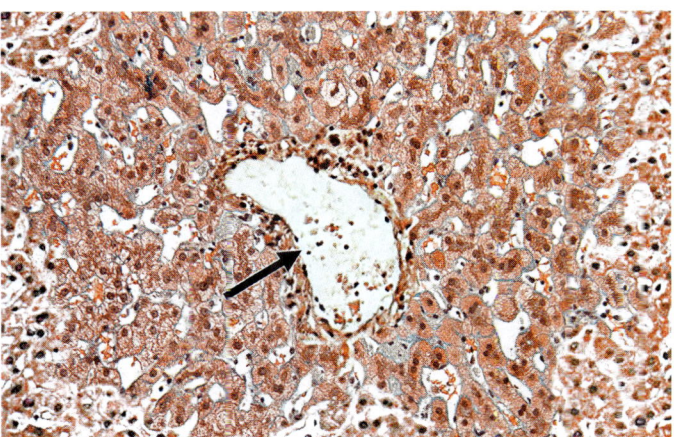

Fig. 3.2: Central venous congestion of liver. It occurs due to a *right-sided* heart failure. Central veins and sinusoids are congested. Hepatocytes at places are showing atrophic changes (arrow) (400X).

include *paroxysmal nocturnal hemoglobinuria, promyelocytic leukemia, protein-C deficiency, protein-S deficiency, antithrombin III deficiency and antiphospholipid autoantibodies* (lupus anticoagulant).

Clinical Features

Patient presents with *ascites, abdominal pain, hepatomegaly*, mild jaundice, edema and eventual hepatic encephalopathy. Acute hepatic failure and death often occur rapidly.

Gross Morphology
Thrombus in the hepatic veins cause obstruction to blood flow to liver leading to venous congestion of the liver (Fig. 3.3).

Light Microscopy
Liver shows severe centrilobular necrosis and hemorrhage as a result of localized obstruction to venous drainage. Rim of hepatocytes in zone 1 shows survival.

CHRONIC VENOUS CONGESTION OF LUNG

Chronic venous congestion of lung is usually caused by *left-sided heart failure*. Left ventricular failure may occur in *acute myocardial infarction, cardiomyopathies, hypertensive, or valvular heart disease (mitral stenosis aortic stenosis in rheumatic heart disease) and left atrial myxoma*. Pulmonary edema refers to intra-alveolar accumulation of fluid. *It is a common complication of left heart failure.*

Pathophysiology

Left ventricular failure causes congestion of alveolar capillaries resulting in rupture and passage of red cells into the alveoli. There is accumulation of transudate in the alveoli. Alveolar macrophages degrade red blood cells and accumulate hemosiderin. These hemosiderin-laden macrophages are called *heart failure cells*. In long-standing congestion, fibrosis of interstitial tissue and hemosiderin deposition result in *brown induration of the lung.*

Light Microscopy
The alveoli in this lung are filled with a smooth to slightly floccular pink material characteristic for pulmonary edema. Capillaries in the alveolar walls are congested with many red blood cells (Figs 3.4 and 3.5).

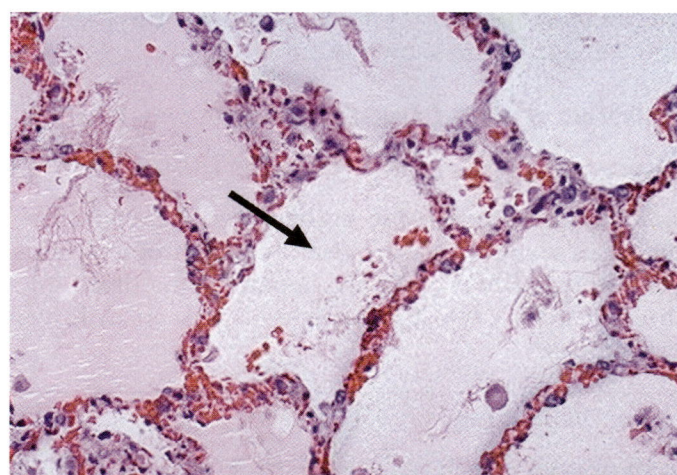

Fig. 3.4: Pulmonary edema. The alveoli in this lung are filled with a smooth to slightly floccular pink material. Alveolar capillaries are congested (arrow) (400X).

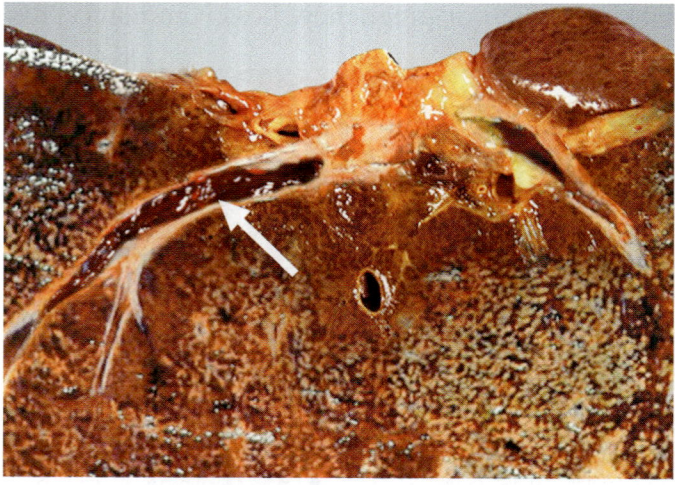

Fig. 3.3: Budd-Chiari syndrome. The liver has been sliced coronally, with the caudate lobe in the middle. Thrombus can be seen in the hepatic veins. This caused obstruction, which resulted in venous congestion of the liver, most marked in the caudate lobe (arrow).

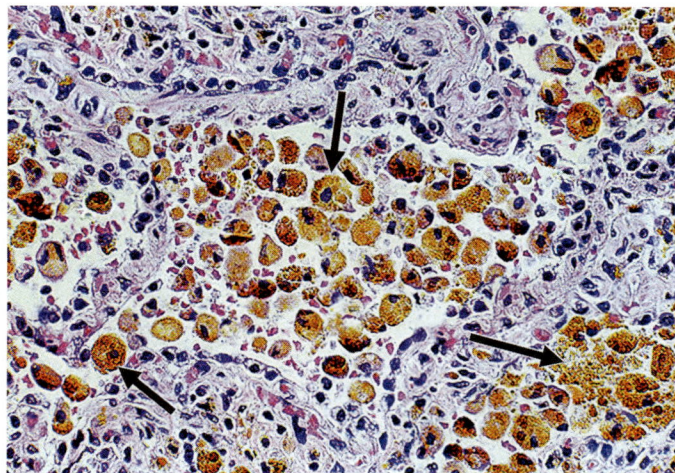

Fig. 3.5: Chronic venous congestion of lung showing heart failure cells laden with hemosiderin due to congestive heart failure (arrows) (400X).

Disorders of Hemostasis

Clinical Features

- *Dyspnea:* Dyspnea is an early symptom from pulmonary congestion. On auscultation, *crackles,* and *wheeze breath sounds are heard.*
- *Orthopnea:* Patient cannot breathe unless sitting up.
- *Cough:* Patient has frothy pink or white sputum.
- *Edema:* Patient develops *pleural effusion* with *hydrothorax.* Reduction in renal perfusion activates renin-angiotensin-aldosterone system and leading to retention of salt and water. Cerebral anoxia is less frequent.
- *Cool moist skin:* Patient has *weak pulse, cool moist skin* as the peripheral vasoconstriction shunts blood to vital organs.

Assay of B-type natriuretic peptide: Assay of B-type natriuretic peptide is elevated in heart failure. Elevated level may aid in the distinction of heart failure from *acute coronary syndrome, bronchial asthma, chronic obstructive pulmonary disease, or pulmonary thromboembolism phenomenon,* which may also present with dyspnea or edema.

CONGESTIVE SPLENOMEGALY

Congestive splenomegaly most often occurs in portal hypertension due to *cirrhosis* and *right-sided cardiac failure with cor pulmonale.* Decreased portal venous drainage in these disorders leads to congestive splenomegaly.

Pathogenesis

The increased portal venous pressure causes *dilatation of sinusoids, with slowing of blood flow from the cords to the sinusoids* that prolongs the exposure of the blood cells to the macrophages, resulting in excessive trapping and destruction (*hypersplenism*). Perivascular hemorrhages result in *organization and formation of Gamna-gandy bodies* (dystrophic calcification).

> **Gross Morphology**
> - Spleen shows irregular tan-white fibrous plaques over the purple capsular surface. This *sugar icing* is termed hyaline perisplenitis.
> - Cut surface of fibrocongestive splenomegaly shows firm and brown fibrotic nodules termed as *Gamna-gandy bodies.*
>
> **Light Microscopy**
> Gamna-gandy body is an organized hemorrhage forming nodule with dystrophic calcification and hemosiderin pigment in spleen (Fig. 3.6).

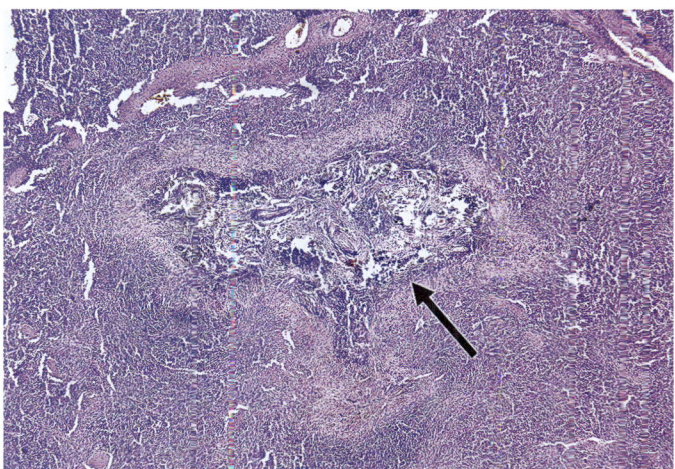

Fig. 3.6: Chronic venous congestion of spleen showing formation of Gamna-gandy bodies as a result of organization of hemorrhage with dystrophic calcification and hemosiderin pigment in spleen (arrow) (400X).

HEMORRHAGE

OVERVIEW

Blood can be released from the circulation to the exterior of the body or into surrounding tissues, hollow organs or body cavities. The most common and obvious cause is trauma. Hematoma and hemorrhage represent extravascular accumulation of blood.

Terminology

- *Erythema:* Erythema is an inflammatory redness of the skin.
- *Purpura:* Purpura is a diffuse superficial hemorrhage in the skin up to 1 cm in diameter.
- *Petechial hemorrhages:* Petechial hemorrhages are *pinpoint hemorrhages* occur in the *skin, mucous membranes (conjunctiva).* These represent the rupture of capillaries or arterioles and occur in conjunction with coagulopathies or vasculitis. In bacterial endocarditis, microemboli from infected cardiac valves may cause rupture of capillaries and arterioles and result in pinpoint hemorrhages under nails known as *Janeway's lesions.*
- *Ecchymosis:* Ecchymosis is a *larger diffuse superficial hemorrhage* in the skin and subcutaneous tissue (a *black and blue* mark). Following hemorrhage, skin shows purple discoloration, turning green and then yellow before resolution. These changes reflect progressive oxidation of bilirubin released from the hemoglobin of degraded erythrocytes. A *black eye* is a good example of an ecchymosis.

- *Hematoma:* Hematoma is localized hemorrhage within a tissue or organ. Hemorrhage into soft tissue; can be merely painful, and fatal, if located in the brain.
- *Hemorrhage in body cavities:* Hemorrhage may occur in the pleural cavity, pericardial sac, peritoneal cavity or a synovial space. Cardiac tamponade occurs when the pressure in the pericardial sac rises to exceed the filling pressure of the heart.
- *Hemopericardium:* Pericardial cavity is filled with hemorrhage due to a ruptured myocardial infarct, dissecting aortic aneurysm due to intimal tear, or trauma. Dissecting aortic aneurysm occurs due to weakening of the aortic media (cystic medial necrosis) or hypertension.
- *Hemarthrosis:* Bleeding into the joint cavity is known as *hemarthrosis*. It is most often caused by hemophilia. Repeated bleeding may cause deformities and may limit the mobility of the joints.
- *Hematemesis:* Hematemesis is presence of blood in vomitus. Massive hematemesis is a frequent cause of death in patients with esophageal varices in alcoholic cirrhosis with portal hypertension. Bleeding occurs due to increased intravascular hydrostatic pressure.
- *Melena:* Melena (black stool) is a symptom of upper gastrointestinal bleeding. Blood from ruptured esophageal varices or a peptic ulcer is partially digested by hydrochloric acid. Hemoglobin is transformed into a black pigment (hematin), which imparts a typical *coffee-ground* color to the stool.
- *Hematochezia:* Hematochezia is passage of bloody stools caused by lower gastrointestinal hemorrhage.
- *Hematobilia:* Hematobilia is bleeding into the biliary passages, as a complication of trauma or neoplasia.
- *Hematocephalus:* Hematocephalus is an intracranial infusion of blood.
- *Hemoptysis:* Hemoptysis is coughing up blood.

EXAMPLES OF HEMORRHAGE

ATHEROMATOUS PLAQUE

Atherosclerosis means hardening (sclerosis) or loss of elasticity of large elastic arteries and medium-sized arteries due to atheromatous plaque formation. Severe atherosclerosis may so weaken the wall of the abdominal aorta that it balloons to form an *aneurysm*, which then may rupture and bleed into the retroperitoneal space. The aneurysms may be demonstrated by ultrasonography and MRI.

MYCOTIC ANEURYSM

Mycotic aneurysm occurs in the *root of aortic arch* and its *descending branches*, due to direct extension from aortic valve endocarditis. Emboli from *infective endocarditis* may involve cerebral blood vessels resulting in hemorrhage into the *basal ganglia*, extending into the *subarachnoid space*.

BERRY ANEURYSM

The most common site of berry aneurysm formation is between the *anterior communicating and the anterior cerebral arteries in the circle of Willis*. These develop as saccular lesions (1.0–1.5) at site of congenital defects in smooth muscle distribution at a branch point of the arterial wall.

These occur in 10 to 15% of patients with adult polycystic kidney disease. Rupture of berry aneurysm causes subarachnoid hemorrhage. Patient presents with history of *severe headache, nuchal rigidity from irritation of the meninges*.

DISSECTING HEMATOMA

Dissecting hematoma of aorta is associated with hypertension or with diseases affecting the vascular media. Risk factors include *hypertension, atheromatous plaque, trauma* to chest, *pregnancy, Marfan's syndrome* (missense mutations of the fibrillin gene 1 located on chromosome 15 causing defective cross linkage), *Ehlers-Danlos syndrome* (defective synthesis of procollagen fibers) and *copper deficiency* (cofactor in lysyl oxidase participating in collagen fibers).

INFECTIONS AND CANCER

Certain infections (e.g. *pulmonary tuberculosis*) and *invasive neoplasms* may erode blood vessels and allow hemorrhage to occur. Malignant tumors that arise in organs (e.g. *ovaries, gastrointestinal tract, or lung*) adjacent to body cavities may shed malignant cells into these spaces. It invariably results in a neoplastic effusion.

VITAMIN C DEFICIENCY

Vitamin C deficiency is associated with capillary fragility and bleeding, owing to a defect in the supporting connective tissue structures.

Vitamin C is essential for *cross linkage of collagen fibrils and gives structural stability to tropocollagen*. Patient presents with bleeding diathesis (e.g. *bleeding into skin and joints*) and poor wound healing.

TRAUMATIC INJURY

Hemorrhage occurs depending on the severity of traumatic injury. Damage to the large blood vessels or heart causes massive hemorrhage with fatal outcome. Blunt trauma to capillaries causes ecchymosis.

Disorders of Hemostasis

LEFT HEART FAILURE

Left ventricular failure leads to congestion of alveolar capillaries resulting in rupture and passage of red cells into the alveoli. There is accumulation of transudate in the alveoli. Alveolar macrophages degrade red blood cells and accumulate hemosiderin. These hemosiderin-laden macrophages are called *heart failure cells*. In long-standing congestion, fibrosis of interstitial tissue and hemosiderin deposition results in brown induration of the lung.

BLEEDING AND COAGULATION DISORDERS

A severe decrease in the number of platelets (*thrombocytopenia*) or deficiency of a coagulation factor (e.g. factor VIII in *hemophilia A*) is associated with spontaneous hemorrhage into various parts of the body without apparent injury.

GASTROINTESTINAL TRACT DISORDERS

A person may exsanguinate into an internal cavity, as in gastrointestinal hemorrhage from a peptic ulcer (*arterial hemorrhage*) or esophageal varices (*venous hemorrhage*). In such cases, fresh blood may fill the entire gastrointestinal tract.

Bleeding into a serous cavity can also result in the accumulation of a large amount of blood, even to the point of exsanguination.

HEMOSTASIS

Hemostasis maintains clot-free blood flow within normal vascular system by *inhibiting activation of platelets, coagulation system and fibrinolytic system*. Interaction of blood vessels, platelets, and coagulation factors induces a rapid and localized hemostatic plug at the site of vascular site.

Thrombosis is opposite to hemostasis. Bleeding and clotting disorders are the result of the failure of hemostatic plug formation mechanisms. Hemostasis as well as thrombosis are regulated by three components: *blood vessel, platelets and coagulation system*. Mechanism of normal hemostasis is described as under.

COMPONENTS OF HEMOSTASIS

VASCULAR ENDOTHELIUM

The blood vessel wall is the first-line of defense in maintaining hemostasis. It is lined by endothelial cells and supported by subendothelial tissue, which maintains the vascular integrity of the structure. *Normal endothelium synthesizes antithrombotic and prothrombotic molecules*. Normal endothelium inhibits aggregation of platelets and coagulation system.

Disruption of normal laminar flow, imbalance between antithrombotic and prothrombotic molecules synthesized by endothelium leads to thrombus formation. Antithrombotic and prothrombotic properties of vascular endothelium are shown in Table 3.2 and Fig. 3.7.

Antithrombotic Properties of Endothelium

Antiplatelet properties: Endothelium *synthesizes prostacyclin* (PGI$_2$), *nitric acid* and *adenosine diphosphatase enzyme*. Prostacyclin (PGI$_2$) and nitric acid are potent vasodilators, which inhibit platelets aggregation. ADP released by platelets play important role in adhesion of platelet to each other.

Endothelium synthesize adenosine diphosphatase enzyme, which degrades ADP resulting in inhibition of platelet adhesion to endothelium.

Synthesis of inhibitors of coagulation: Vascular endothelium synthesizes membrane-associated molecules such as heparin-like molecules, which inhibit coagulation system. *Heparin-like molecules bind to antithrombin III and inactivate thrombin, factor Xa and other clotting factors.*

- *Role of thrombomodulin:* Thrombin is modified by thrombomodulin, found on the surface of endothelial cells. Procoagulant thrombin is converted to anticoagulant thrombin molecule. Modified thrombin activates protein C, which inhibits the activity of V and VIII, so it can no longer convert fibrinogen to fibrin.
- *Role of protein S:* Protein S enhances the activity of protein C resulting in inhibition of the action of factors V and VIII. Tissue factor inhibitor synthesized by endothelium inhibits factor VIIa and factor Xa.

Laminar blood flow: Laminar blood flow dilutes clotting factors and inhibits endothelial cell activation. It increases the inflow of inhibitors of clotting factors.

Prothrombotic Properties of Endothelium

Normal endothelium inhibits platelet adherence and blood clotting. Endothelial injury results in synthesis of prothrombotic molecules such as *von Willebrand factor, tissue factor* and *plasminogen activator inhibitors*.

von Willebrand factor (vWF): It facilitates adhesion of platelets to the underlying subendothelial extracellular matrix.

Table 3.2: Antithrombotic and prothrombotic properties of vascular endothelium

Vascular endothelium	Properties	Molecules	Functions
Antithrombotic factors	Antiplatelet properties	Prostacyclin (PGI$_2$), nitric acid	Potent vasodilator and inhibitor of platelet aggregation
		Adenosine diphosphatase enzyme	Degradation of ADP released by platelets
	Synthesis of inhibitors of coagulation	Heparin-like molecules	Binding to antithrombin III resulting in inactivation of thrombin, factor Xa and other clotting factors
		Thrombomodulin molecules	Conversion of procoagulant thrombin to anticoagulant thrombin molecule that activates protein C
			Protein C inhibits the activity of V, and that can no longer convert fibrinogen to fibrin
	Blood flow	Laminar blood flow	Dilution of clotting factors
			Inhibition of endothelial cell activation
			Increasing the inflow of inhibitors of clotting factors
Prothrombotic factors	Platelets aggregation property	von Willebrand factor (vWF)	Adhesion of platelets to the underlying subendothelial extracellular matrix
	Procoagulant property	Tissue factor (induced by bacterial endotoxins, IL-1 and TNF-α)	Activation of extrinsic coagulation pathway
	Procoagulant property	Plasminogen activator inhibitors	Inhibition of fibrinolytic system

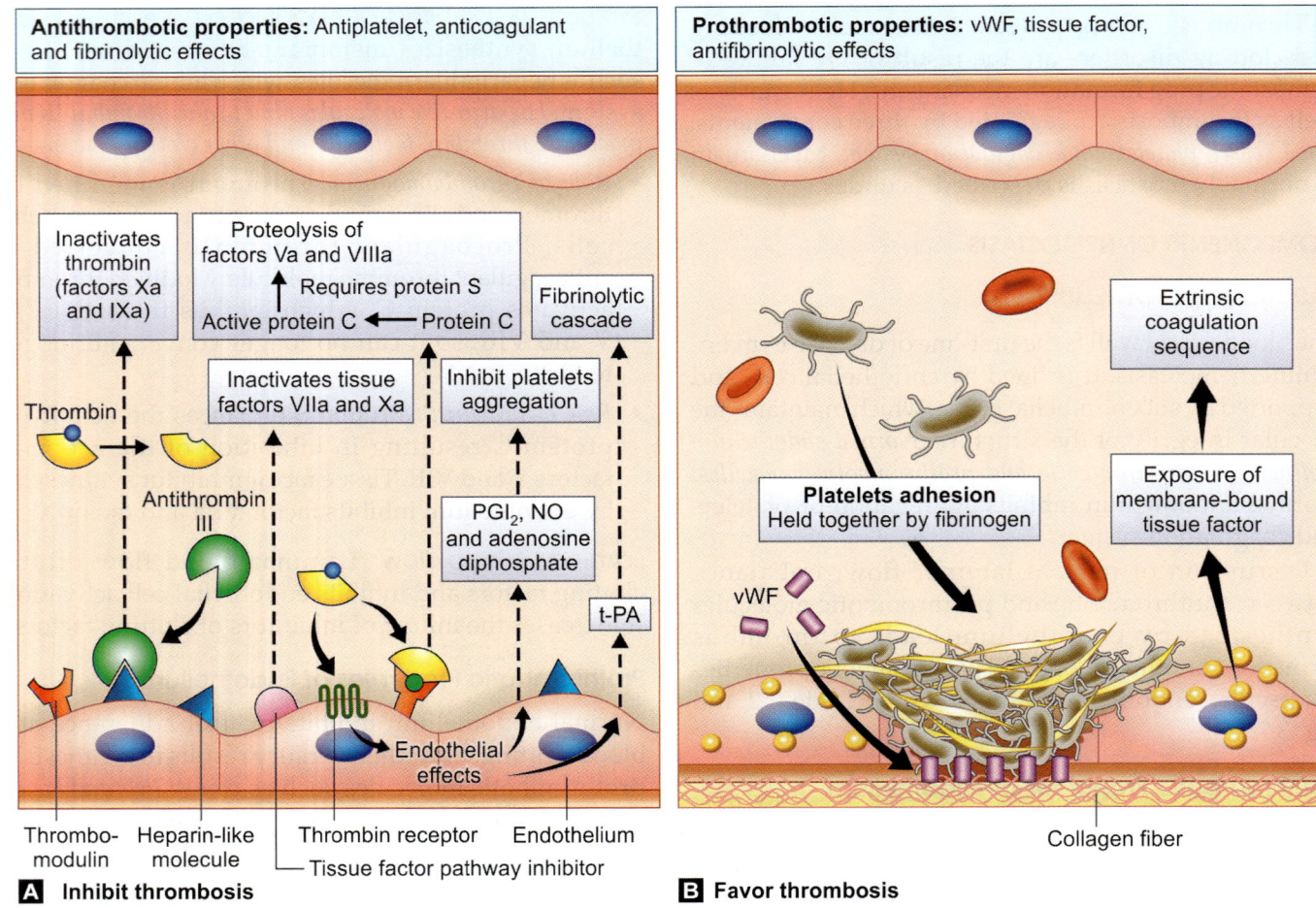

Fig. 3.7: Antithrombotic and prothrombotic properties of vascular endothelium.

Disorders of Hemostasis

Tissue factor: Bacterial endotoxins and cytokines (e.g. IL-1 and tumor necrosis factor-α) stimulate endothelium to synthesize tissue factor resulting in activation of extrinsic coagulation pathway.

Plasminogen activator inhibitors: Endothelium synthesizes inhibitors of plasminogen activator, which inhibits fibrinolytic system leading to thrombus formation.

PLATELETS

Platelets play a central role in normal hemostasis by forming primary hemostatic plug. Platelet structure is shown in Fig. 3.8.

Thrombopoiesis

Thrombopoietin, vitamin B_{12} and folic acid participate in platelet production in bone marrow. These are formed from cytoplasmic fragments of megakaryocyte. They range in size from less than 5 femtoliters (fl) to more than 12 fl; however, the average platelet is about 7.3 fl. *Two-thirds of platelets remain in circulation, while one-third are stored in spleen.*

Structure of Platelets

Platelets are membrane bound porous disc-like structures. These express glycoprotein receptors of the integrin family on their surface. Structure and functions of platelets are shown in Table 3.3.

Plasma Membrane Surface

Plasma membrane surface allows adherence of platelets with the help of fibrinogen.

Cytoskeleton

Beneath plasma membrane, platelets contain actin-myosin filaments that cause the platelets to contract. Microtubules maintain the disc-like shape of platelets.

Platelets' Granules

Platelets contain two types of granules, i.e. α-granules and dense bodies (δ-granules). α-Granules contain fibrinogen, factor V; platelet derived growth factor (PDGF), transforming growth factor β (TGF- β), fibronectin and platelet factor IV. Dense bodies (δ granules) contain ADP, ATP, ionized calcium, serotonin and epinephrine.

Functions

Platelets activate coagulation system through the platelet phospholipid complex. These maintain the physical integrity of the vascular endothelium. These synthesize platelet derived growth factor (PDGF), which repairs injured endothelium.

Platelet Adhesion, Secretion and Aggregation

Reactions involving platelets during hemostasis include adhesion, secretion and aggregation. Platelet function disorders are shown in Table 3.4.

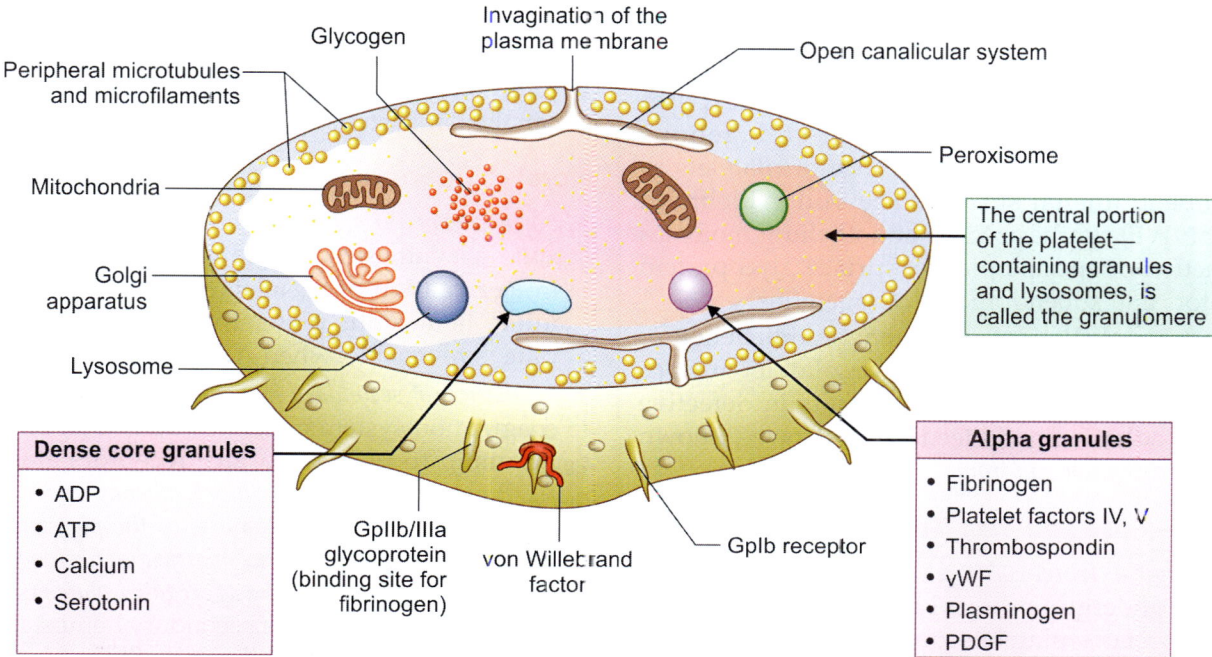

Fig. 3.8: Platelet structure. Platelets contain two types of granules i.e. α-granules and dense bodies (δ-granules). α-granules contain fibrinogen, factors V and VIII; platelet derived growth factor, transforming growth factor β, fibronectin and platelet factor IV. Dense bodies (δ-granules) contain ADP, ATP, ionized calcium, serotonin and epinephrine.

Table 3.3: Structure and functions of platelets

Parameters	Platelet products	Functions
Dense bodies (δ-granules)	ADP	Recruitment of platelets Activation of new platelets resulting in platelets aggregation
	ATP	Agonist for cells other than platelets
	Calcium	Extracellular source for hemostatic reactions
	Serotonin	Vasoconstriction
α-Granules	Fibrinogen	Aggregation and platelets Fibrinogen conversion to fibrin
	Platelet factor IV	Aggregation and platelets
	Thrombospondin	Aggregation and platelets
	Factor V	Adhesion of platelets
	vWF	Inhibition of fibrinolysin
	Plasminogen	Plasminogen conversion to plasmin, that causes fibrinolysis
	PDGF	Repair of smooth muscle cells

Table 3.4: Platelet function disorders

Disorder	Autosomal dominant/recessive	Platelet aggregation	Other features
Glanzmann disease or thrombasthenia	Autosomal recessive	Normal with ADP, epinephrine, collagen, and arachidonic acid Deficient with ristocetin	Severe bleeding and giant platelets in smear
Bernard-Soulier syndrome	Autosomal recessive	Deficient with ADP, epinephrine, collagen, and arachidonic acid Normal with ristocetin	Severe bleeding, small and discrete platelets, defective clot retraction
von Willebrand disease	Autosomal dominant/recessive	Normal with ADP, epinephrine, collagen, and arachidonic acid Deficient with ristocetin	Abnormality of platelets aggregation corrected by cryoprecipitate

Platelets Adhesion

- *Mechanism of adhesion:* Endothelial injury exposes subendothelial collagen or non-collagenous microfibrils resulting in adherence of platelets to the subendothelial surface. The von Willebrand factor (vWF) synthesized by endothelium mediates interaction of specific platelet-surface glycoprotein receptors and subendothelial collagen fibers.
- *Clinical aspect:* Patient with genetic deficiency of von Willebrand factor (vWF) or platelet-surface glycoprotein receptors (GpIb) results in defective platelets adhesion and bleeding tendencies, known as *Bernard-Soulier syndrome.*

Platelets Release Reaction (Secretion)

- *Morphological changes of platelets:* Soon after adhesion, platelets undergo a process known as *release reaction.* In this process platelets undergo morphological changes from a disc shape to a spherical shape.
- *Release of contents of platelets:* Morphological changes are followed by constriction of the microtubules and releasing contents of the granules (primarily ADP, catecholamine, serotonin and PDGF) into the open canalicular system.

Platelets Aggregation

- *Formation of initial hemostatic plug:* ADP and thromboxane A_2 synthesized by platelets play important role in aggregation of platelets results in formation of initial hemostatic platelet plug. Initial hemostatic plug is reversible, when ADP release is minimal.
- *Formation of secondary hemostatic plug:* Activation of coagulation system generates thrombin. Binding of thrombin to platelet surface receptors along with ADP and thromboxane A_2 cause further aggregation. ADP produce conformational changes of the platelets surface GpIIb–IIIa receptors, to which noncleaved fibrinogen binds. Fibrinogen bridges bind the aggregated platelets together resulting in formation of secondary hemostatic plug. The platelet mass is stabilized by fibrin.

Clinical aspect: Therapeutic agent such as GpIIb–IIIa inhibitor is administered following angioplasty to prevent thrombosis. GpIIb–IIIa inhibitor prevents the action of the corresponding platelet surface receptor glycoprotein complex, which is required for formation of fibrinogen bridges between adjacent platelets.

Congenital deficiency of GpIIb–IIIa receptors is known as *Glanzmann disease or thrombasthenia*. Thrombin responsible for thrombus formation is dissolved by thrombolytic agents.

Agonists Promoting Platelets Aggregation

Platelets aggregation is promoted by ADP, thromboxane A_2, epinephrine, collagen, platelet activating factor derived from mast cells and basophils. Thromboxane A_2 is generated from arachidonic acid through cyclooxygenase pathway.

Thromboxane A_2 causes *vasoconstriction* and *promotes aggregation of platelets* by activating guanyl cyclase, which increases intracellular levels of cGMP. *The inhibition of cyclooxygenase by low-dose aspirin is the basis of aspirin therapy for prevention of thrombotic disease.*

Limitation of Platelet Plug Formation

- *Prostacyclin (PGI2) and TxA₂:* Prostacyclin (PGI_2) synthesized by endothelium is a potent vasodilator and prevents platelets aggregation. TxA_2 causes *vasoconstriction and promotes platelets aggregation*. Both prostacyclin and TxA_2 perform balanced function for modulating platelets function.
- *Fibrin degradation products:* Under physiological state, intravascular platelets aggregation is also prevented by fibrin degradation products, but after vascular endothelial injury and formation of hemostatic plug. Leukocytes and RBCs are also present in hemostatic plug. Leukocytes adhere to endothelium and produce inflammatory response.
- *Thrombin:* Thrombin *stimulates leukocytic adhesion* and *cleaves fibrinogen into fibrin*. Fibrin degradation products attract leukocytes (neutrophils and monocytes).

COAGULATION CASCADE

Platelets initially arrest bleeding by forming temporary primary hemostatic plug in severed blood vessels. Formation of clot by activation of coagulation system is necessary to secure the repair of the damaged vessel.

- On activation, platelets undergo *conformational change* in shape resulting in formation of platelet factor 3 derived from *plasma membrane phospholipid of platelets*. It serves as catalytic sites for calcium and coagulation factors in the intrinsic coagulation pathway.
- *Coagulation system comprising* of extrinsic and intrinsic pathways. Reflect how clotting occurs in the test tube during tests. Clotting in the body is initiated in different manner (Fig. 3.9).

Extrinsic Pathway of Coagulation

Extrinsic pathway of coagulation is measured by the prothrombin time.

- *Formation of factor Xa:* Combination of tissue thromboplastin and calcium ions activates factor VII, which acts on factor X leading to formation of factor Xa.
- *Common pathway:* Activated factor X (Xa) proceeds to common pathway of both the intrinsic and extrinsic systems.
- *Formation of thrombin:* Factor Xa binds with factor V, prothrombin. Factor Xa can cleave prothrombin to form thrombin.
- *Formation of fibrin monomers:* Thrombin first splits off fibrinopeptides A and B from fibrinogen, and then form fibrin monomers.
- *Spontaneous polymerization of fibrin:* These fibrin monomers undergo spontaneous polymerization by *hydrogen bonding* to form fibrin network.
- *Stabilization of fibrin network:* It precedes stabilization of fibrin network by factor XIII (fibrin stabilizing factor) resulting in cross-linking of fibrin network. This product is insoluble and resistant to digestion by plasmin.

Clinical aspect: Absence of clotting factors VII, X, V, II, or fibrinogen or presence of inhibitors interferes with conversion of fibrinogen to fibrin. It leads to abnormal prothrombin time. Similarly, abnormalities of fibrinogen and inhibitors of the conversion of fibrinogen to fibrin result in an abnormal thrombin time.

Intrinsic Pathway of Coagulation

Intrinsic pathway of coagulation is measured by activated partial thromboplastin time.

Activation of intrinsic pathway in human: In human, many substances such as collagen, fatty acids, or joint cartilage can activate factor XII.

- *Role of factor XIIa:* Factor XIIa activates factor IX and factor VIII and forms a complex. It leads to activation of factor X. Platelets provide phospholipid in this process.
- *Cleavage of prothrombin to thrombin by factor Xa:* Factor Xa proceeds and forms a link between both extrinsic and intrinsic pathways.

Factor Xa binds with factor V, prothrombin. *Factor Xa cleaves prothrombin to form thrombin*. Thrombin converts fibrinogen into fibrin, which is stabilized by factor XIII.

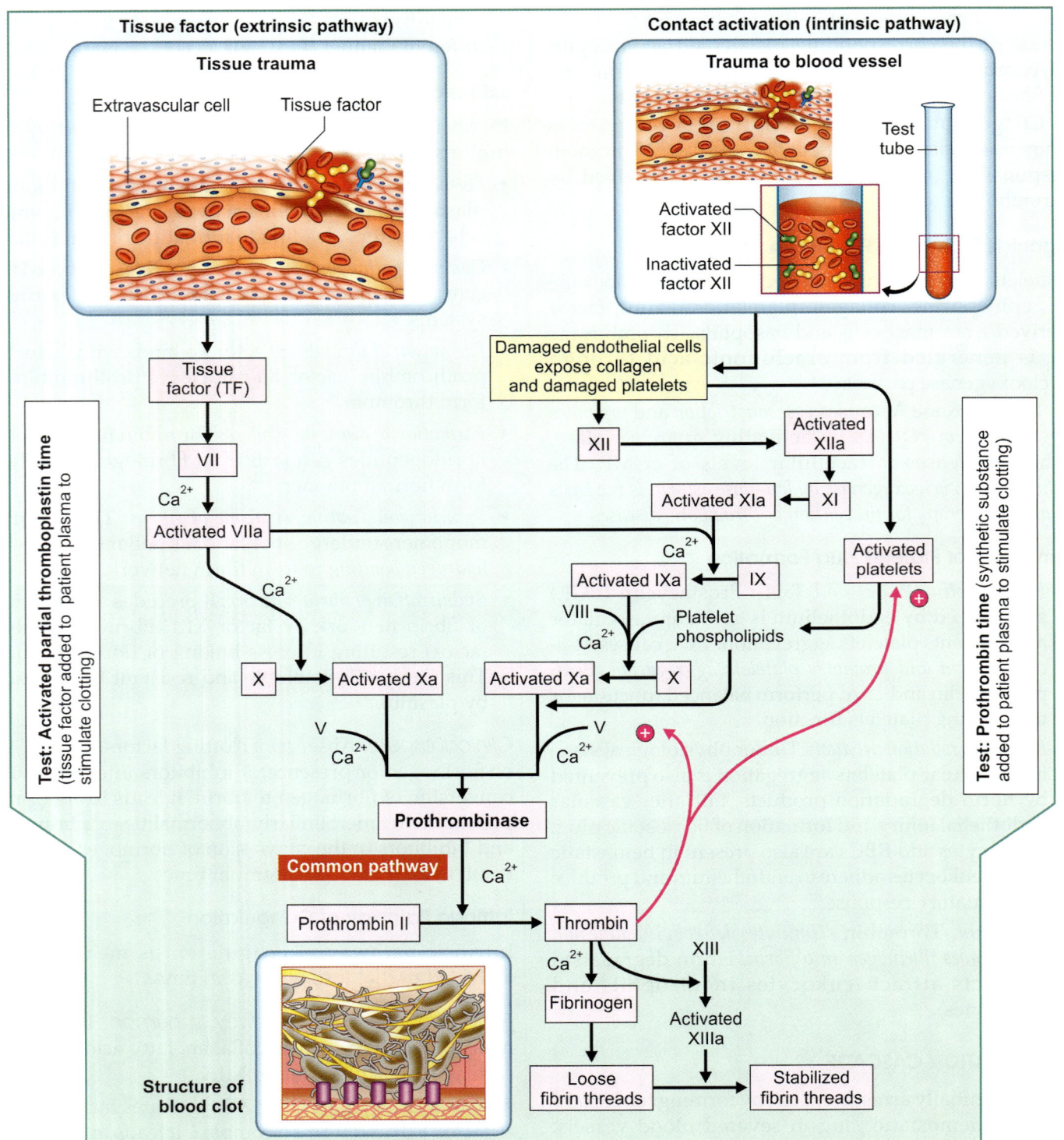

Fig. 3.9: Coagulation pathways. Tissue factor pathway is activated on exposure of clotting factor VIII to tissue factor on extravascular cells. When clotting factor XII contacts collagen fibers or a foreign surface such as glass activates contact activation pathway. Activated factor XII initiates a series of enzymatic reactions. Activated factor VII or factors activated by contact activation pathway, which terminates in the formation of a web of fibrin forming a clot.

- *Abnormal activated partial thromboplastin time:* Abnormalities of any one of the flowing coagulation factors produce an abnormal activated partial thromboplastin time such as factors *XII, IX, X, VII, V, II or prothrombin, kininogen and prekallikrein.*

- *APTT estimation in laboratory:* Intrinsic pathway of coagulation is measured by activated partial thromboplastin time. It measures factors *XII, IX, X, VII, V, II or prothrombin, kininogen and prekallikrein.* Factor XII, kininogen and prekallikrein are essential for normal clotting in the test tube. Activation of factor XII begins, when it is exposed to glass surface in presence of kininogen and prekallikrein. Persons deficient in kininogen and prekallikrein have no significant bleeding disorders.

MECHANISM OF HEMOSTASIS

TRANSIENT VASOCONSTRICTION

Injury to blood vessel causes vasoconstriction due to neural reflex and release of thromboxane A_2 by platelets (Fig. 3.10).

- Vasoconstriction is augmented by endothelin, a chemical mediator derived from endothelium. It immediately reduces the blood flow from the ruptured blood vessel.

- Both local neural reflexes and humoral factors such as TxA_2 released from platelets cause vasoconstriction.
- Vasoconstriction effect is temporary and needs to be supplemented by aggregation of platelets and blood coagulation factors to maintain permanent hemostasis of the injury.

FORMATION OF PRIMARY PLATELET PLUG

Within seconds after vascular injury, vWF is released by endothelium. von Willebrand factor binds to platelet receptors. This phenomenon is responsible for adhesion of platelets to the exposed collagen fibers. Platelets undergo morphologic changes (disc shape to spherical shape) and activation leading to release of *adenosine diphosphate (ADP), serotonin, epinephrine* and *thromboxane A_2. These platelet products such as ADP and TxA_2 attract additional platelets leading to platelets aggregation.* Platelet factor III, a surface phospholipid accelerates clotting by formation of thrombin (Fig. 3.11)

FORMATION OF SECONDARY HEMOSTATIC PLUG

Tissue factor and platelet phospholipids activate coagulation system resulting in formation of secondary hemostatic plug. It is composed of *polymerized fibrin and platelets*. Blood coagulation occurs by intrinsic and extrinsic pathways as a result of vascular injury. Intrinsic pathway begins in blood circulation by activation of circulating factor XII. Extrinsic pathway is activated by cellular lipoprotein known as *tissue factor*. Both these pathways lead to activation of factor X, conversion of prothrombin to thrombin (Fig. 3.12).

- Binding of thrombin to platelet surface receptors along with ADP and thromboxane A_2 cause further aggregation. *ADP produces conformational changes of the platelets surface GpIIb–IIIa receptors, to which noncleaved fibrinogen binds.*

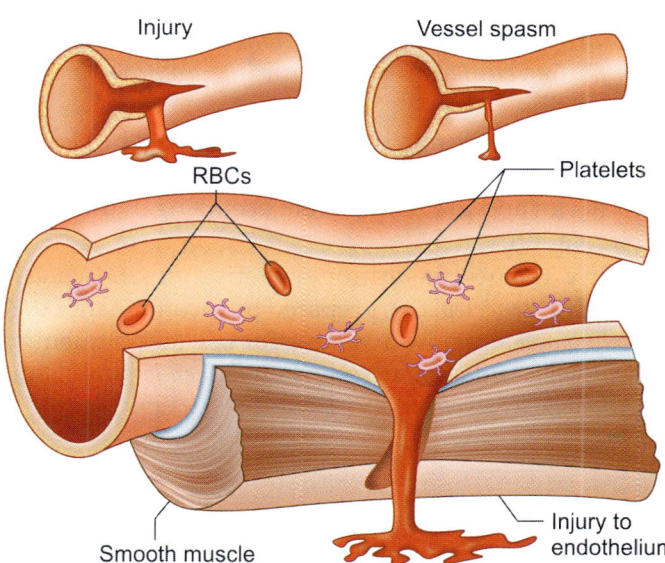

Fig. 3.10: Injury to blood vessel. Vasoconstriction of blood vessel occurs due to neural reflex and release of thromboxane A_2 by platelets resulting in reduction of blood flow.

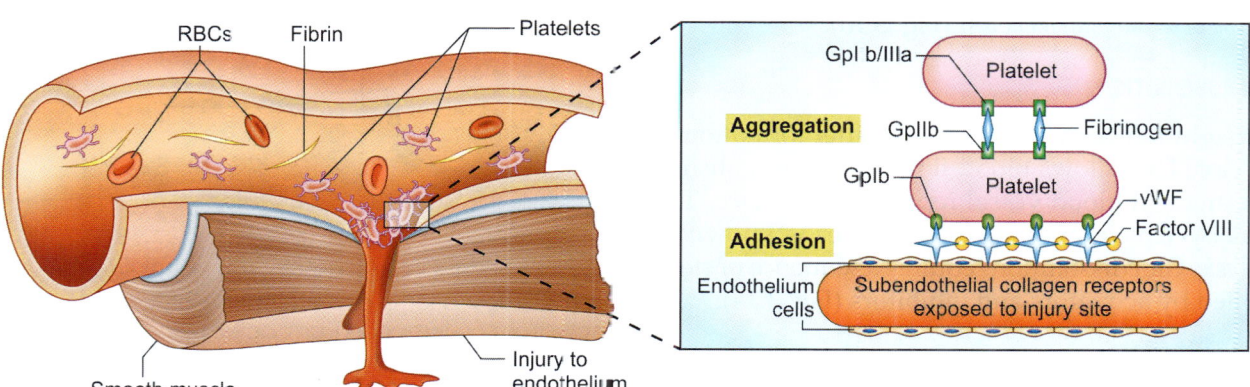

Fig. 3.11: Formation of primary platelet plug. Platelets adhere to be exposed collagen fibers due to binding of von Willebrand factor to platelet receptors. Activated platelets release ADP and TxA_2 resulting in attraction of additional platelets and aggregation.

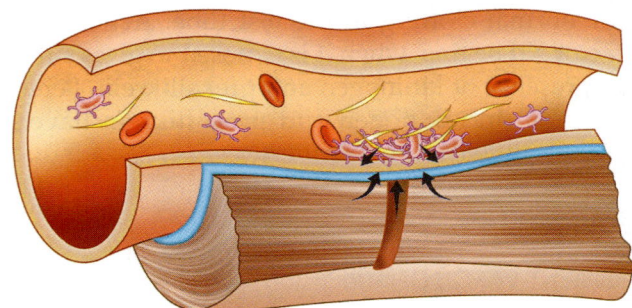
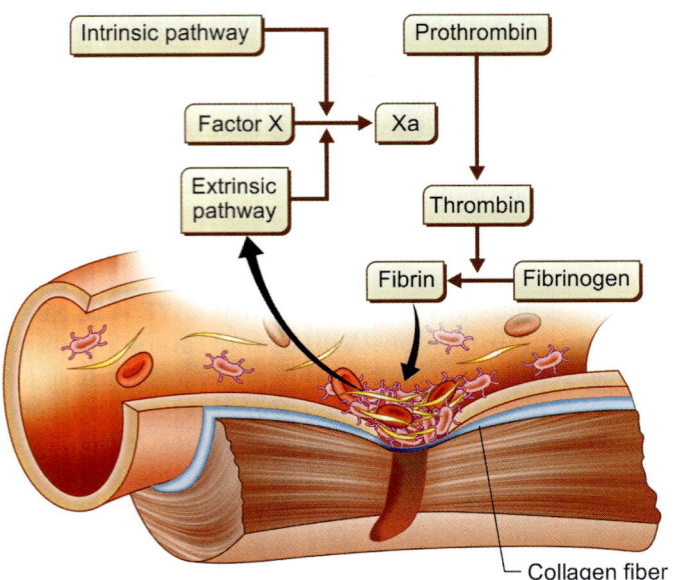

Fig. 3.12: Formation of secondary hemostatic plug. Blood coagulation occurs by intrinsic and extrinsic pathways as a result of vascular injury. Both these pathways lead to activation of factor X, conversion of prothrombin to thrombin. Thrombin converts fibrinogen to fibrin. Fibrin stabilizing factor stabilizes fibrin leading to holding of clot by insoluble fibrin strands.

- *Fibrinogen bridges bind the aggregated platelets* together resulting in formation of secondary hemostatic plug. The platelet mass is stabilized by fibrin. Fibrin strands hold the clot.

CLOT RETRACTION

Clot retraction occurs when platelets are trapped within the enlarging blood clot. It occurs within 20 to 60 minutes after a clot has formed, contributing to hemostasis. *Actin and myosin of platelets pull the clot towards platelets.*

This phenomenon squeezes serum from the blood clot leading to shrinkage of blood clot. *Clot retraction requires large numbers of platelets, and failure of clot retraction is indicative of a low platelet count* (Fig. 3.13).

CLOT DISSOLUTION

Clot dissolution begins immediately after formation of blood clot. This allows blood flow to be reestablished and permanent blood vessel repair to take place. The process by which a blood clot dissolves is known as *fibrinolysis*. Clot dissolution requires a sequence of steps controlled by activators and inhibitors (Fig. 3.14).

Role of Plasminogen

- *Plasminogen participates in clot dissolution*. It is normally present in the blood in its inactive form. *Plasminogen activators formed in the vascular endothelium, liver and kidneys convert plasminogen (inactive form) to plasmin (active form).*
- The *plasmin* formed from plasminogen *digests the fibrin strands of the clot and certain clotting factors such as fibrinogen, factor V, factor VIII, prothrombin, and factor XII.*
- Circulating plasmin is rapidly inactivated by *plasmin inhibitor*, which limits the fibrinolytic process to the local clot and prevents it from occurring in the entire circulation.
- Many tissue plasminogen activators (*alteplase, reteplase, tenecteplase*), prepared by recombinant *DNA technology*, are now available for use in treatment of *acute myocardial infarction, acute ischemic stroke,* and *pulmonary embolism*.

Fig. 3.13: Clot retraction. Within a few minutes after a clot is formed, actin and myosin in the platelets that are trapped in the blood clot begins to contract. As a result, fibrin strands of the clot are pulled towards the platelets, thereby squeezing serum (plasma without fibrinogen) from the clot and causing it to shrink.

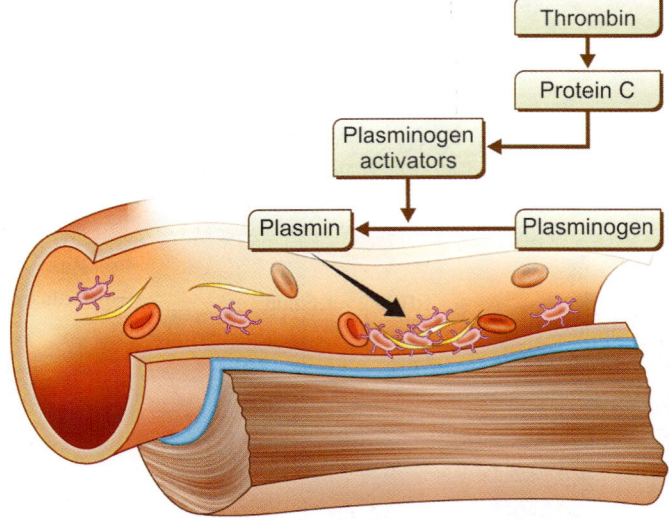

Fig. 3.14: Clot dissolution or lysis. Clot dissolution begins immediately after a clot is formed. This process begins with activation of plasminogen, an inactive precursor of the proteolytic enzyme, plasmin. After the formation of clot, large amounts of plasminogen are trapped in the clot. Tissue plasminogen tissue activator (t-PA) released from injured tissues and vascular endothelium converts plasminogen to plasmin. Plasmin digests the fibrin strands, causing the clot to dissolve.

Disorders of Hemostasis

Role of Thrombomodulin

Thrombomodulin synthesized by *vascular endothelium* has *antithrombotic activity*. It interferes in coagulation pathways. It converts procoagulant thrombin to anticoagulant thrombin molecule that activates protein C. *Protein C inhibits the activity of V and VIII*, that can no longer convert fibrinogen to fibrin.

CONTROL OF HEMOSTASIS

Hemostasis is a self-limited process to the site of endothelial injury. It prevents clotting of the entire vascular system. It is regulated through several mechanisms.

BLOOD FLOW

Normal laminar blood flow dilutes activated clotting factors and results in their removal from clot. It increases the inflow of inhibitors of clotting factors resulting in inactivation of clotting factors.

CONSUMPTION OF PLATELETS AND CLOTTING FACTORS

Platelets and clotting factors are consumed by the clotting process.

PLASMINOGEN-PLASMIN SYSTEM

Plasminogen activator cleaves plasminogen to form enzyme plasmin. Plasmin binds to specific receptors on fibrin strands network and begins degrading the fibrin strands resulting in dissolution of blood clot. Out of these processes, plasminogen-plasmin system and the circulating natural inhibitors of coagulation have clinical significance.

ANTITHROMBIN III

Antithrombin III antagonizes thrombin activity. It also inhibits factors XIIa, XIa, Xa, and IXa. Heparin-like molecules synthesized by endothelium activates antithrombin III. Hence, in clinical practice, *heparin is administered to minimize thrombosis*.

PROTEIN C

Protein C is a vitamin K dependent natural anticoagulant present in circulation. It inhibits factors V and VIII. It is activated by modified thrombin protein. Thrombomodulin synthesized by endothelium modifies thrombin molecule. This modified thrombin protein can no longer convert fibrinogen to fibrin. Protein C also enhances fibrinolysis.

PROTEIN S

Protein S is a vitamin K dependent natural anticoagulant present in circulation. It serves as a cofactor and enhances the activity of protein C resulting in inhibition of factors V and VIII. Protein S does not require activation.

TISSUE FACTOR PATHWAY INHIBITOR

Tissue factor pathway inhibitor (TFPI) is synthesized by endothelium. It binds factor Xa and tissue factor and inactivates them rapidly in circulation, so limiting coagulation.

THROMBOSIS

OVERVIEW

Dysregulation of normal hemostasis results in formation of thrombus formation. *Thrombus is an intravascular coagulation of blood attached to the vessel wall (artery or veins) formed by constituents of blood such as coagulation factors, platelets, and red blood cells.*

Thrombus results in significant interruption of blood flow to organs due to partial or complete occlusion of blood vessels (Fig. 3.15).

- *Thrombi may develop* within *cardiac chambers*, on *cusps*; or in *arteries, veins*, or *capillaries*. These vary in size and shape depending on the site of origin. These occur by *Virchow triad due to endothelial injury, turbulence of blood flow* and *hypercoagulable state*.
- Hemostasis as well as thrombosis is regulated by three components: blood vessel, platelets and coagulation system.

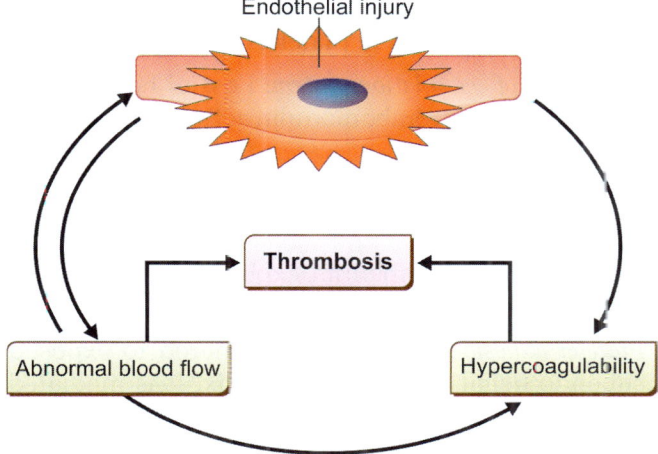

Fig. 3.15: Factors participating in thrombus formation. The most important factor in thrombus is endothelial injury. Abnormal blood flow and hypercoagulable state also play a role in thrombus formation.

PATHOGENESIS OF THROMBOSIS

ROLE OF ENDOTHELIUM

Injury to Endothelium

Endothelial injury is the most important cause of thrombus formation in cardiovascular system, where normally high blood flow rate is *unable to dilute clotting factors* and prevent platelets adhesion. *Thrombi are formed within cardiac chambers following endocardial injury due to myocardial infarction*. These are formed over *ulcerated atheromatous plaques* located in abdominal aorta or site of vasculitis.

Dysfunctional Endothelium

Endothelium is not physically disrupted, but becomes dysfunctional. *Hypercholesterolemia, homocystinuria, cigarette smoking, radiation, and hypertension* are important factors to cause dysfunctional endothelium. It may contribute to development of thrombus formation.

Synthesis of procoagulant factors: Dysfunctional endothelium increases *synthesis of procoagulant factors such as platelets adhesive molecules, tissue factor and plasminogen activator inhibitors*. Expression of platelets adhesion molecules enhances adhesion of platelets. Tissue factor activates coagulation system. Plasminogen activator inhibitors inhibit fibrinolytic system.

Decreased synthesis of antithrombotic molecules: Dysfunctional endothelium synthesizes less amount of antithrombotic molecules such as *prostacyclin (PGI$_2$), nitric acid, adenosine diphosphatase enzyme, heparin-like molecules and thrombomodulin*.

- *Platelets aggregation:* Loss of prostacyclin and nitric oxide promotes platelets aggregation. Loss of adenosine diphosphatase enzyme is not able to degrade ADP results in platelets aggregation.
- *Activation of coagulation system:* Loss of heparin-like molecules and thrombomodulin activate coagulation system.

ROLE OF PLATELETS

Physical loss of endothelium exposes subendothelial extracellular matrix to platelets.

- *Platelet adhesion:* Platelets are adhered to exposed subendothelial extracellular matrix. It is mediated by von Willebrand factor (vWF).
- *Platelets aggregation:* Soon after adhesion; platelets release ADP, catecholamine, serotonin and PDGF into the open canalicular system. Platelets aggregation is promoted by *ADP, thromboxane A$_2$, epinephrine, collagen, platelet activating factor derived from mast cells and basophils*. Platelets aggregation forms initial hemostatic platelet plug. It is reversible, when ADP release is minimal.

TURBULENT BLOOD FLOW

Normal blood flow is laminar, in which platelets circulate in central column separated from endothelium by plasma. Laminar blood flow dilutes clotting factors by fresh blood. It increases the inflow of inhibitors of clotting factors. It inhibits endothelial cell activation.

Turbulent blood flow: Turbulence or stasis of blood flow plays an important role in formation of thrombi in heart, arteries and veins.

- *Effects of turbulent blood flow:* Turbulent blood flow disrupts laminar blood flow *bringing platelets in contact with endothelium*. It prevents *dilution of clotting factors by fresh flowing blood*. It retards *inflow of clotting factor inhibitors* resulting in buildup of thrombi. It *promotes endothelial cell activation* resulting in thrombus formation and leukocytic adhesion.
- *Clinical aspect:* Turbulence and stasis of blood flow occur in many clinical settings such as *ulcerated atheromatous plaques, aneurysms, myocardial infarction* (mural thrombi in left ventricle), and *mitral stenosis in rheumatic heart disease* (mural thrombus in left atrium).

HYPERCOAGULABLE STATE

Hypercoagulable state is less frequent cause of thrombus formation. It may occur in settings of hereditary or acquired disorders (Tables 3.5 and 3.6).

Table 3.5: Hereditary causes of hypercoagulable state

Occurrence	Gene mutations
Common mutations	Factor V gene (factor V Leiden)
	Prothrombin gene
	Methylenetetrahydrofolate gene
Rare mutations	Antithrombin III
	Protein C
	Protein S
Very rare mutations	Fibrinolysin gene

THROMBOTIC DISORDERS

Hereditary thrombophilia is a prothrombotic familial syndrome caused by deficiency of a number of antithrombotic proteins, including antithrombin III, protein C, and protein S. It is characterized by recurrent venous thrombosis and thromboembolism. It most often occurs in adolescents or young women (Table 3.7).

Table 3.6: Acquired causes of hypercoagulable state

Occurrence	Disorders
High risk disorders	Myocardial infarction
	Atrial fibrillation
	Prosthetic valve
	Trauma (surgery, fracture, burns)
	Disseminated intravascular coagulation
	Malignant tumors (mucin secreting tumors)
	Heparin induced thrombocytopenia
	Antiphospholipid antibody syndrome (lupus anticoagulant syndrome)
Low risk disorders	Nephrotic syndrome (urinary loss of antithrombin III)
	Hyperestrogenic state (pregnancy)
	Oral contraceptive use
	Tobacco smoking
	Sickle cell anemia

Table 3.7: Conditions associated with increased risk of thrombosis

Mechanism	Disorders
Hereditary causes	Factor V Leiden mutation (abnormal factor V resists degradation by protein C)
	Prothrombin G20210A transition
	Methylenetetrahydrofolate reductase gene mutation (MTHFRC677T)
	Protein C deficiency or decreased activity
	Protein S deficiency or decreased activity
	Antithrombin III deficiency or decreased activity
	Dysfibrinogenemia
Increased function of platelets (acquired etiology)	Atheromatous plaques
	Diabetes mellitus
	Hyperlipidemia
	Tobacco smoking
	Thrombocytosis
Increased activity of coagulation system (acquired etiology)	Congestive heart failure
	Postsurgical state
	Immobilization
	Use of oral contraceptives
	Pregnancy
	Heparin induced thrombocytopenia
	Antiphospholipid syndrome
	Thrombotic thrombocytopenic purpura
	Nephrotic syndrome (loss of antithrombin III and antiplasmin in urine)
	Myeloproliferative disorders

Indications for investigating thrombophilia: Patient with history of thrombosis at young age, unexplained recurrent episodes of thromboembolic phenomenon, strong family history of thrombosis in the first degree relatives, recurrent abortions and pregnancy associated thrombi in women should be investigated.

HEREDITARY CAUSES

Factor V Leiden Mutation

Mutation of factor V Leiden has been named after the city in Netherlands. It is the most common cause of hereditary thrombophilia. Risk is greatly increased during pregnancy and following oral contraceptive intake.

Molecular Genetics

This abnormal factor V protein is formed due to specific mutation by *substitution of glutamine for normal arginine at position 506*. It alters the cleavage site targeted by APC. This abnormal factor V protein becomes resistant to cleavage by protein C.

As a result, an important antithrombotic counter regulatory mechanism is lost. There is increased prothrombokinase complex and thrombin generation.

Clinical Features

Patient presents with recurrent deep venous thrombosis. This defect predisposes to unchecked thrombosis especially in deep veins of leg.

Laboratory Tests

Laboratory tests for factor V Leiden mutation include activated protein C resistance assay and genetic analysis by polymerase chain reaction.

Prothrombin 20210 Transition

Prothrombin 20210 transition is the secondmost common cause of hereditary thrombophilia. Mutation of prothrombin gene occurs due to a single nucleotide change (G to A) in the 3'-untranslated region at position 20210. It is associated with *elevated plasma prothrombin levels*. Patient has almost three times *increased risk of arterial and venous thrombosis*.

Methylenetetrahydrofolate Reductase Gene Mutation (MTHFRC677T)

Methylenetetrahydrofolate reductase gene mutation (MTHFRC677T) results in mild elevation of homocysteine levels in 5–15% of White and East Asia populations. *Elevated levels of homocysteine inhibit antithrombin III and thrombomodulin. There is increased risk of thrombosis.*

The increased homocysteine can be reduced by dietary supplementation with *folic acid and vitamins B_6 (pyridoxine) and B_{12} (cobalamin)*. This is also associated with an increased risk of neural tube defects and possibly a number of diverse neoplasms.

Increased Levels of Factors VIII, IX, XI, or Fibrinogen

Increased levels of factors VIII, IX, XI, or fibrinogen are also associated with increased venous thrombosis.

Antithrombin III, Protein C and Protein S Deficiency

Vitamin K dependent clotting factors (II, VII, IX and X), protein C and protein S are synthesized by liver. Under physiological state, antithrombin III, protein C and protein S prevent thrombus formation.

Hereditary Deficiency

Hereditary deficiency of antithrombin III and protein C have an autosomal dominant pattern of inheritance with identical clinical manifestations. Approximately, 50% reduction in the plasma concentration of protein C results in *venous thrombosis* and *recurrent thromboembolic pulmonary phenomenon* in adolescents or early life.

Acquired Deficiency

Acquired protein C deficiency is seen in patients with *severe liver disease* and disseminated intravascular coagulation (DIC). Liver is unable to maintain high turnover-rate of protein C. Protein C is rapidly consumed in disseminated intravascular coagulation. *A total lack of protein C is usually associated with death in utero.* Newborns with total absence of protein C suffer from *purpura fulminans neonatalis*. Repeated *infusions of prothrombin complex* help in keeping these *children alive*.

ACQUIRED CAUSES

Antiphospholipid Antibody Syndrome

Antiphospholipid antibody syndrome is associated with high titers of circulating *antibodies (IgG) directed against anionic phospholipids* (cardiolipin) *such as plasma protein epitopes prothrombin.*

- *Lupus anticoagulant syndrome:* Antiphospholipid antibody syndrome having autoimmune disorder etiology such as systemic lupus erythematosus is known as *lupus anticoagulant syndrome*.
- *Clinical features:* Patient presents with *recurrent thrombi* especially in deep veins of legs or *arterial thrombi*. But renal, hepatic, and retinal veins are also susceptible. There is history of *repeated miscarriages, cardiac valvular vegetations, or thrombocytopenia*.
- *Antiphospholipid antibodies:* In vitro these interfere with the assembly of phospholipid complexes and thus inhibit coagulation. However, in vivo, the antibodies induce a hypercoagulable state.

Heparin Induced Thrombocytopenia (HIT) Syndrome

This clinical problem is reduced by administration of low-molecular-weight heparin preparations.

Type I heparin induced thrombocytopenia (HIT) syndrome: Type I HIT syndrome results in a mild to moderate drop in platelets within a day of heparin therapy. It is not immune-mediated disorder. It is not a contraindication to future heparin use.

Type II heparin induced thrombocytopenia (HIT) syndrome: Type II HIT syndrome leads to a severe drop in platelets (often <50% of baseline within 5 to 10 days after heparin therapy.

- Type II HIT syndrome leads to a *severe drop in platelets (often <50% of baseline*. It is immune-mediated disorder. Therapeutic administration of unfractionated heparin induces formation of anti-PF4 antibodies.
- These antibodies *bind to molecular complexes of heparin and platelet factor 4 membrane protein*. These antibodies can also bind to platelets and vascular endothelium resulting in prothrombotic state.
- Once Type II HIT has been diagnosed, further heparin treatment is contraindicated.

Disseminated Intravascular Coagulation

Disseminated intravascular coagulation (DIC) is characterized by widespread clotting with resultant consumption of platelets and coagulation factors, especially factors II, V, and VIII, and fibrinogen. Pathogenesis of disseminated intravascular coagulation is shown in Fig. 3.16. Causes of disseminated intravascular dissemination (DIC) are shown in Table 3.8.

a. DIC occurs as a result of release of tissue thromboplastin (tissue factor) or activation of the intrinsic pathway of coagulation, as well as secondary activation of the fibrinolytic system.

b. Clinical manifestations are thrombotic phenomena in small blood vessels of multiple organs and hemorrhage. Hematological findings include microangiopathic hemolytic anemia with fragmented

Table 3.8: Causes of disseminated intravascular dissemination (DIC)

Cause	Mechanism
Obstetric complications	Toxemia of pregnancy
	Amniotic fluid emboli
	Retained dead fetus
	Abruptio placentae (premature separation of placenta)
Metastatic cancers	Lung carcinoma
	Pancreatic carcinoma
	Prostate carcinoma
	Gastric carcinoma
	Leukemia
Infectious agents	Gram-negative sepsis
	Meningococcal meningitis
	Acute viral infections
	Rickettsial infections (e.g. Rocky Mountain spotted fever)
	Parasitic infections (e.g. malaria)
Trauma or surgery	Chest surgery
	Burns
	Massive trauma
	Surgery involving extracorporeal circulation
	Snakebite
	Heat stroke
Shock	Septic shock
	Severe hypovolemic shock
Immunological mechanism	Immune complex disease
	Hemolytic transfusion reactions

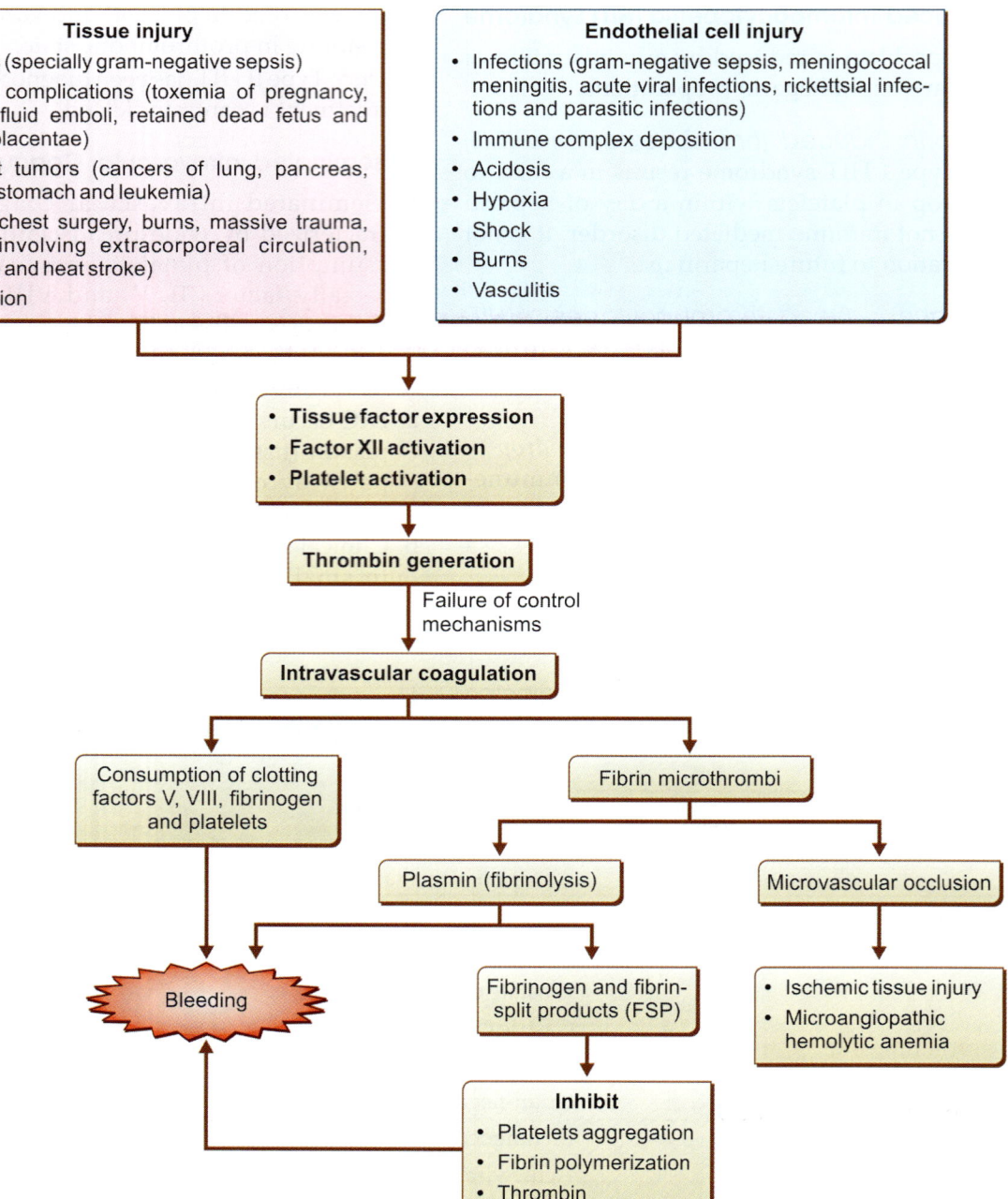

Fig. 3.16: Pathophysiology of disseminated intravascular coagulation. It is triggered by tissue injury, vascular endothelium injury or combination of both these processes. Intravascular coagulation occurs as a result of normal mechanisms controlling hemostasis.

red cells (schistocytes), increased fibrin and fibrinogen degradation (split) products, thrombocytopenia, and prolonged bleeding time, PT, APTT, and thrombin time.

ARTERIAL AND VENOUS THROMBI

Thrombi may be formed in arteries and veins (Table 3.9).

ARTERIAL THROMBI

Arterial thrombi are formed in areas of active blood flow in heart, large elastic and (aorta) muscular arteries (coronary, cerebral arteries) at the site of endothelial injury. These tend to grow in a retrograde direction from the point of attachment. Arterial thromboses typically occur in the cerebral circulation, but coronary, mesenteric, and renal arterial occlusions have also been described.

Thrombi in Heart

Thrombi in left ventricle occur due to a transmural myocardial infarction (mural thrombus). Mitral stenosis of *RHD* is complicated by atrial fibrillation

Disorders of Hemostasis

Table 3.9: Differences between arterial and venous thrombi

Parameters	Arterial thrombi	Venous thrombi
Blood flow	Formed in rapid blood flow in heart chambers or arteries	Formed in slow blood flow in veins (deep veins of leg)
Location	Coronary, cerebral, iliac, femoral arteries and heart chambers in active blood flow	Superficial saphenous veins, deep veins of legs, popliteal veins, femoral veins, hepatic veins, renal veins and dural sinuses in less active blood flow
Pathogenesis	Vascular endothelial injury (atheromatous plaque), turbulent blood flow (e.g. bifurcation of vessel and aortic aneurysm) and hypercoagulable states	Stasis of venous blood especially in immobilized patients, disseminated cancers, pregnancy, antithrombin III deficiency and intravenous cannula
Progression	Growing in a retrograde direction from the point of attachment	Venous thrombi formed in the lower extremities propagating toward the heart may cause pulmonary artery embolization
Occlusion	Partial or complete occlusion of vessels	Occlusive and often creating a long cast of the lumen of vein
Gross morphology	Gray–white friable with alternating pale and red areas	Dark red with a higher concentration of red blood cells along with fair number of platelets and leukocytes
Light microscopy	Lines of Zahn prominent (pale area composed of platelets held together by fibrin; and red areas composed predominantly of RBCs)	Lines of Zahn not prominent or absent
	Inflammatory changes in arteries absent	Inflammatory changes in veins present known as 'thrombophlebitis'
Complications	Infarction of organs such as heart, brain, kidney, spleen, lower limb	Pulmonary thromboembolism, edema, skin ulcers and poor wound healing
Therapy	Aspirin and anticoagulant therapy	Anticoagulants, heparin and warfarin

develop thrombi in left atrium. There is increased risk of development of thrombi in cardiac chambers in *congestive cardiomyopathy*.

- These thrombi usually adhere to the endocardium and termed as mural thrombi. Thrombi may also be formed on cardiac valvular vegetations such as *infective endocarditis* and *nonbacterial thrombotic endocarditis*.
- Patient of systemic lupus erythematosus developing noninfective verucous Libman Sacks vegetations may also develop thrombus formation.

Thrombi in Blood Vessels

Arterial thrombi are usually occlusive. Most common site in descending order includes coronary, cerebral and femoral arteries. Thrombus is usually superimposed on ulcerated atheromatous plaques located in abdominal aorta and medium-sized arteries such as coronary arteries (Fig. 3.17).

These are formed due to turbulence of blood flow at bifurcation of common iliac artery and abdominal aortic aneurysm. These may cause partial or complete occlusion of blood vessel.

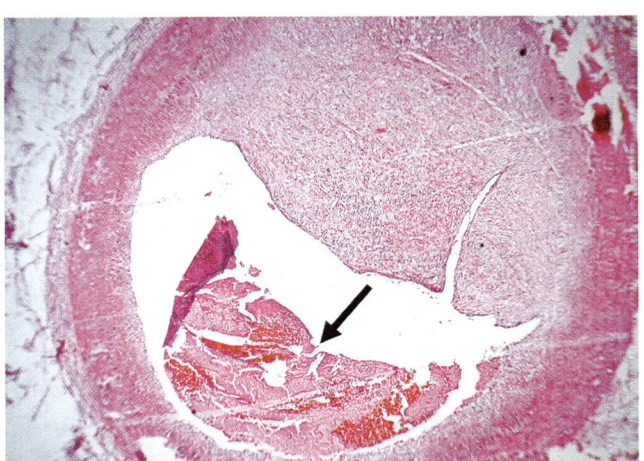

Fig. 3.17: Coronary arteries showing atheromatous plaque with thrombus formation occluding lumen (arrow) (400X).

Morphology of thrombus: Arterial thrombi are gray white and friable. Microscopic examination of mature thrombi demonstrates alternating pale and red areas.

Pale areas are composed of platelets held together by fibrin, while red areas are composed predominantly of RBCs. This layering results in the *lines of Zahn*.

VENOUS THROMBI (PHLEBOTHROMBOSIS)

Venous thrombi are formed in areas of less active blood flow. These are formed due to stasis of venous blood especially in immobilized patients. These extend in the direction of blood flow (i.e. toward heart). Propagating tail of venous thrombi may not be well attached resulting in fragmentation creating an embolus.

Location

Venous thrombi are present in *deep veins in the lower extremities below knee joint (most common in 90%); superior saphenous, periprostatic, ovarian or uterine veins*. Less common sites include hepatic vein, renal veins, and dural sinuses.

Morphology

Venous thrombi are *occlusive*. These often create a long cast of the lumen of vein. These are *dark red* with a *higher concentration of red blood cells* along with fair number of platelets and leukocytes than arterial thrombi. Lines of Zahn are not prominent or are absent.

Deep Vein Thrombosis

Deep vein thrombosis is most common in the deep veins of the calf. It frequently propagates in the femoral and iliac veins, from where it embolizes to the lungs. Venous thrombi may cause venous inflammatory changes. Inflammation of veins with thrombus formation is known as *thrombophlebitis*.

Etiology

Venous thrombi are formed due to stasis of blood. Main causes of deep vein thrombosis include:

- *Immobility:* Sitting for prolonged periods can contribute to deep vein thrombosis. It occurs in clinical settings such as congestive heart failure, severe burns, surgical trauma, and leg fracture.
- *Varicose veins:* There is increased risk of thrombosis in varicose veins. The thrombus formed in the superficial leg veins tends to embolize less frequently than those in the deep veins, known as deep vein thrombosis.
- *Disseminated cancers:* Some cancers can lead to excessive coagulation of blood, either due to changes in the blood.
- *Pregnancy and child birth:* The weight of the fetus on femoral vessels slows blood venous return. Hormonal changes and stress precipitates thrombi formation. Thromboplastin released from amniotic fluid results in activation of coagulation system.
- *Intravenous cannula or catheterization:* There is increased risk of deep vein thrombosis.
- *Hematological disorders:* Polycythemia, anti-thrombin III deficiency, dehydration (increased blood viscosity) may result in deep vein thrombosis.
- *Estrogen therapy:* Hormonal replacement therapy and therapy for carcinoma prostate increase the risk of deep vein thrombosis.
- *Surgery:* Orthopedics surgery (knee or hip replacement, pelvic surgery) or cardiac surgery increase the risk of venous thrombi.

Clinical Features

- *Superficial venous thrombus:* Patient presents with swelling, edema and tenderness along the course of vein in the affected area, ileofemoral venous thrombus is formed during puerperium.
- *Deep vein thrombosis:* Deep vein thrombosis is entirely asymptomatic in 50% cases. Patient presents with pain and distal edema (*Homar's sign*). Such pain and swelling may occur as a result of rupture of gastrocnemius muscle, osteoarthritic cyst (*Baker's cyst*) of knee joint and anterior compartment syndrome (*skin split*).
- *Migratory thrombophlebitis:* Venous thrombi formed in the lower extremities propagate (extend) toward the heart may cause pulmonary artery embolization. These are recognized only after thrombus is embolized.

Differential diagnosis: Pain and swelling in the leg may be due to deep vein thrombosis, ruptured head of gastrocnemius muscle, ruptured osteoarthritic cyst (Baker's cyst) of knee joint and anterior compartment syndrome.

Therapeutic correlation: Anticoagulant therapy with heparin and warfarin prevents formation of venous thrombi.

Postmortem Clots

Postmortem clots appear soon after death. These may be confused for venous thrombi. Postmortem clots are

Disorders of Hemostasis

Table 3.10: Differences between thrombus and postmortem clot

Features	Thrombus	Postmortem clot
Cause	Normal or pathological hemostasis	Dead person, sedimentation and settling down of blood components due to gravity
Location	Present in any vessel in the body	Present in dependent part in relation to the body kept after death
Shape	May or may not fit their vascular contours	Taking the shape of vessels or its bifurcation
Attachment to the vessel wall	Strong attachment of thrombus to vessel wall	Weak/No attachment of postmortem clot to vessel wall
Gross morphology	Dry, granular, firm, and friable	Gelatinous, soft and rubbery; two layers—currant jelly dark appearance in red cell rich lower and a chicken fat appearance in cell—poor upper layer
Light microscopy	Lines of Zahn present	Lines of Zahn absent

gelatinous dark red due to settling down of red cells by gravity giving *red currant jelly* appearance. Yellow chicken fat cell free supernatant resembles melted and clotted chicken.

In contrast to thrombi; these are not attached to the vessel wall. Differences between antemortem thrombus and postmortem clot are shown in Table 3.10.

FATE OF THROMBUS

Fate of thrombus includes resolution, organization, recanalization or embolization to distant organs (Fig. 3.18).

Dissolution

Plasmin is a fibrinolytic enzyme that is formed from plasminogen by tissue plasminogen activator (tPA) synthesized by endothelium in the vicinity of the thrombus. tPA converts plasminogen to plasmin. Plasmin splits fibrin strands (fibrinolysis) and dissolves relatively small thrombus resulting in restoration of blood flow.

Occlusive thrombi can also be dissolved by enzymes, such as streptokinase, that activate plasma fibrinolytic activity. Activation of Hageman factor links the fibrinolytic system, coagulation system, complement system, and kinin system.

Propagation

Propagation implies an increase in size of thrombus. It contains more platelets and fibrin resulting in vessel obstruction.

Organization

Older thrombi undergo organization, characterized by ingrowth of endothelial cells, fibroblasts, smooth muscle cells into the fibrin-rich thrombus.

Contraction of these cells leads to incorporation of smaller thrombus in the subendothelial region of the vessel wall. It is firm and grayish white in color resulting in obliteration of lumen.

Enzymatic Digestion

Occasionally, instead of organization of thrombus, the central portion of thrombus undergoes enzymatic digestion as a result of the release of lysosomal enzymes released by trapped leukocytes and platelets.

It occurs in large thrombi formed in *cardiac chambers* or *abdominal aortic aneurysm*. If the bacterial seeding occurs, it is called as *mycotic aneurysm*.

Recanalization

Formation of new vessels (capillaries) within organized thrombus restores blood flow to organ, at least partially. New capillaries are formed in the thrombus as a result of proliferation of intimal cells, which later fuse to form large vessels.

Embolization

Embolism is caused by fragmentation of the thrombus and resulting in infarction at a distant site such as brain, kidney, intestine and lower limbs.

These emboli may enter coronary arteries resulting in myocardial infarction. Venous thrombi may cause pulmonary embolism with fatal outcome.

Section I: General Pathology

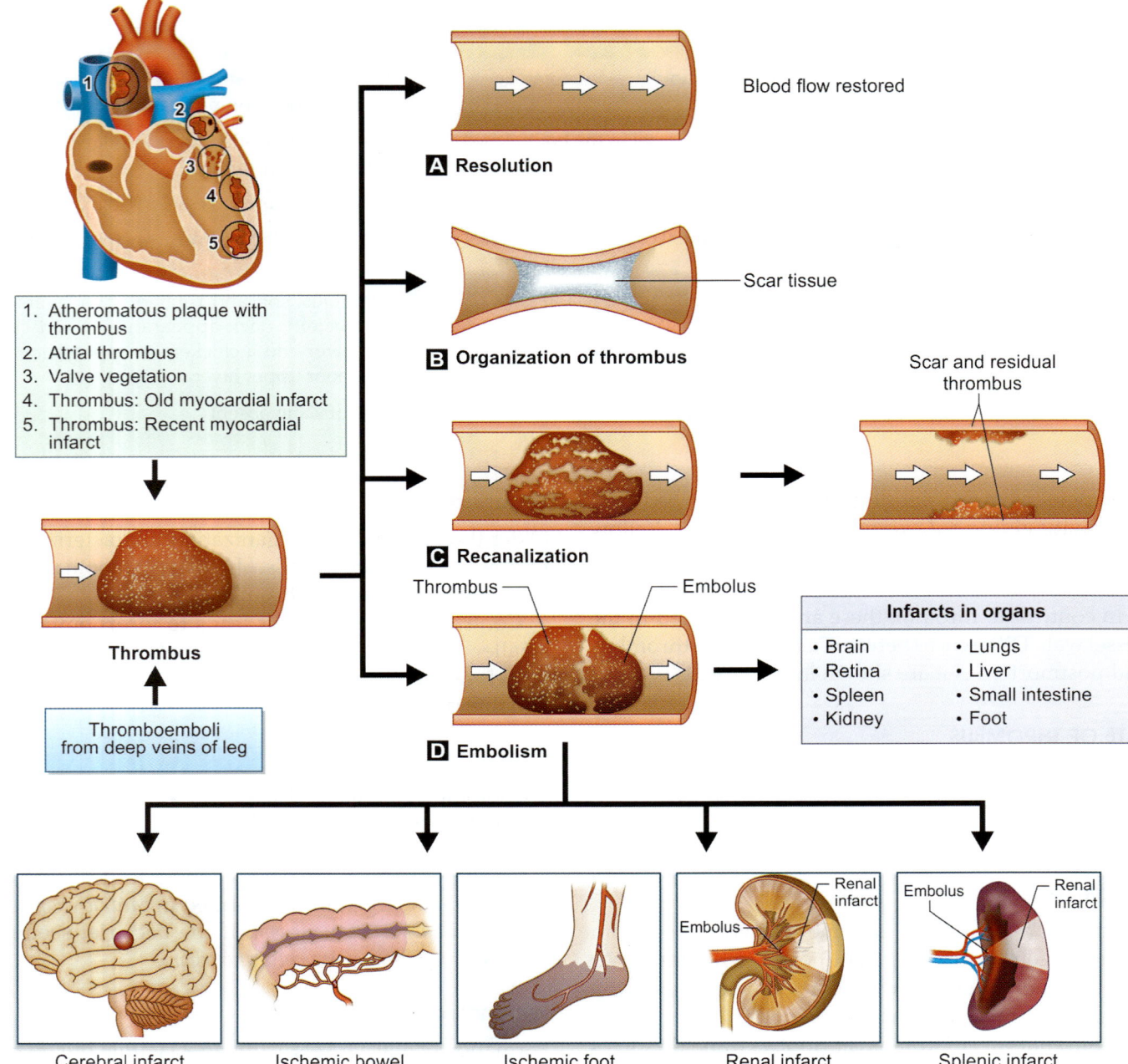

Fig. 3.18: Fate of thrombus showing various outcomes including resolution, organization, recanalization and embolism.

EMBOLISM

OVERVIEW

Embolus is detached mass (e.g. thrombus, fat, gas, amniotic fluid), that is circulating to distant organs and eventual trapping within the vasculature resulting in partial or complete obstruction of vessel. Origin of thrombi causing embolization in various organs is shown in Table 3.11.

Thromboembolism: Detachment of fragments of thrombi originating from veins (deep vein in legs, femoral vein) or heart (cardiac vegetations, myxoma) or atheromatous plaques travel in the arterial system.

One-third of patients with a left atrial or left ventricular myxoma die from tumor embolization to the brain. Emboli obstruct the blood flow and cause ischemic damage of organs.

Types of emboli: These include thromboembolism (pulmonary, systemic and paradoxical emboli), fat embolism, air embolism and amniotic fluid embolism.

Disorders of Hemostasis

Table 3.11: Origin of thrombi causing embolization in various organs

Origin of thrombi	Emboli reaching organs
Thrombi in deep veins of leg	Pulmonary embolism
Mural thrombi in left ventricle	Systemic thromboembolism
Trauma to bone marrow	Fat embolism
Entry of excess air during intravenous fluid infusion, cardiothoracic surgery, delivery and trauma to veins during surgery of head and neck	Air embolism
Divers and ascent during flights	Decompression sickness
Amniotic fluid entry in circulation during delivery	Amniotic fluid embolism
Ulcerated atheromatous plaques	Atheroembolism
Tumor fragments (myxoma heart)	Tumor fragment emboli

THROMBOEMBOLISM

PULMONARY THROMBOEMBOLISM

Pulmonary thromboembolism is most important cause of sudden death. It most often results from thromboembolism *originating from thrombosis in the lower extremity veins* (Fig. 3.19).

Sources of Pulmonary Emboli

These include thrombi in right heart (septal infarction, atrial fibrillation), tumor emboli, air embolism, pelvic veins, thrombi (following pelvic or prostate surgery), fat emboli (fractures long bones) and thrombi in deep veins of lower extremities.

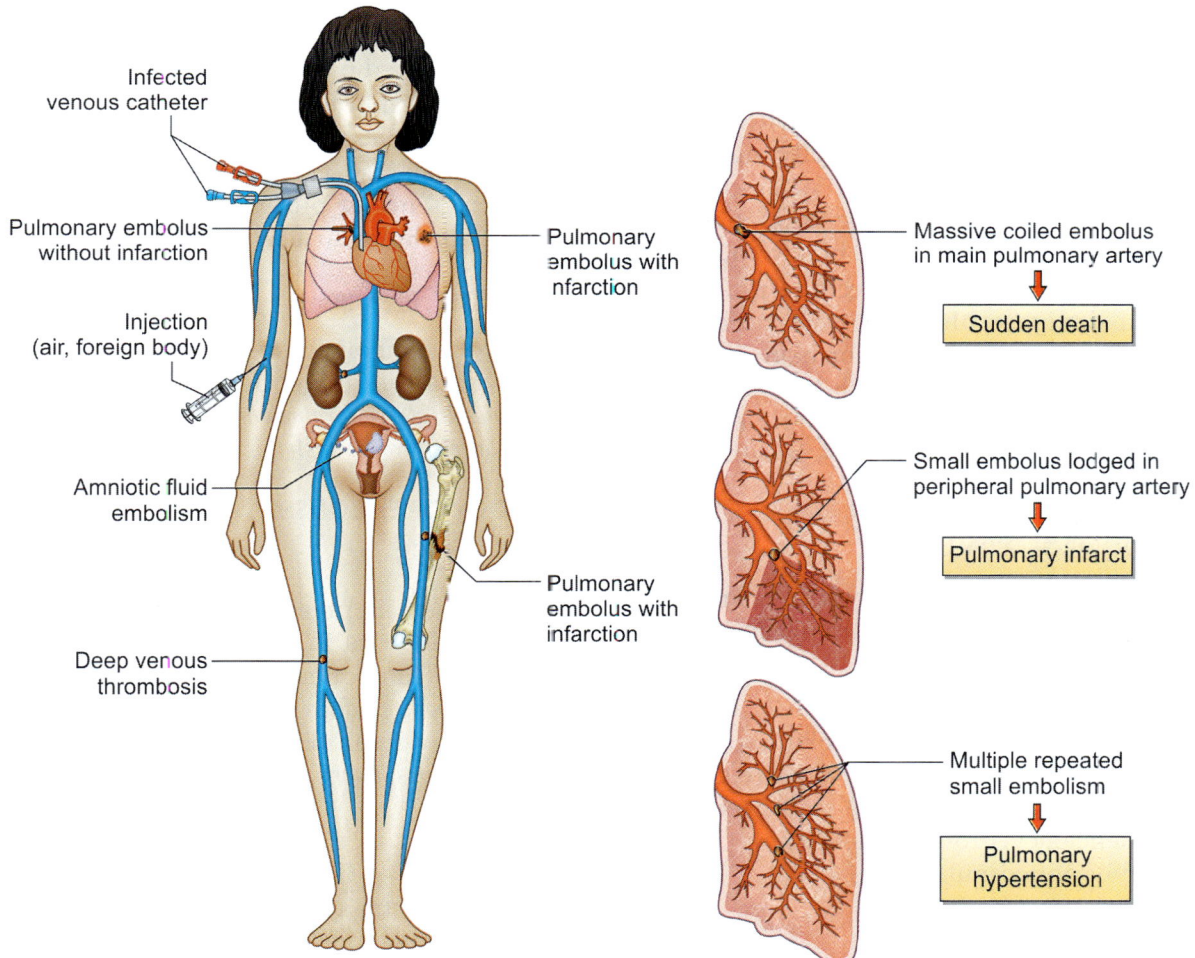

Fig. 3.19: Pulmonary thromboembolism.

Risk Factors

Venous thrombosis is associated with stasis blood flow seen in elderly, debilitated, or chronically bedridden persons, hypercoagulable state and congestive heart failure.

Mechanism

In immobilized patients, thrombi are formed most commonly in the lower extremities (deep veins, femoral vein). Thrombi may also form in pelvic veins or inferior vena cava in some cases. Fragments of thrombi travel through the venous circulation and settle in branches of pulmonary artery.

Size of embolus or emboli: Emboli may differ in size (large saddle thrombus, intermediate or small size). Clinical findings depend on the size of emboli.

Clinical Findings

- *Saddle thrombus:* A large venous embolus occluding the major pulmonary artery branches (bifurcation of the pulmonary artery) is known as *saddle thrombus*, which has sudden fatal outcome.
- *Emboli of intermediate size:* These emboli increase pulmonary artery pressure leading to pulmonary hypertension. Patient may develop *cor pulmonale* (right-sided heart failure).
- *Small emboli:* These are less clinically significant. Patient presents with sudden onset of dyspnea and tachycardia. Auscultation may be normal or there may be few rales and diminished breath sounds.
- *Pulmonary infarction:* Emboli occlude pulmonary artery and decrease blood flow to pulmonary parenchyma and may cause hemorrhagic infarction in less than 10% cases of thromboembolism. It is a *wedge-shaped infarct located just beneath the pleura*. Patient presents with pleural pain, breathlessness and hemoptysis.

SYSTEMIC THROMBOEMBOLISM

Embolus traveling in the arterial system is known as *systemic thromboembolism*. Arterial embolism typically causes infarction.

Risk factors: Injury to endothelial cell (e.g. ulcerated atherosclerotic plaques, cigarette smoking, radiation, and hypertension), stasis of blood flow (e.g. sickle cell anemia) and hypercoagulable states (e.g. antithrombin III deficiency, protein C deficiency, protein S deficiency, lupus anticoagulant).

Sites of Origin of Thrombi

- *Mural thrombi:* Mural thrombi are formed in the left ventricle of patients with *myocardial infarction*. Mural thrombi are formed in the left atrium in *rheumatic heart disease* patients with mitral stenosis and atrial fibrillation.
- *Thrombi in aorta:* Arterial emboli may also arise from fragmentation of cardiac vegetations and *myxoma tumor*. Thrombi formed in *ulcerated atheromatous plaque* and *abdominal aortic aneurysms* may also cause systemic thromboembolism.
- *Thrombi in medium-sized artery:* Thrombi formed at the junction of the internal and external carotid arteries may emboli to produce *brain infarct* (liquefactive necrosis). Ischemia in *brain does not produce coagulative necrosis as it lacks proteins*.

Sites of Lodgment in Organs

- *Brain:* Occlusion of the middle cerebral artery is the most common site of arrest of arterial emboli in branches of the carotid artery resulting in cerebral infarction (liquefactive necrosis as brain lacks proteins). Thrombi at the junction of the internal and external carotid arteries are a cause of thrombotic brain infarcts and can also be a site of origin of emboli.
- *Kidney and spleen:* These emboli obstruct the end arteries supplying kidney and spleen and produce wedge-shaped pale infarcts.
- *Intestine:* Emboli obstructing mesenteric artery supplying intestine produce hemorrhagic infarcts.
- *Leg:* Emboli obstructing arteries of leg leads to sudden pain, absence of pulses, and a cold limb. In some cases, the limb must be amputated.

PARADOXICAL EMBOLI

Paradoxical emboli originate in the venous circulation and bypass the lungs, but gain access through an *incompletely closed foramen ovale* (most common) or *atrial septal defect* into the systemic circulation.

ETIOLOGY OF EMBOLISM

FAT EMBOLISM

Fat embolism is presence of emboli comprising of fat microglobules in the circulation. Fat embolism syndrome is most often a consequence of severe trauma with *long bone fractures* such as femur with abundant fatty marrow. It can also be seen with *extensive trauma to fat laden tissues, burns*, and very rarely with orthopedic procedures.

Pathogenesis

On long bone fracture, bone marrow fatty fragments enter the circulation, lodge in small blood vessels of the lung, skin, kidneys, brain and other organs producing ischemia and hemorrhage. It results in the clinical manifestations. *Fat microglobules* are converted into fatty acids, which damage vascular endothelium resulting in formation of platelet thrombi in areas of injury.

Clinical Features

Patient develops potentially fatal fat embolism syndrome within 24 to 72 hours. It is characterized by pulmonary distress, cutaneous petechial hemorrhages, and various neurologic manifestations.

- *Pulmonary manifestations:* Patient develops *dyspnea* and *tachypnea* is due to presence of fat microglobules in pulmonary capillaries causing hypoxemia.
- *Petechial hemorrhage:* Patient develops petechial hemorrhage over the chest and upper extremities due to thrombocytopenia from platelets adhesion to microglobules of fat.
- *Neurologic manifestations:* Numerous petechial hemorrhages are produced by fat emboli to the brain, particularly in white matter known as *brain purpura*. Patient develops neurologic manifestations such as loss of consciousness, cerebral edema and herniation within a week in less than 10% of cases with fatal outcome (Fig. 3.20).

Laboratory Diagnosis

Bronchoalveolar lavage: It is done to demonstrate fat in alveolar macrophages by staining with fat stains, e.g. Sudan III, Sudan V, Sudan black and Oil red O. In fat embolism, fat microglobules converted into fatty acids are taken by the alveolar macrophages.

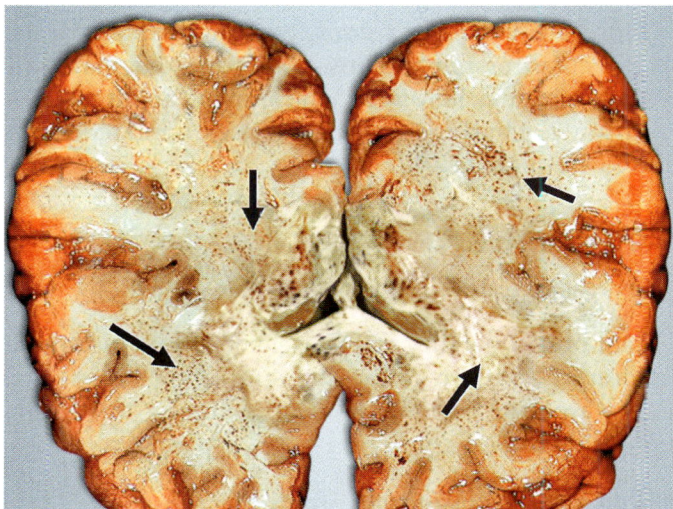

Fig. 3.20: Fat embolus. The patient died due to multiple fractures of both legs in a motorcycle accident. The fat emboli caused petechial hemorrhages in the white matter throughout the brain, resulting in coma and death. The macroscopic appearance of cerebral malaria is identical to this (arrows).

Light Microscopy

In autopsy specimens, frozen section examination reveals fat globules within the pulmonary arterioles by fat stains. Examination of paraffin embedded sections stained with hematoxylin and eosin reveals rounded clear holes due to dissolution of fat during processing in the small pulmonary arterial branch of lung characteristic for fat embolism.

AIR EMBOLISM

Air embolism results from the introduction of excess of air into the circulation leading to vascular flow obstruction. Patient presents with distal ischemic injury, pulmonary gas embolism—sudden death and convulsions and deep coma.

Pathogenesis: Air embolism occurs as a consequence of *penetrating chest injury, clumsily performed criminal abortion, intravenous infusion of fluids* and *deep-sea divers.*

- *Incision of intracranial veins:* Single air embolism occurs when atmospheric air may enter the blood circulation as a result of incision of intracranial vein during head and neck surgery. Inspiration produces a suction effect by causing negative pressure in these veins leading to frothing of blood in right ventricle and impairment of cardiac functions.
- *Penetrating chest injury:* It leads to entry of air into the ruptured vessels resulting in air embolism.
- *Intravenous infusion:* Due to improper monitoring of intravenous infusion, excess of air (more than 100 cc) may result in air embolism.
- *Caisson disease:* Multiple air emboli are formed in sea divers.

Decompression Sickness (Caisson Disease)

Decompression sickness is a form of air embolism observed in *scuba and deep-sea divers* due to sudden change in atmospheric pressure, who return to the surface too rapidly. Insoluble nitrogen coming out of blood forms gas emboli which obstruct blood flow to skeletal system, central nervous system and other tissues.

Clinical Features

Patient presents with musculoskeletal pain in joints, muscle and bones called as *bends*. Obstruction to circulation leads to small infarcts. *Nitrogen has an affinity for adipose tissue;* hence *obese persons* are at increased risk for Caisson disease. *Pneumothorax due to rupture of a preexisting subpleural bleb or pulmonary embolism* are responsible for dyspnea and pleuritic pain. In chronic cases, patients develop aseptic necrosis in bones (e.g. *femur, tibia,* and *humerus*) from bone infarction.

AMNIOTIC FLUID EMBOLISM

Amniotic fluid embolism refers to the entry of amniotic fluid containing fetal squamous cells, lanugo hair, vernix, and mucin following tear in the placental membranes. It may gain access to uterine and cervical veins into the maternal circulation. *It occurs during labor or immediate postpartum period. Patient develops abrupt onset of dyspnea, cyanosis, hypotension and bleeding manifestations* as a result of amniotic fluid emboli contents.

Diagnosis

Amniotic fluid embolism is most often confirmed at autopsy by histopathologic examination. It reveals presence of *squamous epithelial cells, lanugo hair, fat globules, mucinous material, marked pulmonary edema, diffuse alveolar damage* and *fibrin clots* in the systemic circulation (DIC).

Acute Respiratory Distress Syndrome

Diffuse alveolar damage with hyaline membranes is a feature of adult respiratory distress syndrome. Severe damage to alveolar capillary membrane by amniotic fluid emboli contents leads to formation of hyaline membrane and pulmonary edema. Due to impaired exchange of gases across alveolar capillary membrane, patient develops dyspnea and cyanosis. Pulmonary edema in acute respiratory distress syndrome does not resolve, however, it resolves in cases of congestive heart failure.

Disseminated Intravascular Coagulation (DIC)

Amniotic fluid embolism is one of the major obstetric causes of disseminated intravascular coagulation as a result of activation of coagulation system. Patient presents with bleeding manifestations due to consumption of coagulation factors and fibrin (i.e. defibrination syndrome) and results in formation of microthrombi with ischemic changes in various organs. There is sudden onset of cyanosis and shock, followed by coma and death.

EMBOLI FROM ATHEROMATOUS PLAQUE

Atherosclerosis means hardening (sclerosis) or loss of elasticity of large elastic arteries and medium-sized arteries due to atheromatous plaque formation. Emboli of atheromatous plaque material to distant sites may result in infarction (*spleen, kidney, small intestine*).

EMBOLI FROM TUMORS

Embolism may be caused by fragments of tumor such as clear cell carcinoma of kidney, lung carcinoma and malignant melanoma.

MISCELLANEOUS EMBOLI

Various exogenous and endogenous substances may act as emboli. These include fragments from tissue and placenta. Other emboli are formed by parasites, bullets, sutures and barium contrast media.

INFARCTION

OVERVIEW

An infarct is an area of necrosis resulting from ischemia caused by obstruction of arterial or venous blood supply in a particular tissue. Organs involved include myocardium, *brain, lung, kidneys, spleen, bowel, ovaries, testes, and diabetic dry gangrene of lower limb.* Ischemia produces coagulative necrosis in *solid organs rich in proteins such as heart, kidney and spleen.*

Coagulative necrosis refers to light microscopic changes in the dying cells as a result of ischemia. Cellular outlines are maintained but structural details are lost. Widespread tissue necrosis, is called as an *infarction. Liquefactive necrosis* occurs in *brain* (proteins deficient in brain) and *suppurative infections.*

Causes of Infarction

- *Intravascular causes:* Arterial occlusion occurs due to thrombotic or embolic events (99% of all infarcts), local vasospasm and expansion of an atheromatous plaque occluding lumen.
- *Extravascular causes:* These include extrinsic compression of a vessel by tumor, twisting of the vessels: testicular torsion and bowel volvulus, edema inducing ischemia, hernial sac entrapment, and traumatic rupture of the blood vessels. Causes of infarction are shown in Table 3.12.

FACTORS INFLUENCING INFARCTION

ANATOMICAL PATTERN OF ARTERIAL SUPPLY

Extent of tissue injury due to ischemia depends on the anatomical pattern of arterial supply of the organs. There are four patterns of arterial supply to various organs described as under.

Single Arterial Supply without Anastomoses

Some organs such as *kidney, spleen and retina have single arterial supply without significant anastomosis.* Occlusion of arteries supplying these organs produces *white (pale) infarcts.*

Disorders of Hemostasis

Table 3.12: Causes of infraction

Causes	Lesion	Artery involved	Infarct in organ
Arterial causes	Atherosclerosis	Coronary arteries	Myocardial infarction
		Cerebral arteries	Cerebral stroke
		Renal arteries	Renal infarct
	Thromboembolism (originating in heart and blood vessels)	Coronary arteries	Myocardial infarction
		Renal arteries	Renal infarct
		Splenic artery	Splenic infarct
	External pressure on arteries	Arteries of organ	Organ infarct
Venous causes	Strangulated hernia	Mesenteric vessels	Gangrene intestine
	Volvulus intestinal loop	Mesenteric vessels	Gangrene intestine
	Intussusception	Mesenteric vessels	Gangrene intestine
	Torsion testes	Testicular vein	Testicular infarct
Blockage of small vessels	Microthromboemboli (originating from infective endocarditis)	Renal artery branches	Renal infarct
	Sickle cell anemia	Renal peritubular *capillaries in the medulla* due to the low O_2 tension in the medulla	Renal infarct
	Bed sores	Occlusion of small vessels of skin	Gangrene of affected skin
	Decompression sickness	Dissolved gases forming microemboli occluding vessels	Infarcts of organs

Single Arterial Supply with Rich Anastomoses

Intestine supplied by mesenteric artery has multiple anastomoses. *Large bowel* has arterial blood supply from more than one artery. *Splenic flexure and rectosigmoid junction* are the most common sites of infarcts in colon. These are *less vascularized* areas known as *watershed regions*. Watershed regions include *splenic flexure* (junction of the superior and inferior mesenteric arteries) and *rectosigmoid junction* (junction of left colic and sigmoid—superior rectal branches of the inferior mesenteric artery).

Dual Blood Supply

Lungs and liver have dual blood supply, hence less prone to ischemia. Liver receives blood supply from portal vein and hepatic artery. Occlusion of portal vein may produce *red infarct* as liver keeps on receiving arterial supply from hepatic artery.

Lung is supplied by pulmonary and bronchial arteries. Occlusion of pulmonary artery by emboli produces *red infarct*, because lung keeps on receiving blood from bronchial artery.

> **Gross Morphology**
> - Hemorrhagic lung infarct is raised, wedge-shaped area with red blue discoloration that extends to the pleural surface.
> - Majority of infarcts are located in the lower lobes.
> - Perfusion is greater than ventilation in the lower lobes.

Clinical features: Patient presents with dyspnea or pleuritic chest pain on inspiration, expiratory wheezing, tachycardia, productive cough (sputum may be blood-tinged), low-grade fever and pleural effusion (fibrinous exudate).

Parallel Arterial Supply

Forearm is supplied by radial and ulnar arteries running in parallel pattern. Vitality of forearm due to occlusion of one artery is maintained by alternative other artery.

VULNERABILITY OF TISSUES TO HYPOXIA

Ischemic injury depends on the type of cells or tissues undergoing ischemic necrosis. Hypoxia adversely affecting in *descending order includes neurons, myocardium, liver, skeletal muscle and fibroblasts*. Vulnerability of cells (organs) to ischemic irreversible cell injury is shown in Table 3.13.

Nervous system: Complete interruption of blood supply to brain causes *irreversible damage to neurons within 3–5 minutes. Cerebellum's Purkinje cells* and *hippocampus area are more susceptible* to ischemic injury.

Myocardium and liver: Ischemic necrosis of myocardial cells and hepatocytes cause irreversible cell death within 1–2 hours.

Skeletal muscles: Ischemic necrosis of skeletal muscle cells causes irreversible cell death within many hours.

Table 3.13: Vulnerability of cells (organs) to ischemic irreversible cell injury

Organs	Cells/tissue	Duration of irreversible injury
Nervous system	Neurons (cerebellum's Purkinje cells and hippocampus area most susceptible to injury)	3–5 minutes
Heart	Myocardium	20–30 minutes
Liver	Hepatocytes	1–2 hours
Skeletal muscle	Skeletal muscle fibers	Many hours
Fibrous tissue	Fibroblasts	Resistant to ischemic changes

BLOOD OXYGEN CONTENT

Blood oxygen content and cardiovascular system play an important role in maintenance of arterial supply to the tissues. Disorders of blood and cardiovascular system adversely affect the arterial supply to the organs. Various disorders include *blood loss, shock, sickle cell anemia, cardiac failure and atheromatous plaques* in large elastic and medium size arteries. Complete occlusion of arteries produces more severe ischemic necrosis of organs.

RAPID DEVELOPMENT OF INFARCT

Sudden occlusion of arteries produce more severe ischemic tissue injury, because it takes more time for development of collateral blood supply.

TYPE OF INFARCTS

Infarction is gross manifestation of coagulative necrosis. Infarcts are of two types, i.e. *pale infarct and hemorrhagic infarct* depending on the consistency of the tissue. Infarcts are classified based on the color and presence or absence of microbial infection.

Based on the color of infarct: Based on color, there are two types of infarcts, i.e. pale/white infarcts, and hemorrhagic infarcts. *Pale infarcts occur in kidneys, spleen* and *heart.* Differences between pale white and red hemorrhagic infarcts are shown in Table 3.14.

Based on the age of infarct: Infarcts may be recent or healed lesion.

Presence or Absence of Microbial Infection

- *Septic (infective) infarcts:* These occur when bacterial vegetations from a heart valve embolise or when microbes seed an area of necrotic tissue. Such infarcts are converted into abscess with a corresponding greater inflammatory response. These infarcts *get organized*.
- *Bland infarct (non-infective) infarct:* Infarct is *sterile*. No organisms are demonstrated in these infarcts.

WHITE (PALE) INFARCT

White (pale) infarct is secondary to the sudden occlusion of a vessel. It is commonly seen in *solid organs such as heart, kidney*, and *spleen*. Increased density of solid tissue prevents RBCs from diffusing through necrotic tissue.

Table 3.14: Differences between pale white and red hemorrhagic infarcts

Comments	Pale/white infarcts	Red/hemorrhagic infarcts
Arterial circulation	Single arterial supply	Dual arterial supply
Etiology	Occlusion of artery by thrombi, emboli, complicated atheromatous plaque and vasospasm	Occlusion of artery or vein by thromboembolic phenomenon or torsion
Consistency of organ	Solid consistency	Loose texture organs permitting blood
Organs involved	Heart, kidneys, spleen, digits of lower limb (cystic infarct in brain)	Lung, small intestine, testis and ovaries
Morphology of infarcts	Small size infarcts	Large-sized infarcts
	Wedge-shaped with the occluded vessel at the apex and the periphery of the organ forming the base	Well circumscribed, firm and dark red infarcts
Shape of infarct	Zone of hyperemia at the periphery of infarct sharply defines margins	Margin of infarct not well defined. Fibrinous exudates present on serous membrane of organs
Edema in organ	Absent	Present
Light microscopy	Coagulative necrosis in all solid organs except brain*	Coagulative necrosis in all organs involved

*Liquefactive necrosis in brain occurs as brain is deficient in proteins.

Disorders of Hemostasis

Gross Morphology

White infarct produces *wedge-shaped infarct* with apex pointing to the site of obstruction, and the base of infarct at the periphery of the organ.

Light Microscopy

The cellular debris of infarct is degraded by neutrophils, and later by macrophages. Granulation tissue eventually forms, to be replaced ultimately by a scar.

Myocardial Infarct

Myocardial infarct is most often caused by ischemia related to *coronary artery occlusion involving >75% of lumen by atheromatous plaque.*

Major risk factors: Major risk factors for atherosclerosis are hyperlipidemia, hypertension, tobacco smoking and diabetes mellitus.

Vessel involved: The coronary vessels most commonly involved in decreasing order of frequency are *anterior descending branch of left coronary (LAD) 50%, right coronary artery (RCA) 30%* and *left circumflex artery (LCA) (20%)*. Atheromatous plaques are observed in proximal part of anterior descending artery.

Type of myocardial infarcts: Complete coronary occlusion produces *transmural myocardial infarct*. Partial coronary occlusion leads to *subendocardial infarct limited to the interior one-third to inner half of the left ventricle*. Severe reduction of coronary blood flow causes *circumferential myocardial infarct involving* ventricular chamber in circumferential manner (Fig. 3.21).

Kidney Infarct

Renal infarction refers to ischemic necrosis due to occlusion of interlobar or larger branches of the renal artery most often caused as a result of *thromboemboli*. Patient presents with sudden onset of flank pain and hematuria.

Etiology

These *microthrombi* originate from the heart such as mural endocardium, *acute myocardial infarction*, and *infective endocarditis*. Less common causes of renal artery occlusion are severe atheromatous plaque and sickle nephropathy. Sickling of red blood cell may occur in *peritubular capillaries in the medulla* due to the low O_2 tension in the medulla leading to renal ischemia. The glomeruli are conspicuously congested with sickle cells.

Gross Morphology

- Irregular wedge-shaped pale infarcts are present in cortex within one week.
- Old infarcts have a V-shaped appearance due to scar tissue.
- Apex of infarct is pointing towards cortex and base towards medulla.

Light Microscopy

- Histopathological examination of renal infarct shows coagulative necrosis.
- Cellular outlines of renal tubules and glomeruli are maintained with loss of structural details.
- There is presence of polymorphonuclear cells in acute phase followed by macrophages in later phase at the margin of infarct.

Splenic Infarct

Splenic infarction refers to ischemic necrosis due to occlusion of splenic artery and its branches most often caused as a result of *thromboemboli*. These microthrombi originating from the heart such as mural

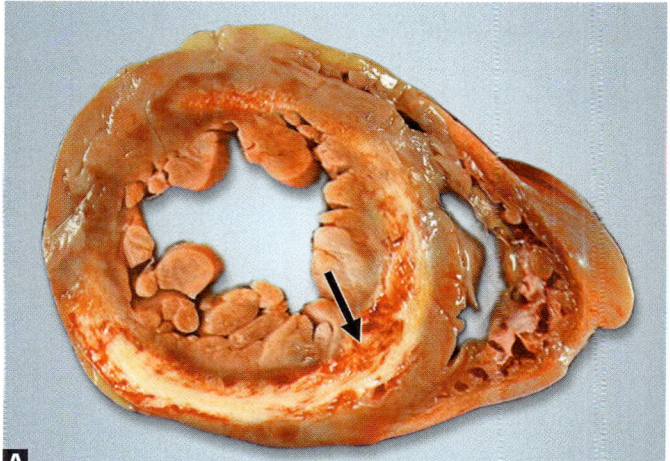
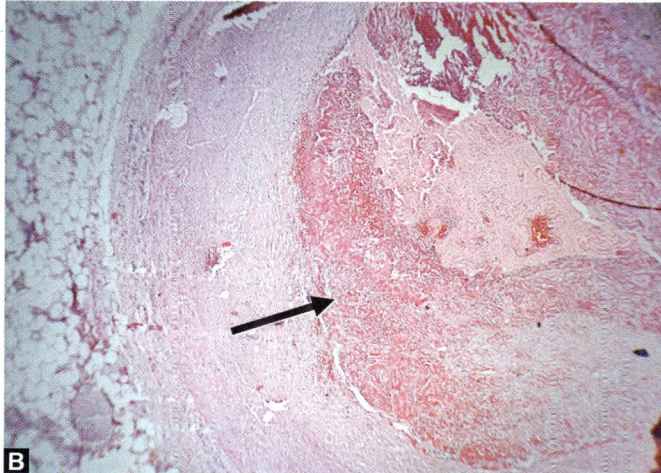

Fig. 3.21: (A) Transmural infarct, (B) complicated atheromatous plaque with thrombus formation and complete occlusion (arrow) (400X).

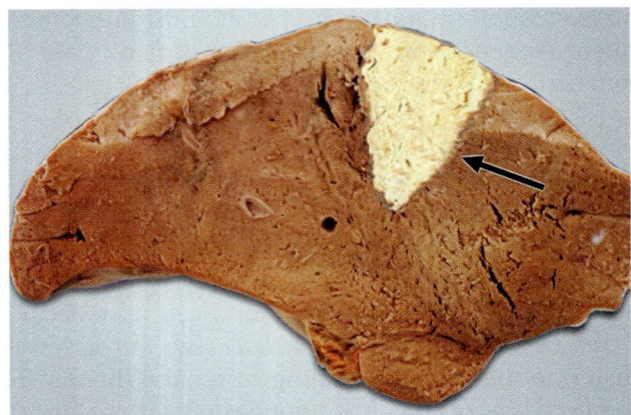

Fig. 3.22: Pale infarct in spleen (arrow).

endocardium, acute myocardial infarction and infective endocarditis occlude splenic artery leading to splenic infarct (Fig. 3.22).

Gross Morphology
Splenic infarcts are most often multiple and wedge shape in appearance.

Light Microscopy
- Histopathological examination of splenic infarct shows coagulative necrosis.
- Cellular outlines are maintained with loss of structural details. There is presence of polymorphonuclear cells in acute phase followed by macrophages in later phase at the margin of infarct.

HEMORRHAGIC (RED) INFARCT

Hemorrhagic (red) infarct may result from *either arterial or venous occlusion*. It occurs principally in the *loose-textured well vascularized organs* such as *lungs, small intestine, ovaries*, and *testis*. Splenic vein occlusion due to thrombosis causes hemorrhagic infarct in spleen. Hemorrhagic infarct allows RBCs to diffuse through necrotic tissue. Gross examination reveals *wedge-shaped hemorrhagic infarct with dark red to purple discoloration extending to the surface of organ*.

Pulmonary Hemorrhagic Infarct

Each lung receives blood supply from pulmonary and bronchial arteries. Pulmonary artery embolism produces *wedge-shaped area of hemorrhagic infarct extending to the pleural surface* (Fig. 3.23). Red infarct area receiving constant blood supply from normal bronchial arteries, allows RBCs to diffuse through necrotic tissue. Gross examination of pulmonary infarct reveals wedge-shaped area of hemorrhage extending to the pleural surface due to embolus in one of the pulmonary artery tributaries.

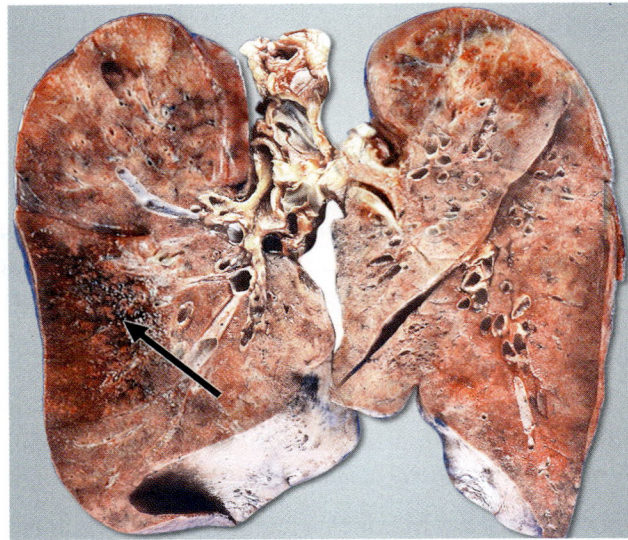

Fig. 3.23: Pulmonary infarction showing wedge-shaped infarct extending to the pleural surface (arrow).

Intestinal Hemorrhagic Infarct

Small intestine has rich blood supply with extensive collateral circulation. Occlusion of mesenteric artery causes hemorrhagic infarct. Volvulus (segment of gut twisting on its mesentery) and strangulated hernial sac cause infarct in small intestine. Red blood cells diffuse through necrotic tissue. On gross examination, red infarcts are sharply circumscribed, firm, and dark red to purple (Fig. 3.24).

Testes or Ovarian Hemorrhagic Infarct

Torsion of testis or ovary and postoperative adhesions may cause venous occlusion which results in red infarcts.

Pale Infarct Undergoing Hemorrhagic Infarct

Myocardial infarct is an example of pale infarct, but a red infarct occurs following spontaneous reperfusion of infarct area due to therapeutically induced lysis of the occluding thrombus.

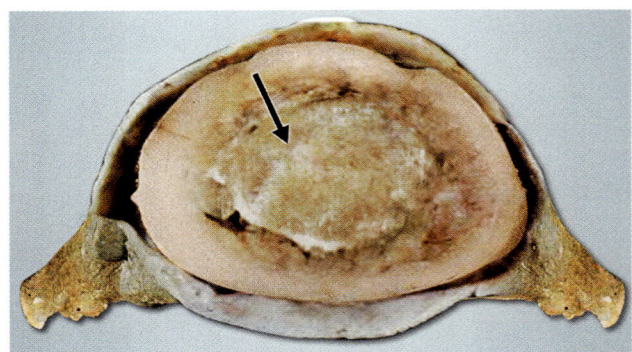

Fig. 3.24: Ischemic bowel disease showing dusky blackish discoloration.

CYSTIC INFARCT IN BRAIN

Cerebrovascular diseases are the most common group of CNS disorders. Complicated atheromatous plaques in arteries supplying brain (bifurcation of carotid arteries), emboli arising from cardiac mural thrombi, vegetations of infected endocarditic valves, clumps of tumor cells, bubbles of air, or droplets of fat into middle cerebral artery cause cerebral ischemia.

Watershed areas: Cerebral infarction occurs in the boundary zone between the territories supplied by middle cerebral and anterior cerebral arteries. Watershed areas are of the arterial territory most remote from the patent arterial stems and thus most vulnerable to the effects of cerebral underperfusion.

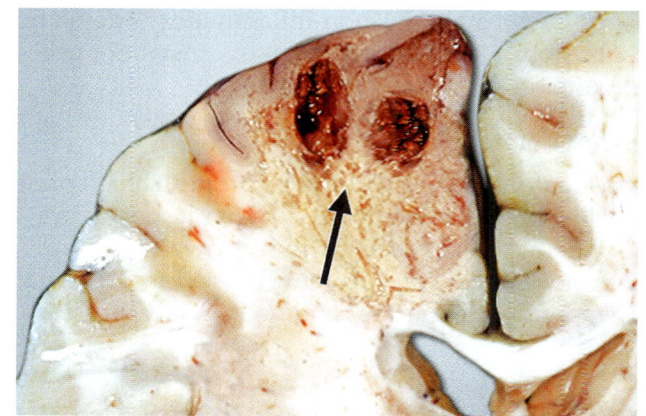

Fig. 3.25: Cerebral infarct in frontal lobe showing liquefactive necrosis with formation of cystic spaces on resolution of infarct (arrow).

Gross Morphology
Brain does not contain proteins, hence ischemia produces liquefactive necrosis resulting in formation of cystic spaces containing creamy liquid necrotic debris by hydrolytic enzymes (Fig. 3.25).

Light Microscopy
Cyst wall is formed by proliferating capillaries, neutrophils, macrophages and proliferating neuroglial cells.

EDEMA

TYPE OF EDEMA FLUID

Abnormal accumulation of fluid in interstitial tissue spaces or body cavities is known as *edema*. Causes of edema are shown in Table 3.15.

TRANSUDATE

A transudate is ultrafiltrate of plasma. It occurs due to alterations in Starling's pressure (hydrostatic pressure or oncotic pressure). Permeability of vascular endothelium

Table 3.15: Causes of edema

Pathogenesis	Mechanism	Disorders
Increased capillary pressure	Increased vascular volume	Heart failure Kidney disease Premenstrual sodium retention Pregnancy Environmental heat stress Thiazolidinedione (e.g. pioglitazone, rosiglitazone) therapy
	Venous obstruction	Liver disease with portal vein obstruction Acute pulmonary edema Venous thrombosis (thrombophlebitis)
	Decreased arteriolar resistance	Calcium channel blocking drug responses
Decreased colloidal osmotic pressure	Increased loss of plasma proteins	Protein-losing kidney diseases Extensive burns
	Decreased production of plasma proteins	Liver disease Starvation, malnutrition
Increased capillary permeability	Inflammation	Allergic reactions (e.g. hives) Malignancy (e.g. ascites, pleural effusion) Tissue injury and burns
Obstruction of lymphatic flow	Obstruction of lymphatic flow	Malignant obstruction of lymphatic structures Surgical removal of lymph nodes

is usually normal. This non-inflammatory edema fluid results from altered intravascular hydrostatic or osmotic pressure.

Composition

Transudate is straw-colored ultrafiltrate of blood plasma with low protein content (<3 g/dl) with specific gravity <1.012. It is composed of mainly water, dissolved electrolytes, and low protein. It produces edema in dependent parts (pitting) and body cavity effusions.

Pathogenesis

Increased vascular hydrostatic pressure: Patient develops pulmonary edema in *left-sided heart failure* (e.g. systemic hypertension, aortic valve stenosis in RHD). Peripheral *pitting edema* occurs in right-sided heart failure. Ascites is seen in portal hypertension in cirrhosis.

Decreased vascular plasma oncotic pressure: Patient develops edema due to malnutrition with *decreased protein intake, cirrhosis with decreased synthesis of albumin, nephrotic syndrome* and *malabsorption syndrome* with decreased absorption of proteins. Patient develops anasarca/generalized edema in nephrotic syndrome.

Renal retention of sodium and water: Decreased glomerular filtration rate in acute renal failure and glomerulonephritis, results in increased renin production, which stimulates liver to synthesize angiotensinogen, which is converted into angiotensin II, which acts on adrenal cortex to synthesize aldosterone, which acts on distal convoluted tubules to absorb sodium and water and increased plasma volume. Hydrostatic pressure is increased due to increased plasma volume. Dilution effect of albumin results in decreased oncotic pressure.

EXUDATE

An exudate occurs due to increased vascular permeability of postcapillary venules during acute inflammatory process. Chemical mediators derived from cells and plasma proteins act on nearby blood vessels result in increased permeability of microvasculature. It produces swelling of tissue but no pitting edema.

Composition

Exudate is rich in plasma proteins (>3 g/dl), fibrinogen/fibrin, immunoglobulins, salts, water and neutrophils. It has a specific gravity exceeding 1.020.

Clinical Correlation

Acute inflammation brings chemical mediators of inflammation into injured site, which acts on nearby blood vessels. It is responsible for *swelling (edema), pain, and impaired function.* Exudates formed in severe burns are life-threatening. *Fibrin formation* in the injured area aids in localizing the *spread of infectious microorganisms.* Exudates *dilute bacterial toxins* and provide *opsonins* (IgG, C3b) to assist in *phagocytosis.* Differences between exudate and transudate are shown in Table 3.16 and formation of transudate and exudate is shown in Fig. 3.26.

Table 3.16: Differences between exudate and transudate

Characteristics	Transudate	Exudate
Cause	Increased hydrostatic pressure or decreased oncotic pressure	Increased permeability of postcapillary venules in inflammation
Pathological state	Congestive heart failure Hypoproteinemia (malnutrition) Nephrotic syndrome (protein loss)	Acute inflammation
Endothelial permeability	Normal endothelial permeability	Altered endothelial permeability
Fluid nature	Ultrafiltrate of blood plasma	Inflammatory extravascular fluid
Composition	Mainly water and dissolved electrolytes	Mainly protein and cellular debris
Endothelial permeability	Normal endothelial permeability	Altered endothelial permeability
Color	Transparent/light straw colored	Yellowish-white opaque appearance
pH	More alkaline (>7.3)	Less alkaline (<7.3)
Specific gravity	<1.012	>1.020 due to raised proteins content in exudate
Proteins content	Low protein fluid (<3 gm/dl)	High protein content, which raises specific gravity
Glucose concentration	Same as that of blood	Low in case of association with infections and cancer
Ratio of LDH levels in fluids and serum	Low (<0.6)	High (>0.6)
Light microscopy	Inflammatory cells absent	PMN cells in acute inflammation Macrophages and lymphocytes in chronic inflammation

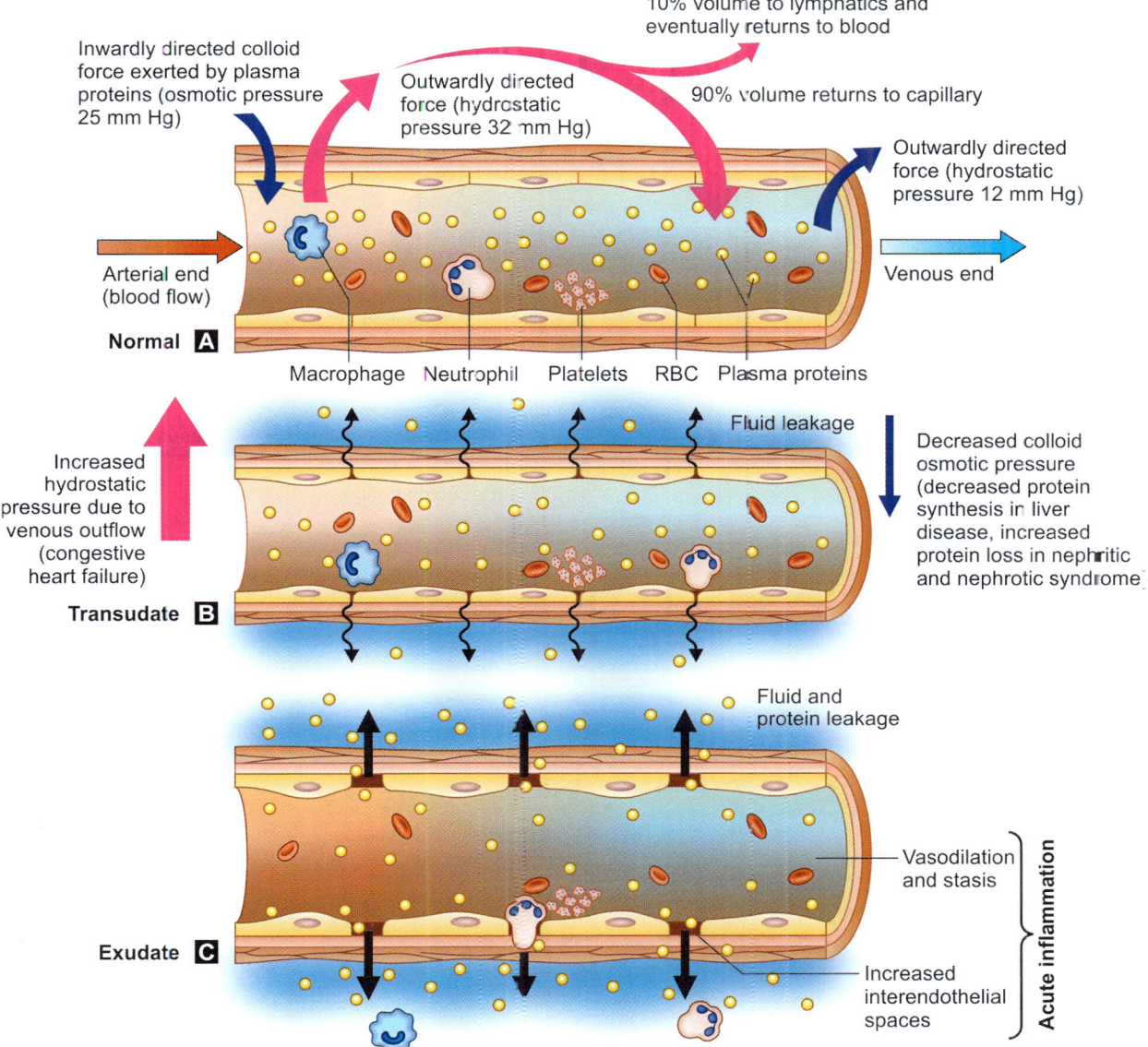

Fig. 3.26: Formation of transudate and exudate. (A) Normal hydrostatic pressure at arterial end of capillary is 32 mm Hg and 12 mm Hg at venous end. Oncotic pressure exerted by plasma proteins is 25 mm Hg. Approximately 90% of fluid is drained back to capillary, while 10% of interstitial fluid drained by lymphatic channels to venous circulation, (B) transudate is formed as a result of increased hydrostatic pressure or decreased oncotic pressure, (C) an exudate is formed due to increased vascular permeability.

LYMPHEDEMA

Lymphedema occurs due to obstruction of lymphatic channels following modified radical mastectomy and radiation. Filariasis due to *Wuchereria bancrofti* causes lymphangitis and ultimately blockage of lymphatic channels. Scrotal and vulvar lymphedema occurs due to lymphogranuloma venereum.

- Breast lymphedema occurs due to blockage of subcutaneous lymphatic channels by malignant cells.
- Lymph nodes are removed in patients with breast cancer undergoing modified radical mastectomy develops edema upper arm due to obstruction of lymphatic drainage.

GLYCOSAMINOGLYCANS

Due to increase in hyaluronic acid and chondroid sulphate, patient develops peritibial nonpitting edema in myxedema and retrobulbar edema in Graves' disease exophthalmos.

CLINICAL TYPES OF EDEMA

Edema may be localized in body cavities, e.g. pleural effusion, pericardial effusion or ascites. Generalized edema in nephrotic syndrome is also known as *anasarca*. Edema formation in congestive heart failure is shown in Fig. 3.27. Differences between cardiogenic edema and non-cardiogenic edema are shown in Table 3.17.

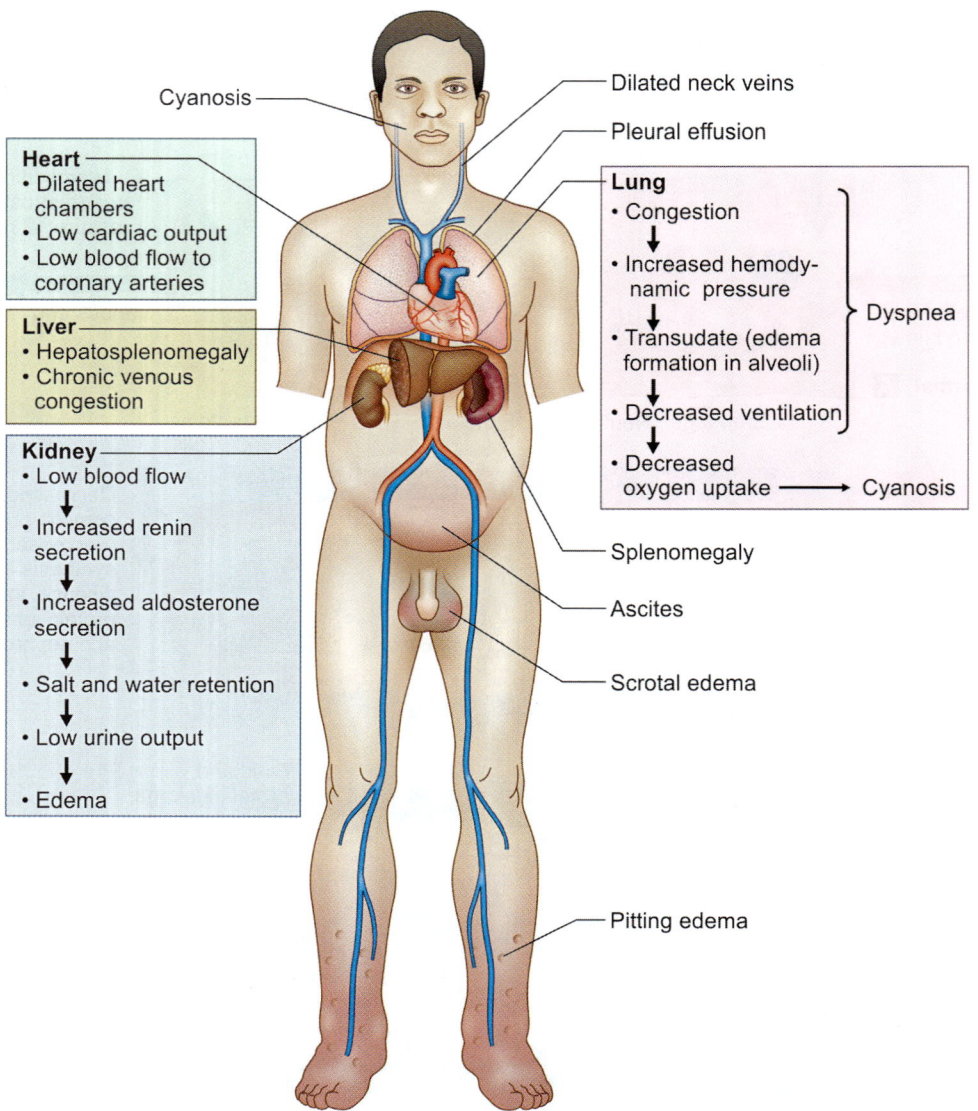

Fig. 3.27: Edema formation in congestive heart failure.

Table 3.17: Differences between cardiogenic edema and non-cardiogenic edema

Parameters	Cardiogenic edema	Non-cardiogenic edema
Etiology	Left ventricular failure	Aspiration of noxious fluids
	Myxoma in left atrium	Ingestion of drugs or poisons
	Mitral valve disease	Inhalation of noxious fluids
	Acute respiratory distress syndrome	Pulmonary infection
	Pulmonary vaso-occlusive disease	Systemic sepsis and trauma
Distribution	Central	More peripheral
Septal lines	More common	Less common
Radiograph	Septal lines common	Septal lines less common
	Peribronchial cuffing common	Peribronchial cuffing less common
	Pleural effusion common	Pleural effusion less common
	Cardiomegaly present	Cardiomegaly absent
	Pulmonary vasculature diversion in upper lobes	No distribution of pulmonary vasculature

PERICARDIAL EDEMA

Pericardial edema is collection of fluid in the pericardial sac beyond the 20–50 ml normally present. Pericardial effusions are caused by pericarditis (e.g. serous, fibrinous, suppurative, hemorrhagic or tubercular), metastatic deposits from lung cancer, breast cancer or lymphomas. Tubercular effusion contains straw-/pale-colored fluid formed by mycobacterial tubercle bacilli.

HYDROTHORAX

Hydrothorax refers to the accumulation of a significant volume of transudate about 200 to 400 ml within the pleural cavities (to be detected by chest radiograph). It is clear, straw-colored fluid with low protein with low specific gravity. Cardiac failure is the most common cause of hydrothorax, which is usually bilateral.

SUBCUTANEOUS EDEMA

Patient develops periorbital edema in nephritic syndrome, because proteinuria varies from mild to moderate <3.5 gm/24 hours. Patient with nephrotic syndrome presents with generalized edema due to massive proteinuria >3.5 gm/24 hours. Dependent edema is seen in congestive heart failure.

ASCITES

Excessive accumulation of serous fluid in the peritoneal cavity is known as *ascites*. Massive proteinuria in nephrotic syndrome and decreased synthesis in chronic liver disease lowers plasma albumin levels which results in ascites. Ascites in liver cirrhosis occurs due to decreased synthesis of albumin by liver, the most significant contributor to plasma oncotic pressure. It is associated with increased sodium and water retention because of stimulation of the renin-angiotensin system. Portal hypertension in cirrhosis results in fluid transudation and increased secretion of hepatic lymph.

PULMONARY EDEMA

Congestive heart failure is most important cause of pulmonary edema. It may also occur in left ventricular failure, mitral valve disease, myxoma in left atrium, acute respiratory distress syndrome and pulmonary vaso-occlusive disease. Non-cardiac edema causes include aspiration of noxious fluids, ingestion of drugs or poisons, inhalation of noxious fluids, pulmonary infection, systemic sepsis and trauma.

Pathogenesis

In patients with congestive heart failure, increased venous hydrostatic pressure leads to congestion of alveolar capillaries which results in accumulation of transudate in the alveoli. Passage of red blood cells into the alveoli are phagocytosed and degraded by macrophages. Hemosiderin-laden macrophages are known as *heart failure cells*.

Clinical Features

Patient presents with shortness of breath (dyspnea) on exertion and when recumbent (orthopnea). Patient may awaken from sleep due to sudden episodes of shortness of breath (paroxysmal nocturnal dyspnea). On auscultation, crackling breath sounds (rales) are heard caused due to expansion of fluid-filled alveoli. Right-sided heart failure reveals distended jugular veins, pitting edema of the lower extremities and an enlarged and tender liver.

CHRONIC VENOUS CONGESTION OF LIVER

In right-sided heart failure, the liver is particularly vulnerable to chronic passive congestion, because the hepatic veins empty into the inferior vena cava. Liver is enlarged and tender.

> **Gross Morphology**
> - Cut surface of chronic venous congestion of liver reveals dark areas of centrilobular congestion alternating with unaffected pale portal areas gives *nutmeg-like appearance*.
> - It resembles a cross-section of a nutmeg.
> - Long-standing chronic passive congestion of liver may produce bridging fibrosis resulting in centrilobular fibrosis and *cardiac cirrhosis* in most extreme cases.
>
> **Light Microscopy**
> - Central veins and sinusoids of hepatic lobules are dilated and congested with blood.
> - Dilation of the sinusoids causes pressure atrophy of the centrilobular hepatocytes.

CEREBRAL EDEMA

Increased intracranial pressure due to cerebral edema leads to herniation of the brainstem or cerebellar tonsils. Patient presents with projectile vomiting, headache and convulsive seizures.

PATHOPHYSIOLOGY OF EDEMA

Normal hydrostatic pressure in capillaries at arterial end is 32 mm Hg and 12 mm Hg at venous end. Osmotic pressure exerted by plasma proteins is 25 mm Hg in capillaries. Due to pressure gradient, hydrostatic blood pressure forces water out of capillaries at the arterial end. At the venous end, 90% of extravasated fluid is drained back in capillaries at venous end due to oncotic pressure exerted by plasma albumin. Remaining 10% fluid in interstitial tissue is drained via lymphatic channels into circulation. When the balance of these forces is altered, the net result is accumulation of fluid in the interstitial spaces (i.e. edema). Edema is classified into five categories described as under.

INCREASED HYDROSTATIC PRESSURE

Increased hydrostatic pressure in vessels exceeds that of plasma oncotic pressure and so water remains in the tissues. It occurs in congestive heart failure.

Clinical Features

Patient develops pulmonary edema in left-sided heart failure due to systemic hypertension, aortic valve stenosis in rheumatic heart disease. Right-sided heart failure results in peripheral edema. Portal hypertension in cirrhosis leads to accumulation of fluid in peritoneal cavity known as *ascites*.

Type of Fluid

Fluid accumulated in these tissues is a transudate, which is straw-colored ultrafiltrate of blood plasma with low protein content with specific gravity less than 1.012. It is composed of mainly water, dissolved electrolytes, and low protein.

INCREASED CAPILLARY PERMEABILITY

Physiological state: The wall of the normal venules is sealed by tight junctions between adjacent endothelial cells. Normally, fluid leaving and entering blood vessels are in equilibrium.

Pathological state: During acute inflammation, chemical mediators widen inter-endothelial space leading to increased vascular permeability of postcapillary venules. Extravasation of inflammatory exudate is accumulated at injury site (edema). It is responsible for swelling (edema), pain, and impaired function. Exudate contains plasma proteins with specific gravity >1020, particularly fibrinogen/fibrin, immunoglobulins, salts, water and neutrophils. Severe injury to microvasculature in severe burns is life-threatening.

DECREASED ONCOTIC PRESSURE

Proteinuria in nephrotic or nephritic syndrome lowers plasma albumin concentration resulting in decreased oncotic pressure. Decreased protein synthesis in liver diseases decreases plasma albumin concentration. Decreased intake of proteins in malnutrition and excessive loss of proteins in malabsorption also decreases oncotic pressure. Fluid accumulated in interstitial tissue is a transudate.

Mechanism

Decreased plasma albumin concentration reduces the plasma oncotic pressure so that water cannot be drained back into the capillary bed at the venous end.

INCREASED SODIUM RETENTION

Primary sodium retention is associated with renal disorders. Secondary sodium retention occurs in congestive heart failure. Decreased cardiac output leads to decreased renal blood flow resulting in activation of renin-angiotensin system. Angiotensin II stimulates adrenal gland to synthesize aldosterone, which acts on renal distal tubule resulting in retention of sodium and water.

BLOCKAGE OF LYMPHATIC CHANNELS

Physiological state: Approximately 90% of extravasated fluid is drained back in capillaries at venous end and remaining 10% fluid in interstitial tissue is drained via lymphatics into circulation.

Pathological state: Lymphatic obstruction prevents drainage of water from the tissues resulting in edema. Breast lymphedema occurs due to blockage of subcutaneous lymphatic channels by malignant cells. Lymphatic system may be obstructed after axillary lymph node dissection for breast cancer.

Radiation also causes lymphatic obstruction. Filariasis due to *Wuchereria bancrofti* causes lymphangitis and ultimately blockage of lymphatic channels. Scrotal and vulvar lymphedema occurs due to lymphogranuloma venereum.

SHOCK

Shock is defined as a clinical state of cardiovascular collapse with resultant reduced perfusion of tissue and impaired oxygenation of tissues. Type and causes of shock are shown in Table 3.18. Pathophysiological findings in hypovolemic, cardiogenic and endotoxic shock are shown in Table 3.19.

Table 3.18: Type and causes of shock

Type of shock	Causes
Hypovolemic shock	Massive acute blood loss
	Severe burns
	Dehydration due to vomiting and diarrhea
	Diabetic precoma state
Cardiogenic shock	Myocardial infarction
	Ventricular arrhythmias
	Cardiomyopathy
	Cardiac tamponade (hemopericardium)
	Acute valve in competence
	Dissecting aortic aneurysm
	Massive pulmonary embolism
Septic shock	Systemic bacterial infections (gram-negative and gram-positive) resulting to vasodilatation
	Systemic fungal infections
Traumatic shock	Severe traumatic injuries
	Surgery induced massive blood loss
	Obstetrical trauma
Neurogenic shock	Spinal administration of anesthetic agent
	Spinal cord injury
	Head injury
Anaphylactic shock	Type I hypersensitivity (excessive histamine resulting to vasodilatation)

Table 3.19: Pathophysiological findings in hypovolemic, cardiogenic and endotoxic shock

Type	Cardiac output	Peripheral vascular resistance	Left ventricle end diastolic pressure
Hypovolemic shock	Decreased	Increased	Decreased
Cardiogenic shock	Decreased	Increased	Increased
Endotoxic shock	Increased	Decreased	Decreased

STAGES OF SHOCK

Stages of shock, etiology, pathogenesis and consequences are shown in Fig. 3.28.

COMPENSATED (INITIAL) SHOCK

Neurohormonal mechanism plays an important role in this stage. Compensatory mechanisms such as baroreceptor reflexes, release of catecholamines by adrenal medulla, activation of renin-angiotensin axis, antidiuretic hormone release and generalized sympathetic stimulation tachycardia, increased peripheral vasoconstriction and conservation of fluid by kidneys lead to maintenance of perfusion of vital organs.

On clinical examination, level of conscious, respiratory rate, blood pressure and urine output are normal. There is mild lactic acidosis.

NONPROGRESSIVE SHOCK

Nonprogressive shock is characterized by persistent hypotension, vasodilatation, tissue hypoperfusion, anaerobic glycolysis, lactic acidosis. Clinical examination reveals low blood pressure, increased pulse rate, increased respiratory rate and decreased urine output.

PROGRESSIVE DECOMPENSATED SHOCK

This stage is characterized by widespread tissue hypoxia, anaerobic glycolysis, excessive production of lactic acid, metabolic lactic acidosis decreased tissue pH, blunting of vasomotor response, peripheral pooling of blood and decreased cardiac output. Compensatory mechanisms are no longer adequate. Clinical examination reveals reduced urine output, drowsy state, increased respiratory rate, increased pulse rate and hypotension.

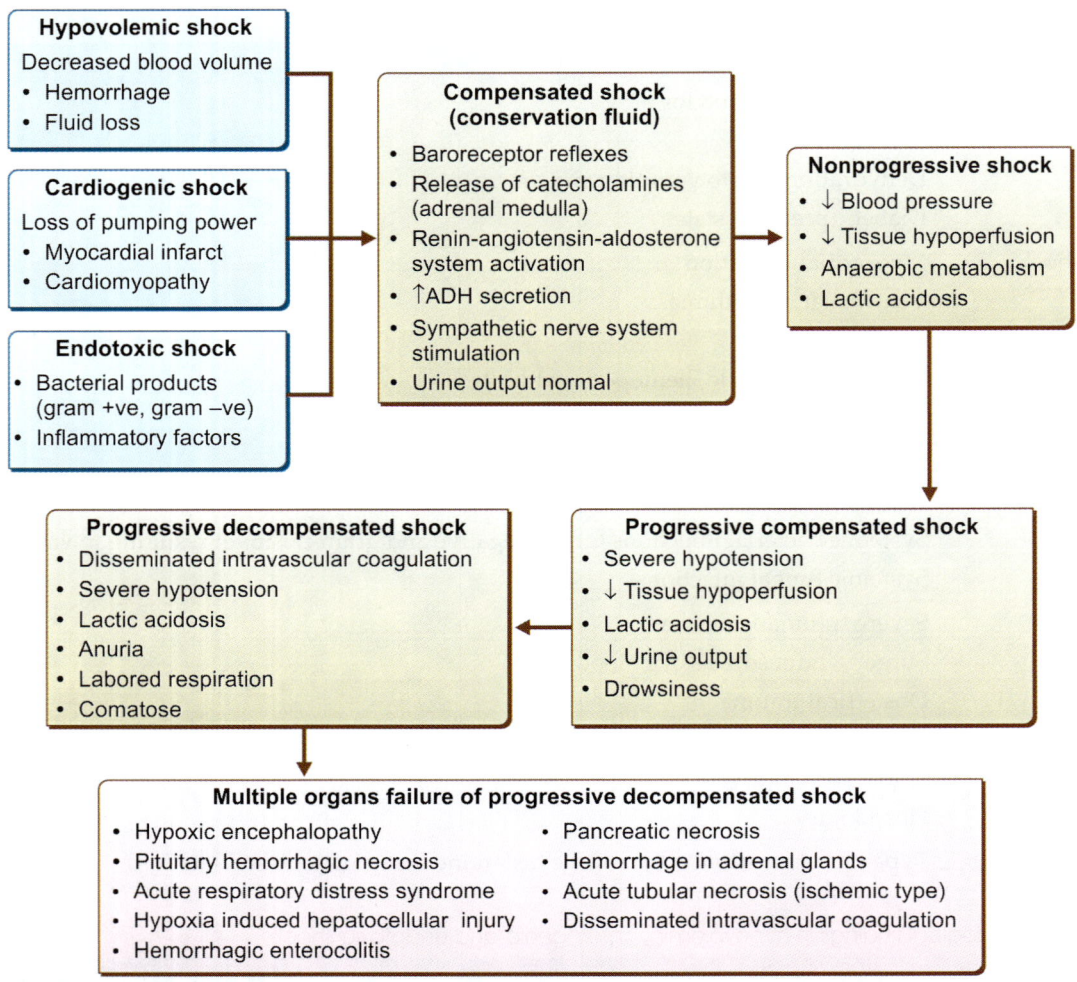

Fig. 3.28: Stages of shock. The illustration shows etiology, pathogenesis and consequences of shock.

IRREVERSIBLE DECOMPENSATED SHOCK

This stage is characterized by anoxic endothelial cell injury, disseminated intravascular coagulation (DIC), widespread tissue anoxia, lysosomal enzyme leakage, aggravation of shock and complete renal shutdown. *Clinical examination reveals anuria, severe hypotension, comatose state, labored respiration, increased pulse rate and lactic acidosis.*

Organ damage and metabolic disturbances are so severe that survival is not possible. Organs involvement in irreversible decompensated shock are shown in Table 3.20 and clinical features of shock are shown in Table 3.21.

TYPES OF SHOCK

HYPOVOLEMIC SHOCK

Hypovolemic shock is characterized by circulatory collapse due to acute reduction of blood volume resulting in circulatory dysfunction and inadequate tissue perfusion.

Table 3.20: Organs involvement in irreversible decompensated shock

Organ	Morphology of organ
Brain	Hypoxic encephalopathy
Pituitary gland	Pituitary hemorrhagic necrosis
Lungs	Acute respiratory distress syndrome
Liver	Hypoxia induced hepatocellular injury
Intestine	Hemorrhagic enterocolitis
Pancreas	Pancreatic necrosis
Adrenal glands	Hemorrhage in adrenal glands
Kidneys	Acute tubular necrosis (ischemic type)
Blood	Disseminated intravascular coagulation

Etiology

Hypovolemic shock is commonly caused by acute blood loss >20% of blood volume or reduction of body fluids. It occurs due to *gastrointestinal bleeding, severe/third degree burns, fluid loss from severe diarrhea or vomiting, intestinal*

Disorders of Hemostasis

Table 3.21: Clinical features of shock

Parameters	Compensated shock	Nonprogressive shock	Progressive decompensated shock	Irreversible decompensated shock
Blood pressure	Normal	Decreased (persistent vasodilatation)	Hypotension	Severe hypotension
Pulse rate	Mild increase	Increased	Increased	Increased
Lactic acidosis	+	+	++	+++
Urine output	Normal	Reduced	Reduced	Anuria
Level of consciousness	Normal	Drowsy	Drowsy	Comatose
Respiratory rate	Normal	Increased respiration	Increased respiration	Labored respiration

obstruction, peritonitis and acute pancreatitis. Shifting of fluid into pleural cavity, pericardial cavity or peritoneal cavity can also cause hypovolemic shock.

Pathophysiology

In hypovolemic shock, body's compensatory mechanism cannot maintain circulation for long. Blood pressure starts declining dramatically.

Compensatory mechanism in initial phase

- In the initial phase, body tries to compensate for fluid loss by *increasing cardiac output, sodium and water retention, synthesis of antidiuretic hormone.*
- Decreased blood supply to kidney leads to *synthesis of rennin, which stimulates liver to release angiotensinogen,* which forms angiotensin I and converted to angiotensin II in lungs. Angiotensin II increases *peripheral resistance* and *stimulates aldosterone production by adrenal cortex.* Aldosterone acts on distal convoluted tubules of kidneys to absorb sodium and water.

Compensatory mechanism in later phase: Compensatory mechanism fails and blood pressure continues dropping, leading to decreased tissue perfusion. Oxygen and nutrient delivery to cells decreases. Cardiac ischemia and arrhythmias may develop (Fig. 3.29).

Clinical Features

Patient has cold, clammy skin due to vasoconstriction, hypotension, and rapid weak pulse due to compensatory response to decreased cardiac output. Patient develops clinical features related to organ involved and finally renal failure. Patient develops metabolic acidosis, cyanosis, cold clammy skin, thready pulse, tachycardia, perspiration, decreased urine output (<25 ml/hour).

Laboratory Findings

- *Blood biochemistry:* It shows increased potassium, blood urea nitrogen and creatinine.

- *Hematological findings:* During hemorrhage, there is no initial effect on hemoglobin and hematocrit concentration. Plasma is replaced first with fluid from interstitial space. Absolute neutrophilic leukocytosis is the first hematologic sign of hemorrhage. RBC production in the bone marrow begins in 5 to 7 days.

CARDIOGENIC SHOCK

Cardiogenic shock is circulatory collapse resulting from pump failure of the left ventricle. It is most commonly caused by *an acute myocardial infarction.* Other causes include *viral myocarditis, pulmonary embolism, cardiac tamponade* and rarely myxoma.

Clinical Features

Patient presents with dyspnea as a result of *pulmonary edema, cold, clammy skin due to vasoconstriction,* hypotension, and rapid weak pulse due to compensatory response to decreased cardiac output. Clinical presentation varies related to organ involved and finally renal failure.

SEPTIC SHOCK

Septicemia (bacteremia) denotes the clinical condition in which bacteria are found in the circulation. Final diagnosis is made by culturing the organisms from the blood.

Etiology

Septicemia with gram-negative organisms (*Escherichia coli*) originating from a urinary tract infection is the most common cause of septic shock. The invading bacteria are responsible for the release of endotoxin, a lipopolysaccharide (LPS).

It may also occur with gram-positive bacteria (*Staphylococcus aureus*). There is increased risk of infection during invasive procedures and immunocompromised patients. Septic shock stages due to synthesis of chemical

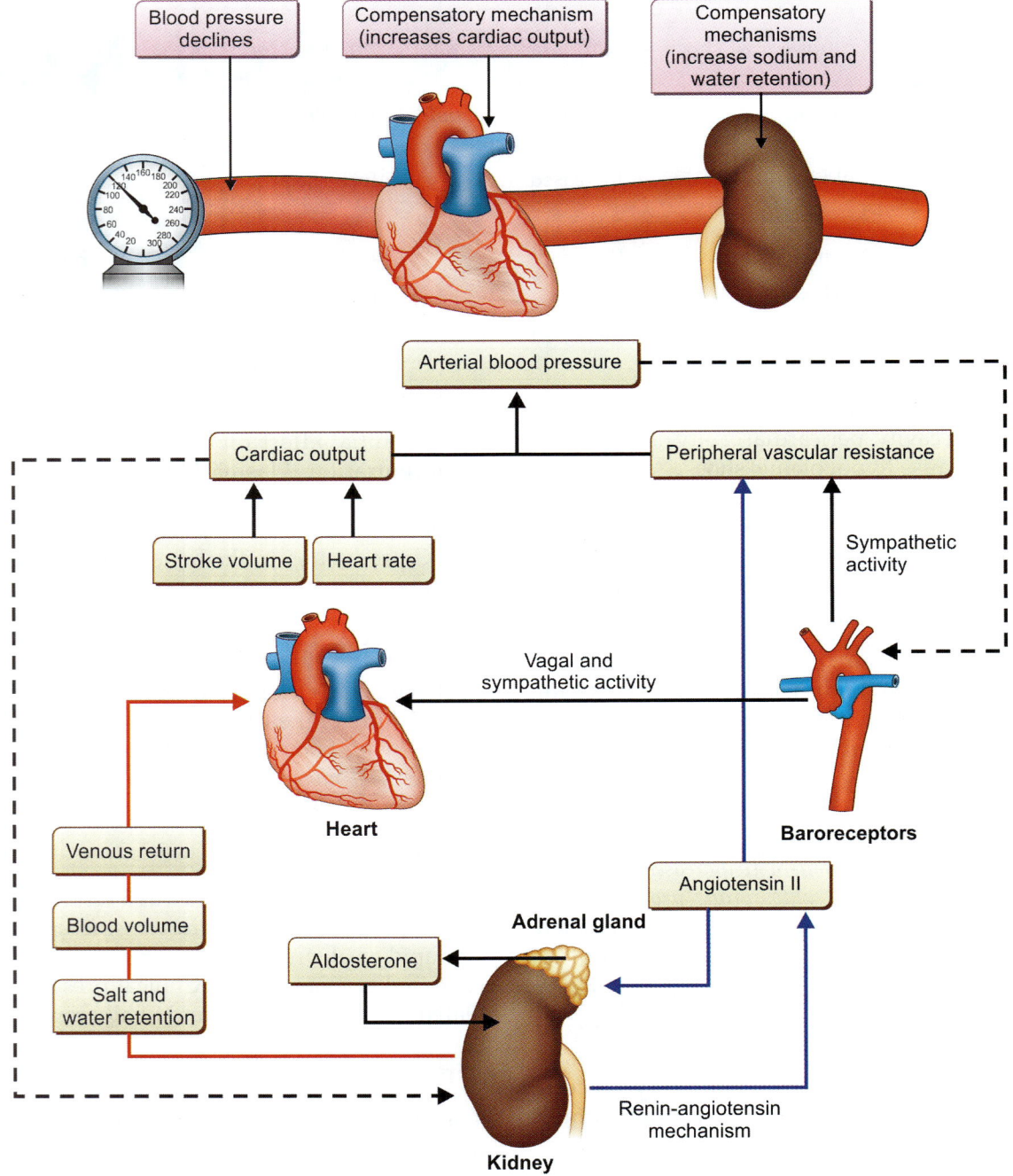

Fig. 3.29: Compensatory mechanism in controlling hypovolemic shock by regulating of blood pressure. The solid lines represent the mechanisms for kidneys and baroreceptor control of blood pressure through changes in cardiac output and peripheral resistance. The dashed lines represent the stimulus for regulation of blood pressure by baroreceptors and kidney.

mediators in varying quantity are shown in Table 3.22 and Fig. 3.30.

SEPTIC SHOCK DUE TO GRAM-NEGATIVE BACTERIA

Pathogenesis

On entry of gram-negative bacteria into the circulation, lipopolysaccharide (LPS) binds to the surface of monocytes/macrophages.

- *Synthesis of cytokines:* CD14 protein molecules expressed on leukocytes recognize LPS and mediate signaling through activation of nuclear transcription factors-kappa B (NF-κB) resulting in increased synthesis of cytokines such as *TNF-α, IL-1, IL-6, IL-8, nitric oxide and platelet activating factor*. These cytokines produce various biologic effects such as local inflammation, systemic inflammation and *septic shock* depending on concentration of cytokines in circulation.

Disorders of Hemostasis 3

Table 3.22: Septic shock stages due to synthesis of chemical mediators in varying quantity

Characteristics	Local inflammation	Systemic effects	Septic shock
Quantity of chemical mediators	Low quantity	Moderate quantity	High quantity
Effects	Activation of neutrophils and monocytes	Fever	Low cardiac output and peripheral resistance
	Activation of endothelial cells and complement	Synthesis of acute phase reactants	Blood vessel injury, thrombosis and disseminated intravascular coagulation
	Activation of complement	Leukocytosis	Acute respiratory distress syndrome

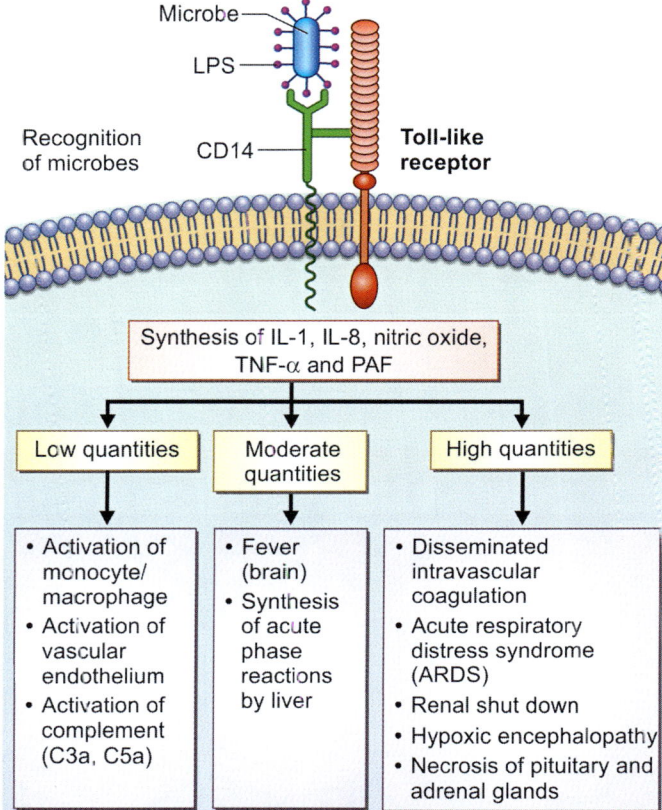

Fig. 3.30: Septic shock stages due to synthesis of chemical mediators in varying quantity.

- *Actions of cytokines:* Cytokines participate in *increasing capillary permeability*. These produce redistribution of circulatory volume into the interstitial tissue. *These activate coagulation pathways, kinin system* and *alternate complement system*. These cause direct toxic injury to vessels resulting in release of vasodilators such as nitric oxide and PGI_2.

Low Concentration of Cytokines

- *Activation of leukocytes and complement:* Low concentration of cytokines in circulation activates monocytes/macrophages, neutrophils and complement resulting in local inflammation.

- *Increased blood flow:* Initially, endothelial injury releases vasodilators such as nitric oxide and PGI_2 which results in increase blood flow. On examination, skin is warm due to vasodilation of skin vessels. Bounding pulse occurs due to increased cardiac output.

Moderate Concentration of Cytokines

Moderate concentration of cytokines in circulation cause fever (effect on brain), synthesis of acute phase reactants by liver and leukocytosis (effect on bone marrow).

High Concentration of Cytokines

- High concentration of cytokines in circulation cause *low cardiac output, low peripheral resistance* (effect on heart), *disseminated intravascular coagulation* (vascular endothelial injury) and *acute respiratory distress syndrome* (damage to alveolar capillary damage).
- Activation of alternate complement pathway stimulates mast cell release of histamine (vasodilator). Significant peripheral pooling of blood from peripheral vasodilation results in relative *hypovolemia and impaired perfusion*.
- Transmigration of neutrophils via pulmonary capillaries into alveoli results in *acute respiratory distress syndrome*. Diffuse alveolar damage with hyaline membranes is a feature of adult respiratory distress syndrome.
- TNF-α increases expression of adhesion molecules resulting in adherence of neutrophils to pulmonary capillaries. Direct cytotoxic endothelial injury can lead to activation of coagulation pathway and to *disseminated intravascular coagulation* (DIC).

SEPTIC SHOCK DUE TO GRAM-POSITIVE BACTERIA

Staphylococcus aureus releases toxic molecules (so-called superantigens) which results in *toxic shock syndrome*. Septic shock causes multiple organ dysfunction syndrome (MODS) characterized by systemic shut down of vital processes and lactic acidosis. It requires major intervention to maintain homeostasis. Multiple organ dysfunction is most common cause of death.

NEUROGENIC SHOCK

Neurogenic shock is most often associated with acute injury to the brain or spinal cord. In high spinal cord injury there is failure of sympathetic outflow and adequate vascular tone (neurogenic shock).

There is loss of function below the site of spinal cord injury. On clinical examination, flaccid paralysis distal to injury site, loss of sympathetic nervous system, relative bradycardia, hypotension, vasodilatation, warm, pink, dry skin, loss of urinary bladder control and priapism.

ANAPHYLACTIC SHOCK

Anaphylactic shock occurs as a consequence of a systemic type I hypersensitivity reaction. *Massive release of histamine may cause circulatory collapse* (anaphylactic shock). Patient develops *hypotension, tachycardia, circulatory failure*, and *shock*.

Immunopathology including Amyloidosis

CHAPTER 4

Learning Objectives

IMMUNE SYSTEM
- Overview
- Types of Immunity
- Components of Immune System
- Lymphoid Organs

NONSPECIFIC (INNATE OR INBORN) IMMUNE RESPONSE
- Host Defenses
- Barriers to Entry of Pathogens

SPECIFIC IMMUNE RESPONSE
- Overview
- Components of Immune System
- Encounter between Antigen and Antibody
- Clonal Selection
- Immune Cells
- Cooperation in Immune Cells and Antigens
- T Cell Response
- B Cell Activation
- Complement System

IMMUNIZATION AND VACCINES
- Immunization
- Vaccines

IMMUNODEFICIENCY DISORDERS
- Primary Immunodeficiency Disorders
- Other Immunodeficiency Diseases
- Acquired Immunodeficiency Syndrome

HYPERSENSITIVITY REACTIONS
- Type I
- Type II
- Type III
- Type IV

IMMUNOLOGIC TOLERANCE
- Overview
- B Cells Immunologic Tolerance
- T Cells Immunologic Tolerance

AUTOIMMUNE DISEASES
- Overview
- Connective Tissue (Collagen Tissue) Diseases

HLA SYSTEM
- Major Classes of HLAs
- Clinical Aspect of HLA System

TRANSPLANTATION IMMUNOLOGY
- Organ Transplantation
- Organ Transplant Rejection
- Graft-versus-host Disease (GVHD)
- Prevention of Transplant Rejection

AMYLOIDOSIS
- Physical Structure of Amyloid
- Chemical Nature of Amyloid
- Organs Involved in Amyloidosis
- Clinical Correlation
- Laboratory Diagnosis

IMMUNE SYSTEM

OVERVIEW

Immunology is the study of immunity, which refers to the development of resistance to infectious agents by white blood cells. Immune system conducts surveillance of the body. The cells and tissues that work to defend the human body against infection are collectively referred to as the immune system. Host defenses comprise physical barriers, cells and chemicals. *There are two fundamental immune responses: nonspecific (innate or inborn) and specific (adaptive) immunity.* Host immune response showing nonspecific and specific immunity is shown in Fig. 4.1.

Pathogenic Organisms

Pathogenic organisms include bacteria, viruses, protozoa, fungi and parasites. Mechanism of diseases caused by these pathogens comprise utilization of host nutritional resources, physical damage to host tissues, production of toxic substances, chromosomal and gene damage resulting in abnormal behavior of body cells.

Overview of Diseases of the Immune System

Hypersensitivity, is an exaggerated, misdirected expression of certain immune responses. There are four types of hypersensitivity reactions. Autoimmunity involves abnormal responses to self-antigens. A deficiency or loss in immune function is called immunodeficiency. Overview of diseases of the immune system is shown in Fig. 4.2.

Types of Immune Response

- *Innate natural defenses:* These are present at birth that provides immediate nonspecific defense against infection. It participates in recruitment of immune cells to the site of infection. *It does not confer long-lasting immunity.* Toll-like receptors on phagocytes play roles in cellular responses to bacterial lipopolysaccharide (LPS, or endotoxin). Phagocytosis and activation of complement are more rapid resulting in destruction of pathogens. Components of innate immune system include anatomical barriers and internal resistance factors.
- *Adaptive immune response:* It is specific and acquired immune response mediated by B and T cells in response to specific antigens. Immune response is not immediate. It takes time for optimal reactivity.

TYPES OF IMMUNITY

Acquired immunity may be natural or artificial. Natural acquired immunity is obtained in course of daily life.

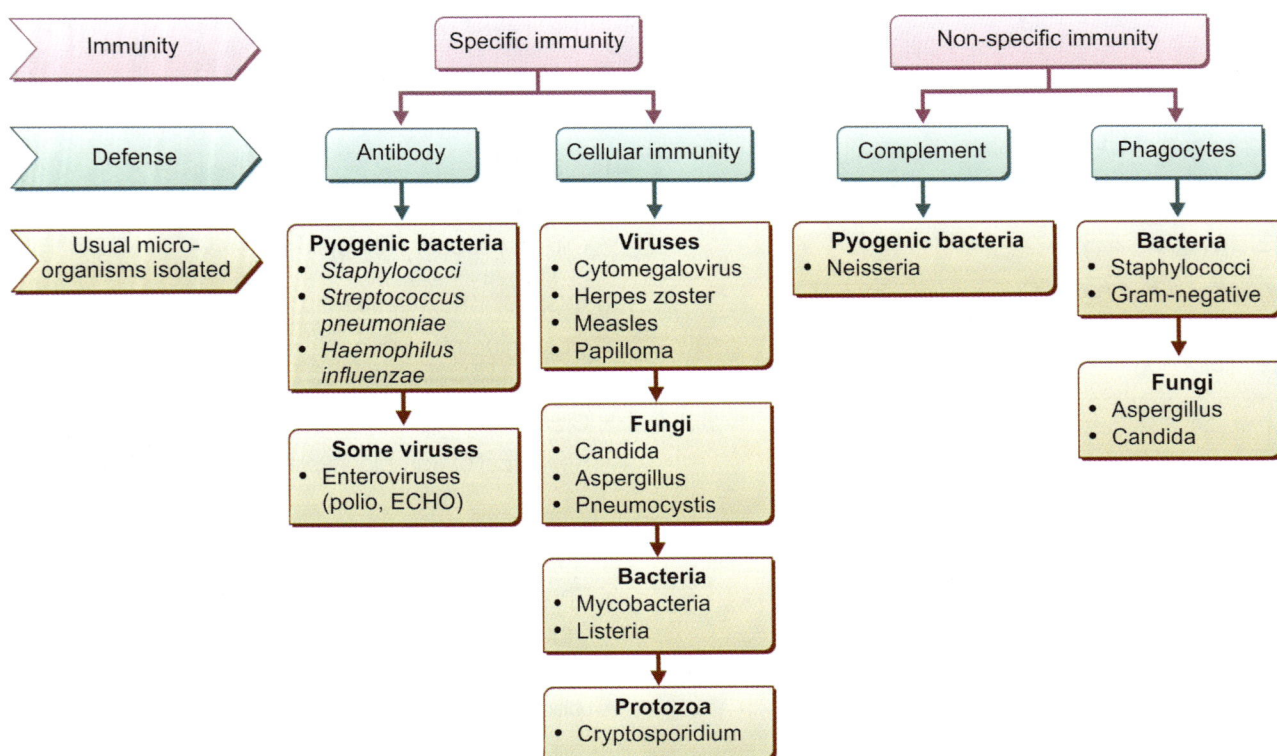

Fig. 4.1: Host immune response showing nonspecific and specific immunity.

4 Immunopathology including Amyloidosis

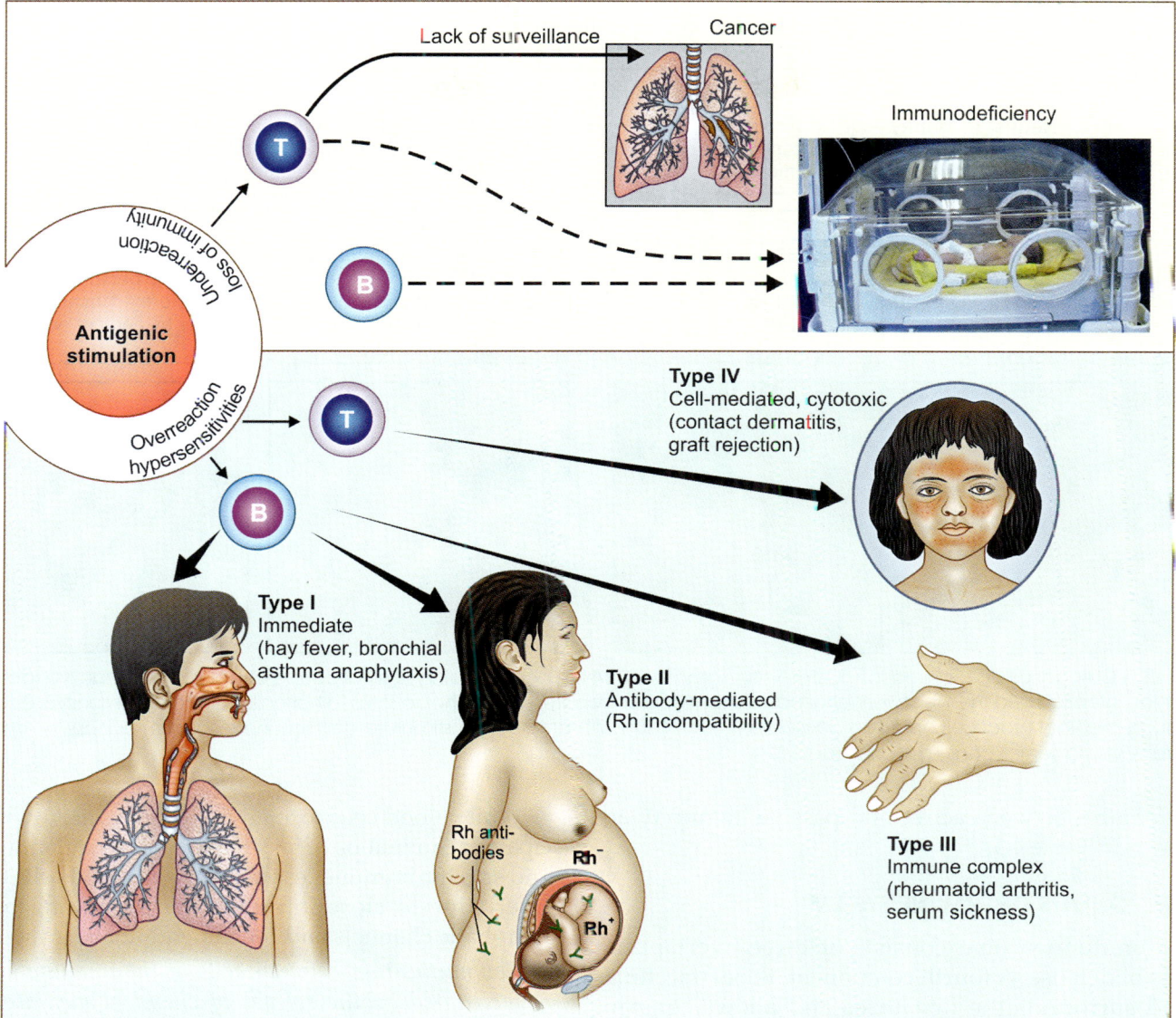

Fig. 4.2: Overview of diseases of the immune system. T and B cells provide necessary protection against infection and disease. Immune system can cause serious and debilitating disorders to immune stimuli. Lack of surveillance of immune system causes immunodeficiency and cancers. Hypersensitivity reactions and autoimmune mechanism cause many diseases.

Artificially acquired immunity is obtained by receiving a vaccine or immune serum. Categories of acquired immunities are shown in Fig. 4.3.

ACTIVE IMMUNITY

Active immunity means immune response caused by a disease agent. Natural active immunity develops as a result of disease process. It creates memory, takes time and is lasting. Artificial active immunity develops as a result of vaccination of person. Vaccines include inactivated toxins, killed microbes, parts of microbes, and viable but weakened microbes. Vaccine stimulates a protective immune response without causing the disease. Active immunity is usually permanent by creating memory.

PASSIVE IMMUNITY

Passive immunity develops, when a patient receives antibodies from another person. Natural passive immunity comes from the mother. *Artificial passive immunity* is acquired through medical procedures such as *administration of human antiserum in patients* (short-lived immunity).

Artificial active immunization is the same as administering a vaccine (long lived-immunity against an infectious agent that may be encountered in the future).

Section I: General Pathology

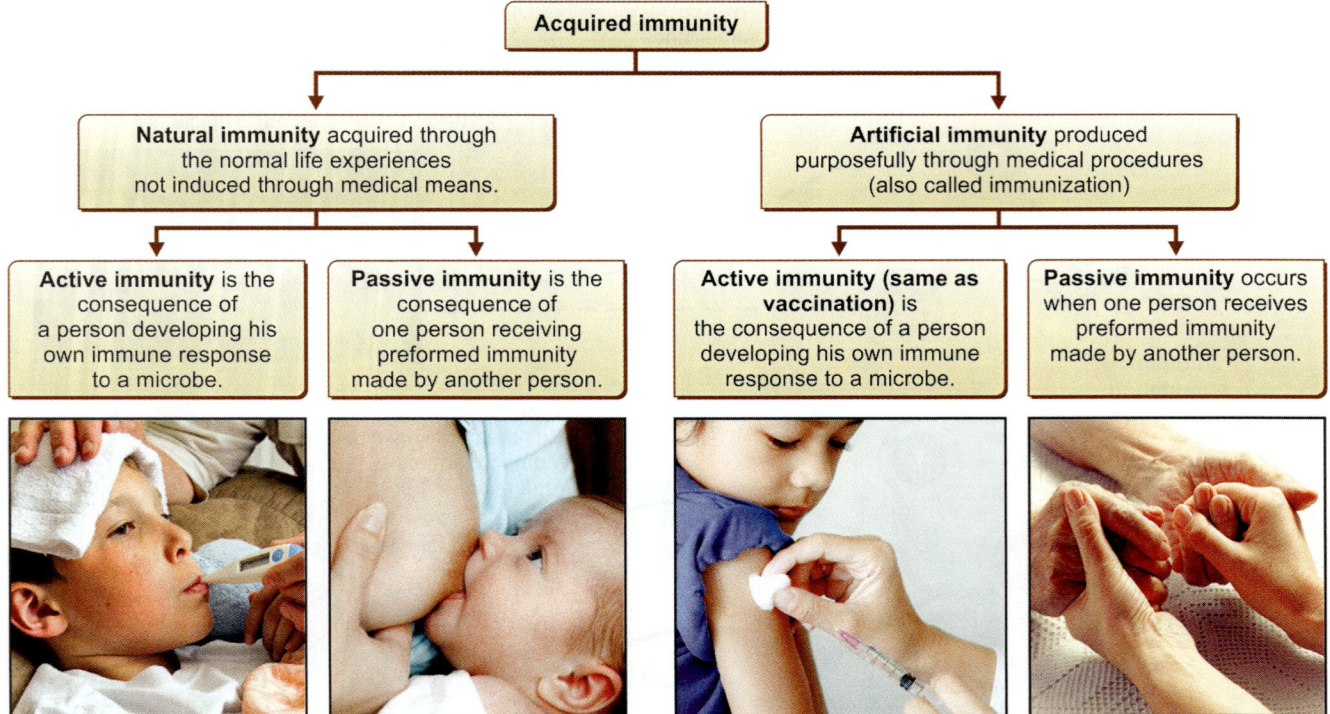

Fig. 4.3: Categories of acquired immunity. Natural immunity, which occurs during normal course of life, are either active (acquired from an infection and then recovering) or passive (antibodies donated by mother to fetus to her child). Artificial immunity is acquired through medical practices and can be active (vaccination with antigen), to stimulate an immune response) or passive (immune therapy with a serum containing antibodies).

Differences between active and passive immunity are shown in Table 4.1.

COMPONENTS OF IMMUNE SYSTEM

The immune system consists of three overlapping lines of defense. A fourth component, the extracellular fluid surrounds the first three and allows constant communication between all areas of the body. Lymph nodes, spleen, and thymus participate in defense mechanisms.

White blood cells formed in the bone marrow participate in elimination of injurious agents by inflammation and specific immune response. White blood cells travel freely due to close interrelationship among blood, lymphatic channels and reticuloendothelial system.

Communication between cells of the immune system is facilitated by the release of chemical mediators by inflammatory cells and injured tissue. Chemical mediators drive inflammatory response, increase blood flow, recruitment of white blood cells to the site of injury,

Table 4.1: Differences between active and passive immunity

Parameters	Active immunity	Passive immunity
Host response	Participating in active immunity	Not participating in passive immunity
Antibodies production	When person comes in contact with living or dead microbes	Ready-made antibodies introduced for immunization
Immune response	Slow immune response because it takes time to generate antibodies	Immediate and quick immune response
Duration of immune response	Long lasting	Short lived
Clinical aspect	Used for prophylaxis to increase resistance (BCG vaccination for prophylaxis of tuberculosis)	Treatment of acute infections
		Breastfeeding (colostrum-rich in abundant IgA)
		Fetus receives some antibodies from mother through placenta during pregnancy

initiate fever and destroy necrotic cells. Complement system acts in nonspecific or specific ways to lyse cells that has been identified as foreign.

Pathogen associated molecular proteins (PAMPs) present on phagocytes recognize pathogens. Neutrophils and macrophages phagocytose and degrade the pathogens.

For purposes of immunologic study, the body is divided into three compartments: *the blood, lymphatic system and the reticuloendothelial system*. Fourth compartment is *extracellular fluid compartment surrounding tissue cells*.

COMMUNICATING BODY COMPARTMENTS

Tissue cells are in direct contact with blood, lymphatic system, reticuloendothelial system and extracellular fluid. Blood cells are formed in the bone marrow by hemopoiesis. It begins early in embryonic development in the yolk sac. Later the function is taken over by liver and lymphatic organs and finally bone marrow. Stem cells in the bone marrow differentiate to produce WBCs, RBCs and platelets. Blood cells are dispersed in the plasma.

BLOOD CELLS

Blood contains both nonspecific and specific defenses. Nonspecific cellular defense includes granulocytes (neutrophils, eosinophils and basophils). Specific immune system consists of lymphocytes. T cells provide cell-mediated immunity. B cells produce specific antibody and provide humoral immunity. Monocytes later differentiate to become tissue macrophages.

LYMPHATIC SYSTEM

The lymphatic system parallels the circulatory system and transports lymph through lymphatic channels to draining lymph nodes. *It returns interstitial tissue fluid to systemic circulation. It drains away excess inflammatory exudate fluid present in inflamed tissue.* It also concentrates and processes invading pathogens and initiates specific immune response through system of phagocytes, lymphocytes and antibodies.

Lymph: Lymph is made up of water, dissolved salts and 2–5% proteins (antibody and albumin). It transports lymphocytes, fats, cellular debris and pathogens.

Lymphatic channels: Lymphatic channels permeate all parts of body except the central nervous system, bone, placenta and thymus gland.

Lymphoid organs and tissues: Lymphatic organs and tissues with immune functions can be classified into primary and secondary. Primary lymphoid organs include *bone marrow* and *thymus gland*. Secondary organs and tissues include *lymph nodes, spleen, MALT* (mucosa associated lymphoid tissues, *SALT* (skin associated lymphoid tissue) and *GALT* (gut associated lymphoid tissue in Peyer's patches).

EXTRACELLULAR FLUID COMPARTMENT

This compartment is extracellular fluid compartment surrounding tissue cells.

LYMPHOID ORGANS

Thymus and bone marrow are primary lymphoid organs. They are sites of maturation for T and B cells, respectively. Lymphoid organs are shown in Table 4.2.

Table 4.2: Lymphoid organs

Categories	Lymphoid organs
Primary lymphoid organs	Bone marrow
	Thymus gland
Secondary lymphoid organs	Lymph nodes
	Spleen
	Mucosa associated lymphoid tissue (MALT)
	Skin associated lymphoid tissue (SALT)
	Gut associated lymphoid tissue (GALT) in Peyer's patches

PRIMARY LYMPHOID ORGANS

Bone marrow and thymus gland are primary lymphoid organs. During embryonic and fetal development, bone marrow stem cells produce B cells and T cells. These undergo further development or maturation at different sites.

- *Maturation of B cells in bone marrow:* B cells mature into stromal cells of bone marrow. B cells, which produce antibodies and T cells, which produce cytokines that mediate and coordinate the entire immune response.
- *Maturation of T cells in thymus:* Immature T cells migrate from bone marrow in the thymus gland (cortex and medulla) for differentiation and maturation.

Clinical aspect: Immediately after birth, thymus is a large organ that nearly fills the region over the midline of the upper thoracic region. In the adults, it becomes small in size. Children born without a thymus suffer from *DiGeorge syndrome* characterized by *severe immunodeficiency disorder*.

SECONDARY LYMPHOID ORGANS

After maturation of B cells in bone marrow and T cells in thymus, these lymphocytes reach the secondary lymphoid organs via circulation. Secondary lymphoid organs comprise lymph node, spleen, tonsils, mucosa of appendix and Peyer's patches of small intestine. Cellular and humoral immune responses occur in the secondary lymphoid organs and tissues; effector and memory cells are generated here.

Lymph nodes: Lymph nodes mount immune responses to antigens in intercellular fluid and in the lymph, absorbed either through the skin (superficial nodes) or from internal viscera (deep nodes). Beneath the collagenous capsule is the subareolar sinus, which is lined by with phagocytic cells. Lymphocytes and antigens from surrounding tissue spaces or adjacent nodes pass into the sinus via the afferent lymphatic system. Lymphocytes enter the node from the circulation through the specialized high endothelial venules in the paracortex.

- *Cortex:* The cortex contains aggregates of B cells forming primary follicles, most of which are stimulated to form secondary follicles.
- *Paracortical region:* The paracortical region contains mainly T cells, many of which are associated with the interdigitating cells (antigen presenting cells).
- *Medulla:* The medulla contains both T and B cells as well as most of the lymph node plasma cells. These are organized into cords of lymphoid tissue. Lymphocytes and antigens from surrounding tissue spaces or adjacent nodes pass into the sinus via the afferent lymphatic system.

Spleen: Spleen is a lymphoid organ which also regulates the destruction of red blood cells. It consists of *white pulp* and *red pulp*. Spleen contributes to the maturation of red blood cells by pitting function. It has ability to remove solid particles from the cytoplasm of red blood cells without causing injury to the cell membrane. *The spleen responds predominantly to blood-borne antigens.* Blood enters the tissue via the trabecular arteries, which give rise to the many-branched central arteries. Some of these end in the white pulp, supplying the germinal centers and mantle zones, but most empty into or near the marginal zones.

- *White pulp:* White pulp is formed by population of numerous macrophages, antigen presenting cells, T cells, slowly circulating B cells, and natural killer cells around splenic arteriole. Dendritic cells present antigens to T cells, where T and B cells interact at the edges of white pulp follicles, generating antibody-secreting plasma cells found mainly within the sinuses of red pulp.
- *Red pulp:* Red pulp consists of capillaries and venous sinuses separated by splenic cords. It stores red blood cells. T cells are distributed in the periarteriolar sheaths of the spleen.

Tonsils, MALT, GALT and SALT: Tonsils, mucosa associated lymphoid tissue (MALT) and gut associated lymphoid tissue in Peyer's patches of small intestine (GALT) respond to antigens that have penetrated the surface mucosal barriers.

- *MALT (mucosa associated lymphoid tissue):* Lymphoid cells stimulated with antigen in Peyer's patches migrate via the regional lymph nodes and thoracic duct into the bloodstream and then to lamina propria of the gut and probably other mucosal surfaces (lungs). Thus, lymphocytes stimulated at one mucosal surface may become distributed throughout the mucosa associated lymphoid tissue.
- *Skin associated lymphoid tissue (SALT):* These respond to antigens that have penetrated the skin barrier.

NONSPECIFIC (INNATE OR INBORN) IMMUNE RESPONSE

Innate immune system is immediate defense system against infection. It defends the host from infection by organisms, in a non-specific manner. It responds to pathogens in a generic way. It does not confer long-lasting or protective immunity.

HOST DEFENSES

The multilevel, intercommunicating network of host protection against pathogen invasion can be organized into three lines of defense. Major components of the host defenses are shown in Fig. 4.4 and Table 4.3.

FIRST LINE OF DEFENSE

First line of defense is an inborn and nonspecific system comprising *anatomical, chemical barriers provided* by skin and mucous membranes. *These barriers prevent entry of pathogens.* There is no creation of memory cells that normally react immediately if same pathogen enters the body in the future.

SECOND LINE OF DEFENSE

Second line of defense comprises phagocytic cells, inflammatory response and antimicrobial proteins such as lysozyme,

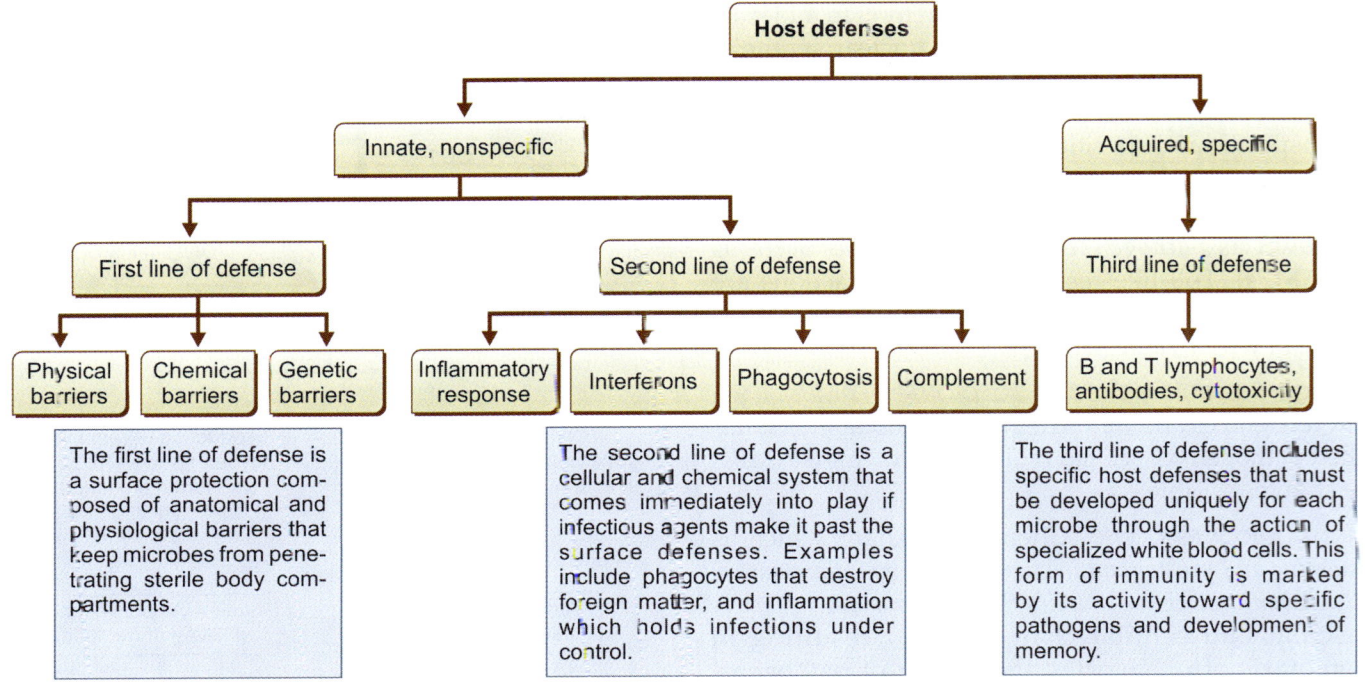

Fig. 4.4: Major components of the host defenses. Defenses are classified into two categories: innate and nonspecific; and acquired and specific. These can be further subdivided into the first, second and third lines of defense. Each of the defense is characterized by a different level and type of protection. The third line of defense is responsible for specific immunity.

Table 4.3: Major components of the host defenses

Line of defense	Function of line of defense	Barriers
Innate host defense (nonspecific response)		
First line of defense	Anatomical and physiological barriers preventing entry of pathogens in body	Physical barriers such as skin, tears, coughing, sneezing
		Chemical barriers such as low pH, lysozyme, digestive enzymes
		Genetic barriers such as resistance inherent in genetic makeup of host (pathogen cannot invade)
Second line of defense	Cellular and chemical system participating in phagocytosis, destruction of pathogens	Inflammatory response
		Interferons
		Phagocytosis
		Complement
Acquired host defense (specific response)		
Third line of defense	Specific host defenses by macrophages and lymphocytes against pathogens	B cells and T cells

interferon and antibodies. This second line of defense does not create memory cells that normally react immediately if same pathogen enters the body in the future. It comprises neutrophils, macrophages and chemical mediators.

Toll-like Receptors (TLRs) on Phagocytes

- Macrophages, neutrophils, dendritic cells, microglial cells, eosinophils, mast cells, endothelial cells, mucosal cells and lymphocytes express *toll-like receptors (TLRs) within wall of phagocytes.*
- TLRs provide defense against invasion by microorganisms. *Phagocytes engulf and degrade pathogens.* Toll-like receptors stimulate innate immune response against microbes. When a molecule specific to a particular class of pathogen is recognized by a receptor, the TLRs merge and bind the foreign molecule.

- TLRs relay signal to the nucleus that foreign molecule has been detected. These activate nuclear synthesis of transcriptional factor resulting in synthesis of *interleukins*. It is the first step to activate both the nonspecific and specific immune response.
- *Currently 10 TLRs are known to exist on human cells.* Each TLR can recognize distinct microbial molecules known as *pathogen-associated molecular patterns* (PAMPs). Toll-like receptors and their actions are shown in Fig. 4.5. Toll like receptors and their ligands are shown in Table 4.4.

Pathogen-associated molecular proteins (PAMPs): Each TLR recognizes and binds distinct microbial molecules called pathogen-associated molecular proteins (PAMPs) are shown in Table 4.5.

Inflammatory response: Chemical mediators such as *histamine and prostaglandins synthesized by inflammatory cells and injured tissue amplify the inflammatory response.* Vascular and cellular changes occur resulting in chemotaxis of phagocytes and killing of pathogens. Inflammatory response is marked by redness, heat, swelling and pain. *Edema swells the tissue, helping prevent the spread of infection.* WBCs, microbes and debris and fluid collect to form pus. Pyrogens may induce fever.

Phagocytosis: Neutrophils and macrophages engage in phagocytosis, engulfing microbes in phagosomes.

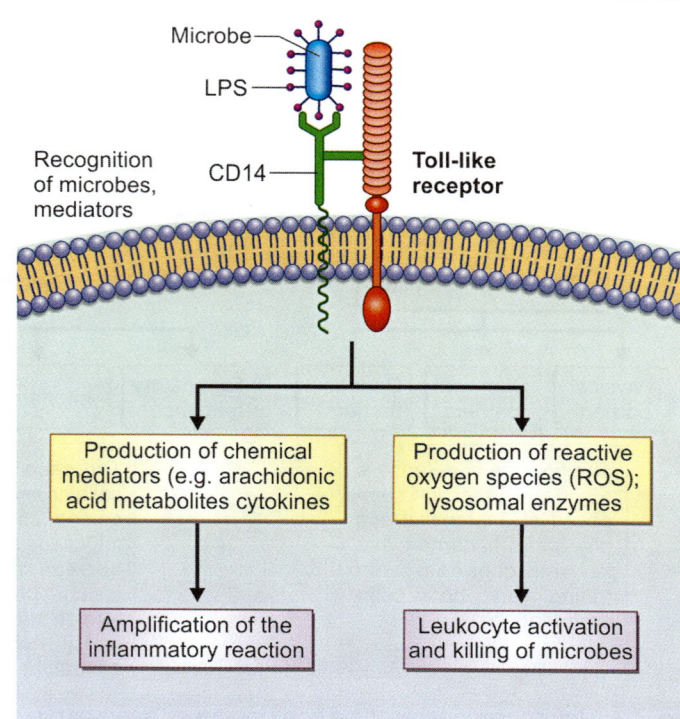

Fig. 4.5: Toll-like receptors and their actions. TLR binds and relays a signal to the nucleus resulting in activation of nuclear synthesis of transcription factors (chemical mediators) such as arachidonic acid metabolites and cytokines amplifying the inflammatory reactions, and production of microbiocidal reactive oxygen species and lysosomal enzymes killing the microbes.

Table 4.4: Toll-like receptors and their ligands

Receptor	Ligand (PAMPs)	Origin of ligand
TLR1	Triacyl lipopeptides Soluble factors	Bacteria and mycobacteria *Neisseria meningitidis*
TLR2	Heat shock protein 70 Peptidoglycan Lipoprotein/lipopeptides HCV core and nonstructural 3 protein	Host Gram-positive bacteria Various pathogens Hepatitis C virus
TLR3	Double-stranded RNA	Viruses
TLR4	Lipopolysaccharides Envelope protein Taxol	Gram-negative bacteria Mouse mammary-tumor virus Plants
TLR5	Flagellin	Bacteria
TLR6	Zymosan Lipoteichoic acid Diacyl lipopeptides	Fungi Gram-positive bacteria Mycoplasma
TLR7	Single-stranded RNA (ssRNA) Imidazoquinoline	Viruses Synthetic compounds
TLR8	Single-stranded RNA (ssRNA) Imidazoquinoline	Viruses Synthetic compounds
TLR9	CpG-containing DNA	Bacteria, malaria and viruses
TLR10	Not determined	Not determined
TLR11	Profilin-like molecule	*Toxoplasma gondii*

Table 4.5: Pathogen-associated molecular proteins (PAMPs)

Pathogens	Pathogen-associated molecular proteins (PAMPs)
Gram-negative bacterial cell wall	Lipopolysaccharides (LPS): endotoxin
Gram-positive bacteria cocci	Peptidoglycans such as lipoprotein, lipotechoic acid
Bacteria with flagella	Flagellin
Viruses	Single-stranded or double-stranded RNA molecules
Fungi	Zymosan

The sequential events in phagocytes include: (i) *toll-like receptors* on phagocyte attaches to microbial molecules known as pathogen-associated molecular patterns (PAMPs), (ii) engulfment, (iii) phagosome digestive vacuole is formed, (iv) phagosome fuses with lysosome results in formation of phagolysosome, (v) enzymes (lysozyme, DNAs, RNAs, proteases, myeloperoxidases) and reactive oxygen products (superoxide, hydrogen peroxide, hydroxyl ions and hypochlorite ions) kill and digest pathogen, and (vi) undigested residual body is released.

Interferon (IFN): Interferon is a family of proteins produced by leukocytes and fibroblasts that inhibit the reproduction of viruses by degrading viral DNA or blocking the synthesis of viral proteins. When a cell is infected with virus, its nucleus is triggered to transcribe and translate the interferon gene. Interferon diffuses out of the cell and binds to interferon receptors on nearby cells, where it induces synthesis of proteins that eliminate viral genes and block viral replication.

Complement system: Complement is a complex defense system that results, in the formation of a membrane attack complex that kills cells by creating holes in their membranes. This system consists of about 20 plasma proteins and their products synthesized by liver present in its inactive form that interact with one another in three distinct enzymatic-activation cascades. These are numbered C1 to C9 (C3 most abundant). *Complement proteins participate in innate and adaptive immunity during inflammation. These cause immune lysis of cells.* Many regulatory proteins expressed by mammals prevent inappropriate activation of complement.

THIRD LINE OF DEFENSE

Third line of defense is an acquired and specific immune response against invader pathogens. It is dependent on the function of T and B cells. Third line of defense also creates memory cells that permit the immune system to immediately react if same pathogen enters the body in the future. Lymphoid organs such as the spleen, lymph nodes, and thymus are intimately involved in these defense mechanisms.

BARRIERS TO ENTRY OF PATHOGENS

Non-specific inborn or innate immunity is present at the time of birth. It provides different types of barriers to entry of the foreign agents in our body. *Patient with severe burns are susceptible to infections.* Blockage in the salivary glands, lacrimal ducts, intestine and genitourinary tract are at greater risk for infection.

Barriers to portal entry of pathogens are shown in Fig. 4.6. Barriers in first and second line of defense in innate immunity are shown in Table 4.6.

PHYSICAL OR ANATOMICAL BARRIERS

The skin and mucous membranes of the respiratory and gastrointestinal tract have several defenses.

- *Skin:* Skin's outermost layer stratum corneum impregnated with *insoluble keratin proteins is highly impervious to most pathogens.* Sweat glands flush out microbes.

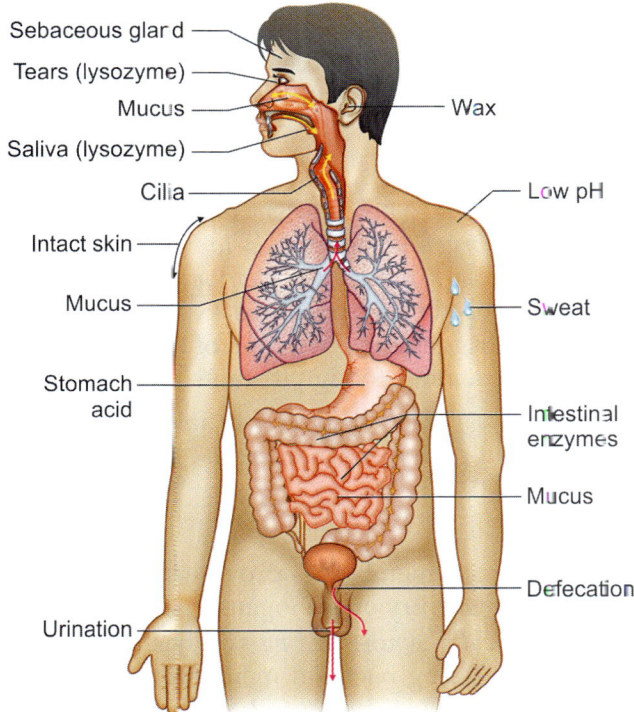

Fig. 4.6: Barriers to portal entry of pathogens

Table 4.6: Barriers in first and second line of defense in innate immunity

Categories of barriers	Characteristics	Organ	Examples of barriers
Anatomical barriers	Preventing the entry of pathogens	Skin	Epidermis
		Nose	Hair and cilia
		Respiratory, gastrointestinal and urogenital passages	Mucous membranes
Chemical barriers	Inhibiting the activity of pathogens (anti-bacterial activity)	Gastrointestinal tract	Hydrochloric acid by parietal cells and enzymes
		Hepatobiliary system	Bile juice (antimicrobial action)
		Saliva	Lysozyme hydrolyzing the peptidoglycan in the wall of bacteria
		Skin	Dermcidin causing lysis of lysing bacterial membranes
		Sweat	High lactic acid and electrolyte concentration
		Eyelids meibonium glands	Secretion lubricating the conjunctiva with an antimicrobial action
		Tears	Lysozyme
		Respiratory tract	Mucus secretion by lining mucosa in respiratory tract (mucociliary apparatus, sneezing and coughing)
		Urogenital system	Semen containing antibacterial secretion Flushing and acidity of urine
		Vagina	Acidic pH (antibacterial action)
		Sebum	Unsaturated fatty acids and hyaluronic acid
Phagocytic barriers	Phagocytic cells	Bone marrow	Macrophages, granulocytes, natural killer cells
		Blood	Monocytes, neutrophils, eosinophils
		Lymph nodes	Tissue macrophages and natural killer cells (NK cells kill cancer cells and virus infected cells)
		Liver	Macrophages (Kupffer cells)
		Spleen	Macrophages and natural killer cells
Chemical mediators	Plasma and cell-derived chemical mediators	Plasma-derived chemical mediators	Kinin system, fibrinolytic system, coagulation system and complement system
		Cells-derived chemical mediators	Preformed chemical mediators include histamine and serotonin

- *Epithelial lining:* The *epithelial lining of the airways* contains a *brush border of cilia to entrap and propel particles upward toward the pharynx.* Sneezing due to irritation of nasal passages expels pathogens. Coughing triggered by irritation of bronchi, trachea and larynx remove foreign irritants.
- *Genitourinary tract:* It gives partial protection by flushing out pathogens in urine.

CHEMICAL DEFENSES

Skin and mucous membranes provide many chemical defenses against entry of pathogens.
- *Skin: Dermcidin synthesized by skin* has antibacterial activity by lysing bacterial membranes. *High lactic acid* and *electrolyte concentration of sweat* and the *skin's acidic pH and fatty acid content* have antibacterial property. Sebaceous secretions have antimicrobial property.
- *Eye:* Meibomian glands of the eyelids lubricate the conjunctiva with an antimicrobial secretion. *Lysozyme enzyme in tears* hydrolyzes the peptidoglycan in the wall of bacteria.
- *Saliva: Lysozyme enzyme in saliva* hydrolyzes the peptidoglycan in the wall of bacteria.
- *GIT: Hydrochloric acid* synthesized by parietal cells of stomach gives protection against many pathogens that are swallowed. Intestinal and bile secretions are also destructive to pathogens.
- *Genital tract:* Semen contains an antibacterial chemical substance. Vagina has a protective acidic pH which maintains normal flora and confers protection against pathogens.

RETICULOENDOTHELIAL SYSTEM

Reticuloendothelial system is network of connective tissue reticular fibers enmeshing each cell inhabitated by macrophages. This network of reticular fibers connects one cell to another within a tissue or organ.

Macrophages attack and phagocytose pathogens that have managed to bypass the first line of defense. Monocytes migrate and differentiate into tissue macrophages, which are diffusely distributed in the connective tissues.

SPECIFIC IMMUNE RESPONSE

OVERVIEW

Overview of the origin of T and B cells and events of adaptive immune responses is shown in Figs 4.7 and 4.8. Acquired specific immunity is a highly specific protection acquired through contact with specific infectious agents due to interrelationship between lymphocytes and macrophages. It has pathogen specificity and memory.

Specific immune system present in human beings is capable of the following features:

- *Recognition of antigen:* Immune system has ability to identify antigen and distinguish between self and non-self.
- *Specific immune response:* Immune system mounts a highly specific response against antigen.
- *Memory:* Some of B cells and T cells become memory cells that recognize the same antigen in the future.

COMPONENTS OF IMMUNE SYSTEM

ANTIGENS

Antigens are foreign proteins or other complex molecules of higher molecular weight that trigger the immune response in the host. *Antigenicity depends on recognition of antigen, size of antigen and complexity of cell or molecule.*

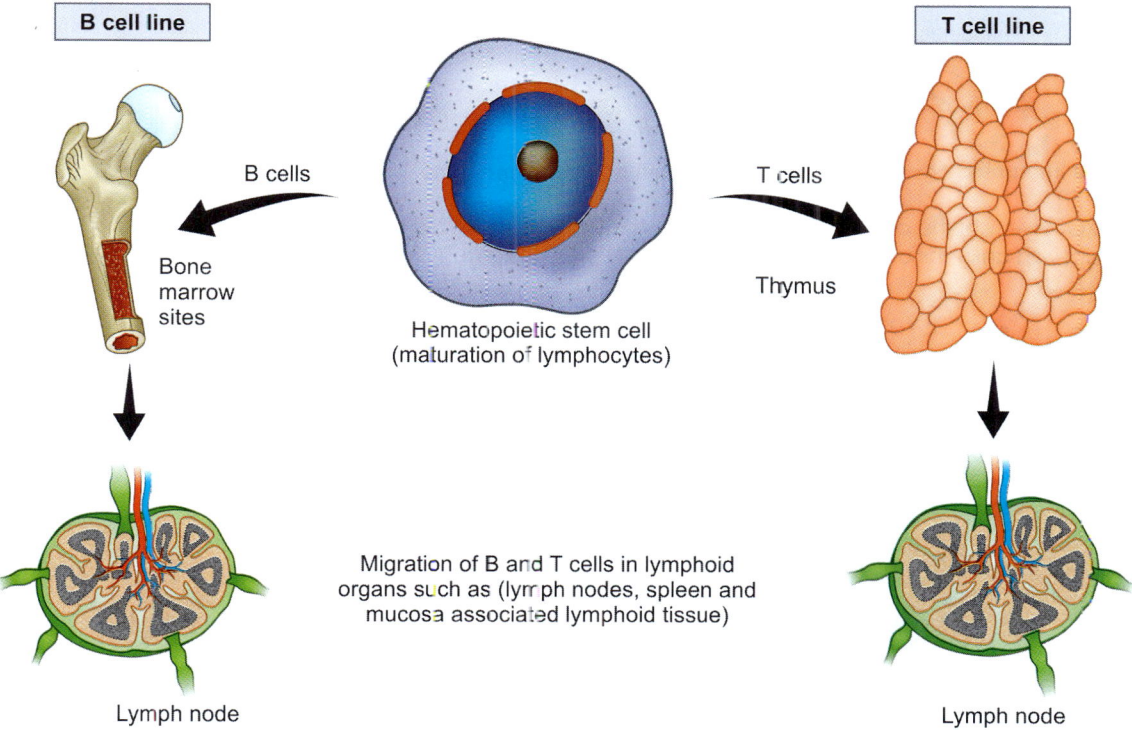

Development of the T lymphocyte and B lymphocyte system
Lymphocytes participates in specific immune response. These originate from hematopoietic stem cells and differentiate into two distinct early T and B cells in the bone marrow. B cells mature in the bone marrow itself. T cells migrate to thymus for maturation. These mature lymphocytes settle in lymphoid organs (lymph nodes, spleen, MALT and GALT) and serve as a constant defense force against pathogens.

Fig. 4.7A: Overview of the origin of T and B lymphocytes and events of adaptive immune responses (humoral and cellular immune response)—development of the T lymphocyte and B lymphocyte system.

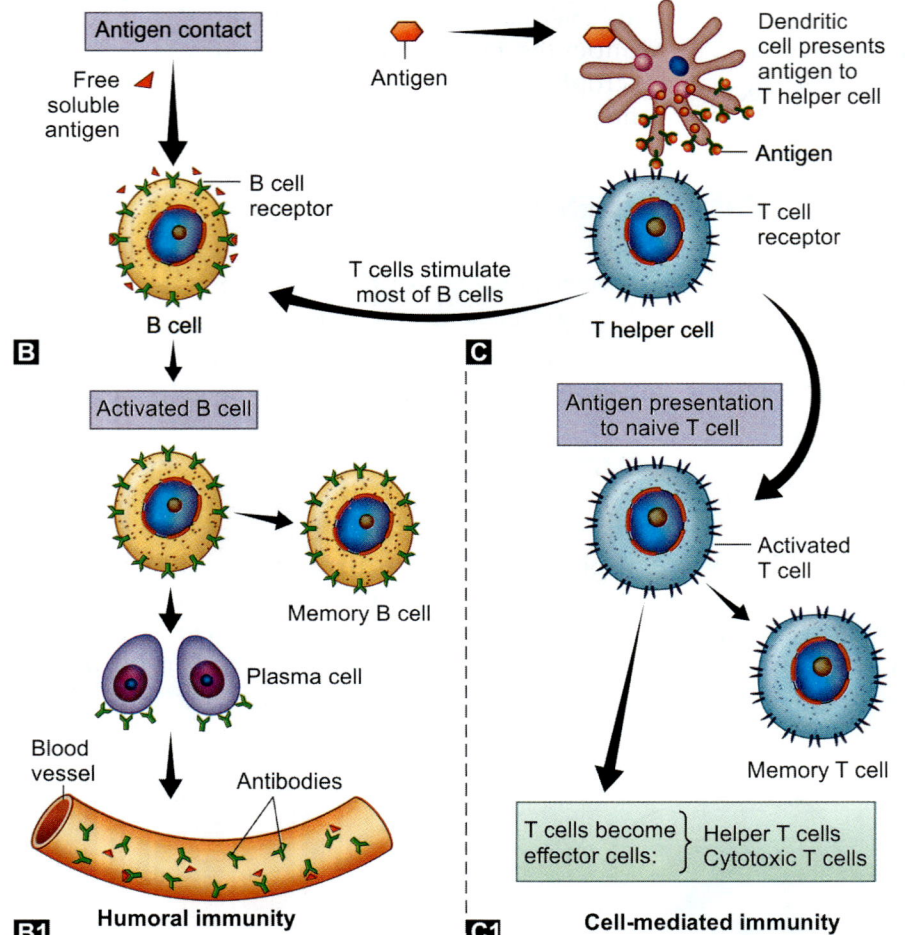

Fig. 4.7B and C: Overview of the origin of T and B cells and events of adaptive immune responses (humoral and cellular immune response): Contact with antigens and presentation by antigen presenting cells. **B1** B cell response and **C1** T cell response.

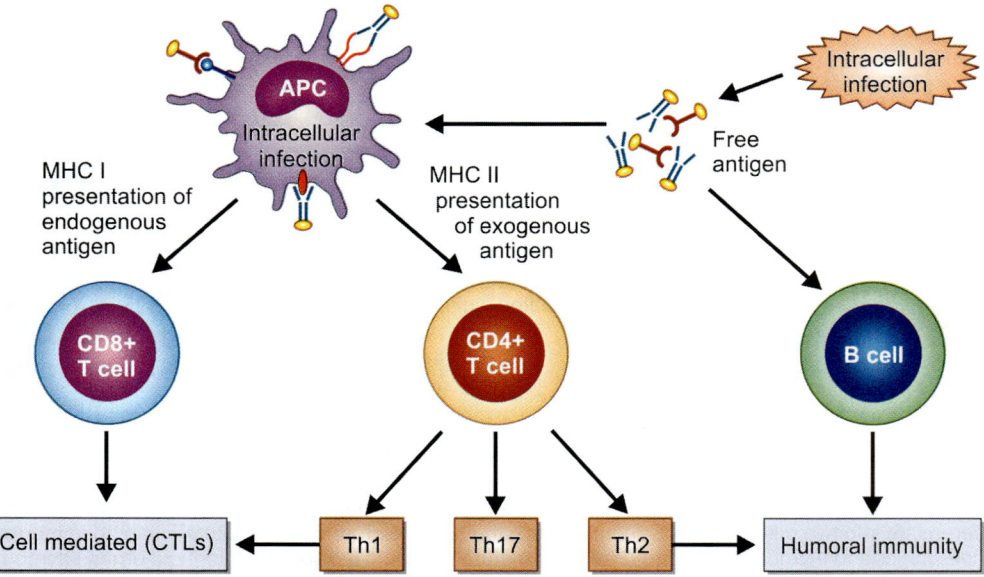

Fig. 4.8: Overview of adaptive immune response: T cell response: When T cells are activated by antigen, these differentiate into helper T cells and memory cells assisting other lymphocytes or cytotoxic T cells that eliminate foreign cells. T cells also synthesize cytokines that regulate cell-mediated immune response. B cell participates in antibody-mediated immune response.

Immunogenicity: Most antigens have high molecular weight in excess of 10,000. Small molecules cannot act as antigen by themselves. Binding of antigen with small carrier produces immune response. *This passenger molecule is known as hapten.* Characteristics of antigens are shown in Fig. 4.9.

- *Hapten:* Hapten is a foreign molecule less than 1,000 MW. It is too small to trigger an immune response alone but can be immunogenic when it attaches to a larger carrier molecule, such as host serum protein. The hapten-carrier phenomenon is shown in Fig. 4.10.

- *Good immunogens:* Microbial cells, foreign human or animal cells and viruses make good immunogens. Complex molecules with several epitopes also make good immunogens. *Epitope* is a small specific portion of antigen that is recognized by lymphocytes. It binds to the receptors of lymphocytes. Cells, viruses and large molecules can have numerous antigenic determinants. A given microorganism has many such isotopes, all of which stimulate individual specific immune response.

- *Poor immunogens:* Poor immunogens include small molecules not attached to carrier molecule. These may be simple, complex and repetitive.

- *Mosaic antigens:* These include *autoantigens, allergens and superantigens.* Autoantigens, allergens cause damage to host tissue as a consequence of the immune response. A small number of antigens can bind to MHC class II proteins without being processed within APCs known as *superantigens.* Superantigens are actually a form of virulence factor present in staphylococci, group A streptococci and Epstein-Barr virus. Exposure of T cells to superantigens produces serious illness. These superantigens can span both MHC II receptors and some antigen receptors (TCRs) on T cells resulting in *release of TNF-α, IL-1 and IL-6.* It leads to massive influx of potent mediators that can cause blood vessel damage, toxic shock syndrome and multiorgan failure.

- *Endogenous antigens:* Many native endogenous antigens present in the host play an important role in both health and disease. These may be classified as *heterologous, analogous and homologous antigens (iso-antigens).*

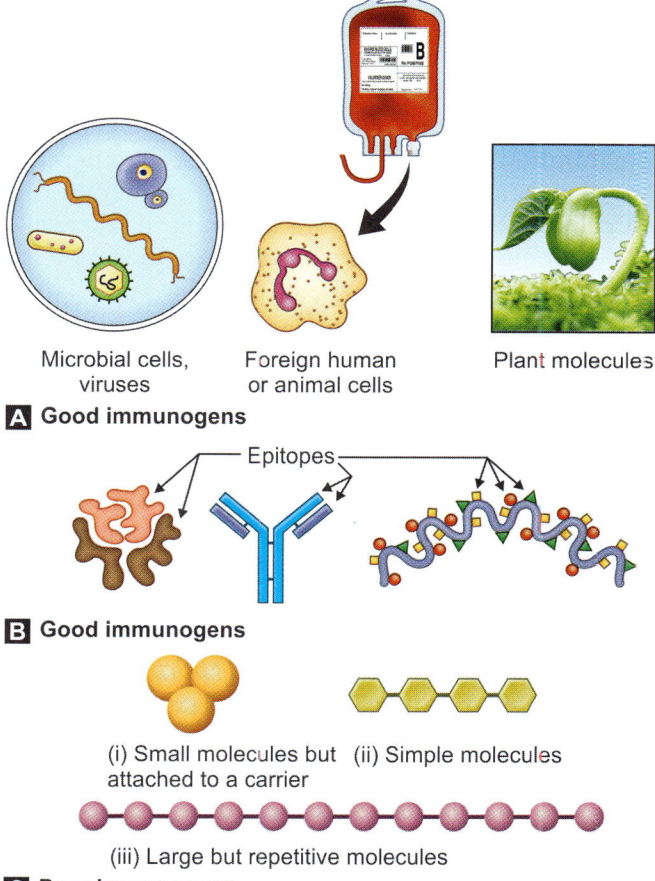

Fig. 4.9: Characteristics of antigens. (A) Microbial cells, foreign human or animal cells and viruses make good immunogens, (B) complex molecules with several epitopes also make good immunogens. Poor immunogens include small molecules not attached to carrier molecule.

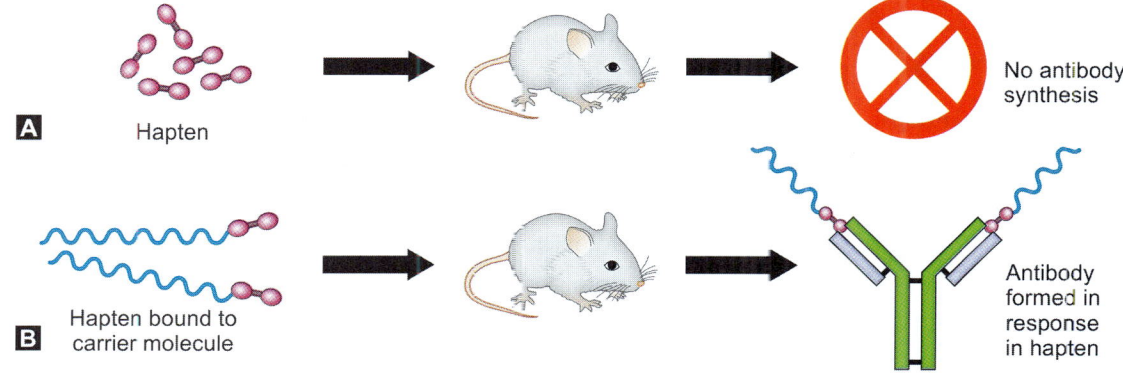

Fig. 4.10: The hapten-carrier phenomenon. (A) Hapten molecule is too small to trigger an immune response, (B) binding of hapten with carrier triggers an immune response.

Endogenous Antigens

- *Heterologous antigens:* These antigens can lead to *cross reaction* resulting in genesis of certain disease. Cross reactivity occurs between M proteins present in certain strain of β-hemolyticus, Streptococcus pyogenes and determinant present in heart and joints resulting in genesis of *acute rheumatic fever*.
- *Analogous antigens:* These antigens are host's own normal constituents. Under many circumstances, these antigens are recognized as *self. These do not elicit immune response*. This state is known as *tolerance*. The disorders associated with *partial breakdown* in the ability to distinguish between self and non-self are known as *autoimmune diseases*.
- *Homologous antigens (iso-antigens):* These homologous antigens (molecules) distinguish the tissue components of one person from another. Their expression is genetically controlled. It can be seen from the mode of inheritance of one important group of such antigens: the *ABO blood group system*.

CELLS OF SPECIFIC (ADAPTIVE) IMMUNE RESPONSE

Cells of specific immune system include *monocytes-macrophages, Langerhans' cells of the skin, dendritic cells of lymphoid tissue, and lymphocytes (B cells and T cells)*. Specific immune response involves the reactions of these cells to foreign proteins or antigens found in pathogens. B cells and T cells develop specific protein receptors for antigen.

CYTOKINES

Cytokines are soluble proteins synthesized by lymphocytes (*lymphokines*), monocytes-macrophages (*monokines*), and NK cells, as well as other cell types. They act as effector molecules influencing the behavior of B cells, T cells, NK cells, monocytes, macrophages, hematopoietic cells, and many other cell types. These include interleukins' growth factors, interferons and tumor necrosis factors. Role of cytokines in specific immune response is shown in Table 4.7.

- *Interleukins' specific immune response:* IL-6 promotes maturation of B and T cells. IL-15 causes proliferation of T cells and B cells. IL-9 causes proliferation of T cells. IL-12 activates T cells and natural killer cells. IL-5 promotes maturation of B cells to plasma cells.
- *Growth factors:* IL-3 acts as a growth factor for hematopoietic stem cells. IL-4 promotes growth of B and T cells; enhances expression of HLA class II antigens. IL-7 acts as a growth factor for bone marrow stem cells.
- *Interferon gamma (IFN-γ):* IFN-γ also activates macrophages and T cells during chronic inflammation. It enhances expression of HLA class II antigens. It participates in differentiation of T cells and B cells. It increases the cytotoxicity of natural killer cells. It activates neutrophils and stimulates diapedesis.
- *Tumor necrosis factors (TNF-α and TNF-β):* Both TNF-α and TNF-β stimulate T cell proliferation and IL-2 production. These are cytotoxic to some tumor cells.

Table 4.7: Role of cytokines in specific immune response

Categories of cytokines	Cytokine	Actions
Interleukins	IL-6	Maturation of B and T cells
	IL-15	Proliferation of T cells and B cells
	IL-9	Proliferation of T cells
	IL-12	Activates T cells and natural killer cells
	IL-5	Maturation of B cells to plasma cells
Growth factors	IL-3	Acts as a growth factor for hematopoietic stem cells.
	IL-4	Promotes growth of B and T cells; enhances expression of HLA class II antigens
	IL-7	Acts as a growth factor for bone marrow stem cells
Interferon	IFN-γ	Activates macrophages and T cells during chronic inflammation
		Enhances expression of HLA class II antigens
		Differentiation of T cells and B cells
		Increases the cytotoxicity of natural killer cells
		Activates neutrophils and stimulates diapedesis
Tumor necrosis factors	TNF-α and TNF-β	Stimulates T cell proliferation
		Synthesis of IL-2
		Cytotoxic to some tumor cells

Immunopathology including Amyloidosis 4

ENCOUNTER BETWEEN ANTIGEN AND ANTIBODY

Introduction of antigen into a host may give rise to one or more of basic reactions such as synthesis of immunoglobulins, clonal proliferation of T cells (cell-mediated immune response) and tolerance. Immunity is categorized into cell-mediated and humoral (antibody)-mediated. Immunity acquired through B cells and T cells can be classified into natural immunity and artificial immunity.

HUMORAL IMMUNITY

When a B cell is activated by antigen and T helper cells, it undergoes cell division resulting in formation of many B cells. These B cells transform into plasma cells that synthesize immunoglobulins circulating in tissue fluids (blood and lymph) providing humoral immunity. *Some of these B cells become memory cells that recognize the same antigen in the future.* B cells activated by antigen give rise to plasma cells that secrete antibodies IgG, IgA, IgM, IgD, IgE, and long-lived memory cells. Antibodies have binding sites that affix tightly to an antigen and hold it in place for agglutination, opsonization, complement fixation, and neutralization.

CELL-MEDIATED IMMUNITY (CMI)

T cells participate in CMI. When T cells are activated by antigen, these differentiate into helper T cells, memory cells assisting other lymphocytes or cytotoxic T cells that eliminate foreign cells. T cells also synthesize lymphokines that regulate cell-mediated immune response. *Cell-mediated hypersensitivity is responsible for graft rejection (heart, eye, liver, and kidney).* It is able to recognize self and non-self. Therefore, immuno-suppression therapy is given lifelong in such cases.

SPECIFIC TOLERANCE

Introduction of antigen to the host during fetal or neonatal life can induce specific tolerance. A second exposure to such antigen is not followed by antibody synthesis or proliferation of sensitized lymphocytes.

CLONAL SELECTION

Both B cells and T cells develop millions of genetically different clones through independent segregation, random reassessment and mutation. B cells have antibody (Ig) receptors and T cells have smaller unrelated glycoprotein molecule T cell receptors (TCRs) called CD markers (Fig. 4.11).

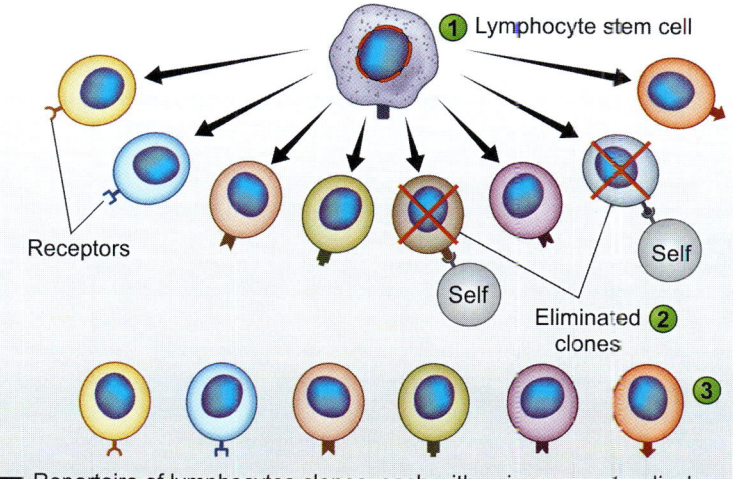

(A) Antigen-independent period
- During development stem cell undergoes rapid cell division to form numerous progeny.

  During this period of cell differentiation, random rearrangements of the genes that code for cell surface protein receptors occur. The result is a large array of genetically distinct cells, called clones, each clone bearing a different receptor that is specific to react with only a single type of foreign molecule or antigen
- Simultaneously lymphocyte clones that develop a specificity for self molecules and could be harmful are eliminated from the pool of diversity this is called immune tolerance.
- The specificity for a single antigen molecule is programmed into the lymphocyte and is set for the life of a given clone. The end result is an enormous pool of mature but naïve lymphocytes that are ready to further differentiate under the influence of certain organs and immune stimuli.

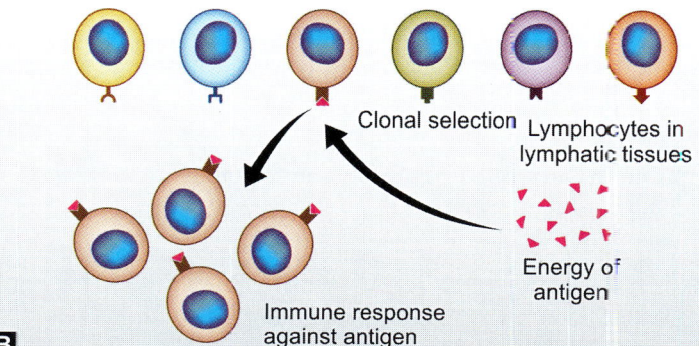

(B) Antigen-dependent period

Lymphocytes come to populate the lymphatic organs, where they will finally encounter antigens. These antigens will become the stimulus for the lymphocytes, final activation and immune function. Entry of a specific antigen selects only the lymphocyte clones the carrier matching surface receptors. This will trigger an immune response, which varies according to the type of lymphocyte involved.

Fig. 4.11: Overview of the clonal selection theory of lymphocytes development and diversity.

Antigen independent period: Hematopoietic stem cells in bone marrow participate in the production of lymphocytes. During development, stem cell undergoes rapid cell division to form numerous progeny.

- *Differentiation and clones formation:* During this period of cell differentiation, random rearrangements of genes encoding cell surface protein receptors take place. Differentiation leads to formation of large array of genetically distinct cells known as *clones*. Each clone bears a different receptors. Each receptor is specific to react with only a single type of foreign antigen.
- *Immune tolerance:* During differentiation, lymphocyte clones harmful to self-molecules formed are eliminated from the pool of diversity known as *immune tolerance*.
- *Differentiation of naïve lymphocytes:* The specificity for a single molecule is programed into the lymphocyte. It is set for the life of a given clone. The net result is an enormous pool of mature but naïve lymphocytes. These cells are ready for further differentiation under the influence of certain immune stimuli.

Antigen-dependent period: Lymphocytes come to populate the lymphatic organs. These will finally encounter antigens. These antigens activate the immune function. Entry of a specific antigen selects only the lymphocyte clones the carrier matching surface receptors. It triggers immune response, which varies according to the type of lymphocyte involved.

IMMUNE CELLS

Immune cells participating in specific immune response comprise monocytes–macrophages, Langerhans' cells of the skin, dendritic cells of lymphoid tissue, and lymphocytes (B cells and T cells). Immune cells are shown in Tables 4.8 to 4.11.

MONOCYTES AND MACROPHAGES

Monocytes constitute 2–8% of white blood cells. Macrophages are largest phagocytes (big eaters) that phagocytose and degrade injurious agent. These possess receptors for IgG and C3b. *These participate in specific-immune reactions.* In addition, they process and present antigen (along with human leukocyte

Table 4.8: Cells of immune response

Cells	Characteristics	Markers	Actions
Natural cytolytic cells	Natural killer cells	Fc receptors for antibody; CD16, CD56, CD57	Kill antibody-decorated cells and virus-infected or tumor cells (no MHC restriction)
Phagocytic cells	Neutrophils, monocytes and tissue macrophages	–	Phagocytosis and killing of bacteria
	Eosinophils	–	Allergic response and parasitic defense
Antibody producing cells	B cells	CD19, CD20, CD21, CD22	Humoral immunity

Table 4.9: Antigen presenting cells (APCs), their characteristics and actions

APCs	Characteristics	Actions
Monocytes, tissue macrophages, Langerhans' cells, dendritic cells, microglial cells, Kupffer's cells	Express class II MHC molecules	Present antigens to CD4+ T cells
Monocytes	Present in blood	Precursors to macrophage-lineage and cytokines release
Tissue macrophages	Possess Fc and C3 receptors	Initiate inflammatory response and also possess antibacterial, antiviral and antitumor properties
Langerhans' cells	Reside in spleen, lymph nodes and other organs. These are activated by interferon-gamma and tumor necrosis factor	Transport antigen to lymph nodes
Dendritic cells	Present in lymph nodes and tissues	Efficient antigen presenting cells
Microglial cells	Present in central nervous system	Produce cytokines
Kupffer's cells	Present in liver	Filter particles (viruses) from blood

Table 4.10: Antigen-responsive T cells

Cells	Characteristics	Markers	Actions
CD4+ T cells	Helper/DTH cells, activation by APCs through class II MHC antigen	CD2, CD3, T cell receptor, CD4	Produce IL-2 and other cytokines. Stimulates T and B cells growth. Promote B cell proliferation, B cell differentiation (class-switching) antibody production
CD8+ T cells (killer cells)	Recognition of antigen presented by class I MHC antigens	CD2, CD3, T cell receptor, and CD8	Kills viral, tumor non-self (transplant). Secretes Th1 lymphokines
CD8+ T cells (suppressor cells)	Recognition of antigen presented by class I MHC antigens	CD2, CD3, T cell receptor, and CD8	Suppress T and B cell response

Immunological markers on T cells are CD1 to CD8

Table 4.11: Antibody producing cells

Cells	Characteristics	Markers	Actions
B cells	Mature in Peyer's patches, bone marrow, large nucleus, small cytoplasm, activation by antigens and T cells antigen	Surface antibody, class II MHC antigens	Produce antibody and present antigen
Plasma cells	Small nucleus, large cytoplasm	–	Terminally differentiated antibody producing cells

antigen (HLA) class II antigens) to CD4+ T cells. These enhance immune response by activation of endothelium (vascular response) and leukocytes (cellular response). *These also participate in delayed hypersensitivity reactions. They may be capable of directly killing tumor cells.*

Origin and differentiation: These originate from a common precursor in the bone marrow monocytes migrate and differentiate into tissue macrophages and dendritic cells. Tissue macrophages are distributed in the connective tissues. Lifespan of tissue macrophage is several months or years. Reticuloendothelial cells distribution in various tissues are shown in Fig. 4.12.

Surface molecules on macrophages: Macrophages possess surface molecules participating in antigen presentation, adhesion, activation of cells and phagocytosis are shown in Fig. 4.13 and Table 4.12.

Lifespan: Half-life of blood monocytes is *one day*, while lifespan of *tissue macrophage is several months or years*. If the injurious agent is eliminated, macrophages eventually disappear either dying off or making their way into the lymphatic channels and lymph nodes.

Activation of macrophages: Cytokines (IFN-γ), endotoxins, chemical mediators, matrix proteins (fibronectin) activate macrophages called epithelioid cells with abundant cytoplasm resulting in formation of epithelioid granulomas and multinucleated giant cells.

Table 4.12: Macrophage surface structures

Parameters	Macrophage surface structures
Antigenic presentation	CD40
Facilitated uptake	Fc receptor for IgG
	Complement receptor for C3b (CR1)
Adhesion molecules	LFA3
	ICAM 1
Bacterial adhesion	LPS receptor
	Toll-like receptor (CD14)
	Mannose receptor
	Scavenger receptor
	Glycan receptor
Cell activation	IFN-γ receptor
	TNF-α receptor
Co-stimulators	B7
	MHC I
	MHC II

Recruitment: Chemotaxis plays key role in migration of circulating monocytes similar to PMNs cells to injured site by chemokines, where these are called tissue macrophages. Chemokines are derived from *mononuclear cells (macrophages, T cells), bacterial products, products derived from injured tissue (e.g. breakdown products of collagen, fibronectin), growth factors*

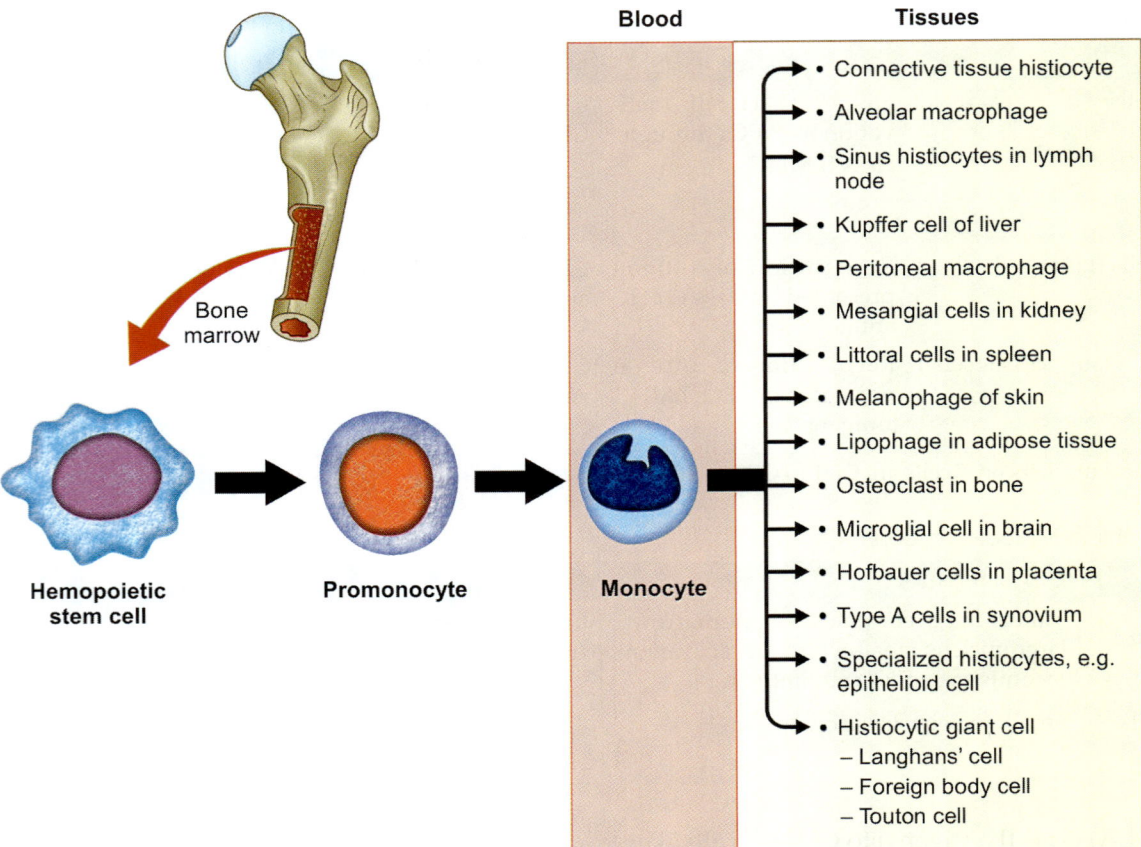

Fig. 4.12: Reticuloendothelial cells distribution in various tissues.

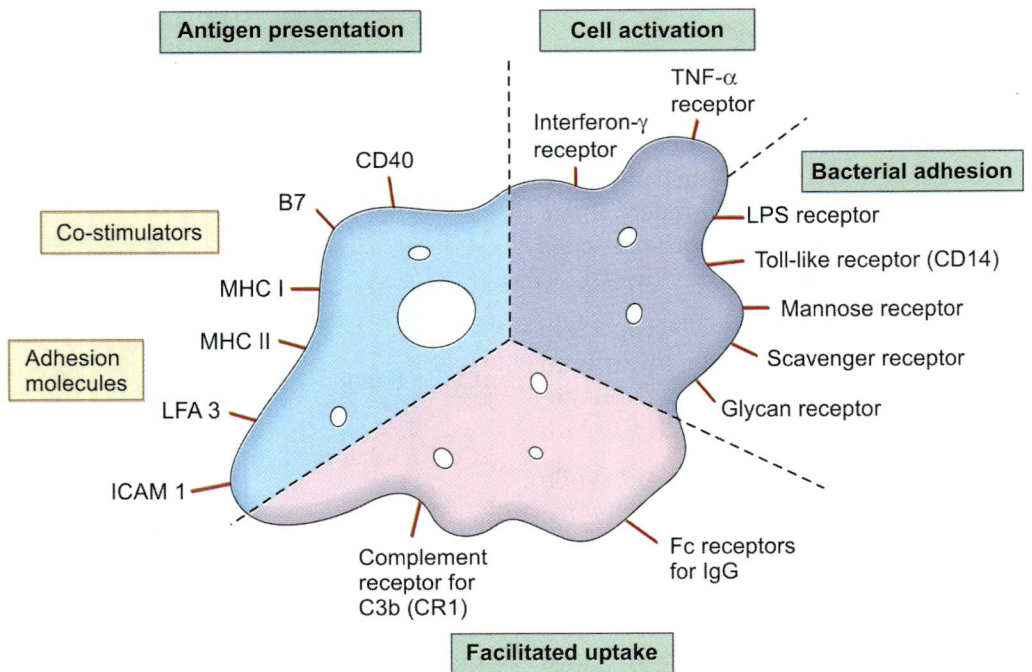

Fig. 4.13: Macrophage surface structures mediate cell function. Bacteria and antigens either bind directly to receptors or bind through antibody or complement receptors (opsonization) and can be phagocytosed; the cell is activated and presents antigen to T cells. The dendritic cell shares many of these characteristics.

(PDGF, TGF-α), *fibrin peptides*, and *complement cascade product* (C5a). Sources of chemokines and their role in chemotaxis of macrophages are shown in Table 4.13.

Table 4.13: Sources of chemokines and their role in chemotaxis of macrophages

Source of chemokines	Examples of chemokines
Blood cells	Macrophage chemotactic protein-I (MCP-I)
Bacteria	Bacterial products
Injured tissue	Breakdown products of collagen fibers and fibronectin
Growth factors	PDGF, TGF-α
Fibrinopeptides	Fibrin degradation products
Complement	C5a

Macrophage's products: Macrophages possess receptors for IgG and C3b, which process antigen, enhance immune response, and participate in phagocytosis of injurious agent. Macrophages synthesize a variety of *cytokines (IL-1 and TNF-α)*, as well as other products such as *acid hydrolases, neutral proteases, oxygen free radicals and prostaglandins*.

TNF-α and IL-1 participate in the recruitment of cells resulting in formation of granulomas in tuberculous and systemic fungal infections. TNF-α inhibitors cause the breakdown of granulomas leading to dissemination of disease. Macrophage products and their actions are shown in Table 4.14.

Opsonin receptors on leukocytes: Macrophages express opsonin receptor (FcR1, CR1 and C1q), scavenger receptors, macrophage integrin receptors MAC1 (CD11 and CD18). FcR1, CR1, C1q receptors recognize microbes coated by IgG, C3 (classical and alternate pathways) and plasma proteins derived mannose binding lectin (MBL). Scavenger receptors bind microbes and modified LDL. Opsonin receptors on leukocytes are shown in Fig. 4.14.

LYMPHOCYTES

Lymphocytes constitute 20–40% of white cells. These include *B cells* (10–20%), *T cells* (60–70%), and *natural killer* (NK) cells (15%) identified by cell-surface glycoproteins specific for both cell type and stage of differentiation. Normal ratio of CD4+ T cells to CD8+ T cells is 2:1. This ratio is altered to 0.5:1 or less in acquired immune deficiency syndrome. T cells participate in specific acquired immunity. Multiple subtypes of lymphocytes are shown in Table 4.15. Differences between B cells and T cells are shown in Table 4.16. Surface markers of human B and T cells are shown in Fig. 4.15.

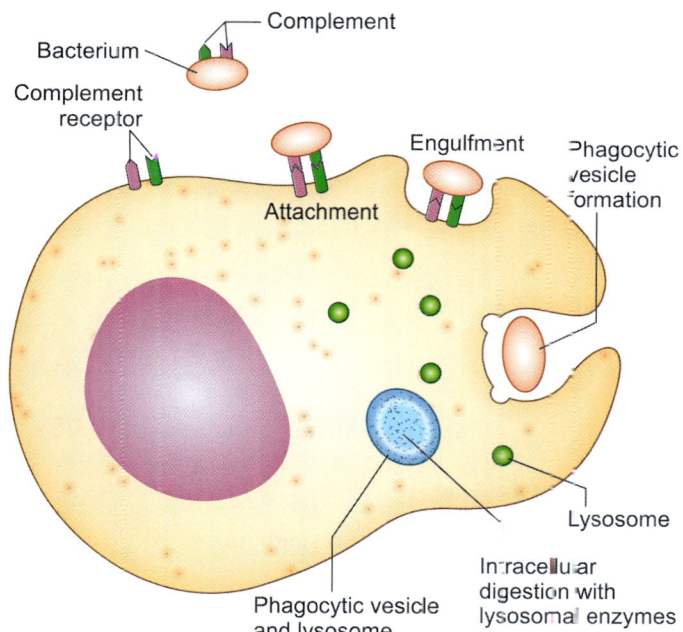

Fig. 4.14: Opsonin receptors on macrophage. One function of the complement is to aid phagocytosis. Complement proteins attract phagocytes to engulf a foreign organism. The organism is enclosed in a phagocytic vesicle, which then merges with a lysosome. Lysosomal enzymes digest the organism.

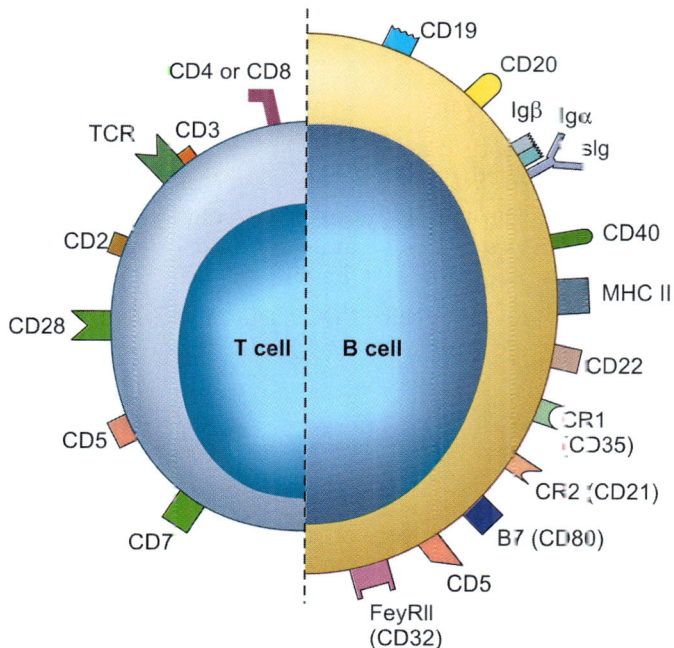

Fig. 4.15: Surface markers of human B and T cells.

T cells: There are two main types of T cells, and each responds to one class of MHC molecule. Features of subsets of T cells are shown in Table 4.17.

- *Helper T (Th) cells:* These have receptors that bind to peptides displayed by the body's class II MHC

Table 4.14: Macrophage products and their actions

Category	Inflammatory mediators	Actions
Cytokines	IL-1, TNF-α	Chemotaxis of inflammatory cells
	IL-6	Synthesis of acute phase reactant by liver
	IL-2	Autocrine action
Chemokines	IL-8	Chemotaxis of inflammatory cells and paracrine action
	MCP-1	
Lysosomal enzymes	Neutral hydrolases	Toxic to extracellular matrix
	Acid hydrolase	Hydrolyzing the muramic acid N-acetylglucosamine bond of bacterial glycopeptides leading to killing of microbes
	Serine protease	
	Metalloproteinases* (MMPs)	Degradation of type III collagen fibers
		Deposition of type I collagen fibers leading to increased tensile strength
Cell derived arachidonic metabolites	Prostaglandins	Platelet aggregation
		Vasodilatation
		Increase vascular permeability with formation of inflammatory exudate
		Modulation of phagocytic activity of leukocytes
		Pain
		Fever
	Leukotrienes	Vasoconstriction
		Increase vascular permeability
		Bronchospasm
Plasminogen activator	–	Cleave plasminogen to form plasmin, that degrades fibrin strands resulting in dissolution of blood clot
Procoagulant activity	–	Activation of coagulation system
Reactive oxygen and nitrogen species	Superoxide, highly reactive hydroxyl molecule and hypochlorous acid (bleach)	Toxic to microbes and host cells
Growth factors, fibrogenic and angiogenic factors	PDGF, FGF, and TGF-β	Fibroblast proliferation
		Collagen deposition
		Angiogenesis

*Metalloproteinases (MMPs) also known as *collagenases synthesized* by macrophages, neutrophils, fibroblasts, synovial cells and some epithelial cells.

Table 4.15: Multiple subtypes of lymphocytes

Lymphocytes	Subtype	Actions
B cell	Plasma cell	Synthesis of antibodies either against persistent antigen to injury site or against altered tissue components in chronic inflammation
T cell	Effector T cells	Delayed hypersensitivity
		Show mixed lymphocytic reactivity
		Cytotoxic killer cells (K cells)
	Regulatory T cells	Activation of CD4+ T cells
		Activation of B cells
Natural killer cells (NK cells)	Cytotoxic cells	Kill tumor cells and virus infected cells by lysing or damaging plasma membrane

Table 4.16: Differences between B cells and T cells

Parameters	T cells	B cells
Origin	Stem cells in bone marrow	Stem cells in bone marrow
Site of maturation	Thymus gland	Bone marrow and lymphoid cells
Distribution in lymph nodes	Paracortical areas of lymph nodes	Cortex (germinal follicles and medullary cords) of lymph nodes
Distribution in spleen	Periarteriolar lymphoid sheaths	Germinal centers of follicles
Differentiation (product of antigenic stimulation)	T helper cells, T suppressor cells, cytotoxic T cells and memory cells	Plasma cells and memory cells
Circulation in blood	High numbers (60–70%)	Low numbers (10–20%)
Immune surface markers	T cell receptor	Immunoglobulin
MHC molecules	MHC I and MHC II	MHC I and MHC II
Fc receptors	Absent	Present
Electron microscopy	Smooth surface	Microvilli present
Requires antigen presenting cells with MHC	Yes, on APCs	No
General functions	Cell function in regulating immune functions killing *foreign cells*, hypersensitivity, synthesize cytokines	Production of antibodies to inactivate, neutralize target antigens
Immunological markers	CD1 to CD8	CD19 to CD22

Table 4.17: Features of subsets of T cells

Types	Primary receptors on T cell	Functions/Important features
T helper cell 1 (Th1)	CD4+ T cells	Activation of other CD4+ T cells Synthesis of IL-2, TNF-α and IFN-γ responsible for delayed hypersensitivity Interacts with MHC II receptors
T helper cell 2 (Th2)	CD4+ T cells	B cell proliferation Synthesis of IL-4 to IL-6, IL-10 Damping of Th1 activity
T cytotoxic cell (Tc)	CD8+ T cells	Requires MHC I for function Destruction of foreign cells Destruction of complex microbes, cancer cells, viral infected cells, graft rejection

molecules. Helper T cells are of two types: helper T cell 1 (activates CD4+ T cell and helper T cell 2. Helper T cell 2 synthesizes cytokines which stimulate B cells to form plasma cells resulting in immunoglobulins synthesis.

- *Cytotoxic T (Tc) cells:* Cytotoxic *T cells provide essential protection against viruses, tumor cells. Cytotoxic T cells can reject grafts.* These have antigen receptors that bind to protein fragments displayed by the body's class I MHC molecules. These participate in cell-mediated immunity. Lymphocytes also act as memory cells, when come across second exposure to the same pathogens. These small killer cells first perforate their targets by perforins with holes followed by enzymatic breakdown, apoptosis and cell death. *The process involves release of perforins and granzymes.*

CD system: Lymphocytes have protein markers on their surfaces that are named using the CD system Subsets of lymphocytes are defined by the CD surface markers that the cells carry. T helper cells express CD4+ T cell. On the other hand T suppressor cells express CD8+ T cell. Markers for T cells include CD1 to CD8+ T cell. Markers for B cells include CD19 to CD22.

B cells: B cells differentiate into plasma cells. Plasma cells synthesize large amounts of *immunoglobulins* (e.g. IgG, IgA, IgM, IgD and IgE). These participate in humoral immunity. CD40 expressed on B cells bind to CD40 L (ligand) of T cells. T cells perform a number of specific cellular responses such as assisting B cells and *killing foreign cells such as mycobacterium tubercle bacilli.* These participate in cell-mediated immunity.

Natural killer cells: Natural killer cells are also known as *large granular lymphocytes*. These contain abundant azurophilic granules and pale granular cytoplasm. These constitute *5–10% of peripheral blood lymphocytes.*

These do not display antigen specificity. Their cytotoxicity is neither MHC restricted nor antibody dependent. *These are identified by CD16 (Fc receptor for IgG) and CD56.*

- *Sites of differentiation:* These cells *differentiate and mature in bone marrow, lymph nodes, spleen, tonsils and thymus.*

- *First line of defense:* Natural killer cells are *first line of defense* against *viruses, fungi and tumor cells.* Fas ligand (Fasl) expressed on the NK cells binds to Fas protein expressed on the surface of *cancer cells, fungi* and *virally infected cells* and kill them by antibody-dependent cell-mediated cytotoxicity (ADCC). These cells release cytokines which contribute to inflammation.

Regulation of functional activity of NK cells: Functional activity of NK cells is regulated by balance between signals from *activating NKG2D family and inhibitory receptors (MHC I).*

- *Activating NKG2D family:* NKG2D receptors recognize surface molecules induced by various kinds of stress like infection and DNA damage.

- *Inhibitory receptors (MHC I):* NK cells inhibitory receptors recognize class I MHC molecules expressed on all healthy cells and prevent killing of normal cells. Viral infection or neoplastic transformation enhances expression of ligands for activating receptors and reduces expression of class I MHC molecules which favors cytotoxicity by NK cells.

ANTIGEN PRESENTING CELLS (APCs)

Antigen presenting cells include dendritic cells of lymphoid tissue and Langerhans' cells of the skin. These express large quantities of cell surface HLA class II molecules. These participate in presenting antigen to lymphocytes. These are poorly phagocytic cells. Antigen presenting cells (APCs) may be either professional or non-professional type. Types of antigen presenting cells (APCs) are shown in Table 4.18.

- *Professional APCs:* These cells express MHC II molecules and interact with native T cells. Examples of professional APCs are *macrophages, dendritic cells, Langerhans' cells of skin* certain activated epithelial cells.

- *Non-professional APCs:* These cells do not express MHC II molecules. These do not interact with native T cells. These are stimulated by interferon. Examples of non-professional APCs are fibroblasts, endothelial cells, thyroid follicular cells, glial cells and β cells of pancreas.

Dendritic cells: Dendritic cells of lymphoid tissue are characterized by dendritic cytoplasmic processes. These are relatives of macrophages and distributed throughout the tissues with reticuloendothelial system. These cells express large quantities of cell surface HLA class II molecules. The most efficient *antigen processing cells* (APCs) are dendritic cells in lymph nodes process and present the antigen to lymphocytes resulting in clonal expansion of lymphocytes. In contrast to macrophages, *dendritic cells are poorly phagocytic*; however, like macrophages, dendritic cells are antigen-presenting cells to lymphocytes.

Langerhans' cells of the skin: Like dendritic cells, Langerhans' cells of the skin express HLA class II molecules. Electron microscopic examination, these cells contain *Birbeck granules* and *tennis racket-shaped cytoplasmic structures.*

NEUTROPHILS

Neutrophils are the dominant players of acute inflammation. These clear debris and begin the process of wound healing. During mild tissue injury, inflammatory exudate is removed resulting in restoration of normal tissue architecture (resolution). Transition to chronic inflammation occurs in cases of persistent injury.

Table 4.18: Types of antigen presenting cells (APCs)

Parameters	Professional APCs	Non-professional APCs
MHC II expression	Present	Absent
Interaction with native T cells	Yes	No
Stimulation by	Not require cytokines	Cytokines (interferon)
Examples	Dendritic cells	Fibroblasts and endothelial cells
	Langerhans' cells of skin	Thyroid follicular cells
	Macrophages	Glial cells
	Certain activated epithelial cells	β cells of pancreas

EOSINOPHILS

Eosinophils are abundant in immune reactions mediated by IgE and in parasitic infections, recruited by chemokine (eotaxin). Eosinophilic granules contain major basic protein, a highly cationic protein that is toxic to parasites but also causes lysis of host epithelial cells.

COOPERATION IN IMMUNE CELLS AND ANTIGENS

Both B and T cells may respond to the same antigen, the way the signal is presented is fundamental.

- *B cells:* B cells can recognize the antigen irrespective of the form it is presented. These cells are capable to bind free antigen in solution, antigens present on the membrane of cells and antigens insolubilized in various ways.
- *T cells:* In contrast, T cells can only bind antigen present on the membrane of cells. Helper T cells bind to antigen that has been processed by antigen presenting cells (with the exception of superantigens). Antigen is presented to macrophages with the help of second signal provided by a glycoprotein on the surface of the antigen presenting cell that is coded for a gene sequence within the MHC (major histocompatibility complex).

Processing of antigen by APCs: Antigen presenting cells (macrophages or dendritic cells) are found in large number in lymphoid tissues. These detect invading foreign antigens (microbes) and present them to T helper cells, which recognize the antigen and initiate the specific immune response.

Cytokines synthesized by APCs: Antigen presenting cells (APCs) synthesize IL-1 that activates T helper cells. T helper cells also synthesize IL-2 that activates B cells and T cells. Activated B cells become plasma cells that produce and secrete antibody. Activated T cells regulate and participate directly in the specific immune response.

Mechanism of T cell activation: APCs and T helper cell cooperate in the formation of a receptor complex that triggers T cell activation. Activation of a helper T cell by a macrophage (antigen presenting cell—APC) is shown in Fig. 4.16.

- *Binding of APC to T cells:* First the MHC I on the APC binds to the T helper cell receptor.
- *Recognition of antigen and MHC receptor:* Next a co-receptor on the T cell (CD4+ T cell) hooks itself to a position on the MHC I receptor. This combination ensures the simultaneous recognition of the antigen (non-self) and the MHC receptor (self).
- *Activation of T cells:* These stimuli provide a signal that is relayed to the T cell genetic material, thus activating T helper cells. The activated T cell is stimulated to release interleukin and to assist other white blood cells such as B cells in their functions.

T CELL RESPONSE

T cells do not synthesize antibodies. These cells can only bind antigen present on the membrane of cells. Helper T cells bind to antigen that has been processed by antigen presenting cells (with the exception of

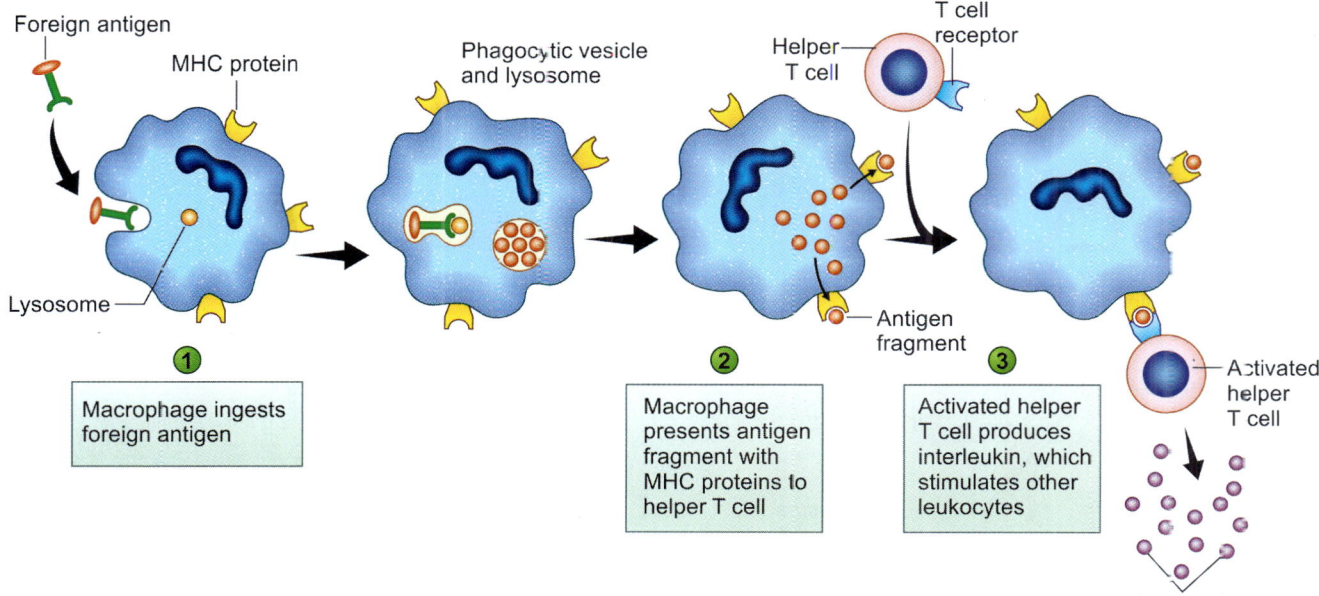

Fig. 4.16: Activation of a helper T cell by a macrophage (antigen presenting cell—APC). An antigen presenting cell (APC) displays digested foreign antigen on its surface along with self-major histocompatibility complex (MHC) antigen. A helper T cell is activated by contact with this complex and synthesizes stimulatory interleukins.

superantigens). Antigen is presented to macrophages with the help of second signal provided by a glycoprotein on the surface of the antigen presenting cell that is coded for a gene sequence within the MHC (major histocompatibility complex).

Functions of T cells: T cells synthesize different cytokines that play diverse roles in the immune response. Each set of T cell synthesizes a distinct set of cytokines that stimulate other lymphocytes providing cell-mediated immunity.

After interacting with the appropriate MHC II receptors, helper CD4+ T cell become *type 1 and type 2 helper cells* that regulate immune functions. CD8+ T cells stimulated by MHC I and antigen can differentiate into cytotoxic T cells that destroy abnormal or foreign cells. *Superantigens are microbial toxins and proteins that overstimulate T cells.* These bind to MHC class II proteins without being processed within APCs.

Exposure of T cells to superantigens produces serious illnesses such as blood vessel damage, toxic shock syndrome and multiorgans failure. It is also suggested that superantigens may be implicated in rheumatoid arthritis.

MHC (MAJOR HISTOCOMPATIBILITY COMPLEX)

Chromosome 6 of mouse contains a *cluster of genes* known as the *major histocompatibility complex,* which in humans is called *human leukocyte antigen (HLA) complex.* All human cells express class I HLA molecules, whereas class II HLAs are displayed primarily on macrophages, dendritic cells, Langerhans' cells, B cells, and some T cells. The two major classes of HLAs are separated on the basis of structure and tissue distribution. Structure of MHC class I showing α and β macroglobulin is shown in Fig. 4.17. Structure of MHC class II proteins is shown in Fig. 4.18.

Class I HLAs

- Class I HLAs include HLA-A, HLA-B, and HLA-C found on *almost all nucleated human cells* in the body. These signal to cytotoxic T cells. These are involved in tissue *graft rejection and cell-mediated killing of virus-infected cells.*
- *Standard serologic techniques are used for identification of HLA-A and HLA-B with the aim to predict the likelihood of long-term graft survival.*

Class II HLAs

- Class II HLAs are chiefly found on immunocompetent (professional) antigen presenting cells such as *macrophages, dendritic cells, Langerhans' cells, B cells, and some T cells (CD4+ T cell).* The products of these genes determine histocompatibility between donor and recipient tissues in transplants.
- The professional APCs present antigen to helper CD4+ T cell, because of their ability to process endocytose antigens and partly possessing cell surface proteins that bind to T cell surfaces. Helper CD4+ T cell become activated to synthesize an array of cytokines.
- Antigens present in class II HLA molecules are HLA-DP, HLA-DQ, and HLA-DR identified by standard serologic techniques or by mixed lymphocyte reactions. The HLA-Ds are identifiable only by mixed lymphocyte reaction.

INTERACTION BETWEEN APCs AND T CELL

Antigen-presenting cells present MHC II antigen peptides to T cell receptor (TCR) expressed on helper CD4+ T cell. These helper CD4+ T cell are activated.

These cells synthesize interleukins resulting in activation of B cells. Interactions between antigen-

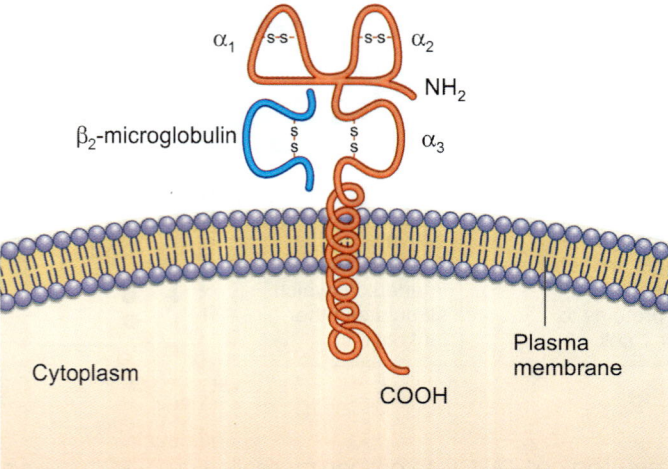

Fig. 4.17: Structure of MHC class I proteins, showing the α-chain and β_2-microglobulin.

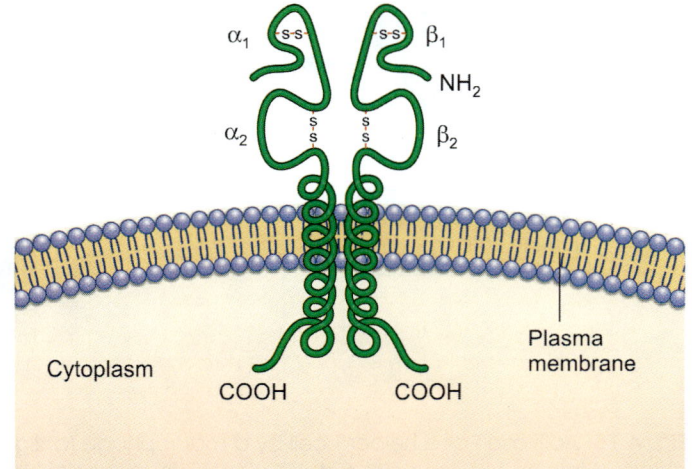

Fig. 4.18: Structure of MHC class II proteins.

presenting cells (APCs) and CD4+ T cell are shown in Fig. 4.19.

PROCESSING OF ANTIGEN

With the exception of superantigens, T cells recognize antigens that have been processed in the same way within antigen presenting cells.

Processing of antigen by MHC class II protein: Processing and presentation of antigen presenting cells (APCs) of antigen in association with MHC class II are shown in Fig. 4.20.

- *Endocytosis of antigen:* It is believed that exogenous antigens (foreign proteins) are endocytosed by APCs.
- *Assembly of MHC class II protein:* α and β-chains of MHC class II protein assemble in the rough endoplasmic reticulum.
- *Binding of MHC class II protein with endocytosed antigen:* Invariant protein synthesized by endoplasmic reticulum directs assembled MHC class II protein in the endosome, where it binds with endocytosed antigen (foreign protein peptide).
- *Folding of MHC class II protein:* Assembling of α and β-chains MHC class II protein complexed with a membrane bound invariate protein dictates the folding of MHC class II molecule and prevents premature binding of proteins to class II molecule before the latter reaches the location of the intracellular processed antigen. In the endosome, there occurs limited proteolysis of antigen (foreign protein peptide) and lysis of invariate protein.
- *Transport of complex to APCs:* Then MHC class II molecule protein is transported along with foreign protein peptide and presented to APCs.

Processing of antigen by MHC class I protein: Processing and presentation of antigen presenting cells (APCs) of antigen in association with MHC class I proteins are shown in Fig. 4.21.

- *Viral coded proteins recognized by T cell receptor:* Viral coded proteins presented on the surface of cells expressing class I MHC coded proteins undergo proteolysis with the formation of peptides, some of which are recognized by T cell receptors.

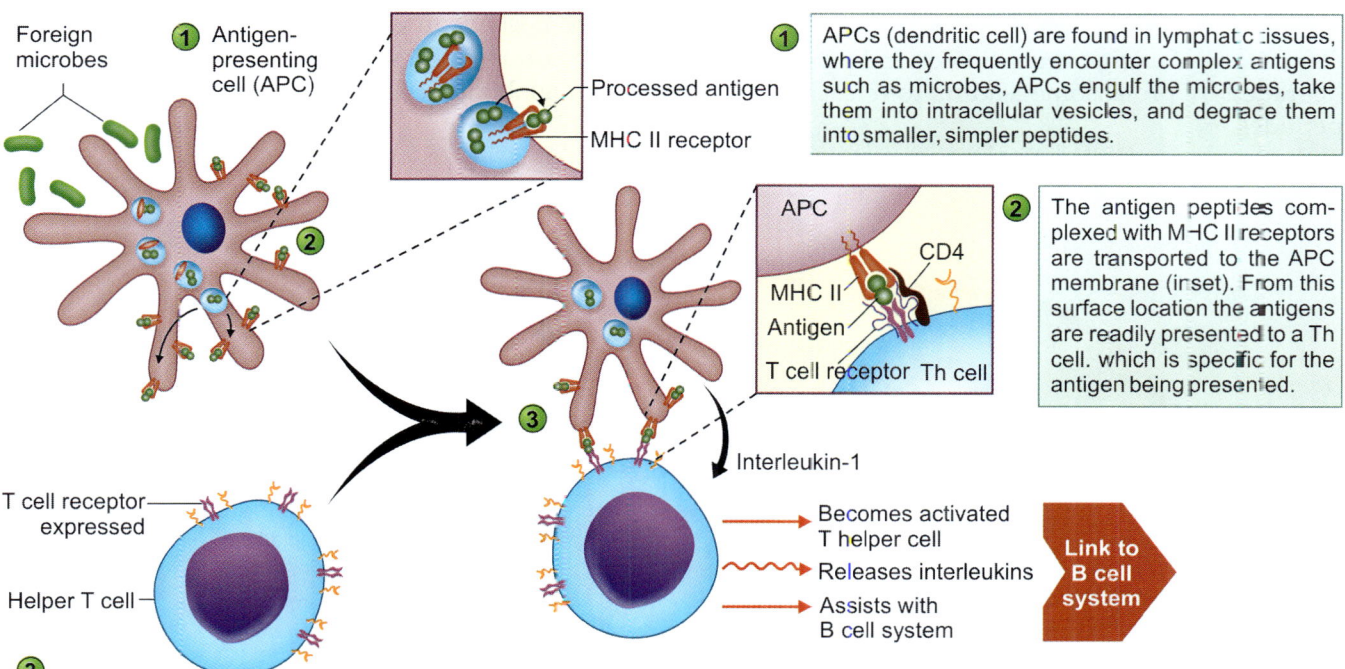

Fig. 4.19: Interactions between antigen-presenting cells (APCs) and CD4+ T cell required T cell activation.

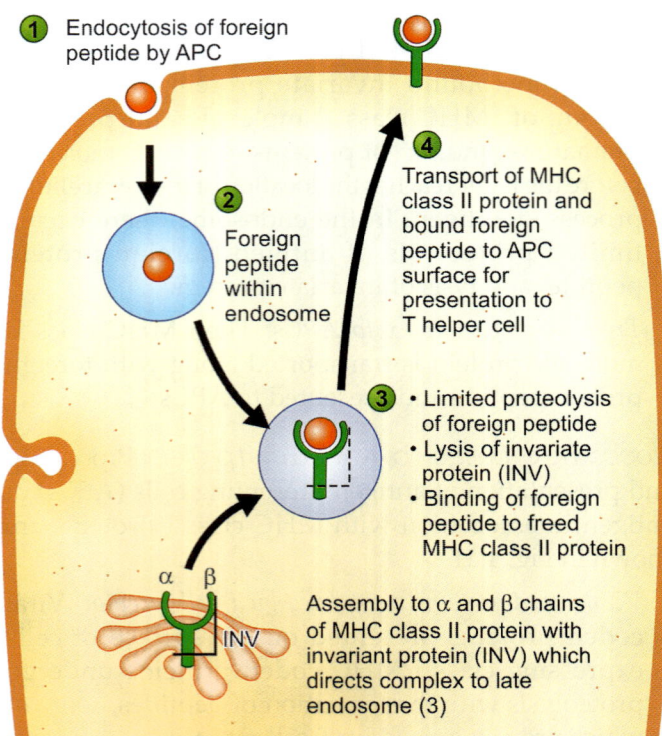

Fig. 4.20: Processing and presentation of antigen presenting cells (APCs) of antigen in association with MHC class II proteins.

- *Degradation of viral proteins:* Some viral proteins are degraded by proteasome leading to release of viral peptides.

- *Complex formation in endoplasmic reticulum:* These viral peptides are transported to endoplasmic reticulum of the infected cell. In the endoplasmic reticulum, viral peptides binds with MHC class I heavy-chains followed by complexing with β-macroglobulin.

- *Presentation of complex to APCs:* MHC class I molecule and viral peptides are transported via Golgi apparatus. Then viral particles are presented on infected surface is association with MHC class I molecule.

T CELL ACTIVATION

Antigen presenting cells present antigenic peptides to T cells bearing either CD4+ T cell or CD8+ T cell markers. CD4+ T cell bind antigen/MHC II complexes on APCs and depending on the type of cytokines released by the APCs. Sequence of events in T cell activation and differentiation into different types of T cells are shown in Fig. 4.22.

Helper CD4+ T cells: Helper CD4+ T cells play dominant role in cell-mediated immune response. *These recognize and select the antigens and epitopes*.

These antigens and epitopes determine which effecter mechanism will be used in the response to the chosen epitopes. These include cytotoxic CD8+ T cells, immunoglobulins, cells (mast cells and eosinophils) and macrophages.

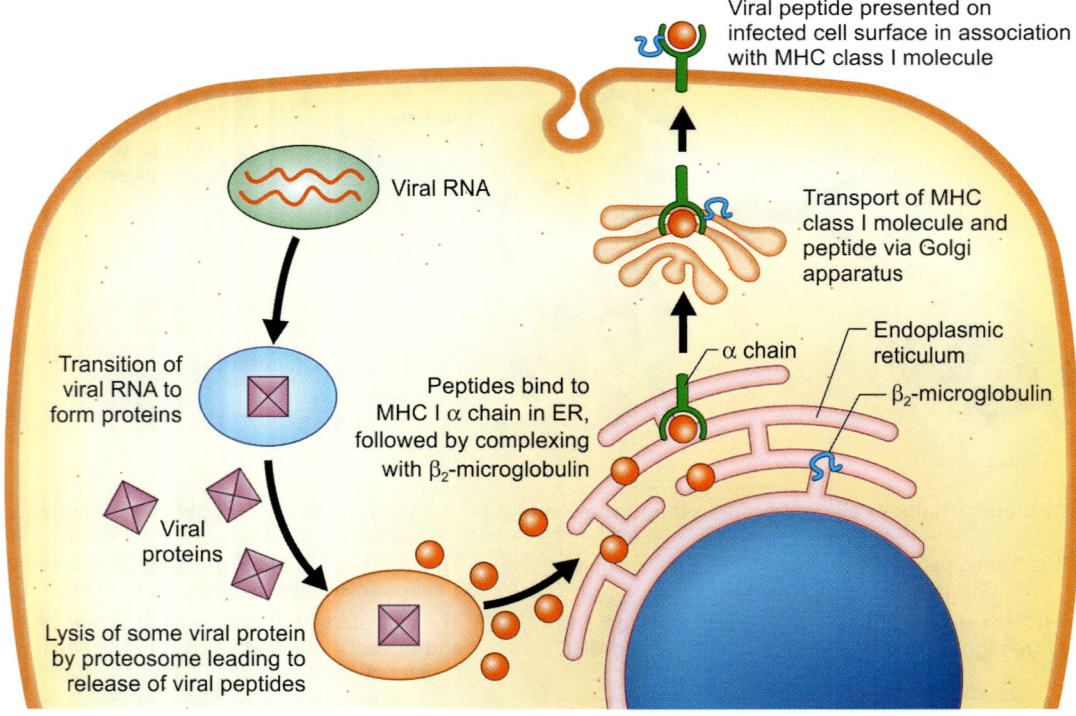

Fig. 4.21: Processing and presentation of antigen presenting cells (APCs) of antigen in association with MHC class I proteins.

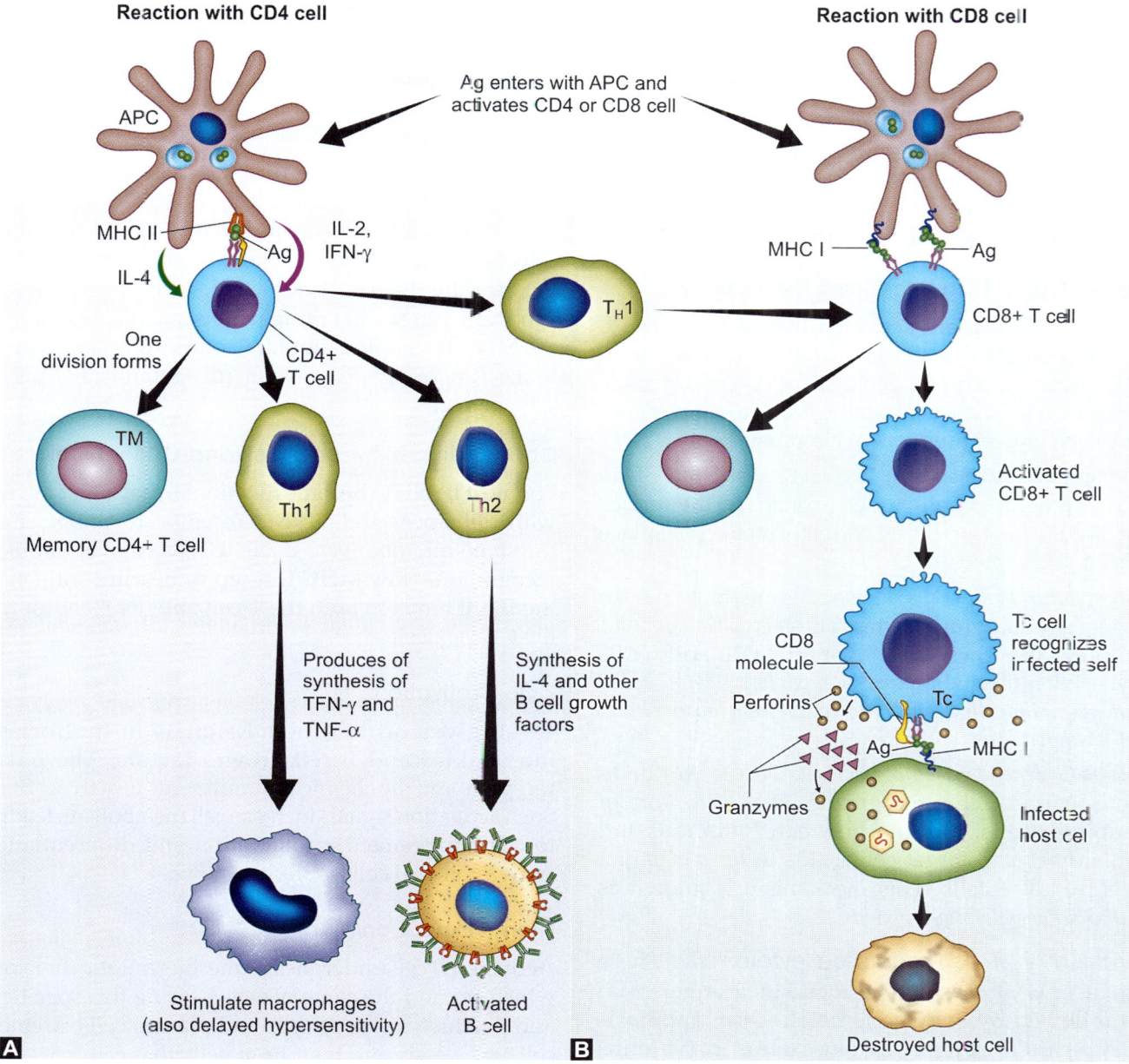

Fig. 4.22: Sequence of events in T cell activation and differentiation into different types of T cells.

Activation of macrophages induces cell-mediated hypersensitivity reaction that occurs in granulomatous inflammation. On stimulation helper CD4+ T cells differentiate to T helper 1 and T helper 2 cells subset. Cytokines synthesized by Th1 and Th2 subsets are shown in Table 4.19.

- *Helper T cell 1 (Th1):* Cytokines IL-1 or IL-12 synthesized by APCs lead to formation of Th1 cells subset. IL-2 synthesized by helper T cell 1 activates suppressor T CD8+ cells and macrophages leading to destruction of ingested microbes.

- *Helper T cell 2 (Th2):* If APCs synthesize another set of cytokines IL-4, IL-5, IL-6. T cell becomes helper

Table 4.19: Cytokines synthesized by Th1 and Th2 subsets

Cytokines	Th1 produced	Th2 produced
IL-2	+	0
IFN-γ	+	0
IL-4	0	+
IL-5	0	+
IL-6	0	+
IL-10	0	+

T cell 2 that secretes cytokines responsible for B cell activation leading to synthesis of immunoglobulins.

Amplification of T Cell Response

Amplification of T cell response is mediated by growth factor IL-2 within hours of activation of T cells following recognition of antigen by T cell receptor. Significance of IL-2 synthesis following antigen rejection is underlined by the effectiveness of drug cyclosporine A. This drug is widely used to prevent rejection of allogenic transplants. Cyclosporine A blocks the transcription of IL-2 gene, which normally follows T cell activation.

Cytotoxic CD8+ T Cells Induced Cytotoxicity

When CD8+ T cells are activated by antigen MHC I, these differentiate into cytotoxic CD8+ T cells. These kill the viruses and tumor cells. These can reject grafts. These cytotoxic T cells also synthesize cytokines. These kill the cells under three sets of circumstances:

- *Killing of virally coded proteins:* MHC restricted CD8+ T cells recognize virally coded proteins on the surface of cells. Binding of virally coded proteins take place via T cell receptor.
- *Role of natural killer cells:* These cells are derived from large granular lymphocytes. These constitute 5% of lymphocytes. These cells express CD16 and CD56 (adhesive molecule). *Expression of class I MHC coded proteins on the cells provide protection from natural killer cell-mediated lysis.*
- *Antibody dependent cytotoxicity (ADCC):* Antibody coated target cell is recognized by Fc receptors of lymphoid cells. Binding between lymphoid and antibody coated target cells leads to lysis of target cells by killer cells. This mechanism is known as *antibody dependent cytotoxicity.*

Mechanism of T cell-mediated cytotoxicity: These cytotoxic CD8+ T cells first perforate their targets with holes followed by enzymatic breakdown, apoptosis and cell death. The process involves release of perforins and granzymes.

- *Perforins:* These are proteins that can punch holes in the membranes of target cells. First the perforins cause ions to leak out of target cells and create a passageway for granzymes to enter.
- *Granzymes:* These are enzymes that can digest proteins. Granzymes induce the loss of selective permeability followed by target cell death through a process called *apoptosis.* The apoptosis is genetically programmed cell death of the infected cell. *It results in destruction of nucleus and complete cell lysis.*

B CELL RESPONSE

B cells can recognize the antigen irrespective of the form it is presented. These cells can bind free antigen in solution, antigen presents on the membrane of cells and antigens insolubilized in various ways. Sequence of events in B cell activation and synthesis of antibodies by plasma cells are shown in Fig. 4.23.

Clonal Selection of B Cells

B cells can independently recognize microbes (for example virus) and their foreign antigens. These can bind them with Ig receptors. This is how the initial selection of the antigen-specific B cell occurs.

Once the microbe is attached, B cell endocytose it, process it into smaller protein units and display these on the MHC II complex (similar to other APCs). This event makes the antigen ready for presentation to specific T helper cells.

Cooperation Between B Cell and CD4+ T Cells

For most B cells to become functional, they must interact with a T helper cells that bears receptors for antigen from the same microbe. Two B and T cells engage in linked recognition. Now MHC II receptor bearing antigen on the B cell binds to both the T cell antigen receptor and the CD4+ T cell.

B Cell Activation

T cell gives off additional signals in the form of interleukins and B cell growth factors. The linked receptors and the chemical stimuli serve to activate B cell. Such activation signals increase cell metabolism, leading to cell enlargement, proliferation and differentiation. Activation of B cells is shown in Fig. 4.24.

Clonal Expansion/Memory Cells

Activated B cell undergoes numerous mitotic divisions, which expand the clone of cells bearing this specificity and produce memory cells and plasma cells. Memory cells are persistent, long-term cells that can react with the antigen on future exposure.

Plasma Cells/Antibodies Synthesis

The plasma cells are short-lived, active secretory cells that synthesize and release antibodies. These antibodies (here IgM) have same specificity as the Ig receptor and circulate in the fluid compartments of the body, where they react with the same antigens and microbes.

Nature of Immunoglobulins

A single immunoglobulin molecule (monomer) is a large Y-shaped protein molecule consisting of four polypeptide chains—two identical light-chains and two identical heavy-chains bound by disulfide bonds. Each chain consists of a variable region (V) and a constant region (C). The

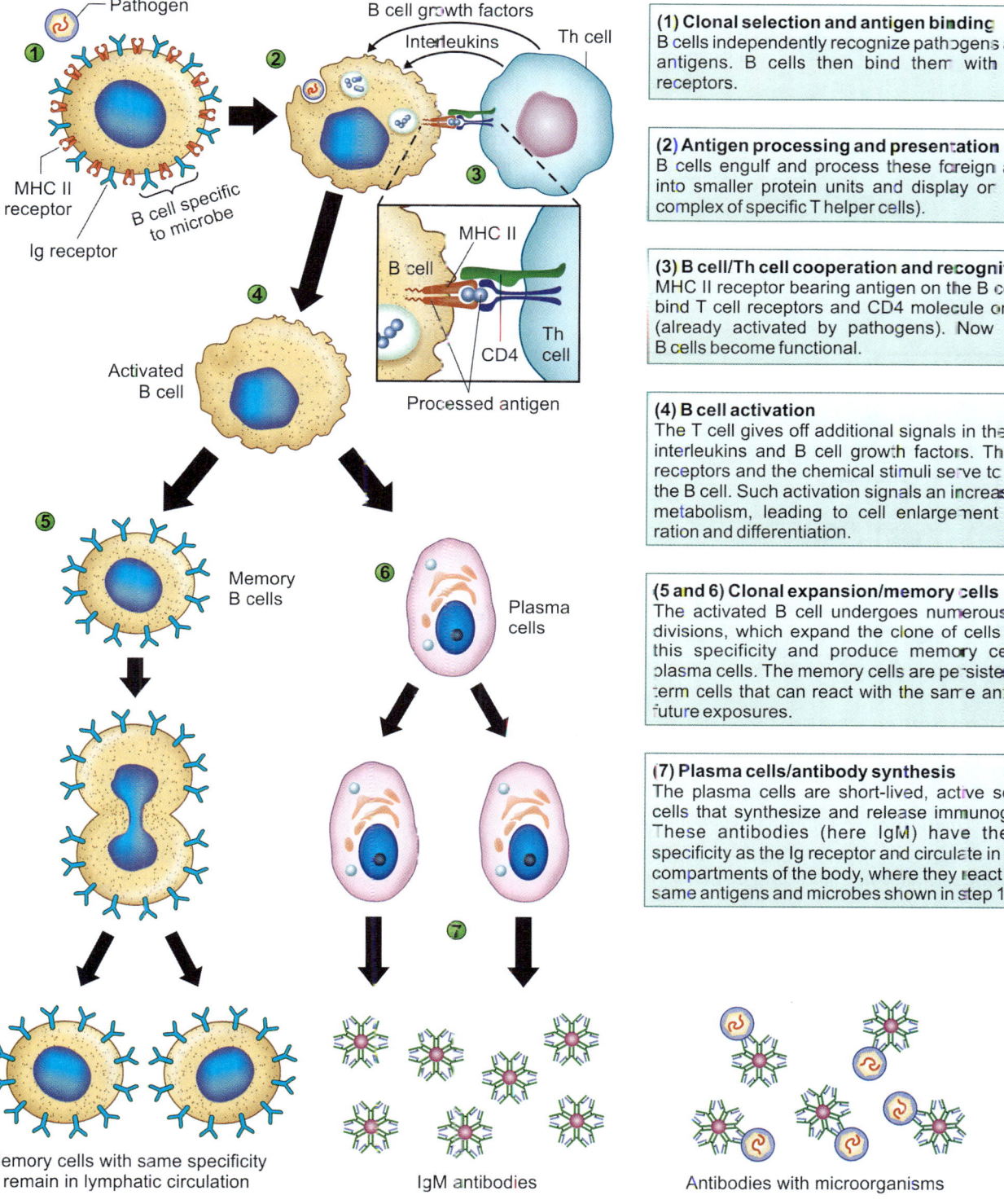

Fig. 4.23: Sequence of events in B cell activation and synthesis of antibodies by plasma cells.

variable regions of light and heavy-chains with ends form the antigen binding fragments (Fabs) that bind with a unique specificity to an antigen. The crystalline fragment (Fc) determines the location and function of the antibody molecule. Working model of immunoglobulin structure is shown in Fig. 4.25.

Class of Immunoglobulins

Plasma cells produce five classes of immunoglobulins (antibodies), which differ in size and function. These include IgG, IgA, IgM, IgD and IgE. Depending on the class of immunoglobulin involved, their operations include: *agglutination and lysis (IgM), opsonization of*

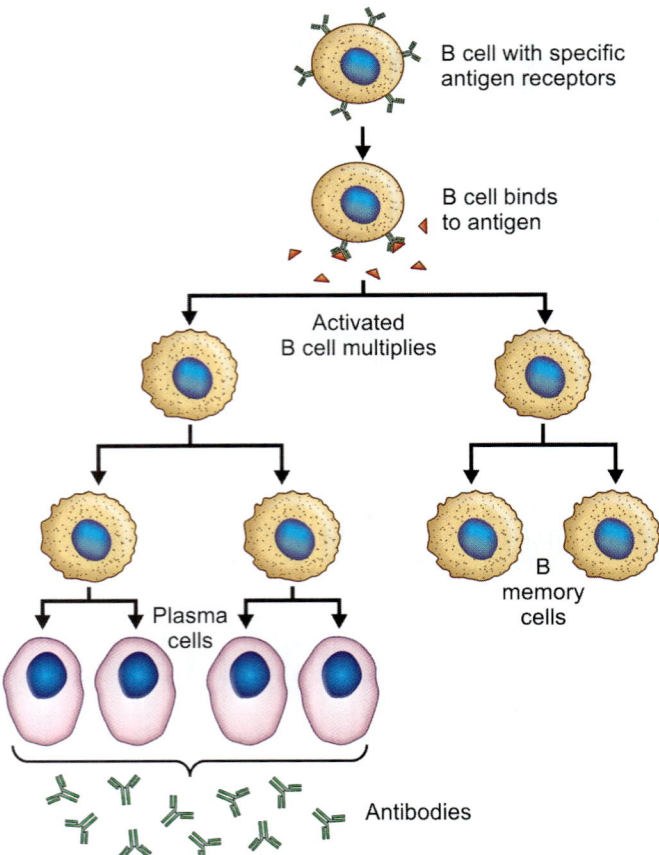

Fig. 4.24: Activation of B cells. The B cell combines with a specific antigen. The cell divides to form plasma cells. Some of the cells develop into memory cells, which protect against infection.

pathogens, activation of complement system by classical pathway, blocking entry of microorganisms from respiratory tract, gastrointestinal tract, eyes and urinary tract (IgA),

killing of infected cells via antibody dependent cell-mediated cytotoxicity and neutralization of bacterial toxins. IgG is present throughout the tissue fluids. It provides long-term immunity. IgA provides protection in body secretions. IgM predominates in plasma. IgD is expressed on B cells as an antigen receptor. IgE binds to tissue cells, producing inflammation. Characteristics of immunoglobulin classes are shown in Table 4.20.

- *IgG:* It has a molecular weight (150,000). It makes up 75% of antibodies in the blood. It is present throughout the tissue fluids. *Of all the immunoglobulins, only IgG can cross placental barrier and provide immunity to fetus.* It provides *long-term immunity.* It is predominant antibody of the secondary response. It has two binding sites, which activate complement.

- *IgA:* It has molecular weight (380,000) with *four antigen binding sites. It provides protection in body secretions.* It is major class of antibody in the mucous membranes in gastrointestinal tract, respiratory tract, saliva and tears. It does not activate complement system.

- *IgM:* It is the first class of antibody to be formed in response to an initial encounter with an antigen (e.g. primary immune response). It has molecular weight (900,000) with 10 antigen binding sites predominantly present in plasma. *It penetrates poorly into the tissues on account of larger size (molecular weight 90,000). It neutralizes microorganisms especially viruses in intravascular compartments aided by its 10 binding sites.* As it has multiple binding sites, resulting in excellent complement activation and lysis of the microorganisms or removal of antigen-antibody complexes by complement receptors on phagocytic cells. It participates in activation of B cells.

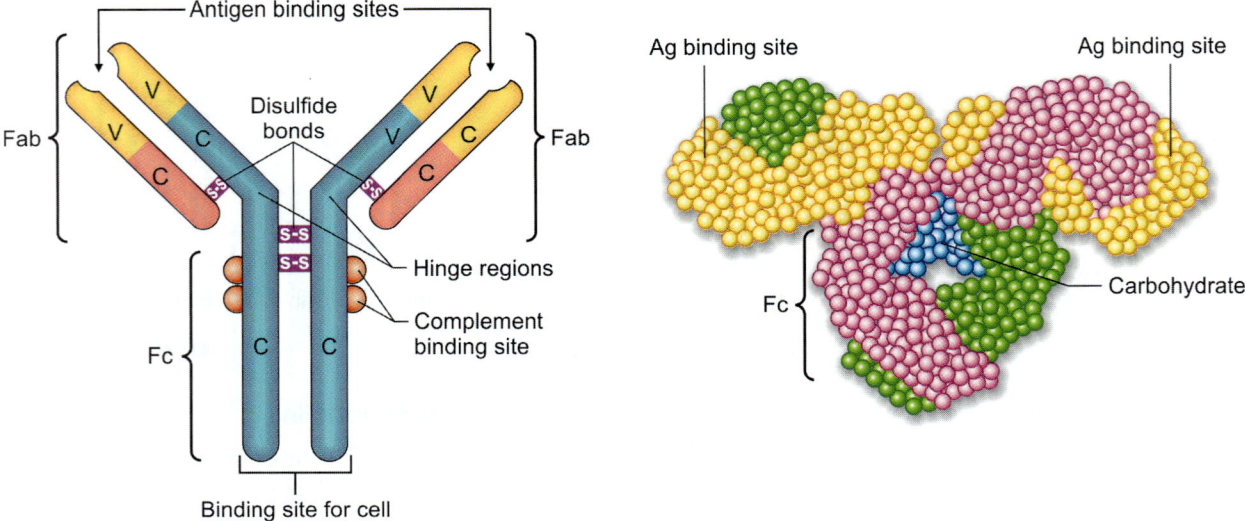

Fig. 4.25: Working model of immunoglobulin structure.

Table 4.20: Characteristics of immunoglobulin classes

Characteristics	IgG	IgA	IgM	IgD	IgE
Composition	Monomer	Dimer, monomer	Pentamer	Monomer	Monomer
Heavy-chains	gamma (γ)	alpha (α)	mu (μ)	delta (δ)	epsilon (ε)
Number of antigen binding sites	2	2 or 4	10	2	2
Molecular weight	150,000	170,000–385,000	900,000	180,000	300,000
Present	Blood, lymph and intestine	Glandular secretions (sweat, tears, saliva, mucus of gut, and digestive juices)	Blood and lymph	Surface of as receptor on B cells	Basophils and mast cells
Total antibody % in serum	80%	13%	6%	0.001%	0.002%
Average lifespan in serum (days)	23	6	5	3	2.5
Crosses placenta or not	Yes	No	No	No	No
Fixation of complement or not	Yes	No	Yes	No	No
Binding of immunoglobulin to various cells	Phagocytes	Epithelial cells	Not applicable	Not applicable	Mast cells and basophils
Biological functions	Long-term immunity memory antibody neutralizing toxins by activating complement and viruses	Secretory antibody on mucous membrane giving local protection against pathogens	First antibody to be secreted synthesized in response to antigen and serving as B cell receptor	Receptor on B cells for antigen recognition	Antibody against allergy and parasitic infections

- *IgD:* It is present in small amount in blood. It is expressed on B cells as an antigen receptor. It participates in activation of B cells.
- *IgE:* It has molecular weight (200,000) with two antigen binding sites. It is present in small amount. It is largely bound to mast cells and to basophils in tissues. Subsequent exposure to antigen leads to release of histamine results in type I hypersensitivity reactions.

Functions of Immunoglobulins

Free immunoglobulins have binding sites that affix tightly to an antigen and hold it in place for *agglutination of bacteria and viruses, opsonization of bacteria to facilitate their subsequent phagocytosis by phagocytes (neutrophils and macrophages), complement fixation (activation of complement cascade), agglutination of foreign cells, and neutralization (block attachment) of viruses and toxins released by bacteria*. Summary of the actions of free immunoglobulins is shown in Fig. 4.26.

- *Opsonization:* Antigen (microbe) is covered with antibodies that enhances its ingestion and lysis by phagocytic cells.
- *Neutralization:* IgG inactivates viruses by binding to their surface and neutralize toxins by blocking their active sites.
- *Agglutination:* Antibodies cause antigens (microbes) to clump together. IgM is more effective that IgG (bivalent). *Agglutination of red blood cells (hemagglutination) is used to determine ABO blood types and to detect influenza and measles viruses.*
- *Complement activation:* Both immunoglobulins (IgG and IgM) trigger the complement system which results in cell lysis and inflammation.
- *Antibody-dependent cell-mediated cytotoxicity:* It is used to destroy worms. Target organism is coated with antibodies and bombarded with chemicals from nonspecific immune cells.

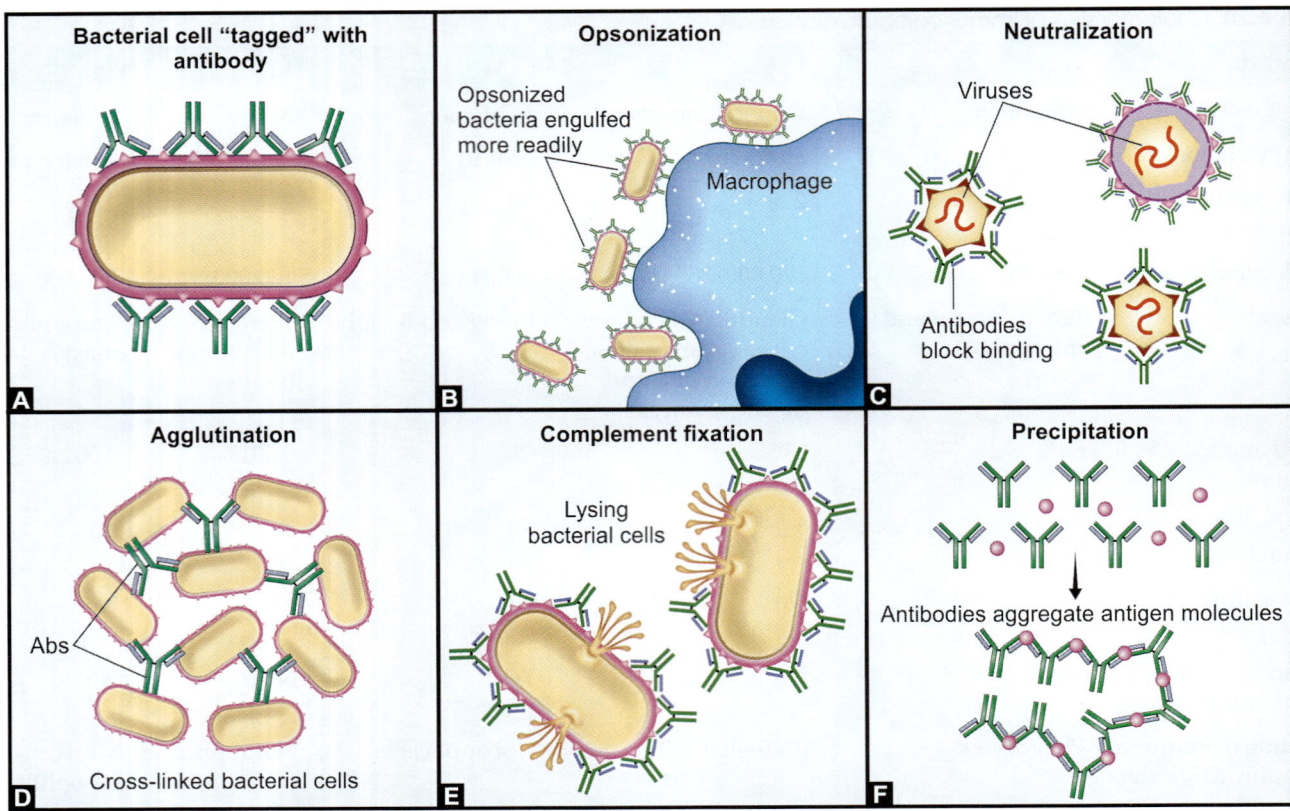

Fig. 4.26: Summary of the actions of free immunoglobulins.

Immunoglobulins in Serum

The first introduction of an antigen to the immune system produces a primary response, with a gradual increase in antibody titer. The second contact with the same antigen produces a secondary or an amnestic response due to primary cells produced during initial response.

Primary and Secondary Immune Response

First exposure to a pathogen produces primary response of low intensity. Subsequent exposure to pathogen elicits a highly intensified secondary response due to the presence of memory of the first encounter. Primary and secondary immune responses are carried out with the help of T cells and B cells.

Primary and secondary responses to antigens are shown in Fig. 4.27 and Table 4.21.

Selected Monoclonal Antibody-based Drugs

Monoclonal antibodies (MABs) are pure forms of immunoglobulins produced in hybridoma cells. They may be tailored to high specifications and have numerous applications in medicine and research.

Monoclonal antibodies can be hybridized with plant or bacterial toxin to form immunotoxin complexes that attach to a target cell and poison it. This type of monoclonal antibody-based drugs is currently employed in the treatment of various cancers such as *breast, colorectal, lung and NHL.* Selected monoclonal

Table 4.21: Differences between primary and secondary response

Primary immune response	Secondary immune response
First exposure to antigen results in synthesis of IgM	Second exposure to same antigen results in synthesis of IgG
Animal takes longer duration to respond	Animal takes shorter duration to respond
Response declines rapidly	Response lasts for longer duration
Immune response feeble	Immune response strong

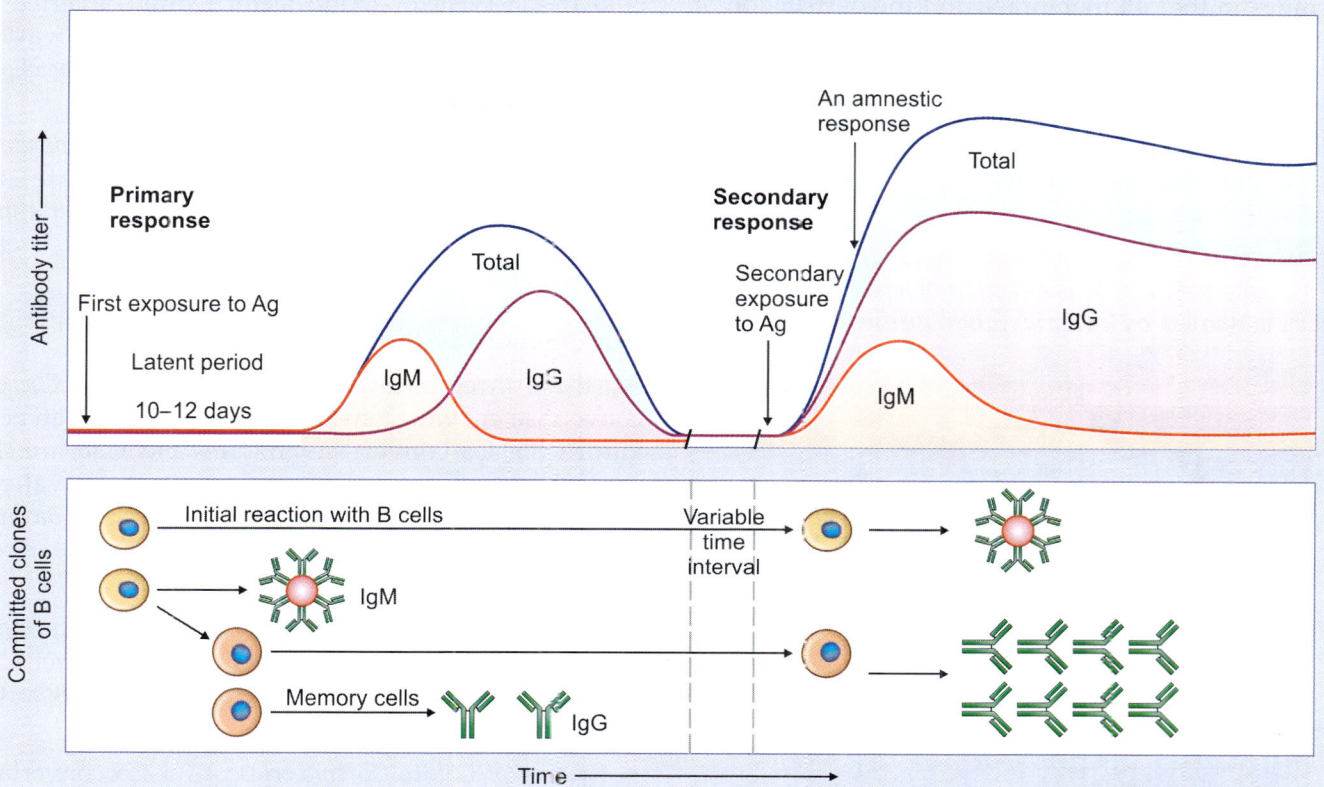

Fig. 4.27: Primary and secondary responses to antigens. The pattern of antibody titer and subclasses as monitored during initial and subsequent exposure (top). A view of the B cell responses that account for this pattern (bottom). Depicted are clonal selection by production of memory cells and the predominant antibody class occurring first and second contact with antigen. Note that residual memory cells remaining from the primary response are ready to act immediately, which produces the rapid rise of antibody levels in the secondary period.

antibody-based drugs used in various disorders are shown in Table 4.22.

COMPLEMENT SYSTEM

Complement system consists of a group of soluble plasma proteins synthesized by liver present in its inactive form that interact with one another in three distinct enzymatic-activation cascades. These are numbered C1 to C9 (C3 most abundant). Complement system cascade and its action is shown in Fig. 4.28 and Table 4.23.

Mechanism of Actions

Complement proteins participate in innate and adaptive immunity during inflammation. These cause immune lysis of cells. Many regulatory proteins expressed by mammals prevent inappropriate activation of complement.

Complement Pathways

Three pathways of complement have different triggers at starting points, but all converge at the same place, C3 convertase. This enzyme begins the formation of tiny

Table 4.22: Selected monoclonal antibody-based drugs used in various disorders

Drug chemical name	Used in treatment of disorder
Trastuzumab	Breast carcinoma
Rituximab	Non-Hodgkin's lymphoma
Bevacizumab	Colorectal carcinoma, lung carcinoma
Gentrumab	Acute myelogenous leukemia
Omalizumab	Bronchial asthma
Infliximab	Crohn's disease
Palivizumab	Respiratory syncytial virus

These names are coded to end in mab-short of monoclonal antibody openings in the cell membrane and the destruction of target pathogen. Three pathways of complement are described as under:

- *Classical pathway:* It is also known as *immunologic pathway*. This pathway involves *fixation of antibodies* (IgG and IgM) and complement (C1). It is rapid and nonspecific. C1q, C1, C1s are converted to form C4, C2, C3.
- *Alternate pathway:* It is *antibody independent pathway*. It is activated by *bacteria, fungi, viruses and parasites and venom*. Factor B and factor D are converted to C3. *Deficiency of C3 affects alternate pathway of complement activation resulting in recurrent infections with fatal outcome, until treated*.
- *MB-lectin pathway:* It is also *antibody-independent pathway*. It binds mannose (carbohydrate) on pathogen surfaces. It is *nonspecific for bacteria and viruses. MBL, MASP-1, MASP-2 are converted to form C4, C2, C3*.

Complement System Activation

All these three pathways converge to form C3. C3 convertase enzyme converts C3 molecule into an activator-C3b. C3 convertase enzyme and C3b are the central features of complement system activation. Activation of complement produces C3a, C5a and C5–9. Mechanism of action of complement is described as under:

- *C3 convertase enzyme:* It activates complement system and splits C3 into two functionally distinct C3a and C3b. C3a is released, while C3b binds to C5 convertase.
- *Binding of C3b to C5 convertase:* C3b–C5 convertase complex cleaves C5 to C5a and C5b. C5a is released, while remaining C5b binds to C5–C9. Other molecules given of C3a, C5a, which are peptide mediators of inflammation. *These participate in chemotaxis of leukocytes and phagocytosis of bacteria*.
- *Binding of C3b to C5–C9:* C5b is a reactive site for the final assembly of an attack complex. C5b fragment polymerizes with complement proteins C6–C9, resulting in the formation of membrane attack complex (MAC). *Insertion of MACs produces hundreds of tiny holes in the lipid bilayer cell membrane and results in cell lysis*.

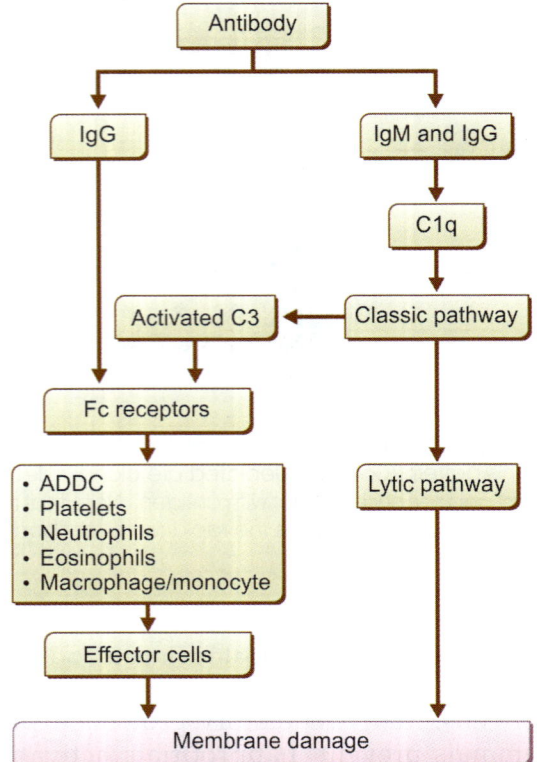

Fig. 4.28: Complement system cascade and its actions.

Table 4.23: Complement system cascade and its actions

Complement system cascade	Actions
C3b	Opsonization of microbes
	Phagocytosis of microbes
C3a and C5a	Increase vascular permeability
C5a	Adhesion of leukocytes
	Transmigration of leukocytes
	Chemotaxis of leukocytes
C3a, C5a and C4	Anaphylactic shock (due to excessive release of histamine)
C5a	Synthesis of arachidonic acid metabolites (lipooxygenase pathway)
C5b–C9 membrane attack complex (MAC)	Degradation of microbes and enhancing arachidonic acid metabolism and producing reactive oxygen metabolites

Defective formation of membrane attack complex (MAC) leads to increased susceptibility to Neisseria organisms.

Complement Actions

Breakdown products of complement system mediate acute inflammation by following mechanisms:

- *Opsonization and phagocytosis:* C3b acts as opsonins, which *coat the bacteria leading to phagocytosis by neutrophils and macrophages.*
- *Increased vascular permeability:* C3a and C5a cause *increased vascular permeability.*
- *Leukocytic adhesion, transmigration and chemotaxis:* C5a fragment is a *chemotactic agent,* which mediates the release of histamine from platelet-dense granules. It *induces the expression of leukocyte adhesion molecules.* It participates in *transmigration and chemotaxis of leukocytes.*
- *Anaphylactic shock:* C3a, C5a and C4 are called *anaphylatoxins.* These stimulate degranulation of mast cells and basophils liberating histamine. Histamine causes *increased vascular permeability, vasodilatation and smooth muscle contraction.* Patient develops *anaphylactic shock.*
- *Synthesis of arachidonic acid metabolites:* C5a fragment activates lipooxygenase enzyme, which acts on membrane of neutrophils and monocytes resulting in synthesis of arachidonic metabolites (lipooxygenase pathway).
- *Membrane attack complex (MAC):* C5b–C9 is a lytic agent for bacteria and target cells. It stimulates arachidonic acid metabolism and produces reactive oxygen metabolites.

Defective formation of membrane attack complex (MAC) leads to increased susceptibility to Neisseria organisms.

IMMUNIZATION AND VACCINES

IMMUNIZATION

Immunization is based on the property of *memory* of the immune system. Edward Jenner showed resistance to the disease because of presence of memory cells in cases of smallpox. It increases herd immunity, protection provided by mass immunity in a population. Boosters (additional doses) are often required. It is performed for therapeutic purpose.

There is no effective vaccine in newly emergent diseases such as HIV/AIDS and malaria. Immunotherapeutic vaccines for diseases such as cancer-critically needed as therapies.

TYPES OF IMMUNIZATION

There are two types of immunization: Active and passive described as under:

- *Active immunization:* It is synonymous with vaccination and provides an antigenic stimulus that does not cause disease but can produce long-lasting, protective immunity.
- *Passive immunization:* Preformed serum globulin and specific immune globulins pooled from donated serum are administered to achieve quick immune response in patients at risk for prevention of infection. Antiserum and antitoxins from animals are occasionally used. Antitoxin are administered against snake venom.

GENETIC ENGINEERING

Genetic engineering techniques include cloning of antigens, recombinant attenuated microbes, and DNA based vaccines. Recombinant DNA technology has allowed the production of antigenic polypeptides of pathogen in bacteria or yeast on large scale, e.g. hepatitis B vaccine. It is prepared from yeast.

VACCINES

VACCINE PREPARATION

Vaccine is a preparation of antigenic proteins of pathogens or inactivated/weakened pathogens, is introduced into the body. The antibodies produced against these antigens would neutralize the pathogen agents during actual infection.

The vaccines also generate memory B and T cells that recognize the pathogen quickly on subsequent exposure. Louis Pasteur worked on cholera and later developed a vaccine against rabies.

Other vaccines developed include *diphtheria, tetanus, pertussis (whooping cough) and tuberculosis (BCG), hepatitis B vaccine.* There is no effective vaccine in newly emergent diseases such as HIV/AIDS and malaria. Immunotherapeutic vaccines for diseases such as cancer are critically needed. Strategies in vaccine design are shown in Fig. 4.29.

Comparison of attenuated vaccine, inactivated vaccine and DNA vaccine is shown in Table 4.24.

- *Killed vaccines:* These are prepared by inactivation of viruses that do not reproduce disease but are antigenic.
- *Live vaccines:* These are prepared by attenuated cells or viruses that are able to reproduce but have lost virulence.

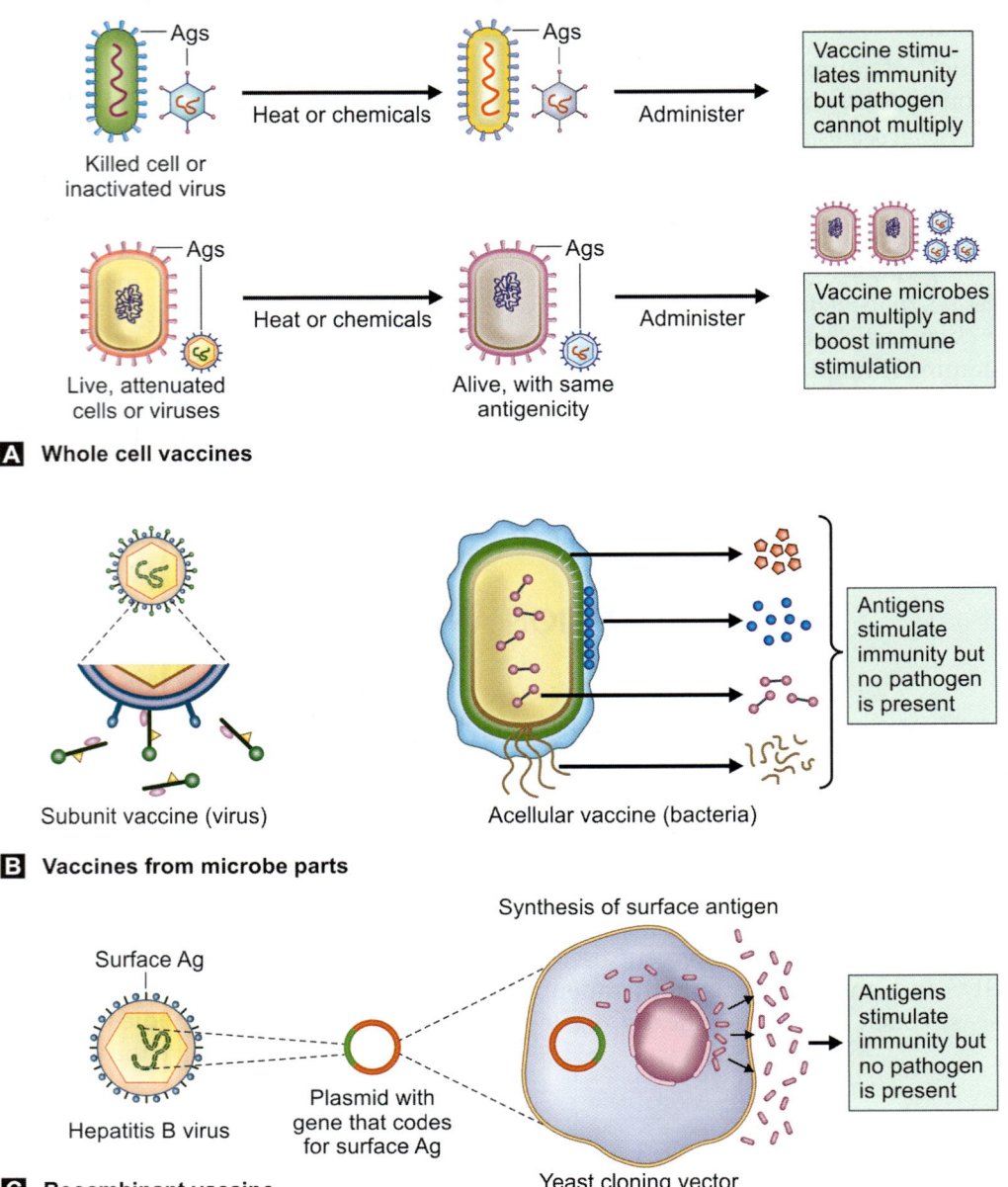

Fig. 4.29: Strategies in vaccine design. (A) Whole cell or viruses are killed or attenuated, (B) a cellular or subunit vaccines are prepared by disrupting the microbes to release various molecules or cell parts that may be isolated and purified, (C) recombinant vaccines are prepared by isolating a gene for the antigen from the pathogen (e.g. hepatitis B virus) and splicing into a plasmid. Insertion of the recombinant plasmid into a cloning host (yeast) leads to increased synthesis of viral surface antigen for vaccine preparation.

Table 4.24: Comparison of attenuated vaccine, inactivated vaccine and DNA vaccine

Characteristics	Attenuated vaccine	Inactivated vaccine	DNA vaccine
Production	Virulent human pathogen cultured through different hosts	Inactivation of virulent pathogen by chemicals, irradiation with gamma-rays	Easily manufactured and purified
Booster dose requirement	Generally requiring only a single booster	Requiring multiple boosters	Single injection of DNA vaccine sufficient
Relative stability	Less stable	More stable	Highly stable
Type of immune response	Humoral and cell-mediated immune response	Mainly humoral response	Humoral and cell-mediated immune response
Reversion tendency	May revert to virulent form	Cannot revert to virulent form	Cannot revert to virulent form

- *Toxoids:* Toxoids are prepared by acellular or subunit components of microbes such as surface antigens or neutralized toxins.
- *DNA vaccine:* There is new approach to immunization and immunotherapy by injecting piece of DNA containing the gene for the antigen of interest. There is generation of desired immune response (T helper cells, T cytotoxic cells and B cells). Global use of DNA vaccines needs population safety.

DNA VACCINE

Vaccines against infectious agents excel at inducing antibodies and provide immune protection against most viruses and bacteria. Exceptions are intracellular organisms such as *Mycobacterium tuberculosis*, malarial parasite, *Leishmania* and HIV-protection depends more on cell-mediated immunity.

Evolution of Vaccine

- *First generation vaccines:* These are prepared by use of live and weakened or killed pathogens. *Examples are smallpox vaccine and polio vaccine.*
- *Second generation vaccines:* These are prepared by use of defined protein antigens or recombinant protein antigens such as *hepatitis B surface antigen*.
- *Third generation vaccines:* Examples are DNA vaccines. There is new approach to immunization and immunotherapy by injecting piece of DNA containing the gene for the antigen of interest. There is generation of desired immune response (T helper cells, T cytotoxic cells and B cells). Global use of DNA vaccines needs population safety.

Manufacture of DNA Vaccine

Direct introduction of a plasmid DNA encoding an antigenic protein is expressed within cells of the host. Naked DNA is simply DNA sequences inserted into bacterial plasmids (simple, extrachromosomal rings of DNA found in bacterial cells) and injected into the host. It is neither a chemical formulation nor a viral coat or envelope structure surrounds it. Preparation of DNA vaccine is shown in Fig. 4.30. Currently approved bacterial and viral vaccines are shown in Tables 4.25 and 4.26.

- *Isolation of DNA:* DNA sequence coding for a specific protein is isolated from the genome of the infectious organism.
- *Eukaryotic promoter and terminator:* Eukaryotic promoter and terminator are added. Bacteria and viruses have different promoters for transcription than do eukaryotes. So, a eukaryotic promoter must be added so that a human cell can begin transcription. A terminator is also necessary—exact sequence for the protein is copied and nothing more.
- *Integration of DNA into plasmid vector:* Gene encoding for antigen of interest is cloned into a bacterial plasmid and engineered to augment the expression of inserted gene in mammalian cells. DNA is integrated into a plasmid vector.
- *Plasmid transformed into bacteria:* Plasmid is transformed into bacteria such as *E. coli*. Plasmid then becomes part of the bacteria's DNA.

Plasmid DNA construct has two major units: (i) plasmid backbone contains origin of replication (*ori*) that delivers adjuvant, mitogenic activity and cloning sites for insertion of genes of interest.

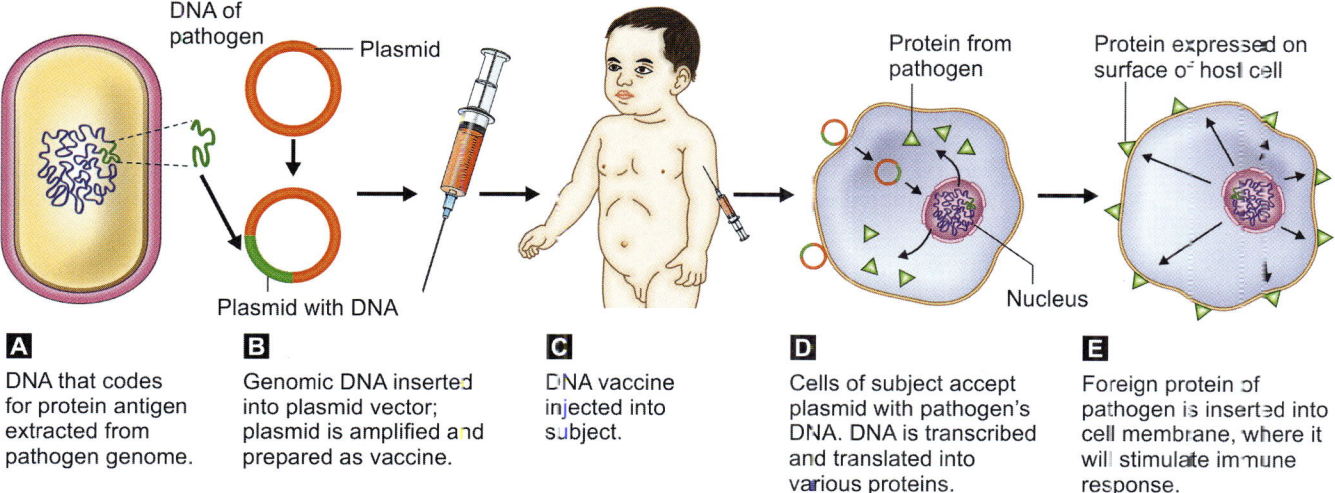

A DNA that codes for protein antigen extracted from pathogen genome.

B Genomic DNA inserted into plasmid vector; plasmid is amplified and prepared as vaccine.

C DNA vaccine injected into subject.

D Cells of subject accept plasmid with pathogen's DNA. DNA is transcribed and translated into various proteins.

E Foreign protein of pathogen is inserted into cell membrane, where it will stimulate immune response.

Fig. 4.30: DNA vaccine preparation.

Table 4.25: Currently approved bacterial vaccines

Disease/vaccine preparation	Obtained from bacteria	Routes of administration	Recommended usage
Contain killed whole bacteria	Cholera	Subcutaneous route	Travelers
	Plague	Subcutaneous route	Travelers
Contain live attenuated bacteria	Tuberculosis (BCG)	Intradermal route	High risk persons
	Typhoid	Oral	Travelers
Acellular vaccines (capsular polysaccharide)	Anthrax	Subcutaneous route	Military persons
	Meningococci (meningitis)	Subcutaneous route	High risk infants and Military persons
	Haemophilus influenzae (meningitis)	Intramuscular route	Infants and children
	Pneumococci (pneumonia)	Intramuscular route/ Subcutaneous route	Immunocompromised persons
	Pertussis (aP) containing recombinant protein	Intramuscular route	Newborn and children
Toxoids (form aldehyde-inactivated bacterial exotoxins)	Diphtheria	Intramuscular route	Children (very effective)
	Tetanus	Intramuscular route	Children (very effective)
	Pertussis	Intramuscular route	Children (very effective)
	Botulism	Intramuscular route	Only in exposed persons working in laboratories

Table 4.26: Currently approved viral vaccines

Disease/vaccine preparation	Obtained from bacteria	Routes of administration	Recommended usage
Contain inactivated whole virus	Poliomyelitis (Salk)	Intramuscular route	Children (administered as first choice)
	Rabies	Intramuscular route	Victims of animal bites
	Influenza	Intramuscular route	High risk persons
	Japanese encephalitis	Subcutaneous route	Endemic areas and laboratory persons
	Hepatitis A	Intramuscular route	Travelers
Contain live attenuated viruses	Adenovirus	Oral route	Military persons
	Measles (rubeola)	Subcutaneous route	Childhood (very effective)
	Mumps	Subcutaneous route	Childhood (very effective)
	Polio (Sabin)	Oral route	Childhood (very effective)
	Rubella	Subcutaneous route	Childhood (very effective)
	Chickenpox (varicella)	Subcutaneous route	Childhood (very effective)
	Rotavirus (Rota Teq)	Oral route	Infants at risk
	Smallpox (live vaccinia virus, not attenuated variola)	Multiple punctures	Since 2003, vaccine administered for voluntary health workers
	Yellow fever	Subcutaneous route	Travelers, military persons
	Influenza	Inhalation route	Same for inactivated
Subunit viral vaccines	Hepatitis B*	Intramuscular route	Children from birth and health workers at risk
	Influenza	Intramuscular route	Same for inactivated
	Human papillomavirus*	Intramuscular route	Prevention of HPV infection
Recombinant	Hepatitis B*	Intramuscular route	Used more than subunit but subunit for same groups
	Pertussis	Intramuscular route	See acellular above

*Hepatitis B and human papillomavirus vaccines are also prepared by recombinant methods

Antibiotic resistance gene confers antibiotic selected growth in *E. coli*. (ii) Transcription unit is viral promoter/enhancer sequences such as antigen cDNA and termination polyadenylation sequences.
- *Bacterial growth:* Many more copies of the plasmid containing the infectious organism's DNA must be produced.
- *Purification of plasmid DNA from bacteria.* Plasmid DNA is purified from the bacteria. All the other bacterial DNA and debris are separated from the plasmid vector. This plasmid can now be used to produce the infectious organism's proteins inside a person.

IMMUNODEFICIENCY DISORDERS

Immunodeficiency disorders occur due to impairment of immune system. It may involve B cells, T cells, phagocytes (neutrophils or macrophages), and complement. Impairment of immune system may result in recurrent infections or cancers. Combined involvement of B cells and T cells leads to severe combined immunodeficiency disease (SCID).

Immunity and cancer: Cytotoxic T cells, NK cells, and macrophages recognize and destroy cancer cells by means of immune surveillance. Failure of immune system results in survival of cancer cells.

Genetic alteration transforms normal cells to cancer cells due to activation of oncogenes or mutation of tumor suppressor genes, irradiation and infection by viruses.

Types of immunodeficiency disorders
- *Primary immunodeficiency disorders:* Congenital defects in inheritance results in functional impairment of B cells, T cells, or combinations of both. There may be impairment of thymus gland.
- *Secondary immunodeficiency disorders:* These are caused by infections, drugs, chemotherapy, radiation and organ damage. The best example is acquired immunodeficiency syndrome (AIDS). T helper cells are the main target. Patient develops numerous opportunistic infections and cancers.

PRIMARY IMMUNODEFICIENCY DISORDERS

Primary immunodeficiency disorders occur due to congenital defects in B cells or T cells or combined (B and T cells). Combined defects in B and T cells lead to severe combined immunodeficiency disease (SCID).

Patient has no adaptive immune response with fatal outcome by two years of age without replacement of bone marrow or gene therapy. Primary immunodeficiency disorders involving lymphocytes are shown in Table 4.27 and Fig. 4.31.

B CELL DISORDERS

X-Linked Agammaglobulinemia of Bruton

Physiological state: B cell tyrosine kinase (Btk) gene located on the long arm of the X chromosome, participates in maturation of pre-B cells to B cells. These B cells transform into plasma cells and resulting in synthesis of immunoglobulins.

Pathological state: Mutation of B cell tyrosine kinase (Btk) gene results in impaired maturation of pre-B cells to B cells. There is an absence of both mature B cells in peripheral blood and plasma cells in lymphoid tissues resulting in failure of synthesis of immunoglobulins. Cell immunity is not affected. Serum analysis reveals absence of immunoglobulins.

Clinical features: This disorder affecting male infants (5 to 8 months of age) usually does not manifest until after the six months of age due to persistence of maternal antibodies.

These patients develop recurrent sinopulmonary infections due to pneumococci, staphylococci, streptococci and *Haemophilus influenzae*. These patients are usually resistant to viral infections except Coxsackievirus and ECHO virus.

> **Light Microscopy**
>
> There is an absence of both mature B cells in peripheral blood and plasma cells in lymphoid tissues. Lymph nodes lack well defined germinal centers. T cells are unaffected.

Common Variable Immunodeficiency

Common variable immunodeficiency is characterized by failure of terminal B cell maturation resulting in decreased number of plasma cells and thus decreased immunoglobulins. Patients are vulnerable to recurrent bacterial infections. Cell immunity is intact.

Table 4.27: Primary immunodeficiency disorders involving lymphocytes

Classification	Defect in lymphocytes	Example	Immune deficiency	Manifestations
B cell deficiency	Defective development in bone marrow	Bruton agammaglobulinemia (X-linked disorder)	Lack of B cells with deficient antibody production	Recurrent life-threatening bacterial infection
	Defects in class switch	Selective IgA deficiency	IgA deficient with normal production of other classes of antibodies	Mild infections of respiratory and gastrointestinal tract
	Failure of terminal B cell maturation (plasma cells not formed)	Common variable immuno-deficiency	Antibodies synthesis absent	Recurrent bacterial infections
	Defects in class switch	Hyper-IgM syndrome (both X-linked as well as autosomal variants)	Increased production of IgM and failure of isotopes switching to IgG, IgA or IgE	Recurrent pyogenic infections
T cell deficiency	Defective development of T cells in thymus	DiGeorge syndrome (thymic hypoplasia)	Lack of T cells	Recurrent life-threatening fungal and viral infections
	Defects in development of cellular immunity against specific antigen	Chronic mucocutaneous candidiasis	Lack of T cell response to Candida	Recurrent and disseminated infections with *Candida albicans*
Combined B and T cells deficiencies	Defective development of both B and T cells in central lymphoid organs	Severe combined immuno-deficiency disease (SCID)	Lack of both B and T cells with a little or no synthesis of antibodies	Recurrent life-threatening infections with many pathogens
	Large variety of defects affecting B and T cells	Wiskott-Aldrich syndrome	Cytoskeletal defect resulting in selective decrease in IgM synthesis	Recurrent infections with select groups of microorganisms with polysaccharide capsules
Complement deficiencies	Defective production in complement cascade	C2, C3, and C5 deficiency	A little or no C2, C3, and C5 production	Recurrent life-threatening bacterial infections
	Defective production of C2 and C4	C2 and C4 deficiency	A little or no C2 and C4 production	Systemic lupus erythematosus due to improper clearance of immune complex
	Defective production of membrane attack complex (MAC)	C5b–C9 (MAC)	A little or no C5b–C9 (MAC) production	Recurrent disseminated infections with Neisseria infections
	Hereditary deficiency of C1 inhibitor (C1 INH)	C1 inhibitor (C1 INH)	Hereditary deficiency of C1 inhibitor	Laryngeal edema
	PIG-A gene mutation encoding phosphatidy-linositol linked membrane proteins	Uncontrolled activation of complement	Complement activation continues	*Paroxysmal nocturnal hemoglobinuria (recurrent bouts of intravascular complement mediated hemolysis)
Phagocyte deficiencies	Defects in production of neutrophils	Severe congenital neutropenia	Lack of neutrophils	Recurrent life-threatening infections
	Defects in bacterial killing	Chronic granulomatous disease (X-linked disorder)	Lack of production of oxygen products (e.g. hydrogen peroxide)	Recurrent infections with bacteria that are sensitive to killing by oxygen-dependent mechanisms

*Flow cytometry demonstrates diminished CD55 and CD59 expression on red blood cells, leukocytes and platelets in paroxysmal nocturnal hemoglobinuria

Immunopathology including Amyloidosis

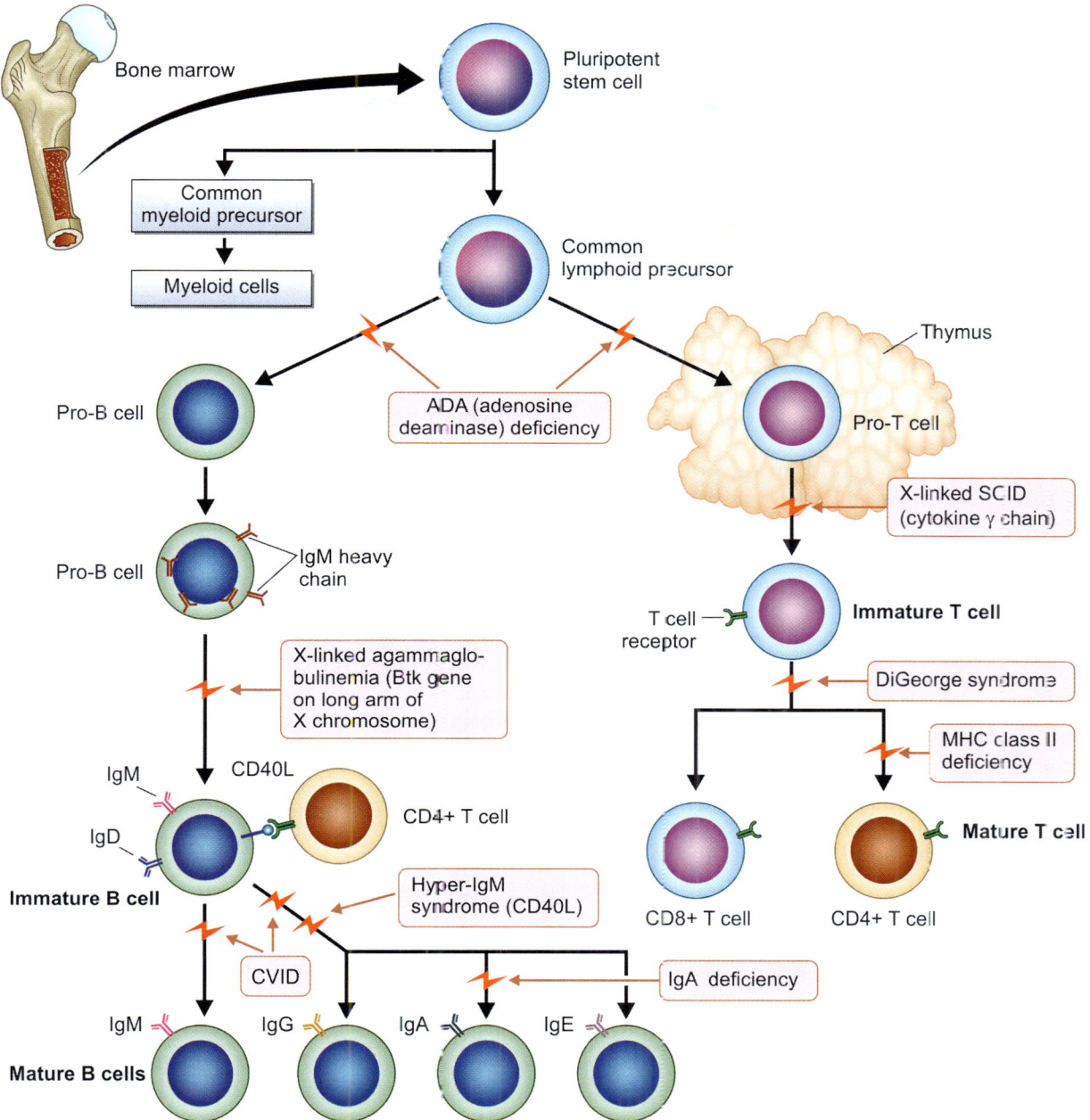

Fig. 4.31: Primary immunodeficiency disorders involving lymphocytes.

Isolated IgA Deficiency

Isolated IgA Deficiency is inherited disorder characterized by inability of IgA secreting B cells to mature into IgA producing plasma cells. Other immunoglobulins are within normal limits.

Clinical features: These patients are usually asymptomatic, but may also be associated with *frequent episodes of diarrhea and recurrent infections especially those involving mucosal surfaces. These patients lacking in IgA may develop anaphylactic reactions to transfused blood due to increased IgE concentration.* This sensitization can result in susceptibility to anaphylaxis on subsequent transfusion.

Hyper-IgM Syndrome

Hyper-IgM syndrome occurs in both X-linked as well as autosomal variants. X-linked is more common than autosomal variant.

It is characterized by normal or increased concentration of IgM, failure of isotopes switching to IgG, IgA or IgE. *These patients are prone to pyogenic infections.*

T CELL DISORDERS

Examples of T cell disorder are DiGeorge and Nezelof's syndromes associated with thymic hyperplasia. There is failure of maturation of T cells without involvement of B cells.

DiGeorge Syndrome and Nezelof's Syndrome

In both DiGeorge syndrome (thymic hypoplasia) and Nezelof's syndrome, there is failure of maturation of T cells, but B cells remain unaffected.

Pathology: In DiGeorge syndrome, aberrant embryonic development of third and fourth branchial arches, results in hypoplasia of thymus and parathyroid glands as well as anomalies of aortic arch, mandible and ear. It can be summed up by *CATCH-22, which denotes cardiac defects, abnormal facies, thymic hypoplasia, cleft palate, hypocalcaemia and microdeletion of chromosome 22q11.* In about 30% of cases, this syndrome is also associated with behavior disorders and psychosis (*bipolar disorder and schizophrenia*) that develop *during adolescence.*

Clinical features: Affected children develop *recurrent infections (bacterial, fungal and viral)* and *tetany* from hypoparathyroidism with hypocalcemia.

COMBINED DEFECTS OF T CELLS AND B CELLS

Severe Combined Immune Deficiency (SCID) Syndrome

Combined deficiency of B and T cells (SCID) manifests as profound lymphopenia and severe defects in both humoral and cell-mediated immunity. Laboratory studies reveal decreased numbers of both B cells and T cells and deficiency of immunoglobulins (agammaglobulinemia). It occurs in both autosomal recessive and X-linked forms.

Pathogenesis: Normally, enzyme adenosine deaminase (ADA) prevents formation of toxic products to lymphocytes in normal individuals. *Approximately 50% of autosomal recessive cases are caused by adenosine deaminase (ADA) deficiency.* It leads to an accumulation of *deoxyadenosine* and *deoxyadenosine 5c-triphosphate,* substances that are toxic to lymphocytes. *These toxic products make the T cells non-functional.*

Clinical features: Patient presents with *failure to thrive* and *increased susceptibility* to bacterial, fungal, and viral infections. There is increased risk for development of cancers. *Graft-versus-host disease occurs as a result of blood transfusions.*

Patient has no adaptive immune response with fatal outcome by two years of age without replacement of bone marrow or gene therapy based on maturation of donor lymphoid progenitor cells.

Anatomic manifestations: These include thymic hypoplasia with absent or greatly reduced thymic lymphoid component, hypoplasia of lymph nodes, tonsils, and other lymphoid tissues.

Gene therapy: Gene therapy is a technique by which faulty gene is replaced by a normal healthy gene. Normal ADA gene is isolated, cloned and inserted into retrovirus vector, which has a packing sequence but no viral genes. *Bone marrow cells of the patient are aspirated, and treated with retrovirus containing ADA gene.*

These treated bone marrow cells are reinjected into the patient. T cells in bone marrow now become fully functional normal ADA gene and hence the immune system. Patient is observed for expression of normal gene. Gene therapy in combined severe immune deficiency syndrome is shown in Fig. 4.32.

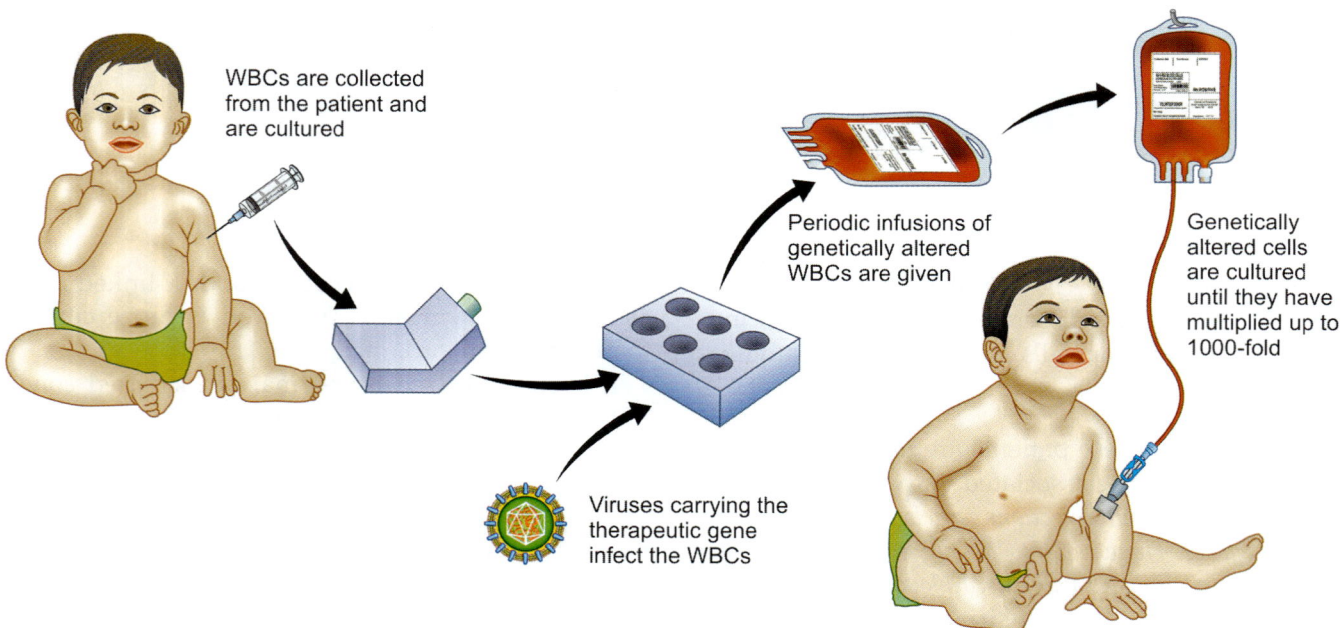

Fig. 4.32: Gene therapy in combined severe immune deficiency syndrome.

Wiskott-Aldrich Syndrome (X-Linked Disorder)

Wiskott-Aldrich syndrome (X-linked disorder) is X-linked disorder associated with defects by both B cell and T cell functions (i.e. humoral and cellular immunity). *It is characterized by low levels of IgM, recurrent infections and eczema. It is caused by the mutation of the gene encoding WASP (Wiskott-Aldrich syndrome protein).*

Molecular defects: Both T cells and platelets show absence of certain surface glycoproteins (CD43), which is ligand for intercellular adhesion molecule 1 (ICAM-1). It has been suggested that a defect of glycosylation especially sialidation of these cell surfaces.

Serum immunoglobulin levels: Serum IgM level is low keeping in view of poor response to polysaccharide antigen. IgA and IgE concentrations are raised. IgG level remains within normal range.

Clinical features: Patient presents with *eczema, thrombocytopenia, bloody diarrhea, recurrent infections and poor antibody response to polysaccharide antigens*. Patient has fatal outcome before six years of age due to bleeding, infection or malignancy (*most often lymphoma*).

Ataxia-telangiectasia

Ataxia-telangiectasia is autosomal recessive trait associated with chromosomal breakages. There is increased risk of development of malignant neoplasm especially *lymphomas*.

Clinical features: Patient presents with triad of features.

- *Cerebellar degeneration and spinocerebellar atrophy:* These lead to appearance of *choreoathetoid movements* in early life.
- *Dilated blood vessels:* Dilated blood vessels are present on the flexor surface of forearms and conjunctiva.
- *Diminished resistance to infection:* Plasma levels of IgA and IgE are decreased. Cell-mediated immunity is also suppressed. Affected patients are prone to recurrent infections of sinuses and respiratory tract resulting in bronchiectasis.

OTHER IMMUNODEFICIENCY DISEASES

Disorders of Complement System

Disorders of complement system cascade are shown in Table 4.28. Patients develop increased susceptibility to infections due to defects in complement proteins, pathological activation and deficiency of regulatory proteins.

Recurrent infections: Patient presents with increased susceptibility to infection due to deficiency of complement components such as C2, C3, and C5. Defective formation of membrane attack complex (MAC) leads to increased susceptibility to Neisseria organisms.

Hereditary angioneurotic edema

a. *Physiological state:* Normally, classical pathway involves fixation antibodies (IgG and IgM) and complement (C1). C1 is inhibited by plasma protein C1 inhibitor (C1 INH).
b. *Pathological state: Hereditary deficiency of C1 inhibitor (C1 INH) causes improper activation of C1 by immune complex* resulting in *excessive breakdown of C4 and C2*. Complement C2 molecule generates vasoactive peptide (bradykinin), which produces *painless non-pitting edema of soft tissues* especially *laryngeal edema, which may be life-threatening.*

Systemic lupus erythematosus: Patient presents with C2 and C4 deficiencies may develop autoimmune disease SLE due to failure to clear immune complexes.

Paroxysmal nocturnal hemoglobinuria

- *Physiological state:* Under physiological state, glycosylphosphatidylinositol (GPI) anchor regulatory proteins such as CD55, CD59, and C8, which are required for the protection of red blood cells, granulocytes, and platelets from complement-mediated lysis. CD55 known as DAF (decay accelerating factor) cleaves C3b. CD59 known as MIRL (*membrane inhibitor reactive lysis*) participates in cleaving C5–9.

Table 4.28: Disorders of complement system cascade

Disorder	Complement system cascade defects
Recurrent infections	C2, C3, and C5 deficiency
Neisseria infections	C5b–C9 defective formation of membrane attack complex (MAC)
Laryngeal edema	Hereditary deficiency of C1 inhibitor (C1 INH)
Systemic lupus erythematosus	C2 and C4 deficiency leading to improper clearance of immune complex
Paroxysmal nocturnal hemoglobinuria	PIG-A gene mutation encoding phosphatidylinositol linked membrane proteins leading to uncontrolled activation of complement resulting in recurrent bouts of intravascular complement-mediated hemolysis
	Flow cytometry demonstrating *diminished CD55 and CD59 expression on red blood cells, leukocytes and platelets*

- *Gene mutation:* PIG-A gene mutation encoding phosphatidylinositol linked membrane proteins leads to uncontrolled activation of complement resulting in recurrent bouts of intravascular complement mediated hemolysis.

- *Clinical manifestations:* The condition is often marked by the *passage of hemoglobin-containing urine on awakening*. During hemolytic episodes, patients develop normocytic or macrocytic anemia, accompanied by an appropriate reticulocyte response. PNH may develop as a primary disorder or evolve from pre-existing cases of aplastic anemia.

- *Laboratory diagnosis:* Flow cytometry demonstrates *diminished CD55 and CD59 expression on red blood cells, leukocytes and platelets*. Traditional diagnostic test was based on hemolysis in sucrose (sucrose hemolysis test) or acidified serum (Ham test) *in vitro*.

Defects in Adhesion of Leukocytes

Leukocytic adhesion is impaired in *diabetes mellitus* and patient on *steroid therapy* and *hemodialysis*.

Under physiological state, β_2 integrins (LFA-1 and Mac-1) expressed on leukocytes participate in adhesion of leukocytes to venular endothelium. Gene mutation of LAD-1 causes deficiency of β_2 integrins resulting in recurrent bacterial infections, delayed wound healing and delayed separation of umbilical cord in newborns. Gene mutation of LAD-2 causes mild disorder.

Defects in Chemotaxis of Leukocytes

Chemotaxis is impaired in *diabetes mellitus, cancer, sepsis, immunodeficiency disorders* and *thermal injuries*.

Defects in Opsonization of Injurious Agents

Defects in opsonization results in *Bruton's agammaglobulinemia*. Opsonization is a process by which injurious stimulus coated by *opsonins, i.e. IgG, C3b and complement mannose binding lectin (MBL)*. It enhances binding of injurious agent to membrane receptors (e.g. FcR1, CR1 and MBL) expressed on activated neutrophils.

Defects in Phagocytosis

Phagocytosis is impaired in leukemias, diabetes mellitus, and malnutrition and neonates. *Chédiak-Higashi syndrome is example of hereditary disorder.*

Defects in phagolysosome formation: Under physiological state, phagocytic vesicle fuses with neutrophilic membrane of lysosome to form phagolysosome. LYST gene located on chromosome 1q42 encodes a protein essential for assembly of microtubules in the cytoplasm.

- *Chédiak-Higashi syndrome:* In *Chédiak-Higashi syndrome*, a defect in microtubule function due to mutation of LYST gene prevents phagolysosome formation. It causes *defective degranulation of neutrophils, impaired microbial killing, and recurrent bacterial infections (Staphylococcus aureus)* forming soft tissue abscess. *Neutrophils contain giant granules due to aberrant organelles*. This order affects other cells such as *platelets (bleeding), melanocytes (albinism), Schwann cells (neuropathy), natural killer cells, and cytotoxic T cells (aggressive lymphoproliferative disorder)*.

- *Albinism:* Impaired membrane fusion of lysosomes with melanosomes in melanocytes causes *albinism*.

ACQUIRED IMMUNODEFICIENCY SYNDROME

Acquired immunedeficiency syndrome (AIDS) caused by the retrovirus human immunodeficiency virus (HIV) is characterized by profound immunosuppression that leads to *opportunistic infections, secondary neoplasms, and neurologic manifestations*.

- This single-stranded RNA (two copies of genomic RNA) retrovirus is transcribed to dsDNA by reverse transcriptase. It integrates into host genome. It has high potential for genetic diversity. It can lie dormant within a cell for many years, especially in resting (memory) CD4+ T cells.

- HIV 1 affects people worldwide pandemic. HIV 2 has been isolated in West Africa, India. HIV 2 causes AIDS much more slowly than HIV 1 but otherwise clinically similar. HIV infection is diagnosed by ELISA test; Western blot and direct assessment of viral RNA.

Basic Defect

CD4+ T cells play a central role in immune response. HIV targets the CD4+ T cells resulting in marked depletion (down to 200 cells/mm^3). Cellular as well humoral immunity is impaired. *These patients are susceptible to opportunistic infections and cancers*. The vast majority of AIDS cases in the United States and Europe are caused by infection with the retrovirus HIV 1.

Structure of HIV

Human immunodeficiency virus (HIV) is 100–140 nm in diameter. The HIV-1 genome consists of two identical 9.7 kb single strands of RNA, reverse transcriptase and other enzymes enclosed within a core of viral proteins. Core is surrounded by *protein capsid*, comprising of protein p24.

Outside the protein coat is a layer composed of another protein called matrix protein p17. Phospholipid bilayer surrounding p17 is studded with virally encoded

Immunopathology including Amyloidosis

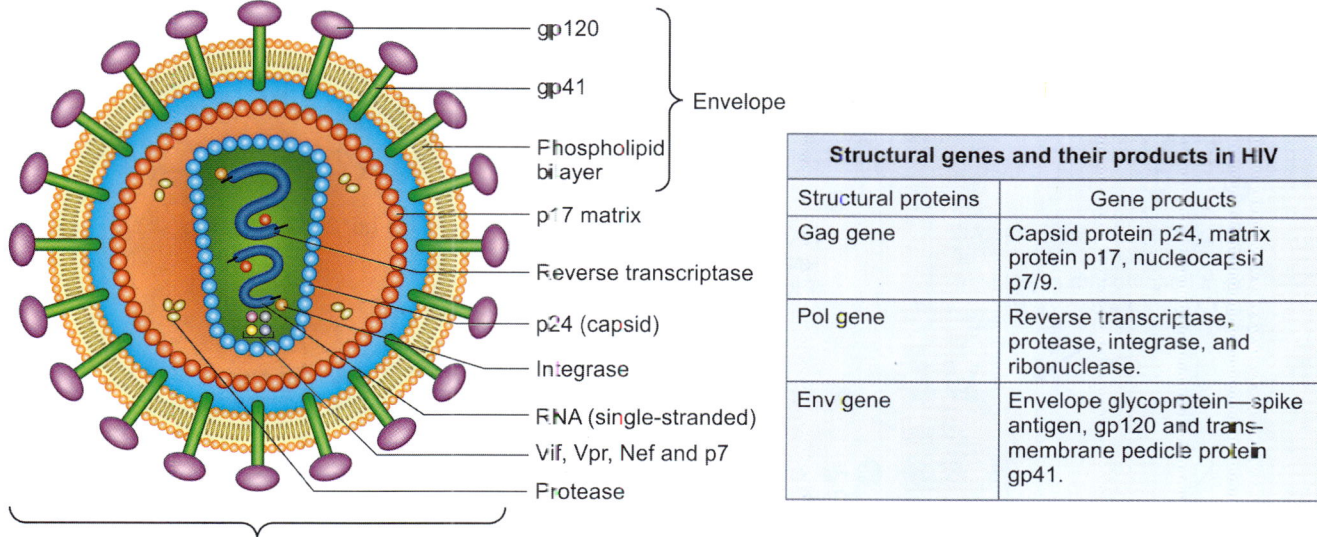

Fig. 4.33: Structure of HIV: Human immunodeficiency virus (HIV), the cause of AIDS (acquired immunodeficiency syndrome). The core contains RNA and reverse transcriptase, plus several other enzymes. The protein coat (capsid) around the core consists of a protein called p24. Outside the protein coat is a layer composed of another protein called p17. The envelope consists of a phospholipid bilayer studded with glycoproteins (gp120 and gp41). These glycoproteins play a vital role when HIV binds to and enters certain target cells.

glycoproteins (gp120 and gp41). Structure of HIV is shown in Fig. 4.33.

Routes of Transmission

High risk population include *homosexual or bisexual men (75%), intravenous drug abusers (15%), multiple blood transfusion recipients (2%), hemophilic patients (1%) and transplacental route for babies of infected mothers.*

- *Sexual transmission:* It is most common mode of transmission of HIV infection. *In more than 75% cases, HIV is carried in the semen, and it enters the recipient's body through abrasion in rectal or oral mucosa or by direct contact with mucosal lining cells.*

- *Parenteral transmission:* HIV transmission occurs in individual's *intravenous drug abusers, random recipients of blood transfusion.* Mechanism of viral transmission includes sharing of needles, syringes and blood transfusion products contaminated with HIV.

- *Vertical transmission:* Mother-to-infant transmission is the major cause of pediatric AIDS. Infected mothers can transmit the infection to their offspring by three routes: (i) *In utero* by transplacental spread, (ii) during delivery through an infected birth canal, and (iii) after birth by ingestion of breast milk.

These transmissions during birth (intrapartum) and in the immediate period thereafter (peripartum) is considered to be the most common mode. Higher risk of transmission is associated with high maternal viral load and low CD4+ T cell counts as well as chorioamnionitis.

Preventive measures: Risk has been greatly diminished by screening donor blood for anti-HIV antibodies, HIV p24 antigen, and HIV 1 RNA. HIV screening and heat inactivation of HIV in factor VIII concentrates have become universal in hemophilic patients.

Targets of HIV

HIV infects many tissues, the two major targets of HIV infection are immune system and CNS. *AIDS primarily affect CD4+ T cells and surviving helper T cells. HIV later affects macrophages, dendritic cells, Langerhans' cells, and microglial cells of the central nervous system.*

Monocytes and macrophages may function as reservoirs for HIV and possibly as vehicles for viral entry into the CNS. HIV may infect neural cells directly by way of CD4+ T cell receptors or may compete (through the gp120) for neural receptor sites for neuroleukin, a neural tissue growth factor.

Life Cycle

Life cycle of HIV comprises binding of HIV to CD4+ T cells, fusion of HIV gp41 to host cell membrane, internalization of HIV into host cell, synthesis of proviral DNA, entry of viral DNA into CD4+ T cells and creating new virus particles virions (Fig. 4.34).

Section I: General Pathology

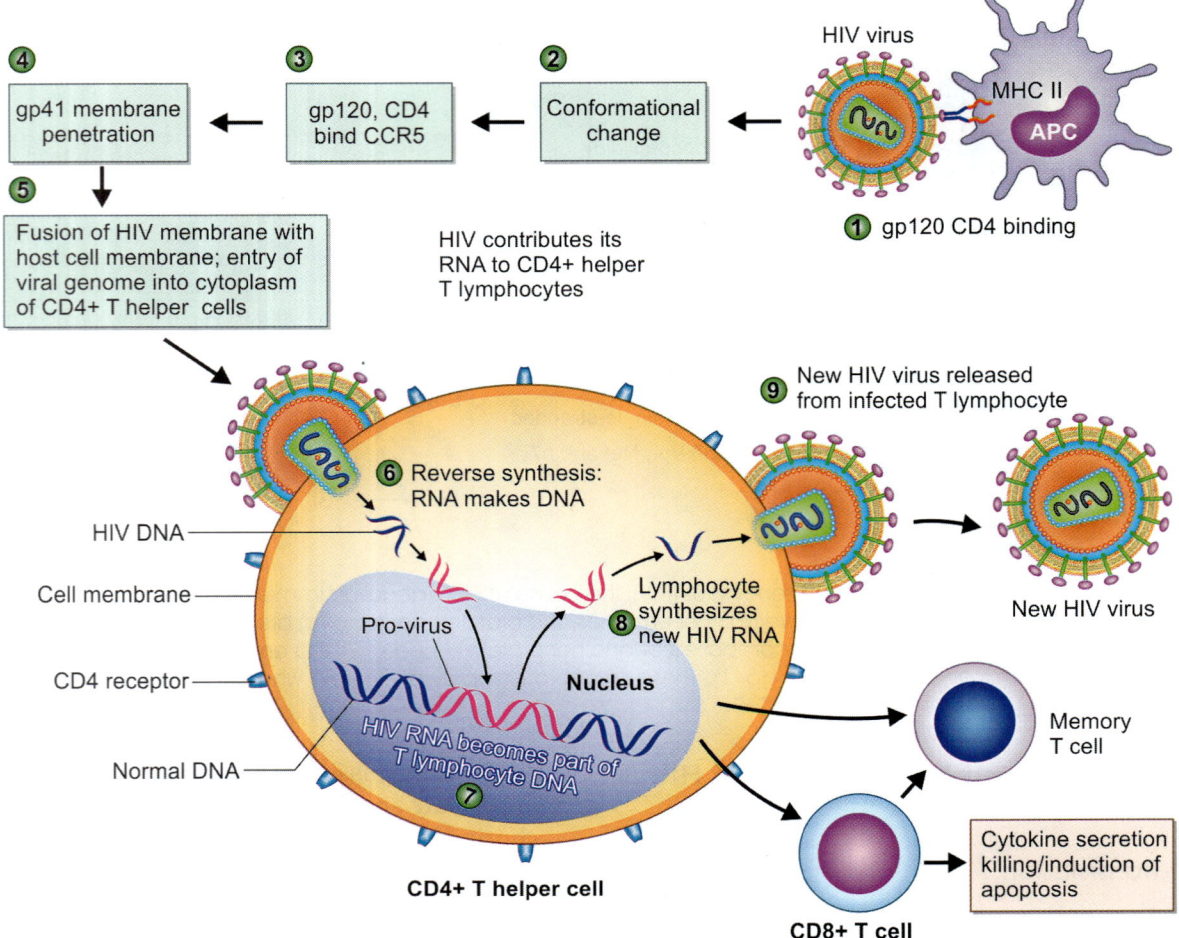

Fig. 4.34: Life cycle of HIV.

Binding of HIV to CD4+ T cells: CD4+ T cell is a co-receptor belonging to immunoglobulin superfamily. HIV 1 cell's envelope surface glycoprotein gp120 uses CD4+ T cell co-receptor for binding to host CD4+ T cells with the help of V3 loop of gp120.

It results in creating a shift in the conformation of HIV 1 cell's surface gp120. It uses chemokines co-receptors such as CCR5 used by macrophage and CXCR4 used by lymphocytes to gain entry of HIV 1 into the host cells.

Fusion of HIV gp41 to host cell membrane: Following a structural change in the viral gp41, HIV inserts a fusion peptide into the host cell that allows the outer membrane of the virus to fuse with the cell membrane.

Internalization of HIV into host cell: After cellular binding of gp120 to CD4+ T cell, viral ribonucleic acid (RNA) is released into the host cell.

Synthesis of pro-viral DNA: The pro-viral RNA is converted into viral deoxyribonucleic acid (DNA) through a process called *reverse transcriptase*.

Reverse transcriptase, an enzyme reads the sequence of pro-viral RNA nucleic acids that have entered the host cell and transcribes the sequence into a complementary DNA sequence.

Entry of viral DNA into CD4+ T cells: HIV enters the body through mucosal tissues and blood and *first infects CD4+ T cells, dendritic cells and macrophages*. Virus integrates itself into the DNA of T cells. The infection becomes established in lymphoid tissues, where it remains latent for long periods until activated by cytomegalovirus or Epstein-Barr virus (EBV).

Active viral replication is associated with more infection of cells and progression to AIDS. HIV does not infect the naïve T cells as it contains an enzyme which inactivates the viral genome. With the activation of T cells, there is upregulation of NF-kB causing cell lysis.

Creating new virus particles: CD4+ T cells begin to make copies of the HIV components. Protease (an enzyme) helps create new virus particles. The new HIV virion (virus particle) is released from the T cell. It is found in *blood, semen, vaginal secretions, breast milk, and saliva*.

Viral Host Interactions

Host mounts HIV-specific immune responses. Cell-mediated is most important. There is antibody-mediated immune response. HIV subverts the immune system by infecting CD4+ T cells that control normal immune responses. Virus integrates into host DNA. It has high rate of mutation. It hides itself in tissue not readily accessible to immune system. It induces a cytokine environment that the virus uses to its own replicative advantage.

Cell-mediated immune response

- *CD8+ cytotoxic T lymphocytes (CTL):* These are critical for containment of intracellular HIV. These are derived from CD8+ T cells. These cells recognize viral antigens in context of MHC class I presentation. These directly destroy infected cells. Their activity is augmented by Th1 response.

- *CD4+ helper T cells:* These play an important role in cell-mediated response. These recognize viral antigens and utilize major histocompatibility complex (MHC) class II molecules. Th1 cells activate CD8+ cells, promoting cell-mediated immunity. Th2 cells activate B cells, promoting antibody-mediated immunity.

Antibody-mediated immune response: Antibodies have many roles in HIV infection. But these antibodies are less effective in controlling HIV infection as compared to cell-mediated immune response by two mechanisms:

- *Neutralization of HIV:* Antibodies formed against proteins on surface of virus block attachment of the virus to the host cell receptor.

- *Antibody-dependent cell-mediated cytotoxicity (ADCC):* Fc portion of antibody binds to NK cell. ADCC stimulates NK cells to destroy infected cells by indirect way.

HIV Evasion Methods

The rapid rate of mutations enable the HIV antigens to escape immune recognition. HIV makes 10 billion copies/day leading to depletion of CD4+ T cells. It integrates into host genome resulting in formation of abnormal proteins. It can remain hidden in resting cells.

There is downregulation of MHC I process, impairment of Th1 response of CD4+ T cell. *HIV infects central nervous system, where antibodies have poor penetration. Disrupted immune system fails to control intracellular infection-like HIV.* These reasons also contribute to the difficulty of HIV vaccine research.

Immune Dysfunction in HIV

Advanced stages of HIV are associated with disruption of lymphoid tissue and maintenance of memory responses. Disrupted immune system fails to respond to new antigen resulting in increased susceptibility to opportunistic infections.

Mechanism of disruption of immune system: HIV causes depletion and dysfunction of CD4+ T cells by direct and indirect mechanisms.

- *Direct mechanism:* HIV eliminates HIV-infected cells by virus-specific immune responses. There is *loss of plasma membrane integrity due to viral budding.* There is *interference with cellular RNA processing.*

- *Indirect mechanism:* HIV causes *syncytium formation in brain, apoptosis and autoimmunity.* Viral gp120 can be found on the surface of infected host cells after fusion of viral envelope and cell membrane, with retention of viral proteins at the cell surface. *Uninfected cells may then bind to infected cells due to viral gp120. This results in fusion of the cell membranes and subsequent syncytium formation. This syncytium formation is highly unstable, and die quickly.*

Mechanism of dysregulation

- *Immune system and viral load:* HIV can manipulate the immune system to its own replicative advantage by increasing viral load. The magnitude of this increased viremia correlates inversely with stage of HIV disease.

- *Role of cytokines:* Immunoregulatory cytokines such as *TNF-α, IL-1, IL-6, IL-10 and IFN-γ activates immune system resulting in upregulation of HIV replication.* There is downregulation of immunoregulatory cytokines such IL-2, IL-12, which are normally essential for modulating effective cell-mediated immune responses such as cytotoxic T cells and NK cells.

Opportunistic Infections in AIDS

Decline in immune status parallels the decline in CD4+ T cells number and function. Loss of these cells results in failure of normal Th1 response and cell-mediated immunity that is necessary for controlling intracellular infections.

Children have a high incidence of opportunistic bacterial infections, such as otitis media, sepsis, chronic salivary gland enlargement, Mycobacterium avium intracellulare complex function, and pneumonias, including lymphoid interstitial pneumonia and Pneumocystis jiroveci pneumonia.

HIV causes direct injury to nervous system (encephalopathy and peripheral neuropathy), kidney (HIV nephropathy), heart (HIV cardiomyopathy), and gonads in both sexes (hypogonadism), and gastrointestinal tract (dysmotility and malabsorption).

HIV causes indirect injury to various organs by opportunistic infections and tumors as a consequence of immunosuppression. Opportunistic infections and cancers associated with AIDS are shown in Fig. 4.35 and opportunistic infections in AIDS are shown in Table 4.29.

Fungal infections: Fungal infections are a major cause for opportunistic pneumonitis in immunocompromised persons. *Gross examination of lungs shows irregular yellowish-gray infiltrate with a granular dry and firm cut surface.* These include *Pneumocystis jiroveci*, Mucor species, Candida, Cryptosporidium, Coccidioides, *Cryptococcus neoformans*, and *Histoplasma capsulatum*.

Bacterial infections: These include Mycobacterium tubercle bacilli both typical and atypical such as *Mycobacterium avium intracellulare*.

Viral infections: Cytomegalovirus is member of the herpes family. It may cause retinitis, blindness, colitis, pneumonia and infection of adrenal glands. Patients are prone to herpes simplex virus, varicella zoster virus, JC virus, Epstein-Barr virus and poxviruses.

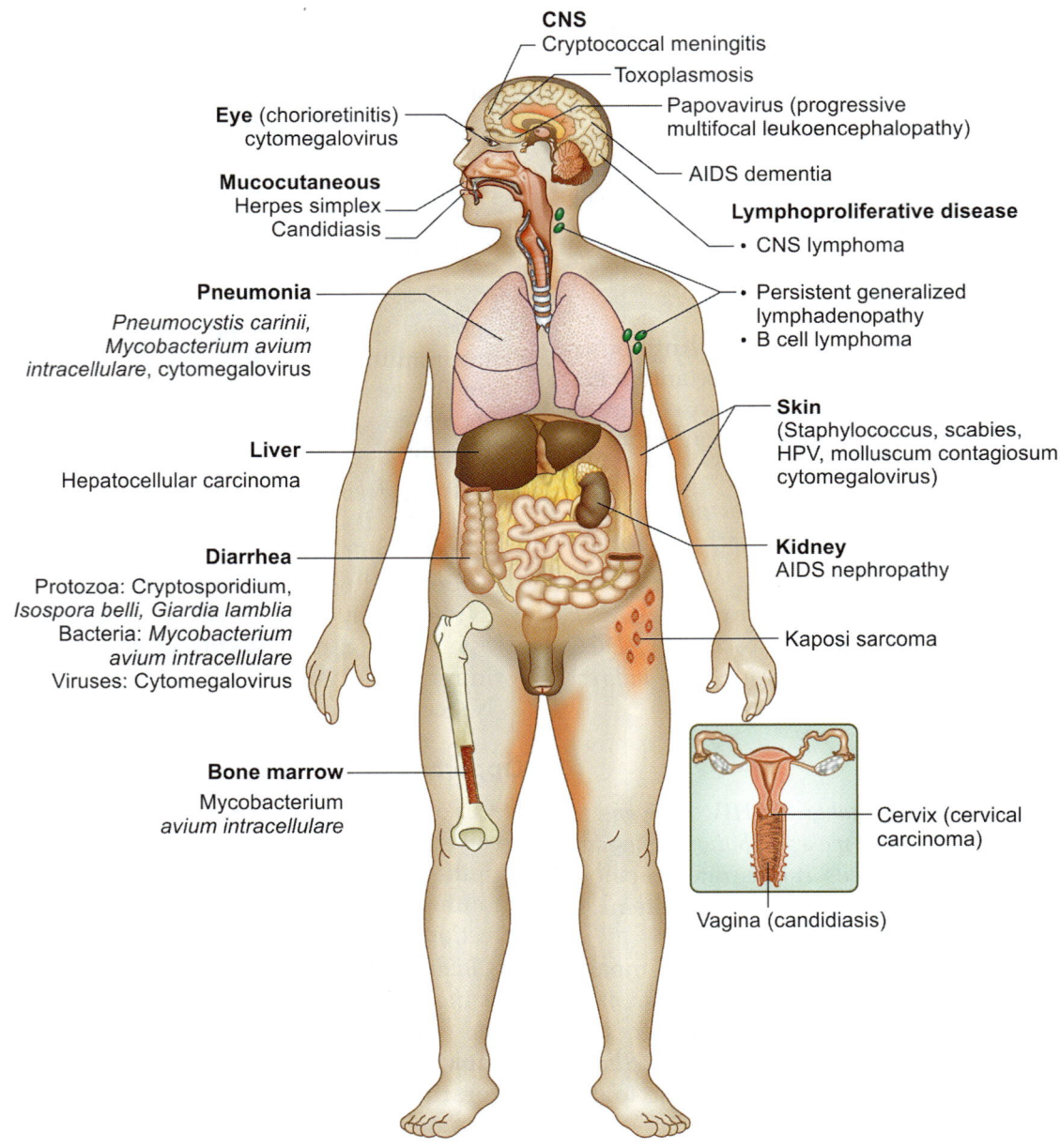

Fig. 4.35: Opportunistic infections and cancers associated with AIDS.

Table 4.29: Opportunistic infections in AIDS

Organs involved	Opportunistic infections
Central nervous system	Cryptococcus (meningitis) Toxoplasma Papovavirus (progressive multifocal leukoencephalopathy) AIDS dementia
Eye (chorioretinitis)	Cytomegalovirus
Mucocutaneous (recurrent aphthous ulcers, angular cheilitis, necrotizing ulcerative gingivitis and periodontitis)	Herpes simplex Herpes zoster Candidiasis Cytomegalovirus Fungal infections (*Candida albicans*, histoplasmosis, cryptococcosis and aspergillosis) Bacterial infections (*Escherichia coli, Enterobacter cloacae, Klebsiella pneumoniae, Pseudomonas aeruginosa*)
Lungs consolidation (pneumonia)	*Pneumocystis Jiroveci* *Mycobacterium avium intracellulare* Cytomegalovirus
Skin (dermatitis, folliculitis and impetigo)	Staphylococcus Scabies Human papillomavirus Molluscum contagiosum Cytomegalovirus
Small intestine (malabsorption syndrome)	Protozoa (Crytospordium, *Isopora belli, Giardia lamblia*) *Mycobacterium avium intracellulare* Virus (cytomegalovirus)
Large colon	Colitis by opportunistic infections
Kidneys	AIDS nephropathy
Vagina	Candidiasis
Bone marrow	*Mycobacterium avium intracellulare*

Protozoal infection: Patient presents with HIV infection may develop giardiasis, leishmaniasis and toxoplasmosis.

Pneumocystis jiroveci: It causes pneumonia in immunocompromised persons. Patient presents with fever, non-productive cough (viscous sputum), dyspnea, weight loss and night sweats. This organism may invade liver, spleen and kidney in minority of cases.

Cancers in AIDS

Decline in immune status parallels the decline in CD4+ T cells number and function. Loss of these cells results in failure of normal Th1 response and cell-mediated immunity that is necessary for controlling cancers. HIV dysregulates immune system, activates cellular genes or proto-oncogenes or inhibit tumor suppressor genes resulting in genetic instability.

HIV may also induce abnormalities of endothelia and epithelial cells resulting in development of cancers. Cancers in AIDS are shown in Table 4.30.

Kaposi sarcoma: Kaposi sarcoma is most often associated with acquired immunodeficiency syndrome (AIDS) especially in male homosexual persons. It is vascular neoplasm involving *mucocutaneous, lymphatic, gastrointestinal tract and lungs.*

- Kaposi sarcoma is caused by *human herpesvirus 8 (HHV-8)* also known as *Kaposi sarcoma herpesvirus* (KSHV). HHV-8 encodes proteins that interfere with the p53 and Rb tumor suppressor pathways.

- Human herpesvirus 8 (HHV-8) and HIV induce angiogenic and inflammatory cytokines responsible for tumor progression.

Table 4.30: Cancers in AIDS

AIDS defined/undefined	Organs	Cancers
AIDS defined cancers	Skin	Kaposi sarcoma (HHV-8), vascular tumor that may involve mucocutaneous, lymphatic, gastrointestinal tract, and pulmonary sites
	CNS	Immunoblastic lymphoma HHV-8
	Lymph nodes	Burkitt's lymphoma (associated with translocations of MYC gene on chromosome 8, surface IgM, CD19, CD20, CD10, and BCL6, phenotype consistent with a germinal center B cell origin involving CNS, jaw and facial bones of orbit)
		Diffuse large B cell lymphoma (CD20 positive, occurs due to dysregulation of BCL6 at chromosome 3q27)
		Primary effusion lymphomas (pleural and peritoneal effusion having clonal IgH gene rearrangements, absence of lymphadenopathy)
		Plasmablastic lymphoma
		Persistent generalized lymphadenopathy
Non-AIDS defined cancers	Cervix	Cervical carcinoma (HPV)
	Anal region	Anal carcinoma (HPV)
	Liver	Hepatocellular carcinoma
	Lymph node	Hodgkin's disease mixed cellularity (EB virus) CD15+, CD30+ in 70% cases
		Hodgkin's disease depletion type (EB virus) CD15+, CD30+
	Conjunctiva	Squamous cell carcinoma of conjunctiva
	Uterus	Leiomyosarcoma (pediatric age group)

Extranodal involvement occurs in central nervous system, liver, bone marrow and gastrointestinal tract.

- Patient presents with *reddish purple macules in distal lower extremities*. AIDS associated Kaposi sarcoma often involves lymph nodes and disseminates widely to viscera early in its course.

Lymphomas associated with HIV: Lymphomas associated with HIV include Burkitt's lymphoma, diffuse large B cell lymphomas (HHV-8), immunoblastic lymphoma (primary CNS), primary effusion lymphomas (pleural and peritoneal effusion having clonal IgH gene rearrangements), plasmablastic lymphoma (advanced stage) and Hodgkin's disease. Extranodal involvement occurs in central nervous system, liver, bone marrow and gastrointestinal tract.

- *Burkitt's lymphoma:* It is associated with translocations of MYC gene on chromosome 8, surface IgM, CD19, CD20, CD10, and BCL6, phenotype consistent with a germinal center B cell origin involving CNS, jaw and facial bones of orbit.

- *Primary effusion lymphoma:* It is malignant large B cell lymphoma associated with pleural or peritoneal effusion in the absence of lymphadenopathy in advanced HIV infection or older adults. The tumor cells are often anaplastic in appearance and typically fail to express surface B or T cell markers, but have clonal IgH gene rearrangements. In all cases, the tumor cells are infected with KSHV/HHV-8, which appears to have a causal role.

- *Plasmablastic lymphoma (PBL):* It is diffuse proliferation of neoplastic cells most of which resemble B immunoblasts affecting AIDS persons of 50 years age group. Immunohistochemistry reveals positivity with CD138, CD38, and IRF4/MUM1. It also shows positivity with CD79a in 50–85% of cases.

- *Hodgkin's disease (mixed cellularity type):* More than 50% of patients present as stage III or IV disease. Males are more affected than females with peak in young adults and again in adults older than 55 years of age. *EB virus plays role in the pathogenesis of Hodgkin's disease.* On histopathological examination of lymph node, it is composed of Reed-Sternberg cells admixed with T lymphocytes, macrophages, plasma cells and eosinophils. *Immunohistochemistry of Reed-Sternberg cells reveals positivity with CD15 and CD30 in 70% of cases.*

- *Hodgkin's disease (lymphocytic depletion type):* It is more common in older males. EB virus plays role in the pathogenesis of Hodgkin's disease. On histopathological examination of lymph node, it is composed of Reed-Sternberg cells and paucity of background reactive cells. Immunohistochemistry of Reed-Sternberg cells reveals positivity with CD15 and CD30. It is more common in older males, HIV-infected individuals, and often presents with advanced disease.

Hepatocellular carcinoma: Patient may develop hepatocellular carcinoma.

Cervical carcinoma: HPV-related carcinomas of cervix and anus.

CNS tumors: Patient may develop lymphoma of central nervous system.

Lymphomatoid granulomatous: Lymphomatoid granulomatous is an angiocentric and angiodestructive lymphoproliferative disease involving extranodal sites composed of EBV positive B cells along with reactive T cells. It has a spectrum of histological grade and clinical aggressiveness, which is related to the proportion of large B cells.

Clinical Features in Primary HIV Infection

HIV disease may be asymptomatic for many years. Before fully developed AIDS occurs, there is acute illness resembling infectious mononucleosis; a long latent phase followed by generalized lymphadenopathy; and a stage marked by chronic fever, weight loss and diarrhea. Manifestation occurs due to damage to immune system.

Initial HIV Infection: HIV seropositivity begins soon after initial HIV infection. Antibodies to the proteins coded by the *genes of retroviral gag, Env and Pol regions* can be demonstrated, especially antibodies to the gp120 and p24 proteins. Initial infection occurs with mild illness in 70% of cases. HIV infection can also be demonstrated by amplification of viral genetic sequences by polymerase chain reaction or by viral culture.

Late stage infection: The late stage, defined as AIDS, is marked by HIV infection complicated by specified secondary opportunistic infection or malignant neoplasms.

HIV Testing for High Risk Persons

Recommended groups for HIV testing include homosexual men, commercial sex workers, unprotected sex, illness or fever without cause, high risk needle sharing, perinatal exposure and patient request. Purpose for HIV testing includes blood safety, donation safety, identification of asymptomatic individuals and diagnosing clinically suspected cases. It is useful for prophylaxis, management and treatment of HIV related illnesses.

WHO Definition of AIDS Patient

An adult or adolescent (>12 years) is considered to have AIDS, if a test for HIV antibody is positive and one or more of the following conditions is/are present. These include *>10% weight loss or cachexia with diarrhea/fever or both, cryptococcal meningitis, pulmonary or extrapulmonary tuberculosis, Kaposi sarcoma, neurological impairment, esophageal candidiasis, life-threatening or recurrent pneumonia with/without known etiology and invasive cervical cancer.*

Laboratory Testing

Blood samples are collected with universal precautions. Samples for testing include blood, serum, plasma, saliva or urine. Approximately 3–5 ml of blood sample may be taken as whole or anticoagulated blood. Additional sample is required if the first comes positive. Specimen should be transported and processed within 24–48 hours. If serum/plasma has been separated then it can be refrigerated at –20 degree for a week.

Window period: The window period in untreated clinical case begins at the time of infection. It can last 4 to 8 weeks. *During this period, infected person is infectious and viremic, with a high viral load and a negative HIV antibody test.* The point when the HIV antibody test becomes positive is called the point of seroconversion. Window period in untreated clinical course is shown in Fig. 4.36.

Reporting procedure: Results are kept confidential.
- *Negative report:* If the initial screen shows non-reactive result.
- *Positive report:* At least 3 screening tests show reactive results concordantly, subsequent sample retested before reporting.
- *Indeterminate report:* Discordant results by 3 screening tests, follow-up samples to retest at 2 weeks, 3 months, 6 months, 12 months before report dispatched. If the

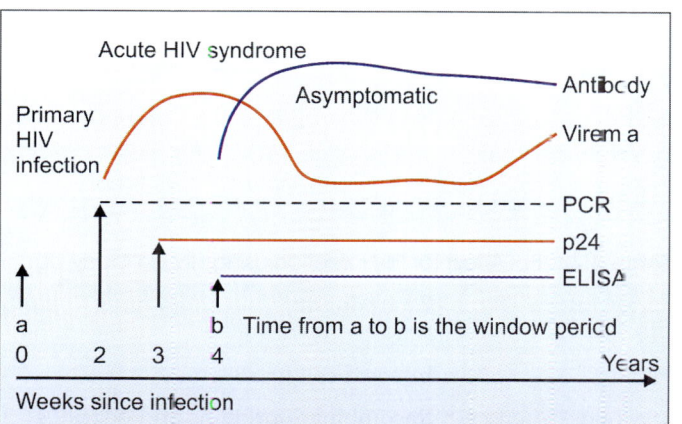

Fig. 4.36: Window period in untreated clinical course.

Section I: General Pathology

Table 4.31: Screening of HIV infection

Testing categories	Analyte detected	Use
ELISA	IgG/IgM	Standard screening using spectrophotometry
Simple ELISA	IgG/IgM	No special equipment required
Rapid ELISA	IgG/IgM	Results obtained in 10–30 minutes
Particle agglutination (PA)	IgG/IgM	ELISA with visual read out of particle clumping
Antigen capture	p24	HIV p24 detection
Immune dissociation	p24	Disrupts p24 antigen-antibody complex permitting capture

result remains indeterminate even after a year, the person is considered to be HIV negative.

Screening of HIV infection: Screening of HIV infection is done by analysis of ELISA, particle agglutination (PA), antigen capture and immune complex deposition. Screening of HIV infection is shown in Table 4.31.

Confirmatory tests for HIV infection: HIV infection is confirmed by Western blot, immunofluorescence, nucleic acid testing, HIV RNA detection and HIV DNA detection (Table 4.32). Testing of body fluids for HIV is shown in Table 4.33.

ELISA test: ELISA test is done for HIV infection. *False positive ELISA test is seen in persons immunized against influenza vaccine up to 3 months before test, presence of rheumatoid factor, chronic alcoholism, HLA DR antibodies in multigravida, autoimmune disorders and hemodialysis.* False negative ELISA test is seen in advanced AIDS and during window period in 6–20% of cases. *Unusual serotypes may give rise to negative results in screening* (Table 4.34).

Particle agglutination assays: Particle agglutination assays are based on the ability of sera containing HIV antibodies to crosslink small particles containing HIV

Table 4.32: Confirmatory tests for HIV infection

Testing categories	Analyte detection	Use
Western blot	IgG	Confirmation of HIV infection
Immunofluorescence (IF)	IgG	Confirmation of HIV infection
Nucleic acid testing (NAT)	HIV RNA	PCR used to detect HIV nuclei acid in donor screening
HIV RNA detection	HIV RNA viral load	Useful in resolving indeterminate cases
HIV DNA detection	HIV DNA	RT-PCR used to detect HIV DNA in neonatal diagnosis

Table 4.33: Body fluids for HIV Testing

Source	ELISA	Rapid ELISA	Western blot	Immunofluorescence (IF)	Nucleic acid testing (NAT)
Whole blood	+	+	–	–	–
Dried blood	+	–	–	–	–
Plasma	+	+	+	+	+
Serum	+	+	+	+	+
Oral fluid	+	–	+	–	–
Urine	+	–	+	–	–

Table 4.34: ELISA test for HIV infection using HIV antibody against immobilized antigens

Generation of ELISA	Component	Approximate window period	Advantages
First	Infected cell lysates	63 days	Laboratory diagnosis of HIV infection
Second	Recombinant proteins and peptides	42 days	Decreases false positive
Third	Sandwich with laboratory antigen	22 days	Short window period
Fourth	p24 antigen sandwich	16 days	Short window period

antigen on the surface. *It has high sensitivity and specificity.* It is easy to perform. Its disadvantages include subject to reader interpretation and no permanent records available.

NAT test: NAT test *is adjunct but not a replacement of serological tests.* Various formats are: *PCR and RT-PCR, NASBA* (nucleic acid sequence based amplification) and *bDNA* (branched chain DNA). *NAT test is best in detecting HIV during seronegative period.* It has a small window period. Its disadvantage is its *high cost.*

Rapid visual test (tri-dot test): Rapid visual test (tri-dot test) *is a visual rapid and sensitive immunoassay for differential detection of HIV 1 and HIV 2 antibodies (IgG) in human serum against antigens (gp41 C terminal of gp120 and gp36. Principle of rapid visual test is based on reaction of immobilized antigens with antibodies present in the serum.* Conjugate binds to the Fc portion of the HIV antibody to give *distinct pinkish purple dot against a white background.* Results are confirmed by confirmatory assay. Assay should be performed on fresh samples.

Immunofluorescence (IF): Immunofluorescence identifies the presence of antibodies by their specific ability to react with antigens on infected cells. Characteristic staining pattern of reactivity provides additional specificity to the interpretation. *Conditions interfering with IF include lipemia, hyperfibrinogenemia, paraproteinemia and autoimmune disease.*

Radioimmunoperception (RIPA): Radioimmunoperception (RIPA) identifies antibodies by their ability to react with radiolabelled antigens. It helps to resolve indeterminate WB in early infection.

CD4+ T cells count: CD4+ T cells count is the best indicator for immediate state of the immune system. Normal CD4+ T cell count (500–1600 IU/L), CD8+ count (375–1100 IU/L), CD4+ T cell/CD8+ T cell ratio ranges from 0.9 to 1.9. It correlates very well with level of immunological tolerance. CD4+ T cell count is performed at every 3–6 months interval. CD4+ T cell count is *most reliable short-term indicator of disease progression.* Changes in CD4+ T cells over the time span of an HIV infection and its relationship to AIDS diagnosis are shown in Fig. 4.37.

HIV RNA determination: HIV RNA determination is *highly sensitive and precise.* It is essential component in monitoring HIV infection. It predicts the outcome of CD4+ T cell counts in future. It provides very important prognostic information. Two most common

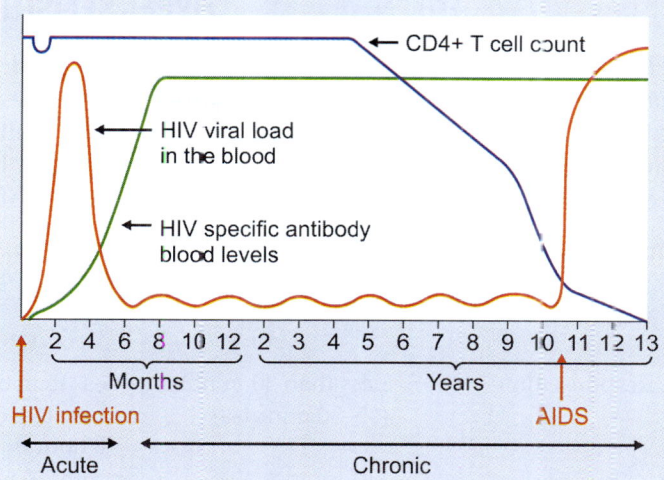

Fig. 4.37: Changes in CD4+ T cells over the time span of an HIV infection and its relationship to AIDS diagnosis.

determinants are RT-PCR and bDNA. During therapy levels of HIV RNA must be measured every 3–4 months.

- *HIV RNA viral loads after infection:* It can be used to assess the viral set point and predict the likelihood of progression to AIDS in the next 5 years. The higher the viral set point, there is rapid fall of CD4+ T cell count and rapid progression of HIV infection to AIDS.

- *Rate of disease progression:* It is determined by the patient's viral load. With levels between 1,000 and 10,000 viral copies, the likelihood of AIDS in 5 years is 8%. At 10,000 to approximately 50,000, the likelihood is 26%. At 50,000 to <100,000 it is 49%. Between 100,000 and 1,000,000 the likelihood is 62% at 5 years.

HIV Vaccines

There are a number of factors that cause development of an HIV vaccine to differ from the development of other classic vaccines. Classic vaccines mimic natural immunity against reinfection generally seen in individuals recovered from infection; there are almost no recovered AIDS patients.

- *Most vaccines protect against disease, not against infection.* HIV infection may remain latent for long periods before causing AIDS. Most effective vaccines are whole-killed or live-attenuated organisms; killed HIV 1 does not retain antigenicity and the use of a live retrovirus vaccine raises safety issues.

- Most vaccines protect against infections through mucosal surfaces of the respiratory or gastrointestinal tract; the great majority of HIV infection is through the genital tract.

4 Section I: General Pathology

HYPERSENSITIVITY REACTIONS

Hypersensitivity reactions are exaggerated or in appropriate immune responses that lead to tissue damage. Four types of hypersensitivity reactions are recognized by Gell and Coombs: types I to IV. Hypersensitivity types I to III reactions require the active production of antibody by plasma cells (terminally differentiated B cells).

Type IV is mediated by the interaction of T cells and macrophages. Comparison of different hypersensitivity reactions is shown in Table 4.35.

Table 4.35: Comparison of different hypersensitivity reactions

Features	Hypersensitivity			
	Type I	Type II	Type III	Type IV
Response time	Less than 30 minutes (15–30 minutes)	Less than 8 hours (minutes to <8 hours)	Less than 8 hours (3–8 hours)	24 to 72 hours (acute cases). More than one week in chronic cases
Antigens	Non-self (heterologous)	Self (autologous cells)	Self or non-self	Self or non-self
Antibody's role	IgE	IgG, IgM	IgG, IgM	T cells (none Ig)
Complement system's role	No	Yes or no	Yes	No
Cells involved in initiation	Mast cells and basophils	None	None	APC, T helper cell 1
Inflammatory cells	Eosinophils	Neutrophils	Neutrophils	Macrophages, T cells, keratinocytes
Mechanism	First allergen exposure results in IgE synthesis that binds to mast cells	IgG, IgM antibodies cause cell injury by three mechanisms	Insoluble antigen-antibody (IgG, IgM) complexes are deposited in vessel wall and serosal surfaces or other tissues	Direct destruction of target antigenic cells by binding of cytotoxic T cells, FAS-related induction of apoptosis, and/or release of perforins and granzymes
	Subsequent exposure to same allergen causes degranulation of mast cells resulting in release of vasoactive amines (histamine) and inflammatory response bronchoconstriction. (Role of platelets and eosinophils is present)	(i) Direct cytotoxicity (ii) Complement-mediated increasing phagocytosis (iii) Autoantibodies blocking or inactivating cell surface receptors	(i) Immune complexes activate complement system resulting in chemotaxis of neutrophils (ii) PMNs cells attempt to phagocytose immune complex resulting in liberation of hydrolytic enzymes and chemical mediators causing tissue damage	(i) T cell cytokine response activation of macrophages resulting in granulomas (IFN-γ and TNF-α) reaction (ii) T cell cytokine response activation of mast cells (IL-3 and IL-5) (iii) T cytokine response activates synthesis of vasoproliferative factors (IL3, IL-8)
Mediators	(i) Early phase (histamine, ECF, PAF, heparin, enzymes) (ii) Late phase (SRS-A, leukotrienes, thromboxane A_2, and prostaglandins)	C3a, C5a, chemotaxis of neutrophil proteases	C3a, C5a, chemotaxis of neutrophil proteases	Monocyte chemotactic factors (MCF), monocyte inhibitory factor (MIF), IFN-γ, TNF-α, IL-3, GM-CSF
Target tissue	Vascular endothelium, bronchial smooth muscle	Blood or tissue cells	Vascular endothelium and epithelial cells	Modified self, infected cells, allografts

Contd...

Table 4.35: Comparison of different hypersensitivity reactions (Contd...)

Features	Hypersensitivity			
	Type I	**Type II**	**Type III**	**Type IV**
Primary responses	Vascular permeability, transudation, erythema, edema, wheal, bronchospasm, wheal and flare	Blood or tissue cell lysis, phagocytosis, inflammation, decreased serum complement	Necrotizing vasculitis (fibrinoid necrosis), vasoconstriction, thrombi, necrosis, decreased serum complement	Erythema, induration, and granuloma formation
Histology	Eosinophils, basophils	Antibody and complement	Complement and neutrophils/macrophages	Monocytes/macrophages Lymphocytes
Beneficial effects	Antiparasitic response and toxin neutralization	Direct lysis and phagocytosis of extracellular bacteria (gram-positive) and other susceptible bacteria and virus neutralization	Acute inflammatory neutrophils recruitment at the site of extracellular microbes and their clear microbes	Protection against fungi, intracellular bacteria (*M. tuberculosis*) and viruses, other intracellular pathogens
Pathological disorders	Bronchial asthma Hay fever Anaphylactic shock	ADCC: *Systemic lupus erythematosus, Hashimoto's thyroiditis, acute rheumatic fever*	Systemic lupus erythematosus, rheumatoid arthritis, immune complex-mediated glomerular diseases, serum sickness, Arthus reaction, polyarteritis nodosa, farmer's lung disease	Contact dermatitis and tuberculin skin test, tumor cell killing; virally infected cell killing Chronic granulomatous diseases (tuberculosis, leprosy and sarcoidosis, and Crohn's disease)

TYPE 1 HYPERSENSITIVITY REACTIONS

Hypersensitivity type I (immediate type) reaction includes: *hay fever (allergic rhinitis), bronchial asthma, urticaria (hives), eczema, food allergy, drug allergy and anaphylaxis (cutaneous and anaphylactic shock)*. It is also referred to as atopy. It is triggered within minutes of exposure to a variety of environmental antigens such as pollen and house dust mite. Immediate hypersensitivity reaction has strong genetic link and caused by an overproduction of IgE. Common allergen classified by portal of entry is shown in Table 4.36.

- *First exposure to allergen:* Mast cells display a high affinity receptor for IgE. Exposure to exogenous antigen (via skin, inhalation or ingestion) leads to synthesis of IgE immunoglobulin resulting in fixation of IgE to Fc receptors on the surface of basophils or tissue mast cells.
- *Subsequent exposure to same allergen:* Subsequent exposure to same antigen causes degranulation with release of histamine, leukotrienes, prostaglandins, platelet activating factor and eosinophilic chemotactic factor, many of which are vasoactive, smooth muscle spasm-inducing, or chemotactic. Examples of type I hypersensitivity reactions include hay fever; allergic asthma; hives; anaphylactic shock.

Table 4.36: Common allergen classified by portal of entry

Portal of entry	Allergens
Inhalation	Pollens, dust mold spores, dander, animal hair, formalin drugs
Ingestion	Food (milk, peanuts, wheat, shellfish, soya beans, nuts, eggs) Food additives Drugs (aspirin, penicillin)
Contact	Drugs, cosmetic, heavy metals, detergents, formalin, rubber, solvents, dyes
Injections	Hymenopterans venom (bee, wasp), drugs, vaccines, serum, enzymes, hormones

CATEGORIES OF TYPE I HYPERSENSITIVITY REACTIONS

Categories of type I hypersensitivity reactions include allergic (atopic) and anaphylaxis (Table 4.37).

Allergic/Atopic Reactions

Allergic reactions include *hay fever (allergic rhinitis), bronchial asthma, urticaria (hives), eczema, food allergy, drug*

Table 4.37: Categories of type I hypersensitivity

Categories	Diseases	Clinical manifestations
Allergic or atopic reactions	Hay fever (allergic rhinitis) seasonal reaction to airborne inhaled plant pollen or molds or house dust	Nasal congestion, sneezing, coughing, profuse mucus secretion, itchy red and teary eyes and mild bronchoconstriction
	Bronchial asthma	Bronchoconstriction and increased mucus secretion
	Urticaria (hives)	Skin hives
	Eczema (atopic dermatitis)	Itchy inflammation of skin characterized by dry scaly lesions on the face, scalp, neck, and inner surfaces of the limbs and trunk
	Food allergy	Vomiting, diarrhea and abdominal pain
	Drug allergy (penicillin, sulphonamides, aspirin, opiates, contrast media)	Affecting 5–10% of hospitalized patients
Anaphylaxis	Cutaneous anaphylaxis (injection of allergen)	Wheal and flare reaction
	Anaphylactic shock (injection of antibiotics or serum administration)	Acute potentially life-threatening characterized by rapidly progressive urticaria, bronchospasm, laryngeal edema, and vascular shock with fatal outcome within a few minutes

allergy. A positive family history of allergy is found in 50% of atopic individuals. Tissue damage and necrosis are present in acute inflammation, while absent in atopic reactions.

Allergic rhinitis (hay fever): Allergic rhinitis is *most common disorder in adults.* It is a seasonal reaction to *airborne inhaled plant pollen or molds or house dust.*
- *Pathogenesis:* Antigens inhaled react with the IgE attached to basophils/basophils in the nasal mucosa, thereby triggering the release of histamine stored in cytoplasmic granules. *Histamine increases the permeability of mucosal vessels, causing edema and sneezing.* The targets are typically *respiratory membranes.*
- *Clinical features:* Patient presents with *nasal congestion, sneezing, coughing, profuse mucus secretion, itchy red and teary eyes* and *mild bronchoconstriction.*

Bronchial asthma: Bronchial asthma is characterized by episodes of impaired breathing due to severe bronchoconstriction. The airways are responsive to minute amounts of inhaled allergens. Thick mucus plugs are present in airways. *Patient presents with shortness of breath, wheezing, cough and ventilatory rales, which may have fatal outcome.*

Atopic dermatitis: Atopic dermatitis is an itchy inflammatory condition of skin, known as eczema. Sensitization occurs through ingestion, inhalation and occasionally skin contact with allergens. It usually begins in infancy with *reddened, vesicular, encrusted skin lesions.* It then progresses in childhood and adulthood to a dry scaly, thickened skin condition. *Lesions can occur on the face, scalp, neck, and inner surfaces of the limbs and trunk.*

Food allergy: Food allergens enter via ingestion, but can affect respiratory tract and skin. Gastrointestinal tract symptoms include vomiting, diarrhea and abdominal pain. In severe cases, young children present with failure to thrive and growth retardation.

Drug allergy: Approximately 5–10% of hospitalized patients may develop drug allergy. Compounds implicated most often are *antibiotics (penicillin), sulphonamides, aspirin, opiates, contrast media* used in imaging techniques. The actual allergen is not the drug itself but a hapten given of when the liver processes the drug. Some forms of penicillin sensitivity are due to the presence of small amounts of drug in meat, milk and other foods. Exposure to penicillium mold in the environment also cause drug allergy.

Anaphylaxis

Clinical types of anaphylaxis seen in human beings include *cutaneous* and *systemic anaphylaxis.*

Cutaneous anaphylaxis is the wheal and flare reaction to the injection of allergen. *Systemic anaphylaxis* is an *acute potentially life-threatening* type I hypersensitivity reaction. The reaction typically occurs *within minutes but can occur up to 1 hour* after re-exposure to the offending antigen.

Clinical features: The allergens and route of entry are variable, i.e. *injection of antibiotics or serum administration.* It is characterized by rapidly progressive urticarial *(vascular swelling in the skin accompanied by itching)*, *bronchospasm, laryngeal edema, and vascular shock with fatal outcome within a few minutes.*

- *Children* are more likely to experience *food-related anaphylaxis*. Children develop severe stomach cramps, nausea, and diarrhea.
- *Adults* are more likely to experience anaphylaxis related to *antibiotics, radio-contrast media, anesthetic agents and insect stings*. Bee venom containing several allergens and enzymes may create sensitivity after exposure.

BRONCHIAL ASTHMA

Bronchial asthma is an example of type I hypersensitivity reaction. It is caused by increased responsiveness of the airways to a variety of stimuli. *Mast cell degranulation release chemical mediators in these patients stimulate bronchial mucus production and bronchoconstriction* (Fig. 4.38). Differences between extrinsic and intrinsic asthma are shown in Table 4.38.

Mast cells play central role in the development of type I hypersensitivity reaction. These are derived from circulating basophils and present near blood vessels and nerves in subepithelial tissue.

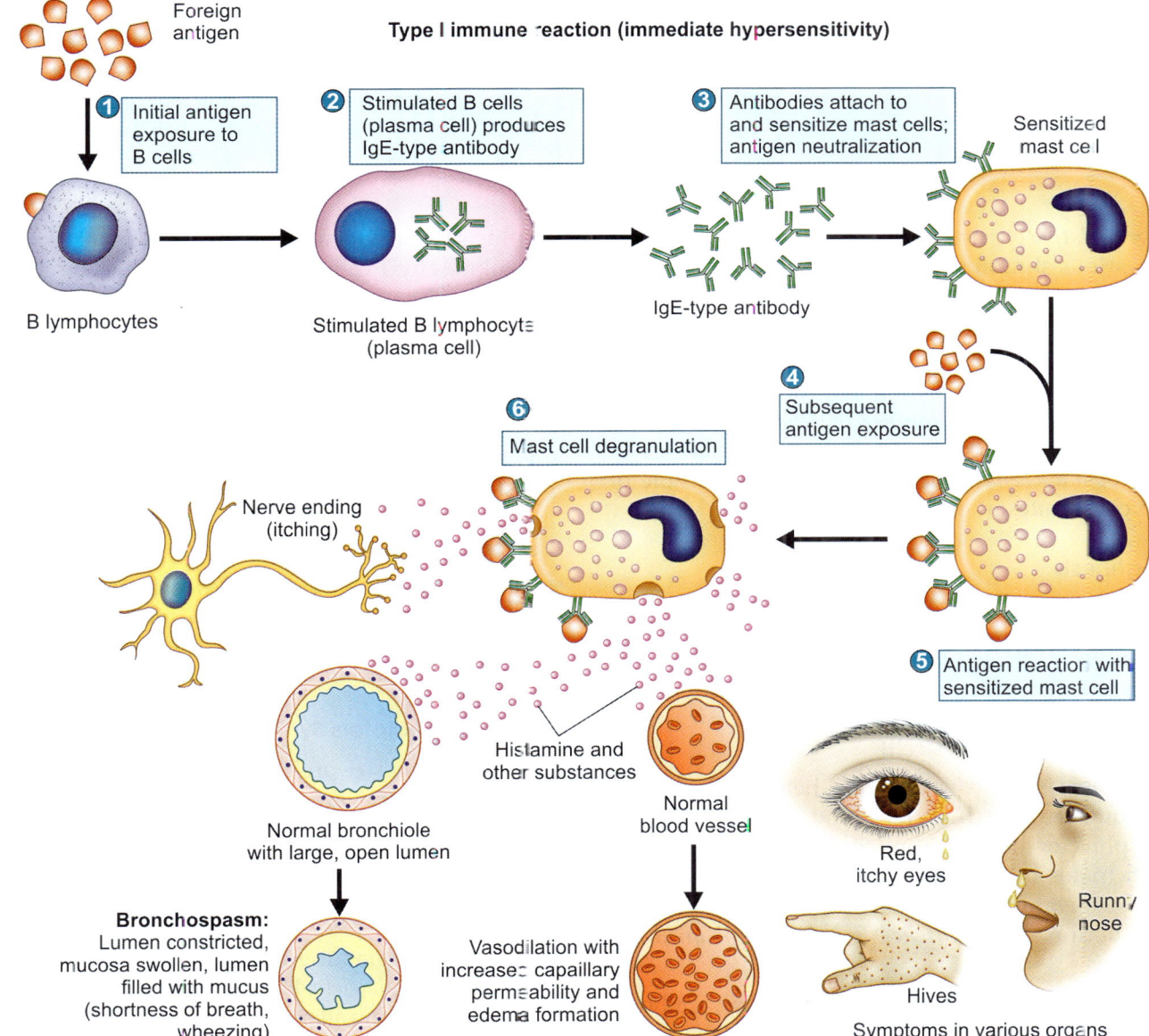

Fig. 4.38: Type I hypersensitivity reactions. Initial exposure to antigen (sensitizing dose) stimulates synthesis of IgE antibody. This IgE binds to surface of mast cells. On subsequent exposure to same antigen (provocative dose), it binds with IgE antibody attached to the mast cells and stimulate mast cells to release cytoplasmic granules containing chemical mediators responsible for itching, bronchospasm, wheezing, shortness of breath and anaphylactic shock.

Table 4.38: Differences between extrinsic asthma and intrinsic asthma

Characteristics	Extrinsic asthma	Intrinsic asthma
Definition	Caused by type I hypersensitivity reaction induced by exposure to an extrinsic antigen	Caused by diverse non-immune mechanisms as a result of intrinsic stimuli
Age of clinical presentation	Childhood	Adult
Family history	Present	Absent
Preceding allergic reactions	It is present in the form of rhinitis, urticaria, and eczema	Absent
Drug hypersensitivity	Absent	Present
Serum IgE level	Increased	Normal
Skin test	Positive skin test	Negative skin test
Emphysema	Unusual	Common
Associated chronic bronchitis	Absent	Present
Miscellaneous	Atopic/allergic asthma	Allergic bronchopulmonary aspergillosis (aspirin ingestion, pulmonary infection especially viral, cold, inhaled irritants, stress, exercise)

- *Degranulation of mast cells and basophils:* It is triggered by various stimuli such as *anaphylatoxins (C4a, C3a, C5a), IL-8, physical stimuli (heat, cold and sunlight), drugs (morphine, codeine), bee venom (malletin, adenine) and calcium ionophores.*
- *Synthesis of chemical mediators:* Mast cells release *preformed and newly synthesized chemical mediators such as histamine, serotonin, leukotrienes and ECF-A (eosinophilic chemoattractant factor A) responsible of clinical manifestations.*

Pathogenesis

First Time Exposure to Antigen (Sensitization)

- *Processing of antigen:* On first exposure with an antigen (allergen), antigen processing cells (macrophages, dendritic cells) process the allergen and present to T helper cells (CD4+ T cell).
- *Synthesis of interleukins and IgE:* T helper cells synthesize interleukins (IL-4, IL-5, and IL-6). IL-5 prime basophils for histamine and leukotriene release. IL-5 participates in maturation, chemotaxis, activation, and survival of eosinophils. IL-6 promotes mucus production. IL-4 switches B cells to IgE antibody synthesis.
- *Binding of IgE to mast cells and basophils:* IgE antibody is then bound to the Fc receptors of tissue mast cells and basophils.
- *Synthesis of cytokines: Tumor necrosis factor-α* synthesized by macrophages activates neutrophils, attracts monocytes and enhances production of other cytokines by T cells.

Subsequent Provocative Exposure to Antigen

Upon subsequent exposure with a provocative dose, the same allergen binds to the IgE-mast cell complex and results in influx of calcium.

- *Preformed chemical mediators:* Mast cells release histamine, serotonin, leukotrienes, prostaglandin, with pharmacological effects such as vasodilation and bronchoconstriction.
- *Newly synthesized chemical mediators:* Mast cells also synthesize new chemical mediators *such as leukotrienes, prostaglandins. Platelets activating factor, adenosine, bradykinin and cyclic nucleotides.*

Chemical Mediators Synthesized by Mast Cells

Mast cells synthesize preformed and newly synthesized chemical mediators are shown in Table 4.39.

Mast Cell's Preformed Products

Mast cells release preformed chemical mediators into the extracellular tissues.

- *Histamine:* Histamine is synthesized by *mast cells, basophils and platelets*. Histamine is the most profuse and fastest-acting allergic chemical mediator. *It causes constriction of the smooth muscle layer of the bronchiole and intestine, thereby causing labored breathing.* Histamine increases mucus secretion and synthesis of *eotaxin*, which attract eosinophils.

Immunopathology including Amyloidosis 4

Table 4.39: Mast cell's preformed and newly synthesized chemical mediators and their actions

Mast cell mediators	Mediators	Pharmacological actions
Preformed products	Histamine	Bronchoconstriction
		Increased mucus secretion
		Synthesis of *eotaxin*, which attracts eosinophils
	Enzymes	Tissue damage
	ECF-A	Chemotaxis of eosinophils
	Kininogenase	Vasodilatation
		Increased vascular permeability and edema
Newly synthesized products	Leukotrienes	LTC-4, LTD-4 and LTE-4 (bronchoconstriction, increase vascular permeability and mucus secretion of respiratory airways)
		LTB-4 (chemotactic for eosinophils, PMN cells, basophils and monocytes)
	Prostaglandins	PGD_2 and $PGF_{2\alpha}$ (bronchoconstriction)
		PGD_2 (histamine release from basophils, edema and pain)
	Platelets activating factor	Bronchoconstriction
		Increased vascular permeability
		Chemotaxis as well as degranulation of eosinophils and neutrophils
	Adenosine	Bronchoconstriction
		Potentiates IgE-induced mast cell mediator release
	Bradykinin	Bronchoconstriction
		Increased vascular permeability
	Cyclic nucleotides	Modulation of immediate hypersensitivity reaction

- *Enzymes:* Mast cells release *neutral protease, chymase, tryptase* and *hydrolytic enzymes*. These enzymes cause tissue damage and proteolysis. These enzymes also synthesize kinins and C3a. *Tryptase is a good marker of mast cell activation.*

- *Eosinophilic chemotactic factor-A (ECF-A):* It participates in *chemotaxis of eosinophils and neutrophils*. Major basic protein synthesized by eosinophils and hydrolytic enzymes by neutrophils cause significant tissue damage/necrosis in the later phases of allergic reactions.

- *Kininogenase:* It causes *vasodilation, vascular permeability and edema*.

Mast cell's newly synthesized products

- *Leukotrienes:* Leukotrienes are 1000 times more potent than histamine, but their actions are similar to histamine. LTC_4 and LTD_4 cause *bronchoconstriction, increase vascular permeability and mucus secretion of respiratory airways*. Leukotriene-B_4 (LT-B_4) is chemotactic for eosinophils, PMN cells, basophils and monocytes.

- *Prostaglandins:* PGD_2 and $PGF_{2\alpha}$ cause *bronchoconstriction*. PGD_2 enhances histamine release from basophils. PGD_2 causes *edema and pain*. PGD_2 inhibits platelets aggregation, whereas $PGF_{2\alpha}$ promotes platelets aggregation.

- *Platelets activating factor:* It causes *bronchoconstriction, increased vascular permeability,* and *chemotaxis* as well as *degranulation* of eosinophils and neutrophils.

- *Adenosine:* It causes *bronchoconstriction*. It potentiates IgE-induced mast cell mediator release.

- *Bradykinin:* It causes *bronchoconstriction and increased vascular permeability*.

- *Cyclic nucleotides:* These *modulate immediate hypersensitivity reaction*.

Phases of Allergic Reactions

Immediate response and late response are phases of allergic reactions (Table 4.40).

- *Immediate response:* Immediate response occurs due to release of histamine, chemotactic factors for eosinophils, and proteases resulting into intense immediate reactions within 5–30 minutes. These mediators produce *tissue swelling by increasing vascular permeability, hypersecretion of bronchial mucosal glands and bronchoconstriction*. Eosinophils are recruited in the tissues, which may be demonstrated by

Table 4.40: Immediate response and late response of allergic reactions

Parameters	Immediate response	Late response
Onset of response	Within 5–30 minutes	Within 2–24 hours and lasts for several days
Chemical mediators	Histamine, chemotactic factors for eosinophils, and proteases	Prostaglandins and leukotrienes
Clinical manifestations	Tissue swelling by increasing vascular permeability, hypersecretion of bronchial mucosal glands and bronchoconstriction	Tissue destruction (mucosal and epithelial tissue)

histopathologic examination of biopsy from reaction site. Peripheral blood shows eosinophilia.

- *Late response:* Late response occurs due to the synthesis and release of *prostaglandins and leukotrienes*. These substances enhance and prolong acute inflammatory reaction. The time interval between the two exposures (i.e. previous and subsequent) can be many years. Allergen enters the body and produces changes within *2–24 hours and lasts for several days. The tissues are infiltrated by eosinophils, neutrophils, monocytes and CD4+ T cells. Tissue destruction (mucosal and epithelial tissue)* occurs.

Actions of Chemical Mediators

Chemical mediators synthesized in type I hypersensitivity reaction participate in bronchoconstriction, increased vascular permeability and chemotaxis of eosinophils. Actions of chemical mediators in type I hypersensitivity reaction are shown in Table 4.41.

- *Smooth muscle spasm:* Histamine, leukotrienes (LTC$_4$, LTD$_4$, and LTE$_4$), PAF, and prostaglandins intensify response by causing *bronchoconstriction*. Leukotrienes also act on alveoli.
- *Vascular changes:* Histamine, LTC$_4$, LTD$_4$, and LTE$_4$, PAF, neutral protease and PGD$_2$ act on blood vessels. Histamine, *prostaglandins* and *bradykinin* increases *vascular permeability* resulting in fluid leakage into alveoli.
- *Cellular infiltration:* IL-4, IL-5, IL-6, TNF-α, LTB$_4$ and ECF-A participate in chemotaxis of eosinophilic and neutrophils.

Table 4.41: Actions of chemical mediators in type I hypersensitivity reaction

Chemical mediators	Actions
Histamine, leukotrienes (LTC$_4$, LTD$_4$, and LTE$_4$), PAF, and prostaglandins	Bronchoconstriction
Histamine, prostaglandins and bradykinin	Increased vascular permeability
IL-4, IL-5, IL-6, TNF-α, LTB$_4$ and ECF-A	Chemotaxis of eosinophils and neutrophils

Light Microscopy

Histopathological changes in bronchial asthma

- *Bronchi/bronchioles changes:* These include bronchial smooth muscle hypertrophy, hyperplasia of goblet cells, thickening and hyalinization of basement membranes.
- *Bronchial wall:* It is infiltrated by eosinophils, mast cells, macrophages and lymphocytes.
- *Bronchial lumen:* Bronchial mucosa shows edema, focal ulceration. Bronchial lumen is occluded with mucus plugs containing whorl-like accumulations of epithelial cells. *Curschmann spirals* and *crystalloids of eosinophils-derived major basic protein* and *cationic proteins* coalesce to form *Charcot-Leyden crystals* demonstrated in the *sputum* of bronchial asthma patients.

Clinical Features

Patient presents with breathlessness and prolonged coughing described as under:

- *Breathlessness:* Bronchial asthma attack may last for hours or even days. Due to narrowing of airways, patient presents with sudden dyspnea, episodic expiratory wheezing (inspiratory in severe cases), and tightness in the chest, nocturnal coughing, and tachypnea with use of accessory muscles for breathing.
- *Prolonged coughing:* After the bronchial asthmatic attack is over, there is prolonged coughing up of tenacious secretions. *Anteroposterior diameter of chest is increased due to air trapping and increase in residual volume.* Initially, patient develops respiratory alkalosis. If bronchospasm is not relieved, patient may develop respiratory acidosis. Such patients need tracheal intubation and mechanical ventilation.

Complications

Patient may develop pneumothorax, pneumomediastinum, status asthmaticus and fatal outcome. When severe acute asthma is unresponsive to therapy, it is referred to as status asthmaticus. Light microscopy of lung in status asthmaticus often shows a bronchus containing a luminal mucous plug, submucosal gland hyperplasia, smooth muscle hyperplasia, basement membrane thickening, and increased numbers of eosinophils.

Therapeutic Agents

Epinephrine, isoproterenol and phenoxybenzamine increase intracellular cAMP and provide relief in bronchial asthma. *Norepinephrine, phenyl-epinephrine, propranolol, acetyl choline and carbacol* decrease intracellular cAMP or stimulate cGMP aggravating these allergic conditions. Relationship between allergic symptoms and cyclic nucleotides are shown in Table 4.42.

Diagnostic Tests

Diagnosis of allergy can be made by skin scratch testing. IgE estimation and histamine release test on basophils.

- *Skin scratch testing:* The forearm or back is mapped and then injected with a selection of allergen extracts. The allergist must be fully aware of potential anaphylaxis attacks triggered by these injections. Approximately 20 minutes after antigenic challenge, histamine-mediated *wheal and flare response* is studied depending on size on a scale of 0 (no reaction) to 4+ (>1.5 cm).
- *Radioallergosorbent test (RAST):* RAST is used to detect *specific IgE antibodies* in serum formed against suspected allergen.
- *Enzyme-linked immunosorbent (ELISA) test:* ELISA test is used to estimate IgE antibodies in an atopic condition. IgE elevation is also seen in *multiple myeloma and helminths infestations*.

Therapeutic Correlation

Various drugs are administered to interrupt allergic response at certain points, i.e. interfering action of histamine, release of chemical mediators from mast cells; and inflammation. Therapeutic agents used to relieve bronchopulmonary symptoms in bronchial asthma are shown in Table 4.43. Strategies for circumventing allergic attacks are shown in Fig. 4.39. The blocking antibody theory for allergic desensitization is shown in Fig. 4.40.

TYPE II HYPERSENSITIVITY REACTIONS

Type II hypersensitivity is also known as *cytotoxic hypersensitivity*. Antigen presenting cells (macrophages and dendritic cells) process cell bound antigen self (intrinsic) or planted (extrinsic usually a drug such as benzyl penicillin or methyldopa) bound to cell membrane or basement membrane; and present to CD4+ T cells resulting in synthesis of antibodies by plasma cells. These antibodies react with cell bound antigen resulting in organ or tissue damage by

Table 4.42: Relationship between allergic symptoms and cyclic nucleotides

Allergic symptoms	Molecular level	Therapeutic agent	Mechanism of action
Improvement of allergic symptoms	Elevation of cyclic-AMP	Epinephrine or isoproterenol	Stimulation of β-adrenergic receptors
		Phenoxybenzamine	Blockage of α-adrenergic receptors
Worsening of allergic symptoms	Lowering of cAMP or elevation of cGMP	Norepinephrine, or phenyl-epinephrine	Stimulation of α-adrenergic receptors
		Propranolol	Blockage of β-adrenergic receptors
		Acetylcholine or carbacol	Stimulation of γ-cholinergic receptors

Table 4.43: Therapeutic agents used to relieve bronchopulmonary symptoms in bronchial asthma

Therapeutic agents	Mechanism of action
Antihistaminic drugs	Blocking receptors expressed on mast cells
Glucocorticoids and disodium chromoglycate	Preventing mast cells degranulation by inhibiting transmembrane influx of calcium ions needed to trigger degranulation
Singulair or accolade agents	Blocking the leukotriene receptors expressed on target cells (leukotrienes cause bronchoconstriction)
Zileuton agent	Preventing synthesis of prostaglandins, TxA_2 and prostacyclin by inhibiting cyclooxygenase pathway
Terbutaline or albuterol agents	Short acting bronchodilators derived from isoproterenol
Theophylline agent	Elevation of cAMP by inhibiting cAMP phosphodiesterase
	Inhibiting intracellular Ca^{++} release
Desensitization therapy	Administration of purified allergens repeatedly to block the primary sensitization process

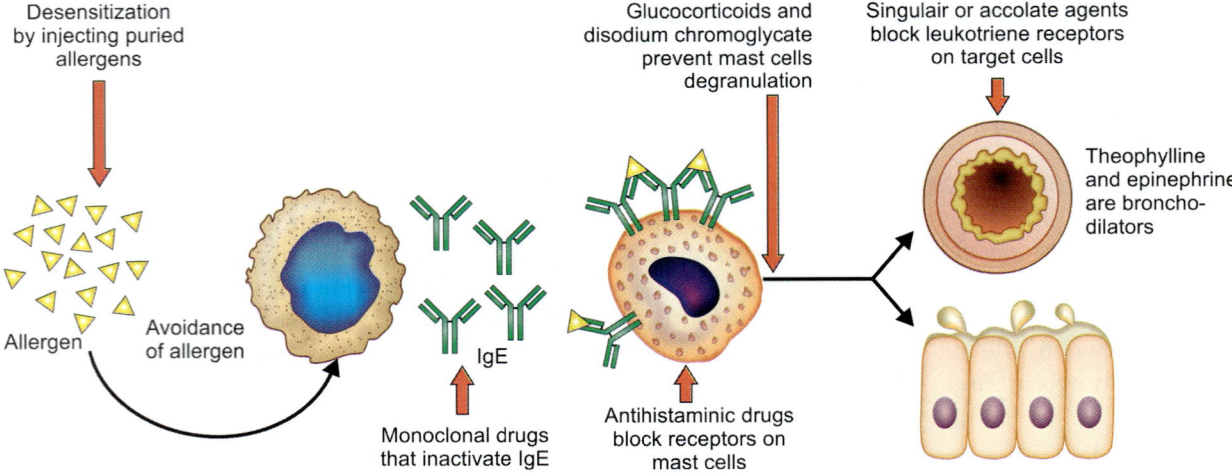

Fig. 4.39: Strategies for circumventing allergic attacks.

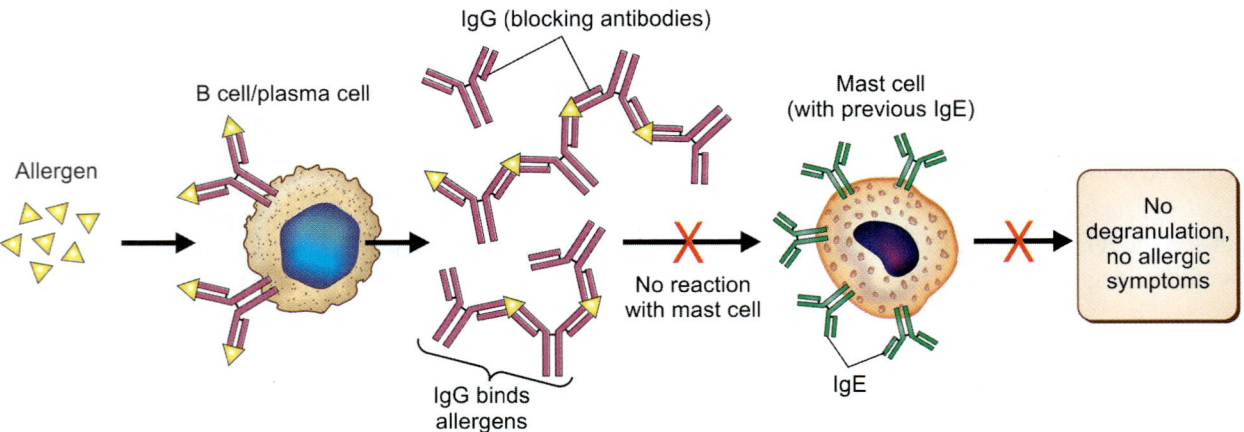

Fig. 4.40: The blocking antibody theory for allergic desensitization. An injection of allergen causes IgG antibodies to be formed instead of IgE; these blocking antibodies cross-link and effectively remove allergen before it can react with IgE in the mast cells.

three mechanisms: *antibody-dependent cell-mediated cytotoxicity, complement-mediated increased susceptibility to phagocytosis and anti-receptor antibodies mediated cytotoxicity*. Pathogenesis of type II hypersensitivity reaction is shown in Fig. 4.41.

ANTIBODY-DEPENDENT CELL-MEDIATED CYTOTOXICITY: TYPE II HYPERSENSITIVITY REACTIONS

Preformed antibodies IgG or IgM in low concentration bind to cell bound intrinsic antigen and coat it. Fc portion of IgG or IgM binds to Fc receptors of cytotoxic leukocytes such as natural killer cells (most important), macrophages, neutrophils and eosinophils.

These cytotoxic leukocytes release hydrolytic enzymes and oxygen-derived free radicals resulting in tissue damage. It does not involve fixation of complement.

Examples of ADCC

Examples include systemic lupus erythematosus, Hashimoto's thyroiditis, and acute rheumatic fever are shown in Table 4.44. Treatment involves anti-inflammatory and immunosuppressive agents.

- *Systemic lupus erythematosus:* Autoantibodies develop to range of nuclear antigens in SLE, and causes non-organ specific autoimmune disease.
- *Hashimoto's thyroiditis:* It often affects HLA-DR5 and HLA-B5 persons. It is an autoantibody-dependent lymphocytic cytotoxicity disorder, in which anti-TSH receptor autoantibody of IgG class to cell surface antigen stimulate natural killer cells, lymphocytes, which destroy sensitized cells. *Circulating autoantibodies (anti-TSH, anti-thyroglobulin, anti-peroxidase, anti-microsomal and anti-iodine receptor autoantibodies) are demonstrated in Hashimoto's thyroiditis.*
- *Acute rheumatic fever:* Autoantibodies develop against streptococcal cell wall (group A streptococcus-β hemolyticus) cross react with myocardial antigens and joints. This multisystem autoimmune disorder affecting periarteriolar connective tissue. *Patient*

Immunopathology including Amyloidosis

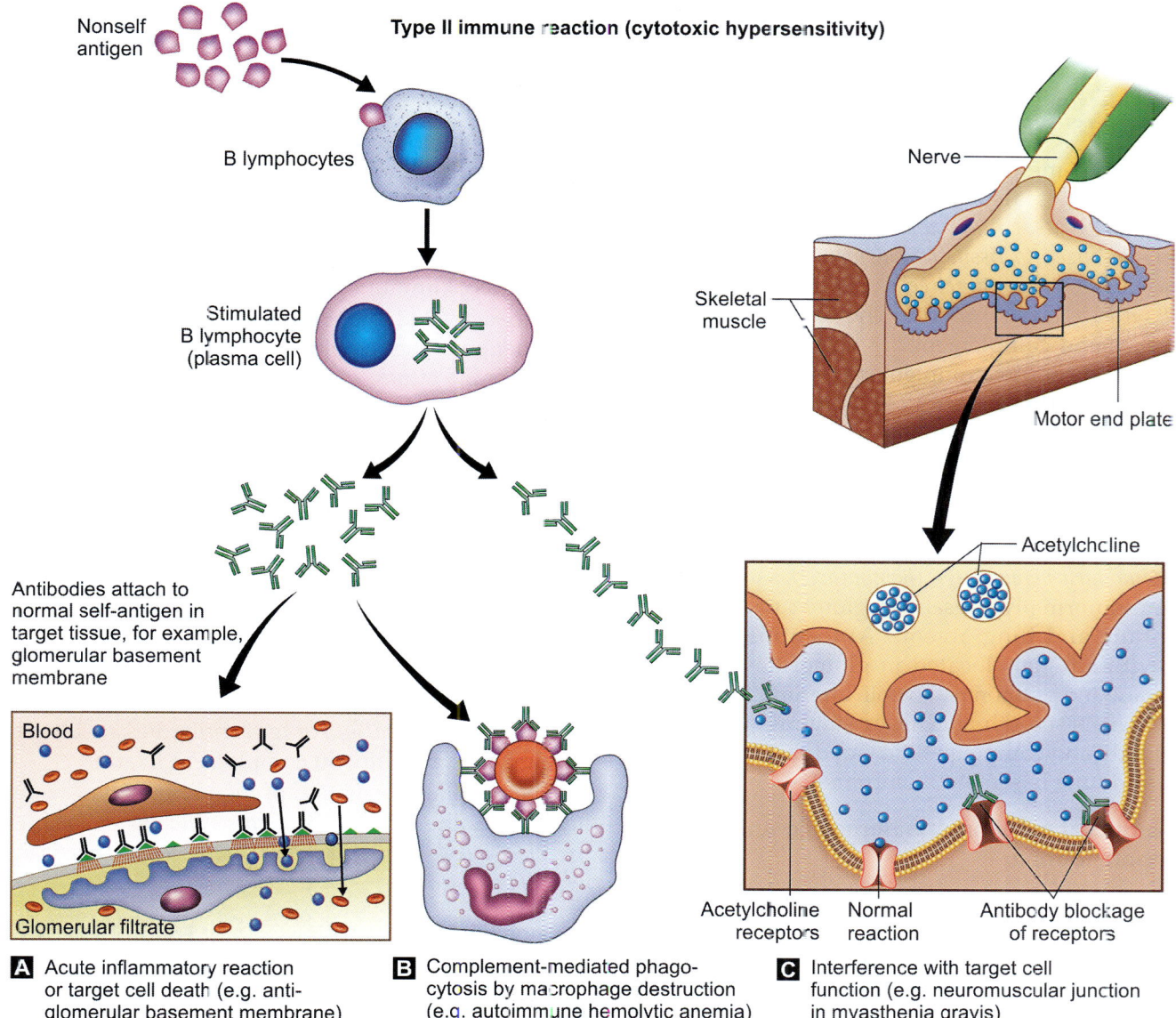

A Acute inflammatory reaction or target cell death (e.g. anti-glomerular basement membrane)

B Complement-mediated phagocytosis by macrophage destruction (e.g. autoimmune hemolytic anemia)

C Interference with target cell function (e.g. neuromuscular junction in myasthenia gravis)

Fig. 4.41: Pathogenesis of type II hypersensitivity reaction. (A) Target tissue inflammation or cell death. Antibodies attach to target antigen, which is destroyed by inflammation (glomerular basement membrane) or phagocytosis (RBCs), (B) complement-mediated phagocytosis by macrophage resulting in tissue damage, (C) interference with target cell function. Antibodies attach to target cell receptors and interfere with function (blockage of signal transmission from nerves to muscle in myasthenia gravis).

Table 4.44: Diseases caused by ADCC mechanism in type II hypersensitivity reaction

Disease	Target antigens	Characteristics
Systemic lupus erythematosus*	Systemic Nuclear antigens (DNA and anti-DNA)	Inflammation of many organs, antibodies against red and white blood cells, platelets, clotting factors, nucleus DNA
Hashimoto's thyroiditis	Thyroid	Destruction of the thyroid follicles
Acute rheumatic fever	Antibodies against streptococcal cell wall cross react with myocardial and joints antigens	Pancarditis and migratory polyarthritis

*Types II and III hypersensitivity reaction participate in the pathogenesis of systemic lupus erythematosus.

develops pancarditis, transient mild migratory polyarthritis, chorea, erythema marginatum and subcutaneous nodules.

Diagnostic Tests

Diagnostic tests include detection of circulating antibody against the tissues involved and the presence of antibody in the lesion (biopsy) by immunofluorescence.

COMPLEMENT-MEDIATED PHAGOCYTOSIS OF TARGET CELLS: TYPE II HYPERSENSITIVITY REACTIONS

Complement-mediated increased susceptibility to phagocytosis is also known as *complement-fixing antibodies mediated. Antibodies (IgG, IgM) bind to fixed antigens localized to tissue basement membranes or blood cell membranes of the target cells resulting in complement activation by classical pathway.* The cells opsonized by antibodies and complement are destroyed by splenic macrophages. Serum complement is characteristically decreased in these patients. Diseases caused by complement-mediated in type II hypersensitivity reaction are shown in Table 4.45.

Goodpasture Syndrome

Goodpasture syndrome is characterized by nephritic syndrome and pulmonary hemorrhage (hemoptysis). Goodpasture antigen is normally present in glomerular basement membrane and lung alveoli. Autoantibodies cross react with antigens located in glomerular basement membrane and pulmonary alveoli. Immunofluorescence study reveals smooth and linear staining pattern due to antibody and complement in Goodpasture nephritis (renal and lung basement membrane).

Drug-induced Autoimmune Hemolytic Anemia or Thrombocytopenia

Sometimes a drug or its metabolite such as *benzyl penicillin may bind firmly to the cell surface to give a highly immunogenic epitope.* Individuals produce IgG cytotoxic autoantibodies to their own drug coated red blood cells or platelets resulting in their destruction, especially in the spleen.

Warm Antibody-mediated Hemolytic Anemia

IgG autoantibody is reactive at 37°C *warm antibody* and causes autoimmune disorders. IgM autoantibody is active at 4°C, which becomes less active at higher temperature; but is still able to bind complement and *agglutinate red cells at the temperature 30° of the peripheral tissues (e.g. hands, feet, nose and ears).* RBCs coated by IgG or IgM autoantibodies become bound to receptors of macrophages because they have receptors for the Fc fragments of immunoglobulins.

Once activated, the complement cascade leads to the destruction of the red blood cells through formation of a membrane attack complex. *IgM antibodies, which are powerful agglutinins, may agglutinate red blood cells in the red pulp of the spleen, resulting in cellular destruction.* IgM may also activate complement, resulting in cellular lysis or promoting to more macrophages. Such autoantibodies are detected by Coombs' test (agglutination test).

Blood Transfusion Reactions

In blood transfusion reactions, humans may become sensitized to special antigens on the surface of the red blood cells of other humans. *The most common type II reactions occur when transfused blood is mismatched to the recipient's ABO type.* IgG or IgM antibodies attach to the foreign cells, resulting in complement fixation.

The resultant formation of membrane attack complexes lyses the donor cells. *Cross-matching of donor and recipient blood is necessary to determine which transfusions are safe to perform.*

Hemolytic Disease of Newborn or Erythroblastosis Fetalis

Hemolytic disease of the newborn most commonly occurs with Rh blood group incompatibility between mother and fetus. It

Table 4.45: Diseases caused by complement-mediated phagocytosis in type II hypersensitivity reaction

Disease	Target antigens	Characteristics
Goodpasture syndrome	Goodpasture antigen in noncollagenous proteins in basement membrane of kidney glomeruli and lung alveoli	Antibodies to basement membrane of glomeruli and alveoli
Drug-induced (benzyl penicillin) autoimmune hemolytic anemia or thrombocytopenic purpura	RBCs or platelets membrane proteins	Antibodies to surface RBCs or platelets Opsonization and phagocytosis of RBCs and platelets
Warm antibody-mediated hemolytic anemia IgG autoantibody is reactive at 37°C	RBCs coated by IgG or IgM autoantibodies become bound to receptors of macrophages because they have receptors for the Fc fragments of immunoglobulins	Antibodies to surface RBCs
Blood transfusion reactions	IgG or IgM antibodies attach to the foreign cells of donor, resulting in complement fixation	The resultant formation of membrane attack complexes lyses the donor cells
Hemolytic disease of newborn or erythroblastosis fetalis	RBCs membrane proteins (Rh blood group antigen, I antigen)	Opsonization and phagocytosis of RBCs results in hemolytic disease of newborn

occurs when the mother is Rh –ve and baby is Rh +ve, having inherited an allele for one of the Rh antigens from the father. An Rh –ve person, if exposed to Rh +ve blood, will form specific IgG antibodies against the Rh antigens. Therefore, Rh group should also be matched before transfusion (Fig. 4.42).

- *During first pregnancy, at birth of newborn:* A small quantity of fetal blood usually leaks across the placenta into the maternal bloodstream. Upon exposure to Rh antigen, the mother's immune system responds by making anti-Rh antibodies. Because the baby is already born, it suffers no damage. Prevention involves therapy with Rh immune globulin after first delivery or abortion.
- *During subsequent pregnancy:* The maternal antibodies cross the placenta into the fetal blood. If the second fetus is Rh +ve, the ensuring antigen–antibody reaction causes hemolysis of fetal RBCs The result

is hemolytic disease of newborn (HDN). *Newborn baby develops severe anemia and jaundice. Development of cardiac failure in newborn is called as erythroblastosis fetalis.*

Direct Coombs' test detects IgG and/or C3b attached to RBCs. Indirect Coombs' test detects antibodies in serum (e.g. anti-D).

ANTI-RECEPTOR ANTIBODY-MEDIATED TYPE II HYPERSENSITIVITY REACTION

In some persons, *autoantibodies are formed against cell surface receptors*. These impair normal cellular functions of receptors without causing cell injury. Examples include *Graves' disease, myasthenia gravis, insulin resistant diabetes mellitus, pernicious anemia, pemphigus vulgaris, Eaton-Lambert syndrome and rheumatoid arthritis* (Table 4.46).

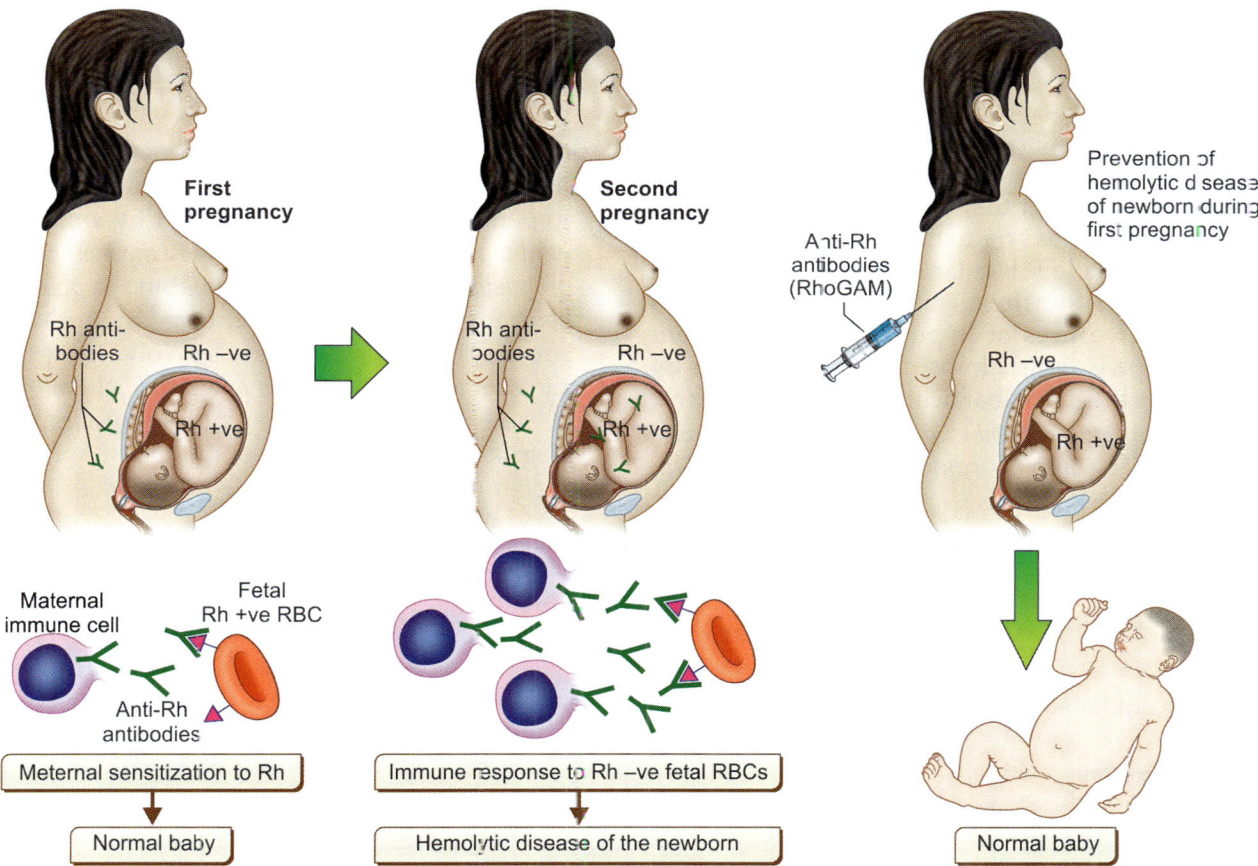

Fig. 4.42: Hemolytic disease of the newborn. Rh factor incompatibility can cause lysis of red blood cells. A naturally occurring red blood cell incompatibility results when a fetus Rh +ve develops within Rh –ve mother, initial sensitization of the maternal immune system occurs when fetal blood passes the placental barrier. In most cases, the fetus develops normally. However, a subsequent pregnancy with Rh +ve fetus results in a severe fetal red blood cells hemolysis. Control of incompatibility is done by administration of anti-Rh antibody (RhoGAM) to Rh –ve mothers during pregnancy to inactivate and remove any Rh factor that may be transferred from the fetus in maternal circulation. In some cases, anti-Rh antibody (RhoGAM) is administered before sensitization occurs.

Table 4.46: Diseases caused by anti-receptor antibody-mediated type II hypersensitivity reaction

Disease	Target antigens	Characteristics
Graves' disease	Thyroid	Antibodies against thyroid-stimulating hormone receptors
Myasthenia gravis	Acetylcholine receptors at neuromuscular junction	Antibodies inhibit acetyl choline binding, down modulates receptors
Insulin-dependent diabetes mellitus	Pancreas	Antibodies cause destruction of insulin secreting cells
Pernicious anemia	Stomach lining	Antibodies against intrinsic factor synthesized by parietal cells prevent transport of vitamin B_{12} resulting in megaloblastic erythropoiesis
Pemphigus vulgaris	Desmoglein-3 proteins in intercellular junctions of epidermis	Antibody-mediated activation of proteases, disruption of intercellular adhesions results in skin vesicles (bullae)
Eaton-Lambert syndrome	Calcium channels	Antibodies to calcium channels formed in patients with Eaton-Lambert syndrome associated with small cell carcinoma of the lung resulting in muscle weakness
Rheumatoid arthritis	Fc portion of IgG	Rheumatoid factor represents multiple antibodies directed against the Fc portion of IgG and is seen in patients with rheumatoid arthritis and many other collagen vascular diseases

DISEASES CAUSED BY ANTI-RECEPTOR ANTIBODY-MEDIATED TYPE II HYPERSENSITIVITY REACTION

- *Graves' disease:* Antibodies to the TSH receptor are seen in patients with Graves' hyperthyroidism—an autoimmune disorder that mimic the action of TSH, but are not regulated by natural negative feedback controls. It leads to follicular glandular hyperplasia and increased synthesis of thyroid hormones resulting in features of hyperthyroidism. Patient also develops exophthalmos due to infiltration by lymphocytes in retrobulbar ocular muscles in 60–90%.

  Circulating autoantibodies demonstrated in Garves' disease are TSI (thyroid-stimulating immunoglobulin mimicking TSH), antimicrosomal and antithyroglobulin. CTL4 or PTPN22 gene mutation increases risk of Graves' disease.

- *Myasthenia gravis:* Myasthenia gravis is a type II hypersensitivity disorder caused by *antibodies that bind to the acetylcholine receptors in the motor end plates of skeletal muscles*. The antibodies bind to postsynaptic receptors and block neurotransmission resulting in progressive muscle weakness involving particularly the *external ocular, eyelids and proximal limb muscles*. It may cause death by respiratory muscles paralysis (Fig. 4.43).

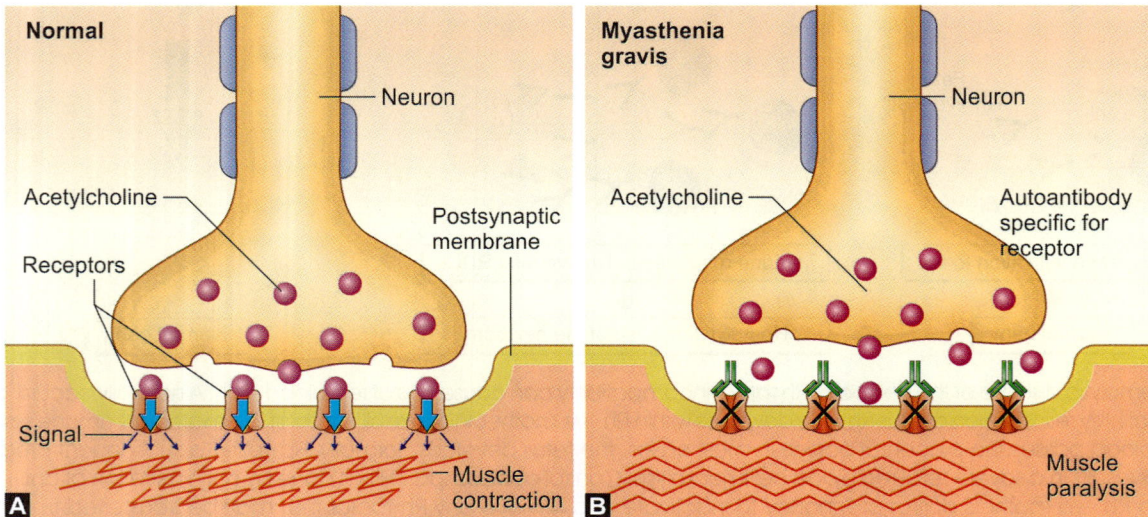

Fig. 4.43: Mechanism for involvement of autoantibodies in myasthenia gravis. (A) Normal neuromuscular junction, (B) in myasthenia gravis, antibodies formed against receptors on the postsynaptic membrane block them so that acetyl choline cannot bind resulting in inhibition of muscle contraction.

- *Insulin resistant diabetes mellitus:* Antibody inhibits binding of insulin to insulin receptors. Patient develops hyperglycemia.
- *Pernicious anemia:* Antibodies are formed against intrinsic factor of gastric parietal cells. Neutralization of intrinsic factor leads to decreased absorption of vitamin B_{12} resulting in megaloblastic erythropoiesis.
- *Pemphigus vulgaris:* Autoantibodies to desmoglein-3 which disrupt intercellular junctions in epidermis are found in patients with pemphigus vulgaris, an autoimmune blistering (vesicles) skin disorder. Immunofluorescence study reveals smooth and linear staining pattern in pemphigus (skin intercellular protein, desmosomes).
- *Eaton-Lambert syndrome:* Antibodies to calcium channels are found in patients with Eaton-Lambert syndrome. *This paraneoplastic syndrome also manifests as muscle weakness but is usually associated with small cell carcinoma of the lung.*
- *Rheumatoid arthritis:* Rheumatoid factor represents multiple antibodies directed against the Fc portion of IgG and seen in patients with rheumatoid arthritis and many other collagen vascular diseases.

TYPE III HYPERSENSITIVITY REACTIONS

Type III hypersensitivity reactions are characterized by immune complex deposition, complement fixation, and localized inflammation. Examples include Arthus reaction, serum sickness, systemic lupus erythematosus, immune complex-mediated glomerular diseases (post-streptococcal glomerulonephritis, membranous glomerulonephritis and lupus nephropathy), and polyarteritis nodosa.

Pathogenesis

Normally, antigen–antibody immune complexes formed in small quantity are cleared by reticuloendothelial system. Pathogenesis of type III hypersensitivity reaction is shown in Fig. 4.44.

- Antibodies (IgG or IgM) formed against soluble antigen (serum or drug) in large quantity are trapped in membranes of various organs (skin, kidney, lung, blood vessels, and joints) in pathological state such as persistent infections, inhaled allergens (farmer's lung) and self-antigens (SLE).
- Immune complex activates the complement system. C3a, C5 attract neutrophils, which release hydrolytic enzymes result in injury. Serum complement level is decreased.
- Injury to endothelium leads to activation of intrinsic coagulation pathway which results in formation of microthrombi in small vessels.
- Activation of the kinin system causes vasodilation and edema.
- Oxygen-derived free radicals, prostaglandins and kinins incite chronic destructive inflammatory response. Macrophages infiltrating in later stages may be involved in the healing process.

Immune complex formation and site of deposition

Immune complexes are trapped in membranes of various organs (skin, kidney, lung, blood vessels, and joints) in pathological state such as persistent infections, inhaled allergens (farmer's lung) and self-antigens (SLE).

Immunofluorescence microscopy reveals immune complex deposits in biopsy specimens. Serum complement level is decreased in these patients. Immune complex formation and site of deposition are shown in Table 4.47. Immune complex deposition induced organs damage are shown in Fig. 4.45.

TYPES OF REACTIONS

There are two kinds of reactions, i.e. localized (Arthus reaction) and systemic in type III hypersensitivity reactions. Diseases caused by type III hypersensitivity reactions are shown in Table 4.48.

Localized Reaction

Arthus reaction is a localized immune complex reaction that occurs when exogenous antigen is introduced, either by injection or by organ transplant, in the presence of an excess of preformed antibodies (usually IgG, but IgM may be involved).

Systemic Reactions

- *Serum sickness:* It is a systemic deposition of antigen–antibody complexes in multiple sites, especially the

Table 4.47: Immune complex formation and sites of deposition

Circumstances	Etiology	Sites of deposition
Persistent infections	Microorganism products	Blood vessels and glomeruli
Inhaled allergens (farmer's lung)	Exposure to thermophilic actinomyces in air	Lungs: IgG class, although IgM may also be involved in the formation of immune complex
Autoimmune disorders	Endogenous (self) antigens	Immune complex deposition in blood vessels, glomeruli and joints in SLE

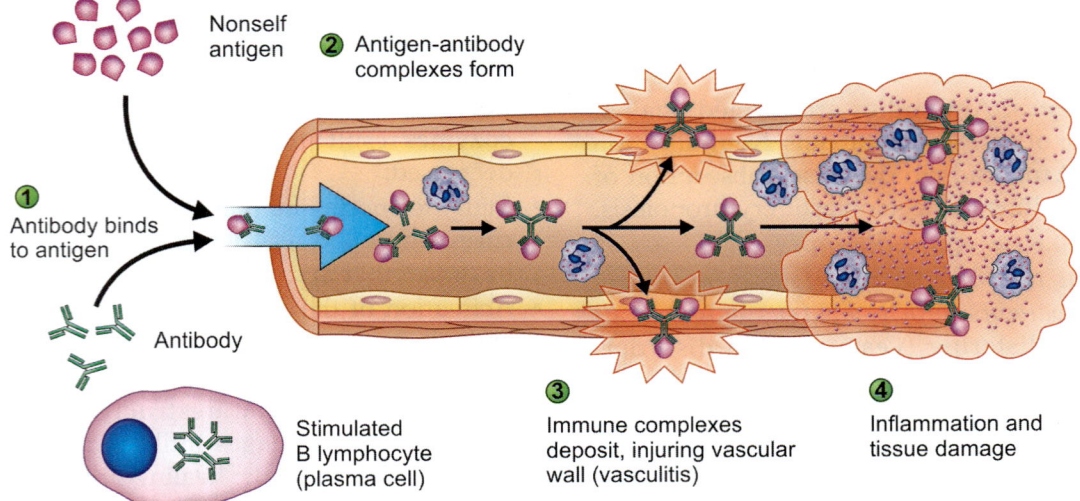

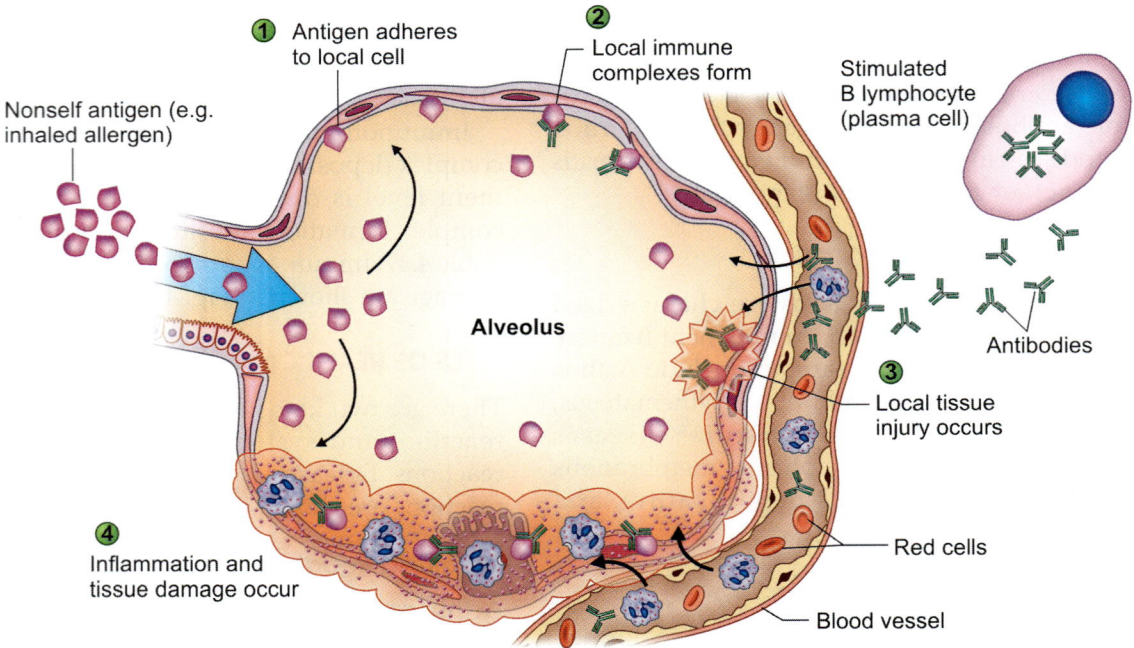

Fig. 4.44: Pathogenesis of type III hypersensitivity reaction. Antigen and antibody bind together to create an immune complex. (A) Systemic immune complex reaction in systemic reactions. Antibody binds to nonself-antigen and enter circulation. Antigen antibody complexes are formed. (B) Local immune complex occurs following injection of antigen or organ transplantation.

heart, joints, and kidneys. In the past, antibody-containing foreign serum (most often horse serum antithymocyte globulin) was administered therapeutically for passive immunization against microorganisms or their toxic products. Because of the danger of serum sickness, this mode of therapy is no longer employed. Differences between serum sickness and Arthus reaction are shown in Table 4.49.

- *Systemic lupus erythematosus:* It is an autoimmune disorder involving multiple systems such as blood vessels, glomeruli and joints. Anti-DNA antibodies are formed against endogenous (self) antigen.
- *Polyarteritis nodosa:* It is systemic vasculitis involving small- and medium-sized arteries due to hepatitis B viral infection.
- *Immune complex-mediated glomerular diseases:* These include post-streptococcal glomerulonephritis, membranous glomerulonephritis, and lupus nephropathy.
- *Farmer's lung:* Inhalation of allergens (exogenous organic dust) involves lungs.

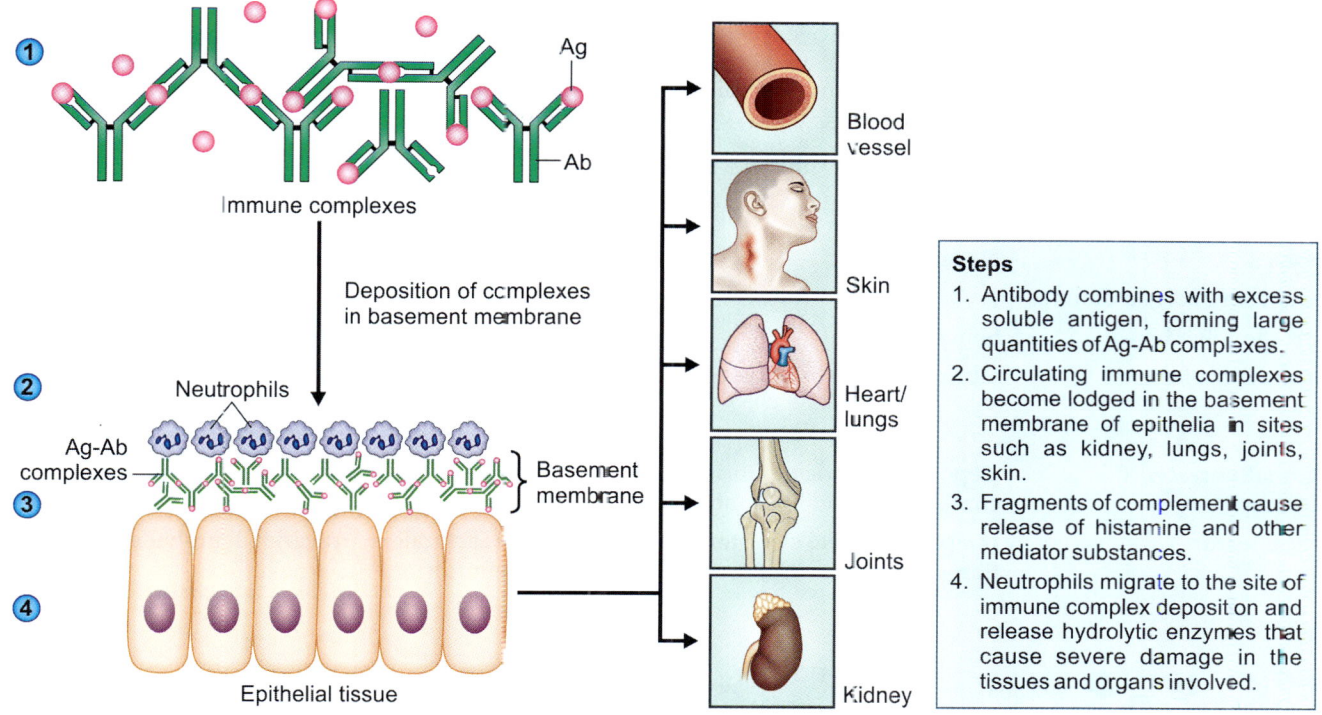

Fig. 4.45: Immune complex deposition induced organs damage.

Table 4.48: Diseases caused by type III hypersensitivity reactions

Localized or systemic reactions	Disease	Target antigens	Characteristics
Localized reaction	Arthus reaction (experimental)	Various foreign proteins	Cutaneous vasculitis (IgG class, although IgM may also be involved)
Systemic reactions	Serum sickness	Various proteins such as foreign serum proteins (horse antithymocyte globulin)	Arthritis, vasculitis, nephritis
	Systemic lupus erythematosus*	Nuclear antigens (DNA and anti-DNA)	Lupus nephritis, skin lesions, arthritis
	Polyarteritis nodosa	Hepatitis B virus antigen	Systemic vasculitis
	Post-streptococcal glomerulonephritis	Streptococcal cell wall antigen, may be planted in glomerular basement membrane	Nephritis
	Farmer's lung	Inhaled allergens (exogenous organic dust)	Lung involvement
	Reactive arthritis	Bacterial antigens (Yersinia)	Acute arthritis

*Types II and III hypersensitivity reactions participate in the pathogenesis of systemic lupus erythematosus.

TYPE IV HYPERSENSITIVITY REACTIONS

Type IV hypersensitivity reaction is antibody-independent T cell-mediated hypersensitivity reaction.

It occurs by two mechanisms: (i) cytotoxic T cell-mediated hypersensitivity, and (ii) delayed type hypersensitivity. Examples of type IV reactions include the tuberculin reaction, contact dermatitis, and mismatched organ transplants (host rejection and GVHD reactions). Pathogenesis of type IV hypersensitivity reaction is shown in Fig. 4.46.

Table 4.49: Differences between Arthus reaction and serum sickness

Characteristics	Arthus reaction	Serum sickness
Disorder	Localized immune complex due to antibody excess	Systemic immune complex disorder due to antigen excess resulting in injury
Onset	4–10 days after exposure to antibody	5–7 days after entry of antigen, e.g. exogenous (horse serum, streptococcal infection) or endogenous (systemic lupus erythematosus)
Subtypes	No subtypes	Acute and chronic serum sickness
Mechanism of organ damage		Complement activation, platelets aggregation
Organs involved	Skin only	Joints, skin, heart, blood vessels, serosal surfaces
Morphology of organs	Fibrinoid necrosis of blood vessels	Immune complex mediated necrotizing vasculitis, fibrinoid necrosis of blood vessels, proliferation of endothelial and mesangial cells
Immunofluorescence microscopy	Deposits comprising fibrinogen, complement and immunoglobulin	Granular deposits of immune complex comprising of immunoglobulin and complement
Clinical features	Dyspnea, flu-like symptoms and lung fibrosis (chronic case)	Fever, arthralgia, urticarial, lymphadenopathy and proteinuria

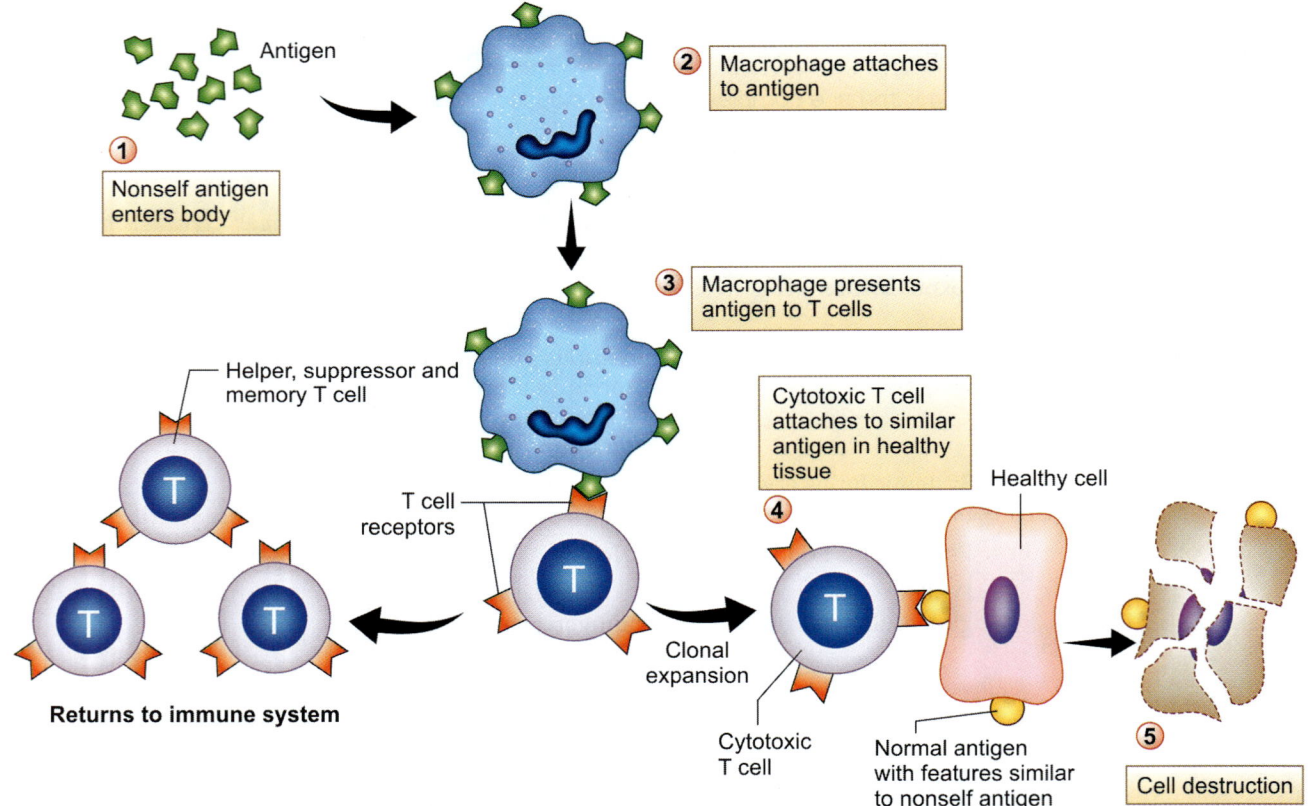

Fig. 4.46: Pathogenesis of type IV hypersensitivity reaction (cell-mediated reaction). Macrophage capture antigen and present to T cells, thus sensitizing these T lymphocytes. Some of these lymphocytes become cytotoxic T cells. These cytotoxic T cells attack the antigen, where present. Other lymphocytes become T helper cells, T-suppressor cells and memory cells.

CD8+ T CELL-MEDIATED CYTOTOXICITY

T cell-mediated cytotoxicity is mediated by cytotoxic CD8+ T cells, which attack specific target cells. These interact with altered MHC-I class antigens present on cancer cells, viral infected cells or donor transplanted cells resulting in cell lysis. These cytotoxic CD8+ T cells synthesize IFN-γ. Cytokines do not participate in this process. T cell-mediated cytotoxicity *kill cancer cells, viral infected cells and transplanted cells* described as under.

Killing of Cancer Cells

Cytotoxic T cells, NK cells, and macrophages recognize and destroy cancer cells by means of immune surveillance. Failure of immune system results in survival of cancer cells. Genetic alteration transforms normal cells to cancer cells due to activation of oncogenes or mutation of tumor suppressor genes, irradiation and infection by viruses.

Viral infected Cells

Cytotoxic T cells also participate in cell-mediated killing of virus-infected cells. The antiviral activity of interferon is shown in Fig. 4.47.

Transplanted Cells

- *Classes of grafts:* The four classes of transplants or grafts are determined by the degree of MHC similarity between graft and host. From most to least similar, these are: *autografts (one part of body to another), isografts (between identical twins), allografts (between two members of same species), and xenografts (between two different species).* All major organs may be successfully transplanted. Allografts require tissue match (HLAs must correspond); rejection is controlled with drugs.

- *Graft rejection:* Reaction of cytotoxic T cells directed against foreign cells of a grafted tissue; involves recognition of foreign human leukocyte antigens (HLAs) by T cells and rejection of tissue.

  Graft rejection can be minimized by tissue matching procedures, immunosuppressive drugs, and use of tissues that do not provoke a type IV response.

DELAYED TYPE HYPERSENSITIVITY-MEDIATED BY CD4+ T CELLS

Delayed type hypersensitivity is mediated by CD4+ T cells. It occurs hours to days after the antigenic challenge. *Interferon-γ is a central mediator of delayed hypersensitivity.* It is a powerful activator of macrophages. It further augments the differentiation of Th1 cells.

T Cells and Macrophages Interaction

Antigenic presenting cells (macrophages, Langerhans' cells/dendritic cells in the epidermis expressing MHC class II molecules) synthesize IL-12, which activates CD4+ T cells and differentiate to Th1 effector cells. These Th1 effector cells synthesize various cytokines such as monocyte chemotactic factor, IL-2, IFN-γ, which recruit macrophages and increase their phagocytic activity. *IL-2 has autocrine and paracrine proliferation of T cells, which accumulate at the site of delayed type hypersensitivity.*

Role of activated macrophages in chronic inflammation is shown in Fig. 4.48 and epithelioid granulomas in tubercular lymphadenitis are shown in Fig. 4.49.

Synthesis of Acute Phase Reactants

One important cytokine is IL-1, which promotes the release of the acute phase reactants of the liver. It increases the proliferation of T cells. It acts on the hypothalamic thermoregulatory centre to induce fever. It is thus responsible for some of the systemic symptoms of delayed type of hypersensitivity.

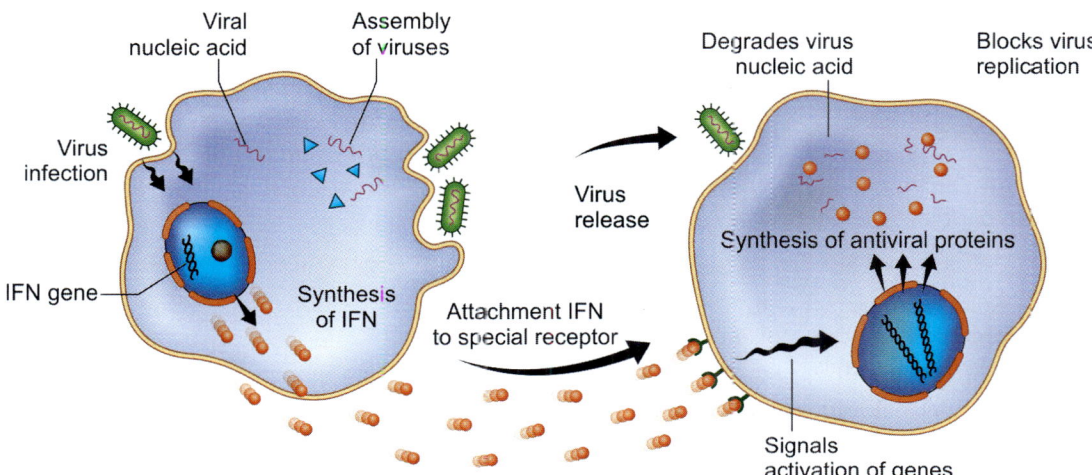

Fig. 4.47: The antiviral activity of interferon. When a cell is infected by a virus, its nucleus is triggered to transcribe interferon (IFN) gene. Interferon diffuses out of the cell and then binds to IFN receptors on nearby uninfected cells, where it induces production of proteins that eliminate viral genes and block viral replication. Note that the original cell is not protected by IFN and that does not prevent viruses from invading the protected cells.

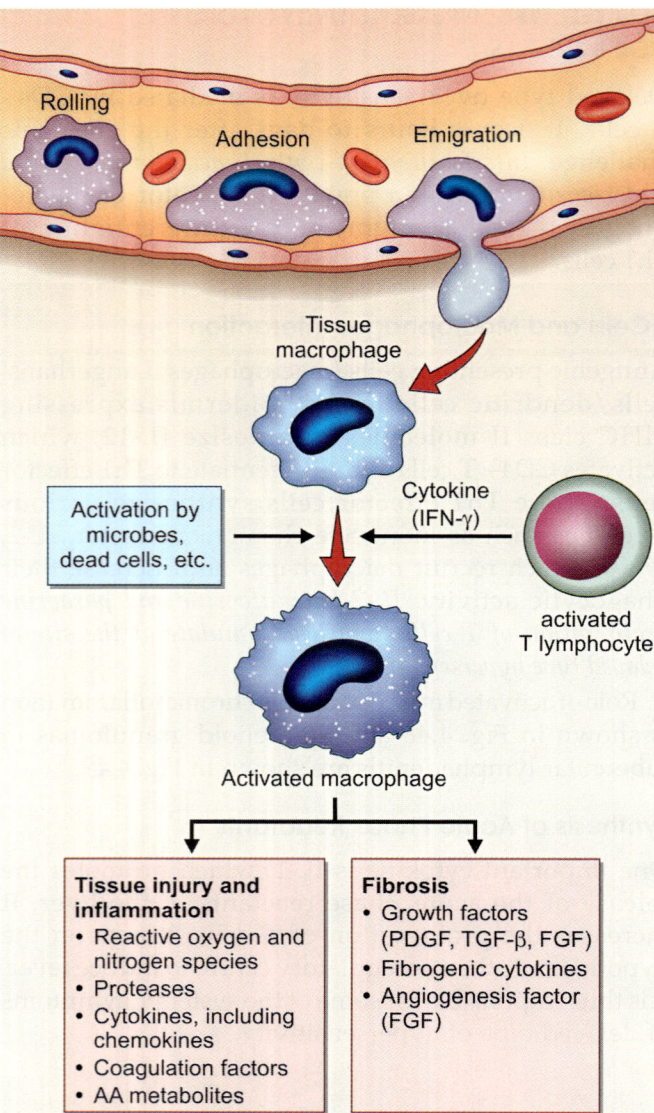

Fig. 4.48: Role of activated macrophages in chronic inflammation. Macrophages are activated by immunological or nonimmunological mechanisms. Various products synthesized by activated macrophages participate in tissue injury and fibrosis.

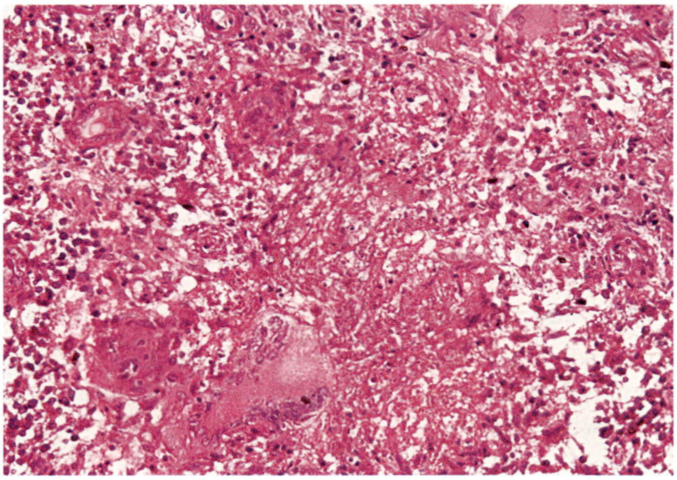

Fig. 4.49: Epithelioid granulomas in tubercular lymphadenitis. Areas of caseous necrosis and Langhan's cells are also seen (100X).

Categories of Delayed Hypersensitivity Reactions

Type IV hypersensitivity can be classified into three categories depending on the time of onset and clinical and histological presentation. These include contact dermatitis, tuberculin reaction and granulomatous hypersensitivity (Table 4.50).

- *Contact dermatitis:* Heavy metals (nickel, chromium), plant (ivy oak), organic chemicals, cosmetics, cyano-acrylate adhesive photographic developer and primula paint absorbed by the skin act as a *hapten-protein complex, which stimulate cell-mediated immune response. Subsequent exposure to these substances induces eczema within 48–72 hours.* Light microscopy reveals lymphocytic infiltration around dermal blood vessels, together with dermal and epidermal edema leading to vesicle formation (Fig. 4.50).

- *Tuberculin reaction:* It is a localized inflammatory reaction developing within 48–72 hours. *It is initiated by the intracutaneous injection of tuberculin.*

Table 4.50: Categories of delayed hypersensitivity reactions

Type	Antigen and site	Reaction time	Clinical appearance	Histology
Contact dermatitis	Epidermal contact with organic chemicals, poison ivy, heavy metals	48–72 hours	Eczema	Lymphocytes followed by macrophages; edema of epidermis
Tuberculin test	Intradermal route (tuberculin or lepromin test)	48–72 hours	Local induration, swelling and swelling with or without fever	Lymphocytes and macrophages
Granulomatous inflammation	Persistent antigen or foreign body presence *Mycobacterium tuberculosis* and leprosy	21–28 days	Hardening	Epithelioid cell granuloma, giant cells with or without necrosis

Immunopathology including Amyloidosis

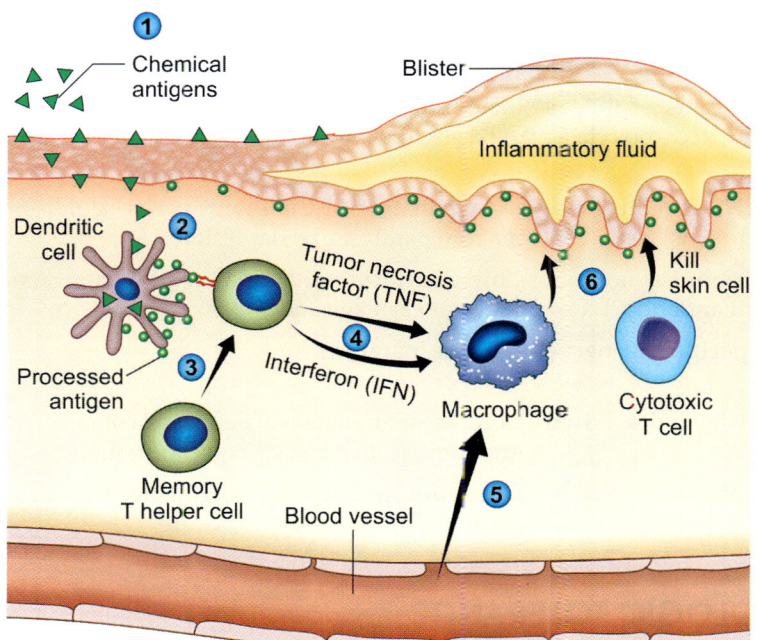

Fig. 4.50: Contact dermatitis. (A) Genesis of contact dermatitis, (B) contact dermatitis from poison oak, showing various stages of involvement: blisters, scales and thickened patches. Lipid-soluble chemicals are absorbed by the skin. Dendritic cells close to epidermis pick up the allergen, process it.

The indurated area resulting in fibrin deposition is marked by accumulation of lymphocytes, monocytes, and small numbers of neutrophils around small blood vessels (i.e. perivascular cuffing).

- *Granulomatous hypersensitivity:* Persistent antigen or foreign body in macrophages leads to granuloma formation as in tuberculosis in more than 3 weeks. *Granuloma is defined as an aggregation of modified macrophages (epithelioid cells) surrounded by lymphocytes and fibroblasts.* Epithelioid cells may differentiate into multinucleate giant cells. Langhans' giant cells show peripherally arranged nuclei seen in tuberculosis.

GRANULOMATOUS T CELL-MEDIATED TYPE IV HYPERSENSITIVITY REACTION

Examples of granulomatous hypersensitivity include tuberculosis, leprosy, syphilis, blastomycosis, histoplasmosis, toxoplasmosis, leishmaniasis, sarcoidosis, Crohn's disease, rheumatoid arthritis, inorganic antigens (zircomin, inert minerals like silica), autoimmune diseases (e.g. diabetes mellitus I, multiple sclerosis, rheumatoid arthritis and Guillain-Barré syndrome). Corticosteroids and other immunosuppressive agents are used in treatment. Examples of granulomatous T cell-mediated hypersensitivity reaction are shown in Table 4.51.

- *Type I diabetes mellitus:* Antigen of pancreatic islets of β cells (e.g. insulin, glutamic acid decarboxylase, others) stimulate cell-mediated immune response. It causes destruction of islets of β cells and results in type I diabetes mellitus.

- *Multiple sclerosis:* Protein antigens in CNS myelin (e.g. basic proteins, proteolytic proteins) stimulate cell-mediated immune response. It results in demyelination in CNS with perivascular inflammation, paralysis, ocular lesions.

- *Rheumatoid arthritis:* Unknown antigens in joint synovium (? type II collagen) stimulate cell-mediated immune response. It resulting in chronic arthritis with inflammation, destruction of articular cartilage and bones.

- *Inflammatory bowel disease (Crohn's disease):* Unknown antigen derived from intestinal microbes stimulates cell-mediated immune response. It causes chronic inflammation of ileum and colon, often with granulomas, fibrosis, and stricture formation.

- *Peripheral neuropathy (Guillain-Barré syndrome):* Protein antigens of peripheral nerve myelin stimulate cell-mediated immune response. It resulting in neuritis and paralysis.

Table 4.51: Granulomatous T cell-mediated hypersensitivity reactions

Disease	Specificity of pathogenic antigen	Clinicopathological manifestations
Type I diabetes mellitus	Antigen of pancreatic islets of β cells (insulin, glutamic acid decarboxylase, others)	Insulitis (chronic inflammation in islets destruction of β cells, diabetes)
Multiple sclerosis	Protein antigens in CNS myelin (basic proteins, proteolytic proteins)	Demyelination in CNS with perivesicular inflammation, paralysis, ocular lesions
Rheumatoid arthritis	Unknown antigens in joint synovium (type II collagen, role of antibody?)	Chronic arthritis with inflammation, destruction of articular cartilage and bones
Peripheral neuropathy (Guillain-Barré syndrome)	Protein antigens of peripheral nerve myelin	Neuritis, paralysis
Inflammatory bowel disease (Crohn's disease)	Unknown antigen may be derived from intestinal microbes	Chronic inflammation of ileum and colon, often with granulomas, fibrosis, stricture formation
Contact dermatitis	Environmental chemicals, i.e. ivy (pentadecylcatechol)	Dermatitis, with itching usually short-lived, may be chronic with persistent exposure

IMMUNOLOGIC TOLERANCE

OVERVIEW

Thymus and bone marrow are sites of maturation for T and B cells respectively them. These cells bind to the foreign antigens and eliminate. These cells are also capable of binding to self-proteins and destroy them. To prevent self-tissue destruction, these cells are eliminated or downregulated in primary and secondary lymphoid organs. This process is called *central and peripheral tolerance*.

Immunologic Tolerance

Immunologic tolerance is the process by which the immune system does not attack an antigen. It occurs in three forms: central tolerance, peripheral tolerance and acquired tolerance. The time of first encounter is critical in determining responsiveness. It contrasts with conventional immuno-mediated elimination of foreign antigen. It can be either natural (self) or induced tolerance.

- *Natural or self-tolerance:* It refers where the body does not mount an immune response to self-antigens. *It enables us to live in harmony with our own cells and tissues.* Normal individuals are tolerant of their own antigens (self-antigen). *Immunologically privileged sites are brain, eye, testis, uterus (fetus).* Immunologic tolerance in pregnancy allows mother to gestate a genetically distinct offspring with an alloimmune response mutated enough to prevent miscarriage.
- *Induced tolerance:* It refers where tolerance to external antigens can be *created by manipulating the immune system.*

Factors Influencing Immunologic Tolerance

These comprise structure of molecule, stage of differentiation when lymphocyte first encounter the epitopes, site of the encounter and nature of the cell presenting the epitopes. Factors influencing immunologic tolerance are shown in Table 4.52.

Classification

Immunologic tolerance is classified into central and peripheral tolerance depending on where the state is originally induced such as bone marrow and thymus. Deficits in central and peripheral resistance cause various autoimmune diseases. Pathogenesis of central and peripheral tolerance is shown in Fig. 4.51.

- *Central tolerance:* It occurs during development of lymphocytes (in bone marrow and thymus). Host immune system is a vast array of TCRs (T cell receptors).

Table 4.52: Factors influencing immunologic tolerance

Factors affecting response	Favoring immune response	Favoring tolerance
Physical form of antigen	Large aggregated complex molecules properly processed	Soluble aggregates-free simple small molecules not processed
Route of administration of antigen	Subcutaneous and sometimes intramuscular route	Oral or sometimes intravenous route
Dose of antigen	Optimum dose	Ranging from small to large dose

Immunologic tolerance of host depends on heredity, age, gender and health.

Immunopathology including Amyloidosis

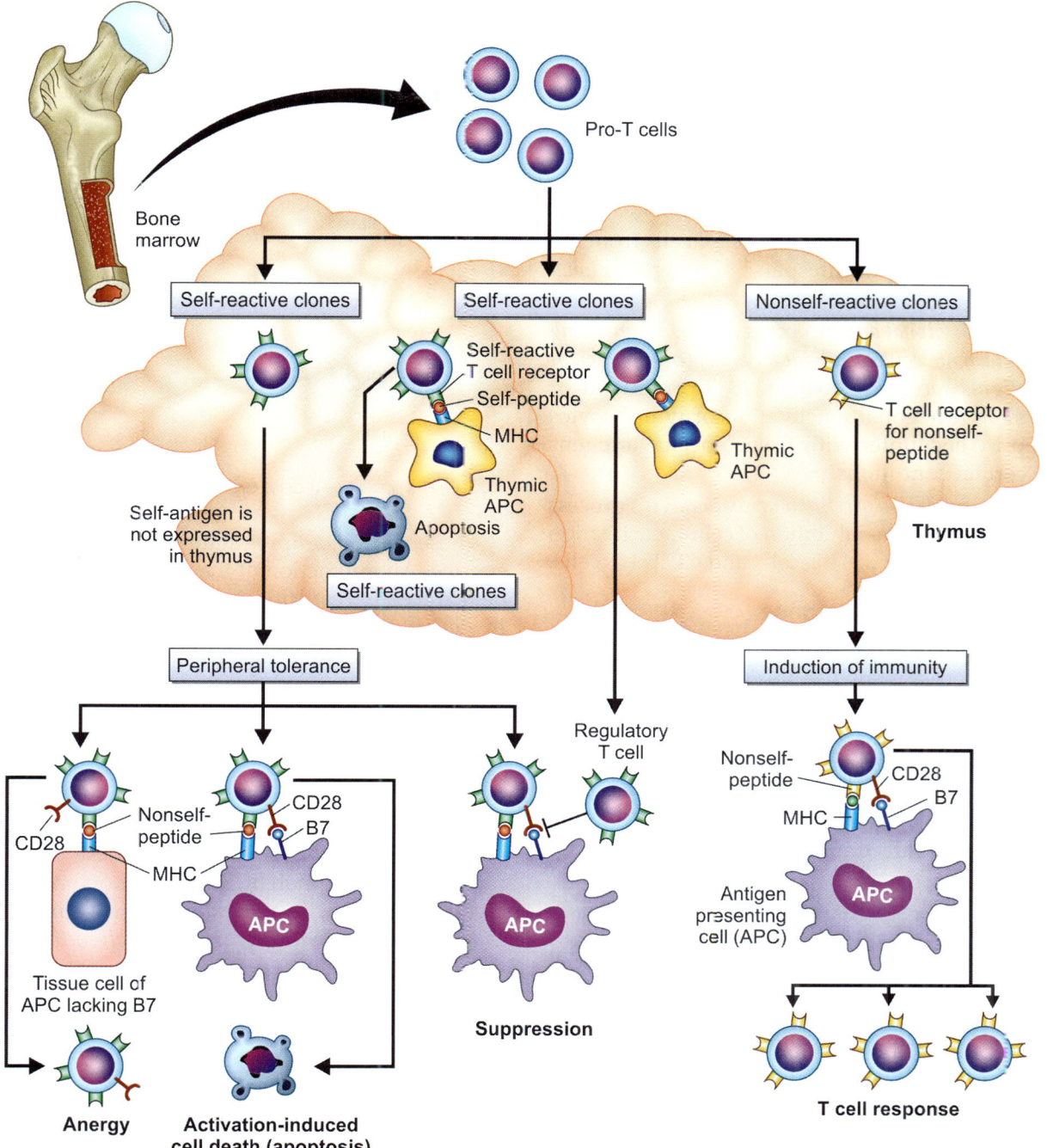

Fig. 4.51: Pathogenesis of central and peripheral tolerance.

T cells function as effector cells as well as regulator cells of immune system. T cells mature in the thymus and dependent on self-MHC for survival. Central tolerance occurs by *clonal deletion of B cells in bone marrow and T cells in thymus*.

- *Peripheral tolerance:* It occurs after lymphocytes leave the primary organs and settle in peripheral lymphoid tissue such as *lymph nodes, spleen, MALT (mucosa associated lymphoid tissue) and SALT (skin associated lymphoid tissue).* It prevents the elimination of lymphocytes by the host system by anergy, cell death and immune *deviation of T and B cells.*

T Cells Development to Various Checkpoints

- *β-chain selection checkpoint:* Only cells with a rearranged β-chain mature from double negative to double positive cells independent of MHC.
- *α selection checkpoint:* Cells expressing an αβ complex must interact with MHC molecules to survive.

- *Lineage commitment checkpoint:* Cells are instructed to repress expression of either CD4+ T cells or CD8+ T cells and to develop into single positive cells.
- *Negative selection checkpoint:* Cells that interact strongly with MHC and antigen in the thymus are deletion.

Possible Ways of Prevention of Self-reactivity

- *Clonal deletion:* Physical elimination of cells from the repertoire during their lifespan is known as *clonal selection*.
- *Clonal anergy: Clonal anergy occurs by down-regulating costimulatory molecules without apoptosis or insufficient second signal for cell activation.* It is prolonged or irreversible functional inactivation of lymphocytes induced by encounter with tissue specific antigens under certain conditions.
- *Suppression–inhibition of cellular activation:* This process involves suppression–inhibition of cellular activation by interaction with CD4+ T cells and CD25+ T cells.

Clinical Application of Tolerance

Induction of immunologic tolerance is done to prevent allogenic grafts, treatment of autoimmune diseases and allergic diseases; and limiting tumor growth.

Termination of Immunologic Tolerance

Termination of immunologic tolerance is done to treat tumor by enhancing first and second signal. It is also performed to treat infectious diseases.

B CELLS IMMUNOLOGIC TOLERANCE

B CELL TOLERANCE TO SELF-ANTIGEN IN BONE MARROW

During B cell development in the bone marrow, complete antigen receptor (IgM) is first expressed on *immature* B cells. If those cells encounter their target antigen in a form which can cross-link their IgM then such cells are programmed to die. The requirement for cross-linking means that the antigen has to be polyvalent. Immature B cell deletion by polyvalent antigens is shown in Fig. 4.52.

B CELL TOLERANCE TO SELF-ANTIGENS IN PERIPHERAL TISSUES

High affinity IgG production by B cells is T cell-dependent. If B cells encounter self-antigen in the absence of specific helper T cells, these are unable to respond to subsequent antigenic stimulation. B cells never express IgG receptors resulting in exclusion from the lymphoid cells undergoing death.

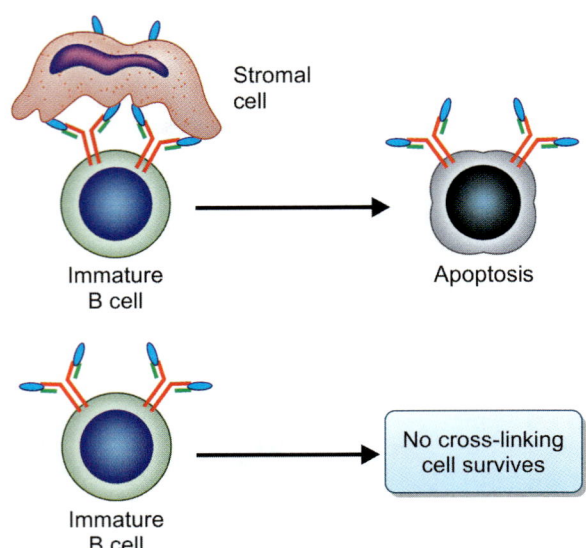

Fig. 4.52: Immature B cells are deleted by polyvalent antigens.

These cells also upregulate FAS molecules on their surface. An interaction of these B cells with Fas-ligand bearing cells resulting in their death via *apoptosis*. In peripheral B cell tolerance, self-reactive cells are removed by negative selection in the spleen in a process that is similar to T cell removal in the thymus.

T CELLS IMMUNOLOGIC TOLERANCE

CENTRAL TOLERANCE

Central tolerance occurs by clonal deletion of auto-reactive lymphocyte clones before these develop into fully immunocompetent B cells in bone marrow and T cells in thymus. *It is the main way, the immune system learns to discriminate self from nonself-antigens.* T cell development involves positive or negative selection and lineage commitment (Fig. 4.53). It depends on expression of TCR repertoire and exposure to MHC molecules. T cells possess high affinity receptors for self-antigens.

Pathogenesis

Random expression of αβTCR repertoire: T cells deletion occurs due to low expression αβTCR on precursor T cells.

Positive selection: T cell with low expression of αβTCR, when exposed to MHC molecules in thymus cortex leads to maturation of T cells. No engagement of T cells with MHC molecules leads to programmed cell death.

Negative selection: Maturation of T cells with high expression of αβTCR occurs in thymus into CD4+ T cell and CD8+ T cell, when there is no interaction with MHC

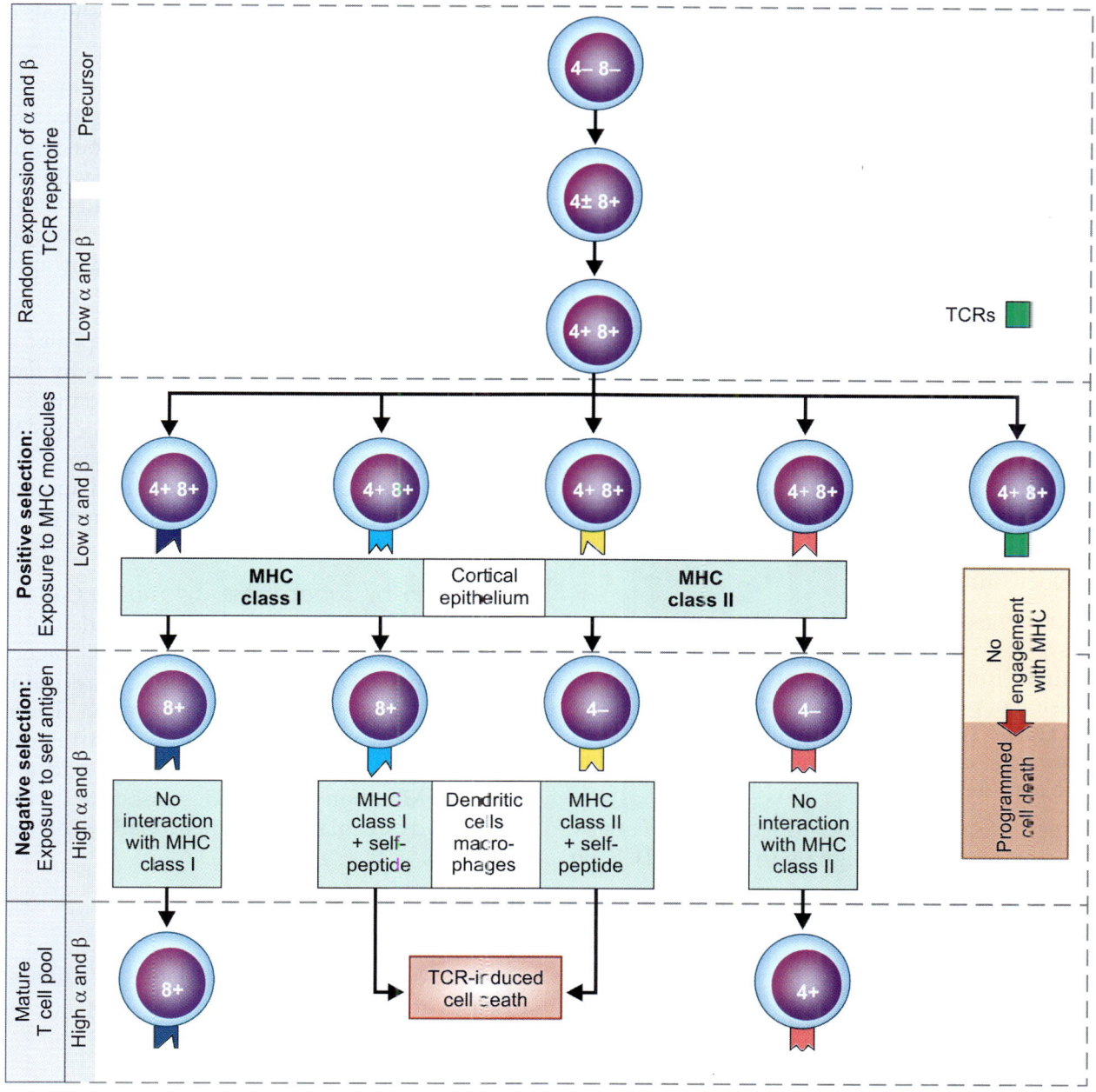

Fig. 4.53: T cell development involves positive or negative selection and lineage commitment.

self-peptides. TCR-induced death occurs when these T cells with high expression of αβTCR to self-antigen, exposed to MHC self-peptides. Autoreactive T cells are eliminated in the thymus following interaction with self-antigen during their differentiation via programmed cell death by mitochondrial pathway.

PERIPHERAL TOLERANCE

Some of the self-reactive T or B cells escape central clone deletion. Several mechanisms silence potentially autoreactive T and B cells in peripheral tissues such as lymph nodes, spleen, mucosa associated lymphoid tissue (MALT) and skin associated lymphoid tissue (SALT). These are best defined for T cells. Summary of peripheral post-thymic mechanisms of tolerance is shown in Fig. 4.54.

Clinical Aspect

Immunologic tolerance prevents over-reactivity of the immune system to various *environmental allergens and gut microbes*. In addition, inducing peripheral tolerance in the local microenvironment is a common survival strategy for a number of *tumors* that prevents their elimination by the host immune system. Failure of peripheral tolerance may occur and produce *autoimmune disorders*.

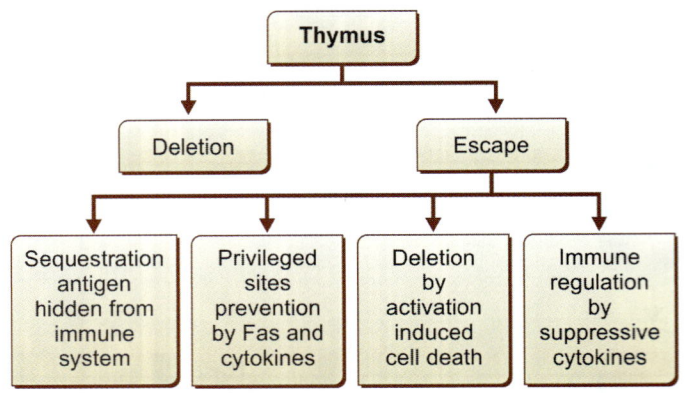

Fig. 4.54: Summary of peripheral post-thymic mechanisms of tolerance.

Pathogenesis

Sequestration of antigens in some tissues: Many self-antigens are effectively kept separate from T cells of immune system. It occurs by sequestration of antigens in areas, where these do not communicate with immune cells in blood and lymph.

Lack of costimulatory signal to T cells: Under physiological state, costimulatory signal CD28 (B7-1 and B7-2) causes functional activation of T cells due to transmission of positive signals. Lack of costimulatory signal CD28 (B7-1 and B7-2) causes functional *inactivation of autoreactive T cells without apoptosis*, when exposed to antigenic peptides.

Transmission of negative signal to T cells: It occurs by transmission of negative signals to T cells. TCR on T cells are unable to trigger biochemical signals due to activation of ubiquitin ligases.

Privileged sites protected by regulatory mechanisms: Some self-antigens are effectively kept separate form immune system. It occurs by sequestration of antigens in areas, where these do not communicate with immune cells in blood and lymph. Immunologically privileged sites are *brain, eye (vitreous humor), testis, uterus (fetus)*. In these sites, lymphocytes are controlled by apoptosis or cytokines such as TNF-β and IL-10.

Clone deletion of T cells by apoptosis: Repeated stimulus to T cells by antigen causes apoptosis by Fas-FasL system. Self-peptide antigens are abundant in body. These are presented by APCs in association with self-MHC to TCR on T cells. APCs also possess B7 ligand, which binds to CD28 of T cells. It results in upregulation of Fas (CD95) receptor, and also expression of FasL on activated T cells.

Regulation by suppressive cytokines: Cells which recognize self-antigens develop into regulatory T cells. Regulatory cells belong to CD4+ T cell lineage. These also express CD25+, α chain of IL-2 receptor and transcription factor of the family Fox p3. These cells may synthesize IL-4, IL-10 and TGF-β resulting in inhibition of lymphocyte activation and effector function. Mutation of Fox p53 is associated with IPEX (immune dysregulation, polyneuropathy, enteropathy, X-linked).

AUTOIMMUNE DISEASES

OVERVIEW

Autoimmune reactions cause disease, when immune system is not able to distinguish self from nonself-antigens. Autoantibodies or host T cells attack against self-antigens in tissues or organs. It may be systemic or organ-specific. Susceptibility to autoimmune disease appears to be influenced by gender and by genes in the MHC. Autoimmune diseases are mediated by types II to IV hypersensitivity reactions. These disorders commonly affect females.

Examples

These include systemic lupus erythematosus, rheumatoid arthritis, Hashimoto's thyroiditis, type I diabetes mellitus, myasthenia gravis, autoimmune hemolytic anemia, Sjögren's syndrome, and multiple sclerosis. Selected autoimmune diseases are shown in Table 4.53. *Molecular mimicry* (tissue antigens cross reactivity with microbial antigen) is shown in Table 4.54 and therapeutic strategies in autoimmune diseases are shown in Table 4.55.

PATHOGENESIS

Mechanism of autoimmune disorders occurs by breakdown of peripheral tolerance. There is no evidence of breakdown of central tolerance. A number of possible mechanisms may mediate autoimmunity. Pathogenesis of autoimmune disease is shown in Fig. 4.55.

GENETIC FACTORS

Susceptibility to autoimmune disease is influenced by genes in the major histocompatibility complex (MHC). Some HLA antigens are associated with increased incidence of certain autoimmune disorders.

For example, there is increased incidence of *Hashimoto's thyroiditis in HLA-DR5 and HLA-B5-positive individuals*.

Table 4.53: Selected autoimmune diseases

Disease	Organ or tissue	Type of hypersensitivity	Characteristics
Endocrine system			
Hashimoto's thyroiditis	Thyroid	II	Destruction of the thyroid follicles
Graves' disease	Thyroid	II	Antibodies against thyroid-stimulating hormone receptors
Type I diabetes mellitus	Pancreas	II	Antibodies cause destruction of insulin secreting cells
Addison disease	Adrenal gland	II	Antibodies against surface antigens on steroid producing cells; microsomal antigens
Male infertility	Testes	II	Antibodies against surface antigens on spermatozoa
Skin			
Pemphigus vulgaris	Skin	II	Antibodies against proteins in intercellular junctions of epidermal cells resulting in bullae formation
Bullous pemphigoid	Skin	II	Antibodies against basement membrane
Vitiligo	Skin surface antigens	II	Antibodies against surface antigens on melanocyte
Neuromuscular system			
Myasthenia gravis	Neuromuscular junction	II	Antibody formed against acetylcholine receptors at neuromuscular junction resulting in inhibiting acetylcholine binding and downregulation of receptors
Multiple sclerosis	Neural tissue	II, IV	T cells and antibodies sensitized to surface antigens on myelin sheath resulting in destroy neurons
Rheumatic fever	Heart	II	Cardiac antigens that cross react with group A streptococci (molecular mimicry)
Eyes			
Sjögren's syndrome	Lacrimal gland	II	Antibodies formed against antigens on lacrimal gland, salivary gland, thyroid gland and nuclei of cells
Gastrointestinal tract and hepatobiliary system			
Pernicious anemia	Gastric parietal cells	II	Antibodies formed against intrinsic factor synthesized by parietal cells prevent transport of vitamin B_{12}
Primary biliary cirrhosis	Liver	II	Antibodies formed against bile duct cells
Connective tissue			
Rheumatoid arthritis	Joints	II, IV	Antibodies formed against collagen IgG (rheumatoid factor)
Ankylosing spondylitis	Joints	II	Sacroiliac and spinal apophyseal joints
Systemic lupus erythematosus	Multiorgans involvement	II, III	Antibodies formed against nuclear antigens (DNA and anti-DNA)
Scleroderma (excess collagen deposition in organs)	Systemic involvement	II	Antibodies formed against many intracellular organelles
Blood vessels			
Vasculitis caused by ANCA	Blood vessels	II	ANCA-induced vasculitis resulting in neutrophil degranulation and inflammation

Contd...

Table 4.53: Selected autoimmune diseases (Contd...)

Disease	Organ or tissue	Type of hypersensitivity	Characteristics
Kidneys and lung			
Goodpasture syndrome	Kidney glomeruli and lung alveoli	II	Antibodies to Goodpasture antigen in non-collagenous proteins in basement membrane of glomeruli and alveoli
Renal system			
Immune complex mediated glomerulonephritis	Kidneys	II, III	Immune complexes formed in excess
Hematological system			
Idiopathic neutropenia	Neutrophils	II	Antibodies formed against surface antigen—present on neutrophils
Idiopathic lymphopenia	Lymphocytes	II	Antibodies formed against surface antigen present on lymphocytes
Autoimmune hemolytic anemia	RBCs	II	Antibodies formed against surface antigen—present on RBCs resulting in hemolysis
Autoimmune thrombocytopenic purpura	Platelets	II	Antibodies formed against platelet membrane proteins

Table 4.54: Molecular mimicry (tissue antigens cross-reactivity with microbial antigen)

Microbial antigen	Tissue self-antigen with similar structure	Disease produced as a result of molecular mimicry
Group A streptococcal antigen	Antigen found in heart and joints	Rheumatic fever
Coxsackie B4 nuclear antigen	Glutamate decarboxylase present in islet cells of pancreas	Insulin-dependent diabetes mellitus
Campylobacter jejuni glycoproteins	Myelin associated gangliosides and glycolipids	Guillain-Barré syndrome

Table 4.55: Therapeutic strategies in autoimmune diseases

Target	Therapeutic strategies
Self-reactive lymphocytes	Inhibition of lymphocyte function (cytotoxic drugs, cyclosporine A, corticosteroids)
	Reinduction of anergy (peptide therapy)
	Removal of co-stimulation (anti-CD28 antibodies)
	Induction of inhibitory T cells (oral feeding of antigen)
Tissue damage	Anti-inflammatory drugs (corticosteroids)
Organ dysfunction	Replacement therapy (joint replacement, renal dialysis, administration of thyroxine in hypothyroidism and insulin in diabetes mellitus)

Environmental factors: Some viruses may initiate autoimmune reactions in genetically susceptible persons. These trigger autoimmune islet cell destruction resulting in type 1 diabetes mellitus.

Exposure of cryptic self and epitope spreading: Cryptic self means hidden epitopes or protein that has not been exposed during embryonic life. Generally each self-protein in the body expresses a few epitopes to T cells during embryonic development. *Thus, these cells are either deleted in the thymus or undergo anergy in the periphery. But sometimes during adult life, the protein may present some uncommon epitopes, which may lead to autoimmune reaction.*

Host antigens recognized as non-self: Host antigens are recognized as non-self, if modified by viral infection, inflammation, and trauma or forming complex with a drug. Examples include *thyroglobulin, lens protein, and spermatozoa.*

A foreign antigen may share a common structure with a host antigen.

Immunopathology including Amyloidosis

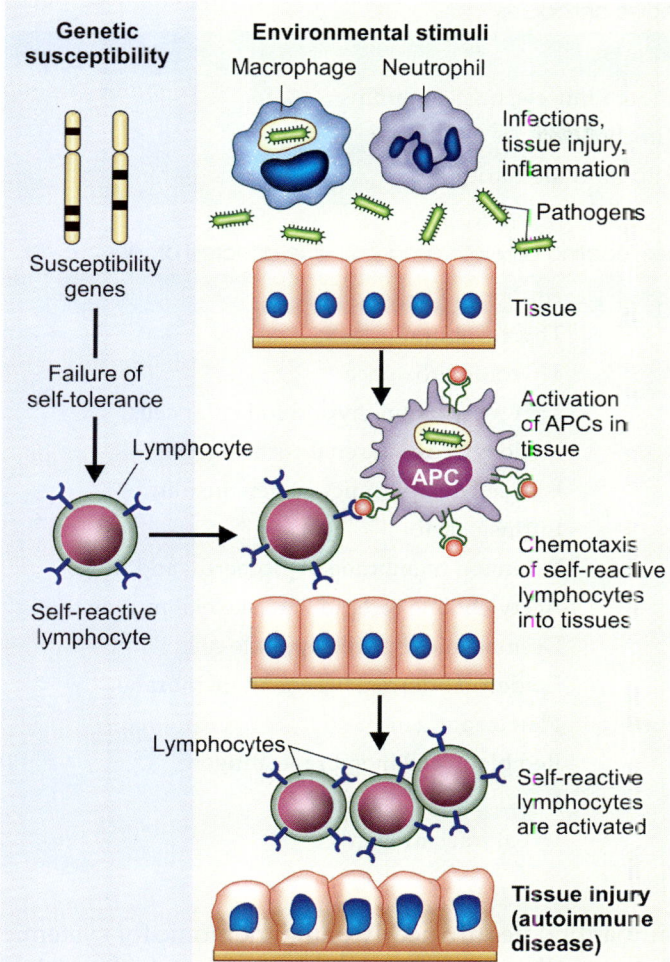

Fig. 4.55: Pathogenesis of autoimmune disease. Autoimmune disease results from susceptibility of genes that may interfere with self-immune tolerance and injurious stimuli leading to influx of lymphocytes into the tissue. Activation of lymphocytes causes tissue damage.

Release of sequestered antigens: Spermatozoa and ocular antigens are completely sequestered during development. These act as foreign bodies, when these come in contact with systemic circulation resulting in immune response.

Autoantibodies: Many autoimmune disorders show presence of autoantibodies directed against host tissue. The demonstration of autoantibodies is presumptive and not entirely conclusive in the diagnosis of autoimmune nature of disorders.

Dysfunctional immunoregulation: Autoimmune disorders are caused by the following mechanisms: (i) there may be increase in helper CD4+ T cells function, or decrease in suppressor CD8+ T cells function, (ii) EB virus may activate B cells resulting in polyclonal antibody synthesis. *Superantigens* (TSST, *Staphylococcus*) activate a large pool of CD+4 T cells in antigen-independent manner without relation to their epitope specificity, (iii) there may be thymic defects of T cell.

Breakdown of T cells anergy: APCs express B7 ligand that synthesize IL-2 that stimulates Th1 cells as in case of multiple sclerosis.

Failure of apoptosis: Failure of apoptosis allows persistence and proliferation of autoreactive T cells in peripheral tissues.

AUTOANTIBODIES AFFECTING ORGANS

Multisystem autoimmune disorders are shown in Table 4.56. Organ specific autoimmune disorders without organ specific antibodies are shown in Table 4.57. Organ specific autoimmune disorders with autoantibodies reacting only with antigens in the affected organs are shown in Table 4.58.

Table 4.56: Multisystem autoimmune disorders

Organ	Disease	Antigen
Exocrine gland	Sjögren's syndrome	Single-stranded RNA (Ro), duct epithelia, mitochondria
Joints	Rheumatoid arthritis	IgG
Kidney	Systemic lupus erythematosus	Double-stranded DNA, single-stranded DNA, histones, Sm (Smith) antigen (ribonuclear antigen), cardiolipin
	Scleroderma	DNA topoisomerase, centromeres
	Mixed connective tissue disease	DNA
Skin	Discoid lupus erythematosus	Nuclear antigens
	Dermatomyositis	Extractable nuclear antigen
	Scleroderma	DNA topoisomerase, centromeres
Muscle	Dermatomyositis	Extractable nuclear antigen

Table 4.57: Organ specific autoimmune disorders without organ specific antibodies

Disease	Antigen
Chronic active hepatitis	Smooth muscle, nuclear lamins
Primary biliary cirrhosis	Mitochondria
Ulcerative colitis	A lipopolysaccharide

Table 4.58: Organ specific autoimmune disorders with autoantibodies reacting only with antigens in the affected organs

Organ	Disorder	Antigen
Thyroid gland	Hashimoto's thyroiditis	Thyroglobulin
	Primary myxedema	Thyroid peroxidase
	Graves' disease	TSH receptor on thyroid follicular cells
Adrenal gland	Addison's disease	Hydoxylase in adrenal cortical cells
Pancreas	Insulin-dependent diabetes mellitus	Islet cell cytoplasmic antigen; insulin
Stomach	Pernicious anemia	Intrinsic factor
Kidney	Goodpasture syndrome	Basement membrane of glomeruli and lungs
Skeletal muscle	Myasthenia gravis	Acetylcholine receptors on skeletal muscle
Skin	Pemphigus vulgaris	Desmosomes between prickle cell
	Pemphigoid	Epidermal-dermal basement membrane
Hematological disorders	Idiopathic thrombocytopenic purpura	Platelet antigen
	Autoimmune hemolytic anemia	Red blood cell membrane antigen
Eye	Phagogenic uveitis	Lens
	Sympathetic ophthalmia	Uveal tract antigen

CONNECTIVE TISSUE (COLLAGEN TISSUE) DISEASES

These encompass a group of loosely related conditions, most of which feature fibrinoid change in connective tissue. They may be of autoimmune origin; antinuclear antibodies (ANAs) and various other autoantibodies are often present.

SYSTEMIC LUPUS ERYTHEMATOSUS (SLE)

Systemic lupus erythematosus (SLE) is an autoimmune chronic inflammatory disease characterized by a generalized dysregulation and hyperactivity of B cells, with production of *autoantibodies to DNA, RNA, and autologous proteins*. The production of autoantibodies leads to immune complex formation.

These immune complexes can be deposited in glomeruli, skin, lungs, joints synovium, mesothelium (serous membranes) and other organs. Renal involvement is most common complication of SLE. It can occur at all ages, but is more common in young women during childbearing age.

Pathogenesis

Antinuclear antibodies: Autoantibodies are formed against double-stranded DNA and soluble nuclear Sm (Smith) antigen part of nucleosome. High titers of these autoantibodies are nearly pathognomonic for systemic lupus erythematosus. Insoluble aggregates of immune complex are deposited in vessel walls, serosal surfaces, and other extravascular sites, and complement is bound.

Tissue damage: The antigen-antibody-complement complexes are highly chemotactic for neutrophils, which release lysosomal enzymes and other mediators of tissue damage (prostaglandins, kinins, and free radicals).

Clinical Features

Patient presents with fever, malaise, lymphadenopathy, and weight loss. Clinical manifestations in systemic lupus erythematosus are shown in Fig. 4.56 and Table 4.59.

Skin manifestations: Patient develops *butterfly rash over the base of the nose and malar eminences*, often is accentuated by sun exposure. When lupus causes superficial blood vessels to become inflamed, patient may develop telangiectasis (spider vein), red lines and painful bumps. *A biopsy of sun-exposed skin that is not involved with a rash will demonstrate immune complex deposition with SLE.*

Ulcers in mucous membranes: Lupus can cause ulcers in the mucous membranes particularly in the nose, throat, and mouth.

Immunopathology including Amyloidosis 4

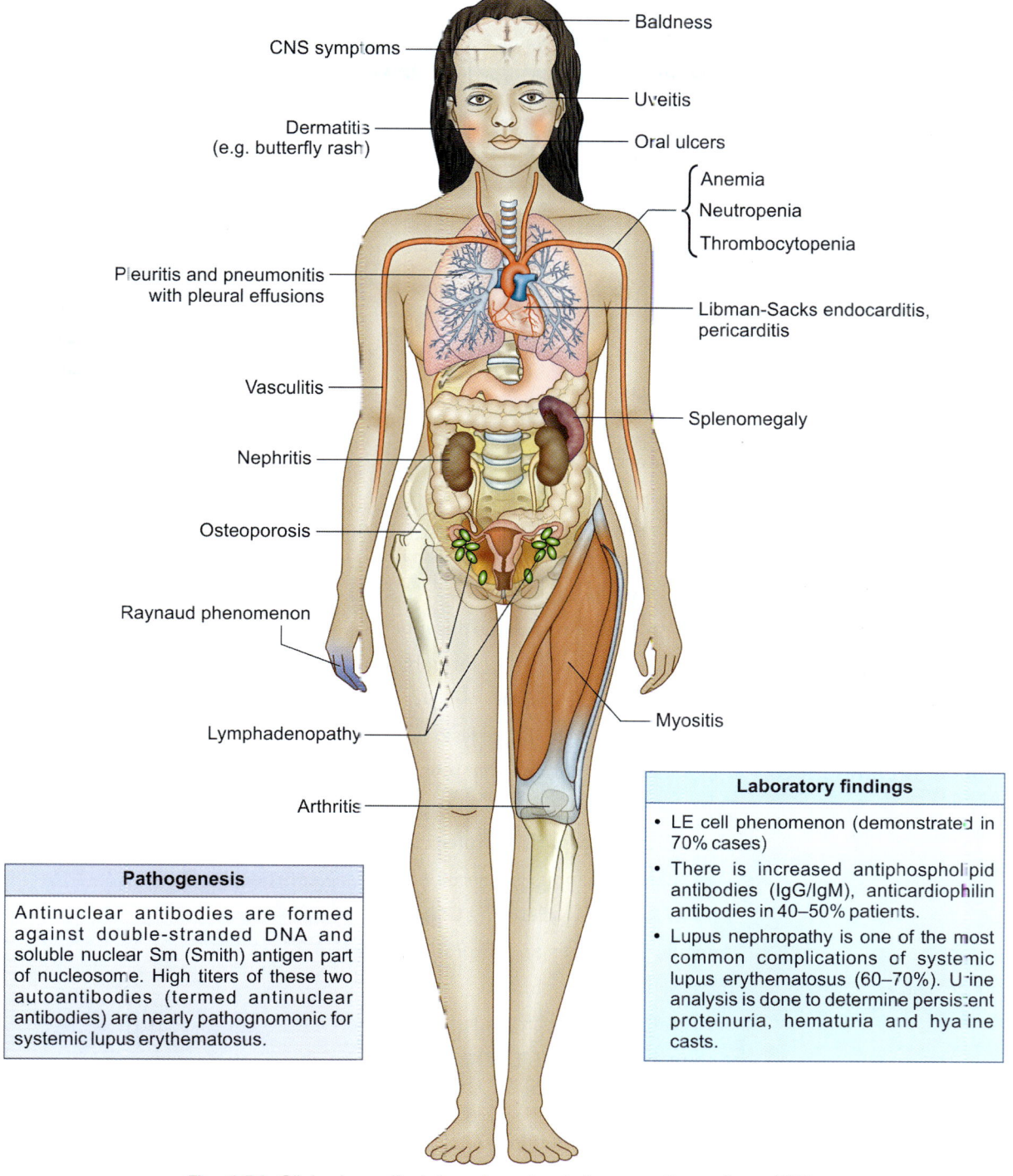

Fig. 4.56: Clinical manifestations in systemic lupus erythematosus (SLE).

Pathogenesis

Antinuclear antibodies are formed against double-stranded DNA and soluble nuclear Sm (Smith) antigen part of nucleosome. High titers of these two autoantibodies (termed antinuclear antibodies) are nearly pathognomonic for systemic lupus erythematosus.

Laboratory findings

- LE cell phenomenon (demonstrated in 70% cases)
- There is increased antiphospholipid antibodies (IgG/IgM), anticardiophilin antibodies in 40–50% patients.
- Lupus nephropathy is one of the most common complications of systemic lupus erythematosus (60–70%). Urine analysis is done to determine persistent proteinuria, hematuria and hyaline casts.

Musculoskeletal system: Most people with lupus develop *painful, swollen*, but nonerosive arthritis. Joints are asymmetrical involved such as *hands, knees* and *seldom spine*. Nonspecific muscle pain is another common symptom.

Raynaud phenomenon: It is manifested by vasospasm of small vessels, most often of the fingers.

Lungs involvement: Patient develops diffuse interstitial pulmonary fibrosis, manifested as interstitial pneumonitis or diffuse fibrosing alveolitis.

Serous membranes: These show inflammation of pericardium and pleura.

Heart: Nonbacterial cardiac vegetations are present on both sides of the mitral valve leaflet (most common)

Table 4.59: Clinical manifestations in systemic lupus erythematosus

Organs involved	Pathological findings
Skin	Butterfly rash over the base of the nose and malar eminences
	Inflammation of superficial blood vessels responsible for telangiectasis (spider vein), red lines and painful bumps
Nose, throat, and mouth	Ulcers in mucous membranes
Musculoskeletal system	Painful, swollen, but non-erosive arthritis of hands, knees and seldom spine
Fingers	Vasospasm of small vessels (Raynaud phenomenon)
Lungs	Diffuse interstitial pulmonary fibrosis
	Pleuritis
Heart	Libman-Sacks endocarditis (mitral valve involvement)
	Pericarditis
Blood vessels	Immune complex-mediated vasculitis
Cervical lymph nodes	Lymphadenopathy
Spleen	Splenomegaly
Female genital system	Repeated spontaneous miscarriages attributable to antibody-mediated inhibition of t-PA activity necessary for trophoblastic invasion of the uterus
Antiphospholipid antibody syndrome (IgG)	Spontaneous abortion
	Recurrent arterial or venous thromboses (deep veins, portal vein, pulmonary artery)
	Prolonged activated partial thromboplastin time (APTT)
Central nervous system	Psychiatric manifestations
Ophthalmic fundus examination	Yellowish, cotton wool-like lesions (cytoid bodies)
Kidneys (lupus nephritis patterns according to WHO)	*Type I:* Lupus nephritis (asymptomatic)
	Type II: Lupus nephritis (focal segmental glomerulosclerosis)
	Type III: Lupus nephritis (proteinuria nephritic range)
	Type IV: Membranous glomerulonephritis: Nephrotic syndrome
	Type V: Advanced sclerosing GN: Chronic renal failure
Blood smear	Anemia, leukopenia and thrombocytopenia
Blood biochemistry	Increased gammaglobulin
	Serum albumin is decreased
	Antinuclear test is positive

Lupus cells may be demonstrated *in vitro*.

and tricuspid valve (less frequent). These are known as *Libman-Sacks endocarditis*.

Blood vessels: Immune complex vasculitis involves vessels of almost any organ.

Spleen: In the spleen, perivascular fibrosis with concentric rings of collagen around splenic arterioles results in a characteristic *onion-skin appearance*.

Respiratory system: Patient develops pleurisy results in pain during inspiration.

Reproductive system: Repeated spontaneous miscarriages are sometimes the first sign of the disease. It is attributable to antibody-mediated inhibition of t-PA activity necessary for trophoblastic invasion of the uterus.

Antiphospholipid antibody syndrome: One-third of patients with systemic lupus erythematosus (SLE) possess elevated concentrations of antiphospholipid antibodies. *Prolonged activated partial thromboplastin time (APTT), recurrent arterial or venous thromboses (deep veins, portal vein, pulmonary artery), and spontaneous abortion are highly suggestive of the antiphospholipid antibody syndrome.* Current treatment includes anticoagulation therapy (aspirin, heparin, and warfarin) and immunosuppression in refractory cases.

CNS and eye changes: Patient develops neurologic and psychiatric manifestations. Ophthalmic fundus examination shows yellowish, cotton wool-like lesions (cytoid bodies).

Lupus nephropathy: *Nephritis is one of the most common complications of systemic lupus erythematosus (60–70%).* Immune complexes (DNA and anti-DNA) may localize in glomeruli by deposition from the circulation, formation *in situ*, or both.

These cause activation of complement system by classical pathway resulting in damage to tubules and interstitium. Decreased serum C3 level correlates with disease activity. Increased immune complex deposits and cellular proliferation indicates more severe form of disease.

Laboratory Findings

LE cell phenomenon: It is performed *in vitro*. It is possibly mediated by an ANA known as *antinucleosome-*specific autoantibody. LE cells are formed in a mixture of mechanically damaged neutrophils and autoantibody-containing patient serum. The LE test is positive in only about 70% of cases and has now been largely replaced by more sensitive determinations.

Immunofluorescence microscopy: It is performed to demonstrate antinuclear antibodies against DNA, histone proteins, non-histone proteins bound to RNA, nucleolar antigens. *Anti-Smith (Sm) antigen antibodies are formed against dsDNA-pathognomonic of SLE.*

Anti-phospholipid antibodies: These are present in 40–50% patients. There is an increase level of IgG/IgM anticardiophilin antibodies. *Lupus anticoagulant antibodies interfere with blood coagulation result in increased clotting time.*

Serum complement: It is often greatly decreased, especially in association with active renal involvement. Immune complexes at dermal-epidermal junction are demonstrable in skin biopsies.

Urine analysis: It is performed to determine persistent proteinuria, hematuria and hyaline casts.

Hematological tests: Reticulocyte count is increased as the patient may develop *autoimmune hemolytic anemia*. Peripheral blood smear shows leukopenia (lymphopenia), and thrombocytopenia. Bleeding time is prolonged.

PROGRESSIVE SYSTEMIC SCLEROSIS (SCLERODERMA)

Scleroderma is an autoimmune disease of connective tissue. *Inflammation stimulates fibroblasts to synthesize excessive collagen fibers.* It frequently occurs in skin, hence the name: sclero (Greek word hard) and derma (Greek word skin). It occurs most frequently in young women (25 to 50 years). It involves widespread fibrosis in *skin, gastrointestinal tract (especially the esophagus), heart, muscle, lung and kidney.*

Types of Scleroderma

Local Scleroderma

It is restricted to skin. The initial edema may last for several weeks or months. Skin thickening develops over a course of 3 years, and then the symptoms gradually stabilize or even reverse. Local scleroderma occurs in two forms:

Morphea scleroderma: Patient presents with discrete oval patches on *trunk, face, or extremities*, where skin is dry and thick. These lesions become pale in center and purplish around the edges.

Linear scleroderma: Patient presents with discolored line or band on *legs, arms or forehead*.

Systemic Sclerosis

It has a slow onset that begins as CREST syndrome, but it may eventually involve internal organs. Tissues most at risk are digestive tract, the heart and circulatory system, kidneys, lungs, musculocutaneous system, especially synovial membranes in joints and around tendons. It can be fatal. It has three major subtypes:

Limited scleroderma: This version begins in CREST syndrome, and it is only progressive.

Systemic scleroderma: It is more sudden onset and earlier involvement of internal organs.

Sine scleroderma: It does not involve the skin at all. It only involves organs.

Clinical Features

Patient initially presents with *skin changes (fixed facial appearance), painful joints, and dysphagia (esophagus involvement).*

Facial expression: Skin involvement results in fixed facial expression. There is thickening, tightening and rigidity of facial skin, with small constricted mouth and narrow lips, in atrophic phase of scleroderma.

Sclerodactyly: Fingers are partially fixed in significant position, *terminal phalanges atrophied,* fingers are pointed and ulcerated.

Esophageal fibrosis: It results in dysphagia. Sclerodactyly is present (claw-like appearance of the hand). Raynaud phenomenon is seen in approximately 75% of patients.

Renal involvement: The kidneys are involved in more than half of patients with scleroderma. They show marked vascular changes, often with focal hemorrhage and cortical infarcts. Among the most severely affected vessels are the interlobular arteries, arcuate arteries and afferent arterioles.

These blood vessels show marked thickening consisting of dense laminated matrix, rich in elastic fibers and small amount of collagen fibers. Early fibromuscular thickening of the subintima causes luminal narrowing, followed by fibrosis. Hypertension often occurs.

Pulmonary involvement: Interstitial fibrosis is a serious complication in scleroderma.

Autoantibodies

Autoantibodies virtually specific for scleroderma include: (i) Scl70 nonhistone nuclear protein topoisomerase in 70% cases, (ii) nucleolar autoantibodies (primarily against RNA polymerase), and (iii) anticentromere antibodies, which are also associated with the "CREST" variant of the disease.

CREST SYNDROME

CREST syndrome is a less severe variant of systemic sclerosis (scleroderma) characterized by calcinosis, Raynaud phenomenon, esophageal dysfunction, sclerodactyly, and telangiectasia.

CREST syndrome stands for:

- **C:** *Calcinosis:* It refers to accumulation of calcium deposits in the skin especially in fingers.
- **R:** *Raynaud's phenomenon:* It is a result of impaired circulation and vascular spasm in the hands.
- **E:** *Esophageal dysmotility:* Refers sluggishness of the digestive tract and chronic gastroesophageal reflux.
- **S:** *Sclerodactyly:* It is hardening of fingers, a result of the accumulation of scar tissue in the hands.
- **T:** *Telangiectasia:* It is discoloration of the skin caused by permanently stretched and damaged capillaries. It is also known as *spider veins*.

SJÖGREN SYNDROME

Sjögren's syndrome is an autoimmune disorder. It is characterized by keratoconjunctivitis sicca and xerostomia in the absence of other connective tissue disease. This disease most often affects women in their late middle age.

Pathogenesis

Antinuclear autoantibodies formed are directed against soluble nuclear nonhistone proteins, especially the *antigens SS-A and SS-B in patients with Sjögren's syndrome.* Autoantibodies to DNA or histones or salivary gland are rare.

Clinical Features

Patient presents with *triad of xerostomia (dry mouth), keratoconjunctivitis sicca (dry eyes) and any one of autoimmune disorders* such as rheumatoid arthritis (most common), scleroderma, Hashimoto's thyroiditis or polymyositis. Bilateral salivary glands show enlargement.

> **Light Microscopy**
>
> Salivary gland shows diffuse infiltration by lymphocytes and plasma cells obscuring the parenchyma. It may mimic lymphoma. In some cases, it can lead to malignant lymphoma.

Laboratory Findings

Serum electrophoresis reveals significant polyclonal hypergammaglobulinemia (a broad-based elevation of serum gammaglobulins). *Antinuclear autoantibodies against soluble nuclear nonhistone proteins SS-B is highly specific, however, against SS-A is less specific in Sjögren's syndrome.*

POLYMYOSITIS

Polymyositis is related to direct muscle cell damage produced by cytotoxic T cells. It involves the proximal muscles of the extremities. Initially, healthy muscle fibers are surrounded by CD8+ T cells and macrophages, followed by degeneration of muscle fibers. *Increased serum creatine kinase and frequent presence of ANAs (anti-Jo-1, an antibody against histidyl-tRNA synthetase) are characteristic.* Light microscopy reveals necrotic muscle cells along with lymphocytic infiltrate.

DERMATOMYOSITIS

Dermatomyositis is an immune-mediated disorder resulting in obliteration of capillaries, ischemic injury and muscle damage. *Involvement of capillaries of skin leads to reddish-purple rash over exposed areas of the face and neck, hence, condition is called dermatomyositis.* When dermatomyositis occurs in a middle-aged man, it is associated with an *increased risk of epithelial cancer*, most commonly *carcinoma of the lung*. Immunofluorescence microscopy demonstrates that the walls of many capillaries contain C5b–9 proteins (i.e. membrane attack complex).

MIXED CONNECTIVE TISSUE DISEASE

Mixed connective tissue disease (MCTD) shares many clinical features with other connective tissue disorders, but renal involvement is uncommon. It most often occurs in women (peak 35 to 40 years). *Patient presents with joints pain, myositis, Raynaud phenomenon and esophageal hypomotility*. There is *increased titer of specific ANAs (anti-nRNP)*. Immunofluorescence microscopy reveals speckled nuclear appearance on morphologic ANA analysis.

POLYARTERITIS NODOSA

Polyarteritis nodosa is immune complex mediated vasculitis. *It is characterized by segmental fibrinoid necrosis of small and medium arteries of many organs*. It most often occurs in men. Vessels undergo ulceration and thrombosis resulting in aneurysms and infarction of organs. Histopathologic changes at different stages of disease process may show acute or chronic or healing stage.

Pathogenesis

This disorder is mediated via type III hypersensitivity, through *antigen–antibody complexes*, in which *anti-neutrophilic cytoplasmic autoantibodies are formed resulting in liberation of hydrolytic enzymes* and *damage to vessels*. Hepatitis B virus (30–40%) and intravenous amphetamines play an important role in its pathogenesis. Drugs such as sulfonamides and penicillin, may form immunogenic hapten–protein complexes.

Organs Involved

These include renal arteries (85%), coronaries (75%), hepatic arteries (75%), mesenteric arteries (60%), musculocutaneous arteries (40%), arteries of central nervous system, peripheral nervous system, retina, pancreas and skin.

Clinical Features

Patient presents with abdominal pain, hypertension, uremia, polyneuritis, allergic asthma, urticaria or rash, splenomegaly, fever, leukocytosis, and proteinuria. Involvement of lungs results in chest pain, cough, dyspnea, and hemoptysis. Severe dyspnea and eosinophilia occur in 20% of patients.

RHEUMATOID ARTHRITIS

Rheumatoid arthritis is a chronic inflammatory auto-immune disorder that primarily attacks *synovium of peripheral joints (interphalangeal and metacarpophalangeal joints)* and the surrounding muscles, tendons, ligaments, and blood vessels. *Subcutaneous nodules are raised, firm, non-tender present in the olecranon bursa and along extensor surface of arm*. The skin slides freely over the nodules. This disorder is three times more common in women than men. It can occur at any age, but the peak onset is ages 30 to 60. It occurs most often in HLA-DR4-positive individuals.

Joints Involved

Knee joints are also involved with formation of subcutaneous nodules. Partial remissions and unpredictable exacerbations mark the course of this potentially crippling disease.

Rheumatoid Factor

Approximately 80% of patients with classic rheumatoid arthritis are positive for rheumatoid factor demonstrated in serum. This factor actually represents multiple antibodies, principally IgM, but sometimes IgG or IgA, directed against the Fc fragment of IgG. Rheumatoid factor is useful in diagnosis. Significant titers of RF are also found in patients with related collagen vascular diseases such as systemic lupus erythematosus, scleroderma, and dermatomyositis.

Morphologic Changes in Joints

Progressive changes include synovial inflammation, hyperplasia, hypertrophy, formation of numerous villi (fronds), formation of pannus (granulation tissue) invading articular cartilage, which results in destruction of joint capsule and subchondral bone. It is followed by fibrous ankylosis and calcification.

- *Stage I:* Synovitis develops from congestion and edema of the synovial membrane and joint capsule. Initially, it shows acute inflammation followed by infiltration by lymphocytes and plasma cells. Synovial cells undergo hyperplasia and hypertrophy and result in formation of numerous villi and frond-like folds.

- *Stage II:* Formation of pannus (thickened layers of granulation tissue), which covers and *invades articular cartilage and subchondral bone*. It eventually erodes and destroys the joint capsule and bone.

- *Stage III:* Fibrous ankylosis refers (fibrous invasion of the pannus and scar formation that occlude the joint space). Bone atrophy and misalignment cause visible deformities and restrict movement, causing muscle atrophy, imbalance, and possibly partial dislocations.

- *Stage IV: Fibrous tissue calcifies, resulting in bony ankylosis (fixation of a joint) and total immobility.* Pain associated with movement may restrict active joint use and cause fibrous or bony ankylosis, soft tissue contractures, and joint deformities. Subcutaneous nodules develop in approximately one-third of patients.

Extra-articular Manifestations

These include effusions (pleura, pericardium), vasculitis, and anemia of chronic disease, neurologic manifestations, lymphadenopathy and secondary reactive amyloidosis.

Clinical Features

Patient presents with fatigue, malaise, anorexia, weight loss, fever, and myalgia, bilateral symmetrical swelling and stiffness of joints especially in the morning or after inactivity. Chronic joint changes occur in proximal interphalangeal and metacarpophalangeal joints of the hands. Patient develops ulnar deviation of fingers resulting from synovitis of ligaments. Minimal radial deviation of the wrist may occur.

GOODPASTURE SYNDROME

Goodpasture syndrome is characterized by nephritic syndrome and pulmonary hemorrhage (hemoptysis). Goodpasture antigen is normally present in glomerular basement membrane and lung alveoli. *Autoantibodies cross react with antigens located in glomerular basement membrane and pulmonary alveoli.* Immunofluorescence study reveals smooth and linear staining pattern due to antibody and complement in Goodpasture nephritis (renal and lung basement membrane). It is complement-mediated type to hypersensitivity reaction resulting in increased susceptibility to phagocytosis.

GRAVES' DISEASE

Antibodies to the TSH receptor are seen in patients with Graves' hyperthyroidism—an autoimmune disorder that mimics the action of TSH, but are not regulated by natural negative feedback controls. It leads to follicular glandular hyperplasia and increased synthesis of thyroid hormones resulting in features of hyperthyroidism. Patient also develops exophthalmos due to infiltration by lymphocytes in retrobulbar ocular muscles in 60–90%. It is type II hypersensitivity reaction (anti-receptor mediated).

MYASTHENIA GRAVIS

Myasthenia gravis is a type-II hypersensitivity disorder caused by *antibodies that bind to the acetylcholine receptors in the motor end plates of skeletal muscles.* The antibodies bind to postsynaptic receptors and block neurotransmission resulting in progressive muscle weakness involving particularly the external ocular, eyelids and proximal limb muscles. *It may cause death by respiratory muscle paralysis.* This is an example of type II hypersensitivity reaction (anti-receptor mediated).

PEMPHIGUS VULGARIS

Autoantibodies formed against desmoglein-3 which disrupts intercellular junctions in epidermis in patients with pemphigus vulgaris, characterized by blistering (vesicles) skin disorder. Immunofluorescence study reveals smooth and linear staining pattern in pemphigus (skin intercellular protein, desmosomes). This is an example of type II hypersensitivity reaction (anti-receptor mediated).

HLA SYSTEM

The HLA system consists of a group of related proteins referred to as HLAs. The genes that code for HLAs are called *histocompatibility genes* and are localized to a region on the short arm of chromo-some 6, known as the *major histocompatibility complex*.

The HLA system is important in organ transplantation, where HLA typing and matching of donor and recipient are now widely used to predict tissue compatibility.

MAJOR CLASSES OF HLAs

All human cells express class I HLA molecules, whereas class II HLAs are displayed primarily on *macrophages, dendritic cells, Langerhans' cells, B cells, and some T cells.*

The two major classes of HLAs are separated on the basis of structure and tissue distribution. Structure of major histocompatibility complex is shown in Fig. 4.57. Molecules of the human major histocompatibility complex are shown in Fig. 4.58. Comparison of class I HLA and class II HLA molecules is shown in Table 4.60.

CLASS I HLAs

These include HLA-A, HLA-B, and HLA-C found on almost all nucleated human cells. *Class I HLAs recognized by cytotoxic CD8+ T cells are involved in tissue graft rejection and cell-mediated killing of virus-infected cells.* Standard

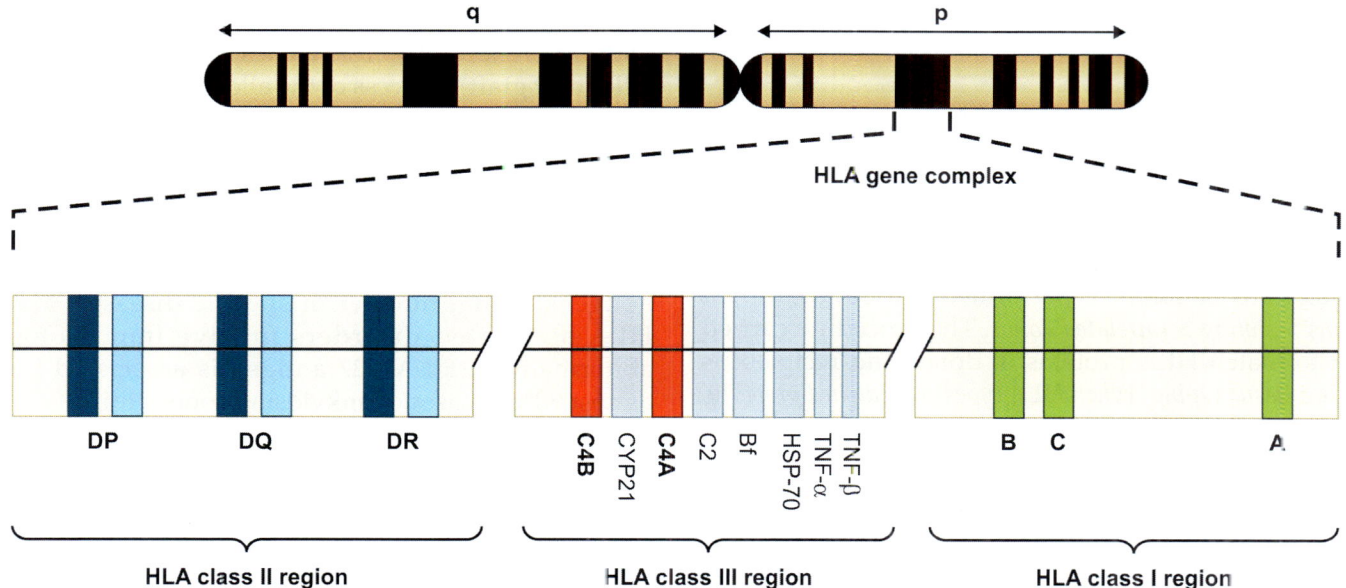

Fig. 4.57: Structure of major histocompatibility complex.

serologic techniques are used for identification of HLA-A and HLA-B antigens with the aim to predict the likelihood of long-term graft survival.

CLASS II HLAs

These are chiefly found on immunocompetent cells such as macrophages, dendritic cells, Langerhans' cells, B cells, and some T cells (CD4+ T cells). The products of these genes determine histocompatibility between donor and recipient tissues in transplants. Class II HLA molecules are recognized by CD4+ T cells, which become activated to synthesize an array of cytokines.

Antigens present in class II HLA molecules are HLA-DP, HLA-DQ, and HLA-DR identified by standard serologic techniques or by mixed lymphocyte reactions.

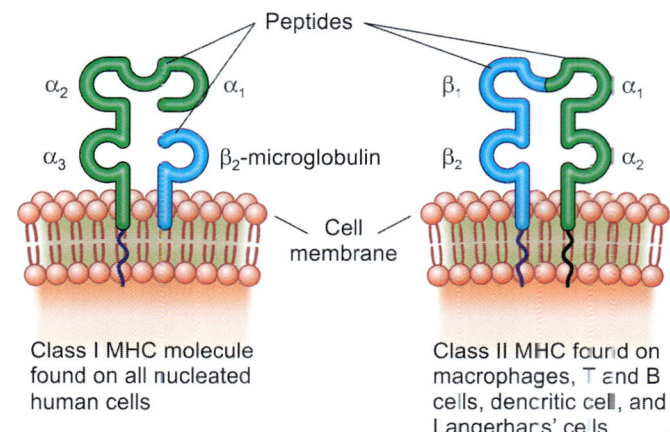

Fig. 4.58: Molecules of the human major histocompatibility complex.

Table 4.60: Comparison of class I HLA and class II HLA molecules

Characteristics	MHC I (class I HLA molecule)	MHC II (class II HLA molecule)
Expression on various cells	All human cells	Macrophages, dendritic cells, Langerhans' cells, B cells, helper CD4+ T cells
Encodes locus or loci in HLA molecule	Three loci HLA-A, HLA-B, HLA-C	One locus HLA-D, which is divided into HLA-DP, HLA-DQ, HLA-DR
Location of peptide binding cleft	Present between α_1 and α_2	Present between α_1 and β_2
Participation	Tissue graft rejection. Killing of virus-infected cells	CD4+ T cells synthesize cytokines
Diagnostic technique	Standard serologic techniques used for identification of HLA-A and HLA-B antigens with the aim to predict the likelihood of long-term graft survival	Standard serologic techniques or mixed lymphocyte reactions used for identification of HLA-DP, HLA-DQ, and HLA-DR antigens. HLA-D antigens identifiable only by mixed lymphocyte reactions

GlyCam-1 facilitates lymphocyte recirculation by providing a receptor for leukocyte attachment to high endothelial venules.

The HLA-Ds are identifiable only by mixed lymphocyte reactions.

CLINICAL ASPECT OF HLA SYSTEM

The array of HLA alleles on a homologue of our chromosome 6 is known as a haplotype. *An individual inherits one HLA haplotype from each parent. Identical twins have the identical haplotype. Therefore, the preference of organ transplantation is performed as follows: identical twins > sibling > unrelated donor.* The procedure carried out to match HLA proteins of donor and recipient is called *tissue typing. When HLA types are matched properly, the survival of transplanted organs increases dramatically.*

TYPE OF ORGAN TRANSPLANTS

Autograft refers to grafting of own tissue from one region to another region (skin graft). Grafts performed between identical twins are known as *isograft*. Grafting performed between individuals of same species but with different MHC/HLA alleles is known as *allograft* (allogenic graft). Success of the allograft depends upon matching and immunosuppressive drugs. Xenograft is referred to graft between animals of different species.

HLA ASSOCIATED DISEASES

There is a significant association of certain HLA antigens with a number of specific diseases. Many HLA associated disorders involve immunologic abnormalities. HLA-B27 antigen is associated with almost 90% of cases of ankylosing spondylitis.

Specific HLA antigens are also associated with insulin-dependent diabetes mellitus, rheumatoid arthritis, uveitis, and Reiter's syndrome (urethritis, conjunctivitis, and arthritis), as well as with many other entities. HLA associated diseases are shown in Table 4.61.

Table 4.61: HLA associated diseases

HLA class	Examples	Diseases
Class I	B-27	Ankylosing spondylitis, psoriatic arthritis, Reiter's syndrome
	B-8	Graves' disease (hyperthyroidism), myasthenia gravis
	CW-6	Psoriasis
	B-21	Behçet disease
Class II	DR-2	Multiple sclerosis, necrolepsy, Goodpasture's syndrome
	DR-3	Type I diabetes mellitus, dermatitis herpetiformis, chronic active hepatitis, Sjögren's syndrome
	DR-4	Pemphigus vulgaris, rheumatoid arthritis, type I diabetes mellitus
	DR-8	Type I diabetes mellitus
	DQ-1	Pemphigus vulgaris
	DQ-2 and DQ-8	Celiac sprue
	DQ-8	Type I diabetes mellitus

TRANSPLANTATION IMMUNOLOGY

ORGAN TRANSPLANTATION

Organ transplantation is the treatment of choice for end stage organ failure. *For a successful graft, donor and recipient must be matched for ABO blood groups and, ideally, for as many HLA antigens as possible.*

Adverse immune responses can be suppressed by immunosuppressant drugs, radiation, or recipient T cell depletion. These processes, however, can result in clinically significant immunodeficiency.

Types of transplants: Organ grafts are of four types: Autografts, isografts, allogenic grafts and xenografts.

- *Autograft:* One's *own tissue* is grafted to another part, e.g. *skin autograft*.
- *Isograft:* Graft between *identical twin*s is known as *isograft*. Donor and recipient are genetically identical.
- *Allograft (allogenic graft):* Graft between individuals of *same species* but with *different MHC/HLA alleles*. Success of the graft depends upon matching and immunosuppressive drug like cyclosporine.
- *Xenograft:* Graft between animals of *different species is* known as *xenograft (e.g. monkey to human)*.

Major histocompatibility complex: Success of organ transplants and skin grafts depends on a proper matching of histocompatibility antigens that occur on all cells of the body. Chromosome 6 of mouse contains a cluster of genes known as *the major histocompatibility complex*, which in humans is called *human leukocyte antigen (HLA) complex*. The alleles of HLA genes are codominant.

- *The products of these genes determine histocompatibility*, i.e. compatibility between donor and recipient tissues in transplants. The array of HLA alleles on a homologue of our chromosome 6 is known as a *haplotype*.
- An individual inherits one HLA haplotype from each parent. The large number of alleles at this locus ensures that only identical twins have the identical haplotype. The best HLA matches would occur within a family. Therefore, the preference order for transplants is as follows: Identical twin > sibling parent > unrelated donor.

Tissue typing: The procedure carried out to *match HLA proteins of donor and recipient is called tissue typing*. When HLA types are matched properly, the *survival of transplanted organs increases* dramatically.

ORGAN TRANSPLANT REJECTION

The graft rejection response is initiated mainly by host cells that recognize the foreign HLA antigens of the graft, either directly (on APCs in the graft) or indirectly (after uptake and presentation by APCs). *There are four mechanisms of graft rejection: hyperacute rejection, acute cellular rejection, acute vascular rejection and chronic rejection.*

Preformed and *de novo* donor-specific antibodies (DSAs) are central to pathogenesis of hyperacute, acute rejection and chronic. Patterns of renal graft rejection are shown in Table 4.62. Comparison of acute and chronic transplant rejection is shown in Table 4.63.

HYPERACUTE ORGAN TRANSPLANT REJECTION

Hyperacute rejection occurs in the presence of pre-existing antibody to donor antigens. These preformed antibodies bind to graft endothelium immediately after transplantation within minutes of transplantation and complement activation. Rejection is a localized Arthus reaction marked by neutrophilic vasculitis, fibrinoid necrosis of small vessels, extensive thrombosis results in ischemic damage and rapid graft failure. Patient

Table 4.62: Patterns of renal graft rejection

Pattern of rejection	Mechanism
Hyperacute graft rejection	Mediated by preformed antibodies in recipient's plasma as a result of ABO incompatibility between donor and recipient
	Type II hypersensitivity reaction resulting in immune complex formation locally and occlusion of small blood vessels in graft
Early acute graft rejection	Antibody-mediated by partly by destruction of renal tubules by CD8+ T cells
Late acute graft rejection (11 days and 6 weeks after organ transplant)	Occurs in patients, who have been immunosuppressed with prednisolone and azathioprine
	Florid vascular damage occurs mediated by antibody resulting in complement
Chronic graft rejection	Fibromuscular hyperplasia of small- and medium-sized arteries with continuing endothelial injury resulting in ischemic necrosis of glomeruli (? immune mechanism)

Table 4.63: Comparison of acute transplant rejection and chronic transplant rejection

Characteristics	Acute transplant rejection	Chronic transplant rejection
Stage of rejection	It is second stage of rejection	It is third stage of rejection
Onset	It occurs within days or suddenly after cessation of immunosuppressive drugs	It occurs over months to years
Components	It consists of two components: (i) Acute cellular component comprises CD4+ T cells and CD8+ T cells, (ii) antibodies-mediated vasculitis	It does not consist of such components It is characterized by progressive dysfunction of the organs
Mechanism	It is mediated by inflammatory cells (CD4+ T cells and CD8+ T cells) and antibodies	It shows presence of macrophages, lymphocytes, plasma cells and eosinophils
Morphology	Acute rejection of kidney transplant shows injury to tubules and endothelium resulting in exfoliation of tubular cells in lumen and necrotizing vasculitis. The blood vessels of kidneys are thrombosed resulting in ischemic changes	Arterioles undergo fibrosis of renal vessels leading to ischemic injury to organ

presents with sudden cessation of urine output, along with fever and pain in the area of the graft site.

ACUTE RENAL TRANSPLANT REJECTION

Acute transplant glomerulopathy develops in 4–10% of allogenic transplant. Blood vessels of graft are destroyed by T cells and antibodies resulting in acute vascular rejection. Recognition of alloantigens in organ graft occurs by direct and indirect pathways. Pathogenesis of acute renal graft rejection by direct and indirect pathways is shown in Fig. 4.59.

Direct Pathway

Donor's class I and class II are recognized by host (recipient) cytotoxic CD8+ T cells and helper CD4+ T cells. Helper CD4+ T cells undergo proliferation and synthesize cytokine IFN-γ.

This cytokine (IFN-γ) activates macrophages resulting in damage to renal tubules. Cytotoxic CD8+ T cells responding to graft antigens differentiate to CTLs that damage graft's blood vessels and tubules. Acute cellular rejection within days to weeks to months after transplantation. Pathogenesis of acute graft rejection by direct pathway is shown in Fig. 4.60.

Clinical features: Patient presents with abrupt onset of azotemia and oliguria, which may be associated with fever and graft tenderness.

> **Light Microscopy**
> Light microscopy of rejected renal graft shows edema, interstitial infiltrates of lymphocytes (CD4+ T cells and CD8+T cells) and macrophages. Tubules show lymphocytic infiltration and tubular necrosis.

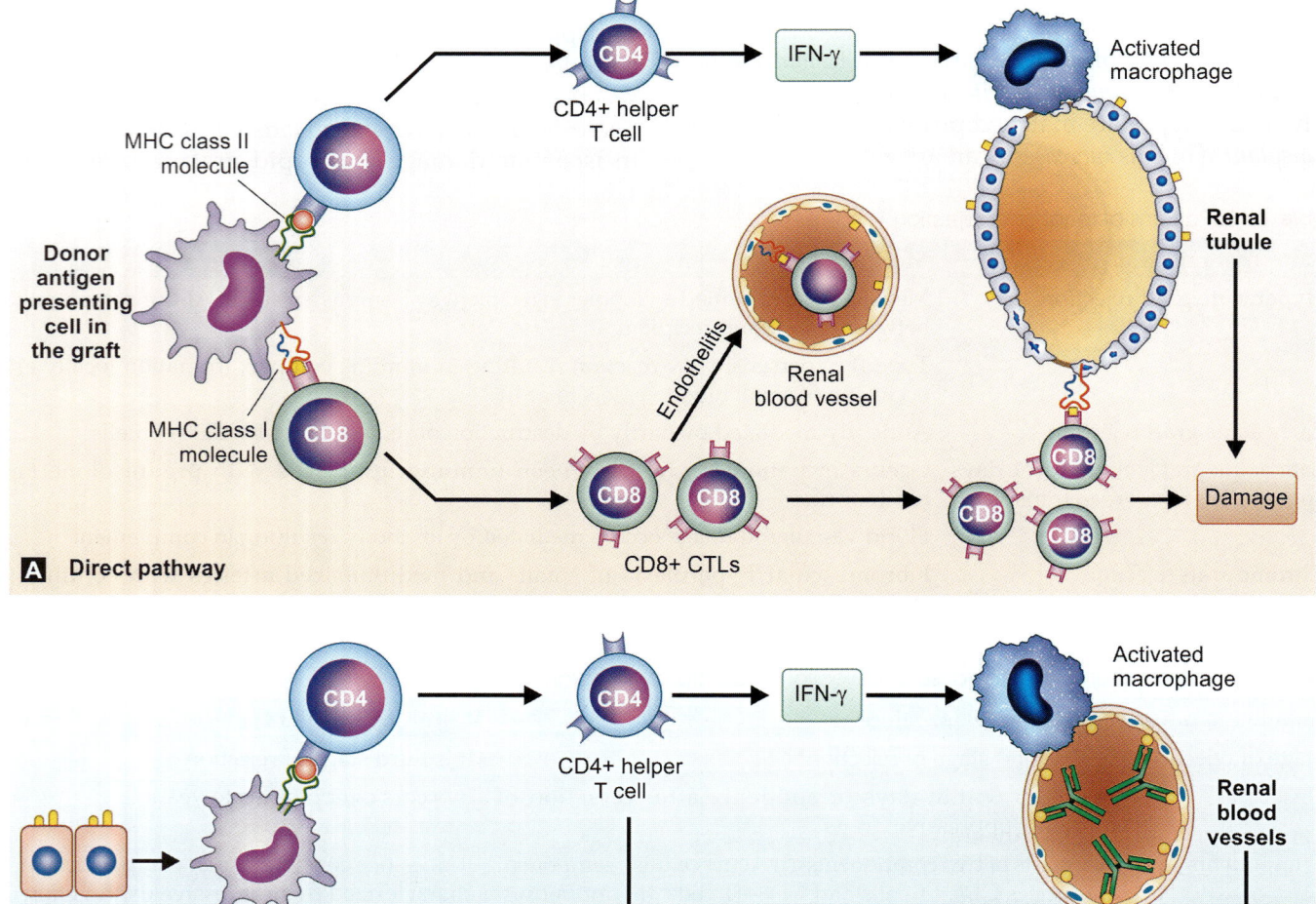

Fig. 4.59: Pathogenesis of renal graft rejection by direct and indirect pathways.

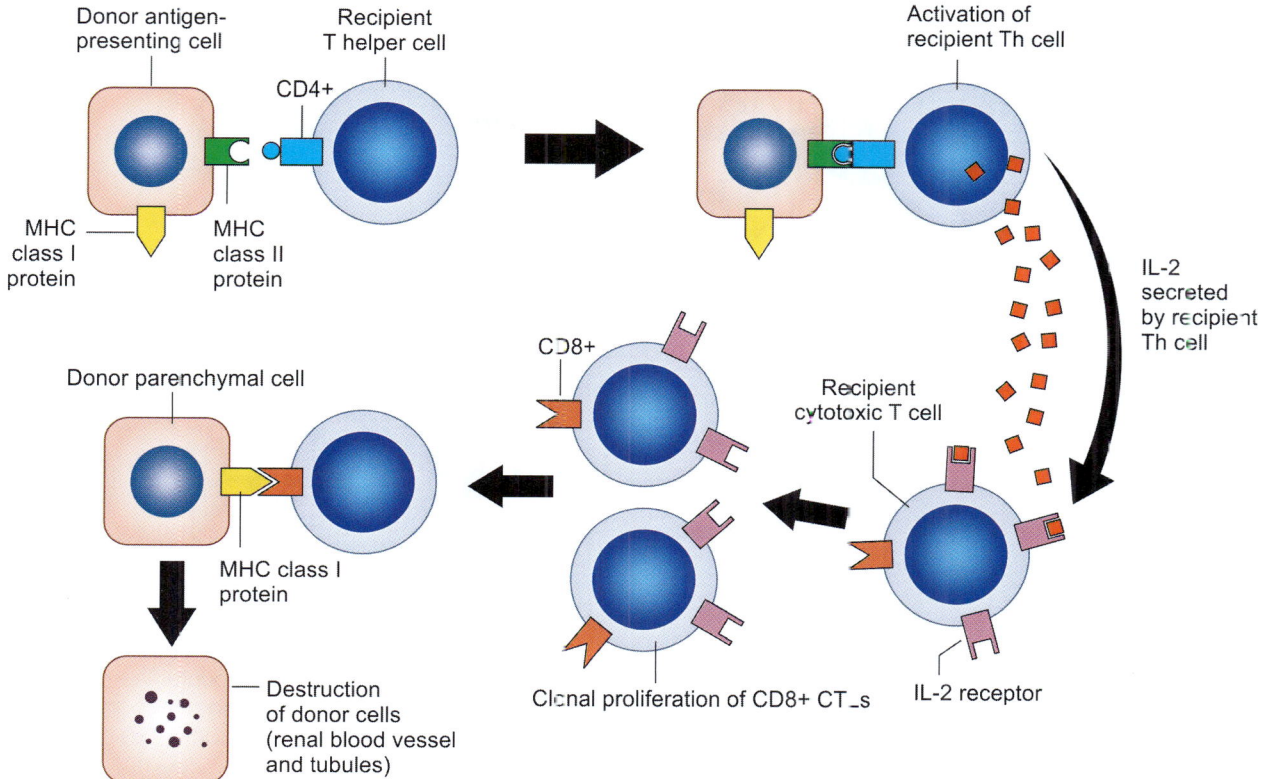

Fig. 4.60: Pathogenesis of acute graft rejection by direct pathway causes damage to blood vessels and tubules of graft in the recipient.

Indirect Pathway

When antibody-mediated mechanisms are prominent, it may show evidence of *arteritis with thrombosis* and *cortical necrosis*. Antibody-mediated rejection of solid transplant is a significant cause of morbidity and mortality. It is difficult to treat these cases. It affects recipients sensitized with pre-transplant donor-specific antibodies (DSAs) to human leukocyte antigens (HLAs) or post-transplant *de novo* HLA or non-HLA antibodies.

Risk factors: Risk factors include younger age, female gender, prior sensitization to OKT3, cytomegalovirus seropositivity, pregnancy, previous blood transfusions, surgical procedures, pre-transplant cardiac support with ventricular assist device and pre- or post-transplant hemodialysis.

Pathogenesis: Recipient antigen processing cells recognize and pick up graft antigens leading to activation of helper CD4+ T cells. These helper CD4+ T cells synthesize IFN-γ, which activates macrophages resulting in damage to renal blood vessels. Helper CD4+ T cells also stimulate B cells to synthesize antibodies. Antibody binding to antigen activates complement via classical pathway which causes endothelial injury of renal vessels. *Immunological detection of capillary C4d deposition in allografts has evolved as a sensitive and specific diagnostic tool for antibody-mediated rejection.*

Diagnosis: Gold standard tissue staining technique for C4d is immunofluorescence (IF) using a monoclonal antibody.

CHRONIC RENAL TRANSPLANT REJECTION

Chronic renal transplant rejection is primarily caused by antibody-mediated vascular damage within months to years after successful organ transplantation.

Rejection is characterized by *arteriosclerosis, glomerulosclerosis, and tubular atrophy*. T cell reaction and synthesis of cytokines induce proliferation of vascular smooth muscle cells especially kidney transplantation.

GRAFT-VERSUS-HOST DISEASE (GVHD)

Graft-versus-host disease is a significant problem, when *bone marrow transplantation* (immunocompetent cells) is performed in *aplastic anemia, acute leukemia and immunological deficiency patients.*

Lymphocytes (CD8+ T cells) from graft directly damage recipient host cells. GVHD can also occur when a patient with *severe combined immunodeficiency disease* (SCID) is transfused with blood containing HLA-incompatible lymphocytes. Potential reactions in organ transplantation are shown in Fig. 4.61.

Billingham described criteria for graft-versus-host disease.

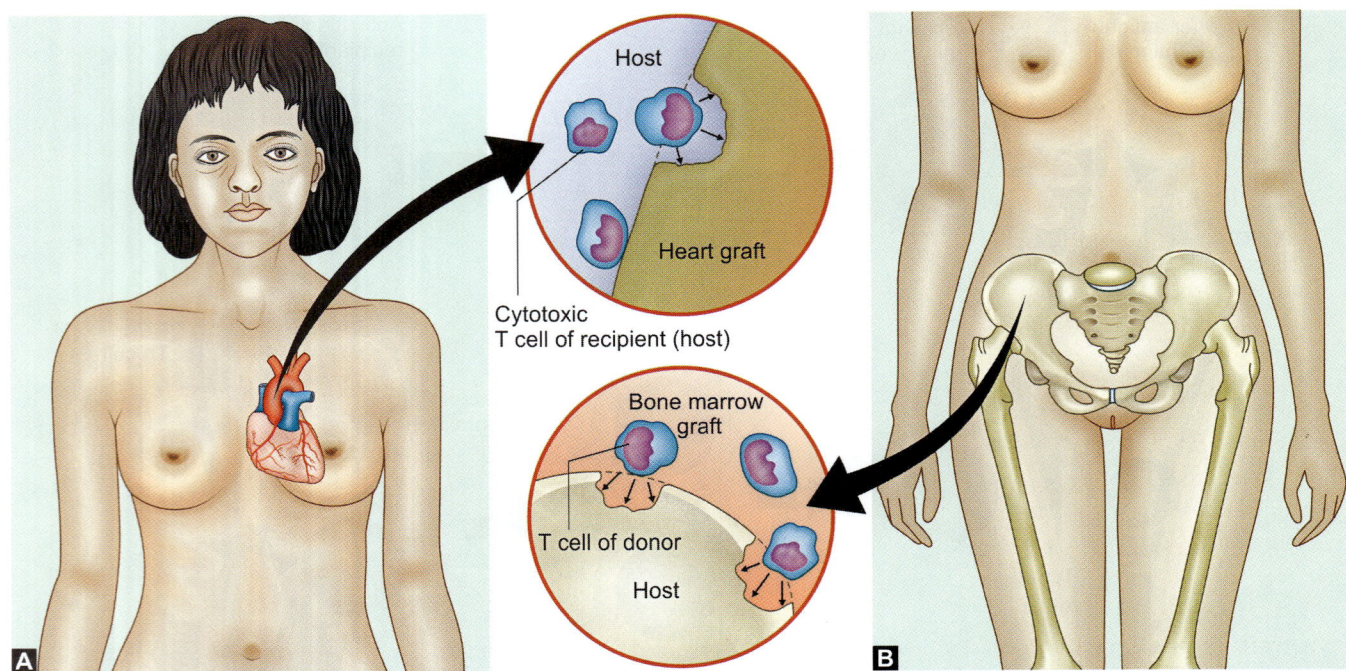

Fig. 4.61: Potential reactions in organ transplantation. (A) Cytotoxic T cells of host immune system encounter the cells of donated organ (heart) and mediate the organ rejection, (B) grafted bone marrow contains endogenous T cells that recognize host's tissues as foreign and mount an attack on many tissues and organs. The recipient will develop symptoms of graft-versus-host disease.

A donor graft has immunocompetent cells. Recipient possesses antigens foreign to graft.

Classification: There are two types of graft-versus-host disease: *Acute GVHD <100 days and chronic >100 days.*

PATHOGENESIS

CD8+ T cells from graft directly damage host epithelial cells of skin, liver and gastrointestinal mucosa. Cytokines from graft CD4+ T cells recruit macrophages, which damage host epithelial cells of skin, liver, and gastrointestinal mucosa (duodenum, ileum and colon).

Acute GVHD

Acute GVHD develops by priming of immune response, activation and expansion of donor; and effector phase.

- *Priming of immune cells:* Immunosuppression causes damage in several tissues including liver and gut. Gut damage is very important in the pathogenesis. Mucosa becomes permeable resulting in synthesis of IL-1 and TNF-α. There is upregulation of adhesion molecules and MHC antigens and increased recognition of host antigens by T cells. Entry of bacterial product (LPS) from systemic circulation aggravates graft-versus-host disease reaction.
- *Donor's cell activation and expansion:* T cells recognize the antigens presented by APCs in the presence of costimulatory molecules (CTLA-4: B7, CD28). Both CD4+ T cells and CD8+ T cells can initiate the GVH reaction. This depends on allogenic component of host.
- *Effector phase:* Along with T cells, NK cells also participate. These secrete cytokines that continue to stimulate other cells and damage tissue. *The Fas/FasL pathway and perforin/granzyme pathway play an important role in this effector phase.*

Chronic GVHD

Pathogenesis of chronic GVHD remains obscure. Role of development of autoantibodies is still not clear. Synthesis of cytokines by Th2 cells play role in the pathogenesis. Immune dysregulation causes immunodeficiency and autoantibodies to several cell-surface and intracellular proteins lead to autoimmunity. Various theories have been proposed in its pathogenesis.

- *Breakage of immune tolerance to self-antigens:* Damage to thymus epithelium dysregulates central tolerance by generation of CD4+ T cells from donor stem cells.
- *CD4+ T cells and CD25 regulatory T cells reduction:* These cells are reported to be reduced in chronic GVHD via synthesis of cytokines such as TGF-β and IL-10.
- *Role of B cells and their antibodies:* Increased level of BAFF drives B cell autoimmunity. There is development of antibodies to minor histocompatibility proteins encoded by Y chromosome in a male recipient receiving transplant from a female. There may be

role in amplification of autoimmune responses and in epitope spreading of autoreactive T cell and B cell.
- *Fibrotic change:* Synthesis of TGF-β and IL-13 produces fibrotic change. Recruitment of macrophages and other cells to the site causes tissue damage. There is C3 deposition at the dermo-epidermal junction in skin.

ORGANS AFFECTED

The major organs affected in GVHD include the skin, gastrointestinal tract, and liver. Clinically, GVHD manifests as *pruritic rash, diarrhea, abdominal cramps, anemia, hepatosplenomegaly and liver dysfunction*. Elevation of *serum bilirubin and liver enzymes* signals the *hepatic involvement*.

Acute GVHD

Acute graft-versus-host reaction occurs within 100 days of transplant. Most commonly seen is a triad involvement of *liver (hepatitis), skin (dermatitis) and duodenum (enteritis)*. Other systems may be involved causing pneumonitis, hemorrhagic cystitis, thrombocytopenia and anemia.

- *Skin involvement:* Patient presents with maculopapular rash, erythema, bullae, and desquamation. Skin epidermal cells are infiltrated by lymphocytes. Duodenal mucosa shows lymphocytic infiltration.
- *Liver involvement:* Patient presents with symptoms related to hepatitis. Liver shows lymphoid cells in portal triad invading and attacking hepatocytes, bile ducts, epithelial cells and vascular endothelial cells.
- *Duodenum involvement:* Patient presents with diarrhea (green, water, mucoid; may contain cells and fecal casts), intestinal bleeding and crampy abdominal pain. Barium studies show increased transit time and loss of haustral folds. Light microscopy reveals single cell necrosis/apoptotic bodies at the base of the crypts or glands.

Chronic GVHD

Chronic graft-versus-host reaction may follow acute GVHD or *de novo*. It is one of the problems affecting the long-term survivors of allogenic graft. It affects *liver and colon*.

Liver shows lymphocytic infiltration in portal triad, fibrosis and loss of bile ducts. Colon shows lymphocytic infiltration, glandular degeneration and mucosal atrophy with loss of glands. Other organs may be involved.

Patient may develop cholestasis, esophageal reflux and strictures, dryness and stenosis of vagina, polymyositis, fasciitis, myasthenia gravis, nephrotic syndrome, and positive autoimmune serology. Organs involved and clinical manifestations in chronic graft-versus-host disease are shown in Table 4.64.

Diagnostic modalities

- Demonstration of donor derived lymphocytes in the areas of tissue destruction in biopsy specimens, viz. dermo-epidermal junction, crypts of gut epithelium and bone marrow.
- DNA polymorphism studies are done using VNTR analysis fingerprinting.
- Polymerase chain reaction (PCR) with donor HLA-DR sequence analyses specific primers.
- Fluorescence *in situ* hybridization (FISH) using Y chromosome specific DNA probe combined with IHC using monoclonal antibodies define cellular phenotypes.
- Demonstration of one-way HLA match between the donor and the recipient is performed.

PREVENTION OF TRANSPLANT REJECTION

The chances of transplant rejection may be reduced by good matching between donor and recipient, and suppression of immune response of the recipient.

Table 4.64: Organs involved and clinical manifestations in chronic graft-versus-host disease

Organs	Clinical manifestations
Gastrointestinal tract	Dysphagia, pain, vomiting, diarrhea, abdominal pain
Skin	Skin rash (lichenoid, sclerodermatous, hyper-/hypopigmented, flaky) and alopecia
Oral and ocular organs	Sjögren's syndrome related to lacrimal gland destruction and reduced tear flow, dry and painful eyes, conjunctivitis, corneal ulcers
Liver	Increased transaminases, hyperbilirubinemia, cirrhosis
Lungs	Bronchiolitis obliterans (BO), bronchiolitis obliterans organizing pneumonia (BOOP)
Hematologic/immune system	Cytopenias and dysfunction
Serous membrane	Pericarditis and pleuritis

IMMUNOSUPPRESSIVE DRUGS

Immunosuppressive drugs are administered to avoid transplant rejections. These include *azathioprine, cyclosporine A, tacrolimus (FK506), rapamycin and biological immunosuppression monoclonal antibodies* (Table 4.65). The action of cyclosporine A in preventing graft rejection is shown in Fig. 4.62.

Adverse Effects of Immunosuppressive Drugs

Adverse effects of immunosuppressive treatment comprise nephrotoxicity, infection, hyperlipidemia, hypertension, and neoplasia risk. Adverse effects of immunosuppressive treatment are shown in Table 4.66.

Table 4.65: Immunosuppressive drugs

Drug	Product	Mechanism
Azathioprine	Azathioprine metabolized to 6-mercaptopurine	Inhibits T cell-mediated transplant rejection
		Interferes with enzyme involved in nucleic acid synthesis
		Inhibiting proliferation of T cells
Cyclosporine A	Fungal product first line of drug used in prevention of allograft rejection	Has no effect on the replicating cells of bone marrow
		Penetrates antigen-sensitive cells in the G_0 and G_1 phase
		Inhibits RNA polymerase leading to blockage of synthesis of IL-2 by T helper cells
Tacrolimus (FK506)	Fungal product	Inhibits synthesis of lymphokines by recipient T helper cells
Rapamycin	Fungal macrolide	Interferes with the intracellular signaling pathways of the IL-2 receptor
Biological immuno-suppression	Monoclonal antibodies	Against T helper (anti-CD4) cells or activated T cells (anti-CD25, the IL-2 receptor)
	Monoclonal antibodies conjugated with toxin such as ricin	Targeted against CD25 molecule expressed on activated T cells
	Lymphokine (IL-2) complexed with diphtheria toxin	Locks onto IL-2 receptors on activated T cells and kills the cells

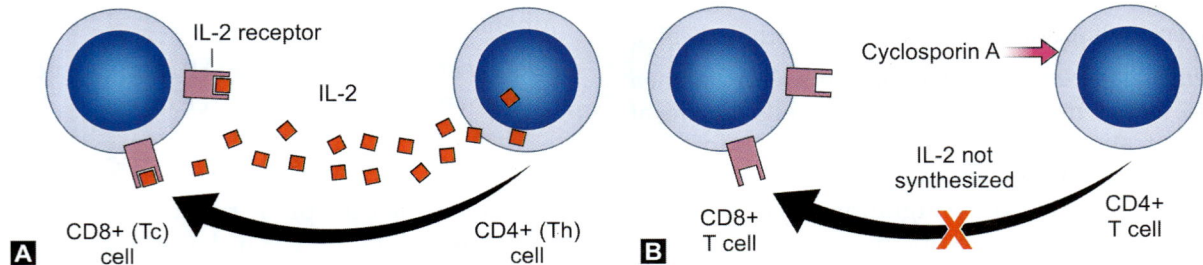

Fig. 4.62: (A) Normally CD4+ (Th) cell synthesizes IL-2 that binds to IL-2 receptor on CD8+ (Tc) cell, (B) the action of cyclosporine A in preventing graft rejection.

Table 4.66: Adverse effects of immunosuppressive treatment

Effects	Findings
Acute nephrotoxicity (cyclosporine A induced)	Vacuoles formation in proximal tubules and hyalinization of arterioles
	Interstitial fibrosis and tubular atrophy
Risk of infection	Cytomegalovirus infection common
Hypertension (cyclosporine A induced)	Hypertension following renal transplant (50% cases) associated with vasoconstriction
Hyperlipidemia	Present in 60% post-transplant cases increases risk of cardiovascular deaths in 30% cases
Post-transplant neoplasia	Squamous cell carcinoma, B cell lymphoma especially associated with Epstein-Barr virus, Kaposi's sarcoma and cervical carcinoma

AMYLOIDOSIS

Amyloidosis is fundamentally a disorder of protein misfolding. More than 20 different proteins result in aggregation to form insoluble fibrils. *These insoluble fibrils are deposited in extracellular tissue in one organ or many organs resulting in tissue damage.* Amyloidosis may be localized or systemic. It is not a single disease entity but rather a diverse group of inherited or acquired disorders.

Mechanisms of Protein Misfolding

Several factors may participate in the protein misfolding, which aggregate to form insoluble fibrils that deposit in extracellular tissues. It occurs by the following mechanisms:

- *Excessive production of proteins:* Misfolding of proteins results in aggregation and formation of amyloid fibrils due to increased concentration in chronic inflammatory conditions.
- *Impaired excretion of proteins:* It occurs in patients on long-term dialysis.
- *Mutation of proteins:* It may give rise to misfolding of proteins in hereditary amyloidosis.
- *Defective or incomplete proteolytic degradation:* Limited proteolysis may generate a protein that forms amyloid fibrils (amyloid associated Alzheimer's disease).

PHYSICAL STRUCTURE OF AMYLOID

Amyloid deposits typically contain three components: amyloid protein fibrils, P component and sulfated glycosaminoglycans (GAGs). Structure of amyloid composed of fibrils arranged in β-pleated sheets is shown in Fig. 4.63.

AMYLOID PROTEIN FIBRILS

Amyloid protein fibrils constitute 90% of the amyloid structure. Regardless of their derivation, all amyloid deposits are composed of nonbranching fibrils, measuring 7.5 to 10 nm in diameter.

Each of these fibrils is made up of two filaments of polypeptide-chains, which are folded in twisted β-pleated sheet fibrils. *These nonbranching fibrils bind to proteoglycans, glycosaminoglycans, heparan sulfate, dermatan sulfate and plasma proteins. Congo red binds to these fibrils and produces a green dichromism (birefringence) under polarized light, which is commonly used to demonstrate amyloid in tissues.*

P COMPONENT

In addition, amyloid protein fibril deposits are intimately associated with the P component (pentagonal globular rod-like structure), a glycoprotein related to normal serum P component. The P component is very similar to serum C reactive protein. *It constitutes 10% of amyloid material.*

SULFATED GLYCOSAMINOGLYCANS

Sulfated glycosaminoglycans (GAGs) are small but constant component, amyloid protein fibrils and P component are closely associated with GAG, complex carbohydrates of connective tissue. The presence of abundant charged sugar groups in these adsorbed proteins give the deposits staining characteristics resembling starch (amylose).

CHEMICAL NATURE OF AMYLOID

Out of more than 20 biochemically distinct forms of amyloid proteins identified, there are two, chemically distinct types of amyloid protein fibrils designated amyloid light-chain (*AL*), and amyloid associated (*AA*). There are several minor types unrelated to AL or AA such as *amyloid-β, transthyretin, $β_2$-microglobulin, procalcitonin.* Classification of amyloidosis is shown in Table 4.67.

AMYLOID LIGHT-CHAIN

Amyloid light-chain (AL) is also known as *immunocyte associated amyloidosis. In the immunocyte associated form, perivascular and vascular localizations are* common. *It occurs in 30% cases of multiple myeloma or B cell lymphomas.* Deposition of AL fibrils associated

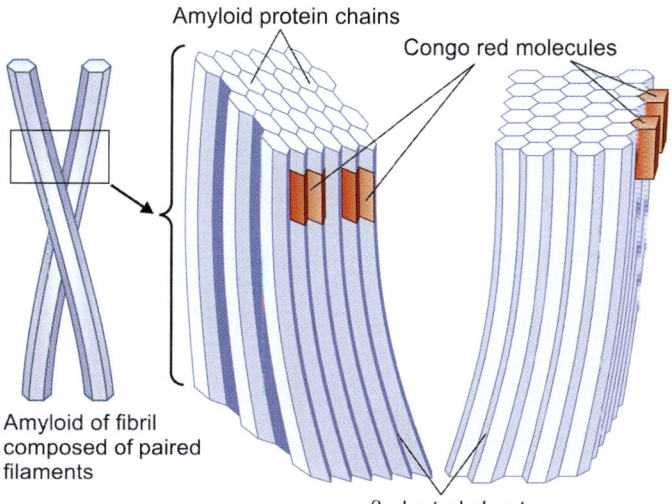

Fig. 4.63: Structure of amyloid showing fibril composed of fibrils arranged in β-pleated sheets.

Section I: General Pathology

Table 4.67: Classification of amyloidosis

Classification of amyloid substances	Associated disorders	Major amyloid substance	Organs involved
Primary amyloidosis	Multiple myeloma, immunoblastic lymphoma	AL (immunoglobulin light-chains or fragments)	Systemic or generalized amyloidosis
Reactive (secondary)	Chronic inflammation, autoimmune diseases and some cancers	AA (serum amyloid protein A an acute phase reactant)	Systemic or generalized amyloidosis
Hemodialysis associated	Chronic renal failure	$A\beta 2M$ (β_2-microglobulin)	Systemic or generalized amyloidosis
Hereditary and familial	Neuropathic	ATTR (transthyretin)	Systemic or generalized amyloidosis
	Familial	AA	Systemic or generalized amyloidosis
Endocrine disorder	Medullary carcinoma thyroid	AF (calcitonin or precursor)	Localized amyloidosis
Senile cerebral	Alzheimer's disease	$A\beta$	Localized amyloidosis
Senile	Heart	Transthyretin	Localized amyloidosis

In addition to major amyloid substance listed, all amyloid deposits also comprise amyloid P glycoprotein as a common constituent

with multiple myeloma is related to monoclonal immunoglobulin either the kappa (κ) or lambda (λ) light-chains synthesized by abnormal plasma cells cause primary amyloidosis. *These light-chains (either kappa or lambda) undergo aggregation, probably because they contain amino acid residue that destabilizes the domain structure.* Pathogenesis of amyloidosis (AL type) is shown in Fig. 4.64.

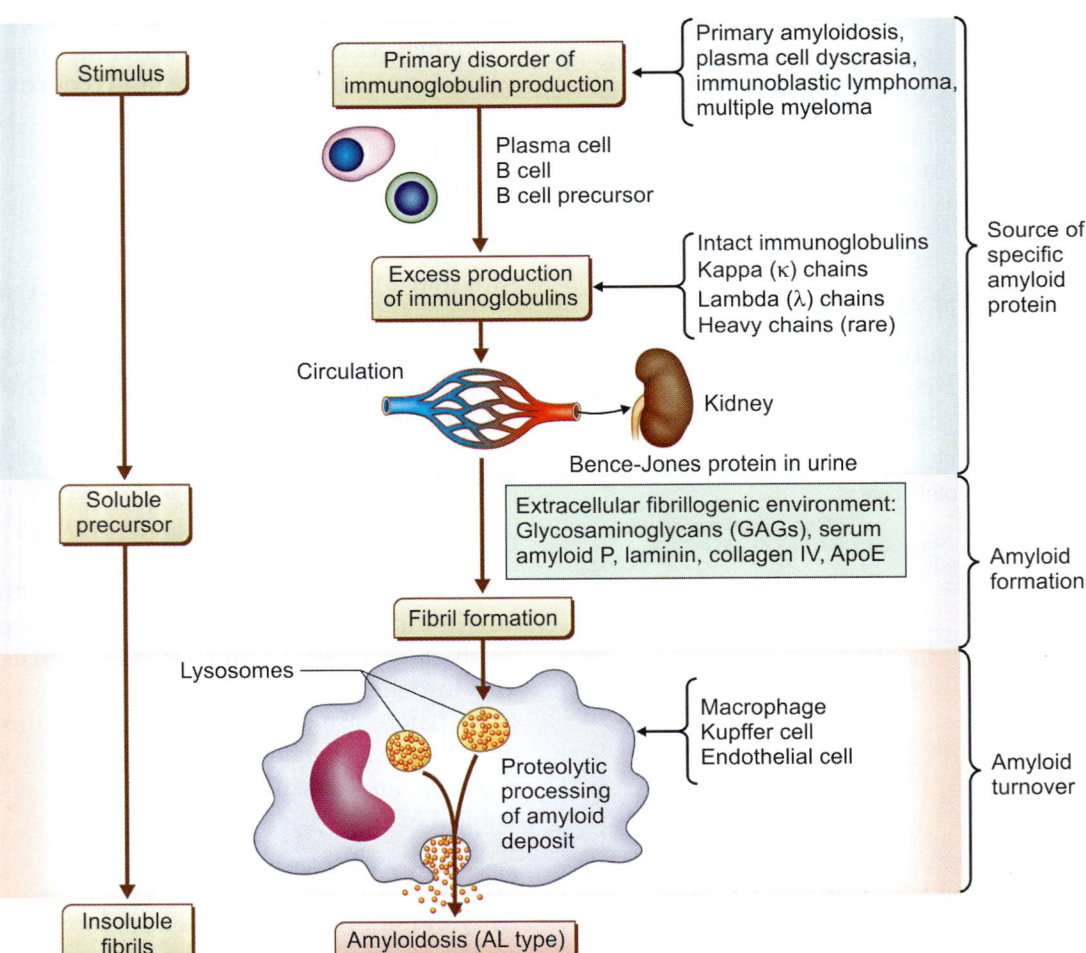

Fig. 4.64: Pathogenesis of amyloidosis (AL type). Primary disorders of B cells/plasma cells such as multiple myeloma leads to synthesis of excessive immunoglobulins. In the extracellular fibrillogenic environment, fibrils are formed. These fibrils are processed by macrophages resulting in amyloid deposition.

Immunopathology including Amyloidosis

Organs Involved

Amyloid light-chain is usually systemic in distribution involving mesodermal tissues most frequently affecting *peripheral nerves, the heart, lung, skin, tongue, thyroid gland, joints* and *intestinal tract*. Localized amyloid 'tumors' may be found in the *respiratory tract*.

AMYLOID ASSOCIATED

Amyloid associated (AA) is also known as *reactive amyloidosis* secondary to chronic inflammatory and autoimmune disorders. Amyloid associated fibril, an acute phase reactant synthesized by liver cells (1,000-fold) under stimulation by interleukin-1 (IL-1) released from activated macrophages is derived from serum amyloid associated (SAA). Denaturing of SAA releases a subunit termed apoSAA, which renders it amyloidogenic. In contrast to AL protein derived from immunoglobulin light-chain, the amino acid sequence of AA proteins is identical in all patients, regardless of the underlying disorder. Pathogenesis of amyloidosis (AA type) is shown in Fig. 4.65.

Causes

Amyloidosis associated occurs in chronic inflammatory diseases, e.g. *tuberculosis, bronchiectasis, chronic*

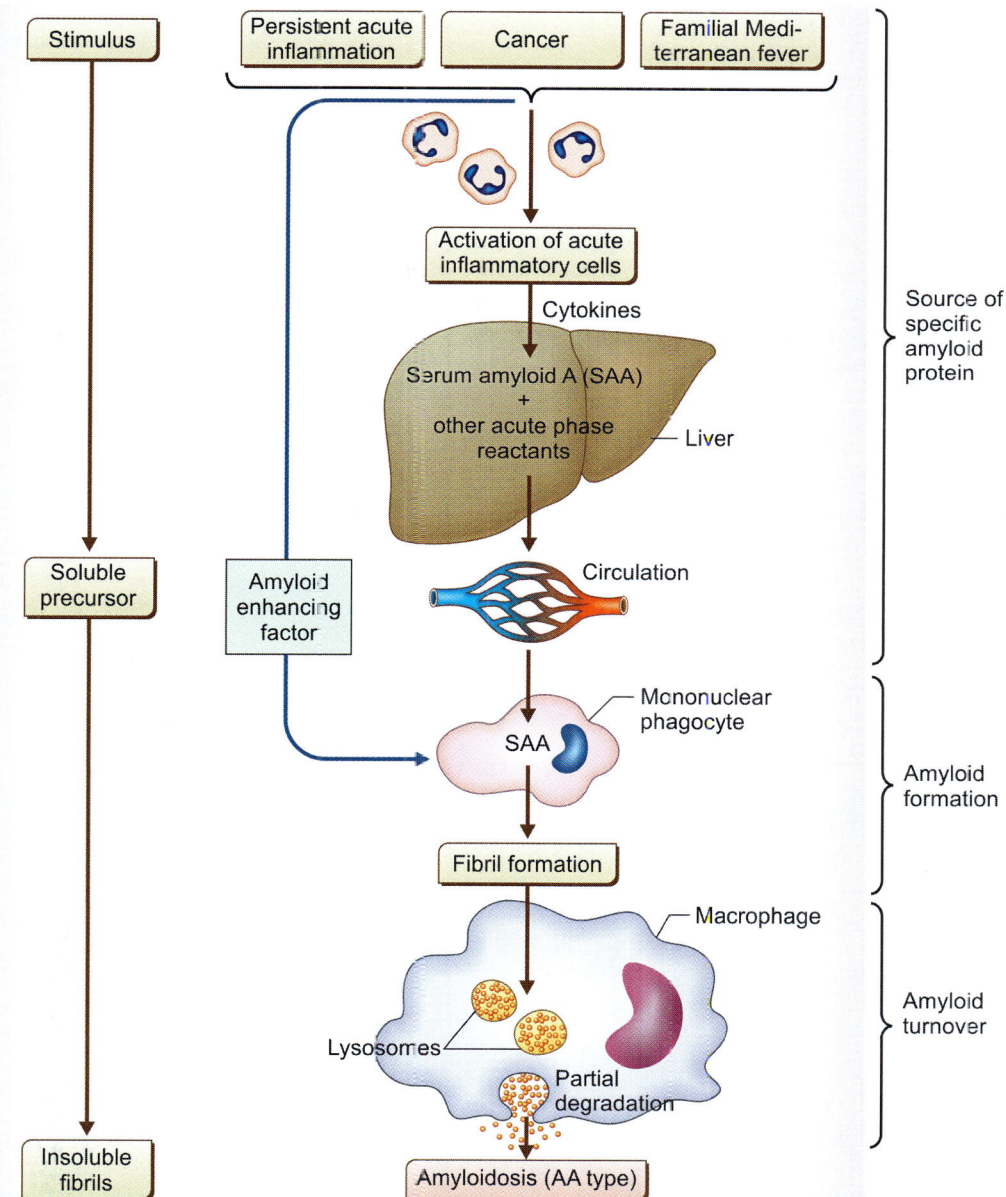

Fig. 4.65: Pathogenesis of amyloidosis (AA type). It is associated with the activation of polymorphonuclear leukocytes and macrophages, which in turn leads to the synthesis and release of acute phase reactants by the liver, including SAA. This SAA is released in association with amyloid-enhancing factor (AEF) by intact macrophages. This released product complexes with glycosaminoglycans and SAP as AA amyloid. The deposit is then processed by macrophages.

osteomyelitis, rheumatoid arthritis, ankylosing spondylitis, dermatomyositis, scleroderma, regional enteritis, ulcerative colitis. It may occur in cases of malignancies, e.g. Hodgkin's disease and renal cell carcinoma.

Mechanism

Normally SAA in chronic inflammation is degraded to soluble end products by the action of monocyte associated serine esterases. When this process is inhibited, insoluble end products form as amyloid material. Defective proteolysis may produce misfolded, incompletely degraded SAA, leading to aggregation and deposition as AA fibrils.

Organs Involved

It involves *liver, spleen, kidney, adrenal glands, and lymph nodes*. However, *no organ system is spared*. Vascular involvement may be widespread. The liver and spleen are often enlarged, firm, and rubbery. The kidneys are usually enlarged. *Sections of the spleen have large, translucent, waxy areas where the normal malpighian bodies are replaced by pale amyloid, producing the sago spleen.* Clinically significant involvement of the heart is rare. Differences between primary and secondary amyloidosis are shown in Table 4.68.

AMYLOID β-PROTEIN (A4 AMYLOID)

Amyloid β-protein is derived from a much larger transmembrane glycoprotein called *amyloid precursor protein* (APP), protein product of chromosome 21. It is deposited in cerebral blood vessels of *Alzheimer's disease*.

Amyloid deposits contain fibrils of β-amyloid (Aβ protein resides on chromosome 21) derived from larger Aβ-protein precursor (AβPP), which is a normal cell membrane constituent.

TRANSTHYRETIN (TTR)

Transthyretin is a normal serum protein that transports thyroxine and retinol. Mutation in the genes encoding transthyretin results in the production of a protein (and its fragments) that aggregates and form deposits. Pathogenesis of amyloidosis (ATTR protein) is shown in Fig. 4.66.

Organs Involved

Amyloid is deposited in peripheral nerves and autonomic nervous system in autosomal dominant familial amyloid polyneuropathy. Amyloid deposits of transthyretin occur in the heart of 8th and 9th decades elderly

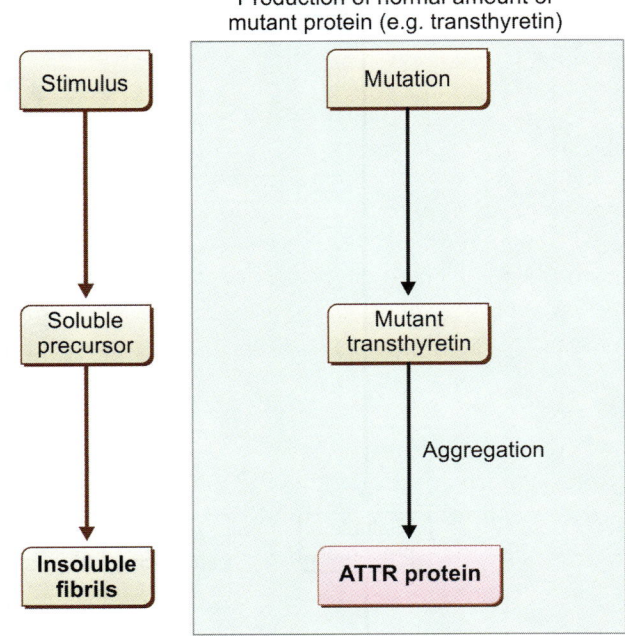

Fig. 4.66: Pathogenesis of amyloidosis (ATTR protein).

Table 4.68: Differences between primary amyloidosis and secondary amyloidosis

Parameters	Primary amyloidosis	Secondary amyloidosis
Etiology	Multiple myeloma, immunoblastic lymphoma	Chronic inflammation (tuberculosis, chronic osteomyelitis, bronchiectasis)
		Autoimmune disorders (rheumatoid arthritis, ulcerative colitis, regional enteritis, dermatomyositis, scleroderma, ankylosing spondylitis)
		Cancers (Hodgkin's disease and renal cell carcinoma)
Chemical nature	AL (amyloid light-chain)	AA (amyloid associated) due to misfolding of AA fibrils as a result of defective proteolysis
Organs involved	Mesoderm derived structures such as peripheral nerves, heart, lung, skin, tongue, thyroid gland, joints and gastrointestinal tract	Parenchymal organs (spleen, liver, kidney, adrenals, and lymph nodes)
	Parenchymal organs also involved (liver, spleen, kidney, heart)	
Frequency	More common	Less common

patients with senile *cardiac amyloidosis* due to increased concentration of mutated transthyretin. In addition, *heart, lungs, pancreas or spleen* may be affected, suggesting that it is a systemic disorder.

HEMODIALYSIS ASSOCIATED AMYLOIDOSIS

The systemic amyloid deposition of β_2 microglobulin, a component of the MHC molecules and a normal serum protein, occurs as a complication of long-term dialysis in patients with chronic renal failure due to increased concentration in serum.

This protein does not pass through conventional dialysis membranes. 60 to 80% of patients on long-term dialysis develop *amyloid deposition in the synovium, joints and tendon sheaths resulting in destructive arthropathy.*

ENDOCRINE ASSOCIATED AMYLOIDOSIS

Microscopic deposits of localized amyloid may be found in certain endocrine lesions, e.g. *medullary carcinoma of the thyroid (amyloid derived from procalcitonin), pheochromocytoma, undifferentiated carcinoma of stomach, islets of Langerhans' in pancreas in type II diabetes mellitus (islet amyloid polypeptides or amylin) and islet tumors of pancreas (islet amyloid polypeptides).* Amyloid deposits in medullary carcinoma thyroid is shown in Fig. 4.67.

AMYLOID OF AGING

Amyloid of aging is also known as senile systemic amyloidosis affecting 8th and 9th decades of elderly persons. Amyloid fibrils derived from mutant form of transthyretin (TTR) are deposited in heart resulting in restrictive cardiomyopathy. In addition to heart, lungs, pancreas or spleen may be affected, suggesting that it is a systemic disorder.

LOCALIZED AMYLOIDOSIS

Sometimes, amyloid deposits are limited to a single organ. The deposits of amyloid are nodular and encountered in the *lungs, larynx, skin, urinary bladder, tongue, and the region about the eyes may be involved.* In some of these cases, infiltrates of plasma cells may be found, and the amyloid is of the AL type.

FAMILIAL AMYLOIDOSIS

Familial amyloidosis is seen in autosomal recessive disorder (Mediterranean fever) and hereditary amyloidosis.

Mediterranean Fever

Mediterranean fever is autosomal recessive disorder characterized by attacks of fever accompanied by *inflammation of pleural, peritoneal and synovial surfaces.* Patient develops widespread tissue involvement such as *kidneys, blood vessels, spleen, and respiratory tract.* It is indistinguishable from reactive systemic amyloidosis.

The amyloid fibril proteins are made up of AA proteins. Normal gene product *pyrin* inhibits neutrophils in acute inflammation. *Mutation of gene product pyrin leads to vigorous tissue damaging inflammatory response due to minor trauma.*

Hereditary Amyloidosis

Hereditary amyloidosis is characterized by *peripheral sensory and motor neuropathy*, often autonomic neuropathy and *cardiovascular and renal amyloid. Carpal tunnel syndrome* and vitreous abnormalities may occur. The fibrils in these familial polyneuropathies are made up of mutant ATTRs.

ORGANS INVOLVED IN AMYLOIDOSIS

RENAL AMYLOIDOSIS

Kidneys are commonly involved in 80% cases of systemic amyloidosis. *Patient presents with proteinuria in nephritic/nephrotic range and ultimately go into chronic renal failure in a span of two years with fatal outcome.* Renal failure is a common cause of death in amyloidosis

Pathogenesis

Amyloid nephropathy occurs due to deposition of amyloid material in primary (AL in multiple myeloma) and secondary amyloidosis (AA in chronic disorders).

- Kappa (κ) or lambda (λ) chains of immunoglobulins synthesized by neoplastic plasma cells are deposited in the *glomerular basement membranes and mesangial*

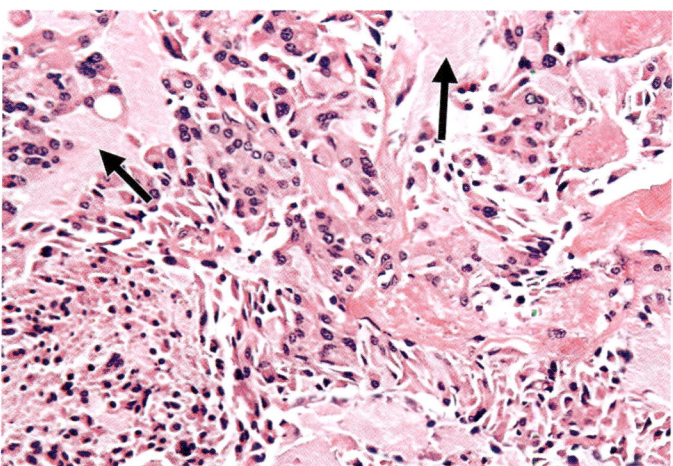

Fig. 4.67: Amyloid deposits in medullary carcinoma thyroid. The tumor is composed of round to polyhedral granular cells arranged in trabecular, glandular, carcinoid-like patterns. The tumor cells are separated by a distinctly fibrovascular stroma containing amyloid material representing deposition of procalcitonin (arrows) (400X).

matrix. These immunoglobulins can be detected in serum or urine by electrophoresis.
- Amyloidosis is a well-known complication of chronic inflammatory disorders such as *tuberculosis,* bronchiectasis, rheumatoid arthritis, or osteomyelitis. It stimulates the production of amyloid from the serum amyloid A (SAA) protein, an acute phase reactant secreted by the liver. The kidneys (80%), liver, spleen, and adrenals are the most common organs involved.

Gross Morphology
Kidneys are enlarged and pale. Cut section of kidneys reveal firm and waxy surface. In advanced cases, the kidneys are contracted and shrunken due to vascular narrowing induced by deposition of amyloid.

Light Microscopy
Renal biopsy shows amyloid deposits primarily affecting glomeruli and renal blood vessels, often causing marked vascular narrowing. Peritubular tissue is also involved. Amyloid nephropathy is shown in Fig. 4.68.
- Glomeruli show thickening of glomerular basement membrane. Amyloid material appears as amorphous, homogenous and eosinophilic in mesangial region, tubular basement membranes, renal vessels and interstitial tissue.
- Expansion of mesangial region obliterates the glomerular capillaries loops rendering the glomerular filter leaky to plasma proteins and impaired renal function. There is no cellular response to the amyloid deposits.

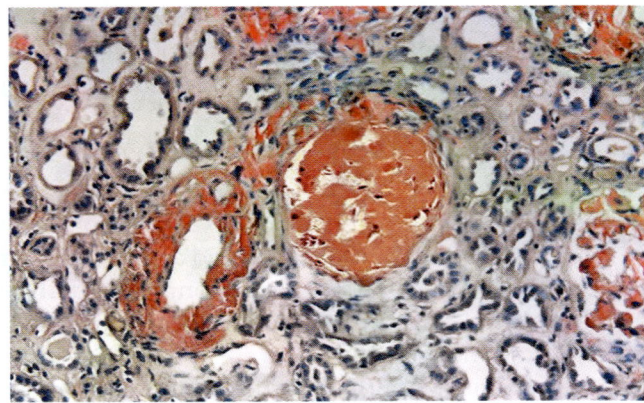

Fig. 4.69: Amyloid nephropathy. Amyloid material is stained by Congo red stain. Nodules in diabetic glomerulosclerosis are PAS positive but negative for Congo red stain (400X).

Electron Microscopy
Electron microscopy reveals deposition of 7–10 mm thick amyloid fibrils in subendothelial region of glomerular basement membrane, mesangial matrix, tubular basement membrane and arterioles.

Amyloid demonstration: Amyloid material in glomerular mesangial matrix, glomerular and tubular basement membrane is demonstrated by *Congo red staining under light microscopy, which reveals characteristic apple-green birefringence (color of a Granny Smith apple) under polarized microscopy.* Amyloid material can also be demonstrated by various other stains, i.e. *thioflavin T, thioflavin-S, methyl violet, crystal violet* (Fig. 4.69).

AA and AL differentiation: Pretreatment of tissue with potassium permanganate stained by Congo red demonstrates AL amyloid only but not AA amyloid.

LIVER AMYLOIDOSIS
Amyloidosis is a well-known complication of chronic inflammatory disorders such as *tuberculosis, bronchiectasis, rheumatoid arthritis, or osteomyelitis.* These disorders stimulate the production of amyloid from the serum amyloid A (SAA) protein, an acute phase reactant secreted by the liver. *The kidneys (80%), liver, spleen, and adrenals are the most common organs involved.*

Gross Morphology
The amyloid liver is usually grossly enlarged (as much as 900 gm), pale, and smooth surface, firm consistency. When sectioned, it has sharp rigid edges.

Light Microscopy
Amyloid material is initially deposited in the *space of Disse* between the hepatocytes and vascular sinusoids. As more amyloid accumulates, it compresses the

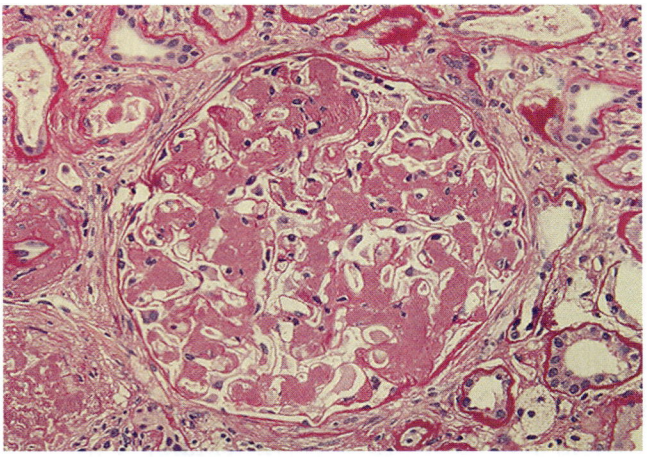

Fig. 4.68: Amyloid nephropathy: initially, amyloid material is deposited in the mesangium and then extending along the inner surface of GBM distorting glomerular lumina. Light microscopy shows amorphous acellular material extending to mesangial matrix and obstructing glomerular lumina (400X).

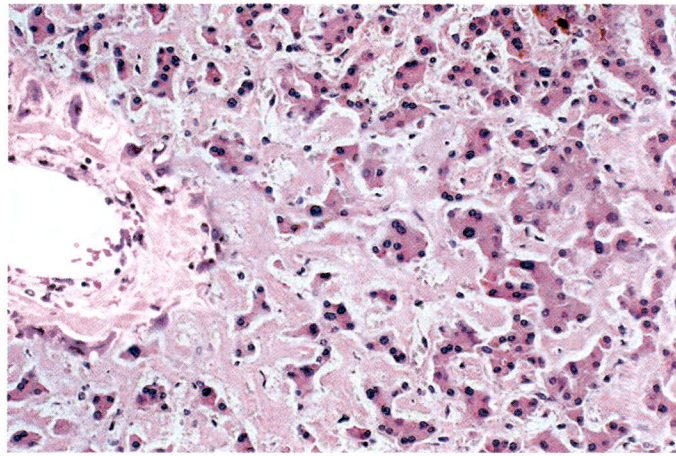

Fig. 4.70: Amyloid liver shows deposition of amyloid material in the space of Disse between the hepatocytes and vascular sinusoids leading to compression of hepatic cords (400X).

hepatic cords and sinusoids. The hepatic cords undergo nutritional and pressure atrophy and become displaced or replaced by bands and nodules of amyloid (Fig. 4.70).

SPLEEN AMYLOIDOSIS

Amyloidosis of the spleen often causes moderate or even marked enlargement (200–800 gm). Amyloidosis of the spleen has two different anatomical patterns such as *sago spleen* or *lardaceous spleen*. In both the patterns, amyloid spleen is firm in consistency, and cut surfaces reveal pale gray, waxy deposits. Amyloid deposit in spleen is shown in Fig. 4.71.

Sago Spleen

Most commonly, the *amyloid deposition is limited to the splenic follicles*, resulting in the gross appearance of a moderately enlarged spleen dotted with tapioca-like gray nodules so-called (sago spleen).

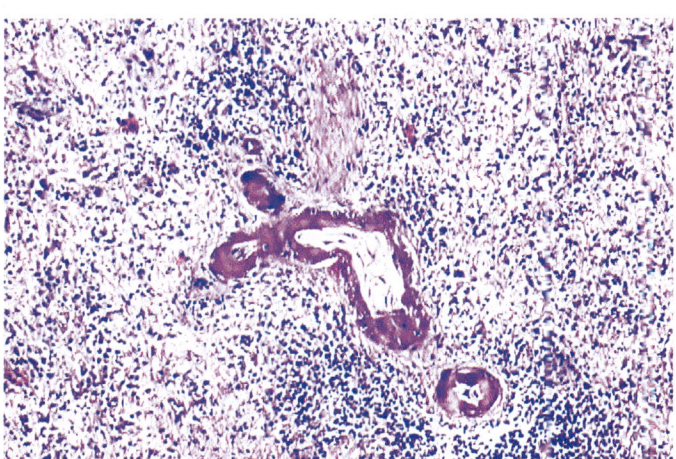

Fig. 4.71: Amyloid deposit in spleen (100X).

Lardaceous Spleen

Alternatively, the amyloid deposits may spare the *follicles and mainly infiltrate the red pulp sinuses*, producing a large, firm spleen mottled with waxy discolorations so-called (lardaceous spleen).

CARDIAC AMYLOIDOSIS

Heart involvement may accompany systemic amyloid deposition usually associated with immunocyte dyscrasias or localized organ involvement (amyloidosis of aging). The amyloid deposits may cause minimal to moderately enlarged heart.

Gross Morphology
Amyloidosis of heart reveals gray-pink dewdrop-like subendocardial elevation, particularly evident in the atrial chambers.

Light Microscopy
Histopathological examination reveals amyloid deposits located between the myocardial fibers eventually causing pressure atrophy or in the walls of the coronary arteries. It reduces the heart's ability to fill with blood in between heartbeats. When amyloidosis affects the electrical system of heart, heart's rhythm may be disturbed.

ADRENAL GLAND AMYLOIDOSIS

In the adrenals, extracellular amyloid deposits encompass, compress, and replace the cortical cells.

GASTROINTESTINAL TRACT AMYLOIDOSIS

The alimentary tract may be involved at any level, from the *tongue to the rectum (submucosa)*. There may be direct involvement of gut or of autonomic nervous system. In amyloidosis of tongue (interstitial tissue) amyloid infiltrates the capillary walls and narrows the lumens of some of them; resulting in macroglossia. Lesions in the gut may cause *obstruction, ulceration, protein loss, malabsorption, diarrhea and hemorrhage*. Biopsy is taken from gingiva and rectum to demonstrate amyloid. Amyloid deposit in rectum is shown in Fig. 4.72.

RESPIRATORY SYSTEM AMYLOIDOSIS

Amyloidosis involves nasal sinuses, larynx, trachea, bronchi and alveolar septa.

SKIN AMYLOIDOSIS

Skin involvement occurs in primary amyloidosis. Patients present with *slightly raised, waxy papules/ plaques* which are usually clustered in the axillae, anal or inguinal regions, which are seldom pruritic. Gentle

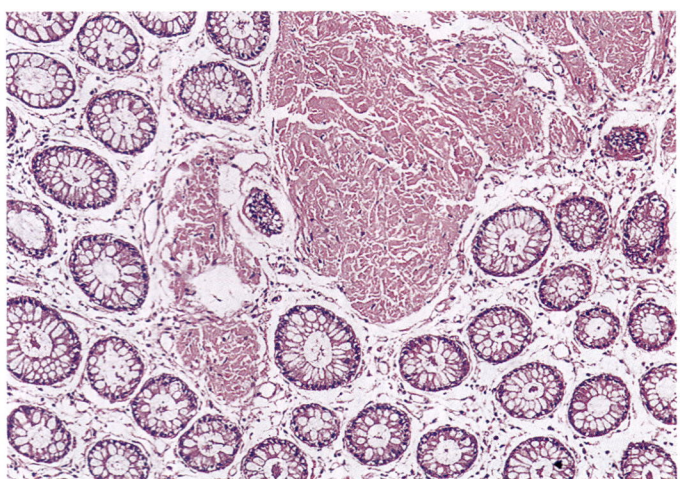

Fig. 4.72: Amyloid deposits in rectum (400X).

rubbing of skin may induce purpuric bleeding into skin. Cutaneous may occur in secondary amyloidosis.

NERVOUS SYSTEM AMYLOIDOSIS

Cranial nerves are generally spared except for those involving pupillary reflexes. Neurologic manifestations include *peripheral neuropathy, postural hypotension, inability to sweat; Adie pupil, hoarseness and sphincter incompetence. 25% of patients suffer from carpal tunnel syndrome due to compression of nerves supplying fingers.* This may cause severe pain especially during night, numbness and tingling of the fingers.

CLINICAL CORRELATION

Patient with amyloidosis may present with minimal to life-threatening manifestations depending upon the organs involved. Initial clinical manifestations include weakness, fatigue, and weight loss. Later manifestations include involvement of various organs such as gastrointestinal tract, heart, liver, spleen, kidney, skin and brain. Patient with renal involvement develops nephrotic syndrome progressing to renal failure. Amyloid deposition in subendocardial region produces restrictive cardiomyopathy resulting in cardiac arrhythmias with fatal outcome. Clinical and laboratory manifestations of amyloidosis are shown in Table 4.69.

LABORATORY DIAGNOSIS

No single set of clinical signs or symptoms points unequivocally to amyloidosis. When one suspects amyloidosis, the diagnosis ultimately rests on its histologic demonstration in *biopsy specimens (heart, liver, skin, kidney, small intestine, sural nerve, rectum, and tongue) and fine needle aspiration of abdominal fat.* Biochemical tests, urine analysis, imaging techniques are also performed. Various stains used to demonstrate amyloid material are shown in Table 4.70.

CONGO RED

Congo red is the most common stain applied on formalin fixed biopsy specimens or aspirates to demonstrate amyloid.

Table 4.69: Clinical and laboratory manifestations of amyloidosis

Organ involvement	Clinical manifestations
Tongue	Macroglossia
Esophagus	Megaesophagus and loss of peristalsis
Stomach	Amyloid deposits in submucosa with loss of gastric rugae Amyloid deposit may be localized to antrum Stomach becomes rigid simulating linitis plastica leading to diminished or absence of stomach peristalsis
Small intestine	Amyloid deposits in diffuse pattern (more common) causing broadened flat undulated mucosal folds (mucosal atrophy) leading to impaired motility Multiple small amyloid deposits causing small bowel dilatation and pseudo obstruction
Colon	Pseudopolyps
Liver	Hepatomegaly
Spleen	Splenomegaly
Heart	Congestive heart failure with cardiomegaly
Kidney	Nephritic/nephrotic syndrome leading to chronic renal failure
Skin	Waxy papules
Brain	Alzheimer's disease (dementia) caused by toxic Aβ deposits in neurons Amyloid precursor protein coded by chromosome 21 associated with Down's syndrome
Bone marrow	Plasmacytosis in multiple myeloma and osteolytic lesions in bones
Serum and urine	Monoclonal Ig and light-chains

Immunopathology including Amyloidosis

Table 4.70: Stains used to demonstrate amyloid material

Amyloid stain	Color imparted
Congo red stain examined under light microscope	Pink
Congo red stain examined under polarizing microscope	Apple green
Fluorescent stains (thioflavin-T, thioflavin S)	Greenish fluorescence
Methyl violet (metachromatic stain)	Rose pink
Crystal violet (metachromatic stain)	Pink
PAS stain (metachromatic stain)	Magenta color
von Gieson stain (metachromatic stain)	Khaki color

Light Microscopy

When the sections stained with Congo red are viewed under light microscopy, amyloid material imparts a pink- or red-colored hyaline-like material.

Polarizing Microscopy

Apple green birefringence is observed under polarized light.

The fibrillary deposits organized in one plane have one color, and those organized perpendicular to that plane have the other color. This reaction is shared by all forms of amyloid and is caused by the crossed β-pleated configuration of amyloid fibrils.

COTTON DYE SIRIUS RED F3B

Cotton dye sirius red F3B stains amyloid red and exhibits apple green birefringence under polarized light.

METACHROMATIC STAINS

Metachromatic stains include methyl violet and crystal violet.

- *Methyl violet stain:* It is best used on frozen sections to demonstrate amyloid. Amyloid stains red purple/violet against a blue background. Addition of ammonium oxalate to methyl violet accentuates the metachromatic effect. Methyl green is used as counter stain in methyl violet method to demonstrate amyloid, which imparts purple red color.
- *Crystal violet stain:* Crystal violet stains amyloid a violet color against a blue background. Formic acid crystal violet method accentuates the metachromatic effect.
- *Periodic Schiff stain:* Amyloid appears magenta pink against background.
- *von Gieson stain:* Amyloid stains Khaki in a yellowish background.

IMMUNOFLUORESCENCE MICROSCOPY

Fluorescein thiocyanate is used for immunofluorescence microscopy. Thioflavin-T stain is not entirely specific to demonstrate amyloid. Thioflavin blue stain demonstrates glycosaminoglycans of amyloid to appear blue. These allow amyloid to fluoresce green.

IMMUNOPEROXIDASE STUDY

Formalin fixed frozen sections are used to differentiate primary from secondary amyloid fibrils. Monoclonal antibodies are prepared to demonstrate different components of amyloid protein fibrils, amyloid-P component and sulfated glycosaminoglycans (GAGs).

ELECTRON MICROSCOPY

Ultrastructurally, all forms of amyloid (AA, AL, ATTR types of amyloid) consist of interlacing bundles of parallel arrays of fibrils, which have a diameter of 7 to 13 nm. The protein in the amyloid fibrils contains a large proportion of crossed β-pleated sheet structure

GROSS MORPHOLOGY STUDY

Iodine solution applied to cut surface of organ. Amyloid typically stains mahogany-brown. Application of dilute sulfuric acid leads to color reaction changes to blue (*starch-like* reaction).

CHAPTER 5

Genetic Disorders

Learning Objectives

HUMAN GENOME
- Overview
- Gene Mutations
- Inheritance of Monogenic Disorders
- Polygenic and Multifactorial Disorders
- Genetic Polymorphism
- Balanced Polymorphism
- Disorders Associated with Genomic Imprinting

CHROMOSOMAL DISORDERS
- Alterations in Chromosomes
- Alterations in Sex Chromosomes
- Autosomal Disorders
- Sex Chromosomal Disorders

SINGLE GENE MUTATION (MENDELIAN DISORDERS)
- Overview
- Autosomal Dominant Disorders
- Autosomal Recessive Disorders
- X-linked Recessive Disorders

DISORDERS OF SEXUAL DIFFERENTIATION
- Hermaphroditism

WORK UP OF GENETIC DISORDERS
- Pedigree Construction
- Barr Bodies
- Y Chromatin
- Karyotyping

HUMAN GENOME

OVERVIEW

Features of person depend on genes inherited from both the parents. Genes are present in DNA of genome. These possess the information from genetic code for the synthesis of genes. Each gene synthesizes specific proteins. *These genes are transmitted from the one generation to the next generation. Study of genes and the laws is known as genetics.* Genome denotes entire set of chromosomes in a cell. Chromosomes in normal cells are present in 23 pairs and thus their genes in the nucleus of each body cell. Half the number of normal chromosomes is called *haploid*. Terminology used by geneticist is shown in Table 5.1.

STRUCTURE OF DNA DOUBLE HELIX MOLECULE

DNA is a pair of molecules joined by hydrogen bonds. It is organized as two complementary strands, head-to-toe, with the hydrogen bonds between them. *Each strand of DNA is a chain of chemical building blocks called nucleotides, of which there are four types: purines (adenine-abbreviated A and guanine-abbreviated G) and pyrimidines (thymine-abbreviated T and cytosine-abbreviated C).* The negatively charged DNA double helix molecule is wrapped around positively charged histone octamer to form a structure called *nucleosome* (10 nm) as shown in Figs 5.1 to 5.3.

- *Nucleosome:* Nucleosome contains 200 base pairs of DNA helix in nucleus. Nucleosomes are seen as *beads*

Genetic Disorders

Table 5.1: Terminology used by geneticist

Term	Description
Genome	Entire set of chromosomes in a human cell
Diploid	Normal pair of 23 chromosomes (diploid or 2 N with 22 autosomes and XX in females and XY in males) in daughter cell
Haploid	Half the number of normal chromosomes (single set of 23 chromosomes in replicating germ cells like ova and sperm) during meiosis
Aneuploidy	Presence of extra copies of chromosome in addition to the normal pair (trisomy seen in Down's syndrome and Klinefelter's syndrome) or deficient in number of chromosome (monosomy seen in Turner syndrome)
Genotype	Representation of an individual's genetic constitution (DNA sequencing) with respect to a single character or a set of characters
Phenotype	Clinical expression of a specific gene or set of genes
Chromosome	Storage units of genes
DNA	Nucleic acid that contains the genetic instructions specifying the biological development of all cellular forms of life
Mitosis	Process by which a cell separates its duplicated genome into two identical halves
Meiosis	Process that transforms one diploid into four haploid cells
Gene	Basic unit of genetic information determining the inherited characters
Locus	Location of a gene/marker on the chromosome. At each locus (except for sex chromosomes) there are 2 genes. These constitute the individual's genotype at the locus
Allele	Representing at least two alternative forms of a gene (each gene consisting of an allelomorphic pair)
	A dominant allele is expressed even if it is paired with a recessive allele
	A recessive allele is only visible when paired with another recessive allele
Codon	Three adjacent base sequences in DNA or RNA, that specifies a particular amino acid
Stop codon	A codon that stops the protein synthesis (examples of stop codon are TGA, TAA, and TAG)
Complete linkage	When two genes located on same chromosome are close to each other, so no crossing takes place
Incomplete linkage	It occurs when crossover takes place in closely located genes. 82% representing parentals, while 18% recombinant
Dominant gene	Dominant gene affecting offspring whose corresponding phenotype expressed in the individual
Mutation	Permanent change in the genetic material of DNA
Point mutation	Replacement of a single DNA base by another
Conservative gene mutation	Replacement of one amino acid with a biochemically similar amino acid
Non-conservative mutation	Replacement of one amino acid with a biochemically dissimilar amino acid
Exon	A region of a gene that codes a particular protein
Intron	A region of a gene that does not code for a particular protein (non-coding region of a gene)
Homozygous	Genotype with two identical alleles of a gene for a single trait
Heterozygous	Genotype with two different alleles of a gene for one trait
Karyotype	Orderly arrangement of photographs of chromosomes from a single cell; used in genetic counseling to identify chromosomal disorders
Chromosomal banding techniques	Demonstration of light and dark strips of chromosomes on staining with Giemsa stain (G banding) and quinacrine fluorescence (Q banding)
Dominant	An allele that influences the appearance of the phenotype even in the presence of an alternative allele
Recessive	An allele that influences the appearance of the phenotype only in the presence of another identical allele
Codominance	Type of dominance in which two versions of a trait are expressed in the same individual

Section I: General Pathology

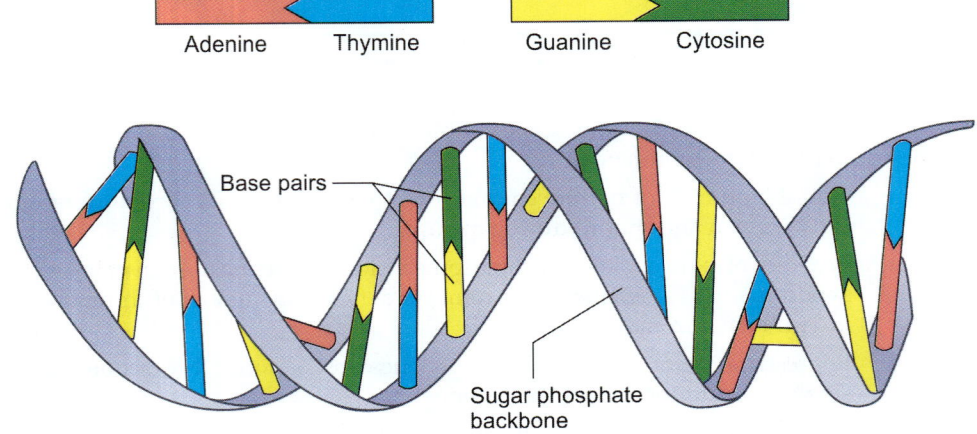

Fig. 5.1: Structure of double-stranded DNA molecule showing base pairs.

on string structure seen under electron microscope at metaphase stage of cell division.

- *Solenoid:* Nucleosomal organization provides a chromatin fiber approximately 10 nm in thickness, which gets further condensed to produce a solenoid of a 30 nm diameter.

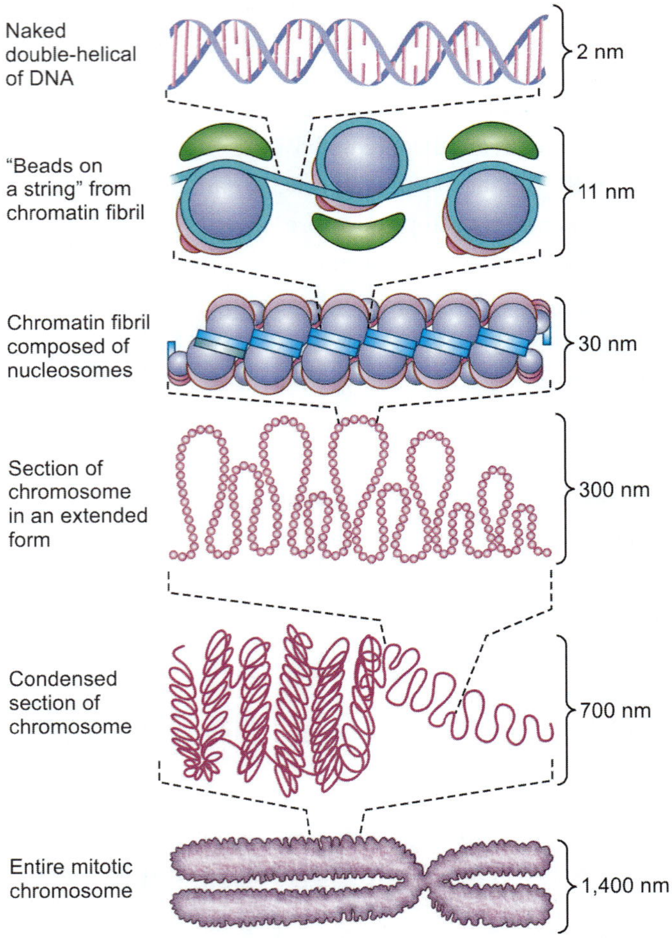

- *Chromatin fibers and chromatid:* The solenoid structures undergo further coiling to produce a chromatin fiber of 200 nm and then a chromatid of 700 nm diameter, which can be seen under electron microscope. The package of chromatin at higher level requires additional set of proteins that are collectively called as *non-histone chromosomal proteins* (NHC proteins).

Chromosomal Proteins

- *Histones:* Histone is a set of positively charged basic proteins comprising amino acids, e.g. *lysine* and *arginine*. Both have positive charge in their side chains. The negatively charged DNA is wrapped around the positively charged histone octamer to form a structure called nucleosome. H1 histone is situated outside the nucleosomal DNA. *Histones are organized to form a unit of eight molecules called histone octamer.*

Fig. 5.2: Structure of chromosome showing negatively charged DNA double helix molecule wrapped around positively charged histone octamer to form a structure called nucleosome (10 nm).

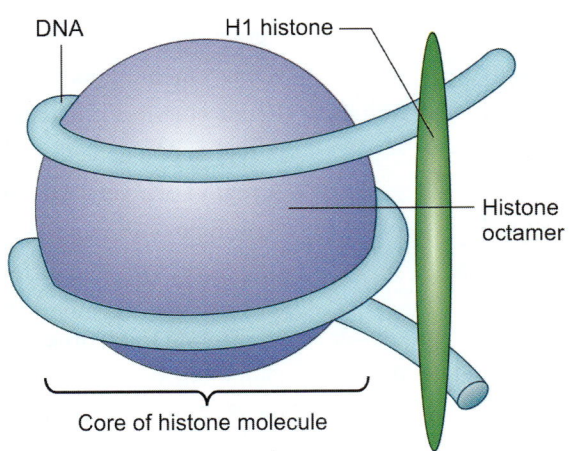

Fig. 5.3: Structure of histone showing a set of positively charged basic proteins comprising amino acids, e.g. 'lysine' and 'arginine'. Both have positive charge in their side chains. The negatively charged DNA is wrapped around the positively charged histone octamer to form a structure called nucleosome.

Genetic Disorders

- **Non-histones chromosomal proteins (NHC proteins):** The package of chromatin at higher level requires additional set of proteins. These are collectively called *non-histone chromosomal proteins (NHC proteins)*.

Nuclear chromatin: Nucleus contains two types of chromatin: euchromatin and heterochromatin. Differences between structure of DNA and RNA are shown in Table 5.2.

RNA (ribonucleic acid): RNA is similar to DNA except that it has one strand instead of two. *It has uracil (also called 5-methyl uracil) instead of thymine. It has ribose instead of deoxyribose.* Messenger RNA (mRNA) carries the genetic information out of the nucleus for protein synthesis.

In RNA, every nucleotide residue has an additional OH group present at 2'-position in the ribose. It is a reactive group and makes RNA labile and easily degradable. Differences between structure of DNA and RNA are shown in Table 5.3.

GENETIC CODE

Genetic code is a process by which genetic information coded in RNA (mRNA) is decoded into a polypeptide. Change in nucleic acids (genetic material) are responsible for change in amino acids in proteins.

Composition: The genetic code consists of 64 triplets of nucleotides. These triplets are called *codons*. Out of 64 codons, 61 codons code for amino acids, while 3 codons do not code for any amino acids; and they function as stop codons. One codon codes for one of the 20 amino acids used in the synthesis of proteins, hence, it is specific and unambiguous.

Functions: Most of the amino acids are coded by more than one codon. One codon signal starts translation and also codes for the incorporation of the amino acid methionine (Met) into the growing polypeptide chain. The code is based on sets of DNA bases and universal from bacteria to human. UUU would code for phenylalanine. Some exceptions to this rule have been found in mitochondrial codons and in some protozoa. *AUG has dual functions: It codes for methionine and acts as initiator codon.*

PROTEIN SYNTHESIS

A gene is defined as the functional unit of inheritance. Genes are located on DNA. DNA sequence coding for t-RNA and r-RNA also define a gene. Normally the genetic information encoded in DNA is transcribed to RNA and translated into amino acids from which the protein is synthesized.

Protein synthesis in human involves three processes: DNA replication, transcription and translation (Fig 5.4). RNA viruses contain reverse transcriptase, an enzyme that produces a DNA transcript of the RNA, this may then

Table 5.2: Differences between euchromatin and heterochromatin

Characteristics	Euchromatin	Heterochromatin
Packing of chromatin	Loosely packed	Densely packed
Staining pattern	Light stained	Dark stained
Protein synthesis	Inactive in protein synthesis	Transcriptionally active protein

Table 5.3: Differences between structure of DNA and RNA

Characteristics	DNA (deoxyribose nucleic acid)	RNA (ribo nucleic acid)
Pentose sugar	Deoxyribose	Ribose
Nitrogen base	Purines: adenine-guanine Pyrimidines: thymine-cytosine	Purines: adenine-guanine Pyrimidines: uracil-cytosine
Number of strands	DNA (double-stranded)	RNA (single-stranded)
Stability provided to DNA	More stable (stability provided by thymine to the genetic material) and less reactive	Less stable and more reactive (due to the presence of 2 OH-group)
Mutations occurrence	Slower rate	Faster rate (viruses have shorter lifespan)
Protein synthesis	DNA dependent on RNA for synthesizing protein	RNA can directly code for the synthesis of proteins. RNA is better for transmission of information
Other functions	DNA being double-stranded and having complementary strand further resists changes by evolving a process of repair	RNA is essential for life processes such as metabolism, translation and splicing, which evolve around RNA

Section I: General Pathology

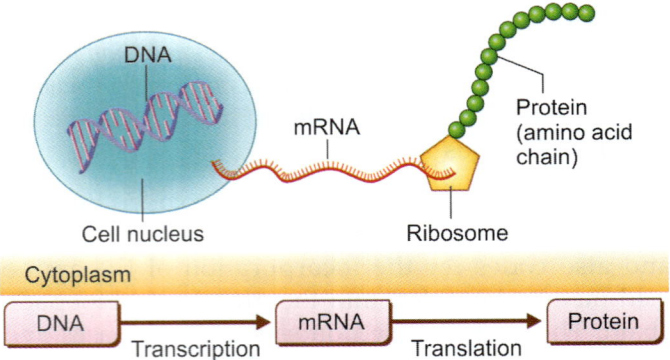

Fig. 5.4: Protein synthesis in human involving DNA replication, transcription and translation.

be incorporated into the genome of the cell, possibly altering permanently its behavior and potentially leading to tumor formation (Fig. 5.5).

Nucleotide sequence in DNA: Sequence of nucleotides present in the double-stranded DNA are transcribed into single strand of messenger RNA. *There are 1200 nucleotides in just one gene in a strand of DNA.* Every three nucleotides will become the instruction for just one amino acid. It means that 400 amino acids will have to be produced to represent one gene in one strand of DNA.

Classes of RNAs: There are three major classes of cellular RNAs based on size, sedimentation, behavior and genetic information.

- *Messenger RNA or mRNA* carries the genetic information out of the nucleus for protein synthesis.
- *Transfer RNA or tRNA:* It is the smallest and decodes the information.
- *Ribosomal RNA or rRNA:* It is the largest and constitutes 50% of a ribosome, which is a molecular assembly involved in protein synthesis. Catalytic RNAs are involved in many reactions in cytoplasm of the cell.

RNA synthesis and its translation into protein: Gene transcription involves binding of RNA polymerase II to the promoter of genes being transcribed with other proteins (transcriptional factors) that regulate the transcriptional rate (Fig. 5.6).

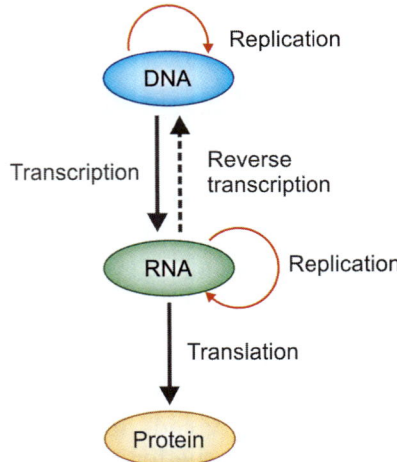

Fig. 5.5: Reverse transcription of DNA from RNA. RNA viruses contain reverse transcriptase, an enzyme that produces a DNA transcript of the RNA, this may then be incorporated into the genome of the cell, possibly altering permanently its behavior and potentially leading to tumor formation.

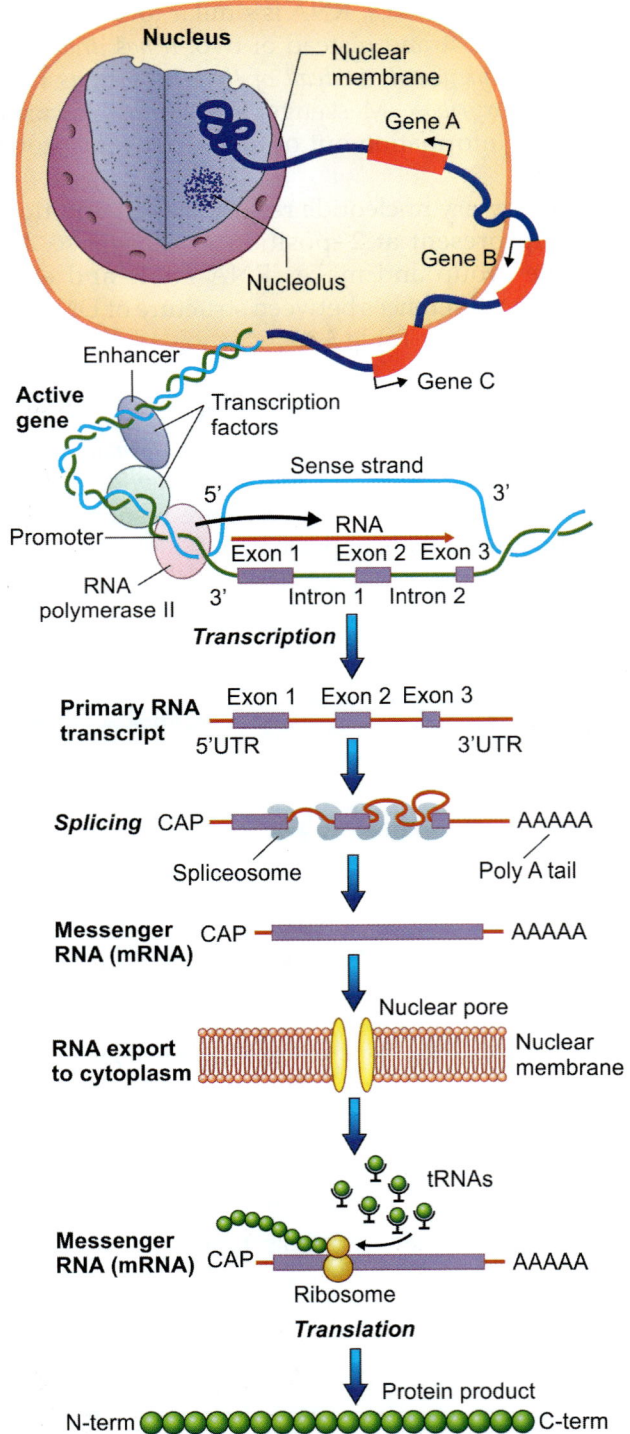

Fig. 5.6: RNA synthesis and its translation into protein.

Genetic Disorders

The primary RNA script is a copy of the whole gene and includes introns and exons. But the introns are removed within nucleus by splicing and the exons are joined to form the messenger RNA (mRNA). Prior to exit from the nucleus, a methylated guanosome nucleotide is added to the 5' end of the RNA (cap) and a string of adenine nucleotides are added to the 3' (poly A tail).

This process protects the RNA from degradation and facilitates transport into the cytoplasm. In the cytoplasm the mRNA binds to ribosomes and forms a template for protein production.

DNA Replication

Replication is the process where DNA makes a copy of itself. DNA replication is semiconservative. The two strands of the double helix separate by breaking the hydrogen bonds between nucleotides. New nucleotides attach at the proper sites and a new strand of DNA is synthesized alongside each of the original strands. Replication doubles the amount of DNA. Thus, each daughter cell contains the normal amount after a somatic cell division. This helps in reduction of number of copy errors (Fig. 5.7).

- *DNA helicases:* These bind to the double-stranded DNA and stimulate the separation of the two strands.
- *DNA gyrase:* This enzyme takes part in unwinding of the strands.
- *DNA single-stranded binding proteins:* These proteins bind to the DNA as a tetramer and stabilize the single-stranded structure that is generated by the action of the helicases. These proteins fasten the replication 100 times.
- *DNA polymerase I and polymerase II:* These detect and excise the wrong bases. 3' to 5' exonuclease takes part in proof-reading activity. 5' to 3' exonuclease takes part in repair. DNA polymerase III participates in elongation of 5' to 3' exonuclease.
- *RNA primase:* RNA primase helps in synthesis of a free 3'-hydroxyl group at the initiation sites.
- *DNA ligase:* Ligase takes part in sealing process. It forms a covalent phosphodiester linkage between 3'-hydroxyl and 5'-phosphate groups. RNA editing may also take place before translation begins. Genetic message carried by mRNA moves out of nucleus into cytoplasm for translation and converts into polypeptide sequence of amino acids.
- *DNA strands:* The strand which supports the continuous DNA synthesis is called *leading or template or sense-coding strand.* The strand which is replicated in a discontinuous manner in short stretches (also known as *Okazaki fragments*) is called *lagging or noncoding antisense strand.*

Transcription

Transcription means RNA is made from DNA. The process of copying genetic information from one strand of DNA into RNA is termed as 'transcription'. Here adenine forms base pair with uracil instead of thymine.

Binding of RNA polymerase II to active genes: Gene transcription involves binding of RNA polymerase II to the promoter of genes being transcribed with transcriptional factors (promoter and terminator) that regulate the transcriptional rate. Promoter at 5' end (upstream of structural gene) defines template and coding strands. A Terminator is located at 3' end downstream of coding strand.

Coding regulatory RNA: The primary RNA script is a copy of the whole gene that comprises protein coding regulatory RNA introns and exons. Exons are coding sequences or expressed sequences that appear in mature or processed RNA. Exons are interrupted by introns. Introns or intermittent sequences do not appear in mature or processed RNA. The introns are removed within nucleus by splicing. The exons are joined to form the messenger RNA (mRNA). Transcription leads to formation of primary RNA transcript.

Non-coding regulatory RNA: Non-coding regulatory RNA regulate gene expression by micro-RNAs and long non-coding RNAs.

- *Micro-RNA (miRNA):* Human genome contains about 1000 micro-RNA constituting 5% of total genome. These micro-RNAs are mature oligomers of 22 nucleotides in length. *These do not code for proteins.* These participate in silencing post-transcriptional genes. All micro-RNAs comprise seed sequence in their

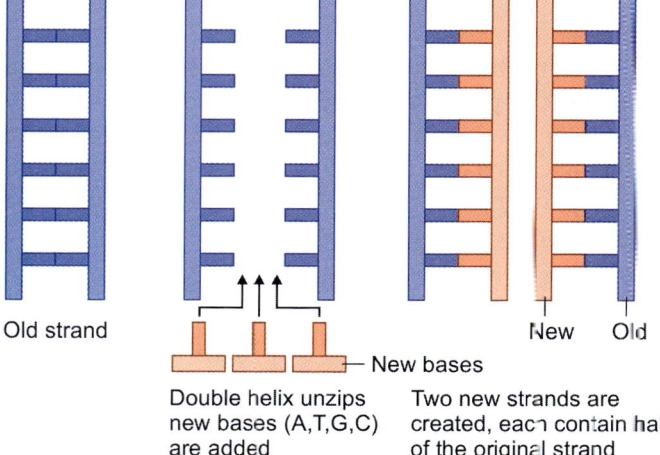

Fig. 5.7: DNA replication showing creation of two new strands.

32 untranslated region (UTR), which determines the specificity of miRNA binding and gene silencing.

- *Long noncoding RNA (LncRNA):* It participates in activation of gene. These inhibit gene transcription. Example of repressive function involves XIST (X inactive specific transcript). *XIST inactivates X chromosomes resulting in Barr body formation. LncRNA stabilizes secondary or tertiary structures that influence gene activity. It is associated with atherosclerosis and cancer.*

Splicing: Prior to export from the nucleus, a methylated guanosome nucleotide is added to the 5' end of the RNA (cap) and a string of adenine nucleotides are added to the 3' (poly A tail). *This protects the RNA from degradation and facilitates transport into the cytoplasm.*

Messenger RNA (mRNA): In the cytoplasm, the mRNA binds to ribosomes and forms a template for protein production.

Translation

Translation refers to the process of polymerization of amino acids to form polypeptides. Amino acids are joined by peptide bonds. Ribosome is the site of protein synthesis. It consists of structural RNAs and 80 different proteins.

GENE MUTATIONS

There are three basic kinds of genes: Dominant (always expressed and mask recessive gene), recessive (only expressed in the absence of dominant gene) and codominant (working together to produce a third trait).

Gene mutation may be at the level of chromosome or point alterations, or involving a single nucleotide pair in DNA. It can be inherited from a parent (hereditary mutations or germline mutations) or acquired during a person's lifetime in the DNA of individual cells caused by environmental factors (acquired or sporadic mutations).

- Acquired mutations in somatic cells cannot be passed onto the next generation, but the germline mutations can do. Penetration refers to percentage of person inheriting mutant gene, which will express the trait.
- Same mutant gene may show variable effects as seen in neurofibromatosis type I. Clinical features in neurofibromatosis type I may range from skin macules to skin tumors and skeletal deformities.
- *Pleotropism refers to single mutant gene producing multiple adverse effects as seen in sickle cell disease. Mutant gene in sickle cell disease produces hemolytic anemia, splenic infarction and bone necrosis.*
- Gene mutations occur due to point mutations, framework and trinucleotide repeat mutations described as under.

POINT MUTATIONS

Missense Gene Mutations

Missense mutation is a change in one DNA base pair that results in the substitution of one amino acid for another in the protein made by a gene. *Example of point mutation is sickle cell disease.* Mutant allele chromosome 11 causes substitution of valine for glutamine at the sixth position in β-chain of globin molecule of hemoglobin due to the single base substitution at the 6th codon of the beta globin gene from GAG to GUG and synthesize *abnormal HbS*. Missense mutation occurs by two mechanisms:

- *Conservative mutation:* There is no significant difference between original and newly synthesized amino acid.
- *Non-conservative mutation:* There is significant difference between original and newly synthesized amino acid.

Nonsense Gene Mutations (Stop Codon)

A nonsense mutation is also a change in one DNA base pair. Instead of substituting one amino acid for another, however, the altered DNA sequence prematurely signals the cell to stop building a protein. This type of mutation results in a shortened protein that may function improperly or not at all. Protein synthesized will be truncated with loss of normal activity as seen in β-*thalassemia*.

INSERTION

An insertion changes the number of DNA bases in a gene by adding a piece of DNA. As a result, the protein made by the gene may not function properly.

DELETION

A deletion changes the number of DNA bases by removing a piece of DNA. Small deletions may remove one or a few base pairs within a gene, while larger deletions can remove an entire gene or several neighboring genes. The deleted DNA may alter the function of the resulting protein(s).

FRAMESHIFT MUTATIONS

Insertions, deletions, and duplications can all be frameshift mutations. Frameshift mutation occurs when the addition or loss of DNA bases changes a gene's reading frame. A reading frame consists of groups of 3 bases that each code for one amino acid. A frameshift mutation shifts the grouping of these bases and changes the code for amino acids. The resulting protein is usually nonfunctional.

EXPANSION OF TRINUCLEOTIDE REPEAT

Normal number of trinucleotide repeats is 29. Expansion of trinucleotide repeat sequences occurs during gametogenesis. Several disorders are associated with the expansion of the number of tandem trinucleotide repeats in certain critical genes. The number of repeats often increases from one generation to another generation and is associated with earlier onset and more severe manifestations in successive generations. This phenomenon is referred to as anticipation. Examples of trinucleotide repeat disorders include *fragile X syndrome, Huntington disease, and myotonic dystrophy.*

Fragile X Syndrome

Fragile X syndrome is an important cause of hereditary mental retardation with *IQ scores varying from 20 to 60*, second in frequency only to Down syndrome. Both males and females can be asymptomatic carriers. *This increased number of repeats is referred to as a premutation. Expansion of premutations in the germline increases in the number of tandem repeats in female carrier.* These increased numbers are referred to as full mutations.

Carrier females can transmit the affected X chromosome to both sons and daughters. *Sons with full mutations exhibit mental retardation and often bilateral macroorchidism (enlarged testes).* Daughters with full mutations may or may not (~50%) exhibit mental retardation.

Pathogenesis: Fragile X syndrome is caused by *expansion of a CGG trinucleotide repeat in the 5'-untranslated (noncoding) region of the familial mental retardation (FMR-1) gene on the long arm of X chromosome during oogenesis.* Expanded CGG repeat silences the FMR-1 gene by methylation of its promoter. Cytogenetic studies reveal a nonstaining gap or chromosomal break.

- Degree of expansion is related to the gender of the parent with the genetic abnormality. Expanded CGG repeat silences the FMR-1 gene by methylation of its promoter.
- The abnormal repeat is associated with an inducible 'fragile site' on the X chromosome, which appears in cytogenetic studies as a nonstaining gap or chromosomal break.

Clinical features: The male newborn afflicted with the fragile X syndrome appears normal. *During childhood, patient presents with increased head circumference, facial coarsening, joint hyperextensibility, enlarged testes, and abnormalities of the cardiac valves. In adult patients with fragile X syndrome have macroorchidism.* A significant proportion of autistic male children carry a fragile X chromosome.

Huntington Disease

In Huntington disease, expansion occurs during spermatogenesis. Even though trinucleotide repeats almost always involve guanine and cytosine (G and C), the third nucleotide is different in two conditions: *CGG in fragile X syndrome and CAG in Huntington disease.*

Myotonic Dystrophy

This disorder demonstrates an *autosomal dominant mode* of inheritance. It is the most common variety of adult onset muscular dystrophy. This disorder is caused by an *increased number of trinucleotide repeats (50–1000) in the myotonin protein kinase gene (normal is less than 30 nucleotides).*

Clinical features: Its primary symptom is *myotonic stiffness or spasm following muscle contraction.* Patient is unable to relax muscles once contracted. It is a progressive disorder that affects *heart, smooth muscles* (gastrointestinal tract), *central nervous system, endocrine glands, testes* (atrophy) and *eyes* (cataract).

INHERITANCE OF MONOGENIC DISORDERS

There are five modes of inheritance of monogenic disorders, i.e. autosomal dominance, autosomal recessive, X-linked recessive, X-linked dominant inheritance and mitochondrial inheritance.

Interaction of genes: When two genes interact, one gene masks or modifies the expression of another non-allelic gene.

- *Epistasis:* It is the interaction between different genes (non-alleles). *Epistasis gene* overrides the expression of other gene. *Hypostasis gene* gets masked by the epistasis gene. Either of the two alleles (recessive or dominance) can bring about the epistasis effect.
- *Dominance:* It refers to interaction between different alleles of the same gene. Inheritance of a character determined by two genes in which one allele is epistatic over the other allele pair.

Mobile genetic elements: Approximately 33% of human genome is composed of *jumping genes.* These can *move within genome.* These participate in regulation of gene and chromatin organization.

Special structural regions of DNA: These are composed of telomeres and centromeres.

AUTOSOMAL DOMINANCE INHERITANCE

In autosomal dominant inheritance, one parent carries a gene and other parent is normal. Only one copy of the gene needs to be inherited for the disease to be expressed in children, thus both homozygous and heterozygous individuals in both sexes are affected. 50% of the children are expected to inherit the gene.

AUTOSOMAL RECESSIVE INHERITANCE

In autosomal recessive inheritance, both the parents carrying abnormal genes need to be inherited for the disease to be expressed in children, thus only homozygous individuals are affected in both sexes. Heterozygous individuals are asymptomatic carriers.

X-LINKED RECESSIVE INHERITANCE

Hemophilia is an example of X-linked disorder. In females, defective gene in hemophilia is located on chromosome X. In females, the other normal X chromosome corrects the abnormality, but females can be asymptomatic carriers. Hemophilia is expressed in males because there is no normal X chromosome to correct the abnormality.

In another setting, only male parent carries abnormal gene and female parent is normal. Their female children inherit the paternal X chromosome and become carriers. But all male children are genotypically and phenotypically unaffected.

X-LINKED DOMINANT INHERITANCE

X-linked dominant inheritance is a rare variant of X-linked inheritance. Hemizygous males as well as heterozygous females phenotypically manifest the disorder.

MITOCHONDRIAL INHERITANCE

Mitochondrial inheritance is mediated through maternal lines (cytoplasmic mitochondrial genes), as mitochondria in the embryo are derived from ovum. *Mitochondrial genes code for enzymes of oxidative phosphorylation.*

Only female parent transmits the trait to all of their children. Transmission of abnormal mitochondrial genes by female parent affects enzymes of oxidative phosphorylation. If an affected male has children, his progeny are unaffected. A mixture of genetically normal and abnormal mitochondria in tissues is termed *heteroplasmy*. Disorders associated with mitochondrial DNA mutations are shown in Table 5.4.

Table 5.4: Disorders associated with mitochondrial DNA mutations

Mitochondrial disorders	System involved	Clinical manifestations
Chronic progressive external ophthalmoplegia	Eye	Progressive weakness of extraocular muscles
Deafness	Ear	Progressive sensorineural deafness often associated with aminoglycoside antibiotics
Kearns-Sayre syndrome	Eye	Progressive weakness of extraocular muscles of early onset, retinal pigmentation
	Heart	Heart block
Leber's optic hereditary neuropathy	Eyes	Painless, subacute visual loss, with central blind spots (scotomata) and abnormal color vision
Leigh disease	Nervous system	Proximal muscle weakness, sensory neuropathy, developmental delay, ataxia, seizures, dementia
	Eyes	Visual pigment degeneration
MELAS	Nervous system (cerebral structural changes)	Mitochondrial encepahlomyopathy (cerebral structural changes), lactic acidosis, and stroke like syndrome, other clinical and laboratory abnormalities; may manifest as diabetes mellitus
MERPF	Nervous system and muscles	Myoclonic epilepsy, ragged red fibers in muscle, ataxia, sensorineural weakness
Myoclonic epilepsy with ragged red fibers	Nervous system and muscles	Myoclonic seizures, cerebellar ataxia, mitochondrial myopathy (muscle weakness, fatigue)

Genetic Disorders

POLYGENIC AND MULTIFACTORIAL DISORDERS

Polygenic disorders are more common than monogenic disorders. Polygenetic disorders are caused by abnormalities of two or more genes regulating their protein products. Environmental factors modulate these genetic disorders. *Common polygenic disorders include ischemic heart disease, diabetes mellitus, hypertension, gout, schizophrenia, bipolar disorder, and neural tube defects.*

GENETIC POLYMORPHISM

Any two persons share 99.9% of their DNA sequences. Variation of DNA sequences between two persons is less than 0.5% (about 15 million base pairs). This variation of DNA sequences is known as *genetic polymorphism*. Example of genetic polymorphism is blood groups. Comparison of mutation and polymorphism is shown in Table 5.5. Genetic variations are of three types described as under.

SINGLE NUCLEOTIDE POLYMORPHISM (SNP)

Two persons possess exactly same DNA sequence in 99.5% of their DNA. Therefore two persons vary in the remaining 0.1% of DNA. Single nucleotide polymorphism (SNP) is the most common variant of genetic polymorphism. It represents variation at single nucleotide per 1000 base pairs. Human genome comprises more than 6 million SNPs. These are present in exons and introns. SNPs occur in the coding regions in <0.1%.

COPY NUMBER VARIATIONS (CNVs)

Human genome contains 5 to 24 million base pair of CNVs. CNVs represent large number of contiguous stretches of DNA from 1000 to millions base pairs. About 50% persons have CNVs in the coding regions. These are the basis of phenotype diversity.

REPEAT LENGTH POLYMORPHISM

Short repetitive sequence of DNA variation is of two types: microsatellites and minisatellites.

BALANCED POLYMORPHISM

Balanced polymorphism refers to the increased incidence of deleterious (usually in homozygotes) alleles among certain populations in environments in which the same allele is associated with a potential survival advantage (usually in heterozygotes). This condition has been observed in both autosomal and X-linked disorders.

HEMOGLOBIN S

Heterozygotes are thought to be relatively resistant to *Plasmodium falciparum* malaria, and homozygotes have sickle cell anemia.

G6PD DEFICIENCY

In this X-linked disorder, hemizygotes manifest drug-related (classically primaquine, an antimalarial) or oxidant-related hemolytic anemia and are also resistant to malaria. In this instance, selection working both positively and negatively clearly represents a manifestation of the balance implied by the term balanced polymorphism.

PHENYLKETONURIA

Unaffected heterozygotes have a lower incidence of spontaneous abortion. It is thought that modestly increased concentrations of phenylalanine exert a protective effect on pregnancy.

TAY-SACHS DISEASE

Patient with Tay-Sachs disease may have protection against tuberculosis.

CYSTIC FIBROSIS

Cystic fibrosis, in which there is an apparent protective effect against cholera. It is thought that the enterotoxin of cholera facilitates the egress of chloride and water from intestinal mucosa by enhanced activity of chloride channels. Both heterozygous carriers and homozygous affected subjects with cystic fibrosis are relatively resistant to this effect, because insufficient chloride channels are available.

DISORDERS ASSOCIATED WITH GENOMIC IMPRINTING

In these hereditary disorders, different phenotypes occur depending on whether an abnormal gene is of maternal or paternal origin. It occurs due to epigenetic changes occurring during gametogenesis, which mark

Table 5.5: Comparison of mutation and polymorphism

Parameters	Mutation	Polymorphism
Gene	Gene directly leads to disorder	Gene confers an increased risk, but does not directly cause disorder
Inheritance	Mendelian pattern of inheritance	No clear inheritance pattern
Population affected	Rare	Common in population

at least some genes. These genes are transmitted to the next generation. Such marking is referred to as genomic imprinting.

- DNA methylation occurring in the female and male gonads, making certain nonactive genes, which are not able to transcribed.
- *Prader-Willi syndrome and Angelman's syndrome have same cytogenetic deletion (15) (q11q13) resulting in differing phenotypes in progeny depending on whether the deletions were transmitted by the mother or the father.*

PRADER-WILLI SYNDROME

Paternal transmission results in the Prader-Willi syndrome. Patient presents with *hypogonadism, hypotonia, mental retardation, behavior problems, and uncontrolled appetite resulting to obesity and diabetes.*

ANGELMAN (HAPPY PUPPET) SYNDROME

Maternal transmission results in the Angelman syndrome. It is sometimes referred to as the *happy puppet syndrome*. Patient presents with *mental retardation, ataxia, seizures,* and *inappropriate laughter.*

CHROMOSOMAL DISORDERS

Normal cells are diploid, containing 46 chromosomes (23 pairs). Out of these, there are 22 pairs of autosomes and 1 pair of sex chromosomes (XX in females or XY in males). Duplication of chromosomes in somatic cell lines involves mitosis. Meiosis is limited to replicating germ cells (ova or sperms). Study of human chromosomal abnormalities is called *cytogenetics.*

Sex determination of individual is shown in Fig. 5.8. Terms associated with chromosomal appearances and abnormalities are shown in Table 5.6.

Lyon's hypothesis: In females, during embryogenesis, inactivation of one of two X chromosomes derived from maternal or paternal is known as *Lyon's hypothesis*. This inactivation is transmitted to all somatic cells except germ cells. Ovaries will always possess active chromosomes.

- In females, the inactive X chromosome in the somatic cells becomes *condensed in the nucleus is called nuclear sexing.*
- Smears stained by *scrapping of oral mucosa* or circulating neutrophils demonstrates *'Barr bodies'*, which appear as *drumstick appendage* attached to *one of the nuclear lobes*. A minimum of 30% cells positive for sex chromatin indicates female genetic constitution.

ALTERATIONS IN CHROMOSOMES

Genetic disorders are inherited as autosomal dominant disorders, in which each child has a 50% chance of inheriting the disorder, or as autosomal recessive disorders, in which each child has a 25% chance of being affected, a 50% chance of being a carrier, and a 25% chance of being unaffected. *Sex-linked disorders almost always are associated with the X chromosome and are predominantly recessive.*

Chromosomal disorders reflect events that occur at the time of meiosis and result from defective movement of an entire chromosome or from breakage of a chromosome with loss or translocation of genetic

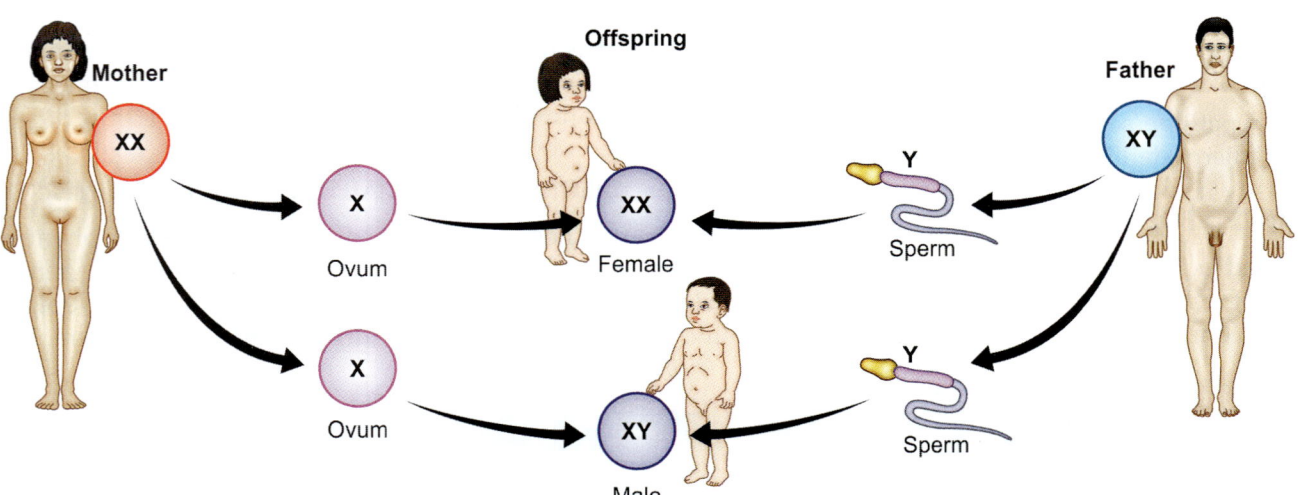

Fig. 5.8: Sex determination of individual. The presence of Y chromosome specifies male sex. In the absence of Y chromosome an individual develops into a female.

Genetic Disorders

Table 5.6: Terms associated with chromosomal appearances and abnormalities

Term	Description
Centromere	The region that connects the two arms of the chromosome
Deletion	Loss of all or part of one chromosomal arm, usually a part toward the end of an arm. An acentric chromosome (without a centromere) is typically lost completely after a few cell divisions. Examples: 46, XX, 4p- or 46, XX, del(13)(q12q14)
Duplication	A segment of chromatin that is repeated on the same or another chromosome. Many are incompatible with life. Example: 46, XY, dup(1)(q11q22)
Fragile site	There is a site on one arm that has a demonstrable fixed break point. Example: 46, fra(X)(q27.3),Y
Insertion	There must be two break points in one chromosome that allow a segment to insert between a break point in another chromosome. Example: 46, XX, ins(11)(p14q23q24)
Isochromosome	The arms of a chromosome are mirror images of each other. Monocentric isochromosomes have two long arms or two short arms. Dicentric isochromosomes have mirrored material between centromeres. Example: 46, X, i(Xq)
Inversion	Two break points in a chromosome allow a 180° turn of a segment with fusion. The inversion is "paracentric" if it only involves one arm, while "pericentric" inversions involve the centromere and parts of p and q arms. Example: 46, XX, inv(8)(p23q22)
Marker	A small extra piece of chromosomal material that travels with the other chromosomes. Example: 46, XY, +mar
Monosomy	Only one of a chromosome pair is present. Autosomal monosomies yield non-viable embryos. Only monosomy X is rarely liveborn. Example: 45, X or 45, XY, –14
Mosaic	Cells with an abnormal karyotype are present along with normal cells. Example: 45,X/46,XX
p arm	The short arm of the chromosome
q arm	The long arm of the chromosome
Ring	Breakage of a chromosome at two points is followed by repair with fusion to a circular chromosome. Example: 46, XX, r(1)(p36q44)
Translocation	There is an exchange of material between arms on different chromosomes. The translocation is "reciprocal" if there is an exchange of two chromosome segments on different (nonhomologous) chromosomes. It is "balanced" if no genetic material is lost. "Unbalanced" translocations involve more breakpoints that lead to loss of genetic material in the exchange. Example: 46, XY, t(9;22)
Triploidy	Three haploid sets of chromosomes are present in a cell. Example: 69, XXY
Trisomy	An extra chromosome is present, making three copies. Extra genetic material reduces viability. Example: 47, XX, +18

material. Changes in chromosome number and structure occurs by various mechanisms described as under.

ALTERATION OF CHROMOSOME STRUCTURE

Alteration of chromosome occurs during cell division: it occurs by deletion, duplication, inversion and translocation.

Deletion of Chromosome

Loss of chromosomal fragment ('p' short arm or 'q' long arm) or entire chromosome during cell division is termed deletion. It leads to the loss of genetic material. Deletions may be terminal or interstitial. The severity of this lost genetic material depends upon the size of the deletion and the nature of the genetic material contained within it. Deletions produce unbalanced meiotic products; thereby resulting in sterility.

Cri du chat syndrome, an example of deletion is characterized by partial loss of the short arm of chromosome 5 is designated as 46,XY, 5p– in males or 46,XX, 5p– in females (Fig. 5.9).

Duplication of Chromosomes

Duplication occurs when a portion of a chromosome is repeated and reattaches to homologous chromosome. Duplication can be random or in reverse order.

Inversion of Chromosome

When a fragment of the chromosome breaks but latter reattaches to original, but in reverse position after rotating by 180°, it results in inversion. As many as 1% of the newborn may carry an inversion that can be detected by G-banded chromosome karyotyping. *Inversions produce unbalanced meiotic products; thereby resulting in sterility.* There are two types of inversion (Fig. 5.10):

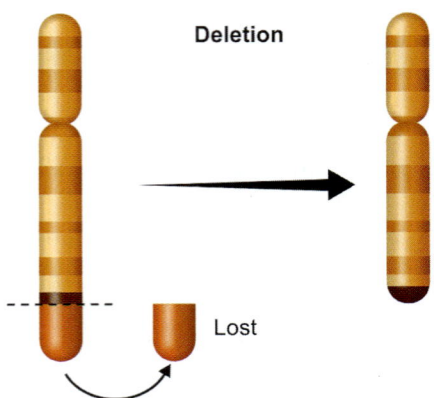

Fig. 5.9: Deletion of fragment of chromosome (long arm or short arm) during cell division leads to loss of genetic material and shortening of the chromosome. Deletion of the chromosome may occur in terminal or interstitial region. Deletions produce unbalanced meiotic products; thereby resulting in sterility.

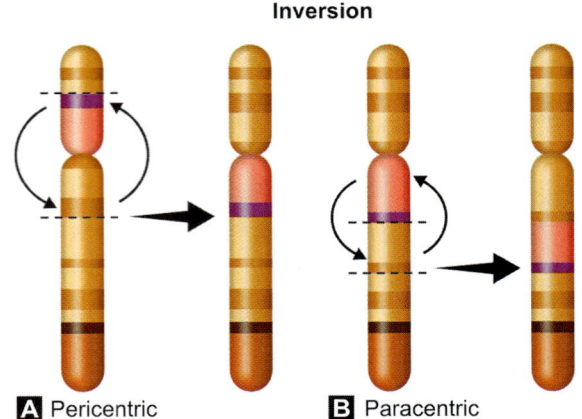

Fig. 5.10: Inversion requires two breaks in a single chromosome.

- *Paracentric inversion:* Centromere is not included in the inverted segment.
- *Pericentric inversion:* Centromere is included in the inverted segment.

Translocation of Chromosome

Exchange of chromosomal segments between nonhomologous chromosomes is called *translocation. Translocation may be balanced (reciprocal translocation in chronic myeloid leukemia without loss of genetic material), or interstitial translocation (loss of segment of chromosome and reattaches to non-homologous chromosome).*

Reciprocal translocation: A 'reciprocal' translocation occurs when there are break points in two chromosomes, with exchange of the fragments between two non-homologous chromosomes, without loss of any portion. Balanced translocation is often clinically silent. *Philadelphia chromosome t (9/22) discovered by Hugo de Vries in chronic myeloid leukemia is an example*

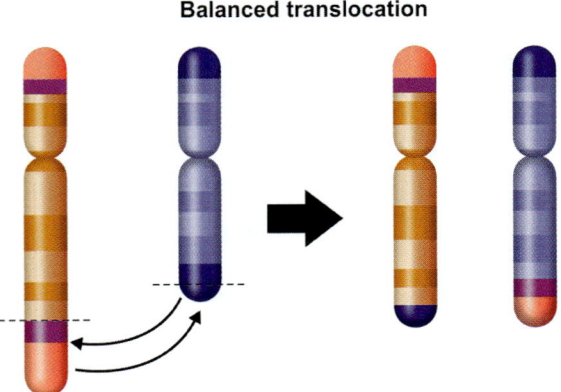

Fig. 5.11: A reciprocal translocation involves two nonhomologous chromosomes, with exchange of the acentric segment.

of reciprocal translocation. Positivity of this Philadelphia chromosome 9/22 indicates good prognosis in these patients (Fig. 5.11).

Robertsonian translocation: Robertsonian translocation is also called *centric fusion*, when two acrocentric chromosomes (with very short 'p' arms) have break points very close to the centromere. There is subsequent fusion of the long arms. It predisposes to *Down's syndrome t (14q; 21q).*

Chromosome 21 is joined to a second acrocentric chromosome, commonly chromosome 14 or 22. The union of a gamete with this translocation with a gamete from an unaffected person can result in trisomy 21. *There is high incidence of spontaneous abortion of such fetuses* (Fig. 5.12).

Ring Chromosome

Ring chromosome is formed by a break at both terminal (telomeric) ends of a chromosome followed by fragments and end to end fusion of fragments. The consequences depend on the amount of loss of genetic material as a result of break (Fig. 5.13).

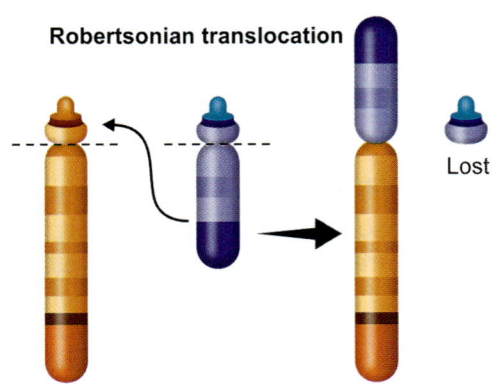

Fig. 5.12: In Robertsonian translocation, two nonhomologous acrocentric chromosomes break near centromeres, after which the long arms fuse to form one large metacentric chromosome.

Genetic Disorders 5

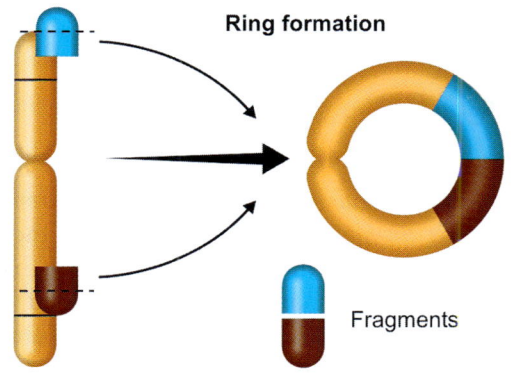

Fig. 5.13: A ring chromosome forms with breaks in both telomeric.

NUMERICAL CHROMOSOMAL ABNORMALITIES

Normal human somatic cell is diploid (46 chromosomes). On the other hand, germ cell is haploid (23 chromosomes). Polyploidy refers to increase in number (a whole set) of chromosomes more than as in diploid. It occurs due to failure of cytokines is after telophase stage of cell division. It can also bring about visible effects on the phenotype.

Triploidy (3X) is three times the haploid number; tetraploidy (4X) is four times the haploid number and so on. Polyploidy is rarely compatible with life and usually results in spontaneous abortion.

Polyploidy

Polyploidy is a term used to denote number of chromosomes multiple of haploid (23). Number of chromosomes present in diploid (46), triploid (69) and tetraploid (92). Polyploidy normally occurs in *megakaryocytes* and *dividing hepatocytes*. Polyploidy occurring in somatic cells of conception leads to *spontaneous abortion*.

Aneuploidy

Failure of segregation of chromatids during cell division cycle resulting in the extra copy (gain) or deficient in number (loss) of a chromosome(s), called aneuploidy. Effects of non-disjunction may result in *trisomy (presence of extra chromosome 2N +1) or monosomy (loss of one chromosome 2N −1)* in the offspring. Non-disjunction is the most common mechanism of aneuploidy. Failure of separation of pair chromosomes or chromatids occurs during cell division (meiosis I, meiosis II and mitosis).

Nondisjunction during meiosis I: There is failure of a pair of homologous chromosomes to separate during first meiotic division during gametogenesis. Therefore, one of the gamete contains both the chromosomes (2N) and other gamete lacks chromosomes. During fertilization, one of the chromosomes is added from the other gamete making it trisomy. Nullisomy is loss of both homologous chromosomes. Examples of aneuploidy are described as under:

- *Trisomy:* It refers to presence of extra copy of chromosome (2N +1). Examples are *Down's syndrome* (gain of extra copy of chromosome 21) and *Klinefelter's* syndrome (gain of chromosome X leading to 47 XXY). Effects of nondisjunction may result in trisomy or monosomy in the offspring (Fig. 5.14).

- *Monosomy:* It refers to loss of one chromosome (2N −1) in Turner's syndrome. Turner's syndrome occurs due to loss of an X chromosome (45, X0) in human females.

- *Nullisomy:* It refers to loss of both homologous chromosomes (2N −2).

Nondisjunction during meiosis II: There is failure of chromatids to separate during meiosis II. During spermatogenesis, each meiotic division is symmetric. Each primary spermatocyte gives rise to 2 secondary spermatocytes after meiosis I, and eventually 4 spermatids after meiosis II. Meiosis II nondisjunction

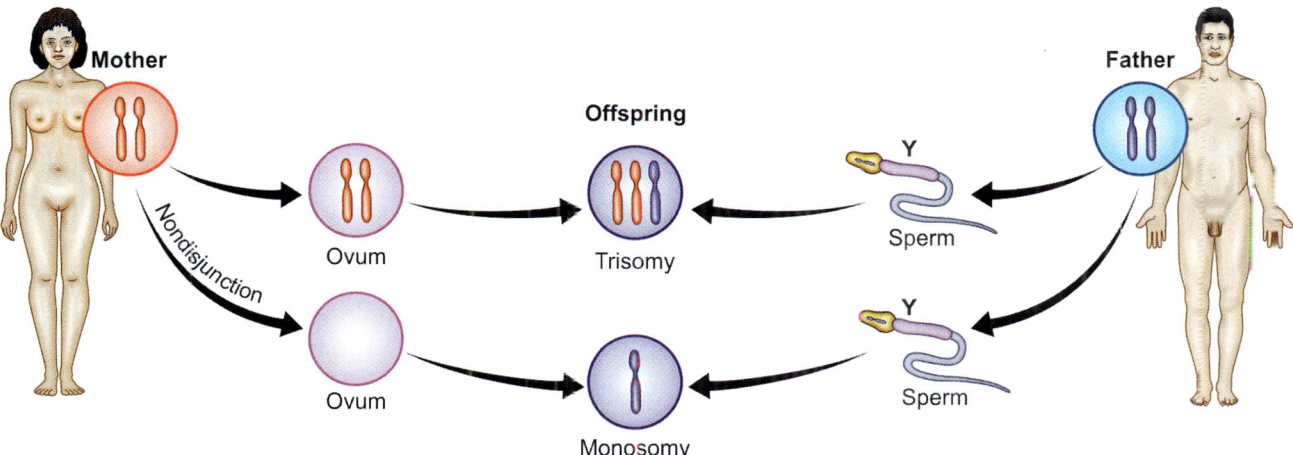

Fig. 5.14: Effects of nondisjunction may result in trisomy or monosomy in the offspring.

may also result in aneuploidy syndromes, but only to a much smaller extent than do segregation failures in meiosis I.

Nondisjunction during mitosis: During early phase of embryogenesis, if somatic cell undergoes nondisjunction during mitosis, it leads to formation of a few somatic cells with normal chromosomes and a few with extra copy (trisomy). It is called *mosaicism*, in which the person has two or more types of cell lines derived from the same zygote. *Mosaicism commonly occurs in cancers as a result of nondisjunction.*

MOSAICISM

Turner's mosaicism: A mosaic person has two lines of cells (one normal chromosome and another with monosomy single residual abnormal chromosome) for the affected chromosome pair due to anaphase lag. *Example is Turner's mosaicism with 45, X0/46, XXor 45, XO/47, XXX. A deletion of the SHOX gene can cause an identical phenotype and may be considered to be a variant of Turner syndrome.*

Confined placental mosaicism: Sometimes the abnormal cell line may appear only in the placenta, while the fetus has a normal karyotype. *This may account for some stillbirths where no fetal abnormality can be found, other than growth retardation.* Such a placenta may be smaller than normal. Conversely, a normal placental karyotype may allow longer survival of a fetus with an abnormal karyotype.

ISOCHROMOSOME FORMATION

Isochromosomes arise from faulty centromere division, which forms two new chromosomes. Each new chromosome consists of either two long arms (iso q) or two short arms as a result of deletion. One of the two isochromosomes, usually the short-arm isochromosome, often is lost. *Example involving isochromosome of*

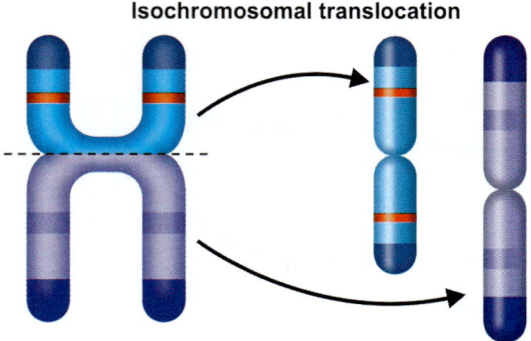

Fig. 5.15: Isochromosomes arise from faulty centromere division, which leads to duplication of the long arm and deletion of the short arm, or the reverse.

X chromosome is demonstrated in 15% cases of Turner's syndrome (Fig. 5.15).

MARKER CHROMOSOME

Appearance of small extra piece of genetic material (chromosomal 'junk') along with a normal set of chromosomes is called marker chromosome. If it arises *de novo*, then there is an increased risk for mental retardation for the fetus. However, if a parent has the marker as well, then it is familial and unlikely to be associated with *mental retardation.*

ALTERATIONS IN SEX CHROMOSOMES

Extreme karyotype deviations in the sex chromosomes are compatible with life; this is believed to be due to X inactivation (lyonization) and the relatively scanty genetic information carried by the Y chromosome.

BARR BODIES

Barr bodies are also known as sex chromatin. These appear as clumps of chromatin in the interphase nuclei of all somatic cells in females. According to the Lyon's hypothesis, each Barr body represents one inactivated X chromosome. One Barr body is present in normal female cells (XX). Barr bodies are absent in males (XY). XXX, XXY cells have two Barr bodies.

The number of Barr bodies is always one less than the number of X chromosomes. Assessment of Barr bodies was considered as diagnostic tool in past. Now it has now been supplemented by more definitive and sophisticated analytic procedures (Fig. 5.16).

X-INACTIVATION

This is the process by which all X chromosomes except one are randomly inactivated at an early stage of embryonic development. It results in all normal females being mosaics, with two distinct cell lines, one with an active maternal X, and another with an active paternal X.

It can be demonstrated if the female is heterozygous for an X-linked gene; if individuals demonstrate inheritable differences that distinguish the protein products of one X chromosome from the other, then members of the two cell lines can be identified.

The X-inactive-specific transcript (XIST) is a large untranslated RNA molecule associated with inactivating of one of the two X chromosomes.

The phenotypic differences between XO, XX, and multiple X genotypes are thought to be caused by residual genes on the X chromosome that escape inactivation.

Genetic Disorders

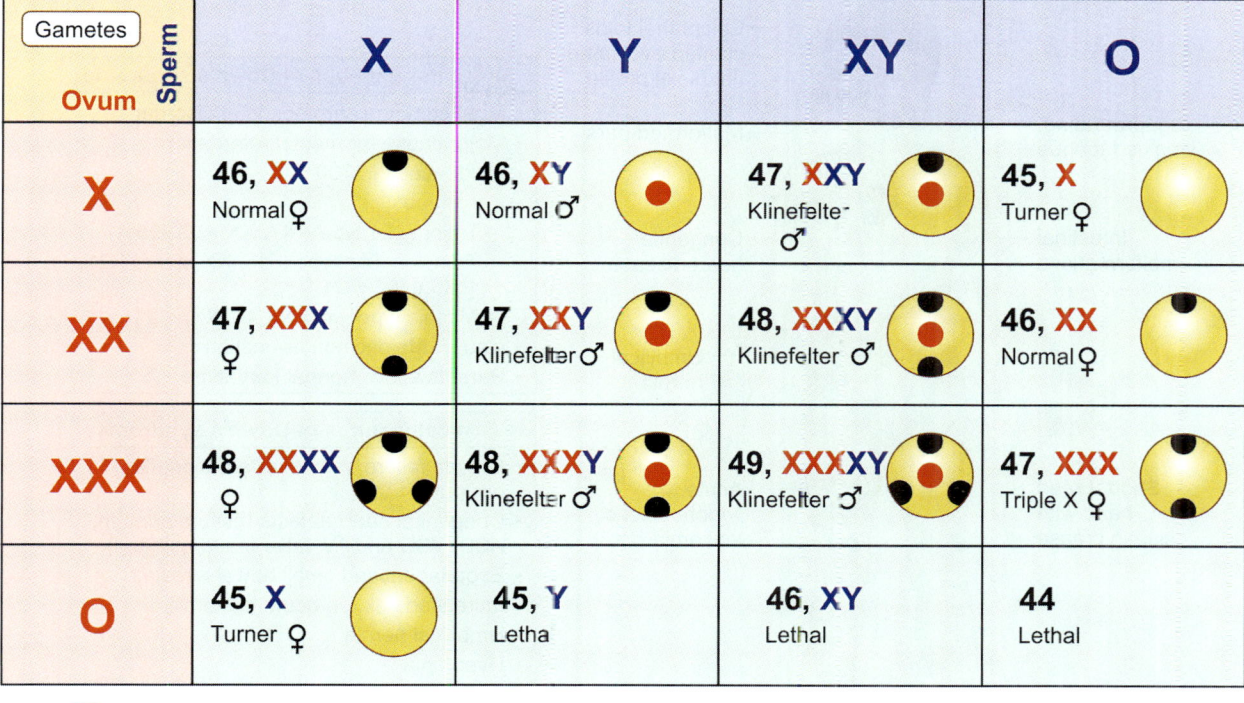

Fig. 5.16: Barr bodies.

AUTOSOMAL DISORDERS

Abnormalities of autosomal chromosomes comprise *Down's syndrome*, *Cri du chat* (5p–, cry of the cat) syndrome, *DiGeorge*/velocardiofacial syndrome, Edward's syndrome (trisomy 18) and *Patau syndrome* (trisomy 13).

DOWN'S SYNDROME

Down's syndrome is most common chromosomal disorder and major cause for mental retardation (Fig. 5.17). It occurs by following mechanisms:

- *Trisomy 21 type:* It shows 47, XX + 21 (95%) pattern. It occurs due to *maternal meiotic nondisjunction of chromosomes*. It accounts for 95% cases of Down's syndrome who have trisomy 21, and the incidence increases with maternal age. When the cause is paternal nondisjunction, there is no relation to paternal age.
- *Translocation:* It shows 46, XX, der (14; 21)(q10;q10), +21 pattern. Translocation of an extra-long arm of chromosome 21 to another acrocentric chromosome causes about 5% of cases of familial Down's syndrome; with significant risk of the syndrome in subsequent children. There is no relation to maternal age.
- *Mosaic pattern:* It shows 46, XX/47, XX, +21 pattern.

Clinical Features

- *IQ:* Mental retardation is always present but is highly variable in degree ranging from 20 to 70.
- *Face:* On examination, patient shows *mongolian idiocy* (flat facial profile, oblique palpebral fissures and epicanthic folds), large forehead, broad nasal bridge, wide-spaced eyes, epicanthal folds, large protruding tongue, small low-set ears and abundant neck skin. Small white spots are present at the periphery of iris known as *Brushfield spots*.
- *Reproduction: Virtually all males are sterile but some females can reproduce.*
- *Musculoskeletal system:* Patient has short, broad hands with curvature of the fifth finger; simian crease, a single palmar crease; and an unusually wide space between the first and second toes.

Complications

- *Congenital heart diseases:* These include congenital heart defects (atrial septal defect, ventricular septal defect) and atrioventricular valve malformations (prolapse).
- *Gastrointestinal disorders:* Patient may develop atresia of *esophagus* and *small bowel*.
- *Hematological malignancy:* Patients with Down's syndrome are at increased risk of acute lymphoblastic leukemia.

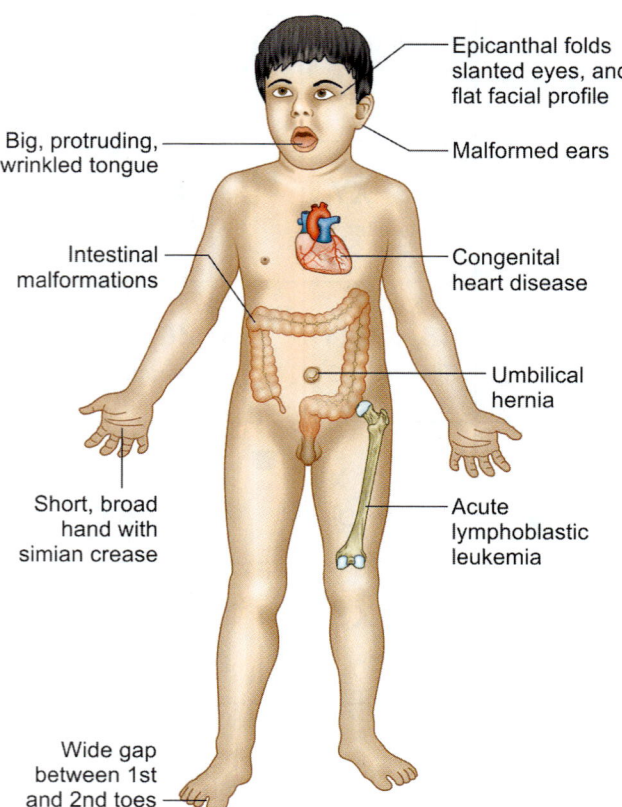

Fig. 5.17: Down's syndrome showing molecular genetic defects and clinical features.

- *Abdominal defects:* Patient may develop *umbilical hernia.*
- *Brain:* In patients surviving into middle age, morphologic changes in the brain *similar to those of Alzheimer's disease.*
- *Susceptibility to infection:* There is increased susceptibility to infection.
- *Mortality:* Approximately *75% of fetuses with Down's syndrome abort spontaneously.* About 20% of patients die before the age of 10 years. Rest may have life expectancy of 60 years.

Maternal Screening of Mothers

- *Hormonal assays:* The mother has *high level* serum *human chorionic gonadotropin (hCG)* and *low levels of α-fetoprotein,* and unconjugated estriol. These assays are referred to as the *triple screen.* When mother has high level of serum inhibin A, it is referred to as the *quadruple screen.* There is also reduced level of pregnancy associated plasma protein A.
- *Imaging technique:* Ultrasonography reveals physical defects such as increased nuchal fold.

CRI DU CHAT (5P–, CRY OF THE CAT) SYNDROME

The cause is the deletion of the short arm of chromosome 5 designated as 46, XY, 5p– in males or 46, XX, 5p– in females. Patient presents with *severe mental retardation, microcephaly, and an unusual cat-like cry.* On examination, patient has *low birth weight, round face, hypertelorism (wide-set eyes), low-set ears, and epicanthal folds.*

DIGEORGE/VELOCARDIOFACIAL SYNDROME

DiGeorge/velocardiofacial syndrome is also known as (microdeletion of 22q11, CATCH22 syndrome). There is failure of maturation of T cells, but B cells remain unaffected.

Pathology: In DiGeorge syndrome, aberrant embryonic development of third and fourth branchial arches, results in hypoplasia of thymus and parathyroid glands as well as anomalies of aortic arch, mandible and ear.

It can be summed up by CATCH22, which denotes *cardiac defects, abnormal facies, thymic hypoplasia, cleft palate, hypocalcemia and microdeletion of chromosome 22q11.* In about 30% of cases, this syndrome is also associated with behavior disorders and psychosis (*bipolar disorder and schizophrenia*) that develop during adolescence.

Clinical features: Affected children develop *recurrent infections (bacterial, fungal and viral)* and *tetany* from *hypoparathyroidism* with *hypocalcemia.*

Genetic Disorders

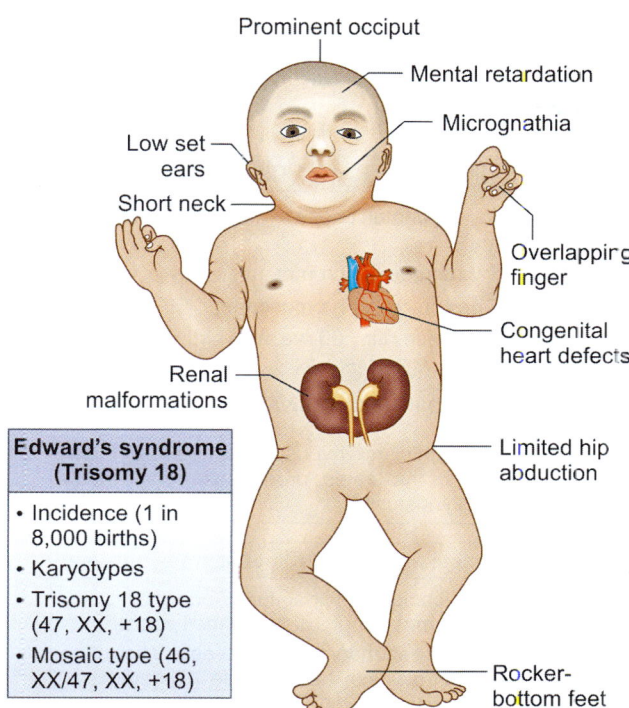

Fig. 5.18: Edward syndrome.

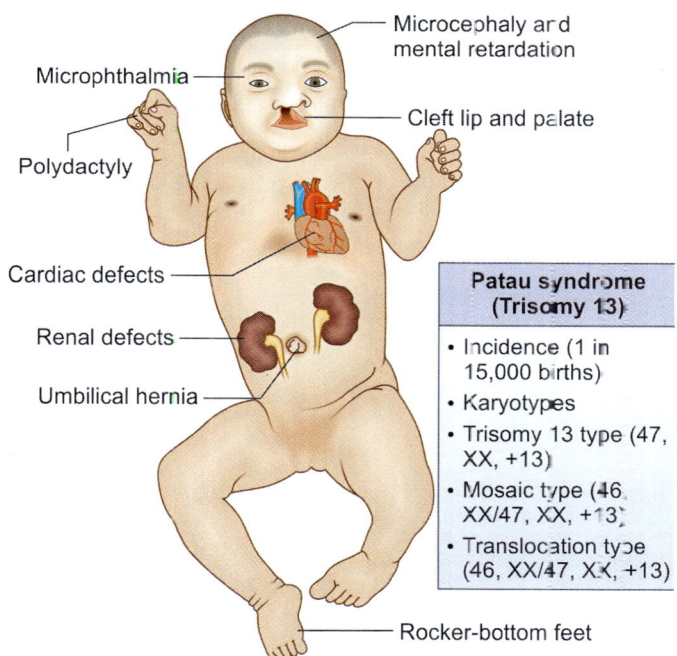

Fig. 5.19: Patau syndrome.

EDWARD'S SYNDROME (TRISOMY 18)

Edward syndrome incidence is 1 in 8000 births. Karyotyping reveals trisomy 18 type (47, XX, +18) and mosaic type (46 XX, 47, XX, +18). *Most frequently, trisomy 18 results from nondisjunction.* On clinical examination, patient shows *mental retardation, prominent occiput, micrognathia (small lower jaw), low-set ears, rocker-bottom feet, flexion deformities of the fingers (index overlapping third and fourth),* and *congenital heart disease* (Fig. 5.18).

PATAU SYNDROME (TRISOMY 13)

Patau syndrome incidence is 1 in 15,000 births. It shows trisomy 13 type (47, XX, +13), translocation type (46 XX, +13 der (13:14) and mosaic type (46XX/47, XX, +13). The disorder is characterized by *mental retardation, microcephaly, microphthalmia, brain abnormalities, cleft lip and palate, polydactyly, rocker-bottom feet,* and *congenital heart disease* (Fig. 5.19).

SEX CHROMOSOMAL DISORDERS

Abnormalities of sex chromosomes comprise Klinefelter's syndrome, Turner syndrome, XYY syndrome, XXX syndrome (47,XXX) and other multi-X chromosome anomalies.

KLINEFELTER'S SYNDROME

Klinefelter's syndrome, or testicular dysgenesis, is related to the presence of one or more X chromosomes in excess of the normal male XY complement (classic pattern 47, XXY karyotype). Variants include additional X chromosomes (e.g. 48 XXXY or 49 XXXXY) and rare mosaic forms.

The additional X chromosome(s) arises as a result of nondisjunction during gametogenesis. The disorder is always manifested by a male phenotype. It is a frequent cause of male infertility. Its incidence is 1 in 1000 births (Fig. 5.20).

Hormonal assays: There are *increased levels of plasma follicular stimulating hormone and luteinizing hormone, plasma pituitary gonadotropin and estradiol. Plasma testosterone level is markedly reduced* in affected males. It is due to loss of feedback inhibition.

Clinical features: Usually, Klinefelter's syndrome is undiagnosed before puberty.

- *Physique:* Patient has *tall stature (abnormal long legs),* due to delayed fusion of epiphyses; and eunuchoid body status appearance.

- *IQ:* These patients have *normal intelligence.* If present, mental retardation is usually mild to moderate, and the extent of retardation increases with increased number of X chromosomes.

- *Sexual characters:* Patient presents with *atrophic testes (sterile)* and *gynecomastia.* Other manifestations include *small penis, cryptorchidism, hypospadias* and *radioulnar synostosis.* There is *lack of secondary male characteristics* such as *deep voice, beard,* and *male distribution of pubic hair.*

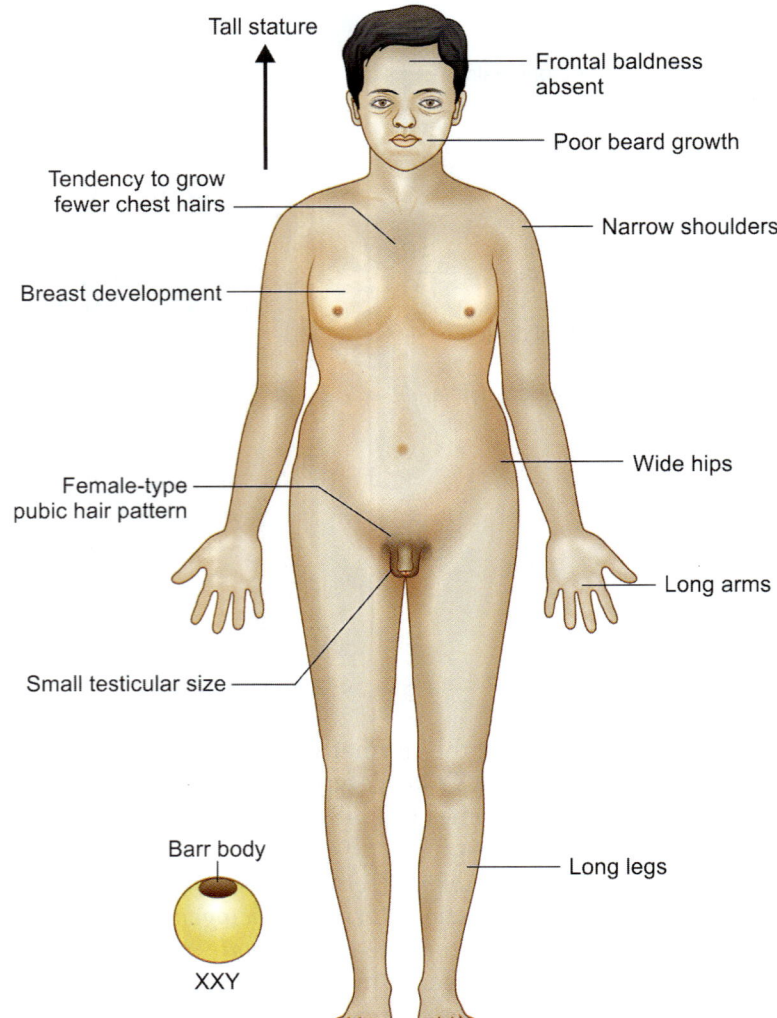

Fig. 5.20: Klinefelter's syndrome showing molecular genetic abnormalities and clinical features.

Barr bodies: Normally, one Barr body is present in normal female cells (XX). Barr bodies are absent in males (XY). *In Klinefelter's syndrome, patient shows Barr bodies (XXY).*

TURNER SYNDROME

Turner's syndrome occurs due to loss of an X chromosome in human females (monosomy). *Ovaries are rudimentary resulting in infertility. Patient somatic growth is normal but lacking menstrual cycle at menarche* (Fig. 5.21).

Karyotyping

- *Classic pattern:* There is complete or partial monosomy of the short arm of X chromosome. An XO karyotype (45, X) is characteristic in 57% cases.
- *Mosaic pattern:* A mosaic person has two lines of cells (one normal chromosome and another with monosomy single residual abnormal chromosome) for the affected chromosome pair due to anaphase lag. Example is Turner's mosaicism with 45,X/46,XX or 45,X/46,XY, 45,X/47,XXX. 45,X/46,X, i(X)(q10). A deletion of the SHOX gene can cause an identical phenotype and may be considered to be a variant of Turner syndrome.
- *Structural abnormalities:* These include 46,X i(Xq) or 46,XXq–, or 46,XXp– or 46,X, r(X) in 14%.

Clinical Features

- *During infancy: Lymphedema* is present *on dorsum of the hand,* foot, and *nape of the neck.*
- *During puberty:* Patient presents with infantile genital organs, inadequate breast development, and a little pubic hair.
- *During adult life:* Adult female has *short stature, shield-like chest* with *widely spaced nipples, bilateral neck webbing,* and wide carrying angle of the *arms,*

Genetic Disorders

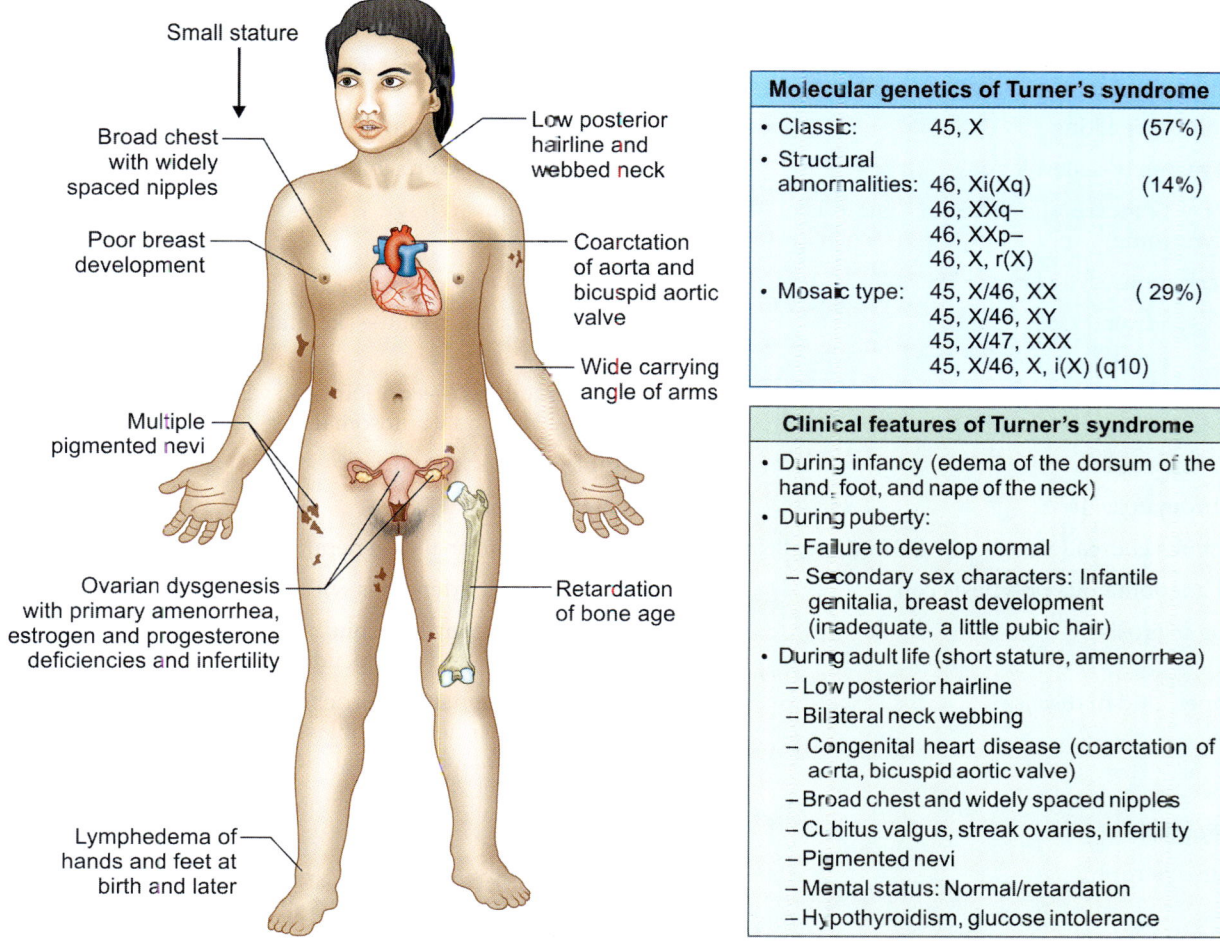

Fig. 5.21: Turner's syndrome showing molecular genetic abnormalities and clinical features.

multiple nevi and *cubitus valgus*. Turner syndrome is also often associated with autoantibody-mediated *hypothyroidism*. Patient may have coarctation of the aorta and *bicuspid valve* malformations.

XYY SYNDROME

XYY syndrome occurs with increased frequency among criminals demonstrating *violent behavior*; the significance of this association is unknown, because only about 2% of XYY individuals display such behavioral abnormalities.

Characteristics include tallness, severe acne, and only rarely mild mental retardation.

XXX SYNDROME (47,XXX) AND OTHER MULTI-X CHROMOSOME ANOMALIES

XXX syndrome may be marked by menstrual irregularities. Additional X chromosomes beyond XXX are marked by progressively increasing mental deficiency, depending on the number of additional X chromosomes.

SINGLE GENE MUTATION (MENDELIAN DISORDERS)

OVERVIEW

Mutation is a permanent change in the DNA sequence that makes up a gene. Mutations range in size from one DNA base to a whole chromosome change. Single gene mutation follows laws of inheritance described by Gregor Mendel in 1856. Mutation of a gene leads to synthesis of abnormal proteins. Therefore, disorders caused by single gene mutation are known as Mendelian disorders. In single-gene disorders, an error occurs at a single gene site on the DNA strand.

An error may occur in the copying and transcribing of a single codon through additions, deletions, or excessive repetitions. Some disorders of single gene mutation and their significance are shown in Table 5.7.

Table 5.7: Some disorders of single gene mutation and their significance

Disorder	Clinical manifestations
Autosomal dominant inheritance	
Adult polycystic kidney	Enlarging cysts replacing kidneys
Familial hypercholesterolemia	Premature atherosclerosis
Hereditary hemorrhagic telangiectasia (Osler-Weber-Rendu syndrome)	Recurrent hemorrhage from skin and mucous membrane telangiectasia
Hereditary spherocytosis	Hemolytic anemia
Marfan's syndrome	Abnormal elastic tissue—skeletal, cardiovascular and ocular disease
Ehlers-Danlos syndrome	Abnormal collagen—skin, joint and vascular effects. Ehlers-Danlos syndrome may show autosomal or sex-linked recessive inheritance
Neurofibromatosis I	Multiple nerve sheath tumor
Neurofibromatosis II	Acoustic neuroma
Huntington's chorea (chromosome 4 mutant allele)	Progressive neuronal degeneration of brain tissue in middle age
Familial adenomatous polyposis coli	Multiple colonic adenomas with malignant potential
Tuberous sclerosis	Multiple hamartomas within brain, face, and kidneys (rhabdomyoma of heart, and subependymal giant cell astrocytoma
von Hippel-Lindau disease	Autosomal dominant disorder characterized by retinal hemangioma, cerebellar hemangioblastoma, adenomas or cysts in liver, kidney, pancreas, and renal clear cell carcinoma (sporadic or familial)
Achondroplasia	Dwarfism
Myotonic dystrophy	Muscle weakness and wasting. These neurological syndromes are known to be the result of inserts of multiple triple repeats
Osteogenesis imperfecta	Brittle bones, fracturing with minimal trauma
Autosomal codominant inheritance	
ABO blood group antigens	Blood group disorders
α-1 antitrypsin deficiency	Inhibitor of trypsin responsible for emphysema
HLA antigens	HLA associated disorders
Autosomal recessive inheritance	
Cystic fibrosis	Abnormal ion-transport protein
Sickle cell anemia	Abnormal hemoglobin
Thalassemia	Decreased synthesis of chain hemoglobin
Glycogen storage disease	*Enzyme deficiency:* Anderson disease (branching enzyme), McArdle disease (phosphorylase V), Hers' disease (phosphorylase VI), Forbes-Cori disease (debranching enzyme), Pompe's disease (lysosomal acid maltase) and von Gierke disease (glucose-6-phosphatase)
Mucopolysaccharidoses	Enzyme deficiency involving liver, spleen, bone marrow, lymph nodes
Lipoidoses	Enzyme deficiency
Phenylketonuria	Deficiency of phenylalanine hydroxylase and impaired brain development
Albinism	Enzyme deficiency
Wilsons' disease	Copper accumulation

Contd...

Genetic Disorders

Table 5.7: Some disorders of single gene mutation and their significance (Contd...)

Disorder	Clinical manifestations
X-linked recessive inheritance	
Hemophilia A	Bleeding tendency due to factor VIII deficiency
Hemophilia B	Bleeding tendency due to factor IX deficiency
Hunter syndrome	Hepatosplenomegaly, joint stiffness, mild mental retardation, retinal degeneration and cardiac lesions
G6PD deficiency	Hemolytic anemia occurs with certain drugs
Duchenne muscular dystrophy	Progressive muscle weakness due to dystrophin deficiency
Becker muscular dystrophy	Relative dystrophin deficiency
Fabry disease	Deficiency of α-galactosidase resulting in accumulation of ceramide trihexoside in skin over the lower trunk, febrile episodes, severe burning pain in the extremities, and cardiovascular and cerebrovascular involvement
X-linked (Bruton) agammaglobulinemia	Decreased gammaglobulins due to B cell maturation
X-linked ichthyosis	Permanently thick scaly skin due to steroid sulfatase deficiency
Fragile X syndrome	Intellectual disability

Autosomal dominant disorders: Affected males and females appear in each generation of the pedigree. *Affected mothers and fathers transmit the phenotype to both sons and daughters.*

Autosomal recessive disorders: The disease appears in male and female children of unaffected parents.

X-linked disorders: Genes for these traits are located only on the X chromosome (not on the Y chromosome). X linked alleles always show up in males whether dominant or recessive because males have only one X chromosome.

Codominant inheritance: Two different versions (alleles) of a gene can be expressed, and each version makes a slightly different protein. *Both alleles influence the genetic trait or determine the characteristics of the genetic condition (e.g. ABO locus).*

Mendelian traits: Mendelian traits are dominant, recessive or codominant. Codominant inheritance is characterized by complete expression of both alleles in a heterozygote as seen in ABO blood group inheritance.

For unknown reasons, on autosomes, one allele may be more influential than another in determining a specific trait. *The more powerful, or dominant, gene is more likely to be expressed in the offspring than recessive, gene.*

Offspring will express a dominant allele when one or both chromosomes in a pair carry it. A recessive allele would not be expressed unless both chromosomes carry identical copies of the allele.

AUTOSOMAL DOMINANT DISORDERS

In single gene disorders, an error occurs at a single gene site on the DNA strand. An error may occur in the copying and transcribing of a single codon through additions, deletions, or excessive repetitions. *Autosomal dominant transmission most often affects male and female offspring equally. Affected males and females appear in each generation of the pedigree. Affected mothers and fathers transmit the phenotype to both sons and daughters.*

Some autosomal dominant disorders of single gene mutation and their significance are shown in Table 5.8.

ADULT POLYCYSTIC KIDNEY DISEASE

Adult polycystic kidney disease is autosomal dominant disorder. Though the genetic defect is present at birth, yet it *manifests between 15 and 30 years of age. It is most often associated with berry aneurysm of the circle of Willis resulting in subarachnoid hemorrhage.*

Patient develops numerous bilateral cysts that replace and ultimately destroy the renal parenchyma resulting in renal enlargement. *Most cases are caused by mutations in the polycystic kidney disease 1 gene, which encodes polycystin.*

The *kidneys are enlarged up to 3 or 4 kg* or more. The affected kidney contains large *fluid-filled cysts with areas of organized hemorrhage.*

Clinical features: Patient presents with sense of heaviness in the loins, bilateral flank and *palpable renal masses, hypertension, blood clots in the urine (hematuria), progression to end-stage renal failure* over a period of

Section I: General Pathology

Table 5.8: Some autosomal dominant disorders of single gene mutation and their significance

Disorder	Clinical manifestations
Adult polycystic kidney	Enlarging cysts replacing kidneys
Familial hypercholesterolemia	Premature atherosclerosis
Hereditary hemorrhagic telangiectasia (Osler-Weber-Rendu syndrome)	Recurrent hemorrhage from skin and mucous membrane telangiectasia
Hereditary spherocytosis	Hemolytic anemia
Marfan's syndrome	Abnormal elastic tissue—skeletal, cardiovascular and ocular disease
Ehlers-Danlos syndrome	Abnormal collagen—skin, joint and vascular effects. Ehlers-Danlos syndrome may show autosomal or sex-linked recessive inheritance
Neurofibromatosis I	Multiple nerve sheath tumor
Neurofibromatosis II	Acoustic neuroma
Huntington's chorea (chromosome 4 mutant allele)	Progressive neuronal degeneration of brain tissue in middle age
Familial adenomatous polyposis coli	Multiple colonic adenomas with malignant potential
Tuberous sclerosis	Multiple hamartomas within brain face, and kidneys (rhabdomyoma of heart, and subependymal giant cell astrocytoma
von Hippel-Lindau disease	Autosomal dominant disorder characterized by retinal hemangioma, cerebellar hemangioblastoma, adenomas or cysts in liver, kidney, pancreas, and renal clear cell carcinoma (sporadic or familial)
Achondroplasia	Dwarfism
Myotonic dystrophy	Muscle weakness and wasting. These neurological syndromes are known to be the result of inserts of multiple triple repeats
Osteogenesis imperfecta	Brittle bones, fracturing with minimal trauma

several years. Secondary polycythemia may occur as a result.

FAMILIAL HYPERCHOLESTEROLEMIA

Familial hypercholesterolemia is an autosomal dominant disorder. *It is caused by mutations of the gene encoding the LDL receptors.* The gene defect affects the uptake of LDL in the liver, causing hypercholesterolemia. It leads to high levels of low density lipoproteins in blood.

Clinical features: Clinically, the disease presents with xanthomas characterized by *raised yellow lesions filled with lipid-laden macrophages,* in the *skin* and *tendons.* Patient develops marked atherosclerosis, ischemic heart disease and peripheral vascular disease.

HEREDITARY HEMORRHAGIC TELANGIECTASIA

Hereditary hemorrhagic telangiectasia (Osler-Weber-Rendu syndrome) is a rare disorder seen with increased frequency in certain populations, such as in *Mormon families of Utah.*

Clinical features: Patient presents with *localized telangiectasia* of the skin and mucous membranes resulting in *recurrent hemorrhage* from these lesions.

HEREDITARY SPHEROCYTOSIS

The normal membrane cytoskeleton of RBCs is composed of spectrin, ankyrin, actin, protein 4.1 and protein 3. These proteins maintain the normal biconcave shape of RBCs.

Hereditary spherocytosis is associated with inherited defects of erythrocyte membrane associated cytoskeleton proteins such as spectrin, ankyrin, actin, protein 4.1 and protein 3.

Mutation of the ankyrin gene is the most common finding, accounting for most cases of autosomal dominant hereditary spherocytosis. *Protein 4.2 deficiency is common in Japan.*

Clinical features: Patient develops hereditary spherocytosis. These spheroidal erythrocytes that are sequestered and *destroyed in the spleen, producing hemolytic anemia.*

MARFAN'S SYNDROME

Marfan's syndrome is an autosomal dominant disorder of connective tissue. It is characterized by changes in *skeleton, eyes* and CVS (Fig. 5.22).

Basic defect: Marfan's syndrome is caused by *missense mutations of the fibrillin gene-1 (FGN-1) on chromosome 15.*

Genetic Disorders

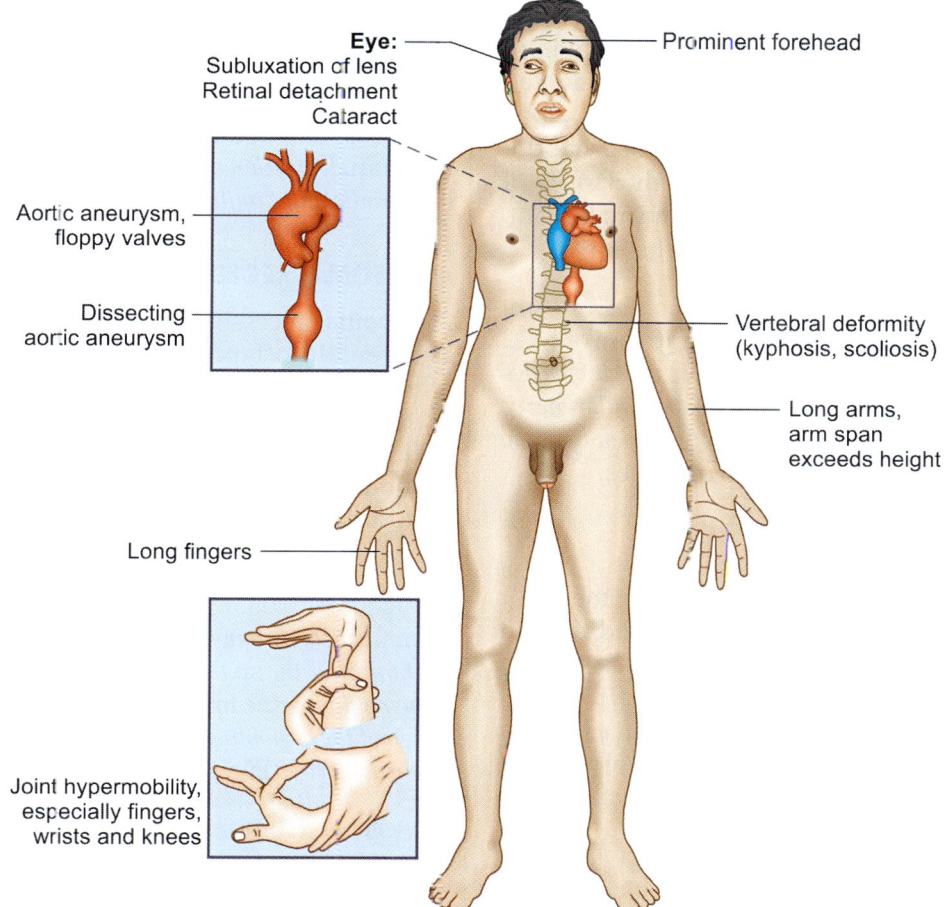

Fig. 5.22: Clinical manifestations of Marfan's syndrome.

Fibrillin is a family of connective tissue proteins analogous to the collagens.

Clinical Features

- *Bone and joints:* Patient presents with thin, tall with long legs and arms, spider-like fingers (arachnodactyly). Joint ligaments of hand and feet lead to hyperextensible joints. Spinal and chest deformities are common such as anterior chest deformity (pectus excavatum), scoliosis and lordosis.
- *Heart and vessels:* Loss of connective tissue support may lead to mitral valve prolapse. Cystic medial necrosis can lead to dilation of the aortic root and aortic regurgitation. *Life-threatening complications are aortic aneurysm and aortic dissection.*
- *Ocular changes:* Dislocation of the ocular lens in both eyes (ectopialentis) is common.

EHLERS-DANLOS SYNDROME

Ehlers-Danlos syndrome is rare autosomal dominant disorder of collagen fibers. There is generalized defect in collagen fibers, molecular structure, synthesis, secretion, and degradation.

Clinical features: Skin, ligaments and joints of person are commonly affected.

- *Skin changes:* Generalized defects in collagen fibers lead to hyperelasticity of skin (stretching of skin to many centimeters). Bleeding diathesis occurs as a result of fragile skin. Dehiscence of surgical incisions is common because sutures do not hold well.
- *Ligaments and joints:* Hypermobility of joints (unusual extension and flexion) is common finding.

NEUROFIBROMATOSIS TYPE I

Neurofibromatosis type I is also known as *von Recklinghausen disease*. It is caused by mutation of NF-1 gene, a tumor suppressor gene. Its protein product neurofibromin is expressed in many tissues. It belongs to family of GTPase-activating proteins (GAPs) that facilitates the conversion of active ras-GTP to inactive ras-GDP.

Loss of GAP activity (in cells acquiring a second hit mutation) permits uncontrolled ras p21 activation, an effect that predisposes to the formation of *benign neurofibromas*.

Clinical Features

Patient presents with disfiguring neurofibromas in skin, skin pigmentation (*café au lait spots*), pigmented lesions of the iris (Lisch nodules), meningioma, optic glioma, pheochromocytoma, Wilms' tumor, rhabdomyosarcoma, and leukemia. Approximately 3 to 5% of patients, benign neurofibromas can become malignant.

NEUROFIBROMATOSIS TYPE II

Neurofibromatosis type II is caused by mutation of *NF-2 tumor suppressor gene on chromosome 22q, which encodes merlin.* Patient presents with *bilateral vestibular nerve schwannomas, meningiomas, astrocytoma* and *ependymoma* as well as posterior subcapsular lens opacities.

TUBEROUS SCLEROSIS

Tuberous sclerosis is caused by mutations in the TSC1 or TSC genes which encode the hamartin and tuberin proteins, respectively. *Tuberous sclerosis is associated with multiple hamartomas within brain (as cortical tubers subependymal hamartomas), face, and kidneys (renal angiomyolipomas in 80% cases).* It may also be associated with rhabdomyoma of heart, and subependymal giant cell astrocytomas.

VON HIPPEL-LINDAU DISEASE

VHL gene is a tumor suppressor gene located on chromosome 3p (3p12 to 3p26). VHL gene mutation is caused by loss of sequences on chromosome 3p, imbalanced translocation (3; 6, 3; 8, 3; 11) and hypermethylation (80%).

VHL gene mutation and associated disorders: von Hippel-Lindau disease is autosomal dominant disorder characterized by retinal hemangioma, cerebellar hemangioblastoma, adenomas or cysts in liver, kidney, pancreas, and renal clear cell carcinoma (sporadic or familial). *Mutation of one allele of VHL gene is seen in 98% of sporadic and familial (2%) renal cell carcinomas.*

AUTOSOMAL RECESSIVE DISORDERS

Autosomal recessive inheritance usually affects male and female offspring equally. If both parents are affected, all their offspring will be affected. If one parent is affected and the other is a carrier, 50% of their children will be affected. Autosomal recessive disorders may occur when there is no family history of the disease. Autosomal recessive disorders are shown in Table 5.9.

SICKLE CELL ANEMIA

Mutant allele chromosome 11 causes substitution of valine for glutamine at the sixth position in b-chain of globin molecule of hemoglobin due to the single base substitution at the 6th codon of the b-globin gene from GAG to GUG and synthesize abnormal HbS (Fig. 5.23).

Genotype: Homozygous genotypes contain abnormal hemoglobin HbSHbS (sickle cell disease). Heterozygous genotypes contain abnormal hemoglobin HbAHbS (sickle cell trait).

Hemolysis of red blood cells: The mutant hemoglobin molecule undergoes polymerization under low oxygen tension causing the change in the shape of the RBC from biconcave to elongated sickle-like structure resulting in

Table 5.9: Autosomal recessive disorders

Disorder	Clinical manifestations
Cystic fibrosis	Abnormal ion-transport protein
Sickle cell anemia	Abnormal hemoglobin
Thalassemia	Decreased synthesis of chain hemoglobin
Lysosomal storage diseases	Tay-Sachs disease (amaurotic familial idiocy), Gaucher's disease, Niemann-Pick disease and Hurler's syndrome
Glycogen storage disease	*Enzyme deficiency:* Anderson disease (branching enzyme), McArdle disease (phosphorylase V), Hers' disease (phosphorylase VI), Forbes-cori disease (debranching enzyme), Pompe's disease (lysosomal acid maltase) and von Gierke disease (glucose-6-phosphatase)
Mucopolysaccharidoses	Enzyme deficiency
Lipoidoses	Enzyme deficiency
Phenylketonuria	Enzyme deficiency (disorders of amino acid metabolism)
Albinism	Enzyme deficiency
Wilsons' disease	Copper accumulation

Genetic Disorders

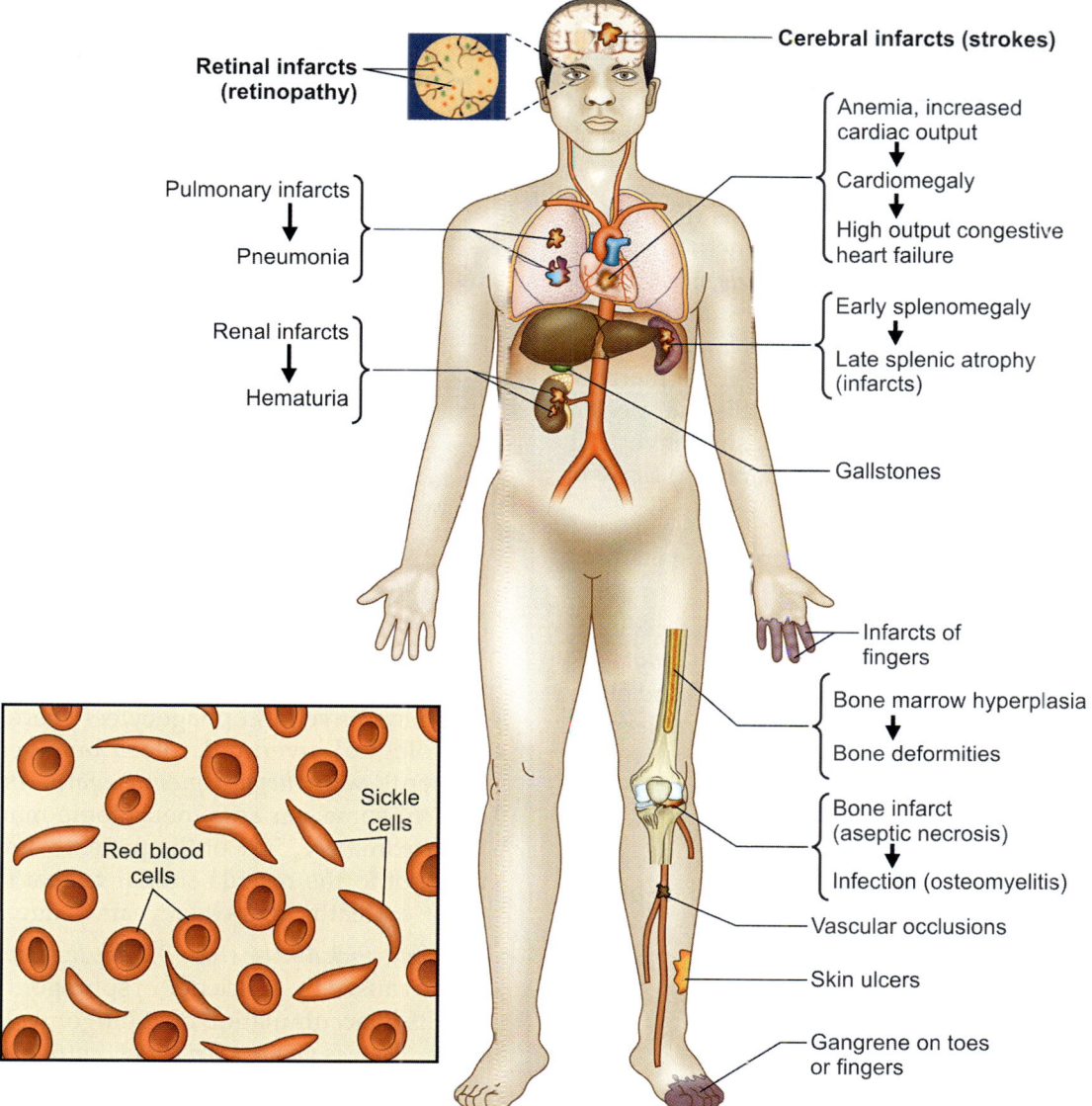

Fig. 5.23: Sickle cell anemia. Clinical and pathological findings, peripheral blood smear shows sickled RBCs. Sickled red cell appears in peripheral blood specimens only in patients with sickle cell disease because all of their hemoglobin is hemoglobin S. Red cells with any amount of hemoglobin S, however, can be induced to sickle as part of a laboratory test for the presence of hemoglobin S.

destruction of RBCs. *The lifespan of RBCs is reduced 10–20 days (normal RBCs lifespan is 100–120 days). Patients suffer from hemolytic anemia.*

LYSOSOMAL STORAGE DISEASES

Lysosomal storage diseases are inborn errors of metabolism characterized by deficiency of a specific single lysosomal enzyme, resulting in an accumulation of abnormal metabolic products.

Tay-Sachs Disease

Tay-Sachs disease is caused by *deficiency of hexosaminidase* resulting in *accumulation of GM2 ganglioside, especially in neurons*. Gene locus is on chromosome 15.

It is an autosomal recessive trait seen in *Ashkenazi* (central European origin) Jewish descent. On average, half of the offspring is expected to be heterozygotes and silent carriers of the gene mutation. It is also known as *amaurotic familial idiocy.*

Clinical features: Patient presents with *severe mental and motor deterioration, CNS degeneration, blindness* and *cherry red spot in the macula.* Children die before 4 years of age.

Gaucher's Disease

Gaucher's disease is autosomal recessive disorder most often seen in *persons of European Ashkenazi* Jewish lineage. It is characterized by *accumulation of glucosylceramide (membrane glycosphingolipids)* derived from the catabolism *of senescent leukocytes,* primarily in the lysosomes of macrophages. The membranes of these cells are rich in the cerebrosides, and when their degradation is blocked by the deficiency of glucocerebrosidase (lysosomal acid β-glucosidase), an intermediate metabolite such as glucosylceramide accumulates.

Diagnostic hallmark: The hallmark of this disorder is the presence of *Gaucher's cells* with a distinctive *cigarette paper-like cytoplasmic appearance and eccentric nuclei, which are lipid-laden macrophages present in the red pulp of the spleen, liver sinusoids (Kupffer cells), lymph nodes, lungs (alveolar macrophages), and bone marrow.* Bone marrow aspiration reveals numerous Gaucher's cells, but specific enzymes (chitotriosidase and angiotensin-converting enzyme markers of macrophage proliferation) assay is required to confirm the diagnosis.

Clinical features: These are variable depending on three variants of Gaucher's disease:

- *Type I, or adult Gaucher's disease:* It accounts for 80% of cases. Patient presents with *hepatosplenomegaly, bone pain* and *fracture due to erosion of femoral head* and other long bones. Mild anemia and thrombocytopenia (easy bruising) are also present. Patient may live a normal lifespan. *Gaucher's cells are demonstrated in the bone marrow, liver, spleen, and lymph nodes.*
- *Type II, or infantile Gaucher's disease:* Infant develops severe CNS involvement with fatal outcome before 1 year of age.
- *Type III, or juvenile Gaucher's disease:* Its onset usually occurs in early childhood. *There is involvement of brain and the viscera.* It is *less severe* than type II Gaucher's disease.

Light Microscopy

- Gaucher's cells are demonstrated in spleen, liver, CNS, bone marrow, tonsil, thymus, Peyer's patches, and lungs. Cytoplasm is fibrillary and crumpled (tissue paper-like).
- Histological examination of liver biopsy shows *Gaucher's cells* with a distinctive cigarette paper-like cytoplasmic appearance and eccentric nuclei, which are lipid-laden macrophages (Fig. 5.24).

Niemann-Pick Disease

Niemann-Pick disease occurs due to *deficiency of sphingomyelinase* leading to *accumulation of sphingomyelin in the lysosomes of phagocytes* especially in *type A and type B.* Diagnostic hallmark is presence of foamy histiocytes containing sphingomyelin in liver, spleen, lymph nodes, skin, bone marrow, tonsil, GIT, lungs. Foam cells show positivity with oil red O and Sudan black on frozen sections.

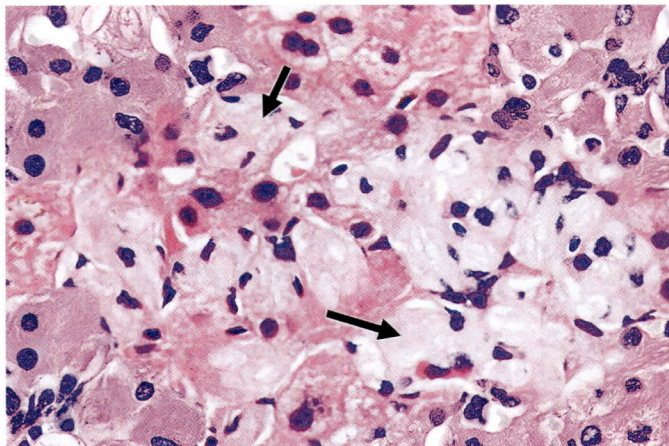

Fig. 5.24: Gaucher's disease shows Gaucher's cells containing cigarette paper-like cytoplasmic appearance and eccentric nuclei, which are lipid-laden macrophages (arrows) (400X).

Types of Niemann-Pick Disease

- *Niemann-Pick disease (type A):* It is *severe disease* affecting infants. It is caused by deficiency of sphingomyelinase which results in accumulation of sphingomyelin in phagocytes. There is extensive neurological, liver and spleen involvement. Child presents with *hepatosplenomegaly, anemia, fever,* and, in some variants, neurologic manifestations. Approximately, 50% of the patients develop cherry red spot in the macula similar to that of Tay-Sachs disease. Death occurs by 3 years of age.
- *Niemann-Pick disease (type B):* It is *less severe disease.* It is also caused by deficiency of sphingomyelinase and results in accumulation of sphingomyelin in phagocytes. *There is no involvement of central nervous system and organs.* Patient survives into adulthood.
- *Niemann-Pick disease (type C):* It is caused by defect in a gene involved in cholesterol transport with cholesterol accumulation within phagocytes.

Light Microscopy

Histological examination of liver biopsy shows *foamy histiocytes* containing sphingomyelin in Kupffer cells (Fig. 5.25).

Hurler's Syndrome

Deficiency of α_1-iduronidase enzyme results in accumulation of mucopolysaccharides, heparan sulfate and dermatan sulfate in the *heart, brain, liver, and other organs.*

Clinical features: Patient presents with *hepatosplenomegaly, progressive mental retardation, dwarfism,* stubby fingers and corneal clouding. Patient has fatal outcome by 10 years of age.

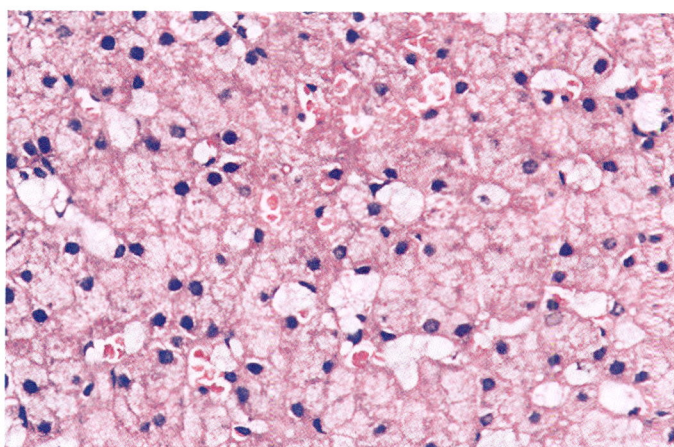

Fig. 5.25: Niemann-Pick disorder. Kupffer cells of liver show foamy histiocytes' containing sphingomyelin (400X).

GLYCOGEN STORAGE DISEASES

Glycogen storage diseases are a group of disorders caused by defects in the synthesis or degradation of glycogen.

von Gierke Disease

von Gierke disease is a glycogen storage disease type I. Deficiency of glucose-6-phosphatase leads to accumulation of glycogen in the liver and kidney. Patient presents with hepatomegaly and sometimes intractable hypoglycemia.

Pompe Disease

Pompe disease is glycogen storage disease type II. It is lysosomal storage disease. Deficiency of α1, 4-glucosidase results in accumulation of glycogen in the liver, heart, and skeletal muscle. Patient presents with cardiomegaly, muscle hypotonia, splenomegaly with intractable hypoglycemia. *Patient has fatal outcome due to cardiorespiratory failure before 3 years of age.*

Forbes-Cori Disease

Forbers-Cori disease is glycogen storage disease type III. It is caused due to deficiency of the debranching enzyme, amylo-1, and 6-glucosidase, resulting in variable accumulation of glycogen in the *liver, heart, or skeletal muscle*. Patient presents with stunted growth, hepatomegaly, and hypoglycemia.

McArdle Syndrome

McArdle syndrome is glycogen storage disease type V. Deficiency of muscle phosphorylase results in accumulation of glycogen in skeletal muscle. It affects persons second decade onwards. *Patient presents with painful muscle cramps and muscle weakness (following exercise).*

Anderson Disease

Anderson disease is glycogen storage disease type VI. It occurs due to deficiency of branching enzyme. Patient presents with *failure to thrive, hypotonia and hepatosplenomegaly.* Liver biopsy reveals findings of cirrhosis.

DISORDERS OF CARBOHYDRATE METABOLISM (GALACTOSEMIA)

Classic Galactosemia

The cause is deficiency of galactose-1-phosphate uridyl transferase, with resultant accumulation of galactose-1-phosphate in many tissues. Patient presents with failure to thrive, infantile cataracts, mental retardation, and progressive hepatic failure resulting in cirrhosis and death. Most of these changes can be prevented by early removal of galactose from the diet.

Galactokinase Deficiency

Galactokinase deficiency is much less frequent than classic galactosemia. The disorder is often marked only by infantile cataracts.

DISORDERS OF AMINO ACID METABOLISM

Phenylketonuria (PKU)

Physiological state: Phenylalanine hydroxylase converts phenylalanine to tyrosine in the liver.

Basic defect: Gene mutation encoding phenylalanine hydroxylase results in failure of conversion of phenylalanine to tyrosine in the liver. *High serum concentrations of phenylalanine are neurotoxic and enter cerebrospinal fluid resulting in progressive cerebral demyelination, mental deterioration* and *seizures by the age of one year.*

Phenylalanine is catabolized into phenylpyruvic acid and phenylacetic acid and excreted in urine in large amounts. Other manifestations include *decreased pigmentation of hair, eyes, skin and musty body odor from phenylacetic acid in urine and sweat.*

Screening test: The concentration of phenylalanine in affected infants is usually normal at birth and increases rapidly during the first days of life. False-negative results are common immediately after birth. *Blood sample for phenylketonuria is usually taken from the infant's heel within 2 to 3 days after birth.*

Therapeutic correlation: Successful treatment is a *phenylalanine-free diet.* If affected mother is not controlled, the infant is at high risk of development of congenital heart disease, growth retardation, microcephaly, and mental retardation.

Alkaptonuria

Due to deficiency of homogentisic oxidase enzyme causes incomplete metabolism of phenylalanine and tyrosine resulting in *accumulation and urinary excretion of homogentisic acid (black pigment). Clinically, this disorder manifests alkaptonuria and ochronosis.* The term alkaptonuria refers to urinary excretion of unmetabolized homogentisic acid imparting a dark color to urine on standing. The term ochronosis refers to pigment deposition in multiple tissues, most prominently in cartilage and connective tissue.

Ochronosis: Homogentisic acid (dark pigment) is deposited in the articular cartilage of vertebral column and later hips, knees and shoulder joints. Cartilage of nose, ears, larynx and bronchi is also affected. Cardiac valves, prostate, and sweat glands may also be involved. Larger joints may be distended by effusion, which is usually non-inflammatory and synovium and is hypertrophied. Light microscopy of the lesion shows granular pigment in chondrocytes and matrix is diffusely stained. Synovium shows evidence of acute or chronic inflammation.

Maple Syrup Urine Disease

Maple syrup urine disease is a rare inborn error of metabolism. Defects in proteins forming branched-chain α-keto acid dehydrogenase (keto acid decarboxylase) results in maple syrup urine disease. Newborns are treated with protein-modified diets.

Clinical features: Patient presents with retardation of physical and mental health along with feeding problems. Untreated newborn may develop mental and physical disabilities with fatal outcome. Urine contains high levels of keto acids of leucine, isoleucine, and valine giving maple syrup odor.

CYSTIC FIBROSIS OF THE PANCREAS

Cystic fibrosis is autosomal recessive disorder of exocrine glands. *Genetic defect of chromosome 7 allele causes failure of chloride ions transport. It leads to abnormally thick secretion in lungs, liver and pancreas. It is a lethal disease among white population* (Fig. 5.26).

Pathogenesis: Normally, transmembrane conductance regulator (CFTr) gene located on long arm of chromosome 7 codes for a membrane protein that participates in the movement of chloride and other ions across membranes. *Mutation of CFTr gene causes malfunction of exocrine glands which results in increased viscosity of mucus and increased chloride concentration in sweat and tears.*

Clinical Features

- *Respiratory system:* Cystic fibrosis has most adverse effects on respiratory system. Patient develops recurrent pulmonary infections.
- *Digestive system:* Digestive system dysfunction can affect both gastrointestinal tract and accessory glands. Warning sign of cystic fibrosis in a newborn

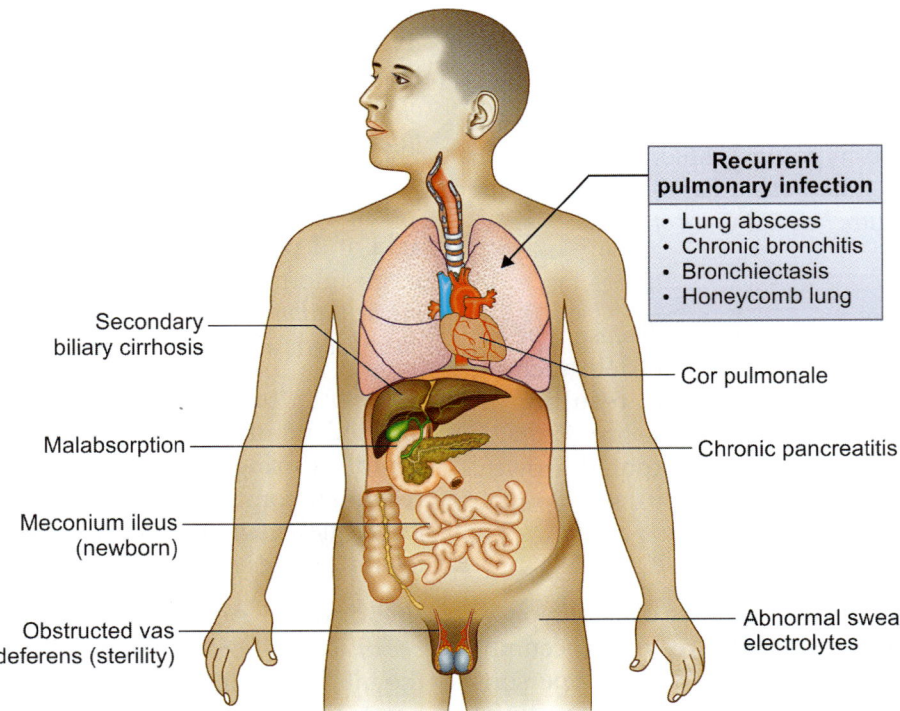

Fig. 5.26: Clinical manifestations of cystic fibrosis.

is intestinal obstruction caused by thick viscous meconium known as meconium ileus.
- *Skin:* Cystic fibrosis affects sweat glands in the skin resulting in abnormally thick salty perspiration. There is increased risk of heat stroke and salt depletion especially in infants.
- *Reproductive system:* Almost all men with cystic fibrosis are *sterile* because epididymis cannot synthesize or incomplete formation of vas deferens. Women with cystic fibrosis often have normal reproductive system and can have successful pregnancies.

Diagnosis

Sweat chloride test is an important diagnostic tool. Secretion by sweat glands of chloride and sodium is normal, but their reabsorption by sweat ducts is impaired. Molecular testing of CFTR gene mutation is another tool. Screening done by using immunoreactive trypsinogen (IrT) assay shows elevated levels in infants with cystic fibrosis.

Treatment: Inhaled bronchodilators reduce resistance in respiratory airways. Inhaled mucolytic agents and saline help in dissolving mucus. Antibiotics are administered to cover infection.

X-LINKED RECESSIVE DISORDERS

Genes for these traits are located only on the X chromosome (not on the Y chromosome). X-linked alleles always show up in males whether dominant or recessive because males have only one X chromosome. X-linked recessive disorders are shown in Table 5.10.

CLASSIC HEMOPHILIA

Classic hemophilia is common X-linked recessive disorder. It is caused by factor VIII gene mutation located on tip of the long arm of the X chromosome. It leads to deficiency of coagulation factor VIII, which is essential for blood clotting.

Heterozygous females are carriers, which transmit the disease to the male progeny. *The family pedigree of Queen Victoria shows a number of hemophilic descendants as she was a carrier of the disease.* In females, the other normal X chromosome corrects the abnormality, but females can be asymptomatic carriers. In males, the disease is expressed because there is no normal X chromosome to correct the abnormality.

Clinical features: Patient presents with hemorrhage from minor wounds and trauma, bleeding from oral mucosa, hematuria, and hemarthroses. Recurrent hemarthroses can lead to progressive crippling deformities.

Therapeutic correlation: These patients need frequent administration of *fresh frozen plasma-rich in factor VIII*.

HUNTER SYNDROME

Hunter syndrome is a lysosomal storage disease. Deficiency of l-iduronosulfate sulfatase results in accumulations of mucopolysaccharide such as heparan sulfate and dermatan sulfate. *It is less severe than Hurler syndrome.* Patient presents with *hepatosplenomegaly, joint stiffness, mild mental retardation, retinal degeneration and cardiac lesions.*

Table 5.10: X-linked recessive disorders

Disorder	Clinical manifestations
Hemophilia A	Bleeding tendency due to factor VIII deficiency
Hemophilia B	Bleeding tendency due to factor IX deficiency
Hunter syndrome	Hepatosplenomegaly, joint stiffness, mild mental retardation, retinal degeneration and cardiac lesions
G6PD deficiency	Hemolytic anemia occurs with certain drugs
Duchenne muscular dystrophy	Progressive muscle weakness due to dystrophin deficiency
Becker muscular dystrophy	Relative dystrophin deficiency
Fabry disease	Deficiency of α-galactosidase results in accumulation of ceramide trihexoside in skin over the lower trunk, febrile episodes, severe burning pain in the extremities, and cardiovascular and cerebrovascular involvement
X-linked (Bruton) agammaglobulinemia	Decreased gammaglobulins due to B cell maturation
X-linked ichthyosis	Permanently thick scaly skin due to steroid sulphatase deficiency

DUCHENNE MUSCULAR DYSTROPHY

This X-linked genetic disorder is the most common and severe variety of the disease due to *deletion of one or many exons in the dystrophin gene (DMD gene) located on the short arm of the X chromosome (Xp21)*.

Dystrophin links the subsarcolemmal cytoskeleton to the exterior of the cell through a transmembrane complex of proteins. Boys with disorder cannot produce dystrophin at all. Dystrophin deficient muscles of *pelvic* and *shoulder girdles* predispose to death of myocytes during contraction. Serum levels of creatine kinase are markedly increased.

Clinical Features

Children fail to walk by 18 months of age due to weakness in the proximal muscles of the extremities, progressing to muscle necrosis, wasting, muscle contracture with fatal outcome in their teens. They develop pneumonia due to weakness of respiratory muscles. *More than 90% of afflicted boys are wheelchair bound by the age of 10 years and bedridden by the age of 15 years.*

Complications

The most common causes of death are complications of respiratory insufficiency caused by muscular weakness or cardiac arrhythmia due to myocardial involvement.

BECKER MUSCULAR DYSTROPHY

Becker muscular dystrophy is *less common and less severe disorder* affecting boys. It is clinically similar to Duchenne muscular dystrophy. In this disease, some dystrophin is produced as a result of segmental deletion of dystrophin gene. It does not cause a coding frame shift.

FABRY DISEASE

Fabry disease is a lysosomal storage disease. It is also known as *angiokeratoma corporis diffusum* universale. Deficiency of α-galactosidase results in accumulation of ceramide trihexoside in body tissues. Patient presents with skin lesions (*angiokeratomas*) *over the lower trunk, febrile episodes,* severe burning pain in the extremities, and cardiovascular and cerebrovascular involvement. *Patient dies of renal failure in early adult life.*

LESCH-NYHAN SYNDROME

Lesch-Nyhan syndrome is caused by deficiency of hypoxanthine-guanine phosphoribosyl transferase (hGPrT), resulting in impaired purine metabolism and excess production of uric acid. Patient presents with gout, mental retardation, choreoathetosis, spasticity, self-mutilation, and aggressive behavior.

DISORDERS OF SEXUAL DIFFERENTIATION

HERMAPHRODITISM

Persons who possess phenotypic features of both males and females are called *hermaphrodites*. True hermaphroditism occurs when genetic sex, gonadal sex, or genital sex of an individual is discordant.

Genetic sex is determined by the presence or absence of a Y chromosome, ovaries or testes. The gene responsible for the development of the testes, the sex-determining region Y gene (SRY gene) is localized to the Y chromosome. Genital sex is based on the appearance of the external genitalia.

TRUE HERMAPHRODITE

True hermaphrodite is characterized by both ovarian and testicular tissues, with ambiguous external genitalia and both X and Y chromosomes. One possible mechanism is the parthenogenetic division of a haploid ova into two haploid ovum, followed by double fertilization and then fusion of the two zygotes in early embryonic development. Patient may show 46,XX (commonest) or 46,XX/46,XY (mosaic) or 46,XY.

PSEUDOHERMAPHRODITE

Pseudohermaphrodite has gonads of only one sex, but the appearance of the external genitalia does not correspond to the gonads present.

Male Pseudohermaphrodite

Male pseudohermaphrodite is congenital disorder also known as *testicular feminization syndrome*. It occurs due to a *congenital deficiency of the androgen receptor*. The cause may be tissue resistance to androgens (testicular feminization), defects in testosterone synthesis, or hormones administered to the mother during pregnancy.

Patient has *cryptorchid testes*, but the *external genital organs appear feminine* or ambiguously female, with signs of virilization. *The condition has also been linked to chromosomal anomalies, such as 46,XY/45,X mosaicism.*

Female Pseudohermaphrodite

The gonads are always ovaries, but the external genitalia are not clearly female.

Genetic Disorders 5

The condition is most often caused by increased androgenic hormones from congenital adrenal hyperplasia, an androgen-secreting adrenal or ovarian tumor in the mother, or hormones administered to the mother during pregnancy. Patient shows 46,XX genotypically normal female.

WORK UP OF GENETIC DISORDERS

Genetic disorders are diagnosed by pedigree construction, demonstration of Barr bodies, Y chromatin, chromosomal analysis (karyotyping), fluorescence *in situ* hybridization, molecular diagnosis and prenatal diagnosis.

PEDIGREE CONSTRUCTION

A pedigree is a diagram that shows the history of a trait as it is passed from one generation to the next. *Study of pedigree construction helps in determining the mode of inheritance of genetic disorder, i.e. autosomal dominant, autosomal recessive or sex-linked. It is useful to identify carriers of genetic disorders and genetic counseling* (Fig. 5.27).

Autosomal dominant disoder: In autosomal dominant disorder, only one copy of abnormal gene is inherited resulting in expression in both homozygous and heterozygous states.

Autosomal recessive disoder: In autosomal recessive disorder, both copies of abnormal gene are inherited resulting in homozygous state. *In heterozygous state, person is a silent carrier.*

X-linked disorder: In X-linked disorder, one of the X chromosomes carrying mutant gene is transmitted to male resulting in *hemophilia*. Because affected males do not have normal X chromosome to correct the abnormality. Heterozygous female is asymptomatic carrier.

BARR BODIES

Lyon's hypothesis: In females, during embryogenesis, random inactivation of one of two X chromosomes is known as *Lyon hypothesis*. This inactivation is transmitted to all somatic cells except germ cells. Ovaries always possess active chromosomes. Inactive X chromosome in the somatic cells becomes condensed in the nucleus called *nuclear sexing*.

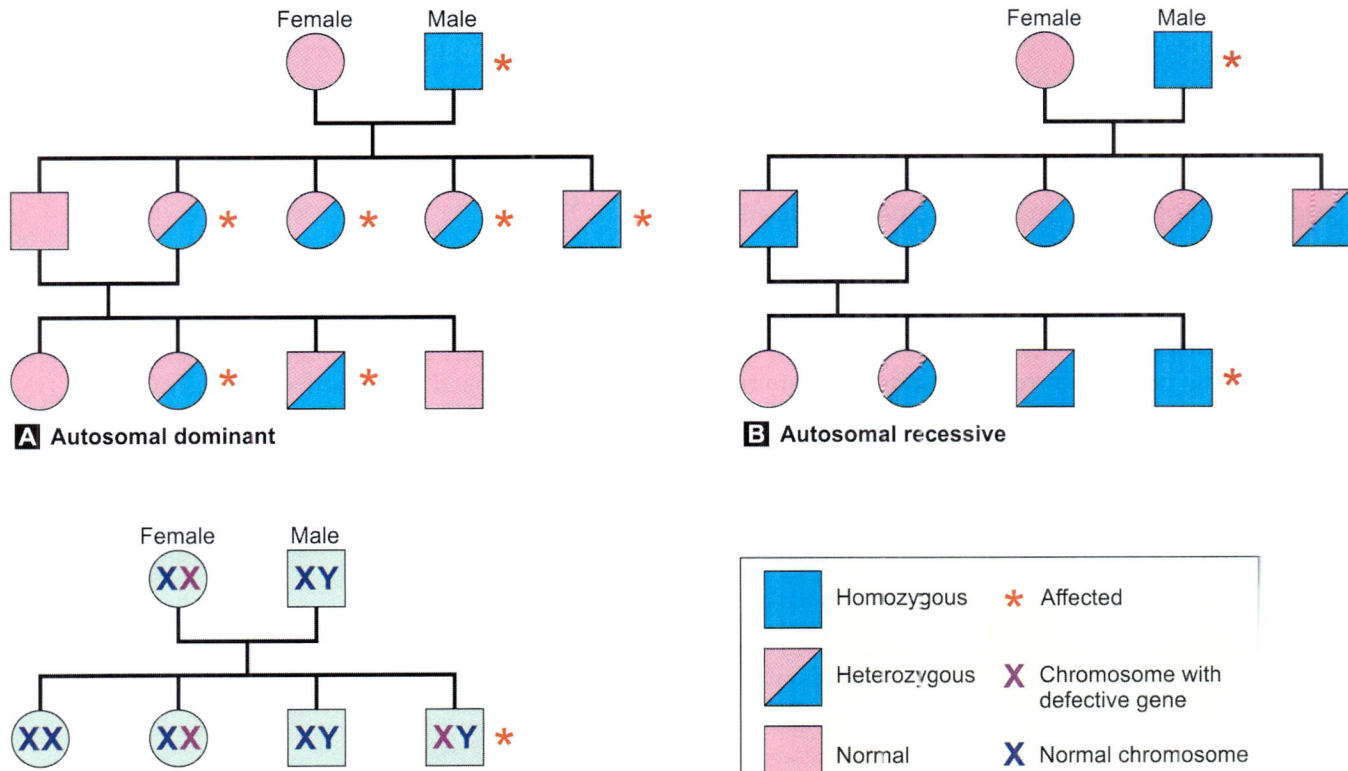

Fig. 5.27: Family pedigrees are used to determine patterns of inheritance (autosomal dominant, autosomal recessive and X-linked disorders) and individual genotypes.

Barr bodies: Barr bodies are also known as *sex chromatin*. These appear as clumps of chromatin in the interphase nuclei of all somatic cells in females. According to the Lyon hypothesis, each Barr body represents one inactivated X chromosome. One Barr body is present in normal female cells (XX). Barr bodies are absent in males (XY). XXXY cells have two Barr bodies.

- The number of Barr bodies is always one less than the number of X chromosomes. Assessment of Barr bodies was considered as diagnostic tool in past. It has now been supplemented by more definitive and sophisticated analytic procedures.
- Smears stained by scraping of oral mucosa or circulating neutrophils demonstrate *Barr bodies*, which appear as drumstick appendage attached to one of the nuclear lobes. *A minimum of 30% cells positive for sex chromatin indicates female genetic constitution.*

Y CHROMATIN

Smears are prepared from oral mucosa. Long arm of Y chromosome exhibits *intense fluorescence with quinacrine dye.* Under ultraviolet light, Y chromatin appears as a *bright dot.* Multiple numerical aberrations of sex chromosome can be demonstrated by immunofluorescence study.

KARYOTYPING

Animal cells contain set of chromosomes, which have constant characteristics, i.e. relative size, number, length, position, secondary constriction and satellite. Photographic representation of the stained preparation of chromosomes is called *karyotyping*.

Chromosomes are studied in any human nucleated cells. *Circulating lymphocytes are most often used for the study done by arresting the dividing cells in metaphase by colchicine.* These cells are spread on slides and stained with Giemsa stain. Distal end of the chromosome is called *telomere*.

Table 5.12: Chromosomal banding techniques

Technique	Staining employed
G-banding	Giemsa stain
Q-banding	Quinacrine fluorescence stain
R-banding	Reverse Giemsa staining
C-banding	Constitutive heterochromatin demonstration

Classification of Chromosomes

Chromosomes are classified based on their length and location of centromere as shown in Table 5.11. According to Denver classification based on the length, chromosomes are classified into seven groups: A to G.

Karyotyping Techniques

Banding techniques: Cells are cultured and a chromosome preparation is made. Chromosomes can be specifically stained by a variety of methods which produce a banding pattern, the most common being Giemsa staining (G-banding). Increasingly, specific DNA probes are being used to analyze the presence of specific chromosomes or chromosome regions. The centromere is a constriction at which the chromatids are joined. *The short arm is designated 'p' (petit) and the long arm* is 'q'. The arms terminate to telomeres rich in repetitive sequences. The dark bands are numbered in order from the centromere to the tip of each arm, sub-bands are preceded by a decimal point. Chromosomal banding techniques are shown in Table 5.12.

Quinacrine banding technique: It allows detection of the region containing repetitive DNA. We get different kinds of bands. Animal karyotyping shows (I, C, G, or R) bands.

FISH and Mc FISH techniques: Fluorescence *in situ* hybridization (FISH) and multilocular fluorescence *in situ* hybridization (Mc FISH) have been widely used in animals. In this DNA probe labeled with radioactive molecules are used to locate the position of special DNA sequence on chromosome. In multilocular fluorescence *in situ* hybridization (Mc FISH), DNA may be labeled

Table 5.11: Classification of chromosomes based on location of centromere

Chromosome	Location of centromere	Chromosome number
Metacentric chromosome	Centromere located exactly in the middle of chromosome	1, 3, 16, 19 and 20
Sub-metacentric chromosome	*Centromere located in sub-terminal region dividing chromosome into short arm (p) and long arm (q)	1 and 3
Acrometric chromosome	Centromere eccentrically located dividing chromosome in very short arm (p) and large long arm (q) capped by a telomere	13, 14, 15, 21, 22 and Y

*French word petit meaning short is used to denote short arm of chromosome as 'p' and long arm as 'q'.

Genetic Disorders

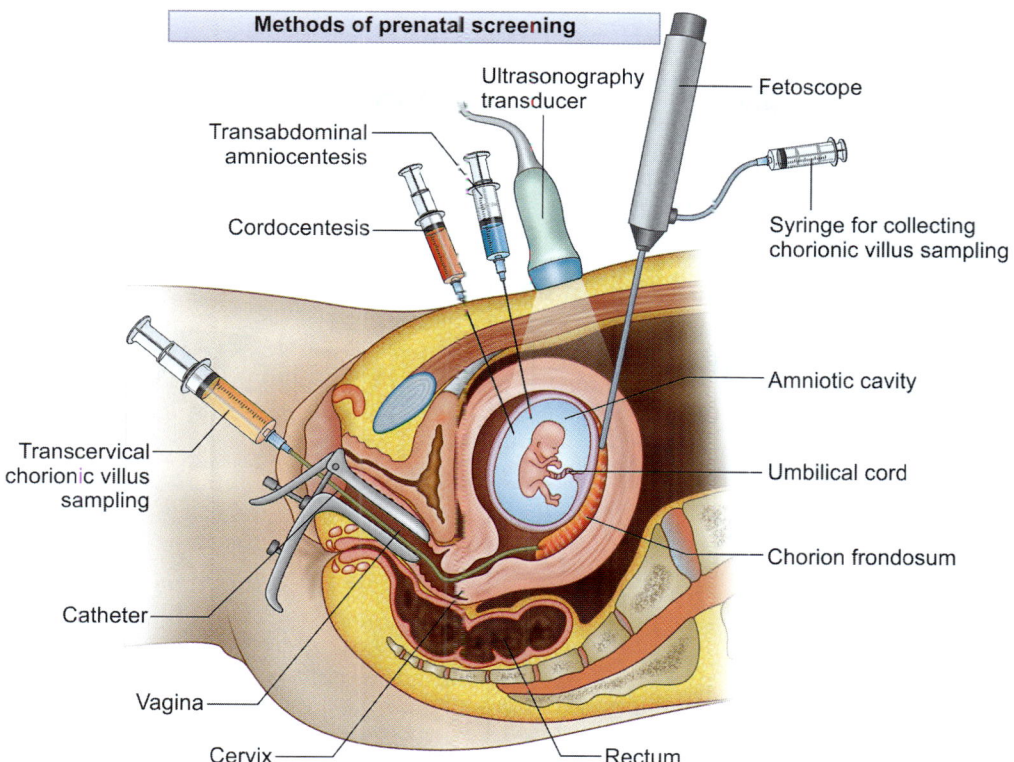

Fig. 5.28: In amniocentesis, a syringe is used to collect amniotic fluid. Ultrasound imaging is used to guide the tip of the syringe to prevent damage to the placenta and fetus. Fetal cells in the collected amniotic fluid can then be chemically tested or used to produce a karyotype of the developing baby.

with fluorochromes to allow the use of one or more colors to locate the position of one or more sequences simultaneously (*refer to Chapter 14 on advanced diagnostic techniques*).

Flow Cytometry: We take suspension of thousands of chromosomes, which are stained with a DNA binding fluorochrome. As these chromosomes are passed through cytometer, the fluorescence is measured for individual chromosome of same size. This technique is so accurate that it allows detection of differences as small as 1.5–4.0 Mbp (mega base pairs). It helps in detection of aneuploidy, duplication and deletion (*refer to Chapter 14 on advanced diagnostic techniques*).

Polymerase chain reaction: Polymerase chain reaction is rapid sensitive diagnostic technique of amplifying specific DNA fragments. *Sampling can be obtained from blood, tissues, saliva or amniotic fluid.* This technique is used in prenatal diagnosis and detection of gene mutations (*refer to chaper 14 on advanced diagnostic techniques*).

Clinical Significance of Karyotyping

Karyotype analysis of chromosomes is usually performed for prenatal diagnosis, or for investigation of conditions in postnatal life.

- *Prenatal diagnosis:* Sonography, first trimester screening, quad screening, amniocentesis, chorionic villi biopsy sampling, and percutaneous umbilical cord blood sampling (PUBS) are important procedures that allow prenatal diagnosis. Karyotype analysis of chromosomes is usually performed for prenatal congenital abnormalities (Fig. 5.28).

- *Postnatal diagnosis:* In postnatal diagnosis, cells are derived from blood lymphocytes, or from biopsy of skin to obtain fibroblasts.

  Karyotype analysis of chromosomes is usually performed for *postnatal diagnosis* of pediatric disorders such as *mental or growth retardation, failure of sexual development at puberty;* obstetric disorders such as *infertility, recurrent abortions, pregnancy in older women;* and oncology disorders such as *leukemia*.

CHAPTER 6

Neoplasia: Molecular Basis, Metastasis, Clinical Oncology and Laboratory Diagnosis

Learning Objectives

NEOPLASIA
- Overview, Oncogenesis, Dysplasia, Carcinoma *in situ*, Invasion and Metastasis

NOMENCLATURE AND CLASSIFICATION
- Benign Tumors, Borderline Tumors, Malignant Tumors, Neuroectodermal Tumors, Blastomas, Mixed Tumors, Teratomas, Hamartomas and Choristoma

CHARACTERISTIC FEATURES OF TUMORS
- Tumor Components, Degree of Differentiation, Nuclear Features, Tumor Development and Growth Rate, Monoclonal Properties of tumors, Telomerase Activity, Tumor Angiogenesis, Tumor Invasion and Dissemination

EPIDEMIOLOGY OF TUMORS
- Incidence, Age and Sex Distribution, Geographical Variables, Occupational Cancers, Racial Factors, Genetic Factors, Alcohol and Tobacco Products, Atmospheric Pollutants, Radiation, Dietary Factors, Sexual Factors and Hormones

CELL CYCLE AND CANCER
- Phases of Cell Cycle, Regulation of Cell Cycle, Check Points of Cell Cycle, Cell Cycle Checkpoint Components and Cell Cycle Inhibitors

GENETIC PREPOSITION OF CANCER
- Overview

ACQUIRED PRENEOPLASTIC LESIONS
- Proliferation of Cells and Chronic Inflammatory State

MOLECULAR BASIS OF CANCER: ROLE OF GENETIC AND EPIGENETIC ALTERATIONS
- Cellular Hallmarks of Cancer, Self-sufficiency in Growth Signal, Oncogenes and Oncoproteins, Insensitivity to Growth-inhibitory Signals, Altered Cellular Metabolism, Evasion of Apoptosis, Limitless Replicative Potential, Angiogenesis, Invasion and Metastasis, Evasion of Host Immune System, Genomic Instability, Cancer-enabling Inflammation, Dysregulation of Genes and Epigenetic Changes

MULTISTEP CARCINOGENESIS
- Overview, Chemical Carcinogenesis, Radiation Carcinogenesis, Viral Carcinogenesis, Bacteria Induced Carcinogenesis, Endoparasites Induced Carcinogenesis, Hormone Induced Carcinogenesis

INVASION AND METASTASIS
- Overview, Epithelial-mesenchymal Transition, Detachment of Tumor Cells, Attachment of Tumor Cells to ECM, Degradation of Extracellular Matrix, Invasion of Lymphatics and Blood Vessels, Tumor Cell Embolization, Extravasation of Tumor Cells, Survival and Growth of Metastatic Deposits, Metabolic Alterations in Tumor Cells

ROUTES OF METASTASIS OF TUMORS
- Local Invasion, Lymphatic Route, Hematogenous Spread, Seeding/Transcoelomic Route and Surgical Implantation

CLINICAL ONCOLOGY
- Clinical Effects on Host, Host Defense Against Cancer, Grading and Staging, Paraneoplastic Syndrome, Tumor Markers, Spontaneous Regression of Tumors, Prognosis of Solid Cancers

LABORATORY DIAGNOSIS
- Overview, History and Physical Examination, Radiographic Techniques, Endoscopy, Laboratory Analysis, Cytological Diagnosis, Histopathological Study, Frozen Section Technique, Electron Microscopy, Immunohistochemistry, Flow Cytometry, DNA Probe Analysis, Southern Blot Analysis, Fluorescence *in situ* Hybridization (FISH), Molecular Diagnosis

NEOPLASIA

OVERVIEW

Neoplasia literally means new growth. Neoplasia is defined as autonomous (uncontrolled) disorderly proliferation of cells that persists in the same excessive manner after cessation of the stimuli which evoked the change (Ancient Greek, *neo*—new and *plasma*—creation). Tumor is composed of cells that deviate from normal program of cell division and differentiation.

Willis definition: Neoplasm is an abnormal mass of tissue, the growth of which exceeds and is uncoordinated with that of normal tissue and persists in the same excessive manner even after cessation of the stimuli which evoked the change.

ONCOGENESIS

Oncogenesis is process of initiation of tumors (*onkos*—mass, *genesis*—birth). Tumors may be sporadic or familial. Neoplasia occurs due to *spontaneous mutations of genes or chromosomal aberrations, exposure to mutagenic agents* such as *chemicals, radiation* (ultraviolet light, X-rays, and gamma radiation), *oncogenic viruses* (DNA and RNA viruses), *microbes, parasites and physical agents*.

Some patients may develop inherited cancer syndromes. Neoplastic cells are relatively or absolutely autonomous, excessive, disorganized. These are unresponsive to extracellular growth factors and regulatory mechanisms operating inside normal tissues.

GENES

Three large groups of genes play an important role in regulating cell functions. These are proto-oncogenes, tumor suppressor genes and DNA repair genes. Neoplasia occurs due to activation of proto-oncogene or inactivation/deletion of tumor suppressor gene. Mutation in single gene is not sufficient to cause cancer. Accumulation of mutation of multiple genes results in cancer. Activation of proto-oncogene occurs as a result of *point mutation, gene amplification, balanced translocation (without genetic loss), deletion, overexpression, chromosomal rearrangement and insertional mutagenesis*. Five groups of genes involved in carcinogenesis are shown in Table 6.1.

Proto-oncogenes

Proto-oncogenes are normal cellular genes of human genome. Their products are involved in the normal growth process and differentiation by growth factors, receptors for growth factors, signal transducing proteins, transcription factors (nuclear regulatory proteins), cyclins and cyclin-dependent kinases (cell cycle regulators). When activated, these are termed c-onc having introns and exons. Proto-oncogenes and normal cell growth control pathway are shown in Fig. 6.1.

Oncogenes

Oncogenes are mutant forms of proto-oncogenes caused as a result of *point mutation, gene amplification, balanced*

Table 6.1: Five groups of genes involved in carcinogenesis

Categories of genes	Examples	Mechanism
Cellular oncogenes	ABL, HER (ERB-B2), MYC, N-MYC, RAS and SIS	Oncogenes code for growth factors, receptors for growth factors, signal-relay and transduction factors
Tumor suppressor genes	APC, BRCA1/BRCA2, RE, TFG-β, TP53, VHL, WT1, NF1 and NF2	Tumor suppressor genes code for factors that down-regulate the cell cycle, promote differentiation and suppress oncogenes from causing cancer
Mutator genes	MLH1, MSH2, MSH6, and PMS2 are caretaker tumor suppressor genes. Mutation of DNA mismatch repair gene leads to accumulation of numerous mismatched errors in DNA replications. Example, mutation of mutator genes is hereditary non-polyposis syndrome (Lynch syndrome)	
DNA repair genes	BRCA1 and BRCA2 proteins also promote DNA repair by binding to RAD51, a molecule that mediates DNA double-strand repair breaks	DNA repair genes participate in the repair of DNA double-stranded breaks
Antiapoptotic genes	BCL2 family of genes (BCL2 and BCL XL)	Increase in anti-apoptotic gene (BCL2) inhibits apoptosis
Apoptotic genes	BAX gene	Increase in apoptotic gene promotes apoptosis

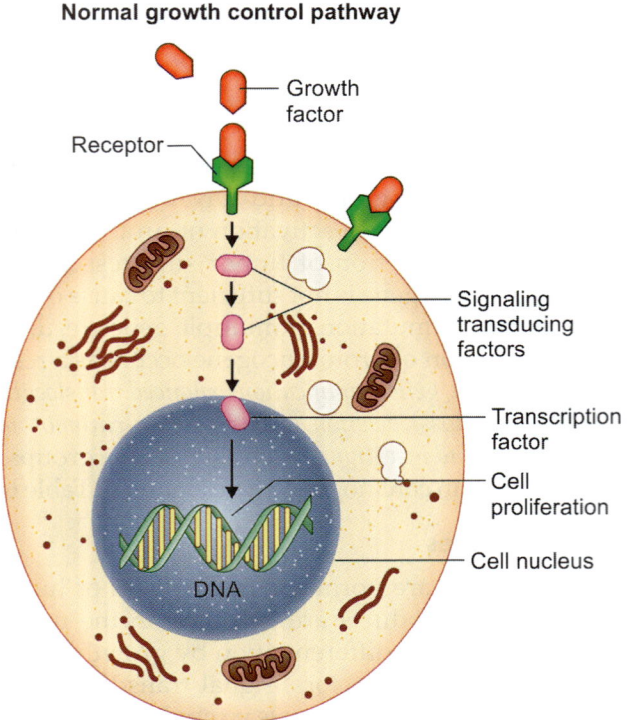

Fig. 6.1: Proto-oncogenes and normal cell growth control pathway.

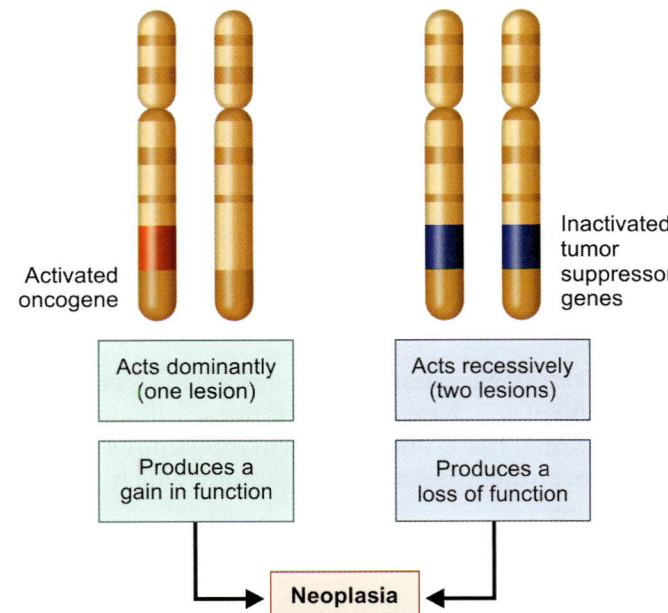

Fig. 6.2: Carcinogenesis by oncogenes and mutated tumor suppressor genes. Loss of single copy of oncogene and both copies of tumor suppressor genes is required for carcinogenesis.

translocation (without genetic loss), deletion, overexpression, chromosomal rearrangement and insertional mutagenesis. Identical genes occur in viruses (v-onc), these have only exons. Single copy of oncogenes is sufficient to result in malignant transformation. On the other hand, loss of both copies of tumor suppressor genes is required for carcinogenesis (Fig. 6.2).

Oncogenes code for growth factors, receptors for growth factors, signal-relay, transduction and transcription disturb protein synthesis and mitosis resulting in cellular alterations and ultimately tumor formation. Examples of cellular oncogenes include *ABL, HER (ERB-B2), MYC, N-MYC, RAS* and *SIS*.

Tumor Suppressor Genes

Tumor suppressor genes' products act passively and apply brakes to cellular proliferation and differentiation (Fig. 6.3). Loss of function by mutation may lead to unrestrained cell growth (Fig. 6.4). These exist in pairs at corresponding gene loci on homologous chromosomes. Loss of both copies of tumor suppressor genes is required for carcinogenesis.

Retinoblastoma follows two-hit model. Examples of tumor suppressor genes are APC, BRCA1/BRCA2, RB, TFG-β, TP53, VHL, WT1, NF1 and NF2. Breast cancer susceptibility genes—BRCA1 and BRCA2 are analyzed by DNA analysis. Gene mutations that disrupt cell function are shown in Table 6.2.

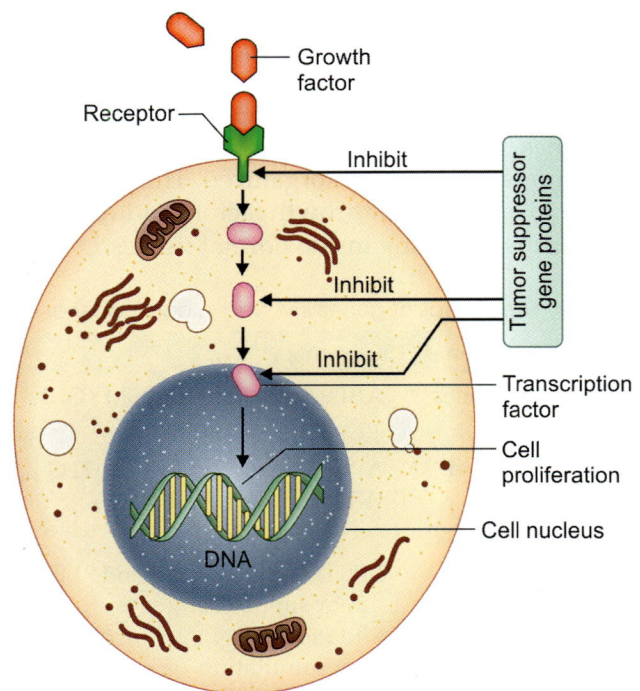

Fig. 6.3: Tumor suppressor gene proteins and normal cell growth control pathway.

Mutator Genes

These comprise MLH1, MSH2, MSH6, and PMS2. Mutation of DNA mismatch repair gene leads to accumulation of numerous mismatched errors in DNA replications. Example, mutation of mutator genes is hereditary nonpolyposis syndrome colon cancer (Lynch syndrome).

Neoplasia: Molecular Basis, Metastasis, Clinical Oncology and Laboratory Diagnosis

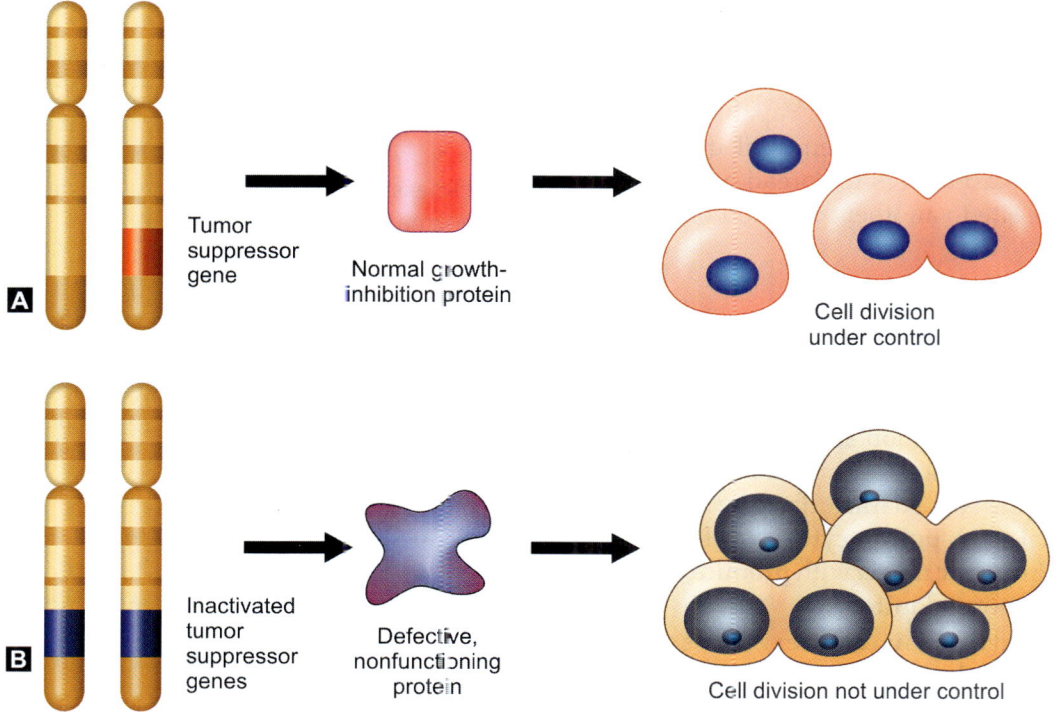

Fig. 6.4: Tumor suppressor gene. (A) Normal protein of tumor suppressor gene participate in controlled cell division, (B) mutated protein of inactivated tumor suppressor gene causes uncontrolled cell division resulting in cancer.

Table 6.2: Gene mutations that disrupt cell function

Gene	Normal function	Malfunction
Proto-oncogene	Promotes normal cell growth	Point mutation, amplification or translocation forms an oncogene, resulting in unrestrained cell growth
Paired tumor suppressor gene	Inhibit cell proliferation	Both genes inactivated in same cell resulting in unrestrained cell proliferation
Paired DNA repair genes	Correct error in DNA	Gene inactivation increases mutation rate

DNA Repair Genes

When DNA is damaged due to radiation, chemicals, or other environmental agents, DNA repair genes regulate processes that monitor and repair any errors in DNA duplication during cell division. BRCA1 and BRCA2 proteins promote DNA repair by binding to RAD51, a molecule that mediates repair of DNA double-stranded breaks.

MLH1, MSH2, MSH6, and PMS2 belong to caretaker tumor suppressor genes also known as *mutator genes*. Their gene products ensure the integrity of the cellular genome by replication and mismatch DNA repairs.

Patient develops *hereditary nonpolyposis colon carcinoma (Lynch syndrome)* due to MLH1, MSH2, MSH6, and PMS2 gene mutations. In Lynch syndrome, errors in DNA repair may cause *hereditary nonpolyposis colon cancer (right colon), xeroderma pigmentosum, Bloom's syndrome, ataxia-telangiectasia and Fanconi anemia*.

Apoptotic Gene

Apoptotic BAX gene proteins promote apoptosis.

Antiapoptotic Genes

Antiapoptotic genes comprise BCL family of genes (BCL2 and BCLXL). Their proteins inhibit apoptosis.

ONCOLOGY

Oncology (Greek *onkos*, tumor + logia) is the study or science of neoplasms, including the etiology and pathogenesis. Some non-neoplastic cellular proliferations such as hyperplasia, metaplasia, and dysplasia must be distinguished from neoplasms.

HISTIOGENESIS

Histiogenesis is a method of **classifying neoplasms** on the basis of the tissue **cell of origin**. Most human organs (except for nervous system) are composed of epithelial or connective tissue cells or both. Benign tumors refer to those tumors incapable of metastasis and having a good prognosis. Malignant tumors are capable of invasive growth and/or metastasis, often fatal if not treated effectively. Metastasis refers to spread of a malignant tumor from one site to another via blood or lymphatic routes.

DYSPLASIA

Dysplasia is usually reversible change, which may transform into malignancy. Morphologic manifestations reveal disorderly maturation and spatial arrangement of cells that are not normal but are not obviously malignant. Dysplasia is characterized by **anisocytosis** (cells of unequal size), **poikilocytosis** (cells of variable shape), **hyperchromatic nucle***i* with **prominent nucleoli** and increased abnormal **mitosis**.

Examples of dysplasia are **cervical squamous intraepithelial neoplasia** and **colorectal region**. Low grade dysplasia does not affect the whole thickness of epithelium. It is reversible if the irritant is removed. On the other hand, high grade dysplasia is precancerous (not reversible). It affects the whole thickness of epithelium.

Cervical Intraepithelial Neoplasia

Squamous dysplasia of the cervix may be graded as mild, moderate, or severe (grade I, grade II and grade III). Severe dysplasia can be distinguished from carcinoma *in situ* (Fig. 6.5).

CARCINOMA *IN SITU*

Carcinoma *in situ* refers to epithelial malignancies confined to just the epithelium without going through the basement membrane. It occurs in epithelia of *breast, bronchi, uterine cervix, vagina and skin*. It involves the full thickness of epithelium by dysplasia and presence of abnormal mitosis.

Tumor cell death in carcinoma *in situ* occurs due to programmed cell death (apoptosis), inadequate blood supply, with consequent ischemia, paucity of nutrients, and vulnerability to specific and nonspecific host defenses. Urinary bladder carcinoma *in situ* is a flat lesion. Light microscopy shows cellular atypia of the entire mucosa of urinary bladder from the basal layer to the surface (Fig. 6.6).

MICROINVASION

Microinvasion is spread of epithelial malignancies just beyond the point of origin through the basement membrane. It is in a position to compromise neighboring tissues and metastasize.

INVASION AND METASTASIS

Malignant tumors disseminate by one of five following pathways: local invasion, lymphatic route, hematogenous route, transcoelomic route, and surgical implantation. Carcinomas most often spread by lymphatic route involving regional lymph nodes, and later by hematogenous spread to distant organs. Sarcomas spread by hematogenous route.

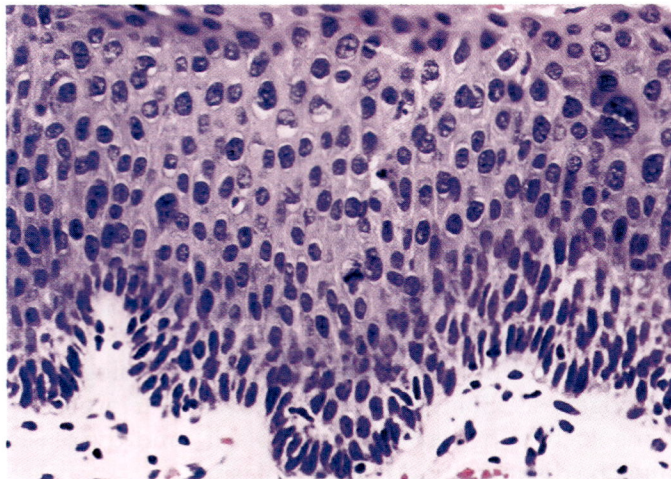

Fig. 6.5: CIN III (cervical intraepithelial neoplasia). This is cervical squamous dysplasia at high magnification extending from the center to the right. The epithelium is normal at the left. Note how the dysplastic cell nuclei are larger and darker, and the dysplastic cells have a disorderly arrangement (400X).

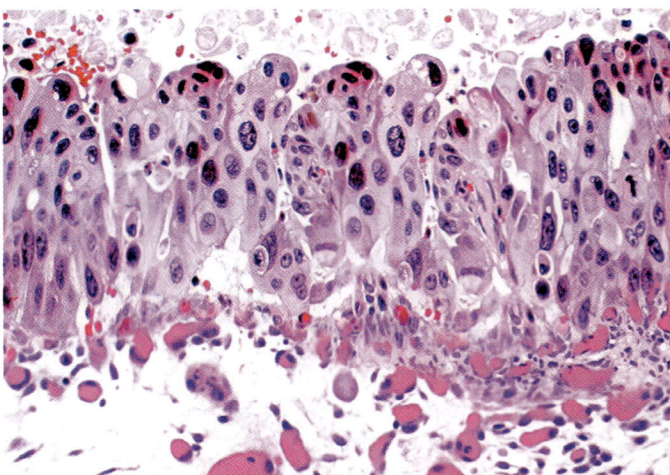

Fig. 6.6: Urinary bladder carcinoma *in situ*. Urothelial atypical cells are pleomorphic with high nucleocytoplasmic ratio, irregular nuclear contours, hyperchromatic nuclei and prominent nucleoli. Cellular polarity is lost. Mitotic figures are atypical. Diagnosis of urothelial carcinoma *in situ* does not require full-thickness involvement. The superficial umbrella cell layer may be intact (400X).

NOMENCLATURE AND CLASSIFICATION

General Considerations

The suffix "-oma" means tumor and usually denotes a benign neoplasm, as in adenoma, papilloma, lipoma, and fibroma. The suffix "-oma" sometimes implies a malignant neoplasm, as with so-called astrocytoma (brain), seminoma (testes), dysgerminoma (ovary) hepatoma, melanoma, lymphoma, and mesothelioma or even a non-neoplastic lesion such as hematoma, granuloma, or hamartoma.

On the basis of their histologic features and presumed cell or tissue origin, neoplasm can be classified as: epithelial tumors (most common) and connective tissue tumors. Tumors of blood cells and lymphocyte are leukemias, non-Hodgkin's lymphomas, multiple myelomas, and Hodgkin's disease. Neuroendocrine tumors may synthesize a number of hormones. Classification of common neoplasms is shown in Table 6.3.

Table 6.3: Classification of common neoplasms

Tissue of origin	Benign tumors	Malignant tumors
Epithelial origin		
Stratified squamous epithelium	Squamous cell papilloma	Squamous cell carcinoma
Basal cell of skin or adnexa	-	Basal cell carcinoma
Epithelial lining of ducts and glands Glandular epithelium	Adenoma	Adenocarcinoma
	Papilloma	Papillary carcinoma
Respiratory passages	Bronchial adenoma	Bronchogenic carcinoma
Renal epithelium	Renal tubular adenoma	Renal cell carcinoma
Liver cell	Liver cell adenoma	Hepatocellular carcinoma
Ovarian surface epithelium	Serous cystadenoma	Serous cystadenocarcinoma
Neuroectoderm (melanocytes)	Mucinous cystadenoma	Mucinous cystadenocarcinoma
	Benign nevus	Malignant melanoma
Urinary tract	Transitional cell papilloma	Transitional cell carcinoma
Placental epithelium	Hydatidiform mole	Choriocarcinoma
Testicular germ cell neoplasms	Benign cystic teratoma (ovary)	Seminoma/dysgerminoma, embryonal carcinoma, yolk sac tumor and choriocarcinoma
Connective tissue origin		
Fibrous tissue	Fibroma	Fibrosarcoma
Adipose tissue	Lipoma	Liposarcoma
Cartilage	Chondroma	Chondrosarcoma
Bone	Osteoma	Osteosarcoma
Muscle origin		
Smooth muscle	Leiomyoma	Leiomyosarcoma
Striated muscle	Rhabdomyoma	Rhabdomyosarcoma
Blood vessels		
Lymphatic channels	Lymphangioma	Lymphangiosarcoma
Blood vessels	Hemangioma	Angiosarcoma
Surface coverings		
Synovium	-	Synovial sarcoma
Mesothelium	Benign fibrous tumor	Malignant mesothelioma
Brain coverings	Meningioma	Invasive meningioma

Contd...

Table 6.3: Classification of common neoplasms (Contd...)

Tissue of origin	Benign tumors	Malignant tumors
Blood cells		
Hematopoietic myeloid cells	-	Myelogenous leukemia
Lymphoid cells	-	Lymphomas (Hodgkin's disease and NHL), malignant thymoma, multiple myeloma, acute lymphoblastic leukemia and chronic lymphocytic leukemia
Histiocytes	-	Histiocytosis X
Primitive mesenchyme	-	Ewing's sarcoma
Mixed tumors usually derived from one germ layer		
Salivary gland	Pleomorphic adenoma	Malignant mixed tumor
Renal analogue	-	Wilms' tumor
Totipotent cells	Benign teratoma	Teratocarcinoma
Nervous system		
Neuroglia	Oligodendroglioma (adults), ependymoma (adults)	Astrocytoma, glioblastoma multiforme
Primitive neuroectodermal cells		Medulloblastoma (children)
		Neuroblastoma (children)
Arachnoid cell	Meningioma	-
Nerve sheaths	Neurilemmoma	Neurofibrosarcoma
Embryonic tissue		
Kidney	-	Wilms' tumor
Liver	-	Hepatoblastoma
Retina	-	Retinoblastoma
Adrenal medulla	-	Neuroblastoma
Secondary tumors		
	-	Carcinoma (epithelial origin)
		Sarcoma (mesenchymal origin)

Tumor eponyms are applied to malignant tumors that cannot be properly classified (e.g. Hodgkin's disease, Wilms' tumor, Ewing's sarcoma, Kaposi's sarcoma, mesothelioma, melanoma, seminoma, dysgerminoma, chordoma and Burkitt's lymphoma).

Classification

Tumors are classified as either benign or malignant (carcinoma or sarcoma), a distinction of great importance in diagnosis, treatment, and prognosis (Table 6.4 and Figs 6.7 and 6.8). These tumors may arise from epithelium or connective tissue.

BENIGN TUMORS

Benign tumors are uncontrolled proliferation of well differentiated cells. These closely resemble the tissue of origin on light microscopy. These are *slow growing, well circumscribed, encapsulated and most often confined to their site of origin*. These do not invade or disrupt surrounding tissues. These do not metastasize **except leiomyoma, cardiac myxoma** and **pleomorphic adenoma salivary gland**. These tumors are designated by attaching suffix '*oma*'. Benign tumors may be derived from epithelial or mesenchymal tissue.

BENIGN EPITHELIAL TUMORS

Benign tumors of epithelial origin arise from ectoderm and endoderm (e.g. adenoma, papilloma and polyp). Shape of epithelium derived benign tumors is sessile, papillary and polypoid growth.

These are usually ovoid or rounded in shape. Cut surface may be solid or cystic lacking hemorrhage and necrosis. Examples of benign epithelial tumors are described as under.

Table 6.4: Principal characteristics of benign and malignant tumors

Feature	Benign tumors	Malignant tumors
Rate of growth	Slow	Relatively rapid
Behavior	Expansile sessile or papillary growth grows locally	Fungating, ulcerated or annular tumors invading surrounding tissue
Direction of growth on skin or mucosal surfaces	Exophytic growth (most often)	Endophytic growth (most often)
Invasion in surrounding tissue	No	Yes
Metastases	Uncommon except leiomyoma, myxoma (heart) and pleomorphic adenoma (salivary gland) may metastasize	Frequent metastases (uncommon in basal cell carcinoma)
Effect on host	Slight harm, due to location or complication	Significant harm, due to invasion and metastasis
Gross morphology		
Border	Often circumscribed or encapsulated	Often poorly defined or irregular
Hemorrhage and necrosis	Rare	Common
Ulceration	Rare	Common on skin or mucosal surfaces
Histopathological examination		
Histological resemblance to normal tissue	Resembles cell of origin (well differentiated)	Most often shows failure of cellular differentiation (may be well differentiated or moderately differentiated)
Cells morphology	Cells are uniform throughout the tumor	Pleomorphic cells vary in shape and size
Ratio of nucleus to cytoplasm	Normal or slightly increased (1:4 or 6)	High nuclear cytoplasmic ratio (1:1)
Nuclear morphology	Often normal	Usually hyperchromatic irregular outlines, multiple nucleoli and pleomorphic
Mitotic activity	A few mitoses (bipolar mitoses)	Many mitoses (some tripolar or quadripolar mitoses)

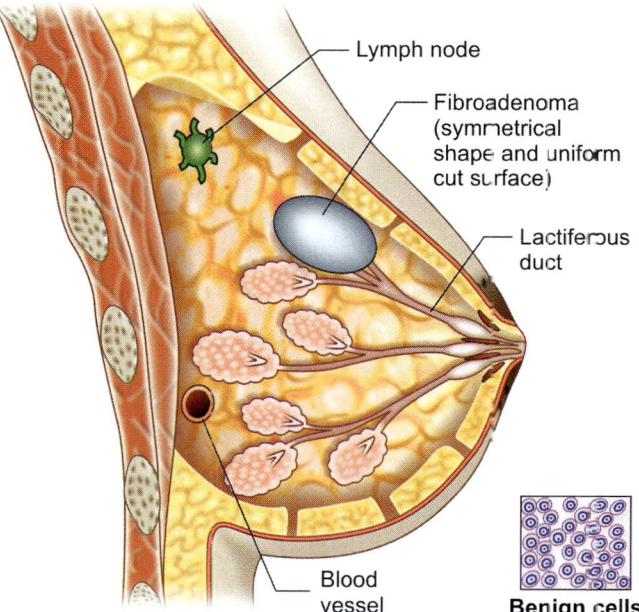

Fig. 6.7: Schematic structure of the adult female breast, showing fibroadenoma (well circumscribed tumor) in young female (*Courtesy:* Dr. Abhijit Das).

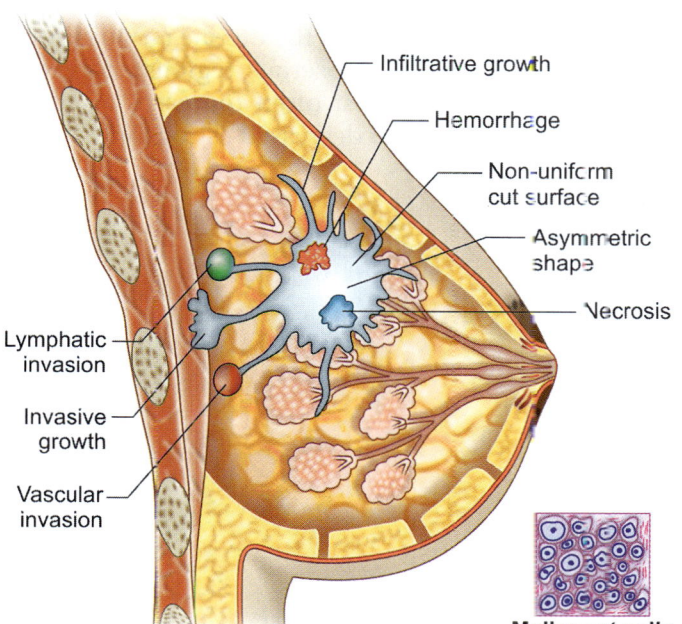

Fig. 6.8: Schematic structure of the adult female breast cancer. It shows invasive duct carcinoma with infiltrating margins and areas of hemorrhage and necrosis (*Courtesy:* Dr. Abhijit Das).

Papilloma

Papilloma has a branching pattern on the surface of the skin or a urinary bladder. It consists of **fibrovascular core** with delicate finger-like projections **lined by epithelial cells**. Squamous cell papilloma occurs in *skin, larynx,* or *tongue*. Transitional cell papilloma is seen in renal pelvis, ureter, or urinary bladder.

Polyps

Polyp is a mass that projects above a mucosal surface to form a macroscopically visible structure. It may be stalked or sessile attached to mucosa of hollow organs. Examples of polyps are *endometrial polyp, fibroepithelial polyp, nasal polyp and intestinal polyps*.

Adenoma

Adenoma is benign epithelial neoplasm producing gland pattern derived from glands but not necessarily exhibiting gland pattern. Examples are cystadenoma ovary and tubular adenoma of breast (Fig. 6.9).

BENIGN MESENCHYMAL TUMORS

Benign tumors of mesenchymal origin are derived from mesoderm and named by the tissue of origin (e.g. lipoma, fibroma, leiomyoma, rhabdomyoma, chondroma, and osteoma). Examples of benign mesenchymal tumors are described as under.

Leiomyoma

Leiomyoma is the most common benign tumor of the uterus, usually arising in women of reproductive age. It originates from smooth muscle cells of the myometrium. It usually occurs in the uterine corpus (intramural, submucous and subserous regions), cervix or uterine ligaments. It most often regresses after the menopause as a result of decreased estrogens.

Leiomyomas can cause **painful menstruation** and contribute to **infertility**. Leiomyomas show clonal abnormalities of 12q/7q and 6p resulting in rearrangement of genes. Gross morphology and light microscopy are shown in Figs 6.10 and 6.11.

Vascular Tumors

Benign vascular tumors include capillary hemangioma, cavernous hemangioma and lymphangioma. Hemangiomas are sometimes considered being a hamartoma rather than a neoplasm. Cavernous hemangioma is large, endothelium-lined spaces in the dermis and subdermis. Benign cavernous or cystic vascular lesion composed of dilated lymphatic channels commonly seen in pediatric age group (first years of life).

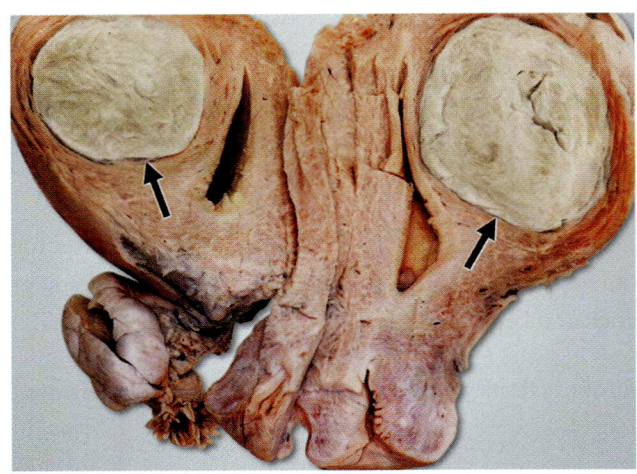

Fig. 6.10: Leiomyoma. Cut surface of intramural leiomyoma reveals whorled pattern reflecting the fact that these are composed of smooth muscle bundles (arrows).

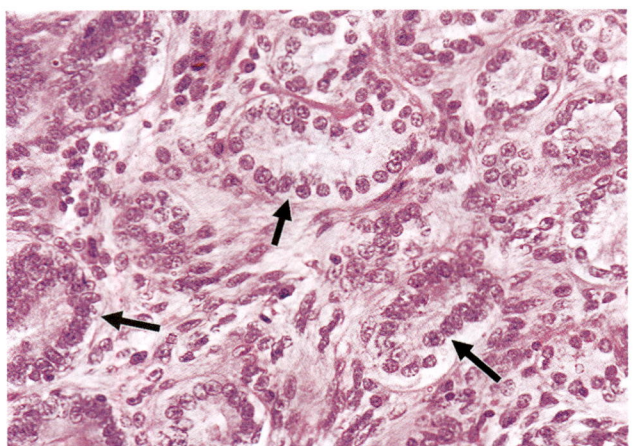

Fig. 6.9: Tubular adenoma of breast shows densely packed uniform round tubules lined by luminal cuboidal epithelial and outer myoepithelial cells without cytological atypia. There is scant intervening stroma without compression of ducts (arrows) (400X).

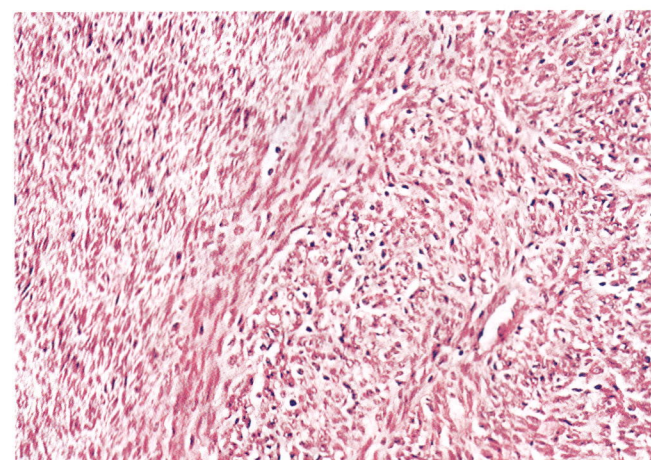

Fig. 6.11: Leiomyoma. Here is the microscopic appearance of a benign leiomyoma. Normal myometrium is at the left, and the neoplasm is well-differentiated so that the leiomyoma at the right hardly appears different. Bundles of smooth muscle are interlacing in the tumor mass (400X).

BORDERLINE TUMORS

The term *borderline* is occasionally used to describe tumors with intermediate behavior, as with some surface epithelial ovarian tumors (serous and mucinous).

SEROUS BORDERLINE TUMOR OF OVARY

This tumor of intermediate malignant potential has a peak incidence in women of 20 to 50 years age group. The tumor cells may shed from the surface and implant on peritoneum, possibly reflecting multifocal origins. S-100 protein is positive in serous borderline tumors of ovary.

MUCINOUS BORDERLINE TUMOR OF OVARY

Like its serous counterpart, this tumor most often occurs in younger women confined to the ovary. It is composed of multilayered atypical epithelial cells, with abundant gland-like or papillary growth with moderate atypia and some mitotic activity, without stromal invasion.

MALIGNANT TUMORS

Malignant tumors are also known as cancers. These occur either due to oncogenes (15–20%) or inactivation of tumor suppressor genes. These show great degree of autonomy. These synthesize growth and angiogenic factors and have ability to escape immune surveillance resulting in clinical cancers. These invade and destroy adjacent structures. These can spread to distant sites.

Origin

Malignant tumors arise from epithelium known as *carcinomas* (squamous cell carcinoma, adenocarcinoma) and mesenchymal tissue known as *sarcomas* (osteosarcoma, chondrosarcoma). Principal characteristics of carcinoma and sarcoma are shown in Table 6.5.

Differentiation

Malignant tumors are usually less differentiated than benign tumors. **Anaplasia** is a term applied to **poorly differentiated carcinoma**. In general, highly anaplastic tumors are very aggressive. Well-differentiated tumors are less aggressive. Most anaplastic tumors often respond well to chemotherapy and radiotherapy, because these modalities are most effective in rapidly dividing cells.

Malignant cells exhibit pleomorphism, hyperchromatic nuclei, high nucleocytoplasmic ratio, and prominent nuclei with coarse **clumped chromatin** reflecting synthetic **mitotic activity**. Mitoses are often numerous and distinctly *atypical tripolar or quadripolar forms*.

Electron Microscopy

Normal Cell

Normally, microfilaments (actin-like protein) participate in binding of cells by exerting a pull on the extracellular organic molecules. Microtubules participate in maintenance of cell shape, intracellular transport,

Table 6.5: Principal characteristics of carcinoma and sarcoma

Parameters	Carcinomas	Sarcomas
Origin	Epithelium	Mesenchymal tissues
Examples	Squamous cell carcinoma, adenocarcinoma	Osteosarcoma, chondrosarcoma, fibrosarcoma
Behavior	Malignant	Malignant
Frequency	Common	Relatively rare
Growth rate	Slow	Rapid
Preferential routes of metastases	Lymphatic route (except renal cell carcinoma, follicular carcinoma thyroid)	Hematogenous route
In situ phase	Yes	No
Age group	>50 years (most often)	<50 years (most often)
Neoangiogenesis (new blood vessels formed)	Confined to carcinomas hence relatively less vascular	Extending from sarcoma in the surround tissue hence more vascular
Light microscopy	Group of cells is separated by connective tissue	Individual cell is separated from adjacent cell by connective tissue
Immunohistochemistry	Keratin expression	Vimentin expression
Electron microscopy	Cells express desmosomes and specialized junctional complexes	Cells do not express desmosomes and specialized junctional complexes
Prognosis	Relatively good	Poor
Carcinomas often exhibit desmosomes and specialized junctional complexes, which are structures that are not typical of sarcomas or lymphomas.		

movement of organelles and chromosomes (cell division). Colchicine drug disrupts and thus no movement of chromosomes occurs.

Cancer Cells

Damage to the cell membrane of malignant cells results in reduced cell adhesions. These cells exhibit increased response to growth factors resulting in increased metabolic demand for nutrients. Cancer cells exhibit free ribosomes, simplification of rough endoplasmic reticulum, pleomorphic mitochondria, and disruption of cytoskeleton (microfilaments, microtubules and intermediate filaments). Differences between normal and cancer cells are shown in Table 6.6.

Invasion and Metastases

Malignant tumors are rapidly growing, poorly circumscribed, and invade surrounding normal tissues and cause destruction. These tumors invade surrounding structures and cause destruction. Malignant tumor cells spread to distant organs by lymphatic, hematogenous or transcoelomic routes with fatal outcome. Basal cell carcinoma of skin rarely metastasizes.

Locally Malignant Tumors

Groups of slow growing malignant tumors spread only locally by direct infiltration. The cells show features of malignancy. Examples are *basal cell carcinoma of skin, osteoclastoma (giant cell tumor of bone), adamantinoma (jaw), bronchial adenoma, carcinoid tumor, astrocytoma in brain and craniopharyngioma* from pituitary gland.

Giant cell tumor of bone is potentially low grade locally aggressive malignant tumor affecting 20 to 45 years of age. It accounts for 20% of all bone tumors and has a monocyte-macrophage lineage. It most often arises in epiphysis mostly **around knee joint** (distal femur or proximal tibia). Tumor gives '**soap bubble** appearance' on **radiograph** (Fig. 6.12) and gross morphology is seen in Fig. 6.13. Tumor is composed of **multinucleated, osteoclastic giant cells** embedded in a supporting spindle-celled stroma (Fig. 6.14).

CARCINOMA

Carcinoma is malignant tumor arising from lining epithelium (e.g. squamous, glandular and transitional epithelium). The epithelia of the body are derived from all three germ cell layers: carcinoma arising from skin (ectoderm), renal cell carcinoma arising from tubular cells (mesoderm) and carcinoma arising from lining

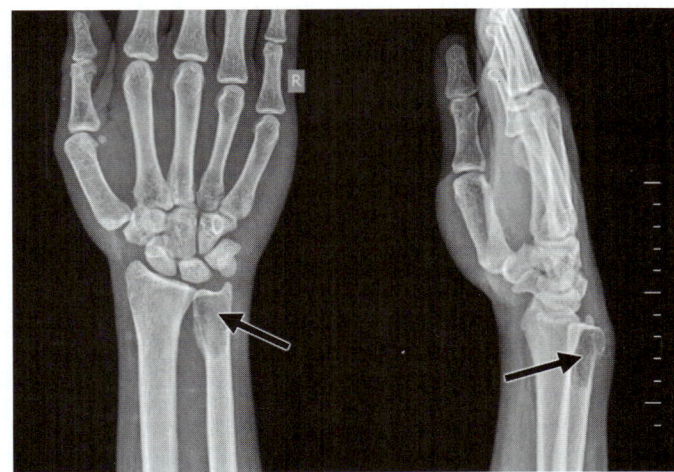

Fig. 6.12: Radiograph of wrist joint showing giant cell tumor of bone. Slightly expansile osteolytic lesion is seen in lower ulna with narrow zone of transition (arrows).

Table 6.6: Differences between normal and cancer cells

Characteristics	Normal cells	Cancer cells
Growth	Regulated	Unregulated
Differentiation	High	Low
Genetic stability	Stable	Unstable
Growth factor dependence	Dependent	Independent
Density dependent	High	Low inhibition
Anchorage dependence	High	Low
Cell-to-cell adhesion	High	Low
Cell-to-cell communication	High	Low
Cell lifespan	Limited	Unlimited
Antigen expression	Absent	May be present
Substance production (protease, hormone)	Normal	Abnormal
Cytoskeleton composition and arrangement	Normal	Abnormal

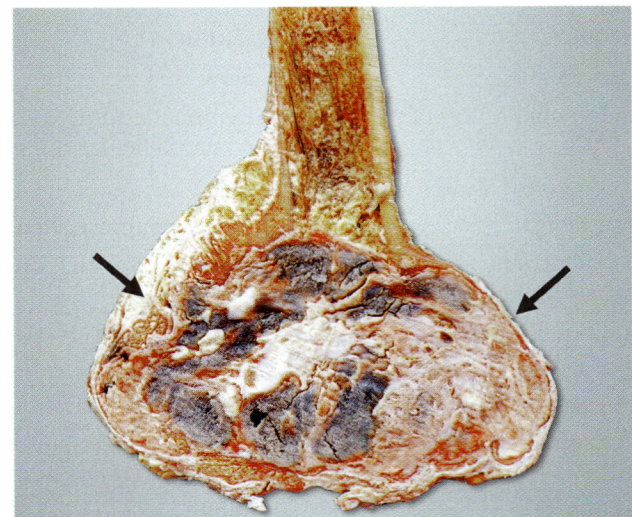

Fig. 6.13: Giant cell tumor in the lower end of the femur. It is a hemorrhagic tumor expanding the lateral condyle and destroying the normal bone (arrows).

Neoplasia: Molecular Basis, Metastasis, Clinical Oncology and Laboratory Diagnosis

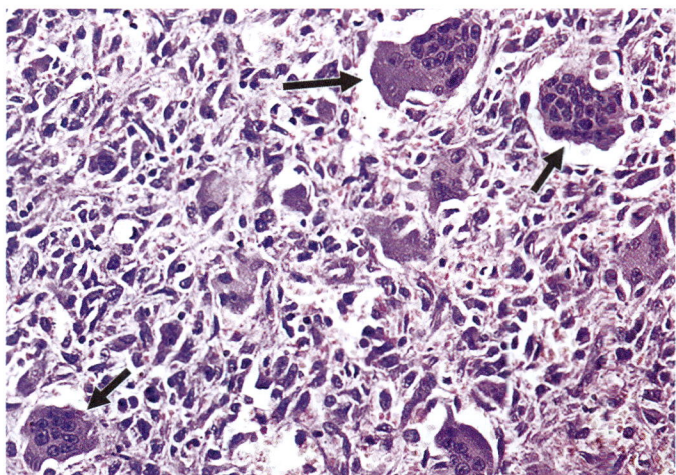

Fig. 6.14: Giant cell tumor of bone. It is composed of mononuclear uniform tumor cells with indistinct cell membrane growing in a syncytium and stromal cells. Multinucleated giant cells containing >100 nuclei are scattered among mononuclear stromal cells. The nuclei of stromal cells have identical features to that of the mononuclear cells (arrows) (400X).

epithelium of gut (mesoderm). *It is evident that mesoderm can give rise to carcinoma (renal cell carcinoma) as well as sarcoma.* Examples of carcinomas are described as under.

Squamous Cell Carcinoma

Common sites of squamous cell carcinoma include skin, oropharynx, esophagus (upper/middle), larynx, areas of squamous metaplasia (bronchi, squamocolumnar junction of the uterine cervix) and vagina (Table 6.7). Common squamous cell carcinoma in India includes cervical carcinoma due to HPV virus. Squamous cell carcinoma of oral cavity and tongue most often occurs due to tabacco chewing. There is increased risk of development of squamous cell carcinoma of lungs in tabacco smokers.

Based on degree of anaplasia and formation of keratin pearls, these are designated as well as differentiated carcinoma (keratin pearls and low anaplasia), moderately differentiated carcinoma (prominent cytoplasmic pearls) and poorly differentiated carcinoma (anaplasia and occasional keratinocytes). Gross morphology and light microscopy of cervical squamous cell carcinoma are shown in Figs 6.15 and 6.16.

Adenocarcinoma

Adenocarcinoma arises from glandular epithelium in various organs (e.g. **stomach, colon, pancreas, breast, endometrium, prostate,** and **lung**). Desmoplasia refers to proliferation of non-neoplastic fibrous connective tissue within a tumor.

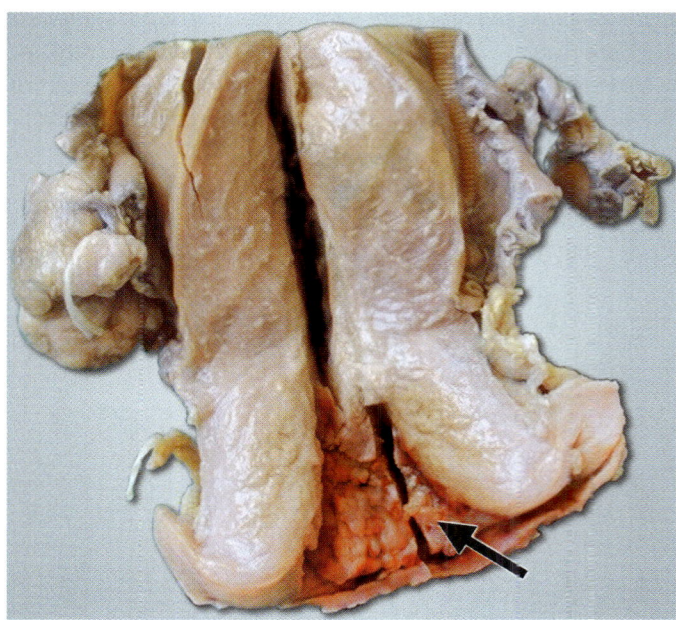

Fig. 6.15: Cervical carcinoma. Growth is seen in cervical region (arrow).

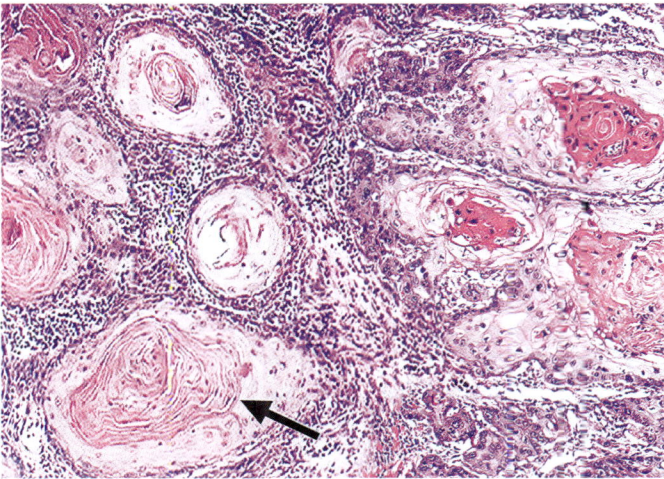

Fig. 6.16: Cervical squamous cell carcinoma. At high magnification, nests of neoplastic squamous cells are invaded through a chronically inflamed stroma. This cancer is well- differentiated, as evidenced by keratin pearls (arrow). However, most cervical squamous carcinomas are non-keratinizing (400X).

Table 6.7: Tissue sites of carcinomas

Histological type of carcinoma	Tissue site
Squamous cell carcinoma	Skin, nasal cavity, oropharynx, esophagus, larynx, lung, cervix
Adenocarcinoma	Stomach, colon, breast, pancreas, lung, prostate, endometrium, ovary and Barrett's esophagus
Other type of carcinomas	Small cell carcinoma and large cell carcinoma of lung, hepatocellular carcinoma, renal cell carcinoma, transitional cell carcinoma urinary bladder.

Desmoplasia is quite common in infiltrating duct carcinoma of *breast (scirrhous type), gastric carcinoma (linitis plastica type), pancreas and prostate*. Gross morphology and light microscopy of classic colorectal adenocarcinoma are shown in Figs 6.17 and 6.18.

Transitional Cell Carcinoma

Transitional cell carcinoma arises from transitional epithelium of the urinary tract (e.g. *urinary bladder, ureter, renal pelvis*).

Risk factors for urinary bladder carcinoma comprise *tobacco smoking, occupational exposure to β-naphthylamine, Schistosoma haematobium infestation, cyclophosphamide* and *analgesics, radiation therapy* (cervical, prostate, or rectal cancer) and *exstrophy of the bladder* (absence of the anterior part of the bladder and abdominal wall).

The earliest sign of bladder cancer is sudden pain less hematuria in urine, which may red or rust colored. In the later stages, the bladder may become irritable, painful urination. Gross morphology of tumor is exophytic (cauliflower-like) or ulcerated lesion. Light microscopy of urinary bladder carcinoma is shown in Fig. 6.19.

SARCOMA

Sarcoma is a malignant tumor of mesenchymal origin. It is often used with a prefix that denotes the tissue of origin of the tumor. Sarcomas are most often **large, bulky** and **necrotic tumor**. *These metastasize by hematogenous route* **except rhabdomyosarcoma**, *which spread by lymphatic channels. Desmin is an intermediate filament protein found in cells of skeletal muscle.* Tissue sites of sarcoma are shown in Table 6.8.

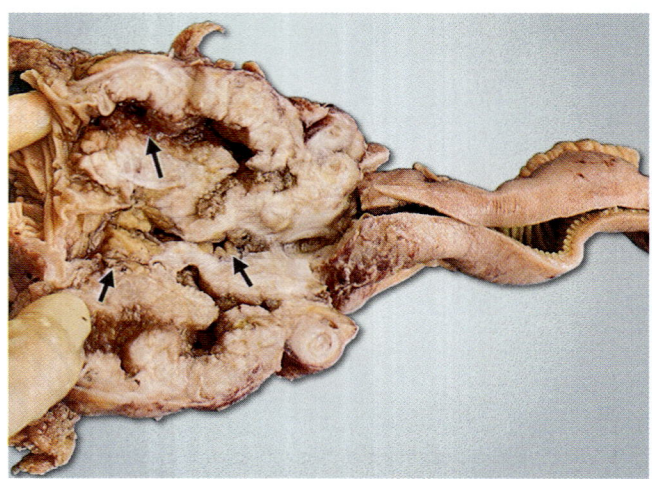

Fig. 6.17: Carcinoma in caecum showing fungating intraluminal growth, tumor is firm with gray white appearance. Cut surface is gray white (arrows).

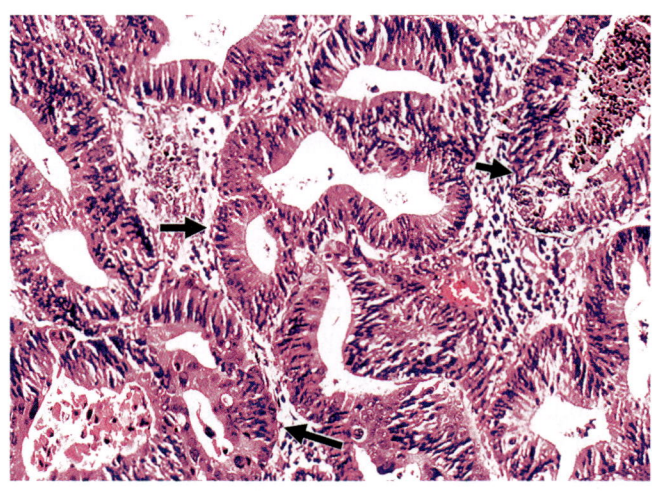

Fig. 6.18: Classic colorectal adenocarcinoma is composed of irregularly distributed tubular structures with intraluminal necrosis (arrows) (400X).

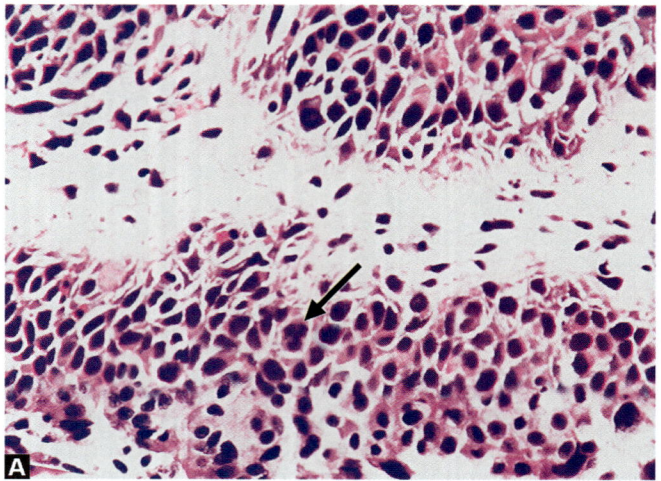

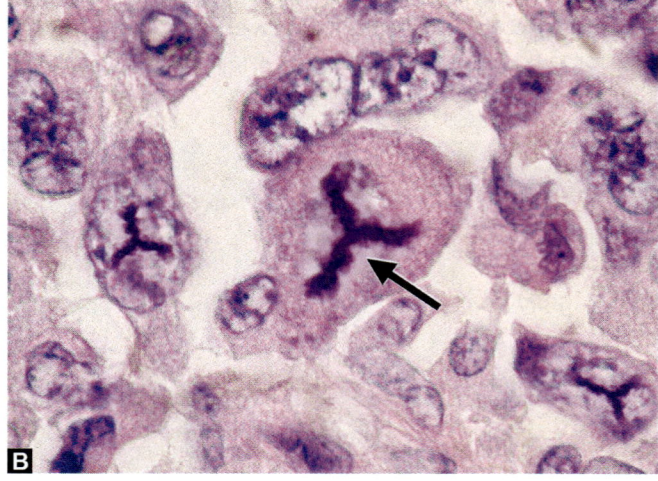

Fig. 6.19: (A) High grade papillary urothelial carcinoma, tumor cells are pleomorphic with hyperchromatic large nuclei and high nuclear to cytoplasmic ratio, (B) mitotic figures are frequent (arrows).

Neoplasia: Molecular Basis, Metastasis, Clinical Oncology and Laboratory Diagnosis

Table 6.8: Tissue sites of sarcomas

Tissue	Sarcoma
Smooth muscle	Leiomyosarcoma
Skeletal muscle	Rhabdomyosarcoma
Cartilage	Chondrosarcoma
Bone	Osteosarcoma
Adipose tissue	Liposarcoma
Fibrous tissue	Fibrosarcoma
Blood vessel	Angiosarcoma

Osteosarcoma

Osteosarcoma is the most common primary malignant tumor of bone. Conventional osteosarcoma most often occurs in 10 to 20 years of age. It constitutes 20% of primary bone cancer. In osteosarcoma, malignant osteoblasts produce variable amount of osteoid collagen and mineralized bone matrix. Depending on the location, osteosarcoma may be **central** (*conventional low grade, telangiectatic osteosarcomas*) or **peripheral** (*parosteal, periosteal, jaw osteosarcomas*). Serum alkaline phosphatase is increased two- to three-fold. Radiograph and light microscopy of osteoblastic osteosarcoma is shown in Figs 6.20 and 6.21.

Chondrosarcoma

Chondrosarcoma is second most common primary malignant bone tumor. It constitutes 15% of all primary malignant bone tumors. These tumors most often originate in the medulla of flat bones such as **pelvic**

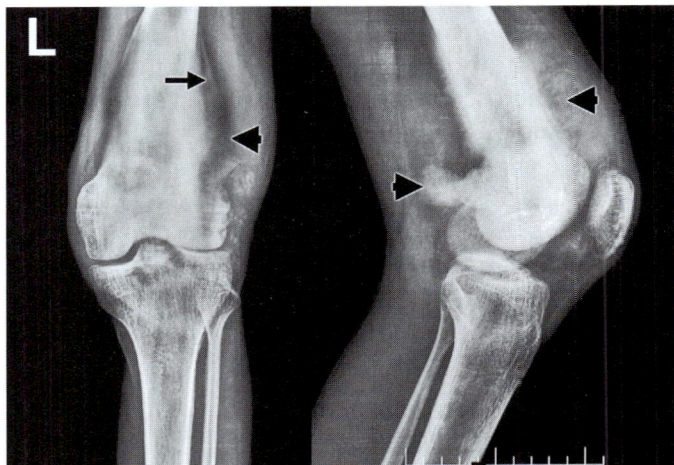

Fig. 6.20: Osteosarcoma arising from lateral femoral condyle. Permeative destruction noted in lateral cortex of lateral femoral condyle with sclerosis in lateral femoral condyle and lower femoral shaft with associated soft tissue swelling showing periosteal elevation forming Codman's triangle (arrow) and ossific densities (arrow heads). Upper tibia and fibula appear normal. Visualized joint spaces are normal.

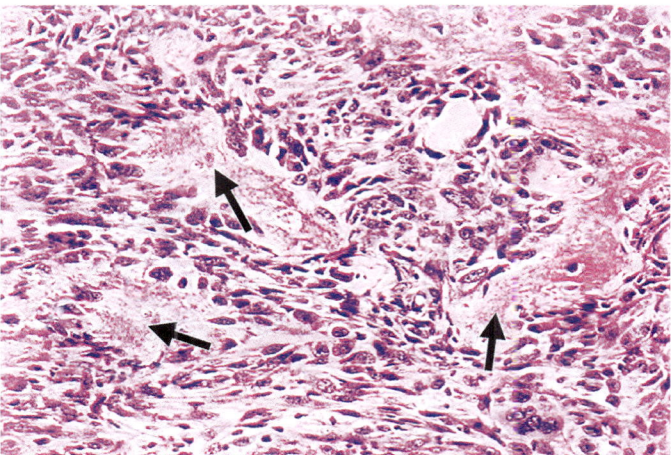

Fig. 6.21: Osteoblastic osteosarcoma. Tumor is composed of pleomorphic polyhedral or spindle shaped neoplastic cells with hyperchromatic nuclei and mitoses. Formation of fine lace-like pattern of neoplastic bone by tumor cells is diagnostic (arrows) (400X).

girdle (25%), **shoulder girdle** (scapula), **ribs**, and **vertebral column**.

Tumor is composed of atypical cells within cartilaginous lacunae. There is increased cellularity showing >2 cells with hyperchromatic nuclei per lacunae. Features of malignancy especially mitoses are best demonstrated at the edge of the tumor (Fig. 6.22).

Leiomyosarcoma

Leiomyosarcoma is a highly malignant tumor of smooth muscle cell origin *de novo*, and unrelated to pre-existing leiomyoma. Diagnostic criteria include the following features on light microscopy: (i) 10 or more mitoses per 10 HPFs; (ii) 5 or more mitoses per 10 HPFs, with nuclear atypia and necrosis; and (iii) myxoid and epithelioid smooth muscle tumors with 5 or more

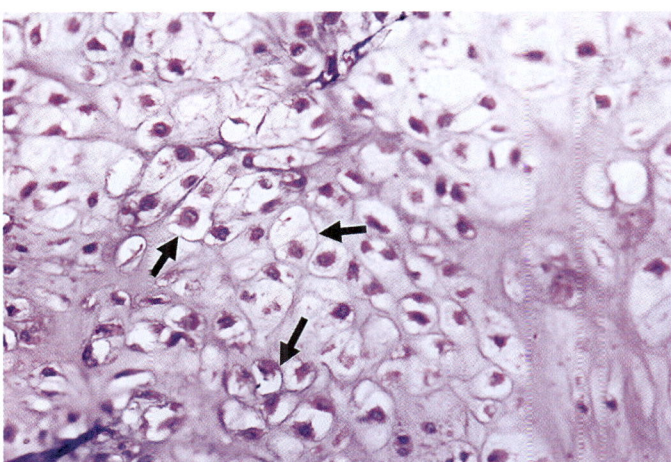

Fig. 6.22: Chondrosarcoma. Tumor is composed of atypical cells within cartilaginous lacunae. Each cartilaginous lacunae contains >2 cells with hyperchromatic nuclei (arrows) (400X).

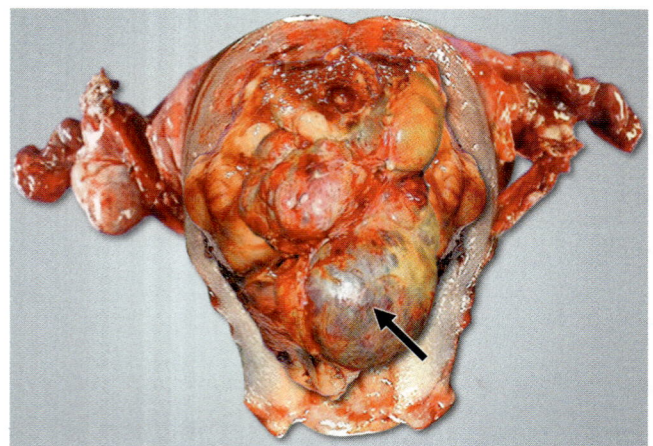

Fig. 6.23: Leiomyosarcoma of the uterus. The uterus is expanded by a massive, fleshy, partly necrotic and hemorrhagic-malignant tumor (arrow).

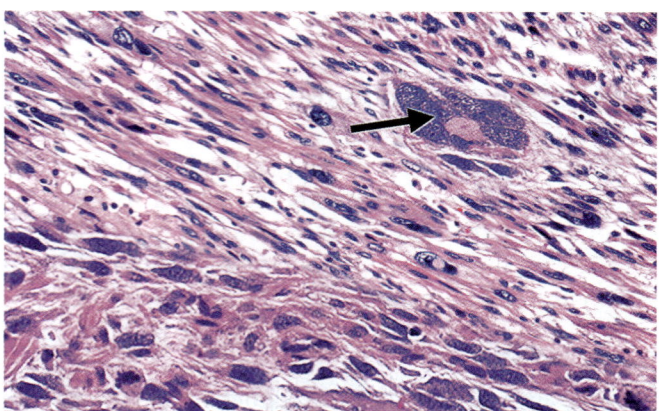

Fig. 6.24: Leiomyosarcoma showing spindle cells. Several mitoses are seen here, just in this one high power field (arrow) (400X).

mitoses per 10 HPFs. Gross and light microscopy are shown in Figs 6. 23 and 6.24.

NEUROECTODERMAL TUMORS

Various types of neuroectodermal malignancies include *glioblastoma multiforme, astrocytoma, ependymoma, medulloblastoma, oligodendroglioma, retinoblastoma, and neuroblastoma*.

Neuroblastoma is a highly malignant catecholamine-producing tumor of neural crest origin (adrenal medulla or sympathetic ganglia). It most often affects children under 5 years with peak incidence in the first 3 years of life. It is composed of neoplastic neuroblasts. Tumor is composed of small round blue tumor cells (neuroblasts) forming characteristic rosette-like structures (*Homer Wright* pseudorosettes) around small vessels (Fig. 6.25).

BLASTOMAS

The suffix *blastoma* denotes a neoplasm of embryonic cells such as **neuroblastoma** (adrenal gland), **retino-blastoma** (retina) and **hepatoblastoma** (liver). These

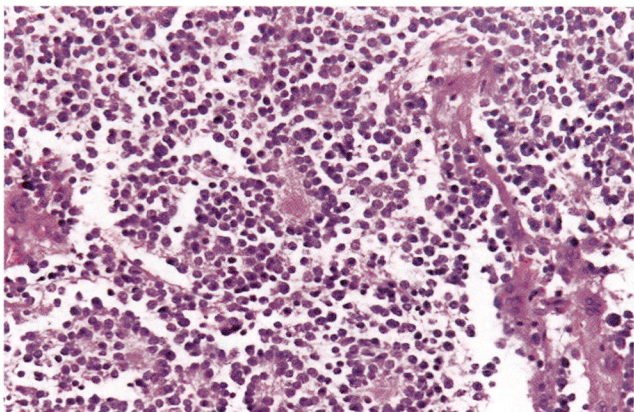

Fig. 6.25: Neuroblastoma showing small round blue tumor cells forming Homer Wright pseudorosettes around small vessels (400X).

tumors composed of immature cells resembling fetal analogue are called *blastomas*.

MIXED TUMORS

Mixed tumors have two different morphologic patterns that are derived from the same germ cell layer, which may be benign (e.g. *fibroadenoma, pleomorphic adenoma of salivary gland*) or malignant (e.g. *carcinosarcoma also called malignant mixed müllerian tumors in uterus, adenosquamous carcinoma and metaplastic carcinoma*). Light microscopy of pleomorphic adenoma is shown in Fig. 6.26.

TERATOMAS

Teratoma is a neoplasm derived from all three germ cell layers (e.g. *ectoderm, mesoderm, and endoderm*). It may contain structures such as skin, bone, cartilage, teeth, and intestinal epithelium. It may be either benign or malignant arising in the **ovaries** or **testes**, **mediastinum** and **pineal gland**. Gross morphology and light microscopy of mature teratoma are shown in Figs 6.27 and 6.28.

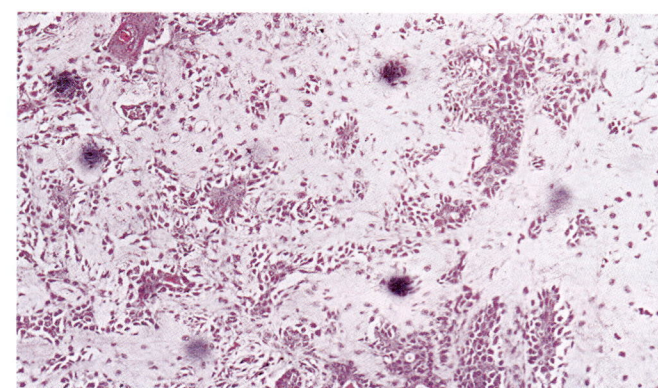

Fig. 6.26: Pleomorphic adenoma is composed of gland-like epithelial component surrounded by a myxomatous stroma often containing foci of bone or cartilage (100X).

Neoplasia: Molecular Basis, Metastasis, Clinical Oncology and Laboratory Diagnosis

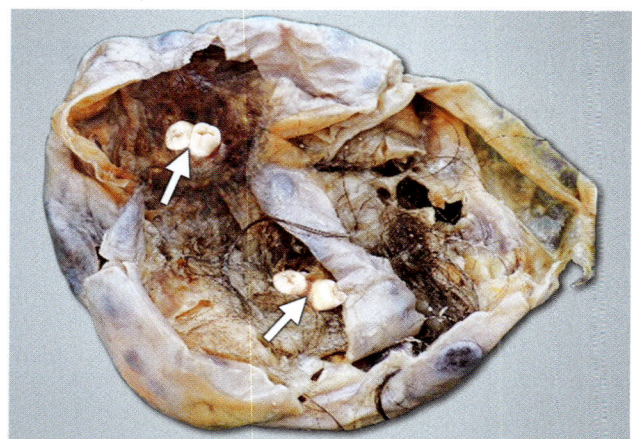

Fig. 6.27: Mature cystic teratoma showing cyst containing teeth and bunch of hair. The radiographic calcifications are highly suggestive of dermoid cyst (arrows).

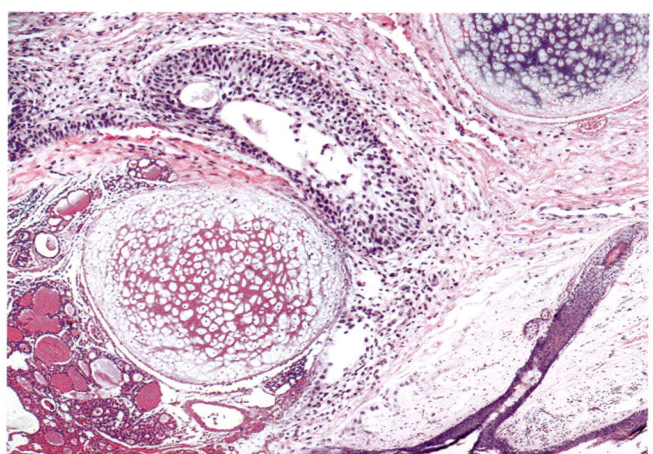

Fig. 6.28: Mature teratoma ovary. Cyst is lined by stratified squamous epithelium, sebaceous glands, hair shafts, other adnexal structures—cartilage, bone, teeth, smooth muscle, and respiratory tract epithelium (400X).

HAMARTOMAS

Hamartoma is disorganized normal tissue found in their normal anatomic location. It contains varying combinations of mature cartilage, ducts or bronchi, connective tissue, blood vessels, and lymphoid tissue. Examples of hamartoma are described below.

Mole (Melanocytic Nevus)

Melanocytic nevus represents an aggregate of pigment cells that are normally dispersed in the skin.

Bronchial Hamartoma

Bronchial hamartoma presents as a nodule composed of cartilage, bronchial epithelium, and smooth muscle cells. It affects adults over 40 years of age, with a peak in the sixth decade of life. It constitutes 10% of coin lesions discovered incidentally on chest radiograph.

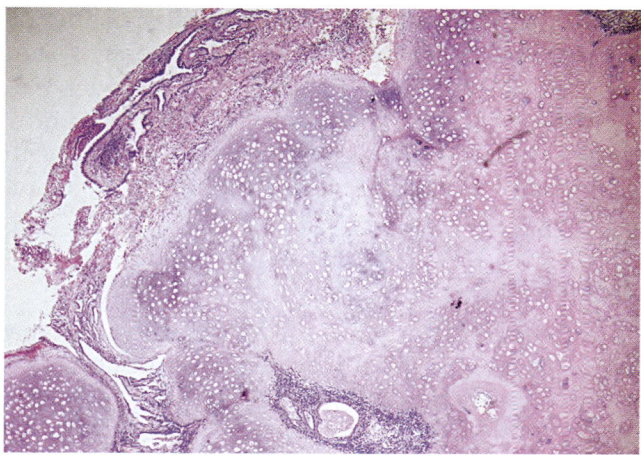

Fig. 6.29: Pulmonary hamartoma is composed of cartilage, bronchial epithelium, and smooth muscle cells (100X). On immunohistochemistry, smooth muscle actin and S-100 are expressed in spindle cells. In males, the cells express ER, FR and androgen receptors (100X).

A characteristic *popcorn* pattern of calcification is often seen by X-ray. Light microscopy is shown in Fig 6.29.

Peutz-Jeghers Syndrome

It is autosomal dominant disorder due to LKB1/STK11 gene in young children 10–15 years of age. Patient presents with **multiple hamartomatous** polyps in *small intestine (most common), stomach* and *colon* in decreasing frequency; *melanotic pigmented macules* (1–5 mm) of *lips, perioral skin, hands* and *genitalia*. There is increased risk of cancers of gastrointestinal tract, thyroid, breast, lung, pancreas, gonads and urinary bladder.

Multiple Bile Duct Hamartomas

Bile duct hamartoma is asymptomatic lesion also known as **von Meyenburg complex**. It shows irregularly

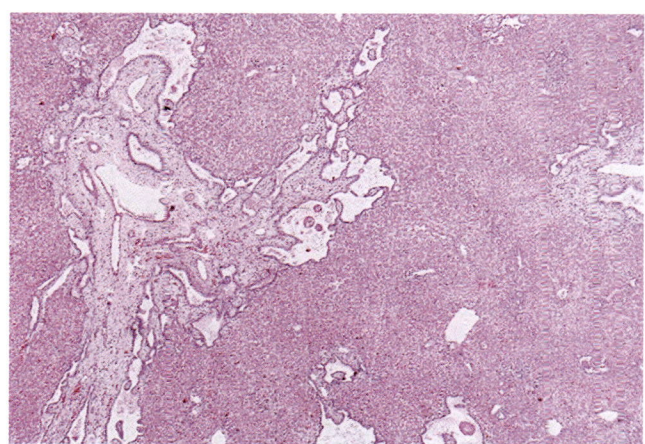

Fig. 6.30: Multiple bile duct hamartomas are also known a von Meyenburg complex. Hamartoma is composed of small disorganized clusters of dilated cystic bile ducts lined by columnar cells enclosed within fibrocollagenous stroma (100X).

dilated bile ducts. It is characterized by multiple bile duct hamartomas and biliary microhamartomas <5 mm.

It is important to distinguish this disorder from multiple hepatic metastases. Women are more affected than men. Histological examination of the hamartomatous nodule shows proliferations of bile ducts (Fig. 6.30).

CHORISTOMA

Ectopic islands of normal tissue are called choristomas. These islands of normal mature tissue are located in another organ (Table 6.9).

Table 6.9: Examples of choristomas

Tissue	Located in another organs
Pancreatic tissue	Wall of stomach
	Wall of intestine
	Liver
Gastric mucosa	Meckel's diverticulum
Adrenal rest	Beneath renal capsule
Ectopic brain tissue	Nasal cavity
Splenic tissue	Peritoneal cavity

CHARACTERISTIC FEATURES OF TUMORS

The gross appearance of neoplasms is highly variable, consistent with the diversity of their origin, size, and biological behavior. Neoplasms may be firm, hard (scirrhous), or soft, homogeneous or heterogeneous in texture, solid or cystic, pale or dark, and discolored by endogenous pigments, hemorrhage, or necrosis. In general, malignant tumors differ from benign tumors in their biological properties as described under.

TUMOR COMPONENTS

All tumors except leukemia are composed of two components: parenchyma and supporting stroma.

TUMOR PARENCHYMA

Parenchyma of tumor is composed of neoplastic cells. It determines the biologic behavior of the tumor from which the tumor derives its name.

TUMOR STROMAL COMPONENT

Stromal component is composed of non-neoplastic host derived supporting connective tissue containing newly formed blood vessels. It carries blood supply and provides support to tumor.

Tumor grows via angiogenesis induced by growth factors. Most infiltrating carcinomas induce production of a dense, fibrous stroma (desmoplasia). Stromal reaction occurs in **breast infiltrating duct carcinoma** and gastric carcinoma (**linitis plastica variant**). On the other hand, medullary carcinoma of breast is soft in consistency.

DEGREE OF DIFFERENTIATION

Differentiation means the extent to which the parenchymal cells of the tumor resemble their normal counterparts morphologically and functionally. Well differentiated neoplasm has close resemblance to tissue of origin. On the other hand, poorly differentiated tumor has a little resemblance to the tissue of origin. Differentiation often predicts responsiveness to certain therapies such as estrogen receptors and tamoxifen in breast cancers.

BENIGN TUMORS

Benign tumors are well differentiated. These closely resemble the tissue of origin.

MALIGNANT TUMORS

Malignant tumors may be well differentiated, moderately differentiated or poorly differentiated (anaplastic tumor).

Well Differentiated Carcinomas

Well differentiated carcinomas synthesize various products. Thyroid follicular carcinoma may synthesize thyroid hormones. Squamous cell carcinoma shows presence of keratin pearls. Bronchogenic carcinoma synthesizes various ectopic hormones such as ACTH, parathyroid-like hormone, insulin and glucagon. Well differentiate squamous cell carcinoma is shown in Fig. 6.31.

Moderately Differentiated Carcinomas

These show intermediate resemblance to normal cells.

Poorly Differentiated (Anaplastic) Carcinomas

Anaplasia refers to tendency of a neoplasm to be composed of less differentiated/mature cells. Anaplasia and metastasis are the *hallmarks* of malignancy. These tumors are rapidly growing tumors invading and destroying surrounding normal tissue and metastasizing

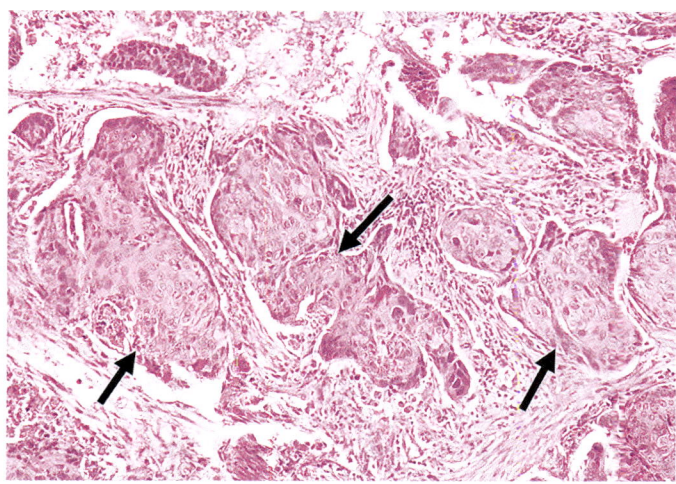

Fig. 6.31: Squamous cell carcinoma lung showing well differentiated polygonal tumor cells with pink cytoplasm with distinct cell borders, intercellular bridges. The nuclei are hyperchromatic and angular with many mitoses (arrows) (400X).

to distant organs. These often contain central ischemic necrosis due to increased oxygen demand by the tumor cells.

Features of anaplasia are pleomorphism, hyperchromatism, prominent nucleoli and increased mitosis with abnormal mitotic figures. Formation of tumor giant cells is demonstrated in some instances.

NUCLEAR FEATURES

BENIGN TUMORS

Nuclear/cytoplasmic ratio of benign tumors is close to the normal cells (ratio 1:4). Mitoses have normal mitotic spindles.

MALIGNANT TUMORS

Histopathological examination shows pleomorphic cells with hyperchromatic nuclei due to abundant DNA content, prominent nucleoli with high nuclear to cytoplasmic ratio (ratio 1:1), atypical mitoses (tripolar or quadripolar) and loss of polarity (disturbed orientation and tendency to form anarchic disorganized growth).

TUMOR DEVELOPMENT AND GROWTH RATE

Growth of the tumors depends on cell cycle, blood supply and hormones. As the epithelial cells have a shorter cell cycle than connective tissue cells, thus tumors of epithelial cells grow more rapidly than do tumors of connective tissue cells. Benign tumors are slow growing, whereas malignant tumors generally grow faster.

BENIGN TUMORS

Most benign tumors have slow growth rate. A few benign tumors have variable growth rate (uterine leiomyomas, pituitary adenoma).

Uterine Leiomyomas

These have variable growth rate depending on estrogen levels. Therapeutic administration of *estrogens increases the size of uterine leiomyomas*. Size of the uterine leiomyomas decreases after menopause due to decreased level of estrogens.

Pituitary Gland Adenoma

It *shrinks in size due to compression of blood vessels* by progressive enlargement of tumor in sella turcica.

MALIGNANT TUMORS

At least 30 doubling times are essential for a tumor to be clinically evident. Malignant tumors continue to grow with further mutations only if available nutrients, oxygen, and blood supply are adequate and the immune system fails to recognize or respond to tumor.

Growth Rate

Growth rate is variable depending on differentiation of malignant tumors. Anaplastic cancers have marked increase in growth rate. Growth rate is faster in leukemias, lymphomas and lung carcinomas. In comparison, slow growth rate is demonstrated in breast carcinomas and colon carcinomas.

Growth Factors

Malignant tumors synthesize own growth factors, which have autocrine effect. There is increased expression of growth factor receptors on the cell membrane of these rapidly growing cancer cells. Increased growth factor and growth factor receptors further enhance cancer cell proliferation.

Management

Chemotherapy is targeted on actively dividing cells. Shifting is done by debulking by surgery or radiotherapy.

MONOCLONAL PROPERTIES OF TUMORS

Benign and malignant tumors are derived from a single precursor cell (monoclonal). On the other hand, non-neoplastic proliferations are derived from polyclonal cells.

Neoplasms are monoclonal; in contrast, polyclonal proliferations are almost always non-neoplastic. Various markers are used to study the monoclonal property of tumors which are described as under.

G6PD MARKER

Monoclonal property is assessed by studying glucose-6-phosphate dehydrogenase (G6PD) in selected neoplasms. Uterine leiomyomas have either G6PD-A or G6PD-B isoenzymes (monoclonal). During pregnancy, some cells of uterus express G6PD-A, while rest cells with G6PD-B isoenzyme indicating polyclonal origin.

HUMAN ANDROGEN RECEPTOR GENE

Human androgen receptor gene is the most common marker used to determine monoclonal property of primary cancers by studying methylation patterns adjacent to high frequency polymorphisms in multiple populations.

MONOCLONAL PROPERTY IN MALIGNANCIES OF B CELL ORIGIN

Markers of monoclonal property in B cell malignancies are assessed by studying immunoglobulin molecules in serum and immunoglobulin chain rearrangement.

Immunoglobulin Chain Rearrangement

It denotes B cell maturation. Neoplastic proliferation of B cell results in production of large numbers of cells.

These cells share immunoglobulin gene rearrangement pattern denoting their common origin from a single cell. Because immunoglobulin heavy-chain rearrangement is limited to B cells, molecular diagnostic techniques demonstrate the B cell origin of a tumor.

MONOCLONAL PROPERTY IN MALIGNANCIES OF T CELL ORIGIN

Markers of monoclonal property in T cell malignancies are assessed by studying surface antigens (markers) on T cells and T cell receptor gene arrangement. Clonal property of lymphoid cell proliferation is shown in Table 6.10.

Surface Antigens (Markers)

These are demonstrated on mature T cells. These include CD4 antigen marking helper T cells, CD8 antigen marking suppressor T cell and cytotoxic T cells.

T Cell Receptor Gene Arrangement

It is analogous to immunoglobulin gene rearrangement. It is used to demonstrate both the T cell origin of a tumor and its monoclonal property.

SPECIFIC TRANSLOCATIONS

Specific translocations (8:14) are used to assess clonal property in certain neoplasm such as *Burkitt's lymphoma*.

TELOMERASE ACTIVITY

Telomerase enzyme adds repetitive sequences to maintain the length of the telomeres by preventing gene loss at the ends of chromosomes after multiple cell divisions. With each round of somatic cell replication, the telomere shortens.

The length of telomeres acts as a *molecular clock* and governs the lifespan of replicating germ cells. Somatic cells do not normally express telomerase. *Telomerase activity is increased in certain malignancies.* Activation of telomerase in malignancy does not lose genetic material after multiple cell divisions.

TUMOR ANGIOGENESIS

Angiogenesis denotes formation of new blood vessels. It is a requirement for the continued growth and survival of cancers, whether primary or metastatic. These vessels are essential for the inflow of nutrients and oxygen into the tumor. In the absence of new vessels, malignant tumors do not grow larger than 1 to 2 mm in diameter. Hypoxia is most important driving force for angiogenesis by inducing hypoxia inducible factor-α (HIF-α) transcriptional factor. It is a balancing act between angiogenic and antiangiogenic factors.

UPREGULATION OF ANGIOGENIC FACTORS

Malignant tumors and host inflammatory cells in the tumor synthesize angiogenic factors (e.g. **VEGF, FGF, TGF-β, angiotensin, platelet activating factor**). Vascular endothelial growth factor is important in the proliferation of blood vessels in a growing tumor. *New vessels in the tumor are torturous, irregular, leaky blood vessels*. Eventually, the tumor outgrows its blood supply, and areas of necrosis appear resulting in slower growth.

Table 6.10: Clonal property of lymphoid cell proliferation

Cell type	Benign lymphoid cells	Malignant lymphoid cells
B cells	Ig light chain heterogeneity	Ig kappa (κ) or lambda (λ) only
Plasma cells	Heterogeneous Ig electrophoresis	Monoclonal Ig spike
T cells	Heterogeneous variable regions	Homogeneous variable regions

DOWNREGULATION OF ANTIANGIOGENIC FACTORS

Various anti-angiogenic factors (**angiostatin, endostatin, vasculostatin,** and **thrombospondin 1**) are also synthesized. These may play an important role in controlling cancer.

TUMOR INVASION AND DISSEMINATION

Invasiveness and metastases are the most reliable feature that distinguishes invasive malignant tumors from benign tumors.

BENIGN TUMORS

Benign tumors most often remain localized to the site of origin. Benign tumors such as **atrial myxoma, uterine leiomyoma** and **pleomorphic adenoma** may *disseminate to distant sites*.

MALIGNANT TUMORS

Malignant tumors are locally invasive later metastasizing to distant organs. *All cancers can metastasize except CNS gliomas and skin basal cell carcinoma.* Basal cell carcinoma rarely disseminate to distant sites. Approximately 30% of newly diagnosed with solid tumors present with clinically evident metastases. Occult (hidden) metastases are seen in 20% of patients at the time of diagnosis. Approximately 30% of newly diagnosed solid tumors present with clinically evident metastases.

EPIDEMIOLOGY OF TUMORS

Many cancers are related to specific environmental and lifestyle factors that predispose a person to develop cancer. Some of these risk factors initiate carcinogenesis, other act as promoters, and some both initiate and promote the disease process.

INCIDENCE

Incidence of cancer varies from country to country and region to region. Many cancers are related to specific environmental and lifestyle factors that predispose a person to develop cancer.

Western Countries

In Western countries like USA and Europe, men are most often affected by cancers of prostate (33%), lung (14%), colorectal region (11%), urinary bladder (6%) and melanoma (4%). Western women develop cancers of breast (32%), lung (12%), colorectal region (11%) and ovaries (4%).

Indian Population

Indian men most often develop cancers of oral cavity, pharynx and lung. Indian women most often are affected by cancers of **cervix** and **breast**. Incidence of cervical cancer is declining due to early detection by exfoliative cytology stained by Papanicolaou stain. Incidence of oropharyngeal cancer is more prevalent in north India, while stomach cancer in south India.

AGE AND SEX DISTRIBUTION

Children younger than 15 years suffer from lethal cancers like *acute lymphoblastic leukemia, Burkitt's lymphoma, Wilms' tumor, cerebellar astrocytoma* of central nervous system, *retinoblastoma, neuroblastoma, yolk sac tumor of the testis, rhabdomyosarcoma and osteosarcoma*. Men develop cancers of prostate, kidney and lung. Women most often develop cancers of breast and cervix. Cancers in females and males are shown in Fig. 6.32.

GEOGRAPHICAL VARIABLES

The geographic variation results mostly from different environmental exposures. Penile cancer is very rare in Muslims and Jews, who undergo circumcision of prepuce. It may be probably smegma that acts as a solvent for environment carcinogens. Penile carcinoma is common in persons with poor hygiene, who suffer from balanitis. Geographical distribution of tumors is shown in Table 6.11.

OCCUPATIONAL CANCERS

Exposure to various occupational carcinogens, workers may develop cancers. Nickel exposure is associated with *cancer of nasal cavity and lungs in mine workers*. Arsenic exposure may cause *squamous cell carcinoma of skin, lung cancer, and liver angiosarcoma*. Heavy exposure to **asbestos** mineral dust may cause **mesothelioma** of the pleural and peritoneal cavities 20 to 40 years after exposure in 2 to 3% cases. There is increased risk for *adenocarcinoma of lung and gastrointestinal cancers*.

Beryllium exposure may cause *bronchogenic carcinoma*. Cadmium used in batteries and metal paintings is associated with prostatic carcinoma. Chromium used in paints, pigments and preservatives is associated with *lung cancer*.

RACIAL FACTORS

Dark skin complexion races have low incidence of melanoma. Persons with blood group A has high incidence of gastric carcinoma. Person with *xeroderma pigmentosum* is prone to squamous cell

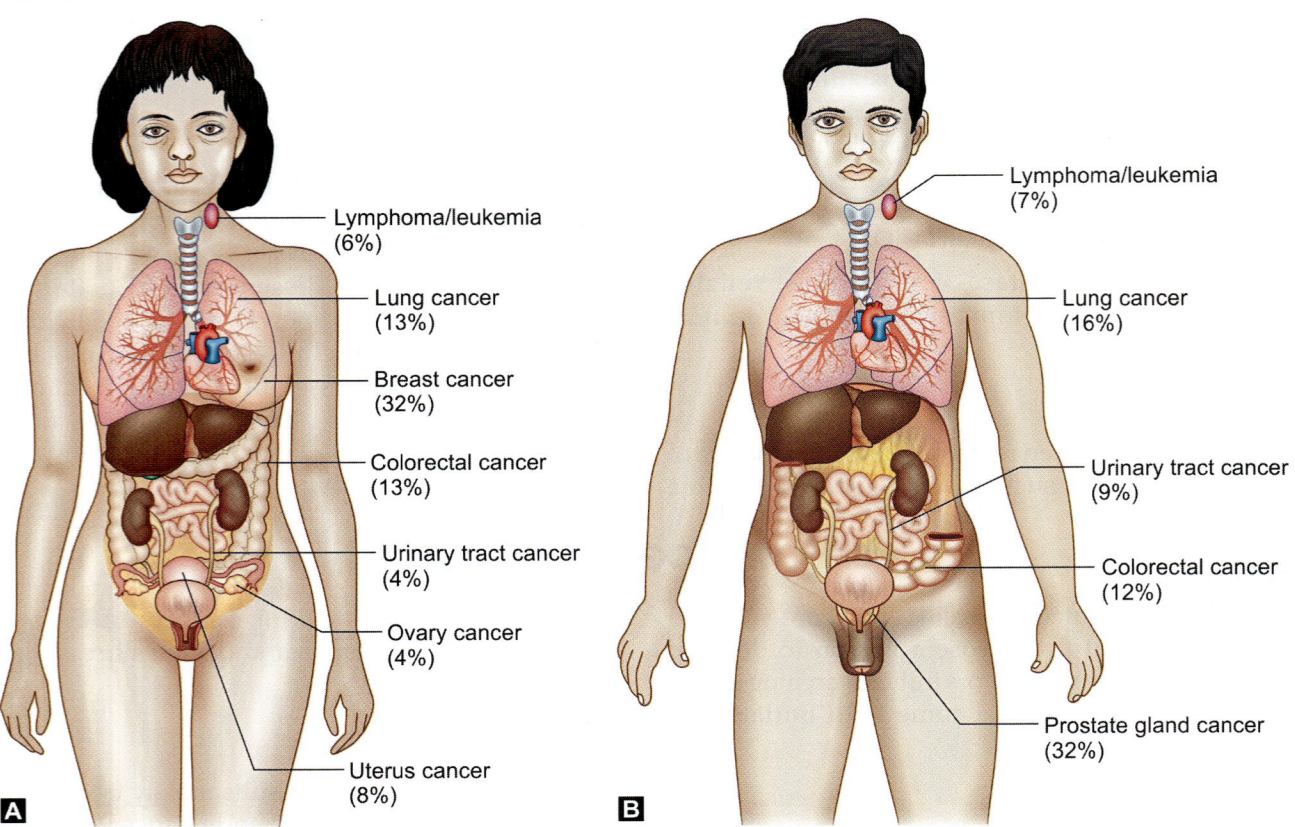

Fig. 6.32: Cancers in females and males. (A) Excluding skin tumors, seven tumors account for 80% cases of malignancy in females, (B) excluding skin tumors, five tumors account for 75% cases of malignancy in males.

Table 6.11: Geographical distribution of tumors

Cancers	Geographical distribution
Malignant melanoma	Worldwide
Oral cancer	Indian population due to consumption of oral betel nut and tobacco chewing France population due to consumption of cidar based liquors
Breast cancer	USA and Europe (incidence is low in Central Asia and Japan)
Gastric carcinoma	Japan due to consumption of smoked fish
Nasopharyngeal carcinoma	China due to Epstein-Barr virus
Hepatocellular carcinoma	African population
Burkitt's lymphoma	African population due to Epstein-Barr virus
Kaposi's sarcoma	African population due to human herpes 8 virus
Hepatocellular carcinoma	South East Asia due to hepatitis B virus and aflatoxin (produced by Aspergillus)
Skin cancer abdominal region	Kashmiri population carry a basket with burning charcoal (*Khangri*) held close to abdomen to keep them warm during winter season
Penile carcinoma	Hindu males due to smegma

carcinoma and basal cell carcinoma. Familial polyposis coli predisposes to colon carcinoma. Women with BRCA1 gene mutation have high risk of *breast carcinoma*.

GENETIC FACTORS

Genotype of an individual plays a role in determining susceptibility to malignant disease as a result of chromosomally determined syndromes or single gene abnormalities. Three chromosomal disorders prone to develop cancers. *Down's syndrome is prone to develop acute lymphoblastic or myeloblastic leukemia.* There is increased risk of breast cancer in males in case of *Klinefelter's syndrome*. Gonadal dysgenesis with male genotype is more likely to develop tumors of gonads.

Person with *xeroderma pigmentosum* is prone to squamous cell carcinoma and basal cell carcinoma. *Familial polyposis coli predisposes to colon carcinoma.* Women with BRCA1 *gene mutation have high risk of breast carcinoma.*

ALCOHOL AND TOBACCO PRODUCTS

Alcohol consumption is commonly associated with cirrhosis of liver, a precursor of *hepatocellular carcinoma*. The risk of breast and colorectal cancers also increases with alcohol consumption. Heavy use of *alcohol and cigarette smoking* synergistically increase the incidence of cancers of the mouth, larynx, pharynx, and esophagus. It is likely that alcohol acts as a solvent for the carcinogenic substances in smoke, thus enhancing their absorption.

Cigarette smoke comprises neutral and acidic fractions. Neutral fraction contains polycyclic hydrocarbons, which bind to nuclear DNA and exert mutagenic effect. Acidic fraction of smoke contains a number of tumor promoting agents. Tobacco smoking increases risk of lung cancer.

ATMOSPHERIC POLLUTANTS

Many outdoor air pollutants such as arsenic, benzene, hydrocarbons, polyvinyl chlorides, and other industrial emissions as well as vehicle exhaust have carcinogenic properties. *Chloromethyl ether is a potent carcinogen causing small cell lung carcinoma.* Combustion of coal and other fossils releases polycyclic aromatic hydrocarbons (benzopyrene) increase risk of lung cancer. Workers involved in the production of dyes, rubber and paint. β-naphthylamine exposure increases risk of urinary bladder carcinoma.

RADIATION

Atom Bomb Explosion

Ionization radiation may cause lung cancer. Japanese are at increased risk of lung cancers (squamous cell carcinoma, adenocarcinoma and small cell carcinoma) after atom bomb explosion in Hiroshima and Nagasaki.

Ultraviolet Radiation

Exposure to ultraviolet radiation, or sunlight, causes genetic mutation in p53 control gene. Ultraviolet sunlight is a direct cause of basal cell carcinoma and squamous cell carcinoma of skin.

Ionizing Radiation

Ionizing radiation (such as prolonged exposure to X-rays) is associated with *acute leukemia, cancers of thyroid, breast, stomach, colon, urinary tract, and multiple myeloma*. Low doses of X-ray radiation can cause DNA mutations and chromosomal abnormalities.

DIETARY FACTORS

Numerous aspects of diet are linked to development of cancer due to high consumption of smoked foods and salted fish or meats and foods containing nitrites. Aflatoxin-β synthesized by *Aspergillus flavus* in stored food grains increases risk of development of hepatocellular carcinoma.

SEXUAL FACTORS

The age of first intercourse and the number of sexual partners are positively correlated with a woman's risk of cervical cancer. Further, there is increased risk of *cervical cancer* in a woman who has had *multiple sexual partners*. The suspected underlying mechanism here involves transmission of *human papillomavirus* (HPV).

HORMONES

Steroid hormones, i.e. estrogen, progesterone, and testosterone have been implicated as promoters of *breast, endometrial, ovarian, or prostatic cancer*. Researchers believe that the hormone sensitizes the cell to the initial precipitating factor, thus promoting carcinogenesis. Breast cancer is more common in women than men, probably due to the greater mammary epithelial volume and to the promoting effects of circulating estrogens.

CELL CYCLE AND CANCER

During cell cycle, series of events that take place in a cell leading to its division and duplication of its DNA to produce two daughter cells. In cell cycle, there are two resting phases (G_1 and G_2) and two active phases (S and M). Cell growth regulated by an internal timer known as *cell cycle*. G_0 phase is the resting phase of stable parenchymal cells. Quiescent cells that have not entered the cell cycle are in the G_0 state.

PHASES OF CELL CYCLE

Cell cycle is divided into four phases: G_1, S, G_2 and M are shown in Fig. 6.33.

G_1 Phase (Pre-synthetic Phase)

G_1 phase (pre-synthetic phase) is characterized by cell growth as a result of synthesis of RNA, protein,

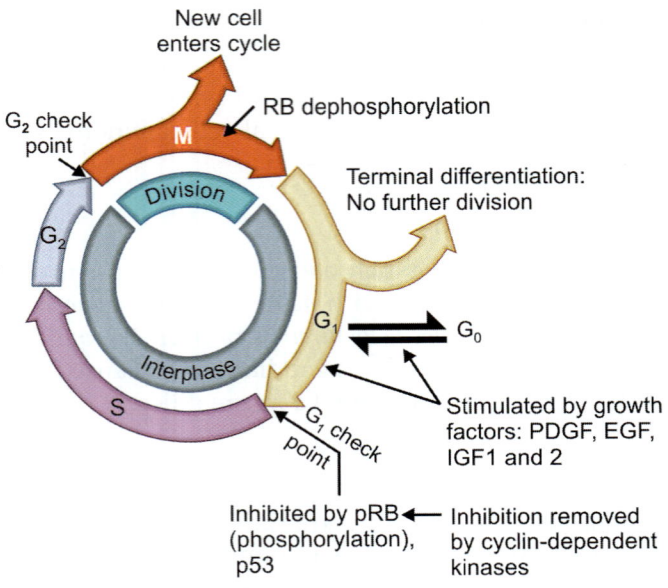

Fig. 6.33: Phases of cell cycle.

organelles and cyclin D. It is the restriction point in which cell enters from G_1 phase to S phase (synthetic phase). The main difference between slowly and rapidly dividing cells is the length of the G_1 phase of cell cycle.

S Phase (Synthetic Phase)

S phase (synthetic phase) is characterized by synthesis of DNA along with RNA, and protein. Labile cells undergo mitosis throughout life. Doubling of DNA occurs in this phase.

G_2 Phase (Pre-mitotic Phase)

After completion of nuclear DNA duplication, cell enters G_2 phase. It is characterized by synthesis of tubulin, which is necessary for formation of mitotic spindle essential for cell division.

M Phase (Mitotic Phase)

M phase describes the interval between the onset of prophase and conclusion of telophase. Two daughter cells are produced in this phase. Division of nucleus is followed by division of cytoplasm resulting in formation of two new daughter cells.

REGULATION OF CELL CYCLE

Growth factors bind to surface receptors on the cell; transmembrane proteins relay information to the cell by signal transduction. Growth factors stimulate cell division. Growth-inhibiting factors inhibit cell division. Normal cells divide only when growth factor and growth-inhibiting factor balance favor cell division. Cancer cells divide without constraint.

Cancer is primarily caused by mutations in growth factor genes and growth factor inhibiting genes, and pathways that inhibit the normal sequence of events associated with apoptosis.

Regulation of the G_1, Checkpoint (G_1 to S) Phase

Regulation of the G_1, checkpoint (G_1 to S) phase is the most critical phase of the cycle. It is controlled by cyclin D and cyclin-dependent kinase 4 (CDK4). Growth factors activate nuclear transcribing proto-oncogenes to produce cyclin D and CDK4. Regulation of cell cycle showing role of cyclins, CDKs, and cyclin-dependent kinase inhibitors is shown in Fig. 6.34.

Binding of Cyclin D to CDK4

Cyclin D binds to CDK4 to form a complex, that causes the cell to enter the S phase by phosphorylation of RB proteins. RB proteins normally arrest the cell in the G_1 phase. CDK4 phosphorylates the RB protein causing the cell to enter the S phase.

TP53 Suppressor Gene

TP53 arrests the cell in G phase by inhibiting CDK4. It prevents RB protein phosphorylation. It may provide time for repair of DNA in the cell.

BAX Apoptotic Gene

When there is excessive DNA damage, BAX gene is activated. *BAX gene inhibits BCL-2 antiapoptotic gene causing release of cytochrome c from the mitochondria and apoptosis of the cell.*

CHECKPOINTS OF CELL CYCLE

Internal controls of cell cycle for DNA repair requires two checkpoints: G_1/S and G_2/M.

G_1/S Checkpoint

G_1/S checkpoint is used for DNA repair after its damage before replication. Failure of DNA leads to either apoptosis or accumulation of mutations responsible for neoplastic transformation. Defect in G_1/S checkpoint is the most important cause of cancers.

G_2/M Checkpoint

G_2/M checkpoint is used for DNA repair after replication. It monitors completion of DNA replication. It also checks cell division (mitosis) into twoseparate chromatids. It is most important checkpoint in cells exposed to ionizing radiation. Chromosomal abnormality occurs due to defects in this checkpoint.

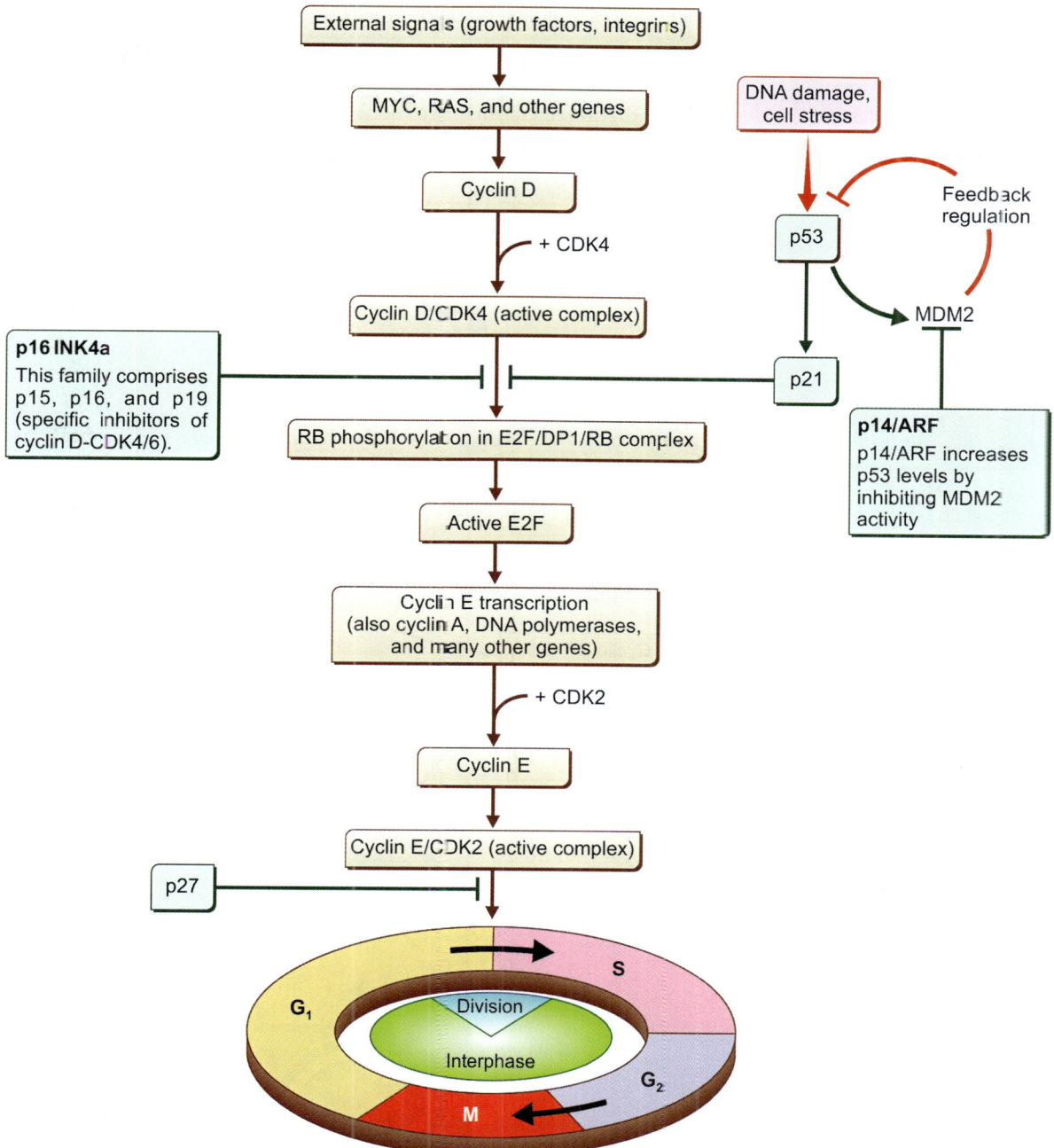

Fig. 6.34: Regulation of cell cycle showing role of cyclins, CDKs, and cyclin-dependent kinase inhibitors. MYC and RAS genes synthesize and stabilize cyclin D leading to formation of cyclin D/CDK active complex. This complex phosphorylates RB located in the E2F/DP1/RB complex in the nucleus. The cell cycle can be blocked by the Cip/Kip inhibitors p21 and p27 and the NK4A/ARF inhibitors p16INK4a.

CELL CYCLE CHECKPOINT COMPONENTS

RB Tumor Suppressor Gene

RB gene is caretaker tumor suppressor gene also known as *Governor of cell cycle*. It was mapped to the long arm of chromosome 13q14. It codes for RB protein, master brake on cell cycle. It inhibits G_1 to S phase by inhibiting nuclear transcription factor. RB protein binds E2F transcription resulting in its hypophosphorylation. It prevents G_1/S transition.

When the Rb gene is phosphorylated, cell division takes place passing through G_1/S transition role of RB as a cell-cycle regulator is shown in Table 6.12 and Fig. 6.35.

Table 6.12: Role of RB gene in cell cycle regulation and its mutation associated with cancers

Gene and locus	Protein	Function	Familial tumors due to gene mutation	Sporadic cancers due to gene mutation
RB gene (locus 13p14)	Retinoblastoma protein	It codes for pRB protein, master brake on cell cycle. It inhibits G_1 to S transition during cell cycle. It inhibits nuclear transcription factor	Retinoblastoma, osteosarcoma	Retinoblastoma, osteosarcoma, cancers of breast, colon, prostate, bladder and lung

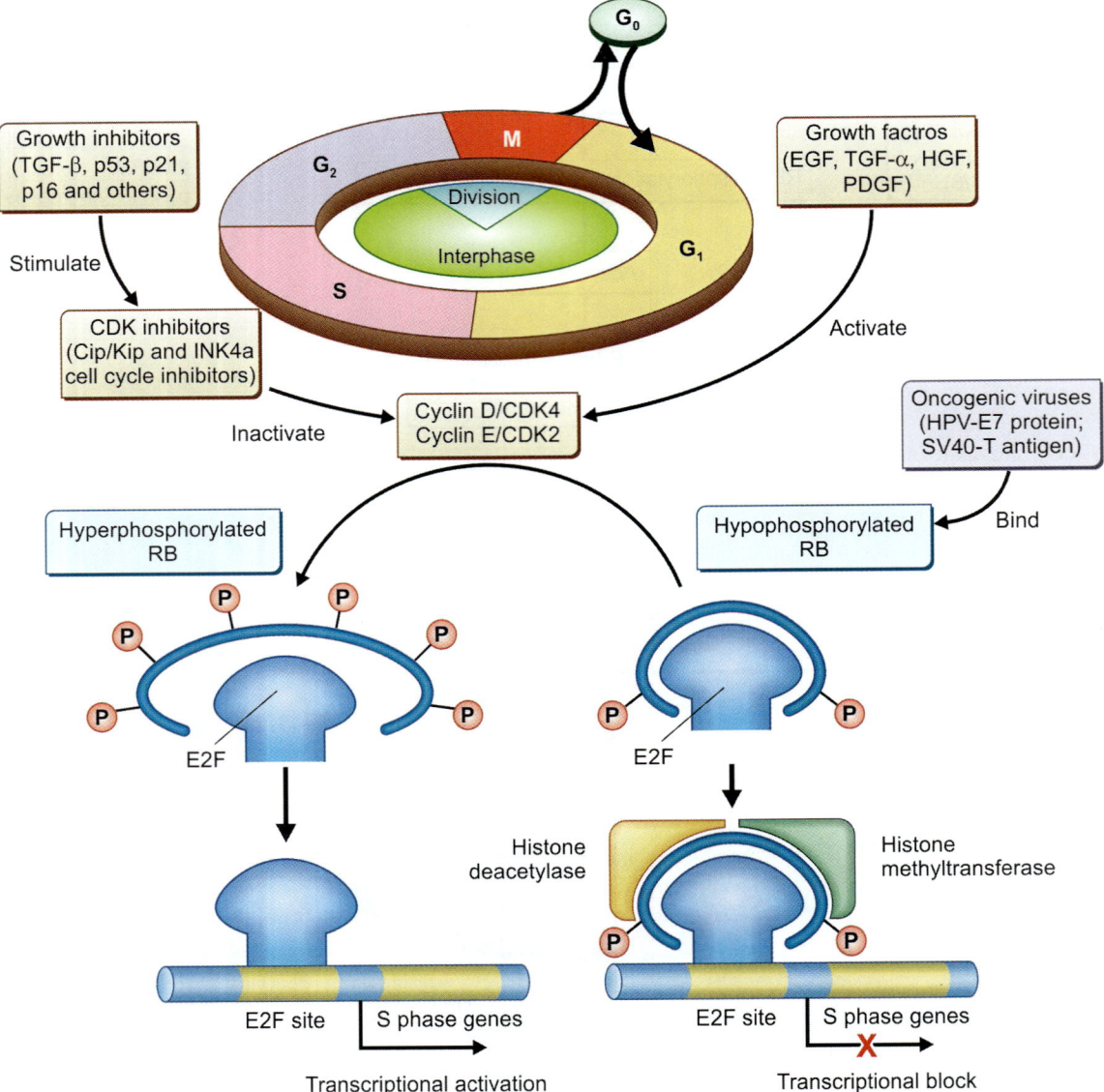

Fig. 6.35: Role of RB as a cell-cycle regulator. Various growth factors promote the formation of the cyclin D-CDK4 complex. This complex transforms active hyperphosphorylated RB to hypophosphorylated inactive state. RB inactivation allows the cell to pass the G_1/S restriction point. Virtually all cancers show dysregulation of the cell cycle.

TP53 Tumor Suppressor Gene

TP53 tumor suppressor gene located on chromosome 17p is known as *guardian of the genome* or molecular policeman. Its gene product p53 prevents G_1/S transition by acting through p21. It also causes apoptosis by inducing the transcription of pro-apoptotic BAX gene. Levels of p53 are negatively regulated by MDM2 through a feedback loop.

p53 gene mutation has been demonstrated in familial and sporadic in more than 50% of human cancers (Table 6.13).

Table 6.13: Role of TP53 in regulation of cell cycle

Gene and locus	Protein	Function	Familial tumors due to gene mutation	Sporadic cancers due to gene mutation
Genomic stability enabler (most important)				
TP53 (locus 17p13.1)	p53	Inhibits cell cycle G_1 to S phase. It repairs DNA. It induces cell suicide (apoptosis) by activating BAX gene	Li-Fraumeni syndrome (cancers of breast and adrenal cortex, sarcoma, leukemia, brain tumors)	>50% of human cancers

CELL CYCLE INHIBITORS

Cell cycle inhibitors are also known as *CDK inhibitors*. These inhibit the activity of cyclin-CDK complexes. There are two classes of cycle cell inhibitors.

Cip/Kip (Cip/WAF Family)

This family comprises p21, p27 and p57. These inhibit all CDKs. p21 is induced by p53 tumor suppressor gene. p27 is induced by TGF-β.

INK4a/ARF Family

This family comprises p16INK4a and p14ARF. P16INK4a comprises p15, p16, p18 and p19.

These specifically inhibit cyclin D-CDK4/6 complex. The p14ARF increases level of p53 tumor suppressor gene by inhibiting MDM2 activity.

GENETIC PREPOSITION OF CANCER

OVERVIEW

Most cancers are sporadic (90%), but some individuals inherit an increased risk of developing certain tumors (10%). Heredity cancers may be autosomal dominant linked to mutation of tumor suppressor gene or autosomal recessive associated with inherited defects in DNA repair. These are transmitted from parents to offspring through defects in the DNA of the egg or sperm cells. These are caused due to loss of a segment of DNA or a change in the coding sequence of DNA. In many cases, there are abnormalities in tumor suppressor genes. Three syndromes associated with malignancy have been described.

Down's syndrome: Down's syndrome is most common chromosomal disorder and major cause for mental retardation. Patient with Down's syndrome is prone to develop *acute lymphoblastic or myeloblastic leukemia.*

Klinefelter's syndrome: Klinefelter's syndrome is related to the presence of one or more X chromosomes in excess of the normal male XY complement (classic pattern 47, XXY karyotype). The disorder is always manifested by a male phenotype. The disorder is a frequent cause of male infertility. There is increased risk of development of *male breast cancer.*

Gonadal dysgenesis: Gonadal dysgenesis with male genotype is more likely to develop tumors of gonads.

Genetic Screening

Extensive history of screening of early development of these cancers is required in the management of these patients. Detection of inherited cancer-causing gene is done by testing the blood cells of family members (inherited changes can be detected in all tissues of the body, in addition to malignant cells).

Examples of Inherited Cancers

These include *retinoblastoma, familial polyposis coli (causing colon carcinoma), breast cancer, Wilms' tumor or renal cell carcinoma.* These inherited cancer syndromes fall into two categories: autosomal dominant and autosomal recessive. Heritable neoplasia syndrome is shown in Table 6.14.

AUTOSOMAL DOMINANT CANCER SYNDROME

Retinoblastoma

Retinoblastoma is a malignant tumor of eye in children. In 40% of cases are inherited. Point mutation inactivates RB tumor suppressor gene on chromosome 3. One gene is inactivated in germ cells, remaining gene is inactivated after birth (*two-hit theory*). These patients also develop *osteosarcoma in adolescence.*

Li-Fraumeni Syndrome

Germline mutations of TP53 tumor suppressor gene cause **Li-Fraumeni syndrome**. Patients may develop multiple cancers such as *breast carcinoma, leukemia, sarcoma, brain tumors, adrenal tumors, laryngeal and lung cancer.*

Cowden Disease

PTEN gene is located on chromosome 10q. Phosphatase and tensin homologue are proteins of PTEN gene. Normally, PTEN gene products inhibit AKT/PI3K

Table 6.14: Heritable neoplasia syndrome

Syndrome	Neoplasia	Genetic defect
MEN syndromes	Multiple tumors in endocrine glands	Mutations on chromosomes 10 and 11
Familial adenomatous polyposis coli	Adenoma and adenocarcinoma of the colon	APC tumor suppressor gene mutation
Li-Fraumeni syndrome	Breast carcinoma, leukemia, sarcoma, brain tumors, adrenal tumors, laryngeal and lung cancer	p53 tumor suppressor gene mutation
Cowden disease	Colon carcinoma	PTEN gene mutation
Xeroderma pigmentosum	Squamous cell carcinoma or basal cell carcinoma	Abnormal DNA repair
Familial retinoblastoma	Malignant tumor of the retina	Absence of Rb tumor suppressor gene
Neurofibromatosis type I	Benign and malignant tumors of peripheral nerves	Abnormal NF1 tumor suppressor gene
Hereditary nonpolyposis colon carcinoma (HNPCC)	Colon carcinoma (may develop cancers of endometrium, urothelium, brain, stomach, and ovaries) occurs in Lynch syndrome	Inactivation of DNA mismatch repair genes (principally MLH1, MSH2, MSH6, and PMS2)

signaling pathway. *PTEN gene mutation* leads to Cowden disease characterized by *fibroadenomas, fibrocystic lesions, ductal epithelial hyperplasia*, and *nipple malformations*. There is increased risk of breast cancer in Cowden disease.

Familial Adenomatous Polyposis Coli

Familial adenomatous polyposis coli occurs due to inactivation of APC tumor suppressor *gene located on long arm of chromosome 5*. It is characterized by multiple polyps in the large intestine, which appears between 10 and 20 years of age. Patient develops colorectal carcinoma as a result of malignant transformation of polyps. By the 40 years, all the patients develop adenocarcinoma, hence need *prophylactic total colectomy*. Gross morphology of familial polyposis coli is shown in Fig. 6.36.

Hereditary Nonpolyposis Colon Cancer

HNPCC (Lynch syndrome) occurs due to inactivation of DNA mismatch repair genes (principally MLH1, MSH2, MSH6, and PMS2), that cannot correct errors in nucleotide pairing. Characteristic finding is alteration in microsatellite nucleotide sequences. Normally, this alteration is absent in normal cells. It predisposes to mutations in other genes more directly related to transformation. There is increased risk of development of cancers in **Lynch syndrome** as described under.

- *Right colon carcinoma:* It is most often preceded by *serrated adenomas*, rather than tubular adenomas seen in the traditional APC tumor pathway.
- *Endometrial carcinoma:* It may be the *first additional malignancy* in these patients.
- *Other cancers:* These patients may develop cancers of urothelium, brain, stomach, and ovaries.
- *Muir Torre syndrome:* A variant that involves a propensity for *sebaceous tumors* of the skin is known as *Muir Torre syndrome*.

BRCA1 and BRCA2 Mutations

Physiological state: Under physiological state, BRCA1 is a tumor suppressor gene located on chromosome 17p21. BRCA2 is also tumor suppressor gene located on chromosome 13q12–13. Both BRCA1 and BRCA2 regulate DNA repair by binding to RAD51, a molecule that mediates repair of double-stranded DNA. These genes encode tumor suppressor proteins involved in checkpoint functions related to progression of the cell cycle into S phase. Gene mutation occurs by methylation.

Pathological state: BRCA1 is responsible for 52% familial breast cancers and 1–2% of all breast cancers. BRCA2 gene mutation is responsible for 32% familial breast cancers and up to 2% of all breast cancers. Risk is increased in age group by 70 years in 30–90% cases. BRAC2 gene mutation is rare in sporadic cases.

- *Familial tumors:* BRCA1 gene mutation may occur in cancers of ovary, male breast, prostate, pancreas

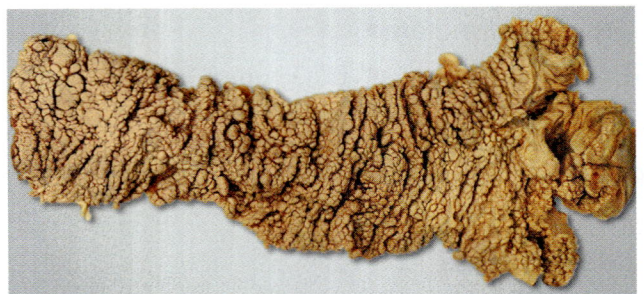

Fig. 6.36: Familial adenomatous coli showing multiple polyps covering virtually the whole of the mucosal surface of the colon >100 tubular adenoma polyps (ranging 500 to 2500).

and fallopian tube; but lower than BRCA2. BRCA2 gene mutation is also demonstrated in *carcinomas of stomach, gallbladder, bile duct, pharynx and melanoma*.
- *Sporadic tumors:* BRCA1 and BRCA2 are rarely demonstrated in *sporadic breast cancers (e.g. medullary carcinoma and metaplastic carcinoma)*.

MEN 1 Tumor Suppressor Gene

Normal MEN 1 protein (menin) regulates transcriptional factor.
- *Familial tumors:* MEN 1 gene mutation results in multiple neoplasia syndrome 1 (MEN 1) characterized by tumors of *pituitary, parathyroid and pancreas)*.
- *Sporadic tumors:* MEN 1 gene mutation has been demonstrated in tumors of *pituitary, parathyroid and pancreas*.

AUTOSOMAL RECESSIVE CANCER SYNDROMES WITH DNA REPAIR DEFECTS

Autosomal recessive cancer syndrome predisposes to DNA instability when exposed to environmental carcinogens.

Xeroderma Pigmentosum

This autosomal recessive disorder is characterized by hypersensitivity to ultraviolet light. There is increased incidence of skin cancers such as *squamous cell carcinoma, basal cell carcinoma and melanoma*. These ultraviolet rays cross-link adjacent pyrimidine dimers and damage DNA. Due to defects in genes function in nucleotide excision repair, UV rays induced pyrimidine (often thymine) dimers neither are removed nor repaired. This condition is more frequently encountered in North Africans. Protection from sunlight, either by suitable clothing or by barrier creams against ultraviolet light may reduce the risk of tumor development.

Chromosome Instability Syndrome

The chromosomes are susceptible to damage by ionizing radiation and drugs. Other syndromes such as *Fanconi syndrome, ataxia-telangiectasia and Bloom syndrome* have increased risk of development of leukemia, lymphoma.

Inherited Ataxia-telangiectasia

Physiological state: ATM gene is a caretaker tumor suppressor gene located on chromosome 11p22. It downregulates tyrosine kinase activity. Patients with *ATM gene mutation* have reduced capacity to repair DNA breaks leading to accumulation of numerous genetic mutations overtime. Patient develops inherited ataxia-telangiectasia characterized by **cerebral ataxia, immunodeficiency** and **dilation of small blood vessels**. There is increased risk of breast carcinoma, gastric carcinoma, leukemia and lymphoma.

ACQUIRED PRENEOPLASTIC LESIONS

Nonhereditary predisposing lesions may lead to development of cancers. There are many acquired clinical conditions, which may undergo malignant transformation in some cases. It occurs due to excessive proliferation of cells and chronic inflammation.

PROLIFERATION OF CELLS

Proliferating cells in regenerating cirrhotic nodules, hyperplasia, metaplasia and dysplasia (CIN III) lead to accumulation of genetic mutations essential for carcinogenesis.

Metaplastic and hyperplastic cells become dysplastic before progressing to cancer. Examples of acquired premalignant lesions and conditions associated with cancers are shown in Table 6.15. Comparison among metaplasia, dysplasia and anaplasia is shown in Table 6.16.

Persistent Regenerative Cell Replication

Squamous cell carcinoma in the margins of a chronic skin fistula or in a long-unhealed skin wound; hepatocellular carcinoma in cirrhosis of liver occurs due to persistent regeneration of cells.

Hyperplastic Proliferations

Atypical epithelial hyperplasia may transform to carcinoma especially in breast and endometrium.

Dysplastic Proliferations

Bronchogenic carcinoma develops in the dysplastic bronchial mucosa of habitual cigarette smokers

Squamous dysplasia of oropharynx, larynx, and uterine cervix may undergo squamous cell carcinoma. Patients with dysplastic nevus may develop malignant melanoma

Glandular Metaplasia

Patients suffering from *Barrett's esophagus* (glandular metaplasia) may develop adenocarcinoma. *Helicobacter pylori* induced gastric glandular metaplasia results in gastric adenocarcinoma.

CHRONIC INFLAMMATORY STATE

Chronic inflammation plays an important role in the pathogenesis of cancer. Synthesis of oxygen derived

Table 6.15: Examples of acquired premalignant lesions and conditions

Organ	Precursor lesion	Cancer
Skin	Acinic (solar) keratosis	Squamous cell carcinoma
	Chronic irritation at sinus orifice	Squamous cell carcinoma
	Third degree burns	Squamous cell carcinoma
	Dysplastic nevus	Malignant melanoma
	Xeroderma pigmentosum	Squamous cell carcinoma
		Basal cell carcinoma
Gastrointestinal tract	Leukoplakia oral cavity (ingestion of tobacco products)	Squamous cell carcinoma
	Dysplasia of oropharynx	Squamous cell carcinoma
	Barrett's esophagus (glandular metaplasia of esophagus)	Adenocarcinoma
	Helicobacter pylori induced chronic atrophic gastritis	Adenocarcinoma, MALT (mucosa associated lymphoid tissue) lymphoma and carcinoid tumors
	Ulcerative colitis	Adenocarcinoma of colon and bile duct
	Villous and tubulovillous adenoma	Malignant transformation
Liver	Regenerative nodule	Hepatocellular carcinoma
	Hepatic cirrhosis	Hepatocellular carcinoma
Respiratory system	Squamous dysplasia of larynx and bronchi	Squamous cell carcinoma
Female genital system	Vaginal adenosis in daughter (diethylstilbestrol during intrauterine life)	Adenocarcinoma (in the daughter)
	Cervical intraepithelial neoplasia (CIN III)	Cervical carcinoma
	Endometrial hyperplasia	Adenocarcinoma
	Hydatidiform mole	Choriocarcinoma
Breast	Mammary ductal atypical hyperplasia	Adenocarcinoma
Blood	Myelodysplastic syndrome	Acute leukemia

Metaplastic and hyperplastic cells become dysplastic before progressing to cancer.

Table 6.16: Comparison among metaplasia, dysplasia and anaplasia

Parameters	Metaplasia	Dysplasia	Anaplasia (cancer)
Definition	The transformation of one mature cell to another mature cell type in response to persistent injury	Alteration in the size, shape and organization of cells due to chronic irritation or inflammation may progress to a neoplasm or revert to normal if the stress is removed	Malignant transformation of cells (autonomous, continue to proliferate even after removal of initiator)
Examples	Squamous metaplasia in bronchi due to smoking	Cervical intraepithelial neoplasia (CIN I, CIN II, CIN III)	Carcinomas and sarcomas
Reversibility	Reversible phenomenon	Reversible in early lesion (CIN I, CIN II)	Irreversible phenomenon
Cell polarity	Normal	Lost	Lost
Nucleus to cytoplasmic ratio	Normal (1:4)	Increased	Markedly increased
Pleomorphism	Absent	Low grade	High grade

free radicals cause genomic instability. Synthesis of cytokines and growth factors participate in proliferation and survival of cells.

Pool of stem cells is adversely affected by mutagens. Chronic inflammatory states associated with cancer are shown in Table 6.17.

Table 6.17: Chronic inflammatory states associated with cancer

Pathological condition	Associated cancers
Asbestosis	Mesothelioma and lung carcinoma
Inflammatory bowel disease (ulcerative colitis/Crohn's disease)	Colorectal cancer
Lichen sclerosis	Vulvar squamous cell carcinoma
Pancreatitis (chronic alcoholism and germline trypsinogen gene mutation)	Pancreatic carcinoma
Chronic cholecystitis with cholelithiasis	Gallbladder carcinoma
Autoimmune diseases (Sjögren syndrome and Hashimoto's thyroiditis)	MALT lymphoma
Reflux esophagitis (Barrett's esophagus)	Esophageal adenocarcinoma
Opsithorchis cholangitis	Cholangiocarcinoma and colon carcinoma
Helicobacter pylori induced gastritis/ulcers	Gastric adenocarcinoma and MALT lymphoma
Hepatitis (HBV, HCV)	Hepatocellular carcinoma
Chronic osteomyelitis (bacterial)	Carcinoma in draining sinuses
Chronic cervicitis (human papillomavirus)	Cervical carcinoma
Chronic cystitis (Schistosomiasis)	Urinary bladder carcinoma

MOLECULAR BASIS OF CANCER: ROLE OF GENETIC AND EPIGENETIC ALTERATIONS

CELLULAR HALLMARKS OF CANCER

Neoplastic cells are relatively or absolutely autonomous, excessive, disorganized. These are unresponsive to extracellular growth factors and regulatory mechanisms operating inside normal tissues. *Malignant cells proliferate, invade tissues and disseminate to distant organs.* These synthesize growth and angiogenic factors and have ability to escape immune surveillance resulting in clinical cancers.

Causes of Neoplasia

Neoplasia is caused by environmental agents and heredity factors. Environmental causes include chemicals, radiation (ultraviolet light, X-rays, and γ-radiation), oncogenic viruses (DNA and RNA viruses) and microbes, parasites and physical agents.

Hallmarks of Cancer

Hallmarks of cancer include sustained proliferating signaling (oncogenes), insensitivity to growth inhibitory signals (tumor suppressor genes), growth promoting metabolic alterations (Warburg effects), evasion of apoptosis, limitless replicative potential (immortality), induction of angiogenesis, escape from host immune system, tumor promoting inflammation, dysregulation of cancer associated genes and epigenetic changes (Table 6.18).

Table 6.18: Hallmarks of cancer

Changes	Mechanism
Self-sufficiency in growth signals	Sustained proliferation of cancer cells as a consequence of oncogene activation without external stimuli
Insensitivity to growth inhibitory signals	Cancer cells insensitive to inhibitory signal due to mutated tumor suppressor genes
Altered cellular metabolism (Warburg effect)	Cancer cells undergoing metabolic switch to aerobic glycolysis (known as *Warburg effect*) needed to synthesize cellular DNA, RNA and proteins for rapid cell growth
Evasion of apoptosis	Cancer cells resistant to programmed cell death
Limitless replicative potential (immortality)	Tumor cells with stem cell like properties possessing unrestrictive proliferative capacity by avoiding senescence
Sustained angiogenesis	Malignant tumors forming new blood vessels for receiving nutrients and oxygen and removal of waste products
Ability to invade and metastasize	Cancer cells invading and metastasizing to distant organs
Ability to escape from host immune system	Cancer cells exhibiting alterations permitting them to escape from host immune system
Dysregulation of cancer associated genes and epigenetic changes	Dysregulation of cancer associated genes and epigenetic changes responsible for malignancy

Role of Oncogenes and Tumor Suppressor Genes

Abnormal expression of oncogenes drive normal cells towards the neoplastic state by dysregulation of cell cycle control or suppression of apoptosis. Loss of tumor suppressor gene enables transformation of normal cells to neoplastic cell by reducing inhibition mechanisms and permitting mutations. These two events simultaneously work together (Fig. 6.37).

Molecular Carcinogenesis

In the molecular carcinogenesis, nonlethal damage to cells occurs due to spontaneous mutations in somatic cells or germ cells. Neoplasms are monoclonal. Polyclonal proliferations are always non-neoplastic. Single genetically damaged progenitor cell (clonal progeny) resulting in tumor is known as *monoclonality*. Genetic damage occurs by regulatory proteins such as growth promoting proto-oncogenes, growth inhibiting tumor suppressor genes, genes regulating apoptosis and DNA repair.

Defective DNA repair predisposing to cancer. In molecular carcinogenesis gene inherited/acquired mutations transform normal cell to cancer cell by

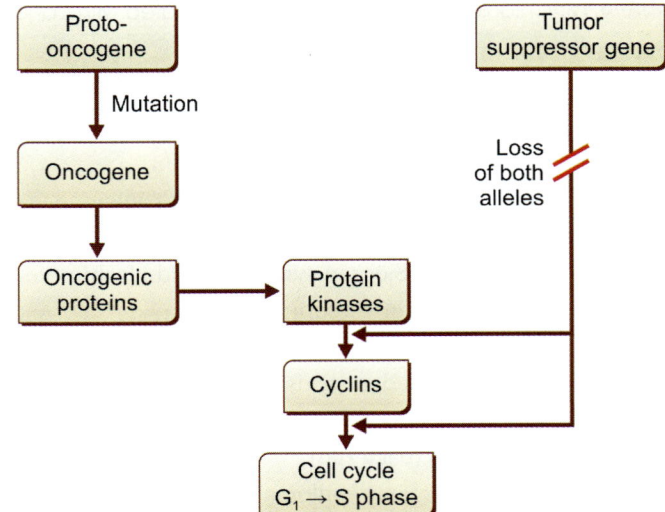

Fig. 6.37: Neoplasia can either results from mutations that turn on the oncogenes or loss of alleles of tumor suppressor genes.

uncontrolled monoclonal proliferation and decreased apoptosis. Tumor progression occurs by additional gene mutations, angiogenesis and escape from host immune response. Cancer cells invade and metastasize to distant organs (Figs 6.38 and 6.39).

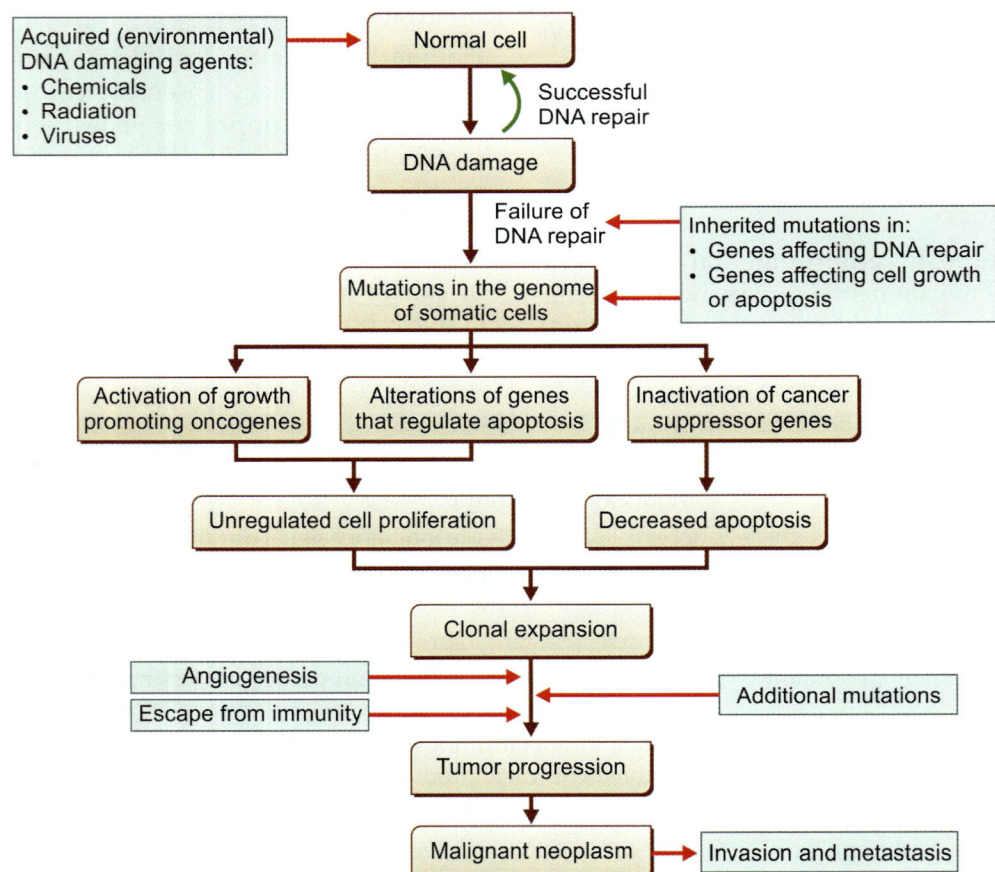

Fig. 6.38: Molecular carcinogenesis shows gene inherited/acquired mutations transforming normal cell to cancer cell by uncontrolled monoclonal proliferation and decreased apoptosis. Tumor progression occurs by additional gene mutations, angiogenesis, escape from host immune response. Cancer cells invade and metastasize to distant organs.

Neoplasia: Molecular Basis, Metastasis, Clinical Oncology and Laboratory Diagnosis

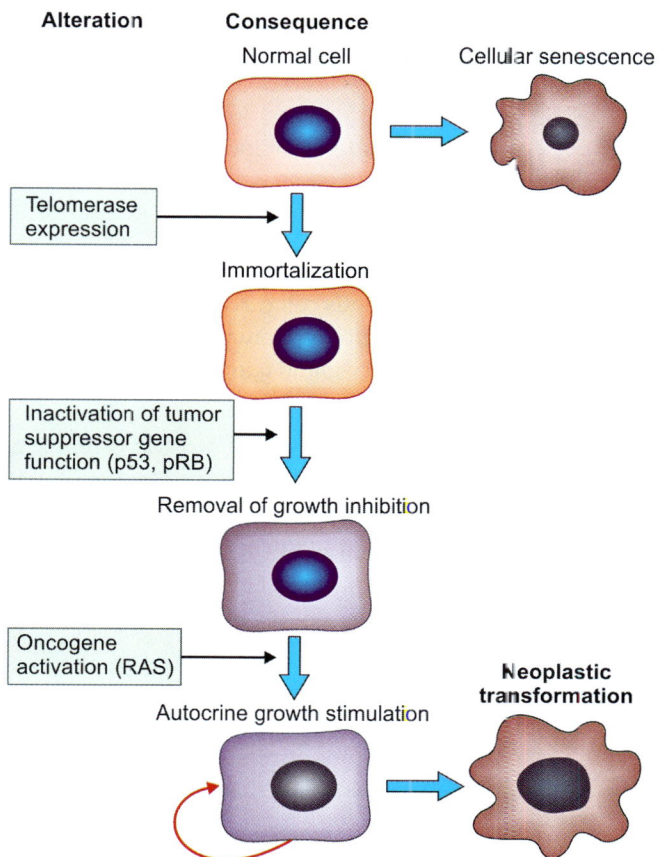

Fig. 6.39: Molecular carcinogenesis showing transformation of normal cell to cancer cells by telomerase expression, inactivation of tumor suppressor genes, oncogenes.

Driver and Passenger Mutations

Carcinogenesis is a multistep process. It results from accumulation of successive mutation of genes. Mutations that contribute to the development of malignant phenotype are known as *driver mutations*. Mutations that have no phenotype consequences are known as *passenger mutations*. In addition to DNA mutations, epigenetic aberrations also contribute to the malignant transformation of cells.

SELF-SUFFICIENCY IN GROWTH SIGNAL

Proto-oncogenes are normal cellular genes whose products promote cell proliferation in controlled manner. These participate in cell proliferation and differentiation. Examples of proto-oncogenes are *growth factors, growth factor receptors, signal transduction proteins, nuclear transcriptional factor and cyclin-dependent kinases (CDKs)*. Mutations transform proto-oncogenes to tumor producing oncogenes.

Carcinogenesis

The cancer cells continue to proliferate in the absence of external stimuli. Neoplasia occurs due to activation of proto-oncogene or inactivation/deletion of tumor suppressor gene. **Mutation in single gene is not sufficient to cause cancer.** Accumulation of mutation of multiple genes (e.g. *growth factors, growth factor receptors, signal transduction, and transcription*) results in cancer.

ONCOGENES AND ONCOPROTEINS

Major classes of oncogenes comprise growth factors, receptors for growth factors, signal transducing proteins, transcription factors (nuclear regulatory proteins), cyclins and cyclin-dependent kinases (cell cycle regulators). Oncogenes, their mode of activation and associated cancers are shown in Table 6.19. Cell surface receptors and their principal signal transduction pathways are shown in Figs 6.40 and 6.41.

Table 6.19: Oncogenes, their mode of activation and associated cancers

Category	Proto-oncogene protein	Mode of activation	Associated malignancies
Growth factors			
PDGF-β chain	PDGFB (*sis*-Simion sarcoma)	Overexpression	Astrocytoma, osteosarcoma
FGF (fibroblast growth factors)	HST1	Overexpression	Osteosarcoma
	FGF3	Amplification	Osteosarcoma, Melanoma, Gastric carcinoma, Breast carcinoma, Urinary bladder carcinoma
	INT2	Increased baseline activity	Breast carcinoma, Melanoma
TGF-α	TGFA	Overexpression	Astrocytoma
HGF (hepatocyte growth factor)	HGF	Overexpression	Hepatocellular carcinoma, Thyroid carcinoma

Contd...

Table 6.19: Oncogenes, their mode of activation and associated cancers (Contd...)

Category	Proto-oncogene protein	Mode of activation	Associated malignancies
Growth factor receptors			
EGF-receptor family	ERBB1 (EGFR) Erb-B1 (avian erythroblastosis)	Amplification	Lung adenocarcinoma
	Erb-B2 (Her2 neu)	Amplification	Breast carcinoma (marker of aggressiveness) Lung carcinoma (adenocarcinoma, squamous cell carcinoma) Ovarian carcinoma Salivary gland carcinoma
FMS-like tyrosine-3 kinase	FLT3	Point mutation	Leukemia
Receptors for neurotrophic factors	RET	Point mutation	*Multiple endocrine neoplasia:* (MEN 2A, MEN 2B familial medullary carcinoma)
PDGF receptor	PDGFRB	Overexpression Translocation	Gliomas Leukemias
Receptor for stem cell factor (KIT ligand)	KIT	Point mutation	Gastrointestinal tumors Seminomas Leukemias
ALK receptor	ALK	Point mutation Translocation/amplification Fused with NPM gene form hybrid NPM–ALK protein	Lung adenocarcinoma Neuroblastoma Anaplastic large cell lymphoma
Proteins involved in signal transduction			
GTP-binding proteins (GTPase)	K-RAS	Point mutation	Colon carcinoma Lung carcinoma Pancreas carcinoma Acute myeloid leukemia (AML)
	H-RAS	Point mutation	Renal cell carcinoma Urinary bladder transitional cell carcinoma
	N-RAS	Point mutation	Melanomas Hematological malignancies
	GNAP	Point mutation	Uveal melanoma
	GNAS	Point mutation	Pituitary adenoma and other endocrine tumors
Non-receptor tyrosine kinase	ABL (Abelson mouse leukemia)	Translocation (9:22) Point mutation	Chronic myeloid leukemia Acute lymphoblastic leukemia
RAS signal transduction	BRAF	Point mutation Translocation	Hairy cell leukemia (100%) Melanoma (60%) Colon carcinoma Dendritic cell tumor Benign nevi
Notch signal transduction	NOTCH1	Point mutation Translocation	Breast carcinoma Leukemia Lymphoma
JAK/STAT signal transduction	JAK2	Translocation	Myeloproliferative disorders Acute lymphoblastic leukemia

Contd...

Table 6.19: Oncogenes, their mode of activation and associated cancers (Contd...)

Category	Proto-oncogene protein	Mode of activation	Associated malignancies
Transcription factors (nuclear regulatory proteins)			
Transcriptional activators	C-MYC	Translocation (8:14)	Burkitt's lymphoma Leukemia Breast carcinoma Gastric carcinoma Lung carcinoma
	N-MYC	Amplification	Neuroblastoma Breast carcinoma
	L-MYC	Amplification	Lung carcinoma
	FOS	Overexpression	Osteosarcoma
	REL	Rearrangement or amplification	Lymphoma
Cyclins and cyclin-dependent kinases (cell cycle regulators)			
Cyclins	CCND1 (cyclin D1)	Translocation Amplification	Mantle cell lymphomas Multiple myeloma Breast carcinoma Esophageal carcinoma
Cyclin-dependent kinase	CDK4	Amplification or point mutation	Glioblastoma multiforme Melanoma Sarcoma

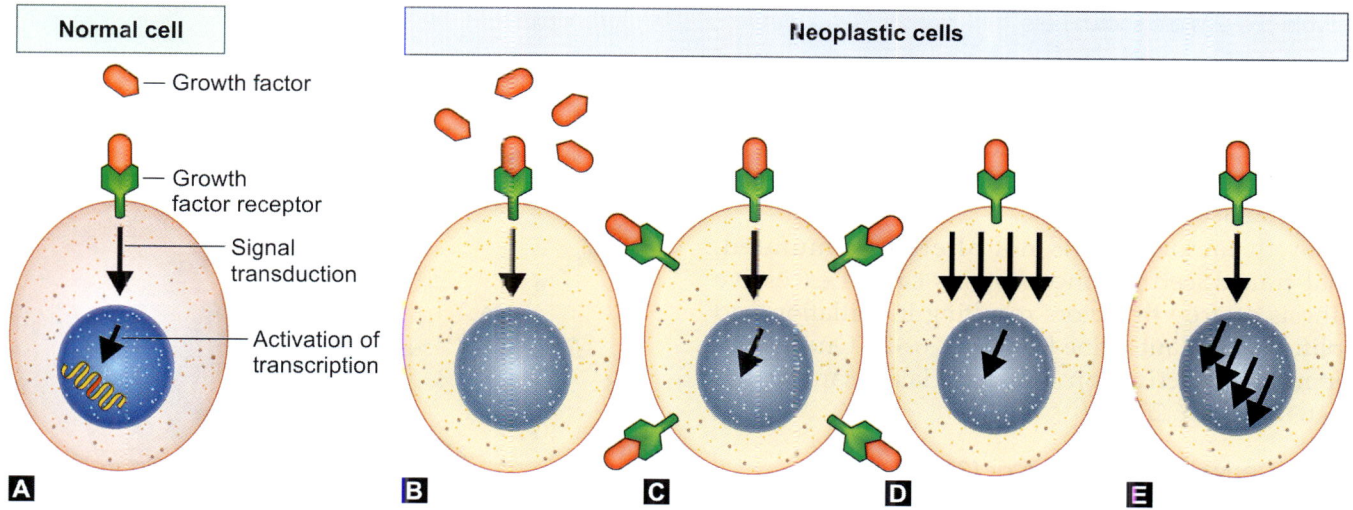

Fig. 6.40: (A) Proliferation of normal cell populations results from a sequence of operations involving the binding of growth factors to receptors, transcription of the growth promoting signal and activation of DNA transcription. The abnormal degree of proliferation in neoplastic cell populations results from the upregulation of one or more than one of these steps, (B) showing increase in growth factors, (C) showing increase in growth factor receptors, (D) showing increased in signal transduction, (E) showing increase in activation of transcription.

GROWTH FACTORS

Growth factors (polypeptides) are synthesized by macrophages, damaged cells and platelets.

Physiological state: Cells need stimulation by growth factors to undergo proliferation. Most soluble growth factors are synthesized by one cell (e.g. macrophage) and act on a neighboring cell (e.g. fibroblast) to stimulate proliferation establishing paracrine action. Paracrine stimulation is common in connective tissue repair of healing wounds and hepatocyte replication during liver regeneration.

Pathological state: Many cancer cells, acquire the ability to synthesize the same growth factors to which they are responsive, generating an autocrine loop. It leads to excessive proliferation of malignant cells.

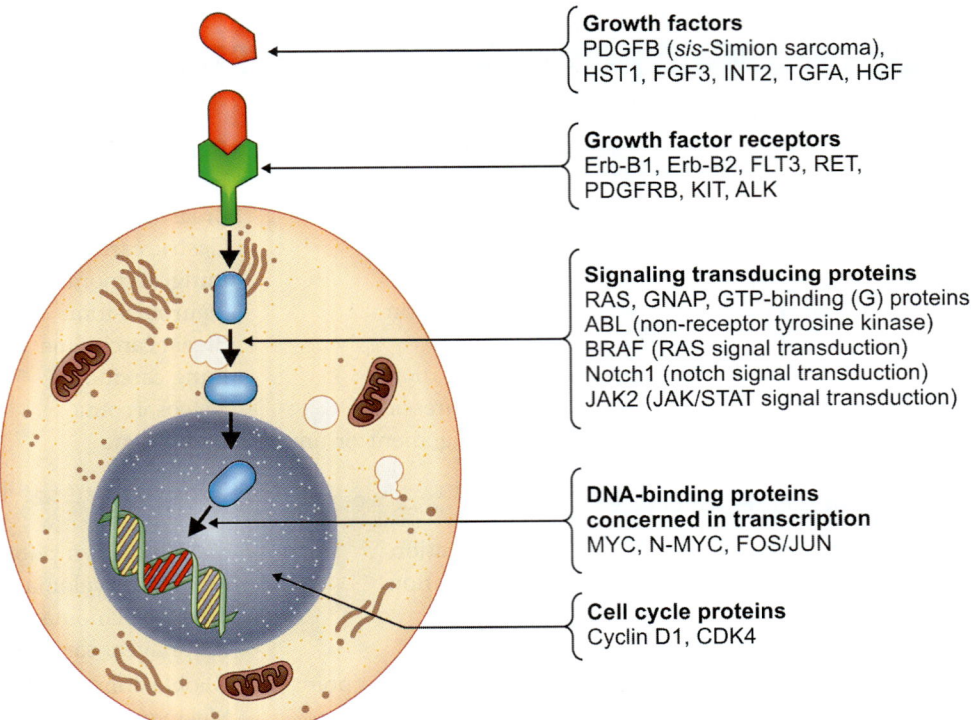

Fig. 6.41: The relation between the gene products of several proto-oncogenes and the operational steps involved in cell division. Examples of growth factors, growth factor receptors, signal transducing proteins, DNA binding proteins involved in transcription and cell cycle proteins are shown here.

Glioblastomas express both PDGF and PDGF receptor kinases. Many sarcomas overexpress both TGF-α and its cognate receptor, epidermal growth factor receptor (EGFR) and another member of the receptor tyrosine kinase family.

Growth factor gene is not altered or mutated. Signal transduced by oncoproteins causes excessive synthesis of growth factors resulting in initiation and amplification of autocrine loop (Fig. 6.42). Oncogenes, their mode of activation and associated cancers are shown in Table 6.20.

Platelet Derived Growth Factor (PDGF)

Platelet derived growth factor is synthesized by *macrophages, smooth muscle cells, endothelial cells, keratinocytes and many tumor cells*. It is *stored in platelet granules* and is *released on platelet activation*. PDGF binds to specific cell surface receptors (transmembrane proteins) and induces tyrosine kinase activity in their intracellular domains resulting in conformational changes. Increased baseline activity of PDGFB is associated with *glioblastoma and breast carcinoma*.

Fibroblast Growth Factors

FGFs are synthesized by *macrophages, T cells, endothelial cells*, and many other cells. These comprise HST1, FGF3 and INT2. Increased baseline activity of HST1 is

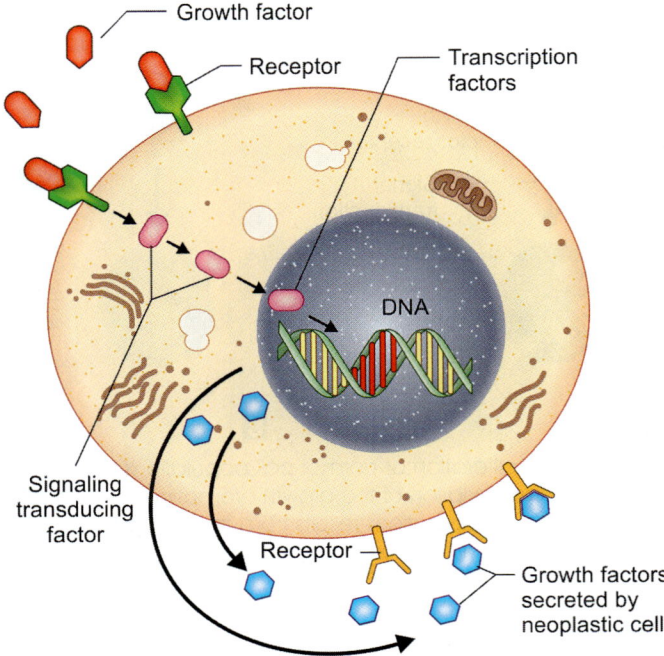

Fig. 6.42: Autocrine signaling in cancer cell showing excessive synthesis of growth factors resulting in initiation and amplification of autocrine loop. There is inhibition of transcription.

associated with *osteosarcomas*. Amplification of FGF3 is associated with *osteosarcoma, stomach cancer, urinary bladder cancer, breast cancer and melanoma*. Increased

Neoplasia: Molecular Basis, Metastasis, Clinical Oncology and Laboratory Diagnosis

Table 6.20: Oncogenes, their mode of activation and associated cancers

Category	Proto-oncogene protein	Mode of activation	Associated malignancies
Growth factors			
PDGF-β chain	PDGFB (sis-Simion sarcoma)	Overexpression	Astrocytoma, Osteosarcoma
FGF (fibroblast growth factors)	HST1	Overexpression	Osteosarcoma
	FGF3	Amplification	Osteosarcoma, Melanoma, Gastric carcinoma, Breast carcinoma, Urinary bladder
	INT2	Increased baseline activity	Breast carcinoma, Melanoma
TGF-α	TGFA	Overexpression	Astrocytoma
HGF (hepatocyte growth factor)	HGF	Overexpression	Hepatocellular carcinoma, Thyroid carcinoma

baseline activity of *INT2* has been demonstrated in *breast carcinoma and malignant melanoma*.

Transforming Growth Factor-α (TGF-α)

Transforming growth factor is synthesized by macrophages, T cells, endothelial cells, platelets. Increased baseline activity of TGF-α oncogene product is associated with **astrocytoma**.

Hepatocyte Growth Factor (HGF)

Hepatocyte growth factors are synthesized by fibroblasts, endothelial cells, and liver mesenchymal cells. It participates in proliferation of hepatocytes, epithelia of biliary tract, lungs, kidney, mammary gland, and skin. Increased baseline activity of HGF oncogene product is associated with *hepatocellular carcinoma and thyroid cancer*.

GROWTH FACTOR RECEPTORS

Binding of a ligand to its receptor induces a series of events by which extracellular signals into the cell leading to expression of genes. A large number of oncogenes encode growth factor receptors. Tyrosine kinase plays an important role in development of cancer.

Physiological state: Receptor's kinase activity is activated transiently by binding of a growth factor to the extracellular domain.

Pathological state: Activated receptor tyrosine kinase residues, which serve as sites for recruitment of many signaling molecules including RAS and P13K. These signaling molecules are key players in receptor tyrosine kinase activity.

Mutant growth factor receptors deliver continuous mitogenic signals to the cell, even in the absence of growth factor in the environment. Growth factor receptors, their mode of activation and associated cancers are shown in Table 6.21.

EGF Receptors

ERBB1: ERBB1 encodes epidermal growth factor receptor (EGFR). Point mutations result in constitutive activation of epidermal growth factor receptor tyrosine kinase. Amplification of ERBB1 is demonstrated in **lung adenocarcinoma**.

ERBB2: ERBB2 encodes a different member of the tyrosine kinase receptor family. Amplification of ERBB-2 (Her2 neu) is demonstrated in cancers of *breast, ovary, lung cancers (adenocarcinoma, squamous cell carcinoma) and salivary gland tumors*. Its expression in cancers is indicative of high grade neoplasm, *invasion of lymph nodes with high rate of recurrence and fatal outcome*. It is demonstrated by immunohistochemistry (monoclonal antibody) on the cell membrane or using *fluorescent in situ hybridization*.

FMS-like Tyrosine-3 Kinase Receptor

Point mutation of FLT3 is associated with **leukemia**.

Receptors for Neurotrophic Factor

Mutant receptors deliver continuous mitogenic signals from mutant proto-oncogene RET to the cells. It is associated with multiple endocrine neoplasia *MEN 2A, MEN 2B and familial medullary carcinoma*.

Table 6.21: Growth factor receptors, their mode of activation and associated cancers

Category	Proto-oncogene protein	Mode of activation	Associated malignancies
EGF receptor family	ERBB1 (EGFR) Erb-B1 (avian erythroblastosis)	Amplification	Lung (adenocarcinoma)
	Erb-B2 (Her2 neu)	Amplification	Breast cancer (marker of aggressiveness) Lung (adenocarcinoma, squamous cell carcinoma) Ovary Salivary gland
FMS-like tyrosine-3 kinase	FLT3	Point mutation	Leukemia
Receptors for neurotrophic factors	RET	Point mutation	Multiple endocrine neoplasia: MEN 2A, MEN 2B Familial medullary carcinoma
PDGF receptor	PDGFRB	Overexpression Translocation	Gliomas Leukemias
Receptor for stem cell factor (KIT ligand)	KIT	Point mutation	Gastrointestinal tumors Seminomas Leukemias
ALK receptor	ALK	Point mutation Translocation/amplification Fused with NPM gene form hybrid NPM–ALK protein	Lung adenocarcinoma Neuroblastoma Anaplastic large cell lymphoma

PDGF Receptors

Overexpression of PDGFRB is associated with *gliomas*. Translocation of PDGFRB is demonstrated in *leukemias*.

KIT Ligand Receptors

Point mutation of KIT is associated with *gastrointestinal tumors, seminoma and leukemias*.

ALK Receptors

Gene rearrangements activate other receptor tyrosine kinases such as ALK. ALK (anaplastic lymphoma kinase) gene is located on chromosome 2. As a result of chromosomal translocation t(2:5), ALK (anaplastic lymphoma kinase) gene is fused with the NPM gene, leading to the production of a hybrid NPM-ALK protein. Patient develops *anaplastic large cell lymphoma* (most important). Translocation/amplification of ALK receptors is seen in *neuroblastoma*. Point mutation of ALK receptors is demonstrated in lung *adenocarcinoma*.

SIGNAL TRANSDUCING PROTEINS

Cell division is regulated by a balance of positive and negative signals. These are GTP binding proteins (tyrosine kinase), non-receptor tyrosine kinase, RAS signal transduction protein, notch signal transduction protein, Wnt signal protein and JAK/STAT signal transduction protein (Fig. 6.43). Signal transduction proteins, their mode of activation and associated cancers are shown in Table 6.22.

GTP Binding Proteins (Tyrosine Kinase Pathway)

The Src protein is a tyrosine kinase. It alters several target molecules by transferring phosphate groups resulting in the transmission of signals to the nucleus that controls the transcription of genes, cellular proliferation differentiation. The phosphate addition/removal process acts like an on/off switch to control the activity of the target molecules. There are two downstream components of the receptor tyrosine kinase signaling pathways described as under.

- *MAP kinase (MAPK) signaling pathway:* MAP kinase signaling pathway is among central signaling pathway that regulates *cell proliferation, cell differentiation and apoptosis*. Adaptor protein GRB2 binds a guanosine triphosphate-guanosine diphosphate (GTP-GDP) exchanger factor called SOS. It acts on the GTP binding protein RAS and catalyzes the formation of RAS-GTP.

  This RAS-GTP product activates MAP kinase pathway stimulates, phosphorylation and synthesis transcriptional factors such as FOS and JUN.

- *MAPK (ERK1/2 type) signaling pathway:* It is a serine/threonine kinase activated by MAPKK via phosphorylation on both threonine and tyrosine

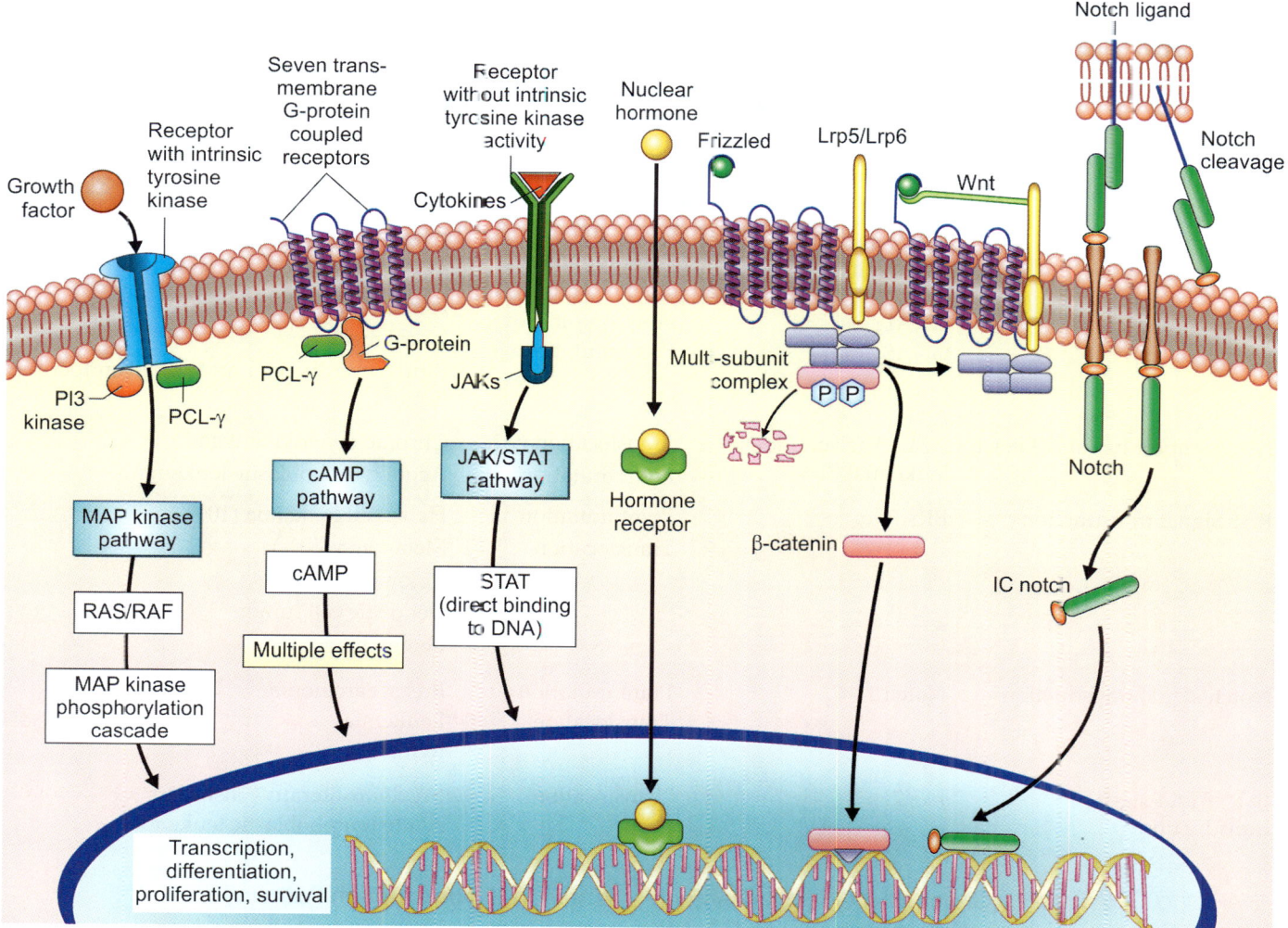

Fig. 6.43: Cell surface receptors and their principal signal transduction pathways show receptors with intrinsic tyrosine kinase activity, seven transmembrane G proteins, and receptors without tyrosine kinase activity. Cyclic adenosine monophosphate (cAMP): Inositol triphosphate (IP3); Janus kinase (JAK); Mitogen activated protein (MAP) kinase; Signal transducers and activators of transcription (STAT). Examples are RAS/MAPK signaling (melanoma, leukemia and colon carcinoma), notch signaling (breast cancer leukemia, and lymphoma), Wnt signaling (colon carcinoma) and Hedgehog signaling (basal cell carcinoma and medulloblastoma).

residues in the TXY sequence. The MAPK family consists of four members, ERK1/2 (also known as *classical MAPK*), JNK/SAPK, p38 and ERK5/BMK1. *These molecules transmit signals from receptors on cell membrane to cytoskeleton and then nucleus of target cells.*

RAS Genes

RAS genes comprise K-RAS (chromosome locus 12p), H-RAS and N-RAS. These participate in intracellular guanosine triphosphate signaling (GTPase). Model for action of RAS genes is shown in Fig. 6.44.

Physiological state: RAS proto-oncogene is a signal transduction protein. To turn 'on' the signal pathway, the RAS protein must bind to a particular molecule (GTP) in the cell. To turn the signal pathway 'off,' the RAS protein must break up the GTP molecule. GTPase activating protein (GAP) activates intrinsic GTPase activity of GTP bound active RAS. It causes hydrolysis of GTP to GDP and returns RAS protein to normal quiescent stage. Stimulation of cells by growth factors activates RAS by exchanging GDP for GTP. Now activated RAS binds to farnesyl transferase resulting in activation of MAP kinase. Active MAP kinase induces mitosis of cells.

Pathological state: RAS oncogene is formed due to point mutation of RAS proto-oncogene. Amplification of RAS no longer breaks up and releases the GTP resulting in turn 'on' the continuous signal pathway. Mutated RAS protein binds to GTPase activating protein (GAP). This process fails to activate intrinsic GTPase activity. This mutant RAS activates mitogen-activating protein (MAP) kinase pathway. The 'on' signal leads to cell growth and proliferation RAS is the most common oncogene mutation responsible for *human cancers in 15–20%.*

Table 6.22: Signal transduction proteins, their mode of activation and associated cancers

Categories	Proto-oncogene protein	Mode of activation	Associated malignancies
GTP-binding proteins (GTPase)	K-ras	Point mutation	Colon carcinoma Lung carcinoma Pancreatic carcinoma AML
	H-ras	Point mutation	Urinary bladder
	N-ras	Point mutation	Renal cell carcinoma Melanomas
	GNAP GNAS	Point mutation Point mutation	Hematologic malignancies Uveal melanoma Pituitary adenoma and other endocrine tumors
Non-receptor tyrosine kinase	ABL (Abelson mouse leukemia)	Translocation (9;22) Point mutation	Chronic myeloid leukemia Acute lymphoblastic leukemia
RAS signal transduction	BRAF	Point mutation Translocation	Hairy cell leukemia (100%) Melanoma (60%) Colon carcinoma Dendritic cell tumor Benign nevi
Notch signal transduction	Notch 1	Point mutation Translocation	Breast carcinoma Leukemia Lymphoma
JAK/STAT signal transduction	JAK2	Translocation	Myeloproliferative disorders Acute lymphoblastic leukemia

GNAP and GNAS gene: GNAP and GNAS are signal transducing proteins. Point mutations of GNAP and GNAS associated with uveal melanoma.

Alterations in Non-receptor Tyrosine Kinase Pathway

The best-known example of an acquired chromosomal translocation in a human cancer is the Philadelphia chromosome, which is found in 95% of patients with *CML*. Reciprocal translocation of ABL (Abelson mouse leukemia on Ch 9) into the BCR site on chromosome 22 creates the *BCR-ABL fusion protein product* in chronic myeloid leukemia.

At the same time, part of the long arm of chromosome 22 is transferred onto the long arm of chromosome 9. The *BCR-ABL fusion protein product* provides a growth factor by virtue of increased non-receptor protein kinase activity, which generates mitogenic and antiapoptotic signals. Point mutation of ABL has also been demonstrated in AML. Treatment of CML has been aimed to develop therapeutic agent that inhibits *BCR-ABL fusion protein product*.

Wnt Signal Transduction Pathway

Wnt signaling controls the level of the key modulator β-catenin for signal transduction through processes involving phosphorylation and ubiquitin-mediated degradation. It is regulated by the cytoplasmic β-catenin destruction complex, that consists of the core proteins AXIN, adenomatous polyposis coli (APC), casein kinase 1 (CK1), and glycogen synthase kinase 3 (GSK3). APC promotes cell migration and adhesion. It binds to cytoskeleton β-catenin. It also acts as oncogene by binding to TGF-β receptor. APC tumor suppressor gene has been mapped on 5q21. Most commonly APC pathway has been presented as a model of tumor progression. APC tumor suppressor gene mutation associated with tumors is shown in Fig. 6.45.

BRAF Increasing RAS Signal Transduction Protein Pathway

BRAF, a member of RAF family is a serine/threonine/ protein kinase. BRAF mutation leads to increased RAS signal transduction. BRAF mutation is demonstrated in *hairy cell leukemias (100%), melanoma (60%), colon cancer, dendritic cell tumor and benign nevi.*

Neoplasia: Molecular Basis, Metastasis, Clinical Oncology and Laboratory Diagnosis

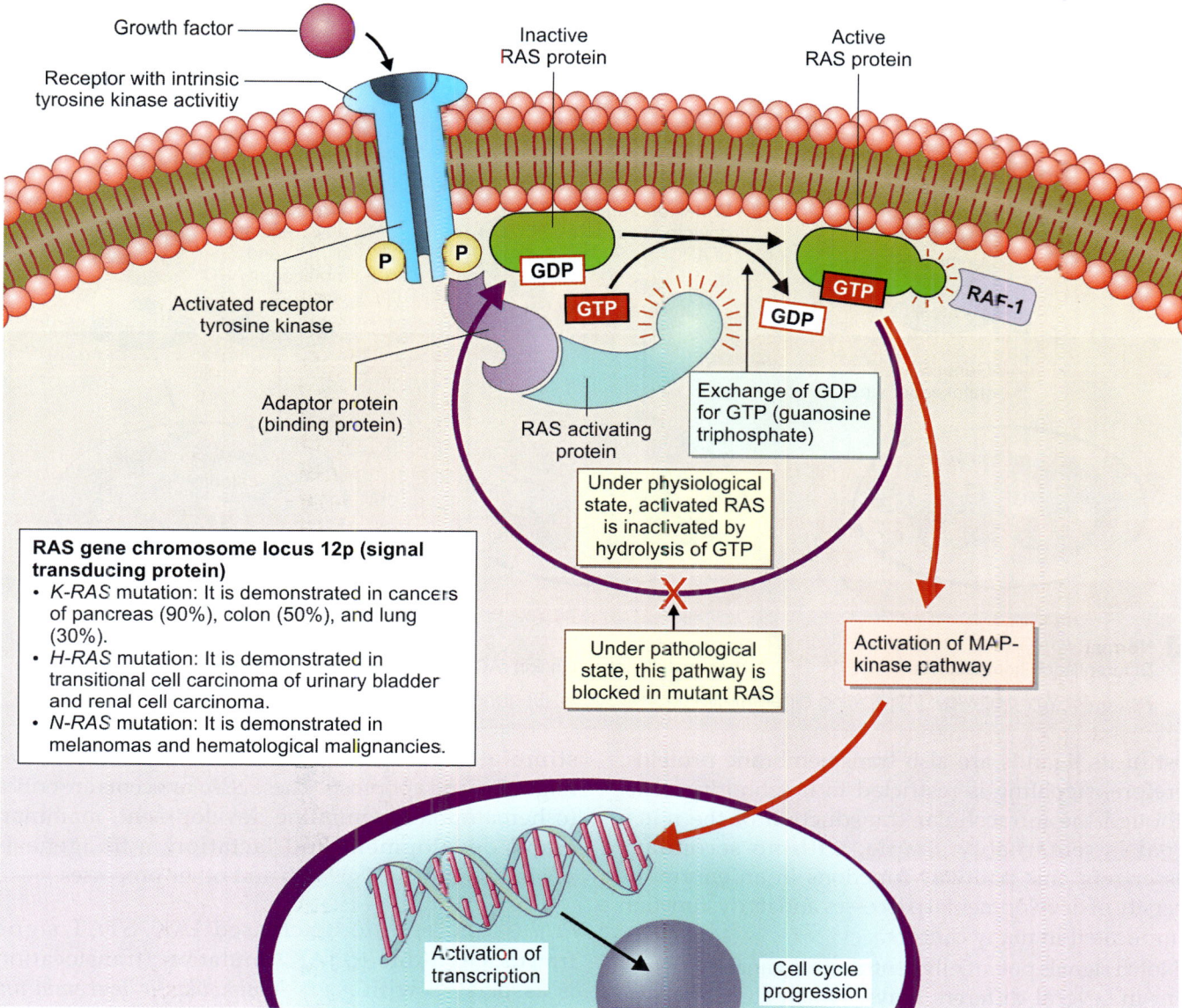

Fig. 6.44: Model for action of RAS genes. When a normal cell is stimulated through a growth factor receptor inactive (GDP-bound) RAS is activated to a GTP-bound state. Activated RAS recruits RAF and stimulates the MAP-kinase pathway to transmit growth-promoting signals to the nucleus. The mutant RAS protein is permanently activated because of inability to hydrolyze GTP, leading to continuous stimulation of cells without any external trigger. The anchoring of RAS to the cell membrane by the farnesyl moiety is essential for its action.

Phosphatidylinositol-3 Kinase (PI3k) Proteins Pathway

PI3K phosphorylates membrane phospholipid resulting in generation of product that activates kinase AKT (also known as *protein kinase B*). Net result is *cell proliferation and survival through inhibiting apoptosis.* Mutation of PI3 kinase family of proteins are common in many cancers. PI3 kinase is recruited by tyrosine kinase activation in plasma membrane associated signaling protein complexes.

Physiological state: PTEN gene is located on chromosome 10q. Phosphatase and tensin homologue are proteins of PTEN gene. Normally, PTEN gene products inhibit AKT/PI3K signaling pathway.

Pathological state: PTEN gene mutation leads to Cowden disease characterized by fibroadenomas, fibrocystic lesions, ductal epithelial hyperplasia, and nipple malformations with increased risk of breast cancer in Cowden disease.

Notch Signal Transduction Protein Pathway

A small number of signaling pathways is used iteratively to regulate cell proliferation and apoptosis. Notch is the receptor in one such pathway, and is unusual in that

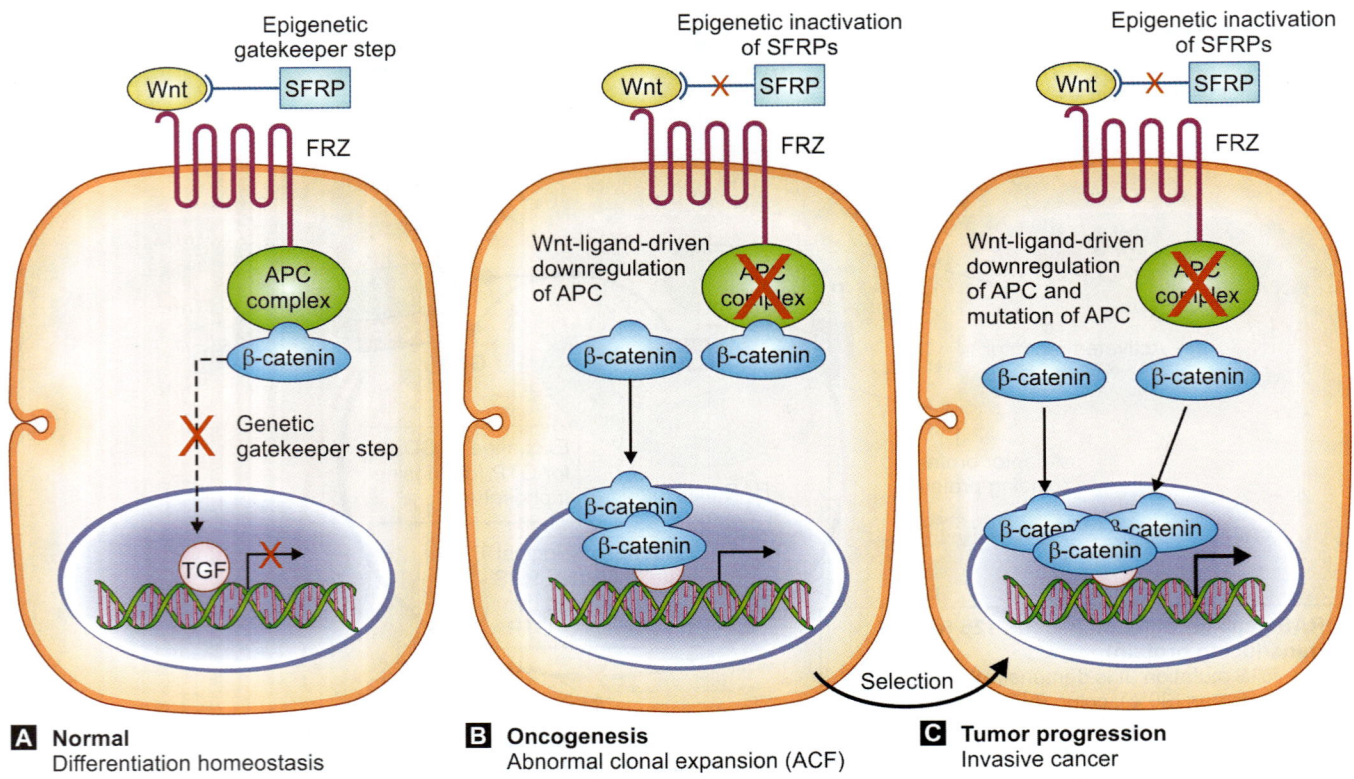

Fig. 6.45: Wnt pathway: (A) showing differentiation homeostasis, (B) abnormal clonal expansion, (C) tumor progression.

most of its ligands are also transmembrane proteins, therefore, signaling is restricted to neighboring cells. Although the intracellular transduction of the notch signal is remarkably simple, with no secondary messengers, this pathway functions in an enormous diversity of developmental processes and its dysfunction is implicated in many cancers.

Notch signals potentially contribute to cancer development in several different ways. Notch signaling was first linked to tumorigenesis through identification of a recurrent t(7;9)(q34;q34.3) chromosomal translocation involving the human notch 1 gene that is found in a small subset of *human pre-T cell acute lymphoblastic leukemias (T-ALL)*. Since this discovery, aberrant notch signaling has been suggested to be involved in a *wide variety of human neoplasms (leukemias, lymphomas and breast carcinomas)*.

JAK/STAT RAS Signal Transduction Protein Pathway

The Janus kinase/signal transducers and activators of transcription (JAK/STAT) pathway is one of a handful of pleiotropic cascades used to transduce a multitude of signals for development and homeostasis in animals, from humans to flies.

Physiological state: In mammals, the JAK/STAT pathway is the principal signaling mechanism for a wide array of cytokines and growth factors. JAK activation stimulates cell proliferation, differentiation, cell migration and apoptosis. These cellular events are critical to hematopoiesis, immune development, mammary gland development and lactation, adipogenesis, sexually dimorphic growth and other processes.

Pathological state: Increased JAK/STAT signal transduction due to JAK2 mutation (translocation) is associated with *acute lymphoblastic leukemia and myeloproliferative disorders*.

TRANSCRIPTION FACTORS

Transcription factors are also known as nuclear regulatory proteins. MYC family comprises C-MYC, N-MYC and L-MYC. MYC protein function acts as a transcription factor.

Physiological state: MYC controls the expression of several genes that are involved in cell growth. It upregulates the expression of rRNA genes and rRNA processing, thereby increasing the assembly of ribosomes required for protein synthesis. It also upregulates gene expression that resulting in metabolic reprograming and Warburg effect. *Besides these functions, MYC is considered master transcriptional regulator of cell growth. It upregulates expression of telomerase that has endless replicative capacity of cancer cells.*

Neoplasia: Molecular Basis, Metastasis, Clinical Oncology and Laboratory Diagnosis

Table 6.23: Transcription factors (nuclear regulatory proteins), their mode of activation and associated cancers

Category	Proto-oncogene protein	Mode of activation	Associated malignancies
MYC transcriptional factor	C-MYC	Translocation (8;14)	Burkitt's lymphoma Leukemia Breast carcinoma Gastric carcinoma Lung carcinoma
	N-MYC	Amplification	Neuroblastoma Breast carcinoma
	L-MYC	Amplification	Lung carcinoma
	FOS	Overexpression	Osteosarcoma
	REL	Rearrangement or amplification	Lymphoma

Pathological state: MYC family is activated by gene rearrangement or amplification. Gene rearrangements involve the breakage and re-sealing of chromosomes. *All signaling pathways transform cells in part through upregulation of MYC.* Examples are *RAS/MAPK signaling (melanoma, leukemia and colon carcinoma), notch signaling (breast cancer, leukemia, and lymphoma), Wnt signaling (colon carcinoma) and Hedgehog signaling (basal cell carcinoma and medulloblastoma).* Transcription factors (nuclear regulatory proteins), their mode of activation and associated cancers are shown in Table 6.23.

CYCLINS AND CYCLIN-DEPENDENT KINASES

Cyclins (CCND1/cyclin D1) and cyclin-dependent kinase (CDK4) act as cell cycle regulatory proteins and control the expression of several genes. Cyclin D binds to CDK4 to form a complex; that causes the cell to enter the S phase by phosphorylation of RB proteins. *RB proteins normally arrest the cell in the G_1 phase.* CDK4 phosphorylates the RB protein causing the cell to enter the S phase. Cell cycle is inhibited by CIK/PIK family (p21 and p27) and INK/ARF family. Downregulation of cell cycle inhibitors promotes progression of cell cycle.

Cell Cycle Checkpoints

There are main two cell cycle checkpoints, one at G_1/S and other at G_2/M transition. Each of these checkpoints is tightly regulated by synthesis of growth promoting, growth suppressing factors in balanced manner and sensors of DNA damage. When DNA damage occurs, there is arrest of cell cycle progression until damage is repaired. If DNA of cell is not repaired, it undergoes apoptosis. Defect in G_1/S checkpoint is more important in cancer. TP53 arrests the cell in G phase by inhibiting CDK4. It prevents RB protein phosphorylation. It may provide time for repair of DNA in the cell. Two most important tumor suppressor genes such as RB and TP53 encode proteins that inhibit G_1/S progression.

Table 6.24: Dysregulation of cyclins and cyclin-dependent kinase associated tumors

Cyclins and cyclin-dependent kinase	Cancers
Cyclins (CCND1/cyclin D1)	Mantle cell lymphoma Multiple myeloma Breast carcinoma Esophageal cancer Hepatocellular carcinoma
Cyclin-dependent kinase (CDK4)	Glioblastoma Melanoma Sarcoma

Gene Mutations

Translocation and amplification activate cyclins (CCND1/cyclin D1). Cyclin-dependent kinase (CDK4) is activated by amplification or point mutation. Dysregulation of cyclins and cyclin-dependent kinase associated tumors are shown in Table 6.24.

OTHER MOLECULES

BCL2 normal protein blocks cell suicide (lymphoma). BCL1 codes for cyclin D1, stimulatory protein of the cell cycle (breast, neck, head cancers). MDM2 codes for antagonist of p53 (sarcomas).

INSENSITIVITY TO GROWTH INHIBITORY SIGNALS

Under physiological state, tumor suppressor genes prevent cancer by inhibiting mitosis (controlling G_1 to S phase cell cycle). These act like a pedal by inhibiting receptor for growth factor, signaling enzymes and transcription factors. The cancer cells are insensitive to tumor suppressor genes.

Mutation of tumor suppressor genes fail to *inhibit proliferation and differentiation of cells resulting in malignant transformation.* Tumor suppressor genes, their subcellular location and associated human neoplasms are shown in Tables 6.25 and 6.26.

Table 6.25: Tumor suppressor gene mutations and associated cancers

Gene and locus	Protein	Function	Familial tumors due to gene mutation	Sporadic cancers due to gene mutation
Mitogenic signaling pathway inhibitors				
APC (locus 5p22.2)	APC protein	Inhibits Wnt signaling activator pathway, thus prevents nuclear transcription. It degrades catenin	Familial polyposis coli and carcinoma	Cancers of colon, stomach, pancreas, thyroid and melanoma
NF1 (locus 13p11)	Neurofibrinin protein 1	Inhibits RAS/MAP-kinase signaling activator pathway	Neurofibromatosis type 1 (neurofibroma and increased risk of malignant peripheral nerve tumors)	Juvenile myeloid leukemia, neuroblastoma and schwannoma
NF2 (locus 22q)	Merlin	Stabilization of cytoskeleton membrane linkage	Neurofibromatosis type 2 (acoustic schwannoma and meningioma)	Schwannomas and meningioma
PTCH1	Patched	Inhibits Hedgehog signaling pathway	Gorlin's syndrome (basal cell carcinoma, medulloblastoma and other benign tumors)	Basal cell carcinoma and medulloblastoma
SMAD2 SMAD4	SMAD-2 and SMAD-4	Both inhibit TGF-β Signaling pathway, repress CDK4 and MYC and induce expression of CDK inhibitor	Juvenile polyposis	Cancers of pancreas and colon
PTEN	Phosphatase and tensin homologue	Inhibits AKT/PKB signaling pathway	Cowden syndrome (cancers of breast, endometrium and thyroid gland)	Lymphoid neoplasms Carcinomas
Cell cycle progression inhibitors				
CDKN2A	P16/INK4a and P14ARF	P16 inhibits CDK. P14 indirectly activates p53 tumor suppressor gene.	Familial melanoma	Cancers of breast, pancreas and esophagus
RB gene (locus 13p14)	Retinoblastoma protein	It codes for pRB protein, master brake on cell cycle. It inhibits G_1 to S transition during cell cycle. It inhibits nuclear transcription factor	Retinoblastoma, osteosarcoma	Retinoblastoma, osteosarcoma, cancers of breast, colon, prostate, bladder and lung
Angiogenesis inhibitors genes				
VHL (locus 3p25)	von Hippel-Lindau (VHL) protein	It inhibits hypoxia inducible factor (HIF1a). It regulates nuclear transcription.	von Hippel-Lindau syndrome (cerebellar hemangioblastoma, retinal angiomas, renal cell carcinoma (bilateral and pheochromocytoma)	Renal cell carcinoma

Contd..

Table 6.25: Tumor suppressor gene mutations and associated cancers (Contd...)

Gene and locus	Protein	Function	Familial tumors due to gene mutation	Sporadic cancers due to gene mutation
SDHB, SDHD	Succinate dehydrogenase subunits of B and D	These participate in TCA cycle and oxidative phosphorylation	Paraganglioma	Paraganglioma
STK11	Liver kinase B1 (LKB1) or STK11	It activates AMPK family of kinases. It suppresses cell growth when cell nutrients and energy levels are low	Peutz-Jeghers syndrome (cancers of GIT, pancreas)	Diverse carcinomas in 5–20% cases
CDH1	E-cadherin	Participates in cell adhesion. It inhibits cell motility	Gastric carcinoma	Gastric carcinoma Breast lobular carcinoma
Genomic stability enabler (most important)				
TP53 (locus 17p13.1)	p53	Inhibits cell cycle G_1 to S phase. It repairs DNA. It induces cell suicide (apoptosis) by activating BAX gene	Li-Fraumeni syndrome (cancers of breast and adrenal cortex, sarcoma, leukemia, brain tumors)	More than 50% of human cancers
DNA repair genes				
BRCA1 (locus 17)	BRCA1	It binds RAD51 molecule that mediates repair of double-stranded breaks in DNA	Cancers of ovary, breast, prostate, pancreas and fallopian tube	Rare mutated in medullary and metaplastic carcinomas of breast
BRCA2 (locus 13)	BRCA2	It binds RAD51 molecule that mediates repair of double-stranded breaks in DNA	Cancers of stomach, gallbladder, bile duct, pharynx and melanoma	Fanconi anemia
MLH1, MSH2, MSH6, and PMS2	MLH1, MSH2, MSH6, and PMS2 proteins	Accumulation of numerous mismatched errors in DNA replications	Hereditary nonpolyposis syndrome (Lynch syndrome) increased risk of development of carcinoma of endometrium (first most common cancer), ovary and right colon carcinoma	Unknown
Functions of genes by various mechanisms				
WT1 [(WT1) on 11p13]	Wilms' tumor 1 Nonsense mutation	Transcriptional factor	Familial Wilms' tumor	Wilms' tumor and certain leukemias
MEN 1	Menin	Transcriptional factor	Multiple neoplasia syndrome 1 (MEN 1: Tumors of pituitary, parathyroid and pancreas)	Tumors of pituitary, parathyroid and pancreas
DPC4 (MADH4/SMAD4) locus 18q21.1	DPC4	It codes for relay molecule in cell division inhibitory pathway	Rare	Cancer of pancreas (most common), breast and ovaries

Contd..

Table 6.25: Tumor suppressor gene mutations and associated cancers (Contd...)

Gene and locus	Protein	Function	Familial tumors due to gene mutation	Sporadic cancers due to gene mutation
ATM	ATM (locus 11p22) Mutation by deletion	Unknown/tyrosine	Ataxia-telangiectasia, breast cancer, stomach cancer, leukemia, and lymphoma	Unknown
p16	p16 (locus 9p21) Mutation by deletion and nonsense	It inhibits nuclear cyclin D dependent kinase activity	Familial melanoma	Mesotheliomas, carcinoma pancreas, melanoma, astrocytoma
TGF-β (locus 19q)	TGF-β	It inhibits G_1 to S phase	–	Cancers of pancreas and colorectal region
CHEK2 (locus 22q12.1)	CHEK2	CHEK2 induces cell cycle arrest. It repairs damaged DNA. It activates BRCA1 and p53 tumor suppressor genes by phosphorylation	Breast carcinoma (5%)	Cancers of breast prostate, thyroid, and kidney especially after radiation

Table 6.26: Selected tumor suppressor genes, their subcellular location and associated human neoplasms

Subcellular location	Gene	Function	Tumors associated with inherited mutations	Tumors associated with somatic mutations
Cell surface	TGF-β receptor	Growth inhibition	Unknown	Colon carcinoma
	E-cadherin	Cell adhesion	Familial gastric carcinoma	Gastric carcinoma
Inner surface of plasma membrane	NF1 (locus 13p11)	Inhibition of RAS/MAP signal transduction and of p21 cell cycle inhibitor	Neurofibromatosis type 1 and sarcoma	Neuroblastoma, juvenile myeloid leukemia and schwannoma
Cytoskeleton	NF2 (locus 22q)	Cytoskeleton stability	Neurofibromatosis type 2 (acoustic schwannomas and meningioma)	Schwannoma and meningioma
Cytosol	APC/β-catenin (locus 22p) Inhibition of Wnt signal transduction, nuclear transcription causes degradation of catenin	Familial adenomatous polyposis coli/colon carcinoma	Carcinoma of stomach, colon, pancreas, thyroid and melanoma	
	PTEN	Inhibition of AKT/PKB signal transduction	Cowden syndrome (cancers of breast, endometrium and thyroid)	Carcinoma of endometrium and prostate
	SMAD2 and SMAD4	TGF-β signal transduction	Juvenile polyposis	Carcinoma of colon and pancreas
Nucleus	RB (locus 13p14)	Regulation of cell cycle (master brake inhibiting G_1 to S transition and nuclear transcription)	Retinoblastoma, osteosarcoma	Retinoblastoma, osteosarcoma; carcinomas of breast, colon, lung
	TP53 (locus 17p13.1)	Cell cycle arrest, apoptosis in response	Li-Fraumeni and multiple cancers	Most human cancers such as pancreas, lung, colon and breast

Neoplasia: Molecular Basis, Metastasis, Clinical Oncology and Laboratory Diagnosis

Functional Categories of Tumor Suppressor Genes

There are two functional categories of tumor suppressor genes: gatekeeper and caretaker genes. Functional categories of tumor suppressor genes and associated cancers are shown in Table 6.27.

- *Gatekeeper genes:* These inhibit the proliferation of cells with damaged DNA and also promote the death of these cells. Examples of gatekeeper genes are **TP53 gene, RB1** and **APC gene**.
- *Caretaker genes:* These maintain the integrity of the genome by repairing DNA damage. Examples of caretaker genes are BRCA1, BRCA2, MLH1, MSH2, MSH6, PMS2, FAMC, and Xp.

Hypermethylation of Tumor Suppressor Genes

Physiological state: Tumor suppressor gene performs its functions due to lack of methylation of DNA. But addition of cytosines (Cs) in the DNA (methylation of DNA promoter(s) of the gene) shuts down expression of the gene. Hypermethylation can inactivate normal p53 tumor suppressor gene. Hypermethylation of many tumor suppressor and DNA repair genes has been demonstrated in human tumors.

Mutation of Allele/both Alleles

- *Mutation of one allele:* Mutant allele of tumor suppressor gene behaves as a recessive, that is, as long as the cell contains one normal allele, tumor suppression continues. It is known as *heterozygous state*.
- *Mutation of both alleles:* Mutation of both alleles of tumor suppressor genes is essential for carcinogenesis, because *heterozygous state (single allele) has adequate tumor suppressor activity*. Mutation of second allele of tumor suppressor gene leading to carcinogenesis

Table 6.27: Functional categories of tumor suppressor genes and associated cancers

Gene	Function	Tumor susceptibility if germline mutation	Comment
Gatekeeper genes			
TP53 gene	Transcriptional factor responds to DNA damage	Li-Fraumeni syndrome (cancers of breast and adrenal cortex, sarcoma, leukemia, brain tumors)	Mutated in 50% of human cancers
RB1 gene	Transcriptional regulator controls cell cycle G_1/S checkpoint	Retinoblastoma, osteosarcoma	Retinoblastoma, osteosarcoma, cancers of breast, colon, prostate, bladder and lung
APC gene	Inhibits Wnt signaling activator pathway, thus prevents nuclear transcription. Degrades β-catenin	Familial polyposis coli and carcinoma	Cancers of colon, stomach, pancreas, thyroid, and melanoma
Caretaker genes			
BRCA1 gene	DNA repairs—ds breaks	Cancers of ovary, female breast, male breast, prostate, pancreas and fallopian tube	Rarely mutated in breast cancers
BRCA2 gene	DNA repairs—ds breaks	Breast, prostate and pancreatic cancer	Homozygous mutation with Fanconi anemia
MSH2 gene	DNA repairs—mismatch repair pathway	Hereditary nonpolyposis colorectal cancer (Lynch syndrome)	Defective mismatch repair permits mismatch mutation (? mutator phenotype)
MSH1 gene	DNA repairs—mismatch repair pathway		
FAMC gene	DNA repairs—Fanconi anemia repair pathway	Fanconi anemia	Defective DNA repair pathway permits cross link mutations and tumor formation
XP gene	DNA repairs—nucleotide excision repair pathway	Xeroderma pigmentosum	Defective nucleotide excision repair pathway permits UV mutation and tumor formation

is known as *loss of heterozygosity*. Oncogenes, by contrast, behave as dominants; one mutant, or overactive, allele can predispose the cell to tumor formation. It is known as *homozygous state*. Some cancers show deletions of specific sites on tumor repressor genes that normally inhibit cell growth and division of cancer cells in *breast, colon, and lung*.

MITOGENIC SIGNALING PATHWAY INHIBITORS

Gene products of various tumor suppressor genes such as APC, NF1, NF2, PTCH, SMAD2, SMAD4 and PTEN inhibit nuclear transcription.

APC Tumor Suppressor Gene

Under physiological state, APC is a gatekeeper tumor suppressor gene located on long (q) arm of chromosome 5 in band q22.2. APC inhibits Wnt signaling activator pathway, thus prevents nuclear transcription by degrading catenin. APC mutation occurs by deletion and nonsense. Germline APC gene mutation associated with familial and sporadic tumors is shown in Table 6.28.

NF1 Tumor Suppressor Gene

Under physiological state, NF1 gene located on chromosome 13p11 codes for protein that inhibits a stimulatory GTPase (RAS) protein. NF1 gene mutation (deletion) associated with familial and sporadic tumors (Table 6.29).

NF2 Tumor Suppressor Gene

Under physiological state, NF2 is located on chromosome 22q codes for cytoskeleton membrane linkage. NF2 gene mutation (deletion and nonsense) associated with familial and sporadic tumors is shown in Table 6.30.

PTCH Tumor Suppressor Gene

Physiological state: PTCH gene inhibits Hedgehog signaling pathway. PTCH gene mutation associated with familial and sporadic tumors is shown in Table 6.31.

SMAD2 and SMAD4 Tumor Suppressor Genes

Under physiological state, SMAD4 is located on chromosome 18q. It is also known as *DPC4*. SMAD2 and

Table 6.28: APC tumor suppressor gene mutation associated with tumors

APC gene	Function	Familial tumors	Sporadic tumors
APC gene locus on long (q) arm of chromosome 5 in band q22.2.	Regulates β-catenin function in Wnt pathway	Familial adenomatous polyposis Colon carcinoma	Colorectal cancer (most often) Gastric cancer Thyroid cancer Melanoma Gardner syndrome*

*Gardner syndrome is characterized by polyposis coli, with osteomas, epidermal cysts, and fibromatosis.

Table 6.29: NF1 gene mutation and associated tumors

Gene and locus	Protein	Function	Familial tumors due to gene mutation	Sporadic cancers due to gene mutation
NF1 (locus 13p11)	Neurofibrinin protein 1	Inhibits RAS/MAP-kinase signaling activator pathway	Neurofibromatosis type 1 (neurofibroma and increased risk of malignant peripheral nerve tumors)	Juvenile myeloid leukemia Neuroblastoma Schwannoma

Table 6.30: NF2 gene mutation and associated familial and sporadic tumors

Gene and locus	Protein	Function	Familial tumors due to gene mutation	Sporadic cancers due to gene mutation
NF2 (locus 22q)	Merlin	Stabilization of cytoskeleton membrane linkage	Neurofibromatosis type 2 (acoustic Schwannoma and meningioma)	Schwannoma Meningioma

Table 6.31: PTCH gene mutation and associated familial and sporadic tumors

Gene	Protein	Function	Familial tumors	Sporadic cancers
PTCH1	Patched	Inhibits Hedgehog signaling pathway	Gorlin's syndrome (basal cell carcinoma, medulloblastoma and other benign tumors)	Basal cell carcinoma Medulloblastoma

Neoplasia: Molecular Basis, Metastasis, Clinical Oncology and Laboratory Diagnosis

Table 6.32: SMADA2 and SMADA4 gene mutations associated with familial and sporadic tumors

Gene	Protein and locus	Function	Familial tumors	Sporadic cancers
SMAD2 SMAD4	SMAD2 and SMAD4	Both proteins inhibit TGF-β signaling pathway, repress CDK4 and MYC, and induce expression of CDK inhibitor	Juvenile polyposis	Pancreas (55%) Colon

Table 6.33: PTEN gene mutations associated with familial and sporadic tumors

Gene	Protein	Function	Familial tumors due to gene mutation	Sporadic cancers due to gene mutation
PTEN	Phosphatase and tensin homologue	Inhibits AKT/PKB signaling pathway	Cowden syndrome (cancers of breast, endometrium and thyroid gland)	Lymphoid neoplasms Carcinomas

SMAD4 normally inhibit cell division by inhibiting TGF-β signaling pathway resulting in suppression of growth. These also promote apoptosis. These repress CDK4 and MYC. These also induce expression of CDK inhibitor. SMADA2 and SMADA4 gene mutations associated with familial and sporadic cancers are shown in Table 6.32.

PTEN Tumor Suppressor Gene

Under physiological state, phosphatase and tensin homologue is a protein encoded by PTEN. It inhibits AKT/PI3K signaling pathway. PTEN gene mutation associated with familial and sporadic cancers is shown in Table 6.33.

CELL CYCLE PROGRESSION INHIBITORS

Gene products of CDKN2A and RB tumor suppressor genes inhibit progression of cell cycle.

CDKN2A Tumor Suppressor Gene

Under physiological state, P16/INK4a inhibits CDK and P14ARF, thus indirectly activates p53 tumor suppressor gene. CDKN2A gene mutation associated with familial and sporadic tumors is shown in Table 6.34.

RB Tumor Suppressor Gene (Two-hit Mutation Model of Retinoblastoma)

Knudson postulated a **two-hit** model for retinoblastoma disease: Hit 1 (germline inherited mutation in allele 1) and hit 2 (somatic event involving remaining normal allele).

Two mutations are required for the development of **retinoblastoma** (familial or sporadic) are shown in Fig. 6.46.

Physiological state: Retinoblastoma caretaker tumor suppressor gene is also known as *Governor of cell cycle*. It was mapped to the long arm of chromosome 13q14. Normal people have two alleles of the Rb gene. It encodes for RB protein which acts as master brake on cell cycle. It inhibits G_1 to S phase by inhibiting nuclear transcription factor. Dephosphorylated Rb gene inhibits cell division. When the Rb gene is phosphorylated, cell division takes place passing through G_1/S transition (Fig. 6.47).

Pathological state: Retinoblastoma occurs due *to loss of heterozygosity*. It means that both normal RB alleles at chromosome 13q14 must be inactivated (two hits) for development of retinoblastoma.

Retinoblastoma occurs in two forms: familial and sporadic. Onset of familial retinoblastoma is earlier than sporadic form. Function of RB is affected by gene amplification of CDK4 and cyclin D genes and loss of CDK inhibitors (p1/INK4a). E7 oncoprotein of HPV inhibits RB gene and E6 degrades p53 (Fig. 6.48).

- *Familial retinoblastoma:* Familial retinoblastoma constitutes 40% of retinoblastoma cases. Infant develops retinoblastomas in both eyes in the first weeks of infancy. It occurs when the fetus inherits from one of its parents, a chromosome (13q14) that has its RB locus deleted (or otherwise mutated).

Table 6.34: CDKN2A gene mutation associated with familial and sporadic tumors

Gene	Protein and locus	Function	Familial tumors	Sporadic cancers
CDKN2A	P16/INK4a and P14ARF	P16 inhibits CDKP14 indirectly activates p53 tumor suppressor gene	Familial melanoma	Breast Pancreas Esophagus

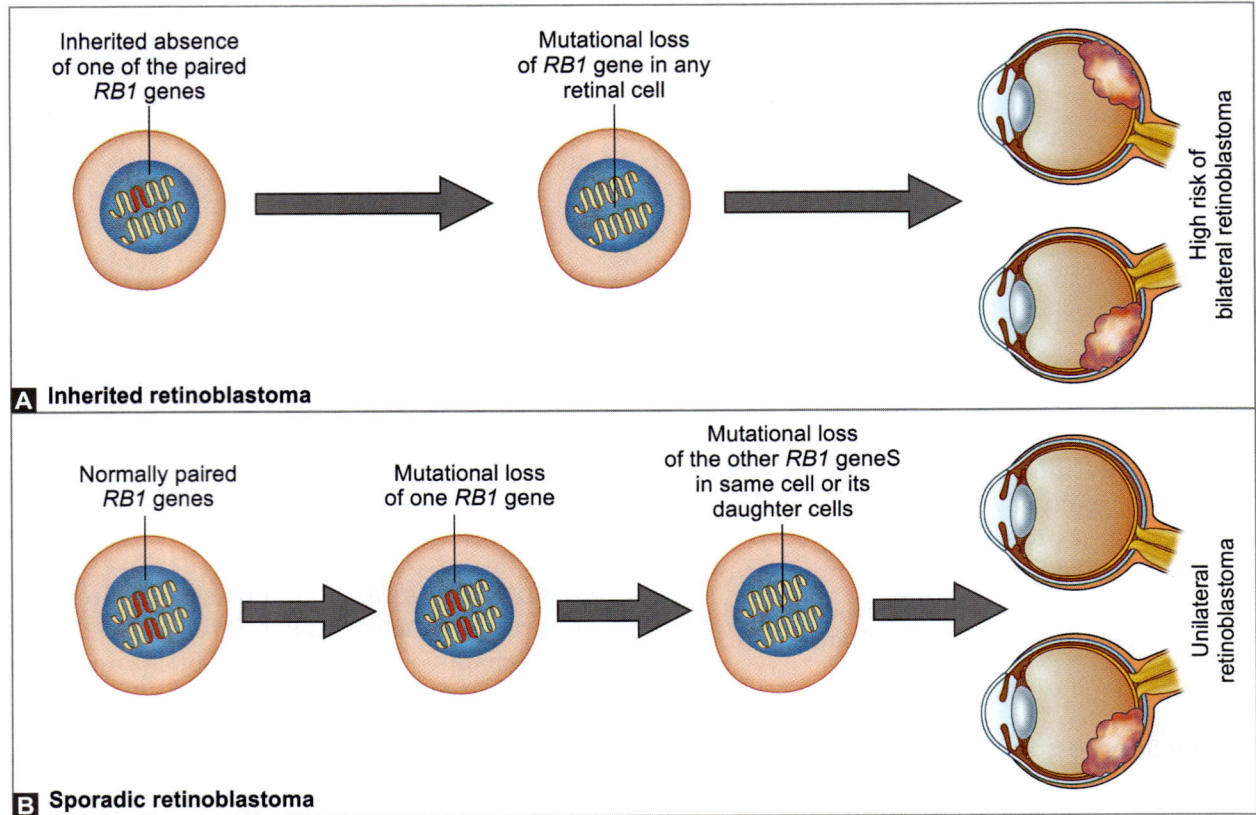

Fig. 6.46: Retinoblastoma is a tumor suppressor gene located on long arm of chromosome 13. Mutation of RB1 gene predisposes to increased risk of development of retinoblastoma. (A) Germline mutation in one of the paired alleles of the RB1 is required to develop inherited bilateral retinoblastoma, (B) normal individuals without an inherited germline mutation of the RB1 gene have a low incidence of sporadic unilateral retinoblastoma.

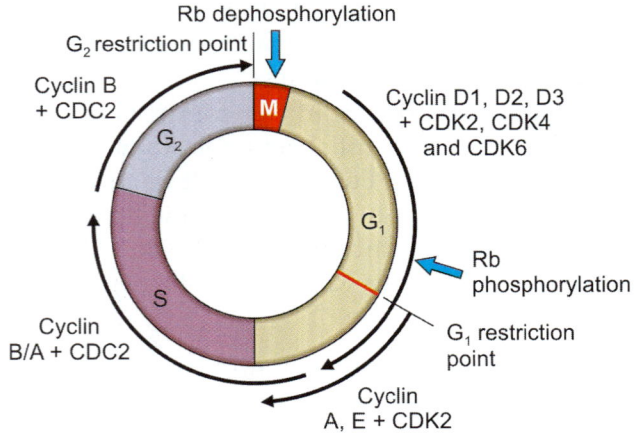

Fig. 6.47: RB phosphorylation and dephosphorylation in cell cycle.

The normal Rb protein prevents mitosis. Child starts with heterozygous alleles (RB/RB+). Only one mutation is required to produce disease (RB/RB). Mutations resulting in loss of heterozygosity (LOH) occur in rapidly dividing cells, responsible for multiple tumors including bilateral retinoblastoma.

- *Sporadic retinoblastoma:* Sporadic retinoblastoma constitutes 60% of retinoblastoma cases. It develops in children with no family history. A single tumor appears in one eye sometime in early childhood before the retina is fully developed and mitosis in it ceases. Child starts with two wild type alleles (RB+/RB+). Both alleles must mutate to produce the disease (RB/RB). Probability of both mutations occuring in the same cell is low, resulting in unilateral retinoblastoma. RB gene mutation associated with familial and sporadic tumors is shown in Table 6.35.

Light Microscopy

- Tumor is composed of small round cells with hyperchromatic nuclei and scant cytoplasm, numerous mitoses and formation of **Flexner-Wintersteiner rosettes.**
- These rosettes show central lumen lined by pink material with nuclei away from lumen (Fig. 6.49).

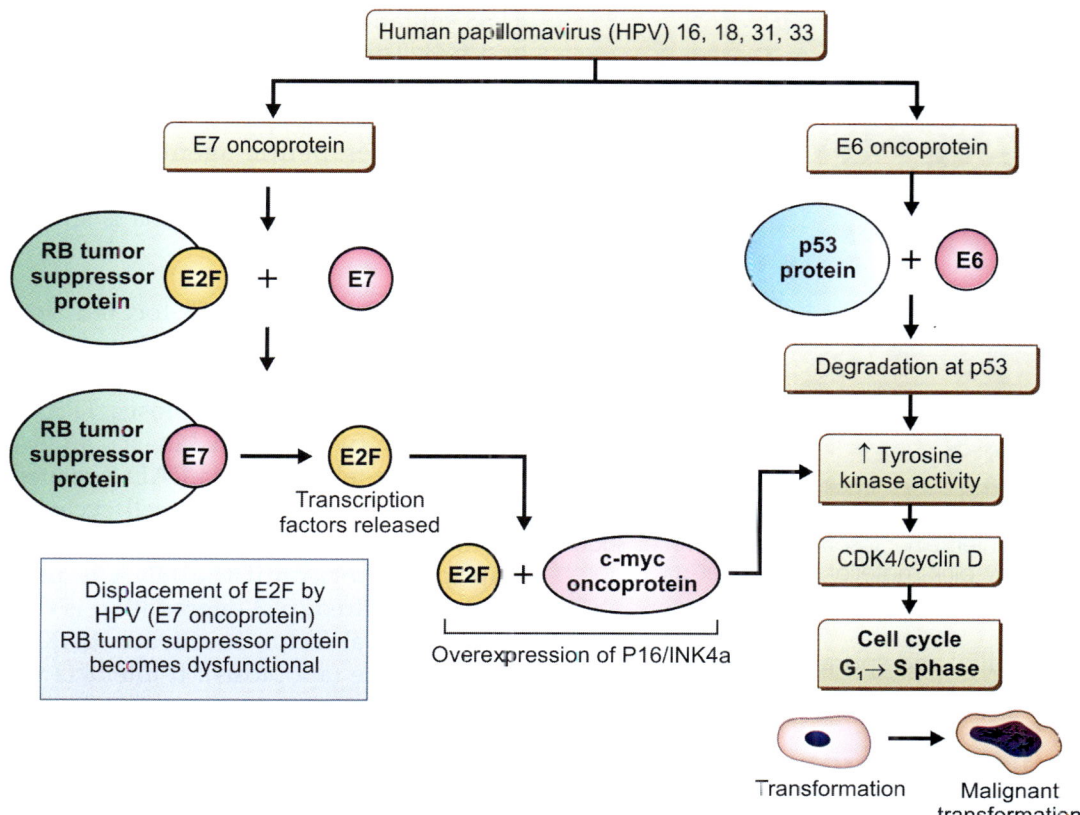

Fig. 6.48: Principles of HPV E6/E7 oncogene activity in cancer. E7 protein of HPV inhibits RB gene.

Table 6.35: RB gene mutation associated with familial and sporadic tumors

Gene and locus	Protein	Function	Familial tumors due to gene mutation (deletion and nonsense)	Sporadic cancers due to gene mutation (deletion and nonsense)
RB gene (locus 13p14)	Retinoblastoma protein	It codes for pRB protein, master brake on cell cycle. It inhibits G_1 to S transition during cell cycle. It inhibits nuclear transcription factor	Retinoblastoma Osteosarcoma	Retinoblastoma Osteosarcoma Breast carcinoma Colon carcinoma Prostatic carcinoma Urinary bladder carcinoma Lung carcinoma

ANGIOGENESIS INHIBITORS GENES

VHL, SDHB, SDHD and STK11 tumor suppressor gene products inhibit angiogenesis in cancers.

VHL (von Hippel-Lindau) Tumor Suppressor Gene

VHL (von Hippel-Lindau) protein is located on chromosome 3p25. It inhibits hypoxia inducible factor-α (HIF-α). It regulates nuclear transcription. VHL gene mutation associated with familial and sporadic tumors is shown in Table 6.36.

SDHB and SDHD Tumor Suppressor Genes

Succinate dehydrogenase subunits of B and D participate in TCA cycle and oxidative phosphorylation. SDHB and SDHD gene mutations associated with familial and sporadic tumors are shown in Table 6.37.

STK11 Tumor Suppressor Gene

Liver kinase-B1 (LKB1) or STK11 activates AMPK family of kinases. It suppresses cell growth when cell nutrients and energy levels are low. STK11 gene mutation

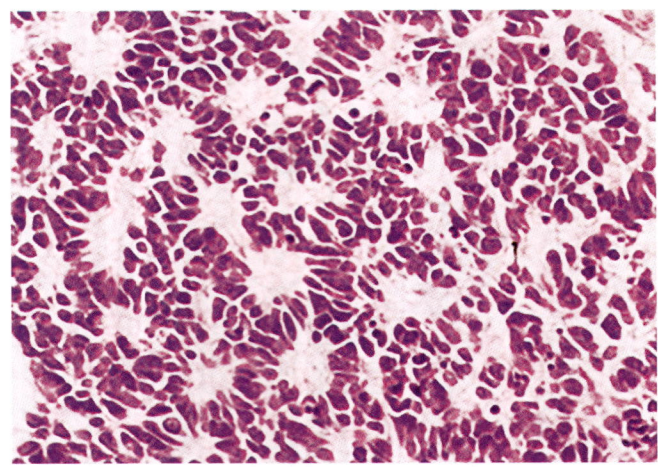

Fig. 6.49: Retinoblastoma shows small round cells with hyperchromatic nuclei and scant cytoplasm, numerous mitoses and formation of Flexner-Wintersteiner rosettes. These rosettes show central lumen lined by pink material with nuclei away from lumen (400X).

GENOMIC STABILITY ENABLER (MOST IMPORTANT)

TP53 Tumor Suppressor Gene

TP53 tumor suppressor gene located on chromosome 17p is known as *guardian of the genome* or molecular policeman. More than 50% of cancers show TP53 mutation. Other family members comprise p63 and p73. This p63 gene participates in differentiation of stratified squamous epithelia. On the other hand, p73 gene causes apoptosis of damaged cells as a result of chemotherapeutic agents. Role of TP53 tumor suppressor gene product p53 protein in maintaining integrity of the human genome is shown in Figs 6.50 and 6.51.

Physiological state: TP53 located on 17q13 is the guardian of the genome. Its p53 protein product senses DNA damage and slows the cycle to allow repair. If repair fails it induces apoptosis. TP53 sensors DNA damage by two protein kinases such as ATM and ATR (ataxia-telangiectasia RAD-3 related). TP53 gene product (p53 protein) halts cell cycle in G_1/S checkpoint for DNA repair by inhibiting nuclear transcription factor, until the DNA is repaired. When DNA is repaired, p53 degradation is done by MDM2 transcriptional factor. It activates BAX gene resulting in cell suicide (apoptosis). It interacts with at least 17 cellular and viral proteins.

Pathological state: TP53 gene product (p53 protein) is inactivated by viral oncoproteins like E6 protein of HPV. Anoxia, inappropriate signaling by mutated oncoproteins and DNA damage activate p53. TP53 gene mutation associated with familial and sporadic tumors is shown in Table 6.39.

Table 6.36: VHL tumor suppressor gene mutation associated with familial and sporadic tumors

Gene and locus	Protein	Function	Familial tumors due to gene mutation by deletion	Sporadic cancers due to gene mutation by deletion
VHL (locus 3p25)	von Hippel-Lindua (VHL) protein	In inhibits hypoxia inducible factor (HIF1a). It regulates nuclear transcription	von Hippel-Lindau syndrome (cerebellar hemangioblastoma, retinal angiomas, renal cell carcinoma (bilateral, and pheochromocytoma)	Renal cell carcinoma

Table 6.37: SDHB and SDHD gene mutations associated with familial and sporadic tumors

Gene	Protein and locus	Function	Familial tumors due to gene mutation	Sporadic cancers due to gene mutation
SDHB, SDHD	Succinate dehydrogenase subunits of B and D	These participate in TCA cycle and oxidative phosphorylation	Paraganglioma Pheochromocytoma	Paraganglioma

Table 6.38: STK11 gene mutation associated with familial and sporadic tumors

Gene	Protein	Function	Familial tumors due to gene mutation	Sporadic cancers due to gene mutation
STK11	Liver kinase B1 (LKB1)	It activates AMPK family of kinases. It suppresses cell growth when cell nutrients and energy levels are low	Peutz-Jeghers syndrome (cancers of GIT, pancreas)	Diverse carcinomas in 5 to 20% of cases

Neoplasia: Molecular Basis, Metastasis, Clinical Oncology and Laboratory Diagnosis

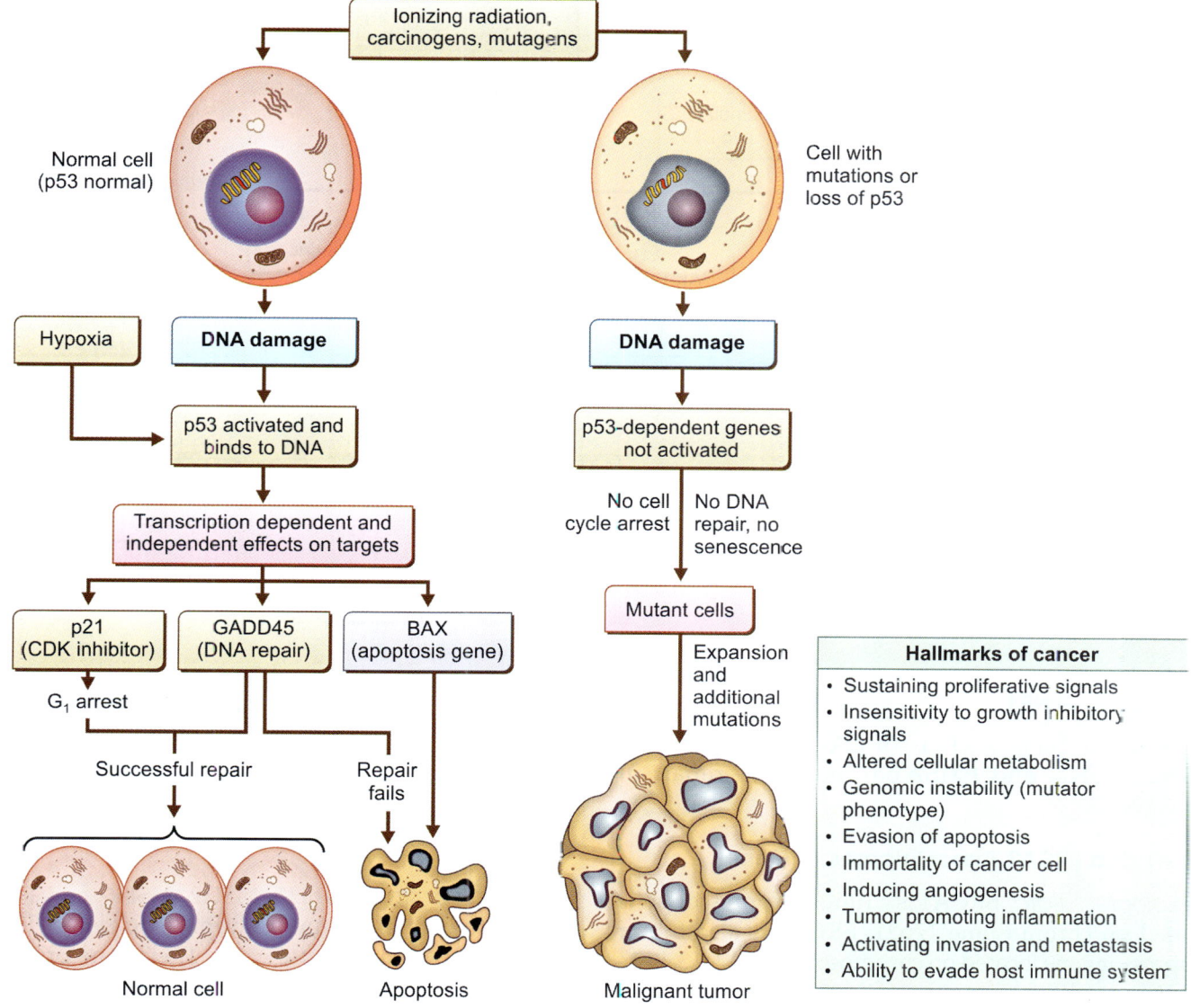

Fig. 6.50: Role of TP53 tumor suppressor gene product, p53 protein in maintaining integrity of the human genoma. In the presence of normal p53 gene, cells with mutation resulting in carcinogenic stimulus are arrested in G_1 of cell cycle by upregulation of cyclin-dependent kinase inhibior CDKN1A (p21) and GADD45 genes until either the DNA mutation is repaired in mild damage or undergoing apoptosis in severe damage. If p53 is defective, carcinogen induced damaged cell proceeds to S phase. Such mutation is propagated to duaghter cells, possibly leading to malignant tumor formation.

Table 6.39: TP53 tumor suppressor gene mutation associated with familial and sporadic tumors

Gene	Protein	Function	Familial tumors	Sporadic cancers
TP53 (locus 17p13.1)	p53	Inhibits cell cycle G_1 to S phase Repairs DNA Induces cell suicide (apoptosis) by activating BAX gene	Li-Fraumeni syndrome (carcinoma breast and adrenal cortex, sarcoma, leukemia, brain tumors)	Pancreatic carcinoma (50–70%) Breast carcinoma Lung carcinoma Colon carcinoma

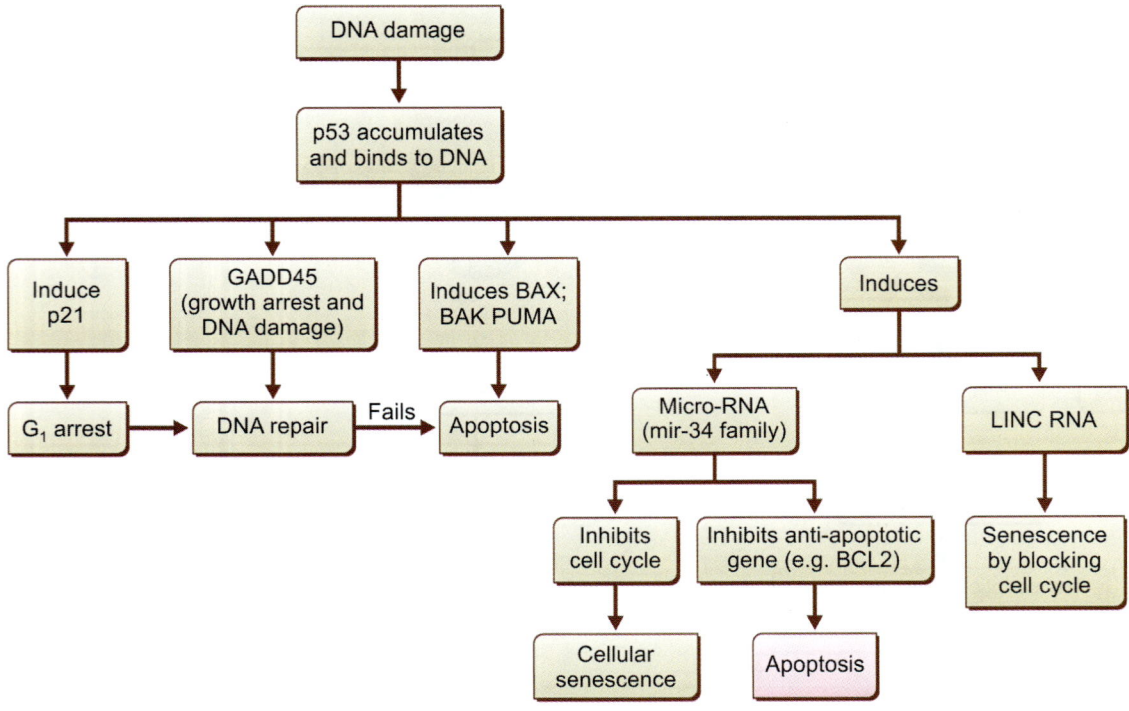

Fig. 6.51: p53 Guardian of human genome.

DNA REPAIR GENES

DNA repair genes such as BRCA1, BRCA2, MLH1, MSH2, MSH6, and PMS2 participate in repair of damaged DNA.

BRCA1 and BRCA2 Tumor Suppressor Genes

Physiological state: BRCA1 is a tumor suppressor gene located on chromosome 17p21. BRCA2 is also tumor suppressor gene located on chromosome 13q12–13. Both BRCA1 and BRCA2 regulate DNA repair by binding to RAD51, a molecule that mediates repair of double-stranded DNA. It encodes tumor suppressor proteins involved in checkpoint functions related to progression of the cell cycle into S phase.

Pathological state: Gene mutation of BRCA1 and BRCA2 occurs by methylation. BRCA1 is responsible for 52% familial breast cancers and 1–2% of all breast cancers. BRCA2 gene mutation is responsible for 32% familial breast cancers and up to 2% of all **breast cancers**.

Risk is increased in age group by 70 years in 30–90% cases. BRCA2 gene mutation is rare in sporadic cases (Table 6.40).

MLH1, MSH2, MSH6, and PMS2 Tumor Suppressor Genes

Physiological state: MLH1, MSH2, MSH6, and PMS2 belong to caretaker tumor suppressor genes. These are also known as *mutator genes*. Their gene products ensure the integrity of the cellular genome by replication and mismatch DNA repairs. DNA blood tests are now available for evaluation of all four genes.

Pathological state: Mutation of DNA mismatch repair gene leads to accumulation of numerous mismatched errors in DNA replications. Patient develops *hereditary nonpolyposis syndrome colon carcinoma*.

Hereditary nonpolyposis colon cancer (Lynch syndrome): Lynch syndrome occurs due to inactivation

Table 6.40: BRAC1 and BRAC2 gene mutations associated with familial and sporadic tumors

Gene	Protein	Function	Familial tumors	Sporadic cancers
BRCA1 (locus on 17)	BRCA1 protein	It binds RAD51 molecule that mediates repair of double-stranded breaks in DNA	Cancers of ovary, breast, prostate, pancreas and fallopian tube	Rare mutated in breast, medullary and metaplastic carcinomas
BRCA2 (locus on 13)	BRCA2 protein	It binds RAD51 molecule that mediates repair of double-stranded breaks in DNA	Cancers of stomach, gallbladder, bile duct, pharynx and melanoma	Fanconi anemia

of DNA mismatch repair genes (principally MLH1, MSH2, MSH6, and PMS2). These mutator genes are unable to correct errors in nucleotide pairing. Extensive history of screening of early development of these cancers is required in the management of these patients.

- *Associated tumors:* There is increased risk of development of carcinoma of *endometrium (first most common cancer)*, ovary and right colon carcinoma. Right colon carcinoma is often preceded by serrated adenomas, rather than tubular adenomas seen in the traditional APC tumor pathway.

- *Other cancers:* There is increased risk of development of cancers of urothelium, brain and stomach in these patients. Microsatellite instability is seen in 90% of the tumors that develop in these patients. A variant that involves a propensity for *sebaceous tumors of the skin* is known as *Muir-Torre syndrome*.

FUNCTIONS OF GENES BY VARIOUS MECHANISMS

Tumor suppressor genes functioning by different mechanisms associated with familial and sporadic tumors are shown in Table 6.41.

WT1 Tumor Suppressor Gene

WT1 tumor suppressor gene is located on chromosome 11p13. It regulates nuclear transcriptional factor. Nonsense WT1 gene mutation results in *familial Wilms' tumor, sporadic Wilms' tumor and certain leukemias*.

MEN 1 Tumor Suppressor Gene

MEN 1 protein (menin) regulates transcriptional factor. MEN 1 gene mutation is associated with familial multiple neoplasia syndrome 1 (*tumors of pituitary, parathyroid and pancreas*) and sporadic tumors of pituitary, parathyroid and pancreas.

DPC4 (MADH4/SMAD4) Tumor Suppressor Gene

DPC4 is located on chromosome 18q21.1. It codes for relay molecule in cell division inhibitory pathway. DPC4 gene mutation rarely causes familial tumors. Gene mutation is demonstrated in sporadic cases such as *cancers of pancreas (most common), breast and ovaries*.

ATM Tumor Suppressor Gene

ATM is a caretaker tumor suppressor gene located on chromosome 11p22. It may downregulate tyrosine activity. Patients carrying ATM gene mutation have a

Table 6.41: Tumor suppressor genes functioning by different mechanisms associated with familial and sporadic tumors

Gene	Protein	Function	Familial tumors	Sporadic cancers
WT1 [(WT1) on 11p13.]	Wilms' tumor 1, nonsense mutation	Transcriptional factor	Familial Wilms' tumor	Wilms' tumor Certain leukemias
MEN 1	Menin	Transcriptional factor	Multiple neoplasia syndrome 1 (MEN 1: Tumors of pituitary, parathyroid and pancreas)	Tumors of pituitary, parathyroid and pancreas
DPC4 (MADH4/SMAD4) locus 18q21.1	DPC4	It codes for relay molecule in cell division inhibitory pathway	Rare	Cancer of pancreas (most common), breast and ovaries
ATM (locus 11p22)	ATM	Unknown/tyrosine	Ataxia-telangiectasia, breast cancer, stomach cancer, leukemia	Unknown
p16 (locus 9p21)	p16	It inhibits nuclear cyclin D dependent kinase activity	Familial melanoma	Mesotheliomas, carcinoma pancreas, melanoma, astrocytoma
TGF-β (locus 19q)	TGF-β	It inhibits G_1 to S phase	-	Cancers of pancreas, colorectal region
CHEK2 (locus 22q12.1)	CHEK2	CHEK2 induces cell cycle arrest. It repairs damaged DNA. It activates BRCA1 and p53 tumor suppressor genes by phosphorylation	Breast carcinoma (5%)	Cancers of breast prostate, thyroid, and kidney especially after radiation

reduced capacity to repair DNA breaks and are prone to accumulating numerous genetic mutations overtime. Mutation of ATM (deletion) has been demonstrated in *inherited ataxia-telangiectasia, leukemia, lymphoma, breast and stomach cancers*. Ataxiatelangiectasia is characterized by cerebellar ataxia, immunodeficiency, and dilations of small blood vessels. Sporadic tumors are unknown.

Tumor p16 Suppressor Gene

Tumor suppressor p16 gene is located on chromosome 9p21. It inhibits cyclin D dependent kinase activity. Patient with gene mutation develops *familial melanoma*. In sporadic tumors, it is most frequently inactivated tumor suppressor genes in carcinoma of pancreas in 90% of cases. Mutation of p16 (deletion and nonsense) has also been demonstrated in *mesotheliomas, carcinoma, pancreas, melanoma, and astrocytoma*.

TGF-β Tumor Suppressor Gene

TGF-β tumor suppressor gene is located on chromosome 19q. It inhibits G_1 to S phase of cell cycle. In sporadic cases, mutation of TGF-β has been demonstrated in *pancreatic and colorectal cancers*. Familial tumors are unknown.

CHEK2 Tumor Suppressor Gene

CHEK2 a tumor suppressor gene is located on chromosome 22q12.1. CHEK2 induces cell cycle arrest. It repairs damaged DNA. It activates BRCA1 and p53 tumor suppressor genes by phosphorylation. Gene mutation is responsible f or 5% of *familial breast carcinomas*. Approximately 70–80% of breast cancers are ER positive. In sporadic cases, CHEK2 gene mutation increases risk of breast *cancer in 10–20% cases by 70 years of age especially after radiation exposure*. Gene mutation is also demonstrated in cancers of prostate, thyroid and kidney.

ALTERED CELLULAR METABOLISM

Malignant cells preferentially utilize glucose by glycolysis for energy purpose rather than more energy efficient mitochondrial oxidative phosphorylation pathways. This phenomenon is known as *Warburg effect* or aerobic glycolysis. Aerobic glycolysis provides glucose to the rapidly dividing cancer cells for synthesis of cellular components such as DNA, RNA, and proteins required before cell division, whereas oxidative mitochondrial phosphorylation pathway does not. Oxidative phosphorylation yields abundant ATP for the synthesis of cellular components. This metabolic reprogramming is produced by signaling cascade downstream of growth factor receptors.

EVASION OF APOPTOSIS

Physiological state: Normally, apoptosis occurrs by extrinsic death receptor pathway, and intrinsic mitochondrial pathway.

The extrinsic pathway is activated by signal such as Fas ligand (Fasl), that on binding to the Fas receptor, forming a death-inducing complex by joining the Fas-associated death domain (FADD) to the death domain of the Fas receptor.

Intrinsic pathway is activated by injurious stimuli such as reactive oxygen species and DNA damage that induce the release of mitochondrial cytochrome c into the cytoplasm. Both pathways of apoptosis differ in their

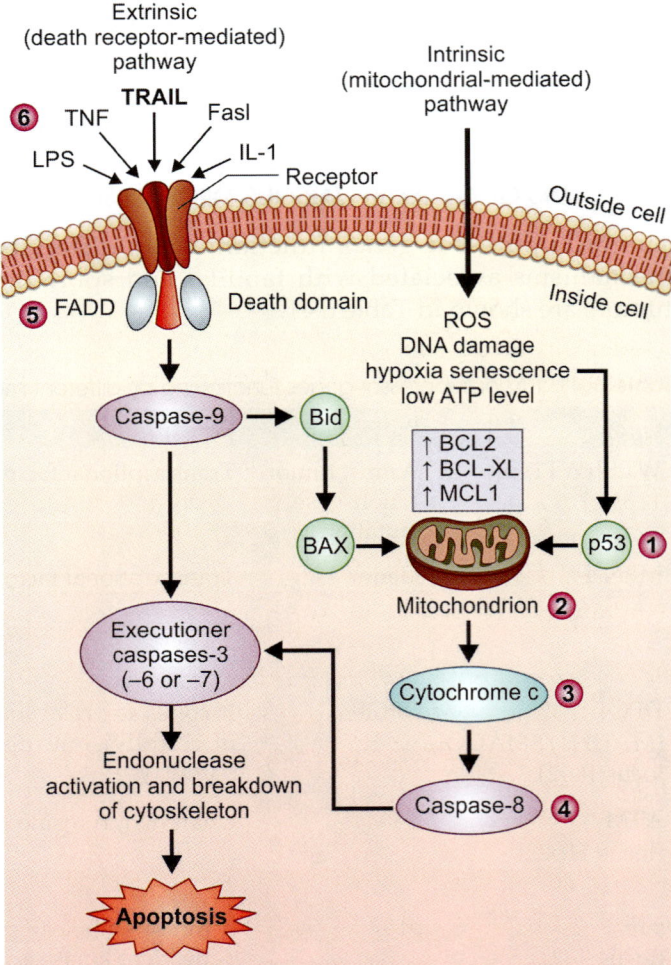

Fig. 6.52: Intrinsic and extrinsic pathways of apoptosis and mechanisms used by tumor cells to evade programmed cell death. (1) Loss of p53 leads to reduced function of pro-apoptotic factors such as BAX. (2) Reduced egress of cytochrome c from mitochondria as a result of upregulation of anti-apoptotic factors such as BCL2, B3CLX and MCL1. (3) Loss of apoptotic peptidase activating factor 1 (APAF1). (4) Upregulation of inhibitors of apoptosis (AP). (5) Reduced CD95 level in hepatocellular carcinoma. (6) Inactivation of death-induced signaling complex FADD (Fas associated via death domain).

induction and regulation. Both pathways culminate in the activation of 'executioner' caspases.

Pathological state: The cancer cells continue to proliferate without undergoing apoptosis. Some tumors have high level of protein that binds to death inducing signals complex and that prevents the activation of caspase 8.

BCL2 activation in **Burkitt's lymphoma** in the translocation of chromosome t(14;18) helps in protecting lymphocytes from apoptosis. CD95 is reduced in hepatocellular carcinoma. Downregulation of apoptotic gene products (BAX gene) and upregulation of antiapoptotic gene products (BCL2) are responsible for promotion of tumorigenesis.

Intrinsic apoptotic pathway (mitochondrial pathway) is most often disabled in cancers. Intrinsic and extrinsic pathways of apoptosis and mechanisms used by tumor cells to evade programmed cell death are shown in Fig. 6.52. Mechanism of evasion of apoptosis is described as under.

DOWNREGULATION OF BAX APOPTOTIC GENES

BAX Apoptotic Gene Product

Under physiological state, BAX apoptotic gene protein participates in programmed cell death after a limited lifespan. It inactivates BCL2 antiapototic gene. When DNA damage occurs, TP53 gene product activates BAX gene. Mutation of BAX gene contributes immortalization of cancer cells.

TP53 Tumor Suppressor Gene Product

Under physiological state, TP53 gene product inhibits cell cycle G_1 to S phase. It repairs DNA. It induces cell suicide (apoptosis) by activating BAX apoptotic gene. It interacts with at least 17 cellular and viral proteins. TP53 gene mutation renders the BAX gene inoperative, which prevents apoptosis. Mutation of BAX apoptotic gene may contribute to immortalization of cancer cells.

Loss of apoptotic peptidase activating factor (APAF1) and upregulation of inhibitors of apoptosis (IAP) promote immortalization of cancer cells.

UPREGULATION OF ANTIAPOPTOTIC GENES

BCL Family

BCL family comprises BCL2, BCL XL and MCL1. BCL2 gene family located on chromosome 18 produces gene products that prevent mitochondrial leakage of cytochrome c (signal for apoptosis). Upregulation of BCL family prevents apoptosis leading to immortalization of malignant cells.

Physiological state: Normally cytochrome c leaving mitochondria and entering into the cytosol activates caspases and initiate apoptosis. Protein product of antiapoptotic BCL2 gene prevents cytochrome c from leaving mitochondria.

Pathological state: Translocation t(14;18) causes overexpression of the BCL2 protein product, which prevents apoptosis of B-lymphocytes causing *B cell follicular lymphoma and chronic lymphocytic leukemia.* Lymphoma cells do not die but accumulate in the **lymph nodes, bone marrow**, and the **blood circulation**. Overexpression of MCL1 (a BCL2 member) plays an important role in drug resistance of tumors.

LIMITLESS REPLICATIVE POTENTIAL

The cancer cells have limitless replicative potential. More than 90% of tumors show **increased telomerase activity**. Cancer cells overcome these limitations by reactivating telomerase activity. Telomerase is a DNA polymerase expressed in germ cells and somatic cells. **Telomerase activity** is **maximum** in **germ cells.** Telomerase is not active in somatic cells (Fig. 6.53).

Physiological state: Most normal human cells have a capacity of 60–70 doubling, after the cell enters nonreplicative senescence resulting in shortening of telomeres at the end of chromosome. Loss of telomeres beyond a certain point will lead to massive chromosomal abnormalities and death.

Chromosomal telomeres progressively shorter with each cell division until DNA replication can no longer proceed. Shortened telomeres are demonstrated by DNA repair machinery as *double-stranded breaks* causing cell cycle halt via p53 and RB gene resulting in cellular senescence.

Pathological state: In order to develop tumor, maintenance of cells and avoid cell senescence is done by upregulation of telomerase enzyme. Uncontrolled cell division progression takes place in cancers. Mutations of RB gene and p53 gene activate non-homologous end joining (NHEJ) resulting in fusion of shortened ends of two chromosomes.

This inappropriate DNA repair forms dicentric chromosomes, which break during anaphase to form new round of double-stranded breaks. This genetic instability of repeated cycles of bridge-fusion breakage leads to mitotic catastrophe and cell death.

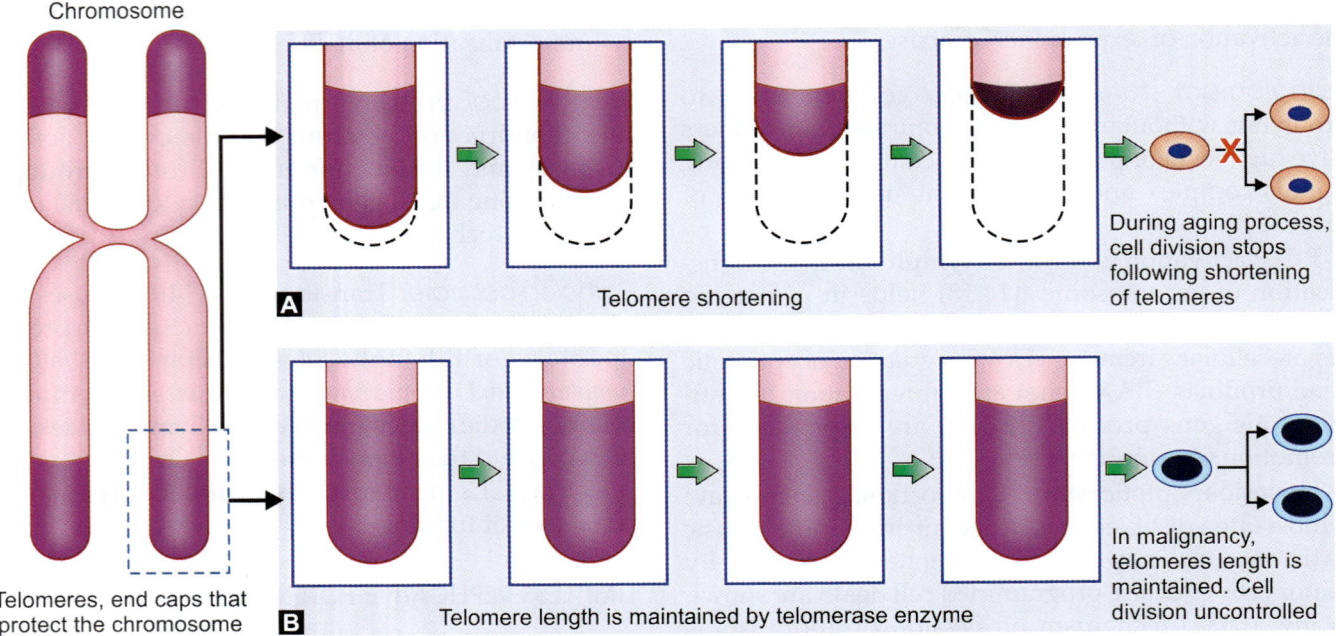

Fig. 6.53: Telomeres are the caps at the end of chromosomes that shorten as aging process continues. (A) During aging process, cell division stops following shortening of telomeres, (B) in malignancy, length of the telomeres is maintained by telomerase enzyme. Uncontrolled cell division takes place in cancers.

ANGIOGENESIS

Angiogenesis denotes formation of new blood vessels. It occurs as a result of imbalance between angiogenic and anti-angiogenic factors synthesized by the tumor and inflammatory cells (Table 6.42). It is essential for the *continued growth and survival of cancers, whether primary or metastatic*. In the absence of new vessels to supply the nutrients and removal of waste products; malignant tumors do not grow >1 to 2 mm in diameter.

Hypoxia induces synthesis of hypoxia inducible factor-α (HIF-α) transcriptional factor resulting in formation of new blood vessels. TP53 inhibits angiogenesis by stimulation of anti-angiogenesis molecules. VEGF is under the control of RAS oncogene. Proteases are involved in regulating angiogenic and anti-angiogenic factors.

UPREGULATION OF ANGIOGENIC FACTORS

Malignant tumors and host inflammatory cells in the tumor synthesize angiogenic factors (e.g. **VEGF, FGF, TGF-β, angiotensin, platelet activating factor**). Vascular endothelial growth factor is important in the proliferation of blood vessels in a growing tumor. New vessels in the tumor are **torturous, irregular, leaky** blood vessels. Eventually, the tumor outgrows its blood supply, and areas of necrosis appear resulting in slower growth. *VEGF inhibitors are used to treat advanced cancers.*

DOWNREGULATION OF ANTI-ANGIOGENIC FACTORS

Anti-angiogenic factors may play an important role in controlling cancer. Downregulation of anti-angiogenic factors (**angiostatin, endostatin, vasculostatin, and thrombospondin 1**) occurs in cancer.

INVASION AND METASTASIS

Invasion and metastasis constitute important hallmark of malignant tumors. Tumor cells invade basement membrane and stromal extracellular matrix. After invading the interstitial tissue, cancer cells penetrate lymphatic or vascular channels. *In the lymph nodes, communications between the lymphatic channels and venous tributaries allow malignant cells access to the systemic circulation.*

Table 6.42: Angiogenic and anti-angiogenic factors

Factors in relation to angiogenesis	Examples
Angiogenic factors	VEGF
	FGF
	TGF-β
	Angiotensin
	Platelet activating factor
Anti-angiogenic factors	Angiostatin
	Endostatin
	Vasculostatin
	Thrombospondin 1

Neoplasia: Molecular Basis, Metastasis, Clinical Oncology and Laboratory Diagnosis

Table 6.43: Tumor cells expressing various types of tumor antigens

Categories of mutated protein	Examples of mutated protein
Mutated products of oncogene	RAS
	BCR/ABL fusion
Mutated products of tumor suppressor gene	p53
Mutated self-protein	Mutant protein in carcinogen
	Mutant protein in melanoma
Overexpression or aberrantly expressed self-protein	Tyrosinase (gp 100) and MART
Oncogenic viral antigen	E6, E7 protein of HPV in cervical carcinoma
	EBNA proteins in EB virus induced lymphoma

EVASION OF HOST IMMUNE SYSTEM

Tumor antigens are derived from mutated proto-oncogenes and tumor suppressor genes or oncogenic viruses (Table 6.43). MHC1 molecules present tumor antigen to CD8+ cytotoxic T cells. Apoptosis of CD8+ T cells occurs as a result of tumor cell FasL expression. Immune system can recognize and destroy tumor cells by cell-mediated mechanism (Fig. 6.54).

The cancer cells continue to proliferate and escape themselves from immune system by the following mechanisms.

Selective Outgrowths of Antigenic Negative Tumor Variants

Immune system fails to recognize tumors lacking antigens due to selective outgrowths of antigenic negative variant of tumors. Cancer cells express different types of tumor antigens. These tumor antigens include oncogenic mutated products (RAS or BCR/ABL fusion proteins), mutated p53 protein of tumor suppressor gene, mutated radiation induced self-protein, overexpression of aberrantly expressed self-protein such as tyrosinase (gp 100, MART1), cancer testis antigens (MAGE, BAGE), mutated proteins of E6, E7 of HPV in cervical cancer and EBNA proteins in EBV induced lymphoma. Immune evasion by tumor due to lack of recognition T cells is shown in Fig. 6.55.

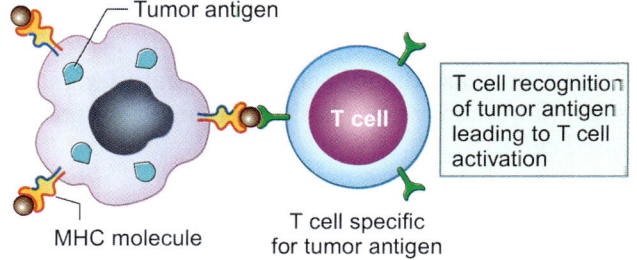

Fig. 6.54: Anti-tumor immune response showing recognition of tumor antigen by T cells.

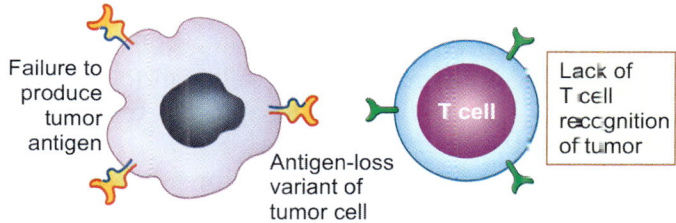

Fig. 6.55: Immune evasion by tumor due to lack of recognition T cells.

Loss or Decreased Expression of MHC1 Molecules

Normally, MHC 1 molecules present tumor antigen to CD8+ cytotoxic T cells. Loss or decreased expression of MHC1 molecules leads to escape of tumor cells from immune system. Immune evasion by tumor due to mutations in MHC genes needed for antigen processing is shown in Fig. 6.56.

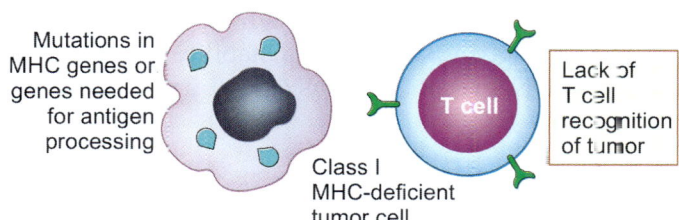

Fig. 6.56: Immune evasion by tumor due to mutations in MHC genes needed for antigen processing.

Synthesis of Immunosuppressive Factors by Cancer Cells

Tumor cells synthesize TGF-β, PD1 ligands (programmed cell death) and galectins leading to suppression of immune system. Immunosuppressed persons are at increased risk of development of cancer by oncogenic DNA viruses (HPV and Epstein-Barr virus). Immune evasion by tumor due to synthesis of immunosuppressive proteins (TGF-β) is shown in Fig. 6.57.

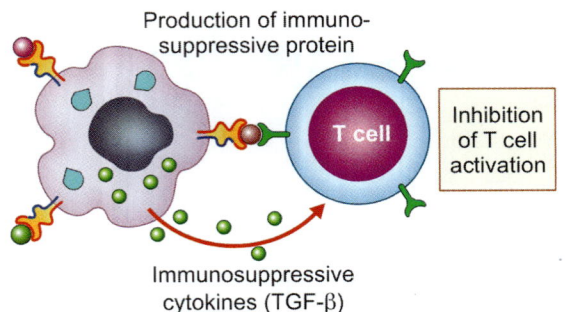

Fig. 6.57: Immune evasion by tumor due to synthesis of immuno-suppressive proteins (TGF-β).

Lack of Expression of Co-stimulatory Molecules

Tumor cells may downregulate expression of co-stimulatory molecules on antigen presenting cells inducing anergy. These antigen presenting cells fail to activate stimulatory CD28 and instead activate inhibitory receptor CTLA4 on effector T cells.

Cancer cells may upregulate the expression of PDL1 and PDL2 receptors on T cells. In advanced cancer, antibodies are administered to inhibit receptors such as PD1 and CTLA4 expressed on T cells in clinical practice.

Tumor Antigen Masking

Tumor antigens are masked as a result of increased synthesis of glycocalyx on tumor cells.

GENOMIC INSTABILITY

DNA repair genes maintain genomic stability by correcting errors in nucleotide pairing and excising pyrimidine dimmers in ultraviolet-damaged skin. Mutations of DNA repair proteins allow cells with lethal damage to proliferate, which increases the risk of carcinogenesis (genomic instability syndromes). Defects of DNA repair proteins occur by the following mechanisms.

MISMATCH REPAIR

Mismatch repairs (e.g. MSH2, MSH1) are spellchecker to correct errors in multiple genes including tumor proto-oncogenes and tumor suppressor genes. Mismatch repair is reflected by microsatellite instability. Variations of microsatellite length are a hallmark of mismatch repair defects.

Under physiological state, microsatellites are tandem repeats of one to six nucleotides throughout genome with constant length. Example of mismatch repair is *hereditary nonpolyposis colon carcinoma*.

NUCLEOTIDE EXCISION REPAIR DEFECTS

Nucleotide excision repair genes are essential to correct ultraviolet induced pyrimidine dimer formation. Example of nucleotide excision repair genes is **xeroderma pigmentosum**. There is increased risk of development of *skin carcinoma* in patient with xeroderma pigmentosum.

RECOMBINATION REPAIR DEFECTS

Defects in homologous recombination occur in ataxia-telangiectasia, Fanconi syndrome, Bloom syndrome and BRCA genes.

Ataxia-telangiectasia

Under physiological state, ATM gene encodes a helicase that participates in DNA repair by homologous recombination. Helicase that repairs DNA by homologous recombination.

Fanconi Anemia

Fanconi anemia is a rare autosomal recessive disorder. It is caused by defects in multiprotein defects that required for DNA repair. Patient develops bone marrow suppression and multiple congenital anomalies such as hypoplasia of bones of thumbs or radius, kidney or spleen. Person with Fanconi anemia shows BRCA2 mutations.

BRCA1 and BRCA2 Tumor Suppressor Genes

These participate in the repair of double-stranded DNA by homologous recombination. Mutations of these genes are responsible for 25% of cases of *familial breast cancer*. BRCA1 mutation is demonstrated in *cancers of ovary and prostate*. Defective germline BRCA2 increases cancers of *ovary, prostate, pancreas, stomach, bile ducts and melanocytes*.

CANCER-ENABLING INFLAMMATION

Invading cancers evoke chronic inflammatory reactions resulting in systemic manifestations such as *anemia* as a result of *downregulation of erythropoietin*. Inflammatory cells also modify the local microenvironment to enable many of the hallmarks of cancer. Proposed cancer-enabling effects of inflammatory cells and resident cells are described as under.

Synthesis of Growth Factors by ECM

EGF and proteases synthesized extracellular matrix cause inflammatory cells infiltration and activation of stromal cells.

Degradation of Adhesion Molecules

Proteases synthesized by inflammatory cells degrade adhesion molecules and suppress cell-cell and cell-ECM interactions.

Enhanced Resistance to Cell Death

Tumor associated macrophages participate in enhanced resistance to cell death called *amoikis* by expression adhesion molecule integrins. The integrins mediate physical interactions with cancer cells. This sustained stromal cell–cancer cell interactions enhance resistance of cancer cells to chemotherapeutic agents by activating signal pathways that promote cancer cell survival.

Inducing Angiogenesis

VEGF family comprises VEGF-C and VEGF-D. VEGF synthesized by inflammatory cells participate in angiogenesis in malignant tumor via three tyrosine kinase receptors.

Promoting Invasion and Metastasis

TGF-β synthesized by *macrophages, T cells, endothelial cells and platelets* promotes epithelial–mesenchymal transitions, which are considered to be key event in the invasion and metastasis of cancer cells. EGF is synthesized by *macrophages, keratinocytes,* and other inflammatory cells. Amplification of EGFR1 occurs in *glioblastoma and cancers of the lung, head and neck,* and breast.

Evading Immune Destruction of Cancer Cells

TGF-β synthesized by macrophages, T cells, endothelial cells and platelets favor recruitment of immunosuppressive T regulatory cells resulting in suppression of functions of CD8+ cytotoxic T cells. Various cytokines synthesized by activated macrophages participate in angiogenesis, proliferation of fibroblasts and ECM deposition.

DYSREGULATION OF GENES

Chromosomal changes and epigenetic changes (e.g. DNA methylation) may induce malignant transformation.

CHROMOSOMAL CHANGES

Proto-oncogenes are transformed into oncogenes by the following mechanisms: point mutation, gene amplification, balanced translocations without loss of genetic material, deletions with loss of genetic material, overexpression of gene activity and chromosomal rearrangements.

Point Mutation

Point mutation is the most common type of mutation, in which a single base substitution in the DNA resulting in a miscoded protein. Point mutation of genes associated cancer is shown in Table 6.44.

Table 6.44: Point mutation of genes associated cancers

Point mutation of gene	Cancers
RAS gene	Pancreas carcinoma Colon carcinoma Lung carcinoma
FLT3 gene	Leukemia
RET gene	MEN 2A MEN 2B
KIT gene	Gastric carcinoma Colon carcinoma Seminoma Leukemia
GNAP gene	Uveal melanoma
GNAS gene	Pituitary adenoma and other endocrinal tumors

Deletion

Deletion of genes occurs with loss of genetic material. Deletion most often occurs in non-hematopoietic solid tumors and T cell ALL. Deletion on chromosome 5 produces an oncogenic *EML4-ALK fusion oncogene* demonstrated in *lung adenocarcinoma*. Deletion on chromosome 1 produces TAL1 oncogene resulting in *T cell acute lymphoblastic leukemia*. Deletion of genes associated with cancers is shown in Table 6.45.

Table 6.45: Deletion of genes associated with cancers

Deletion of gene	Cancers
EML4-ALK fusion oncogene	Lung adenocarcinoma
TAL1 oncogene	T cell acute lymphoblastic leukemia

Gene Amplification

Amplification and reduplication of DNA sequences forming multiple copies of gene play an important role in carcinogenesis. *Gene amplification is indicative of more aggressive behavior of malignant tumors.* Cytological analysis of gene amplification reveals homogenous staining regions (HSRs) and abnormal banding regions on chromosomes stained with special stains, and double minutes recognized as small, paired cytoplasmic bodies. Gene amplification are associated cancers are shown in Table 6.46.

Chromosomal Rearrangements

Chromosomal rearrangements occur by translocation and deletions. These form new gene complexes, in which one gene acts as the promoter for the other

Table 6.46: Gene amplification and associated cancers

Gene amplification	Cancers
N-MYC gene	Neuroblastoma (25–30% cases)
FGF3 gene	Osteosarcoma Melanoma Breast carcinoma Gastric carcinoma Urinary bladder transitional cell carcinoima
ERBB1 gene	Lung adenocarcinoma
ERBB2 gene	Breast carcinoma (20% cases)

genes. Chromosomal rearrangements associated cancers are shown in Table 6.47. Examples of chromosomal rearrangement are described as under.

Chronic Myeloid Leukemia

The best-known example of an acquired chromosomal translocation in a human cancer is the Philadelphia chromosome, which is found in 95% of patients with CML.

Reciprocal translocation of ABL (Abelson mouse leukemia on chromosome 9) into the BCR site on chromosome 22 creates the *BCR-ABL fusion protein product* in 90% cases of chronic myeloid leukemia. At the same time, part of the long arm of chromosome 22 is transferred onto the long arm of chromosome 9.

The *BCR-ABL fusion protein product* provides a growth factor by virtue of increased non-receptor protein kinase activity which may amplify normal proliferative signals (Fig. 6.58).

Burkitt's Lymphoma t(8;14)

Translocation of C-MYC oncogene from chromosome 8 to an immunoglobulin heavy gene locus on chromosome 14 results in expression of C-MYC gene. The immunoglobulin gene acts as a promoter for the C-MYC gene. This chromosomal rearrangement is the basis of malignant transformation of lymphocyte in Burkitt's lymphoma (Fig. 6.59).

Ewing's Sarcoma

Translocation involving chromosomes 11 and 22 distinguishes this tumor from neuroblastoma, which may resemble on light microscopy. Approximately 90% of Ewing's sarcomas have a reciprocal translocation between chromosomes 11 and 22(11;22), which result in the fusion of the amino terminus of the EWS1 gene to the FLI1 gene, which encodes a nuclear transcription factor to drive cellular proliferation. Approximately 5–15% of these tumors have q22; q12 translocation. Occasionally translocation (21; 22) may also be seen.

Follicular Center Cell Lymphoma

Follicular center cell lymphoma shows abnormalities in the control of apoptosis. It displays chromosomal translocation t(14;18) in which the BCL2 gene is brought under the transcriptional control of the immunoglobulin light-chain gene promoter, resulting in expression of BCL2 gene inhibiting apoptosis. As a result of the antiapoptotic properties of BCL2, the neoplastic clone accumulates in lymph nodes.

Pediatric Renal Cell Carcinoma

It often demonstrates translocations involving Xp11, with t(X; 17).

Table 6.47: Chromosomal rearrangements associated cancers

Cancers	Chromosomal rearrangements	Effects
Chronic myeloid leukemia	t(9;22) (q34,q11) known as *Philadelphia chromosome*	Fusion oncogene BCR-ABL increases tyrosine kinase activity
Ewing's sarcoma	t(11;22) (q24;q21)	Fusion of FLI1 gene from chromosome 11 with EWS on chromosome 22 leads to fusion protein increased transcription activity
Burkitt's lymphoma	t(8;14) (q24;q32)	Fusion of c-MYC on chromosome 8 with IgH from chromosome 14 leads to c-MYC expression
Follicular center cell lymphoma	t(14;18) (q32;q21)	IgH gene from chromosome 14 fuses to BCL2 gene on chromosome 21 leading to prevention of apoptosis of malignant cells
Synovial sarcoma	t(X;18) (p11;q11)	SYT gene from chromosome 18 is fused to SSX1 and SSX2 gene located on X chromosome. Possible ectopic expression of SSX1 and SSX2 products
Alveolar rhabdomyosarcoma	t(2;13) (q35;14)	PAX3 gene from chromosome 2 is fused with FKHR gene on chromosome 13 leads to a fusion protein with increased transcription factor activity

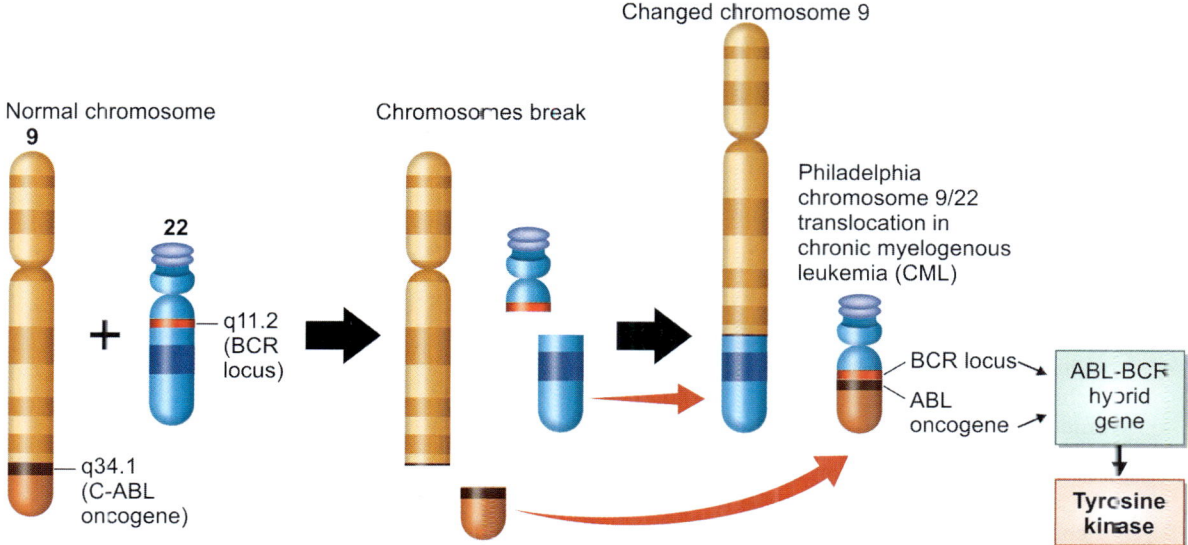

Fig. 6.58: Chronic myeloid leukemia. Reciprocal translocation of ABL (Abelson mouse leukemia on chromosome 9) into the BCR site on chromosome 22 creates the 'BCR-ABL fusion protein product' in 90% cases of chronic myeloid leukemia.

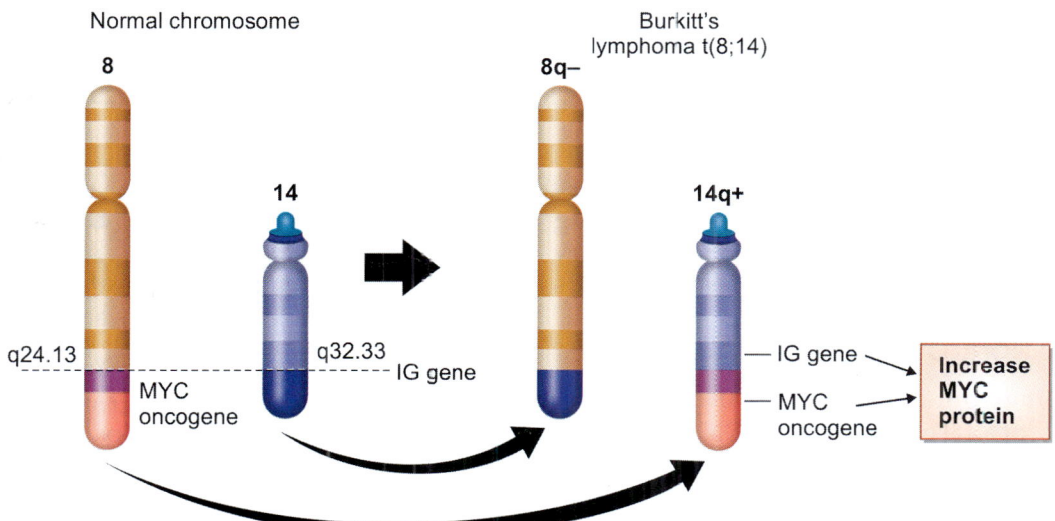

Fig. 6.59: Burkitt's lymphoma t(8;14). Translocation of C-MYC oncogene from chromosome 8 to an immunoglobulin heavy gene locus on chromosome 14 results in expression of C-MYC gene.

Alveolar Soft Part Sarcoma

This translocation (Xp11 with t(X; 17)) is also seen in alveolar soft part sarcoma. But it lacks specificity of translocations in some instances.

Synovial Sarcoma

This translocation t(X; 18) is seen in synovial sarcoma.

Insertional Mutagenesis

This form of oncogene activation occurs due to insertion of a viral gene into the mammalian DNA, resulting in genetic dysregulation. The best example of such an event may be found in hepatitis virus-infected human liver cells resulting in **hepatocellular carcinoma**.

CHROMOTHRIPSIS

Chromothripsis means shattering of chromosomes. It is also known as *dramatic chromosome catastrophe*. Chromosomal breaks are followed by haphazard repair by activating oncogenes and inactivating tumor suppressor genes. Shattering of chromosomes is demonstrated in **osteosarcomas** and **gliomas**. Chromothripsis has been seen to cause oncogene amplification, amplification of oncogene containing regions and the loss of tumor suppressors.

EPIGENETIC CHANGES

Post-translational acetylation of histones and DNA methylation (hyper/hypo) in the absence of primary

Table 6.48: Epigenetic regulatory genes and associated cancers

Genes	Functions	Frequency of mutations in tumors
DNMT3A	DNA methylation	Acute myeloid leukemia (20%)
MLL1	Histone methylation	Acute leukemia in infants (90%)
MLL2	-	Follicular lymphoma
ARIDIA	Nucleosome positioning or chromatin remodeling	Ovarian carcinoma (60%)
SNF5	Nucleosome positioning or chromatin remodeling	Malignant rhabdoid tumor (100%)
PBRM1	-	Renal cell carcinoma
CREBBP/EP300	Histone acetylation	Diffuse large B cell lymphoma (40%)

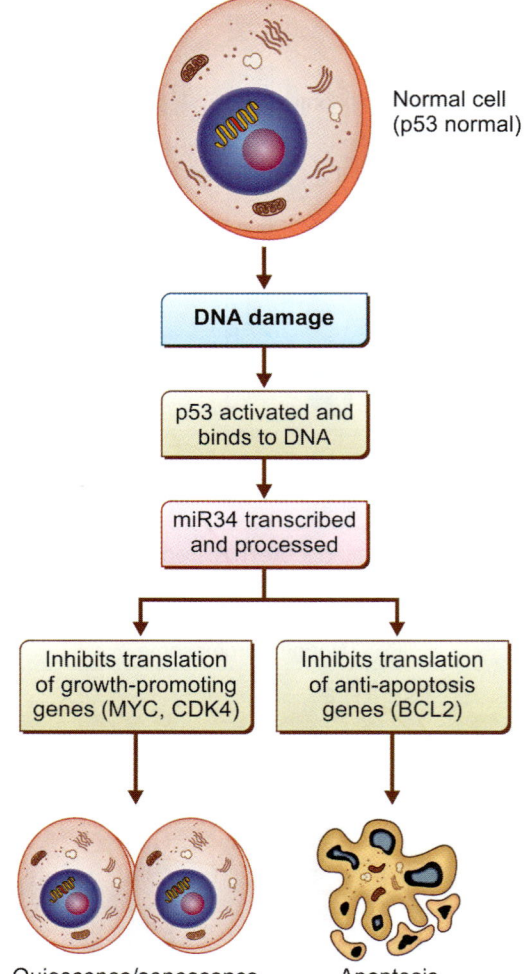

Fig. 6.60: Role of p53 gene repression by activating transcription of miRNAs. This p53 activates transcription of the miR34 family of miRNAs. This activated miR34 represses translation of both proliferative genes such as cyclins and BCL2 anti-apoptotic genes. Repression of these genes can promote their quiescence or senescence as well as apoptosis.

DNA sequences can influence expression of gene including silencing of tumor suppressor genes. Epigenetic changes play role in expression of genes, control of differentiation and self-renewal; drug sensitivity and drug resistance. Epigenetic regulatory gene and associated cancers are shown in Table 6.48.

CANCERS AND NONCODING RNAs (MICRO-RNAs)

Human genome contains about 1000 micro-RNA constituting 5% of total genome. Micro-RNAs are small noncoding single-stranded RNAs with 22 nucleotides. These do not code for proteins. These participate in silencing post-transcriptional genes by inhibiting messenger RNA (mRNA) translation.

All Micro-RNAs comprise seed sequence in their 32 untranslated region (UTR), which determines the specificity of miRNA binding and gene silencing. Role of p53 gene repression by activating transcription of miRNAs is shown in Fig. 6.60.

Micro-RNA in Cancer

In cancer, miRNAs function as regulatory molecules, acting as oncogenes or tumor suppressors.

Amplification or overexpression of miRNAs can downregulate tumor suppressor genes. Amplication of MiRNAs now act as oncogenes resulting in cellular proliferation, angiogenesis ad invasion of tissues.

Similarly, miRNAs can downregulate different proteins with oncogenic activity, i.e. they act as tumor suppressors. More than half of the miRNAs genes are located in cancer associated genomic regions or in fragile sites. The loss of function of a miRNA could be due to several mechanisms, including genomic deletion, mutation, epigenetic silencing, and/or miRNA processing alterations.

On the other hand, miRNAs can act as oncogenic micro-RNAs by targeting mRNAs encoding tumor suppressor proteins. Role of miRNAs in tumorigenesis is shown in Fig. 6.61.

Tumor Suppressive Micro-RNA

Decreased expression of tumor suppressive micro-RNAs enhances translation of oncogenic RNAs.

Examples of tumor suppressive micro-RNA are miR-15 and miR16. Deletion of miR15 and miR16 upregulate *anti-apoptotic BCL2 protein in* **chronic lymphocytic leukemia.**

Neoplasia: Molecular Basis, Metastasis, Clinical Oncology and Laboratory Diagnosis

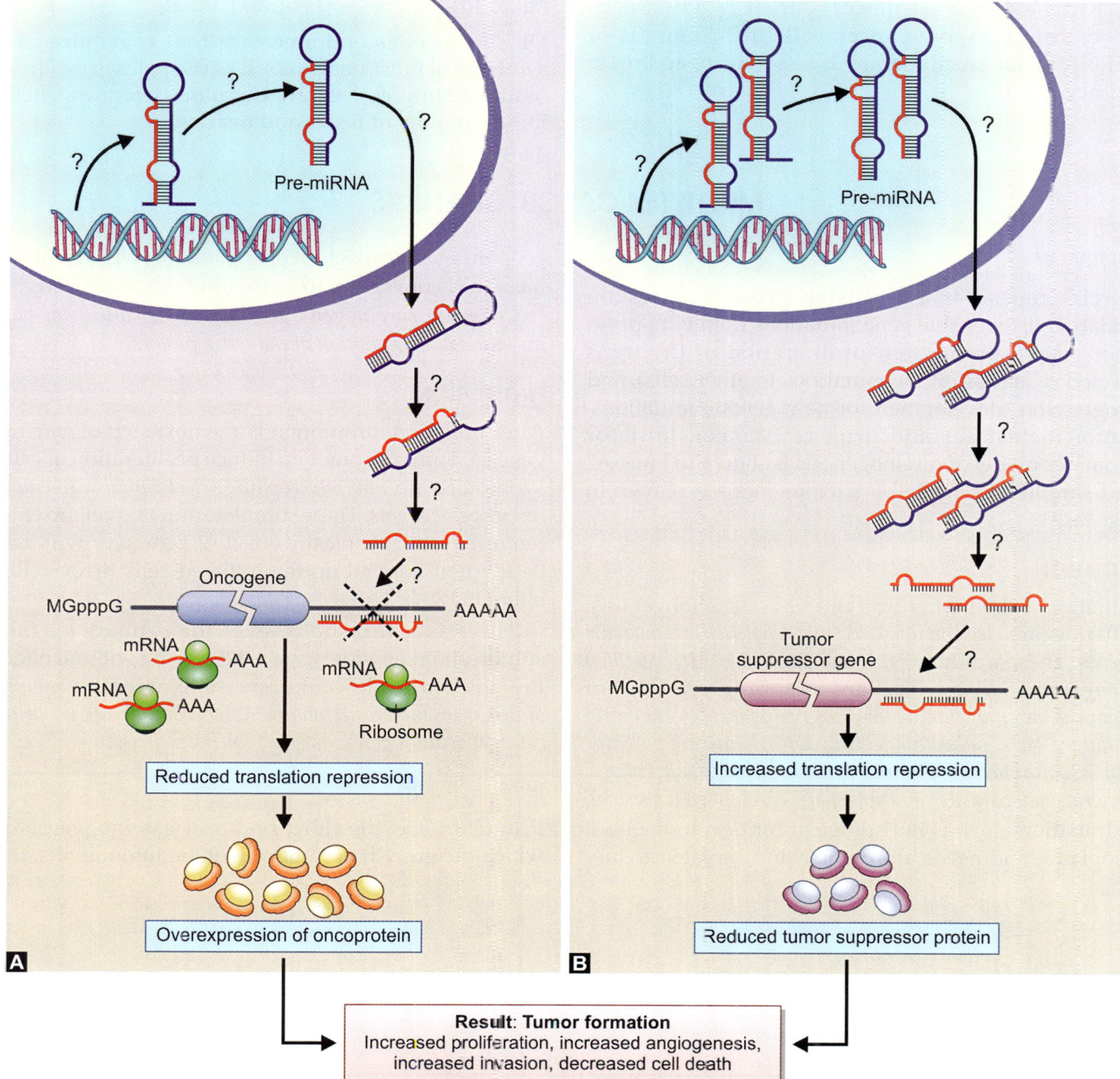

Fig. 6.61: Role of miRNAs in tumorigenesis. (A) Reduced activity of a miRNA that inhibits translation of an oncogene leads to an excess of oncoproteins, (B) overactivity of a miRNA that targets a tumor suppressor gene reduces the production of the tumor suppressor protein. Question marks in (A) and (B) denote unknown mechanism of changes in the level or activity of miRNA.

Onco-micro-RNA

Increased expression of onco-micro-RNA inhibits tumor suppressor genes. Examples of onco-micro-RNAs are miR155 and miRNA200.

Onco-micro-RNA (miRNA155)

Overexpression of miR155 upregulates MYC (a nuclear transcriptional factor) results to **B cell lymphoma**.

Onco-micro-RNA (miRNA200)

Overexpression of miRNA200 participates in invasiveness and metastases by *promoting epithelial-mesenchymal transition*.

Onco-micro-RNA (miRNA221)

Onco-miR221 is significantly overexpressed in triple-negative primary breast cancer. Oncosuppressor p27Kip1, a validated miR221 target is downregulated in aggressive cancer cell lines. Benefit of miRNA replacement therapy is less toxicity and more efficacy.

Micro-RNA Processing Factor (DICER)

DICER encodes endonuclease that is required for synthesis of functional miRs. It participates in synthesis of tumor suppressive miR. Germline defects in DICER induce **tumors of testes and ovaries.**

MULTISTEP CARCINOGENESIS

OVERVIEW

Carcinogenesis is a multistep process involving initiation (irreversible gene mutations involving proto oncogenes), promotion (proliferation of the trans formed cells pass on the mutations to other cells), and progression (development of new genetic mutations, tumor metastases and drug resistance). Initiator promoter model of carcinogenesis is shown in Fig. 6.62 and simplified scheme of carcinogenesis is shown in Fig. 6.63.

INITIATION

Initiation is the first critical process of carcinogenesis. Initiators are *electrophilic (electron deficient) carcinogenic agents*. These produce *rapid and permanent (irreversible) changes in DNA* by exposure to appropriate dose of *chemical carcinogenic agent (DNA alkylating), ionizing radiation (free radicals affecting DNA), ultraviolet rays 280–320 nm affecting pyrimidine dimers), oncogenic viruses, bacteria, endoparasites and epigenetic carcinogen (asbestos).*

Initiation alone is not sufficient for development of neoplasia, and needs a promoter. Incomplete carcinogens are agents capable of only initiation, which requires metabolic conversion to form ultimate carcinogens.

Complete carcinogens possess the capability of both initiation and promotion of inducing tumors.

PROMOTION

After initiation, promotion is the next step of carcinogenesis. Tumor promoters induce proliferation of cells. Promoters are *non-electrophilic (electron-rich and non-carcinogenic agents.* These stimulate mutated cells to enter the cell cycle. Neoplastic effect of promoter will only be there, if applied on the initiated cells (irreversibly altered DNA).

There is a threshold level for promoters, thus subthreshold or widely spaced doses are without effect. Promotion is a slow and reversible process. *Examples of tumor promoters are phorbol esters (croton oil), hepatitis, estrogens, androgens, and Epstein-Barr virus.*

PROGRESSION

Progression is the third phase of carcinogenesis in which the growth of tumor becomes autonomous. It is

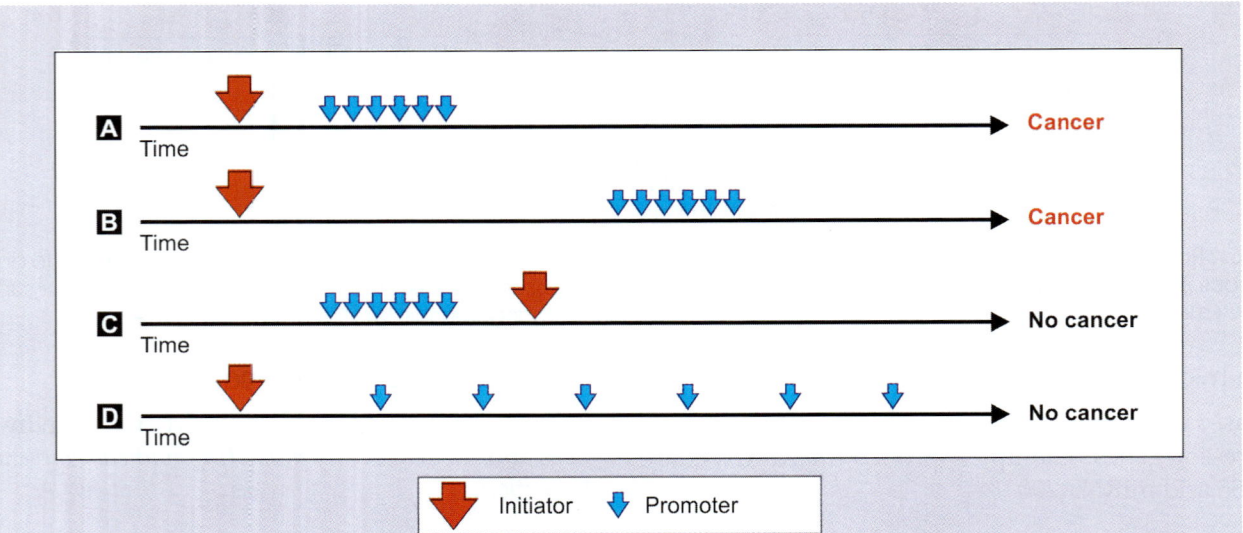

Fig. 6.62: Initiator-promoter model of carcinogenesis developed by Berenblum and Shubik by painting polycyclic aromatic hydrocarbons and croton oil on mouse skin. (A) Simultaneously exposure to initiator and then promotor leads to cancer, (B) exposure initiator and then promoter after long time also causes cancer, (C) exposure first to promoter and then initiator does not cause cancer, (D) exposure to initiator then promoter at wide intervals does not cause cancer.

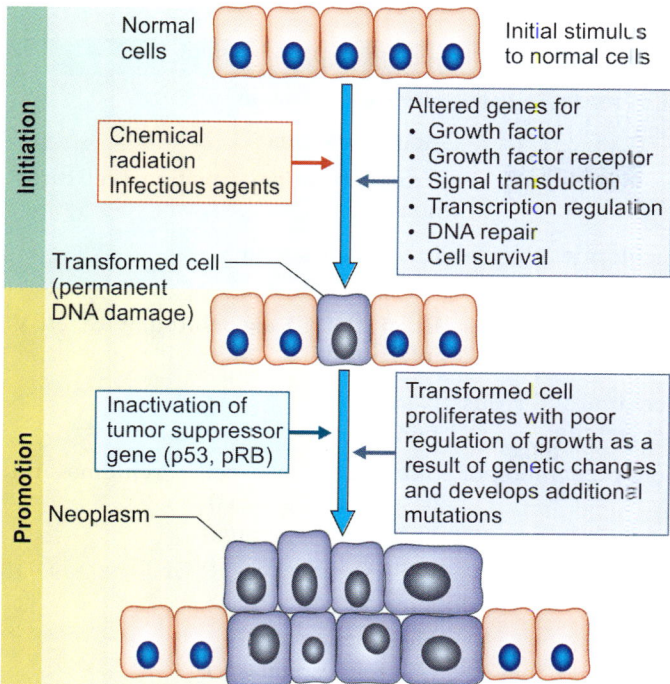

Fig. 6.63: Simplified scheme of carcinogenesis. Exposure to chemical agents, radiation and infectious agents and altered genes cause damage to DNA of normal cell resulting in transformed cells. Additional mutations and inactivation of tumor suppressor genes participate in promotion process by clonal proliferation of cells.

characterized by accumulation of new mutations with development of sub-clones of autonomous neoplastic cells, angiogenesis, and development of detectable cancer, invasion or metastases to distant organs.

CHEMICAL CARCINOGENESIS

Chemical carcinogens play an important role in pathogenesis of cancer by causing point mutations. Upon exposure to chemical carcinogen, the body makes an attempt to eliminate it through a process called biotransformation. Though this process makes the carcinogen more water-soluble so that it can be removed from the body, yet it can also convert a less toxic carcinogen into a more toxic carcinogen. When body is not able to eliminate it, the ultimate chemical carcinogen's electron deficient (electrophilic) molecules possessing memory reacts with cellular electron-rich DNA in nucleus, RNA and proteins, results in apoptosis of damaged DNA.

If the programmed cell death pathway is damaged, the cell cannot prevent itself from becoming a cancer cell. It takes a long latent period before a neoplasm develops. It is thought that altered cells are primed but require a second change to bring about molecular genetic changes expressed as neoplasia. Chemical carcinogens associated with cancers are shown in Table 6.49.

Table 6.49: Chemical carcinogens associated with cancers

Chemical carcinogen	Examples	Associated cancers
Direct acting carcinogens associated with cancers		
Alkylating agents	Nitrogen mustard, cyclophosphamide, chlorambucil, nitrosoureas, β-propiolactone, dimethyl sulphate, diepoxybutane	Lymphomas (Hodgkin's disease and NHL) Leukemia Ovary
Acylating agents	1-Acetyl-imidazole, dimethylcarbamyl chloride	Squamous cell papilloma Squamous cell carcinoma
Indirect acting carcinogens associated with cancers		
Polycyclic hydrocarbons	Consumption of smoked meat and fish and cigarette smoke	Cancers of oral cavity, esophagus (middle and distal), pancreas, lung cancer and renal pelvis, and urinary bladder
Aromatic amines	Aniline dye and rubber industries (β-naphthylamine, Benzidine-O, Anisidine-O, toluidine) (unlike polycyclic hydrocarbons, aromatic amines produce no local carcinogenic effect)	Urinary bladder (transitional cell carcinoma)
Nitrosamines	Nitrates and nitrites are widely used as fertilizers and as food additives. These are converted to nitrosamines by gut bacteria in hypochlorhydria	Gastrointestinal tract
Azo dyes derivatives of aromatic amines	Dimethylaminoazobenzene, known as *butter yellow* imparts an appetizing yellow color to margarine	Liver

Contd...

Table 6.49: Chemical carcinogens associated with cancers *(Contd...)*

Chemical carcinogen	Examples	Associated cancers
Aromatic hydrocarbons	Benzene present in crude oil (petrochemical), Benz(a) anthracene, Benz(a) pyrene	Hodgkin's disease Acute leukemia Urinary bladder (transitional cell carcinoma)
Organohalogen compounds	Polyvinyl chloride, carbon tetrachloride, chloroform, hexachlorobenzene, trichloroethylene	Liver angiosarcoma
Natural carcinogens	Aflatoxin-β_1 synthesized by fungus *Aspergillus flavus* in growing stored grains, nuts and peanut	Liver (HCC) associated with HBV infection
Occupational carcinogens	Nickel used in nickel plating ceramics, ferrous alloys, batteries and stainless steel welding	Nasal cavity Lung
	Arsenic used in alloys, medication, preparation of fungicides and herbicides	Skin (squamous cell carcinoma and basal cell carcinoma) Liver (angiosarcoma) Lung
	Asbestos used in building material	Lung Mesothelioma Gastrointestinal tract
	Beryllium and its compounds used in missile fuel, nuclear reactors, aerospace application and light weight alloys	Lung
	Cadmium used in batteries and metal paintings	Prostate
	Chromium used in paints, pigments and preservatives	Lung
	Uranium mine workers	Lung

Direct or Indirect Acting Carcinogens

- *Direct acting carcinogens*: These do not require metabolic conversion to become carcinogenic agents. Chemotherapeutic alkylating agents cause DNA mutation.
- *Indirect acting carcinogens:* These require metabolic conversion to become carcinogens by cytochrome P450 oxidases. Examples are polycyclic hydrocarbons, benzopyrene and nitrosamines.

Complete or Incomplete Carcinogens

- *Complete carcinogens:* Complete carcinogens possess the capability of both initiation and promotion of inducing tumors. Exposure to chemical carcinogen, procarcinogen is transformed into ultimate carcinogen that interacts with macromolecules. Covalent binding of carcinogen to DNA occurs with formation of adducts.

  Fixation of carcinogen to DNA initiates carcinogenesis. It induces errors in transcription. Binding of carcinogen to oncogenes that code for cell growth and differentiation may result in cell transformation. Binding of carcinogen to tumor suppressor genes leads to apoptosis.

- *Incomplete carcinogens:* These are agents *capable of only initiation*. Most chemical carcinogens require metabolic conversion into active carcinogens.

Main Groups of Chemical Carcinogens

These three groups cause cancers by direct or indirect mechanisms.

- *Genotoxic:* Chemical carcinogen causes direct damage to DNA by forming chemical DNA adducts that are prone to damage in replication or resistant to DNA repair mechanisms.
- *Mitogenic:* Chemical carcinogen binds to receptors or in cells and stimulate mitosis by activation of tyrosine kinase activity without causing direct DNA damage.
- *Cytotoxic:* Chemical carcinogen causes tissue damage leading to hyperplasia with cycles of tissue regeneration. Chemical carcinogen can act as mitogen factor.

Steps in carcinogenesis comprise biotransformation, initiation (covalent binding to DNA), fixation (mutation stabilized by mitosis), gene expression, transformation, neoplastic growth, proliferation, progression, local effects, and metastasis. Mechanism of chemical carcinogenesis is shown in Fig. 6.64.

Neoplasia: Molecular Basis, Metastasis, Clinical Oncology and Laboratory Diagnosis

DNA-adduct Formation

Since most chemical carcinogens react with DNA and are mutagenic, interactions with DNA have been viewed as the most important reactions of these agents. The principal reaction products of the nitrosamines and similar alkylating agents with DNA are N7 and O6 guanine derivatives. Reactions also occur with other DNA bases.

Consequences of DNA-adduct Formation

Polycyclic hydrocarbon double-helical DNA by frame-shift mutation during DNA replication. Alkylated bases in DNA can mispair with the wrong base during DNA replication. There is loss of bases due to induction of instability in the glycosidic bond between the purine base and deoxyribose. Some carcinogens cause conformational transition of DNA from its usual double-helical B form to a Z-DNA form. Multistep carcinogenesis showing morphologic and molecular

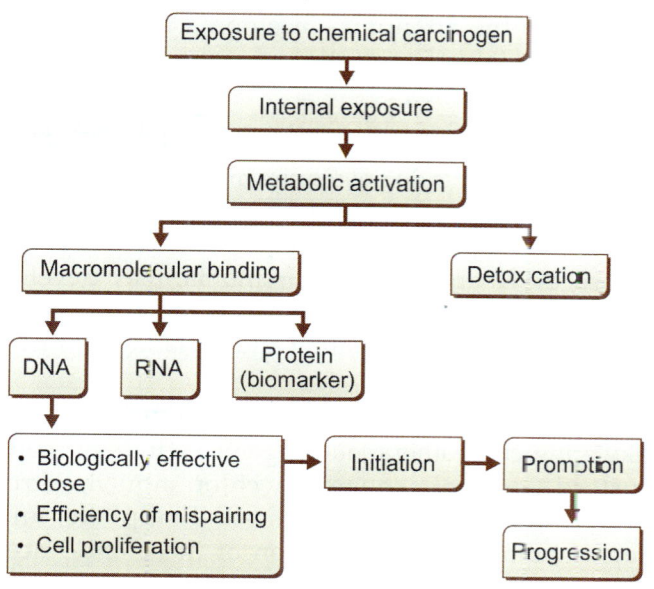

Fig. 6.64: Mechanism of chemical carcinogenesis.

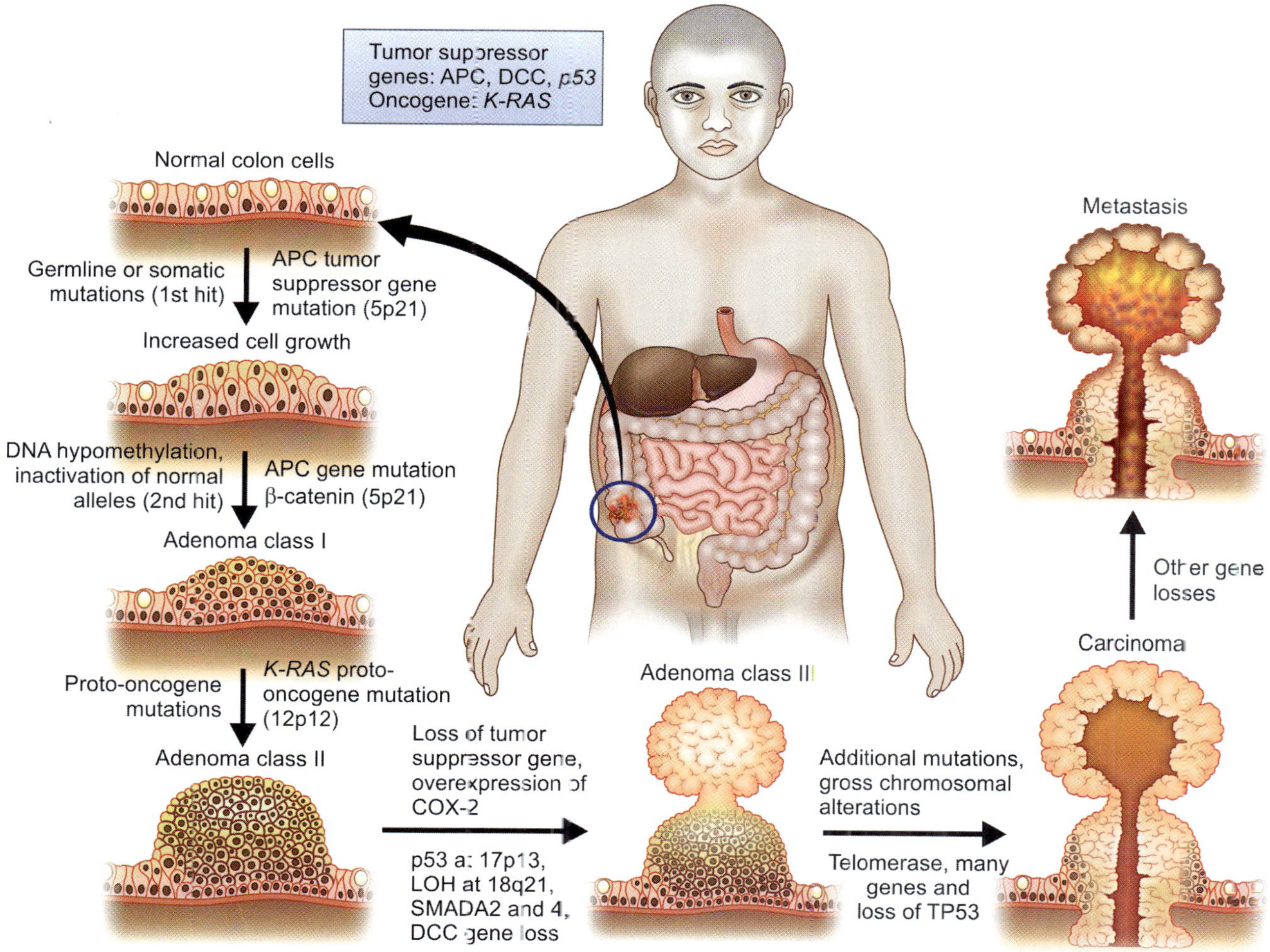

Fig. 6.65: Multistep carcinogenesis showing morphologic and molecular changes in the adenoma–carcinoma sequence. It is postulated by Knudson's hypothesis that losses of normal copy of tumor suppressor APC gene occurs early in life. This is the first hit. Loss of intact copy of APC gene follows (second hit). Other gene mutations include K-RAS, losses at 18q21 involving SMAD2 and SMAD4 and inactivation of tumor suppressor p53 gene. It leads to the emergence of colorectal carcinoma and metastases, in which additional gene mutations occur.

changes in the adenoma–carcinoma sequence are depicted in Fig. 6.65.

DIRECT ACTING CARCINOGENS

Direct acting agents do not require metabolic conversion to become carcinogen. Therapeutic administration of alkylating agents in cancer patients in Hodgkin's disease, NHL and ovarian carcinoma, may develop another cancer such as leukemia. Direct acting chemical carcinogens include alkylating and acylating agents.

Alkylating Agents

Alkylating chemotherapeutic agents include nitrogen mustard—cyclophosphamide, chlorambucil, nitrosoureas, β-propiolactone, dimethyl sulphate, and diepoxybutane. Administration of these anticancer therapeutic agents in *Hodgkin's disease*, NHL and ovarian carcinoma may evoke later a second form of cancer, usually leukemia.

Acylating Agents

Acylating agents include dimethylcarbamyl chloride, dichloroacetyl chloride (DCAC) and ethyl chloroformate (ECF). Exposure to these agents causes squamous cell papilloma or squamous cell carcinoma.

INDIRECT ACTING CARCINOGENS

Most chemical agents require metabolic conversion from procarcinogen to active ultimate carcinogen. It occurs by hydroxylation by aryl carbohydrate hydroxylase in microsomal fraction of endoplasmic reticulum with cytochrome P450 dependent monooxygenase. Hydroxylating enzymes (e.g. aryl carbohydrate hydroxylase) are ubiquitous in human tissues and readily induce cancer in susceptible individuals. Various indirect acting carcinogens are described below.

Polycyclic Hydrocarbons

Polycyclic hydrocarbons are aromatic hydrocarbons originally derived from coal tar, are among the most extensively studied carcinogens. These are also derived from animal fat by process of broiling of meats (e.g. smoked meat and fish) and tobacco smoking.

Polycyclic hydrocarbons present in tobacco smoke via circulation reach liver and activates cytochrome P450. Benzo (a) pyrene gets converted to benzopyrene epoxide resulting in formation of vicinal-diol-epoxide (unstable compound). This unstable product is further converted to carbonium ion (nucleophilic compound), that binds to DNA resulting in *lung cancer* (local site) and *cancers renal cell carcinoma and bladder cancer* (distant sites).

Ingestion of Smoked Meat and Fish

Polycyclic hydrocarbons in smoked fish undergoes hydroxylation in liver forming *epoxides* covalent adducts. These bind to cellular DNA, RNA and proteins and alter the genome. These are associated with cancers of *oral cavity, esophagus* (upper- and middle-third) and *pancreas*.

Aromatic Amines

Incidence of transitional cell carcinoma of urinary bladder is increased in aniline dye workers heavily exposed to β-naphthylamine (aromatic amines). Product of azo dyes β-naphthylamine undergoes hydroxylation in liver and converted to 1-hydroxy-2-naphthylamine (water-soluble active carcinogenic metabolite) in the liver. This active carcinogenic metabolite combines with glucuronic acid in liver and excreted in the urinary tract. This molecule is deconjugated by bladder mucosal enzyme glucuronidase, thus exposing the urothelium to the active carcinogen results in *bladder cancer* (Fig. 6.66).

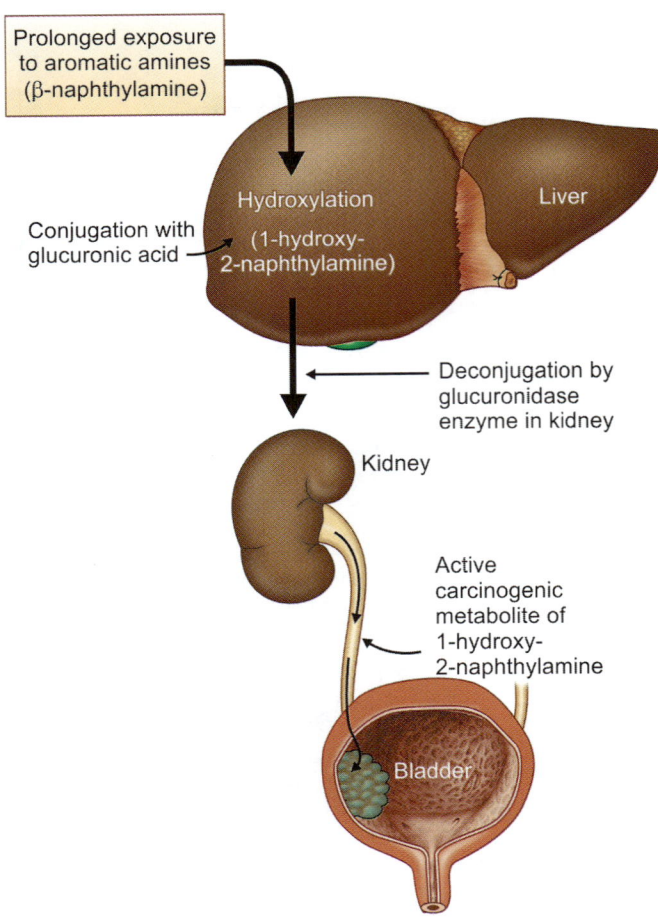

Fig. 6.66: Role of β-naphthylamine (aromatic amines) in the pathogenesis of urinary bladder carcinoma.

Nitrosamines

Nitrates are used widely as fertilizers (contaminating drinking water) and food additives. During hypochlorhydria, overgrowth of commensal bacteria in stomach convert nitrates into secondary amines and amides (carcinogen) resulting in *gastric carcinoma*.

Azo Dyes Derivatives of Aromatic Amines

Azo dyes are derivatives of aromatic amines. Dimethylaminoazobenzene, known as *butter yellow* impart an appetizing yellow color to margarine causes hepatocellular carcinoma.

Aromatic Amines

Workers in benzene chemical and petrochemical industries are associated with *leukemia and Hodgkin's disease*.

Organohalogen Compounds

Polyvinyl chloride (PVC) exposure has been associated with **hepatic angiosarcomas**.

Natural Carcinogen

Aflatoxin-β_1 is potent natural carcinogen synthesized by *Aspergillus flavus* grown on peanuts and grains stored in hot humid conditions. Like the polycyclic aromatic hydrocarbons, consumption of aflatoxin-β_1 reach the liver and activates cytochrome P450 resulting in formation of aflatoxin-2, 3-epoxide. This carcinogenic compound binds to guanine of DNA and causes specific point mutations in the p53 gene resulting in hepatocellular carcinoma in Asian and African population.

Occupational Carcinogens

Exposure to various occupational carcinogens such as nickel, arsenic, asbestos, beryllium, cadmium, chromium and uranium produces cancers in workers (Table 6.50).

RADIATION CARCINOGENESIS

Radiations contain energies greater than that present in chemical bonds. Therefore, chemical bonds can be broken by radiation. Energy is released from atomic particles (X-rays), ultraviolet (UV) light and visible light. Approximately, 2% of cancer deaths are caused by radiation.

Ionizing radiation (X-rays, radon gas, radioactive material) can cause leukemia and thyroid cancer. It depends of the type of ultraviolet radiations (UV-α, UV-β, UV-γ or neutron), magnitude of exposure, penetration and capacity to cause ionization in tissues. Survivors of atomic bombs dropped in World War II develop leukemia and other cancers.

Types of Radiation

Excessive exposure to ultraviolet radiation, X-rays, and γ-radiation, generally is carcinogenic. Neutron radiation produced inside nuclear reactors can produce secondary radiation through nuclear transmutation. Both X-rays and ultraviolet (UV) radiation cause DNA damage. Low energy waves on the electromagnetic spectrum are generally non-carcinogenic, including radio waves, microwave radiation, infrared radiation and visible light.

Table 6.50: Occupational cancers

Chemical carcinogen	Examples	Associated cancers
Nickel	Nickel used in nickel plating ceramics, ferrous alloys, batteries and stainless steel welding	Nasal cavity Lung
Arsenic	Arsenic used in alloys, medication, preparation of fungicides and herbicides	Skin (squamous cell carcinoma or basal cell carcinoma) Liver (angiosarcoma) Lung
Asbestos	Asbestos used in building material	Lung Mesothelioma Gastrointestinal tract
Beryllium	Beryllium and its compounds used in missile fuel, nuclear reactors, aerospace application and light weight alloys	Lung cancer
Cadmium	Cadmium used in batteries and metal paintings	Prostate cancer
Chromium	Chromium used in paints, pigments and preservatives	Lung cancer
Uranium	Uranium mine workers	Lung cancer

EXPOSURE TO ULTRAVIOLET RAYS

UV radiation is a low-energy emission and does not penetrate deeply. Hence, the skin absorbs most of the radiation and is the primary carcinogenic target. When cells are exposed to UV light in the 240 to 300 nm range, nucleic acid–bases acquire excited energy states, producing photochemical reactions between DNA bases.

The principal products in DNA at biologically relevant doses of UV light are cyclobutane dimers formed between two adjacent pyrimidine bases in the DNA chain. Both thymine-thymine and thymine–cytosine dimers are formed.

Xeroderma Pigmentosum

Patient with this autosomal recessive disorder characterized by failure of DNA excision repair mechanisms. There is increased risk of development of *skin cancers*.

Sporadic Cancers

Exposure to UV-B (290–320 nm) radiation (sunlight) is associated with *basal cell carcinoma, squamous cell carcinoma and melanoma of skin*.

EXPOSURE TO IONIZING RADIATION

Exposure to ionizing radiation produces various cancers is shown in Table 6.51.

VIRAL CARCINOGENESIS

Both RNA and DNA oncogenic viruses play an important role in pathogenesis of cancer by disrupting cellular genes in the host especially young persons. Oncogenic viruses typically integrate their genomes into host cells and enter a period of *latency*.

Approximately, 20% of all human cancers are caused by one of 5 viruses: *Epstein-Barr virus, hepatitis B, hepatitis C, HTLV-1 and human papillomaviruses*. Oncogenic RNA and DNA viruses and associated cancers are shown in Table 6.52. Comparison between RNA and DNA oncogenic viruses is shown in Table 6.53. Oncogenes, functions and their products are shown in Table 6.54.

Types of viral carcinogenesis: These are two types of viral carcinogenesis to activate oncogenes.

- *Slow-transforming viruses:* These insert viral-derived DNA into the genome randomly. Insertion of

Table 6.51: Radiation-induced cancers

Neoplasm	Association
Thyroid carcinoma	Thymic radiation, atom bomb
Leukemia (AML, CML) and not lymphoid cancers	Atom bomb, radiologists
Breast carcinoma	Atom bomb, radiotherapy, mammography
Skin (basal cell carcinoma, squamous cell carcinoma and melanoma)	Ultraviolet radiation* (UV-B: 290–320 nm) in xeroderma pigmentosum and sporadic cases
Hepatocellular carcinoma	Thorium dioxide
Lung carcinoma	Uranium miners (low doses of radiation can cause or enhance DNA mutations and chromosomal abnormalities)
Osteosarcoma	Radium dial painters

*Ultraviolet radiation causes p53 gene mutation. TNF-α released by exposed skin diminishes immune response. It induces dimer formation between neighboring thymine pairs in DNA.

Table 6.52: Oncogenic RNA and DNA viruses and associated cancers

Viruses	Associated cancer	Mechanism of action of virus
RNA oncogenic viruses		
HCV	Hepatocellular carcinoma	HCV is small (65–65 nm in size) enveloped positive sense single-stranded RNA virus. It is the cause of hepatitis C and lymphomas in humans HCV produces post-necrotic necrosis and results in hepatocellular carcinoma *Mechanism:* HCV causes mutation of HBx protein results in transcriptional activation of growth promoting genes responsible for hepatocellular carcinoma
HTLV-1 (retrovirus)	T cell leukemia Primary effusion lymphoma	HTLV-1 activates TAX gene and also neutralizes growth inhibitory signals by p53 tumor suppressor genes and CDKN2A/Alp16 genes leading to leukemia. Additional mutations result in T cell malignancies

Contd...

Table 6.52: Oncogenic RNA and DNA viruses and associated cancers (Contd...)

Viruses	Associated cancer	Mechanism of action of virus
DNA oncogenic viruses		
EB virus	CNS lymphoma in AIDS Nasopharyngeal carcinoma Hodgkin's disease (mixed cellularity) Burkitt's lymphoma	EB virus causes CNS lymphoma in AIDS EB virus is important cause of this cancer EB virus protects RS cells from apoptosis. It also protects RS cells from killer T cells. EB virus causes mutation of p53 tumor suppressor gene Translocation (8;14) Activation of oncogene (c-MYC) Stimulates proliferation of B cells
	Extranodal marginal zone B cell NHL	Occurs in mucosa associated lymphoid tissue (MALT) and in the settings of Hashimoto's thyroiditis, *Helicobacter pylori* associated gastritis and Sjögren syndrome Molecular genetics: Trisomy 18, t(11;18), t(1;14); latter create MALT1-IAP2 and BCL10-IgH fusion genes, respectively
HBV	Hepatocellular carcinoma	HBV activates proto-oncogenes and inactivates TP53 tumor suppressor gene
HHV 8 (human herpesvirus 8)	Kaposi's sarcoma in AIDS	HHV 8 is active only when immune system is suppressed It encodes proteins that interfere with the p53 and Rb tumor suppressor pathways
HPV (types 16, 18)	Squamous cell carcinoma of cervix, vulva, vagina, anus (associated with sexual inter-course), larynx and oropharynx	E6 gene product of HPV inhibits TP53 tumor suppressor gene and responsible for 10% cases of cancers

Table 6.53: Comparison between RNA and DNA oncogenic viruses

Parameters	RNA oncogenic virus	DNA oncogenic virus
Prototype virus	Rous sarcoma virus	S40
Genome	ssRNA	dsDNA
Reverse transcriptase	Present	Absent
Interaction with host genome	First RNA is transcribed into dsDNA and then integrates into host genome	Linear DNA genome forms a double-stranded circle within infected cell and then covalently integrated into the host genome
Name of gene	src	Early region of A gene
Name of protein	src protein	T-antigen
Functions of proteins	Protein kinase that phosphorylate tyrosine—disturbs the growth control process	Protein kinase, ATPase binding to DNA and stimulation of DNA synthesis
Location of protein	Plasma membrane	Primarily nuclear, but sometimes in plasma membrane
Required for viral growth	No	Yes
Genes have cellular homologue	Yes	No

Remember: Protein products from both DNA and RNA oncogenic viruses are required for cell transformation

viral DNA next to a proto-oncogene may cause neoplasia.
- *Acute transforming viruses:* These viruses contain a viral oncogene. When viral-derived DNA is inserted into the host genome, the transcribed viral oncogene is expressed resulting in neoplasia.

RNA ONCOGENIC VIRUSES

RNA viruses are also known as *retroviruses*. Retrovirus is a single-stranded RNA virus that replicates via double-stranded DNA intermediate. RNA is converted to cDNA by reverse transcriptase. These show CD4+

Table 6.54: Oncogenes, functions and their products

Viral oncogene	Human cellular proto-oncogene	Location	Function of oncoprotein	Tumor in natural host
V-ABL (Abelson mouse leukemia)	C-ABL	9	It acts via non-receptor protein-tyrosine kinase activity	Chronic myeloid leukemia
V-MYC (Chicken myelomatosis)	C-MYC	8	It binds to DNA, directly stimulating synthesis	Myelomatosis
V-SIS (Simian sarcoma)	C-SIS	22	It is a growth factor (platelet derived growth factor)	Sarcoma
V-ras (Rat sarcoma)	C-ras	11	It acts on intracellular signaling (cyclic nucleotides)	Sarcoma
Erb-B2 (Avian erythroblastosis)	Erb-B2	-	It is receptor-like kinase for epidermal growth factor	Breast carcinoma

T cell tropism. These are transmitted via blood products, sexual contact and breastfeeding. The range of following infections with oncogenic retrovirus is shown in Fig. 6.67.

- *Isolation:* F. Peyton Rous in 1910 isolated retrovirus from a chicken tumor later named the Rous sarcoma virus. Non-oncogenic retroviruses possess no oncogenes and hence direct their own life cycle.

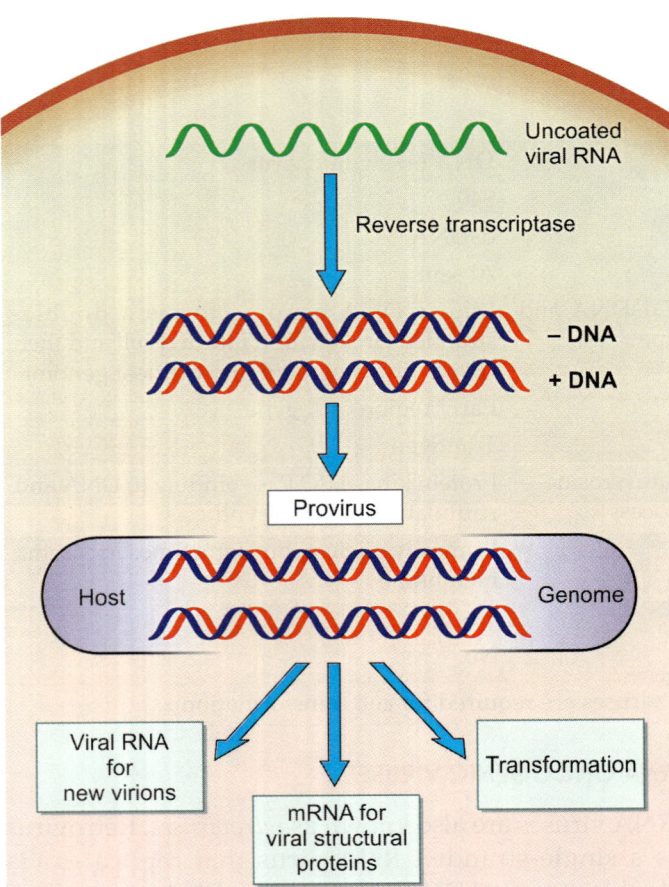

Fig. 6.67: The range of following infections with oncogenic retrovirus.

For example, HIV infects T-helper cells (CD4+ T cell) and destroys them.

- *Transduction:* Retroviral oncogenes are formed from proto-oncogenes (cellular genes), which cause cancer. The process is called transduction. Genomic DNA sequences in retroviruses are known as viral oncogenes (v-oncs), genomic DNA sequences in human beings are known as *cellular oncogenes* (c-oncs).
- *Genes in RNA viruses:* These are three types of genes in most retroviruses: (i) *gag* (group antigen): codes the protein core, (ii) *pol* (polymerase): codes reverse transcriptase and an enzyme for proviral integration, and (iii) *env* (envelope): codes envelope glycoproteins.
- *Entry of retrovirus:* Oncogenic retroviruses (v-onc) enter the host cell by reverse transcriptase and mutate genome. Proviral DNA and host chromosome DNA crossover and are joined by recombination.
- *Transcription:* Host RNA polymerase transcribes proviral DNA and produces viral mRNAs required for the virus life cycle. Proviral promoters can activate transcription of nearby genes.
- *Mechanism:* Oncogenic retroviruses are also called transducing viruses. Most transducing viral oncogenes are defective and cannot replicate independently. Viral encoded TAX protein causes cancer by following mechanisms. It *inactivates p6/INK4a* and *enhances cyclin deactivation* resulting in increased cell replication. It *interferes with DNA repair mechanism* resulting in *genomic instability*. It also activates NF-Kb transcriptional factor to form monoclonal tumor cells.
- *Malignant transformation:* Malignant transformation may occur if the nearby gene is an oncogene (c-MYC) or disruption of tumor suppressor genes. It leads to permanent activation of cellular signal transduction cascades and disruption of cell cycle regulation resulting in cancer. Oncogenic RNA viruses associated with cancers are described as under.

Hepatitis C Virus

HCV is small (65–65 nm in size) enveloped positive sense single-stranded RNA virus. It is transmitted by blood-borne parental route, sexual contact, transplacental infection of the fetus and co-infection with HCB. It causes mutation of HBx protein leading to transcriptional activation of growth promoting genes responsible for post-necrotic cirrhosis progressing to **hepatocellular carcinoma. HCV also causes lymphoma** (Fig. 6.68).

HTLV 1 (Human T-Lymphotropic Virus Type 1)

HTLV 1 causes *adult T cell leukemia and primary effusion lymphoma in Japan*. It infects many T cells. Viral encoded *TAX protein* stimulate T cell proliferation and also neutralizes growth inhibitory signals by p53 tumor suppressor genes and CDKN2A/Alp16 genes leading to leukemia. Additional mutations result in T cell malignancies.

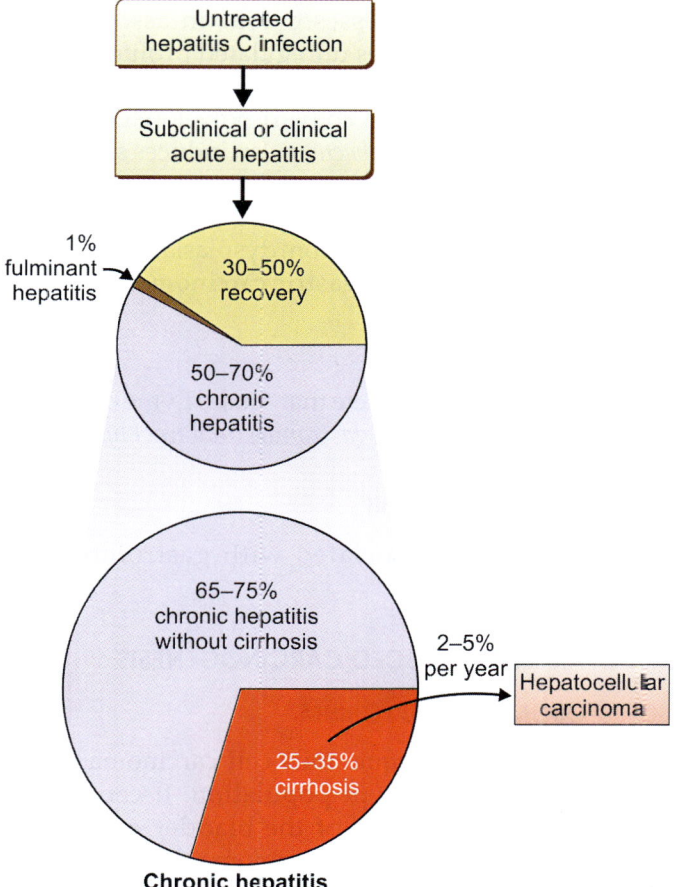

Fig. 6.68: Outcome of untreated hepatitis C infection. The most serious consequences of chronic HCV infection are progressive liver fibrosis leading to cirrhosis over 10 to 30, end-stage liver disease, and hepatocellular cancer.

DNA ONCOGENIC VIRUSES

Oncogenic DNA viruses do not carry oncogenes, but induce cancer by activity of viral gene products on the host genome of cell. DNA viruses integrate viral DNA into host genomes, perhaps resulting in host cell expression of viral mRNA coding for specific proteins. These produce proteins that target key cellular regulatory proteins (tumour suppressor proteins. Rb and p53). DNA viruses causing human cancers include *human papillomavirus, Epstein-Barr virus, hepatitis B virus,* and *herpesvirus 8.*

Epstein-Barr Virus Associated Cancers

EB virus is a herpesvirus. It infects B cells through CD21 (CR-2; complement receptor 2). It causes inactivation of immune system. It is responsible for infectious mononucleosis. It inactivates immune system resulting in malignant transformation of cells. B cells infected by EB viral genes (LMP-1 and EBNA-2) become immortal. Latent membrane protein 1 (LMP-1) activates NF-Kb and JAK/STAT pathways resulting in proliferation and survival of B cells. EMBNA-2 encodes a nuclear protein that activates cyclin D and proto-oncogenes. Cancers associated with EB virus are described as under.

Burkitt's Lymphoma

EB virus promotes polyclonal B cell proliferation, which increases risk of translocation (8;14). It activates oncogene (c-MYC). It stimulates proliferation of B cells. Burkitt's lymphoma is high grade germinal center B cell lymphoma but curable disorder. Most patients present with extranodal tumors (**maxilla, mandible or abdomen**) that emerge in a short period of time and respond to aggressive chemotherapy. African variant is strongly associated with EB virus. Molecular genetic alterations demonstrated are t(8;14), t(2;8) and t(8;22).

Hodgkin's Disease

Epstein-Barr virus has been demonstrated in **Reed-Sternberg** cells of Hodgkin's disease (mixed cellularity) in 50% cases. It may actually protect the Reed-Sternberg cell from apoptosis and immune response of killer T cells. It may also cause a mutation in the p53 gene. Hodgkin disease is a malignant neoplasm of lymph node with involvement of single lymph node or multiple nodes. Diagnostic criteria include demonstration of neoplastic Reed-Sternberg cells derived from B cells. Reed-Sternberg cells develop as a result of this genetic rearrangement and constitute 1–10% of cell population in Hodgkin's disease.

Extranodal Marginal Zone B Cell NHL

Extranodal marginal zone B cell lymphoma occurs in mucosa-associated lymphoid tissue (MALT). It also occurs in the settings of Hashimoto's thyroiditis, *Helicobacter pylori* associated gastritis in pyloric region and Sjögren's syndrome.

Nasopharyngeal Carcinoma

Epstein-Barr virus is also responsible for nasopharyngeal carcinoma.

CNS Lymphoma in AIDS

EB virus causes CNS, non-Hodgkin's lymphoma.

Hepatitis B Virus Associated Carcinoma

Approximately 70–85% of **hepatocellular carcinomas** are due to HBV and HCV infections worldwide. HBV infection is most often associated with hepatocellular carcinoma. HBV causes immune mediated chronic inflammation of hepatocytes. HBV activates proto-oncogene. It encodes a regulatory HBx that inactivates TP53 suppressor gene resulting in hepatocellular carcinoma.

Human Papillomavirus Associated Lesions

Human papillomavirus: HPV (16, 18) causes cervical carcinoma. HPV (6, 11) cause **genital warts.** HPV (1, 2, 4, 7) may cause squamous papilloma which regresses spontaneously. A few human papillomaviruses are associated with human cancers such as cervix, penis, anus, vagina, vulva, mouth and oral cavity. Vaccines against some of human papillomavirus are available. **HPV 16, 18** infect immature epithelial basal cells at the squamocolumnar junction. These viruses do not infect the mature superficial squamous cells that cover the ectocervix, vagina, or vulva.

Pathogenesis

Gene products of HPV 16, 18 viruses inactivate tumor suppressor proteins. Once inside the cells of their host, human papillomavirus (16, 18) synthesizes a protein designated E7 and another designated E6. Oncoproteins encoded by the E6 and E7 genes of HPV 16 bind p53 and Rb tumor suppressor genes. The virus can infect only the immature squamous cells, replication of HPV occurs in the maturing squamous cells and resulting in a cytopathic effect, "koilocytic atypia," consisting of nuclear atypia and a cytoplasmic perinuclear halo.

- *E7 oncoprotein:* It increases activity of CDK4/cyclin D by inactivating CDK inhibitors (p21 and p27). It binds to the RB protein and displaces transcription factor E2F. Now E2F is free to bind to the promoters of genes (like c-MYC) that cause the cell to enter the cell cycle. Therefore, inhibition of p21 and RB-E2F causes increased activity of CDK4/cyclin D resulting in genome instability.

- *E6 oncoprotein:* It degrades p53 protein. It stimulates the expression of TERT, the catalytic subunit of telomerase resulting in increased tyrosine kinase activity. These changes cause genome instability. The host cells enter the cell cycle resulting in increased proliferation (*see* Fig. 6.48).

BACTERIA INDUCED CARCINOGENESIS

HELICOBACTER PYLORI

World Health Organization has designated *Helicobacter pylori,* a potential human carcinogen. *Helicobacter pylori* is strongly associated with *gastric adenocarcinoma (lower portion of gastric region) and low grade B cell NHL of the mucosa-associated lymphoid tissue (MALT) type.*

Pathogenesis

Helicobacter pylori expresses cytotoxin associated A (Cag A) gene that induces unregulated proliferation of hepatocytes. These bacteria stimulate reactive T cells to synthesize cytokines that convert polyclonal B cells to monoclonal B cells. *Helicobacter pylori* induces sequential changes in stomach such as chronic gastritis, gastric atrophy, intestinal metaplasia, sustained epithelial proliferation, genomic mutation, dysplasia, early gastric carcinoma and advanced **gastric carcinoma.**

BORRELIA BURGDORFERI

This organism is a spirochete that causes Lyme disease. It has been associated with *gastrointestinal tract lymphoma.*

CAMPYLOBACTER JEJUNI

This organism is associated with gastrointestinal lymphoma.

ENDOPARASITES INDUCED CARCINOGENESIS

SCHISTOSOMA HAEMATOBIUM

The parasite causes squamous cell carcinoma of the urinary bladder in Egypt population. It causes foci of squamous metaplasia of the bladder epithelium resulting in squamous cell carcinoma of the bladder. The earliest sign of bladder cancer is sudden painless hematuria in urine, which may red or rust colored. In the later stages, the bladder may become irritable, painful urination. Gross morphology of tumor is *exophytic (cauliflower-like) or ulcerated lesion.*

CLONORCHIS SINENSIS (LIVER FLUKE)

The parasite is transmitted through consumption of raw or undercooked vegetables. It resides in the biliary tree and may result in cholangiocarcinoma in far east population. It also causes **hepatocellular carcinoma** and **pancreatic carcinoma**.

OPISTHORCHIS VIVERRINI

The parasite causes cholangiosarcoma of the bile ducts.

FASCIOLA HEPATICA

The parasite causes cholangiocarcinoma. Pathogen induced carcinogenesis is shown in Table 6.55.

HORMONE INDUCED CARCINOGENESIS

Hormones such as estrogen, progesterone, and testosterone have been implicated as promoters of **breast, endometrial, ovarian,** or **prostatic cancers**. Hormones induced carcinogenesis are shown in Table 6.56.

ORAL CONTRACEPTIVES

Patient on long-term oral contraceptives may develop carcinomas of *breast and endometrium*.

DIETHYLSTILBESTROL (DES)

Clear cell adenocarcinoma is a rare vaginal tumor found in young daughters whose mothers take **diethylstilbestrol (DES)** during pregnancy. Patient initially develops vaginal adenosis characterized by mucosal columnar epithelium-lined crypts in areas normally lined by stratified squamous epithelium. **Vaginal adenosis** is thought to be a precursor of **clear cell adenocarcinoma**.

ANDROGEN

Androgen is associated with prostatic carcinoma.

Table 6.55: Pathogens induced carcinogenesis

Category of pathogens	Pathogen	Associated carcinoma
Bacteria	*Helicobacter pylori*	Gastric carcinoma (lower half of stomach)
		Low grade B cell NHL of the mucosa-associated lymphoid tissue (MALToma)
	Borrelia burgdorferi	Gastrointestinal tract lymphoma
	Campylobacter jejuni	Gastrointestinal tract lymphoma
Viruses	HCV (RNA)	Hepatocellular carcinoma
	HTLV-1 (RNA)	T cell leukemia/lymphoma
	EB virus (DNA)	CNS lymphoma in AIDS
		Nasopharyngeal carcinoma
		Hodgkin's disease (mixed cellularity)
		Burkitt's lymphoma
		Extranodal marginal zone B cell NHL
	HBV (DNA)	Hepatocellular carcinoma
	HHV 8 (human herpesvirus 8) (DNA)	Kaposi's sarcoma in AIDS
	HPV (types 16, 18) (DNA)	Squamous cell carcinoma of vulva, vagina, anus (associated with sexual intercourse), larynx and oropharynx
Parasites	*Schistosoma haematobium*	Squamous cell carcinoma of the urinary bladder
	Clonorchis sinensis (liver fluke)	Hepatocellular carcinoma
		Cholangiocarcinoma (bile duct carcinoma)
		Pancreatic carcinoma
	Opisthorchis viverrini	Cholangiocarcinoma (bile duct carcinoma)
	Fasciola hepatica	Cholangiocarcinoma (bile duct carcinoma)
Fungus	*Aspergillus flavus* (aflatoxin-β_1 product)	Hepatocellular carcinoma

Table 6.56: Hormones induced carcinogenesis

Hormones	Associated carcinoma
Oral contraceptives	Breast carcinoma
	Endometrial carcinoma
Diethylstilbestrol (DES)	Clear cell adenocarcinoma of vagina occurs in daughters of patients who received DES during pregnancy

INVASION AND METASTASIS

OVERVIEW

Invasion and metastasis constitute important hallmark of malignant tumors. The first event in tumor cell invasion is breach of the basement membrane and stromal extracellular matrix. After invading the interstitial tissue, malignant cells penetrate lymphatic or vascular channels.

In the lymph nodes, communication between the lymphatic channels and venous tributaries allows malignant cells access to the systemic circulation. Outline of operational steps involved in metastases is shown in Fig. 6.69. Sequence of events of metastatic cascade is shown in Table 6.57.

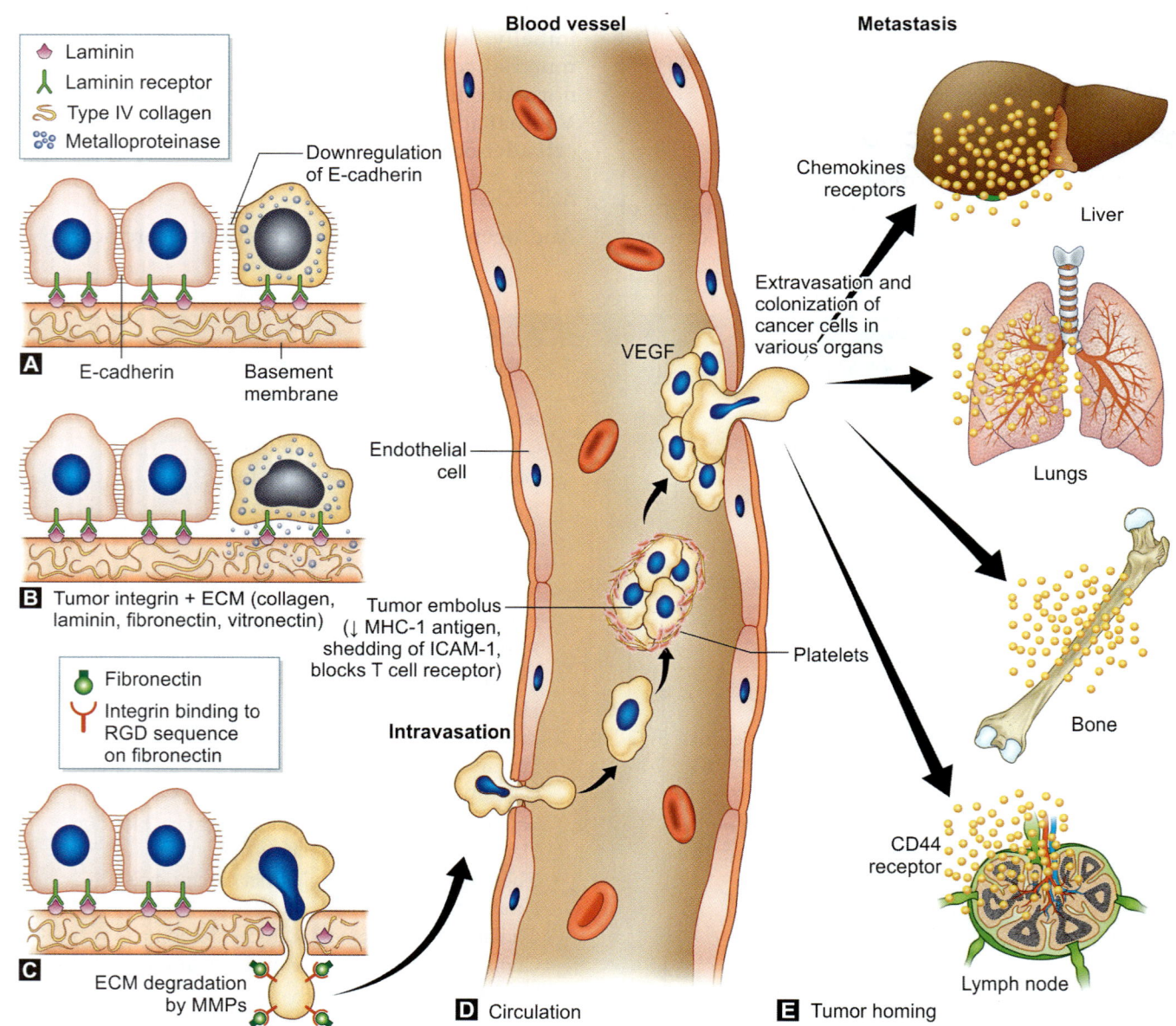

Fig. 6.69: Outline of operational steps in involved in metastases mediated by tumor–host interactions. (A) Penetration through basement membranes by tumor cells is preceded by adhesion to basement membrane components. Tumor cells express receptors for the basement membrane protein laminin and their ligand receptor interaction between laminin and its receptor on tumor cells is an important mechanism mediating binding, (B and C) binding to connective tissue matrix proteins is followed by proteolytic breakdown of these matrices and detachment of tumor cells, which then move through the breaches created by matrix protein-breakdown, (D) intravasation cancer cells, (E) extravasation of cancers and metastases to distant organs.

Table 6.57: Sequence of events of metastatic cascade

Process	Possible mediators	Consequences
Detachment of cancer cells	Downregulation of E-cadherins	Migration of individual cancer cells
Invasion of tissue boundaries	Metalloproteinases synthesis Downregulation of inhibitors of metalloproteinases Upregulation of integrin expression	Erosion of tissue boundaries
Intravasation	Metalloproteinases synthesis Downregulation of inhibitors of metalloproteinases	Access of cancer cells to vascular routes of dissemination
Evasion of host defense in circulation	Reduced expression of MHC class I antigen Shedding of ICAM-1 blocks T cell receptor	Survival of cancer cells against host defenses
Adherence of cancer cells to vascular endothelium	Binding of CD44 to endothelial ligand	Arrest of movement by adhesion to endothelium
Extravasation of cancer cells	Integrin Laminin receptor	Colonization of site of metastases

Steps of Metastases

These include detachment of cells, attachment of tumor cells to extracellular matrix (ECM), degradation of ECM, migration of tumor cells into blood vessels, tumor cell embolization, and extravasation of tumor cells from blood vessels to distant organs.

Regulation of Metastasis

Metastasis is regulated by *metastasis signature genes*. It is prevented by *metastasis suppressor genes*.

- *Metastasis signature genes:* These include Ezarin, miR10b, SNAIL and TWIST genes. Ezarin gene is involved in metastases of *rhabdomyosarcoma and osteosarcoma*. SNAIL and TWIST genes are involved in metastases of *breast carcinoma*.
- *Metastasis suppressor genes:* These include miR226, miR335, NM23, KAI-1, KiSS and NM23. KAI-1 is involved in metastases of *prostate carcinoma*. KiSS participates in metastases of *melanoma*.

EPITHELIAL-MESENCHYMAL TRANSITION (EMT)

In order to develop this migratory behavior, epithelial cancer cells acquire properties that come close to the mesenchymal cells. Consequently, this phenomenon has been called *epithelial-mesenchymal transition* (EMT).

Physiological state: Normal epithelial cells are characterized by strong intercellular adhesive interaction, structurally reflected in the existence of adherence intercellular junctions. Epithelial cells form continuous sheets. On the other hand, mesenchymal cells do not form continuous sheets, but do make connections by forming loose network of extracellular matrix.

Pathological state: Epithelial cells undergo morphological and behavioral changes in cancers.

SNAIL and TWIST genes promote epithelial-mesenchymal transition (EMT).

- SNAIL-1 and SNAIL-2 are central regulators of EMT. SNAIL-1 participates in downregulation of E-cadherin and reduction of cell adhesion. SNAIL-2 participates in activation of cytoskeleton, migration, rearrangement of focal adhesion and increased migration.
- In EMT, carcinoma cells downregulate epithelial marker (e.g. E-cadherin) and upregulate mesenchymal markers (e.g. vimentin and smooth muscle actin). These changes transform tumor cells to promigratory phenotype, which is essential step for metastases to distant organs.
- Drug developers are using cystatin C to inhibit EMT in breast cancer. Cellular modifications associated with epithelial-mesenchymal transition (EMT) are shown in Table 6.58.

DETACHMENT OF TUMOR CELLS

Physiological state: Cadherins are calcium-dependent transmembrane glycoproteins that mediate cell-cell adhesion. Cadherins suppress invasion and metastasis.

Pathological state: Expression of E-cadherin is reduced in most carcinomas. The detachment of cancer cells from

Table 6.58: Cellular modifications associated with epithelial-mesenchymal transition (EMT)

Proteins	Examples
In vitro morphology and function	Stellate or spindle shape Increased migration Invasion into collagen matrix
Downregulated proteins	E-cadherin Cytokeratin Occludin Claudin
Upregulated proteins	N-cadherin Vimentin SNAIL-1 SNAIL-2 TWIST MMPs (2, 3, 9) Integrin α2β2
Activated proteins	ILK GSK-3b Rho
Nuclear expression of proteins	β-catenin SMADA (2, 3) SNAIL-1 SNAIL-2

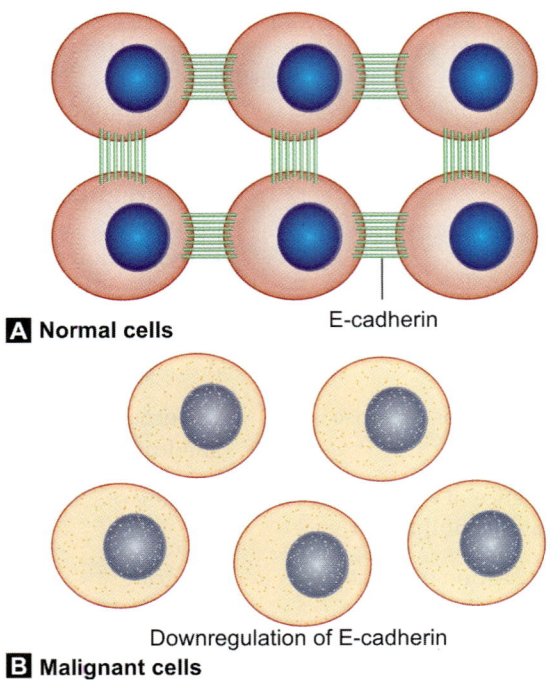

Fig. 6.70: E-cadherin molecule. (A) E-cadherin expression in normal cells, (B) cancer cells showing downregulation of E-cadherin.

the tissue of origin occurs due to loss of E-cadherin and catenin; diminished number of cell junctions; and other alterations in surface membrane structures. E-cadherin molecule is shown in Fig. 6.70.

ATTACHMENT OF TUMOR CELLS TO ECM

Tumor cells express integrin that helps attachment of tumor cells to extracellular matrix components (e.g. collagen fibers, laminin, fibronectin, vitronectin) promoting tumor cells migration. Laminin is a matrix glycoprotein. It appears to participate in the process of tissue invasion by binding to tumor cells and forms a bridge with tissue collagen type IV fibers. Some invasive tumor cells have an increased number of laminin receptors on their surface.

Degradation of Extracellular Matrix

ECM degradation is required for migration of tumors. It is carried by families of proteases: invading malignant cells and surrounding stromal cells synthesize metalloproteinases (MMPs), urokinase-type plasminogen activator (u-PA), elastase, cathepsins. These cause breakdown of basement membrane matrix (collagenous and noncollagenous matrix). MMP-9 plays important function in metastatic cascade. It induces VEGF resulting in angiogenesis.

Degradation of Collagenous Matrix

Metalloproteinases (type IV collagenase) cleave (dissolve) basement membrane collagen type IV fibers.

Degradation of Non-collagenous Matrix

Plasminogen activator activates elastase and cathepsins, which cleave non-collagenous matrix of basement membrane matrix. Plasminogen activator converts serum plasminogen to plasmin, a serine protease that degrades laminin. Plasminogen activator also stimulates cancer cells to synthesize collagenases in abundance (autocrine action). In some tumors, proteolytic enzymes are released in the stroma by *cooperating* host cells such as macrophages.

ROLE OF CLEAVAGE PRODUCTS

Cleavage products of matrix components derived from collagen fibers and proteoglycans have growth promoting (basic fibroblast growth factor), angiogenic (vascular endothelial growth factor) and chemotactic activities. Changes in the expression of u-PA, the u-PA receptor, and PA inhibitors have been reported in different cancers.

INVASION OF LYMPHATICS AND BLOOD VESSELS

The malignant cells become motile and invade into the region where the matrix has been broken down. These malignant cells have capacity to proliferate resulting in formation of progeny cells. Finally, malignant cells invade lymphatic or blood vascular channels (capillaries and venules).

TUMOR CELL EMBOLIZATION

After ECM migration, tumor cells enter into the lumen of lymphatic channels or capillaries and venules. Tumor emboli are formed covered with fibrin, platelets and leukocytes. Small number of embolized cells is apparently able to establish metastatic lesions. The survival and growth of metastatic cells is not a random process but depends upon the selection of cancer cells possessing specific properties needed for metastatic growth.

EXTRAVASATION OF TUMOR CELLS

Adhesion of Tumor Emboli to Endothelium

Tumor emboli adhere to the vascular endothelium. CD44 adhesion molecules expressed on the tumor cells bind to the endothelial venules in the lymph nodes. Some tumors express chemokine receptors that bind to the endothelia of venules present in lymph nodes. Some tumors express chemokine receptors that bind to CXC4 and CCR7 ligands expressed on the vascular endothelium in breast cancer.

Tumor Emboli Extravasation

The process of extravasation of tumor emboli occurs by the following mechanisms: cancer cells attach to the endothelial surface and induce retraction of endothelial cells. Cancer cells migrate through the breach, dissect and degrade the vascular basement membrane leading to migration out of the vascular compartment to form metastatic tumor. Within a primary cancer, there is marked cellular heterogeneity of metastatic potential.

Factors Establishing Tumor Metastases

Factors which influence the establishment of tumor metastases are: (i) genetic instability of the tumor cells; (ii) enzymatic degradation of basement membrane collagen; (iii) ability to withstand rheologic trauma; (iv) size of the tumor cell embolus; (v) interaction with cytotoxic T cells, natural killer cells, and macrophages; (vi) entrapment by fibrin or platelets; and (vii) surface properties (glycoproteins). These favor the ability of variant tumor cells to reach and colonize specific organs.

Evasion of Immune Surveillance

Tumor cells can be recognized by immune system. Tumor antigens may be mutated proto-oncogenes or tumor suppressor genes.

Tumor antigens are also produced by oncogenic viruses. MHC class I molecules process and present tumor cells to CD8+ cytotoxic T cells. There is increased risk of development of cancers in immunocompromised persons.

Tumor cells escape from immune system in immunocompetent patients by the following mechanisms: selective outgrowth of antigen negative variant of tumor cells, loss of MHC-I molecules, immunosuppression due to synthesis of TGF-β, PD1 ligands and galectins by tumor cells, tumor antigen masked by enhanced synthesis of glycocalyx on tumor cells and apoptosis of CD8+ cytotoxic T cells.

SURVIVAL AND GROWTH OF METASTATIC DEPOSITS

Extravasation of tumor emboli invades organs at distant sites. Formation of platelet-tumor aggregates may enhance tumor cell survival due to poor host immune response. Dissemination of malignant tumors occurs in *liver, lungs, brain, adrenal glands, lymph nodes, and bone marrow.*

METABOLIC ALTERATIONS IN TUMOR CELLS

Malignant cells preferentially utilize glucose by glycolysis for energy purpose rather than more energy efficient mitochondrial oxidative phosphorylation pathways. This phenomenon is known as *Warburg effect* or aerobic glycolysis.

ROUTES OF METASTASIS OF TUMORS

Preferential routes of metastasis vary with specific neoplasms. Carcinomas of kidney, thyroid (follicular carcinoma), and prostate metastasize initially to regional lymph nodes via lymphatic channels and later by hematogenous route to **lungs, liver, bones, and brain**. Gastrointestinal carcinomas most often metastasize to liver. Sarcomas metastasize by hematogenous route to lungs. Ovarian cancers most often involve peritoneum. Tumors rarely metastasizing include basal cell carcinoma and gliomas. Malignant tumors disseminate by one of five pathways (Fig. 6.71).

LOCAL INVASION

Local invasion is growth of the tumor into surrounding tissues. It is the first step in metastasis. It follows line of least resistance. It damages surrounding tissue. It

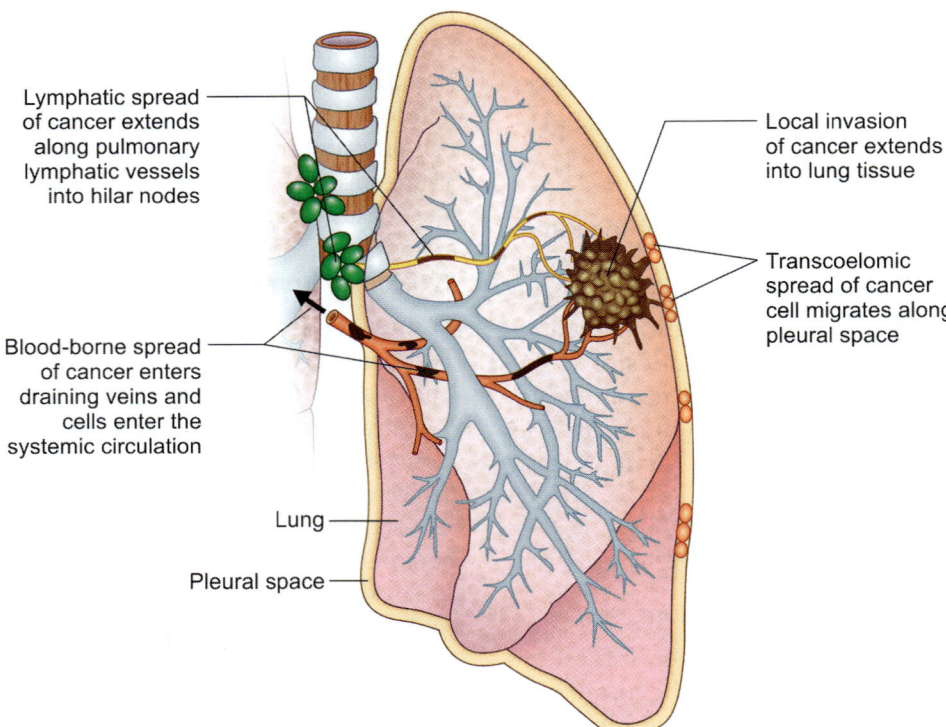

Fig. 6.71: Metastases of primary lung carcinoma showing by local invasion, lymphatic, hematogenous and transcoelomic routes.

exerts mechanical pressure on the surrounding cells and tissues, which eventually die as a result of interruption of blood supply. It causes pain as a result of nerve invasion.

Cancers of liver, colon, cervical, lung, pancreas, ovary and astrocytoma metastasize by direct extension. Invasion of *lung cancer* forms *bronchopleural fistula*. Invasion of *cervical cancer may form vesicovaginal fistula*. *Pancreatic carcinoma invades celiac plexus* resulting in severe pain. *Ovarian cancer* involves *peritoneum*.

LYMPHATIC ROUTE

Lymphatic spread is usual mechanism of dissemination of carcinomas followed by hematogenous spread to distant organs. *Breast cancer in outer quadrant involves axillary lymph nodes.* Breast cancer present in *inner quadrant metastasizes to internal mammary lymph nodes.* Lung cancer metastasizes to *perihilar tracheobronchial and mediastinal lymph nodes. Colorectal carcinomas metastasize first to mesenteric lymph nodes.*

Mechanism

Tumor cells become trapped in the first lymph node, it encounters. Presence of tumor cells within lymph node leads to its enlargement. Localized immune reaction to the tumor cells, limit their further spread. The cells that escape can enter the blood from the lymphatic circulation through plentiful connections between the venous and lymphatic systems.

Sentinel Node

The first lymph node involved in a regional lymphatic drainage is called sentinel lymph node, which can be identified by injecting blue dye. If the sentinel lymph node is involved, the patient needs extensive surgery or *vice versa*. Sentinel lymph node mapping is done in cancers of **breast** and **colon.**

Sinus Histiocytosis

Necrotic products of the neoplasm and tumor antigens often evoke reactive changes in the lymph nodes such as enlargement and hyperplasia of the lymphoid follicles, proliferation of macrophages in the subcapsular sinuses (sinus histiocytosis).

Skipped Metastases

Metastases to regional draining lymph nodes may be bypassed (skipped metastases) because of involvement of venous-lymphatic anastomoses by inflammation or irradiation resulting in obliteration of these channels.

HEMATOGENOUS SPREAD

Hematogenous spread is usual mechanism of dissemination for sarcomas. However, some carcinomas (e.g. renal cell carcinoma, hepatocellular carcinoma, follicular carcinoma of thyroid, prostatic carcinoma) may also metastasize by this route. **Renal cell carcinoma** often invades the renal vein to grow in a **snake-like fashion** up the inferior vena cava sometimes reaches the right side of the heart.

- *Mechanism:* Tumor cells invade the blood vessels (e.g. capillaries and venules). These are carried by blood to distant sites (e.g. liver, lung, bones). Conversely, skeletal muscles, although rich in capillaries, are rare site of secondary deposits by this route. Cancer cells reaching venous tributaries of the inferior vena cava flow to the right side of the heart and reach the lungs, whereas cancer cells via portal vein drainage metastasize to the liver. Systemic arterial routes carry malignant tumor cells to distant sites.
- *Preferential site of metastases:* Metastases irrespective of anatomic localization of the neoplasm and natural pathways of venous drainage: occurs by the following ways. Prostatic cancer preferentially spreads to bone. **Bronchogenic carcinomas** involve the **adrenals** and the **brain**. **Neuroblastoma** spreads to the **liver** and **bones**.
- *Distant metastases:* Distant metastases may reach lungs, liver, bones and brain.

Metastases in Lungs

Pulmonary metastases are more common than primary lung cancers. In one-third of all fatal cancers, pulmonary metastases are evident at autopsy.

Blood-borne metastases from *breast (most common), kidney, colon, thyroid and testes cancers* reach the lungs via systemic venous circulation to right side of heart. Other cancers from *salivary glands, thyroid gland, uterus, ovaries, urinary bladder and prostate* may metastasize to the lungs.

On imaging study, metastases are most often multiple and sharply circumscribed lacking cavitation. Calcification is unusual except metastases from osteosarcoma and chondrosarcoma.

Metastases in Liver

Liver is the commonest site of blood-borne metastases via portal vein from *gastrointestinal tract, lung cancers, breast and kidney including malignant melanoma*. Tumor emboli obstructing portal vein may produce portal hypertension, splenomegaly, and ascites.

Patient presents with **massive hepatomegaly** with nodules at the free edges, jaundice at a later stage as a result of massive liver involvement and obstruction of major hepatic ducts.

There is unexplained increase in the serum concentration of alkaline phosphatase. Metastases in liver in adults and children are shown in Figs 6.72 and 6.73. Liver metastases from breast carcinoma are shown in Fig. 6.74.

Metastases in Bones

Batsons' paravertebral venous plexus has connection with the vena cava and vertebral venous system.

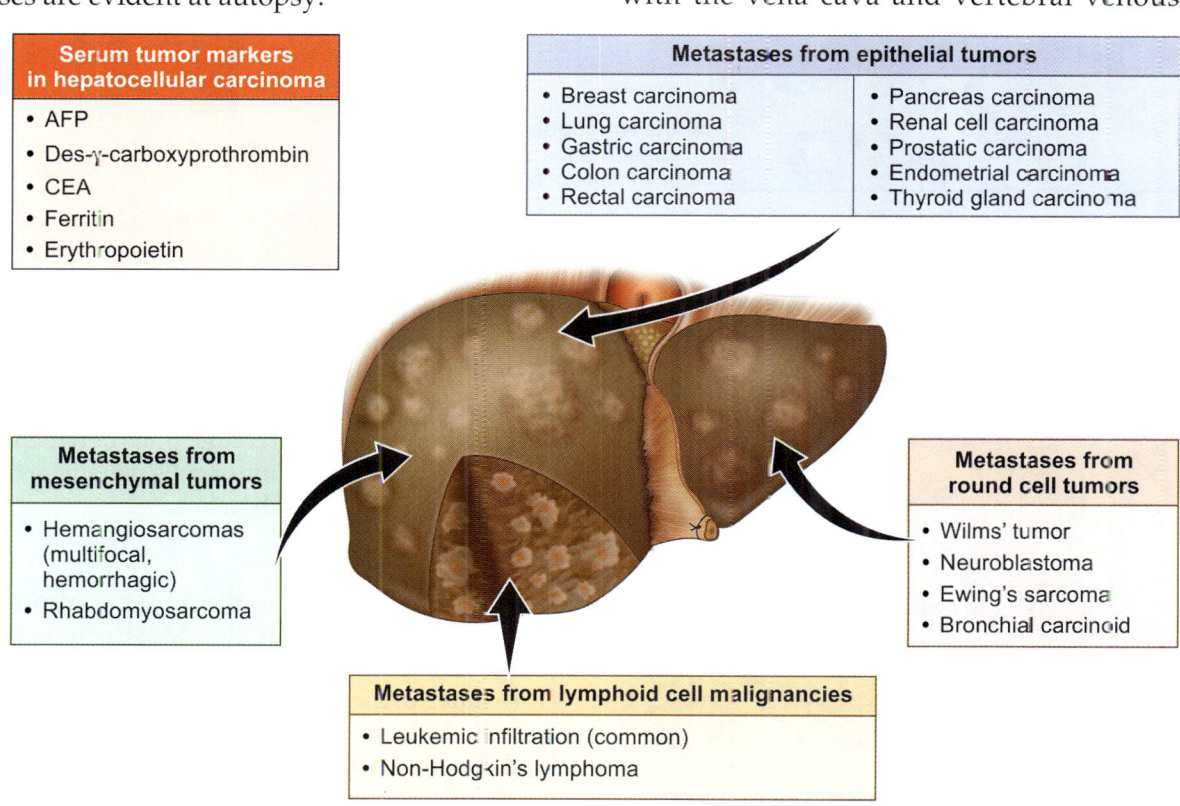

Fig. 6.72: Metastases in liver. Metastases from epithelial, mesenchymal tumors and round cell tumors.

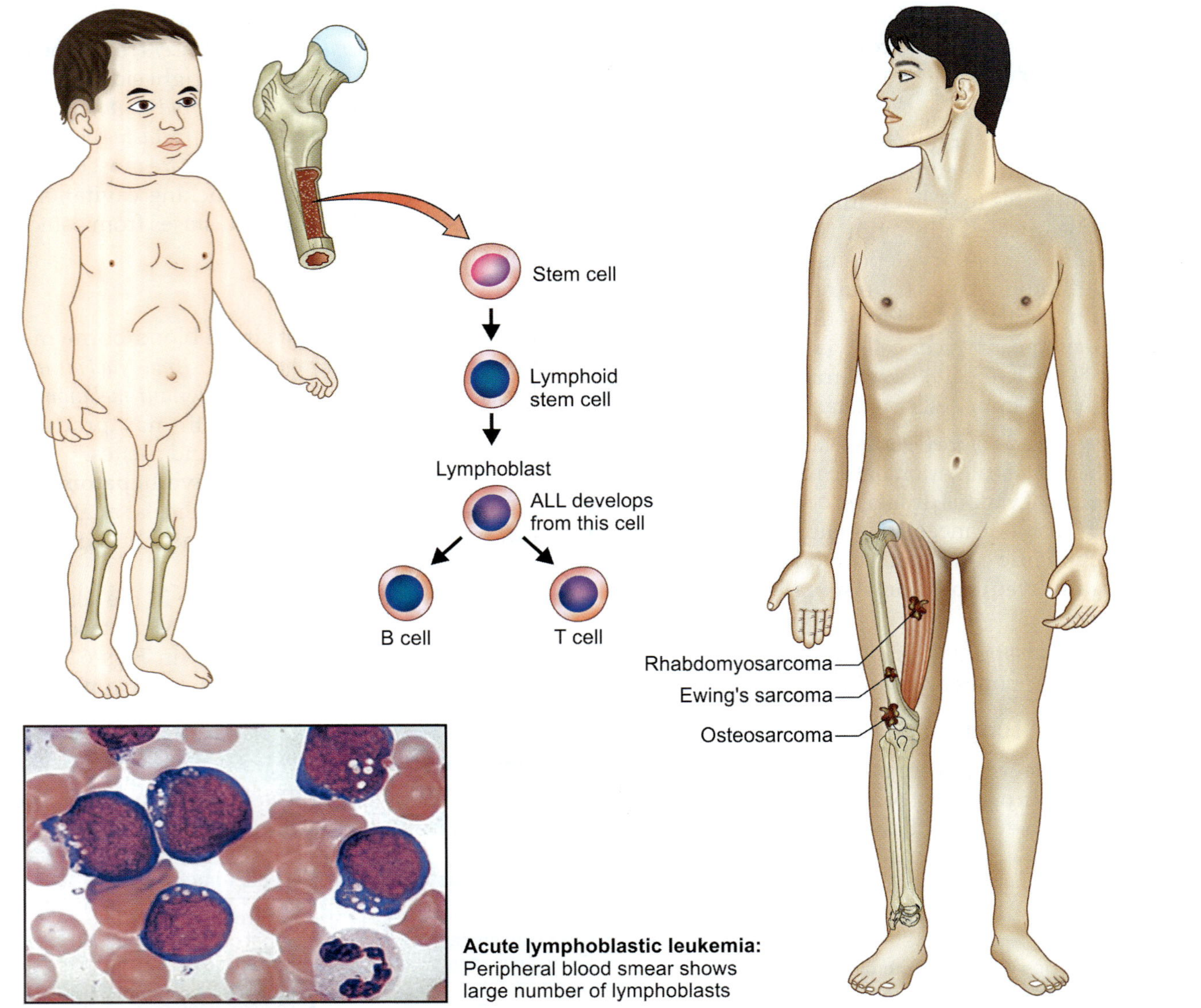

Section I: General Pathology

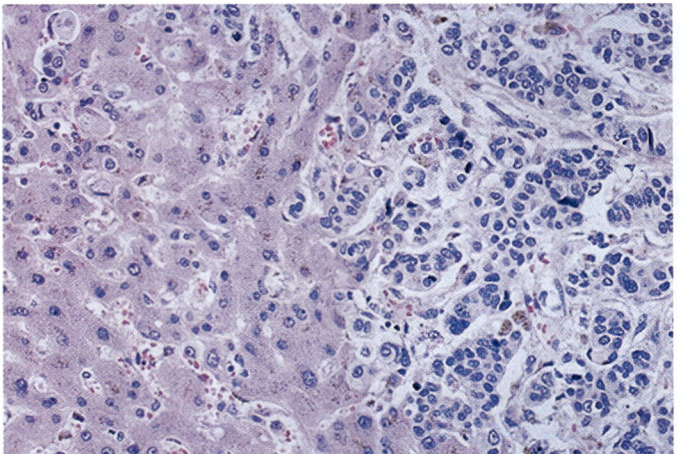

Acute lymphoblastic leukemia: Peripheral blood smear shows large number of lymphoblasts

Fig. 6.73: Common brain metastases in children and young adults from acute lymphoblastic leukemia, Ewing's sarcoma, osteosarcoma and rhabdomyosarcoma.

Fig. 6.74: Microscopically, metastatic infiltrating ductal carcinoma from breast is seen on the right, with normal liver parenchyma on the left (400X).

Vertebral venous system is extensive and valveless, and has **constant connection** to *breast, thyroid, lung,* and *prostate*. In addition, the plexuses are connected to dural sinuses and vasa vasorum of humerus and femur. There are numerous interconnections between vascular and lymphatic system. Tumor cells usually arrive in the bone by way of the bloodstream.

Age Group

Metastatic carcinoma is the most common tumor of bone after 40 years of age. Most common tumors metastasizing to the bones in adults include cancers of prostate, urinary bladder, breast, lung (small cell variant), kidney, gastrointestinal tract and thyroid gland. In children, metastatic tumors of bone include neuroblastoma, embryonal rhabdomyosarcoma, and retinoblastoma.

Site of Metastases

Vertebral column is the most common site of metastases in hematopoietic bone marrow; followed by pelvis, ribs, skull and proximal long bones. Skeletal metastases are uncommon below knee or elbow joints. Basal cell carcinoma, gliomas and soft tissue sarcomas except embryonal rhabdomyosarcoma rarely metastasize to bone. Bone metastases in adults and children are shown in Table 6.59.

Type of Bone Metastases

There may be osteolytic or osteoblastic lesions. **Breast cancer** may produce either *osteolytic* or *osteoblastic lesion*.

Clinical Features

Patients with metastatic deposits to bone present with pain, swelling, deformity, encroachment of hemopoietic tissue in the bone marrow, compression of spinal cord or nerve roots and pathological fractures.

Table 6.59: Bone metastases in adults and children

Age group	Tumors metastasizing to bones
Adults	Prostatic carcinoma
	Transitional cell carcinoma of urinary bladder
	Small cell carcinoma of lung
	Renal cell carcinoma
	Gastric carcinoma
	Colorectal carcinoma
	Thyroid carcinoma
Children	Neuroblastoma
	Retinoblastoma
	Embryonal rhabdomyosarcoma

Metastases in Brain

Metastatic tumors are more common than primary intracranial tumors of the CNS. These occur in adults (30%

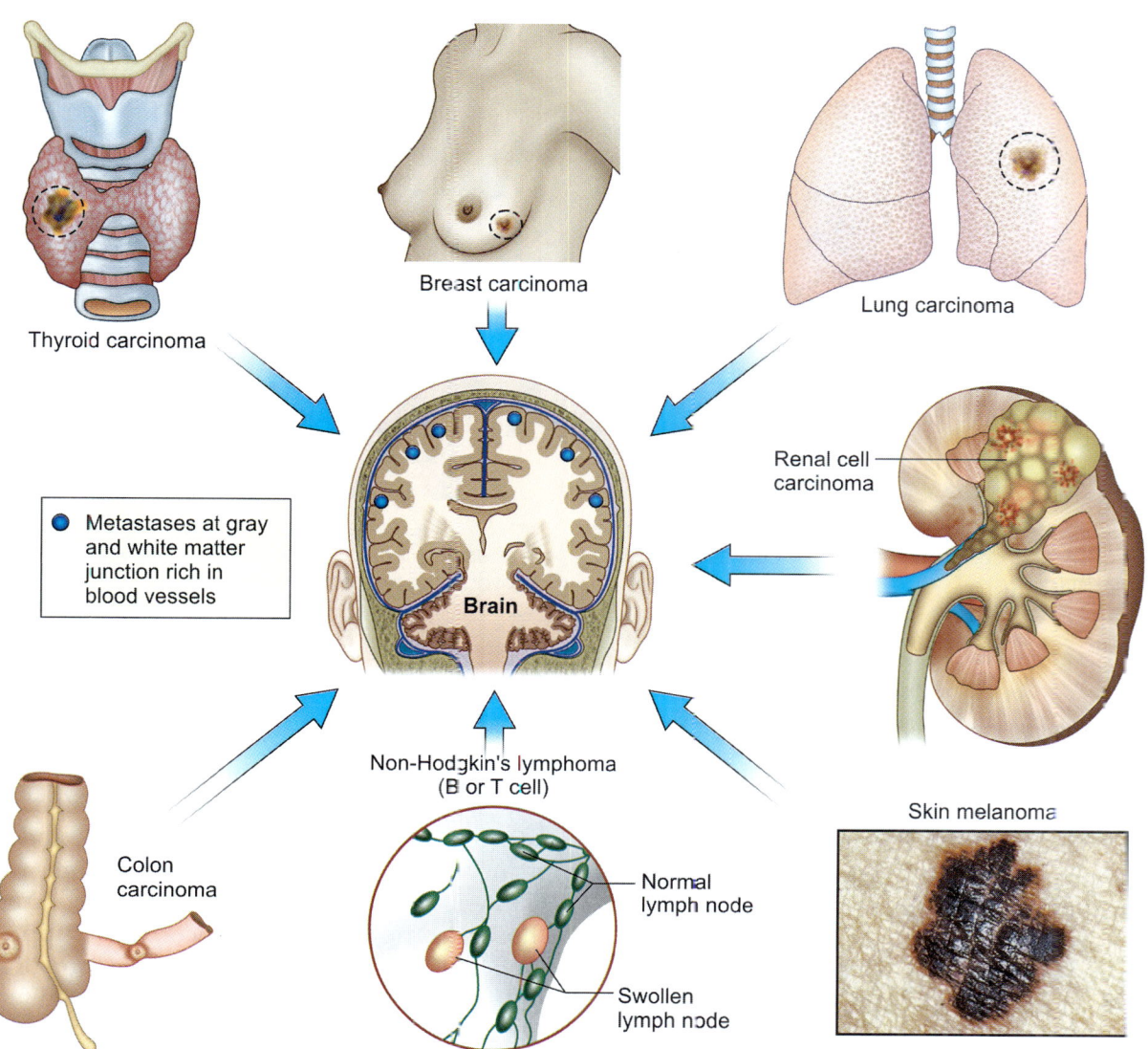

Fig. 6.75: Common brain metastases in adults from thyroid, breast, lung, kidney, colon, skin melanoma and NHL.

cases) and children (6–10% cases). Common sources of metastases in adults and children are shown in Fig. 6.75.

SEEDING/TRANSCOELOMIC ROUTE

Malignant tumors that arise in organs (e.g. ovaries, gastrointestinal tract, or lung) adjacent to body cavities may shed malignant cells into these spaces. It invariably results in a neoplastic effusion.

Peritoneal Cavity

Primary carcinoma of stomach, colon and breast may involve the peritoneum and then metastasize to ovaries, known as **Krukenberg tumor**, which refers to bilateral ovarian neoplasms composed of malignant, mucin containing, signet-ring cells.

Peritoneal seeding is common in patients with ovarian *serous cystadenocarcinoma*. The tumor cells (*mucinous cystadenocarcinoma*) secreting large amount of mucinous material in filling the abdominal cavity, known as *pseudomyxoma peritonei*. Gross morphology and light microscopy are shown in Figs 6.76 and 6.77.

Pleural Cavity

Breast cancer and peripherally located lung cancer and commonly seeds pleural surfaces leading to pleural effusion. Malignant cells may be demonstrated in pleural fluid examination.

Subarachnoid Space

Glioblastoma multiforme, medulloblastoma and **ependymoma** of CNS commonly seed the CSF causing spread to brain and spinal cord.

SURGICAL IMPLANTATION

Accidental spillage of neoplastic cells from one serous or mucous surface to another by direct contact may occur during the course of surgery via surgical instruments. It is significant **potential hazard during cancer surgery.**

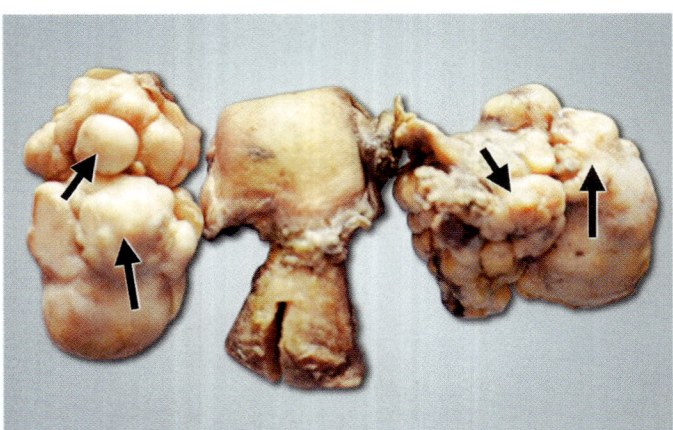

Fig. 6.76: Krukenberg's tumor: Both ovaries show involvement as a result of metastases from primary cancers of stomach or colon or breast (arrows).

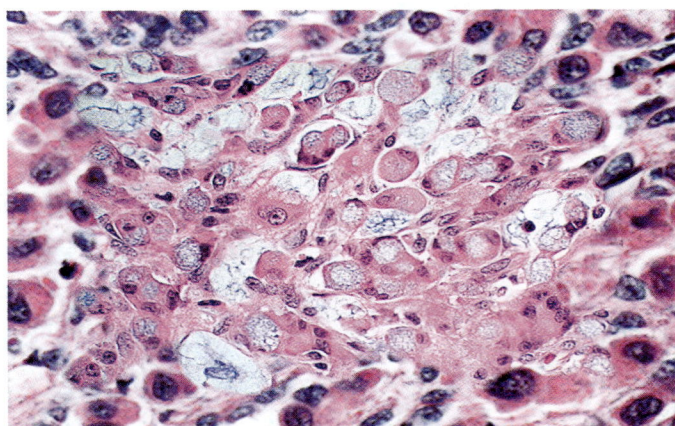

Fig. 6.77: Krukenberg's tumor shows nests of mucin-filled "signet-ring" epithelial cells with eccentric nuclei within a cellular stroma derived from the ovary (400X).

CLINICAL ONCOLOGY

CLINICAL EFFECTS ON HOST

Tumors cause atrophy of surrounding cells, obstruction of the lumen or organs, invasion, ulceration or destruction of adjacent structures, metabolic effects due to appropriate or unexpected neoplastic cell products; and effects due to metastases if the tumor is malignant. Most of the cancer cells entering circulation are destroyed by immune system. Clinical effects of cancer in host are shown in Fig. 6.78.

Cachexia

Cachexia means loss of body fat as well as muscular mass. Patient presents with progressive weakness, weight loss (>20%), anorexia, anemia, and infection. It occurs due to ubiquitin proteasome pathways. Tumor necrosis factor-α (TNF-α) synthesized by host macrophages and cancer cells suppresses the appetite center and decreases β-oxidation of fatty acid for fuel. Loss of appetite is common manifestation in

Neoplasia: Molecular Basis, Metastasis, Clinical Oncology and Laboratory Diagnosis

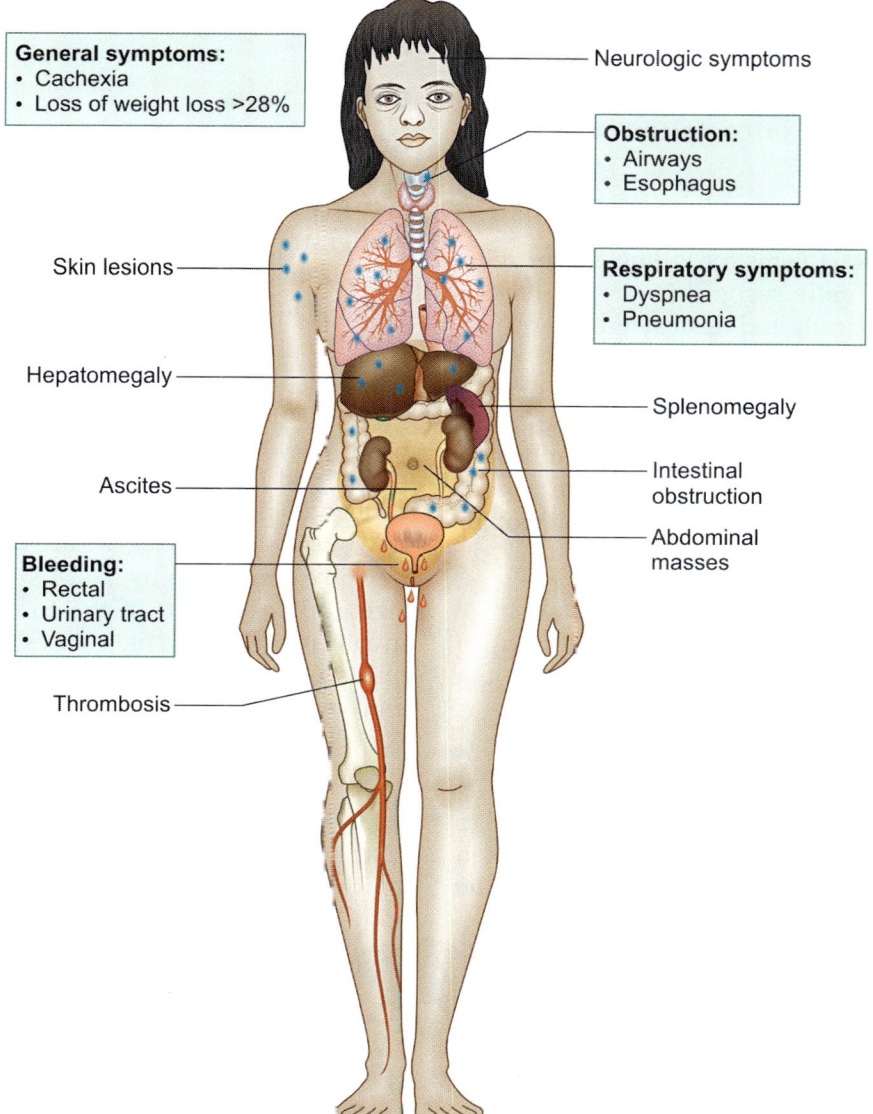

Fig. 6.78: Clinical effects of cancer in host (*Courtesy:* Dr. Abhijit Das).

cancers. **Malabsorption** may occur in association with **medullary carcinoma of thyroid.**

Anemia

Patient develops microcytic hypochromic anemia due to blood loss (e.g. GIT blood loss—colorectal cancer) from various sites. Macrocytic anemia occurs due to folate deficiency from rapid tumor growth; and bone marrow metastases (e.g. immature hemopoietic elements in peripheral blood known as *myelopthisic anaemia*).

Fever

Patient develops fever due to *infections* (e.g. gram –ve sepsis from *Escherichia coli* or *Pseudomonas aeruginosa*. Patient may develop pneumonia or urinary tract infection.

Ulceration and Bleeding

Cancers of colon, stomach and kidney may lead to ulceration and bleeding.

Rupture

Cancers of colon, ovarian and bladder may rupture.

Tumor Impingement on Nearby Structures

Pancreatic carcinoma may obstruct bile duct resulting in obstructive jaundice.

Leukopenia and Thrombocytopenia

Leukopenia and thrombocytopenia occur due to tumor invasion of bone marrow, chemotherapy or radiation.

HOST DEFENSE AGAINST CANCER

Humoral Immunity
Antibodies to tumor cells are important for antibody-dependent cell mediated or complement mediated cytotoxicity.

Type IV Cellular Immunity
It is most efficient mechanisms for killing cancer cells. Cytotoxic (CD8+) T cells recognize altered class I antigens on neoplastic cells and destroy them.

Natural Killer Cells
These cells have innate antitumor activity and kill cancer cells without previous sensitization. Lymphokine activated killer cells (LAKs) are even more potent than natural killer cells, which kill cancer cells through type II hypersensitivity reaction.

Macrophages
These cells are also part of the nonspecific natural immune response to tumor cells. These are activated by interferon-γ (IFN-γ).

GRADING AND STAGING
Both staging and grading (Fig. 6.79) systems are used to classify malignant neoplasms for prognostic evaluation and planning of clinical management. In general, the higher the stage or the higher the grade, the worse the prognosis.

Grading
Grading is based on histological cellular and differentiation/anaplasia of cancers along with nuclear atypia and invasiveness. It may be well differentiated or moderately differentiated or poorly differentiated (anaplastic) tumor. Prognosis is better in well differentiated than poorly differentiated cancers.

Staging
Staging is based on size, extent of spread of tumor invading surrounding tissue and disseminating to lymph nodes and distant metastases. It generally correlates better with prognosis than does histopathologic grading; however, both approaches are useful.

It is exemplified by TNM system. It evaluates the size and the extent of the tumor (T), lymph nodes involvement (N) and metastases (M) refers to extranodal metastases (e.g. *liver, lung and bone*). The most commonly employed staging guidelines are those laid out by the American Joint Committee on Cancer (AJCC).

PARANEOPLASTIC SYNDROME
Malignant tumors may synthesize hormones and produce remote clinical manifestations, collectively

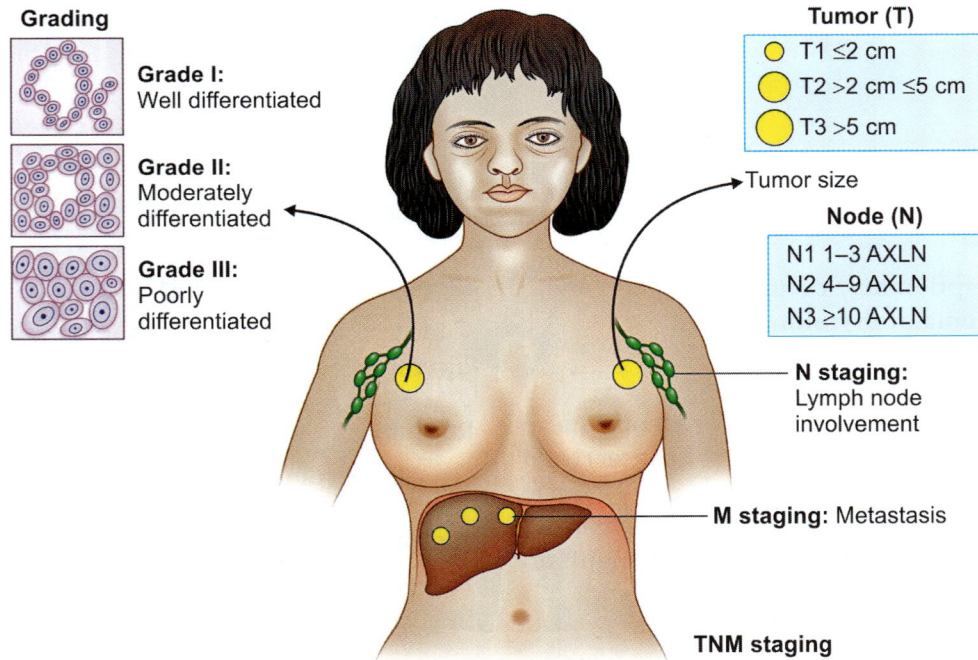

Fig. 6.79: Grading and staging in breast cancer. TNM stands for tumor, lymph node metastases and distant metastases. Grading and staging of breast carcinoma: grading classifies tumor according to their light microscopic characteristics. Staging is a clinical exercise that classifies tumors according to their size, invasiveness and spread. Tumors are staged according to the TNM system (T, tumor size, N, lymph node involvement, M. metastases to distant organs). Schemes for TNM classification vary according to tumor type and organ involved (*Courtesy* Dr. Abhijit Das).

termed paraneoplastic syndromes in 10–15% cases. It may represent the earliest manifestation of an occult neoplasm.

These clinical manifestations may even be lethal. Paraneoplastic syndromes are classified, i.e. *endocrinal, hematological, neuromuscular,* and *dermatologic.* Paraneoplastic syndromes are shown in Table 6.60.

ENDOCRINAL MANIFESTATIONS

Endocarinal manifestations are caused by ectopic production of hormones or chemically unrelated substances inducing effects similar to those of a given hormone. Endocrinal manifestations are described as under.

Table 6.60: Paraneoplastic syndromes

Syndrome	Underlying cancers	Mechanism by synthesis of molecules
Endocrinopathies manifestations		
Cushing's syndrome	Small cell carcinoma of lung Pancreatic carcinoma Medullary carcinoma of thyroid	ACTH or ACTH-like
Hypercalcemia	Squamous cell carcinoma of lung Breast carcinoma Renal cell carcinoma Ovarian carcinoma	Parathormone related protein, TGF-α, TNF, IL-1
Hypocalcemia	Medullary carcinoma of thyroid	Calcitonin
Syndrome of inappropriate antidiuretic hormone (SIADH) resulting in hyponatremia	Small cell carcinoma of lung (most common) Prostatic carcinoma Thymoma Gastrointestinal tract carcinoma Non-Hodgkin's lymphoma (NHL) Hodgkin's disease	ADH
Polycythemia	Renal cell carcinoma Hepatocellular carcinoma Cerebellar hemangioma	Erythropoietin
Hypoglycemia	Fibrosarcoma Ovarian carcinoma	Insulin or insulin-like hormone
Hypocalcemia	Medullary carcinoma of thyroid	Calcitonin
Bone changes		
Hypertrophic osteoarthropathy and clubbing of fingers	Bronchogenic carcinoma Thymoma	Occurs due to periosteal reaction of distal phalanx (often associated with clubbing of nails)
Antibody mediated disorders		
Lambert-Eaton syndrome (characterized by myasthenia gravis like weakness)	Bronchogenic carcinoma Thymoma	Autoantibodies formed against presynaptic voltage gated channels in the neuromuscular junction
Stiff-Person syndrome	Breast carcinoma Small cell carcinoma of lung	Anti-amphiphysin and anti-GAD antibodies formed
Opsoclonus	Neuroblastoma Small cell carcinoma of lung	Formation of anti-Ri and anti-Hu antibodies
Carcinoid syndrome		
Carcinoid syndrome	Gastric carcinoma Pancreatic carcinoma Bronchial adenoma	Serotonin

Contd...

Table 6.60: Paraneoplastic syndromes (Contd...)

Syndrome	Underlying cancers	Mechanism by synthesis of molecules
Dermatologic manifestations		
Seborrheic keratosis	Gastric carcinoma	Develops sudden appearance of numerous pigmented seborrheic keratosis (Leser-Trélat sign)
Dermatomyositis	Bronchogenic carcinoma Breast carcinoma	Immunologic mechanism
Acanthosis nigricans (black verrucoid-appearing lesions)	Lung carcinoma Gastric carcinoma Uterine cancers	Immunologic mechanism (synthesis of epidermal growth by these tumors)
Hematologic and vascular manifestations		
Disseminated intravascular coagulation	Acute myelocytic leukemia Prostatic carcinoma	Tumor products activate coagulation
Trousseau syndrome (superficial migratory thrombophlebitis results in venous thrombosis)	Bronchogenic carcinoma Pancreas carcinoma	Tumor products like mucin activate clotting
Renal manifestations		
Nephrotic syndrome	Renal cell carcinoma Lung carcinoma Colon carcinoma Lymphomas	Tumor derived antigen combine with antibody to form immune complexes deposited in glomeruli leading to glomerular injury
Male breast manifestation		
Gynecomastia	Choriocarcinoma of testis	β-HCG

Cushing Syndrome

It is caused by production of ACTH-like substances by small cell (oat cell) carcinoma of the lung and medullary carcinoma thyroid.

Inappropriate Secretion of Antidiuretic Hormone

It is most commonly caused by small cell carcinoma of the lung. Serum sodium level is decreased.

Hypercalcemia

Squamous cell carcinoma of lung, breast carcinoma and ovarian carcinoma synthesize PTH-related protein that causes bone resorption resulting in hypercalcemia.

Osteoclast activating factor synthesized by multiple myeloma leads to hypercalcemia.

Hypoglycemia

It is caused by secretion of insulin-like substances by hepatocellular carcinomas, mesotheliomas, and leiomyosarcomas.

Hyperthyroidism

It is caused by production of substances such as thyroid-stimulating hormone by hydatidiform moles, choriocarcinomas, and some lung tumors.

Carcinoid Syndrome

It is caused by synthesis of serotonin by bronchial adenoma, pancreatic carcinoma and gastric carcinoma.

HEMATOLOGIC AND VASCULAR EFFECTS

Thrombosis

There is increased risk for vessel thrombosis due to thrombocytosis, increased synthesis of coagulation factors (e.g. fibrinogen, factor V and factor VII); release of procoagulants from cancer cells.

Polycythemia

Polycythemia is caused by synthesis of erythropoietin by renal cell carcinoma, hepatocellular carcinoma, uterine leiomyomas, and cerebellar hemangioblastoma.

Migratory Thrombophlebitis

Pancreatic adenocarcinoma synthesizes thromboplastin-like substance develops superficial migratory thrombophlebitis **(Trousseau syndrome).**

Disseminated Intravascular Coagulation

Tumor products of acute myelocytic leukemia and prostate carcinoma may cause disseminated intravascular coagulation.

Autoimmune Hemolytic Anemia

It occurs due to synthesis of cold autoantibodies by lymphomas.

ANTIBODY MEDIATED DISORDERS

Lambert-Eaton Syndrome

This is characterized by myasthenia gravis like weakness in **bronchogenic carcinoma** and **thymoma** as a result of autoantibodies formed against presynaptic voltage gated channels in the neuromuscular junction.

Stiff-Person Syndrome (SPS)

This is a rare acquired neurological disorder characterized by progressive muscle stiffness (rigidity) and repeated episodes of painful muscle spasms. It occurs due to formation of **anti-amphiphysin** and **anti-GAD antibodies** in patients with **breast carcinoma** and **small cell carcinoma** lung.

Opsoclonus–Myoclonus Syndrome

This is also known as *opsoclonus–myoclonus–ataxia* (OMA). It occurs due to formation of anti-Ri and anti-Hu antibodies in patient with **neuroblastoma** and **small cell carcinoma lung**. Patient presents with rapid involuntary conjugate fast eye movements, twitching of a muscle or group of muscles, cerebellar atxia, aphasia, and mutism.

DERMATOLOGIC MANIFESTATIONS

Acanthosis Nigricans

Patient with gastric carcinoma synthesizes epidermal growth factor (EGF) results in hyperkeratosis and pigmentation of the axilla, neck, intertriginous areas, flexures, and anogenital region known as *acanthosis nigricans*. Approximately 50% patients with acanthosis nigricans have gastric carcinoma.

Dermatomyositis

Patient with visceral malignancies may develop dermatomyositis. Leser-Trélat sign is sudden appearance of multiple seborrheic keratoses.

MISCELLANEOUS MANIFESTATIONS

Hypertrophic Osteoarthropathy

Patient with bronchogenic carcinoma of lung may develop hypertrophic osteoarthropathy due to periosteal reaction of distal phalanx (often associated with clubbing of nails).

Nonbacterial Thrombotic Endocarditis

Patient with mucus secreting pancreatic and colorectal carcinoma may develop sterile vegetations on mitral valve known as *nonbacterial thrombotic endocarditis*.

TUMOR MARKERS

Tumor markers are biological substances synthesized and released by cancer cells. Tumor products include cell surface antigens, cytoplasmic proteins, enzymes and hormones. These can be detected in cells or body fluids before they become symptomatic.

Evaluation of tumor markers has utility to confirm the diagnosis. These tumor markers fall into following categories: oncofetal antigens, hormones, isoenzymes, specific proteins, viruses, mucins and glycoproteins. Carcinoembryonic antigen represents dedifferentiation process of cancer. Her2 neu and prostate-specific antigen (PSA) reflect increased cellular proliferation.

Some tumor markers such as β-HCG and α-fetoproteins are estimated to monitor the response to therapy in germ cell tumors of testes. An ideal tumor marker has high sensitivity, specificity and low price. Potential use of tumor markers is population screening, diagnosis, establishing prognosis, staging, evaluation in postoperative cases, monitoring treatment response, surveillance for recurrence, and targets for therapeutic intervention.

FUNCTIONAL CLASSIFICATION

Oncofetal Antigens

Carcinoembryonic antigen (CEA) and α-fetoprotein (AFP) are normally expressed during fetal development but do not occur normally in the tissues or sera of children and adults. Expression of oncofetal proteins by neoplastic cells is considered a manifestation of dedifferentiation.

The undifferentiated neoplastic cells tend to resemble their embryonic counterparts. CEA is increased in cancers of colon, pancreas, lung, stomach and breast. Tumor marker α-fetoprotein (AFP) is increased in **hepatocellular carcinoma** and **yolk sac** tumor (endodermal sinus tumor) of testis and ovary. AFP is also increased in fetal anencephaly and other neural tube defects.

Proteins Occurring in Epithelial Cells

CA 19-9, CA 125, and CA 15-3 proteins are elevated in various cancers.

Polypeptide Hormones

β-chain of human chorionic gonadotropin (β-hCG), and specific enzymes such as the placental isoform of alkaline phosphatase (ALP) are elevated in the serum of patients with specific tumors. Tumor markers are shown in Table 6.61 and Figs 6.80 to 6.82.

Table 6.61: Tumor markers

Categories	Serum tumor markers	Associated malignancies
Oncofetal antigens	Alpha fetoprotein (AFP)	Hepatocellular carcinoma
		Yolk sac tumor
	Carcinoembryonic antigen (CEA)	Nonseminomatous germ cell testicular tumors
		Colon carcinoma
		Gastric carcinoma
		Pancreatic carcinoma
		Lung carcinoma
		Breast carcinoma
		Also increased in hepatitis, pancreatitis, benign nodular hyperplasia prostate and hemolytic anemia
Hormones	Human chorionic gonadotropin (β-hCG)	Choriocarcinoma
		Seminoma/dysgerminoma with trophoblastic element
		Also increased during pregnancy
	Calcitonin	Medullary carcinoma thyroid
	Adrenocorticotropin (ACTH) ectopic hormone	Small cell carcinoma of lung
		Pancreatic carcinoma
		Neural tumors
	Antidiuretic hormone/atrial natriuretic hormone (ADH/ANH)	Small cell carcinoma of lung (most common)
		Thymoma
		Prostatic carcinoma
		Intracranial neoplasms
		Hodgkin's disease
		Non-Hodgkin's Lymphoma (NHL)
		Gastrointestinal tract carcinomas
	Parathyroid hormone related protein (PTHrP)	Small cell carcinoma of lung
		Breast carcinoma, ovarian carcinoma, renal cell carcinoma
		Adult T cell lymphoma
		Prostatic carcinoma
		Hepatocellular carcinoma
		Tumors with neuroendocrine differentiation
	Insulin ectopic hormone	Fibrosarcoma
		Mesenchymal sarcoma
		Hepatocellular carcinoma
	Thyroid hormones	Struma ovarii (germ cell tumor variant of teratoma)
	Erythropoietin ectopic hormone	Renal cell carcinoma
		Cerebellar hemangioma
		Hepatocellular carcinoma
	Catecholamine and metabolites	Pheochromocytoma
	Serotonin	Bronchial adenoma
		Pancreatic carcinoma
		Gastric carcinoma
	Ferritin	Hepatocellular carcinoma
		Acute leukemia
		Hodgkin's disease
		Multiple myeloma
		Malignant lymphoma
		Hepatocellular carcinoma
		Prostatic carcinoma

Contd...

Table 6.61: Tumor markers (Contd...)

Categories	Serum tumor markers	Associated malignancies
Isoenzymes	Prostatic acid phosphatase (PAP)	Prostatic carcinoma Also increased in benign nodular hyperplasia prostate and prostatitis
	Neuron-specific enolase (NSE) and chromogranin	Small cell carcinoma of lung Neuroblastoma
	Lactate dehydrogenase (LDH)	Seminoma Ewing's sarcoma Also increased in hepatitis and cirrhosis
Specific proteins	Immunoglobulins	Multiple myeloma and other gammopathies
	β2 microglobulin	Multiple myeloma
	Prostate specific antigen (PSA)	Prostatic carcinoma
	Thyroglobulin	Thyroid carcinoma (well differentiated)
	Insulin-like growth factor binding protein-2 (IGFBP-2)	Prostatic carcinoma
	Human epididymis protein-4 (HE-4)	Ovarian carcinoma
	Nuclear matrix protein-22 (urine)	Urothelial carcinoma
	Cytokeratin fragment 21.1 (CYFRA 21.1)	Non-small cell carcinoma of lung
	Synaptophysin (synaptic vesicle membrane protein)	Neuroendocrine tumors Small cell carcinoma of the lung
	Calretinin	Mesothelioma
	Urinary peptides in urine	Endometrial carcinoma
Mucins and glycoproteins	CA 125	Ovarian cancer Endometrial carcinoma
	CA 19.9	Pancreatic carcinoma Colon carcinoma
	CA 72.4	Gastric carcinoma Colon carcinoma
	CA 15.3	Breast carcinoma
	CA-27.29	Breast carcinoma
	Cytokeratin fragment 21.1 (CYFRA 21.1)	Non-small cell lung cancer
Viruses	Human papillomavirus (HPV)	Cervical carcinoma
	EBV-DNA	Burkitt's lymphoma Nasopharyngeal carcinoma Some lymphoproliferative disorders
Other products	Chromogranin A	Neuroendocrine tumors Insulinoma (episode of hypoglycemia) Gastrinoma (Zollinger-Elison syndrome: peptic ulcer disease)

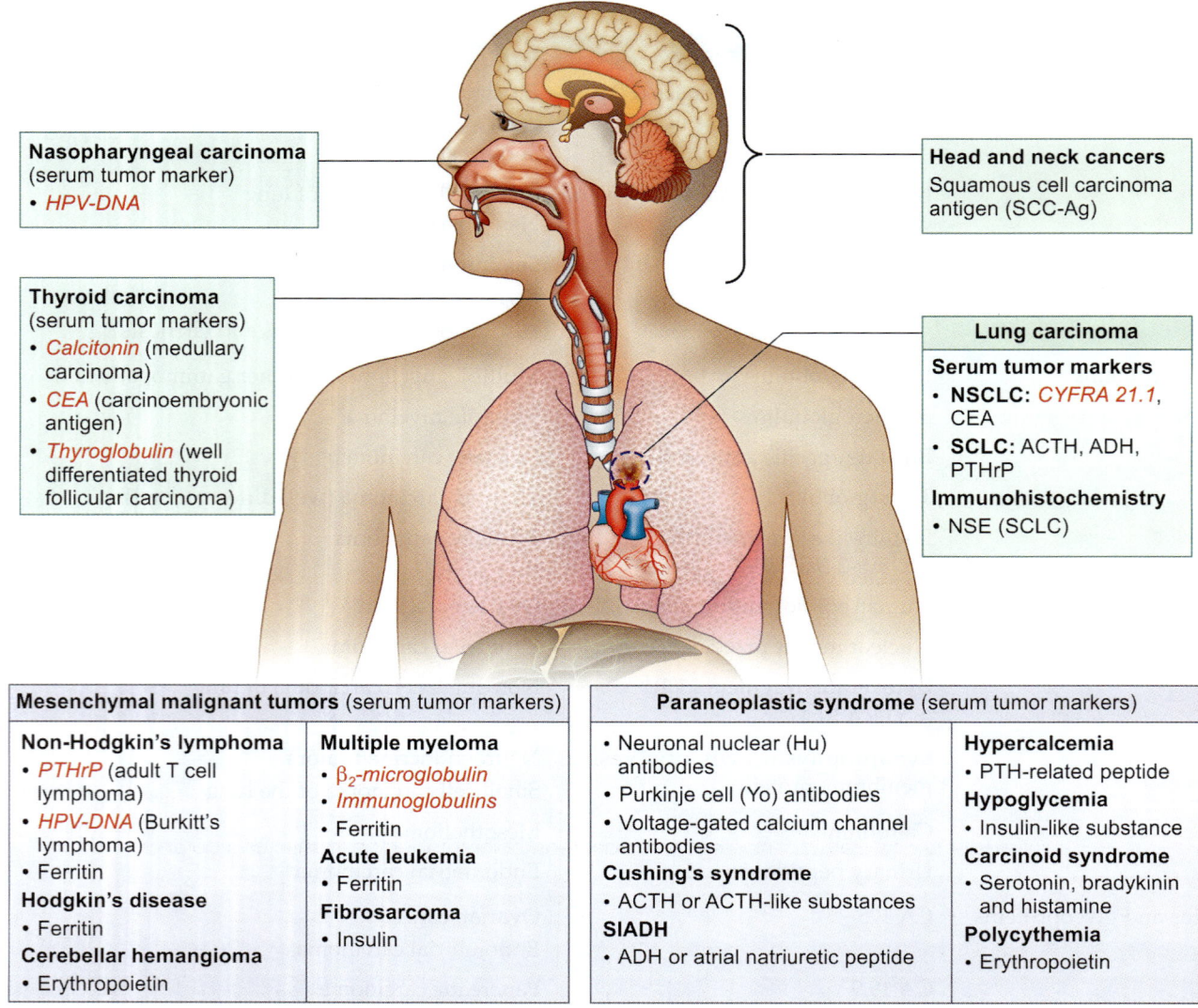

Fig. 6.80: Tumor markers in cancers of head and neck, lung, mesenchymal and paraneoplastic syndromes.

TREATMENT

Targets for Cancer Suppression

Targets for cancer suppression are to reduce cell proliferation and promoting apoptosis of cancer cells. Administration of tyrosine kinase inhibits block signal pathways that cause cells to proliferate; upregulate pathways that cause apoptosis. Angiogenesis inhibitors are administered to cutoff blood supply of cancer cells. Site-specific cancer treatments are shown in Table 6.62.

Surgery

Surgical excision of cancerous growth along with draining lymph nodes is performed. Mastectomy includes breast cancer along with axillary lymph nodes.

Radiation

Radiotherapy is used in treatment of various cancers. Radiation may be external, internal or systemic.

Chemotherapeutic Agents

Monoclonal antibodies kill cancers, interfere with angiogenesis, suppress local growth factors and stimulate immune system. These monoclonal antibodies can be hybridized with plant or bacterial toxin to form immunotoxin complexes that attach to a target cell and poison it. The most exciting prospect of this therapy is that it can target a specialized cancer cell and no normal cells. This type of monoclonal antibody-based drugs is currently employed in the treatment of various cancers such as breast, colorectal and NHL. Selected monoclonal antibody-based drugs used in various cancers are shown in Table 6.63.

Neoplasia: Molecular Basis, Metastasis, Clinical Oncology and Laboratory Diagnosis

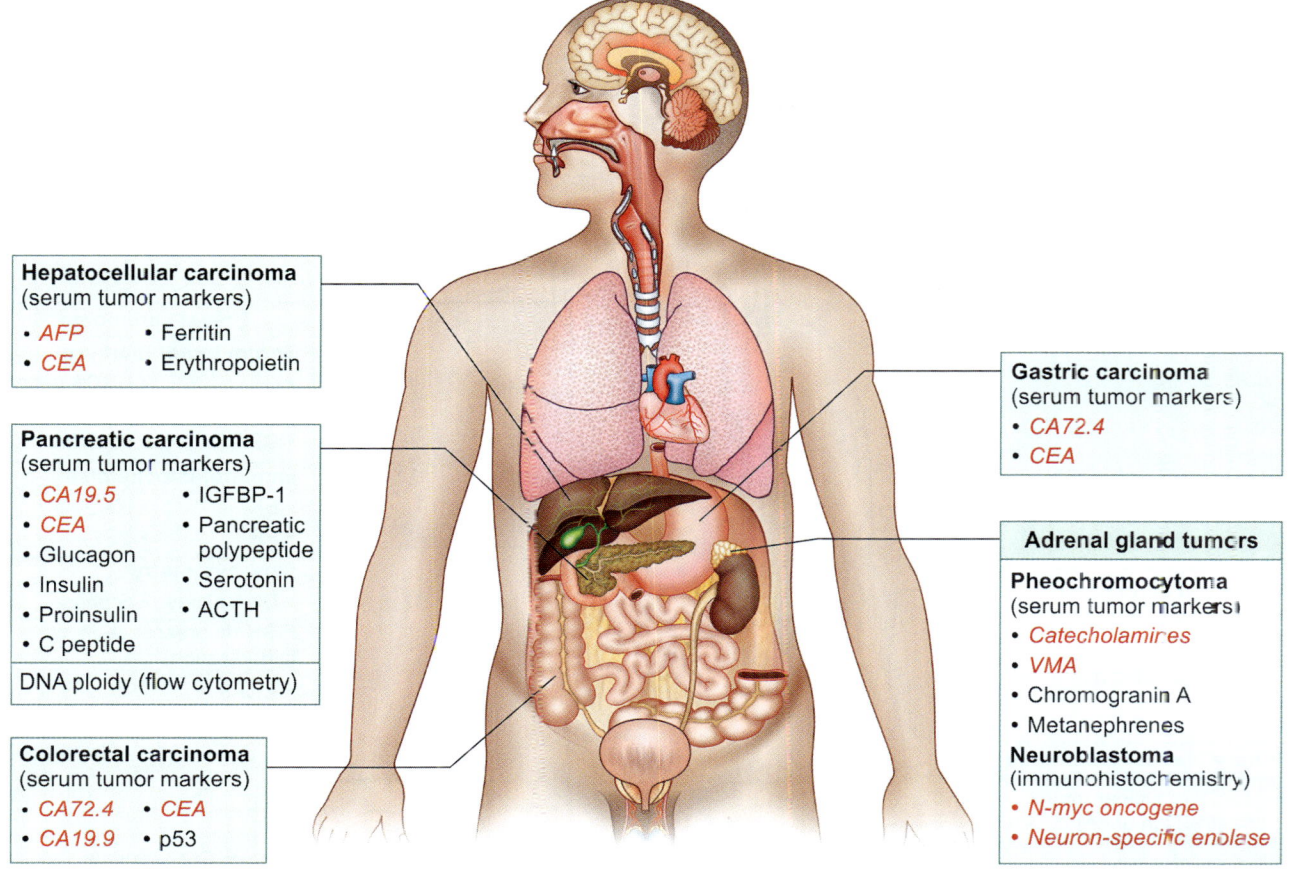

Fig. 6.81: Tumor markers in cancers of liver, pancreas, colorectal region, gastric and adrenals.

Table 6.62: Site-specific cancer treatments

Treatment	Method	Aim of treatment	Site of cancer
Surgery	Excision of tumor along with lymph nodes	Surgical excision of cancerous growth along with draining lymph nodes is performed	Breast, thyroid gland, lung, colon, ovary, uterus, and skin
Radiation	External radiation	Radiation source is outside body. Beam of radiation is focused on the malignant growth of brain	Breast, lung, uterus, cervix, lymphoma (many cancers need combined surgery and radiation therapy)
	Internal radiation	Radiation source is inside body. Radioactive material (capsule, needles or seeds) is placed in prostate gland to treat prostatic carcinoma	
	Systemic radiation	Radioactive substance (radioactive iodine) is absorbed by thyroid cancers. It binds and acts on malignant cells in thyroid gland	
Biologic therapy (immunotherapy)	Administration of synthetic monoclonal antibodies or vaccination with tumor antigen	Synthetic monoclonal antibodies are administered to target cancer cells. Vaccination with tumor antigen is performed to stimulate immune system. For example 'rituximab' is a manufactured monoclonal antibody (mab) used to treat NHL, which targets CD20 of B cells.	Breast, ovary, leukemia, lymphoma, and melanoma

Hormone therapy is given in cancers of breast and prostate. Bone marrow transplant is performed in leukemia, multiple myeloma, and lymphoma

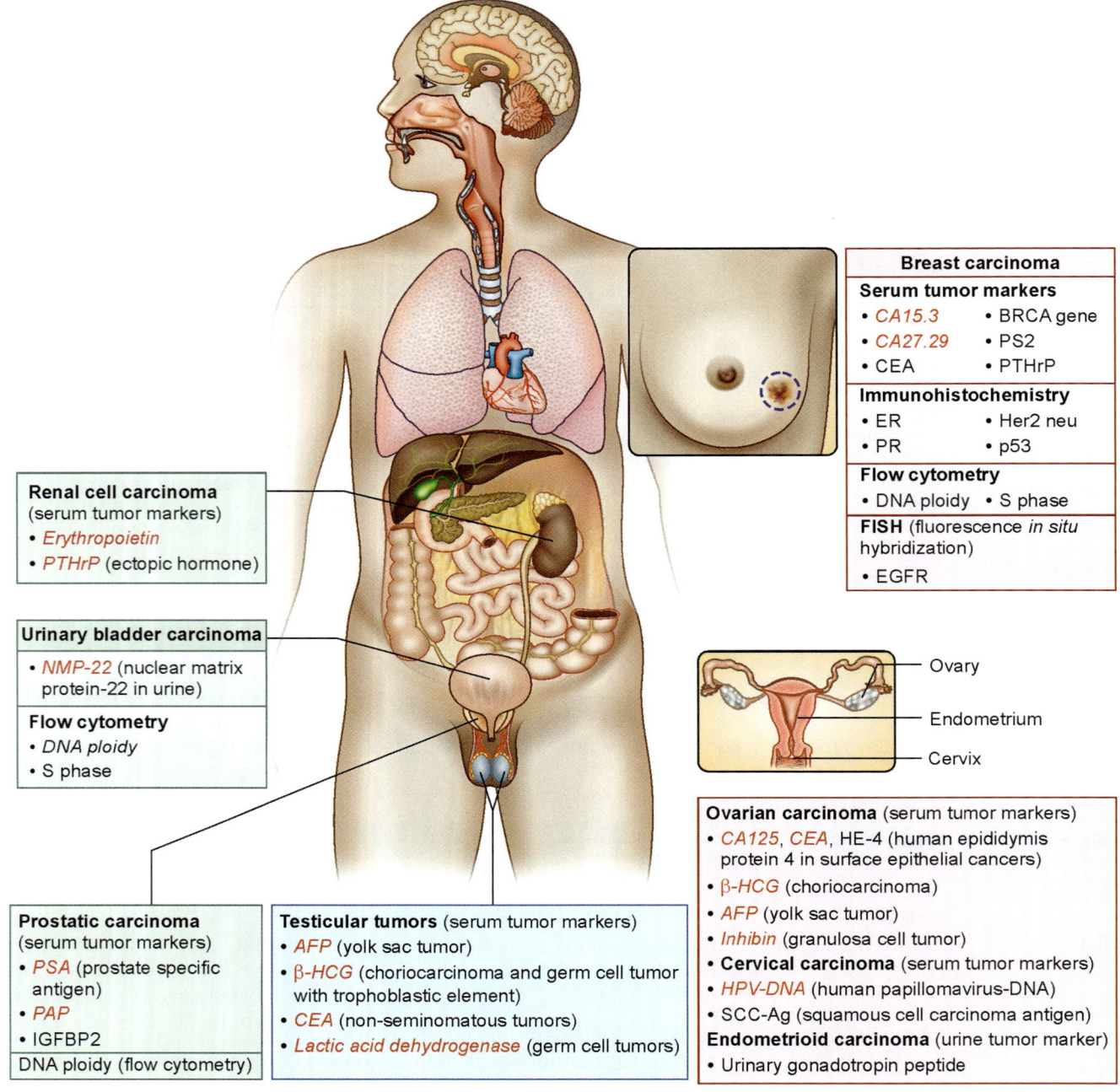

Fig. 6.82: Tumor markers in cancers of breast, kidney, urinary bladder, prostate, testes, ovaries, endometrium, and cervix.

SPONTANEOUS REGRESSION OF TUMORS

The spontaneous regression of pathologically confirmed human cancers, including those with metastases, is extremely rare but is documented for some malignant tumors of infancy and childhood and also of adults. Some tumors may regress spontaneously. These include **renal cell carcinoma, neuroblastoma, retinoblastoma, malignant melanoma, leukemias,** **lymphomas, choriocarcinoma, hepatocellular carcinoma, cholangiocarcinoma** and **osteosarcoma.**

Notable in this regard is neuroblastoma of infants and childhood. This tumor originates from neuroblasts of the adrenal medulla and usually has a highly malignant course but, remarkably, in a small proportion of cases regresses by *maturation*/differentiation to a benign ganglioneuroma or disappears.

Table 6.63: Selected monoclonal antibody-based drugs used in various cancers

Agent	Target	Process targeted	Cancer type
Monoclonal antibody (MAB)			
Bevacizumb	Vascular endothelial growth factor (VEGF)	Angiogenesis	Colorectal carcinoma (metastatic) Lung carcinoma
Cetuximab	Epidermal growth factor receptor	Growth factor signaling	Colorectal carcinoma
Trastuzumab	Her2 neu growth factor receptor	Growth factor signaling	Breast carcinoma
Rituximab	CD20 receptor	Induction of cell death	Non-Hodgkin's B cell lymphoma
Gentrumab			Acute myelogenous leukemia
Small molecule inhibitors			
Imatinib	BCL-ABL fusion protein; kit	Growth factor signaling (tyrosine kinase inhibitor)	Chronic myeloid leukemia Gastrointestinal stromal tumors
Erlotinib	Epidermal growth factor receptor	Growth factor signaling	Non-small cell lung carcinoma
Bortezomib	Proteosome	Multiple processes affected	Multiple myeloma

Note that these names are coded to end in mab—short of monoclonal antibody.

PROGNOSIS OF SOLID CANCERS

Prognosis of solid tumors varies depends on origin in various organs (Table 6.64).

PREVENTION MODALITIES OF CANCERS

Lifestyle Modifications

Cigarette smoking is usually associated with lung cancer. In smokers, there is also increased incidence of cancers of oral cavity and urinary bladder. Alcohol abstinence reduces squamous cell carcinoma of orophaynx and upper/middle esophagus, pancreatic and hepatocellular carcinomas.

Increased adipose tissue increases aromatase conversion of *androgens to estrogens*. Increased estrogen increases risk for *endometrial and breast carcinoma*. Therefore, reduction of weight decreases endometrial and breast cancer.

Hepatitis B Vaccination

Immunization against HBV decreases the risk of **hepatocellular carcinoma** due to hepatitis B induced post-necrotic cirrhosis.

Screening Procedures

Cervical Papanicolaou (Pap) smear examination detects cervical dysplasia (preneoplastic lesion), which can be surgically removed. Colonoscopy detects numerous polyps that are precancerous.

Table 6.64: Prognosis of solid tumors

Prognosis	Solid tumors
Good prognosis	Seminoma testes
	Basal cell carcinoma
Intermediate prognosis	Breast carcinoma
	Colorectal carcinoma
	Laryngeal carcinoma
	Uterus cancer
	Melanoma
	Teratoma testes
	Osteosarcoma
Poor prognosis	Carcinomas of lung
	Pancreatic carcinoma
	Stomach carcinoma
	Esophageal carcinoma
	Hepatocellular carcinoma
	Malignant mesothelioma

Mammography detects non-palpable masses in breasts. **Prostate-specific antigen** detects prostatic cancer, but lacks specificity as it is increased in benign hyperplasia of prostate.

Treatment of Conditions that Predispose to Cancer

Eradication of *Helicobacter pylori* decreases the risk for developing malignant lymphoma and adenocarcinoma of the stomach. Treatment of **gastroesophageal reflux** decreases the risk for developing **adenocarcinoma** arising from Barrett's esophagus.

LABORATORY DIAGNOSIS

OVERVIEW

Useful tests for early detection and staging of tumors include *screening tests, X-rays, radioactive isotope scanning (nuclear medicine imaging), computed tomography (CT) scanning, endoscopy, ultrasonography, and magnetic resonance imaging (MRI)*. Several sampling approaches exist for the diagnosis of tumors including excision, biopsy, fine needle aspiration, and cytologic smears.

Early Detection

Early diagnosis of cancer can be achieved in *skin cancer, cervical cancer* by Pap smear, *colon cancer* by colonoscopy and *breast cancer* by mammography.

Histopathological Examination

Early diagnosis is difficult in *liver, lung, brain, pancreatic cancer*. The singlemost important diagnostic tool is the biopsy for direct histologic study of the tumor tissue.

Immunohistochemistry and Flow Cytometry

Immunohistochemistry and flow cytometry help in the diagnosis and classification of tumors, because distinct protein expression patterns define different entities (*refer* to Chapter 14).

Serum Tumor Markers

Proteins released by tumors into the serum such as PSA, can be used to screen populations for cancer and to monitor recurrence by the following treatment.

Molecular Analyses

Molecular analyses are used to determine diagnosis, prognosis, the detection of minimal residual disease, and the diagnosis of hereditary predisposition to cancer (*refer* to Chapter 14).

Molecular profiling of tumors by cDNA arrays can determine expression of large segments of the genome at once and can be useful in molecular stratification of otherwise identical tumors for the purpose of treatment. Methods used for detection of gene mutations are shown in Table 6.65. Techniques used to analyze DNA, RNA and proteins are shown in Table 6.66.

HISTORY AND PHYSICAL EXAMINATION

Signs and symptoms such as weight loss, fatigue, and pain may be present. A mass may be palpable or visible.

RADIOGRAPHIC TECHNIQUES

The use of *plain films* (X-rays), *computed tomography* (CT), *magnetic resonance imaging* (MRI), *mammography*, and *ultrasonography* (US) may be very helpful to detect the presence and location of mass lesions. These methods may aid in staging and determination of therapy. X-rays are most commonly ordered to identify and evaluate changes in **tissue densities.** *Ultrasonography* uses high frequency sound waves to detect changes in the density of tissues, thus helps to differentiate cysts from solid tumors.

Table 6.65: Methods used for detection of gene mutations

Technique	Principle	Type of gene mutation detection
Cytogenetic analysis	Unique visual appearance of various chromosomes	Numerical structural abnormalities in chromosomes
Fluorescence *in situ* hybridization (FISH)	Hybridization to chromosomes with fluorescent labeled probes	Numerical structural abnormalities in chromosomes
Southern blot	Hybridization with genomic probe or cDNA probe after digestion of high molecular DNA	Detection of large deletion, insertion, and rearrangement
Polymerase chain reaction	Amplification of DNA	Expansion of triplet repeats, variable number of tandem repeats (VNTR), gene rearrangement, and translocation
Reverse transcriptase PCR (RT-PCR)	Reverse transcription, amplification of DNA segment, absence or reduction of mRNA transcription	Analyze expressed mRNA (cDNA) sequence detects loss of expression
DNA sequences	Direct sequencing of PCR products. Sequencing of DNA segment cloned into plasmid vectors	Point mutation, small deletions and insertions
Restriction fragment length polymorphism	Detection of altered restriction pattern of genome: DNA Southern blot or PCR products	Point mutation, small deletion and insertion

Table 6.66: Techniques used to analyze DNA, RNA and proteins

Technique	Sample analyzed	Gel used	Purpose
Southern blot	DNA	Yes	Detection of DNA changes
Northern blot	RNA	Yes	Analysis of mRNA amount and size
Western blot	Protein	Yes	Analysis of protein content
Allele-specific oligonucleotides	DNA	No	Detection of DNA mutations
Microarray	RNA or cDNA	No	Measurement of many mRNA at one time
ELISA	Protein or antibodies	No	Detection of proteins (antigens) or antibodies

Radioactive isotope scanning provides a view of organs and regions within an organ that cannot be seen with a simple X-ray. *CT scanning* evaluates successive layers of tissue to provide a cross-sectional view of the structure. It also can reveal different characteristics of tissues within a solid organ.

ENDOSCOPY

Endoscopy provides a direct view of a body cavity or passage way to detect abnormalities. During endoscopy, the medical professionals can *excise small tumors, aspirate fluid, or obtain tissue samples for histological examination.*

LABORATORY ANALYSIS

General findings such as *anemia, enzyme abnormalities* (such as an increased *alkaline phosphatase*), and *hematuria or positive stool* **occult blood** are helpful to suggest further workup. More specific testing such as measurement of prostate specific antigen levels, may help to determine the presence of specific neoplasms, but such tests are not perfect screening tools in a general population. Detection of specific genes (such as **BRCA1 for breast cancer**) may suggest an increased risk for some malignancies.

CYTOLOGICAL DIAGNOSIS

Methods of obtaining cells for cytological examination are simple, cost effective and minimally invasive. Cells shed naturally into body fluids, e.g. *sputum, urine, fluid in pleural and peritoneal cavities.*

Exfoliative Cytology

Cancers involving or protruding from the surface of organs continuously shed cells into the surrounding space. These cells are known as **exfoliative cells**. The cells are obtained from *cervix (cervical cancer), sputum (lung cancer), pleural fluid (lung cancer), peritoneal fluid (various cancers), cerebrospinal fluid (brain tumors)* and *urine (transitional cell carcinoma).* Smears are prepared and stained by Papanicolaou stain and examined under light microscopy. Immunohistochemistry is performed on these smears.

Scrap Smears

These are prepared with endoscope from cervix and gastrointestinal tract lesions and studied.

Fine Needle Aspiration Cytology (FNAC)

It is commonly done to aspirate lymph nodes and solid tumors, e.g. (breast, thyroid, and pancreas). Smears are stained by *May-Grünwald-Giemsa stain (MGG)*. Immunocytochemistry plays an important role in diagnosis of tumors.

HISTOPATHOLOGICAL STUDY

Needle Biopsy

Needle biopsy is used with a cutting needle to sample any lesion, including those in brain. Small size biopsy measuring 1–2 mm wide and 2 cm long biopsy can make histological interpretation difficult.

Endoscopic Biopsy

Small forceps are used to sample lesions often via *endoscopic techniques.* It is applied to lesions in gastrointestinal, respiratory, genital and urinary tracts.

Incisional Biopsy

Scalpel is used to biopsy from a lesion. Sample is variable in size depending on nature of lesion. It is applied to surgically accessible lesions only.

Excision Biopsy

Whole abnormal lesion is surgically removed and fixed in 10% buffered formalin to obtain paraffin sections. Sampling of large specimen would include tumor (for histogenetic pattern of differentiation, staging

Table 6.67: Common stains used for histopathological study

Stains used	Name of the stain
Fat stain	Sudan III, Sudan IV, Sudan B, Oil red O and Osmic acid
Bile salts	Hall stain
Tubercular bacilli	Ziehl-Neelsen stain (20% acid)
Lepra bacilli	Fite-Faraco stain
Reticulin stain	Silver methenamine
Calcium	von Kossa Alzarin red
Fibrous tissue	von Gieson stain
Fungi	PAS stain Silver methinamine
Helicobacter pylori	Modified Giemsa
Amyloid	Methyl violet (metachromatic stain) Crystal violet (metachromatic stain) Congo red with polarizing microscopy Fluorescent stains (Thioflavin T, Thioflavin S) von Gieson stain PAS stain
Hemosiderin	Perl's reaction (Prussian reaction) using acidified $K_4Fe(CN)_6$
Melanin	Fontana-Masson silver stain
Lipofuscin	Ziehl-Neelsen stain
Copper	Rhodamine stain
Glycogen, neutral mucin, fungus, glycoproteins, glyoclipids, amyloid and basement membrane	PAS
Acidic epithelial mucin	Mucicarmine stain
Acid mucopolysaccharide	Alcian blue at pH 2.5
Highly acidic mucin (sulphated mucin)	Alcian blue at pH 1

and grading), resection margins, lymph nodes and background tissue. Hematoxylin and eosin stained sections are studied by light microscopy. Freshly prepared 2% **buffered glutaraldehyde** is recommended for fixation of tissues for **electron microscopy**. Prompt refrigeration is required for study of hormone receptors. Common stains used for histopathological study are shown in Table 6.67.

FROZEN SECTION TECHNIQUE

Frozen section is used for rapid diagnosis of malignancy. It should be used only in the following circumstances, i.e.
- Confirmation of a cytological diagnosis of malignancy before proceeding to definite surgery
- Assessment of excision margins for a wide local excision to ensure complete excision
- Assessment of draining lymph nodes to identify patients who are node negative and who require only a limited dissection.

Tissues are quickly frozen, sectioned, mounted on slides, stained and interpreted within a few minutes, which enable surgeon to take appropriate decisions about the extent of surgery.

ELECTRON MICROSCOPY

Electron microscopy plays significant role in the diagnosis of poorly differentiated cancers, e.g. *carcinoma, sarcoma or lymphoma*, whose classification is difficult by

Neoplasia: Molecular Basis, Metastasis, Clinical Oncology and Laboratory Diagnosis

routine light microscopy. Desmosomes and specialized junctional complexes are demonstrated in carcinoma, while *absent in mesenchymal tumors and lymphomas*. Carcinoma exhibits short microvilli, blunt *with terminal* web, while microvilli of lymphoid and mesenchymal tumors do not show a terminal web.

Cells of *ectodermal* origin often have *many cilia*. Epithelial tumors show presence of bundles of tonofilaments; whereas slender microfilamemts are common in *mesencymal tumors*. Malignant melanoma shows presence of melanosomes. Small membrane-bound granules with dense core are features of endocrine neoplasms.

IMMUNOHISTOCHEMISTRY

Monoclonal antibodies are used directed against specific antigens located in cell membrane, cytoplasm and nuclear membrane. The immune complex formed is demonstrated by the **peroxidase–antiperoxidase** method. It is used to differentiate **carcinomas** and **sarcomas**, T and B lymphomas. It is also used to diagnose **round cell tumors** and **metastatic disease** in bone marrow and lymph nodes.

It is now frequently applied in the diagnosis of tumors, particularly when small samples of tissues are submitted for diagnosis. Monoclonal antibodies directed against specific proteins (e.g. *intermediate filaments*) can be used to stain slides, aiding identification of the cell of origin of a lesion.

Immunocytochemistry in conjunction with immunofluorescence is a useful diagnostic tool in the identification and classification of tumors arising from T and B cells and from mononuclear phagocytic cell. Monoclonal antibodies have diagnostic significance in the classification of undifferentiated tumors. Immunohistochemistry as diagnostic tool in cancers is shown in Table. 6.68 (*refer* to Chapter 14).

FLOW CYTOMETRY

Flow cytometry is performed to quantify different types of cells according to their membrane antigen character and DNA content used in classification of lymphomas and leukemias. **DNA is extracted from the tumors** and studied, which has prognostic significance. Cells are made to flow in laminar flow in an isotonic fluid under pressure. Monoclonal antibodies are used to differentiate different hematological lineages. **Aneuploidy** is associated with **poor prognosis** in early stage of breast, lung, colorectal and urinary bladder cancers (*refer* to Chapter 14).

DNA PROBE ANALYSIS

Probes are copies of complementary DNA (cDNA). Two probes are prepared: one from the tumor and another from normal tissue. The tumor (cDNA) is now tagged with red color fluorochrome. Normal DNA probe is tagged with green color fluorochrome. DNA of the cells is digested by one or more restriction enzymes (bacterial enzymes). Base pair of DNA is identified and cut. DNA fragments are separated by **gel electrophoresis**, then denatured and transferred to nitrocellulose membrane and then DNA probe is applied resulting in hybridization. (*refer* to Chapter 14).

Table 6.68: Immunohistochemistry as diagnostic tool in cancers

Intermediate filaments	Tissue origin of tumor	Tumors
Cytokeratin	Epithelial tissue	Squamous cell carcinoma (skin), Renal cell carcinoma, Mesothelioma
Vimentin	Mesenchymal tissue	Sarcoma
Desmin	Skeletal muscle	Rhabdomyosarcoma
	Smooth muscle	Leiomyoma
Neurofilament	Neurons	Neuronal tumors of brain (e.g. ganglioglioma, gangliocytoma and neurocytoma)
	Neural crest derivatives	Neuroendocrine tumors, e.g. neuroblastoma, pheochromocytoma and small cell carcinoma of lung
GFAP (glial fibrillary acidic protein)	Glial cells	Glial tumors of brain
		Breast carcinoma

Renal cell carcinoma expresses both cytokeratin and vimentin.

SOUTHERN BLOT ANALYSIS

T and B cells neoplasms can be identified on the basis of clonal rearrangement of their receptor genes by applying Southern blot analysis (*refer* to Chapter 14).

FLUORESCENCE *IN SITU* HYBRIDIZATION (FISH)

FISH is most often performed to study translocation in **CML t(9;22)** and amplification of **N-MYC in neuroblastoma** and other cancers (*refer* to Chapter 14). FISH is a cytogenetic diagnostic technique that uses fluorescent probes that bind to only those parts of the chromosome with a high degree of sequence complementarity.

MOLECULAR DIAGNOSIS

Polymerase chain reaction (PCR) is used to amplify DNA, generating thousands to millions of copies of a particular sequence. PCR is currently used in biomedical research laboratories for the diagnosis of hereditary and infectious diseases.

It is performed to assess minute translocation such as **BCR-ABL in chronic myeloid leukemia**. K-RAS mutation is studied in stool sample to assess minimal residual disease in previously treated colonic cancer. Demonstration of K-RAS indicates recurrence of disease (*refer* to Chapter 14).

CHAPTER 7

Nutritional and Infectious Diseases

Learning Objectives

NUTRITIONAL DISEASES
- Protein–Calorie Malnutrition
- Obesity Associated Disorders
- Vitamins

BACTERIAL INFECTIONS
- Tuberculosis
- Leprosy (Hansen Disease)
- *Actinomyces israelii*
- *Salmonella typhi*

VIRAL INFECTIONS
- Molluscum Contagiosum
- Varicella (Chickenpox)
- Rabies Virus
- Poliovirus
- Herpes II Virus
- Human Papillomavirus
- Cytomegalovirus
- Hepatotropic Viruses
- HIV Infection
- Arbovirus

FUNGAL INFECTIONS
- Superficial Fungal Infections
- *Candida albicans*
- *Aspergillus flavus*
- *Cryptococcus neoformans*
- *Histoplasma capsulatum*
- Coccidioiodomycosis
- Mucormycosis

PARASITIC DISEASES
- *Entamoeba histolytica*
- *Giardia lamblia*
- *Trichomonas vaginalis*
- Malarial Parasite
- *Echinococcus granulosus*
- *Strongyloides stercoralis*
- *Wuchereria bancrofti*
- *Ancylostoma duodenale*
- *Enterobius vermicularis*

NUTRITIONAL DISEASES

PROTEIN–CALORIE MALNUTRITION

Protein–energy malnutrition (PEM) or protein–calorie malnutrition refers to a form of malnutrition where there is inadequate calorie or protein intake.

In developing countries, protein–calorie malnutrition occurs in two forms—*marasmus and kwashiorkor*. Kwashiorkor refers to predominant protein malnutrition and marasmus as a result of deficiency in calorie intake.

Differences between kwashiorkor and marasmus are shown in Table 7.1.

Diagnosis

Protein–calorie malnutrition is diagnosed by measurement of body weight for given height with standard tables (weight <80% of normal), evaluation of fat stores (thickness of skin folds), muscle mass (mid-arm

Table 7.1: Differences between kwashiorkor and marasmus

Characteristics	Kwashiorkor	Marasmus
Age group	2–5 years	Less than one year
Deficiency of nutrients	Protein deficiency marked	Protein and calories deficiency
Loss of protein in compartment	Depletion of liver proteins stores	Depletion of protein stores in somatic tissues
Etiology	Weaning of child at early age without protein supplement	Weaning of child at early age without protein as well as carbohydrates, and chronic diarrhea
Skeletal muscle	Relatively spared	Loss of skeletal mass due to catabolism
Serum proteins levels	Markedly reduced	Normal or slightly decreased
Immune status	Immunodeficiency with secondary infection	Immunodeficiency with secondary infection
Subcutaneous fat	Spared	Mobilized for energy purpose
Extremities	Edematous due to decreased serum albumen level	Emaciated
Skin folds and mid-arm circumference	Relative spared	Reduced skin fold, and decreased mid-arm circumference
Growth retardation	Present but less	Present but more severe
Skin lesions	Skin-flaky paint appearance	No characteristics skin and hair changes
	Hair loss of color, alternating bands of pale and dark hair, loss of scalp attachment	No characteristics skin and hair changes
Hepatomegaly	Fatty change present	Fatty change absent
Small bowel changes	Mucosa is atrophic, loss of villi, and decreased mitotic index in crypts of glands	No such change
Bone marrow	Hypoplastic with decreased erythropoiesis	Hypoplastic with decreased erythropoiesis
Thymic and lymphoid atrophy	More marked	Less marked
Brain changes	Usually absent	Brain—cerebral atrophy, reduced no. of neurons, impaired myelination of white matter
Associated nutritional deficiency	Present	Present

circumference), serum proteins (albumin), decreased mid-arm circumference (marasmus) and decreased serum proteins (kwashiorkor).

MARASMUS

Marasmus is caused by widespread deficiency of almost all nutrients, notably *protein and calories*. It often coexists with vitamin deficiencies.

It typically occurs in *children younger than 1 year* of age who are not breastfed and do not have an adequate intake of substitute nutrients. Chronic diarrhea is also underlying cause. Weight for age is <60% of expected normal.

Clinical Features

Patient presents with retarded growth due to *depletion of protein stores in tissues and emaciated extremities. Loss of subcutaneous fat (wasting away)* occurs due to mobilization of fat for energy purpose. Child is prone to recurrent infection due to immunosuppression. On clinical examination, there is no edema (Fig. 7.1).

KWASHIORKOR (EDEMATOUS MALNUTRITION)

Kwashiorkor is caused by protein deficiency but with adequate calorie intake. It usually affects children older than 1 year of age who are no longer breastfed and receive a starch-rich, protein-poor diet. It has 50–60%

Nutritional and Infectious Diseases 7

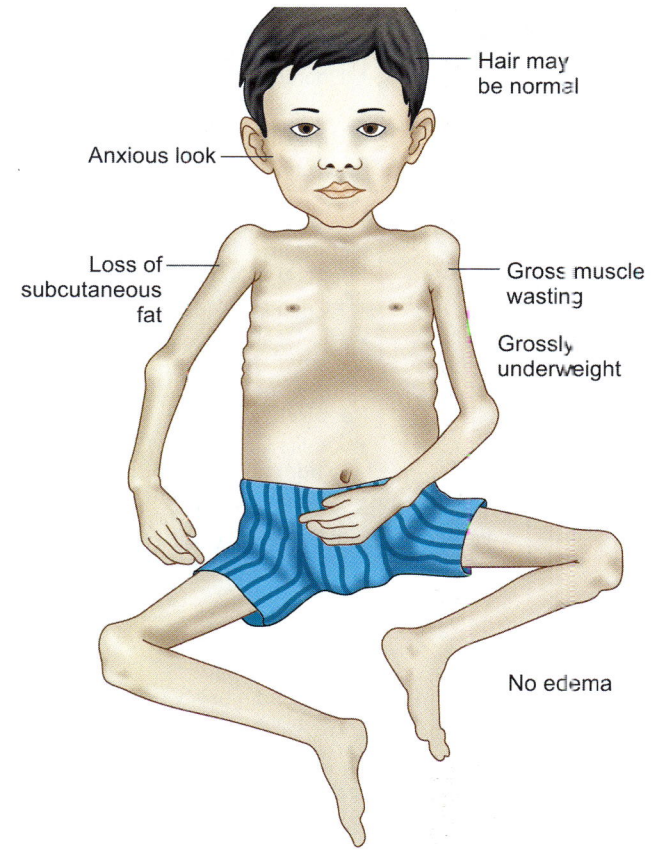

Fig. 7.1: Marasmus is caused by lack of proteins and calories resulting in emaciated extremities, loss of subcutaneous fat, muscle wasting, retarded growth but no edema.

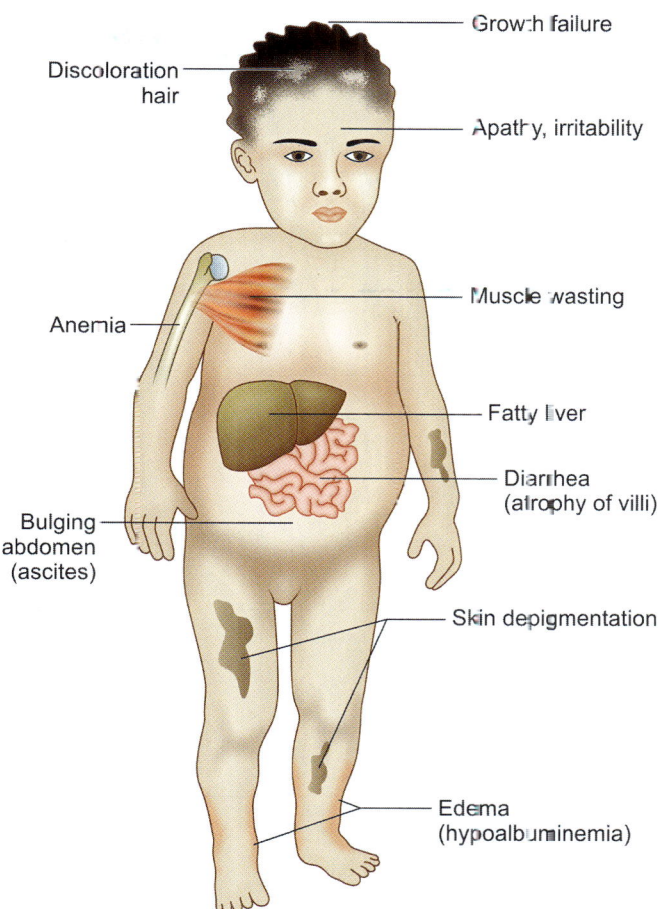

Fig. 7.2: Kwashiorkor is caused by lack of proteins resulting in edema, ascites, anemia, skin pigmentation, muscle wasting, fatty liver and growth failure.

mortality rate. Serum proteins are markedly reduced. There is suppression of bone marrow and thymus. Child is underweight with edema showing electrolyte abnormalities.

Clinical Features

Patient presents with retarded growth and muscle wasting due to inadequate protein intake, but with preservation of subcutaneous fat. Kwashiorkor is distinguished from marasmus by the presence of the following abnormalities: *fatty liver, severe edema due to protein deficiency and decreased oncotic pressure, anemia, malabsorption* as result of atrophy of the small intestinal villi depigmented bands with pale streaking in the hair or skin (Fig. 7.2).

OBESITY ASSOCIATED DISORDERS

Obesity is independent risk factor for development of venous thromboembolic disease. Adipose tissue has endocrine role by synthesizing *adipokines responsible for inflammation*.

These adipokines have been implicated in the development of *atherosclerosis, cancer and thrombosis*. Obesity is also associated with increased risk of *type 2 diabetes mellitus, hypertension, gallstones, and osteoarthritis* (Fig. 7.3).

Assessment of obesity by BMI: Obesity is commonly assessed by BMI, which is calculated by weight in kilograms divided by the square of the height in meters (kg/m^2) World Health Organization classification system for BMI defines obesity as a BMI >30 with further subcategories shown in Table 7.2.

Table 7.2: WHO classification of obesity

BMI (kg/m^2)	Alternative commonly used terminology	WHO classification
<18.50	Underweight	Underweight
18.50–24.99	Normal	Normal range
25–29.99	Overweight	Overweight
30.00–34.99	Obese	Obese class I
35.00–29.99	Obese	Obese class II
≥40.00	Morbid obesity	Obese class III
≥50.00	Superobesity	
≥60.00	Super-superobesity	

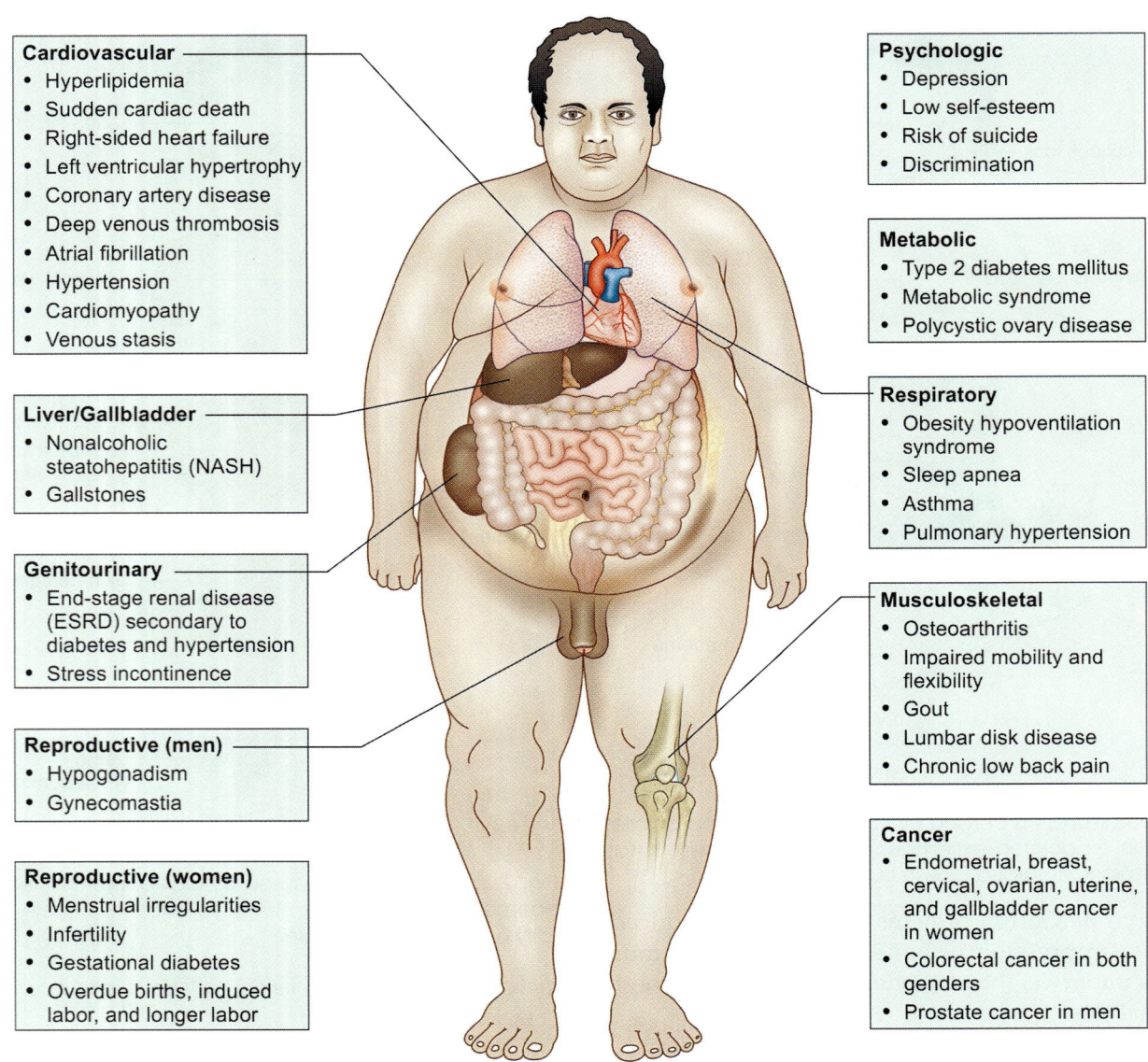

Fig. 7.3: Obesity associated health problems.

Pathogenesis

Leptin gene is most often defective in obesity. Mutation of leptin gene inhibits leptin release by adipositis. Obesity is related to synthesis of leptin, an antiobesity hormone produced by adipocytes.

Neuropeptide Y, pro-obesity is synthesized by the hypothalamus in response to leptin deficiency. Pathogenesis of obesity is shown in Figs 7.4 and 7.5.

- Leptin synthesis increases when adipose stores are increased. It decreases food intake via hypothalamus and increases energy expenditure.
- On the other hand, leptin synthesis decreases when adipose stores are decreased in tissues.

RESPIRATORY SYSTEM DISORDERS

Obesity causes obstructive sleep apnea, obesity hypoventilation syndrome, bronchial asthma, cor pulmonale (pulmonary hypertension and right ventricular hypertrophy).

Obstructive sleep apnea: Obstructive sleep apnea refers to recurrent episodes of apnea (interrupted airflow) due to obstruction of the upper airway during sleep followed by transient awakening to restore airway patency.

This condition occurs due to accumulation of fat in neck region. *Recurrent apneas cause chronic alveolar hypoxia resulting in pulmonary hypertension and cor pulmonale.* The condition is confirmed by polysomnography. This condition is exacerbated by *smoking, sedative drugs and alcohol consumption.*

Nutritional and Infectious Diseases

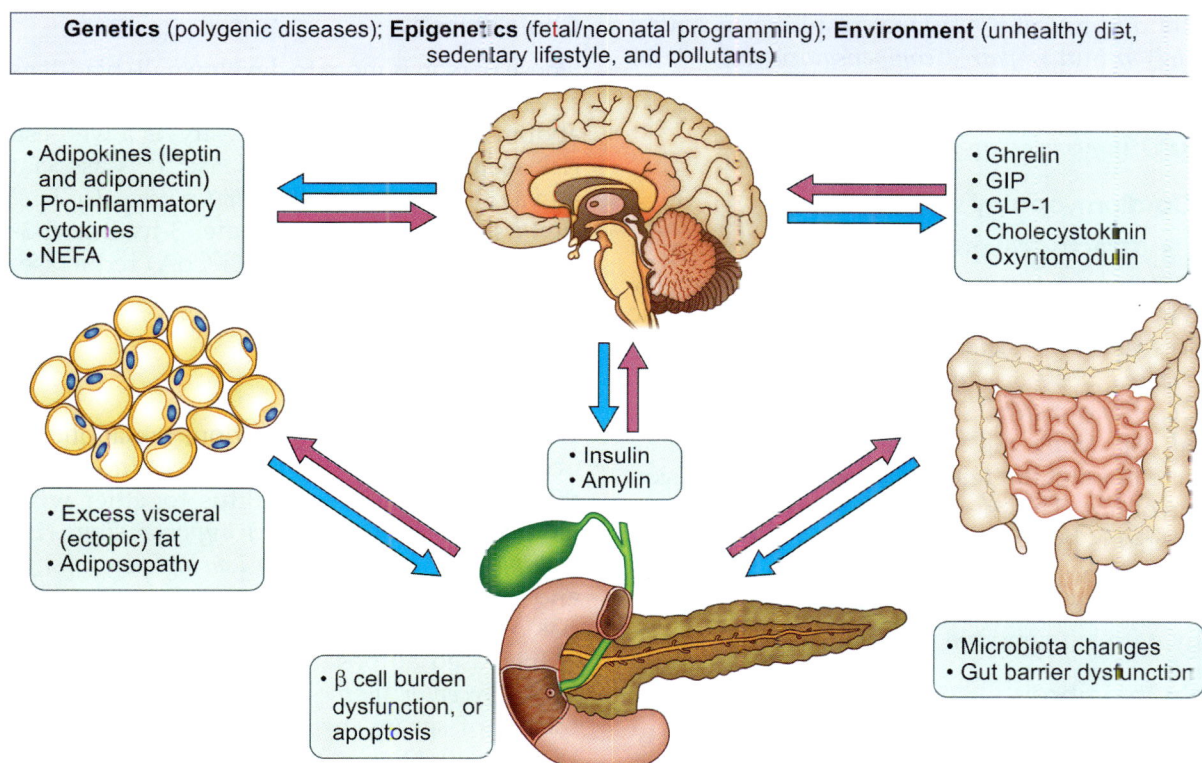

Fig. 7.4: Pathogenesis of obesity. Leptin gene is most often defective in obesity. Mutation of leptin gene inhibits leptin release by adipositis. Obesity is related to synthesis of leptin, an antiobesity hormone produced by adipocytes. Neuropeptide Y, pro-obesity is synthesized by the hypothalamus in response to leptin deficiency.

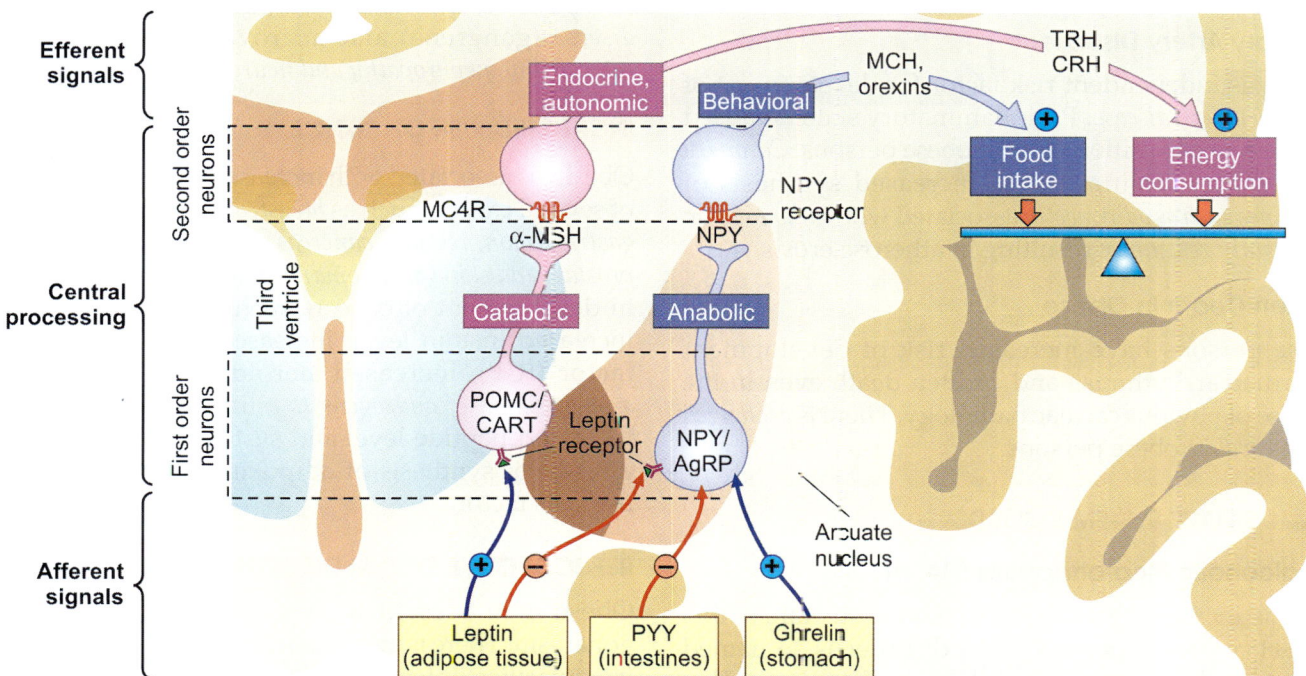

Fig. 7.5: Neurohumoral circuits in the hypothalamus that regulate energy balance.

Obstructive sleep apnea is independent *risk factor for congestive heart failure, hypertension, myocardial infarction, cardiac arrhythmias and sudden cardiac death.*

Obstructive hypoventilation syndrome: Obstructive hypoventilation syndrome is also known as *pickwickian syndrome* comprising *hypoventilation, daytime hypercapnia and hypoxemia* ($PaCO_2$ >45 mm Hg and PaO_2 <10 mm Hg). *The diagnostic test for obstructive hypoventilation syndrome is daytime arterial blood gas.* This disease has a high mortality rate.

It occurs due to *leptin resistance* resulting in *central hypoventilation* and *impaired compensatory response* to acute hypercapnia.

CARDIOVASCULAR DISORDERS

Obesity Cardiomyopathy

Obesity is directly responsible for alterations in the structure and function of the heart. Obesity cardiomyopathy is multifactorial involving *metabolic disturbances (insulin resistance, increased free fatty acid levels, increased levels of adipokines), activities of angiotensin aldosterone system, sympathetic nervous system, myocardial remodeling and small vessel disease*. Plasma insulin increases sodium retention leading to expansion of plasma volume. This mechanism causes *hypertension* in obese persons leading to obesity cardio myopathy. *Thickness of left ventricle wall is >10 mm.* It should be differentiated from a genetic disorder dilated cardiomyopathy with left ventricle wall thickness <10 mm.

Deep Vein Thrombosis

Obesity is independent risk factor for development of *deep vein thrombosis*. Pathogenesis of thromboembolic phenomenon in obese is complex potentially involving a number of *hormones, cytokines, growth factors synthesized by adipose tissue such as leptin*.

Coronary Artery Disease

Obesity is independent risk factor for development of *coronary artery disease*. Proinflammatory state is caused by excess of deposition of fat in obese persons. *Coronary artery disease* occurs due to increased synthesis of *adipokines such as adiponectin* associated with *inflammation* and *insulin resistance* resulting in atherosclerosis.

Sudden Death in Obese

Obese persons have increased risk of development of cardiac arrhythmias and sudden death even in the absence of obvious cardiac pathology. There is *prolonged QT interval* in obese persons.

HEPATOBILIARY SYSTEM DISORDERS

Nonalcoholic Steatohepatitis (NASH)

There is increased risk of nonalcoholic steatohepatitis (NASH) in obese persons. This disorder is so named because it closely resembles alcoholic fatty liver. This condition represents a spectrum of liver injuries that initially display steatosis, with or without hepatitis. This disorder may progress to bridging fibrosis and cirrhosis of liver. It is consistently associated with metabolic syndrome (*central obesity, type 2 diabetes mellitus, dyslipidemia, and microalbuminuria*).

Cholelithiasis

Obese person is more to develop gall-bladder stones as a result of supersaturation of fat. Obesity, particularly abdominal or centripetal obesity, is a well-established risk factor for gallstone disease. It is associated with an *increased activity of the rate-limiting step in cholesterol synthesis*, the hepatic enzyme, 3-hydroxyl-3-methyl-glutaryl co-enzyme A (HMG-CoA) reductase, leading to *increased cholesterol synthesis in the liver*, its secretion *into bile* and *storage in the gallbladder*.

METABOLIC DISORDERS

According to WHO definition, metabolic syndrome occurs due to insulin resistance, impaired glucose tolerance or diabetes mellitus together with at least two of the following: (i) *hypertension*, (ii) *obesity*, (iii) *high triglycerides and or low high density lipoproteins*, and (iv) *microalbunemia*. Metabolic syndrome increases risk of cardiovascular disease.

Increased adipose tissue in the body *downregulates insulin receptor synthesis* resulting in increased concentration of serum insulin and thus diabetes mellitus. Weight reduction increases insulin receptor synthesis. Uncontrolled diabetes mellitus is associated with increased risk of life-threatening complications, i.e. macrovascular diseases (*atherosclerosis*) such as *coronary artery disease, cerebral vascular disease, peripheral vascular disease* (gangrene) and microvascular diseases like *retinopathy, nephropathy and neuropathy*.

INCREASED RISK OF CANCERS

Obesity is associated with increased risk of development of several cancers such as *breast, endometrium, esophagus, gastric, colon, rectum, pancreas, liver, biliary tract, kidney, prostate and skin (melanoma)*. Various factors participate in development of cancers such as insulin resistance, increased insulin level, increased insulin-like growth factor (IGF), increased steroid level as a result of *aromatization of androgens to estrogens in adipose tissue*, increased peptide level and systemic inflammation as a result of synthesis of adipokine (leptin) and tumor necrosis factor.

REPRODUCTIVE SYSTEM DISORDERS

Obese men present with gynecomastia and hypogonadism. There is increased development of menstrual irregularities, infertility, gestational diabetes, overdue child birth, induced labor and prolonged labor in obese women.

GENITOURINARY SYSTEM DISORDERS

Obese persons are more prone to develop end stage renal disease as a result of hypertension and diabetes mellitus.

Nutritional and Infectious Diseases

End stage renal disease refers to GFR <5% of normal. It is the terminal stage with uremic manifestations. Renal biopsy shows marked glomerular sclerosis, tubular atrophy with thyroidization, intestinal fibrosis and vascular thickening.

MUSCULOSKELETAL SYSTEM DISORDERS

There is increased risk of osteoarthritis, impaired mobility, gout, prolapse lumbar intervertebral discs and chronic low back pain in obese persons. Osteoarthritis is a slowly progressive destruction of the articular cartilage. Articular cartilage loses its elasticity results to fragmentation, which floats into synovial fluid. Floating cartilage erodes bone, which exhibits polished and ivory-like appearance (eburnation). It is accompanied by new bone formation (osteocytes) subchondrally and at the margins of the affected joint.

VITAMINS

Fat-soluble vitamins include A, E, D and K. Vitamin B_{12} (cyanocobalamin), folic acid, vitamin B_1 (thiamine), vitamin B_2 (riboflavin), vitamin B_6 (pyridoxine) and vitamin C are all water-soluble vitamins. Beriberi occurs due to deficiency of *thiamine*. Vitamin C deficiency results in scurvy. Vitamin B_{12} and folic acid deficiency often manifests with megaloblastic anemia. Vitamin B_6 (pyridoxine) deficiency can manifest with convulsions. Niacin deficiency results in pellagra. Major functions of vitamins and deficiency syndrome are shown in Table 7.3.

Table 7.3: Major functions of vitamins and deficiency syndrome

Nutrient	Functions	Deficiency syndrome
Fat-soluble vitamins		
Vitamin A	Visual pigment regulating cell growth	Night blindness, xerophthalmia, keratomalacia, metaplasia of columnar epithelium in ducts. Immune deficiency
Vitamin D	It facilitates calcium and phosphates absorption from small intestine. It maintains plasma facilitates calcium and phosphates levels	Rickets in children, osteomalacia in adults and hypocalcemic tetany
Vitamin E	Antioxidant maintaining nervous system	Spinocerebellar syndrome
Vitamin K	Acts as cofactor for hepatic carboxylation of prothrombin; VII, IX and X, protein C and protein S	Bleeding diathesis
Water-soluble vitamins		
Thiamine (B_1)	Thiamine pyrophosphate functions as a coenzyme essential for maintaining nervous system	Wet beriberi, dry beriberi and Wernicke-Korsakoff syndrome
Riboflavin (B_2)	Acts as cofactor for enzyme including FMN and FAD	Ariboflavinosis, cheilosis, glossitis, dermatitis, keratitis
Niacin	Component of coenzyme NAD and NADF	Pellagra, dementia, diarrhea and dermatitis
Pyridoxine (B_6)	Forms pyridoxal-5-phosphate, a coenzyme in many reactions	Cheilosis, glossitis, dermatitis and peripheral neuropathy
Pantothenic acid	Component of coenzyme A and acyl carrier proteins	Recognized only under experimental conditions: Constitutional and gastrointestinal symptoms, paresthesia, cramps, impaired coordination
Biotin	Acting as cofactor in several carboxylation reactions	Deficiencies extremely rare. Patient presenting with anorexia, dermatitis, atrophic glossitis, myalgia, ECG changes, hypothermia and mild anemia
Folate	Acting as coenzyme in transfer and utilization of 1-carbon units, essential step in nucleic acid synthesis	Megaloblastic anemia
Cyanocobalamin (B_{12})	Participates in utilization of folate in nucleic acid synthesis	Megaloblastic anemia
	Essential for maintenance of nervous system	Subacute combined degeneration of spinal cord in midthoracic region
Vitamin C	Acting as cofactor in hydroxylation and amidation reactions	Scurvy

FAT-SOLUBLE VITAMINS

Deficiency of fat-soluble vitamins (vitamins A, D, E, and K) can occur in malnutrition, and malabsorption syndromes as a result of pancreatic exocrine insufficiency, or biliary obstruction. Excess intake of vitamins A and D may cause toxic effects.

Vitamin A

Vitamin A is a fat-soluble vitamin. Sources of vitamin A include: liver, fish, eggs, milk, butter, yellow and green leafy vegetables (carrots, sweet potatoes, pumpkins, mangoes, and spinach). Vitamin visual cycle is shown in Fig. 7.6.

Structure

Retinol is a most active alcohol. Oxidation of retinol leads to formation of aldehyde, retinal and retinoic acid compounds. Retinyl esters are storage form of vitamin A.

Functions

Vitamin A is essential for the maintenance of mucus-secreting epithelium. A derivative, retinol, is a component of the photoprotective visual pigment rhodopsin. *This visual pigment rhodopsin present in cones is sensitive in reduced light. Iodopsin in cones is responsive in bright light.*

Vitamin A participates in hormonal regulation of cell growth, i.e. epithelial cell differentiation. It acts as an antioxidant agent, hence prevents oxidant-induced mutagenic effect. It has anticarcinogenic effect through epithelial regulatory function. It acts through immunity-enhancing function.

Wald's Visual Cycle

Retinal, a component of the photoprotective visual pigment rhodopsin presents in cones is sensitive in reduced light. Rhodopsin visual pigment present in cones is sensitive in reduced light. Iodopsin in cones is responsive in bright light (Fig. 7.7).

- Retinol is transported to retina via circulation. Retinol moves into retinal pigment epithelial cells and gets esterified to form retinyl esters and stored.
- When needed, retinyl esters are hydrolyzed and isomerized to form 11-*cis*-retinol. 11-*cis*-retinol shuttles to rod cells of retina, where it binds to protein called opsin to form visual pigment, rhodopsin (also known as *visual purple*).

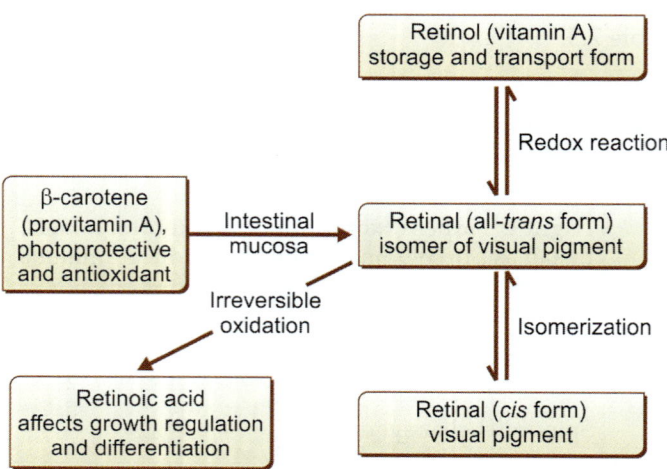

Fig. 7.6: Vitamin visual cycle. Oxidation of retinol leads to formation of aldehyde, retinal and retinoic acid compounds. A derivative, retinol, is a component of the photoprotective visual pigment rhodopsin. This visual pigment rhodopsin present in cones is sensitive in reduced light. Iodopsin in cones is responsive in bright light.

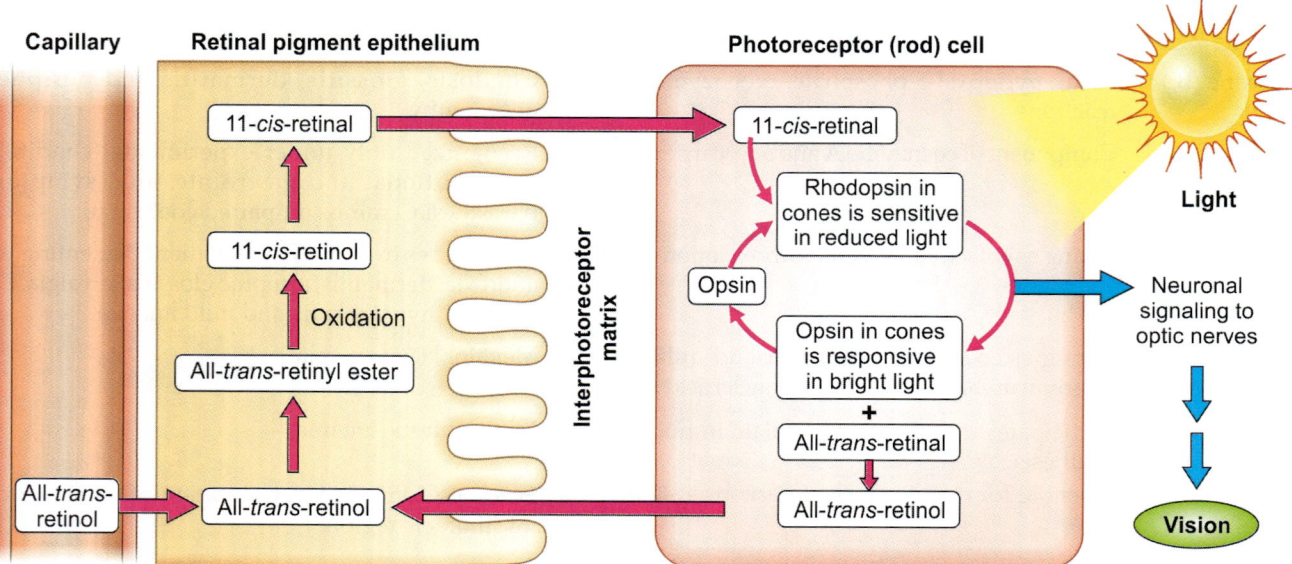

Fig. 7.7: Wald's visual cycle.

Nutritional and Infectious Diseases

- Absorption of a photon of light converts 11-*cis*-retinal to all-*trans*-retinal by isomerization resulting in its release.
- This isomerization triggers generation of electrical signal to optic nerves. The nerve impulse generated by optic nerve is transmitted to the brain, where it is interpreted as vision.
- Once released, all-*trans*-retinal is converted to all-*trans*-retinol. The all-*trans*-retinol is transported across the interphotoreceptor matrix to the retinal epithelial cell to complete the visual pigment.

Deficiency

Vitamin A deficiency leads to *night blindness, xerophthalmia (dry eye), Bitot's spots, keratomalacia, squamous metaplasia of columnar epithelium* lining respiratory, urinary system and glandular ducts, *secondary pulmonary infections, urinary lithiasis, follicular papillary dermatosis,* and *immune deficiency* (Fig. 7.8).

Hypervitaminosis A

Hypervitaminosis A is most often caused by excessive intake of vitamin A preparations. It is manifested by *alopecia, hepatocellular damage and bone changes*.

Vitamin D

Vitamin D is derived from skin exposed to sunlight and dietary source. After absorption, vitamin D is metabolized by liver and kidneys.

Sources of Vitamin D

- *Skin and gastrointestinal tract:* 7-dehydrocholesterol is derived from diet and ultraviolet irradiation of skin. Vitamin D is absorbed through gastrointestinal tract and skin.
- *Metabolism in liver and kidneys:* Vitamin D (7-dehydrocholesterol) enters blood and reaches liver. Liver enzyme D-25-hydroxylase converts 7-dehydrocholesterol to vitamin 25-OH-D. Now vitamin 25-OH-D reaches the kidney and converted to vitamin 1, 25.(OH)2D (active metabolite) with the help of renal enzyme α_1-hydroxylase (Fig. 7.9).

Functions

Vitamin 1, 25 (OH)2D acts on gastrointestinal tract and helps in absorption of calcium and phosphorus and maintains normal plasma levels of calcium and phosphorus. Calcium and phosphorus participate in *bone mineralization*. It collaborates with parathormone in mobilization of calcium from bone. It facilitates parathormone dependent reabsorption of calcium in the distal renal tubules. It is requisite for normal mineralization of cartilage and bone.

Deficiency

Vitamin D deficiency leads to *rickets in children, osteomalacia in adults* and *hypocalcemic tetany*.

- *Rickets:* During infancy, head and chest sustain the greatest stresses. Child presents with rickets and with *craniotabes, frontal bossing, rachitic rosary, Harrison's groove, pigeon shaped chest, deformities of pelvic bones and spine*. These clinical manifestations occur as a result of inadequate calcification of cartilage and replacement of cartilage by osteoid matrix on inadequately mineralized cartilaginous remnants. It leads to projection of distorted, irregular masses of cartilage into marrow cavity

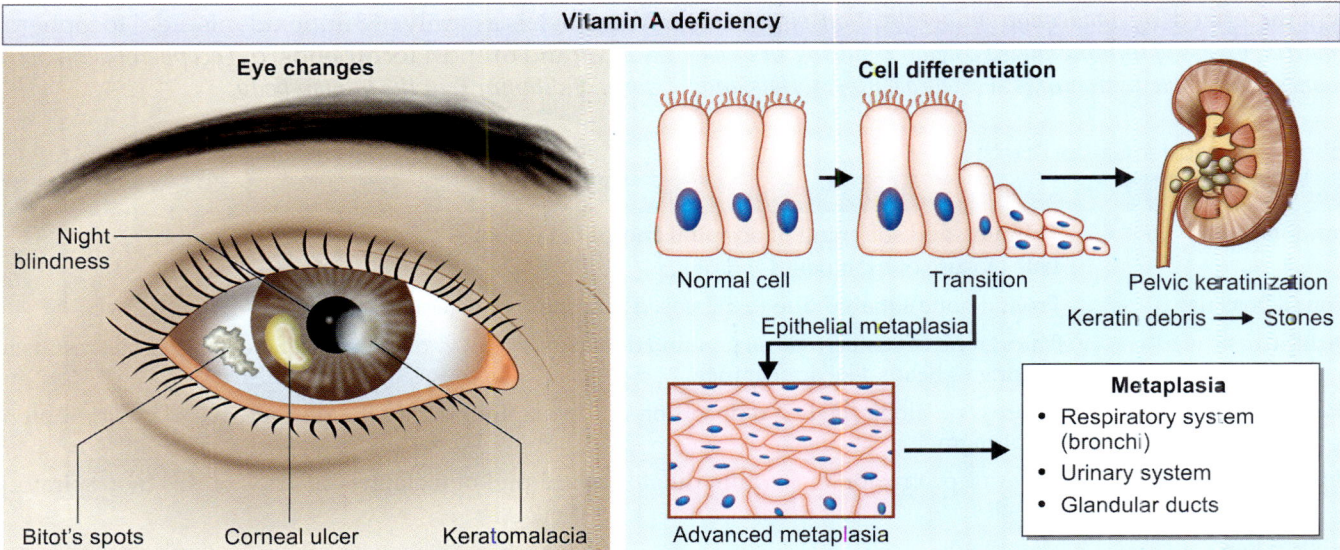

Fig. 7.8: Vitamin A efficiency. Showing Bitot's spots, night blindness, corneal ulcer, keratomalacia and squamous metaplasia of epithelium lining bronchi, urinary system and glandular ducts.

Section I: General Pathology

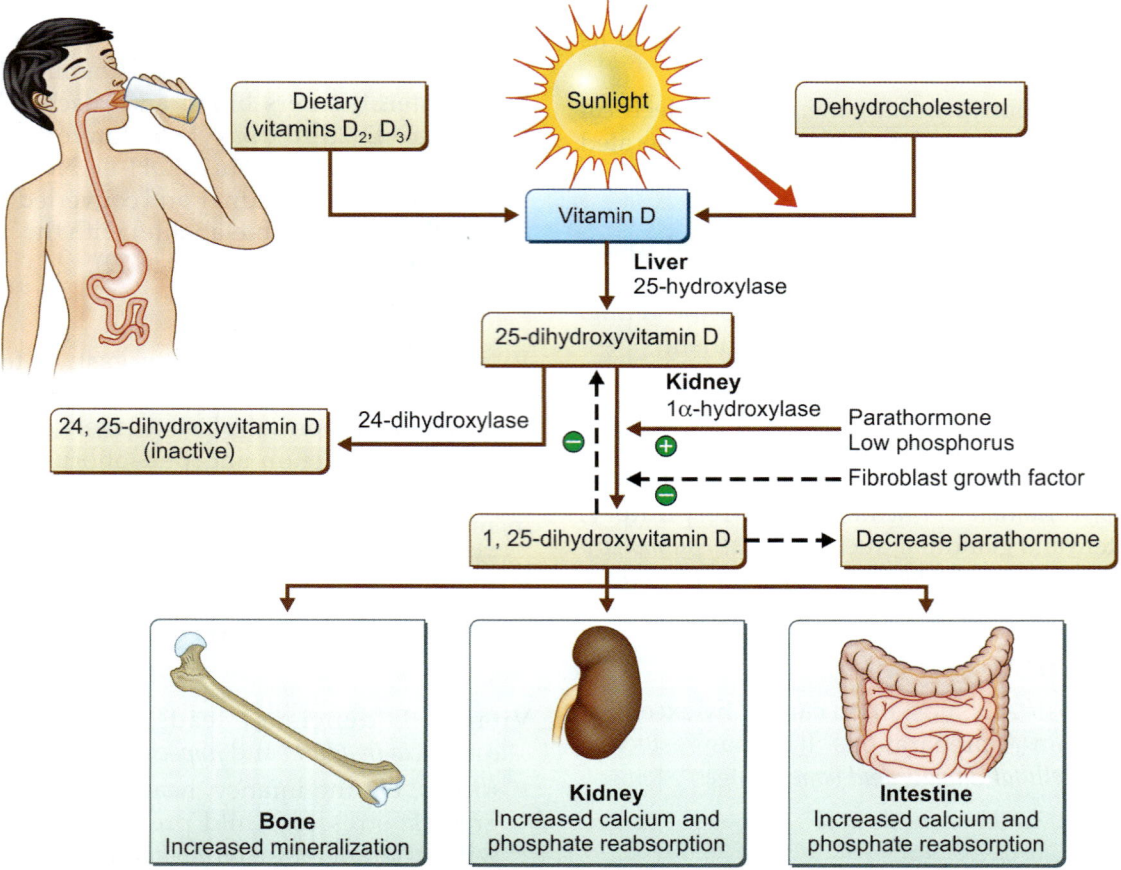

Fig. 7.9: Vitamin D metabolism. Vitamin D is synthesized from 7-dehydrocholesterol in the skin. Vitamin D is also derived from dietary source. Vitamin D is metabolized in the liver and kidney.

and enlargement and lateral expansion of the osteochondral junction. Clinical features of rickets are shown in Table 7.4.

- *Osteomalacia (soft bones):* Osteomalacia means loss of skeletal mass or too little bone (osteopenia). It is characterized by *inadequate mineralization of osteoid matrix, excess of unmineralized osteoid resulting in weak bones vulnerable to fractures (vertebrae, hips, wrists and ribs) in 25% cases.* Patient may develop kyphoscoliosis. There is apparent loss of bone density and cortical thickness, visualized by radiographically.

Vitamin E

Vitamin E is a family of 8 antioxidants, i.e. 4 tocopherols (α, β, γ and δ) and 4 tocotriends. α-Tocopherol is the active form of vitamin E in the human body.

Table 7.4: Clinical features of rickets

Clinical findings	Mechanism
Craniotabes	Thinning and softening of occipital and parietal bones Late closure of fontanelles
Frontal bossing	Frontal bone squared due to increased formation of osteoid
Rachitic rosary	Thickening of costochondral junction due to overgrowth of cartilage and osteoid tissue results in a string of beads-like appearance
Harrison's groove	Depression along the line of insertion of the diaphragm into the rib cage due to inward pull of diaphragm
Pigeon-shaped chest	Anterior protrusion of sternum due to inward pull of metaphyseal areas of ribs by respiratory muscles
Pelvis bones	Deformed
Spine deformity	Lumbar lordosis in ambulatory child

Dietary source: Vitamin E is derived from vegetable oils, almonds, peanuts, avocado, spinach and carrots (least).

Functions: Vitamin E participates in *maintenance of nervous system*. It acts as *antioxidant* and participates in *maintenance of cell membranes*. It intercepts free radicals and prevents *destruction of cell membrane* by modulation of lipid peroxidation. It protects the fat in LDL from oxidation. It *inhibits platelets aggregation*. It enhances vasodilatation. It inhibits the activity of protein kinase C.

Causes of deficiency: These include malnutrition, genetic defects affecting transfer protein of α-tocopherol, malabsorption syndrome.

Clinical features: Patient develops *spinocerebellar syndrome*, characterized by neurological symptoms (impaired coordination and muscle weakness due to degenerations of axons in posterior columns). There is *loss in sensory nuclei of trigeminal, auditory and vagus nerves*. There is increased risk of cardiovascular diseases in adults, and hemolytic anemia (premature destruction of red blood cells) in children.

Therapeutic significance: Vitamin E is administered to prevent cardiovascular disease, diabetes mellitus, cancer, dementia, and to boost immunity.

Toxicity of vitamin E: Excess of vitamin E may cause impaired blood clotting leading to increased risk of bleeding in some persons. It is recommended that vitamin E supplements to be stopped one month before elective surgery.

Vitamin K

Glutamyl carboxylation is required for synthesis of γ-carboxyglutamyl residues of active serine proteases (e.g. *clotting factors II, VII, IX, and X*).

Sources: Bacteria in large intestine produce vitamin K_2 and 40–50% of human requirement. Dietary sources include: vegetables, almonds, peanuts, avocado, broccoli, spinach, lettuce, and parsley (raw).

Functions of vitamin K: Vitamin K is needed for production of vitamin K dependent coagulation factors in the liver. *Vitamin K is a cofactor for hepatic carboxylation of prothrombin; factors VII, IX, and X; and protein C and protein S*.

Vitamin K deficiency: Vitamin K deficiency leads to bleeding diathesis. It is uncommon in adults, except in those with severe liver disease and on oral anticoagulants. Deficiency occurs exclusively in breastfed and premature babies, because human milk is low in vitamin K, and their gut is not yet colonized with bacteria. *Hemorrhagic disease of the newborn is a serious threat to life*. Routine *vitamin K administration is administered prophylactically*.

WATER-SOLUBLE VITAMINS

Water-soluble vitamins include the B complex vitamins, B_1 (thiamine), B_2 (riboflavin), B_3 (niacin), B_6 (pyridoxine), and B_{12} (cyanocobalamin); folic acid; and vitamin C (ascorbic acid). Biotin and pantothenic acid deficiencies are extremely rare. These found in numerous foods and also are synthesized by intestinal bacteria. *Biotin deficiency may occur with prolonged antibiotic therapy and ingestion of raw eggs*. Toxicity from excessive intake is rare, because excess of these vitamins are excreted in the urine. *In general, deficiencies of vitamin B complex are often marked by glossitis, dermatitis, and diarrhea*.

Dietary sources: B complex vitamins (except vitamin B_{12}) are present in *whole grain cereals, green leafy vegetables, fish, meat, and dairy foods*. Vitamin B_{12} is derived from foods of animal origin only. Folic acid is derived from leafy vegetables, cereals, fruits, and a number of animal products. Vitamin C is derived from fruits (especially citrus fruits and tomatoes), vegetables, various meats, and milk.

Storage: Water-soluble vitamins are not stored in the body except for vitamin B_{12}. That is the reason that regular intake is essential. *Vitamin B_{12} is stored in the liver in large quantities*.

Functions: Water, soluble vitamins participate in the release and storage of energy especially in tissues with active metabolism.

Thiamine (Vitamin B_1)

Dietary requirement of thiamine is proportional to the caloric intake of the diet and ranges from 1.0 to 1.5 mg/day for normal adults.

Functions: Thiamine is rapidly converted into thiamine pyrophosphate (active form) in the brain and liver by thiamine diphosphotransferase enzyme. Thiamine pyrophosphate is essential as cofactor for the reactions of the *pentose phosphate pathway for maintaining nervous system*

Causes of deficiency: Vitamin B_1 (thiamine) deficiency is most often associated with *severe malnutrition and alcoholism*. Other causes include: increased demand (malaria and AIDS) and excessive loss (hemodialysis and diuretics). *Anti-thiamine factors in diet such as tea and coffee retard thiamine absorption. Thiaminases found in raw fish, raw shellfish and silkworms retard thiamine absorption*.

Clinical features: Thiamine is used for treatment of *congestive heart failure and Alzheimer's disease* as well as in *cancer prevention*. Deficiency of thiamine causes dry beriberi, wet beriberi and Wernicke-Korsakoff syndrome.

- *Dry beriberi:* Patient with severe thiamine deficiency presents with *peripheral neuropathy* resulting in *atrophy*

of the muscles of the extremities. Peripheral neuropathy occurs due to fragmentation of myelin sheath, axons of extremities. There is also *involvement of vagus nerve.*
- *Wet beriberi:* It is characterized by congestive heart failure associated with dilated cardiomyopathy. Congestive heart failure occurs due to peripheral dilation of arterioles and capillaries.
- *Wernicke-Korsakoff syndrome:* It is characterized by *impairment of symmetric motor and sensory reflexes, involvement of extraocular muscles (ophthalmoplegia), confusion, ataxia and marked memory loss.* Degenerative changes occur in the brainstem and diencephalon, with hemorrhagic lesions of cortical and bilateral paramedian masses of gray matter and the mamillary bodies.

Riboflavin (Vitamin B_2)

Riboflavin (B_2) is obtained from eggs, meat, and cereals. It acts as cofactor in several enzymes. Component of FAD (flavin adenine dinucleotide) and FMN (flavin mononucleotide) is essential in a variety of oxidation–reduction processes.

Causes: Deficiency is more common in chronic alcoholics due to poor dietary habits. Riboflavin decomposes when exposed to visible light especially in newborns treated by phototherapy.

Clinical features: Patient presents with *glossitis, angular stomatitis, cheilosis* (skin fissures, crust at angle of mouth), *seborrheic dermatitis* (nasolabial folds, scrotum, or vulva), *keratitis* (vascularization of cornea, photophobia) and *pure red cell hypoplasia* of bone marrow.

Niacin (Vitamin B_3)

Niacin (nicotinic acid) can be synthesized from the essential amino acid tryptophan with the help of pyridoxine. It is a component of the nicotinamide adenine dinucleotides (NADs and NADP). Niacin is essential for glycolysis, the citric acid cycle, and other oxidative metabolic processes.

Causes of deficiency: Hartnup disease, malignant carcinoid syndrome and isoniazid can lead to niacin deficiency. In large doses, niacin lowers plasma cholesterol but it elevates blood glucose and uric acid levels. So it is not recommended with diabetes mellitus and gout.

Clinical features: Patient with severe niacin deficiency develops *pellagra*, which is characterized by the *three Ds*: **d**ementia, **d**ermatitis (keratotic scaly lesions on exposed area such as face, neck, dorsum of hands and feet), and **d**iarrhea. There is presence of red ulcerated oral mucosa, thickening of colon wall with atrophy of crypts and demyelination of posterior and lateral columns of spinal cord as well as cerebrum.

Pyridoxine (Vitamin B_6)

Pyridoxine is widely available in diet. Daily requirement is 0.5–2.0 mg. It forms pyridoxal-5-phosphate, acts as coenzyme in many reactions essential for catabolism of the amino acids, glycogenolysis, and synthesis of porphyrin niacin from tryptophan. It converts glutamic acid to γ-aminobutyric acid.

Causes of deficiency: Pyridoxine deficiency occurs due to *chronic alcoholism* and therapeutic administration of *INH* (isonicotinic acid hydrazide) and *penicillamine*. INH reacts as competitive inhibitors for pyridoxine binding sites.

Clinical features: Patient presents with *cheilosis, glossitis; dermatitis, microcytic hypochromic anemia* (reduced heme synthesis), *convulsions in infants and neurologic dysfunction. Neonatal convulsions* occur due to decreased activity of pyridoxal-dependent glutamate decarboxylase, which leads to *deficient production of γ-aminobutyric acid (GABA), a neurotransmitter*. Clinical manifestations are similar to those of vitamin B_2 (riboflavin) deficiency.

Pantothenic Acid

Pantothenic acid is a component of coenzyme A and acyl carrier protein. It is recognized only under experimental conditions, constitutional and gastrointestinal symptoms, paresthesia, cramps, impaired coordination.

Biotin

Biotin is a cofactor in several carboxylation reactions. Deficiency is extremely rare. Patient may develop lassitude, anorexia, dermatitis, atrophic glossitis, myalgia, ECG changes, hypothermia and mild anemia.

Cyanocobalamin (Vitamin B_{12})

Cyanocobalamin (B_{12}) is derived from animal source. It is absorbed by small intestine. *Deficiency is common in strict vegetarians*, pernicious anemia, Crohn's disease, blind loop syndrome, *Diphyllobothrium latum* (giant fish tapeworm) infestation and prolonged antibiotic treatment.

Functions

Vitamin B_{12} acts as cofactor for enzymes required for the catabolism of fatty acids, and the conversion of homocysteine to methionine. *High homocysteine in blood is a risk of ischemia heart disease and cerebral stroke.* Vitamin B_{12} plays role in utilization of folate in nucleic acid synthesis. It is essential for maintenance of nervous system.

Megaloblastic Anemia

Deficiency causes *megaloblastic anemia and subacute combined degeneration of spinal cord in midthoracic region.*

- *Hematological findings:* Peripheral blood smear shows *microcytes, leukopenia, thrombocytopenia and hypersegmented neutrophils*. Bone marrow shows megaloblastic erythropoiesis.
- *Peripheral neuropathy:* Patient develops demyelination of peripheral nerves leading to sensorimotor disturbances.

Physiological state: Normally methylcobalamin converts homocysteine to methionine, which acts as a donor in the synthesis of choline containing phospholipids an important component of myelin. Normally deoxyadenosylcobalamin converts methylmalonyl CoA into succinyl CoA. *Deficiency of methylcobalamin results in decreased synthesis of choline required for myelin synthesis.*

Pathological state: Vitamin B_{12} deficiency results in *accumulation of methylmalonyl CoA, which is converted into methylmalonate and propionate. It leads to increased production of abnormal fatty acids, which incorporate into neuronal lipids. Myelin sheath breakdown occurs. Posterior and lateral white columns of midthoracic spinal cord involved. Patient develops total paralysis of lower legs.*

Subacute Combined Degeneration of Spinal Cord

Subacute combined degeneration of spinal cord occurs in mid-thoracic and cervical region.
- *Morphology of spinal cord:* Spinal cord shows pale areas of demyelination in the posterior columns and the lateral corticospinal tracts.
- *Clinical features:* Patient develops *spastic paraparesis, sensory ataxia and marked paresthesia leading to total paralysis of trunk and lower limbs*. Associated lesions include: optic atrophy and axonal peripheral neuropathy.
- *Light microscopy:* Spinal cord shows *swollen myelin sheath* with *disintegration and axonal degeneration*.

Folic Acid

Folic acid is obtained from yeast and leafy vegetables as well as animal liver. Animals cannot synthesize folate, thus it must come from diet. Deficiency occurs due to less intake, intestinal malabsorption and alcoholism, increased demand during pregnancy and hemolytic anemia; and chemotherapeutic agents containing folic acid antagonists.

Functions: Folate acts as a coenzyme in transfer and utilization of 1-carbon units, essential step in nucleic acid synthesis.

Clinical features: Folic acid deficiency does not cause neurologic changes (in contrast to vitamin B_{12} deficiency). Its deficiency causes megaloblastic anemia and neural tube defects *in utero*. It is used for treatment of chronic hemolytic anemia. Differences between vitamin B_{12} and folic acid are shown in Table 7.5.

Table 7.5: Differences between vitamin B_{12} and folic acid

Parameters	Vitamin B_{12}	Folic acid
Contents in foods	Liver, meat, dairy products	Raw vegetables, fresh fruits, whole grain cereals, diet rich in meat and liver
Loss due to cooking	10–30%	70–100%
Daily requirements	2 µg	100 µg
Daily intake	5–30 µg	500–800 µg
Site of absorption	Ileum	Duodenum and jejunum
Body stores	2–5 mg	5–10 mg

Laboratory Diagnosis of Megaloblastic Anemia

Peripheral smear examination
- *RBCs:* Anisocytosis, poikilocytosis, macrocytes (macrocytes are oval in megaloblastic anemia, while round in shape in normoblastic anemias in hemolytic anemia and post-hemorrhagic anemia). Macrocytosis and increased MCV may be seen in alcoholic patients, reticulocytosis results to polychromasia.
- *WBCs:* Leukopenia, hypersegmented neutrophils 8–9 lobes (>5/100 neutrophils) are demonstrated.
- *Platelets:* Moderate thrombocytopenia is present.

Bone marrow examination: Bone marrow shows megaloblastic erythropoiesis.

Vitamin C (Ascorbic Acid)

Vitamin C is derived from fruits, vegetables, milk, liver and fish. It is not synthesized endogenously. It is stored in the body (normal range 1.5 to 4.0 gm). L-ascorbic acid is converted to dehydroxy-ascorbic acid. It participates in oxidation and reduction reactions. *It participates in the synthesis of collagen and reticulin fibrils from mucopolysaccharide ground substance in wound healing.*

Physiological state: Vitamin C participates in the *synthesis of collagen and reticulin fibrils from mucopolysaccharide ground substance in wound healing*. It is required for *hydroxylation of proline and lysine*, which are essential for collagen synthesis in coats of blood vessels. It is required for *hydroxylation of dopamine* in synthesis of norepinephrine. It enhances maintenance of reduced state of other metabolically active agents, such as iron and FH4 (activated tetrahydrofolate). It has *antioxidant property* by scavenging free radicals. It acts indirectly by regenerating the antioxidant form of vitamin E.

Causes: Vitamin C deficiency is observed in elderly individuals, persons, alcoholics, hemodialysis patients and infants on processed milk.

Clinical features: Ascorbic acid deficiency results in scurvy, which is characterized by defective formation of mesenchymal tissue and osteoid matrix. Patient presents with bleeding gums, subperiosteal hemorrhage; and perifollicular petechial hemorrhages, defective wound healing; hemorrhagic phenomena. Hemorrhages and healing defects occur in both children and adults (Fig. 7.10).

- *Bleeding (hemorrhages):* Defective connective tissue also leads to fragile capillaries, resulting in abnormal bleeding. Infants and children present with *hemorrhages in mucocutaneous* and *muscles along fascial planes* at mechanical stress points due to loosened endothelial cells from capillaries especially in nail beds, *subperiosteal hematomas, bleeding into spaces: joints, retrobulbar, subarachnoid*, and *intracerebral hemorrhages*. In adults, ulceration and hemorrhage in gums occur due to loosening of teeth.
- *Skeletal changes:* Bone changes in scurvy are secondary to defective osteoid matrix formation. Insufficient production of osteoid matrix results in *cartilaginous overgrowth, widening of epiphysis, bowing of the long bones and chest deformity*. Osteoporosis is seen especially at the *metaphyseal ends of bone*.
- *Other changes:* Patient presents with *gingival swelling and periodontal infection, impaired wound healing, impaired localization of focal infections* and anemia.

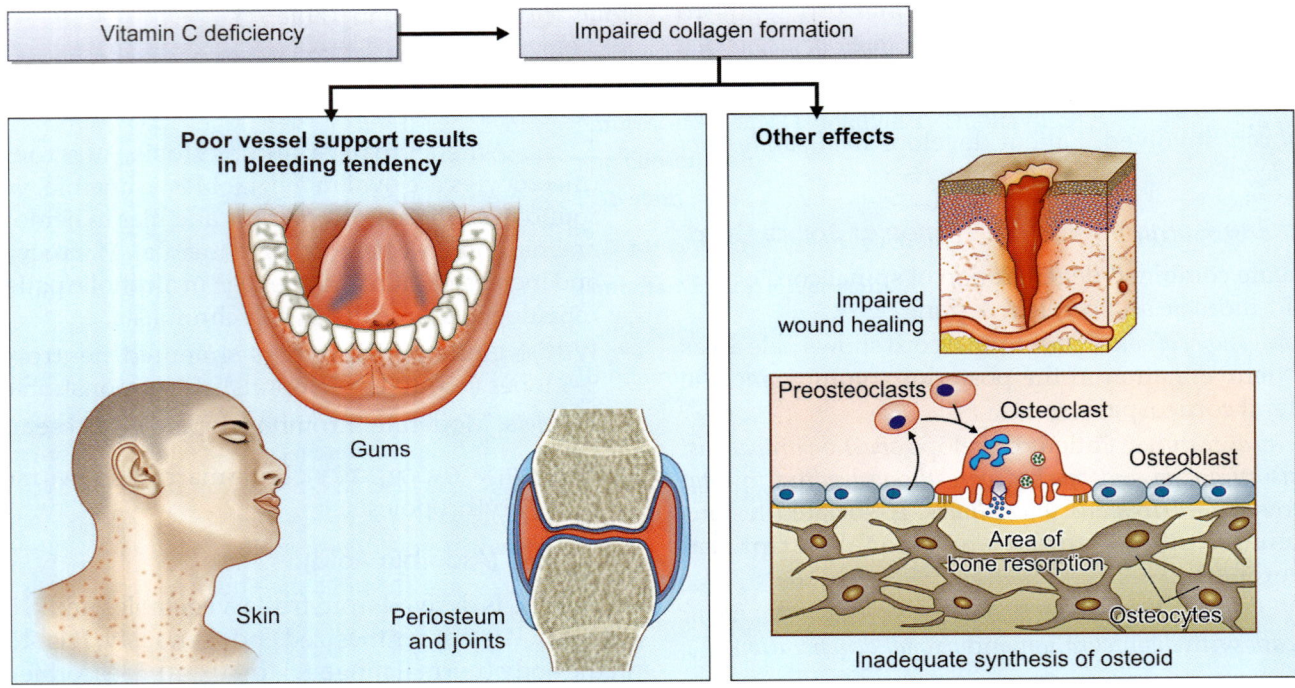

Fig. 7.10: Vitamin C deficiency causes impaired synthesis of collagen fibers leading to bleeding gums, hemorrhages in mucocutaneous, muscles along fascial planes, retrobulbar, subarachnoid, and intracerebral regions and bone changes.

BACTERIAL INFECTIONS

TUBERCULOSIS

Tuberculosis is worldwide health problem caused by Mycobacterium tubercle bacilli (homis strain). It is transmitted by *inhalation of droplets (most common)*, ingestion of infected milk and skin inoculation (handling infected specimens). It may involve multiple systems.

Mycobacterium Tubercle Bacillus

- *Acid-fast organism:* Mycobacterium tubercle bacillus is strict aerobe. It is acid-fast due to presence of mycolic acid in its cell wall and stained by Ziehl-Neelsen staining (decolorized by 20% H_2SO_4).
- *Composition:* Acid-fast bacilli contain large quantity of *hydrophobic waxes and fatty acids* of high molecular weight, which prevents entry of Gram's stain.
- *Virulence:* Virulence of bacillus depends on presence of *cord factor* (a sulphated glycolipid), *which prevents fusion of phagosomes with lysosomes* and thus favors intracellular revival of AFB in macrophages. If cord factor is extracted, AFB becomes avirulent.

- *Viability:* Bacillus is viable for months in dry or wet sputum. Single AFB is potentially infective in immunocompromised persons.

Risk factors: There is increased risk of tuberculosis in persons, who is in *close contact with a newly diagnosed tuberculosis case (sputum smear positive)*, history of *previous tuberculosis exposure* and immunocompromised individuals (*AIDS and corticosteroids therapy*), history of silicosis, diabetes mellitus, malnutrition, cancer, Hodgkin's disease, or leukemia, gastrectomy, chronic renal failure and alcoholism increases the risk of developing tuberculosis.

Tubercular infection: Tubercular infection refers to a positive TB skin test (Mantoux test or tuberculin test or PPD test) with no evidence of active disease. Purified protein derivative (PPD) is injected by intradermal route on forearm. Area of induration is demonstrated after 48–72 hours in immunocompetent individuals after exposure to tubercle bacilli after 2–4 weeks. Positive tuberculin test does not distinguish infection (inactive disease) from active disease.

Tuberculous disease: Tuberculous disease refers to cases that have positive acid-fast smear or culture for *Mycobacterium tuberculosis* or radiographic and clinical presentation of tuberculosis. *Children below 2 years of age are more susceptible.* Patients with silicosis and immunosuppression are more susceptible to tuberculosis.

Pathogenesis: Mycobacterium tubercle bacillus antigens plays important role in cell-mediated immunity and type IV hypersensitivity reaction. To study the virulence of Mycobacterium tubercule bacilli, virulence and bacterial factors have been devised, which are associated with intracellular survival, and genotype differences in the community prevalence of clinical strains. Virulence and bacterial factors in Mycobacterium tubercle bacilli are shown in Table 7.6.

- *Pathogenesis of tuberculosis <3 weeks duration:* Mycobacterium tubercle bacilli's mannose capped glycolipid (lipoarabinomannan) binds to mannose receptors expressed on alveolar macrophages leading to engulfment of AFB. *Cord factor synthesized by these organisms prevent fusion of phagosomes with lysosomes.* Hence, unchecked proliferation of tubercle bacilli continues inside alveolar macrophages.
- *Pathogenesis of tuberculosis >3 weeks duration:* Macrophages are antigen presenting cells, which transmit Mycobacterium tubercle bacilli antigen to T-helper cells. Macrophages synthesize IL-12, which takes part in differentiation of T-helper cells in lungs and lymph nodes.
  - ♦ **Bactericidal activity of immune system:** T cells synthesize interferon-g (IF-g), which stimulates nitrogen synthase enzyme resulting in synthesis of nitrogen intermediates (NO, NO_2 and HNO_3) and free radicals. These cause oxidative destruction of AFB.
  - ♦ **Formation of epithelioid granulomas:** Macrophages synthesize *tumor necrosis factor* and chemokines participate in *recruitment of monocytes and sensitization of T cells*. This process leads to formation of epithelioid granulomas composed of macrophages and surrounded by lymphocytes. Granulomas prevent spread of infection by confining bacteria within a compact collection of activated macrophages and lymphocytes. Mechanism of formation of granuloma is shown in Fig. 7.11.

Table 7.6: Virulence and bacterial factors in Mycobacterium tubercle bacilli

Characteristics	Name	Actions
Virulence factors	*Cord factor composed of glycolipids, mycolic acid and trehalose dimycolate	Cord factor preventing fusion of phagosomes with lysosomes thus favoring intracellular revival of AFB in macrophages
		Cord factor eliciting granulomas formation
	Catalase-peroxidase and lipoarabinomannan (LAM)	Resisting the host cell oxidative response
	Sulfatides and trehalose dimycolate	Triggering toxicity in animal models
	Lipoarabinomannan (LAM)	Induction of cytokines and resist host oxidative stress
Bacterial factors	Nonreplicating persistent (NRP1) state	Under aerophilic conditions with increased glycine dehydrogenase activity
	Nonreplicating persistent (NRP2) state	Under anaerobic conditions with decreased glycine dehydrogenase activity
	A sigma factor	Unknown
	α-crystallin-like heat shock protein (acr)	Unknown

*If cord factor is extracted, AFB becomes avirulent

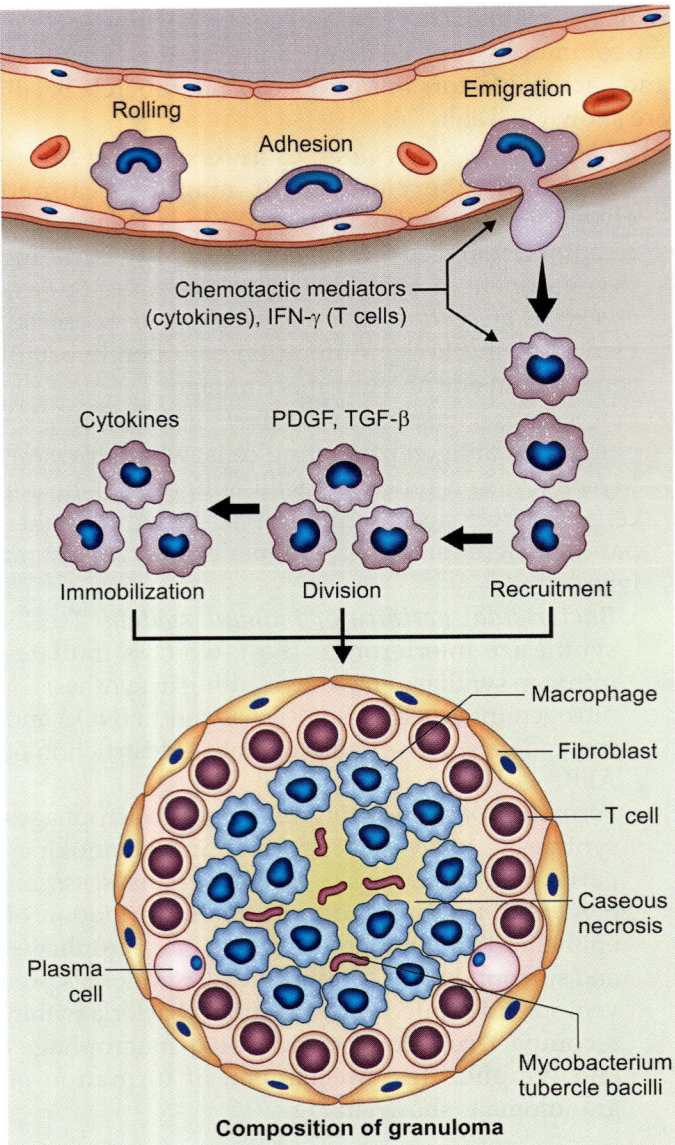

Fig. 7.11: Mechanism of formation of granuloma.

- **Caseous necrosis:** CD8+ T cells cause destruction of macrophages by *Fas independent* mechanism. On the other hand, CD4+ and CD8+ T cells cause destruction of macrophages by *Fas dependent* mechanism resulting in caseous necrosis.

Tissue susceptibility: Lungs are the most common site of *tuberculosis in children and adults*. Most common organs involved in *children* include *lungs, lymph nodes, spleen and meninges*. Lungs, adrenal glands, kidneys, liver, spleen, bone, meninges, serous membranes, fallopian tubes, epididymis and lymph nodes are involved in adults. Tissues rarely involved include *cardiac muscle, skeletal muscle, stomach, thyroid gland, and pancreas*.

Light Microscopy
Histopathological examination of lesion shows epithelioid cell granulomas, caseous necrosis and Langhans' giant cells (Figs 7.12 and 7.13).

Drug resistance: Patient develops drug *resistance due to mutations involving mycolic acid, catalase* and *peroxidase enzyme*. Catalase enzyme is required to activate isoniazid.

Categories: Tuberculosis is divided into two categories: pulmonary (85% cases) and extrapulmonary tuberculosis (15% cases). Active disease develops in 5 to 15% of those infected with *M. tuberculosis*. Pulmonary tuberculosis has two distinct phases, i.e. primary tuberculosis (children) and secondary tuberculosis (adults). Organs involved in primary, secondary and miliary tuberculosis are shown in Fig. 7.14.

PRIMARY TUBERCULOSIS (PRIMARY COMPLEX)

Primary tuberculosis is also known as *Ghon's complex* caused by Mycobacterium tubercle bacillus. *It is demonstrated in lung, tonsil, ileocecal region* and skin. It usually does not progress to clinically evident disease. Granuloma in tuberculosis is known as *tubercle. Histological examination* reveals caseous necrosis, epithelioid granulomas, Langhans' giant cells.

Mode of transmission: Mycobacterium tubercle bacilli are transmitted by *droplet infection, ingestion of infected milk products, skin inoculation and vertical transmission*.

- *Droplet infection:* Infection is most common contracted by droplet infection from open case of pulmonary tuberculosis (cavities lung).

- *Ingestion of infected milk:* Ingestion of unpasteurized milk containing AFB produces Ghon's focus in *tonsils* and *ileocecal region*. Acid-fast bacilli produce circumferential *ulcers perpendicular to long axis of small intestine*. Fibrosis in this region is responsible for *stricture formation*.

- *Skin inoculation:* Primary cutaneous inoculation with AFB occurs in person *handling infected specimens*. Patient develops painless nonhealing papule (Ghon's focus) in 2 to 4 weeks after inoculation, which forms cold abscess resulting to discharging sinuses after several weeks.

- *Vertical transmission:* Placental transmission of tuberculosis from mother to fetus shows lesions in *liver* and *portal lymph nodes seen at birth*.

Nutritional and Infectious Diseases

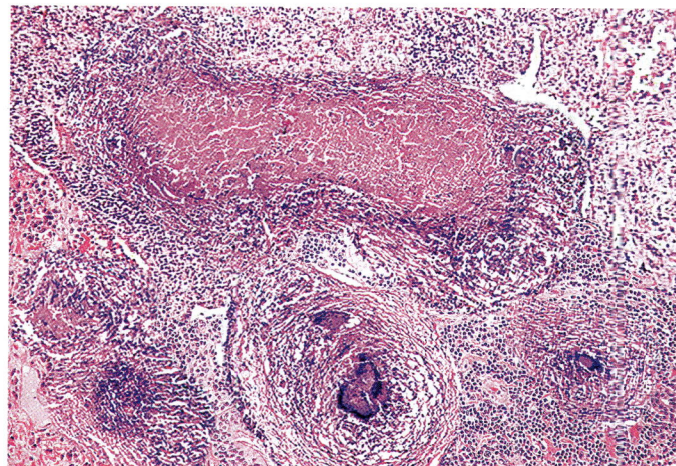

Fig. 7.12: Tuberculosis lung shows epithelioid granulomas, Langhans' giant cells and caseous necrosis (400X).

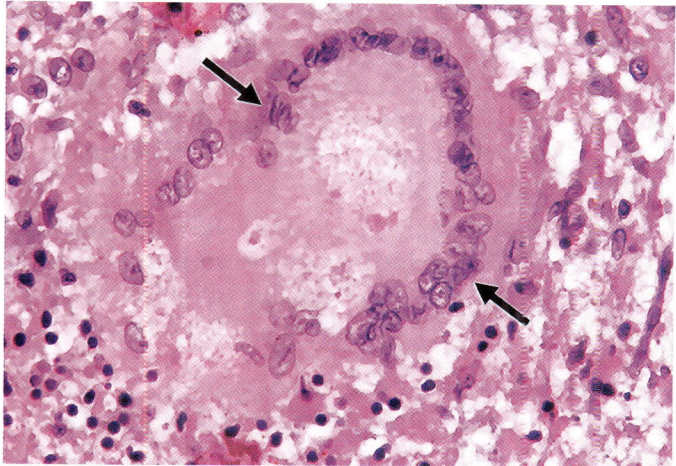

Fig. 7.13: Langhans' giant cells in a case of tuberculosis (arrows) (400X).

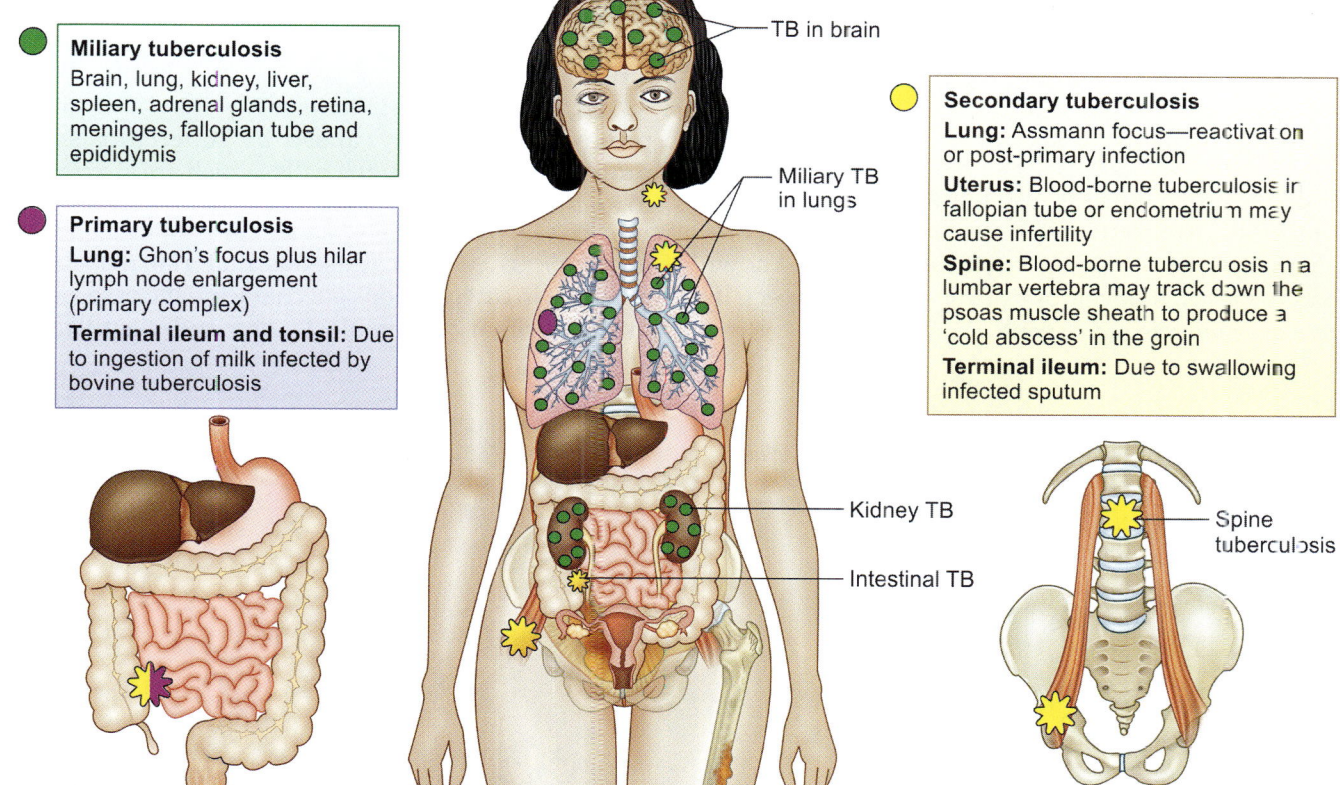

Fig. 7.14: Organs involved in primary, secondary and miliary tuberculosis. Primary tuberculosis produces a subpleural midzone lesion in lung. In secondary tuberculosis, lesion is located in apical region of lung. Miliary tuberculosis shows tubercles in various organs.

Pulmonary Ghon's Complex Lesion

Pulmonary Ghon's complex lesion is caused by *Mycobacterium tuberculosis* especially in children. The lesion can retain viable bacteria responsible for reactivation of the disease in later life. Ghon's complex consists of Ghon's focus in lung, lymphatic channel and draining lymph nodes involvement (Fig. 7.15).

Pulmonary lesion

- *Location:* Primary tuberculosis produces a small midzone subpleural focus of consolidation near with interlobar fissure, involvement of lymphatic channels and hilar lymph nodes.
- *Dystrophic calcification:* The lesion most often heals by fibrosis and dystrophic calcification in 95% cases.

The calcified lesion known as *Ranke's complex* is often visible on radiography.

- *Lung lesions:* Approximately 5% of immunocompromised children develop symptomatic infection (cavities, bronchopneumonia, pleural effusion or miliary tuberculosis).
- *Nidus for secondary tuberculosis:* Because acid-fast bacilli persisting in dormant form in old necrotic calcified lesions are still capable of initiating lesion, and thus a nidus for secondary tuberculosis.

Lymphatic channels involvement: Lymphatic channels are laden with Mycobacterium tubercle bacilli without producing lesion.

Draining lymph nodes: Lymph nodes draining Ghon's focus shows caseous necrosis. Lymph nodes are enlarged, i.e. lungs (hilar region), tonsils (cervical region), GIT (ileocecal region) and skin (cutaneous region). *Nodal lesions of tuberculosis take longer time to regress hence remain a potential source of reinfection.*

SECONDARY TUBERCULOSIS

Secondary tuberculosis is also known as post-primary pulmonary tuberculosis or reactivation disease. Pulmonary lesion in secondary tuberculosis is known as *Simon's focus*. It develops during adult life especially in *immunocompromised persons*.

It occurs either due to *inhalation of Mycobacterium tubercle bacilli* or *reactivation of dormant lymph node and old calcified healed parenchymal lesion*. It causes extensive tissue destruction (caseous necrosis) by the action of cytokines synthesized by memory T cells. Morphology of lung in tuberculosis is shown in Fig. 7.16.

Pulmonary Morphology in Tuberculosis

Simon's focus in apical region: Initially, the tubercular lesion is 2.0 cm, *diffuse solid, gray white to yellowish, with poorly defined margins and central areas of caseous necrosis.* The lesion is located in the apical region of upper lobes of posterior segments *high oxygen tension and paucity of macrophages due to decreased blood supply.*

Growth of Mycobacterium tubercle bacilli is inhibited at pH <6.5. Some patients may develop tubercular cavities, which are *highly contagious*. Large cavities are associated with hemoptysis. Hilar lymphadenopathy is prominent. The lesion frequently ruptures into the bronchi.

Aspergilloma: Aspergillus species may also grow in pre-existing cavities caused by tuberculosis. They proliferate to form fungus balls, which are also referred to as *aspergillomas or mycetomas*.

Tuberculous cavities: Caseous material may liquefy resulting in cavity lesions is a characteristic of secondary, but not primary tuberculosis. The cavity is filled with

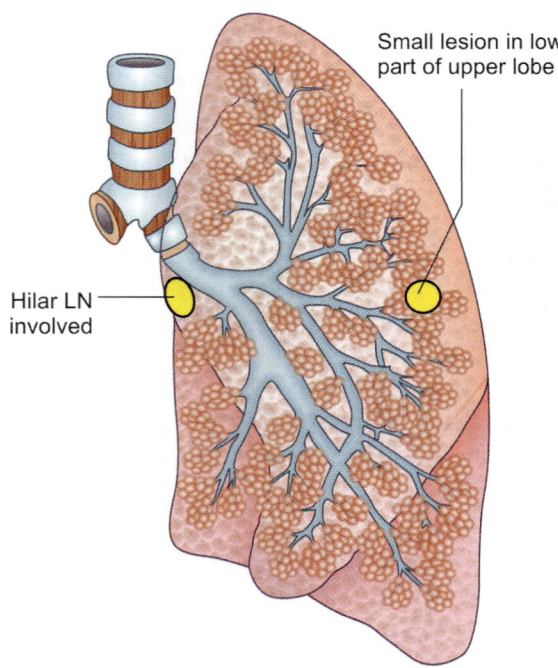
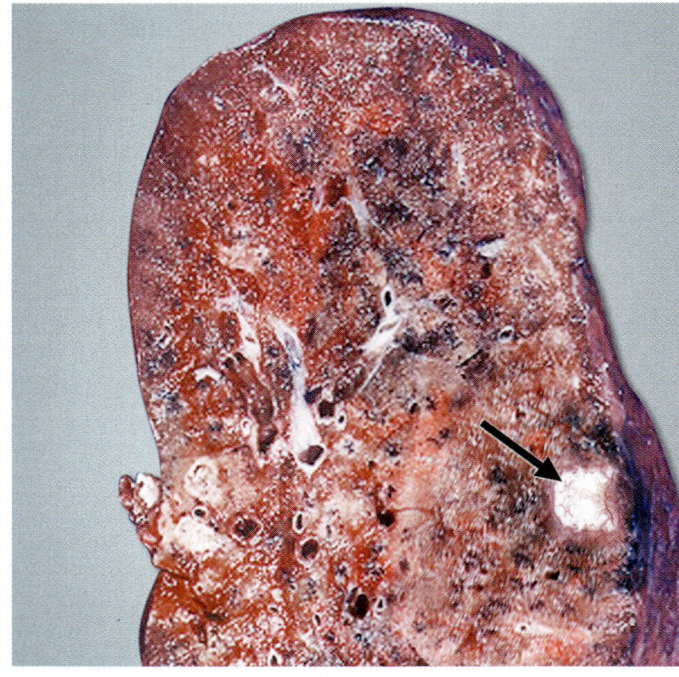

Fig. 7.15: Primary tuberculosis showing subpleural midzonal Ghon's focus and hilar lymph node enlargement. Gross examination of lung showing subpleural midzonal Ghon's focus (arrow).

Nutritional and Infectious Diseases

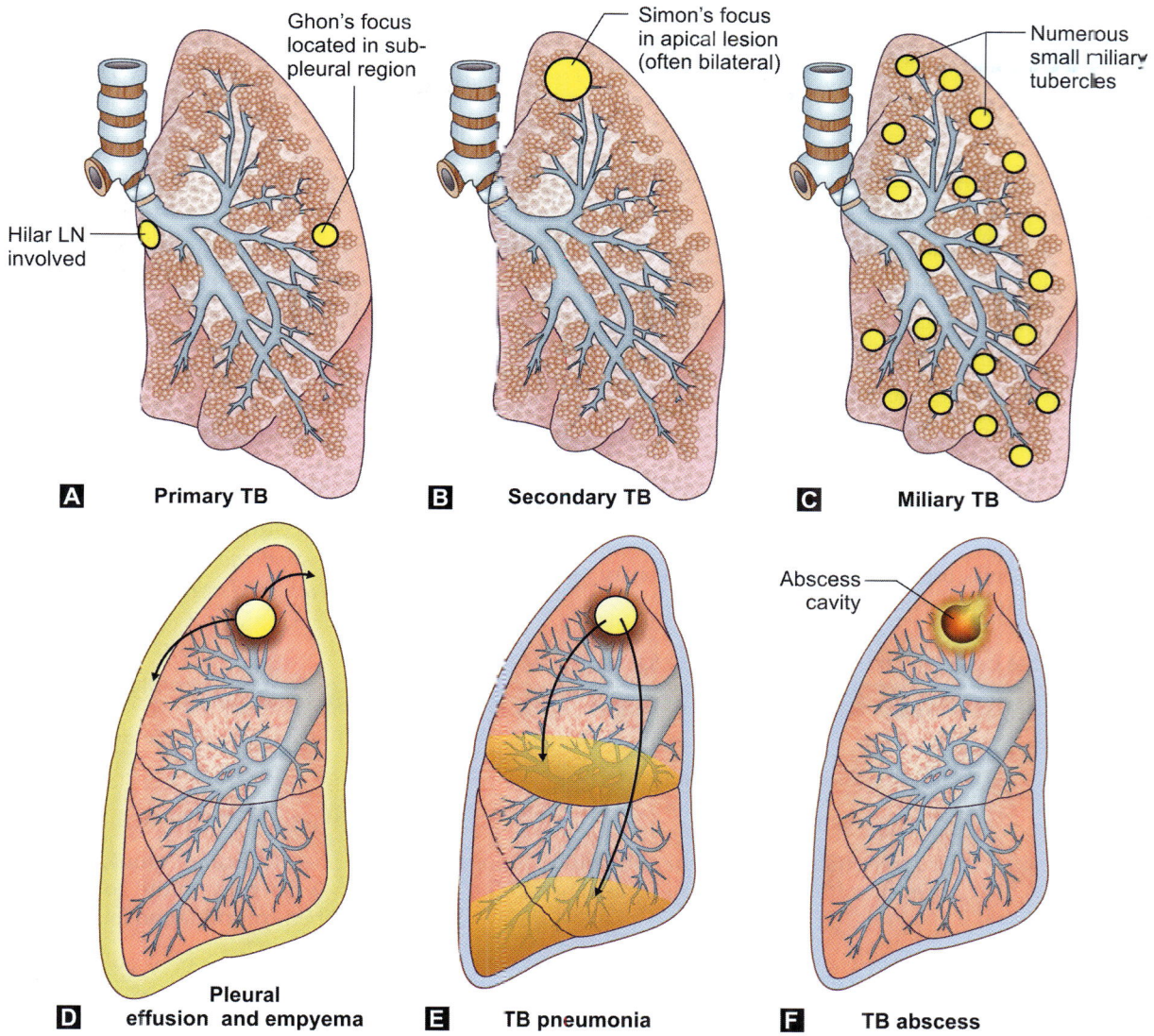

Fig. 7.16: Morphology of lung in tuberculosis. (A) Primary tuberculosis shows subpleural midzone and lesion hilar lymph node enlargement, (B) apical lesion is seen in secondary tuberculosis, (C) small miliary tubercles are demonstrated in lung, (D to F) pleural effusion, empyema, consolidation (pneumonia) and abscess are complications of tuberculosis.

yellow-grayish caseous material more or less surrounded by fibrous tissue. AFB can easily be demonstrated in open cavities. Tubercular lesion may *erode into airways*. Patient may develop empyema, *hemoptysis,* and *sputum* becomes positive for AFB. Causes of hemoptysis are shown in Table 7.7.

Lung consolidation: Immunocompromised young children and elderly persons may develop *tubercular bronchopneumonia or lobar pneumonia.* These patients are very infectious. Patients have a high fever and productive cough.

Tubercular pleuritis and effusion: Tubercular pleuritis with effusion usually develops soon after initial infection. Tuberculous focus located at the edge of the lung ruptures into the pleural space causing pleurisy and pleural effusion. Patient presents with *dyspnea and sharp chest pain that worsens with a deep breath* (pleurisy). Tuberculosis pleurisy generally resolves without treatment. *Differences between primary and secondary tuberculosis* are shown in Table 7.8 and *differences between tuberculosis and sarcoidosis* are shown in Table 7.9.

Outcome of Pulmonary Tuberculosis

Outcome of pulmonary tuberculosis is lung fibrosis, lung cavitation, miliary tuberculosis and other lesions described as under:

- *Fibrosis:* Healing of secondary pulmonary tuberculosis occurs by fibrosis in favorable conditions.
- *Lung cavitation:* In some patients, tubercular lesion continues to progress for months and years resulting

Table 7.7: Causes of hemoptysis

Etiology	Disorders
Inflammatory lesions	Tuberculosis*
	Bronchiectasis*
	Pneumonias*
Neoplastic lesions	Primary lung cancers*
	Metastatic lung cancers*
	Bronchopulmonary adenoma
Other lesions	Pulmonary embolism and infarction*
	Mitral stenosis
	Left ventricular failure
	Anticoagulant therapy
	Bronchial adenoma
	Idiopathic pulmonary hemosiderosis

*Most common causes of hemoptysis are tuberculosis, bronchiectasis, pneumonias, bronchogenic carcinoma, pulmonary embolism and infarction

in further pulmonary damage. It leads to *cavity formation, lobar pneumonia, fibrocaseous tuberculosis* and *miliary tuberculosis* (Fig. 7.17).

- *Airways involvement:* Endobronchial and endotracheal spread of tuberculosis cause laryngeal tuberculosis of vocal cords. Erosion of airways reveals AFB in sputum.
- *Miliary tuberculosis:* Secondary tuberculosis may disseminate via hematogenous route resulting in multiple small innumerable small *millet seed-like lesions, tubercular granulomas* known as *miliary tuberculosis*. Mycobacterium tubercle bacilli may disseminate via systemic circulation to seed distant organs such as *bone marrow, liver, spleen, adrenal glands, retina, meninges, kidneys, fallopian tubes, and epididymis*. Mycobacterium tubercle bacilli reach the lungs via pulmonary arteries. *Chest radiograph reveals very small nodules throughout the lungs that look like millet seeds.* It occurs shortly after

Table 7.8: Differences between primary and secondary (post-primary) tuberculosis

Parameters	Primary tuberculosis	Secondary tuberculosis
Exposure to AFB	First time	Reactivation or second time exposure
Age group	Children/younger age group	Any age group
Consolidation	Solitary lesion	Multifocal lesions (poorly defined)
Location	Midzone (Ghon's focus in subpleural lesion), other sites (tonsils, ileocecal region and skin)	Upper lobes (apical region), Simon's focus in lungs: 2 cm gray white to yellowish well circumscribed consolidation in apical regions of one or both lungs
		Sputum for AFB positive
Lymphadenopathy	Common	Rare
Severity of lesion	Less severe, healing by fibrosis and dystrophic calcification	More severe progressing to cavitation, lobar pneumonia, extension in lumen of bronchi, trachea, and larynx with vocal cord involvement
Pleural effusion	Common	Empyema
Cavitation	Rare	Common
Miliary tuberculosis	Yes (lung, liver, bone marrow, spleen, adrenal glands, meninges, kidneys, fallopian tubes, and epididymis)	Yes (lung, liver, bone marrow, spleen, adrenal glands, meninges, kidneys, fallopian tubes, and epididymis)

Table 7.9: Differences between tuberculosis and sarcoidosis

Characteristics	Tuberculosis	Sarcoidosis
Etiology	Mycobacterium tubercle bacilli	Unknown etiology
Granuloma	Caseating granuloma	Noncaseating granulomas
Cytoplasmic inclusions in giant cells	Absence of Schaumann's bodies, asteroid bodies and birefringent crystals	Presence of Schaumann's bodies, asteroid bodies and birefringent crystals
Steroid therapy	Worsens the disease	Improves the patient
Diagnosis	Acid-fast bacilli present	Excluding causes of granulomatous lesions

Nutritional and Infectious Diseases

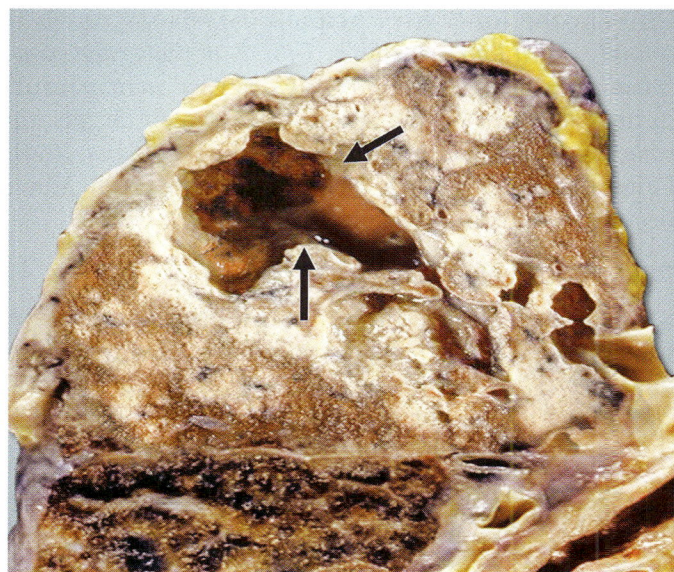

Fig. 7.17: Lung showing cavity in a case of secondary tuberculosis (arrows).

primary infection in immunocompromised persons (Fig. 7.18).

- *Other complications:* Patient may develop tubercular laryngitis, bronchopleural fistula, bronchiectasis, vertebral tuberculosis (Pott's disease), amyloidosis, scar carcinoma lung and granulomatous hepatitis.

Clinical features: Patient presents with *cough, expectoration, hemoptysis* (blood-tinged sputum) *night sweats,* and *evening rise of temperature, anorexia, loss of weight, lassitude and chest pain. Fever* is probably caused by the absorption of toxic products from the site of infection and synthesis of cytokines (*TNF-α* and *IL-1*) by macrophages.

Clinical examination: On clinical examination, *percussion note is dull* over the affected area. On auscultation, one can *hear bronchial breath sounds, crepitant crackles* and *wheeze.* Sound is heard through stethoscope, when the patient whispers, it is known as *whispered pectoriloquy.*

TUBERCULOSIS IN HIV CASES

Mycobacterium avium intracellulare (MAC) complex is a progressive systemic disorder, often occurring in patients who have AIDS. Approximately 33% of all patients develop overt disease due to depletion of CD4+ T cells cripples the immune response.

CD4+ T cells count <200/cu mm

- Immunosuppression is more severe. Consolidation occurs in lower and middle lobes of lungs. Lymphadenopathy occurs in 50% cases. This pneumonia is characterized by an extensive infiltrate of macrophages.
- Lesions range from epithelioid granulomas containing a few organisms to loose aggregates of foamy macrophages.
- Clinical presentation associated with *Mycobacterium avium intracellulare* disease resembles that of tuberculosis.

CD4+ T cells count >300/cu mm: Immunosuppression is less severe. Apical regions of lungs are affected. Extrapulmonary organs involvement occurs in 15% of cases.

EXTRAPULMONARY TUBERCULOSIS

Extrapulmonary tuberculosis occurs primarily in immunocompromised patients. Examples of extrapulmonary tuberculosis include: *tubercular meningitis, Pott's disease of the spine, paravertebral abscess, or psoas abscess.* Other organs involved include: kidney, adrenal glands, fallopian tubes, peritoneum, pericardium, breast, larynx and lymph node.

Tubercular Meningitis

Tuberculous meningitis has insidious onset and may last for weeks or months. It is secondary to tuberculous infection occurring elsewhere in the body. It has a *predilection for the base of the brain.* Basal cisterns and the lateral sulci that contain gelatinous whitish gray material.

Inadequately treated tuberculous meningitis results in meningeal fibrosis, communicating hydrocephalus and vasculitis. Inflammation of striate arteries results in cerebral infarcts. Patient may develop focal mass in the brain known as *tuberculoma.* Patient presents with *headache, neck rigidity, drowsiness* and *focal neurological symptoms.*

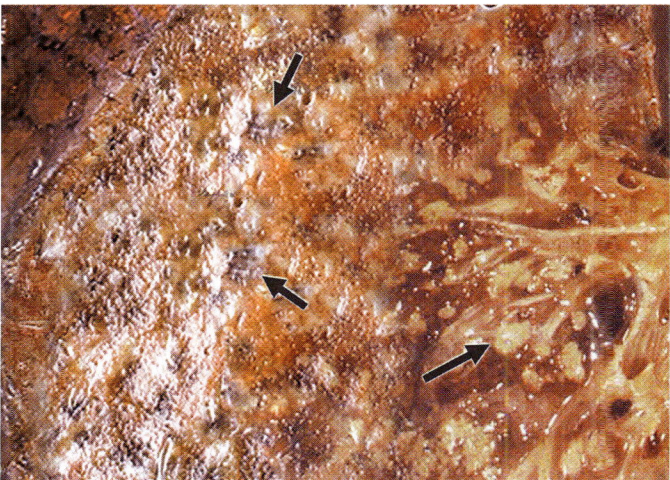

Fig. 7.18: Miliary tuberculosis. Lung showing millet-like seedlings of tuberculosis (arrows).

CSF findings: Lumbar puncture reveals increased pressure yielding *straw-colored CSF*. *Protein's content is markedly increased*. Light microscopy of CSF shows *numerous lymphocytes*. Acid-fast bacteria may be grown on culture media. CSF findings in tubercular meningitis are shown in Table 7.10.

Instestinal Tuberculosis

Mycobacterium tubercle bacilli reach the intestine either ingestion of infected sputum or ingestion of unpasteurized milk. The tubercular lesions begin in the Peyer's patches (lymphoid follicles) and spread through lymphatic channels resulting in tubercular ulcer in terminal ileum especially in ileocecal region.

> ### Gross Morphology
> - Intestinal tuberculosis produces *circumferential ulcers perpendicular to long axis of small intestine*. Fibrosis in this region is responsible for *stricture formation*.
> - Draining lymph nodes of small intestine are enlarged and matted with caseous necrosis known as *tabes mesenterica*. It most often *heals by fibrosis and dystrophic calcification*.
> - *Hyperplastic ileocecal tuberculosis* is a variant of intestinal tuberculosis characterized by *thickening of terminal ileum, cecum* and *ascending colon with mucosal ulceration*.
> - On clinical examination, hyperplastic ileocecal tuberculosis is palpable and mistaken for cecal carcinoma. Stricture formation in the intestine is shown in Fig. 7.19.
>
> ### Light Microscopy
> Light microscopy reveals caseating epithelioid granulomas with Langhans' giant cells.

Tubercular Osteomyelitis

Tubercular osteomyelitis most commonly occurs secondary to hematogenous extension from a primary focus in the lung. It principally *targets the vertebral column, called Pott's disease in 1 to 3% of people and paraspinal cold abscess*. Vertebral body destruction may result in impingement on the spinal cord. It also targets *hip bone, long bones (femur, tibia) and small bones (hands, feet)*. Patient presents with fever, fatigue, bone pain, some tissue swelling and discharging sinuses.

Tubercular Pyelonephritis

Kidneys are most common extrapulmonary site in tuberculosis. This can cause asymptomatic pyuria (white blood cells in the urine). Tubercular pyelonephritis can spread to the reproductive organs and affect reproduction. In men, tubercular epididymitis may occur.

> ### Gross Morphology
> Kidneys are enlarged. Cut surface reveals caseous material filling the renal pelvis (Fig. 7.20).
>
> ### Light Microscopy
> Histopathological examination shows caseous necrosis, epithelioid cell granulomas and Langhans' giant cells.

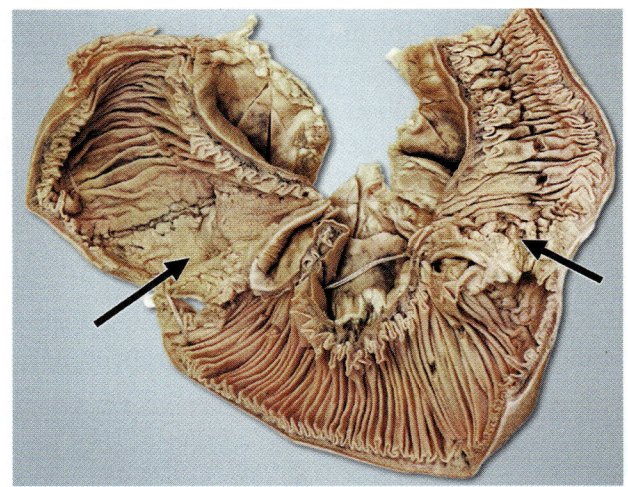

Fig. 7.19: Tubercular stricture of intestine (arrows).

Table 7.10: CSF findings in tubercular meningitis

Features	Tubercular meningitis	Normal CSF
Causative organism	Mycobacterium tubercle bacillus	No organisms
CSF pressure	Increased	80 to 180 cm of H_2O (20 drops/minute)
Color	Straw colored	Clear, colorless
CSF proteins	Increased due to vascular permeability	Normal 15–40 mg%
CSF sugar	Normal range	50–80 mg%
CSF white blood cells	Lymphocyte count increased	0–4 lymphocytes/mm^3
CSF culture	Bacterial growth on LJ medium	Sterile
ZN staining	Acid-fast bacteria demonstration	Organisms absent, hence insignificant

Adrenal Gland Tuberculosis

Tuberculosis of the adrenal glands can lead to adrenal insufficiency characterized by inability to increase steroid production in times of stress, resulting in weakness and collapse.

Tubercular Breast Abscess

Breast tuberculosis usually occurs due to *extension from a rib in females.* Patient presents with breast abscess and fever. Breast abscess contains caseous material. Light microscopy reveals epithelioid granulomas, caseous necrosis and Langhans' type of giant cells.

Laryngeal Tuberculosis

Laryngeal tuberculosis is extremely infectious as it affects larynx or the vocal cords.

Tubercular Salpingitis

Tubercular salpingitis occurs as a result of extension of tubercular infection endometrium. Spread of tubercular infection through intraluminal route causes *adhesions of lining epithelium, which is important cause of infertility.* On histopathological examination, fallopian tube shows epithelioid cell granulomas, Langhans' giant cells and caseous necrosis.

Tubercular Peritonitis

Mycobacterium tuberculosis can involve the outer linings of the intestines and the linings inside the abdominal wall, producing increased fluid, as in tuberculosis peritonitis. Increased fluid leads to abdominal distension and pain.

Tubercular Pericarditis

Tubercular pericardial effusion impairs functioning of the heart. It may progress to constrictive pericarditis.

Tubercular Lymphadenitis

Lymph nodes contain macrophages that capture the bacteria (Fig. 7.21). Any lymph node can harbor uncontrolled replication of bacteria, causing the lymph node to become enlarged. The infection can develop a fistula from the lymph node to the skin.

LABORATORY DIAGNOSIS

Smear Examination

Smears are prepared from specimens, i.e. sputum for three consecutive days, laryngeal, bronchoalveolar and gastric lavage. Smears are prepared and stained with ZN staining, *auramine* and *rhodamine O* for examination by immunofluorescence microscopy.

- *Sputum collection:* Sputum should be collected for three consecutive days to demonstrate acid-fast bacilli.
- *Laryngeal swab:* By laryngoscope, two swabs are collected and put in 10% H_2SO_4 in test tube for 5 minutes for killing contaminants. Then transfer these swabs to another test tube containing 2% NaOH for 5 minutes. NaOH kills other bacilli.
- *Bronchoalveolar lavage:* Smears are prepared and stained with ZN staining.
- *Gastric lavage:* It is indicated in *children and older patients, who are unable to cough out sputum.* Specimen is collected by Ryle's tube and processed immediately to avoid the effect of gastric secretions and processed immediately to avoid the effect of gastric secretions.

Neutralize the gastric contents with N/10 NaOH and put in refrigerator for 15 minutes. Remove

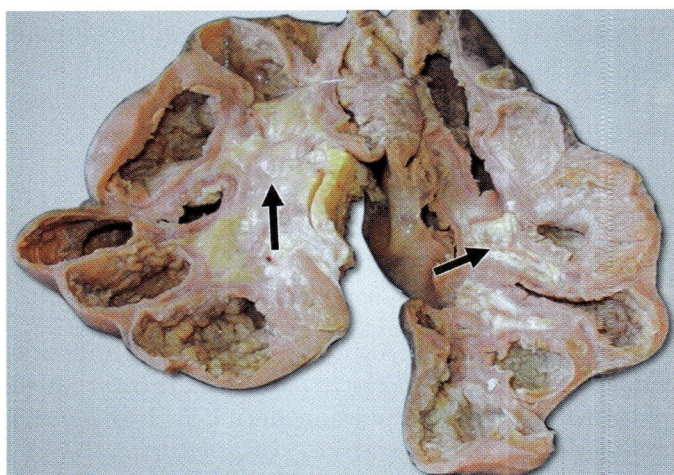

Fig. 7.20: Tubercular pyelonephritis. Fibrous-walled abscess cavity filled with caseous material is shown on cut surface. This patient had a previous well-established history of pulmonary tuberculosis. Section from the patient's nephrectomy specimen shows a tuberculous granuloma, with central caseating necrosis and peripheral scarring (arrows).

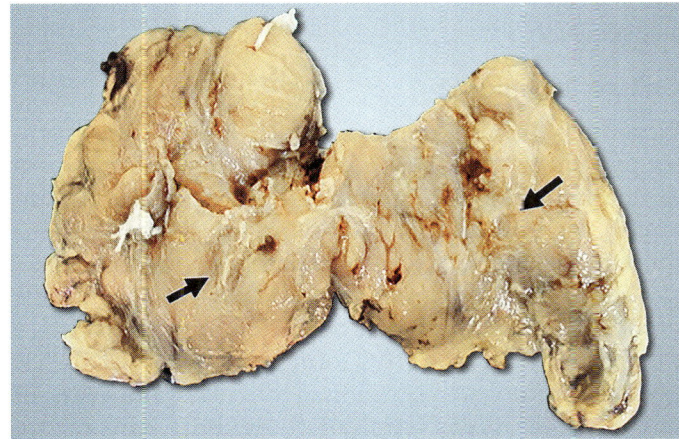

Fig. 7.21: Tubercular lymphadenitis showing cheesy appearance on cut surface (arrows).

the supernatant and centrifuge at 3000 rpm for 15 minutes. Smears are made from deposits.

Stains for AFB

Tubercle bacilli can be demonstrated by Ziehl-Neelsen stain and fluorescent like stains such as auramine O and rhodamine stain. Grading of AFB is done as follows:
- Grade I: 3–9 AFB in entire smear.
- Grade II: 10 or more AFB in entire smear.
- Grade III: 10 or more AFB in most oil immersion fields of smear.

Imaging Techniques

Chest X-ray: It reveals *cavitation, calcification* (healed disease), and *nodes in the upper lobes*, but cannot confirm the diagnosis.

Computed tomography (CT): It is *more sensitive than chest radiography for detection of cavities, lymphadenopathy, miliary disease,* bronchiectasis, bronchial stenosis, bronchopleural fistula, and pleural effusion.

Magnetic resonance imaging: It is *preferred for* diagnosis of extrapulmonary disease, such as *skeletal and intracranial tuberculosis.*

Fine Needle Aspiration Cytology

Smears are stained with May Grunwald-Giemsa stain. Microscopic examination reveals epithelioid granulomas, caseous necrosis and Langhans' giant cells. Acid-fast bacilli are demonstrated by ZN staining.

Histopathological Examination

Biopsy is done to establish diagnosis. It consists of epithelioid granulomas, caseous necrosis and Langhans' giant cells.

Fluid Examination

Fluid examination is done in extrapulmonary tuberculous, i.e. *cerebrospinal fluid, pleural fluid, peritoneal fluid and synovial fluid.*

Culture Techniques

Liquid media based culture takes 2 weeks. *Lowenstein-Jensen culture medium takes 10 weeks.* Drain off excess of fluid and inoculate in two test tubes of Lowenstein-Jensen medium. Aeration is done for every week for more than 8 weeks to remove water of condensation.

Growth starts appearing in 10–14 days. Human strains of Mycobacterium tubercle bacilli (eugonic) grow more than bovine strains (dysgonic). Addition of 0.75% glycerol promotes the growth of human strains without any effect on bovine strain. After culture, smears are made from colonies and stained with Ziehl-Neelsen stain.

Gas Chromatographic Method

Gas chromatographic method is useful diagnostic tool to demonstrate *tuberculostearic acid,* when AFB is not demonstrated.

Nucleic Acid Amplification (Gene Probes)

Direct tests of nucleic acid amplification (NAA) are rapid, widely available, and can be performed in a day (within 2–7 hours). The amplified *Mycobacterium tuberculosis* direct test (gene-probe) targets mycobacterial ribosomal RNA by transcription-mediated amplification. *The test uses DNA probes that are highly specific for M. tuberculosis species.* It is best used (and only approved for use) in patients in whom acid-fast bacilli smears are positive and cultures are in process. *In contrast, the nucleic acid amplification tests (NAATs) are highly specific for Mycobacterium tuberculosis.* Specificity is greater than 95% in either smear negative or smear positive samples.

Polymerase Chain Reaction (PCR) Testing

PCR testing technique amplifies even very small portions of a predetermined target region of *M. tuberculosis*-complex DNA. The test uses an automated system that can rapidly detect as few as one organism from sputum, bronchoalveolar lavage, blood, cerebrospinal fluid, pleural fluid, or other fluid and tissue samples and has shown sensitivity and specificity of nearly 90% in pulmonary disease.

LEPROSY (HANSEN DISEASE)

Leprosy is known since ancient times and remains a major public health problem in many developing countries including India. It is rare in developed countries. It is caused by *Mycobacterium leprae* with spectral clinical presentation determined by the host. It affects all the systems except central nervous system, heart and ovaries.

Mycobacterium leprae: Mycobacterium leprae are slender rod shaped weakly acid-fast bacilli. These are not grown on culture medium or cell culture. *These can be grown only in aramadillo (ant-eating mammal).*

Mode of transmission: Although mode of transmission is still uncertain, yet *Mycobacterium leprae* are transmitted by oronasal route. Incubation period is 2 to 7 years (average 3–5 years).

Sites of involvement: After entering body, *Mycobacterium leprae* spread through circulation and reach *cooler parts* of body such as skin of *extremities, peripheral nerves, mouth and eyes.* These organisms may be demonstrated in bone marrow, liver, spleen and lymph nodes.

CLASSIFICATION

According to Indian classification, leprosy is classified into five categories: indeterminate, tuberculoid, borderline, lepromatous and pure neuritic. According to WHO system of working classification, leprosy is classified into paucibacillary (PB) and multibacillary (MB) because they entail different treatment regimens. *According to Myrid classification, leprosy is classified into two categories: immunological stable (lepromatous and tuberculoid, and immunological unstable (indeterminate and borderline).* The most widely accepted scheme of classification is Ridley-Jopling classification.

Ridley-Joppling Classification

The most widely accepted scheme of classification is Ridley-Jopling classification (Fig. 7.22). It is based on a combination of *clinical findings, bacteriological index (BI), immunological reactivity (lepromin test) and the histological findings*. This classification ranges from a spectrum of high- to low-resistance pattern.

Leprosy is classified into two polar clinically stable categories: *TT (tuberculoid leprosy)* and *LL (lepromatous leprosy)*. Borderline group includes *BT (borderline tuberculoid), BB (borderline leprosy)* and *BL (borderline lepromatous leprosy)*.

- *TT (tuberculoid leprosy):* It is characterized by presence of immunological response against *Mycobacterium leprae*. Patient develops large macular *lesions on cooler parts especially nose, outer ears, testes and superficial nerve endings*. There is presence of *cell-mediated immune response. Infectivity is low in tuberculoid leprosy* (Fig. 7.23).

- *LL (lepromatous leprosy):* It has least capacity to mount immunological response against *Mycobacterium leprae*. Patient develops *extensive erythematous macules, papules or nodules with extensive destruction of skin*. Immune response is severely depressed. There is high infectivity in lepromatous leprosy (Fig. 7.24).

- *Borderline leprosy:* Majority of leprosy patients have variable immunological response. *These do not fall into polar group*. BT (borderline tuberculoid) tends to be more towards TT (tuberculoid leprosy) and BL (borderline lepromatous leprosy) towards LL (lepromatous leprosy).

Indian Classification

According to Indian classification, leprosy is classified into five categories: indeterminate, tuberculoid, borderline, lepromatous and pure neuritic.

WHO System of Working Classification

According to WHO system of working classification, leprosy is classified into paucibacillary (PB) and multibacillary (MB) because they entail different treatment regimens.

- *Paucibacillary (PB) leprosy:* It is characterized by *1–5 skin lesions, one nerve involvement* and *slit skin smear negative for AFB*.

- *Multibacillary (MB) leprosy:* It is characterized by *6 or more skin lesions, involvement of more than two nerves* and slit skin *smear positive for AFB*.

Myrid Classification

According to Myrid classification, leprosy is classified into two categories: *immunological stable (lepromatous and*

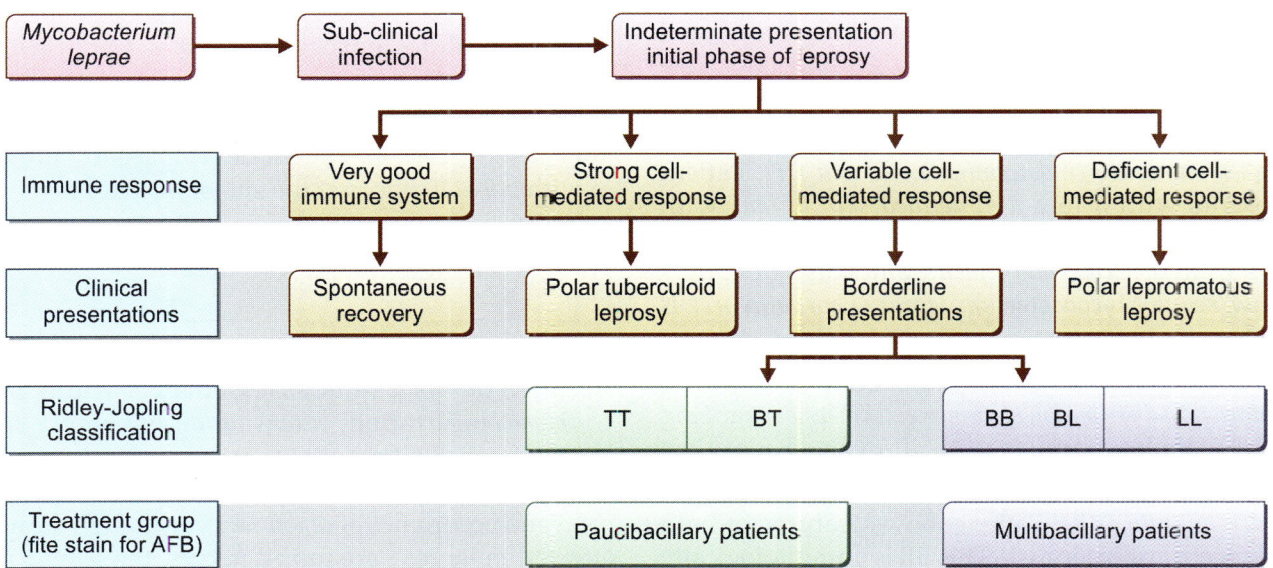

Fig. 7.22: Ridley-Jopling classification of leprosy.

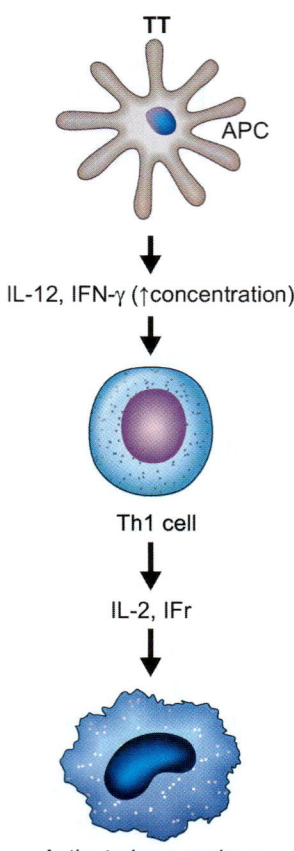

Fig. 7.23: Genesis of cell-mediated immunity in TT (tuberculoid leprosy). It induces good immune response. Infectivity is low in TT.

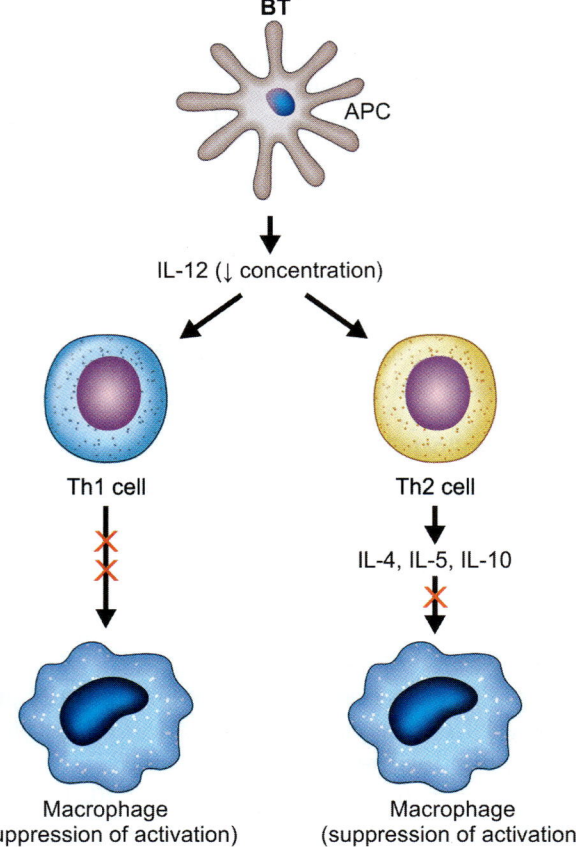

Fig. 7.24: Genesis of cell-mediated immunity in LL (lepromatous leprosy). It induces poor immune response. Infectivity is high in lepromatous leprosy.

tuberculoid) and *immunological unstable* (indeterminate and borderline).

IMMUNE STATUS

Cell mediated and humoral immunity have been implicated in leprosy. T cells participate in cell-mediated immunity. Increased titers of IgG, IgA and IgM have been demonstrated in these patients. These antibodies are not protective.

- *Higher immunity (indeterminate, TT and BT):* Patient presents with a few *well-defined skin lesions* with regular borders with asymmetrically distribution pattern and *nerve enlargement*. Slit skin smear may show *scant Mycobacterium leprae. Lepromin test is positive.*

- *Lower immunity (BL and LL):* Patient presents with *symmetrical distribution of numerous skin lesions* ranging from macules–papules with ill-defined margins. These skin lesions may be *hypoanesthetic*.

- *Mid immunity (BB):* Patient shows features of both the spectrums of leprosy. This BB is immunologically unstable, and hence *prone to reactions*.

LEPROMIN TEST

Lepromin test is used to demonstrate immune status in leprosy patients. Antigenic extract obtained from *Mycobacterium leprae* is administered by intradermal route. Delayed hypersensitivity is demonstrated in TT (tuberculoid leprosy). *Lepromin test is negative in LL (lepromatous leprosy).* Lepromin positive reaction is of two types described as under.

- *Fernandez reaction:* Patient develops skin induration within 24–48 hours at the site of injection.
- *Mitsuda reaction:* Granulomatous lesion appears after 3–4 weeks at the site of injection.

CLINICAL FEATURES

Activity of disease is assessed by various signs: *erythema*/infiltration, *extension or appearance of new lesions*, extension/new appearance of *anesthesia, paresis and paralysis, tenderness and pain in nerves, morphological index* and occurrence of reaction. Even though the nerves affected in leprosy are mixed nerves, the *sensory loss is more marked compared to motor dysfunction*.

Nutritional and Infectious Diseases

- *Indeterminate leprosy:* The initial cutaneous manifestations of leprosy are subtle and not specific. Initially erythematous patch, which in darker-skinned individuals appears pale; most cases resolve, some advance into more severe disease (Fig. 7.25).
- *Tuberculoid leprosy:* Patients present with one or multiple erythematous or scaly, well circumscribed macules or patches; usually *hypoanesthetic or anesthetic*. All patients have *nerve involvement*. Inflammation of Schwann cells leads to *thickening of peripheral nerves*. Course is generally benign. Clinical features of borderline tuberculoid leprosy are shown in Fig. 7.26.
- *Lepromatous leprosy:* Papular and nodular lesions are *symmetrically distributed*. These lesions often start on *nose* and *ears*, later involve *hands, arms, buttocks*. Facial lesions can be markedly swollen with loss of eyebrows (*Lucio sign*). *Nasal secretions rich in organisms*.

  Complications include orchitis, facial mutilation, neurotrophic ulcers, flexion contractures of hands, foot drop. Clinical features of lepromatous leprosy are shown in Fig. 7.27.

  Differences between tuberculoid and lepromatous leprosy are shown in Table 7.11.

DIAGNOSTIC APPROACH

Diagnostic approach includes clinical examination of skin patches with definite sensory impairment, peripheral nerves enlargement, skin biopsy and positive skin smears for AFB. Involvement of nerves is seen in 100% patients.

The type C fibers which mediate sensations towards heat and cold or different temperatures are lost first before loss of pain or light touch fibers.

HISTOPATHOLOGICAL EXAMINATION

Histopathological examination of skin biopsy is performed. Fite stain is done to demonstrate leprae bacilli.

Tuberculoid Leprosy (TT)

Well-formed granulomas: Skin biopsy from patient with tuberculoid leprosy shows discrete non-caseating epithelioid granulomas surrounded by zone of lymphocytes. Langhans' giant cells are demonstrated. Borderline tuberculoid leprosy is shown in Fig. 7.28.

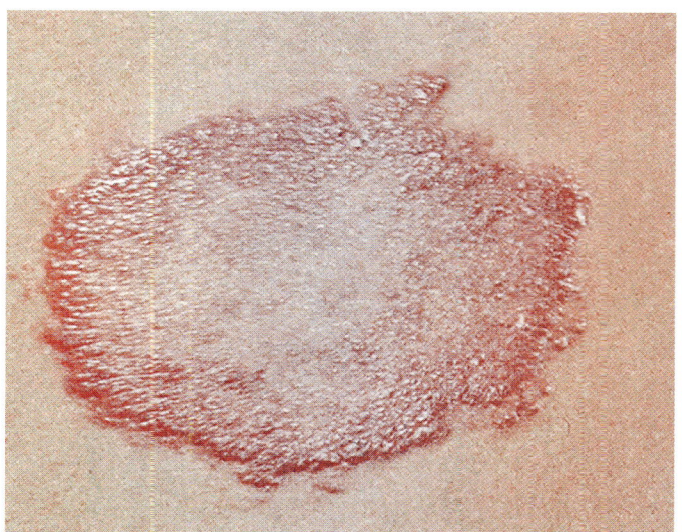

Fig. 7.26: Borderline tuberculoid leprosy. It shows more widespread and less sharply defined lesions than in tuberculoid form. These are usually symmetrical on trunk but may be asymmetric on face. These are less likely to have scale. Nerve involvement is less prominent.

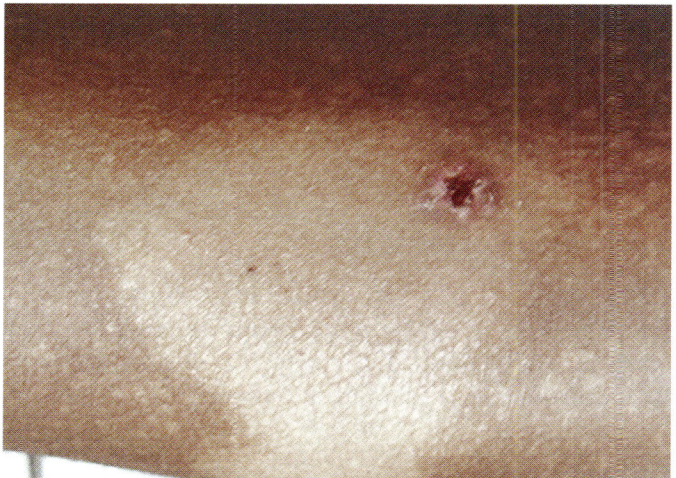

Fig. 7.25: Indeterminate leprosy: The initial cutaneous manifestations of leprosy are subtle and not specific. Initially erythematous patch, which in darker-skinned individuals appears pale; most cases resolve, some advance into more severe disease.

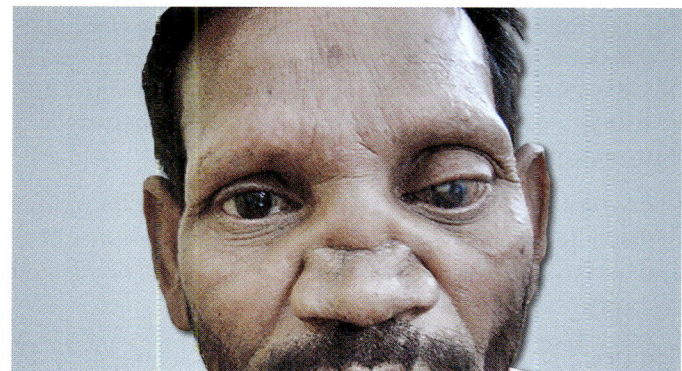

Fig. 7.27: Lepromatous leprosy. Facial lesions can be markedly swollen (leonine facies) with loss of eyebrows (Lucio sign).

Table 7.11: Differences between tuberculoid and lepromatous leprosy

Characteristics	Tuberculoid leprosy	Lepromatous leprosy
Host resistance	Present	Absent
T cell immunity	Present	Absent
Lepromin test	Strongly positive	Negative
Fernandez reaction (24–48 hours)	Positive	Negative
Mistuda reaction (3–4 weeks)	Positive	Negative
Skin lesions	Macular lesions with central depressed areas and hypopigmented margins	Macular/papular/nodular lesions on hand and face (leonine face)
	Asymmetrical lesions not involving both sides	Symmetrical lesions involving both sides
Touch sensation	Hypoanesthetic/anesthetic lesions	Absent (anesthetic patches)
Clinical appearance	Disfigurement minimal	Disfigurement maximum (leonine facies, claw hands and pendulous ear lobes)
Nerves involved	Ulnar, facial and peroneal nerves	Ulnar and peroneal nerves
Other organs	Other organs not involved	Anterior chamber eye, upper respiratory tract, testes lymph nodes, liver, spleen and gynecomastia in males
Infectivity	Low	Very high
Skin histology	Epidermis non-atrophic	Epidermis atrophic
	Rete ridges present	Rete ridges absent
	Dermal papillae normal	Dermal papillae flattened
	Clear zone between epidermis and dermis is absent	Clear zone between epidermis and dermis is present
	Epithelioid cell granulomas present	Epithelioid cell granulomas absent
	CD4+ T cells: present at the periphery of granulomas	CD4+ T cells are absent
	CD8+ T cells: very few at the center of lesion	CD8+ T cells are present in large number in diffuse manner
	Fite stain: AFB (*M. lepare* bacilli) few (4–5) in macrophages	Fite stain: AFB (*M. lepare* bacilli) abundant in macrophages
Complications	These are related to nerve damage like paralysis, distinct sensory losses	Antigen–antibody complex mediated erythema nodosum, leprosum, vasculitis, glomerulonephritis besides nerve related
Prognosis	Milder disease, hence good prognosis	Extensive progressive disease, hence poor prognosis

Absence of Grenza zone (clear zone): There is absence of clear zone at the junction of epidermis and dermis in tuberculoid leprosy. Clear zone is demonstrated in lepromatous leprosy.

Perineural inflammation: Histopathological examination of dermal nerve twigs shows infiltration by lymphocytes and macrophages. It indicates destruction of nerves responsible for sensory loss.

Fite stain: Mycobacterium leprae are usually negative.

Lepromatous Leprosy (LL)

Epidermis and dermis: Epidermis shows atrophy. There is loss of rete ridges of epidermis. Dermal papillae are flattened. There is loss of dermal appendages. Borderline lepromatous histology is shown in Fig. 7.29.

Grenza zone (clear zone): Clear zone is demonstrated at the junction of epidermis and dermis in lepromatous leprosy.

Nutritional and Infectious Diseases 7

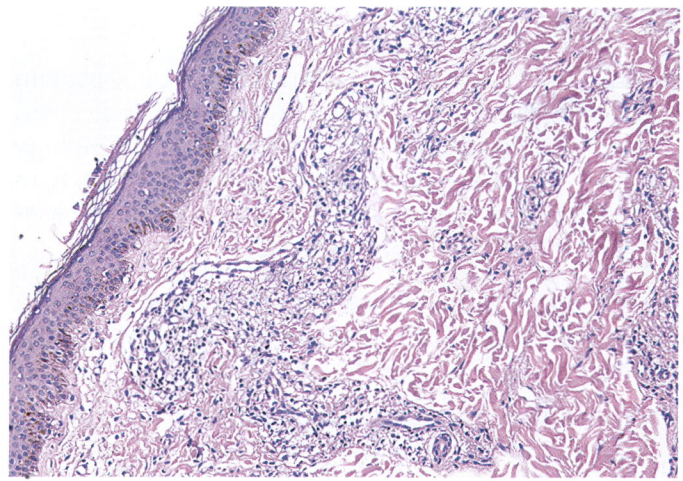

Fig. 7.28: Borderline tuberculoid leprosy showing formation of epithelioid granulomas (400X).

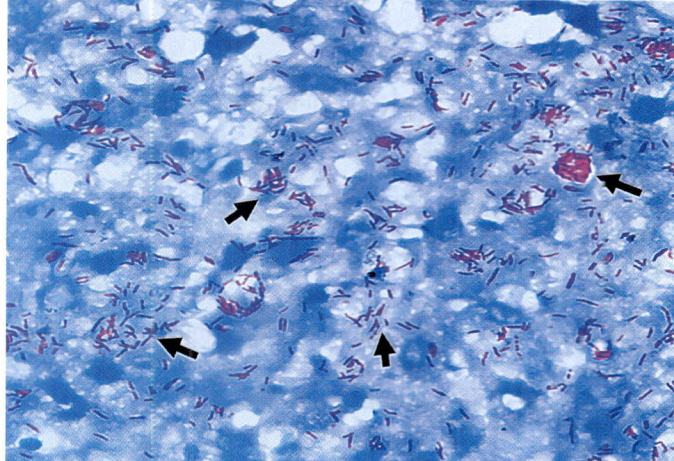

Fig. 7.30: Lepromatous leprosy. Fite stain showing macrophages laden with leprae bacilli (arrows) (400X).

ACTINOMYCES ISRAELII

Actinomyces israelii is a gram-positive anaerobic filamentous bacteria no longer classified as a fungus. *It is a normal colonizer of the vagina, colon, and mouth.* It is an opportunistic pathogen. Infection is established first by a breach of the mucosal barrier during various procedures (dental, gastrointestinal), aspiration, or *diverticulitis*.

Clinical Features

Patient develops *chronic abscess* with *sinus tract* formation in *cervicofacial, pulmonary, abdominal* (colon and appendix) and *skin. Lower genital tract infection* may be associated *with intrauterine device*.

Histopathological Examination

Light microscopy shows exudates containing sulfur granules, yellow clumps of the organism.

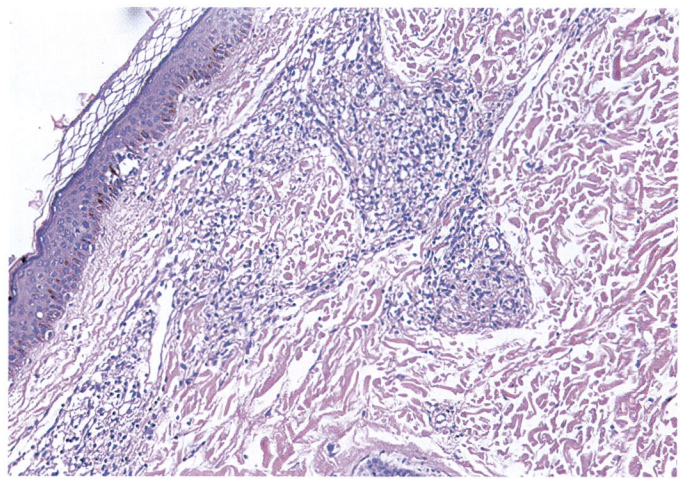

Fig. 7.29: Borderline lepromatous leprosy (400X).

Foamy macrophages: Dermis shows collection of macrophages arranged in nodular or diffuse patterns.

Fite stain: Macrophages in dermis are laden with *Mycobacterium leprae* (Fig. 7.30).

TREATMENT

Many different agents available for treating leprosy. Current WHO recommendations:

- *Tuberculoid leprosy:* Dapsone 100 mg daily and rifampicin 600 mg monthly for 6–9 months are administered in these patients.
- *Lepromatous leprosy:* Dapsone 100 mg daily; clofazimine 150 mg, and rifampicin 600 mg monthly for 12–18 months are administered in these patients.

SALMONELLA TYPHI

Typhoid fever is a systemic disease caused by *Salmonella typhi* bacilli. It has three *antigenic structures: O antigens, H antigens* and *Vi antigens*. The organism is transmitted by *feco-oral route*. There is involvement of mononuclear phagocytic system with nodule formation in the *Peyer's patches of lower ileum*. Patient may present with *step-ladder rise of fever* during *first week* and *continued during second and third stages*, relative bradycardia, headache, nausea, vomiting, abdominal tenderness, rose spots (2–4 mm on trunk) and hepatosplenomegaly.

VIRAL INFECTIONS

Viruses are infectious particles lacking organelles. A virus particle comprises nuclei acid core either DNA or RNA and not both. It is surrounded by a protein shell, or capsid. Combination of nuclei acid and capsid is called nucleocapsid. Basic types of viral morphology may be complex, enveloped or naked shown in Table 7.12. Important human viruses induced diseases are shown in Table 7.13.

Multiplication of enveloped virus in animal cell: Virus enters animal cell leading to formation of complete viral particles is shown in Fig. 7.31.

- *Adsorption:* Enveloped virus attaches to its host wall by specific binding of its spikes to cell receptors.
- *Penetration and uncoating:* It is engulfed into a vesicle leading to uncoating of its envelope and freeing the virus RNA into the cells cytoplasm.

Table 7.12: Basic types of viral morphology

Basic type of virus	Examples
Complex viruses	Poxvirus (large DNA virus)
	Flexible-tailed bacteriophage
Enveloped viruses	With a helical nucleocapsid (e.g. mumps virus and rhabdovirus)
	With an icosahedral nucelocapsid (e.g. herpes virus and HIV)
Naked viruses	Helical capsid (e.g. plum pox virus)
	Icosahedral capsid (e.g. poliovirus and papillomavirus)

Table 7.13: Important human viruses induced diseases

Nucleic acid type	Common name of genus members	Name of diseases
DNA viruses	Variola and vaccinia	Smallpox, cowpox
	Herpes simplex 1 (HSV-1)	Fever, blister, cold sores
	Herpes simplex 2 (HSV-2)	Genital herpes
	Varicella zoster virus	Chickenpox
	Human cytomegalovirus	CMV infections
	Human adenovirus	Adenovirus infections
	Human papillomaviruses	Several type of warts
	JC virus	Progressive multifocal leukoencephalopathy
	Hepatitis B virus (HBV or Dane particle)	Serum hepatitis
	Parvovirus B19	Erythema infectiosum
RNA viruses	Poliovirus	Poliomyelitis
	Cocksackievirus	Hand-foot-mouth disease
	Hepatitis A virus	Short-term hepatitis
	Human adenovirus	Common cold, bronchitis
	Norwalk virus	Viral diarrhea, Norwalk vial syndrome
	Yellow fever virus	Yellow virus
	Rubella virus	Rubella (German measles)
	Dengue fever virus	Dengue virus
	Ebola, Marbung virus	Ebola virus
	Human rotavirus	Rotavirus gastroenteritis
	Influenza type A virus	Influenza or flu
	Mumps virus	Mumps
	Measles virus	Measles
	Rabies virus	Rabies (hydrophobia)
	Human T cell leukemia virus (HTLV)	T cell leukemia
	HIV (human immunodeficiency virus 1 and virus 2)	Acquired immunodeficiency syndrome (AIDS)
	SRAS virus	Severe acute respiratory syndrome

Nutritional and Infectious Diseases

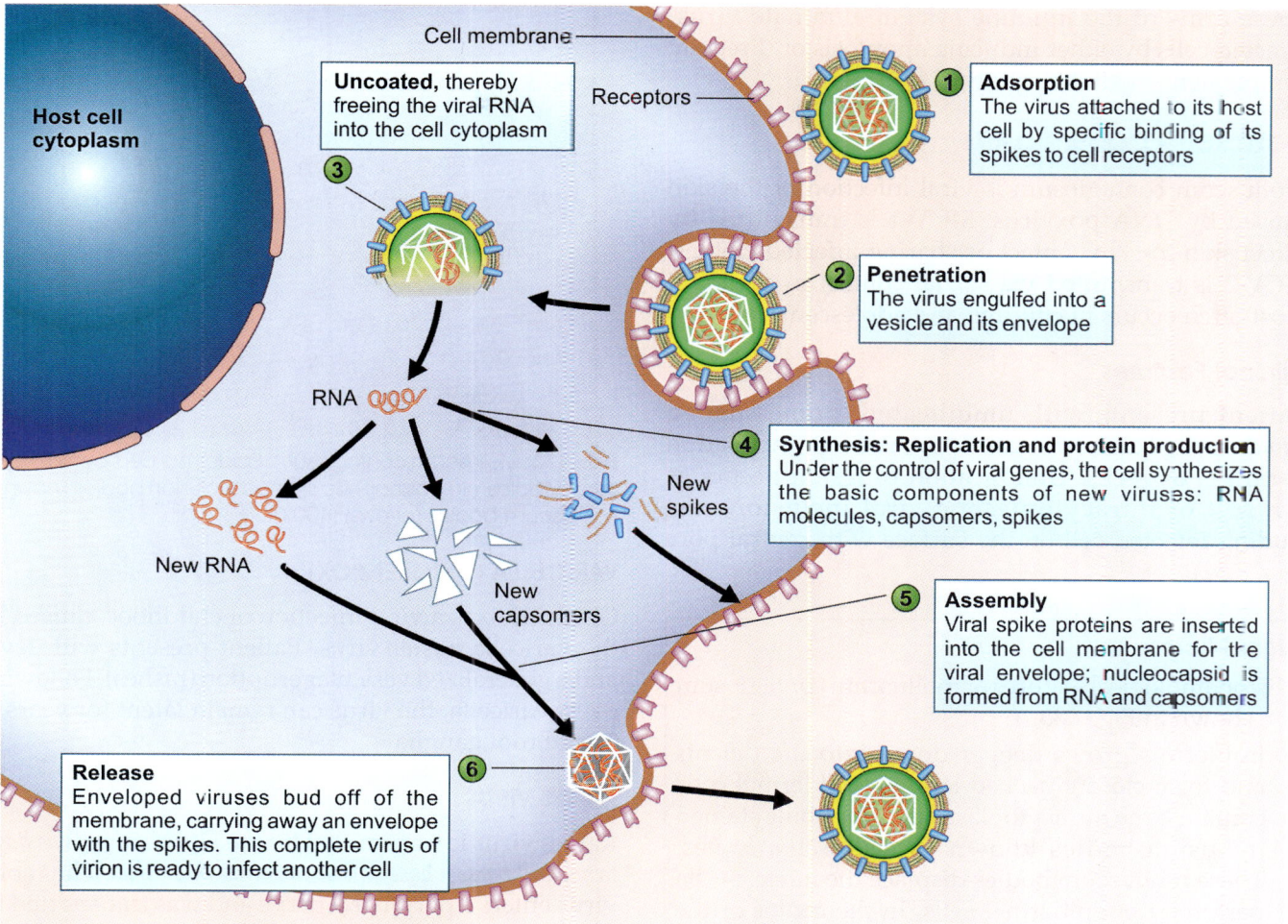

Fig. 7.31: Major event in the multiplication cycle of an enveloped RNA virus in human.

- *Replication and protein synthesis:* Under the control of viral genes, the cell synthesizes the basic components of new viruses such as RNA molecules, capsomers and spikes.
- *Assembly:* Viral spike proteins are inserted into the cell membrane for the envelope. Nucleocapsid is formed from RNA and capsomers.
- *Release:* Released complete virus is ready to infect another cells.

- *Cytopathic changes:* Released virus infects another cells and produce cytopathic changes (Table 7.14).

Protection of animal cells: Both humoral and cellular arms of the immune system protect against the harmful effects of viral infections.

Presentation of viral proteins to the immune system immunizes the body against the invader and elicits both killer cells and the production of antiviral antibodies.

Table 7.14: Cytopathic changes in selected virus infected animal cells

Virus	Shape of animal cell	Inclusions in cytoplasm or nucleus
Smallpox virus	Cell round	Cytoplasm
Herpes simplex virus	Cells fuse to form multinucleated syncytium	Nucleus
Adenovirus	Clumping of cells	Nucleus
Poliovirus	Cell enlarged	Absent
Influenza virus	Cell round	Absent
Rabies virus	No change in cell shape	Cytoplasm (Negri bodies)
Measles virus	Multinucleated cell forming syncytium	Absent
Cytomegalovirus	Cell enlarged	Nucleus (owl eye inclusion)

These arms of the immune system eliminate virus-infected cells by either inducing apoptosis or directing complement-mediated cytolysis.

MOLLUSCUM CONTAGIOSUM

Molluscum contagiosum is viral infection of the skin caused by DNA poxvirus. MCV-1 is transmitted by direct skin-to-skin contact or sharing infected clothes. MCV-2 is transmitted via sexual contact in adults. It most often occurs in children and adolescents.

Clinical Features

Patient presents with umbilicated, dome-shaped *papules over body, arms and legs.* Average incubation period is 6 weeks. Umbilication of lesion occurs as a result of intracytoplasmic viral inclusions extruding infected cell on the surface with central pore (Fig. 7.32).

> ### Light Microscopy
> Histopathological features of molluscum contagiosum are shown in Fig. 7.33.
> - Epidermis grows deeper down into the dermis and form closely packed lobules. Epidermal cells contain large intracytoplasmic eosinophilic stained inclusion bodies known as *molluscum bodies*. These molluscum bodies displace the nuclei at the periphery of epidermal cells. In the center of the lesion, stratum corneum disintegrates and release the molluscum bodies together with keratinous debris resulting to formation of central crater.
> - Dermis shows prominent acute and chronic inflammatory infiltrate and foreign body giant cells.

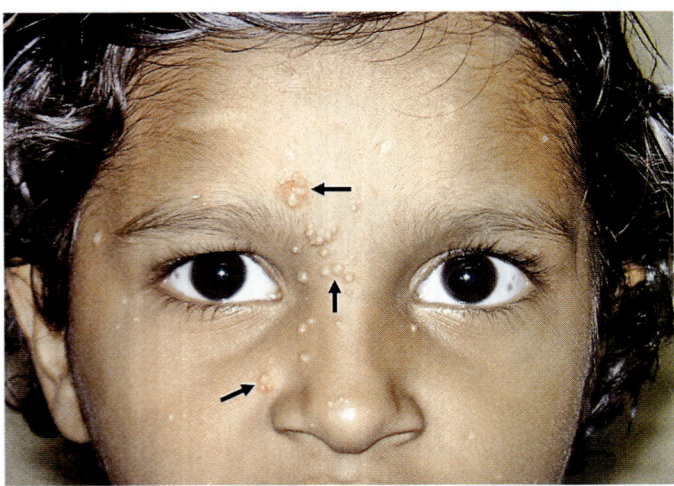

Fig. 7.32: Molluscum contagiosum. This is a typical distribution of lesions on a child's face. Note the eyelid lesions (arrows).

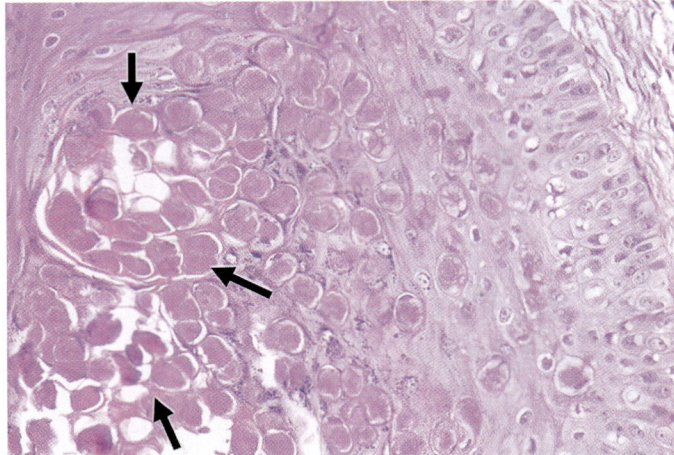

Fig. 7.33: Molluscum contagiosum. Epidermal cells contain large intracytoplasmic eosinophilic stained inclusion bodies known as molluscum bodies (arrows) (400X).

VARICELLA (CHICKENPOX)

Chickenpox is a viral infection of childhood caused by the varicella zoster virus. Patient presents with fever and a generalized vesicular eruption (rashes). Following overt varicella, the virus can remain latent for years in dorsal root ganglia.

RABIES VIRUS

Rabies virus is transmitted by the *bite of animals as dogs, foxes and bats, whose saliva contains this virus.* The rabies virus enters a peripheral nerve and was transported by retrograde axoplasmic flow to the spinal cord and brain. The inflammation is centered in the brainstem and spills into the cerebellum and hypothalamus.
- *Clinical features:* Patient presents with *hydrophobia (fear from water)* characterized by *violent muscle contractions* and *convulsions.*
- *Light microscopy:* Brain shows eosinophilic *intracytoplasmic inclusions (Negri bodies)* in the *hippocampus* and *Purkinje cells of the cerebellum.* Brainstem and spinal cord shows neuronal degeneration, perivascular accumulations of mononuclear cells.

POLIOVIRUS

Brainstem nuclei are affected by poliovirus. Poliomyelitis is characterized by degeneration and necrosis of anterior horn cells of the spinal cord.

HERPES II VIRUS

Herpes simplex encephalitis is most common in teenagers and young adults. Herpes simplex targets the *temporal lobes* by binding on the plasma membranes of CNS cells. The virus has ability to remain latent or selective replication in distinct intracellular microenvironments.

Nutritional and Infectious Diseases

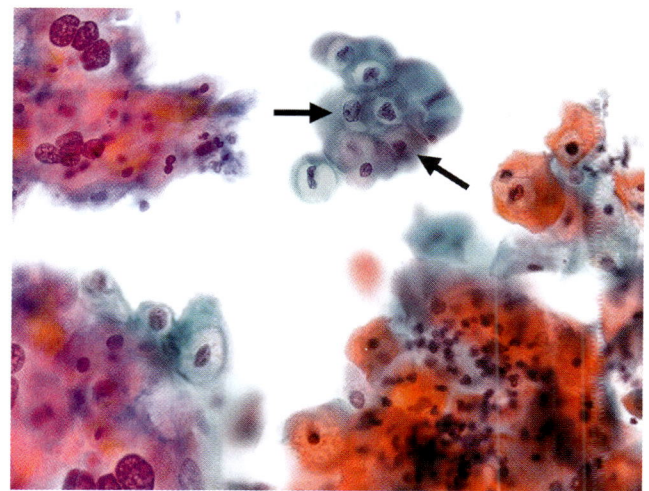

Fig. 7.34: Photomicrograph from a smear showing koilocytosis, the typical appearance of cervical squamous cell infected by human papilloma virus (HPV). There is a 'halo' of cleared cytoplasm surrounding an enlarged nucleus (arrows) (400×).

HUMAN PAPILLOMAVIRUS

Human *papillomavirus* (6, 11) causes vulvar wart known as *condyloma acuminatum* on vagina and cervix. *Koilocytes (intracytoplasmic vacuolation) are indicative of HPV-infected epithelial cells.* These are apparent in cytopathologic (Papanicolaou smear) and histopathologic preparations (Fig. 7.34). It may contribute to the pathogenesis of squamous cell carcinoma of vulva and vagina.

CYTOMEGALOVIRUS

Cytomegalovirus affects lungs, kidneys (tubules and glomerular endothelial cells), gastrointestinal tract (epithelial lining), brain (neurons) and eye. It is transmitted via droplets, saliva, sexual contact (vaginal discharge) and transplacental route (mother to fetus).

Congenital CMV infection: Vertical transmission of cytomegalovirus (mother to fetus) causes *intrauterine growth retardation*. Lesion in proximity to third ventricle and aqueduct cause hydrocephalus. *Neonate presents* with *jaundice, hepatosplenomegaly, encephalitis, chorioretinitis, anemia,* and *thrombocytopenia*.

Postnatal CMV infection: Postnatal CMV infection most often occurs in *immunocompromised persons*. It causes *encephalomyelitis*. It affects *lungs, kidneys, liver* and *salivary glands*.

> **Light Microscopy**
>
> The organ affected shows mononuclear cells infiltration with mild edema. The infected cells are large with *prominent large deep blue inclusion in nuclei* surrounded by a clear space giving an *owl eye appearance*. Necrosis and calcification are seen.
> - *Histochemistry:* Cytomegalovirus is highlighted by PAS and silver methenamine stain.
> - *Immunohistochemistry:* Monoclonal antibodies to cytomegalovirus are used for diagnosis.

HEPATOTROPIC VIRUSES

Hepatotropic viruses infecting liver include *HAV, HBV, HCV, HDV* and *HEV*. Acute viral hepatitis shows similar morphology irrespective of their precise etiology. *HAV infection has a direct cytopathic effects.* Incubation period is the period from the time of infection and the first symptoms appear. Acute hepatitis has three phases: preicteric phase (prodromal phase), icteric phase (jaundice) and recovery phase (convalescence phase).

Liver cell injury occurs due to attack by cytotoxic T and killer cells followed by antibodies formed against viral neoantigens expressed on virally infected hepatocytes. The mechanisms of injury have been most closely studied in HBV. It is thought that the extent of inflammation and necrosis depends on the person's immune response. Clinical course following viral hepatitis is shown in Table 7.15.

- *Prompt immune response:* A prompt immune response during the acute phase of the infection may cause liver cell injury but at the same time eliminate the virus.
- *Marginal immune response:* People with marginal immune response and fewer symptoms are less likely to eliminate the virus, and hepatocytes expressing the viral antigens persist, leading to the chronic or carrier state.

Table 7.15: Clinical course following viral hepatitis

Clinical pattern of disease	Viruses
Asymptomatic (most often with HAV infection)	HAV, HBV, HCV, HDV and HEV
Acute hepatitis without jaundice (anicteric hepatitis)	HAV, HBV, HCV, HDV and HEV
Acute hepatitis with jaundice (icteric jaundice)	HAV, HBV, HCV, HDV and HEV
Massive liver necrosis with acute liver failure (rare)	HAV, HBV, HCV, HDV and HEV
Chronic hepatitis	HBV, HCV and HDV
Chronic career state	HBV, HCV and HDV

- *Accelerated immune response:* Fulminant hepatitis would be explained in terms of an accelerated immune response with severe liver necrosis.

HIV INFECTION

HIV may affect the brain, spinal cord, or peripheral nervous system before the onset of immunodeficiency syndrome. Reticuloendothelial cells are vehicles for viral entry into the nervous system. HIV infection results in AIDS dementia complex, characterized by impairment of memory, coordination of balance and motor functions with progressive dementia. Patient is prone to opportunistic bacterial and fungal infections.

ARBOVIRUS

Arbovirus may cause encephalitis: St. Louis encephalitis (mild to severe), Eastern equine encephalitis (high mortality) and Western equine encephalitis (less severe). Person contracts infection from reservoirs such as horses, birds and mosquitoes.

FUNGAL INFECTIONS

Important fungal diseases include: Candida, mucormycosis, Aspergillus, Cryptococcus, histoplasmosis, chromomycosis and rhinosporidiosis. Rhinosporidiosis mainly involve the mucosa of nose, nasopharynx and conjunctiva. Classification of pathogenic fungi, cutaneous mycoses, subcutaneous infective fungi and systemic fungal infections involving organs is shown in Tables 7.16 to 7.19.

SUPERFICIAL FUNGAL INFECTIONS

Superficial fungal infections are primarily by dermatophytes growing in the soil and on animals. These are often *confined to the stratum corneum, hair and nails*. The genera most often causing dermatophytosis include: *Epidermophyton, Microsporum,* and *Trichophyton*. They can produce a number of diverse and characteristic clinical lesions according to the area involved. Tinea corporis is commonly referred to as *ringworm*, a term used by laypersons, to describe practically any annular or ring-like eruption on the body. It may spread from other infected humans, or it may be autoinoculated from other areas of the body that are infected by tinea such as tinea pedis or tinea capitis.

A scraping with KOH mount can be utilized to identify these fungi. Fungal cell walls are rich in mucopolysaccharides and stained with PAS resulting to bright pink to red appearance. Involved areas of skin and nails may fluoresce under ultraviolet light.

Table 7.16: Classification of pathogenic fungi

True/opportunistic fungi	Categories	Species
True pathogens	*Cutaneous infective fungi also called *dermatophytoses*	Trichophyton
		Epidermophyton species
		Microsporum species
	Subcutaneous infective fungi (acquired through traumatic injury)	*Actinomadura medurae*
		Cladosporium
		Medurella grisea
		Sporothrix schenckii
	Systemic infective fungi	*Blastomyces dermatitidis*
		Coccidioiodes immitis
		Histoplasma capsulatum
		Paraccocidioides brasiliensis
Opportunistic pathogens	Invading multiple organs	*Aspergillus fumigatus*
		Cryptococcus neoformans
		Candida albicans
		Absidia corymbifera
		Rhizomucor pusillus
		Rhizopus oryzae

*Cutaneous mycoses use keratin as a source of nutrition.

Table 7.17: Cutaneous mycoses

Disease	Fungi responsible	Cutaneous lesions
Tinea pedis (athlete foot)	*Trichophyton rubrum* *Trichophyton mentagrophytes* *Epidermophyton floccosum*	Area between toes spreading to nails
Tinea corporis (ringworm)	*Epidermophyton floccosum* *Trichophyton species* *Microsporum*	Most often on nonhairy areas of the trunk, but any area may be affected Active site of growth of fungi in the periphery of lesion
Tinea capitis (scalp ringworm)	*Trichophyton species* *Microsporum*	Scalp lesions with hair loss
Tinea cruris (jock itch)	*Epidermophyton floccosum* *Trichophyton rubrum*	Skin lesions in moist areas such as upper thighs and genitalia
Tinea unguium	*Trichophyton rubrum*	Nails thickened and brittle

Table 7.18: Subcutaneous infective fungi (acquired through traumatic injury)

Disorder	Fungus	Clinical manifestations
Sporotrichosis	*Sporothrix schenckii*	Granulomatous ulcer at punctured site Secondary lesions along draining lymphatics
Chromomycosis	*Phialophora* and *Cladosporium* species	Wart nodules Crusty abscess along draining lymphatics
Mycetoma (madura)	*Actinomadura medurae, Madurella grisea* and *Cladosporium*	Localized abscess on feet discharging sinuses with pus, serum and blood Colored grains (black, white, red or yellow) from discharging sinuses

Table 7.19: Systemic fungal infections involving organs

Systemic fungi	Possible sites of infection
Blastomyces dermatitidis	Skin, bone and genitourinary system
Coccidioides immitis	CNS and bone
Histoplasma capsulatum*	Liver, spleen, spleen and bone marrow (demonstrated in macrophages)
Paracoccidioides brasiliensis	Mucosa of mouth and nose

*Histoplasma capsulatum occurs in immunocompromised states like HIV infection, corticosteroid therapy and immunosuppression therapy.

DEEP FUNGAL INFECTIONS

CANDIDA ALBICANS

Candida albicans causes vulvovaginitis affecting 10% of women. *Candida albicans is a normal vaginal flora. Infection is commonly associated with pregnancy, diabetes mellitus, broad-spectrum antibiotic therapy, oral contraceptive use, and immunosuppression resulting in fungal growth.* In immunocompromised patients, invasive form produces blood-borne dissemination leading to abscess formation in lungs, kidneys, renal liver and endocardium. *Patient presents with white curd-like vaginal discharge that may cause intense itching.* Per vaginal examination shows white patches on the mucosal surface of vagina covered with vaginal discharge. Diagnosis is best made microscopically on wet mounts on Pap smear showing fungal hyphae.

ASPERGILLUS FLAVUS

Invasion of blood vessels and tissue infarcts are common in *Aspergillus flavus* infection. Aspergillus species may also grow in pre-existing cavities caused by tuberculosis or bronchiectasis. Invasive form of aspergillosis has predilection for growth into vessels, with consequent widespread hematogenous dissemination. *The fungus proliferates to form fungus balls, which are also referred to as aspergillomas or mycetomas in patients* with a previous history of cavitating pulmonary disease such as pulmonary tuberculosis. The organisms generally do not invade the lung parenchyma. Lung shows focal yellow areas of consolidation. There are *three different types of pulmonary aspergillosis,* namely *allergic bronchopulmonary aspergillosis, aspergillomas,* and *invasive aspergillosis.*

CRYPTOCOCCUS NEOFORMANS

Pneumonia results from the inhalation of spores of *Cryptococcus neoformans.* The main reservoir for this fungus is pigeon droppings. *Cryptococcus almost exclusively affects persons with impaired cell-mediated immunity.* It has a proteoglycan capsule, which is essential for pathogenicity. It primarily affects the *meninges and lungs.* The organisms appear as faintly stained, basophilic yeast with a clear, 3–5 μm thick mucinous capsule. It stains positively with a mucicarmine stain or Indian ink for capsular polysaccharides.

HISTOPLASMA CAPSULATUM

Histoplasma capsulatum occurs in immunocompromised states like HIV infection, corticosteroid therapy and immunosuppression therapy. It causes multiple pulmonary lesions with late calcification. Disseminated form, marked by multisystem involvement with infiltrates of macrophages filled with fungal yeast forms.

COCCIDIOIDOMYCOSIS

Coccidioides immitis occurs in primary and disseminated forms. Fungal spherules contain endospores found within granulomas.

MUCORMYCOSIS

There are *three principal forms of mucormycosis, namely rhinocerebral, pulmonary, and subcutaneous.* It can produce necrotizing opportunistic infections that begin in the nasal sinuses or lungs. Pulmonary mucormycosis is usually fatal. The hard palate or nasal cavity is typically covered by a black crust, and the underlying tissues become friable and hemorrhagic. The fungal hyphae grow into arteries, causing devastating and rapidly progressive septic embolic infarctions.

Microscopic examination shows a purulent arteritis with thrombi composed of hyphae. Mucormycosis should be suspected in patients who present with a paranasal sinusitis unresponsive to antibiotic treatment, particularly those who also have an underlying chronic disease (e.g. diabetes or leukemia).

PARASITIC DISEASES

Parasite is an organism that lives in or on another and takes its nourishment from that other organism. Parasitic diseases include infections that are due to protozoa and helminths.

Parasites include *protozoa* and *helminths.* Cysticercosis, malaria, filariasis and hydatid cysts are common in India. Clinically important protozoa and helminths are shown in Tables 7.20 and 7.21.

Table 7.20: Clinically important protozoa

Site of infection	Pathogenic protozoa	Mode of locomotion	Site of infection
Intestinal protozoa	*Entamoeba histolytica* (amoeba)	Move by cytoplasmic projections	Colon and secondary liver involvement
			Cysts demonstrated in stool
	Giardia lamblia (flagellates)	Move by rotating whip-like flagella	Duodenum (infection with drinking contaminated water)
			Foul smelling watery diarrhea
			Trophozoites and cysts demonstrated in stool
	Cryptosporidium parvum (sporozoan)	Nonmotile adult form	Small intestine
			Parasite intracellular in intestinal villus epithelium
			Infection by drinking contaminated water
			Duodenum involved (foul smelling diarrhea)
			Stool examination showing trophozoites and cysts

Contd...

Table 7.20: Clinically important protozoa (Contd...)

Site of infection	Pathogenic protozoa	Mode of locomotion	Site of infection
Urogenital system	Trichomonas vaginalis (flagellates)	Move by rotating whip-like flagella	Vagina, vulva and cervix in women Urethra, seminal vesicle and prostate in men Higher than normal pH favoring growth
Blood and tissues	Plasmodium species (sporozoan)	Nonmotile adult form	Sprozoites introduced by mosquito bite
	Toxoplasma gondii (sporozoan)	Nonmotile adult form	Sprozoites entering liver becoming merozoites infecting red blood cells
	Trypanosoma species (flagellates)	Move by rotating whip-like flagella	Cardiomyopathy in Americans by Trypanosoma cruzi Sleeping sickness in African by Trypanosoma brucei CNS by Trypanosoma bruceigambiense
	Leishmania species (flagellates)	Move by rotating whip-like flagella	Phlebotomus (sand fly) bite Liver, spleen, lymph nodes and bone marrow (parasite infecting macrophages and migrating to these organs) LD bodies demonstrated in tissue

Table 7.21: Clinically important helminths

Groups	Examples
Cestodes (tapeworms)	Echinococcus granulosus (dog tapeworm) produces hydatid cyst in liver, lung and brain Taenia solium (pork tapeworm) produces cysticercosis diagnosed by CT and histopathological examination Taenia saginata (beef tapeworm) Diphyllobothrium latum (broad fish tapeworm)
Trematodes (flukes)	Schistosoma haematobium (blood fluke) Schistosoma mansoni (blood fluke) Clonorchis sinensis (Chinese or oriental liver fluke) Paragonimus westermani (lung liver fluke)
Nematodes (roundworms)	Ancylostoma duodenale (hookworm in intestine) Ascaris lumbricoides (giant roundworm in intestine) Enterobium vermicularis (small roundworm or threadworm in intestine) Trichinella spiralis (intestine) Trichuris trichiura (whipworm in intestine) Wuchereria bancrofti (filarial worm) causing tissue infection Oncocerca volvulus (filarial worm) causing tissue infection Loa loa (filarial worm or African eye worm) causing tissue infection Brugia malayi causing tissue infection Dracunculus medinensis causing tissue infection Toxocara canis (dog worm) causing tissue infection

ENTAMOEBA HISTOLYTICA

Entamoeba histolytica resides in the colon of infected persons and is transmitted by fecal-oral contact. The trophozoites invade submucosal veins of the colon, enter the portal circulation, and gain access to the liver leading to *amoebic liver abscess*. The amebae kill hepatocytes, producing a slowly expanding, necrotic cavity. The abscess is filled with a dark brown material that resembles anchovy paste. *An amebic liver abscess can rupture and extend into the peritoneal cavity.*

Clinical features: Patient with amoebic liver abscess presents with abrupt onset of *fever* and *dull aching abdominal pain* in the right upper quadrant or epigastrium, usually lasting less than 10 days. Jaundice is unusual.

GIARDIA LAMBLIA

Giardiasis is an infestation of the small intestine by the flagellated protozoan *Giardia lamblia*. The organism can be acquired from contaminated water or food. Patient presents with *abdominal cramping and nonbloody diarrhea*. The gastrointestinal symptom usually resolves in 1 to 4 weeks, but chronic giardiasis may lead to malabsorption, weight loss, and growth retardation. It does not induce significant villus architectural changes. The organisms are recovered from stool specimens, duodenal aspirates, or luminal surface of normal appearing mucosa of intestinal biopsies. The parasite is mistaken as cytoplasmic debris. *Giemsa stain and trichrome stain* highlight the parasite.

TRICHOMONAS VAGINALIS

Trichomonas vaginalis is the second most common cause of vaginitis. It is commonly transmitted by sexual contact. Patient presents with a profuse opaque or creamy-colored frothy discharge with fishy smell. Discharge may cause vulvar irritation and burning micturition due to urethral inflammation. These flagellated protozoa are best diagnosed in freshly prepared wet mounts (i.e. smears of unfixed vaginal discharge, in which the protozoa keep moving). *Trichomonas vaginalis* is also demonstrated as flagellated motile organisms in wet mounted smear.

MALARIAL PARASITE

Plasmodium is a wide distribution in many tropical or subtropical regions of the world. Malarial parasite comprises *Plasmodium vivax, Plasmodium falciparum, Plasmodium ovale* and *Plasmodium malariae*. All of these organisms infect erythrocytes, but *Plasmodium falciparum* causes the most severe disease due to ischemic injury to the brain leading to range of symptoms, including somnolence, hallucinations, behavioral changes, seizures, and even coma. The liver, spleen, and lymph nodes are darkened by macrophages that are filled with hemosiderin and malaria pigments.

Life cycle: Asexual life cycle occurs in human and sexual life cycle in mosquito. Infected mosquito bites and injects sporozoites. These sporozoites infect the hepatocytes resulting in release of merozoites. These merozoites infect red blood cells and develop into trophozoites, schizont and gametocytes. The trophozoites multiply and produce merozoites leading to cause infection of other red blood cells. Rupture of infected red blood cells liberates gametocytes. The female mosquito picks up gametocytes from an infected human. Sexual cycle occurs in the mosquito leading to fomation of sporozoites.

ECHINOCOCCUS GRANULOSUS

Hydatid cyst is caused by *Echinococcus granulosus*. Adult parasites are found in dogs and sheep. Humans are infected after ingestion of eggs. *Right lobe of liver is the commonest site of hydatid cyst followed by lung.* When the lungs are affected, protoscolices might be found in sputum or bronchial washings. Liver contains multiple cysts of variable size invading surrounding tissue. Color of the cysts resembles white of boiled egg.

Echinococcosis is diagnosed mainly with imaging techniques such as ultrasonography, radiology, magnetic resonance imaging (MRI) or CT scanning, supported by serology.

Cytological smear examination: Cytological smear examination shows laminated membranous structures resembling ectocyst of hydatid cyst. PAS stain highlights the laminated membranous structures as magenta-colored structures.

Gomori methenamine stains laminated membranous structures black. Claw-like refractile hooklets are demonstrated in the background by Ziehl-Neelsen stain as bright purple. Accidental spillage during fine needle aspiration may cause anaphylactic shock.

> ### Light Microscopy
>
> On histopathological examination, cyst wall consists of endocyst and ectocyst surrounded granulation tissue (pericyst).
>
> Serological tests used in humans include enzyme-linked immunosorbent assay (ELISA), indirect immunofluorescence, indirect hemagglutination, immunoblotting and latex agglutination.

STRONGYLOIDES STERCORALIS

Strongyloidiasis is a human disease caused by nematode roundworm called *Strongyloides stercoralis*. It most often infects small intestine and rarely colon. The parasite is *diagnosed by demonstration of larvae, eggs and adult worms embedded in the crypts*. Eosinophils, sometimes with Charcot-Leyden crystals may be present. Gastric strongyloidiasis may occur in association with human T-lymphotropic virus causing adult T cell lymphoma.

WUCHERERIA BANCROFTI

Infective form is third stage larva of *Wuchereria bancrofti* responsible for lymphatic filariasis. It enters through skin inoculation by mosquito bite. It localizes in the lymphatic system especially inguinoscrotal region. Microfilariae are demonstrated in small number in circulating blood during the day and peak density at night between 10 pm and 2–4 am. It is due to feeding habit of mosquitoes at night. In subperiodic form, microfilariae are demonstrated between noon and 8 pm. It occurs due to feeding habit of mosquitoes during daytime.

Pathogenesis: Adult worm and developing larva incites an inflammatory reaction in the lymphatic system lymphangitis. The reaction products of growing larvae are highly allergenic producing urticaria, *fugitive swellings* and lymphedema. Intensity and type of host immune response may reflect range of clinical manifestations. Immune response varies by stage of infection. *Elephantiasis is relatively a late complication of filariasis characterized by swelling of limbs, scrotum, breasts or vulva with dermal hypertrophy.* Impairment of the circulation leads to secondary bacterial and fungal infections in the regions. Chronic lymphedema leads to hyperplasia of connective tissue, infiltration by eosinophils, macrophages and plasma cells.

Clinical features: Initially, patient is asymptomatic. Later patient presents with fever and symptoms due to inflammation and obstruction of lymphatic channels (limbs, breasts, and scrotum), lymphadenitis (femoral, inguinal, axillary and epitrochlear nodes), orchitis, lymphocoel, hydrocele and elephantiasis.

Laboratory diagnosis: It is frequently made on clinical grounds in endemic regions but demonstration of microfilariae in circulating blood is the key. Where more than one species of filarial infection occurs, it needs well stained slides for morphological identification of microfilariae.

- *Conventional method:* Thick stained blood smear is examined to demonstrate parasite.
- *Concentration technique:* It is done by nucleospore filtration or Knott's concentration, detection of circulating filarial antigen by rapid format card test/ immunochromatographic card test (ICT).
- *Serodiagnosis:* It is PCR-based assays for DNA analysis.
- *Imaging studies:* High frequency ultrasound, lymphoscintigraphy is performed.
- *Light microscopy: Adult worm lodges in the lymph node leading to lymphangitis and lymph varices.* The endothelium of the vessels is occupied by the parasite leading to obliterative endolymphangitis and occlusion of the lymphatic channels. There is infiltration of monocyte, macrophage and giant cells killing the worm and replacing the lymph node with fibrous tissue eventually.

LEISHMANIASIS

Leishmaniae are protozoans that are transmitted to humans through insect bites. They cause a spectrum of clinical syndromes, ranging from indolent self-resolving cutaneous ulcers to fatal disseminated disease. *Leishmaniasis is transmitted by the bite of phlebotomus sandflies, which acquire infections from feeding on infected animals.* Three distinct clinical entities are recognized: Localized cutaneous leishmaniasis, mucocutaneous leishmaniasis, and visceral leishmaniasis.

Clinical features: Patient with *visceral leishmaniasis* presents with *persistent fever, progressive weight loss, hepatosplenomegaly, anemia, thrombocytopenia,* and *leukopenia*. Light-skinned persons develop darkening of the skin. If untreated, the disease is fatal.

ANCYLOSTOMA DUODENALE

Ancylostoma duodenale (hookworm) is an intestinal nematode that infects the small bowel. A duodenale molts within the duodenum and attaches to the mucosa. With extensive infections, particularly with hookworm, considerable blood loss results in iron deficiency anemia.

ENTEROBIUS VERMICULARIS

Enterobius vermicularis (pinworm) is an intestinal nematode. It is encountered worldwide but is more common in temperate zones. Individuals can be infected at any age, but parasitism is more common in children. Most people complain of pruritus caused by migrating worms.

Section II

Hematology

8. Red Blood Cells
9. White Blood Cells
10. Bleeding Disorders
11. Coagulation Disorders
12. Blood Groups and Blood Transfusion
13. Lymph Nodes, Spleen and Thymus
14. Advanced Diagnostic Techniques

CHAPTER 8

Red Blood Cells

Learning Objectives

HEMATOPOIESIS
- Site of Hematopoiesis
- Erythropoiesis
- Leukopoiesis
- Thrombopoiesis
- Bone Marrow Aspiration
- Trephine Bone Biopsy

RED BLOOD CELL, HEMOGLOBIN AND CLASSIFICATION OF ANEMIAS
- Red Blood Cell
- Reticulocyte Count
- Hemoglobin Synthesis
- Anticoagulants Used in Laboratory
- Romanowsky Stains
- Anemia

IRON DEFICIENCY ANEMIA
- Iron Metabolism
- Iron Deficiency Anemia

MEGALOBLASTIC ANEMIA: VITAMIN B_{12} AND FOLIC ACID DEFICIENCY
- Classification
- Folic Acid (Pteroylglutamic Acid) Deficiency
- Vitamin B_{12} Deficiency
- Pernicious Anemia

RED BLOOD CELLS DESTRUCTION AND CLASSIFICATION OF HEMOLYTIC ANEMIA
- Overview
- Clinical Manifestations
- Compensatory Mechanisms

HEREDITARY SPHEROCYTOSIS, OVALOCYTOSIS AND STOMATOCYTOSIS

THALASSEMIAS
- Overview
- β-Thalassemias, α-Thalassemia Trait
- Hereditary Persistence of Fetal Hemoglobin

SICKLE CELL DISORDERS AND OTHER HEMOGLOBINOPATHIES
- Overview
- Sickle Cell Disease and Sickle Cell Thalassemia Syndrome
- Hemoglobin C and E Disorders

HEMATOPOIESIS

SITE OF HEMATOPOIESIS

Process of formation of blood cells is called *hematopoiesis*. Hematopoiesis during intrauterine life and postnatal period is shown in Fig. 8.1 and Table 8.1.

Hematopoiesis during intrauterine life: During embryonic life, hematopoiesis begins in the 2 weeks embryo. Liver takes over this function in 8 weeks embryo and continues until a few weeks before birth. Spleen starts hematopoiesis during 3–7 months of intrauterine period.

Thymus gland and lymph nodes participate in production of lymphocytes. Bone marrow also participates in hematopoiesis during intrauterine life.

Hematopoiesis during postnatal period: At birth until first 2–3 years after birth, all bones contain red marrow

Table 8.1: Hematopoiesis during intrauterine life and postnatal period

Period	Site	Hematopoiesis in organs	Major type of Hb
During embryonic and fetal life	Yolk sac	2 weeks up to 2 months	Embryonic Hb (Hb Gower I, Hb Gower II, Portland)
	Liver	8 weeks to 4 months until a few weeks before birth	HbF (α_2, γ_2)
	Spleen	3–7 months	HbF (α_2, γ_2)
	Bone marrow	4–9 months	HbF (α_2, γ_2)
	Thymus gland	Lymphopoiesis	Lymphocytes
	Lymph nodes	Lymphopoiesis	Lymphocytes
At birth until first 2–3 years after birth	All bones	Red bone marrow	HbF (α_2, γ_2) is replaced by HbA (α_2, γ_2)
During adult life in red marrow of flat bones	Axial skeleton (cranial bones, vertebrae, sternum and ribs) Pelvic girdle (iliac bones) Epiphyseal ends of long bones such as humerus and femur	Red marrow is gradually replaced by yellow (fatty) marrow by the age of 18–22 years in most bones except axial skeleton, pelvic girdles and epiphyseal ends of humerus and femur	HbA (α_2, γ_2)

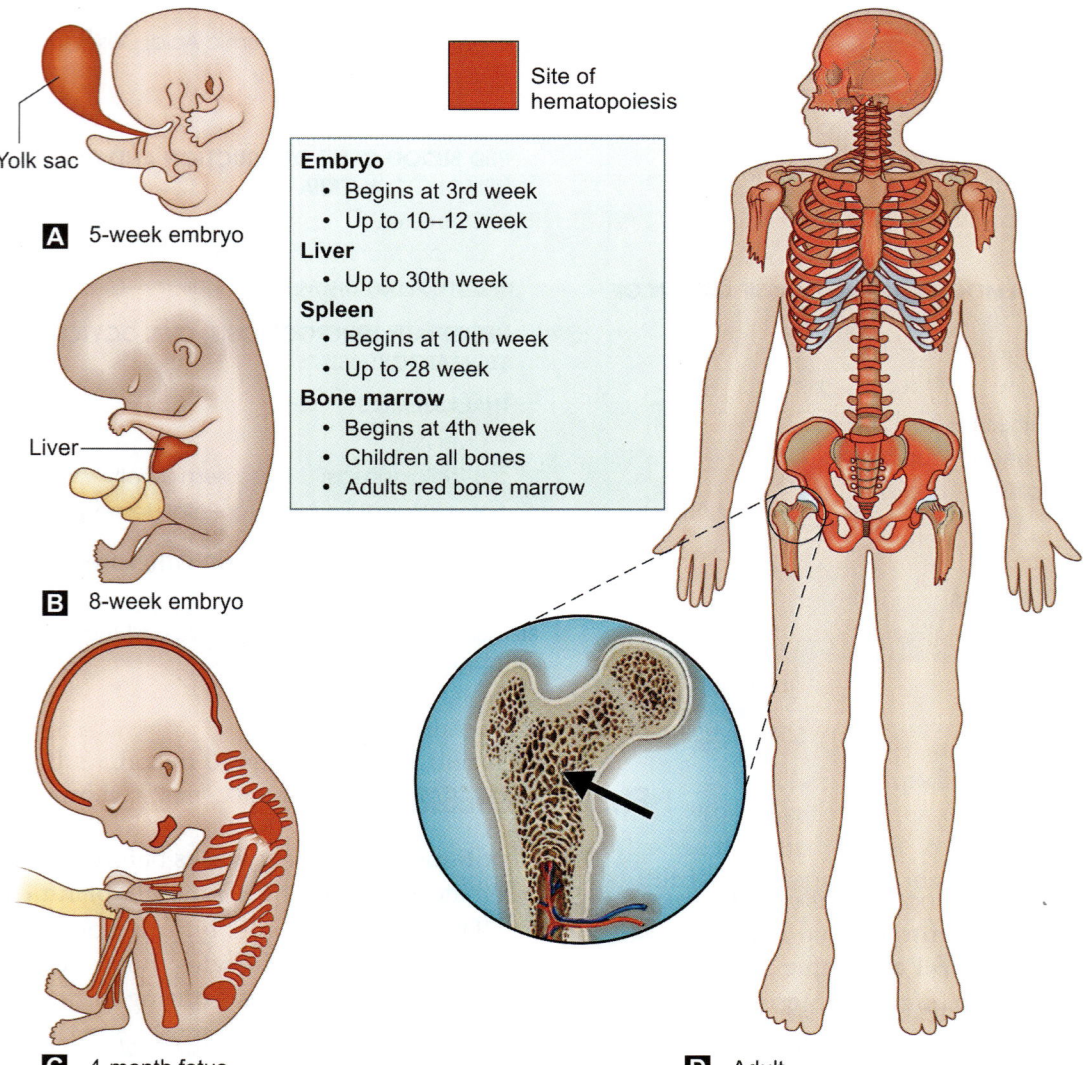

Fig. 8.1: Hematopoiesis during intrauterine life and postnatal period.

involved in hematopoiesis. During adult life by the age of 18–22 years, hematopoiesis occurs in cranial bones, vertebrae, sternum and ribs, iliac bones and upper ends of femur and humerus.

HEMATOPOIETIC MICROENVIRONMENT

Hematopoietic microenvironment comprises two types of cells: hematopoietic cells and non-hematopoietic cells. Hematopoietic microenvironment is shown in Fig. 8.2.

Hematopoietic Cells

Hematopoietic cells comprise hematopoietic stem cells (CD34+), progenitor cells (committed cells) and mature cells (RBCs, WBCs and platelets). Self-renewal is an important property of hematopoietic stem cells. Some of the stem cell disorders are shown in Table 8.2.

Lineages: Hematopoietic stem cells have the potential to self-replicate and differentiate into committed progenitors of trilineage myeloid and lymphoid cells (B cells, T cells and NK cells). Trilineage emyeloid cell gives rise to erythroid/megakaryocytic, eosinophilic, and granulocytic/macrophage pathways. Progenitor cells are multipotent stem cells derived from hematopoietic stem cells.

These are committed to one cell lineage such as myeloid, erythroid, megakaryocyte or lymphoid cells. Late progenitor cells differentiate and undergo maturation forming red cells, white blood cells, platelets and lymphocytes.

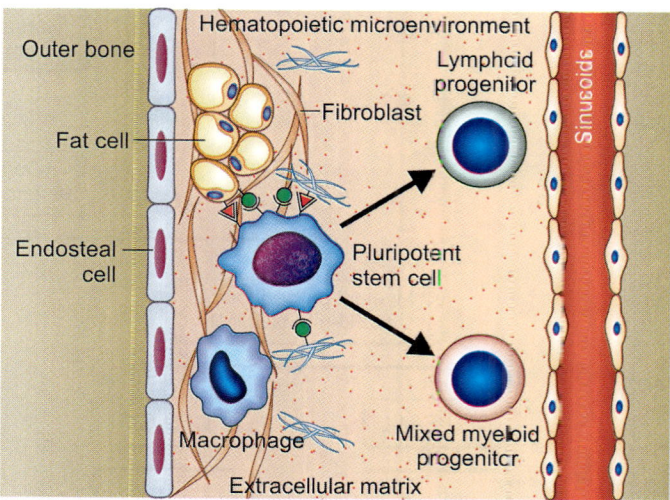

Fig. 8.2: Bone marrow hematopoietic microenvironment.

Colony forming units: Committed stem cells have been grown *in vitro* by cell culture techniques on semisolid media of agar or methylcellulose, with the production of colonies of differentiated progeny. Colony consists of 40 to a few hundred cells.

Thus, the committed stem cells have been called colony forming units (CFU), e.g. CFU-G/M, CFU-Eo and CFU-E/M. Cluster consists of 3–40 cells. *During bone marrow transplantation, administration of G-CSF, GM-CSF and IL-1 act on bone marrow microenvironment and cause migration of bone marrow stem cells to peripheral blood.* Colony forming units are shown in Table 8.3 and Fig. 8.3.

Table 8.2: Hematopoietic stem cell disorders

Hematopoietic stem cell (HSC)	Disorder
Proliferation and differentiation of HSC	Chronic myeloid leukemia Polycythemia vera Essential thrombocythemia
Proliferation with nil or minimal differentiation of HSC	Acute myeloid leukemia Acute lymphoblastic leukemia
Failure of proliferation with somatic mutation of HSC	Paroxysmal nocturnal hemoglobinuria
Proliferation with abnormal differentiation and apoptosis of HSC	Myelodysplastic syndrome
Failure of proliferation of HSC	Aplastic anemia

Table 8.3: Colony forming units

Colony forming unit	Production of cells
CFU-GEMM or CFU-MIX	Earliest units giving rise to granulocytic, erythroid, monocytic and megakaryocytic cells
CFU-GM	Unit of progenitor cells giving rise to granulocytic–monocytic series
CFU-Eo	Colonies of eosinophilic myeloid cells
CFU-BAS	Colonies of basophilic myeloid cells
CFU-MG	Colonies of megakaryocytic myeloid cells
BFU-E (Bursa forming units)	Earliest progenitor erythroid cells
CFU-E	More differentiated cells of erythroid progenitors

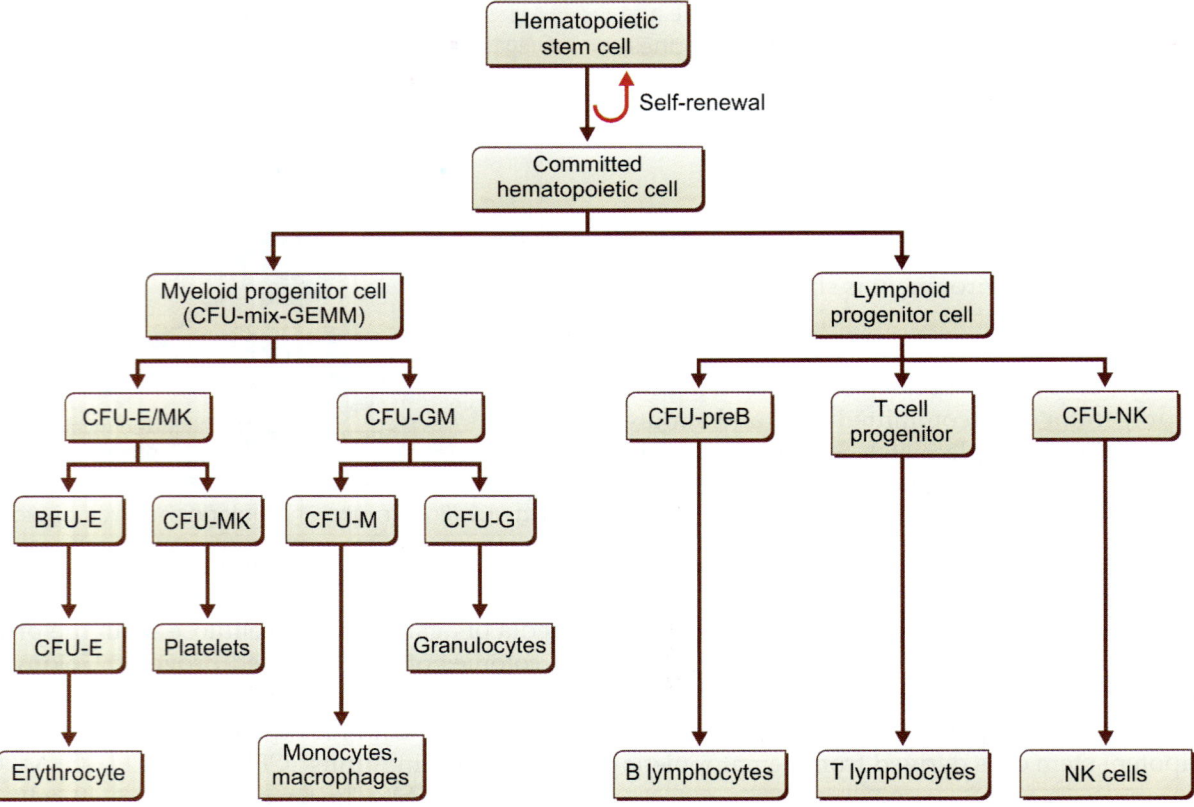

Fig. 8.3: Hematopoiesis showing stages of development of cells.

Non-hematopoietic Cells

Non-hematopoietic cells comprise stromal cells, macrophages, fibroblasts and endothelial cells. These synthesize growth factors, which stimulate hematopoiesis.

REGULATION OF HEMATOPOIESIS

Hematopoiesis is regulated by erythropoietin, thrombopoietin and cytokines. Inhibitory mechanisms and apoptosis regulate hematopoiesis. Substances stimulating hematopoietic microenvironment are shown in Table 8.4.

Erythropoietin: Erythropoietin synthesized by *juxtaglomerular cells of kidneys* participates in erythropoiesis. These cells are sensitive to oxygen tension in blood. It is essential for the survival of early erythroid progenitor cells by inhibition of default apoptosis pathway. Thus, erythropoietin rescue these erythroid precursor cells from apoptosis. It also participates in the differentiation of erythroid precursors.

Thrombopoietin: Thrombopoietin synthesized by the liver and kidneys stimulates megakaryopoiesis.

Growth factors: Hematopoietic growth factors are cytokines that act on stromal cells to synthesize colony forming units (E-CSF, GM-CSF and M-CSF). IL-7 acts as a growth factor for bone marrow stem cells. IL-13 synthesized by T cells acts as a growth factor for bone marrow stem cells.

G-CSF synthesized by T cells participates in differentiation and activation of neutrophils. G/M-CSF synthesized by bone marrow fibroblasts acts on CFU-G/M to produce granulocyte/macrophage colonies. IL-3 or multi-CSF is a growth factor for the trilineage myeloid stem cell. It stimulates the more committed precursors.

Role of hormones in erythropoiesis: TSH, thyroid hormones, ACTH, corticosteroids and human growth hormone also stimulate erythropoietin synthesis. Polycythemia is often a feature of Cushing's syndrome. However, very high doses of steroid hormones seem to inhibit erythropoiesis. Androgens stimulate and estrogens, which depress the erythropoiesis (Table 8.5).

PATHWAYS INVOLVED IN HEMATOPOIESIS

Bone marrow stem cells give rise to myeloid, lymphoid and erythroid precursor cells, which differentiate to form mature cells under the influence of colony stimulating factors, cytokines and erythropoietin. Bone marrow stromal cells can synthesize local hormones participating in hemopoiesis. Erythrocytes normally lose their nuclear material prior to entering the blood

Table 8.4: Important hematopoietic factors

Growth factors	Source	Site of action
Kit ligand	Bone marrow and stromal cells	Pluripotent hematopoietic stem cells
Erythropoietin	Liver and kidneys (juxtaglomerular cells)	Erythropoiesis, differentiation of erythroid precursors and survival by inhibiting apoptosis
Thrombopoietin	Liver and kidneys	Megakaryopoiesis
IL-13	T cells	Hematopoietic stem cells
G-CSF (granulocyte colony stimulating factor)	Monocyte/macrophages, T cells, fibroblasts, vascular endothelium	Differentiation and activation of neutrophils
G/M-CSF (granulocyte/macrophage colony stimulating factor)	T cells, fibroblast, endothelial cells, monocytes	Acts on CFU-G/M to produce granulocyte/macrophage colonies, platelets and red blood cells
Macrophage colony stimulating factor	Monocytes, endothelial cells, fibroblasts	Monocytes
Stem cell factor	Exact source unknown	Pluripotent stem cells
IL-3 or multi-CSF	T cells	Stimulate hematopoietic trilineage stem cells and more committed precursors
IL-5	T cells	Eosinophils
IL-6	T cells, monocytes, fibroblasts	Differentiation of B and T cells
		Proliferation of plasma cells
		Hematopoietic stem cells
IL-7	Stromal cells in bone marrow, dendritic cells, hepatocytes, keratinocytes, neurons, epithelial cells	Hematopoietic stem cells
IL-13	T cells	Stimulates hematopoietic stem cells
FLT-3 ligand	T cells	Stimulates hematopoietic stem cells

Table 8.5: Dietary requirements for red blood cell production

Dietary element	Role in red blood cell production
Amino acids	Synthesis of chains of globin
Iron	Hemoglobin synthesis
Vitamin B_{12} and folic acid	Nucleic acid synthesis of erythroid precursors
Vitamin B_6	Functions as coenzyme in amino acid metabolism and synthesis of ALA in haem synthesis
Vitamin C	Required for folate metabolism and to facilitate the absorption of iron
Vitamin E	Maintenance of red blood cell integrity
Copper	Participates in transfer of iron for maintenance of red blood cell integrity
Thyroid hormones, corticosteroids, human growth hormone and androgens	Stimulate erythropoietin synthesis

circulation. Platelets are formed from megakaryocytes. Pathways involved in hematopoiesis are shown in Fig. 8.4

Composition of blood: Human blood is composed of plasma (55%) and formed elements (45%). *Blood formed elements include RBCs, WBCs and platelets.*

Plasma contains water and solutes such as plasma proteins, nutrients, vitamins, hormones, glucose, respiratory gases O_2 and CO_2, bilirubin, inorganic constituents such as sodium, potassium, calcium chloride, carbonate, and bicarbonate; and waste products like urea and creatinine (Fig. 8.5).

8　Section II: Hematology

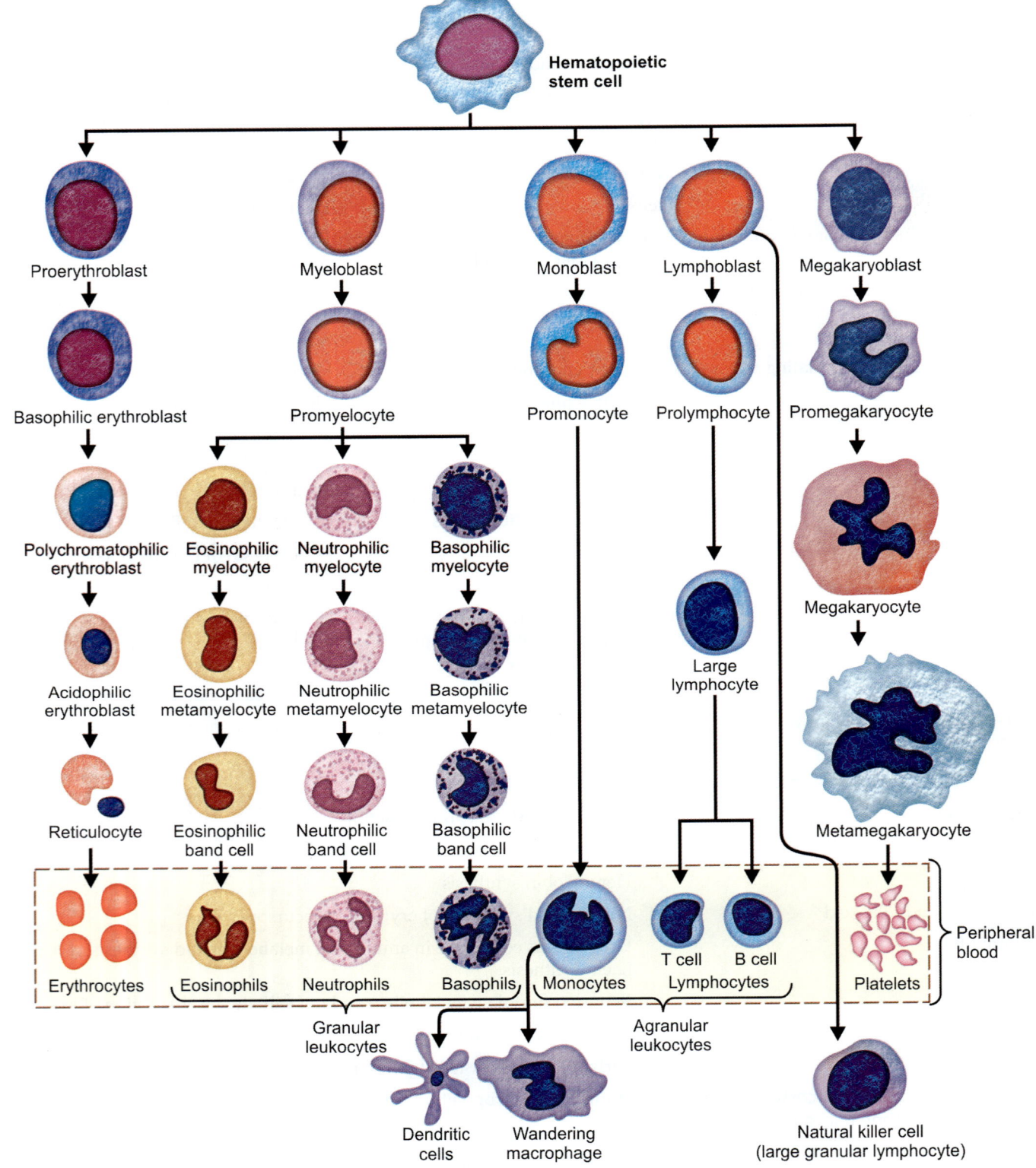

Fig. 8.4: Pathways involved in hematopoiesis.

ERYTHROPOIESIS

The production of RBCs is referred to as erythropoiesis. Hemocytoblasts give rise to erythrocytes. Erythropoietin synthesized by juxtaglomerular cells of kidneys participates in erythropoiesis. It is essential for the differentiation of erythroid precursors. It is released in response to hypoxia in renal arterial blood supply. Patients suffering from *erythropoietin secreting tumors, e.g. leiomyoma, renal cell carcinoma, hepatocellular carcinoma, and cerebral hemangioblastoma* develop secondary polycythemia.

Red Blood Cells

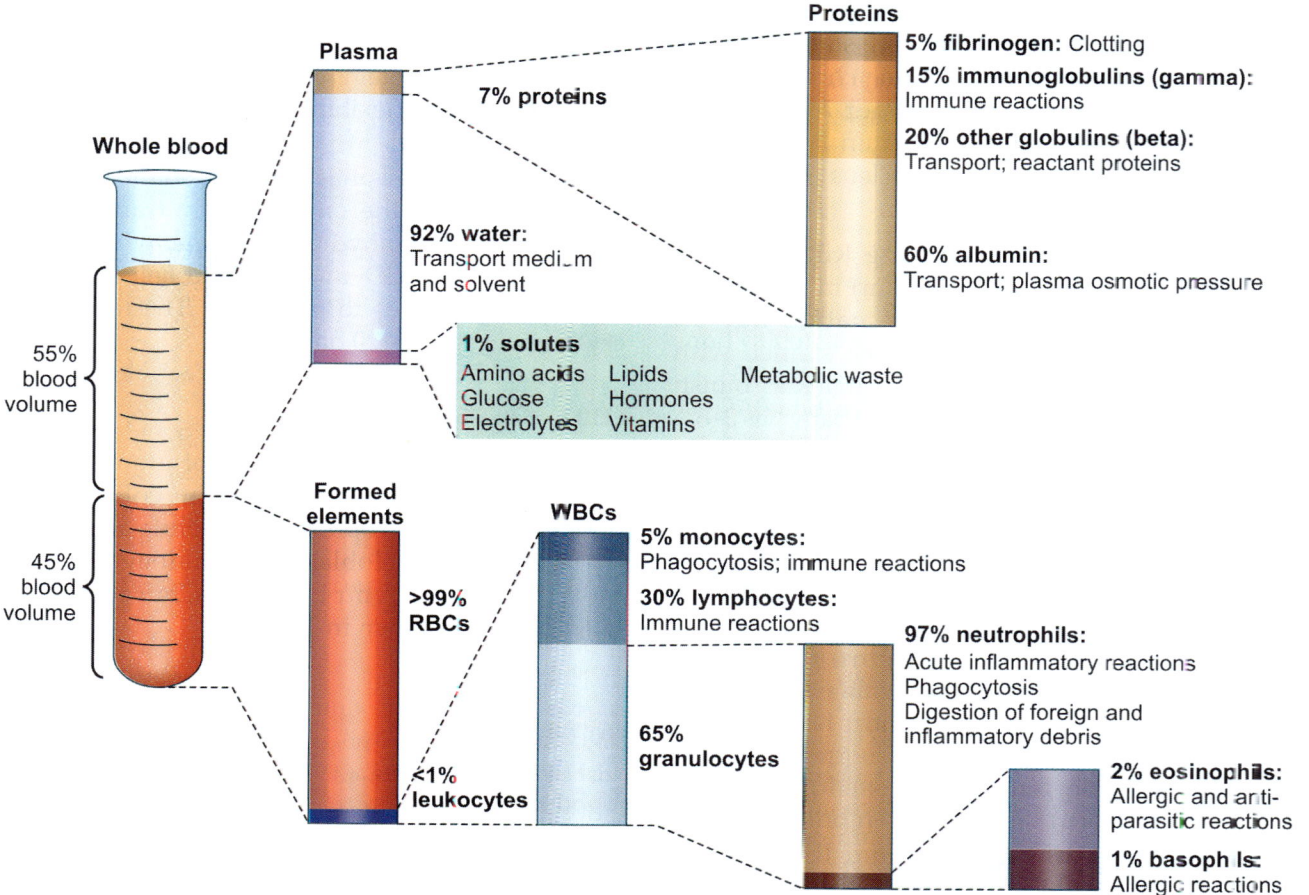

Fig. 8.5: Composition of blood showing plasma and formed elements.

Dyserythropoiesis: This term refers to production of abnormal cells resulting in their destruction in the bone marrow prior to their release into blood circulation. These developing normoblasts may show *nuclear budding, abnormal mitosis, fragmentation of nuclei, basophilic stippling* and *Howell-Jolly bodies.* These Howell-Jolly bodies may also be demonstrated in the red blood cells.

Ineffective erythropoiesis: This term ineffective erythropoiesis refers to erythroid hyperplasia in the bone marrow, but the patient is anemic. Ineffective erythropoiesis develops in megaloblastic anemia and myelodysplastic syndrome. Reticulocyte count is normal or low in these cases. Erythroid hyperplasia in hemolytic anemia is associated with increased reticulocyte count.

DEVELOPMENT OF RED BLOOD CELLS

During RBCs development, there is gradual reduction in size of cells, loss of mitochondria, disappearance of ribonucleic acid (RNA), extrusion of nuclei and gradual appearance of hemoglobin. Stages of development of RBC are shown in Table 8.6.

Table 8.6: Stages of development of RBC

Cell	Size (μ)	Nucleus	Cytoplasm
Proerythroblast	15–20	Large with immature chromatin, usually a single nucleolus	Blue
Early erythroblast	12–16	Fine chromatin clumps, nucleolus barely visible	Deep blue due to high RNA
Intermediate erythroblasts	12–15	Smaller size, chromatin clumps coarse	Polychromatic due to beginning of hemoglobinization
Late erythroblast	8–12	Small, dense, pyknotic and eccentric	Polychromatic
Reticulocytes	8–10	No nucleus	Polychromatic, remnants of RNA visible as a network on supravital staining
Erythrocyte	7–8	No nucleus	Pink

Stages of development: Proerythroblasts undergo 3 to 4 mitotic cell divisions, so that each stem cell gives rise to 8 or 16 cells of basophilic, polychromatic and orthochromatic erythroblasts in about 7 days. Iron is required for haem synthesis. Vitamin B_{12} and folic acid are needed for maturation of nucleus of erythroid precursors.

Reticulocyte: Reticulocyte, a young RBC contains network of ribonucleic acid (reticulum) in cytoplasm. It normally takes about 4 days to mature into an erythrocyte in blood circulation. When stained with new methylene blue, the RNA precipitates as bluish filaments and their cytoplasm. Newborn baby has 2–6% circulating reticulocytes. Reticulocyte count is 0.5–1.5% in adults.

Mature red blood cells: RBCs are biconcave discs, anucleate, and essentially without organelles. These are filled with water content 97% hemoglobin (Hb), a protein that functions in gas transport. Biconcave shape of RBCs possesses huge surface area to volume, and thus contributes to its gas transport function.

Cytoskeleton proteins present in RBC membrane give erythrocytes, their flexibility, and allows them to change shape as necessary.

ATP is generated anaerobically, so the erythrocytes do not consume the oxygen, they transport. RBCs contain carbonic anhydrase enzyme, which catalyzes reaction between CO_2 and H_2O and helps in transport of CO_2 from tissues to the lungs. The lifespan of an erythrocyte is 100–120 days.

LEUKOPOIESIS

White blood cells are composed of granulocytes and agranulocytes. Granulocyte is the collective name designated to neutrophils, eosinophils and basophils derived from myeloblast. Agranulocytes comprise monocytes and lymphocytes. Characteristics of leukocytes are shown in Table 8.7.

Table 8.7: Characteristics of leukocytes

Cell type	Prevalence	Morphology	Primary function	Comments
Neutrophils (12–15 μm)	50–70%	Nucleus 2–5 lobed. Cytoplasm contains small purple granules rich in digestive enzymes	Essential blood phagocytes, engulf and kill bacteria	Lifespan of 2 days with only 4–10 hours in the circulation
Eosinophils (12–15 μm)	1–4%	Bilobed nucleus with large coarse orange-colored granules containing toxic proteins, inflammatory mediators and digestive enzymes	Destroy worms and fungi. Participate in allergies and other inflammatory reactions	Found in much large numbers in the spleen and bone marrow
Basophils (10–12 μm)	0–1%	Constricted nuclei with dark blue to black granules in cytoplasm	Participate in inflammatory and allergic reactions	Cytoplasmic granules contain histamine, prostaglandins and other chemical mediators of allergic response
Monocytes (12–20 μm)	2–8%	Largest size cells with large nuclei often indented. Granules are not visible on light microscopy	Participate in phagocytosis followed by final differentiation into macrophages and dendritic cells. Dendritic cells are relatives of macrophages responsible for processing foreign matter and presenting to lymphocytes	Monocytes also secrete several chemicals that moderate the functions of the immune system
Lymphocytes (7–10 μm) or (10–14 μm)	20–40%	Small spherical cells with uniformly staining dark round nuclei	Participate in specific acquired immunity	T cells are responsible for cell-mediated immunity and assisting B cells. B cells differentiate into plasma cells and participate in humoral immunity. Natural killer cells are related to T cells but display no antigen specificity. These cells are active against cancer cells and virally infected cells

Red Blood Cells

Granulocytes

Granulocytes are derived from same committed cells called as myeloblasts. During development through various stages such as myeloblast, promyelocyte, myelocyte, metamyelocyte, band form and mature granulocyte (Table 8.8). There is progressive condensation and lobulation of nuclei, development of cytoplasmic granules, loss of RNA and mitochondria. Red marrow also contains a large reserve of mature granulocytes. Mature granulocytes pass actively across endothelial lining of bone marrow sinusoids. Turn out of granulocytes is very high. Stages of maturation of myeloid cells are shown in Fig. 8.6.

Neutrophils: Neutrophils measure 12–15 μm in diameter. These constitute 50–70% of leukocytes. These have 2–5 lobed nucleus. Cytoplasm contains small purple granules rich in digestive enzymes. These remain in circulation for 4–10 hours. Lifespan of neutrophils is 2 days. These cells are recruited to the site of injury within first 24 hours of inflammation.

Eosinophils: Eosinophils measure 12–15 μm in diameter. These constitute 1–4% of leukocytes. These have bilobed nucleus. Cytoplasm contains large coarse orange-colored granules. Eosinophilic granules contain highly cationic *major basic protein* (MBP) that kills only invasive helminthes. Eosinophils are recruited by chemokine

Table 8.8: Stages of maturation of myeloid cells

Cell	Size (μ)	Nucleus	Cytoplasm
Myeloblast	15–20	Nucleus is large, immature, fine dispersed chromatin with 2–5 nucleoli	Cytoplasm is scanty, light blue
Promyelocytes	16–20	Similar to myeloblast	Azurophil granules appear
Myelocytes	14–16	Chromatin condensed, no nucleoli	Specific and azurophil granules present. Specific granules predominate
Metamyelocytes	14–18	Indented or kidney shaped; peripheral clumping of chromatin	Specific numerous pink granules and fine faint pink azurophil granules
Band form	14–16	U-shaped or band-like nucleus with heavily clumped chromatin	Specific numerous pink granules and fine faint pink azurophil granules
Neutrophils	12–15	2–5 lobes joined by chromatin strands	Specific numerous pink granules and fine faint pink azurophil granules

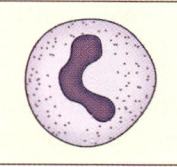

'Band' cell or 'stab' cell. An immature form. Present in increased proportion in the presence of bacterial infection.

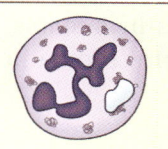

'Toxic' granulation. Coarse, increased granulation. Often with neutrophil leukocytosis, in bacterial sepsis. A Döhle body (bluish, peripheral inclusion body) is also present.

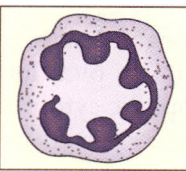

Hypersegmented form (more than 6 lobes). A large cell with an increased of nuclear lobes. Present in megaloblastic anemia.

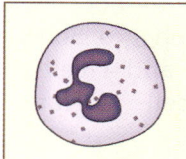

Hypogranular form. Present in myeloid leukemias and myelodysplasia.

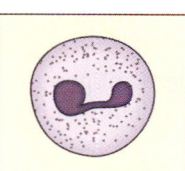

Pelger form. Majority of neutrophils have bilobed nucleus and hypogranular cytoplasm. Present in myelodysplasia or as a congenital variant.

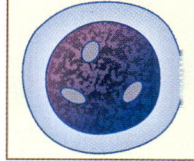

Blast cell. An immature leukocyte, with a few or no cytoplasmic granules and prominent nuclei. Present in acute leukemias.

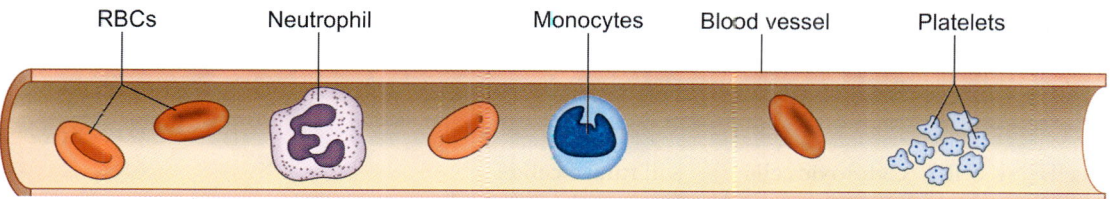

Fig. 8.6: WBCs qualitative anomalies.

(*eotaxin*) at injury site in IgE-mediated allergic reactions. Eosinophilic red granules contain crystalline material in cytoplasm, which become *Charcot-Leyden crystals* in the *sputum of asthmatic patients.*

Basophils: Basophils measure 10–12 µm in dimeter. These constitute 0–4% of leukocytes. These have pale staining constricted nucleus. Cytoplasm contains dark blue to black granules. Basophils possess coarse granules rich in *histamine.*

WBCs qualitative anomalies

- *May-Hegglin anomaly:* May-Hegglin anomaly is autosomal disorder due to *mutation of MYH9 gene.* This disorder is characterized by basophilic inclusions (Döhle body-like) in neutrophils, anemia, thrombocytopenia and giant platelets.

- *Alder-Reilly anomaly:* It is autosomal recessive disorder associated with several genetic mucopolysaccharidoses. There is deficiency of lysosomal enzymes required for breakdown of mucopolysaccharides. There is presence of liliac inclusions with clear halo in neutrophils stained with Giemsa stain. These granules are also demonstrated with toluidine blue.

- *Peggler-Huet anomaly:* Peggler-Huet anomaly is autosomal dominant disorder due to *mutation of lamin B receptor (LBR) gene.* It is characterized by lack of segmentation of neutrophils. Nuclei are dumble shaped in >70% of neutrophils. Chromatin is coarse. Two lobes of the nuclei are joined by thin chromatin bridge.

Agranulocytes

Agranulocytes comprise monocytes and lymphocytes. Monocytes differentiate into tissue macrophages. Bone marrow participates in production of B and T cells. B cells mature in the bone marrow. T cells migrate to thymus gland for maturation. Multiple subtypes of lymphocytes are shown in Table 8.9. Comparison between B cells and T cells is shown in Table 8.10.

Monocytes: Monocytes are derived from monoblasts in the bone marrow. These have lifespan of 12 hours. Monocyte contains reinform, lobulated or indented nuclei with open chromatin without nucleoli. Cytoplasm is pale blue. Monocytopoiesis is regulated by GM-CSF.

T cells: T cells participate in cell mediated immunity. Activated macrophages display antigens to T cells. Macrophages synthesize IL-12 that stimulates T cell responses. Activated T cells recruit monocytes from the circulation with IFN-γ, a powerful activator of macrophages.

B cells: B cells, when stimulated with antigen, become plasma cells and secrete immunoglobulins (e.g. *IgG, IgA, IgM, IgD* and *IgE*). Plasma cells participate in humoral immunity.

Natural killer cells: These kill tumor cells and virus infected cells by lysing or damaging plasma membranes.

THROMBOPOIESIS

Platelets are produced in the bone marrow by a process termed as thrombopoiesis. Platelets production is regulated by thrombopoietin synthesized from liver. Megakaryocytes derived from the bone marrow stem cells known as megakaryoblasts mature in about 10 days.

Megakaryoblast: Megakaryoblast measures 15–30 µ in diameter. It has high nucleus to cytoplasmic ratio. It contains basophilic cytoplasm with granules.

Promegakaryocyte: Promegakaryocyte measures 20–30 µ in diameter. It contains oval lobulated and elongated nucleus with basophilic cytoplasm.

Table 8.9: Multiple subtypes of lymphocytes

Lymphocytes	Subtype	Actions
B cell	Plasma cell	Synthesis of antibodies either against persistent antigen to injury site or against altered tissue components in chronic inflammation
T cell	Effector T cells	Delayed hypersensitivity
		Showing mixed lymphocytic reactivity
		Cytotoxic killer cells (K cells)
	Regulatory T cells	Helper T cells
		Suppressor T cells
Natural killer cells (NK cells)	Cytotoxic cells	Kill tumor cells
		Virus infected cells by lysing or damaging plasma membranes

Table 8.10: Comparison between B cells and T cells

Parameters	B cells	T cells
Origin	Stem cells in bone marrow	Stem cells in bone marrow
Site of maturation	Bone marrow and lymphoid cells	Thymus gland
Distribution in lymph nodes	Cortex (germinal follicles and medullary cords) of lymph nodes	Paracortical areas of lymph nodes
Distribution in spleen	Germinal centers of follicles	Periarteriolar lymphoid sheaths
Differentiation (product of antigenic stimulation)	Plasma cells and memory cells	T-helper cells, T-suppressor cells, cytotoxic T cells and memory cells
Circulation in blood	Low numbers (10–20%)	High numbers (60–70%)
Lifespan	Short-lived (weeks to a few months)	Long lived (2–4 years)
Fc receptors	Present	Absent
Electron microscopy	Microvilli present	Smooth surface
Requires antigen presenting cells with MHC	No	Yes on APCs
General functions	Production of antibodies to inactivate, neutralize target antigens	Cell function in regulating immune functions killing *foreign cells*, hypersensitivity, synthesize cytokines
MHC molecules	MHC-I and MHC-II	MHC-I and MHC-II
Immune surface markers	Immunoglobulin	T cell receptor
Immunological markers	CD19 to CD22	CD1 to CD8

Platelets: Platelets are 3–4.5 microns in diameter. These possess 2 membrane glycoproteins. Normal platelet count is 150,000–400,000/cu mm.

Platelets are formed by pinching off cytoplasm of magakaryocytes which are situated close to marrow sinusoids circulation. It is known as *platelet budding*. Platelets have normal lifespan of 8 to 10 days. They are destroyed by macrophages, mainly in the spleen and also in the liver.

Platelet consists of dense bodies and α-granules. These contain primary inflammatory mediators. Platelets regulate vascular permeability and proliferation of mesenchymal cells in chronic inflammation. Platelets participate in surveillance of blood vessel continuity, formation of primary and secondary hemostatic plugs, and healing of injured tissue. Structure and functions of platelets are shown in Fig. 8.7 and Table 8.11.

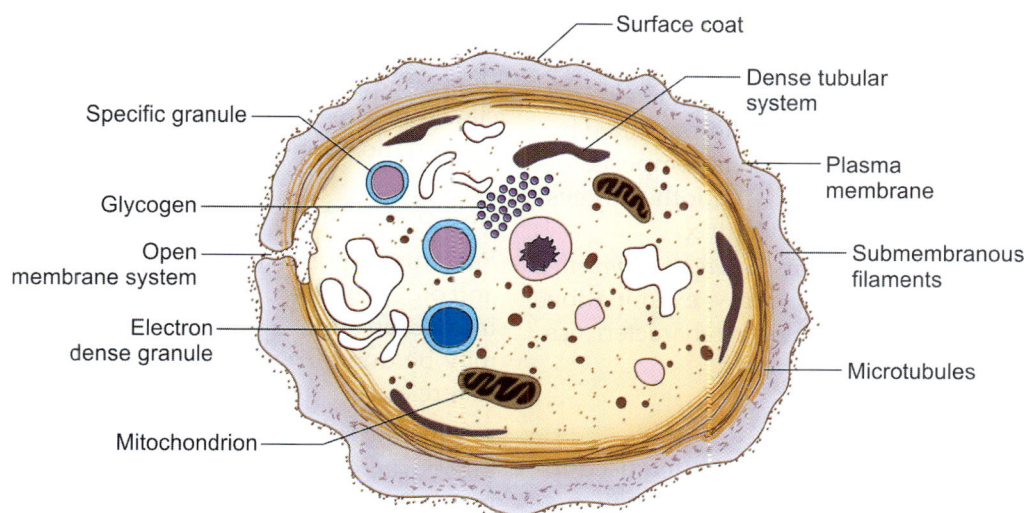

Fig. 8.7: Structure of platelet. Platelet consists of outer glycocalyx layer and inner plasma membrane. Cytoskeleton maintains discoid shape. It consists of dense and α-granules.

Table 8.11: Structure and functions of platelets

Parameters	Functions
Platelet membrane	
Glycocalyx	Outermost coat comprising glycolipids, glycoproteins and mucopolysaccharide
	Negative charge due to sialic acid residue of proteins and lipids
Plasma membrane	Composed of glycolipids, cholesterol and glycoproteins
	Lipoprotein layer containing platelet factor III involved in blood coagulation
Membrane glycoproteins (acting as receptors for cell-cell and ligand-cell interaction)	
Glycoprotein IIb/IIIa	Cross-linking of IIb/IIIa to vWF and fibrinogen leading to platelets aggregation
Glycoprotein Ib–IX	In Bernaurd-Soulier syndrome, deficiency of GP Ib–IX results in bleeding diathesis
Cytoskeleton	
Short actin filament	Present under plasma membrane involved in maintaining discoid shape
Actin microfilament network	Present in cytoplasm
Microtubules	Present in peripheral part of cytoplasm involved in maintaining discoid shape
Dense granules	
ADP	Recruits platelets and activates new platelets result in platelets aggregation
ATP	Agonist for cells other than platelets
Calcium	Extracellular source for hemostatic reactions
Serotonin	Vasoconstrictor
α-granules	
Fibrinogen	Causes aggregation and platelets
	Fibrinogen itself gets converted to fibrin
Platelets factor IV	Promotes aggregation of platelets
Thrombospondin	Promotes aggregation of platelets
Factor V	Participates in adhesion of platelets
vWF	Inhibits fibrinolysin
Plasminogen	Plasminogen gets converted to plasmin. Plasmin participates in fibrinolysis
PDGF	Promotes repair of smooth muscle cells

BONE MARROW ASPIRATION

Bone marrow is composed of network of blood vessels, hematopoietic cells, stroma, nerves and reticuloendothelial cells. Venous sinusoids are lined by endothelial cells. Bone marrow stroma is composed of cells (fibroblasts, stromal cells, fat cells, endothelial cells and macrophages) and extracellular matrix.

Extracellular matrix comprises *collagen, laminin, fibronectin* and *proteoglycans*. Bone marrow examination gives more information and morphological characteristics are better defined in stained blood films.

Marrow Aspiration Needles

Klima needle and Salah needle are most often used to aspirate bone marrow. Islam needle is used in patients either with osteosclerotic bone or osteoporotic bone. The needles are stout wide bore with short bevel, a stellate and adjustable guard, which prevents overpenetration. Bone marrow aspiration needles (Fig. 8.8) must be sterilized in a hot air oven or autoclaved before being used. Indications of bone marrow examination are shown in Table 8.12.

Sites of Aspiration

Posterior superior iliac crest site is preferred in adults and older children. *Calcaneum* is site of choice in *infants*. In children under 2 years of age, bone marrow aspiration may be done from medial aspect of tibia below tibial tubercle.

Midline of sternum at the height of the second intercostal space provides best representative material in adults, but the patient is more apprehensive when aspiration is done from this site. No attempt should be made to aspirate bone marrow from below the second

Red Blood Cells

Procedure

Under aseptic conditions and local anesthesia by adjusting guard the needle is inserted with a boring and slight rotating motion in bone marrow and applying a strong vacuum pressure via an attached syringe.

Preparation of Smears

Bone marrow fragments are aspirated and smears are prepared, stained with Romanowsky stains and examined under low power. The ideal area for examination of smear is one in which the hematopoietic cells constitute a monocellular layer and the red blood cells exhibit pink stained morphology.

The cellularity of marrow varies with the age of the patient. In early childhood, the marrow contains a little fat. In adults, the marrow usually has about 50% fat cells, while 75% fat in elderly persons.

Staining of Smears

Smear is stained with Romanowsky stain One smear is used for iron stain. CD markers used for hematolymphoid neoplasms are shown in Table 8.13.

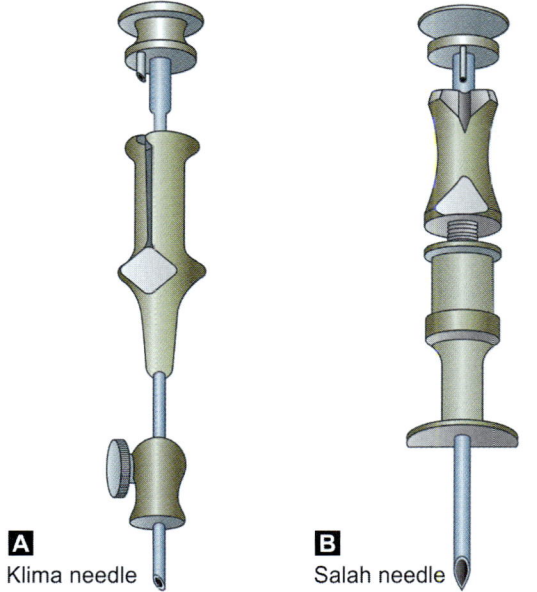

Fig. 8.8: Bone marrow aspiration needles.
A: Klima needle
B: Salah needle

intercostal space, because if the inner cortical layer is perforated, the great vessels and the right atrium located below this space may be damaged.

Table 8.12: Indications of bone marrow examination (diagnostic significance)

Disorders	Examples
Red blood cell disorders	Megaloblastic anemia Pure red cell aplasia Iron deficiency anemia to assess iron stores in bone marrow Sideroblastic anemia to assess iron in sideroblasts
White blood cell disorders	Subleukemic leukemia Acute myeloid leukemia Acute lymphoblastic leukemia
Myeloproliferative disorders	Chronic myeloid leukemia Polycythemia rubra vera Idiopathic thrombocythemia
Megakaryocytic disorders	Idiopathic thrombocytopenic purpura Other thrombocytopenic purpura
Plasma cell disorders	Multiple myeloma Waldenström's macroglobulinemia
Storage disorders	Gaucher's disease Niemann-Pick disease
Metastases in bone marrow	*Adults:* Cancers of prostate, urinary bladder, breast, lung (small cell type), kidney, gastrointestinal tract and thyroid gland. Hodgkin's disease involves bone marrow in stage IV. Non-Hodgkin's lymphoma also involves bone marrow *Children:* Neuroblastoma, embryonal rhabdomyosarcoma, and retinoblastoma
Parasites	*Leishmania donovani* bodies in kala-azar Malarial parasites
Histiocytic disorders	Langerhans' histiocytosis Hemophagocytic syndrome

Table 8.13: CD markers used for hematolymphoid neoplasms

Hematology cells	Immunophenotyping markers on flow cytometry
RBCs	Glycophorin A
Megakaryocytes	CD41, CD61
WBCs	CD45 (leukocyte common antigen)
Blasts	CD34, TdT, HLA-DR
Myeloid cells	Anti-MPO, CD13, CD33, CD14, CD117
B cells	CD19, CD20, CD10, FMC7, CD23, CD79a, Ig, IgM

EVALUATION OF BONE MARROW ASPIRATE

Bone marrow smears are screened for bone marrow fragments under scanner objective. Most of the bone marrow particles are present in the tail of smears.

Cellularity: Cellularity of bone marrow is assessed by visualization of marrow particles. Number, cellularity of fragments and cellular details are observed. Bone marrow is more cellular in children than adults. Bone marrow is reported as hypercellular, hypocellular or normocellular.

Erythropoiesis: Type of erythropoiesis, normoblastic or megaloblastic. Activity and maturity of erythroid precursors are observed. Largest number of bone marrow cells is erythroid cells.

Leukopoiesis: Maturity, abnormal granules, atypical cells, lymphocytes and plasma cells are observed.

Myeloid to erythroid ratio: At least 500 marrow cells are counted. Ratio of normal fat to hematopoietic cells is 1:1 in adults. Normal myeloid to erythroid ratio is 3:1 in adults. Normal fat to erythroid cells ratio is 4:1 in adults.

Megakaryopoiesis: Megakaryocytes are examined in marrow particles near tail of marrow smears. It is important to look for budding of platelets from megakaryocytes. Relative number of promegakaryoblasts and megakaryocytes is also observed.

Other bone marrow cells: Plasma cells, lymphocytes and reticulum cells are observed. Differential cell count in adult bone marrow aspirate is shown in Table 8.14.

Abnormal cells: One must look for metastases, LD bodies, malarial parasite and *Histoplasma capsulatum*. Granulomas are demonstrated in bone marrow due to tuberculosis, sarcoidosis, *Histoplasma capsulatum* and *Cryptococcus neoformans*, systemic lupus erythematosus and infectious mononucleosis. Microorganisms demonstrated in bone marrow are shown in Table 8.15.

Table 8.14: Differential cell count in adult bone marrow aspirate

Bone marrow cells	Percentage of cells
Myeloid cells*	
Myeloblasts	0–3
Promyelocytes	3–10
Neutrophilic myelocytes	4–10
Metamyelocytes	3–8
Neutrophils including band form	25–45
Erythroid cells	
Proerythroblasts	0–1
Early/basophilic normoblasts	1–5
Intermediate/polychromatic normoblasts	5–20
Late/orthochromatic normoblasts	5–15
Lymphoid cells	
Lymphocytes	5–10
Plasma cells	0–2
Monocyte/macrophages	
Monocytes	1–3
Macrophages	0–1
Megakaryocytic cells	
Megakaryocytes	0–2

*Normal myeloid to erythroid ratio ranges 3:1 to 15:1

Table 8.15: Microorganisms demonstrated in bone marrow

Microorganisms demonstrated in bone marrow in immunocompromised persons	
Parasites	*Leishmania donovani* bodies (LD bodies) Malarial parasite
Bacteria	Mycobacterium tubercle bacilli Mycobacterium lepra bacilli
Fungi	*Cryptococcus neoformans* *Histoplasma capsulatum*
Virus	Cytomegalovirus

BONE MARROW IRON CONTENT

By means of a cytochemical stain, the amount of stainable iron in the bone marrow can be visualized and quantitatively assessed. It has *diagnostic role* in diagnosing *iron deficiency anemia*, *β-thalassemia*, and *sideroblastic anemia*.

Principle

The test is based on the Prussian blue reaction (Perl's reaction). Ionic iron reacts with acid potassium ferricyanide solution (2% potassium ferricyanide + N/5 HCl) to produce a blue color. Smears are counter stained by 1% *nuclear fast* or 0.1% *neutral red* to stain nuclei as red.

Interpretation

Iron granules appear as bright blue or blue-green aggregates not exceeding 1 μ in diameter in the cytoplasm of nucleated (sideroblasts) or non-nucleated (siderocytes) precursors contrasting sharply with the pink stained background.

Normally, 25–50% of normoblasts will show 1–4 small granules. Often, iron granules can also be seen in the reticuloendothelial cells of the bone marrow, and they may be spherical or irregularly shaped. When the granules surround the erythroid nuclei, they constitute the so-called ring sideroblasts. Grading of iron stores on bone marrow aspirate is shown in Table 8.16.

Pathological Disorders

Bone marrow is deficient in iron deficiency anemia. Bone marrow iron is increased in thalassemia. Iron granules scattered throughout cytoplasm surrounding nuclei occur in sideroblastic anemia. Excess of iron is deposited in reticuloendothelial cells in dyserythropoietic anemia and anemia secondary to inflammation. Demonstration of iron granules in normoblasts under oil immersion lens is shown in Table 8.17.

TREPHINE BONE BIOPSY

Trephine bone biopsy should be performed when the marrow obtained by aspiration is inadequate for examination in cases of aplastic anemia or myelofibrosis.

Needles

The procedure is done with a biopsy needle, such as Jamshidi-Swaim needle or Islam needle or Osgood biopsy needle. The preferred site is the posterior superior iliac spine. Sternal site is always avoided due to danger of penetrating heart.

Procedure

Under aseptic conditions and anesthetizing the area, the sterile trephine biopsy needle is inserted in bone marrow by to and fro rotation clockwise and anticlockwise at least 10 times.

Fixation

The material is aspirated and put in 2 ml of *Helly's fluid* for fixation. Helly's fluid consists of potassium dichromate (2.5 g); mercuric chloride (5.0 g); 40% formaldehyde (5 ml); dissolved in 100 ml of water. The biopsy is stained with hematoxylin and eosin. The preparation allows for optimal evaluation of bone marrow cells with bony trabeculae. It is helpful in evaluating extrinsic features such as metastatic tumor or fibrosis in the marrow.

Indications

Trephine bone biopsy is performed in cases of aplastic anemia, metastases in bone marrow, myelofibrosis, aleukemic leukemia, hypoplastic acute myeloid leukemia (AML-M7), miliary tuberculosis involving marrow, malignant lymphomas, myelodysplastic syndrome and chronic lymphoproliferative disorders. Grading of iron in trephine biopsy is shown in Table 8.18.

Table 8.16: Grading of iron stores on bone marrow aspirate

Grade	Interpretation	Iron content in marrow cells
Grade 0	Iron stores—nil	Absence of iron granules
Grade 1	Diminished iron stores	Small granules in reticulum cells observed under oil immersion lens
Grade 2	Normal iron stores	Presence of iron granules with low power lens
Grade 3	Normal iron stores	Numerous small granules present in all marrow particles
Grade 4	Increased iron stores	Presence of large granules in clumps
Grade 5	Increased iron stores	Presence of dense clumps of granules
Grade 6	Increased iron stores	Very large granules present obscuring marrow cells

Table 8.17: Demonstration of iron granules in normoblasts under oil immersion lens

Erythroid cells	Iron granules
Late normoblasts	1–3 pinpoint granules
Abnormal sideroblasts (late and intermediate normoblasts) seen in megaloblastic anemia	1–10 pinhead granules
Ring sideroblasts (sideroblastic anemia)	>5 coarse granules surrounding nucleus

Table 8.18: Grading of iron in trephine biopsy

Grade	Iron content
Grade 0	Absence of granules
Grade 1	Fine iron granules in every 3–4 HPF
Grade 2	Heavy iron granules in every 2–3 HPF
Grade 3	Iron granules in every HPF in ≥1 cell
Grade 4	Massive iron granules present in clumps

RED BLOOD CELL, HEMOGLOBIN AND CLASSIFICATION OF ANEMIAS

RED BLOOD CELL

Red blood cell measures 7–8 μ in diameter with lifespan of 100–120 days. It contains hemoglobin. The normal red blood cell membrane cytoskeleton of RBCs comprises spectrin, ankyrin, actin, protein 4.1 and protein 3. Together, these proteins maintain the normal biconcave shape of RBCs. Patient develops heredity spherocytosis due to deficiency of any of these membrane cytoskeleton proteins.

RED CELL INDICES

Hematocrit values are basically the measures of red blood cells size and their hemoglobin content. These give valuable information in diagnosing anemia. Automated cell counters provide these data on each sample. These values vary slightly between laboratories. Mean corpuscular volume (MCV), mean corpuscular hemoglobin (MCH) and mean corpuscular hemoglobin concentration (MCHC) are calculated as under.

Mean Corpuscular Volume (MCV)

MCV is the index used to measure the average volume of a red blood cell. MCV categorizes RBCs according to their size. Cells with normal size are called *normocytic*, smaller cells are termed microcytic, and larger cells are referred to as macrocytic. Normal MCV is 82–96 femtoliters. MCV is decreased in iron deficiency anemia (<80 femtoliters). MCV is increased in megaloblastic anemia (>100 femtoliters).

Mean Corpuscular Hemoglobin (MCH)

MCH is the index used to measure average hemoglobin content per red blood cell. It is calculated by dividing hemoglobin concentration (g/dl) by red blood cells concentration/liter. Normal value of MCH is 26–33 pg. MCH is decreased in iron deficiency anemia and increased in megaloblastic anemia.

Mean Corpuscular Hemoglobin Concentration (MCHC)

It measures the average concentration is a given volume of packed cell volume of red cells. Normal MCHC value is 33–37 g/dl. MCHC is decreased in iron deficiency anemia and increased in hereditary spherocytosis. MCHC remains normal in megaloblastic anemia.

Red Blood Cell Distribution Width (RDW)

RDW is the index to measure degree of anisocytosis (various in size of red blood cells). Normal value is 11.5 to 14.5. RDW is increased in iron deficiency anemia, megaloblastic anemia and immune hemolytic anemia. RWD remains within normal range in thalassemia.

Table 8.19: Cut off points for anemia according to WHO

Subject	Hemoglobin (%)	MCHC
Children (6 months to 6 years)	11 g/dl	34%
Children (>6–14 years)	12 g/dl	34%
Women (during pregnancy)	11 g/dl	34%
Women (non-pregnant)	12 g/dl	34%
Men	13 g/dl	34%

Hematocrit or Packed Cell Volume (PCV)

It is the index to measure blood volume proportion occupied by red blood cells. Normal range in males is 40–52% and 36–48% in females. Increase in number of red blood cells will increase hematocrit or packed cell volume except in thalassemia and megaloblastic anemia.

Hemolysis in thalassemia increases production of number of red blood cells, but with small size red cells and decreased hematocrit value. Patient of megaloblastic anemia shows macrocytic red blood cells size but decreased hematocrit value. Cut off points for anemia according to WHO are shown in Table 8.19.

RETICULOCYTE COUNT

Approximately 50,000 reticulocytes are produced daily. These circulate for about one day to form mature red blood cells. Reticulocyte count is used to assess the capacity of the bone marrow to increase RBC production in response to increased demand.

Supravital New Methylene Blue

Reticulocytes are demonstrated by supravital stains such as new methylene blue (best stain) and brilliant cresyl blue. Heinz bodies are demonstrated by supravital stains (Table 8.20).

Conditions with Increased or Decreased Reticulocyte Count

Reticulocyte count is increased following massive bleeding, acute hemolysis, and response to specific therapy in nutritional anemia and even after voluntary blood donation. Peripheral blood examination under these conditions shows red cell polychromasia and increased reticulocyte count. *Reticulocyte count is decreased in aplastic anemia, pernicious anemia, bone marrow metastases* and *congenital dyserythropoietic anemia*.

Table 8.20: Composition of new methylene blue reagent

Stain constituents	Quantity
New methylene blue	0.5 g
Potassium oxalate	0.6 g
Distilled water	100 ml

HEMOGLOBIN SYNTHESIS

Hemoglobin is tetrameric protein composed of haem and globin chains (4 polypeptide chains). Embryonic hemoglobin exists up to 8 weeks of intrauterine life. Fetal hemoglobin is synthesized after 8 weeks of intrauterine life. Fetal hemoglobin level is attained <2% by 7 months of intrauterine life. HbA2 synthesis begins by 35 weeks of intrauterine life. Switch over from fetal to adult hemoglobin starts at 30 weeks of intrauterine life. Adult hemoglobin synthesis is completed by 38 weeks at the time of birth of newborn.

Significant time for switching over synthesis from fetal hemoglobin to adult starts at 30 weeks of intrauterine life. Adult hemoglobin synthesis is completed by 38 weeks at the time of birth of newborn. After one year of life and in adults, normal fetal hemoglobin (HBF) is <1% and HbA_2 is <3%. Steps of haem synthesis are shown in Fig. 8.9.

Nomenclature of Hemoglobin

The various forms of hemoglobin are named according to the types of globin chains present. Some of these hemoglobins are present in adults, while others may be found only *in utero* or early in infancy.

Embryonic hemoglobin exists up to 8 weeks of intrauterine life. Fetal hemoglobin is synthesized after 8 weeks of intrauterine life. Hemoglobin synthesis during intrauterine period and adults is shown in Table 8.21.

Genetic Control

Hemoglobin consists of pairs of globin chains. A variety of globin chains can be present. Normally, α and β (and to a lesser extent δ) globin chains form adult hemoglobin. In fetal life (γ, ε, and ζ) chains are present. The globin chains of hemoglobin are synthesized independently and are under separate genetic control. *The α chain and*

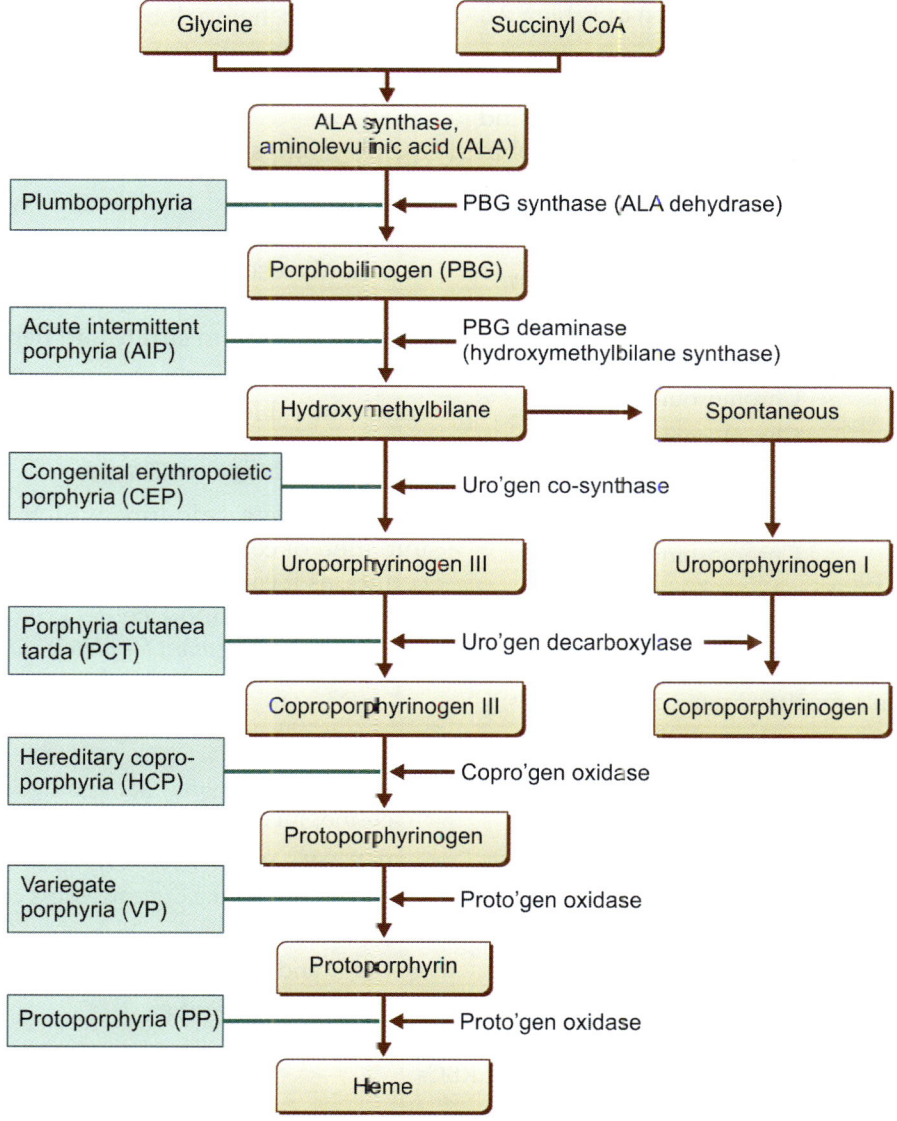

Fig. 8.9: Steps in haem synthesis.

Table 8.21: Hemoglobin synthesis during intrauterine period and adults

Nomenclature of hemoglobin	Polypeptide globin chains	Hemoglobin	Percentage
Hemoglobin A	α_2, β_2	Adult	97% of normal adult hemoglobin
Hemoglobin A$_2$	α_2, δ_2	Adult	1–3% of normal adult hemoglobin
Hemoglobin F	α_2, γ_2	Fetal—neonatal period	<1% of normal fetal hemoglobin in adults
Hemoglobin Gower 1	ζ_2, ε_2	Embryonic Hb	Synthesis up to 8 weeks of intrauterine life
Hemoglobin Gower 2	α_2, ε_2	Embryonic Hb	Synthesis up to 8 weeks of intrauterine life
Hemoglobin Portland 1 (HbE Portland 1)	γ_2, ζ_2	Embryonic Hb	Synthesis up to 8 weeks of intrauterine life
Hemoglobin Portland 2 (HbE Portland 2)	γ_2, ζ_2	Embryonic Hb	Synthesis up to 8 weeks of intrauterine life

After one year of life and in adults, normal fetal hemoglobin (HBF) is <1% and HbA$_2$ is <3%.

ζ chain are under genetic control on chromosome 16. Rest globin chains (β chain, γ chain, δ chain, and ε chain) are under genetic control on chromosome 11. Globin chains and their locus on chromosomes are shown in Table 8.22.

Hemoglobin Disorders

Hemoglobin disorders are of two types—qualitative and quantitative hemoglobinopathies. These hemoglobin disorders lead to hemolytic anemias. Qualitative hemoglobinopathies occur due to defect in abnormal structure of hemoglobin without change in their quantity of synthesis (HbS, HbC, HbD and HbE. Quantitative hemoglobinopathies occur due to decreased synthesis of hemoglobin affecting quantity of chains without defect in structure of hemoglobin. Examples are α-thalassemia and β-thalassemia.

ANTICOAGULANTS USED IN LABORATORY

Most often blood is collected by venepuncture into collection tubes containing anticoagulant. Most commonly used anticoagulants are tripotassium and trisodium salts of ethylenediaminetetra-acetic acid (EDTA), trisodium citrate and heparin.

Anticoagulants, mechanism of action and uses are shown in Table 8.23.

EDTA and Trisodium Citrate

These remove calcium, which is essential for the initiation of coagulation. EDTA is often used for blood counts, as it causes minimal morphologic and physical effects on the blood cells. Trisodium citrate is the preferred *anticoagulant for platelets and coagulation studies*.

Table 8.22: Globin chains and their locus on chromosomes

Globin chain	Location of gene
α chain	Chromosome 16
β chain	Chromosome 11
γ chain	Chromosome 11
δ chain	Chromosome 11
ε chain	Chromosome 11
ζ chain	Chromosome 16

Hemoglobin α chain and ζ chain are under genetic control on chromosome 16. Rest hemoglobin globin chains ($\beta, \gamma, \delta, \varepsilon$ chains) are under genetic control on chromosome 11.

Table 8.23: Anticoagulants, mechanism of action and uses

Anticoagulant	Mechanism of action	Uses
EDTA	Chelates calcium and removes thus prevents blood coagulation	Hb estimation, platelet count, RBCs count, absolute eosinophil count, estimation of HbF, Hb electrophoresis
Trisodium citrate	Binds with calcium and form complex	ESR estimation by Westergren's pipette method (4:1) Prothrombin time done to assess coagulation study (9:1)
Heparin	Acts against thrombin	Assess osmotic fragility for spherocytosis, RBCs enzymes, G6PD and pyruvate kinase
Ammonium–potassium mixture (2:3)	Ammonium causes swelling of RBCs, whereas potassium leads to shrinkage of RBCs resulting in maintaining size of RBCs	Used instead of EDTA
Sodium fluoride	Inhibits glycolysis	Best anticoagulant to estimate blood sugar

Red Blood Cells

Heparin

Heparin acts by forming complex with *antithrombin III* in the plasma to prevent thrombin formation. Heparin causes a *bluish coloration of the background when a smear is stained with Wright-Giemsa stain*. Heparin is often used for *red cell testing, osmotic fragility testing and functional or morphological analysis of leukocytes*.

ROMANOWSKY STAINS

Routine stain for peripheral smear and bone marrow examination is a family of Romanowsky stains: May-Grunwald stain, Leishman stain, Giemsa stain, Wright's stain and Jenner's stain. These stains also highlight Howell Jolly bodies. Basophilic stippling and Cabot's ring. Romanowsky stain cannot stain *Heinz bodies*. Comparison of Leishman and Giemsa stain is shown in Table 8.24. Composition of buffered water (Sorenson's phosphate buffer) is shown in Table 8.25.

ANEMIA

Anemia is fefined as decrease in whole body red cell mass, a definition that precludes relative decreases in red blood cell count, hemoglobin, or hematocrit, which occur when the plasma volume is increased. Anemia of pregnancy is not anemia but rather is a manifestation of increased plasma volume. A practical working definition of anemia is decrease in red blood cell count, hemoglobin, or hematocrit; all are commonly measured red cell parameters.

Table 8.24: Comparison of Leishman and Giemsa stain

Parameters	Leishman stain	Giemsa stain
Stain powder	Leishman powder: 1 g	Giemsa stain powder: 1 g
Methanol	Methanol (acetone-free): 500 ml	Methanol (acetone-free): 66 ml
Glycerol	Nil	Glycerol: 66 ml

Table 8.25: Composition of buffered water (Sorenson's phosphate buffer)

Solution	Salt
Solution A	Potassium dihydrogen phosphate: 9.08 g/L
Solution B	Dibasic hydrogen phosphate: 9.47 g/L

Preparation of buffer water with 6.8 pH: Solution A 50.8 ml + Solution B 49.2 ml = 100 ml

CAUSES OF ANEMIA

Anemia may be caused by two major mechanisms: decreased production or destruction of red blood cells (hemolytic anemia). Iron plays role in haem synthesis. Vitamin B_{12} and folic acid are essential in DNA synthesis during hematopoiesis. Decreased red cell production results from damage to hematopoietic stem cells or deficiency of nutrients such as iron, vitamin B_{12} and folic acid. Classification of anemia is shown in Figs 8.10 and 8.11.

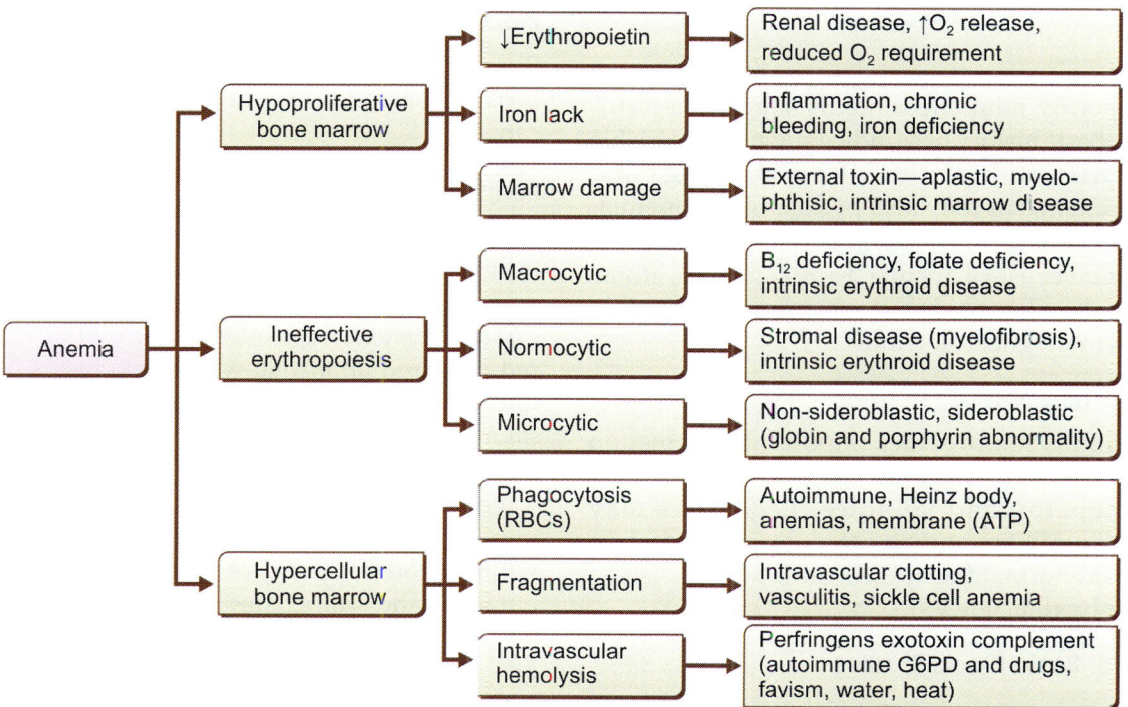

Fig. 8.10: Classification of anemia according to hypoproliferative, ineffective or hypercellular (hemolytic process) erythropoiesis.

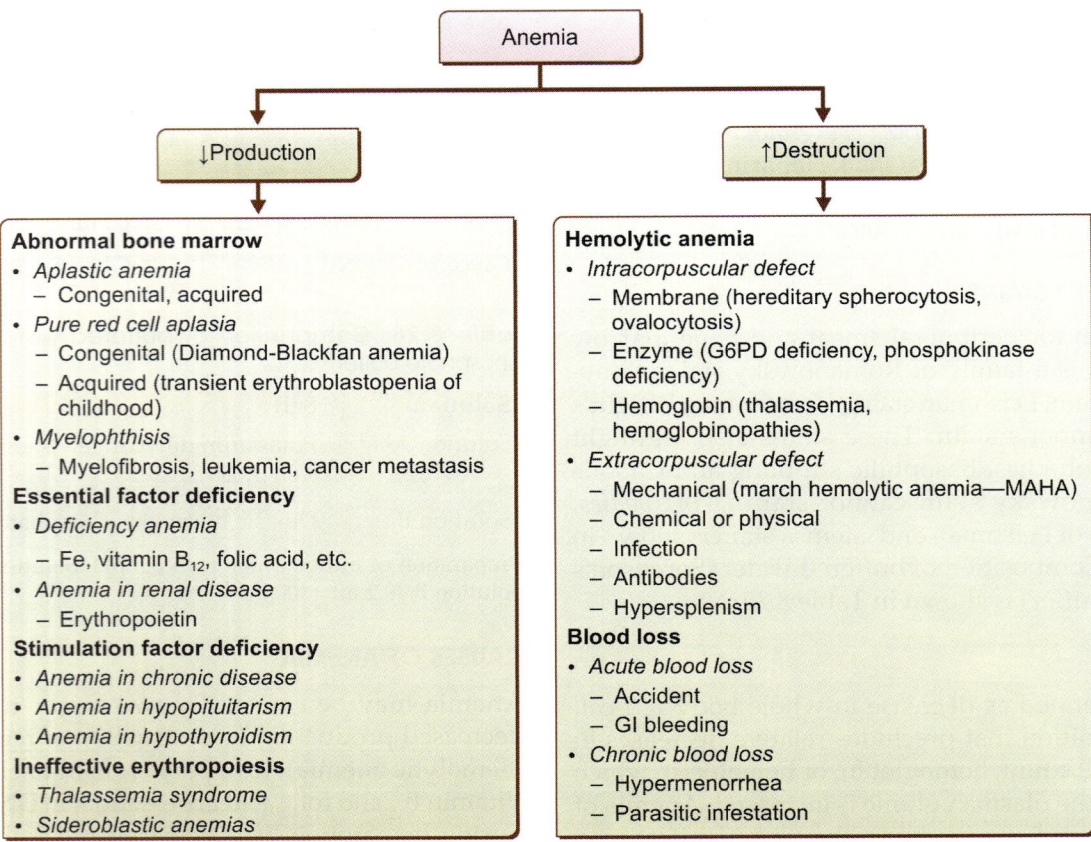

Fig. 8.11: Classification of anemia according to decreased production or increased destruction of red blood cells.

DIAGNOSTIC APPROACH

Anemia is diagnosed by incorporating information obtained from the clinical history, physical examination and laboratory evaluation.

History

Anemia in poorly nourished infants suggests a nutritional cause. Basic history of jaundice suggests a possible hemolytic process. Ingestion of certain drugs and exposure to chemicals may also predispose to anemia.

History of chronic blood loss in females and males is most important cause of anemia. Family history, ethnic and geographical considerations provide valuable information in diagnosis anemias.

Physical Examination

Physical examination provides important information such as pallor, bruising, shock, palpable spleen, lymphadenopathy and jaundice. Leg ulcers may occur in sickle cell anemia and thalassemia. Residual neurological abnormalities are seen in sickle cell disease and vitamin B_{12} deficiency.

Evaluation of Basic Blood Studies

Basic blood studies include hemoglobin, PCV, reticulocyte count and examination of peripheral blood smears. MCV, MCH and MCHC are measured by blood cell count. Main hematologic parameters are shown in Table 8.26.

Biochemical Parameters

Biochemical parameters include analysis of serum ferritin, serum iron and serum total iron binding capacity.

Peripheral Blood Smear Examination

Blood smear examination provides valuable information in studying anemias, leukemias and platelets disorders and demonstration of parasites (e.g. *microfilaria, Plasmodium* and *trypanosomes*). Scanning for nucleated red cells and abnormal white blood cells can be done under high power (40X). *In a normal well-prepared blood smear, one may see 1–3 leukocytes, 10–15 platelets and 200 red blood cells in each high power field.*

Finally, blood film should be examined under oil immersion to study the morphology of red blood cells, white blood cells and platelets. Presence of malarial parasites and spirochetes should be carried out.

Red Blood Cells Morphology

One should look for anisocytosis, poikilocytosis of RBCs, hypochromia, polychromasia, presence of

Red Blood Cells

Table 8.26: Main hematologic parameters

Hematologic parameter	Calculations	Normal range	Interpretations
Hematocrit	The ratio of RBC to serum expressed in percentage It is measured by centrifuging whole blood in a calibrated capillary tube	Men (39–49%) Women (33–43%)	Hematocrit value is low Hematocrit value is high in polycythemia
MCV of RBCs	The average calculated volume of a single RBC (hematocrit/erythrocyte count)	82–6 femtoliters	MCV is decreased in iron deficiency anemia (<80 femtoliters) MCV is increased in megaloblastic anemia (>100 femtoliters)
MCH	The average content of hemoglobin in each RBC (hemoglobin/RBC count)	26–33 pg	MCH is decreased in iron deficiency anemia and increased in megaloblastic anemia
MCHC	The average concentration of hemoglobin in a given volume of packed RBCs (hemoglobin/hematocrit)	33–37 g/dL	MCHC is decreased in iron deficiency anemia and increased in hereditary spherocytosis MCHC remains normal in megaloblastic anemia
Red blood cell distribution width (RDW)	RDW is the index to measure degree of anisocytosis (various in size of red blood cells)	11.5 to 14	RDW is increased in iron deficiency anemia, megaloblastic anemia and immune hemolytic anemia RWD remains within normal range in thalassemia

abnormal cells like target cells, burr cells, acanthocytes, fragmented red cells (schistocytes), sickle cells, spherocytes. One should also look for red cell inclusions like nuclear fragments (Howell-Jolly bodies), aggregated ribosomes (stippling) or malarial parasites. Abnormal RBCs morphology and interpretations are shown in Table 8.27 and Fig. 8.12.

Inclusions in Red Blood Cells

- *Howell-Jolly bodies:* Howell-Jolly bodies are nuclear remnants (aggregates of chromatin material) present in the RBCs and intermediate normoblasts. These are demonstrated by examination of Romanowsky stained smear in postsplenectomy/hyposplenism, megaloblastic anemia and acute hemolytic anemia.
- *Basophilic stippling:* Basophilic stippling is also known as punctate basophilia due to precipitated ribosomal RNA. Periphery of RBCs display small blue-black dots in Romanowsky stained blood films. These are demonstrated by examination of Romanowsky stained smear in lead poisoning, β-thalassemia, megaloblastic anemia, myelodysplastic syndrome and alcoholism.
- *Siderotic nodules/Pappenheimer bodies:* Siderotic nodules are aggregates of ferritin located close to the cell membrane appear as pale blue; which can be demonstrated by examination of Prussian blue stained smear in sideroblastic anemia, megaloblastic anemia, hemolytic anemia and postsplenectomy.
- *Hemoglobin H inclusions:* Hemoglobin H inclusions are β-chains appearing as golf ball shaped inclusions in red blood cells. These are demonstrated by supravital stains on peripheral blood smear in α-thalassemia and some cases of myelodysplastic syndrome.
- *Heinz bodies:* Heinz bodies are denatured globin located close to the cell membrane. These are demonstrated by examination of supravital stained smear in G6PD deficiency, poisons with oxidative agents, some hemoglobinopathies, hyposplenism.
- *Cabot's ring:* Cabot's ring is circular or figure of eight probably formed as a result of damage to RBCs stromal lipoproteins. These are demonstrated in megaloblastic anemia and lead poisoning.
- *Hemoglobin C inclusions:* Hemoglobin C inclusions are tetragonal in shape and are birefringent in a polarized light seen as a result of crystallization of hemoglobin C in 10% of RBCs following splenectomy in homozygous hemoglobin C disease.

Other Abnormalities of RBCs

- *Rouleaux formation:* RBCs are aggregated resembling a stack of coins known as *rouleaux* as a result of increased gammaglobulins in cases of multiple myeloma, kala-azar, Waldenstörm macroglobulinemia and chronic inflammatory disease.
- *Polychromasia:* Reticulocytes appear as bluish red in Romanowsky stained blood film.

Table 8.27: Abnormal RBCs morphology and interpretations

Abnormal red blood cells	Interpretations
Macrocytes	Megaloblastic anemia, liver disease, myelodysplasia
Microcytes	Iron deficiency anemia, thalassemia, sideroblastic anemia
Microspherocytes	Hereditary spherocytosis, immune hemolytic anemia, HbC disease, splenectomy, stored blood, burns
Ovalocytes (elliptocytes)	Hereditary elliptocytes, thalassemia, pernicious anemia, iron deficiency anemia, myelofibrosis
Sickle cells (drepanocytes)	Hb sickle cell disease (Hb SS), other sickle cell disease
Target cells	Hemoglobinopathy, liver disease, iron deficiency anemia, splenectomy
Schistocytes (fragmented red blood cells)	Microangiopathic hemolytic anemia, thalassemia, drug induced hemolytic anemia, mechanical hemolytic anemia, disseminated intravascular coagulation
Hypochromia	Iron deficiency anemia, thalassemia, sideroblastic anemia, chronic renal failure (sometimes)
Polychromasia	Hemolytic anemia, hypoxia, megaloblastic anemia, acute blood loss
Basophilic stippling	Lead poisoning, thalassemia
Howell-Jolly bodies (nuclear remnants)	Hemolytic anemia, megaloblastic anemia, splenectomy
Cabot ring (loop like figure of 8)	Megaloblastic anemia, lead poisoning
Heinz body (denatured globin located close to the cell membrane)	G6PD deficiency, drug/toxin induced injury, unstable hemoglobin, HbH, splenectomy
Pappenheimer's bodies (iron deposits in siderocytes or sideroblasts)	Sideroblastic anemia, myelodysplasia, splenectomy, sickle cell disease
Acanthocytes (spiny projections of the surface due to defect within the lipid bilayer of the red cell membrane may be associated with hemolysis)	Chronic liver disease (increased free cholesterol is deposited within the cell membrane), abetalipoproteinemia, splenectomy
Poikilocytes (tear shaped red cells)	Megaloblastic anemia, thalassemia, myelosclerosis, micro-angiopathic hemolytic anemia, iron deficiency anemia
Burr cells (ethinocytes)	Uremia
Stomatocytes (slit or mouth-like area)	An artifact, alcoholism, stomatocytosis
Leptocytes (RBCs with thin ring of membrane due to grossly deficient hemoglobin)	Iron deficiency anemia, thalassemia
Helmet cells	Disseminated intravascular coagulation, thrombotic thrombocytopenic purpura
Bite cells	G6PD deficiency

These appear as fine reticular network in supravital staining in cases of hemorrhage, hemolysis and response to hematinic replacement.

BONE MARROW EXAMINATION

Bone marrow aspiration is usually performed on the back of hip bone or posterior iliac crest. Bone marrow examination gives more information and morphological characteristics are better defined in Romanowsky stained blood films. Bone marrow examination study is done to diagnose iron deficiency anemia, megaloblastic anemia, leukemias, ITP, multiple myeloma, Gaucher's disease, Niemann-Pick disease, metastatic deposits and parasites. *Iron content is demonstrated by Perl's stain.*

Red blood cell abnormalities	Causes	Red blood cell abnormalities	Causes
Normal	—	Spherocyte	Hereditary spherocytosis, autoimmune hemolytic anemia, septicemia
Microcytic	Hypochromic anemia, e.g. iron deficiency, thalassemia	Fragments	DIC, microangiopathy, HUS, TTP, burns, cardiac valves
Macrocytic	Liver disease, alcoholism, oval in megaloblastic anemia	Elliptocyte	Hereditary elliptocytosis
Target cell	Iron deficiency, liver disease, hemoglobinopathies, postsplenectomy	Tear drop poikilocyte	Myelofibrosis, extramedullary hemopoiesis
Stomatocyte	Liver disease, alcoholism	Bite cell	Oxidant damage, e.g. G6PD deficiency, unstable hemoglobin
Pencil cell	Iron deficiency	Howell-Jolly body cell	Hyposplenism, postsplenectomy
Ecchinocyte	Liver disease, postsplenectomy	Basophilic stippling	Hemoglobinopathy, lead poisoning, myelodysplasia, hemolytic anemia
Acanthocyte	Liver disease, abetalipoproteinemia, renal failure	Malarial parasite	Malaria: Other intraerythrocytic parasites include *Bartonella bacilliformis*, babesiosis
Sickle cell	Sickle cell anemia	Siderotic granules (Pappenheimer bodies)	Disordered iron metabolism, e.g. sideroblastic anemia, postsplenectomy

Fig. 8.12: Abnormal RBCs morphology and interpretations.

IRON DEFICIENCY ANEMIA

Iron deficiency is the most common nutritional disorder across world. It is frequent cause of hypochromic microcytic anemia.

Decreased dietary iron, increased demand, decreased iron absorption, or blood loss lead to iron deficiency anemia.

IRON METABOLISM

Iron metabolism participates in various chemical reactions and maintains homeostasis of iron at both the systemic and cellular levels. A well-balanced diet contains sufficient iron. Normal diet contains 10–20 mg of dietary iron each day. Iron present in the ferrous form (Fe^{2+}) is mainly absorbed in the duodenum and upper jejunum. This is sufficient to balance the 1.0 to 2.0 mg daily losses from desquamation of epithelia of gastrointestinal tract and skin. Iron absorption is enhanced by citrate and ascorbate present in citrus fruits and acidic pH, while decreased by tannates (tea), phytates, tetracycline, milk and alkaline pH.

REGULATION OF IRON ABSORPTION

Heme iron derived from animal products like liver and meat is more readily absorbed. Non-heme iron (inorganic iron) derived from raw vegetables and cereals is first reduced to ferrous (Fe^{2++}) form inside enterocytes of duodenum via cytochrome B. Regulation of iron metabolism is shown in Fig. 8.13.

Binding of Fe^{2++} with DMT 1

Ferrous (Fe^{2++}) form binds to apical transporter called DMT1 (divalent metal transporter-1) encoded by SLC11A2 gene. DMT1 also participates in transfer of iron from endosomes into the cytosol of developing erythroid precursors. Mutation of SLC11A2 gene encoding DMT1 (divalent metal transporter-1) causes severe microcytic hypochromic picture in newborns. Serum ferritin level in these newborns is decreased due to defective release of iron into the blood. Patient's transferrin saturation % is increased.

Iron Transport Across Enterocytes

Absorbed iron is transported by ferroprotein and hephaestin across basolateral membrane of enterocytes. These transporter proteins convert ferrous (Fe^{2++}) to ferric (Fe^{3+++}) form. Intracellular mucosal ferritin in the enterocytes is subsequently lost during sloughing of epithelia. Iron absorption in enterocytes in duodenum is shown in Fig. 8.14.

Master Regulator

Hepcidin is main regulator of iron absorption also known as *liver expressed antimicrobial peptide* or LEAP1, encoded by the *HAMP gene*. It decreases iron absorption by degrading ferroprotein. Decrease in hepcidin level increases ferroprotein expression leading to increased iron absorption. Hepcidin also blocks the release of important source of iron from macrophages required for heme synthesis during erythropoiesis.

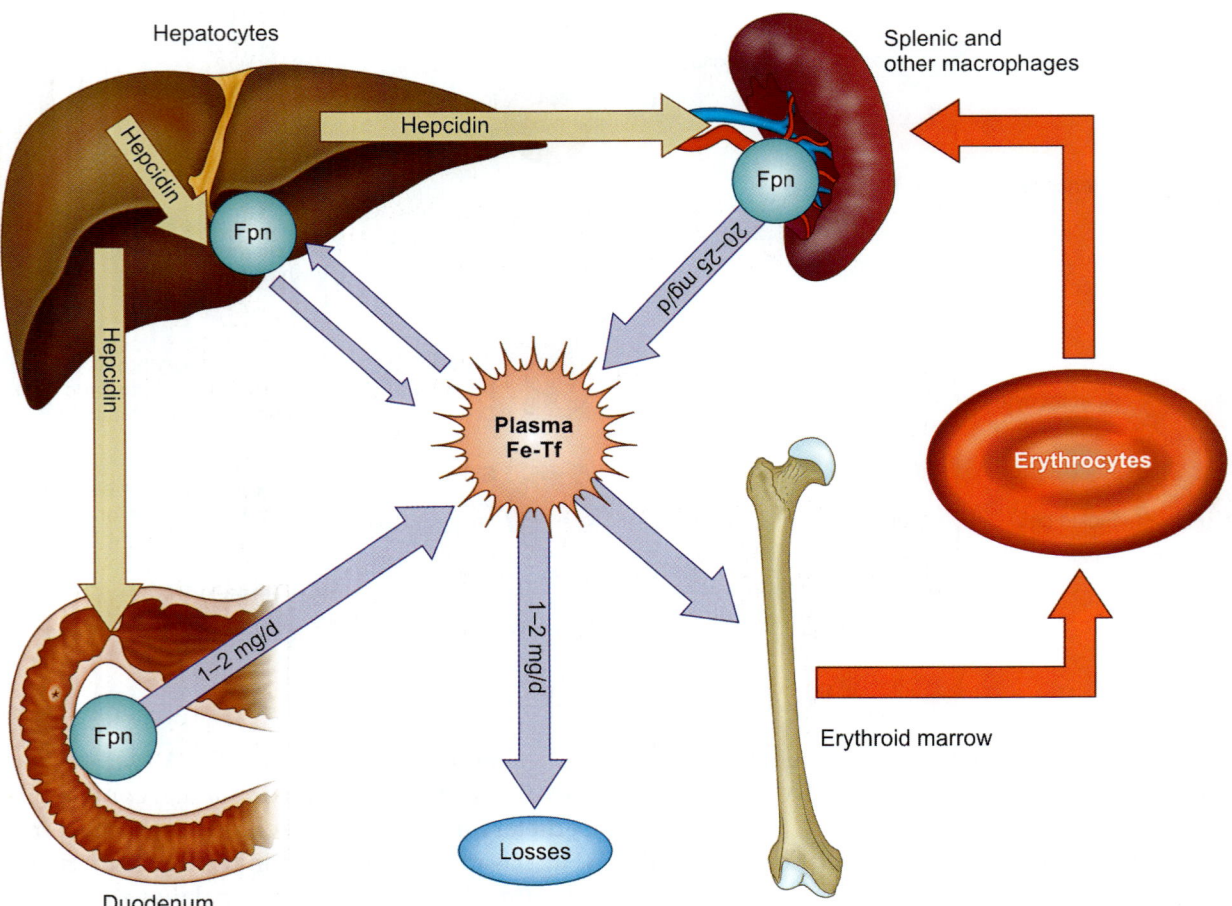

Fig. 8.13: Regulation of iron metabolism. Hepcidin (also known as LEAP1) encoded by HAMP gene is the main regulator of iron metabolism. It degrades ferroprotein (protein involved in iron absorption). It blocks ferroprotein carrying iron to spleen. It blocks iron release from macrophages required for heme synthesis during erythropoiesis.

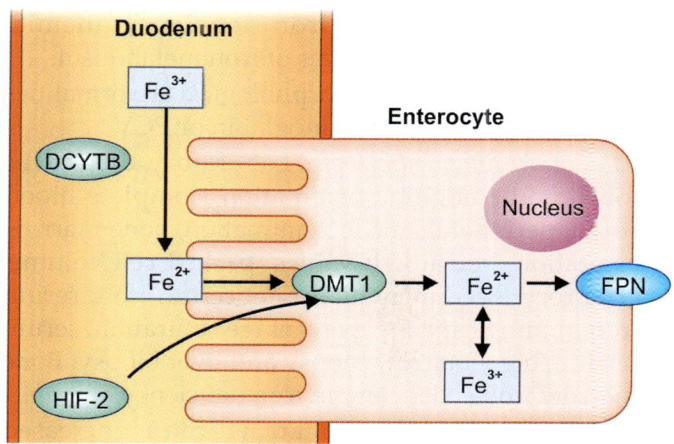

Fig. 8.14: Iron absorption in enterocytes in duodenum.

Transport in Plasma

Absorbed iron is carried in the bloodstream by the glycoprotein named transferrin. Normally, about 20 to 45% of transferrin binding sites are filled (the percent saturation). Familial atransferrinemia causes microcytic hypochromic anemia.

Storage of Iron

Serum iron (Fe^{3++}) is mainly stored in the *liver* (33%), *spleen* (33%), *bone marrow* (33%) and skeletal muscle. Iron is initially stored as ferritin, but ferritin can be incorporated by phagolysosomes to hemosiderin. Distribution of iron in adults is shown in Table 8.28. Differences between ferritin and hemosiderin are shown in Table 8.29.

Utilization of Iron

Most absorbed iron (Fe^{3++}) is utilized in bone marrow for erythropoiesis. About 10 to 20% of absorbed iron goes into a storage pool, which is also being recycled into erythropoiesis, so there is a balance of storage and use.

IRON DEFICIENCY ANEMIA

Iron deficiency anemia occurs due to dietary deficiency, increased demand during reproductive period in women, decreased absorption and chronic blood loss.

ETIOPATHOGENESIS

Dietary Deficiency

Dietary deficiency is rare except in infants, because human milk is low in iron. Newborn iron stores are depleted within the first 6 months unless it is replaced by dietary supplementation. Iron deficiency anemia is common infants within the first 12 months of life, who are non-breastfed and supplemented with cow's milk, rather than iron-fortified formula. Other uncommon causes include poor economic status, anorexia in pregnancy, poor dentition and financial constraints.

Increased Demand

During reproductive period, women require more iron due to menstrual blood loss. During pregnancy 0.5 g of extra iron is needed for growing fetus. Growth spurt during childhood requires more iron.

Decreased Absorption

Diseases that could impair iron absorption include celiac disease, achlorhydria, partial or total gastrectomy. Absorption of iron is decreased by tanrates (tea), phytates, tetracycline, milk and alkaline pH.

Chronic Blood Loss

Chronic blood loss is most common cause iron deficiency anemia in adults due to pathological disorders. Gastrointestinal bleeding may occur due to *peptic ulcer disease, GIT, carcinomas, hemorrhoids, chronic use of aspirin, hookworm disease*. Bleeding from respiratory tract occurs

Table 8.28: Distribution of iron in adults

Iron	Sites	Values [total body iron (3.0–5.0 g)]
Functional iron	Hemoglobin Essential/functional/nonavailable iron	1.5–3.0 g Myoglobin: 0.3 g Enzymes of cellular respiration: 0.05 g
Storage/available tissue iron	Ferritin, hemosiderin	1.2–2.0 g
Plasma iron	Transferrin bound iron for transport	3–4 mg

Table 8.29: Differences between ferritin and hemosiderin

Parameters	Ferritin	Hemosiderin
Color	Colorless (unstained smear)	Golden yellow (unstained smear)
Solubility in water	Water soluble	Water insoluble
Iron content	Contains less iron	Contains more iron
Storage sites	Bone marrow, liver and spleen	Storage: bone marrow, liver and spleen

due to hemoptysis and recurrent epistaxis. Renal pathology may lead to hematuria and hemoglobinuria.

Chronic blood loss in women may occur due to dysfunctional uterine bleeding, early onset of menarche, postmenopausal bleeding and cervical malignancy. Of course, hemorrhage will increase the iron need to replace lost RBCs. Hookworm infestation is a common cause of iron deficiency anemia.

CLINICAL FEATURES

Patient presents with pallor, fatigue, or dyspnea on exertion. Fatigue appears first than abnormal laboratory findings. Latent iron deficiency refers to deficient iron stores but hemoglobin remains within normal range. In severe iron deficiency anemia, associated features may include glossitis, gastritis, koilonychia (spooning of the nails) due to loss of essential iron containing enzymes (Fig. 8.15 and Table 8.30).

Plummer-Vinson Syndrome

Plummer-Vinson syndrome also known as *Paterson-Kelly syndrome* is a triad, i.e. chronic iron deficiency anemia, dysphagia due to partially obstructing postcricoid webs in esophagus and glossitis. Postcricoid esophageal web may undergo squamous cell carcinoma.

LABORATORY DIAGNOSIS

If during initial evaluation of peripheral blood smear, pathologist finds microcytic hypochromic picture, he must consider common causes of microcytic hypochromic anemia such as iron deficiency anemia, thalassemia and abnormalities of iron metabolism.

- *PCV analysis:* Extent of morphological abnormalities depend on the level of hemoglobin or PCV.
- *Laboratory diagnostic tools:* Laboratory diagnostic tools are hemoglobin estimation, complete blood count, peripheral smear examination, bone marrow aspiration, hematocrit values, packed cell volume, erythrocyte sedimentation rate, serum iron, serum iron binding capacity, percentage saturation, serum ferritin, bone marrow biopsy and liver biopsy. Bone marrow iron is deficient in iron deficiency anemia.
- *Bone marrow iron:* Bone marrow iron is increased in thalassemia and other hemoglobinopathies. In sideroblastic anemia, bone marrow evaluation reveals sideroblasts and increased iron. Hemoglobin electrophoresis is normal in iron deficiency and sideroblastic anemia.

Peripheral Smear Examination

RBCs show anisocytosis, poikilocytosis, microcytes, hypochromic red cells (central pallor area > half), ring cells, target cells, pencil cells, elliptical cells. Complete blood count will also give an indirect measure of iron stores, because the mean corpuscular volume (MCV) is decreased with iron deficiency.

Microcytic hypochromic anemia is also observed in thalassemia major, thalassemia trait, thalassemia intermedia, HbE thalassemia and HbH disease. RDW is <15% in thalassemia trait and >15% in iron deficiency anemia (Fig. 8.16).

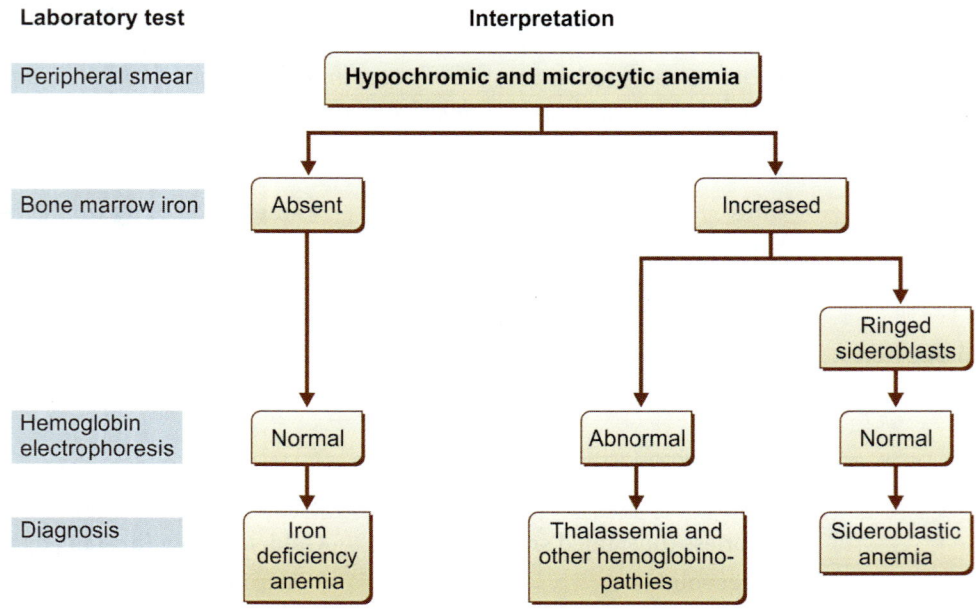

Fig. 8.15: Scheme for investigating patients with microcytic hypochromic anemia. This figure represents a convenient approach to the diagnosis of this form of anemia.

Table 8.30: Laboratory investigations of iron deficiency anemia

Laboratory method	Reference range	Iron deficiency anemia
Complete blood count and peripheral smear examination		
RBC count	Male 4.6–6 million/mm^3 Female 4.2–5 million/mm^3	Decreased
Hemoglobin	Male 13–16 g/dl Female 12–15 g/dl	Male <13 g/dl Female <12 g/dl
MCV	80–98 femtoliter (fl)	<79 femtoliter (fl)
MCH	27–32 pg	<26 pg
MCHC	32–36 g/dl	<30 g/dl
RDW-CV	11.5–14.5%	Increased
Mentzer index (children): It is used as a rough guide to differentiate between iron deficiency anemia (>13) and thalassemia trait (<13)		>13
RBC morphology	Normocytic normochromic anemia	Microcytic hypochromic cells, anisocytosis, poikilocytosis (ring cells, target cells, pencil cells, elliptical cells)
Serum ferritin	Male 20–500 µg/L Female 10–200 µg/L	<15 µg/L <10 µg/L
Serum iron	50–150 µg/dl	<30 µg/dl
Serum TIBC	250–435 µg/dl	>400 µg/dl
Serum TIBC % saturation: It is calculated by serum iron × 100/TIBC	20–45%	<16%
Bone marrow iron stores: It is graded by Galle's bone marrow aspirate smear iron grading (0–6+). Iron is demonstrated by Prussian blue reaction/Perl's reaction	1–3	0
Bone marrow sideroblasts %	40–60%	<10%
RBC-free protoporphyrin level	30–50 µg/dl	>200 µg/dl (increased)
Serum soluble transferrin receptor (sTfR)	4–9 µg/L	Increased
Flow cytometric analysis of reticulocytes: Reticulocyte hemoglobin content (CHr) and percentage of hypochromic reticulocytes		

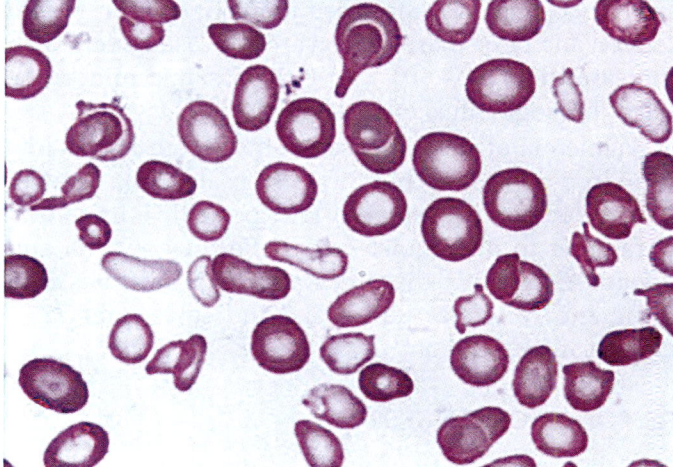

Fig. 8.16: Peripheral blood smear showing microcytic hypochromic anemia. There is central pallor area of erythrocytes. Erythrocytes show anisocytosis and poikilocytosis. RBCs are elongated known as pencil cells.

Bone Marrow Examination

Bone marrow examination is a diagnostic tool for differentiating iron deficiency from other causes of hypochromic anemia. By definition, iron deficiency anemia means that the bone marrow has no iron stores.

This lack of iron is most often determined by an iron stain. Iron granules appear as bright blue or blue-green aggregates contrasting sharply with pink stained background. Bone marrow smear shows following features (Fig. 8.17).

- *Cellularity:* Bone marrow shows hypercellular marrow as a result of erythroid hyperplasia.
- *Erythroid series:* Erythroid hyperplasia shows micronormoblastic erythropoiesis. Predominant cells are polychromatic (late) normoblasts with fraying of cell borders.
- *Myeloid series:* Myelopoiesis is normal.

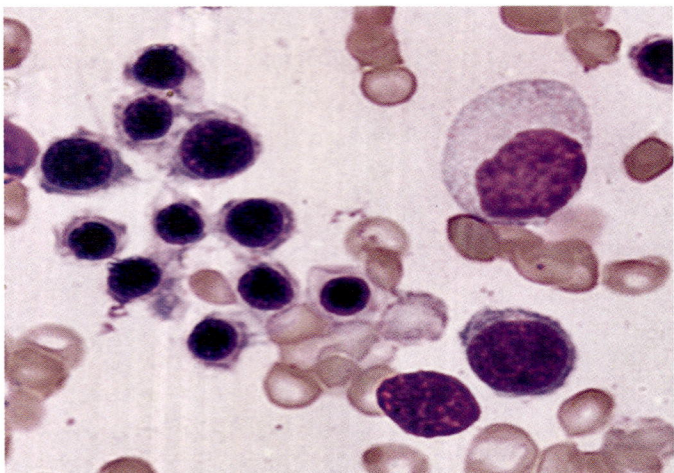

Fig. 8.17: Bone marrow aspiration showing micronormoblastic erythropoiesis.

- *Myeloid/erythroid ratio:* Myeloid/erythroid ratio is decreased due to erythroid hyperplasia.
- *Megakaryocytic series:* Megakaryopoiesis is normal.

Bone Marrow Iron

Bone marrow store study is another reliable method for estimating iron stores, but drawback is invasive technique. The amount of storage iron for erythropoiesis can be quantified by performing an iron stain (Prussian blue reaction/Perl's reaction) on a bone marrow aspiration.

Potassium ferrocyanide combines with iron forming potassium ferroferricyanide complex giving bluish coloration. Iron stores are depleted in iron deficiency anemia. Excessive iron stores can be determined by bone marrow and by liver biopsies.

Biochemical Markers

Biochemical markers comprise serum ferritin, serum iron, TIBC, % saturation of transferrin, serum transferrin receptors.

- *Serum ferritin:* Ferritin is largely derived from the storage pool of iron. Serum ferritin is the most sensitive indicator of body iron stores in iron deficiency anemia and iron overload. In normal adults, serum ferritin concentration is in the range of 150–3000 µg/dl. Concentration of serum ferritin in children is low. Serum ferritin estimation lacks specificity. It can also be elevated despite absence of iron stores in patients with liver disease, inflammatory conditions, and malignant neoplasms.
- *Serum iron:* Serum iron test gives indirect indication of iron stores. Normal serum iron concentration is the range of 60–150 mg/dl. Its concentration is below normal in iron deficiency anemia. Its concentration is increased in cases of thalassemia, hemoglobinopathy, sideroblastic anemia and history of multiple blood transfusions.
- *Serum total iron binding capacity:* Serum total iron binding capacity (TIBC) measurement may provide useful in information about iron stores. Normal range of TIBC is 250–450 µg/dl and its saturation is 33%. Measurement of TIBC is based on saturating plasma with iron and removal of excess of unbound iron by adsorbing onto chemical agent and then estimation of iron in the iron-saturated serum.
- *Hemoglobin electrophoresis:* HbA_2 and HbF determinations are very useful for differentiating thalassemia from abnormal use of iron. HbA_2 and HbF are increased in patients with β-thalassemia. Hemoglobin electrophoresis is not useful in α-thalassemia. Therefore, demonstration of HbH in RBCs on smear stained by brilliant cersyl blue is useful in α-thalassemia.
- *Other tests:* RBC's protoporphyrin level is increased due to nonavailability of iron for synthesis of heme (normal range 20–40 µg/dl). Osmotic fragility is increased.

Differential Diagnosis

Iron deficiency anemia must be distinguished from other causes of hypochromic microcytic anemia such as β-thalassemia major/minor and anemia of chronic disease. Free erythrocyte protoporphyrin level is increased in iron deficiency anemia and anemia of chronic disease; but normal in thalassemia.

In iron deficiency anemia, serum ferritin is markedly reduced (<15 µ/L) and bone marrow iron is very low or absent. In β-thalassemia major/minor, serum ferritin and bone marrow iron are increased along with increased HbF (20–90%). In β-thalassemia minor, the HbA_2 hemoglobin is increased.

In anemia of chronic disease, the serum iron is low as in iron deficiency, but the TIBC is also low. Ratio of serum transferrin receptors (sTfR) to ferritin is important parameter to distinguish iron deficiency anemia and anemia of chronic disease. Ratio >1.5 indicates iron deficiency anemia. Ratio <1.5 indicates anemia of chronic inflammation.

RESPONSE TO IRON THERAPY

Oral iron preparations in the form of ferrous salts containing 100–200 mg of elemental iron is given per day for 3–6 months in severe iron deficiency anemia. Patients may be treated by administering injectable iron–dextran or iron–sorbitol citrate.

Subjective Symptoms

Iron supplement therapy leads to improvement in symptoms due to synthesis of iron containing enzymes and globin. *Iron containing enzymes are cytochrome B, catalase, ferrochelatase countase and ribonucleotide reductase.*

Reticulocyte Count

Response to iron therapy is evaluated by reticulocyte count on day 7 of therapy. There is increase in the reticulocyte count within 7–10 days after iron therapy.

Hemoglobin Content

Hemoglobin estimation is the most accurate measure of degree of iron deficiency anemia. Hemoglobin level achieves normal range within 2 months after iron therapy. Atrophic gastritis disappears. Koilonychia (spooning of the nails) due to loss of essential iron containing enzymes disappears by 3–6 months after iron therapy.

IRON OVERLOAD

Excessive iron can accumulate acutely or chronically.

Acute Iron Poisoning

Acute iron poisoning is mainly seen in children following ingestion of 20 mg of elemental iron per kg of body weight. It occurs when free iron not bound to transferrin appears in the blood. This free iron can damage blood vessels resulting in vasodilation with increased vascular permeability, hypotension and metabolic acidosis.

In addition, excessive iron damages mitochondria and causes lipid peroxidation, manifest mainly as renal demage and hepatic damage. Early signs of iron poisoning include vomiting and diarrhea, fever, hyperglycemia, and leukocytosis. Later signs include hypotension, metabolic acidosis, lethargy, seizures, and coma. Hyperbilirubinemia and elevated liver enzymes suggest liver injury, while proteinuria and appearance of tubular cells in urine suggest renal injury.

Chronic Iron Overload

This can occur in patients who receive multiple transfusions for anemias caused by anything other than blood loss. Patients with congenital anemias may require numerous transfusions for many years. Each unit of blood has 250 mg of iron.

MEGALOBLASTIC ANEMIA: VITAMIN B_{12} AND FOLIC ACID DEFICIENCY

CLASSIFICATION

MACROCYTIC ANEMIA WITH MEGALOBLASTIC ERYTHROPOIESIS

Megaloblastic macrocytic anemia occurs due to deficiency of vitamin B_{12} and or folic acid. It is characterized by decreased DNA synthesis, with a consequent delay in DNA replication and nuclear division.

Cytoplasmic maturation is relatively unimpeded. Bone marrow shows megaloblastic erythropoiesis and manifests as nuclear-cytoplasmic asynchrony of large erythroid precursor cells with an open, loose-appearing chromatin pattern. Peripheral blood smear shows oval macrocytes, leukopenia, hypersegmented neutrophils, and decreased platelets. Major functions of folate and vitamin B_{12} and deficiency syndrome are shown in Table 8.31. Differences between vitamin B_{12} and folic acid are shown in Table 8.32.

MACROCYTIC ANEMIA WITH NORMOBLASTIC ERYTHROPOIESIS

Normoblastic macrocytic anemia occurs due to liver disease, alcoholism, hypothyroidism, postsplenectomy, pregnancy, hemolytic anemia, posthemorrhagic anemia, aplastic anemia, hypothyroidism, cytotoxic therapy, chronic myeloproliferative neoplasm (erythroleukemia), myelodysplastic syndrome and chronic obstructive pulmonary disease.

FOLIC ACID (PTEROYLGLUTAMIC ACID) DEFICIENCY

Megaloblastic anemia due to folate deficiency is similar to vitamin B_{12} deficiency. But no neurological

Table 8.31: Major functions of folate and vitamin B_{12} and deficiency syndrome

Nutrient	Functions	Deficiency syndrome
Folate	Acts as coenzyme in transfer and utilization of 1-carbon units, essential step in nuclei acid synthesis	Megaloblastic anemia
Cyanocobalamin (B_{12})	Participates in utilization of folate in nucleic acid synthesis. Essential for maintenance of nervous system	Megaloblastic anemia. Subacute combined degeneration of spinal cord in midthoracic region

Table 8.32: Differences between vitamin B_{12} and folic acid

Parameters	Vitamin B_{12}	Folic acid (folates)
Contents in foods	Dairy products Other dietary products	Liver Meat Raw vegetables, fresh fruits, and whole grain cereals
Effect of cooking	10–30% loss	70–100%
Daily requirements	2.0 μg	50–100 μg
Daily intake	5–30 μg	500–800 μg
Site of absorption	Ileum	Duodenum and jejunum
Body stores	2–5 mg	5–10 mg
Storage sites	Liver (main site), kidney, heart and brain	Liver
Functions	Participates in utilization of folate in nucleic acid synthesis Essential for maintenance of nervous system	Acts as coenzyme in transfer and utilization of 1-carbon units, essential step in nuclei acid synthesis
Central and peripheral nervous system involvement	Involved due to vitamin B_{12} deficiency (subacute combined degeneration of spinal cord in mid-thoracic region and peripheral neuropathy)	Not involved due to folic acid deficiency
Serum assays	Serum B_{12} decreased	Serum folate decreased RBCs folate level decreased

abnormalities and gastric atrophy occur due to folate deficiency in contrast to vitamin B_{12} deficiency. Folate deficiency results in megaloblastic anemia in approximately 20 weeks.

Deficiency occurs due to less intake, intestinal malabsorption and alcoholism, increased demand during pregnancy and hemolytic anemia; and chemotherapeutic agents containing folic acid antagonists. Causes of megaloblastic anemia due to folic acid deficiency are shown in Table 8.33.

SOURCE, ABSORPTION AND STORAGE

Folates are derived from leafy vegetables, fresh fruits, whole grain cereals, and dairy products. Heating and boiling of food stuffs destroy 90–95% of folic acid. Goat's milk is lower in folate than cow's milk. Daily requirement is 50–100 μg.

Daily intake is 500–800 μg. During cooking, 70–100% of folates are lost. Folate is present in diet in the form of polyglutamate. It is broken down to monoglutamate. It is absorbed in duodenum and jejunum and stored in the liver (capacity of 5–10 mg).

FUNCTIONS

Physiological state: Under physiological state, folate acts as a coenzyme in transfer and utilization of 1-carbon units, essential step in nucleic acid synthesis. Folate is taken into cells as N^5-methyl-tetrahydrofolate (THF). Reduction to tetrahydrofolate derivative is essential for folate to participate in metabolic reactions. Tetrahydrofolate must be demethylated before conjugation can occur. Demethylation is mediated by cobalamin.

Table 8.33: Causes of megaloblastic anemia due to folic acid deficiency

Mechanism	Etiology
Decreased intake	Malnutrition, elderly persons
Increased demand	Pregnancy, infancy, cancers, hemolytic anemia (hyperplasia of bone marrow)
Impaired absorption	Malabsorption syndrome, oral contraceptives, diphenylhydantoin (antiepileptic drug), alcoholism and cirrhosis
Impaired utilization	Folic acid antagonists such as anticancer drug (methotrexate, 6-mercaptopurine, 5-fluorouracil, cytosine arabinoside and vinca alkaloids)
Increased loss	Steatorrhea or tropical sprue, hemodialysis

Pathological state: If cobalamin supply is inadequate, demethylation does not occur. If N^5-THF is not conjugated, it will leak out of the cell again. Normally, dUMP is entirely converted to dTMP. Deoxyuridine gets converted to deoxyuridylate and then thymidylate. Thymine is necessary for DNA synthesis. Due to folate deficiency, dUMP is not converted to dTMP. As a consequence, dUTP concentration rises and begins to replace dTTP in DNA synthesis. It leads to impairment of DNA synthesis.

CLINICAL FEATURES

Folic acid deficiency does not cause neurological changes in contrast to vitamin B_{12} deficiency. Its deficiency causes megaloblastic anemia and neural tube defects *in utero*. It is used for treatment of chronic hemolytic anemia.

LABORATORY FINDINGS

Peripheral blood smear shows oval macrocytes, leukopenia, hypersegmented neutrophils, and decreased platelets. Normal schilling test (vitamin B_{12} absorption) indicates folic acid deficiency. Serum folate assay may be variable and should be carried out with a RBC folate assay.

VITAMIN B_{12} DEFICIENCY

Vitamin B_{12} deficiency is reflected by impaired DNA synthesis in developing precursors in the bone marrow and defective fatty acid degradation leading to excessive demyelination. Vitamin B_{12} therapeutic administration gives excellent response. Vitamin B_{12} occurs in three forms: dehydroxyadenosylcobalamin form present in diet, methyl cobalamin form in plasma and hydroxocobalamin used for therapeutic purpose (Fig. 8.18).

VITAMIN B_{12} METABOLISM

Most dietary dehydroxyadenosylcobalamin are derived from animal products. Peptic digestion releases cobalamins from the dietary vitamin B_{12}.

Binding to Salivary R Protein

Deoxyadenosylcobalamin binds with salivary R protein known as *haptocorrin* temporarily.

Release by Pancreatic Enzymes

Cobalamin is liberated in duodenum by pancreatic enzymes.

Binding with IF

Cobalamins combine with intrinsic factor synthesized by parietal cells of stomach, which becomes resistant to proteolysis.

Absorption

IF vitamin B_{12} complex binds to IF receptors (cubilin) on mucosal epithelium of ileum. Vitamin B_{12} is absorbed in ileum, which is facilitated by calcium at pH >6.

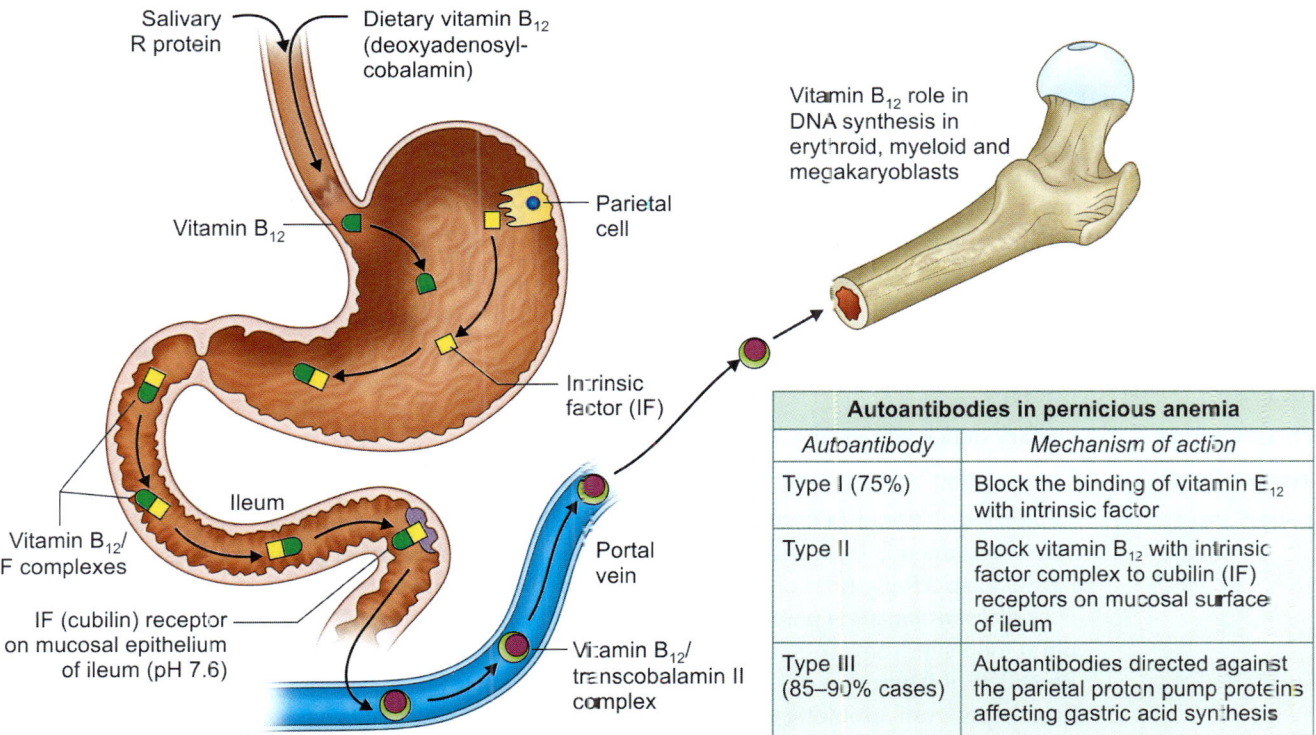

Autoantibodies in pernicious anemia	
Autoantibody	Mechanism of action
Type I (75%)	Block the binding of vitamin B_{12} with intrinsic factor
Type II	Block vitamin B_{12} with intrinsic factor complex to cubilin (IF) receptors on mucosal surface of ileum
Type III (85–90% cases)	Autoantibodies directed against the parietal proton pump proteins affecting gastric acid synthesis

Fig. 8.18: Vitamin B_{12} absorption. It also shows autoantibodies demonstrated in pernicious anemia.

Transport

Methylcobalamin form is present in plasma. Vitamin B_{12} is present in the form of methylcobalamin in plasma. It is transported by transcobalamin II (β-globulin) synthesized by liver. Congenital deficiency of transcobalamin II results in severe megaloblastic anemia.

Storage Sites

Vitamin B_{12} is mainly stored in liver in the form of dehydro adenosylcobalamin. Other storage sites are kidneys, heart and brain. Intrinsic factor synthesized by parietal cells of stomach is required for absorption of vitamin B_{12}.

CAUSES OF VITAMIN B_{12} DEFICIENCY

Deficiency of vitamin B_{12} most often occurs in strict vegetarian and chronic alcoholism and impaired absorption. Most common cause of vitamin B_{12} is impaired absorption. Causes of megaloblastic anemia due to vitamin B_{12} deficiency are shown in Table 8.34.

Increased Demand

Vitamin B_{12} deficiency may also occur due to increased demand during pregnancy or disseminated cancer; and decreased absorption due to gastrectomy or malabsorption syndromes affecting terminal ileum.

Gastric Causes

In achlorhydria, vitamin B_{12} is not released from salivary R binding proteins. Gastrectomy causes loss of synthesis of intrinsic factor by parietal cells in the gastric fundus, the clinical picture is the same as in pernicious anemia.

Pernicious anemia is the most common form of vitamin B_{12} deficiency megaloblastic anemia. It is immune-mediated disorder associated with formation of autoantibodies against intrinsic factor essential for vitamin B_{12} absorption.

Intestinal Causes

Vitamin B_{12} is not absorbed in patient, who has undergone resection of ileum. Bacterial overgrowth in a surgically induced intestinal blind loop results in the depletion of vitamin B_{12}. Broad-spectrum antibiotic therapy can result in intestinal bacterial overgrowth with vitamin B_{12} depletion. The giant fish tapeworm (*Diphyllobothrium latum*) of man, acquired by ingestion of freshwater fish, inhabits the intestine and causes vitamin B_{12} depletion.

ROLE OF VITAMIN B_{12} AND FOLIC ACID IN DNA SYNTHESIS

Vitamin B_{12} and folic acid are essential for maturation of nuclei of developing precursors in bone marrow. Deficiency of vitamin B_{12}/folic acid causes megaloblastic erythropoiesis due to decreased DNA synthesis. The nuclear maturation of developing precursors lags behind than maturation of cytoplasm. All the developing precursors in the bone marrow show abnormalities. Peripheral blood smear shows macrocytosis, hypersegmented neutrophil and thrombocytopenia.

Patient with vitamin B_{12} deficiency develops subacute combined demyelination of posterolateral columns of spinal cord in midthoracic region. Role of vitamin B_{12} and folic acid in DNA synthesis is shown in Fig. 8.19.

Role of Vitamin B_{12} in DNA Synthesis

Vitamin B_{12} (methylcobalamin) is indirectly required for DNA synthesis. It converts homocysteine to methionine and forms tetrahydrofolate, which is then converted to polyglutamate used for DNA synthesis. Vitamin B_{12} is also required for conversion of methylmalonyl CoA to succinyl CoA. Due to deficiency of vitamin B_{12}, these reactions do not take place.

Role of Folic Acid in DNA Synthesis

5,10-methylene TH_4 is required for conversion of deoxyribose uracil monophosphate (uUMP) to deoxyribose

Table 8.34: Causes of megaloblastic anemia due to vitamin B_{12} deficiency

Mechanism	Etiology
Decreased intake	Dietary deficiency, strict vegetarians
Increased demand	During pregnancy, disseminated malignancies
Impaired absorption	Achlorhydria (vitamin B_{12} not released from salivary R binding proteins) Pernicious anemia (autoantibodies against intrinsic factor essential for vitamin B_{12} absorption) Partial gastrectomy (loss of parietal cells synthesizing intrinsic factor) *Diphyllobothrium latum* parasite (inhibiting vitamin B_{12} absorption) Blind loop syndrome (depletion of vitamin B_{12} due to overgrowth of bacteria) Resection of ileum Broad-spectrum antibiotic therapy (depletion of vitamin B_{12} due to bacterial overgrowth)

Neurologic symptoms develop in vitamin B_{12} deficiency, secondary to degeneration of the posterior and lateral columns of the spinal cord

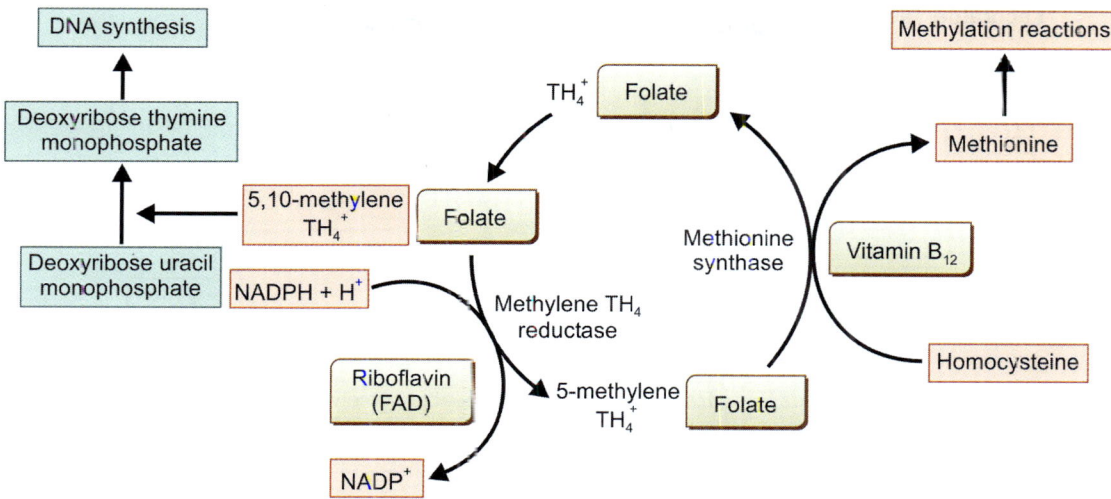

Fig. 8.19: Role of vitamin B_{12} and folic acid in DNA synthesis. 5,10-methylenetetrahydrofolate (TH_4) is required for the formation of methionine from homocysteine. Methionine, in the form of S-adenosylmethionine is required for many biological reactions including DNA methylation. Methylene TH_4 reductase is a flavin-dependent enzyme required to catalyze the reduction of 5,10-methylene TH_4 to 5-methylene TH_4.

thymine monophosphate (dTMP). Thus, deficiency of folic acid hinders synthesis of DNA.

Physiological state: Histidine is metabolized to form formiminoglutamic acid (FIGLU), which combines with tetrahydrofolate.

Pathological state: Deficiency of folic acid leads to accumulation of formiminoglutamic acid and excreted in urine. FIGLU test is performed to diagnose folic acid deficiency.

PATHOPHYSIOLOGY OF MEGALOBLASTIC ANEMIA DUE TO VITAMIN B_{12} DEFICIENCY

Megaloblastic anemia occurs due to decreased DNA synthesis, ineffective erythropoiesis and mild hemolysis as a result of intramedullary death of bone marrow precursors especially erythroid precursors. Patient may have mild jaundice due to increased serum bilirubin.

CLINICAL FEATURES

Patient presents with pallor, glossitis, central nervous system manifestations and peripheral neuropathy. Patient with peripheral neuropathy presents with spastic paraparesis, sensory ataxia and marked paresthesia leading to total paralysis of trunk and lower limbs. There is ataxic gait, hyperreflexia with extensor plantar reflexes, and impaired position and vibration sensation. There may also be associated optic atrophy and axonal peripheral neuropathy. Mechanism of neuropathy is described as under.

Peripheral Neuropathy

Physiological state: Methylcobalamin converts homocysteine to methionine, which acts as a donor in the synthesis of choline containing phospholipids, an important component of myelin. Deficiency of methylcobalamin results in decreased synthesis of choline required for myelin synthesis. Normally deoxyadenosylcobalamin converts methylmalonyl CoA into succinyl CoA.

Pathological state: Vitamin B_{12} deficiency leads to accumulation of methylmalonyl CoA, which is converted into methylmalonate and propionate. It leads to increased production of *abnormal fatty acids* like methylmalonic acid and propionic fatty acids. These fatty acids *incorporate into neuronal lipids* and cause *breakdown of myelin sheath*.

Subacute Combined Degeneration of Spinal Cord

Subacute combined degeneration of spinal cord occurs in midthoracic and cervical region. Spinal cord shows pale areas of demyelination in the posterior columns and the lateral corticospinal tracts. On histopathological examination, *spinal cord* shows *swollen myelin sheath with disintegration* and *axonal degeneration*.

LABORATORY DIAGNOSIS

Patient with macrocytic anemia should be investigated by examination of peripheral blood smear, bone marrow, reticulocyte count and therapeutic response (Fig. 8.20).

Peripheral Smear Examination

Peripheral smear examination reveals anemia, leukopenia and mild thrombocytopenia. Hypersegmented neutrophils may be demonstrated (Fig. 8.21).
- *Red blood cells:* Large number of oval macrocytes MCV >100 femtoliters is present. RBCs are normochromic

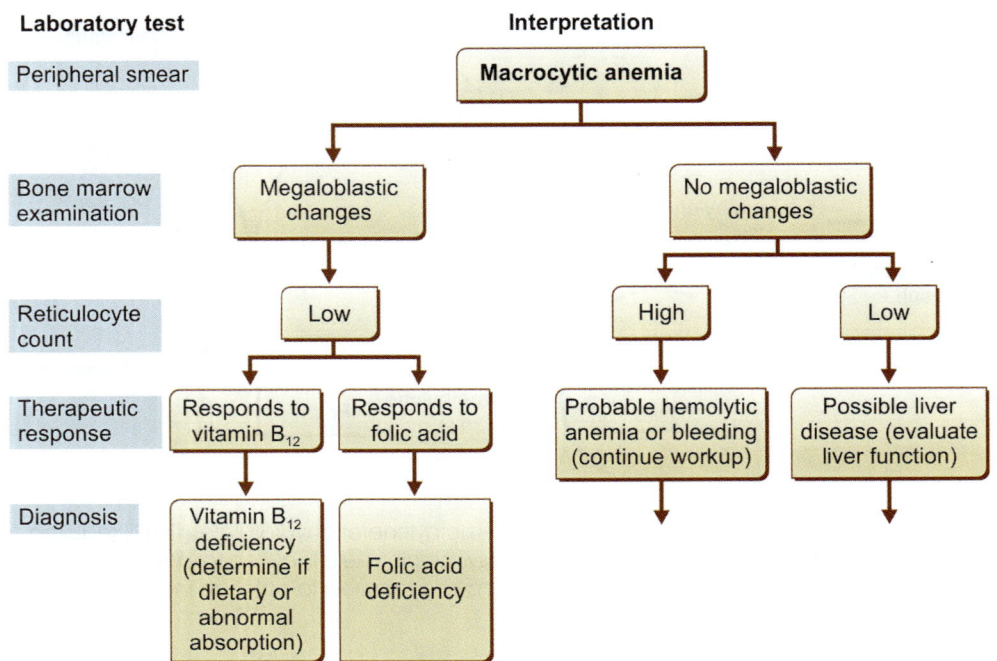

Fig. 8.20: Scheme for investigating patients with macrocytic anemia. It represents a convenient approach to this form of anemia by peripheral blood smear and bone marrow examination, reticulocyte count, therapeutic response to administration of vitamin B_{12} or folic acid.

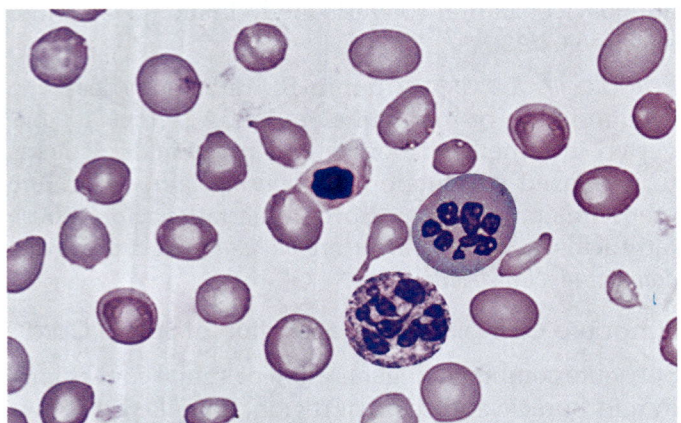

Fig. 8.21: Peripheral blood smear showing anisocytosis, poikilocytosis with macrocytosis and a tear drop cell. Hypersegmented neutrophils with >5 lobes are also present.

and show polychromasia, anisocytosis and poikilocytosis. Macrocytes are oval in megaloblastic anemia, while round macrocytes in normoblastic macrocytic anemia. Presence of tear drop cells, Howell-Jolly bodies, basophilic stippling and Cabot's rings indicate dyserythropoiesis.

- *White blood cells:* Total leukocyte count is decreased. Hypersegmented neutrophils constitute >5% of all neutrophils. These should have >5 lobes and even one neutrophil has >6 lobes. This finding indicates *shift-to-the-right* in megaloblastic anemia.
- *Platelets:* Moderate thrombocytopenia with giant platelets is seen.

- *Reticulocyte count:* Reticulocyte count is decreased as a result of dyserythropoiesis in megaloblastic anemia. Post-therapeutic response should be assessed by demonstration of increased reticulocyte count on the sixth day. Reticulocytes are round with polychromasia in peripheral blood smear.

Bone Marrow

Vitamin B_{12} and folic acid are essential for maturation of nuclei developing precursors in bone marrow. Deficiency of either of the two results in megaloblastic erythropoiesis due to decreased DNA synthesis. Abnormalities will be observed in all the developing cells in the bone marrow. Bone marrow smears show changes at all stages of RBCs development. Maturation of the nuclei of erythroid, myeloid and megakaryocytes lags behind and thus chromatin of these cells remains open *sieve-like*. Megaloblastic erythropoiesis is shown in Fig. 8.22.

Cellularity: Bone marrow becomes hypercellular with reversal of myeloid to erythroid ratio (M:E ratio 1:1) due to erythroid hyperplasia. Normal myeloid to erythroid ratio is 4:1. Ineffective erythropoiesis leads to intramedullary hemolysis of erythroid precursors. Bone marrow iron store increased due to dyserythropoiesis.

Erythroid precursors
- *Dyserythropoiesis:* Erythroid precursors show hyperplasia. Erythroid precursors are extremely large

Red Blood Cells

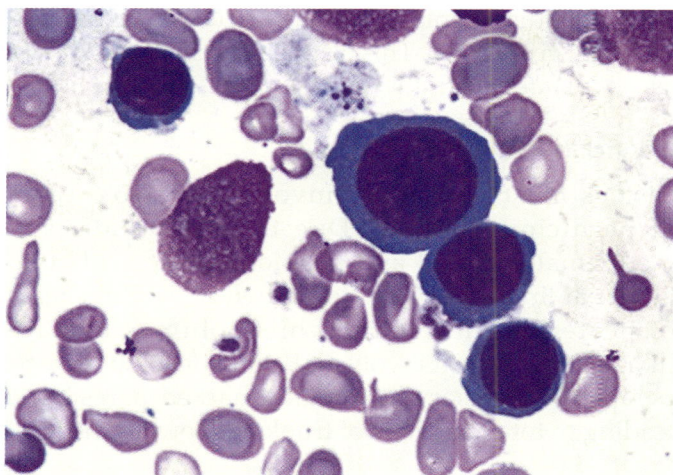

Fig. 8.22: Megaloblastic erythropoiesis. There is preponderance of early and intermediate normoblasts showing stippled nuclear chromatin (open sieve-like).

called *megaloblastic cells*. Early megaloblasts do not mature to late normoblasts. Intermediate and late erythroid precursors (megaloblasts) undergo ineffective apoptosis in the bone marrow. It is known as *dyserythropoiesis*.

- *Erythroid precursors %:* Promegaloblasts and basophilic megaloblasts constitute 50% of population indicate maturation arrest. Polychromatic megaloblasts are well marked, while orthochromatic megaloblasts are less common.
- *Morphology:* Megaloblasts show nuclear budding, irregular dumble shaped nuclei, irregular mitosis and Howell-Jolly bodies. Megaloblasts are extremely large erythroid precursors. Chromatin remains open and arranged in a fine reticular fashion to give stippled appearance. Although some of the megaloblasts are well hemoglobinized, the nucleus is still present suggesting nuclear/cytoplasmic developmental asynchrony. Oval macrocytes may also be demonstrated.

Leukopoiesis: Presence of giant band form and metamyelocytes in bone marrow give a clue megaloblastic anemia. Many myeloid precursor cells die within marrow and rest develop into giant stab forms and hypersegmented neutrophils.

Megakaryopoiesis: Megakaryocytes demonstrate nuclear hypersegmentation with open *sieve-like* nuclear chromatin. Maturation of the cytoplasm of these cells is normal. The size of these cells remains large. Most of these cells die with in bone marrow.

Other Tests

- *Serum bilirubin:* Serum bilirubin is increased due to short lifespan of macrocytes. Imbalanced nuclear and cytoplasmic maturation of erythroid precursors results in hemolysis.
- *Serum vitamin B_{12} assay:* Normal serum vitamin B_{12} is 160–900 ng/L. Serum vitamin B_{12} is decreased to <100 ng/L in vitamin B_{12} deficiency.
- *Serum folate assay:* Serum folate level is decreased in folic acid deficiency. It is determined by isotope dilution and microbial chemiluminiscence methods.
- *Striking reticulocyte response to vitamin B_{12} therapy:* Reticulocyte count is increased in megaloblastic anemia due to vitamin B_{12} deficiency, when the patient is given vitamin B_{12}.
- *Striking neurological improvement to vitamin B_{12} therapy:* Patient shows neurological improvement in response to vitamin B_{12} therapy.
- *Urinary analysis:* Methyl malonic acid level is raised in vitamin B_{12} deficiency.
- *FIGLU excretion in urine:* FIGLU test is performed to diagnose folic acid deficiency. Normally, histidine is metabolized to form formiminoglutamic acid (FIGLU), which combines with tetrahydrofolate. Deficiency of folic acid leads to accumulation of formiminoglutamic acid and excreted in urine.

TREATMENT

Shotgun therapy of may be used where the etiology is unclear. Folate, then vitamin B_{12} must be attempted to make the patient well. Intramuscular hydroxycobalamin daily for a week. Regime will depend on the cause of the anemia.

THERAPEUTIC RESPONSE

Therapeutic response to vitamin B_{12} and folic acid in patients with megaloblastic anemia is dramatic described as under.

Relief from Clinical Manifestations

Patient starts recovering from sore throat and glossitis in a day or two after therapy. Tongue becomes normal within 2 weeks.

Hemoglobin

Hemoglobin starts increasing within one week after the therap.

Bone Marrow

Megaloblastic erythropoiesis returns to normal within 10 hours of therapy.

Peripheral Blood Smear

Macrocytic anemia picture returns to normocytic morphology within 4 to 8 weeks after therapy. Platelet count returns to normal within a week.

Reticulocyte Count

Decreased platelet count in megaloblastic anemia returns to normal within 2 to 3 weeks after therapy.

PERNICIOUS ANEMIA

Pernicious anemia, an autoimmune disorder causes megaloblastic anemia. Immunoreactive T cells cause autoimmune gastritis. Autoantibodies formed adversely affecting intrinsic factor that is essential for vitamin B_{12} absorption. Demonstration of autoantibodies is highly specific for pernicious anemia. Atrophic glossitis is common finding in pernicious anemia characterized by shiny red and glazed tongue.

EPIDEMIOLOGY

Pernicious anemia is more prevalent in European persons. It is rare in India and South Asia. Females are more affected than males.

PATHOGENESIS

Pernicious anemia is considered autoimmune disorder. Its association with Hashimoto's thyroiditis and type I diabetes mellitus and Addison's disease is well established. Three types of autoantibodies are shown in Table 8.35.

CLINICAL FEATURES

Patient presents with anemia, paresthesia, glossitis, recurrent diarrhea, anorexia, weight loss, abdominal pain, mental disturbance and visual disturbance.

Atrophic Glossitis

Tongue becomes shiny red and glazed in pernicious anemia.

Chronic Atrophic Gastritis

Sections from gastric biopsy of fundus region shows features of chronic atrophic gastritis due to antiparietal autoantibodies. Replacement of parietal cells by mucin-secreting goblet cells. This histological change is known as *gastric intestinalization*.

Central Nervous System

CNS is most commonly involved in >75% cases of pernicious anemia. Due to incorporation of methylmalonic acid and propionic fatty acids into neuronal lipids, there is breakdown of myelin sheath of posterior and lateral white columns of mid-thoracic spinal cord involved. Patient develops spastic paraparesis, sensory ataxia and marked paresthesia leading to total paralysis of trunk and lower limbs.

LABORATORY DIAGNOSIS

Peripheral smear examination: peripheral blood smear shows oval macrocytes, leukopenia, hypersegmented neutrophils and thrombocytopenia.

Bone Marrow

Bone marrow shows megaloblastic erythropoiesis. It shows reversal of myeloid to erythroid ratio.

Serum Assays

Serum B_{12} levels are low. Due to diminished thymidine and methionine synthesis, serum concentration of homocysteine and methylmalonic acid is increased.

Therapeutic Response

Diagnosis of pernicious anemia is confirmed by increased reticulocyte count, following parental administration of vitamin B_{12}.

Schilling Test

Schilling test is done to establish the diagnosis of pernicious anemia. Injectable dose of vitamin B_{12} is given to saturate body vitamin B_{12} stores. Oral dose of radioactive vitamin B_{12} is given. If intrinsic factor is intact, then vitamin B_{12} is absorbed otherwise not. Its excretion is estimated in urine. Normally, >8% of oral radioactive vitamin B_{12} is demonstrated in urine. But in pernicious anemia and malabsorption syndrome, its excretion will be decreased depending upon the severity of the disease. Now oral dose of radioactive vitamin B_{12} combined with intrinsic factor is given to the patient with pernicious anemia, its excretion is within normal range. In patient with chronic renal failure not suffering from pernicious anemia, Schilling test is false positive due to impaired renal functions.

Table 8.35: Autoantibodies in pernicious anemia

Autoantibody	%	Mechanism of action
Type I blocking autoantibodies	75–80	Block binding of vitamin B_{12} with intrinsic factor
Type II autoantibodies	50	Block vitamin B_{12} with intrinsic factor (IF) complex to cubilin receptors on mucosal surface of ileum
Type III autoantibodies	85–90	Autoantibodies directed against the parietal proton pump proteins affecting gastric acid synthesis

RED BLOOD CELLS DESTRUCTION AND CLASSIFICATION OF HEMOLYTIC ANEMIA

OVERVIEW

Hemolytic anemia is produced by an increased rate of destruction of red blood cells that cannot be compensated by hematopoiesis in bone marrow. The RBC destruction may be due to intrinsic defects within red cells or extrinsic etiology. Intracorpuscular hemolytic anemia is marked by defects, most often genetically determined, in the red cell itself. Extracorpuscular hemolytic anemia is marked by defects, most often acquired such as circulating antibodies or splenomegaly. Normal lifespan of red blood cells is 100–120 days. But in hemolytic anemia, lifespan of red blood cells may be reduced to as low as 15 days. Classification of hemolytic anemias is shown in Table 8.36. Differences between extravascular hemolysis and intravascular hemolysis are shown in Table 8.37.

Red blood cells destruction may occur in the extravascular or intravascular compartments. Clinical data on the patient give clue to the diagnosis; such data include a family history of hemoglobinopathies or hereditary spherocytosis, a recent blood transfusion, malaria or splenectomy or malignant tumor.

In addition to the basic symptoms of anemia, splenomegaly and jaundice may be present. There is presence of reticulocytes higher than normal in the blood. These immature red blood cells cannot carry as much as oxygen as the fully developed red blood cells.

CLINICAL MANIFESTATIONS

Clinical manifestations of hemolytic anemia depend on duration and severity of red blood cells destruction. Clinical findings include anemia, jaundice, cholelithiasis, leg ulcers, dark or red-colored urine, cortical bone thinning, extramedullary hematopoiesis and splenomegaly.

Pallor

Depending on the severity of hemolysis, patient presents with anemia. Pallor is demonstrated in conjunctiva and tongue.

Jaundice

Hemolytic jaundice occurs due to rapid destruction of red blood cells resulting in production of excess of

Table 8.36: Classification of hemolytic anemias

Hereditary/acquired hemolytic anemia	Characteristic features
Hereditary hemolytic anemia	
Defects in red blood cell membrane	Hereditary spherocytosis, hereditary elliptocytosis, hereditary stomatocytosis, hereditary pyropoikilocytosis, hereditary xerocytosis, abetalipoproteinemia (acanthocytosis)
Defects in globin synthesis	Thalassemia (β, α and intermedia), sickling syndrome, HbD, HbC, HbE, unstable hemoglobin disease
Enzyme deficiency of glycolytic pathway	G6PD deficiency
Enzyme deficiency of red blood cell nucleotide metabolism	Pyrimidine 5'-nucleotidase, pyruvate kinase
Acquired hemolytic anemia	
Immune mediated hemolytic anemia	Autoimmune hemolytic anemia due to warm and cold antibodies, cold agglutinin disease and paroxysmal nocturnal hemoglobinuria Alloimmune hemolytic anemia (hemolytic disease of newborn)
Fragmentation syndrome (microangiopathic hemolytic anemia)	Thrombotic thrombocytopenic purpura, disseminated intravascular coagulation, malignant hypertension, severe burns, eclampsia/pre-eclampsia, diffuse metastatic tumor, severe renal disease, hemolytic-uremic syndrome, prosthetic cardiac valves, march hemoglobinuria, severe aortic valvular disease
Drugs	Methyldopa, penicillin, oxidant drugs, primaquine, dapsone
Chemicals	Naphthalene, nitrites, nitrates
Thermal injuries	Severe burns
Severe infections	*Clostridium welchii* septicemia, *Vibrio cholerae*, bartonellosis
Miscellaneous	Hypersplenism, snake venoms, celiac disease, vitamin E deficiency

Table 8.37: Differences between extravascular hemolysis and intravascular hemolysis

Feature	Extravascular hemolysis	Intravascular hemolysis
Site of hemolysis	Reticuloendothelial cells (spleen, bone marrow)	Inside blood circulation
Examples	Red blood cell membrane defect, HbS, thalassemia	Fragmentation syndrome, mismatched blood transfusion, *Clostridium welchii* sepsis, paroxysmal nocturnal hemoglobinuria
Clinical features	Anemia, jaundice	Anemia, jaundice
Splenomegaly	Present	Absent
Serum bilirubin (unconjugated)	Increased (++)	Increased (+)
Serum haptoglobin	Normal	Decreased
Serum methemalbumin	Absent	Present
Plasma hemoglobin	Absent	Present
Serum LDH	Increased (+)	Increased (++)
Urine hemoglobin	Absent	Present
Urine hemosiderin	Absent	Present
Body iron stores in spleen, bone marrow, liver	Increased	Decreased

Morphologically changes in both types of hemolysis are identical, except for the fact that erythrophagocytosis in extravascular hemolysis causes hypertrophy of the mononuclear phagocytic system, and this may lead to splenomegaly.

bilirubin. Liver is not able to conjugate excess of bilirubin. Most hemoglobinopathies are characterized by mild jaundice. Patient with hereditary spherocytosis or G6PD deficiency develop moderate to severe jaundice.

Splenomegaly

In chronic hemolytic anemia, patient presents with vague abdominal discomfort. Splenomegaly is appreciated on clinical examination.

Pigment Gallstones

Chronic intravascular hemolysis is the most common cause of pigment stones. Pigment stones are commonest and associated with hemolysis and cirrhosis. These are confined to the gallbladder. Bile is sterile.

These stones consist of large amounts of polymerized degradation product of oxidized bilirubin. Patient presents sudden pain in right upper quadrant that may radiate to scapular region, lasts for 2–4 hours following ingestion of fatty meals, alcohol, and caffeine. It is associated with nausea and vomiting.

Skeleton Abnormalities

Skeleton abnormalities occur in congenital hemolytic anemias such as thalassemia major. Erythroid hyperplasia leads to widening of dipole of skull bones (parietal and frontal bones) and maxilla. Clinical examination reveals *frontal bossing, eminent cheek bones* and *widening of teeth*. Radiograph of skull shows *crewcut appearance* as a result of widening of diploë and formation of new bone especially in young patients.

Leg Ulcers

Patient suffering from hereditary spherocytosis or thalassemia may develop leg ulcers as a result of *thrombosis of small blood vessels* and necrosis of skin. Leg ulcers are demonstrated on medial and lateral malleoli.

COMPENSATORY MECHANISMS

Hematopoiesis is increased as a consequence of hemolytic process to compensate RBCs destruction. Compensatory mechanisms are erythroid hyperplasia and reticulocytosis.

Evidence of Erythroid Hyperplasia

Increased erythropoiesis compensates in part for the shortened red cell survival in hemolytic anemia. It shows normoblastic erythroid hyperplasia in bone marrow.

There is increased number of circulating reticulocytes (newly formed red cells identified by residual stainable RNA). Because reticulocytes are larger than other red cells, the MCV may be modestly increased (up to about 105 fl). Peripheral blood smear shows nucleated red blood cells, polychromasia (large red blood cells) and leukocytosis.

Reticulocytosis

Reticulocyte count is increased following massive bleeding, acute hemolysis, and response to specific therapy in nutritional anemia and even after voluntary blood donation.

Reticulocyte count is used to assess the capacity of the bone marrow to increase RBC production in response to increased demand. Reticulocytes are demonstrated by supravital stains such as new methylene blue (best stain) and brilliant cresyl blue.

PERIPHERAL BLOOD SMEAR FINDINGS

Peripheral blood smear examination provides valuable information about hemolytic anemia. Red blood cells exhibit polychromasia and increased reticulocyte count. Normoblasts are demonstrated in peripheral blood smear following moderate to severe hemolysis. One must look for spherocytes, sickle cells, target cells, fragmented red cells and acanthocytes. Neutrophilia with shift to left with myelocytes and metamyelocytes is seen. Thrombocytosis is demonstrated in acute hemolysis.

EXTRAVASCULAR RBCs DESTRUCTION

After 100–120 days, RBCs are destroyed by reticuloendothelial system and liberate hemoglobin, which dissociates to form heme (porphyrin and iron) and globin.

Iron goes to iron storage sites for further utilization. Globin goes to amino acid pool. Iron goes to iron storage (e.g. bone marrow, spleen and liver) for reutilization. Metabolic products of porphyrin such as urobilinogen and stercobilinogen are excreted via urine and stool respectively. Total normal bilirubin level is 0.3–1.0 mg/dl. Simplified pathway of bilirubin metabolism is shown in Fig. 8.23.

Serum Bilirubin

Absence of jaundice does not exclude hemolytic anemia. Increased red cell destruction results in liberation of hemoglobin or its degradation products. Hemolytic anemia is not accompanied with pruritus. Hyperbilirubinemia may lead to pigment-containing gallstones as a late complication.

Clinical jaundice is not apparent until the serum bilirubin exceeds 40 micromol per liter. Urine contains increased level of urobilinogen. Aqueous diazotized sulphanilic acid's reacts only with conjugated bilirubin, giving red color.

Addition of alcohol (methanol) frees the albumin, hence, rest of the unconjugated bilirubin reacts with the reagent. Bilirubin is destroyed by direct sunlight or ultraviolet light including fluorescent light.

Increased Excretion of Urobilinogen

Extravascular red blood cell destruction leads to increased excretion of urobilinogen in urine giving high-colored urine.

Increased Excretion of Stercobilinogen

Extravascular red blood cell destruction leads to increased excretion of stercobilinogen exhibiting dark-colored stool.

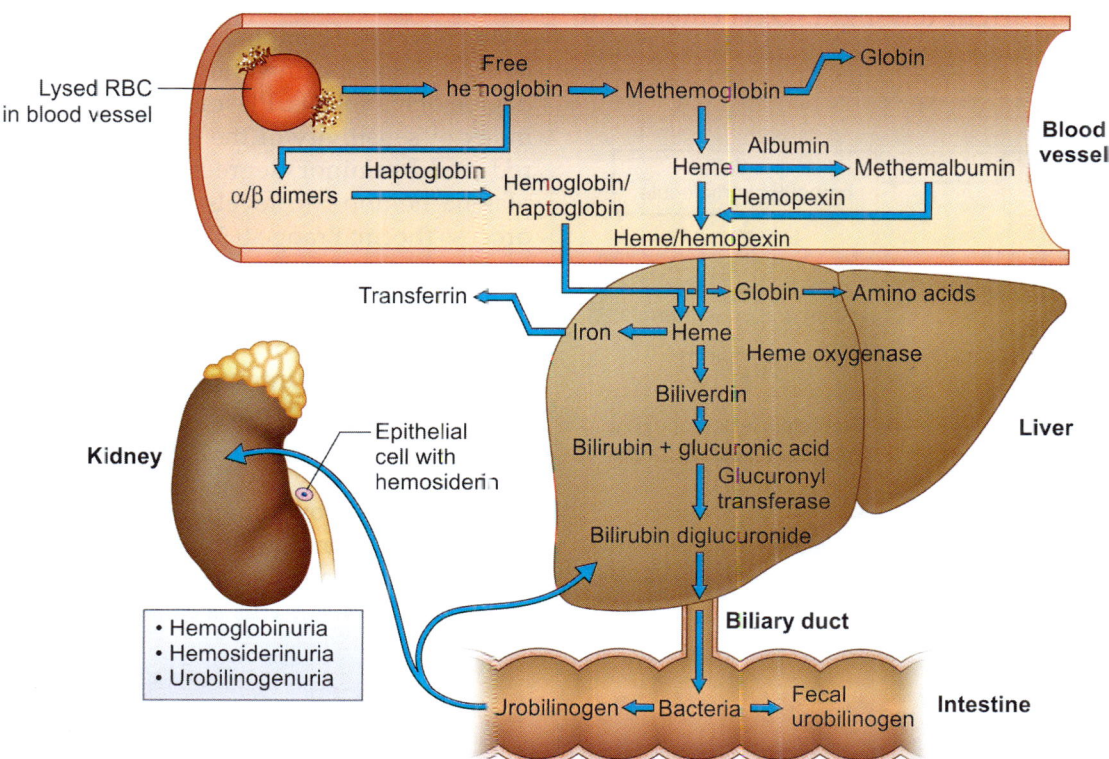

Fig. 8.23: Simplified pathway of bilirubin metabolism. Hemolytic anemia leads to increased biliary excretion of bilirubin.

Increased Iron Stores

Hemolytic anemia due to extravascular etiology leads to excess release and deposition of iron in tissues.

INTRAVASCULAR RBCs DESTRUCTION

Estimation of serum haptoglobin, hemopexin and methemalbumin provide good indicators of severity of intravascular hemolytic process. Indicators of intravascular hemolytic anemia are shown in Fig. 8.24.

BIOCHEMICAL ALTERATIONS

Hemoglobinemia

Normal free hemoglobin in plasma is 0.6 mg/dl. When free hemoglobin is markedly raised, the color of the plasma becomes pink or red. When rise of free hemoglobin is moderate, the color is lacking due to low hemoglobin concentration. Hemoglobin in plasma is detected by benzidine test.

Presence of other pigments such as bilirubin gives yellow color and methemoglobin exhibits brownish color. Methemoglobin is dark brown in acidic urine, while oxyhemoglobin is bright red in alkaline urine.

Hemoglobinuria

Hemoglobinuria occurs in severe intravascular hemolysis. Hemoglobin in urine is demonstrated by spectroscopy in bright day light. Oxyhemoglobin appears in the yellow-green, while methemoglobin in the red. It must be distinguished from hematuria.

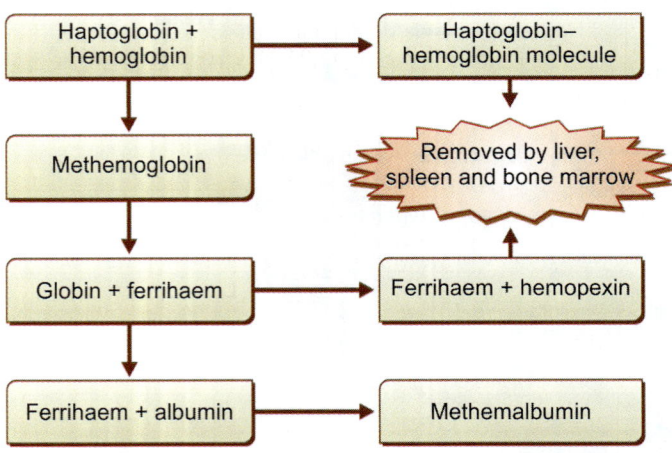

Fig. 8.24: Indicators of intravascular hemolytic anemia.

In hematuria, intact RBCs are seen in freshly voided specimens. *In vitro* lysis of the red blood cells in hematuria results in artificial hemoglobinuria.

Hemosiderinuria

Hemosiderinuria is a valuable sign for chronic hemolytic process. It persists for several weeks after a hemolytic episode. Examination of urinary sediment stained by Prussian blue reaction demonstrates iron-containing renal tubular cells.

Decreased Haptoglobin Level in Serum

Haptoglobin is α_2 glycoprotein synthesized by liver. It combines with any hemoglobin in plasma and prevents its excretion in urine. Haptoglobin–hemoglobin molecule is removed by liver, spleen and bone marrow. Hence, plasma haptoglobin levels are decreased with episode of hemolysis, which come to normal within 3 days. Decreased levels of plasma haptoglobin are very sensitive indicator of mild hemolytic process (normal range 0.5–1.5 g/L).

Plasma Hemopexin

Hemopexin is a glycoprotein synthesized by liver. It does not bind hemoglobin rather binds only ferrihaem. When hemolysis occurs, hemoglobin liberated is reduced to methemoglobin, which splits into ferrihaem and globin.

Globin goes to amino acid pool for further utilization. While ferrihaem combines with hemopexin and cleared by liver. Hemopexin value is decreased only in severe degree of hemolysis. Plasma hemopexin level is a good index of sensitivity of the hemolytic process as it not reduced by minor degrees of hemolysis. Decreased plasma hemopexin levels indicate severe hemolytic process (normal range 0.5–1.0 g/dl).

Plasma Methemalbumin

Methemalbumin occurs in hemolytic anemia, especially when hemolysis is intravascular. Methemalbumin has a characteristic absorption in the red band (at 624 nm) which may be seen by means of spectroscope. Now cover the sample with a layer of ether, and add 1/10th of saturated yellow ammonium sulphide and mix. It leads to formation of an ammonium hemochromatogen, a more intense band can be seen in the green part of the spectrum (588 nm). This is called *Schumm's test*.

HEREDITARY SPHEROCYTOSIS, OVALOCYTOSIS AND STOMATOCYTOSIS

HEREDITARY SPHEROCYTOSIS

Physiological state: Normal biconcave shape and flexibility of red blood cells are maintained by the presence of cytoskeleton proteins composed of spectrin, ankyrin, actin, protein 4.1 and protein 3 (Fig. 8.25).

Pathological state: Hereditary deficiency of these cytoskeleton proteins leads to reduced membrane stability, loss of lipid bilayer membrane and microspherocytes formation. These microspherocytes fail to pass through interendothelial fenestrations of sinusoids and get trapped in spleen.

Due to accumulation of lactic acid in these microspherocytes disrupts sodium pump resulting in sequestration in the spleen and chronic extravascular hemolysis. Lifespan of red blood cells is decreased to 10–20 days. Hereditary spherocytosis is autosomal dominant (more common and less severe) or recessive disorder (less common but more severe). Pathophysiology of hereditary spherocytosis is shown in Fig. 8.26.

GENE MUTATIONS

Isolated or combined mutation of spectrin and ankyrin genes account for most cases. Isolated mutation occurs in band 3 or band 4.2. Glycophorin is not involved in the pathogenesis of hereditary spherocytosis. Hereditary spherocytosis (HS) and inherited defects of cytoskeleton proteins are shown in Table 8.38.

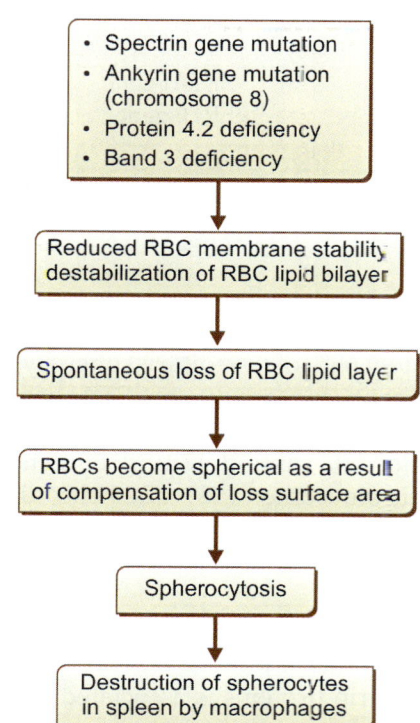

Fig. 8.26: Pathophysiology of hereditary spherocytosis.

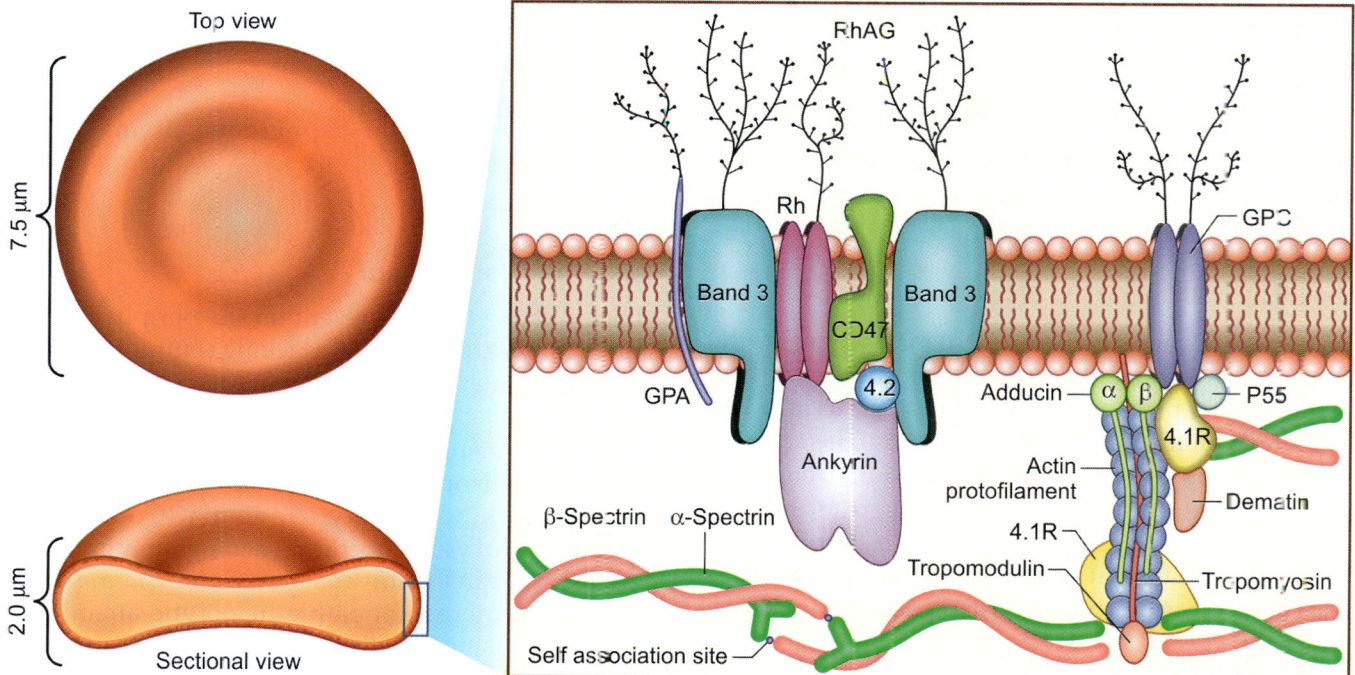

Fig. 8.25: Cross-sectional side view of the biconcave structure of red blood cell. Diagram shows cytoskeleton and flexible spectrin, ankyrin, actin, protein 4.1 and protein 3. Vertical interaction proteins include spectrin, ankyrin, protein 4.2 and band 3. Horizontal interaction proteins include actin, protein 4.1 and adducin.

Table 8.38: Hereditary spherocytosis (HS) and inherited defects of cytoskeleton proteins

Encoding proteins	Gene	Location on chromosome	Autosomal dominant/recessive hereditary spherocytosis	Percentage
Spectrin	SPTAI gene SPTB gene	1q22–q23 14q23–q24.1	Autosomal dominant Autosomal dominant	65% cases 30% cases
Ankyrin	ANK1 gene	8p11.2	Autosomal dominant	Majority of cases
Band 3 (anion channel)	SLC4A1	17q21	Autosomal dominant	25%
Band 4.2	EPB42	15q15–q21	Autosomal recessive	3% (common in Japan)

Spectrin Proteins

Approximately 65% of hereditary spherocytosis/autosomal dominant cases are due to SPTAI gene mutation located on chromosome 1q22–q23 encoding spectrin proteins, and 30% cases due to SPTB gene mutation located on chromosome 14q23–q24.1 encoding spectrin proteins. α-Spectrin mutation correlates with severity of hemolysis and osmotic fragility.

Ankyrin Proteins

ANK1 gene mutation located on chromosome 8p11.2 encoding ankyrin proteins is associated with majority of hereditary spherocytosis (autosomal dominant). It is most common mutation.

Band 3 (Anionic Channel)

Band 3 is ionic transport protein. SLC4A1 gene mutation located on chromosome 17q21 encoding *band 3* (anion channel) accounts for 25% of hereditary spherocytosis (autosomal dominant).

Band 4.2 Proteins (Pallidin)

EPB42 gene mutation located on chromosome 15q15–q21 encoding *band 4.2* accounts for 3% of hereditary spherocytosis/autosomal recessive. Protein 4.2 deficiency is common in Japan.

CLINICAL FEATURES

Due to chronic hemolysis of microspherocytes in the spleen, patient presents with intermittent jaundice, splenomegaly, pigmented gallstones (50%), mild to moderate anemia and chronic leg ulcers. The severity of the disease is quite variable among individuals.

Patient may develop aplastic crisis due to bone marrow depression by Parvovirus B19 infection. Splenectomy is the treatment of choice. Microspherocytes persist in blood circulation in postsplenectomy patients.

Age and Sex

Hereditary spherocytosis manifests in neonates, children and adults affecting both sex groups.

Anemia

Patient presents with mild to moderate anemia. Severe anemia rarely occurs. Aplastic crisis occurs due to bone marrow depression by Parvovirus B19 infection. Majority of patients present with moderate anemia showing 15–30 microspherocytes/HPF and splenomegaly.

Jaundice

Intermittent jaundice is the most common presentation in children. Pregnancy, fatigue and infection may aggravate jaundice.

Splenomegaly

Mild to moderate splenomegaly is most common findings in hereditary spherocytosis as a result of trapping of microspherocytes in the red pulp of the spleen.

Gallstones

Pigment stones are most often demonstrated during first to second decade in 50 to 75% of cases.

Leg Ulcers

Patient with hereditary spherocytosis may rarely develop leg ulcers.

LABORATORY DIAGNOSIS

Peripheral Blood Smear

Microspherocytes are present on the peripheral blood smear. These are small RBCs lacking central pallor area. Normocytic normochromic anemia and polychromasia are seen. Platelet count is within normal range (Fig. 8.27).

Hereditary spherocytosis should be differentiated from other disorders showing spherocytosis. These include immune hemolytic anemia (Coombs' test positive), paroxysmal nocturnal hemoglobinuria, G6PD deficiency, transfusion reactions, *Clostridium sepsis*, snakebites, microangiopathic hemolytic anemia and malarial parasitic infection.

Hemoglobin

Hemoglobin is low depending on degree of hemolysis.

Red Blood Cells

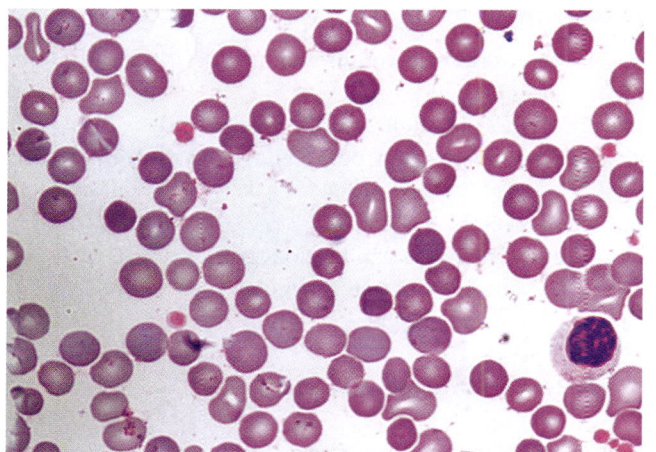

Fig. 8.27: Hereditary spherocytosis showing darkly stained microspherocytes lacking central pallor.

Reticulocyte Count
Reticulocyte count is increased (>8%).

Hematocrit Values
MCHC is often increased. MCH is within normal range. MCV is decreased.

Bone Marrow
Bone marrow is hypercellular due to normoblastic erythroid hyperplasia. Myelopoiesis and megakaryopoiesis are within normal range.

Serum Bilirubin
There is increase in indirect (unconjugated) serum bilirubin, but not direct (conjugated). The jaundice is acholuric (no bilirubin in the urine, so bilirubinuria would not be expected).

Osmotic Fragility
Osmotic fragility is most reliable diagnostic test for hereditary spherocytosis. It is performed to measure the erythrocyte's resistance to hemolysis by osmotic stress. It mainly depends on volume of the cell, surface area and membrane function. Osmotic fragility test on human red blood cells is shown in Fig. 8.28.

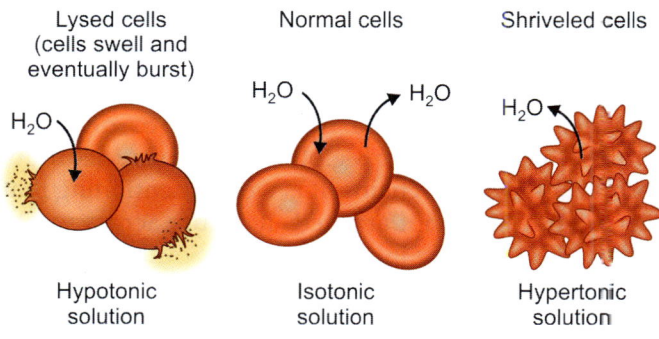

Fig. 8.28: Osmotic fragility test on human red blood cells.

Physiological state: Normal cells begin to hemolyze at 0.5% NaCl concentration. Hemolysis is complete at about 0.3%. There is increased erythrocyte osmotic fragility to hypotonic saline.

Pathological state: Red blood cells are incubated in varying concentrations of hypotonic NaCl solution. The erythrocytes take in water in an effort to achieve osmotic equilibrium. Further uptake of water by red blood cells results in rupture of membrane. Osmotic fragility curve demonstrates a shift-to-the-right in hereditary spherocytosis, and autoimmune hemolytic anemia.

Coombs' Test
Spherocytes present in the peripheral blood smear and along with family history, strongly suggest a diagnosis of hereditary spherocytosis. Spherocytes are also observed in warm antibody autoimmune hemolytic anemia and G6PD deficiency. Coombs' test is negative in hereditary spherocytosis, but positive in autoimmune hemolytic anemia.

Flow Cytometry Test
Flow cytometry is based on eosin-5-maliemide test.

HEREDITARY OVALOCYTOSIS
Hereditary ovalocytosis (elliptocytosis) is an autosomal dominant disorder affecting assembly of membrane associated cytoskeleton horizontal proteins band 3 (anion channel) and band 4.1. It is characterized by elongated, oval red cells in peripheral blood smears. It is found in some populations residing in Melanesia. There may be mild hemolysis during infancy. Homozygous persons may rarely develop chronic hemolytic anemia. It does not cause anemia in most of the cases.

GENE MUTATIONS
Hereditary ovalocytosis occurs due to gene mutations encoding band 3 or band 4.1. Hereditary ovalocytosis and inherited defects of cytoskeleton proteins are shown in Table 8.39.

Band 3 (Anion Channel)
SLC4A1 gene mutation (polymorphic mutation-deletion of 9 amino acids) located on chromosome 17q21 encoding band 3 (anion channel) is associated with autosomal dominant ovalocytosis in South-East Asia. The patients are clinically symptomatic and resistant to *Plasmodium falciparum*.

Band 4.1
EPB41 gene mutation located on 1p33–p34.2 encoding band 4.1 accounts for 5% cases. Severe hemolysis occurs in homozygotes but no hemolysis in heterozygotes (Table 8.40).

Table 8.39: Hereditary ovalocytosis and inherited defects of cytoskeleton proteins

Encoding proteins	Gene	Location on chromosome	Disorder	Percentage and comments
Band 3 (anion channel)	SLC4A1	17q21	Autosomal dominant	Polymorphic deletion of 9 amino acids. South-East Asian persons are asymptomatic and resistant to *Plasmodium falciparum*
Band 4.1	EPB41	1p33–p34.2	Autosomal dominant	5% cases. Severe hemolysis in homozygotes. No hemolysis in heterozygotes

Table 8.40: Hereditary stomatocytosis and inherited defects of cytoskeleton proteins

Encoding proteins	Gene	Location on chromosome	Disorder	Percentage and comments
Band 3 (anion channel)	SLC4A1	17q21	Hereditary stomatocytosis	Certain specific missense mutations shift protein function from anion exchanger to cation conductance

HEMATOLOGICAL FINDINGS

Hemoglobin, MCV, MCH, MCHC and osmotic fragility are within normal range. Anemia is seen in a few patients. Peripheral blood smear examination shows ovalocytes constituting 20–90% of red blood cells (Fig. 8.29).

HEREDITARY STOMATOCYTOSIS

SLC4A1 gene mutation located on 17q21 encoding band 3 (anion channel) causes shift protein function from anion exchanger to cation conductance leading to stomatocytosis.

It provides protection against malarial infection. Hereditary stomatocytosis and inherited defects of cytoskeleton proteins are shown in Table 8.40.

Peripheral Blood Smear

Peripheral blood smear examination shows stomatocytes with central slit shaped area (Fig. 8.30).

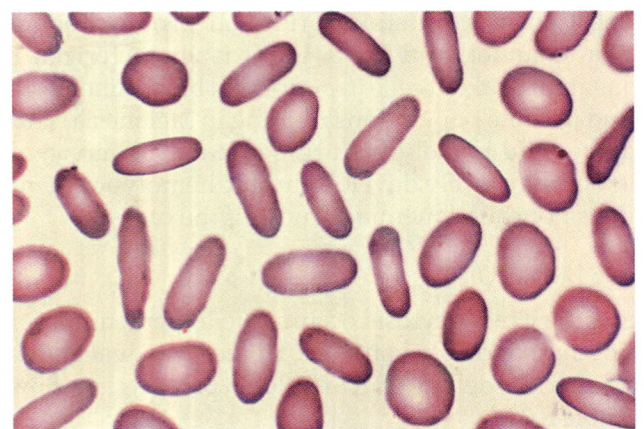

Fig. 8.29: Hereditary ovalocytosis showing large number of ovalocytes.

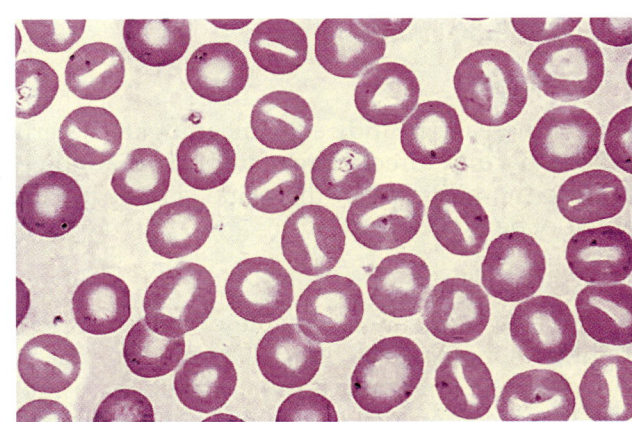

Fig. 8.30: Hereditary stomatocytosis showing stomatocytes with central slit shaped area. These stomatocytes are also demonstrated in liver disease.

THALASSEMIAS

OVERVIEW

Physiological state: A normal hemoglobin molecule contains four globin chains, consisting of two α- and two β-chains. Three normal variants of hemoglobin are encountered, based on the nature of the non-α-chains. Hemoglobin A (α_2, β_2) accounts for 95 to 98% of the total hemoglobin in adults; only minor amounts of HbF (α_2, γ_2) and HbA$_2$ (α_2, δ_2) are present.

Pathological state: Thalassemia is group of genetic disorders characterized by complete or deficient synthesis of either α- or β-globin chains of structurally normal hemoglobin chains. It is worth mentioning that haem synthesis is not affected. It occurs across world with high frequency in Africa, India, South-East Asia, and the Mediterranean area.

Classification: This disease is classified according to the type of chains that are missing. If the α-chains are not synthesized, it is called α-*thalassemia*; if the β-chains are missing, it is called β-*thalassemia*. Homozygous β-thalassemia is a more serious disease and silent carrier for α-thalassemia is asymptomatic. Thalassemia intermedia is double heterozygotes and less severe.

Classification of thalassemias is shown in Fig. 8.31 and Table 8.41.

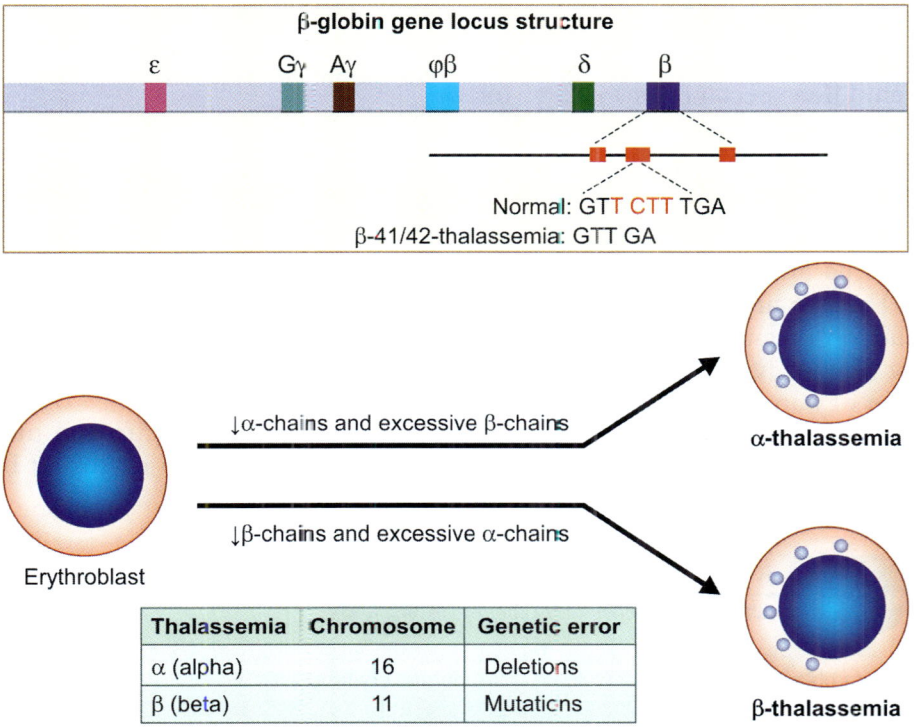

Fig. 8.31: Classification of thalassemias.

Table 8.41: Classification of thalassemias

Clinical disease	Globin chains present	Features
β-thalassemia variants		
Thalassemia major	Homozygous β_0/β_0 Homozygous β^+/β^+	Microcytic hypochromic anemia due to severe hemolysis Hepatosplenomegaly Bone marrow hyperplasia Blood transfusion dependent Skeletal abnormalities Iron overload due to repeated blood transfusion
Thalassemia minor	Heterozygous β^+/β_0 Heterozygous β_0/β	Mild anemia with hypochromic cells Moderate reduction of HbA Increased HbA_2
Thalassemia intermedia	Double heterozygotes	Moderate severe hemolytic anemia Not blood transfusion dependent
α-thalassemia variants		
Silent carrier	Deletion of single α-gene on chromosome 16	Asymptomatic but no abnormality
α-thalassemia trait	Deletion of two α-genes on chromosome 16	Asymptomatic but mild hemolytic anemia with some microcytic red blood cells
Hemoglobin H disease (β_4)	Deletion of three α-genes on chromosome 16	Moderate hemolytic anemia with microcytic hypochromic HbH is derived from tetramers of β-chains
Hydrops fetalis	Deletion of four α-genes on chromosome 16	Lethal *in utero*

8 Section II: Hematology

β-THALASSEMIA MAJOR

β-thalassemia major is also known as *Mediterranean anemia* or *Cooley anemia*. In transfusion-dependent anemia, morbidity and mortality occur due to cardiac failure as a result of expansion of plasma volume and iron overload. It is a serious disease which often results in death during childhood unless frequent blood transfusions are given. Life expectancy is 15–25 years with or without treatment death occurs by 5 years of age.

PATHOPHYSIOLOGY

The lack of β-chains leads to accumulation of unpaired α-chains (which are free and uncombined) within developing red cells. These chains aggregate and result in premature destruction of maturing erythroblasts within bone marrow (ineffective erythropoiesis) and premature destruction of abnormal mature red cells in the spleen (hemolysis). Serum ferritin and serum iron levels are increased. Excess of iron is deposited in liver, heart, spleen, hypothalamus and endocrine glands (pituitary, islets of Langerhans' and parathyroid glands). Pathophysiology of β-thalassemia major is shown in Fig. 8.32.

Point Mutations

β-thalassemia occurs due to various point mutations on the globin gene clusters. Suppression of β-globin occurs as a consequence of single nucleotide substitution in the promoter region or messenger RNA processing region.

Gene mutation at terminator region causes β-thalassemia characterized by absence of synthesis of β-chains. On the other hand, gene mutation in the splicing region cause $β_1$ thalassemia characterized by some synthesis of β-chains. Diagrammatic representation of the β-globin gene is shown in Fig. 8.33.

Bone Marrow Changes

Development of anemia stimulates erythropoietin synthesis resulting in erythroid hyperplasia in bone

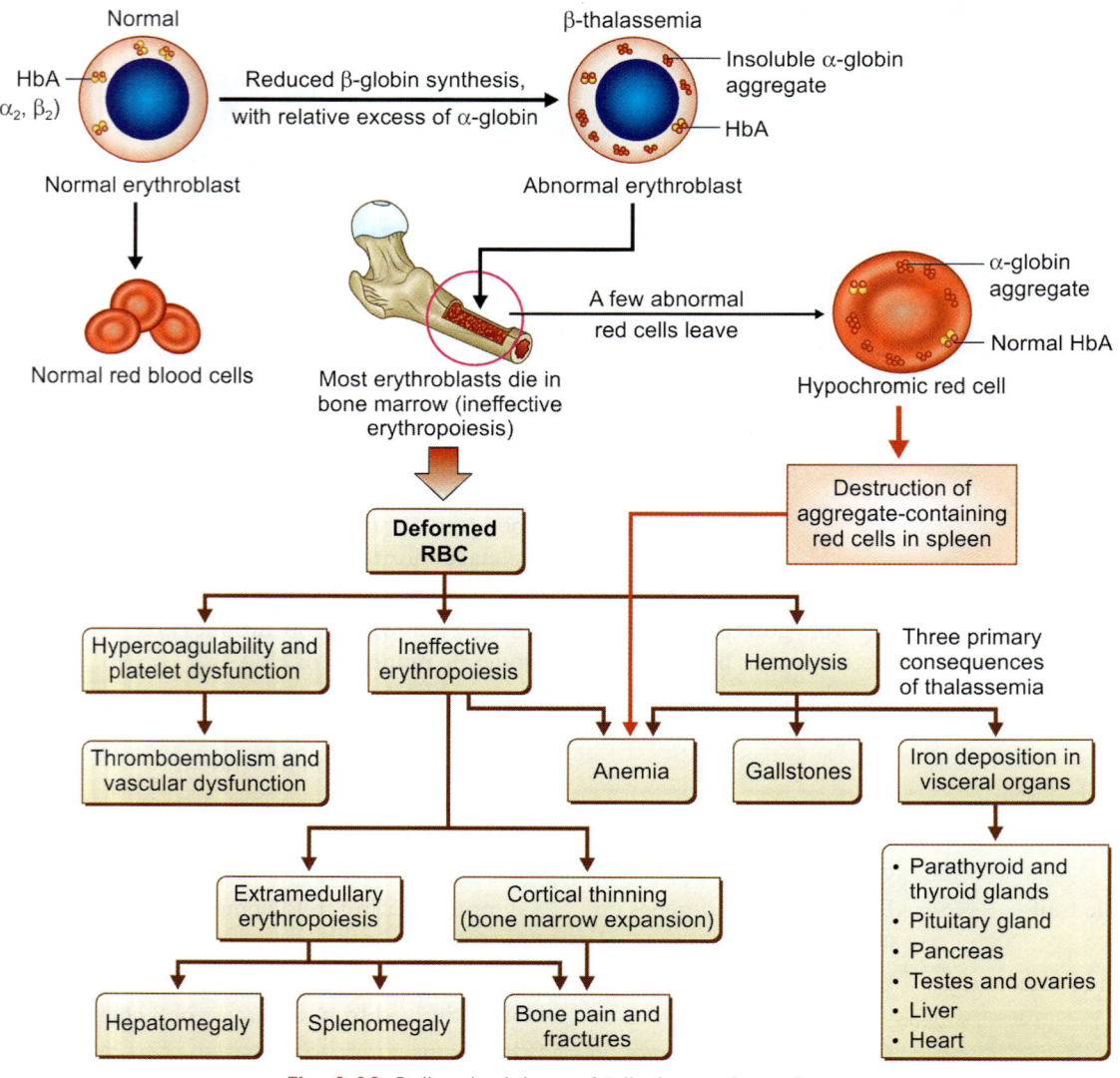

Fig. 8.32: Pathophysiology of β-thalassemia major.

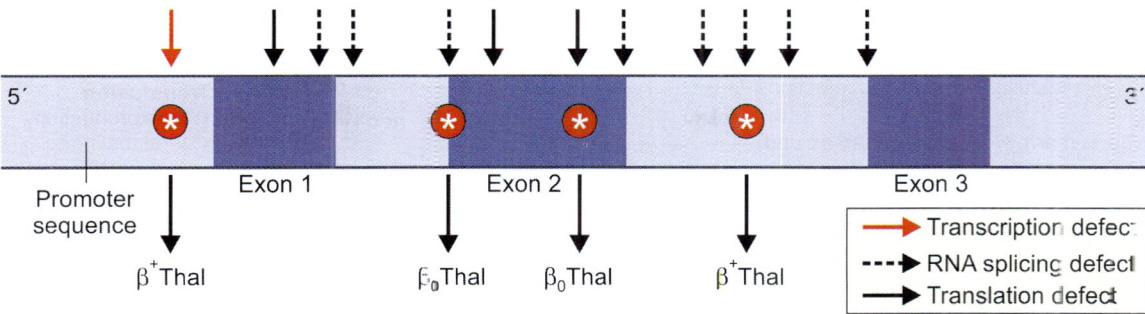

Fig. 8.33: Diagrammatic representation of the β-globin gene. Arrows denote sites where point mutations give rise to thalassemia have been identified.

marrow. Expansion of bone marrow leads to widening of diploë of the skull and other bones. Skull radiograph shows *hair-end-on* appearance.

Extramedullary Hematopoiesis

Extramedullary hematopoiesis occurs in liver and spleen.

Synthesis of HbF

Synthesis of γ-chains continues even after 6 months of age. These γ-chains combine with α-chains resulting in synthesis of HbF (α_2, γ_2) varying from 20 to 90%.

CLINICAL FEATURES

Clinical manifestations begin in child after attaining 6–9 months of age as hemoglobin synthesis switch from HbF to HbA. Bone marrow transplantation is the only curative therapy. Clinical manifestations of β-thalassemia major are shown in Fig. 8.34.

Severe Anemia

Anemia becomes obvious within first year of life. Anemia results from decrease in hemoglobin synthesis, marked shortening of red cell lifespan due to aggregation of insoluble excess α-chains, ineffective erythropoiesis and relative folate deficiency. Severe anemia leads to cardiac dilatation.

Failure to Thrive

If untreated, the disease often results in failure to thrive. Impairment of growth results in short stature, diarrhea and recurrent infections.

Bone Marrow Expansion

Increased oxygen affinity of hemoglobin F and the underlying anemia impair oxygen delivery and lead to marked bone marrow erythroid hyperplasia. Expansion of erythroid bone marrow causes facial and cranial bone deformities results in *Mongoloid face*. These changes are demonstrated by X-rays in skull, long bones, small bones of hands and feet. Pathological fractures and bone pain may occur.

Marked Splenomegaly

Child develops marked splenomegaly by the age of 3. It occurs due to sequestration, intramedullary destruction of red cells and extramedullary hemopoiesis.

Hepatomegaly

Child develops moderate to marked hepatomegaly as a result of iron overload and extramedullary hemopoiesis. Excessive absorption of iron due to ineffective erythropoiesis and repeated blood transfusion cause iron overload.

Spinal Cord Compression

Extramedullary hemopoiesis in vertebrae causes compression of the spinal cord.

Generalized Hemosiderosis

Excess iron deposition in tissues is a major cause of morbidity and mortality in these patients. Extravascular hemolysis together with repeated transfusions, creates iron overload. Excessive iron is deposited in *bone marrow, liver* (Kupffer's cells), *myocardium, pituitary gland, hypothalamus, pancreas* (islets of Langerhans) and *parathyroid glands*. Hemochromatosis is rare, if occurs, patient may develop bronze diabetes comprising of cirrhosis, diabetes mellitus and pericarditis.

Septicemia

Septicemia is cause of mortality.

LABORATORY DIAGNOSIS

Hemoglobin

Patient suffers from moderate to severe anemia. Hemoglobin level ranges between 3 and 8 g/dl.

Routine Investigations

Hemoglobin, MCH, MCHC and MCV are decreased. Serum bilirubin is slightly increased. Reticulocyte count is increased. Osmotic fragility is decreased.

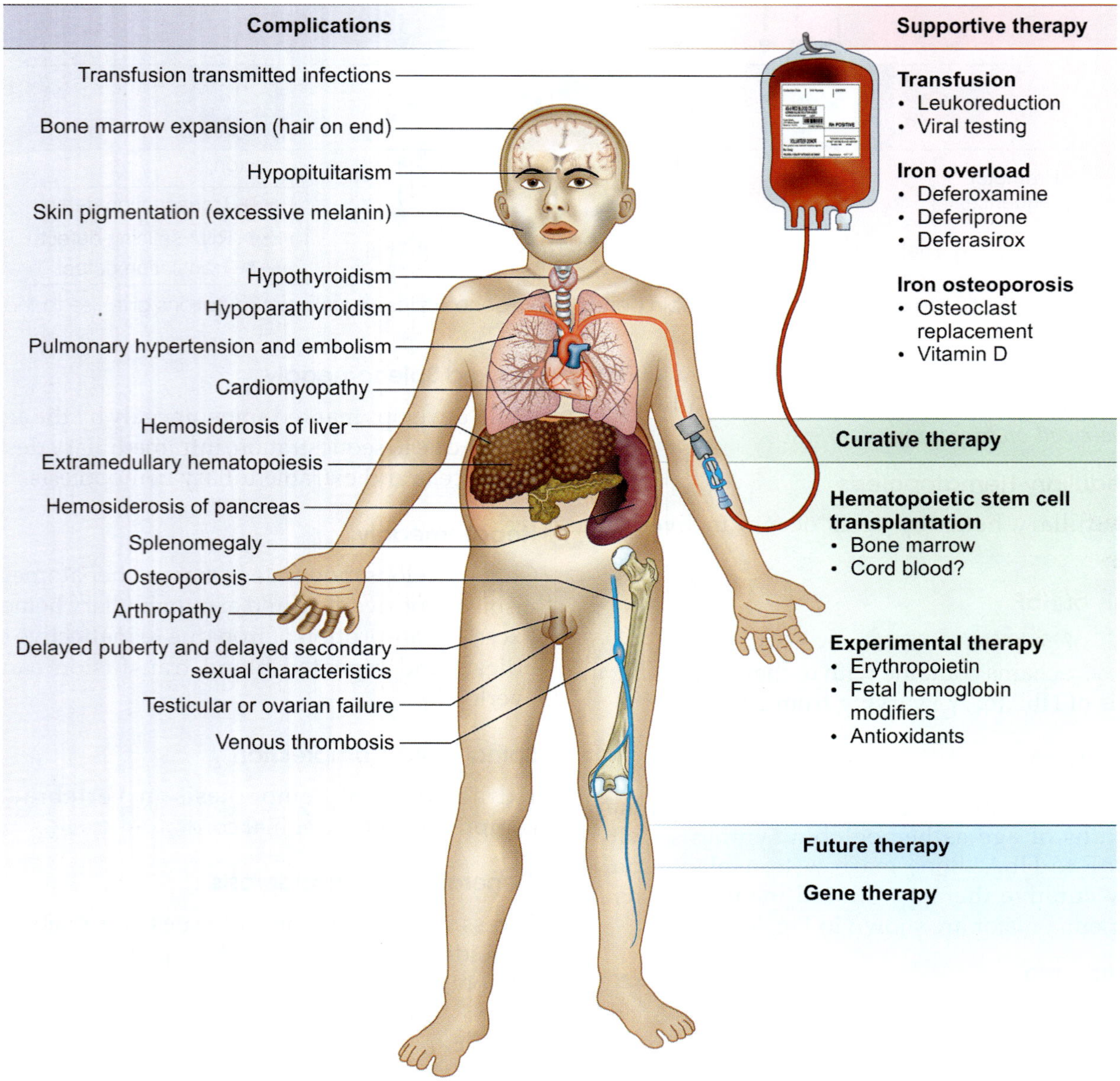

Fig. 8.34: Clinical manifestations of β-thalassemia major.

Peripheral Blood Smear

Peripheral blood smear findings are shown in Fig. 8.35.
- *RBCs morphology:* RBCs show marked anisocytosis, poikilocytosis with microcytic hypochromic picture. Presence of target cells is characteristic finding. Basophilic stippling is constant findings. Normoblasts range between 5 and 40/100 WBCs. There is presence of tear drop cells, inclusion bodies in red blood cells (aggregation of α-chains), and fragmented red blood cells.
- *WBCs morphology:* TLC normal or increased. DLC shows slight shift-to-the-left with presence of some myelocytes and metamyelocytes.
- *Platelets:* Platelet count is normal but may be decreased due to sequestration of platelets in cases showing splenomegaly.

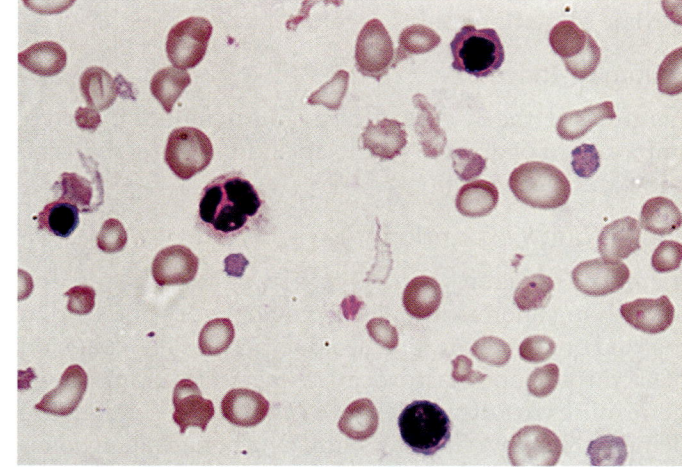

Fig. 8.35: β-thalassemia major of peripheral blood smear shows anisopoikilocytosis, many target cells and a few normoblasts.

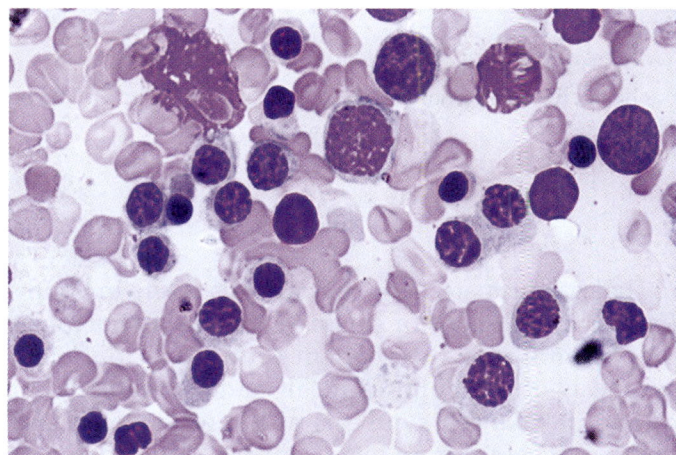

Fig. 8.36: β-thalassemia major. Bone marrow shows erythroid hyperplasia.

Reticulocyte Count

Reticulocyte count is increased to 3–10%. Brilliant cresyl blue stain is used for reticulocyte count.

Bone Marrow Examination

Bone marrow of β-thalassemia major is shown in Fig. 8.36.

- *Cellularity:* Bone marrow is hypercellular as a result of erythroid hyperplasia.
- *Erythroid series:* Erythroid hyperplasia with micro-normoblastic erythropoiesis (e.g. basophilic and polychromatic normoblasts) is seen. Siderotic nodules are commonly seen in developing normoblasts. Some normoblasts demonstrate dyserythropoiesis with irregular nuclear borders.
- *Myeloid series:* Myeloid precursors are within normal range. Myeloid hyperplasia occurs due to infection.
- *Myeloid erythroid ratio:* M:E ratio is decreased.
- *Megakaryocytes:* Megakaryocytes are normal.

Bone Marrow Iron

Iron stores are increased in bone marrow due to hemolysis and multiple blood transfusions, demonstrated by Perl's reaction/Prussian blue reaction. Iron study in iron deficiency and thalassemia is shown in Table 8.42.

Table 8.42: Iron study in iron deficiency and thalassemia

Iron study	Iron deficiency	Thalassemia
Serum iron	Decreased	Normal/increased
Serum ferritin	Decreased	Normal/increased
TIBC	Increased	Normal/increased
Percent saturation	Decreased	Increased
Storage iron	Absent	Increased
FEP (free erythrocyte protoporphyrin)	Increased	Normal

Serum Iron, TIBC and % Saturation

Serum iron level and % saturation are increased. Serum iron is above 200 µg%. Serum ferritin is increased above 1000 µg%.

NESROFT Test (Naked Eye Single Tube Red Cell Osmotic Fragility Test)

NESROFT test is most common screening test for thalassemia in India and across world. Normal saline (0.35%) is added to the test tube containing blood sample. Keep it for 30 minutes. A plain white paper with a black line is placed behind the test tube. Black line is visible in normal person as a result of hemolysis. On the other hand, black line is not visible in blood sample of thalassemia patient, because red blood cell membranes are relatively stable and resistant to hemolysis.

Fetal Hemoglobin

Fetal hemoglobin is high ranging between 30 and 90% especially in β-thalassemia estimated by alkali denaturation test. HbF may also be demonstrated by acid elution test. These RBCs containing HbF are well stained. Red blood cells containing HbA appear as ghost cells.

Hemoglobin Electrophoresis

Diagnosis of β-thalassemia major is confirmed by hemoglobin electrophoresis with increased level of HbF in range of 30–90%. HbA_2 is also increased in these patients. Synthesis of HbF (α_2, γ_2) continues throughout life even after 6 months of age. These γ-chains combine with α-chains result in formation of fetal hemoglobin. In β-thalassemia, HbF and HbA_2 are present but no HbA.

High Performance Liquid Chromatography (HPLC)

HPLC is one of the commonest laboratory investigations performed for the identification of abnormal hemoglobin.

Mutation Studies

DNA analysis is carried out to demonstrate gene mutations.

β-THALASSEMIA MINOR (TRAIT)

In this condition, a single aberrant β-globin gene is present on one chromosome 11. The result is mild anemia, or no anemia at all. Heterozygotes are usually asymptomatic due to sufficient synthesis of β-globin. These patients have protection against malaria. Differences between thalassemia minor and iron deficiency anemia are shown in Table 8.43.

Peripheral blood smear: Peripheral blood smear examination shows minimal hypochromic microcytic anemia, target cells, basophilic stippling.

Table 8.43: Differences between thalassemia minor and iron deficiency anemia

Parameters	Thalassemia minor	Iron deficiency anemia
Peripheral blood smear	Microcytic hypochromic picture	Microcytic hypochromic picture
RDW	Normal	Increased
Mentzer's index calculated by dividing MCV by RBCs	<13	>13

Hematocrit values: RBCs have reduced MCV and MCH.

Hemoglobin electrophoresis: Increased HbA_2 (α_2, δ_2) level between 3 and 6% is diagnostic for thalassemia minor. It demonstrates double the normal amount of hemoglobin A_2 (α_2, δ_2), about 3 to 6%, and up to 5% fetal hemoglobin (α_2, γ_2).

This finding is useful in distinguishing β-thalassemia minor from iron deficiency anemia and the anemia of chronic disease.

β-THALASSEMIA INTERMEDIA

β-thalassemia intermedia is of less severity. There is sufficient quantity of HbA. Insoluble α-globin chain aggregates are absent. These patients are anemic. They become transfusion dependent later during adulthood. Complications are not as severe as for β-thalassemia major. These patients are diagnosed between 15 and 30 years of age. Hemolysis and increased iron absorption result in increased iron stores.

Thalassemia intermedia is double heterozygotes due to interaction of α, β with HbD, HbE and HbS. HbE. The clinical presentation is intermediate between thalassemia major and thalassemia minor. Hemolysis and increased iron absorption result in increased iron stores.

Clinical Features

Patient presents with pallor, mild to moderate splenomegaly, skeleton changes (many cases), leg ulcers and infections.

Laboratory Investigations

- *Peripheral blood smear:* Peripheral blood smear shows microcytic hypochromic anemia, moderate degree of anisocytosis, poikilocytosis, target cells and tear drop cells.
- *Hemoglobin and hematocrit values:* Hemoglobin varies between 7 and 10 g/dl. MVC, MCH, and MCHC are decreased.
- *Bone marrow:* Bone marrow examination shows erythroid hyperplasia with increased iron stores.
- *Fetal hemoglobin:* HbF ranges between 10 and 30% in comparison to thalassemia major with HbF 40–90%.

α-THALASSEMIAS

α-Thalassemias are most common disorders in South-East Asia. Deletions of single or more α-globin genes on chromosome 16 result in reduced or deficient synthesis of α-globin. Clinical manifestations occur due to imbalanced synthesis of α- and non-α-chains such as γ-chain during infancy and β- and δ-chains at 6 months of age.

Classification

These are classified on the basis of the number and position of the α-globin genes deleted: silent career, α-thalassemia trait, hemoglobin H disease (β_4) and hydrops fetalis.

SILENT CARRIER

Silent carrier occurs due to *deletion of single α-gene* on chromosome 16. These patients are asymptomatic without development of anemia.

α-THALASSEMIA TRAIT

α-Thalassemia trait occurs due to deletion of *two α-genes on one chromosome 16* (Asians) or two α-genes (one each on chromosome) in Africans. Peripheral blood smear examination shows absence or minimal anemia showing some microcytic red blood cells. These patients are asymptomatic without physical signs and clinical findings identical to β-thalassemia minor (microcytic hypochromic).

HEMOGLOBIN H DISEASE (β_4)

Hemoglobin H disease occurs due to deletion of three α-genes on chromosome 16. It leads to formation of unstable tetramers of β-globin (β_4) known as HbH are formed. These tetramers are nonfunctional in oxygen transport, so anemia is disproportionate to hemoglobin level.

Clinical Features

Patient develops moderate hemolytic anemia. It resembles β-thalassemia intermedia.

Laboratory Findings

Hemoglobin level is decreased. Peripheral blood smear shows microcytic hypochromic picture, target cells and Heinz bodies with anisocytosis and poikilocytosis. Hematocrit values (MCV, MCH, and MCHC) are decreased. Reticulocyte count is increased.

HYDROPS FETALIS

Hydrops fetalis occurs due to *deletion of all four α-globin chains*. Due to absence of α-chains, fetus synthesizes excess of γ-globin chains forming tetramers known as *hemoglobin Bart* (γ_4). During intrauterine life, this hemoglobin Bart (γ_4) is unable to deliver the oxygen to tissues. Without intrauterine transfusions, the fetus invariably dies. Newborn is either stillborn or death occurs immediately after birth from pulmonary hypoplasia or cardiac failure. It is the most common cause for hydrops fetalis in persons of South-East Asian ancestry.

Clinical Features

The fetus shows pallor, generalized edema and massive hepatosplenomegaly.

Peripheral Blood Smear

Peripheral blood smear examination shows macrocytic hypochromic anemia, marked anisocytosis, poikilocytosis, with numerous normoblasts. MCV is more than 110 femtoliter. MCH is decreased.

Reticulocyte Count

Reticulocyte count is increased.

Hemoglobin Electrophoresis

Hemoglobin electrophoresis will reveal affected fetuses or neonates to have about 80% hemoglobin Bart (γ_4, a tetramer of γ-chains) and about 20% hemoglobin Portland (γ_2, ζ_2) or sometimes hemoglobin Gower 1 ($\zeta_2 \varepsilon_2$) normally present only in embryonic life in the first trimester. There is absence of adult hemoglobin.

HEREDITARY PERSISTENCE OF FETAL HEMOGLOBIN

Hereditary persistence of fetal hemoglobin (HPFH) is characterized by continuous synthesis of fetal hemoglobin in significant quantity since postnatal to adulthood life.

It occurs due to mutation of β-globin gene cluster. Fetal hemoglobin concentration ranges between 10 and 100%. These patients are most often asymptomatic and detected during screening.

SICKLE CELL DISORDERS AND OTHER HEMOGLOBINOPATHIES

OVERVIEW

Every person has 2 genes responsible for hemoglobin synthesis. Persons having one normal (HbA) gene and one sickle (HbS) gene known as heterozygous (sickle cell trait) having HbA (60%) and HbS (20–40%). These patients are asymptomatic because sufficient HbA prevents polymerization of HbS.

Person having both sickle cell genes is known as *homozygous*. Such person has 85–95% of HbS. Sickle cells are demonstrated in the peripheral blood smear in sickle cell anemia in contrast to sickle cell trait. Double heterozygote state occurs as a result of interaction of HbS with thalassemia (α, β), HbC, HbD and HbE.

SICKLE CELL DISEASE

Sickle cell disease is autosomal recessive disorder. It most often affects African and Mediterranean populations. Approximately 7% of African Americans carry the *hemoglobin S gene*. It confers resistance to *Plasmodium falciparum* malarial infection.

Prenatal diagnosis of HbS can be performed on amniotic cells or on chorionic villus samples. Hemoglobin percentage in normal adult person is shown in Table 8.44.

Table 8.44: Hemoglobin percentage in normal adult person

Hemoglobin type	Chains	Percentage
Hemoglobin A	α_2, β_2	97%
Hemoglobin A_2	α_2, δ_2	1–3%
Hemoglobin F	α_2, γ_2	<1%

BASIC DEFECT

Sickle cell disease occurs due to partially missense point mutation in codon 6 of the β-globin gene resulting in substitution of valine for glutamic acid in the β-globin gene (Fig. 8.37). Consequently, sickle cell hemoglobin (HbS) replaces normal adult HbA in the red blood cells. HbS causes polymerization of hemoglobin leading to formation of needle like insoluble crystals within RBCs. Therefore, RBCs take shape of crescentic or holly leaf-like or boat shape.

These are called as sickle cells or drepanocytes. Solubility of HbS is altered by nonpolar (water insoluble) valine without affecting its structure, function and/or stability.

CLINICAL MANIFESTATIONS

Clinical manifestations of sickle cell disease are shown in Fig. 8.38 and Table 8.45.

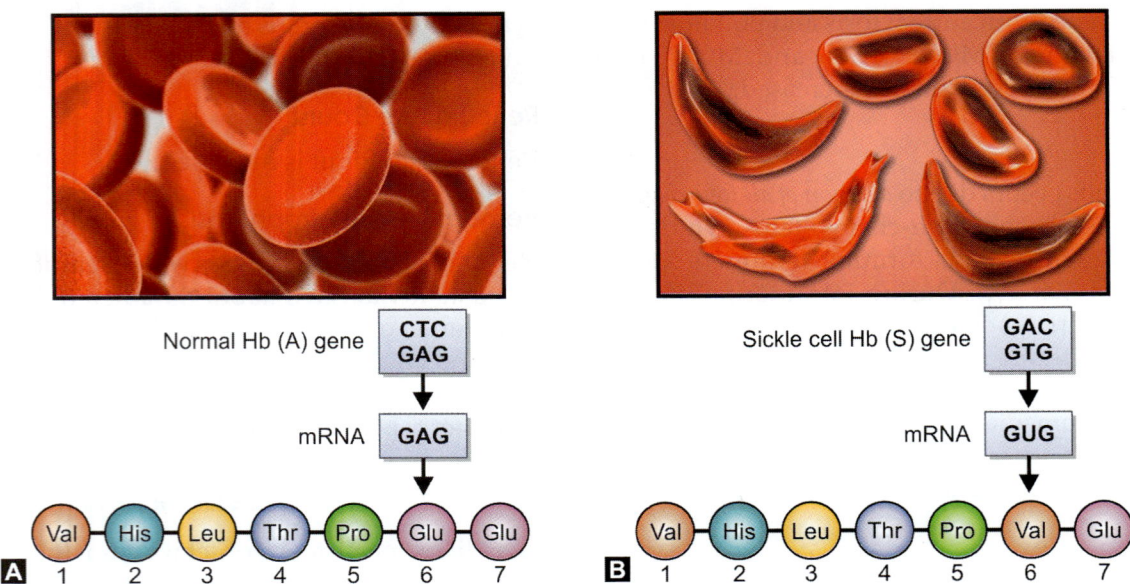

Fig. 8.37: (A) HbA peptide shows synthesis of normal hemoglobin; (B) HbS peptide shows synthesis of HbS as a result of replacement of glutamic acid (polar) by valine (non-polar) in codon 6 of the β-globin gene.

Table 8.45: Systemic complications of sickle cell disease

Organs	Clinical manifestations
Hepatobiliary system	Jaundice, pigmented gallstones and anemia. Pigment stones occur due to hemolysis. Secondary hemosiderosis occurs due to overload of transfused patients
Retina	Blindness caused by small vessel occlusion and ischemic retinopathy
Brain	Cerebral infarction due to vascular occlusion
Lungs	Pulmonary infarction, lobar pneumonia, development of acute chest syndrome, characterized by decreased pulmonary function, which may be fatal
Kidneys	Papillary necrosis caused by vascular occlusion in vasa recta due to hypoxia and hyperosmolarity in the renal medulla creates an environment for sickling in the vasa recta
Bones	Aseptic bone necrosis Salmonella osteomyelitis (predisposed by small infarcts in bone caused by vascular occlusion)
Priapism	Prolonged painful penile erection due to venous occlusion as a result sickling is common, often requiring surgical decompression
Immune system	Autosplenectomy or hyposplenism increases susceptibility to bacterial infection
Bone marrow	Human Parvovirus B19, suppresses erythrocyte production results in aplastic crises in 80% cases with a high mortality
Legs	Chronic leg ulcers around the malleoli (ankles) and both sides of lower legs due to stagnant blood flow caused by sickled red blood cells

Severe Hemolytic Anemia

Deoxygenated HbS is 50 times less soluble in blood than deoxygenated HbA. Under low oxygen tension in capillaries, deoxygenated HbS comes out of solution forming long parallel fibers (crystals) called *tactoids* which distort the red cells to assume sickle or crescent shaped.

- *Hemolysis:* Repeated episodes of sickling lead to destruction of red blood cells and obstruction of the microvasculature. These cells are then susceptible to premature destruction resulting in a lifespan of only 10–20 days as opposed to a normal 120 days. This causes a chronic hemolytic anemia with hemoglobin of around 5–8 g/dl.
- *Sickle cell crisis:* This leads to cell death and tissue infarction at the site of obstruction. This is termed a sickle cell crisis. Apart from hypoxia, acidosis irrespective of the prevailing oxygen tension is important reason for most sickling occurring in the venous circulation. Therapeutic agent is administered to increase HbF levels in these patients.

Red Blood Cells

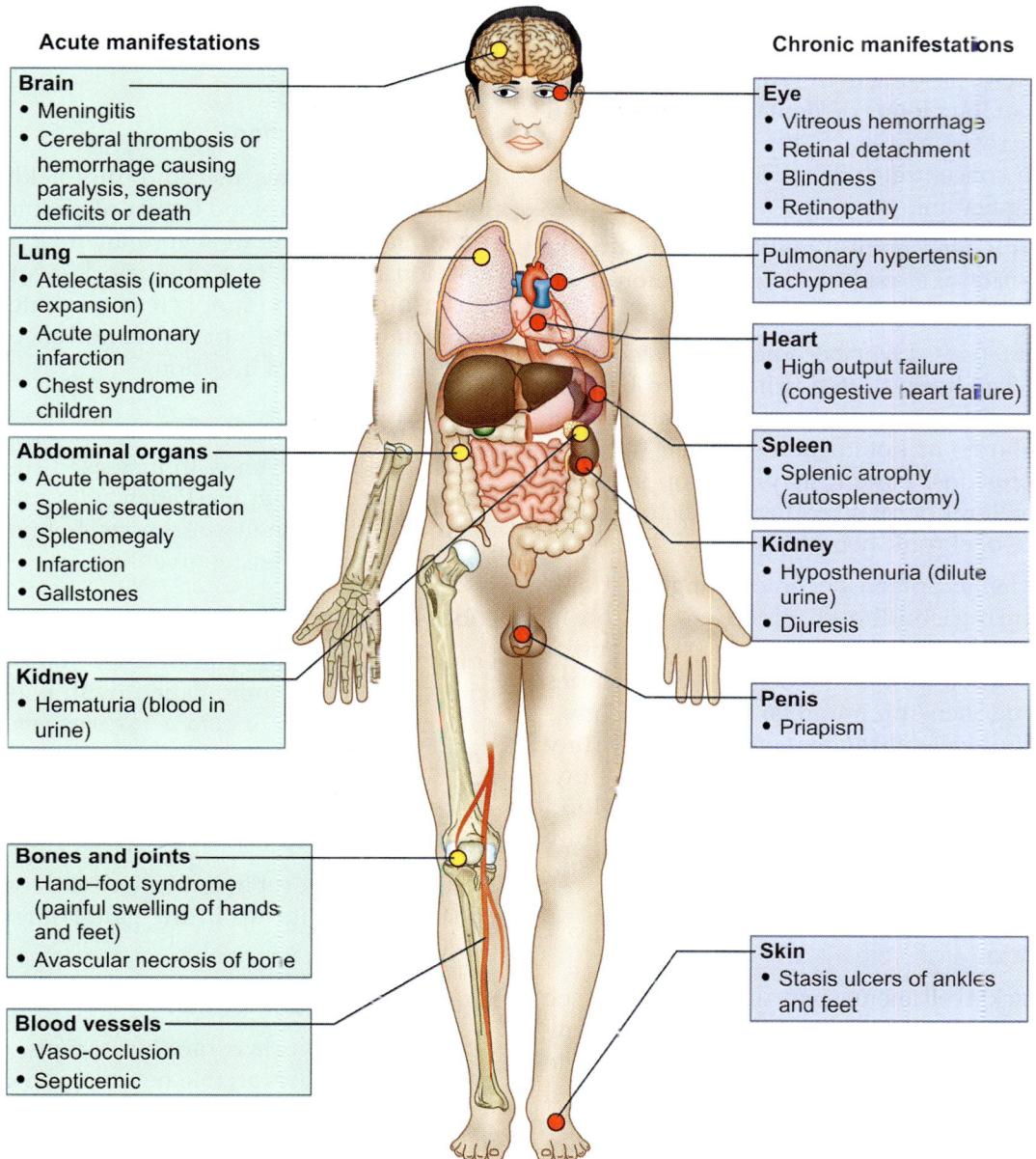

Fig. 8.38: Clinical manifestations of sickle cell disease.

Vascular-occlusive Episodes

Vascular-occlusive episodes occur at about 6 months of age after the reduction in fetal hemoglobin (HbF) which initially acts as a protective mechanism. Vascular-occlusive phenomenon is often precipitated by infection or dehydration. Patient develops infarction of bones, lungs, brain, renal papillae, lungs, spleen, and liver resulting in pain lasting a few minutes or several days.

- *Hand and foot syndrome:* Patient develops *hand and foot syndrome* (dactylitis of small bones of hands and feet) in first 2 years of life.
- *Avascular necrosis of femoral head:* Avascular necrosis of the femoral head often cripples sickle cell patients. Aseptic necrosis is also referred to as osteonecrosis. Pain, tenderness and disability are frequently signs of avascular necrosis.
- *Bone and joint crises:* Vascular occlusion of vertebrae, long bones such as femur, tibia, fibula and humerus undergo infarction. This can cause permanent damage to hips, shoulders or knees. Fish mouth vertebrae are demonstrated due to vaso-occlusive phenomenon. Skull shows *crewcut appearance* on radiographs. It occurs due to expansion of bone marrow leading to bone resorption and new bone formation.
- *Acute chest syndrome:* Repeated vascular-occlusive episodes result in pulmonary infarction and impaired lung functions. Patient presents with classical features of the *acute chest syndrome* characterized by dyspnea, cough, pleuritis (chest pain) and hemoptysis.

- *Renal papillary necrosis:* The relative hypoxia and hyperosmolarity in the renal medulla create an environment for sickling in the vasa recta. It leads to destruction of long loops of Henle resulting in renal papillary necrosis and renal failure. The kidney loses its ability to concentrate urine. Hematuria is also a complicating feature.
- *Priapism:* Prolonged painful penile erection due to venous occlusion as a result sickling is common, often requiring surgical decompression.
- *Liver manifestations:* Liver becomes congested with sickle cells. The liver is often firm and can become tender. Liver failure may supervene as a result of multiple infarcts or hemosiderosis from frequent blood transfusions. Patient may develop jaundice (yellow discoloration of sclera) and gallstones as a consequence of chronic hemolysis.
- *Autosplenectomy:* Spleen becomes congested and enlarged during childhood. Blood circulation in spleen is slow. Deoxygenation promotes sickling of red blood cells resulting in blockage of capillaries in spleen and ischemic infarcts. Later it becomes progressively smaller through repeated multiple tiny infarcts and fibrosis resulting in autosplenectomy. In autosplenectomy patients, peripheral blood smear shows numerous target cells, Howell-Jolly bodies, marked anisocytosis, poikilocytosis and thrombocytosis.

Aplastic Anemia

Patients with sickle cell anemia may undergo an aplastic crisis in 80% cases due to infection of the bone marrow by human Parvovirus B19, which suppresses erythrocyte production. It is characterized by a precipitous fall in hemoglobin concentration. Bone marrow failure (aplastic crisis) also occurs with a high mortality.

Sequestration Crisis

Sequestration crisis is most severe crisis in infants and children. There is massive entrapment of sickle cells in spleen. Patient presents with painful splenomegaly and hypovolemic shock. There is acute fall in hemoglobin usually secondary to infection induced hemolysis or an acute sequestration syndrome in the spleen. Blood transfusion is often essential. Gamna-Gandy bodies are demonstrated in the spleen due to organization of splenic hemorrhages. There is deposition of calcium and hemosiderin in Gamna-Gandy bodies.

Chronic Leg Ulcers

Patient is susceptible to chronic leg ulcers particularly around the malleoli (ankles) and both sides of lower legs. It is due to stagnant blood flow caused by sickled red blood cells. The ulcers are often complicated by trauma and poor hygiene.

Splenic Sequestration

Spleen participates in removing sickled red cells. Sudden pooling of blood in the spleen known as *splenic sequestration* results in severe anemia, shock, loss of consciousness with fatal outcome. Repeated sickling in spleen impairs blood supply results in autosplenectomy. Impairment of the normal function of the spleen increases the risk of infection.

Osteomyelitis

Damage to the spleen with increased susceptibility to infections occurs with age. Patient with autosplenectomy is prone to Salmonella infections. Salmonella is most often implicated in osteomyelitis.

Lobar Pneumonia and Meningitis

Lobar pneumonia is extremely common in children with sickle cell anemia. Patient with poor functioning spleen is prone to *Streptococcus pneumoniae* infection. These children frequently develop meningitis due to pneumococci and Haemophilus bacteria.

Gallstones

Accumulated bilirubin in the liver can concentrate into crystals that build up in the gallbladder resulting in cholelithiasis.

Neurological Manifestations

Acute brain syndrome is rare but serious, characterized by confusion with variable neurological defects. There is an increased risk of subarachnoid hemorrhage, retinal hemorrhage (partial or complete blindness) and deafness.

LABORATORY DIAGNOSIS

Following tests are useful to complement the clinical history and examination.

Hemoglobin

Normal hemoglobin level excludes sickle cell disease.

Peripheral Blood Smear

Person with sickle cell disease has mostly HbS. Peripheral blood film shows sickle cells, some target cells, nucleated red cells, Howell-Jolly bodies and sideroblasts. Patients with sickle trait are usually fit and healthy. Peripheral blood film may show a few sickle cells in sickle cell trait (Fig. 8.39).

Red Blood Cells

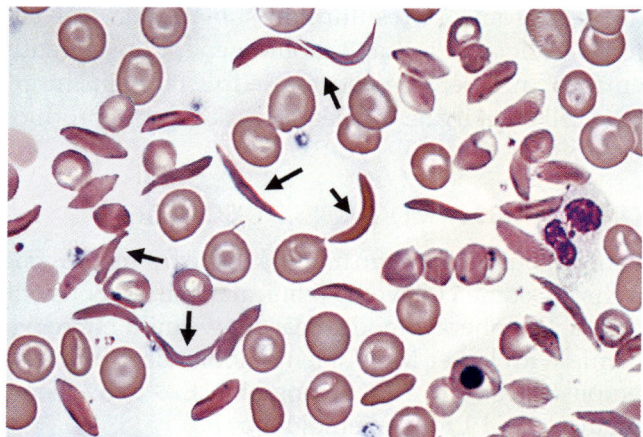

Fig. 8.39: Peripheral blood smear showing sickling (arrows).

Erythrocyte Sedimentation Rate

ESR is most often increased in all anemias except sickle cell anemia. Rouleax formation does not occur in sickle cell anemia.

Serum Bilirubin

Unconjugated bilirubin may be raised in the blood as a result of the hemolytic anemia.

Sickling Test

Sickling test is a screening test for sickle cell anemia. Mixing blood with the reducing agent, sodium metabisulphite on a sealed slide, will induce sickling in susceptible sickle cells. The test is simple and quick.

The results can be viewed under light microscope after 20 minutes. The sickle cell preparation is positive whenever hemoglobin S is present (e.g. sickle cell anemia, sickle cell trait, sickle C disease, sickle cell thalassemia). Sickling test is shown in Fig. 8.40.

High Performance Liquid Chromatography (HPLC)

HPLC is one of the commonest laboratory investigations performed for the identification of globin chain

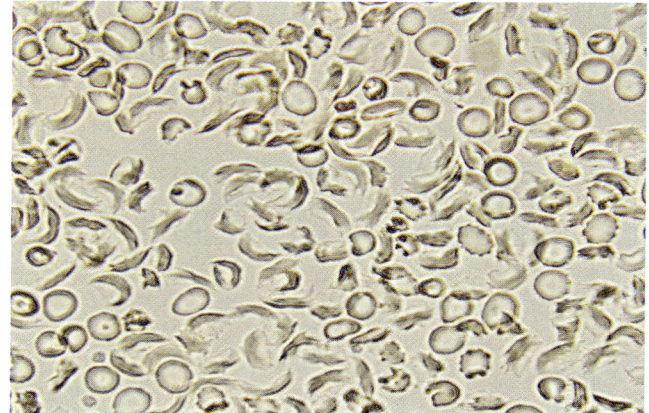

Fig. 8.40: Sickling test performed by mixing blood with the reducing agent, sodium metabisulphite on a sealed slide.

synthesis. It estimates quantity of normal and abnormal hemoglobins. It is the investigation of choice to confirm diagnosis of sickle cell anemia.

Hemoglobin Electrophoresis

Hemoglobin electrophoresis is the second best method for diagnosing sickle cell disease. HbA moves faster than HbS towards anode. HbS moves faster than HbA towards cathode. Formation of 1 band indicates sickle cell anemia. Formation of 2 band is suggestive of sickle cell carrier.

Hemoglobin moves in the *S region* on hemoglobin electrophoresis (alkaline pH). HbD, HbC, HbQ India and HB Lepore are also demonstrated in the same *S region* on hemoglobin electrophoresis. It differentiates between homozygous and heterozygous conditions. In the absence of electrophoresis, a positive sickling test associated with normal hemoglobin concentration indicates a patient with sickle cells disease.

Kidney Function Tests

Blood urea, serum creatinine and electrolytes are done to assess renal function to rule out renal papillary necrosis.

Cardiovascular System

ECG is performed to look for evidence of cardiac damage.

SICKLE CELL THALASSEMIA SYNDROME

Sickle cell thalassemia syndrome results from coinheritance of hemoglobin S gene and a thalassemic variant of the β-globin gene (compound heterozygosity). Clinical picture resembles thalassemia intermedia. Prognosis is better than sickle cell anemia and thalassemia.

HEMOGLOBIN C DISORDERS

Hemoglobin C disorder primarily affects 2–3% of African lineage. HbC disorder occurs due to point mutation in codon 6 of the β-globin gene on chromosome 11 resulting in substitution of lysine for glutamic acid in the β-globin gene. Consequently, hemoglobin C replaces normal adult hemoglobin (HbA) in the red blood cells. But it does not lead to sickling, but produces *target cells*.

HOMOZYGOUS HEMOGLOBIN C DISORDER

Homozygous person with mutation of two β-globin genes on chromosome 11 develops clinical manifestations such as anemia varying in severity, episodes of abdominal and joint pain, splenomegaly, and mild jaundice.

Laboratory Diagnosis

Serum bilirubin (indirect) concentration is increased. Peripheral blood smear examination shows many target cells and occasionally elongated hexagonal crystals in red blood cells particularly in splenectomized persons. Hemoglobin electrophoresis reveals 80–90% of HbC and 1 to 7% HbF. When hemoglobin C is present, the amount of hemoglobin A_2 is difficult to assess, as these two hemoglobins are hard to distinguish by electrophoresis.

HETEROZYGOUS (HBS/HBC) DISORDER

Heterozygous person develops disorder, when HbC and HbS are inherited together. Patient presents with sickling-related complications at about half the rate of patients homozygous sickle cell disease. The patient is prone to avascular necrosis of the bone and proliferative retinopathy.

HEMOGLOBIN E DISORDERS

Hemoglobin E disorders are prevalent in South-East Asia. Clinical and laboratory manifestations are similar to those of hemoglobin C disorders. HbE occurs due to point mutation in codon 26 of the β-globin gene on chromosome 11 resulting in substitution of lysine for glutamic acid in the β-globin gene. Consequently, hemoglobin E replaces normal adult HbA in the red blood cells. But it does not lead to sickling, but produces microcytosis.

HOMOZYGOUS HEMOGLOBIN E DISORDER

Homozygous person with mutation of two β-globin genes on chromosome 11 develops clinical manifestations mild anemia. Peripheral blood smear shows mild microcytic anemia with lower MCV. Hemoglobin electrophoresis demonstrates 90 to 95% hemoglobin E, 3 to 5% hemoglobin A_2, and 1 to 5% hemoglobin F.

HETEROZYGOUS HBE DISORDER

Heterozygous person with mutation of single β-globin gene on chromosome 11 has no clinical manifestations. Peripheral blood smear shows microcytes with decreased MCV. Hemoglobin electrophoresis demonstrates 30 to 40% hemoglobin E and 60 to 70% hemoglobin A.

GLUCOSE-6-PHOSPHATE DEHYDROGENASE DEFICIENCY AND PYRUVATE KINASE DEFICIENCY

GLUCOSE-6-PHOSPHATE DEHYDROGENASE DEFICIENCY

G6PD deficiency is an X-linked recessive disorder affecting males that causes a hemolytic anemia characterized by abnormal sensitivity of red cells to oxidative stress (Fig. 8.41).

Major hemolysis is extravascular, while minor component as intravascular. It is the most common form of enzyme deficiency hemolytic anemia. G6PD should not be assessed during hemolytic episode, because reticulocytes contain normal G6PD. It should be assessed when reticulocyte count is within normal range.

Age and Sex Predilection

Full expression of G6PD deficiency is seen only in males, with females being asymptomatic carriers. Affected persons are also more prone to infection.

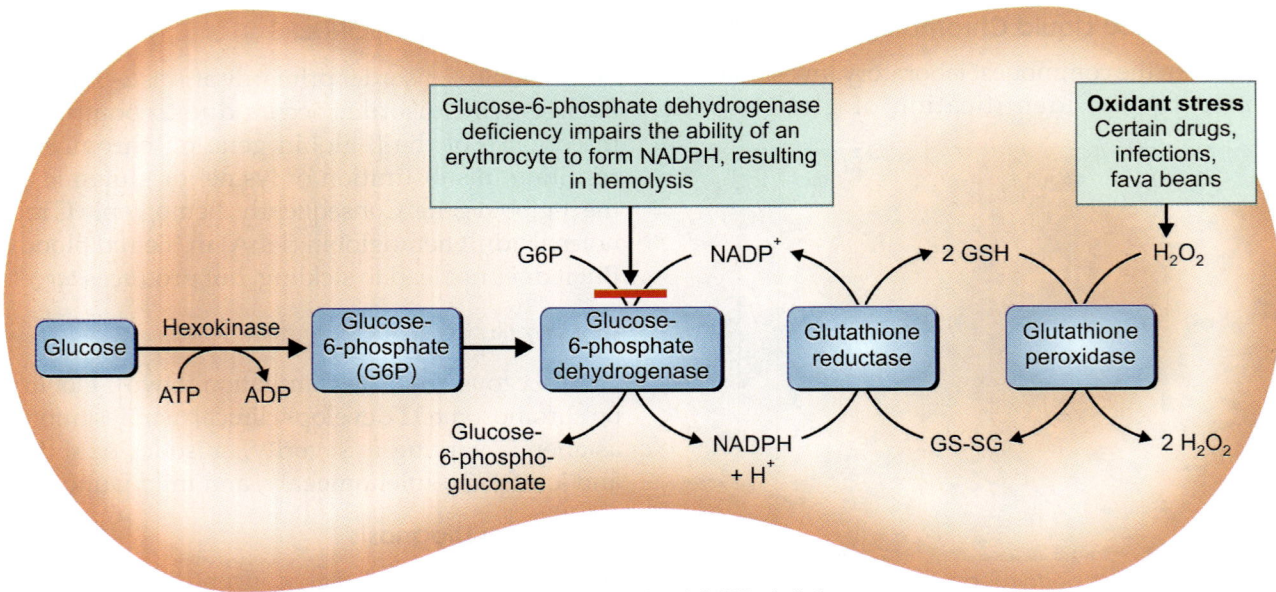

Fig. 8.41: Pathogenesis of G6PD deficiency.

Prevalence

The highest prevalence is in Africa and the Mediterranean region in 10% population. G6PD deficiency gives protection against malarial parasitic infection.

Etiology

Drugs that cause oxidative stress (e.g. primaquine, chloroquine, phenacetin, nitrofurantoin, sulfonamides drugs) result in intravascular hemolytic anemia in subjects (most often male) with G6PD deficiency. Viral hepatitis, pneumonia and typhoid fever cause oxidative stress. Ingestion of fava beans causes oxidative stress in people in Mediterranean region. Disease is termed as favism.

PATHOPHYSIOLOGY

Physiological state: Under physiological state, G6PD enzyme is involved in the hexose monophosphate shunt pathway. G6PD reduces nicotinamide adenine dinucleotide phosphate (NADP) to NADPH. This NADPH reduces glutathione within RBCs. This reduced glutathione aids in protecting cells against oxidant injury.

Pathological state

- *Gene mutations:* Red blood cells deficient in G6PD are less resistant to oxidant injury. Mutant gene on X-chromosome results in either impaired G6PD enzyme synthesis or impaired enzyme stability due to loss of normal folding of G6PD proteins.

    The unfolding form of G6PD proteins undergo proteolytic degradation. Any exposure to oxidants results in hemolysis. Hemolysis mainly occurs in the older red blood cells due to reduced amount of G6PD, hence prone to hemolysis. WHO mutant G6PD isoenzymes are shown in Table 8.46.

- *Oxidant stress:* Under oxidant stress, inadequate G6PD activity leads to oxidation of sulfhydryl groups of hemoglobin resulting in precipitation of denatured hemoglobin known as *Heinz bodies*.

    Heinz bodies can cause direct injury to RBCs. Cell rigidity and increased membrane permeability cause erythrocyte injury leading to intravascular and extravascular hemolysis in spleen. Splenic macrophages remove Heinz bodies and form *bite cells* demonstrated in peripheral blood smear.

CLINICAL FEATURES

Red blood cells are more prone to hemolysis. It is manifested by acute self-limited intravascular hemolytic anemia with hemoglobinemia and hemoglobinuria caused by oxidative stress. Patient may present with malaise, severe lethargy, nausea, vomiting, abdominal pain, fever with chills. Due to intermittent hemolysis, there is no splenomegaly and cholelithiasis.

LABORATORY DIAGNOSIS

Peripheral Blood Smear

Peripheral blood smear examination shows *bite cells*, Heinz bodies and polychromasia, fragmented RBCs. When RBCs containing Heinz bodies pass through the spleen, reticuloendothelial cells of spleen take a bite of red blood cells and removes Heinz bodies and result in formation of bite cells (Fig. 8.42).

Supravital Staining

Heinz bodies are inclusions of denatured hemoglobin present near cell membrane demonstrated by supravital staining (brilliant cresyl blue or methylene blue) and not with Romanowsky stains. Failure of disposal of

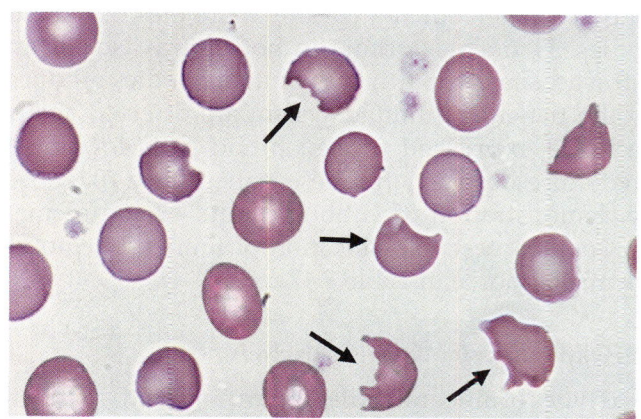

Fig. 8.42: Peripheral blood smear showing bite cells (arrows).

Table 8.46: WHO classification of mutant G6PD isoenzymes

Class	G6PD	Hemolysis
I	Severely deficient G6PD seen in African–American population (<10%)	Chronic hemolysis is self-limited course because younger RBCs are not affected
II	Mediterranean form with severely deficient G6PD	More severe acute episode of hemolysis. Patients are protective against *Plasmodium falciparum*
III	Mild to moderate deficient (10–60%)	Acute hemolysis (episodic)
IV	Mild to normal deficient	Hemolysis absent
V	Increased G6PD	Hemolysis absent

oxygen derived free radicals converts hemoglobin to methemoglobin results in condensation to form Heinz bodies.

Fluorescent spot test: Principle of the test is based on generation of NADPH by normal G6PD in the lysate of red blood cells to fluorescence under ultraviolet light. In G6PD deficiency, no fluorescence is observed as a result of lack of generation of NADPH.

Reticulocyte count: Reticulocyte count is increased (8–10%).

Serum bilirubin: Serum bilirubin is increased (indirect bilirubin) due to hemolysis.

Serum haptoglobin: Haptoglobin is α_2 glycoprotein synthesized by liver. It combines with any hemoglobin in plasma and prevents its excretion in urine. Haptoglobin–hemoglobin molecule is removed by liver, spleen and bone marrow. Hence, plasma haptoglobin levels are decreased with episode of hemolysis, which come to normal within 3 days.

Serum LDH: Values of plasma lactic dehydrogenase are increased in hemolytic anemia (normal range is 125–270 microliter).

PYRUVATE KINASE DEFICIENCY

Pyruvate kinase is the second most common enzyme deficiency hemolytic anemia. This autosomal recessive disorder is characterized by hereditary non-spherocytic hemolytic anemia.

In contrast to the more common G6PD deficiency, in which the anemia is episodic and self-limited, the anemia is chronic and sustained. Peripheral blood smear shows acanthocytes (Fig. 8.43).

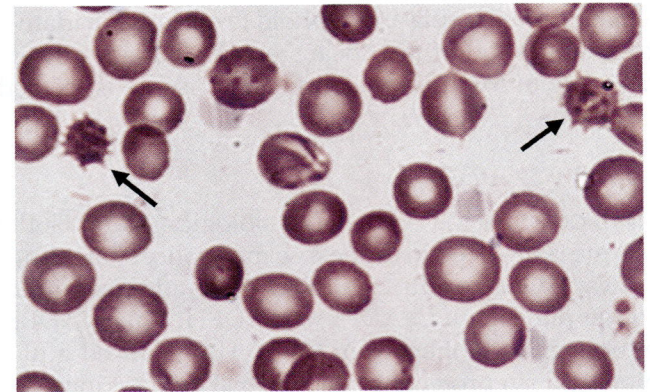

Fig. 8.43: Peripheral blood smear showuing acanthocytes in pyruvate kinase deficiency (arrows).

IMMUNE HEMOLYTIC ANEMIA

In immune hemolytic anemias, hemolysis of red blood cells is mediated by autoantibodies or alloantibodies. Hemolysis occurs in both intravascular and extravascular compartments. Autoantibodies produced by the patient's immune system are directed against antigens expressed on red blood cells leading to premature destruction. These patients are diagnosed by demonstration of antibodies and or complement by Coombs' test. Classification of immune hemolytic anemia is shown in Table 8.47.

AUTOIMMUNE HEMOLYTIC ANEMIA

Two types of autoantibodies (warm and cold) react with antigens expressed on cells leading to their destruction by spleen. Warm autoantibodies (IgG) being active at 37°C bind to antigens expressed on red blood cells without activation of complement leading to their destruction by splenic macrophages.

On the other hand, cold autoantibodies (IgM) being active at 30°C bind to antigens expressed on red blood cells and activates complement leading to RBCs destruction by splenic macrophages. These splenic macrophages possess Fc receptor for Fc fragment of immunoglobulin. Comparison of warm and cold antibodies is shown in Table 8.48. Pathogenesis of immune hemolytic anemia is shown in Fig. 8.44.

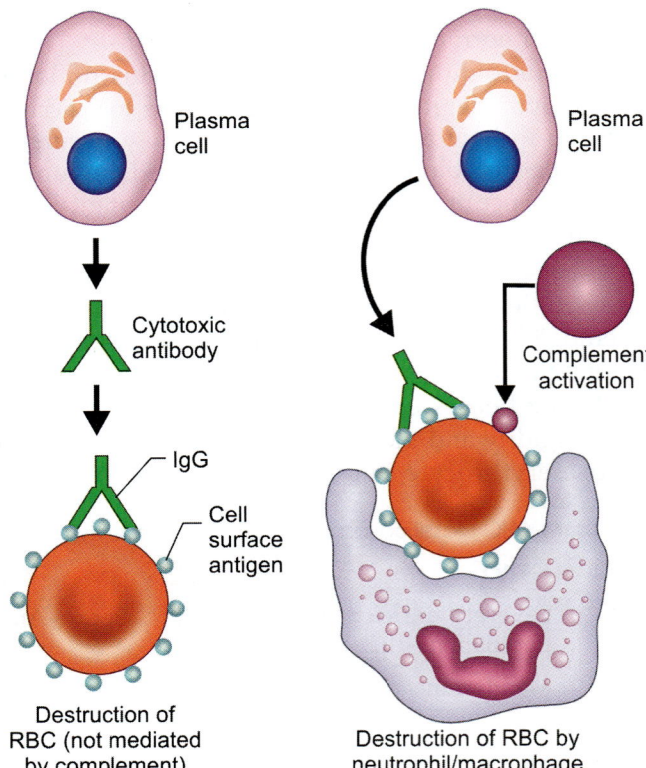

Fig. 8.44: Pathogenesis of immune hemolytic anemia by type II hypersensitivity reaction complement mediated phagocytosis by macrophage resulting in RBCs destruction by spleen.

Table 8.47: Classification of immune hemolytic anemia

Immune hemolytic anemia	Mechanism	Examples
Autoimmune hemolytic anemia		
Warm antibody-mediated immune hemolytic anemia	RBCs coated by IgG (most common) or IgM autoantibodies bind to Fc receptors of macrophages in spleen at 37°C leading to RBCs hemolysis in spleen	Primary or idiopathic (50%) Chronic lymphocytic leukemias Systemic lupus erythematosus Viral infections Drug-induced hemolysis (benzylpenicillin, α-methyldopa and quinidine)
Cold agglutinin disease	IgM class antibody agglutinate RBCs at 0–4°C (<37°C) leading to extravascular destruction of RBCs in spleen by macrophages	Primary disorder Lymphoma-related *Mycoplasma pneumoniae* Paroxysmal cold hemoglobinuria Infectious mononucleosis
Drug induced (benzyl penicillin) autoimmune hemolytic anemia	Antibodies directed against surface antigens on RBCs. Opsonization and phagocytosis of RBCs and platelets	Benzylpenicillin, cephalosporins and quinidine
Alloimmune hemolytic anemia		
Hemolytic disease of newborn	Antibodies directed against RBCs membrane proteins (Rh blood group antigen, I antigen) leading to opsonization and phagocytosis and destruction of red blood cells in newborn	Hemolytic disease of newborn (rhesus incompatibility)
Hemolytic mismatch blood transfusion	IgG or IgM antibodies attach to the foreign cells of donor, resulting in complement fixation leading to formation of membrane attack complex lysing the donor cells	Hemolytic transfusion reactions

Table 8.48: Comparison of warm and cold antibodies

Parameters	Warm antibodies	Cold antibodies
Immunoglobulins	IgG, rarely IgM or IgA	IgM (except PCH-IgG)
Reacts at temperature	Reacts at 37°C	Reacts below 30°C
Hemolysis	Extravascular hemolysis in spleen	Both extravascular and intravascular hemolysis

WARM ANTIBODY-MEDIATED HEMOLYTIC ANEMIA

Warm antibody-mediated hemolytic anemia is the most common form of immune hemolytic anemia. It is mediated by IgG class antibodies that react with red cell surface antigens (often Rh antigens) at 37°C. IgM autoantibody is active at 4°C, which becomes less active at higher temperature; but is still able to bind complement and agglutinate red cells at the temperature 30°C of the peripheral tissues (e.g. hands, feet, nose and ears). Sometimes, this disorder is mediated by IgA.

Etiology

This disorder is idiopathic (primary) in majority of patients. Secondary disorder is associated with systemic lupus erythematosus, rheumatoid arthritis, chronic lymphocytic leukemia, Hodgkin disease, or non-Hodgkin lymphomas and drugs hypersensitivity.

Pathogenesis

RBCs coated by IgG or IgM autoantibodies bind to receptors of macrophages because they have receptors for the Fc fragments of immunoglobulins. Once activated, the complement cascade leads to the destruction of the red blood cells through formation of a membrane attack complex.

IgM antibodies, which are powerful agglutinins, may agglutinate red blood cells in the red pulp of the spleen, resulting in cellular destruction. IgM may also activate complement, resulting in RBCs lysis or promoting to more macrophages. Such autoantibodies are detected by Coombs' test (agglutination test).

Clinical Features

Patient presents with progressive anemia, jaundice and mild splenomegaly. Disease is manifested by anemia and reticulocytosis, often with spherocytosis. History of drug intake such as benzylpenicillin, cephalosporins, methyldopa and quinidine should be taken into consideration.

Laboratory Diagnosis

Hemoglobin: Hemoglobin and PCV become low.

Peripheral blood smear examination: Peripheral blood smear shows polychromasia and spherocytes. Spherocytosis is due to progressive loss of membrane protein by serial passage of antibody-coated red cells through the spleen (Fig. 8.45).

Reticulocyte count: Reticulocyte count is increased between 5 and 20%. Higher reticulocyte count is demonstrated in acute hemolytic process.

Serum bilirubin: There is mild to moderate increase in unconjugated serum bilirubin.

Serum lactic acid dehydrogenase: Hemolysis of red blood cells increases serum LDH level.

LE cell phenomenon: LE cell test is significant in immune hemolytic anemia induced by systemic lupus erythematosus.

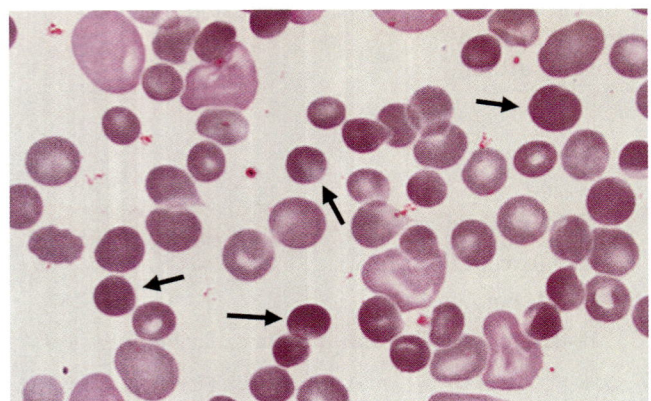

Fig. 8.45: Peripheral blood smear from a case of autoimmune hemolytic anemia showing polychromasia and spherocytes (arrows).

Coombs' test: Positive direct Coombs' test (also known as *direct antiglobulin test* or DAT) is reflecting the binding of IgG autoantibody to the red cell surface (Table 8.49).

COLD AGGLUTININ DISEASE

Cold agglutinin disease is caused by IgM antibodies, which agglutinate RBCs at low temperature (0° to 4°C). It is also known as *cold agglutinin syndrome*. It is mediated by IgM antibodies optimally active at low temperatures at 4°C against the red blood cells *I antigen*. These antibodies cause agglutination of red blood cells at low temperature at especially during winter season in the capillaries of nose and fingers.

Complement coated RBCs are phagocytozed by macrophages in spleen leading to extravascular hemolysis.

Etiology

This disorder occurs due to formation of anti-I antibodies in EB virus associated infectious mononucleosis. These anti-I antibodies frequently complicate *Mycoplasma pneumoniae* infection. This disorder also occurs in patient with HIV infection. Chronic hemolysis may primary or associated with B cell neoplasms.

Clinical Features

Patient presents with chronic hemolytic anemia exacerbated by cold weather, episodes of jaundice, sometimes with hemoglobinemia and hemoglobinuria. It is self-limited course. It rarely induces significant hemolysis.

Laboratory Diagnosis

Peripheral blood smear examination: The peripheral blood smear from this patient shows clumped red cells caused by cold agglutinins during especially winter. During winter, it is difficult to prepare peripheral blood smear, because agglutination occurs at low temperature (Fig. 8.46).

Table 8.49: Direct and indirect Coombs' Test

Parameters	Coombs' test	
	Direct antiglobulin test (DAT)	Indirect Coombs' test
Principle	Detects antibodies or complement bound to surface of RBCs antigens *in vivo*	Detects *in vitro* antigen–antibody reactions or antibodies in serum
Utility in clinical practice	Immunomediated hemolytic anemia	Detection of low concentration of antibodies in patient's blood prior to blood transfusion
	Drug-induced hemolytic anemia	Detection of antibodies in antenatal women that may cause hemolytic disease of newborn
	Hemolytic disease of newborn	Compatibility testing in blood banking
	ABO hemolytic disease of newborn	RBC phenotyping
		Identification of antibody in mother's serum
	Mismatched blood transfusion	Titration studies

Red Blood Cells

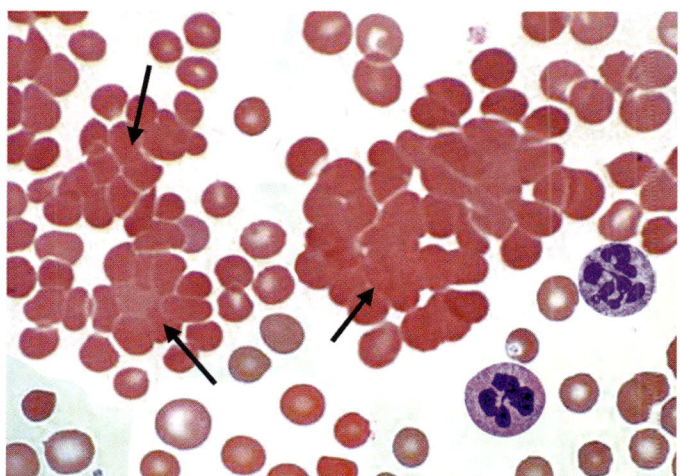

Fig. 8.46: Cold agglutinin disease. Peripheral blood smear examination shows agglutination of red blood cells (arrorws).

Hematocrit values: MCH and MCHC values are very high due to agglutination of red blood cells. Red blood cell value is very low.

PAROXYSMAL COLD HEMOGLOBINURIA

Paroxysmal cold hemoglobinuria (PCH) most often occurs in children associated with viral infections. IgG autoantibodies are formed against P antigen on surface of RBCs at low temperature. These antibodies fix complement and induce intravascular hemolysis. IgG antibodies are also known as *Donath-Landsteiner antibody*.

Hemoglobinuria: Hemoglobin in urine is demonstrated by benzidine test.

Hemosiderinuria: Hemosiderin is demonstrated by Prussian blue reaction.

Hemoglobinemia: Presence of hemoglobin in the plasma gives red discoloration. It is demonstrated by benzidine test.

DRUG-INDUCED HEMOLYTIC ANEMIA

Most antigens have high molecular weight in excess of 10,000. Small molecules cannot act as antigen by themselves. Binding of antigen with small carrier produce immune response. This passenger molecule is known as *hapten*. Hapten molecule is too small (MW <1000) to trigger an immune response alone but can be immunogenic when it attaches to a larger carrier molecule such as host serum protein. Drug-induced hemolytic anemia occurs by two mechanisms: antigenic drugs and tolerance-breaking drugs. The hapten-carrier phenomenon is shown in Fig. 8.47.

Antigenic Drugs

These are benzylpenicillin, cephalosporins and quinidine. These drugs bind to the surface of RBCs leading to formation of antibodies against drug. These antibodies react with drugs and form complex on the surface of RBCs leading to hemolysis.

Tolerance Breaking Drugs

Example, α-methyl dopa drug. This drug induces antibodies against intrinsic antigens.

ALLOIMMUNE HEMOLYTIC ANEMIA

HEMOLYTIC DISEASE OF NEWBORN

Hemolytic disease of newborn most commonly occurs with Rh blood group incompatibility between mother and fetus. It occurs when the mother is Rh −ve and baby is Rh +ve, having inherited an allele for one of the Rh antigens from the father (Fig. 8.48).

During First Pregnancy

At birth, a small quantity of fetal blood usually leaks across the placenta into the maternal bloodstream. Upon exposure to Rh antigen, the mother's immune system

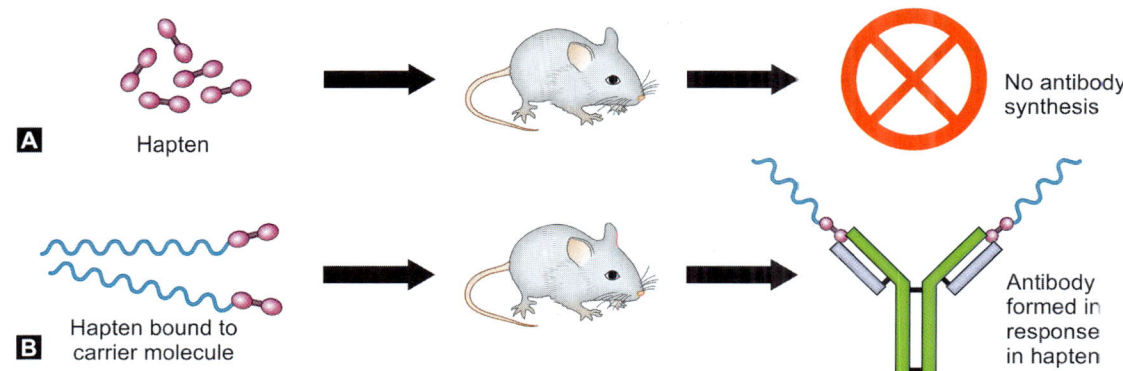

Fig. 8.47: The hapten-carrier phenomenon. (A) Hapten molecule is too small to trigger an immune response, (B) binding of hapten with carrier triggers an immune response.

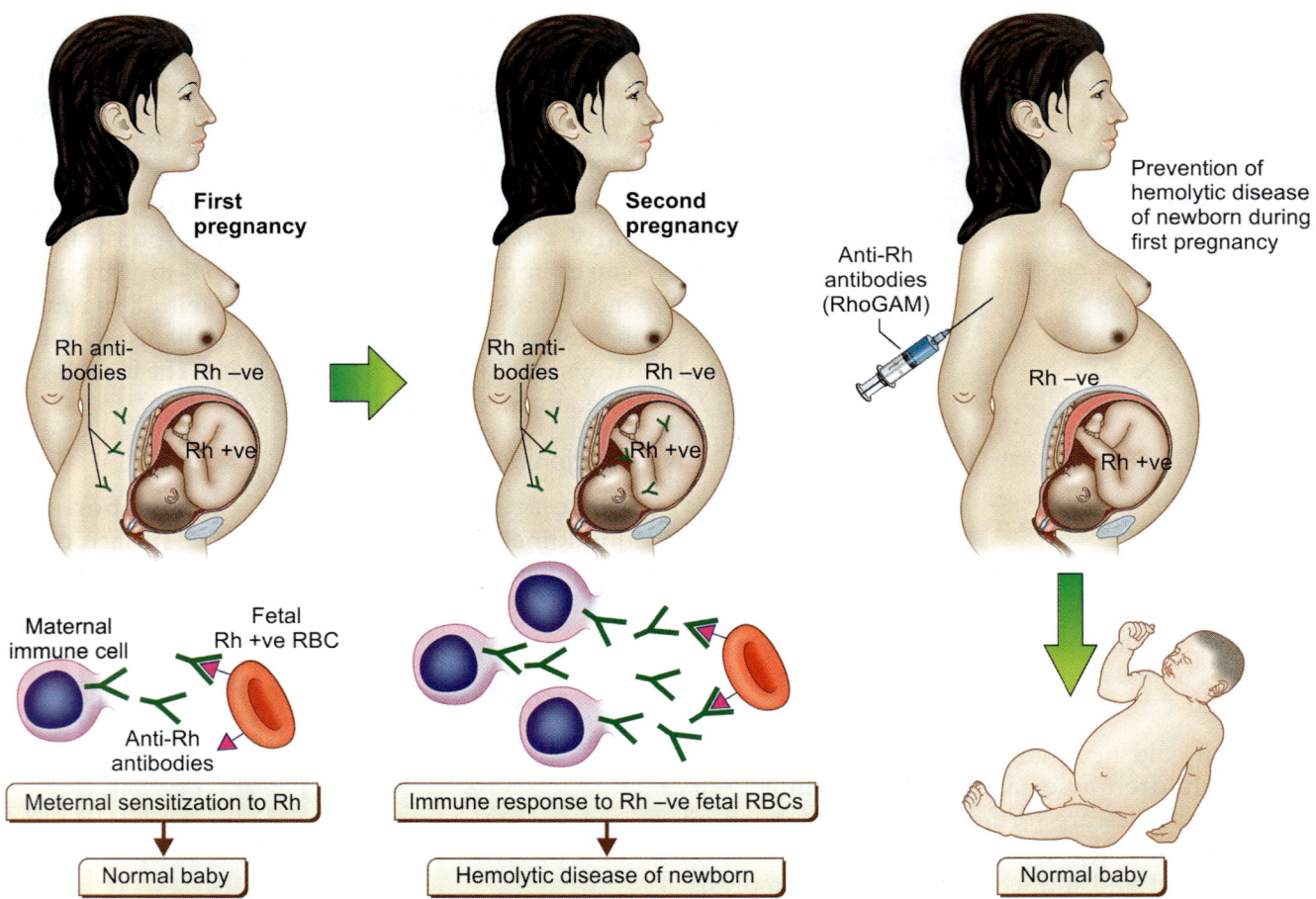

Fig. 8.48: Hemolytic disease of newborn. Rh factor incompatibility can cause lysis of red blood cells. A naturally occurring red blood cell incompatibility results when a fetus Rh +ve develops within Rh –ve mother. Initial sensitization of the maternal immune system occurs when fetal blood passes the placental barrier. In most cases, the fetus develops normally. However, a subsequent pregnancy with Rh +ve fetus results in a severe fetal red blood cells hemolysis. Control of incompatibility is done by administration of anti-Rh antibodies (RhoGAM) to Rh –ve mothers during pregnancy to inactivate and remove any Rh factor that may be transferred from the fetus in maternal circulation. In some cases, anti-Rh antibody (RhoGAM) is administered before sensitization occurs.

responds by making anti-Rh antibodies. Because the baby is already born, it suffers no damage.

During Subsequent Pregnancy

The maternal antibodies cross the placenta into the fetal blood. If the second fetus is Rh +ve, the ensuring antigen–antibody reaction causes hemolysis of fetal RBCs. The result is hemolytic disease of newborn (HDN).

Clinical Features

Newborn develops anemia, jaundice, hepatosplenomegaly, cardiac failure and kernicterus (staining of the basal ganglion and other structures of CNS by unconjugated bilirubin). Kernicterus with resultant neurological damage is the most significant long-term consequence of hemolytic disease of newborn. In addition, consequences include stillbirth or in hydrops fetalis, fetal heart failure with massive generalized edema.

Management

Administration of anti-D antiserum to a D-negative mother at the time of delivery of a D-positive child prevents maternal alloimmunization by removing fetal red cells from the maternal circulation.

Preventive Measures

Routine administration of anti-D IgG antiserum to D-negative mothers at 28 weeks gestation and at the time of first delivery (or at the time of termination of pregnancy) of a D-positive child results in the antibody-mediated removal of fetal red cells from the maternal circulation, preventing maternal alloimmunization.

Laboratory Investigations

Cord blood hemoglobin and bilirubin, bilirubin binding reserve of albumin are estimated by hydroxy benzene azobenzoic acid dye test and indirect Coombs' test. The peripheral blood smear displays erythroid precursors.

HEMOLYTIC TRANSFUSION REACTIONS

In ABO mismatch blood transfusion, preformed IgM antibodies present in the serum of recipient are active at 37°C. These antibodies and complement coat red blood cells and activate complement system resulting in intravascular hemolysis.

PAROXYSMAL NOCTURNAL HEMOGLOBINURIA

PNH may develop as a primary disorder or evolve from pre-existing cases of aplastic anemia. During hemolytic episodes, patient develops normocytic or macrocytic anemia, accompanied by an appropriate reticulocyte response. Patient of PNH may transform to acute myeloid leukemia (AML) or myelodysplastic syndrome.

PATHOGENESIS OF PNH

Physiological state: PIG-A gene converts PI to GPI (glycosylphosphatidylinositol) anchor regulatory proteins. These anchor regulatory proteins bind to various red blood cell membrane proteins like MIRL (CD59), DAF (CD55), CD8, CD14, CD16a and CD52 required for the protection of red blood cells, granulocytes, and platelets from complement-mediated lysis. DAF (decay accelerating factor) cleaves C3b. MIRL (membrane inhibitor reactive lysis) participates in cleaving C5–9. These complement regulatory proteins are required for the protection of red blood cells, granulocytes, and platelets from complement-mediated lysis.

Pathological state: PIG-A gene mutation leads to deficient expression of glycosylphosphatidylinositol (GPI)-linked membrane proteins (CD55, CD59, CD8, CD14, CD16a and CD52). Acidic pH causes uncontrolled activation of complement pathway to form *membrane attack complex* (C5b–9). C5b–9 attacks RBCs, granulocytes and platelets. It leads to recurrent bouts of intravascular complement mediated hemolysis. In normal persons, *membrane attack complex* (C5b–9) formation is neutralized by CRP (complementary regulatory proteins). Pathogenesis of paroxysmal nocturnal hemoglobinuria is shown in Fig. 8.49.

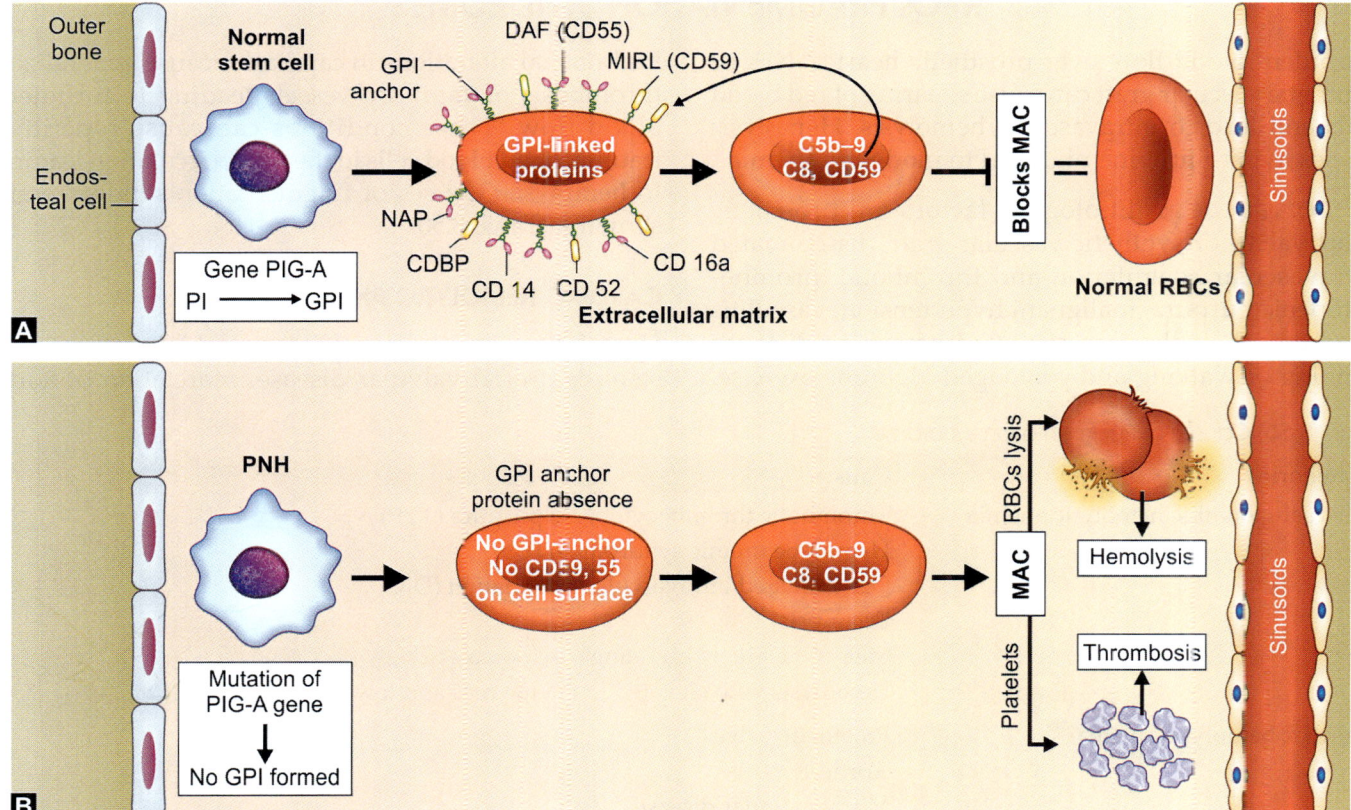

Fig. 8.49: Pathogenesis of paroxysmal nocturnal hemoglobinuria. (A) Under physiological state, PIG-A gene encoding GPI membrane anchoring proteins, which bind to CD55, CD59, CD8, CD14, CD16a and CD52 resulting in maintenance of red blood cell membrane, (B) under pathological state, PIG-A gene mutation causes deficiency of membrane anchoring proteins leading to red blood cell destruction.

CLINICAL FEATURES

The condition is often marked by the passage of hemoglobin-containing urine on awakening. Patient presents with recurrent bouts of intravascular complement mediated hemolysis, mild jaundice, abdominal pain and pancytopenia. There is increased risk of thrombosis in the portal vein, hepatic veins and cerebral veins. Most common cause of death is thrombosis in portal vein and hepatic veins. PNH may be associated with aplastic anemia and myelodysplastic syndrome progressing to acute myeloid leukemia.

LABORATORY DIAGNOSIS

Hematological findings: Hemoglobin and hematocrit values are decreased. Reticulocyte count is increased. Peripheral smear examination shows normocytic normochromic anemia with polychromasia. Bone marrow examination reveals erythroid hyperplasia. NAP score is decreased. Hemoglobinemia and hemoglobinuria are demonstrated by benzidine test. Serum bilirubin is raised with decrease in serum haptoglobin.

Flow cytometry: Flow cytometry demonstrates diminished CD55 and CD59 expression on red blood cells, leukocytes and platelets.

CD55 and CD59: Modified gel diffusion of the red blood cell membrane proteins is used to confirm the diagnosis. DAF and MIRL are markedly reduced on the red blood cells in PNH.

Ham's test: Ham's test (*in vitro*) is the best screening test for PNH. Acidic pH activates complement pathway leading to RBCs lysis.

Sucrose hemolysis test: Sucrose hemolysis test (*in vitro*) is also screening test for PNH. Sucrose reduces pH and thus activates complement pathway leading to RBCs lysis.

FLAER (fluorescent aerolysin) test: FLAER test is a diagnostic tool to demonstrate clones of neutrophils and monocytes.

MANAGEMENT

These patients are managed by blood transfusions, oral anticoagulants and antibiotics. Bone marrow transplantation is curative.

RBCs FRAGMENTATION SYNDROMES

Turbulent blood flow over prosthetic heart valves or synthetic vascular graft can cause shearing of red blood cells and lead to intravascular hemolysis. Hemolysis causes hyperbilirubinemia, mild to moderate anemia.

Etiopathogenesis: Etiological factors are prosthetic heart valves or synthetic vascular graft, disseminated intravascular coagulation and thrombotic thrombocytopenic purpura, malignant hypertension, vasculitis syndrome, hemolytic uremic syndrome, long-distance running or walking and prolonged vigorous exercise.

Endothelial alterations in capillaries cause generalized thrombosis of capillary vessels leading to turbulent blood flow. These conditions can cause repetitive trauma to red blood cells in the microcirculation leading to hemolysis. Causes of fragmentation syndrome are shown in Table 8.50.

CARDIAC HEMOLYTIC ANEMIA

Hemolytic anemia occurs due to prosthetic valve, aortic stenosis, mitral valvular disease, coarctation of aorta

Table 8.50: Causes of fragmentation syndrome

Categories	Causes
Microangiopathic hemolytic anemia	Thrombotic thrombocytopenic purpura (TTP) Hemolytic uremic syndrome (HUS) Disseminated intravascular coagulation (DIC) Eclampsia Metastatic mucin-secreting carcinoma Hemolysis with elevated liver enzymes and low platelets (HELLP)
Cardiac hemolytic anemia	Prosthetic valve Aortic stenosis Mitral valvular disease Coarctation of aorta Ruptured chordae tendineae
March hemoglobinuria	Athletes and soldiers

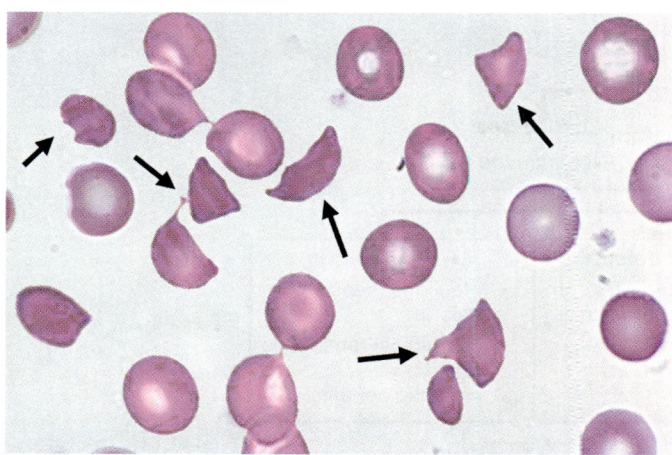

Fig. 8.50: Red blood cells are showing fragmentation (arrows) from a case mitral valvular disease.

and ruptured chordae tendineae. Turbulence of blood flow in cardiovascular system causes mechanical injury to erythrocytes.

LABORATORY DIAGNOSIS

Peripheral smear examination: Periheral blood smear examination shows fragmented triangular shaped red blood cells known as schistocytes or helmet cells (Fig. 8.50).

Reticulocyte count: Reticulocyte count is increased.

Serum bilirubin: Serum bilirubin level is increased.

MICROANGIOPATHIC HEMOLYTIC ANEMIA

Red blood cells undergo destruction, when these pass through arterioles, capillaries and venules in cases of hemolytic-uremic syndrome, thrombotic thrombocytopenic purpura, mucin secreting metastatic carcinoma and eclampsia.

HEMOLYTIC-UREMIC SYNDROME

Hemolytic-uremic syndrome is a triad characterized by acute renal failure, microangiopathic hemolytic anemia and thrombocytopenia. Bacterial toxins play role in the pathogenesis of HUS. These toxins cause endothelial damage resulting in activation of coagulation system.

Clinical Features

Patient presents with bloody diarrhea, anemia, jaundice, oliguria, hemoglobinuria and proteinuria.

Hematological Findings

Hematological findings are low hemoglobin, microcytic hypochromic picture with fragmented red blood cells, increased serum bilirubin, increased blood urea and serum creatinine.

Urine Analysis

Urine analysis shows oliguria, hemoglobinuria and proteinuria.

THROMBOTIC THROMBOCYTOPENIC PURPURA

Thrombotic thrombocytopenic purpura may affect young adults. There is widespread thrombi formation in arterioles, capillaries and venules. Patient presents with fever, central nervous system manifestations and renal failure. There are three variants of TTP: congenital, primary and secondary.

Pathogenesis

Congenital and primary TTP occur due to deficiency of ADAMTS 13. The disorder is initiated as a result of endothelial injury resulting in release of von Willebrand factor and other procoagulant substances.

Deficient cleaving protease activity causes accumulation of vWF multimers resulting in platelets aggregation and microthrombi formation in microcirculation.

MARCH HEMOLYTIC ANEMIA

March hemolytic anemia is seen in athletes and soldiers following strenuous exercise and marching. Mechanical destruction of red blood cells occurs in the microvessels of the feet. There is transient hemoglobinemia and hemoglobinuria persisting for a few days.

DIAGNOSTIC APPROACH OF HEMOLYTIC ANEMIA

Hemolytic anemia is produced due to increased red blood cell destruction that cannot be compensated by bone marrow. RBCs destruction may be due to defects within red blood cells or due to extrinsic causes.

Family history of hemoglobinopathy or hereditary spherocytosis, recent blood transfusions, malaria and drug intake provide clues to proper diagnosis. Diagnostic approach of hemolytic anemia is shown in Fig. 8.51.

PERIPHERAL BLOOD SMEAR

Peripheral blood smear should be examined for the presence of *microspherocytes*, fragmented red blood cells and malarial parasite. Hemolytic anemia in which spherocytes are not present include G6PD deficiency, hemoglobinopathies (other than HbC and thalassemia), unstable hemoglobin, drugs, snakebite and malaria. RHAG gene located on chromosome 6p21.1–p11 encodes *rhesus antigen*. RHAG gene mutation causes

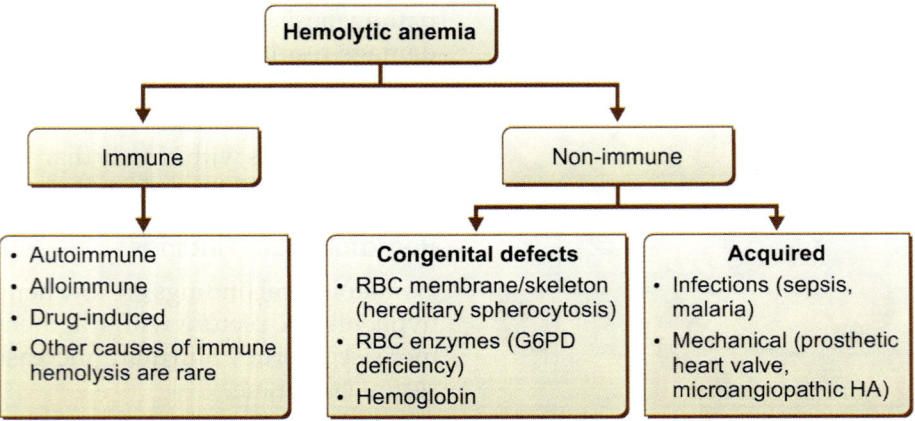

Fig. 8.51: Diagnostic approach of hemolytic anemia.

total loss of all *rhesus antigens* leading to chronic nonspherocytic hemolytic anemia.

Microspherocytes: These red blood cells appear small dense and spherical. These are demonstrated in *hereditary spherocytosis* and *immune hemolytic anemia*. These are also demonstrated in HbC and hypersplenism. When hereditary spherocytosis is considered as a possible cause, peripheral blood smear obtained from family members supports the diagnosis.

Presence of microspherocytes and numerous target cells are highly suggestive of hemoglobin C disease. Hemoglobin electrophoresis should be performed to establish hemoglobin C. Hereditary spherocytosis is diagnosed by osmotic fragility and acidified glycerol tests.

Ovalocytes: These are demonstrated in hereditary ovalocytosis.

Acanthocytes: These are demonstrated in pyruvate kinase deficiency.

Fragmented RBCs: Presence of fragmented red blood cells (burr cells, schistocytes and helmet cells) indicate microangiopathic hemolytic anemia.

Sickle cells: These are demonstrated in cases of sickle cell disease and trait.

Bite cells: These are demonstrated in G6PD deficiency. The diagnosis of G6PD is done by methemoglobin reduction test and fluorescent assay.

PLASMA HAPTOGLOBIN

Haptoglobin is a glycoprotein that is synthesized in the liver. It consists of two pairs of α-chains and β-chains. With hemolysis, free hemoglobin readily dissociates into dimers of α- and β-chains.

These bind with haptoglobin in plasma or serum. The complex is removed by liver. Plasma haptoglobin level is decreased in hemolytic anemia.

PLASMA HEMOPEXIN

Hemopexin is a $β_1$ glycoprotein of molecular weight 70,000, synthesized in the liver. In severe intravascular hemolysis, when haptoglobin is depleted, hemopexin is low or absent and elevated plasma methemalbumin. With less severe hemolysis, although haptoglobin is likely to be reduced or absent, hemopexin may be normal or only slightly lowered.

PLASMA HEMOGLOBIN

In this method, the catalytic action of haem-containing proteins brings about the oxidation of benzidine by H_2O_2 give a green color, which changes to blue and finally to reddish violet. The intensity of reaction may be compared in a spectrophotometer with that produced by solutions of known hemoglobin. When the plasma hemoglobin is >50 mg/L, it can be measured as hemoglobin cyanide (HiCN) or oxyhemoglobin by a spectrometer at 540 nm.

HEMOSIDERIN IN URINE

Hemosiderinuria is a sequel to the presence of hemoglobin in the glomerular filtrate. It is a valuable sign of intravascular hemolysis because the urine will be found to contain iron-containing granules even if there is no hemoglobinuria at the time.

However, hemosiderinuria is not found in the urine at the onset of a hemolytic attack even if this is accompanied by hemoglobinemia and hemoglobinuria because the hemoglobin has first to be absorbed by the cells of the renal tubules. The intracellular breakdown of hemoglobin liberates iron, which is then re-excreted. Hemosiderinuria may persist for several weeks after a hemolytic episode.

SICKLING TEST

Hemoglobin S is less soluble in a reducing agent than other forms of hemoglobin. Mixing blood with the reducing agent, sodium metabisulphite on a sealed slide, will induce sickling in susceptible sickle cells. The test is simple and quick. The results can be viewed under light microscope after 20 minutes. The sickle cell preparation is positive whenever hemoglobin S is present (e.g. sickle cell anemia, sickle cell trait, sickle C disease, sickle cell thalassemia). False positivity is seen in exceptionally high hematocrit, unstable hemoglobin, elevated plasma proteins and lipids.

ANTIHUMAN GLOBIN TEST (COOMBS' TEST)

Direct Coombs' test also known as *antihuman globin test* is performed to detect autoantibodies. Patient's RBCs are mixed with antibodies directed against human immunoglobulin or complement Presence of RBCs agglutination indicates positive Coombs' test. Test detects antibodies or complement bound to surface of RBCs antigens *in vivo*. It is performed in immune mediated hemolytic anemia, hemolytic disease of newborn, mismatched blood transfusion. Drug-induced hemolytic anemia may also be associated with direct Coombs' test. If the test is negative in the presence spherocytes, one should consider hereditary spherocytes as a possible cause of hemolysis.

Indirect Coombs' test is performed to detect *in vitro* antigen–antibody reactions or antibodies in serum. It detects low concentration of antibodies in patient's blood prior to blood transfusion and antenatal Rh –ve with Rh +ve fetus. It is also performed for compatibility testing in blood banking, and RBCs phenotyping (Fig. 8.52).

HEMOGLOBIN ELECTROPHORESIS

Hemoglobin electrophoresis is a diagnostic tool to measure different types of hemoglobin in the blood. It is performed in suspected disorder associated with abnormal hemoglobin sickle cell anemia and thalassemia.

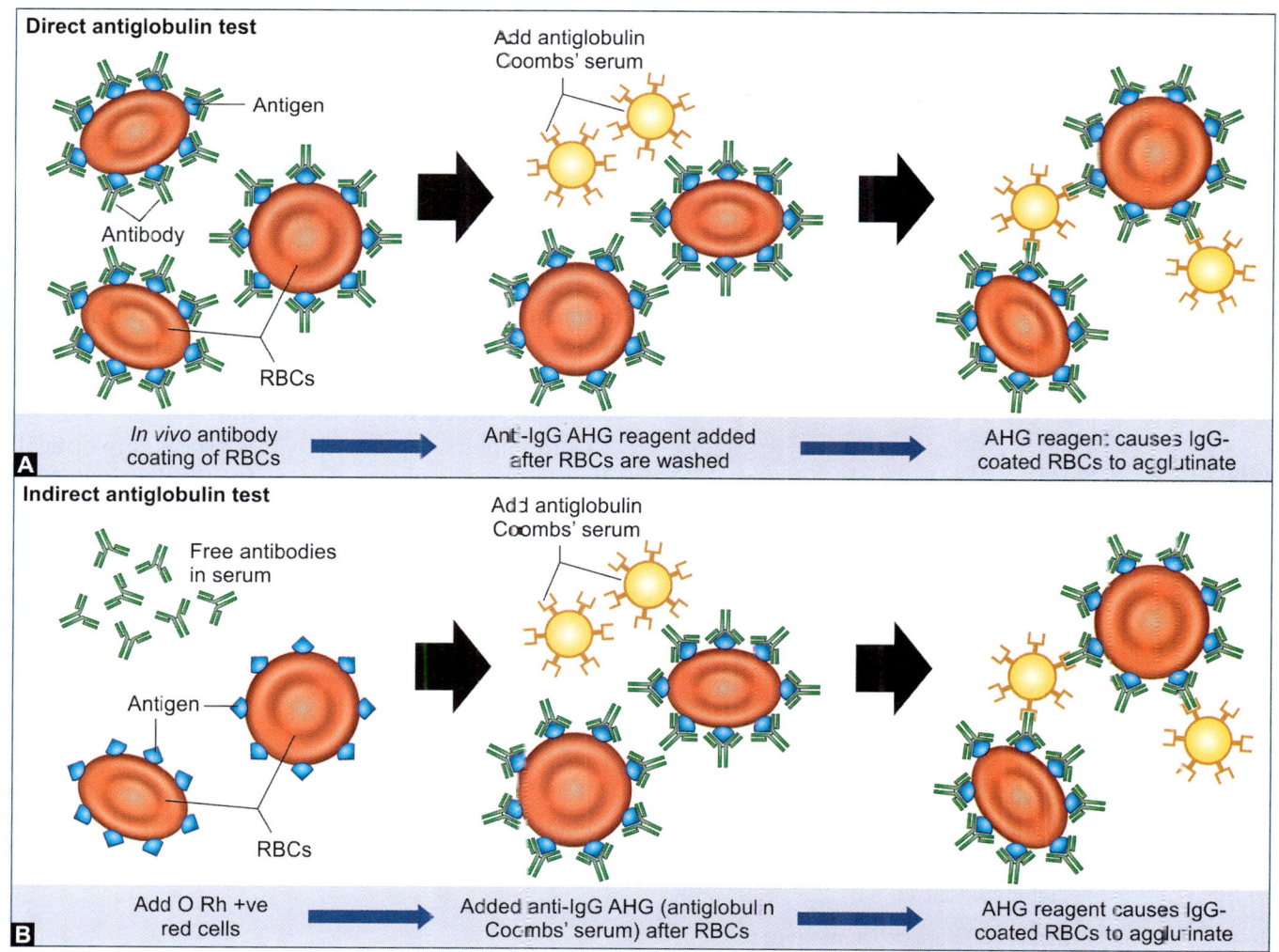

Fig. 8.52: Coombs' test.

Principle: The principle behind electrophoresis is that when proteins are exposed to a *charge gradient*, they separate from each other by forming *bands* that separate toward one end or the other end in the electric field. Cellulose acetate membrane, starch gel, agarose gel, citrate agar gel and filter paper are the commonly used mediums. *Cellulose acetate electrophoresis* is performed at alkaline pH of 8.2–8.6. Citrate agar or agarose gel electrophoresis is done in acidic pH of 6.0–6.2. HPLC is rapidly taking its place in many laboratories.

Blood Sampling

Blood transfusions within the previous 12 weeks may alter test results. Hemoglobin electrophoresis is performed on venous blood samples taken in anticoagulant EDTA container. Red cell lysate is prepared using a lysing reagent (Na_4EDTA and KCN).

Interpretation

Each of the major hemoglobin types has an electrical charge of a different degree. Hemoglobin electrophoresis separates and measures normal and abnormal hemoglobin. The components then move away from each other at different rates, and when separated form a series of distinctly *pigmented bands*.

Table 8.51: Hemoglobin electrophoresis pattern in normal persons

Age group	Hemoglobin	Percentage
Adults	HbA_1	95–98%
	HbA_2	2–3%
	HbF	0.8–2.0%
	HbS	0%
	HbC	0%
Children	HbF (newborn)	50–80%
	HbF (6 months age)	8%
	HbF (>6 months age)	1–2%

These bands are then compared with those of a normal sample. Each band is further assessed as a % of the total hemoglobin, thus indicating the severity of any abnormality. Description of hemoglobin (Hb) is comprised of many different types, the most common being HbA_1, HbA_2, HbF, HbS, and HbC. Normal reference values can vary by laboratory but are generally within the following ranges.

Hemoglobin Electrophoresis Patterns

In normal adults, HbA_1 is the major component of hemoglobin in the normal red blood cell. HbA_2 is a minor component of normal hemoglobin, comprising approximately 2–3% of the total. In children, HbF is the major hemoglobin component in the fetus, but usually exists only in minimal quantities in the normal adult.

Levels of HbF greater than 2% in patients over three years of age are considered abnormal. Hemoglobin electrophoresis pattern in normal persons and hemoglobin disorders is shown in Tables 8.51 and 8.52.

HIGH PERFORMANCE LIQUID CHROMATOGRAPHY

High performance liquid chromatography (HPLC) is one of the commonest laboratory investigations performed for the identification of globin chain synthesis.

Principle: Cation exchange HPLC is a process by which mixture of hemoglobins with net positive charge are separated by their adsorption onto a negatively charged *stationary phase* in a chromatography column. This process is then followed by their elution by a liquid *mobile phase* containing increasing concentrations of cations flowing through the column.

Hemoglobins separated by this process are optically identified in the eluate. The quantification is done by computing the area under the corresponding peak in the elution profile.

Table 8.52: Hemoglobin electrophoresis pattern in hemoglobin disorders

Hemoglobin	Hemoglobin disorder	Percentage
HbA_2	β-thalassemia	4.00–5.8%
	HbH disease	<2%
HbF	β-thalassemia major	10–90%
	β-thalassemia minor	2–5%
	Homozygous hereditary persistence of fetal hemoglobin (HPFH)	100%
	Heterozygous hereditary persistence of fetal hemoglobin (HPFH)	5–35%
	Heterozygous HbS	15%
HbS	Sickle cell disease (homozygous)	70–98%
HbC	Hemoglobin C disease (homozygous)	90–98%

Table 8.53: Retention times of common normal and variant hemoglobins

Window	Retention time (minutes)	Hemoglobins that appear in the window
–	Peak within first minute	HbH, Bart's hemoglobin, bilirubin, acetylated HbF
F	1.10	HbF
A	2.50	HbA, glycosylated S
A_2	3.60	HbA_2, D—Iran, E, Lepore
D	4.10	D—Punjab
S	4.50	S
C	5.10	C—constant spring

Interpretation

Different hemoglobins have different affinity for the stationary phase. Hemoglobin with strong positive charge has higher affinity for stationary phase and appears in elute later than other hemoglobins.

Retention time is the time taken by normal and variant hemoglobin to appear in the eluate. Retention times of normal and variant hemoglobins are shown in Table 8.53.

Advantages of HPLC: HPLC is performed on very small venous sample. It estimates quantity of normal and abnormal hemoglobins. It is used to estimate quantity of HbA_2 in diagnosing β-thalassemia trait. Overall has more advantages than electrophoresis and routinely performed in many laboratories.

Disadvantages of HPLC: HPLC instrument and its reagents are very costly.

ISOELECTRIC FOCUSING (IEF)

Isoelectric focusing is a technique for separating different molecules by differences in their isoelectric point. Hemoglobins in isoelectric focusing (IEF) are separated in agarose gel according to their isoelectric points at which these have no net charge.

Bands in IEF are sharper as compared to electrophoresis. But this diagnostic toll is more expensive than electrophoresis.

MICROCOLUMN CHROMATOGRAPHY

Microcolumn chromatography is an anion exchange chromatography used to estimate quantity of HbA_2 in α-thalassemia.

IMMUNOASSAY

Immunoassay is used to evaluate various hemoglobins by commercially available kits such as hemocards for specific hemoglobins.

KLEIHAUER-BETKE TEST (ACID ELUTION TEST)

Kleihauer test (acid elution test) is a blood test to measure the amount of fetal hemoglobin transferred from a fetus to a mother's bloodstream. Test is based on principle that red cells containing HbF is resistant to lysis as compared to red cells containing HbA. It is most often performed on Rh –ve mothers to determine the required dose of Rho (D) immune globulin (RhIg) to inhibit formation of Rh antibodies in the mother and prevent Rh disease in future Rh positive children.

FLOW CYTOMETRY

Flow cytometry is done by using fluorochrome conjugated monoclonal antibody to HbF.

2,6-DICHLOROPHENOLINDOPHENOL TEST (DCIP)

Hemoglobin E is an abnormal hemoglobin with a single point mutation in the β-chain due to change in the amino acid, from glutamic acid to lysine at position 26. This disorder is very common in South-East Asia but has a low frequency amongst other ethnicities. HbE can be detected on electrophoresis. 2,6-dichlorophenolindophenol test (DCIP) is used to screen patient with HbE.

SUPRAVITAL STAINING

Supravital staining is used to demonstrate HbH inclusions. Smears are stained with brilliant cresyl blue. This stain acts as a mild oxidant and precipitates HbH.

GLOBIN CHAIN ELECTROPHORESIS

DL-dithiothreitol and urea added to red cell lysate to dissociate heme and globin chains. Electrophoresis then carried out on cellulose acetate membrane with both acid and alkaline buffer systems. This method permits the distinction between α- and β-chain abnormalities.

BONE MARROW FAILURE SYNDROMES

Bone marrow participates in hematopoiesis. Bone marrow failure is characterized by marrow hypoplasia leading to pancytopenias (erythroid, myeloid and megakaryocytes) and decreased reticulocyte count as a result of failure of bone marrow precursor cells. Bone marrow failure occurs due to inherited or acquired causes.

APLASTIC ANEMIA

Aplastic anemia is pluripotent stem cell disorder results in bone marrow failure. It affects erythroid, myeloid and megakaryocytic series. Bone marrow shows variably reduced cellularity, depending on the clinical stage of the disease.

CLASSIFICATION

Bone marrow pluripotent stem cell failure occurs due to primary or secondary causes. Primary aplastic anemia occurs in 65% of cases. Four inherited aplastic anemia syndromes include Fanconi anemia, dyskeratosis congenita, Shwachman-Diamond syndrome and congenital megakaryocytic thrombocytopenia. Fanconi anemia is characterized by pancytopenia, congenital abnormalities and increased risk of cancers.

PATHOGENESIS

Secondary aplastic anemia may be caused by total body irradiation, drugs, chemicals, viral infections, and Fanconi anemia.

Physical agent: Ionizing radiation causes aplastic anemia.

Exposure to chemicals: Bone marrow suppression due to drugs and chemicals may be dose related (e.g. benzene, alkylating agents, vincristine).

Exposure to drugs: Drugs causing bone marrow suppression in unpredictable manner (idiosyncrasy) are streptomycin, chloramphenicol and chlorpromazine.

Viruses: Aplastic anemia may be caused by human Parvovirus B19 or HCV.

Hematological disorders: Aplastic anemia can occur in the course of hereditary spherocytosis or sickle cell anemia. Some cases of paroxysmal nocturnal hemoglobinuria is associated with aplastic anemia, while some may progress to myelodysplastic syndrome resulting in acute myeloid leukemia.

Fanconi anemia is inherited disease due to defects in telomerase activity.

LABORATORY DIAGNOSIS

Peripheral blood smear: Peripheral blood smear shows anemia, pancytopenia, thrombocytopenia, and reticulocytopenia. In severe aplastic anemia, patient shows neutrophils (less than 500 µl), platelets (less than 20,000/µl) and reticulocytes (less than 1%).

Reticulocytes count: The lack of an appropriate reticulocytes response to the anemia indicates decreased or ineffective hematopoiesis as the mechanism for the pancytopenia.

Bone marrow: Hematopoietic elements are replaced by fat cells lacking normal hematopoietic activity. There is relative increase in lymphocytes and plasma cells.

As the cellularity decreases, there is a corresponding increase in bone marrow fat. One must look for metastatic deposits in bone marrow (Fig. 8.53).

CLINICAL FEATURES

Patients with aplastic anemia present with weakness, fatigue (progressive anemia), infection (neutropenia), and bleeding tendencies (thrombocytopenia). Withdrawal of potential inciting agent may sometimes lead to recovery.

TREATMENT

Bone marrow transplantation is recommended in these cases.

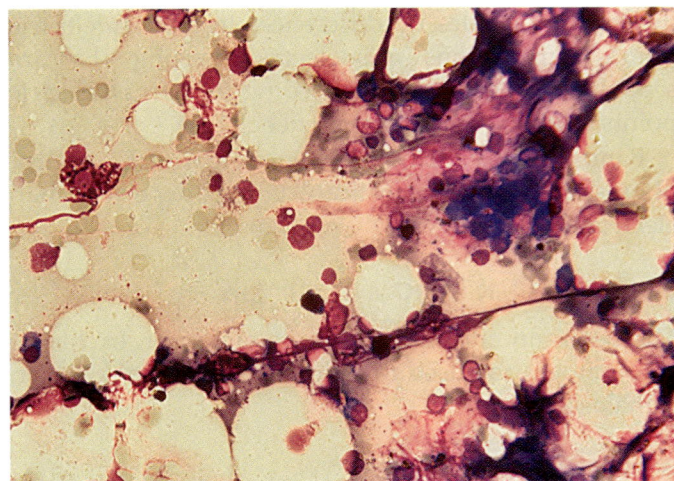

Fig. 8.53: Bone marrow in aplastic anemia showing marked reduction in the erythroid, myeloid and megakaryocytic precursor cells with increased adipose cells.

PURE RED CELL APLASIA (ERYTHROBLASTOPENIA)

Pure red cell anemia (PRCA) is used to describe this disorder in adults, whereas Diamond-Blackfan anemia (DBA) and transient erythroblastopenia with normal myelopoiesis and megakaryopoiesis of childhood (TEC) are used for the congenital and acquired forms respectively.

CLASSIFICATION

Pure red cell aplasia may be congenital or acquired. Congenital pure red cell aplasia may be inherited (Diamond-Blackfan anemia) or non-herited (Pearson syndrome). Diamond-Blackfan anemia belongs to one of the rare group of genetic disorders known as the *inherited bone marrow failure syndromes (IBMFSs)*. These disorders share a predilection to bone marrow failure, birth defects, and cancer are characterized by *proapoptotic hematopoiesis*. Acquired pure red cell aplasia is shown in Table 8.54.

PATHOGENESIS

In some cases, the IgG seems to be cytotoxic to CFU-E in the presence of complement; in others, its inhibitory activity is independent of the presence of complement but its presence is continuously required during the 7-day period of maturation of CFU-E to erythroblasts.

Stage of arrest: The arrest occurs at *any level between CFU-E and basophilic erythroblasts*. The stage of erythropoiesis at which the arrest occurs has been studied by assaying PRCA marrow cells in semisolid media for erythroid progenitors.

CLINICAL FEATURES

Adult patients present with symptoms of anemia that at the time of diagnosis may be quite severe.

Complete arrest of erythropoiesis leads to a decline of red cell count averaging about 1% a day, so the development of anemia is slow and progressive, allowing for physiologic compensatory changes. Physical examination in primary PRCA is usually negative except for pallor and signs of anemia. In secondary cases, patients may have physical findings related to the underlying disease. *Hepatosplenomegaly and lymphadenopathy are not findings consistent with primary PRCA.*

LABORATORY DIAGNOSIS

Hemogram: Peripheral smear examination shows normochromic and normocytic. *The white cell count and the differential count are normal.* Occasionally, mild leukopenia, lymphocytosis, and/or eosinophilia may be present. There is a complete absence of polychromatophilic red cells on the smear, and the reticulocyte count is between 0 and 1%.

Bone marrow: The hallmark of PRCA is the absence of erythroblasts from an otherwise normal marrow. The cellularity of the marrow is normal or slightly increased. High cellularity with elimination of fat spaces should lead away from the diagnosis of PRCA. In typical cases, the erythroblasts are either totally absent, or they constitute <1% on the marrow differential count. The myeloid cells and the megakaryocytes in the marrow are normal and exhibit full maturation.

An increased number of lymphocytes on marrow smear, or an increased number of lymphoid aggregates in marrow biopsy, or a mild increase in plasma cells, eosinophils, or mast cells may be seen.

Iron stores: Iron stores are increased and normally distributed, *but during recovery or the phase of ineffective erythropoiesis, a few ring sideroblasts may be seen.*

Table 8.54: Acquired pure red cell aplasia

Acquired disorder	Causes
Primary PRCA	Diamond-Blackfan syndrome
Secondary PRCA	Thymoma (T cell-mediated suppression of erythropoiesis)
	Autoimmune disorders
	Hematologic malignancies (B cell CLL PRCA is 6% and T cell CLL)
	Solid tumors
	Parvovirus 19 infection* in children (sickle cell disease and immunocompromised) cytotoxic to CFU-E growth and development
	Chronic hemolytic anemias
	Collagen vascular disorders
	Drugs (phenytoin, procainamide and anti-tubercular drugs)
	Chemicals

*Parvovirus 19 infection affects erythroid precursors in bone marrow, showing a few giant proerythroblasts. These cells are large with basophilic cytoplasm and intranuclear inclusions in sieve like nuclear chromatin.

Table 8.55: Classification of sideroblastic anemia

Hereditary/acquired	Disorders
Hereditary causes	X-linked recessive disorder (most common)
	Autosomal recessive disorder (a few cases)
Acquired causes	Hematological disorders (leukemia, multiple myeloma, polycythemia vera and myelodysplastic syndrome)
	Drugs (isoniazid, chloramphenicol)
	Toxic agents (alcohol and lead) blocking at mitochondrial level of hemosynthesis
	Vitamin deficiency (pyridoxine deficiency) in antitubercular therapy, celiac disease, alcoholism
	Autoimmune disorders (systemic lupus erythematosus and rheumatoid arthritis)
	Miscellaneous causes (porphyria and iron overload)

SIDEROBLASTIC ANEMIA

Sideroblastic anemias (SA) are heterogeneous group of disorders characterized by presence of ringed sideroblasts in the bone marrow, ineffective erythropoiesis, increased levels of tissue iron and microcytic hypochromic picture. Sideroblastic anemia may be hereditary or secondary (more common). Classification of sideroblastic anemia is shown in Table 8.55.

Sideroblasts: Sideroblasts are erythroblasts containing aggregates of iron which are demonstrable by prussian blue reaction. There are three types of sideroblasts: normal sideroblast, abnormal sideroblast and ring sideroblast (Fig. 8.54). Types of siderblasts according to WHO are shown in Table 8.56.

Pathogenesis: Normally, iron present in mitochondria combines with protoporphyrin to synthesize heme in erythroid precursors. Under pathological state, iron present in mitochondria fails to bind with protoporphyrin affecting heme synthesis. Iron remains in the mitochondria and forms ring sideroblasts. These ring sideroblasts do not mature into RBCs leading to sideroblastic anemia. Ineffective erythropoiesis increases iron overload.

HEREDITARY SIDEROBLASTIC ANEMIA

Hereditary sideroblastic anemia may be X-linked affecting males or autosomal recessive disorder. It occurs due to defective ALA synthatase resulting in defective synthesis of hemoglobin.

Clinical features: Patient presents with anemia, hepatomegaly, splenomegaly, failure to thrive and cardiac arrhythmias.

Hematological findings

Peripheral blood smear: Hemogram shows anisopoikilocytosis and microcytic hypochromic anemia. Leukocytes and platelets are within normal ranges.

Hematocrit values: MCH and MCHC are decreased.

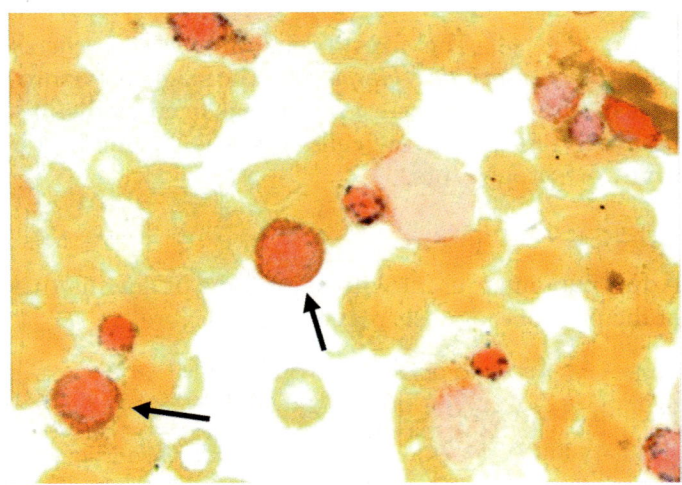

Fig. 8.54: Bone marrow aspirate showing ring sideroblasts.

Table 8.56: Types of sideroblasts according to WHO

Type according to WHO	Features	Iron contents demonstrated by Prussian blue reaction
Type 1	Intermediate or late normoblasts in bone marrow	1–2 pinpoint size iron granules in normoblasts randomly distributed
Type II	Intermediate or late normoblasts in bone marrow	1–5 pinpoint size iron granules in normoblasts seen in megaloblastic anemia and thalassemia
Type III	Intermediate or late normoblasts in bone marrow	Non-ferritin iron, pinpoint-sized granules forming partial or complete ring seen in primary/secondary sideroblastic anemia

Bone marrow: Bone marrow shows erythroid hyperplasia and dyserythropoiesis. Megakaryocytes are normal. Bone marrow iron stores are increased demonstrated by Prussian blue reaction. Serum iron and ferritin levels are increased.

ACQUIRED SIDEROBLASTIC ANEMIA

Acquired sideroblastic anemia occurs more frequently affecting adults than hereditary type. It occurs due to reduction in ALA synthatase resulting in decreased haem synthesis. Ineffective erythropoiesis leads to iron overload.

Clinical features: Patient presents with progressive anemia, signs of congestive heart failure and mild hepatosplenomegaly.

Hematological findings

- *Peripheral blood smear:* Hemogram shows dimorphic picture comprising of both microcytic hypochromic and macrocytic anemia. RBCs show basophilic stippling and target cells. RBCs also show iron deposits known as *Pappenheimer bodies* demonstrated by Perl's Prussian blue reaction. RDW is increased.
- *Bone marrow:* Bone marrow is hypercellular showing ringed sideroblasts demonstrated by Perl's Prussian blue reaction. Dyserythropoiesis is characterized by nuclear budding. Howell-Jolly bodies are demonstrated in the normoblasts. Megakaryopoiesis is normal.
- *Biochemical tests:* Serum iron, serum ferritin, % transferrin saturation and free protoporphyrin are increased. TIBC is decreased.

CONGENITAL DYSERYTHROBLASTOPOIETIC ANEMIA (CDA)

Congenital dyserythropoietic anemia is a heterogeneous disorder characterized by markedly ineffective erythropoiesis with dysplastic multinucleated erythroblasts and reduced reticulocyte count. These CDAs are designated as types I to III defined by the presence of distinctive morphologic abnormalities in erythroblasts demonstrated by light and electron microscopy. Dyserythropoiesis refers to abnormalities in the morphology or function or both of erythroid precursors.

TYPE I CONGENITAL DYSERYTHROBLASTIC ANEMIA

This is autosomal recessive disorder characterized by megaloblastic erythropoiesis. On electron microscopy, erythroblasts in bone marrow show spongy nuclear chromatin giving *Swiss-cheese* appearance. A few patients with CDA type I have been treated with interferon-α_2, with a good response.

TYPE II CONGENITAL DYSERYTHROBLASTIC ANEMIA

This is most common autosomal recessive disorder. It occurs due to mutation of CDAN2 gene located on chromosome 20q11.2. Geographic distribution—higher frequency of the gene in North-West Europe, Italy and North Africa. Both sexes are equally affected. CDA II patients suffer from lifelong anemia.

Pathogenesis: This diorder results from a combination of the death of erythroblasts in the bone marrow (ineffective erythropoiesis) and an increased breakdown of released red cells (peripheral hemolysis). The red cell glycosylation defects are responsible for both mechanisms.

Clinical features: Present during infancy or early childhood with anemia, jaundice and hepatosplenomegaly. There may be evidence of extramedullary hematopoiesis.

Laboratory diagnosis: This disorder is defined by serological abnormalities. It is also known as *hereditary multinuclearity* with a positive acid serum lysis test (HEMPAS), because RBCs most often show positive result on the acidified serum lysis test. RBCs membrane show marked reduction in membrane glycoprotein and band 3 detected by sodium dodecyl sulfate polyacrylamide gel electrophoresis (SDS-PAGE). On electron microscopy, RBCs show double cytoplasmic membrane.

TYPE III CONGENITAL DYSERYTHROBLASTIC ANEMIA

This is autosomal dominant disorder. Erythroblasts show multiple nuclei up to 12.

ANEMIA OF CHRONIC DISEASE

Anemia of chronic disease can be secondary to acute and chronic inflammation, viral infections including HIV, hematologic solid tumors, autoimmune diseases (rheumatoid arthritis, systemic lupus erythematosus, inflammatory bowel disease, and sarcoidosis), chronic rejection of solid organ transplantation and chronic renal disease. This common form of anemia is second in incidence to iron deficiency anemia. It occurs due to impaired utilization of iron from macrophage stores in the bone marrow. It is a functional iron deficiency, although storage iron is normal or even increased.

PATHOGENESIS

In chronic inflammation, activated macrophages synthesize cytokines like IL-6, IL-1 and TNF-α. IL-6 activates synthesis of master regulator of iron protein hepcidin by liver. Hepcidin inhibits release of iron from storage sites resulting in decreased erythropoiesis. These cytokines inhibit CFU-E (colony forming units-erythroid) leading to decreased red blood cells. Anemia with chronic kidney disease shares some of the characteristics of anemia of chronic disease, although the decrease in the production of erythropoietin, mediated by renal insufficiency and the antiproliferative effects of accumulating uremic toxins, contribute importantly.

Interleukin I: IL-1 synthesized by activated macrophages inhibits synthesis of erythropoietin by kidney. IL-1 also increases uptake of iron by reticuloendothelial cells.

Tumor necrosis factor-α: Tumor necrosis factor-α synthesized by activated macrophages participates in phagocytosis and degradation of red blood cells.

Interferon-γ: IFN-γ synthesized by lymphocytes inhibits erythropoiesis and increases uptake of iron by reticuloendothelial cells.

Pro-inflammatory cytokines: Erythropoiesis may be decreased by infiltration of bone marrow by microorganisms and tumor cells. Tumor cells can produce pro-inflammatory cytokines and free radicals that damage erythroid progenitor cells.

Hematological findings: Peripheral blood smear shows mild to moderate microcytic hypochromic picture (Fig. 8.55). However, in contrast to iron deficiency anemia, TIBC is characteristically decreased. Serum iron levels tend to be reduced. Anemia in chronic renal disease is often normochromic and normocytic. When associated with liver disease, it may be moderately macrocytic.

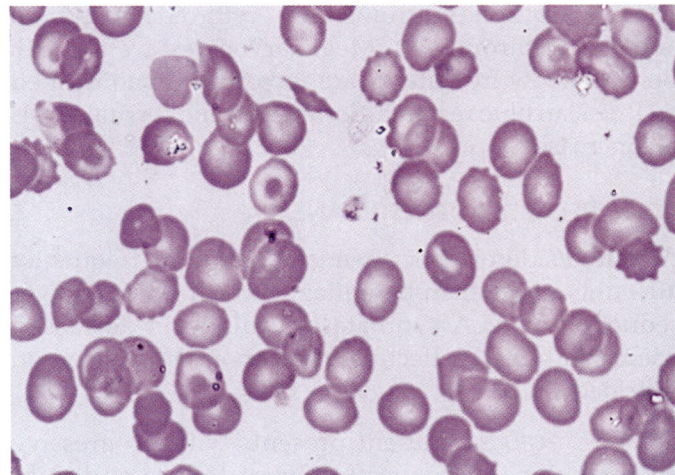

Fig. 8.55: Anemia of chronic disease. Peripheral blood smear shows mild to moderate microcytic hypochromic picture.

MYELOPHTHISIC ANEMIA

Myelophthisic anemia occurs due to infiltration of bone marrow by metastases (most common), granulomatous lesions, leukemia, lymphomas or hairy cells leukemia. It leads to suppressed hematopoiesis. Metastatic deposits from cancers of breast, prostate, lung, stomach, kidney and thyroid replace bone marrow elements, thereby bone marrow failure and myelophthisic anemia.

Peripheral blood smear: Peripheral blood smears show severe anemia, immature myeloid and erythroid precursors (leukoerythroblastosis).

Bone marrow: Bone marrow examination may demonstrate metastatic deposits from carcinomas or granulomatous lesions or lymphoma deposits.

CHAPTER 9

White Blood Cells

Learning Objectives

LEUKOCYTES AND THEIR QUANTITATIVE AND QUALITATIVE DISORDERS
- Leukopoiesis
- Quantitative Alterations in DLC
- Qualitative Alterations in WBC
- Infectious Mononucleosis

ACUTE LEUKEMIAS
- General Considerations
- Acute Lymphoblastic Leukemia (ALL)
- Acute Myeloid Leukemia
- Distinct Forms of AML

MYELODYSPLASTIC SYNDROMES/MYELOPROLIFERATIVE NEOPLASMS
- Myelodysplastic Syndrome
- MDS/Myeloproliferative Disorders

MYELOPROLIFERATIVE NEOPLASMS
- Chronic Myelogenous Leukemia
- Polycythemia Vera
- Essential Thrombocythemia
- Primary Myelofibrosis

CHRONIC LYMPHOPROLIFERATIVE DISORDERS
- Chronic Lymphocytic Leukemia (CLL)
- Hairy Cell Leukemia
- B-Prolymphocytic Leukemia (PLL)
- Adult T Cell Leukemia/Lymphoma (ATLL)
- NHL—Spillover in Blood
- Hodgkin's Disease
- Mantle Cell Lymphoma—Spillover in Blood
- Splenic Lymphoma with Villous Lymphocytes

MULTIPLE MYELOMA AND WALDENSTRÖM MACROGLOBULINEMIA
- Multiple Myeloma
- Waldenström Macroglobulinemia
- Benign Monoclonal Gammopathy

DISORDERS OF MONONUCLEAR PHAGOCYTIC SYSTEM
- Storage Histiocytosis

HEMATOPOIETIC STEM CELL TRANSPLANTATION
- Sources of Stem Cells
- Selection of Donor
- Recipients

LEUKOCYTES AND THEIR QUANTITATIVE AND QUALITATIVE DISORDERS

LEUKOPOIESIS

Hematopoietic cells comprise hematopoietic stem cells (CD34+), progenitor cells (committed cells) and mature RBCs, WBCs and platelets (Table 9.1). Self-renewal is an important property of hematopoietic stem cells.

Neutrophils are predominant cells in the first few weeks in the newborn. Lymphocytes are predominant cells in the postnatal period between 4 weeks and 4 years. After 4 years of age, neutrophils are predominant cells.

Table 9.1: Normal and differential white blood cell count

White blood cells	Percentage	Absolute values
Neutrophils	40–75	$25–75 \times 10^6/L$
Eosinophils	2–6	$0.04–0.4 \times 10^6/L$
Basophils	0–2%	$0.01–0.1 \times 10^6/L$
Lymphocytes	20–40	$1.5–3.5 \times 10^9/L$
Monocytes	2–10	$0.2–0.8 \times 10^9/L$

NEUTROPHILS

G-CSF derived from *monocyte/macrophages, T cells, fibroblasts, vascular endothelium* participates in **differentiation** and **activation** of neutrophils. Neutrophils measure 12–15 µm in dimeter. These constitute 50–70% of leukocytes. These have 2–5 lobed nucleus.

Cytoplasm contains small purple granules rich in digestive enzymes. These remain in circulation for 4–10 hours. Lifespan of neutrophils is 2 days. These cells are recruited to the site of injury within first 24 hours of inflammation.

EOSINOPHILS

Eosinophils measure 12–15 µm in dimeter. These constitute 1–4% of leukocytes. These have bilobed nucleus. Cytoplasm contains large coarse orange-colored granules. IL-5 derived from T cells participates in regulation of eosinophils.

Eosinophilic granules contain highly cationic **major basic protein** (MBP) that kills only invasive helminthes. Eosinophils are recruited by **chemokine (eotaxin)** at injury site in IgE-mediated allergic reactions. Eosinophilic red granules contain crystalline material in cytoplasm, which becomes *Charcot-Leyden crystals* in the *sputum* of asthmatic patients.

BASOPHILS

Basophils measure 12–15 µm in dimeter. These constitute 0–4% of leukocytes. These have pale staining constricted nucleus. Cytoplasm contains dark blue to black granules. Basophils possess coarse granules rich in histamine.

MONOCYTES

Monocytopoiesis is regulated by GM-CSF and macrophage colony-stimulating factors. Monocytes are derived from monoblasts in the bone marrow. These have lifespan of 12 hours.

Monocyte contains reinform, lobulated or indented nuclei with open chromatin without nucleoli. Cytoplasm is pale blue.

LYMPHOCYTES

IL-6 derived from *T cells, monocytes, fibroblast* participates in **differentiation** of B and T cells and proliferation of plasma cells.

T cells

T cells participate in cell-mediated immunity. Activated macrophages display antigens to T cells. Macrophages synthesize IL-12 that stimulates T cell responses. Activated T cells recruit monocytes from the circulation with IFN-γ, a powerful activator of macrophages.

B cells

B cells, when stimulated with antigen, become plasma cells and secrete immunoglobulins (e.g. IgG, IgA, IgM, IgD and IgE). Plasma cells participate in humoral immunity.

Natural Killer Cells

These kill **tumor cells** and **virus infected cells** by lysing or damaging plasma membranes.

QUANTITATIVE ALTERATIONS IN DLC

Leukocytosis is defined as increase in the white blood cell count (>11000/µl) in adults. It most often occurs due to increase in the neutrophils. But leukocytosis may also occur as a result of increase in the number of lymphocytes or monocytes.

NEUTROPHILIA

Neutrophilia is defined as an increase in the absolute neutrophil count $>7.5 \times 10^9/L$. During pregnancy and parturition, neutrophil count is raised.

Causes of neutrophilia due to pathological disorders are shown in Table 9.2. Polymorphonuclear leukocytosis is shown in Fig. 9.1.

LYMPHOCYTOSIS

Lymphocytosis is defined as an increase in the number of lymphocytes $>4 \times 10^9/L$ in adults, $>7 \times 10^9/L$ in

Table 9.2: Causes of neutrophilia due to pathological disorders

Etiological categories	Clinical conditions
Acute bacterial infections	Lobar pneumonia Bronchopneumonia Pyogenic meningitis Acute appendicitis Infected burns Diphtheria
Acute stress state	Acute myocardial infarction Post-hemorrhagic state Post-surgery state
Myeloproliferative state	Chronic myeloid leukemia Polycythemia vera
Miscellaneous disorders	G-CSF therapy induction Corticosteroid therapy Rheumatoid arthritis Gout Leukemoid reactions

White Blood Cells

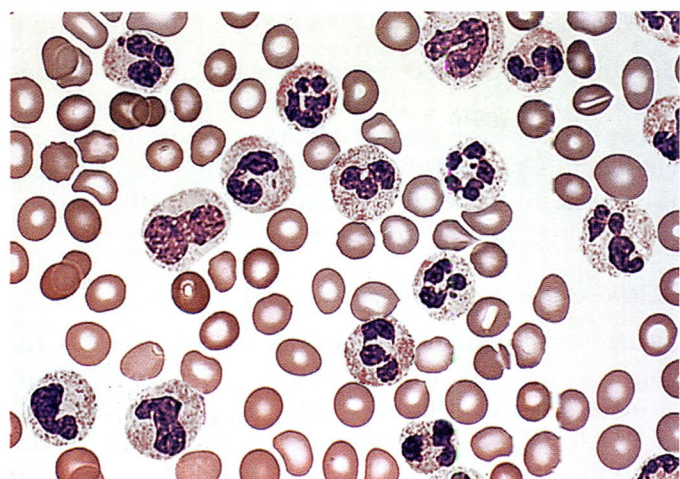

Fig. 9.1: Polymorphonuclear leukocytosis shows toxic granules in neutrophils.

children and $>9 \times 10^9/L$ in neonates. Lymphocytosis in peripheral blood smear is shown in Fig. 9.2. Causes of lymphocytosis are given in Table 9.3.

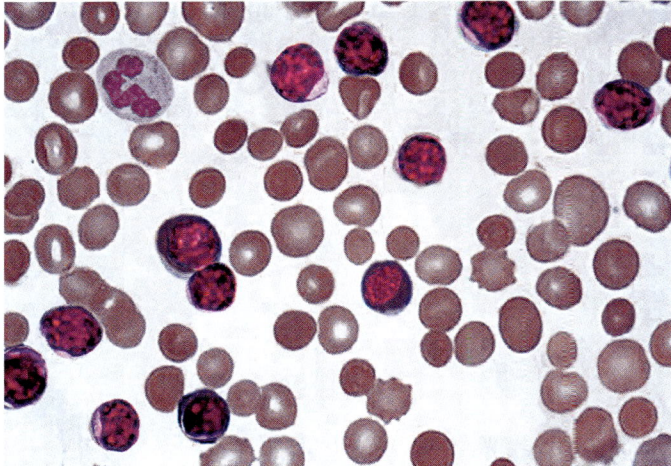

Fig. 9.2: Lymphocytosis in peripheral blood smear.

Table 9.3: Causes of lymphocytosis

Etiological categories	Causes
Chronic inflammation	Tuberculosis Syphilis Brucellosis
Hematological malignancies	Chronic lymphocytic leukemia Spillover of NHL Adult T cell leukemia/lymphoma Prolymphocytic leukemia Hairy cell leukemia
Acute viral infections	Infectious mononucleosis Mumps Measles Chickenpox Cytomegalovirus

EOSINOPHILIA

Eosinophilia is defined as an increase in the absolute eosinophil count above $0.4 \times 10^9/L$. Eosinophil count may be increased above $30 \times 10^9/L$ in allergic disorders.

Hypereosinophilic syndrome is *characterized* by *persistent eosinophilia* for 6 months in blood ($\geq 1.5 \times 10^9/L$), increased eosinophils in **bone marrow** and **organ infiltration**.

Clonal eosinophilia occurs due to gene mutations of *PDGFRA, PDGFRB and FGFR1 seen in acute leukemia and myeloproliferative disorders*. Eosinophilia in peripheral blood smear is shown in Fig. 9.3. Causes of eosinophilia are shown in Table 9.4.

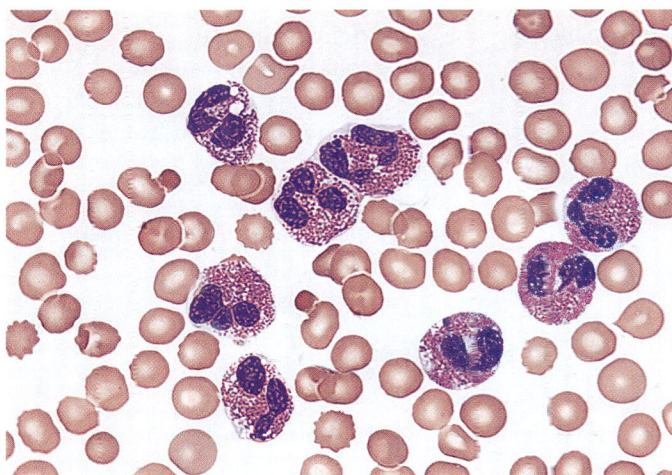

Fig. 9.3: Eosinophilia in peripheral blood smear.

Table 9.4: Causes of eosinophilia

Etiological categories	Causes
Allergic state	Bronchial asthma, urticaria, hay fever, allergic rhinitis
Primary eosinophilia	Chronic myeloid leukemia Chronic eosinophilia Mastocytosis AML Idiopathic chronic eosinophilic pneumonia Acute eosinophilic pneumonia with respiratory failure
Parasitic infestations	Hookworm infestation, roundworm infestation, filariasis, trichinosis, *Ascaris lumbricoides*
Skin disorders	Eczema, pemphigus, psoriasis, bullous pemphigoid, dermatitis herpetiformis
Miscellaneous disorders	Tropical eosinophilia, pulmonary eosinophilia, hypereosinophilic syndrome, Hodgkin's disease, eosinophilic granuloma

MONOCYTOSIS

Absolute monocytosis is defined as an increase in the monocyte count $>1 \times 10^9/L$ in adults and $1.2 \times 10^9/L$ in neonates. Causes of monocytosis are shown in Table 9.5.

Table 9.5: Causes of monocytosis

Etiological categories	Causes
Infections	Tuberculosis Syphilis Bacterial endocarditis Brucellosis Kala-azar Trypanosomiasis
Hematological malignancies	AML (M4 and M5) Hodgkin's disease Chronic myeloid leukemia Chronic myelomonocytic leukemia Myelodysplastic syndrome
Autoimmune disorders	Ulcerative colitis Crohn's disease Systemic lupus erythematosus Rheumatoid arthritis Sarcoidosis

BASOPHILIA

Basophilia is defined as an increase in the number of basophils $>0.1 \times 10^9/L$. It most often occurs in chronic myeloid leukemia, basophilic leukemia, Hodgkin's disease, polycythemia vera, hypothyroidism, IgE mediated allergic reactions, ulcerative colitis, mastocytosis and tuberculosis.

NEUTROPENIA (AGRANULOCYTOSIS)

Neutropenia is defined as decrease in the neutrophil count $<1.5 \times 10^9/L$ in adults and $<2.5 \times 10^9/L$ in children. Neutropenia occurs due to suppression of myelopoiesis, destruction of neutrophils in the peripheral blood or pooling in the peripheral regions. Patient with neutropenia presents with sore throat, recurrent infections and delayed wound healing. Causes of neutropenia are shown in Table 9.6.

LYMPHOCYTOPENIA

Lymphocytopenia is defined as decrease in the lymphocyte count $<1 \times 10^9/L$ in adults and $<2 \times 10^9/L$ in the peripheral blood. It is observed in patients following therapeutic administration of **corticosteroid** and

Table 9.6: Causes of neutropenia

Etiological categories	Causes
Bacterial infections	Typhoid fever Endotoxic shock (gram –ve) Tuberculosis
Viral infections	Human immune deficiency virus Papovavirus B19 Epstein-Barr virus Hepatitis B virus
Drug induced	Anti-inflammatory drugs (phenylbutazone, ibuprofen) Anti-thyroid drugs (thiouracil, carbimazole) Antibacterial drugs (penicillin, gentamycin, doxycycline, ciprofloxacin, cephalosporins, cotrimoxazole) Anti-epileptic drugs (phenytoin, trimethadione, volproic acid)
Autoimmune disorders	Systemic lupus erythematosus Blood transfusion reactions Felty syndrome
Congenital disorders	Severe congenital neutropenia Chronic benign neutropenia Cyclic neutropenia
Miscellaneous disorders	X-ray irradiation Hypersplenism Splenomegaly Megaloblastic anemia Myelodysplastic syndrome Aplastic anemia Chronic autoimmune neutropenia

Table 9.7: Causes of lymphocytopenia in pathological state

Etiological categories	Causes
Drug-induced lymphocyte destruction	Cytotoxic drugs Corticosteroid therapy Anti-thymocyte globin administration
Miscellaneous disorders	Miliary tuberculosis Systemic lupus erythematosus Acquired immunodeficiency syndrome Radiation therapy Rheumatoid arthritis Sarcoidosis Ataxia-telangiectasia Myasthenia gravis Severe combined immune deficiency Malnutrition

cytotoxic drugs, radiation induced and viral infections. Causes of lymphocytopenia in pathological state are shown in Table 9.7.

QUALITATIVE ALTERATIONS IN WBC

PELGER-HUËT ANOMALY

Pelger-Huët anomaly is autosomal dominant disorder due to **mutation of lamin B receptor (LBR) gene**. It is characterized by **lack of segmentation of neutrophils**. Nuclei are dumble shaped in >70% of neutrophils. Chromatin is coarse. Two lobes of the nuclei are joined by thin chromatin bridge.

ALDER-REILLY ANOMALY

Alder-Reilly anomaly is autosomal recessive disorder associated with several genetic mucopolysaccharidoses. There is deficiency of lysosomal enzymes required for breakdown of mucopolysaccharides. There is presence of **liliac inclusions with clear halo in neutrophils** stained with Giemsa stain. These granules are also demonstrated with toluidine blue.

MAY-HEGGLIN ANOMALY

May-Hegglin anomaly is autosomal disorder due to **mutation of MYH9 gene**. This disorder is characterized by basophilic inclusions (Döhle body-like) in neutrophils, anemia, thrombocytopenia and giant platelets.

CHÉDIAK-HIGASHI SYNDROME

Chédiak-Higashi syndrome is an example of defects in *phagolysosome formation* and defective degranulation of neutrophils.

Under physiological state, LYST gene located on chromosome 1q42 encodes a protein essential for assembly of microtubules in the cytoplasm. Mutation of

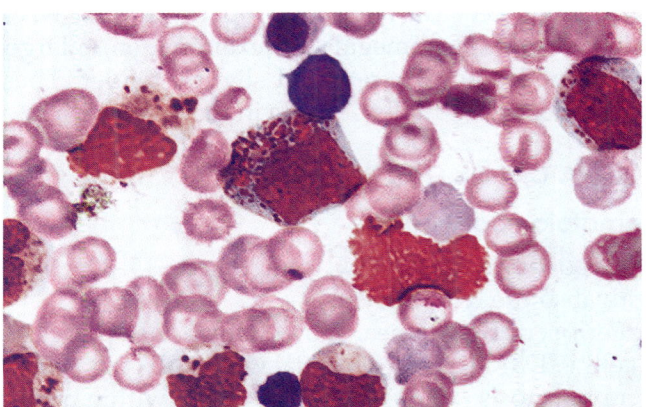

Fig. 9.4: Chédiak-Higashi syndrome. Neutrophils contain giant granules due to aberrant organelles.

LYST gene leads to defect in assembly of microtubules in neutrophils. This disorder is characterized by *defective degranulation of neutrophils, impaired microbial killing, and recurrent bacterial infections (Staphylococcus aureus)* forming soft tissue abscess. Neutrophils contain giant granules due to aberrant organelles (Fig. 9.4).

CHRONIC GRANULOMATOUS DISEASE OF CHILDHOOD

Defect in NADPH oxidase activity in neutrophils causes X-linked disorder *chronic granulomatous disease of childhood*. This disorder is characterized by phagocytic cells that ingest but unable to kill certain microorganisms.

Nitroblue tetrazolium (NBT) slide test is used for screening defects in NADPH oxidase. The number of neutrophils with dark cytoplasmic granules of reaction product is counted. Normally, >95% of the granulocytes containing NADPH oxidase are positive for nitroblue tetrazolium (NBT). **In the abnormal NBT test in chronic granulomatous disease, <5% of neutrophils are stained.**

INFECTIOUS MONONUCLEOSIS

Infectious mononucleosis is caused by Epstein-Barr virus. Incubation period is 1–2 months. Infection is contracted through **oropharyngeal secretions** and close contact. This acute infection is characterized by *fever, sore throat, splenomegaly* and presence of *transformed lymphocytes* in the peripheral blood.

EB virus infects B cells and induces humoral and cellular response. Cellular response occurs as a result of proliferation of cytotoxic (CD8) cells, which appear as transformed lymphocytes.

Clinical Features

Onset of infectious mononucleosis disease is abrupt. It most often occurs between 5 and 30 years of age affecting both males and females. Patient presents with fever, sore throat, cervical lymphadenopathy in first week, skin rash and splenomegaly. On examination, enlarged lymph nodes are discrete and slightly tender. These lymph nodes gradually subside in the second week.

LABORATORY DIAGNOSIS

Hematological Findings

Total leukocyte count: TLC is increased $>15–30 \times 10^9/L$ with absolute lymphocytosis.

Peripheral blood smear shows transformed polyclonal T cells (CD8) >10%. Differential white cell count shows lymphocytosis (>50%). Platelet count is within normal range. Morphological variations in lymphocytes in infectious mononucleosis are shown in Fig. 9.5. Morphology of transformed T cells is shown in Table 9.8.

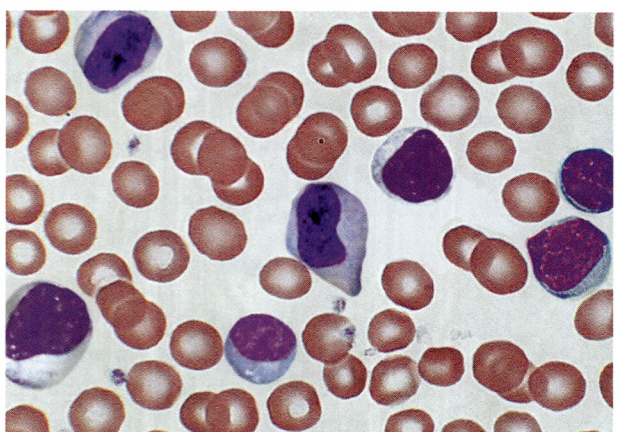

Fig. 9.5: Morphological variations in lymphocytes in infectious mononucleosis.

Bone marrow: Bone marrow is performed to rule out leukemia. Bone marrow shows infiltration by transformed lymphocytes.

Heterophilic IgM Antibodies

Heterophilic IgM antibodies are formed due to Epstein-Barr infection. These are demonstrated in the second to third week of infection. *These antibodies agglutinate horse red blood cells.* These may also react with guinea pig kidney.

Paul-Bunnell test: Sheep red blood cells are used to demonstrate heterophilic antibody. Serial dilution of patient's serum is mixed with sheep red blood cells. Agglutination is observed. *Normal level of hetrophilic antibody is 1:28 titre.*

Titre heterophilic antibody >1:256 has **diagnostic** significance. This heterophilic antibody test is positive in the second and third weeks of infection. Test remains positive up to 4–8 weeks. *Heterophilic antibody test may be positive* in *leukemias* and *lymphomas*.

Rapid slide test (monospot test): In monospot slide test, ox red cells and guinea pig kidney are used.

Enzyme immunoassay: Solid phase enzyme immunoassay is used to demonstrate heterophilic antibody.

Epstein-Barr Virus Specific Antibodies

During acute phase of EB virus infection, antibodies are formed against viral antigen and membrane antigen. EBV specific antibodies are formed against EBV specific antigens (viral capsid antigen, early antigen, EBV nuclear antigens). Presence of antibodies against viral capsid antigen is diagnostic of acute infection. Antibodies formed against EB virus antigen and membrane appear after 1–2 months, which persist throughout life.

Molecular Techniques

EBV DNA is demonstrated by polymerase chain reaction and *in situ* hybridization in specimens such as **tissues, body fluids** and **peripheral blood.**

COMPLICATIONS

Complications of infectious mononucleosis are immune hemolytic anemia, immune-mediated thrombocytopenia, hemophagocytic syndrome, secondary bacterial sore throat, meningoencephalitis, Gullain-Barré syndrome, and splenic rupture (rare). *EB virus*

Table 9.8: Morphology of transformed T cells

Parameters	Plasmacytoid cells (type I)	Monocytoid cells (type II)	Blastoid cells (type III)
Nuclear chromatin	Condensed chromatin giving cartwheel appearance with basophilic cytoplasm	Kidney shaped nucleus with open chromatin	Open chromatin with thin cytoplasm

associated disorders are Burkitt's lymphoma, nasopharyngeal carcinoma, Hodgkin's disease, body cavity lymphoma (HIV/AIDS patients) and X-linked lymphoproliferative disease (Duncan's syndrome).

ACUTE LEUKEMIAS

GENERAL CONSIDERATIONS

Hematopoietic stem cells (HSCs) and their progenitors maintain normal hematopoiesis during life-time of an individual. *HSCs differentiate into myeloid and lymphoid cell lines.* Origin of bone marrow myeloid malignancies is shown in Fig. 9.6. Hematopoietic stem cell myeloid and lymphoid neoplasms are shown in Table 9.9 and Fig. 9.7.

Leukemia

Leukemia is a **stem cell disorder** characterized by a neoplastic proliferation of either lymphoid or myeloid cell in the bone marrow.

It results in accumulation of immature nonfunctional leukocytes in bone marrow and circulation. Failure of normal production of red cells, leukocytes and platelets results in anemia, recurrent infection and thrombocytopenia. *Leukemic cells infiltrate liver, spleen, lymph nodes and other organs.*

Table 9.9: Hematopoietic stem cell myeloid and lymphoid neoplasms

HSCs neoplasms	Examples
Myeloid neoplasms	Acute myeloid neoplasm Myelodysplastic syndrome Myeloproliferative neoplasms
Lymphoid neoplasms	Acute lymphoid leukemia (B or T cell) Chronic lymphoproliferative disorders (B or T cell) Lymphomas (Hodgkin's disease or NHL)

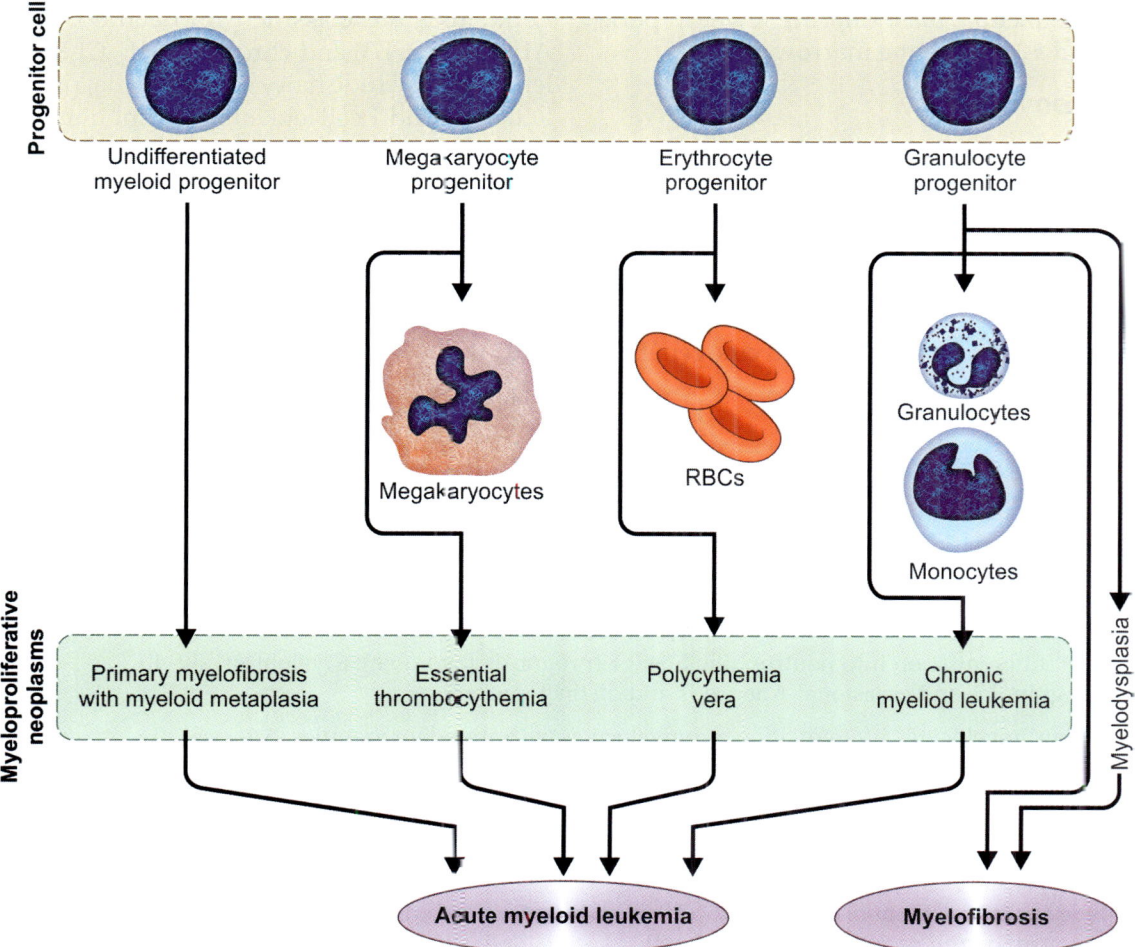

Fig. 9.6: Origin of bone marrow myeloid malignancies. Each malignant disorder is derived from particular type of myeloid progenitor cell.

Section II: Hematology

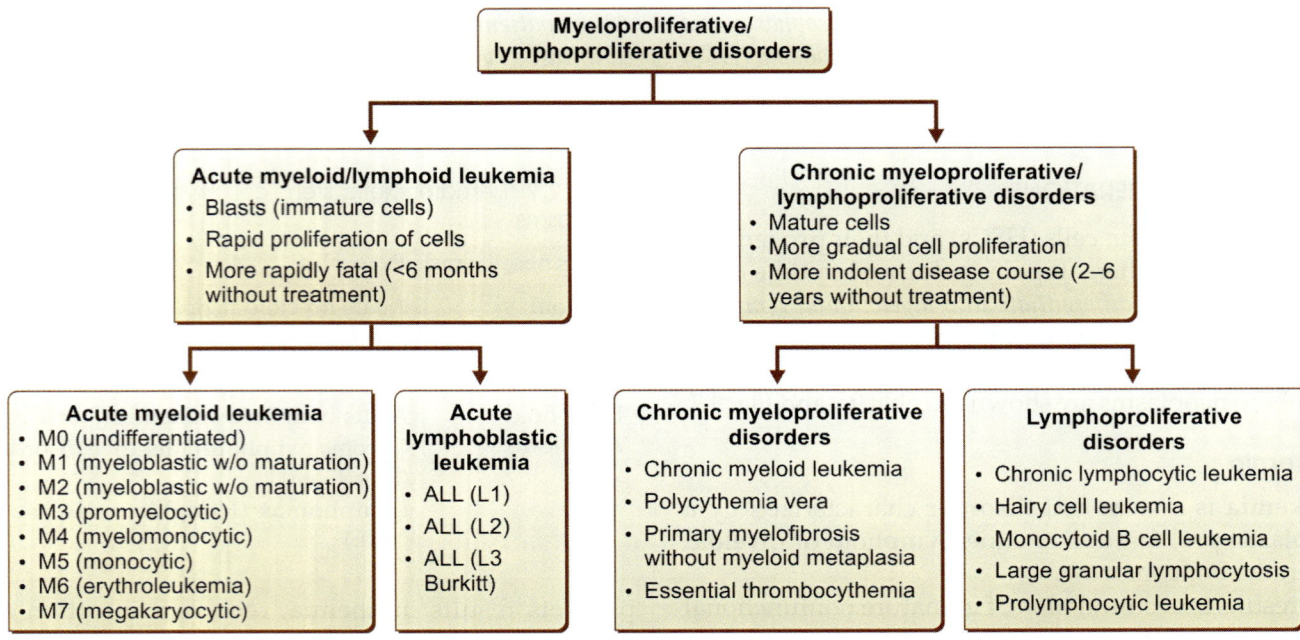

Fig. 9.7: Hematopoietic stem cell myeloid and lymphoid neoplasms.

Subleukemic Leukemia

In subleukemic leukemia, blast cells are fewer in peripheral blood, and >20% in bone marrow.

Aleukemic Leukemia

Aleukemic leukemia refers to low total leukocytes count (<4 × 10^9/L) with absence of blasts in the peripheral smear. However, bone marrow shows >20% blasts.

CLASSIFICATION

Classification of leukemia is based on morphology, cytochemistry, immunophenotyping and cytogenetics.

FAB Classification

Leukemias are classified into acute (AML: M0–M7, ALL: L1, L2, L3) and chronic (CML, CLL) types. Other leukemias include hairy cell leukemia, prolymphocytic leukemia and T cell leukemia/lymphoma. According to FAB classification, acute leukemias contain more than 30% blasts in bone marrow and peripheral blood. FAB classification of ALL is based on cell size, cytoplasm, nuclear chromatin, nuclear shape, nucleoli, color and vacuolation of cytoplasm. Acute lymphoblastic leukemia has three types: L1, L2 and L3. FAB classification of AML and ALL is shown in Table 9.10.

Table 9.10: FAB classification of AML and ALL

FAB	Morphology	Incidence (%)
Acute myeloid leukemia		
M0	Minimal differentiation expressing myeloid lineage	2–3
M1	AML without maturation (prognosis favorable). Myeloblast with faint granules and occasional Auer rods and distinct nucleoli	20
M2	AML with differentiation into neutrophilic lineage (prognosis favorable). Myeloblast with faint granules and occasional Auer rods and distinct nucleoli	30–40
M3	AML with promyelocytic differentiation, promyelocytes with abundant granules, Auer rods and folded (cottage-loaf) nuclei (commonly associated with DIC due to release of thromboplastin-like substance)	5–10
M4	Myelomonocytic leukemia showing myelocytic and monocytic differentiation (>20% monocytoid cells involving) gums, skin or CNS involved)	15–20
M5a	Monocytic leukemia. Monoblasts without differentiation (extramedullary disease of the gums, skin, lymph node and CNS involved)	10%
M5b	Monocytic leukemia (monoblasts with differentiation)	

Contd...

Table 9.10: FAB classification of AML and ALL (Contd...)

FAB	Morphology	Incidence (%)
M6a	Acute erythroblastic leukemia showing dysplastic erythroblasts (>50%) and myeloblasts (>20%)	Uncommon
M6b	Acute erythroblastic leukemia showing dysplastic erythroblasts (>80%)	
M7	Acute megakaryocytic leukemia showing abnormal megakaryocytes (common in Down's syndrome and myelofibrosis)	<1%
Acute lymphoblastic leukemia		
L1	Lymphoblasts (uniform, homogenous scant basophilic cytoplasm with regular nuclei and nucleoli inconspicuous)	>80% (children with good prognosis)
L2	Lymphoblasts (large heterogenous, with irregular, clefting, indentation of nuclei and prominent nucleoli)	10–50% (adults with poor prognosis)
L3	Lymphoblasts (large homogenous with round to oval nucleus, finely stippled chromatin, prominent nucleoli, and abundant basophilic vacuolated cytoplasm)	<3–4% (adults with poor prognosis)

WHO Classification 2016

Cut off percentage of blasts is >20% (WHO classification). **PML-RARA molecular abnormality** is the **diagnostic** feature of **AML-M3**. WHO classification 2016 of acute myeloid leukemia and related neoplasm is discussed in AML and ALL.

EPIDEMIOLOGY

AML most often affects young adults. ALL is a disorder of children. Both ALL and AML more commonly affect males than females. ALL is most often seen in white population.

PATHOGENESIS

Various factors are believed to participate in the pathogenesis of acute leukemia. These include *genetic disorders, ionization radiation, chemotherapeutic agents, chemicals, virus (HTLV-1)* and *acquired hematological disorders*. Hereditary and acquired disorders associated with increased risk of leukemia are shown in Table 9.11.

Chemotherapy-induced Leukemias

Chemotherapy may cause somatic mutations resulting in AML. Administration of these anticancer therapeutic alkylating agents in Hodgkin's disease, NHL and ovarian carcinoma may evoke later a second form of cancer, usually leukemia. Chromosomal abnormalities observed in these patients are monosomy 5, monosomy 7, 5p and 11q23. Alkylating agents comprise nitrogen mustard—cyclophosphamide, chlorambucil, nitro-soureas, β-propriolactone, dimethyl sulphate, and dieproxibutane.

Ionizing Radiation

Ionizing radiation pose a potential worldwide threat in this nuclear age. Low doses of ionization radiation can cause DNA mutations and chromosomal abnormalities results in cancer. Large doses of radiation can inhibit cell division. Survivors of atomic blasts in **Hiroshima and Nagasaki** are developing **AML or CML** (*but not lymphoid leukemia*). **Radiologists** may develop **myeloid leukemia.**

Table 9.11: Hereditary and acquired disorders associated with increased risk of leukemia

Hereditary/acquired disorder categories	Examples
Hereditary disorders	Down's syndrome (AML or ALL) Fanconi anemia (AML) Bloom syndrome Ataxia-telangiectasia (ALL or NHL) Wiscott-Aldrich syndrome Diamond-Blackfan syndrome Klinefelter's syndrome
Acquired hematological disorders	Myelodysplastic syndrome (AML) Chronic myeloproliferative disorders (AML) Aplastic anemia Paroxysmal nocturnal hemoglobinuria (AML and rarely ALL) HTLV-1 (acute T cell leukemia)

Occupational Exposure

Workers in benzene chemical petrochemical industries (aromatic hydrocarbons) are associated with leukemia and Hodgkin's disease.

Viruses

Human T-lymphotropic virus type 1 (HTLV-1) causes adult T cell leukemia or NHL in Japan. HTLV-1 activates TAX gene that causes proliferation of T cells. Activated TAX gene also neutralizes growth-inhibitory signals by affecting p53 and CDKN2A/Alp16 genes. Additional gene mutations lead to T cell leukemia.

Bone Marrow Failure

Bone marrow failure syndrome increases risk of leukemia due to *Fanconi syndrome, Diamond-Blackfan, ataxia-telangiectasia* and *familial aplastic anemia*.

Oncogenes

Pathogenesis of acute leukemia is shown in Figs 9.8 and 9.9. Oncogenes activation and associated leukemias are shown in Table 9.12.

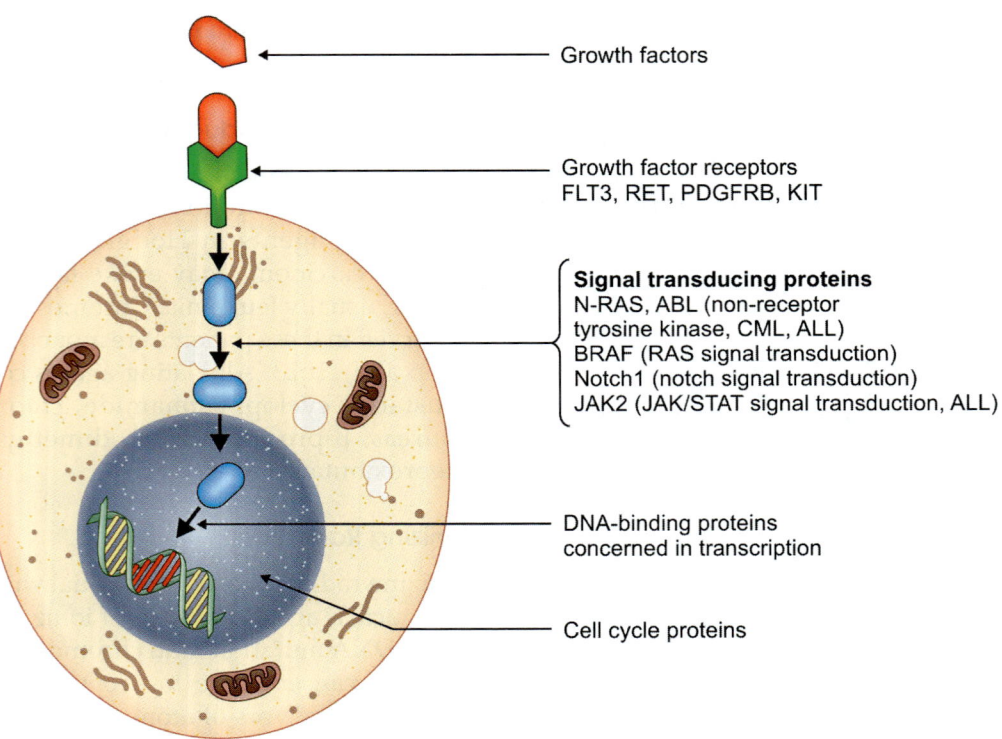

Fig. 9.8: Pathogenesis of acute leukemia.

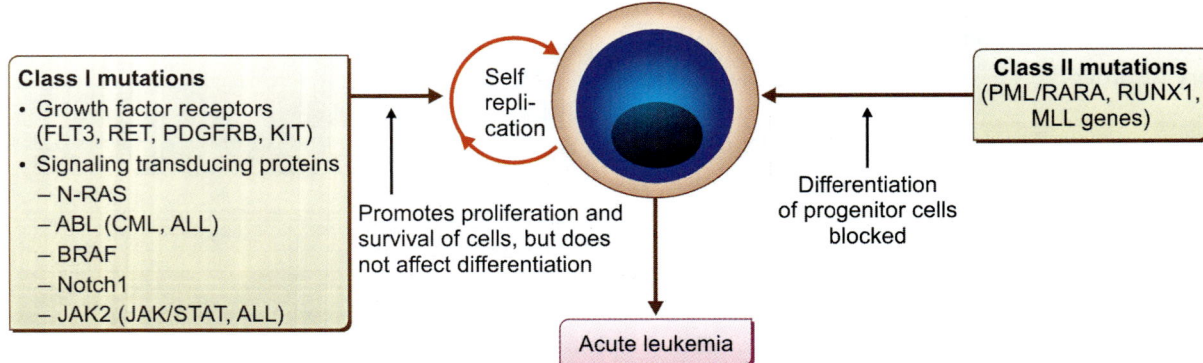

Fig. 9.9: Pathogenesis of acute leukemia. Class I mutations of growth factors and signaling transducing proteins act on hematopoietic stem cell that replicates. Class II mutations block the differentiation of progenitor cells.

Table 9.12: Oncogenes activation and associated leukemias

Category	Proto-oncogene	Mode of activation	Associated malignancies
Growth factor receptors			
FMS-like tyrosine 3 kinase	FLT3	Point mutation	Leukemia
PDGF receptor	PDGFRB	Overexpression Translocation	Gliomas Leukemia
Receptor for KIT ligand	KIT	Point mutation	Gastrointestinal tumors Seminomas Leukemia
Signal-transducing proteins			
Non-receptor tyrosine kinase	ABL (Abelson mouse leukemia)	Translocation (9:22) Point mutation	Chronic myeloid leukemia Acute lymphoblastic leukemia
RAS signal transduction	BRAF	Point mutation Translocation	Melanoma Leukemia Colon carcinoma
Notch signal transduction	Notch1	Point mutation Translocation	Breast carcinoma Leukemia Lymphomas
JAK/STAT signal transduction	JAK2	Translocation	Myeloproliferative disorders Acute lymphoblastic leukemia

CYTOCHEMICAL ANALYSIS

Cytochemical analysis includes demonstration of myeloperoxidase, Sudan black, nonspecific esterase, chloracetate esterase, acid phosphatase and periodic acid–Schiff. Sudan black B stains granules of neutrophils, eosinophils and monocytes.

Myeloblasts show positivity with *Sudan black*. Lymphoblasts are negative for Sudan black. Myeloblasts are also peroxidase positive, which may also be used to confirm their lineage. Cytochemistry in ALL and AML is shown in Table 9.13.

IMMUNOCYTOCHEMISTRY

Monoclonal antibodies are useful to differentiate AML and ALL in case inconclusive on cytochemistry. Patients with AML express HLA-DR, cAnti-MPO (cytoplasmic anti-MPO), CD13, CD33 and CD65. HLA-DR, CD10, CD19, CD20 are positive in ALL (B cell) and T-ALL cases are positive with CD2, CD3, CD5 and CD7.

Monocyte is CD14 positive. **AML (M6)** is positive with **glycophorin A**. *AML (M7)* is positive for *CD33, CD61, vWF, GpIIb/IIIa and glycophorin A*. Immunophenotyping of AML, ALL (B cell) and ALL (T cell) is shown in Table 9.14.

Table 9.13: Cytochemistry in ALL and AML

Cytochemical stain	ALL	AML
Myeloperoxidase	Negative	Positive
Sudan black B	Negative	Positive
Non-specific esterase	Negative	Positive (M4 and M5)
PAS	Positive	Negative
Acid phosphatase	Positive in T-ALL	Negative
Erythroblasts in AML (M6) are positive for PAS (diffuse)		

Table 9.14: Immunophenotyping of AML, ALL (B cell) and ALL (T cell)

Characteristics	AML	ALL (B cell)	ALL (T cell)
HLA-DR	Positive	Positive	-
CD13	Positive	-	-
CD33	Positive	-	-
CD65	Positive	-	-
cAnti-MPO (cytoplasmic anti-MPO)	Positive	-	-
CD2	-	-	Positive
CD3	-	-	Positive
CD5	-	-	Positive
CD7	-	-	Positive
CD10	-	Positive	-
CD19	-	Positive	-
CD20	-	Positive	-

ACUTE LYMPHOBLASTIC LEUKEMIA (ALL)

ALL is more common in children between 2 and 7 years than adults. Boys are more affected than girls. This malignant neoplasm arises from lymphoid precursor B cells (80%) and precursor T cell (20%) in the bone marrow resulting in leukocytosis in peripheral blood. Patients are most responsive to therapy with good prognosis.

CLINICAL FEATURES

Bone marrow progenitor cells (erythroid, myeloid and megakaryocytes) do not mature normally resulting in anemia, neutropenia (recurrent infection) and thrombocytopenia (bleeding tendencies). Patient with ALL presents with **bone pain, cervical lymphadenopathy** and **splenomegaly**.

Generalized Lymphadenopathy

Patients with ALL present with lymphadenopathy in 75% cases. On examination, cervical *lymph nodes* are enlarged, *discrete* and *firm* in consistency. Generalized lymphadenopathy is associated with high white blood cells resulting in fatal outcome.

Organomegaly

Patient with ALL presents with **splenomegaly** (more common) and hepatomegaly.

Mediastinal Mass

Patient presenting with mediastinal mass has poor prognosis.

CNS and Testes Involvement

ALL most often involves testes and CNS in 1–2% cases. Central nervous system involvement results in increased intracranial pressure and nerve palsies in 5% of cases.

TERMINAL DEOXYRIBONUCLEOTIDYL TRANSFERASE (TDT)

Terminal deoxyribonucleotidyl transferase (TdT) is a specialized DNA polymerase expressed only by pre-B and pre-T lymphoblasts in >95% of ALL cases. The demonstration of TdT activity suggests that a leukemic blast is of lymphoid rather than myeloid lineage.

CLASSIFICATION

Further classification (FAB or WHO classification) into a number of subgroups is based on differences in morphology, cytogenetic changes, antigenic cell–surface markers, or rearrangement of the immunoglobulin heavy-chain or T cell receptor genes.

According to FAB classification, acute lymphoblastic leukemias are of three types: L1, L2 and L3. Acute lymphoblastic leukemias (FAB subtypes) are shown in Table 9.15. WHO classification of B-ALL/lymphoma (2016) is shown in Table 9.16.

B-ALL/LYMPHOMA WITH RECURRENT GENETIC ABNORMALITIES

B-lineage ALL shows immunoglobulin gene rearrangement. T-lineage ALL shows TCR gene rearrangement and presents with mediastinal mass. Genetic alterations include hyperploidy (>50 chromosomes); polyploidy;

Table 9.15: Acute lymphoblastic leukemias (FAB subtypes)

Features	ALL (L1)	ALL (L2)	ALL (L3)
Frequency	70–75% (most common)	20–30%	1–2% (rare)
Class	Childhood ALL (B-ALL and T-ALL)	Adult ALL (mostly T-ALL)	B-ALL (equivalent to Burkitt's type ALL)
Cell size	Small cells predominate (twice size of red blood cell)	Large with variation in size—heterogeneous	Large blasts homogeneous in size
Nuclear shape	Regular, occasional clefting or indentation	Irregular, clefting and indentation common	Regular, oval to round
Nuclear chromatin	Homogeneous	Heterogeneous	Finely stippled and homogeneous
Nucleoli	Small or inconspicuous	Prominent (one or more)	Prominent (one or more)
Amount of cytoplasm	Scanty	Moderate	Moderate to abundant
Cytoplasmic basophilia	Slight or moderate	Variable	Very deep
Cytoplasmic vacuolation	None or few	Variable	Prominent (positive with oil red O)
Cytochemistry	PAS positive	PAS negative	PAS usually negative
	Acid phosphatase +ve/–ve	Acid phosphatase +ve/–ve	Acid phosphatase +ve/–ve
Prognosis	Good prognosis	Worse prognosis	Poor prognosis

White Blood Cells

Table 9.16: WHO classification of B-ALL/lymphoma (2016)

B-ALL/lymphoma	Recurrent genetic abnormalities
B-ALL/lymphoma, NOS	-
B-ALL/lymphoma	B-ALL/lymphoma with: t(9;22)(q34.1;q11.2); BCR-ABL1 t(v;11q23.3); KMT2A rearranged t(12;21)(p13.2;q22.1); ETV6-RUNX1 Hyperdiploidy Hypodiploidy t(5;14)(q31.1;q32.3); IL3-IGH t(1;19)(q23;p13.3); TCF3-PBX1
	Provisional entity B-ALL/lymphoma with BCR-ABL1-like
T-ALL/lymphoma	Provisional entity early T cell precursor lymphoblastic leukemia
Natural killer cell lymphoblastic leukemia/lymphoma	Provisional entity natural killer cell lymphoblastic leukemia/lymphoma

and translocations including t(9; 22), t(12; 21), t(4;11), TEL-AML1, t(1;19), 11q23 rearrangements and hypo-ploidy. These sometimes predict prognosis. The salient features of various B-ALL/lymphoma with recurrent genetic abnormalities are shown in Table 9.17.

LABORATORY DIAGNOSIS

White Blood Cell Count

WBC count is markedly increased ranging between $20 \times 10^9/L$ and $200 \times 10^9/L$. Some patients with subleukemic/aleukemic leukemia may show pancytopenia with a few blasts. Lower the white blood cell count, there is

Table 9.17: Salient features of B-ALL/lymphoma with recurrent genetic abnormalities

Genetic abnormality	Epidemiology	Clinical features	Morphology	Immunophenotype	Aberrant antigen	Prognosis
t(9;22)(q34;q11.2); BCR-ABL1	Adults	Organomegaly	No unique morphologic features	CD10, CD19, TdT, CD25	CD13, CD33	Worst prognosis
t(v;11q23); MLL rearranged	Infants <1 year	Very high TLC, frequent CNS involvement	No unique morphologic features	CD19, CD15+ CD10, CD24– Chondroitin sulfate, proteoglycan neural glial antigen 2 (NG2)+	-	Poor prognosis
t(12;21)(p13;q22); TEL-AML1	Children	Similar to other ALL	No unique morphologic features	CD19, CD10, CD34+	CD13	Very favourable prognosis
Hyperdiploidy (more than 50 to 66 chromosomes)	Children	Similar to other ALL	No unique morphologic features	CD19, CD10, CD34+	-	Very favourable prognosis
Hypodiploidy (less than 45 chromosomes)	Children and adults	Similar to other ALL	No unique morphologic features	CD19, CD10+	-	Poor
t(5;14)(q31;q32); IL3-IGH	Children and adults	Asymptomatic eosinophilia	Increase in circulating eosinophils	CD19, CD10+	-	Uncertain
t(1;19)(q23;p13.3); E2A-PBX1	Children	Similar to other ALL	No unique morphologic features	CD19, CD10+, cytoplasmic μ (cμ) heavy chain +, CD9+	-	Better with intensive therapy

increased chances of remission. Red blood cell and platelets count are decreased resulting in anemia and thrombocytopenia.

Peripheral Blood Smear

Peripheral blood smear shows lymphoblasts >40% up to 95%. Lymphoblasts are cells with high nucleocytoplasmic ratio, coarse chromatin and 1–2 nucleoli. Platelet count is <30,000/cu mm. It shows neutropenia and normocytic normochromic picture.

Bone Marrow

ALL results in a highly cellular marrow. Lymphoblasts constitute >30–100%. Leukemic cells virtually replace or suppress normal hematopoiesis affecting other progenitor cells. There is a near-absence of adipocytes in bone marrow.

Cut off value of blasts is >20% (WHO) and >30% as per FAB classification. In aleukemic leukemia, there are no circulating blasts in peripheral blood but bone marrow shows >20% blasts. *In subleukemic leukemia, peripheral blood smear shows a few blasts and bone marrow shows >20% blasts.*

ALL (L1)

This acute lymphoblastic leukemia (B-ALL or T-ALL) most often occurs in children. It constitutes 75–80% of cases. Lymphoblasts are small with regular nucleoli, homogenous chromatin, and scanty cytoplasm. Cells are block positive with **PAS stain**. Prognosis is good in these patients (Fig. 9.10).

ALL (L2)

This acute lymphoblastic leukemia constitutes 20–30% of cases (mostly T-ALL) with poor prognosis. Lymphoblast

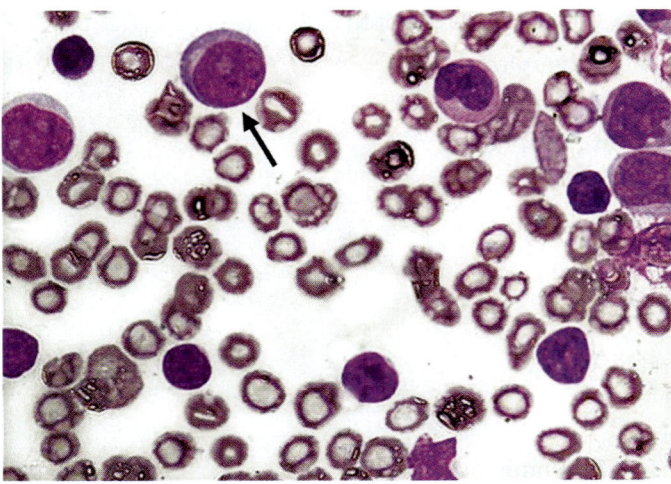

Fig. 9.11: Peripheral blood smear in a case of ALL (L2) showing lymphoblasts of variable size with high nucleocytoplasmic ratio, slightly opened up chromatin, prominent nucleoli and mild to moderate cytoplasm (arrow).

size is variable. These contain irregular indented nuclei with moderate amount of cytoplasm. PAS staining is negative (Fig. 9.11).

ALL (L3)

This acute lymphoblastic leukemia constitutes 1–2% of cases with poor prognosis. Lymphoblasts are large homogenous with regular chromatin, prominent nucleoli and moderate vacuolated cytoplasm (Fig. 9.12).

CYTOCHEMISTRY

Approximately 5–10% of B-ALL and T-ALL show positivity for Sudan black B. However, Burkitt's lymphoma (ALL-L3) shows Sudan black B positivity in the vacuoles. Cytochemistry in ALL is shown in Table 9.18.

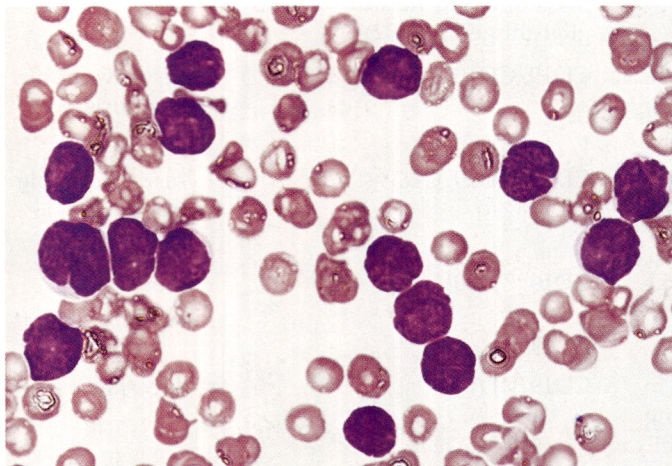

Fig. 9.10: Peripheral blood smear in a case of ALL (L1) showing lymphoblasts with high nucleocytoplasmic ratio, coarse chromatin, inconspicuous nucleoli and scant cytoplasm.

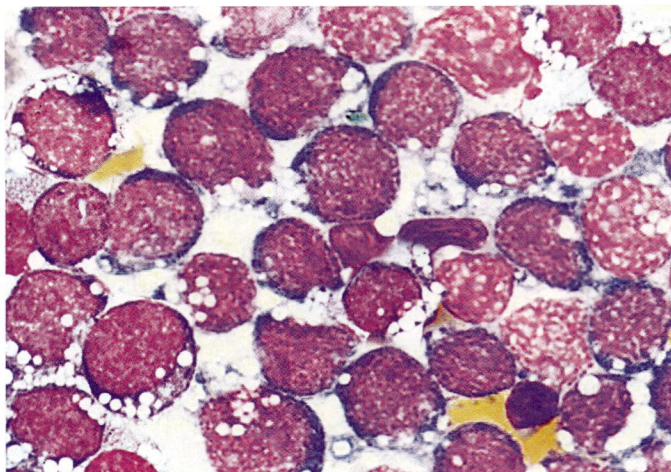

Fig. 9.12: Peripheral blood smear in a case of ALL (L3) showing large lymphoblasts with basophilic vacuolated cytoplasm. These lymphoblasts are similar to those seen in Burkitt's lymphoma.

Table 9.18: Cytochemistry in ALL

Cytochemical stain	ALL
PAS	Positive
Acid phosphatase	Positive in T-ALL
Myeloperoxidase	Negative
Sudan black B	Negative
Non-specific esterase	Negative

B CELL AND T CELL LINEAGE MARKERS

B cell lineage markers include cCD79a/cCD22. These cells show also positivity with CD10 (CALLA), CD19, and CD22. ALL with CD10 positive is most frequent and most amenable to therapy. Thus, **CD10 is a favorable prognostic marker of this disease.** T cell lineage expresses cCD3 marker. It also demonstrates CD2, CD3, CD4, CD5, CD7 and TdT.

Immunophenotype of ALL is shown in Table 9.19. Differences between B-ALL and T-ALL are shown in Fig. 9.13 and Table 9.20.

PROGNOSIS

Patient with CD10 positive marker, hyperdiploidy, and t(12;21)/TEL-AML1 rearrangement has been associated with good prognosis. *Patient has poor prognosis showing chromosomal t(9;22), t(1;19), 11q23 rearrangements and hypodiploidy.* Prognostic factors in acute lymphoblastic leukemia (ALL) are shown in Table 9.21.

Table 9.19: Immunophenotype of ALL (lineage markers of lymphoblasts)

Cytochemical stain	ALL
ALL (B cell)	ALL (T cell)
cCD79a	cCD1
cCD22	CD2
CD10* (CALLA)	CD3
CD19	CD4
CD22	CD5
HLA-DR	CD7
TdT	TdT

*CD10 (CALLA) is favorable prognostic marker and most amenable to therapy.

RESPONSE TO TREATMENT

Approximately >90% ALL achieve complete remission with treatment. Relapse is common in 75% of cases without prophylactic intrathecal chemotherapy. ALL in adults has worse prognosis and requires bone marrow transplantation as well as chemotherapy.

ACUTE MYELOID LEUKEMIA

Acute myeloid leukemia is a stem cell disorder characterized by neoplastic proliferation of myeloblasts in the bone marrow. It results in accumulation of immature nonfunctional leukocytes in bone marrow and circulation. Failure of normal production of red cells,

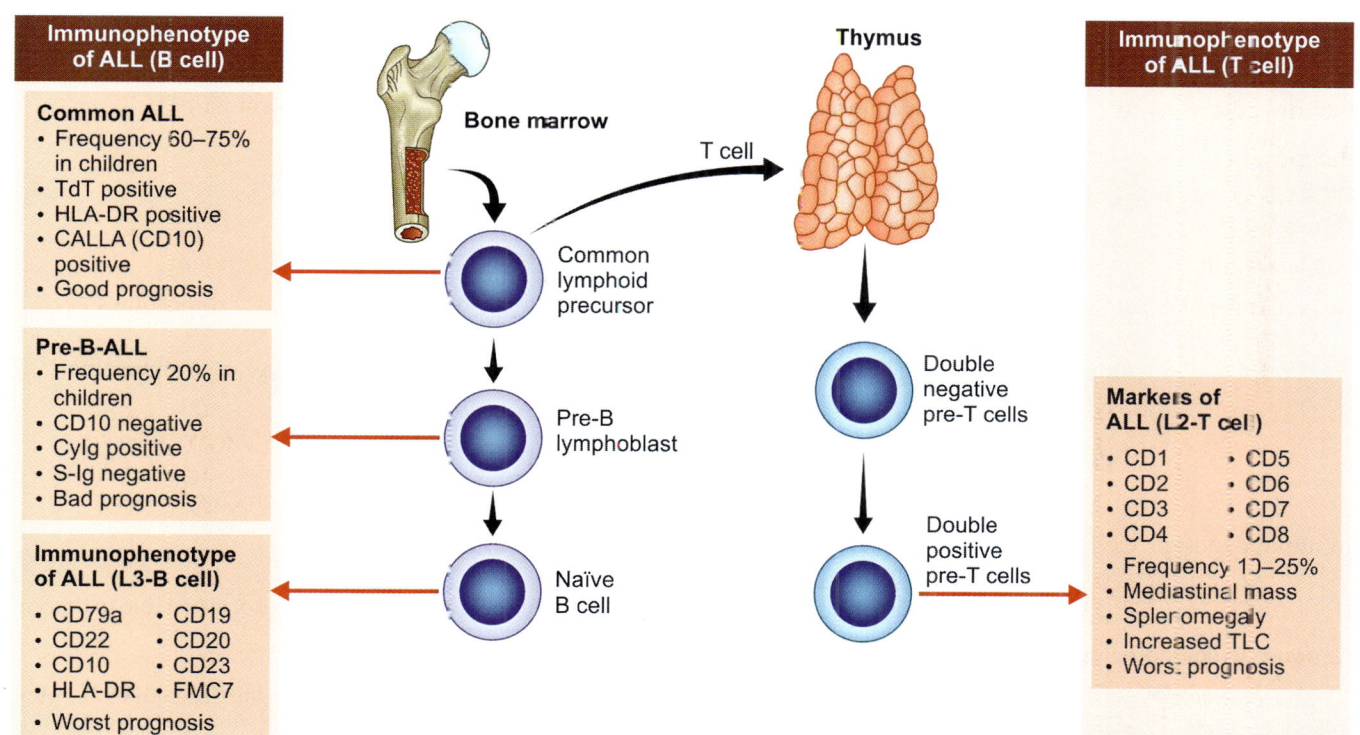

Fig. 9.13: Immunophenotype of acute lymphoblastic leukemia.

Table 9.20: Differences between ALL (B cell) and ALL (T cell)

Parameters	ALL (B cell)	ALL (T cell)
Age group	2–5 years	13–17 years
Frequency in India	80%	20%
Tumor load	Low	High
Clinical presentation	Extensive bone marrow and peripheral blood involvement	Mediastinal lymphadenopathy
Molecular pathogenesis	Hyperploidy >50 chromosomes most common Hypoploidy <50 chromosomes PAX5, E2A or EBF gene mutations Balanced translocations t(12;21) involving genes ETV6 and RUNX1	Gain of function mutation of Notch1
Immunophenotype (lineage markers of lymphoblasts)	CD10 (CALLA—most favorable prognostic marker amenable to therapy) CD79a CD22 CD19 HLA-DR TdT	CD1 CD2 CD3, CD5 CD4 CD7 TdT
Prognosis	Good	Poor

Table 9.21: Prognostic factors in acute lymphoblastic leukemia (ALL)

Characteristics	Favorable prognosis	Adverse prognosis
Age	2–10 years of age	<1 year and >10 years of age
Gender	Females	Males
Race	White	Black
FAB classification	ALL (L-1)	ALL (L2), ALL (L3)
Cell types	Early pre-B-ALL Common ALL antigen	Pre-B-ALL (bad prognosis) Pre-T-ALL (bad prognosis) B-ALL (worse prognosis)
Extramedullary involvement (CNS, mediastinum, testis)	Absent or minimal involvement	Extensive involvement
TLC	<10,000/cu mm	>50,000/ cu mm
Hemoglobin	>10 gm/dl	<7 gm/dl
Platelets count	More than 100,000/cu mm	Less than 30,000/cu mm
Molecular genetics	Hyperploidy >50 chromosomes Trisomy 4, 7, 10 t(12; 21)/TEL-AML1 rearrangement	Hypoploidy <50 chromosomes - t(9;22): Philadelphia chromosome t(4,11) t(8,14) t(1;19) 11q23 rearrangements
Immunophenotype CD10	Early pre-B-ALL CALLA positive CD10 positive. It is the most amenable to therapy	Pre-B-ALL Mature B-ALL CD10 negative (not amenable to therapy)
Response to chemotherapy	Response—good	Unresponsive
Translocation t(9;22) seen in ALL is cytogenetically identical but molecularly distinct from the one typically seen in CML. Minor breakpoint region is more commonly involved in ALL. But in CML, major breakpoint region is typically involved. In childhood ALL, a BCR/ABL fusion protein, P190, is produced		

leukocytes and platelets results in anemia, recurrent infection and thrombocytopenia.

FAB CLASSIFICATION OF AML

According to FAB (French-American-British) classification, acute leukemias are classified into M0–M7 based on blast cell count and morphology on bone marrow and peripheral smear examination.

WHO CLASSIFICATION

According to WHO classification cut-off percentage of blasts is more than 20%. WHO classification of AML with recurrent genetic alterations is shown in Table 9.22.

AML WITH RECURRENT GENETIC ABNORMALITIES

This group has AML with balanced translocations inversions which have prognostic significance. Most common ones such as t(8;21), t(15;17), t(6;16) are considered acute leukemias even if the blast counts are <20%. Cytogenetic analysis and RT-PCR are used to diagnose these recurrent genetic abnormalities. AML with recurrent genetic abnormalities are shown in Table 9.23.

CLINICAL FEATURES

Acute myeloid leukemia most often occurs in the adults. It may occur at any age. Symptoms are related to anemia, neutropenia (recurrent upper respiratory tract infections) and thrombocytopenia (bleeding tendencies). Bone tenderness is common.

Physical examination reveals mild to moderate hepatomegaly and splenomegaly. Clinical course is short marked by anemia, infection, and hemorrhage, and death occurs within 6 to 12 months. These are less responsive to therapeutic intervention.

Fever

Patient becomes febrile as a result of neutropenia (recurrent upper respiratory tract infections).

Bleeding Tendencies

Patient presents with bleeding tendencies as a result of depletion of megakaryocytes in the bone marrow. Common sites of bleeding are *gums and skin* (purpuric spots, ecchymosis). *Disseminated intravascular coagulation is common in AML (M3) leukemia.*

Table 9.22: WHO classification of AML (2016)

AML	Recurrent genetic abnormalities
AML with recurrent genetic abnormalities	AML with t(8;21)(q22;q22.1); RUNX1-RUNX1T1 AML with inv(16)(p13.1q22) or t(16;16)(p13.1;q22); CBFB-MYH11 APL with PML-RARA AML with t(9;11)(p21.3;q23.3); MLLT3-KMT2A AML with t(6;9)(p23;q34.1); DEK-NUP214 AML with inv(3)(q21.3q26.2) or t(3;3)(q21.3;q26.2); GATA2, MECOM AML (megakaryoblastic) with t(1;22)(p13.3;q13.3); RBM15-MKL1 Provisional entity: AML with BCR-ABL1 AML with mutated NPM1 AML with biallelic mutations of CEBPA provisional entity: AML with mutated RUNX1
AML with myelodysplasia related changes	Not applicable
Therapy related myeloid neoplasms	Not applicable
Acute myeloid leukemia (not otherwise specified)	AML with minimal differentiation AML without maturation AML with maturation Acute myelomonocytic leukemia Acute monoblastic and monocytic leukemia Pure erythroid leukemia Acute megakaryoblastic leukemia Acute basophilic leukemia Acute panmyelosis with myelofibrosis
Myeloid sarcoma	Not applicable
Myeloid proliferations related to Down syndrome	Not applicable

Table 9.23: AML with recurrent genetic abnormalities

AML with recurrent genetic abnormality	Secondary genetic defects	Age	Clinical features	Similarity to FAB type	Morphology in peripheral blood and bone marrow	Immuno-phenotype	Aberrant markers	Prognosis
AML with t(8;21)(q22;22) RUNX1-RUNX1T1	(–Y), del 9q	Young age group	Myeloid sarcoma may be present at presentation	M2	Large blasts with abundant basophilic cytoplasm with numerous azurophilic granules. Pseudogranules (Chédiak-Higashi) in a few blasts. Variable dysplasia in myeloid series in the form of pseudo-Pelger-Huët nuclei, homogenous pink cytoplasm. Single long sharp Auer rods. Eosinophilic recursors are frequently increased	CD34, HLA DR, CD13, MPO (strong) CD33 (weak) Maturation asynchrony (co-expression of CD15 and CD34)	CD19, PAX5, CyCD79a	Good response to chemotherapy. CD56 and KIT mutations (poor prognosis)
AML with t(16;16)(p13.1;q22) or Inv(16)(p13.1;q22) CBFB-MYH11	+22, +8, del 7q, +21	Young age group	Myeloid sarcoma may be present at presentation	M4	AMML with variable number of eosinophils in BM. Promyelocytes and myelocytes have immature eosinophilic granules. Naphthol-ASD-chloracetate esterase is positive in eosinophils	Multiple blast populations CD34, CD117 blasts with granulocytic differentiation (CD13, CD33, 65, MPO). Blasts with monocytic differentiation (CD14, CD11b, CD11c, CD64, CD36, lysozyme)	CD2	+22 (good prognosis) KIT (poor prognosis)
AML with t(15;17)(q22;q12); PML-RARA	+8, FLT3-ITD	Adults	DIC	M3, M3v	Promyelocytes with kidney/bilobed nucleus and large bright pink/purple granules. Faggot cells. Large Auer rods	CD33 homogenous, CD13 heterogenous HLA-DR and CD34 negative	CD2	Good prognosis if treated optimally with ATRA. CD56 (poor prognosis)
AML with t(9;11) p22;q23. MLLT3-MLL	+8	Children	DIC, gingival infiltration	M4, M5	Monoblasts and promonocytes predominate	CD33, CD65, HLA-DR strong. CD13, CD34, CD14 weak	-	Intermediate survival

Contd...

Table 9.23: AML with recurrent genetic abnormalities (Contd...)

AML with recurrent genetic abnormality	Secondary genetic defects	Age	Clinical features	Similarity to FAB type	Morphology in peripheral blood and bone marrow	Immuno-phenotype	Aberrant markers	Prognosis
AML with t(6;9) (p23;q34) DEK-NUP	FLT3:ITD	Children and adults	Pancytopenia or anemia with thrombocytopenia	M2, M4	Blasts of any FAB except M3 and M7 Multilineage dysplasia Basophilia >2% Pancytopenia Ringed sideroblasts	MPO, CD13, CD33, CD38, HLA-DR+	TdT positive	Poor prognosis
AML with Inv (3) q21;q26.2 or t(3;3) (q21;q26.2) RPN1-EVI1	Monosomy 7, del 5q	Adults	Arise *de novo* or from MDS hepatomegaly, splenomegaly	M1, M4, M7	Blasts any FAB except M3, normal or increased platelets Increased atypical megakaryocytes Multilineage dysplasia	CD13, CD33, HLA DR, CD34, CD38+ CD41 and CD61 in a subset of blasts	CD7	Aggressive disease
AML with t(1;22) (p13;q13) RBM15-MKL1	-	Infants and young children	Hepatomegaly, splenomegaly in children <3 years	M7	Small and large megakaryoblasts admixed with blasts similar to lymphoblasts	No dysplasia	CD41, CD61, CD42+, CD13, CD33±, CD34, HLA-DR, CD45 negative	Good response to intensive chemotherapy

Organs Involved

Patient with AML (M4 or M5) presents with widespread infiltration gums (hypertrophy), liver, spleen, lymph nodes, diffuse erythematous skin rashes and central nervous system.

CNS Involvement

Approximately 10% patients with AML (M4 or M5) show central nervous system involvement. There may be involvement of V and VII cranial nerves.

Pancytopenia and Marrow Fibrosis

AML (M7) results in pancytopenia and marrow fibrosis.

HEMATOLOGICAL FINDINGS

Blood Counts

Hemoglobin: Low, TLC is increased except in subleukemic leukemia. Platelet count is markedly reduced.

Peripheral Blood Smear

Total leukocyte count is increased varying from $20 \times 10^9/dl$ to $100 \times 10^9/dl$. Peripheral blood smear shows large **immature myeloblasts (>20%)** with fine chromatin in nuclei and *multiple nucleoli*. Myeloblasts contain linear red **Auer rod** composed of crystallized azurophilic granules. There may be increase in monocytes, eosinophils and basophils. **Thrombocytopenia** is marked.

Normocytic normochromic anemia with nucleated red blood cells is seen. *Auer rods are present in myelodysplastic syndrome, AML-M2, AML-M3 and blast crisis of CML.* Differences between myeloblast and lymphoblast are shown in Table 9.24. Comparison between cytochemistry, immunocytochemistry of AML and ALL is shown in Table 9.25.

Bone Marrow

Bone marrow is hypercellular with high myeloid to erythroid ratio. Myeloblasts are present >30% (FAB classification) or >20% as per WHO classification. Myeloid to erythroid ratio is increased. Normal hematopoiesis

Table 9.24: Differences between myeloblast and lymphoblast

Characteristics	Myeloblast	Lymphoblast
Nuclear membrane	Very fine	Relatively dense
Size	Larger	Smaller
Cytoplasm	Scant to moderate	Scant
Nucleoli	3–5	1–2
Auer rods	Present	Absent
Myeloperoxidase staining	Positive	Negative
Sudan black B	Positive	Negative
PAS staining	Negative	Positive
Acid phosphatase	Negative	Positive
Nonspecific esterase	Negative/positive in M4/M5	Negative

Table 9.25: Comparison between cytochemistry, immunocytochemistry of AML and ALL

Characteristics	AML	ALL
Age group	15–39 years	<10 years mostly <15 years
Peripheral blood and bone marrow findings	Myeloblasts and other myeloid cells	Lymphoblasts
Cytochemistry		
Myeloperoxidase: blue granules in cytoplasm	Positive staining in M1–M6 Auer rods are present	Negative staining
Sudan black B (black granules in cytoplasm due to membrane phospholipids	Positive staining	Negative staining
Nonspecific esterase (dark red granules)	Positive staining in M4, M5	Negative staining
Chloracetate esterase	Positive	Negative
Acid phosphatase	Positive in M4, M5	Negative (T-ALL+)
PAS staining (magenta granules)	Negative staining (faint staining)	Positive staining (coarse staining)
TdT (terminal deoxynucleotidyl transferase)	Negative	Positive
Immunocytochemistry of leukemias		
Immunocytochemistry (monoclonal antibodies are useful to differentiate AML and ALL in case inconclusive on cytochemistry)	CD13 cAnti-MPO (cytoplasmic anti-MPO) CD33 CD61 (M7)	CD10 CD19 HLA-DR T-ALL (cCD3)
Therapeutic response and prognosis		
Chemotherapeutic agents	Cytosine Arabinoside Anthracyclin 6-Thioguanine	Vincristine Anthracyclin Prednisolone L-asparaginase
Response to therapy	Remission rate is low Duration of remission is short	High remission rate Duration of remission prolonged
Median survival	12–18 months	Children with CNS prophylaxis are 5 years Adults survive for 8–12 months

Table 9.26: Cytochemistry of AML (FAB)

FAB	Differentiation	Cytochemistry
AML (M0)	Minimal differentiation	Myeloperoxidase negative
AML (M1)	AML without maturation	Myeloperoxidase Sudan black B Chloracetate esterase
AML (M2)	AML with differentiation into *neutrophilic lineage*	Myeloperoxidase Sudan black B Chloracetate esterase
AML (M3)	AML with promyelocytic differentiation (commonly associated with DIC due to release of thromboplastin like substance)	Myeloperoxidase Sudan black B Chloracetate esterase
AML (M4)	Myelomonocytic leukemia	Myeloperoxidase positive Nonspecific esterase positive Acid phosphotase
AML (M5a)	Monoblastic without differentiation	Myeloperoxidase positive Nonspecific esterase positive Acid phosphatase
AML (M5b)	Monoblastic with differentiation	
AML (M6a)	Dysplastic erythroblasts and myeloblasts	PAS stain and myeloperoxidase stain positive
AML (M6b)	Dysplastic erythroblasts	
AML (M7)	Acute megakaryocytic leukemia	-

is reduced by replacement (**myelophthisic process**) or as a result of suppression of stem cells division. Megakaryopoiesis is diminished.

Cytochemical Analysis

Cytochemistry of AML (FAB) is shown in Table 9.26.

Lineage Markers

Lineage markers of AML while analyzing on flow cytometric analysis include: Anti-MPO cytoplasmic is lineage marker of AML.

Table 9.27: Lineage markers of AML analyzing on flow cytometry

Parameters	Lineage markers of AML
AML	Anti-MPO cytoplasmic is lineage marker of AML CD13 CD41 CD33 CD68 CD117
Markers of immaturity	CD34
Monocytic differentiation	CD14 CD64
Megakaryocytic differentiation	CD41 CD61
Erythroid differentiation	CD235A Glycophorin A

Table 9.28: Laboratory diagnosis of AML

Parameters	Findings
Clinical findings	Anemia, recurrent infections, bleeding tendencies and organs involvement
Myeloblasts in bone marrow	>20%
Auer rods in myeloblasts	Present
Bone marrow trephine biopsy	Indicated in dry bone marrow tap
Flow cytometry	Useful when cytochemistry is negative

Other markers include CD13, CD33 and CD117. Lineage markers of AML analyzing on flow cytometry are shown in Table 9.27.

Bone Marrow Biopsy

Bone marrow biopsy is performed in cases of dry bone marrow tap in AML with pancytopenia. Bone biopsy examination shows sheets of blast cells and fibrosis.

Immunohistochemistry is performed using anti-MPO, CD13, CD41, CD68 to confirm diagnosis. Laboratory diagnosis of AML is shown in Table 9.28.

PROGNOSTIC FACTORS

Prognostic factors of AML (FAB classification) are shown in Table 9.29.

Table 9.29: Prognostic factors of AML (FAB classification)

Characteristics	Favorable prognosis	Adverse prognosis
Age group	<40 years	<2 years and >60 years in AML (M0, M6, M7)
Disorder	*De novo*	Therapy induced or myelodysplastic syndrome associated
Infection	Absent	Present in AML (M5)
Total leukocyte count	<25,000/cu mm	>100,000/cu mm
Serum LDH		>400 IU/L
Extramedullary involvement	Absent	Present
CNS involvement	Absent	Present
Sex predilection	Females	Males
Other hematological disorders	Absent	Present
Cytogenetics	AML (M2) t(8;21) AML (M3) t(15;17) AML (M4) inversion (16q)	AML (M2) t(6;9) AML (M5) translocation or deletion of chromosome 5
Molecular prognostic factors	NPM1 gene mutation (5q35)	FLT3-ITD (13q12)
	Biallelic CEBPA gene mutation (19q13.1)	WT1 mutation (11p13) KIT mutation (4q11–q12) BAALC overexpression (8q22.3) ERG overexpression (21q22.3) EVI1 overexpression (3q26) MN1 overexpression (22q12.1)
Immunophenotype	Negative for CD34, CD14 and HLA-DR	Positive for CD34 and HLA-DR

Markers are studied in bone marrow smears and bone marrow trephine biopsy. Other parameters such as angiogenesis and proliferative index are also studied.

DISTINCT FORMS OF AML

AML with Minimal Differentiation (FAB-M0)

AML (M0) lacks evidence of myeloid differentiation on light microscopy or cytochemical analysis. Most patients are either infants or older adults. Patient presents with evidence of bone marrow failure. Blasts in M0 are medium in size with round or slightly indented nuclei and one or two nucleoli and agranular cytoplasm (Fig. 9.14).

Cytochemistry

Blasts are negative for MPO, Sudan black B, naphthol-ASD-chloracetate esterase. However, <3% blasts are positive for these stains.

Immunophenotype

CD34, CD38, HLA-DR are expressed by the blasts. CD13, CD117, CD33 are expressed in some blasts. Myeloid and monocyte maturation associated antigens are not expressed such as CD11b, CD15, CD14, CD64 and CD65 (Table 9.30).

AML without Maturation (FAB-M1)

AML (M1) is characterized by presence of >90% blasts in peripheral blood and bone marrow with <10% maturing

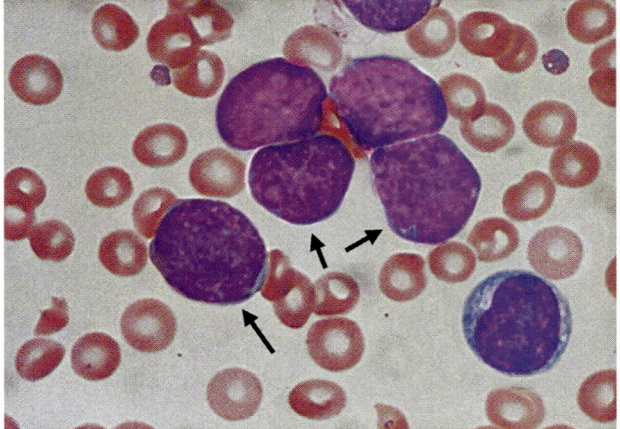

Fig. 9.14: Giemsa stain on peripheral blood shows blasts in AML with minimal differentiation. The blasts are large with scant amount of cytoplasm, high nucleocytoplasmic ratio, fine nuclear chromatin and 2–4 prominent nucleoli (arrows).

cells of neutrophil lineage. 3% or more of the blasts show MPO or Sudan black B positivity. AML (M1) occurs more commonly in adults. Patient presents with anemia, thrombocytopenia and neutropenia.

Blasts Morphology

Blasts resemble myeloblasts in some cases with presence of azurophilic granules and Auer rods. In some cases

White Blood Cells

Table 9.30: Immunophenotype in AML (M0)

Immunophenotype	Expression
CD34	Positive
CD38	Positive
HLA-DR	Positive
CD13	Positive (some cases)
CD117	Positive (some cases)
CD33	Positive (some cases)

Myeloid and monocyte maturation associated antigens are not expressed such as CD11b, CD15, CD14, CD64 and CD65.

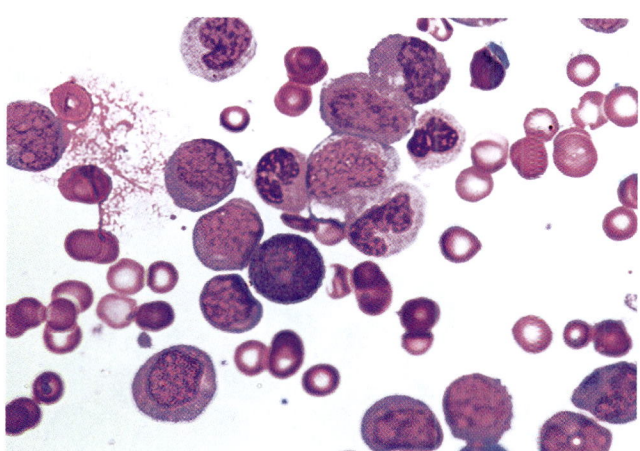

Fig. 9.15: Peripheral smear showing blasts in AML (M1) with maturation. The blasts show opened up chromatin with high nucleocytoplasmic ratio, 2–4 prominent nucleoli and moderate amount of cytoplasm.

resemble lymphoblasts. Myeloperoxidase stain is positive in blasts. Peripheral blood smear showing blasts in AML (M1) with maturation is depicted in Fig. 9.15.

Immunophenotype

Blasts show positivity for CD13, CD33, CD117, HLA-DR and CD34 (Table 9.31).

Table 9.31: Immunophenotype in AML (M0)

Immunophenotype	Expression
CD13	Positive
CD33	Positive
CD117	Positive
HLA-DR	Positive
CD34	Positive

AML with Maturation (FAB-M2)

AML (M2) is characterized by presence of >20% blasts in peripheral blood and bone marrow with >10% maturing cells of neutrophil lineage. It occurs in all age groups. Patient presents with anemia, thrombocytopenia and neutropenia.

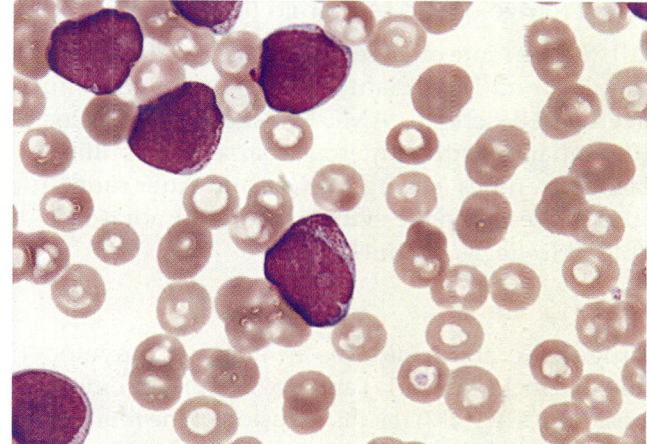

Fig. 9.16: AML (M2). Myeloblasts with promyelocyte, myelocyte and band forms of polymorphonuclear cells showing evidence of maturation.

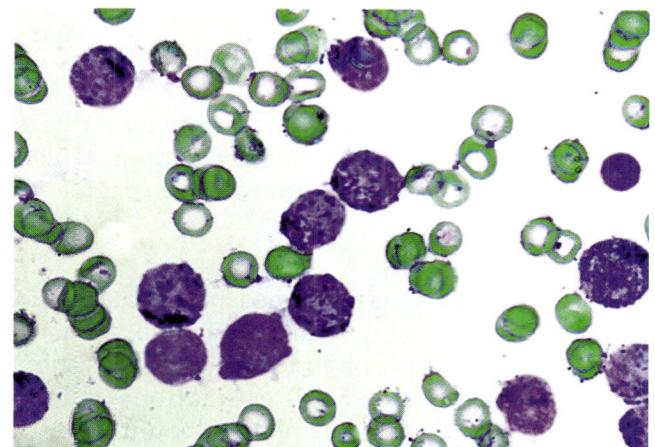

Fig. 9.17: AML (M2). Peripheral smear showing MPO (myeloperoxidase) positive in AML with maturation.

Blasts Morphology

Myeloblasts with Auer rods and azurophilic granules are seen along with promyelocytes, myelocytes and mature neutrophils comprising up to 10% of bone marrow cells (Fig. 9.16). Myeloblasts show positivity with myeloperoxidase stain (Fig. 9.17).

Immunophenotype

Myeloblasts express positivity for CD13, CD33, CD65, CD11b and CD15 (Table 9.32).

Table 9.32: Immunophenotype in AML (M0)

Immunophenotype	Expression
CD13	Positive
CD33	Positive
CD65	Positive
CD11b	Positive
CD15	Positive

Acute Promyelocytic Leukemia (M3 and M3V)

AML (M3) is more often seen in adults. AML-M3 (hypergranular) and its variant AML-M3V (hypogranular) have been described. AML-M3 shows promyelocytic differentiation with numerous coarse azurophilic cytoplasmic granules (**strong MPO+**) and **Auer rods**. Auer rods are present in the cytoplasm and tumor cells have a folded (*cottage-loaf*) nuclei.

Molecular Genetics

Cytogenetic abnormalities in acute promyelocytic leukemia include t(15;17) and t(q22;q12). Chromosomal translocation t(15;17) results in fusion of the retinoic acid receptor-α (RAR-α) gene on chromosome 17 with the PML gene on chromosome 15, resulting in blockage of myeloid differentiation at the promyelocytic stage. It is demonstrated by FISH. Currently AML *(M3) is classified under AML with recurrent genetic abnormalities.*

Clinical Features

Senescent leukemic cells degranulate and release thromboplastin like substance into the peripheral blood and can cause disseminated intravascular coagulation.

Hemostatic Function Tests

Hemostatic function tests performed include coagulation studies, clotting time, prothrombin time, activated partial thromboplastin time, fibrinogen levels, fibrin degradation products (FDP) estimation, platelets studies (bleeding time and platelet count), plasma LDH level, lysozyme levels in serum and urine. Hematological findings in AML (M3) are shown in Table 9.33.

Peripheral Blood Smear

Peripheral blood smear shows hypergranular or hypogranular promyelocytes, neutropenia and monocytosis (Figs 9.18 and 9.19).

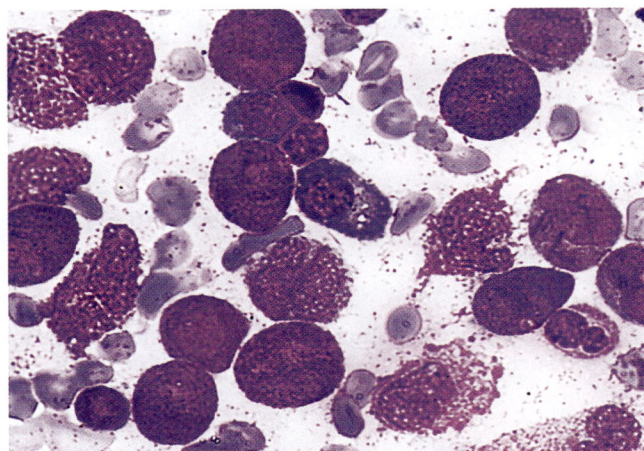

Fig. 9.18: AML (M3). Acute promyelocytic leukemia showing coarse granules (hypergranularity).

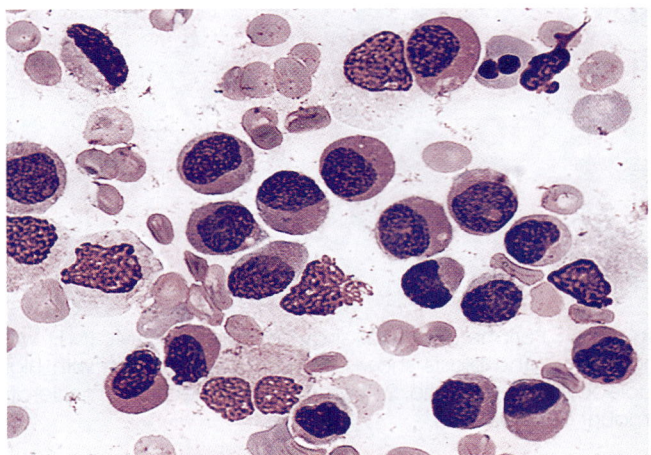

Fig. 9.19: AML (M3V). Acute promyelocytic leukemia showing fine sparse granules (hypogranularity).

Remission

Remission is obtained by administration of **oral all-*trans* retinoic acid**, a vitamin A analogue (ATRA), a form of *differentiation* therapy that overcomes the maturation arrest.

Table 9.33: Hematological findings in AML (M3)

Parameters	Hematological findings
Hemoglobin	Low
Hematocrit values	Decreased (MCV, MCH, MCHC and RDW)
ESR	Increased
TLC	Increased
Peripheral blood smear	AML (M3) hypergranular AML (M3V) hypogranular Neutropenia and monocytosis Normocytic normochromic picture with nucleated erythroid cells
Bone marrow	Hypercellular marrow with high M/E and predominant promyelocytes
Cytochemistry	Myeloperoxidase positive

White Blood Cells

Treatment

All variants of AML except promyelocytic leukemia are treated by continuous infusion of cytarabine for 7 days and a 3-day course of daunorubicin followed by autologous hematopoietic stem cell transplant (HSCT) and allogeneic HSCT.

Acute Myelomonocytic Leukemia (FAB-M4)

AMML is a leukemia characterized by **both neutrophil** and **monocytic precursor proliferation.** It occurs more commonly in **older** individuals. Patient presents with anemia and thrombocytopenia.

Peripheral Blood Smear

Peripheral blood or bone marrow shows >20% blasts including promonocytes along with neutrophil and their precursors and monocytes (Fig. 9.20).

Immunophenotype

Several population of blasts are seen variably expressing myeloid antigens and some markers of monocytic differentiation.

Acute Monoblastic and Monocytic Leukemia (FAB-M5)

There are two subtypes of AML-M5: AML-M5A (monoblastic with >80% blasts), AML-M5B (monocytic with <80% blasts). M5A is more common in young individuals whereas M5B is seen more commonly in adults.

Clinical Features

Patient with AML-M5 presents with gum hypertrophy due to infiltration by leukemic cells. Similar infiltrates can be seen in *skin, lymph nodes, meninges* and *lungs.*

PBF and Bone Marrow

- *AML (M5A):* AML (M5A) shows predominantly monoblasts in peripheral blood. Monoblasts are large cells with abundant basophilic cytoplasm with pseudopod formation and scattered fine azurophilic granules and vacuoles (Fig. 9.21).
- *AML (M5B):* More mature forms of monocytic series are demonstrated in peripheral blood in M5B. Promonocytes predominate with delicately convoluted nucleus, less basophilic cytoplasm and more obvious azurophilic granules (Fig. 9.22).

Bone Marrow

Bone marrow examination shows more monoblasts and promonocytes. It is essential to evaluate both peripheral blood smear and bone marrow for subtyping AML (M5).

Immunophenotype

Tumor cells variably express CD13, CD33, CD15 and CD65. At least two markers of monocytic differentiation are positive such as CD14, CD11b, CD64, CD68, CD36 and lysozyme (Table 9.34).

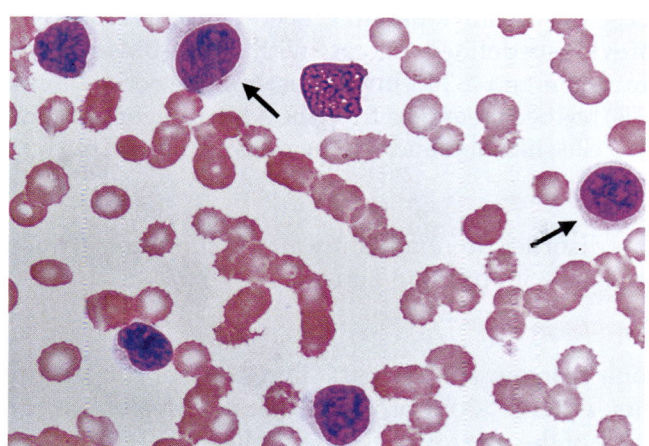

Fig. 9.21: Giemsa stained peripheral smear showing monoblasts with rounded nuclei with 1–2 prominent nucleoli and abundant lacy chromatin (marked by arrows), this case was diagnosed as acute monoblastic leukemia (AML-M5A).

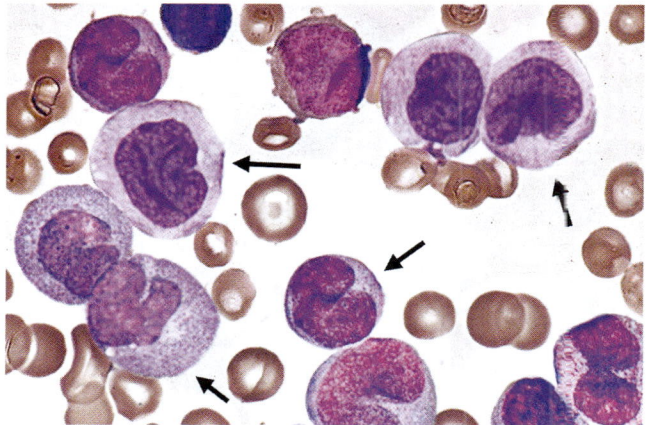

Fig. 9.20: AML (M4). Acute myelomonocytic leukemia shows cells of monocytic series (arrows).

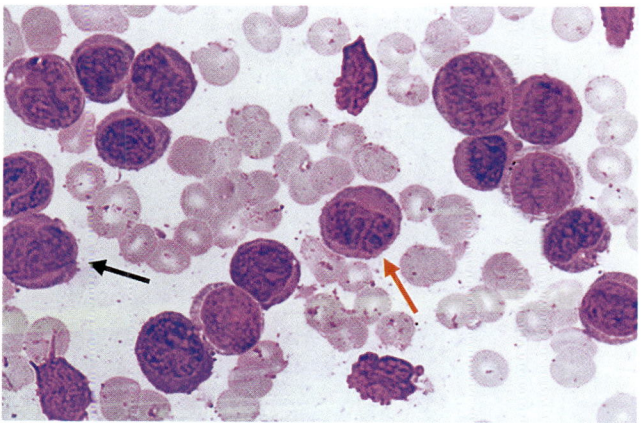

Fig. 9.22: AML (M5B). Acute monocytic leukemia (AML-M5B) shows presence of promonocytes (black arrow) and monoblasts (red arrow).

Table 9.34: Immunophenotype of AML (M5)

Immunophenotype	Expression
CD13	Positivity (variable)
CD33	Positivity (variable)
CD15	Positivity (variable)
CD65	Positivity (variable)
CD14	Positive
CD11b	Positive
CD64	Positive
CD68	Positive
CD36	Positive
Lysozyme	Positive

Acute Erythroblastic Leukemia (FAB-M6)

AML (M6) was of two subtypes: AML-M6A (erythroleukemia) and AML-M6B (pure erythroid leukemia) as per WHO 2008 classification have subcategory of acute erythroid leukemia, erythroid/myeloid type (previously defined as a case with ≥50% BM erythroid precursors and ≥20% myeloblasts among non-erythroid cells) has been removed from the AML category in WHO 2016 classification and will be classified as MDS.

Clinical Features

This disorder predominantly affects the adults. Patient presents with profound anemia.

Bone Marrow

Bone marrow shows >80% immature erythroid precursors with >30% proerythroblasts. Myeloblasts are <20% of the marrow nucleated cells (Fig. 9.23).

Prognosis

Prognosis is associated with an aggressive clinical course.

Acute Megakaryoblastic Leukemia (FAB-M7)

AML (M7) demonstrates >20% blasts, out of which at least 50% are of megakaryocyte lineage. Patient presents with thrombocytopenia and sometimes with increased platelets count. Liver and spleen are usually not enlarged. Prognosis is very poor.

Peripheral Blood Smear

Peripheral blood smear shows micromegakaryocytes, fragments of megakaryocytes, dysplastic large platelets. Blasts may show vacuolation (Fig. 9.24).

Bone Marrow

Bone marrow aspirate smear shows poorly differentiated blasts and maturing dysplastic megakaryocytes. It may show a dry tap due to varying degree of fibrosis.

Immunophenotype

Cells show positivity for **CD41** and **CD61** demonstrated by *immunocytochemistry* and *flow cytometry*.

Myeloid Sarcoma

Myeloid sarcoma arises from hematopoietic stem cell affecting adults. It occurs in 5–15% cases of AML. Tumor is composed of myeloblasts with or without maturation present in tissues outside bone marrow such as **bone (periosteum) orbit, paranasal sinuses, skin, breast, gastrointestinal tract, mediastinum, pleura, ovary** and **lymph nodes.**

It can occur *de novo* or initial manifestation of relapse in a patient previously diagnosed as AML or blastic transformation of MDS and MPN.

> **Light Microscopy**
> Myeloid sarcoma is composed of myeloblasts with or without promyelocytic or neutrophilic maturation that effaces the tissue architecture (Fig. 9.25).

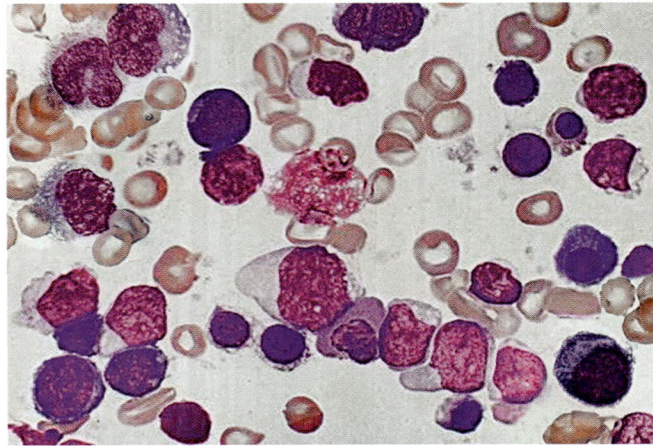

Fig. 9.23: AML (M6). Erythroleukemia. Smear shows myeloblast, promyelocyte and normoblasts with evidence of dyserythropoiesis.

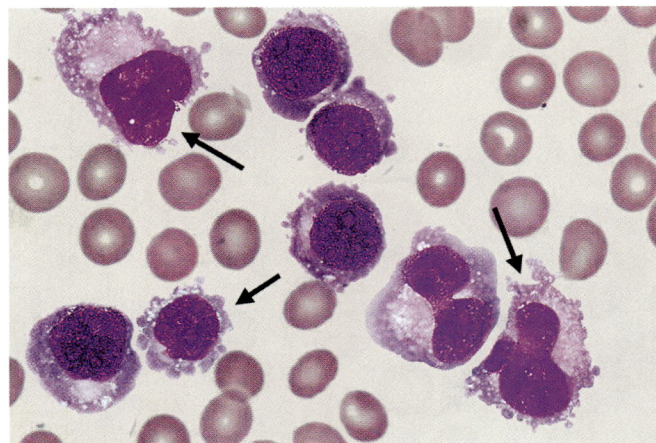

Fig. 9.24: AML (M7). Blasts are variable in size. Some blasts are showing cytoplasmic budding (arrows).

White Blood Cells

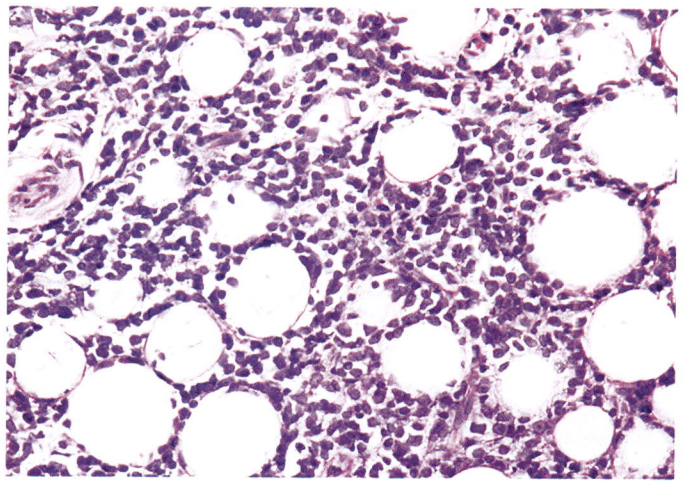

Fig. 9.25: Orbital biopsy from a case of myeloid sarcoma orbit showing sheets of atypical cells infiltrating into surrounding adipose tissue (hematoxylin and eosin 100X).

Cytochemistry
These tumor cells show positivity for myeloperoxidase.

Table 9.35: Immunophenotype of myeloid sarcoma

Immunophenotype marker	Expression
CD68	Positive
anti-cMPO (anti-cytoplasmic MPO)	Positive
CD117	Positive
CD99	Positive
CD34	Positive
Lysozyme	Positive
TdT	Positive

Immunophenotype
Tumor cells are positive for CD68, anti-cMPO (anti-cytoplasmic MPO), CD117, CD99, CD34, lysozyme and TdT (Table 9.35).

Prognosis
Untreated patients develop acute myeloid leukemia. Myeloid sarcoma patients are managed similar to AML cases.

MYELODYSPLASTIC SYNDROMES/MYELOPROLIFERATIVE NEOPLASMS

MYELODYSPLASTIC SYNDROME

Myelodysplastic syndrome (MDS) is clonal stem cell disorder of bone marrow affecting middle-aged and elderly persons. It involves 2 or more than 2 hematopoietic cells lines.

MDS is characterized by paucity of peripheral blood elements (cytopenia) and marked hyperplasia in the bone marrow with features of dysplasia of hematopoietic cell lines, impairment of proliferation and differentiation of hematopoietic cells. There is increased risk of malignant transformation to AML in 30–50% of patients.

CLASSIFICATION

Primary myeloproliferative syndrome originates *de novo*. Secondary myelodysplastic syndrome most often occurs due to administration of **chemotherapeutic alkylating drugs** or **radiotherapy** for treatment of various cancers. Chronic myelomonocytic leukemia has been included in WHO classification in the category of myelodysplastic disorders. FAB classification of myelodysplastic syndrome is shown in Table 9.36. Classification of myelodysplastic syndrome according to WHO (2016) is shown in Table 9.37.

Table 9.36: FAB classification of myelodysplastic syndrome

Subtypes of MDS	Peripheral blood findings	Bone marrow findings	Prognosis
Refractory anemia	Blasts <1% WBC count (normal to mild leukopenia) Macrocytic anemia	Blasts <5% Ring sideroblasts <15% Dyserythropoiesis	Favorable
Refractory anemia (RA) with ring sideroblasts	Blasts <1% WBC count (normal to mild leukopenia) Dimorphic anemia	Blasts <5% Ring sideroblasts >15% Dyserythropoiesis	Favorable
Refractory anemia with excess blasts	Blasts ≤5% WBC count low (trilineage cytopenia)	Blasts >5–19% (may show Auer rods) Dysplastic change	Unfavorable
Refractory anemia with excess blasts in transformation (RAEB-t)	Blasts >5% WBC count—low	Blasts 21–29%	Unfavorable
Chronic myelomonocytic leukemia (with marked splenomegaly)	Blasts <5% ≥1 × 10⁹/L monocytes WBC count—high	Blasts 1–20%	Unfavorable

Table 9.37: Classification of myelodysplastic syndrome according to WHO (2016)

Disorder	Lineage involved	Peripheral blood smear findings	Bone marrow findings	Prognosis
Refractory cytopenia with unilineage dysplasia (RUCD)	Unilineage erythroid or granulocytic or megakaryocytic	Unicytopenia/bicytopenia (Bi) Blast nil/rare	Unidysplasia ≥ 10 cells in one myeloid lineage, <5% blasts and <15% sideroblasts	Good
Refractory anemia with ring sideroblasts (RARS)	Unilineage or erythroid lineages	Anemia	Erythroid hyperplasia with dyserythropoiesis	Good
Refractory cytopenia with multilineage dysplasia (RCMD)	Two or more myeloid lineages	Bi/pancytopenia, monocytes <1 × 10⁹/L Blasts rare	Dysplasia seen in ≥ of 3 hematopoietic cells lines Blasts<5%	Intermediate
Refractory anemia with ring sideroblasts	Unilineage or erythroid lineages	Blasts nil/rare	>5% Ring sideroblasts <10%	Intermediate
Refractory anemia with excess blasts 1 (RAEB-1)	Unilineage or multi-lineages	Bi/pancytopenia Blasts <5%	Dysplastic changes in ≥ 1 hematopoietic cell line Blasts 5–9%	Intermediate
Refractory anemia with excess blasts 2 (RAEB-2)	Unilineage or multi-lineages	Cytopenia Blasts 5–9%	Myelodysplasia in ≥ 1 hematopoietic cell line 10–19%	Unfavorable
Myelodysplastic syndrome unclassified (MDS-U)	Unilineage or multi-lineages	Cytopenia Blasts nil	Dysplasia of granulocytic or megakaryocytic series Blasts <5%	Unfavorable
Myelodysplastic syndrome with isolated del (5q)	Erythroid, myeloid and megakaryocyte	Anemia with normal or raised platelet count Blasts <5%	Megakaryocytes with hypolobated nuclei increased or normal Blasts <5%	Good
Childhood myelodysplastic syndrome (refractory cytopenia of childhood)	Unilineage or multi-lineages	Dysplastic changes in >10% neutrophils Blasts <2%	Dysplastic changes in >10% erythroid and granulocytic series with dysmegakaryopoiesis	-

ETIOPATHOGENESIS

MDS may be either primary (*de novo*) or secondary (therapy related). Secondary MDS occurs following chemotherapy (alkylating agent) or radiotherapy in cancer patients after 5–7 years. Exposure to tobacco smoking, benzene exposure and viruses predispose to secondary MDS.

Other causes of secondary MDS are stem cell disorders, congenital disorders, gene mutations and genetic. Causes of secondary myelodysplastic syndrome (MDS) are shown in Table 9.38.

Table 9.38: Causes of secondary myelodysplastic syndrome (MDS)

Categories	Causes
Chemotherapy or radiotherapy administered in cancer patients	Alkylating agent (busulfan), DNA topoisomerase inhibitors, therapeutic radiation
Exposure to agent	Benzene, tobacco smoke, viruses
Stem cell disorders	Paroxysmal nocturnal hemoglobinuria
	Aplastic anemia
Congenital disorders	Neurofibromatosis, Shwachman-Diamond syndrome, Kostmann agranulocytosis
Genetic predisposition	Down's syndrome (trisomy 21), trisomy 8, trisomy 11, monosomy 5, monosomy 7, Deletion 7q, 11q, 12q, 13q, 20q, 17q, 17p, Loss of Y chromosomes, DNA repair defects (Fanconi anemia, ataxia-telangiectasia)
Gene mutations	N-RAS gene mutation, p53 gene mutation, IRF-1 gene mutation, BCL2 gene mutation

CLINICAL FEATURES

Patient presents with anemia, fatigue, recurrent infections and bleeding (thrombocytopenia) as a result of cytopenias due to apoptosis of hematopoietic cells. Synthesis of TGF-β and PDGF cause marrow fibrosis, with pancytopenia, extramedullary hematopoiesis, and massive splenomegaly (>1000 gm and 15 cm long) with secondary hypersplenism. MDS patients may develop AML in 40–50% in advanced cases. Philadelphia chromosome does not occur in MDS.

5q Syndrome

This syndrome occurs due to deletion of chromosome 5 affecting elderly patients. Peripheral blood smear shows macrocytic anemia and increased platelets. Bone marrow examination shows decreased erythropoiesis with monolobate/bilobate forms of megakaryocytes.

Monosomy 7

This cytogenetic abnormality is demonstrated in MDS patients between 6 months and two years of age. Children are prone to recurrent infection due to impaired neutrophilic functions.

MORPHOLOGICAL FINDINGS

Morphological findings suggestive of myelodysplastic syndrome include unexplained persistent pancytopenia (low hemoglobin and TLC high monocytes) and bone marrow showing dysplastic features such as 5–15% blasts, >15% ringed erythroblasts, micromegakaryocytes and nuclear hypersegmentation.

Peripheral Blood Smear

RBCs show dimorphic anemia, **basophilic stippling, Howell-Jolly bodies** and a few nucleated red blood cells (with sieve-like nuclei).

White blood cells: WBCs show refractory neutropenia with hypogranular neutrophils.

Platelets: Majority of patients develop large platelets lacking granules. Thrombocytosis is demonstrated in isolated MDS with 5q deletion.

Table 9.39: Abnormal features of erythroid precursors, myeloid precursors and megakaryocytes

Bone marrow precursors	Morphology
Dyserythropoiesis	Erythroblasts show nuclear budding, multinucleation
	Howell-Jolly bodies
Dysmyelopoiesis	Myeloid hyperplasia
	Myeloblasts increased (normal <5%)
	Myelocytes and metamyelocytes (hypogranular)
Dysmegakaryopoiesis	Megakaryocytes decreased
	Micromegakaryocytes with vesicular monolobate/bilobate nuclei

NAP score: NAP score is decreased in myelodysplastic syndrome.

Bone Marrow

Bone marrow in majority of cases is hypercellular showing **dyserythropoiesis** with **ring sideroblasts, dysmyelopoiesis** and **dysmegakaryopoiesis.** Iron stores are most often increased due to ineffective erythropoiesis. Ring sideroblasts are characteristic features of refractory anemia. Reticulin stain shows slight increase in the reticulin fibers.

Bone marrow biopsy examination shows presence of blasts in the central region of marrow. Abnormal features of erythroid precursors, myeloid precursors and megakaryocytes are shown in Table 9.39.

MDS/MYELOPROLIFERATIVE DISORDERS

JUVENILE MYELOMONOCYTIC LEUKEMIA (WHO, 2016)

Juvenile myelomonocytic leukemia constitutes 2% of childhood leukemias. It affects younger children >4 years. Philadelphia chromosomal abnormality is negative. Diagnostic criteria for juvenile myelomonocytic leukemia is shown in Table 9.40.

Table 9.40: Diagnostic criteria for juvenile myelomonocytic leukemia (WHO 2016)

Diagnostic criteria	Features
Clinical and hematologic features (all features mandatory)	Peripheral blood monocyte count $>1 \times 10^9/L$, blast percentage in peripheral blood and bone marrow <20% and splenomegaly
Genetic studies (1 finding sufficient)	Somatic mutation in PTPN11 or KRAS or NRAS, clinical diagnosis of NF1 or NF1 mutation, germline CBL mutation and loss of heterozygosity of CBL
For patients without genetic features, besides the clinical and hematologic features criteria mentioned must be fulfilled	Monosomy 7 or any other chromosomal abnormalities or at least 2 of the following criteria: hemoglobin F increased for age, myeloid or erythroid precursors on peripheral blood smear, GM-CSF hypersensitivity in colony assay, hyperphosphorylation of STAT5

Clinical Features

Patient presents with **hemorrhagic tendencies, lymphadenopathy** and **skin rashes**. Marked splenomegaly less frequent. It has poor response to therapy with fatal outcome.

Peripheral Blood Smear

Peripheral blood smear shows leukocytosis, monocytosis (>1000/μl) and thrombocytopenia. Blasts and promonocytes constitute <5%. Thrombocytopenia is present unlike adult CML. Nucleated red blood cells may be present. Neutrophil alkaline phosphatase score is low.

Bone Marrow

Bone marrow is hypercellular with increased blasts (<20%), immature and mature monocytes. Megakaryocytes are decreased. Approximately 50% cases show low hemoglobin and decreased NAP score. Poor prognostic factors include thrombocytopenia and increased fetal hemoglobin.

CHRONIC MYELOMONOCYTIC LEUKEMIA (CMML)

Chronic myelomonocytic leukemia is a **clonal stem cell disorder**. Monocyte count is >1000/μl. Monocytosis is persistent for >3 months without any identifiable cause. There is absence of Philadelphia chromosomal abnormality. Patient presents with **pallor** and generalized weakness and **hepatosplenomegaly**. Diagnostic criteria of chronic myelomonocytic leukemia are shown in Table 9.41.

ATYPICAL CHRONIC MYELOID LEUKEMIA

Atypical chronic myeloid leukemia (aCML) shares clinical and laboratory features of CML, but lacks the BCR-ABL1 fusion. *Molecular genetic analysis reveals somatic alteration of SETBP1 encoding a protein Gly870 Ser.* Individuals with mutation have higher white blood cell count with worse prognosis.

Hematological Findings

Total white blood cell count is increased (20000–50000/cu mm) with blasts <5% and monocytosis. Immature white blood cells are <10%. Blasts and promonocytes constitute <20%. Myeloid/monocyte lineage shows dysplasia.

Table 9.41: Diagnostic criteria of chronic myelomonocytic leukemia

Diagnostic criteria	Features
Peripheral blood smear	Persistent monocytosis ≥ 1 ×10⁹/L (monocyte count >10% at least 3 months) Blasts and promonocytes <20% showing Auer rods Blasts <5% in CMML1 Blasts <10% in CMML2
Bone marrow	Blasts and promonocytes <20% showing Auer rods Blasts < 5% in CMML-1 Blasts < 10% in CMML-2 Dysplasia in one or more myeloid lineages
Not meeting WHO criteria	BCR-ABL1 positive CML Primary myelofibrosis Polycythemia vera Essential thrombocythemia
No evidence	PDGFRA PDGFRB FGFR1 rearrangement PCM1-JAK2

MDS/MPN WITH RING SIDEROBLASTS WITH THROMBOCYTOSIS (MDS/MPN-RS)

MDS/MPN-RS is a rare myelodysplastic/myeloproliferative neoplasm proposed by WHO in 2008. It is characterized by **refractory anemia** with **ring sideroblasts** and **essential thrombocytosis**. The higher risk of thrombotic events in this disorder suggests that anti-platelet therapy might be considered in this subset of patients. *Prognosis of RARS-1 is worse than essential thrombocytosis.*

Peripheral Smear and Bone Marrow

Anemia associated with erythroid lineage dysplasia with or without multilineage dysplasia, ≥15% ring sideroblasts, <1% blasts in peripheral blood and <5% blasts in the bone marrow. Persistent thrombocytosis with platelet count ≥450 × 10⁹/L.

MYELOPROLIFERATIVE NEOPLASMS

Myeloproliferative neoplasms are **clonal hematopoietic stem cell disorders** characterized by *proliferation of one or more of the myeloid lineages and differentiation to form white blood cells, red blood cells and platelets. Myeloproliferative neoplasms originate from pluripotent stem cells.*

CLASSIFICATION

Classification of myeloproliferative neoplasms is based on hyperplasia of cell line. Chronic myelogenous leukemia is characterized by proliferation of myeloid cells marked by release of nonfunctional immature cells into the peripheral blood. In polycythemia vera, there is excessive production of erythroid cells resulting in excessive release of red blood cells into peripheral blood.

Essential thrombocythemia is characterized by hyperplasia of megakaryocytes resulting in excessive release of platelets in the blood circulation. In primary myelofibrosis, there is proliferation of granulocytes and megakaryocytes. WHO (2016) classification of myeloproliferative neoplasms and myelodysplastic diseases is shown in Table 9.42.

SALIENT FEATURES

Salient features of myeloproliferative neoplasms comprise increased white blood cell count with shift-to-the-left, bone marrow hyperplasia, splenomegaly, bone marrow fibrosis of variable degree, Many patients with polycythemia rubra vera, agnogenic myeloid metaplasia and essential thrombocythemia have mutations in the gene for the Janus 2 signaling protein. **Cell lines show JAK2V617F positive.** BCR-ABL is demonstrated in CML. Myeloproliferative neoplasms may transform to acute leukemia. Genetic and molecular changes in myeloproliferative neoplasms are shown in Table 9.43.

INTERRELATION

Clinical and morphological features are variable. These are interrelated disorders, one disorder may transform to another disorder. Patient with polycythemia vera may transform to CML terminating in myelofibrosis. Patient with CML may develop acute leukemia in 25% cases (AML, ALL, acute megakaryocytic crisis or mixed phenotype acute leukemia).

Table 9.43: Genetic and molecular changes in myeloproliferative neoplasms

Genetic and molecular changes	Myeloproliferative neoplasms
BCR-ABL	Chronic myelogenous leukemia
JAK2	Polycythemia *rubra vera* Agnogenic myeloid metaplasia Essential thrombocythemia Primary myelofibrosis
Calreticulin	Primary myelofibrosis

CHRONIC MYELOGENOUS LEUKEMIA

Chronic myelogenous leukemia constitutes 15–20% of all leukemias. It is malignant disorder of pluripotent bone marrow stem cell affecting all three lines (myeloid, erythroid cells and megakaryocytes).

CML always involves the blood and bone marrow, as well as the spleen (massive splenomegaly) and liver. Bone marrow shows proliferation of myeloid cells with full range of maturation and prominent neutrophilic leukocytosis.

AGE AND SEX PREDILECTION

Peak incidence is in middle age (35 to 50 years) but can be seen in any age group, even in children. It is twice as frequent in men as in women.

CLINICAL FEATURES

Replacement of the bone marrow by neoplastic cells causes anemia and thrombocytopenia and a predisposition to infections. The initial symptoms are nonspecific and include weakness, malaise, fever, bone pain, sternal tenderness and splenomegaly. In most cases, *CML terminates in an accelerated phase followed by blast crisis* marked by increased numbers of primitive blast cells and promyelocytes.

Table 9.42: WHO (2016) classification of myeloproliferative neoplasms and myelodysplastic diseases

Categories	Disorders
Myeloproliferative neoplasms	Chronic myelogenous leukemia (CML) Chronic neutrophilic leukemia Chronic eosinophilic leukemia, NOS Polycythemia vera (PV) Essential thrombocythemia (ET) Myeloproliferative disorders—unclassified Mast cell disease
Myeloproliferative diseases	Chronic myelomonocytic leukemia (CMML) Atypical chronic myelogenous leukemia (aCML) Juvenile myelomonocytic leukemia (JMML) MDS/MPN unclassified

Patient in **blast crisis** presents with refractory total leukocyte count, *chloromas, splenomegaly, sudden bone pains,* involvement of CNS and *lymph nodes*. Unusual symptoms include spinal cord compression, vision disturbance (blindness), cerebral stroke and priapism in males (hyperviscosity).

PHYSICAL EXAMINATION

Physical examination reveals anemia, massive splenomegaly and hepatomegaly. *Splenomegaly correlates with magnitude of leukocytosis.* Splenic infarct is common. *Sternal tenderness localized to mid body sternum is reliable sign of disease.*

MOLECULAR CHANGES

Philadelphia chromosome is an acquired chromosomal abnormality t(9;22) found in 95% cases of CML associated with good prognosis. It was named after the city where it was first recorded. Translocation of a portion of the q arm of chromosome 22 to the q arm of chromosome 9, is designated t(9;22). Chronic myelogenous leukemia **showing balanced reciprocal translocation 9/22** known as *Philadelphia chromosome* is shown in Fig. 9.26. Pathogenesis of chronic myelogenous leukemia is shown in Fig. 9.27.

BCR-ABL HYBRID (FUSION) GENE

The c-ABL proto-oncogene (Abelson leukemia virus) on chromosome 9 is transposed to an area on chromosome 22, adjacent to an oncogene referred to as BCR (breakpoint cluster region), forming a new BCR-ABL hybrid or fusion gene.

The hybrid BCR-ABL fusion gene encodes a fusion protein, p210 with tyrosine kinase activity. Tyrosine kinase activates signal transduction pathways, promotes growth through nuclear stimulation leading to uncontrolled cell growth. This finding suggests the clonal origin of CML from the myeloid cells. There is no block in the maturation of leukemic stem cells.

PHILADELPHIA CHROMOSOME

Philadelphia chromosome can be demonstrated in all blood cell lineages in **bone marrow** (erythroblasts, granulocytes, monocytes, megakaryocytes, B cell and T cell progenitors). Philadelphia is not demonstrated in the majority of circulating B cells or T cells. Philadelphia chromosome is demonstrated in various myeloproliferative neoplasms (Table 9.44).

- *Major breakpoint region:* In CML, the major breakpoint region is most commonly involved, whereas in ALL the minor breakpoint region is usually involved.

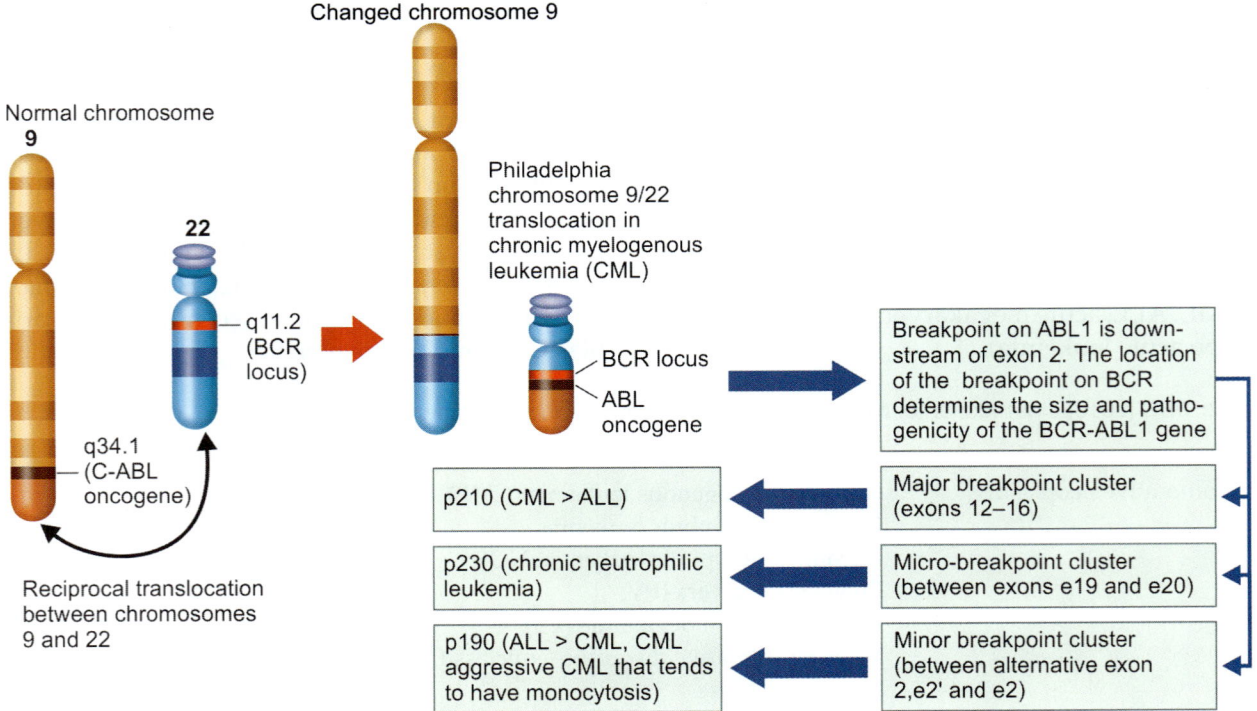

Fig. 9.26: Chronic myelogenous leukemia showing balanced reciprocal translocation 9/22 known as *Philadelphia chromosome*. A reciprocal translocation involves two nonhomologous chromosomes, with exchange of the acentric segment. There is exchange of a segment between two non-homologous chromosomes. Balanced reciprocal translocation 9/22 known as *Philadelphia chromosome* is seen in chronic myeloid leukemia. Positivity of this Philadelphia chromosome indicates good prognosis. In interstitial translocation, a segment of a chromosome is lost and reattaches to non-homologous chromosome.

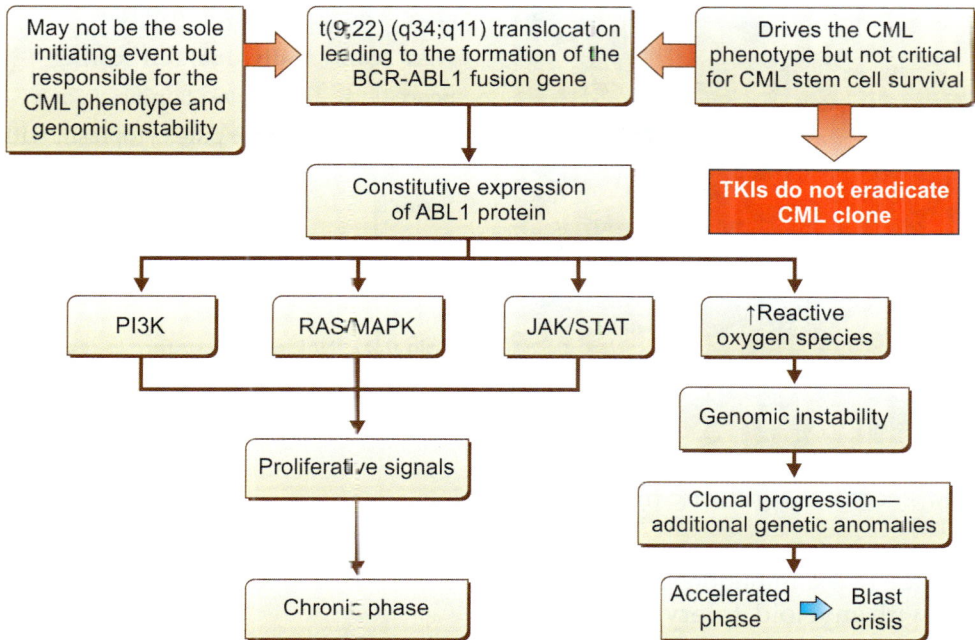

Fig. 9.27: Pathogenesis of chronic myelogenous leukemia.

Table 9.44: Philadelphia chromosome in various hematological disorders

Variant	Philadelphia chromosome
Chronic myelogenous leukemia	Positive
Juvenile CML (adult variant)	Positive
Acute lymphoblastic leukemia	Positive
Acute myeloid leukemia	Negative
Acute myelomonocytic leukemia	Negative
Acute basophilic leukemia	Negative
Acute eosinophilic leukemia	Negative
Polycythemia rubra vera	Negative
Myelofibrosis with myeloid metaplasia	Negative
Myelofibrosis without myeloid metaplasia	Negative

Table 9.45: Differential leukocyte count in CML (chronic phase)

Differential white blood cells	Percentage
Myelocytes	15–30%
Myeloblasts	1–10% (chronic phase)
Promyelocytes	2–8%
Metamyelocytes	15–25%
Band forms	5–15%
Neutrophils	40–70%
Monocytes	2–10%
Basophilia (2–10%)	Basophil count increased
Eosinophilia (a few cases)	Eosinophil count increased

Myeloblasts are demonstrated in bone marrow and peripheral blood during chronic phase (1–10%), accelerated phase (11–20%) and blast crisis (>20).

- *Additional chromosomal changes:* When blast crisis occurs, then additional chromosomal changes may occur, which affect the morphology and number. A relatively common occurrence is the appearance of more than one Philadelphia chromosomes.

HEMATOLOGICAL FINDINGS

This diagnosis is often made incidentally, when an elevated white blood cell is noticed in a routine blood workup. A bone marrow will establish the diagnosis.

The white blood count may be extremely high. An evaluation of blood and bone marrow under microscope will lead to a diagnosis. In chronic phase, CML shows the following findings:

- *Hemoglobin:* It is decreased.
- *Total leukocyte count:* It ranges $50 \times 10^9/L$ to $500 \times 10^9/L$.
- *Peripheral blood smear:* Differential leukocyte count shows leukemic myeloid cells of all stages of maturation, from myeloblasts to neutrophils. RBCs show normocytic normochromic picture. Thrombocytosis is demonstrated in 50% of cases. Platelets may be large irregular and dysfunctional due to absence of granules. Megakaryocytes are seen in the peripheral smear in 25% of cases. Differential leukocyte count in CML (chronic phase) is shown in Table 9.45

BONE MARROW ASPIRATE

Bone marrow smear showing chronic myelogenous leukemia is depicted in Fig. 9.28.

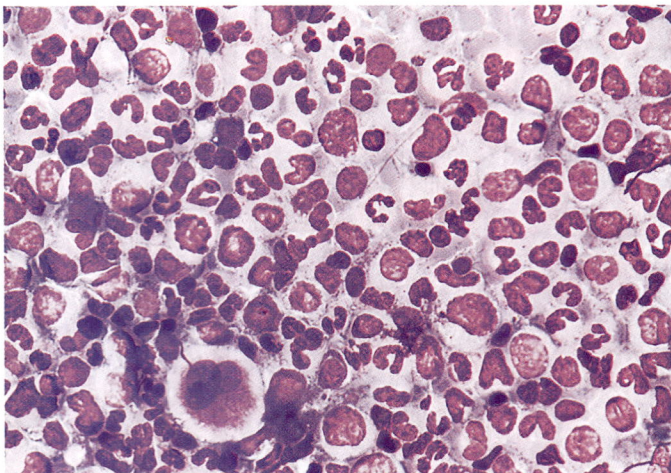

Fig. 9.28: Bone marrow smear showing chronic myelogenous leukemia (chronic phase).

- *Cellularity:* Bone marrow examination shows hypercellular marrow with myeloid to erythroid ratio >10:1.
- *Myeloid series:* There is marked increase in granulocytic cells myeloblasts to neutrophils. Myelocytes are relatively increased in number admixed with promyelocytes and neutrophils. Myeloblasts are present in small numbers in the chronic phase, but increase in number when blast transformation occurs.
- *Erythroid series:* Erythroid precursors are relatively suppressed due to expansion of myeloid precursors.
- *Megakaryocytic series:* Megakaryocytes are numerous.

Immunohistochemistry

Immunohistochemistry in blast crisis: Myeloblasts are most often negative for myeloperoxidase. Diagnosis is confirmed by immunohistochemistry (CD13, CD33, anti-MPO).

Immunohistochemistry of chronic myelogenous leukemia.

Marker	Expression
CD13	Positive
CD33	Positive
Amto-MPO	Positive

NAP Scoring System

A useful test to help distinguish CML from leukemoid reaction is the NAP score, which should be low with CML in 95% cases and high with a leukemoid reaction. Neutrophil alkaline phosphatase is present in specific granules in neutrophils.

Based on number of granules and intensity of staining; individual cells are scored as 0–4. At least 100 consecutive cells are counted and sum of their scores

Table 9.46: Scoring system of NAP

NAP score	Individual cell scoring
Score 0	Negative staining
Score 1	Diffuse pale cytoplasm with occasional granules
Score 2	Moderate blue granules
Score 3	Unevenly distributed blue granular precipitate
Score 4	Uniform, strongly positive

Table 9.47: NAP scoring system in disorders

NAP scoring system	Disorders
Low NAP score	Chronic myeloid leukemia (middle age) Atypical CML (elderly adults) Juvenile CML (infantile variant <5 years) Juvenile CML (adult variant >5 years) Paroxysmal nocturnal hemoglobinuria Hereditary hypophosphatasia
High NAP score	Leukemoid reactions Myelofibrosis Polycythemia rubra vera Idiopathic thrombocythemia Chronic neutrophilic leukemia

is determined. Normal range in adults is 25–100 and children 150–300. Scoring system of NAP is shown in Table 9.46. NAP scoring system in disorders is shown in Table 9.47.

Serum Vitamin B_{12} Levels

Serum vitamin B_{12} levels are increased due to production of binding proteins by the granulocytic series.

STAGING OF CML

The best indicators for this purpose are stages of the illness: chronic phase, accelerated phase and blast crisis. Patients who do not develop blast crisis may go into bone marrow failure.

Chronic Phase

Leukemic cells are confined to bone marrow and spleen. Bone marrow and blood contain <10% myeloblasts. Patient is **stable** in this phase. Patient presents with anemia, sternal tenderness, massive splenomegaly and discomfort in left upper quadrant of abdomen.

Increasing splenomegaly and **not responding** to **therapy** suggests the *progression of chronic phase* of *CML to accelerated and blast crisis*. Chronic phase of CML is shown in Fig. 9.29.

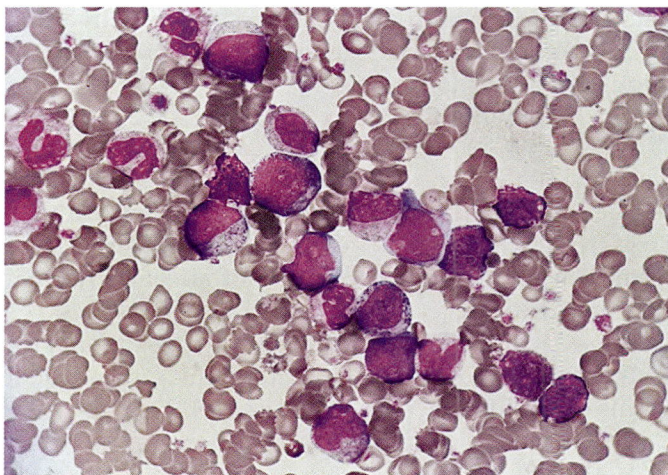

Fig. 9.29: Chronic myelogenous leukemia showing chronic phase in peripheral blood smear.

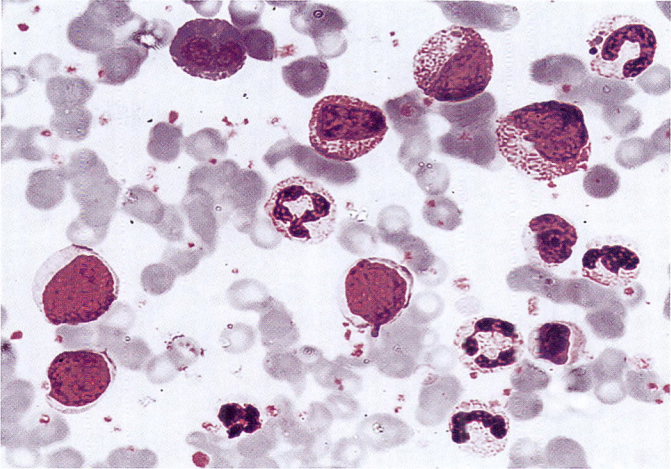

Fig. 9.30: Chronic myelogenous leukemia showing accelerated phase in peripheral blood smear.

Accelerated Phase

Accelerated phase occurs due to failure to response to treatment. **Leukemia** involves organs **outside bone marrow** and spleen.

Criteria for accelerated phase include blasts (11–20%) in peripheral blood and bone marrow, basophils (>20%), persistent thrombocytopenia (platelet count less than 100,000/cu mm) unrelated to treatment, cytogenetic abnormality in addition to a single Philadelphia chromosome and marrow fibrosis (Fig. 9.30).

Additionally the updated WHO (2016) classification includes a *provisional* response-to-TKI criteria. Criteria for accelerated phase of CML (BCR-ABL positive) are shown in Table 9.48.

Blast Crisis

Peripheral and bone marrow show >20% blasts. Patient develops extramedullary blast chloromas. *CML is pluripotent stem cell disorder, and thus capable of myeloid, lymphoid and megakaryocytic differentiation.* Secondary genetic abnormalities occur in 70–80% patients in blast crisis include *second Philadelphia chromosome, trisomy, isochromosome 17 and 19*. Blast crisis in chronic myelogenous leukemia and associated findings is shown in Fig. 9.31 and Table 9.49.

CHEMOTHERAPY

Chemotherapy causes lowering of WBCs, reduction of symptoms, and reversal of symptomatic splenomegaly.

Table 9.48: Criteria for accelerated phase of CML (BCR-ABL positive)

One or more of hematologic/cytogenetic criteria	Parameters	Findings
Hematologic criteria	WBC count	Persistent or increasing WBC (>10 × 10⁶/L), unresponsive to therapy
	Splenomegaly	Persistent or increasing splenomegaly unresponsive to therapy
	Platelet count	Persistent thrombocytosis (>1000 × 10⁹/L), unresponsive to therapy
	Basophils count	Basophils in peripheral blood (>20%)
	Blasts	Blasts in bone marrow and peripheral blood (10–19%)
	Clonal chromosomal abnormalities	Philadelphia chromosome, trisomy 8, trisomy 19, i17q and 3q26.2
	New clonal chromosomal abnormalities in Philadelphia positive cells	Following therapy
Provisional response-to-TKI criteria	First TKI response	Hematologic resistance
	Second sequential TK response OR	Hematologic and cytogenetic resistance
	Two or more mutations	BCR-ABL1 during TKI therapy

Section II: Hematology

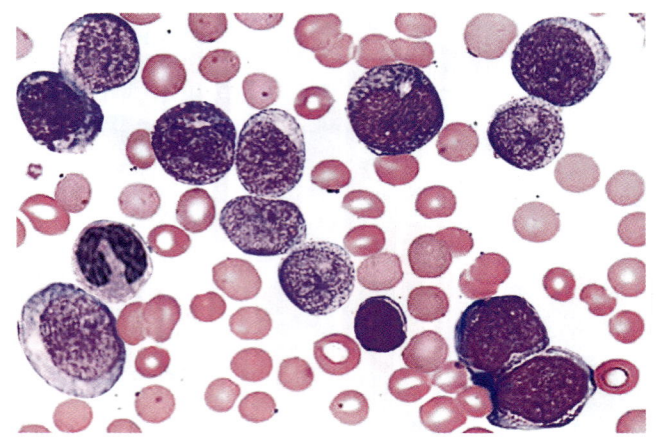

Fig. 9.31: Blast crisis in a case of chronic myelogenous leukemia.

Tyrosine kinase inhibitors like imatinib are used successfully to treat CML. Patients who transform into blast crisis are treated with proper acute leukemia regimens. Leukemic subclones that develop resistance to imatinib are treated with second generation compounds like nilotinib and dasatinib.

Therapeutic Trial

Development of antisense oligomers (short DNA segments), may be useful in blocking formation of BCR-ABL hybrid gene, resulting in suppression of formation of leukemic cells and not affecting normal bone marrow cells.

These techniques may lead to future treatments for CML. Bone marrow transplantation results are excellent in this condition.

DIFFERENTIAL DIAGNOSIS

Chronic myeloid leukemia has to be differentiated from atypical chronic myeloid leukemia and leukemoid reactions on the following criteria (Tables 9.50 and 9.51).

Table 9.49: Blast crisis in chronic myelogenous leukemia and associated findings

Blast crisis (>20%) in bone marrow and blood	Parameters	Findings
Myeloblastic crisis	Development of acute myelogenous leukemia (70%)	AML (M1, M2, M4, M6, M7)
		AML (M7) associated with marrow fibrosis
	Cytochemistry	Sudan black negative
		Myeloperoxidase positive
	Basophil count	Basophilia
	Immunocytochemistry	AML (M7), CD61/CD41 positive
Lymphoblastic leukemia	Development of acute lymphoblastic leukemia (20%)	ALL (L1 or L2)
	Immunocytochemistry	T cell lineage
Megakaryoblastic crisis	Development of acute megakaryoblastic leukemia (5–10%)	Approximately 5–10% cases develop mixed blasts or acute megakaryoblasts crisis

A few patients show blasts having immunophenotype of MPAL (mixed phenotypic acute leukemia).

Table 9.50: Comparison of CML and atypical CML (aCML)

	Characteristics	CML	aCML
Cytogenetic abnormalities	Philadelphia chromosome	Present	Absent, but other cytogenetic abnormalities are seen such as trisomy 8, t(5;12) and t(5;10)
Age predilection	Elderly age group	Mean 53 years	Mean 65–72 years
Clinical findings	Anemia and thrombocytopenia	Less common	More common
Peripheral blood	Blasts	<2%	>2%
	Immature granulocytes	>20%	10–20%
	Basophils	>2%	<2%
	Eosinophilia	More common	Less common
	Monocytes	<3%	>3–10% (usually <10% immature)
	Dysplasia	Absent	Present
Bone marrow	Myeloid:Erythroid	>10:1	<10:1
	Blasts	<5%	Increased but <20%
	Megakaryocytes	Normal or increased	Decreased
	Dysplasia	Absent	Present

aCML has similar clinical presentation and has a low NAP score. aCML also terminates in blast crisis which is usually myeloid but occasional lymphoid crises have been seen.

White Blood Cells

Table 9.51: Comparison of chronic myeloid leukemia and leukemoid reactions

	Chronic myeloid leukemia	Leukemoid reactions
Age group	25–60 years (peak 30–40 yeras)	Any age
Etiology	Clonal malignant disorder	Infections
Clinical features	Massive splenomegaly	Clinical features of causative disorder often obvious
TLC	>50 × 10⁹/L (marked increase)	<50 × 10⁹/L (moderate increase)
Proportion of immature cells	Usually numerous (myelocytes 20–50%)	Usually small or moderate. Myelocytes seldom exceeds 5–15% and myeloblasts 5%
White cell morphology	Cells often atypical as well as immature	Cells are typical
WBC toxic granules	Toxic changes uncommon	Toxic changes may be seen in infective cases
NAP score	Low or absent	High
Döhle's bodies	Absent	Present
Anemia	Usually present and progressive more than 30% cases	May occur but often slight or absent in 5–10% cases
Nucleated red cells	Less frequent	Frequent in leukoerythroblastic anemia due to marrow infiltration
Platelets	Decreased except in chronic myeloid leukemia	Mainly normal or increased, but reduced in intravascular coagulation
Bone marrow	Hyperplastic with potentially large proportion of immature cells	White cell hyperplasia may be present but seldom to same degree as in leukemia
Philadelphia chromosome	Present	Absent
Course	Progressive	Transient
Autopsy	Leukemic infiltration of organs and tissues	Infiltration of organs and tissue absent

A leukemoid reaction is typically a transient but exaggerated bone marrow response to inflammatory cytokines such as IL-1 and TNF-α, which stimulate bone marrow progenitor cells.

CHRONIC NEUTROPHILIC LEUKEMIA

Chronic neutrophilic leukemia is characterized by increase in total leukocyte count ≥ 25000/μl.

Patient develops **hepatosplenomegaly**. To differentiate it from leukemoid reaction, **monoclonality** of the neutrophils need to be **established**. Blast transformation occurs in about 20% of the cases, especially with follow up cases of myelodysplastic syndrome

Peripheral Blood Smear

Peripheral blood smear shows neutrophils containing coarse granules (>80%), myeloblasts (<1%) and promyelocytes, myelocytes and metamyelocytes.

Bone Marrow

Bone marrow examination shows hyperplasia of neutrophils with normal maturation and blasts <5% of nucleated cells. Philadelphia chromosomal abnormalities are absent. Diagnostic criteria of chronic neutrophilic leukemia are shown in Table 9.52.

CHRONIC EOSINOPHILIC LEUKEMIA

Diagnosis of chronic eosinophilic leukemia is made by excluding other secondary causes of eosinophilia.

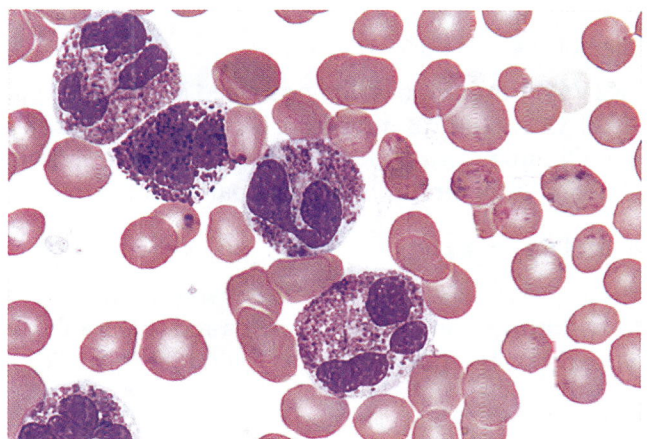

Fig. 9.32: Peripheral blood smear shows chronic eosinophilic leukemia.

Predominant cell population are eosinophils in peripheral blood and less than 20% eosinophilic blasts in bone marrow (Fig. 9.32).

Absolute eosinophil count should be >1500/μl. Monoclonality of the eosinophils needs to be established. Cytogenetic abnormalities include t(5;12), t(8;13), monosomy 7, trisomy 8, trisomy 15.

Patient presents with hepatosplenomegaly, lymphadenopathy, cardiac injury and other tissue damages

Table 9.52: Diagnostic criteria for chronic neutrophilic leukemia

Hematological parameters	Peripheral blood smear and bone marrow findings
TLC	$\geq 25 \times 10^9/L$
DLC	Neutrophils containing coarse granules (>80%) Myeloblasts <5% Promyelocytes, myelocytes and metamyelocytes <10%
Bone marrow	Hyperplasia of neutrophils with normal maturation Myeloblasts <5% of nucleated cells
Not meeting WHO criteria for *BCR-ABL1* positive *CML, PV, ET* or *PMF*	
No rearrangement of *PDGFRA, PDGFRB* or *FGFR1*, or *PCM1-JAK2*	
Presence of *CSF3R T618I* or other activating *CSF3R* mutation	
In the absence of a CSFR3R mutation, persistent neutrophilia (at least 3 months), splenomegaly and no identifiable cause of reactive neutrophilia including absence of a plasma cell neoplasm or, if present, demonstration of clonality of myeloid cells by cytogenetic or molecular studies	
Philadelphia chromosomal abnormalities are absent	

due to release of eosinophilic granules. Mean survival of patient is short.

POLYCYTHEMIA VERA

Polycythemia vera (primary polycythemia) is one of the myeloproliferative syndromes. It is characterized by prominent erythrocytosis (Hb >18 gm/dl), moderate granulocytosis, thrombocytosis, decreased erythropoietin and splenomegaly. Hematocrit value is >55% with normal oxygen saturation. WHO (2106) criteria for polycythemia vera (PV) are shown in Table 9.53.

Molecular Genetics

JAK2V617F mutation is demonstrated in polycythemia vera. JAK2 exon 12 mutation is also demonstrated. Polycythemia vera 1 (PRV-1) receptor gene is overexpressed in neutrophils in these patients.

Clinical Features

Patient presents with headache, visual disturbances, ruddy skin, red conjunctiva, pruritus and splenomegaly. Hyperviscosity and sludging of blood results in deep vein thrombosis, hemorrhagic phenomena and cerebral stroke.

Polycythemia vera most often progresses to bone marrow fibrosis, anemia and extramedullary hematopoiesis in liver and spleen. About 3% of these patients terminate in acute leukemia, not CML, who have received antimitotic drugs or radiation therapy.

The spleen is moderately enlarged, and its cut surface is uniformly dark red, with expansion of the red pulp and obliteration of the white pulp. *Most patients have fatal outcome due to vascular complications.*

Erythropoietin Level

Patient with polycythemia vera has normal or decreased erythropoietin level. Conditions associated with increased erythropoietin level are shown in Table 9.54. Comparison between polycythemia vera and secondary polycythemia is shown in Table 9.55.

Blood Viscosity and Peripheral Blood Smear

Blood viscosity is 4–7 times than normal. Red blood cell count, red blood cell mass and hemoglobin are raised.

Table 9.53: WHO (2016) criteria for polycythemia vera (PV)

Major/minor criteria	Parameters	Findings
Major criteria	Hemoglobin	>16.5 g/dl in men >16.0 g/dl in women
	Hematocrit values	>49% in men >48% in women
	Bone marrow biopsy	Hypercellular (due to proliferation of erythroid, myeloid and megakaryocytes) Pleomorphic, mature megakaryocytes
	Gene mutations	Presence of JAK2V617F or JAK2 exon 12 mutation Polycythemia vera 1 (PRV-1) receptor gene overexpression
Minor criteria	Erythropoietin level	Subnormal serum erythropoietin level

Platelet count is increased. There is mild leukocytosis with neutrophilia.

Bone Marrow

Bone marrow shows hyperplasia of hematopoietic cells, trilinear maturation and increased megakaryocytes. In the later phase (spent phase), bone marrow undergoes fibrosis with increased marrow reticulin. ESR is decreased with high NAP score.

Differential Diagnosis

Polycythemia vera should be differentiated from secondary polycythemia, Gaisbock syndrome (also known as *chronic relative polycythemia* or *spurious* or *stress erythrocytosis*) and relative polycythemia (also known as *pseudopolycythemia* with increased hemoglobin due to reduced fluid intake or excessive fluid loss resulting in hemoconcentration).

Table 9.54: Secondary polycythemia associated with increased erythropoietin level

Categories	Disorders
Chronic hypoxia	Pulmonary disease
	Congenital heart disease
	Heavy tobacco smoking
	High altitudes
Tumors and tumor-like conditions	Renal cell carcinoma
	Hepatocellular carcinoma
	Cerebellar hemangioma
	Pheochromocytoma
	Adrenal adenoma with Cushing syndrome
	Adult polycystic kidney disease
Therapeutic hormone	Androgen therapy

ESSENTIAL THROMBOCYTHEMIA

Essential thrombocythemia is an uncommon **clonal disorder** of hematopoietic stem cells. It is characterized by uncontrolled proliferation of megakaryocytes in bone marrow.

Platelet counts in excess of $1,000,000/\mu l$ are common (normal value is $150,000$ to $350,000/\mu l$). Additional features include bleeding and thrombosis.

WHO (2016) DIAGNOSTIC CRITERIA

WHO (2016) **diagnostic criteria** require a *sustained platelet count above* $>450 \times 10^9/L$ and prominent megakaryocytic proliferation in the bone marrow.

There is no evidence of reactive thrombocytosis. Diagnosis of essential thrombocytosis requires all four major criteria or first three major criteria and minor criterion (Table 9.56).

MOLECULAR GENETICS

JAK2 mutation is demonstrated in essential thrombocytosis.

CLINICAL FEATURES

Patient presents with thrombosis and hemorrhagic manifestations. Platelets coagulant activity is increased due to loss of PGD_2 receptors.

Storage pool defects in platelets promotes hemorrhagic tendency.

HEMATOLOGICAL FINDINGS

Peripheral Blood Smear

Peripheral blood smear shows platelet count $>450 \times 10^9/L$.

Table 9.55: Comparison between polycythemia vera and secondary polycythemia

Parameters	Polycythemia vera	Secondary polycythemia
Etiology	Hematopoietic stem cell disorder	Various causes
Hypoxia association	Absent	Present
Erythropoietin (EPO) levels	Low	High
O_2 saturation (arterial blood)	Normal	Normal or low
Red blood cell mass	Increased	Normal
Bone marrow cellularity	Increased (trilineage hyperplasia with predominance of erythroid precursors)	Normal
Spleen size	Splenomegaly present	No splenomegaly
JAK2 gene mutation	Present	Absent
NAP score	Increased	Normal
Serum uric acid	Increased	Normal
Serum LDH	Increased	Normal

Table 9.56: Diagnostic criteria for essential thrombocythemia according to WHO classification 2016

Major/minor criteria	Parameters	Hematological findings
Major criteria	Platelet count	Platelet count >450 × 10^9/L
	Bone marrow biopsy	Proliferation of megakaryocyte lineage
		Megakaryocytes increased with hyperlobulated nuclei
		No significant increase or left-shift in neutrophil granulopoiesis or erythropoiesis
		Rare increase in reticulin fibers (grade 1)
	Not meeting the WHO criteria for BCR-ABL1+	CML, PV, PMF, myelodysplastic syndromes, or other myeloid neoplasms
	Gene mutations	JAK2, CALR or MPL gene mutation
Minor criterion	Clonal marker or absence of reactive thrombocytosis	Presence of clonal marker or absence of evidence for reactive thrombocytosis

Bone Marrow

Bone marrow shows normal cellularity or hypocellularity. It shows hyperplasia of megakaryocytes. These megakaryocytes are present in clusters. Majority of megakaryocytes are large (giant megakaryocytes) and functional.

Differential Diagnosis

Essential thrombocythemia should be differentiated from reactive thrombocytosis, cellular phase of myelofibrosis and CML. Reactive thrombocytosis occurs due to infections, iron deficiency, splenomegaly, surgical procedures, metastatic cancers and lymphoproliferative disorders.

PRIMARY MYELOFIBROSIS

Primary myelofibrosis is also known as *agnogenic myeloid metaplasia*. Myelofibrosis replaces normal hematopoietic cells. It is characterized by **extensive extramedullary hematopoiesis** in **liver** and **spleen** and sometimes the **lymph nodes.**

WHO (2016) CRITERIA

WHO criteria comprise presence of megakaryocytic proliferation and atypia, accompanied by reticulin or collagen fibrosis. JAK2V617F or other clonal markers (CALR, MPL W515K/L) are positive. Diagnosis of pre-PMF requires meeting all three major criteria, and at least one minor criterion (Table 9.57). WHO (2016) criteria for overt primary myelofibrosis (PMF) are shown in Table 9.58.

PATHOGENESIS

Megakaryocytic proliferation may be the primary abnormality. Platelet-derived growth factor (PDGF) and transforming growth factor-β (TGF-β) synthesized by platelets and megakaryocytes simulate marrow fibroblasts resulting in deposition of reticulin/collagen fibers known as *myelofibrosis*. This late manifestation is often preceded by marrow hypercellularity.

Table 9.57: WHO (2016) criteria for prefibrotic/early primary myelofibrosis (pre-PMF)

Major/minor criteria	Parameters	Hematological findings
Major criteria	Bone marrow	Megakaryocytic proliferation and atypia
		Without reticulin fibrosis > grade 1
		Increased age-adjusted BM cellularity, granulocytic proliferation and often decreased erythropoiesis
	Not meeting the WHO criteria for BCR-ABL1+	CML, PV, ET, myelodysplastic syndromes, or other myeloid neoplasms
	Gene mutations	Presence of JAK2, CALR or MPL mutation or in the absence of these mutations, presence of another clonal marker or absence of minor reactive BM reticulin fibrosis
Minor criterion	Presence of at least one of the following, confirmed in two consecutive determinations	Anemia not attributed to a comorbid condition
		Leukocytosis >11 × 10^9/L
		Palpable splenomegaly
		LDH increased to above upper normal limit of institutional reference range

White Blood Cells

Table 9.58: WHO (2016) criteria for overt primary myelofibrosis (PMF)

Major/minor criteria	Parameters	Hematological findings
Major criteria	Bone marrow	Presence of megakaryocytic proliferation and atypia, accompanied by either reticulin and/or collagen fibrosis grades 2 or 3
	Not meeting the WHO criteria for BCR-ABL1+	CML, PV, ET, myelodysplastic syndromes, or other myeloid neoplasms
	Gene mutations	Presence of JAK2, CALR or MPL mutation or in the absence of these mutations, presence of another clonal marker or absence of minor reactive BM reticulin fibrosis
Minor criterion	Presence of at least one of the following, confirmed in two consecutive determinations	Anemia not attributed to a comorbid condition Leukocytosis >11 × 10^9/L Palpable splenomegaly LDH increased to above upper normal limit of institutional reference range Leukoerythroblastosis

CLINICAL FEATURES

Patient presents with anemia, weakness, moderate hepatomegaly and massive splenomegaly.

HEMATOLOGICAL FINDINGS

Peripheral Blood Smear

Peripheral blood smear shows leukoerythroblastic blood picture with many tear drop cells (Fig. 9.33).

Bone Marrow

Bone marrow aspirate is dry due to fibrosis. Therefore, bone biopsy is essential to establish diagnosis. There are three phases of primary myelofibrosis: early cellular phase, fibrosis phase and osteomyelofibrosis phase.

- *Early cellular phase:* Bone marrow shows granulocytic hyperplasia and megakaryocytic proliferation with dysplasia.

- *Fibrotic phase:* Megakaryocytes are spared in the marrow fibrotic process. Increase in megakaryocytic number results in prominent bone marrow megakaryocytosis and peripheral blood thrombocytosis. Reticulin and collagen fibers are increased and demonstrated by Massons' trichome stain, megakaryocytes lining dilated sinusoids (Fig. 9.34).

- *Osteomyelofibrosis phase:* There is formation of new bone in the marrow results in decreased cellularity.

DIFFERENTIAL DIAGNOSIS

Secondary myelofibrosis occurs due to metastases in bone marrow, tuberculosis, sarcoidosis, fungi, osteopetrosis, hairy cell leukemia, Hodgkin's disease (bone marrow) and T-NHL. Bone marrow in autoimmune myelofibrosis occurs due to autoantibodies and shows lymphoid aggregates.

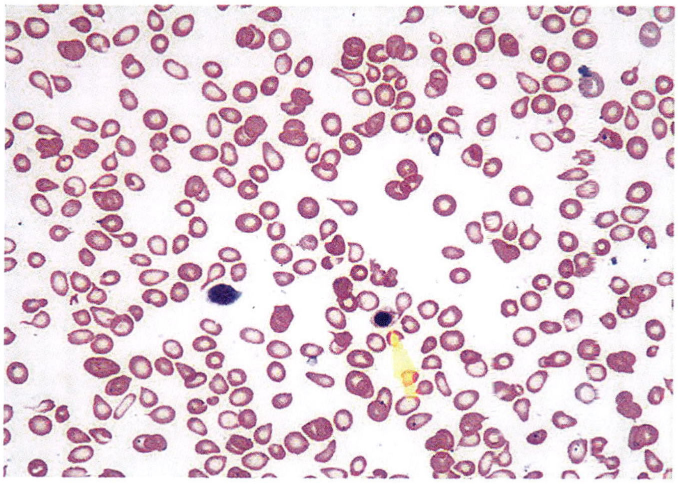

Fig. 9.33: Peripheral blood smear in a case of primary myelosclerosis showing tear drop cells and immature cells.

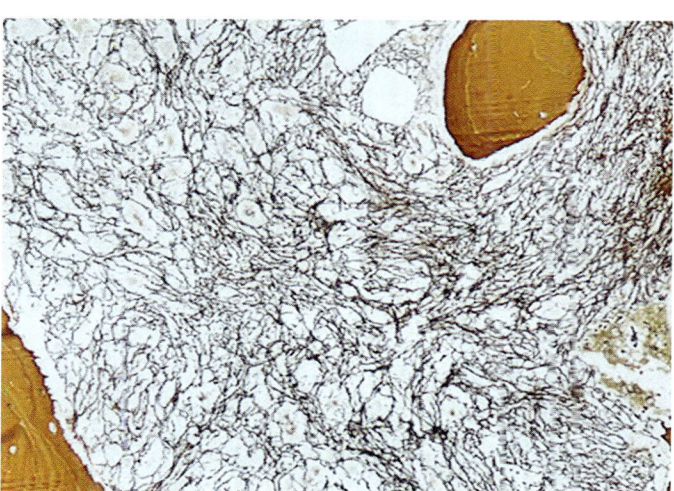

Fig. 9.34: Reticulin stain on bone marrow biopsy in a case of myelofibrosis.

CHRONIC LYMPHOPROLIFERATIVE DISORDERS

Chronic lymphoproliferative disorders are a heterogeneous group of disorders with involvement of bone marrow and blood variable clinical course. TNF-α, IL-2, IL-4 and IL-13 play an important role in pathogenesis of chronic lymphoproliferative disorder by either promoting cell proliferation or inhibiting apoptosis.

Classification: Chronic lymphoid leukemias are mature B or T cell neoplasms. Differences between chronic myeloid leukemia and chronic lymphocytic leukemia– are shown in Table 9.59.

- *B cell lineage (95%):* It comprises chronic lymphocytic leukemia, prolymphocytic leukemia, hairy cell leukemia, plasma cell leukemia and leukemia–lymphoma syndromes.
- *T cell lineage (5%):* It comprises large granular lymphocytic leukemia, T-prolymphocytic leukemia, adult T cell leukemia–lymphoma and Sézary syndromes.

CHRONIC LYMPHOCYTIC LEUKEMIA (CLL)

According to WHO classification in 2008, chronic lymphocytic leukemia (CLL), a clonal disorder has been placed under *mature B cell neoplasm*. It constitutes 25% of leukemias. It occurs due to **monoclonal proliferation of small mature appearing lymphocytes in the bone marrow, lymph nodes**, and **spleen,** with an expression in the peripheral blood. It most often occurs in older than 50 years of age. Men are more affected than women. Guidelines for diagnostic criteria of CLL according to international workshop in 2008 are shown in Table 9.60. Subtypes of chronic lymphocytic leukemia according to FAB classification are shown in Table 9.61.

CLL (B CELL LINEAGE)

Leukemic cells (lymphocytes) appear mature, but are actually arrested at an early stage of B cell development. These are less capable of differentiating into antibody-producing plasma cells. When >15% lymphocytes contain nuclei with clefts or lobulation or mixed; it is termed as *atypical CLL.*

MOLECULAR GENETICS

Approximately 50% show abnormal karyotype **trisomy chromosome 12, chromosomal abnormalities**

Table 9.59: Differences between chronic myeloid leukemia and chronic lymphocytic leukemia

Characteristics	Chronic myeloid leukemia	Chronic lymphocytic leukemia
Age group	20–60 years and juvenile CML in less than 3 years	50–60 years
Male:female ratio	1:1	2:1
Cytogenetics	Philadelphia chromosome t(9;22) in 75–90% except juvenile CML	Trisomy of 12, 14 in 30%
Organomegaly	Massive splenomegaly, hepatomegaly in adults In juvenile CML	Lymphadenopathy
Clinical features	Bone tenderness, dragging sensation in abdomen, left upper quadrant pain due to splenic infarct	Patient usually asymptomatic
Cell type	Increased myeloid cells	Increased lymphocytes
NAP score	Decreased or absent	Normal range
Other manifestations	Vitamin B_{12} decreased	Immunoglobulin decreased

Table 9.60: Guidelines for diagnostic criteria of CLL according to international workshop in 2008

Parameters	Findings
Peripheral blood smear	Clonal proliferation of abnormal B cells in blood for >3 months $\geq 5 \times 10^9$/L (B cells) <55% (atypical/immature lymphocytes)
Bone marrow	>30 lymphoid cells
Monoclonal lymphocytes should have CLL immunophenoptype	CD19 positive CD20 positive CD5 positive CD23 positive Weak surface immunoglobulins such as IgG, IgM with κ or λ Lack of pan T cell markers other than CD5

White Blood Cells

Table 9.61: Subtypes of chronic lymphocytic leukemia according to FAB classification

Subtypes	Features
CLL	Lymphocytes (majority) Prolymphocytes (<10%)
CLL-PLL (CLL-prolymphocytic leukemia)	Prolymphocytes (11–55%)
PLL (prolymphocytic leukemia)	Prolymphocytes (>55%)

of **13q, 14 and 16**. Patients showing trisomy have *poor prognosis*.

CLINICAL FEATURES

Patient is asymptomatic for many years. Later, patient presents with **generalized lymphadenopathy** (80%), **hepatomegaly** (50–60%), splenomegaly (less marked), **pallor, weakness, fatigue** and **dyspnea**. Purpura and hemorrhagic manifestations occur at a later stage.

Physical examination reveals generalized lymphadenopathy in cervical, axillary and inguinal regions; and not attached to skin.

HEMATOLOGICAL FINDINGS

In chronic lymphocytic leukemia, monoclonal proliferation of lymphocytes replacing bone marrow occurs over a period of a few years. Therefore, the patient develops anemia, neutropenia and thrombocytopenia in late stage of the disorder.

Hemoglobin

Hemoglobin is markedly reduced to <10 gm/dl in the later stage of disorder.

Red Blood Cells

RBCs are normocytic normochromic.

Total Leukocyte Count

Approximately 50% cases show increased WBC count in the range of $20 \times 10^9/L$ to $50 \times 10^9/L$. Some patients show WBC count $>50 \times 10^9/L$. Total leukocyte count is $100 \times 10^9/L$ to $200 \times 10^9/L$ up to $500 \times 10^9/L$.

Differential Leukocyte Count

Lymphocytosis is the hallmark of CLL. Lymphocyte count $>15 \times 10^9/L$ is diagnostic.

Peripheral blood smear shows >50% of lymphocytes of white blood cells. The leukemic cells closely resemble mature lymphocytes (monotonous appearances) with thin rim of cytoplasm and **fragile chromatin.** The cells are susceptible to mechanical disruption during preparation of blood smear. Therefore, these appear on the peripheral blood smear as *smudge* or *smear* cells (Fig. 9.35).

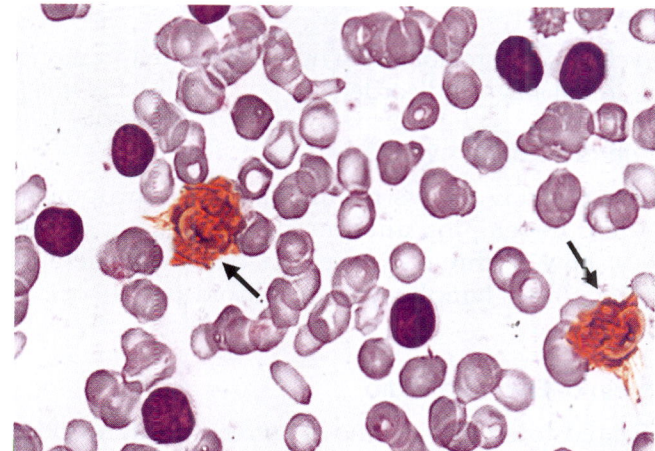

Fig. 9.35: Chronic lymphocytic leukemia. Peripheral blood smear shows large number of lymphocytes with smudge cell (arrows).

Platelet Count

Initially in the early stage of disorder, platelet count may be normal. But in the later stage, patient develops thrombocytopenia with platelet count $<100 \times 10^9/L$.

BONE MARROW

Cellularity

Bone marrow is **hypercellular** due to monoclonal proliferation of lymphocytes in the bone marrow. **Lymphocytes constitute >30% of nucleated cells in the marrow.** There is gradual replacement of bone marrow erythroid, myeloid and megakaryocyte by neoplastic lymphocytes over a few years. Therefore, the patient develops anemia, neutropenia and thrombocytopenia (Fig. 9.36).

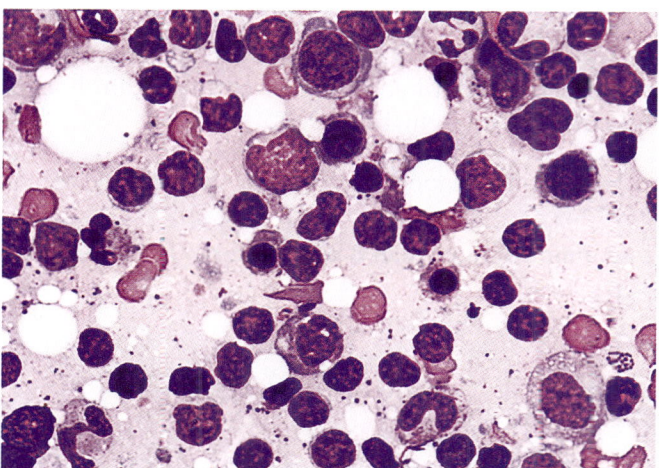

Fig. 9.36: Chronic lymphocytic leukemia. Bone marrow shows increased lymphocytes replacing erythroid, myeloid and megakaryocytic cell lines.

Myeloid Series

Myeloid cells are normal in number and maturation in the initial stage of disorder.

Erythroid Series

Bone marrow shows normoblastic erythropoiesis. Patient developing autoimmune hemolytic anemia may show erythroid hyperplasia. Due to proliferation of neoplastic lymphocytes, erythroid precursors are suppressed.

Myeloid/Erythroid Ratio

Myeloid to erythroid ratio is increased due to clonal proliferation of lymphocytes and decreased erythroid cells.

Megakaryopoiesis

Megakaryopoiesis is normal in the initial stage of disorder. In the later stage, megakaryopoiesis is suppressed resulting in thrombocytopenia.

COOMBS' TEST

Some patients of CLL may develop autoimmune hemolytic anemia in 10–20% of cases, Therefore, direct Coombs' test is carried out in all cases.

IMMUNOPHENOTYPING

Activation of BCL-2 proto-oncogene leads to decreased apoptosis resulting in increased accumulation of monoclonal B cells. *Leukemic pan B cell markers express clonal Ig gene rearrangements* and possess immunoglobulins (IgM, IgD), expression of single chain (κ/λ) on lymphocytes indicates their monoclonality.

Monoclonal immunoglobulin is displayed on cell surfaces, but there is unlikely to be a marked increase in circulating immunoglobulin. CLL cells show positivity for CD19, CD20, CD23 and CD5 (C5 is also T cell marker). Immunophenotying of chronic lymphocytic leukemia is shown in Table 9.62.

Table 9.62: Immunophenotyping of chronic lymphocytic leukemia

Immunophenotype (pan B cell markers)	Expression
CD5*	Positive
CD23	Positive
CD19	Positive
CD20	Positive
Clonal Ig gene arrangements	Positive

*CD5 (T cell marker) is expressed by CLL cells. It is negative on normal B cells.

CLINICAL COURSE

Recurrent Infections

Patient develops **recurrent infections** in early course of the disease (respiratory tract, sinuses, ears, skin, and kidney) due to absence of immunoglobulins (IgG), neutropenia and steroid therapy. **Herpes zoster infection** of skin results in pruritus, vesiculobullous and popular eruptions.

Autoimmune Hemolytic Anemia

Patient may develop warm antibody autoimmune hemolytic anemia. It may be accompanied by immuno-mediated thrombocytopenic purpura.

Richter Syndrome

In a minority of cases (3–5%), CLL (B cell) transforms to high grade B cell large cell lymphoma (Richter syndrome). Patient with this complication presents with rapid onset of fever, abdominal pain, and progressive lymphadenopathy and hepatosplenomegaly. *Richter syndrome is aggressive and refractory to therapy, with a mean survival of 2 months.*

Secondary Malignancy

Chronic lymphocytic leukemia may transform to secondary malignant disorders such as Hodgkin's disease, prolymphocytic leukemia, multiple myeloma and acute lymphoid leukemia in 1% case.

GIT Involvement

Leukemic infiltration in gastrointestinal tract results in anorexia and occasionally intestinal obstruction.

Mikulicz Syndrome

Patient may develop tonsillar enlargement along with Mikulicz's syndrome (lacrimal and salivary gland enlargement).

DIFFERENTIAL DIAGNOSIS

Chronic lymphocytic leukemia should be differentiated from NHL, prolymphocytic leukemia, Waldenström's macroglobulinemia, Sézary syndrome and lymphocytosis (Table 9.63).

PROGNOSIS

The mean survival is 5 to 10 years after diagnosis, although much longer symptom-free survivals are quite common. A subset of patients experience a more rapid course with death within 2 to 3 years of diagnosis.

Table 9.63: Differential diagnosis of chronic lymphocytic leukemia

Disorders	Features
Leukemia phase of NHL (mantle cell lymphoma, marginal zone lymphoma)	Positivity with CD5, cyclin D1 and CD21 CD23 is negative
Prolymphocytic leukemia	Larger cells with eccentric nucleus and punched out nucleolus
Waldenström's macroglobulinemia	Peripheral blood smear shows moderate lymphocytosis with plasmacytoid lymphocytes
Sézary syndrome	Circulating T cells have cleaved and clefted nuclei
Lymphocytosis	Multiple causes

PROGNOSTIC FACTORS

Prognosis is **worse** in patients with CLL expressing CD38, soluble CD23 levels, ZAP-70, IgVH mutation, soluble serum β-microglobulin, trisomy 12, 11q23, t(11;14), deletion 17, Rai staging system (stage 3 and stage 4) and Binet stage C.

Poor prognostic factors of chronic lymphocytic leukemia are shown in Table 9.64. Rai and Binet staging systems are shown in Tables 9.65 and 9.66.

HAIRY CELL LEUKEMIA

Hairy cell leukemia is chronic B cell lymphoproliferative disorder affecting **elderly persons** during 40–85 years age group. It most often occurs in men than women. It arises from post-germinal center memory mature B cell in marginal zone of lymph node. *It involves bone marrow, spleen, and liver.*

It is associated with **pancytopenia** and **splenomegaly**. Myelofibrosis caused by leukemic cells infiltration in

Table 9.64: Poor prognostic factors of chronic lymphocytic leukemia

Parameters	Poor prognosis
Lymphocyte doubling time	Doubling time <12 months
Rai staging system	Stage 3 and stage 4
Binet staging system	Stage C
Plasma β-microglobulin	Higher levels
Molecular genetics	p53 gene mutations, ZAP 70 gene mutations, 13q deletion, trisomy 12 cases, 11q23 mutation, t(11;14), Notch1 mutations (poor response to therapy), SF_83 mutations (poor response to therapy)
Bone marrow trephine biopsy	High tumor load due to diffuse lymphocytic infiltration
CD38 expression surrogative marker of IgVH	

Table 9.65: Rai staging system for chronic lymphocytic leukemia

Stage	Features	Prognosis
Stage 0	Lymphocytosis alone	Good (no treatment but monitoring essential)
Stage 1	Lymphocytosis with lymphadenopathy	Intermediate
Stage 2	Lymphocytosis, hepatomegaly and or splenomegaly and lymphadenopathy	Intermediate
Stage 3	Lymphocytosis and hemoglobin (<11 g/dl)	Unfavorable
Stage 4	Lymphocytosis, low platelet count (<100 × 10^9/L), anemia (+/−)	Unfavorable

Table 9.66: Binet staging system of CLL

Stage	Hb and platelet count	Lymph nodes	Survival
A	Normal (Hb and platelet count)	<3 lymph nodes. Liver and spleen are enlarged	100 months
B	Normal (Hb and platelet count)	<3 lymph nodes. Liver and spleen are enlarged	80 months
C	Hb <10 gm/dl or platelet count <100,000/cu mm	Lymphadenopathy and organs involvement	20 months

bone marrow and pooling of blood cells in spleen are responsible for pancytopenia. Most cases show BRAF gene mutation encoding threonine kinase.

CLINICAL FEATURES

Patient presents with *moderate to* **massive splenomegaly** (due to pooling of blood) and **pancytopenia** (anemia, leukopenia, and thrombocytopenia) due to bone marrow involvement. Patient may develop *secondary hypersplenism due to increased splenic sequestration of peripheral blood cells in spleen.*

Patient less often develops slight hepatomegaly, rarely lymphadenopathy. Constitutional symptoms are weakness, weight loss and fever. Spleen and liver show diffusely infiltrative and rarely necrotic or hemorrhagic areas on abdominal scan. **Leukemic infiltrates** are demonstrated in the **red pulp of spleen** unlike other lymphoproliferative disorders involving white pulp.

HEMATOLOGICAL FINDINGS

Pancytopenia is most important findings in majority of cases. Monocyte count is most often decreased in these patients. Peripheral blood smear shows pancytopenia with very scanty leukemic cells (abnormal B cells) known as *hairy cells*.

Hairy Cells

These neoplastic hairy cells are small- to medium-sized (15 to 25 μ) mononuclear cells with round to kidney shaped nuclei, finely stippled chromatin, moderate pale blue cytoplasm with circumferential cytoplasmic **hairy projections.**

Electron microscopy study reveals presence of hairy processes (microvilli) and rod shaped structures (ribosomal lamellar complexes) in the cytoplasm (Fig. 9.37).

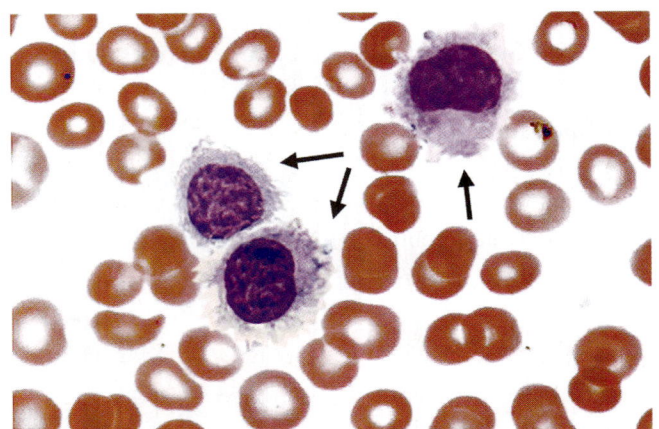

Fig. 9.37: Hairy cell leukemia. Peripheral blood smear neoplastic cells with round to kidney cell nucleus and circumferential cytoplasmic *hairy projections* (arrows).

BONE MARROW ASPIRATE

Bone marrow aspiration results in a *dry tap* due to extensive bone marrow fibrosis by leukemic cells. Bone marrow biopsy is essential diagnostic tool showing *honeycomb* appearance.

BONE MARROW TREPHINE BIOPSY

Bone marrow trephine biopsy demonstrates infiltration of marrow by leukemic cells exhibiting *honeycomb* appearance. These leukemic cells contain round to oval nuclei surrounded by clear halo. Each nucleus resembles *fried egg*. There is moderate to marked decrease in hematopoiesis involving erythroid, myeloid and megakaryocytic series.

DIAGNOSTIC CRITERIA

Diagnostic criteria of hairy cell leukemia include pancytopenia, moderate to marked splenomegaly, presence of hairy leukemic cells in blood and bone marrow.

Bone marrow aspirate is dry tap due to marrow fibrosis. Trephine biopsy shows honeycomb appearance.

Cytochemistry

Neoplastic hairy cells show **positive** red staining with **tartrate-resistant acid phosphatase** (TRAP).

Immunophenotyping

The neoplastic hairy cells usually express pan B cell markers CD19 and CD20, surface IgH, CD11c, CD25, and CD103. BRAF gene mutation encoding threonine kinase is demonstrated in most cases.

DIFFERENTIAL DIAGNOSIS

Hairy cell leukemia should be differentiated from splenic lymphoma, with villous lymphocytes, prolymphocytic leukemia and large granular lymphocytic leukemia. Bone marrow aspirate is dry only in hairy cell leukemia.

Hairy cells show positivity with TRAP (tartrate-resistant acid phosphatase), but negative in other disorders.

THERAPEUTIC CORRELATION

Hairy cell leukemia often has an indolent course, and chemotherapy often produces long-lasting remission. These patients show dramatic long-term response to therapeutic agents such as α-interferon, 2-chlorodeoxyadenosine, and deoxycoformycin.

B-PROLYMPHOCYTIC LEUKEMIA (PLL)

Some patients with chronic lymphocytic leukemia may develop B-prolymphocytic leukemia. It most often affects older age group. Presence of >55% prolymphocytes in the peripheral blood smear is diagnostic criteria of prolymphocytic leukemia. Bone marrow shows nodular or interstitial pattern of involvement.

CLASSIFICATION

According to FAB classification, taking prolymphocytes into consideration, chronic lymphocytic leukemia is classified as: CLL with <10% prolymphocytes, CLL with 11–55% prolymphocytes and CLL with >55% prolymphocytes.

Prolymphocytes are larger than lymphocytes. These leukemic cells contain abundant basophilic cytoplasm with round nucleus, condensed chromatin and prominent nucleolus. Total leukocyte count is increased.

CLINICAL FEATURES

Patient presents with moderate to massive and **splenomegaly.** Anemia and thrombocytopenia are demonstrated in 50% of cases. Patient with prolymphocytic leukemia has **worse prognosis**.

IMMUNOPHENOTYPING

Prolymphocytes express B cell antigens such as CD19, CD20, CD79a and FMS7.

ADULT T CELL LEUKEMIA/LYMPHOMA

Adult T cell lymphoma is prevalent in **Japan** and **Central Africa** affecting adults. It is caused by HTLV-1 virus. It occurs in three forms: acute, chronic and lymphomatous forms. The lymphoma cells are large containing nucleus with homogenous condensed chromatin and nucleoli. Some cells contain convoluted clover leaf-like nuclei.

CLINICAL FEATURES

Patient presents with lymphadenopathy, hepatosplenomegaly, skin rashes (50%) and raised serum calcium levels (increased osteoclastic activity).

LABORATORY DIAGNOSIS

Total leukocyte count: Total leukocyte count is increased due to spillover in blood.

Peripheral blood smear: Leukemic cells medium- to large-sized lymphoid cells with prominent pleomorphic nuclei resembling clover leaf.

Bone marrow: Bone marrow shows patchy infiltration. Osteoclastic activity increases serum calcium levels.

Immunophenotyping: These cells are **strongly positive** with **CD25**.

NHL—SPILLOVER IN BLOOD

Bone marrow may be involved due to spillover of non-Hodgkin's lymphomas. Low grade NHL most often involves bone marrow in 60–80% cases as compared to high grade NHL in 30–40%. Presence of NHL spillover in blood indicates bone marrow involvement (stage IV).

BONE MARROW

Bone marrow shows deposits of NHL. Atypical lymphoma cells contain lobulated and notched nuclei. NHL deposits in bone marrow demonstrated in diffuse pattern is associated with poor prognosis.

Deposits of follicular center cell lymphoma are demonstrated in paratrabecular pattern.

FLOW CYTOMETRY

This diagnostic tool is used to differentiate B and T cells origin.

HODGKIN'S DISEASE

Hodgkin's disease is a malignant neoplasm of lymph node. It is important to determine whether the patient has only a single lymph node region involved, multiple node regions, or extranodal involvement.

Diagnostic criteria include demonstration of neoplastic **Reed-Sternberg** cells derived from B or T cells admixed with inflammatory cells in background as a result of cytokines produced by them.

MODE OF SPREAD

Initially Hodgkin's disease involves adjacent lymph nodes then other nodes via lymphatic route in continuous and predictable fashion. Later it spreads via the blood and involves the spleen, liver and bone marrow. Spleen is practically always involved. *Liver is involved if splenic hilum and retroperitoneal lymph nodes are involved.* Bone marrow is involved in Hodgkin's disease depletion type.

MANTLE CELL LYMPHOMA—SPILLOVER IN BLOOD

Mantle cell lymphoma occurs in the middle and elderly persons. It resembles small cell lymphoma except slightly different cellular details. It most often occurs in **older men**. It is disseminated, moderately aggressive incurable disease. It is derived from the **naïve B cell of lymphoid follicles in mantle zone of lymph node.**

ORGANS INVOLVED

Mantle cell lymphoma involves bone marrow in most cases. About 20% cases are associated with leukemia. It has *tendency to involve gastrointestinal tract* with submucosal polypoid nodules.

MOLECULAR GENETICS

Neoplastic cells show **t(11;14) with fusion of the cyclin D1 gene on chromosome 11 to the immunoglobulin heavy-chain (IgH)** promoter/enhancer region on chromosome 14. Fusion product leads to increased cyclins (CCND1/cyclin D1) expression with loss of cell cycle regulation.

> **Light Microscopy**
> - Mantle cell lymphoma comprises hyalinized blood vessels and scattered epithelioid histiocytes giving 'starry sky' appearance.
> - Classic cells are small with irregular indented nuclear contours. These cells may have blastoid or pleomorphic anaplastic morphology.
> - Blastoid form of mantle cell lymphoma and sometimes classic cells may be accompanied by involvement of blood, bone marrow and spleen.

Table 9.67: Immunophenotyping of mantle cell lymphoma

Immunophenotyping markers	Expression
CD5	Positive
CD20	Positive
CD22	Positive
CD43	Positive
Cyclin D1 (BCL1, PRAD)	Positive
t(11;14)	Positive
CD10	Negative
CD25	Negative
CD23	Negative
CD11C	Negative

IMMUNOPHENOTYPING

Immunophenotyping of mantle cell lymphoma is shown in Table 9.67.

SPLENIC LYMPHOMA WITH VILLOUS LYMPHOCYTES

Splenic lymphoma with villous lymphocytes is characterized by pallor and **splenomegaly**. It involves bone marrow in patchy manner and then spillover in blood. Leukemic cells show a few short villi in one direction. These leukemic cells are negative for CD11 and CD103.

MULTIPLE MYELOMA AND WALDENSTRÖM MACROGLOBULINEMIA

Plasma cell dyscrasias are monoclonal B cell lymphoid neoplasms showing expansion of a single clone of immunoglobulin secreting plasma cells. These include multiple myeloma, Waldenström macroglobulinemia, and benign monoclonal gammopathy, primary amyloidosis and heavy-chain (Franklin) disease.

Most often, these clonal proliferations show malignant behavior. These most often occur in >40–50 years of age.

M Component

The monoclonal immunoglobulin in the blood is known as an *M component*, in reference to myeloma. Complete M components are restricted largely to circulating plasma and extracellular fluid.

They may also appear in the urine, in case of glomerular damage with heavy proteinuria.

Diagnostic Criteria According to International Myeloma Working Group (2011)

International myeloma working group (2011) diagnostic criteria is shown in Table 9.68. Comparison among multiple myeloma, smoldering myeloma and monoclonal gammopathy of undetermined significance (MGUS) is shown in Table 9.69.

MULTIPLE MYELOMA

Multiple myeloma is a malignant tumor of plasma cells (derived from postgerminal center B cells) involving bone marrow. The neoplastic cells can easily be identified by bone marrow biopsy or aspiration smears. It most often affects older adults with median age of 65 years. It rarely affects under 40 years of age.

There is increased risk with **radiation exposure**. *Benzene, solvents, pesticides, insecticides* may play some role in its pathogenesis.

DIAGNOSTIC CRITERIA

Multiple myeloma is diagnosed by presence of increased plasma cells in the bone marrow, osteolytic lesions and M protein synthesis. In multiple myeloma, neoplastic plasma cells synthesize IgG or IgA immunoglobulin of

White Blood Cells

Table 9.68: International myeloma working group (2011) diagnostic criteria

Plasma cell dyscrasias	Diagnostic criteria
Plasma cell myeloma	M protein in serum and/or urine (no level of M protein in serum or urine included): M protein in most cases is >30 g/L or IgG >25 g/L or IgA >10 g/L of urine light chain in 24 hours Bone marrow: It shows >10% monoclonal plasma cells or biopsy proven plasmacytoma Myeloma-related organ or tissue impairment: **CRAB** stands for raised serum **c**alcium (>11.5 mg), **r**enal insufficiency (>1.96 mg/dl), **a**nemia (Hb <10 gm/dl) and **b**one lesion (osteolytic lesion or osteoporosis)
Monoclonal gammopathy of undetermined significance (MGUS)	M protein in serum <30 g/L Bone marrow clonal plasma cells <10% No evidence of other B cell proliferative disorders No myeloma-related organ or tissue impairment
Asymptomatic myeloma (smoldering myeloma)	M protein in serum ≥30 g/L and/or bone marrow clonal plasma cells ≥10% No myeloma-related organ or tissue impairment (no end organ damage, including bone lesions) or symptoms

Table 9.69: Comparison among multiple myeloma, smoldering myeloma and MGUS

Parameters	Multiple myeloma	Smoldering myeloma	MGUS (monoclonal gammopathy of undetermined significance)
Osteolytic lesions	Present	Absent	Absent
Myeloma related organs damage	Present	Absent	Absent
Monoclonal plasma cells in bone marrow	>30%	10–30%	<10%
M protein (IgG)	>35 g/L	>30 g/L	<30 g/L
Excretion of light chains κ or λ in urine	>3 g/24 hours	1–3 g/24 hours	>1 g/24 hours

either κ or λ light-chain specificity resulting in increased concentration in serum. **Serum electrophoresis** reveals monoclonal protein **M spike**.

Bence Jones protein refers to excretion of either κ or λ light-chain class in urine in these cases. Their assays are used for monitoring therapeutic response and prognostic outcome. **Death is often caused by renal insufficiency caused by myeloma kidney.** Diagnostic criteria of multiple myeloma according to Salmon and Durie and international myeloma working group are shown in Tables 9.70 and 9.71.

MOLECULAR GENETICS

Cytogenetic abnormalities may include t(4;14), which juxtaposes the IgH locus on 14q32 with the fibroblast growth factor receptor 3 (FGFR3) gene on chromosome 4p16. Tumor cells synthesize cytokines such as MIP1a

Table 9.70: Diagnostic criteria of multiple myeloma (Salmon and Durie)

Diagnostic criteria	Parameters	Findings
Major criteria	Histopathological examination Bone marrow Serum electrophoresis or Urine excretion of light chains (κ or λ)	Plasmacytoma on biopsy Plasma cells (>30%) Monoclonal immunoglobulin peak IgG (>3.5 g/dl) or IgA (>2 gm/dl) Excretion of κ or λ light chain in urine (≥1 g/24 hours)
Minor criteria	Bone marrow Serum electrophoresis Bone lesion Immunoparesis	Plasma cells (10–30%) Monoclonal immunoglobulin spike showing IgG (<3.5 g/dl) or IgA (<2 g/dl) Osteolytic lesion Residual normal IgM (<0.5 g/dl), IgA (<1 g/dl) or IgG (<0.6 g/dl)

Table 9.71: Diagnostic criteria of multiple myeloma (international myeloma working group)

Parameters	Findings
M proteins	Present in serum and urine
Clonal plasma cells in bone marrow or biopsy proven	≥10%
Myeloma related organ dysfunction	Serum calcium >11.5 mg/5 Renal insufficiency (serum creatinine >1.96 mg%) Bone lesions (osteolytic or osteoporosis) Anemia (Hb <10 g/dl)
In the absence of end organ damage	Clonal plasma cells in bone marrow

and the receptor activator of NF-κB ligand (RANKL), which serve as an *osteoclast-activating factor*. Cytogenetic abnormalities in multiple myeloma are shown in Table 9.72.

PATHOGENESIS

Survival of plasma cells depends on synthesis of IL-6 by plasma cells and stromal cells of bone marrow. Cytokine IL-1 acts as growth factor and antiapoptotic factor.

Role of IL-6

IL-6 synthesized by myeloma cells has autocrine effect. IL-6 synthesized by bone marrow stromal cells acts on JAK stat and RAS-MAP pathways. Activation of JAK pathway prevents apoptosis of myeloma cells. Activation of RAS-MAP pathway acts through transcriptional factor causes proliferation of myeloma cells. Osteoclastic activating factor synthesized by monoclonal plasma cells causes osteolytic lesions. (Fig. 9.38).

Table 9.72: Cytogenetic abnormalities in multiple myeloma

Oncogenes/tumor suppressor genes	Cytogenetic abnormalities	Prognosis
FGRF3	t(4;14)	Poor prognosis
p53	Deletion p53	Poor prognosis
C-maf	t(14;16)	Poor prognosis
Cyclin D1	t(11;14)	Good prognosis

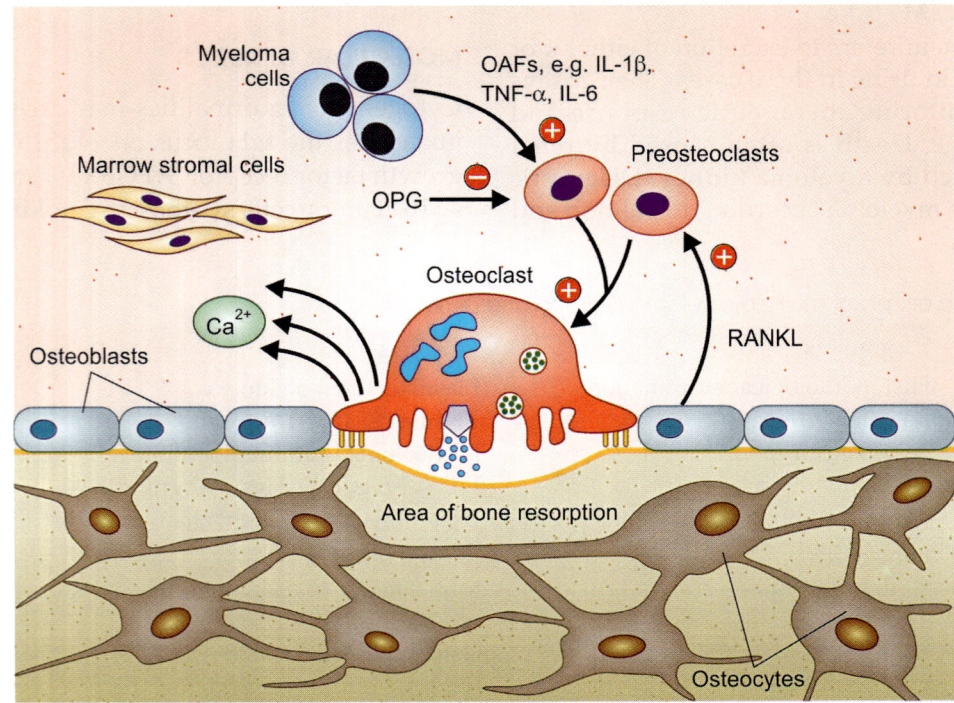

Fig. 9.38: Pathogenesis of bone disease in multiple myeloma as a result of synthesis of osteoclastic activating factors.

Rearrangement Involving IgH

There is diverge rearrangements involving IgH. It is associated with prominent serum and urinary protein abnormalities. Widespread **punched-out lytic bone lesions** in a patient in the older age group (median age 65) are highly suggestive of multiple myeloma.

TERMINOLOGY OF MULTIPLE MYELOMA

Terminology of multiple myeloma is shown in Table 9.73.

Secretory Myeloma

Clonal proliferation of plasma cells synthesizing immunoglobulins (paraproteins) is known as *secretory myeloma*. IgG or IgA *M proteins* are almost always found in multiple myeloma. IgM myeloma is very uncommon.

Non-secretory Myeloma

M proteins are **absent** in **serum** and/or **urine** with immunodiffusion in these patients. Bone marrow shows clonal plasma cells 10% or plasmacytoma. Some cases of multiple myeloma do not secrete M proteins (non-secretory MM) and hence not demonstrated in serum and urine.

Solitary Plasmacytoma

Solitary plasmacytoma, either occurs in **bone** or **soft tissues (oropharynx)**. Single area of bone destruction occurs due to clonal plasma cells. There is no M protein in serum and/or urine. Bone marrow examination is not consistent with multiple myeloma. There is no end organ damage other than solitary bone lesion. Most cases of solitary plasmacytoma involving bone evolve into multiple myeloma. *Extraosseous myeloma is commonly seen in IgD myeloma*.

Smoldering Myeloma (Asymptomatic Myeloma)

Diagnostic criteria of smoldering myeloma are M proteins in serum ≥ 30 g/L and or bone marrow shows clonal plasma cells ≥ 10–30%. Patients have no myeloma related organ or tissue impairment (no end organ damage including bone). Smoldering myeloma occurs in 15–20% cases of multiple myeloma. These patients progress to multiple myeloma within 1–3 years of age.

Covert Myeloma

Patient with covert myeloma does not develop tumor, but synthesize abnormal paraprotein resulting in amyloidosis.

Osteosclerotic Myeloma

Osteoclastic myeloma occurs in young persons. POEMS (**P:** polyneuropathies, **O:** organomegaly, **E:** endocrinopathy, **M:** myeloma protein, **S:** skin changes is seen in rare cases of osteosclerotic multiple myeloma. Patient presents with **hepatosplenomegaly and lymphadenopathy**.

CLINICAL MANIFESTATIONS

Clinical features of multiple myeloma are shown in Fig. 9.39.

Bone Involvement

Osteolytic Lesions

Osteoclastic activating factor synthesized by monoclonal plasma cells cause osteolytic lesions. The lesions begin in the medullary cavity, erode cancellous bone and progressively destroy the bony cortex. Bone lesions are associated with bone pain and spontaneous fractures.

Vertebral column is the most common site especially in lumbar region. Other bones affected in decreasing frequency include **ribs, sternum, skull, pelvis, femur, clavicle,** and **scapula**. IgG and Bence Jones myeloma

Table 9.73: Terminology of multiple myeloma

Terminology	Characteristic features
Secretory myeloma	*M proteins* (IgG or IgA) almost present, but IgM uncommon
Non-secretory myeloma	No synthesis of *M proteins* hence absent in serum or urine
Solitary plasmacytoma	Bone (osteolytic) or soft tissues (oropharynx with raised IgD) No organ damage except osteolytic lesion
Smoldering (asymptomatic) myeloma	M proteins in serum ≥ 30 g/L and or bone marrow shows clonal plasma cells ≥ 10% CRAB absent (no impairment of myeloma related organ or tissue including bone
Covert myeloma	No tumor formation, but synthesis of abnormal paraprotein resulting in amyloidosis
Osteosclerotic myeloma (young age group)	Development of **POEMS** in a few cases (P: polyneuropathies, O: organomegaly, E: endocrinopathy, M: myeloma protein, S: skin changes). Patient presents with hepatosplenomegaly and lymphadenopathy

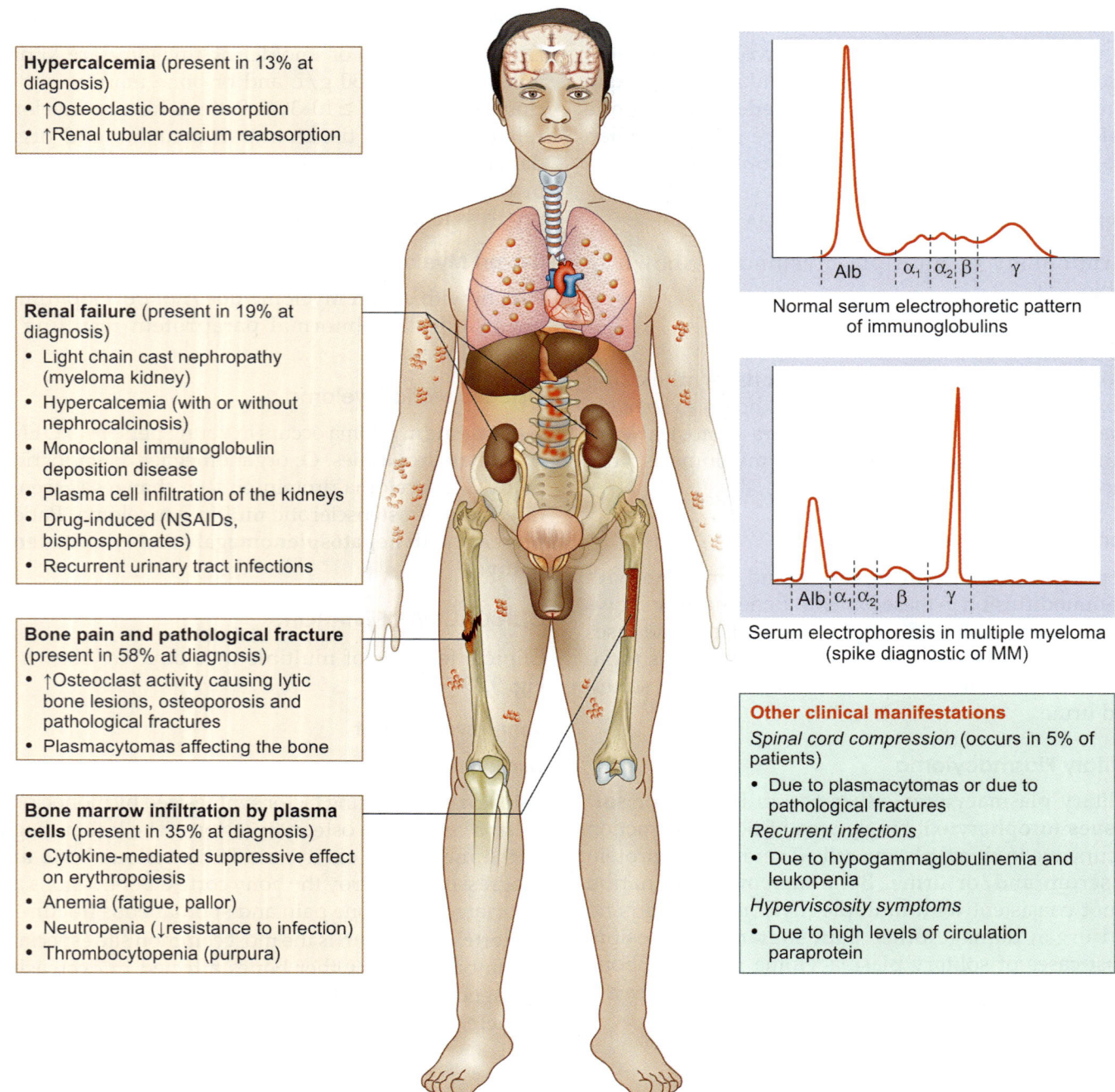

Fig. 9.39: Clinical features of multiple myeloma. Protein electrophoresis shows 'M-band' in the gamma region of a patient with multiple myeloma.

produce osteolytic lesions. IgD myeloma produces extraosseous lesions.

Pathological Fractures and Neurological Symptoms

Bone pain is aggravated by movement in 65% of cases, sometimes with an associated loss of height from vertebral collapse. Such lesions can produce bone pain aggravated by movement and less at rest. Patient is prone to **pathological fractures**, spinal cord compression due to compressed vertebral fractures and diffuse osteopenia.

Increased Serum Calcium

Serum calcium levels are increased in multiple myeloma (IgG, IgA, IgD and Bence Jones). Hypercalcemia causes confusion, weakness, lethargy, constipation, polyuria, and contributes to renal disease.

White Blood Cells

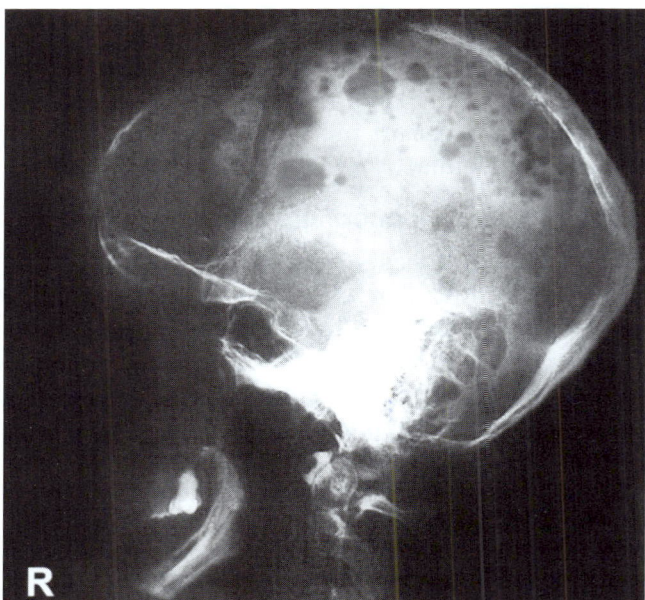

Fig. 9.40: Multiple myeloma. Radiograph of skull shows multiple punched-out osteolytic lesions.

Radiograph of Bones

Radiograph study of bones reveals rounded *punched-out defects* measuring 1 to 4 cm in diameter and diffuse osteopenia occurs in an older adult (Fig. 9.40).

Recurrent Infections

Patients with IgG myeloma lead to decreased synthesis of normal immunoglobulins which resulting in recurrent infections with *Streptococcus pneumoniae, Staphylococcus aureus, Escherichia coli* and *Haemophilus influenzae*. Cellular immunity is relatively unaffected. Recurrent infections are less common with IgA myeloma.

Manifestations due to M Proteins

Bleeding Abnormalities

M proteins coat platelets resulting in bleeding tendencies from gums, gastrointestinal tract and respiratory tract.

Coagulation Abnormalities

M proteins combine with factors I, II, V, VII, and VIII resulting in coagulation abnormalities.

Cryoglobulinemia

In some patients, M proteins behave like cryoglobulins resulting in tingling sensation and numbness, and skin rashes.

Hyperviscosity Syndrome

Hyperviscosity syndrome is not common in multiple myeloma. Patient presents with symptoms related to central nervous system and cardiovascular symptoms.

Easy Fatigue/Anemia

Patient presents with easy fatigue/anemia due to bone marrow infiltration, production of inhibitory factors, hemolysis, decreased red cell production and decreased erythropoietin levels.

Amyloidosis

The excessive light-chain production may lead to the AL form of amyloidosis, with deposition of amyloid in **kidneys, liver, spleen, lymph nodes.** It may involve any organ.

Amyloid deposition in organs is overt in 3% and subclinical up to 35%. Renal amyloidosis occurs in Bence Jones myeloma, IgG and IgA myelomas. IgD myeloma cases produce heavy proteinuria.

Myeloma Kidney

Paraproteins form **casts** in tubules with **giant cells** reaction. *The renal functions are impaired due to blockage of tubules by these casts.*

Visceral Involvement

Lymph node, liver and spleen may be involved in multiple myeloma.

BLOOD FINDINGS

Hemoglobin

Hemoglobin ranges between 6 and 10 gm/dl.

Bleeding Time and Clotting Time

Bleeding time and clotting time are prolonged in multiple myeloma cases. These occur due to coating of platelets by paraprotein.

Erythrocyte Sedimentation Rate

Erythrocyte sedimentation rate is increased.

Peripheral Blood Smear

Peripheral blood smear shows rouleaux formation of red blood cells, leukopenia (chemotherapy or relative suppression of white cell precursors) or leukocytosis (recurrent infections) and thrombocytopenia.

Platelets coated by paraprotein become functionally abnormal. A bluish background tint is seen due to excessive paraprotein on the slide. Leukoerythroblastic picture is seen in 10% of cases. Peripheral blood smear shows **red blood cells forming rouleaux formation** is shown in Fig. 9.41.

Plasma Cell Leukemia

Patient rarely develops plasma cell leukemia. Presence of >20% of WBC count and absolute plasma cell count

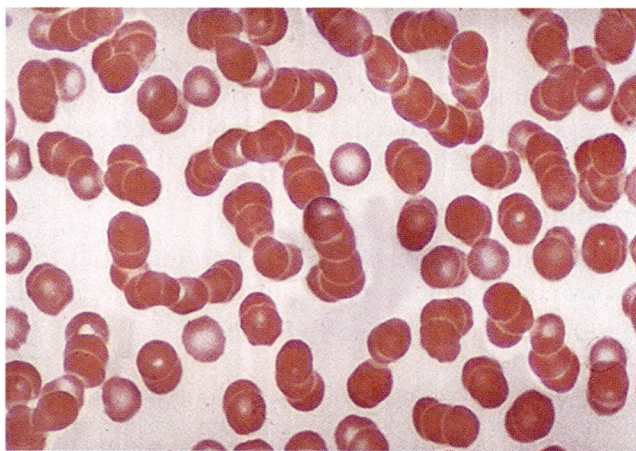

Fig. 9.41: Multiple myeloma. Peripheral blood smear shows red blood cells forming rouleaux formation.

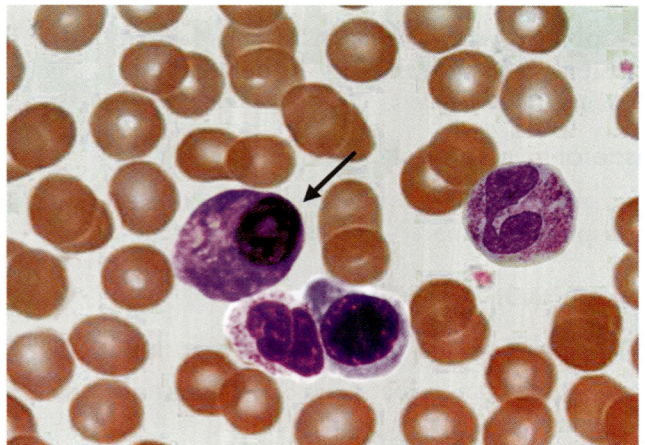

Fig. 9.42: Plasma cell leukemia. Peripheral blood smear shows spillover of myeloma cells in peripheral blood (arrow).

exceeds 2×10^9/L. in peripheral blood is termed as plasma cell leukemia. Organomegaly is common with unfavorable prognosis (Fig. 9.42).

Plasmacytosis

Peripheral blood plasmacytosis occurs in the following conditions—viral infections, typhoid, bacterial endocarditis, streptococcal infections, serum sickness, sarcoidosis, kwashiorkor, severe burns and Waldenström's macroglobulinemia.

Serum β_2 Microglobulin

Increased level of serum β-microglobulin is not specific for diagnosis of multiple myeloma. But its levels are used as **prognostic factor** in multiple myeloma.

Lactic Dehydrogenase and CRP Levels

Increased levels of these parameters not specific for diagnosis of multiple myeloma. But LDH and CRP are used as prognostic factors in these cases.

Serum Proteins

The marked serum immunoglobulin increase is often initially detected by laboratory screening as increased total protein with an increase in serum globulin (hyperglobulinemia).

Serum and Urine Electrophoresis

Serum electrophoresis demonstrates monoclonal immunoglobulin (κ or λ light-chain class or single heavy-chain) **M-spike in the γ-zone in 80% and occasionally α or β zones.** It indicates presence of a specific immunoglobulin (paraprotein) such as IgG (50%) or IgA (25%) or IgD (10%) and rarely IgM or IgE. **Urine electrophoresis** is **essential** to demonstrate κ or λ **light chains** irrespective of serum electrophoresis study.

Urine Analysis

The urine often contains significant quantities of free immunoglobulin light chains, either κ or λ light-chain class, which is referred to as Bence Jones protein in 60–70% cases. These **light chains** are **toxic to renal tubules**, and can lead to tubular injury with renal failure. On heating urine specimen Bence Jones proteins appear between 50° and 60°C. These disappear below 50°C and above 60°C temperature.

Renal Function Tests

The excessive light-chain production may lead to the AL form of amyloidosis, with deposition of amyloid in kidneys. Paraproteins form casts in tubules with giant cell reaction. The renal functions are impaired due to blockage of tubules by these casts. Renal function tests must be performed to rule out renal involvement.

BONE MARROW ASPIRATE

Bone marrow is hypercellular. It shows >30% of neoplastic mature or immature myeloma (plasma) cells. Myeloid, erythroid and megakaryocytic series are relatively decreased (Fig. 9.43).

Morphology of Myeloma Cells

Mature Myeloma Cells

Mature myeloma cells are 20–30 micron in diameter with abundant cytoplasm and eccentric nuclei, condensed chromatin giving *cartwheel appearance*.

Immature Myeloma Cells

Immature myeloma cells have nucleus with fine chromatin clear cytoplasmic droplets due to aggregation of immunoglobulin known as *Russel bodies*. Morphology of neoplastic plasma cells is indistinguishable from normal plasma cells except by their increased numbers. *Presence of immature plasma cells indicates bad prognosis.*

White Blood Cells

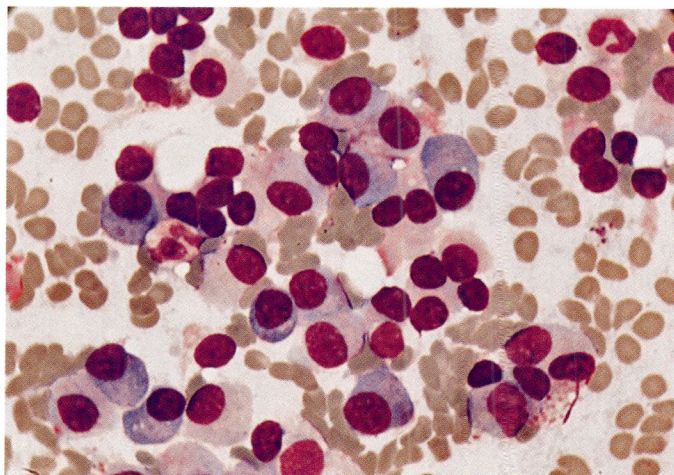

Fig. 9.43 Multiple myeloma. Bone marrow aspirate shows infiltration by myeloma cells. These cells have eccentric nucleus and perinuclear halos. A few binuclear plasma cells are also seen.

Plasmablastic Myeloma Cells

Plasmablastic myeloma cells have large nucleus and reticular chromatin and prominent nucleus with high nucleocytoplasmic ratio. Plasma cell grading system is shown in Table 9.74.

Staining Technique of Plasma Cells

Plasma cells can be stained by methyl green pyronine, which stains cytoplasm as red (pyronine) and nucleus as blue green (methyl green). Other stains are toluidine blue and azures.

Conditions Associated with Increased Plasma Cells

Bone marrow rarely shows >10% plasma cells due to metastatic carcinomas producing osteolytic lesions, Hodgkin's disease, sarcoidosis, systemic lupus erythematosus, rheumatoid arthritis, tuberculosis, syphilis, cirrhosis and aplastic anemia.

Table 9.74: Plasma cell grading system

Monoclonal plasma cell's type	Findings
Mature monoclonal plasma cells	Cells with dense clumped chromatin. Nuclei eccentrically placed with abundant cytoplasm
Immature monoclonal plasma cells	Cells with diffuse chromatin. Nuclei large eccentrically placed with prominent nucleolus
Plasmablastic cells	Cells with central large immature nucleus with reticular chromatin and prominent nucleolus

BONE MARROW TREPHINE BIOPSY

The tumor is soft, red tumor with a gelatinous consistency typically filling the bony defects. On light microscopy, tumor shows sheets of plasma cells that are very similar to normal plasma cells, with eccentric nuclei and abundant pale purple cytoplasm. In some cases, the myeloma cells may also be poorly differentiated.

Immunohistochemistry	
Monoclonal plasma cells show positivity for **CD38** and **CD138**.	
Marker	Expression
CD38	Positive
CD138	Positive

POOR PROGNOSTIC AND PREDICTIVE FACTORS

Prognosis is poor in advanced clinical stage, increased serum levels (β_2 microglobulin, LDH, CRP, serum free light-chain assay and ratio of κ or λ chairs) and diffuse bone marrow involvement, plasmablastic morphology, high plasma cell proliferative activity, cytogenetics t(4;14), t(14;20), t(14;16), deletion 17p/TP53 and stage III of Durie and Salmon.

Favorable cytogenetics include **hyperdiploidy, t(11;14), t(6;14)**. Plasma cell myeloma is incurable with median survival of 3–4 years. *Death is often caused by renal insufficiency due to myeloma kidney.* Median survival is 6 months without treatment (Table 9.75).

DIFFERENTIAL DIAGNOSIS

Multiple myeloma should be differentiated from reactive plasmacytosis, smoldering myeloma, Waldenström macroglobulinemia, tuberculosis, cirrhosis.

MANAGEMENT

Patients of multiple myeloma are treated by administration of chemotherapy, radiotherapy and stem cell transplantation.

WALDENSTRÖM MACROGLOBULINEMIA

Waldenström macroglobulinemia is a rare B cell lymphoproliferative disorder. It is characterized by proliferation of lymphoplasmacytic cells in the bone marrow. These cells synthesize excessive IgM.

Approximately 80% of patients with Waldenström macroglobulinemia present with a monoclonal IgM spike on serum electrophoresis (>3 g/dl). It can also occur without protein production. Many of the clinical symptoms are associated with hyperviscosity of the blood.

Table 9.75: Poor prognostic and predictive factors in multiple myeloma

Parameters	Findings
Durie and Salmon staging	Stage III (high tumor load)
	Stage II (intermediate tumor load)
	Stage II (low tumor load)
Myeloma variant	Plasmablastic myeloma
Serum creatinine	High levels indicating renal impairment
Serum IL-6 levels	High levels
Bone marrow involvement	Diffuse involvement by monoclonal plasma cells
Serum β_2 microglobulin	High levels
Serum LDH	High levels
Serum CRP	High levels
Serum free light-chain assay and ratio of κ or λ chains	High levels
Cytogenetics abnormalities	t(4;14), t(14;20), t(14;16), deletion 17p/TP53
Favorable cytogenetics include hyperdiploidy, t(11;14), t(6;14)	

DEFINITIVE CHARACTERISTICS

Serum IgM immunoglobulin of either κ or λ specificity is occurring as M protein. Plasmacytoid lymphocytes infiltrate in the blood, bone marrow, lymph nodes, and spleen. Bence Jones proteinuria is demonstrated in about 10% of cases. There is **absence of bone lesions.**

CLINICAL FEATURES

Most frequently seen in men older than 50 years of age. Slowly progressive course, often marked by generalized lymphadenopathy, mild anemia, Raynaud phenomenon and retinal hemorrhages.

Sometimes, emergency plasmapheresis is required to prevent blindness. Neurological symptoms such as headache, vertigo and ataxia are common. Approximately 50% cases present with mucosal bleeding. Abnormal bleeding, which may be due to vascular and platelet dysfunction secondary to the serum protein abnormality.

HEMATOLOGICAL FINDINGS

Peripheral blood smear examination shows **rouleaux formation of red blood** cells and lymphocytosis.

BONE MARROW ASPIRATE

Bone marrow examination shows large number of lymphoplasmacytoid cells with slightly eccentric nucleus and moderate basophilic cytoplasm. These cells show positivity with CD19, CD20 and CD22. These monoclonal cells show positivity with markers for κ and λ chains.

MANAGEMENT

These patients are treated by chemotherapy and plasmapheresis.

BENIGN MONOCLONAL GAMMOPATHY

Benign monoclonal gammopathy (monoclonal gammopathy of undetermined significance, or MGUS) occurs in 5–10% of otherwise healthy older persons.

A monoclonal M protein spike of <2 g/100 ml, minimal or no Bence Jones proteinuria, <5% plasma cells in the bone marrow, and no decrease in concentration of normal immunoglobulins is characteristic. MGUS is most often without clinical consequence.

DISORDERS OF MONONUCLEAR PHAGOCYTIC SYSTEM

In immunology, mononuclear phagocytic system is a part of immune system, that consists of monocytes and macrophages. Mononuclear phagocytes are derived from a common precursor in the bone marrow, which gives rise to monocytes. Blood monocytes migrate and differentiate into tissue macrophages known as *reticuloendothelial cells* diffusely distributed in the connective tissues in various organs (Table 9.76).

Disorders of mononuclear phagocytic system include storage histiocytosis and Langerhans' cell histiocytosis. Examples of storage histiocytosis are Gaucher's disease, Niemann-Pick and Sea blue histiocytosis.

Langerhans' histiocytosis comprise Letterer-Siwe disease (acute disseminated LCH), Hand-Schüller disease (multifocal LCH) and eosinophilic granuloma (unifocal LCH).

White Blood Cells

Table 9.76: Reticuloendothelial cell distribution in various tissues

Tissue	Reticuloendothelial cells
Blood	Monocytes
Connective tissue	Macrophages
Lung	Alveolar macrophages
Peritoneum	Peritoneal macrophages
Kidney	Mesangial cells
Liver	Kupffer's cells
Lymph nodes	Sinus histiocytes
Spleen	Littoral cells
Placenta	Hofbauer cells
Skin	Melanophages
Brain	Microglial cells
Synovium	Type I (type A cells)
Bone	Osteoclasts
Adipose tissue	Lipophage
Specialized histiocytes	Epithelioid cells, histiocytic giant cells, Langhans' giant cells, foreign body giant cells, touton giant cells

STORAGE HISTIOCYTOSIS

GAUCHER'S DISEASE

Gaucher's disease is autosomal recessive disorder most often seen in persons of European (Ashkenazic) Jewish lineage. It is characterized by accumulation of glucosylceramide (membrane glycosphingolipids) derived from the catabolism of senescent leukocytes, primarily in the lysosomes of macrophages.

The membranes of these cells are rich in the cerebrosides, and when their degradation is blocked by the deficiency of glucocerebrosidase (lysosomal acid β-glucosidase), an intermediate metabolite such as glucosylceramide accumulates.

Diagnostic Hallmark

The hallmark of this disorder is the presence of *Gaucher's cells* with a distinctive cigarette paper-like cytoplasmic appearance and eccentric nuclei, which are lipid-laden macrophages.

These are demonstrated in spleen, liver, CNS, bone marrow, tonsil, thymus, Peyer's patches, and lungs. Cytoplasm is fibrillary and crumpled (tissue paper-like).

Clinical Features

Clinical features are variable depending on three variants of Gaucher's disease as shown in Table 9.77.

Bone Marrow Aspirate

Bone marrow aspiration reveals numerous Gaucher's cells, but specific enzyme (chitotrioxidase and angiotensin-converting enzyme markers of macrophage proliferation) assay is required to confirm the diagnosis.

Gaucher's cells with a distinctive **cigarette paper-like** cytoplasmic appearance and **eccentric nuclei**, which are lipid-laden macrophages present in liver sinusoids (Kupffer cells) and bone marrow. Gaucher's cells are demonstrated in bone marrow and trephine biopsy (Figs 9.44 and 9.45).

NIEMANN-PICK DISEASE

Niemann-Pick disease occurs due to **SMPD1 gene** mutation encoding protein resulting in accumulation of sphingomyelin in the lysosomes of phagocytes. There are three subtypes of disorder (types A, B and C). Type C differs from types B and C.

Patient with Niemann-Pick disease (type C) is unable to metabolize cholesterol and other lipids leading to deposition in **liver, spleen** and **central nervous system.** Comparison among three types of Niemann-Pick disease is shown in Table 9.78.

Table 9.77: Comparison among three types of Gaucher's disease

Parameters	Adult Gaucher's disease (type I)	Infantile Gaucher's disease (type II)	Juvenile Gaucher's disease (type III)
Age group	Adults (more prevalent among Ashkenazi Jews)	Infants	Early childhood
Frequency	80% (commonest)	Uncommon	Uncommon
Organs involved	Liver, bone, bone marrow, spleen and lymph nodes	Central nervous system	Brain and visceral organs
Clinical features	Splenomegaly, hepatomegaly, mild anemia, thrombocytopenia, bone fracture of femoral head	Failure to thrive	Myoclonic fits
Prognosis	Normal lifespan	Fatal by one year of age	Less severe disorder

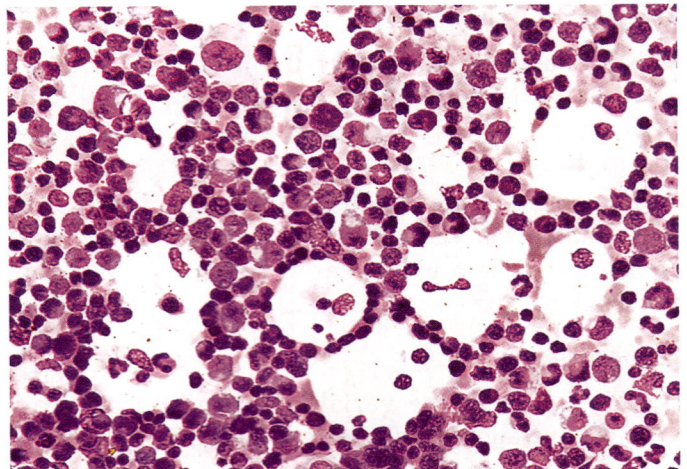

Fig. 9.44: Gaucher's disease. Bone marrow shows Gaucher's cells containing cigarette paper-like cytoplasmic appearance and eccentric nuclei, which are lipid-laden macrophages.

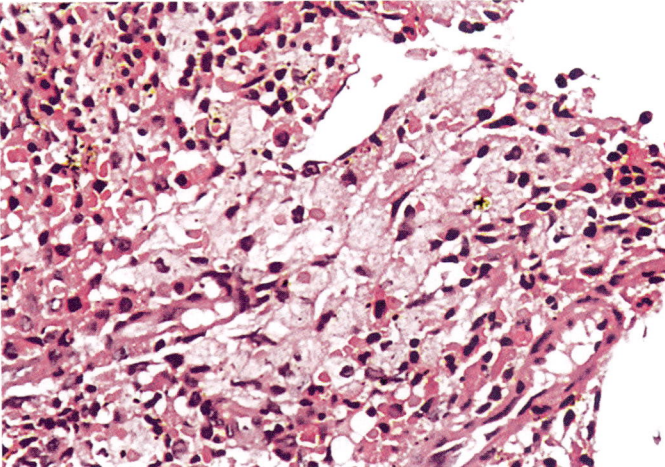

Fig. 9.45: Gaucher's disease. Bone marrow trephine biopsy shows Gaucher's cells containing cigarette paper-like cytoplasmic appearance and eccentric nuclei, which are lipid-laden macrophages (400X).

Table 9.78: Comparison among three types of Niemann-Pick disease

Parameters	Niemann-Pick disease (type A)	Niemann-Pick disease (type B)	Niemann-Pick disease (type C)
Age group	Infants (severe disorder)	Adults (less severe)	-
Basic defect	Accumulation of sphingomyelin in the lysosomes of phagocytes	Accumulation of sphingomyelin in the lysosomes of phagocytes	Unable to metabolize cholesterol and other lipids and deposited in liver, spleen and CNS
Clinical features	Hepatosplenomegaly, anemia, fever, neurologic manifestations and cherry red spots (50%)	Central nervous system, liver and spleen	Hepatomegaly and splenomegaly
Prognosis	Death occurs by three years of age	Survives into adulthood	-

Diagnostic Hallmark

Diagnostic hallmark is presence of *foamy histiocytes* containing sphingomyelin in liver, spleen, lymph nodes, skin, bone marrow, tonsil, GIT, and lungs.

Bone Marrow

Bone marrow aspirate shows Niemann-Pick cells. These are large 25–100 μm in size with eccentric nuclei and foamy cytoplasm. Foam cells show positivity with **oil red O** and **Sudan black B** (Fig. 9.46).

SEA BLUE HISTIOCYTOSIS

Sea blue histiocytosis may be hereditary or acquired. Acquired sea blue histiocytosis occurs due to *thalassemia major, chronic myeloid leukemia* and *idiopathic thrombocytopenia.*

Hereditary sea blue histiocytosis is autosomal recessive disorder due to **APOE gene mutation.** Patient with hereditary sea blue histiocytosis presents with **splenomegaly** and **thrombocytopenia.**

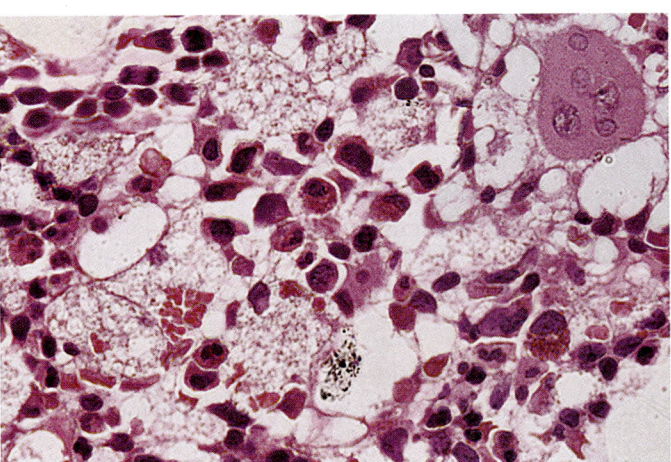

Fig. 9.46: Bone marrow showing Niemann-Pick disease.

Bone Marrow Aspirate

Bone marrow aspirate shows numerous histiocytes with granules and sea blue cytoplasm on Giemsa stain (Fig. 9.47). These granules are demonstrated by PAS stain.

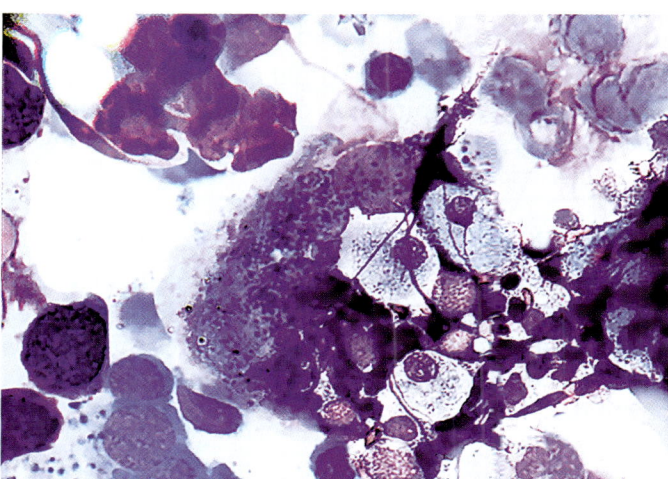

Fig. 9.47: Sea blue histiocytosis. Histiocytes with sea blue-colored granules are demonstrated.

LANGERHANS' CELL HISTIOCYTOSIS

Langerhans' cells participate in immunity by presenting antigen to T cells. Langerhans' cell histiocytosis is clonal disorder characterized by proliferative disorders of histiocytic cells that closely resemble the Langerhans' cells of the epidermis.

Langerhans' cell histiocytosis includes Letterer-Siwe disease, Hand-Schüller-Christian disease and eosinophilic granuloma. Clinical manifestations range from involvement of single site (bone or lymph node) in 75% to an aggressive systemic disorder involving multiple organs (25%).

Molecular Genetics

BRAF gene mutation has been demonstrated in 50% cases.

Diagnostic Features

Langerhans'-like cells are tennis racket-shaped containing *Birbeck granules*. These cells express distinctive surface antigens. These contain various enzymes such as acid phosphatase, α-naphthyl acetate esterase and α-naphthyl butyrate esterase. These cells show positivity with S-100, CD1a and langerin.

LETTERER-SIWE DISEASE (ACUTE DISSEMINATED LCH)

Letterer-Siwe disease is acute disseminated Langerhans' cell histiocytosis affecting **infants** and **small children.** Disease is **rapid aggressive course** with fatal outcome. Light microscopy reveals lack of lipids in histiocytes. Foci of necrosis are present.

Clinical Features

Patient presents with painless, yellow brown maculopapular skin lesions scattered over face, especially around eyes, mouth, truck, perineum, axillae; and recurrent infection as a result of widespread histiocytic proliferation. Physical examination reveals hepatosplenomegaly, lymphadenopathy, pulmonary involvement (honeycomb appearance, spontaneous pneumothorax and pleural effusion).

Hematological Findings

Peripheral blood smear examination shows pancytopenia as a result of replacement of bone marrow elements due to accumulation of histiocytosis.

Bone Marrow

Bone marrow aspirate shows numerous histiocytes with abundant cytoplasm admixed with a few lymphocytes and eosinophils. These cells are laden with cholesterol. Birbeck granules may be demonstrated on electron microscopy.

HAND-SCHÜLLER-CHRISTIAN DISEASE (MULTIFOCAL LCH)

Hand-Schüller-Christian disease is acute onset followed by chronic progressive histiocytosis affecting infants to elderly persons. It most often presents before 5 years of age. It has a **better prognosis** than Letterer-Siwe disease. Light microscopy shows histiocytic proliferation mixed with inflammatory cells in bone, especially the skull, liver, spleen, and other tissues.

Clinical Features

Disorder has classic triad: **bone lesions, diabetes insipidus** and **exophthalmos**. *Bone lesions* are demonstrated in the *orbit, tooth-bearing area of mandible and mastoid bone*. Diabetes insipidus occurs due to destruction of sella turcica.

Exophthalmos is caused by involvement of the orbit. Other lesions may occur such as femur, pelvis, ribs, humerus (end of shaft), spine, lung, skin and mucosa. Hepatosplenomegaly and lymphadenopathy may occur in 25–50% of cases.

Light Microscopy

Light microscopy demonstrates numerous histiocytes admixed with eosinophils.

EOSINOPHILIC GRANULOMA

Eosinophilic granuloma constitutes 75% of all cases. It is a localized, usually self-limited disorder affecting older children and young adults. This disorder has the **best prognosis** within the group. The lesion sometimes heals without treatment.

Organs Involved

Patient most often has a solitary bone lesion in **head, ribs, femur, ramus of mandible, vertebral bodies** and **orbit.** *Head and femur are affected in children, while ribs in adults.*

Light Microscopy

The lesion is composed of proliferation of histiocytes admixed with inflammatory cells, including ordinary macrophages, lymphocytes, and many eosinophils is characteristic.

Clinical Features

Patient with lung lesion affects young males with sudden onset, and has cough, weight loss, dyspnea and pneumothorax. Lesion in gastrointestinal tract is solitary, which may simulate polyps, gastric carcinoma or duodenal ulcer.

HEMATOPOIETIC STEM CELL TRANSPLANTATION

Hematopoietic stem cells constitute major bone marrow component. These are positive for CD34 (most widely used), CD90, and CD123, but negative for HLA-DR. Hematopoietic stem cells differentiate into cells of two lineages: lymphoid and myeloid. These cells then form the progenitor cells, which are committed to form a particular cell lineage, which then differentiates into mature cells in the peripheral blood.

Stem cell transplantation is the term now used in preference for bone marrow transplantation (BMT). Healthy hematopoietic stem cells are administered to restore normal hematopoiesis in patients suffering from hematological disorders. Source of graft may be autologous (grafting of own cells), allogenic (graft from donor to recipient with *different MHC/HLA alleles*) or syngeneic (graft between *identical twins*). In autologous stem cell transplantation, patient's own marrow cells are used for graft. Stem cell transplantation is done for chemotherapy or radiotherapy resistant leukemias and multiple myeloma.

Allogenic grafts have low relapse rate and graft-versus-host disease. Success of the graft depends upon matching and immunosuppressive drug-like cyclosporine. Indications for stem cell transplantation are shown in Table 9.79. Overview of hematopoietic stem cell transplantation is shown in Figs 9.48 and 9.49.

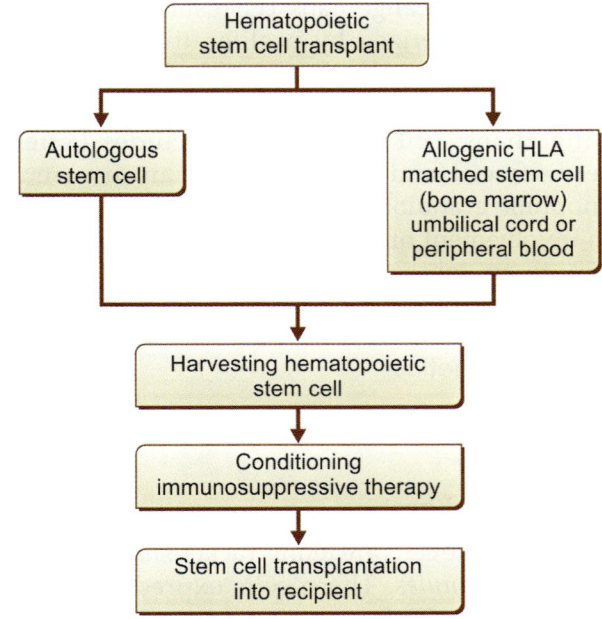

Fig. 9.48: Hematopoietic stem cell transplantation.

Table 9.79: Indications for stem cell transplantation

Hematological malignancies	Nonmalignant hematological disorders
Acute myeloid leukemia	Aplastic anemia
Acute lymphoblastic leukemia	Thalassemia
Chronic lymphatic leukemia	Sickle cell anemia
Multiple myeloma	Paroxysmal nocturnal hemoglobinuria
Non-Hodgkin's lymphoma	Fanconi's anemia
Hodgkin's disease	Diamond-Blackfan anemia
Myelodysplastic syndrome	Glanzmann thrombasthenia
Myeloproliferative disorders	Severe combined immunodeficiency

White Blood Cells

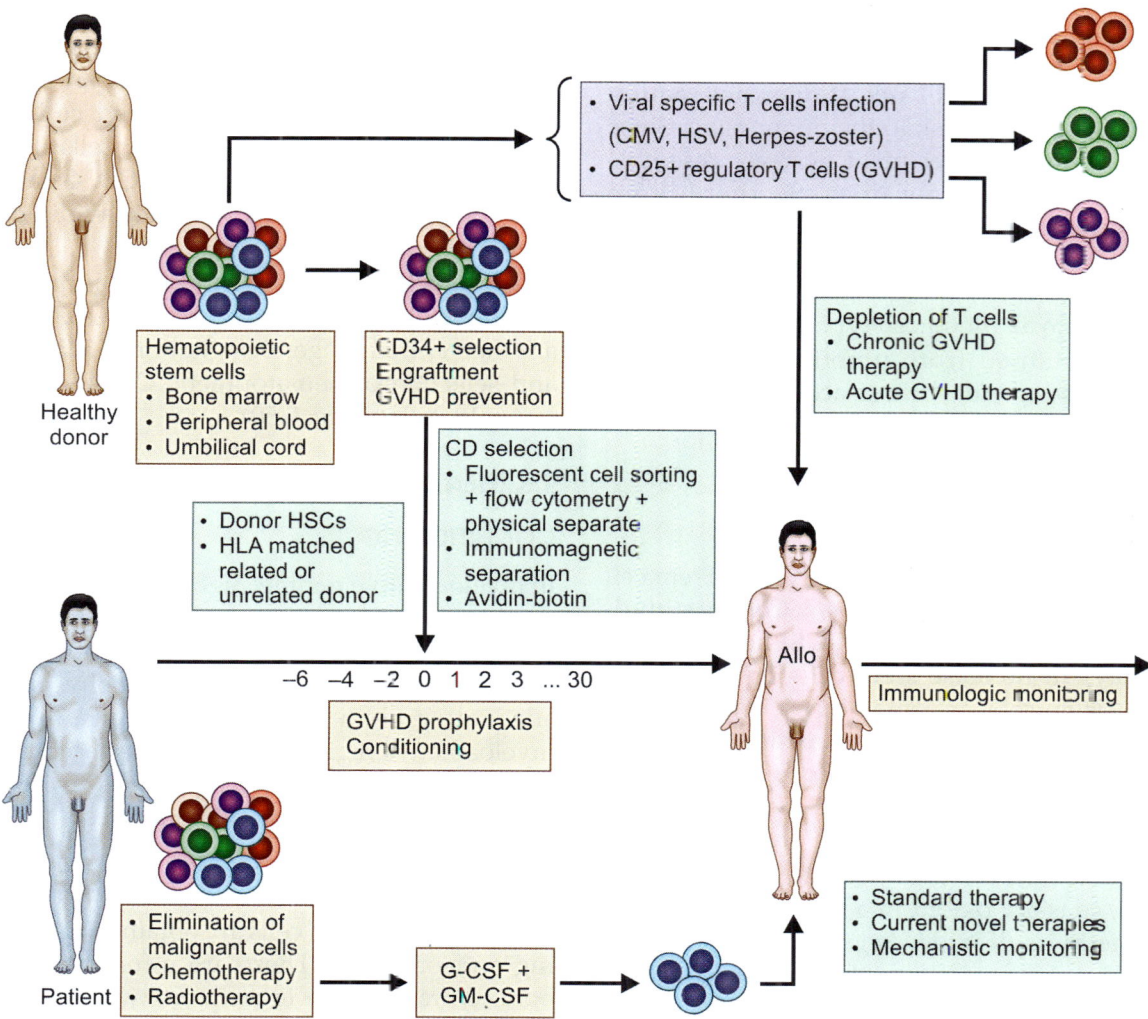

Fig. 9.49: Overview of hematopoietic stem cell transplantation.

SOURCES OF STEM CELLS

Cancer patients, whose bone marrow is destroyed by chemotherapy often require stem cell transplants. Stem cells may be obtained from bone marrow, peripheral blood, umbilical cord blood and amniotic fluid (Table 9.80).

BONE MARROW HARVESTING

Bone marrow is obtained by surgical procedure from **pelvis** and **sternum**. Bone marrow is filtered to remove debris. Bone marrow may be administered fresh or preserved cryoprecipitate. There may be risk of infection. It requires HLA typing. Patient may develop **graft-versus-host disease**.

Table 9.80: Comparison among stem cells obtained from umbilical cord blood versus bone marrow

Characteristics	Umbilical cord blood	Bone marrow
Obtaining stem cells	Obtained immediately after baby birth and stored in blood bank	Obtained by surgical procedure
Risk	No risk to the donor baby Lower risk to the recipient	Risk of infection to donor More risk to recipient
HLA typing	Not require HLA typing	Requires HLA typing
Time taken by engraftment	Longer period (delayed)	Shorter period
Graft-versus-host disease	Immature T cells reduce risk of GVHD	May develop GVHD

UMBILICAL CORD BLOOD HARVESTING

Cord blood is easily obtained immediately after baby birth and stored in a blood bank. **It does not require HLA typing.** There is no risk to the donor baby. Since cord blood is immature, recipient's tissues resemble as closely as bone marrow does. So there is **no chance of graft-versus-host disease** in the recipient. Harvesting umbilical cord can save lives. Like bone marrow, umbilical cord contains stem cells capable of differentiating into all blood cell types.

Stem cells obtained from umbilical cord blood offers some advantages over those acquired from bone marrow. There is **low risk of contamination with cytomegalovirus.**

STEM CELLS FROM PERIPHERAL BLOOD

Peripheral blood contains 0.1% of stem cells. Stem cell count is more than umbilical cord blood. **Colony stimulating factors such as G-CSF and GM-CSF administered for 4 to 5 days to increase stem cells in peripheral blood.** These stem cells are obtained by venipuncture and separated in separator. After processing, these cells are cryopreserved in the vapor phase of liquid nitrogen for later infusion. Granulocytes do not survive during cryopreservation.

To allow survival of granulocyte during cryopreservation, cells are placed in a medium containing 7.5–10% **dimethyl sulfoxide.** *Engraftment of peripheral blood stem cells is more rapid than obtained from umbilical cord. There is higher risk of acute and chronic graft-versus-host reactions.*

SELECTION OF DONOR

HLA matched identical sibling is the ideal donor. Sibling identical in HLA-A, HLA-B, DRB1, DQB1 loci are considered identical. ABO compatibility is not essential for bone marrow transplantation.

Donor evaluation is done for the safety of the stem cells of the donor and recipient. History of vaccination and previous blood transfusions is taken. Approximately 7 days prior to stem cell collection, each donor should be tested for HIV, HBV, HCV and CMV.

METHODS OF HEMATOPOIETIC CD34+ STEM CELLS SELECTION

CD34+ stem cells selection is done by the following methods. Fluorescent-activated cell sorting combines flow cytometry with physical separator segregates individual cells based on expression of molecules.

In immunoadsorption systems, CD34+ stem cells are magnetically retained and removal of unwanted cells by passive deletion and tumor cells are magnetically retained and collection of desired cells by active selection. In Avidin-biotin selection, cells are incubated with biotin labelled antibody to CD34+ antigen and processed over a column containing avidin-conjugated beads.

The labelled CD34+ stem cells bind to the beads and unlabeled cells wash through. CD34+ stem cells are then eluted by gentle agitation. Method of culture and selection of hematopoietic CD34+ stem cells for transplantation (Fig. 9.50).

RECIPIENTS

CONDITIONING

In myeloablative regime, high dosage of chemotherapy and radiotherapy is given to achieve three goals: elimination of malignant cells, immunosuppression to allow engraftment and creation of physical space for adequate growth of donor stem cells. Alternative to myeloablative regimen, fludarabine based antiglobulin is administered in elderly patients to lower tumor burden in hematological malignancies.

INFUSION OF HEMATOPOIETIC STEM CELLS

Hematopoietic stem cells are obtained in a bag containing anticoagulant. These are infused through large-bore central catheter in recipient within a few hours of collection. Engrafting is considered as established, when peripheral blood neutrophil count reaches $>0.5 \times 10^9/L$ on 3 successive days.

SUPPORTIVE CARE

High dosage of chemotherapy and radiotherapy induces **pancytopenia** in recipients may lead to infections. Therefore, **antibiotics** are administered to combat bacterial and fungal infections. Number of CD34+ stem cells required for hematopoietic recovery is $2.5–5.0 \times 10/kg$. Blood components therapy is given, Hematopoietic growth factors such as G-CSF or GS-CSF are administered to stimulate myelopoiesis.

COMPLICATIONS

In allogenic hematopoietic stem cell transplantation, GVHD is a significant complication. Since the disease process is mediated by host reactive T cells, therefore, strategies are employed to deplete T cells to lower the severity of GVHD. Treatment with cyclosporine or

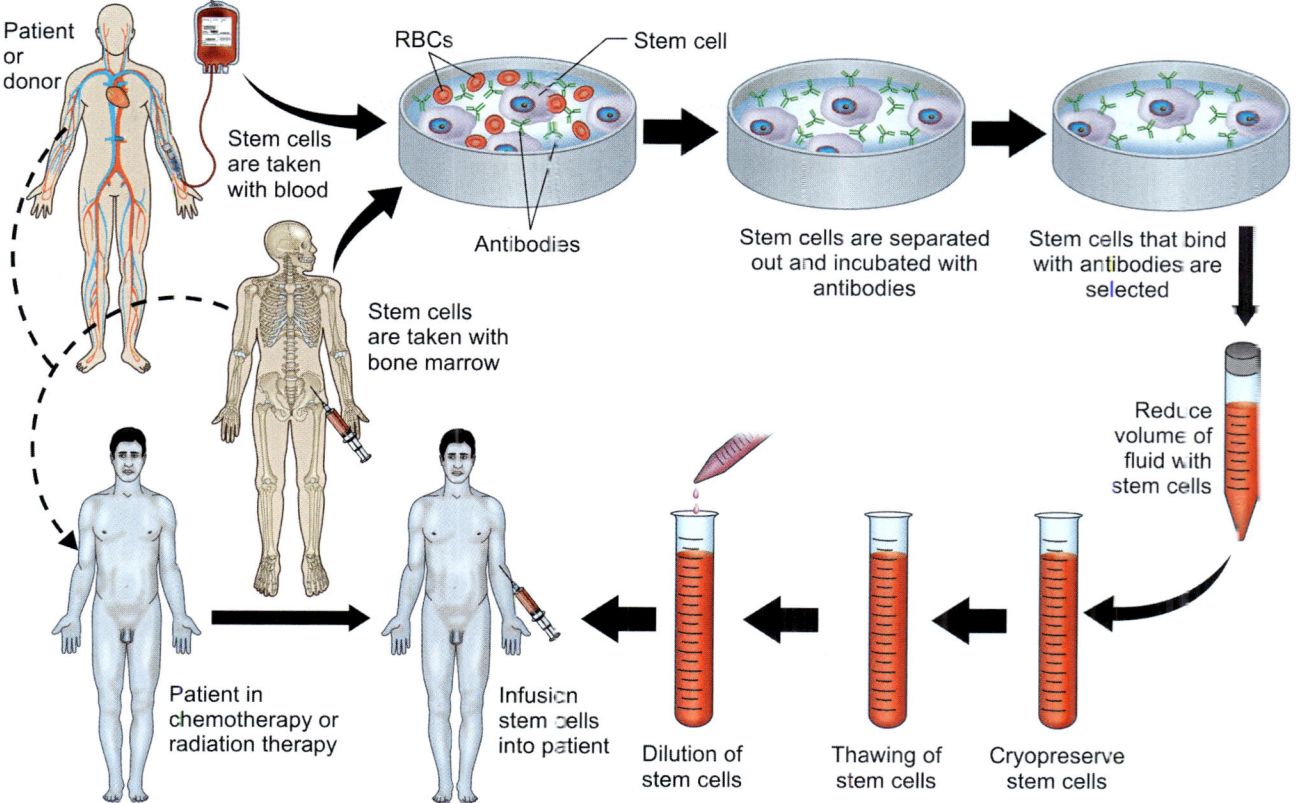

Fig. 9.50: Method of culture and selection of hematopoietic CD34+ stem cells for transplantation.

methotrexate should be administered to prevent graft-versus-host disease.

Acute Graft-versus-host Disease

Acute graft-versus-host disease occurs due to immunological event involving activation and clonal activation of donor's effector T cells. It occurs in first 100 days of bone marrow transplantation. There is involvement of skin, gastrointestinal tract and liver.

Chronic Graft-versus-host Disease

Chronic graft-versus-host disease occurs after acute GVHD/*de novo* after 100 days of bone marrow transplantation. Progressive GVHD evolving from acute GVHD has worst prognosis. There may be limited involvement of skin and liver. Extensive disease causes oral infections, hepatic dysfunction, eyes lesions and skin lesions.

Infections

Infections may occur 2–4 weeks prior to engraftment. During early post-engraftment, impaired cellular and humoral immunity leads to viral infections (CMV, herpes simplex virus and herpes zoster) and fungal infections.

During late post-engraftment, prolonged T cell dysfunction may cause infections with *Streptococcus pneumoniae*, *Haemophilus influenzae* and *Neisseria meningitidis*. Patient may develop diffuse or interstitial pneumonias.

Failure of Engraftment

Failure of engraftment occurs due to inadequate stem cell number, infections, graft-versus-host disease and high risk unrelated donor and HLA mismatch.

CHAPTER 10

Bleeding Disorders

Learning Objectives

NORMAL AND DISORDERS OF HEMOSTASIS
- Normal Hemostasis

PLATELET DISORDERS
- Overview

THROMBOCYTOPENIAS
- Idiopathic Thrombocytopenic Purpura
- Secondary Thrombocytopenia

PLATELET FUNCTION DISORDERS

VASCULAR PURPURA

NORMAL AND DISORDERS OF HEMOSTASIS

NORMAL HEMOSTASIS

Normal laminar blood flow dilutes activated clotting factors. It also increases the inflow of inhibitors of clotting factors resulting in inactivation of clotting factors. Hemostasis is the maintenance of blood flow within vascular system *inhibiting activation of platelets, coagulation system and fibrinolytic system.*

It involves the interaction of the blood vessels, platelets, coagulation factors leading to formation of hemostatic plug at the site of vascular site. Bleeding and clotting are the result of the failure of hemostatic mechanisms.

Normal endothelium synthesizes antithrombotic and prothrombotic molecules (Table 10.1 and Fig. 10.1).

Table 10.1: Antithrombotic and prothrombotic properties of vascular endothelium

Vascular endothelium	Properties	Molecules	Functions
Antithrombotic properties	Antiplatelet properties	Prostacyclin (PGI$_2$), nitric oxide	Potent vasodilators and inhibitors of platelets aggregation
		Adenosine diphosphatase enzyme	Degradation of ADP released by platelets
	Synthesis of inhibitors of coagulation	Heparin-like molecules	Binding to antithrombin III resulting in inactivation of thrombin, factor Xa and other clotting factors
		Thrombomodulin molecules	Conversion of procoagulant thrombin to anticoagulant thrombin molecule that activates protein C
			Protein C inhibits the activity of V, and that can no longer convert fibrinogen to fibrin
	Blood flow	Laminar blood flow	Dilution of clotting factors
			Inhibition of endothelial cell activation
			Increasing the inflow of inhibitors of clotting factors

Contd...

Table 10.1: Antithrombotic and prothrombotic properties of vascular endothelium (Contd...)

Vascular endothelium	Properties	Molecules	Functions
Prothrombotic factors	Platelets aggregation property	von Willebrand factor (vWF)	Adhesion of platelets to the underlying subendothelial extracellular matrix
	Procoagulant property	Tissue factor (induced by bacterial endotoxins, IL-1 and TNF-α)	Activation of extrinsic coagulation pathway
	Procoagulant property	Plasminogen activator inhibitors	Inhibition of fibrinolytic system

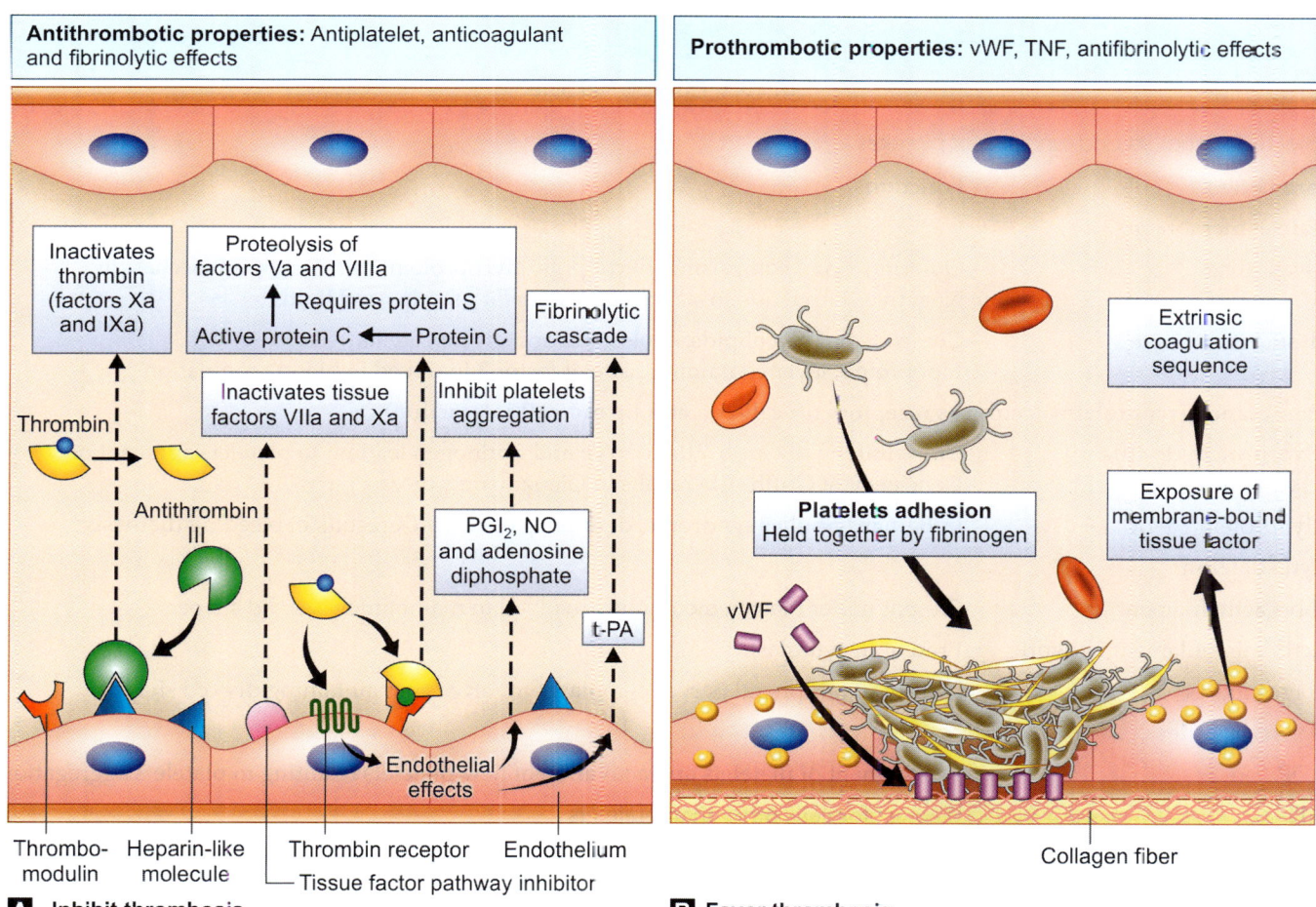

Fig. 10.1: Antithrombotic and prothrombotic properties of vascular endothelium.

VASCULAR COMPONENT

Vascular system is composed of vessels, that carry blood and lymph throughout the body. The blood vessel wall is the first line of defense for normal hemostasis. It is supported by subendothelial tissue, which maintains the integrity of structure. It is lined by endothelium. Laminar blood flow dilutes clotting factors and inhibits endothelial cell activation. It increases the inflow of inhibitors of clotting factors.

PLATELETS

Platelets play a central role in normal hemostasis by forming primary hemostatic plug. Platelets are membrane bound porous disc-like structures ranging from <5 to 12 femtoliter. These maintain the physical integrity of the vascular endothelium. These synthesize platelet derived growth factor (PDGF), which repairs injured endothelium. Structure and functions of platelets are shown in Fig. 10.2 and Table 10.2.

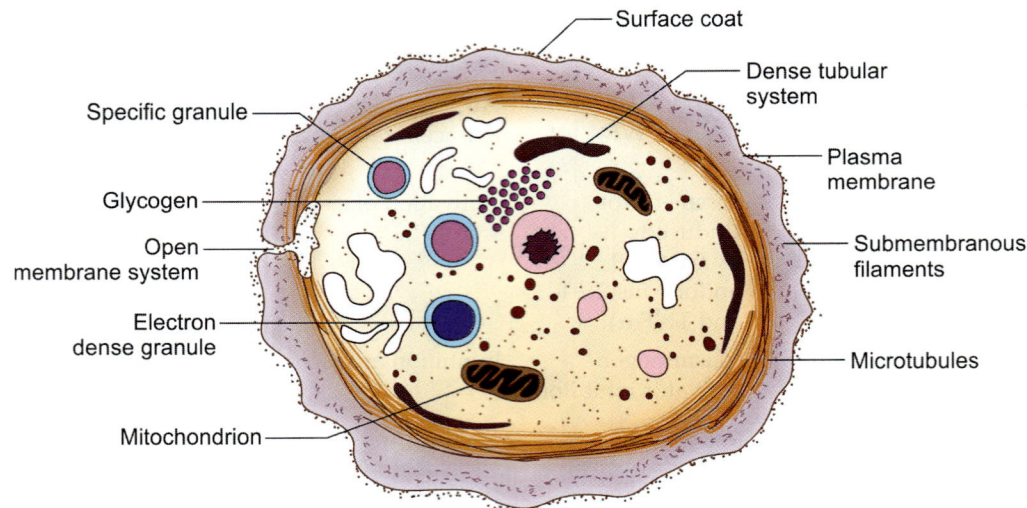

Fig. 10.2: Platelets structure.

Table 10.2: Structure and functions of platelets

Parameters	Functions
Platelet membrane	
Glycocalyx	Outermost coat comprising glycolipids, glycoproteins and mucopolysaccharide Negative charge due to sialic acid residue of proteins and lipids
Plasma membrane	Composed of glycolipids, cholesterol and glycoproteins Lipoprotein layer containing platelet factor 3 involved in blood coagulation
Membrane glycoproteins (acting as receptors for cell-cell and ligand-cell interaction)	
Glycoprotein IIb/IIIa	Cross-linking of GpIIb/IIIa to vWF and fibrinogen leading to platelets aggregation Deficiency of GpIIb/IIIa results in Glanzmann's disease
Glyoprotein 1b–IX	In Bernard-Soulier syndrome, deficiency of GP1b-IX results in bleeding diathesis
Cytoskeleton	
Short actin filament	Present under plasma membrane involved in maintaining discoid shape
Actin microfilament network	Present in cytoplasm
Microtubules	Present in peripheral part of cytoplasm involved in maintaining discoid shape
Dense granules	
ADP	Recruitment of platelets and activation of new platelets resulting in platelets aggregation
ATP	Agonist for cells other than platelets
Calcium	Extracellular source for hemostatic reactions
Serotonin	Vasoconstrictor
α-granules	
Fibrinogen	Aggregation of platelets Fibrinogen itself gets converted to fibrin
Platelet factor IV	Aggregation of platelets
Thrombospondin	Aggregation of platelets
Factor V	Adhesion of platelets
vWF	Inhibits fibrinolysin
Plasminogen	Plasminogen gets converted to plasmin. Plasmin participates in fibrinolysis
PDGF	Promotes repair of smooth muscle cells

10
Bleeding Disorders

Thrombopoiesis

Thrombopoietin, vitamin B_{12} and folic acid participate in platelets production in bone marrow. Platelets are formed by precursor cells called megakaryocytes that reside within bone marrow by a process called endomitosis where each megakaryocyte gives rise to approximately three thousand platelets. Two-thirds of platelets remain in circulation, while one-third are stored in spleen. These express glycoprotein receptors of the integrin family on their surface. Lifespan of platelets is 8–14 days.

Formation of Primary Hemostatic Plug

Platelets adhesion: Exposure of subendothelial tissue activates platelets, which change their shape by producing pseudopodia. These adhere to subendothelial tissue via receptor sites, which interact with von Willebrand factor (vWF).

This vWF is multimeric proteins synthesized by endothelial cells and megakaryocytes. The vWF binds with coagulation factor VIII in the plasma (Fig. 10.3).

Platelets aggregation: Platelets interact with each other via receptor sites, which utilize fibrinogen as an intercellular bridge. *Platelets contract and release granules, which contain substances participating in platelets aggregation.* These substances include ADP, 5-hydroxytryptamine, fibrinogen, and vWF.

Cell membrane of platelets synthesizes metabolic arachidonic product such as thromboxane A_2, which also promotes platelets aggregation in addition to vasoconstriction (Fig. 10.4). *Deficiency of GpIIb/IIIa results in Glanzmann's disease.* Platelet functions *in vivo* are shown in Fig. 10.5.

Fibrin generation: Exposure of tissue factor activates extrinsic coagulation system. Thrombin generation augments the platelet activation. These activated platelets provide phospholipid, which is an essential cofactor at several points in the coagulation.

COAGULATION CASCADE

Formation of secondary hemostatic plug occurs by intrinsic and extrinsic pathways as a result of vascular injury. Both these pathways lead to activation of factor X, conversion of prothrombin to thrombin. Thrombin converts fibrinogen to fibrin. *Fibrin stabilizing factor stabilizes fibrin resulting in holding of clot by insoluble fibrin strands.* Coagulation system comprises two pathways: *extrinsic and intrinsic.* These systems

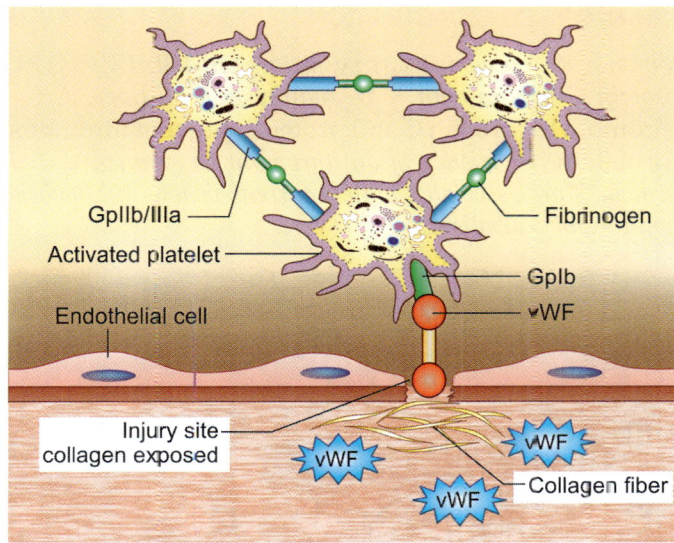

Fig. 10.4: Platelets aggregation participating in primary hemostatic plug.

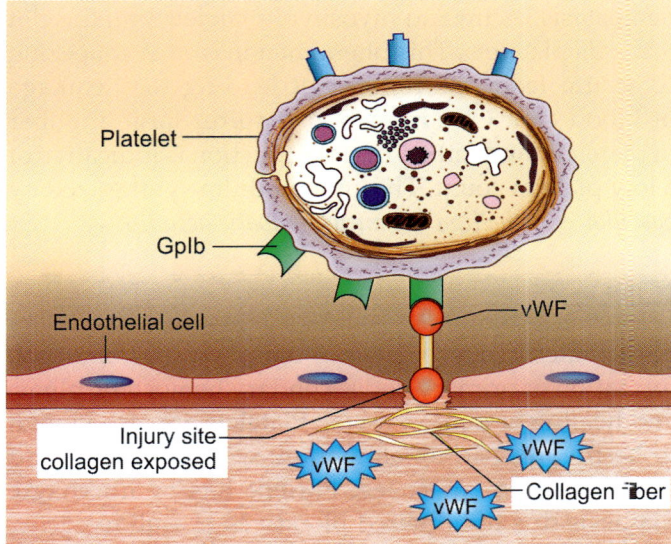

Fig. 10.3: Platelets adhesion participating in primary hemostatic plug.

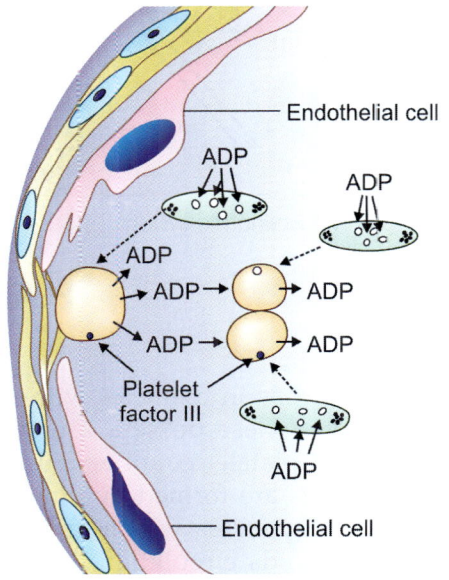

Fig. 10.5: Platelet functions *in vivo*.

reflect how clotting occurs in the test tube during tests. Clotting in the body is initiated differently.

FIBRINOLYTIC SYSTEM

Plasminogen activator cleaves plasminogen to form enzyme plasmin. *Plasmin binds to specific receptors on fibrin strands network and begins degrading the fibrin strands resulting in dissolution of blood clot.* Plasmin also degrades fibrinogen, factor V, factor VIII, prothrombin, and factor XII.

Dissolution of blood clot restores normal blood flow. Plasmin action is limited to the site of injury and formation of thrombus or clot. Systemic action of plasmin does not occur. Fibrinolytic system is shown in Fig. 10.6.

INHIBITORS OF COAGULATION

Vitamin K dependent clotting factors (II, VII, IX and X), protein C and protein S are synthesized by liver. Antithrombin III, protein C and protein S prevent thrombus formation. *Deficiency of antithrombin III, protein C and protein S are associated with recurrent venous thrombosis and thromboembolism.*

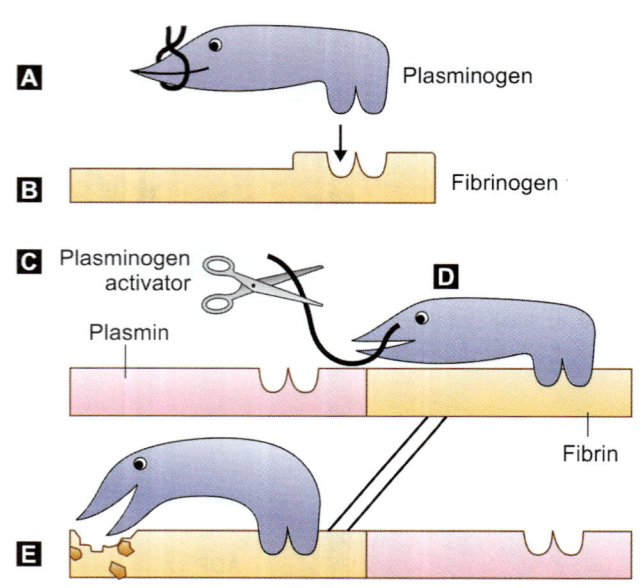

Fig. 10.6: Fibrinolytic system.

Antithrombin III

Antithrombin III antagonizes thrombin activity. It also inhibits factors XIIa, XIa, Xa, and IXa. Heparin-like molecules synthesized by endothelium activates antithrombin III. Hence, in clinical practice, *heparin is administered to minimize thrombosis.*

Protein C

Protein C is a vitamin K-dependent natural anticoagulant presents in circulation. It inhibits factors V and VIII. It is activated by modified thrombin protein. *Thrombomodulin synthesized by endothelium modifies thrombin molecule.* This modified thrombin protein can no longer convert fibrinogen to fibrin. Protein C also enhances fibrinolysis. Protein C deficiency is the most common cause of inherited thrombophilia.

Protein S

Protein S is a vitamin K dependent natural anticoagulant present in circulation. It serves as a cofactor and enhances the activity of protein C resulting in inhibition of factors V and VIII. Protein S does not require activation.

TISSUE FACTOR PATHWAY INHIBITOR

Tissue factor pathway inhibitor (TIFI) is synthesized by endothelium. It binds factor Xa and tissue factor and inactivates them rapidly in circulation, so limiting coagulation.

CLOT RETRACTION

Clot retraction occurs when platelets are trapped within the enlarging blood clot. It occurs within 20 to 60 minutes after a clot has formed, contributing to hemostasis. Actin and myosin of platelets pull the clot towards platelets. This phenomenon causes squeezing of serum from the blood clot leading to shrinkage of blood clot. Clot retraction requires large number of platelets, and failure of clot retraction is indicative of a low platelet count. Thrombomodulin synthesized by *vascular endothelium has antithrombotic activity.*

PLATELET DISORDERS

OVERVIEW

Platelets are 3–4.5 microns in diameter with normal lifespan of 4–10 days. These possess 2 membrane glycoproteins. Normal platelet count is $150 \times 10^9/L$ to $400 \times 10^9/L$. Platelets are formed by pinching off cytoplasm of megakaryocytes which are situated close to marrow sinusoids circulation. *Platelets are regulated by thrombopoietin synthesized from liver.* Platelet participates in surveillance of blood vessel continuity, formation of primary and secondary hemostatic plugs, and healing of injured tissue. Platelets are also known to be involved in inflammation, wound healing and cardiovascular diseases. Patient has hemorrhagic diathesis due to impaired blood vessel wall integrity, platelet deficiency or dysfunction, derangement in the coagulation mechanism and combination of the factors.

Table 10.3: Classification of thrombocytopenic purpura

Mechanisms	Causes
Decreased platelet production	
Bone marrow suppression	Drugs (chlorthiazide and ethanol), irradiation, viral infection, chemicals, alcohol
Ineffective thrombopoiesis	Megaloblastic anemia
Thrombopoietin deficiency	Disorders of thrombopoietic control
Increased platelet destruction	
Immunologic mechanisms	*Autoimmune process:* It may be primary or secondary (infections, pregnancy, collagen vascular disorders, and drugs)
	Alloimmune process: Neonatal purpura and post-transfusion purpura
Nonimmunologic mechanisms	*Thrombotic microangiopathies:* DIC (diffuse), TTP (diffuse), hemolytic uremic syndrome (localized)
	Hematological disorders: Acute leukemia and aplastic leukemia
	Prosthetic valves: Platelets are damaged by abnormal vascular surfaces (prosthetic valves)
	Drugs: Cyclophosphamide, busulphan and 6-mercaptopurine
	Miscellaneous: Infection, burns, drugs, hypothermia, cryopathy, hyperbaric exposure
Pooling of platelets (abnormal platelet distribution)	
Disorders of spleen	Splenomegaly (hyperfunctioning of phagocytic cells)
Massive blood transfusions	Dilution of platelet count
Low temperature	Hypothermia
Miscellaneous	Malignancy, pregnancy and HIV infection

THROMBOCYTOPENIA

Thrombocytopenia occurs when platelet count falls below $<100 \times 10^9/L$. *Patient presents with bleeding into skin, mucous membranes, gastrointestinal tract and genitourinary tract.* Bleeding may also occur following traumatic injury. Platelet count may fall due to decreased production in bone marrow, increased destruction in blood and pooling of platelets. Classification of thrombocytopenic purpura is shown in Table 10.3.

PATHOPHYSIOLOGY

Thrombocytopenic purpura occurs due to decreased production, ineffective maturation, increased destruction and pooling of platelets.

Decreased Platelet Production

Decreased production of platelets may be due to marrow hypoplasia, replacement of marrow by metastatic deposits, immune-mediated damage, drugs and idiopathic.

Ineffective Maturation

Ineffective maturation of platelets in the cytoplasm of megakaryocytes occurs due to *megaloblastic anemia, myelodysplastic syndrome and myeloproliferative disorders.*

Increased Platelet Destruction

Increased platelet destruction occurs due to *immune-mediated mechanism, splenomegaly* or *hypersplenism* and *heparin therapy.*

Pooling of Platelets

When the spleen is enlarged, it can pool without destroying a disproportionate amount of the circulating platelets. This pooling results in lowering of the platelet count in the peripheral blood.

THROMBOCYTOPENIAS

IDIOPATHIC THROMBOCYTOPENIC PURPURA

Idiopathic thrombocytopenic purpuras (ITP) are of two variants: acute ITP and chronic ITP. Acute thrombocytopenic purpura is of <6 months duration, while chronic ITP is >6 months duration. *Chronic ITP responds to steroid therapy.* Comparison between acute and chronic ITP is shown in Table 10.4.

ACUTE IDIOPATHIC THROMBOCYTOPENIC PURPURA

Acute ITP (acute idiopathic thrombocytopenic purpura) in *children* typically appears *after a viral illness* during winter and spring season. It most often affects *children* and *young adults.*

Spontaneous recovery can be expected in more than 80% of cases within 6 months. Diagnosis of ITP should be made only after exclusion of other causes of thrombocytopenia.

Pathophysiology

Acute ITP is a quantitative disorder of platelets caused by antibodies (IgG, IgA) directed against platelet membrane glycoproteins (GpIIb/GpIIIa (or) GpIb–IX antigens or megakaryocytic antigens. Platelets are opsonized by autoantibodies.

Opsonized platelets bind to Fc receptors of macrophages and are rapidly destroyed in spleen. T cell mediated cytotoxicity plays a role in platelet destruction. In adults with acute ITP, the platelet count is typically $<20 \times 10^9/L$.

Clinical Features

Patient presents with petechial hemorrhages, ecchymosis, bleeding from the gums and nose, melena, hematuria, excessive menstrual flow, subarachnoid hemorrhage, and intracerebral hemorrhage. There is no significant splenomegaly. Acute idiopathic thrombocytopenic purpura resolves spontaneously. Platelet count and clinical manifestations are shown in Table 10.5.

Hematological Findings

The peripheral blood smear in ITP exhibits reduced platelets, and the bone marrow shows a compensatory increase in megakaryocytes.

Clinical Course

Acute idiopathic thrombocytopenic purpura resolves spontaneously. *Bone marrow aspiration is not indicated in acute ITP.* Approximately 7–28% cases develop chronic ITP.

Table 10.5: Platelet count and clinical manifestations

Platelet count	Severity of bleeding
$>50 \times 10^9/L$	No spontaneous bleeding
$10–50 \times 10^9/L$	Spontaneous bleeding in skin and mucous membrane Post-traumatic bleeding
$<10 \times 10^9/L$	Genitourinary bleeding Gastrointestinal bleeding Intracranial bleeding

Table 10.4: Comparison between acute ITP and chronic ITP

Feature	Acute ITP	Chronic ITP
Age	2–6 years	20–40 years
Sex predilection	1:1	3:1
Antecedent viral infection	Common (1–3 weeks prior to acute or ITP)	Uncommon
Onset	Abrupt	Gradual
Duration	2–8 weeks	Months or years
Spontaneous remission	85–90% cases	Uncommon
Progression	Self-limited	Not so
Hemorrhagic bullae	Common in severe form	Uncommon
Platelet count	$<20 \times 10^9/L$	$40 \times 10^9/L$ to $100 \times 10^9/L$
Eosinophilia and lymphocytosis	Common	Rare
Response to corticosteroids	Variable	Common
Response to splenectomy	Variable	Common

CHRONIC IDIOPATHIC THROMBOCYTOPENIC PURPURA

Chronic idiopathic thrombocytopenic purpura is >6 months duration. It most often affects *women <40 years*. Ratio of female to male is 3:1. Diagnosis is made by excluding platelet deficiency due to systemic lupus erythematosus, AIDS, heparin and drugs.

Pathogenesis

Autoantibodies (mostly IgG) are formed against platelet membrane glycoproteins (GpIIb/IIIa) mostly in the spleen. Opsonized platelets are phagocytosed by monocytes/macrophages. Approximately, 75–85% of patients respond to splenectomy.

Clinical Features

Patient presents with bleeding into the skin (petechial, ecchymosis) and mucosal surface. *Most often there is a long history of easy bruising, epistaxis, bleeding gums and extensive soft tissue hemorrhages* from relatively minor trauma. Patient may also present with malena, hematuria or excessive menstrual flow.

Blood Findings

Hemoglobin is low due to blood loss. In chronic adult ITP, the platelet count varies from a few thousand to $100 \times 10^9/L$. The peripheral blood smear in chronic ITP exhibits few *large platelets* and *microcytic hypochromic picture* (Fig. 10.7). Mean platelet volume is increased in large platelets. Platelet width increases.

Bleeding and Coagulation Parameters

Bleeding time is increased with normal clotting time. Clot retraction is decreased. Prothrombin and activated thromboplastin time is within normal range.

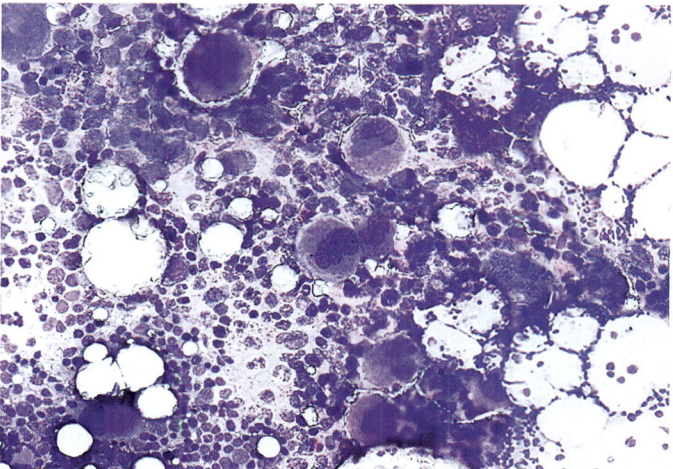

Fig. 10.8: Chronic idiopathic thrombocytopenia. Bone marrow aspirate shows marked hyperplasia of megakaryocytes. Borders of megakaryocytes are smooth indicating nonfunctional megakaryocytes.

Bone Marrow

Bone marrow shows increased cellularity due to compensatory hyperplasia of megakaryocytes (immature and mature) and accelerated thrombopoiesis and abnormal megakaryocytes.

Normoblastic or micronormoblastic erythropoiesis is seen. Myelopoiesis is normal. Iron stores are depleted with severe bleeding demonstrated by Perl's stain (Fig. 10.8).

Other Tests

Glycoprotein immobilization assays are performed for antiplatelet antibodies. Plasma level of glycocalicin is high. Thrombopoietin is not increased. *Evans' syndrome is characterized by thrombocytopenia, autoimmune hemolytic anemia and positive Coombs' test.*

Management

Patient with platelet count $>20 \times 10^9/L$ need no treatment. *Corticosteroids are first choice of treatment.* Immunosuppressive drugs are administered in patients not responding to corticosteroid therapy.

Administration of immunoglobulin temporarily enhance platelet counts. Elective splenomegaly is beneficial in patients, who do not respond to corticosteroid therapy.

SECONDARY THROMBOCYTOPENIA

Secondary thrombocytopenia occurs in the course of systemic disorders such as systemic lupus erythematosus, drug induced, hypoplasia of megakaryocytes, splenomegaly, abnormal pooling of platelets and thrombotic thrombocytopenic purpura.

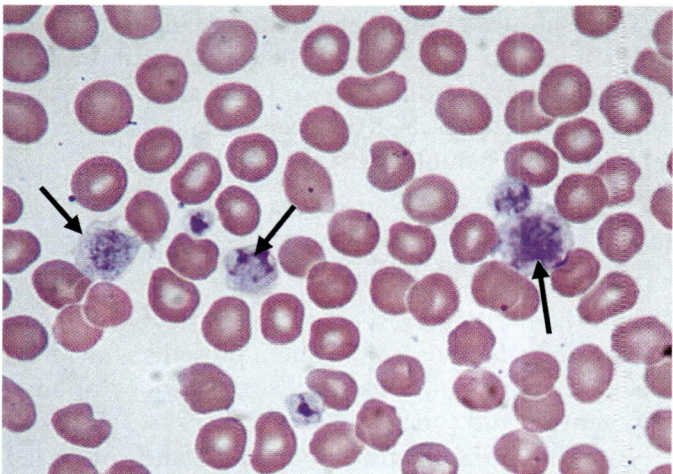

Fig. 10.7: Thrombocytopenia. Peripheral blood smear shows lack of platelets and a few giant platelets (arrows).

SYSTEMIC LUPUS ERYTHEMATOSUS

Systemic lupus erythematosus is an autoimmune disorder involving multiple systems such as blood vessels, glomeruli and joints. *Anti-DNA antibodies are formed against endogenous (self) antigen.* Antibodies coat the platelets and cause destruction resulting in secondary thrombocytopenia.

DRUG INDUCED THROMBOCYTOPENIA

Sometimes a drug or its metabolite such as *benzylpenicillin may* bind firmly to the cell surface to give a highly immunogenic epitope.

Individuals produce IgG cytotoxic autoantibodies to their own drug coated platelets resulting in their destruction in the spleen. Various drugs inducing secondary thrombocytopenia are *quinine, chlorothiazide and heparin therapy* (10%).

HEPARIN INDUCED THROMBOCYTOPENIA SYNDROME

HIT Syndrome (Type I)

Heparin induced thrombocytopenia syndrome (type I) *results in a mild to moderate drop in platelets within a day of heparin therapy.* It is not immunomediated disorder. Heparin induced thrombocytopenia syndrome is reduced by administration of low-molecular-weight heparin preparations.

HIT Syndrome (Type II)

Heparin induced thrombocytopenia syndrome (type II) leads to a *severe drop in platelets (often <50% of baseline) within 5 to 10 days after heparin therapy.* It is immuno-mediated disorder.

Therapeutic administration of unfractionated heparin induces formation of anti-PF4 antibodies, *which bind to molecular complexes of heparin and platelet factor IV membrane protein.* These antibodies can also bind to platelets and vascular endothelium resulting in prothrombotic state. Once type II HIT has been diagnosed, further heparin treatment is contraindicated.

ABNORMAL POOLING OF PLATELETS

When the spleen is distinctively enlarged, it can pool without destroying a disproportionate amount of circulating platelets. This pooling of platelets in the enlarged spleen results in lowering of the platelets count in the peripheral blood.

HYPOPLASIA OF MEGAKARYOCYTES

Hypoplasia of megakaryocytes may occur due to drugs, toxic chemical agents and following viral infection. Bone marrow is deficient in megakaryocytes, but shows normal erythropoiesis and myelopoiesis.

THROMBOTIC THROMBOCYTOPENIC PURPURA

Thrombotic thrombocytopenic purpura is a rapidly fulminating disorder. Bacteria induced endothelial injury causes release of von Willebrand factor resulting in *widespread thrombosis in the arterioles* and capillaries leading to tissue and organ ischemia.

An enzyme disintegrin-like and metalloproteinase with thrombospondin motifs 13(ADAMTS 13) has been involved in its pathogenesis by cleavage of vWF. Binding of vWF to platelets are prevented by ADAMTS 13. Acquired TTP is seen in >99% cases.

Clinical Features

Patient presents with fever, bleeding manifestations, pain abdomen, impairment renal functions, seizures and subsequent coma. It is important cause of flea bitten kidney.

Hematological Findings

Platelet count ranges between $5 \times 10^9/L$ and $100 \times 10^9/L$. Peripheral blood smear shows *schistocytes*. Reticulocyte count is increased. Urine analysis shows *proteinuria* and *hematuria*. Coombs' test is negative.

HEMOLYTIC UREMIC SYNDROME

Hemolytic uremic syndrome (HUS) is characterized by *hemolytic anemia* (anemia caused by destruction of red blood cells), *acute kidney failure (uremia), and a low platelet count*. Ingestion of contaminated food with *Shiga toxin strain of Escherichia coli* is most important cause of hemolytic uremic syndrome.

Toxin induced endothelial injury leads to thrombi formation in arterioles and capillaries. Patient presents with hemorrhagic diarrhea and rapidly progressive renal failure. Comparison between thrombotic thrombocytopenia and hemolytic uremic syndrome is shown in Table 10.6.

DENGUE HEMORRHAGIC FEVER

Dengue hemorrhagic fever is caused by flavivirus transmitted by Aedes mosquito. Patient presents with fever, bleeding manifestations due to thrombocytopenia, hypotension and shock.

There is impaired thrombopoiesis and increased platelet destruction in these cases. *Diagnosis is confirmed by dengue hemagglutination inhibition antibody titre.*

Hematological Findings

Platelet count is low ranging between $5 \times 10^9/L$ and $80 \times 10^9/L$. Peripheral blood smear shows many transformed lymphocytes and giant platelets.

Management

Dengue hemorrhagic fever is treated by platelets transfusion, intravenous fluids and hydrotherapy.

Immature platelet fraction (IPF) that contains RNA particles are assessed by automated counters. Immature platelet fraction is decreased in hypoplastic bone marrow and increased in active bone marrow. IPF % can be used to evaluate the recovery of platelets in patients with dengue. It can be used as a guide for decisions concerning platelet transfusions.

Table 10.6: Comparison between thrombotic thrombocytopenia and hemolytic uremic syndrome

Features	Thrombotic thrombocytopenia (TTP)	Hemolytic uremic syndrome (HUS)
Age predilection	Adults (20–40 years)	Children <5 years of age
Etiology	Severe deficiency of ADAMTS 13	Infection by *Escherichia coli* O157:H7 (in typical HUS)
Thrombocytopenia	Present	Absent
Microangiopathic hemolytic anemia	Present	Absent
Renal manifestations	Uncommon Mild renal dysfunction	Common Acute renal failure
Neurologic abnormalities	Common Severe CNS symptoms	Uncommon Mild CNS symptoms
Fever	Present	Absent
Bloody diarrhea	Absent	Present
Coagulation tests	Normal	Normal
Management	Plasma exchange	Supportive

PLATELET FUNCTION DISORDERS

Dysfunction of platelets leads to defective hemostatic plug. The dysfunction of platelets may be either acquired or inherited is shown in Table 10.7. Inherited platelet function disorders are shown in Table 10.8.

Table 10.7: Classification of platelet function disorders

Categories	Examples
Inherited platelet function disorders	
Defects in platelet membrane	Bernard-Soulier syndrome Thrombasthenia (Glanzmann's disease)
von Willebrand factor defect	von Willebrand disease
Storage organelle deficiency	Storage pool disease, Chédiak-Higashi syndrome, gray platelet syndrome
Acquired platelet function disorders	
Drugs	Aspirin (inhibits prostaglandins synthesis) Nonsteroidal anti-inflammatory drugs (indomethacin, butazolidin and sulfinpyrazone) Miscellaneous platelet function inhibitors (carbenicillin, dipyridamole, phenothiazines, tricyclic antidepressants) Plasma expanders (dextran or hydroxyethyl starch) coat platelets
Dysproteinemias	Multiple myeloma (paraproteins coat platelets) Waldenström's syndrome (paraproteins coat platelets)
Myeloproliferative disorders/MDS	Chronic myelogenous leukemia, polycythemia vera and myelofibrosis
Miscellaneous hematological disorders	Disseminated intravascular coagulation Hemolytic uremic syndrome Thrombotic thrombocytopenic purpura

Table 10.8: Inherited platelet function disorders

Disorder	Autosomal dominant/recessive	Platelets aggregation	Other features
Bernard-Soulier syndrome	Autosomal recessive	Deficient with ADP, epinephrine, collagen, and arachidonic acid. Normal with ristocetin	Severe bleeding, small and discrete platelets, defective clot retraction
Glanzmann's disease (thrombasthenia)	Autosomal recessive	Normal with ADP, epinephrine, collagen, and arachidonic acid. Deficient with ristocetin	Severe bleeding and giant platelets in smear
von Willebrand disease	Autosomal dominant/recessive	Normal with ADP, epinephrine, collagen, and arachidonic acid. Deficient with ristocetin	Abnormality of platelets aggregation corrected by cryoprecipitate

BERNARD-SOULIER SYNDROME

Patient with inherited *deficiency of von Willebrand factor (vWF)* or platelet-surface glycoprotein receptors (GpIb) results in defective platelets adhesion and bleeding tendencies, known as *Bernard-Soulier syndrome*. It is autosomal recessive disorder. Patient presents with bruising, epistaxis and gingival bleeding at an early age.

Hematological Findings

Peripheral blood smear shows mild thrombocytopenia and giant platelets. There is defective clot retraction. Platelets aggregation studies demonstrate defective aggregation with ristocetin, but normal with ADP, epinephrine, collagen, and arachidonic acid.

THROMBASTHENIA (GLANZMANN'S DISEASE)

Congenital deficiency of GpIIb–IIIa receptors is known as *Glanzmann disease* or *thrombasthenia*. It is an autosomal recessive disorder. *Normally, GpIIb–IIIa act as receptor for fibrinogen bridging between adjacent platelets resulting in aggregation of platelets.* Patient presents with bleeding tendencies like gum bleeding and petechiae hemorrhages. Platelet count and morphology are essentially normal.

Hematological Findings

Platelets aggregation studies demonstrate defective aggregation with ristocetin, but normal with ADP, epinephrine, collagen, and arachidonic acid.

VON WILLEBRAND DISEASE

This autosomal dominant/recessive disorder occurs due to *deficiency of vWF resulting in defective aggregation of platelets to collagen. It is corrected by cryoprecipitate.* Factor VIIIc is also decreased. Patient presents with *mucosal bleeding* with hemophilia like coagulation defect. *Platelets aggregation studies demonstrate defective aggregation with ristocetin, but normal with ADP, epinephrine, collagen, and arachidonic acid.*

WISKOTT-ALDRICH SYNDROME

Wiskott-Aldrich syndrome is X-linked disorder associated with defects of both B cell and T cell functions. Wiskott-Aldrich syndrome protein (WASP) gene mutation encoding WASP expressed on cells of hematopoietic system. T cells and platelets show absence of certain surface glycoproteins (CD43), which are ligand for intercellular adhesion molecule ICAM-1. *Patient has low IgM level* due to poor response to polysaccharide antigen. IgA and IgE concentrations are raised. IgG level remain within normal range. Half-life of platelets is reduced.

Clinical Features

Patient presents with *eczema, thrombocytopenia, bloody diarrhea, recurrent infections* and *poor antibody response to polysaccharide antigens*. Patient has *fatal outcome before six years of age* due to bleeding, infection or malignancy (*most often lymphoma*).

Management

These patients have WASP gene mutation encoding WASP protein. These patients may be treated by stem cell transplantation.

DRUGS INDUCED PLATELET DYSFUNCTION

Many drugs induce platelet dysfunction. *Aspirin, indomethacin, butazolidin and sulfinpyrazone inhibit platelets aggregation by inhibiting platelet thromboxane A_2 and $PGE2_\alpha$ by blocking cyclooxygenase pathway.* Administration of low dose of aspirin prevents platelets aggregation lasting for 3–4 days.

Plasma expander dextran interferes with platelet function, probably by coating the platelets. Miscellaneous platelet function inhibitor includes carbenicillin, dipyridamole, clofibrate, phenothiazine, tricyclic antidepressants and certain general anesthetics.

DYSPARAPROTEINEMIAS AND UREMIA

Acquired platelet dysfunction has been most often associated with dysproteinemias such as multiple myeloma and Waldenstrom's macroglobulinemia, which coat the platelets resulting in platelet dysfunction. Metabolic products accumulated in uremia also impair platelet function.

MYELODYSPLASTIC SYNDROMES/DISORDERS

Thrombocytosis is defined as platelet count >450 × 100^9/L. When the thrombocytosis represents a primary disorder of bone marrow, it is known as thrombocythemia. Platelet count in thrombocythemia is >1000 × 100^9/L.

Platelet production in these cases are autonomous. Thrombocythemia may be part of chronic myelogenous leukemia, polycythemia vera and myelofibrosis. Patient with thrombocythemia presents with both arterial or venous thrombotic problems as well as hemorrhagic complications due to defective platelet function.

VASCULAR PURPURA

Vascular purpuras are congenital or acquired disorders of blood vessels resulting in bleeding. These disorders should be differentiated from thrombocytopenic purpura and platelet function disorders.

Classification of vascular purpuras is shown in Table 10.9.

SCURVY

Vitamin C participates in the synthesis of collagen and reticulin fibrils from mucopolysaccharide ground substance in wound healing. Deficiency of vitamin C is known as *scurvy*, in which there is defective formation of mesenchymal tissue and osteoid matrix.

Clinical features: Patient presents with *hemorrhages in mucocutaneous and muscles along fascial planes due to capillary fragility*. Insufficient production of osteoid matrix results in cartilaginous overgrowth, *widening of epiphysis, bowing of the long bones* and chest deformity.

Osteoporosis is seen especially at the metaphyseal ends of bone. Other findings are gingival swelling and periodontal infection, impaired wound healing, impaired localization of focal infections and anemia.

HENOCH-SCHÖNLEIN PURPURA

Henoch-Schönlein purpura is the most common type of childhood immune complex-mediated vasculitis in the age group 4–11 years. The glomerular lesion is identical with that of IgA nephropathy.

Etiopathogenesis

This disorder may be precipitated by exogenous antigens such as *drugs, foods, or upper respiratory infections*. IgA deposition occurs in vessel of skin often similar to IgA nephropathy in >50% cases.

Clinical Features

Patient presents with *nephritic syndrome and skin rashes on extensor surfaces of the arms, legs, and buttocks, painful joints, gastrointestinal involvement (colicky abdominal pain with malena)*. Most patients do well, but a few progress to end stage renal disease. In adults, a rapidly progressive (crescentic) glomerulonephritis can occur.

SENILE PURPURA

Senile purpura occurs in elderly persons. There is atrophy of collagen fibers in the dermis with advancing

Table 10.9: Classification of vascular purpuras

Etiology	Disorders
Inherited etiology	Hereditary hemorrhagic telangiectasia, Ehlers-Danlos syndrome, Marfan's syndrome, osteogenesis imperfecta, Fabry's syndrome
Infections	Bacteria, viruses and rickettsiae
Allergic	Henoch-Schölein syndrome, drugs, food
Atrophic collagenous tissue	Senile purpura, Cushing's syndrome, corticosteroid therapy, and scurvy purpura
Miscellaneous	Simple easy bruising, autoerythrocytic sensitization, fat embolism, dysproteinemia

age. Patient presents with purpura, ecchymosis on the back of neck, extensor aspect of forearms and legs.

SIMPLE BRUISING

Simple bruising is most often demonstrated in the women on arms and legs.

These purpuras resolve rapidly. Hemostatic tests are within normal range.

HEREDITARY HEMORRHAGIC TELANGIECTASIA

Ataxia hemorrhagic telangiectasia is *autosomal recessive* trait associated with *chromosomal breakages.* There is increased risk of development of malignant neoplasm especially lymphomas.

Patient presents with epistaxis, bright red spots on the face, lips, nose, flexor surface of forearms and conjunctiva, cerebellar degeneration and spinocerebellar atrophy (choreoathetoid movements) and recurrent infections of respiratory tract. Plasma levels of IgA and IgE are decreased. Bleeding from these malformed blood vessels in gastric mucosa may cause gastrointestinal hemorrhages resulting in iron deficiency anemia.

MARFAN'S SYNDROME

Marfan's syndrome is an autosomal dominant disorder of connective tissue. It is characterized by changes in skeleton, eyes and CVS. It occurs due to *missense mutations of the fibrillin gene 1 (FGN1)* on chromosome 15. Fibrillin is a family of connective tissue proteins analogous to the collagens.

Patient presents with *hyperflexibility of joints due to elastic tissue abnormality, dislocation of the ocular lens in both eyes and life-threatening complications are aortic aneurysm and aortic dissection.*

EHLERS-DANLOS SYNDROME

Ehlers-Danlos syndrome may show *autosomal dominant* or *sex-linked recessive* inheritance of collagen fibers. There is generalized defect in collagen fibers, molecular structure, synthesis, secretion, and degradation.

Patient presents with symptoms due to *abnormal collagen in the skin, joint and blood vessels.* Bleeding diathesis occurs as a result of fragile skin. *Hypermobility of joints is common finding.*

CHAPTER 11

Coagulation Disorders

Learning Objectives

INHERITED AND ACQUIRED COAGULATION DISORDERS
- Overview of Coagulation Factors
- Hemophilia A
- Hemophilia B
- von Willebrand Disease
- Disseminated Intravascular Coagulation
- Hemorrhagic Disease of Newborn
- Coagulation Disorders in Hepatic Disease

THROMBOPHILIA (HYPERCOAGULABLE STATE)
- Hereditary Hypercoagulable State
- Acquired Hypercoagulable State

CLINICAL ASPECTS OF BLEEDING DIATHESIS
- Platelet Function Tests

INHERITED AND ACQUIRED COAGULATION DISORDERS

OVERVIEW OF COAGULATION FACTORS

Vitamin K is essential for synthesis of coagulation factors II, VII, IX and X by liver. These coagulation factors are present in inactive form. *Liver enzyme reductase converts inactive coagulation factors to active form. On the other hand, enzyme epoxide has opposite function by converting active to inactive coagulation factors.*

Oral anticoagulants inhibit reductase enzyme in liver, thus active vitamin K is not available to synthesize II, VII, IX and X protein C and protein S. Coagulation factors are shown in Table 11.1.

CALCIUM

The binding of calcium to vitamin K-dependent II, VII, IX, X factors is required for normal clotting. *Without attached calcium, these factors will not bind phospholipids and thus rate of activation will be sharply reduced.* Inactive precursor coagulation factor contains glutamyl residue.

This precursor coagulation factor becomes functional by addition of carboxyl group from HCO_3 with the help of carboxylase enzyme. Calcium binds glutamyl residue if carboxyl group is added to the functional factor.

HEMOPHILIA A

Normal factor VIII is essential for blood clotting. Gene encoding *factor VIII* is located on tip of the long arm of the *X chromosome*. Hemophilia A is an *X-linked recessive disorder* of blood clotting. It results from mutation in the gene encoding factor VIII. *Patient* presents with *spontaneous bleeding into joints, muscles, and internal organs.*

INHERITANCE

As males have only one X chromosome. Hence, defective VIII gene leads to decreased synthesis of factor VIII resulting in hemophilia. *Heterozygous females are carriers, which transmit the disease to the male progeny.* It is clinically indistinguishable from hemophilia B (factor IX deficiency). *The family pedigree of Queen Victoria shows a number of hemophilic descendents as she was a carrier of the disease.* In females, the other normal X chromosome corrects the abnormality, but females can be asymptomatic carriers. *In males, the disease is expressed because there is no normal X chromosome to correct the abnormality.* Family trees in a case of hemophilia are shown in Figs 11.1 and 11.2.

Table 11.1: Coagulation factors

Factor	Synonyms	Site of synthesis in body	Inheritance incidence	Deficiency affects	Therapy and half-life of infused factor
I	Fibrinogen	Liver	Autosomal recessive (rare)	Both sexes	Cryoprecipitate, fresh frozen plasma, fibrinogen (96–144 hours)
II	Prothrombin	Liver (vitamin K dependent)	Autosomal recessive (rare)	Both sexes	Fresh frozen plasma, factors II, VII, IX, X concentrate (50–80 hours)
III	Tissue extract (thromboplastin)	-	-	-	-
IV	Calcium	-	-	-	-
V	Labile factor	Liver (vitamin K dependent)	Autosomal recessive	Both sexes	Fresh frozen plasma (24 hours)
VI	Not assigned	-	-	-	-
VII	Stable factor	Liver (vitamin K dependent)	Autosomal recessive	Both sexes	Factors II, VII, IX, X concentrate in plasma (4–6 hours)
VIII	Antihemophilic globulin A	Liver, spleen, kidneys	Sex-linked recessive	Male affected (1 in 3000) (female career)	Factor VIII concentrate, cryoprecipitate, fresh frozen plasma (12 hours)
IX	Christmas factor (antihemophilic factor B)	Liver (vitami K dependent)	Sex-linked recessive (1 in 20,000)	Male affected (female career)	Factors II, VII, IX, X concentrate (20–30 hours)
X	Stuart-Prower factor	Liver (vitamin K dependent)	Autosomal recessive (rare)	Both sexes	Factors II, VII, IX, X concentrate in plasma
XI	Plasma thromboplastin antecedent, (antihemophilic factor C)	Unknown	Autosomal dominant (rare)	Both sexes	Plasma (40–84 hours)
XII	Hageman factor	Unknown	Autosomal recessive (rare)	Both sexes	Treatment not required
XIII	Fibrin stabilizing factor	Unknown	Autosomal recessive? (rare)	Both sexes	Plasma (150 hours)
-	von Willebrand factor (factor vWF antigen assay)	Endothelial cells	Autosomal dominant	Both sexes	DDAVP, cryoprecipitate, fresh frozen plasma, whole blood (24 hours)

Prekallikrein: Fletcher factor
Kininogen (high MW): Fitzerald factor

FACTOR VIII (ANTIHEMOPHILIC GLOBULIN)

Factor VIII gene encoding factor VIII glycoprotein is located on X chromosome. Factor VIII gene comprises A1, A2, B, A3, C1 and C2 domains. First 19 amino acids of protein sequence comprise secretory leader peptide of precursor factor VIII. Factor B domain is cleaved off during activation. *Most of the 23 cysteine residues of mature factor VIII are located in A and C domains.*

POSSIBLE SITES OF SYNTHESIS

Possible sites of synthesis of factor VIII are *liver, spleen, bone marrow and kidney*. Its concentration in plasma is 0.1 mg/dl with half-life of 5–12 hours. On starch electrophoresis, it migrates as α-globulin. Factor VIII solvents of high ionic strength such as NaCl and $CaCl_2$ form high MW fractions (VIIIAg and vWF) and low MW (VIIIc).

Coagulation Disorders 11

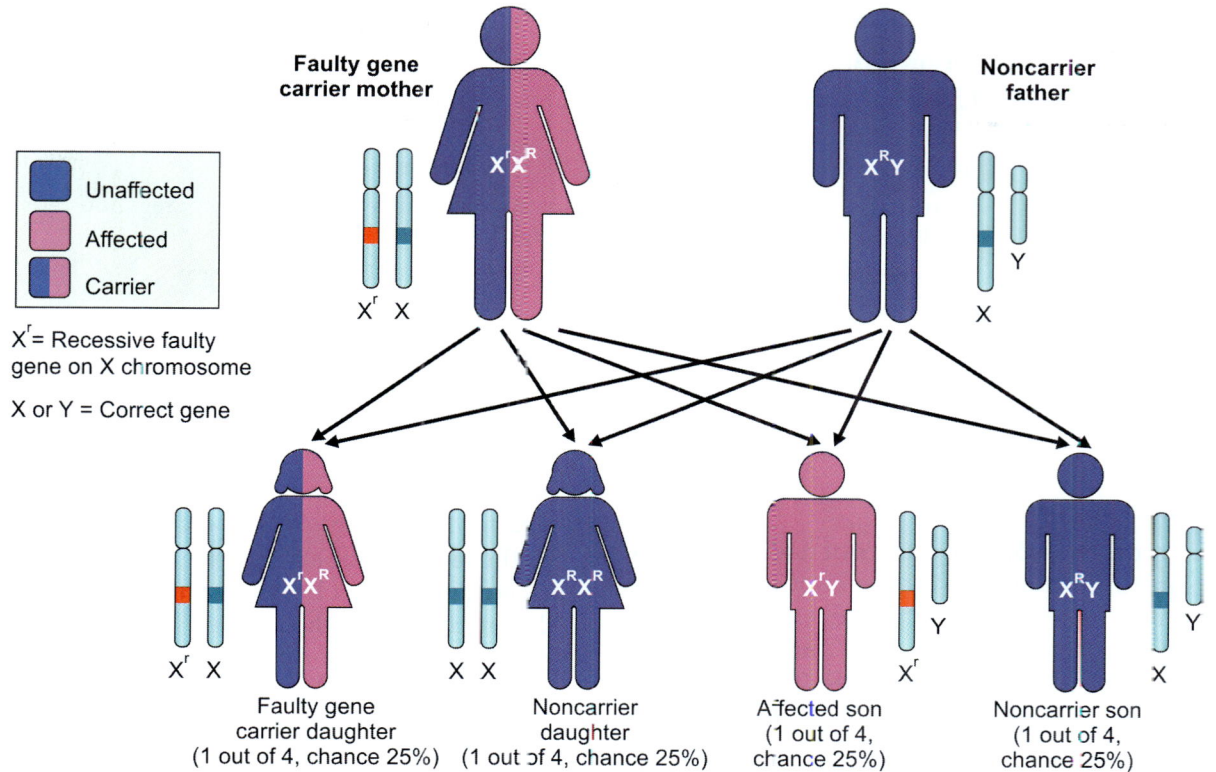

Fig. 11.1: Family tree in a case of hemophilia, where mother is faulty gene carrier and noncarrier father. Chances of hemophilia in their children are shown.

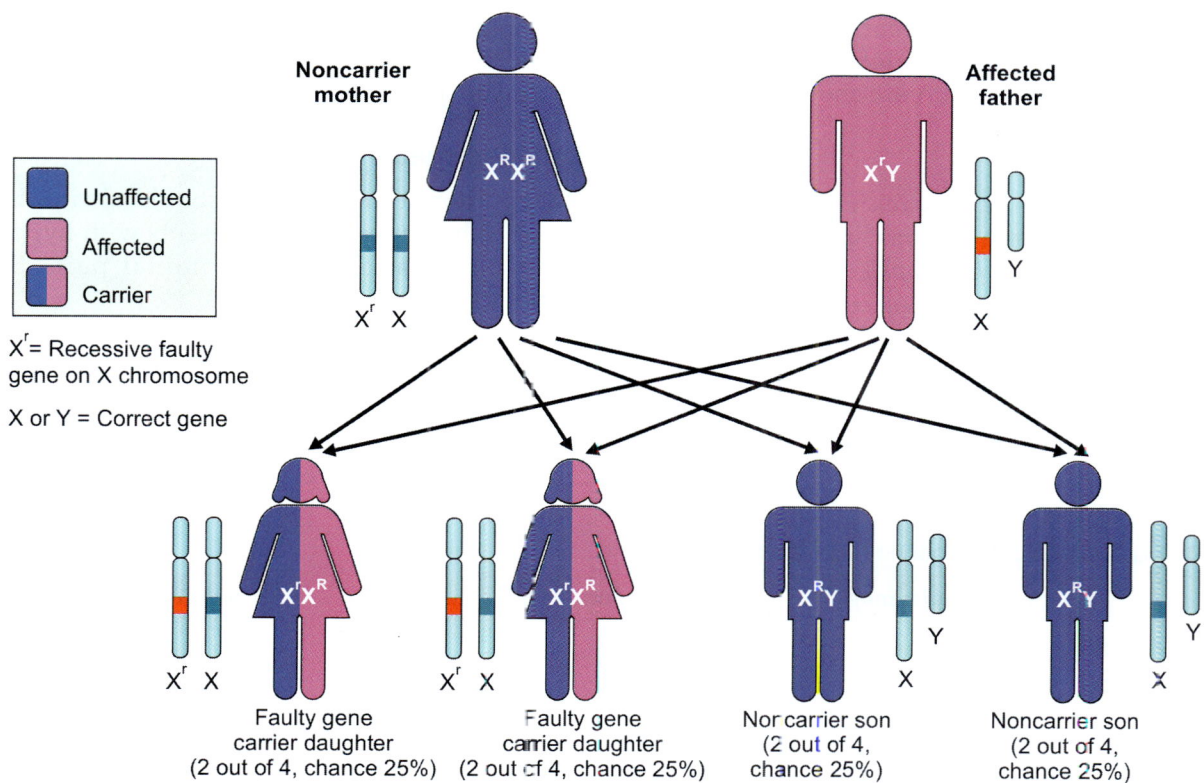

Fig. 11.2: Family tree in a case of hemophilia, where mother is noncarrier and father with faulty gene carrier. Chances of hemophilia in their children are shown.

Table 11.2: Comparison of subunits factor VIII (VIIIc and vWF)

Parameters	Factor VIIIc	vWF
Possible sites of synthesis	Liver (most common site), spleen, bone marrow and kidney	Endothelial cells and megakaryocytes
Gene control	X-linked gene	Chromosome 12
Function	Participates in intrinsic coagulation pathway resulting in formation of hemostatic plug	Platelets adhesion (aggregation by ristocetin *in vitro*)
Deficiency	Hemophilia	von Willebrand disease

Normal plasma adsorbed with barium salts removes factor IX and not VIII, which will correct APTT. Serum contains factor IX but not VIII. Comparison of subunits factor VIII (VIIIc and vWF) is shown in Table 11.2.

Severity of Hemophilia A

Depending on the concentration of factor VIII in comparison to normal activity, hemophilia A cases are categorized as severe factor VIII level deficiency of (<1%), moderate factor VIII level (1–5%) and mild factor VIII level (6–25%) of hormonal range. Classification of hemophilia A depending on severity is shown in Table 11.3.

CLINICAL FEATURES

Patient presents with hemorrhage from minor wounds and trauma, bleeding from oral mucosa, hematuria, and bleeding into joints. Recurrent hemarthroses can lead to progressive crippling deformities. Clinical manifestations of hemophilia A are shown in Fig. 11.3.

Hemarthrosis

Hemarthrosis is the most common event, which can be spontaneous or with trauma. *Joints involved* in hemophilia include *knee, elbow, ankle, wrist, shoulder, hip* and *temporomandibular joints*. Repeated bouts of bleeding lead to the joint destruction resulting in *deformities in weight-bearing joints*.

Joints are swollen, tender and painful. Approximately 400 units of factor VIII are administered by intravenous route.

Soft Tissue Bleeding

Soft tissue bleeding is the second most bleeding manifestation occurring *between fascial planes* such as *retropharyngeal region, oral cavity* and between *two heads of gastrocnemius muscles. To avoid pain, the patient hyperextends the ankle to shorten the gastrocnemius muscles.*

If these patients are not treated, gastrocnemius muscles deformities becomes chronic and the patient walks on the toes of the affected legs. *The classic Equine gait is often the first orthopedics event.* Approximately 300–400 units of factor VIII are administered by intravenous route.

Genitourinary System Bleeding

Nontraumatic spontaneous *genitourinary bleeding without a structural lesion* is encountered in hemophilics. *Epsilon aminocaproic* acid is usually administered in hemophilic to prevent lysis of blood clots. But this drug is *contraindicated in patients with genitourinary bleeding for the fear of causing obstructive uropathy from blood clots.*

Retroperitoneal Hemorrhage

Retroperitoneal hemorrhage should always be considered in hemophilic, who presents with hypotension, tachycardia and mild abdominal pain. Surgical exploration is not indicated.

Gastrointestinal Tract Bleeding

Gastrointestinal tract bleeding is associated with a *structural lesion* in contrast to genitourinary bleeding. Traumatic bleeding occurs following tonsillectomy

Table 11.3: Classification of hemophilia A depending on severity

Parameters	Severe deficiency	Moderate deficiency	Mild deficiency
Factor VIII activity	<1%	1–5%	6–25%
Frequency	15%	15%	70%
Onset	Newborn	Children	Adolescents and young persons
Clinical features	Spontaneous frequent episodes of severe bleeding especially in joints	Bleeding episodes on slight injury with joint bleeding in some cases	Post-surgical severe bleeding (joint involvement rare)

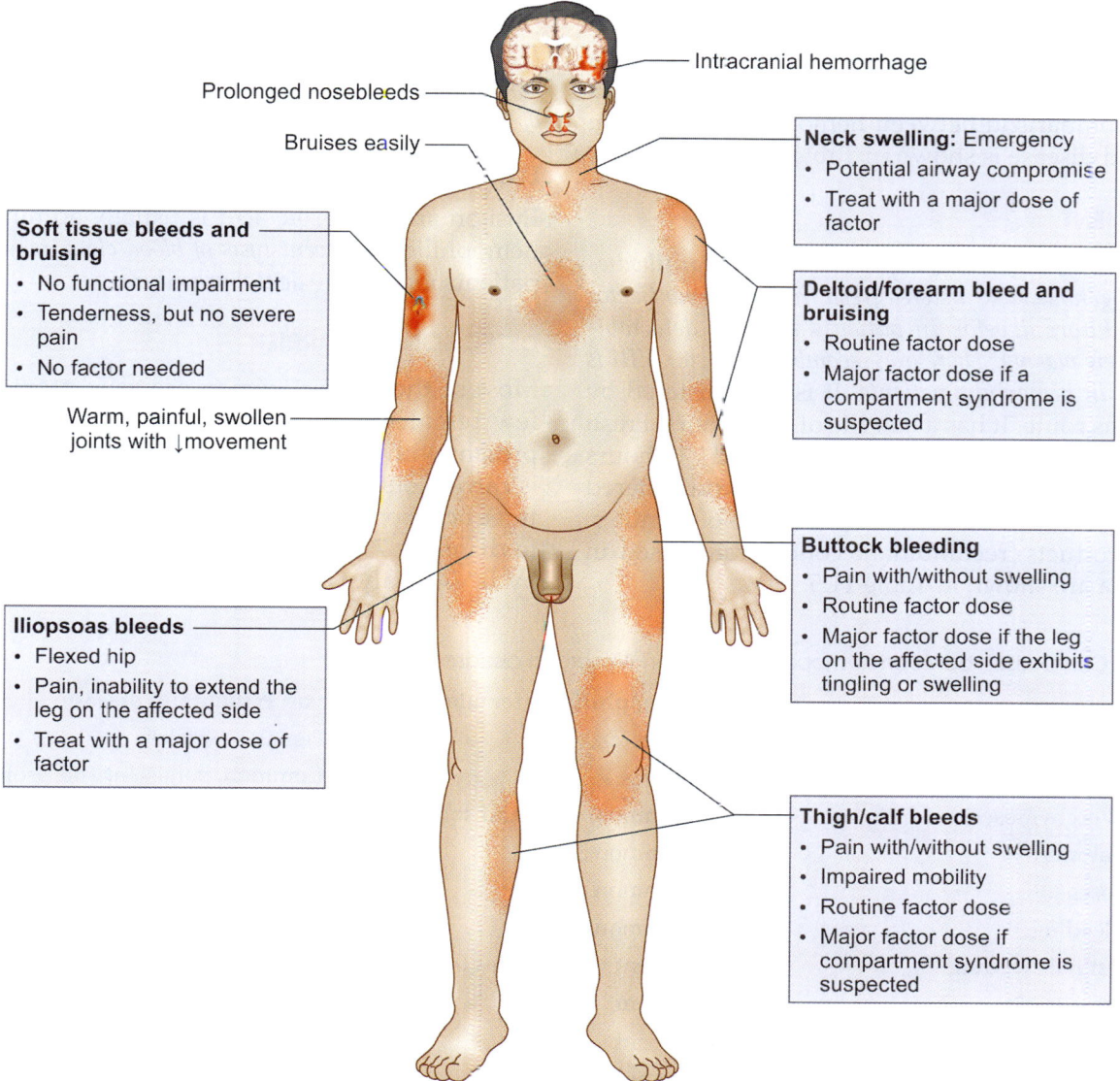

Fig. 11.3: Clinical manifestations of hemophilia A.

and tooth extraction. Approximately 300–400 units of factor VIII are administered by intravenous route.

Delayed Wound Healing

Delayed wound healing occurs due to intermittent bleeding and infection.

Dental Procedures

In normal persons, bleeding persists for 12 hours after dental procedures. But bleeding persists for 3 days in hemophilic patients. Factor VIII should be administered to control bleeding.

LABORATORY DIAGNOSIS

Bleeding and prothrombin time are within normal range. Platelet count and functions are normal.

Clotting Time and APTT

Clotting time is prolonged. In both forms of hemophilia, *activated partial thromboplastin time (APTT) is prolonged.* Mixing of a patient's blood with that of a normal donor normalizes the APTT.

Normal APTT is 30–35 seconds. APTT measures intrinsic pathway of coagulation based on factors XI, IX, VIII, X, V, prothrombin and fibrinogen. Phospholipid is added to plasma and clotting is observed. Phospholipid is a part of thromboplastin. Therefore, test is known as *activated partial thromboplastin time.*

Factor VIII Assay

Factor VIII assay is analyzed to assess severity of disease.

DIFFERENTIAL DIAGNOSIS

Hemophilia A should be differentiated from hemophilia B (factor IX deficiency) and severe von Willebrand disease. Comparison between hemophilia A and von Willebrand disease is shown in Table 11.4.

MANAGEMENT

Approximately, 6–12% hemophiliacs develop antibodies against exogenous administered fresh frozen plasma (factor VIII). Inhibitors develop in patients with no detectable factor in their plasma. Therefore, recombinant factor VIII is being used in hemophilic patients. It is administered by intravenous route. It has a half life of 8–12 hours. Fresh frozen plasma is prepared from fresh blood <12 hours old. It is stored at –20°C for one year. It is administered in the dose 7–15 ml/kg body weight for 30–60 minutes. Plasma products/recombinant concentrates used in hemophilia are shown in Table 11.5.

DDAVP

DDAVP (D-amino-delta-D-arginine vasopressin) hormone preparation is administered *to enhance activity of factor VIII in mild hemophilic patients.*

Epsilon Aminocaproic Acid (EACA)

Epsilon aminocaproic acid is usually administered in hemophilic to *prevent lysis of blood clots* in hemophilic patients *undergoing dental procedures.*

DETECTION OF CARRIER

Most of the carrier women are asymptomatic. Only few females with very low factor VIII levels may present with menorrhagia. Accurate family tree study is carried out. Clotting profile should be estimated on three occasions by analyzing factors VIII, IX and VWAg to diagnose 75% cases. Exact detection is carried out by DNA analysis. Heterozygous women carriers are

Table 11.4: Comparison between hemophilia A and von Willebrand disease

Finding	Hemophilia A (female carrier)	von Willebrand disease
Sex	Males	Females > males
Skin and mucous membrane bleeding	Rare	Common, persistent and profuse
Superficial ecchymoses	Common; large and solitary	Small and multiple
Deep hematoma	Common	Rare
Hemarthroses	Common	Rare
Delayed bleeding	Common	Rare
Gastrointestinal bleeding	Present with GIT lesions	Present
Hematuria	Present	Present
Epistaxis	Present	Present
Gingival bleeding	Present	Present
Excessive bleeding after tooth extraction	Present	Present
Intracranial bleeding	Present	Present
Bleeding time	Normal	Increased
Clotting time	Increased	Increased
Prothrombin time	Normal	Normal
APTT	Increased	Increased
Factor VIII assay	Decreased	Normal or decreased
vWF ristocetin cofactor assay	Normal	Decreased

Table 11.5: Plasma products/recombinant concentrates used in hemophilia

Plasma products/recombinant concentrates	Indications for use
Human factor VIII	Hemophilia A, von Willebrand disease
Human factor VIII (high purity)	Hemophilia A especially with HIV infection
Recombinant factor VIII	Hemophilia A
Porcine factor VIII	Factor VIII inhibitors
Activated prothrombin complex concentrates	Factor VIII inhibitors

diagnosed by PCR-RFLP or Southern blotting to detect intron 12 inversion.

HEMOPHILIA B

Hemophilia B is also known as *Christmas disease*. Hemophilia B is an *X-linked recessive disease* caused by *mutations in the F9 gene encoding factor IX*. It affects 1 in 40,000 males. It accounts for 15% of hemophilia cases. One-third of all cases represent new mutations. It is clinically indistinguishable from hemophilia A (factor VIII deficiency).

CLINICAL FEATURES

Patient presents with mild clinical manifestations such as hemarthrosis during 5–15 years of age.

LABORATORY DIAGNOSIS

In both forms of hemophilia A and B, the activated partial thromboplastin time (APTT) is prolonged. Mixing of a patient's blood with that of a normal donor normalizes the APTT. Prothrombin time is within normal range. *Activated plasma thromboplastin time is increased (normal 30–40 seconds)*. Thromboplastin generation time is performed to differentiate factor VIII from factor IX deficiency.

VON WILLEBRAND DISEASE

von Willebrand disease is an *autosomal dominant disorder* associated with *reduced quantity of circulating vWF*. It is a common hereditary bleeding disorder in humans. It has *three types (I, II, III). Type I von Willebrand* disease is the *most common variant (70% cases)* disorder. Majority inherited as incompletely dominant autosomal trait with variable penetrance. One subtype is autosomal recessive. Variants of von Willebrand's disease are shown in Table 11.6.

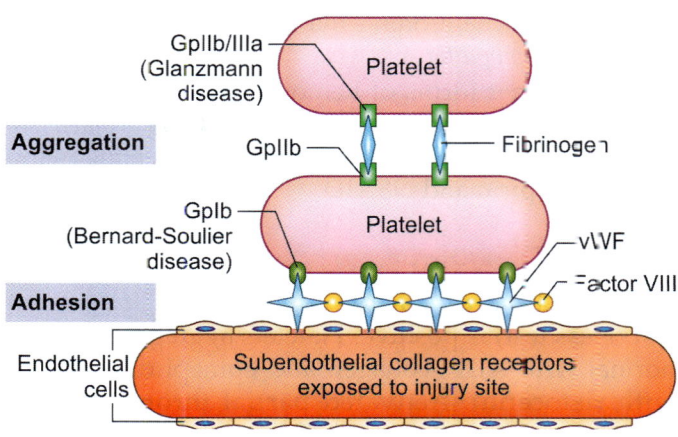

Fig. 11.4: vWF and factor VIII complex showing platelets aggregation on exposed subendothelial tissue.

SYNTHESIS OF vWF AND FACTOR VIII

von Willebrand factor is synthesized by *endothelial cells (major source)* and megakaryocytes under control of gene on chromosome 12. Coagulation factor VIII is synthesized in the liver under control of gene located on tip of the long arm of the X chromosome.

vWF and Factor VIII Complex

Both factors VIII (10%) and vWF (90%) form complex and circulate in the plasma to promote blood clotting and the interaction with vessel wall and platelets resulting in *hemostatic plug. vWF serves as a carrier for factor VIII. vWF stabilizes half-life of factor VIII in the circulation for 12 hours*. If patient has deficient vWF, half-life of factor VIII is reduced to 2–4 hours (Fig. 11.4).

CLINICAL FEATURES

Patient with von Willebrand disease presents with mild to severe spontaneous bleeding from mucous membranes, excessive bleeding from wounds and menorrhagia.

Table 11.6: Variants of von Willebrand's disease

Features	vWF disease (type I)	vWF disease (type II)	vWF disease (type III)
Genetics	Autosomal dominant	Autosomal dominant	*Autosomal recessive* (associated with gene deletions and mutations)
vWF quantitative or qualitative	Quantity disorder (levels reduced)	Qualitative defect due to multimer assembling	Quantity disorder (extremely low levels)
Frequency	1–2%	Rare	1 in 250,000
Bleeding	Commonest variant with mild to moderate bleeding	Second more common with mild to moderate bleeding	Severe bleeding
Response to vWF concentrate	Good	Good	Good

It is worth mentioning that *hemarthroses are rare in contrast to hemophilia A*.

Unlike other forms of hemophilia, *von Willebrand disease is not X-linked disorder, so men and women are affected equally*. Clinical manifestations worsen following intake of aspirin and NSAID.

LABORATORY FINDINGS

Factor VIII and vWF levels are decreased. Tourniquet test (Hess test) is positive. Platelets aggregation test is normal with ADP, collagen and epinephrine (absent with ristocetin). Activated partial thromboplastin time is normal or decreased. Template bleeding time, platelets count, prothrombin time, thrombin time and fibrinogen lysis tests are within normal range (Table 11.7).

DISSEMINATED INTRAVASCULAR COAGULATION

Disseminated intravascular coagulation (DIC) is characterized by widespread clotting due to consumption of platelets and coagulation factors, especially factors II, V, and VIII, and fibrinogen. DIC occurs as a result of release of tissue thromboplastin (tissue factor) or activation of the intrinsic pathway of coagulation, and fibrinolytic system.

The history is typical of amniotic fluid embolism, one of the major obstetric causes of disseminated intravascular coagulation (DIC).

ETIOPATHOGENESIS

Neoplastic causes include tumors of the lung, pancreas, prostate, and stomach, and *FAB M3 acute myeloblastic (promyelocytic hypergranular) leukemia*. Tissue damage can result from lung surgery, *hemolysis or hemolytic transfusion reactions, gram-negative sepsis* and immune complex disease. Pathophysiology of disseminated intravascular coagulation is shown in Fig. 11.5.

Activation of both intrinsic and extrinsic coagulation pathways leads to wide systemic thrombi formation in small vessels. Entrapment of platelets in the thrombi causes thrombocytopenia in addition due to marked reduction of coagulation factors (consumptive coagulopathy).

Tissue factor inhibitor mechanism having anticoagulant property is disabled in DIC. Proteins C and S having anticoagulant properties are reduced due to consumption in DIC.

CLINICAL FEATURES

Clinical manifestations are *thrombotic phenomena* in small blood vessels of *multiple organs* and hemorrhages.

Table 11.7: Laboratory findings in von Willebrand disease

Parameters	Results
Tourniquet test (Hess test)	Positive
Template bleeding time	Normal
Platelet count	Normal
Platelets aggregation test	Normal with ADP, collagen and epinephrine (absent with ristocetin)
Factor VIII assay	Decreased
vWF assay	Decreased
Prothrombin time	Normal
Thrombin time	Normal
Activated partial thromboplastin time	Normal or increased
Fibrinolysis test	Normal

Patient presents with abrupt onset of *bleeding* in the form of *petechiae or ecchymosis*. There may be bleeding from gums. Patient develops *hypotensive shock, intracranial bleeding* and *pulmonary hemorrhages*.

HEMATOLOGICAL FINDINGS

Hematological findings in DIC include microangiopathic hemolytic anemia with fragmented red cells (schistocytes), increased fibrin and fibrinogen degradation (split) products, thrombocytopenia, and prolonged bleeding time, PT, APTT, and thrombin time.

Euglin lysis time measures fibrinolytic activity in DIC. FDP-dimer test is specific diagnostic test for DIC. D-dimer assay can be measured by commercially available latex agglutination, ELISA or immunodilution-based D-dimer assay kits. Hematological findings in disseminated intravascular coagulation are shown in Table 11.8.

MANAGEMENT

Patient with DIC manifestations is treated by heparin therapy, platelets transfusion, replacement therapy with coagulation factors and fresh frozen plasma.

HEMORRHAGIC DISEASE OF NEWBORN

Vitamin K is needed for production of vitamin K-dependent coagulation factors in the liver. *Vitamin K is a cofactor for hepatic carboxylation of prothrombin, factors VII, IX, and X, protein C and protein S. Vitamin K deficiency leads to serious life-threatening hemorrhagic disease of the newborn.*

Coagulation Disorders

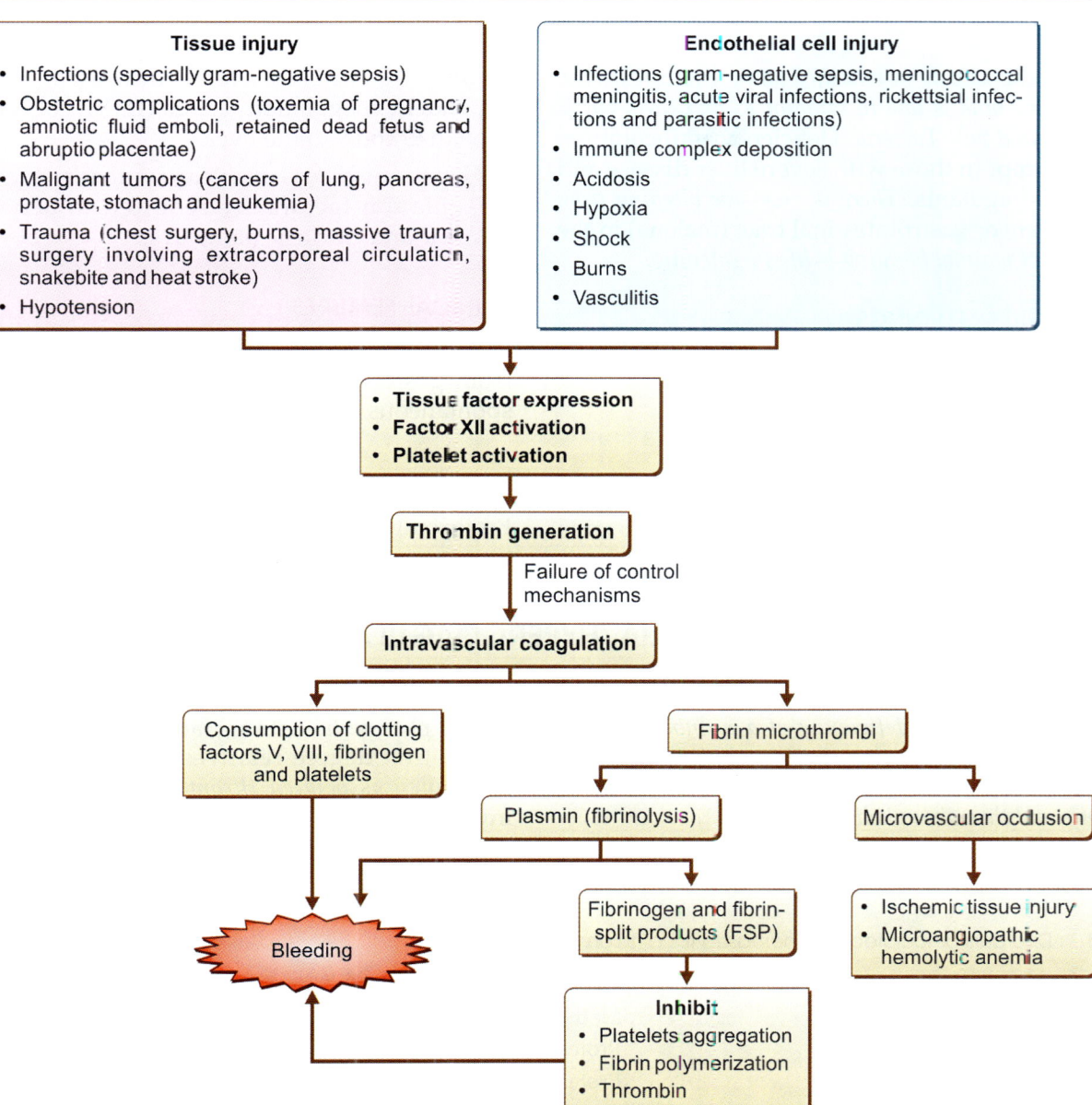

Fig. 11.5: Pathophysiology of disseminated intravascular coagulation. It is triggered by tissue injury, vascular endothelium injury or combination of both these processes. Intravascular coagulation occurs as a result of normal mechanisms controlling hemostasis.

Table 11.8: Hematological findings in disseminated intravascular coagulation

Parameters	Findings
Peripheral blood smear	Anemia and thrombocytopenia
Platelet count	Low
Fibrinogen	Low
Prothrombin time	Increased due to decreased fibrinogen
Activated partial thromboplastin time	Increased due to decreased fibrinogen
Thrombin time	Increased due to decreased fibrinogen
Fibrin and fibrinogen degradation products	Increased
Antithrombin III, protein C and protein S levels	Low
INR	Increased due to consumptive coagulopathy

Euglin lysis time measures fibrinolytic activity in DIC. FDP-dimer test is specific diagnostic test for DIC.

ETIOLOGY

Deficiency is exclusively in breastfed and premature babies, because human milk is low in vitamin K, and their gut is not yet colonized with bacteria. Deficiency is uncommon in adults, except in those with severe liver disease and on oral anticoagulants. *There is excessive bleeding from umbilical stump* or gastrointestinal tract (malena) in the newborn. *Intracranial bleeding is life-threatening.*

HEMATOLOGICAL FINDINGS

Prothrombin time and activated partial thromboplastin time are prolonged.

MANAGEMENT

Liver of the newborn is not mature to synthesize vitamin K dependent coagulation factors. Routine *vitamin K is administered prophylactically.*

COAGULATION DISORDERS IN HEPATIC DISEASE

Vitamin K is needed for synthesis of vitamin K-dependent coagulation factors (II, VII, IX and X) and protein C and S in the liver.

Hepatic disease is unable to synthesize these factors. Coagulation factors are required to activate both intrinsic and extrinsic pathways.

CLINICAL FEATURES

Patient with hepatic disease presents with bleeding from gastrointestinal tract; a few patients develop spontaneous superficial hemorrhage.

HEMATOLOGICAL FINDINGS

Prothrombin time and activated partial thromboplastin time are prolonged. INR is increased.

THROMBOPHILIA (HYPERCOAGULABLE STATE)

Hereditary thrombophilia is a prothrombotic familial syndrome caused by *deficiency of a number of antithrombotic proteins, including antithrombin III, protein C, and protein S.* It is characterized by *recurrent venous thrombosis and thromboembolism.*

It most often occurs in *adolescents or young women.* Patient with history of thrombosis at young age, unexplained recurrent episodes of *thromboembolic phenomenon*, strong family history of thrombosis in the first degree relatives, *recurrent abortions* and *pregnancy associated thrombi* in women should be investigated.

Disorders associated with increased risk of thrombosis are shown in Table 11.9.

Table 11.9: Disorders associated with increased risk of thrombosis

Mechanism	Disorders
Hereditary causes	Methylene tetrahydrofolate reductase gene mutation (MTHFRC677T)
	Protein C deficiency or decreased activity
	Protein S deficiency or decreased activity
	Antithrombin III deficiency or decreased activity
	Dysfibrinogenemia
Increased function of platelets (acquired etiology)	Atheromatous plaques
	Diabetes mellitus
	Hyperlipidemia
	Tobacco smoking
	Thrombocytosis
Increased activity of coagulation system (acquired etiology)	Congestive heart failure
	Postsurgical state
	Immobilization
	Use of oral contraceptives
	Pregnancy
	Heparin induced thrombocytopenia
	Antiphospholipid syndrome
	Thrombotic thrombocytopenic purpura
	Nephrotic syndrome (loss of antithrombin III and antiplasmin in urine)
	Myeloproliferative disorders

Coagulation Disorders

HEREDITARY HYPERCOAGULABLE STATE

ANTITHROMBIN III DEFICIENCY

Antithrombin III is synthesized by liver. It prevents thrombus formation by inhibiting the activity of thrombin, Xa, IXa and XIa. *Gene for antithrombin III is located on chromosome 1, band q23.1–23.9.*

Hereditary deficiency of antithrombin III is an autosomal dominant disorder. Approximately, 50% reduction in the plasma concentration of antithrombin III results in *venous thrombosis and recurrent thromboembolic pulmonary phenomenon* in adolescents or early life.

Clinical Aspects

In clinical practice, heparin is most often administered to prevent thrombus formation. Heparin combines with antithrombin III. In patient with hereditary deficiency of antithrombin III, antithrombotic action of heparin is markedly reduced.

Acquired deficiency of antithrombin III occurs in nephrotic syndrome due to its loss in urine along with massive proteinuria.

Assessment of Antithrombin III

Assessment of antithrombin III is done by chromogenic and coagulation assays.

PROTEIN C DEFICIENCY

Vitamin K is required to synthesize protein C. It prevents thrombus formation. Thrombin, factor Xa and protein C activating enzyme convert protein C into activated form. Normally, activated protein C along with protein S degrade factors Va and VIIIa. Protein C enhances clot lysis.

Clinical Manifestations

Hereditary deficiency of protein C is an *autosomal dominant disorder*. Approximately, 50% reduction in the plasma concentration of protein C results in *venous thrombosis* and *recurrent thromboembolic pulmonary phenomenon* in adolescents or early life.

A total lack of protein C is usually associated with *death in utero*. Repeated *infusions of prothrombin complex* help in keeping these *children alive*. Deficiency of protein C may occur in liver disease.

PROTEIN S DEFICIENCY

Vitamin K is required to synthesize protein S. It prevents thrombus formation. Normally, activated protein C along with protein S degrade factors Va and VIIIa.

Hereditary deficiency of proteins is an autosomal dominant disorder due to PROS1 gene. Hereditary deficiency of protein S is associated with arterial and venous thrombi.

Protein C activity is measured by ELISA, functional and antigenic assays.

ACTIVATED PROTEIN C RESISTANCE (FACTOR V LEIDEN)

Mutation of factor V Leiden has been *named after the city in Netherlands*. It is the most common cause of *hereditary thrombophilia*. Pregnancy and oral contraceptive intake increases risk of hypercoagulable sate.

Molecular Genetics

This abnormal factor V protein is formed due to specific mutation by *substitution of glutamine for normal arginine at position 506*. It alters the cleavage site targeted by APC. *This abnormal factor V protein becomes resistant to cleavage by protein C. As a result, an important antithrombotic counter regulatory mechanism is lost.* There is increased generation of prothrombokinase-thrombin complex.

Clinical Features

Patient presents with cerebral and *recurrent deep venous thrombosis in legs*. Arterial thrombi are rare. There is increased *risk of abortions during second trimester of pregnancy*.

Laboratory Tests

Laboratory tests for factor V Leiden mutation include activated protein C resistance assay and genetic analysis by polymerase chain reaction.

PROTHROMBIN G20210A MUTATION

Prothrombin G20210A transition is the second most common cause of hereditary thrombophilia. Mutation of prothrombin gene occurs due to a single nucleotide change (G to A) in the 3'-untranslated region at position 20210. It is associated with *elevated plasma prothrombin levels*. Patient has almost three times *increased risk of arterial and venous thrombosis*.

HYPERHOMOCYSTINEMIA

Methylenetetrahydrofolate reductase gene mutation (MTHFRC677T) results in mild elevation of homocysteine levels in 5–15% of White and East Asia populations. *Elevated levels of homocysteine inhibit antithrombin III and thrombomodulin.* There is increased risk of thrombosis.

The increased homocysteine can be reduced by dietary supplementation with *folic acid and vitamins B_6 (pyridoxine) and B_{12} (cobalamin)*. This is also associated with an increased risk of *neural tube defects* and possibly a number of diverse neoplasms.

ACQUIRED HYPERCOAGULABLE STATE

ANTIPHOSPHOLIPID SYNDROME

Antiphospholipid antibody syndrome has underlying etiology of *systemic lupus erythematosus*. It is associated with high titers of circulating *antibodies (IgG) directed against anionic phospholipids* (cardiolipin) *such as plasma protein epitopes prothrombin*.

Pathogenesis

Lupus anticoagulant is an IgG or IgM. It binds to phospholipid used in activated partial thromboplastin time resulting in prolonged APTT (normal 30–40 seconds).

In vivo, these antibodies induce a hypercoagulable state by activating platelets, interfering in protein C activity and inhibiting synthesis of PGI_2 by endothelial cells.

Clinical Features

Lupus anticoagulant is associated with *recurrent venous thrombosis* in deep veins of legs or *arterial thrombi*. But renal, hepatic, and retinal veins are also susceptible. There is history of *repeated miscarriages due to inhibition of tissue plasminogen activator required for trophoblastic invasion of uterus*. There is increased risk of cardiac valvular vegetations or thrombocytopenia. Anticardiolipin antibodies are associated with arterial thrombi.

Laboratory Investigations

In vitro these antibodies interfere with the assembly of phospholipid complexes and thus inhibit coagulation. APTT is prolonged. Prothrombin time, thrombin time and fibrinogen level are within normal range. Confirmatory tests include kaolin clotting time, platelet neutralizing test and Russell viper venom time test.

CLINICAL ASPECTS OF BLEEDING DIATHESIS

Investigations of hemostatic function is essential if patient has history of excessive bleeding following injury or dental extractions, menorrhagia, hematuria, poor healing of superficial lacerations, easy bruising, hemarthrosis, incidental abnormal hemostatic test; and past or family history of excessive bleeding or bruising. *Four steps of investigating hemostatic function are complete history, physical examination, screening tests of hemostasis and special tests.*

Clinical manifestations in vascular, platelet and coagulation disorders are shown in Table 11.10.

COMPLETE HISTORY

Patient may present with easy bruising, development of purpura, epistaxis, heavy menstruation with passage of blood clots, excessive bleeding following dental procedures, passage of red-colored urine, painful joints or muscles and delayed wound healing. Exposure to

Table 11.10: Clinical manifestations in vascular, platelet and coagulation disorders

Finding	Vascular disorders	Platelet disorders	Coagulation disorders
Petechial hemorrhages	Common	Common	Rare
Bleeding superficial cuts and scratches	Persistent; often profuse	Persistent; often profuse	Minimal
Superficial ecchymosis	Small and multiple	Small and multiple	Common; large and solitary
Deep hematoma	Rare	Rare	Common
Hemarthrosis	Rare	Rare	Common
Delayed bleeding	Rare	Rare	Common
Gastrointestinal bleeding	Absent	Present	Present with GIT lesions
Hematuria	Absent	Present	Present
Epistaxis	Absent	Present	Present
Gingival bleeding	Absent	Present	Present
Excessive bleeding after tooth extraction	Absent	Present	Present
Intracranial bleeding	Absent	Present	Present
Sex	More common in females	More common in females	80–90% of inherited forms occur only in male patients
Family history	Rare (except vWD and HHT)	Rare (except vWD and HHT)	Common

Coagulation Disorders 11

drugs or toxins and family history of bleeding should be enquired.

PHYSICAL EXAMINATION

Patient may have evidence of bleeding such as petechial hemorrhages, purpura and ecchymosis, bleeding from mucous membranes, hemarthroses, muscle hematoma, gastrointestinal bleeding, renal hematuria or epistaxis. One must look for hepatosplenomegaly, jaundice, fever, joint abnormalities.

Clinical summary of bleeding disorders is shown in Table 11.11. Clinical findings and diagnostic possibilities in thrombotic disease in various age groups are shown in Table 11.12.

BLOOD EXAMINATION

Complete blood counts, hemoglobin or packed cells volume, WBC count, platelet count, erythrocyte sedimentation rate and peripheral blood smear examination to rule out macrocytic anemia, aplastic anemia and acute leukemia for underlying cause of thrombocytopenia. Interpretation of routine tests in bleeding disorders is shown in Fig. 11.6. Comparison between platelets and coagulation defects is shown in Table 11.13.

Table 11.11: Clinical summary of bleeding disorders

Observations	Diagnostic possibilities
History observations	
History of bleeding/bruising since childhood	Congenital defect
Recent history of bleeding/bruising since childhood	Acquired defect
Sudden onset of bleeding/bruising, poorly healing cuts	Acquired defect, probably drug induced
Physical examination	
Small hemorrhages from skin, mucous membrane especially in females. Persistent bleeding from superficial lesions	Abnormalities of the blood vessels or low platelet count or impaired platelet function
Delayed bleeding, hemarthrosis, hematomas, joint deformities, bleeding following trauma, bleeding from GIT and renal hematuria, epistaxis in males with positive family history	Defects in coagulation
Bleeding from only one organ	Probably not caused by hemostatic defect

Table 11.12: Clinical findings and diagnostic possibilities in thrombotic disease in various age groups

Age group	Clinical findings	Possible causes
Birth to 45 years	Family history with migratory or recurrent thrombi	Hereditary hypercoagulable state (deficiency of antithrombin III, protein C and protein S) and homocystinuria
	Smoking and hormones (estrogen, progesterone and oral contraceptives)	Aggravate these conditions
10–45 years	Migratory or recurrent thrombi	Acquired hypercoagulable state (lupus inhibitor)
	Multiple organs failure, massive purpura (severely ill patients)	Disseminated intravascular coagulation and hemolytic uremic syndrome
>45 years	Localized sudden onset thrombi without recurrence	Acquired thrombosis associated with infection/inflammation, trauma, venous stasis and drug reaction
	Arterial occlusion	Atherosclerosis, hyperlipidemia, diabetes mellitus and protein S deficiency
	Weight loss, anorexia, weakness	Underlying malignancy (lung, pancreas, prostate, stomach and AML—acute myelomonocytic leukemia) AML (M3) is commonly associated with DIC due to release of thromboplastin-like substance)
	Fever, infection (localized or systemic)	Underlying infection or inflammation
	Severe or massive trauma	Disseminated intravascular coagulation
	Deep vein thrombosis or thrombophlebitis, emboli	Any thrombotic disease

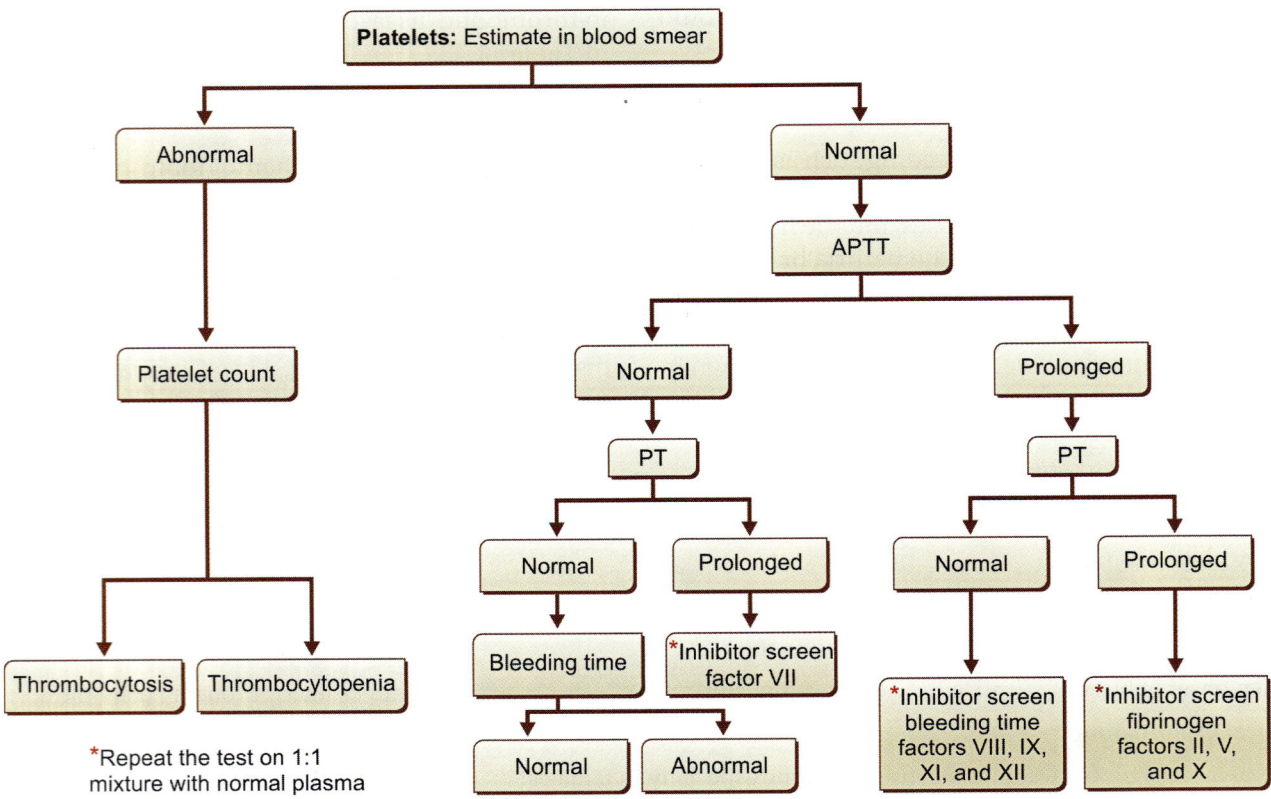

Fig. 11.6: Interpretation of routine tests in bleeding disorders.

Table 11.13: Comparison between platelet and coagulation defects

Feature	Platelet defects	Severe coagulation defects
Purpura (petechiae)	Very common	Absent
Spontaneous bleeding	Common	Uncommon
Application of local pressure	Bleeding does not stop quickly	Bleeding stops quickly
Bleeding from superficial cut	Present	Absent
Family history	Absent	Possible
Mucosal bleeding from mouth and gut	Usually present	Relatively uncommon except urinary tract
Hemarthroses (bleeding in joints)	Absent	Very common in severe coagulation defect
Muscle hematomas	Present in response to trauma	Spontaneous even without trauma
Bleeding after trauma or surgery	Immediate for short time	Often delayed, after several more than 48 hours

PLATELET COUNT

Platelets normally clump in groups of 2 to 5. Normal value is 4–8 platelets per 100 red blood cells. A reasonable estimate of platelet number can be obtained by counting platelets present in relation to 500 red blood cells. If platelet count is low, one should rule out secondary causes of thrombocytopenia before establishing acute or chronic ITP. *Giant platelets are demonstrated in Bernard-Soulier syndrome, myeloproliferative disorders and May-Hegglin anomaly.*

PLATELET FUNCTION TESTS

Platelets aggregation test with ADP, collagen, epinephrine and ristocetin should be performed to rule out various platelet function disorders.

In *Bernard-Soulier syndrome, platelets aggregation is deficient with ADP,* epinephrine, and collagen, but normal with ristocetin.

In *Glanzmann disease* and von Willebrand disease, *platelets aggregation* is normal with ADP, epinephrine, and collagen, but deficient with ristocetin.

Coagulation Disorders

BLEEDING TIME

The bleeding time measures vascular and platelet integrity. It is estimated by Ivy method and Template method. In general, 95% of all values are <4 minutes. If the bleeding time is >4 minutes, abnormality should be considered.

COAGULATION PROFILE

Prothrombin Time

Prothrombin time is the time required for plasma to clot after tissue thromboplastin and optimum amount of calcium chloride is added. Incubate plasma at 37°C in a water bath for five minutes. Add 0.2 ml thromboplastin and 0.1 ml of calcium chloride to the test tube. Record the time for formation of blood clot every second. End point is identified by formation of fibrin strand attached to the wire hook.

Prothrombin time is measured to diagnose bleeding diathesis, monitoring patients on anticoagulant therapy and prior to liver biopsy. Normal range is between 11 and 16 seconds. Procedure of one stage prothrombin time is shown in Fig. 11.7.

Interpretation of prothrombin time: Prothrombin time *measures extrinsic procoagulant pathway.* It is prolonged in disseminated intravascular coagulation, vitamin K deficiency, deficiency of one or more of clotting factors (fibrinogen, prothrombin, V, VII or X), liver disease and oral coagulant therapy.

Activated Partial Thromboplastin Time (APTT)

This test (APTT) measures the intrinsic procoagulant activity of plasma. Partial thromboplastin is a substitute for platelet factor III. Contact activation is standardized by adding an activator (kaolin) to the reagent.

This test does not measure activities of factors VII and IX. *Activated partial thromboplastin time is prolonged in hemophilia A, hemophilia B, disseminated intravascular coagulation and von Willebrand disease. Normal range is between 30 and 40 seconds.* Procedure of activated partial thromboplastin time is shown in Fig. 11.8. Interpretation of tests of hemostasis function in normal and abnormal patients is shown in Table 11.14.

Thrombin Time

Thrombin time measures fibrinogen concentration. *Normal thrombin time is between 15 and 19 seconds.* It is prolonged in *disseminated intravascular coagulation* and *fibrinogen deficiency.*

Fibrinogen Degradation Products D-Dimer

FDP D-dimer is demonstrated in disseminated intravascular coagulation.

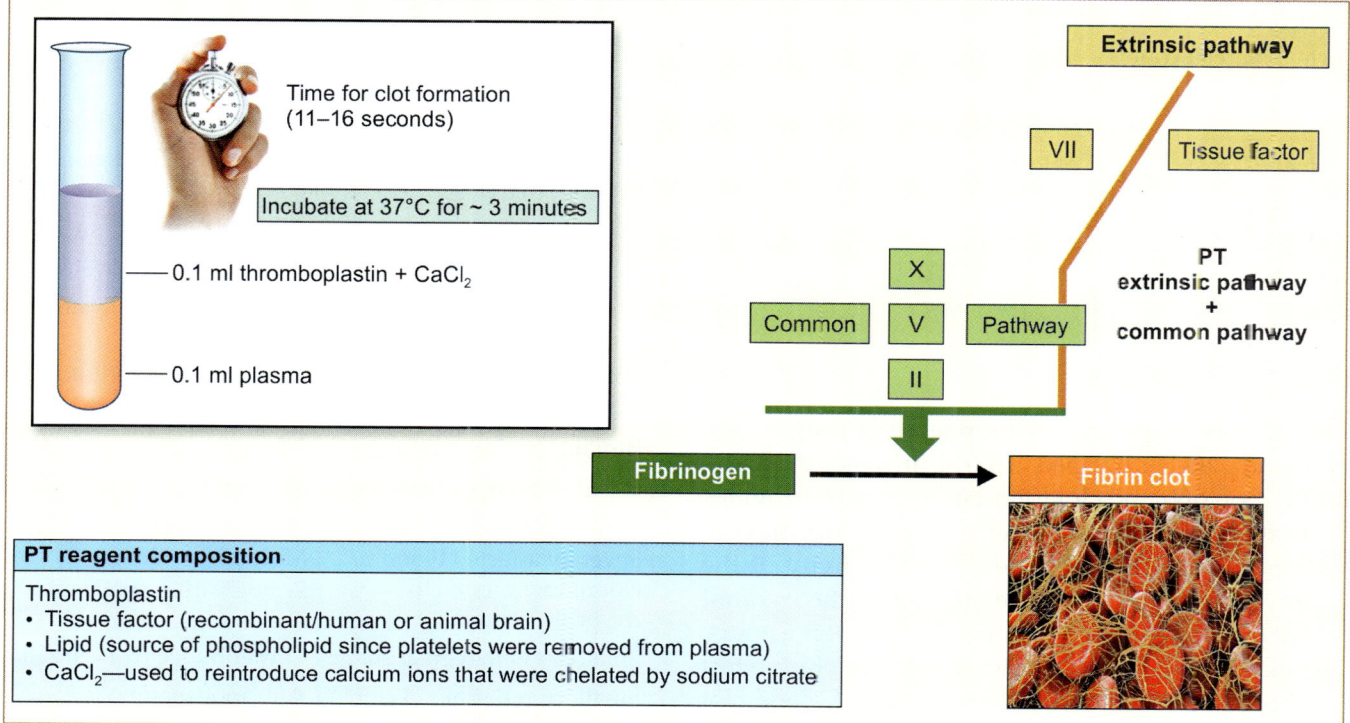

Fig. 11.7: Procedure of one stage prothrombin time.

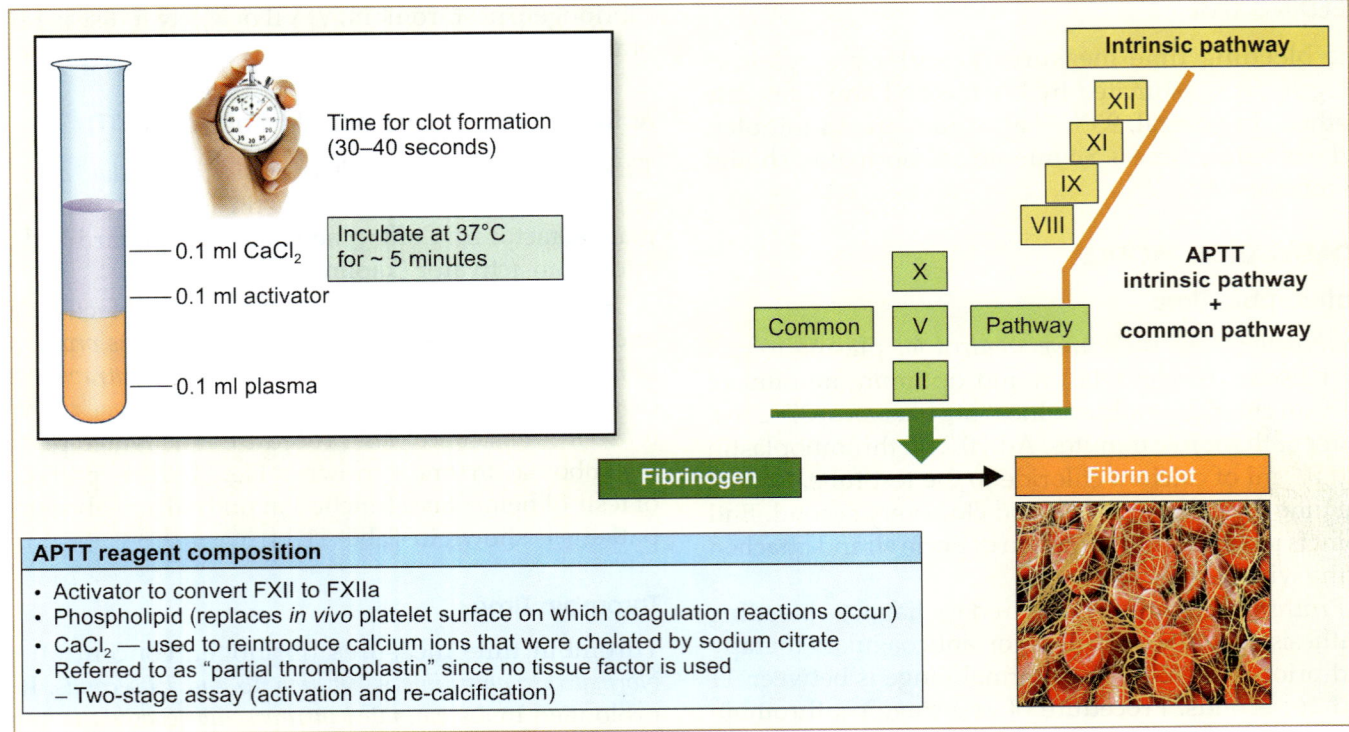

Fig. 11.8: Procedure of activated partial thromboplastin time.

Table 11.14: Interpretation of tests of hemostasis function in normal and abnormal patients

Tests and results		Conclusion
Platelet count	Bleeding time	Interpretation
Normal platelet count	Normal	Normal result (platelets are related to bleeding disorders, so suspect coagulation defect in case of bleeding diathesis)
Low platelet count	Prolonged	Low platelet count (thrombocytopenia)
Normal platelet count	Prolonged	Abnormal platelet function
Prothrombin time (PT)	Activated partial thromboplastin time (APTT)	Interpretation
Normal PT	Normal APTT	Normal function of coagulation system (suspect platelet or vascular defect)
Abnormal PT	Abnormal APTT	Defects in common pathway of coagulation system
Normal PT	Abnormal APTT	Defects in the intrinsic pathway of coagulation system
Abnormal PT	Normal APTT	Defects in the extrinsic pathway of coagulation system

Clot Retraction Test

Clot retraction depends on the release of coagulation factors and platelets trapped in the fibrin mesh of the clot. Examination of blood clot found in a test tube provides information regarding concentration of fibrinogen, number and function of platelets; and activity of the fibrinolytic system. Test tube containing anticoagulant free blood is placed in water bath at 37°C for three hours. In normal persons, 30% of the total volume in the test tube should be blood clot. Interpretation of blood clot retraction in various hematological disorders is shown in Figs 11.9 and 11.10 and Table 11.15.

Table 11.15: Blood clots observed in various hematological disorders

Blood clot structure	Disorders
Large clot with weak structure	Thrombocytopenia Thrombasthenia
Severely affected blood clot retraction due to dysproteinemias	Multiple myeloma Waldenström syndrome
Small clot with regular shape	Low fibrinogen concentration
Small irregular blood clot digested by enhanced fibrinolysis	Afibrinogenemia Disseminated intravascular coagulation

Coagulation Disorders

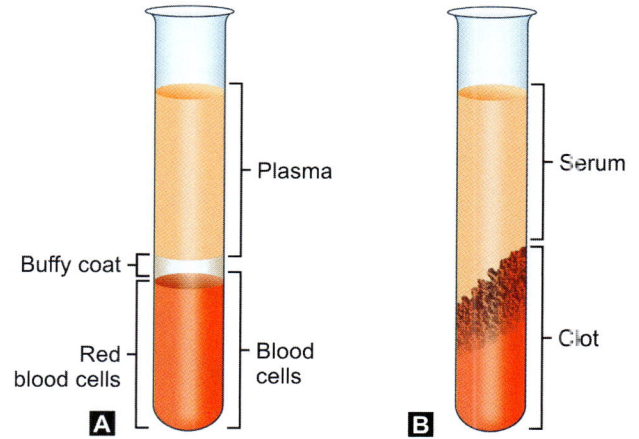

Fig. 11.9: (A) Unclotted whole blood with anticoagulant showing blood cells, plasma and buffy coat after centrifuge, (B) clotted whole blood without adding anticoagulant showing blood clot and serum.

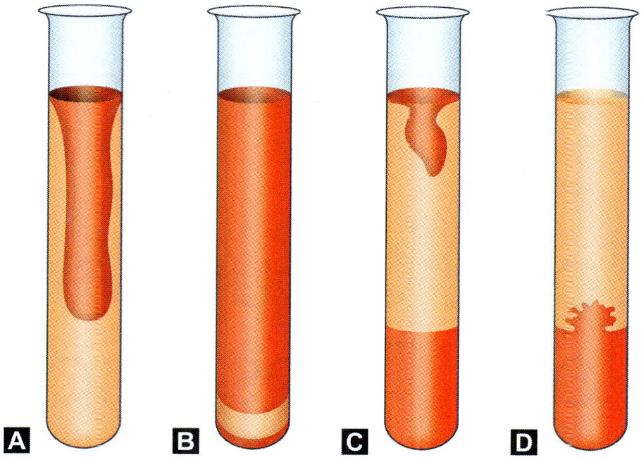

Fig. 11.10: Blood clots observed in normal persons and patients with coagulation disorders. (A) Blood clot in normal person, (B) blood clot in thrombocytopenia and thrombasthenia, (C) blood clot formed due to low fibrinogen concentration, (D) blood clot formed due to enhanced fibrinolysis in disseminated intravascular coagulation.

Euglobulin Lysis Test

Euglobulins are proteins that precipitate when plasma is diluted in water. Precipitate contains plasmin, plasminogen and fibrinogen. Euglobulins are redissolved and fibrin clotted with thrombin.

Activated thrombin activates plasminogen to plasmin. Time required for the plasmin to lyse fibrin is the euglobulin lysis time. Interpretation of euglobulin lysis time is shown in Table 11.16.

Table 11.16: Interpretation of euglobulin lysis time

Time	Interpretation of results
<2 minutes	Severe fibrinolysis, explaining severe bleeding
2–10 minutes	Moderate fibrinolysis, explaining postoperative or post-traumatic bleeding
10–30 minutes	Mild fibrinolysis, but not explaining bleeding
30 minutes to 2 hours	Physiological enhanced fibrinolysis
2–4 hours	Normal
>4 hours	Possibly defective fibrinolysis

CHAPTER 12

Blood Groups and Blood Transfusion

Learning Objectives

BLOOD GROUP SYSTEMS
- ABO Blood Group System
- Antigens of ABO Blood Group System
- Rh Blood Group System
- Other Blood Group Systems

BLOOD COLLECTION, PROCESSING AND STORAGE

BLOOD GROUPING

BLOOD CROSS-MATCHING (COMPATIBILITY TEST)

BLOOD COMPONENTS THERAPY
- Whole Blood Transfusion, Packed Cells Transfusion, Plasma Transfusion, Platelets Transfusion
- Leukocytes Reduced Blood Component
- Fresh Frozen Plasma
- Cryoprecipitate
- Factor VIII and Factor IX Concentrates, Prothrombin Complex Concentrates
- Immunoglobulins

AUTOLOGOUS BLOOD TRANSFUSION AND PLASMA EXCHANGE

ADVERSE BLOOD TRANSFUSION REACTIONS

BLOOD GROUP SYSTEMS

ABO blood group system follows mendelian law. H gene locus located on chromosome 19p locus is occupied by one of the 3 allelic genes, i.e. A, B, or O. Most of the blood group genes are expressed in a codominant manner. *Two allelic genes are inherited equally and expressed in heterozygous state.* No gene or allele is dominant over another gene or allele. The particular *alleles* at a specific gene locus in a person constitute genotype, and their outward expression is known as *phenotype.*

ABO and Rh blood group systems are most important in the blood transfusion in clinical practice. Red cell antigens (A, B and RhD) elicits strong humoral immune response. Alloantibodies formed can cause destruction of transfused red blood cells. ABO antigens are also significant in organ transplantation.

ABO BLOOD GROUP SYSTEM

ABO blood group system comprises four blood major groups: A, B, AB and O identified based on presence or absence of A and/or B antigens on red blood cells. According to Landsteiner's law, anti-A and/or anti-B antibodies are always present in the plasma of persons, who lack corresponding antigen(s).

In ABO blood group system, person lacking an antigen has corresponding anti-A and/or anti-B antibodies. Both A and B genes are dominant, while O gene is recessive. ABO blood group system is shown in Table 12.1.

Blood group O: Large amounts of H antigen are present on blood group O red blood cells. Genotype of persons with blood group 'O' is OO. Their plasma contains anti-A and anti-B antibodies of IgG nature in their plasma. IgG can cross placenta and induce hemolytic disease of newborn.

Blood group A: Genotype of persons with blood group A is AA (homozygous) or AO (heterozygous). These persons have both A and H antigens on their red blood cells. Plasma of person with blood group A plasma contains anti-B antibodies of IgM nature in their plasma.

Blood Groups and Blood Transfusion 12

Table 12.1: ABO Blood group system

Blood group	Genotype	Quantity of H antigen on RBCs	Antigen(s) on RBCs	Plasma antibodies	Reacts with antiserum	Indian frequency
A	AA (homozygous) AO (heterozygous)	++	A	Anti-B (IgM)	Anti-A	27%
B	BB (homozygous) BO (heterozygous)	++	B	Anti-A (IgM)	Anti-B	31%
AB	AB (heterozygous)	+	AB	None	Anti-A, anti-B	8%
O	OO	++++	None	Anti-A and anti-B (IgG hence crosses placenta leading to HDN)	None	34%

Large amounts of H antigen are present on blood group O red blood cells. AB blood group has least amount of antigens on red blood cells.

There are two subgroups of blood group A: A1 (80%) and A2 (20%).

Blood group B: Genotype of persons with blood group B is BB (homozygous) or BO (heterozygous). These persons contain both B and H antigens on their red blood cells. Plasma of persons with blood group B contains anti-A antibodies of IgM in nature.

Blood group AB: Genotype of persons with blood group AB has antigens A and B. Their red blood cells contain small amount of H antigen. Plasma of persons with AB blood group lacks anti-A and anti-B antibodies.

ANTIGENS OF ABO BLOOD GROUP SYSTEM

Red blood cells of ABO blood group system contain various antigens: A (A1, A2), B and H. These antigens comprise glycolipids, glycoproteins or glycosphingolipids. In addition to red blood cells, these antigens are also present in body fluids and body tissues. White blood cells and platelets contain least amount of these antigens.

Formation of ABH Antigen

H gene synthesizes fucosyltransferase enzyme, which converts precursor substance (oligosaccharides) presents on the red blood cells to H substance by addition of L-fucose to glycoproteins backbone.

Genes A and B located on chromosome 9 synthesize N-acetylgalactosaminyltransferase enzyme and D-galactosyl transferase, resulting in conversion of H substance into A and B antigens on red blood cells, respectively (Figs 12.1 to 12.3).

Blood group A: Subsequent addition of N-acetylglucosamine to H substance creates *A antigen* to form blood group A.

Blood group B: Subsequent addition of galactose to H substance creates *B antigen* to form blood group B.

Blood group AB: Presence of both *A and B transferases* forms *AB blood group.*

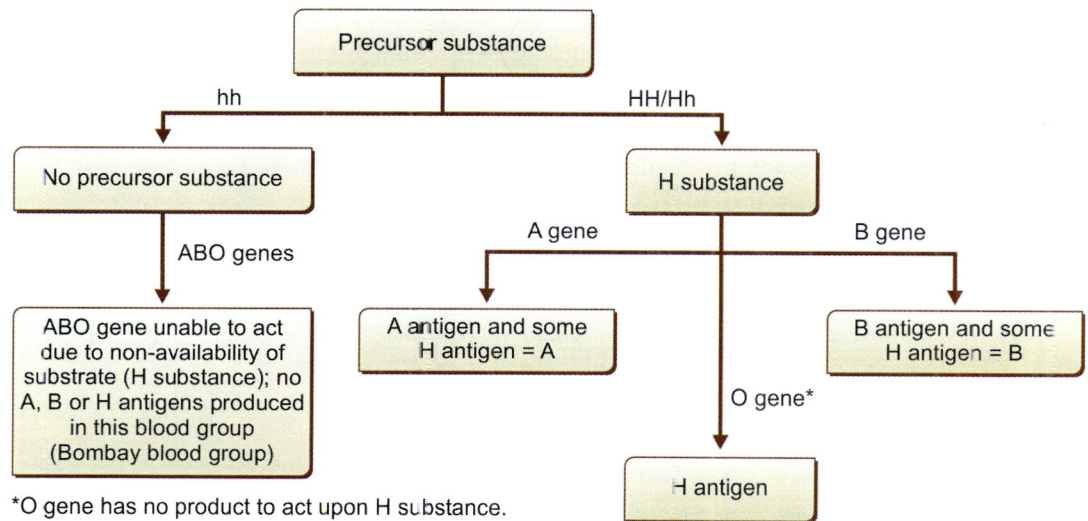

*O gene has no product to act upon H substance.

Fig. 12.1: Formation of ABO and Bombay blood groups.

Section II: Hematology

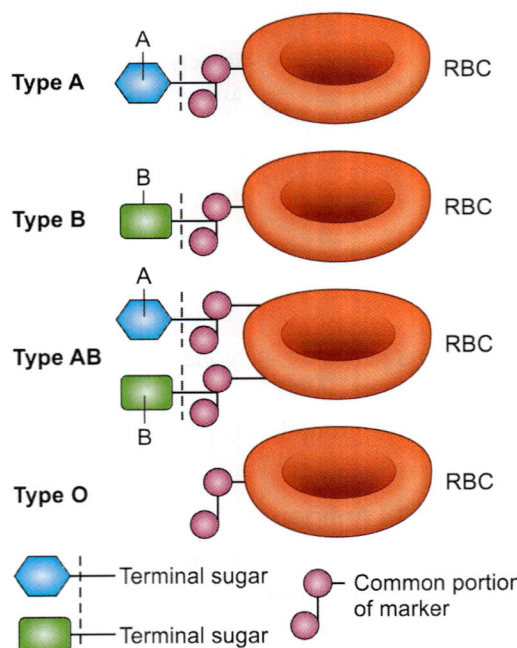

Fig. 12.2: Genetic or molecular basis for the A and B antigens (receptors) on the red cells. In general, persons with blood group A, B and AB inherit a gene for the transferase enzyme that adds a certain terminal sugar to the basic RBC receptor. Blood group O persons do not have such an enzyme and lacks terminal sugar.

Blood group O: The *O gene* synthesizes an inactive transferase resulting in unchanged H antigen. Blood group O has large amount of H antigen.

Bombay Blood Group (Oh)

Some persons do not inherit H antigen (genotype hh) and thus cannot produce H substance. Therefore, these persons may inherit A and B genes without their expression due to their inability to synthesize H substance. Such persons are said to have Bombay phenotype or Bombay blood group *Oh Bombay blood group* was first reported by Dr YM Bhende in 1952 with 1:7600 incidence in India.

Bombay blood group is autosomal recessive pattern of inheritance due to mutation of *H gene* on chromosome 19 that leads to synthesis of non-functional H-glycosyl transferase. Such persons lack A, B and H antigens on the red blood cells. Serum contains anti-A, anti-B and anti-H antibodies, which react with all O blood groups. These persons are non-secretors and hence not demonstrated in body fluids.

Para-Bombay Blood Group

Person with Para-Bombay blood group synthesizes H-determinants in secretory epithelia but not in erythroid cells. Person is homozygous for null alleles at H locus. At least 1 functional SE allele is present (Table 12.2).

Rh BLOOD GROUP SYSTEM

Landsteiner and Wiener in 1941, injected rhesus monkey red blood cells into the rabbits and guinea pigs resulting

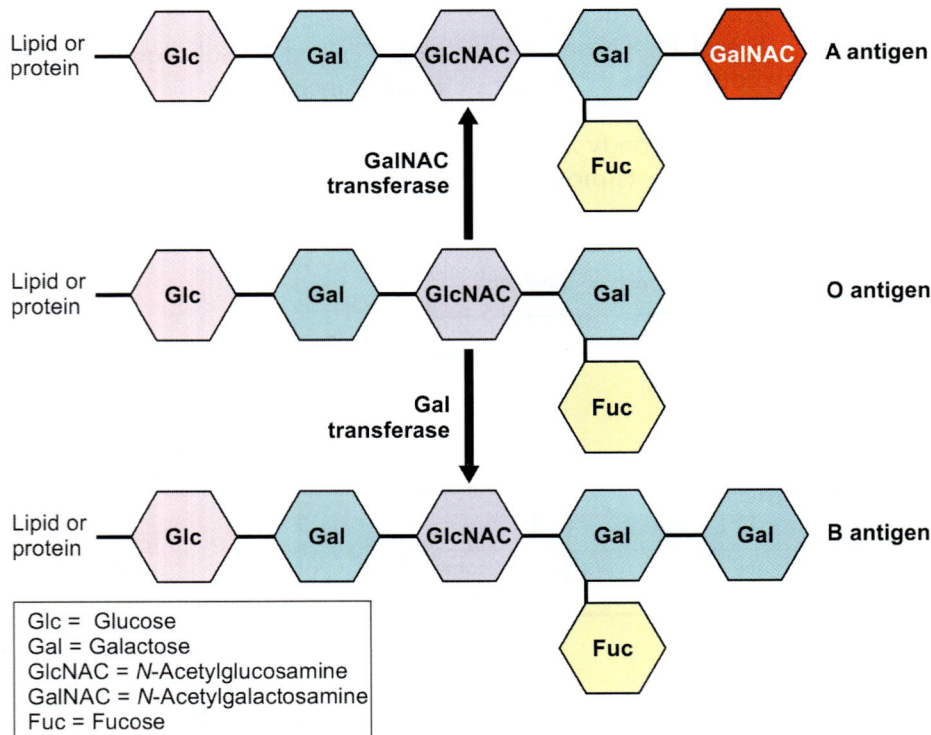

Fig. 12.3: ABO antigen specificity. ABO antigens are different by just one sugar at the antigen terminus. Only the carbohydrate portion of the antigen is demonstrated here.

Blood Groups and Blood Transfusion

Table 12.2: Differences between secretors and non-secretors

Parameters	Secretors	Non-secretors
Frequency	80%	20%
Quantity of secretion of A, B and H substances	Abundant depending on blood group in plasma, gastric juice, saliva, tears, semen and human milk	Traces depending on blood group
Genotype	Sese/Sese	Not applicable

in increased antibodies titre. Red blood cells of rhesus monkey and human (White residents of New York City) have similar antigens. Antigen involved was called Rh factor. In 1939, Levin and Steven later discovered anti-D antibody that is responsible for hemolytic disease of newborn.

ANTIGENS OF RH SYSTEM

Rh system consists of about 40 antigens. Most important antigens are C, D, E, c, and e (d absent). The genes encoding Rh proteins determine the phenotype of person. A related protein, the Rh glycoprotein is essential for assembly of the Rh protein complex in the erythrocyte membrane and for expression of Rh antigens. CDE (Fisher-Race) and Dr Alexander Wiener nomenclature systems are employed for Rh blood group inheritance.

CDE (Fisher Race) Nomenclature System

According to Fisher-Race nomenclature system, three closely linked loci located on chromosome 1 are inherited from each parent. The alleles occupying these loci are known as C, D, E, c, d and e. Out of these, D gene is dominant over d. On the other hand, loci such as C, c, E and e are codominant. Each gene except d codes for a specific antigen on red blood cells. Each person inherits one haplotype from each parent making 8 possible genotypes (Fig. 12.4).

Dr Alexander Wiener Nomenclature System

According to Dr Alexander Wiener nomenclature system, single Rh gene having multiple alleles is inherited from each parent. R1 gene codes for one Rh1 antigen comprising three factors, which correspond with C, D and e of Fisher-Race nomenclature system. Similarly, R2 gene codes for one Rh2 antigen comprising factors, which correspond with of Fisher-Race nomenclature system (Fig. 12.5).

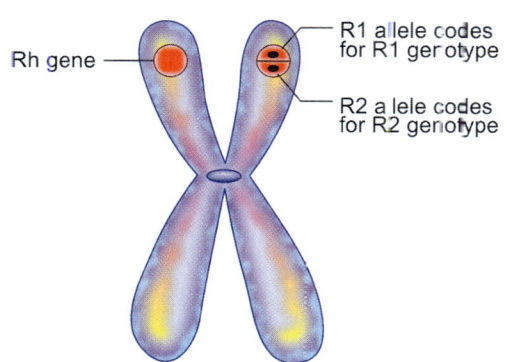

Fig. 12.5: Dr Alexander Wiener system of nomenclature of Rh blood group inheritance.

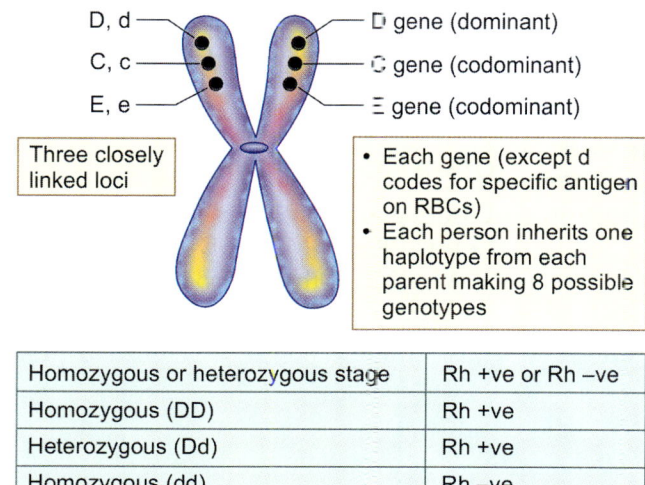

DCe	dCe
DcE	dCE
Dce	dcE
DCE	dce

- There are 8 gene complexes at the Rh locus
- Fisher-Race uses DCE as the order
- Others alphabetize the genes as CDE

Fig. 12.4: CDE (Fisher-Race) system of nomenclature of Rh blood group inheritance.

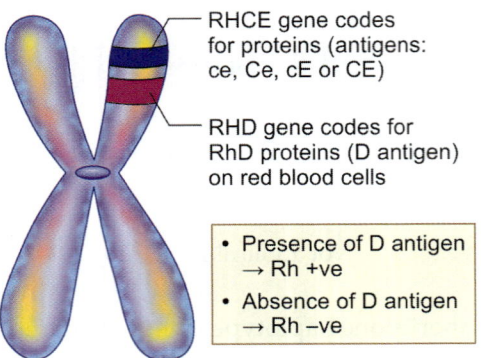

Fig. 12.6: Current genetic analysis shows two genes (RHCE and RHD) located on chromosome 1. These genes differ by 32 to 35 amino acids.

Current Genetic Analysis Nomenclature System

According to current genetic analysis, RHCE and RHD genes are located on chromosome 1. RHD gene synthesizes D antigen.

Presence of D gene makes the person Rh positive, while Rh negative lack D antigen. RHCE gene can synthesize C or c, Ce, CE, and ce (Fig. 12.6).

RH FACTOR INCOMPATIBILITY DURING PREGNANCY

Rh factor incompatibility can cause lysis of red blood cells known as hemolytic disease of newborn. A naturally occurring red blood cell incompatibility results when a Rh +ve fetus develops within Rh –ve mother. Initial sensitization of the maternal immune system occurs when fetal blood passes the placental barrier.

In most cases, the fetus develops normally. However, a subsequent pregnancy with Rh +ve fetus results in a severe fetal red blood cell hemolysis. Pathogenesis of hemolytic disease of newborn and its prevention is shown in Fig. 12.7.

ANTI-D ANTIBODY (RHOGAM) ADMINISTRATION

Routine antenatal prophylaxis to infuse 500 IU anti-D antibody (RhoGAM) to Rh negative mothers at 28 weeks and 34 weeks of pregnancy to inactivate and remove any Rh factor that may be transferred from the fetus in maternal circulation.

Post-delivery anti-D Ig must be given to Rh negative, mother if infant is Rh positive. If the screening for fetal cells shows >4 ml additional anti-D Ig should be given.

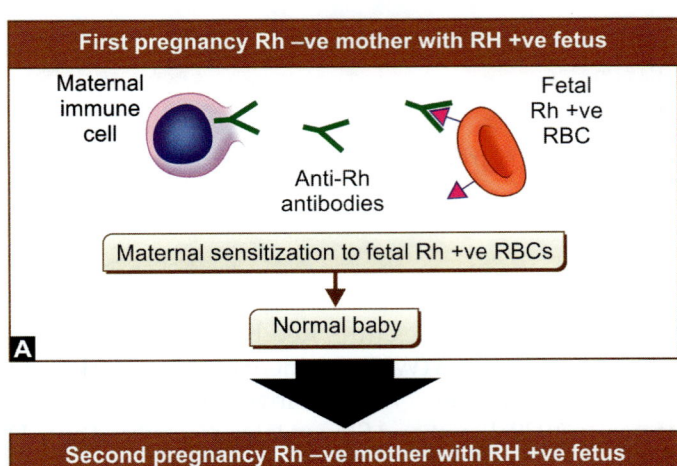
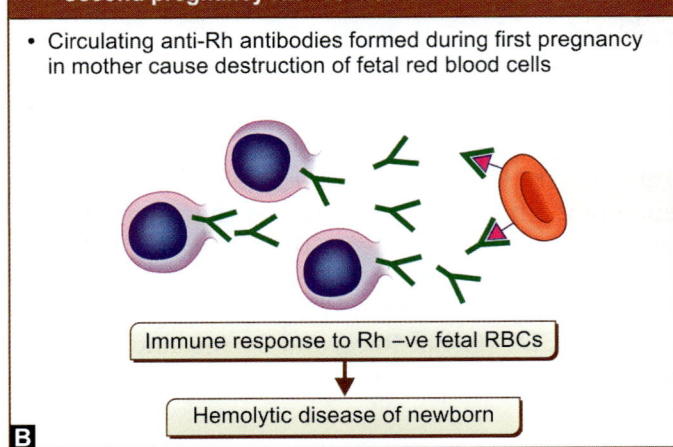
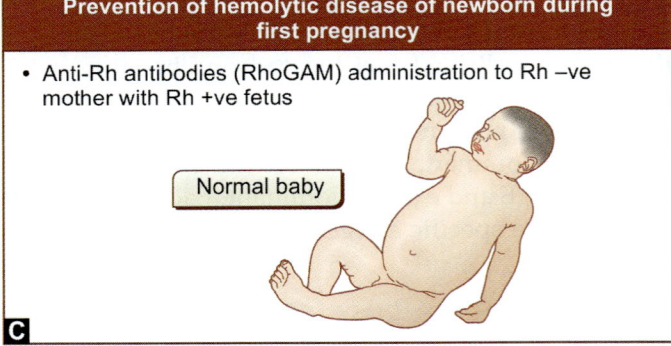

Fig. 12.7: Pathogenesis of hemolytic disease of newborn and its prevention.

OTHER BLOOD GROUP SYSTEMS

Blood group system other than ABO and Rh are Lewis, Kell, MNS, Duffy, P and Kidd systems (Table 12.3). Other blood group systems are Lutherean, Yt, Bombrok, Giego, Colton, Indian, XG, Landsteiner-Wiener and John Milton Hagen systems.

Table 12.3: Blood group systems other than ABO and Rh

Blood group systems	Gene locus	Antigens	Antibodies	Comments
Lewis system	Le gene on FUT3 on chromosome 19 codes for fucosyl-transferase	Lea and Leb located on glycosphingolipids (integral part of RBC membrane)	IgM (natural occurring) not crossing placenta, hence HDN absent	Lewis antigens are passively adsorbed from plasma on RBCs
Kell system	Kell locus on chromosome 7 (7q23)	Kell antigens (for synthesis of Kell antigens, additional gene on locus at KX on X chromosome required)	IgG (crosses placenta hence HDN present)	Some persons express weak Kell antigens resulting in McLeod syndrome characterized by acanthocytes, progressive cardiomyopathy, muscle wasting and neurological disorders
MNS system	-	Consists of 43 antigens (M and N situated on glycophorin A; while S, s and U on glycophorin B of RBC membrane)	IgM (reactive at low temperature)	M and N antigens testing is significant in paternal testing. Antibodies against S, s are formed following sensitization to transfusion and detected by indirect Coombs' test
Duffy (Fy) system	-	Fya (FY1) and Fyb (FY2) found in Caucasians	IgG (crosses placenta hence HDN present)	IgG crosses placenta resulting in hemolytic disease of newborn. *Plasmodium vivax* enters RBCs at the Duffy antigen site, hence persons lacking Fya (FY1) and Fyb (FY2) are resistant to *Plasmodium vivax*
P system	-	P+, P−, P1, P2 and Pk antigens (P1 and P2 most important)	IgG and IgM	P negative (p) persons are resistant to Parvovirus 19 infection. Auto-anti-P occurs in paroxysmal nocturnal hemoglobinuria
Kidd system	-	JKa and JKb	IgG	Antibody causes delayed hypersensitivity reaction and mild hemolytic disease of newborn

BLOOD COLLECTION, PROCESSING AND STORAGE

In India, blood collection, processing, storage and preparations of blood components are regulated by Food and Drug Administration (FDA). Blood donors may be voluntary, professional and replacement by relative of patient.

Donor must have hemoglobin ≥12 gm/dl. There should be interval of at least three months between two donations. Donor must be rejected showing positivity with HBV, HCV, HIV, history of drug abuse, bisexual and suffering from serious illnesses. Screening of donor's blood must be carried out for infections.

PRECAUTIONS

Flow of blood should be uninterrupted and continuous >8 minutes to draw is unsuitable for preparation of platelet concentrate, fresh frozen plasma and cryoprecipitate.

Blood bag should be stored at 20–25°C within 6–8 hours of collection for harvesting platelets. Triple pack system is used to prepare red cells, platelet concentrate and FFP. Quad packs system is used to prepare red cells, platelet concentrate and cryoprecipitate. Double bags are used to prepare red cells and plasma only.

PRESERVATIVE USED IN BAGS

Bag consists of acid-citrate-dextrose (ACD) preservative. Blood bag with citrate-phosphate-dextrose (CPD) preservative can be stored up to 21 days. Citrate-phosphate-dextrose with adenine-1 (CPDA-1) preservative blood bags can be stored up to 35 days.

Dextrose provides nutrition to red blood cells. Adenine provides ATP to blood cells. Citrate prevents coagulation by chelating calcium. Phosphate buffer is used to maintain pH.

BLOOD GROUPING

ABO BLOOD GROUPING

ABO blood grouping is performed by two methods: cell grouping (forward grouping) and serum grouping (reverse grouping). Blood grouping is done by three methods: slide test, tube test and microplate test.

Cell (Forward) Blood Grouping

In cell grouping, red blood cells are tested to demonstrate the presence of A and B antigens by employing known specific anti-A and anti-B. Sometimes, anti-A and anti-B sera are also used. ABO antisera used for blood grouping are anti-A (blue-colored), anti-B (yellow-colored) and anti-A, B (colorless). *Sodium azide* is used to prevent bacterial growth. These are stored at 4–6°C. Routinely, anti-A and anti-B sera are used for blood grouping.

Serum (Reverse) Blood Grouping

In serum group testing, serum is used to demonstrate the anti-A and anti-B antibodies by employing known group A and group B red blood cells. Forward grouping using anti-A and anti-B sera are shown in Table 12.4.

PROCEDURE FOR ABO BLOOD GROUPING

Slide Test

In slide test, red blood cells from blood sample are reacted with antisera (anti-A and anti-B). Demonstration of agglutination of red blood cells indicates presence of corresponding antigen on red blood cells (Fig. 12.8).

One drop of anti-A and one drop of anti-B are placed different area on slide ensuring that these are not mixed. Now add one drop of blood sample to be tested to each drop of antiserum and then mixed by using stick.

Agglutination is observed in both areas of slide. Results of slide tests are always confirmed by cell and serum grouping by test tube method.

Tube Test

Tube method is more reliable than slide test. Red blood cells of blood sample are washed with saline and then mixed with known antiserum in the test tube. Mixture is incubated at room temperature and centrifuged.

Following centrifugation, cell button formed is dislodged gently by tapping the base of the tube and examined for agglutination. Agglutination of red blood cells is graded from 1+ to 4+ observed with naked eye. Blood grouping using tube test is shown in Fig. 12.9.

Microplate Method

Microplate is composed of polystyrene. It consists of 96 microwells of either V or U shape. Blood grouping performed by microplate method is sensitive.

Rh BLOOD GROUPING

Both D and ABO antigens are immunogenic. Therefore, red blood cells for D antigen is routinely performed. Depending on the presence or absence of D antigen, persons are called *Rh positive* or *Rh negative*. Transfusion of Rh positive blood group to especially Rh negative mother will develop anti-RhD antibodies.

These antibodies can cross placenta during pregnancy and cause destruction of fetal red blood cells. Newborn will develop hemolytic disease of newborn. In Rh blood grouping, person's red blood cells are mixed with anti-RhD reagent.

Table 12.4: Forward grouping using anti-A and anti-B sera

Parameters	Forward grouping using anti-A serum	Forward grouping using anti-B serum
Color code	Blue	Yellow
Nature of antibody	IgM	IgM
Amount of antiserum required	2 drops	2 drops

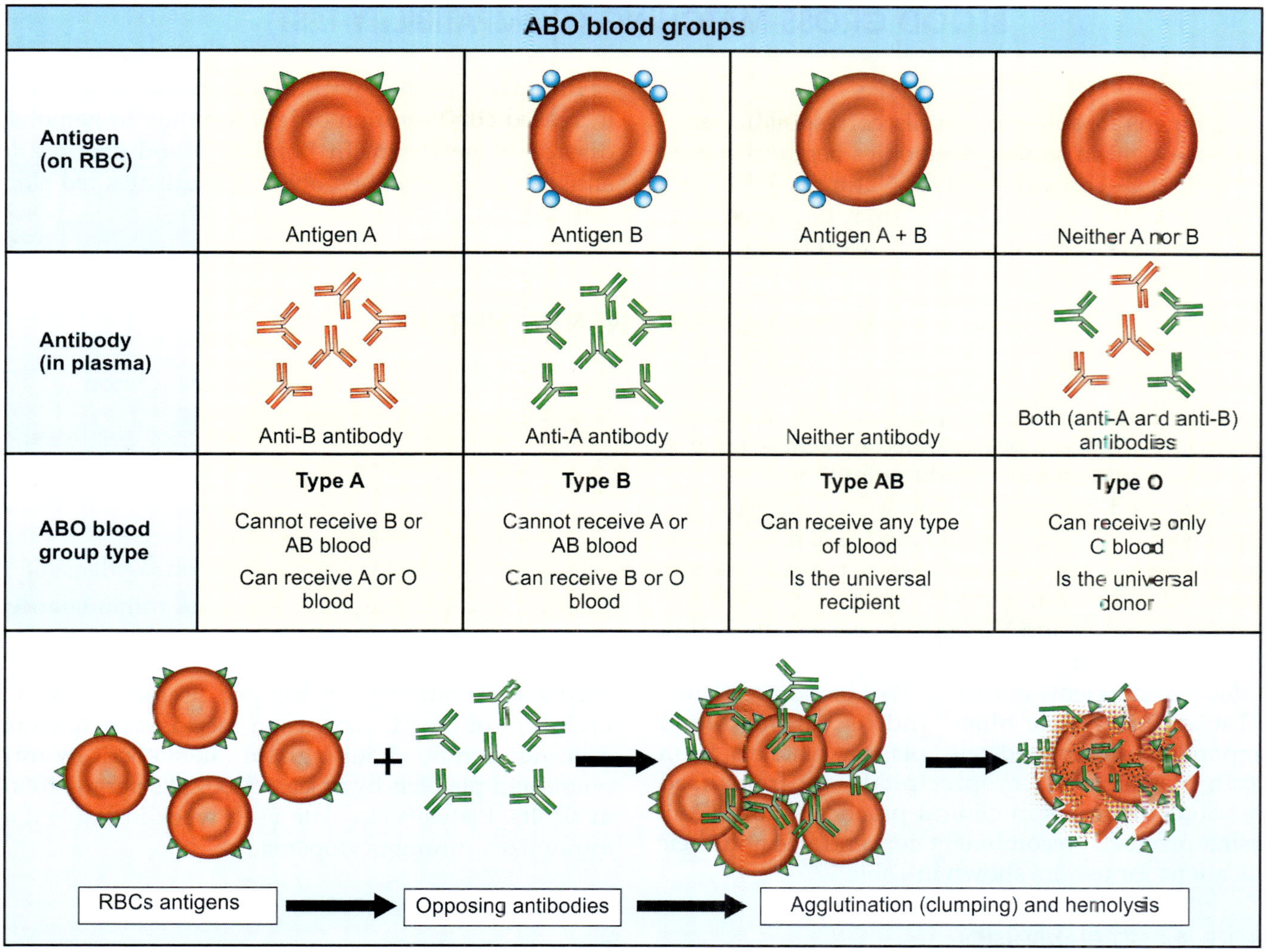

ABO blood groups
Antigen (on RBC)
Antigen A
Antigen B
Antigen A + B
Neither A nor B
Antibody (in plasma)
Anti-B antibody
Anti-A antibody
Neither antibody
Both (anti-A and anti-B) antibodies
ABO blood group type
Type A
Cannot receive B or AB blood
Can receive A or O blood
Type B
Cannot receive A or AB blood
Can receive B or O blood
Type AB
Can receive any type of blood
Is the universal recipient
Type O
Can receive only O blood
Is the universal donor
RBCs antigens
Opposing antibodies
Agglutination (clumping) and hemolysis

Fig. 12.8: Blood grouping using slide test.

Patient serum
Donor RBCs
2 drops
1 drop (5%)
Incubation 37°C, 1 hour
3 Washes
2 drops AHG mix properly
Centrifuge
No agglutination = compatible
Agglutination = incompatible

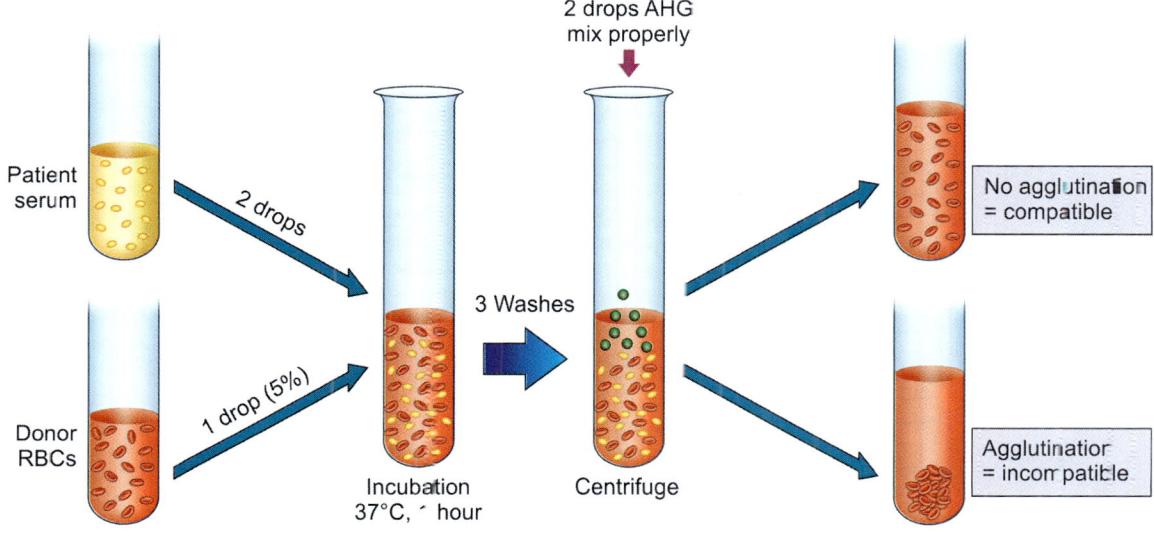

Fig. 12.9: Blood grouping using tube test.

BLOOD CROSS-MATCHING (COMPATIBILITY TEST)

ANTIBODIES OF ABO SYSTEM

Once antigens are absent from cells, corresponding antibody is present in serum. Antibodies begin to appear during first 3–4 months of life. Naturally occurring anti-A and anti-B mostly IgM, IgG may be present. IgG is more commonly present in *blood group O* individuals.

Pregnant mother with blood group O develops increased concentration of IgG resulting in hemolytic disease of newborn. In Bombay blood group alloantibody appears as hemolysin agglutinates red blood cells at 37°C.

BLOOD COMPONENTS THERAPY

Blood consist of plasma and cellular components (Fig. 12.10). Due to different specific gravity of cellular components, they can be separated by centrifuging at different centrifugal force for different time.

Refrigerated centrifuge rotor speed and duration of spin is critical. Each unit of blood (450 ml) contains 65 gm of hemoglobin, 225 mg of iron, platelets, factors V and VIII. When refrigerated, RBCs are viable up to 6 weeks. Factors V and VII begin to deteriorate within hours of collection.

Blood components in each unit of blood are shown in Table 12.5. Whole blood and its various blood components, e.g. packed cells, plasma, platelets, fresh frozen plasma, and cryoprecipitate are transfused in various disorders in clinical practice (Table 12.6). Plasma products/recombinant concentrates and their indications for use are shown in Table 12.7.

Table 12.5: Blood components in each unit of blood

Component	Value/characteristics
Hemoglobin	65 gm
Iron	225 mg
Platelets	6×10^9/L
RBCs	Viable up to 6 weeks in refrigerator
Factors V and VIII	Begin to deteriorate within hours of collection

used in the treatment of hemolytic disease of newborn. Each unit of blood transfusion increases hemoglobin concentration by about 1 gm/dl, hematocrit by three points and platelets by at least 5000 cells per microliter in adults. Platelets circulate for a week in stable non-immunized thrombocytopenia.

PACKED CELLS TRANSFUSION

Packed cells (RBCs) transfusion permits restoration of oxygen carrying capacity with less risk of volume overload.

WHOLE BLOOD TRANSFUSION

Whole blood is used in medical and surgical emergencies during excessive bleeding. Whole blood replacement is

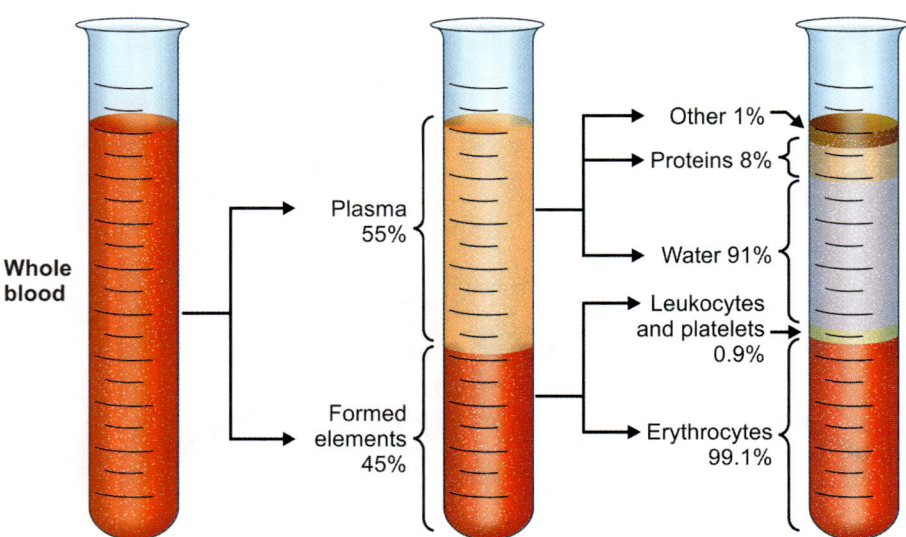

Fig. 12.10: Composition of blood showing plasma and cellular components.

Table 12.6: Blood components used in clinical practice

Components	Composition	Quantity	Indications
Whole blood	RBC, WBC, platelets, plasma deficiency in factors V, VIII	500 ml	Increase red cells and plasma volume
Red blood cells	RBC, WBC, some platelets, reduced plasma	250 ml	Increase red cell mass in chronic blood loss and symptomatic anemia
Leukocyte reduced red blood cells	RBCs >85% with low WBCs	225 ml	Reducing FNHTR (febrile non-hemolytic transfusion reaction) Useful in prevention of febrile reactions Prevention of HLA immunization before transplantation Reducing CMV transmission
Washed red blood cells	RBCs, with low WBCs (no plasma)	180 ml	Transfusion reaction to plasma proteins (use within 24 hours)
Gamma irradiated red blood cells	RBCs	180 ml	Prevention of transfusion associated with graft-versus-host disease (used within 24 hours)
Platelet concentrates	Platelets 5.5×10^{10} a few RBCs, WBCs and plasma	50 ml	Thrombocytopenia (primary or secondary) and Glanzmann disease (functional defect)
Fresh frozen plasma (FFP)	Plasma having all coagulation factors	220 ml	Coagulation disorders with prothrombin time >18 seconds, and APTT >60 seconds
Cryoprecipitate	Factors VIII, XIII, vWF, fibrinogen	15 ml	Hemophilia A von Willebrand disease Deficiency of fibrinogen
Plasma	Plasma, stable clotting factors, no platelets	220 ml	Stable clotting factor deficiency

Sterility testing of blood components should be carried out

Table 12.7: Plasma products/recombinant concentrates and their indications for use

Plasma products/recombinant concentrates	Indications for use
Human factor VIII	Hemophilia A von Willebrand disease
Human factor VIII (high purity)	Hemophilia A especially with HIV infection
Recombinant factor VIII	Hemophilia A
Porcine factor VIII	Factor VIII inhibitor
von Willebrand factor	von Willebrand disease
Factor IX (high purity)	Hemophilia B
Recombinant factor IX	Hemophilia B
Prothrombin complex concentrates	Congenital deficiency of factors II and X Oral anticoagulant overdose Factor VIII inhibitors Severe liver disease
Activated prothrombin complex concentrates	Factor VIII inhibitors
Factor VII	Congenital deficiency of factor VII Oral anticoagulant overdose Severe liver disease
Recombinant factor VIIa	Congenital deficiency of factor VII Inhibitors
Factor XI	Congenital deficiency of factor XI with history of cardiovascular disease

Contd...

Table 12.7: Plasma products/recombinant concentrates and their indications for use (Contd...)

Plasma products/recombinant concentrates	Indications for use
Factor XIII	Congenital deficiency of factor XIII
Fibrinogen	Congenital deficiency of fibrinogen/dysfibrinogenemia
Fibrin sealant glues	Congenital or acquired hemostatic disorders to promote local hemostasis
Antithrombin	Congenital deficiency (in selected cases)
Protein C	Congenital deficiency of protein C
C1 esterase inhibitor	Hereditary angioedema
$\alpha 1$ antitrypsin	Hereditary α_1 antitrypsin deficiency (emphysema and cirrhosis)
Immunoglobulins	Passive prophylaxis, congenital agammaglobulinemia, chronic lymphocytic leukemia, immunomediated thrombocytopenic purpura

PLASMA TRANSFUSION

Burns patient lose lot of plasma. Plasma transfusion is used in cases of burns.

PLATELETS TRANSFUSION

Platelets transfusion usually controls bleeding in thrombocytopenic patients, either due to suppressed platelets production in leukemias, chemotherapy, radiotherapy; or dilutional thrombocytopenia after massive transfusions. Platelets circulate for a week in stable non-immunized thrombocytopenic patients.

LEUKOCYTES REDUCED BLOOD COMPONENT

Febrile reactions are common in sensitized patients, who receive components $>5 \times 10^8$ leukocytes and alloimmunization to the HLA antigens of residual lymphocytes may occur when $>10^6$ lymphocytes are transfused.

FRESH FROZEN PLASMA

Fresh frozen plasma is prepared from fresh blood within 8 hours of collection by avoiding clotting. It is stored at $-20°C$ for one year. It contains factor VIII and factor IX. It is used in coagulation disorders by transfusing 7–15 ml/kg body weight via intravenous route for 30–60 minutes. Its disadvantage is allergic reaction.

Approximately, 6–12% hemophilic patients develop antibodies against factor VIII after therapy following fresh frozen infusion. Therefore, recombinant factor VIII is being used in hemophilic patients.

Fresh *frozen plasma is valuable in patients with thrombotic thrombocytopenic* purpura. It can also be used in reversal of the effects of oral anticoagulant therapy associated with bleeding occurring due to depletion of coagulation factors. Plasma fractionation pathways are shown in Fig. 12.11.

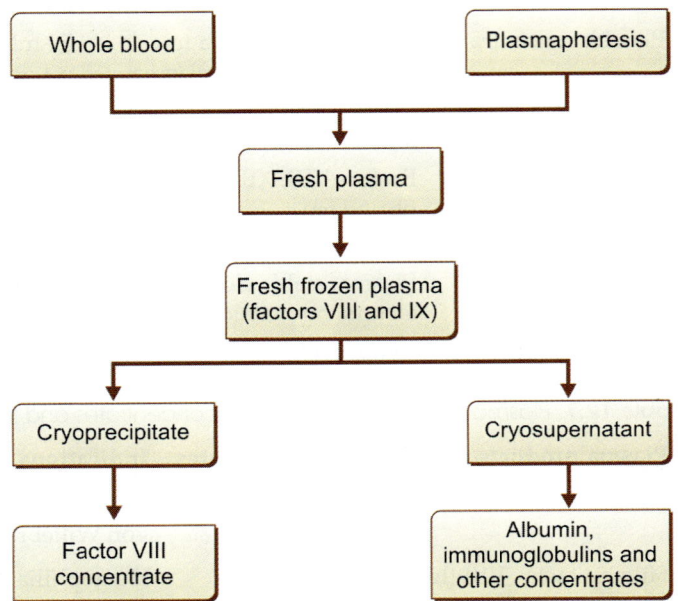

Fig. 12.11: Plasma fractionation pathways.

CRYOPRECIPITATE

Cryoprecipitate is used in coagulation disorders. It is prepared from fresh frozen plasma. It contains factor VIII, fibrinogen, von Willebrand factor, and factor XIII. Bag containing 200 units of factor VIII is *stored at –90°C*.

Thawing is performed at 4°C. It is administered by intravenous route. It is used to promote hemostasis in various acquired coagulation disorders. Its advantage is exposure of the recipients to a few donors. Blood products are costly and limited worldwide. Excessive administration of factor VIII is not beneficial to the patients.

FACTOR VIII CONCENTRATE

Factor VIII concentrate is the product of choice for patients with hemophilia A. It has a short half-life about

12 hours *in vivo*. High purity factor VIII concentrate is administered continuously during surgery.

FACTOR IX CONCENTRATE

High purity factor IX concentrate is used for patients with hemophilia B also known as *Christmas disease*.

PROTHROMBIN COMPLEX CONCENTRATES

Prothrombin complex concentrates contain coagulation factors IX, X, II and sometimes factor VII. These are more effective than fresh frozen plasma. These are used to treat hemophilia A, who have circulating antibody (inhibitor) to factor VIII.

IMMUNOGLOBULINS

Specific immunoglobulins are obtained from donors, who have high concentration of IgG. These are administered in patients for passive prophylaxis against infectious agents. Anti-D is administered to the Rh –ve mother having Rh +ve fetus in the prevention of hemolytic disease of newborn.

AUTOLOGOUS BLOOD TRANSFUSION AND PLASMA EXCHANGE

AUTOLOGOUS BLOOD TRANSFUSION

Autologous blood transfusion refers to collection of blood from the patient prior to surgery for whom the transfusion is used later. Benefits of autologous transfusion are to avoid transfusion transmitted infectious disease, immunological effects. Autologous transfusion is safe and useful in patients with rare blood group and with multiple alloantibodies.

THERAPEUTIC APHERESIS

Therapeutic apheresis refers to removal of blood or red blood cells, platelets or white blood cells from the body for clinical purpose. Techniques of apheresis are automated apheresis and centrifugal devices.

Red Blood Cells Removal (Erythropheresis)

Simple venesection and manual exchange are employed for treatment of *polycythemia vera, sickle cell crisis* and severe **hemolytic disease** of newborn.

Platelets Removal (Thrombopheresis)

Platelets are removed to lower platelet count in patients with myeloproliferative disorders and platelet count >1000 × 10^9/L in patients with polycythemia vera, thrombocythemia and chronic granulocytic leukemia. Main aim is to prevent the development of thrombotic or hemorrhagic complication before conventional chemotherapy.

White Blood Cells Removal (Leukopheresis)

White cells are removed in leukemia to prevent vascular occlusion in the microcirculation by increased white blood cell count. Leukocytapheresis can rapidly reduce white blood cell count and viscosity.

PLASMAPHERESIS/PLASMA EXCHANGE

Plasmapheresis/plasma exchange is the selective removal of small volumes (<600 ml) of plasma, which requires replacement by an appropriate fluid to maintain homeostasis (Table 12.8).

Table 12.8: Diseases in which plasma exchange is beneficial

Disease	Pathogenetic factors
Waldenstörm's macroglobulinemia (hyperviscosity syndrome) and multiple myeloma	Monoclonal immunoglobulins
Acute myasthenia gravis	Anti-ACh receptors
Cryoglobulinemia	Cryoglobulin
Hemophilia with inhibitors	Anti-factor VIII inhibitor
Cold agglutinin hemolytic anemia	Cold agglutinin
Neonatal hyperbilirubinemia (HDN)	Rh incompatibility not responding to phototherapy
Acute Gullain-Barré syndrome	Anti-ganglioside
Goodpasture's syndrome	Anti-glomerular basement membrane
Thrombotic thrombocytopenic purpura	Unknown
Poison (mushroom)	α-amanitin
Drugs	Digoxin, parathion methyl

Possible complications of exchange blood transfusions are hyperglycemia, hyperkalemia, air embolism, thrombocytopenia, coagulation factor deficiency.

ADVERSE BLOOD TRANSFUSION REACTIONS

Blood transfusion is a lifesaving procedure in clinical practice. Recipients are at high risk of developing adverse blood transfusion reactions such as circulatory overload, bronchopneumonia, hemolytic reactions, thrombophlebitis (if blood transfusion given at one site for >12 hours), air embolism, transmission of diseases and transfusion hemosiderosis (Table 12.9).

HEMOLYTIC TRANSFUSION REACTION

Acute Hemolytic Transfusion Reactions

Acute hemolytic transfusion reactions result from transfusion of ABO mismatched blood to the recipient due to technical error. Donor RBCs are destroyed by recipient's blood containing IgM. Antigen-antibody activates complement system resulting in RBCs hemolysis in circulation. Intravascular hemolysis leads to hemoglobinuria, hypotension, acute renal failure and oliguria.

Laboratory findings are hemoglobinemia, hemoglobinuria, fragmented red blood cells in peripheral smear, direct positive Coombs' test and increased serum bilirubin. In anesthetized patients, hypotension and bleeding are the only findings.

Delayed Hemolytic Transfusion Reactions

Delayed reactions patients, who have been sensitized to red blood cell antigen during pregnancy or prior blood transfusion. Patient develops delayed hemolytic transfusion reactions *4 days to 2 weeks* after blood transfusion due to extravascular destruction of red blood cells by IgG.

Laboratory findings are raised serum bilirubin, anemia, spherocytosis and positive direct Coombs' test. Comparison between acute and delayed hemolytic transfusion reactions is shown in Table 12.10.

TRANSMISSION OF INFECTIONS

Various viruses can be HIV, HBV, HCV, HDV, cytomegalovirus and parvovirus B_{19}. It is essential to screen donor's blood before transfusing in recipients. Normally blood is stored at *20–25°C*. Pseudomonas is capable to grow even at 1–6°C. Malarial parasite survives at 4°C.

Tests used for screening donor for HCV are by anti-HCV antibody test and polymerase chain reaction. Infectious agents transmitted by blood transfusion is shown in Table 12.11. Infectious disease testing performed on blood donations is shown in Table 12.12.

Table 12.9: Adverse reactions of blood transfusion

Complications	Characteristics
Hemolytic transfusion reactions	*Immediate reactions:* Donor RBCs are destroyed by recipient's blood containing IgM. Intravascular hemolysis leads to hemoglobinuria, acute renal failure and oliguria *Delayed reactions:* These occur 4 days to 2 weeks after blood transfusion due to extravascular destruction of RBCs
Transmission of infections	*Viral diseases:* HIV, HBV, HCV, HDV, cytomegalovirus, parvovirus B_{19} *Bacterial:* Pseudomonas grow at 1–6°C (blood is stored at 20–25°C) *Parasite:* Malarial parasite survives at 4°C
Febrile reactions	Fever, chills and rigors due to sensitization of donor WBCs within one hour of transfusion
Allergic reactions (anaphylaxis)	Urticaria, bronchospasm and rarely anaphylactic shock
Circulatory overload	Acute pulmonary edema with impaired cardiac functions
Transfusion related acute lung injury	Acute respiratory distress syndrome occurs within six hours of transfusion due to antibodies formed against RBC antigens and phagocytes
Air embolism	Occurs when bottle transfusion is given
Thrombophlebitis	Occurs in patients with indwelling catheters
Transfusion hemosiderosis	Occurs due to multiple blood transfusions, so chelating agents are administered
Transfusion associated graft-versus-host disease	When immunocompetent T cells of donor are transfused to immunodeficient recipients recognize HLA as foreign and cause acute graft-versus-host reaction

Table 12.10: Comparison between acute and delayed hemolytic transfusion reactions

Parameters	Acute hemolytic transfusion reactions	Delayed hemolytic transfusion reactions
Clinical features appearance following transfusion	Fever, chills, acute renal failure within minutes after transfusion	Fever, mild jaundice and anemia within 4 days to 2 weeks after transfusion
Site of hemolysis of red blood cells	Intravascular hemolysis	Extravascular hemolysis
Antibody responsible for hemolysis	Anti-ABO Natural occurring antibody	Anti-Kidd Antibody formed due to immune response

Table 12.11: Infectious agents transmitted by blood transfusion

Infectious agent	Examples
Viruses	Plasma-borne (HIV-1, HIV-2, HBV, HCV, HDV, parvovirus B19 Cell associated viruses (cytomegalovirus, Epstein-Barr virus, HTLV-I, HTLV-II)
Bacteria	*Treponema pallidum* Brucellosis Pseudomonas (occasional) Salmonella (occasional)
Parasites	Malarial parasite *Trypanosoma cruzi* *Toxoplasma gondii* *Leishmania donovani* *Babesia microti*

Table 12.12: Infectious disease testing performed on blood donations

Infection	Tests designated to detect
Hepatitis B	Hepatitis B surface antigen (ELISA) IgM antibody and IgG antibody to hepatitis B core antigen HBV-DNA (nucleic acid testing)
Hepatitis C	IgG antibody to hepatitis C peptides Hepatitis C virus RNA (ELISA) Polymerase chain reaction
HIV-1 and HIV-2	IgM and IgG antibody to HIV-1 and HIV-2 (ELISA) HIV-RNA
HTLV-I and HTLV-II (human T cell lymphotropic virus)	IgG antibody to HTLV-I and HTLV-II
Syphilis	IgM and IgG antibody to *Treponema pallidum* antigens (VDRL and TPHA)

FEBRILE NON-HEMOLYTIC TRANSFUSION REACTIONS

Febrile non-hemolytic transfusion reactions are observed in 1% cases following especially multiple blood transfusions. Recipient presents with fever, chills and rigors due to sensitization of donor WBCs within one hour of transfusion.

Antibodies in the recipients react with antigens on donor leukocytes and platelets and activate complement system resulting in release of pyrogenic cytokines. Fever may also occur as a result of release of pyrogenic cytokines from white cells of stored blood used. Febrile transfusion reactions are also observed in acute hemolytic transfusion reaction, bacterial contamination of donor unit, transfusion associated lung injury and delayed transfusion reactions.

ALLERGIC REACTIONS (ANAPHYLAXIS)

Recipient may develop skin rashes, bronchospasm and rarely anaphylactic shock. Anaphylactic shock occurs in IgA deficient recipients, whose antibodies react with donor plasma IgA leading to activation of complement and formation of anaphylatoxin.

CIRCULATORY OVERLOAD

Following excessive blood transfusion, patient may develop acute pulmonary edema with impaired cardiac function as a consequence of congestive heart failure. This complication can be prevented by giving slow blood transfusion. Infusion of red blood cells concentrate is helpful in these patients.

TRANSFUSION RELATED ACUTE LUNG INJURY

Transfusion related acute lung injury (TRALI) is the most common cause of major morbidity and death after transfusion. It presents as an acute respiratory distress syndrome (ARDS) either during or within 6 hours of transfusion due to antibodies formed against RBCs antigens and phagocytes. It occurs due to multiple blood transfusions.

Hypoxemia, dyspnea, cyanosis, fever, tachycardia and hypotension result from non-cardiogenic pulmonary edema. Radiograph shows bilateral pulmonary infiltration, a characteristic finding of pulmonary edema.

AIR EMBOLISM

Air embolism results from the introduction of excess of air (>100 cc) into the circulation leading to vascular flow obstruction. It occurs when bottle transfusion is given. It may also occur due to improper monitoring of intravenous infusion.

THROMBOPHLEBITIS

Thrombophlebitis occurs in patients with indwelling catheters. This complication is not serious but very painful. It is not uncommon to see cellulitis extending from wrist to the elbow.

TRANSFUSION ASSOCIATED GRAFT-VERSUS-HOST DISEASE

Blood unit contains red blood cells, granulocytes, platelets and immunocompetent T cells. When such blood unit is transfused into immunodeficient recipients, the donor's immunocompetent T cells undergo multiplication and recognize HLA antigen as foreign resulting in acute graft-versus-host disease within 1–2 weeks.

Patient presents with fever, erythematous lesions beginning centrally progressing to hands and feet, and bloody diarrhea. Patient may later develop leukopenia due to bone marrow suppression leading to recurrent infections.

POST-TRANSFUSION THROMBOCYTOPENIA

Multiple blood transfusions may cause dilutional thrombocytopenia within 7–10 days after blood transfusion. It is observed in patients, who have been immunized earlier as a result of platelets transfusion. Patient presents with fever, chills and generalized purpura. Post-transfusion thrombocytopenia is self-limited entity.

TRANSFUSION HEMOSIDEROSIS

Transfusion hemosiderosis occurs due to multiple blood transfusions, so chelating agents are administered.

CHAPTER 13

Lymph Nodes, Spleen and Thymus

Learning Objectives

DISORDERS OF LYMPH NODE
- Organization of Lymph Nodes
- Non-neoplastic Disorders of Lymph Nodes
- Cervical Lymphadenopathy
- Malignant Lymphoid Neoplasms

HODGKIN'S DISEASE
- Overview
- Morphologic Subtypes

NON-HODGKIN'S LYMPHOMA
- Overview
- Precursor B Cell NHL

- Mature B Cell NHL
- Mature T Cell and NK Cell HNL

SPLEEN
- Structure
- Functional Disorders
- Reactive Splenic Disorders
- Non-neoplastic Infiltrative Disorders
- Neoplastic Disorders

THYMUS GLAND
- Overview
- Immunodeficiency Disorders
- Thymic Neoplasms

DISORDERS OF LYMPH NODE

ORGANIZATION OF LYMPH NODES

Lymph nodes are collections of lymphoid tissue widely distributed within the lymphoreticular system. Beneath the collagenous capsule is the subareolar sinus, which is lined by phagocytic cells. Lymphocytes and antigens from surrounding tissue spaces or adjacent nodes pass into the sinus via the afferent lymphatic system.

ORGANIZATION

On histopathological examination, lymph nodes show four compartments: cortex showing primary and secondary follicles containing B cells found near capsule, paracortex containing T cells surrounding follicles, medullary region and sinuses. T cells in the cortex are associated with the interdigitating antigen presenting cells.

ARTERIAL SUPPLY AND VENOUS DRAINAGE

Each lymph node has its own arterial supply and venous drainage. Lymphocytes enter the node from the circulation through the specialized high endothelial venules in the paracortex. The medulla contains both T and B cells as well as most of the lymph node plasma cells are organized into cords of lymphoid tissue. Lymphocytes can leave the node through the efferent lymphatic vessel. Tissue sampling and histological slide preparation are shown in Table 13.1.

Table 13.1: Tissue sampling and histological slide preparation

Sampling	Utility
Wet touch preparation	Hematoxylin and eosin (fixed in formalin) Papanicolaou staining (fixed in 95% alcohol)
Air dried touch smears	Myeloperoxidase stain Nonspecific esterase FISH (fluorescence *in situ* hybridization) for cytogenetics
Rapid frozen tissue	Immunohistochemistry Cytochemistry Genetic analysis
Fresh tissue in RPMI 1640 medium or saline	Flow cytometry
Sterile fresh tissue	Microbial culture
Paraffin embedded	Hematoxylin and eosin Giemsa stain PAS Masson's trichome
Thin shaved tissue	Electron microscopy (fixed in glutaraldehyde)

NON-NEOPLASTIC DISORDERS OF LYMPH NODES

These reactions include acute and chronic nonspecific lymphadenitis occurring in response to a number of infectious agents or immune stimuli.

LYMPHOID HYPERPLASIA

Lymphoid hyperplasia is enlargement of lymphoid follicles (principally in the cortex of the lymph node), which consist of B cells. Reactive follicular hyperplasia of lymph nodes represents a response to infections, inflammation, or tumors. Hyperplasia of the secondary follicles, germinal centers, and increased plasma cells in medullary cords indicates B cell immune response. Hyperplasia of the deep cortex or paracortex (diffuse hyperplasia in interfollicular region) is characteristic of T cell response.

SINUS HISTIOCYTOSIS

Necrotic products of the neoplasm and tumor antigens often evoke reactive changes in the lymph nodes such as enlargement and hyperplasia of the lymphoid follicles, proliferation of macrophages in the subcapsular sinuses (sinus histiocytosis).

INFECTIOUS MONONUCLEOSIS

This benign, self-limited disorder is caused by Epstein-Barr virus (EBV), which has an affinity for B cells. It occurs frequently in young adults. Circulating atypical reactive CD8+ T cells are characteristic. The disorder is marked by a number of serum anti-EBV antibodies and heterophil antibodies (heterophil agglutinins) directed against sheep erythrocytes.

Patient presents with prominent sore throat, fever, generalized lymphadenopathy, and hepatosplenomegaly. The spleen is especially susceptible to traumatic rupture. Heterophil-negative infectious mononucleosis is most often associated with cytomegalovirus infection.

SUPPURATIVE LYMPHADENITIS

Suppurative lymphadenitis occurs in the lymph nodes that drain a site of acute bacterial infection. The lymph nodes rapidly become enlarged due to edema and hyperemia and are tender due to distension of the capsule.

Light microscopy reveals polymorphonuclear leukocytic infiltration in lymph node sinuses and stroma associated with prominent follicular hyperplasia.

GRANULOMATOUS LYMPHADENITIS

Granulomatous lymphadenitis is characterized by formation of epithelioid granulomas in the lymph nodes. Caseating granulomas with central necrosis and caseation are demonstrated in *Mycobacterium tuberculosis*. Acid-fast bacilli are stained by Ziehl-Neelsen stain appearing as bright red, slender and beaded rods.

Mycobacterium leprae and histoplasmosis are other examples of caseating lymphadenitis. Noncaseating granulomas are seen in sarcoidosis composed of epithelioid histiocytes with scattered multinucleated giant cells. This type of noncaseating epithelioid granulomas can be demonstrated in draining lymph nodes in Crohn's disease.

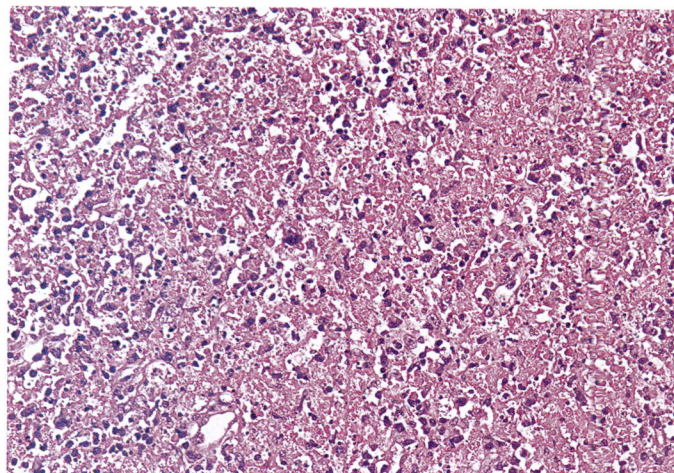

Fig. 13.1: Kikuchi disease showing necrotizing lymph node (100X).

KIKUCHI DISEASE

Kikuchi disease is characterized by generalized necrotizing lymphadenopathy. It is a benign disorder affecting young more often women than men. Patient presents with recurrent necrotizing lymphadenitis often associated with other systemic inflammatory disorders such as systemic lupus erythematosus, tuberculosis, HIV and papovavirus B19 (Fig. 13.1).

KIMURA'S DISEASE

Kimura's disease is characterized by angiolymphoid proliferation of lymph nodes predominantly in the head and neck region forming eosinophilic abscess, involvement of subcutaneous tissue and eosinophilia. Salivary gland involvement, glomerulonephritis, nephrotic syndrome, eosinophilia and increased IgE are more common in Kimura's disease than Kikuchi disease.

CASTLEMAN DISEASE

Castleman disease is also known as *angiofollicular lymph node hyperplasia* or *giant lymph node hyperplasia* or *angiomatous lymphoid hamartoma*. It may be localized or multicentric lymph nodes involvement in mediastinum. It most often affects adults but less prevalent in children.

Clinical Features

Patient presents with dyspnea and radiograph reveals widening of mediastinum due to solitary or multicentric lymph node enlargement. It may be associated with Kaposi sarcoma, mantle cell lymphoma, and diffuse large cell lymphoma.

Histological Variants

Hyaline-vascular variant: Hyaline-vascular variant is unicentric and asymptomatic disease. Patient presents with anemia, night sweats, weight loss, elevated sedimentation rate and hypergammaglobulinemia. Histopathological examination shows increased lymphoid follicles in cortex and medulla. Follicles contain hyalinized and sclerosed blood vessels resembling white pulp of spleen.

Plasma cell variant: Plasma cell variant is multicentric disease. Patient presents with generalized lymphadenopathy. Histopathological examination exhibits proliferation of blood vessels surrounded by mature plasma cells. There is distension of lymph node sinuses. Children have good prognosis with corticosteroid therapy. It is associated with HHV8 infection, with an accumulation of HHV8+ lymphocytes in mantle zone leading to dissolution of the germinal center.

CERVICAL LYMPHADENOPATHY

The most common swellings in cervical region are enlarged lymph nodes. These are caused by *bacterial or viral infections, lymphomas* and *metastatic deposits*. Inflammatory lymphadenopathy is most often painful, firm and mobile. Malignant lymph nodes are painless and hard.

These may be located in the midline or lateral side of neck. **Delphin lymph nodes** located along thyrohyoid membrane are enlarged in *thyroid cancer*. LD bodies in the lymph node aspirate are shown in Fig. 13.2. Metastatic deposits in lymph nodes are shown in Figs 13.3 and 13.4. Lymphadenopathy may be generalized or localized (Table 13.2). Differential diagnosis of cervical lymphadenopathy is shown in Table 13.3.

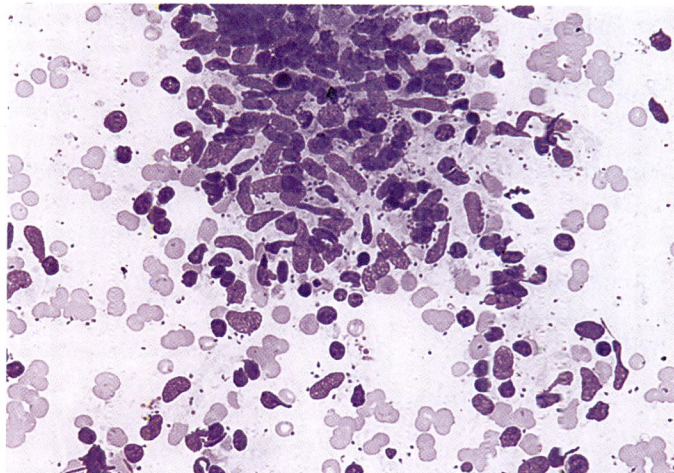

Fig. 13.2: *Leishmania donovani* bodies are demonstrated in the lymph node aspirate. Epithelioid granuloma is also seen (400X).

Table 13.2: Causes of lymphadenopathy

Categories	Causes
Generalized lymphadenopathy	
Lymphomas	Hodgkin's disease Non-Hodgkin's lymphoma
Leukemias	Acute lymphoblastic leukemia Chronic lymphocytic leukemia
Infections	Tuberculosis Brucellosis Syphilis *Toxoplasma gondii* Sarcoidosis
Autoimmune disorders	Systemic lupus erythematosus Rheumatoid arthritis
Hypersensitivity	Serum sickness
Lipid storage diseases	Gaucher's disease Niemann-Pick disease
Drug	Phenytoin
Miscellaneous	Sarcoidosis Pseudolymphoma
Localized lymphadenopathy	
Infections	Acute or chronic infections
Metastatic cancers	Breast carcinoma Lung carcinoma Kidney carcinoma Head and neck

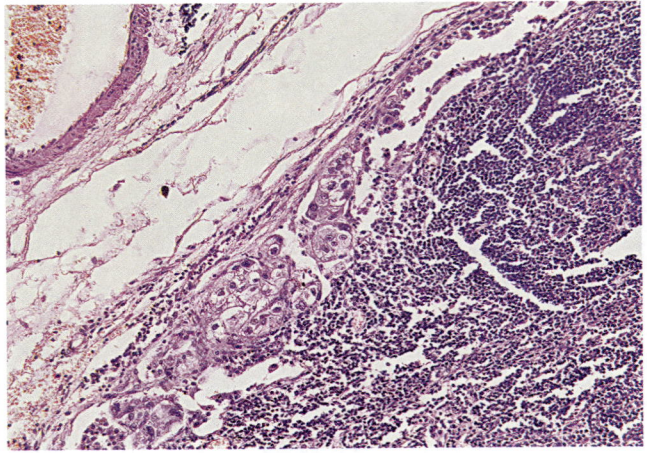

Fig. 13.3: Metastatic deposits from carcinoma are seen in subcapsular area of lymph node (400X).

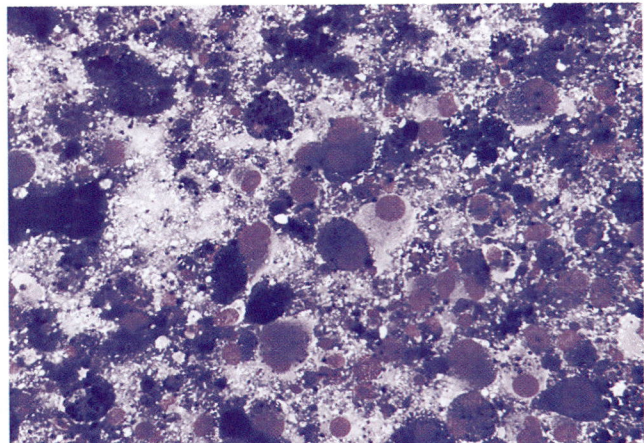

Fig. 13.4: Fine needle aspirate from lymph node showing deposits from melanoma (400X).

Table 13.3: Differential diagnosis of cervical lymphadenopathy

Lymph node groups	Areas drained by lymph node group	Categories of etiology	Differential diagnosis
Preauricular or posterior cervical lymph nodes	Scalp and skin	Infections	Tubercular lymphadenitis
		Cancers	Squamous cell carcinoma skin (head and neck regions) Hodgkin's disease Non-Hodgkin's lymphoma
Supraclavicular nodes	Gastrointestinal tract, pulmonary and genitourinary systems	Infections	Tubercular lymphadenitis Fungal infections
		Cancers	Cancers of thorax, abdomen, thyroid and larynx
Submandibular or anterior lymph nodes	Oral cavity	Infections	Tubercular lymphadenitis Dental or upper respiratory tract infections Infectious mononucleosis Toxoplasma Cytomegalovirus Rubella
		Cancers	Squamous cell carcinoma of head and neck Leukemia Lymphomas (Hodgkin's and NHL)

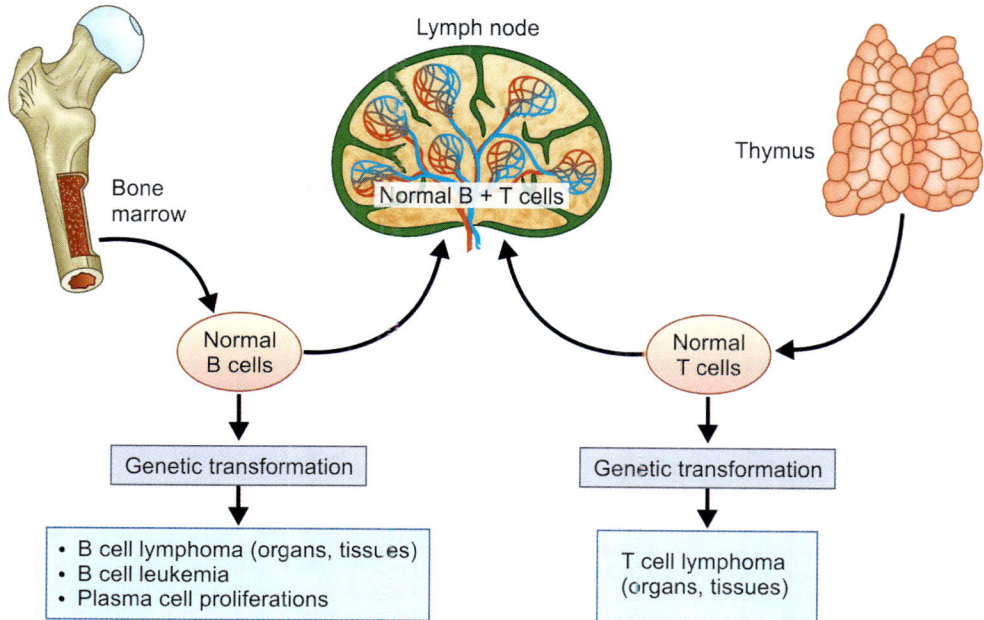

Fig. 13.5: Development of lymphoid malignancies.

MALIGNANT LYMPHOID NEOPLASMS

Malignant lymphoid neoplasms arise from T or B cells and their precursor cells. Patient presents with localized lymphadenopathy characterized by formation of gross tumor nodules.

Conversely, neoplastic proliferation of lymphocytes with diffuse and systemic involvement from their inception are categorized as leukemias. Malignant lymphoid neoplasms can be divided into two major categories—Hodgkin's disease and non-Hodgkin's lymphoma.

WHO CLASSIFICATION

WHO Classification of Non-Hodgkin's Lymphomas

High-grade non-Hodgkin's lymphoma (NHL) may involve a single lymph node, a localized group of lymph nodes, or an extranodal site.

Low-grade NHL tends to involve multiple lymph nodes at multiple sites, whereas **high-grade** NHL tends to be more **localized**. B cell NHLs are more common than T cells. WHO classification of non-Hodgkin's lymphoid neoplasms is based on origin from B or T cells—precursor cells or mature cells.

Development of lymphoid malignancies is shown in Fig. 13.5. Pathway of B cells differentiation within and without follicle center is shown in Fig. 13.6. Normal and abnormal counterparts of B cell progeny are shown in Fig. 13.7. Normal T cell progeny is shown in Fig. 13.8.

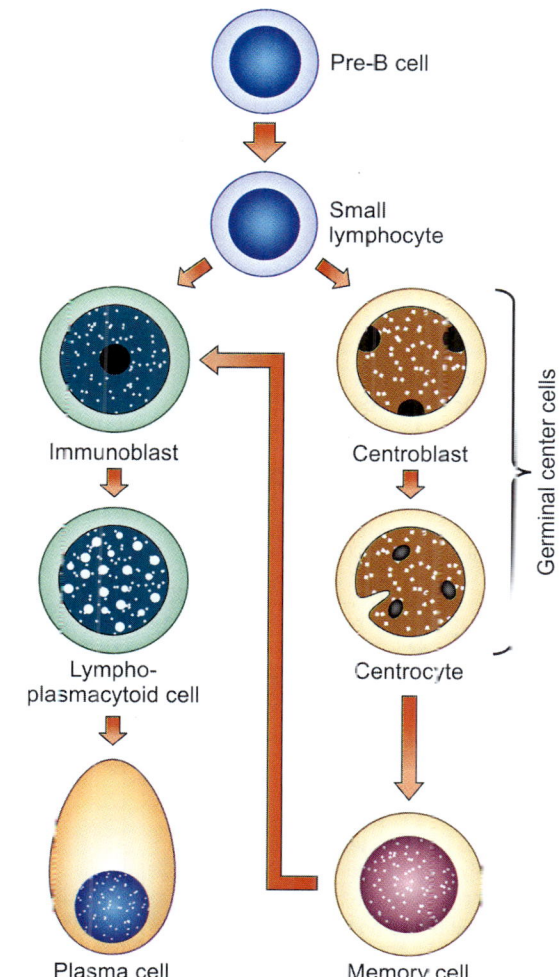

Fig. 13.6: Pathway of B cells differentiation within and without follicle center. Clones of malignant cells may arise any stage differentiation.

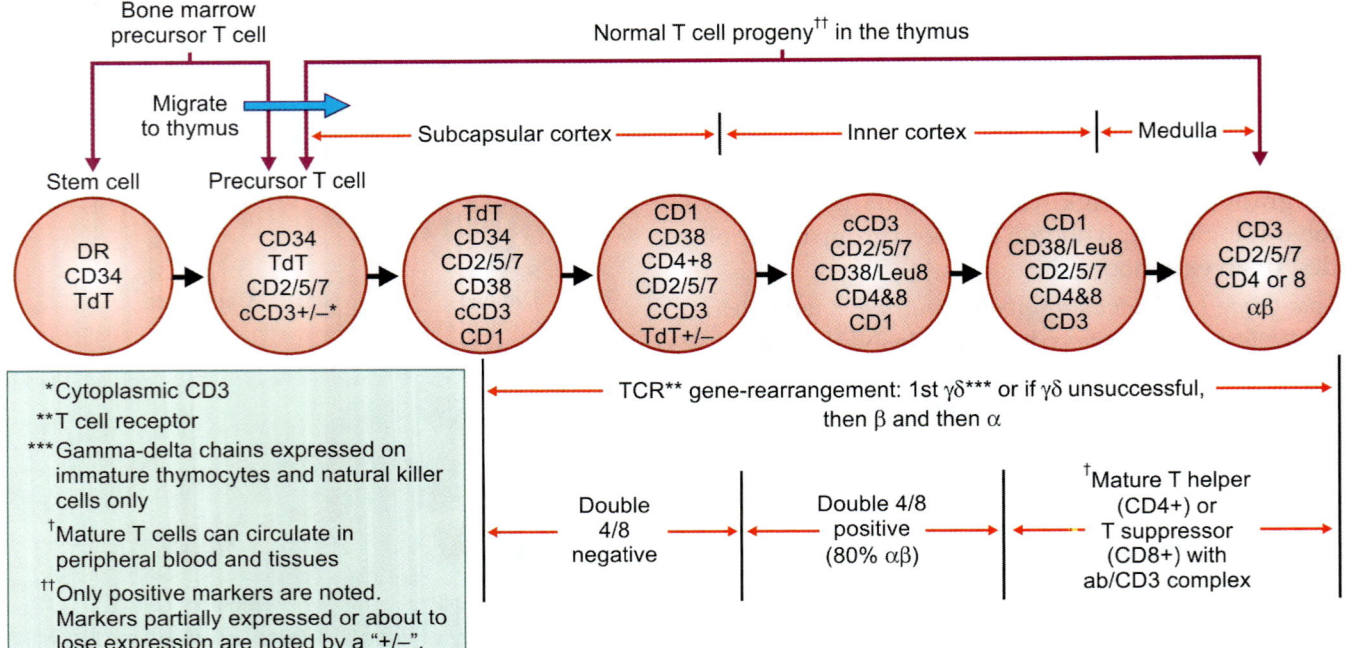

Fig. 13.7: Normal and abnormal counterparts of B cell progeny.

Fig. 13.8: Normal T cell progeny.

Who Classification of Hodgkin's Lymphomas

Diagnostic criteria of Hodgkin's disease are demonstration of **Reed-Sternberg cells** in the lymph nodes. The World Health Organization (WHO) classification identifies a number of disease variants: *classic variants* (lymphocytic-rich, lymphocytic depletion, nodular sclerosis and mixed cellularity) and nodular lymphocytic-histiocytic predominant. Differences between Hodgkin's disease and non-Hodgkin's lymphoma are shown in Table 13.4.

PATHOGENESIS

Molecular Genetics

Physiological state: BCL family comprises BCL-2, BCL-XL and MCL-1. BCL-2 gene family located on chromosome 18. This family produces gene products that prevent mitochondrial leakage of cytochrome-c (signal for apoptosis). Normally cytochrome-c leaving mitochondria and entering into the cytosol activates caspases and initiate apoptosis. Protein products of antiapoptotic genes prevent cytochrome-c from leaving mitochondria.

Pathological state: Translocation t(14;18) causes overexpression of the BCL-2 protein product, which prevents apoptosis of B cells causing B cell **follicular lymphoma** and **chronic lymphocytic leukemia**. Lymphoma cells do not die but accumulate in the lymph nodes, bone marrow, and the blood circulation.

Chemical Carcinogen-induced Lymphomas

Alkylating agents and aromatic amines participate in pathogenesis of lymphomas (Table 13.5).

PATHOGEN-INDUCED LYMPHOMAS

Bacteria and viruses participate in the pathogenesis of lymphomas (Table 13.6).

Table 13.4: Differences between Hodgkin's disease and non-Hodgkin's lymphoma

	Hodgkin's disease	Non-Hodgkin's lymphoma
Cell derivation	Mostly B cells	B cells (90%), T cells (10%)
Stage/grade	Begins in one lymph node then spread to other lymph nodes. In some cases, grade may be significant, but it is mostly unremarked	Systemic disease and grade influences prognosis and therapy more than stage
Source of mass	Neoplastic Reed-Sternberg cells are usually <1% of the total population of other benign inflammatory cells	Majority of the lymphoid cells are malignant
Lymph nodes involvement	Localized to single axial group of nodes (cervical, mediastinal, para-aortic) lymph nodes	Frequent involvement of multiple peripheral nodes
GI mesenteric/Waldeyer's involvement	Rarely involved	Commonly involved
Extranodal involvement	Uncommon (10% cases)	Common (40% cases)
Immune deficiency	Cell-mediated immunity impaired in all classic variants except nodular sclerosis. Mycobacterial, fungal, viral and protozoal infections	Humoral immunity impaired. Recurrent bacterial infections
Bone marrow involvement	Common (significant)	Uncommon (bone marrow involvement in some cases)
Architecture of lymph node	Effaced	Effaced
Other autoimmune disease	Uncommon	Common
Constitutional symptoms	Common	Uncommon
Chromosomal defects	Aneuploidy	Translocation and deletion
Spread	Ordinarily contiguous spread	Non-contiguous spread
Treatment	Radiotherapy (mild localized lesion)	Chemotherapy and radiotherapy (systemic disorder)
Prognosis	Good	Poor

Table 13.5: Chemical carcinogens and associated with cancers

Chemical carcinogens	Examples	Associated cancers
Direct acting chemical carcinogens and associated with cancers		
Alkylating agents	Nitrogen mustard, cyclophosphamide, chlorambucil, nitrosoureas, β-propiolactone, dimethyl sulphate and diepoxibutane are chemotherapeutic agents	Hodgkin's disease Non-Hodgkin's lymphoma Leukemias Ovarian carcinoma
Indirect acting chemical carcinogens and associated with cancers		
Aromatic hydrocarbons	Benzene present in crude oil (petrochemical), Benz (a) anthracene and Benz(a) pyrene	Acute leukemia Hodgkin's disease Urinary bladder carcinoma

Table 13.6: Pathogens induced carcinogenesis

Pathogens	Associated tumors
Bacteria	
Helicobacter pylori	Gastric carcinoma (lower half of stomach) Low grade B cell NHL of the mucosa-associated lymphoid tissue (MALToma)
Borrelia burgdorferi	Gastrointestinal tract lymphoma
Campylobacter jejuni	Gastrointestinal tract lymphoma
Viruses	
HTLV-1 (RNA)	T cell leukemia/lymphoma
EB virus (DNA)	CNS lymphoma in AIDS Nasopharyngeal carcinoma Hodgkin's disease (mixed cellularity) Burkitt's lymphoma Extranodal marginal zone B cell NHL
Molecular genetics in extranodal marginal zone NHL: Trisomy 18, t(11;18), t(1;14); latter create MALT1-IAP2 and BCL10-IgH fusion genes, respectively	

HODGKIN'S DISEASE

OVERVIEW

Hodgkin's disease is a malignant neoplasm of lymph node. It is important to determine whether the patient has only a single lymph node region involved or multiple node regions, or extranodal involvement. After therapy, about 5% of patients develop myelodysplastic syndromes, acute myelogenous leukemia, or carcinomas, particularly of the lung. Hodgkin's disease has bimodal age distribution with a peak at 15–40 years and second small peak during seventh decade.

DIAGNOSTIC CRITERIA

Diagnostic criteria include demonstration of neoplastic Reed-Sternberg cells in the lymph nodes. Reed-Sternberg cells are derived from B cells admixed with inflammatory cells in background as a result of cytokines synthesis such as IL1, IL-4, IL-5, IL-6, TNF-α, GM-CSF, and TGF-β. Reed-Sternberg cells develop as a result of this genetic rearrangement and constitute 1–5% of cell population. Background lymphocytes are usually T cells.

REED-STERNBERG CELLS

Mystery of the origin of Reed-Sternberg cells in Hodgkin's disease was solved by molecular studies that relied on single cell of Reed-Sternberg cells, coupled with amplification of RNA and genomic DNA by polymerase chain reaction. These techniques established that Reed-Sternberg cell arises from germinal center or post-germinal center B cells. *These cells usually have clonal somatically mutated IgG rearrangements indicative of B cell origin.* Some reports suggest that classic Reed-Sternberg cells can be of T cell origin, where T cell markers are expressed on these cells.

Growth and survival: Growth and survival of classic Reed-Sternberg cells are closely related to the activation of the nuclear factor kappa B (NF-κB) transcription factor-signaling pathway. The consecutive nuclear activity of NF-κB can both prevent apoptosis and promote cell proliferation. Epstein-Barr virus (EBV), which is found in the Reed Sternberg cells expresses viral proteins such as LMP1 leading to NF-κB activation. Morphology of Reed-Sternberg cells is described as under.

Role of EBV in pathogenesis: Approximately 40% cases of Hodgkin's disease (classic or lymphocytic depletion) are associated by Epstein-Barr virus detected in Reed Sternberg cells. *EB virus plays an important role in the pathogenesis* of Hodgkin's disease. It protects Reed Sternberg cell from apoptosis and immune killer T cells, which would ordinarily destroy the abnormal cells. It may cause *mutation in the p53 tumor suppressor gene.* Epstein-Barr virus is demonstrated by *EBV-LMP1 by immunohistochemistry or EBV encoded early RNA (EBER) in situ hybridization.*

Pathogenesis of Hodgkin's disease is shown in Fig. 13.9. Cellular interactions in the Hodgkin's disease and Reed-Sternberg cells microenvironment are shown in Fig. 13.10.

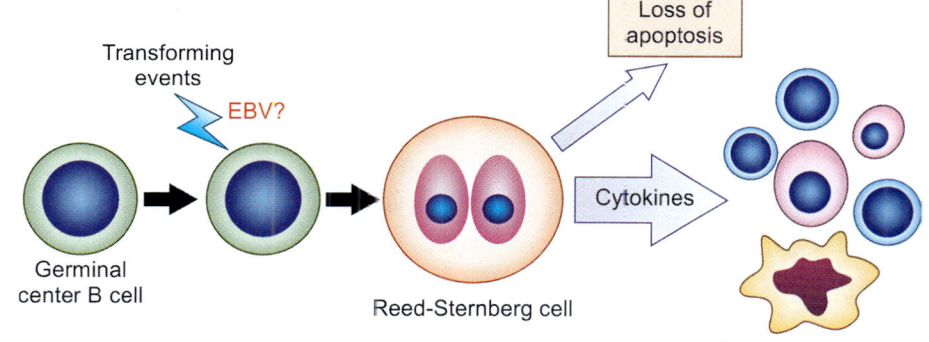

Fig. 13.9: Pathogenesis of Hodgkin's disease.

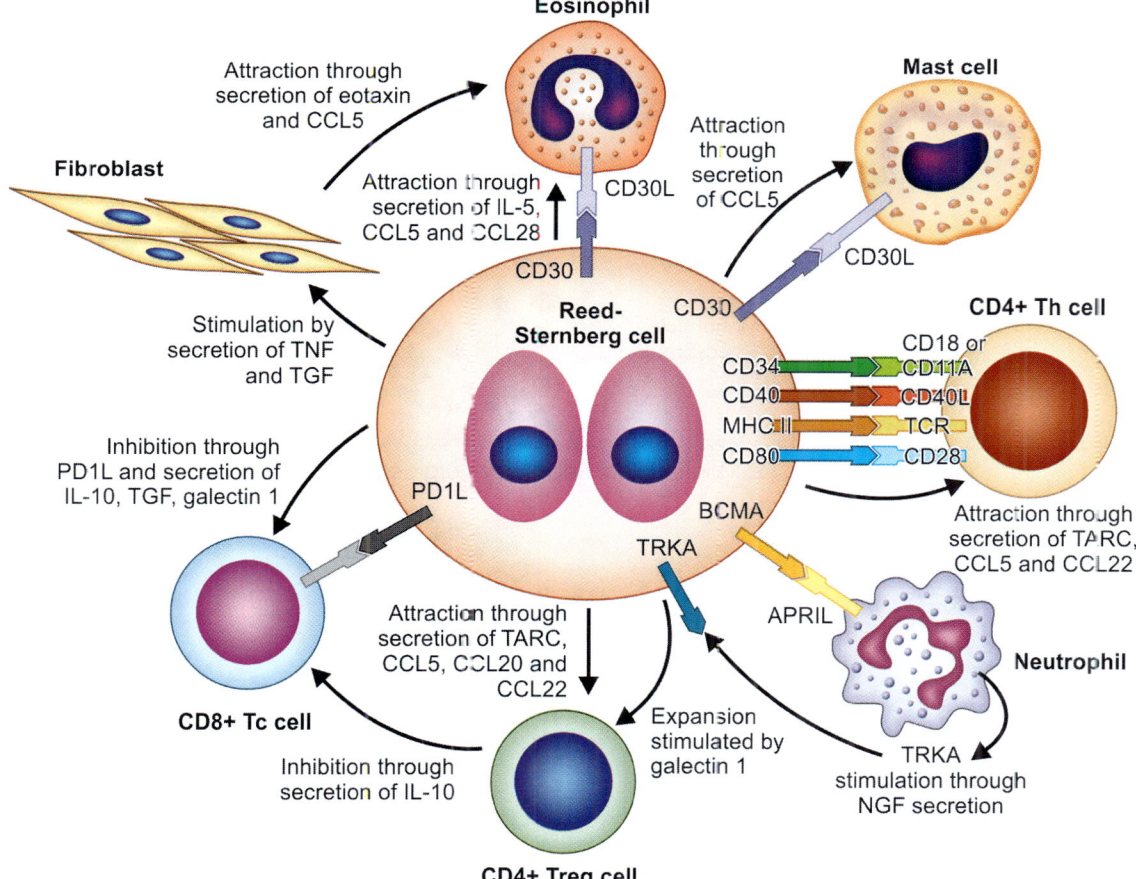

Fig. 13.10: Cellular interactions in the Hodgkin's disease and Reed-Sternberg cells microenvironment.

Classical Reed-Sternberg Cells

Classical Reed-Sternberg cells are large and binucleate or bilobed, with **two halves** often appearing as **mirror images** of each other resembling *owl eyes* from prominent nucleoli. These measure 20–50 μm in diameter with amphophilic cytoplasm. Nuclear membrane is thick and sharply defined. These are seen in mixed cellularity variant of Hodgkin's disease (Fig. 13.11).

Mononuclear Reed-Sternberg Cells

These may be seen in any type of Hodgkin's disease but are encountered in mixed cellularity disease (Fig. 13.12).

Pleomorphic Reed-Sternberg Cells

Pleomorphic Reed-Sternberg cells are larger than other type of Reed-Sternberg cells. These contain hyperchromatic large nuclei. These are seen in **lymphocytic depletion variant** of Hodgkin's lymphoma (Fig. 13.13).

Lacunar Reed-Sternberg Cells

Lacunar Reed-Sternberg cells are predominantly seen in the nodular sclerosis variant. These have more delicate folded or solitary nuclei surrounded by abundant pale cytoplasm in histological sections that can retract during processing (Fig. 13.14).

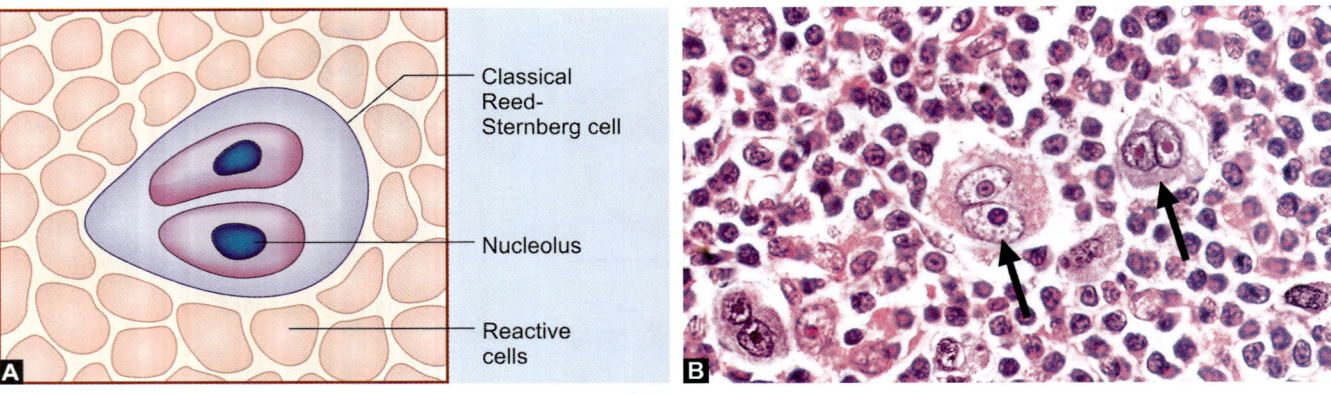

Fig. 13.11: Classical Reed-Sternberg cells (arrows).

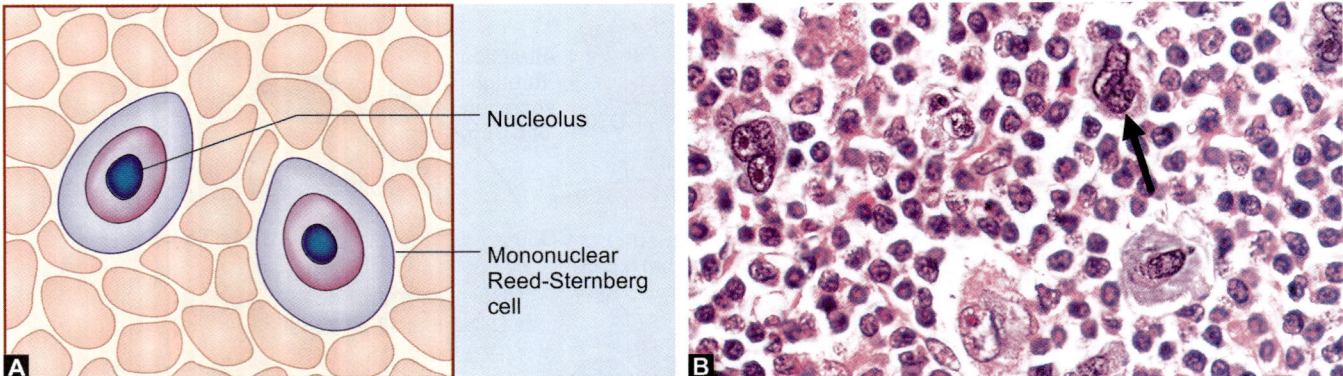

Fig. 13.12: Mononuclear Reed-Sternberg cells (arrow).

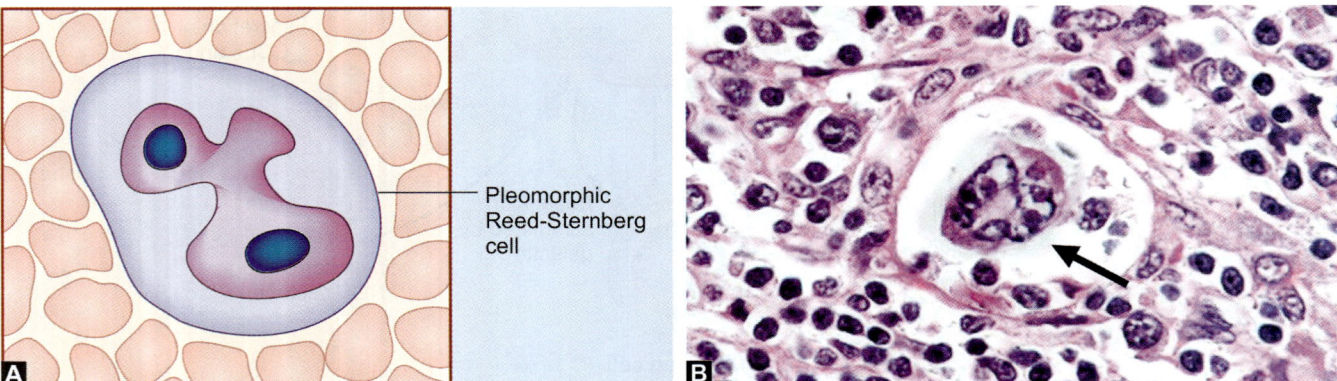

Fig. 13.13: Pleomorphic Reed-Sternberg cells (arrow).

Lymph Nodes, Spleen and Thymus

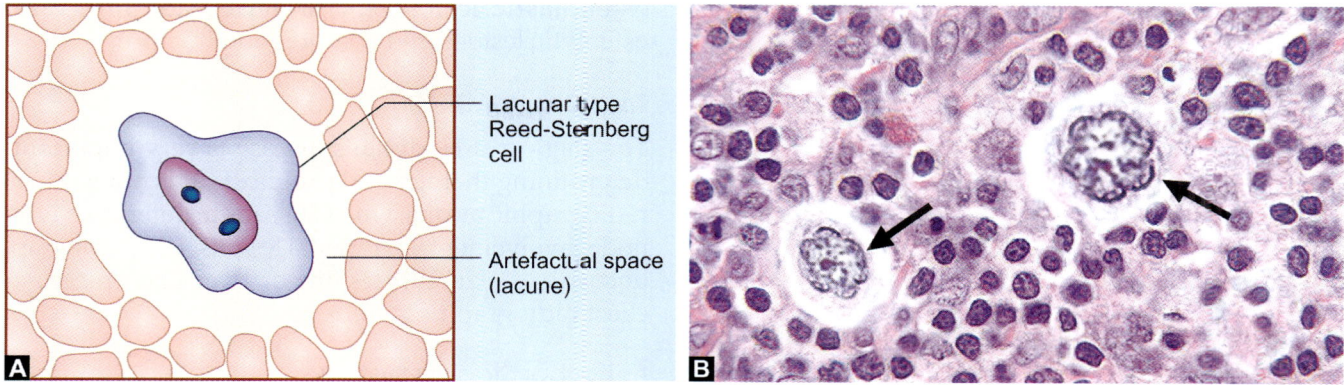

Fig. 13.14: Lacunar type Reed-Sternberg cells (arrows).

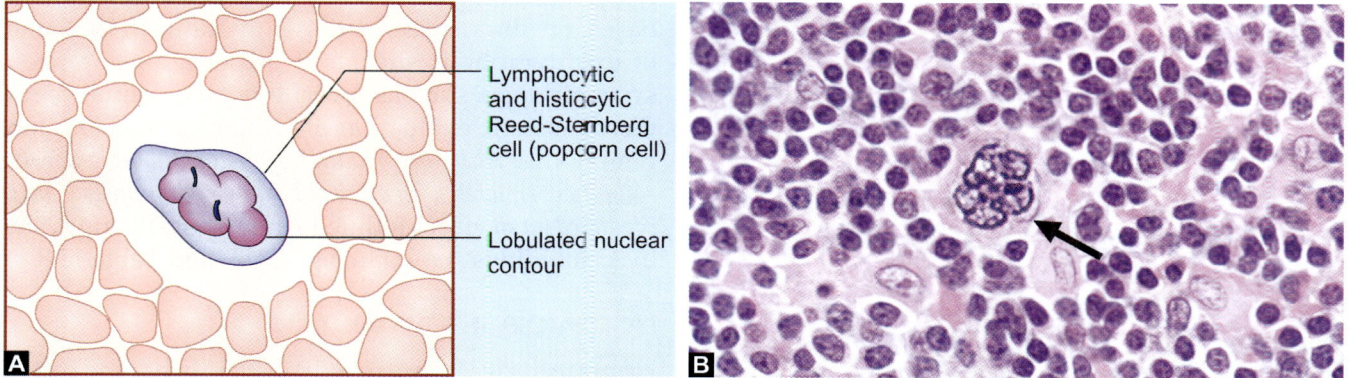

Fig. 13.15: Lymphocytic-histiocytic Reed-Sternberg cells (arrow).

Lymphocytic-Histiocytic Reed-Sternberg Cells

Lymphocytic-histiocytic (L&H) Reed-Sternberg cells are sometimes called *popcorn cells* seen in nodular lymphocyte predominant disease. **Popcorn cells** have **bubbly outline of nucleus** (Fig. 13.15).

REED-STERNBERG-LIKE CELLS

Reed-Sternberg-like cells should be differentiated from multinucleated cells in lymph node. Megakaryocyte can simulate closely in hematoxylin and eosin stained sections. *Megakaryocytes are strongly positive* for factor *VIII related* antigen and ***CD61***.

Immunoblasts in infectious mononucleosis are morphologically similar to Reed-Sternberg cells. Reed-Sternberg-like cells are demonstrated in peripheral T cell lymphoma, anaplastic large cell lymphoma, infectious mononucleosis and reactive viral lymphadenitis. Differences between Reed-Sternberg cells and Reed-Sternberg-like cells are shown in Table 13.7.

CLINICAL FEATURES

Patient presents with *painless lymphadenopathy* most often in upper half of body in *cervical or mediastinal* regions, but occasionally in the axilla or inguinal-femoral region. Constitutional symptoms such as *fever, night sweats*, and *weight loss* are observed in 40–50% cases. *Pruritus* is present in some cases.

Ingestion of alcohol may cause pain at involved sites. Patients of Hodgkin's disease are categorized into two grades: *Grade B* with one or more of these symptoms and *grade A lacking these symptoms*. On clinical examination, the **lymph nodes** are enlarged **discrete, rubbery, painless** and **mobile**.

Table 13.7: Differences between Reed-Sternberg cells and Reed-Sternberg-like cells

Parameters	Reed-Sternberg cells	Reed-Sternberg-like cells
Cell morphology	Reed-Sternberg cells in Hodgkin's disease	Pleomorphic immunoblast in infectious mononucleosis
Nucleolus	Acidophilic, regular with clear halo and more centrally placed	Basophilic, irregular and adjacent to nuclear membrane
Cytoplasm	Usually acidophilic and variable	Amphophilic with usual strong pyroninophilic
Surrounding cells	Lymphocytes and histiocytes	Mononuclear immunoblasts and plasmacytoid cells

CHEST RADIOGRAPHS

Chest radiographs demonstrate mediastinal lymphadenopathy in 40%; with associated lower cervical lymphadenopathy in Hodgkin's disease.

MODE OF SPREAD

Hodgkin's disease spreads by following routes.

Direct Extension

Direct extension of Hodgkin's disease involves adjacent lymph nodes, skin, skeletal muscle; while mediastinal lymph nodes invade large vessels, lung and chest wall in nodul or sclerosis variant.

Lymphatic Route

Initially Hodgkin's disease involves other nodes via lymphatic route in continuous and predictable fashion.

Hematogenous Route

Later it spreads via the *blood and involves the spleen, liver and bone marrow. Spleen is practically always involved. Liver is involved if splenic hilum and retroperitoneal lymph nodes are involved. Bone marrow is involved in Hodgkin's disease depletion type.* Other organs like lung, GIT, skin and CNS may also be involved. **Bone involvement** is often asymptomatic but may produce *pain* with vertebral osteoblastic lesions (*ivory* vertebrae) and, rarely, osteolytic lesions and compression fracture.

CLINICAL STAGING

The staging of Hodgkin's disease is very important in determining therapy and prognosis. It is often done by radiographic means, with CT scans to determine lymph node involvement, extranodal lesions. Ultrasonography determines size and lesions of liver and spleen, and chest radiograph.

Ann Arbor Staging System

Ann Arbor staging system is the basis for most Hodgkin's lymphoma staging. This system of classification is based on the degree of dissemination, involvement of extralymphatic sites, and presence or absence of systemic signs such as fever. It is an essential part of the diagnostic evaluation of patients with Hodgkin's lymphoma. *Although grading of histopathologic variants roughly correlates with clinical behavior, prognosis is better predicted by staging.* Modified Ann Arbor staging system by Costwold is shown in Fig. 13.16 and Table 13.8.

LABORATORY INVESTIGATIONS

Hematological abnormalities may be caused by extensive bone marrow involvement with the Hodgkin's

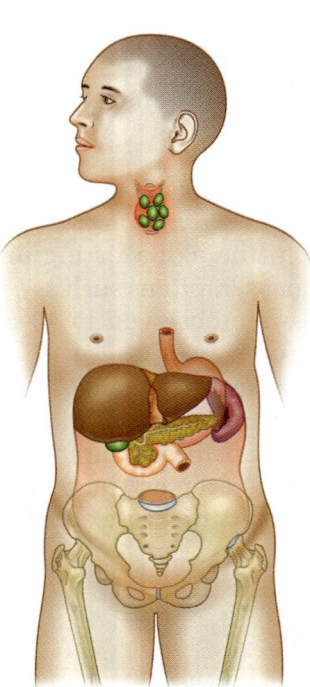
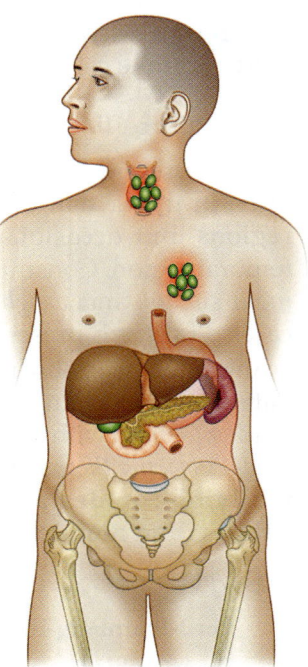
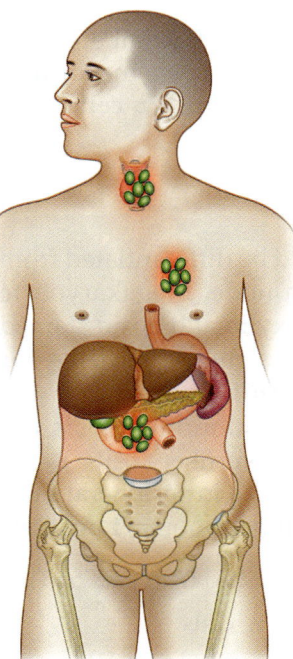
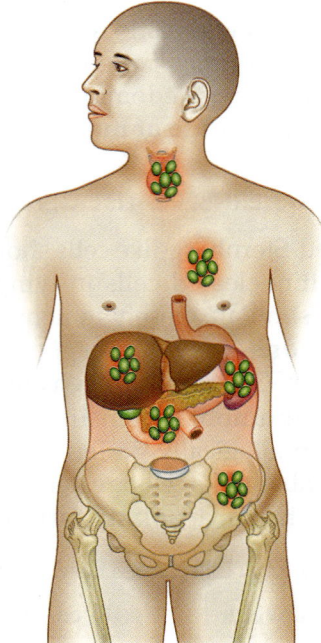

Stage I
Involvement of single lymph node or group of lymph nodes

Stage II
Involvement of >2 lymph nodes on same side of diaphragm invading mediastinum

Stage III
Involvement of lymph nodes on both sides of diaphragm including spleen

Stage IV
Widespread extralymphatic involvement (liver, bone marrow, lung and skin)

Fig. 13.16: Staging of Hodgkin's diseases.

Table 13.8: Modified Ann Arbor staging system by Costwold

Stage	Organs involved
Stage I	Single lymph node or lymphoid structures (spleen, thymus, Waldeyer's ring)
Stage II	Two or more lymph nodes on the same sides of the diaphragm
Stage III	Lymph nodes involved on both sides of the diaphragm Stage III$_1$ (with or without splenic, hilar, celiac or portal nodes) Stage III$_2$ (with para-aortic, iliac or mesenteric nodes)
Stage IV	Involvement of extranodal site(s) beyond those designated E

The stages can also have a designation of 'A' for asymptomatic or 'B' for constitutional symptoms (weight loss >10%, drenching sweats, fever).

disease. Hypersplenism may appear, but mainly in patients with marked splenomegaly. Elevated serum alkaline phosphatase levels usually indicate bone marrow or liver involvement or both.

Indicators of Active Disease

Increase in leukocyte alkaline phosphatase, serum haptoglobin, ESR, serum copper, and other acute phase reactants usually reflect active disease.

Anemia and Iron Parameters

Anemia, often microcytic, usually develops with advanced disease. Defective iron reutilization is characterized by low serum iron, low iron-binding capacity, and increased bone marrow iron.

Total and Differential WBCs

Slight-to-moderate polymorphonuclear leukocytosis may be present. Lymphocytopenia may occur early and become pronounced with advanced disease. Eosinophilia is present in about 20% of patients, and thrombocytosis may be observed.

Erythrocyte Sedimentation Rate

The erythrocyte sedimentation rate is commonly *elevated* in patients with *active disease* and sometimes may be the only evidence that the disease has been *inadequately treated* or that clinical recurrence is imminent.

Bone Marrow Aspiration

Bone marrow involvement can only rarely be demonstrated by the usual marrow aspirate technique and examination of marrow smears. The involvement is focal, often associated with fibrosis. It may be found with increasing frequency as the disease is or becomes more widespread with systemic symptoms and is often associated with an elevated serum alkaline phosphatase, radiologic evidences of bone involvement and unexplained pancytopenia.

Histopathological Examination

Hodgkin's disease can be definitively diagnosed by lymph node biopsy that reveals Reed-Sternberg cells in a characteristic histologic setting.

Differential Diagnosis

Hodgkin's disease may be difficult to differentiate from lymphadenopathy caused by infectious mononucleosis, toxoplasmosis, cytomegalovirus, NHL, or leukemia. The clinical picture can also be simulated by lung carcinoma, sarcoidosis, TB, and various diseases in which splenomegaly is the predominant feature.

Preferred Biopsy Sites

Hodgkin's disease is very rare in the absence of lymphadenopathy. Lymph node biopsy must be taken from **cervical region, axillary region, splenic hilum** and **retroperitoneal region**. Biopsy specimens then can be obtained from bone marrow, liver, or other parenchymal tissue. *Mesenteric and inguinal lymph nodes are usually spared, hence should not be biopsied* for histological diagnosis.

Fixation of Sample

Excised lymph node should be fixed in 10% buffered formalin or Zenker's fixative.

Gross Morphology

Cut surface of involved lymph node is uniform. Capsule is rarely involved, hence not invading surrounding fat.

Histopathological Examination

Sections stained with hematoxylin and eosin are examined by light microscopy. On histological examination, one finds difficulty in differentiating *granulocytic leukemia* and *large cell lymphoma*, hence imprint smears are helpful in differentiating these entities.

Immunohistochemistry

- Reed-Sternberg cells in classic variants of Hodgkin's disease express B cell markers such as CD15 (Leu M-1), CD30 (Ki-1) and PAX5.
- On the other hand, nodular lymphocytic-histiocytic variants of Hodgkin's disease show positivity for CD15 (Leu M-1), CD30 (Ki-1) and PAX5, CD20, 45 and epithelial membrane antigen (EMA).

CD30 expression: CD30 expression is demonstrated by Reed-Sternberg cells in *Hodgkin's disease*, immunoblasts in *infectious mononucleosis*, peripheral *T cell NHL*, *embryonal carcinoma* and *pancreatic carcinoma*.

MORPHOLOGIC SUBTYPES

There are two morphologic subtypes of Hodgkin's disease: classic (lymphocyte-rich, lymphocyte depletion, nodular sclerosis and mixed cellularity) and nodular lymphocytic-histiocytic predominant variant with or without histiocytes. Nodular sclerosis and nodular lymphocyte predominant variants arise from B cells. Rest variants are of T cell origin. Morphologic subtypes of Hodgkin's disease are shown in Table 13.9. Histological variants of classic Hodgkin's disease are shown in Table 13.10.

LYMPHOCYTE-RICH VARIANT

Lymphocyte-rich variant constitutes about 5 to 10% of patients. It is a slow growing disease associated with excellent prognosis. This variant is more common in men than in women under 35 years of age. There is an association with EBV infection in 40% of cases.

Clinical Features

Patient usually presents with solitary enlarged lymph node usually in *cervical* or *inguinal regions*. It never involves liver, spleen and bone marrow except when it changes to more aggressive histologic pattern. The clinical course is moderately aggressive.

Table 13.9: Morphologic subtypes of Hodgkin's disease

Hodgkin's disease variant	Immunophenotype	Reed-Sternberg cells	Prognosis
Classic variant			
Lymphocyte-rich variant (T cell markers)	CD30+ (Ki-1) specific marker CD15+ (Leu M-1)	Popcorn RS cells (lymphocytic-histiocytic cells)	Good prognosis
Lymphocyte-depleted variant (T cell markers)	CD30+ (Ki-1) specific marker CD15+ (Leu M-1)	Many RS cells with diffuse fibrosis	Worst prognosis
Nodular sclerosis variant (B cell markers)	CD30+ (Ki-1) specific marker CD15+ (Leu M-1) CD20+ CD79a+ CD5+ CD3+ IgM+ IgD+	Lacunar RS cells with bands of collagen fibers	Best prognosis
Mixed cellularity variant (T cell markers)	CD30+ (Ki-1) specific marker CD15+ (Leu M-1)	Classic RS cells with heterogeneous population of reactive cells	Commonest variant in India with fair prognosis
Nodular lymphocytic-histiocytic predominant variant with or without benign histiocytes (L&H cells)			
Nodular lymphocytic-histiocytic predominant with L&H cells (pan-B markers)	CD19+ CD20+ CD22+ CD45RA+ CD45RB (LCA)+ CD74+ CDw75+ EMA+	Lymphocytic-histiocytic cells (L&H cells)	Good prognosis

All are classic variants of Hodgkin's lymphoma except nodular lymphocytic-histiocytic predominant variant.

Table 13.10: Histological variants of classic Hodgkin's disease

Characteristics	Nodular sclerosis	Mixed cellularity	Lymphocyte-rich	Lymphocyte-depletion
Origin	B cells	T cells	T cells	T cells
Frequency	Most frequent type (75%)	Overall second most frequent (25%)	Uncommon (6%)	Uncommon (4%)
Age group	Young age group	Young adults and older persons (more than 55 years), bimodal peak	Young age group	Older age group
Sex predilection	Female predominance	Males predominance	Males predominance	Males predominance
EB virus association	No association	Associated with EB virus	No association	Associated with EB virus
Clinical features	Mediastinal mass, lower cervical, supraclavicular lymphadenopathy	Lower cervical and supraclavicular	Axillary lymphadenopathy (mediastinal uncommon)	Patient is associated with HIV infection having disseminated disease
Light microscopy	Lacunar Reed-Sternberg cells with bands of collagen fibers divide the lymph node in multiple nodules	Classic and mononuclear Reed-Sternberg cells admixed with many reactive cells	A few popcorn Reed-Sternberg cells	Many Reed-Sternberg cells with diffuse fibrosis
Immunophenotype	*Reed-Sternberg cells:* CD30 (Leu M-1) and CD15 (Ki-1)	*Reed-Sternberg cells:* CD30 (Leu M-1) and CD15 (Ki-1)	*Reed-Sternberg cells:* CD30 (Leu M-1), CD15 (Ki-1) and CD20	*Reed-Sternberg cells:* CD30 (Leu M-1) and CD15 (Ki-1)
Stage	Most are stage I or II	Most are stage III or IV (>50%)	Most are stage I or II	Most are stage III or IV
Prognosis	Best prognosis	Fair prognosis	Good prognosis	Worst prognosis

Light Microscopy

Lymphocyte-rich variant is composed of mature lymphocytes admixed with Reed-Sternberg cells, i.e. *popcorn* or *elephant's foot cells* which have excessively lobulated nuclei.

Immunohistochemistry

- The Reed-Sternberg cells have same immunophenotype as in other subtypes of classical Hodgkin's lymphoma.
- These show positivity for T cell markers such as CD30 (Leu M-1) and CD15 (Ki-1).
- These are constantly negative for pan-B markers such as CD19, CD20, CD22, 45RA, 45RB (LCA), CD74, CDw75, CD20 or CD45.
Immunohistochemistry of lymphocyte-rich variant of Hodgkin's disease

Marker	Expression
CD30 (Leu M-1)	Positive
CD15 (Ki-1)	Positive

Prognosis

This slow growing variant has best prognosis.

LYMPHOCYTE-DEPLETION VARIANT

Lymphocyte-depletion variant is least common constituting 4% of Hodgkin's disease with worst prognosis. *It is most often associated with Epstein-Barr virus.* It most often affects elderly persons *associated with HIV infection.*

Clinical Features

This lymphocyte-depletion variant is usually not diagnosed until the disease is widespread involving **liver** (60%), **bone marrow** (40%), **spleen** and **retroperitoneal lymph nodes**. Advanced stage and systemic symptoms are frequent. Pancytopenia is occasionally caused by bone marrow invasion, usually by the lymphocyte-depletion type.

Light Microscopy

- Lymphocyte-depletion variant can easily be confused with non-Hodgkin's lymphoma.
- *It should only be diagnosed when anaplastic large cell lymphoma has been excluded.*
- On histopathological examination, it may show any of two patterns: diffuse fibrosis and reticular pattern.

Diffuse fibrosis: This shows diffuse fibrosis, a few lymphocytes and polypoid Reed-Sternberg cells. Diffuse fibrosis is demonstrated by collagen fibers non-birefringent in polarizing microscopy.

Reticular pattern: This shows reticular pattern with sheets of bizarre Reed-Sternberg cells and areas of necrosis. *Reticular pattern needs to be differentiated from large cell NHL.*

Prognosis

This variant has the poorest prognosis among all the variants of Hodgkin's disease.

NODULAR SCLEROSIS VARIANT

Nodular sclerosis is most common variant of Hodgkin's disease constituting 60 to 75% of all cases. *This variant involves* B cells (*all other types of Hodgkin's disease involve T cells*). Presence of large bundles of collagenous connective tissue that separates the node into nodules. Most nodular sclerosis cases are of lower stage I or II (Fig. 13.17).

Age and Sex Predilection

This usually affects adolescents and young adults between 20 and 30 years of age. Females are more affected than males.

Clinical Features

The patient presents with lymphadenopathy in **upper mediastinum** (50%), **supraclavicular** or **lower cervical regions**. There is rarely an association with EBV infection. Patient may have recurrent laryngeal paralysis due to compression of recurrent laryngeal nerves. Neuralgic pain follows nerve root compression. Lymphadenopathy in thorax compresses respiratory tract (trachea and bronchi) resulting in cough, chest pain and severe dyspnea.

Hematological Findings

Hematological findings are anemia, leukocytosis, and an elevated erythrocyte sedimentation rate.

Gross Morphology

- This shows enlarged, firm, fleshy lymph node with irregular nodules separated by bands of firmer, fibrotic tissue.
- Fibrosis is caused by cytokines synthesized by neoplastic lacunar cells, i.e. IL-5 (attracting eosinophils), IL-4, TNF-α and GM-CSF.

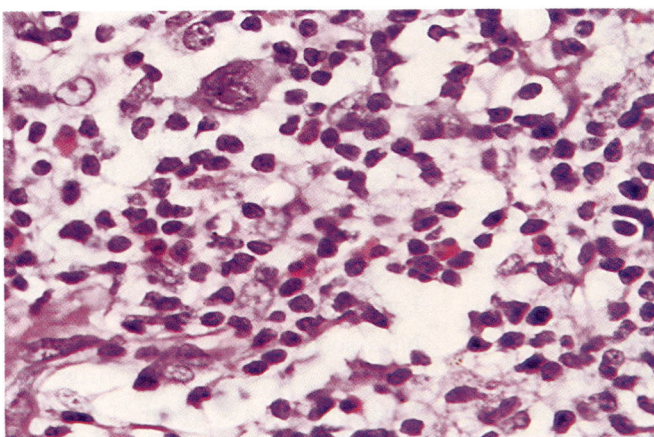

Fig. 13.17: Nodular sclerosis variant of Hodgkin's disease (400X).

Light Microscopy

- Histopathological examination shows broad bands of pink-staining birefringent collagen fibrous tissue on polarizing microscopy.
- There is presence of lacunar Reed-Sternberg cells and reactive cells.
- *Lacunar cells:* Lacunar cells contain more delicate folded or solitary nuclei surrounded by abundant clear or pale eosinophilic cytoplasm in histological sections that can retract during processing. It is an artifact of formalin fixation.
- *Cytokines synthesized by Reed-Sternberg cells are currently believed* to cause progressive attraction of T cells, histiocytes, plasma cells and eosinophils.
- Nodular sclerosis has cellular phase and syncytial phase. Syncytial phase is more aggressive in clinical behavior.

Immunohistochemistry

- The Reed-Sternberg cells have same immunophenotype as in other subtypes of classical Hodgkin's lymphoma. Reactive component consists of small lymphocytes bearing phenotype of mantle B cells.
- These B cells show positivity for *CD30* (Leu M-1), *CD15* (Ki-1), *CD20, CD79a, CD5, CD3, IgM* and *IgD*. Immunohistochemistry of nodular sclerosis variant of Hodgkin's disease.

Marker	Expression
CD30 (Leu M-1)	Positive
CD15 (Ki-1)	Positive
CD20	Positive
CD79a	Positive
CD5	Positive
CD3	Positive
IgM	Positive
IgD	Positive

Prognosis

The prognosis of this variant is relatively good. Patients respond to locoregional treatment with radiation and have an **excellent prognosis**. Cell-mediated immunity is often reduced, as evidenced by anergy with skin testing.

MIXED CELLULARITY VARIANT

Mixed cellularity variant of Hodgkin's disease constitutes 5 to 25% of all cases. *This variant is most common in India.* It is associated with EBV infection in 70% of cases. Although >50% cases progress to stage III or IV, yet prognosis is still good.

Age and Sex Predilection

This variant most often affects elderly men and women. It may affect immunocompromised children.

Clinical Features

Patient presents with *multiple painless, rubbery discrete lymph node groups*. **Spleen, liver** and **bone marrow** may be involved. Reed-Sternberg cells synthesize powerful cytokines such as IL-1, IL-6 and TNF-α, which cause local pain, fever, night sweats and weight loss exceeding 10% of body weight. *Pruritus indicates with progression of the disease.* Clinical course of moderately aggressive but curable.

> **Gross Morphology**
> - Lymph nodes are enlarged with diffuse involvement.
> - Cut surface is fleshy, gray tan lymph node without well-defined nodules or fibrosis.
>
> **Light Microscopy**
> - Histopathological examination shows classic **Reed-Sternberg** cells admixed with reactive inflammatory cells such as **eosinophils, plasma cells, small lymphocytes, histiocytes** in the background.

- Cytokine IL-5 synthesized by Reed-Sternberg cells and exotoxin released by fibroblasts participate in attraction of eosinophils.
- Patches of necrosis and fibrosis may be present.
- Presence of noncaseating **epithelioid granulomas** in Hodgkin's disease indicates **good prognosis** is shown in Fig. 13.18.

Reed-Sternberg cells: Classic Reed-Sternberg cells constitute 1–10% of total population of cells. These are large and binucleate or bilobed, with two halves often appearing as mirror images of each other resembling owl eyes. These measure 20–50 μm in diameter with amphophilic cytoplasm.

Nuclear membrane is thick and sharply defined. Mononuclear Reed-Sternberg cells are also encountered in mixed cellularity disease. These synthesize IL-5, IL-4, TNF-α and GM-CSF.

Immunohistochemistry

- The Reed-Sternberg cells have same immunophenotype as in other subtypes of classical Hodgkin's lymphoma.
- These show positivity for T cell markers such as CD30 (Leu M-1) and CD15 (Ki-1). These are constantly negative for pan-B markers such as CD19, CD20, CD22, 45RA, 45RB (LCA), CD74, CDw75 or CD45.
- Immunohistochemistry of mixed cellularity variant of Hodgkin's disease is shown as under.

Marker	Expression
CD30 (Leu M-1)	Positive
CD15 (Ki-1)	Positive

NODULAR LYMPHOCYTIC-HISTIOCYTIC PREDOMINANT VARIANT

Nodular lymphocytic-histiocytic predominant variant is distinct entity from classic Hodgkin's disease. It constitutes 5% of all Hodgkin's disease cases. It most often affects young males involving cervical or axillary adenopathy with long history. Rarely, mediastinal or bone marrow may be involved. It has indolent behavior, but higher recurrence rate than classical Hodgkin's disease.

Clinical Course

Patients with stage I/II have excellent prognosis with 10-year survival of 80–90% of cases. Recurrence is frequent and associated with progressive transformation of germinal centers with infiltration by small lymphocytes. Approximately 3–5% transform to diffuse large B cell lymphoma. *Bone marrow involvement is associated with aggressive disease.*

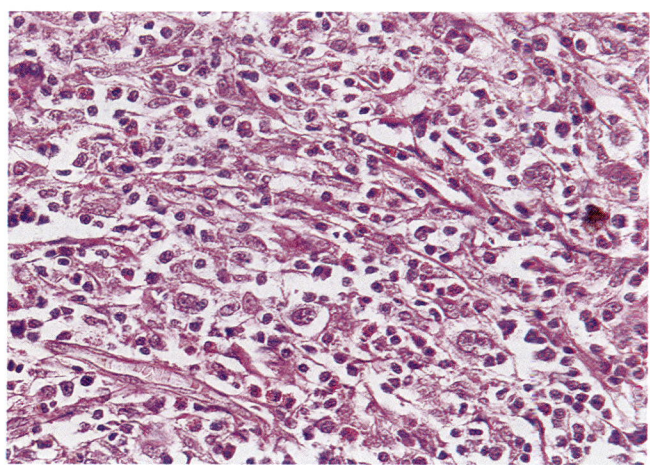

Fig. 13.18: Mixed cellularity variant of Hodgkin's disease (40CX).

Gross Morphology
Lymph node architecture is completely effaced with formation of vague nodules of small lymphocytes.

Light Microscopy
- Nodular lymphocytic/histiocytic-predominant variant is composed of small B cells with or without accompanying population of benign appearing histiocytes.
- Eosinophils, plasma cells and foci of fibrosis are scanty or absent. Endothelium of postcapillary venules may be prominent.

Immunohistochemistry
Reed-Sternberg cells of nodular lymphocytic/histiocytic variant of Hodgkin's disease show positivity for pan-B markers such as CD19, CD20, CD22, 45RA, 45RB (LCA), CD74, CDw75 and EMA. These are constantly negative for T cell markers such as CD15 (Ki-1) and CD30 (Leu M-1).

Immunohistochemistry of lymphocytic/histiocytic variant of Hodgkin's disease.

Marker	Expression
CD19	Positive
CD20	Positive
CD22	Positive
45RA	Positive
45RB (LCA)	Positive
CD74	Positive
CDw75	Positive
EMA	Positive

NON-HODGKIN'S LYMPHOMA

OVERVIEW
Non-Hodgkin's lymphomas arise from lymphoid cells or other cells native to lymphoid tissue. They originate most frequently within lymph nodes or in other lymphoid areas. Tumor involvement of the para-aortic lymph nodes is frequent. The seriousness of lymphoma depends on which type of cell has undergone mutation, and how quickly it replicates. WHO classification of non-Hodgkin's lymphoid neoplasms is based on origin of B or T cells: precursor lymphoid neoplasms and mature B cell neoplasms are shown in Table 13.11. Origin of lymphoid neoplasms is shown in Fig. 13.19.

Table 13.11: WHO classification of lymphoid neoplasms

Precursor lymphoid neoplasms	
• B lymphoblastic leukemia/lymphoma, NOS	
• B lymphoblastic leukemia/lymphoma with recurrent genetic abnormalities	
• T lymphoblastic leukemia/lymphoma	
Mature B cell neoplasms	**Mature T cell and NK cell neoplasms**
• Chronic lymphocytic leukemia/small lymphocytic leukemia	• T cell prolymphocytic leukemia
• B cell prolymphocytic leukemia	• T cell large granular cell leukemia
• Splenic marginal zone lymphoma	• Aggressive NK cell leukemia
• Hairy cell leukemia	• Adult T cell leukemia/lymphoma
• Lymphoplasmacytic lymphoma	• Extranodal NK/T cell lymphoma nasal type
• Plasma cell neoplasms	• Enteropathy associated T cell lymphoma
• Extranodal marginal zone lymphoma	• Mycosis fungoides
• Nodal marginal zone lymphoma	• Sézary syndrome
• Follicular lymphoma	• Angioimmunoblastic T cell lymphoma
• ALK positive large B cell lymphoma	• Anaplastic large cell lymphoma, ALK positive
• Plasmablastic lymphoma	• Anaplastic large cell lymphoma, ALK negative
• Primary effusion lymphoma	
• Burkitt's lymphoma	
• Diffuse large B cell lymphoma (NOS)	

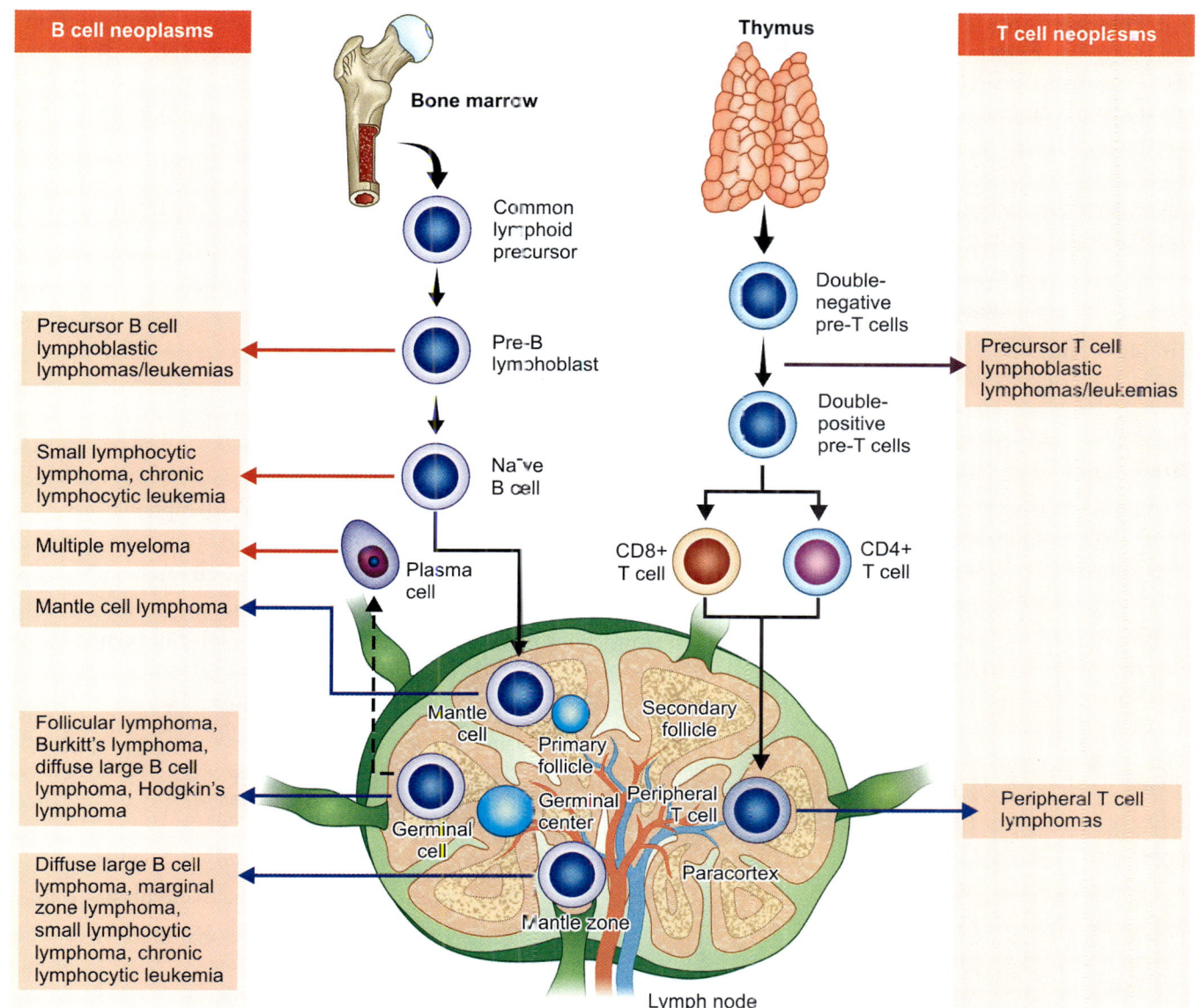

Fig. 13.19: Origin of lymphoid neoplasms.

GRADES OF NHL

The disease is sometimes described by the behavior of its cells: low-grade, intermediate grade and high-grade (Table 13.12).

Low-grade NHL tends to involve multiple lymph nodes at multiple sites, whereas *high-grade NHL* tends to be *more localized*. Low-grade NHLs are *slow growing* and responsive to treatment.

Table 13.12: Grades of NHL and clinical course

Grades of NHL	Examples of NHLs	Features
Low-grade or indolent NHL*	Small lymphocytic lymphoma Follicular (nodular) lymphoma Mantle cell lymphoma Marginal zone B cell lymphoma	Slow growing and responsive to treatment
High-grade NHL	Burkitt's lymphoma Diffuse large B cell lymphoma	Rapidly growing, aggressive but may be resistant to treatment

*Low-grade or indolent NHL may change to a more aggressive form later.
Intermediate NHLs are rapidly growing, aggressive but responsive to treatment.

Intermediate grade NHLs are rapidly growing, aggressive but responsive to treatment. High-grade NHLs are rapidly growing, aggressive but may be resistant to treatment.

APPROACH TO LYMPHOMA WORK UP

Antigen markers useful in delineating and sub-classifying lymphoid malignancies are shown in Table 13.13.

The work up of lymphoma is done by evaluation of disease specific markers such as cyclin D1 and anaplastic large lymphoma kinase (ALK-1), which can only be evaluated by immunohistochemistry in tissue sections.

PRECURSOR B CELL NHL

Precursor B cell neoplasms arise in from precursor B cell in the bone marrow. Examples are precursor

Table 13.13: Antigen markers used in subclassification of non-Hodgkin's lymphoma

Examples of markers	Cellular distribution
Leukocyte marker	
CD45 (known as *common leukocyte antigen*)	All leukocytes
Markers of immaturity	
TdT (terminal deoxynucleotidyl transferase, a specialized DNA polymerase)	Nuclear expression in pre-B and pre-T lymphoblasts
CD34	Pluripotent hematopoietic stem cells and progenitor cells of many lineages
CD10 (CALLA—common acute lymphoblastic leukemia antigen)	Bone marrow pre-B cells and mature follicular center B cells
CD22	Pre-B cells
cμ heavy chains	Cytoplasmic μ heavy chains
Primary B cell associated markers	
CD19	Bone marrow pre-B cells, mature B cells (not on plasma cells)
CD20	Bone marrow pre-B cells, mature B cells (not on plasma cells)
CD79a	Bone marrow pre-B cells, mature B cells and plasma cells
CD22 (transmembrane molecule)	Bone marrow pre-B cells (cCD22) and mature B cells
Markers helpful in sub-classifying mature B cell lymphomas	
CD5	T cells, small subsets of B cells, neoplastic CLL and mantle cell lymphoma cells
CD10	Immature B cells in germinal centers and mature granulocytes
CD11c	Monocytes/macrophages, natural killer cells, granulocytes, subsets of B and T cells
CD23	Activated mature B cells
CD38	Mature B cells and plasma cells
CD43	All leukocytes except resting B cells, also demonstrated in B cell lymphoma
BCL-6	Germinal center lymphocytes in normal lymph node
BCL-2	T cells and normal mantle B cells, also expressed in aberrantly B cell lymphomas
Cyclin D1 (cell regulatory protein)	Rearranged through t(11;14) in mantle cell lymphoma, weakly expressed in hairy cell leukemia and plasma cell dyscrasias
CD138 (Syndecan-1)	Myelomas, but also present in carcinomas

Contd...

Table 13.13: Antigen markers used in subclassification of non-Hodgkin's lymphoma (Contd...)

Examples of markers	Cellular distribution
Markers of clonality	
κ or λ immunoglobulins	Multiple myeloma
Primarily T cell and NK cell associated markers	
CD1	Thymocytes and Langerhans' cell histiocytosis
CD2	T cells in thymus and peripheral blood and NK cells
CD3	Lineage specific marker for T cells and cytoplasmic form expressed in NK cells
CD5	All T cells and subsets of B cells
CD7	All T cells and subsets of myeloid precursor cells
CD8	Cytotoxic T cells, subset of peripheral T cells, thymocytes and NK cells
CD16	NK cells and granulocytes
CD56	NK cells, subset of T cells and myeloma cells
TIA (cytoplasmic granule associated RNA binding protein)	NK cells and cytotoxic T cells
Flow cytometry	
κ or λ immunoglobulins	B cell neoplasms, clonality of T cell neoplasms can be demonstrated by molecular or genetic analysis
Southern blot analysis	
Clonal immunoglobulin heavy chain (IgH) or TCR rearrangements	Southern blot targets TCRb detects additional band in B cell and T cell malignancies (normal T cells rearrange TCR genes such as α, β, γ and δ)
PCR (polymerase chain reaction)	
TCRg gene	T cell malignacies
Cytogenetic analysis	
Conventional karyotyping	Acute leukemias
FISH	B cell, T cell and NK cell malignancies

B-lymphoblastic lymphoma/leukemia and small lymphocytic leukemia. Lymphoid neoplasms of precursor B and T cells are shown in Table 13.14.

MATURE B CELL NHL

Mature B cell lymphomas are categorized into low-grade and high-grade NHLs. Low-grade NHLs are small lymphocytic lymphoma, follicular (nodular) lymphoma, mantle cell lymphoma and marginal zone B cell lymphoma.

Examples of high-grade lymphomas are Burkitt's lymphoma and *diffuse large B cell lymphoma*. Chromosomal abnormalities in B cell NHLs are shown in Table 13.15. Characteristic features of various B cell leukemias/lymphomas are shown in Table 13.16.

BURKITT'S LYMPHOMA

Burkitt's lymphoma is **high-grade** germinal center B cell lymphoma but curable disorder. BCL-2 gene rearrangements are often seen, suggesting a potential germinal center origin. There is a close relationship to B-ALL (acute lymphoblastic leukemia of late-stage B cell origin), which is called Burkitt's cell leukemia in the WHO classification.

Most patients present with extranodal tumors (maxilla, mandible or abdomen) that emerge in a short period of time and respond to aggressive chemotherapy.

Variants

African (endemic) variant: African variant is strongly associated with EB virus in Central African children.

Section II: Hematology

Table 13.14: Lymphoid neoplasms of precursor B and T cells

Disorder	Origin	Age group	Clinical features	Genotype	Immunophenotype
B cell acute lymphoblastic leukemia or lymphoma	Precursor B cells in bone marrow	Children	Recurrent infections, anemia and bleeding related to pancytopenia	Diverse chromosomal translocation t(12;21) involving RUNX1 and ET16	CD19, CD79a, CD22, CD10, CD22, CD24 and PAX5
T cell acute lymphoblastic leukemia or lymphoma	Precursor B cells in thymus	Adolescents	Mass in thymus, variable bone marrow involvement with aggressive clinical course	Diverse chromosomal translocation, NOTCH mutations in 50–70% cases	Tdt, CD1a, CD2, CD3 (specific), CD4, CD5 and CD8

Table 13.15: Chromosomal abnormalities in B cell NHLs

Histological variant of lymphoma	Cytogenetic abnormality	Oncogene	Juxtaposed gene
*Burkitt's lymphoma (tropical and nontropical)	t(8;14) t(8;22) t(2;8)	c-MYC c-MYC c-MYC	Ig heavy chain Ig κ chains Ig λ chains
Centroblastic/centrocytic lymphoma	t(14;18)	BCL-2	Ig heavy chain
Centrocytic (intermediate cell) mainly in mantle zone	t(11;14)	BCL-2 (PRAD 1)	Ig heavy chain
Small lymphocytic B cell lymphoma	Trisomy 12	-	-
B cell chronic lymphocytic leukemia	t(14;19)	BCL-3	Ig heavy chain
Centroblastic/centrocytic large cell type	t(3;22)	-	Ig λ chains

*In Burkitt's lymphoma, t(8q24) is always involved.

Table 13.16: Characteristic features of various B cell leukemias/lymphomas

Disease	Origin	Clinical presentation	Morphology	Immunophenotype	Genetics
CLL/SLL	Naïve B cell or memory B cells	Weakness, autoimmune hemolytic anemia, enlargement of lymph nodes, liver and spleen	Small mature appearing lymphocytes cells involving bone marrow	Bright staining (CD5, CD19), weak staining (CD20, CD22, CD23, CD19, IgD, CD79a, CD43)	Favorable prognosis t(13q14) Poor prognosis (deletion of 17p and TP53), Trisomy 12, deletions (11q22–23) and rearrangement of IgH (50–60%)
Prolymphocytic leukemia	B cells in marginal zone of lymph node	Market splenomegaly without lymphadenopathy, rapidly rising lymphocyte count (>100 × 10^9/L)	PB: Medium-sized cells with round nucleus, moderately condensed chromatin, and prominent central nucleolus	CD20 (bright), CD19, IgM, CD22, CD79a, FMC7, CD23 typically absent, CD5 present in 30% cases	Complex karyotypes are common, abnormalities of TP53 in ~50%, IgH clonally rearranged
Hairy cell leukemia	Memory B cell	Predominantly middle-aged men, splenomegaly, pancytopenia with monocytopenia	Hairy cells in peripheral blood, bone marrow virtually always involved, and spleen infiltration (red pulp)	CD19, CD20, CD22 (bright), CD79a, CD11c (bright), CD25 (bright), CD103, TRAP, DBA in tissue sections	Activating FRAF mutations, rearrangement of IgH

Contd...

Table 13.16: Characteristic features of various B cell leukemias/lymphomas (Contd...)

Disease	Origin	Clinical presentation	Morphology	Immunophenotype	Genetics
Splenic marginal zone B cell lymphoma	B cell in spleen	Splenomegaly, sometime associated with autoimmune thrombocytopenia or anemia, peripheral lymphadenopathy uncommon	*PB:* Small- to medium-sized cells with polar villi (villous lymphocytes) *Spleen:* Both white pulp and red pulp infiltration	CD19, CD20, CD79a, IgM, and IgD, no expression of CD10, CD5, CD23, and CD43	Allelic loss of chromosome 7q21–32 in 40% of cases, trisomy 3 in rare cases, IgH clonally rearranged
Extranodal marginal zone B cell lymphoma (MALT lymphoma)	Naïve B cell	GI tract most common site of involvement	Small lymphocytes with ample cytoplasm	CD19, CD20, CD79a, IgM, no expression of CD5, CD23, CD10	t(11;18), t(14;18), t(14;18) creating API2-MALT1, BCL10-IgH fusion genes, respectively
Nodal marginal zone B cell lymphoma	B cell	Localized or generalized lymphadenopathy	Marginal zone and interfollicular areas infiltrated by centrocyte-like B cells, monocytoid B cells, or small lymphocytes; plasma cell differentiation may be present	CD19, CD20, CD79a, IgM, no expression of CD5, CD23, CD10	The translocations associated with extranodal MZL are not detected; IgH clonally rearranged
Follicular lymphoma	Germinal center B cell	Widespread peripheral and central lymphadenopathy, infiltration in liver (portal tract), spleen (white pulp) and bone marrow (85%)	Neoplastic cells with variable morphology forming closely packed neoplastic follicles	CD19, CD20, CD22, CD79a, BCL-6, BCL-2, CD10	t(14;18) (q23;q21) → rearrangement of BCL-2 gene leading to overexpression of the BCL-2 protein and survival advantage of malignant cells; IgH clonally rearranged
Mantle cell lymphoma	Naïve B cell	Lymphadenopathy, most common extranodal site is the GI tract (multiple lymphomatous polyposis)	Small neoplastic lymphocytes with nuclei showing clefts	CD19, CD20, CD5, FMC-7, CD43, cyclin-D1, lack of expression of CD23, CD10, BCL-6	t(11;14) creating cyclin D1-IgH fusion gene
Diffuse large B cell lymphoma (DLBCL)	Germinal center or post-germinal center B cell	Rapidly enlarging, often symptomatic mass, often disseminated disease	Variable morphology (centroblastic, immunoblastic, anaplastic cells) with round to oval nucleus, prominent nucleoli and frequent mitosis	CD19, CD20, CD22, CD79a, CD10, BCL-6	Diverse chromosomal rearrangement, BCL6 (30%), BCL-2 (10%) and MYC (5%)

Contd...

Table 13.16: Characteristic features of various B cell leukemias/lymphomas (Contd...)

Disease	Origin	Clinical presentation	Morphology	Immunophenotype	Genetics
Mediastinal (thymic) large B cell lymphoma	B cell in thymus	Mostly women in their third to fifth decade, large anterior mediastinal mass, sometimes with impending superior vena cava syndrome	Large cells with associated delicate interstitial fibrosis causing compartmentalization, possible thymic remnants, biopsy samples often small and obscured by profuse sclerosis and crush artifact	CD19, CD20, CD30 (weak) IgH and HLA class I and II expression is often absent	IgH clonally rearranged; hyperdiploid-karyotype gains in chromosome 9p
Burkitt's lymphoma	Germinal center B cell	African variant (EB virus related tumor in maxilla, mandible), Western variant (abdominal lymph nodes around ileocecal region in children), and lymphoma in HIV patients	Medium-sized cells with basophilic vacuolated cytoplasm and regular nuclei with several small nucleoli, tangible-body macrophages imparting "starry-sky" appearance	CD19, CD20, CD22, CD38, CD10, CD79a, BCL-6, BCL-6, Ki-67 index (100%)	IgH clonally rearranged; t(8;14) in most cases, t(2;8) and t(8;22) rare

Patient presents with swelling in the **maxilla** or **mandible**. It is associated with EB virus. EB virus activates oncogene (c-MYC). It stimulates proliferation of B cells. It increases opportunity for translocation of N-RAS gene t(8;14).

Western (sporadic variant): Patient presents with **abdominal lymph node mass around and ileocaecal mucosa**. It is not strongly associated with EB virus. It mainly affects children and young adults in the Western world, where it accounts for 1 to 2% of all lymphomas.

Immunodeficiency (Burkitt-like lymphoma) variant: Immunodeficiency-associated Burkit-like lymphoma mainly occurs in **HIV-infected persons**.

Molecular Genetics

Burkitt's lymphoma is associated with t(8;14) in 75% cases, t(2;8) in 5% cases and t(8;22) in 10% cases. Epstein-Barr virus promotes polyclonal B cell proliferation. It increases risk of translocation (8;14). EB virus activates c-MYC proto-oncogene located on chromosome 8, which is transposed to a site adjacent to the immunoglobulin heavy-chain locus on chromosome 14. Pathogenesis of Burkitt's lymphoma is shown in Fig. 13.20.

Proximity of regulatory sequences of the immunoglobulin heavy chain gene results in increased expression of the c-MYC gene. This chromosomal rearrangement is the basis of malignant transformation of lymphocyte

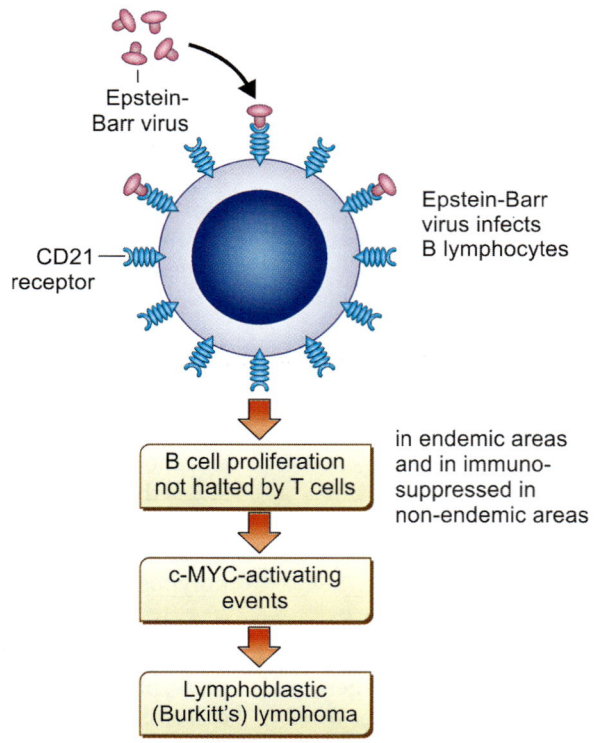

Fig. 13.20: Pathogenesis of Burkitt's lymphoma.

in Burkitt's lymphoma. In endemic areas, translocation t(8;14) occurs in the pre-B cell, but in nonendemic areas at later stage of B cell development. Burkitt's lymphoma associated with t(8;14) is shown in Fig. 13.21.

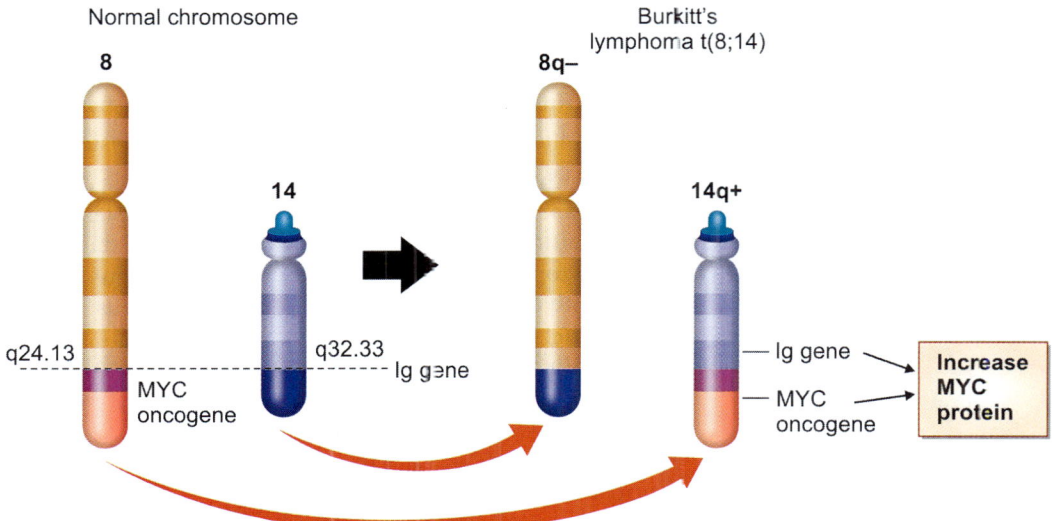

Fig. 13.21: Burkitt's lymphoma showing t(8;14) in which c-MYC proto-oncogene located on chromosome 8 is transposed to a site adjacent to the immunoglobulin heavy-chain locus on chromosome 14.

Light Microscopy

The cellular debris of apoptotic tumor cells is cleared by numerous non-neoplastic macrophages, whose scattered appearance is termed *starry-sky*. It is worth mentioning that this appearance can be seen in any highly proliferative lymphoid tumor (Fig. 13.22).

Immunohistochemistry

Neoplastic cells express CD10, CD19, CD20, CD22, BCL-6, and CD38. Nearly 100% of cells are positive for Ki-67 (Table 13.17).

Prognosis

Burkitt's lymphoma is highly aggressive but potentially curable. Even patients with advanced stage disease including bone marrow and CNS involvement can be cured with high intensity chemotherapy.

DIFFUSE LARGE B CELL LYMPHOMA (DLBCL)

Diffuse large B cell lymphoma is high-grade lymphoma but curable disorder. It affects all ages but most

Table 13.17: Immunohistochemistry of Burkitt's lymphoma

Marker	Expression
CD10	Positive
CD19	Positive
CD20	Positive
CD22	Positive
CD38	Positive
BCL-6	Positive
Ki-67	Positive (100% cases)

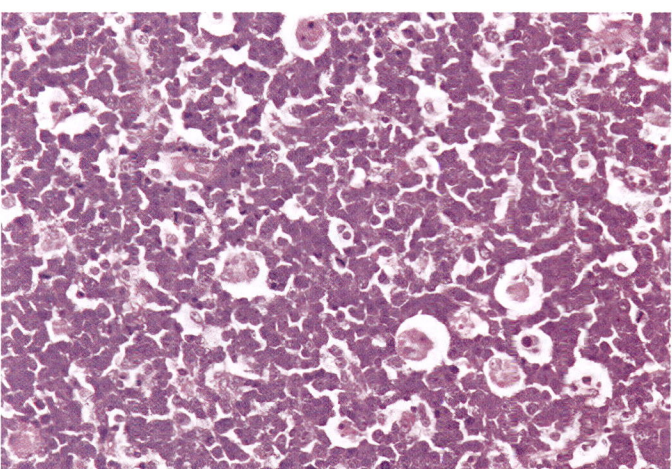

Fig. 13.22: Burkitt's lymphoma shows starry-sky appearance (400X).

common in adults. It most often occurs in older persons; however, age range is wide affecting children. It arises from germinal center or post-germinal center B cell. BCL-2 gene rearrangements are often seen, suggesting a potential germinal center origin.

Diffuse large B cell lymphoma has three variants: centroblastic, immunoblastic and anaplastic NHLs (Table 13.18).

Transformation

Diffuse large B cell lymphoma may arise by transforming low-grade B cell large cell lymphoma (Richter syndrome). *Richter syndrome* is characterized by *rapid onset of fever, abdominal pain,* and *progressive lymphadenopathy* and *hepatosplenomegaly.*

Richter syndrome is aggressive and refractory to therapy, with a mean survival of 2 months. Follicular

Table 13.18: Three variants of diffuse large B cell lymphoma

Parameters	Centroblastic variant	Immunoblastic variant	Anaplastic variant
Architecture	Diffuse	Diffuse	Diffuse in some cases
Sinus involvement	Obliteration	Obliteration	Distension
Cell population	Centroblasts (10–100%) admixed with centrocytes Cytoplasm scanty Nucleus vesicular with several nucleoli near nuclear membrane	Centroblasts (10%) admixed with plasmablasts with plasmacytoid features Cytoplasm moderate to abundant with deep staining Nucleus solitary centrally placed with prominent nucleus	Anaplastic cells Cytoplasm to abundant with deep staining Nucleus large with prominent nucleus
Mitotic activity	Low	High	High

lymphoma, marginal zone lymphoma or nodular lymphocyte predominant Hodgkin's lymphoma (NLPHL) can transform into DLBCL.

Molecular Genetics

Diverse chromosomal aberrations are seen in 30% cases. These tumors show activation of BCL-2 gene, amplification of cREL, t(14;18), point mutations and DNA breakage of BCL-6 regulatory regions.

Organs Involved

These include lymph nodes, Waldeyer ring of oropharyngeal lymphoid tissues, tonsils and adenoids, liver (portal tracts), spleen, gastrointestinal tract, skin, and brain. Bone marrow involvement occurs late in the course, leukemia is rare.

> **Light Microscopy**
>
> Three common morphological variants have been recognized centroblastic, immunoblastic, anaplastic variants.
> *Cell morphology:* The tumor cells are large 4–5 times diameter of small lymphocytes. These have round to oval nucleus, with either 2–3 nucleoli located adjacent to the nuclear membrane or a single nucleolus centrally placed and moderate pale or basophilic cytoplasm. Mitoses are frequent.
>
> *Arrangement:* These are arranged in diffuse pattern. More anaplastic tumors may contain multinucleated Reed-Sternberg-like cells with large, inclusion-like nucleoli, and these may be termed immunoblastic lymphoma. Variants of diffuse large B cell lymphoma are shown in Table 13.19.

Subtypes of DLBCL

These are histiocyte-rich large B cell lymphoma, primary DLBCL of the CNS, primary cutaneous DLBCL of leg, and EBV positive DLBCL of the elderly. Light microscopy of diffuse large B cell lymphoma is shown in Fig. 13.23.

Differential Diagnosis

Diffuse large B cell lymphoma should be differentiated from metastatic carcinomas. The presence of cell surface monoclonal immunoglobulin by immunohistochemistry would help to confirm this lesion as a malignant lymphoma.

Table 13.19: Variants of diffuse large B cell lymphoma

Parameters	Centroblastic variant	Immunoblastic variant	Anaplastic variant
Architecture	Diffuse	Diffuse	Diffuse in some cases
Sinus involvement	Obliteration	Obliteration	Distension
Centroblasts	10–100%	<10%	Absent
Background cells	Centrocytes	Plasmablast with plasmacytoid features	Absent
Cytoplasm	Scanty	Moderate to abundant	Abundant
Nuclear features	Vesicular nuclei with several nucleoli	Solitary nucleus with prominent nucleolus	Large nucleus with prominent nucleus
Mitotic activity	Low	High	High

Lymph Nodes, Spleen and Thymus

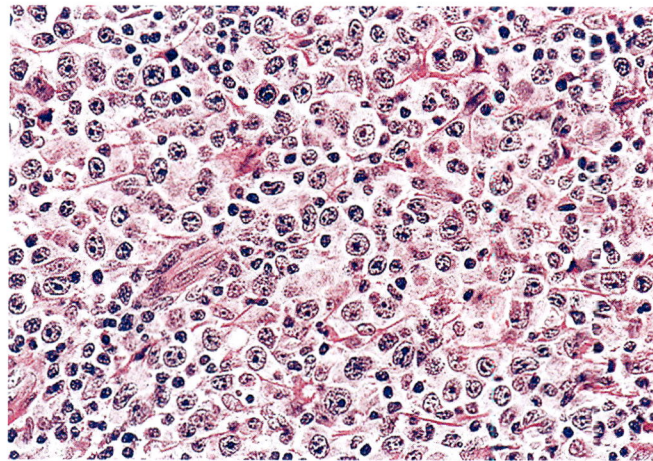

Fig. 13.23: Diffuse large B cell lymphoma (400X)

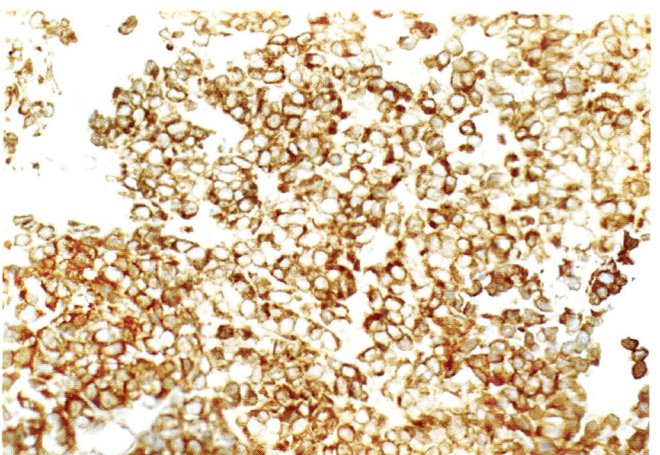

Fig. 13.25: Diffuse large B cell lymphoma shows positivity for BCL-2 (400X).

Immunohistochemistry

The neoplastic cells often mark with CD19, CD20, CD22 and CD79a. Most express surface immunoglobulin. Expression of CD10, BCL-6, and IRF4/MUM1 varies. All are –ve for TdT (Table 13.20, Figs 13.24 and 13.25).

Table 13.20: Immunohistochemistry of diffuse large B cell lymphoma

Marker	Expression
CD19	Positive
CD20	Positive
CD22	Positive
CD79a	Positive
Surface immunoglobulins	Positive

Clinical Features

Patient presents with rapidly growing single large nodal mass confined to local region. It has greater propensity to be extranodal disseminating to various organs than the low-grade NHL.

Immunodeficiency associated large B cell lymphoma: Large B cell lymphoma occurs in end stage of HIV infection, severe combined deficiency and organ transplantation (bone marrow or solid organs). Tumor B cells are infected with Epstein-Barr virus, which may play critical role in its pathogenesis.

Body cavity large cell lymphoma: Patient develops malignant pleural or ascetic effusions especially in advanced HIV infection. The tumor cells are infected with KSHV (most often) or HHV 8 in cases, which may play role in its pathogenesis.

Complications

Diffuse large B cell lymphoma can be associated with immunocompromised state and another with Kaposi sarcoma herpesvirus (KSHV).

SMALL LYMPHOCYTIC LYMPHOMA/CLL

Small lymphocytic lymphoma/chronic lymphocytic leukemia arises from *naïve B cell or post-germinal center memory B cell.* About 10% of cases transform to a diffuse large B cell lymphoma. An autoimmune hemolytic anemia appears in about one-sixth of CLL/SLL cases.

Chronic lymphocytic leukemia: A diagnosis of CLL is made if bone marrow and peripheral blood are primarily involved. Peripheral blood smear shows neoplastic small lymphocytes (smudge cells due to fragile chromatin), autoimmune hemolysis and thrombocytopenia in a minority.

Small lymphocytic lymphoma: If the tumor cells give rise to lymphadenopathy or solid tumor masses, the term small lymphocytic lymphoma is used. Both disorders most often affect older persons.

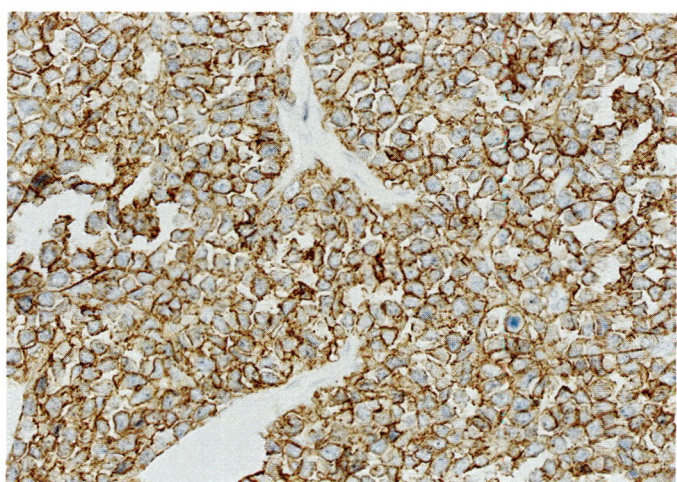

Fig. 13.24: Diffuse large B cell lymphoma shows positivity for CD20 (400X).

Molecular Genetics

Chromosomal translocations are rare in CLL/SLL. Chromosomal aberrations occur such as trisomy 12, deletions of 11q, 13q, and 17p. In some cases, immunoglobulin genes are somatically hypermutated, and there may be a small immunoglobulin 'spike' in the serum.

Organs Involved

Neoplastic cells infiltrate many organs. **Liver (portal tracts), spleen (white and red pulp)**, and **lymph nodes** may become enlarged, although organ function is often not markedly diminished.

Light Microscopy

- Architecture of lymph node is diffusely obliterated.
- Neoplastic cells completely surround benign germinal center and form inverse follicular pattern.
- These neoplastic cells may completely surround benign follicles as third layer and form marginal zone pattern.
- Neoplastic cells are mature appearing lymphocytes measuring 6 to 12 µm in diameter replacing the lymph node and extending through the capsule of the node and into the surrounding adipose tissue.

Neoplastic lymphocytes: These are small round containing irregular nuclei with condensed chromatin and scanty cytoplasm. There is scant mitotic activity.
Presence of prolymphocytes: Neoplastic cells are admixed with prolymphocytes with prominent mitotic activity. Presence of prolymphocytes is pathognomonic for CLL/SLL (Fig. 13.26).

Immunohistochemistry

The neoplastic cells express surface immunoglobulin and pan-B cell markers such as CD19, CD20, CD22, CD5, CD79a, CD23 and CD43 (Table 13.21, Figs 13.27 and 13.28).

Prognosis

Mean survival rate of small lymphocytic lymphoma is 4–6 years. The presence of deletions of 11q and 17p correlates with higher-stage disease and worse prognosis.

FOLLICULAR LYMPHOMA

Follicular lymphoma is the most common slowly progressive B cell NHL with fatal outcome. It arises from angulated grooved cells present in germinal center B cell. It most often affects older age group. About 30–50% of cases may transform to diffuse large B cell lymphoma.

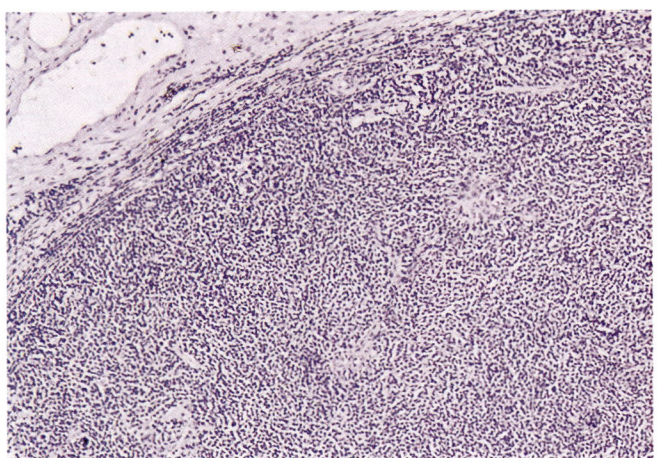

Fig. 13.26: Small lymphocytic lymphoma/chronic lymphocytic leukemia (100X).

Table 13.21: Immunohistochemistry of small lymphocytic lymphoma/chronic lymphocytic leukemia

Marker	Expression
IgM (either κ or λ light chain)	Positive
IgG (either κ or λ light chain)	Positive
CD19	Positive
CD20	Positive
CD22	Positive
CD5	Positive
CD79a	Positive
CD23	Positive
CD43	Positive

Neoplastic cells are negative for CD11c, CD10, FMC7 and CD79b

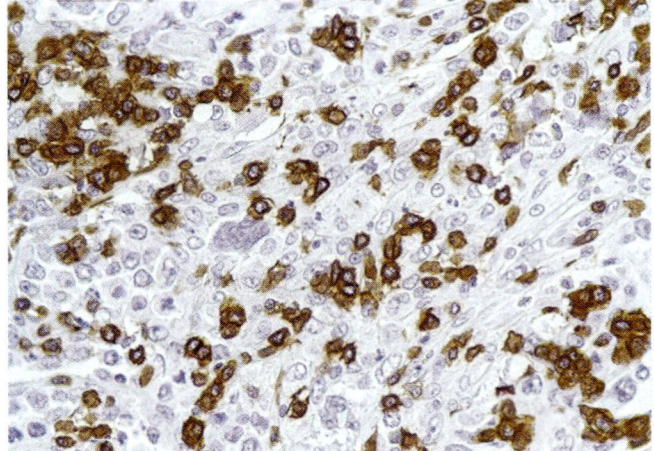

Fig. 13.27: Small lymphocytic lymphoma/chronic lymphocytic leukemia shows positivity for CD5.

Molecular Genetics

Physiological state: Normally cytochrome-c leaving mitochondria and entering into the cytosol activates

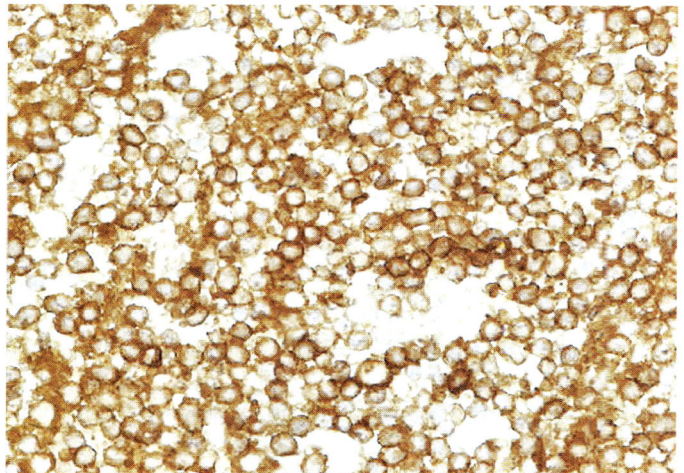

Fig. 13.28: Small lymphocytic lymphoma/chronic lymphocytic leukemia shows positivity for CD23.

Light Microscopy
- Neoplastic cells invade the lymph node capsule and extend into the surrounding adipose tissue
- It shows numerous irregularly shaped follicles in cortex and medulla with loss of corticomedullary distinction and giving nodular appearance.
- It comprises small cells (majority of small cleaved cells with scant cytoplasm known as *centrocytes with scant cytoplasm*) and large cells (referred as centroblasts—large cells with open chromatin with several nuclei and moderate cytoplasm). Light microscopy of follicular lymphoma is shown in Figs 13.29 and 13.30.

Immunohistochemistry
Neoplastic cells show positivity with CD10, CD20 and BCL-2.

Marker	Expression
CD10	Positive
CD20	Positive
BCL-2	Positive

caspases initiating apoptosis. Protein products of anti-apoptotic genes prevent cytochrome-c from leaving mitochondria. BCL-2 gene family (chromosome 18) produces gene products that prevent mitochondrial leakage of cytochrome-c (signal for apoptosis).

Pathological state: Translocation t(14;18) causes over-expression of the BCL-2 protein product, which prevents apoptosis of B cells causing B cell follicular lymphoma and chronic lymphocytic leukemia.

Lymphoma cells do not die but accumulate in the lymph nodes, bone marrow, and the blood circulation. All follicular lymphomas also express BCL-6, a transcriptional repressor that regulates germinal center B cell development.

Clinical Features
Older adults present with *painless generalized lymphadenopathy* and *marrow involvement*. Involvement of gastrointestinal tract, central nervous system or testes is uncommon. Overall median survival is 3–5 years. However, majority of patients cannot be cured.

Organs Involved
Neoplastic cells involve lymph nodes, liver (portal tracts), splenic white pulp and bone marrow (85%). Lymphoma cells are present in paratrabecular pattern in the bone marrow.

Gross Morphology
- In contrast to metastases, lymph nodes involved by lymphoma tend to have a little necrosis and only focal hemorrhage.
- Cut surface is sold, fleshy tan appearance.

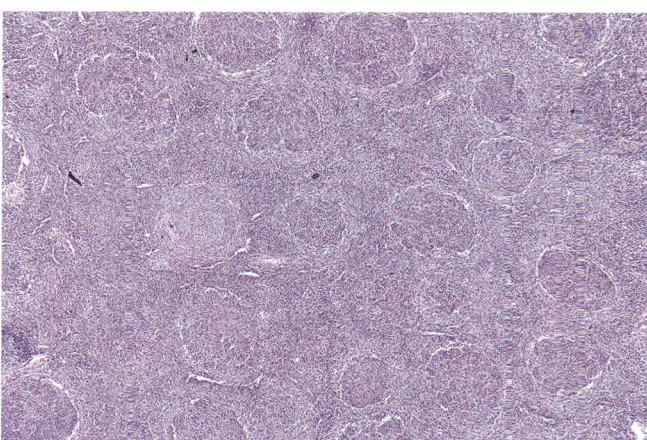

Fig. 13.29: Follicular lymphoma (100X).

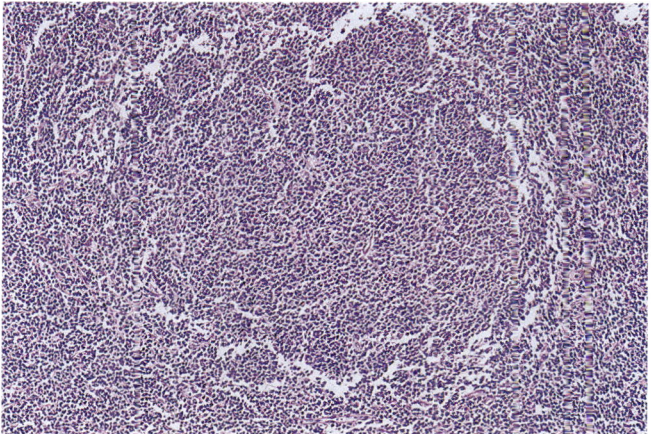

Fig. 13.30: Follicular lymphoma (200X).

Table 13.22: Grading of follicular lymphoma based on number of centroblasts/histopathological findings

Grade	Histopathological findings
Grade I	Centroblasts (0–5/high power field)
Grade II	Centroblasts (6–15/high power field)
Grade III	Centroblasts (>15/high power field)

Grading (Mann and Berard)

Follicular lymphomas are graded as I, II and III based on number of centroblasts (Table 13.22). Comparison between reactive hyperplasia and follicular lymphoma is shown in Table 13.23.

Histochemistry

Reticulin stain shows condensation of reticulin fibers at the periphery of the neoplastic follicles.

Immunohistochemistry

In addition to positive pan-B cell markers, CD19, CD20 CD10 (CALLA), naïve B cells express CD5 and CD23 CD79a and BCL-2. But these are negative for CD5, CD10, CD23 and CD43.

Immunohistochemistry of follicular lymphoma.

Marker	Expression
CD19	Positive
CD20	Positive
CD22	Positive
CD10 (CALLA)	Positive
CD5	Positive
CD79a	Positive
CD23	Positive
BCL-2	Positive

Translocation t(14;18) is demonstrated in follicular lymphoma.

MANTLE CELL LYMPHOMA

Mantle cell lymphoma is also known as *intermediate lymphocytic, mantle zone, centrocytic* and *diffuse small cleaved lymphoma.* It most often affects middle and elderly persons.

Light Microscopy

- Mantle cell lymphoma is composed of small cells with irregular and intended nuclear contours. There are three histological variants—blastoid (classic form) and anaplastic (pleomorphic).
- Blastoid form may be accompanied by involvement of blood, bone marrow and spleen, hence termed as mantle cell leukemia.
- There is presence of hyalinized blood vessels and scattered epithelioid histiocytes sometimes resembling *starry-sky appearance* (Fig. 13.31).

Immunohistochemistry

Mantle cell lymphoma shows positivity with CD5, CD20, CD22, CD43, cyclin D1 (BCL-1, PRAD) and BCL-2. Neoplastic cells are negative for CD10, CD25, CD23 and CD11c (Table 13.24). Positivity of mantle cell lymphoma for CD5 and cyclin D1 is shown in Fig. 13.32.

Table 13.24: Immunohistochemistry of mantle cell lymphoma

Marker	Expression
CD5	Positive
CD20	Positive
CD43	Positive
Cyclin D1 (BCL-1, PRAD)	Positive
BCL-2	Positive

Translocation t(11;14) creating cyclin D1-IgH fusion gene is demonstrated in mantle cell carcinoma

Table 13.23: Comparison between reactive hyperplasia and follicular lymphoma

Characteristics	Reactive hyperplasia	Follicular lymphoma
Architecture	Architecture not effaced	Architecture effaced
Subcapsular sinuses obliteration	Absent	Present
Presence of follicles	Cortex	Cortex and medulla
Reactive centers demarcation	Sharply demarcated	Poorly demarcated
Follicles appearance	Pleomorphic	Monomorphic
Condensation of reticulin fibers	These are slightly altered around follicles	These may be condensed at periphery of follicles
Macrophages	Macrophages contain debris	Macrophages inconspicuous
Mitotic figures	Frequent	Scarce

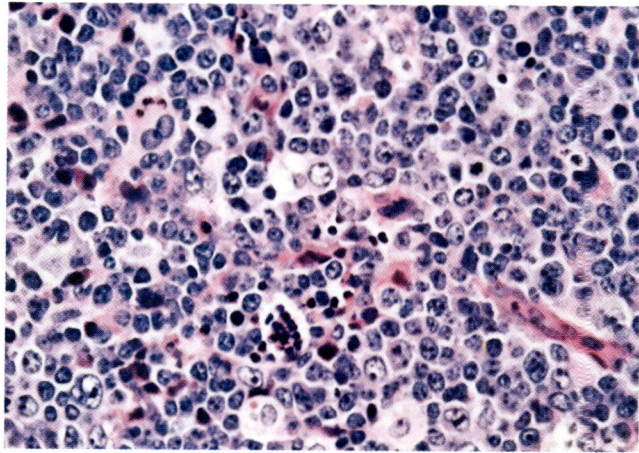

Fig. 13.31: Mantle cell lymphoma (400X).

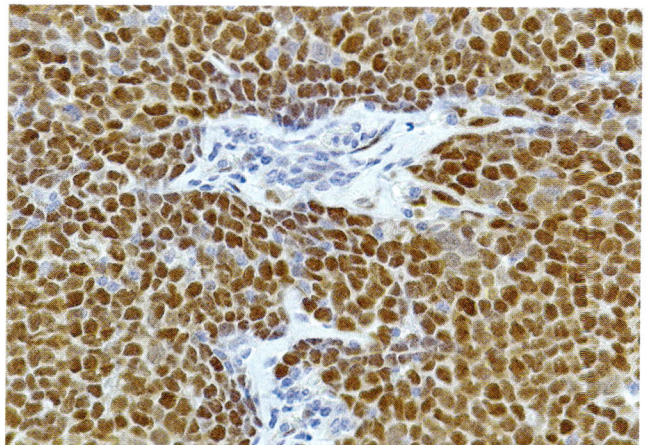

Fig. 13.32: Mantle cell lymphoma shows positivity for cyclin D1.

MARGINAL ZONE LYMPHOMA

There are three types of marginal zone lymphoma: nodal type, extranodal MALT type and splenic type NHLs.

NODAL MARGINAL ZONE LYMPHOMA

Nodal marginal zone lymphoma (NMZL) occurs without evidence of extranodal or splenic disease. It arises from mature B cells in marginal zone of lymph node.

Light Microscopy

Lymph node shows tumor cells surrounding reactive follicles and expanding the interfollicular zone. Tumor cells are composed of centrocyte like B cells, monocytoid B cells, plasma cells and transformed B cells.

Immunohistochemistry

Tumor cells express CD19, CD20, and CD22 along with CD5, CD23, CD10, and BCL-6. Cyclin D1 is negative. BCL-2 is positive in most of the cases.

Marker	Expression
CD19	Positive
CD20	Positive
CD22	Positive
CD5	Positive
CD23	Positive
CD10	Positive
BCL-6	Positive
BCL-2	Positive in most of the cases

Prognosis: About 60–80% of patients survive more than 5 years. Transformation to large B cell lymphoma may occur.

EXTRANODAL MARGINAL ZONE LYMPHOMA

Extranodal marginal zone lymphoma most often involves gastric mucosa. Patient develops mucosa-associated lymphoid tissue (MALT) lymphoma. MALT lesion often arises in *Helicobacter pylori* associated chronic gastritis, Hashimoto's thyroiditis and sialadenitis with Sjögren's syndrome. These MALT lesions are indolent. These may regress after elimination of predisposing stimulus. These may be surgically excised. It arises from mature B cells in marginal zone of lymph node.

Molecular genetics: Trisomy 18, t(11;18), t(1;14), latter create MALT1-IAP2 and BCL-10 IgH fusion genes, respectively.

Light Microscopy

- Extranodal marginal zone lymphoma shows small- to medium-sized round to irregular lymphocytes admixed with plasma cells present in the marginal zone of lymphoid follicles.
- Some of these cells show plasmacytoid appearance.
- The cells tend to invade gastric epithelium as small nests producing lymphoepithelial lesions.

Immunohistochemistry

Tumor cells are positive for CD20, CD79a, CD21 and CD35. These are negative for CD10, CD23, and CD11c.

Immunohistochemistry of extranodal marginal zone of lymph node.

Marker	Expression
CD20	Positive
CD79a	Positive
CD21	Positive
CD35	Positive

Prognosis: MALT lymphomas have indolent course and are slow to disseminate. Antibiotic therapy induces remission in *Helicobacter pylori* associated gastric MALT lymphoma whereas cases with t(11;18) are resistant to antibiotic therapy.

SPLENIC MARGINAL ZONE LYMPHOMA

Splenic marginal zone lymphoma (SMZL) is a specific low-grade small B cell lymphoma. It is characterized by splenomegaly, moderate lymphocytosis with villous morphology involving various organs, especially bone marrow. It has relatively indolent course in most of the cases except blastic form with aggressive behavior. Therapeutic options include treatment abstention, splenectomy, splenic irradiation, and chemotherapy. Mild neutropenia ($<1 \times 10^9/L$) occurs due to a combination of splenic sequestration and bone marrow infiltration in 5% cases.

PLASMABLASTIC LYMPHOMA

Plasmablastic lymphoma arises from B cell that corresponds to the differentiation stage between B immunoblast and plasma cell. It is highly aggressive neoplasm. In immunocompetent persons, this neoplasm involves lymph nodes and extranodal sites.

> **Light Microscopy**
>
> Tumor is composed of large cells with vesicular nuclei, centrally located nucleoli with abundant cytoplasm and paranuclear hof. Neoplastic cells are monomorphic and admixed with immature plasma cells.
>
> **Immunohistochemistry**
>
> Neoplastic cells show positivity with CD138 and MUM1.

HAIRY CELL LEUKEMIA

Hairy cell leukemia arises from activated small mature B memory cells. It most often affects middle and elderly persons. It most often involves peripheral blood, bone marrow and splenic red pulp.

Clinical Features

Most patients present with splenomegaly, pancytopenia, weakness, fatigue, pain in left upper quadrant, fever and bleeding. Bone marrow is virtually always involved. Hairy cells are demonstrated in the peripheral blood by the presence of cytoplasmic projections, hence named as hairy cell leukemia. Hairy cell leukemia is resistant to conventional chemotherapy. Sometimes hairy cells may invade spleen.

> **Light Microscopy**
> - Hairy cells are small- to medium-sized lymphoid cells with bean shaped nucleus with ground glass chromatin, absent or inconspicuous nucleoli and abundant pale blue cytoplasm with circumferential hairy projections.
> - The abundant cytoplasm and prominent cell borders produce fried egg appearance in bone marrow biopsies.

Cytochemistry

Hairy cells are tartrate-resistant acid phosphatase (TRAP) positive.

Immunophenotype

Hairy cells express CD20, CD22, CD11c, CD103, CD25, CD123, T-bet, Annexin A1 and DBA 44 (Table 13.25).

Table 13.25: Immunohistochemistry of hairy cell lymphoma

Marker	Expression
CD20	Positive
CD22	Positive
CD11c	Positive
CD103	Positive
CD25	Positive
CD123	Positive
T-bet	Positive
Annexin A1	Positive
DBA 44	Positive

Flow cytometry: Hairy cells show positivity with pan-B antigens CD19 and CD20. In addition, these neoplastic cells coexpress CD11c, CD25, CD103 and FMC7.

Prognosis

Complete remissions are achieved with purine analogs or α-interferon. Overall 10-year survival exceeds 90%. There is an increased risk of second cancers such as Hodgkin's disease, NHL and thyroid cancer.

B CELL PROLYMPHOCYTIC LEUKEMIA

B cell prolymphocytic leukemia arises from B cells in marginal zone in lymph node. It is difficult to distinguish from mantle cell lymphoma (MCL) and chronic lymphocytic leukemia (CLL). B-PLL cases may show translocation t(11;14). It is discussed with chronic lymphoproliferative neoplasms.

MULTIPLE MYELOMA

Multiple myeloma is malignant tumor of plasma cells resulting in synthesis of monoclonal light-chain and heavy-chain immunoglobulins.

Multiple myeloma or solitary plasmacytoma arises from post-germinal center B cell. There is diverge rearrangements involving IgH. It most often affects older adults. Proliferation and survival of these cells depend on elaboration of IL-6 by plasma cells and marrow stromal cells.

Clinical Features

Patient presents with osteolytic bone lesions, pathologic fractures, hypercalcemia, renal failure, and primary amyloidosis.

Bones Involved

In decreasing frequency, these include **vertebral column** 66% (especially lumbar regions); **ribs**, 44%; **skull** 41%; **pelvis**, 28%; **femur**, 24%; **clavicle**, 10%; and **scapula**, 10%. The lesions begin in the medullary cavity, erode cancellous bone and progressively destroy the bony cortex (osteolytic lesions).

Patient is prone to pathological fractures and vertebral compressed fractures. Radiograph study reveals rounded *punched-out defects*, of 1 to 4 cm in diameter in an older adult. Such lesions can produce bone pain. Hypercalcemia and an elevated serum alkaline phosphatase are common laboratory findings. Most cases of solitary plasmacytoma involving bone evolve into multiple myeloma.

Molecular Genetics

Cytogenetic abnormalities may include t(4;14), which juxtaposes the IgH locus on 14q32 with the fibroblast growth factor receptor 3 (FGFR3) gene on chromosome 4p16. Tumor cells synthesize cytokines such as MIP1a and the receptor activator of NF-κB ligand (RANKL), which serves as an osteoclast-activating factor.

Serum Electrophoresis

Serum protein electrophoresis shows monoclonal immunoglobulin (light-chain class or single heavy-chain) *spike* of M protein indicates increased level of IgG (50%) or IgM (25%). There is no increase in circulating immunoglobulin is <1% of cases.

Urinary Findings

In 60–70% of cases, increased light chains (either κ or λ), known as *Bence Jones protein*, are synthesized and excreted in the urine termed as *Bence Jones proteinuria*. These light chains are toxic to renal tubules, and can lead to tubular injury with renal failure.

Bone Marrow Aspirate

Bone marrow aspirate shows >30% of neoplastic plasma cells. These plasma cells well-differentiated with eccentric nuclei and perinuclear halo (clear cytoplasm

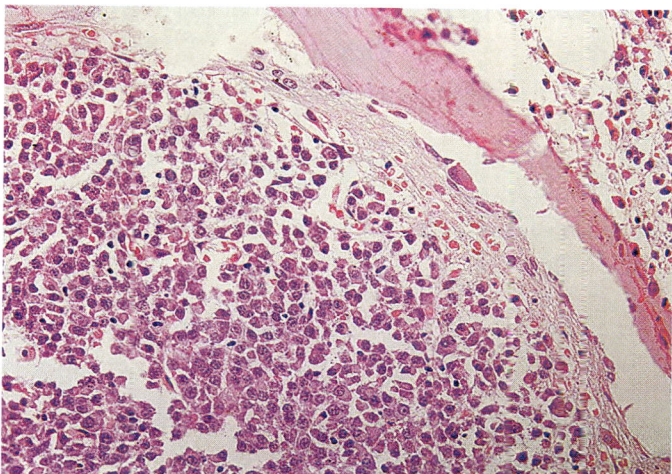

Fig. 13.33: Trephine bone biopsy showing sheets of plasma cells with eccentric nuclei and abundant pale purple cytoplasm (400X).

representing the Golgi apparatus). Clear cytoplasmic droplets contain immunoglobulin. Morphology of neoplastic plasma cells is indistinguishable from normal plasma cells except by their increased numbers. Patient rarely develops plasma cell leukemia.

Trephine Bone Biopsy

Tumor shows sheets of plasma cells that are very similar to normal plasma cells, with eccentric nuclei and abundant pale purple cytoplasm. In some cases, the myeloma cells may also be poorly differentiated (Fig. 13.33).

Recurrent Infection

The diminished amount of normal circulating immunoglobulin increases the risk for infections, particularly with bacterial organisms such as *Streptococcus pneumoniae, Haemophilus influenzae, Staphylococcus aureus,* and *Escherichia coli*.

Amyloidosis

The excessive light-chain production may lead to the AL form of amyloidosis, with deposition of amyloid in many organs. Renal failure due to amyloid deposition is most common cause of death.

MATURE T CELL AND NK CELL NHL

Lymphoid neoplasms of mature T cells and NK cells are shown in Table 13.26.

ADULT T CELL LEUKEMIA/LYMPHOMA

Adult T cell leukemia/lymphoma arises from peripheral CD4+ T cells (regulatory cells). It is caused by human

Table 13.26: Lymphoid neoplasms of mature T cells and NK cells

Disorder	Origin	Age group	Clinical features	Genotype
Adult T cell leukemia/lymphoma	Helper T cell	Adults	Cutaneous lesions, bone marrow involvement and hypercalcemia	HTLV-1 provirus demonstrated in neoplastic cells
Peripheral T cell lymphoma	Helper or cytotoxic T cell	Elderly persons	Lymphadenopathy with aggressive behavior	No specific chromosomal abnormalities
Anaplastic large cell lymphoma	Cytotoxic T cell	Children and young adults	Lymphadenopathy and soft tissue involvement with aggressive behavior	Rearrangement of ALK (anaplastic large cell kinase) in a subset
Extranodal NK cell/T cell lymphoma	NK cell (common) or cytotoxic T cell (rare)	Adults	Destructive extranodal masses (most common in sinunasal region) with aggressive course	EBV-associated without specific chromosomal abnormality
Mycosis fungoides	Helper T cells	Adults	Cutaneous lesions, and generalized erythema	No specific chromosomal abnormality
Sézary syndrome	Helper T cells	Adults	Cutaneous lesions, and generalized erythema	No specific chromosomal abnormality
Large granular lymphocytic leukemia	Cytotoxic T cells or NK cells	Adults	Anemia, splenomegaly, neutropenia, anemia accompanied by autoimmune disorder	

T cell leukemia virus type 1 (HTLV-1). It is endemic in several regions of the world.

Clinical Feature

Patient presents with widespread lymph node and peripheral blood involvement. Skin is the most common extralymphatic site involved. Several clinical variants have been described: acute, lymphomatous, chronic and smoldering.

- *Acute variant:* It is most common and characterized by leukemic phase.
- *Lymphomatous variant:* It is characterized by lymphadenopathy.
- *Chronic variant:* It is characterized by exfoliative skin rash.
- *Smoldering variant:* It is characterized by skin or pulmonary lesions with normal TLC and >5% circulating neoplastic cells.

Light Microscopy

- Several morphologic variants have been described such as pleomorphic small, medium and large cells with anaplasia.
- Multiple indentations of clefts are evident in most nuclei.
- Mutinucleated giant cells may be present simulating Reed-Sternberg cells. Mitotic activity is very high (Fig. 13.34).

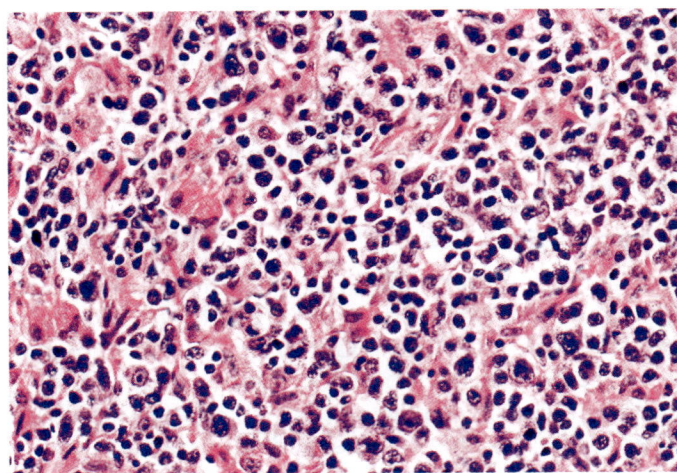

Fig. 13.34: Peripheral T cell lymphoma (400X).

Immunophenotype

Most cases are CD4+ T cell lymphomas. There is loss of normal pan-T cell markers such as CD2, CD3, and CD5.

Prognosis

The acute and lymphomatous variants have shorter survival. Death is due to infectious complications such as *Pneumocystis pneumoniae*, Cryptococcus, herpes zoster.

ANAPLASTIC LARGE T CELL LYMPHOMA (ALK POSITIVE)

Anaplastic large T cell lymphoma is derived from cytotoxic T cells. It is also known as *Ki-1 lymphoma*. Primary anaplastic large cell lymphoma originates *de novo* in lymph node or skin. Secondary anaplastic large cell lymphoma represents transformation of another lymphoma such as mycosis fungoides to anaplastic large cell lymphoma. It has bimodal age distribution with one peak in children and a second in older persons.

Molecular Genetics

ALK (anaplastic lymphoma kinase) gene is located on chromosome 2. As a result of chromosomal translocation t(2;5), it is fused with the NPM (nucleophosphin) gene, resulting in the production of a hybrid NPM–ALK protein. It is demonstrated by ALK-1 (p80) monoclonal antibody. This translocation is seen in majority of children and young adults. These patients have a relatively good prognosis.

Variants

Anaplastic large B cell lymphoma has been categorized based on ALK expression (Table 13.27).

Table 13.27: Categories of anaplastic large B cell lymphoma

Parameters	ALK positive	ALK negative
Age group	Children and young persons	Elderly persons
Prognosis with treatment	Good	Poor outcome

Clinical Features

Large T cell lymphoma involves lymph nodes, bone marrow, bone, respiratory tract, skin, soft tissue disease and gastrointestinal tract.

Light Microscopy

- Histopathological examination reveals large, pleomorphic cells showing sinusoidal pattern of infiltration, often with horseshoe-shaped or doughnut-shaped nuclei (hallmark cells).
- They may mimic poorly differentiated carcinoma.
- Morphologic variants are small cell and lymphohistiocytic (Fig. 13.35).

Immunohistochemistry

Anaplastic large cell lymphoma shows positivity for CD30 (Ki-1), anaplastic lymphoma kinase (ALK), T cell phenotype, EMA, clustrin, cadherin and galectin (Table 13.28). Distinction of ALTCL is done by absence of B cell transcription factor PAX2, which is positive in Hodgkin's disease.

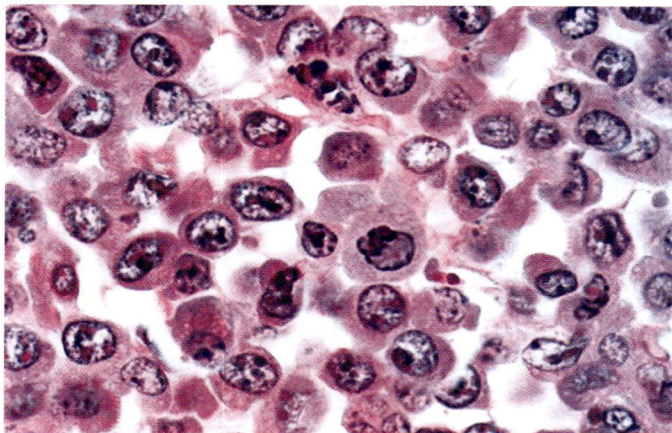

Fig. 13.35: Anaplastic large T cell lymphoma (400X).

Table 13.28: Immunohistochemistry of anaplastic large T cell lymphoma

Marker	Expression
CD30 (Ki-1)	Positive
EMA (epithelial membrane antigen)	Positive
IL-2 receptor	Positive
Clustrin	Positive
Cadherin	Positive
Galectin	Positive

Prognosis

ALCLs have good prognosis with 75% cure rate with chemotherapy. Immunohistochemistry in common T cell lymphoma is shown in Table 13.29.

EXTRANODAL NK CELL/T CELL LYMPHOMA

Extranodal NK cell/T cell lymphoma arises from activated NK cell and less commonly cytotoxic T cell. It is most often *associated with Epstein-Barr virus*. It is more prevalent in Asians and affects adults. Survival rate is very poor (30–40%).

Table 13.29: Immunohistochemistry in common T cell lymphoma

Marker	Anaplastic large T cell lymphoma	Peripheral T cell lymphoma	T lymphoblastic lymphoma
CD3	Positive/negative	Positive	Positive/negative
CD30	Positivity (sheets of cells)	Positive (focal cells)	Negative
EMA	Positive	Negative	Negative
ALK1	Positive	Negative	Negative
CD99	Positive/negative	Negative	Positive
Tdt	Negative	Negative	Positive

Clinical Features

Patient presents as a destructive nasopharyngeal mass with involvement of skin, soft tissue, GI tract and testis being the other extranodal sites of involvement. Patient presents with epistaxis and nasal obstruction.

> ### Light Microscopy
> The mucosa shows ulceration with diffuse and permeative lymphomatous infiltrate. An *angiocentric* and *angiodestructive* growth pattern is commonly seen. The tumor cells may be small-, medium-sized, large, anaplastic. Cells have irregularly folded nuclei, granular chromatin, and inconspicuous nucleoli with pale cytoplasm containing azurophilic granules.

Immunophenotype

The atypical cells are CD2, CD3 and CD5 positive. EBV encoded RNA (EBER) *in situ* hybridization shows presence of EBV in all lymphoma cell (Table 13.30).

Table 13.30: Immunohistochemistry of extranodal NK cell/T cell lymphoma

Marker	Expression
CD2	Positive
CD3	Positive
CD5	Positive

MYCOSIS FUNGOIDES

Mycosis fungoides is the most common form of cutaneous lymphoma arising from mature skin homing CD4+ T cell. The disease is always limited to the skin. It most often occurs in adults/elderly. Patients with limited disease have excellent prognosis.

Clinical Features

Patient presents with cutaneous patches, ranging from plaques or nodules, or generalized erythematous rashes. These cutaneous patches may remain localized to the skin for many years. Later, neoplastic cells eventually disseminate to lymph nodes and internal organs. Clinical stage is the most important prognostic factor.

> ### Light Microscopy
> The histology of the skin lesions varies with the stage of the disease (Fig. 13.36).
> - *Early patch stage:* Band-like or lichenoid infiltrates of lymphocytes and histiocytes are demonstrated. Atypical cells are small- to medium-sized with cerebriform nuclei present mainly in the basal layer of epidermis.
> - *Plaque stage:* Epidermotropism is prominent with intraepidermal atypical cell collections called *Pautrier microabscesses*.
> - *Tumor stage:* Dermal infiltrates of neoplastic cells are more diffuse with prominent nuclei. Intradermal atypical cell collection is less.

Immunophenotype

Tumor cells express CD2, CD3, TCRβ, CD5, and CD4+ T cell. Cutaneous lymphocyte antigen (CLA) is expressed in most of the cases.

SÉZARY SYNDROME

Sézary syndrome is defined by the triad of erythroderma, generalized lymphadenopathy and presence of clonally related neoplastic T cells with cerebriform nuclei (Sézary cells). Leukemic cells from skin lesion in mycosis fungoides most often *involve bone marrow* and lymph nodes.

Sézary syndrome presents with generalized exfoliative erythroderma and an associated leukemia of *Sézary cells*. Adults are more commonly involved. Sézary syndrome is an aggressive disease with poor overall 5-year survival.

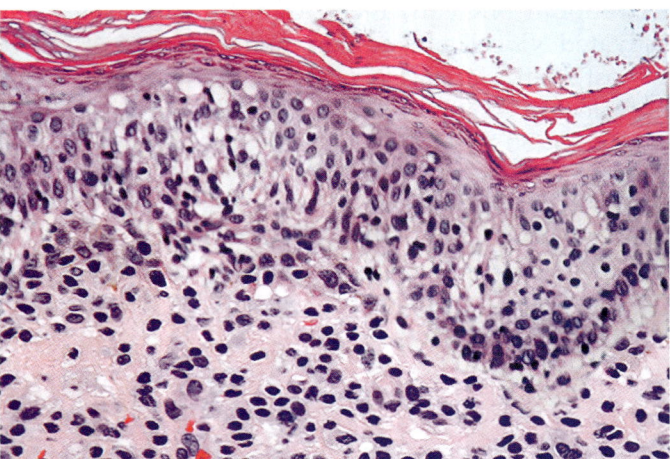

Fig. 13.36: Cutaneous T cell lymphoma (400X).

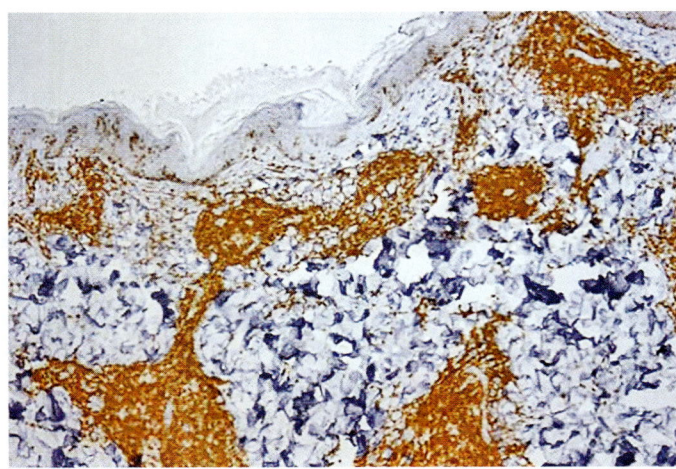

Fig. 13.37: Cutaneous T cell lymphoma shows positivity for CD3.

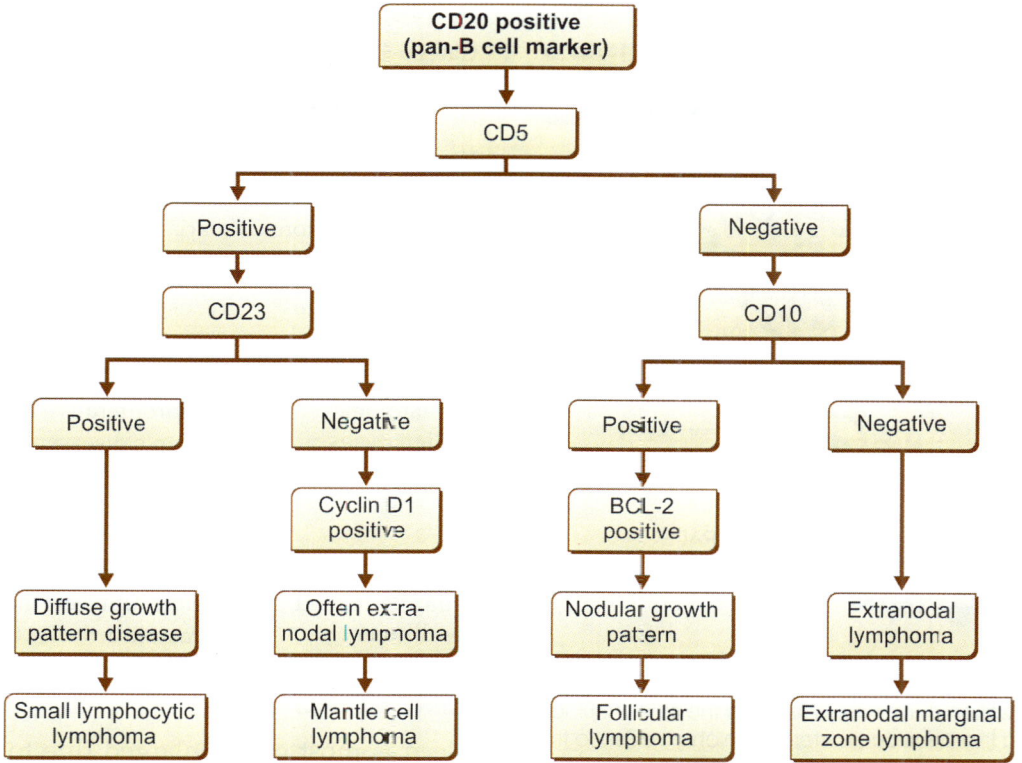

Fig. 13.38: Interpretation of various non-Hodgkin's lymphomas.

Light Microscopy

Peripheral blood examination shows *Sézary-Lutzner cells* with deep-clefted, cerebriform nucleus. Late in the course of this disease, transformation to a large T cell lymphoma often occurs.

Immunophenotype

Tumor cells express CD2, CD3, CD5, TCRβ, CD4, CLA and skin homing receptor CCR4 (Fig. 13.37). Interpretation of various non-Hodgkin's lymphomas is shown in Fig. 13.38.

SPLEEN

STRUCTURE

Spleen is the largest lymphoid organ. In normal adults, it weighs 50–200 gm.

It contributes to the maturation of red blood cells by pitting function. It has ability to remove solid particles from the cytoplasm of red blood cells without causing injury to the cell membrane. Normal red blood cells squeeze through slit pores in the sinusoids, but red blood cells with membrane defect (spherocytosis or elliptocytes) and sickle cells cannot squeeze resulting in destruction in spleen termed extravascular hemolysis.

Spleen is divided into white pulp and red pulp, separated by an ill-defined interface known as *marginal zone*. Organization of lymphoid tissue in the spleen is shown in Fig. 13.39.

WHITE PULP

The white pulp contains periarteriolar lymphoid sheath (PALS) containing germinal follicles. It is surrounded by the marginal zone, which contains numerous macrophages, antigen presenting cells, slowly recirculating B cells, and natural killer cells. T cells are located in the periarteriolar lymphoid nodules. B cells are distributed in the lymphoid follicles. In routine hematoxylin and eosin stained sections, white pulp appears basophilic due to dense heterochromatin in lymphocytes nuclei.

RED PULP

The red pulp contains venous sinuses separated by splenic cords. It participates in the storage of red blood cells, white blood cells and platelets. When

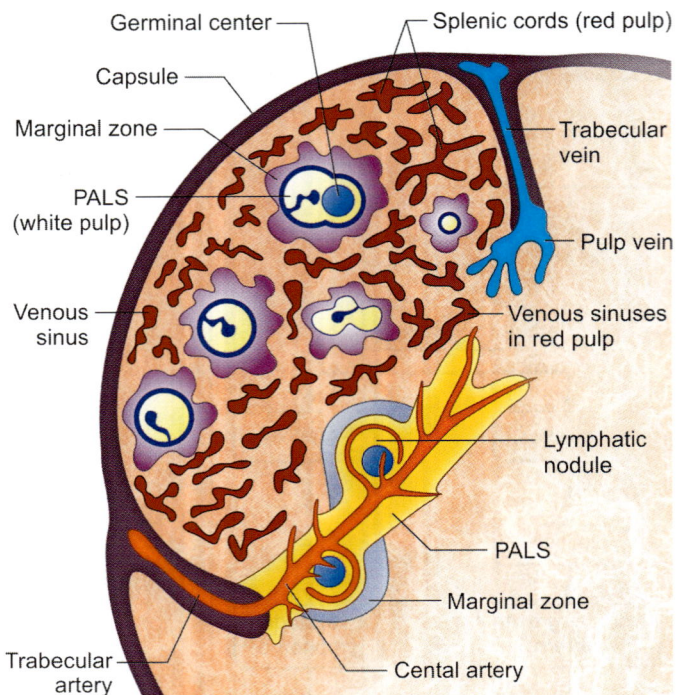

Fig. 13.39: Organization of lymphoid tissue in the spleen. Blood enters the tissue via the trabecular arteries, which give rise to the many-branched central arteries. Some of these end in the white pulp, supplying the germinal centers and mantle zones, but most empty into or near the marginal zones (PALS—periarteriolar lymphoid sheath).

Table 13.31: Conditions associated with splenomegaly

Categories	Conditions
Bacterial infections	Infectious endocarditis, tuberculosis, syphilis
Viral infections	Infectious mononucleosis, cytomegalovirus
Parasitic infection	Malaria
Fungal infection	Histoplasmosis
Congestive states	Cirrhosis Congestive heart failure Splenic vein thrombosis
Hematologic malignancies	Myeloproliferative disorders, Hodgkin's disease, non-Hodgkin's lymphoma, hepatosplenic T cell lymphoma, splenic marginal B cell lymphoma, mantle cell lymphoma, hairy cell leukemia, multiple myeloma
Immune-related conditions	Systemic lupus erythematosus, rheumatoid arthritis, Gaucher's disease

splenomegaly occurs, excessive pooling of these cells may cause fall in the peripheral blood count. Special endothelial cells that express both reticular cells and histiocytic markers are known as *Littoral cells*.

Blood enters into the tissue via the trabecular arteries, which give rise to the many-branched central arteries. Some of these end in the white pulp, supplying the germinal centers and mantle zones, but most empty into or near the marginal zones. The splenic venous outflow is drained into the portal vein, adding as rich supply of antibodies to the portal blood entering the liver.

FUNCTIONAL DISORDERS

SPLENECTOMY

Therapeutic splenectomy is performed in idiopathic thrombocytopenic purpura, chronic myeloproliferative disorders, Hodgkin's disease and non-Hodgkin's lymphoma. Following splenectomy, children under the age of three years are susceptible to infection, i.e. pneumococci, streptococci group A, enteric group and *Haemophilus influenzae*, therefore, resulting in septicemia, meningitis and disseminated intravascular coagulation.

SPLENOMEGALY

Spleen is most often enlarged due to infections and congestive state. *Red pulp congestion is most common finding*. Massive splenomegaly occurs due to chronic myeloid leukemia, myelofibrosis, kala-azar, malaria, Gaucher's disease and hepatosplenic T cell lymphoma. Conditions associated with splenomegaly are shown in Table 13.31.

FIBROCONGESTIVE SPLENOMEGALY

Congestive splenomegaly most often occurs in portal hypertension due to cirrhosis and right-sided cardiac failure with cor pulmonale. Decreased portal venous drainage in these disorders leads to congestive splenomegaly.

Pathogenesis: The increased portal venous pressure causes dilation of sinusoids, with slowing of blood flow from the cords to the sinusoids that prolongs the exposure of the blood cells to the cordal macrophages, resulting in excessive trapping and destruction (hypersplenism). Perivascular hemorrhages result in organization and formation of Gamna-Gandy bodies (dystrophic calcification).

Gross morphology: Spleen shows irregular tan-white fibrous plaques over the purple capsular surface.

This *sugar icing* is termed hyaline perisplenitis. Cut surface of fibrocongestive splenomegaly shows firm and brown fibrotic nodules termed as *Gamna-Gandy bodies*.

Light microscopy: Gamna-Gandy body is an organized hemorrhage forming nodule with dystrophic calcification and hemosiderin pigment in spleen (Fig. 13.40).

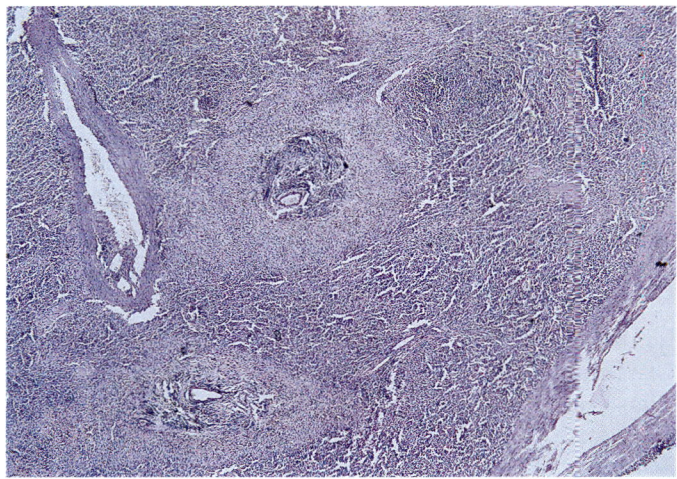

Fig. 13.40: Chronic venous congestion of spleen showing formation of Gamna-Gandy bodies as a result of organization of hemorrhage with dystrophic calcification and hemosiderin pigment in spleen (400X).

HYPERSPLENISM

Hypersplenism refers to destruction of one or more blood cell lines by the spleen. It is characterized by *splenomegaly, anemia, leukopenia, thrombocytopenia, bone marrow hyperplasia.*

Cytopenias occur due to sequestration of blood elements in the spleen. These findings are corrected by splenectomy. Diagnostic criteria for hypersplenism include cytopenia of one or more cell lines, bone marrow hyperplasia, splenomegaly and correction of cytopenias following splenectomy. Disorders associated with hypersplenism are shown in Table 13.32.

AUTOSPLENECTOMY

Sickle cell disease is important cause of autosplenectomy. It leads to susceptibility to disseminated infection with encapsulated bacteria such as pneumococci, meningococci, and *Haemophilus influenzae*.

HYPOSPLENISM

Hyposplenism refers to absence of functioning of spleen following splenectomy. Findings suggestive of hyposplenism are presence of Howell-Jolly bodies, poikilocytosis, target cells, acanthocytes, and nucleated red blood precursor cells. Other causes of hyposplenism are Fanconi anemia and sickle cell disease, infiltrative disorders and old age.

SPLENOSIS

Splenosis refers to splenic implants of splenic tissue over the peritoneal surface, pleural surface, and lung parenchyma following trauma or surgical splenectomy.

SPLENIC RUPTURE

Splenic rupture results most often from blunt force injury with abdominal trauma. The hemorrhage can extend into the peritoneal cavity to produce hemoperitoneum. Spontaneous rupture of spleen following minor trauma may occur due to malaria, infectious mononucleosis, subacute bacterial endocarditis, lymphoid neoplasms and typhoid fever.

Table 13.32: Disorders associated with hypersplenism

Mechanism	Disorders
Abnormal sequestration of blood cells with intrinsic defects in normal spleen	Inherited disorders (hereditary spherocytosis and elliptocytosis), malaria, autoimmune hemolytic anemia, autoimmune thrombocytopenia and/or neutropenia
Sequestration of normal blood cells in abnormal spleen	Gaucher's disease Niemann-Pick disease Langerhans' cell histiocytosis Chronic congestive splenomegaly Malignant infiltrative disorders (CML, AML, splenic marginal B cell lymphoma, mantle cell lymphoma, hairy cell leukemia, hepatosplenic T cell lymphoma, Hodgkin's disease, plasma cell dyscrasias, metastatic carcinoma) Extramedullary hematopoiesis (severe hemolytic states, chronic idiopathic myelofibrosis) Chronic infections (tuberculosis and brucellosis) Vascular tumors Splenic cysts Hamartomas
Miscellaneous conditions	Hypogammaglobulinemia, hypothyroidism, progressive multifocal leukoencephalopathy

HEMOSIDEROSIS

Thalassemia major is important cause of hemosiderin deposition in spleen, liver, pancreas, myocardium, adrenal glands and pituitary gland. The hemosiderin is deposited as refractile granular golden brown pigment in macrophages lining sinusoids in spleen.

REACTIVE SPLENIC DISORDERS

GRANULOMATOUS INFLAMMATION

Granuloma in spleen is focal benign process ranging from lipogranulomatous inflammation to caseating and noncaseating inflammation. Caseating granulomas occur due to Mycobacterium tubercle bacilli, fungal infection and X-linked chronic granulomatous disease. Noncaseating granulomas are most often seen in sarcoidosis.

SPLENIC INFARCT

Splenic infarct occurs as a consequence of systemic arterial embolization in a patient with an infective endocarditis involving either aortic or mitral valve.

Wedge-shaped Infarct

Most splenic infarcts are due to emboli that arise from thrombi in the heart, either vegetations on valves or mural thrombi. Emboli from infective endocarditis lead to septic infarct in kidney. These emboli reach the spleen via splenic artery and obstruct splenic branches resulting in ischemic infarct with base *towards capsule, pale, and wedge-shaped.*

The remaining splenic parenchyma appears dark red. This wedge-shaped infarct gets replaced by granulation tissue resulting into fibrous scar. Patient presents with left upper quadrant pain and splenic enlargement.

Non-wedge-shaped Infarcts

Non-wedge infarcts are most often occur in essential thrombocythemia and myelofibrosis. Less common causes are paroxysmal nocturnal hemoglobinuria, sickle cell anemia, aplastic anemia, polyarteritis nodosa and splenic artery aneurysm.

NON-NEOPLASTIC INFILTRATIVE DISORDERS

GAUCHER'S SPLEEN

The enlarged spleen is pale and has a firm feel. It is an autosomal recessive disorder error of metabolism with lack of the enzyme glucocerebrosidase, resulting in accumulation of storage product in cells of the mononuclear phagocyte system.

Hallmark of Disorder

The hallmark of this disorder is the presence of *Gaucher's cells* with a distinctive **cigarette paper-like cytoplasmic appearance and eccentric nuclei**, which are lipid-laden macrophages present in the red pulp of the **spleen, liver sinusoids** (Kupffer cells), **lymph nodes, lungs** (alveolar macrophages), and **bone marrow**.

Enzymes in Gaucher's Cells

Gaucher's cells contain specific enzymes such as chitotriosidase and angiotensin-converting enzyme. These markers of macrophage proliferation assay are required to confirm the diagnosis.

Clinical Variants

Gaucher's disease has three variants: adult type (normal lifespan), infantile type (fatal disease) and juvenile type (less severe).

SPLEEN IN AMYLOIDOSIS

Deposition of amyloid in spleen results in splenomegaly. Gross examination shows diffuse *lardaceous pattern* or the nodular *sago pattern* due to amyloid deposition (AL or AA) in white pulp.

NEOPLASTIC DISORDERS

Considering its size and blood flow, the spleen is uncommon site of either primary hematologic (leukemias) of metastatic malignancies (extranodal Hodgkin's disease and NHL). It is due to immunological role of spleen. Spleen in Hodgkin's and NHL shows multiple nodular pale deposits.

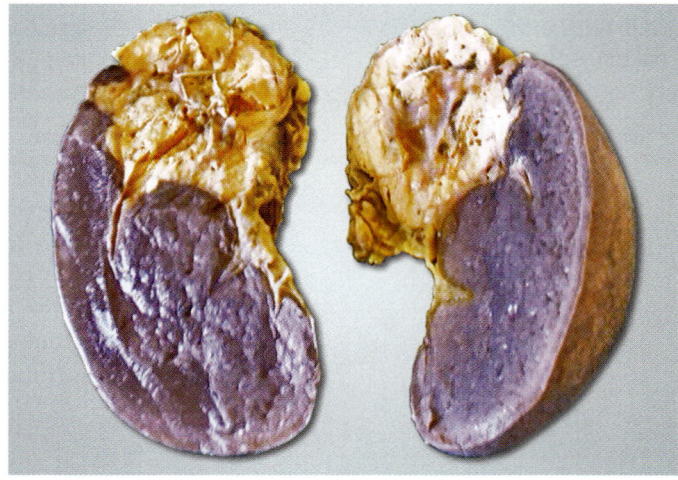

Fig. 13.41: Carcinoma metastasizing to spleen.

Lymph Nodes, Spleen and Thymus

Table 13.33: Neoplastic disorders of spleen

Disorder	Origin	Spleen morphology	Other characteristics
Primary splenic lymphoma			
Primary splenic lymphoma	B or T cells	Diffuse large B cell lymphomas (origin germinal center or post-germinal center B cell) with single or multiple nodules of varying size	Diverse chromosomal rearrangement. BCL-6 (30%), BCL-2 (10%) and MYC (5%)
Secondary splenic lymphomas			
Hodgkin's disease (classic variant)	B cells Reed-Sternberg cells are CD30+ (Ki-1) specific marker, CD15+ (Leu M-1)	Splenomegaly	Prognosis varies depending on variants and staging
Low-grade non-Hodgkin's lymphoma	B or T cells	Splenomegaly (single or multiple nodules)	50% cases show splenomegaly and splenic lymph nodes involvement
Lymphomas presenting with prominent lymphadenopathy			
Splenic marginal B cell lymphoma	B cells	Massive splenomegaly (infiltration in both red and white pulp)	Allelic loss of chromosome 7q31–32 in 40% of cases, trisomy 3 in rare cases, IgH clonally rearranged Peripheral cytopenias
Mantle cell lymphoma	Naïve B cell	Prominent splenomegaly	t(11;14) creating cyclin D1-IgH fusion gene
Hairy cell leukemia	Memory B cell	Prominent splenomegaly	Activating BRAF mutations, rearrangement of IgH
Hepatosplenic T cell lymphoma	T cell	Triad of peripheral cytopenias, sinusoidal tropism and massive splenomegaly (>3000 gm)	Isochrome 7q10 and trisomy 8 strong genetic abnormality
Myeloid neoplasms			
Chronic myeloid leukemia with blast crisis	Pluripotent stem cell	Leukemic cells are confined to bone marrow and spleen. Bone marrow and blood contain <10% myeloblasts. Anemia, massive splenomegaly and hepatomegaly. Splenomegaly correlates with magnitude of leukocytosis	Philadelphia chromosome t(9;22)
Acute myeloid leukemia	Myeloid cell	Anemia, neutropenia (recurrent upper respiratory tract infections) and thrombocytopenia (bleeding tendencies), bone tenderness, mild to moderate hepatomegaly and splenomegaly	AML with recurrent genetic alterations
Mast cell disease with systemic mastocytosis	Mast cell	Spleen frequently involved (both red and white pulp involved)	Flow cytometry helpful in establishing diagnosis

Splenic masses are more likely due to hematopoietic diseases rather than metastases. Neoplastic disorders of spleen are shown in Table 13.33.

METASTASES IN SPLEEN

Despite its size, the spleen is a rare site of metastases from non-hematological malignancies. Melanomas are aggressive neoplasms that can often be widely metastatic. Most of these masses are tan, but some have brown-black pigmentation from the melanin elaborated by the neoplastic cells.

The most common epithelial malignancies metastasizing to spleen are carcinomas of breast and lung origin. Sarcomas involving the spleen tend to be of dendritic/histiocytic or vascular lineage. Carcinoma metastasizing to spleen is shown in Fig. 13.41.

ANGIOSARCOMA OF SPLEEN

Angiosarcoma is malignant proliferation of primitive mesenchymal cells with vascular differentiation.

THYMUS GLAND

OVERVIEW

Anterior compartment is most common site for mediastinal masses in >50%. Primary tumors of the mediastinum include thymoma, neurogenic tumors, germ cell tumors and lymphoma. Primary lung cancer can invade mediastinum. Summary of mediastinal masses is shown in Table 13.34.

ANATOMY

Thymus gland situated in the anterior mediastinum of the chest is prominent during third trimester (late fetal life), infancy and childhood. It is populated with T cells. During late fetal life, progenitor cells of bone marrow origin migrate to the thymus and give rise to mature T cells that are exported to the peripheral lymphoid organs. Thymus undergoes atrophy during adulthood.

Table 13.34: Summary of mediastinal masses

Mediastinum compartment	Pathological disorders
Anterior mediastinum	Thymic tumors, retrosternal thyroid mass, germ cell tumors, lymph nodes (lymphomas), cystic hygroma, aortic aneurysm, hernia (Morgagni), pericardial cysts, sternal masses
Middle mediastinum	Lymph nodes (sarcoidosis, tuberculosis, lymphomas, metastases), aortic aneurysm, mediastinal paraganglioma, carcinoma bronchus, fatty mediastinal tumors, mediastinal lipomatosis, hiatal hernia
Posterior mediastinum	Myeloma, metastases, aortic aneurysm, sympathetic ganglion cell tumors, lateral thoracic meningocele, paravertebral abscess, extramedullary hematopoiesis, pancreatic pseudocyst

HISTOLOGY

On histological examination, it consists of cortex and medulla. Cortex consists of large cells with prominent nucleoli in the superficial zone. In the deeper zone, the cells are small with less prominent nucleoli. Medulla consists of spindle cells with densely stained nuclei and inconspicuous nucleoli. Hassall corpuscles composed of epithelial cells are in the center of the medullary regions. These become keratinized on enlargement. Thymus also consists of macrophages, dendritic cells, a few B cells; rare neutrophils and eosinophils.

THYMUS HYPERPLASIA

Normally, adult thymus is composed mostly of adipose tissue, with a few clusters of lymphocytes and residual Hassall corpuscles. Approximately 75% of patients diagnosed with myasthenia gravis have thymic hyperplasia composed of lymphoid cells associated with autoantibody production. These **autoantibodies bind to acetylcholine receptor** and diminish the receptor

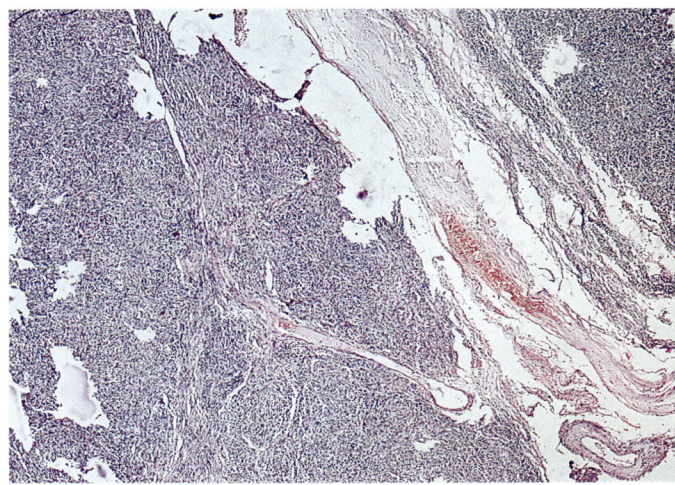

Fig. 13.42: Thymic hyperplasia (100X).

function in the skeletal muscle motor end plates, resulting in onset of **muscular weakness**, particularly with repetitive muscular contraction (Fig. 13.42).

IMMUNODEFICIENCY DISORDERS

DIGEORGE SYNDROME

In DiGeorge syndrome, there is failure of maturation of T cells, but B cells remain unaffected. Thymus gland shows hypoplasia. In DiGeorge syndrome, aberrant embryonic development of third and fourth branchial arches, results in hypoplasia of thymus and parathyroid glands as well as anomalies of aortic arch, mandible and ear. It can be summed up by CATH22, which denotes **cardiac defects, abnormal facies, thymic hypoplasia, cleft palate, hypocalcemia** and **microdeletion of chromosome 22q11**. In about 30% of cases, this syndrome is also associated with behavior disorders and psychosis (bipolar disorder and schizophrenia) that develop during adolescence.

Clinical Features

Affected children develop recurrent infections (bacterial, fungal and viral) and tetany from hypoparathyroidism with hypocalcaemia.

WISKOTT-ALDRICH SYNDROME (X-LINKED DISORDER)

Wiskott-Aldrich syndrome is X-linked disorder associated with defects of both B cell and T cell functions (humoral and cellular immunity). It is associated with thymic hypoplasia, eczema, thrombocytopenia, bloody diarrhea, recurrent infections and poor antibody response to polysaccharide antigens. Patient has fatal outcome before six years of age due to bleeding, infection or malignancy (most often lymphoma).

> **Light Microscopy**
> Thymus gland shows hypoplasia characterized by absence of thymocytes. A few Hassall corpuscles, and only epithelial components may be present.

THYMIC NEOPLASMS

Neoplasms of the thymus gland are thymoma, thymic carcinoma and neuroendocrine tumors including thymic carcinoid.

THYMOMA

Thymoma is the most common mediastinal tumor located in anterior mediastinum. It tends to maintain overall variable degree of architecture and mixture of cells normally present in thymus gland. It most often has multilobular growth pattern with presence of fibrous bands that enclose epithelial islands. It varies in behavior from benign (70%) to malignant (30%).

Reliable indicator of malignancy is capsular invasion. There is some correlation between WHO classification histologic variants having aggressive behavior with invasive features. WHO classification of thymomas (A, B1, B2, B3, AB and C system) is shown in Table 13.35.

Clinical Features

Clinical syndrome associated with thymoma is myasthenia gravis (50%), symptoms related to mediastinal tumor mass (40%) and non-myasthenic paraneoplastic syndrome.

Table 13.35: WHO classification of thymomas (A, B1, B2, B3, AB and C system)

Categories	Histopathologic features	Frequency (%)	Invasiveness (%)
A	Ovoid to spindle cells arranged in diffuse or hemangiopericytoma-like pattern Lymphocytes absent	8	10
B1	Morphology similar to normal thymus Immature thymocytes with epithelial cells with or without Hassall's corpuscles	15	45
B2	Large polygonal epithelial cells forming lobules and separated by immature T thymocytes	28	70
B3	Large polygonal epithelial cells arranged in sheets with minimal lymphocyte component Cells are showing mild atypia raising the possibility of thymic carcinoma	11	35
AB	Lobules of mixed pattern A (lymphocytic rich) and B (lymphocytic poor)	31	40
C	Any pattern of carcinoma with squamous, lymphoepithelial, clear cell, mucoepidermoid, basaloid, sarcomatoid, papillary and mucinous features	5	5

Approximately 65–75% patients are often associated with myasthenia gravis due to autoantibodies against acetylcholine receptors in the motor end plates of skeletal muscles (type II hypersensitivity reaction). The antibodies bind to postsynaptic receptors and block neurotransmission resulting in progressive muscle weakness involving particularly the external ocular, eye lids and proximal limb muscles. It may cause death by respiratory muscles paralysis.

Thymectomy may reduce the plasma concentrations of autoantibodies and improve clinical picture. Some patients of thymomas are associated with pure red cell anemia, Graves' disease and hypoglobulinemia.

Gross Morphology
- Tumor is well circumscribed, encapsulated and firm. Invasive thymoma has poorly defined edges and tend to ensheath blood vessels and neighboring organs within the mediastinum.
- Average weight of tumor is 150 gm. It may weigh up to several kilogram.

Light Microscopy
- Tumor consists of epithelial neoplastic element. Histopathologic features depend on morphology of cells based on categories A, B1, B2, B3, AB and C.
- Histological variants such as types B2 and B3 are most invasive. Thymic carcinoma or type C is regarded as separate distinct category of thymoma (Fig. 13.43).

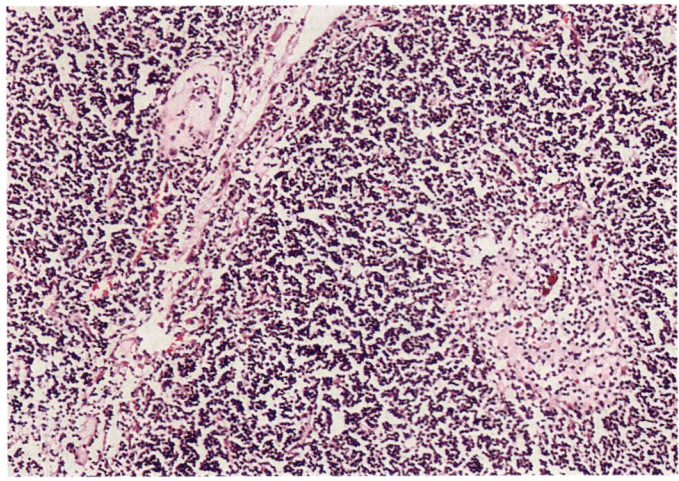

Fig. 13.43: Thymoma.

Immunohistochemistry

Immunohistochemistry of thymoma is shown in Table 13.36.

Clinicopathologic staging of thymoma according to Masaoka is shown in Table 13.37.

Management

Diagnosis and treatment are best achieved by complete excision of thymus gland along with tumor.

THYMIC CARCINOMA

Thymic carcinoma is a rare but highly aggressive neoplasm, easily metastasizing cancer derived from thymic epithelial cells. It constitutes ≤5% of all primary neoplasms of thymus gland. It occurs most frequently in adults between 30 and 60 years of age. It arises *de novo* in the thymus.

The tumor presents as multilocular cyst. Unlike thymoma, which is usually found because it is associated with paraneoplastic syndrome, thymic carcinoma is almost always found at an advanced stage because patients often have atypical symptoms. Thymoma on imaging technique is shown in Fig. 13.44. Gross morphology of thymic carcinoma is shown in Fig. 13.45.

Table 13.36: Immunohistochemistry of thymoma

Marker	Thymoma according to WHO (ABC system)	Expression
CK7	Type A	Positive
CD15	Type A	Positive
BCL-2	Type A and C	Positive
CK5, CK6 and CK7 are positive in both thymoma and thymic carcinoma		
CK18, CD5, CD117, MUC1 and GLUT-1 are positive in thymic carcinoma		

Table 13.37: Clinciopathologic staging of thymoma according to Masaoka

Stage	Qualifying features	5-year survival (%)
I	Completely encapsulated tumor without invasion of capsule	95–100
II	Gross invasion into surrounding soft tissues or mediastinal pleura and or microscopic invasion into capsule	80–85
III	Gross invasion into pericardium, lung and great vessels (intraoperative biopsy obtained for confirmation)	60–70
IVa	Dissemination to pericardium and/or pleura without contiguous spread as in stage III	40–50
IVb	Distant metastases to lung, liver, bone and skin	25–30

Lymph Nodes, Spleen and Thymus

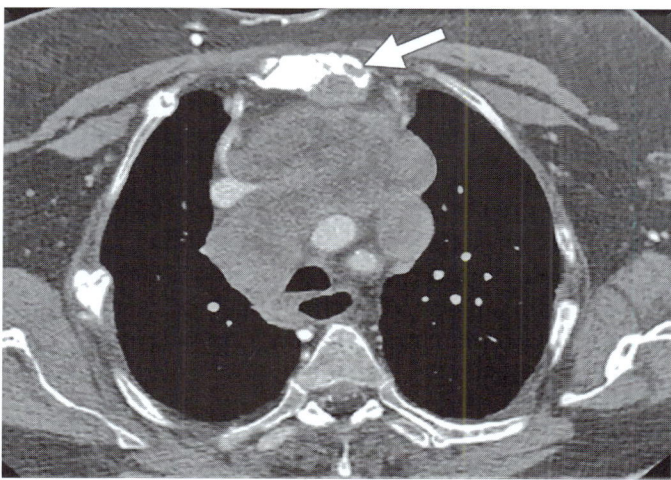

Fig. 13.44: Thymoma on imaging technique.

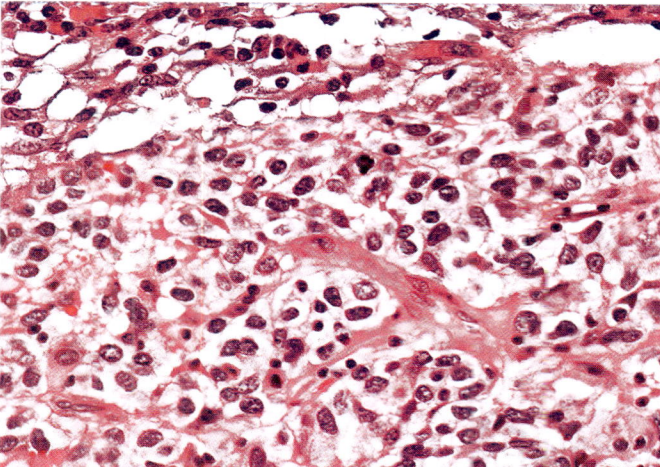

Fig. 13.46: Thymic carcinoma (400X).

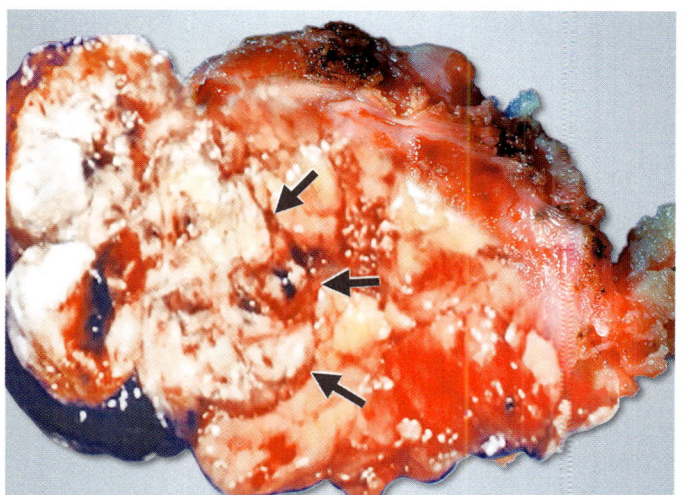

Fig. 13.45: Gross morphology of thymic carcinoma (arrows).

Light Microscopy

- Most common histological variant of tumor is composed of undifferentiated neoplastic cells with or without squamous differentiation.
- There may diverse histopathologic features such as basaloid, adenoid cystic, papillary, clear cell, lymphoepithelial-like or adenocarcinoma type (Fig. 13.46).

Immunohistochemistry

Immunohistochemistry of thymic carcinoma is shown in Table 13.38. Differential diagnosis of atypical thymoma, thymic carcinoma and lung carcinoma is shown in Table 13.39.

Table 13.38: Immunohistochemistry of thymic carcinoma

Marker	Expression
BCL-2	Positive
CK5	Positive
CK6	Positive
CK7	Positive
CK18	Positive
CD5	Positive
CD117	Positive
MUC1	Positive
GLUT-1	Positive

CK5, CK6 and CK7 are positive in both thymoma and thymic carcinoma.

Table 13.39: Differential diagnosis of atypical thymoma, thymic carcinoma and lung carcinoma

Immunophenotype	Atypical thymoma	Thymic carcinoma	Lung carcinoma
CK7	Positive	Positive	Positive/negative
CD5	Negative	Positive	Negative
CD117	Negative	Positive	Negative
CD1a	Positive in immature thymocytes	Negative	Negative
TTF-1	Negative	Negative	Positive
CD205	Positive	Positive	Positive/negative
FOXN1	Positive (nuclear staining)	Positive (nuclear staining) or negative	Negative

Management

Complete resection of the tumor is the mainstay of treatment and leads to the best survival rate for patients. However, the complete resection rate is only approximately 50% and the recurrence rate after complete resection is high, up to 40%.

CHAPTER 14

Advanced Diagnostic Techniques

Learning Objectives

FROZEN SECTION TECHNIQUE
- Cryostat

ELECTRON MICROSCOPY AND POLARIZING LIGHT MICROSCOPY
- Electron Microscopy
- Polarizing Light Microscopy

HISTOLOGY AND HISTOCHEMICAL STAINS
- Fixatives
- Decalcification
- Surgical Specimens
- Special Stains

IMMUNOHISTOCHEMISTRY
- Overview
- Detection Systems
- Immunohistochemistry Protocol

IMMUNOFLUORESCENCE MICROSCOPY

CHEMILUMINESCENCE VS CHEMIFLUORESCENCE

FLOW CYTOMETRY
- Components of Flow Cytometer

CYTOGENETIC ANALYSIS
- Traditional Cytogenetic Analysis
- Metaphase Fluorescence *in situ* Hybridization

- Multiplex Metaphase FISH
- Comparctive Genomic Hybridization (CGH)
- Microarray Analysis

FLUORESCENCE *IN SITU* HYBRIDIZATION
- Overview
- Advantages and Limitations
- Development of FISH Test for Clinical Use

ENZYME-LINKED IMMUNOSORBENT ASSAY (ELISA)
- Overview
- Types of ELISA

METHODS FOR DNA SEQUENCES
- Polymerase Chain Reaction
- Southern Blot Technique
- Northern Blot Technique

TISSUE MICROARRAY
- Tissue Microarray Technique

HIGH PERFORMANCE LIQUID CHROMATOGRAPHY (HPLC)
- HPLC Technology

ELECTROPHORESIS
- Hemoglobin Electrophoresis
- Gel Electrophoresis

FROZEN SECTION TECHNIQUE

Frozen section is used for rapid diagnosis of malignancy. It determines the presence or absence of cancer at the resected margins during surgery. It is used to demonstrate fat, enzymes and also IgG, IgM, IgA and complement in kidney biopsies in various types of glomerulonephritis by immunofluorescence microscopy. The piece(s) of tissue to be studied are snap frozen in a cold liquid or cold environment ($-20°$ to $-70°C$). Freezing makes the tissue solid enough to section with a microtome.

CRYOSTAT

Frozen sections are performed with an instrument called a *cryostat*. The cryostat is just a refrigerated box containing a microtome. The temperature inside the cryostat is about −20° to −50°C. The freezed tissue sections are cut and picked up on a glass slide. The sections are then ready for staining. This technique is much faster than traditional histology technique. Cryosections can also be used in immunohistochemistry as freezing tissue does not alter or mask its chemical composition as much as preserving it with a fixative.

STAINING

Frozen sections are stained normally, because this is faster for one or a few individual sections. The toludine blue stain generally used is a *progressive* stain in which the section is left in contact with the stain until the desired tint is achieved. The oil red O (ORO) stain can identify neutral lipids and fatty acids in smears and tissues.

Fresh smears or cryostat sections of tissue are necessary because fixatives containing alcohols, or routine tissue processing with clearing, will remove lipids. The oil red O stain is a rapid and simple stain. It can be useful in identifying fat emboli in lung tissue or clot sections of peripheral blood. Other fat stains are Sudan black, Sudan III and Sudan IV. Examples of fresh frozen section evaluation are shown in Table 14.1.

Table 14.1: Examples of fresh frozen section evaluation

Anatomic sites	Indication	Comments
Skin	Squamous cell carcinoma (eyelid, nose or ear) Basal cell carcinoma (eyelid, nose or ear) for evaluation of margins	Not indicated for melanoma skin
Breast	Breast carcinoma	Evaluation of margins is sometimes required
Lymph nodes	Metastases of breast carcinoma in lymph nodes (sentinel node)	Sensitivity (60%)
Thyroid	Papillary carcinoma of thyroid (imprint smear cytology for nuclear groove)	Not suitable for follicular neoplasms
Female genital system	Intraoperative ovarian neoplasm (most important)	Not suitable for cervical carcinoma
Pancreas	Intraoperative pancreatic carcinoma to look for margins	Accuracy 98%

ELECTRON MICROSCOPY AND POLARIZING LIGHT MICROSCOPY

ELECTRON MICROSCOPY

Electron microscope (EM) was invented by Ernst Ruska in 1933, for which he was awarded the Nobel Prize in Physics in 1986. Electron microscopes are scientific instruments that use a beam of energetic electrons to examine objects on a very fine scale. It was developed due to the limitations of resolution power of light microscope that is limited by physics of light.

Electron microscopes are basically of two types: transmission electron microscopy (TEM) and scanning electron microscopy (SEM). Principle of light microscopy, transmission electron microscopy and scanning electron microscopy is shown in Fig. 14.1.

TRANSMISSION ELECTRON MICROSCOPY (TEM)

Source is a beam of high velocity electrons accelerated under vacuum, focused by condenser lens (electromagnetic bending of electron beam) onto specimen. This causes loss and scattering of electrons by individual parts of specimen. Emergent electron beam is focused by objective lens. Final image is formed on a fluorescent screen for viewing. Standard transmission electron microscopes have a resolving power to about 15 to 30 angstroms. Magnified images are typically from 1000X to 50,000X. By using fine grain photographic film, it is possible for further enlargements from 150,000X to 1,000,000X.

SCANNING ELECTRON MICROSCOPY

Scanning electron microscopy (SEM) differs from standard transmission electron microscopy in that the electrons are bounced off the surface of an object with SEM, not passed through it. The major advantages of SEM are the great depth of field (more of the specimen can be in focus at once) and simple specimen preparation.

Principle: The basic principle is that a beam of electrons is generated by a suitable source, typically a tungsten filament or a field emission gun. The electron beam is accelerated through a high voltage and pass through a system of apertures and electromagnetic lenses to produce a thin beam of electrons. Then the beam scans

Advanced Diagnostic Techniques

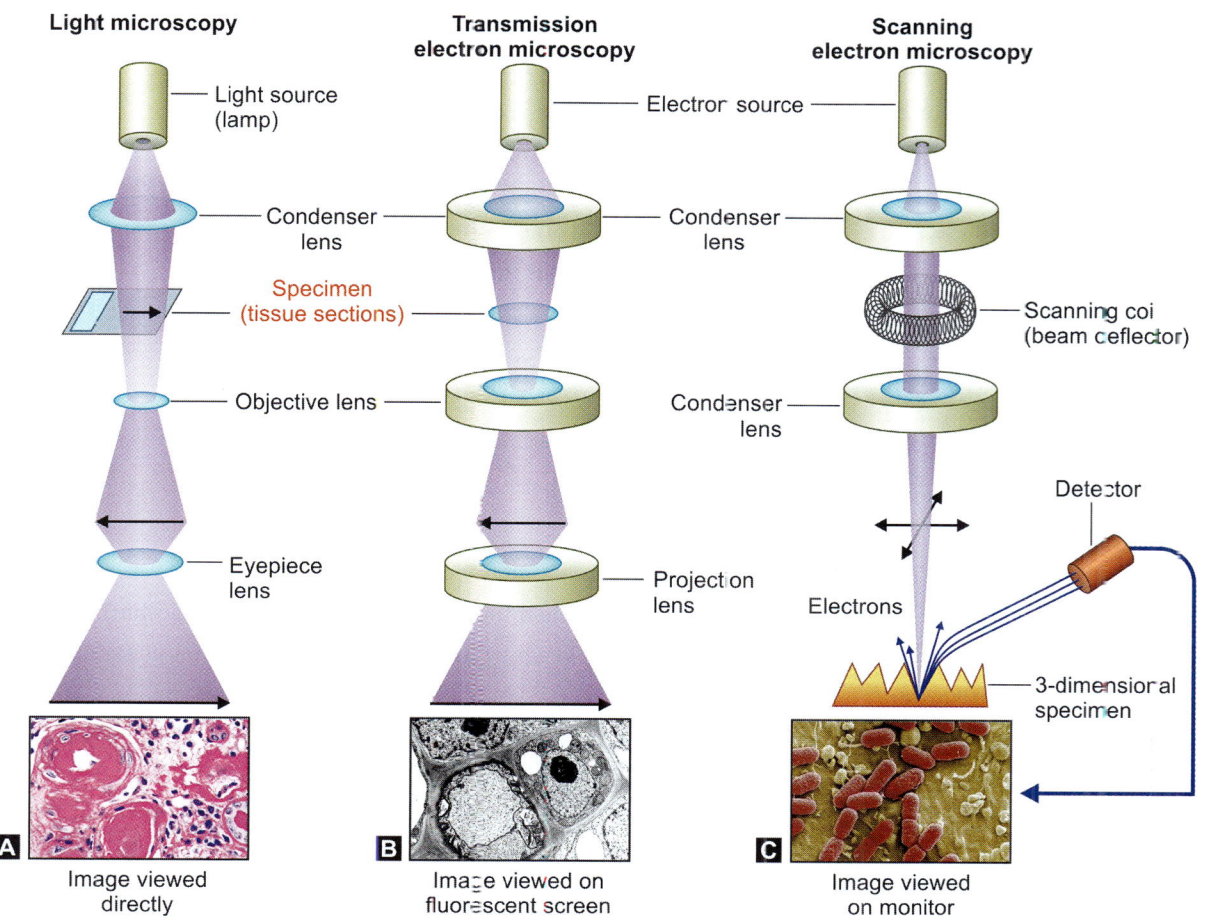

Fig. 14.1: Principle of light microscopy, transmission electron microscopy and scanning electron microscopy.

the surface of the specimen. Electrons are emitted from the specimen by the action of the scanning beam and collected by a suitably positioned detector.

Comparison between light microscope and electron microscope is shown in Table 14.2. Comparison between transmission and scanning electron microscopy is shown in Table 14.3.

Applications in surgical pathology: Electron microscopy is a useful diagnostic technique to supplement morphologic, immunohistochemical, cytogenetic and molecular analysis of tissues, although immunoperoxidase techniques have largely replaced EM for tumor diagnosis in surgical pathology. Electron microscopy is used to diagnose alcoholic liver disease, genetic disorders, neoplasms, glomerulonephritis and identification of microorganisms.

Diagnostic utility of electron microscopy in various disorders is shown in Table 14.4.

Table 14.2: Comparison between light microscope and electron microscope

Light microscope	Electron microscope
Small and portable	Very large and operated in a special room
Resolution is 200 nm	Resolution is 0.4 nm (in SEM) or 0.5 Å (in TEM)
Magnification is 1000X	Magnification is 2 million (in SEM) or 50 million (in TEM)
It is unaffected by magnetic fields	It is affected by magnetic fields
Preparation of material is quick and simple	Preparation of material is lengthy and requires expertise
Preparation rarely distorts the material	Preparation may distort the material
Cheap to purchase and operate	Expensive to purchase and operate
Natural color of object is observed	Images are in black and white

Table 14.3: Comparison between transmission electron microscopy and scanning electron microscopy

Transmission electron microscopy	Scanning electron microscopy
TEM is based on transmitted electrons	SEM is based on scattered electrons
Electrons are directly pointed towards the sample in TEM	The scattered electrons in SEM produce the image of sample after the microscope collects and counts the scattered electrons
It shows the sample as a whole	It shows the sample bit by bit
It has up to 50 million magnification	It has up to 2 million magnification
It provides a 2-dimensional image	It provides a 3-dimensional image
The resolution in TEM is 0.5Å (1 Å = 10^{-10} m)	The resolution in SEM is 0.4 nm (1 nm = 10^{-9} m)

Table 14.4: Diagnostic utility of electron microscopy in various disorders

Subcellular features in cell or tissue	Diagnostic setting
Genetic disorders	
Cilia in epithelial cells	Primary ciliary dyskinesis
Lysosomes in neurons	Demonstration of lipids and mucopolysaccharides
Absence of peroxisomes in liver and kidneys	Zellweger syndrome and neonatal adrenoleukodystrophy
Acquired non-neoplastic disorder	
Increased number of peroxisomes in hepatocytes	Alcoholic liver disease, chronic venous congestion, oral contraceptives
Siderosomes in mitochondria	Sideroblastic anemia
Neoplasms	
Intercellular junctions in epithelial and lymphoma	Distinction between carcinoma and lymphomas (intercellular junctions present in carcinomas and absent in lymphomas)
Intracellular or intercellular in glandular epithelium	Diagnosis of adenocarcinoma
Microvillous core rootlets in glandular epithelium of intestines	Diagnosis of metastatic gastrointestinal origin carcinoma
Cytoplasmic tonofibrils in squamous epithelium	Diagnosis of squamous differentiation of epithelial neoplasms
Premelanosomes and melanosomes in melanotic cells	Diagnosis of melanoma
Neurosecretory granules in neuroendocrine and neuroectodermal cells	Diagnosis of neuroendocrine and neuroectodermal neoplasms
Birbeck granules in Langerhans' cells	Diagnosis of Langerhans' cell histiocytosis
Miscellaneous	
Viruses and parasites in solid tissues, fecal specimens and body fluids	Identification of infectious agents
Electron dense deposits in glomeruli	Identification and classification of glomerulonephritis
Electron dense deposits present adjacent to vascular smooth muscle	Cerebral autosomal-dominant arteriopathy with subcortical infarcts and leukoencephalopathy (CADASIL) syndrome

POLARIZING LIGHT MICROSCOPY

Some materials such as crystals or fibers have the property of *birefringence* which is the ability to pass light in a particular plane. Such materials are called *anisotropic* because of this property.

Normally, most materials are *isotropic* because any light that passes through them will be scattered in all directions.

When viewed under polarized light, however, anisotropic materials will be brightly visible in one plane (*birefringent*), but will be dark in a plane turned 90°. Principle of polarizing microscope is shown in Fig. 14.2.

CATEGORIES OF BIREFRINGENCE

The birefringence is categorized into positive or negative based on the property of birefringence in which rays

Advanced Diagnostic Techniques

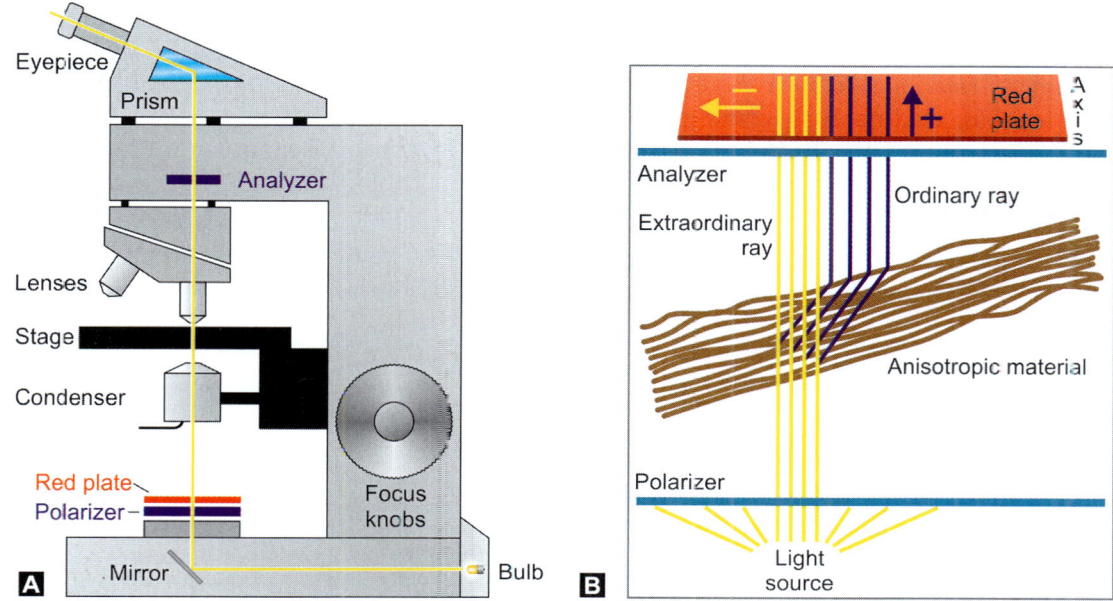

Fig. 14.2: Principle of polarizing microscope.

of light travelling through the anisotropic material in perpendicular planes (at right angles) will travel at different velocities through the material.

REFRACTIVE INDEX

Birefringent material has two refractive indices: High for fast rays and small for slow rays. Fast rays travel in parallel with the crystalline structure of the birefringent material than the *extraordinary's low rays* traverses the material. Negative birefringence occurs when the *ordinary* ray becomes the *slow* ray when it is reflected and travels across the crystalline structures.

POLARIZER AND ANALYZER

There are two polarizing filters made of glass or plastic material in polarizing microscope: polarizer and analyzer. These filters pass light in only one plane.

APPLICATIONS

Exogenous crystalline material (most common example is talc crystals found in subcutaneous injection site, in lungs, and in organs of the mononuclear phagocyte system of persons engaging in injection drug use). Applications of polarizing microscopy are shown in Table 14.5.

Table 14.5: Applications of polarizing microscopy

Disorders	Characteristics
Sodium urate crystals gout	Negative birefringence
Calcium pyrophosphate crystals	Positive birefringence
Amyloid deposits in various organs	Apple green birefringence
Silicosis in organs	Insignificant finding in lungs and lymph nodes
Formalin-heme pigment (artefact of poor fixation)	Bright white birefringence
Collagen: Collagen fibrils	Dull yellow-white

HISTOLOGY AND HISTOCHEMICAL STAINS

FIXATIVES

Fixatives preserve tissues in their natural state and fixes all components by denaturing or precipitating proteins. The ideal fixative would prevent autolysis and bacterial decomposition.

Microorganisms are also fixed and killed during fixation. Most fixatives act by denaturing or precipitating proteins which then form a sponge or meshwork tending to hold the other cell constituents. Formaldehyde is fixative of choice.

Classification: Fixatives are classified according to mechanism of action: *aldehydes (formaldehyde and glutaraldehyde), mercurials, alcohols, oxidizing agents and picrates* (Table 14.6), routine 10% formalin saline fixative (Table 14.7), routine 10% buffered formalin fixative (Table 14.8), composition of Zenker's fixative (mercurial fixative) (Table 14.9), Schaudinn's *sublimated alcohol* fixative (mercurial fixative) (Table 14.10), composition of Carnoy's fluid (alcohol fixative) (Table 14.11), Orth's fluid fixative (chromate fixative) (Table 14.12) and Regaud's (Moller's) fluid (chromate fixative) (Table 14.13).

Table 14.6: Fixatives used in histopathology

Categories of fixatives	Examples	Advantages	Disadvantages
Aldehyde fixatives	Neutral formalin (10%)	Immunoperoxidase techniques	Formol-heme pigment
	Buffered formalin (10%)	Immunoperoxidase techniques. Prevents formol-heme pigment	Nil
	Buffered glutaraldehyde (%)	Electron microscopy	Not good for immunoperoxidase techniques
Mercurial fixatives	Zenker's fixative	Hematopoietic and reticulo-endothelial tissues, i.e. lymph nodes, spleen, thymus, and bone marrow	Marked shrinkage and hardness of tissues. It reduce the amount of demonstrable glycogen
Alcohol fixatives	Carnoy's fluid	Suitable for small biopsies giving nuclear details. Preserves glycogen	Causes lysis of RBCs, dissolution of lipid and myelin; and shrinkage of tissue
Chromate fixatives	Helly's fluid	Used to demonstrate chromaffin tissue (adrenal medulla), mitochondria and preservation of phospholipids	Glycogen preservation poor
Picrate fixatives	Bouin's fluid fixative (40% formalin, picric acid and glacial acid)	Testicular, gastrointestinal tract, and endocrine tissue biopsies	Makes tissue hard and brittle
		Gives yellow color to the tissue and gives good nuclear details	Lysis red cells, reduce amount of demonstrable ferric iron

Table 14.7: Routine 10% formalin saline fixative

Constituents	Composition
Formalin	100 ml
Water	900 ml
Sodium chloride	8.5 gm

Disadvantage: Routine 10% formalin saline fixative forms formol-heme pigment giving black discoloration to tissues.

Table 14.8: Routine 10% buffered formalin fixative

Constituents	Composition
Formalin	100 ml
Water	900 ml
NaH_2PO_4	3.5 gm
Na_2HPO_4	6.5 gm

Advantage: 10% buffered formalin prevents formation of formol-heme pigment.

Table 14.9: Composition of Zenker's fixative (mercurial fixative)

Constituents	Composition
$HgCl_2$	50 gm
Potassium dichromate	25 gm
Sodium sulfate	10 gm
Distilled water	1000 ml

Mercurial fixatives are used to fix lymph nodes, spleen, thymus, and bone marrow.

Table 14.10: Schaudinns *sublimated alcohol* fixative (mercurial fixative)

Constituents	Quantity
$HgCl_2$	3 gm
Distilled water	50 ml

Schaudinn's *sublimated alcohol* fixative is most useful fixative for making smears of loose cells on a slide.

Table 14.11: Composition of Carnoy's fluid (alcohol fixative)

Constituents	Quantity
Absolute ethyl alcohol	60 ml
Chloroform	30 ml
Glacial acetic acid	10 ml

Table 14.12: Orth's fluid fixative (chromate fixative)

Constituents	Composition
Potassium dichromate (2.5%)	100 ml
Formalin solution	10 ml

Formalin solution is added just before using as fixative. Chromate fixatives are used to demonstrate chromaffin tissue (adrenal medulla), mitochondria, Golgi apparatus and mitotic figures.

Table 14.13: Regauds (Moller's) fluid (chromate fixative)

Constituents	Composition
Potassium dichromate (3%)	80 ml
Formalin	20 ml

Formalin solution is added just before using as fixative. Chromate fixatives are used to demonstrate chromaffin tissue (adrenal medulla), mitochondria, Golgi apparatus and mitotic figures.

Factors affecting fixation: There are a number of factors that will affect the fixation process: *volume, buffering, penetration, temperature, concentration and time interval.* Fixation is best carried out close to neutral pH, in the range of 6–8. Commercial formalin is buffered with phosphate at a pH of 7. Factors affecting fixation of tissue are shown in Table 14.14.

DECALCIFICATION

Bone and other tissues containing calcified areas and calcium deposits which are extremely firm and which will not section properly with paraffin embedding owing to the difference in densities between calcium and paraffin. This calcium must be removed prior to embedding to allow sectioning. Mineral acids (nitric acid and hydrochloric acid), organic acids (acetic acid and formic acid), EDTA, and electrolysis are used to decalcify such tissues.

STRONG ACIDS

Strong acids, i.e. nitric acid and hydrochloric acid are used to decalcify dense cortical tissue at a rapid rate; but also damage cellular details. These are not recommended for delicate tissues such as bone marrow.

ORGANIC ACIDS

On the other hand, organic acids such as acetic acid and 10% formic acid are better suited to bone marrow, because they act more slowly on dense cortical bone. Formic acid in a 10% concentration is the best all-around decalcifier.

EDTA

EDTA can remove calcium slowly but is expensive in large amounts. Electrolysis removes calcium slowly, hence not suited for routine purpose.

COMMERCIAL DECALCIFYING SOLUTIONS

Commercial solutions comprising formic acid with formalin is available to decalcify tissues

Table 14.14: Factors affecting fixation of tissue

Parameters	Characteristics
Volume	10–20 times of tissue sample
Agitation of specimen	Enhances fixation
Buffers	Neutral buffered formalin prevents excessive acidity and formation of formalin-heme pigment Common buffers (phosphate, bicarbonate, cacodylate and veronal)
Penetration	Formalin and alcohol fixatives best Glutaraldehyde (worst penetration) Mercurial fixatives somewhat in between Sectioning of specimen 2–3 mm enhances fixation
Temperature	Increasing temperature of formalin increases the speed of fixation
Concentration of fixative	Formalin 10% used for fixation Glutaraldehyde 0.25 to 4% used for electron microscopy
Time interval between fixation and removal of tissue	Tissue should be fixed faster and removed within 6–8 hours. Longer fixation leads to nuclear shrinkage and loss of organelles

SURGICAL SPECIMENS

Under normal circumstances, the specimens are received in 10% neutral buffered formalin. Fixation process prevents autolysis and decomposition of specimen. Gross processing comprise description of size, shape, color and overall appearance. The tissues placed in cassettes are designated number. When a malignancy is suspected, then the specimen is often covered with ink in order to mark the margins of the specimen.

TISSUE PROCESSOR

This multistep process is done by an automatic machine which has multiple jars containing different chemicals, i.e. formalin, ascending series of alcohols, xylene and paraffin through which tissue is passed on a preset time scale. Tissue processor with digitally programmed schedule is shown in Table 14.15.

PARAFFIN EMBEDDING

Properly fixed and processed tissue in the tissue processor are embedded in the molds containing paraffin with melting point 54–62°C to prepare them for cutting in microtome. During embedding, the tissue is oriented with the surface placed down in the mold becoming the face of tissue block.

MICROTOMY

Tissue embedded in paraffin can be sectioned at 4 to 8 microns with a microtome having thick metallic knife. Tissue ribbon is then floated on warm water bath at a temperature 6 to 8°C below the melting point of paraffin. This aids in mounting sections on a glass slide properly labelled for light microscopy.

Thin sections for electron microscopy are best done with a diamond knife which is very expensive. After embedding tissues in epoxy resin, a microtome equipped with a glass or diamond knife is used to cut very thin sections (typically 60 to 100 nm). Sections are stained and examined with a transmission electron microscope.

HEMATOXYLIN AND EOSIN STAINING

The staining process makes use of a variety of dyes that have been chosen for their ability to stain various cellular components of tissue. Hematoxylin and eosin (H&E) stain is routinely done. Hematoxylin is derived from the log of wood tree in the past. Eosin at pH 4.6 to 5.0 has high affinity for positively charged tissue protein group. However, *special stains* are employed in specific situations according to the diagnostic need.

Commercially ripened synthetic hematoxylin is commonly used due to less availability of logwood tree. Hematoxylin is the oxidized/ripened product of the logwood tree known as *hematein*. Hematoxylin, a basic dye has an affinity for the nucleic acids of the cell nucleus. Eosin, an acidic dye has affinity for cytoplasmic components of the cell. Problem with eosin may occur due to overstaining of decalcified tissues. Routine of hematoxylin and eosin staining technique is shown in Table 14.16.

Table 14.15: Tissue processor (histokinette) with digitally programmed schedule

Jar No.	Chemical used	Time variable depending on convenience and fixation of tissues	Step
1.	70% alcohol	½ hour	
2.	95% alcohol	½ hour	
3.	100% alcohol	1 hour	
4.	100% alcohol	1 hour	Dehydration of tissue is done to replace fixative and water by a dehydrating fluid
5.	100% alcohol	1 hour	
6.	100% alcohol	1 hour	
7.	100% alcohol	1 hour	
8.	100% alcohol + xylene	1 hour	Clearing is performed to replace dehydrating fluid with a medium totally miscible with embedding medium (molten paraffin wax)
9.	Xylene	1 hour	
10.	Xylene	2 hour	
11.	Molten paraffin wax	2 hour	A vacuum can be applied inside the tissue processor to assist penetration of the embedding paraffin agent. This process replaces water content of tissue and clearing agent by paraffin wax used in molten state
12.	Molten paraffin wax	2 hour	

Advanced Diagnostic Techniques

Table 14.16: Routine of hematoxylin and eosin staining technique

Sequences	Chemical used	Time	Steps
Deparaffinization and hydration	Xylene	2–3 minutes	Deparaffinize the section with xylene, followed by two changes of absolute alcohol to remove xylene and hydration through graded alcohol to water
Staining	Hematoxylin	10–20 minutes ≤5 minutes	Staining with hematoxylin Wash well in running tap water until section becomes 'blue'
Differentiation	1% acid alcohol	5–10 seconds 10–15 minutes	Differentiate in 1% acid alcohol Wash well in tap water until section again becomes 'blue'
Blueing	Alkaline solution (ammonia water)	5 minutes	Blue by dipping in alkaline solution Tap water wash
Counter stain	1% eosin Y	10 minutes 1–5 minutes	Stain in 1% eosin Y Wash in running tap water
Dehydration	95% alcohol	2 minutes	Dehydrate in 95% and absolute alcohol, two changes of 2 minutes each or until excess eosin is removed
	100% alcohol	2 minutes	
Clearing	Xylene	2 minutes	Clear in xylene, two changes of 2 minutes each
Mounting	DPX		Mount in DPX

Mordant: Hematoxylin will not directly stain tissues, but needs a *mordant* or link to the tissues, i.e. metal cation iron, aluminum, or tungsten. Depending on the mordant used, there is variety of hematoxylins, which vary in intensity.

Progressive staining: Hematoxylin stains are either *progressive* or *regressive*. With a progressive stain the slide is dipped in the hematoxylin until the desired intensity of staining is achieved such as with a frozen section. This is simple for a single slide, but lends itself poorly to batch processing.

Regressive stain: With a regressive stain, the slides are left in the solution for a set period of time and then taken back through a solution such as acid alcohol that removes part of the stain. This method works best for large batches of slides to be stained and is more predictable on a day-to-day basis.

SPECIAL STAINS

Commonly used stains in histopathology are shown in Table 14.17. Carbohydrate classification is shown in Table 14.18. Mucin types and their origin are shown in Table 14.19.

Table 14.17: Commonly used stains in histopathology

Stain	Use	Result
Hematoxylin and eosin stain	Routine stain	Nucleus blue, cytoplasm pink, bone blue, mucoid and cartilaginous area pale blue, RBC and eosinophil granules orange red
Stains for carbohydrates		
Periodic acid–Schiff's stain	Glycogen	Red
	Fungi	Red
	Neutral mucin	Red
	Amyloidosis	Red
	Basement membrane	Red
	Glycoproteins	Red
	Glycolipids	Red

Contd...

Table 14.17: Commonly used stains in histopathology (*Contd...*)

Stain	Use	Result
Periodic acid–Schiff's with diastase stain	Neutral mucin	
Alcian blue stain at pH 2.5	All acidic mucopolysaccharides Sulphated mucin	Blue Blue
Mucicarmine stain	Acidic epithelial mucin Cryptococcus capsule	Blue Blue
Colloidal iron stain pH 1	Prussian blue reaction (Perl's reaction) to demonstrate hemosiderin	Blue
Congo red	Amyloid	Pink under light microscope Green birefringence for under polarizing microscope
Methyl violet (metachromatic stain)	Amyloid	Rose pink
von Gieson stain	Amyloid	Khaki color
Crystal violet (metachromatic stain)	Amyloid	Pink
Thioflavin T and thioflavin S	Amyloid	Yellow to yellow green under immunofluorescent microscopy
Stains for microorganisms		
Gram stain after use of crystal violet	Gram-positive bacteria	Blue
Gram stain after use of basic fuschin	Gram-negative bacteria	Red
Ziehl-Neelsen stain (decolorized with 1% acid aloocohol, 20% H_2SO_4)	Mycobacterium tubercle bacilli	Red
Fite's stain (decolorized with 5% H_2SO_4)	*Mycobacterium leprae* bacilli	Red
Modified Giemsa stain	*Helicobacter pylori*	Blue
Steiner's stain	*Helicobacter pylori*	Black
Gomori's methenamine silver stain	Fungi	Black in light green background
PAS stain (most useful when counterstain of light green used)	Fungi in tissue	Magenta pink
Warthin-Starry stain	Spirochetes	Black color against yellow to pale brown background
Stains for connective tissue		
Reticulin stain (used to highlight outlines of parenchyma of organs and highlighting growth pattern of neoplasia)	Reticulin fibers	Black against clear background
Jones methenamine silver stain	Similar to reticulin stain	
Masson's trichrome stain (used in chronic active hepatitis with hepatocytes collapse, cerebral abscess and scleroderma with fibrosis of gastric submucosa)	Elastic fibers Collagen fibers Background	Black Red Yellow
VVG (used to outline arteries)	Elastic fibers	Black
PTAH (Zenker's fixative)	Fibrin Cross striations in muscle fibers	Deep purple Deep purple

Contd...

Table 14.17: Commonly used stains in histopathology (Contd...)

Stain	Use	Result
Pentachrome stain	Elastic fibers	Black
	Collagen fibers	Red
	Fibrin	Red
	Muscle	Red
	Mucin	Red
Oil red O	Fat stain	Red
Stains for nervous system		
Bielschowsky's stain	Nerve endings, neuron fibrils, tangles and plaques	Black
Luxol fast blue	Myelin	Blue
Pigments and minerals		
Prussian blue reaction (used in hemochromatosis)	Iron	Blue
Hall's bile	Bile pigments	Emerald green
von Kossa stain	Calcium	Black
Alzarin red S (pH 4.8)	Calcium	Red
Rhodamine stain	Copper	Red to orange
Gomori's stain	Urate crystals	Black
Masson-Fontana stain (used in melanoma)	Melanin	Black
Churukian-Scherik stain	Argyrophil granules	Black

PAS reactive tissue components are glycogen, starch, mucin, α_1-antitrypsin, fungal capsule, pancreatic zymogen granules, thyroid, colloid, corpora amylacea and plasma cell of Russel bodies.

Table 14.18: Carbohydrate classification

Parameters	Simple carbohydrates	Glycoconjugates
Composition	Composed of pure carbohydrate	Composed of carbohydrates and other molecules such as protein and lipid
Examples	Monosaccharides (glucose, mannose, galactose) Oligosaccharides (sucrose, maltose) Polysaccharides (glycogen, starch)	Proteoglycans Mucins Other glycoproteins

Table 14.19: Mucin types and their origin

Parameters	Neutral mucins	Acidic simple non-sulfated epithelial mucins (sialomucins)	Acidic complex or sulfated epithelial mucins (sulfomucins)	Acidic simple mesenchymal mucins contain hyaluronic acid	Acidic complex, connective tissue mucins
Location of mucin	Surface epithelia of gastric mucosa, Brunner's glands and prostatic epithelia	Bronchial submucous glands Salivary glands Goblet cells	Bronchial mucous glands	Sarcomas	Tissue stroma, cartilage, and bone (chondroitin sulfate or keratan sulfate)
PAS stain	Positive	Positive	Positive	Positive	Negative
Alcian blue at pH	Negative	Positive (pH 2.5)	Positive (pH 1)	Negative	Selectively positive at pH 0.5
Colloidal iron	Negative	Positive	Positive	Negative	Negative
Mucicarmine	Negative	Positive	Positive	Negative	Negative
Metachromatic stain	Negative	Positive	Positive	Negative	Negative

PAS stain is used to demonstrate mucin and glycogen. Mucicarmine stain is specific for epithelial mucins. Acidic sulfomucins resist hyaluronidase digestion.

IMMUNOHISTOCHEMISTRY

OVERVIEW

Immunohistochemistry (IHC) is the most powerful and widely used ancillary methods in surgical pathology to detect antigens in tissue sections by use of labeled antibody through antigen–antibody reactions. These are visualized by using fluorescent dye, enzyme, radioactive element or colloidal gold.

Immunofluorescence is still used in the evaluation of medical renal biopsies. Currently, antigens are detected in formalin fixed paraffin embedded tissue sections by immunoperoxidase technique.

INDICATIONS

Common indications for immunohistochemistry are characterization of neoplasms, detection of infectious organisms and evaluation of prognostic or predictive factors.

FIXATION OF TISSUE

Tissue should be fixed in neutral pH formalin for 12 to 48 hours at room temperature. It is worth mentioning that formalin induces crosslinks that may mask some epitopes resulting in loss of immunoreactivity. Decalcification of bone samples also reduces immunoreactivity.

TISSUE SECTION USED

Unstained tissue sections are cut from paraffin block. These are placed on charged slides coated with poly-L-lysine or gelatin or albumin. Immunostaining should be performed immediately because unstained sections exposed to air for prolonged time may lose antigen immunoreactivity.

FROZEN SECTION

If the unfixed tissue is frozen, the sections obtained may need to be used for immunoassays.

- *Advantage:* Tissue antigens in these sections are not altered.
- *Disadvantage:* Tissue sections may fall off the slides.

PARAFFIN EMBEDDED SECTION

If the tissue is paraffin embedded, deparaffinize first (it removes the infiltrated paraffin wax by using organic solvents). The section then needs to be rehydrated by sequential immersion in graded alcohols (100%, 70%, 50% and then PBS, i.e. phosphate buffered saline). The deparaffinized section may need to be treated to expose buried antigenic epitopes with either proteases or by heating in low pH citrate buffer or high pH EDTA buffer (*antigen retrieval*).

CLASSIFICATION OF ANTIBODIES

Antibodies can also be classified as primary or secondary.

PRIMARY ANTIBODY

Primary antibody is an immunoglobulin molecule that binds to the target antigen in the tissue sections. Antibodies used for specific detection can be monoclonal derived via the hybridoma technique or polyclonal obtained from an antiserum (Table 14.20). Primary antibodies are unconjugated antibodies. In general, monoclonal antibodies are considered to exhibit greater specificity than polyclonal antibodies.

SECONDARY ANTIBODY

Secondary antibodies are raised against primary antibodies. These secondary antibodies recognize immunoglobulin of a particular species. These are not visible with standard microscopy, hence labeled with fluorochrome (fluorescein, rhodamine), enzymes (horseradish peroxidase, alkaline phosphatase). Labeling is done in such a manner that it does not interfere with their binding specificity. For electron microscopy study, scattering compounds such as ferritin and colloidal gold are used.

BACKGROUND STAINING

Background staining occurs due to binding of non-specific antibody or endogenous enzymes to the chromogenic substrate. Therefore, working dilution of primary antibody must be performed, that yields

Table 14.20: Comparison between polyclonal antibody and monoclonal antibody

Parameters	Polyclonal antibody	Monoclonal antibody
Synthesis	Mixture of synthesis of different antibodies to a single antigen	Synthesis by single clone commonly raised in mice
Specificity	Multiple epitopes	Single epitope

greatest contrast between specific staining and background staining. Endogenous enzymes present in normal cells such as *red blood cells, neutrophils, eosinophils, monocytes/macrophages and neoplastic cells* yield background staining. Endogenous peroxidase activity can be blocked by incubation with hydrogen peroxide.

DETECTION SYSTEMS

The principle of immunohistochemistry is to localize antigens in tissue sections by the use of labeled antibodies as specific reagents through antigen–antibody interactions that are visualized by a marker such as fluorescent dye, enzyme, radioactive element or colloidal gold.

DIRECT CONJUGATE-LABELED ANTIBODY METHOD

Direct method is one step staining method. In this method, the label such as peroxidase or fluorescein is linked to primary antibody. The labeled antibody reacts directly with the antigen in the tissue sections. This technique utilizes only one antibody. This procedure is short and quick. Disadvantages of this technique include requirement of large amount of antibody for labeling and lack of signal amplification. It gives quick results, however, labeling intensity is low. It is used for kidney or *skin biopsies* (Fig. 14.3).

INDIRECT OR SANDWICH METHOD

In indirect or sandwich method, the primary antibody is unlabeled (first layer). Secondary antibody carrying a label such as fluorescent dye or peroxidase enzyme (second layer) reacts against primary unlabeled antibody. This method is more sensitive due to signal amplification through several secondary reactions with different antigens. In addition, it is also economical since one labeled second layer antibody can be used with many first layer antibodies to different antigens (Fig. 14.4).

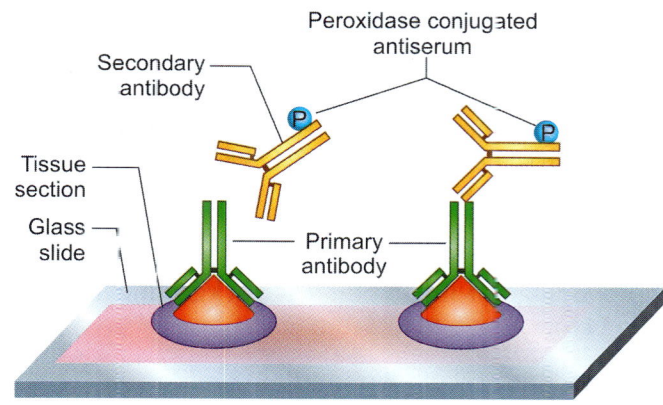

Fig. 14.4: Two-step indirect method. Enzyme labeled secondary antibody reacts with primary antibody bound to tissue antigen, if the primary antibody is prepared in rabbit or mouse, the secondary antibody must be directed against rabbit or mouse immunoglobulins, respectively.

Peroxidase-Antiperoxidase (PAP) Method

Unlabeled antibody technique is also known as *peroxidase-antiperoxidase* (PAP) method. This method uses an unlabeled primary antibody, an unlabeled bridge antibody and an antiperoxidase antibody and peroxidase molecule. Unlabeled bridge antibody directed against both primary antibody and the antiperoxidase antibody links the primary antibody to tissue antigen via signal generated by peroxidase.

The sensitivity is about 100 to 1000 times higher since peroxidase molecule is not chemically conjugated with anti-IgG. Though peroxidase molecule is immunologically bound, yet it does not lose its enzymatic activity. It also permits much higher dilution of primary antibody resulting in elimination of many unwanted antibodies and reducing nonspecific background staining (Fig. 14.5).

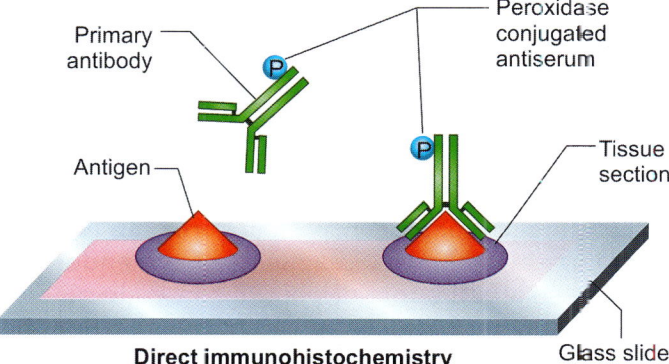

Fig. 14.3: Direct method. Enzyme-labeled primary antibody reacts with tissue antigen.

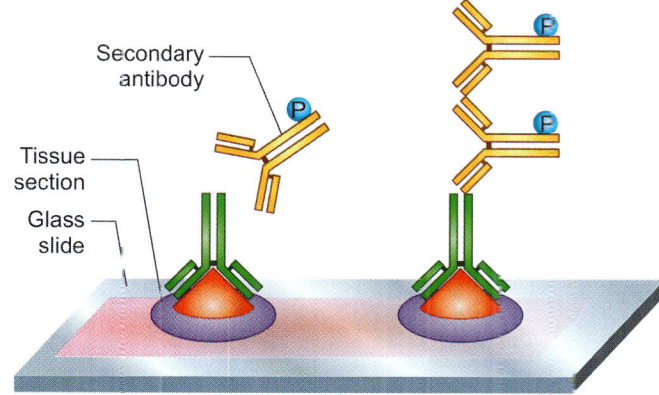

Fig. 14.5: Peroxidase-antiperoxidase (PAP) method. In this three-step indirect method, enzyme labeled tertiary antibody reacts with enzyme-labeled secondary antibody. Three-step indirect method provides a simple way to further increase the staining intensities compared to the two previous techniques.

Avidin-Biotin Complex (ABC) Method

A biotinylated secondary antibody is used to recognize primary antibody. Avidin complexed with biotinylated peroxidase is then bound to secondary antibody. The peroxidase is then developed by DAB or other substrate to produce different calorimetric end products. This reaction delivers several peroxidase molecules to the primary antibody sites and boosts its sensitivity. Disadvantage of this method is background staining (Fig. 14.6).

Labeled Streptavidin-Biotin (LSAB) Method

Streptavidin derived from Streptococcus avidin is recent substitute of avidin. A biotinylated secondary antibody is used to recognize primary antibody. Streptavid incomplexed with biotinylated peroxidase is then bound to secondary antibody. This technique is similar to standard avidin-biotin complex method. This reaction delivers several peroxidase molecules to the primary antibody sites and boosts its sensitivity. The enzyme is then visualized by application of the substrate chromogen solutions to produce different calorimetric end products. Streptavidin-Biotin method has decreased background staining (Fig. 14.7).

Alkaline Phosphatase and Antiphosphatase Method

Enzyme alkaline phosphatase and anti-alkaline phosphatase instead of peroxidase is widely used nowadays. It gives most sensitive results and can be applied on paraffin, cryostat sections or on smears (Fig. 14.8).

IMMUNOHISTOCHEMISTRY PROTOCOL

In order to visualize enzyme-substrate reactions, various chromogens which get converted into visible colored end-products, are used. Commonly used chromogens are diaminobenzidine (DAB), 3-amino-

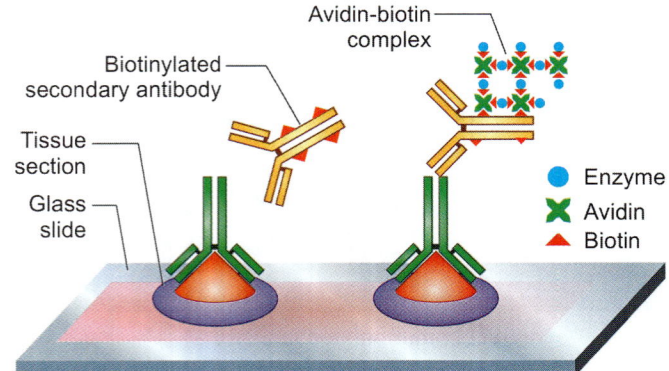

Fig. 14.6: Indirect ABC immunohistochemistry method: In the ABC technology, the avidin or streptavidin-biotin enzyme complex reacts with the biotinylated secondary antibody.

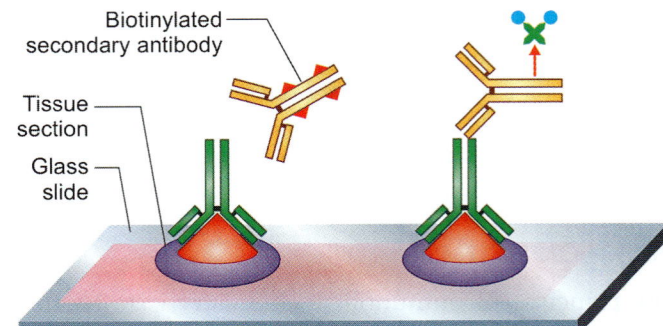

Fig. 14.7: Indirect LAB or LSAB immunohistochemistry method: labeled streptavidin-biotin (LSAB) method. Labeled streptavidin reacts with biotinylated secondary antibody.

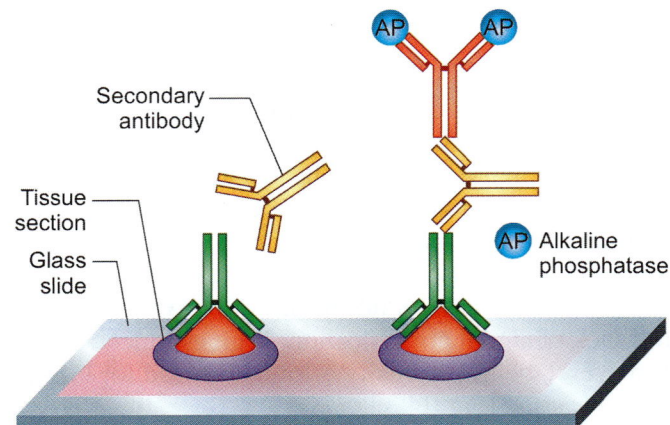

Fig. 14.8: Indirect APAAP immunohistochemistry method: alkaline phosphatase and antiphosphatase method.

9-ethylcarbazole (AEC) and 4-chloro-1-naphthol (CN) producing brown, red and dark blue colors, respectively. Immunohistochemistry protocol is shown in Table 14.21.

CONTROLS

Positive control is to test for a protocol or procedure used. It will be ideal to use the tissue of known positive as a control. *Negative control* is to test for the specificity of the antibody involved.

APPLICATIONS

Immunohistochemistry is used for detection of intercellular antigens (e.g. immunoglobulins of the kidney, glomerular basement membrane), cell surface antigens, tissue antigen for diagnosing autoimmune diseases, soluble antigens of the cell, protein hormones in histopathological diagnosis, diagnosis of the endocrine tumors, small amounts of peptides in endocrine or neuroendocrine cells, immunodeposits and tumoral markers and tumor typing. Panel of monoclonal antibodies in various malignancies is shown in Table 14.22.

Advanced Diagnostic Techniques

Table 14.21: Immunohistochemistry protocol

Protocol	Steps	Procedure
Tissue preparation	Fixation Sectioning	Immersion or perfusion fixation (neutral formalin, paraformaldehyde and Bouin's solution) Microtome for paraffin blocks; cryostat for frozen tissue and vibratome for fixed hard tissue
Pre-incubation steps	Deparaffinization of tissue section Removing the fixative Neutralization of endogenous peroxidase Blocking Blocking the surface tension	Paraffin is removed from section Washing in buffer solutions (phosphate buffer, tris-HCl buffer, HEPES, i.e. hydroxyethyl piperazine-ethane-sulfonic acid buffer, etc.) Endogenous peroxidase is removed Covering the non-immunological sticky sites on tissues (bovine serum albumin, non-immune normal serum, gelatin, milk) Triton X-100 and NaCl are used
Incubation	Primary antibody Secondary antibody	Used in a solution at different dilutions with the blocking agent. The incubation time changes according to the properties of the antigen or antibody as well as depending on the temperature Must be raised in the species other than the species of which the cells or tissues are taken or the primary antibody is raised. It should specifically recognize the immunoglobulin of the species in which the primary antibody is raised
Labelling	Labeling of antibody	Immunoenzyme, immunofluorescence, immunogold
Microscopical analyses	Microscopic study of tissue section	Slides are examined under microscope

Table 14.22: Panel of monoclonal antibodies in common malignancies

Malignancies	Monoclonal antibodies
Female genital system	
Breast carcinoma	ER, PR, Her2 neu, CK7, GCDFP-15 mammoglobin, Ki-67, p53 (negative prognostic factor), CK5, NY-BR1 (highly specific marker for undifferentiated breast carcinoma) and E-cadherin (negative in lobular carcinoma) *Infiltrating lobular carcinoma:* ER (+), PR (+), Her2 neu (–) and reduced or absent E-cadherin expression *Medullary carcinoma and metaplastic carcinoma:* Triple negative, i.e. ER (–), PR (–) and Her2 neu (–)
Endometrial carcinoma	*Endometrial carcinoma type 1:* ER, PR and PTEN *Endometrial carcinoma type 2:* p53
Ovarian surface neoplasms	*Serous cystadenocarcinoma:* B72.3, CEA, Ber-EP4, PAX8, PLAP *Mucinous cystadenocarcinoma:* CA125, CK7 *Clear cell carcinoma:* CA125, CEA, PAX8, CK7, CAM, EMA, CD15 (Leu-M1), vimentin, BCL-2, p53, ER and PR *Brenner tumor:* Keratin, EMA, CEA
Ovarian germ cell tumors	*Dysgerminoma:* PLAP, CD117, OCT4 *Embryonal carcinoma:* Pankeratin, CD30, OCT3/4, SALL4 *Yolk sac tumor:* AFP, α_1-antitrypsin, pankeratin *Choriocarcinoma:* hCG (most specific), keratin 7, LK26 (a folate-binding protein) *Carcinoid tumor:* NSE, chromogranin, 5-HT
Ovarian granulosa cell tumors	Calretinin (most sensitive than inhibin), inhibin, melan-A (mart-1, clone A103), ER, PR

Contd...

Table 14.22: Panel of monoclonal antibodies in common malignancies (*Contd...*)

Malignancies	Monoclonal antibodies
Respiratory system	
Lung carcinoma	*Squamous cell carcinoma:* p40, cytokeratin, CEA, EMA, p63, cytoplasmic and intranuclear surfactant *Adenocarcinoma:* EMA, CK7, TTF1, napsin, B.72.3, CD15 (Leu-M) *Small cell carcinoma:* NSE, synaptophysin, chromogranin, CD57, NCAM (CD56) and CK *Bronchopulmonary carcinoid tumors:* NSE, synaptophysin, chromogranin, CD57, NCAM (CD56) and CK (CDX2 is negative, but positive in GIT carcinoids)
Malignant mesothelioma	Calretinin, WT1, cytokeratin 5/6
Endocrine system	
Thyroid carcinoma	TTF1, TG, CA125, cell surface glycoprotein *Medullary thyroid carcinoma:* Calcitonin, synaptophysin, chromogranin, CEA
Adrenal tumors	*Adrenocortical carcinoma:* Calretinin, inhibin, melan-A, vimentin *Pheochromocytoma:* Chromogranin, synaptophysin, S-100 and non-specific enolase (NSE)
Salivary glands	
Adenocystic carcinoma	CEA, cytokeratin, S-100, muscle specific protein and Kit-67
Polymorphous low-grade adenocarcinoma	CEA, EMA, cytokeratin, vimentin, S-100, GFAP, galectin 3 and BCL-2
Gastrointestinal tract	
Gastric carcinoma	CK, EMA, CEA
Colorectal carcinoma	CK20, CDX2 (poor prognostic marker), CEA, β-catenin, SAT2, p53, CK7
Gastrointestinal stromal tumors	DOG-1, CD117, PDGFR-α
Gastrointestinal carcinoids	NSE, synaptophysin, chromogranin, CD57, NCAM (CD56), CK, CDX2 and PAX8
Gastric MALT lymphoma	DD20, CD79a, CD21, CD35
Hepatobiliary and pancreas	
Pancreatic carcinoma	Vimentin, α_1-antitrypsin and α_1-antichymotrypsin
Hepatocellular carcinoma	Hep Par-1, α_1-antitrypsin (75%), AFP (60–80%) and CEA (30%)
Hepatoblastoma	AFP, Hep Par-1, hCG, keratin, CEA, glycipan 3, EMA and vimentin
Cholangiocarcinoma	CK7 and CK19
Hematologic and lymph nodes	
NHL B cell	CD10, CD19, CD20
NHL T cell	CD3
Acute lymphoblastic leukemia	*B cell lineage:* cCD79a/cCD22 *T cell lineage:* cCD3, CD2, CD3, CD4, CD5, CD7 and TdT
Classic Hodgkin's disease	CD15, CD30
Central nervous system	
CNS tumors	*Astrocytoma:* GFAP *Ependymoma:* GFAP, S-100, vimentin *Medulloblastoma:* Synaptophysin or nestin, NSE *Meningioma:* EMA, PR, Ki-67 (atypical meningioma) *Retinoblastoma:* GFAP, S-100, NSE, synaptophysin and MBP *Hemangioblastoma:* CD31, CD34, CD56, S-100, vimentin, NSE, inhibin-α
Chordoma	NSE, S-100, EMA
Male genitourinary system	
Renal cell carcinoma	Co-expression of EMA and vimentin
Prostate carcinoma	PSA, PSAP, EMA, NXK31, prostein, p63

Contd...

Table 14.22: Panel of monoclonal antibodies in common malignancies (Contd...)

Malignancies	Monoclonal antibodies
Testicular tumors	*Seminoma:* LIN28 (RNA binding protein), SALL4 (+ nuclei), PLAP, c-kit (CD117), OCT4, vimentin, LDH, podoplanin *Embryonal carcinoma:* LIN28, SALL4 (+ nuclei), PLAP, OCT4, CD30 *Yolk sac tumor:* LIN28, SALL4 (+ nuclei), PLAP
Round cell tumors	
Round cell tumors	*Wilms' tumor:* WT1, WT2 Neuroblastoma (NSE, neurofilament, chromogranin, synaptophysin) *Ewing's sarcoma:* CD99 (MIC2 specific marker), vimentin, NSE *Bronchial carcinoid:* NSE, chromogranin, synaptophysin, cytokeratin *Alveolar rhabdomyosarcoma:* Desmin, myogenin, vimentin, myoglobin, MyoD1
Skeletal system and soft tissues	
Osteosarcoma	Vimentin
Soft tissue sarcoma	*Rhabdomyosarcoma:* Desmin, myogenin, vimentin, myoglobin, MyoD1 *Leiomyosarcoma:* SMA, vimentin, S-100 *Fibrosarcoma:* Vimentin and nonspecific SMA *Synovial sarcoma:* Vimentin, CD99, CK, EMA, S-100 *Liposarcoma:* S-100 *Angiosarcoma:* CD31, CD34, FXIII related antigen
Skin	
Skin melanoma	HMB45, MART-1 (melan-A), tyrosinase, Ki-67 (excellent marker), S-100 and CAM 5.2
Miscellaneous category	
Paraganglioma	Chromogranin, synaptophysin, neuron-specific enolase, CD56 and CD57

Abbreviation: ER (estrogen receptor), PR (progesterone receptor), Her2 (human epidermal growth factor receptor 2), CK (cytokeratin), GCDFP-15 (gross cystic disease fluid protein-15), EMA (epithelial membrane antigen), TTF-1 (thyroid transcription factor-1), TG (thyroglobulin), NSE (neurone-specific enolase), CEA (carcinoembryonic antigen), NCAM (neural cell adhesion molecule), DOG-1 (detected on GIST-1), PDGFR-α (platelet derived growth factor receptor-α), Hep-Par-1 (hepatocyte paraffin-1), AFP (α-fetoprotein), hCG (human chorionic gonadotrophin), PSA (prostate specific antigen), PSAP (prostate specific acid phosphatase), PTEN (phosphatase and tensin), HMB-45 (human melanoma black-45), Mart-1 (melanoma antigen recognized by T cells 1), TdT (terminal deoxynucleotydyl transferase), GFAP (glial fibrillary acidic protein), MBP (major basic protein), PLAP (placental alkaline phosphatase), LDH (lactate dehydrogenase), 5-HT (5-hydroxytryptamine), SMA (smooth muscle actin), WT (Wilms' tumor).

IMMUNOFLUORESCENCE MICROSCOPY

Immunofluorescence (IF) is a powerful technique that utilizes fluorescent labeled antibodies to detect specific target antigens. Fluorescein dye emits greenish fluorescence under UV light. It can be tagged to immunoglobulin molecules.

Sometimes, this technique is used to make viral plaque more readily visible to human eye. Immunofluorescent labeled tissue sections are studied using a fluorescent microscopy. It is very sensitive method.

Disadvantages are expensive equipment and its reagents, cross reactivity and non-specific immunofluorescence.

PRINCIPLE

Principle involves usage of fluorescein isothiocyanate labeled-immunoglobulin to detect antigens or antibodies according to test systems under a fluorescent microscope.

The second layer antibody can be labeled with fluorescent dye such as FITC, rhodamine or texas red in indirect immunofluorescence method.

TYPE OF IMMUNOFLUORESCENCE

There are two types of immunofluorescence: direct and indirect (Fig. 14.9). Immunofluorescence technique by using probe is shown in Table 14.23.

Table 14.23: Differences between direct and indirect immunofluorescence

Parameters	Direct immunofluorescence	Indirect immunofluorescence
Time	Shorter procedure, single labeling step	Longer procedure, double labeling step
Cross reactivity	Minimized	May cross react with other than the target
Sensitivity	Less	High due to amplification of signal
Cost	Expensive	Relatively inexpensive

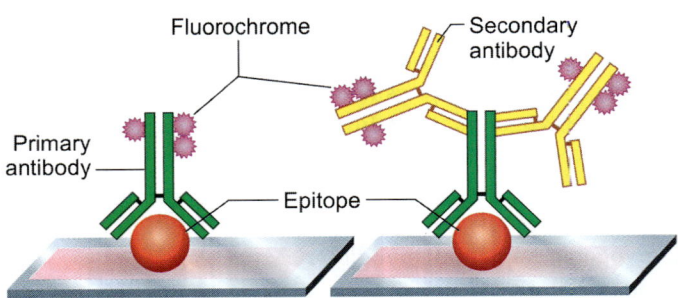

Fig. 14.9: Direct and indirect immunofluorescence.

Direct Immunofluorescence Microscopy

Direct immunofluorescence microscopy is a simple and very common procedure. Antigen is fixed on a slide and fluorescein labeled antibodies is layered over it. Then the slides are washed to remove unattached antibodies and examined under UV light in a fluorescent microscope. The site where the antibody attaches to its specific antigen shows apple green fluorescence. It is used for direct detection of pathogens or their antigens in tissue or in pathological samples.

Indirect Immunofluorescence Microscopy

Indirect immunofluorescence microscopy utilizes a two-step procedure to detect antigens. In the first step, a primary unlabeled antibody is used to bind and detect antigen. Then a second fluorescent labeled antibody binds the Fc portion of the primary antibody. This technique is more sensitive because multiple secondary antibodies can bind to a single primary antibody, thus amplifying the signal strength. Clinical applications of immunofluorescence are shown in Table 14.24.

Table 14.24: Clinical applications of immunofluorescence microscopy

Type of immunofluorescence	Sampling	Systems involved	Applications in diagnosing disorders
Direct immunofluorescence microscopy	Tissue sample	Skin and mucosa	Bullous pemphigoid Pemphigus vulgaris Dermatitis herpetiformis Discoid lupus
		Kidney (evaluation with fluorescein isothiocyanate—FITC conjugated method against IgG, IgM, IgA, C3, C1q, fibrinogen, albumin, κ and λ)	Glomerulonephritis
		Kidney (evaluation of C4d)	Humoral renal transplant rejection
		Lung (evaluation of C4d)	Humoral lung transplant rejection
Indirect immunofluorescence microscopy	Blood sample without anticoagulant (serum dilutions is removed and applied to an epithelial substrate together with fluorescein-labeled IgG)	Skin lesions	Pemphigus vulgaris Paraneoplastic pemphigus Bullous and/or cicatricial pemphigoid

Other applications of immunofluorescence are to detect viruses (herpes, varicella, zoster, cytomegalovirus, influenza, HIV), bacteria (Mycobacterium tubercle bacilli and *Treponema pallidum*), and *Entamoeba histolytica*.

Advanced Diagnostic Techniques

CHEMILUMINESCENCE VS CHEMIFLUORESCENCE

Traditionally, radioisotopic protocols have been used in the laboratory. Keeping in view of high cost of isotopes and difficulty in their disposal, many scientists are turning to non-isotope methods as a substitute to isotopes. Currently, chemiluminescence and chemifluorescence are used in the laboratories.

CHEMILUMINESCENCE

Chemiluminescence is non-isotope method. It is based on chemical reaction occuring between an enzyme such as horseradish peroxidase (HRP) and chemiluminescence such as luminol resulting in light emission. The light emission is detected by CCD, X-ray film, PMT based detectors. This method is more sensitive than calorimetric methods.

The antibody based systems provide target specificity. Enzyme component provides signal amplification. This has now become a protocol for substituting radioisotopes worldwide. Schematic of chemiluminescence reaction is shown in Fig. 14.10. Applications of chemiluminescence are shown in Table 14.25.

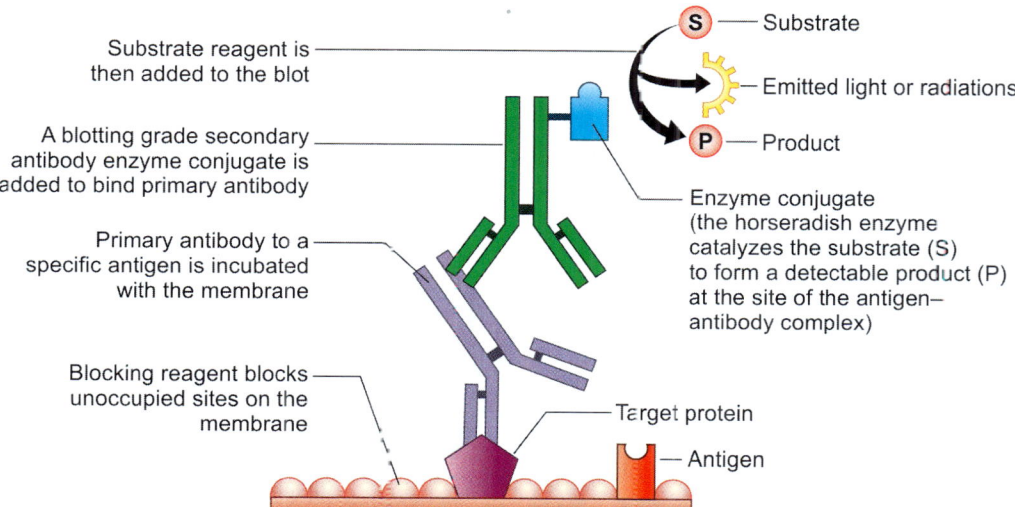

Fig. 14.10: Schematic of chemiluminescence reaction.

Table 14.25: Applications of chemiluminescence

Categories	Uses
Chemiluminescence immunoassay	It provides a sensitive, high throughput alternative to conventional colorimetric methodologies. Principle is same as ELISA and uses a chemiluminescent substrate for detection of: • *Hormones:* Insulin, thyroxin, estradiol, testosterone, progesterone • *Vitamin:* Vitamin B_{12} • *Tumor markers:* Bone morphogenic protein-2, carcinoembryonic antigen (CEA), α-fetoprotein (AFP) and human β-chorionic gonadotropin (β-hCG) • *C-reactive protein and tumor necrosis factor:* During inflammation
DNA hybridization detection	This hybridization technique uses specific chemiluminescent detecting reagents containing H_2O_2 and luminol for the following uses: • Identifying DNA in crime case • Paternal dispute • Classify DNAs of various organisms
Western blotting	Western blotting (or protein immunoblotting) is a technique widely used to detect specific proteins in samples of tissue, cell lysates, cell culture supernatants or body fluids
Food analysis	Chemiluminescence is used to determine N-nitrosocompounds, sugar, anabolic hormone, metabolites, food oxidations, metals and other interesting compounds
Forensic science	Chemiluminescence is used by criminalists to detect traces of blood at crime scene. Tiny amount of iron from hemoglobin in blood serves as catalyst for the chemiluminescence reaction that causes chemiluminescent reagent luminol to glow

CHEMIFLUORESCENCE

Chemifluorescence is an alternative method used for molecular study. It combines fluorescence and chemiluminescence. Difference between chemiluminescence and chemifluorescence is based on detection mechanism. In chemiluminescence, light is generated based on enzymatic reaction. In chemifluorescence, fluorescent molecule is attached to either secondary or tertiary antibody, which requires excitation via laser or some other high intensity light source. Excitation of fluorescent molecule generates a light emission collected by CCD or PMT based detector.

This method provides greater sensitivity, targeted specificity and amplification of signal as compared to calorimetric methods as well as chemiluminescence. Comparison between chemiluminescence and chemifluorescence is shown in Table 14.26. Schematic of chemifluorescence is shown in Fig. 14.11.

Table 14.26: Comparison between chemiluminescence and chemifluorescence

Parameters	Chemiluminescence	Chemifluorescence
Detection system	CCD, X-ray film, PMT based detectors	CCD, PMT based detector
Excitation	None	Required
Detection levels	Femtogram	Femtogram
Shelf life	Up to one year	<1 month
Cost	Inexpensive	Expensive

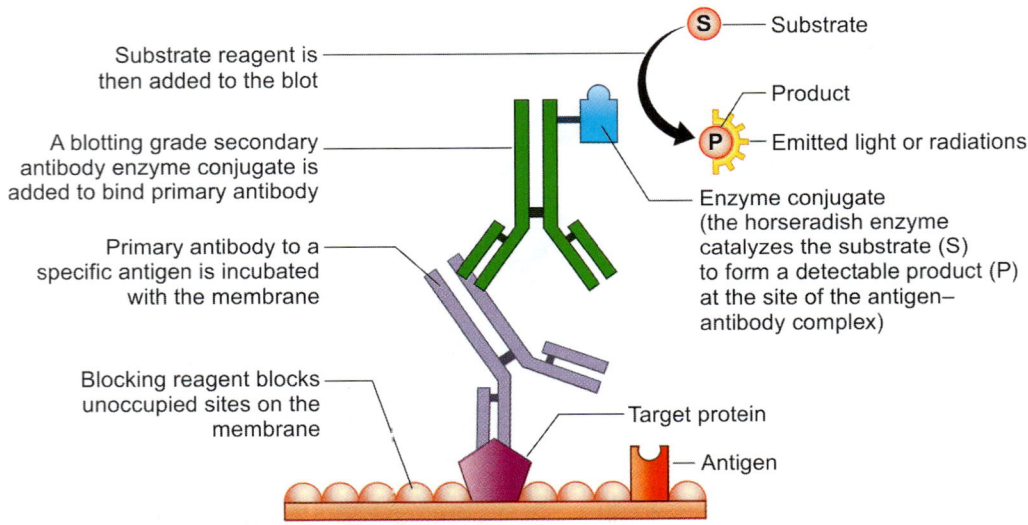

Fig. 14.11: Schematic of chemifluorescence.

FLOW CYTOMETRY

Flow cytometry simultaneously measures and analyzes multiple suspended cells ranging from 0.2 to 150 µm, as they flow in a fluid stream through a beam of light. Peripheral and bone marrow aspirate specimens can be studied by forming represent a suspension of cells.

Samples are prevented clotting by adding anticoagulant such as disodium EDTA, sodium citrate or heparin. Concentration of white blood cells is enhanced by lysis of red blood cells by addition of ammonium chloride. Cells can also be obtained from solid tissue and converted into suspension for flow cytometric analysis suspensions.

COMPONENTS OF FLOW CYTOMETER

The flow cytometer is composed of a flow system, optical system and electronic system. The flow system transports cells in a stream to the laser beam for analysis. The optical system consists of lasers to illuminate the cells in the sample stream and optical fibers to direct the resulting light signals to the appropriate detectors. The electronic system converts light signals into electronic signals that are processed by the computer (Fig. 14.12). Flow cytometry is used in classifying leukemias and DNA analysis.

Advanced Diagnostic Techniques 14

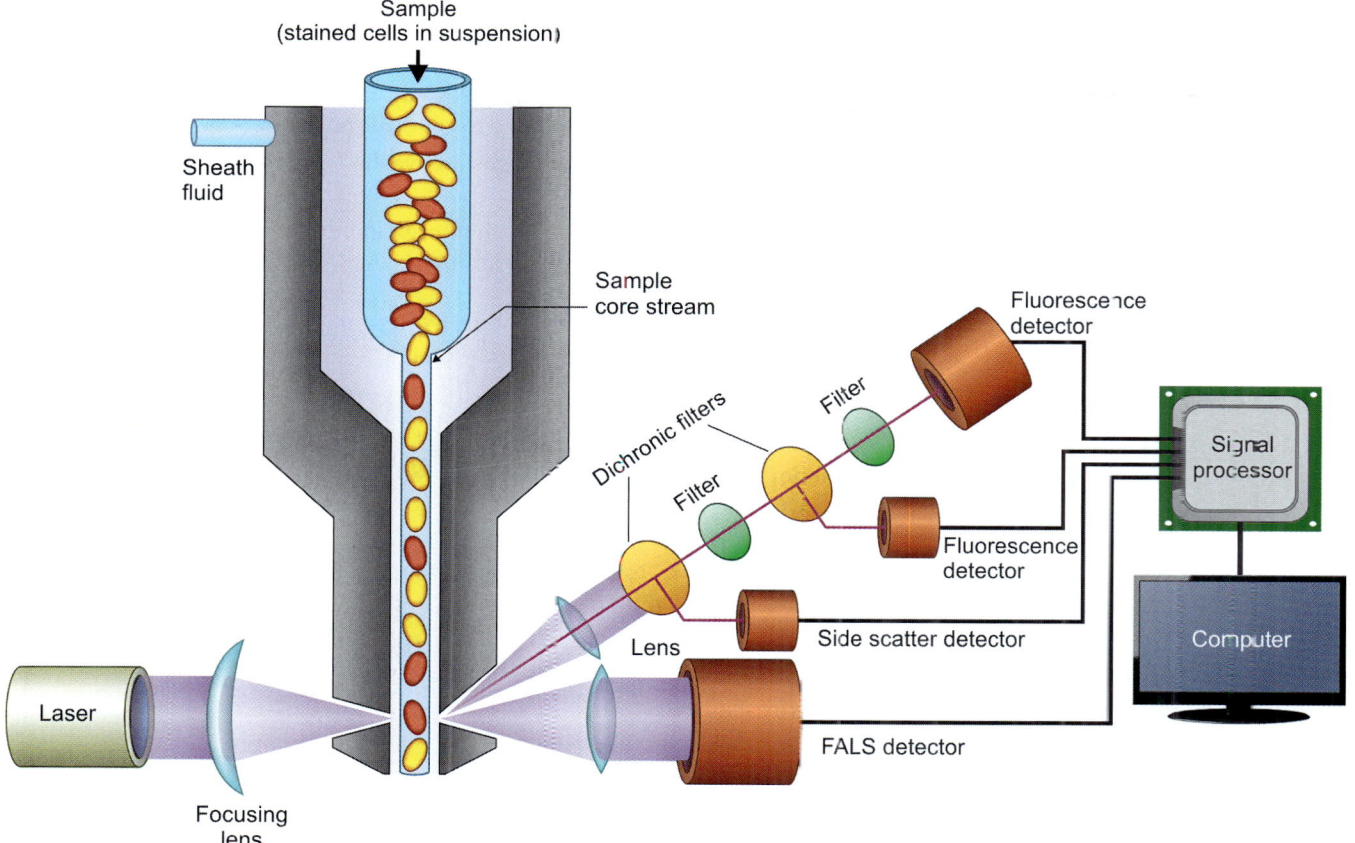

Fig. 14.12: The flow cytometer is composed of a flow system, optical system and electronic system.

FLOW SYSTEM

Sample obtained from peripheral blood and bone marrow aspirate or solid tissue suspension mixed with anticoagulant are injected into a stream of sheath. Cell particles are forced into center of the stream enabling transporting of single cell. Higher flow rate is used for the immunophenotyping of cells. Lower flow rate is used for DNA analysis.

OPTICAL SYSTEM

Optical system consists of light scattering and fluorescence. Lasers participate in illumination of particles in the sample stream. Filters direct the generated light signals to the appropriate detectors. Most flow cytometers have Argon ion laser as source of light. The light signals are generated when laser beam strikes the cells. A system comprising optical mirrors and filters direct the specialized wavelength of light to the designated photodetectors.

Light Scattering

Light scattering occurs when cell deflects laser light. Leukocytes can be separated into different subpopulations of cells using forward light scattering (FSC) and side light scattering (SSC) are shown in Table 14.27. Neutrophils contain granular cytoplasm and complex nuclei, therefore, show both high forward and a side scatter. On the other hand, lymphocytes lack cytoplasmic granules and hence show both a low forward and a low side scatter.

Fluorescence

Conjugation of fluorescent dyes to monoclonal antibodies directed toward antigens on a particular cell subset help in identification of subpopulations. There

Table 14.27: Type of light scattering

Type of light scattering	Characteristics
Forward light scattering (FSC)	Collected in the line with laser light beam
	Analyzes measurement of the cell surface size
Side light scattering (SSC)	Collected perpendicular to the laser light beam
	Analyzes internal complexity of a cell

Table 14.28: Type of fluorescence staining procedures

Steps	Direct fluorescence staining procedure	Indirect fluorescence staining procedure
First incubation	Incubation of cells with single fluorescence staining	Incubation of cells with a non-fluorescence staining directed towards specific antigen
Washing	Incubated cells are washed to remove non-specific bound antibodies	Incubated cells are washed remove non-specific bound antibodies
Second incubation	Not required	Required with fluorescent dye directed against monoclonal antibody

Table 14.29: Comparison between fluorescein isothiocyanate (FITC) and phyoerythrin (PE)

Parameters	Fluorescein isothiocyanate (FITC)	Phyoerythrin (PE)
Range of absorption of light and then fluoresces	460 to 510 nm	448 to 555 nm
Then fluoresces	510 to 560 nm giving green fluorescence	480 to 565 nm giving red fluorescence

Staining pattern of subpopulation of cells and percentage are defined.

are two types of fluorescence staining procedures: direct and indirect (Table 14.28). Argon ion lasers are most common lasers used in most flow cytometers because 488 nm light emitted may be absorbed by more than one fluorochrome. Fluorescent dyes such as fluorescein isothiocyanate (FITC) and phyoerythrin (PE) are used to conjugate with monoclonal antibodies (Table 14.29).

ELECTRONIC SYSTEM

Photodetectors convert the generated forward and side scattered cells, and fluorescent light signals into electrical impulses. There are two types of photodetectors in flow cytometer: photomultiplier tubes (PMTs) and photodiodes.

Photomultiplier tubes (PMTs) amplify the electric current generated from light signals. Long amplifiers are used to negative from dim positive signals from cells stained with fluorochrome-labeled antibodies. Linear amplifiers are used to detect forward and side scatter signals. Photodiodes are used to detect strong FSC signals. The intensity of the electronic impulses derived from the photodetectors is analyzed by digital converter.

USES OF FLOW CYTOMETER

Classification of Leukemias

Flow cytometry is an ancillary method for classification of acute leukemias and lymphomas. Monoclonal antibodies specific to nuclear, cytoplasmic and surface antigens and characteristic of particular cell subsets are used in flow cytometer. These are organized as clusters of differentiation (CD) antigens, which differentiate hematopoietic malignancies and lymphomas.

In cases of acute leukemias, it is essential to know the myeloid or lymphoid lineage. It is required to

Table 14.30: Immunophenotying of ALL (B cell) and ALL (T cell)

Characteristics	ALL (B cell)	ALL (T cell)
HLA-DR	Positive	-
cCD1	-	Positive
CD2	-	Positive
CD3	-	Positive
CD5	-	Positive
CD7	-	Positive
CD10 (CALLA)*	Positive	-
CD19	Positive	-
CD20	Positive	-

*CD10 (CALLA) is favorable prognostic marker and most amenable to therapy.

know the prognosis and line of treatment in those cases in which routine cell morphology and cytochemistry fail to subtype or assign proper lineage in acute leukemias.

Immunophenotyping using flow cytometry improves the diagnosis of acute lymphoblastic leukemia and differentiate B cell ALL and T cell ALL (Table 14.30).

Lineage markers of AML while analyzing on flow cytometric analysis include anti-MPO cytoplasmic, CD13, CD33 and CD117. Immunophenotyping of AML is shown in Table 14.31. Immunophenotyping of chronic lymphocytic leukemia is shown in Table 14.32.

DNA Content Analysis

Flow cytometry can also be used in analyzing DNA content of a cell by using fluorescent stains, which target different DNA bases within double helix.

Fluorescent stains: Fluorescent stains such as HOECHST 33342 or 4′,6-diamino-2-phenylindole (DAPI) are specific for the adenine/thymine base pairs. Mithramycin and

Table 14.31: Lineage markers of AML analyzing on flow cytometry

Parameters	Lineage markers of AML
AML	Anti-MPO cytoplasmic is lineage marker of AML CD13 CD33 CD117
Markers of immaturity	CD34
Monocytic differentiation	CD14 CD64
Megakaryocytic differentiation	CD41 CD61
Erythroid differentiation	CD235A Glycophorin A

Table 14.32: Immunophenotyping of chronic lymphocytic leukemia

Immunophenotype (pan-B cell markers)	Expression
CD5*	Positive
CD23	Positive
CD19	Positive
CD20	Positive

*CD5 is positive in normal B cell and T cell.

chromomycin A3 are target guanine/cytosine base pairs. Propidium iodide stains all double-stranded nucleic acids, hence it is used in conventional cytometers with low power argon lasers because it absorbs light at 488 nm. DNA content analysis helps in differentiating normal cells from aneuploid malignant cells. The histograms from malignant tumors show abnormal peaks than normal cells.

Cell Cycle Analysis

Cell cycle shows G_0 (resting phase), G_1 (pre-synthetic phase), G_2 (synthetic phase), S and M (mitotic) phases. Cells of G_2 have finished DNA synthesis with double the amount of DNA. In M phase, two daughter cells are formed. G_1/S and G_2/M are checkpoints of cell cycle. The cell cycle can be plotted as a histogram with the number of cells per channel on the Y axis and fluorescence intensity of the cells stained for DNA content on the X axis.

CYTOGENETIC ANALYSIS

TRADITIONAL CYTOGENETIC ANALYSIS

There milestones in the history of clinical cytogenetics comprise preparation of chromosomes from blood cultures. Chromosomal spread is enhanced by development of hypotonic methods. Discovery of fluorescent quinacrine compounds helped in the demonstration of unique banding pattern for each human chromosome.

Cytogenetic analysis is commonly used in the evaluation of congenital disorders, diagnosing syndrome associated with chromosomal abnormality, screening karyotypic abnormalities in patients with multiple birth defects and prenatal diagnosis. In surgical pathology, cytogenetic analysis recognizes cytogenetic abnormalities in patients with leukemias, lymphomas and soft tissue sarcomas. Cytogenetic analysis in cancers has aided targeted therapy, prognosis, and risk-based stratification of intensive therapy.

ADVANTAGES

Conventional cytogenetic analysis has ability to evaluate entire genome without any foreknowledge of the chromosomal regions involved in the disease process.

LIMITATIONS

Conventional cytogenetic analysis is performed on viable tissue specimens that contain proliferating cells. It is only suited for detection of numerical abnormalities and gross structural abnormalities. This technique lacks sensitivity to detect mutations such as deletions, amplifications, single base substitutions and so on.

BASIC LABORATORY PROCEDURES

Overall scheme for the production of metaphase chromosomes for conventional cytogenetic analysis is shown in Fig. 14.13.

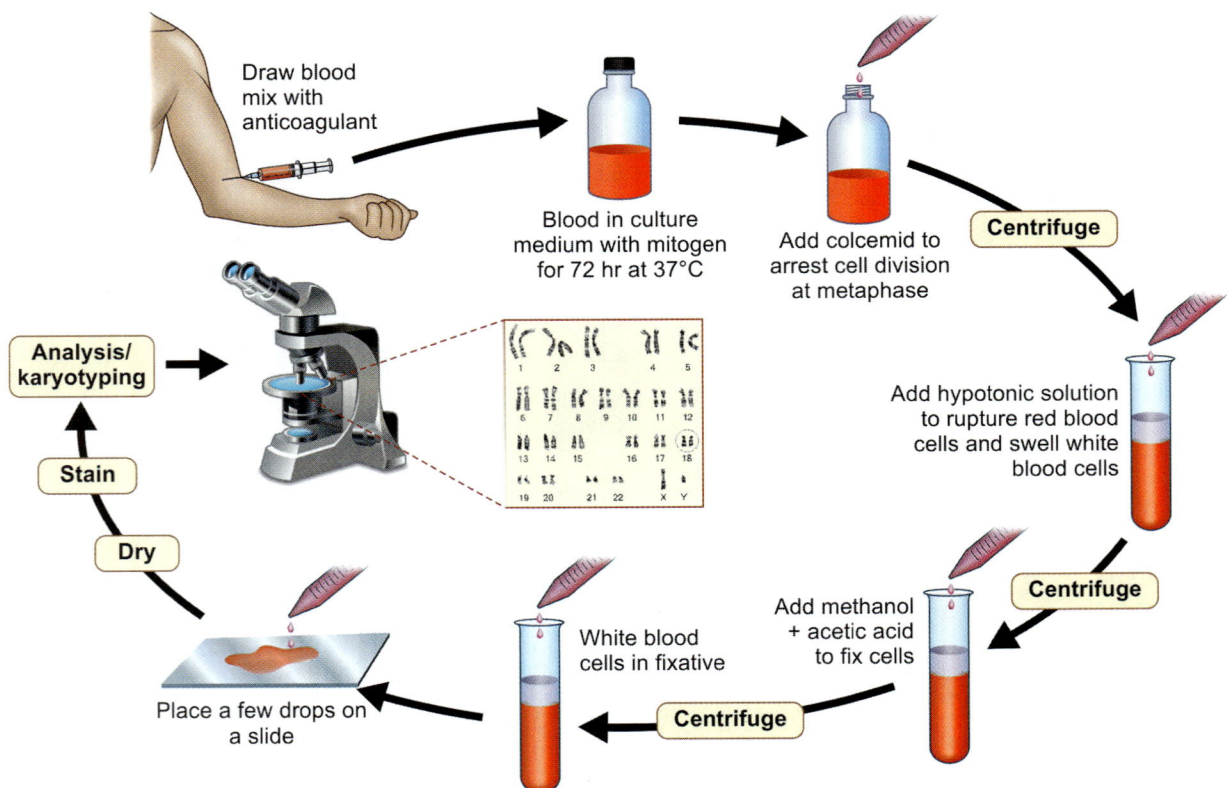

Fig. 14.13: Overall scheme for the production of metaphase chromosomes for conventional cytogenetic analysis.

CULTURE INITIATION

Blood sample is withdrawn and mixed with anticoagulant. Blood is kept in culture bottle with mitogen for 72 hours at 37°C. Different specimens are collected for traditional cytogenetic analysis as shown in Table 14.33. Bone marrow and sold tumor consist of cells, which proliferate at slow rate. Therefore, mitogen is added to enhance proliferation (Table 14.34).

Table 14.33: Specimen requirements for traditional cytogenetic analysis

Type of sample	Sample collection
Peripheral blood	Blood sample with anticoagulant kept in refrigerator or at room temperature
Bone marrow aspirate	Bone marrow aspirate with anticoagulant kept at room temperature
Solid tissue from tumor	Viable tumor sample kept in sterile container containing broad spectrum antibiotics to prevent microbial overgrowth and autolysis
	Sterile container is transported on ice

CULTURE MAINTENANCE

The length of *in vitro* culture depends on cell type is shown in Table 14.35.

Table 14.34: Mitogens used to enhance proliferation of cells of bone marrow and solid neoplasms

Mitogen	Cell proliferation in culture
Phytohemagglutinin (PHA)	T cells
Lipopolysaccharide (LPS)	B cells
Protein A	B cells
12-O-tetradecanoyl phorbol-13-acetate (TPA)	B cells
Epstein-Barr virus	B cells
Synthetic oligonucleotides	B cells
Pokewood mitogen	B cells

Table 14.35: Time required for proliferation of cells in culture medium

Cell proliferation	Time required
Peripheral blood cells	72 hours
Bone marrow cells	24 to 48 hours
Solid neoplasms	≥2 weeks

Advanced Diagnostic Techniques

CELL HARVESTING

Colcemid is added to the bottle to arrest cell division at metaphase. Colcemid, a synthetic analogue of colchicine (an alkaloid derived from the bulb of Mediterranean plant colchicine) prevents separation of sister chromatids. It blocks proliferation of cells in metaphase stage. Since cell cycle is asynchronous *in vitro*.

Cells are obtained in acceptable mitotic index by addition of thymidine followed by dethymidine to obtain normal DNA replication. Alternately, 5-fluoro-deoxyuridine may be used to stall cells at G1/S boundary, addition of thymidine leads to release the block.

Next steps: The blood is now centrifuged in test tube. Then add hypotonic solution to the test tube to rupture red blood cells and swelling of white blood cells. Again centrifuge the test tube. Then add methanol and acetic acid to the test tube to fix cells. Then centrifuge the test tube containing fixed white blood cells. Place a few drops on glass slide. Dry the smear and then stain. The slide is analyzed for karyotyping. Quinacrine banding technique allows detection of the region containing repetitive DNA.

BANDING

Techniques used to stain metaphase chromosome are shown in Table 14.36.

MICROSCOPIC ANALYSIS

Bright field microscopy or fluorescence microscopy is used to visualize chromosomes. Electronic imaging system is used to capture the images.

ASSAY FAILURE

Assay failure occurs due to sampling from necrotic tumor, overgrowth of microbes, overgrowth of non-representative clone of tumor cells, post-culture failure and wrong interpretation of results.

METAPHASE FLUORESCENCE *IN SITU* HYBRIDIZATION

All metaphase chromosomes *in situ* hybridization analysis is performed by using probes labeled with fluorophores. Metaphase FISH technique is a modified Southern blot in which the target DNA comprises chromosomes rather than membrane bound DNA. This technique has four steps as shown in Table 14.37. Type of probes used in metaphase *in situ* hybridization is shown in Table 14.38.

Table 14.36: Techniques used to stain metaphase chromosome

Staining technique	Staining patterns
Technique producing specific alternating bands along each chromosome	
Giemsa banding (G-banding)	Dark bands are AT-rich Light bands are CG-rich
Quinacrine banding (Q-banding)	Bright regions are AT-rich
Reverse banding (R-banding)	AT rich regions stain lightly (dull fluorescence) CG-rich regions staining darkly (bright fluorescence)
4,6-Diamidino-2-phenylindole (DAPI) staining	DAPI binds AT-rich regions produces a pattern similar to C-banding (bright regions are AT-rich)
Technique staining selective chromosome regions	
Constitutive heterochromatin banding (C-banding)	Stains heterochromatin (α-satellite DNA) around the centromere Used to demonstrate some inherited polymorphisms
Telomere banding (T-banding)	Technical variation of R-banding used to stain telomeres
Silver staining for nuclear organizer regions (NOR staining)	Stains the NORs (which contain rRNA genes) on the satellite stalks of acrocentric chromosome
Fluorescence *in situ* hybridization (FISH)	Staining pattern dependent on the probe

Table 14.37: Four steps of metaphase fluorescence *in situ* hybridization

Steps	Procedure
Step 1	Denaturing of probe and metaphase target by high temperature and formamide
Step 2	Hybridization of probe to the chromosomal target
Step 3	Removal of unbound post-hybridization probe by washing
Step 4	Detection of bound probe by fluorescent microscopy

Table 14.38: Type of probes used in metaphase in situ hybridization

Characteristics	Repetitive sequence probes	Unique sequence probes	Whole chromosome probes (WCPs) also known as painting probe
Basis of development of probe	Differences in α-satellite sequences of centromeres	Derived from genomic clones or cDNA by using vectors such as bacterial artificial chromosomes (BACs) and yeast artificial chromosomes (YACs)	Probes isolated through flow sorting of specific chromosomes, micro-dissection of specific chromosomes accompanied by PCR amplification
Use	Most widely used to detect repetitive sequence	Used to detect sequences present on given chromosome	Used to identify chromosomal rearrangements

MULTIPLEX METAPHASE FISH

Multiplex metaphase FISH is also known as *multicolor FISH*. Special karyotyping (SKY) is related technique. In both techniques, metaphase chromosome spreads are hybridized with a combination of probes labeled with different fluorophores. Five different fluorophores can produce different color combinations to uniquely labeled WCPs to visualize 24 different human chromosomes, X and Y chromosomes in one hybridization.

ADVANTAGES

Multiplex FISH and special karyotyping (SKY) are used to detect aneuploidy, interchromosomal rearrangements and marker chromosome (extrachromosomal material of unknown origin).

DISADVANTAGES

Multiplex FISH and special karyotyping (SKY) do not provide direct information on the involved chromosomal bands. Both techniques do not detect intrachromosomal rearrangements such as inversions. These do not provide information on regions with repetitive DNA.

MODIFICATIONS OF MULTIPLEX FISH AND SKY

Multiplex FISH and special karyotyping (SKY) are modified by mixing with partial chromosome paints. These modified techniques detect translocation breakpoints and interchromosomal rearrangements.

COMPARATIVE GENOMIC HYBRIDIZATION (CGH)

Comparative genomic hybridization (CGH) has higher sensitivity than conventional cytogenetic analysis.

METAPHASE CGH

Metaphase CGH technique is a variation of metaphase FISH. It is used to survey entire genome for chromosomal deletions and amplifications. For a typical CGH test, genomic DNA extracted from tumor is labeled with red fluorophore, and genomic DNA from a paired normal issue is labeled with green fluorophore. Both red and green probes are now mixed and used in single hybridization.

The relative difference in DNA content between the normal and specimen DNA is represented by a difference in the green: red fluorescence ratios. Conventional chromosomal CGH is shown in Fig. 14.14.

ARRAY CGH (aCGH)

Array CGH technique utilizes a microarray comprising an orderly arrangement of DNA molecules linked to a solid matrix support. The labeled probe mixture is hybridized to the microarray. Ratio of green to red fluorescent signals is measured for each feature. Genomic microarrays are currently employed to detect genomic copy number changes, copy neutral changes and loss of heterozygosity. Comparative genomic hybridization *vs* conventional cytogenetic analysis is shown in Table 14.39.

Table 14.39: Comparative genomic hybridization *vs* conventional cytogenetic analysis

Parameters	Comparative genomic hybridization (CGS)	Conventional cytogenetic analysis
Sensitivity	High sensitivity	Low sensitivity
Sample obtained	DNA extraction from fixed as well as fresh tumor	Peripheral blood, bone marrow aspirate and solid tumor
Utility	Genomic wide scan for structural alterations	Genomic wide scan for structural alterations is not possible

Advanced Diagnostic Techniques 14

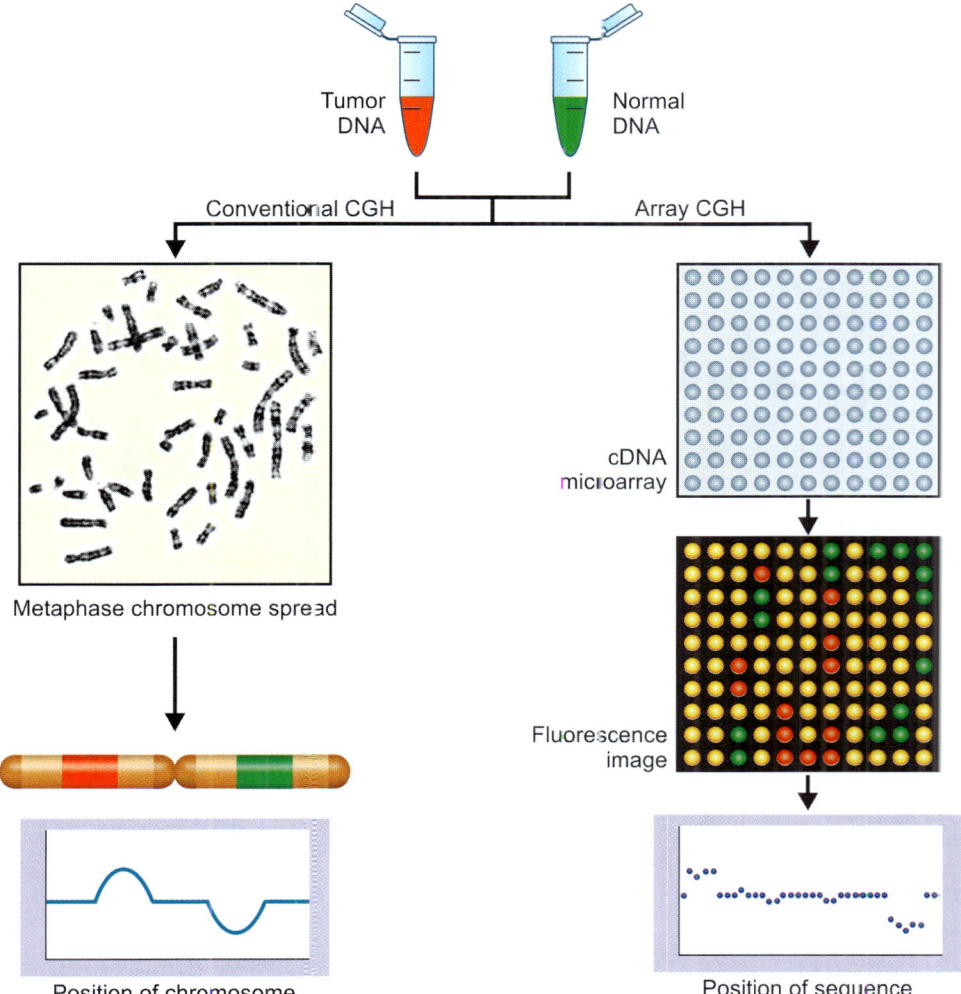

Fig. 14.14: Conventional chromosomal CGH: in conventional chromosomal CGH, the ratio of fluorescence intensities along each chromosome is analyzed. Increased DNA copy number in the tumor sample will be detected by increased red fluorescence, whereas decreased copy number will allow more binding of the normal DNA and increased green fluorescence. On the right, a similar hybridization to a cDNA array permits measurement of copy number at a higher resolution.

Advantages: The major advantage of CGH in tumor studies is that the actual chromosome preparations from the study tissue are not needed. Retrospective studies on archived samples can be conducted using DNA extracted from formalin-fixed material. It does not require prior knowledge of the chromosome imbalance involved.

MICROARRAY ANALYSIS

Microarray analysis is used to evaluate patients with genomic imbalance especially in diagnostic testing for congenital anomalies, developmental delay and intellectual disabilities. However, this technique is not widely used in diagnosis of cancers especially of solid tumors.

It depends on the nucleic acid composition of the array (probe) and the test material (target) that is hybridized to it. Microarray application and technology are shown in Fig. 14.15. SNP array procedures are shown in Fig. 14.16.

MICROARRAY APPLICATION AND TECHNOLOGY

CGH Array

In CGH array, fragments of genomic DNA are spotted as probes onto the microarray surface using robotics. Genomic DNA from the patient's tissue and germline are then co-hybridized to the array to identify regions of chromosomal gain or loss.

SNPs/re-sequencing: SNPs are evaluated by comparing signal intensities from the assay substrate derived from DNA of patient. Alternatively, genomic DNA sequence can be used to computationally design oligonucleotide probes that detect specific alterations in DNA samples (either germline or tissue) for either SNP genotyping or DNA sequencing studies. Comparison between SNP and oligo arrays is shown in Table 14.40.

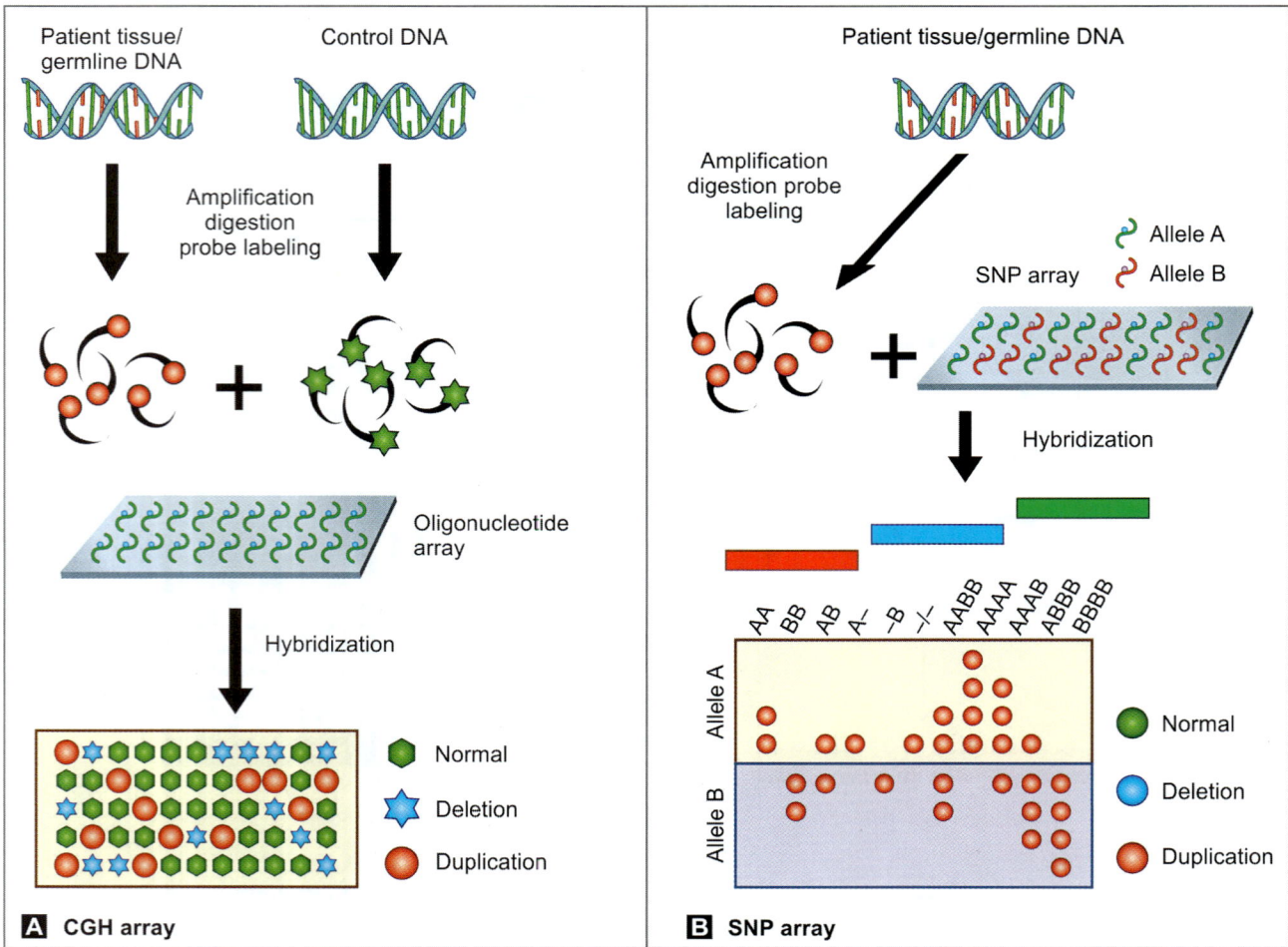

Fig. 14.15: Microarray application and technology. Microarray technology can be used in many different applications depending on the nucleic acid composition of the array (probe) and the test material (target) that is hybridized to it. (A) CGH array: in CGH array, fragments of genomic DNA are spotted as probes onto the microarray surface using robotics. Genomic DNA from the patient's tissue and germline are then co-hybridized to the array to identify regions of chromosomal gain or loss, (B) SNPs/re-sequencing: alternatively, genomic DNA sequence can be used to computationally design oligonucleotide probes that detect specific alterations in DNA samples (either germline or tissue) for either SNP genotyping or DNA sequencing studies.

Table 14.40: Comparison between SNP and oligo arrays

Array attribute	Single nucleotide polymorphism (SNP) arrays	Oligonucleotide arrays
Method of assessment of copy number imbalance	Probe signal intensities derived from patient's sample compared to a silico-reference mode	Patient's sample is directly hybridized against control DNA to detect relative gains or loss
Detection of balanced chromosomal rearrangements	No	No
Detects number of markers	1,000,000 markers	<2000,000 markers
DNA input requirement	200–500 ng	1–5 µg
Type of probe	SNP and oligo probes	Oligo probes
Limits of resolution	<10–20 kb	As low as 10–20 kb
Threshold for detection of mosaicism	As low as 5%	20–30%
Ability to detect copy of neutral LOH	Yes	No
Ability to detect uniparental disomy	Yes	No
Ability to detect consanguinity	Yes	No

Advanced Diagnostic Techniques

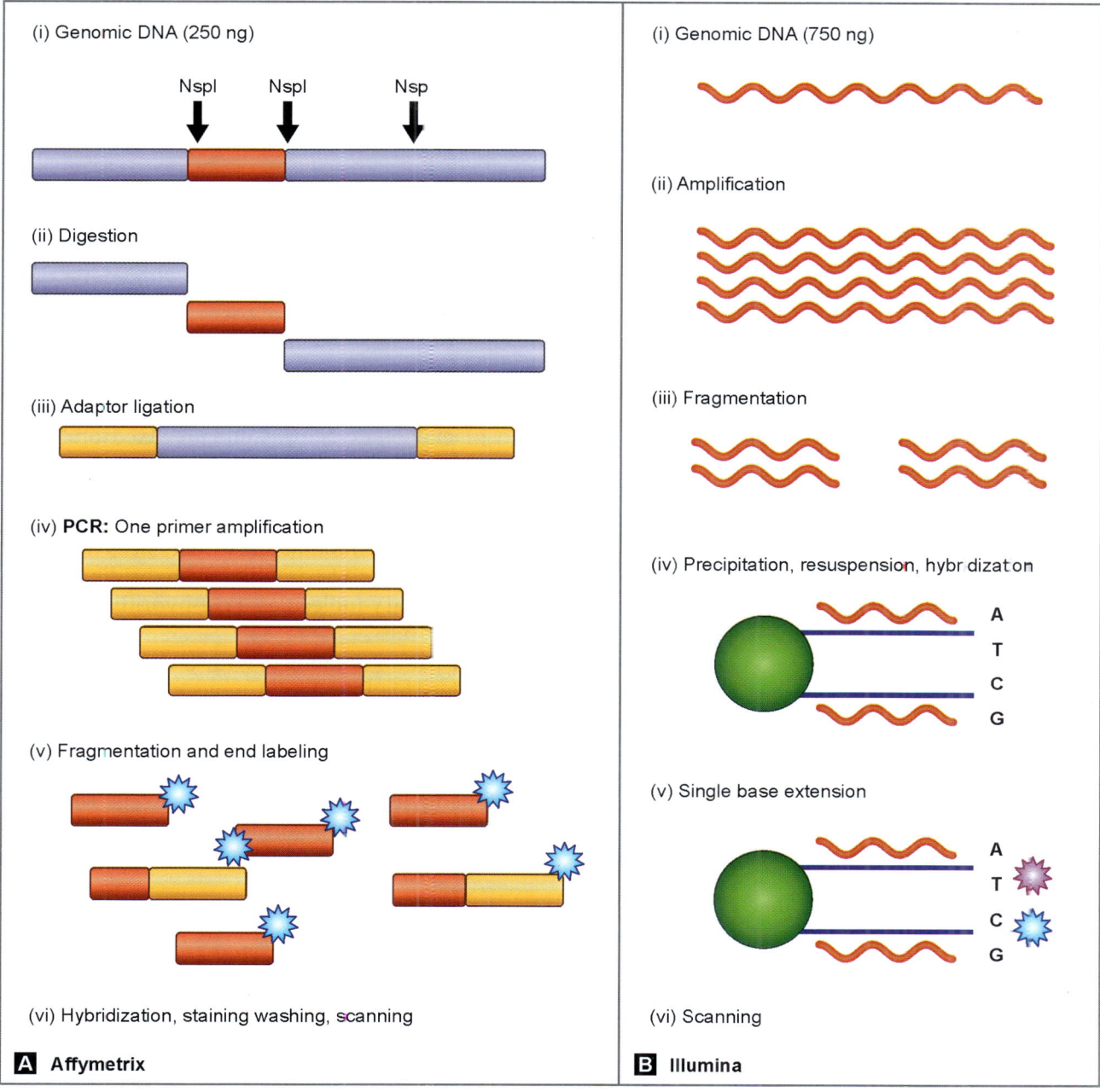

Fig. 14.16: SNP array procedures. (A) Affymetrix platform: genomic DNA is digested with NspI restriction enzyme. The resulted DNA fragments are ligated to adaptors and subsequently amplified. Amplification products are end-labeled and hybridized to the array. (B) Illumina platform: the entire genome is amplified and then hybridize to a bead array; allelic discrimination is achieved by single base extension reaction. In both platforms, the probe intensity is measured and compared with a silicoreference to evaluate DNA copy number.

ADVANTAGES OF MICROARRAY ANALYSIS

Microarray analysis has markedly increased resolution of chromosomal analysis. It does not require cell viability since DNA serves as the starting material. The technique is employed on samples such as peripheral blood lymphocytes, bone marrow aspirates, lymph nodes, formalin-fixed paraffin embedded tissue, aminocytes, products of conception and buccal cells.

LIMITATIONS OF MICROARRAY ANALYSIS

The technique can detect copy number changes. Microarray analysis has certain limitations. It cannot detect chromosomal rearrangements, balanced translocations, insertions and inversions. It also cannot analyze segmental duplication and repetitive sequences. Low level of mosaicism may not be detectable. LOH is demonstrated only by SNP-based platforms.

FLUORESCENCE IN SITU HYBRIDIZATION (FISH)

OVERVIEW

FISH is a technique that hybridizes a DNA nucleic acid probe to a target chromosomal-specific DNA sequence of interest contained within a cell nucleus. The technique permits identification of both structural and numeric aberrations characteristics of certain hematopoietic and non-hematopoietic cancers in many clinical settings (Table 14.41).

FISH can be performed on non-dividing (interphase) cells on air-dried or formalin fixed specimens. It can detect molecular abnormalities in cancers with low proliferative rates such as multiple myeloma. This technique detects aneusomes/deletions, gene amplification and chromosomal translocations.

On the other hand, conventional cytogenetic analysis has ability to evaluate entire genome for detection of numerical abnormalities and gross structural abnormalities. Conventional cytogenetic analysis lacks sensitivity to detect mutations such as deletions, amplifications, and single base substitutions.

A variety of specimen types can be analyzed using FISH. The intact cells are attached to a microscope slide using standard cytogenetic methods. It allows one to look at multiple genomic changes within a single cell, without destruction of the cellular morphology.

Probe: Probe is a nucleic acid that can be labeled with a marker which hybridizes to another nucleic acid on the basis of base complementarity allowing identification and quantitation. Various types of labeling are used—direct and indirect, radioactive (^{32}P, ^{35}S, ^{14}C, ^{3}H), fluorescent (FISH: fluorescent *in situ* hybridization) and biotinylated (avidin-streptavidin).

Direct method: Fluorescent dye binds directly to DNA probe using polymerase enzymes and labelled nucleoside triphosphates.

Indirect method: DNA probe is tagged with a hapten (biotin/digoxigenin) and detected by antibody tagged with fluorescent dye. It gives easy amplification of signal.

Multicolor FISH can provide *colorized* information relative to chromosome rearrangements, especially useful in specimens where chromosome preparations are less than optimal for standard cytogenetic banding analysis.

FISH PROCEDURE

Sample is fixed in Carnoy's fixative (3:1 methanol and glacial acetic acid). Cells are fixed on the slide. Denaturation is done by formamid at 42°C. Hybridization of probe and target DNA is performed. Nucleic acid hybridization is the formation of a duplex between two complementary sequences. *Annealing* is another term used to describe the hybridization of two complementary molecules. Post-hybridization washes are carried out.

DNA probe is labeled with a colored fluorescent molecule. This fluorescent molecule remains attached to the DNA during the hybridization process. The molecule emits a particular color when viewed through a fluorescence microscope in the dark room that is equipped with the appropriate filter sets. Technique of fluorescence *in situ* hybridization (FISH) is shown in Figs 14.17 and 14.18.

ADVANTAGES AND LIMITATIONS

Specimen Type Applicable to FISH

Fluorescent *in situ* hybridization is applicable to various specimens including cytology smears, buccal smears, fresh/frozen specimens and formalin

Table 14.41: Diagnostic tests by FISH to detect various disorders

Diagnostic tests	Disorders
Prenatal testing	Trisomy 13, 18, 21 XY aneusomes
Microdeletion syndromes	Cri du chat (5p) Prader-Willi/Angelman (15q) DiGeorge syndrome
Transplant pathology	XY FISH on sex mismatched organ transplant Disease relapse using known genetic alterations in primary tumor
Oncology (diagnostic, predictive and prognostic markers)	Chromosomal aneusomes Gene locus/locus deletions Gene amplifications Translocations

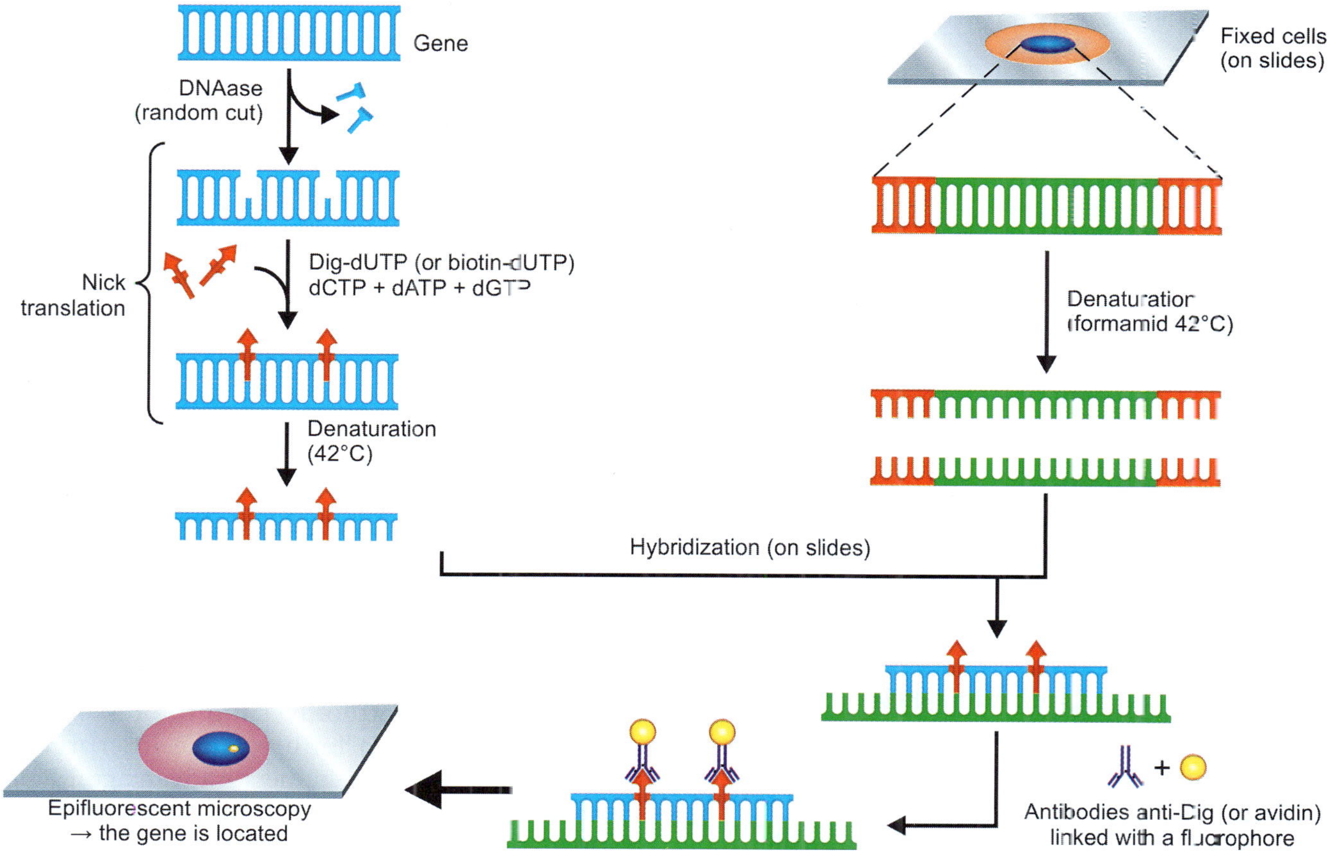

Advanced Diagnostic Techniques

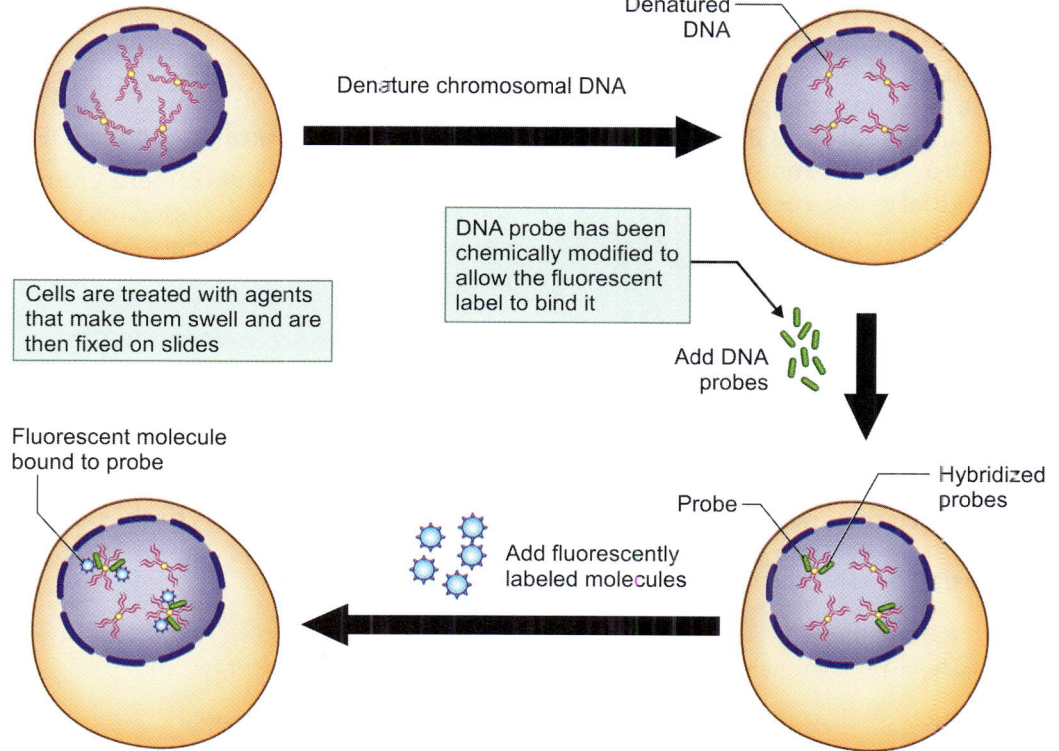

Fig. 14.17: Technique of fluorescence *in situ* hybridization (FISH).

Fig. 14.18: Technique of fluorescence *in situ* hybridization (FISH).

Table 14.42: Specimens analyzed by fluorescence *in situ* hybridization

Categories	Characteristics
Peripheral blood and bone marrow aspirate	Rapid analysis required
Cytology specimens	Body fluids, urine, pleural effusions Intraoperative cytology smears Cell culture preparations
Buccal smears	Used for sex determination
Fresh/frozen tissue	Fresh/frozen tissue analysis
Formalin fixed paraffin-embedded (FFPE) tissues	Thin sections obtained (4–6 µm) Disaggregated nuclei Archived unstained sections Previously stained sections (e.g. negative immunohistochemistry control)

fixed paraffin-embedded (FFPE) tissues specimens (Table 14.42).

FISH Versus Cytogenetic and Other Molecular Techniques

Fluorescent *in situ* hybridization (FISH) can be performed on non-dividing (interphase) cells. It can be performed on air-dried or formalin-fixed specimens. It detects molecular abnormalities in neoplasms with low proliferation rates such as multiple myeloma. It detects deletions, gains, chromosomal translocations and amplifications.

FISH is more sensitive and quicker than conventional karyotyping. It provides targeted approach for alterations, which have been identified by various global techniques such as classic cytogenetics, loss of heterozygosity (LOH), screening, comparative genomic hybridization (CGH), array CGH (aCGH), array single nucleotide polymorphism (SNP) and gene expression profiling. Minimal residual disease or early recurrences are better detected by polymerase chain reaction.

TISSUE MICROARRAY-FISH

Tissue microarray-FISH technology has advantage over multiple specimen paraffin blocks tissue microarrays. It is constructed from hundreds of 0.6 to 2.0 nm neoplastic, non-neoplastic and tissue cores of interest. The technique reduces data acquisition time, probe, reagents and storage space requirement space. Tissue microarray-FISH technique is excellent for validation of new probe, proficiency testing and quality control.

DISADVANTAGES AND PITFALLS

Artifacts due to underestimation of copy number, aneuploidy or hyperploidy, auto-fluorescence and partial hybridization failure make interpretation difficult. Signal fading is another disadvantage. Minimal residual disease or early recurrences are better detected by polymerase chain reaction (PCR). Permanent record is not possible unless CISH (chromogenic *in situ* hybridization) is used. Differences between FISH and CISH (chromogenic *in situ* hybridization) are shown in Table 14.43.

FISH PROBES AND PROBE DEVELOPMENT

Centromere Enumerating Probes (CEPs)

Initially developed centromere enumerating probes remain ideal for detection of gains and losses of whole chromosomes such as monosomy, trisomy and other polysomies.

A Whole Chromosome Paint (WCP)

A whole chromosome paint probe consists of a cocktail of DNA fragments that targets all the non-repetitive DNA sequences of an entire chromosome. As WCP covers large region, it produces a diffuse signal in interphase nuclei. WCP probes are not often used

Table 14.43: Differences between FISH and CISH (chromogenic *in situ* hybridization)

FISH	CISH
Fluorescence fades quickly, so photographic record is required	CISH provides permanent record
Modern expensive fluorescence microscope with filters is used	Bright field microscope is used
Morphological features are difficult to visualize	Histological analysis is similar to immunohistochemistry

Advanced Diagnostic Techniques

in interphase FISH. These are primarily utilized in advanced cytogenetic applications.

Locus Specific Identifier (LSI) Probes (Most Versatile)

These versatile probes target distinct chromosomal regions of interest. These utilize single copy rather than repetitive DNA sequences. Assortment of locus specific is now commercially available. Various cloning vectors such as bacterial artificial chromosomes (BACs), P1 artificial chromosome (PACs) and yeast artificial chromosome (YACs) are important sources of development of FISH probes.

Clinical Applications

Clinical applications of FISH include detection of chromosomal microdeletion, gene arrangements, breakpoint mapping of chromosomes and interphase chromosome. Clinical applications of fluorescence *in situ* hybridization (FISH) in detection of cancer associated alterations are shown in Table 14.44.

Table 14.44: Clinical applications of fluorescence *in situ* hybridization (FISH) in detection of cancer associated alterations

Systems involved	Malignant neoplasms	Alterations	Diagnostic/predictive/prognostic significance
Aneusomes and deletions			
Nervous system	Glioblastoma multiforme Oligodendroglioma Medulloblastoma Meningioma Malignant peripheral nerve sheath tumor	+7, −10 1p− with 19q− 17q−, 17q+ (i17q) NF2 (22q−) NF1 (17q−)	Diagnostic significance Diagnostic/predictive/prognostic significance Diagnostic significance Diagnostic significance Diagnostic significance
Hematologic system	Chronic lymphocytic leukemia Leukemia/myelodysplastic syndrome Diagnostic/prognostic significance Multiple myeloma	13q−, 11q−, 17q− Diagnostic/prognostic significance +8, +12; −5, −7 RB1 (−13q), TP53 (17p−)	Diagnostic/prognostic significance Diagnostic/prognostic significance Diagnostic significance
Respiratory system	Lung carcinoma	+17p, 7, or 17; 9q−	Diagnostic significance
Urogenital system	Urothelial carcinoma	+3, 7 or 17; 9p−	Diagnostic significance
Soft tissue	Malignant rhabdoid tumor Atypical rhabdoid tumor	INI1/Hsnf5 (22q−)	Diagnostic significance Diagnostic significance
Gene amplifications			
Nervous system	Glioblastoma multiforme Medulloblastoma Neuroblastoma	EGFR c-MYC N-MYC	Diagnostic significance Diagnostic/prognostic significance Diagnostic/prognostic significance
Breast	Breast carcinoma	Her2 neu	Diagnostic/predictive significance
Gastrointestinal tract	Gastric carcinoma	Her2 neu	Diagnostic/predictive significance
Translocations			
Soft tissue	Synovial sarcoma Alveolar rhabdomyosarcoma Desmoplastic round cell tumor Myxoid round cell liposarcoma Inflammatory myoblastic tumor (IMT)	SYT-SSX, SYT-BA PAX3-FKHR, FKHR-BA EWS-WT1, EWS-BA CHOP-BA ALK-TPM3, ALK-TPM4, ALK-CARS, ALK-BA	Diagnostic significance Diagnostic significance Diagnostic significance Diagnostic significance Diagnostic/prognostic significance

Contd...

Table 14.44: Clinical applications of fluorescence *in situ* hybridization (FISH) in detection of cancer associated alterations (*Contd...*)

Systems involved	Malignant neoplasms	Alterations	Diagnostic/predictive/prognostic significance
Skeletal system	Ewing's sarcoma/primitive neuroectodermal tumors	EWS-FLI1, EWS-BA	Diagnostic significance
Hematologic lymphoid system	Acute myeloid leukemia	AML1-ETO, CBFB-BA, PML-RARA, RARA-BA, MLL-BA, BCR-ABL	Diagnostic/predictive/prognostic significance
	Acute lymphoblastic leukemia	TEL-AML1, BCR-ABL, MLL-BA	Diagnostic/predictive/prognostic significance
	Chronic myelogenous leukemia	BCR-ABL	Diagnostic/predictive significance
	Myeloid and lymphoid neoplasms with eosinophilia	PDGFRA, PGDFRB, FGFR1, FIP1L1-PDGFRA IGH-CCND1, IGH-FGFR3, IGH-BA	Diagnostic minimal residual disease/ predictive/ prognostic significance
	Multiple myeloma	MYC-OGH, MYC-BA	Diagnostic significance
	Burkitt's lymphoma	IGH-BCL-2	Diagnostic significance
	Follicular lymphoma	IGH-CCND1	Diagnostic significance
	Mantle cell lymphoma	ALK-BA	Diagnostic significance
	Anaplastic large cell lymphoma MALT lymphoma	AP12-MALT1, IGH-MALT1, MALT1-BA	Diagnostic/predictive/prognostic significance
	BCL, unclassified with features in between diffuse large B cell lymphoma and Burkitt's lymphoma	IGH-BCL-2, MYC-IGH, MYC-BA	Diagnostic significance

Aneusomes and Deletions

Aneusomes represent gains or losses of whole chromosomes. Deletions refer to losses of distinct chromosomal regions, varying in size from loss of a specific gene or portion of a gene to entire chromosomal arm.

Gene Amplifications

Gene amplification occurs in one of two patterns demonstrated by FISH. Presence of amplified gene on extrachromosomal segments is known as double minutes and demonstrated numerous individual signal on FISH. Gene amplification consisting of numerous contiguously arranged gene of copies within single chromosomal region gives abnormal globular signals on fluorescence *in situ* hybridization. Her2 neu amplification is demonstrated in breast carcinoma in 20–35%. Herceptin administration is beneficial in breast carcinoma patients with Her2 neu positivity.

MYCN and c-MYC amplifications have been demonstrated in medulloblastoma.

Chromosomal Translocations

Tumor-associated chromosomal translocations demonstrated by FISH are useful diagnostic aid in primitive appearing hematopoietic and soft tissue malignancies.

Reliable probes are commercially available for most common translocations. Three types of strategies are employed to demonstrate translocations as shown in Table 14.45.

DEVELOPMENT OF FISH TEST FOR CLINICAL USE

Development on the frequencies of various translocations and breakpoints, FISH-F, FISH-BA, FISH-ES, D-FISH or combination of strategies can be designated. Newly developed FISH tests are useful to demonstrate cytogenetic abnormalities such as chromosomal gain or loss, deletion of gene or locus, gene amplification and translocation, diagnostic, prognostic and predictive response or lack of response to patient therapy.

Table 14.45: Comparison among three types of strategies to demonstrate translocations

Parameters	FISH-F	FISH-BA	FISH-ES
Probe used	Two loci-specific probes with different fluors (color tags) targeting two different partners (BCR on 22q and ABL on 9q)	Two probes localizing just proximal and distal to one of two breakpoints of interest (c-MYC at chromosome 8q24 can fuse with IGH at 14q32 in Burkitt's lymphoma)	One large probe that spans a breakpoint region demonstrated in minimal residual disease in patients with CML

Advanced Diagnostic Techniques

ENZYME-LINKED IMMUNOSORBENT ASSAY (ELISA)

OVERVIEW

Enzyme-linked immunosorbent assay (ELISA) is a sensitive plate-based assay immunochemical technique. It is also called *solid-phase enzyme immunoassay* as it employs an enzyme-linked antigen or antibody as a marker for the detection of specific protein (antigen or antibody). It is used to assess the presence of specific protein (antigen or antibody) in the given sample and its quantification. Antigen–antibody reaction is immuno-mediated reaction.

Enzyme used acts on colorless substrate and converts into colored (chromogenic) product. Color intensity of the colored product generated by enzyme is measured.

PRINCIPLE

An enzyme conjugated with an immunoglobulin reacts with a colorless substrate to generate a colored reaction product. A number of enzymes employed for ELISA, include alkaline phosphatase, horseradish peroxidase, and β-galactosidase.

Signals are developed by the action of hydrolyzing enzyme on chromogenic substrate and the optical density measured by microplate reader. General procedure of ELISA is shown in Fig. 14.19.

CLINICAL APPLICATIONS OF ELISA

Clinical applications of ELISA is shown in Table 14.46.

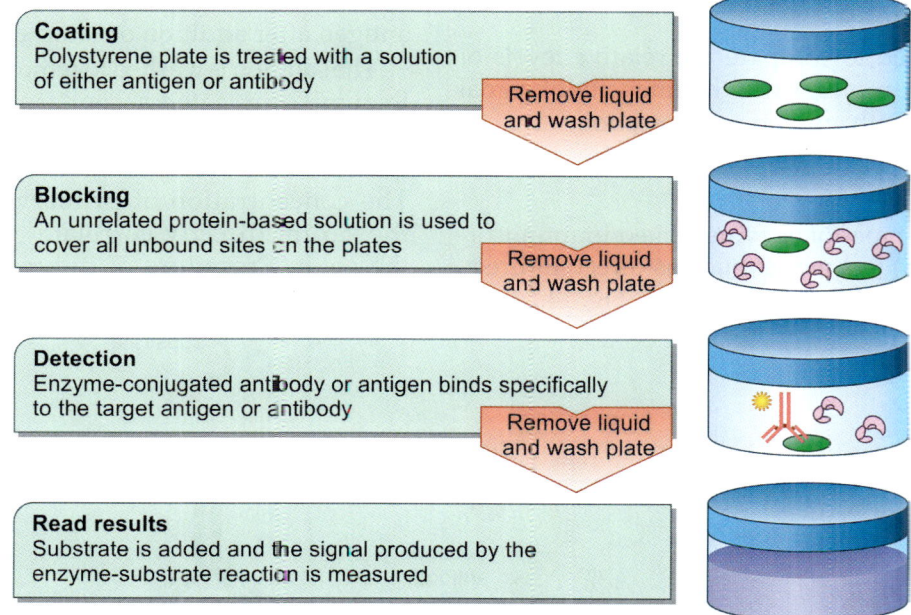

Fig. 14.19: General procedure of ELISA.

Table 14.46: Clinical applications of ELISA

Sample	Disease
Serum immunoglobulin concentrations	Clinical settings
Serum markers	Hepatitis B virus infection
Blood hormones	Pregnant women
Blood sample for antibody to infectious agents	Human immunodeficiency virus Mycobacterium tubercle bacilli *Treponema pallidum* infection (syphilis) *Vibrio cholerae* (cholera) Bird flu Lyme disease Pernicious anemia Toxoplasmosis Varicella-zoster virus (chickenpox)
Feces	Rotavirus

ELISA DATA INTERPRETATION

Enzyme-linked immunosorbent assay yields three different types of data output.

Quantitative Data

ELISA data can be interpreted in comparison to a standard curve (a serial dilution of a known, purified antigen) in order to precisely calculate the concentration of antigen in various samples.

Qualitative Data

ELISAs can also be used to achieve a yes or no answer indicating whether a particular antigen is present in a sample, as compared to a blank well containing no antigen or an unrelated control antigen.

Semiquantitative Data

ELISAs can be used to compare the relative levels of antigen in assay samples, since the intensity of signal will vary directly with antigen concentration.

TYPES OF ELISA

There are various types of enzyme-linked immunosorbent assay (ELISA) techniques such as direct, indirect, sandwich and competitive are shown in Fig. 14.20.

DIRECT ELISA

Direct ELISA uses directly labeling antibody itself. Sample of antigen is applied to the surface, often in the well of a microtiter plate. The antigen is fixed to the surface to render it immobile. The plate well and other surfaces are then coated with a blocking buffer. Antibody labeled by an enzyme (detecting antibody), usually diluted in buffer, is applied to the plate for binding to the antigen coated on plate.

INDIRECT ELISA

The indirect ELISA detects the presence of antibody in a sample. The protein antigen to be tested for is added to each well of ELISA microtiter plate; where it is given time to adhere to the plastic through charge interactions. Primary antibody present in the sample binds to the antigen after addition of sample.

The solution is washed to remove unbound antibodies. Enzyme conjugated secondary antibodies are added to the solution. The substrate for enzyme is added to quantify the primary antibody through a color change. The concentration of primary antibody present in the serum directly correlates with the intensity of the color. Procedure of indirect ELISA is shown in Fig. 14.21.

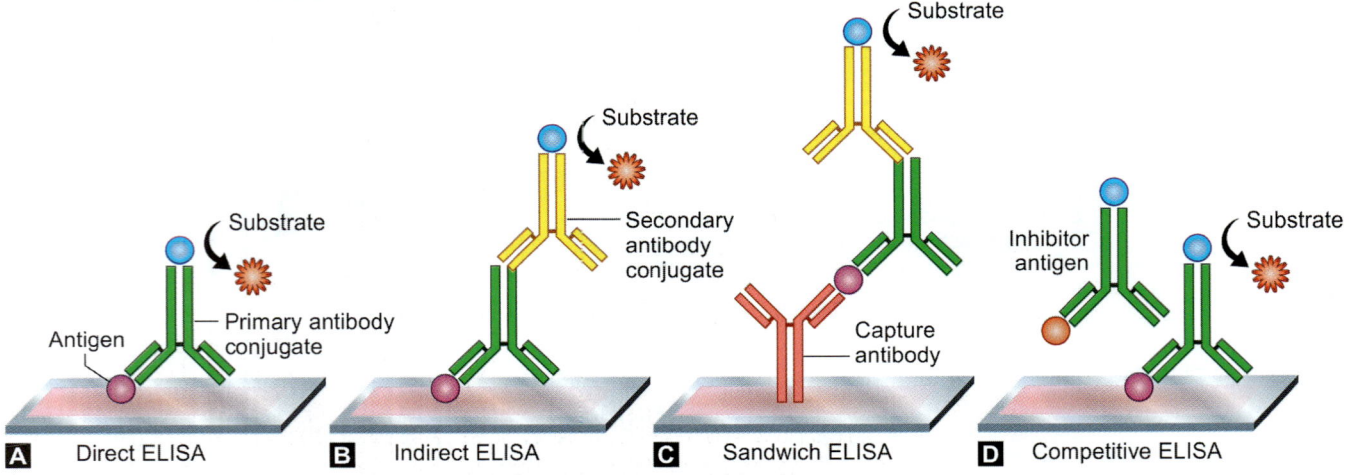

Fig. 14.20: Types of enzyme-linked immunosorbent assay (ELISA).

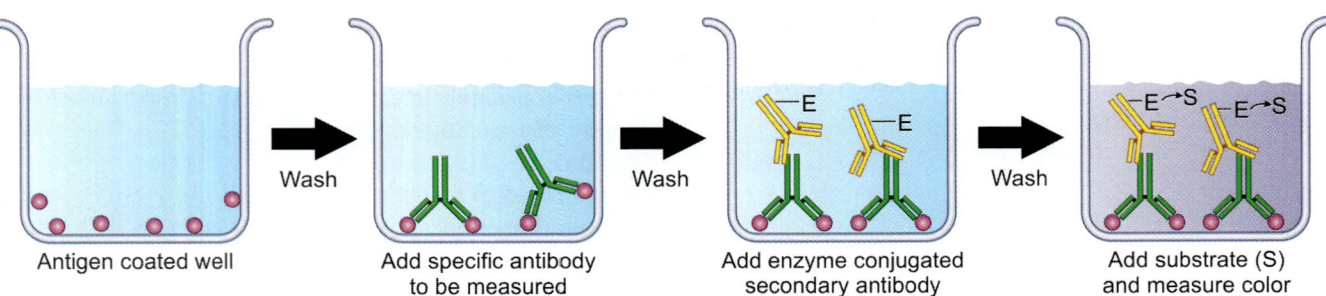

Fig. 14.21: Procedure of indirect ELISA.

Advantages

A wide variety of labeled secondary antibodies is now available commercially. The technique is versatile because many primary antibodies can be prepared in one species and the same labeled secondary antibody can be used for detection. Maximum immunoreactivity of the primary antibody is retained because it is not labeled. Sensitivity is increased because each primary antibody contains several epitopes that can be bound by the labeled secondary antibody, permitting for signal amplification.

Disadvantages

Cross reactivity may occur with the secondary antibody resulting in nonspecific signal. An extra incubation step is required in the procedure. Comparison between direct ELISA and indirect ELISA is shown in Table 14.47.

SANDWICH ELISA

The ELISA plate is coated with antibody to detect specific antigen. Any nonspecific binding sites on the surface are blocked by using bovine serum albumin. Antigen-containing sample is applied to the plate. Unbound antigen is removed by washing. Enzyme-linked primary antibodies are applied as detection antibodies which also bind specifically to the antigen. Then the unbound antibody-enzyme conjugates are removed by washing. A chemical substance is added which is converted by the enzyme into a colored product, absorbency of which is measured to determine the presence and quantity of antigen. Sandwich ELISA technique is shown in Fig. 14.22.

Advantages

Sandwich ELISA technique is highly specific because antigen/analysate is specially captured and detected. It is suitable for complex (or crude/impure) samples as the antigen does not require purification prior to measurement. It is flexible and sensitive, both direct and indirect detection methods can be used.

COMPETITIVE ELISA

Competitive ELISA technique is highly sensitive technique even when the specific detecting antibody is present in relatively small amounts. The technique depends on the competitive reaction between the sample antigen and antigen bound to the wells of microtiter plate with the primary antibody. Antigen and antibody are labeled with enzyme and allowed to compete with unlabeled ones (in patient's serum) for binding to the

Table 14.47: Comparison between direct ELISA and indirect ELISA

ELISA	Direct ELISA	Indirect ELISA
Advantages	Quick as only one antibody and fewer steps are used Cross reactivity of secondary antibody is eliminated	A wide variety of labeled secondary antibodies are available commercially Maximum immunoreactivity of primary antibody is retained because it is not labeled Increased sensitivity allowing signal amplification, as each primary antibody contains many epitopes bound by labeled secondary antibody Different visualization markers can be used with the same primary antibody
Disadvantages	Immunoreactivity of primary antibody may be adversely affected by labeling with enzymes or tags Minimal signal amplification occurs Labeling primary antibody for each specific ELISA system is time-consuming and expensive	Cross reactivity might occur with secondary antibody resulting in nonspecific signals Extra incubation step is required in the procedure

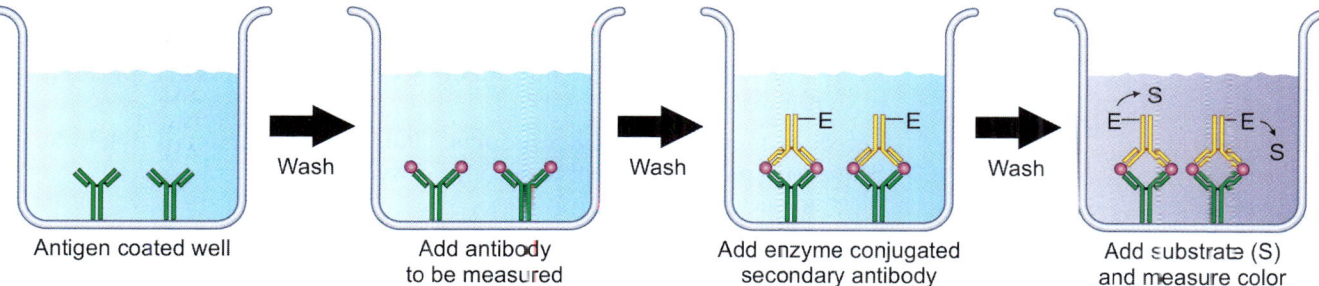

Fig. 14.22: Sandwich ELISA technique.

same target. Hydrolysis signal from Ag–Ab complex (enzyme-labeled) is measured. Antigen or antibody in serum is then calculated.

There is no need to remove the excess/unbound Ag or Ab from the reaction plate or tubes. Concentration of color is inversely proportional to the amount of antigen presents in the sample. Competitive ELISA technique is shown in Fig. 14.23.

NONCOMPETITIVE ELISA

Excess/unbound Ag or Ab must be removed before every step of reactions. It can be of various types—direct ELISA, indirect ELISA, sandwich ELISA and Ab capture ELISA (similar to sandwich ELISA but in first step, anti-IgM or IgG is coated on the plate and then antibodies in patient serum are allowed to capture in next step).

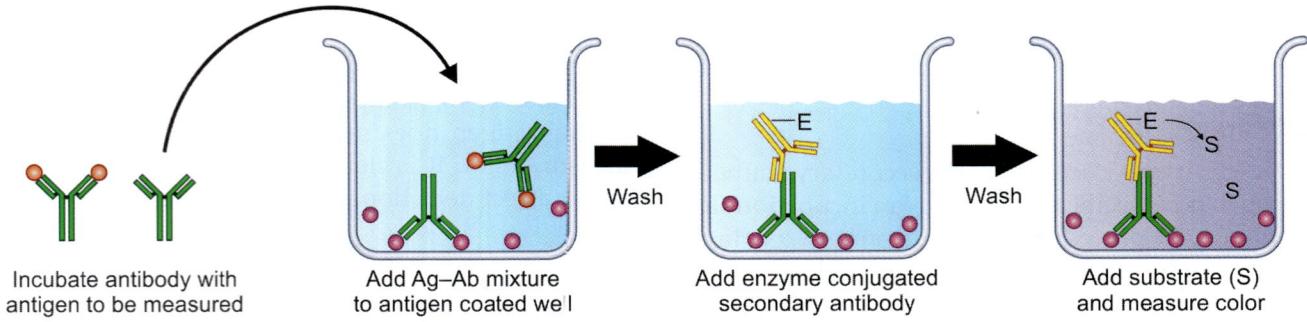

Fig. 14.23: Competitive ELISA technique.

METHODS FOR DNA SEQUENCES

Molecular analyses are used to determine *diagnosis, prognosis,* the detection of minimal residual disease, and the diagnosis of hereditary predisposition to cancer. Molecular profiling of tumors by cDNA arrays can determine expression of large segments of the genome at once and can be useful in molecular stratification of otherwise identical tumors for the purpose of treatment. Methods used for detection of gene mutations are shown in Table 14.48. Techniques used to analyze DNA, RNA and proteins are shown in Table 14.49.

POLYMERASE CHAIN REACTION

Most molecular tests performed in surgical pathology focus on somatic or acquired DNA variations in the cells of the disease process. These tests provide information of diagnostic, prognostic and predictive indicators.

Table 14.48: Methods used for detection of gene mutations

Technique	Principle	Type of gene mutation detection
Cytogenetic analysis	Unique visual appearance of various chromosomes	Numerical structural abnormalities in chromosomes
Fluorescence *in situ* hybridization (FISH)	Hybridization to chromosomes with fluorescent labeled probes	Numerical structural abnormalities in chromosomes
Southern blot technique	Hybridization with genomic probe or cDNA probe after digestion of high molecular DNA	Detection of large deletion, insertion, rearrangement
Polymerase chain reaction	Amplification of DNA	Expansion of triplet repeats, variable number of tandem repeats (VNTR), gene rearrangement, translocation
Reverse transcriptase PCR (RT-PCR)	Reverse transcription, amplification of DNA segment, absence or reduction of mRNA transcription	Analyze expressed mRNA (cDNA) sequence detect loss of expression
DNA sequences	Direct sequencing of PCR products. Sequencing of DNA segment cloned into plasmid vectors	Point mutation, small deletions and insertions
Restriction fragment length polymorphism (RFLP)	Detection of altered restriction pattern of genome: DNA Southern blot or PCR products	Point mutation, small deletions and insertions

Table 14.49: Techniques used to analyze DNA, RNA and proteins

Technique	Sample analyzed	Gel used	Purpose
Southern blot	DNA	Yes	Detection of DNA changes
Northern blot	RNA	Yes	Analysis of mRNA amount and size
Western blot	Protein	Yes	Analysis of protein content
Allele specific oligonucleotides	DNA	No	Detection of DNA mutations
Microarray	RNA or cDNA	No	Measurement of many mRNA at one time
ELISA	Protein or antibodies	No	Detection of proteins (antigens) or antibodies

Polymerase chain reaction is quick, reliable and sensitive technique. It has become a central diagnostic toll in clinical molecular genetic testing.

SPECIMENS REQUIRED

Nuclear acids are used for molecular testing by PCR. Specimen requirements are dictated by the disease process. Sources of nucleic acids are peripheral blood, bone marrow aspirate, fresh or frozen tissue stored at −200° to −700°C, formalin-fixed paraffin-embedded tissue (FFPE), cytology specimens, enriched population of cells from flow cytometry.

Transport of these specimens on ice reduces cell lysis, minimizes nuclease activity and reduces nucleic acid degradation. Peripheral blood and bone marrow aspirate are added anticoagulants. Samples for molecular cytogenetic testing are shown in Table 14.50.

TISSUE MICRODISSECTION

Microdissection enables the targeted collection of cells or tissues from slide-mounted cytologic specimens or frozen or FFPE tissues sections. After that sample tissues may be treated for nucleic acids or protein extraction. Microdissection is carried out by *dissecting microtome* (simplest method) and *laser capture microdissection* (LCM) requiring a specialized microscopy. It is primarily a research application but also is useful in surgical pathology practice.

NUCLEIC ACID EXTRACTIONS

Extraction of nucleic acids from pathology samples involves cell lysis followed by selective DNA or RNA isolation and a quantitative or qualitative assessment. Pathology samples used for molecular analysis include *tissue samples* (fresh or formalin-fixed, paraffin-embedded, i.e. FFPE); *body fluids* (amniotic fluid, saliva, stools, urine); buccal and cervical scrapes; fine needle aspirates; peripheral blood, cell cultures and hair root.

DNA Extraction Methods

Classic methods are time-consuming (about 3 days) and require relatively large quantities of tissues (100 mg to 1 g). Numerous extraction kits are now available that use glass-fiber filters that selectively bind DNA after tissue treatments with a protease and chaotropic buffers (which disrupt protein and DNA secondary structures). With these kits, pure DNA recovery from diverse pathology samples is possible within several hours. Nowadays, automated DNA extraction platforms are available for the processing of multiple patient samples.

Table 14.50: Samples for molecular cytogenetic testing

Prenatal/postnatal period and cancer genetic sampling	Sample
Prenatal period	Amniotic fluid Chorionic villus (fresh or formalin-fixed) Fetal cord blood
Postnatal period	Peripheral blood Product of conception (fresh or formalin-fixed) Skin biopsy fresh or formalin-fixed)
Cancer cytogenetic sampling	Bone marrow Oncology blood Solid tumor Lymph node Core biopsy Pleural effusion

RNA Extraction Methods

Classic methods cause rapid homogenization of large quantities of fresh tissues in protease and guanidinium thiocyanate solution to denature ubiquitous endogenous RNases. Current methods allow relatively rapid (1 day) recovery of RNA, again after tissue homogenization in a chaotropic guanidinium salt solution that leaves RNA contained in an aqueous phase and protein and DNA in an organic phase.

Other Characteristics

Extraction from fresh tissue specimens gives high-integrity nucleic acids. Next best option is preservation of extraction from tissues in liquid nitrogen (commercially available storage reagents, e.g. RNA later, ambion). DNA and RNA extracts from FFPE block tissues tend to be degraded with block age. The concentration and purity of extracted nucleic acids are assessed spectrophotometrically (*NanoDrop spectrophotometer*). Nucleic acid integrity can be estimated by comparing nucleic acid fragment size against a molecular weight ladder after agarose gel electrophoresis.

Nucleic Acids Storage

DNA is generally stored at 4°C for assays performed within 1 week to 1 month of extraction and in aliquots at −20°C or −80°C for long-term storage. Repeated freeze-thawing may lead to DNA degradation. RNA is more labile than DNA and is susceptible to degradation by RNases. RNA is stored at −20°C for short-term use and at −80°C or under liquid nitrogen for long-term use.

PCR Technique

Polymerase chain reaction (PCR) generates thousands to millions of copies of a particular sequence. It is currently used in biomedical research laboratories for the diagnosis of hereditary and infectious diseases. Essential ingredients of PCR are shown in Table 14.51. It is a method for the *in vitro* amplification of DNA involving automated cycles of denaturation, annealing, and extension or synthesis performed in a thermocycler.

Basic Steps of PCR

Basic steps of PCR are denaturation, annealing and extension (Table 14.51, Figs 14.24 and 14.25).

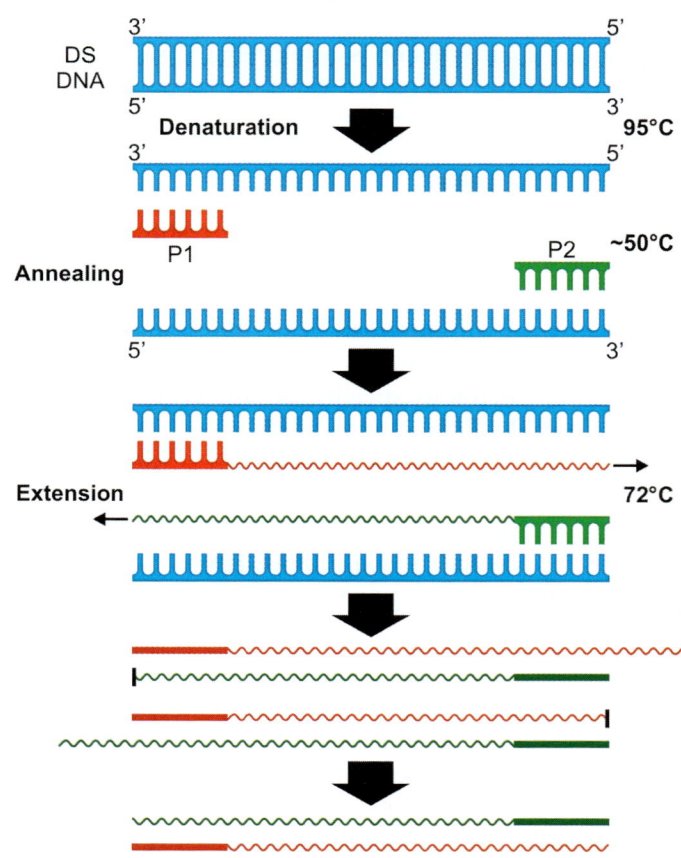

Fig. 14.24: Polymerase chain reaction showing denaturation, annealing and extension.

Table 14.51: Essential ingredients of PCR

Essential ingredients	Characteristics
Buffer	pH is typically maintained using a Tris-HCl-based buffer Other ingredients include KCl (aid primer template annealing), bovine serum albumin (BSA) and nonionic detergents (aid Taq DNA polymerase enzyme stability)
DNase or RNase free pure water	Final PCR reaction volumes vary from 10 to 50 μl
Magnesium cations (Mg^{2++})	Stabilizes the interaction between the oligonucleotide primer, template DNA and Taq DNA polymerase enzyme
dNTP (deoxyribonucleoside triphosphate)	-
Oligonucleotide primers	18 to 25 bases in length
Template DNA	Sample amount in a reaction can range from 1 ng to 1 μg
Thermostable DNA polymerase enzymes	Taq DNA polymerase extracted from Thermus aquaticus isolated from a hot-springs dwelling bacterium of the Deinococcus-Thermus phylum

Advanced Diagnostic Techniques

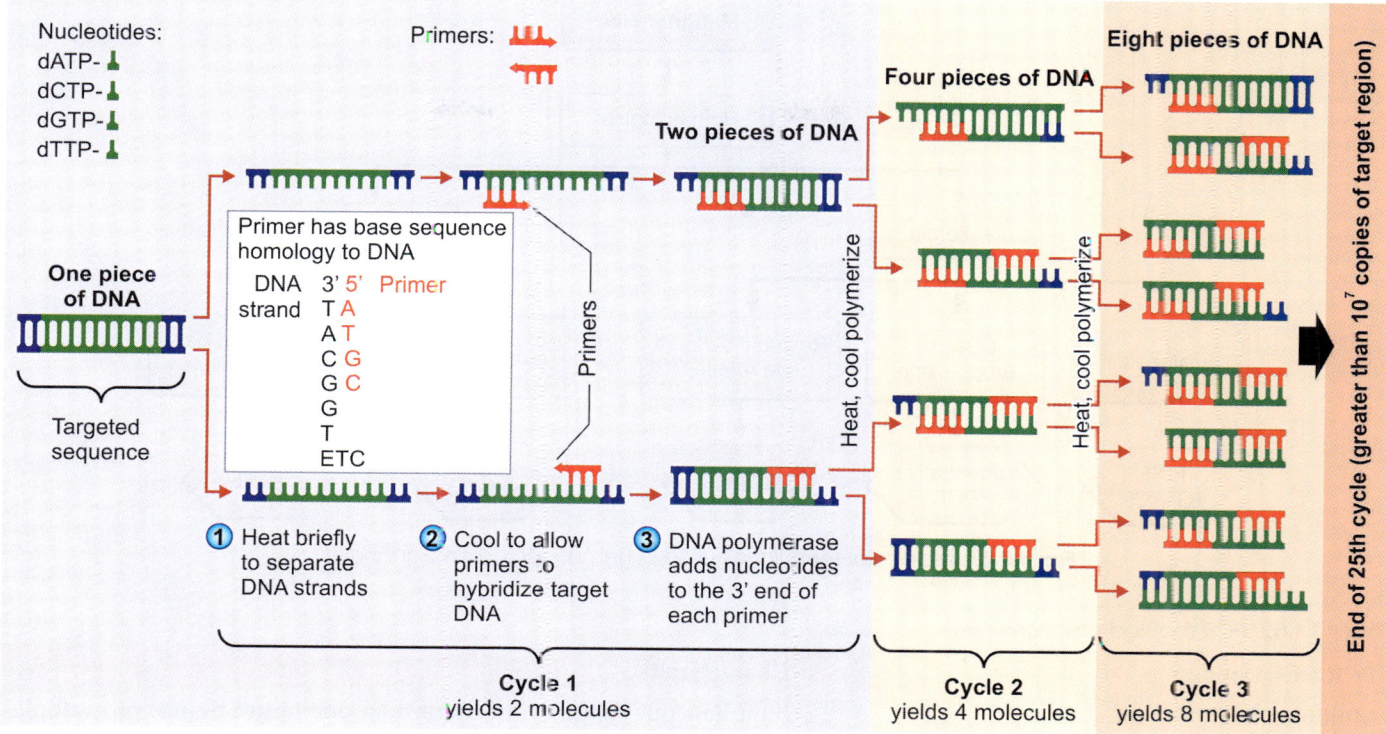

Fig. 14.25: Polymerase chain reaction technique.

Denaturation step: Sample specimen DNA is rendered single-stranded by heating to 94° to 98°C.

Annealing step: In this step, oligonucleotide primers hybridize with the target sequences. The annealing temperature depends on deoxyribonucleoside triphosphate (dNTP) composition of the primers and is typically in the range of 40° to 60°C.

Extension step: The extension step (72°C) leads to DNA synthesis (5'→3') by thermostable DNA polymerase of a new DNA strand. DNA amplification is accomplished by repetitive cycle (30 to 50 times) of the denaturation, annealing, and extension steps.

The time period for each of the denaturation, annealing and extension steps can vary from 10 seconds to more than 1 minute. It depends on reaction volume size, amplicon base composition and length, thermostable DNA polymerase activity (about 1000 bp are extended per minute) and hardware specifications.

PCR Tests in Pathology

PCR tests are performed to detect genetic disorders, BCR-ABL translocation in CML, gene fusion detection (EWS/FLI1) in Ewing's sarcoma, hereditary nonpolyposis colorectal cancer (HNPCC) mutation analysis and detection of circulating tumor or pathogen.

Molecular techniques used in non-hematological and hematological malignancies are shown in Figs 14.26 and 14.27.

VARIATIONS OF PCR

PCR method variations are shown in Table 14.52.

Other Nucleic Acids Amplification Methods

Other nucleic acids amplification methods are shown in Table 14.53.

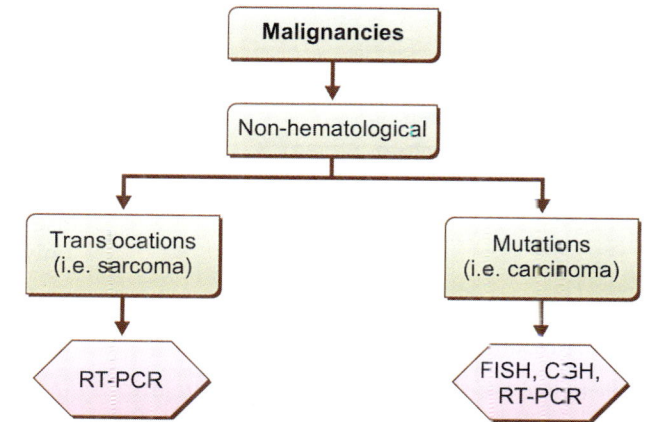

Fig. 14.26: Molecular techniques used in non-hematological malignancies.

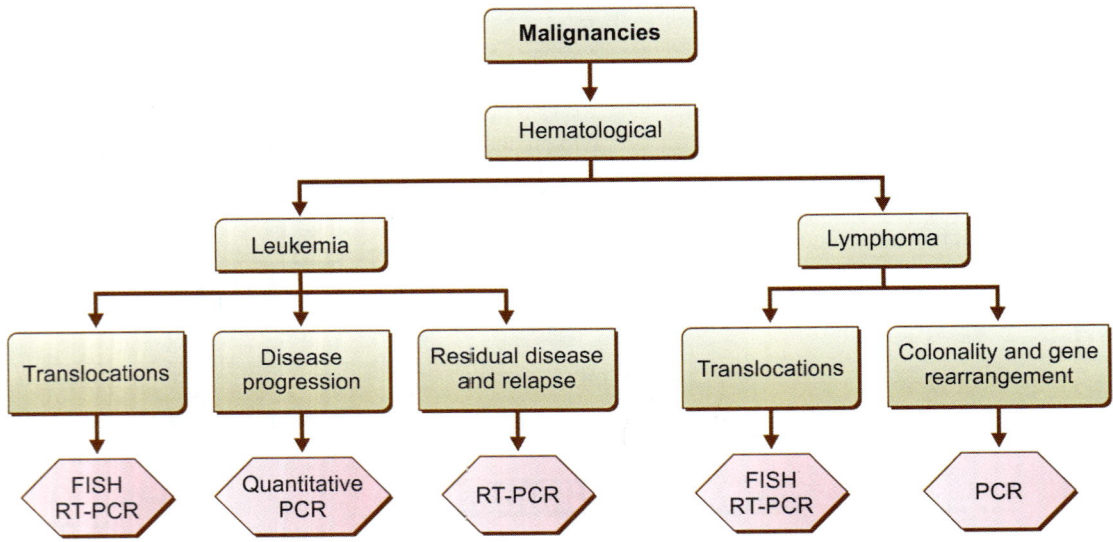

Fig. 14.27: Molecular techniques used in hematological malignancies.

Table 14.52: PCR method variations

PCR variations	Characteristics
Multiplex PCR	Simultaneous detection of more than one target by use of multiple primer pair sets
Consensus PCR	Used to amplify a single target that has variable sequences or multiple targets that have similar (common) sequences
Degenerate PCR	Also used in the amplification of a variable sequence target
Nested PCR	Used for improved PCR sensitivity and specificity
Reverse transcription PCR (RT-PCR)	For investigation of RNA expression through PCR, first step is conversion of total RNA or mRNA into single-stranded complementary DNA (cDNA) as thermostable DNA polymerases require DNA as a substrate
Real-time quantitative PCR (qPCR)	Used for the accurate quantification of a DNA or RNA and cDNA target in a sample (note: In standard PCR/end-point PCR, final product is obtained after 30 to 50 cycles. Although end-point PCR can be semiquantitative, it is essentially a qualitative assay)
Allele-specific PCR (AS-PCR)	Allows direct detection of any point mutation in human DNA by analyzing PCR products in an ethidium bromide stained agarose or ployacrylamide gel
PCR amplification of specific alleles (PASA)	Generally applicable technique for detection of known point mutations, small deletions, insertions and polymorphisms
Long and accurate PCR (LA-PCR)	Allows the amplification of sequences 5 to >20 kb in length
Amplification refractory mutation system (ARMS)	Simple method for detecting any mutation involving single base change, uses sequence-specific primers that allow amplification of test DNA only when the target allele is contained within the sample

Signal Amplification Techniques

Previously described techniques directly amplify target nucleic acid sequences to a threshold of detection. Alternative strategy is to employ amplification technology at the level of detection, where a nonamplified nucleic acid is targeted using a probe and an amplified signal is generated from the probe.

These techniques are less susceptible to false positive data and used in *multiple ligation-dependent probe amplification* (MLPA) and hybrid capture (Table 14.54).

Table 14.53: Other nucleic acids amplification methods

Amplification methods	Description	Applications
Transcription-mediated amplification (TMA)	Amplification of RNA targets, including species-specific rRNA sequences	Detection of *Chlamydia trachomatis*, *Neisseria gonorrhoeae*, *Mycobacterium tuberculosis* and hepatitis C virus (HCV)
Nucleic acid sequence-based amplification (NASBA)	Isothermal amplification of a DNA or RNA target, identical to TMA but uses a separate RNase H enzyme and fluorescence resonance energy transfer (FRET) based detection technology	Detection of CMV and human immunodeficiency virus (HIV) RNA
Strand displacement amplification (SDA)	Requires a DNA polymerase that has *strand displacement* activity	Detection of *Chlamydia trachomatis*, *Neisseria gonorrhoeae*, and *Legionella pneumophila*
Ligase chain reaction (LCR)	Involves cycles of DNA denaturation and annealing and uses a thermostable DNA ligase	Detection of *Chlamydia trachomatis* and *Neisseria gonorrhoeae*

Table 14.54: Signal amplification techniques

Techniques	Description	Applications
Multiple ligation-dependent probe amplification (MLPA)	Involves ligation of two oligonucleotides hybridized immediately adjacent to each other at the target of interest. The ligation product is then amplified by PCR	Detection of familial cancers (*BRCA1* and *BRCA2* testing, colon polyposis (APC), retinoblastoma, Wilms' tumor); prenatal and postnatal screening; syndromes (Turner and Klinefelter syndromes)
Hybrid capture	Involves an *in vitro* solution hybridization of a target DNA sequence with an RNA probe, followed by a signal amplification step	Screening of 13 high-risk HPV genotypes (16, 18, 31, 33, etc.); detection and quantitation of CMV, *Chlamydia trachomatis*, *Neisseria gonorrhoeae*, HBV and herpes simplex virus (HSV)

SOUTHERN BLOT TECHNIQUE

Southern blot technique was developed by *Dr EM Southern* in 1975 as a method for transferring DNA out of an agarose slab gel onto a solid support like a nitrocellulose or nylon membrane.

The method involves the use of *restriction endonucleases* which cut or restrict genomic DNA into differently sized fragments. These fragments are size-fractionated by gel electrophoresis. After transfer, the membrane is hybridized with a labeled probe specific to the target sequence of interest. The technique generally requires relatively large quantities of high-molecular-weight DNA (Fig. 14.28).

APPLICATIONS

Southern blotting can be used to detect chromosomal rearrangements, DNA amplifications, deletions and loss of heterozygosity. It can be used in combination with PCR. This technique is mostly used in RFLP (*restriction fragment length polymorphism*) analysis.

Clinical applications of Southern blot technique are mentioned as under:
- Autosomal dominant ataxia evaluation
- Myotonic dystrophy evaluation
- Epstein-Barr virus clonality assay
- Beckwith-Wiedemann syndrome
- Fragile X syndrome
- Hemophilia A analysis for inversion, deletion, and carrier
- Ig gene rearrangement detection in B cell lymphoma and minimal residual disease
- T cell receptor gene rearrangement
- *MLH1, MSH2, MSH6* deletion/duplication screening
- Partial Duchenne muscular dystrophy (DMD) deletion/duplication assay.

ADVANTAGES

Southern blot technique has advantages over PCR when available sequence data are insufficient to design PCR primers specific to the site of a chromosomal

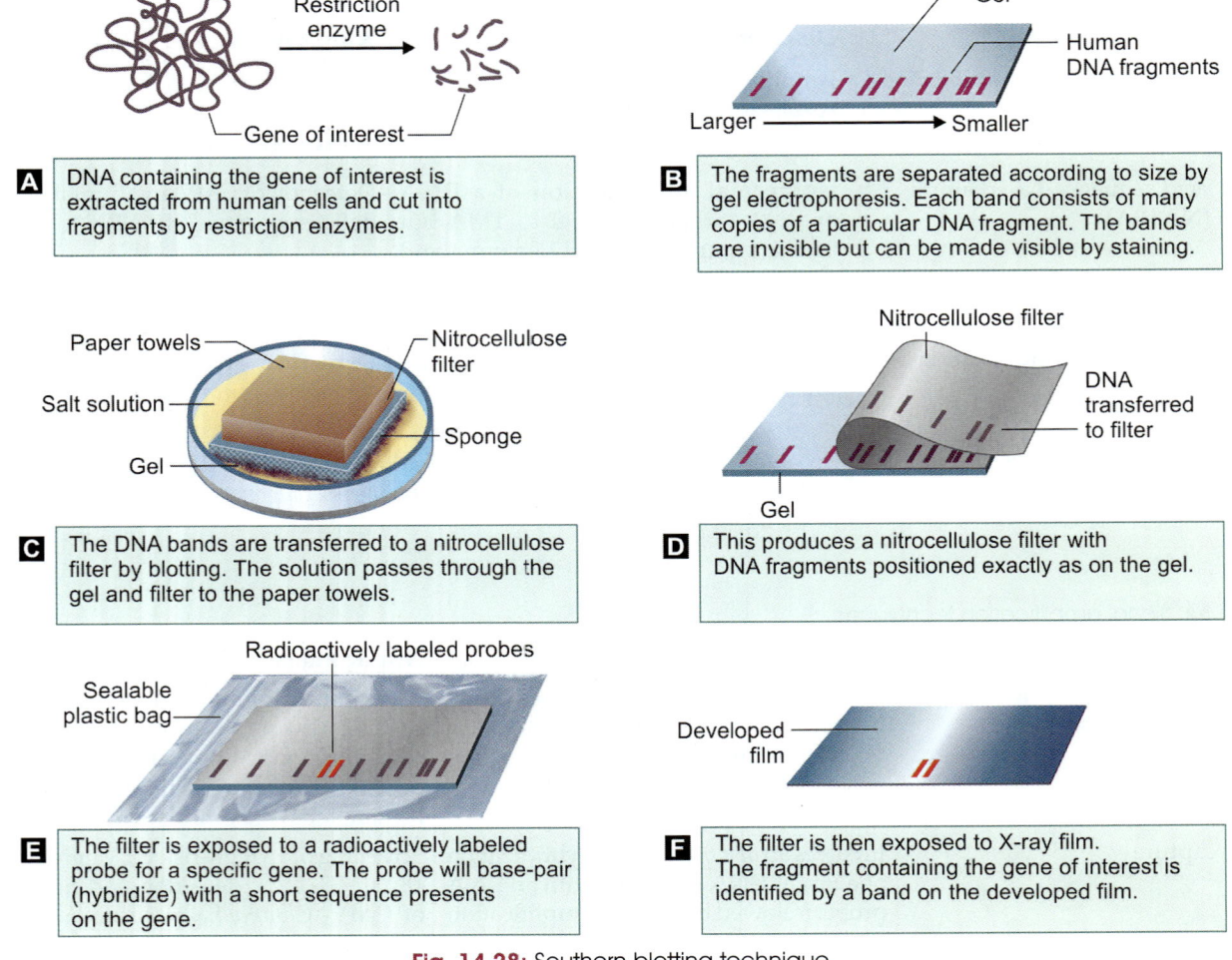

Fig. 14.28: Southern blotting technique.

rearrangement. Comparison between PCR and Southern blotting is shown in Table 14.55.

DISADVANTAGES

Southern blot technique requires large quantities of DNA. It is a time-consuming process.

NORTHERN BLOT TECHNIQUE

Northern blot technique is used in the analysis of mRNA expression. The mRNA constitutes up to 5% of the total cellular RNA.

Table 14.55: Comparison between PCR and Southern blotting

Features	PCR	Southern blot
DNA amount	≤1 μg	At least 30 μg per probe
Restriction enzyme digestion	Not needed	Required
DNA quality and size	Can be severely degraded and 100–300 bp DNA	High quality DNA and at least 20 kb
Gel electrophoresis	Polyacrylamide gel required	Agarose gel required
Detection methods	Fluorescence dye, silver stain, chemiluminescence radioactivity	Usually radioactivity, less often chemiluminescence
Time	1–2 days	1–2 weeks
False negative results	Common for B cell lymphomas, but uncommon in T cell lymphomas	Rare
Sensitivity	1 cell per 1000 cells	1–5% of total DNA

PROCEDURE

Extracted mRNA is denatured with formaldehyde or glyoxal to prevent the formation of secondary RNA structures. The RNA digestion into smaller fragments is not required as native mRNA fragment sizes range from about 300 to 12,000 nucleotides (average size is 1,000 to 3,000 nucleotides). After agarose gel electrophoresis, RNA is transferred to a membrane by a capillary, vacuum, or electrotransfer process, and then the membrane is hybridized with a labeled probe to the gene target. The resulting data indicate whether a gene is overexpressed or underexpressed or if an abnormally sized transcript is expressed.

DISADVANTAGES

Northern blotting is time-consuming technique. The method requires relatively large amounts of high-integrity RNA. The technique requires a high level of laboratory skill. Differences between Southern blotting and Northern blotting are shown in Table 14.56.

Table 14.56: Differences between Southern blotting and Northern blotting

Features	Southern blotting	Northern blotting
Naming of blotting	Named after inventor Southern	It is a misnomer
Separation	DNA	RNA
Denaturation step	Required	Not required
Membrane used	Nitrocellulose filter membrane	Amino benzyloxymethyl filter paper
Hybridization	DNA-DNA	RNA-DNA

TISSUE MICROARRAY

TISSUE MICROARRAY TECHNIQUE

Tissue microarray technology involves core needle biopsies of multiple tissues constructed in the same paraffin embedded tissue block by inserting tissue core from the donor's block and inserted into recipient's block. It is a new method used to analyze several hundred tissues, especially tumor samples at a single slide by *in situ* technology. Difficulty with paraffin-embedded tissues is due to antigenic changes in proteins and mRNA degradation induced by the fixation and embedding processes.

It allows rapid visualization of morphology and molecular targets (DNA/RNA/protein) in thousand's of tissue specimens at a time. It correlates gene and protein expression patterns in intact tissues with clinical outcomes. Tissue microarray technology is shown in Fig. 14.29. Tissue microarray is described under the following headings.

SELECTION OF DONOR'S BLOCK

Primary donor paraffin-embedded tissue block may be obtained from surgical pathology, autopsy or research material. Ideally donor block should contain 2–3 mm thickness of target tissue to permit large number of histological sections (usually 100–300 sections) from it. A morphologically representative area of interest within the donor block is identified under microscope using a hematoxylin and eosin stained section on a glass slide as a guide.

CREATION OF NEW PARAFFIN-EMBEDDED TISSUE BLOCK

The tissue cores are removed from the donor and inserted into a *recipient* paraffin block. Using a precise spacing pattern, tissues can be inserted at high density, with up to 1,000 tissue cores in a single paraffin block.

CUTTING TISSUE SECTIONS

Sections from this block that are cut with a microtome are placed onto standard glass slides that can then be used or *in situ* analysis. Depending on the overall depth of tissue remaining in the donor blocks, tissue arrays can generate between 100 and 500 sections.

RECORDING OF SOURCE DATA

Recording of source tissue data comprises clinical history, metastatic disease, staging, treatment history, tumor gross description such as size, shape, infiltration of margins and core tissue.

TISSUE PROCESSING

Marked slide and paraffin wax block are transferred to the person who will make the array. Then the core biopsies from selected tissue are taken either manually or by automated arrays: first generation, second generation and third generation. TMA cores of 0.6 mm diameter are taken and intercore space of 0.8 mm is kept.

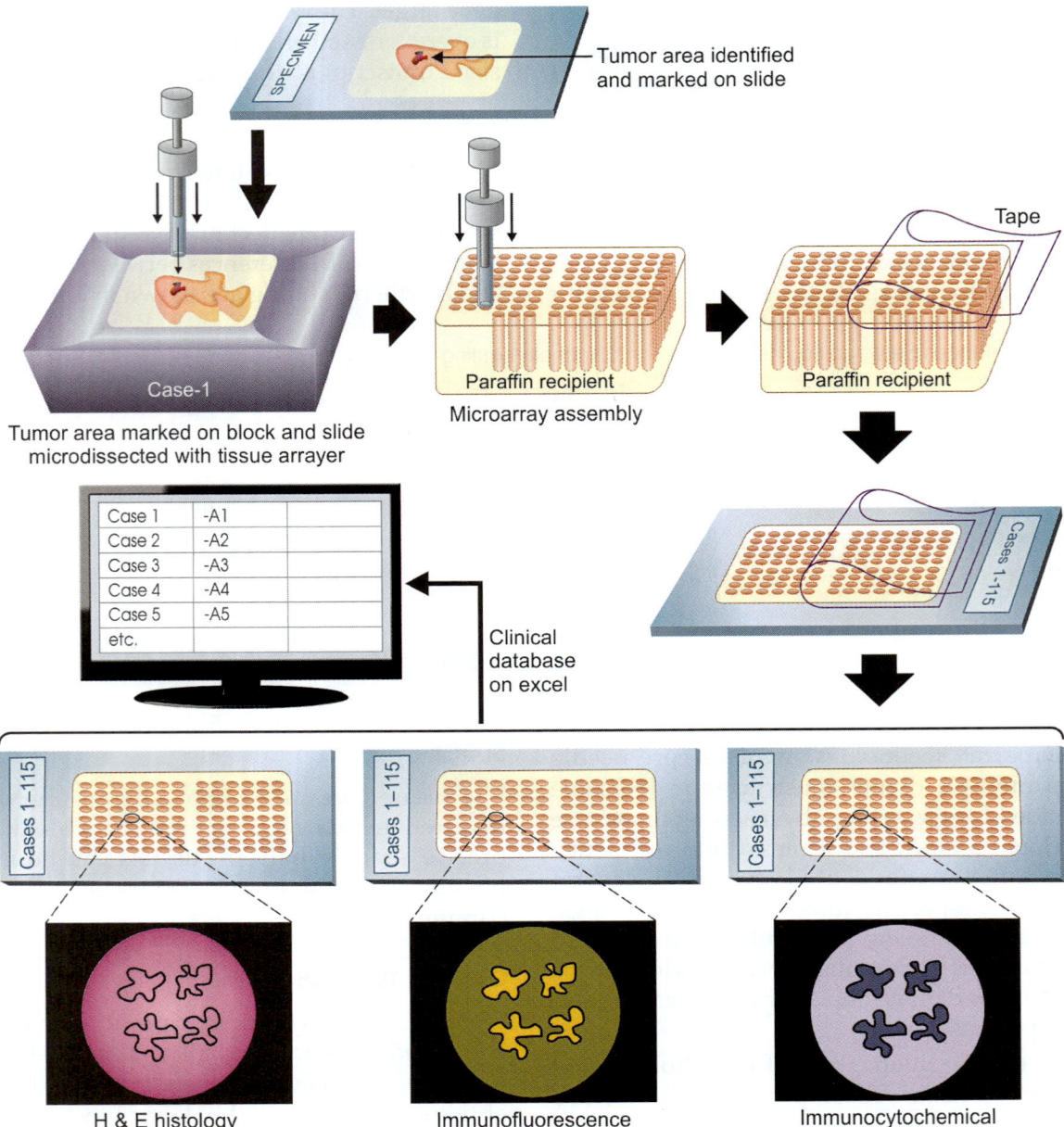

Fig. 14.29: Tissue microarray technology.

This size just fills the field of 40X objective. The core thickness should be 2–3 mm uniformly, if this is variable some sections of the block face will have empty spaces.

ARRAY DESIGN

The cores are placed in X-Y axis positioning. While scoring TMA microscopically, it is easy to loose place when >10 cores in either axis. In such cases, sub arrays of 5 rows and 5 columns can be made with empty spaces between arrays. Histological sections/blocks can be stored for 70 years at room temperature as antigenicity of most tissues stored in paraffin wax is retained. However, form RNA ISH sections stored up to 1 year are best.

SECTIONING OF ARRAYS

Most TMA cores are slip fit into recipient block holes without any bonding material between cores and wax. Thus, sections cut from block face have nothing to hold cores in place. Ideally melting temperature and hardness of donor and recipient block's paraffin wax should match.

HEMATOXYLIN AND EOSIN STAINING

This stain permits visualization of morphology of area of interest from different donor blocks in one slide. Also since morphology of tissues may change with more sections from the TMA; 1st and every

50th section of TMA block may be stained with H&E to monitor morphology and representability of the specimens.

ANALYSIS OF TISSUE SECTIONS

Once constructed tissue microarrays can be used with a wide range of techniques including histochemical staining, immunohistochemical/immunofluorescent staining or *in situ* hybridization or *in situ* hybridization for either DNA or mRNA.

IMAGE CAPTURING

Regular bright field microscope can be used for analysis and scoring TMA slides. It can image 8–10 slides on a single run in each of bright field, dark field and 3 color fluorescent mode if needed and view them simultaneously. It can also do morphometric analysis of these images.

APPLICATIONS OF TMA

TMA is an emerging tool for research which has high throughput, uniform reaction conditions and experimental uniformity. It does not destroy the original block for diagnosis and economizes the use of reagents. Tissue microarray also facilitates data recording and linking to clinical data. Main application of TMA is understanding tumor biology.

There are different types of tissue microarrays: multi-tumor TMA, progression TMA and prognosis TMA. In multi-tumor TMA, samples obtained from multiple tumors are analyzed for role of newly identified genes in normal and neoplastic tissues. Progression TMA is used to study molecular changes in different stages of one particular tumor type. Prognosis TMA comprises samples from tumors with available clinical follow-up data.

> **Immunohistochemistry**
>
> Immunohistochemistry measures the detection of protein antigens. One IHC experiment can give quantitative (fluorescence intensity value) and semiquantitative (pathologist's score) data.

FISH

FISH is used for analysis of genetic alterations. A single hybridization provides visualization of specific gene change in up to 1,000 tissues.

mRNA *in situ* Hybridization

This detects mRNA transcripts in multiple different tissues.

DNA Microarray

DNA microarray can be used along with TMA to generate information regarding DNA in different solid tissue cancers.

HIGH PERFORMANCE LIQUID CHROMATOGRAPHY (HPLC)

HPLC TECHNOLOGY

High performance liquid chromatography (HPLC) is one of the commonest laboratory investigations done for the identification of globin chain synthesis. It is a separation technique that involves the injection of a small volume of liquid sample into a tube packed with tiny particles (3 to 5 μm in diameter called the stationary phase). Here individual components of the sample move down the packed tube (column) with a liquid (mobile phase) forced through the column by high pressure delivered by a pump.

Schematic of high performance liquid chromatography is shown in Fig. 14.30.

PRINCIPLE

Cation exchange HPLC is a process in which a mixture of hemoglobins with net positive charge are separated by their adsorption onto a negatively charged stationary phase in a chromatography column followed by their elution by a liquid mobile phase containing increasing concentrations of cations flowing through the column.

APPLICATIONS

Hemoglobins separated by this way are optically identified in the eluate. The quantification is done by computing the area under the corresponding peak in the elution profile. Different hemoglobins will have different affinity for the stationary phase. Hemoglobins with strong positive charge have higher affinity for stationary phase and appear in the elute later than other hemoglobins.

Retention time is the time taken by normal and variant hemoglobins to appear in the eluate. Retention times known for many of the normal and variant hemoglobins are shown in Table 14.57.

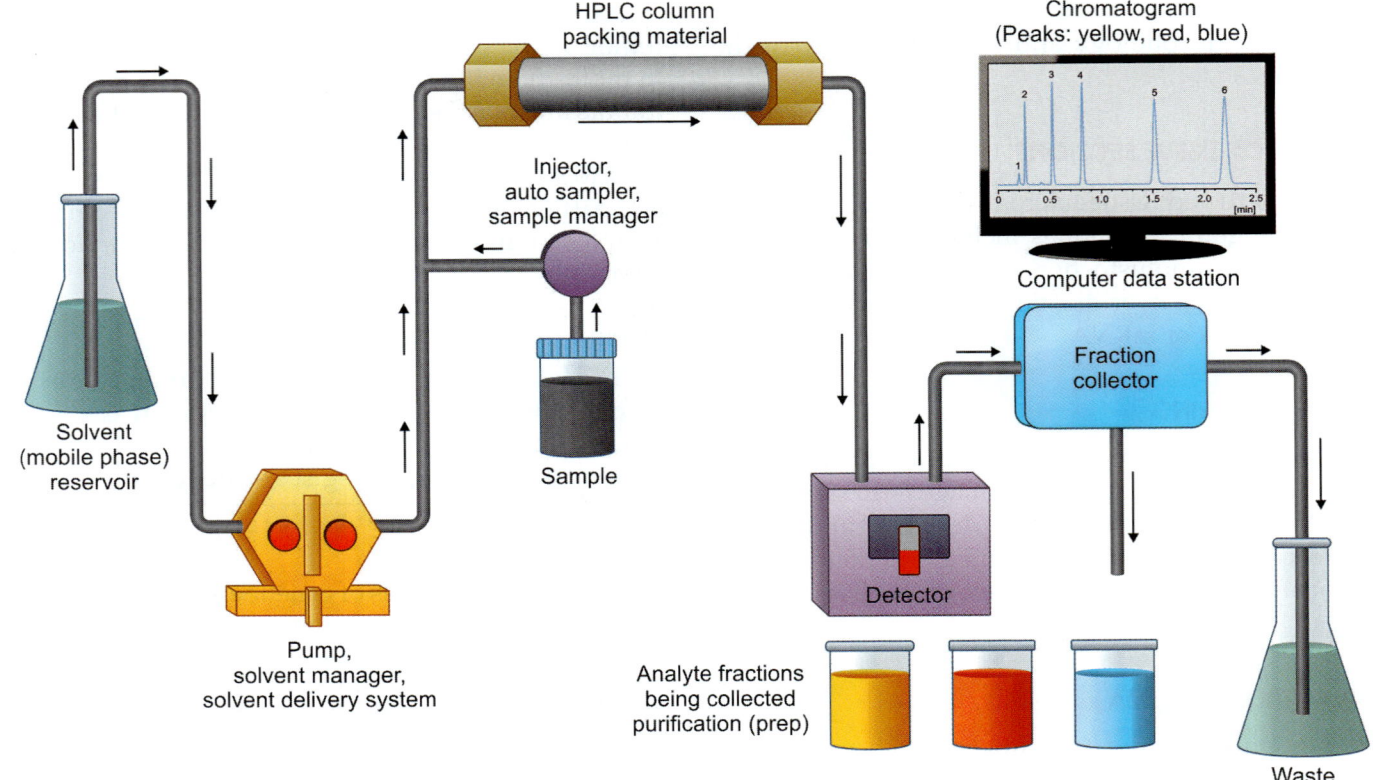

Fig. 14.30: Schematic of high performance liquid chromatography.

Table 14.57: Retention times of common normal and variant hemoglobins

Window	Retention time (minutes)	Hemoglobins that appear in the window
	Peak within first minute	HbH, Bart's hemoglobin, bilirubin, acetylated HbF
F	1.10	HbF
A	2.50	HbA, glycosylated S
A2	3.60	HbA_2, D—Iran, E—lepore
D	4.10	D—Punjab
S	4.50	S
C	5.10	C: Constant spring

ADVANTAGES OF HPLC

HPLC can be performed on very small venous sample. It is performed to estimate quantity of normal and abnormal hemoglobins. It is used to diagnose β-thalassemia trait by quantification of HbA_2. Many variant hemoglobins are identified by this technique.

DISADVANTAGES OF HPLC

Cost of equipment and reagents is more. Overall HPLC has more advantages than electrophoresis and routinely performed in many laboratories.

ELECTROPHORESIS

HEMOGLOBIN ELECTROPHORESIS

Hemoglobin electrophoresis is a diagnostic tool to measure different types of hemoglobin in the blood. It is performed in suspected disorder associated with abnormal hemoglobin sickle cell anemia and thalassemia.

The most common ones are HbA, HbA_2, HbF, HbS, HbC and HbE.

PRINCIPLE

The principle behind electrophoresis is that when proteins are exposed to a charge gradient, they separate

Advanced Diagnostic Techniques

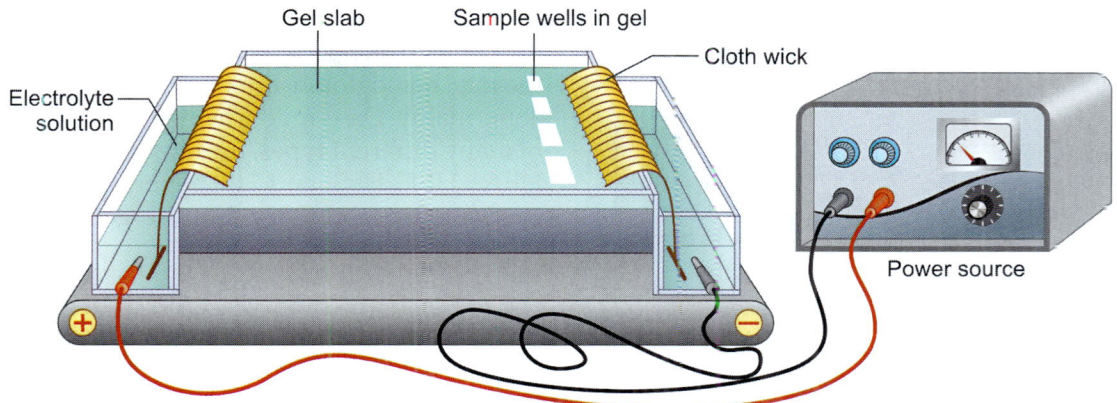

Fig. 14.31: Principle of hemoglobin electrophoresis.

from each other by forming *bands* that separate toward one end or the other end in the electric field. The hemoglobins are separated on a variety of supporting media on the basis of electric charge differences. The commonly used mediums are cellulose acetate membrane, starch gel, agarose gel, citrate agar gel and filter paper.

Cellulose acetate electrophoresis is performed at alkaline pH of 8.2–8.6. Citrate agar or agarose gel electrophoresis is done in acidic pH of 6.0–6.2. HPLC is rapidly taking its place in many laboratories. Principle of hemoglobin electrophoresis is shown in Fig 14.31.

BLOOD SAMPLING

Blood transfusions within the previous 12 weeks may alter test results. Hemoglobin electrophoresis is done on venous blood samples taken in anticoagulant EDTA container. Red cell lysate is prepared using a lysing reagent (Na_4 EDTA and KCN).

TYPE OF ELECTROPHORESIS

Cellulose acetate electrophoresis at pH 6.8 is the method of choice in most clinical laboratories. In this technique, there is overlapping of bands of hemoglobins S, D, G and lepore. Agar gel electrophoresis using a citrate buffer at pH 6.0 is useful in supplementing technique that helps in getting separate hemoglobin S band (Fig. 14.32).

Cellulose Acetate Electrophoresis (pH 8.6)

Cellulose acetate electrophoresis is the primary screening procedure used to detect variant of abnormal hemoglobins. The major portion of normal adult Hb is HbA. In addition, up to 3.5% HbA_2 is normally present, along with less than 2% HbF. The more common mutant Hbs are S, C, E, D, G, and lepore.

Principle: In an alkaline pH (8.2–8.6), Hb is a negatively charged molecule and will migrate toward the anode

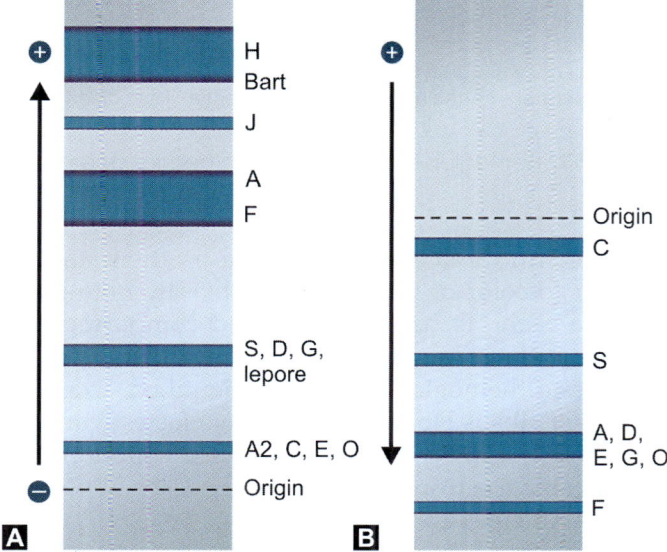

Fig. 14.32: (A) Schematic representation of electrophoretic mobility of normal and abnormal hemoglobins on cellulose acetate at pH 8.6, (B) agar gel at pH 6.

(+). The various Hbs move at different rates depending on their net negative charge.

Procedure: The red cell hemolysate (red blood cell membranes are destroyed to free the Hb molecules for testing) is placed in a cellulose acetate membrane, which is positioned in an electrophoresis tray with the inoculated hemolysate near the cathode (–).

One end of the cellulose acetate strip is immersed in the buffer (pH 8.2–8.6) on the cathode side and the other end is placed in the buffer on the anode (+) side. An electric current of specific voltage is allowed to run for a timed period. During electrophoresis, the hemoglobin molecules migrate toward the anode because of their negative charge.

The difference in the net charge of the hemoglobin molecule determines its mobility and manifests itself by the speed with which it migrates to the positive pole.

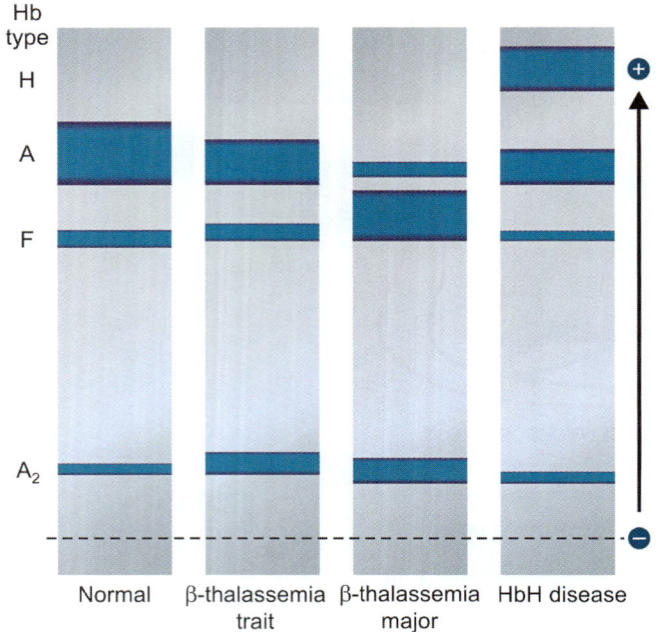

Fig. 14.33: Hemoglobin electrophoresis (cellular acetate at pH 8.6).

The cellulose acetate membrane is then stained in order to color of the proteins (Hbs). By noting the distance each Hb has migrated and comparing this distance with the migration distance of known controls, the types of hemoglobins may be identified. Example of the fast Hbs is Hb Bart and the two fastest variants HbH and I, while HbC is the slowest common Hb. Hemoglobin electrophoresis (cellular acetate at pH 8.6) is shown in Fig. 14.33.

Citrate Agar Electrophoresis (pH 6)

Citrate agar electrophoresis separates hemoglobin fractions that migrate together on cellulose acetate agar. All Hb specimens that show an abnormal electrophoretic pattern in alkaline media (cellulose acetate agar) should undergo electrophoresis on an acid citrate agar. Citrate agar electrophoresis is used to confirm variant Hbs and further differentiates HbS from HbD and G and HbC from HbE, O_{Arab}, and C_{Harlem}. The procedure should not be used as a screening procedure because many abnormal Hbs migrate with HbA.

INTERPRETATION

Each of the major hemoglobin types has an electrical charge of a different degree. Hemoglobin electrophoresis separates and measures normal and abnormal hemoglobins. The components then move away from each other at different rates, and when separated from a series of distinctly *pigmented bands*.

These bands are then compared with those of a normal sample. Each band is further assessed as a % of the total hemoglobin, thus indicating the severity of any abnormality. Description: hemoglobin (Hb) is comprised of many different types, the most common being HbA_1, HbA_2, HbF, HbS, and HbC. Normal reference values can vary by laboratory, but are generally within the following ranges.

Hemoglobin electrophoresis patterns: In normal adults, HbA_1 is the major component of hemoglobin in the normal red blood cell. HbA_2 is a minor component of normal hemoglobin, comprising approximately 2–3% of the total. In children, HbF is the major hemoglobin component in the fetus, but usually exists only in

Table 14.58: Hemoglobin electrophoresis pattern in normal persons

Hemoglobin	Percentage
Adults	
HbA_1	95–98%
HbA_2	2–3%
HbF	0.8–2.0%
HbS	0%
HbC	0%
Children	
HbF (newborn)	50–80%
HbF (6 months age)	8%
HbF (>6 months age)	1–2%

Table 14.59: Hemoglobin electrophoresis pattern in hemoglobin disorders

Hemoglobin	Hemoglobin disorder	Percentage
HbA_2	β-Thalassemia	4.00–5.8%
	HbH disease	<2%
HbF	β-thalassemia major	10–90%
	β-thalassemia minor	2–5%
	Homozygous hereditary persistence of fetal hemoglobin (HPFH)	100%
	Heterozygous hereditary persistence of fetal hemoglobin (HPFH)	5–35%
	Heterozygous HbS	15%
HbS	Sickle cell disease (homozygous)	70–98%
HbC	Hemoglobin C disease (homozygous)	90–98%

minimal quantities in the normal adult. Levels of HbF >2% in patients over three years of age are considered abnormal. Hemoglobin electrophoresis pattern in normal persons and hemoglobin disorders is shown in Tables 14.58 and 14.59.

GEL ELECTROPHORESIS

Gel electrophoresis is a method for separating, identifying or purifying nucleic acids. Nucleic acids are negatively charged at neutral pH (due to phosphate in the sugar-phosphate backbone of DNA or RNA). In the presence of an electrical field, nucleic acids migrate from the cathode to the anode. This migration through a sieving matrix (gel) depends on the size of the nucleic acid molecule, its conformation (secondary folding), pore size of the gel and the net charge (dependent on the pH of the gel buffer).

Two basic forms are agarose gel electrophoresis and polyacrylamide gel electrophoresis. Other variations on these methods include pulsed-field gel electrophoresis (PFGE), capillary gel electrophoresis (CGE), denaturing gradient gel electrophoresis (DGGE) and temperature gradient gel electrophoresis (TGGE). Commonly used electrophoresis methods are described in Table 14.60.

Table 14.60: Various types of electrophoresis

Electrophoresis	Description
Agarose gel electrophoresis	Agarose composed of multiple linked repeat units of disaccharide agarobiose (d-galactose and 3, 6-anhydro-l-galactose) is manufactured from seaweed such as Rhodophyta *Applications:* Analysis of end-point PCR or RT-PCR assays; analysis of restriction fragment length polymorphism (RFLP) assays; routinely used in molecular biology for the analysis of recombinant DNA experiments and can also be used for the purification of probes for ISH
Polyacrylamide gel electrophoresis (PAGE)	Polyacrylamide is produced from monomers of acrylamide in a reaction initiated by free radicals generated by reduction of ammonium persulfate; higher the concentration of acrylamide, the finer the resolution of DNA fragments The advantage of polyacrylamide over agarose is that size differences at the base-pair level can be distinguished *Applications:* End-point PCR fragment analysis where fragment size differences are slight; for sequencing assays and for microsatellite marker-based assays using autoradiography or fluorescence-labeled fragments
Pulsed-field gel electrophoresis (PFGE)	Used for improved resolution (accomplished by alternating the direction of the electrical field) of high-molecular-weight DNA *Applications:* Identification of microorganism strains such as *Escherichia coli* O157:H7, Salmonella, Shigella, Listeria, or Campylobacter species; evaluation of autosomal dominant ataxia
Capillary gel electrophoresis	It supports automated DNA sequencing and fragment analyses *Applications:* Widely used for sequencing and microsatellite assay

Index

A

α₁-antitrypsin deficiency 38, 46, 302, 883, 879, 1104
α-actin 4 protein (ACTN4) 1162
α-fetoprotein (AFP) 405
α-hydroxylase deficiency (vitamin D resistant rickets) 1456
α-methylacyl-CoA racemase enzyme 1281
α-smooth muscle actin 1361, 1375
α-tocopherol 426
Abetalipoproteinemia 991
Abnormal folding of proteins by reactive oxygen species 22
Abnormal pooling of platelets 604
ABO blood group antigens 302
ABO blood group system 626
ABO blood grouping 632
Acanthosis nigricans 405, 1578
Accelerated phase of chronic myeloid leukemia 567
Accelerated phase of CML (BCR-ABL positive) 567
Accessory nipple 1401
Acetaminophen induced hepatocellular injury 1080
Achalasia 962
Achondroplasia 302, 1513
Acid–base equilibrium imbalance 1198
Acid elution test 527
Acid hydrolase 99, 196
Acid phosphatase 543
Acid serum lysis test 531
Acne 1579
Acquired atelectasis of lung 900
Acquired cystic renal disease 1229
Acquired hypercoagulable state 149, 620
Acquired hyperlipidemia 750
Acquired immunodeficiency syndrome 220
Acquired sideroblastic anemia 531
Acral lentiginous melanoma 1572

Actin filaments 37
Actinic keratosis 13, 1565, 1567
Actinomyces israelii 445, 868
Activated partial thromboplastin time (APTT) 556, 613, 623
Activated prothrombin complex concentrates 635
Activation of leukocytes 64
Active hyperemia 134
Active immunity 179
Acute appendicitis 1029
Acute bacterial endocarditis 812
Acute chest syndrome in sickle cell disease 511
Acute cholecystitis 1127, 1135
Acute cystitis 1245
Acute disseminated encephalomyelitis 1617
Acute endocarditis 812
Acute endometritis 1310
Acute erosive gastritis 970
Acute erythroblastic leukemia 558
Acute fatty liver of pregnancy 1107
Acute fibrinous pericarditis 791
Acute gouty arthritis 1522
Acute graft-versus-host disease (GVHD) 270, 595
Acute Guillain-Barré syndrome 637
Acute heart failure 827
Acute icteric hepatitis 1071
Acute idiopathic thrombocytopenic purpura 602
Acute inflammation 53
Acute iron poisoning 487
Acute lymphangitis 769
Acute lymphoblastic leukemia (ALL) 544, 552
Acute mastitis 1364
Acute megakaryoblastic leukemia 558
Acute myasthenia gravis 637

Acute myeloid leukemia (AML) 547, 550, 552
Acute myocardial infarction 734, 785, 787, 789, 791, 794–797
Acute necrotizing ulcerative gingivitis 933
Acute nephritic syndrome 1187
Acute oophoritis 1346
Acute otitis media 847
Acute pancreatitis 1134, 1140
Acute pericarditis 823
Acute peritonitis 1034
Acute phase reactants 94, 247, 306
Acute promyelocytic leukemia 556
Acute pyelonephritis 1183, 1209, 1421
Acute renal failure 1208, 1209
Acute renal transplant rejection 268
Acute respiratory distress syndrome 160, 886, 887
Acute rheumatic heart disease 802
Acute rhinosinusitis 836
Acute salpingitis 1306
Acute sialadenitis 939
Acute thyroiditis 1431
Acute tubular necrosis 1206, 1207
Acute urate nephropathy 1214
Acute viral hepatitis 1062
Acylating agents 384
Adamantinoma bone 1508
Addison's disease 255, 933, 1461
Adenocarcinoma esophagus 993
Adenocarcinoma gallbladder 1138
Adenocarcinoma lung 918, 966
Adenocarcinoma of extrahepatic bile ducts 1139
Adenocarcinoma—various sites 327
Adenoid cystic carcinoma of salivary gland 947
Adenoma gallbladder 1137
Adenoma of the nipple 1376
Adenoma various sites 324
Adenomatoid odontogenic tumor 953

Adenomatoid tumor of fallopian tube 1307
Adenomatoid tumor of testicular adnexa 1271
Adenomatous polyps of colon 1019
Adenomyosis uteri 1312
Adenosine 235
Adenosine deaminase 218
ADH deficiency 1469
Adhesive pericarditis 825, 826
Adipocytes 419
Adipocytic tumors 1526
ADP 142
Adrenal cortex 1457
Adrenal cortical insufficiency 1461
Adrenal hyperfunction 1459
Adrenal virilism 1462
Adrenocortical adenoma 1465
Adrenocortical carcinoma 1465
Adrenogenital syndrome 1462
Adult and infantile fibrosarcoma 1531
Adult Gaucher's disease (type 1) 1106
Adult polycystic kidney 302, 1226
Adult stem cells 112
Adult T cell leukemia/lymphoma 579, 673
Advanced gastric carcinoma 979
Adverse reactions of blood transfusion 638
Aflatoxin B_1 385, 1117
Agar gel electrophoresis 735
Agenesis of corpus callosum 1619
Agenesis of kidney 13
Air embolism 157, 159, 640
AKT/PI3K signaling pathway 363
Alagille syndrome 1057
Albinism 220, 302, 1569
Alcian blue stain 697 925
Alcohol fixative 692
Alcoholic (Laënnec) cirrhosis 1082, 1098
Alcoholic liver disease 1094
Alder-Reilly anomaly 468, 537
Aleukemic leukemia 540
Alexander Wiener nomenclature blood group system 629
ALK receptors 352
Alkaline phosphatase 698, 1048
Alkaptonuria 310
Alkylating chemotherapeutic agents 384
Allergic polyps 837
Allergic reactions 231, 639
Allergic rhinitis 232
Allogenic grafts 592
Alloimmune hemolytic anemia 519
Alport's syndrome 1162
Alternate pathway of complement activation 210
Alveolar rhabdomyosarcoma 844, 1533
Alveolar soft part sarcoma 377, 1537
Ameloblastic carcinoma 955
Ameloblastic fibroma 953
Ameloblastic fibrosarcoma 956
Ameloblastic odontoma 954
Ameloblastoma 954
Amenorrhea 1309

Amniotic fluid embolism 157, 160, 1355
Amoebic colitis 1014
Amoebic encephalitis 1589
Amoebic liver abscess 1078
Amorphous ground substance 124
Amyloid adrenal gland 279
Amyloid associated 275
Amyloid gastrointestinal tract 279
Amyloid heart 279
Amyloid laboratory diagnosis 280
Amyloid light-chain 273
Amyloid liver 278, 1106
Amyloid nephropathy 277, 1183
Amyloid nervous system 280
Amyloid of aging 277
Amyloid P component 273
Amyloid respiratory system 279
Amyloid skin 279
Amyloid spleen (lardaceous and sago) 279, 680
Amyloid stains 281, 1107, 1185
　Congo red stain examined under light microscope 281
　Congo red stain examined under polarizing microscope 281
　crystal violet (metachromatic stain) 281
　fluorescent stains (thioflavin-T, thioflavin-S) 281
　methyl violet (metachromatic stain) 281
Amyloid β-protein 276
Amyloidosis 47, 273, 933
Amylopectin 1105
Anaerobic glycolysis 20, 21
Anal fissure 1032
Analgesic induced nephropathy 1215
Analogous antigens 190
Anaphylactic shock 176, 211
Anaphylatoxins (C3a, C5a) 81
Anaphylaxis 232, 639
Anaplastic astrocytoma 1599
Anaplastic dysgerminoma 1334
Anaplastic large T cell lymphoma 674
Anaplastic seminoma 1260
Anatomical barriers to pathogens 185
Anatomical dead space refers 860
ANCA glomerulonephritis 1168
Ancylostoma duodenale 455
Anderson disease 309
Androblastoma (Sertoli cell tumor) of testis 1269
Androblastoma—ovary 1343
Androgen induced prostatic carcinoma 391
Anemia of chronic disease 531
Anencephaly 1618
Aneuploidy 295
Aneurysm of sinus of Valsalva 759
Aneurysmal bone cyst 952, 1510
Aneurysms 755, 756, 759, 760
Angelman (happy puppet) syndrome 292
Angina pectoris (>12 hours) in AMI 795
Angina pectoris 783
　stable (typical) angina 784

　unstable (crescendo/pre-infarction) angina 784
　variant (Prinzmetal) angina 784
Angiodysplasia 1016
Angiogenesis 127, 372
Angiogenic factors 334, 372
Angiomyolipoma 771
Angiosarcoma 682, 771
Angiosarcoma breast 1395
Angiosarcoma liver 1123
Angiostatin 335
Angiotensin 334
Angiotensin aldosterone system 422
Angular stomatitis 428
Anionic-sialoglycoproteins 1159
Anitschkow cells 800
Ankylosing spondylitis 255, 1520, 1521
Ankyrin proteins in RBC membrane 500
Annular pancreas 1140, 1409
Anorectal fistula 1032
Anterior cerebral artery occlusion 1611
Anterior pituitary gland 1467
Anti-angiogenic factors 335, 372
Antiapoptotic genes 319
Antibodies induced glomerular injury 1168
Antibodies of ABO system 634
Antibody-dependent mediated cytotoxicity 238
Anticardiolipin antibodies 620
Anticoagulants 476, 477
Anti-D antibody (RhoGAM) administration 630
Antidiuretic hormone (ADH) 1153
Anti-DNA antibody 1049
Anti-DNAase 799
Anti-DNAase-B titer 1192
Anti-DNase-B/anti-hyaluronidase titer 805
Anti-GBM-mediated glomerulonephritis 1164
Antigen presenting cells (APCs) 198
Antigen-responsive T cells 193
　CD4+ T cells 193
　CD8+ T cells (natural killer cells) 193, 402, 534
　CD8+ T cells (suppressor cells) 193
Antigens 187
Antigens ABO blood group system 627
Antigens of Rh system 629
Anti-HBc (both IgG and IgM) in serum 1069
Anti-HBs antibody marker in serum 1069
Anti-HDV IgM in serum 1073
Anti-hyaluronidase titer 1192
Anti-inflammatory agents 85, 94
Anti-mitochondrial antibody 1049
Anti-nuclear antibody 1049
Antinuclear autoantibodies against SS-B 262
Antiphospholipid antibodies 150, 261
Antiphospholipid antibody syndrome 150, 620
Anti-receptor antibody-mediated type II hypersensitivity reaction 241

Anti-smooth muscle antibody 1049
Antistreptolysin-O (ASO) titer 799, 805, 1192
Antistreptozyme test 805
Antithrombin III 147, 148, 150, 600, 619
Antithrombotic properties of endothelium 139, 140
Aortic coarctation 834
Aortic stenosis 820
Aortic valve insufficiency/regurgitation 820
APC tumor suppressor gene 362
APC/β-catenin pathway 1025
Aphthous stomatitis 934
Aplasia of bone marrow 14
Aplastic anemia 528, 512, 541
Apocrine breast carcinoma 1394
Apocrine metaplasia in fibrocystic disease 1368
Apolipoprotein L-1 gene (APOL1) 1162
Apoptosis 16, 32, 33
Apoptotic gene 319
Appendicular osteoporosis 1482
Applications 691
Aqueduct of Sylvius 1582
Arachidonic acid metabolite pathways 82, 84
Arias-Stella reaction 1312
Armanni-Ebstein lesions in tubules 1421
Arnold-Chiari malformation 1619
Aromatase inhibitors 1407
Aromatic amines 384, 385
Array CGH technique 712
Arrhinencephaly 1618
Arrhythmogenic right ventricular cardiomyopathy 811
Arterial thrombi 152
Arteriovenous fistula 760, 1614
Arthritis of metabolic origin 1521
Arthroscopy 1518
Arthus reaction 243
Asbestosis 887, 893, 908
Ascaris strongyloidiasis 994
Ascending cholangitis 1134
Aschoff's nodule 800, 803
Ascites 169, 829, 1047, 1089
Aspergilloma 434
Aspergillus flavus 385, 451
Aspergillus fumigatus 868
Aspirin (NSAIDs) 83
Assay of B-type natriuretic peptide 827, 904
Asterixis (flapping tremors) 1046
Astrocytes 1581
Astrocytic tumors 1598
Astrocytomas 1598
Asymptomatic acute prostatitis 1277
Asymptomatic/silent gallstones 1132
Ataxia hemorrhagic telangiectasia 608
Ataxia-telangiectasia 219, 343, 374, 541, 1379
Atelectasis neonatorum 900
Atelectasis or lung collapse 900

Atheroembolism due to atherosclerosis 157
Atherosclerosis 45, 138, 743, 744, 747, 748, 751, 752, 754, 778, 1419
Atherosclerotic aneurysms 756
ATM tumor suppressor gene 369
Atopic dermatitis 232
ATP 142
ATP7B gene 1048, 1103
ATPase 20
Atrial myxoma 830
Atrial natriuretic factor 1153
Atrial septal defects 833
Atrial thrombi 793
Atrophy—various organs 4, 6
Atypical alveolar hyperplasia 921
Atypical chronic myeloid leukemia (aCML) 562
Atypical ductal hyperplasia 1369, 1379
Auer rods in myeloblasts 553
Auspitz sign in psoriasis 1562
Austin Flint murmur in syphilitic aortitis 756
Autoantibodies in liver disorders 1049
Autocrine signaling 118, 119
Autoimmune disorders 255, 297
Autoimmune enteropathy 990
Autoimmune hemolytic anemia 256, 405, 516
Autoimmune hepatitis (lupoid hepatitis) 1075
Autoimmune oophoritis 1346
Autoimmune pancreatitis 1143
Autoimmune pericarditis in AMI 794
Autoimmune sialadenitis 939
Autoimmune thrombocytopenic purpura 256
Autologous blood transfusion 637
Autonomic nervous system neuropathy 1423
Autosomal codominant inheritance 302
Autosomal dominant inheritance 290, 302, 303
Autosomal recessive inheritance 290, 302, 303, 306
Autosplenectomy 512, 679
AV node conduction system heart 782
Avascular necrosis of femoral head in sickle cell disease 511
Axial osteoporosis 1482
Axillary lymph nodes 1359, 1395, 1396, 1402
Azathioprine immunosuppressive drug 272
Azo dyes derivatives of aromatic amines 385

B

β-hCG 1268
β-microglobulin 577
B cell lymphoma (DLBCL) 663
B cell prolymphocytic leukemia 672

B cells 534
B cells dysfunction role in diabetes mellitus 1416
Bacillary angiomatosis 771
Bacteria induced carcinogenesis 390
Bacterial cervicitis 1297
Bacterial liver infections 1077
Bacterial meningitis 1584, 1586
Bacterial orchitis 1273
Bacterial pneumonias 862
Bacterial products 195
Bacterial vaginosis 1291
Bactericidal permeability increasing protein 69
Balanced polymorphism 291
Ballooning angioplasty 787
Ballooning degeneration 1061
Band 3 (anionic channel) in RBC membrane 500
Band 4.1 in RBC membrane 501
Band 4.2 proteins (pallidin) in RBC membrane 500
Barium enema 1029
Barr bodies 296, 313
Barrett esophagus 961
Barriers to pathogens 185
Bartholin glands 1290
Basal cell carcinoma of skin 326, 1568
Basaloid carcinoma 1033
Basilar artery occlusion 1611
Basophilia 536
Basophilic stippling 465, 479, 480, 561
Basophils 534
BCL family 371
BCL-1 cell cycle regulatory gene 1382
BCR-ABL hybrid (fusion) protein product 376, 564
Becker muscular dystrophy 303, 312, 1543
Beckwith-Wiedemann syndrome (BWS) 1232
Bellini duct renal cell carcinoma 1240
Benign Brenner tumor—ovary 1333
Benign epithelial tumors 322
Benign mesenchymal tumors 324
Benign monoclonal gammopathy 588
Benign nephrosclerosis 1223
Benign phyllodes tumor—breast 1372
Benign surface epithelial tumors—ovary 323
Benign tumors 906
BER-EP4 monoclonal antibody 925
Bernard-Soulier syndrome 142, 606, 622
Berry aneurysm 138, 755, 758, 1614
Berylliosis 895
Bilateral renal agenesis 1229
Bile canalicular antibody 1049
Bile canaliculi 1043
Bile duct disorders 1107
Bile duct hamartoma 1115
Bile juice composition 1129
Biliary adenocarcinoma 1139
Biliary atresia 1056

Biliary cholestasis 1061
Biliary cirrhosis 1107, 1082
Biliary intraepithelial neoplasia 1137
Bilirubin pigment 39
Biological immunosuppression 272
Biological therapy in breast carcinoma 1407
Biotin 428
BIRADS system used for reporting mammograms 1403
Bite cells 480, 515,524
Bitot's spots in eyes 425
Bland infarct (non-infective) infarct 162
Blast crisis in CML 566, 567, 568
Bleeding diathesis 427, 620, 621, 622, 623
Bleeding into vitreous 1423
Bleeding time 623
Blood components therapy 631, 634, 635
Blood cross-matching 634
Blood culture 806
Blood group A 626
Blood group AB 627
Blood group B 627
Blood group O 626
Blood group systems 626
Blood group systems other than ABO and Rh 631
Blood sampling 526, 735
Blood transfusion reactions 240, 638
Blood–brain barrier 1581
Bloom syndrome 541
Blue bloaters tolerate hypoxia 882
Blue nevus 1570
Boerhaave's syndrome 963
Bombay blood group (Oh) 628
Bone and joint crises in sickle cell disease 511
Bone forming tumors 1487
Bone fracture healing 121
Bone marrow 575, 579
Bone marrow aspirate 472, 565, 578, 588
   abnormal cells 472
   cellularity 472
   erythropoiesis 472
   leukopoiesis 472
   megakaryopoiesis 472
   myeloid to erythroid ratio 472
   other bone marrow cells 472
Bone marrow aspiration needles 470
   Klima needle 470
   Salah needle 470
Bone marrow failure syndromes 528
Bone marrow harvesting 593
Bone marrow hyperplasia 10
Bone marrow stem cells 112
Bone marrow stromal cells (MSCs) 113
Bone marrow trephine biopsy 578, 587
Bone metastases 1509
Bone scan in malignancy 1404
Bone tumors 1484
Borderline Brenner tumor 1333
Borderline endometrioid tumors 1324
Borderline phyllodes tumor 1373

Borderline serous tumors of low malignant potential of ovary 1327
Borderline serous tumors with micro-invasion 1327
Borderline surface epithelial tumors of ovary 1323
Borrelia burgdorferi 390, 982
Botryoid rhabdomyosarcoma 1254, 1294, 1534
Bouin's fluid fixative 692
Bouveret's syndrome 1136
Bowen disease of penis 1282
Bowen disease of the vulva 1288
Bowenoid papulosis 1282
Bowman's capsule 1159, 1160
B-prolymphocytic leukemia (PLL) 578
Brachial plexus injury induced by Pancoast tumor 918
Bradykinin 81
BRAF increasing RAS signal transduction protein pathway 354
Brain purpura 902, 1615
Branchial cyst 853
BRCA1 tumor suppressor gene 342, 368, 1325, 1378, 1381
BRCA2 tumor suppressor gene 342, 368, 1145, 1379, 1381
Breast carcinoma 1376
Breast carcinoma—prognostic and predictive factors 1397
Breast lumps 1362
Breast lumps frequency 1360
Breast sarcoidosis 1365
Breast tuberculosis 439, 1365
Breasts during pregnancy 10
Brenner tumor of ovary 1332
Bridging necrosis liver 1047, 1061
Brilliant cresyl blue stain 474, 515
Broad group of cells 111
Brodie abscess 1478
Bromsulphthalein excretion 1056
Bronchial adenoma 906
Bronchial asthma 232, 233, 877, 884
Bronchial biopsy 925
Bronchial hamartoma 331
Bronchial papilloma 906
Bronchiectasis 876, 877, 882
Bronchiolitis 877
Bronchioloalveolar carcinoma 920, 921
Bronchoalveolar lavage 439, 925
Bronchopneumonia 862, 866, 867
Bronchopulmonary carcinoids 907
Bronze diabetes 41, 1102
Brown atrophy of organs 6
Brown tumor of hyperparathyroidism 956
Brucellosis 535
Brudzinski's sign 1586
Bruton's agammaglobulinemia 67
Budd-Chiari syndrome 135, 1111
Bullous pemphigoid 255, 1563
Bundle of His and its branches of heart 782
Burkitt's lymphoma 376,389, 546, 661, 664

Burr cells 480
Byssinosis 897

C

C peptide levels 1411
C5a 195
C5a 63
Cabot's ring 479, 480
Cachexia 6, 400
Cadherins 126
CagA effector molecules 968
Calcific aortic stenosis 821
Calcification 42
Calcifying epithelial odontogenic tumor 953
Calcifying odontogenic cyst 952
Calcinosis 42, 262
Calcitonin 1451, 1452
Calcium 142, 609
Calcium and phosphate disturbances 1200
Calcium metabolism 1452
Calcium oxalate stones—kidney 1219
Calcium phosphate stones—kidney 1219
Calcium pump 20
Calcium stones—kidney 1219
Calcospherites 1601
Call-Exner bodies in granulosa cell tumor of ovary 1341
Calretinin 843, 925
CAM 5.2 843
Cambium layer 1294
Campylobacter jejuni 390, 982, 992
Cancer testis antigens 373
Cancers in AIDS 225
Candida albicans 451, 868, 934
Capillary hemangioma 770,154
Capillary microaneurysms 760
Capsular drop in diabetic nephropathy 1183, 1421
Caput medusae in portal hypertension 1089
Carbon tetrachloride induced liver injury 1081
Carbuncle 1290
Carcinoembryonic antigen (CEA) 405, 925, 1406, 1451
Carcinogenesis 347
Carcinoid heart disease 1000
Carcinoid syndrome 404, 1000
Carcinoid tumor 985, 1031, 1149, 1338
Carcinoma *in situ* 320
Carcinoma of penis 1282
Carcinosarcoma (malignant mixed müllerian tumor) of ovary 1334
Carcinosarcoma of salivary gland 950
Cardiac arrhythmias in AMI 422, 791
Cardiac cirrhosis 135, 1110
Cardiac enzymes in AMI 796
Cardiac hemolytic anemia 522
Cardiac hypertrophy 7, 777, 829
Cardiac imaging techniques in AMI 797

Cardiac muscle stem cells 114
Cardiac rhabdomyoma 831
Cardiac tamponade 822
Cardiac transplantation 809
Cardiac troponins (Tn I and Tn T) in AMI 796
Cardiac tumors 830
Cardiac valves 818
Cardiac vegetations 812, 813
Cardiac vegetations—comparison 817
Cardiogenic shock 171, 173, 791
Cardiomyopathies 807, 808
Carnitine palmityl transferase deficiency 1547
Carnoy's fluid fixative 692
Carotid angiography 855
Carotid body tumor 855
Carprofen drug 85
Cartilaginous tumors 1495
Caseating granulomas 106
Caseous necrosis 26, 28, 432
Caspases and apoptosis 35
Castleman disease 643
Catalase 25
Cataracts 1423
Catarrhal inflammation 73
Categories of birefringence 690
Categories of delayed hypersensitivity reactions 248
Caterpillar cells 800
Cathepsin D 20, 968, 1004, 1400, 1400
Cauliflower ear 846
Causes of valvular diseases 818
Cavernous hemangioma 324, 770, 1614
CD15 (LeuM1) 925
CD2 associated proteins 1159
CD31 62
CD55 522
CD59 522
CDE (Fisher-Race) nomenclature system 629
CDKN2A tumor suppressor gene 363
Celiac disease 988
Cell (forward) blood grouping 632
Cell adhesion proteins 125
Cell cycle 114
Cell cycle inhibitors 341
Cell injury 15
Cell-mediated immunity (CMI) 191
Cell surface receptors 119
Cells in epidermis 1552
Cellular aging 48
Cellular changes in acute inflammation 61
Cellular proteins in blood 19
Cellulose acetate electrophoresis 735
Cementifying fibroma 956
Cementoma 954
Central core (nucleocapsid) 1067
Central core disease 1546
Central diabetes insipidus 1470
Central giant cell granuloma 956
Central nervous system 1580

Central tolerance 250, 252
Centriacinar emphysema 880
Centrilobular emphysema 1041
Centrilobular necrosis liver 1045
Centromere enumerating probes (CEPs) 718
Centromere protein H (CENP-H) 925
Cerebral abscess 1589
Cerebral edema 169
Cerebral hemangioblastoma 464
Cerebral infarction 1611
Cerebral malaria 1589
Cerebral parenchymal compartment 1582
Cerebral strokes 748
Cerebral toxoplasmosis 1589
Cerebral vascular disease 1420
Cerebrospinal fluid 1582
Ceruloplasmin 25, 1048
Cerumic gland adenoma 846
Cervical biopsy 1305
Cervical carcinoma 1300
Cervical intraepithelial dysplasia 12
Cervical intraepithelial neoplasia (CIN) 1299
Cervical intraepithelial neoplasia 320, 1299
Cervical lymphadenopathy 643
CFTr gene 7, 883
Chancroid 1293
Charcot joints 1589
Charcot-Leyden crystals in sputum 455, 534, 884
Chédiak-Higashi syndrome 38, 67, 93, 220, 537
Cheilosis 428
CHEK2 tumor suppressor gene 370, 1381
Chemical carcinogens 381
Chemical defenses against pathogens 186
Chemical mediators 73, 235
Chemifluorescence 705
Chemilumiescence 705
Chemokines 195, 431
Chemotactic factors 63
Chemotaxis 61, 63
Chemotherapeutic agents 408
Chemotherapy 567, 1407
Chemotherapy-induced leukemias 541
Cherry hemangioma 1576
Cherubism 956
Chest radiographs 652
Chest wall invasion by Pancoast tumor 918
Chlamydia trachomatis 1292
Cholangiocarcinoma 1122
Cholangitis and liver abscess 1080
Cholecystitis 1127
Choledochal cyst 1129
Cholelithiasis (gallstone disease) 1129
Cholestasis 1050, 1051
Cholesteatoma 847
Cholesterol gallstones 1132
Cholesterol granuloma 847
Cholesterolosis (strawberry gallbladder) 45, 1128

Chondroblastoma 1497
Chondrocalcinosis (pseudogout) 1522
Chondroid syringoma 1576
Chondroma 1495
Chondromyxoid fibroma 1497
Chondronectin 129
Chondrosarcoma 329, 1498
Chordoma 1505
Choreoathetoid movements 508
Chorioamnionitis 1356
Choriocarcinoma 1268, 1339
Choroid plexus 1582
Choroid plexus papilloma 1602
Chromogranin-A 843
Chromophobe variant of renal cell carcinoma 1233
Chromosomal banding techniques 314
C-banding 314
G-banding 314
Giemsa stain 314
Q-banding 314
R-banding 314
Chromosomal disorders 292
Chromosomal rearrangements 375
Chromosome instability syndrome 343
Chromothripsis 377
Chronic active hepatitis 1064, 1071
Chronic active myocarditis 807
Chronic bronchitis 876, 877
Chronic carriers in hepatitis 1071
Chronic cervicitis 1297
Chronic cholecystitis 1127
Chronic cystitis 1246
Chronic endometritis 1310
Chronic eosinophilic leukemia 569
Chronic gastritis type A, B and AB 970, 971
Chronic glomerulonephritis 1197
Chronic graft-versus-host disease (GVHD) 270, 595
Chronic granulomatous disease of childhood 68, 537, 883
Chronic granulomatous inflammation 103
Chronic heart failure 827
Chronic hepatitis 1071
Chronic idiopathic thrombocytopenic purpura 603
Chronic interstitial cystitis 1247
Chronic ischemic heart disease 798
Chronic lobular hepatitis 1063
Chronic lymphocytic leukemia (CLL) 574, 662
Chronic lymphocytic leukemia 517, 667
Chronic lymphoproliferative disorders 574
Chronic myeloid leukemia 376, 563
Chronic myeloid leukemia *vs* leukemoid reactions 569
Chronic myelomonocytic leukemia 562
Chronic myeloproliferative disorders 541
Chronic neutrophilic leukemia 569, 570
Chronic obstructive pulmonary disease 876, 908
Chronic obstructive sialadenitis 939

Chronic otitis media 847
Chronic pancreatitis 824, 1142
Chronic prostatitis 1277
Chronic pyelonephritis (CPN) 1212
Chronic recurrent parotitis 940
Chronic renal transplant rejection 269
Chronic rheumatic heart disease 803
Chronic salinities 1306
Chronic sinusitis 837
Chronic urate nephropathy 1214
Chronic venous congestion of liver 135, 1110
Chronic venous congestion of lung 136
Chronic viral hepatitis 1063
Churg-Strauss syndrome 766
Chylothorax 928
Chylous effusion 769
Cip/Kip (Cip/WAF family) 341
  INK4a/ARF family 341
Circulatory overload 639
Circumferential myocardial infarct 784
Cirrhosis 1082
Citrate agar electrophoresis 736
Classes of RNAs 286
Classic dysgerminoma 1334
Classic galactosemia 309
Classic hemophilia 311
Classic seminoma 1260
Classical Reed-Sternberg cells 650
Classification of antibodies 698
Classification of common neoplasms 321
Classification of diabetes mellitus 1414
Classification of hemolytic anemias 495
Classification of soft tissue tumors 1525
Classification of the vasculitides 761
Clear cell adenocarcinoma 1294
Clear cell carcinoma 1332
Clear cell odontogenic carcinoma 955
Clear cell sarcoma of soft tissue 1538
Clear cell variant of renal cell carcinoma 1233
Cleft palate 932
Clinical features in primary HIV infection 227
Cloaca 1478
Clonal deletion 252
Clonal energy 252
Clonal selection 191
Clone deletion of T cells by apoptosis 254
Clonorchis sinensis (liver-fluke) 391
Closed comedon 1579
Closed pneumothorax 898
Clostridium difficile 992
Clot dissolution 146
Clot retraction 146, 600
Clot retraction test 624
Clotting time 613
CML vs atypical CML (aCML) 568
C-MYC oncogene 1382
CNS cells vulnerable to hypoxia 1611
CNS lymphoma in AIDS 390
CNS tumors 1590

Coagulation cascade 143
Coagulation disorders in hepatic disease 618
Coagulation factors 610
Coagulation profile 623
Coagulation system 75, 599
Coagulative necrosis 26
Coal dust 42
Coal worker's pneumoconiosis 892, 887
Coarctation of aorta 834
Cobblestone appearance of mucosa 1013
Cobweb turbidity in CSF 1588
Coccidioides immitis 452, 868
Coding regulatory RNA 287
Codman triangle in osteosarcoma 1490
Codominant inheritance 303
Co-infection in hepatitis 1073
COL1A1 gene 1513
COL1A2 gene 1513
Cold agglutinin disease 518
Cold agglutinin hemolytic anemia 637
Collagen fibers 123
Collagen fibers breakdown products 195
Collagen IV and V 1158
Collagen matrix deposition 1205
Collagen vascular diseases 897
Collagenous colitis 1015
Collagenous sprue 990
Collecting duct carcinoma in renal medulla 1233
COLLIA1-PDGFB fusion protein 1531
Colloid breast carcinoma 1391
Colloidal iron 697
Colonoscopy 1029, 1038
Colorectal carcinoma 1022
Colposcopy 1305
Columnar metaplasia in Barrett's esophagus 11
Combined gallstones 1130
Comedocarcinoma—breast 1385
Common variable immunodeficiency 215, 991
Commonly used stains in histopathology 695, 696
Communicating hydrocephalus 1619
Comparative genomic hybridization (CGH) 712
Compensatory mechanisms 496
Competitive ELISA 723
Complement actions 211
Complement classical pathway 210
Complement-mediated phagocytosis of target cells 240
Complement system 76, 77, 209, 210
Complement system defects 93
Complete carcinogens 382
Complete hydatidiform mole 1351
Complete resolution 32, 69
Complex adenoma 1376
Complex (adenomatous) endometrial hyperplasia with atypia 1311
Complex (adenomatous) endometrial hyperplasia without atypia 1311

Complex odontoma 954
Complications of acute myocardial infarction 795
Component 273
Composite pheochromocytoma 1463
Compound odontoma 954
Compound papillae 1152
Compression atelectasis 900
Condyloma acuminatum 1288
Confined placental mosaicism 296
Congenital dyserythroblastopoietic anemia (CDA) 531
Congenital epulis 933
Congenital heart diseases 831
Congenital hydrocephalus 1619
Congenital hypoplasia of the breast 1401
Congenital lactase deficiency 991
Congenital lip pits 933
Congenital myopathies 1546
Congenital nephrotic syndrome 1162
Congenital pyloric stenosis 985
Congestion 134
Congestive cardiomyopathy 808
Congestive heart failure 791, 826
Congestive heart failure in AMI 791
Congestive splenomegaly 137, 678
Congo red stain 281
Congo red stain for amyloid 280, 1201
Conization of cervix 1305
Connective tissue mucins 925
Constrictive pericarditis 439, 825
Constrictive pericarditis—clinical features 825
Contact dermatitis 248, 250
Contraction atelectasis 900
Conventional osteosarcoma 1490
Coombs' test 501, 517, 525, 576
Corbovinum 756
Cord factor 431
Core biopsy 1404
Coronary artery bypass graft (CABG) 787
Coronary artery disease 422
Coronary care units 787
Cor pulmonale 830
Corpus luteal cysts 1348
Corticotropic adenoma 1473
Councilman bodies 34, 1045, 1061
Covert myeloma 583
Cowden disease 1379
Cowden syndrome 1019
Cranial nerve disorders 1423
Craniopharyngioma 1474
Craniotabes in rickets 425
C-reactive proteins 94, 797
Creatine kinase-MB (CK-MB) 796
Creeping fibrosis 1107
Crescentic glomerulonephritis 1163
CREST syndrome 262, 962
Cretinism (thyroid dwarf) 1431
Cri du chat syndrome 293, 298
Cribriform breast carcinoma 1395
Crigler-Najjar syndrome 1054, 1055

Crohn's disease 104, 249, 1012
Cronokite-Canada syndrome 1022
Cryoglobulinemia 637, 1072
Cryoglobulinemia vasculitis 766
Cryoprecipitate 635, 636
Cryostat 687, 688
Cryptococcus neoformans 452, 472, 868
Cryptorchidism 1273
Crystal violet (metachromatic stain) 281
CST3 gene 1244
Current genetic analysis nomenclature system 630
Curschmann spirals 884
Cushing's syndrome 404, 1459
Cutaneous infections 1558, 1559
Cutaneous metastases 1577
Cw6 gene 1562
Cyanocobalamin 428
Cyclic nucleotides 235
Cyclin D and Cdk-4 synthesis 115
Cyclins and cyclin-dependent kinase 357, 1382
Cyclooxygenase pathway 82, 93
Cyclosporine A immunosuppressive drug 272
Cylindrical aneurysm 755
Cystatin aasay in renal diseases C 1244
Cystic diseases of kidney 1226
Cystic fibrosis of pancreas 291, 302, 310, 837, 883, 1143
Cystic hygroma 770
Cystic infarct in brain 165
Cysticercosis 452
Cystine kidney stones 1220
Cystinuria 1216
Cystitis glandularis 1247
Cystoscopy 1221
Cytochemistry in ALL and AML 543
Cytogenetic aberrations in soft tissue sarcomas 1525
Cytogenetic analysis 709–715
Cytokeratin 925
Cytokines 86, 190
Cytokine receptors 65
Cytomegalovirus 449, 472, 868
Cytoskeleton abnormalities 37
Cytoskeleton filaments 23

D

2,6-dichlorophenolindophenol test (DCIP) 527
DAF (decay accelerating factor) 521
Dane particle 1067
DDAVP (desmopressin 1-sesamino-8 arginine vasopressin) 614
Decalcification 693
Decalcifying solutions 693
Decay accelerating factor (DAF) 521
Decompression sickness 157, 159
Decreased erythropoiesis 806
Decreased platelet production 601

Dedifferentiated pleomorphic liposarcoma 1528
Deep vein thrombosis 422, 768, 1355
Defensins 69
Degenerative joint disease 1521
Delayed wound healing 613
Deletion of chromosome 288
Delphin lymph nodes 643
Dementia 428
Demyelinating disorders 1616
Dendrites 1581
Dendritic cells 198
Dengue hemorrhagic fever 604
Dental caries 950
Dental procedures 613
Dentigerous cyst 951
Denys-Drash syndrome (DDS) 1232
Deoxyadenosylcobalamin 489
Dermal dendritic cells 1553
Dermatitis 428
Dermatitis herpetiformis 1564
Dermatofibroma 1573
Dermatofibrosarcoma protuberans 1530, 1574
Dermatomyositis 257, 262, 405
Dermatopathy 1434
Dermis 1553
Desmoglein-1 (Dsg-1) 1550
Desmoglein–desmocollin 1550
Desmoid/deep-seated fibromatosis 1530
Desquamative interstitial pneumonia (DIP) 868
Destructive bone disease 43
Detection of carrier of hemophilia A 614
Detection systems of immunochemistry 699
Dexamethasone suppression test 1473
Diabetes insipidus 1469
Diabetes mellitus 751, 1412
Diabetes mellitus pathophysiology 1417
Diabetic glomerulosclerosis 1421
Diabetic ketoacidosis 1415, 1417
Diabetic nephropathy 1181
Diabetic retinopathy 1423
Diabetic vascular disease 766
Diagnosis of allergy 237
Diagnostic criteria—hairy cell leukemia 578
Diagnostic features—Langerhans' cell histiocytosis 591
Diagnostic utility of serum autoantibodies in liver disorders 1049
Dialysis principle 1201
Diamond-Blackfan syndrome 541
Diethylstilbestrol (DES) 391
Diffuse alveolar damage (DAD) 891
Diffuse and nodular glomerulosclerosis 1421
Diffuse cortical necrosis 1221
Diffuse glomerulonephritis 1163
Diffuse glomerulosclerosis 1182, 1421

Diffuse hyperplasia liver 1117
Diffuse infiltrative type gastric adenocarcinoma 981
Diffuse large B cell lymphoma (DLBCL) 665, 1002
Diffuse linear staining of GBM 1205
Diffuse malignant mesothelioma 929, 1035
Diffuse proliferative glomerulonephritis 1162
Diffuse pulmonary fibrosis 908
DiGeorge/velocardiofacial syndrome 218, 298, 683, 1456
Digital mammography 1402
Dihydrotestosterone (DHT) 1278
Dilutional hyponatremia 1418
Dilutional thrombocytopenia 640
Dipalmitoyl-phosphatidyl-choline 858
Direct acting carcinogens 382
Direct Coombs' test 525
Direct immunofluorescence microscopy 704
Disaccharidase deficiency 991
Discoid lupus erythematosus 257
Disorders of complement system 79, 219
  hereditary angioneurotic edema 79
  recurrent infections 79
  systemic lupus erythematosus 80
Disorders of complement system cascade 93
Disorders of intermediate filaments 38
Disorders of microtubules 38
Disrupted atheromatous plaque in AMI 787
Dissecting hematoma 138, 755, 757, 777
Disseminated intravascular coagulation (DIC) 95, 151, 160, 404, 549, 616
Distal adenocarcinomas 1139
Distal (paraseptal) emphysema 880
Divalent metal transporter-1 (DMT-1) 482
Diversion colitis 1015
Diverticulitis 1006
Diverticulum 1005
DMT-1 (divalent metal transporter-1) 482
DNA content of the tumor 1398
DNA defects 48
DNA double helix molecule 282
DNA gyrase 287
DNA helicases 287
DNA ligase 287
DNA oncogenic viruses 389
DNA polymerase 287, 1067
DNA probe analysis 415
DNA repair genes 319, 368
DNA replication 287
DNA sequences methods 724–730
DNA single-stranded binding proteins 287
DNA strands 287
DNA-adduct formation 383
Double contrast barium enema 1038
Down's syndrome 295, 297, 541
DPC4 (MADH4/SMAD4) tumor suppressor gene 369

Dressler's syndrome 794
Driver mutations 347
Drug-induced acute tubulointerstitial diseases 1214
Drug-induced autoimmune hemolytic anemia 240
Drug-induced hemolytic anemia 519
Drug-induced hepatitis 1057
Drug-induced platelet dysfunction 606
Drug-induced thrombocytopenia 240, 604
Drug-induced vasculitides 766
Drugs and toxins induced liver injury 1080
Drugs associated with interstitial fibrosis 895
Dry beriberi 427
Dry gangrene 31
Dubin-Johnson syndrome 1055
Duchenne muscular dystrophy 303, 312, 1542
Duct ectasia 1367
Ductal carcinoma of breast 1385
Ductal epithelial hyperplasia of fibrocytic disease 1369
Ductus arteriosus 834
Duodenal atresia 997
Duodenal peptic ulcer 972
Duplication of small intestine 987
Durck's granuloma 108
D-Xylose test in malabsorption 1039
Dyserythropoiesis 561
Dysfunctional leukocytes 38
Dysfunctional uterine bleeding 1309
Dysgerminoma 1334
Dysmegakaryopoiesis 561
Dysmenorrhea 1309
Dysmyelopoiesis 561
Dysparaproteinemias and uremia 607
Dysphagia 959
Dysplasia 12, 320
Dysplasia in bronchial epithelium 13
Dysplasia liver 1116
Dysplastic nevus 1570
Dysplastic proliferations 343
Dystrophic calcification 32, 42, 433
Dystrophin gene 312, 1543

E

E selectins 126
Early gastric carcinoma 979
Eaton-Lambert syndrome 241, 243
E-Cadherins 1382
Ecchymosis 137
Echinococcus granulosus 454, 1079
Echocardiography two-dimensional 797
Ectopic kidneys 1229
Ectopic pregnancy 1307
Ectopic thyroid tissue 1449
Eczematous dermatitis 1556
Edible shellfish 1065
EDNRB gene 1003
EDTA (ethylene diamine tetra acetic acid) 476

Edward's syndrome (trisomy 18) 299
Effacement of visceral epithelial foot processes 1175
Efferocytosis 36
Ehlers-Danlos syndrome 302, 305, 608, 757
Electrocardiogram 805
Electrocardiogram (12 leads) in AMI 795
Electron dense immune complex deposits 1205
Electron microscopy (EM) 414, 688–690
    comparison of light and electron microscope 689
    scanning electron microscopy 688
    transmission electron microscopy 688
Electrophoresis 734–737
    cellular acetate electrophoresis 725
    citrate agar electrophoresis 726
    gel electrophoresis 737
Elephantiasis 455
ELISA (enzyme-linked immunosorbent assay) 237, 721–724
Emboli from tumors 160
Embolism 156
Embryonal carcinoma 1263, 1335
Embryonal rhabdomyosarcoma 1532
Embryonic stem cells 112
Emery-Dreifuss muscular dystrophy 1545
Emigration 60
Emphysema 876, 877, 879
Empty-sella syndrome 1469
Empyema 928
Empyema gallbladder 1127, 1135
Encephalitis 1588
Enchondromatosis 1496
End stage renal disease 1198
Endocarditis 802, 811
Endocarditis in intravenous drug abuse 815
Endocarditis in prosthetic valves 815
Endocarditis in rheumatic heart disease 816
Endocarditis of carcinoid syndrome 817
Endocervical curetting 1305
Endocervical polyp 1298
Endocrine associated amyloidosis 277
Endocrine pancreas 1409
Endocrine signaling 119
Endodermal sinus tumor 1266
Endogenous antigens 189
Endogenous melanin 933
Endogenous pigmentation 933
Endometrial hyperplasia 10, 1310, 1311
Endometrial stromal tumor 1318
Endometrioid adenocarcinoma 1330
Endometriosis 1313
Endometriosis (chocolate cysts) 1349
Endometritis 1310
Endoparasites induced carcinogenesis 390
Endophytic papilloma 839
Endoscopic retrograde cholangiography (ERCP) 1137
Endostatin 335
Endothelial adhesion molecule 62
    CD4 62
    E selectin 62

GlyCam-1 62
PECAM (CD31) 62
P selectin 62
VCAM-1 (Ig family) 62
Endotoxic shock 171
Entamoeba histolytica 454
Enterobius vermicularis 455
Enterochromaffin cells 999
Enzymatic glycosylation mechanism 1419
Enzyme-linked immunosorbent assay (ELISA) 237, 721–724
Eosinophilia 535
Eosinophilic chemotactic factor-A (ECF-A) 235
Eosinophilic cystitis 1247
Eosinophilic gastroenteritis 991
Eosinophilic granuloma 592, 897, 1504
Eosinophilic myocarditis 807
Eosinophilic peritonitis 1034
Eosinophilic pneumonia 897
Eosinophils 534
Ependymal cells 1581
Ependymomas 1601
Epidermal growth factor (EGF) 116, 753
Epidermal growth factor (EGF) receptors 351
Epidermal inclusion cyst 1577
Epidermis 1550
Epidermis stem cells 113
Epidermoid carcinoma 1033
Epidermophyton 1561
Epidural hematoma 1615
Epidural space 1582
Epigenetic changes 377
Epiphrenic diverticulum 962
Epispadias 1283
Epistasis 289
Epithelial mucins 925
Epithelial-mesenchymal transition (EMT) 393
Epithelioid granulomas 431
Epithelioid sarcoma 1538
Epsilon aminocaproic acid (EACA) 614
Epstein-Barr virus 538
Epstein-Barr virus associated cancers 389
Equine gait in hemophilia 612
ER and Her2 neu negative molecular pathway in breast carcinoma 1384
ERBB2 (Her2 neu) oncogene 1325, 1381
ERCP (endoscopic retrograde cholangiography) 1137
Erythema 137
Erythema marginatum 805
Erythema multiforme 933, 1564
Erythematous macule 1557
Erythroblastosis fetalis 240
Erythroplasia of Queyrat 1282
Erythropoiesis 464
Erythropoietin 462, 1153
Erythropoietin secreting tumors 464
    cerebral hemangioblastoma 464
    hepatocellular carcinoma 464

leiomyoma 464
renal cell carcinoma 464
Esophageal diverticulum 962
Esophageal dysmotility 262
Esophageal stricture 963
Esophageal varices 767, 963, 1088
Essential hypertension 773
Essential thrombocythemia 571
Essential thrombocytosis 562
ESWL (extracorporeal shock wave lithotripsy) 1221
Etiology of large hepatic vein thrombosis 1111
Etiopathogenesis 616
Euglin lysis time 616
Euglobulin lysis test 625
Evasion of apoptosis of cancer 370
Evasion of immune surveillance in cancer 395
Evolution of cervical carcinoma 1302, 1303
Ewing's sarcoma/primitive neuroectodermal tumors (PNET) 376, 1499
Exchange of gases 858
Executioner caspases 36
Exfoliative cytology 413, 1305
Exocrine glands atrophy 7
Exocrine tumors 1145
Exophthalmos 1434
Exophytic carcinomas of gastric carcinoma 979
Exophytic papillomas of nasal cavity 838
Expansion of myocardial infarct area in AMI 795
Expansion of trinucleotide repeat 289
Expiratory reserve volume 860
Exposure to chemicals 908
Exposure to ionizing radiation 908
Exstrophy of urinary bladder 1247
External hemorrhoids 1031, 1089
External hydrocephalus 1619
Extracellular accumulations 47
Extracorporeal shock wave lithotripsy (ESWL) 1221
Extrahepatic jaundice 1058
Extramammary Paget's disease of vulva 1289
Extranodal marginal zone B cell lymphoma 390, 663, 671
Extranodal NK cell/T cell lymphoma 675
Extrapulmonary tuberculosis 437
Extravascular RBCs destruction 497
Extrinsic (death receptor) pathway 35
Extrinsic pathway of coagulation 143
Exudate 57, 166
Exudative diarrhea 993
Exudative effusions 928
Exudative pharyngitis 934

F

11β-hydroxylase gene 774
24 hours fecal fat test in malabsorption syndrome 1039
FAB classification of leukemias 540

Fabry disease 303, 312, 1162
Facial clefts 932
Facioscapulohumeral muscular dystrophy 1545
Factor IX (high purity) 635
Factor IX concentrate 637
Factor V 142
Factor V Leiden 148, 150, 619
Factor VII 635
Factor VIII (antihemophilic globulin) 610
Factor VIII and VWF synthesis 610
Factor VIII assay 613
Factor VIII concentrate 636
Factor XI 635
Factors influencing infarction 160
Failure of engraftment 595
Familial adenomatous polyposis (FAP) 302, 342, 978, 1021
Familial amyloidosis 277
Familial glomerulopathy 1162
Familial hypercholesterolemia 302, 304
Familial hyperlipidemia 750
Familial medullary carcinoma of thyroid 1446
Fanconi anemia 374, 528, 541
Fanconi's syndrome 1216
Farmer's lung 244
Fasciola hepatica 391
Fasting blood glucose level 1412
Fat embolism 157, 158, 1615
Fat embolism syndrome 902
Fat necrosis 26, 29, 1364
Fat necrosis of breast 1364
Fat stairs 1097, 1201
Fate of thrombus 155
Fat-soluble vitamins 423, 424
Fatty change liver (steatosis) 17, 1095, 1424, 1844
Fatty cysts liver 1097
Fatty streaks 743
FDP D-dimer 623
Febrile non-hemolytic transfusion reactions 639
Feces examination 1038
Felty syndrome 1519
Female genital system 1285
Female pseudohermaphrodite 312
Fenton reaction 22
Fernandez reaction 442
Ferritin 25, 483
Fetal alcohol syndrome 1619
Fetal hemoglobin 507
FGF3 (fibroblast growth factor 3) 1251, 1381
Fiberoptic bronchoscopy 925
Fibrillary deposit 1205
Fibrillin 608
Fibrin cap in glomeruli 1183, 1421
Fibrin generation 599
Fibrin stabilizing factor 599
Fibrinogen 63, 142, 556
Fibrinogen degradation product (FDP D-dimer) 195, 556, 623

Fibrinoid necrosis 26, 31, 743, 776, 1224
  Henoch-Schönlein purpura 31
  lupus erythematosus 31
  polyarteritis nodosa 31
  malignant hypertension 31
Fibrinolysin gene 148
Fibrinolytic system 74, 600
Fibrinous inflammation 71
Fibrinous or serofibrinous pericarditis 779, 791, 823
Fibroadenoma—breast 1370
Fibroblast growth factor (FGF) 99, 196, 334, 350, 753
Fibroblast growth factor 3 (FGF3) 1251, 1381
Fibroblastic growth factor-β 117
Fibroblasts 1159, 1553
Fibrocongestive splenomegaly 678
Fibroepithelial polyp 1577
Fibrohistiocytic tumors 1532
Fibrolamellar variant of hepatocellular carcinoma 1120
Fibroma 1342
Fibroma group lesions 956
Fibromatosis colli 1529
Fibronectin 63, 123, 129, 195, 1159
Fibrosarcoma 1507, 1531
Fibrosis of peritoneum 1034
Fibrous (fibroblastic) meningioma 1607
Fibrous dysplasia 956, 1511
Fibrous dysplasia of bone 933
Fibrovascular polyps 964
FIGLU test 493
Firm adhesion 61
First line of host defense 182
FISH and Mc FISH techniques 314
FISH probes and probe development 718
FISH procedure 716
Fistulous tract 1013
Fite stain 445
Fixatives 691
FLAER (fluorescent aerolysin) test 522
Flapping tremors in liver failure 1091
Flat mucosal lesions 979
Flexible sigmoidoscopy 1037
Flow cytometry 315, 415, 501, 522, 527, 579, 706
Fluorescein 698
Fluorescence in situ hybridization (FISH) 314, 716, 719
Fluorescent like stains 440
Fluorescent spot test 516
Fluorescent stains (thioflavin-T, thioflavin-S) 281
Focal glomerulonephritis 1163
Focal liver necrosis 1045
Focal nodular hyperplasia liver 1116
Focal proliferative glomerulonephritis 1162
Focal segmental glomerulosclerosis 1162, 1175
Folic acid 429, 487
Folic acid in DNA synthesis 490

Follicular carcinoma of thyroid 1443
Follicular center cell lymphoma 376
Follicular cysts 1346
Follicular lymphoma 663, 668, 670
Food poisoning 992
Foramen of Luschka and Magendie 1582
Forbers-Cori disease 309
Fordyce's granules 933
Foreign body granuloma 106
Formaldehyde 691, 692
Formation of ABH antigen 627
Formulated peptides 63
Fractional curettage 1305
Fragile X syndrome 289, 303
Frameshift mutations 288
Freckle (ephelis) 1569
Free radical injury 48
Fresh frozen plasma 635, 636
Friedler's myocarditis 807
Friedreich ataxia 809
Frontal bossing in rickets 425
Frozen section technique 414, 687, 688, 1405
Frustrated (regurgitated) phagocytosis 69
Fulminant acute hepatitis with massive hepatic necrosis 1071
Fulminant hepatitis 1066
Fulminant liver necrosis 1046
Fulminant myocarditis 807
Function of insulin 1411
Functional (acalculus) gallbladder disease 1132
Functional residual capacity 860
Functional zones of liver acinus (lobule) 1041
Functions of placenta 1286
Fungal infections 838
Fungal meningitis 1587
Fungal pneumonias 862
Fungal sinusitis 838
Fusiform aneurysm 755

G

G6PD deficiency 291, 303, 514
Galactokinase deficiency 309
Galectin 3 1382, 1400, 1406
Gallbladder 1126
Gallstone ileus 997
Gallstones 1130
Gallstones in sickle cell disease 512
Gamma irradiated red blood cells 635
Gamna-gandy bodies 137, 678, 829
Ganglioneuroma 1610
Gangrene 31
Gangrenous inflammation 73
Gangrenous necrosis 26, 30
Gardner's syndrome 1021
Gardnerella vaginalis 1292
Gas gangrene 31
Gastric adenocarcinoma 976, 981
Gastric adenocarcinoma—intestinal types 979
Gastric carcinoma (linitis plastica variant) 332
Gastric lavage 439
Gastric MALT lymphoma 982
Gastric peptic ulcer 71, 972
Gastrinoma 1149
Gastroesophageal reflux disease (GERD) 960
Gastrointestinal stromal tumors (GIST) 984, 1001
Gastrointestinal tract bleeding 612
Gaucher's cells 680, 1106
Gaucher's disease 307, 480, 589, 680, 1106
GBM replication 1205
GBM thickening 1205
Gel electrophoresis 737
Gene amplification 375
Gene mutation 288, 515
Generalized lymphadenopathy 644
Genetic code 285
Genetic predisposition 798
Genetic variations 291
Genetics terminology 283
Genitourinary system bleeding 612
Genomic stability 374
Germ cell tumors 1334
Germinoma 1609
Gestational choriocarcinoma 1352
Gestational diabetes 422
Gestational diabetes mellitus 422, 1355, 1417
Gestational trophoblastic tumors 1349
GFAP (glial fibrillary acidic protein) 1361
Ghon's focus 432, 873
Giant Aschoff's bodies in rheumatic fever 801
Giant cell tumor (osteoclastoma) of bone 326, 1501, 1502
Giant cell tumor of soft tissue 1532
Giant cells seen in bone tumors and tumor-like conditions 1503
Giardiasis 454, 994
Giemsa stain 477
Gilbert's syndrome 1053
Gingival cyst 952
Glandular metaplasia 343
Glandular odontogenic cyst 952
Glanzmann disease (thrombasthenia) 142, 622
Glaucoma 1423
Gleason system of grading of prostatic carcinoma 1280
Glial fibrillary acidic protein (GFAP) 1361, 1375, 1406
Glioblastoma multiforme 1599
Glisson's capsule 1046
Global glomerulonephritis 1162, 1163
Globin chain electrophoresis 527
Globulomaxillary cyst 952
Glomangioma 770
Glomerular basement membrane (GBM) 1158, 1205
Glomerular capillaries 1157
Glomerular filtrate rate (GFR) 1160
Glomerular filtration pressure 1161
Glomerular permeability barriers 1160
Glomerulonephritis 1164
Glomerulus 1157
Glomus tumors 1536
Glucagonoma 1148
Glucocerebrosidase 680
Glucocorticoid-remediable aldosteronism 774, 1460
Glucocorticoids 85, 94
Glucose tolerance test 1425
Glucuronyl transferase 1051
Glutamyltranspeptidase 1048
Glutaraldehyde 692
Glutathione peroxidase (GPX) 25
Glycocalyx 598
Glycogen storage disease 37, 46, 302, 309, 1105
Glycoprotein IIb/IIIa 598
Glycosaminoglycans 124, 127, 167
Glycosylated hemoglobin (HbA1c) 751, 1425
GNAS1 gene 1512
Goblet cell carcinoid 999
Goiter 1436
Gomori methenamine stain 454, 1080
Gonadal dysgenesis 1325
Gonadoblastoma 1344
Gonococcal arthritis 1523
Good immunogens 189
Goodpasture's syndrome 240, 256, 264, 637, 897, 1194
Gouty arthritis 1521
Gouty tophus 1522
Grades of NHL 659
Grading and staging 402, 1398
Graft rejection 247
Graft-versus-host disease (GVHD) 269, 593
Grain leather-like appearance—kidney 1223
Granular cell tumor 967
Granular lumpy bumpy deposits in glomeruli 1205
Granulation tissue 102
Granuloma formation 105
  breakdown of granuloma 105
  maintenance of granuloma 105
Granuloma inguinale 1287
Granuloma pyogenicum 937, 1578
Granulomatous cervicitis 1298
Granulomatous cystitis 1247
Granulomatous inflammation 103, 248, 249, 680
Granulomatous liver abscess 1078
Granulomatous lymphadenitis 642
Granulomatous mastitis 1365
Granulomatous orchitis 1273
Granulomatous prostatitis 1277
Granulomatous salpingitis 1306
Granulomatous serositis 1034

Index

Granulomatous T cell-mediated hypersensitivity reactions 250
Granulosa cell tumor of ovary 1341
Granzyme B protease 36
Graves' disease 241, 242, 255, 264, 1433
Grenza zone 444
Grocott's methenamine silver stain 838
Growth factors 116
Growth hormone insensitivity (Laron syndrome) 1469
Guillain-Barré syndrome 249, 250, 637, 1617
Gumma syphilis 1589
Gummatous necrosis 31
Gut associated lymphoid tissue (GALT) 181
Gynecomastia 1047, 1407

H

Haber-Weiss reaction 22
Hairy cell leukemia 577, 662, 672
Hairy cells 578
Hallmarks of cancer 345
Halogenase 1427
Ham's test 522
Hamartoma 331
Hamartomatous polyps 976
Hamazaki-Weissenberg bodies 42
HAMP gene 482
Hand and foot syndrome in sickle cell 511
Hand-Schüller-Christian disease 591, 1503
Happy puppet (Angelman) syndrome 292
Hapten 189
Haptoglobin 498, 524
Harelip 932
Harrison's groove in rickets 425
Hartnup disease 428, 1216
Hashimoto's thyroiditis 104, 255, 1427
Hassall corpuscles in thymus 682
HbA1c (glycated hemoglobin) 1412
HbE thalassemia 484
HBeAg 1069
HbH disease 484
HBV-DNA 1069
Head injuries 1615
Healing by primary intention 131
Healing of bone fractures 121
Heart anatomy and physiology 782
Heart failure 136, 827
Heart failure cells 136
Heat shock protein 27, 1400, 1406
Heinz bodies in RBCs 479, 480, 515
Helicobacter pylori 390, 968
Helicobacter pylori tests 1039
Helly's fluid fixative 692
Helmet cells 480
Hemangioblastoma 844, 1609
Hemangioendothelioma 771, 1115
Hemangioma 1114, 1540, 1575
Hemangiopericytoma 771
Hemarthrosis 138, 612, 615
Hematemesis 138
Hematin pigment 41

Hematobilia 138
Hematocele 1275
Hematocephalus 138
Hematochezia 138
Hematocrit values 474
Hematogenous spread of cancer 396
Hematological findings in AML (M3) 556
Hematological findings of CLL 575
Hematological findings of CML 565
Hematoma 138
Hematopoiesis 459, 496
Hematopoietic CD34+ stem cells infusion 594
Hematopoietic growth factors 462
Hematopoietic microenvironment 461, 462
Hematopoietic stem cell transplantation 592
Hematopoietic stem cells (HSCs) 112, 461, 533, 539, 592
Hematoxylin and eosin stain 694, 1201
Hemifacial hypertrophy 933
Hemochromatosis 41, 933, 1100
Hemochromatosis induced cirrhosis 1082
Hemodialysis 1201
Hemodialysis associated amyloidosis 277
Hemoglobin C inclusions 479
Hemoglobin E disorders 514
Hemoglobin electrophoresis 507, 513, 525, 526, 734
Hemoglobin H inclusions 479, 508
Hemoglobin S 291
Hemoglobin synthesis 475, 476, 524
Hemoglobinemia 498
Hemoglobinuria 498
Hemolytic anemia 240, 495
Hemolytic disease of newborn 240, 519
Hemolytic jaundice 40, 495, 1058
Hemolytic transfusion reaction 521, 638
Hemolytic uremic syndrome 523, 604, 1195
Hemopericardium 138, 822
Hemopexin 498, 524
Hemophilia A 303, 609
Hemophilia B 303, 615
Hemophilia with inhibitors 637
Hemoptysis 138
Hemorrhage 137, 138
Hemorrhagic (red) infarct 27, 164
Hemorrhagic cystitis 1247
Hemorrhagic disease of newborn 427, 616
Hemorrhagic inflammation 73
Hemorrhagic lung infarct 901
Hemorrhagic pericarditis 823
Hemorrhoids 1031, 1089
Hemosiderin pigment 40
Hemosiderinuria 498, 524
Hemosiderosis 41, 680
Hemostasis 139
Hemothorax 928
Henoch-Schönlein purpura 607, 766, 1194
Heparin 477
Heparin anticoagulant 477
Heparin induced thrombocytopenia (HIT) syndrome 151, 604

Heparin-like molecules 596
Hepatic encephalopathy 1047, 1090
Hepatic sinusoids 1043
Hepatic vasculature 1041
Hepatitis 1058
Hepatitis A virus (HAV) 1064
Hepatitis B core antigen (HBcAg) 1067
Hepatitis B surface antigen (HBsAg) 1067
Hepatitis B virus (HBV) 1067
Hepatitis B virus associated carcinoma 390
Hepatitis Be antigen (HBeAg) 1067
Hepatitis C virus (HCV) 1071
Hepatitis C virus 389
Hepatitis D virus 1073
Hepatitis E virus 1074
Hepatitis G virus (HGV) 1074
Hepatoblastoma 1122
Hepatocellular adenoma 1113
Hepatocellular carcinoma 464, 1117
Hepatocellular hyperplasia 1116
Hepatocellular jaundice 1058
Hepatocellular necrosis 1061
Hepatocyte growth factor (HGF) 117, 351
Hepatocyte membrane antibody 1049
Hepatocytic embryonic stem cells 112
Hepatomegaly 829
Hepatomegaly due to malaria 1080
Hepatoportal sclerosis 1112
Hepatorenal or von Gierke disease type I 46
Hepatorenal syndrome 1093
Hepatotropic viruses 449, 1058, 1064
Hepatotropic viruses comparison 1076
Hepcidin 482
Her2 neu enriched molecular pathway 1384
Hereditary amyloidosis 277
Hereditary angioneurotic edema 79, 219
Hereditary hemorrhagic telangiectasia 302, 304, 608, 770
Hereditary hyperbilirubinemia 1052
Hereditary hypercoagulable state 148, 619
Hereditary nonpolyposis colorectal cancer (HNPCC) 342, 977, 1022
Hereditary ovalocytosis 501
   band 3 (anion channel) 501
   band 4.1 501
Hereditary sideroblastic anemia 530
Hereditary spherocytosis 302, 304, 499
   ankyrin proteins 500
   band 3 (anionic channel) 500
   band 4.2 proteins (pallidin) 500
   gallstones 500
   jaundice 500
   leg ulcers 500
   spectrin proteins 500
   splenomegaly 500
Hereditary stomatocytosis 502
Hereditary thrombophilia 148, 618
Hermaphroditism 312
Herpes simplex encephalitis 448
Herpes simplex virus 934, 1283, 1560
Herpetic dermatitis 1560

Herring-bone pattern in fibro-
　　sarcoma 1508, 1531
Heterologous antigens 190
Heterophilic IgM antibodies 538
Heterotropic gastric mucosa 987
HFE gene 1100, 1103
Hiatus hernia 962
Hibernoma 1527
High grade surface osteosarcoma 1494
High performance liquid chromatography
　　(HPLC) 52, 507, 513, 733, 734
High resolution MRI 797
Highly reactive hydroxyl molecule 68
Hippel-Lindau disease 306
Hirschsprung's disease 1003
Histamine 80, 234, 235
Histiocytic tumors 1503
Histochemical stains 691–697
Histological classification of ovarian
　　tumors 1321
Histological patterns of liver necrosis 1046
Histoplasma capsulatum 452, 472, 868
HIV evasion methods 223
HIV testing for high risk persons 227
HIV vaccines 229
HLA antigens 302
HLA classes (class I and class II) 200
HLA system 264
　　Class I HLAs 264
　　Class II HLAs 265
　　HLA associated diseases 266
　　organ transplants 266
HMGA2 1526
Hodgkin's disease 389, 517, 579, 648
Hodgkin's disease—morphologic sub-
　　types 654
Holoprosencephaly 1618
Homar's sign 1355
Homogentisic acid 41
Homologous antigens (ISO-antigens) 190
Hormone induced carcinogenesis 391
Hormone therapy 1407
Hormones and breast development 1360
Horner's syndrome 918
Horseradish peroxidase 698
Horseshoe kidneys 1230
Host defenses 182
Hourglass deformity and pyloric
　　stenosis 975
Howell-Jolly bodies 465, 479, 480, 561
HPV E6/E7 oncogene activity in cancer 365
H-RAS signal-transducing proteins 1251
HTLV 1 (human T-lymphotropic virus
　　type 1) 389
Human chorionic gonadotropin
　　(hCG) 1339
Human factor VIII 635
Human factor VIII (high purity) 635
Human genome 282
Human leukocyte antigen 265
Human papillomavirus 390, 449, 1287, 1301
Humoral immunity 191

Hunter syndrome 303, 311
Huntington disease 289
Huntington's chorea 302
Hurler's syndrome 37, 308
Hutchinson melanotic 1570
Hutchinson-Gilford progeria 49
Hyaline arteriolosclerosis 742, 1183, 1421
Hyaline change 17, 18
Hyaluronidase 799
Hydatid cyst 454, 1078
Hydrocele 1274
Hydrocephalus 1618
Hydrogen peroxide 22
Hydromyelia 1618
Hydronephrosis 1217
Hydropericardium 822
Hydropic change 18
Hydrops fetalis 509
Hydrothorax 169, 928
Hydroxyl radicals 22
Hyperacute graft rejection 267
Hyperaldosteronism 1459
Hypercalcemia 404
Hyperemia 134
Hyperestrinism in women 1093
Hyperhomocystinemia 619, 797
Hyper-IgM syndrome 217
Hyperlipidemia 749
Hyperosmolar hyperglycemia state in
　　DM 1417
Hyperparathyroidism 1453
Hyperplasia 4, 9
Hyperplastic arteriolitis 743
Hyperplastic arteriolosclerosis 776, 1224
Hyperplastic ileocecal tuberculosis 438, 995
Hyperplastic polyps 975, 1017
Hyperplastic (regenerative) polyps 986
Hypersensitivity pneumonitis 868, 897
Hypersensitivity reactions 230–249
　　type I hypersensitivity reactions 231
　　type II hypersensitivity reactions 237
　　type III hypersensitivity reactions 243
　　type IV hypersensitivity reactions 245
Hypersensitivity reactions—
　　comparison 230
Hypersplenism 679
Hypertension 772
　　benign hypertension 772
　　cardiovascular disorders 774
　　cardiovascular manifestations 777
　　cerebral hemorrhage 777
　　CNS disorders 775
　　determinants of hypertension 772
　　endocrine disorders 774
　　essential hypertension 772
　　liver manifestations 780
　　malignant hypertension 772
　　peripheral edema 780
　　renal manifestations 780
　　renovascular hypertension 774
　　retinopathy 777
　　role of hormones 774

　　secondary hypertension 772
　　toxemia of pregnancy 775
Hyperthyroidism 404, 1433
Hypertrophic cardiomyopathy 809
Hypertrophic osteoarthropathy 405, 1523
Hypertrophy 4, 7
Hypertrophy of endoplasmic reticulum 37
Hyperviscosity syndrome 585
Hypervitaminosis D 43
Hypochlorous acid 22
Hypochlorous acid (bleach) 99
Hypoglycemia 404
Hypoplasia 14
Hypoplasia of megakaryocytes 604
Hypoplastic left heart syndrome 835
Hypospadias 1283
Hyposplenism 679
Hypothyroidism 1431
Hypovolemic shock 171, 172
Hypoxia inducible factor (HIF) 92

I

Iatrogenic hypopituitarism 1469
ICAM (intercellular adhesion mole-
　　cule-1) 752
Idiopathic giant cell myocarditis 807
Idiopathic pulmonary fibrosis 896
Idiopathic thrombocytopenic purpura 602
Idiosyncrasy 1080
IL-1 and TNF-α 117
Ileofemoral venous thrombus 1355
Imaging techniques 805
Immature platelet fraction (IPF) 605
Immature teratoma 1337
Immotile cilia syndrome 38
Immune complex mediated glomerulo-
　　nephritis 256, 1162
Immune dysfunction in HIV 223
Immunity 178
Immunoassay 527
Immunofluorescence microscopy 261,
　　703, 704
Immunoglobulin classes 207
　　IgA 207
　　IgD 207
　　IgE 207
　　IgG 207
　　IgM 207
Immunohistochemistry 415, 698–703
　　immunohistochemistry protocol 700,
　　　　701
　　panel of monoclonal antibodies in
　　　　common malignancies 701
Immunologic tolerance 250–254
　　central tolerance 252
　　peripheral tolerance 253
Immunological mediated granulomas 106
Immunophenotyping of chronic lympho-
　　proliferative disorders 576
Immunosuppressive drugs 272
　　azathioprine 272
　　biological immunosuppression 272

cyclosporine A 272
rapamycin 272
tacrolimus (FK506) 272
Impetigo 1557
In situ anti-glomerular membrane disease 1161
In situ (noninvasive) breast carcinoma 1377
Inactivation of free radicals 25
Inappropriate secretion of antidiuretic hormone 404
Inclusions in red blood cells 479
   basophilic stippling 479
   Cabot's ring 479
   Heinz bodies 479
   hemoglobin C inclusions 479
   hemoglobin H inclusions 479
   Howell-Jolly bodies 479
   siderotic nodules/Pappenheimer bodies 479
Incomplete carcinogens 382
Incomplete hydatidiform mole 1352
Increased cellularity of glomeruli 1201
Increased extracellular material 1201
Increased platelet destruction 601
Increased vascular permeability 56, 211
Indeterminate leprosy 443
Indian childhood cirrhosis 1107
Indications for stem cell transplantation 592
Indirect acting carcinogens 382
Indirect Coombs' test 525
Indirect ELISA 722
Indirect immunofluorescence microscopy 704
Infantile embryonal carcinoma 1266
Infantile Gaucher's disease (type 2) 1106
Infantile polycystic kidney disease 1227
Infarction 160
Infections 595
Infectious mononucleosis 538, 642
Infective endocarditis 811, 813
Infertility 422
Inflammation and infection 836
Inflammatory bowel disease 1007
Inflammatory bowel disease (Crohn's disease) 250
Inflammatory carcinoma 1390
Inflammatory dermatoses terminology and examples 1555
Inflammatory fibroid polyp 976
Inflammatory myopathies 1546
Inflammatory polyps 964, 1018
Infusion of hematopoietic stem cells 594
Ingestion of smoked meat and fish 384
Inguinal hernia 997
Inheritance of monogenic disorders 289
Inherited ataxia-telangiectasia 343, 1379
Inherited cancer syndromes 977
Inhibitors of coagulation 600
Initiator caspases in apoptosis 36
Insertion 288
Insertional mutagenesis 377

Inspiratory reserve volume 860
Insulin receptor substrate molecules 1412
Insulin resistant diabetes mellitus 241, 243
Insulin-like growth factor 117, 422
Insulinoma 1148
INT2 oncogene 1381
Integrin family 59, 62, 126
   β1 integrin 126
   β2 integrin (LeuCAMs) 126
   β3 integrin (cytoadhesions) 126
Integrin receptors 120
Intercellular adhesion molecule-1 (ICAM-1) 752
Interferon-α (IFN-α) 88
Interferon-β (IFN-β) 88
Interferon-γ (IFN-γ) 88
Interleukins 99
Intermediate filaments 38
Internal carotid artery occlusion 1611
Internal hemorrhoids 1032, 1089
Internal hydrocephalus 1619
Interpretation 526
Interstitial emphysema 881
Interstitial pneumonia 862, 866
   gross morphology 867
   hypersensitivity pneumonitis 867
   light microscopy 867
   lymphocytic interstitial pneumonia 867
   mycoplasma pneumoniae 867
   viral pneumonias 867
Intestinal epithelium stem cells 114
Intestinal hemorrhagic infarct 164
Intestinal intussusception 997
Intestinal tuberculosis 438
Intestinal type gastric adenocarcinoma 979
Intracanalicular pattern in fibroadenoma 1371
Intracellular accumulations 44
Intracellular microbial killing 6, 68
Intracoronary stenting 787
Intracranial compartments 1582
Intraductal papilloma 1374
Intramembranous deposits in glomeruli 1203, 1204
Intrathoracic manifestations of bronchial carcinoma 913
Intrauterine toxoplasma infection 42
Intravascular RBCs destruction 498
   plasma haptoglobin level 498
   plasma hemoglobinemia 498
   hemoglobinuria 498
   hemosiderinuria 498
   plasma hemopexin 498
   plasma methemalbumin 498
Intraventricular space 1582
Intrinsic factor 490
Intrinsic mitochondrial pathway 35
Intrinsic pathway of coagulation 143
Invasion and metastases 326, 392
Invasive breast carcinoma 1378
Invasive carcinoma of penis 1282

Invasive ductal carcinoma breast 1385, 1387, 1408
Invasive hydatidiform mole 1352
Invasive lobular carcinoma 1386
Invasive micropapillary breast carcinoma 1393
Invasive squamous cell carcinoma 1567
Invasive urothelial neoplasms 1250
Involucrum formation in osteomyelitis 1477
Iron deficiency anemia 483, 484, 486
Iron metabolism 481, 482
Irregular (fluffy) deposits in glomeruli 1205
Irregular emphysema lung 879, 880
Irreversible cell injury 15, 18
Ischemic infarct 27
Ischemic/reperfusion injury 15
Islet β cells hyperplasia of the pancreas 10
Islet cell tumors 1148
Isochromosome formation 296
Isoelectric focusing (IEF) 527
Isolated gonadotropin deficiency 1469
Isolated IgA deficiency 217
Ito cells in liver 1043

J

JAK/STAT RAS signal transduction protein pathway 356
JAK2 mutation 571
Janeway's lesions in acute bacterial endocarditis 814
Jaundice 1050
Jaundice—differential diagnosis 1057
Jaw lesions 950
Jenner's stain 477
Jensen's score 1255
Jones diagnostic criteria in rheumatic fever 801, 805
Jones methenamine silver impregnation stain 1201
Jugular venous pressure 829
Junctional nevus 1569
Juvenile (aggressive) ossifying fibroma 956
Juvenile adenoma 1376
Juvenile coli 1022
Juvenile Gaucher's disease (type 3) 1106
Juvenile hypertrophy of the left breast 1401
Juvenile myelomonocytic leukemia 561
Juvenile onset insulin-dependent type 1 diabetes mellitus 1415
Juvenile papillomatosis breast (Swiss cheese disease) 1373
Juxtacrine signaling 119
Juxtaglomerular apparatus 1151
Juxtaglomerular cells 1151

K

Kallikrein (kinin) 63, 74
Kallmann syndrome 1469
Kaposi sarcoma 771, 936, 1541

Kartagener's syndrome 38, 837
Karyolysis 26
Karyorrhexis 26
Karyotyping 314, 315
Karyotyping techniques 314
Kawasaki disease 764
Kayser-Fleischer ring eye 1083, 1103
Keloid 1529, 1578
Keratinization 1552
Keratoacanthoma 1566
Keratomalacia 425
Ketoacidosis 1415
Kidney infarct 163
Kikuchi disease 643
Killed vaccine 211
Killing of cancer cells 247
Kimmelsteil-Wilson disease in diabetes nephropathy 1421
Kimura's disease 643
Kininogenase 235
KIT ligand receptors 352
KIT mutations 1001
Kleihauer-Betke test (acid elution test) 527
Klinefelter's syndrome 299, 541
Köhler bone disease 1514
K-RAS signal-transducing proteins 1145
Kreberg's stain 925
Krukenberg's tumor of ovaries 400, 981, 1323
Kupffer cells 1043, 1061, 1106
Kwashiorkor 418

L

L selectin (CD62L) 62, 126
Labile cells 111
Laboratory diagnosis of AML 553
Laboratory testing in HIV 227
Lack of costimulatory signal to T cells 254
Lactalbumin 1406
Lactate dehydrogenase (LDH) 796
Lactating adenoma 1375
Lactiferous ducts and sinuses 1362
Lactoferritin 25, 69
Lactotrope adenoma (prolactinoma) 1471
Lacunar type Reed-Sternberg cells 651
Lambert-Eaton syndrome 405, 1547
Laminar blood flow 597
Laminin 124, 129, 1158
Langerhans' cell histiocytosis 591
Langerhans' cells (dendritic cells) 198, 1552
Langerhans' cells of the skin 198
Langhans' giant cells 438
Lardaceous spleen in amyloidosis 47, 279
Large bowel infarction 1015
Large cell carcinoma lung 921
Large regenerative nodules liver 1116
Large-sized vessel vasculitis 1225
Laron syndrome 1469
Laryngeal edema 79
Laryngeal swab 439
Laryngeal tuberculosis 439

Larynx lesions 856
Lateral periodontal cyst 951
LE cell phenomenon 261
Lectins 126
Left heart failure 139, 827, 830
Left ventricular hypertrophy 829
Left-sided colorectal cancer 1027
Leg ulcers in sickle cell disease 512
Leg vein thrombosis 793
Legg-Calvé-Perthes disease 1514
Leiomyoma 324, 464, 966, 1319, 1535
Leiomyosarcoma 329, 1295, 1320, 1535
Leishman stain 477
Leishmania donovani bodies 472
Leishmaniasis 455, 472
Lentigo maligna melanoma 1570
Lentigo simplex 1569
Lepromatous leprosy 443, 444
Lepromin test 442
Leprosy 440
Leptin 420
Leptocytes 480
Leptomeningeal venulitis 1585
Lesch-Nyhan syndrome 312
Letterer-Siwe disease 1503
Leukemia 539
Leukemoid reaction 95
Leukemoid reactions 569
Leukocyte adhesion 211
Leukocyte adhesion receptors 62
Leukocyte chemotaxis 211
Leukocyte reduced red blood cells 635
Leukocyte transmigration 211
Leukocytes induced injury 69
Leukocytes reduced blood component 636
Leukocytosis 95
Leukoplakia 937
Leukoplakia of vulva 1288
Leukopoiesis 466, 533
Leukotrienes (LTC4, LTD4 and LTE4) 83, 84, 99, 196, 235
Leydig (interstitial) cell tumor 1269
Libman-Sacks endocarditis in SLE 815
Lichen planus 933, 1565
Lichen sclerosis 1291
Licorice 774
Liddle syndrome 774
Li-Fraumeni syndrome 978, 1379
Light chain cast nephropathy in multiple myeloma 1215
Limb-girdle dystrophy 1545
Limitations of microarray analysis 715
Limiting plates of liver 1041
Lineage markers of AML analyzing on flow cytometry 553
Lingual thyroid 1449
Linitis plastica variant 332
Lipid deposition 20
Lipid peroxidation 23
Lipoarabinomannan 431
Lipofuscin pigment 41
Lipogranulomas 1365

Lipoidoses 302
Lipoma 1526
Lipooxygenase pathway 83
Liposarcoma 1527
Lipoxins (LXA4, LXB4) 84
Liquefactive necrosis 26, 27, 28
Liquefactive necrosis in brain 28
Liquefactive necrosis in lungs 28
Lissencephaly 1618
Lithopodion 42
Live vaccines 211
Liver abscess 1077
Liver acinus (lobule) 1041, 1061
Liver amyloidosis 47
Liver cell necrosis 1061
Liver metastases 1124
Liver necrosis—histological patterns 1046
Liver regeneration 121
Liver stem cells 113
Lobar pneumonia 512, 862, 863, 867
  congestion 863
  grey hepatization 865
  organization (carnification) 865
  pathogenesis 863
  red hepatization 863
  resolution 865
  risk factors 863
Lobular carcinoma breast 1385
Lobular carcinoma *in situ* (LCIS) 1386
Lobular disarray 1061
Local scleroderma 261
Localized amyloidosis 277
Localized lymphadenopathy 644
Localized reaction 243
Localized tenosynovial giant cell tumor 1532
Locally malignant tumors 326
Location of stem cells 113
  canals of Hering 113
  hair follicle bulge 113
  hematopoietic stem cells 113
  marrow stem cells 113
  satellite cells 113
  subventricular zone (SVZ) dentate nuclei 113
Locus specific identifier (LSI) probes 719
Long noncoding RNA 288
Looser's zones 1480
Low grade central osteosarcoma 1490, 1493
Lowenstein-Jensen culture medium 440
Ludwig angina 934
Lumpectomy 1407
Lumpy bumpy deposits in glomeruli 1204
Lung abscess 869
Lung capacities 859
Lung consolidation 435
Lung consolidation in tuberculosis 874
Lung tumors 906
Lung volumes and capacities 860
Lungs 857
Lupoid hepatitis 1075
Lupus anticoagulant 620

Lupus anticoagulant syndrome 150
Lupus nephritis 1185
Lyme disease 1523
Lymph nodes 182, 641
Lymphangiectasia 991
Lymphangioma 1541
Lymphangioma liver 1115
Lymphatic spread 396
Lymphatic system 769
Lymphedema 167, 769
Lymphoblast 552
Lymphoblastic leukemia 568
Lymphocyte-depletion variant of Hodgkin's disease 655
Lymphocyte-rich variant of Hodgkin's disease 654
Lymphocytes 534
Lymphocytic-histiocytic Reed-Sternberg cells 651
Lymphocytopenia 536
Lymphocytosis 534, 535
   brucellosis 535
   syphilis 535
   tuberculosis 535
Lymphogranuloma venereum 1287
Lymphoid hyperplasia 642
Lymphoid organs 181
   bone marrow 181
   gut associated lymphoid tissue (GALT) in Peyer's patches 181
   lymph nodes 181
   mucosa associated lymphoid tissue (MALT) 181
   skin associated lymphoid tissue (SALT) 181
   spleen 181
   thymus gland 181
Lymphomatoid granulomatosis 767
Lysosomal dysfunction 37
Lysosomal enzyme 69, 81
Lysosomal hydrolytic enzymes 66
Lysosomal storage disease 307, 1105
LYST gene 93, 220

M

B72.3 monoclonal antibody 925
M spike in multiple myeloma 581
Macronodular cirrhosis 1083
Macrophage chemotactic protein-I (MCP-I) 99, 195
Macrophage inhibitory factor (MIF) 888
Macrophage products 99, 196
Macrovesicular steatosis liver 1096
Macula densa kidney 1151
Magnesium ammonium phosphate stones 1219
Magnetic resonance cholangiopancreatography (MRCP) 1137
Major basic proteins 69
Major diagnostic criteria 801
Major histocompatibility complex 200, 265
Major molecular pathways in evolution of breast carcinoma 1382
Malabsorption syndrome 987
Malacoplakia 1247
Malarial parasite 454, 472
Male hypogonadism 1272
Male impotence 1272
Male infertility 255, 1275
Male pseudohermaphrodite 312, 1274
Male sterility 38
Malignant Brenner tumor 1333
Malignant fibrous histiocytoma 1508
Malignant lymphoid neoplasms 645
Malignant melanoma 1570
Malignant mixed müllerian tumor 1334
Malignant nephrosclerosis 1223, 1224
Malignant peripheral nerve sheath tumor (MPNST) 1540
Malignant phyllodes tumor 1373
Malignant surface epithelial tumors 1324
Malignant tumors 325
Mallory hyaline 38
Mallory's Denk hyaline inclusions 1098
Mallory-Weiss syndrome 963, 1092
Malrotation of small intestine 987
Maltese-cross pattern 1173
Mammaglobin 1406
Mammalian sirtuin system 49
Mannose-binding lectin (MBL-2) 798
Mantle cell lymphoma 663, 670
Mantoux test 870
Marasmus 418
March hemolytic anemia 523
Marfan's syndrome 302, 304, 608, 757
Marginal zone lymphoma 671
Margination of leukocytes 57, 60, 61
Marker chromosome 296
Massive (fulminant) liver necrosis 1046
Massive splenomegaly 1089
Masson's trichrome stain 1201
Mast cells 233, 235
Mature callous formation in bone fracture 121
Mature cystic teratoma of testis 1336
Mature solid teratoma of testis 1337
Mature T cell and NK cell NHL 673
Maturity onset diabetes mellitus of the young (MODY) 1416
May-Grunwald stain 477
May-Grunwald-Giemsa stain 440
May-Hegglin anomaly 468, 537
MB-lectin pathway of complement 210
McArdle syndrome 37, 46, 309
McBurney's point abdomen 1030
McCallum plaque in RHD 803
McCune-Albright syndrome 1511
MDS/myeloproliferative disorders 561
Mean corpuscular hemoglobin (MCH) 474
Mean corpuscular hemoglobin concentration (MCHC) 474
Mean corpuscular volume (MCV) 474
Mechanism of apoptosis 33
Meckel's diverticulum 986
Meconium ileus 997
Median palatal cyst 952
Mediastinal (thymic) large B cell lymphoma 664
Mediterranean fever 277
Medium-sized vessel vasculitis 1225
Medullary breast carcinoma 1390
Medullary carcinoma thyroid 1444–1447
Medullary sponge kidney 1229
Medulloblastoma 1604
Megakaryoblastic crisis in CML 568
Megaloblastic anemia 423, 428, 487, 489
Megaloblastic macrocytic anemia 487
Meigs' syndrome 1342
Melanin pigment 39
Melanocytes 1552
Melanocytic nevus 331, 1569
Melanocytic tumors 1569
Melanoma 843, 1295
Melanoma of sinonasal region 843
Melena 138
Meloxicam drug 85
Membranoproliferative glomerulonephritis 1180
Membranous glomerulonephritis 1177
MEN 1 tumor suppressor gene 343, 369
MEN IIa syndrome (Sipple syndrome) 1463
MEN IIb syndrome 1463
Mendelian traits 303
Ménétrier disease 977, 985
Meningeal tumors 1606
Meningioma 1606, 1607
Meningiomas grade II (atypical meningiomas) 1607
Meningiomas grade III (anaplastic meningioma) 1607
Meningitis 512, 1584–1588
   bacterial meningitis 1584
   tubercular meningitis 1586
   viral meningitis 1587
Meningocele 1617
Meningoepithelial (syncytial) meningioma 1607
Meningomyelocele 1617
Menstrual cycle 1308
Mercaptans 1092
Mercurials 692
Merkel cell carcinoma of skin 1575
Merkel cells in epidermis 1552
Mesangial cells 1160
Mesangial deposits in glomeruli 1204
Mesenteric granulomatous lymphadenitis 1030
Mesothelioma 930
Messenger RNA (mRNA) 286, 288
Metabolic acidosis 1413
Metabolic bone disease 1479
Metachromatic stain 281, 697
Metalloproteinases (MMPs) 99, 129, 196
Metaphase CGH technique 712
Metaphase FISH technique 711

Metaphase fluorescence *in situ* hybridization 711
Metaphyseal fibrous defect (nonossifying fibroma) 1512
Metaplasia 5, 11, 1034
Metaplasia in neoplasm 12
Metaplastic breast carcinoma 1393
Metastases in bones 397
Metastases in brain 399
Metastases in liver 397
Metastases in lungs 397
Metastases in spleen 682
Metastases in testes 1271
Metastasis signature genes 393
Metastasis suppressor genes 393
Metastatic calcification 43, 1454
Methemalbumin 498
Methods for DNA sequences 724
Methyl green pyronine stain 587
Methyl violet (metachromatic stain) 281
Methylene blue stain 515
Methylenetetrahydrofolate gene 148
Microalbuminuria 1160
Microangiopathic hemolytic anemia 523
Microarray analysis 713, 715
Microcolumn chromatography 527
Microglia 1581
Microglia cells 1581
Microinvasion 320
Micronodular cirrhosis 1083
Microorganisms invading bone marrow 472
Microplate method 632
Micro-RNA (miRNA) 287
Micro-RNA in cancer 378
Microscopic polyarteritis 766
Microspherocytes 480
Microsporum 1561
Microtomy 694
Microtubules 38
Microvesicular steatosis 1096
Microvillus inclusion disease 991
Mid-diastolic murmur 819
Middle cerebral artery occlusion 1611
Midzonal necrosis–liver 1045
Migratory polyarthritis in rheumatic fever 801
Migratory thrombophlebitis 404, 1355
Mikulicz syndrome 576
Miliary tuberculosis 436, 875
Milk alkali syndrome 43
Milk fat globule membrane antigen 1406
Milroy disease 769
Minimal change disease of glomeruli 1174
Mirizzi's syndrome 1136
MIRL (membrane inhibitor reactive lysis) 521
Missense gene mutations 288
Mitochondrial dysfunction 21, 37, 1095
Mitochondrial inheritance 290
Mitochondrial myopathies 1546
Mitogenic signaling pathway inhibitors 1251
Mitral valve insufficiency 819
Mitral valve prolapse 820
Mitral valve stenosis 819
Mitsuda reaction in leprosy 442
Mixed cellularity variant of Hodgkin's disease 657
Mixed connective tissue disease 257, 263
Mixed gall calculi 1130
Mixed germ cell tumors 1268, 1340
Mixed germ cell tumors of ovary 1340
Mixed germ cell tumors of testis 1268
Mixed somatotroph–lactotroph adenoma 1473
Mixed teratoma of testis 1265
Mixed tumors of various organs 330
MLH1, MSH2, MSH6, and PMS2 tumor suppressor genes 368
Mode of spread of cancer 579, 652
Modes of cell signaling 119
Modifications of multiplex FISH and SKY 712
Modified radical mastectomy 1407
Molecular carcinogenesis 346
Molecular cytogenetic testing 725
Molecular genetics 574, 580, 581, 591, 910
Molecular genetics in osteosarcomas 1492
Molluscum bodies 448
Molluscum contagiosum 448, 1558
Monckeberg's medial calcific sclerosis 742
Monoclonal antibodies therapy in malignancies 701
Monoclonal antibody-based drugs 208
Monoclonal hypothesis of atherosclerosis 751
Monoclonal property of neoplasia 334
Monocyte chemotactic protein-1 (MCP-1) 196
Monocytes 534
Monocytosis 536
Monomorphic adenoma of salivary gland 945
Mononuclear Reed-Sternberg cells 650
Monosomy 295
Monostotic fibrous dysplasia of bone 1511
Monostotic lesion in Paget's disease of bone 1483
Montelukast 94
Morphological changes in AMI 790
Mosaic antigens 189
Mosaicism 296
MRCP (magnetic resonance cholangio-pancreatography) 1137
Mucicarmine stain 925, 697
Mucin types and their origin 697
Mucinous borderline tumors of ovary 1323, 1329
Mucinous bronchioloalveolar carcinoma 921
Mucinous cystadenocarcinoma of ovary 1329
Mucinous cystadenoma of ovary 1329
Mucinous surface epithelial tumors of ovary 1328
Mucocele 940
Mucocele of appendix 1031
Mucocele of gallbladder 1129, 1135
Mucoepidermoid carcinoma 945
Mucopolysaccharides 302
Mucormycosis 452, 1424
Mucosa associated lymphoid tissue (MALT) 181
Müllerian ducts 1284
Multibacillary (MB) leprosy 441
Multicystic mesothelioma 1035
Multinodular goiter 1438
Multiple endocrine neoplasia 1 (MEN 1) 973, 1149
Multiple myeloma 580, 672, 1504
Multiple myeloma terminology 583
Multiple neuromas 1610
Multiple sclerosis 249, 255, 1616
Multiplex metaphase FISH 712
Multistep carcinogenesis 380
Multisystem autoimmune disorders 257
    dermatomyositis 257
        discoid lupus erythematosus 257
        mixed connective tissue disease 257
        rheumatoid arthritis 257
        scleroderma 257
        Sjögren's syndrome 257
        systemic lupus erythematosus 257
Mumps orchitis 1273
Munro microabscesses 1562
Mural thrombi 793, 794
Mutant ALK receptor 1464
Mutator genes 318
Myasthenia gravis 242, 255, 264, 683, 1546
Mycoplasma pneumonias 862
Myocardial rupture in AMI 792
Myocardial embryonic stem cells 112
Mycobacterium avium intracellulare 437
Mycobacterium lepra bacilli 472
Mycobacterium tubercle bacilli 472, 870
Mycobacterium tuberculosis 28
Mycosis fungoides 676
Mycotic aneurysm 138
Mycotic aneurysms 759
Myelin figures 17
Myeloblast 552
Myeloblastic crisis in chronic myeloid leukemia 568
Myelodysplastic syndrome (MDS) 541, 559
Myelofibrosis 563
Myeloid metaplasia 12
Myeloid sarcoma 558
Myeloma kidney 585, 1505
Myeloperoxidase 543
Myeloperoxidase stain 555
Myeloproliferative diseases 563
    atypical chronic myelogenous leukemia 563
    chronic myelomonocytic leukemia 563
    juvenile myelomonocytic leukemia 563
    MDS/MPN unclassified 563

Index

Myeloproliferative neoplasms 562, 563
    chronic eosinophilic leukemia 563
    chronic myelogenous leukemia 563
    chronic neutrophilic leukemia 563
    essential thrombocythemia 563
    mast cell disease 563
    polycythemia vera (PV) 563
Myocardial infarct 163
Myocardial infarction 149
Myocarditis 806
Myocardium disorders 802
Myometrium 1319
Myotonic dystrophy 289, 302
Myotonic muscular dystrophy 1545
Myotonin protein kinase gene 289
Myxedema 1432
Myxofibrosarcoma 1531
Myxoid liposarcoma 1527
Myxopapillary ependymoma 1602

N

Na^+/K^+ pump 20
Nail disorders 1553
NAP scoring system 566
Nasal adenocarcinoma 844
Nasal plasmacytoma 844
Nasopalatine duct cyst 952
Nasopharyngeal angiofibroma 844
Nasopharyngeal carcinoma 390, 841
Natriuretic peptide B type assay 827, 904
Natural carcinogen 385
Natural killer cells 193, 402, 534
Naxos syndrome 811
Necroptosis 16
Necrosis 26
Negative selection 252
Negri bodies in brain of rabies 1589
Neisseria infections 79
Nelson syndrome 1469
Nemaline myopathy 1546
Neonatal amniotic fluid aspiration syndrome 1355
Neonatal cholestasis 1056
Neonatal hepatitis of unknown etiology 1057
Neonatal hyperbilirubinemia (HDN) 637
Neoplasms of thyroid gland 1439
Neoplastic urothelial lesions 1248
Nephrin molecules 1159
Nephrocalcinosis 1216
Nephrogenic diabetes insipidus 1470
Nephrolithiasis 1218
Nephrolithotomy 1221
Nephrosialidosis 1162
Nephrotic syndrome 1171
NESTROFT test 507
Neural defects 1617
Neural stem cells in brain 113
Neural tumors 1539
Neuregulin gene 1003
Neurilemmocytes 1581

Neurilemmoma 1539, 1608
Neuroaxis 1580
Neuroblastoma 330, 1464
Neurocysticercosis 1589
Neurodermatitis 1557
Neuroectodermal malignancies 330
Neuroendocrine (carcinoid) tumors 999
Neuroendocrine cells 999
Neuroepithelial tumors 1598
Neurofibroma 1539, 1574
Neurofibromatosis 302, 303, 306, 933, 1610
Neurogenic shock 176
Neuroglial cells in CNS 1581
Neuroglial cells in peripheral nervous system 1581
Neurological manifestations in sickle cell disease 512
Neuromuscular abnormalities in lung carcinoma 912
Neuromuscular disturbances 1201
Neuronal cell bodies 1581
Neuronal tumors 1610
Neurons 1581
Neuron-specific enolase (NSE) 843, 925
Neuropeptide Y 420
Neuropeptides (substance P) 91
Neuropil 1581
Neurotensin 1120
Neutral hydrolases 99, 196
Neutropenia (agranulocytosis) 536
Neutrophilia 534
Neutrophils 534
New methylene blue stain 474
Nezelof's syndrome 218
NF1 tumor suppressor gene 362
NF2 tumor suppressor gene 362
NHL-spillover in blood 579
Niacin 428
Niemann-Pick disease 45, 308, 480, 589, 1105
Nil disease 1174
Nipple and areola eczema 1402
Nipple discharge 1362
Nipple retraction 1362, 1387
Nitric oxide 89
Nitroblue tetrazolium (NBT) slide test 68
Nitrosamines 385
N-MYC nuclear regulatory proteins 1464
Nocardiosis 868
Nodal marginal zone lymphoma 671
Nodular fasciitis 1530
Nodular glomerulosclerosis in diabetic nephropathy 1182, 1421
Nodular hidradenoma 1576
Nodular hyperplasia of prostate 1277
Nodular lymphocytic-histiocytic predominant variant HD 657
Nodular melanoma 1572
Nodular regenerative hyperplasia 1112
Nodular sclerosis variant of Hodgkin's disease 656

O

Obesity 419
Obliterative endarteritis 756
Obstructive atelectasis 900
Obstructive hypoventilation syndrome 421
Obstructive jaundice 1134
Obstructive sleep apnea 420
Obstructive uropathy 1217
Occult (hidden) metastases 335
Occult blood 1038
Occupational carcinogens 385
Occupational exposure 908
Ochronosis 1522
Oculopharyngeal muscular dystrophy 1545
Odontogenic carcinoma 955
Odontogenic keratocyst 951
Odontogenic myxoma 954
Odontogenic tumors 952
Odontoma 954
Odynophagia 959
Olfactory neuroblastoma 843
Oligodendrocytes 1581
Oligodendroglial tumors 1601
Oligodendroglioma 1601
Oliguria 1191
Omega-3 fatty acid 85, 94
Oncocytic papillomas 840
Oncocytoma 944
Oncofetal antigens 405
Oncogenes 317
Oncogenesis 317
Onco-micro-RNA (miRNA155, 200, 221) 379
Onco-micro-RNA 379
Open biopsy 925, 1405
Open comedone 1579
Open pneumothorax 898
Opisthorchis viverrini 391
Opportunistic infections in AIDS 223
Opportunistic pulmonary infections 868
Opsoclonus–myoclonus syndrome 405
Opsonin receptors on leukocytes 65
Opsonin receptors on macrophage 195
Opsonization 66, 211
Oral anticoagulants 609
Oral cavity disorders 932, 933
    cleft palate 932
    facial clefts 932
    Fordyce's granules 933
    harelip 932
    hemifacial hypertrophy 933
Oral contraceptives 391
Oral glucose tolerance test (OGTT) 1412
Oral lesions in systemic disorders 933
Orchidometer 1275
Organ transplantation 266
Organohalogen compounds 335
Organs involved 580
Origin 910
Osgood-Schlatter disease 1514
Osler's nodes 814

Osler-Weber-Rendu syndrome 302, 304
Osmoreceptors 1153
Osmotic fragility 501
Osseous metaplasia 11
Osseous metaplasia in myositis ossificans 12
Ossifying fibroma 956
Osteitis deformans 1482
Osteitis fibrosa cystica 1481
Osteoarthritis 423, 1521
Osteoblastic lesions 1510
Osteoblastoma 1489
Osteoblasts 1476
Osteochondroma (exostosis) 1496
Osteoclastic activating factor 582, 583
Osteoclasts 1476
Osteogenesis imperfecta 302, 1513
Osteoid osteoma 1488
Osteolytic lesions 1505, 1510
Osteoma 1488
Osteomalacia 426, 1480
Osteomyelitis in sickle cell disease 512
Osteonecrosis (avascular necrosis) 1514
Osteonectin 129
Osteophytes (bony spurs) 1521
Osteoporosis 1481
Osteosarcoma 329, 1489, 1490
Osteosclerotic myeloma 583
Other blood group systems 630
Other viral infections 934
Otosclerosis 848
Outcome of acute inflammation 69
Outcome of necrosis 32
Ovalocytes 480
Ovarian cysts 1346
Ovarian tumors—histological classification 1321
Overt albuminuria 1160
Oxidant stress 515
Oxidized LDL molecule 754
Oxygen derived free radicals 21, 89
Oxygen-dependent intracellular microbial killing 68
Oxygen-independent microbial killing 69

P

β-pleated sheets of amyloid 273
P selectins 126
p53 tumor suppressor gene mutation 1379
Pacemaker cells of Cajalin GIST 984
Pachygyria 1618
Packed cell volume (PCV) 474
Packed cells transfusion 634
Paget's disease of bone (osteitis deformans) 1482
Paget's disease of breast 1388
Pale (ischemic) infarct 27
Pale infarct undergoing hemorrhagic infarct 164
Palmar erythema 1093
Panacinar emphysema 880
Pancarditis 802

Pancoast tumor of lung 918
Pancreas 1139
Pancreatic amylase 1140
Pancreatic chymotrypsin 1140
Pancreatic duct adenocarcinoma 1145
Pancreatic enzymatic fat necrosis 29
Pancreatic heterotropic rests 986
Pancreatic juice 1140
Pancreatic lipase 1140
Pancreatic trypsin 1140
Pancreatic tumors 1145
Pancreatitis 975, 1140
Pancreatoblastoma 1148
Panel of monoclonal antibodies in common malignancies 701
Papillary breast carcinoma 1392
Papillary carcinoma 1441
Papillary hidradenoma 1288
Papillary necrosis—kidney 1183, 1421
Papillary polypoid (bullous) cystitis 1247
Papillary variant of renal cell carcinoma 1233
Papilloma of various organs 324
Pappenheimer's bodies 479, 480
Para-Bombay blood group 628
Paracrine signaling 118, 119
Paradoxical emboli 158
Paraesophageal hernia 962
Paraffin embedding 694
Parafollicular cells or C cells of thyroid gland 1426
Paraganglioma 855
Paraneoplastic syndrome 402, 684
Paraneoplastic syndromes in lung cancer 912
Paraovarian or paratubal cysts 1348
Paraphimosis 1283
Parasitic encephalitis 1589
Parathormone (PTH) 1452
Parathyroid adenoma 1456
Parathyroid carcinoma 1457
Parietal epithelial cells of Bowman's capsule 1160
Parkinson disease 38
Parosteal osteosarcoma 1490
Paroxysmal cold hemoglobinuria 519
Paroxysmal nocturnal hemoglobinuria 79, 80, 219, 521, 541
Paroxysmal nocturnal hemoglobinuria (PNH)—pathogenesis 521
Partial pressure of gas 859
PAS stain (metachromatic stain) 281, 543, 697, 925, 1201
Passenger mutations 347
Passive immunity 179
Passive venous congestion 134
Patau syndrome (trisomy 13) 299
Patchy atelectasis 900
Patent ductus arteriosus (PDA) 833
Pathogen-associated molecular proteins (PAMPs) 65, 184
Pathological atrophy 6

Pathological calcification 42
Pathological hyperplasia 10
Pathological hypertrophy 7
Pathophysiology of diabetes mellitus 1417
Pavementing of leukocytes 57, 60, 61
PCR (polymerase chain reaction) 3, 15, 440, 724, 1258
Peau d' orange skin 1362, 1402
Pediatric renal cell carcinoma 376
Pedigree construction 313
Peggler-Huet anomaly 468, 537
Peliosis hepatitis 1112
Pelvic bones deformities in rickets 425
Pelvic inflammatory disease (PID) 1296
Pemphigus vulgaris 241, 243, 255, 264, 933, 1562
Peptic ulcer disease 971
Percutaneous transhepatic cholangiography (PTC) 1137
Perforated gallbladder 1135
Perforin 36
Perfusion scintigraphy 797
Pericanalicular pattern of fibroadenoma 1371
Pericardial edema 169
Pericardial effusion 821
Pericarditis 822
Pericarditis complications 804
Pericardium 821
Periductal mastitis 1364
Perihilar adenocarcinomas of extrabiliary duct 1139
Periodic acid–Schiff stain (PAS stain) 543, 697, 925, 1201
Periodontal disease 951
Periorbital puffiness (edema) 1191
Periosteal osteosarcoma 1490, 1494
Peripheral neuropathy (Guillain-Barré syndrome) 250
Peripheral neuropathy 491, 1423
Peripheral tolerance 251, 253
Peripheral vascular disease 748
Periportal area 1041
Periportal necrosis 1045
Periportal piecemeal necrosis 1047
Perisinusoidal endothelial cells 1084
Perisinusoidal stellate cells (Ito cells) 1043
Peritoneal dialysis 1201
Perivascular tumors 1536
Perl's stain 40, 480
Permanent cells in brain, cardiac and skeletal muscle 111
Pernicious anemia 241, 243, 255, 494, 977
Peroxidase enzyme 1427
Peroxidase-antiperoxidase (PAP) method 699
Peroxynitrite 22
Persistence of urachal sinus 1248
Petechial hemorrhages 137
Peutz-Jeghers syndrome 331, 933, 978, 1019
Peyronie disease 1283
Phagocytes 66

Index

Phagocytic receptors 65
Phagocytosis 61, 211
Phagolysosome 66
Pharynx disorders 856
Phases of acute renal failure 1209
Phenylketonuria (PKU) 291, 302, 309
Pheochromocytoma 1462
Philadelphia chromosomal t(9/22) 294, 561, 564, 565
Phimosis 1283
Phlebotomus sandflies 455
Phosphatidyl inositol-3 kinase (PI3k) proteins pathway 355
Phospholipase 20, 968
Photomultiplier tubes 708
PHOX2B gene 1003
Phyllodes tumor of breast 1372
Physiologic atrophy 6
Physiological calcification 42
Physiological hyperplasia 9
Physiological hypertrophy 7
Physiological jaundice 1051
Piecemeal necrosis 1063
PIG-A gene mutation 521
Pigeon-shaped chest in rickets 425
Pigment gallstones 1133
Pigmentation disorders 1569
Pigments 38
Pilocytic astrocytomas 1598
Pilomatrixoma 1576
Pilonidal sinus 1032
Pinealoblastoma 1603
Pink puffers do not tolerate hypoxia 882
Pitocin 1159
Pitting edema 828
Pituitary adenomas 1470
Pituitary gland 1467
PKHD1 gene 1057
Placenta accreta 1357
Placenta increta 1357
Placental abnormal attachments 1356
Placental alkaline phosphatase 1262
Placental site trophoblastic tumor 1353
Plasma 635
Plasma cell leukemia 585
Plasma exchange 637
Plasma products/recombinant concentrates 635
Plasma transfusion 636
Plasmablastic lymphoma 672
Plasmacytoma 844
Plasmacytoma testes 1271
Plasmacytosis 586
Plasmapheresis/plasma exchange 637
Plasminogen 142, 146, 598
Plasminogen activator 394, 600
Plasminogen-plasmin system 147
Platelet activating factor (PAF) 63, 91, 235, 334
Platelet concentrates 635
Platelet count 622
Platelet derived growth factor (PDGF) 63, 99, 116, 142, 195, 196, 350, 597, 753
Platelet derived growth factor (PDGF) receptors 352
Platelet disorders 142, 600, 605
Platelet factor IV 142
Platelet function tests 622
Platelet neutralizing test 620
Platelet products 142
Platelets 141, 597
Platelets adhesion 142, 148, 599, 787
Platelets aggregation 142, 148, 599, 787
Platelets pooling 601
Platelets release reaction 142, 787
Platelets removal 637
Platelets transfusion 636
Platelets' granules 141
Pleomorphic adenoma 942
Pleomorphic liposarcoma 1528
Pleomorphic Reed-Sternberg cells 650
Pleomorphic rhabdomyosarcoma 1534
Pleural effusion 828, 927
Pleural fibrosis 929
Pleuritis 927
Plummer-Vinson syndrome 484
Pneumocystis jiroveci 868
Pneumonias 860, 861, 862,
Pneumonias in immunocompromised persons 862
Pneumothorax 898
Point mutation 288, 375
  missense gene mutation 288
  non-missense gene mutation 288
Polarizing light microscope 281, 690, 691
Polarizing microscopy 691
Poliomyelitis 448
Polyanionic-proteoglycans in glomeruli 1159
Polyarteritis nodosa 263, 764
Polychromasia 479
Polycyclic hydrocarbons 384
Polycystic ovaries (Stein-Leventhal syndrome) 1348
Polycythemia 404
Polycythemia vera 570, 571
Polygenic and multifactorial disorders 291
Polymerase chain reaction (PCR) 315, 440, 724, 1258
Polymerized human serum albumin (PHSA) 1068
Polymicrogyria 1618
Polymyositis 262
Polyostotic fibrous dysplasia 1511
Polyostotic lesions 1483
Polyp 324
Polyploidy 295
Polyps in fundal region 976
Pompe disease type II 37, 46, 309
Poor immunogens 189
Porcelain gallbladder 1135
Porcine factor VIII 635
Portal hepatitis 1063
Portal hypertension 1036
Portal tract 1041, 1061
Portosystemic shunts 1088
Positive D-dimer 902
Positive selection 252
Positron emission tomography 924
Post-cricoid webs in iron deficiency anemia 963
Posterior cerebral artery occlusion 1611
Posterior pituitary gland 1467
Postmortem autolysis 31
Postnatal diagnosis 315
Post-necrotic cirrhosis 1082
Post-streptococcal glomerulonephritis 1187
Post-transfusion thrombocytopenia 640
Prader-Willi syndrome 292
PRCC gene 1233
Preauricular sinus 846
Precursor lesions 909
Pregnancy luteoma 1344
Prenatal diagnosis 315, 509
Presbycusis 848
Preservative used in transfusion bags 632
Prevention of transplant rejection 271
Priapism in hematological disorders 512, 1283
Primary aldosteronism 1460
Primary biliary cirrhosis 255, 1107
Primary CNS lymphoma 1609
Primary CNS tumors 1590
Primary complex 432, 872
Primary diabetes mellitus 1414
Primary glomerular diseases 1161
Primary gout 1522
Primary hemochromatosis 41, 1100, 1101
Primary hyperparathyroidism 43, 1453
Primary hypopituitarism 1467
Primary hypothyroidism 1432
Primary immunodeficiency disorders 215
Primary intestinal tuberculosis 994
Primary myelofibrosis 572
Primary neoplasms 830
Primary osteoporosis 1482
Primary other CNS tumors 1590
Primary platelet plug 145
Primary pleural effusion lymphoma 930
Primary pneumothorax 898
Primary pulmonary malignant tumors 907
Primary sclerosing cholangitis 1109
Primary tuberculosis (primary complex) 432, 872, 873
Primary viral myocarditis 807
Primitive neuroectodermal tumors (PNETs) 1603
Prinzmetal angina 784
Proctoscopy 1036
Professional APCs 198
Prognosis of solid tumors 411
Prognostic and predictive factors of breast carcinoma 1397
Prognostic factors of AML (FAB classification) 554

Prognostic factors of synovial sarcoma 1537
Progressive staining 695
Prolactinoma 1471
Proliferative fibrocystic changes 1367
Proliferative glomerulonephritis 1164
Proliferative retinopathy 1423
Prolonged immobilization 43
Prolymphocytic leukemia 662
Proptosis 17
Prostacyclin (PGI$_2$) 83, 84, 596
Prostaglandins 83. 84, 99, 196, 235
Prostate-specific antigen (PSA) 1281
Prostatic adenocarcinoma 1279
Prostatic hyperplasia 10
Prosthetic valve endocarditis 815
Protease (cathepsin D) 20, 968, 1400
Protein C 147, 148, 150, 600, 619
Protein S 147, 148, 150, 600, 619
Protein synthesis 285
Protein–energy malnutrition 417
Proteins associated with podocytes 1159
Proteins in epithelial cells 405
Proteinuria 1173
Proteoglycans 124, 127
Prothrombin 20210 transition 150
Prothrombin complex concentrates 635, 637
Prothrombin G20210A mutation 619
Prothrombin gene 148
Prothrombin time 556, 623, 1050
Prothrombotic factors 140
Prothrombotic properties of endothelium 139
Proto-oncogenes 317
Prussian blue staining 1101
Pseudoarthrosis 1523
Pseudochylous effusion 928
Pseudogout 1522
Pseudohermaphrodite 312
Pseudohypoparathyroidism 1456
Pseudomembranous colitis 1013
Pseudomembranous inflammation 73
Pseudomyxoma peritonei 1035
Pseudo-obstruction syndrome 1005
Psoriasis 10, 1562
Psoriatic arthritis 1521
PTCH tumor suppressor gene 362
PTEN tumor suppressor gene 363, 1382
Pulmonary alveolar proteinosis (PAP) 898
Pulmonary angiogram 902
Pulmonary artery embolization 1355
Pulmonary edema 169, 903
Pulmonary embolism 157
Pulmonary hamartoma 906
Pulmonary hemorrhagic infarct 164
Pulmonary hypertension 902
Pulmonary manifestations 779
Pulmonary stenosis 821
Pulmonary thromboembolism 157, 900
Pulmonary tuberculosis 432
Pulmonary valve stenosis 821
Pulmonary vascular disorders 900
Pulmonary vasculitis 904

Pulmonary volumes 859
Pure gall calculus 1130
Pure Leydig cell tumor 1343
Pure red cell anemia 529
Pure red cell aplasia (erythroblastopenia) 529
Pure teratoma 1265
Purkinje fibers 782
Purpura 137
Purpura fulminans neonatalis 150
Purulent exudate 823
Purulent or suppurative inflammation 72
Purulent or suppurative pericarditis 823
Pyelonephritis 1209
Pyknosis nucleus 25
Pyogenic bacterial liver abscess 1077
Pyogenic granuloma 770
Pyogenic meningitis—CSF findings 1586
Pyogenic osteomyelitis 1477
Pyothorax 928
Pyothorax effusion lymphoma 931
Pyridoxine 428
Pyruvate kinase deficiency 516

Q

Quinacrine banding technique 314

R

Rabies virus 448
Racemose/cirsoid aneurysm 755
Rachischisis 1618
Radiation carcinogenesis 385
Radiation colitis 1015
Radiation induced interstitial lung disease 896
Radiation therapy 1407
Radical hysterectomy (Wertheim's hysterectomy) 1305
Radicular cyst 952
Radioactive iodine uptake and thyroid imaging 1450
Radioallergosorbent test (RAST) 237
Radiological findings in bone lesions 1515
Radionuclide scan 902, 1441
Radionuclide scanning (99mTc) stannous pyrophosphate 797
Ramsay Hunt syndrome 846
Rapamycin immunosuppressive drug 272
Rapidly progressive glomerulonephritis (RPGN) 1195
RAS proto-oncogene 353, 1382
Raynaud's phenomenon 262, 766
RB tumor suppressor gene 339, 363, 1381
RBCs cast in urine 1191
RBCs fragmentation syndromes 522
Reaction to injury hypothesis 751
Reactive hyperplasia 670
Reactive oxygen species 22
Reciprocal translocation 294
Recombinant factor IX 635

Recombinant factor VIIa 635
Recombinant factor VIII 635
Rectal prolapse 1032
Recurrent infections 79, 219
Recurrent jaundice during pregnancy 1052
Recurrent myocardial infarction 794
Red blood cells 635
Red blood cells removal 637
Red cell indices 474
    hematocrit or packed cell volume (PCV) 474
    mean corpuscular hemoglobin (MCH) 474
    mean corpuscular hemoglobin concentration (MCHC) 474
    mean corpuscular volume (MCV) 474
    red blood cell distribution width (RDW) 474
Red infarct 27, 164
Red pulp spleen 677
Reed-Sternberg cells 647, 648
Reed-Sternberg-like cells 651
Refractive index 691
Refractory sprue 990
Regenerative changes 1061
Regressive stain 695
Regulation by suppressive cytokines 254
Regulation of apoptosis 36
Regulation of cell cycle 114
Regurgitation during feeding 69
Reinke crystalloid 1343
Relapsing polychondritis 846
Remodeling of callus formation in bone fracture 121
Renal amyloidosis 47
Renal angiomyolipoma 1240
Renal atrophy 7
Renal blood flow 1152
Renal cell carcinoma (RCC) 464, 1233
Renal cell carcinoma—systemic manifestations 1237
Renal infarction 1222
Renal lesions in diabetic nephropathy 1421
Renal osteodystrophy 1200, 1481
Renal stones (nephrolithiasis and urolithiasis) 1218
Renal tubular functional disorders 1216
Renin-angiotensin-aldosterone system 1153
Repair by fibrosis 32
Repair phase of bone fracture 121
Reperfusion injury in AMI 789
Residual volume 860
Residual volume of urine 1211
Resorption of necrotic tissue 32
Respiratory disorders 859
Respiratory distress syndrome in the infants 889
Respiratory system—anatomy 856, 857
Restricrtive cardiomyopathy 811
Restrictive pulmonary diseases 886, 889

Index

Reticulocyte 466
Reticulocyte count 474
Reticuloendothelial cells distribution 97, 98, 194
Reticuloendothelial system 187
Retinoblastoma 330, 1603
Retinoic acid receptor-α (RAR-α) gene 556
Retinoids 25
RET-PTC oncogene 1442
Retroperitoneal hemorrhage 612
Revascularization procedures in AMI 787
Reversible cell injury 15, 17
Reye syndrome 1107
Rh blood group system 628
Rh blood grouping 632
Rh factor incompatibility during pregnancy 630
Rhabdomyolysis 1547
Rheumatic fever and RHD 798
Rheumatoid arthritis 241, 243, 249, 250, 255, 257, 263, 517, 897, 1518
Rheumatoid factor 255, 263
Rhinorrhea 837
Rhinoscleroma 845
Rhinosporidiosis 845
Rhinosporidium seeberi 845
Rhodamine 698
Rhodopsin 424
Riboflavin 428
Ribosomal RNA or rRNA 286
Richardson Grading System 1398
Richter syndrome 576, 665
Rickets 425, 1480
    craniotabes in rickets 425
    deformities of pelvic bones in rickets 425
    frontal bossing in rickets 425
    Harrison's groove in rickets 425
    pigeon-shaped chest in rickets 425
    rachitic rosary in rickets 425
    spine deformity in rickets 425
Riedel's thyroiditis 1430
Right heart failure 827
Right ventricular hypertrophy 830
Right-sided colorectal carcinoma 1027
Ring chromosome 294
Ring sideroblasts 561
Risk factors of AMI 785
RNA oncogenic viruses 387
RNA primase 287
Robertsonian translocation 294
Role of platelets in AMI 787
Rolling of leukocytes 61
Romanowsky stains 477
Rota virus 992
Roth's retinal hemorrhages 814
Rotor's syndrome 1056
Rouleaux formation of RBCs 479
Rugger Jersey appearance 1481
RUNX3 gene promoter 1266
Russell bodies in plasma cells 586
Russell viper venom time test 620

S

S-100 protein 1004, 1361, 1375
SA node in heart 782
Saccharopolyspora rectivirgula 897
Saccular aneurysm 755
Saddle embolus 901
Sago spleen in amyloidosis 47
Salivary gland disorders 938
Salmonella typhi 992
Salmonella typhimurium 992
Salpingitis isthmica nodosa 1307
Sandwich ELISA 723
Saponification 29
Sarcoidosis 896
Sarcoma of various organs 328
Sarcoptes scabiei 1557
Satellite cells in liver 1581
Satellite granuloma 107
Scabies 1557
Scanning electron microscopy (SEM) 688
Schatzki ring 963
Schaumann's bodies 436
Schiller's test 494, 1305
Schiller-Duval bodies in endodermal sinus tumor 1339
Schistosoma haematobium 390
Schistosomiasis liver 1080
Schneiderian sinonasal papillomas 838
Schwann cells 1581
Schwannoma (neurilemmoma) 1539, 1608
Sclerodactyly 262
Scleroderma 255, 257, 261, 897, 962
Sclerosing adenosis 1368
Sclerosing lymphocytic lobulitis 1366
Sclerosing odontogenic carcinoma 955
Sclerotherapy 1088
Scoring system of NAP 566
Scurvy 430, 607, 1483
SDHB and SDHD tumor suppressor genes 365
Sea blue histiocytosis 590
Seborrheic dermatitis 428
Seborrheic keratosis 1565
Second line of host defense 182
Secondary aldosteronism 1460
Secondary biliary cirrhosis 1108
Secondary diabetes mellitus 1414
Secondary glomerular diseases 1162
Secondary gout 1522
Secondary hemochromatosis 41, 1103
Secondary hemostatic plug 145
Secondary hyperparathyroidism 43, 1455
Secondary hypertension 774
Secondary hypothyroidism 1432
Secondary intestinal tuberculosis 994
Secondary messenger systems 1400
Secondary myelofibrosis 573
Secondary neoplasms 830
Secondary osteoporosis 1482
Secondary pneumothorax 899
Secondary polycythemia 571
Secondary pulmonary malignant tumors 922
Secondary thrombocytopenia 603
Secondary tuberculosis 434, 873
Secretory breast carcinoma 1394
Secretory diarrhea 993
Secretory myeloma 583
Seeding/transcoelomic route of carcinomas 400
Segmental glomerulosclerosis 1162, 1163
Selected autoimmune diseases 255
Selectin family 61, 126
    E selectins 61
    L selectins 61
    P selectins 61
Selectins 61, 59, 126, 752
Selection of donor 594
Selective proteinuria 1160
Semen analysis 1275
Seminoma with syncytiotrophoblastic element 1260
Seminoma with yolk sac element 1259
Senile purpura 607
Sentinel lymph node 396, 1396, 1405
Septic (infective) infarcts 152
Septic shock 95, 173
Sequestration crisis 512
Sequestration of antigens 254
Sequestrum formation in osteomyelitis 1477
Serine protease 99, 196
Serofibrinous pericarditis 779, 802, 823
Serotonin 81, 142
Serous borderline tumors of ovary 1323
Serous cystadenocarcinoma of ovary 1328
Serous cystadenoma of ovary 1326
Serous inflammation 71
Serous pericarditis 823
Serous surface epithelial tumors of ovary 1326
Serpentine aneurysm 755
Sertoli cell tumor (androblastoma) of testis 1269
Sertoli-Leydig cell tumor of testis 1343
Serum (reverse) blood grouping 632
Serum alkaline phosphatase 1281
Serum amyloid associated (SAA) level 94
Serum ceruloplasmin 1048
Serum des-gamma carboxyprothrombin 1120
Serum ferritin 486, 1103
Serum fibrinogen 94
Serum iron 486
Serum prostatic acid phosphatase 1281
Serum sickness 243
Serum total iron binding capacity (TIBC) 486
Serum TSH, T4 and T3 levels 1449
Serum α-fetoprotein 1266, 1335
Serum β-microglobulin 586
Sessile serrated adenomas 1021

Seven α-helical transmembrane G-protein coupled receptors 64
Seven transmembrane G-protein coupled receptors 119
Severe acute respiratory syndrome (SARS) 890
Severe biliary colic 1134
Severe combined immune deficiency (SCID) syndrome 218
Sex chromosomal disorders 299
Sex cord stromal tumors of ovary 1340
Sex cord-gonadal stromal tumors of testis 1269
Sézary syndrome 576, 676
Sheehan's syndrome 1356, 1468
Shigella sonnei 992
Shock 170
Sialyl-Lewis X PSGL-1 62
Sickle cell disease 302, 306, 480, 509, 512, 513
Sickle cell nephropathy 1222
Sickle cell thalassemia syndrome 513
 heterozygous (HBS/HBC) disorder 514
 homozygous hemoglobin C disorder 513
Sickling test 480, 513, 524
Sideroblastic anemias 530
Siderotic nodules 479
Sigmoidoscopy 1029
Silicone breast implants 1365
Silicosis 887, 892
Silo filler's disease 897
Silver methenamine stain 1179
Simond's disease 1468
Simon's focus 434
Simple bone cyst 952
Simple bruising 608
Simple cystic endometrial hyperplasia 1311
Simple papillae of kidney 1152
Single cell or group of cells necrosis 1046
Single nucleotide polymorphism (SNP) 291
Sinonasal undifferentiated carcinoma 840
Sinonasal papillomas 838
Sinus histiocytosis 396, 642
Sinusoidal obstruction syndrome 1112
SIP1 gene 1003
Sipple syndrome 1463
Size-dependent barrier of glomeruli 1160
Sjögren's syndrome 255, 257, 262, 939, 1519
Skeletal muscle atrophies 1542
Skeletal muscle atrophy 7
Skeletal muscle dystrophies 1542
Skeletal muscle hypertrophy 1547
Skeletal muscle stem cells 114
Skeletal muscle tumors 1532
Skin associated lymphoid tissue (SALT) 181
Skin barrier to pathogens 1552
Skin biopsy 1405
Skin dysplasia 13
Skin histology 1550–1552
Skin scratch testing 237

Skip metastases 396, 1396
Skipping lesions of Crohn's disease 1013
Slide test for blood grouping 632
Sliding hiatal hernia 962
SMADA4 tumor suppressor gene 1145, 1325
Small bowel infarction 998
Small cell lung carcinoma (SCLC) 909, 913
Small cell osteosarcoma 1494
Small lymphocytic lymphoma 667
Small lymphocytic lymphoma/CLL 667
Small-sized vessel vasculitis 1225
Smoldering (asymptomatic) myeloma 583
Smooth muscle tumors 1535
SNAIL and TWIST genes 393
Sodium dodecyl sulfate polyacrylamide gel electrophoresis 531
Soft tissue bleeding 612
Soft tissue tumors 1524
Solitary plasmacytoma 583
Solitary renal cyst 1228
Somatotropic adenoma 1471
Sources of stem cells 593
Southern blot technique 729
Space of Disse in liver 1043
Special form of granuloma 107
Special stains 695
Specific tolerance 191
Spectrin proteins in RBC membrane 500
Spermatocele 1275
Spermatocytic seminoma 1262
Spermatogenesis 1255
Spider nevi 1093
Spider telangiectasis 769
Spikes and domes appearance in MGN 1179
Spina bifida cystica 1617
Spina bifida occulta 1617
Spine deformity in rickets 425
Spinocerebellar syndrome 427
Spitz nevus 1570
Spleen 677
 angiosarcoma of spleen 682
 autosplenectomy 679
 fibrocongestive splenomegaly 678
 Gaucher's spleen 680
 granulomatous inflammation 680
 hemosiderosis 680
 hypersplenism 679
 hyposplenism 679
 metastases in spleen 682
 red pulp 677
 spleen in amyloidosis 680
 splenectomy 678
 splenic infarct 680
 splenomegal 678
 white pulp 677
Spleen amyloidosis 47
Splenectomy 678
Splenic infarct 163, 680
Splenic lymphoma with villous lymphocytes 580

Splenic marginal zone B cell lymphoma 663
Splenic marginal zone lymphoma 672
Splenomegaly 678, 829
Spontaneous regression of tumors 410
Sporadic medullary carcinoma of thyroid 1446
Sporadic renal angiomyolipoma 1240
Sporadic Wilms' tumor 1231
Squamous cell carcinoma 327, 843, 934, 950, 964
Squamous cell carcinoma *in situ* (Bowen's disease) 1566
Squamous cell carcinoma lung 915
Squamous cell carcinoma of vagina 1294
Squamous cell carcinoma of vulva 1288
Squamous cell papilloma 934
Squamous metaplasia 11
Squamous odontogenic tumor 953
Squamous papilloma 849, 964
Stable (typical) angina 784
Stable cells 111
Staging of CML 566
Staging of Wilms' tumor 1232
Steatohepatitis 1097
Stein-Leventhal syndrome 1348
Stellate (Ito) cells of liver 1084
Stem cell therapy 112
 β cells embryonic stem cells 112
 hepatocytic embryonic stem cells 112
 myocardial embryonic stem cells 112
Stem cell transplantation 592
Stem cells 111, 114, 594
Stem cells in canals of Hering 113
Stem cells in dentate nuclei 113
Stem cells in hair follicle bulge 113
Stem cells in subventricular zone (SVZ) 113
Stercoral ulcer 1015
Steroid receptors 120
Stiff-Person syndrome (SPS) 405
Still disease (juvenile rheumatoid arthritis) 1519
STK11 tumor suppressor gene 365
Stomatocytes 480
Stomatostatinoma 1149
Storage histiocytosis 589
Storiform pattern 1508
Strawberry capillary hemangioma 1576
Strawberry gallbladder 45, 1128
Stress response proteins 27 (Srp27) 27, 1400, 1406
Stricture in Crohn's disease 1013
Stricture in intestinal tuberculosis 438
String sign in Crohn's disease 1013
Strongyloides stercoralis 455
Structural fibrous glycoproteins 123
Structure and functions of platelets 598
Structure of HIV 220
Struma ovarii 1338
Sturge-Weber syndrome 1540, 1576
Subacute bacterial endocarditis 812
Subacute combined degeneration of spinal cord 428, 491

Subacute endocarditis 813
Subacute granulomatous thyroiditis 1430
Subacute painless lymphocytic thyroiditis 1430
Subcellular and cellular alterations 15
Subcellular hypertrophy of liver organelles 8
Subcellular response to injury 37
Subcutaneous edema 169
Subcutaneous necrosis of newborn 32
Subcutaneous nodules 805
Subdural hematoma 1615
Subdural space 1582
Subendocardial infarct 789, 795
Subendocardial myocardial infarct 784, 789
Subendothelial deposits 1203, 1204
Subleukemic leukemia 540
Submassive liver necrosis 1046
Sucrose hemolysis test 522
Sudan black B stain 543
Sudden cardiac death in AMI 791
Sulfated glycosaminoglycans 273
Superantigens 1189
Superficial fibromatosis 1530
Superficial fungal infections 450, 1561
    epidermophyton 450
    microsporum 450
    trichophyton 450
Superficial spreading melanoma 1572
Superinfection 1073
Superoxide anion 22
Superoxide molecule 99, 196
Suppurative fistula 71
Suppurative lymphadenitis 642
Suppurative thrombosis of portal vein 1080
Supravital staining 527
Surface epithelial inclusion cysts 1348
Surface markers of human B and T cells 195
Surfactant phosphatidylcholine (lecithin) 900
Surgical emphysema 899
Surgical implantation 400
Surgical specimens 694
Swan-neck fingers in rheumatoid arthritis 1519
Swiss cheese disease (juvenile papillomatosis breast) 1373
Sydenham's chorea (St. Vitus dance) 805
Symptomatic gallstones disease 1132
Synaptophysin 843
Syndrome of inappropriate ADH (SIADH) secretion 1470
Synovial joints 1518
Synovial sarcoma 377, 1536
Synthesis of insulin 1411
Synthesis of VWF and factor VIII 610, 615
Syphilis 535, 1293
Syphilitic (luetic) aneurysm 756
Syphilitic orchitis 1273
Syringomyelia 1618
Systemic effects of hypertension 777
Systemic effects of inflammation 94

Systemic lupus erythematosus 79, 219, 255, 257, 258, 517, 897
Systemic sclerosis 261
Systemic thromboembolism 157, 158
Systemic venous thrombosis in AMI 795

T

T cells 534
Tabes dorsalis 1589
Tacrolimus (FK506) immunosuppressive drug 272
Takayasu arteritis 763
Tamm-Horsfall proteins 1207
Target cells 480
Tattooing 42
Tay-Sachs disease 291, 307
TCF7L2 gene 1416
Telangiectasia 262
Telangiectatic osteosarcoma 1490, 1494
Telomerase activity 334
Temporal (cranial/giant cell) arteritis 763
Tension pneumothorax 899
Teratocarcinoma 1266
Teratoma 330, 1265, 1336
Terminal deoxyribonucleotidyl transferase (TdT) 544
Terminal duct lobular unit (TDLU) 1358
Tertiary hyperparathyroidism 1456
Tertiary syphilis 31
Testicular atrophy 1274
Testicular lymphoma 1270
Testicular torsion 1274
Tetany 1456
Tetrahydrofolate 488
Tetralogy of Fallot 834
TFE 3 gene 1233
TGF-β tumor suppressor gene 370
Thalassemia 302, 502, 504, 505, 507, 508
    α-thalassemia 508
    α-thalassemia trait 494, 508
    β-thalassemia intermedia 484, 508
    β-thalassemia major 484, 504, 505
    β-thalassemia minor 507
Theca luteal cysts 1349
Thecoma ovary 1342
Theories of aging 48
Therapeutic advances in AMI 787
Thermophilic actinomyces 897
Thiamine 427
Thin membrane disease of kidney 1163
Thioflavin-S 281
Thioflavin-T 281
Third line of host defense 185
Thoracic vena cava syndrome 768
Thrombasthenia (Glanzmann's disease) 606
Thrombi in blood vessels 153
Thrombi in heart 152
Thrombin time 623
Thromboangiitis obliterans 764
Thromboasthenia 142, 622
Thrombocytopenia 601, 602

Thrombocytosis 565
Thromboembolism 157, 1555
Thrombomodulin 147
Thrombomodulin molecules 596
Thrombophilia 618
Thrombophlebitis 640, 815
Thrombopoiesis 141, 468
Thrombopoietin 462
Thrombosis 404
Thrombospondin 142, 335, 598
Thrombotic microangiopathy 1224
Thrombotic thrombocytopenic purpura 523, 604, 637
Thromboxane A2 (TxA2) 34
Thymic carcinoma 684
Thymoma 683
Thymus hyperplasia 682
Thyroglobulin 1451
Thyroglossal duct cyst 854, 1448
Thyroid adenoma 1439
Thyroid anaplastic carcinoma 1448
Thyroid binding globulins 1427
Thyroid follicular cells 1426
Thyroid function tests 1449
Thyroid gland 1425
Thyroid gland anomalies 1448
Thyroid gland hyperplasia 10
Thyroid hormone binding proteins (TBP) 1450
Thyroid hormones in circulation and tissues 1427
Tidal volume 860
Tinea corporis 1561
Tissue factor pathway inhibitor 600
Tissue fibrosis 103
Tissue microarray (TMA) 731, 732, 733
Tissue microarray—FISH 718
Tissue processor 694
Tissue typing 267
Tobacco smoking 908
Toll-like receptors (TLRs) on leukocytes 64, 183, 184
Toluidine blue 587
TORCH complex 1618
Total anomalous pulmonary venous return 835
Total lung capacity 860
Toxemia of pregnancy 1225, 1553
Toxic nodular goiter 1433
Toxic shock syndrome 1291
TP53 tumor suppressor gene 340, 366, 1381
Trachea disorders 857
Tracheoesophageal fistula 959
Traction diverticulum 962
Traditional cytogenetic analysis 709
Transaminases 1048
Transbronchial biopsy 925
Transcription factors 356
Transcription of RNA to DNA 287
    coding regulation of RNA 287
    non-coding RNA 287
Transfer RNA or tRNA 286
Transferrin 483

Transforming growth factor-α
    (TGF-α) 63, 116, 196
Transforming growth factor-β
    (TGF-β) 99, 195, 334, 351
Transforming growth factor-β 117, 753
Transfusion associated graft-versus-host
    disease 640
Transfusion hemosiderosis 640
Transfusion related acute lung injury 640
Transient ischemic attacks (TIA) 1614
Transient jaundice 1051
Transitional (mixed) meningioma 1607
Transitional cell carcinoma 328, 1252
Translocation of chromosome 294
Transmigration (diapedesis) 61, 63
Transmission electron microscopy
    (TEM) 688
Transmission of infections 638
Transmission of negative signal to
    T cells 254
Transmural infarct 795, 789
Transmural myocardial infarct 784, 789
Transplant rejection prevention 271
Transplantation immunology 266
    acute renal graft rejection 268
    chronic renal transplant rejection 269
    graft-versus-host disease (GVHD) 269
    hyperacute organ transplant
        rejection 267
    immunosuppressive drugs 272
    organ transplant rejection 267
    organ transplantation 266
Transplanted cells 247
Transport proteins 25
    ceruloplasmin 25
    ferritin 25
    lactoferritin 25
    transferrin 25
Transposition of the great vessels 835
Transthyretin 276
Transudate 57, 165
Transudative effusions 928
Traumatic neuroma 1574
Tree bark appearance in syphilis 756
Trephine bone biopsy 473
Trichobezoar 986
Trichomonas vaginalis 454, 1292
Trichophyton 1561
Tricuspid insufficiency 821
Trilateral retinoblastoma 1603
Triple assessment 1404
Trisodium citrate 476
Trisomy 295
Tropical sprue 993
Troponins (Tn I and Tn T) in AMI 796
TRPC6 (transient receptor potential
    calcium channel-6) gene 1162
True hermaphrodite 312
Truncus arteriosus communism 835
Tubal endometriosis 1307
Tube test 632

Tubercular arthritis 1523
Tubercular effusion 874
Tubercular granulomas 875
Tubercular infection 431
Tubercular intestinal ulcer 994
Tubercular lymphadenitis 439
Tubercular osteomyelitis 438, 1479
Tubercular pericardial effusion 439
Tubercular peritonitis 439
Tubercular pleuritis 435
Tubercular pyelonephritis 438, 1214
Tubercular salpingitis 439
Tuberculin test 248, 870
Tuberculoid leprosy 443
Tuberculosis 430, 535, 870, 871
Tuberculosis in HIV cases 876
Tuberculous cavities 874
Tuberculous disease 431
Tuberculous epididymitis 1273
Tuberculous meningitis 437, 1586
Tuberous sclerosis 302, 306, 1022
Tuberous sclerosis syndrome 1620
Tubular adenoma 1019, 1375
Tubular breast carcinoma 1391
Tubulointerstitial nephritis 1209
Tubulovillus adenomas 1020
Tumor angiogenesis 334
Tumor antigen masking 374
Tumor cell embolization 395
Tumor emboli extravasation 395
Tumor fragment emboli 157
Tumor impingement on nearby
    structures 401
Tumor markers 405
Tumor markers of breast carcinoma 1406
Tumor necrosis factor 88, 431
Tumor necrosis factor-α (TNF-α) 99
Tumor p16 suppressor gene 370
Tumor suppressive micro-RNA 378
Tumor suppressor genes 318
Tumors of blood vessels 769, 770, 771
    angiomyolipoma 771
    angiosarcoma 771
    bacillaryangiomatosis 771
    capillary hemangioma 770
    cavernous hemangioma 770
    cystic hygroma 770
    glomangioma 770
    hemangioendothelioma 771
    hemangiopericytoma 771
    hereditary hemorrhagic telangiec-
        tasia 770
    Kaposi sarcoma 771
    pyogenic granuloma 770
    spider telangiectasis 769
Turcot's syndrome 1021
Turner's mosaicism 296
Turner's syndrome 295, 300
Two-hit hypothesis of Knudson 1603
Tympanosclerosis 847
Type I diabetes mellitus 249, 250

Type I hypersensitivity reactions 231
Type II hypersensitivity reaction 237, 798
Type III hypersensitivity reaction 243
Type IV hypersensitivity reaction 245, 799
Type of electrophoresis 735
Type of immunofluorescence 703
Type of metastases 1510
Typhoid fever 445, 995
Typhoid intestinal ulcers 995
Tyrosinase 373
Tyrosine kinase pathway 352

U

Ulcerated carcinoma 979
Ulcerative colitis 104, 1011
Ultrasound or CT-guided percutaneous
    needle biopsy 925
Umbilical cord blood 594
Umbilical cord blood harvesting 594
Umbilical hernia 998
Undifferentiated pleomorphic
    sarcoma 1538
Unilateral renal agenesis 1229
Unstable (crescendo/pre-infarction)
    angina 784
Urachal diverticulum 1248
Uranium exposure 908
Urate nephropathy 1214, 1522
Urease 968
Uremic medullary cystic renal disease 1228
Ureter anomalies 1230
Uric acid stones 1220
Urinary tract obstruction 1213
Urine electrophoresis 586
Urinothorax 928
Urolithiasis 1218
Urothelial carcinoma *in situ* 1248
Urothelial carcinoma of renal pelvis 1241
Urothelial dysplasia 1248
Uses of flow cytometer 708
Uterine endometrial hyperplasia 10
Uterus muscle hyperplasia during preg-
    nancy 10

V

VacA exotoxin 968
Vaccines 211
Vaginal intraepithelial neoplasia 1293
Variant (Prinzmetal) angina 784
Varicella (chickenpox) 1561
Varicocele 768, 1275
Varicose veins in legs 767
Various types of electrophoresis 737
Vascular cell adhesive molecule I
    (VCAM I) 752
Vascular changes in hypertension 775, 776
Vascular endothelial growth factor
    (VEGF) 117, 334
Vascular endothelium 139
Vascular events in inflammation 55

Vascular purpura 607
Vascular-occlusive episodes in sickle cell disease 511
    acute chest syndrome 511
    autosplenectomy 512
    avascular necrosis of femoral head 511
    bone and joint crises 511
    hand and foot syndrome 511
    priapism 512
    renal papillary necrosis 512
Vasculitis 760, 763
    Churg-Strauss syndrome 766
    cryoglobulinemia vasculitis 766
    diabetic vascular disease 766
    drug-induced vasculitides 766
    Henoch-Schönlein purpura 766
    Kawasaki disease 764
    lymphomatoid granulomatosis 767
    microscopic polyarteritis 766
    polyarteritis nodosa 764
    Raynaud's phenomenon 766
    temporal (cranial/giant cell) arteritis 763
    thromboangiitis obliterans 764
    Wegener's granulomatosis 765
Vasculitis involving kidneys 1225
Vasculostatin 335
Vasoactive amines 80
Vasoactive intestinal peptide tumor 1149
Vasoconstriction 55
Vasodilation 55
Vater's syndrome 963
Veins 767
Vena cava syndrome 768, 769
Veno-occlusive disorder 1112
Venous thrombi 154
Ventral hernia 998
Ventricular aneurysm in AMI 794
Ventricular mural thrombi 793
Ventricular septal defects 833
Verocay bodies 1539
Verruca vulgaris (common wart) 1559
Vesicoumbilical fistula 1248
Vesicoureteral reflux 1210, 1211, 1213
vHL (von Hippel-Lindau) tumor suppressor gene 365, 1235
Vibrio cholerae 992
Villus adenomas 1019
Vim Silverman needle biopsy 1050
Vincent angina 933
Viral carcinogenesis 386
Viral cervicitis 1298
Viral encephalitis 1588
Viral infected cells 247
Viral meningitis 1587
Viral sialadenitis 939
Visceral epithelial cells of Bowman's capsule 1159
Vital capacity 860
Vitamin A 424
Vitamin B_{12} deficiency 489, 491
Vitamin B_{12} in DNA synthesis 490

Vitamin C (ascorbate) 25, 429
Vitamin D 425, 1453, 1480
Vitamin D resistant rickets 1456
Vitamin E (α-tocopherol) 25, 426
Vitamin K 427
Vitiligo 255, 1569
VLA-4 integrin 62
Vocal cord nodule 849
Volvulus 1007
von Gierke disease 37, 146, 309
von Gieson stain 281
von Hippel-Lindau disease 302
von Hippel-Lindau syndrome 306, 1235, 1540, 1576
von Willebrand disease 142, 606, 615
von Willebrand factor 142, 635
Vulnerability of tissues to hypoxia 161

W

WAGR syndrome 1231
Wald's visual cycle 424
Waldenströrm's macroglobulinemia 576, 587, 637
Warburg effect 395
Warm antibody-mediated hemolytic anemia 240, 517
Warthin's tumor salivary gland 943
Warts 1560
Washed red blood cells 635
Water and electrolytes imbalance 1198
Waterhouse-Friderichsen syndrome 1461
Watershed regions 1015
Water-soluble vitamins 427
WBCs qualitative anomalies 468
    Alder-Reilly anomaly 468
    May-Hegglin anomaly 468
    Peggler-Huet anomaly 468
Wegener's granulomatosis 765, 837, 1194
Well differentiated liposarcoma 1527
Well differentiated papillary mesothelioma 1034
Werner syndrome 49
Wernicke-Korsakoff syndrome 427, 428
Wertheim's hysterectomy 1305
Wet beriberi 428
Wet gangrene 31
Whipple disease (tropical sprue) 993
White (pale) infarct 162
White blood cells removal 637
White sponge nevus 933
WHO classification 645
WHO classification of AML (2016) 549
WHO classification of lung tumors 910
WHO classification of lymphoid neoplasms 658
WHO definition of AIDS patient 227
Whole blood 635
Whole blood transfusion 634
Whole chromosome paint (WCP) 718
Willebrand disease 622
Williams-Campbell syndrome 883
Wilms' tumor 1230

Wilms' tumor in familial syndromes 1231
Wilson disease 302, 1103
Wilson's disease induced cirrhosis 1083
Window period 1069
Wire loop lesion in glomeruli in SLE 1186
Wiscott-Aldrich syndrome 219, 541, 606, 683
WNT signal transduction pathway 354
Wound contraction 129
Wound healing by primary intention 10
Wright's stain 477
WT1 tumor suppressor gene 369
Wuchereria bancrofti 455

X

Xanthine stones kidney 1220
Xanthogranulomatous pyelonephritis 1214
Xanthomas 45, 1578
Xeroderma pigmentosum 343, 386
Xerophthalmia 425
X-inactivation 296
X-linked (Bruton) agammaglobulinemia 303
X-linked agammaglobulinemia of Bruton 215, 303
X-linked disorders 303
X-linked dominant inheritance 290
X-linked ichthyosis 303
X-linked recessive disorders 311
X-linked recessive inheritance 290, 303
    Becker muscular dystrophy 303
    Duchenne muscular dystrophy 303
    Fabry disease 303
    Fragile X syndrome 303
    G6PD deficiency 303
    hemophilia A 303
    hemophilia B 303
    Hunter syndrome 303
Xp11 translocation renal cell carcinoma 1233
XXX syndrome (47, XXX) and other multi-X chromosome anomalies 301

Y

Y chromatin 314
Yersinia enterocolitica 1030
Yolk sac tumor of ovary 1339
Yolk sac tumor of testis 1266

Z

Zenker's diverticulum 962
Zenker's fixative 692
Zenker's necrosis 32
Ziehl-Neelsen stain 440
Zileutin drug 94
Zollinger-Ellison syndrome 973
Zona fasciculata of adrenal cortex 1457
Zona glomerulosa of adrenal cortex 1457
Zona reticularis of adrenal cortex 1457
Zonal liver necrosis 1045
Zones of prostate 1277

Textbook of
Pathology
VOLUME II

Textbook of Pathology
VOLUME II

Chief Editor

Vinay Kamal
Director Professor of Pathology
Maulana Azad Medical College
Bahadur Shah Zafar Marg
New Delhi (India)

Editors

Anubhav MD

Vigyat MD

Illustrations by

Ram Murti Senior Graphic Artist

Volume I contains: General Pathology, Hematology including Recent Diagnostic Techniques
Volume II contains: Systemic Pathology

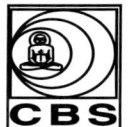

CBS Publishers & Distributors Pvt Ltd
New Delhi • Bengaluru • Chennai • Kochi • Kolkata • Mumbai
Hyderabad • Jharkhand • Nagpur • Patna • Pune • Uttarakhand

Disclaimer
Science and technology are constantly changing fields. New research and experience broaden the scope of information and knowledge. The editors have tried their best in giving information available to them while preparing the material for this book. Although, all efforts have been made to ensure optimum accuracy of the material, yet it is quite possible some errors might have been left uncorrected. The publisher, the printer and the editors will not be held responsible for any inadvertent errors, omissions or inaccuracies.

Textbook of
Pathology
Volume II

ISBN: 978-93-86478-39-9

Copyright © Author and Publisher

First Edition: 2017

All rights reserved. No part of this book may be reproduced or transmitted in any form or by any means, electronic or mechanical, including photocopying, recording, or any information storage and retrieval system without permission, in writing, from the editors and the publisher.

Published by Satish Kumar Jain and produced by Varun Jain for

CBS Publishers & Distributors Pvt Ltd
4819/XI Prahlad Street, 24 Ansari Road, Daryaganj, New Delhi 110 002, India.
Ph: 23289259, 23266861, 23266867   Website: www.cbspd.com
Fax: 011-23243014   e-mail: delhi@cbspd.com; cbspubs@airtelmail.in.

Corporate Office: 204 FIE, Industrial Area, Patparganj, Delhi 110 092
Ph: 4934 4934   Fax: 4934 4935   e-mail: publishing@cbspd.com; publicity@cbspd.com

Branches

- **Bengaluru:** Seema House 2975, 17th Cross, K.R. Road,
  Banasankari 2nd Stage, Bengaluru 560 070, Karnataka
  Ph: +91-80-26771678/79   Fax: +91-80-26771680   e-mail: bangalore@cbspd.com

- **Chennai:** 7, Subbaraya Street, Shenoy Nagar, Chennai 600 030, Tamil Nadu
  Ph: +91-44-26680620/26681266 Fax: +91-44-42032115   e-mail: chennai@cbspd.com

- **Kochi:** Ashana House, No. 39/1904, AM Thomas Road, Valanjambalam, Ernakulam 682 016, Kochi, Kerala
  Ph: +91-484-4059061–65   Fax: +91-484-4059065   e-mail: kochi@cbspd.com

- **Kolkata:** 6/B, Ground Floor, Rameswar Shaw Road, Kolkata-700 014, West Bengal
  Ph: +91-33-22891126, 22891127, 22891128   e-mail: kolkata@cbspd.com

- **Mumbai:** 83-C, Dr E Moses Road, Worli, Mumbai-400018, Maharashtra
  Ph: +91-22-24902340/41   Fax: +91-22-24902342   e-mail: mumbai@cbspd.com

Representatives

• **Hyderabad**	0-9885175004	• **Jharkhand**	0-9811541605	• **Nagpur**	0-9021734563
• **Patna**	0-9334159340	• **Pune**	0-9623451994	• **Uttarakhand**	0-9716462459

Printed at: Thomson Press India Ltd., Faridabad, Haryana, India

Eminent worthy teachers, our promising students and esteemed faculty members for enduring inspiration
and
My loving soulmate Dr (Mrs) Manita Kamal, dear Dr Spriha Arun, Dr Mansi Dhende, Dr Anubhav and Dr Vigyat for always being there with me. This book could be completed due to their outstanding support and encouragement at every step.

Contents

Preface — xi
Foreword by Dr Meera Sikka — xiii
Foreword by Dr Rajeev Sen — xiv
Foreword by Dr Ezhil Arasi N — xv
Foreword by Dr Nita Khurana — xvi
Foreword by Dr Sunita Sharma — xvii
Foreword by Dr Kuldeep Kumar Kaul — xviii
Foreword by Dr Syed Besina Yasin — xix
Foreword by Dr Sujata Kanetkar — xx
Foreword by Dr Hansa Goswami — xxi

Section I: General Pathology

1. **Cellular Adaptations, Cell Injury, Apoptosis, Pigments Calcification, Cellular Accumulations and Aging** — 3
   Cellular Adaptations 4
   Cell Injury 14
   Apoptosis 32
   Subcellular Response to Injury 37
   Pigments 38
   Calcification 42
   Intracellular Accumulations 44
   Extracellular Accumulations 47
   Cellular Aging 48

2. **Inflammation, Tissue Healing and Repair** — 51
   Acute Inflammation 53
   Chronic Inflammation 96
   Tissue Healing and Repair 110

3. **Disorders of Hemostasis** — 134
   Hyperemia and Congestion 134
   Hemorrhage 137
   Hemostasis 139
   Thrombosis 147
   Embolism 156
   Infarction 160
   Edema 165
   Shock 170

4. **Immunopathology including Amyloidosis** — 177
   Immune System 178
   Nonspecific (Innate or Inborn) Immune Response 182
   Specific Immune Response 187
   Immunization and Vaccines 211
   Immunodeficiency Disorders 215
   Hypersensitivity Reactions 230
   Immunologic Tolerance 250
   Autoimmune Diseases 254
   HLA System 264
   Transplantation Immunology 266
   Amyloidosis 273

5. **Genetic Disorders** — 282
   - Human Genome 282
   - Chromosomal Disorders 292
   - Single Gene Mutation (Mendelian Disorders) 301
   - Disorders of Sexual Differentiation 312
   - Work up of Genetic Disorders 313

6. **Neoplasia: Molecular Basis, Metastasis, Clinical Oncology and Laboratory Diagnosis** — 316
   - Neoplasia 317
   - Nomenclature and Classification 321
   - Characteristic Features of Tumors 332
   - Epidemiology of Tumors 335
   - Cell Cycle and Cancer 337
   - Genetic Preposition of Cancer 341
   - Acquired Preneoplastic Lesions 343
   - Molecular Basis of Cancer: Role of Genetic and Epigenetic Alterations 345
   - Multistep Carcinogenesis 380
   - Invasion and Metastasis 392
   - Routes of Metastasis of Tumors 395
   - Clinical Oncology 400
   - Laboratory Diagnosis 412

7. **Nutritional and Infectious Diseases** — 417
   - Nutritional Diseases 417
   - Bacterial Infections 430
   - Viral Infections 446
   - Fungal Infections 450
   - Parasitic Diseases 452

Section II: Hematology

8. **Red Blood Cells** — 459
   - Hematopoiesis 459
   - Red Blood Cell, Hemoglobin and Classification of Anemias 474
   - Iron Deficiency Anemia 481
   - Megaloblastic Anemia: Vitamin B_{12} and Folic Acid Deficiency 487
   - Red Blood Cells Destruction and Classification of Hemolytic Anemia 495
   - Hereditary Spherocytosis, Ovalocytosis and Stomatocytosis 499
   - Thalassemias 502
   - Sickle Cell Disorders and Other Hemoglobinopathies 509
   - Glucose-6-Phosphate Dehydrogenase Deficiency and Pyruvate Kinase Deficiency 514
   - Immune Hemolytic Anemia 516
   - Paroxysmal Nocturnal Hemoglobinuria 521
   - RBCs Fragmentation Syndromes 522
   - Diagnostic Approach of Hemolytic Anemia 523
   - Bone Marrow Failure Syndromes 528

9. **White Blood Cells** — 533
   - Leukocytes and their Quantitative and Qualitative Disorders 533
   - Acute Leukemias 539
   - Myelodysplastic Syndromes/Myeloproliferative Neoplasms 559
   - Myeloproliferative Neoplasms 562
   - Chronic Lymphoproliferative Disorders 574
   - Multiple Myeloma and Waldenström Macroglobulinemia 580
   - Disorders of Mononuclear Phagocytic System 588
   - Hematopoietic Stem Cell Transplantation 592

10. **Bleeding Disorders** — 596
    - Normal and Disorders of Hemostasis 596
    - Platelet Disorders 600
    - Thrombocytopenias 602
    - Platelet Function Disorders 605
    - Vascular Purpura 607

11. **Coagulation Disorders** — 609
    - Inherited and Acquired Coagulation Disorders 609
    - Thrombophilia (Hypercoagulable State) 618
    - Clinical Aspects of Bleeding Diathesis 620

12. **Blood Groups and Blood Transfusion** — 626
    - Blood Group Systems 626
    - Blood Collection, Processing and Storage 631
    - Blood Grouping 632
    - Blood Cross-matching (Compatibility Test) 634
    - Blood Components Therapy 634
    - Autologous Blood Transfusion and Plasma Exchange 637
    - Adverse Blood Transfusion Reactions 639

13. **Lymph Nodes, Spleen and Thymus** — 641
    - Disorders of Lymph Node 641
    - Hodgkin's Disease 648
    - Non-Hodgkin's Lymphoma 658
    - Spleen 677
    - Thymus Gland 682

14. **Advanced Diagnostic Techniques** — 687
    - Frozen Section Technique 687
    - Electron Microscopy and Polarizing Light Microscopy 688
    - Histology and Histochemical Stains 691
    - Immunohistochemistry 698

Immunofluorescence Microscopy 703
Chemiluminescence *vs* Chemifluorescence 705
Flow Cytometry 706
Cytogenetic Analysis 709
Fluorescence *in situ* Hybridization 716
Enzyme-linked Immunosorbent Assay (ELISA) 721

Methods for DNA Sequences 724
Tissue Microarray 731
High Performance Liquid Chromatography (HPLC) 733
Electrophoresis 734

Index I–XXV

Section III: Systemic Pathology

15. **Blood Vessels** 741
    Arteriosclerosis 742
    Atherosclerosis 744
    Aneurysms 755
    Vasculitis 760
    Veins 767
    Lymphatic System 769
    Tumors of Blood Vessels 769
    Hypertension 772

16. **Heart** 781
    Ischemic Heart Disease 783
    Rheumatic Fever and RHD 798
    Myocardium 806
    Endocardium 811
    Cardiac Valves 818
    Pericardium 821
    Congestive Heart Failure 826
    Cardiac Hypertrophy 829
    Cardiac Tumors 830
    Congenital Heart Diseases 831

17. **Nasal Cavity, Nasopharynx, Paranasal Sinuses, Ear, Larynx and Neck** 836
    Inflammation and Infections 836
    Neoplastic Disorders 838
    Miscellaneous Disorders 845
    Ear 845
    Larynx 849
    Neck 851

18. **Lung** 856
    Pneumonias 860
    Lung Abscess 869
    Tuberculosis 870
    Chronic Obstructive Pulmonary Disease 876
    Restrictive Pulmonary Diseases 886
    Pneumothorax and Atelectasis Lung 898
    Pulmonary Vascular Disorders 900
    Lung Tumors 906
    Pleural Diseases 927

19. **Oral Cavity and Salivary Glands** 932
    Oral Cavity 932
    Salivary Glands 938
    Jaw 950

20. **Gastrointestinal Tract** 957
    Esophagus 959
    Stomach 967
    Small Intestine 986
    Large Intestine 1002
    Appendix 1029
    Anus and Perianal Region 1031
    Peritoneum 1034
    Investigations of Gastrointestinal Disorders 1036

21. **Liver, Gallbladder and Exocrine Pancreas** 1040
    Liver 1041
    Jaundice and Cholestasis 1050
    Hepatitis 1058
    Bacterial and Parasitic Infections of Liver 1077
    Cirrhosis 1082
    Metabolic Liver Diseases 1094
    Bile Duct Disorders 1107
    Vascular Disorders 1110
    Liver Tumors 1113
    Gallbladder 1126
    Common Neoplasms and Precursor Lesions of Gallbladder 1137
    Pancreas 1139
    Pancreatitis 1140
    Pancreatic Tumors 1145

22. **Kidney and Ureter** 1150
    Anatomy 1150
    Physiology 1153
    Glomeruli 1157
    Glomerulonephritis 1161
    Nephrotic Syndrome 1171
    Acute Nephritic Syndrome 1187
    Chronic Glomerulonephritis 1197
    Evaluation of Renal Biopsy 1201
    Diseases of the Tubules 1205

Tubulointerstitial Disorders 1209
Obstructive Uropathy and Hydronephrosis 1217
Renal Stones (Nephrolithiasis and Urolithiasis) 1218
Vascular Disorders 1221
Cystic Diseases of Kidney 1226
Congenital Anomalies of the Urinary Tract 1229
Neoplasms of the Kidney 1230
Laboratory Diagnosis 1242

23. Urinary Bladder and Male Reproductive System — 1245
Urinary Bladder 1245
Testes 1255
Prostate Gland 1276
Penis 1282

24. Female Reproductive System — 1284
Vulva 1287
Vagina 1291
Cervix 1297
Fallopian Tubes 1306
Endometrium 1308
Ovary 1321
Gestational Trophoblastic Tumors 1349
Pregnancy Associated Diseases 1353

25. Breast — 1358
Female Breasts 1358
Inflammatory Disorders 1364
Fibrocystic Disease 1366
WHO Classification: Breast Tumors 1370
Breast Carcinoma 1376
Male Breasts 1407

26. Endocrine System: Pancreas, Thyroid, Parathyroid, Adrenal and Pituitary Glands — 1409
Endocrine Pancreas 1409
Diabetes Mellitus 1412
Thyroid Gland 1425
Parathyroid Glands 1452
Adrenal Glands 1457
Pituitary Gland 1467

27. Bones and Joints — 1475
Bones 1475
Osteomyelitis 1477
Metabolic Bone Diseases 1479
Bone Tumors 1484
Joints 1517

28. Soft Tissue Tumors and Skeletal Myopathies — 1524
Soft Tissue Tumors 1524
Skeletal Muscles 1542

29. Skin — 1549
Normal Skin 1550
Inflammatory Disorders 1555
Cutaneous Infections 1558
Autoimmune Disorders 1562
Nonmelanocytic Lesions and Tumors 1565
Pigmentation Disorders and Melanocytic Tumors 1569
Fibrous and Fibrohistiocytic Tumors 1573
Neural and Neuroendocrine Tumors 1574
Vascular Tumors 1575
Tumors of Cutaneous Appendages 1576
Cutaneous Metastases 1577
Miscellaneous Disorders 1577

30. Nervous System — 1580
CNS Infections 1584
CNS Tumors 1590
Reaction of CNS to Injury 1611
Cerebrovascular Diseases 1611
Head Injuries 1615
Demyelinating Disorders 1616
Congenital Disorders 1617

Index — 1621

Preface

The study of pathology is essential for safe clinical practice. In modern era, tremendous growth is in progress in diagnostic pathology with recent advances in molecular methods, cytogenetics and immunohistochemistry. Rapidly changing hematology needs integration of recent guidelines and diagnostic criteria of hematological disorders.

I joined India's premier institution in Department of Pathology, Maulana Azad Medical College, New Delhi. I puzzled over the fact that the students admitted of very high caliber still had problems in grasping the teaching material. I interacted with students and eminent faculty members across country. I discussed problems faced by the students in reproducing text. I analyzed their inputs and then started working on Textbook of Pathology in 2007. Primary aim of this book is to discuss complex topics in a straightforward, clear and organized manner.

All the chapters have been shared with the eminent teachers and young budding residents across country. Their valuable opinion on various aspects has been taken positively during drafting of the chapters to meet the need of the young generation of pathologists. Each chapter focuses on the essentials necessary to build a broad fundamentals backed up with numerous colored figures, gross morphology, light microscopy, photographs, tables and flow diagrams.

I trust you will enjoy reading this book. I have spent a great deal of time and energy ensuring easy grasp and retaining the topics. I am inviting your comments, valuable suggestions and criticism.

Chief Editor
Vinay Kamal
Email: vinaykamal@hotmail.com
Mobile: 09818001202

Foreword

The *Textbook of Pathology* by Dr Vinay Kamal, Director Professor, Department of Pathology, Maulana Azad Medical College, New Delhi, covers various aspects of pathology in a systematic manner. The book includes several strong points such as a reader-friendly font size of text and the simple language used in the text making it easy to understand.

The text is very well illustrated in the form of gross and microscopic pictures. An attempt has been made to include the recent advances specially the current WHO classifications wherever applicable. Key points have been placed separately in a box to facilitate quick revision by the students. The clinical features of disease along with their pathologic basis have also been included which will greatly help the students. The flow diagrams provided along with the text will aid in understanding. The text is accompanied by several tables particularly useful for the professional examination. All these features reflect the author's vast experience as a teacher. I am sure the students will find the book easy to read and comprehend.

Dr Meera Sikka
Director Professor and Head
Department of Pathology
University College of Medical Sciences
and
GTB Hospital, New Delhi

Foreword

I have known Dr Vinay Kamal, ever since I joined the then Govt Medical College, Rohtak, on December 31st, 1983, with deepening bond of friendship between us. I have been witness to his commitment to the undergraduate and postgraduate students and his evolution as a teacher. He would deliver a lecture in a lucid fashion, yet will ensure that it is conceptually comprehensible.

I have seen glimpses of the *Textbook of Pathology* comprising of high resolution figures, numerous tables and recent WHO classifications with clinicopathological correlation. It holds a wealth of information for undergraduate students, postgraduate scholars and practicing pathologists.

It connects from basic understanding learnt by a medical student in preclinical courses to genesis of diseases, its manifestations and contemporary practice of the science of clinical pathology using bridge of contemporary knowledge.

Without prejudice of our friendship, I am sure that this textbook is going to provide answers to most of the questions, a medical student is seeking in pathology.

Dr Rajeev Sen
Senior Professor and Head
Department of Pathology
Post Graduate Institute of Medical Sciences
Rohtak (Haryana)

Foreword

It gives me immense pleasure and privilege for having given me the opportunity to contribute to the publication of *Textbook of Pathology* by Dr Vinay Kamal, Director Professor, Department of Pathology, Maulana Azad Medical College, New Delhi. He has covered recent concepts of pathology in a systemic manner in easy language. Book contains recent WHO classification whereever applicable, clinicopathological correlation, diagnostic approach, numerous colored figures, gross morphology, light microscopy and flow diagrams.

The book will be of a great source of enlightenment to the students reflecting the zeal and enthusiasm of the author. I wish him all the success in his endeavor and sincerely pray that the book will be of much help to the budding doctors all over the nation and abroad.

Dr Ezhil Arasi N
Vice Principal (Administration)
Professor and Head
Department of Pathology
Osmania Medical College
Hyderabad (Telangana)

Foreword

I feel pleased and honored to be given an opportunity to write the foreword for the first edition of the *Text book of Pathology* written by Dr Vinay Kamal, Director Professor, Department of Pathology at India's premier medical institute, Maulana Azad Medical College, New Delhi. I have known him since 1990 when I joined MAMC as a postgraduate student. He connects with the students and takes keen interest in their learning and tries to help them out in all their personal and academic problems. A similar helpful attitude towards staff with all help extended to them has been his nature at all times.

I have reviewed all the chapters of this *Textbook of Pathology*. From its inception the book was intended to fulfill the needs of the medical students to understand the basic principles of pathology in a simple language and concise format. I convey my heartfelt appreciation for the hard work done by Dr Vinay Kamal for conceptualizing and executing this body of work.

The author with his more than three decades of teaching experience has put the essential elements of the subject in a student-friendly format complete with high resolution of 1533 figures and 1097 tables, inclusion of up-to-date recent advances and recent diagnostic techniques. Emphasis has been kept on the section on hematology and hematolymphoid disorders so that the students use this book as a complete package.

The enormous time and effort put into creating tables and key points so as to clarify the subject and help in distinguishing closely related terms and disorders particularly useful to undergraduate student and ready resource for the postgraduate students. The chapters of this textbook have been shared with the eminent teachers and young budding residents across country. Their valuable opinion on various aspects has been taken positively during the drafting of the chapters to meet the need of the young generation of pathologists. This positive attitude towards suggestions for betterment was greatly appreciated by the colleagues and students alike. This Herculean task is the result of many months of sleepless nights and hard work.

The experience and enthusiasm of the author to help the learning of the student is evident in the simple format and comprehensive information provided in a context necessary to translate knowledge of pathology into clinical practice.

I hope the students and pathologists will enjoy the book and it will be a ready tool for updating knowledge for the postgraduates and teachers alike. The balance of detail and brevity and integrated coverage of clinical information and pathology will serve its intended purpose of building a solid foundation in pathology for the future doctors to better serve their patients.

Dr Nita Khurana
Director Professor
Department of Pathology
Maulana Azad Medical College
New Delhi

Foreword

It is a proud moment for me to write a brief review of the first edition of the *Text book of Pathology* written by Dr Vinay Kamal. It provides a comprehensive coverage to all the diseases. Each chapter starts with learning objectives. This textbook contains 1533 illustrations and 1097 tables, recent WHO classification, recent concepts in pathology, recent diagnostic techniques, gross morphology, light microscopy and flow diagrams. These have simplified the subject in making the concepts easily understandable. I convey my heartfelt appreciation for the hard work done by Dr Vinay Kamal for conceptualizing and executing this body of work. I hope that the students will enjoy reading this book and will find pathology a much easier and interesting subject.

Dr Sunita Sharma
Director Professor and Head
Department of Pathology
Lady Hardinge Medical College
New Delhi

Foreword

I have been associated with Dr Vinay Kamal, Director Professor, Department of Pathology, Maulana Azad Medical College, New Delhi, for the last two decades. We have been together as examiners on various occasions. His positive attitude towards students, clear and honest thoughts impressed me. We had long discussions on many academic topics and the problems faced by the students in their examinations.

Our department had an opportunity to review many of the chapters of the forthcoming *Textbook of Pathology*. He shared these chapters with senior faculty and postgraduates across country to seek their opinion. He used to analyze their suggestions and incorporated relevant matter in the book.

Highlights of this *Textbook of Pathology* include recent WHO classification, 1533 figures, 1097 tables, recent concepts in pathology, immunohistochemistry, molecular biology, recent diagnostic techniques and clinicopathological correlation. For a quick revision, the tables, pictures and diagrams are given in such a nice way, which reflects that the author has taken due care of all these areas that makes the book a unique.

Hence, it is an ideal comprehensive *Textbook of Pathology* for undergraduates, postgraduates, consultants and clinicians. I am confident that his contribution in pathology shall be remembered forever.

Dr Kuldeep Kumar Kaul
Professor and Head
Department of Pathology
Govt Medical College, Jammu
Jammu and Kashmir

Foreword

Good teachers are the reason why ordinary students dream to do extraordinary things. Dr Vinay Kamal, Director Professor, Department of Pathology, besides being a pathologist par excellence is a dedicated teacher for whom the welfare of students is of prime importance.

I have known him for the last 15 years. What has impressed me most is his sincerity, honesty and desire to help others. He has played a pivotal role in getting the MD pathology degrees recognized both at Govt Medical College, Srinagar as well as Sher-I-Kashmir Institute of Medical Sciences, Srinagar. Credit goes to him in enhancement of postgraduates intake in these institutions. His contributions in the specialty of pathology as a teacher, educator and consultant is praiseworthy.

Now as an author he has this prestigious *Textbook of Pathology* to his credit. Our department has reviewed his chapters. He has worked hard to complete the project in 11 years. *Textbook of Pathology* is well written with 1533 high resolution figures and 1097 tables. Latest WHO classifications and recent advances have been incorporated appropriately. It holds a wealth of information for undergraduate students, postgraduate scholars and practicing pathologists. I congratulate him for this phenomenal effort. I am sure reading this book will enrich all the readers.

Dr Syed Besina Yasin
Additional Professor and Head
Department of Pathology
Sher-I-Kashmir Institute of Medical Sciences
Srinagar, Jammu and Kashmir

Foreword

Dr Vinay Kamal, Director Professor, Department of Pathology, has illustrious teaching career of 35 years. His *Textbook of Pathology* is a fruit of his tireless, meticulous efforts for quality, simplicity and standardization. The author shared some topics and illustrations with me.

The topics have been covered in such a way to make things easy to understand as well as assure success in various competitive examinations. This textbook is rich with high resolution 1533 illustrations as well as 1097 tables, which provide key points for better understanding. It covers all the recent updates in the medical field. I am confident that it will be appreciated and will be useful for both undergraduates and postgraduates in pathology.

Dr Sujata Kanetkar
Professor and Head
Department of Pathology
Krishna Institute of Medical Sciences
Satara, Karad, Maharashtra

Foreword

I have been interacting with Dr Vinay Kamal on various occasions on the subject of pathology for the last 15 years. The undaunted association with teaching undergraduates and postgraduates at premier institution as Director Professor, Department of Pathology, Maulana Azad Medical College, New Delhi since many years, distinguishes him from many other academicians by way of his integrated innovative approach, to make the subject of pathology simple and easy. He has vast teaching experience of more than three decades.

I have reviewed some of the chapters of forthcoming *Textbook of Pathology* by Dr Vinay Kamal. Salient features of textbook include comprehensive knowledge of pathology with recent WHO classification, recent concepts in pathology, 1533 figures and 1097 tabulated data analysis, molecular pathology, immunohistochemistry, recent advanced techniques, clinicopathological correlation, gross morphology, light microscopy and flow diagrams This book will go long away in making students understand pathology and its relevance, significance and importance in medicine. This book is the eventual result of his immense passion of teaching students, without compromising quality. I wish great success to his new endeavor.

Dr Hansa Goswami
Professor and Head
Department of Pathology
BJ Medical College
Ahmedabad, Gujarat

Acknowledgments

Foremost acknowledgement is gratefulness to Almighty for guiding me all time during preparation of first edition of *Textbook of Pathology*. I express my gratitude to Mr Satish Kumar Jain CHAIRMAN and Mr Varun Jain MANAGING DIRECTOR of CBS Publishers & Distributors Pvt. Ltd. for extending their whole hearted support at every step in completion of book.

I am grateful to Mr YN Arjuna VICE PRESIDENT—PUBLISHING, EDITORIAL AND PRODUCTION, Mrs Ritu Chawla ACM and Dr Krishna Garg. I express my gratitude to Mr Sunil Dutt PROMOTION MANAGER, who has been main guiding force behind in completion of the book.

Credit goes to the outstanding team comprising of Mr Ram Murti SENIOR GRAPHIC ARTIST, Mrs Sunita Rautela SENIOR DTP OPERATOR and Mr Ananda Mohanty SENIOR PROOF READER for their devotion and excellent work in the book. Mr Ram Murti and Mrs Sunita Rautela deserve special mention in preparation of layout of the book. Mr Ram Murti put sincere efforts in finalizing 1533 figures.

The magnitude of the work pertaining to first edition of *Textbook of Pathology* has been possible for outstanding support and cooperation from friends, well-wishers, my departmental colleagues and especially residents, the backbone of department across the country.

The chapters of this textbook have been shared with the eminent teachers and young budding residents across country. Their valuable opinion on various aspects has been taken positively during the drafting of the chapters to meet the need of the young generation of pathologists. This positive attitude towards suggestions for betterment was greatly appreciated by the colleagues and students alike.

I express my gratitude especially to Dr Meera Sikka, Dr Rajeev Sen, Dr Ezhil Arasi N, Dr Nita Khurana, Dr Sunita Sharma, Dr Kuldeep Kumar Kaul, Dr Hansa Goswami, Dr Syed BesinaYasin, Dr Sandeep Mathur, Dr Narender Kumar Mogra, Dr SS Surana, Dr Surender Pal, Dr Archna Buch, Dr Seema Rao, Dr Uday, Dr Abhijit Das, Mr GD Manoj and Mr Rajiv Aggarwal for extending whole hearted support and advice.

Andhra Pradesh
Sidhartha Medical College, Vijayawada
Professor of Pathology
Dr Venkata Rama Reddy Bollareddy

Bihar
Govt Medical College, Patna
Assistant Professor of Pathology
Dr Pallavi Agrawal

All India Institute of Medical Sciences, Patna
Senior Resident/Tutor of Pathology
Dr Iffat Jamal

Chandigarh (Union Territory)
Post Graduate Institute, Chandigarh
Assistant Professor of Hematology
Dr Prashant Sharma

Senior Resident of Pathology
Dr Chandni Garg

Post Graduate Residents of Pathology
Dr Archana Sundram, Dr Shilpi Thakur, Dr Debajyoti Chatterji

Govt Medical College, Chandigarh
Professor of Pathology
Dr RPS Punia

Senior Resident of Pathology
Dr Garima Rakheja

Former Senior Resident of Pathology
Dr Vidhu Jaswal Wadhwa

Post Graduate Resident of Pathology
Dr Nayan Koul

Delhi

Maulana Azad Medical College, New Delhi
Former Director Professor and Head of Pathology
Dr Tejinder Singh

Former Professors
Dr Nita Kumar, Dr DK Shome, Dr Sonu Nigam

Director Professor of Pathology
Dr Nita Khurana

Director Professor of Community Medicine
Dr GK Ingle

Director Professor of Microbiology
Dr Surinder Kumar

Professor of Pathology
Dr Sarika Singh

Associate Professors of Pathology
Dr Richa Gupta, Dr Sharmana Mandal

Assistant Professors of Pathology
Dr Prerna Arora, Dr Reena Tomar, Dr Meeta Singh, Dr Nidhi Verma, Dr Varuna Mallya Ashwin, Dr Priyanka Saxena, Dr Ritika Walia

Senior Residents of Pathology
Dr Surekha Yadav, Dr Latika Gupta, Dr Barkha Maheswari, Dr Nishant Sagar, Dr Sushil Kumar Sharma, Dr Ashutosh Rath, Dr Dimple Chaudhary, Dr Radhika Agarwal, Dr Vishal Singh

Post Graduate Residents of Pathology
Dr Usha Rani, Dr Neelam Singh, Dr Gunjan Nain, Dr Jyotsna Ranjan, Dr Lalnunsangi Saila, Dr Pritika Kushwaha, Dr Sneha Goswami, Dr Kirti Balhara, Dr Neelakashi Goyal, Dr Rabish Kumar

Alumni Post Graduate Residents of Pathology since 1990
Dr Neelam Sood, Dr Rajeev Bajaj, Dr Promila Gautam, Dr Rajiv Sharma, Dr Pooja Sakhuja, Dr Sangita Sarkar Basu, Dr Sandhya Bajaj, Dr Anand Verma, Dr Debadutt Basu, Dr Sangita Lamba, Dr Sangita Saigal, Dr Sunanda, Dr Meenakshi Gupta, Dr Sangita Sonkar, Dr Nita Khurana, Dr Anju Goyal, Dr Rupa Sarma, Dr Jyotika, Dr Rekha Aggarwal, Dr Ira Gulati, Dr Neerja Vajpayee, Dr Meena Sidhu, Dr Nakhat, Dr Anju Jain, Dr Ramona Chopra, Dr Renu Das, Dr Dinesh Rakheja, Dr Nilanjana, Dr Sonu Nigam, Dr Deepali Gupta, Dr Shobini Rajan, Dr Shikha Gupta, Dr Sameer Gupta, Dr Haimanti Sarin, Dr Meenashi Sidar, Dr Pragati Narula Kumar, Dr Naveen Sharma, Dr Payal Kapur, Dr Pradeep Suri, Dr Som Pal Singh, Dr Archana, Dr Ruma Pahwa, Dr Deepali Verma, Dr Deepika Sharma, Dr Kirti Sharma, Dr Niti Singhal, Dr Sandeep Singhal, Dr Ritesh Sachdeva, Dr Divya Chhabra, Dr Abha Goel, Dr Prashant Sharma, Dr Sanjeev Gupta, Dr Samhita Bhattacharya, Dr Shyam Sunder, Dr Ruchika Aggarwal, Dr Parul Jain, Dr Reema Gulati, Dr Shubhita Bhatnagar, Dr Kajal Puneet Phull, Dr Deepti Mahajan, Dr Deepak Kumar Singh, Dr Nidhi Goyal, Dr Sukriti Singhal, Dr Prerna Arora, Dr Kavita Kohli, Dr Namarta Setia, Dr Somak Roy, Dr Vijay Saroha, Dr Debpriya Ghosh, Dr Doris Zaultei, Dr Meeta Singh, Dr Ankur Garg, Dr Akhila Lakshmikantha, Dr Vibha Chhabra, Dr Nidhi Mahajan, Dr Nivedita Ghosh, Dr Pallavi Aggarwal, Dr Ashumi Gupta, Dr Swapnil Agarwal, Dr Jyotsna Nigam, Dr Rachna Khera, Dr Sangita Tripathi, Dr Parul Sobti, Dr Alphy Sara Verghese, Dr Ruchi Jha, Dr Reema Dahiya, Dr Poonam Rani, Dr Divya Sharma, Dr Jenna Bhattacharya, Dr Devi Subarayan, Dr Amita Jain, Dr Bembem Khuraijam, Dr Barkha Maheshwari, Dr Parul Gautam, Dr Annapurna Saxena, Dr Chandni Garg, Dr Vasudha Goyal, Dr Parth Desai, Dr Prasad S Dange, Dr Roopali Rathi, Dr Garima Rakheja, Dr Suniti Pahwa Sikund, Dr Vikram Raj Gopinathan, Dr Ashna Mittal, Dr Ashu Singh, Dr Sushil Kumar Sharma, Dr Nishant Sagar, Dr Uday, Dr Darilin, Dr Vijaya Vaishnav, Dr Radhika Aggarwal, Dr Dimple Chaudhary, Dr Kamal Wadhwa, Dr Vishal Chauhan, Dr Anusha S Bhat, Dr Chetna Mehrol, Dr Shubhra Narayan, Dr Pomilla Singh, Dr Saumya Pandey, Dr Tushar Kalonia, Dr Babita Khangar

Former Senior Residents of Pathology
Dr Rashmi Jain, Dr Sabita Basu, Dr Kachnar Verma, Dr Neha Singh, Dr Garima Goyal, Dr Rekha Boyal, Dr Sharmana Mandal, Dr Sangita Sonkar, Dr Arun Kumar Thakran, Dr Ankita Jaswal

Technical Staff of Pathology
Mr Ashok Aggarwal, Mr Vinod Sharma, Mr Ramesh Kumar, Mr Rajan, Mr Narender Singh, Mr Rakesh Kumar, Mrs Sudha Roy, Mrs Promila, Mrs Ranjana, Mrs Bindu, Mrs Aji, Mrs Soffie, Mrs Neelam, Mrs Geeta Verma

Photography Section of Pathology
Mr Subhankar Ghosh

Office of Pathology
Mrs Bimla Devi

Avni Book Depot, MAMC, New Delhi
Mr Varis Sharma

Photocopy Center
Mr Narender Kumar

University College of Medical Sciences, New Delhi
Director Professor and Head of Pathology
Dr Meera Sikka

Director Professors/Professors
Dr Satinder Sharma, Dr VK Arora, Dr Sonal Sharma, Dr Mrinalini Kotru

Lady Hardinge Medical College, New Delhi
Director Professor and Head of Pathology
Dr Sunita Sharma

Director Professors/Professors of Pathology
Dr Manjula Jain, Dr Monisha Chaudhary, Dr Kiran Aggarwal, Dr Shilpi Aggarwal, Dr Selja Shukla

Assistant Professors of Pathology
Dr Vandana Puri Tiwari, Dr Lalita Jyotsna Prakhya, Dr Shivali Sehgal

All India Institute of Medical Sciences, New Delhi
Professor of Pathology
Dr Sandeep Mathur

Acknowledgments

Assistant Professor of Internal Medicine
Dr Arvind Kumar

Assistant Professor of Hematoncology
Dr Sanjiv Gupta

Assistant Professors of Pathology
Dr Shipra Goel, Dr Seema Kaushal

DM Residents Hematology
Dr Uday, Dr Prasad S Dange

Senior Resident of Pathology
Dr Vikram Raj Gopinathan

Vardhman Medical College, New Delhi
Director Professor/Professor of Pathology
Dr Ashish Kumar Mandal, Dr Rashmi Arora

Senior Resident of Pathology
Dr Tanvi Aggarwal

Intern Trainee
Dr Sugandha Bansal

Ambedkar Medical College, Rohini
Assistant Professors of Pathology
Dr Bembem Khuraijam, Dr Divya Sharma

PGIMER, Ram Manohar Lohia Hospital, New Delhi
Director Professor of Orthopedics
Dr Anil Mehtani

Professor of Dermatology
Dr Kabir Sardana

Senior Resident Anesthesiology
Dr Monika Chandra

North DMC Hindu Rao Medical College, New Delhi
Professor of Pathology
Dr Raj Bala Yadav

Consultant Pathologist
Dr Som Pal Singh

Chacha Nehru Bal Chikitsalaya, Geeta Colony
Assistant Professor of Pathology
Dr Nidhi Mahajan

Sir Ganga Ram Hospital, Rajinder Nagar
Consultant Pathologist
Dr Seema Rao

Central Govt Health Scheme, New Delhi
Consultant Pathologist
Dr Ila Tyagi

Janakpuri Super Speciality Hospital, New Delhi
Director
Dr MM Mehandiratta

Assistant Professor of Pathology
Dr Abhijit Das

Institute of Human Behaviour and Allied Sciences, New Delhi
Professor of Pathology
Dr Sujata Chaturvedi

Gujarat
BJ Medical College, Ahmedabad
Professor and Head of Pathology
Dr Hansa Goswami

Professors of Pathology
Dr HA Oza, Dr Smita Shah, Dr Nandita Mehta, Dr Manesh Patel, Dr Sanjay Dhotre, Dr Ina Shah

Associate Professor of Pathology
Dr Hemina Desai, Dr Ami Shah, Dr Monika Kohli

Assistant Professor of Pathology
Dr Meena Patel, Dr Purvi Patel, Dr Sakera Baji, Dr Hetal Jani, Dr Ami Shah, Dr Uvri Parikh, Dr Vashali Anand, Dr Hitender Baro

Tutors of Pathology
Dr Prabha Rathod, Dr Bharat Pateliya, Dr Shivani Dixit, Dr Bhavesh Faldu, Dr Pooja Dave, Dr Garshma Jobanpura, Dr Neelam Mehta, Dr Amit Satosiya, Dr Kajal Parikh, Dr Priyanka Gohel, Dr Mital Chokshi, Dr Binal Vagh, Dr Taruna Hadiya

Post Graduate Residents of Pathology
Dr Hiralben Patel, Dr Ruchira Wadhwa, Dr Devanshi Gosai, Dr Nishith Thakor, Dr Pratibha Vyas, Dr Mehul Kumar Patel, Dr Varsha Dhuliya, Dr Shalibhadra Shah, Dr Hiren Mandiyo, Dr Triputi Sonawan, Dr Ritesh Gohail, Dr Komalben Joshi, Dr Jaymalakumari Solanki, Dr Aritra Aash, Dr Juhi Khanna, Dr Ronnak Jain, Dr Neeraja Barve, Dr Vivek Kumar, Dr Ruchi Patel, Dr Sneha Patel, Dr Dhruvi Patel, Dr Neetal Desai, Dr Mital Yadav, Dr Yamini Rana, Dr Kajal Parikh, Dr Taruna Hidiya, Dr Binal Vaghani, Dr Bharat Pateliya, Dr Prabha Rathod, Dr Garishma Jobanputra, Dr Sonali Tirvaniya, Dr Siddhartha Ghelani, Dr Payal Malviyo, Dr Jaimin Manek, Dr Vaibhavi Dhimmar, Dr Avani Oza, Dr Dhaval Vachela, Dr Niraj Maiyad, Dr Khushali Parikh, Dr Shreya Solanki, Dr Nikita Patel, Dr Hemangi Mehta, Dr Alisha Mody, Dr Ajay Devraniya, Dr Akash Thakkar

NHL Medical College, Ahmedabad
Associate Professor of Pathology
Dr Anjali Goyal

GCS Medical College, Ahmedabad
Professor and Head of Pathology
Dr Deepak Joshi

PDU Medical College, Rajkot
Associate Professor of Pathology
Dr Amit Agravat

Post Graduate Resident of Pathology
Dr Rashi Garg

GMERS Medical College, Himmat Nagar
Associate Professor of Pathology
Dr Atul Shrivastav

Haryana
Post Graduate Institute of Medical Sciences, Rohtak
Former Senior Professors of Pathology
Dr Uma Singh, Dr SK Mathur

Senior Professor and Head of Pathology
Dr Rajeev Sen

Senior Professor of Pathology
Dr Sunita Singh

Professors of Pathology
Dr Nisha Marwah, Dr Rajnish Kalra, Dr Sanjay Kumar, Dr Veena Gupta, Dr Meenu Gill, Dr Sant Parkash, Dr Sumiti Gupta, Dr Sonia Chhabra

Associate Professor of Pathology
Dr Gajender Singh

Assistant Professors of Pathology
Dr Monika Gupta, Dr Promil Gupta, Dr Shivani Dua Batra, Dr Renuka Verma

Senior Residents of Pathology
Dr Hemant, Dr Padam, Dr Deepika, Dr Neha Singh, Dr Richa, Dr Sonu, Dr Pansi, Dr Sucheta, Dr Gauri, Dr Dimple, Dr Shivani, Dr Mansi, Dr Shilpi, Dr Divya, Dr Nitika

Post Graduate Residents of Pathology
Dr Mega, Dr Suma, Dr Tapsya, Dr Vasundhra, Dr Komal, Dr Saurav, Dr Ajay, Dr Neha, Dr Namita, Dr Yashika, Dr Sweta, Dr Shruti, Dr Vikas, Dr Sakshi, Dr Manpreet, Dr Gurupriya, Dr Nitish, Dr Roomi, Dr Madhulika, Dr Deepshika, Dr Meena, Dr Ritesh, Dr Gurjeet, Dr Nidhi, Dr Bharti, Dr Vipul, Dr Lalit, Dr Aayushi, Dr Reeti, Dr Himadri, Dr Aardhna, Dr Sandeep, Dr Manish, Dr Raman Kapil

SHKM Govt Medical College, Nalhar
Principal
Dr Sansar Sharma

Professor and Head of Pathology
Dr Shivani Kalhan

Associate Professor of Pathology
Dr Pawan Singh Bodwal

BPS Govt Medical College, Khanpur, Sonepat
Associate Professor of Pathology
Dr Kulwant Singh

Post Graduate Resident of Pathology
Dr Kanika Makkar

ESIC Medical College, Faridabad
Assistant Professor of Pathology
Dr Nimisha Sharma

Maharishi Markandeshwar University, Mullana, Ambala
Professors of Pathology
Dr Sanjay Bedi, Dr Prem Singh Madhan

Shanti Diagnostic Center, Faridabad
Managing Director
Dr Satya Pal Jayant

Maharishi Dayanand University, Rohtak
Professor and Head of Music Department
Dr (Mrs) Vimal Dinesh

Himachal Pradesh
Indira Gandhi Medical College, Simla
Professor and Head of Pathology
Dr Vijay Kaushal

Professor of Pathology
Dr Kavita Mardi

Maharishi Markandeshwar University, Solan
Professor and Head of Pathology
Dr Manohar Lal Gupta

Jammu & Kashmir
Govt Medical College, Jammu
Former Professor and Head of Pathology
Dr Yudhvir Gupta

Professor and Head of Pathology
Dr Kuldeep Kumar Kaul

Professors of Pathology
Dr Kuldeep Singh, Dr Subhash Bhardwaj, Dr Jyotsna Suri

Associate Professors of Pathology
Dr Surender Atri, Dr Ruchi Khajuria, Dr Deepti Mahajan, Dr Sindhu Sharma, Dr Rupali Bargotra

Lecturers of Pathology
Dr Deepa Hans, Dr Ameet Kaur, Dr Teepulsher, Dr Navneet Naaz

Senior Residents of Pathology
Dr Vidhu Mahajan, Dr Anu Gupta, Dr Mansi Sharma, Dr Deepti Gupta, Dr Akhtar Salaria, Dr Sunil Raina, Dr Sailja Kotwal, Dr Gousia Rather, Dr Poonam Sharma, Dr Virender Rana, Dr Ritu Bhagat, Dr Megha Sharma, Dr Sharoly Singh, Dr Bahrti Thaker, Dr Jagriti, Dr Suby Singh

Post Graduate Residents of Pathology
Dr Neha Bharti, Dr Chiterlekha Bhasin, Dr Anu Mangoch, Dr Sonia Nagyal, Dr Bhavneet Kour, Dr Priyanka, Dr Navkiran Kaur, Dr Anjali Saini, Dr Shelly Singh, Dr Isha Sharma, Dr Sunali Gupta, Dr Shweta Bhagat, Dr Usha Kiran, Dr Monika Pangotra, Dr Shabnam Sarfaraz, Dr Sovia Anand, Dr Madhubala, Dr Aashna Gupta, Dr Sonika Rukhwal, Dr Chhavi Gupta, Dr Himanshu Rana, Dr Abhishek Dogra, Dr Faiza Hafiz, Dr Wasim-Ul-Shafi, Dr Shazia Khatana, Dr Saba Mustaq, Dr Faisal Bashir, Dr Rashmi Aithmia

Govt Medical College, Srinagar
Professor and Head of Pathology
Dr Ruby Reshi

Professor of Pathology
Dr Riyaz Ahmad Tasleem

Associate Professors of Pathology
Dr Bilal Sheikh, Dr Lateef A Wani, Dr Mehnaaz Sultan

Assistant Professors of Pathology
Dr Salma Bhat, Dr Sheema Sheikh, Dr Shazia Handoo

Lecturers of Pathology
Dr Adil Sidique, Dr Nusrat Baseer

Assistant Surgeons of Pathology
Dr Ruksana, Dr Nazia Quyoom, Dr Bilal Banday

Demonstrators of Pathology
Dr Summiya, Dr Baba Iqbal Khaliq, Dr S Imtiyaz, Dr Jibrna, Dr Suhail, Dr Nusart Ali, Dr Manzoor, Dr Shaheen, Dr Irfan

Post Graduate Residents of Pathology
Dr Farooq, Dr Aijaz Amin, Dr Farzana, Dr Arshi, Dr Saymah

Sher-I-Kashmir Institute of Medical Sciences, Srinagar
Former Professors and Heads of Pathology
Dr KM Baba, Dr Parveen Shah

Acknowledgments

Former Professors of Pathology
Dr Nassima Chanda, Dr GN Sofi

Additional Professor and Head of Pathology
Dr Syed Besina Yasin

Additional Professors of Pathology
Dr Rumana Makhdooni, Dr Mohd Iqbal Lone

Associate Professor of Pathology
Dr Zubaida Rasool

Senior Residents of Pathology
Dr Danish Khan, Dr Tazeen Jeelani, Dr Suhail Mushtaq, Dr Nuzhat Samoon, Dr Sumat Khursheed, Dr Imza Feroz, Dr Ozma Masoodi, Dr Duri Mateen, Dr Huzaifa Tak, Dr Nazia Bhat, Dr Naheena Bashir, Dr Mir Wajahat

Post Graduate Residents of Pathology
Dr Shaziya Ashraf, Dr Farhat Abbas, Dr Sagir Akhtar, Dr Zarka Nabi, Dr Faizan Mir, Dr Salma Gull, Dr Prabhleen Kaur, Dr Nazia Tabassum, Dr Majid Khan, Dr Salma Yaseen, Dr Ishrat Younis, Dr Muneera Gul, Dr Asima Aijaz, Dr Mehak Shafat, Dr Subuh Parvez Khan, Dr Fiza Parvez khan, Dr Barqul Afaq, Dr Showkat Ahmed, Dr Shazieya Akhtar, Dr Noor Jahan

Former Post Graduate Residents of Pathology
Dr Sumaira Qadri, Dr Iram Naaz

SKIMS Medical College, Srinagar
Professor and Head of Pathology
Dr Rasheed Khan

Associate Professors of Pathology
Dr Afiya Shafi, Dr JB Singh

Acharya Shri Chander College of Medical Sciences, Jammu
Professor and Head of Pathology
Dr Arvind Khajuria

Professor of Pathology
Dr KC Gosain

Associate Professor of Pathology
Dr Mahima Sharma

Assistant Professor of Pathology
Dr Nitin Gupta

Karnataka
Sri Devraj Urs Medical College, Kolar
Professor of Pathology
Dr CSBR Prasad

VIMS, Bellary
Post Graduate Resident of Pathology
Dr Prachi Singhal

Sapthagiri Institute of Medical Sciences, Bangalore
Executive Director
Mr GD Manoj

Professor and Head of Pathology
Dr Vijaya C

Associate Professors of Pathology
Dr Aparana Narasimha, Dr AH Nagarajappa, Dr Amoolya Bhat, Dr Arachana C Shetty

Assistant Professors of Pathology
Dr Smita S Massamatti, Dr Padma Priya Kasukurti, Dr Suraksha Rao B

Madhya Pradesh
Mahatma Gandhi Memorial Medical College, Indore
Professor and Head of Pathology
Dr CV Kulkarni

Bundelkhand Medical College, Sagar
Professor and Head of Pathology
Dr Bharat Jain

Index Medical College, Indore
Professor and Head of Pathology
Dr Shri Kant Nema

Professors of Pathology
Dr Sanjeev Narang, Dr Anil Kapoor, Dr Arjun Singh

Assistant Professors of Pathology
Dr Anjali Singh, Dr Parul Dargar, Dr Priyanka Sachdeva

Post Graduate Residents of Pathology
Dr Akanchha, Dr Harmeet Choudhary, Dr Radhika Rathi, Dr Randeep Kaur Bal, Dr Saniya Sharma, Dr Snehil Agrawal, Dr Somendra Dhariwal, Dr Surekha Sharma, Dr Aditya Tignath, Dr Apurrva Malhotra, Dr Awani Jain, Dr Himani, Dr Jai Singh, Dr Neelambara Bidwai, Dr Rahul Krode, Dr Shahar Bano Khan, Dr Vikas Mishra, Dr Atul Partap Singh, Dr Prachi Mehla, Dr Priya Roy, Dr Pulkit, Dr Rajesh, Dr Ranu Yadav, Dr Rohit Sangtani, Dr Shipra Yadav, Dr Vinitha Jose

All India Institute of Medical Sciences, Bhopal
Professor and Head of Pathology
Dr Neelkamal Kapur

Assistant Professor of Pathology
Dr Garima Goyal

Netaji Subhash Chandra Bose Medical College, Jabalpur
Post Graduate Resident of Pathology
Dr Amita Gupta

Sri Aurobindo Institute of Medical Sciences, Indore
Post Graduate Resident of Pathology
Dr Priyanka Kiyawat Jain

Maharashtra
Seth GS Medical College and KEM Hospital, Mumbai
Associate Professor of Pathology
Dr Rachna Chaturvedi

Post Graduate Resident of Pathology
Dr Pranav Patwardhan

Grant Medical College and Sir JJ Group of Hospitals, Mumbai
Associate Professor of Pathology
Dr Kalpana Anand Deshpande

Tata Memorial Hospital, Mumbai
Associate Professor of Pathology
Dr Asawari Patil

Dr DY Patil Medical College, Navi Mumbai
Medical Director and Trustee
Dr Priya Darshini

Mahatma Gandhi Mission Medical College, Navi Mumbai
Dean
Dr GS Narshetty

Professor and Head of Pathology
Dr Rita Dhar

Professors of Pathology
Dr Ujwala Maheshwari, Dr BD Bolker

Alumni of the Institution
Dr Akshun Kalia, Dr Anubhav, Dr Harman Preet Chinna, Dr Manan Dave, Dr Amit Sharma, Dr Anurag Tiwary, Dr Saurabh Kumar

Mahatma Gandhi Mission Medical College, Aurangabad
Professor and Head of Pathology
Dr Bhale

Professor of Pathology
Dr Smita Mulay

Dr DY Patil Medical College, Pune
Former Vice Chancellor
Dr Amarjit Singh

Dean
Dr Jitender Bhowalkar

Professor and Head of Pathology
Dr Harsh Kumar

Professors of Pathology
Dr SS Chandanwale, Dr Charusheela Gore, Dr Archna Buch, Dr Pagaro Pradhan

Associate Professors of Pathology
Dr Rupali Bavikar, Dr Shruti Vimal, Dr Arpana Dharwadkar, Dr Tushar Kamble, Dr Iqbal Banymme

Lecturers of Pathology
Dr Vidya Vishvanathan, Dr Sushama Kulkarni, Dr Yamini Ingale, Dr Shubhangi Tayade, Dr Yogesh Tayade, Dr Dadaso Baravkar

Demonstrators of Pathology
Dr Anjali Deshpande, Dr WC Raut, Dr AJ Nagarkar, Dr Monali Kadam, Dr Kamini Masul, Dr Sharad Pole

Post Graduate Resident of Surgery
Dr Mansi Dhende

Post Graduate Resident of Pediatrics
Dr Udit Sihag

Alumnus of Ophthalmology
Dr Spriha Arun

Bhartiya Vidyapeeth Medical College, Pune
Principal
Dr Vivek Saoji

Professor and Head of Pathology
Dr NS Mani

Professors of Pathology
Dr Manjiri Karandikar, Dr Ravinder C Nimbargi

Krishna Institute of Medical Sciences, Krar
Former Professor and Head of Pathology
Dr Sushma Desai

Medical Superintendent of Krishna Hospital
Dr Ashok Yadavrao Kshirsagar

Professor and Head of Pathology
Dr Sujata Kanetkar

Professor of Pathology
Dr Jyotsna Wadar

Assistant Professor of Pathology
Dr Dhiraj Shukla

MPV Vasantrao Medical College, Nasik
Professor and Head of Pathology
Dr Preeti Bajaj

ESI Post Graduate Institute of Medical Sciences, Mumbai
Professor and Head of Pathology
Dr Madhuri Kate

Odisha

Kalinga Institute of Medical Sciences, Bhubaneshwar
Professor and Head of Pathology
Dr Urmila Senapati

Professors of Pathology
Dr Jayasree Rath, Dr Kanakalata Dash, Dr Amit Kumar Adhya

Associate Professors of Pathology
Dr Ranjita Panigrahi, Dr Ranjana Giri

Assistant Professors of Pathology
Dr Sarojini Raman, Dr Nageshwar Sahu, Dr Pranati Misra, Dr Prajna Das, Dr Madhusmita Mohanty, Dr Rajni Sharma, Dr Prita Pradhan

Post Graduate Residents of Pathology
Dr Soma Pradhan, Dr Malvika Mgadhi, Dr Monideepa Chattopadhyay, Dr Rituparna Ghosh, Dr Sandhya Biswal, Dr Chinmayee Panigrahi, Dr Pallavi Mishra

MKCG Medical College and Hospital, Berhampur
Post Graduate Residents of Pathology
Dr Chandan Bajad, Dr Kamal Kant

Pondicherry

JIPMER, Pondicherry
Professors of Pathology
Dr Bhawana Ashok Badhe, Dr Debdatta Basu, Dr N Siddaraju, Dr Surendra Kumar Verma, Dr Rakhee Kar

Aarpaddai Veedu Medical College, Kirumampakkam
Assistant Professor of Pathology
Dr Ashu Singh

Punjab

Govt Medical College, Amritsar
Former Professor and Head of Pathology
Dr SK Kahlon

Professor and Head of Pathology
Dr Surender Pal

Professors of Pathology
Dr Amarjit Singh, Dr Kuldeep Singh Chahal

Associate Professors of Pathology
Dr Vijay Mehra, Dr Permeet Kaur Bagga

Acknowledgments

Assistant Professors of Pathology
Dr Jagdeep, Dr Ram Krishan Sharma, Dr Navjot Kaur, Dr Mandeep Randhawa, Dr Jaspreet Singh

Senior Residents of Pathology
Dr Poonam Katru, Dr Harkirat Kaur, Dr Sofia, Dr Neeraj Bisht, Dr Rekha, Dr Sanjeev Kohli, Dr Vinay Sharma, Dr Hardeep Sethi, Dr Jagpal Kaur

Post Graduate Residents of Pathology
Dr Sonal Aggarwal, Dr Swati Sharma, Dr Navpreet Kaur, Dr Vrinda Aggarwal, Dr Moninder Kaur, Dr Krishma Goyal, Dr Gaurav, Dr Supreet Kaur, Dr Babita Rani, Dr Shweta Mahajan, Dr Utkarshni, Dr Gurpal Kaur, Dr Anamika Sharma, Dr Nidhima Aggarwal, Dr Megha Bansal, Dr Dikshi Aneja, Dr Neha Saini, Dr Kanika Wadhwa, Dr Saloni Saini, Dr Gurinderpal Kaur

Dayanand Medical College, Ludhiana
Former Professor and Head of Pathology
Dr Vinita Malhotra

Former Professor of Pathology
Dr BS Shah

Professor and Head of Pathology
Dr Neena Sood

Professor
Dr Harpreet Kaur

Christian Medical College, Ludhiana
Professors of Pathology
Dr Roma Issac, Dr Rupinder Kaur

Govt Medical College, Patiala
Professor and Head of Pathology
Dr Ramesh Kundal

Assistant Professor of Pathology
Dr Chetan Dass

Adesh Medical College, Bhatinda
Professor and Head of Pathology
Dr Vijay Suri

Senior Resident of Pathology
Dr Saumya Bhagat

Sri Guru Ramdas Medical College, Amritsar
Professor and Head of Pathology
Dr Mridu Manjiri

Associate Professor of Pathology
Dr Manisha Sharma

Assistant Professor of Pathology
Dr Neha Sharma

Punjab Institute of Medical Sciences, Jalandhar
Professor and Head of Pathology
Dr Usha Bandish

Port Blair Union Territory
Andaman and Nicobar Islands Institute of Medical Sciences, Port Blair
Assistant Professors of Pathology
Dr Jyotsna Nigam, Dr Jitender Nigam

Rajasthan
Geetanjali Medical College, Udaipur
Professor and Head of Pathology
Dr Narender Kumar Mogra

Assistant Professor of Pathology
Dr Tarang Patel

Pacific Medical College, Udaipur
Professor of Pathology
Dr SS Surana

Pacific Institute of Medical Sciences, Udaipur
Professor of Pathology and Medical Superintendent
Dr DR Mathur

RNT Medical College, Udaipur
Professor and Head of Pathology
Dr Sunita Bhargav

Post Graduate Resident of Pathology
Dr Pupul Bose

SMS Medical College, Jaipur
Professor and Head of Pathology
Dr Ajay Yadav

Associate Professor of Pathology
Dr Ranjana Solanki

Assistant Professor of Pathology
Dr Subhash Sharma, Dr Vidhi Sharma

Jawahar Lal Nehru Medical College, Ajmer
Professor and Head of Pathology
Dr Geeta Pachauri

Sardar Patel Medical College, Bikaner
Professor and Head of Pathology
Dr Neelu Gupta

Associate Professor of Biochemistry
Dr Anita Verma

SN Medical College, Jodhpur, Rajasthan
Professor of Pathology
Dr Ajay Malviya

Senior Resident of Pathology
Dr Praveen Verma

Medical College, Kota
Professor of Pathology
Dr Rajeev Saxena

National Institute of Medical Sciences, Jaipur
Professor of Pathology
Dr Vineet Choudhary

Mahatma Gandhi Medical College, Jaipur
Post Graduate Resident of Pathology
Dr Shubhi Saxena

All India Institute of Medical Sciences, Jodhpur
Senior Resident of Pathology
Dr Parul Gautam

Tamil Nadu

SRM Medical College, Kuttankuathur, Chennai
Professor and Head of Pathology
Dr John Jaison

Chettinad Medical College, Chennai
Assistant Professor of Pathology
Dr Devi Subbarayan

Telangana

Osmania Medical College, Hyderabad
Vice Principal-cum-Professor and Head of Pathology
Dr Ezhil Arasi N

Associate Professor of Pathology
Dr BS Nithyanand

Gandhi Medical College, Secunderabad
Professor and Head of Pathology
Dr O Sharvan Kumar

Bhaskar Medical College, Moinabad, Hyderabad
Principal-cum-Professor of Pathology
Dr Narsing Rao

Professor of Pathology
Dr Vijay Sreedhar

Govt Medical College, Mehboob Nagar
Associate Professor and Head of Pathology
Dr Devojee Nayak

Rajiv Gandhi Institute of Medical Sciences, Adilabad
Professor and Head of Pathology
Dr Chandra Shekhar

Mallareddy Women Institute of Medical Sciences, Surram, Hyderabad
Professor and Head of Pathology
Dr Jijiya Bai

Mallareddy Institute of Medical Sciences, Surram, Hyderabad
Professor and Head of Medicine
Dr EA Ashok Kumar

MNR Medical College, Fasalwadi
Professor and Head of Pathology
Dr Asoka RS Kumar

Shadan Institute of Medical Sciences, Perranchuru
Professor of Pathology
Dr Salma Mahajbeen

Kamineni Institute of Medical Sciences, Narkatpally
Professor and Head of Pathology
Dr V Sathyanarayana

Uttar Pradesh

SN Medical College, Agra
Professor and Head of Pathology
Dr Atul Gupta

King George Medical University, Lucknow
Professors of Pathology
Dr Suresh Babu, Dr Uma Shankar Singh

Assistant Professor of Pathology
Dr Chanchal Rana

MLN Medical College, Allahabad
Professor of Pathology
Dr Kachnar Varma

Post Graduate Resident of Pathology
Dr Faheema Hasan Younus

Rohilkhand Medical College, Bareilly
Professor and Head of Pathology
Dr Parbodh Kumar Kakkar

Professor
Dr Ranjan Aggarwal

Hind Institute of Medical Sciences, Safedabad
Assistant Professor of Pathology
Dr Sangita Tripathi

Sharda Medical College, Noida
Professor and Head of Pathology
Dr Geeta Desmukh

Muzaffarnagar Medical College, Muzaffarnagar
Professor
Dr Anupam Varshney

Uttarakhand

All India Institute of Medical Sciences, Rishikesh
Director
Padma Shree Dr Ravi Kant

Jolly Grant Medical College, Dehradun
Assistant Professor of Pathology
Dr Ankita Katara Pandey

All India Institute of Medical Sciences, Dehradun
Assistant Professor of Pathology
Dr Neha Singh

West Bengal

Vivekanand Institute of Medical Sciences, Kolkata
Professor and Head of Pathology
Dr Debashish Bandopadhyaya

Section III

Systemic Pathology

15. Blood Vessels
16. Heart
17. Nasal Cavity, Nasopharynx, Paranasal Sinuses, Ear, Larynx and Neck
18. Lung
19. Oral Cavity and Salivary Glands
20. Gastrointestinal Tract
21. Liver, Gallbladder and Exocrine Pancreas
22. Kidney and Ureter
23. Urinary Bladder and Male Reproductive System
24. Female Reproductive System
25. Breast
26. Endocrine System: Pancreas, Thyroid, Parathyroid, Adrenal and Pituitary Glands
27. Bones and Joints
28. Soft Tissue Tumors and Skeletal Myopathies
29. Skin
30. Nervous System

CHAPTER 15

Blood Vessels

Learning Objectives

ARTERIOSCLEROSIS
- Histological Variants

ATHEROSCLEROSIS

ANEURYSMS
- Atherosclerotic Aneurysms
- Syphilitic (Luteic) Aneurysms
- Dissecting Hematoma
- Berry Aneurysms
- Mycotic Aneurysms
- Aneurysm of Sinus of Valsalva
- Arteriovenous Fistula
- Capillary Microaneurysms

VASCULITIS
- Large Vessel Vasculitides
- Medium-sized Vasculitides
- Small Vessel Vasculitides

VEINS
- Varicose Veins
- Deep Vein Thrombosis
- Thoracic Vena Cava Syndrome

LYMPHATIC SYSTEM
- Acute Lymphangitis
- Lymphedema
- Chylous Effusion

TUMORS OF BLOOD VESSELS
- Benign Tumors
- Malignant Tumors

HYPERTENSION
- Determinants of Hypertension
- Essential (Primary) Hypertension
- Secondary Hypertension
- Vascular Changes in Benign Hypertension
- Vascular Changes in Malignant Hypertension
- Complications of Hypertension

ANATOMY AND PHYSIOLOGY

- Arterial system is composed of:
  - Large or elastic arteries (e.g. aorta, innominate arteries, subclavian arteries, origin of common carotid arteries and origin of pulmonary arteries).
  - Medium-sized/muscular arteries (e.g. radial artery, renal artery and mesenteric artery).
  - Small-sized arterioles <2 mm present within substance of tissues and organs (peripheral resistance vessels).
- Arterioles transport blood from heart, maintain blood pressure and regulate peripheral resistance through vasoconstriction and vasodilation.
- Capillaries participate in exchange of gases and nutrients between blood and interstitial tissue.
- Venules transport blood from capillary beds toward the heart.
- Vein is composed of tunica intima, thinner tunica media and tunica adventitia. Its lumen is larger than arteries. Veins participate in transport of blood from venules to the heart (Table 15.1).

Table 15.1: The structure and function of blood vessels

Blood vessel	Structure	Function
Artery	Tunica intima, thick tunica media and tunica adventitia	Transports blood from heart
	Contractility and elasticity	Maintenance of blood pressure
Arteriole	Tunica intima, tunica media and tunica adventitia	Transports blood from heart and maintenance of blood pressure
	Lumen smaller than artery	Regulation of peripheral resistance through vaso-constriction and vasodilation
Capillary	Microscopic size vessel with single-layered wall of endothelium	Exchange of gases and nutrients between blood and interstitial tissue
Venule	Tunica intima, tunica media and tunica adventitia and gradually enlarge as reaching near the heart	Transports blood from capillary beds toward the heart
Vein	Tunica intima, thinner tunica media and tunica adventitia with larger lumen than artery	Transports blood from venules to the heart
	Presence of valve aids in the unidirectional blood flow towards the heart	

ARTERIOSCLEROSIS

Arteriosclerosis is defined as thickening and loss of elasticity (hardening) of arterial walls. It is responsible for morbidity and mortality via narrowing and weakening of arteries. There are three variants of arteriosclerosis described as under.

HISTOLOGICAL VARIANTS

MONCKEBERG'S MEDIAL CALCIFIC SCLEROSIS

It is age-related clinically insignificant entity seen in >50 years of age. Calcium deposited in the media of arteries in a ring-like fashion resulting in stiff *pipe stem* arteries. Blood vessels are often palpable. These lesions can be demonstrated on radiological examination. This form of arteriosclerosis may coexist with atheromatous plaques, but it is distinct and unrelated to it (Fig. 15.1).

Blood Vessels Involved

It involves the media of medium-sized muscular arteries, i.e. *radial, ulnar, femoral and uterine arteries*. These calcific deposits do not encroach the lumen of blood vessels; hence blood supply to tissues is not impaired.

ARTERIOLOSCLEROSIS

Arteriolosclerosis is characterized by hyaline thickening or proliferative changes of small arteries and arterioles, especially in the kidneys. It is usually associated with diabetes mellitus, hypertension, or normotensive elderly persons.

In the kidneys, it is called **malignant nephrosclerosis** associated with malignant hypertension. Renal arterioles exhibit two patterns: hyperplastic arteriolosclerosis or fibrinoid necrosis, i.e. necrotizing arteriolitis.

Hyaline Arteriolosclerosis in Benign Hypertension

Hyaline arteriolosclerosis is characterized by hyaline thickening of arteriolar walls. Light microscopy reveals eosinophilic glassy appearance in hematoxylin and eosin sections (Fig. 15.2).

Mechanism

- The increased intraluminal pressure imposed on the arteriolar walls drives proteins into the vessel, which get deposited in the vessel wall and occlude

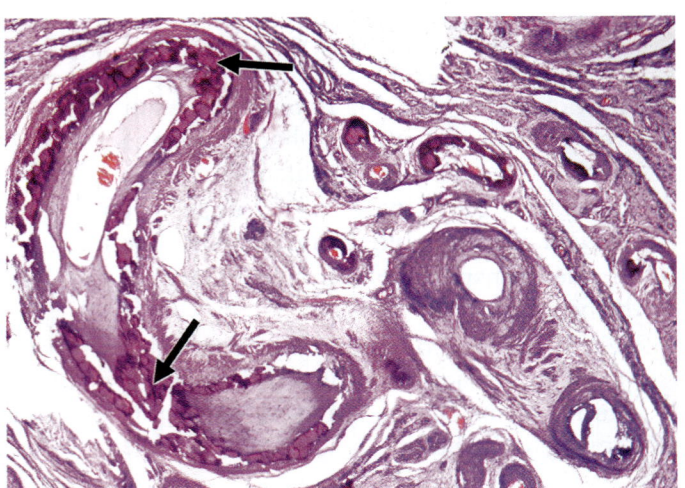

Fig. 15.1: Monckeberg calcific sclerosis (arrows).

Blood Vessels

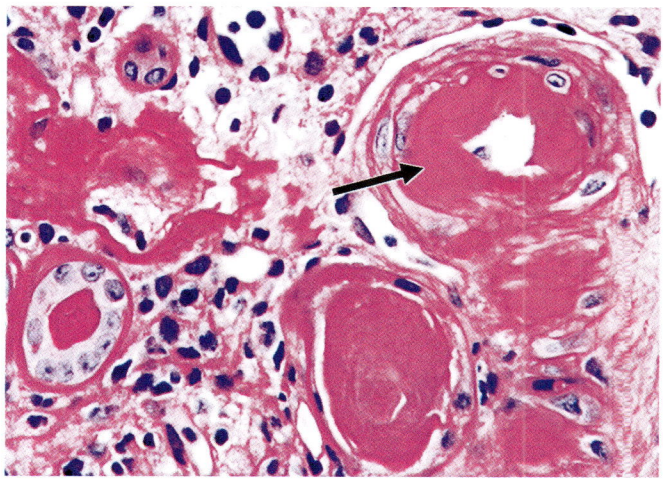

Fig. 15.2: Hyaline arteriolosclerosis (arrow) (400X).

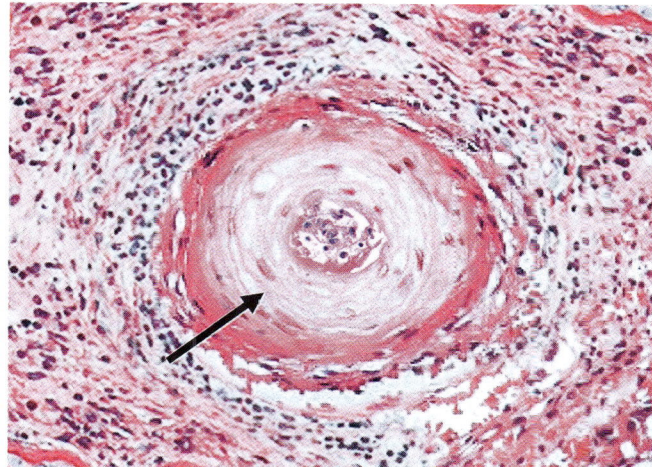

Fig. 15.3: Hyperplastic arteriolosclerosis—blood vessel shows proliferation of intimal and smooth muscle cells arranged in concentric laminated pattern exhibiting an *onion-skin* pattern (arrow) (400X).

the lumen. It leads to progressive loss of nephrons and renal atrophy.

- In *diabetes mellitus,* nonenzymatic glycosylation (glucose attached to amino acids) of the basement membrane of the vessels renders arterioles permeable to proteins.

Hyperplastic Arteriolitis in Malignant Hypertension

Hyperplastic arteriolitis is characterized by proliferation of intimal and smooth muscle cells arranged in concentric laminated pattern exhibiting an *onion-skin* pattern. There is subsequent marked narrowing of the lumen of arterioles. This change occurs in malignant hypertension and progressive systemic sclerosis. It may be accompanied by necrotizing arteriolitis (Fig. 15.3).

Fibrinoid Necrosis in Malignant Hypertension

Fibrinoid necrosis is most often associated with malignant hypertension, with diastolic blood pressure >120 mm Hg. It is characterized by *intramural deposition of fibrinoid material in arterioles with vascular necrosis and inflammation.* There may be focal hemorrhage. The lumen of the arterioles is narrow and fixed. The surrounding tissue may demonstrate focal ischemia or infarction. It leads to impairment of renal functions (Fig. 15.4).

ATHEROSCLEROSIS

Atherosclerosis is a progressive disease characterized by the formation of atheromatous plaques in the intima of large- and medium-sized blood vessels including abdominal aorta, proximal coronary arteries, carotid arteries, vertebral arteries, iliac arteries, anterior tibial and posterior tibial arteries.

It is most frequent cause of morbidity and mortality caused by vascular pathology across world. It is more common in males than in females.

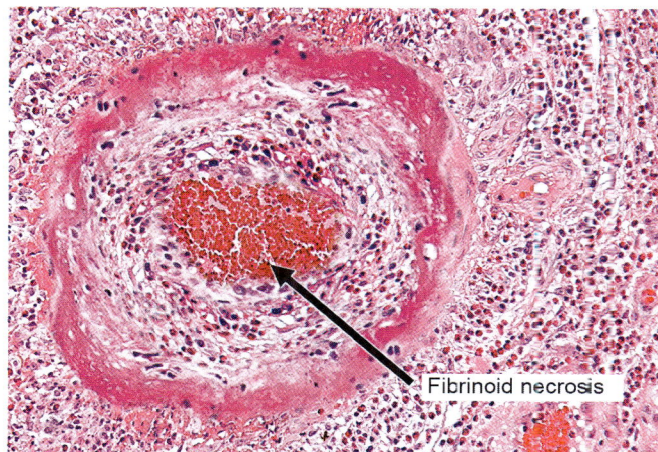

Fig. 15.4: Fibrinoid necrosis. Malignant hypertension leads to fibrinoid necrosis of small arteries as shown here. The damage to the arteries leads to formation of pink fibrin, hence the term *fibrinoid* (arrow) (400X).

Deaths from myocardial infarction (20–25% of all deaths) are mostly related to underlying atherosclerosis.

Evolution

During its evolution, it progresses from fatty streaks to atheromatous plaques resulting in various complications.

These include *narrowing or occlusion of blood vessels, dystrophic calcification, ulceration and rupture, thrombus formation, embolization, aneurysm formation and bleeding* in atheromatous plaque.

Fatty Streaks

Fatty streaks in coronary arteries may represent the initial precursor to atherosclerotic plaque. However, all fatty streaks are not precursor of atherosclerotic plaques. *Virtually these are present in aortas of children older than 10 years.* These do not cause any disturbance in blood flow.

> **Gross Morphology**
> Fatty streaks begin as multiple, minute yellow elongated slightly raised spots (1 cm long or more and 0.1 cm in diameter) in thoracic aortas of infants and younger children.
>
> **Light Microscopy**
> - Fatty streaks are characterized by *focal accumulation of lipid-laden foam cells in the intima.*
> - Lipoproteins bind to the constituents of the extracellular matrix, i.e. glycosaminoglycans (Fig. 15.5).

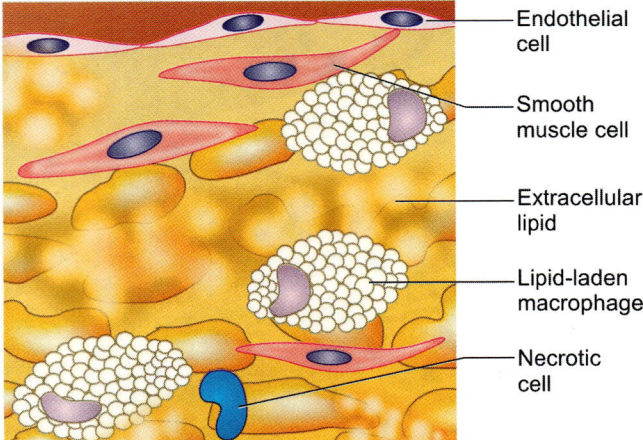

Fig. 15.5: Fatty streaks show macrophages laden with lipid.

ATHEROSCLEROSIS

GENERAL CONSIDERATIONS

Atherosclerosis means hardening (sclerosis) or loss of elasticity of large elastic arteries and medium-sized arteries due to atheromatous plaque formation. These lesions are usually eccentric lesions due to vascular hemodynamic stress at branching points and posterior wall of aorta susceptible to atheromatous plaque.

Locations

Atheromatous plaques affecting blood vessels in decreased frequency are described as under:
- Large elastic arteries (abdominal aorta, carotids, iliac).
- Large- to medium-sized muscular arteries (coronary, popliteal, anterior tibial, posterior tibial, ostea of mesenteric and renal arteries, circle of Willis) (Fig. 15.6).

Vessels Spared

Internal mammary arteries and upper extremities are spared. That is the reason that internal mammary arteries are used as graft in coronary bypass surgery.

Critical Areas

Critical areas of atheromatous plaque formation in arteries of various organs include brain, heart, kidneys, abdominal aorta, lower limb and intestine described as under (Table 15.2):

- *Brain:* Chronic ischemia leads to mental deterioration. Acute occlusion results in cerebral infarction. Rupture of atheromatous plaque leads to cerebral hemorrhage.
- *Coronary arteries:* Involvement of coronary arteries due to atheromatous plaques may cause clinical manifestations. Intermittent ischemia causes angina

Table 15.2: Critical areas of atheromatous plaques

Organs	Site of atheromatous plaque	Clinical manifestations
Brain	Chronic ischemia of cerebral vessels	Mental deterioration and syncope
	Acute occlusion	Cerebral infarct or rupture
Coronary arteries	Intermittent ischemia	Angina pectoris
	Acute occlusion	Myocardial infarction
	Chronic ischemia	Myocardial fibrosis
Kidneys	Extrarenal stenosis	Hypertension
	Intrarenal atherosclerosis	Hypertension and uremia
Abdominal aorta	Aneurysm just below renal vessels	Pressure symptoms
	Rupture of aortic aneurysm	Double barrel aorta, hemopericardium and bleeding in thorax
Peripheral blood vessels	Stenosis	Ischemia leads to leg gangrene
Mesenteric arteries	Occlusion	Gangrene gut; ischemic bowel disease

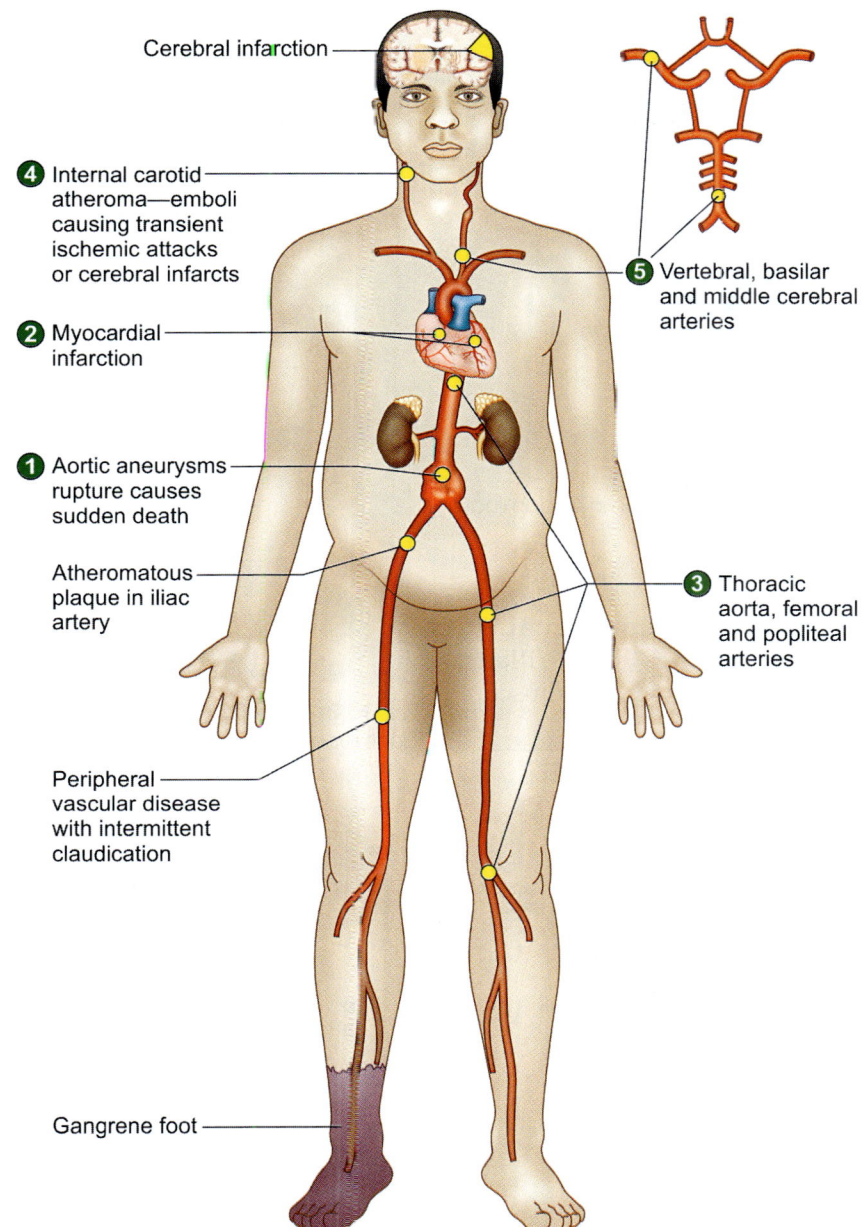

Fig. 15.6: Atheromatous plaques. Locations in order of frequency and clinical manifestations.

pectoris. Acute occlusion leads to myocardial infarction. Chronic ischemia results in myocardial fibrosis.
- *Renal vessels:* Atherosclerotic plaques in renal arteries cause hypertension. Atheromatous plaques in branches of renal blood vessels within renal substance lead to hypertension and uremia.
- *Abdominal aorta:* Atherosclerotic plaques in abdominal aorta cause aneurysm resulting in rupture.
- *Peripheral vessels in leg:* Atherosclerotic plaques in blood vessels supplying lower limb resulting in gangrene.
- *Mesenteric vessels:* Atherosclerotic plaques in blood vessels supplying intestine cause gangrene gut.

Gross Morphology

Atheromatous lesion begins as an elevated white to yellowish fibrous or fibrofatty patchy lesion in intima (0.3–1.5 cm to large in size) protruding toward lumina (Figs 15.7 and 15.8).

Light Microscopy

The fibrous cap separates the lumen from the central necrotic core of atheromatous plaque. Peripheral portion of lesion near normal intima is known as *shoulder* (Fig. 15.9).

Atheromatous
plaques

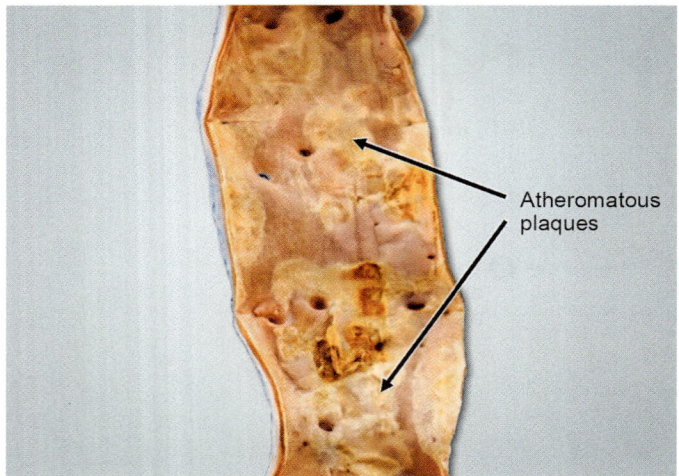

Fig. 15.7: Atheromatous plaques. These are shown in abdominal aorta (arrows).

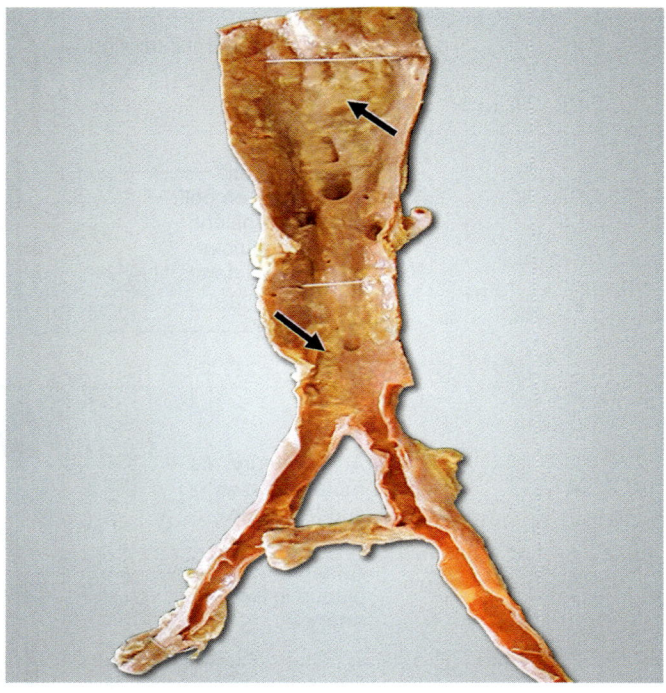

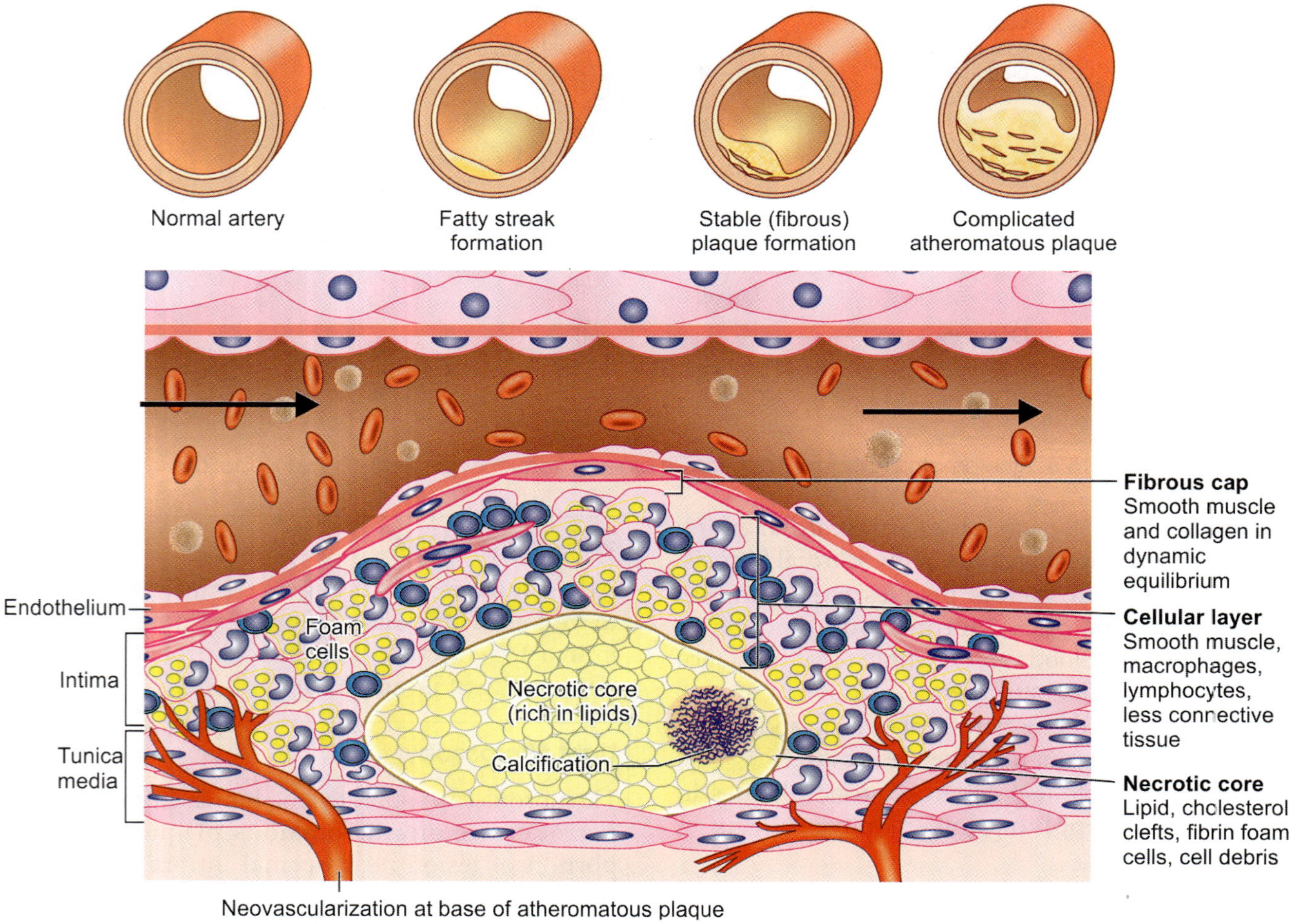

- *Central core:* Atheromatous plaque contains cholesterol and cholesterol esters, lipid-filled macrophages (foam cells), necrotic smooth muscle cell debris and calcium.

Fig. 15.8: Atheromatous plaques. These are shown in abdominal aorta and iliac arteries (arrows).

Normal artery
Fatty streak formation
Stable (fibrous) plaque formation
Complicated atheromatous plaque
Fibrous cap
Smooth muscle and collagen in dynamic equilibrium
Cellular layer
Smooth muscle, macrophages, lymphocytes, less connective tissue
Necrotic core
Lipid, cholesterol clefts, fibrin foam cells, cell debris
Endothelium
Intima
Tunica media
Foam cells
Necrotic core (rich in lipids)
Calcification
Neovascularization at base of atheromatous plaque

Fig. 15.9: Key components of atheromatous plaque. It consists of central lipid core and fibrous cap.

- *Fibrous cap:* Central necrotic core of atheromatous plaque is covered by a subendothelial fibrous cap. It is composed of smooth muscle cells, foam cells, fibrin, and extracellular matrix materials, such as collagen, elastin, glycosaminoglycans, and proteoglycans. Endothelium over the surface of the fibrous cap frequently appears intact. Shoulder of fibrous cap reveals presence of macrophages, T cells and smooth muscle cells.

Organisms in Atheromatous Plaque

Various organisms (e.g. *Chlamydia pneumoniae, herpesvirus, cytomegalovirus, Helicobacter pylori*) in atheromatous plaques have been demonstrated by immunocytochemistry. The organisms may play a role in development of atherosclerosis by initiating and enhancing the inflammatory response.

COMPLICATIONS

As the advanced atheromatous plaque increases in size, it produces significant morbidity and mortality. Patients become symptomatic, if vessels consisting of atherosclerotic plaque encroach on the lumen of the artery occluding >75% of lumen. Complications of atheromatous plaque are described as under (Fig. 15.10).

Narrowing or Occlusion

Atheromatous plaque causes narrowing/occlusion of lumen leading to organ ischemia.

Dystrophic Calcification

The atheromatous plaques get calcified (dystrophic calcification) and the affected blood vessels become hard. Due to vasospasm, the lesion may rupture.

Bleeding in AS Plaque

Newly formed blood vessels in atherosclerotic plaque may rupture and cause sudden enlargement of atheromatous plaque leading to organ infarction.

Ulceration and Rupture

Ulceration of atheroma induces thrombus formation. Cracking, ulceration, rupture usually occurs at the edge of intima of atheromatous plaque. Entry of blood through ulcerated site causes sudden acute enlargement of atheromatous plaque leads to occlusion of lumen and organ infarction.

Thrombus Formation

Turbulent blood flow and ulceration of atheromatous plaque exposes subendothelial connective tissue resulting in platelets aggregation and thrombus formation. Thrombotic occlusion may manifest as myocardial infarction (coronaries), cerebral stroke (internal carotid and middle cerebral artery), or gangrene of intestinal loops or lower extremities (popliteal, anterior and posterior tibial arteries).

Embolization

Emboli of atheromatous plaque material to distant sites may result in infarction (spleen, kidney, small intestine).

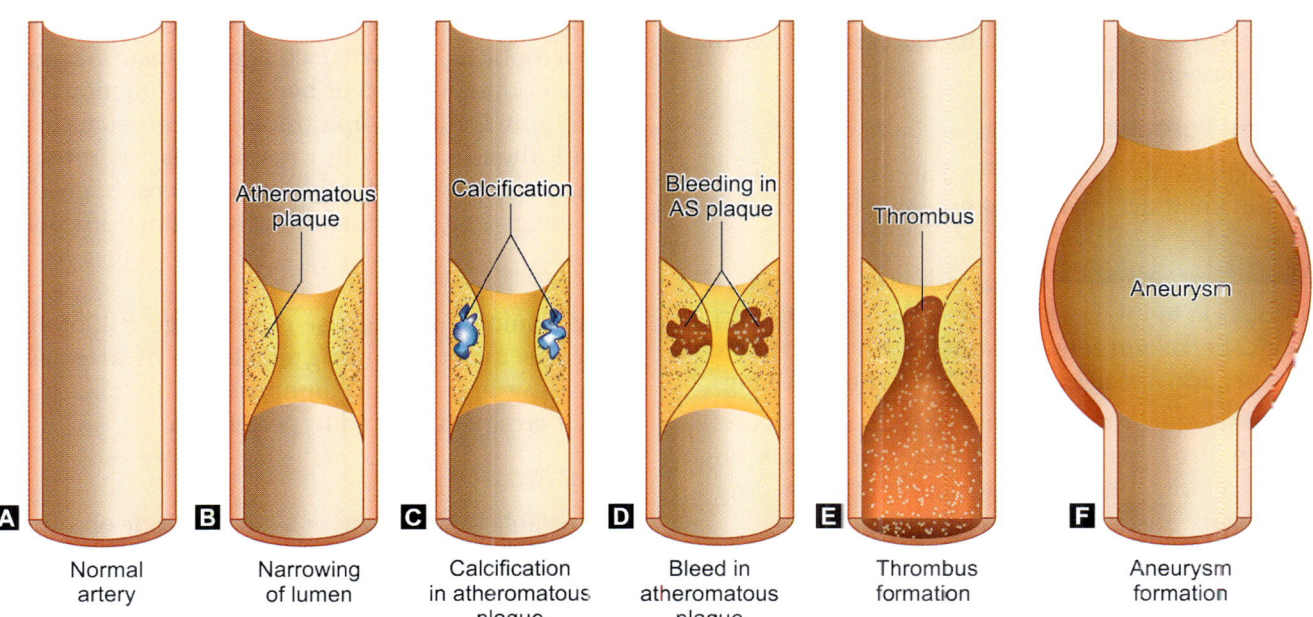

Fig. 15.10: Complications of atheromatous plaque. These are narrowing of lumen, calcification, bleeding, thrombus formation and aneurysm.

Aneurysm Formation

- Encroachment by atheromatous plaque weakens vessel wall of abdominal aorta, which undergoes aneurysm and rupture.
- The shapes of aneurysms may be saccular, fusiform or cylindrical. The patient presents with mass abdomen, pressure symptoms, rupture in cavities, and thromboembolism.
- The aneurysms may be demonstrated by ultrasonography and MRI.

CLINICAL MANIFESTATIONS

Major complications resulting from ischemia due to atherosclerosis include myocardial infarction leading to heart attack and cerebral infarction leading to strokes. Less common complications include peripheral vascular disease, aneurysmal dilatation due to weakened arterial wall, chronic ischemic heart disease, ischemic encephalopathy and ischaemic bowel disease.

Angina and Acute Myocardial Infarction

Atheromatous plaque in coronary arteries may cause angina, acute myocardial infarction and cardiac failure. Patients become symptomatic if atherosclerotic plaque involves >75% of vessel lumen.

Cerebral Vascular Disease (Cerebral Strokes)

Cerebral vascular disease refers to diseased arteries in the brain. Partial blockage may result in temporary reductions of blood supply to a part of the brain (transient ischemic attack). A complete loss of blood supply to an area of the brain due to clogging or breaking of a blood vessel results in a cerebral vascular accident (cerebral stroke).

Peripheral Vascular Disease

Atheromatous plaque in popliteal arteries, anterior and posterior tibial arteries develops peripheral vascular disease.

- *Partial or complete blockage* adversely affects the circulation to lower extremities. Patient with partial blockage of vessels presents with intermittent claudication (cramps, pain in legs when walking).
- *Complete vessel blockage* causes gangrene foot and is made worse in patient with diabetes mellitus through the development of diabetic neuropathy, leading to propensity for injury.

Aortic Aneurysms

Abdominal aortic atheromatous plaque may undergo aneurysms below the origin of renal arteries leading to rupture and sudden death.

Small Bowel Ischemia

Atheromatous plaques in superior mesenteric artery may cause small bowel infarction.

Hypertension

Atheromatous plaques in renal artery may cause renal ischemia. Patient may develop hypertension due to activation of renin-angiotensin-aldosterone system.

> **High Yield Facts—C-reactive Protein Analysis**
> - Estimation of C-reactive protein synthesized by liver is an important marker in inflammation and disrupted atheromatous plaque with superimposed thrombosis.
> - Its level is increased in patients with disrupted atheromatous plaque with superimposed thrombosis in acute myocardial infarction, cerebral stroke and peripheral vascular disease.

CATEGORIES OF RISK FACTORS

Modifiable Major Risk Factors

Major Risk Factors

- *These are hyperlipidemia* (familial/acquired), hypertension, diabetes mellitus and tobacco smoking. These cause chronic endothelial injury resulting in dysfunctional endothelium. It leads to increased vascular permeability to lipids and macrophages. Lipids modified by malondialdehyde enzyme get oxidized to form oxidized lipid molecule.
- Foam cells are formed due to accumulation of lipids in macrophages. Growth factors participate in migration of smooth muscle cells beneath dysfunctional endothelium. Oxidized lipid molecule causes necrosis of endothelium, smooth muscle cells, chemotaxis of macrophages and inhibition of macrophages. These changes lead to formation of atheromatous plaque.

Sedentary Lifestyle

Regular moderate exercise reduces the risk of atherosclerosis by maintaining elasticity of arteries and increasing high density lipoproteins, reduces the risk of diabetes mellitus and hypertension.

Minor Risk Factors

Less established minor risk factors include obesity, lack of exercise, 'type A' personality with stress factors in lifestyle, increased homocysteine level (>100 μmol/L), hyperuricemia, increased serum ferritin level, methylene tetrahydrofolate reductase mutation, lipoprotein A, hormonal replacement therapy in postmenopausal women, and infectious agents (*Chlamydia pneumoniae*, herpesvirus, and cytomegalovirus).

Non-modifiable Risk Factors

Genetic Factors

Hereditary genetic derangements of lipoprotein metabolism predispose the individuals to high blood lipid level and familial hypercholesterolemia. Genetic constitution of person is one of the factors of development of atherosclerosis.

Familial Predisposition

Coronary artery disease definitely runs in some families. A family history of premature coronary artery disease is a major risk factor.

Racial Factors

Blacks have less severe atherosclerosis than Whites.

Gender

Both men and women develop atheromatous plaques at the age of 45 in men and 55 in women. This reflects shift in hormones that occur after menopause. In premenopausal women, high levels of estrogens and high-density lipoproteins have probably anti-atherogenic influence.

Advancing Age

The incidence of development of atheromatous plaques rises with age, but it is not a disease exclusively in elderly. It begins in the young, but clinically significant lesions usually appear in 40s and beyond.

MAJOR RISK FACTORS

HYPERLIPIDEMIA

Hyperlipidemia (familial or acquired) is correlated with the early onset of atherosclerosis. It is characterized by excess levels of cholesterol, triglycerides, and lipoproteins in the blood. Lipoproteins act as *fat shuttles*, transporting cholesterol through the bloodstream (Figs 15.11 and 15.12).

Bad Cholesterol

LDL and IDL are bad cholesterol and directly related to the risk of atherosclerosis, which is the total cholesterol concentration.

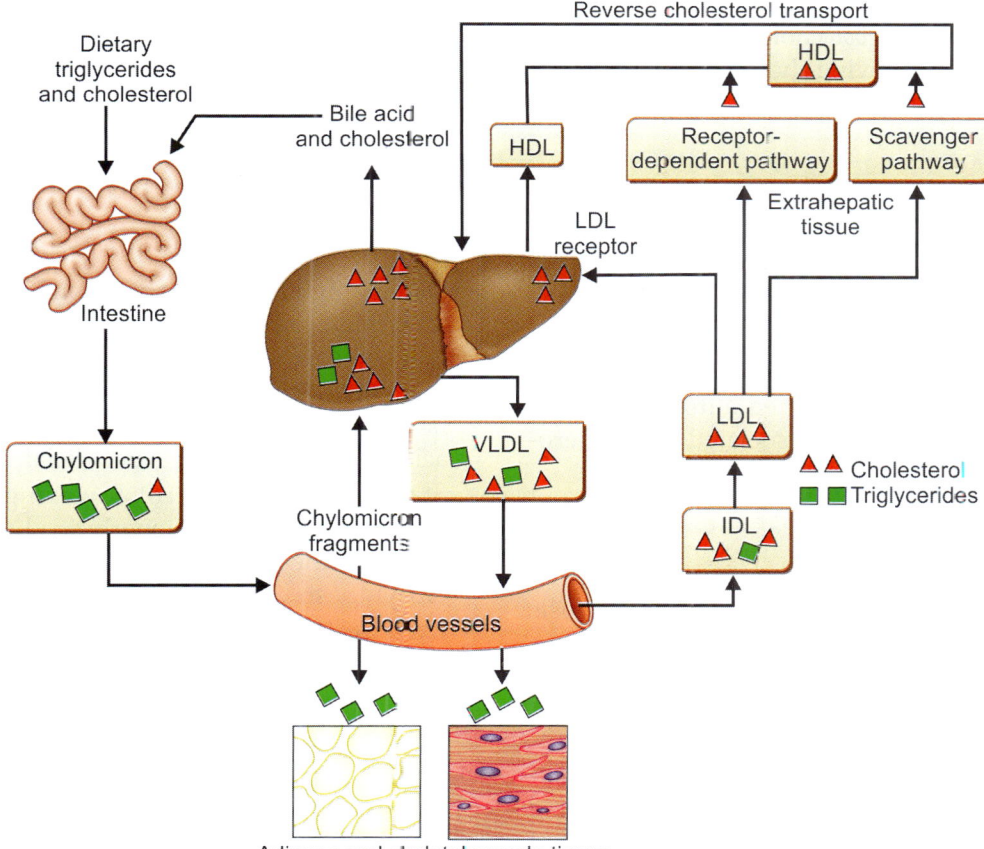

Fig. 15.11: Schematic representation of the exogenous and endogenous pathways for triglyceride and cholesterol transport. The relationship between circulating LDL, LDL receptors, and synthesis of cholesterol. Excess of cholesterol in the cell is esterified to cholesteryl esters and stored.

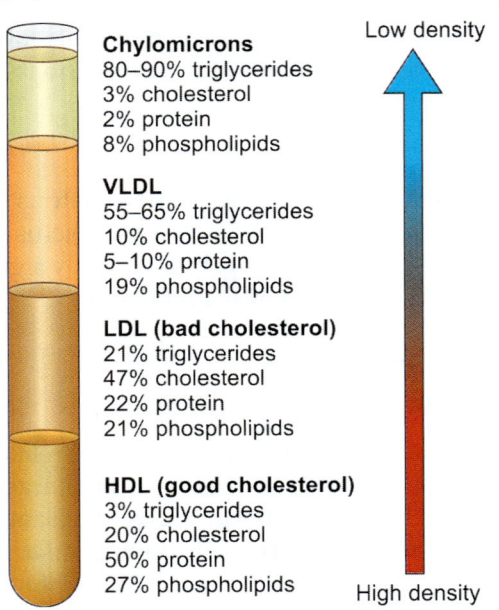

Fig. 15.12: Lipoproteins are named based on their protein content, which is measured in density. Lipoprotein includes HDL, LDL, VLDL and chylomicrons. Because fats are less dense than proteins, as the proportion of triglycerides decreases, the density increases.

Good Cholesterol

On the other hand, HDL is *good* cholesterol, which exerts its protective effect by removing cholesterol from tissues and from atherosclerotic plaques.

Clinical Correlation

Relative concentration of lipoprotein fractions are used as clinical predictors of atherosclerotic plaque formation. Ideally, the ratio between LDL and HDL cholesterol should be 4:1.

Familial Hyperlipidemia

Familial hyperlipidemia is inherited autosomal recessive or dominant trait disorder associated with atherosclerosis.

Physiological State

The LDL receptor is a cell surface glycoprotein that regulates plasma cholesterol by mediating endocytosis and recycling of apolipoprotein E. Capillary lipoprotein lipase participates in degradation of lipids.

Pathological State

- *Gene mutations of apolipoproteins, hepatic lipoprotein receptors and capillary lipoprotein lipase lead to hyperlipidemia.* It is due to defective assembly of lipid with apolipoproteins, defective internalization of lipids and degradation of lipids respectively.
- Lacking LDL receptor function, high levels of LDL in circulation, are taken up by tissue macrophages, and accumulate to form occlusive arterial plaques (atheromas) and papules or nodules of lipid-laden, foamy macrophages (xanthomas).

Acquired Hyperlipidemia

Dietary Factors

- Dietary fat (cholesterol and saturated fats) intake greater than 40% of total calories; saturated fat intake greater than 10% of total calories (egg, animal fat, milk and butter) adversely affect cholesterol profile.
- Saturated fatty acids in butter and animal fat consist of single bond with high melting point, hence more stable and deposited under skin.
- On the other hand, unsaturated fatty acids in ground nut consist of double bond with low melting point, hence less stable and not deposited under skin.

Diseases

Patients suffering from diabetes mellitus, nephrotic syndrome and hypothyroidism frequently have increased cholesterol, triglyceride and decreased HDL.

Obesity and Smoking

These decrease plasma HDL levels.

Progesterone Therapy

It increases plasma levels of LDL, cholesterol, and triglyceride and decreases HDL.

Lipids Lowering Agents

- Dietary regulation and administration of cholesterol-lowering drugs have beneficial effect on reducing the risk of ischemic heart disease.
- Low cholesterol and or higher ratio of polyunsaturated fats in diet lower blood cholesterol. Omega-3 fatty acid present in fish oil is beneficial.
- Statins are cholesterol lowering drugs. These inhibit hydroxymethoxyglutaryl CoA reductase, which is rate limiting enzyme in hepatic cholesterol biosynthesis.
- Exercise, loss of weight, ethanol intake, and estrogen increase HDL level.

HYPERTENSION

Uncontrolled hypertension is a major risk factor of premature atherosclerosis. Persistent high blood pressure causes chronic mechanical injury to the arterial endothelium resulting in atheromatous plaque formation in arteries.

DIABETES MELLITUS

Diabetes mellitus is associated with premature atherosclerosis. Atherosclerotic peripheral vascular occlusive disease, often leading to gangrene of the lower extremities, is common in diabetic patients.

Diagnostic Criteria

These include fasting blood sugar >126 mg/dl or random >200 mg/dl. Two-hour plasma glucose level after 75 gm glucose challenge is at or above 200 mg/dl. One of the preceding three criteria must be present on a subsequent day to confirm the diagnosis of diabetes mellitus.

Pathogenesis

Increased level of glucose combines with apolipoproteins and other proteins to form Schiff's base (reversible reaction). Schiff's base is converted to early glycosylated products [(amadori products), reversible reaction], and then advanced glycosylated end products (irreversible reaction). Advanced glycosylated end products act on macrophages, which synthesize chemotactic IL-1 and tumor necrosis factor.

- *Glycosylation:* It is a process that affects lipoproteins, circulating proteins and proteins component of the arterial wall.
- *Glycosylated collagen fibers:* Advanced glycosylated end products bind and trap LDL, which increase arterial wall stiffness, activate macrophages and stimulates lipoprotein adherence.
- *Glycosylated LDL:* It is less susceptible to oxidation and thus delivers cholesterol to blood vessels. It stimulates platelets aggregation and forms covalent bonds with the proteins of the arterial wall.
- *Glycosylated HDL:* It is rapidly degraded. It blocks cholesterol efflux from the cells.
- *Glycosylated proteins:* These bind to circulating immune complexes that will lead to other arterial lesions.

Glycosylated Hemoglobin (HbA1C)

Hemoglobin A1C is an indicator of long-term blood glucose control in diabetes mellitus. In the normal individual, about 3–6% of adult hemoglobin is glycosylated. The percentage of glycosylated hemoglobin is increased depending upon the degree of hyperglycemia. A value more than 6.5 is diagnostic of diabetes. It is directly related to the average concentration of glucose in the blood. Its estimation evaluates long-term glycemic control.

TOBACCO SMOKING

Tobacco smoking is associated with higher risk of atherosclerosis, ischemic heart disease and sudden cardiac death.

Pathogenesis

- *Endothelial dysfunction:* Tobacco smoking causes endothelial dysfunction.
- *Hyperlipidemia:* It causes deranged lipids, i.e. raised LDL due to decreased degradation in lysosomes and decreased HDL.
- *Platelet activation:* It causes increased platelet adhesiveness due to activation of platelets liberating ADP and TXA_2.
- *Nervous system stimulant:* Nicotine in tobacco smoke stimulates sympathetic nervous system resulting in vasoconstriction.
- *Vessel hypoxia:* Tobacco smoke causes arterial wall hypoxia due to accumulation of carbon monoxide in the blood.

THEORIES OF ATHEROSCLEROSIS

Lipid Insudation Hypothesis

Virchow in 1852 stated it is a low grade inflammation of blood vessel. Imbibing of lipids from the blood causes cellular proliferation of the intimal cells.

Encrustation (Thrombogenic) Hypothesis

Rokitansky in 1852 stated that incorporation of small thrombus results in atheromatous plaque formation.

Monoclonal Hypothesis

- It was proposed that atherosclerosis is a neoplastic lesion. Presence of only two forms of G6PD enzymes supported this monoclonal hypothesis.
- Exogenous injurious agents such as cigarette smoke or endogenous metabolites like lipoproteins or some viruses like herpesvirus cause mutations which result in monoclonal proliferation of smooth muscle cells in atherosclerosis.

Reaction to Injury Hypothesis

- Earlier known as *lipid theory* is now called *response to injury hypothesis* and is the most widely accepted theory. According to original theory described by the author in 1973, initial event is endothelial injury followed by smooth muscle cell proliferation in atherogenesis.
- Later in 1993, author modified the theory and described lipoprotein entry into the intima as the initial event followed by lipid accumulation in the

macrophages known as *foam cells*, which according to modified theory are the dominant cells in early lesions.
- LDL and monocytes entering beneath dysfunctional endothelium play key role in formation of atheromatous plaques.
- There is increased adhesion of monocytes, T cells and platelets on dysfunctional endothelium. These cells release cytokines, which cause migration and proliferation of smooth muscle cells followed by recruitment of lipid into the atherosclerotic plaque.

Evolution of Atheromatous Plaque

- *Major components of atheromatous plaques include:* (i) Cells (smooth muscle cells, WBCs), (ii) ECM (collagen, elastin, and proteoglycans), and (iii) accumulation of cholesterol in macrophages.
- The fibrous atheromatous plaque is the basic lesion of clinical atherosclerosis. It is characterized by the accumulation of intracellular and extracellular lipids, proliferation of vascular smooth muscle cells, and formation of scar tissue.

PATHOGENESIS

CHRONIC ENDOTHELIAL INJURY

Etiology

Hyperlipidemia, hypertension, diabetes mellitus, cigarette smoking, increased serum homocysteine, hemodynamic disturbances (ostea, branching points and posterior wall of abdominal aorta), immune complexes, toxins, infectious agents cause chronic endothelial injury of large elastic and muscular arteries. Injured endothelium becomes dysfunctional, which is now more permeable to lipoproteins and monocytes (Fig. 15.13).

Role of Hyperlipidemia

- Hyperlipidemia may initiate endothelial injury, promote foam cell formation, act as a chemotactic factor for monocytes, inhibit macrophage motility, or injure smooth muscle cells. Hyperlipidemia can directly impair endothelial cell function by following mechanisms.
- Lipids increase local production of reactive oxygen species, which decays nitrous oxide, the vasodilator synthesized by endothelium. These increase local shear stress.

These increase endothelial permeability to LDL and monocytes. These enhance expression of adhesive molecules on dysfunctional endothelium. Dysfunctional endothelium has thrombotic potential.

ADHERENCE OF BLOOD CELLS TO DYSFUNCTIONAL ENDOTHELIUM

Circulating monocytes, T cells and platelets migrate from central column of blood and then adhere to the dysfunctional endothelium via adhesive molecules such as VCAM-I, ICAM and selectins (E and P selectins). Expression of these adhesion molecules is enhanced by cytokines synthesized by macrophages, lymphocytes and endothelium.

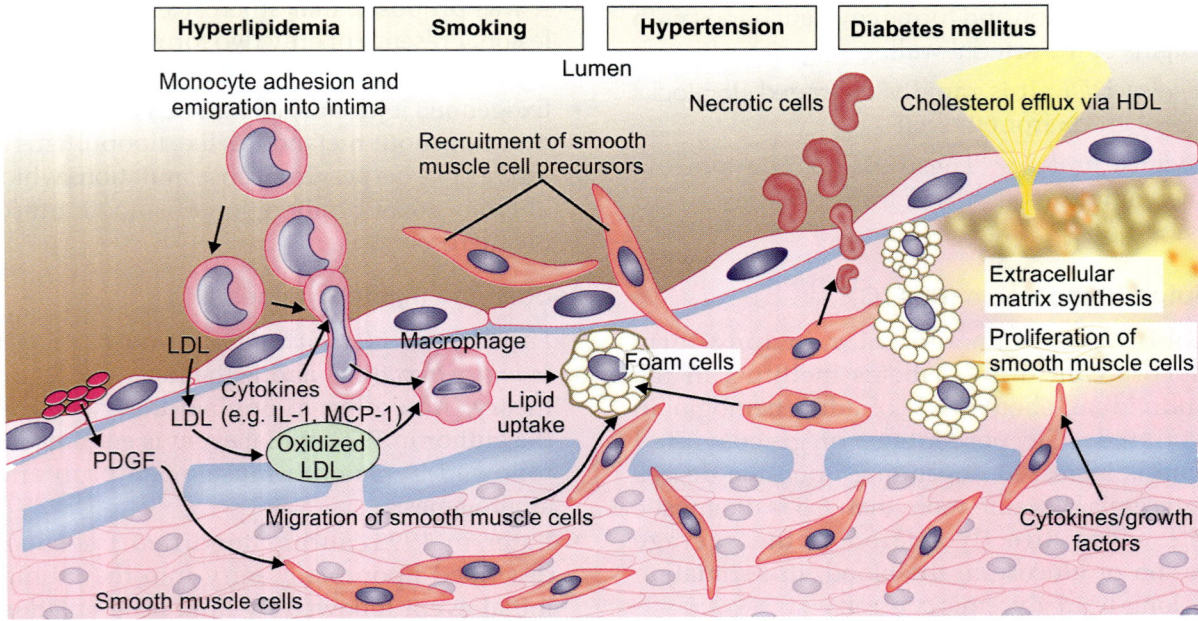

Fig. 15.13: Pathogenesis of atheromatous plaque.

INFLUX OF LDL AND MONOCYTES

Dysfunctional endothelium of vessel becomes permeable to LDL, monocytes (now called macrophages), and T cells, which enter beneath dysfunctional endothelium. Cytokines stimulate macrophages and endothelium to synthesize MCP-1 (monocytes chemoattractant-1), which participate in chemotaxis of monocytes.

ROLE OF GROWTH FACTORS

Source

- *Macrophages:* Activated macrophages synthesize platelet derived growth factor. These also synthesize IL-1, TNF-α and TGF-β, which act on smooth muscle cells and endothelial cells to synthesize platelet derived growth factor.
- *Smooth muscle cells:* These directly synthesize platelet derived growth factor, which has autocrine effect.
- *Platelets:* These synthesize PDGF, EGF, TGF-α, TXA_2 and thrombin. Thrombin stimulates protease activated receptors, which give signal for migration, proliferation of smooth muscle cells and extracellular production of matrix.
- *T cells:* These synthesize IL-1, IFN-γ, TNF-α and TGF-β (Fig. 15.14).

Mode of Action

- Growth factors such as *platelet derived growth factor, fibroblast growth factor, epidermal growth factor, and transforming growth factor-β* are released from platelets and perhaps also from monocytes.
- Smooth muscle cells also synthesize PDGF, which has autocrine effect. Simultaneously, there is decreased synthesis of growth inhibitors such as heparin and TGF-α synthesized by T cells and endothelium.
- These growth factors (PDGF, FGF, EGF, and TGF-β) induce proliferation and migration of smooth muscle cells into the intima, with the production of connective tissue matrix proteins (collagen, elastin, glycosaminoglycans, and proteoglycans).

ROLE OF CYTOKINES

IL-1 and TNF-α

These increase the expression of adhesive molecules on dysfunctional endothelium. These stimulate the synthesis of growth factors, i.e. PDGF, EGF, TGF-α. These participate in proliferation, migration of smooth muscle cells, matrix proliferation and neovascularization in intima of atheromatous plaque.

IL-1, TNF-α, and IFN-γ

These activate macrophages, which synthesize metalloproteinases, resulting in degradation of collagen fibers in the atheromatous plaque.

MCP-1 and M-CSF

These participate in recruiting additional leukocytes, activating leukocytes in the media, resulting in recruitment and proliferation of smooth muscle cells.

ROLE OF OXIDIZED LDL MOLECULE

Monocytes and smooth muscle cells phagocytose lipid and contribute to the deposition of lipid into lesions.

Modification of LDL Molecule by Platelets

Platelets synthesize malondialdehyde, which converts LDL to modified LDL molecule in subintimal region. Plasma LDL on entry into the intima undergoes oxidation.

Synthesis of O_2 Reactive Species

Macrophages and dysfunctional endothelium synthesize O_2 reactive species, which converts LDL into toxic oxidized LDL molecules, potent enhancer of the atherosclerotic process.

Uptake of Oxidized LDL Molecules

- Monocytes express receptors such as β-VLDL receptor and scavenger receptor, which bind modified LDL. Lipid-laden macrophages are called *foam cells*. Smooth muscle cells also imbibe LDL.
- Lipid is accumulated in the intracellular as well as extracellular compartments.
- Accumulation of cholesterol in foam cells leads to mitochondrial dysfunction, apoptosis, and necrosis, with resultant release of cellular proteases, inflammatory cytokines, and prothrombotic molecules.

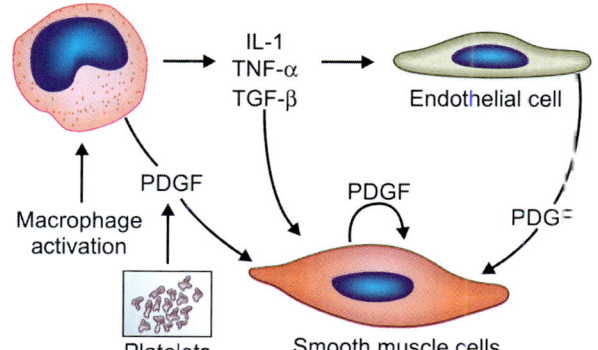

Fig. 15.14: Cellular interactions in the progression of atheromatous plaque that promotes proliferation of smooth muscle cells.

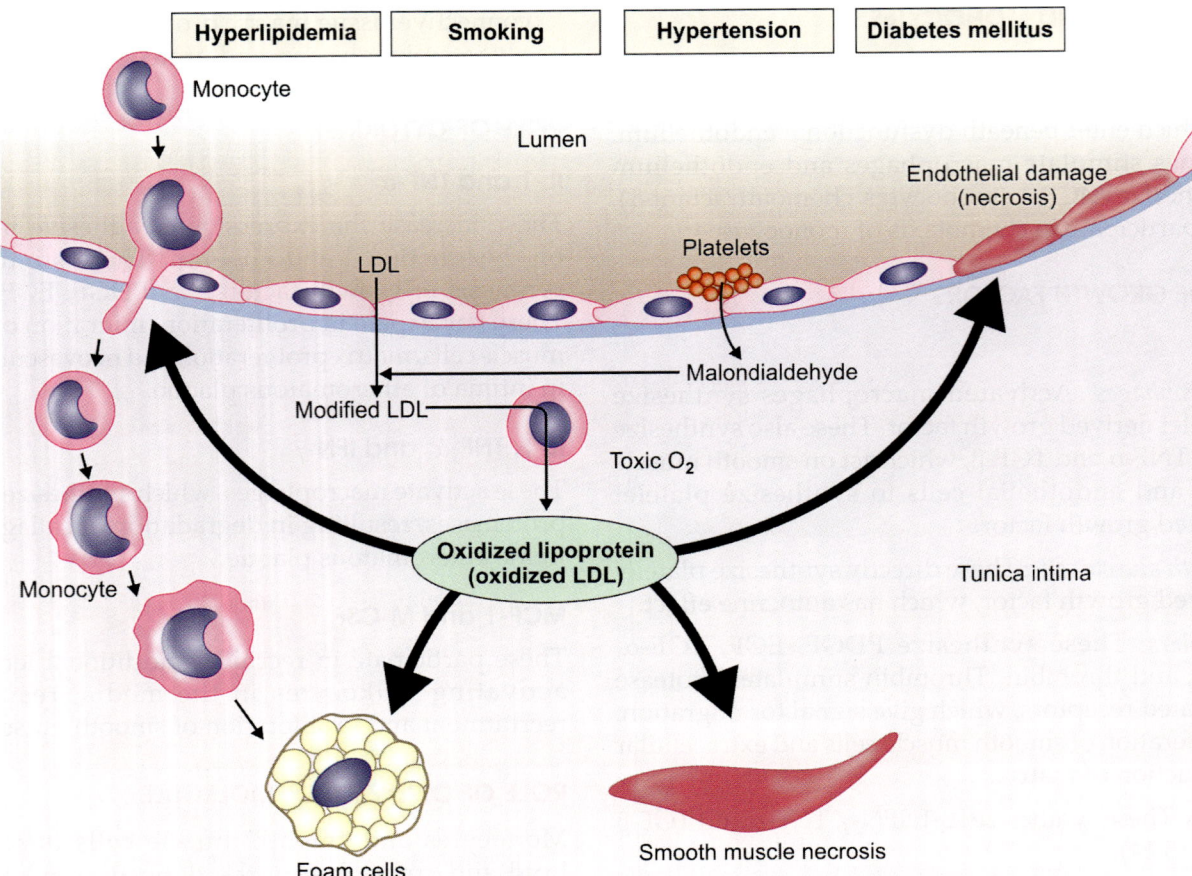

Fig. 15.15: Role of oxidized LDL molecule in the pathogenesis of atherosclerosis.

Toxic Effect of Oxidized LDL Molecule

- *Introduction:* Oxidized LDL molecule imbibed by macrophages (e.g. foam cells) and smooth muscle cells plays key role in formation of atheromatous plaque.
- *Necrosis of cells:* Oxidized LDL molecule causes necrosis of smooth muscle cells and endothelium. Lipids released from necrotic foam cells accumulate to form the lipid core of unstable plaques.
- *Chemotaxis:* It attracts additional macrophages with the help of monocyte-binding protein synthesized by endothelium. It is chemoattractant for smooth muscle cells from the media. Toxic LDL molecule inhibits migration of macrophages recruited (Fig. 15.15).

SYNTHESIS OF EXTRACELLULAR MATRIX

Smooth muscle cells release cytokines that produce extracellular matrix. Matrix components include collagen, proteoglycans and elastin. ECM subsequently produces fibrous plaques. Connective tissue synthesis determinates stiffness, calcium fixation and further enlargement of atheromatous plaque.

ROLE OF THROMBUS

Thrombin induces fibrin generation. It stimulates protease activated receptors, which give signal for migration, proliferation of smooth muscle cells and extracellular production of matrix.

THERAPEUTIC AGENTS

- Cholesterol management drugs include reductase inhibitors and bile sequestration drugs.
- Hypertension is controlled by antihypertensive drugs, including β-blockers, calcium channel blockers, angiotensin converting enzyme inhibitors. Anticoagulants including aspirin are used to prevent thrombus formation. Anti-angina drug nitroglycerine is administered in patients with coronary artery disease.

ANEURYSMS

Definition

Aneurysms are localized, abnormal permanent dilatation of cardiovascular tree that results from weakening of the wall of artery or vein. It can erode adjacent structures and cause pressure symptoms, pain, edema, rupture resulting in hypotensive shock and gangrene. Common sites of aneurysm are shown in Table 15.3.

Table 15.3: Most common site of aneurysms and their etiology

Site of aneurysm	Etiology
Ascending aorta	Hypertension, syphilis
Descending aorta especially below the origin of renal arteries	Atherosclerosis
Aortic arch of aorta	Atherosclerosis
Popliteal artery	Atherosclerosis

Aneurysm is more common in splenic artery than hepatic artery.

Classification

Aneurysms may be congenital or acquired. These may be true or false. False occurs due to trauma to intima and media. Aneurysms may take various shapes, i.e. saccular, fusiform, cylindrical, berry aneurysms, racemose/cirsoid (scalp), serpentine (torturous), arteriovenous fistula, and dissecting hematoma.

Shape

- *Saccular aneurysm:* These most often occur in abdominal or thoracic aorta. The aortic wall bulges like a rounded sac-like structure. It throbs and pushes against surrounding structures. Mural thrombus is most often found within aneurysmal sac of saccular aneurysm.
- *Fusiform aneurysm:* It is most common type of aortic aneurysm assuming round and more tubular shape. The aorta is widened like a sausage for a few inches.
- *Cylindrical aneurysm:* Aorta aneurysm assumes cylindrical shape due to atherosclerosis (Figs 15.16 and 15.17).
- *Berry aneurysm:* It is small aneurysm located in the arteries of brain.
- *Dissecting hematoma:* It is not a true aneurysm and least common, but most painful type of aortic damage. Increased blood pressure and weakened wall split the layers of the aorta between the tunica intima (innermost) and the tunica media (muscular layer). It is possible to have a dissecting hematoma of aorta without aneurysm.
- *Racemose/cirsoid aneurysm:* It is most often seen in scalp.
- *Serpentine aneurysm:* Aneurysm may assume serpentine (torturous) shape.

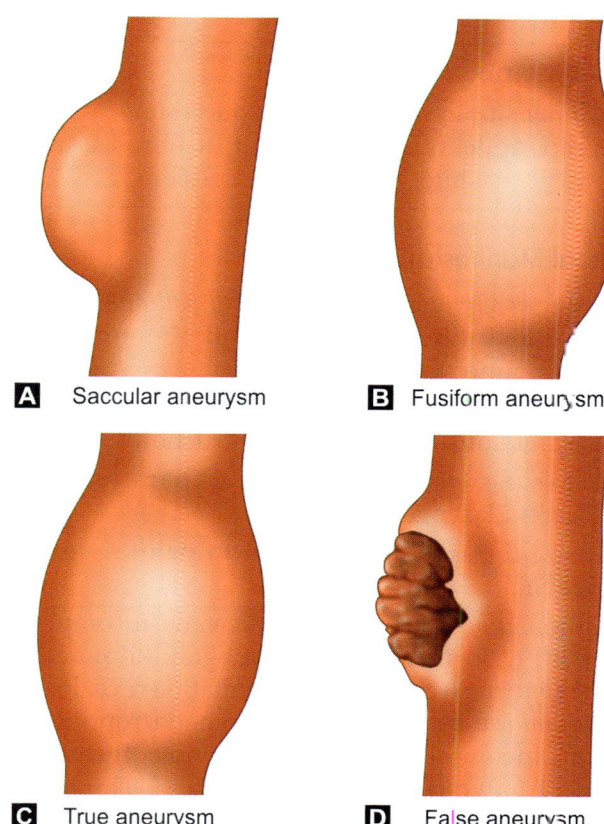

Fig. 15.16: Shape of aneurysms.

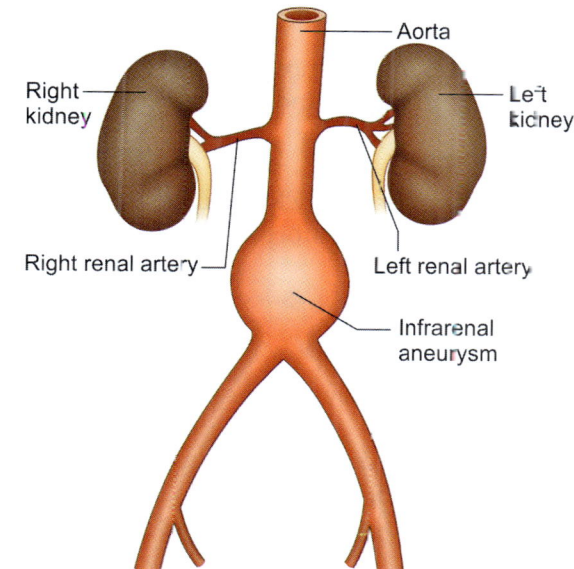

Fig. 15.17: Aneurysm in abdominal aorta due to atheromatous plaque.

- *Arteriovenous fistula:* Arteriovenous fistulas are often secondary to trauma. Arteriovenous (AV) fistulas are abnormal communications (direct shunt) between arteries and veins.

Etiology

Several factors participate in the development of aneurysms. These include atheromatous plaques, smoking, congenital weakness of arterial wall (Marfan's syndrome or Ehlers-Danlos syndrome), inflammation (bacterial endocarditis), untreated syphilis and trauma.

ATHEROSCLEROTIC ANEURYSMS

Aneurysm of the abdominal aorta is associated with atherosclerosis. Major risk factors include hyperlipidemia, hypertension, diabetes mellitus and tobacco smoking. Males are more affected than females above 50 years of age.

Locations and Morphology

These occur in descending order, i.e. abdominal aorta below the origin of renal arteries (most common site), common iliac arteries and rarely aortic arch. It may take any shape, i.e. fusiform, cylindrical or saccular. Most abdominal aortic aneurysms are fusiform in shape extending to involve common iliac arteries. Femoral or popliteal aneurysms are relatively uncommon.

Clinical Features

Patient presents with lower abdominal pain and dull backache, pulsatile abdominal mass, pressure symptoms, massive retroperitoneal hemorrhage and thromboembolism.

Imaging Technique

These aneurysms are diagnosed by imaging techniques such as ultrasonography and MRI.

Blood Biochemistry

Serum C-reactive peptide (CRP) is increased in patients with disrupted (inflammatory) atheromatous plaques.

SYPHILITIC (LUTEIC) ANEURYSMS

Etiology

Syphilitic (luteic) aneurysm is associated with tertiary syphilis. It typically affects the ascending arch of thoracic aorta resulting in dilation and aortic valve insufficiency (Fig. 15.18).

Pathogenesis

- Lesion shows obliterative endarteritis and periarteritis of the vasa vasorum.

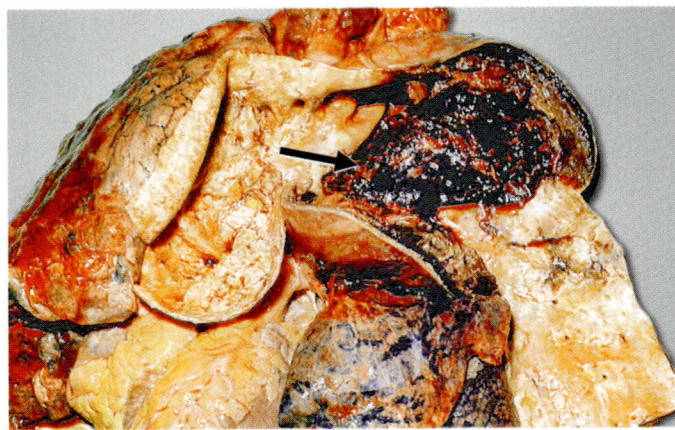

Fig. 15.18: Syphilitic aneurysm of the arch of aorta. The aortic wall shows thickening and numerous wrinkled whitish plaques on the intimal surface. Patient may die due to rupture of the aneurysm (arrow).

- Vasa vasorum penetrate the outer- and middle-third of the aorta. In syphilitic aortitis, the vasa vasorum are surrounded by lymphocytes, plasma cells, and macrophages.
- Obliteration of the vasa vasorum causes focal necrosis, scarring of the media, and calcification. It results in disruption and disorganization of the elastic lamellae.

Table 15.4 shows differences between atherosclerotic aneurysm and sphilitic aneurysm.

> **Gross Morphology**
>
> The inner surface of the affected aorta shows a typical *tree bark* appearance as a result of fibrosis. Intima shows gray white, and gelatinous lesions.

Clinical Manifestations

- *Blood vessels involved: Treponema pallidum* involves aortic arch (most common) and abdominal aorta (less common).
- *Bronchial obstruction:* It may cause superior mediastinal compression and bronchial obstruction.
- *Hoarseness of voice:* It is due to paralysis of left recurrent laryngeal nerve.
- *Vertebral erosion:* It may lead to painful vertebral erosion.
- *Cor bovinum:* It may cause aortic valve incompetence resulting in massive cardiomegaly known as *cor bovinum* (most common). Auscultation reveals *Austin Flint murmur* due to excessive blood dropping back from incompetent aortic valve onto the anterior mitral valve leaflet during diastole. This finding indicates the need for aortic valve replacement (Fig. 15.19).

Table 15.4: Differences between atherosclerotic aneurysm and syphilitic aortitis

Parameters	Atherosclerotic aneurysm	Syphilitic aneurysm
Etiology	Hyperlipidemia Hypertension Diabetes mellitus Smoking	*Treponema pallidum* (tertiary syphilis)
Age group	More common >50 years	Young >20 years
Sex predilection	Males > Females	Males and females equally affected
Site of blood vessel involved	Abdominal aorta below origin of renal arteries	Aortic arch of thoracic aorta
Morphology	Fibrofatty plaques measuring 0.3–1.5 cm in blood vessel affecting lumen	Obliterative endarteritis of vasa vascrum leads to necrosis of aortic media. Healing lesion in aorta gives tree bark appearance in intima due to fibrosis.
Consequences	Ulceration Thrombus formation Embolism Calcification Pressure symptoms on surrounding structures Atherosclerotic aneurysm rupture leads to fatal outcome	Superior mediastinal compression Bronchial obstruction Aortic valve incompetence Massive cardiomegaly occurs known as cor bovinum Vertebral compression Recurrent laryngeal nerve paralysis of left site

DISSECTING HEMATOMA

Dissecting hematoma of aorta is associated with hypertension or with diseases affecting the vascular media, most notably Marfan's syndrome (Figs 15.20 to 15.22).

Location

It usually occurs due to longitudinal tear in thoracic aorta and major branches; within 10 cm of the aortic valve. Type A aneurysms (most common and worst type) involve the ascending aorta, while type B aneurysms begin below the subclavian artery. Blood dissects aorta proximally and/or distally under arterial pressure through the areas of the weakness.

Risk Factors

- *Hypertension:* It is the single most important factor responsible for aortic dissecting hematoma.
- *Atheromatous plaques:* Severe atheromatous plaque in abdominal aorta weakens aortic wall.
- *Traumatic injury:* Trauma to chest may cause tear in aorta.
- *Pregnancy:* Accumulation of proteoglycans rich extracellular matrix in aorta and increased blood volume weaken aortic wall in pregnant women.
- *Marfan's syndrome:* It is an autosomal dominant disorder caused by missense mutations of the fibrillin gene-1 (FGN 1) located on chromosome 15. Fibrillin is a family of connective tissue proteins analogous to the collagens. Defective cross-linkage collagen fibers weaken aortic wall. Mucin stain of the wall of the aorta demonstrates cystic medial necrosis.
- *Ehlers-Danlos syndrome:* Genetic defect in the synthesis of procollagen fibers in Ehlers-Danlos syndrome weakens the aortic wall. Mutation of lysyl hydroxylase gene is seen in patients with Ehlers-Danlos syndrome.
- *Advancing age:* Blood vessels may undergo myxoid degeneration in advancing age.
- *Copper deficiency:* Copper is cofactor in lysyl oxidase, which takes part in collagen synthesis. Its deficiency leads to defective collagen synthesis which weakens the blood vessel.
- *Coarctation of aorta (wall stress):* It may result in aortic tear.

Pathological Effects

Dissecting hematoma may egress proximally and distally. It causes vascular occlusion of branches arising from thoracic arch (i.e. loss of peripheral pulses), hemopericardium (i.e. retrograde spread), formation

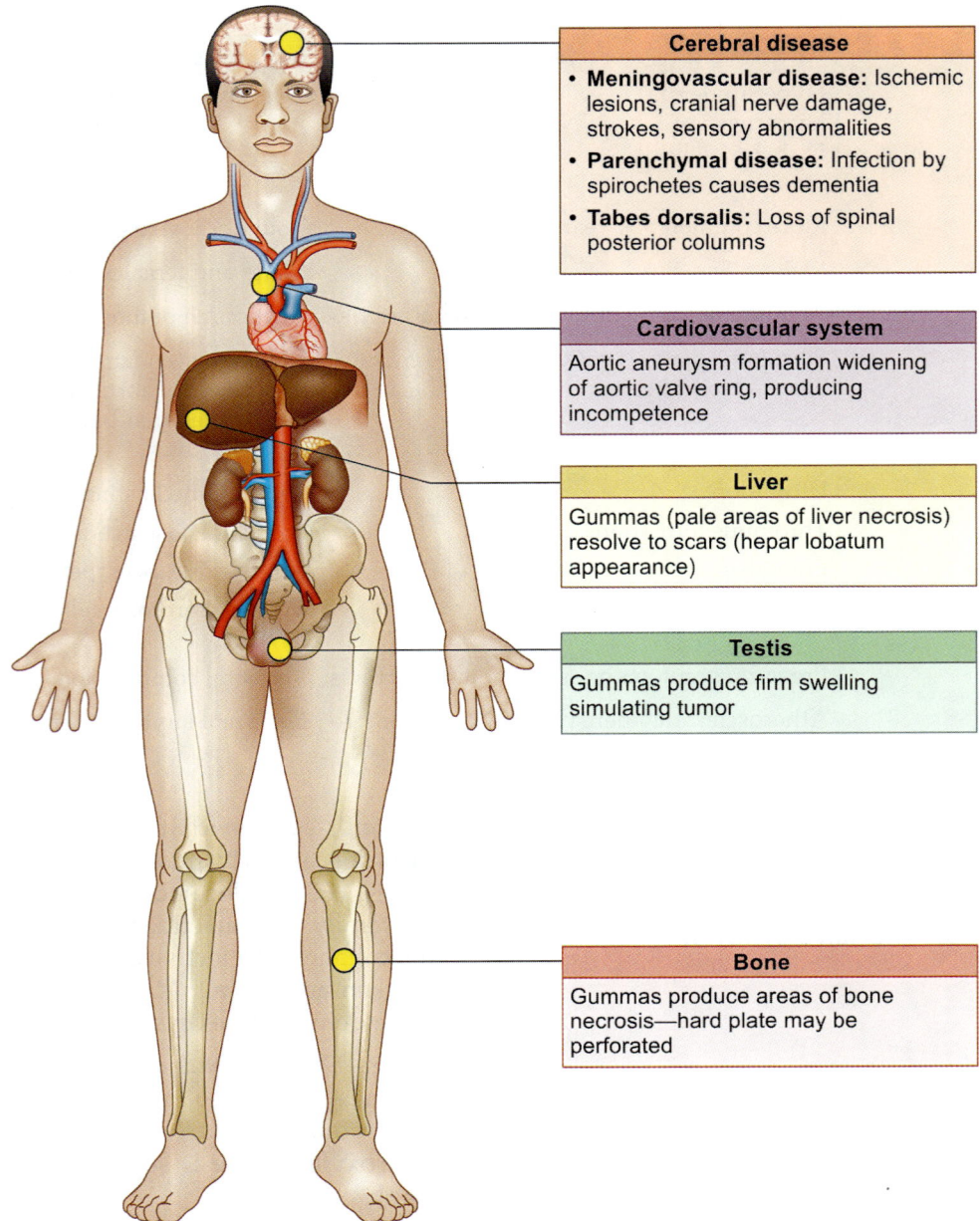

Fig. 15.19: Organs involved in tertiary syphilis.

of second arterial lumen within the media (double-barreled aorta) and external rupture (retroperitoneal and mediastinal hemorrhage).

Clinical Features

- *Retrosternal pain:* Patient presents with severe tearing retrosternal chest pain often radiating into the back. It may be clinically confused with acute myocardial infarction. Abnormal electrocardiogram, increased serum troponin I and serum myocardial enzymes such as CK-MB and LDH indicate AMI.
- *Absence of pulse in subclavian artery:* There is absence of pulse due to compression of the subclavian artery.
- *Cerebral stroke:* It occurs due to carotid dissection.
- *Cardiac tamponade:* Aortic dissection resulting in cardiac tamponade has fatal outcome.

Imaging Techniques

The mediastinum is often widened by radiographic examination. Retrograde arteriography is a gold standard test diagnostic tool.

BERRY ANEURYSMS

The most common site of berry aneurysm formation is between the anterior communicating and the anterior

Blood Vessels

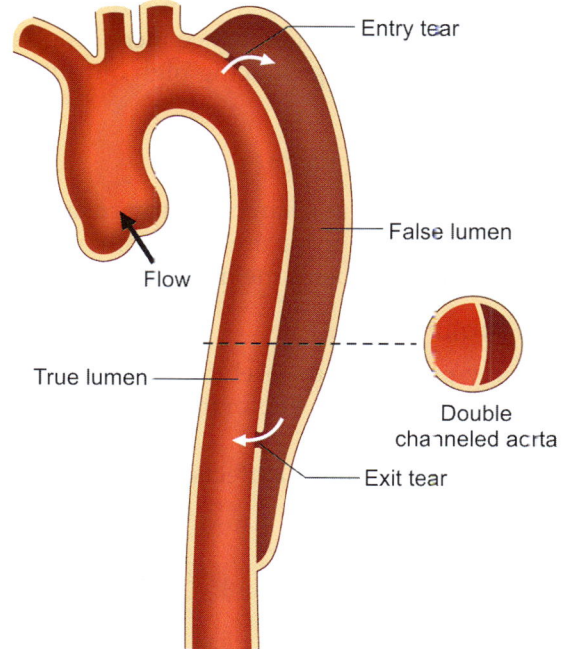

Fig. 15.20: Dissecting hematoma. Illustration shows splitting of aortic intima, entry of blood in false lumen and forming double barrel aorta.

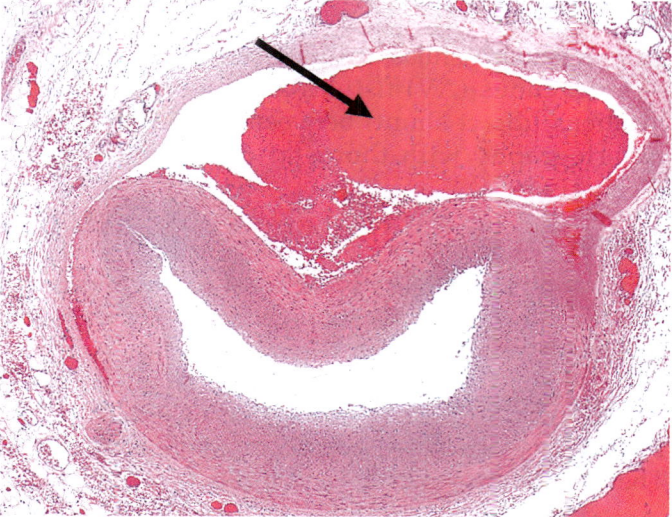

Fig. 15.22: Aortic dissection shows dissection extending into the muscular wall. Blood dissecting up around the great vessels can close off the carotids. Blood can dissect down to the coronaries and shut them off.

Risk Factors
Risk factors include hemodynamic stress, hypertension and coarctation of aorta.

Clinical Features
Rupture of these aneurysms is the most common cause of subarachnoid hemorrhage. Patient presents with history of severe headache, nuchal rigidity from irritation of the meninges.

MYCOTIC ANEURYSMS

Etiology
These occur in the root of aortic arch and its descending branches, due to direct extension from aortic valve endocarditis.

Clinical Features
Emboli from infective endocarditis may involve cerebral blood vessels resulting in hemorrhage into the basal ganglia, extending into the subarachnoid space.

ANEURYSM OF SINUS OF VALSALVA

Etiology
It occurs due to lack of continuity between aortic media and fibrous ring of aortic valve resulting into thin paper-like aneurysm. It may be congenital or acquired.

Clinical Features
Patient presents with chest pain, heart failure, coarse murmur and thrill bounding pulse with fatal outcome. Arteriography establishes the diagnosis.

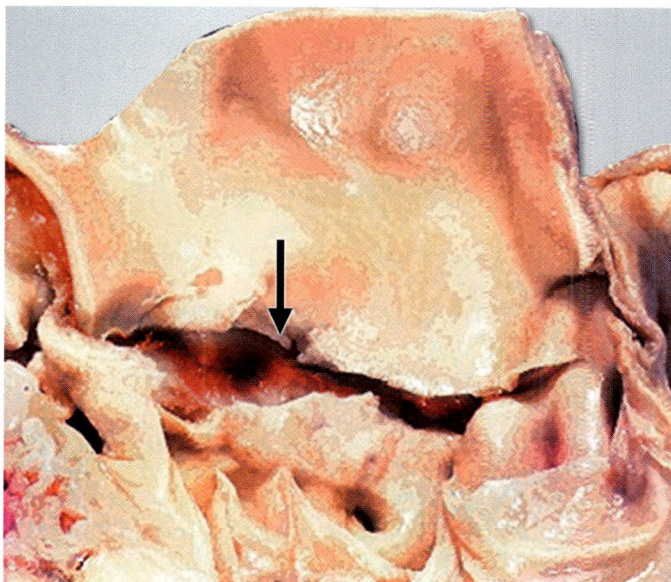

Fig. 15.21: This aortic dissection occurred just above the aortic root. The tear extends across the aorta. Hemopericardium with tamponade occurred within minutes of this event (arrow).

cerebral arteries in the circle of Willis. These are not present at birth.

Shape
These develop as saccular lesions (1.0–1.5) at site of congenital defects in smooth muscle distribution at a branch point of the arterial wall. These occur in 10 to 15% of patients with adult polycystic kidney disease.

ARTERIOVENOUS FISTULA

Arteriovenous fistulas are often secondary to trauma. Arteriovenous (AV) fistulas are abnormal communications (direct shunt) between arteries and veins. Arteriography with thorostat dye establishes the diagnosis.

Etiology

Penetrating knife injury is the most common cause of arteriovenous fistula. Most common sites are scalp, arm and leg vessels. Veins are arterialized.

Clinical Features

Patient develops increased circumference of the limbs. There is presence of bruits and thrills.

Large AV fistulas reduce systemic resistance and by pass the microcirculation, hence increasing venous return to the heart and producing high output cardiac failure.

CAPILLARY MICROANEURYSMS

These are also known as Charcot-Bouchard aneurysms. These are formed in intracerebral capillaries due to hypertension and diabetes mellitus.

Clinical Features

Patient may present with cerebral hemorrhage due to hypertension or retinal hemorrhage due to diabetic retinopathy.

Table 15.5 shows clinical effects of aneurysms.

Table 15.5: Clinical effects of aneurysms

Types	Site and mechanism	Clinical effects
Atherosclerotic aneurysm	Thinning and fibrous replacement of media affecting lower abdominal aorta and iliac arteries	Pulsatile abdominal mass Lower limb ischemic Rupture with massive retroperitoneal hemorrhage
Aortic dissection	Aortic and major branches	Loss of peripheral pulses (e.g. radials) Hemopericardium External rupture (retroperitoneal hemorrhage)
Berry aneurysm	Congenital defect(s) in elastic lamina/media Circle of Willis	Subarachnoid hemorrhage
Microaneurysms (Charcot-Bouchard)	Intracerebral capillaries	Intracerebral hemorrhage associated with hypertension
Syphilitic aneurysm	Inflammatory destruction of media and fibrous replacement affecting ascending and arch of aorta	Aortic incompetence
Mycotic (infective)	Destruction of wall by root of aorta (direct extension from aortic valve endocarditis) Any vessel	Thrombus or rupture causing cerebral infarction or hemorrhage

VASCULITIS

OVERVIEW

Vasculitis is usually immune-mediated disorder affecting arteries, arterioles, capillaries or venules. These are multisystem disorders with a predilection for highly vascular tissue such as skin, renal glomerulus, synovium and eye.

Classification of the vasculitides is described in Table 15.6.

Etiological Classification

- *Immune-mediated vasculitis:* It is mediated by immune complex formation and complement activation. Examples are polyarteritis nodosa, Wegener's granulomatosis, systemic lupus erythematosus and rheumatoid arthritis.
- *Infective vasculitis:* It occurs due to bacteria (pyogenic bacteria, *Neisseria meningitidis*, *Neisseria gonorrhoeae*, fungi (Candida, Aspergillus, and Mucormycosis), viruses (HBV, HCV, rubella, herpes zoster), and *Rickettsia rickettsii*.
- *Metabolic disorder:* Diabetic vascular disease occurs in uncontrolled diabetes mellitus.
- *Unknown etiology:* These include cranial or giant cell (temporal) arteritis, Takayasu's arteritis (pulseless disease), thromboangiitis obliterans (Buerger's disease).

Table 15.6: Classification of the vasculitides

Examples	Diagnostic features	Light microscopy	Clinical features
Large vessel vasculitides			
Giant cell (temporal) arteritis	**Three of five diagnostic criteria:** Age >50 years, recent localized headache, temporal artery tenderness, ESR 50 mm/hour and biopsy temporal artery shows vasculitis	Transmural granulomatous inflammation and giant cells	Recent localized headache, temporal artery tenderness
Takayasu arteritis (pulseless disease)	Aortic arch carotid, subclavian arteries (most common), pulmonary arteries and abdominal aorta involved in 50% cases in >90% women under 30 years	Granulomatous inflammation	Absence of pulses in carotid, radial or ulnar arteries, visual disturbances
Medium-sized vasculitides			
Polyarteritis nodosa	Necrotizing vasculitis weakens wall, aneurysm formation resulting in rupture associated with HBV (30–40%), intravenous amphetamines, sulfonamides and penicillin	Necrotizing vasculitis of medium-sized or small arteries, segmental involvement with partial circumferential not associated with glomerulonephritis	Renal artery (85%), coronaries (75%), hepatic artery (75%), mesenteric arteries (65%), skeletal muscles arteries (40%), cerebral arteries, arteries supplying nerves, pancreas, and eye
Kawasaki disease	Large, medium-sized or small arteries (especially coronaries)	Acute necrotizing inflammation vasculitis similar to polyarteritis nodosa	Febrile illness of childhood, self-limited acute vasculitis syndrome associated with mucocutaneous lymph node syndrome
Thromboangiitis obliterans	Tibial and radial arteries in heavy smokers. Segmental involvement with thrombus formation, sometimes involving nerves and veins of extremities	Vessel shows acute and chronic inflammation	Pain on claudication
Small vessel vasculitides (ANCA-positive)			
Wegener's granulomatosis (ANCA-positive)	Necrotizing vasculitis of arteries, capillaries and venules due to autoantibodies PR3-antineutrophilic cytoplasmic antibody (c-ANCA) against proteinase 3, and MPO-ANCA perinuclear ANCA (p-ANCA) against myeloperoxidase	Destructive nasal lesions, lung and renal lesions	Clinical features related to organs involved

Contd...

Table 15.6: Classification of the vasculitides (Contd...)

Examples	Diagnostic features	Light microscopy	Clinical features
Microscopic polyangiitis (ANCA-positive)	Necrotizing vasculitis of capillaries, venules and arterioles involving glomeruli and lungs Immune complex deposits (a few or absent)	Necrotizing vasculitis of glomeruli and lungs	Lung and renal manifestations
Churg-Strauss syndrome (ANCA-positive)	Bronchial asthma, granuloma and eosinophilia	Granulomatous inflammation	Asthmatic attacks
Drug induced small vessel vasculitides involving skin (ANCA-positive)	Dermal post-capillary venules inflammation due to administration of penicillin or phenylbutazone	Acute or chronic inflammation	Skin rash 1–3 weeks after the drug therapy
Henoch-Schölein purpura (ANCA-negative)	IgA deposition occurs in vessel of skin often similar to IgA nephropathy. Other antigens may include drugs or foods	Vasculitis	Nephritic syndrome and skin rashes on extensor surfaces of the arms, legs and buttocks, painful joints, gastrointestinal involvement (colicky abdominal pain with melena)
Cryoglobulinemia vasculitis (ANCA-negative)	Necrotizing vasculitis involving arterioles, capillaries, and venules. Glomeruli and small vessels of skin are involved in elderly population infected with hepatitis C infection. Serum cryoglobulin (IgM) is increased	Necrotizing vasculitis	Purpura of skin, arthralgia, and glomerulonephritis. Renal involvement can be life-threatening
Diabetic vascular disease (ANCA-negative)	Microangiopathy in uncontrolled diabetes **Etiology:** Hyperglycemia produce premature atherosclerosis, and microangiopathy resulting to kidneys, nerves and retina	Atheromatous plaque in large- and medium-sized arteries	Gangrene foot, renal failure and blindness
Raynaud's phenomenon (ANCA-negative)	Arterial insufficiency of the digital vessels secondary to systemic lupus erythematosus and progressive systemic sclerosis. Raynaud's phenomenon may also occur in thromboangiitis obliterans, Takayasu's arteritis, cryoglobulinemia, ergot poisoning, thoracic outlet syndrome, and cold agglutinin diseases (IgM)	Vasculitis	Extreme cold temperatures and emotional stress may trigger color changes of the fingers from white to blue to red

LARGE VESSEL VASCULITIDES

TEMPORAL (CRANIAL/GIANT CELL) ARTERITIS

Temporal (cranial/giant cell) arteritis is the most frequent form of granulomatous vasculitis. It primarily involves branches of the carotid artery, particularly the temporal artery. Involvement of the ophthalmic branch of the external carotid can lead to blindness. Aorta, its major branches and coronaries may also be affected.

Three of five diagnostic criteria: Age >50 years, recent localized headache, temporal artery tenderness, ESR 50 mm/hour and biopsy temporal artery shows vasculitis.

Etiopathogenesis

Exactly etiology is unknown, but type IV cell hypersensitivity mediates this form of vasculitis.

Clinical Features

Patient presents with unilateral headache (most common) or claudication of the jaw, painful, palpably enlarged, tender temporal artery, morning stiffness in the neck and fever. Temporary or permanent impaired vision occurs due to involvement of ophthalmic artery.

> **Light Microscopy**
> - Biopsy shows transmural granulomatous inflammation of vessel, giant cells, thrombus formation, organization and intimal fibrosis, disrupted elastic lamellae, and marked intimal edema.
> - Neovascularization in media is a useful indicator of previous inflammation. It can be quite focal, requiring serial sections even of a small biopsy.

Laboratory Diagnosis

The erythrocyte sedimentation rate (ESR) is the screening test of choice (>100 mm/hour) in conjunction with tender temporal artery is highly suggestive of cranial or giant cell arteritis (temporal arteritis).

Treatment

Treatment is immediate institution of corticosteroid therapy to prevent blindness.

TAKAYASU ARTERITIS (PULSELESS DISEASE)

Takayasu arteritis involves the vessels of the aortic arch, i.e. carotid, subclavian arteries, pulmonary arteries and abdominal aorta involved in 50% cases. It is characterized by chronic progressive granulomatous inflammation and stenosis of aortic arch and its branches (carotid, subclavian arteries), producing aortic arch syndrome (Fig. 15.23).

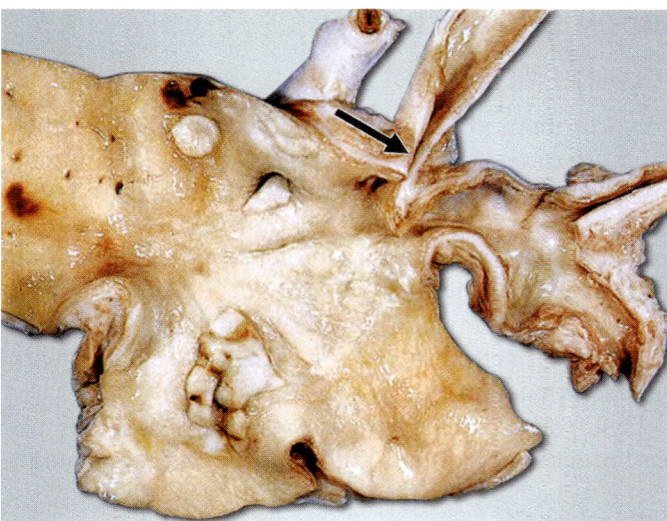

Fig. 15.23: Takayasu's arteritis. It is common in Japan with unknown etiology. The aortic wall is thickened. Intima shows thick plaques. The walls of the innominate and common carotid arteries show thickening and narrowing. Consequences of occlusions lead to *pulseless disease*. Gross morphology and histopathological appearances are identical to syphilitic aortitis (arrow).

Age and Sex Predilection

More than 90% of patients are women under 30 years of age. It may affect middle-aged women of Asian descent.

Pathogenesis

Type IV hypersensitivity reaction is mainly responsible for the formation of this form of vasculitis.

Clinical Features

Patient presents with absence of pulse in carotid, radial or ulnar arteries, visual disturbances, myocardial infarction (coronary arteries) and hypertension (renal artery). Constitutional symptoms include fever, night sweats, malaise, myalgia, arthritis, and arthralgia, eye problems; and painful skin nodules.

> **Gross Morphology**
> On gross examination, the aorta is thickened, and the intima exhibits focal, raised plaques.

> **Light Microscopy**
> Blood vessel shows granulomatous inflammation.

Diagnosis

Arteriography is a diagnostic tool.

Therapeutic Correlation

Patient is treated by bypass surgery.

MEDIUM-SIZED VASCULITIDES

POLYARTERITIS NODOSA (PAN)

Polyarteritis nodosa is systemic necrotizing vasculitis of medium-sized or small arteries, segmental involvement or partial circumferential associated with glomerulonephritis. It leads to marked destruction of media and internal elastic lamella of arteries resulting in aneurysm formation.

Vessels undergo thrombosis, ulceration and infarction of organs. Affected blood vessel is firm and nodular with beaded appearance.

Histopathological changes at different stages of disease process may show acute, chronic or healing stage.

Pathogenesis

- PAN is mediated via type III hypersensitivity through antigen–antibody complexes, in which antineutrophilic cytoplasmic autoantibodies are formed resulting to liberation of hydrolytic enzymes and damage to vessels.
- Hepatitis B virus (30–40%) and intravenous amphetamines play an important role in its pathogenesis. Drugs, such as sulfonamides and penicillin may form immunogenic hapten–protein complexes.

Clinical Features

Patient presents with clinical manifestations due to involvement of renal artery (85%), coronaries (75%), hepatic artery (75%), mesenteric arteries (65%), and arteries supplying skeletal muscles (40%), brain, nerves, pancreas and eyes (Table 15.7).

Laboratory Findings

These include peripheral neutrophilic leukocytosis and eosinophilia, positive antineutrophil cytoplasmic antibodies with perinuclear staining (p-ANCA), and renal abnormalities (hematuria with RBC casts).

Diagnosis

Arteriography or biopsy of palpable nodulations in the skin or organ involved is confirmatory.

Therapeutic Significance

Untreated, the disease is progressive, but most patients improve with corticosteroids and or cytotoxic drug therapy.

KAWASAKI DISEASE

Kawasaki disease is also known as mucocutaneous lymph node syndrome. It involves the coronary arteries. It is an acute febrile self-limited illness of children under the age of 10 in Japan. It is characterized by acute necrotizing vasculitis of small- and medium-sized vessels.

Clinical Features

Patient presents with fever, desquamating skin rash, mucosal inflammation (conjunctivae, lips, and oral mucosa) and cervical lymphadenopathy. Coronary artery vasculitis results in coronary thrombosis and aneurysm formation with fatal outcome.

> **Light Microscopy**
>
> It shows similar morphology as seen in polyarteritis nodosa, i.e. acute, chronic and fibrosis stages.

THROMBOANGIITIS OBLITERANS

Thromboangiitis obliterans also known as *Buerger's disease* is acute disorder seen in young men especially in Jewish populations.

Blood Vessels Involved

It involves arteries of extremities such as tibial, popliteal, and radial, extending to adjacent veins and nerves, i.e. *neurovascular compartment*.

Table 15.7: Clinical manifestations of polyarteritis nodosa

Blood vessels affected	Percentage of cases	Clinical manifestations
Renal arterioles and glomeruli	85%	Renal hypertension
		Acute renal failure due to microinfarcts
Coronary arteries	75%	Ischemic heart disease
		Congestive heart failure
Mesenteric arteries	65%	Gut microinfarcts and mucosal ulceration, nausea, vomiting, or abdominal pain
Skeletal muscle arteries	40%	Skeletal muscle fibers necrosis resulting in myalgia, weakness, arthralgia, or arthritis
Cerebral arteries	Few cases	Focal infarcts with focal neurological symptoms

Pathology

The vessels undergo thrombosis resulting in painful gangrenous toes and fingers due to ischemia. It is precipitated by heavy cigarette smoking. Blood vessels show thrombosis and microabscesses formation. Distal gangrene often requires below knee amputation.

SMALL VESSEL VASCULITIDES

Pathogenesis

Immunologic mechanism is responsible for most cases of vasculitis (not all). Identification of these autoantibodies in serum is used in diagnostic evaluation of patients with possible vasculitis.

- *Antineutrophilic cytoplasmic autoantibodies (c-ANCA):* Anti-proteinase-3 autoantibodies are formed against proteinase-3 antigen of cytoplasmic component of polymorphonuclear cells. It leads to subsequent release of hydrolytic enzymes and toxic free radicals. Immunofluorescence study reveals a cytoplasmic pattern, which correlates with anti-proteinase-3 (anti-PR3 antibody). It is more indicative of Wegener's granulomatosis.

- *Perinuclear antineutrophilic cytoplasmic autoantibodies (p-ANCA):* Immunofluorescence study reveals a perinuclear pattern of staining, which correlates anti-myeloperoxidase antibody (anti-MPO. It strongly suggests microscopic polyarteritis. This pattern may also appear in other vasculitis as well as crescentic glomerulonephritis.

- *Antinuclear autoantibody:* Antinuclear antibody test is helpful in diagnosis of autoimmune disorder, i.e. systemic lupus erythematosus.

WEGENER'S GRANULOMATOSIS (ANCA-POSITIVE)

Wegener's granulomatosis is a systemic necrotizing granulomatous vasculitis of unknown etiology. It involves blood vessels of respiratory tract such as nose, sinuses and lungs (90–95%).

Patient develops destructive nasal, lung and renal lesions. It mainly affects 50–60 years of age group. Males are more affected than females. It is usually positive for ANCA (Fig. 15.24).

Etiopathogenesis

It is caused due to inhalation of some infectious agent. PR3-antineutrophilic cytoplasmic antibody (c-ANCA) against proteinase 3, and MPO-ANCA perinuclear ANCA (p-ANCA) against myeloperoxidase are formed. Immune complexes formed are deposited in small vessels of upper and lower respiratory tract, kidneys and other organs, resulting in necrotizing vasculitis.

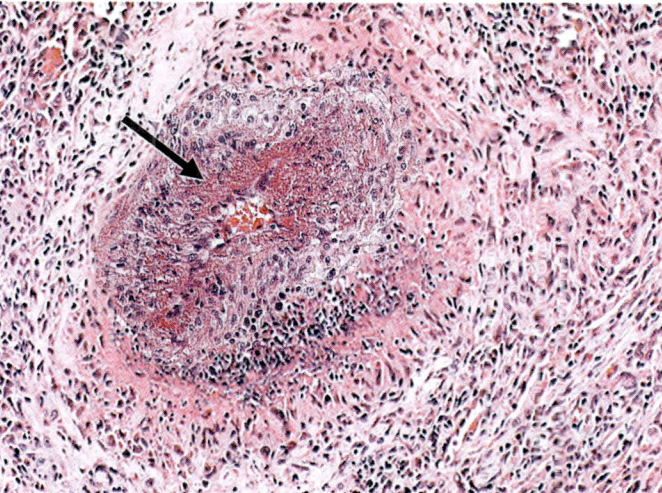

Fig. 15.24: Wegener's granulomatosis. Blood vessel shows granulomatous inflammation (arrow) (100X).

Clinical Features

Many organ systems are involved. It usually involves upper and lower respiratory tract in 90–95%. Patient develops chronic sinusitis (95%), saddle nose deformity, nasopharyngeal ulcers or pneumonias. Patient may also develop necrotizing glomerulonephritis (70%) resulting renal failure, arthralgia due to joints involvement (60%), heart (40%), skin, eyes, and ears (Table 15.8).

Table 15.8: Clinical manifestations of Wegener's granulomatosis

Location	Lesions
Upper respiratory tract	Ulcerative lesions of nose, sinuses and pharynx
Lower respiratory tract	Necrotic areas and cavitation in lungs, cough, dyspnea, hemoptysis and chest pain

Chest Radiograph

Chest radiograph may demonstrate bilateral nodular infiltrates or cavitary lesions.

> **Light Microscopy**
> - Biopsy shows fibrinoid necrosis of small arteries and veins, early infiltration by neutrophils, subsequent macrophage cell infiltration, and fibrosis.
> - Fibrosis occurs with chronic lesions.
> - Granuloma formation with giant cells is prominent.

Treatment

Cyclophosphamide plus corticosteroids are useful in treating these patients. In untreated patients, outcome is fatal within one year.

MICROSCOPIC POLYANGIITIS (ANCA-POSITIVE)

Microscopic polyarteritis is necrotizing vasculitis involving glomeruli and pulmonary capillaries. It occurs most often in old age. Immune complex deposits are a few or absent.

> **Light Microscopy**
> - Histological features are similar to polyarteritis nodosa.
> - Immune deposits in the involved vessels are not common, but may be demonstrated only in a few cases. The p-ANCA is often positive.

CHURG-STRAUSS SYNDROME (ANCA-POSITIVE)

Churg-Strauss syndrome is necrotizing vasculitis also known as allergic granulomatous angitis. It involves pulmonary, artery, coronary and skin vessels.

Pathogenesis

Types I, III, and IV hypersensitivity reactions contribute to the formation of this form of vasculitis.

Clinical Features

Patient develops bronchial asthma and peripheral eosinophilia.

DRUG-INDUCED VASCULITIDES INVOLVING SKIN (ANCA-POSITIVE)

Etiology

Administration of penicillin or phenylbutazone produces vasculitis involving post-capillary venules of skin.

Pathology

Dermal post-capillary venules show infiltration by polymorphonuclear cells, nuclear dusts due to karyorrhexis of neutrophils and leakage of RBCs leading to purpura. In some cases, blood vessels are mainly infiltrated by lymphocytes.

Clinical Features

Patient develops skin rash 1–3 weeks after the drug therapy.

HENOCH-SCHÖNLEIN PURPURA (ANCA-NEGATIVE)

Etiology

Henoch-Schönlein purpura may be precipitated by exogenous antigens, such as drugs, foods, or infectious organisms. It follows an upper respiratory infection post-streptococcal in origin.

Pathology

IgA deposition occurs in vessel of skin often similar to IgA nephropathy. Other antigens may include drugs or foods.

Clinical Features

Patient presents with nephritic syndrome and skin rashes on extensor surfaces of the arms, legs, and buttocks, painful joints, gastrointestinal involvement (colicky abdominal pain with melena).

CRYOGLOBULINEMIA VASCULITIS (ANCA-NEGATIVE)

Etiology

Cryoglobulinemia vasculitis is a necrotizing vasculitis involving arterioles, capillaries, and venules. Glomeruli and small vessels of skin are involved in elderly population infected with hepatitis C.

Clinical Features

Patient presents with purpura of skin, arthralgia, and glomerulonephritis. Renal involvement can be life-threatening.

Laboratory Findings

Serum cryoglobulin (IgM) concentration is increased. It precipitates at 4°C and redissolves at 37°C. Complement C4 is decreased, while C3 is normal.

DIABETIC VASCULAR DISEASE (ANCA-NEGATIVE)

Etiology

Hyperglycemia produces premature atherosclerosis, and microangiopathy involving vessels of kidneys and retina.

Complications

These include gangrene, renal failure and blindness.

Management

Effective control of diabetes reduces the incidence of renal, and retinal disease.

RAYNAUD'S PHENOMENON (ANCA-NEGATIVE)

Raynaud's phenomenon (ANCA-negative) is arterial insufficiency of the digital vessels.

Etiology

- It is most often secondary to systemic lupus erythematosus, progressive systemic sclerosis. It may also occur in thromboangiitis obliterans, Takayasu's arteritis, cryoglobulinemia, ergot poisoning, thoracic outlet syndrome, and cold agglutinin disease (IgM).
- Extreme cold temperatures and emotional stress may trigger color changes of the fingers from white to blue to red.
- The CREST syndrome is a limited variant of progressive systemic sclerosis. It is associated with calcinosis of the fingertips.

Patient develops Raynaud's phenomenon, esophageal motility disorder, sclerodactyly, telangiectasia, and a positive anti-centromere antibody.

Age and Sex Predilection

It most often affects young, healthy women.

Clinical Features

Patient presents with recurrent vasospasm of small arteries and arterioles, with resultant pallor or cyanosis, most often in the fingers and toes.

LYMPHOMATOID GRANULOMATOSIS

Lymphomatoid granulomatosis is a rare granulomatous vasculitis characterized by infiltration by atypical lymphocytoid and plasmacytoid cells.

Blood Vessels Involved

It most often involves pulmonary vasculature but also has a predilection for vessels of the central nervous system, skin, liver, and kidneys.

Predisposing Factors

It usually arises in the setting of immunosuppression. It is associated with infection with Epstein-Barr virus. At present, it is thought to represent a B cell neoplasm with an exuberant T cell response.

VEINS

Varicose veins and venous thrombosis together account for 90% of clinical venous disorders.

Physiological State

- Superficial saphenous veins drain into deep saphenous veins) via communicating branches.
- Valves prevent blood flow from the deep into the superficial venous system except around the ankles, where blood flow is normally in that direction.
- Muscle contraction in the legs reduces hydrostatic pressure in the veins below the resting pressure, hence increasing the return of blood to the heart.

VARICOSE VEINS

A varicose vein is an enlarged and tortuous blood vessel. Varicose veins may occur in leg, esophagus (esophageal varices), anorectal region (hemorrhoids) and spermatic cord (varicocele).

VARICOSE VEINS IN LEGS

Location

It most often affects superficial veins of the lower extremities due to prolonged increased intraluminal pressure and loss of vessel wall support. Superficial varicosities of the leg veins, usually in the saphenous system, are among the most common ailments of humans due to our upright posture.

- *Predisposing factors:* Prolonged standing in certain occupations, pregnancy, obesity, and inflamed deep vein thrombosis increase the venous pressure up to 10 times of normal resulting in varicose veins.

  Defective venous wall development is responsible for varicosity in approximately 20% of general population. Individuals with normal veins may develop pedal edema (simple orthostatic edema) during prolonged standing or during journey.
- *Morphology:* Varicose veins are dilated and tortuous. Cut opened affected veins reveal thrombus in lumen.

  Histological examination shows variations in thickness as a result of hypertrophy of smooth muscle and subintimal fibrosis. Spotty dystrophic calcification is also demonstrated.
- *Clinical features:* Patient develops venous stasis, congestion, edema, pain, venous thrombosis, stasis dermatitis, ulceration, rupture, poorly healing wounds and superadded infections.

ESOPHAGEAL VARICES

Esophageal varices are dilated tortuous veins in the submucosa of the lower esophagus in patients with cirrhosis developing portal hypertension.

Esophageal varices commonly cause massive upper gastrointestinal hemorrhage (hematemesis-vomiting of blood), requiring emergency care to control hemorrhage and prevent hypovolemic shock.

Hemorrhoids

Hemorrhoids are dilations of veins of the rectum and anal canal, which may occur inside or outside the anal sphincter. Condition is aggravated by repeated pregnancy, straining at defecation and venous obstruction by rectal tumors.

Thrombosis of hemorrhoids is exquisitely painful, may result in ulceration. Internal hemorrhoids typically bleed without pain, whereas external hemorrhoids typically cause pain but do not bleed.

VARICOCELE

A varicocele is a varicose dilatation of the veins draining the testis.

Physiological State

Normally veins draining testis and epididymis form the pampiniform plexus resulting in drainage into testicular veins. Left testicular vein directly opens into left renal vein, and the right into the inferior vena cava.

Clinical Features

Most patients develop varicocele on the left side due to obstruction of testicular venous drainage due to spread of left-sided renal cell carcinoma into left renal vein.

Patient presents with dragging discomfort. On palpation, with patient standing, the varicose plexus feels like a bag of worms.

DEEP VEIN THROMBOSIS (THROMBOPHLEBITIS)

Venous thrombosis occurs most often in the deep veins of the lower extremities due to stasis of venous blood especially in immobilized patients. Inflammation of veins with thrombus formation is known as *thrombophlebitis*.

Predisposing Factors

- Cardiac failure, pregnancy, prolonged bed rest, or varicose veins cause venous circulatory stasis results in venous thrombus formation.
- Patient with cancers of pancreas, colon, or lung may develop venous thrombosis at one site and then disappear to be followed by thrombosis in other veins, is known as *migratory thrombophlebitis* (Trousseau sign).
- Pregnant women develop thrombosis in ileofemoral vein (painful white leg). Gravid uterus and hypercoagulable state during pregnancy initiates inflammation of thrombus with painful swelling. It is also known as *plegmasia alba dolens*.

Location

- Venous thrombi are present in deep veins in the lower extremities below knee joint (most common in 90%); superior saphenous, periprostatic, pelvic (ovarian or uterine) veins.
- Less common sites include hepatic vein, renal veins, and dural sinuses (due to meningitis).

Clinical Features

- Patient presents with pain, tenderness and distal edema. In some cases, forced dorsiflexion of the foot resulting in pain is known as *Homan sign*.
- Deep vein thrombosis is entirely asymptomatic in 50% of affected patients. It is recognized only after thrombus is embolized to lung results in pulmonary hemorrhagic infarcts.

Therapeutic Correlation

Anticoagulant therapy with heparin and warfarin prevents formation of venous thrombi.

THORACIC VENA CAVA SYNDROME

It occurs due to compression of superior vena cava or inferior vena cava.

Depending on the location of vena cava, these are categorized into superior or inferior vena cava syndrome described as under.

SUPERIOR VENA CAVA SYNDROME

Etiology

Superior vena cava obstruction is caused by bronchogenic carcinoma in 90% of cases. Mediastinal lymphoma and cervical rib are less common causes.

Clinical Features

- Patient presents with dusky cyanosis, marked dilatation of veins of the face, arms, and shoulders giving purple discoloration.
- Compression of pulmonary veins may result in respiratory distress.
- Involvement of nerves results in neurologic manifestations.
- Visual disturbances occur due to congestion of retinal veins.
- The jugular veins are visibly distended.

INFERIOR VENA CAVA SYNDROME

Etiology

It may be caused by compression of inferior vena cava by a tumor, or propagation of thrombus from the iliofemoral vein, or growing of renal cell carcinoma as well as hepatocellular carcinoma into inferior vena cava, and occasionally into the right atrium.

Clinical Features

Due to obstruction of inferior vena cava, patient presents with marked pedal edema, distension of the superficial collateral veins of the lower abdomen.

Involvement of renal vein may result in massive proteinuria.

LYMPHATIC SYSTEM

Lymphatic vessels have an incomplete basement membrane, hence predisposing them to infection and tumor invasion.

Drainage of infected material to regional lymph nodes leads to reactive hyperplasia with enlarged, tender nodes.

Lymphatic drainage of tumor emboli first occurs in the subcapsular sinus.

ACUTE LYMPHANGITIS

Etiology

Acute lymphangitis is inflammation of the lymphatics (*red streak*). It is most commonly secondary to group A β-hemolyticus streptococci in majority of cases and *Staphylococcus aureus* to a lesser degree.

Affected lymphatics are dilated and filled with inflammatory exudate, which extends through the wall and produce cellulites or focal abscess.

Clinical Features

Patient presents with painful red streaks in subcutaneous region along the course of inflamed lymphatic channels; and painful lymphadenopathy.

Septicemia occurs due to spillage of bacteria into venous system.

LYMPHEDEMA

Physiological State

Under normal circumstances, more fluid is filtered into the interstitial spaces than reabsorbed into the vascular bed. This excess interstitial fluid is removed by the lymphatics. Thus, obstruction to the lymphatic flow leads to localized edema formation.

Pathological State

Lymphedema is an abnormal interstitial collection of lymphatic fluid due to obstruction to lymphatic flow. Increased concentration of proteins in lymphedema gives fibrogenic stimulus resulting in dermal fibrosis in chronic lymphedema. Lymphedema usually occurs due to secondary causes.

Variants of Lymphedema

- *Secondary lymphedema:* Lymphatic channels can be obstructed by (i) malignant neoplasms, (ii) fibrosis resulting in inflammation, filariasis (elephantiasis) or irradiation, and (iii) surgical ablation (axillary dissection of radical mastectomy).

  Breast cancer cells obstructing lymphatic channels produce peau d'orange of the breast (inflammatory carcinoma).

- *Primary lymphedema:* It occurs due to congenital defect of lymphatic channels. It is known as *Milroy disease* or *heredofamilial lymphedema*.

  Third form of primary lymphedema known as *lymphedema praecox* affects females of 10–25 years.

  Females develop slow onset edema feet extending to trunk resulting in superimposed infection or ulcerations.

CHYLOUS EFFUSION

Chylous effusions are collections of lymphatic fluid (chylomicrons plus lymphocytes) in a body cavity.

These are caused by rupture of obstructed lymphatic channels due to invasion by an infiltrating malignant lymphoma (most common) or trauma.

TUMORS OF BLOOD VESSELS

BENIGN TUMORS

These are usually not true neoplasms but are better characterized as malformations or hamartomas.

Spider Telangiectasis

It is small benign arteriovenous communication commonly located on the skin of face and upper thorax.

It is associated with hyperestrinism as seen during normal pregnancy and patient with cirrhosis.

Hereditary Hemorrhagic Telangiectasis

It is an autosomal dominant condition also known as *Osler-Weber-Rendu syndrome*. It involves venules and capillaries of the skin and mucous membranes. These small vessels are dilated (aneurysms). It commonly produces epistaxis or gastrointestinal bleeding often leading to iron deficiency.

Hemangioma

Capillary hemangioma is composed of masses of vascular channels filled with blood (Fig. 15.25).

Capillary Hemangioma

Capillary hemangioma is also known as *strawberry hemangioma*. It is composed of closely packed mature capillary channels. It commonly seen on the skin in 10% of newborns and regress with age without treatment. It may also occur in the lips, liver, spleen, or kidneys (Fig. 15.26).

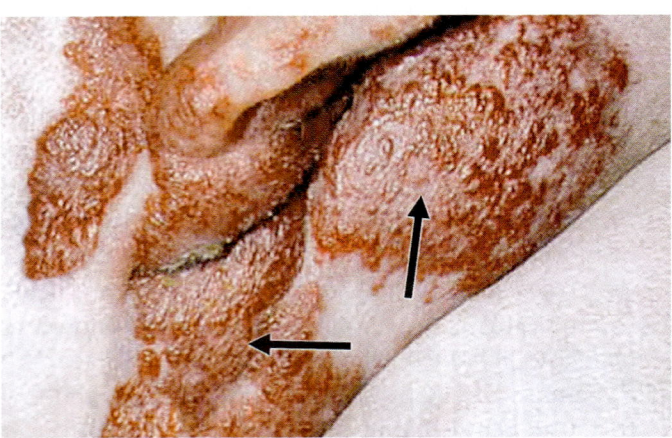

Fig. 15.25: Cutaneous hemangioma (arrows).

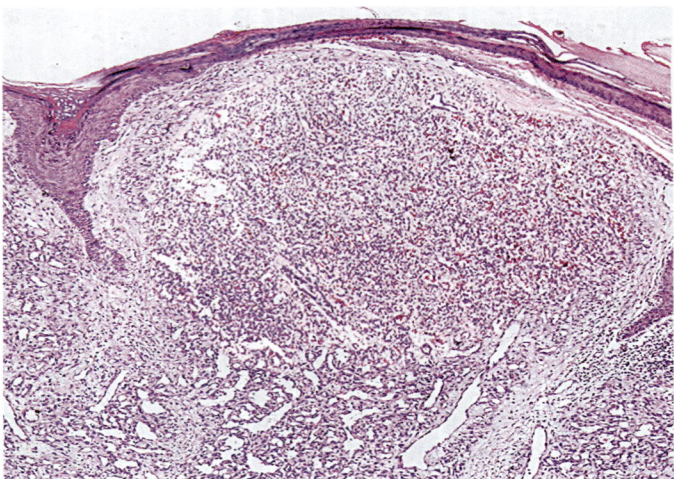

Fig. 15.26: Capillary hemangioma (100X).

Cavernous Hemangioma

Cavernous hemangioma consists of large vascular spaces located on skin, especially head and neck region, mucosal surfaces, and in internal organs, i.e. liver, pancreas, spleen, placenta and brain.

It can undergo a variety of changes, including thrombosis and fibrosis, cystic cavitations, and intracystic hemorrhage. It can also occur in infant as portwine stain, von Hippel-Lindau (vHL) disease and Sturge-Weber syndrome.

- *Portwine stain:* It is the most common flat pink, red, or purple benign lesion of infancy. It consists of large vascular channels frequently interspersed with small capillary type vessels. It occurs primarily in the skin of face, where it is termed as portwine stain.
- *von Hippel-Lindau (vHL) disease:* It is an autosomal disorder, characterized by hemangioblastomas of the cerebellum, brainstem, retina, adenomas and cysts of the liver, kidneys, pancreas, and an increased risk of renal cell carcinoma.
- *Sturge-Weber syndrome:* It is characterized by facial portwine stain, leptomeningeal venous angiomas, and neurological manifestations.

Glomangioma

Glomangioma is also known as glomus tumor. It is a benign tumor of the glomus body. Glomus bodies are normal neuromyoarterial receptors that are sensitive to temperature and regulate arteriolar blood flow.

> **Gross Morphology**
> Glomangioma is small less than 1.00 cm in diameter painful elevated red-blue nodular lesion beneath the nailbed of finger or toe.
>
> **Light Microscopy**
> Histopathological examination reveals branching vascular channels in connective tissue stroma and aggregates of specialized glomus cells.

Cystic Hygroma

Cystic hygroma is benign cavernous lymphangioma (possibly hamartomas). It develops during embryogenesis and present at birth as a cystic mass (cystic hygroma) in the neck and axilla. It is associated with Turner syndrome (Fig. 15.27).

Pyogenic Granuloma

Pyogenic granuloma is highly vascular benign lesion located in the gingival region. Its incidence is increased

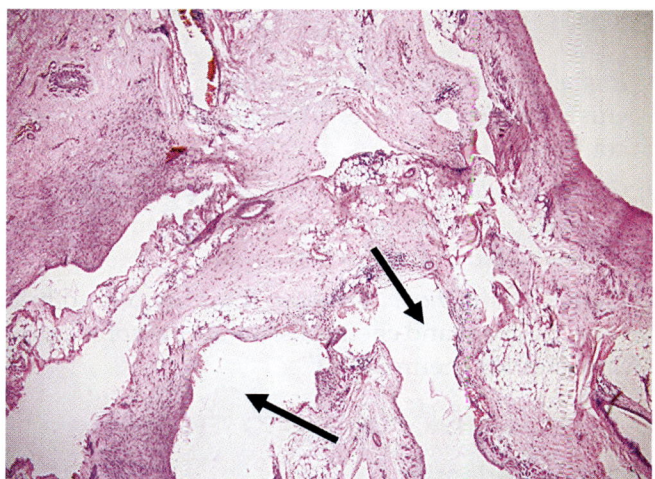

Fig. 15.27: Lymphangioma (arrows) (100X).

during pregnancy. This lesion bleeds easily as a result of trauma.

Angiomyolipoma

Angiomyolipoma is hamartomatous tumor composed of blood vessels, muscle, and mature adipose tissue that are most commonly found in the kidneys of patients with tuberous sclerosis.

Bacillary Angiomatosis

Bicillary angiomatosis is caused by *Bartonella hensalae* or *Bartonella quintana* infectious agent. It is most common in AIDS patients. Histologically, it simulates Kaposi's sarcomas. Silver stains can identify the organisms in tissue.

MALIGNANT TUMORS

Hemangioendothelioma

Hemangioendothelioma is intermediate in behavior between a benign and a malignant tumor.

Hemangiopericytoma

Hemangiopericytoma arises from pericytes and varies in behavior from benign to malignant.

Angiosarcoma

Angiosarcoma is rare highly malignant tumor arising from the vessel endothelium.

Locations

It occurs in the skin, liver, musculoskeletal system and following radiation in breast. It is associated with exposure to toxic substances such as radioactive diagnostic agent thorium dioxide (thorostast).

Etiology

Exposure to polyvinyl chloride is risk factor for developing liver angiosarcoma. It may develop in soft tissue, or as a complication of chronic lymph-edema.

> **Light Microscopy**
>
> Histopathological examination reveals distinct vascular elements to undifferentiated tumor with marked nuclear pleomorphism, and frequent mitosis.

Kaposi Sarcoma

Kaposi sarcoma is a malignant tumor most likely arising from endothelial cells. It exists in several forms—classic, endemic (or African) and epidemic (or immunodeficiency variant).

All forms are associated with a virus known as *human herpesvirus 8* (HHV 8), also called *Kaposi sarcoma herpesvirus* (KSHV).

Variants

- *Classic variant:* It occurs in elderly men of Jewish/Mediterranean origin. It commonly affects lower extremities.
- *Endemic (or African) variant:* It is noted in young African men and children. It accounts for approximately 10% of all malignancies in Africa.
- *Epidemic (or immunodeficiency) variant:* It is most common cancer in AIDS (35%). Prolonged immuno-suppressive therapeutic agents increase risk of Kaposi sarcoma.

Clinical Features

- Patient presents with solitary to multiple red purple lesions. These lesions appear flat that progresses to a plaque to nodule and later results in ulceration.
- These lesions are located on skin, oropharynx, lungs and gastrointestinal tract. Lung involvement is most common cause of death.

> **Light Microscopy**
>
> Tumor is composed of spindle cells (neoplastic element) with increased mitotic activity surrounding slit-like spaces with protuberances into the lumen filled with blood.

HYPERTENSION

OVERVIEW

Hypertension is intermittent or sustained elevation of systolic blood pressure >139 mm Hg or diastolic blood pressure >89 mm Hg. It occurs as essential (primary) hypertension or as secondary hypertension. Normal blood pressure is <120/80 mm Hg. Optimal blood pressure is <115/80 mm Hg (Table 15.9).

Organs Damage

Patient with blood pressure <120–139/80–89 mm Hg is prone to develop hypertension. Hypertension can cause damage to multiple organs such as brain, eyes, cardiovascular system, lungs, kidneys and liver.

Adverse Effects

If left untreated, essential hypertension can cause retinal changes, left ventricular hypertrophy, cardiac failure, and benign nephrosclerosis. It can predispose to ischemic heart disease or cerebral stroke.

Clinical Features

Patient presents with bruits over abdominal aorta or carotid, renal and femoral arteries, dizziness, confusion, fatigue, blurred vision, nocturia, and edema.

Table 15.9: Blood pressure (BP) criteria

Category	Systolic BP (mm Hg)	Diastolic BP (mm Hg)
Optimum	<120	<80
Pre-hypertension	122–139	80–89
Hypertension (stage I)	140–159	90–99
Hypertension (stage II)	>160	>100
Isolated hypertension	>140	>90

CLASSIFICATION

Hypertension is classified according to etiology and severity described as under.

ETIOLOGICAL CLASSIFICATION

Essential Hypertension

Essential hypertension is a multifactorial disease of unknown etiology. It accounts for 95% of all diagnosed cases of hypertension.

Secondary Hypertension

It represents 5% cases of hypertension due to temporary complication of various disorders:

- *Renovascular hypertension:* It occurs due to renal artery stenosis.
- *Endocrinal hypertension:* Primary aldosteronism, Cushing's syndrome, pheochromocytoma, oral contraceptive.
- *Cardiovascular system and blood disorders:* Coarctation of aorta, polyarteritis nodosa, polycythemia vera and excessive blood transfusions.
- *Increased intracranial pressure:* It occurs due to brain tumors, drugs and chemicals, notably amphetamines and steroids (neurologic).

CLASSIFICATION ACCORDING TO SEVERITY

Benign Hypertension

Benign hypertension involves diastolic pressure that rises slowly and remains over prolonged period. Untreated cases produce vascular changes in kidneys known as *benign nephrosclerosis*.

Malignant Hypertension

Malignant hypertension can occur in essential or secondary hypertension. It involves diastolic pressure that rises quickly over weeks or months. It causes severe damage to circulatory system resulting in cerebral strokes and papilloedema. It produces vascular changes (hyperplastic arteriolosclerosis and fibrinoid necrosis) in kidneys known as *malignant nephrosclerosis*.

DETERMINANTS OF HYPERTENSION

Blood pressure depends on the cardiac output and peripheral resistance. Blood pressure may result from increasing the cardiac output or peripheral resistance.

Factors increasing cardiac output: Increased heart rate (hyperthyroidism). Water and sodium retention (aldosterone and ANF). Aldosterone and atrial natriuretic factor/cardionatrin have opposite actions.

- *Aldosterone:* It increases blood volume by enhancing absorption of sodium and water by kidneys. Increased blood volume causes distension of both atria resulting in synthesis of atrial natriuretic factor/cardionatrin by atria.
- *Atrial natriuretic factor/cardionatrin:* It participates in decreasing blood volume by increasing excretion of sodium and water by kidneys. It decreases synthesis of renin and aldosterone. It also decreases venous return.

Factors affecting peripheral resistance

- *Introduction:* Changes in the arteriolar bed causing increased total peripheral resistance depends on neutral α-adrenergic effect on arterioles, catecholamines and renin-angiotensin-aldosterone system.

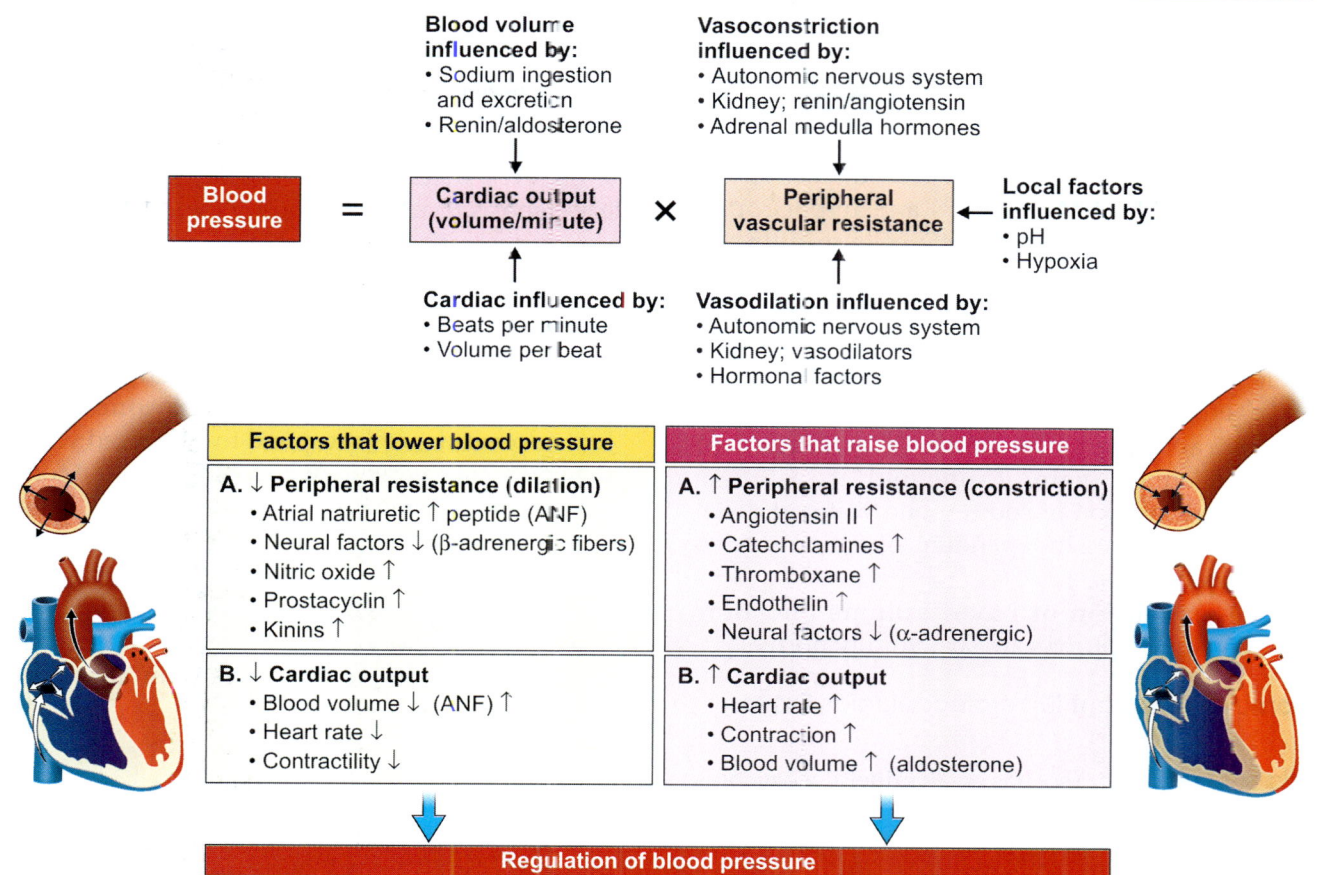

Fig. 15.28: The regulation of blood pressure. Blood pressure is a product of cardiac output (volume of blood flow) and peripheral vascular resistance. Multiple factors influence blood pressure.

Increased arteriolar thickening by genetic factors and increased arteriolar tone by overactivity of sympathetic nervous system (α-adrenergic effect) lead to increased total arteriolar peripheral resistance. Abnormal renin release results in formation of angiotensin II, which constricts the arterioles and increases blood volume.

- *Renin-angiotensin-aldosterone system:* Kidneys release renin into the bloodstream. Renin participates in conversion of angiotensinogen to angiotensin I in liver. Angiotensin I is converted to angiotensin II (a potent vasoconstrictor) in lungs by angiotensin converting enzyme (ACE). Angiotensin II increases arteriolar peripheral resistance and expansion of blood volume. Angiotensin II causes vasoconstriction resulting to increased peripheral resistance.

It stimulates adrenal cortex to synthesize aldosterone, which acts on distal tubules resulting in absorption of sodium and water by kidneys, and thus plasma expansion. It also stimulates sympathetic nervous system and thus causes vasoconstriction. It causes proliferation of smooth muscle cells and thickening (Fig. 15.28).

ESSENTIAL (PRIMARY) HYPERTENSION

Essential hypertension accounts for 95% of cases of hypertension. It is of unknown etiology. It represents an interaction of predisposing determinants with a number of exogenous factors such as family history of hypertension, ethnicity (Africans), stress, obesity, smoking, advancing age, sedentary lifestyle, high intake of sodium and saturated fats. Pathogenesis of essential hypertension is discussed below.

Increased Release of Vasoconstrictors

There is increased release of vasoconstrictors (e.g. renin, catecholamines and endothelin) in persons resulting in hypertensive state.

Environmental Factors

In some areas, people salt intake is more thus prone to hypertension.

Obesity and Stress

Obese persons under stress and strain are more prone to develop hypertension.

Genetic Defect of Calcium Transport

Genetic defect of calcium transport in vascular smooth muscle cells leads to increased intracellular concentration of calcium, myosin phosphorylation and ATP production. It leads to increased reactivity of blood vessels to vasoconstrictors and hypertrophy of smooth vascular smooth muscle cells resulting in increased peripheral resistance and hypertension.

Liddle Syndrome

- Liddle syndrome is autosomal dominant disorder due to gene mutation chromosome 16.
- It is characterized by sustained activation of sodium channels (gain of function). It results to increased absorption of sodium and water at distal convoluted tubules independent of action due to mineralocorticoids.
- There is expansion of blood volume and thus hypertension. Nephrons are structurally normal.

Syndrome of Apparent Mineralocorticoids Excess (AME)

Physiological state: Cortisol has weak mineralocorticoids activity. 11β-hydroxysteroid dehydrogenase converts cortisol into cortisone in tubules.

Pathological state: Gene mutation controlling this 11β-hydroxysteroid dehydrogenase results to accumulation of cortisol. It leads to expansion of blood volume due to sodium and water retention and thus hypertension. Licorice containing glycyrrhetinic acid also inhibits 11β-hydroxysteroid dehydrogenase, thus causes hypertension.

Glucocorticoid-Remediable Aldosteronism (GRA)

Glucocorticoid-remediable aldosteronism is autosomal dominant disorder.

Physiological state: Aldosterone synthetase gene and 11β-hydroxylase gene are present on chromosome 8. Aldosterone synthetase acts on zona glomerulosa to synthesize aldosterone hormones. 11β-hydroxylase gene controls the synthesis of cortisol by zona fasciculata of adrenal glands.

Pathological state: Mutations of aldosterone-synthetase gene and 11β-hydroxylase gene present on chromosome 8 form hybrid genes resulting into ectopic production of aldosterone by zona fasciculata of adrenal cortex. It leads to expansion of blood volume and thus hypertension.

SECONDARY HYPERTENSION

Secondary hypertension accounts of 5% cases of all diagnosed cases of hypertension.

RENOVASCULAR HYPERTENSION

It is most important cause of secondary hypertension as a result of increased plasma renin activity. Renal arteriogram reveals narrowing of the ostia due to atherosclerosis. Renal parenchymal diseases and renal artery stenosis result in secondary hypertension. Renal artery stenosis is caused due to atherosclerosis, giant cell arteritis and Takayasu arteritis.

Mechanism

- Renal hypertension occurs through stimulation of the renin-angiotensin-aldosterone system. Juxtaglomerular cells respond to decreased vascular tone by secreting renin, which facilitates the conversion of angiotensinogen to angiotensin I in liver, which is further converted to angiotensin II in lungs by angiotensin converting enzyme.
- Angiotensin II promotes hypertension by acting both as a vasoconstrictor and as an activator of aldosterone secretion. Aldosterone promotes sodium and water retention (Fig. 15.29).

Clinical Features

Patient presents with severe uncontrollable hypertension, epigastric bruit (e.g. sound is due to turbulence of blood flow through the narrow renal artery).

ROLE OF HORMONES

- Testosterone and estrogens stimulate renin-angiotensin system resulting into expansion of blood volume and vasoconstriction.
- Testosterone and estrogens also increase plasma insulin level, which enhances the synthesis of catecholamines. Insulin increases the peripheral resistance by vasoconstriction of blood vessels.
- Increased plasma insulin stimulates smooth muscle cells proliferation thus increase peripheral resistance and thus hypertension.

ENDOCRINE DISORDERS

Endocrine disorders, such as Conn syndrome, pheochromocytoma, or acromegaly, represent the next most common cause. Conn syndrome is an endocrine disorder most commonly caused by an adrenal cortical adenoma or bilateral adrenal hyperplasia. Aldosterone secreted by the adrenal cortical tumor causes hypertension, hypernatremia, and hypokalemia.

CARDIOVASCULAR DISORDERS

Coarctation of the aorta is a frequent cause of hypertension limited to the upper extremities.

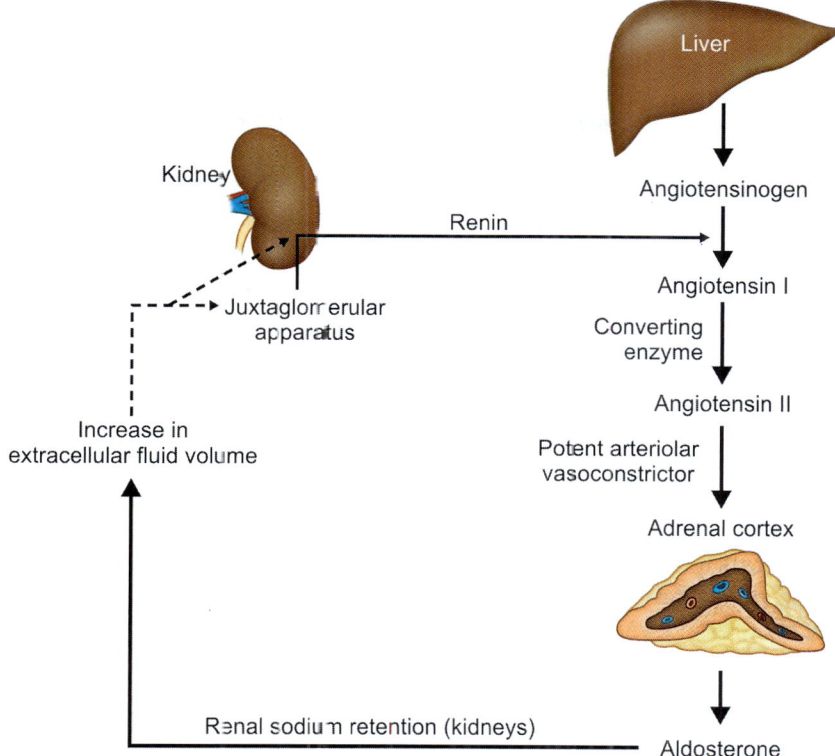

Fig. 15.29: Renin-angiotensin-aldosterone system role in renovascular hypertension.

TOXEMIA OF PREGNANCY

Pre-eclampsia refers to the triad of hypertension, proteinuria, and edema, complicating the third trimester of pregnancy. When these features are complicated by convulsions, the term eclampsia is applied. Abnormal placentation leads to decreased perfusion. Vasoconstriction causes damage to endothelial cells. Immunohistochemistry reveals nonspecific deposits of IgG, IgM and fibrin.

Light Microscopy

Histopathologic examination of renal biopsy reveals diffuse uniform enlargement of glomeruli and the endothelial cells are swollen (endotheliosis), an appearance that results in an apparently bloodless glomerular tuft. Patient blood pressure returns to normal in postpartum period.

Clinical Features

Patient presents with hypertension, proteinuria, and edema usually in the third trimester. Pre-eclampsia is defined as the development of hypertension with proteinuria and generalized edema after 20 weeks gestation. Eclampsia is diagnosed when seizures occur in the setting of pre-eclampsia.

CNS DISORDERS

Hypertension occurs due to increased intracranial pressure due to brain tumors, drugs and chemicals, notably amphetamines and steroids (neurologic).

VASCULAR CHANGES IN BENIGN HYPERTENSION

Pathogenesis

Hypertensive nephrosclerosis is identified in approximately 15% of patients with benign hypertension. Even mild-to-moderate hypertension causes hypertensive nephrosclerosis.

Pathology

Due to benign hypertension, persons develop increased permeability of vessels resulting into deposition of plasma proteins in subintimal regions of blood vessels. Lumen of the blood vessels is decreased leading to ischemic changes in organs.

Vascular Changes

Vascular changes in benign hypertension include hyaline arteriosclerosis and reduplication of elastic lamina. Similar changes are also seen in elderly persons (normal and hypertensive) and diabetes mellitus. Renal changes in benign hypertension are known as *benign nephrosclerosis*.

Light Microscopy

In benign nephrosclerosis, renal arterioles exhibit concentric hyaline thickening of the wall with narrowing of lumen. It shows tubular atrophy, interstitial fibrosis replacing nephrons and lymphocytic infiltration.

Gross Morphology

In benign nephrosclerosis, kidneys are symmetrically reduced in size due to ischemia. External surface of the kidneys is finely granular giving grain leather like appearance. V-shaped infarcts may be seen due to occlusion of medium-sized renal vessels. On cut section, cortex is thinned out.

VASCULAR CHANGES IN MALIGNANT HYPERTENSION

- Malignant hypertension refers to a severely elevated blood pressure (diastolic blood pressure >130 mm Hg). It results to rapidly progressive vascular disease. It most often occurs in young African-American males.
- It affects the brain (cerebral stroke), heart (left ventricular hypertrophy and failure), kidney (renal failure) and retina (focal retinal hemorrhages and papilloedema). It can be a complication of either essential (primary) or secondary hypertension (Table 15.10).

Blood Vessels Morphology

Malignant hypertension causes necrotizing arteriolitis and glomerulitis with *fibrinoid necrosis* and hyperplastic arteriolosclerosis *onion skin* appearance.

Consequence

Poor perfusion of the kidneys stimulates the release of renin, which serves to elevate systemic blood pressure even further by activation of renin-angiotensin-aldosterone system resulting in renovascular hypertension.

Renal Changes

Renal changes in malignant hypertension are known as malignant nephrosclerosis. Renal arterioles and glomeruli rupture, resulting in *flea-bitten* kidney, multiple pinpoint petechial hemorrhages on the external surface of kidney.

Light Microscopy

Renal tubules are atrophic. Tubules contain eosinophilic material known as *thyroidization of tubules*. There is tubular loss in relation to sclerosed glomeruli present. Renal arterioles show *fibrinoid necrosis* and hyperplastic arteriolosclerosis *onion skin* appearance. Patients develop chronic renal failure with manifestations of uremia.

- *Hyperplastic arteriolosclerosis:* Acute vascular injury is followed by smooth muscle proliferation with an increase in concentric layers of smooth muscle cells that yield the so-called *onion skin* appearance. Smooth muscle hyperplasia occurs as a result of growth factors derived from platelets and inflammatory cells at the site of vascular injury.
- *Fibrinoid necrosis:* Malignant hypertension injures endothelial cells and causes increased vascular permeability, which leads to the insudation of plasma proteins into the vessel wall. Severe endothelial injury causes intravascular coagulation and rupture of blood vessels. Lumen becomes narrow and fixed resulting into ischemia. This morphologic change in renal arterioles is known as *fibrinoid necrosis*.

Table 15.10: Vascular changes in benign and malignant nephrosclerosis

Parameters	Benign nephrosclerosis	Malignant nephrosclerosis
Etiology	Benign hypertension	Malignant hypertension
Injury to blood vessels	Mild to moderate injury	Severe injury
Vascular lesions	Hyaline arteriolosclerosis	Hyperplastic arteriolosclerosis gives onion skin appearance
	Reduplication of elastic lamina	Fibrinoid necrosis
Pathogenesis	There is increased permeability of vessels	Hyperplastic arteriolosclerosis results in ischemia
	Plasma proteins are deposited in subintimal regions. It leads to decreased vascular lumen resulting to organs ischemia	Severe endothelial injury leads to intravascular coagulation and rupture of blood vessels resulting to fibrinoid necrosis. Blood vessel lumen is fixed
Renal changes	External surface shows fine granularity giving grain leather appearance. Cut surface shows decrease in renal cortex and medulla thickness	Hemorrhages are demonstrated on external surface due to rupture of renal arterioles and glomeruli known as flea bitten kidney

Clinical Features

Patient develops renal failure, vascular stress that may present as myocardial infarct, congestive heart failure, or cerebral strokes, and increased intracranial pressure, which often produces symptoms such as siezures, headache, nausea, vomiting, visual impairment, and coma.

Physical Examination

Blood pressure is very high >160/110 mm Hg, pounding heartbeat, and bulging optic disc papilledema.

COMPLICATIONS OF HYPERTENSION

- Hypertension is most called as silent killer. Initially, patient presents with shortness of breath after mild exercise, headache or dizziness, swelling of the ankles during day time, excessive sweating and anxiety.
- Long standing hypertension causes organs damage resulting in various other manifestations such as coronary artery disease, cerebral stroke, congestive heart failure, end stage renal disease and peripheral vascular disease.
- These complications may be prevented by treating hypertensive patients by salt restriction, exercise, vasodilators, calcium channel blockers, ACE inhibitors, angiotensin blockers, diuretics, β-blockers and α-blockers (Table 15.11 and Fig. 15.30).

CEREBRAL HEMORRHAGE

Patient may develop cerebral hemorrhages in basal ganglia especially putamen—thalamus region (65%), pons (15%) and cerebellum (10%). Cerebral stroke is common in persons with berry aneurysms undergoing rupture due to hypertension. Cerebral thrombus or embolism may also cause cerebral stroke (Fig. 15.31).

RETINOPATHY

Chronic hypertension results in narrowing of retinal arterioles and hemorrhages in retina producing papilledema giving *cotton wool spots* appearance on fundus examination (Fig. 15.32).

CARDIOVASCULAR MANIFESTATIONS

- *Concentric cardiac hypertrophy:* Chronic hypertension results in marked concentric cardiac hypertrophy of left ventricle with decrease in size of left ventricular chamber (Fig. 15.33).
- *Dissecting hematoma (aortic dissection):* Chronic hypertension may tear the intima of aorta. Blood enters and dissects aortic media. External rupture

Table 15.11: Systemic effects of hypertension

Organ	Systemic effects
Brain	*Cerebral hemorrhages:* Basal ganglia (especially putamen)—thalamus (65%), pons (15%) and cerebellum (10%)
	Cerebral thrombosis
	Rupture of berry aneurysms
	A mass effect with midline shift, often with secondary edema, may lead to herniation.
Eyes	*Retinopathy:* Hemorrhages in retinal vessels produce *cotton wool* spots and papilloedema.
Cardiovascular system	*Atherosclerosis:* Large elastic and medium-sized arteries
	Concentric left ventricular hypertrophy: The myocardial fibers have undergone hypertrophy.
	Left heart failure: It leads to congestive heart failure
	Fibrinous pericarditis: Bread and butter pericarditis. *Friction rub* on auscultation
	Dissecting hematoma (aortic dissection): External rupture occurs in thoracic cavity. Retrograde rupture leads to hemopericardium with fatal outcome. Internal rupture leads to form double channeled aorta
Lungs	Passive congestion of lungs (pulmonary edema)
Kidneys	*Benign nephrosclerosis:* Grain leather surface
	Malignant nephrosclerosis: Flea-bitten kidneys
Liver	*Chronic venous congestion of liver:* Cut surface of liver gives nutmeg appearance

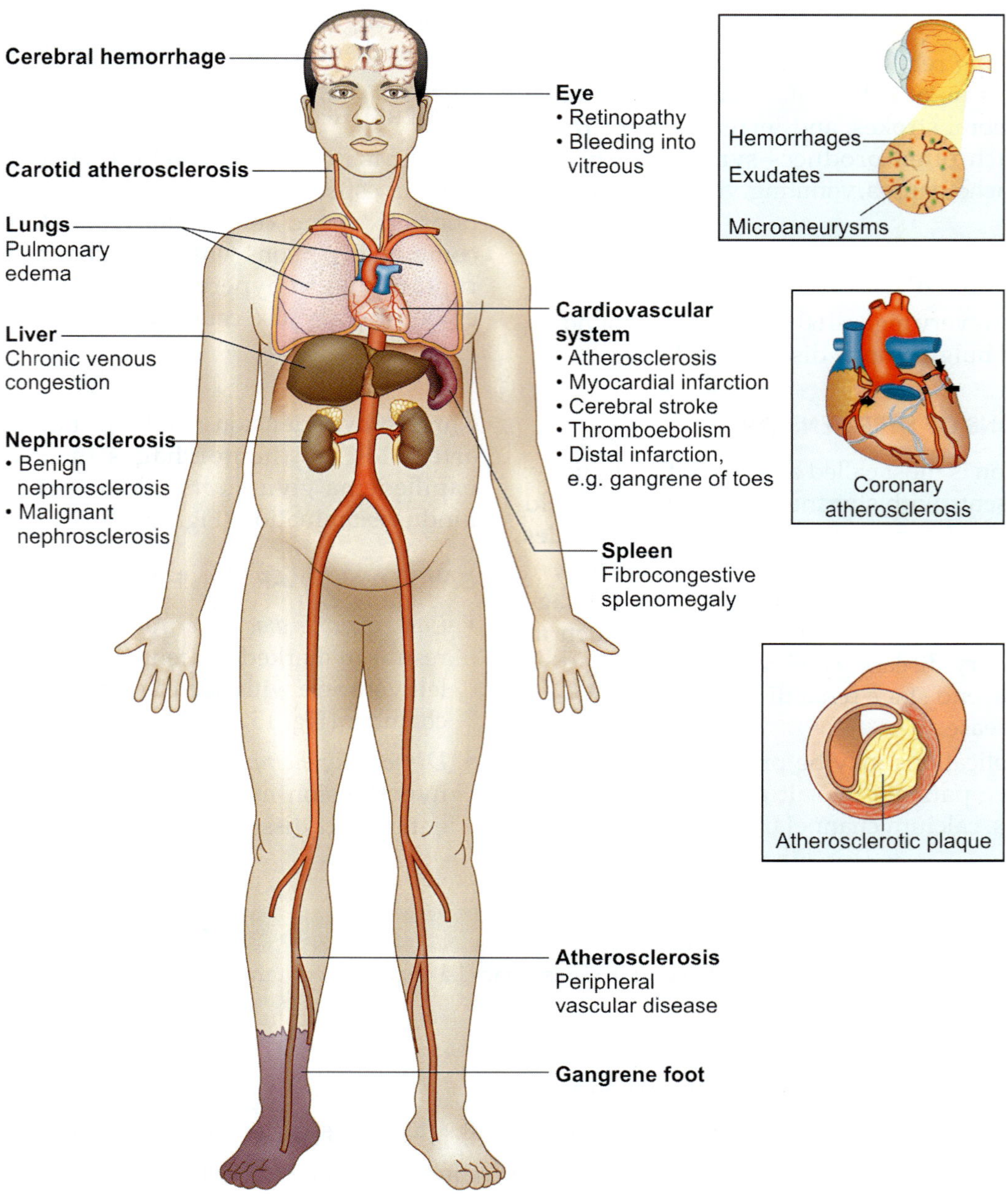

Fig. 15.30: Complications of hypertension. Hypertension is a major risk factor for atherosclerosis.

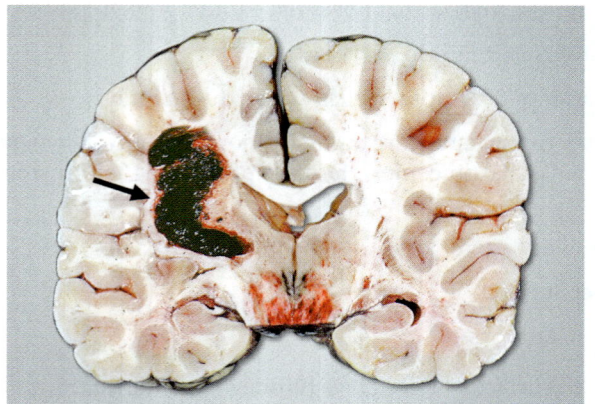

Fig. 15.31: Hemorrhages involving the basal ganglia area (the putamen in particular) tend to be non-traumatic.

results in massive hemorrhage into the thoracic cavity. Retrograde rupture results in massive hemorrhage into the pericardial cavity. Rarely, internal rupture dissects the aortic wall and reopens at distal region producing double-channeled aorta (Fig. 15.34).

- *Atherosclerosis:* Chronic hypertension is a major risk factor of atherosclerosis in large elastic and medium-sized arteries. Atheromatous plaques consist of central core of lipids covered by fibrous plaques. These may undergo various complications such as ulceration, thrombus formation, embolism, bleeding due to rupture of new vessels formed in AS plaque, calcification and aneurysm.

Blood Vessels

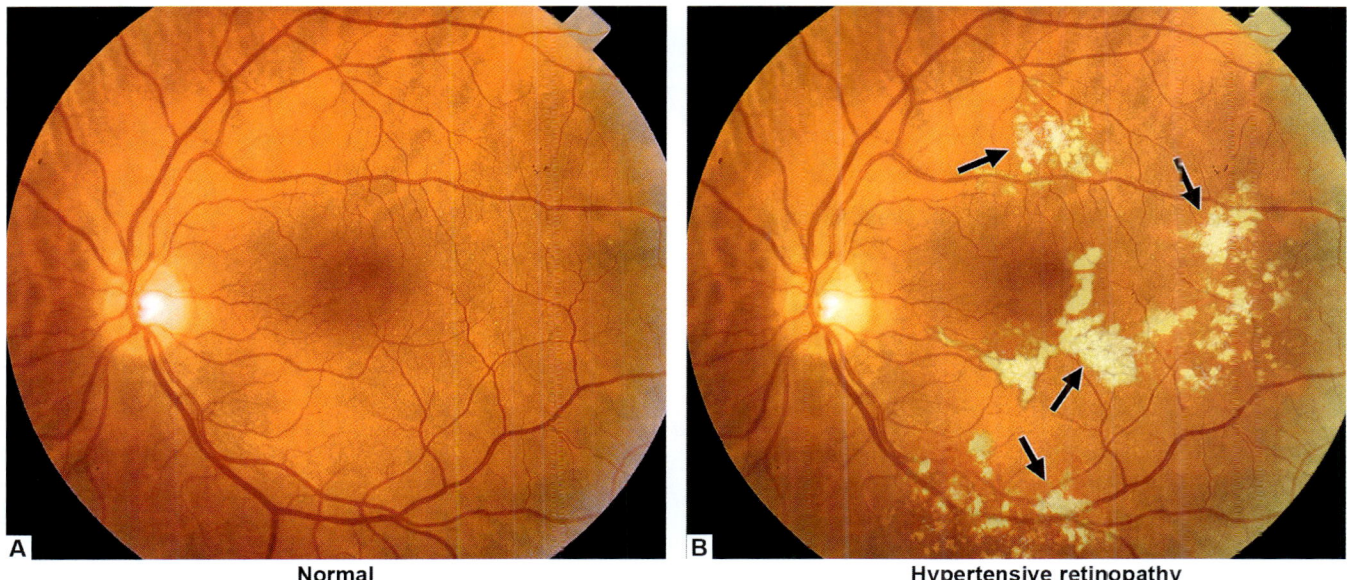

Fig. 15.32: Hypertensive retinopathy. There is arteriolar narrowing and *cotton wool* spots. Additional findings can include hemorrhages into the nerve fiber layer and papilledema.

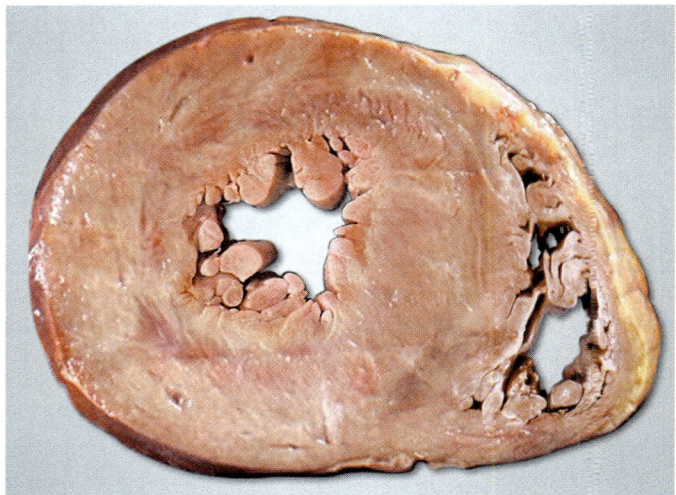

Fig. 15.33: The left ventricle is markedly thickened in this patient with severe hypertension that was untreated for many years. The myocardial fibers have undergone hypertrophy.

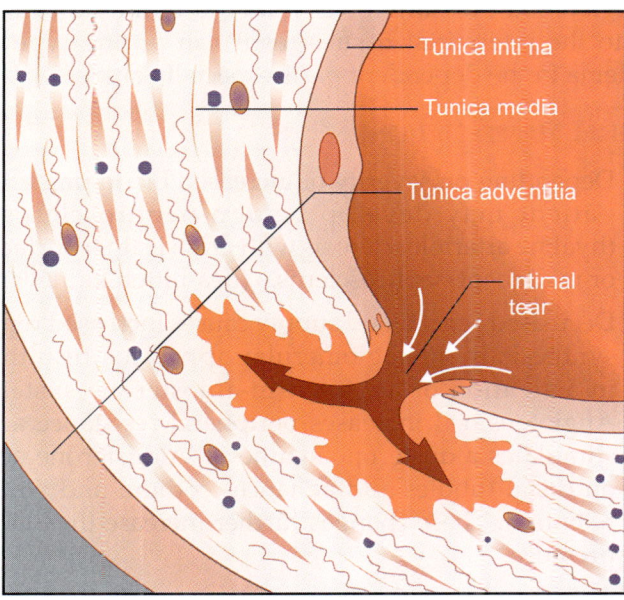

Fig. 15.34: This aortic dissection occurred in patient with uncontrolled hypertension.

Atheromatous plaques in coronary arteries may cause angina, acute myocardial infarction or chronic ischemic disease (Fig. 15.35).

- *Fibrinous pericarditis:* Chronic hypertension results in deposition of fibrin between visceral and parietal layers of pericardium known as *fibrinous pericarditis*. Keeping apart of pericardial layers gives *bread and butter* appearance.

On auscultation, friction rub is appreciated. It is worth mentioning that fibrinous pericarditis may also occur in acute myocardial infarction and chronic renal failure.

PULMONARY MANIFESTATIONS

Chronic hypertension leads to pulmonary edema. Lungs show passive congestion in alveolar capillaries resulting in accumulation of fluid in the alveoli exhibiting slightly floccular pink material along with *heart failure cells* (Fig. 15.36).

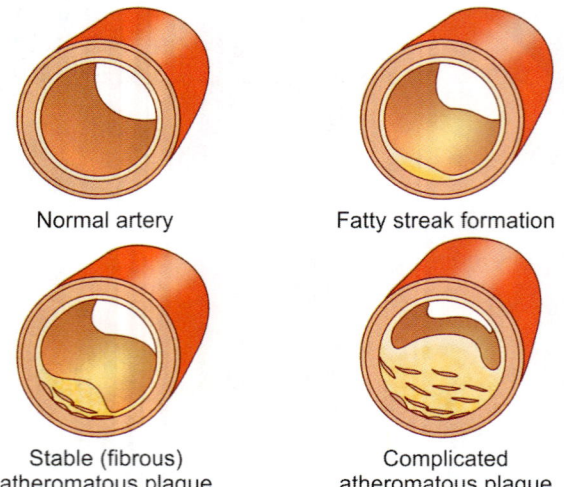

Fig. 15.35: Atheromatous plaques. Uncontrolled hypertension is major risk factor for atherosclerotic plaques in large elastic and medium-sized arteries.

PERIPHERAL EDEMA

High blood pressure forces fluid out of the capillaries into the interstitial tissues results in pitting type of edema in the dependent parts especially ankles.

RENAL MANIFESTATIONS

- Depending on severity of increased blood pressure, patient may develop benign nephrosclerosis (hyaline arteriolosclerosis with grain leather surface) or malignant nephrosclerosis (flea-bitten kidneys).
- Decreased renal blood supply causes increased renin synthesis by juxtaglomerular apparatus resulting in activation of angiotensin-aldosterone system. Angiotensin II increases peripheral resistance and stimulates aldosterone synthesis. Aldosterone acts on distal tubules and enhances sodium and water retention. These changes further increase the blood pressure.

LIVER MANIFESTATIONS

In long-standing hypertension, patient may also develop right-sided heart failure. Jugular venous pressure is increased. Liver shows chronic passive congestion of sinusoids, atrophy of hepatocytes, dilation of central veins and ischemic changes in zone 3 of lobule. Long-standing case of chronic venous congestion may develop cirrhosis, known as *cardiac cirrhosis* (Fig. 15.37).

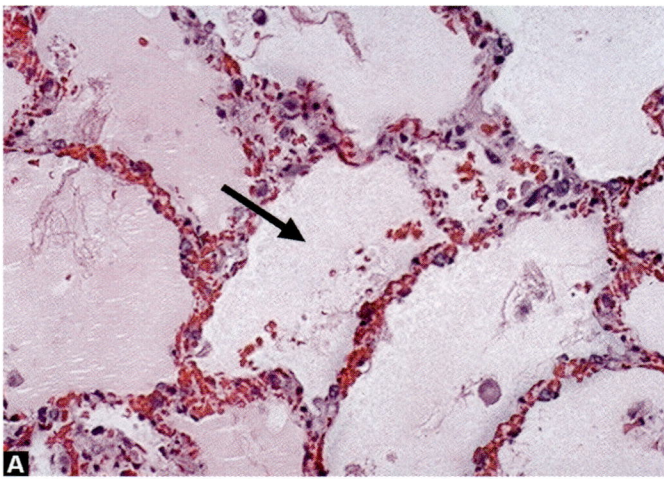

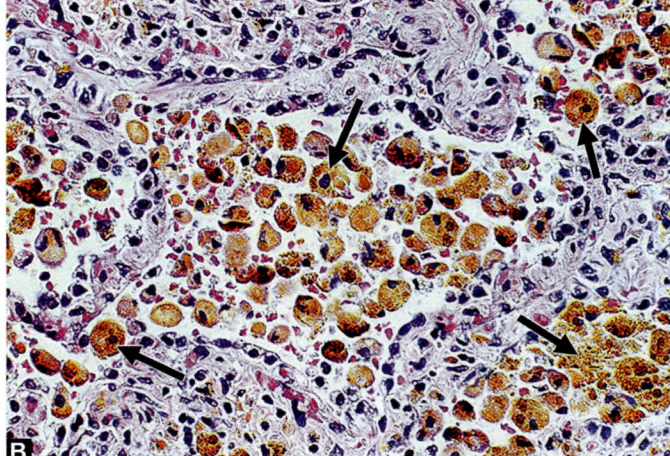

Fig. 15.36: Pulmonary edema. (A) The alveoli in this lung are filled with a smooth to slightly floccular pink material. Alveolar capillaries congested (arrow) (400X), (B) pulmonary edema with heart failure cells (arrows).

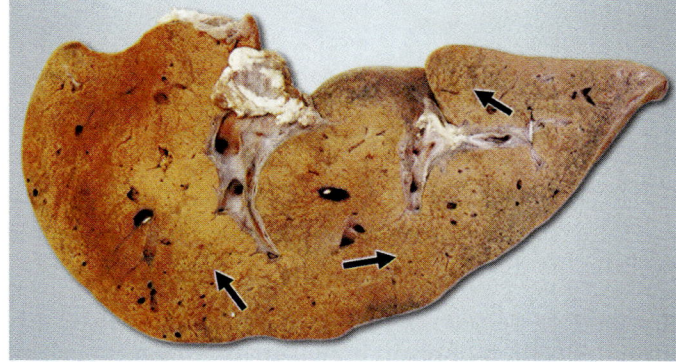

Fig. 15.37: Chronic venous congestion in liver. Cut surface shows nutmeg appearance (arrows).

CHAPTER 16

Heart

Learning Objectives

ISCHEMIC HEART DISEASE
- General Considerations
- Angina Pectoris
- Acute Myocardial Infarction
- Chronic Ischemic Heart Disease

RHEUMATIC FEVER AND RHD
- General Considerations
- Pathogenesis
- Aschoff's Nodule
- Jones Diagnostic Criteria
- Laboratory Diagnosis
- Management

MYOCARDIUM
- Primary Viral Myocarditis
- Cardiomyopathies

ENDOCARDIUM
- Infective Endocarditis
- Endocarditis in Prosthetic Valves
- Endocarditis in Intravenous Drug Abuse
- Libman-Sacks Endocarditis
- Nonbacterial Thrombotic Endocarditis
- Endocarditis in Rheumatic Heart Disease
- Endocarditis of Carcinoid Syndrome

CARDIAC VALVES
- Mitral Valve Stenosis
- Mitral Valve Prolapse
- Aortic Stenosis
- Aortic Valve Insufficiency/Regurgitation
- Calcific Aortic Stenosis
- Tricuspid Insufficiency
- Pulmonary Stenosis

PERICARDIUM
- Anatomy and Physiology
- Hydropericardium
- Hemopericardium
- Cardiac Tamponade
- Pericarditis

CONGESTIVE HEART FAILURE
- Left Heart Failure
- Right Heart Failure

CARDIAC HYPERTROPHY
- Left Ventricular Hypertrophy
- Right Ventricular Hypertrophy

CARDIAC TUMORS
- Atrial Myxoma
- Cardiac Rhabdomyoma

CONGENITAL HEART DISEASES
- Overview
- Atrial Septal Defects
- Ventricular Septal Defects
- Patent Ductus Arteriosus (PDA)
- Coarctation of Aorta
- Tetralogy of Fallot
- Truncus Arteriosus Communis
- Malformations

ANATOMY AND PHYSIOLOGY

Normal heart weighs 300–350 gm (male) and 250–300 gm (female). Cardiomegaly has a critical weight of 500 gm termed as *cor bovinum* in tertiary syphilis. Normal ventricular thickness is 1.2–1.5 cm on the left and 0.3–0.5 cm on the right measured at the base of papillary muscles. Heart is composed of three layers: epicardium, muscular myocardium and endocardium. Pericardium comprises serous and visceral layers of pericardium and coronary arteries.

> **Light Microscopy**
> Normal myocardium is composed of functional syncytium of myocardial fibers with centrally placed nuclei. Numerous capillaries are present in the interstitial tissue between myocardial fibers.

CARDIAC VALVES

Heart consists of atrioventricular valves (mitral and tricuspid). These comprise an annulus, leaflets, chordae tendiniae and papillary muscles. The semilunar valves of aorta and pulmonary artery comprise three cusps, which meet at commissures.

BLOOD SUPPLY

Both coronary arteries arising from root of aorta supply blood to heart during diastole. The principal veins of heart are the cardiac vein and the coronary sinus. Most abundant blood supply goes to the myocardium of the left ventricle. Site of infarct depends on level of occlusion in coronary arteries.

Left Coronary Artery

Occlusion of left coronary artery at origin site causes produces *massive anterolateral acute myocardial* infarction. Left coronary artery divides into left anterior descending (LAD) and left circumflex artery (LCA).

- *Left anterior descending branch of left coronary artery (LAD):* It runs in anterior interventricular sulcus. It supplies *anterior portion of left ventricle including apex, anterior two-thirds interventricular septum, and adjacent area of right ventricle.* Stenosis of LAD leads to infarction of anterior part of the left ventricle along with anterior two-thirds of the interventricular septum in 40% to 50%.
- *Left circumflex artery (LCA):* It runs in coronal sulcus is a transverse groove present between the atria and ventricles. It supplies blood to the lateral free wall of the left ventricle. Stenosis of LCA leads to infarction in the lateral wall of the left ventricle in 15–20% cases.

Right Coronary Artery

- Right coronary artery runs in posterior interventricular sulcus. It nourishes the entire right ventricle, postero-inferior wall of the left ventricle including the posteromedial papillary muscle, and posterior one-third of the interventricular septum. It also supplies 90% of the blood to the SA node (sinoatrial node) and AV node (atrioventricular node).
- Stenosis of right coronary causes infarction in the right ventricle, posterior–inferior wall of left ventricle, along with posterior one-third of the interventricular septum in 30–40%.

CONDUCTION SYSTEM

The conduction system is comprised of specialized myocytes, with fewer intercalated discs and higher glycogen content. The conduction system is demonstrated by *Masson trichrome, Verhoeff-van Gieson* and *alcian blue*.

Sinoatrial (SA) Node

SA node measures 0.3 mm and located in the upper right atrial wall near the opening of the superior vena cava. It initiates cardiac action potentials at a velocity of 0.3 *m/second*, which sets basic pace for heart rate and conduction throughout both atria. It possesses high concentration of sodium ions in the extracellular fluid and negative charge inside the nodal fibers.

Atrioventricular (AV) Node or Node of Tawara

AV node is located in posterior wall of right atrium along the lower part of interatrial septum. It receives action potentials, from SA node.

Bundle of His and its Branches

It is located in superior portion of interventricular septum and divides into left and right branches. It receives action potentials from atrioventricular (AV) node and passes to myofibers through right and left bundle branches.

Conduction Myofibers (Purkinje Fibers)

These are located in ventricular septum—Purkinje fibers extend out to the papillary muscles and lateral walls of ventricles. These receive action potentials from bundle branches and pass them to ventricular myocardium.

ISCHEMIC HEART DISEASE

GENERAL CONSIDERATIONS

Clinical Manifestations
These are comprising of: (i) angina pectoris (e.g. stable angina, Prinzmetal angina, unstable angina), (ii) acute myocardial infarction, (iii) sudden cardiac death and (iv) chronic ischemic heart disease with congestive heart failure.

Acute Coronary Syndrome
It comprises angina pectoris, acute myocardial syndrome and sudden cardiac death.

Salient Features
Ischemic heart disease is caused by partial or complete interruption of arterial blood flow to the myocardium. Most important cause is atheromatous narrowing of the coronary arteries, sometimes aggravated by superimposed thrombosis or vasospasm which resulting in occlusion. Patients become symptomatic, if atherosclerotic plaque is involving >75% of coronary artery lumen.

Site of Infarct
The coronary vessels most commonly involved in decreasing order of frequency are *anterior descending branch of left coronary 50%, right coronary artery (RCA) 30% and left circumflex artery (LCA) 20%*. Atheromatous plaques are observed in proximal part of anterior descending artery (Fig. 16.1).

Clinical Correlation
Myocardial ischemia may be clinically silent or present as angina pectoris, acute myocardial infarction or chronic ischemic heart disease.

Risk is increased in persons with hyperlipidemia, hypertension, diabetes mellitus (insulin resistance), tobacco smoking, obesity, and genetic predisposition.

Prognosis
Approximately 25% of patients either succumb to a terminal ventricular arrhythmia prior to reaching the hospital (sudden cardiac death) or suffer a similar event while in the critical care unit.

ANGINA PECTORIS
Angina pectoris is episodic chest pain or discomfort in substernal area caused by inadequate oxygenation of the myocardium.

Myocardial ischemia occurs as a result of occlusive atheromatous plaque (90% of all cases), coronary arteries vasospasm (5%) and aortic valve disease (aortic stenosis or regurgitation).

Incidence
Angina pectoris is most common in middle-aged and elderly males. Females are usually affected after menopause.

Approximately 10–20% of patients develop unstable angina or acute myocardial infarction within one year of diagnosis of angina pectoris.

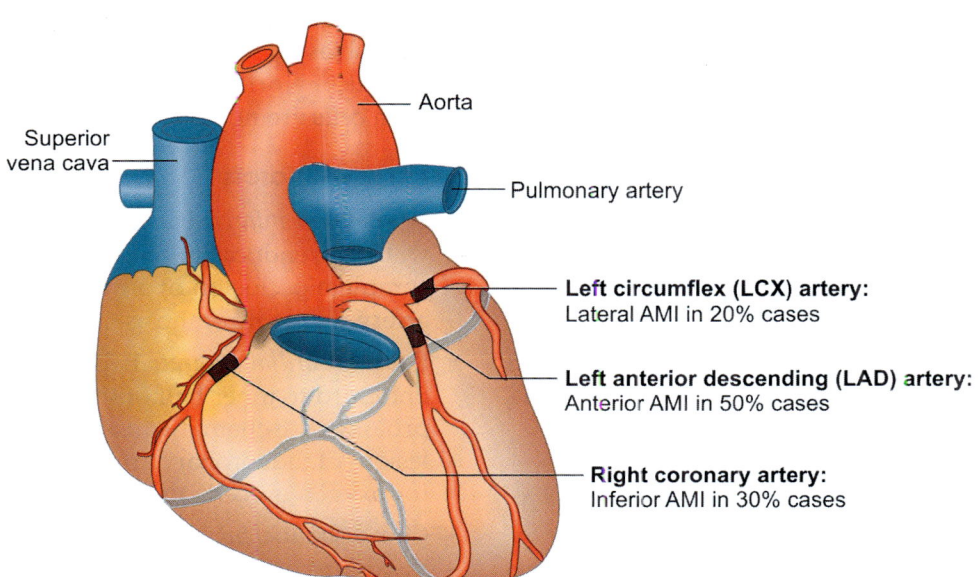

Fig. 16.1: Location of blockage in coronary arteries 50%, right coronary artery (RCA) 30% and left circumflex artery (LCA) (20%).

Patterns of Angina Pectoris

There are three patterns of angina pectoris: stable, unstable and Prinzmetal. Myocardial cell necrosis is only present in unstable angina.

STABLE (TYPICAL) ANGINA

Pathogenesis

Stable angina is most common variant of angina pectoris results from severe narrowing of atherosclerotic coronary vessels (>70% stenosis). It leads to decreased blood supply to subendocardial region of heart. Coronary occlusion may be demonstrated by coronary angiography.

Clinical Features

It is the most common variant of angina pectoris. Patient presents with sudden onset of exercise induced chest pain in substernal region, lasting 30 seconds to 30 minutes. Pain is relieved on rest or vasodilator sublingual intake of nitroglycerin. Risk factors of atherosclerosis include hyperlipidemia, hypertension, diabetes mellitus, cigarette smoking and family history of coronary artery disease.

ECG Study

Stress test reveals ST-segment depression (inversion) >1 mm. Inverted T-wave correlates with areas of ischemia at the periphery of the infarct.

UNSTABLE (CRESCENDO/PRE-INFARCTION) ANGINA

Pathogenesis

Unstable angina is generally caused by disruption of an atheromatous plaque with superimposed thrombosis. It may also be caused by vasospasm or emboli reaching coronary vessels. It results in ischemia of myocardium. It may be accompanied by focal myocyte necrosis, which is repaired by fibrosis.

Clinical Features

Patient presents with prolonged frequent intermittent chest pain at rest or with minimal exertion. Patient is prone to myocardial infarction.

VARIANT (PRINZMETAL) ANGINA

Pathogenesis

Coronary vasospasm occurs due to thromboxane A_2 or decreased synthesis of endothelin (vasodilator) by vascular endothelium. It leads to decreased blood flow to heart.

Clinical Features

Patient presents with intermittent chest pain at rest with or without superimposed coronary artery atherosclerotic plaque. It is generally considered to be caused by vasospasm. Patient responds well to vasodilator (nitroglycerin) and calcium-channel blocker.

ECG Study

During the attack, stress test electrocardiogram (ECG) shows a transient ST segment elevation (e.g. transmural ischemia). ST segment elevation correlates with injured myocardial cells surrounding the area of necrosis.

ACUTE MYOCARDIAL INFARCTION

GENERAL CONSIDERATIONS

Myocardial infarction is the most important cause of morbidity and mortality from ischemic heart disease. Most myocardial infarcts are seen in left ventricle and interventricular septum, as these areas receive blood supply from both coronaries.

Occlusion of coronary arteries by atheromatous plaque with superimposed thrombosis involving >90% of vessel lumen resulting in coagulative necrosis of myocardium. It can be averted by immediate thrombolytic therapy.

Changes During Evolution

Myocardial infarction is followed by a series of progressive gross and microscopic changes of the heart. Cardiac enzymes and troponins are released into the circulation as a result of altered membrane permeability of necrotic myocardial cells. Neutrophils, macrophages and fibroblasts participate in the evolution of myocardial infarct. It is worth mentioning that lymphocytes and plasma cells are not involved in evolution of AMI.

Patterns of Infarcts

- *Transmural infarct:* It involves the entire ventricular wall from endocardium to epicardium. It results from complete occlusion of a major extramural coronary artery due to thrombosis.
- *Subendocardial infarct:* It is limited to the interior one-third to inner half of the left ventricle. It reflects prolonged ischemia caused by partially occluding lesions of the coronary arteries when the requirement for oxygen exceeds the supply.
- *Circumferential infarct:* It involves ventricular chamber in circumferential manner. It occurs due to severe reduction of coronary blood flow (Figs 16.2 to 16.4).

Heart

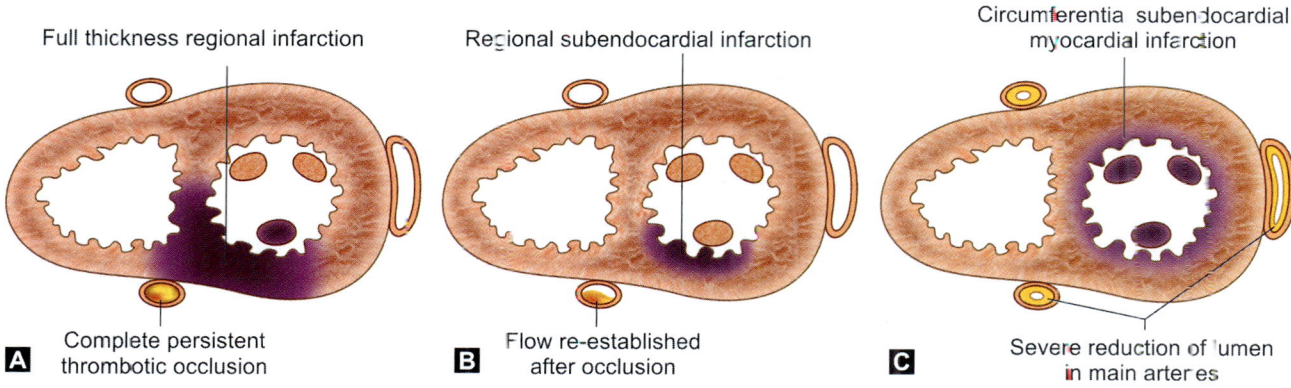

Fig. 16.2: Patterns of myocardial infarcts. (A) Transmural infarct occurs due to complete persistent thrombotic phenomenon, (B) regional subendocardial infarct occurs as a result of reestablishment of blood flow after occlusion, (C) circumferential subendocardial infarct occurs due to severe reduction of lumen in main coronary arteries.

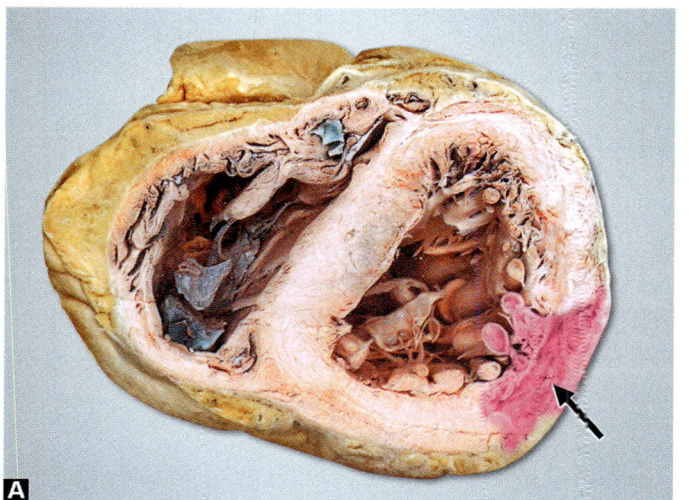
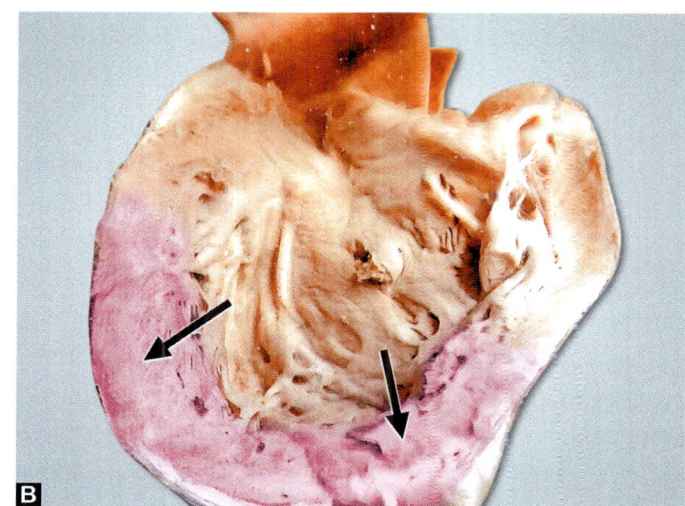

Fig. 16.3: Transmural infarct.

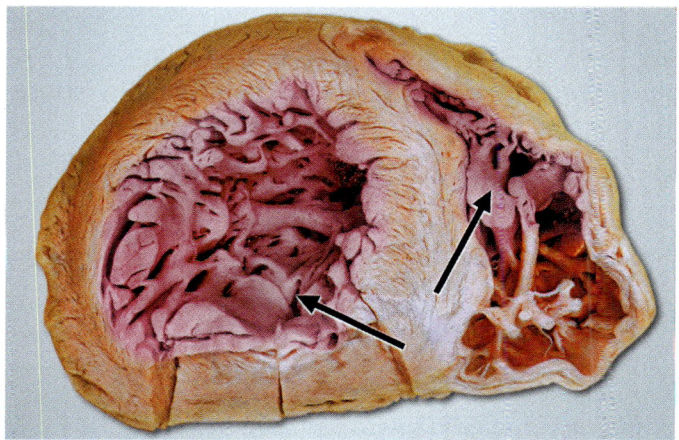

Fig. 16.4: Subendocardial infarct.

Complications

Patient may develop various complications such as arrhythmias (most common cause of mortality in first several hours), cardiac failure, mitral incompetence due to papillary muscle rupture, and hemopericardium due to myocardial rupture within first 4–7 days, mural thromboembolism phenomenon and ventricular aneurysm.

RISK FACTORS

Risk factors for acute myocardial infarction may be non-modifiable and modifiable. Modifiable major risk factors include hyperlipidemia, hypertension, diabetes mellitus, tobacco smoking, sedentary lifestyles and other factors.

Non-modifiable risk factors include genetic factors, familial predisposition, racial factors, gender and advancing age (Table 16.1). Desirable lipid fractions are given in Table 16.2.

INCIDENCE IN PRESENT SCENARIO

Incidence of coronary artery disease is decreasing due to various diagnostic and therapeutic advances in present scenario.

Table 16.1: Risk factors for atherosclerosis

Risk factors	Comments
Modifiable risk factors	
Hyperlipidemia	*Acquired hyperlipidemia:* High lipid diet and nephrotic syndrome increases risk of atherosclerosis.
Hypertension	Persistent high blood pressure causes endothelial dysfunction
Diabetes mellitus	Diagnostic criteria: Fasting blood sugar >126 mg/dl or random blood sugar >200 mg/dl. Advanced glycosylated end products formed participate in pathogenesis of atheromatous plaque
Tobacco smoking	Tobacco smoking causes endothelial dysfunction, deranged lipids (increased LDL and decreased HDL), platelets activation synthesizing ADP and TXA_2, platelets adhesion and arterial wall hypoxia due to accumulation of carbon monoxide in the blood
Sedentary lifestyle	Regular moderate exercise reduces the risk of atherosclerosis by increasing HDL
Minor risk factors	Type 'A' personality with stress factors in lifestyle
	Increased homocysteine level (>100 µmol/L)
	Hyperuricemia
	Increased serum ferritin level
	Methylene tetrahydrofolate reductase mutation
	Lipoprotein 'a' mutation
	Hormonal replacement therapy in postmenopausal women
	Infectious agents demonstrated in atheromatous plaque (*Chlamydia pneumoniae*, herpesvirus and cytomegalovirus)
Non-modifiable risk factors	
Genetic factors	*Familial hyperlipidemia:* Defective LDL receptor inhibits cholesterol uptake by the liver.
Familial predisposition	A family history of premature coronary artery disease
Racial factors	Blacks have less severe atherosclerosis than Whites
Gender	Women >45 and men >55 years (↑ Risk)
	High levels of estrogens and HDL have anti-atherogenic influence in premenopausal women
Advancing age	Peak incidence after age of 60 in men and after age of 70 in women

Table 16.2: Desirable lipid fractions

Parameters	Lipid fraction range
Cholesterol	<200 mg/dl
Triglycerides	<150 mg/dl
LDL	<100 mg/dl
HDL	>60 mg/dl
LDL cholesterol : HDL cholesterol ratio	4:1

Modification of major risk factors

Stoppage of cigarette smoking and controlling hyperlipidemia, hypertension and diabetes mellitus reduce the incidence of myocardial infarction.

Diagnostic advances

Most of the coronary care units equipped with diagnostic facilities to diagnose coronary artery disease (Table 16.3).

Table 16.3: Diagnostic advances

Diagnostic advances	Comments
Coronary angiography	Detection of blockage in coronaries
Electrocardiogram: 12-lead	Diagnostic in majority of cases
Echocardiography: 2-dimensional	Detection of motion of cardiac chambers
Radionuclide scanning	Location of infarct area
Cardiac troponins level	Definite evidence of myocardial necrosis
Cardiac enzymes (CK-MB, LDH)	Diagnostic markers in AMI
Non-specific indexes of tissue injury (leukocytosis)	Nonspecific evidence of AMI

Coronary Care Units

These are well equipped with modern facilities to control arrhythmias in patients with acute myocardial infarction.

Therapeutic Advances

- *Statins:* These are cholesterol lowering drugs. Drawback is risk of development of cholesterol stones in gallbladder.
- *Prophylactic use of aspirin:* Aspirin inhibits platelets aggregation. Excessive use of aspirin causes ulcers in gastrointestinal tract. Patient hospitalized with acute myocardial infarction treated with anticoagulants may bleed from GIT ulcers in such patients on aspirin therapy.
- *Thrombolytic agents:* Administration of thrombolytic agents such as streptokinase or tissue plasminogen activator (TPA) cause lysis of recently formed thrombus to reestablish the coronary blood flow. It can at least help to reduce further myocardial damage.

Revascularization Procedures

- *Ballooning angioplasty:* It is percutaneous transmural coronary angioplasty. Balloon angioplasty dilates and ruptures the atheromatous plaque. Its disadvantage is re-stenosis of coronary arteries.
- *Intracoronary stenting:* Intracoronary stents decrease the rate of restenosis of coronary vessels. During procedure, most common early complication is a *localized dissection* with *thrombosis.*
- *Coronary artery bypass graft (CABG):* It is used for *multi-vessel coronary artery atherosclerosis.* Internal mammary artery is always spared from atheromatous plaque. Therefore, internal mammary artery graft is best. This graft has longer life in comparison to saphenous vein graft.

Saphenous vein graft undergoes adaptive arterialization of the vessels and reparative changes. Atheromatous plaques in saphenous vein grafts are formed in 5–10 years that is indistinguishable from those found in native coronary arteries, a process referred to as atherosclerotic *restenosis.*

PATHOGENESIS

Disrupted Atheromatous Plaque

Disrupted atheromatous plaque in coronary arteries and platelets play most important role in the pathogenesis of acute myocardial infarction. It leads to occlusion of coronary arteries (stenosis >90%) (Fig. 16.5). Concentric and eccentric atheromatous plaques and their clinical significance are given in Fig. 16.6.

Role of Platelets

- *Platelets adhesion:* Sudden disruption of atheromatous plaque leads to exposure of subendothelial collagen and non-collagenous microfibrils to platelets and clotting factors. It results in adherence of platelets to the subendothelial surface. The von Willebrand factor (vWF) synthesized by endothelium mediates interaction of specific platelet surface glycoprotein receptors and subendothelial collagen fibers.
- *Platelets release reaction:* Soon after adhesion, platelets undergo a process known as *release reaction.* Platelets undergo morphological changes from a disc shape to a spherical shape. Platelets containing microtubules undergo constriction resulting in release of contents stored in granules into the open canalicular system, such as ADP, catecholamine, serotonin and PDGF.
- *Platelets aggregation:* ADP and thromboxane A_2 synthesized by platelets play an important role in aggregation of platelets. Activation of coagulation system generates thrombin. Binding of thrombin, along with ADP and thromboxane A_2 to platelet surface receptors result in further aggregation. ADP produces conformational changes of the platelets surface GpIIb-IIIa receptors, to which noncleaved fibrinogen binds. Thus, fibrinogen forms bridges between platelets resulting in formation of secondary hemostatic plug.

Less Common Causes

- *Nonatherosclerotic lesions:* These include polyarteritis nodosa, Kawasaki disease, and systemic lupus erythematosus and syphilitic aortitis.
- *Embolization of coronary arteries:* Emboli from left-sided mural thrombus, infective vegetative endocarditis or paradoxical emboli from right side of heart through a patent foramen ovale may block the coronary blood flow leading to acute myocardial infarction.
- *Thrombotic syndromes:* Antithrombin III deficiency and polycythemia are less common causes of acute myocardial infarction.
- *Vasospasm of coronary arteries:* Vasospasm of coronary vessels with or without coronary atherosclerosis and possible association with platelets aggregation and release of thromboxane A_2 may cause myocardial infarction. In cocaine drug abuse, cocaine may cause sudden vasospasm resulting in acute myocardial infarction.
- *Homodynamic alteration:* Patient undergoing surgery under spinal anesthesia developing hypotensive shock may lead to acute myocardial infarction.

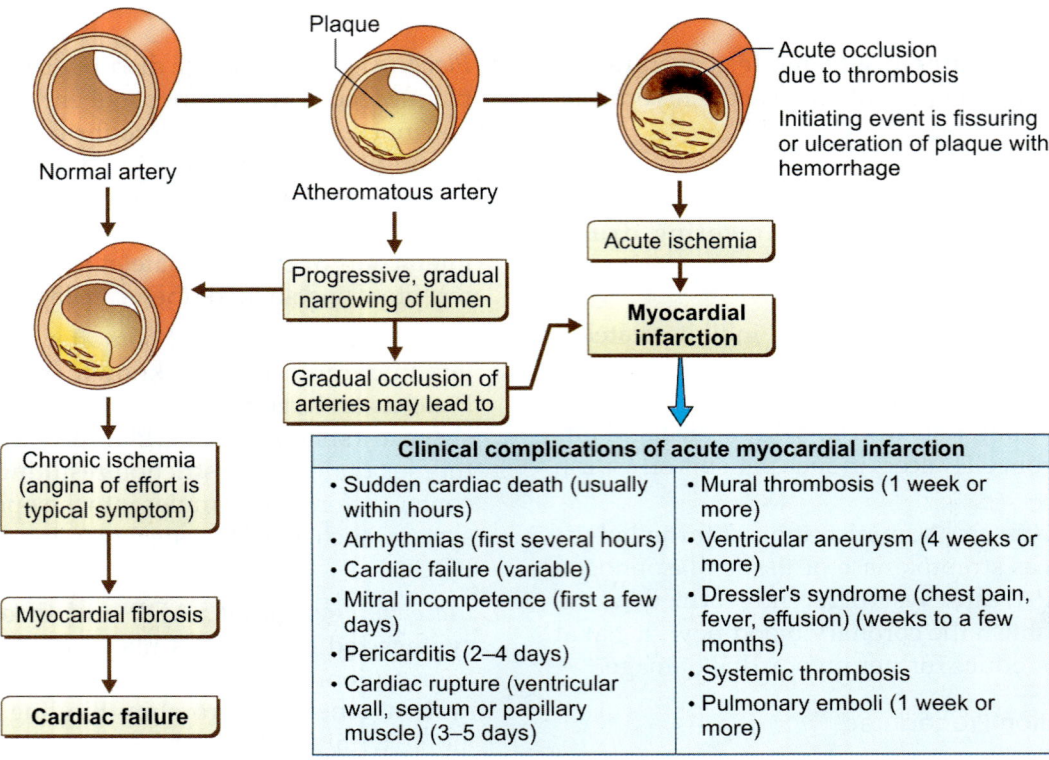

Fig. 16.5: Sequence of events of acute myocardial infarction and its complications.

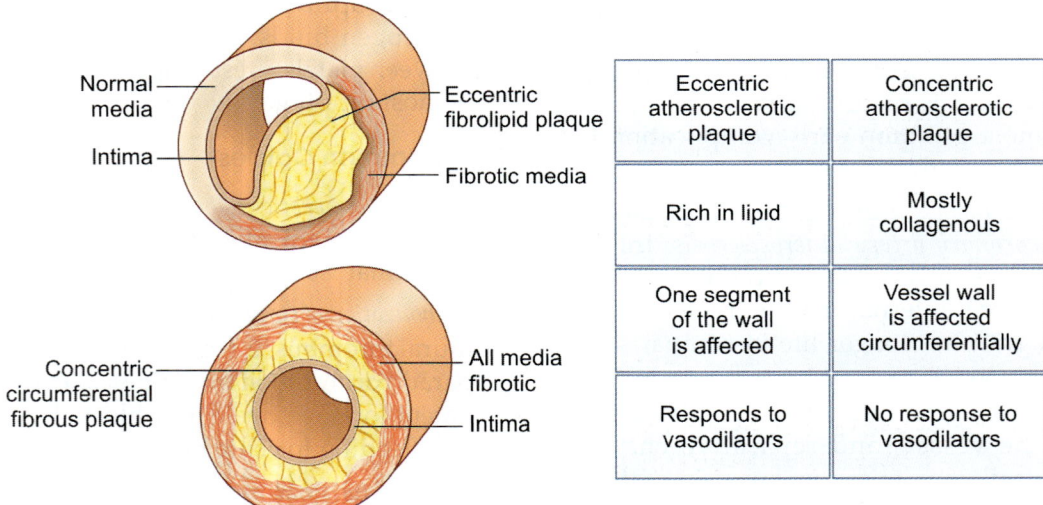

Fig. 16.6: Coronary arteries show eccentric or concentric lesion and their clinical correlation.

- *Congenital abnormal origin of LAD:* Abnormal origin of left anterior descending artery may cause acute myocardial infarction.
- *Dissecting hematoma of aorta:* It may ascend and cause compression of coronary arteries at site of origin resulting in acute myocardial infarction.
- *Trauma to coronary arteries:* Direct trauma to coronaries during accident may cause acute myocardial infarction.

TYPES OF MYOCARDIAL INFARCT

- Gross morphology of myocardial infarct depends on extent of involvement of myocardium. There are three types of myocardial infarcts (transmural, subendocardial and circumferential infarcts).
- ECG is diagnostic of AMI in 75–80% cases (appearance of new Q wave). Appearance of new Q wave on ECG is more dependent on the volume of infarct area rather than transmural tissue infarction. That is the

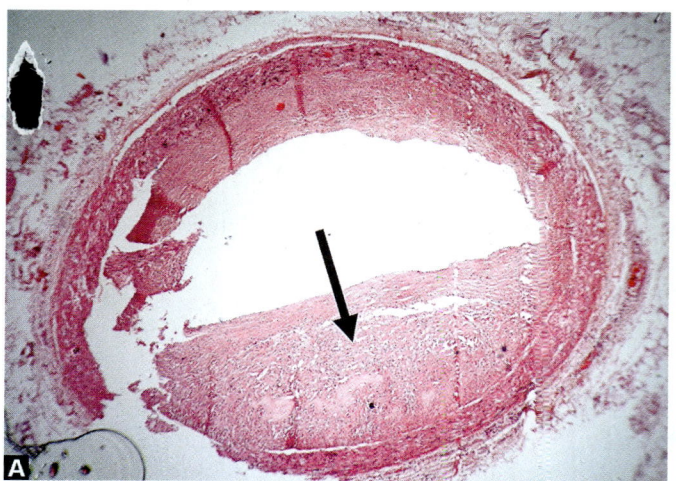 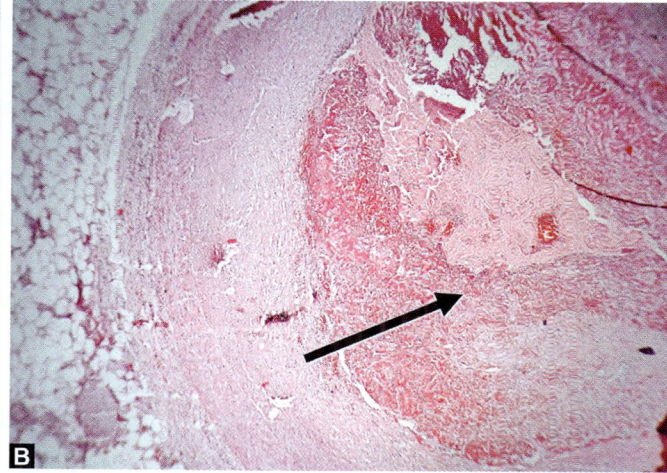

Fig. 16.7: Coronary arteries. (A) Shows atheromatous plaque partial occlusion (arrow) (400X) and (B) shows complicated atheromatous plaque with thrombus formation and complete occlusion (arrow) (400X).

reason that ST segment study is important, which differentiates transmural and subendocardial infarcts.

Transmural Infarct

Transmural infarction involves the entire ventricular wall from endocardium to epicardium including involvement of interventricular septum.
- *Pathogenesis:* It is caused by disrupted atheromatous plaque with superimposed thrombus. Blood supply to the heart is not restored after ischemia. In a small number of cases, transmural infarct is related to thromboemboli or vasospasm.
- *ECG study:* It reveals ST segment elevation (STEMI) and appearance of new Q wave. ST segment elevation indicates area of injury and loss of normal myocardial cell membrane ion pumps. Appearance of new Q wave indicates extent of myocardial infarct.
- *Therapeutic correlation:* These patients require emergency treatment to reopen the obstructed coronary artery either by coronary angioplasty or drugs that activate the plasminogen system to lyse thrombosis in coronary arteries.

Subendocardial Infarct

Under physiologic state, subendocardium region of myocardium receives oxygen and nutrients by diffusion directly from the circulating blood in the ventricular cavity.

Subendocardial infarct involves inner one-third to inner half of the left ventricular wall or sometimes right ventricle. It exhibits multi-focal areas coagulative necrosis. Isolated infarcts of right ventricle and right atrium are extremely rare.
- *Pathogenesis:* Typically, subendocardial infarct occurs as a result of decreased perfusion of myocardium in hypotensive shock, and blood supply to heart is restored.
- *ECG study:* It reveals absence of ST segment elevation (NSTEMI) as well as appearance of new Q wave. In minority of cases, ECG study reveals absence of ST segment elevation and appearance of new Q wave.
- *Diagnostic correlation:* These patients require estimation of cardiac troponins for establishing diagnosis.

REPERFUSION INJURY

Reperfusion of the myocardial infarct by therapeutic administration of thrombolytic agents may cause further injury to heart by synthesis of oxygen derived free radicals.

Oxygen-derived Free Radicals

- Initially, ischemia produced cellular damage results in generation of oxygen derived free radical species.
- Subsequently, reperfusion by thrombolytic agents provides abundant molecular oxygen (O_2) to generate more oxygen derived free radical species through the xanthine oxidase pathway in activated neutrophils.
- These oxygen derived free radicals injure viable myocytes.

Histological Alterations

Reperfusion histologically alters irreversibly damaged cells. It produces contraction band necrosis of myofibrils in dying cells due to influx of calcium into the cytosol.

Removal of Necrosed Myocytes

Removal of irreversibly damaged myocytes improves short- and long-term function and survival. It prevents any further damage to myocardial cells. It limits the size of the infarction.

MORPHOLOGICAL CHANGES

Gross Morphology
- No gross changes are evident within 24 hours of myocardial infarction. In autopsy specimen, myocardial infarct area can be appreciated by applying triphenyl tetrazolium chloride (TTC) to slices of infarct heart (2–3 hours old). Due to depletion of dehydrogenase enzyme, infarct area of myocardium remains unstained.
- Normal myocardium is rich in dehydrogenase enzyme, hence gives uniform brownish discoloration to the dye TTC.

Light Microscopy
Irreversible injury occurs in 20–40 minutes. It shows wavy myocardial fibers within 1–3 hours of myocardial infarction. There may be eosinophilia of myocardial fibers.

- *Acute inflammatory changes:* Neutrophils accumulate at the peripheral zone and then infiltrate the necrotic tissue within 18–24 hours. Two days after myocardial infarction, the affected heart muscle will show coagulative necrosis with loss of cross striations, contraction bands, edema, and hemorrhage. Neutrophils are replaced by macrophages.
- *Healing stage:* Proliferation of fibroblasts results in fibrosis of infarct area. Myocardial cells being terminally differentiated permanent cells are unable to regenerate and healing occur by fibrosis. However, the patient may die due to electrical disturbances before the infarct heals. Examination of the heart in such cases at autopsy will reveal the typical macroscopic features of an infarct at various stages of evolution and/or healing (Figs 16.8, 16.9 and Table 16.4).

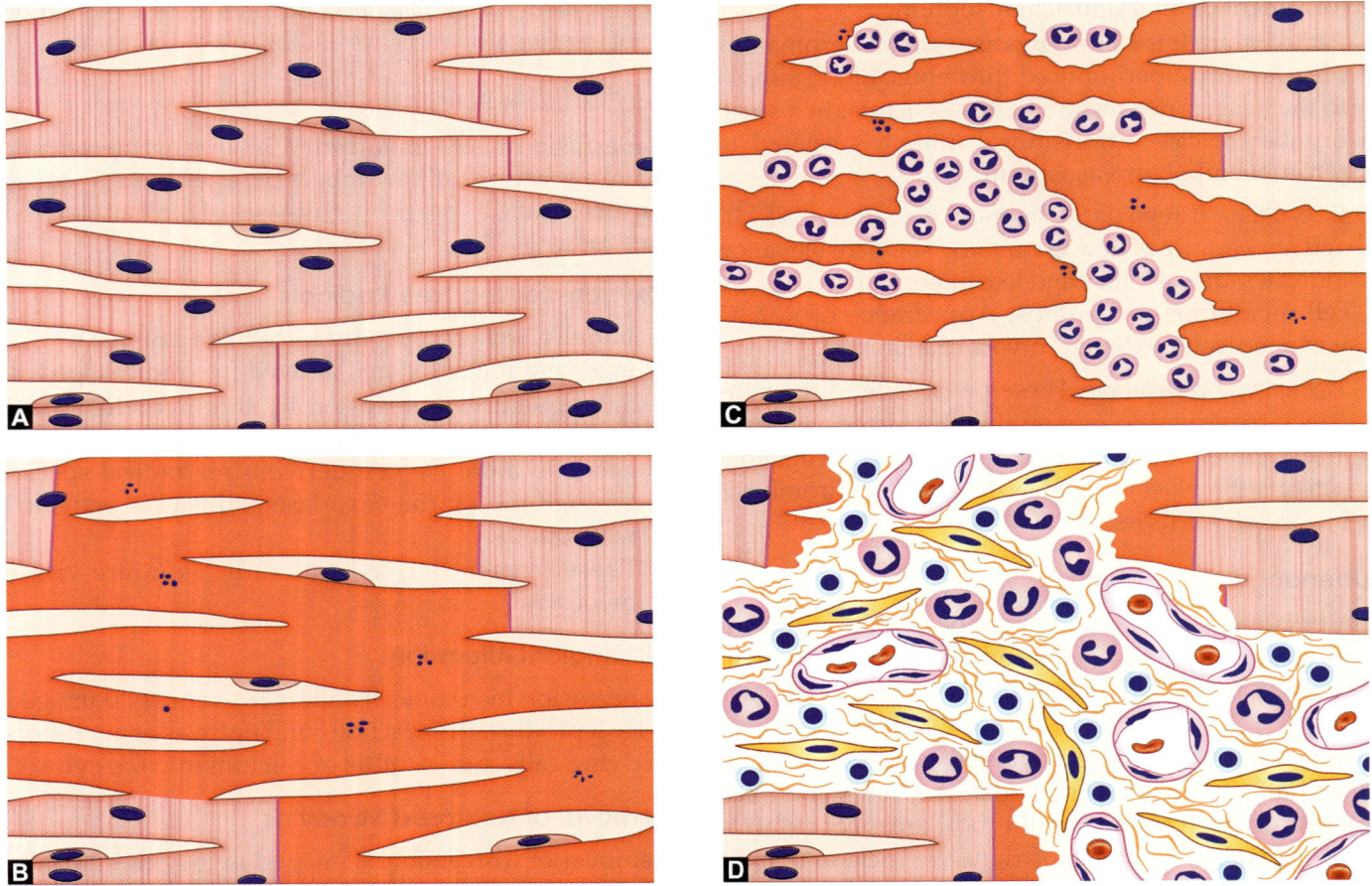

Fig. 16.8: Morphological changes in acute myocardial infarction. (A) Normal heart muscles, (B) coagulative necrosis of acute myocardial infarct (AMI) after 12 to 18 hours, (C) PMN cells about 24 hours after acute myocardial infarct (AMI), (D) granulation tissue after about 3 weeks of acute myocardial infarct (AMI).

Heart

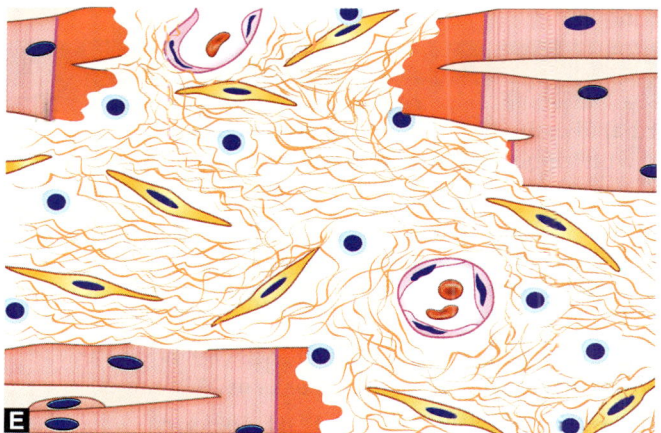

Fig. 16.8E: Morphological changes in acute myocardial infarction—after 3 months or more, the infarct myocardium has been replaced by scar tissue.

CLINICAL COMPLICATIONS

Clinical manifestations of acute myocardial infarction depend upon the size and location of the infarction, as well as pre-existing myocardial damage. Arrhythmia is the most common cause of death in early 0–4 hours of AMI. Risk of myocardial rupture is greatest complication within first 3–7 days. Ventricular aneurysm is common in scarred area after 7 weeks of AMI.

Cardiogenic Shock

Cardiogenic shock is commonly associated with large infarcts. It occurs in the first 24 hours in 10–15% cases. Weakening of the myocardium leads to *cardiac failure*. Revascularization improves survival.

Cardiac Arrhythmias

- Arrhythmias account for half of all deaths within the first 24 hours after an acute myocardial infarction. The risk of arrhythmia is greatest within the first 6 hours after myocardial infarct.
- Acute infarction is often associated with premature ventricular beats, ventricular tachycardia, complete heart block (anterior or posterior region), ventricular fibrillation and cardiogenic shock with fatal outcome within 2 days of acute myocardial infarction.

Sudden Cardiac Death

Most often, sudden cardiac death occurs due to ventricular arrhythmia and other electrical disturbances. It occurs within an hour of onset of symptoms in acute myocardial infarction. It occurs more frequently in the morning hours, when hypercoagulability is at its peak.

- *Pathogenesis:* Disrupted atheromatous plaque releases thromboplastin, which initiates thrombus formation in affected coronary artery. It results in complete occlusion of the coronary artery with superimposed thrombus (>80% lumen occlusion) resulting in ischemia. Ventricular arrhythmia is the cause of death in these patients.
- *Autopsy findings:* Most patients have severe, fixed atherosclerotic coronary artery disease involving one or more coronary arteries. However, a grossly obvious coronary thrombosis or acute changes in the myocardium (coagulative necrosis) are not usually present.

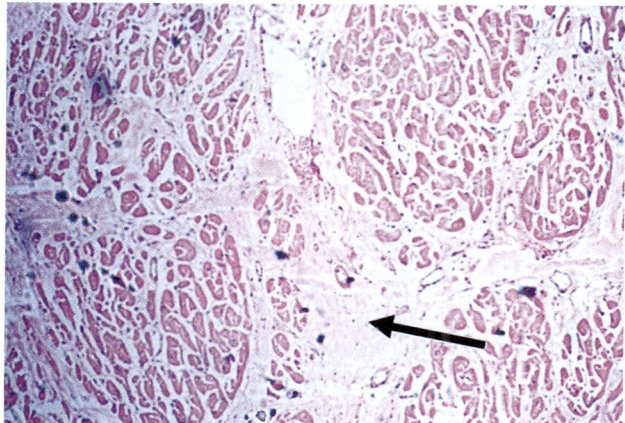

Fig. 16.9: Healed myocardium after infarction (arrow).

Congestive Heart Failure

Congestive heart failure usually occurs within the first 24 hours. Patient develops breathlessness as a result of pulmonary edema.

Fibrinous Pericarditis with or without Effusion

- Acute fibrinous pericarditis occurs with a transmural infarction usually within 2–10 days. It occurs as a result of increased vessel permeability in the pericardium with pouring of fibrinous exudate in the pericardium (Fig. 16.10).

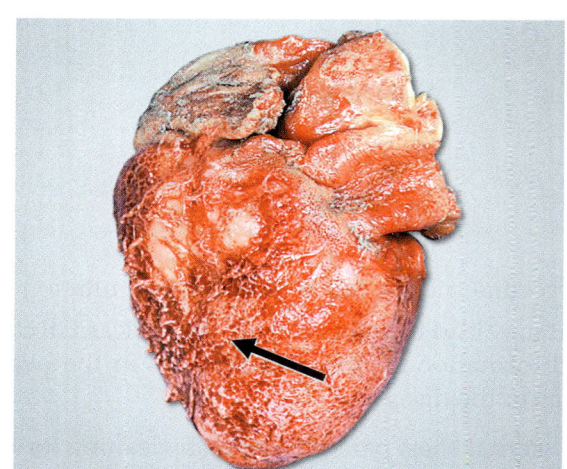

Fig. 16.10: Fibrinous pericarditis (arrow).

Table 16.4: Progressive morphological changes in myocardial infarction

Time post-AMI	Gross morphology	Microscopic examination	Laboratory findings
0–4 hours	No change	Wavy myocardial fibers Staining defect with triphenyl tetrazolium chloride in 2–3 hours	No change
4–12 hours	No change	Coagulative necrosis begins with loss of cross striations, contraction bands, edema, hemorrhage and early neutrophilic infiltrate	CK-MB (4–8 hours) LDH (10 hours) AST (6–12 hours)
12–24 hours	Early pallor of myocardium due to coagulative necrosis	Continued coagulative necrosis with nuclear pyknosis, marginal contraction bands, loss of cardiac striations with eosinophilic cardiac fibers and neutrophilic infiltrate in interstitial tissue. Cytoplasm displays affinity for acidophilic dyes	CK-MB (4–8 hours) and peaks in 24 hours LDH (10 hours) AST (6–12 hours)
1–3 days (24–72 hours)	Definite pallor of the infarct area with zone of hyperemia	On second day, total loss of striations and nuclei along with heavy neutrophilic infiltrate. Some macrophages start appearing in the infarct area	CK-MB starts disappearing LDH flip peaks in 2–3 days AST peaks 1–2 days
3–7 days	On 4th day, central yellow infarct area with well demarcated hyperemic border. There is maximum softness and danger of rupture	On 4th day, there is influx of macrophages from hyperemic area, which slowly replace neutrophils and remove the dead myocardial cells At end of first week, it shows fibrovascular response with formation of granulation tissue surrounding area of infarct	LDH starts disappearing
7–10 days	Same findings as seen in 1–3 days. Central yellow area and well demarcated hyperemic border. There is maximum softness and danger of rupture	By the end of first week, neovascularization marks the beginning of granulation tissue formation, i.e. repair with collagen synthesis. Macrophages infiltration is present	CK-MB is absent, as it disappears by 3–4 days LDH disappears in 5–9 days AST disappears
10–21 days	Maximum yellow and soft central area with vascular margins by third week (21 days)	During second week, fibrovascular response begins to form granulation tissue to replace the yellow necrotic myocardium By third week, granulation tissue slowly transforms into a fibrous scar, i.e. repair. Phagocytosis of necrotic debris by macrophages is complete. Inflammatory infiltrate recedes	No enzyme or cardiac troponins are detected in blood after 2 weeks
7 weeks	White fibrosis	Infarct tissue is replaced by white, patchy and non-contractile scar tissue by sixth week Ventricular aneurysm may occur in scarred area	No enzyme or cardiac troponins are detected in blood after 2 weeks

- Precordial friction rub is heard on auscultation.
  It may lead to obliteration of the pericardial cavity and formation of fibrous adhesions in the healing stage of the disease.
- Substernal chest pain is relieved by leaning forward and aggravated by leaning backward.

Myocardial Rupture

Rupture of the heart occurs within 3–7 days after myocardial infarction, when the necrotic area has the least tensile strength. It occurs in transmural due to *softening* of the necrosed myocardium by increased neutrophil activity before organization is established (Figs 16.11 and 16.12).

Heart

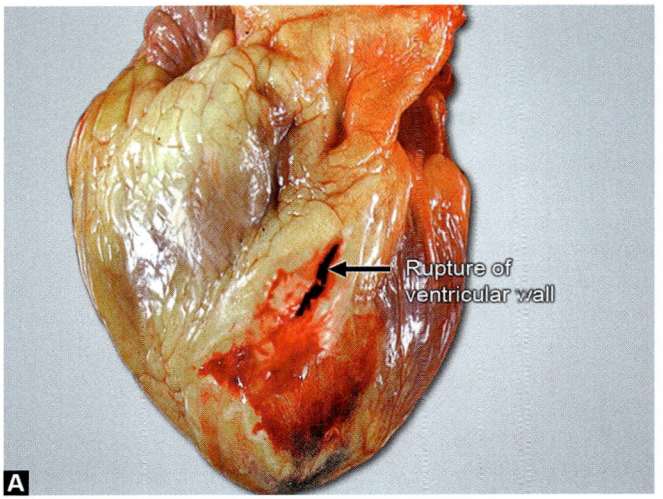
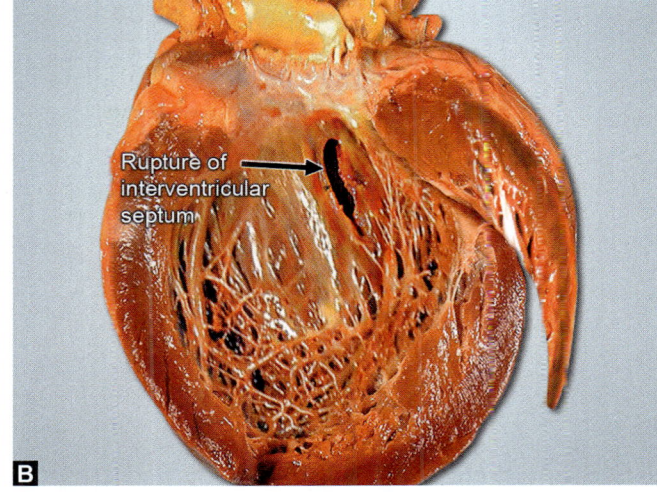

Fig. 16.11: Acute myocardial infarction. (A) Shows rupture of ventricular wall and (B) shows rupture of interventricular septum.

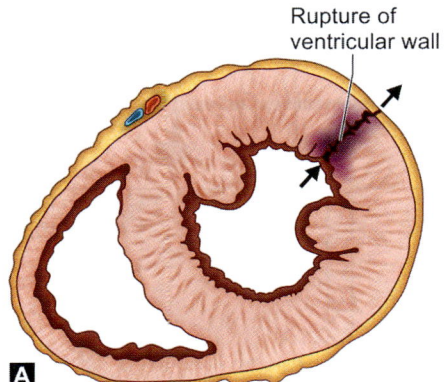
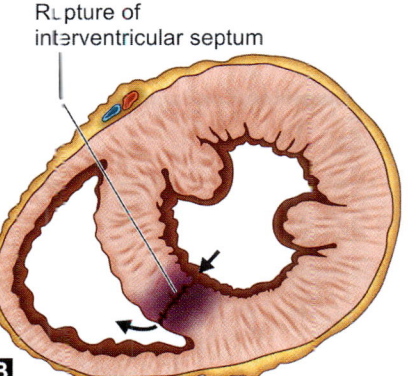
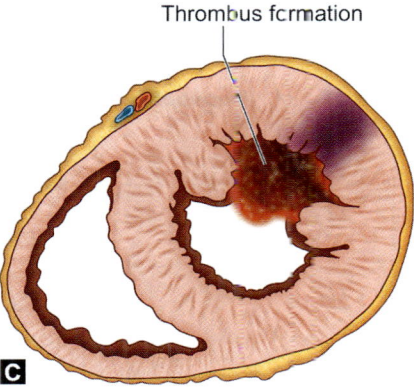

Fig. 16.12: Acute myocardial infarction. (A) Shows rupture of ventricular wall, (B) shows rupture of interventricular septum, and (C) shows thrombus formation.

- *Rupture of anterior wall of left ventricle:* The anterior wall of the heart is the most frequent site of rupture, usually resulting in fatal *cardiac tamponade*. It occurs in transmural infarct.

  High pressure in left ventricle blows out the necrotic myocardium resulting in rupture of anterior wall. Rupture permits escape of massive blood into the pericardial cavity called hemopericardium. Patient dies of *cardiac tamponade*.

- *Posteromedial papillary muscle necrosis/dysfunction:* It is most often associated with right coronary artery thrombosis and inferior myocardial infarction.
- Since the damaged papillary muscle cannot contract, this typically causes acute onset of *mitral valve insufficiency/regurgitation* resulting left ventricular failure.
- *Interventricular septum rupture:* It is most often associated with anterior descending branch of left coronary artery thrombosis. Rupture of interventricular septum produces a left-to-right shunt resulting in right heart failure and pulmonary hypertension. There is increased O_2 saturation and pressure in right ventricle.

Mural Thrombi with Possible Embolization

Patient with acute myocardial infarction may develop thrombi in left ventricle, left atria and leg veins (Fig. 16.13).

- *Ventricular mural thrombi:* These are formed during first week of acute myocardial infarction as a result of left anterior descending artery (LAD) disease.

  Thrombi are attached to endocardium overlying infarct area of left ventricle. These thrombi have the potential for embolization to brain, intestine, kidney and lower limbs.

- *Atrial thrombi:* These develop in atrial appendages, especially if atrial rhythm is disturbed due to irregular blood flow inside the dilated and irregularly contracting left atrium, i.e. *atrial fibrillation* and *atrial flutter*.

- *Leg vein thrombosis:* It may develop due to prolonged bed rest and venous stasis. Patient presents with pain and swelling in the affected leg. Patient may have pulmonary embolism with fatal outcome

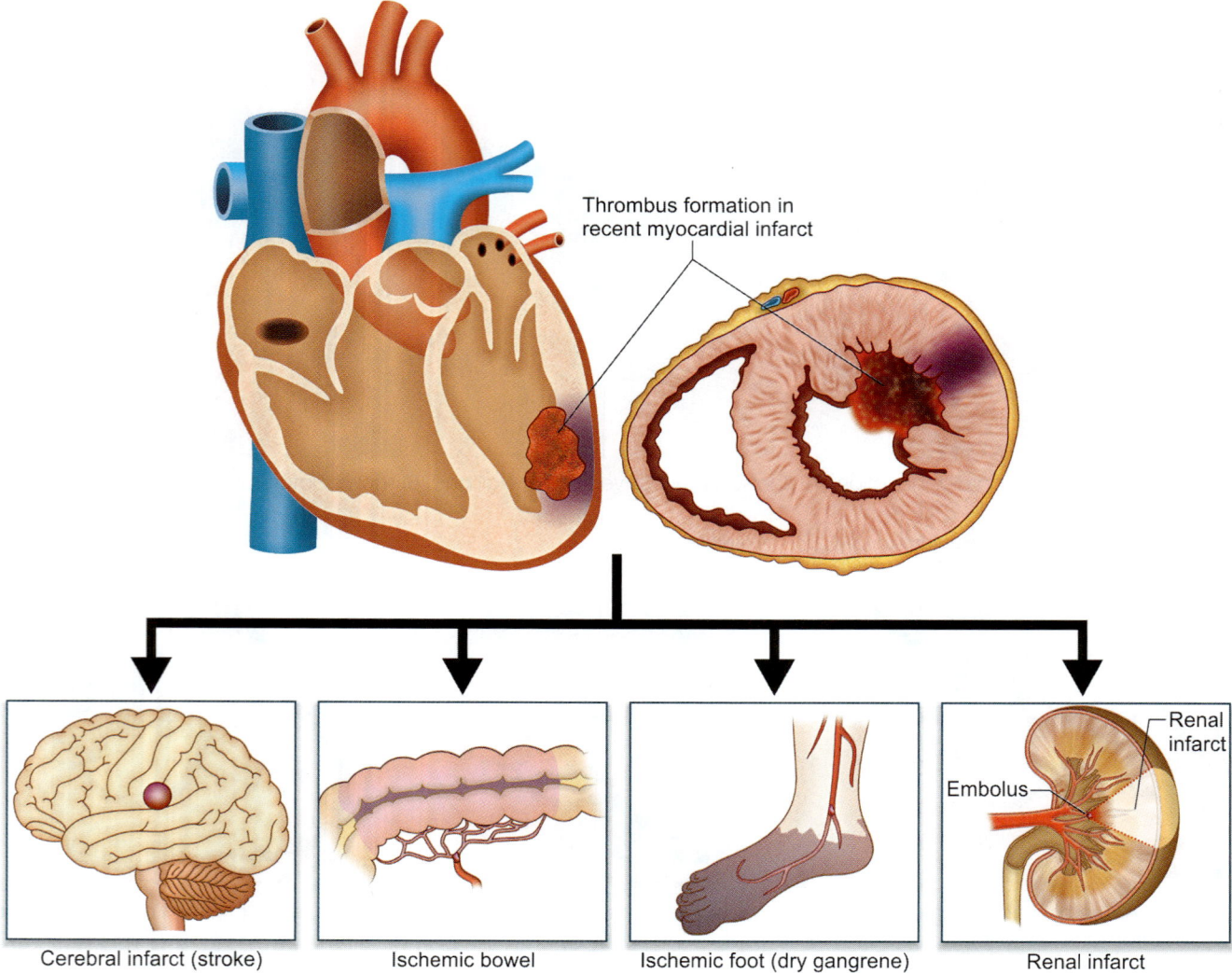

Fig. 16.13: Myocardial infarction. Thromboembolism phenomenon produces infarcts in vital organs.

Autoimmune Pericarditis

- Dressler's syndrome is a complication of transmural myocardial infarct after 2–10 weeks, clinically presenting with pericardial pain associated with pleural effusion, joints and fever (i.e. symptoms suggestive of serum sickness).
- Autoantibodies formed against pericardial proteins released from the necrotic cells results in pericarditis.
- Cortisone treatment is beneficial, also supporting an immunologic explanation.
- Other causes of immune-mediated pericarditis include systemic erythematosus, scleroderma and rheumatic heart disease.

Ventricular Aneurysm

- Ventricular aneurysms may develop in the large myocardial fibrotic scar within 3–6 months after myocardial infarct in 10–15% cases. During each systole, healed myocardial scar does not contract, and actually bulges out resulting in ventricular aneurysm.
- Mural thrombi also form over ventricular aneurysms, which are found at the site of a healed transmural myocardial infarct resulting in embolization. Rupture is uncommon as scar tissue has good tensile strength.

Right Ventricular AMI

Right ventricular infarcts occur in one-third of patients in the inferior region. It is associated with right coronary artery thrombosis. It is clinically significant in 30% of cases. Patient presents with hypotension, right heart failure and preserved left ventricular function.

Recurrent Myocardial Infarction

Recurrent myocardial infarction is characterized by the reappearance of CK-MB in blood after 3 days of acute myocardial infarction.

Table 16.5: Clinical complications of acute myocardial infarction

Complications	Interval	Mechanism
Sudden cardiac death	Usually within hours	Often ventricular fibrillation
Arrhythmias	First several hours	Pump failure results in hypotensive shock
Persistent pain	12 hours to a few days	Progressive myocardial necrosis (extension of infarcts)
Angina pectoris	Immediate or delayed (weeks)	Ischemia of non-infarcted cardiac muscle
Cardiac failure	Variable	Ventricular dysfunction occurs following muscle necrosis and arrhythmias
Mitral valve incompetence	First few days	Papillary muscle dysfunction, necrosis or rupture
Pericarditis	2–4 days	Transmural infarct with inflammation of pericardium
Cardiac rupture (ventricular wall, septum or papillary muscle)	3–5 days	Weakening of wall following muscle necrosis and acute inflammation
Mural thrombosis	1 week or more	Abnormal endothelial surface following infarction
Ventricular aneurysm	4 weeks or more	Stretching of newly formed collagenous scar tissue
Dressler's syndrome (chest pain, fever, effusion)	Weeks to a few months	Autoimmune mechanism
Pulmonary emboli	1 week or more	Deep venous thrombosis in lower limb

Expansion of Infarct Area

Patient may develop expansion of infarct area.

Systemic Venous Thrombosis

Patient may develop systemic venous thrombus formation.

Angina Pectoris (>12 hours)

Patient may present with symptoms of angina after 12 hours of myocardial infarction.

CLINICAL FEATURES

Patient with acute myocardial infarction may be symptomatic (majority cases) or asymptomatic (silent). Silent acute myocardial infarction occurs due to high pain threshold or problems with nervous system in diabetes mellitus and elderly persons.

Chest Pain

Patient presents with sudden onset of severe crushing substernal chest pain of long duration for 30 to 45 minutes in central portion of chest, which is not relieved by nitroglycerin. It is often precipitated by exertion. It occurs most often in the morning hours (catecholamine burst after awakening). It radiates down the left arm in 30% to the shoulders or to the jaw or epigastrium or beneath xiphoid process or occipital region. It never radiates below umbilicus.

Constitutional Symptoms

Patient develops breathlessness, fever, discomfort, giddiness. Severe distress is marked by symptoms such as nausea, sweating and vomiting.

Clinical Findings

Patient shows pallor and cold extremities, tachycardia (sympathetic overactivity), bradycardia (parasympathetic overactivity), apical pulse difficult to palpate, apical systolic murmur due to mitral regurgitation (due to papillary muscle necrosis) pericardial friction rub—fibrinous pericarditis and raised jugular venous pressure due to right heart failure.

LABORATORY DIAGNOSIS

The prognosis depends on the degree of left ventricular dysfunction. The electrocardiogram (ECG), cardiac enzymes (CK-MB), and cardiac-specific troponin I assays are the main diagnostic tools in confirming an AMI.

Electrocardiogram (12 Leads)

ECG (12 leads) gives a good guide as to which coronary artery is narrowed and the extent of myocardial damage.

It is diagnostic of AMI in 75–80% cases during the first 2 days of onset of the infarction. Acute infarcts are now classified according to presence or absence of ST-segment elevation and appearance or absence of Q wave on ECG.

- *Transmural infarct:* ECG shows ST elevation (STEMI) along with appearance of new Q wave in 75–80% cases of myocardial infarction. It is more dependent on the volume of infarct area rather than transmural infarction (Fig. 16.14).
- *Subendocardial infarct:* ECG shows absence of ST segment elevation (NSTEMI), as well as appearance of new Q wave (Q wave absent). These patients require estimation of troponins for diagnosis.

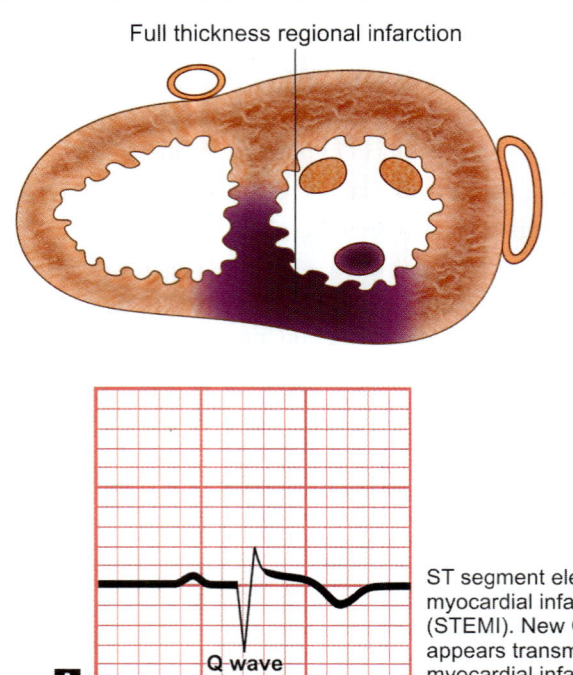
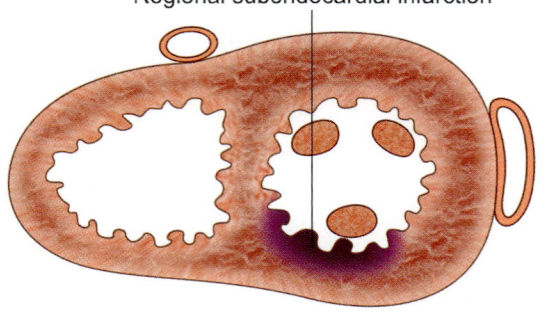
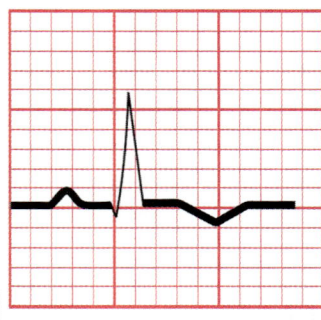

Fig. 16.14: Acute myocardial infarction.

Serum Cardiac Enzymes

Cardiac enzymes like creatine kinase-MB (CK-MB), lactic dehydrogenase (LDH) and aspartate aminotransferase (AST) are estimated to diagnose myocardial infarction (Table 16.6).

- *Creatine kinase-MB (CK-MB):* It exists in two isoforms, i.e. CK-MB1 and CK-MB2 with sensitivity 95%. If ratio of these two isoforms (CK-MB1:CK-MB2) is 1.5 or more, it is an excellent indicator for early acute myocardial infarction. Its half-life is 16 hours; it appears within 4 to 8 hours, peaks at 24 hours and disappears within 1.5 to 4 days. Serial testing for a period of 9 to 12 hours after myocardial infarction will provide a pattern to determine whether CK-MB is rising, indicative of myocardial injury. Subsequent elevation of serum CK-MB after 4 days of acute myocardial infarction is indicative of recurrent re-infarction.
- *Lactate dehydrogenase (LDH):* It is an excellent indicator for myocardial infarction. Its half-life is 54 hours. It begins to rise within 12–24 hours, peaks at 2–3 days and disappears within 7 to 14 days due to its more half-life. It exists in two isoforms, i.e. LDH-1 and LDH-2.

  Ordinarily, ratio of LDH-2 to LDH-1 is >1. But in acute myocardial infarction, this pattern is *flipped* and ratio of LDH-1 to LDH-2 becomes higher.
- *Aspartate aminotransferase (AST):* Aspartate aminotransferase (AST) first appears in 6–12 hours, peaks in 1–2 days, and disappears within 3–4 days (half-life 20 hours). This test is not performed to diagnose acute myocardial infarction.

Cardiac Troponins (Tn I and Tn T)

Cardiac troponins (Tn I and Tn T) are structural components of cardiac muscle, which regulate calcium mediated contractions.

- *Cardiac troponins:* Following acute myocardial infarction, cardiac troponins are released into the bloodstream within 3 to 12 hours. Its level attains peak

Table 16.6: Serum estimation of cardiac enzymes in acute myocardial infarction

Cardiac enzymes	Half-life	Rise	Peak	Baseline
CK-MB enzyme (ratio of MB-1 to MB-2 is >1.5)	16 hours	4–8 hours	24 hours (18–36 hours)	(1.5–4 days) except recurrent myocardial infarction sensitivity 95%
SGOT (AST) aspartate aminotransferase	20 hours	8 hours	18–36 hours	3–4 days
LDH-1:LDH-2 ratio is >1 (Normally LDH-2 > LDH-1)	54 hours	It appears within 12–24 hours of AMI	2–3 days	LDH disappears within 7–14 days

Troponin I and CK-MB elevations are highly characteristic of myocardial infarction.

at 24 hours disappear within 7–10 days. Troponin I (Tn I) is more specific indicator of myocardial injury. Troponin T lacks some specificity because elevations can also appear in skeletal myopathies and with renal failure.

- *Serial testing:* Serial testing of troponin I (Tn I) in blood is a diagnostic tool in these patients. Its sensitivity is 84–96% and specificity is 80–95%. False positive results are usually related to ischemia in patients with unstable angina. CK-MB is used in conjunction in cardiac troponins I (Tn I) to diagnose myocardial infarction. CK-MB detects re-infarction, while troponins do not (Fig. 16.15).

Cardiac Imaging Techniques

- *Echocardiography two-dimensional:* This technique is useful for demonstrating abnormally contracting parts of ventricular myocardium and visualizing thrombi or ruptures in the wall of the myocardium. It is difficult to differentiate between acute myocardial infarct and old myocardial infarct. Doppler echocardiography is done to detect VSD and mitral valve regurgitation due to myocardial infarction.
- *High resolution MRI:* A standard imaging agent *gadolinium* is administered. As normal myocytes are tightly packed, hence agent does not penetrate. But the agent penetrates into the expanded intercellular junction of infarct zone.
- *Radionuclide scanning (^{99m}Tc) stannous pyrophosphate:* It is performed 2–5 days after AMI. It is a chemical which emits radioactive γ-rays (similar to X-rays) after intravenous dose or oral dose. More active cells of organs take up more of the radionuclide hence, emit radioactive γ-rays as (*hot spots*) on the picture on the computer monitor. Poor blood flow to organs, emit low levels of γ-rays may be shown as blue *cold spots*.
- *Perfusion scintigraphy:* Thallium 201 or Tc 99m sestamibi is administered. It is concentrated in viable myocardium. It is difficult to differentiate acute myocardial infarct from old myocardial infarct.

Other Important Parameters

- *Hyperhomocystinemia:* Serum homocysteine level >100 μm/L is associated with increased risk of coronary arterial disease and peripheral vascular disease.
- *C-reactive proteins:* C-reactive proteins (CRP) synthesized by liver cause opsonization of bacteria and activation of complement. Its level is increased in patients with disrupted coronary atheromatous plaques resulting in acute myocardial infarction. It may be a strong predictor of cardiovascular events,

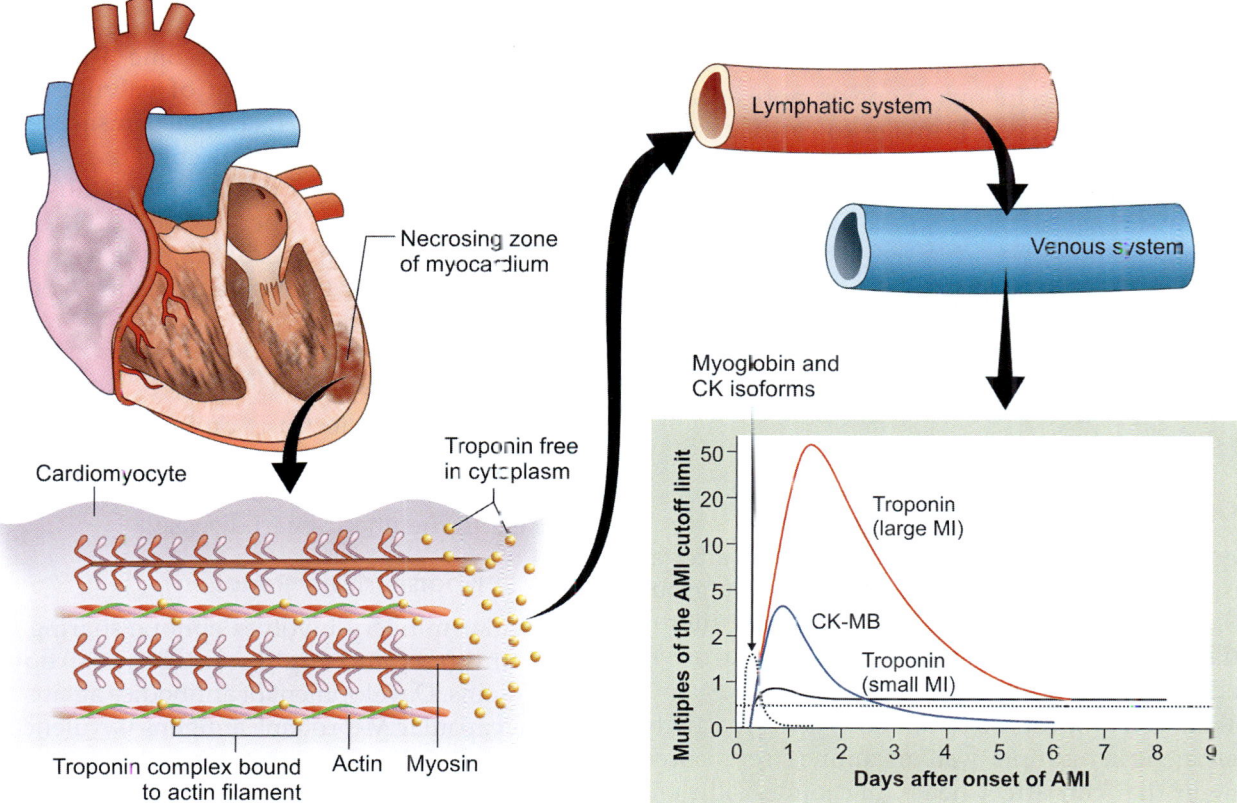

Fig. 16.15: Acute myocardial infarction (AMI)—CK-MB and cardiac troponins.

e.g. acute myocardial infarction, stroke and peripheral vascular disease than serum LDL level.

Nonspecific indexes of tissue necrosis: Leukocytosis (neutrophilia) occurs within 6 hours and persists for 3–7 days. Patient has fever 39°C before Q wave appears and persists for a week. ESR rises more slowly and persists for 1–2 weeks.

CHRONIC ISCHEMIC HEART DISEASE

Chronic ischemic damage to myocardial tissue resulting in progressive congestive heart failure. Focal replacement of myocardium resulting in non-contractile scar tissue. Myocardial fibrosis tends to be progressive, reflecting the progression of atheromatous plaque. Loss of myocardium in scar tissue is accompanied by increased oxygen demand.

Clinical Features

Patient presents with symptoms related to congestive heart failure and coronary artery insufficiency. Patient may develop congested cardiomyopathy.

RHEUMATIC FEVER AND RHD

GENERAL CONSIDERATIONS

Rheumatic Fever

Rheumatic fever is a multisystem autoimmune disorder affecting periarteriolar connective tissue. It usually occurs 1–4 weeks after an episode of exudative pharyngitis caused by Group A *Streptococcus* β-*haemolyticus*. Patient develops pancarditis, transient mild migratory polyarthritis, chorea, erythema marginatum and subcutaneous nodules.

Rheumatic Heart Disease (RHD)

Rheumatic heart disease comprises spectrum of lesions from pericarditis, myocarditis, and valvulitis during acute rheumatic fever (ARF), to chronic valvular lesions that evolve over years following one or more episodes of acute rheumatic fever. Damage to cardiac valves may be chronic and progressive, resulting in cardiac decompensation.

AGE GROUP

Rheumatic fever most often affects children between 5 and 15 years of age (80%). It may affect 20% adults. It rarely affects <4 years and adults >40 years. Poverty and overcrowding contribute to increased incidence in under developed countries.

ETIOLOGY

- Rheumatic fever usually occurs 1–4 weeks after an episode of exudative pharyngitis caused by group A *Streptococcus* β-*haemolyticus*. An elevated titer of antistreptolysin-*O* (ASO) is evidence of a recent streptococcal infection.
- It is believed to be caused by antibody cross-reactivity, as antigens in multiple systems mimic streptococcal antigen that can affect heart, big joints, skin and brain.

MULTIPLE SYSTEMS INVOLVED

Shortly after the infection, signs appear within 2–3 weeks (1–5 weeks) in the heart (pancarditis), joints (migratory polyarthritis; most common), skin (erythema marginatum), basal ganglia (Sydenham's chorea) and subcutaneous nodules in soft tissues.

PATHOGENESIS

The pathogenesis of rheumatic fever, RHD and complications is known to involve molecular mimicry and genetic predisposition (Fig. 16.16).

Genetic Predisposition

HLA-DR7 located on chromosome 6 is most often associated with development of valvular lesions in rheumatic heart disease. Exact mechanism is unknown. It is suggested that HLA molecules may play role in presenting antigens to T cell receptors, thus triggering an immune response. There is increased expression of TNF-α cytokine in HLA-DR7 patients, which may exacerbate valvular tissue inflammation, contributing to RHD pathogenesis.

Mannose-binding Lectin (MBL-2)

Mannose-binding lectin is an inflammatory protein involved in pathogen recognition. Increased synthesis of mannose binding protein is associated with mitral stenosis in rheumatic heart disease.

Type II Hypersensitivity Reaction

Molecular mimicry involves epitope sharing between host antigens and highly antigenic streptococcal M-proteins. Development of antibodies against streptococcal capsular M-proteins antigens (virulence factor), cross react with some proteins in human connective tissue (e.g. heart-myosin, joints, skin, brain, arteries), and induce cytokine release resulting in tissue destruction

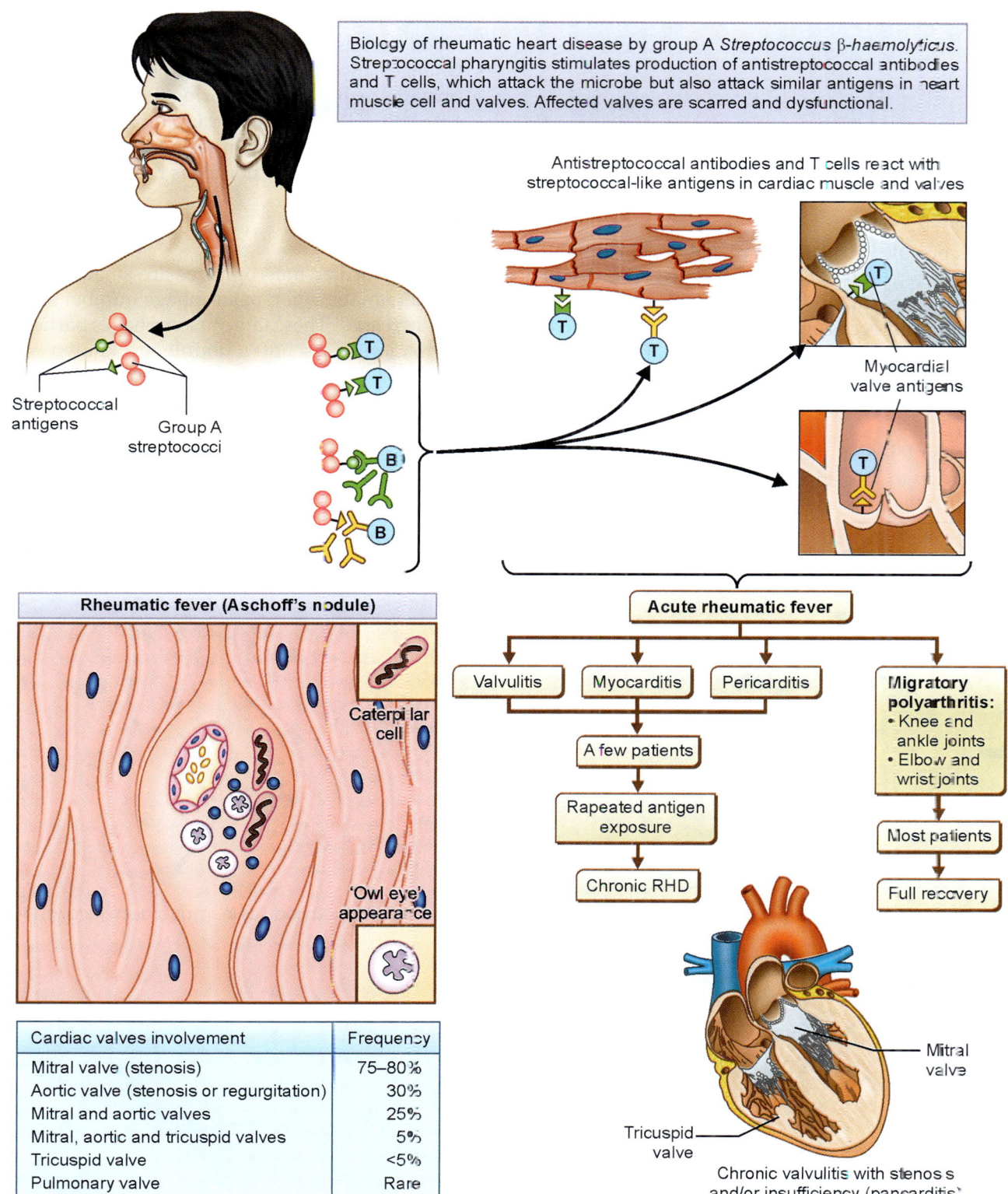

Fig. 16.16: Pathogenesis of rheumatic fever and heart disease and clinical manifestations.

in rheumatic fever. Antistreptolysin-O (ASO), anti-DNAase and hyaluronidase are estimated to establish streptococcal etiology of this disease. An elevated antistreptolysin-O (ASO) titer is a proof of a previous streptococcal infection.

Type IV Hypersensitivity Reaction

Type IV hypersensitivity reaction has been implicated in pathogenesis of rheumatic fever, as valvular lesions predominantly contain CD4+ T cells and macrophages. Rheumatic valves display increased expression of

VCAM-1, a protein that mediates the adhesion of CD4+ T cells.

ASCHOFF'S NODULE

Aschoff's nodule is the classic lesion of rheumatic fever. It develops after several weeks after the onset of symptoms.

Composition

Aschoff's nodule is composed of swollen eosinophilic collagen fibers, central fibrinoid necrosis surrounded by macrophages (Anitschkow myocytes'), lymphocytes, plasma cells and occasional multinucleated giant cells, demonstrated on light microscopy. It is globular, elliptic, or fusiform microscopic structure (Figs 16.17 and 16.18).

Phases

- *Early phase:* It is also known as exudative phase, which persists up to the 4th week of rheumatic fever. It is characterized by swelling of collagen fibers around blood vessels.
- *Granulomatous phase:* It is also known as proliferative phase, which is evident during the 4th to 13th weeks of the disease. It assumes granulomatous appearance.
- *Late phase:* It is also known as fibrous or healing phase. Eventually Aschoff's nodule is replaced by a nodule of scar tissue.

Anitschkow Cells

Normally, cardiac macrophages are small in number. But in rheumatic fever, macrophage number as well as size is increased. These large macrophages participating in formation of Aschoff's nodule are known as *Anitschkow cells*. Nuclei of these *Anitschkow cells* contain a central band of clumped chromatin, that gives *caterpillar-like appearance* in longitudinal sections (also called as caterpillar cells); and *owl-eyed* appearance in cross sections (Fig. 16.19).

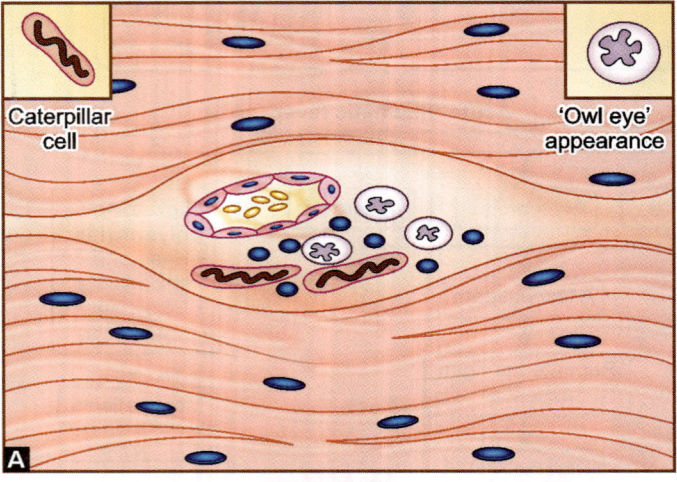

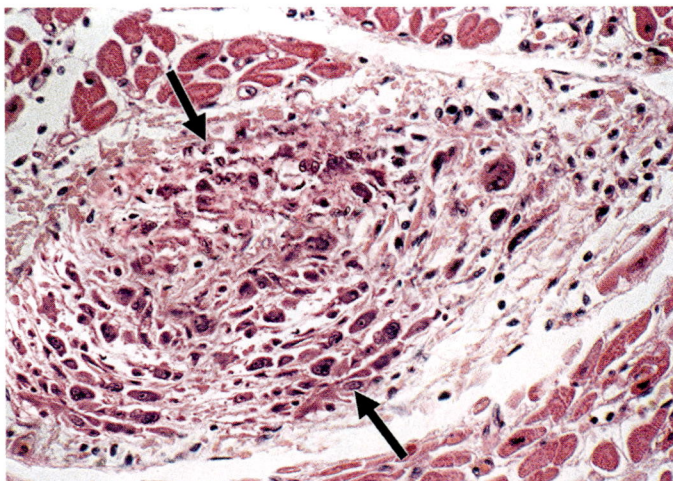

Fig. 16.18: Aschoff nodules in myocardium (arrows) (400X).

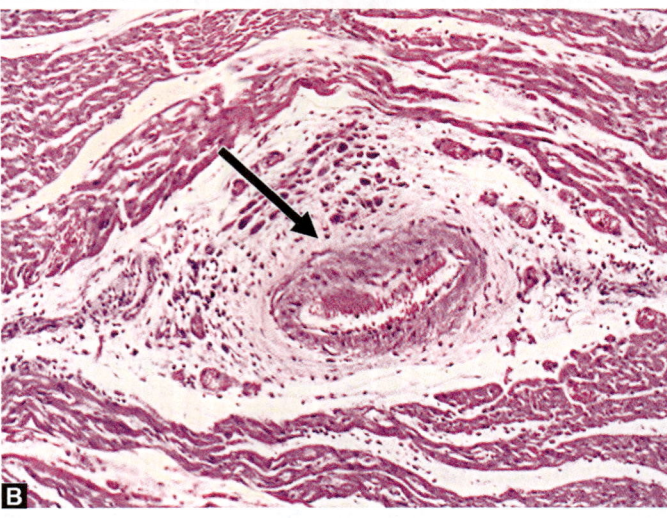

Fig. 16.17: (A) Aschoff nodules schematic, (B) Aschoff nodules in myocardium—these are centered in interstitium around vessels as shown here. The myocarditis may be severe enough to cause congestive heart failure (arrow) (100X).

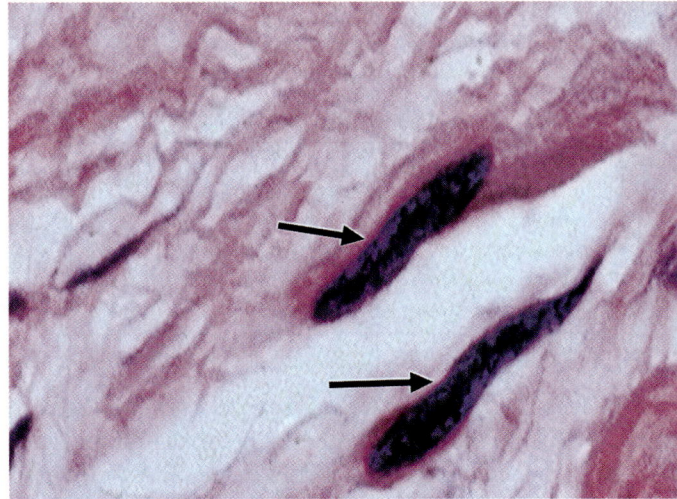

Fig. 16.19: Anitschkow/caterpillar cell in myocardium (arrows) (400X).

Giant Aschoff's Bodies

Fusion of multiple Aschoff's nodules produces giant Aschoff's bodies, located over bony prominences and tendons in subcutaneous regions.

Location

In acute rheumatic fever, Aschoff's nodules can be seen in periarteriolar tissue of any layer of the heart (most common in myocardium) and hence called *pancarditis*. Occasionally, these are present in the pericardium. These have also been described in the adventitia of the aorta.

Nature and Lesions

As Aschoff's nodules in big joints are *more exudative* and less proliferative in nature, thus inflammatory changes in the joints completely resolve and hence no residual effect like joint deformity. On the other hand, Aschoff's nodules in heart are more proliferative and less exudative type, resulting into fibrosis of cardiac valves (stenosis/incompetence of valves).

JONES DIAGNOSTIC CRITERIA

Diagnostic criteria was first published in 1944 by T. Duckett Jones. According to revised Jones criteria by American Heart Association, the diagnosis of rheumatic fever can be made when two of the major criteria, or one major criterion plus two minor criteria, are present along with evidence of streptococcal infection: elevated or rising antistreptolysin-*O* titer or DNAase. Exceptions are chorea and indolent carditis, each of which by itself can indicate rheumatic fever.

Major Diagnostic Criteria

- *Migratory polyarthritis (up to 75%):* It is a temporary migrating inflammation of the large joints, usually starting in the legs and migrating upwards.
- *Pancarditis (up to 35%):* Inflammation of the heart muscle (myocarditis) which can manifest as congestive heart failure with shortness of breath, pericarditis with a rub, or a new heart murmur.
- *Subcutaneous nodules (up to 10%):* Patient develops painless, firm collections of collagen fibers over bony prominences or tendon. They commonly appear on the back of the wrist, the outside elbow, and the front of the knees.
- *Skin rashes (erythema marginatum):* Skin rashes have bathing suit distribution (up to 10%). A long-lasting reddish rash that begins on the trunk or arms as macules, which spread outward and clear in the middle to form rings, which continue to spread and coalesce with other rings, ultimately taking on a snake-like appearance. This rash typically spares the face and is made worse with heat.
- *Sydenham's chorea:* It is known as *St. Vitus dance* (up to 10%). A characteristic series of random rapid involuntary movements without purpose of the face and arms. This can occur very late in the disease for at least three months from onset of infection.

Minor Diagnostic Criteria

- *Fever:* Patient has 38.2–38.9°C (101–102°F)
- *Arthralgia:* Patient presents with joint pain without swelling. It cannot be included if polyarthritis is present as a major symptom.
- *Increased acute phase reactants:* There is raised ESR and C-reactive protein values.
- *Total leukocyte count:* Peripheral smear examination shows leukocytosis: neutrophilia.
- *ECG study:* It shows features of first degree heart block, such as a prolonged PR interval. This minor cannot be included if carditis is present as a major symptom.
- *Past history:* Previous episode of rheumatic fever or inactive rheumatic heart disease.

OTHER SIGNS AND SYMPTOMS

There is preceding streptococcal infection: Recent scarlet fever raised antistreptolysin-O or other streptococcal antibody titer, or positive throat culture. Supportive evidence of streptococcal infection is absent up to 10% cases.

SYSTEMIC MANIFESTATIONS

MIGRATORY POLYARTHRITIS

Incidence

Migratory polyarthritis is most common initial presentation of acute rheumatic fever up to 75% cases.

Clinical Features

Patient develops temporary migrating inflammation of the large joints, usually starting in the lower extremities (knees and ankles) and migrating upwards in the upper extremities, i.e. elbows and wrists. It reaches maximum severity in 12–24 hours. Affected joints are painful, swollen, warm, erythematous, and limited in their range of motion.

Resolution

Articular cartilage and synovial membrane are never involved; hence there is no permanent joint deformity. As the Aschoff's nodules in big joints are *more exudative* and less productive in nature, thus inflammatory changes in the joints completely resolve and hence no residual effect like joint deformity occurs.

Therapeutic correlation: Aspirin improves symptoms in affected joints and prevents further migration of the arthritis. Complete resolution of the symptoms typically occurs with improvement in 1–2 weeks and full recovery in 2–3 months.

PANCARDITIS

Pancarditis is the most common and serious complication of rheumatic fever (50%). It involves all three layers of heart.

- Degree of involvement of cardiac valves depends on severity of the initial attack and number of recurrent episodes by streptococcal bacteria.
- If heart murmur is not cleared within three weeks time after an episode of rheumatic fever; prognosis is poor due to valve deformity. New or changing murmurs are considered necessary for a diagnosis of rheumatic valvulitis.
- Echo-Doppler evidence of mitral valve insufficiency in association with aortic valve involvement may be sufficient for a diagnosis of carditis.

Myocarditis

- Myocardium is first to be involved in acute rheumatic fever. During early stage of acute rheumatic fever, myocarditis may lead to congestive heart failure with fatal outcome.
- Aschoff's nodules are present in periarteriolar interstitial tissue of myocardium.
- These usually heal and transform into fibrous scar. Spread of inflammation results into serofibrinous pericarditis and endocarditis.

Serofibrinous Pericarditis

- Inflammation may cause a serofibrinous pericardial exudate described as *bread-and-butter* pericarditis due to deposition of fibrin giving *shaggy appearance* (Fig. 16.20).
- Patient presents with precordial pain. On auscultation, friction rub can be heard.
- Other causes of serofibrinous pericarditis include uremic pericarditis, systemic lupus erythematosus, acute myocardial infarction, uremia and chest radiation.
- Resolution of serofibrinous pericarditis is uncommon. It most often gets organized and resulting in constrictive pericarditis.

Endocarditis

- Endocarditis leads to valvular damage. Usually left-sided cardiac valves are inflamed, i.e. mitral valve

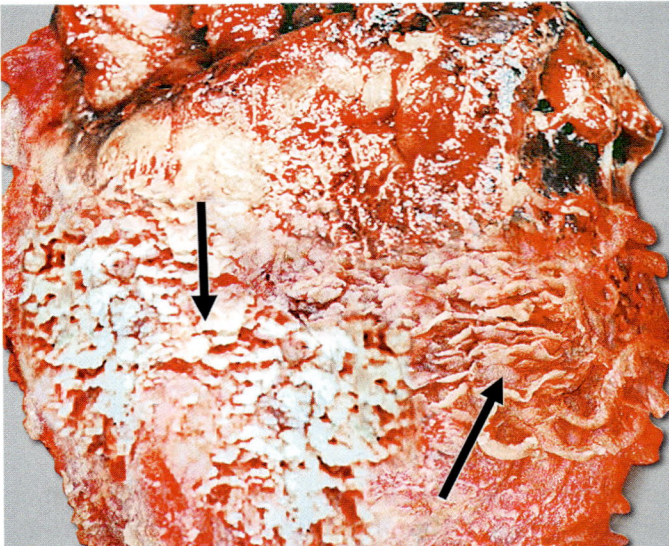

Fig. 16.20: Fibrinous pericarditis (arrows).

(75–80%), aortic valve (30%), mitral and aortic (25%), and tricuspid (<5%).

- Residual effects occur in mitral and aortic valves. Mitral stenosis is marked by high diastolic pressure in the left atrium than in the left ventricle.
- The aortic valve is affected most often along with the mitral valve. Aortic valve can be affected by stenosis or insufficiency.
- The tricuspid valve is affected along with the mitral valve and aortic valves (trivalvular involvement) in approximately 5% of cases of rheumatic heart disease. The pulmonary valve is rarely involved (Table 16.7).

Table 16.7: Cardiac valves involvement in acute rheumatic fever and RHD

Cardiac valves involvement	Frequency
Mitral valve (stenosis)	75–80%
Aortic valve (stenosis or regurgitation)	30%
Mitral and aortic valves	25%
Mitral, aortic and tricuspid valves	5%
Tricuspid	<5%
Pulmonary valve	Rare

Acute Rheumatic Heart Disease

Acute inflammation

In acute stage of the disease, all the valves and chordae tendineae are swollen due to inflammation. Mitral valve regurgitation occurs in acute phase, while mitral valve stenosis in chronic phase.

Cardiac vegetations

- Fibrin-rich exudate forming tiny, warty, bead-like, rubbery sterile vegetations measuring 1–2 mm in

Heart 16

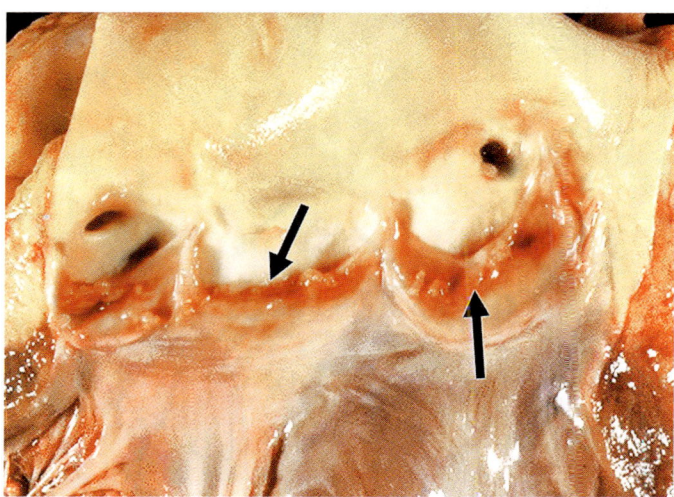

Fig. 16.21: Acute rheumatic endocarditis. Small verrucous vegetations measuring a few mm are seen along the closure line of this mitral valve (arrows).

size are present along the line of opposition of valvular cusps and chordae tendineae; but never present behind cusps.

- These vegetations are nonfriable and hence not a source of peripheral emboli. These valvular changes resolve with minimal fibrosis (Figs 16.21 to 16.23).

McCallum plaque

- McCallum plaque is a healed lesion located in posterior wall of left atrium.

- Blood regurgitation jets result in subendocardial thickening known as *McCallum plaque*.

Chronic Rheumatic Heart Disease

Nature of Aschoff's nodules in heart

- Aschoff's nodules in heart are more proliferative and less exudative type, and lead to valvular leaflet fibrosis, commissural fusion, thickening and shortening of the chordae tendineae.
- Aschoff's nodules are replaced by fibrosis hence not demonstrated on light microscopy.

Mitral stenosis: Buttonhole stenosis of valves with dystrophic calcification results in fish mouth appearance of affected valve (Fig. 16.24).

Clinical features

- These changes are accompanied by murmurs that can be heard on auscultation (Table 16.8).
- In advanced cases, patients may manifest as congestive heart failure, dyspnea, mild-to-moderate chest discomfort, pleuritic chest pain, edema, cough, or orthopnea or a new heart murmur.

Development of infective endocarditis

- Residual fibrinous cardiac vegetations often become infected with even low virulent bacteria and known as *subacute infective endocarditis*.
- Superimposed infection may cause ulceration of the cusps, perforation of valves, and rupture of chordae tendineae. The infected cardiac vegetations are more

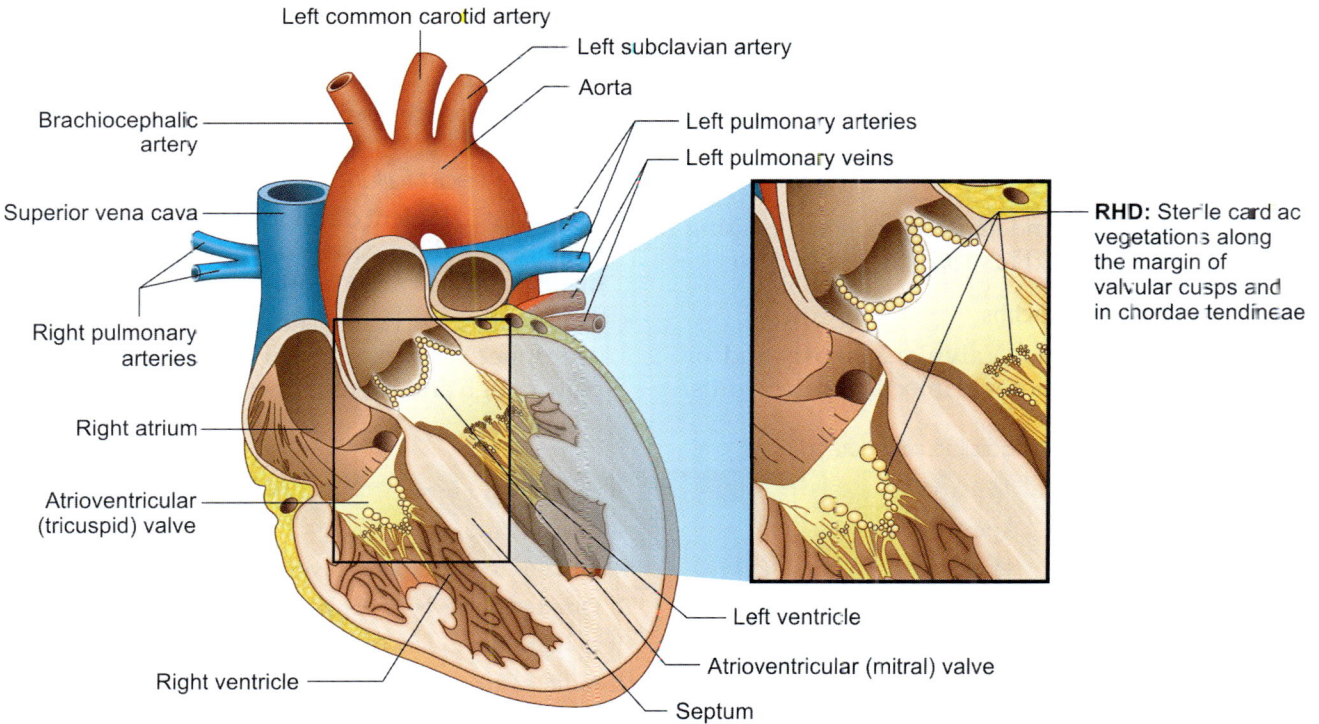

Fig. 16.22: Cardiac vegetations in rheumatic heart disease.

16 Section III: Systemic Pathology

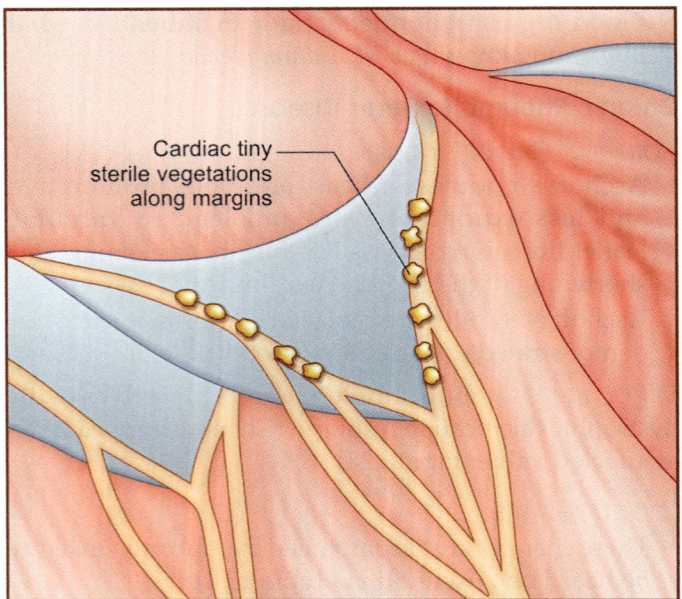

Fig. 16.23: Cardiac vegetations in rheumatic heart disease.

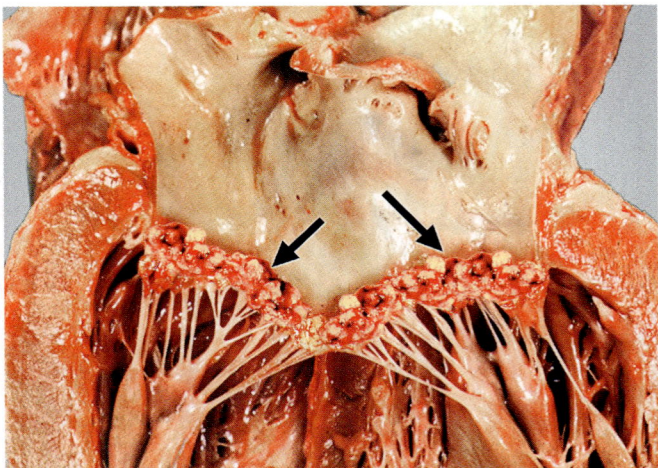

Fig. 16.25: Development of endocarditis in rheumatic heart disease (arrows).

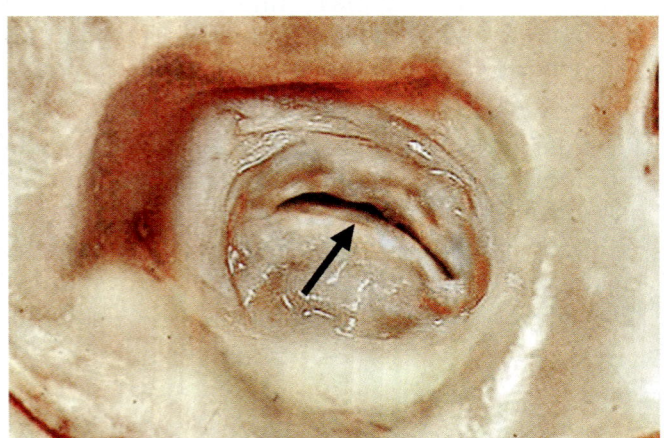

Fig. 16.24: Severe mitral stenosis in RHD showing fish mouth appearance. Cusps are rigid, fibrotic and calcified with narrowing of orifice.

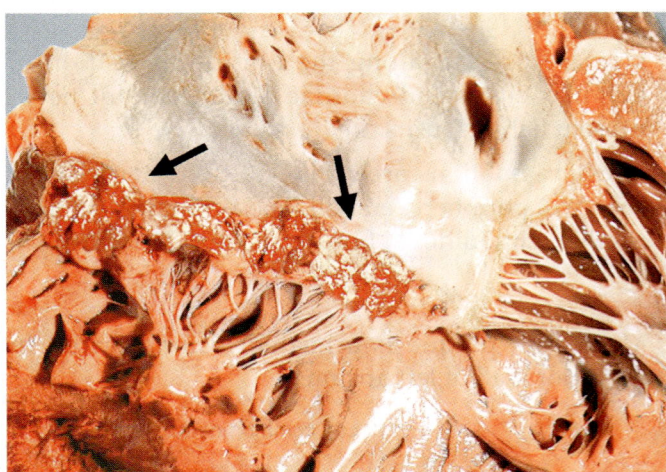

Fig. 16.26: Vegetations on the mitral valve in subacute bacterial endocarditis. These are also a source of peripheral emboli.

likely to be detached and cause embolism resulting in infarction of organs (Figs 16.25 and 16.26).

Complications of Pancarditis

Long-term complications: Valvular stenosis and or incompetence and predisposes to infective endocarditis.

Congestive heart failure
- *Pathogenesis:* Patient develops congestive heart failure in long-standing cases secondary to severe valve insufficiency or myocarditis.
- *Clinical features:* Patient may present with dyspnea, orthopnea, and peripheral edema, pleuritic chest pain, cough and rheumatic pneumonitis.

Table 16.8: Sites of radiation of cardiac murmurs

Cause	Primary site	Radiation of murmer
Mitral stenosis	Apex	It does not radiate
Mitral regurgitation	Apex	It radiates to left axilla beneath left scapula
Aortic stenosis	Apex	It radiates towards upper right sternal edge over carotids
Aortic regurgitation	Left sternal edge	It radiates down left sternal edge towards apex
Ventricle septal defect	Left sternal edge	It radiates all over precordium
Pulmonary stenosis	Left sternal edge in upper part	It radiates towards left clavicle beneath left scapula

- *Clinical examination:* On examination, patient with right heart failure shows signs of raised jugular venous pressure and hepatomegaly and peripheral edema.
- *Imaging findings:* Right ventricular hypertrophy is very common in mitral stenosis, and left ventricular hypertrophy seen in aortic regurgitation.

Arrhythmias-atrial fibrillation: Patient may develop atrial fibrillation, tachycardia, and arrhythmias.

Thromboembolism: Mural thrombi are very common in left atrium. Patient is prone to thromboembolism with infarction of affected organs.

Constrictive pericarditis
- There is deposition of fibrinous exudate between two layers of pericardium giving shaggy appearance. It is known as *bread-and-butter* pericarditis. Its resolution is uncommon.
- It most often gets organized results in constrictive pericarditis. Patient presents with precordial pain. On auscultation, friction rub can be heard.

Other organs involvement: Blood vessels and lungs may be involved in rheumatic fever, i.e. coronary arteries, renal arteries, mesenteric arteries, cerebral arteries, aorta, pulmonary arteries and lungs (pneumonitis and pleuritis). A few patients may develop abdominal pain and nose bleeds.

SUBCUTANEOUS NODULES

Subcutaneous nodules are formed due to fusion of multiple Aschoff's nodules.

Clinical Feature

Patient develops a few mm to 1–2 cm size firm, painless subcutaneous nodules, over bony prominences or tendon in adults, i.e. *wrists, elbows, scapula, ankles, knees, patella margins, scalp and spinous processes of thoracic and lumbar vertebrae* especially in adults in 10–60% cases.

SKIN RASHES (ERYTHEMA MARGINATUM)

Skin rashes exhibit bathing suit distribution (up to 10%): Patient presents with development of 1–3 cm ring shaped reddish rashes as macules/papules on the trunk and extremities (*bathing suit distribution*), which coalesce to exhibit snake-like appearance. These rashes typically spare the face and are made worse with heat.

SYDENHAM'S CHOREA (ST. VITUS DANCE)

Sydenham's chorea is delayed manifestation of rheumatic fever. This can occur at least 3 months from onset of infection up to 10% cases.

Clinical Features

Patient presents with series of random rapid involuntary purposeless muscular movements of the face and arms. Patient has difficulty in writing, drawing, hand work, and talking.

Physical Examination

Patient develops hyperextension of joints, hypotonia of muscles, diminished deep tendon reflexes, and relapsing grip (e.g. alternate increase and decrease in tension).

Complete Resolution

Patient starts improving in 1–2 weeks, and full recovery occurs in 2–3 months. CSF examination reveals no pathological findings.

LABORATORY DIAGNOSIS

JONES DIAGNOSTIC CRITERIA

Rheumatic fever is diagnosed clinically using Jones criteria, which are divided into two groups: major and minor manifestations. The diagnosis is established when two major and one minor or one major and two minor criteria are present.

ANTISTREPTOCOCCAL O TITER (ASO TITER)

- ASO titer is estimated in patient with rheumatic fever. Peak level is achieved at 4–5 weeks after streptococcal infection. High titers are supportive but not diagnostic.
- ASO titer is expressed in Todd units. ASO titers more than >400 Todd units in adults and >300 Todd units in children >5 years of age are significant.

ANTI-DNASE-B/ANTI-HYALURONIDASE TITER

It is less reliable than ASO titer. It is raised in cases of Sydenham's chorea.

ANTISTREPTOZYME TEST

- Antistreptozyme test is very sensitive in recent rheumatic fever.
- Hemagglutination test value >200 units/ml associated with polyarthritis suggests acute rheumatic fever.

ELECTROCARDIOGRAM

ECG study shows prolonged PR interval.

IMAGING TECHNIQUES

Echocardiography is done to visualize cardiac motion. Chest radiograph is done to evaluate heart and lungs.

BLOOD CULTURE

- Blood culture is done to diagnose or rule out infective endocarditis in these patients. Blood culture is positive in 95% cases due to presence of bacterial colonies not covered by fibrin (Fig. 16.27).
- Presence of deep seated bacterial colonies covered by fibrin leads to negative blood culture (Fig. 16.28).

ACUTE PHASE REACTANTS

Serum complement, mucoproteins, α_2-globulin and β-globulin levels are increased. Peripheral blood smear examination shows leukocytosis. Erythrocyte sedimentation rate and C-reactive proteins (CRP) levels are raised in polyarthritis.

DECREASED ERYTHROPOIESIS

Chronic inflammatory changes suppress erythropoiesis leading to anemia.

MANAGEMENT

Aspirin

Aspirin is the drug of choice for treatment of migratory polyarthritis by reducing inflammation.

Antibiotics

Patients with positive throat cultures should be treated with antibiotics.

Corticosteroids

These are reserved for cases where there is evidence of pancarditis. Use of corticosteroids prevents further scarring of tissue and development of mitral stenosis. Unlike normal heart failure, rheumatic heart failure responds well to corticosteroids.

Long Acting Penicillin

Basic aim of monthly injections of long acting penicillin is to prevent development of infective endocarditis. It must be given for a period of five years in patients having one attack of rheumatic fever. If there is evidence of carditis, the length of long acting penicillin therapy may be continued up to 40 years of age.

ACE Inhibitors, Diuretics, β-blockers, and Digoxin

These drugs are used for treatment of carditis, which manifests as congestive heart failure.

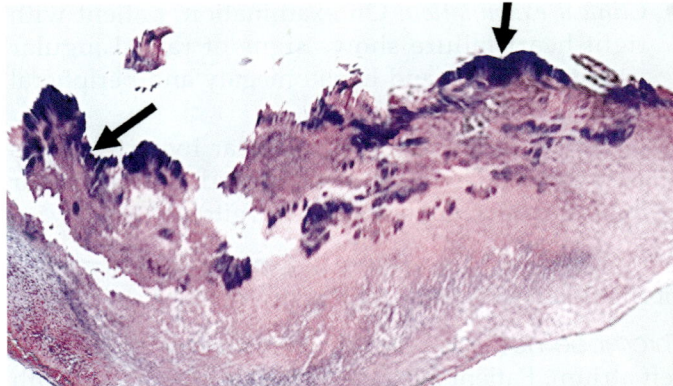

Fig. 16.27: Infective endocarditis. Valves are relatively avascular, so high dose antibiotic therapy is needed to eradicate the infection. Blue bacterial colonies are extending into the pink fibrin, platelets and connective tissue of the valve. Blood culture is positive (arrows) (400X).

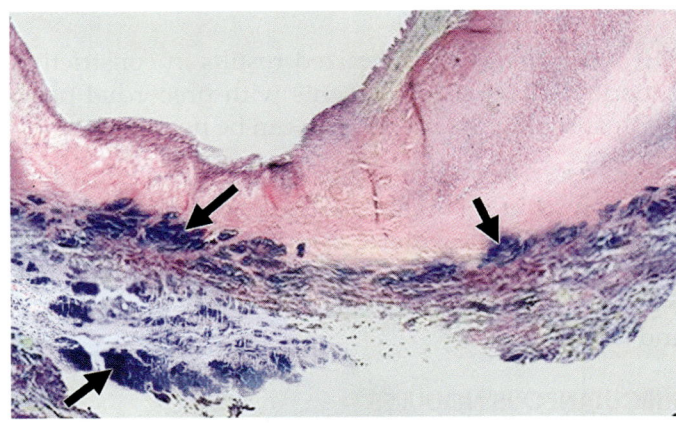

Fig. 16.28: Infective endocarditis. Valves are relatively avascular, so high dose antibiotic therapy is needed to eradicate the infection. Blue bacterial colonies are extending into the pink fibrin, platelets and connective tissue of the valve. Blood culture is negative (arrows) (400X).

MYOCARDIUM

MYOCARDITIS

Myocarditis is focal or diffuse inflammation of the myocardium affecting any age group. Myocarditis constitutes 10% cases of new onset cardiac dysfunction. If myocarditis is not fatal, it often progresses to dilated cardiomyopathy. There are many causes of myocarditis, including viral infections, autoimmune disorders, environmental toxins and adverse reactions to medications.

Diagnosis of active myocarditis is based on inflammatory infiltrate usually lymphocytes and myocyte necrosis not of ischemic etiology.

Clinical Features

Patient presents with the classical findings of congestive heart failure, tachypnea, peripheral edema, and hepatomegaly. Atrial or ventricular arrhythmias are common with fatal outcome.

Electrocardiogram

ECG may show low voltage QRS complex, ST elevation, or heart block. Serial 24-hour Holter recordings should be obtained in all patients.

Imaging Techniques

Chest X-ray shows pulmonary edema. Echocardiography is extremely useful in excluding congenital structural defects; pericardial effusion with cardiac tamponade should also be excluded.

Diagnosis

Cardiac catheterization with endomyocardial biopsy remains the gold standard for the diagnosis of myocarditis.

PRIMARY VIRAL MYOCARDITIS

Primary viral myocarditis is most common often caused by Coxsackie B virus. It may be caused by HIV, EB virus, poliovirus, cytomegalovirus. Infectious organism triggers an autoimmune, cellular, and humoral reaction resulting in myocarditis.

Primary viral myocarditis has four clinicopathological manifestations described as under.

Fulminant Myocarditis

Patient with fulminant myocarditis develops ventricular dysfunction without dilatation within 2 weeks of infection.

Complete histological and functional recovery occurs. Some patients die within 2 weeks.

Light Microscopy

Histopathological examination shows multiple foci of active inflammation (lymphocytes) and necrosis (Fig. 16.29).

Chronic Active Myocarditis

Patient has an indistinct onset with moderate dysfunction. Patient may develop restrictive cardiomyopathy within 2–4 years of clinical manifestations.

Light Microscopy

Histopathological examination shows active or borderline myocarditis.

Eosinophilic Myocarditis

Eosinophilic myocarditis is attributed to allergic reactions. It leads to left ventricular dysfunction. It is linked to treatment with methyldopa, penicillin, para-aminosalicylic acid, streptomycin, anticonvulsants and antidepressants.

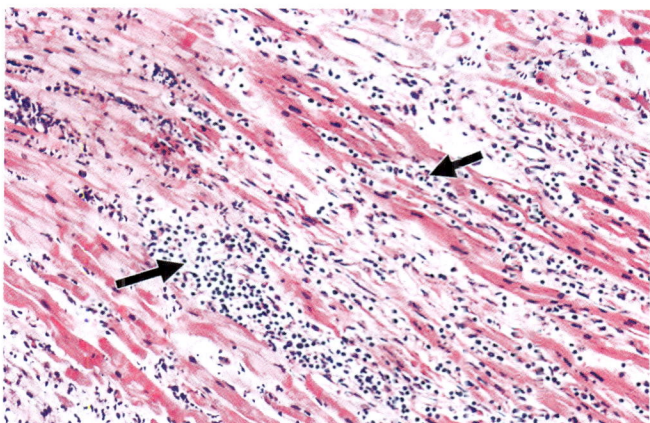

Fig. 16.29: Viral myocarditis. It is caused by Coxsackie B virus showing heavy but focal increase of lymphocytes in the interstitial tissue of the myocardium. Outcome is subclinical or fatal (arrows) (100X).

Light Microscopy

- Histopathological examination shows myocarditis infiltrated by eosinophils and occasional giant cells.
- There is presence of a little myocardial necrosis and infiltration by lymphocytes and histiocytes around blood vessels. In a few cases, inflammation is present in subendocardium with poorly formed granulomas.

Idiopathic Giant Cell Myocarditis

It is also known as *Friedler's myocarditis*. It is associated with autoimmune diseases such as inflammatory bowel disease. It affects young adults.

Light Microscopy

- Histopathological examination shows infiltration by lymphocytes, macrophages, and multinucleated giant cells in the absence of granulomas.
- Giant cells have immunohistochemical profile of histiocytes.

CARDIOMYOPATHIES

Definition

Cardiomyopathy refers to non-inflammatory diseases of myocardium. It is diagnosed by exclusion of all cases of hypertension, ischemic heart disease, valvular diseases and congenital heart diseases. It is characterized by unexplained ventricular dysfunction unresponsive to digitalis.

Classification

Primary cardiomyopathies include congestive (dilated), hypertrophic and restrictive types. Secondary

Table 16.9: Comparison of cardiomyopathies

Parameters	Congestive CMP	Hypertrophic CMP	Restrictive CMP
Etiology	Alcohol toxicity Peripartum postviral genetic mutation	Autosomal dominance beta heavy chain on chromosome 14 (50%) ++++ Troponin T gene on chromosome 1 (15%) Alpha-tropomyosin gene on chromosome 15 (3–5%)	Unknown in majority of cases Amyloid deposition in sub-endocardial region Hemosiderin deposition in sub-endocardial region
Age	Any age	Young age	Infants, children
Valves motion	Normal motion	Anterior motion of mitral valve during systole	Normal motion
Heart wall and chambers	All chambers are dilated and congested	Left ventricle is hypertrophied	Endocardial thickening is marked
Heart contraction	Poor	Marked	Poor due to heart rigid
CHF	Slow onset	Rapid onset	Rapid onset
Cardiomegaly	++++ (marked)	++ (moderate)	+ (less)
Arrhythmias	++	Absent	++++ (marked)
Atrial fibrillation	Absent	++++ (marked)	Absent
Thrombus	Common	Common	Absent
Infective endocarditis	Absent	Present	Absent
Prognosis	Poor	Poor	Poor

cardiomyopathies occur due to specific causes (e.g. hemochromatosis, amyloidosis, and alcohol and thiamine deficiency). Diagnostic evaluation of cardiomyopathies is based on history, clinical examination, imaging tools, ECG, cardiac catheterization and cardiac biopsy examination (Table 16.9).

CONGESTIVE CARDIOMYOPATHY

Congestive cardiomyopathy is most common form and also known as *dilated cardiomyopathy*. Damage to cardiac muscle fibers results in poor contraction. The resulting loss of muscle tone dilates all four chambers of the heart, resulting in cardiomegaly (>500 gm) giving the heart, a globular shape (Figs 16.30 and 16.31).

Patient is prone to thrombus formation and arrhythmias (atrial and ventricular). Mural thrombi may fragment and enter circulation in the form of emboli. Emboli from left side of heart are carried to brain, kidney, coronary arteries and peripheral tissues resulting in interruption of blood supply. Emboli from

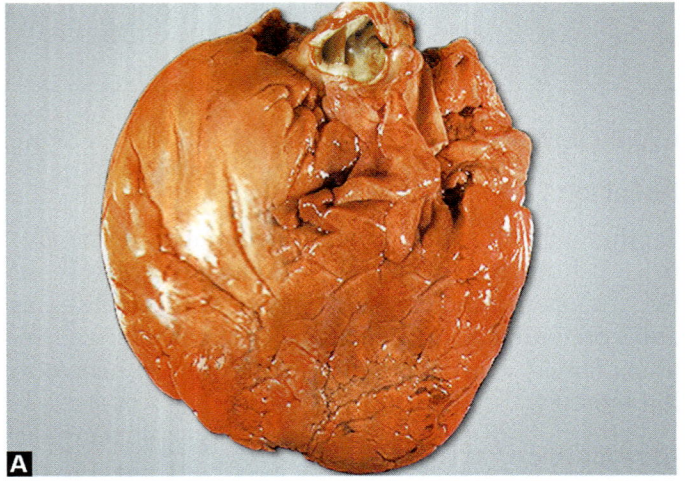
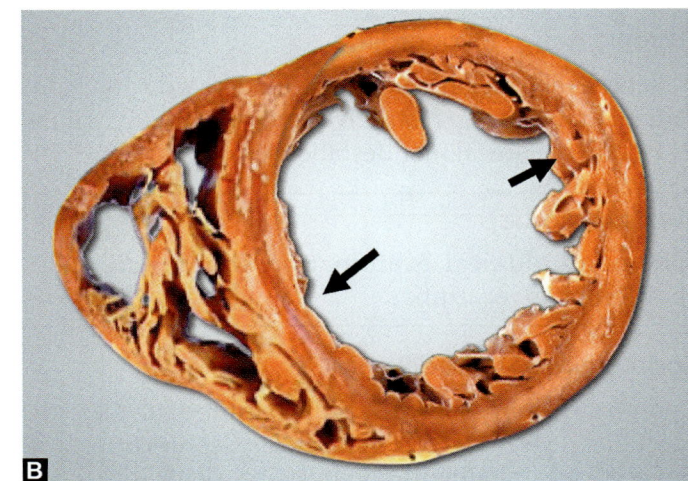

Fig. 16.30: Congestive cardiomyopathy. (A) Heart has a globoid shape because all of the chambers are dilated, (B) heart is very flabby, large and the myocardium is poorly contractile (arrows).

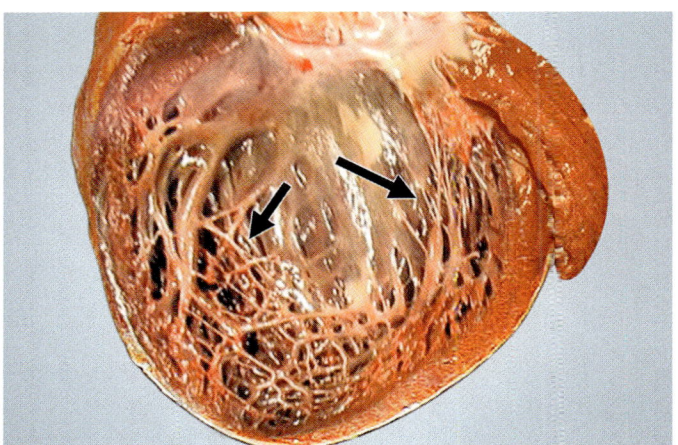

Fig. 16.31: Congestive cardiomyopathy. Cut opened chamber is showing marked dilatation. Heart is very flabby, large and the myocardium is poorly contractile (arrows).

right-sided heart reach pulmonary artery resulting in pulmonary infarction.

Etiology

Etiology is most often unknown. In some cases, it is associated with chronic alcoholism, thiamine deficiency (beriberi heart), peripartum period (last trimester or within 6 months in postpartum period), and end stage of viral myocarditis, myxedema, drug toxicity (e.g. doxorubicin, daunorubicin, cocaine) and rare disease Friedreich ataxia. Some cases are associated with mutant cytoskeletal proteins (i.e. dystrophin or desmin), sarcomeric proteins (troponin), such as cardiac myosin heavy chain; and other muscle proteins, such as actin. Mutations in mitochondrial genes have also been implicated.

Light Microscopy
- Normal myocytes are filled with myofibrils, hence exhibit a uniform pink cytoplasm.
- Damaged myocytes undergo loss of myofibrils in myocytes, hence exhibit empty spaces within cytoplasm. There is presence of focal myocyte necrosis, interstitial fibrosis, and infiltration by T cells and macrophages (Fig. 16.32).

Clinical Features

Patient develops slow onset congestive heart failure, shortness of breath, orthopnea, dyspnea on exertion, fatigue and dry cough at night.

Physical Examination

Physical examination reveals jugular vein distention, peripheral edema, hepatomegaly, peripheral cyanosis, irregular pulse and tachycardia.

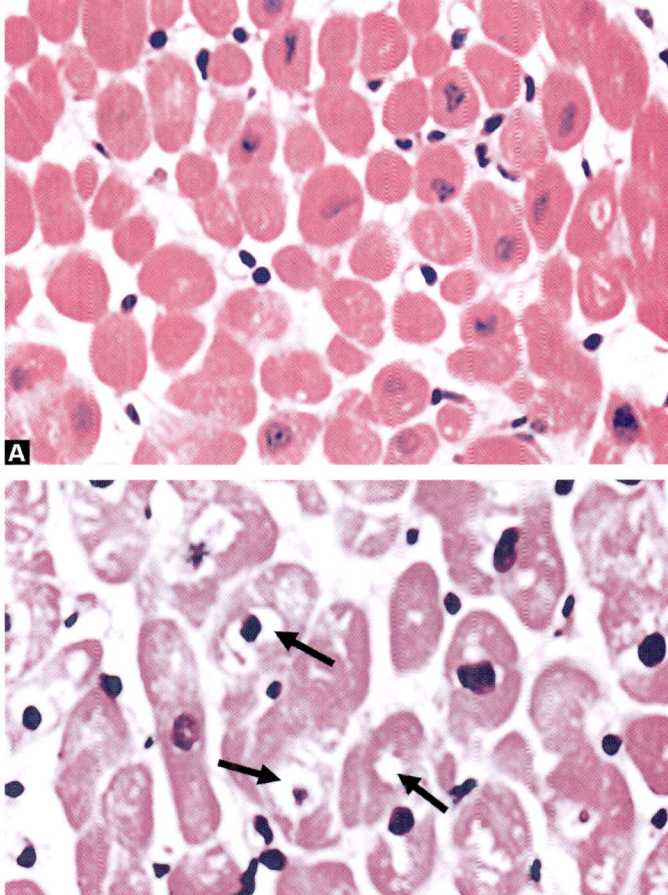

Fig. 16.32: (A) Each normal myocyte in cross section has a uniform pink cytoplasm owing to the majority of the cell being filled by myofibrils, (B) congestive cardiomyopathy. The myocytes have lost myofibrils and empty spaces have appeared within the cytoplasm (arrows).

Auscultation

Dilated congested heart weakens papillary muscles resulting in mitral and tricuspid valve insufficiency. On auscultation, pansystolic murmur is heard.

Clinical Course

Prognosis is very poor. Death occurs within 2 years from onset of symptoms.

Therapeutic Correlation

Cardiac transplantation is recommended.

HYPERTROPHIC CARDIOMYOPATHY

Hypertrophic cardiomyopathy is also known as *idiopathic hypertrophic subaortic stenosis* (IHSS). It is transmitted as an autosomal dominant trait in 50%. It is most common form of cardiomyopathy with hypercontracting heart affecting younger adults.

Genetic Basis

More than 50% cases are inherited as an autosomal dominant trait. Gene mutations implicated in this disorder include gene coding for β-*myosin heavy chain on chromosome 14* (most common and severe form in 50%), cardiac troponins T and I (less severe form in 15%), α-tropomyosin gene on chromosome 15 (less severe in 3–5%), myosin-binding protein C, and myosin light chain.

Gross Morphology
- Heart shows hypertrophy of all the chamber walls especially asymmetric interventricular septum hypertrophy.
- It becomes stiff and noncompliant. It is unable to relax during ventricular filling.
- Lumen of the left ventricle is markedly reduced assuming banana shaped chamber (Fig. 16.33).

Light Microscopy
The myocytes in normal myocardium are arranged in parallel, and within the myocyte myofibrils. But in hypertrophic cardiomyopathy, the cells are arranged in disoriented tangled criss-cross whorls losing their normal parallel arrangement (Figs 16.34 and 16.35).

Pathophysiology

In patient, asymmetrical hypertrophy of the interventricular septum is responsible for subaortic stenosis resulting in obstruction to blood flow and systolic motion of anterior leaflet of mitral valve toward the

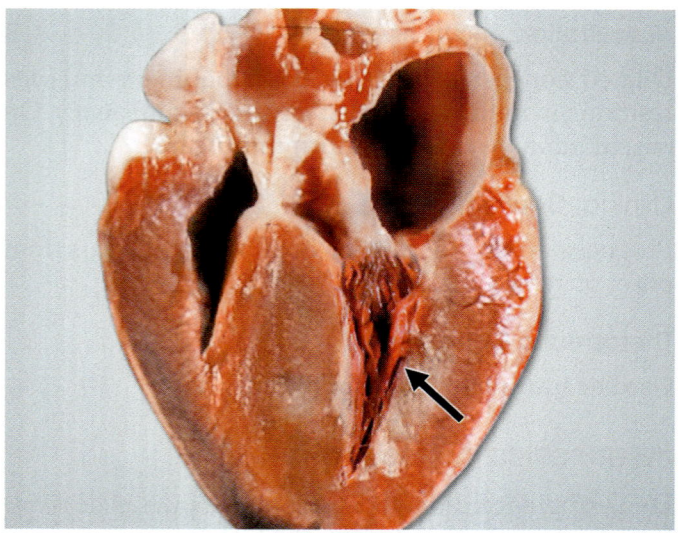

Fig. 16.33: Hypertrophic cardiomyopathy. Left ventricular hypertrophy with asymmetrical septal hypertrophy, systolic anterior motion of mitral valve, banana-shaped left ventricular chamber and hypercontracting heart (arrow).

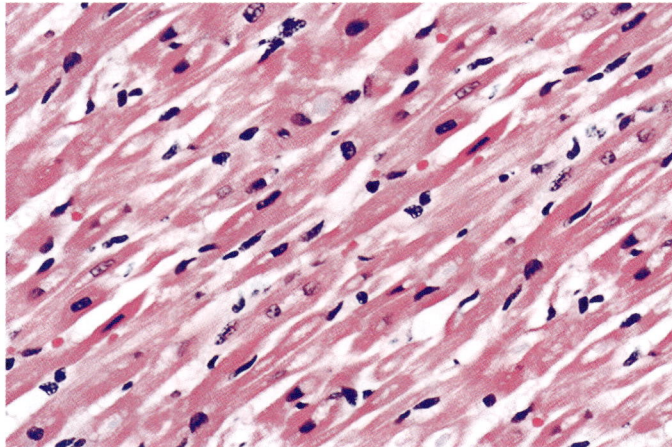

Fig. 16.34: Normal cardiac muscle biopsy. The myocytes in normal myocardium are arranged in parallel, and within the myocyte myofibrils (400X).

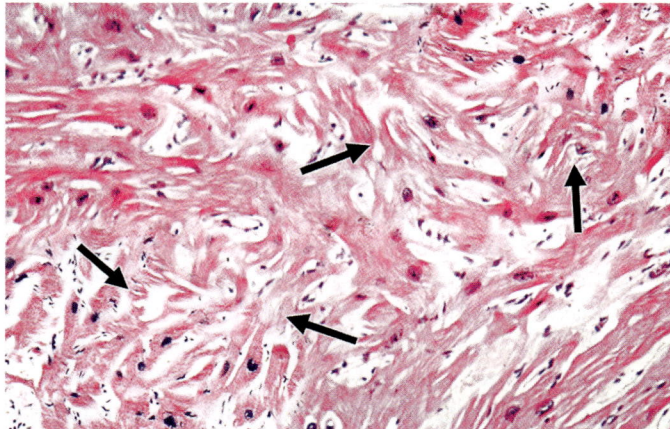

Fig. 16.35: Hypertrophic cardiomyopathy. The cells arranged in whorls around foci of connective tissue. Higher power magnification shows the myofibrils within the cell criss-cross whorls losing their normal parallel arrangement (arrows) (400X).

interventricular septum. It impairs ventricular filling resulting in increased pressure in left atrium and pulmonary veins. It causes unexpected death in young athletes.

Clinical Features

Patient presents with breathlessness on exertion, dizziness, fainting, precordial pain, and arrhythmias. The obstruction to blood flow from the left ventricle increases the ventricle's work, and harsh systolic ejection murmur may be heard along the left sternal border and at the apex. Patient develops abrupt arterial pulse, irregular pulse (atrial fibrillation).

Complications

Patient may develop arrhythmia (most common), atrial fibrillation, infective endocarditis, congestive heart failure and thrombus formation with fatal outcome.

RESTRICTIVE CARDIOMYOPATHY

- Restricrtive cardiomyopathy is least common but serious disorder. It affects infants and children.
- Infiltration of extraneous material in the ventricles cause left ventricular hypertrophy with decreased ventricular chamber lumen and endocardial fibrosis.
- This stiffness reduces the ventricle's ability to relax and fill during diastole. The rigid myocardium fails to contract completely during systole. As a result, cardiac output falls.

Etiology

In adults, cardiac amyloidosis and hemochromatosis cause restrictive cardiomyopathy. It is characterized by reduced diastolic filling and right-sided heart failure. Infiltration of the conduction system by amyloid material can result in arrhythmias or sudden cardiac death.

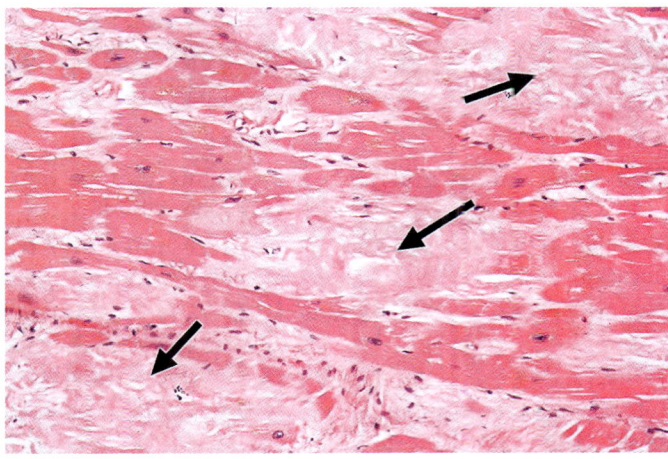

Fig. 16.36: Restrictive cardiomyopathy. Pale, pinkish, amorphous material is deposited between myocardial fibers due to amyloid deposition. Arrhythmias occur during surgery (arrows).

> **Light Microscopy**
> - Amyloid appears amorphous, glassy, and eosinophilic material in extracellular compartment.
> - It is readily documented using a Congo red stain, which demonstrates green birefringence when viewed under polarized light.
> - Prussian blue staining is done to demonstrate iron in hemochromatosis involving heart (Fig. 16.36).

Clinical Features

Patient develops congestive heart failure and arrhythmias during surgery as a result of enlarged atria and impairment of ventricular filling during diastole. Patient presents with dyspnea, orthopnea and chest pain. Physical examination reveals peripheral edema, hepatomegaly, peripheral cyanosis, pallor. Auscultation reveals S3 or S4 gallop rhythm.

ARRHYTHMOGENIC RIGHT VENTRICULAR CARDIOMYOPATHY

It is rare autosomal dominant disorder due to defective molecules in desmosomes. It is characterized by right-sided heart failure and arrhythmias. Right ventricular muscle is severely thinned out and gradually replaced by adipose tissue. Patient develops arrhythmias. It may cause sudden death in athletes. *Osteoglycan (OGN) gene is associated with left ventricular hypertrophy*

Naxos syndrome is associated with mutations of the genes encoding the *desmosome-associated protein plakoglobin*. It is characterized by arrhythmogenic right ventricular cardiomyopathy and hyperkeratosis of plantar and palmar skin surfaces. Comparison of cardiomyopathies is given in Table 16.9.

ENDOCARDIUM

OVERVIEW

ENDOCARDITIS

Depending on etiology, endocarditis is categorized in two groups—infective or non-infective endocarditis.

Infective Endocarditis

Acute endocarditis affects normal heart due to highly virulent bacteria. Subacute endocarditis occurs in previously diseased heart due to even low virulent bacteria.

Non-infective Endocarditis

Examples are Libman-Sacks endocarditis (SLE), non-bacterial thrombotic endocarditis (mucin secreting carcinoma of colon and pancreas) and small sterile verrucous vegetations in rheumatic heart disease.

INFECTIVE ENDOCARDITIS

Definition

Infective endocarditis is an infection of the endocardium, cardiac valvular surfaces, or cardiac prosthesis resulting from bacterial (most common) or fungal invasion. Infective endocarditis may be acute or subacute. There are, however, no strict criteria for separating clinically acute bacterial endocarditis from subacute bacterial endocarditis (Table 16.10 and Fig. 16.37).

Section III: Systemic Pathology

Table 16.10: Differences between acute and subacute bacterial endocarditis

Characteristics	Acute bacterial endocarditis	Subacute bacterial endocarditis
Heart status	Previously normal	Previously diseased
Onset	Rapid	Gradual
Pathogen's virulence	Highly virulent organisms, e.g. *Staphylococcus aureus*	Less virulent organisms β-hemolytic streptococci
Cardiac vegetations size and location	More bulky and friable, present along edges of cusps	Less bulky and present along edges of cusps myocardium
Nature of lesions	More erosive and destructive lesions result in perforation of cusps (quite common) and chordae tendineae	Less erosive and destructive lesions may cause perforation of cusps (less common)
Myocardial involvement	Myocardium microabscesses ++++	Myocardium microabscesses ++
Clinical features	Fever high grade with chills and arthralgia ++	Fever slight (flu-like syndrome)
Physical examination	Splenomegaly present	No splenomegaly
	Splinter hemorrhages due to microemboli beneath nails known as Janeway's lesions	No splinter hemorrhages beneath nails (Janeway's lesions absent)
Auscultation	Cardiac murmurs are quite common	Cardiac murmurs may be present

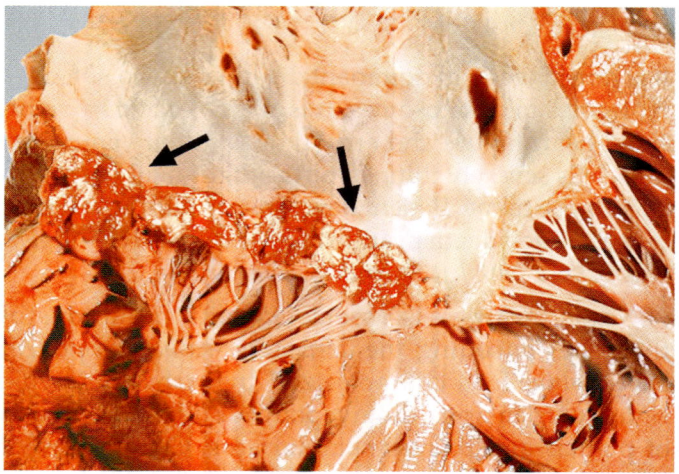

Fig. 16.37: Infective endocarditis. Large friable vegetations are seen along the margin of cusps and chordae tendineae of mitral valve. Patient presents with a 4-week history of fever, fatigue and weight loss. Physical examination revealed petechial hemorrhages and clubbing of fingers (arrows).

Cardiac Valves Affected

Mitral valve is most frequently involved, followed by the aortic, tricuspid, and the pulmonary valve. The mitral valve along with the aortic valve is involved in about 40% of cases. The tricuspid valve is involved in >50% of cases of endocarditis due to intravenous drug use, in whom endocarditis is most often caused by staphylococcal infection.

Risk Factors

Infective endocarditis is most commonly secondary to bacterial pathogens. Predisposing factors include dental procedures, immunodeficiency, intravenous drug addicts, surgery, tooth extractions, venous access devices, such as central or peripheral catheters and artificial heart valves.

Source of Infections

Organisms reach the endocardium by hematogenous spread route from oropharynx flora (dental procedures), skin flora, gastrointestinal tract flora, and genitourinary procedure and lung infections.

- *Highly virulent bacteria:* *Staphylococcus aureus* produces abscess at multiple sites in >30% cases.
- *Low virulent bacteria:* These include Streptococci group A and B (55%), oropharyngeal flora HACEK (e.g. Haemophilus, Actinobacillus, Cardiobacterium, Eikenella, Kingella), enterococci-penicillin resistant (6%) by genitourinary manipulations. *Streptococcus viridans* and Staphylococcus may be indolent with minimal symptoms.

ACUTE ENDOCARDITIS

Etiology

Acute endocarditis is caused by highly virulent bacteria. *Staphylococcus aureus* produces an *acute* bacterial endocarditis in previously normal heart in 50% of cases. This type of endocarditis is often secondary to infection occurring elsewhere in the body.

Cardiac Vegetations

These are large, bulky, destructive, and extremely friable on the valve cusps that can extend onto the chordae tendineae, hence predisposing to systemic embolization producing infected infarcts in various organs.

Clinical Features
The symptoms are more pronounced and develop much rapidly. Fever is most consistent sign in 95% of cases.

Blood Cultures
Blood cultures are positive in 95% of cases. Negative blood culture is either due to deep seated organisms covered by fibrin, or prior antibiotic therapy and organisms like fungus, Coxiella or Chlamydia.

SUBACUTE ENDOCARDITIS

Etiology
Subacute endocarditis is caused by low virulent bacteria *Streptococcus viridans* more than 50% of cases) or fungi (e.g. Candida and Aspergillus).

Predisposing Factors
This type of endocarditis tends to occur in patients with congenital heart disease or pre-existing valvular heart disease or acquired. Congenital heart diseases include ASD, VSD, patent ductus arteriosus, coarctation of aorta tetralogy of Fallot, and mitral valve prolapse.

Acquired causes include chronic rheumatic endocarditis, prosthetic valve, syphilitic aortitis, calcific aortic stenosis, arteriovenous fistula and degenerative heart disease.

Cardiac Vegetations
These are smaller, less fragile, and associated with fewer destructive lesions. Thrombus formation and septic embolization can subsequently occur.

Clinical Features
These patients present with gradual onset of nonspecific symptoms such as slight fever (flu-ike syndrome).

COMPLICATIONS OF INFECTIVE ENDOCARDITIS
Complications of infective endocarditis include destruction of cardiac valves, dissemination of bacteria, embolization and immune complex formation (Figs 16.38 and 16.39). Remote embolic complications of infective endocarditis are given in Table 16.11.

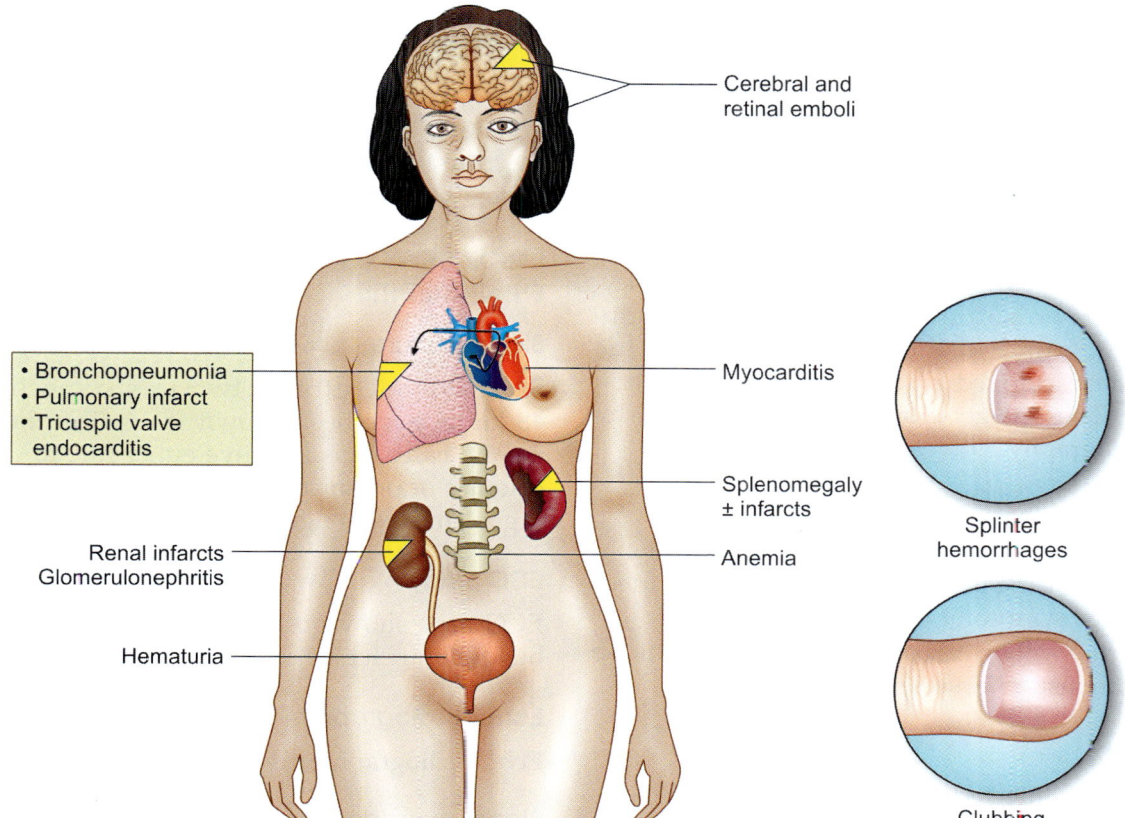

Fig. 16.38: Complications of infective endocarditis. Septic emboli may lodge in various organs causing infarcts, bronchopneumonia and splinter hemorrhages (*Courtesy:* Dr. Abhijit Das).

Table 16.11: Remote embolic complications of infective endocarditis

Organs	Clinical manifestations
Brain	Infarction of brain with secondary hemorrhage from embolus to anterior cerebral arteries, small infarcts of basal ganglion
Retina	Embolus in ocular fundus with retinal infarction and petechial hemorrhages
Hands skin and fingers	Multiple petechial hemorrhages of skin and clubbing of fingers
Mucous membrane	Petechial hemorrhages of mucous membrane
Kidneys	Petechial hemorrhages
Spleen	Mycotic aneurysms of splenic arteries and infarct of spleen. It shows splenomegaly

Embolization is a serious complications of infective endocarditis

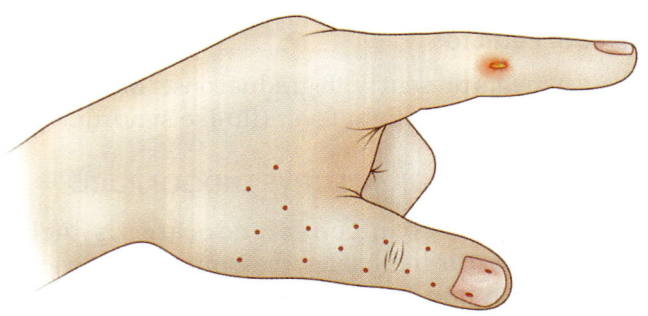

Fig. 16.39: Complications of infective endocarditis. It shows splinter hemorrhage.

Destruction of Cardiac Valves

- Endocarditis may impede the blood flow and cause turbulence reflecting murmurs. As the disease advances, bacteria may destroy parts of the valve, cause perforation, rupture of chordae tendineae, or abscesses at the base of the cusps.
- All these pathologic chances adversely affect the function of the valve and may cause insufficiency. Stenosis may also develop, even though more often it is found in the healing stages of the disease, characterized by fibrosis and calcification of cusps. These vegetations are demonstrated by echocardiography.

Dissemination of Bacteria

- The entry of bacteria into the circulation results in bacteremia causing bronchopneumonia. The patient typically has symptoms of sepsis.
- Blood culture will reveal bacteria as the cause of these relatively nonspecific symptoms.

Embolization

- Fragments of infected endocardial vegetations are carried by the blood, lodging in terminal arteries.
- Such microemboli interrupt the blood supply to the affected areas and cause septic infarcts in various organs, i.e. brain (cerebral strokes), retina, spleen, kidney (glomerulonephritis and renal infarct) and digits.
- Thromboemboli from tricuspid valve endocarditis may result in bronchopneumonia and pulmonary infarcts.

Immune Complexes Deposition

- Antibodies are formed against bacterial antigens released in the infected endocardial vegetations. These immune complexes circulate in the blood and are deposited in the wall of *glomeruli and small blood vessels* resulting to rupture.
- Patients develop *Roth's retinal hemorrhages, Osler's nodes (painful nodules on pads of the fingers and toes), glomerulonephritis and Janeway's lesions.*
- Janeway's lesions are *splinter hemorrhages (linear red streaks) on palms, soles beneath nails;* due to rupture of small vessels by microemboli.

LABORATORY DIAGNOSIS OF INFECTIVE ENDOCARDITIS

Blood Culture

Serial blood cultures two to six specimens over 48 hours have been shown to confirm the diagnosis in 95% cases. It is negative either due to deep seated colonies of organisms, or prior antibiotic therapy and organisms like fungus, Coxiella or Chlamydia.

ECG Study

ECG may show prolongation of the P-R interval or bundle branch block.

Echocardiography

Echocardiography is done to localize the lesion in heart.

Blood Investigations

Peripheral smear shows leukocytosis and anemia. ESR is raised.

ENDOCARDITIS IN PROSTHETIC VALVES

Prosthetic valve endocarditis accounts for approximately 20% of all clinically diagnosed cases of endocarditis. Aortic valve is commonly affected along the suture of prosthetic valve. It occurs in two forms, i.e. early onset and late onset.

Early Onset Endocarditis

Early onset endocarditis occurs within the first within 60 days of heart valve surgery (i.e. plastic, metal and bioprosthesis of animal origin) in 2 or 3% of patients either due to contamination during surgery or with drug resistant pathogens in postoperative period. *Staphylococcus aureus* and *Staphylococcus epidermidis* account for >50% of infections, gram-negative bacteria and fungi (Candida, Aspergillus).

Late Onset Endocarditis

Late onset endocarditis occurs after 60 days of valve replacement in 0.5% patients. It is usually related to transient bacteremias. It is most often caused by *Staphylococcus* (50%) and *Streptococcus viridans* (40%).

Complications

The most important complications include thromboembolism, paravalvular leaks, mechanical malfunction, mechanical deterioration (rupture and calcification of valves), microangiopathic hemolytic anemia with hemoglobinuria and mechanical dysfunction with heart failure. The thrombi that develop on the artificial valves may also become infected.

ENDOCARDITIS IN INTRAVENOUS DRUG ABUSE

Intravenous drug abuse persons develop endocarditis by *Staphylococcus aureus* (50%), streptococci (15%), enterococci and opportunistic fungal infections, i.e. Candida and Aspergillus. Tricuspid valve (55%) is most often affected in drug addicts followed by bicuspid valve (20%) and aortic valve (25%) (Fig. 16.40)

Clinical Features

Patient may develop cellulitis, thrombophlebitis and embolic episodes in femoral arteries and lungs. It is worth mentioning that tricuspid valve may also be affected in patients with indwelling catheters, cardiac surgery, ventricular septal defects and carcinoid tumors.

LIBMAN-SACKS ENDOCARDITIS

In patients with systemic lupus erythematosus, endocarditis is the most striking cardiac lesion, termed Libman-Sacks endocarditis in 10–30% of patients.

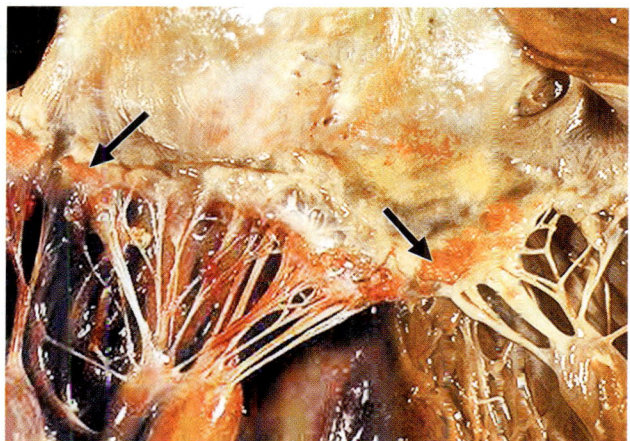

Fig. 16.40: Libman-Sacks endocarditis in SLE. The verrucous 1 to 2 mm, multiple, sterile widely spaced vegetations along margins of the mitral valve and less commonly tricuspid valve in 30–50% of cases of systemic lupus erythematosus. These vegetations usually heal without residual effect (arrows).

Pathogenesis

Immune complex-mediated injury of the valvular endocardium results in formation of sterile vegetations.

Locations

- These vegetations are 1–4 mm in size widely spaced, seen on the undersurface of the mitral valve (most common) close to the origin of the leaflets from the valve ring (Libman-Sacks endocarditis). These are less often present in tricuspid valve and adjacent endocardium.
- Mitral valve deformity and regurgitation may occur. There is fibrinoid necrosis of small vessels with focal degeneration of interstitial tissue. These vegetations can be identified in living patients by echocardiography.

Clinical Correlation

It is not a serious complication during the course of the disease. These vegetations usually heal without residual effect, hence are clinically of limited significance.

NONBACTERIAL THROMBOTIC ENDOCARDITIS

Nonbacterial thrombotic endocarditis, also known as marantic endocarditis, refers to the presence of sterile vegetations on apparently normal cardiac valves, almost always in association with metastatic cancer or debilitating disorders. The principal danger is embolization to distant organs.

Pathogenesis

The cause of marantic endocarditis is poorly understood, but it has been attributed to increased blood coagulability and immune complex deposition.

- *Mechanical injuries:* Thrombi are formed on sites of minute mechanical injuries of the endothelium due to intracardiac procedures, turbulent blood flow, deformed valves, and old scars in chronic rheumatic heart disease.
- *Malignant tumors:* They may develop as part of a paraneoplastic syndrome in malignancies associated with procoagulant effect of circulating mucin secreting tumors of colon or pancreas or lung.
- *Cachexia:* In debilitated people, i.e. cancer and chronic infection normal repair mechanisms are defective. Small thrombi formed are not removed by plasminogen and fibrinolytic substances grow and transform into large excrescences.

Cardiac Vegetations

- These are composed of fibrin, platelets, and red blood cells, resemble thrombi. These are sterile, measuring 1–5 mm in size, non-destructive (single or multiple) loosely attached randomly (Fig. 16.41).
- These are present on superior surface of aortic, mitral, tricuspid and pulmonary valves as a result of mild inflammation and associated surface endothelial damage (Fig. 16.42).

Complications

These sterile vegetations may cause peripheral embolization to brain, heart, lungs and kidneys.

Therapeutic Significance

Since NBTE vegetations require treatment with anticoagulants which are contraindicated in bacterial infective endocarditis. It is important to distinguish these two diseases. Administration of anticoagulants in infective endocarditis may result in fragmentation of cardiac vegetations and embolization to distant organs.

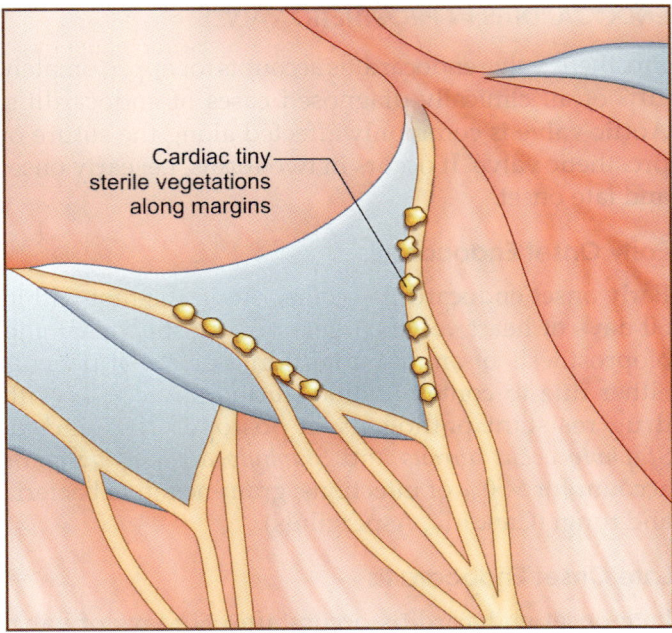

Fig. 16.42: Cardiac vegetations in rheumatic heart disease. These are tiny sterile vegetations present along the margin of mitral valve.

ENDOCARDITIS IN RHEUMATIC HEART DISEASE

Cardiac Vegetations

These are sterile vegetations measuring 1–2 mm in diameter, present along the line of opposition of cusps and chordae tendineae. These are never present behind cusps (Fig. 16.43).

Cardiac Valve Involved

Frequency of cardiac valves involved includes mitral valve (75–80%), aortic (30%), mitral and aortic

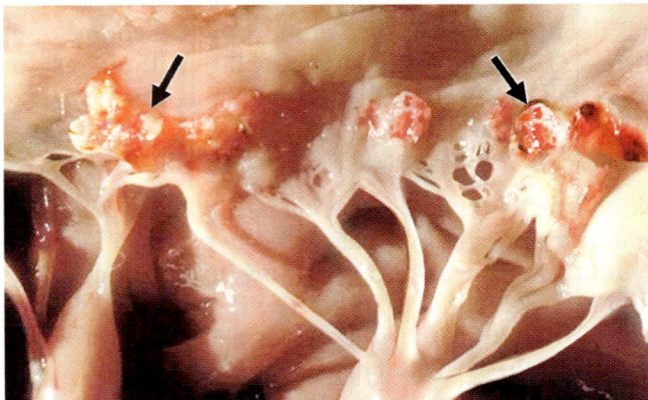

Fig. 16.41: Nonbacterial thrombotic endocarditis—sterile large vegetations are loosely attached along margins of normal cardiac valves on both sides. These are associated with cancer and wasting diseases. There is principal risk of bacterial endocarditis and embolization to brain, heart, lungs and kidneys (arrows).

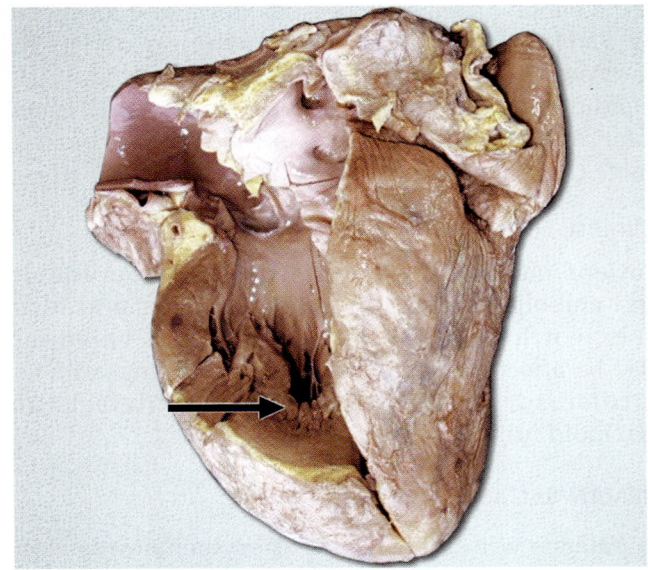

Fig. 16.43: Rheumatic heart disease. Sterile vegetations are seen along margin of mitral valve (arrow).

valves (25%), mitral valve, tricuspid valve (<5%) and pulmonary valve (rare). These vegetations with super added infection lead to subacute bacterial endocarditis.

ENDOCARDITIS OF CARCINOID SYNDROME

Etiology

Endocarditis of carcinoid syndrome is caused by secretory products of intestinal carcinoid tumors, i.e. vasoactive amines (serotonin) and vasoactive peptide hormones (somatostatin and glucagon).

Pathogenesis

- These secretory products of non-metastasizing intestinal carcinoid tumor are inactivated and metabolized in liver as well as lungs.
- In case of metastases of carcinoid tumor to liver, these secretory products enter circulation and cause tricuspid regurgitation and pulmonary trunk stenosis.
- The valves on the left side of the heart are rarely involved, because serotonin and other carcinoid secretory products are detoxified in the lung. These valvular lesions heal by fibrosis.

Clinical Correlation

Patient presents with cutaneous flushing, diarrhea, and valvular disease (tricuspid regurgitation and pulmonary trunk stenosis).

Comparison of cardiac vegetations is given in Table 16.12 and Fig. 16.44.

Table 16.12: Comparison of cardiac vegetations

Parameters	Rheumatic fever	Non-bacterial thrombotic endocarditis	Libman-Sacks endocarditis (SLE)	Infective endocarditis
Etiology	Group A *Streptococcus pyogenes*	Hypercoagulable state, mucin secreting carcinoma of colon and pancreas	Autoimmune disorder	Infective agents
Mechanism	Type II and Type IV hypersensitivity reaction (molecular mimicry)	Non-inflammatory disorder	Immune complex mediated by DNA-anti-DNA autoantibody	Acute inflammation
Size	1–2 mm size firm and warty	1–5 mm single/multiple friable results in embolism	1–4 mm single or multiple widely spaced	Large, friable bulky loosely attached to valves
Nature	Sterile, non-destructive	Sterile non-destructive	Sterile small and non-destructive	Infective, destructive
Composition	Aschoff's nodule	Fibrin, platelets, and RBCs	Fibrin platelets and RBCs	Acute inflammation PMN with bacteria
Location	Along the lines of closure of valvular cusps	Along the lines of closure of cusps or both side of valvular cusps	Present on both sides of mitral valvular cusps. Most common on inferior surface. Pocket of valves. Less common on mural endocardium	Upper surface of valvular cusps. It can extend to the chordae tendineae
Valves affected	Mitral valve (75–80%), aortic valve (30%), mitral valve and aortic valve (25%), tricuspid valve and pulmonary valve <5%	Any cardiac valve	Mitral valve (most common), tricuspid valve +	Tricuspid valve (most common)
Chances of embolization	Low incidence	High incidence	Absent	High incidence
Blood test	Antistreptolysin-O titer raised	Not diagnostic	LE cells preparation	Blood culture positive (95%)

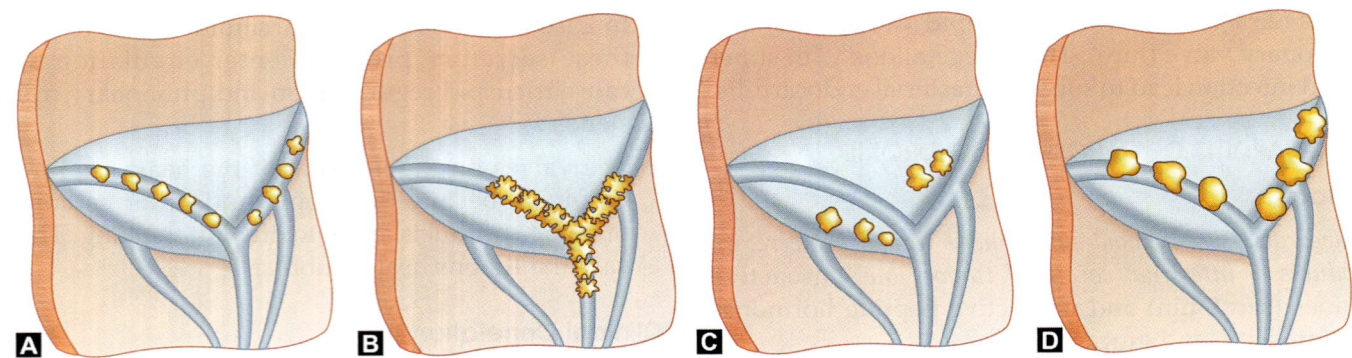

Fig. 16.44: Cardiac vegetations. (A) Cardiac vegetation in RHD, (B) infective endocarditis (IE), (C) Libman-Sacks endocarditis (LSE), (D) non-bacterial thrombotic endocarditis (NBTE).

CARDIAC VALVES

OVERVIEW

Cardiac valvular diseases most often occur as a result of advanced rheumatic heart disease. Valves may be affected secondary to various inflammatory processes. Prosthetic valves are the site of thrombus formation or infective endocarditis.

These cause mechanical disruption of red blood cells which result in hemolytic anemia with formation of schistocytes. Causes of valvular diseases are described in Table 16.13.

Pathological causes and clinical features of mitral and aortic valvular lesions are given in Table 16.14.

Table 16.13: Causes of valvular diseases

Mitral valve stenosis	
Rheumatic heart disease	
Mitral valve insufficiency	
Rheumatic heart disease	Hypertrophic obstructive cardiomyopathy
Mitral valve prolapse	Acute myocardial infarction (papillary muscle necrosis)
Mitral valve prolapse	
Marfan's syndrome (90%)	
Tricuspid valve insufficiency	
Bacterial endocarditis in intravenous drug abuse (most common)	
Rheumatic heart disease (5%)	
Aortic valve stenosis	
Rheumatic heart disease	
Aortic valve insufficiency	
Acute aortic insufficiency: Endocarditis, chest trauma, prosthetic valve malfunction, acute ascending aortic dissection and cystic medial necrosis.	
Chronic aortic insufficiency: Systemic hypertension, chronic rheumatic heart disease, Marfan's syndrome, ankylosing spondylitis, syphilis and ventricular septal defect.	
Calcific aortic valve stenosis	
Rheumatic disease	
Senile calcific stenosis	
Congenital aortic stenosis	
Pulmonary stenosis	
Tetralogy of Fallot	
Carcinoid heart disease	
Rheumatic heart disease (rare)	

Heart

Table 16.14: Pathological causes and clinical features of mitral and aortic valvular lesions

Valvular lesion	Pathological cause	Clinical features
Mitral stenosis	Rheumatic fever	Pulmonary hypertension Left atrial and right ventricular hypertrophy Opening snap and diastolic murmur
Mitral incompetence	Rheumatic fever, dilatation of mitral valve annulus, papillary muscle fibrosis and dysfunction and mucoid degeneration of valve cusps (mitral valve prolapse)	Variable hemodynamic effects Pansystolic murmur Mid-systolic click and late systolic murmur in mitral valve prolapse
Aortic stenosis	Calcific degeneration and rheumatic fever	Ejection systolic murmur Left ventricular hypertrophy leading to left ventricular failure Angina pectoris, syncope or sudden cardiac death
Aortic incompetence	Rheumatic fever, dilatation of aortic root (age related or syphilitica ortitis), rheumatoid arthritis or ankylosing spondylitis	Diastolic murmur, wide pulse pressure, collapsing pulse Left ventricular failure Angina pectoris

MITRAL VALVE STENOSIS

Mitral valve is most commonly affected in chronic rheumatic heart disease. It undergoes fibrosis and dystrophic calcification, with fusion of the commissures resulting in stenosis (*fish mouth appearance*) (Fig. 16.45).

Consequences

Mitral valve stenosis hampers normal blood flow from left atrium to left ventricle during diastole. It leads to hypertrophy of the left atrium, pulmonary congestion and brown induration; and right ventricle hypertrophy (cor pulmonale).

Clinical Features

The patient presents with breathlessness, orthopnea and hemoptysis secondary to pulmonary congestion; dysphagia for solids owing to left atrial enlargement. Mural thrombi in left atrium result in systemic embolization dislodged by atrial fibrillation.

Auscultation

Turbulent blood flow through the mitral stenosis presents with a mid-diastolic murmur heard best at apex.

MITRAL VALVE INSUFFICIENCY

Etiology

- Mitral valve insufficiency usually occurs as a result of rheumatic heart disease. It can also result from mitral valve prolapse, hypertrophic obstructive cardiomyopathy, damage to papillary muscle from myocardial infarction, ruptured chordae tendineae and transposition of great arteries.
- It can be secondary to left ventricular dilation, with stretching of the mitral valve ring. Blood from the left ventricle flows back into the left atrium during systole, causing the atrium to enlarge to accommodate the backflow. Patient eventually leads to left-sided and right-sided heart failure.

Clinical Features

Patient presents with exertional dyspnea, paroxysmal nocturnal dyspnea, orthopnea, weakness, fatigue and palpitations. Physical examination reveals peripheral edema, jugular vein distention, ascites, and hepatomegaly (right-sided heart failure)

Auscultation

On auscultation, crackles and a loud S1 or opening snap and a holosystolic murmur are heard at the apex.

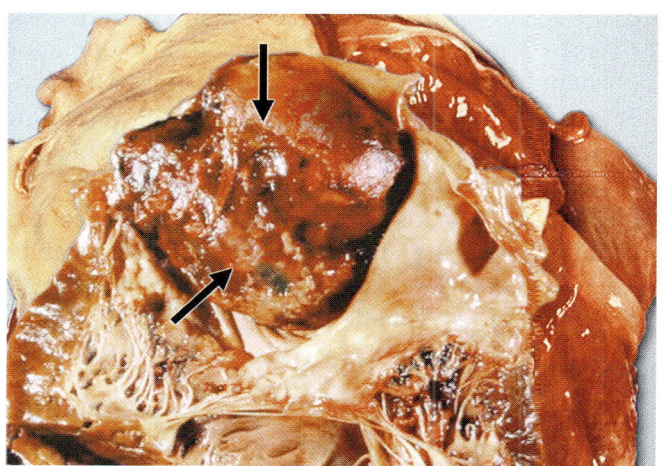

Fig. 16.45: Mitral valve stenosis. Ball thrombus (arrows) in the left atrium is complication in mitral stenosis and atrial fibrillation.

MITRAL VALVE PROLAPSE

Mitral valve prolapse is the most frequent valvular lesion resulting in mitral valve insufficiency. Under physiological state, mitral valve closes during systole. It commonly affects young women. It is common in patients with Marfan's syndrome (90%) (Fig. 16.46).

Pathogenesis

Valve shows myxoid degeneration of ground substance due to stromal accumulation of glycosaminoglycans. Architecture of the valve is maintained. It shows elongation and thinning of chordae tendineae of valve. It leads to stretching of the posterior valve leaflet resulting in *floppy cusp,* i.e. parachute deformity with prolapse into the left atrium during systole.

Consequences

Regurgitation of the blood across the incompetent mitral valve leads to reflux of blood from left ventricle into left atrium. Back pressure is transmitted to lungs resulting in pulmonary congestion and the right-sided heart chambers.

Clinical Features

Patient presents with pulmonary symptoms, i.e. breathlessness and cough occurring late in the disease.

Auscultation

Regurgitation of the blood across the incompetent mitral valve presents with *pansystolic murmur* radiating into the axilla heard best at the apex and increases in intensity on expiration. Mid-systolic click can be heard in mitral valve prolapse.

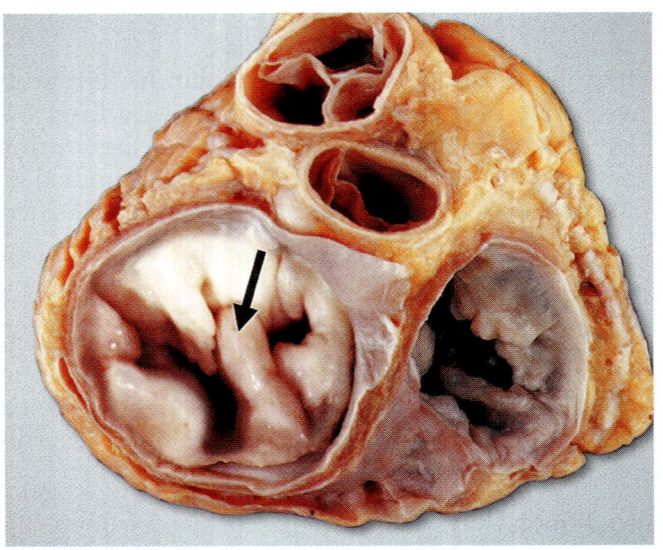

Fig. 16.46: Mitral valve prolapse. Many patients are asymptomatic. There is increased risk of cerebral embolism (arrow).

Complication

Mitral valve prolapse is often associated with arrhythmias. Infectious endocarditis with arterial embolization is a possible consequence of this very common lesion. Antibiotic prophylaxis for dental procedures is recommended.

AORTIC STENOSIS

Aortic valve along with the mitral valve is frequently involved in rheumatic heart disease. Under physiological state, aortic valve is closed during diastole. Aortic stenosis prevents the outflow of blood from left ventricle into the aorta during systole.

Etiology

Aortic stenosis may result from rheumatic fever, idiopathic aortic valve fibrosis and calcification of aortic valve in old age >60 years and congenital aortic bicuspid valve.

Consequence

Aortic stenosis increases blood pressure inside the left ventricle resulting in *concentric hypertrophy* associated with decreased chamber size. Patient develops *left ventricular failure* leading to pulmonary congestion. Patient ultimately develops *core pulmonale.*

Clinical Features

Patient presents with breathlessness, cough, syncope, chest pain (angina) or sudden death.

Auscultation

Patient develops *high-pitched ejection systolic murmur.*

AORTIC VALVE INSUFFICIENCY/REGURGITATION

- Aortic valve insufficiency is the incomplete closure of the aortic valve. During diastole, blood from aorta flows back into the left ventricle resulting in dilatation of chamber and eccentric myocardial hypertrophy.
- Stroke volume is increased often >100 ml. Widening of pulse pressure leads to hyperdynamic circulation, i.e. *water-hammer pulse.*
- Ultimately, it leads to left-sided heart failure and pulmonary edema. Aortic valve insufficiency can be acute or chronic and is usually caused by scarring or retraction of valve leaflets.

Etiology

- *Acute aortic insufficiency:* It is caused by endocarditis, chest trauma, prosthetic valve malfunction, acute ascending aortic dissection and non-dissecting aneurysm due to cystic medial necrosis.

- *Chronic aortic insufficiency:* It occurs due to hypertension, chronic rheumatic heart disease, Marfan's syndrome, ankylosing spondylitis, syphilitic aortitis and ventricular septal defect.

Clinical Features

Patient develops left-sided heart failure and pulmonary congestion. Patient presents with dyspnea, orthopnea, paroxysmal nocturnal dyspnea, fatigue, palpitation and exercise intolerance. Auscultation reveals S3 heart sound and high-pitched blowing *diastolic murmur* at left sternal border.

CALCIFIC AORTIC STENOSIS

Calcific aortic stenosis refers to a narrowing of the aortic valve orifice as a result of the deposition of calcium in the valve cusps and ring (Fig. 16.47).

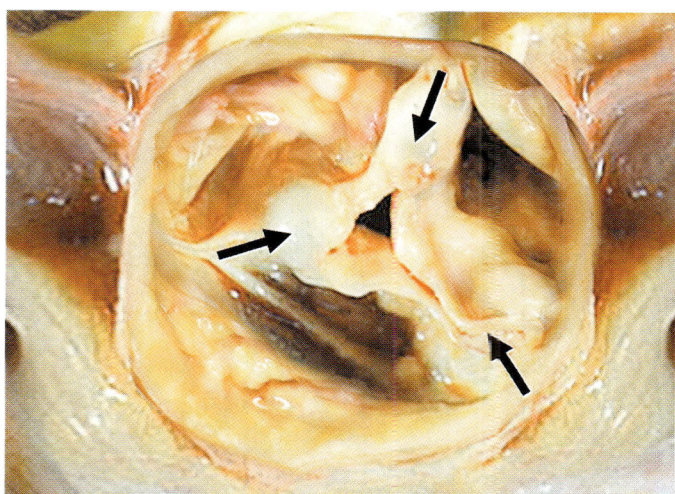

Fig. 16.47: Calcific aortic stenosis. A 75-year-old man presented with history of recurrent syncope underwent surgery for aortic valve disease. Valve was markedly deformed and calcified (arrows).

Pathogenesis

Causes of calcific aortic stenosis are rheumatic disease, senile calcific stenosis, and congenital aortic stenosis. It is related to the cumulative effect of years of trauma due to turbulent blood flow around the valve. It becomes progressively narrowed with some degrees of regurgitation.

TRICUSPID INSUFFICIENCY

Tricuspid insufficiency secondary to bacterial endocarditis is one of the most common complications of intravenous drug abuse. It may be involved together with the mitral and aortic valves in 5% of cases of rheumatic heart disease. The cardiac lesions consist of plaque-like deposits of dense fibrous tissue on the tricuspid and pulmonary valves.

Clinical Features

- Patient develops tricuspid insufficiency and pulmonary valve stenosis in carcinoid heart disease due to release of active tumor products, characterized by diarrhea, flushing, bronchospasm, and skin lesions.
- Elevated levels of 5-HIAA (5-hydroxyindole acetic acid), a metabolite of serotonin, are diagnostic of carcinoid syndrome.

PULMONARY STENOSIS

Pulmonary valve stenosis usually occurs due to congenital malformations occurring either alone or in the tetralogy of Fallot. It may be involved in the *carcinoid syndrome*.

Carcinoid Heart Disease

The cardiac lesions in *carcinoid syndrome* consist of plaque-like deposits of dense fibrous tissue on the tricuspid and pulmonary valves in the *carcinoid syndrome*. Pulmonary valve is rarely involved in rheumatic heart disease.

PERICARDIUM

ANATOMY AND PHYSIOLOGY

Pericardium consists of outer parietal and inner visceral layers, which are intimately related to the myocardium. Pericardial cavity contains 20–50 ml of fluid, which provides protection to the heart and prevents intracardial pressure changes associated with postural variation and respiration.

Pericardium minimizes friction of pericardial layers. It facilitates atrial filling during ventricular systole. It prevents sudden dilatation of chambers during exercise and increased blood volume. It prevents displacement of heart and kinking of the blood vessels. It prevents spread of infection from lung and pleura to heart.

PERICARDIAL EFFUSION

Definition

Pericardial effusion is sudden collection of fluid in the pericardial sac without chamber enlargement beyond the 20–50 ml normally present. There is filling of the retrosternal space, and effacement of the normal cardiac borders giving a *water bottle configuration*. Causes of transudative pericardial effusion include cardiac surgery, congestive heart failure, uremia, myxedema and collagen vascular diseases.

Etiology

Pericardial effusions are caused by pericarditis (e.g. serous, fibrinous, suppurative, hemorrhagic or tubercular), metastatic deposits from lung cancer, breast cancer or lymphomas. Tubercular effusion is straw/pale-colored fluid formed by Mycobacterium tubercle bacilli.

Laboratory Diagnosis

Laboratory diagnosis includes imaging techniques, i.e. X-ray chest (e.g. water bottle configuration), echocardiography (to demonstrate amount of fluid), complete urine analysis for proteins and sugar, liver function tests, kidney function tests, blood sugar, and fluid cytology.

HYDROPERICARDIUM

Accumulation of serous transudate in the pericardial space is known as hydropericardium. It is caused by congestive heart failure and hypoproteinemia. Malnutrition, chronic liver disease and nephrotic syndrome are important causes of hypoproteinemia.

HEMOPERICARDIUM

Accumulation of blood in the pericardial cavity is known as hemopericardium. It may cause cardiac tamponade with fatal outcome.

Etiology

Hemopericardium occurs due to traumatic perforation of the heart or dissecting aortic hematoma, myocardial rupture associated with acute myocardial infarction or neoplasm. As the first part of the aorta (root) lies within the pericardial sac, rupture of the aortic wall due to aortic dissection may cause intrapericardial bleeding.

CARDIAC TAMPONADE

Rapid accumulation of excessive fluid or blood in pericardial cavity leads to cardiac tamponade, resulting in interference in cardiac filling (Figs 16.48 and 16.49).

It is characterized by cardiogeneic shock (hypotension), reduced cardiac output and raised jugular venous pressure. Pulsus paradoxus, the hallmark of cardiac tamponade is >10 mm fall in systolic blood pressure during inspiration.

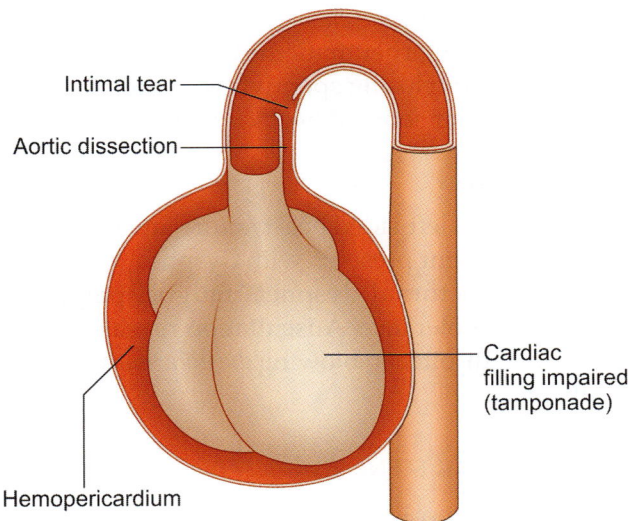

Fig. 16.48: Hemopericardium—pericardial cavity is filled with blood.

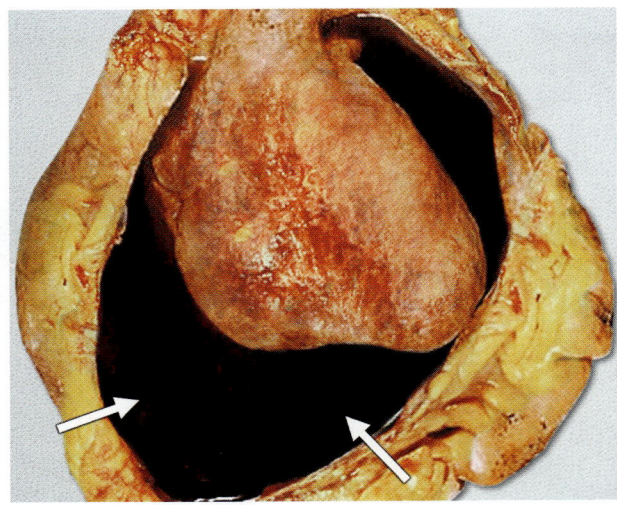

Fig. 16.49: Hemopericardium—aortic dissection may lead to hemopericardium when blood dissects through the media proximally. Such a massive amount of hemorrhage can lead to cardiac tamponade (arrows).

PERICARDITIS

Pericarditis is inflammation of the pericardium. In most instances, it is mild and unrecognized.

Acute pericarditis can be fibrinous exudate, purulent, serous, or hemorrhagic exudate. Chronic constrictive pericarditis is characterized by dense, fibrous pericardial thickening. Common symptoms of pericarditis are pain at the sternum and shallow, rapid respirations.

Etiological Classification

- *Infectious causes:* These include bacteria (e.g. pyogenic bacteria, Mycobacterium tubercle bacilli, *Treponema pallidum*), viruses and fungi. Infection may occur after cardiac surgery.

- *Non-infectious causes:* Fibrinous pericarditis known as *bread and butter pericarditis* is associated with uremia, acute myocardial infarction (Dressler syndrome), and rheumatic fever. Other causes include high dose radiation to mediastinum, or metastasis (lung, breast or lymphomas), sarcoidosis, myxedema and chylopericardium.
- *Immunologic causes:* These include acute rheumatic pancarditis, rheumatoid arthritis, systemic lupus erythematosus (very common), scleroderma and drugs (e.g. procainamide and hydralazine).

Pathogenesis

- Pericardial tissue damaged by injurious agent releases chemical mediators of inflammation into the surrounding tissue. Friction occurs as the inflamed pericardial layers rub against each other.
- Various chemical mediators such as histamines increase vessel permeability resulting in leakage of inflammatory exudate. Neutrophils, macrophages begin to phagocytose and degrade the injurious agent, remove necrotic tissues and dead inflammatory cells. These products are eventually reabsorbed into healthy tissue.

Clinical History

Patient presents with sharp sudden pain at the sternum radiating to the neck, shoulders, and arms; shallow, rapid respiration, mild fever, dyspnea and orthopnea.

Physical Examination

Patient may develop congestive heart failure, i.e. elevated jugular pressure, hepatomegaly and peripheral edema. Patient develops Beck's triad (e.g. hypotension, elevated jugular venous pulse, and muffled distant heart sounds). Friction rub is appreciated on auscultation. Apex pulse may vanish. Dullness beneath angle of left scapula is known as *Ewart's sign*.

ACUTE PERICARDITIS

Acute pericarditis is characterized by rapid accumulation of fluid or exudate in the pericardial cavity known as *pericardial effusion*. It is usually diagnosed with echocardiography. Several pathologic forms of pericarditis are described below.

Serous Pericarditis

Serous pericarditis is associated with viral infections, rheumatic heart disease and systemic lupus erythematosus. Pericardial sac contains clear, straw-colored, protein-rich exudate containing small numbers of inflammatory cells. These patients may develop chest pain due to pericardial effusion (Fig. 16.50).

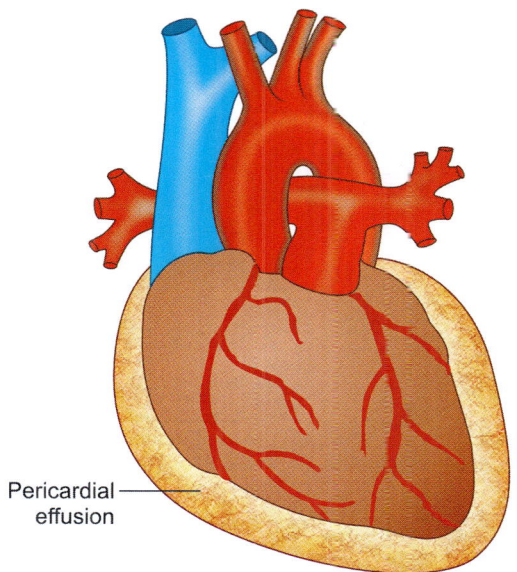

Fig. 16.50: Pericardial effusion shows accumulation of serous fluid in pericardial cavity.

Fibrinous or Serofibrinous Pericarditis

Fibrinous or serofibrinous pericarditis is characterized by a fibrin-rich exudate due to increased vascular permeability. It may be caused by chronic renal failure (uremia), myocardial infarction, or acute rheumatic fever or systemic lupus erythematosus. Fibrin deposited in pericardium exhibits *bread and butter appearance*. Friction rub is heard on auscultation. Fibrinous debris may be removed by fibrinolysis and macrophages resulting in restoration of normal tissue structure. When fibrinogen is not removed, there is danger of obliteration of pericardial cavity due to fusion of parietal and visceral layers (Figs 16.51 and 16.52).

Purulent or Suppurative Pericarditis

Pus or purulent exudate accumulates in the pericardial cavity. It is almost always caused by bacterial infection as a consequence of direct spread from a subjacent lung infection caused by *Staphylococcus aureus* or *Streptococcus pneumoniae*. Pericardium exhibits yellowish microabscesses. On histopathological examination, microabscess consists of blue bacterial colonies and is surrounded by acute inflammatory cells (Fig. 16.53).

Hemorrhagic Pericarditis

Accumulation of bloody inflammatory exudate in the pericardial cavity is known as hemorrhagic pericarditis. It usually results from tumor invasion of the pericardium, i.e. lung cancer, esophageal cancer, breast cancer or lymphomas in 5–10% cases. Surface of the epicardium shows pale white-tan nodules of metastatic tumor. Cardiac surgery and tubercular etiology may also result in hemorrhagic pericarditis (Fig. 16.54).

Section III: Systemic Pathology

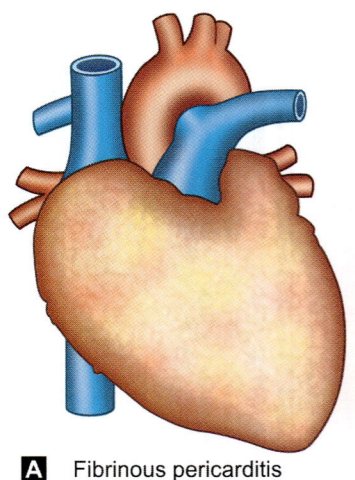
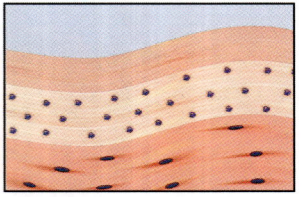

A Fibrinous pericarditis | Fibrinous pericarditis (microscopy)

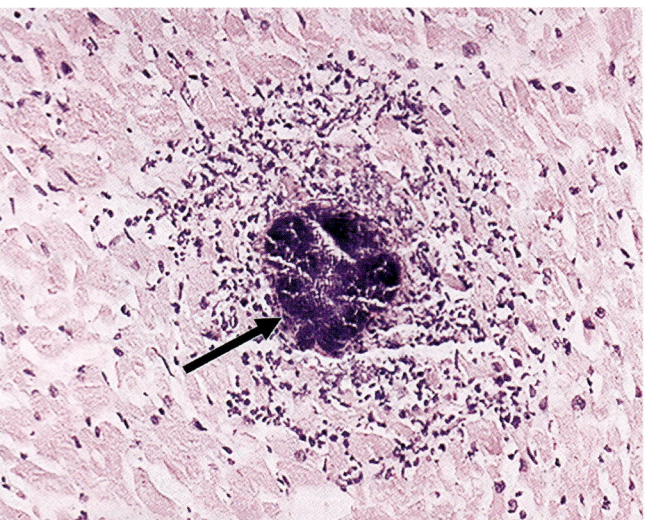

Fig. 16.53: Purulent or suppurative pericarditis. Yellowish purulent exudate is visible on the surface of pericardium. Bacterial clonies are shown (arrow).

Fig. 16.51: Fibrinous pericarditis after acute myocardial infarction (arrow).

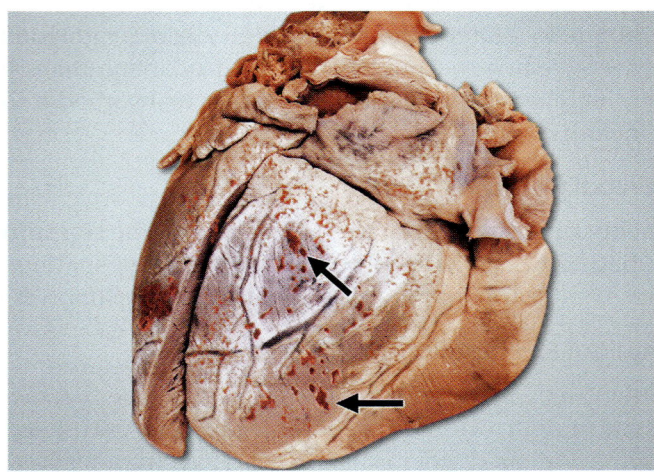

Fig. 16.54: Petechial hemorrhages on epicardium. It occurs due to low platelets count and sudden hypoxia (arrows).

CHRONIC PERICARDITIS

Patient develops chronic pericarditis, when fluid or fibrinous exudate is not removed from pericardial sac. Patient develops obliteration of pericardial sac due to fusion of parietal and visceral layers, known as constrictive pericarditis.

Pathology

Chronic pericarditis is characterized by thickening and scarring of the pericardium with resultant loss of elasticity. Proliferation of fibrous tissue with occasional small foci of calcification is marked. This prevents the pericardium from stretching and thus interferes with cardiac function and venous return, often mimicking the signs and symptoms of right-sided heart failure.

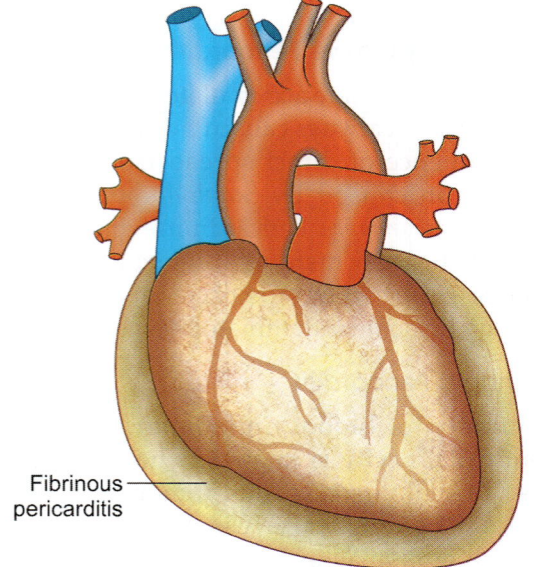

Fig. 16.52: Fibrinous pericarditis shows deposition of fibrin in pericardial sac.

CONSTRICTIVE PERICARDITIS

Constrictive pericarditis represents a chronic phase of fibrous scarring, pericardial thickening and obliteration of the pericardial cavity. It can result in restriction of diastolic cardiac filling. Acute pericardial injury and exuberant healing response by forming granulation tissue leads to fusion of parietal and visceral layers of pericardium (Fig. 16.55).

Etiopathogenesis

- Pericarditis may be caused by bacteria, viruses, or fungi. Previous radiation therapy to the mediastinum and cardiac surgery account for one-third of the cases.
- Tuberculosis is the most common cause of constrictive pericarditis. Stiffness of the pericardium is often enhanced by dystrophic calcification.
- Constrictive pericarditis restricts the heart's ability to pump effectively. The return of venous blood to the right heart is also compromised. Thickened pericardium compresses epicardial coronary artery resulting to under perfusion of the heart. Constrictive pericarditis should be differentiated from angina pectoris.

Clinical Features

Patient presents with chest pain, cough, exertional dyspnea and orthopnea. Elevated systemic venous pressure results in raised jugular venous pressure, hepatomegaly, marked ascites and peripheral edema. Reduced cardiac output causes fatigue and tachycardia (Table 16.15).

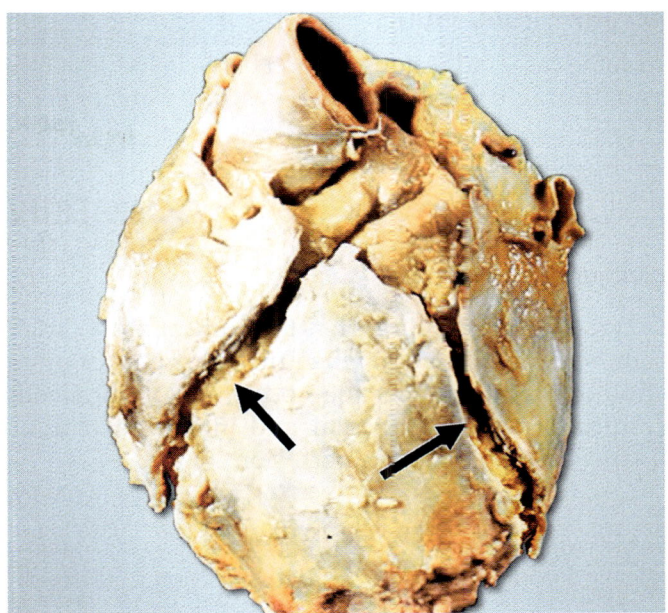

Fig. 16.55: Constrictive pericarditis in a case of tuberculosis. Patient presents with dyspnea, chest pain and abdominal discomfort. Physical examination revealed hepatomegaly, ascites and pitting edema. Cardiac auscultation revealed pericardial rub, respiratory crackles in both lungs and bases (arrows).

CT/MRI Techniques

Constrictive pericarditis is characterized by pericardial thickening, i.e. 4 mm, pericardial calcification, reduced right ventricular volume, a dilated right atrium, superior vena cava, inferior vena cava, hepatomegaly and ascites.

Table 16.15: Clinical features of constrictive pericarditis

Systemic changes	Clinical features
Reduced cardiac output	Fatigue, hypotension, reflex tachycardia
Elevated systemic venous pressure	Jugular venous distension, hepatomegaly with marked ascites, peripheral edema
Pulmonary venous congestion	Exertional dyspnea, cough and orthopnea
Chest pain typical of angina may be related to under perfusion of the coronary arteries or compression of an epicardial coronary artery by the thickened pericardium	Because the most impressive physical findings are often the insidious development of ascites of hepatomegaly and ascites, such patients are often mistakenly thought to suffer from hepatic cirrhosis or an intra-abdominal tumor. It is only after a careful inspection of the jugular veins that a cardiac source is identified

Table 16.16: Differences between constrictive and adhesive pericarditis

Parameters	Constrictive pericarditis	Adhesive pericarditis
Etiology	Bacteria, viruses, parasites and fungi	Bacteria, viruses, parasites and fungi
	Rheumatic fever, AMI, uremia and SLE causing fibrinous pericarditis leads to constrictive pericarditis	Rheumatic fever, AMI, uremia and SLE causing fibrinous pericarditis leads to adhesive pericarditis
Pathology	Parietal and visceral layers are fused	Adhesions between pericardium and thoracic cage
Clinical effects	It restricts the heart's ability to pump effectively	Cardiac hypertrophy results to cardiomegaly

ADHESIVE PERICARDITIS

In some cases, adhesions formed between pericardium and thoracic cage leads to systolic retraction of thoracic cage and cardiac hypertrophy (cardiomegaly demonstrated by X-ray). Differences between constrictive and adhesive pericarditis are shown in Table 16.16.

CONGESTIVE HEART FAILURE

OVERVIEW

Congestive heart failure refers to failure of left ventricle, right ventricle, or both, when the heart cannot pump enough blood to meet the body's metabolic needs, resulting into intravascular and interstitial volume overload and poor tissue perfusion.

Pateint presents with dyspnea and/or edema. Causes of left- or right-sided heart failure are described in Table 16.17. Clinical manifestations of heart failure are described in Fig. 16.56.

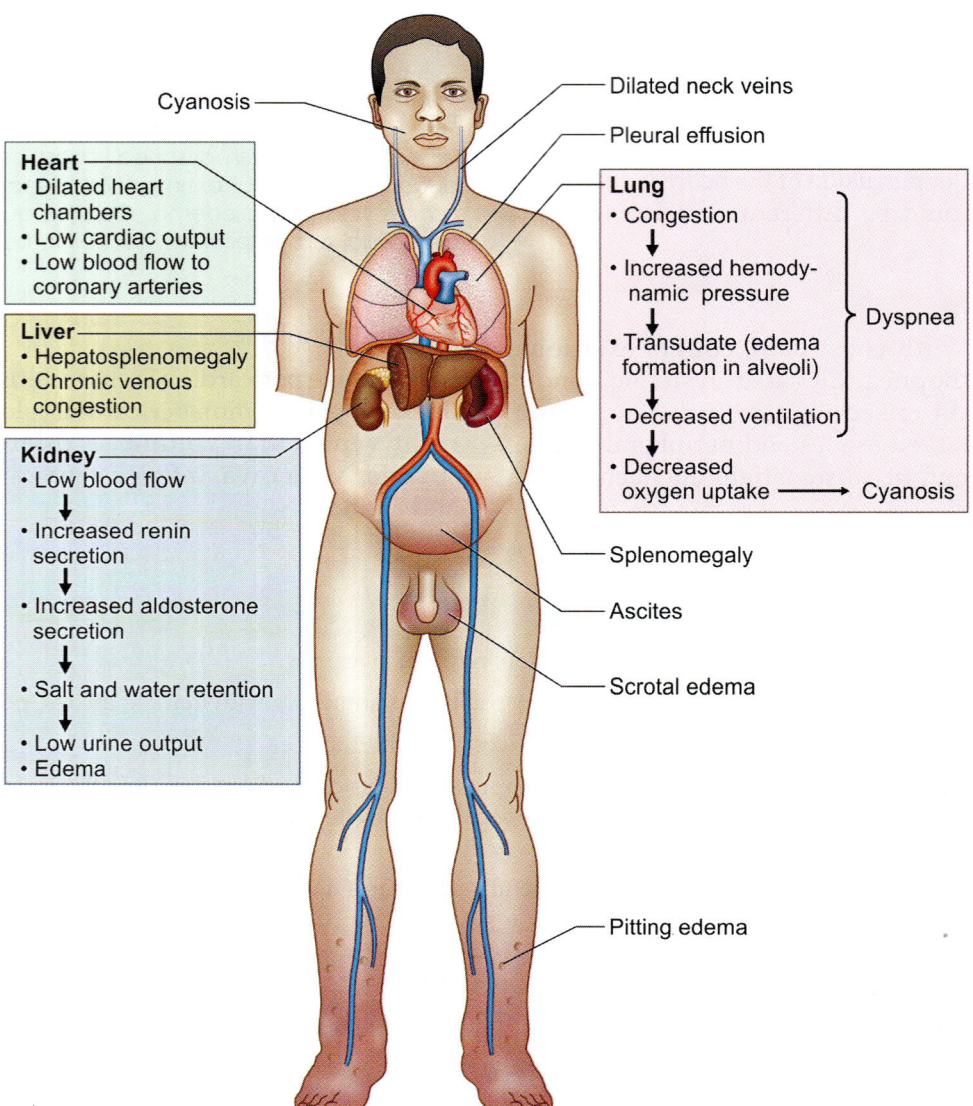

Fig. 16.56: Clinical manifestations in heart failure. Left heart failure is associated with retention of salt and water, pulmonary congestion, dyspnea, cyanosis, generalized edema, ascites, hydrothorax and scrotal edema. Right heart failure is associated with systemic venous congestion, peripheral pitting edema over ankles and hepatosplenomegaly.

Table 16.17: Causes of heart failure in adults

Left-sided heart failure	Right-sided heart failure
Ischemic heart disease	Left-sided heart failure (most common cause)
Hypertension	Pulmonary hypertension
Aortic valvular disease	Tricuspid valvular disease
	Pulmonary valvular disease
Mitral valvular disease	Mitral stenosis
Myocardial diseases: Myocarditis and cardiomyopathies	*Myocardial diseases:* Myocarditis and cardiomyopathies

Heart Failure in Adults

- *Acute heart failure:* It follows acute myocardial infarction when direct damage to the heart's contracting ability has occurred.
- *Chronic heart failure:* It occurs in patients with hypertension, when the ventricles pump against chronically increased pressure.

Heart Failure in Children

In children, heart failure occurs mainly as a result of congenital heart defects. Therefore, treatment guidelines are directed toward the specific cause.

Assay of B-type Natriuretic Peptide

Assay of B-type natriuretic peptide is elevated in heart failure. Natriuretic peptide elevation may aid in the distinction of heart failure from other disorders such as acute coronary syndrome, bronchial asthma, chronic obstructive pulmonary disease, or pulmonary thromboembolism phenomenon, which may also present with dyspnea or edema.

Signs and Symptoms

Signs and symptoms of heart failure come from basic two mechanisms:

- The heart is unable to pump enough blood to meet the metabolic demands of the body.
- The kidney's compensatory mechanism of abnormal retention of sodium and water to compensate for the decreased cardiac output. This increases blood volume and venous return, which cause further pulmonary congestion.

LEFT HEART FAILURE

Etiology

Left heart failure occurs due to ischemic heart disease, hypertension, aortic valvular disease, mitral valvular disease and myocardial diseases, i.e. myocarditis and cardiomyopathies.

Pathophysiology

- Blood pools in the ventricle and atrium and eventually backs up into the pulmonary veins and capillaries. Rising capillary pressure pushes sodium (Na) and water (H_2O) into the interstitial space, causing pulmonary edema.
- Because the left ventricle cannot handle the increased venous return, fluid pools in the pulmonary circulation, and worsening pulmonary edema. Decreased breath sounds, dullness on percussion, crackles, and orthopnea.
- The right ventricle may now become stressed because it is pumping against greater pulmonary vascular resistance and left ventricular pressure.

Clinical Features

- *Dyspnea:* It is an early symptom from pulmonary congestion. On auscultation, crackles, wheeze breath sounds are heard. Pulmonary vascular congestion and proteinaceous pink staining intra-alveolar fluid can be seen in this manifestation of left-sided heart failure (Fig. 16.57).
- *Orthopnea:* Patient cannot breathe unless sitting up.
- *Cough:* Patient has frothy pink or white sputum.
- *Edema:* Pleural effusion with hydrothorax most often occur. Reduction in renal perfusion activates renin-angiotensin-aldosterone system and leading to retention of salt and water, is less frequent. Cerebral anoxia is less frequent.
- *Cool moist skin:* Patient has weak pulse, and cool moist skin as the peripheral vasoconstriction shunts blood to vital organs.

RIGHT HEART FAILURE

Etiology

Right heart failure is caused by left-sided heart failure (most common cause), mitral stenosis, pulmonary hypertension, myocardial diseases (myocarditis and

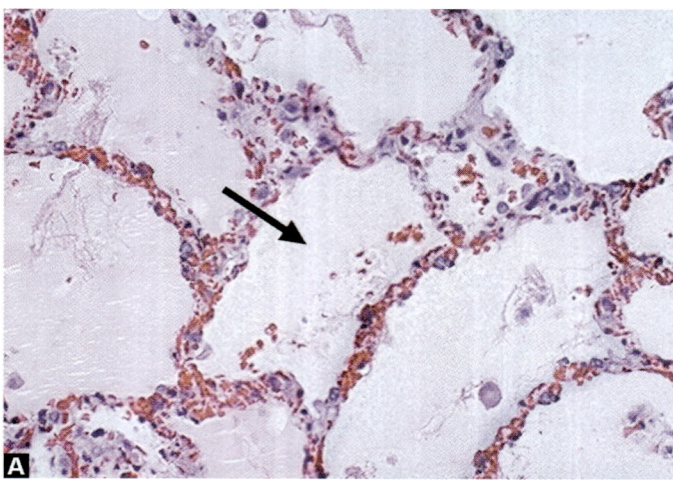
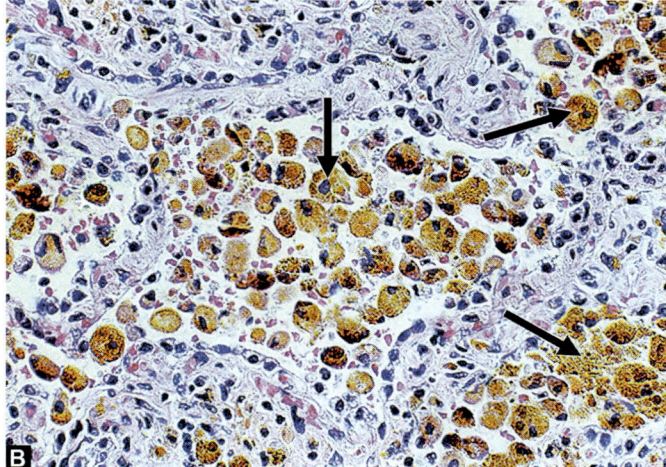

Fig. 16.57: Pulmonary edema. (A) The alveoli in this lung are filled with a smooth to slightly floccular pink material. Alveolar capillaries (arrow) congested (400X), (B) pulmonary edema with heart failure cells (arrows) (400X).

cardiomyopathies), tricuspid and pulmonary valvular disease. Causes of heart failure are described.

Pathophysiology

- The stressed right ventricle is enlarged. Blood pooling occurs in the right ventricle and right atrium. Increased back pressure causes congestion in the vena cava and systemic circulation.
- Backed-up blood distends the visceral veins, especially the hepatic vein. As the liver and spleen become engorged, their functions are impaired.
- Rising capillary pressure forces excess fluid from the capillaries into the interstitial space.

Clinical Features

- *Pitting edema of the ankles:* Left heart failure causes renal hypoxia that activates renin-angiotensin-aldosterone system resulting in greater retention of fluid and peripheral pitting edema of the ankles.
- *Pleural effusion:* Patient may develop pleural effusion. On clinical examination, percussion note is dull.

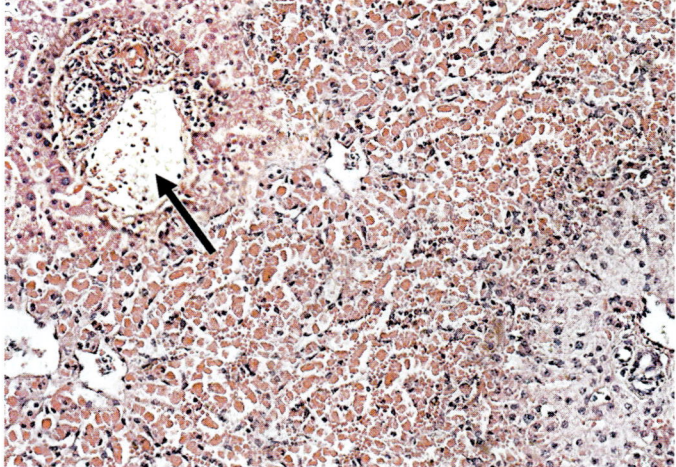

Fig. 16.59: Chronic venous congestion in liver shows congestion of central vein and hepatocytes. The hepatocytes at places have become atrophic (arrow) (400X).

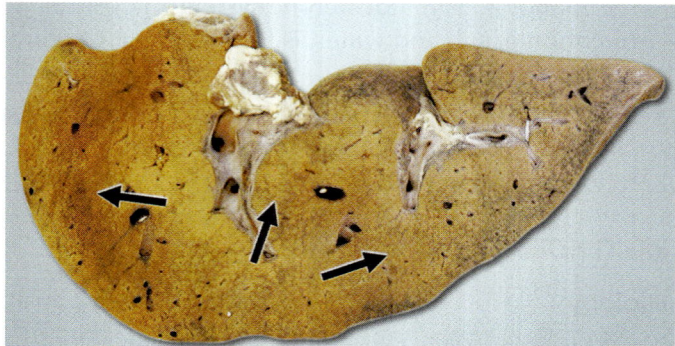

Fig. 16.58: Chronic venous congestion in liver. Cut surface shows nutmeg appearance (arrows).

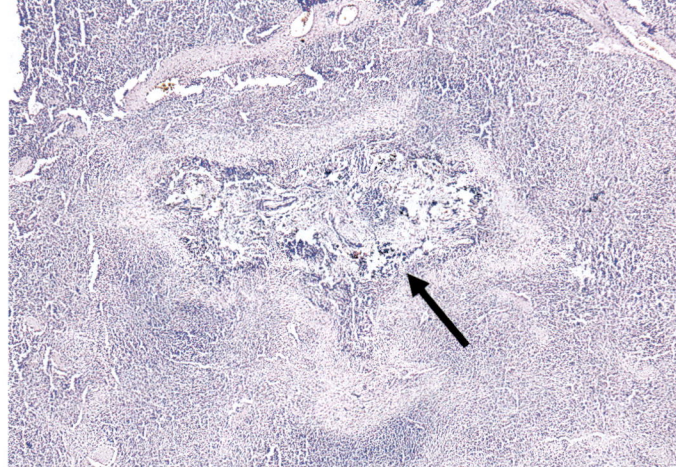

Fig. 16.60: Chronic venous congestion in spleen showing Gamna-Gandy bodies (arrow) (400X).

- *Ascites:* Patient may develop ascites. Ascitic fluid is demonstrated by shifting dullness.
- *Hepatomegaly:* Patient presents with hepatomegaly due to chronic passive congestion. Chronic passive congestion of the centrilobular veins of the liver surrounded by relatively pale, sometimes fatty, peripheral regions leads to a *nutmeg pattern* (Figs 16.58 and 16.59).
- *Splenomegaly:* Perivascular hemorrhages result in organization and formation of *Gamna-Gandy bodies* (dystrophic calcification). Cut surface of fibrocongestive splenomegaly shows firm brown fibrotic nodules termed as *Gamna-Gandy bodies* (Fig. 16.60).
- *Raised jugular venous pressure:* Patient with right-sided heart failure shows distention of the neck veins.

CARDIAC HYPERTROPHY

OVERVIEW

Hypertrophy is enlargement of a cell without cell division due to an increased workload. It can result from normal physiologic or abnormal pathologic conditions.

Cardiac Hypertrophy

- Hypertrophy of the left ventricle most often occurs due to systemic hypertension and aortic or mitral valvular disease. Congestive heart failure is the most common cause of death in untreated hypertensive patients. The overall weight of the heart increases, exceeding 375 gm in men and 350 gm in women.
- Right ventricular hypertrophy is caused by left ventricular failure, chronic lung disease, mitral valve disease and congenital heart disease with left-to-right shunt.

LEFT VENTRICULAR HYPERTROPHY

- Heart pumps out blood against resistance in patients with chronic hypertension and valvular disease (aortic or mitral valve).
- Increased oxygen demand is met by enlargement of the muscle cells, as myocardium is composed of terminally differentiated myocytes.
- Left ventricle shows concentric hypertrophy, characterized by increase in thickness of left ventricular wall and decrease in size of ventricular chamber (Figs 16.61 and 16.62).

  Differences between concentric and eccentric hypertrophy are given in Table 16.18.

Mechanism

- Mechanical stretch induces production of growth factors, i.e. TGF-β, FGF, insulin-like growth factor-1 and vasoactive agents, i.e. angiotensin II and endothelin.
- These bind to G-protein coupled receptors, induce signal to increase synthesis of contractile proteins, cardiac actin, atrial natriuretic factors and growth

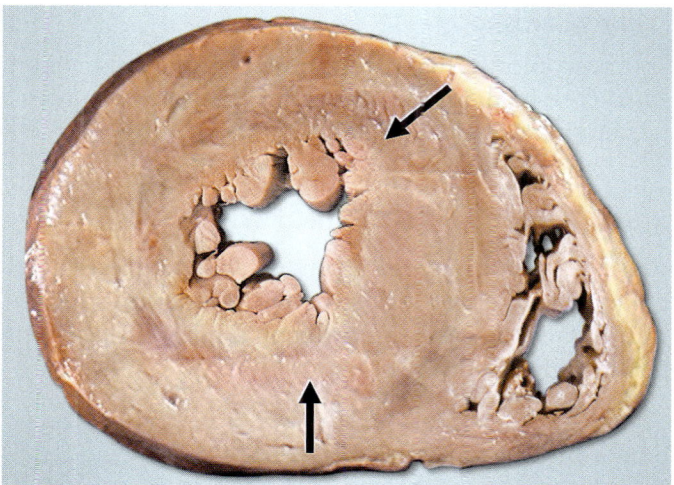

Fig. 16.61: Left ventricular hypertrophy. The left ventricle is markedly thickened in this patient with severe hypertension that was untreated for many years. The myocardial fibers have undergone hypertrophy. Normal thickness of wall of left ventricle is 1.2–1.5 cm (arrows).

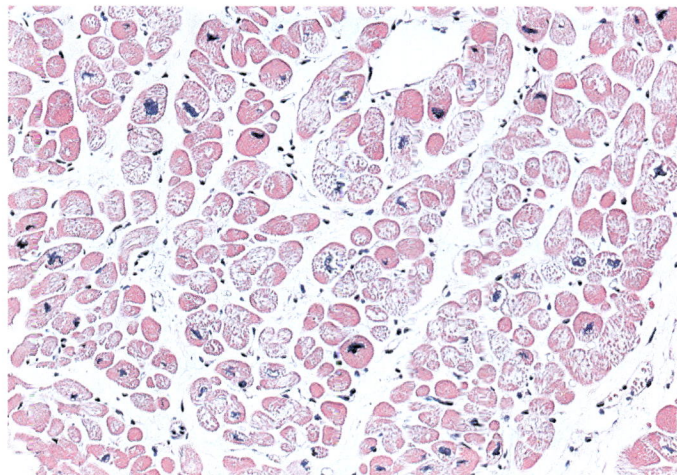

Fig. 16.62: LM—myofiber degeneration, marked hypertrophy of the cardiac myocytes + focal interstitial fibrosis (100X).

factors. Hypertrophy resulting in from transcriptional regulation increases of mRNA, rRNA, and protein. These increase the strength and work capacity of heart. Cardiac muscle shows increased cytosol, number of organelles and DNA content.

Table 16.18: Differences between concentric and eccentric cardic hypertrophy

Type	Concentric hypertrophy	Eccentric hypertrophy
Pathophysiology	Pressure overload	Volume overload
Definition	Deposition of the sarcomeres is parallel to the long axis of the cells	Dilatation with increased ventricular diameter
Cause	• Aortic stenosis • Hypertension	• Valvular regurgitation (mitral/aortic) • Thyrotoxicosis • Severe anemia

> **Light Microscopy**
>
> Microscopically, hypertrophic myocardial cells exhibit an increased diameter with enlarged, hyperchromatic, rectangular (*boxcar*) nuclei.

RIGHT VENTRICULAR HYPERTROPHY

Right ventricular hypertrophy is caused by left ventricular failure, chronic obstructive pulmonary disease, mitral valve disease and congenital heart disease with left-to-right shunt.

Left heart failure enhances pressure in pulmonary circulation that creates overload on right side of the heart. Most common cause of isolated right-sided heart failure is severe pulmonary hypertension.

Cor Pulmonale

Cor pulmonale is defined as right ventricular hypertrophy and dilation secondary to lung disease as a result of smoking (emphysema frequent cause) or pulmonary vasculature disease (pulmonary hypertension). Pulmonary stenosis is a rare cause of cor pulmonale.

CARDIAC TUMORS

CLASSIFICATION

Cardiac tumors are classified into primary (benign or malignant) and secondary tumors. Myxoma is the most common primary cardiac tumor in adults. Secondary tumors are more common than primary.

Primary Neoplasms

- *Benign tumors:* These include atrial myxoma and rhabdomyoma. Myxoma of the left atrium is most common primary benign tumor of heart. Other tumors include papillary fibroelastoma and fibroma.
- *Malignant tumors:* These are extremely rare. These include angiosarcoma and mesothelioma.

Secondary Neoplasms

These are more common than primary tumors of heart. Tumors metastasizing to heart include lung cancer, breast cancer and malignant melanoma. Epicardial surface is covered by pale white-tan multiple nodules of metastases. Metastases may lead to a hemorrhagic pericarditis (Fig. 16.63).

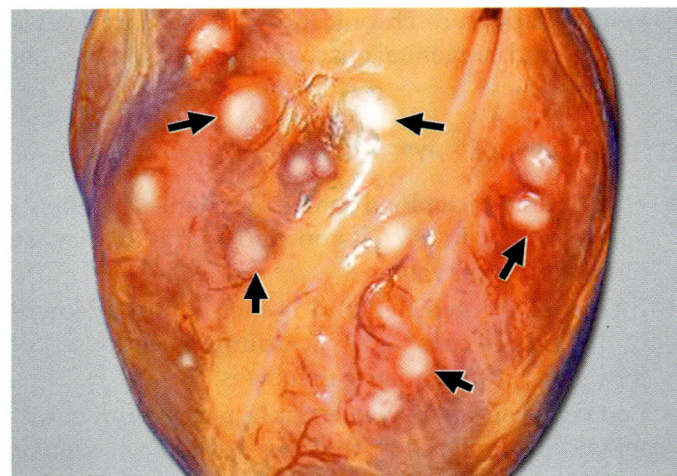

Fig. 16.63: Metastatic tumors to heart. It shows multiple metastatic pale, white-tan deposits on the pericardium (arrows).

ATRIAL MYXOMA

Atrial myxoma is most common benign primary cardiac neoplasm. It accounts for >50% of all primary tumors. Most myxomas are sporadic, but some occur as part of Carney syndrome characterized by skin tumors and schwannomas (Fig. 16.64).

Origin

Cardiac myxoma arises from multipotent mesenchymal cells exhibiting endothelial and neural differentiation.

Location

It is most often found in left atrium (90%). It arises from the left atrial septal wall around the fossa ovalis (80%), on valves and in ventricles.

Pathology

Most tumors are pedunculated. But some are broad based and sessile. The size varies, between 5 mm to 5 cm. *Ball-valve* effect of myxoma partially obstructs mitral valve intermittently, which prevents diastolic filling of the left ventricle simulating mitral valve stenosis.

Clinical Features

Patient presents with episodes of syncope, and non-specific symptoms (e.g. fever, anemia and elevated ESR). Tumor may fragment and give rise to arterial emboli to the brain.

Gross Morphology
On gross examination, myxomas appear gelatinous (*myxoid*).
Light Microscopy
Myxoma is composed of spindle-shaped cells with scant pink cytoplasm surrounded by loose myxoid matrix containing chondroid sulphate and hyaluronic acid.
Immunohistochemistry
Tumor cells show positivity for *vimentin, calretinin, CD31, CD34, and α-antitrypsin.*

Diagnosis

Echocardiography is the most useful technique for visualizing myxoma. The left atrium is located in posterior region of heart.

CARDIAC RHABDOMYOMA

Cardiac rhabdomyoma is second most common primary tumor of the heart in infants and children. It is associated with tuberous sclerosis in adults. It arises from striated muscle of myocardium. At autopsy, a large firm, white tumor mass is found filling much of the left ventricle.

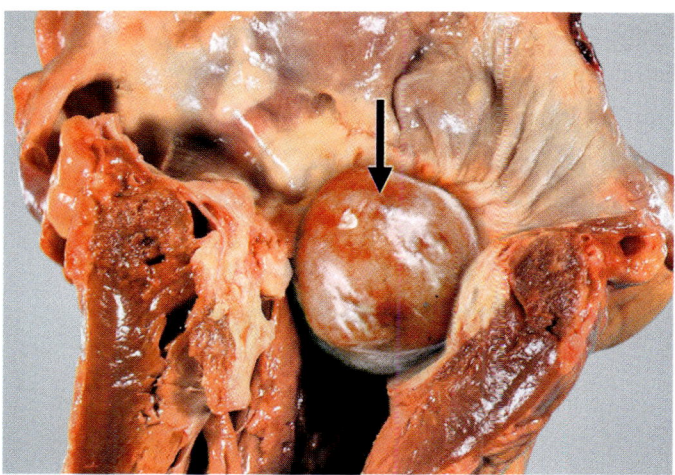

Fig. 16.64: Cardiac myxoma. 'Ball valve' effect of myxoma is partially obstructing mitral valve intermittently. It is diagnosed by echocardiography (arrow).

CONGENITAL HEART DISEASES

OVERVIEW

- Developmental anomalies of the heart and the major blood vessels are seen in 6–8 per 1000 newborns. Some congenital defects become clinically apparent at birth or in infancy, others are recognized in early childhood. Patients with mitral valve prolapse are diagnosed in early adulthood.
- Most common congenital heart diseases are ventricular septal defect (30%), tetralogy of Fallot (10%), atrial septal defect (8%), patent ductus arteriosus (8%), coarctation of the aorta (6%) and transposition of the great arteries (5%).
- The most common acyanotic heart disease is ventricular septal defect, whereas the most common cyanotic heart disease is tetralogy of Fallot (Table 16.19).

Etiology and Associations

- *Chromosomal disorders:* Patients with chromosomal disorders are associated with congenital heart disease. Child with Down's syndrome is associated with atrial and ventricular septal defects. Turner syndrome has been associated with coarctation of aorta.
- *Genetic predisposition:* Due to multifactorial inheritance, tetralogy of Fallot can cluster in families.
- *High altitude:* There is increased incidence of patent ductus arteriosus in persons living at high altitude,

suggesting an association with decreased supply of oxygen to fetus.

- *Rubella infection (German measles):* Intrauterine exposure to rubella virus during the first trimester of pregnancy is important cause of congenital heart disease. Newborn develops congenital rubella syndrome, characterized by cardiovascular defects, microcephaly with mental retardation, deafness, cataracts, and growth retardation. Cardiovascular defects include ventricular septal defect, aortic stenosis, patent ductus arteriosus, valvular stenosis and tetralogy of Fallot. It is mandatory to determine mother's immune status to rubella. Presence of antirubella IgM antibodies indicates recent primary infection, and IgG antibodies indicate past infection.

Gene defects associated with congenital heart diseases are shown in Table 16.20.

Functional Abnormalities of CHD

- *Noncyanotic diseases (left to right shunt):* These include atrial septal defect (ASD), ventricular septal

Table 16.19: Major groups of congenital heart disease

Functional abnormalities	Examples
Noncyanotic diseases (left to right shunt)	ASD
	VSD
	PDA
Cyanotic diseases (right to left shunt)	Tetralogy of Fallot
	Transposition of the great vessels
Malformations	Hypoplastic left heart syndrome
	Total anomalous pulmonary venous return

Table 16.20: Gene defects associated with congenital heart diseases*

Disorder	Gene	Gene product function
Nonsyndromic		
ASD or conduction defects	NKX2.5	Transcription factor
ASD or VSD	GATA4	Transcription factor
Tetralogy of Fallot	ZFPM2 or NKZ2.5	Transcription factor
Syndromic*		
Alagille syndrome: Pulmonary artery stenosis or tetralogy of Fallot	JAG1 OR N0TCH2	Signaling proteins or receptors
Char syndrome: PDA	TFAP2B	Transcription factor
CHARGE syndrome: ASD, VSD, PDA, or hypoplastic right side of the heart	CHD7	Helicase-binding protein
DiGeorge syndrome: ASD, VSD, or outflow tract obstruction	TBX1	Transcription factor
Holt-Oram syndrome: ASD, VSD, or conduction defect	TBX5	Transcription factor
Noonan syndrome: Pulmonary valve stenosis, VSD, or hypertrophic cardiomyopathy	PTPN11, KRAS, S0S1	Signaling proteins

ASD—atrial septal defect, VSD—ventricular septal defect, PDA—patent ductus arteriosus, CHARGE—posterior coloboma, heart defect, choanal atresia, retardation, genital and ear anomalies.

*Different mutations can cause the same phenotype, and mutations in some genes can cause multiple phenotypes (e.g. NKX2.5). Many of these congenital lesions also can occur sporadically, without specific genetic mutation.

**Only the cardiac manifestations of the syndrome are listed; the other skeletal, facial, neurologic and visceral changes are not.

defect (VSD) and patent ductus arteriosus. In atrial septal defects, both pressure and oxygen saturation may be equalized between the two atria.

- *Cyanotic diseases (right to left shunt):* These include tetralogy of Fallot and transposition of the great vessels.
- *Malformations without left to right shunt:* These include hypoplastic left heart syndrome, coarctation of aorta and total anomalous pulmonary venous return.

ATRIAL SEPTAL DEFECTS

Atrial septal defects account for 10% of all congenital heart diseases. Normally, the left atrial pressure keeps the foramen ovale closed. Fossa ovalis represents the remnant of foramen ovale on right interatrial septum. Patent foramen ovale is usually clinically insignificant. Depending on the location, there are three types of defects.

Septum Secundum

- *Incidence:* It accounts for 90% of all atrial septal defects. It is a true defect and should not be confused with patent foramen ovale.
- *Location:* Defect occurs in the middle portion of septum varying in size to involve entire fossa ovalis. It is most common disease usually diagnosed in adult life.
- *Consequence:* Large defects cause dilation and hypertrophy of the right atrium and ventricle resulting in pulmonary hypertension. The defect may allow a thrombus from right atrium to left atrium known as *paradoxical embolus,* so-called because a thromboembolus arising from the venous circulation can end in the systemic circulation.
- *Lutembacher syndrome:* It is characterized by atrial septal defect with mitral stenosis.

Septum Primum

Large defect in the lower part of septum is known as *septum primum.* It may be associated with deformities of atrioventricular valves.

Sinus Venosus

Defect in the upper part of the septum near the entrance of the superior vena cava is known as *sinus venosus.*

Complications of ASDs

These include cyanosis, atrial arrhythmias, right ventricular hypertrophy, right heart failure, bacterial endocarditis, and paradoxical emboli.

VENTRICULAR SEPTAL DEFECTS

The interventricular septum usually closes down spontaneously in the first 2 years of life. VSD is within the membranous (80%) or muscular (20%) portions of interventricular septum that produces a left-to-right shunt. Ventricular septal defect may vary in size.

Small VSDs

These constitute 50% of cases, these may close spontaneously. These are recognized by *high-pitched holosystolic murmur.*

Large VSDs

These produce more severe disease. Left to right shunt may lead to pulmonary hypertension and eventual right-sided heart failure. Reversal of the shunt occurs when the pulmonary hypertension exceeds the pressure in the aorta (Eisenmenger syndrome) leads to cyanosis. Patient now develops left ventricular hypertrophy and dilatation.

PATENT DUCTUS ARTERIOSUS (PDA)

During intrauterine life, ductus arteriosus permits the blood from the venous system to bypass the lungs. During fetal life, its patency is maintained by combined effects of low oxygen tension and prostaglandin synthesis. Patent ductus arteriosus normally closes soon after birth. *If the ductus arteriosus remains open, a left-to-right shunt develops* (Fig. 16.65).

Clinical Correlation

Failure of closure of the fetal ductus arteriosus leads to pulmonary hypertension and right ventricular

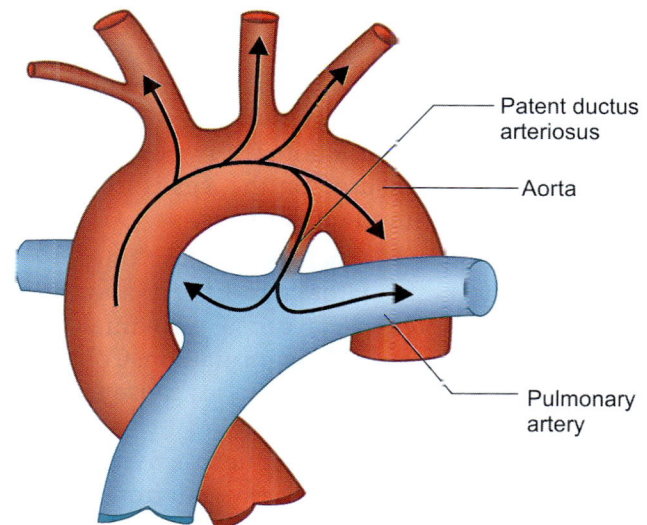

Fig. 16.65: Patent ductus arteriosus. There is persistence of patency of duct communicating aorta and pulmonary trunk.

hypertrophy. This left-to-right shunt is associated with a *loud machinery murmur* during systole and diastole.

Therapeutic Correlation

PDA can be closed surgically or pharmacologically treated with injection indomethacin (prostaglandins inhibitor).

COARCTATION OF AORTA

- Aortic coarctation is common, accounting for 6% of all cases of congenital heart disease. It is localized narrowing of the aortic lumen leading to outflow obstruction. It usually occurs in the thoracic portion of the descending aorta, distal to the take off of the left subclavian artery at the site of the ductus arteriosus.
- The cardinal physical finding is diminution or absence of femoral pulses and hypertension in the upper extremities. It occurs in two types—infantile and adult (Fig. 16.66).

Infantile Type

Infantile form constitutes 70% of cases. Ascending aorta as well as aortic arch is markedly narrowed with persistence of ductus arteriosus.

- *Clinical features:* Newborns are symptomatic at birth. The head and the upper extremities are hypoxic, whereas the lower parts of the body receiving the blood through the open ductus arteriosus are cyanotic.
- *Prognosis:* Most infants do not survive without surgical correction of the defect.

Adult Type

- *Location:* Narrowing of the aorta is distal to the origin of the subclavian arteries.
- *Clinical features:* Hypertension is limited to the upper extremities and cerebral vessels. The parts of the body below the obstruction are hypoxic, and the blood pressure measured on the legs is lower than the pressure measured on the arms.
- *Consequences:* There is increased risk of developing dissecting aortic hematoma and berry aneurysms in the cerebral vessels. It causes proximal aortic dilation resulting in aortic regurgitation. Collaterals that involve the intercostals arteries cause notching of the ribs seen on X-ray.
- Diastolic hypertension occurs due to activation of the renin-angiotensin-aldosterone system from reduced blood flow.

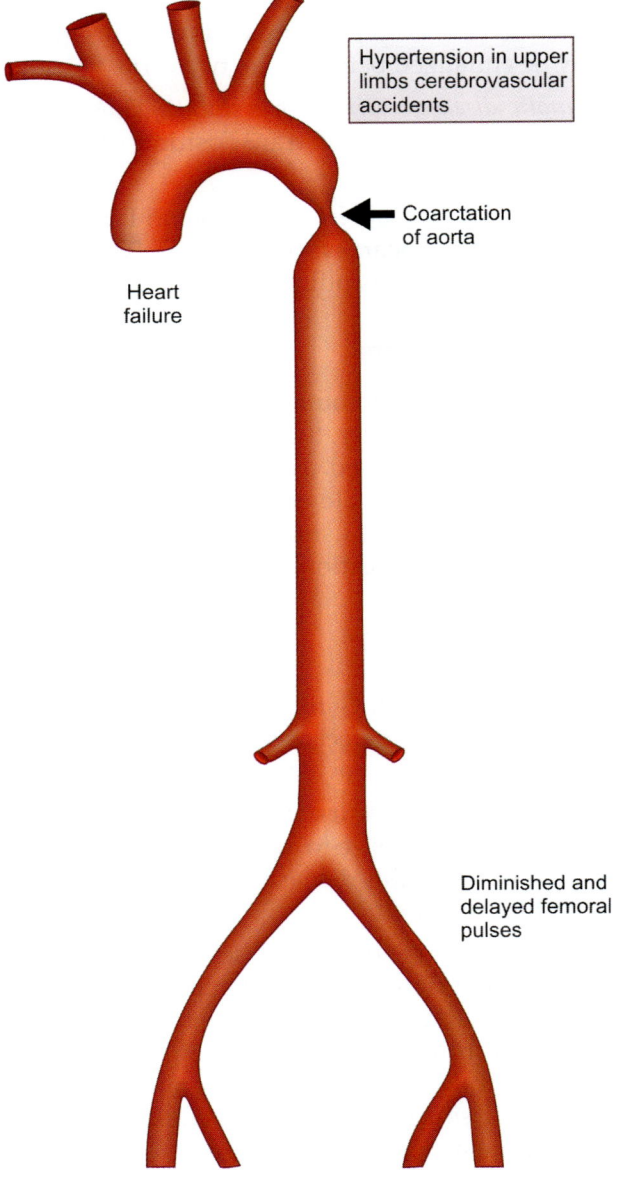

Fig. 16.66: Coarctation of aorta leads to diminished blood flow to lower extremities.

TETRALOGY OF FALLOT

Tetralogy of Fallot is the most common cyanotic disease in newborn.

Components

Tetralogy of Fallot comprises four pathologic findings, i.e. (i) ventricular septal defect (membranous type), (ii) overriding aorta sitting over the ventricular septal defect, (iii) pulmonary artery stenosis (below pulmonary valve), and (iv) right ventricular hypertrophy (Fig. 16.67).

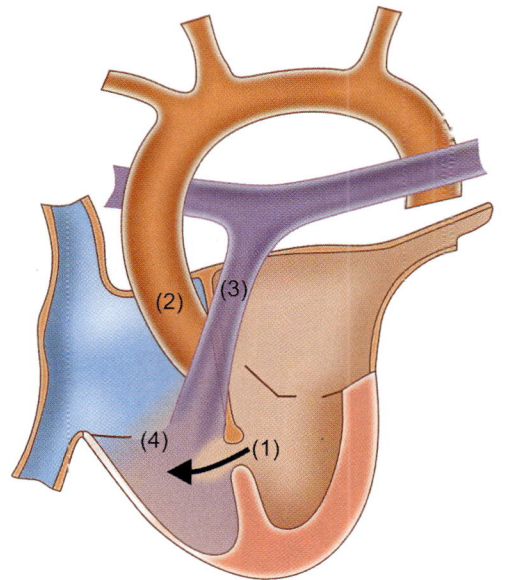

Fig. 16.67: Tetralogy of Fallot comprises four pathologic findings, i.e. (1) ventricular septal defect, (2) overriding aorta sitting over the ventricular septal defect, (3) pulmonary artery stenosis results in, (4) right ventricular hypertrophy.

Pathophysiology

- The obstruction to right ventricular outflow creates a right-to-left shunt that leads to cyanosis from birth.
- Pulmonary artery stenosis does not permit entry of venous blood into the lungs for oxygenation.
- Overriding aorta sitting over the ventricular septal defect receives blood from both ventricles results in cyanosis.

Clinical Features

Newborn develops bluish discoloration of the skin and mucosa, i.e. cyanosis at birth. In most children, cyanosis is evident by the age of 4 months. Children develop hypoxemic spells, i.e. faint or loss of consciousness, retarded growth, squatting position and clubbing of fingers.

Prognosis

Some children may die in the first year of life. Death occurs due to hypoxia, infections and cerebrovascular accidents related to thromboembolism. Surgery is recommended as the treatment of choice for most cases. But it is associated with a 3–15% mortality rate.

TRUNCUS ARTERIOSUS COMMUNIS

Truncus arteriosus communis refers to a common trunk for the origin of the aorta, pulmonary arteries, and coronary arteries.

Pathology

It occurs due to incomplete separation of the aortic and pulmonary outflows and forming single vessel overriding both ventricles during development. It allows mixing of oxygenated and deoxygenated blood with right-to-left shunting.

MALFORMATIONS

Transposition of the Great Vessels

The aorta arises from the right ventricle, and the pulmonary artery arises from the left ventricle. There is right-to-left shunting. It accounts up to 5% of congenital heart disease. Its incidence is increased in maternal diabetes mellitus. Compensatory anomaly such as patent ductus arteriosus is necessary for survival.

Hypoplastic Left Heart Syndrome

There is varying degree of hypoplasia or atresia of the aortic and mitral valves, along with a small to absent left ventricular chamber.

Total Anomalous Pulmonary Venous Return

The pulmonary veins do not directly connect to the left atrium, but drain into left innominate vein, coronary sinus, or some other sites, leading to possible mixing of blood and right-sided overload.

CHAPTER 17

Nasal Cavity, Nasopharynx, Paranasal Sinuses, Ear, Larynx and Neck

Learning Objectives

INFLAMMATION AND INFECTION
- Acute Rhinosinusitis
- Chronic Sinusitis
- Wegener's Granulomatosis
- Allergic Polyps
- Fungal Infections

NEOPLASTIC DISORDERS
- Schneiderian Sinonasal Papillomas
- Sinonasal Undifferentiated Carcinoma (SNUC)
- Nasopharyngeal Carcinoma
- Squamous Cell Carcinoma
- Melanoma
- Olfactory Neuroblastoma
- Nasopharyngeal Angiofibroma
- Alveolar Rhabdomyosarcoma
- Nasal Plasmacytoma
- Nasal Adenocarcinoma
- Hemangioblastoma

MISCELLANEOUS DISORDERS
- Rhinosporidiosis
- Rhinoscleroma

EAR
- Anatomy
- External Ear
- Cauliflower Ear
- Chondrodermatitis Nodularis Chronica
- Malignant Neoplasm
- Middle Ear
- Inner Ear
- Presbycusis
- Toxic Damage from Drugs
- Acoustic Neuroma

LARYNX
- Anatomy
- Inflammatory Diseases
- Tumors and Tumor-like Diseases

NECK
- Neck Swellings
- Cervical Lymphadenopathy
- Thyroglossal Duct Cyst

INFLAMMATION AND INFECTIONS

ACUTE RHINOSINUSITIS

Upper respiratory tract infections are most common cause of sinusitis. These occur as a result of extension of nasal cavity or dental infection. Blockage of sinuses results in accumulation of inflammatory exudates in ethmoid sinus in children and maxillary sinus in adults.

Acute rhinosinusitis is caused by bacteria (*Streptococcus pneumoniae*, staphylococci, or *Haemophilus influenzae*), viruses (adenovirus) and allergy (allergens).

Acute rhinosinusitis caused by bacteria may be superimposed on acute viral or allergic rhinitis by injury to mucosal cilia.

Adenovirus causes coryza (runny nose), sneezing, nasal congestion, and mild sore throat. Allergic rhinosinusitis is characterized by nasal discharge and peripheral eosinophilia.

Respiratory epithelium is infiltrated by necrotic material, apoptotic neutrophils and nuclear debris. Diagnostic modalities include bacterial culture of sinus aspirate, sinus radiographs and CT scan (most sensitive).

CHRONIC SINUSITIS

Predisposing factors of chronic rhinosinusitis include allergy, upper respiratory tract infections, cystic fibrosis, and immotile cilia syndrome (Kartagener's syndrome) especially secondary to obstruction of paranasal sinuses outflow. It commonly affects children. Submucosa is infiltrated by lymphocytes, plasma cells and eosinophils. Complications are superadded bacterial infection and inflammatory polyp.

WEGENER'S GRANULOMATOSIS

Wegener's granulomatosis is autoimmune disorder. It shares some features with lethal midline granuloma. Both diseases are characterized by necrotizing, ulcerated, mucosal lesions of upper respiratory tract. Lethal midline granuloma is a sign of underlying lymphomas. Wegener's granulomatosis is characterized by necrotizing vasculitis (fibrinoid necrosis) involving arterioles, small arteries and veins. The lesions are not limited to the upper respiratory tract; they also involve the lungs and the kidneys.

Clinical Features

Patient presents with rhinorrhea, sinusitis, headache, nasal obstruction and symptoms due to eustachian tube obstruction. More than 90% of patients with Wegener granulomatosis exhibit antineutrophil cytoplasmic antibody (ANCA).

> ### Light Microscopy
> Histopathological examination of lesion shows chronic inflammatory infiltrate, granulomas and necrotising vasculitis.

ALLERGIC POLYPS

Allergic polyps are most common polyps in nasal cavity. Long standing chronic allergic rhinitis causes non-neoplastic mucosal and submucosal projections forming nasal polyps.

These most often affect adults. In case of nasal polyps in children, sweat test must be done to rule out cystic fibrosis.

Clinical Features

Patient presents with nasal obstruction and rhinorrhea. Unilateral or bilateral multiple polyps arise from lateral nasal wall or ethmoid recess. These polyps may cause deviated nasal septum, destruction of bone and rarely extend to nasopharynx (Fig. 17.1).

> ### Gross Morphology
> Polyps may measure up to several centimeters. These are boggy, gelatinous, and translucent with broad base (Fig. 17.2).

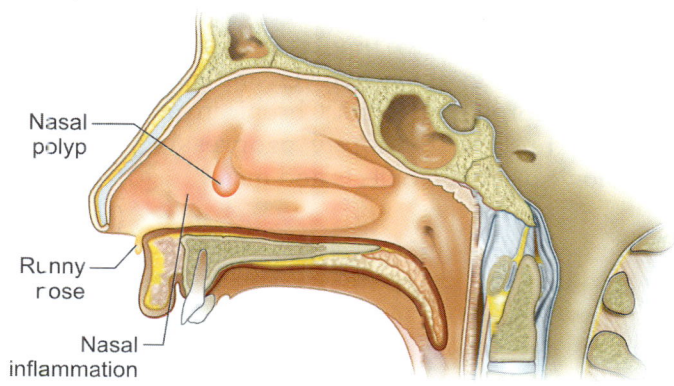

Fig. 17.1: Nasal polyp.

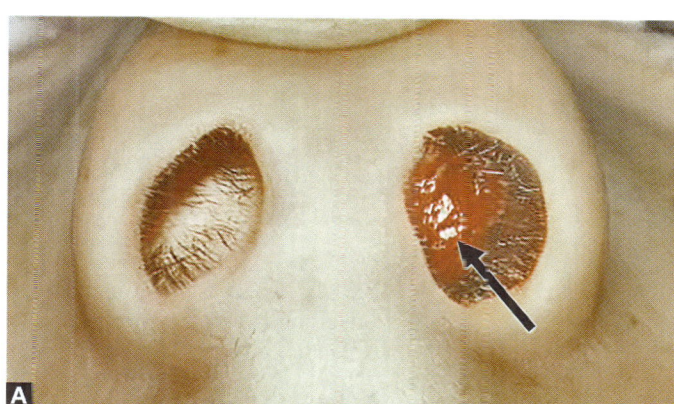

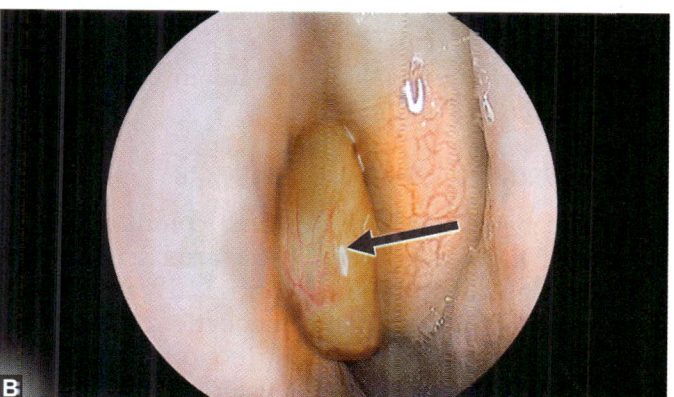

Fig. 17.2: Nasal polyp (arrows).

> **Light Microscopy**
> - Histopathological examination of polyps reveals intact respiratory epithelium, edematous, myxomatous stroma, infiltrated by lymphocytes, plasma cells and eosinophils.
> - There is absence of seromu-cinous glands (Fig. 17.3).

FUNGAL INFECTIONS

Fungi may cause noninvasive or invasive sinusitis. Patient with noninvasive fungal sinusitis presents with polyps formation involving single or multiple paranasal sinuses.

Patient with invasive fungal acute sinusitis presents with severe acute sinusitis, fever, and nasal discharge, ocular or neurologic deficits. Chronic invasive sinusitis is characterized by slowly progressive sinusitis neurologic or orbital defects and mass.

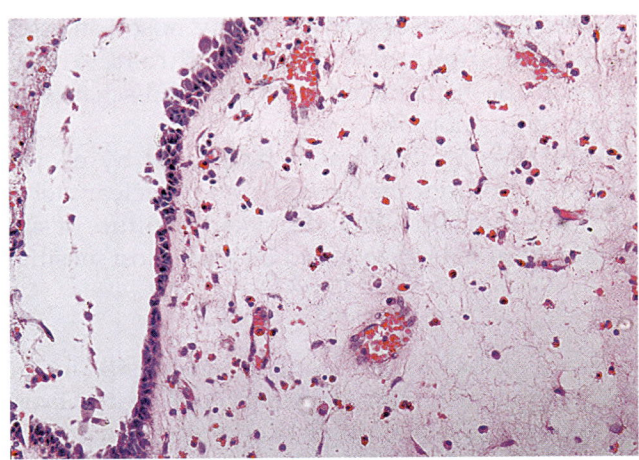

Fig. 17.3: Allergic nasal polyp. It shows dense eosinophilic infiltrate (400X).

Fungi are demonstrated by *Grocott's methenamine silver stain*. Features of fungal sinusitis are shown in Table 17.1.

Table 17.1: Features of fungal sinusitis

Entity	Clinical manifestations	Light microscopy	Causative organism
Noninvasive fungal sinusitis			
Fungal sinusitis	Allergic polyps involving multiple sinuses	Eosinophils, Charcot-Leyden crystals and hyphae	Bipolaris, Curvularia, Alternaria, *Aspergillus dematiaceous*, Cladosporium
Mycetoma (fungal ball)	Non-allergic polyps, involving single sinus	Fungal hyphae	Mycetoma
Invasive fungal sinusitis			
Acute invasive fungal sinusitis	Severe acute sinusitis, fever, nasal discharge, ocular or neurologic deficits	Fungal hyphae in blood vessels, granulomas, necrosis	Mucor, Rhizopus, Absida, Cumuinghammella *Asperigillus dematiaceous* (uncommon)
Chronic invasive sinusitis	Slowly progressive sinusitis onset, neurologic or orbital defects, mass	Fungal hyphae in blood vessels, granulomas, necrosis	*Aspergillus dematiaceous*

NEOPLASTIC DISORDERS

A wide variety of neoplasms occurs in the sinonasal region (Table 17.2 and Fig. 17.4).

SCHNEIDERIAN SINONASAL PAPILLOMAS

Sinonasal papillomas are the most common benign tumors of the nasal cavity. These are derived from schneiderian membrane. Histological variants are exophytic, endophytic and oncocytic. Histopathological examination is essential due to their different clinical behavior and risk of development of invasive carcinomas.

EXOPHYTIC PAPILLOMA

Exophytic papillomas most often arise from nasal septum in 20–50 years males. These are solitary and discrete. Human papillomavirus (6 and 11) has been demonstrated in large number of cases.

Clinical Features

Patient presents with epistaxis, unilateral nasal obstruction or symptomatic nasal mass. Recurrence of exophytic papilloma is common after surgery. There is no risk of development of carcinoma in these patients.

Nasal Cavity, Nasopharynx, Paranasal Sinuses, Ear, Larynx and Neck 17

Table 17.2: Classification of tumors of nasal cavity and paranasal sinuses

Benign tumors	Malignant tumors
Exophytic papillomas, endophytic papillomas, oncocytic papillomas, nasopharyngeal fibroma	*Nasopharyngeal carcinoma:* Keratinizing squamous cell carcinoma (WHO-1), nonkeratinizing differentiated carcinoma (WHO-2a), nonkeratinizing undifferentiated carcinoma (WHO-2b) and basaloid squamous cell carcinoma (WHO-3)
	Squamous cell carcinoma (keratinizing or nonkeratinizing), malignant melanoma, olfactory neuroblastoma, alveolar rhabdomyosarcoma, nasal plasmacytoma, nasal adenocarcinoma, hemangiopericytoma

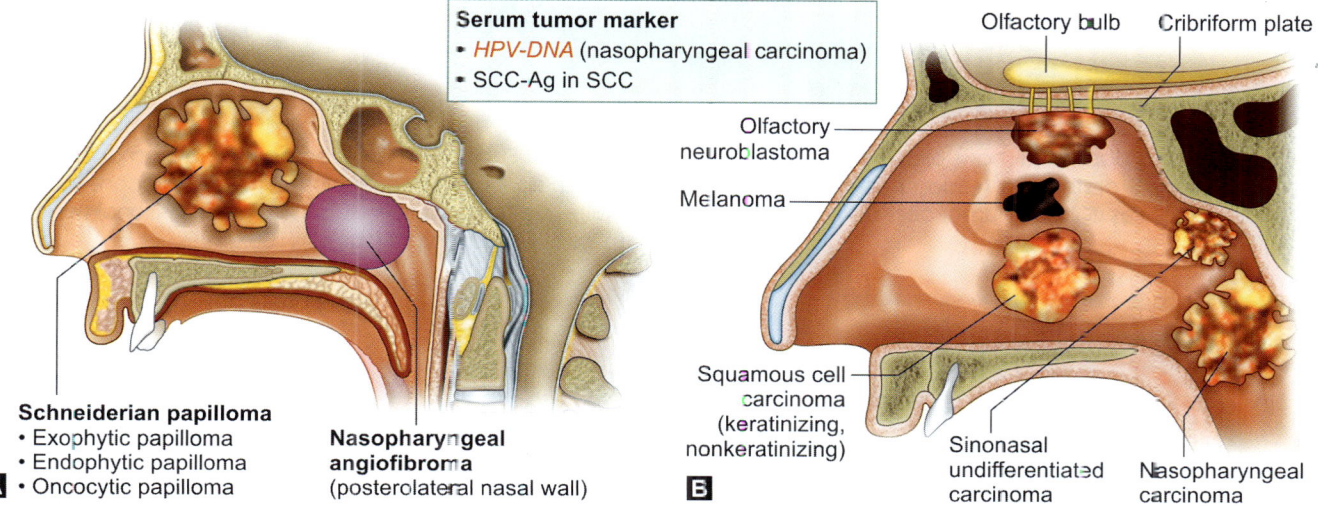

Fig. 17.4: Tumors of nasal cavity and paranasal sinuses—(A) benign tumors, (B) malignant tumors.

Gross Morphology

Tumor is gray pink, translucent mass with broad base (Fig. 17.5).

Light Microscopy

- Tumor is composed of exophytic papillary fronds lined by thickened epithelium (squamous to respiratory or transitional or features of both).
- Scattered mucin secreting cells are also present.
- Neutrophil collections are present in epithelial fronds. Surface keratinization is absent except in rare case.
- Tumor cells do not show atypia (Fig. 17.6).

ENDOPHYTIC PAPILLOMA

Endophytic papilloma most often occurs in 40–70 years adults. It arises from lateral nasal wall in the region of middle turbinate and ethmoid recesses. It may also arise from nasal septum in 8% cases. Human papillomavirus (6 and 11) has been demonstrated in 50% cases.

Clinical Features

Patient presents with unilateral nasal obstruction or symptomatic nasal mass. Recurrence is common in 5–20% of cases after surgery.

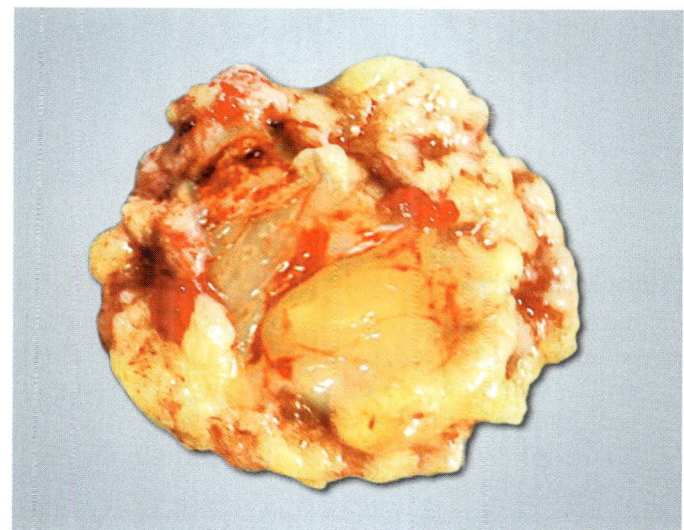

Fig. 17.5: Exophytic papilloma. Tumor is gray pink, translucent mass with broad base.

There is risk of development of carcinoma in 10–15% of cases.

Gross Morphology

Tumor is fleshy pink tan with papillary or polypoid (Fig. 17.7).

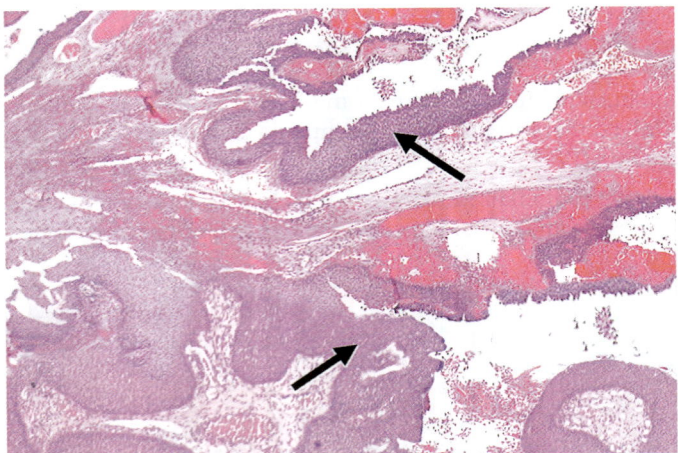

Fig. 17.6: Exophytic papilloma shows exophytic papillary fronds lined by thickened epithelium (squamous to respiratory or transitional or features of both). Tumor cells do not show atypia (arrows) (100X).

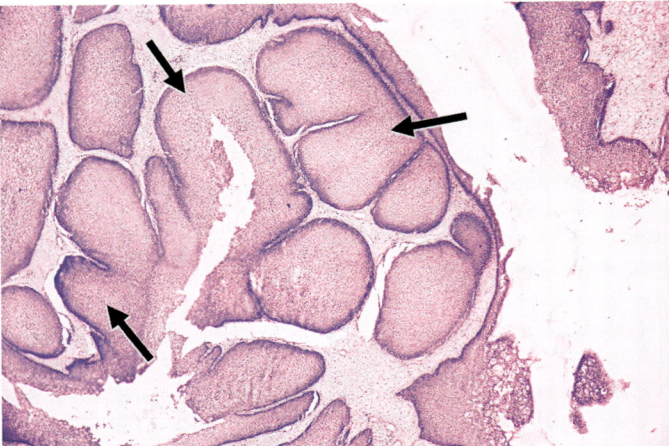

Fig. 17.8: Endophytic (inverted papilloma). Tumor is composed of numerous basement-enclosed, rounded ribbons of thickened epithelium ranging from squamous to transitional with minimal mitoses without atypia (arrows) (100X).

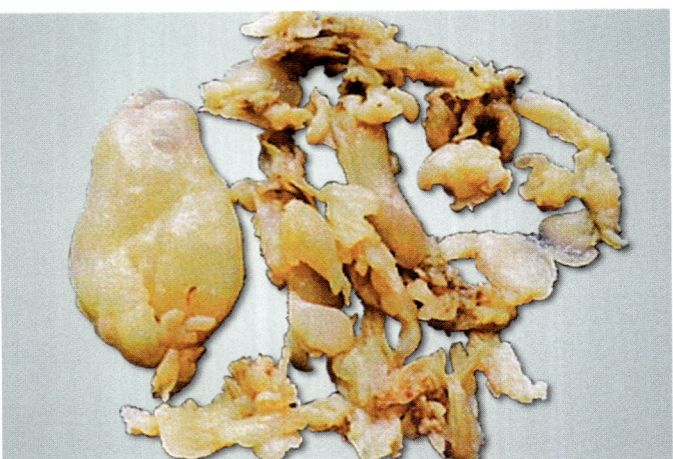

Fig. 17.7: Inverted papilloma.

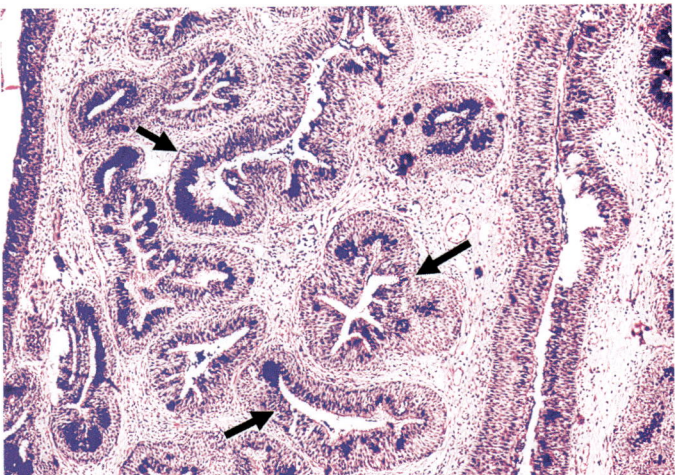

Fig. 17.9: Endophytic (inverted papilloma) shows numerous rounded ribbons of thickened epithelium ranging from squamous to transitional with minimal mitoses without atypia (arrows) (200X).

Light Microscopy
- Tumor is composed of numerous basement membrane enclosed, rounded ribbons of thickened epithelium ranging from squamous to transitional with minimal mitoses without atypia.
- Neutrophils are present in the epithelium (Figs 17.8 and 17.9).

ONCOCYTIC PAPILLOMA

Oncocytic papillomas are least common. These equally affect men and women. HPV has not been demonstrated in these lesions.

Clinical Features

Patient presents with unilateral nasal obstruction or symptomatic nasal mass. Recurrence is common after surgery. There is risk of development of carcinoma in 5–15% of cases.

Light Microscopy

Tumor is composed of exophytic and endophytic nests of columnar, oncocytic cells with abundant, granular eosinophilic cytoplasm; intraepithelial neutrophils and microcysts (Fig. 17.10). Features of schneiderian sinonasal papillomas are shown in Table 17.3.

SINONASAL UNDIFFERENTIATED CARCINOMA (SNUC)

Sinonasal undifferentiated carcinoma is aggressive form of sinonasal carcinoma. It most often occurs in elderly persons in their 6th decade. It arises from superior region of nasal cavity or maxillary or ethmoid sinuses.

Table 17.3: Features of scineiderian sinonasal papillomas

Histologic variants	Common location	Pathology	Behavior after surgical excision	Malignant transformation to invasive carcinoma
Exophytic papilloma	Nasal septum	Exophytic fronds of squamous or transitional, epithelium containing neutrophils	Local recurrence	No risk of malignancy
Inverted papilloma	Lateral nasal wall; paranasal sinuses	Endophytic fronds of squamous or transitional, epithelium containing neutrophils	Local recurrence	10–15%
Oncocytic papilloma	Lateral nasal wall; paranasal sinuses	Exophytic and endophytic nests of columnar, oncocytic cells with abundant, granular eosinophilic cytoplasm; intraepithelial neutrophils and microcysts	Local recurrence	5–15%

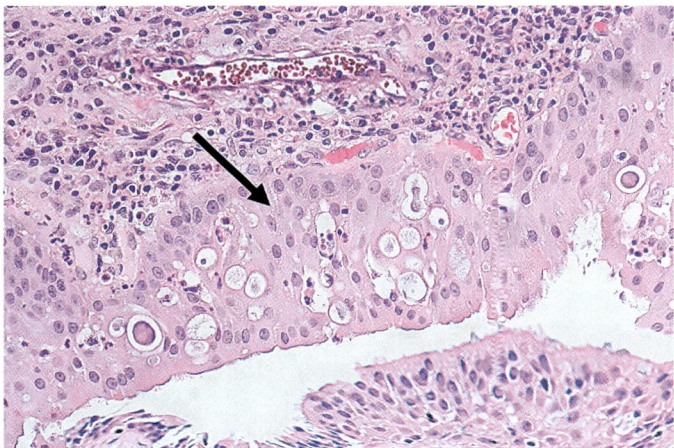

Fig. 17.10: Oncocytic papilloma. Tumor is composed of nests of oncocytic cells with abundant, granular eosinophilic cytoplasm; and intraepithelial neutrophils (arrow) (400X).

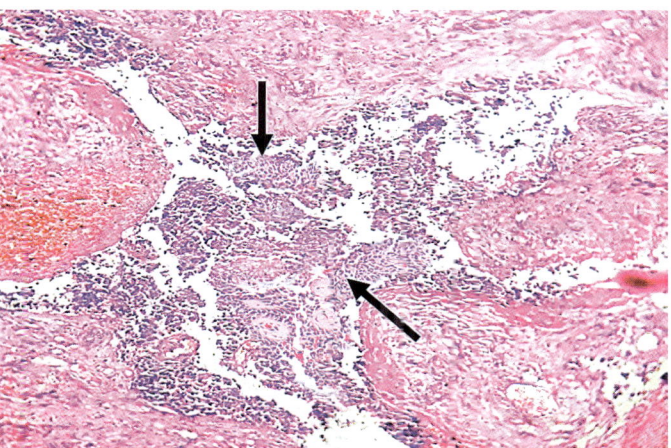

Fig. 17.11: Sinonasal undifferentiated carcinoma shows atypical cell with hyperchromatic nuclei and prominent nucleoli arranged in nests (arrows) (100X).

Clinical Features

Patient presents with nasal obstruction, epistaxis, orbital or cranial nerve deficits.

Gross Morphology
This bulky tumor has no unique gross features.

Light Microscopy
- Tumor is composed of small- to moderate-sized uniform cells with hyperchromatic to vesicular nuclei and prominent nucleoli.
- Tumor cells are arranged in nests, lobular or trabeculae pattern.
- There is abundant apoptosis, mitoses and necrosis in the tumor (Fig. 17.11).

Immunohistochemistry
Panel of markers is employed on histological sections obtained from tumor (Table 17.4).

Table 17.4: Immunohistochemistry of SNUC

Markers	Expression
Pancytokeratin (7, 8, 19)	Positive
Epithelial membrane antigen (EMA)	Positive
Neuron-specific enolase (NSE)	Positive (30% cases)

Neuroendocrine markers: Tumor expresses NSE, but negative for chromogranin A and synaptophysin

NASOPHARYNGEAL CARCINOMA

Nasopharyngeal carcinoma is most common tumor of nasopharynx. It is associated with Epstein-Barr virus (EB virus). It is more prevalent in males especially in Chinese and African population. It metastasizes to cervical lymph nodes. Most patients have anti-EBV IgA in their serum.

Clinical Features

Patient presents with sinonasal mass, nasal obstruction, epistaxis and serous otitis media due to blockage of eustachian tube. Infrequently, primary may be asymptomatic with neck metastases.

Gross Morphology

Tumor is gray white to tan. Cut surface is gray white with areas of hemorrhage (Fig. 17.12).

Light Microscopy

WHO classification of nasopharyngeal carcinoma is shown in Table 17.5. EB virus is strongly related the oncogenesis of nonkeratinizing nasopharyngeal carcinoma (types WHO-2a and 2b).

- *Keratinizing squamous cell carcinoma (WHO-1):* It has morphology similar to keratinizing squamous cell carcinoma elsewhere in head and neck and graded as well to poorly differentiated carcinoma (Fig. 17.13).
- *Nonkeratinizing differentiated carcinoma (WHO-2a):* It has surface disease with stratified cells that have similar morphology to that of urothelial carcinoma of urinary bladder.
- *Nonkeratinizing undifferentiated carcinoma (WHO-2b):* It is the most common variant of nasopharyngeal carcinoma. It is composed of tumor cells arranged in sheets/syncytial aggregates. Tumor cells contain eosinophilic cytoplasm, large vesicular nuclei and prominent nuclei. These tumor cells are admixed with chronic inflammatory cells (Fig. 17.14).
- *Basaloid squamous cell carcinoma (WHO-3):* It is least common variant of nasopharyngeal carcinoma. It has similar morphology that occurs in head and neck.

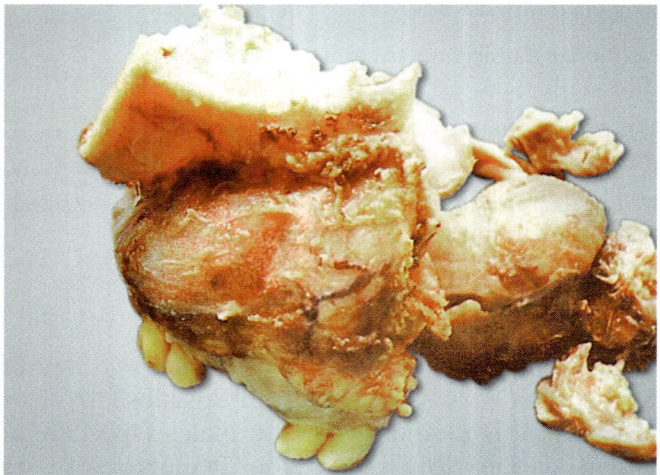

Fig. 17.12: Squamous cell carcinoma. Tumor is arising from maxillary sinus.

Table 17.5: WHO classification of nasopharyngeal carcinoma

Histological variants	Type
Keratinizing squamous cell carcinoma	1
Nonkeratinizing differentiated carcinoma	2a
Nonkeratinizing undifferentiated carcinoma	2b
Basaloid squamous cell carcinoma	3

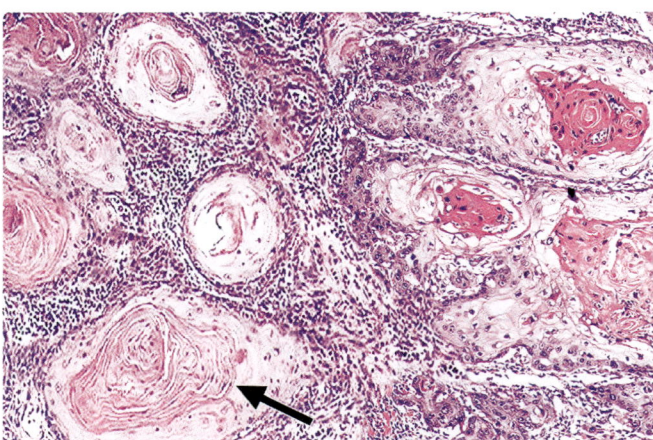

Fig. 17.13: Keratinizing squamous cell carcinoma (WHO-1). Tumor shows areas of keratinization (arrow) (400X).

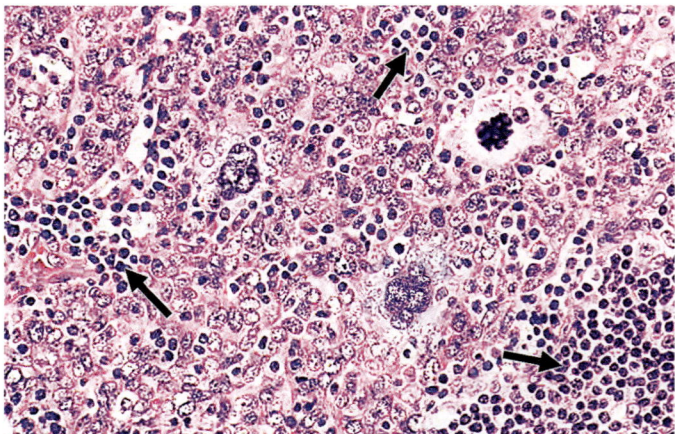

Fig. 17.14: Nonkeratinizing undifferentiated carcinoma most common variant (WHO-2b)—tumor cells contain eosinophilic cytoplasm, large vesicular nuclei and prominent nuclei, arranged in sheets syncytial aggregates and admixed with chronic inflammatory cells (arrows) (100X).

Immunohistochemistry

These are immunoreactive with antibodies to cytokeratins.

Clinical Course

- *Nonkeratinizing nasopharyngeal carcinoma:* It most often metastasizes to cervical lymph nodes in posterior triangle (level 5). These tumors respond well to systemic therapy. Radiotherapy is the first line of treatment. Surgery is reserved for salvage therapy.

- *Keratinizing nasopharyngeal squamous cell carcinoma:* Patient most often presents with localized disease. It does not respond to systemic therapy.

SQUAMOUS CELL CARCINOMA (KERATINIZING/NONKERATINIZING)

Squamous cell carcinoma is the most common tumor in head and neck. It constitutes 65% of carcinomas in the nasal cavity and paranasal sinuses.

Histological Variants

- *Keratinizing squamous cell carcinoma:* It is associated with tobacco smoking, exposure to nickel, textile dusts and chlorophenols.
- *Nonkeratinizing squamous cell carcinoma:* It has papillary configuration. Tumor is composed of ribbons of pleomorphic cells lacking keratinization. It has been associated with HPV. This variant has better prognosis.

MELANOMA

Primary malignant melanoma of sinonasal region constitutes 1% of all melanomas. It occurs in the nasal cavity and paranasal sinuses especially middle or inferior turbinate in patients over 50 years.

The tumor may be sessile/polypoidal with mucosal ulceration and heavily pigmented (brown or black). It metastasizes to sinonasal region. Prognosis of melanoma is poor.

Light Microscopy

- Melanoma has a wide range of morphological features. It is composed of high grade epithelioid cells. Some tumors are composed of mixture of epithelioid cells and spindle cells.
- There is also presence of junctional component with pagetoid spread of melanocytes in the intact mucosa.

Immunohistochemistry

Panel of markers is employed on histological sections obtained from tumor (Table 17.6).

Table 17.6: Immunohistochemistry of melanoma

Markers	Expression
S-100	Positive
HMB-45	Positive
Melan-A	Positive
CAM 5.2	Positive
Ki-67	Positive

OLFACTORY NEUROBLASTOMA

Olfactory neuroblastoma most often occurs in older men between 30 and 40 years unlike pediatric neuroblastoma, which most often occurs in the adrenals/abdomen of infants and young children.

Origin

Tumor arises from olfactory mucosa of the cribriform plate in the upper nasal cavity wall and superior turbinate.

Clinical Features

Patient presents with unilateral polypoid mass in nasal cavity causing to nasal obstruction and epistaxis.

Light Microscopy

- Tumor is comprised of small round blue cells set in a neurofibrillary matrix.
- Tumor cells contain round uniform nuclei with uniform delicate stippled chromatin (Fig. 17.15).

Immunohistochemistry

Panel of markers is used on histological section to demonstrate expression by tumor cells (Table 17.7).

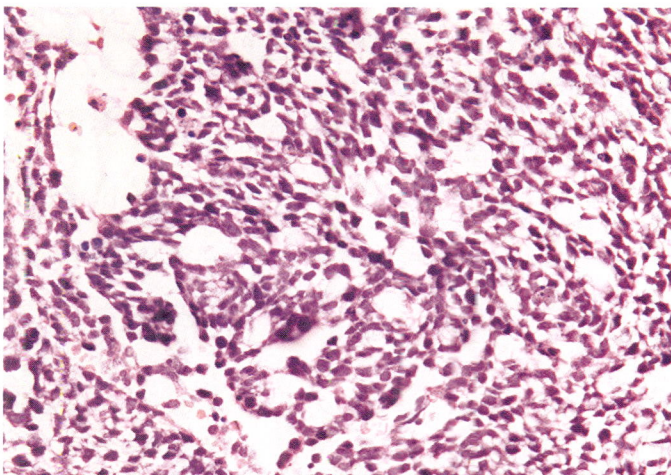

Fig. 17.15: Olfactory neuroblastoma (diffuse pattern) with neurofibrillary background (100X).

Table 17.7: Immunohistochemistry of olfactory neuroblastoma

Tumor markers	Expression
Synaptophysin	Positive
Chromogranin-A	Positive
Neuron-specific enolase (NSE)	Positive
Calretinin	Positive
CAM 5.2	Positive

NASOPHARYNGEAL ANGIOFIBROMA

Nasopharyngeal angiofibroma is a rare vascular neoplasm. It arises from fibrovascular nidus in the *posterolateral nasal wall adjacent to the sphenopalatine foramen*. It may occur in maxilla and ethmoid bones in elderly females.

It most often affects adolescent males between 10 and 20 year. It is histologically benign but locally aggressive. It may *destroy nearby bone and extend in cranial cavity*.

Clinical Features

Patient presents with nasopharyngeal mass bulging in nasopharynx and cause to *nasal obstruction and epistaxis*.

Gross Morphology

Tumor is gray white to tan, smooth with lobulated appearance. Cut surface is homogenous.

Light Microscopy

- Tumor is composed of vascular channels of variable size dispersed in collagenized stroma containing scattered spindle and stellate cells.
- Vascular channels are lined by flat to plump endothelial cells without cytologic atypia. Stromal cells contain vesicular nuclei with vesicular chromatin without cytologic atypia (Fig. 17.16).

Immunohistochemistry

- Vascular endothelium is positive with **CD31** and **CD34**.
- Fibroblastic component expresses cytoplasmic **vimentin**.

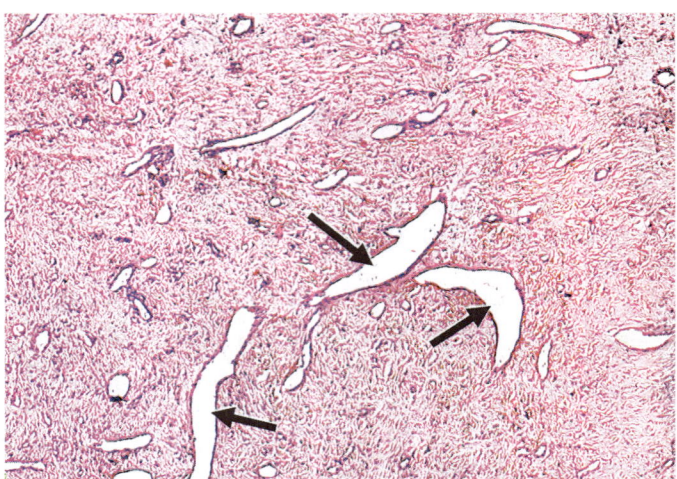

Fig. 17.16: Nasopharyngeal angiofibroma shows vascular channels lined by flat to plump endothelial cells of variable size dispersed in collagenized stroma (arrows) (100X).

ALVEOLAR RHABDOMYOSARCOMA

Alveolar rhabdomyosarcoma is an aggressive mesenchymal malignancy most common in young children. It is always characterized by two characteristics translocations.

Translocation (1;13) leading to PAX7-FKHR fusion transcription factor in 20% of cases is associated with better prognosis only in setting of metastatic disease. Translocation (2;13) causes PAX3-FKHR fusion transcription factor in 80% of cases.

Gross Morphology

Tumor has fleshy to firm tan-gray appearance.

Light Microscopy

- Tumor is composed of small- to medium-sized cells with hyperchromatic nuclei and scant eosinophilic cytoplasm.
- Tumor cells are arranged in loosely cohesive sheets separated by fibrous septa.

Immunohistochemistry

Panel of markers is used on histological section to demonstrate expression by tumor cells (Table 17.8).

Table 17.8: Immunohistochemistry of alveolar rhabdomyosarcoma

Tumor markers	Expression
Desmin	Positive
Muscle-specific actin	Positive
Myoglobin	Positive
MyoD1	Positive

NASAL PLASMACYTOMA

Plasmacytoma is a plasma cell neoplasm in its extraosseous form, it produces tumors in the upper respiratory tract. It lacks radiographic or morphologic evidence of bone marrow involvement.

Tumor is composed of plasma cells and their precursors at various stages of development. Accordingly, immunohistochemical reactivity for **CD138** or **CD38** can be useful to confirm the diagnosis.

NASAL ADENOCARCINOMA

Nasal adenocarcinoma accounts for 5% of malignant tumors of the nose and throat, includes intestinal-type and nonintestinal-type cases.

HEMANGIOBLASTOMA

Hemangioblastoma is a benign tumor of nose. It is treated by surgical excision. This vascular tumor is composed of fascicles of spindle cells with indistinct borders arranged around blood vessels. Tumor may exhibit storiform pattern or whorled appearance.

MISCELLANEOUS DISORDERS

RHINOSPORIDIOSIS

Rhinosporidiosis is caused by *Rhinosporidium seeberi*.

Clinical Features

Patient presents with polypoidal masses containing sporangia in the nose (most common site), larynx, trachea, skin and ear.

> **Light Microscopy**
> - Nasal mucosa may undergo squamous metaplasia. Thick-walled sporangia containing numerous endospores are present beneath epithelium.
> - Sporangia are surrounded by mixed inflammatory cells with numerous eosinophils.
> - These sporangia may rupture resulting in formation of thick hyalinized wall (Fig. 17.17).

Histochemistry

Sporangia are demonstrated by *PAS* and *silver methenamine stains*.

RHINOSCLEROMA

Rhinoscleroma is caused by gram-negative *Klebsiella rhinoscleromatis* by droplet infection. It most often occurs in nose may extend to pharynx and upper respiratory tract.

Clinical Features

Patient presents with tumor mass in the nasal cavity protruding from the nostril and extending in the nasopharynx.

> **Light Microscopy**
> - Rhinoscleroma is composed of large foamy histiocytes laden with organisms known as *Mikulicz cells*.
> - These cells are admixed with numerous plasma cells (Fig. 17.18).

Histochemistry

The organisms are demonstrated by Giemsa, PAS and silver impregnation stains.

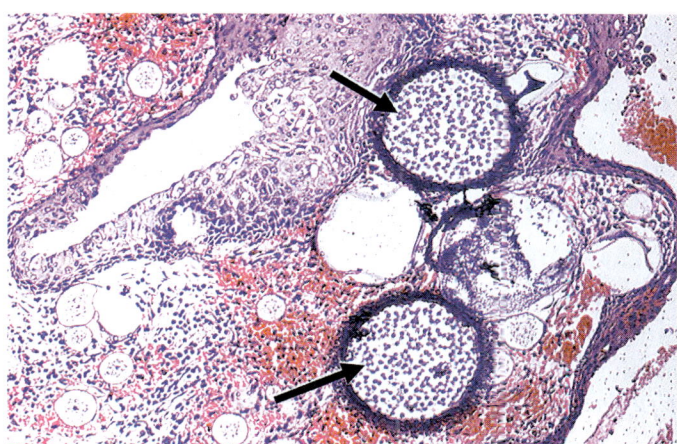

Fig. 17.17: Rhinosporidiosis shows many sporangia containing spores (arrows) (100X).

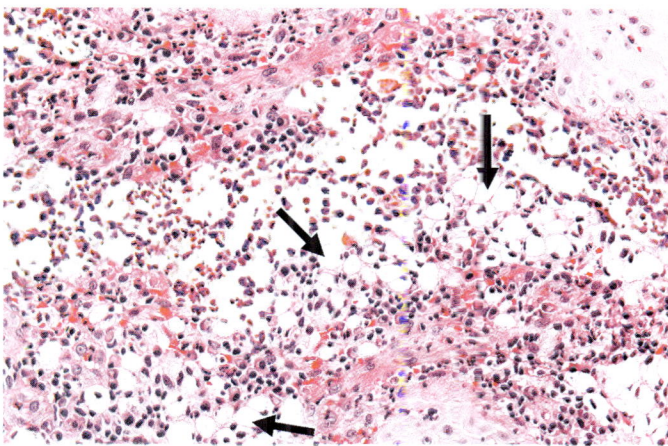

Fig. 17.18: Rhinoscleroma is composed of large foamy histiocytes laden with organisms known as *Mikulicz cells* (arrows) (400X).

EAR

ANATOMY

Ear is composed of external, middle and internal portions. External ear consists of auricle, external auditory canal, and eardrum (tympanic membrane).

The external auditory meatus extends up to the tympanic membrane. It is lined by wax secreting sebaceous glands.

Middle ear consists of the auditory (eustachian tube), ossicles (malleus, incus and stapes), oval window and round window. Sound waves travel down the external auditory canal and strike tympanic membrane. Vibrations from eardrum pass to three tiny bones of the middle ear called *ossicles*. Eustachian tube or the auditory tube connects the middle ear cavity with the nasopharynx. It helps in equalizing the pressures on either sides of the eardrum. Inner ear consists of bony labyrinth, membranous labyrinth and vestibular apparatus. Common diseases affecting ear are shown in Fig. 17.19.

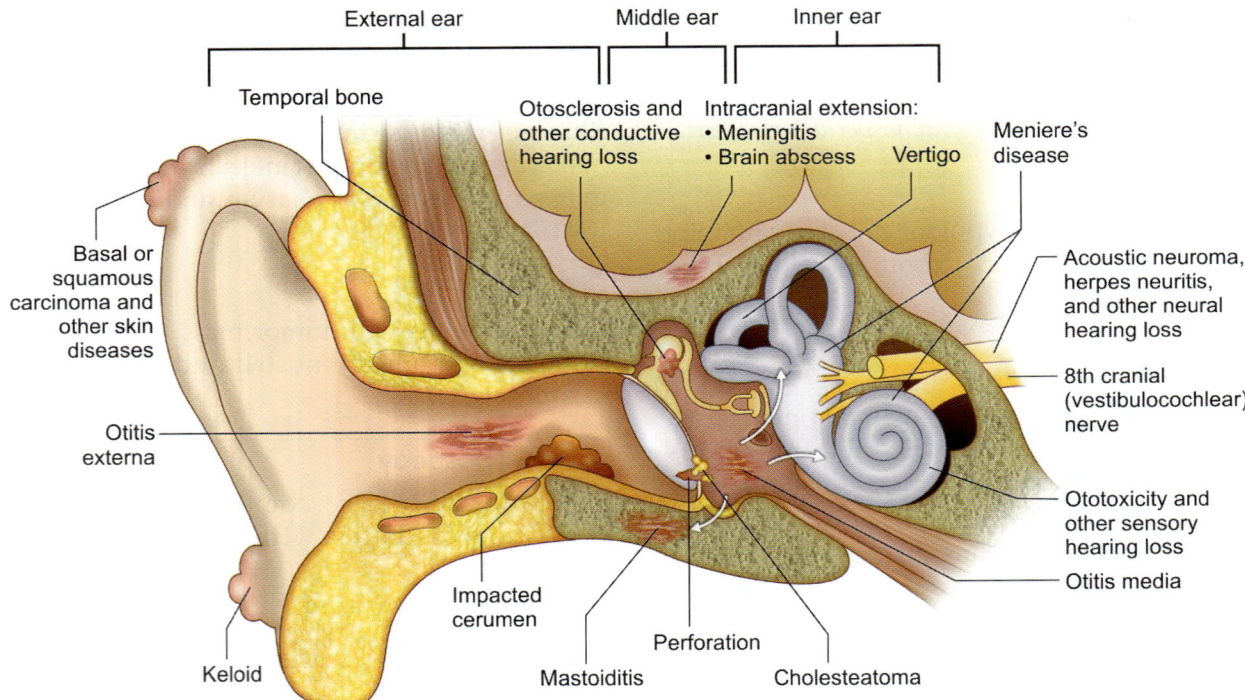

Fig. 17.19: Common diseases of the external, middle and internal ear.

EXTERNAL EAR

PREAURICULAR SINUS

Preauricular sinus, commonest disorder arising as a result of abnormal fusion of facial folds. It leads to formation of blind-ending track opening on the skin just anterior to the external auditory meatus. Obstruction of this opening results information of keratin-filled epidermal cyst. Sinus tract may undergo superadded infection resulting in abscess formation.

DIAGONAL EAR LOBE CREASE

Some persons show a crease of the ear lobe running downwards from the external auditory meatus. There is increased risk of development of cerebrovascular disease, most notably ischemic heart disease.

CAULIFLOWER EAR

Cauliflower ear is characterized by thickening of the pinna due to partial organization of repeated hematoma resulting from trauma. It is commonly seen in boxers.

CHONDRODERMATITIS NODULARIS CHRONICA

This order is characterized by painful nodule on the superior portion of the helix. Skin ulceration extends to cause degenerated eosinophilic cartilage associated with inflammation of the perichondrium. Trauma is considered to be underlying etiology.

RELAPSING POLYCHONDRITIS

Relapsing polychondritis is characterized by involvement of cartilage, eye and heart. Patient presents with reddening, swelling and painful pinna followed by atrophy and destruction of cartilage. It is considered to be of autoimmune disorder related to autoimmune vasculitis.

INFLAMMATION OF PINNA AND EXTERNAL AUDITORY MEATUS

Inflammation may affect pinna and external auditory meatus caused by bacteria, viruses or fungi. *Pseudomonas aeruginosa* produces very severe otitis externa. Herpes simplex 1 and 2 produce painful blisters in the auditory canal and meatus.

Varicella zoster lying dormant in ganglion involves pinna and meatus. Occasionally varicella zoster may involve 8th cranial nerve ganglion leading to disturbances in hearing and balance known as *Ramsay Hunt syndrome*. Foreign bodies within tissues of the external ear produce non-infective inflammatory disease.

CERUMINOUS GLAND ADENOMA

Cerumic gland adenoma most often presents with blockage of the external auditory canal and unilateral deafness.

MALIGNANT NEOPLASM

Malignant neoplasms are rare in external ear.

MIDDLE EAR

ACUTE SEROUS OTITIS MEDIA

Acute otitis media is common in children most often associated with bacterial infection, i.e. *Streptococcus pneumoniae* and *Haemophilus influenzae* at the orifice of the eustachian tube. It may be precipitated by viruses, allergens or sudden changes in atmospheric pressure during flying in an aircraft or deep-sea diving resulting in obstruction of the eustachian tube.

Clinical Features

Repeated bouts of otitis media in early childhood often contribute to unsuspected hearing loss due to residual sterile fluid in the middle ear. Acute suppurative otitis media is unlikely without fever.

Complications

In untreated cases, infection may spread to mastoid air spaces within bone. Infection from mastoid air spaces further leads to meningitis, encephalitis or brain abscess.

CHRONIC OTITIS MEDIA

Chronic otitis media most often develops without a preceding acute phase. It is usually caused by Proteus, Pseudomonas.

Pathogenesis

Mastoid cells and tubotympanic region of the middle ear are most commonly involved. Chronic inflammation leads to formation of abundant granulation tissue that protrudes through tympanic membrane perforation as a polypoid mass, i.e. aural polyp. This process triggers scarring and new bone formation. *Cholesteatoma and cholesterol granulomas are not associated with chronic otitis media*.

Clinical Features

Patient presents with persistent earache, conduction deafness and chronic discharge from the external auditory meatus.

CHOLESTEROL GRANULOMA

Cholesterol granuloma most often occurs as a consequence of previous hemorrhage. The lipid is being derived from cell membrane. Patient develops yellow nodules within tympanic membrane and mastoid. Light microscopy shows chronic inflammatory cells, foreign body giant cells.

TYMPANOSCLEROSIS

Tympanosclerosis is special form of scarring associated with chronic otitis media. It is characterized by laying down of large amounts of dense hyalinized collagen fibers within the middle ear lining adversely affecting tympanic membrane and crura of stapes. There is presence of spotty calcification and new bone formation within plaques of fibrous tissue.

OTITIS MEDIA WITH EFFUSION (OR GLUE EAR)

Otitis media with effusion is common cause of hearing loss in children. It is characterized by thick effusion in the middle ear behind non-perforated tympanic membrane. As the drainage via eustachian tube is impaired, this order is treated by insertion of groomets through the tympanic membrane

CHOLESTEATOMA

Cholesteatoma refers to formation of actively growing, keratinizing, stratified squamous epithelium in the external ear canal resulting in extension into the middle ear through perforated eardrum and mastoid air cells. The keratin mass frequently becomes infected and shields the bacteria from antibiotics. It is a complication of chronic suppurative otitis and a rupture of the eardrum. Cholesteatoma may exist either as a *closed* cystic mass or in the form of *open* form, in which patient presents with keratin squames discharge into the middle ear cavity.

Classification

- *Congenital cholesteatoma:* It arises from an epithelial rest in the developing middle ear. Most common site of congenital cholesteatoma is, where middle ear epithelium joins eustachian tube.
- *Acquired cholesteatoma:* It most often occurs in the upper and posterior portion of middle ear filling most of middle ear cavity.

Consequences

Clinical significance of cholesteatoma is erosion of bony structures such as ossicles or the labyrinth and surrounding soft tissue especially facial nerve.

> ### Light Microscopy
>
> Cholesteatoma is identical to epidermal inclusion cysts surrounded by granulation tissue and fibrosis. It is worth mentioning that squamous cell carcinoma rarely occurs in the ear (Fig. 17.20).

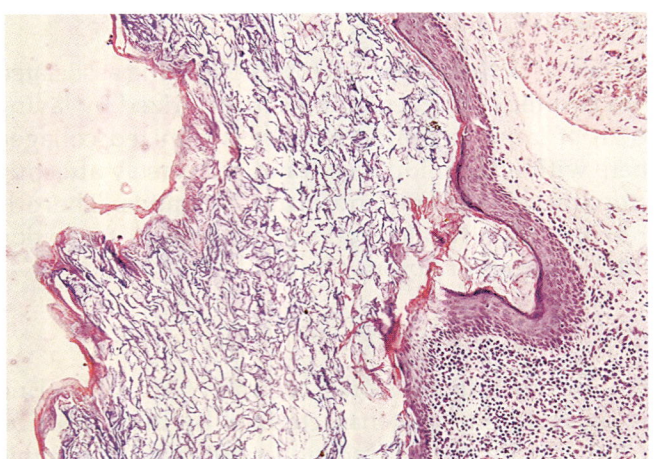

Fig. 17.20: Cholesteatoma is surrounded by granulation tissue and fibrosis. It is worth mentioning that it is identical to epidermal inclusion cysts. Squamous cell carcinoma rarely occurs in the ear (400X).

OTOSCLEROSIS

Otosclerosis is commonest disorder affecting the cochlea and the footplates of stapes. This autosomal dominant disorder affects young and middle-aged adults in the United States. Approximately 90% of cases are asymptomatic.

Pathogenesis

Otosclerosis is characterized by formation of new spongy bone about the stapes and the oval window, resulting in progressive conductive deafness. Fixation of stapes leads to failure of transmission of sound vibrations.

> **Light Microscopy**
> - Stapedectomy specimen shows similar morphology resembling Paget's disease.
> - It shows foci of woven bone rather than normal lamellar bone and numerous *cement lines*.

Electron Microscopy

Stapedectomy specimen shows structure resembling measles virus, and nucleocapsid antigen.

PARAGANGLIOMA (GLOMUS JUGULARE TUMOR)

Paraganglioma is the *commonest tumor* of the middle ear. It is a slow growing vascular tumor that bleeds freely on surgical excision. It may invade the petrous temporal bone reaching the intracranial region in some cases.

Origin

Paraganglioma arises from paraganglionic tissue in the wall of the jugular bulb in majority of cases. It tends to invade the petrous bone. Paraganglioma arising from paraganglion located near the middle ear surface of the promontory and remains localized to the middle ear.

Clinical Features

Patient presents with red mass either behind tympanic membrane or protruding out in the auditory canal. Metastases are very rare. Recurrence is common after surgical resection.

> **Light Microscopy**
> - Paraganglioma has similar morphology in all sites.
> - Tumor is composed of well-defined nests of catecholamine-containing cells.
> - These tumor cells are separated by highly vascular fibrous tissue septa.
> - Tumor cells are surrounded by sustentacular cells.
>
> **Immunohistochemistry**
> Tumor cells do not contain catecholamine but react with monoclonal antibodies against the nuclear marker **S-100**.

INNER EAR

Patient with disorders of inner ear presents with hearing loss, tinnitus and or vertigo.

VIRAL LABYRINTHITIS

Mumps is the most common cause of deafness in 80% of cases among the postnatal viral infections. By contrast, prenatal infection of the labyrinth with rubella is usually bilateral, with permanent loss of cochlear and vestibular function.

A number of other viruses are suspected to cause labyrinthitis, i.e. influenza and parainfluenza viruses, Epstein-Barr virus, herpesviruses, and adenoviruses. Temporal bone specimens of such cases reveal severe damage to the organ of Corti, with almost total loss of both inner and outer hair cells.

PRESBYCUSIS

Presbycusis is the commonest cause of sensorineural hearing loss with aging. There is loss of outer hair cells at the base of lower end of the cochlea.

MENIER'S DISEASE

Menier's disease is characterized by both hearing loss and balance disturbance. Patient presents with episodic deafness, tinnitus and vertigo.

TOXIC DAMAGE FROM DRUGS

Inner ear damage may be caused by genticin, loop of diuretics, salicylates, quinine and cisplatin. Patient presents with sensorineural deafness.

ACOUSTIC NEUROMA

Acoustic neuroma arises from the Schwann cells of 8th cranial nerve. Most patients develop unilateral acoustic neuroma. Patient presents with sensorineural deafness. Bilateral acoustic neuromas are characteristic of neurofibromatosis-2 characterized by deletion of 22 chromosome.

LARYNX

ANATOMY

Larynx is composed of several cartilaginous structures such as thyroid, cricoid and arytenoid. Epiglottis guards the opening of the larynx, which prevents food from entering the larynx. Glottis refers to the vocal cords from the edge of the ventricle to the free edge of the vocal cords. Larynx is lined by mixture of squamous and pseudostratified ciliated columnar epithelium. True cords are covered by squamous epithelium.

INFLAMMATORY DISEASES

Laryngitis is caused by viruses or bacteria, irritants, or overuse of the voice resulting in inflammation and edema of the vocal cords, with resultant hoarseness. Acute epiglottitis is usually caused by *Haemophilus influenzae* that may be life-threatening in young children. Acute laryngotracheobronchitis is acute inflammation of the larynx, trachea, and epiglottis most often caused by viral infection. It is potentially life-threatening in infants. Infant presents with harsh cough and inspiratory stridor.

TUMORS AND TUMOR-LIKE DISEASES

VOCAL CORD NODULE

Vocal cord nodule is also known as *singer's nodule*. It is small *reactive benign laryngeal polypoidal lesion* usually induced by chronic irritation and localized to the true vocal cords.

Pathogenesis

Vocal cord nodule has been associated with *excessive use of the voice and heavy cigarette smoking*. Chronic cigarette smoke and excessive voice abuse injures, disrupts basement membrane and superficial layer of lamina propria resulting in hemorrhage in the stroma. Healing occurs by fibrosis and fibrin deposition.

> **Gross Morphology**
> Macroscopically, it appears as gray or white broad-based nodule or polyp.

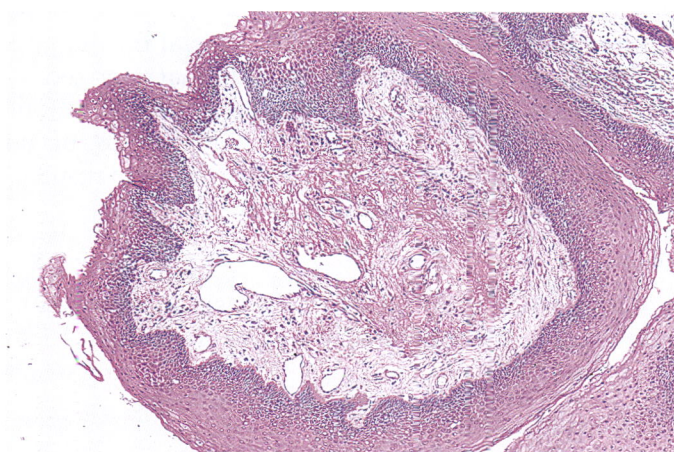

Fig. 17.21: Vocal nodule showing hyperplastic squamous epithelium surrounding fibrovascular core composed of pinkish fibrin deposits, plump proliferating fibroblasts and blood vessels. Stroma is infiltrated by chronic inflammatory cells (100X).

> **Light Microscopy**
> - Vocal nodule is lined by hyperplastic squamous epithelium surrounding fibrovascular core composed of pinkish fibrin deposits, plump proliferating fibroblasts and blood vessels.
> - Stroma is infiltrated by chronic inflammatory cells.
> - *Telangiectic variant* is chiefly composed of dilated blood vessels.
> - *Gelatinous variant* shows fibrin deposits and thin blood vessels (Fig. 17.21).

SQUAMOUS PAPILLOMA

Squamous papilloma arises around the true vocal cords. It is most often associated with low-risk HPV (6 and 11) infections. Children and adolescents may develop multiple lesions, i.e. juvenile laryngeal papillomatosis, that may extend into the trachea and bronchi causing life-threatening state. Recurrence after resection is common. It may rarely undergo malignant change.

> **Gross Morphology**
> Tumor is exophytic, granular, friable, pink-red lesion.

Light Microscopy

Tumor is composed of arborizing papillary fronds of squamous epithelium with some hyperplasia of the basal cells. Cells in the midlayer most often have cytoplasmic clearing.

INTRAEPITHELIAL NEOPLASIA (CARCINOMA *IN SITU*)

Intraepithelial neoplasia is usually seen at the margins of invasive laryngeal carcinoma. It is characterized by variations in size and shape of dividing cells with mitotic activity arranged in disordered fashion with loss of cell maturation as cells progress to the surface, as a result of chronic irritation or inflammation.

Etiology

Tobacco smoking produces dysplasia in respiratory epithelium. It is potentially reversible if the patient stops smoking.

Diagnostic Criteria

Criteria for diagnosing intraepithelial neoplasia is the presence of atypia involving the epithelial covering of the vocal cord.

Clinical Features

Patient may present with hoarseness of voice as a result of slight reddening of vocal cords.

SQUAMOUS CELL CARCINOMA

Approximately 90% of malignant tumors of larynx are squamous cell carcinoma. Tumor most often arises from true vocal cords affecting 50–70 years of age. Men are more affected than women. Most cases involve the glottis or supraglottic region. Glottis tumors manifest earliest. Carcinoma of larynx arising from the vocal cord is shown in Fig. 17.22.

Risk Factor

Tobacco smoking appears to be main risk factor for development of laryngeal carcinoma. Alcohol consumption is another risk factor.

Clinical Features

Patient presents with persistent hoarseness of voice, often associated with cervical lymphadenopathy.

Gross Morphology

- Gross morphology of laryngeal squamous cell carcinoma is variable ranging from fungating, exophytic to endophytic, ulcerated tumors with raised edges (Fig. 17.23).

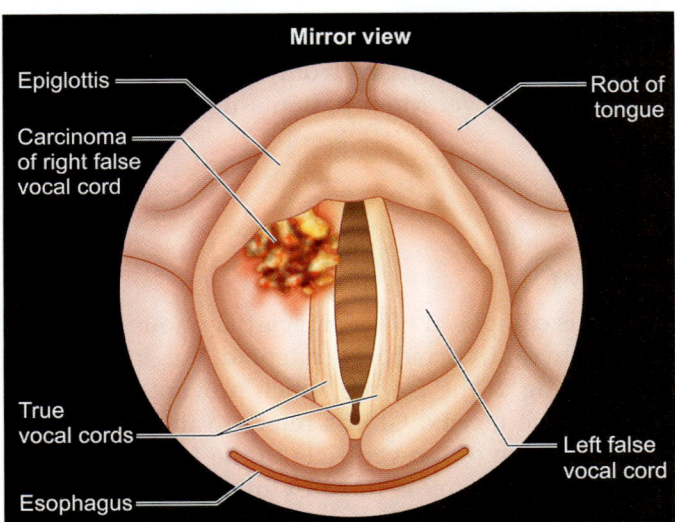

Fig. 17.22: Carcinoma of larynx arising from the vocal cord.

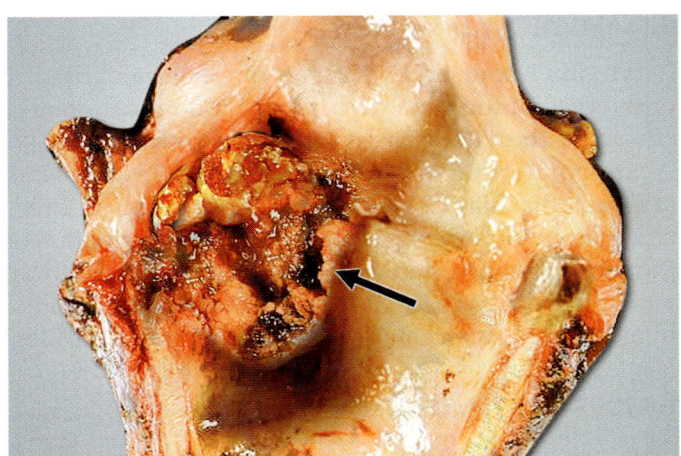

Fig. 17.23: Laryngeal carcinoma showing fungating growth with ulceration (arrow).

Light Microscopy

- *Keratinizing squamous cell carcinoma:* It is composed of round to oval cells with abundant eosinophilic cytoplasm and prominent nucleoli arranged in nests and sheets showing keratin pearls (Fig. 17.24).
- *Moderately differentiated tumor:* It comprises pleomorphic cells with high nucleocytoplasmic ratio and moderate eosinophilic cytoplasm.
- *Poorly differentiated tumor:* It is composed of small cells with less cytoplasm arranged singly or forming nests with marked mitotic activity.
- *Verrucous carcinoma:* It is well differentiated non-metastasizing variant of squamous cell carcinoma. Tumor appears as well as *circumscribed, warty exophytic growth with broad base white granular and friable mass.*

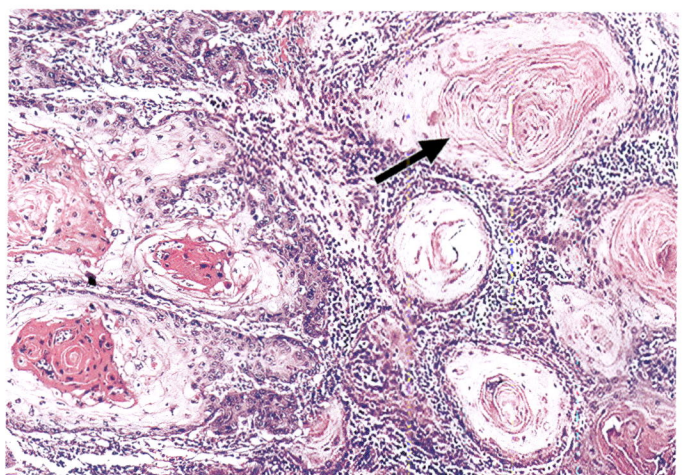

Fig. 17.24: Laryngeal keratinizing well differentiated squamous cell carcinoma showing keratin pearls formation (arrow) (400X).

- Tumor is composed of thick club-shaped papillae with broad pushing bases. There is *absence of cytologic atypia and mitotic activity. Prognosis* of this variant is *excellent.*

- *Spindle cell carcinoma:* It is poorly differentiated carcinoma adopting *spindle or sarcomatoid* pattern. Patient develops *polypoid mass with smooth ulcerated surface.*

  Tumor is composed of sheets of spindle cells mimicking fibrosarcoma or malignant fibrous histiocytoma. There is presence of mitotic activity and necrosis.

- *Basaloid squamous cell carcinoma:* It is a variant squamous cell carcinoma. On gross examination, tumor shows central ulceration with thickening at edges. On histopathological examination, tumor is composed of small basaloid cells.

Classification

Classification of laryngeal carcinoma is based on the location (Table 17.9).

Prognosis

Prognosis is *excellent in carcinoma arising from true vocal cord.* Patient with carcinoma involving supraglottis and subglottis is less common but poor prognosis.

Table 17.9: Classification of laryngeal carcinoma

Location	Frequency	Clinical behavior	5-year survival rate
Glottic region	60–65%	Originating true vocal cords (anterior portion) localized for long duration. Cervical lymph node metastases late. Treated by irradiation or surgical removal of vocal cords curative	80%
Supraglottic region	30–35%	Tumor involving false vocal cord, laryngeal ventricle and epiglottis (33%). Surgical removal of tumor possible without permanent loss of voice. Cervical lymph node metastases in 40% of cases	65%
Transglottic region	<5%	Tumor crossing laryngeal ventricle. Cervical lymph nodes frequently involved. Total laryngectomy together with prophylactic cervical lymph node dissection curative	50%
Subglottic region	<5%	Tumor arising from true vocal cord extending 1 cm or more into the subglottis region. Thyroid gland and cricoid cartilage involved. Cervical and paratracheal lymph nodes involved in 50% of cases	40%

NECK

NECK SWELLINGS

There are many causes of swellings in the neck region. These include lymphadenopathy, cysts, vascular masses, thyroid gland masses and salivary gland masses. The most common swellings are enlarged lymph nodes. Neck swelling may be congenital or acquired, solid or cystic, single or multiple, benign or malignant.

Primary and secondary tumors in the neck are shown in Fig. 17.25. Lateral neck swellings are shown in Table 17.10. Midline neck swellings are shown in Table 17.11.

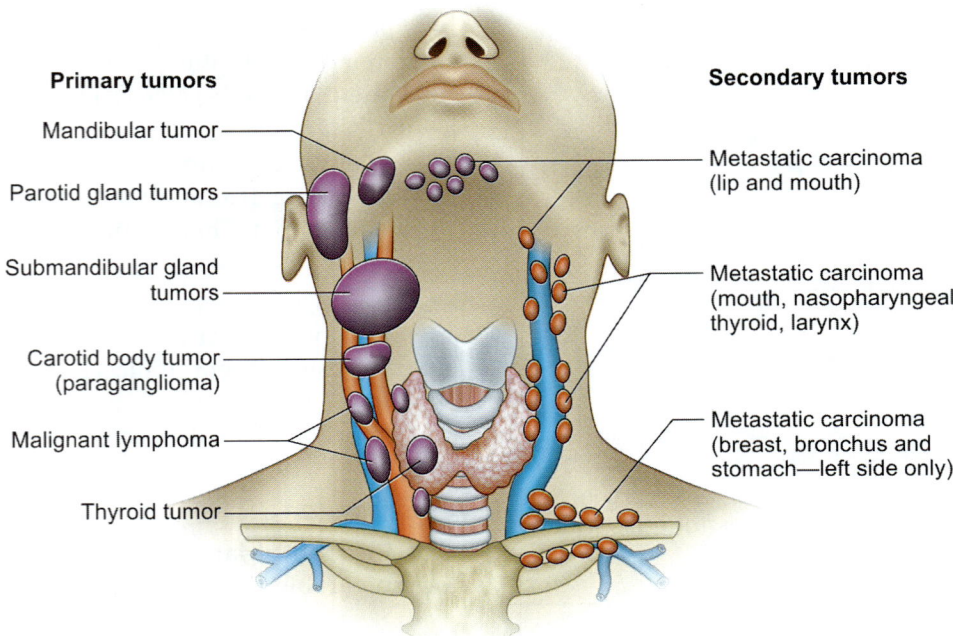

Fig. 17.25: Primary and secondary tumors in the neck.

Table 17.10: Lateral neck swellings

Nature of swelling		Differential diagnosis
Solid swelling	Glands	Lymph nodes (commonest) Salivary glands (thyroid, submandibular and tail of parotid)
	Blood vessels	Carotid body tumor Glomus jugulare
	Subcutaneous tissue	Lipoma
	Nerves	Schwannoma Neurofibroma
	Sternocleidomastoid muscle	Organized hematoma (infants) Fibrosarcoma
	Bone	Cervical rib
Cystic swelling	Fluid	Thyroglossal duct cyst Branchial cyst Sebaceous cyst Cystic hygroma (lymphangioma in children)
	Air	Pharyngeal diverticulum Laryngocele Pneumatocele
	Abscess	Cold abscess (tubercular lymphadenitis) Parapharyngeal abscess Parotid abscess
	Blood vessels	Hemangioma Carotid artery aneurysm Subclavian artery aneurysm

17 Nasal Cavity, Nasopharynx, Paranasal Sinuses, Ear, Larynx and Neck

Table 17.11: Midline neck swellings

Nature of swelling		Differential diagnosis
Solid swelling	Glands	Lymph nodes (submental, prelaryngeal or pretracheal) Thyroid gland isthmus nodule Median ectopic thyroid tissue
	Subcutaneous tissue	Lipoma of Burn's space (suprasternal notch)
Cystic swellings	Fluid	Thyroid gland cyst in isthmus Thyroglossal cyst Dermoid cyst (sublingual or suprasternal) Sebaceous cyst Subhyoid bursa
	Abscess	Cold abscess (tubercular lymphadenitis) Pyogenic abscess
	Blood vessels	Hemangioma Aneurysm of innominate artery

Age Group

Neck swellings occur in various age groups. In children, neck swellings are most likely of infective or development anomaly.

In young adults, neck swellings occur due to infections, leukemia or lymphomas. In elderly persons, neck swellings occur due to primary or secondary malignant diseases.

History of a Neck Lump

History of duration of lump is most important. Seven days duration indicates infection resulting in reactive lymphadenitis. There is long history of seven weeks to months in patient with tumor. Congenital or development swellings have seven years of duration.

Past History

Past history of thyroid cancer, irradiation and pervious scar must be enquired.

Imaging Techniques

Neck swellings are assessed by imaging techniques. These include plain radiograph of neck (AP and lateral view), barium studies, sialography, laryngogram, carotid angiography and MRI studies.

Endoscopic Biopsy

Endoscopic biopsy is oral cavity, nose and nasopharynx.

CERVICAL LYMPHADENOPATHY

The most common swellings are enlarged lymph nodes. These are caused by bacterial or viral infections, lymphomas and secondary metastatic deposits. Inflammatory lymphadenopathy is most often painful, firm and mobile.

Malignant lymph nodes are painless and hard. These may be located in the midline or lateral side of neck. Delphin lymph nodes located along thyrohyoid membrane are enlarged in thyroid cancer.

Cervical lymph nodes showing draining areas and enlargement due to various disorders are shown in Fig. 17.26. Cervical lymph node swellings are shown in Table 17.12.

BRANCHIAL CYST

Branchial cyst is also known as *lymphoepithelial cyst*. It is present as a solitary nodule anterior to sternocleidomastoid muscle. It is considered to arise from remnants of second branchial arch It most often occurs in young adults.

On clinical examination, cyst measures 2–5 cm in diameter. Similar lesions may be encountered in parotid gland or oral cavity beneath tongue. It may rarely undergo malignant transformation.

Gross Morphology
- Cyst is well circumscribed measuring 2–5 cm in dimeter.
- Cut section of cyst may contain clear, watery, mucoid or granular debris.

Light Microscopy
- Fibrous cyst wall is lined by stratified epithelium or pseudostratified columnar epithelium.
- Cyst wall contains lymphoid tissue forming germinal centers.

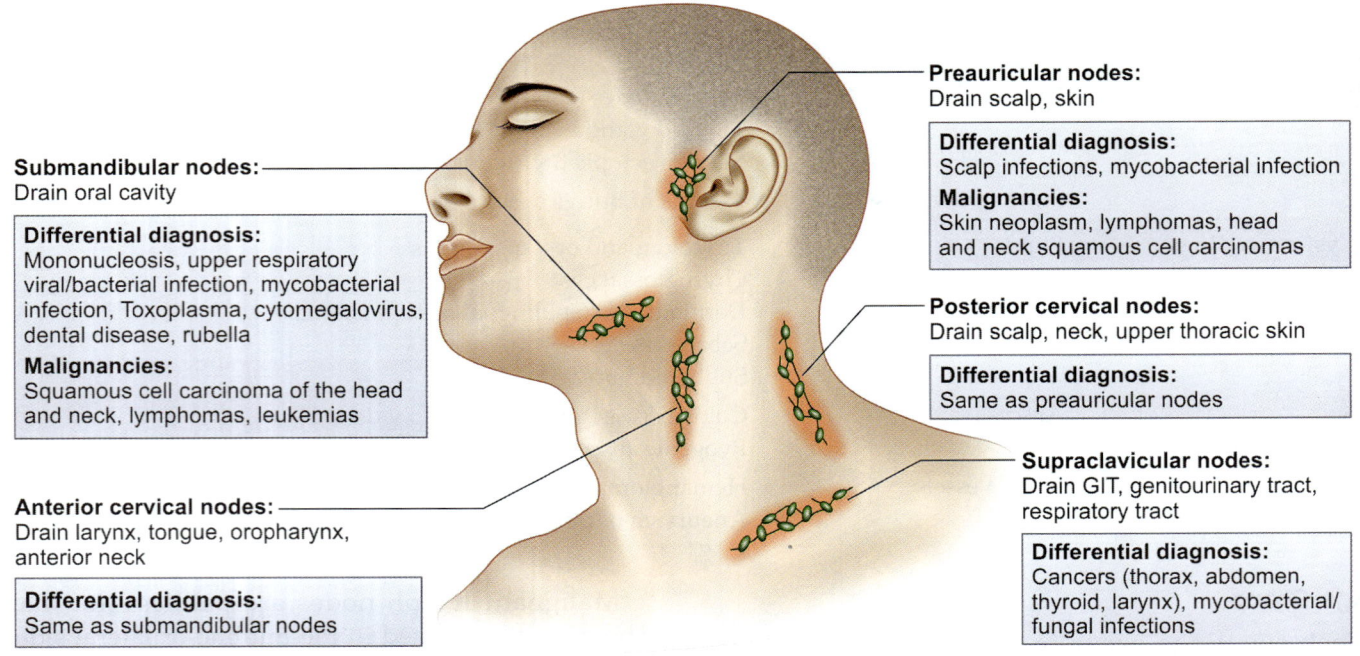

Fig. 17.26: Cervical lymph nodes showing draining areas and enlargement due to various disorders.

Table 17.12: Cervical lymph node swellings

Lymph node groups	Areas drained by lymph node group	Differential diagnosis
Preauricular nodes	Scalp and skin	Scalp infections, mycobacterial infections
		Skin neoplasms, Hodgkin's disease, NHL, SCC of head and neck
Posterior cervical nodes	Scalp, neck skin, thoracic skin	Scalp infections, mycobacterial infections
		Skin neoplasms, Hodgkin's disease, NHL, SCC of head and neck
Supraclavicular nodes	Gastrointestinal tract, pulmonary and genitourinary systems	Cancers of thorax, abdomen, thyroid and larynx
		Tubercular lymphadenitis
		Fungal infections
Submandibular nodes	Oral cavity	Infectious mononucleosis, upper respiratory tract infections, tubercular lymphadenitis, toxoplasma, cytomegalovirus, rubella, dental disease
		Squamous cell carcinoma of head and neck, leukemia, lymphomas
Anterior cervical nodes	Larynx, tongue, oropharynx, anterior neck	Infectious mononucleosis, upper respiratory tract infections, tubercular lymphadenitis, Toxoplasma, cytomegalovirus, rubella, dental disease
		Squamous cell carcinoma of head and neck, leukemia, lymphomas

THYROGLOSSAL DUCT CYST

A thyroglossal cyst occurs due to persistent thyroglossal duct. During its normal development, the thyroid gland descends from the base of the tongue to its final position in the neck. Thyroglossal cyst, a remnant of the thyroglossal duct is the most common thyroid anomaly. It may occur anywhere along the path of descent. It is midline cystic swelling that is close to or within the hyoid bone.

Failure to resect hyoid bone often results in persistence of thyroglossal duct cyst.

Clinical Features

Patient presents with dysphonia, sore throat and midline swelling evident during adolescence and pregnancy. Patient does not develop endocrine complications. Surgery with removal of the proximal duct along with hyoid bone cures it.

> ### Light Microscopy
> - Because thyroglossal duct cysts develop from a hollow tube, most of them do not show thyroid tissue on histopathological examination.
> - Thyroid tissue in sample is demonstrated in 5% of cases and 40% in serial sectioning. Otherwise, the lesion is lined by squamous or respiratory type of epithelium without a muscular wall.

PARAGANGLIOMA (CAROTID BODY TUMOR)

Paraganglia are clusters of neuroendocrine cells associated with sympathetic or parasympathetic nervous system.

Paraganglioma is a painless slow growing tumor arising from the carotid body in the adventitia of the posteromedial aspect of the carotid bifurcation. There is higher incidence in persons residing at higher altitude. It most often occurs in 50 years persons.

Clinical Features

Patient presents with firm, rubbery, mobile side to side and pulsatile tumor. It may decrease in size with carotid compression. Tumor recurs after incomplete surgical resection. Despite its benign nature, it may metastasize to regional lymph nodes and distant organs.

Imaging Techniques

Carotid angiography shows widening of carotid bifurcation. CT scan and MRI determine the extent of tumor.

> ### Gross Morphology
> Tumor is well circumscribed mass with a fibrous pseudocapsule measuring 1–6 cm in diameter. Cut surface reveals gray-tan to pale brown color.

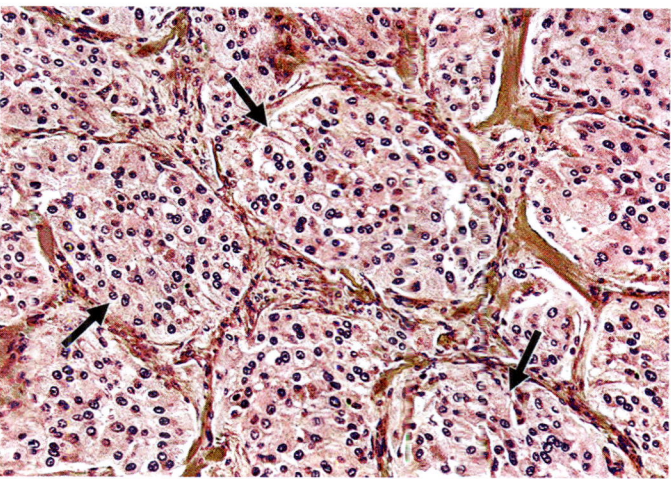

Fig. 17.27: Paraganglioma (carotid body tumor) showing clusters of large eosinophilic tumor cells separated by stroma containing elongated sustentacular cells (400X).

> ### Light Microscopy
> - Tumor is composed of uniform pale staining cytoplasm with and finely granular nuclear chromatin surrounded by fibrovascular network.
> - Compressed spindle-shaped cells are present at the periphery of nests of tumor cells (Table 17.27).
>
> ### Immunohistochemistry
> Panel of markers is used to analyze expression in paraganglioma (chief cells) on histopathological sections (Table 17.13).

Table 17.13: Immunohistochemistry of paraganglioma

Tumor markers	Expression in chief cells
Chromogranin	Positive
Synaptophysin	Positive
Neuron-specific enolase	Positive
CD56	Positive
CD57	Positive

Compressed spindle-shaped cells at the periphery of nests of tumor cells show S-100 protein positivity.

CHAPTER 18

Lung

Learning Objectives

PNEUMONIAS
- Overview
- Lobar Pneumonia
- Bronchopneumonia
- Interstitial Pneumonia
- Opportunistic Pulmonary Infections

LUNG ABSCESS

TUBERCULOSIS
- Mycobacterium Tubercle Bacillus
- Primary and Secondary TB

CHRONIC OBSTRUCTIVE PULMONARY DISEASE
- Overview

RESTRICTIVE PULMONARY DISEASES
- Acute Restrictive Pulmonary Diseases
- Chronic Restrictive Pulmonary Diseases

PNEUMOTHORAX AND ATELECTASIS LUNG
- Pneumothorax
- Atelectasis or Lung Collapse

PULMONARY VASCULAR DISORDERS
- Pulmonary Thromboembolism
- Fat Embolism syndrome
- Pulmonary Hypertension
- Pulmonary Edema
- Pulmonary Vasculitis

LUNG TUMORS
- Benign Tumors
- Primary and Secondary Pulmonary Malignant Tumors

PLEURAL DISEASES
- Pleural Effusion
- Pleuritis
- Pleural Fibrosis
- Malignant Pleural Tumors

ANATOMY

Respiratory system comprises nose, pharynx, larynx, trachea, bronchi, bronchioles, terminal bronchioles and lungs. Major functions of the lungs are to supply oxygen (O_2) and remove carbon dioxide (CO_2) from blood.

The respiratory epithelium is derived from endoderm. With the exception of the pharynx, epiglottis and vocal cords, the respiratory tract is lined by specialized ciliated mucus secreting epithelium. *Structure of respiratory tract is shown in Fig. 18.1.*

Nose

Nose warms, moistens, and filters air and functions in olfaction and speech. Newborn with choanal atresia cannot breathe through the nose. *Allergic polyps* are most common polyps in nasal cavity. In children with nasal polyps, *sweat test* must be done to rule out *cystic fibrosis*.

Pharynx

Pharynx comprises nasopharynx, oropharynx, and laryngopharynx lined by mucous membrane. *The nasopharynx participates in respiration.* The oropharynx and laryngopharynx function both in digestion and in respiration.

Larynx

Larynx contains the *thyroid cartilage* (*Adam's apple*). The epiglottis guards the opening of the larynx, which

Lung

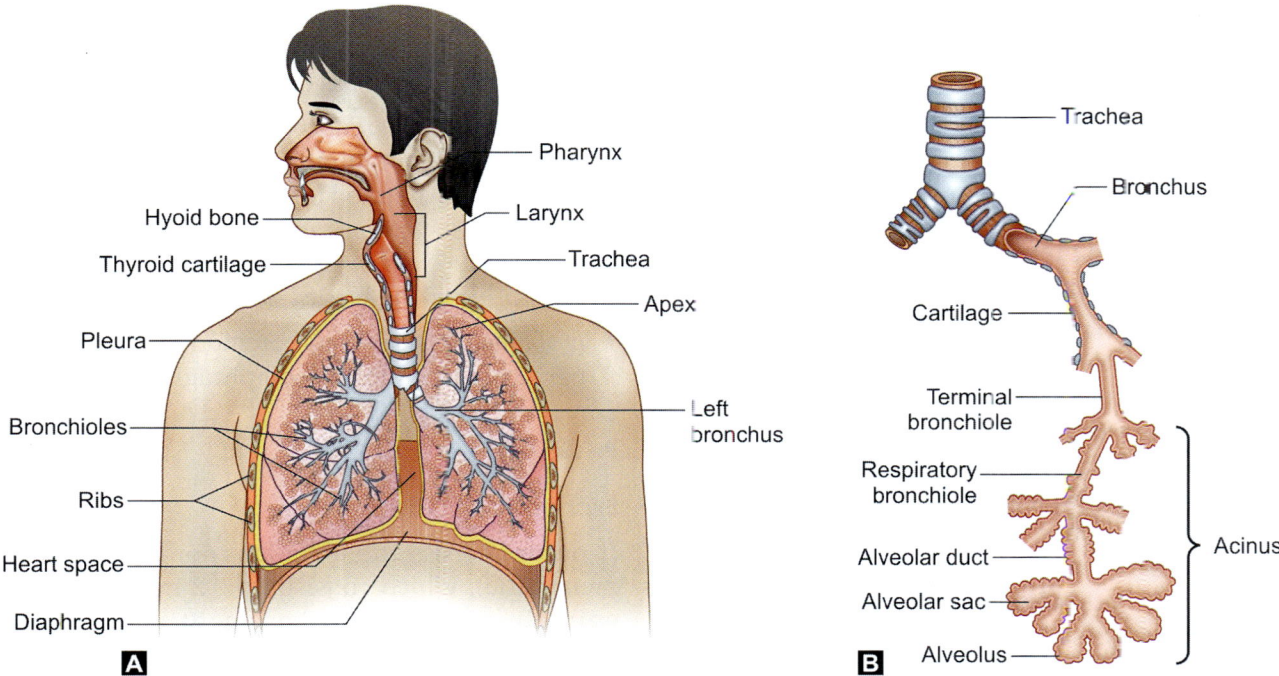

Fig. 18.1: Structure of respiratory tract.

prevents food from entering the larynx; the cricoid cartilage, which connects the larynx and trachea; and the *paired arytenoids, corniculate, and cuneiform cartilages*.

Trachea

Trachea measures *12 cm in length and 2.5 cm in diameter.* Presence of incomplete (C-shaped) ring of *hyaline cartilage prevents collapsing of trachea.* It is lined with *pseudo-stratified ciliated columnar epithelium. The carina is in located at approximately the T4 level.*

Two methods of bypassing obstructions in the airways are *tracheostomy by* making opening into trachea and *intubation by putting tube into trachea.*

Bronchi

The bronchial tree consists of the *primary bronchi, secondary bronchi, tertiary bronchi, bronchioles, and terminal bronchioles.*
- The walls of bronchi contain discontinuous foci of cartilage. Bronchi also have seromucinous glands. Walls of bronchi contain plates of decreasing cartilage and increasing smooth muscles.
- *Right bronchus is more vertical than left bronchus;* hence *foreign body* enters more frequently in right bronchus.
- *Bronchogram* is a radiograph of the bronchial tree after introduction of an *opaque contrast medium* usually containing iodine.

Bronchioles

Bronchioles lack cartilage and submucous glands. These are lined by ciliated epithelium. These contain Clara cells participating in synthesis of proteinaceous fluid. Terminal bronchiole leads to the respiratory bronchiole and finally to the alveolar ducts and delicate alveoli.

Lungs

The lungs are a pair of organs surrounding mediastinum and in close proximity to the heart and major blood vessels. The lungs extend from above the clavicles to T1, T2 vertebral level with full inspiration. The right lung has 3 lobes, whereas the left lung has 2 lobes.

- *Pleura:* Pleural membrane covering lungs consists of outer parietal pleura and the deep visceral pleura derived from mesoderm. Pleural cavity contains pleural fluid.
- *Root (hilum):* Root of lung consists of *primary bronchus, pulmonary artery, two pulmonary veins* and corresponding lymphatic channels. Each lung has a dual blood supply *via* the pulmonary and the bronchial arteries. *Bronchial arteries protect lungs from infarction.* Dyspnea and tachypnea are common symptoms in a case of pulmonary infarction.
- *Bronchopulmonary segment:* It is the smallest functional unit of the lungs. *Left lung consists of 8 broncho-pulmonary segments and 10 in the right lung.* A single bronchopulmonary segment can be resected when disease is confined to that one segment. Each bronchopulmonary segment consists of lobules, which contain lymphatic channels, veins, arterioles, terminal bronchioles, respiratory bronchioles, alveolar ducts, and alveoli.

- *Alveoli:* Each lung consists of approximately 150 million alveoli. Alveolar walls consist of thin, delicate type 1 alveolar cells, i.e. pneumocytes lined by squamous cells, type 2 pneumocytes, and alveolar macrophages. Type 2 pneumocytes secrete surfactant *dipalmitoyl-phosphatidylcholine*, which decreases the surface tension exerted by alveolar fluid. Alveolar macrophages present in lungs participate in phagocytosis. There are no lymphatic channels in the alveoli.

- *Pulmonary lymphatic drainage:* Each lung consists of *superficial beneath visceral pleura and deep lymphatic plexuses located within the submucosa of the bronchi.* The two plexuses communicate at the hilum, ending in bronchopulmonary nodes which drain to tracheobronchial nodes which in turn drain to the left subclavian vein.

  Lung cancers generally spread by the lymphatics to the hilar and mediastinal lymph nodes and then out of the thorax *via* the supraclavicular cervical lymph nodes. Axillary lymph nodes are generally not involved in lung cancer due to their lymphatic range.

- *Nerve supply:* The lungs are innervated by the sympathetic and parasympathetic supply.

Applied Anatomy

- *Compression of structures:* Direct extension of a tumor itself or enlargement of adjacent lymph nodes may compress structures in close proximity to the lungs.

- *Hoarseness of voice:* Lung cancer usually involves recurrent laryngeal nerve supplying left vocal cord leading to hoarseness of voice.

- *Horner's syndrome:* Pancoast tumor (usually squamous cell carcinoma of lung) involves sympathetic chain/ganglion leading to Horner's syndrome.

  Horner's syndrome is characterized by drooping of upper eyelid, sunken eyes, constriction of pupil and loss of sweating on the affected side.

- *Diaphragm paresis:* Lung carcinoma involving phrenic nerve may lead to hemidiaphragm paresis.

PHYSIOLOGY

Exchange of Gases

It occurs across the alveolar-capillary (respiratory membrane); which consists of 0.2 mm thick alveolar epithelium, epithelial basement membrane, thin interstitial space, capillary basement membrane, capillary endothelial membrane. Gas exchange occurs across the alveolar-capillary (respiratory) membranes.

Alveoli are the primary sites of exchange of O_2 and CO_2 gases. Exchange of gases also occurs between blood and tissues by simple diffusion based on pressure/concentration gradient.

Solubility of the gases as well as the thickness of the membranes involved in diffusion are also important

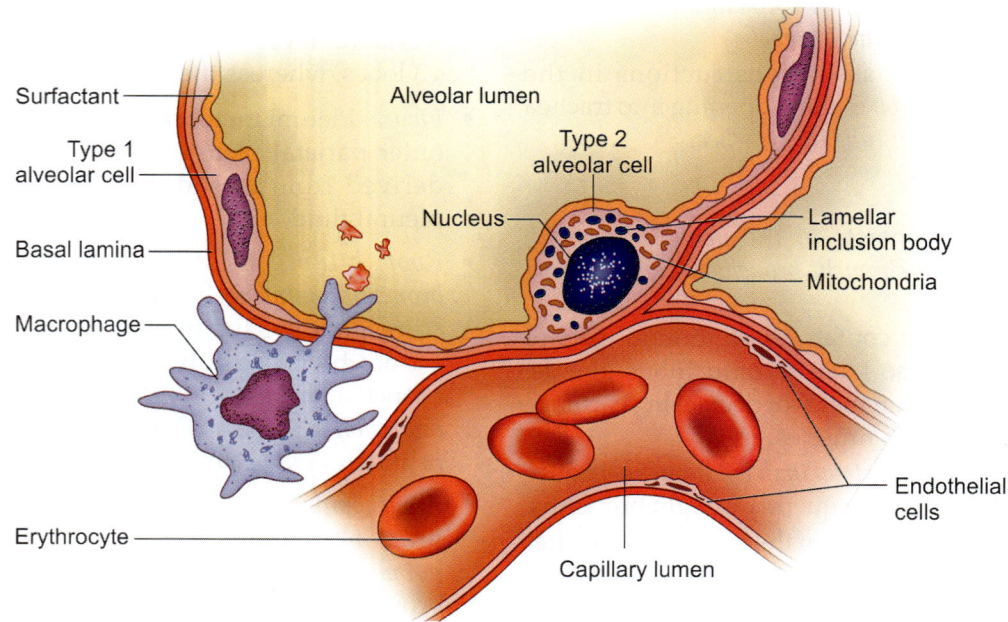

Fig. 18.2: Structure of alveolar-capillary respiratory membrane. Alveolus is lined by epithelial cells. Alveolar basement membrane is thin on one side and widened where it is continuous with the interstitial space. Gas exchange occurs across the alveolar-capillary (respiratory) membranes.

Lung

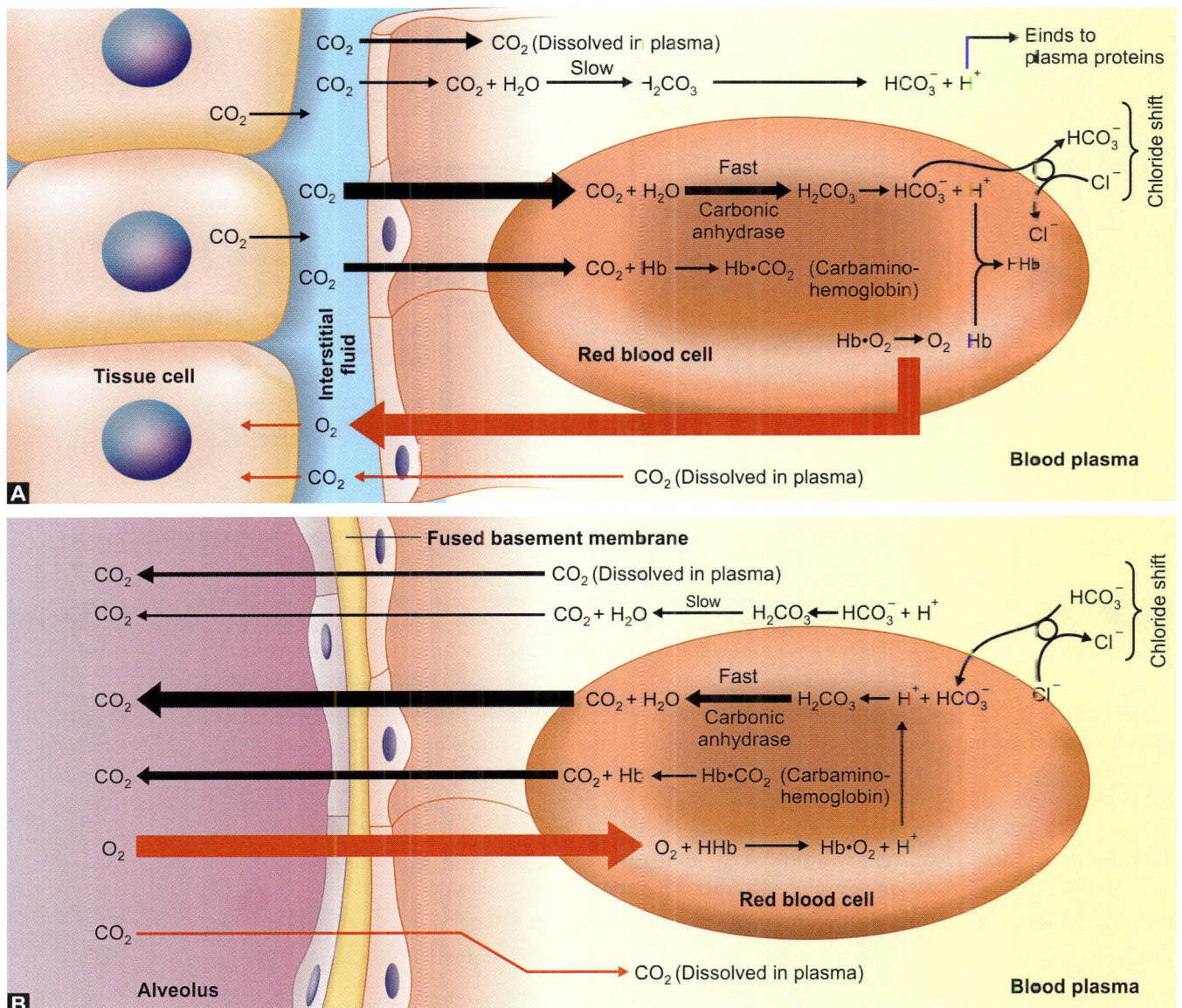

Fig. 18.3: Exchange of gases in lung and tissue. It includes pulmonary ventilation, gas exchange in the lungs, transport of O_2 gas by the blood to tissues, gas exchange in the tissues. Transport of CO_2 gas by the blood to the heart and then to the lungs for oxygenation.

factors that can affect the rate of diffusion. The solubility of CO_2 is 20–25 times higher than that of O_2 (Figs 18.2 to 18.4).

Partial Pressure of Gas

The partial pressure of a gas is the pressure exerted by that gas in a mixture of gases. It is represented as pO_2, pCO_2 and pN_2 for oxygen, carbon dioxide and nitrogen, respectively. Arterial blood pO_2 and pCO_2 is equal to the alveolar pO_2 and pCO_2.

Pulmonary Volumes

Spirometer is an instrument used to measure volume of air in lungs. Alveolar ventilation is the volume of inspired air that reaches the alveoli.

Lung Capacities

These are the sum of two or more volumes that include inspiratory, functional, residual, vital and total lung capacity. Lung capacities are shown in Table 18.1.

Respiratory Disorders

Respiratory disorders are caused by cystic fibrosis, α_1-antitrypsin deficiency, smoking, air pollution, pneumoconiosis and infectious agents. These disorders affect the respiratory airways, interstitial tissue and vasculature of lungs. Patient develops chronic obstructive diseases, acute lung injury, pulmonary infections, diffuse interstitial tissue infiltrative disorders, and lung tumors.

18   Section III: Systemic Pathology

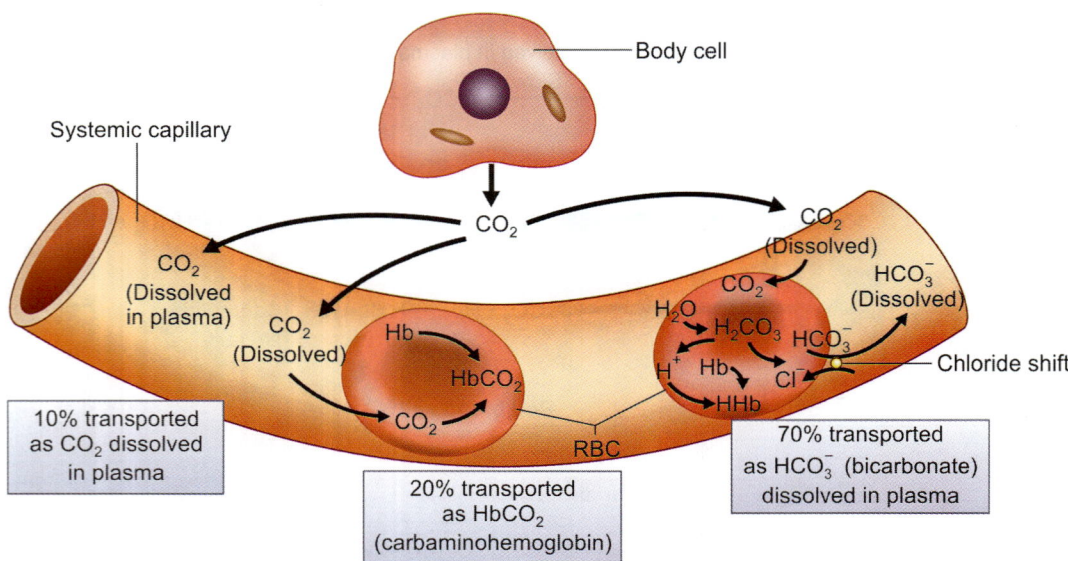

Fig. 18.4: Transport of CO_2 in blood. CO_2 circulates in blood vessel in three forms. Approximately 10% of CO_2 is dissolved in plasma, 20% transported by red blood cells in the form of carbaminohemoglobin and 70% as bicarbonate dissolved in plasma.

Table 18.1: Lung volumes and capacities

Volume	Definition	Average volumes (ml)
Tidal volume	It is the amount of air moved in and out of the lungs in quite, relaxed breathing	500
Residual volume	The amount of air that remains in the lungs after maximum exhalation	1200
Inspiratory reserve volume	The additional amount of air that can be inhaled in by force after a normal inhalation	2500–3000
Expiratory reserve volume	The additional amount of air that can be exhaled by force after a normal exhalation	1100–1200
Vital capacity	The volume of air that can be breathed out from the lungs by maximum exhalation after maximum inhalation	4000
Functional residual capacity	The amount of air remained in the lungs after normal exhalation	2500
Total lung capacity	The total volume of air that can be contained in the lungs after maximum inhalation	5200
Anatomical dead space refers to amount of air present in respiratory tract not participating in exchange of gases.		

PNEUMONIAS

OVERVIEW

Pneumonia is an inflammatory process of the lungs commonly caused by infectious agents (i.e. bacteria, viruses, fungi or *Pneumocystis jiroveci*), chemicals, and inhalation of secretions and aspiration of material.

Source of Infection

Pneumonias are classified as community acquired or nosocomial (hospital acquired pneumonias) or aspiration pneumonia.

- *Community acquired pneumonia:* It is the most common form of pneumonia caused by bacterial infection or a complication of flu.

- *Nosocomial or hospital acquired pneumonias:* Hospital acquired pneumonias are often fatal, in hospitalized patients suffering from serious, debilitating diseases. Patient develops infection within 48 hours being hospitalized or other health care settings.

  Respirator is most common source of *Pseudomonas aeruginosa* causing nosocomial pneumonia. *Escherichia coli* and *Staphylococcus aureus* may also be underlying cause. Endotoxins produced by these organisms play an important role in pulmonary infection.

- *Aspiration pneumonia:* This infection occurs, when a person accidentally inhales food, liquid or vomitus into the lungs. There is increased risk of aspiration pneumonia in persons with dysphagia or with a weakened cough reflex. Chest radiograph is gold standard for diagnosing pneumonia.

Predisposing Factors

Predisposing factors include loss of suppression of the cough reflex (i.e. cerebral stroke, dementia, Parkinson's disease), injury to mucociliary apparatus (i.e. tobacco smoking), interference in the phagocytosis and bactericidal activity of alveolar macrophages, pulmonary congestion (i.e. heart diseases, chronic pulmonary obstructive disease), accumulation of secretions, frequent suction, immunosuppression, liver cirrhosis, diabetes mellitus and recent respiratory tract infections (Table 18.2).

ANATOMICAL CLASSIFICATION

Pneumonias are classified according to etiology (i.e. bacteria, viruses, fungi) and involvement of the pulmonary lobes (i.e. lobar, bronchopneumonia and interstitial pneumonias). More than one type of pathogen may be present that makes diagnosis and treatment, a challenge. There are three morphological and clinical patterns: lobar pneumonia, bronchopneumonia, and interstitial pneumonia (Fig. 18.5).

Table 18.2: Type of immune deficiency determining the organisms responsible for pneumonia

Defects	Organisms
Neutrophil defects	Klebsiella Aspergillus
Antibody defects	*Haemophilus influenzae* Pneumococci
Cell mediated immune defects	Fungi *Pneumocystis carinii* Mycobacterium tubercle bacilli Measles virus Herpesvirus Cytomegalovirus

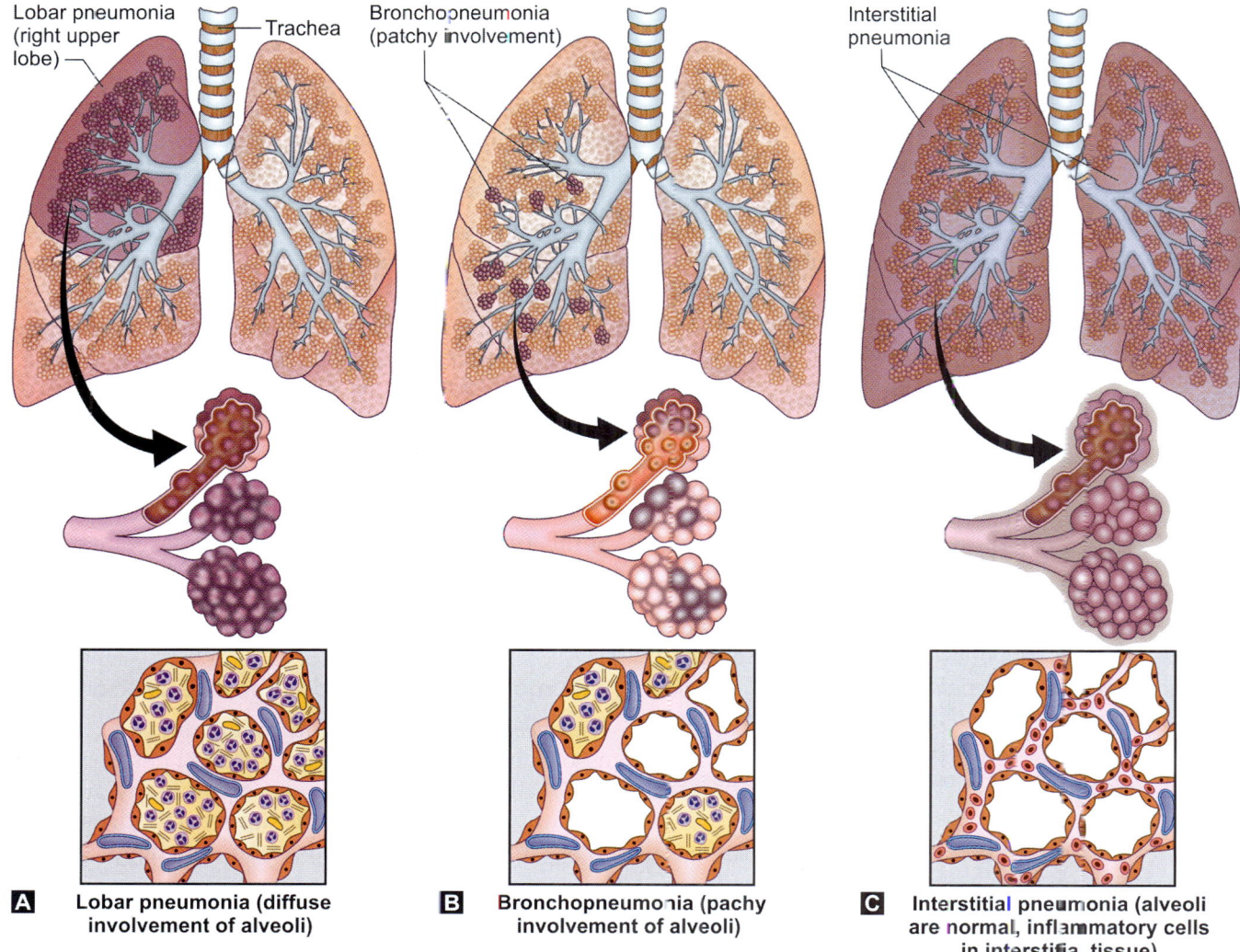

A. Lobar pneumonia (diffuse involvement of alveoli)
B. Bronchopneumonia (pachy involvement of alveoli)
C. Interstitial pneumonia (alveoli are normal, inflammatory cells in interstitia tissue)

Fig. 18.5: There are three morphologic and clinical patterns: Bronchopneumonia, lobar pneumonia, and interstitial pneumonia.

- *Lobar pneumonia:* It is restricted to one lobe of the lungs. Eventually, the whole lobe may be affected.
- *Bronchopneumonia:* It starts as *bronchial inflammation and extends to surrounding alveoli involving one or more lobules.* It shows patchy and focal reddish-gray consolidation in relation to bronchi or bronchioles filled with pus (microabscesses) at the base of both lungs. Consolidation at the base of lungs occurs because of the tendency of secretions to gravitate into the lower lobes or right middle lobe. It usually occurs in infancy and old age.
- *Interstitial pneumonia:* It is also called as primary atypical pneumonia. It shows diffuse, patchy inflammation localized to interstitial areas of the alveolar walls. It involves one or more lobes.

Clinical features: Patient presents with fever, chills, productive cough, blood-tinged or rusty sputum, pleuritic pain, hypoxia with shortness of breath, and sometimes cyanosis. If bacterial etiology it is most characteristically associated with neutrophilic leukocytosis with an increase in band neutrophils with *shift-to-the-left*.

ETIOLOGICAL CLASSIFICATION

Bacterial Pneumonias

Streptococcus pneumoniae: Streptococcus pneumoniae is the most common cause of *lobar pneumonia* especially in *immunocompromised persons*. Capsule of *Streptococcus pneumoniae* prevents phagocytosis by inflammatory cells. This pathogen synthesizes copious mucoid secretion resulting in lobar pneumonia.

Staphylococcal pneumonia: It accounts for only 1% of bacterial pneumonias especially in *intravenous drug abusers* associated with bacterial endocarditis. These persons develop lung *abscess* and empyema. Hematogenous dissemination leads to abscess formation in distant organs such as *brain* and *kidney*.

Klebsiella pneumoniae: Klebsiella pneumoniae is most common cause of bacterial pneumonia in *debilitated hospitalized patients*, diabetics or chronic alcoholic and elderly persons. The organism produces *viscid capsular polysaccharide responsible for thick gelatinous sputum*. Such individual may have difficulty in coughing up. The organism causes alveolar damage, necrosis and abscess formation.

Pseudomonas aeruginosa: Pseudomonas aeruginosa causes pneumonia in patients with *extensive burns*, immunosuppression, and mechanical ventilation. The bacteria invade blood vessels with consequent extrapulmonary spread with fatal outcome within days. Light microscopy shows coagulative necrosis of lung parenchyma and vasculitis.

Hemophilus influenzae: Capsule of *Haemophilus influenzae* prevents opsonization and phagocytosis by host cells. It can cause *life-threatening pneumonias in infants and children*. It may also affect debilitated adults with chronic obstructive pulmonary disease. Patient develops lobular or patchy pneumonia, but may involve entire lung.

Legionella pneumophila: Legionella pneumophila is a gram-negative bacillus transmitted by inhalation of aerosol from contaminated *water storage systems*. It produces *bilateral bronchopneumonia*.

- *Clinical features:* Patient presents with cough, dyspnea, and chest pain with myalgia, headache, confusion, nausea, vomiting and diarrhea.
- *Light microscopy:* On histopathological examination, the alveoli are packed with fibrinous exudate, neutrophils and red blood cells.

Alveolar capillaries are dilated and congested. The exudates may organize resulting in interstitial fibrosis with permanent loss of lung function.

Moraxella catarrhalis: Moraxella catarrhalis constitutes one of the three most common causes of *otitis media*. The pathogen causes pneumonia in elderly persons.

Viral Pneumonias

Viral infections account for *50% of pneumonia cases*. *Influenza* and *respiratory syncytial* viruses are the most common culprits.

Other viruses include adenovirus, cytomegalovirus and herpes simplex. The incubation period is 1–3 days. Viral pneumonias most often affect *children*. Clinical course of viral pneumonia is short-lived and not serious in nature.

Fungal Pneumonias

Some fungi that are endemic are associated with pneumonia. These include *Coccidioides, Histoplasma capsulatum, Blastomyces dermatitidis, Aspergillus fumigatus and phycomycetes*.

Pneumonias in Immunocompromised Persons

Pneumocystis jiroveci is an infection almost exclusively associated with immunocompromised persons such as HIV/AIDS, patients receiving radiotherapy or chemotherapy for cancer, immunosuppressive drugs given in organ transplant persons or nonfunctional spleen.

Mycoplasma Pneumonias

Mycoplasma is smallest free living bacteria responsible for *Mycoplasma pneumonia* after incubation period of

1 to 4 weeks. It is *less serious pneumonia* than due to bacteria or viruses. This type of pneumonia is also known as *walking pneumonia* or *atypical pneumonia*. *Mycoplasma pneumonia* responds well to antibiotics.

LOBAR PNEUMONIA

Lobar pneumonia refers to diffuse consolidation of entire lung due to acute inflammatory exudate within the alveoli without bronchial involvement. There is abrupt demarcation at the interlobar fissure. Lobular pneumonia involves portion of a lung resulting in consolidation. Purulent exudate is observed in bacterial pneumonia (Fig. 18.6).

Etiology

Streptococcus pneumoniae is the most common cause of lobar pneumonia in young healthy adults between 20 and 50 years of age especially in immunocompromised persons. Capsule of *Streptococcus pneumoniae* prevents phagocytosis by inflammatory cells. This pathogen synthesizes *copious mucoid secretion* resulting in lobar pneumonia. However, *Klebsiella pneumoniae* typically affects elderly, diabetics and alcoholics persons.

Risk Factors

Lobar pneumonia occurs due to impairment of normal defense mechanisms. Spleen plays important role in degradation of *Streptococcus pneumoniae*. Risk factors are described as under.

- *Respiratory diseases:* These include atelectasis, bronchiectasis, or cystic fibrosis, lung cancer and tracheostomy patients.
- *Immunosuppression disorders:* These include malnutrition, immunosuppressive therapy, chronic illness, diabetes mellitus, chronic alcoholism and premature birth.
- *Inhalation of toxic gases and cigarette smoke:* These play important role in pathogenesis of lobar pneumonia.
- *Hematological disorder:* Sickle cell disease is a predisposing risk factor for lobar pneumonia.

Pathogenesis

The streptococci reach the alveoli and cause inflammation by pouring of exudates into the lung alveolar spaces. White blood cells migrate to alveoli. The alveoli are filled with exudates resulting in consolidation of lungs. It leads to occlusion of alveoli causing decrease in alveolar oxygen content. Venous blood reaching the affected areas is not oxygenated and returned to systemic circulation. It leads to arterial hypoxemia and even death due to interference with ventilation.

STAGES OF PNEUMONIA

In this antibiotics era, full blown lobar consolidation is infrequent. Untreated patients may morphologically evolve through four stages: congestion, red hepatization, gray hepatization and resolution (Fig. 18.6).

Stage of Congestion (12–24 Hours)

The first stage lasts for about 24 hours. Congestion correlates with the onset of the illness described as typical pneumonias.

Gross Morphology
Affected lung is heavy, edematous and red.
Light Microscopy
Alveolar capillaries are congested. Increased alveolar capillaries permeability results to outpouring of protein-rich fluid with a few neutrophils (inflammatory exudate) and numerous bacteria into alveolar spaces.

Red Hepatization (2–4 Days)

This second stage of red hepatization lasts for 2–4 days. There is progressive disintegration of red blood cells with persistent fibrinosuppurative exudate.

Gross Morphology
The lung is brick red, solid and airless, with a consistency resembling fresh liver (Fig. 18.7).
Light Microscopy
• Alveolar capillaries are congested, and the alveolar spaces are completely filled with fluid and polymorphonuclear cells, i.e. inflammatory exudates.
• Alveoli often show presence of many bacteria and RBC.
• Overlying pleura bears fibrinous exudates (Fig. 18.8).

Clinical features: These occur due to presence of inflammatory exudate. Onset of lobar pneumonia is usually abrupt. Patient presents with high grade fever 40°C with chills, productive 'rusty' sputum containing flecks of blood and occasionally patients may have hemoptysis. Acute pleuritic chest pain on deep respiration reflects involvement of pleura. The clinical findings are dramatically modified on by administration of antibiotics.

- *Inspection:* There is increased respiratory rate, guarding and lag on affected side. Children show sternal retraction and nasal flaring.
- *Palpation:* Chest expansion is decreased on affected side. Tactile fremitus is increased, if bronchus is patent, decreased if bronchus is obstructed.

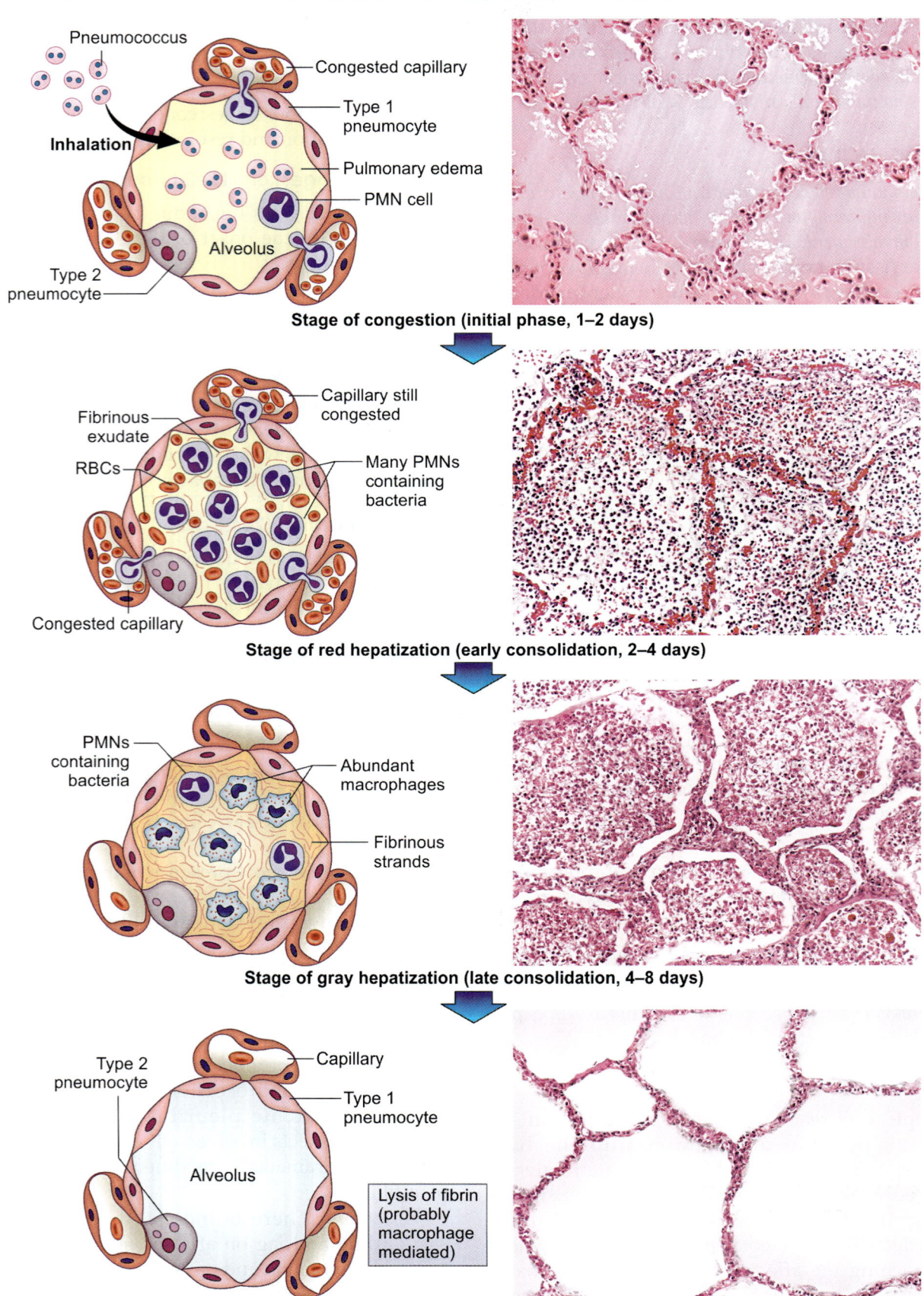

Fig. 18.6: Stages of lobar pneumonia.

Lung 18

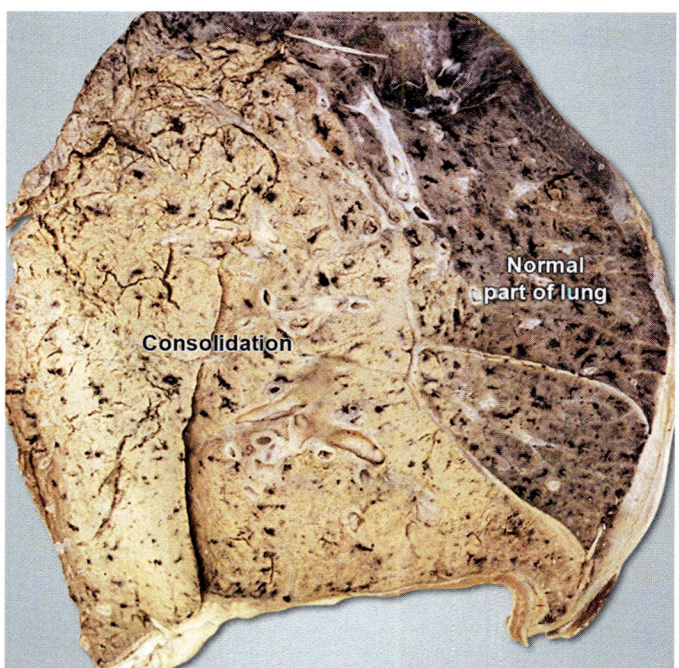

Fig. 18.7: Lobar pneumonia showing consolidation in major portion with small portion of normal lung.

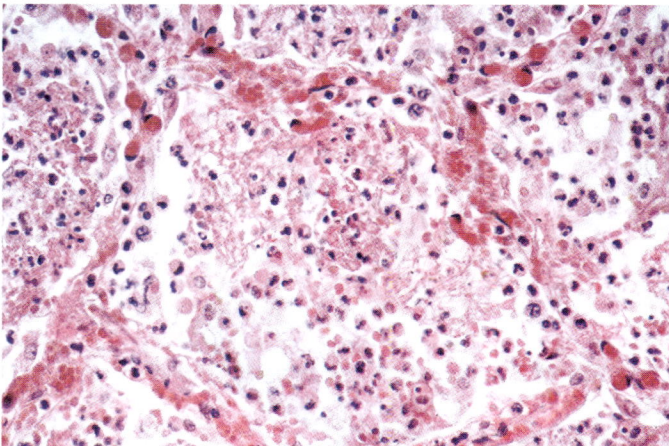

Fig. 18.8: Bacterial lobar pneumonia showing alveoli filled with exudate containing neutrophils. The surrounding alveolar walls having dilated capillaries filled with red blood cells. The exudate in alveoli gives rise to the productive cough of purulent yellow sputum (400X).

- *Percussion:* Percussion note is dull over lobar pneumonia, which recedes with resolution.
- *Auscultation:* Breath sounds are louder with patent bronchus as if coming from larynx. Voice sounds have increased clarity. Bronchophony, egophony and whispered pectoriloquy are present. Late inspiratory crackles of fine to medium size are heard.

Grey Hepatization (4–8 Days)

From red to gray hepatization, there is progressive disintegration of red blood cells. There is persistent fibrinosuppurative exudate which resulting in consolidation of lung. It lasts for 4–8 days.

> **Gross Morphology**
>
> On cut section, lung appears gray brown and consolidated. Compression of alveolar capillaries by inflammatory exudates in alveoli reduces the pulmonary blood flow, thus giving this appearance.
>
> **Light Microscopy**
>
> The alveoli are filled with fibrinopurulent exudates and the capillaries in the alveolar walls appear compressed and contain less blood than in red hepatization.

Resolution (8–10 Days)

Stage of resolution is characterized by granular, semifluid debris, which represents enzymatic digestion of inflammatory debris, ingested by macrophages with preservation of the underlying alveolar wall architecture.

Organization (Carnification)

Carnification of lung is also called organization of lobar pneumonia. When lobar pneumonia fails to resolve, it gets organized by formation of granulation tissue and finally fibrosis. Lung parenchyma becomes hard in consistency.

COMPLICATIONS OF LOBAR PNEUMONIA

- *Pleuritis:* Patient develops pleuritis as a result of extension of inflammation to the pleural surface.
- *Lung abscess:* Pulmonary abscess is a focal suppurative destructive necrosis within the lung parenchyma. It is most often caused by Staphylococcus, Pseudomonas, Klebsiella, or Proteus, often in combination with anaerobic organisms.
- *Empyema:* It refers to collection of pus in pleural cavity. It follows the spread of bacterial infection to the pleural space.
- *Bacterial dissemination (sepsis):* It results in endocarditis, pericarditis, meningitis, suppurative arthritis, abscesses in kidneys and spleen.

LABORATORY DIAGNOSIS

- *Imaging techniques:* Chest radiograph is gold standard diagnostic tool with 50–80% sensitivity to diagnose pneumonias. Bronchopneumonia shows patchy/focal opacities, whereas lobar pneumonia shows radiopaque infiltrate involving entire lobe.

- *Sputum examination:* Gram stained sputum examination shows presence of neutrophils containing numerous lancet shaped diplococci with tapered ends pointing to each other establishes evidence of pneumonia due to streptococcal pneumoniae. But it must be remembered that *Streptococcus pneumoniae* is a part of normal flora and may give false positive results.
- *Blood culture:* The identification of the causative microorganism and the subsequent determination of its antibiotic sensitivity are the key notes to appropriate therapy. During early phase of illness, blood culture is positive in 20 to 30% of persons with pneumonia. Whenever possible, antibiotic sensitivity must be done.

BRONCHOPNEUMONIA

Bronchopneumonia is characterized by patchy distribution of inflammation that generally involves more than one lobe.

- This pattern results from *extension of initial infection of bronchi or bronchioles* extending into *surrounding alveoli* involving one or more lobules.
- Inflammatory pulmonary focus shows patchy reddish-gray consolidation (e.g. microabscesses) with pus filled bronchi or bronchioles.
- The infection is often bilateral and basal because of the tendency of secretions to gravitate into the lower lobes or right middle lobe. It usually occurs in infancy and old age especially immunosuppression state.

Etiopathogenesis

Bronchopneumonia is acute suppurative inflammation caused by *Staphylococcus aureus, Haemophilus influenzae, Klebsiella pneumoniae, Pseudomonas aeruginosa* and *Streptococcus pyogenes*. Other predisposing factors include whooping cough, measles, chronic bronchitis, malnutrition and cancer.

Clinical Features

Patient often becomes septicemic and toxic with fever and decreased consciousness.

> **Gross Morphology**
> Consolidated region of lungs shows acute suppurative inflammation. Cut surface shows dry, granular, and grey-red to yellow patchy consolidation with poorly defined margins. Pleural involvement is less common than lobar pneumonia (Fig. 18.9 and Table 18.3).

> **Light Microscopy**
> Histopathological examination shows focal suppurative exudate filling the bronchioles and surrounding alveolar spaces (Fig. 18.10).

INTERSTITIAL PNEUMONIA

Interstitial pneumonia is also called as primary atypical pneumonia. Unlike *typical* acute pneumonias, sputum production is modest. There is absence of physical

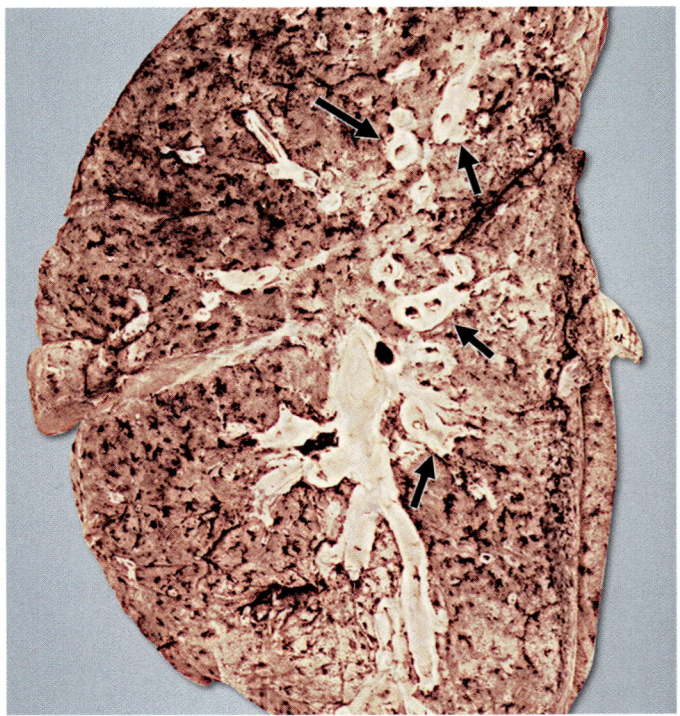

Fig. 18.9: Bronchopneumonia shows tan yellow patchy consolidation. The areas of consolidation are more firm than the surrounding lung (arrows).

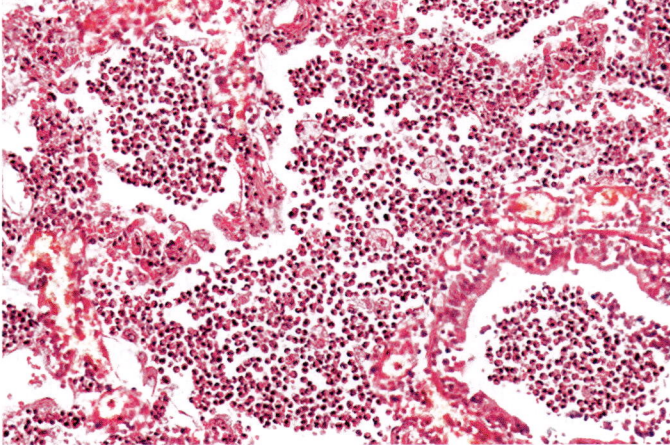

Fig. 18.10: Bronchopneumonia showing alveoli filled with neutrophilic exudate corresponding to the areas of consolidation seen on grow examination. Focal suppurative exudate filling the bronchioles involving surrounding alveolar spaces (100X).

Table 18.3: Differences between bronchopneumonia and lobar pneumonia

Parameters	Lobar pneumonia	Bronchopneumonia
Definition	Acute respiratory tract infection involving alveoli	Acute respiratory tract infection involving bronchioles and extending to alveoli
Age group	Adults	Infants, old persons
Immunity status	Previously healthy persons	Immunocompromised persons
Organisms	Pneumococci, streptococccal pneumococci, *Haemophilus influenzae, Klebsiella pneumoniae*	Staphylococcus, streptococci, pneumococci, *Haemophilus influenzae, Pseudomonas aeruginosa* coliforms
Opportunistic infection	Absent	May be present
Pathology	Lung alveoli filled with exudate	Bronchitis/bronchiolitis involving lung alveoli
Consolidation lung	Diffuse consolidation	Patchy consolidation
Lobes involved	Part of lobe or entire lobe	Multiple lobe, often bilateral
Lung lobe involved	Upper or lower lobe or whole lung	Basal portion of lower lobe due to secretions
Stages of inflammation	Early congestion (1–2 days), red hepatization (2–4 days), gray hepatization (4–8 days) and resolution (7–21 days)/organization	Not clearly defined
Exudation seen on light microscopy	More exudate	Less exudate
Severity	More severe	Less severe
Sputum	Initially scanty, watery. Later on thick, purulent, hemorrhagic	Purulent
Complications	Uncommon, organization, pleural effusion, empyema, lung abscess	Uncommon, organization, pleural effusion, empyema, lung abscess and bronchiectasis

findings of consolidation. Bacteria and viruses are not isolated.

Gross Morphology
Lung shows diffuse, patchy inflammation localized to interstitial areas of the alveolar walls. It involves one or more lobes. It occurs as a result of droplet infection.

Light Microscopy
- Inflammatory reaction is confined to the interstitium of lung.
- Alveolar spaces are usually free of exudates.
- The alveolar septa are widened and edematous, infiltrated by lymphocytes, macrophages and occasionally plasma cells.

Clinical Features
Patient has insidious onset of low grade fever, non-productive cough, and chest pain, flu-like symptoms, i.e. pharyngitis, laryngitis, myalgia, and headache. Patient's lungs show no signs of consolidation.

Etiopathogenesis
- *Mycoplasma pneumoniae* is most common cause of atypical pneumonia, i.e. interstitial pneumonia with insidious onset. It usually occurs in children and young adults. It usually follows a mild self-limited course.
- *Viral pneumonias:* Viruses most often cause pneumonia in children. These include influenza virus, adenovirus, rhinovirus, and respiratory syncytial virus, rubeola (measles) or varicella (chickenpox). Cytomegalovirus produces a characteristic interstitial pneumonia with marked enlargement of infected cells containing intranuclear inclusions. Measles virus produces giant cell pneumonia and marked by numerous giant cells.
- *Lymphocytic interstitial pneumonia:* It is often associated with Sjögren's syndrome and HIV infection. Clinical course of the disease varies from an indolent condition to one of those progresses to end-stage lung disease and respiratory failure.
- *Hypersensitivity pneumonitis:* It occurs in response to repeated exposure to a variety of organic materials (e.g. pigeon bird droppings, feathers, mushrooms, and tree bark). Inhalation to pigeon bird droppings is known as pigeon breeder lung. Light microscopy of lung lesion shows poorly formed granulomas.
- *Usual interstitial pneumonia:* It is of unknown etiology in majority of cases. It occurs in various clinical

settings including collagen vascular disease, chronic hypersensitivity pneumonitis, and drug toxicity.

- *Nonspecific interstitial pneumonias (NIP):* It is associated with collagen vascular disease, hypersensitivity pneumonitis, drug reaction). Patient develops diffuse, temporarily uniform proliferative and fibrosing changes. Prognosis is better than usual interstitial pneumonias with five-year survival in more than 80% cases.
- *Desquamative interstitial pneumonia (DIP):* It is a chronic fibrosing interstitial pneumonitis of unknown etiology. Lungs show minimal fibrosis with preservation of lung architecture. It primarily occurs in smokers. Prognosis is better than usual interstitial pneumonias with 10-year survival from 70 to 100%. The pathologic changes can regress following smoking cessation.
- *Hypersensitivity pneumonitis:* It is caused by thermophilic actinomyces, molds, animal proteins and rarely exposure to drugs such as methotrexate and amiodarone.

OPPORTUNISTIC PULMONARY INFECTIONS

Immunocompromised patients may develop pneumonias due to opportunistic infectious agents.

Pneumocystis Jiroveci

It is most common pathogen causing pneumonia in acquired immune deficiency syndrome. This organism has been reclassified as a fungus.

- *Light microscopy:* Lung lesion shows interstitial infiltrate of plasma cells and lymphocytes, diffuse alveolar damage, and hyperplasia of type 2 pneumocytes. The alveoli contain foamy exudate. The organisms appear as small bubbles in a background of proteinaceous exudates.
- *Bronchoalveolar lavage:* Specimen obtained by bronchoalveolar lavage impregnated with silver shows a cluster of cysts. The cysts appear as round or indented (crescent moon) bodies measuring 2–3 µm in diameter.

Candida Albicans

In immunocompromised patients, invasive form produces blood-borne dissemination. Pulmonary, renal, and hepatic abscesses and vegetative endocarditis.

Cytomegalovirus

It is now well recognized in immunocompromised persons. CMV causes marked enlargement of infected cells, which contain typical intranuclear and often cytoplasmic inclusions. Diagnosis is by morphologic demonstration of the organism in biopsy or bronchial washing specimens.

Nocardiosis

Nocardia are gram-positive aerobic, filamentous, weakly acid-fast bacteria closely related to *Actinomyces israelii*. Typically opportunistic infection may disseminate to the brain and meninges.

Aspergillus Fumigatus

Invasion of blood vessels and tissue infarcts are common in *Aspergillus fumigatus* infection. Aspergillus species may also grow in pre-existing cavities caused by tuberculosis or bronchiectasis. They proliferate to form fungus balls, which are also referred to as aspergillomas or mycetomas. Lung shows focal yellow areas of consolidation.

Cryptococcus Neoformans

Pneumonia results from the inhalation of spores of *Cryptococcus neoformans*, an organism frequently encountered in pigeon droppings. Most serious cases occur in immunocompromised persons. Cryptococcus stains positively with a mucicarmine stain or Indian ink for capsular polysaccharides.

Histoplasma Capsulatum

It results in multiple pulmonary lesions with late calcification. Disseminated form, marked by multisystem involvement with infiltrates of macrophages filled with fungal yeast forms.

Aspergillosis

Invasive form has predilection for growth into vessels, with consequent widespread hematogenous dissemination.

Coccidioidomycosis

Coccidioidomycosis occurs in primary and disseminated forms. Fungal spherules contain endospores found within granulomas.

Actinomyces Israelii

Actinomyces israelii is a gram-positive anaerobic filamentous bacteria no longer classified as a fungus. It is a normal colonizer of the vagina, colon, and mouth. It is an opportunistic pathogen. Infection is established first by a breach of the mucosal barrier during various procedures (dental, gastrointestinal), aspiration, or diverticulitis. Patient develops abscess and sinus tract formation. Light microscopy shows exudates containing sulfur granules, yellow clumps of the organism.

LUNG ABSCESS

Lung abscess is a focal suppurative process within the lung characterized by necrosis of lung parenchyma. It is most often caused by Staphylococcus, streptococci, Pseudomonas, Klebsiella, or Proteus, often in combination with anaerobic organisms.

Pathogenesis

Lung abscess most often occurs due to aspiration of oropharyngeal and gastric material, superior segment, right lower lobe is most common site for aspiration. Other causes include bronchial obstruction (often by tumor), or complication of bacterial pneumonias, septicemias and penetrating lung injury.

- *Aspiration:* Person with decreased cough reflex due to alcohol or drug overdose, general anesthesia or neurological disorders may aspirate infected oropharyngeal material, tonsillitis, sinusitis or gingivodental sepsis, that localize in the lung depending on the posture of patient.

  Person in sitting or standing posture, aspirated material is located in the posterobasal segment of the right lower lobe. In the supine posture, superior segment of the right lower lobe is affected. In right-sided posture, it is localized in the right middle lobe or the posterior segment of the right upper lobe.
- *Bronchial obstruction:* It occurs due to centrally located squamous cell carcinoma lung in 10–15%, bronchopulmonary carcinoid tumor, and foreign body.
- *Pneumonias:* Lung abscess occurs in patients suffering from pneumonias caused by streptococci, *Staphylococcus aureus*, pneumococci, *Klebsiella pneumoniae*, and anaerobic bacteria.
- *Septicemia:* Septic emboli in case of infective endocarditis, thrombophlebitis and puerperal sepsis by pyogenic organisms seed the lung *via* hematogenous route.
- *Direct penetrating lung injury:* It may cause lung abscess.

Gross Morphology
- Lung abscess varies in size and location depending on underlying cause.
- Aspiration of infected oropharyngeal material is located in the superior segment of right lung due to vertical course of right bronchus.
- Distribution of lung abscess is shown in Fig. 18.11 and Table 18.4.

Light Microscopy
Necrotic material obtained from lung abscess shows inflammatory cells. Necrotic area is surrounded by granulation tissue and fibrosis (Fig. 18.12).

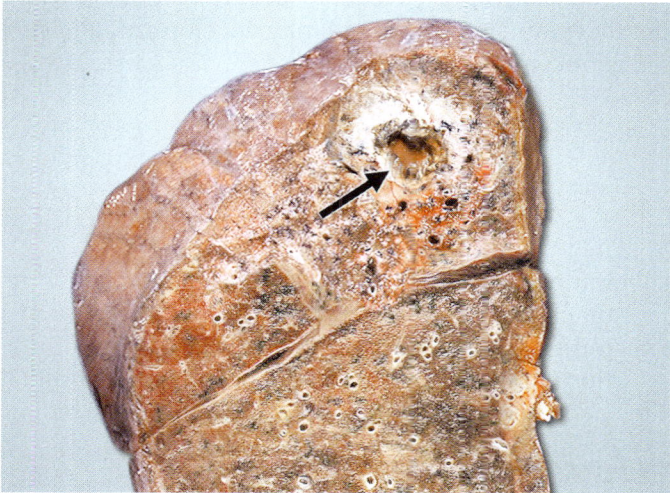

Fig. 18.11: Lung abscess present in apical region.

Table 18.4: Distribution of lung abscess

Causes of lung abscess	Gross morphology
Aspiration sitting or standing posture	Posterobasal segment of the right lower lobe
Aspiration supine posture	Superior segment of the right lower lobe
Aspiration right-sided posture	Right middle lobe or the posterior segment of the right upper lobe
Pneumonia	Multiple abscesses
Septic emboli	Multiple abscesses
Bronchiectasis	Base of the lung

Clinical Features

Patient presents with productive cough (foul smelling sputum), chest pain and fever of spiking pattern. Chest radiograph shows cavitation with an air-filled level.

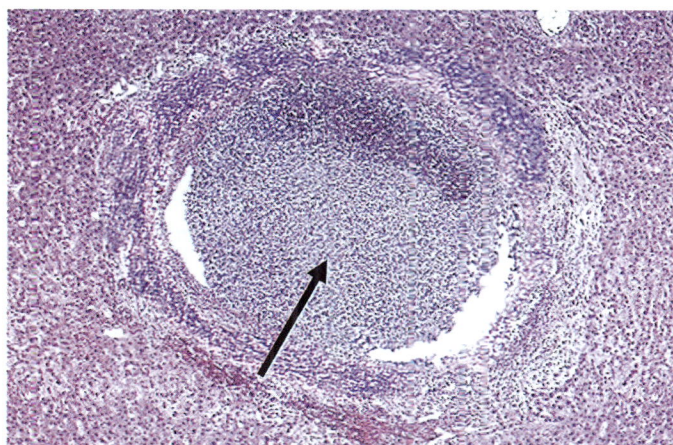

Fig. 18.12: Lung abscess showing collection of neutrophils (arrow) (100X).

Complications

Lung abscess may spread to pleura, mediastinum, meninges, and bones. Patient may develop amyloidosis and septicemia.

Treatment

Most acute abscesses resolve with appropriate antibiotic therapy (clindamycin) and postural drainage. In a few cases, imaging guided, tube is inserted to drain the abscess. Bronchoscopy is done if lung abscess does not resolve.

TUBERCULOSIS

Tuberculosis is worldwide health problem caused by Mycobacterium tubercle bacilli (homis strain). It is transmitted by inhalation of droplets (most common), ingestion of infected milk and skin inoculation (handling infected specimens). It may involve multiple systems.

MYCOBACTERIUM TUBERCLE BACILLUS

- *Acid-fast organism:* Mycobacterium tubercle bacillus is strict aerobe. It is acid-fast due to presence of mycolic acid in its cell wall and stained by Ziehl-Neelsen staining (decolorized by 20% sulfuric acid).
- *Composition:* It contains large quantity of hydrophobic waxes and fatty acids of high molecular weight, which prevents entry of Gram's stain.
- *Virulence:* Virulence of bacillus depends on presence of cord factor (a sulfated glycolipid), which prevents fusion of phagosomes with lysosomes and thus favors intracellular survival of AFB in macrophages. If cord factor is extracted, AFB becomes avirulent.
- *Viability:* Bacillus is viable for months in dry or wet sputum. Single AFB is potentially infective in immunocompromised persons (Table 18.5).

RISK FACTORS

There is increased risk of tuberculosis in person, who is in close contact with a newly diagnosed open case of pulmonary tuberculosis case (sputum smear positive), history of previous tuberculosis exposure and immunocompromised individuals (AIDS and corticosteroids therapy), history of silicosis, diabetes mellitus, malnutrition, cancer, Hodgkin's disease, or leukemia, gastrectomy, chronic renal failure and alcoholism.

TUBERCULAR INFECTION AND DISEASE

Tubercular Infection

Tubercular infection refers to a positive TB skin test, i.e. Mantoux test or tuberculin test or PPD test with no evidence of active disease. Purified protein derivative (PPD) is injected by intradermal route on forearm. Area of induration is demonstrated after 48–72 hours in immunocompetent individuals after exposure to tubercle bacilli after 2–4 weeks. Positive tuberculin test does not distinguish infection, i.e. inactive disease from active disease.

Tuberculosis Disease

It refers to cases that have positive acid-fast smear or culture for *Mycobacterium tuberculosis* or radiographic and clinical presentation of tuberculosis. Children below 2 years of age are more susceptible. Patients with silicosis and with immunosuppression are also more susceptible to tuberculosis.

PATHOGENESIS

Mycobacterium tubercle bacillus antigens play important role in cell mediated immunity and type 4 hypersensitivity reaction. Virulence and bacterial factors in tubercle bacilli are shown in Table 18.6.

Table 18.5: Nontuberculous mycobacteria: four groups

Group	Example	Pathologic lesions
Group I: Photochromogens	Mycobacterium kansasii	Koch's chest in adults Cervical lymphadenopathy in children
Group II: Scotochromogens	Mycobacterium scrofulaceum	Cervical lymphadenopathy in children, rarely involving lungs
Group III: Non-photo-chromogens	Mycobacterium intracellulare Mycobacterium avium	Koch's chest in adults Cervical lymphadenopathy in children Osteomyelitis may affect any age group
Group IV: Rapid growers	Mycobacterium fortuitum	Koch's chest rare (organism present in fresh salty water and swimming pools)

Table 18.6: Virulence and bacterial factors in tubercle bacilli

Characteristics	Name	Functions
Virulence factors	Cord factor composed of glycolipids, mycolic acid and trehalose dimycolate	Cord factor prevents fusion of phagosomes with lysosomes and thus favors intracellular survival of AFB in macrophages. If cord factor is extracted, AFB becomes avirulent. Cord factor can elicit granulomas formation in the tissue
	Catalase-peroxidase and lipoarabinomannan (LAM)	These resist the host cell oxidative response
	Sulfatides and trehalose dimycolate	It can trigger toxicity in animal models
	Lipoarabinomannan (LAM)	It can induce cytokines and resist host oxidative stress
Bacterial factors	Nonreplicating persistent (NRP1) state	Under aerophilic conditions with increased glycine dehydrogenase activity
	Nonreplicating persistent (NRP2) state	Under anaerobic conditions with decreased glycine dehydrogenase activity
	A sigma factor	
	α-Crystallin-like heat shock protein (acr)	Unknown

Pathogenesis of Tuberculosis <3 Weeks Duration

Mycobacterium tubercle bacilli's mannose capped glycolipid (lipoarbinomannon) binds the mannose receptors expressed on alveolar macrophages. These macrophages engulf these organisms. Cord factor synthesized by these organisms prevent fusion of phagosomes with lysosomes. Hence, unchecked proliferation of tubercle bacilli continues inside alveolar macrophages.

Pathogenesis of Tuberculosis >3 Weeks Duration

Macrophages are antigen presenting cells, which transmit mycobacterium tubercle bacilli antigen to T-helper cells. Macrophages synthesize IL-12, which takes part in differentiation of T-helper cells in lungs and lymph nodes.

- *Bactericidal activity of immune system:* T-helper cells synthesize interferon-γ (IFN-γ), which stimulates *nitrogen synthase* enzyme resulting in synthesis of *nitrogen intermediates* (NO, NO_2 and HNO_3) and free radicals causing oxidative destruction of AFB.
- *Formation of epithelioid granulomas:* Macrophages synthesize tumor necrosis factor and chemokines participate in recruitment of monocytes and sensitization of T cells. This process leads to formation of epithelioid granulomas comprised of macrophages and surrounded by lymphocytes. Granulomas prevent spread of infection by confining bacteria within a compact collection of activated macrophages and lymphocytes.
- *Caseous necrosis:* CD8+ T cells cause destruction of macrophages by *fas dependent* mechanism resulting in caseous necrosis.

TISSUE SUSCEPTIBILITY AND DRUG RESISTANCE

Tissue Susceptibility

Most common organs involved in children include *lungs, lymph nodes, spleen* and *meninges*. In adults, most common organs involved comprises lungs, adrenal glands, kidneys, liver, spleen, bone, meninges, serous membranes, fallopian tubes, epididymis and lymph nodes. *Lungs are the most common site of tuberculosis in children and adults.* Tissues rarely involved include cardiac and skeletal muscle, stomach, thyroid gland, and pancreas.

Drug Resistance

Patient develops resistance due to mutations involving *mycolic acid, catalase* and *peroxidase enzyme*. Catalase enzyme is required to activate isoniazid.

CATEGORIES

Tuberculosis is divided into two categories—pulmonary (85% cases) and extrapulmonary tuberculosis (15% cases). Active disease develops in 5 to 15% of those infected with Mycobacterium tuberculosis. Pulmonary tuberculosis has two distinct phases, i.e. primary tuberculosis and secondary tuberculosis. Organs involved in primary, secondary and miliary tuberculosis are shown in Fig. 18.13.

Light Microscopy

Histopathological examination of lesion shows epithelioid cell granulomas, caseous necrosis and Langhan's giant cell (Fig. 18.14).

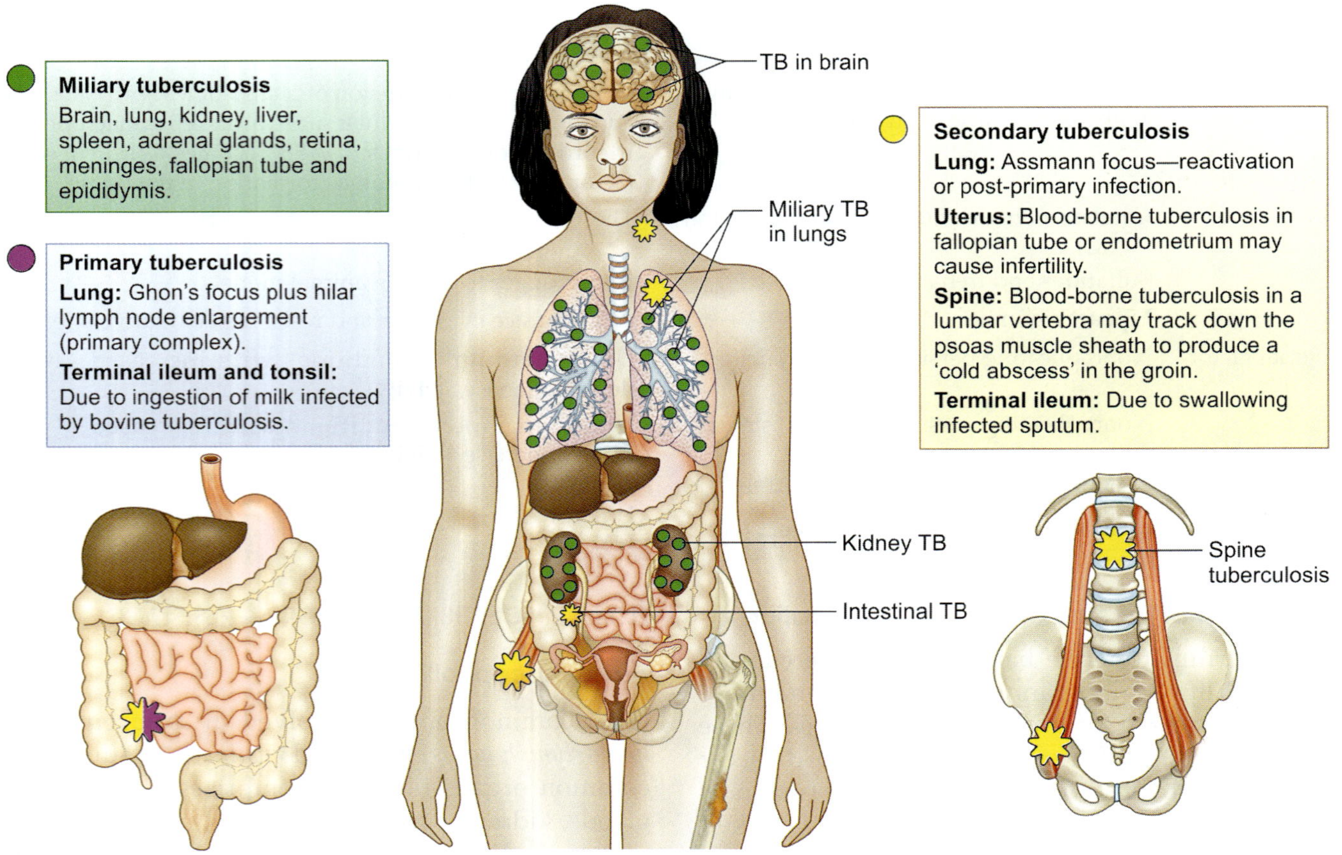

18 Section III: Systemic Pathology

Miliary tuberculosis
Brain, lung, kidney, liver, spleen, adrenal glands, retina, meninges, fallopian tube and epididymis.

Primary tuberculosis
Lung: Ghon's focus plus hilar lymph node enlargement (primary complex).
Terminal ileum and tonsil: Due to ingestion of milk infected by bovine tuberculosis.

Secondary tuberculosis
Lung: Assmann focus—reactivation or post-primary infection.
Uterus: Blood-borne tuberculosis in fallopian tube or endometrium may cause infertility.
Spine: Blood-borne tuberculosis in a lumbar vertebra may track down the psoas muscle sheath to produce a 'cold abscess' in the groin.
Terminal ileum: Due to swallowing infected sputum.

Fig. 18.13: Organs involved in primary, secondary and miliary tuberculosis. Primary tuberculosis produces a subpleural mid-zone lesion in lung. In secondary tuberculosis, lesion is located in apical region of lung. Miliary tuberculosis shows tubercles in various organs.

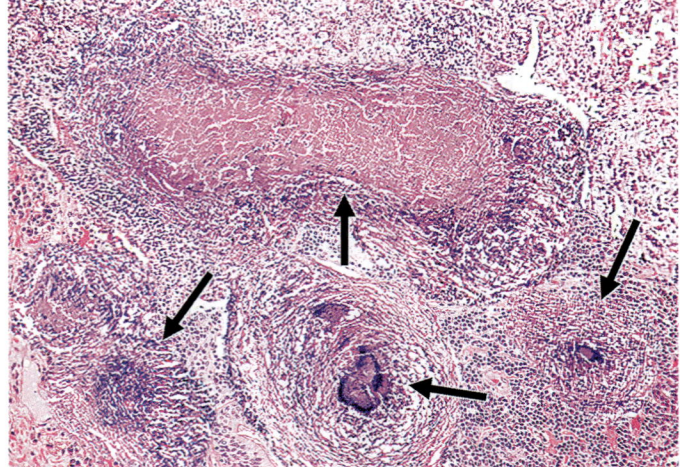

Fig. 18.14: Tuberculosis lung shows epithelioid granulomas, Langhan's giant cells and caseous necrosis (arrows) (400X).

PRIMARY TUBERCULOSIS (PRIMARY COMPLEX)

Primary tuberculosis is also known as *Ghon's focus* caused by tubercle bacillus. It is demonstrated in lung, tonsil, ileocecal region and skin. It usually does not progress to clinically evident disease. Granuloma formation in tuberculosis is known as *tubercle*.

Mode of Transmission

- *Lung:* Infection is most common contracted by droplet infection from open case of pulmonary tuberculosis with cavities lung. Initial exposure to tubercle bacilli produce clinically insignificant nonspecific alveolitis. Patient is asymptomatic at this stage.

- *Tonsils and intestine:* Ingestion of infected milk produces Ghon's focus in tonsils and ileocecal region. Tubercle bacilli reach the intestine either by ingestion of infected sputum or ingestion of unpasteurized milk and affects terminal ileum and most often ileocecal region. It produces circumferential ulcers perpendicular to long axis of small intestine. Fibrosis in this region is responsible for *stricture formation*.

  Light microscopy reveals caseating epithelioid cell granulomas with Langhan's giant cells. Crohn's disease also produces stricture formation, in which segmental involvement of intestine with skip areas is demonstrated, thickened wall in Crohn's disease resembles pipe-like and show irregular linear ulcers in the mucosa.

- *Skin inoculation:* Primary cutaneous inoculation with AFB occurs in person handling infected specimens.

Patient develops painless non-healing papule (primary focus) in 2 to 4 weeks after inoculation, which forms cold abscess resulting in discharging sinuses after several weeks.

- *Vertical transmission:* Placental transmission of tuberculosis from mother to fetus shows lesions in liver and portal lymph nodes seen at birth.

Primary Tuberculosis (Ghon's Complex in Lung)

Ghon's complex consists of Ghon's focus in organ (lung, tonsil, ileocecal region and skin), lymphatic channel and draining lymph nodes involvement.

Ghon's Focus in Lung

- *Location:* Primary tuberculosis produces a small mid-zone subpleural focus of consolidation near the interlobar fissure with involvement of lymphatic channels and hilar lymph nodes.
- *Dystrophic calcification:* The lesion most often heals by fibrosis and dystrophic calcification in 95% cases. The calcified lesion known as *Ranke's complex* is often visible on chest radiograph.
- *Lung lesions:* Approximately 5% of immunocompromised children develop symptomatic infection (cavities, bronchopneumonia, pleural effusion or miliary tuberculosis).
- *Nidus for secondary tuberculosis:* Because, acid-fast bacilli persisting in dormant form in old necrotic calcified lesions is still capable of initiating lesion, and thus a nidus for secondary tuberculosis.

Lymphatic Channels Involvement

Lymphatic channels are laden with Mycobacterium tubercle bacilli without producing lesion.

Draining Lymph Nodes

Lymph nodes draining Ghon's focus show caseous necrosis. Lymph nodes are enlarged in hilar region in pulmonary tuberculosis. Cervical lymphadenopathy occurs in tonsillar tuberculosis. Intestinal tuberculosis involves ileocecal lymph nodes. Cutaneous lymph nodes are involved in skin tuberculosis. Nodal lesions of tuberculosis take longer time to regress, hence remain a potential source of reactivation (Fig. 18.15).

SECONDARY TUBERCULOSIS

Secondary tuberculosis is also known as *post-primary pulmonary tuberculosis or reactivation disease*. Lung lesion in secondary tuberculosis is known as *Simon's focus*. It develops during adult life especially in immunocompromised persons. It occurs either due to inhalation of Mycobacterium tubercle bacilli or reactivation of dormant lymph node and old calcified healed parenchymal lesion. It causes extensive tissue destruction producing caseous necrosis by the action of cytokines synthesized by memory T cells.

Location

- Reactivation of tubercular focus produces cavitary lesions in the apical regions or posterior segments of the upper lobes either unilateral or bilateral. Hilar

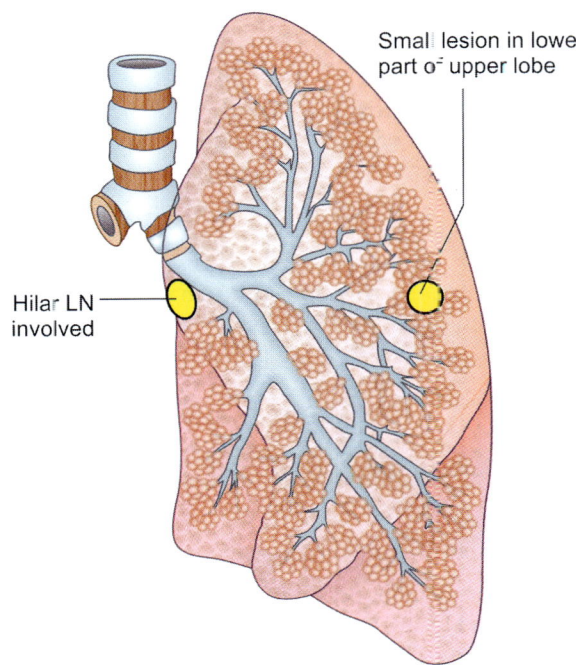
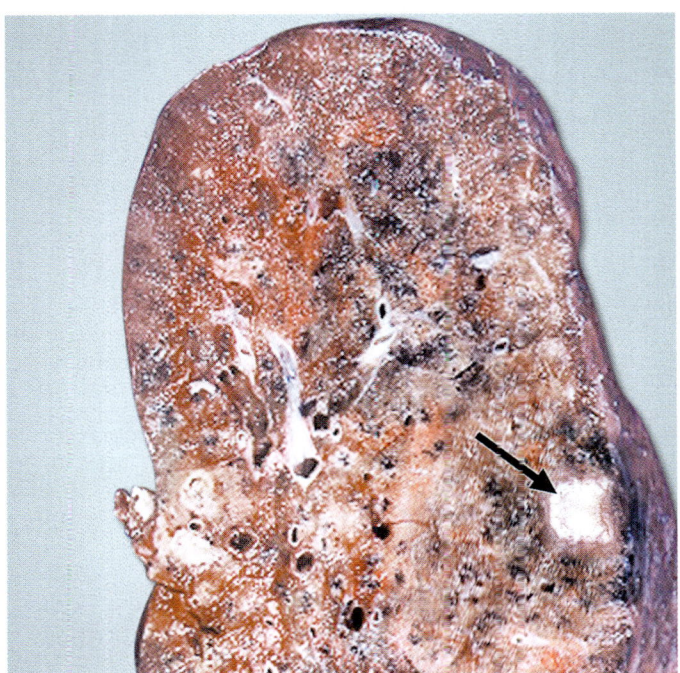

Fig. 18.15: Primary tuberculosis showing subpleural mid-zonal Ghon's focus and hilar lymph node enlargement. Gross examination of lung showing subpleural mid-zonal Ghon's focus (arrow).

lymph node involvement is also common. Apical lesions occur due to *high oxygen tension and paucity of macrophages due to decreased blood supply.*
- Growth of Mycobacterium tubercle bacilli is inhibited at pH <6.5. Large cavities are associated with hemoptysis.
- Aspergillus species may also grow in pre-existing cavities caused by tuberculosis. They proliferate to form fungus balls, which are also referred to as *aspergillomas or mycetomas.*

Morphology

Initially, the tubercular lesion is 2.00 cm, solid, gray-white to yellowish, with poorly defined margins and central areas of caseous necrosis. Some patients may develop tubercular cavities, which are *highly contagious.* The lesion frequently ruptures into the bronchi.

- *Tuberculous cavities:* Caseous material may liquefy resulting in cavitary lesions in secondary, but not primary tuberculosis. The cavity is filled with *yellow-grayish caseous material* more or less surrounded by fibrous tissue. AFB can easily be demonstrated in open cavities. Tubercular lesion may erode into airways. Patient may develop empyema and *hemoptysis, and sputum* becomes positive for AFB.
- *Lung consolidation:* Immunocompromised young children and elderly persons may develop tubercular bronchopneumonia or lobar pneumonia. These patients are very infectious. Patients have high fever and productive cough.
- *Tubercular pleuritis and effusion:* These usually develop soon after initial infection. Tuberculous focus located at the edge of the lung ruptures into the pleural space causing pleurisy and pleural effusion.

Patient with pleurisy presents with dyspnea and sharp chest pain that worsens with a deep breath (pleurisy). Tubercular pleurisy generally resolves without treatment. Morphology of lung in tuberculosis is shown in Fig. 18.16, differences between primary and secondary tuberculosis are shown in Table 18.7 and differences between tuberculosis and sarcoidosis are shown in Table 18.8.

Table 18.7: Differences between primary and secondary (post-primary) tuberculosis

Parameters	Primary tuberculosis	Secondary tuberculosis
Exposure to AFB	First time	Reactivation or reinfection
Age group	Children/younger age group	Any age group
Consolidation	Solitary lesion	Multifocal lesions (poorly defined)
Location	Mid-zone (Ghon's focus in subpleural lesion), other sites (tonsils, ileocecal region, skin)	*Upper lobes (apical region), Simon's focus in lungs:* 2 cm gray-white to yellowish well circumscribed consolidation in apical regions of one or both lungs
Lymphadenopathy	Common	Rare
Severity of lesion	Less severe, healing by fibrosis and dystrophic calcification	More severe progressing to cavitation, lobar pneumonia, extension in lumen of bronchi, trachea, and larynx with vocal cord involvement. Sputum positive for AFB in these persons
Pleural effusion	Common	Empyema
Cavitation	Rare	Common
Miliary tuberculosis	Yes (lung, liver, bone marrow, spleen, adrenal glands, meninges, kidneys, fallopian tubes, epididymis)	Yes (lung, liver, bone marrow, spleen, adrenal glands, meninges, kidneys, fallopian tubes, epididymis)

Table 18.8: Differences between tuberculosis and sarcoidosis

Characteristics	Tuberculosis	Sarcoidosis
Etiology	Mycobacterium tubercle bacilli	Unknown etiology
Granuloma	Caseating granuloma	Noncaseating granulomas
Cytoplasmic inclusions in giant cells	Absence of Schaumann bodies, asteroid bodies and birefringent crystals	Presence of Schaumann bodies, asteroid bodies and birefringent crystals
Steroid therapy	Worsens the disease	Improves the patient
Diagnosis	Acid-fast bacilli demonstration	Excluding causes of granulomatous lesions

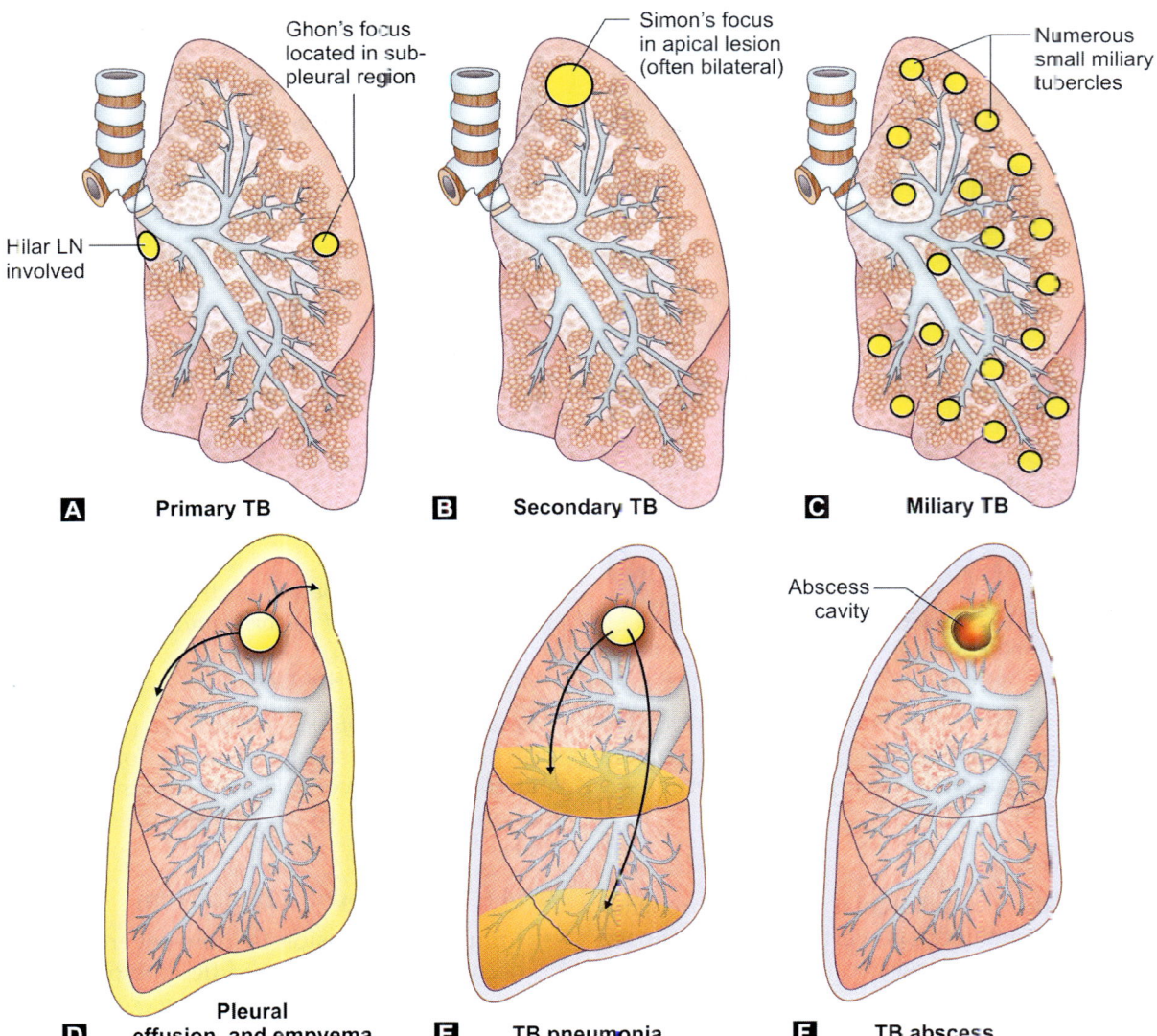

Fig. 18.16: Morphology of lung in tuberculosis. (A) Primary tuberculosis shows subpleural mid-zonal region and lesion hilar lymph node enlargement, (B) apical lesion is seen in secondary tuberculosis, (C) small miliary tubercles are demonstrated in lung, (D to F) pleural effusion, empyema, consolidation (pneumonia) and abscess are complications in tuberculosis.

Complications

These are lung fibrosis, lung cavitation, miliary tuberculosis and other lesions described as under.

Fibrosis

Healing of secondary pulmonary tuberculosis occurs by fibrosis in favorable conditions.

Lung Cavitation

In some patients, tubercular lesion continues to progress for months and years results in further pulmonary damage. It leads to cavity formation, lobar pneumonia, fibrocaseous tuberculosis and miliary tuberculosis (Fig. 18.17).

Airways Involvement

Endobronchial or endotracheal spread of tuberculosis may cause laryngeal tuberculosis with involvement of vocal cords. Erosion of airways reveals AFB in sputum.

Miliary Tuberculosis

Tuberculosis may disseminate via hematogenous route resulting in multiple small innumerable small *millet seed-like tubercular granulomas* known as *miliary tuberculosis*.

Mycobacterium tubercle bacilli may disseminate via systemic circulation to seed distant organs such as bone marrow, liver, spleen, adrenal glands, retina, meninges, kidneys, fallopian tubes, and epididymis. Mycobacterium tubercle bacilli reach the lungs via pulmonary arteries.

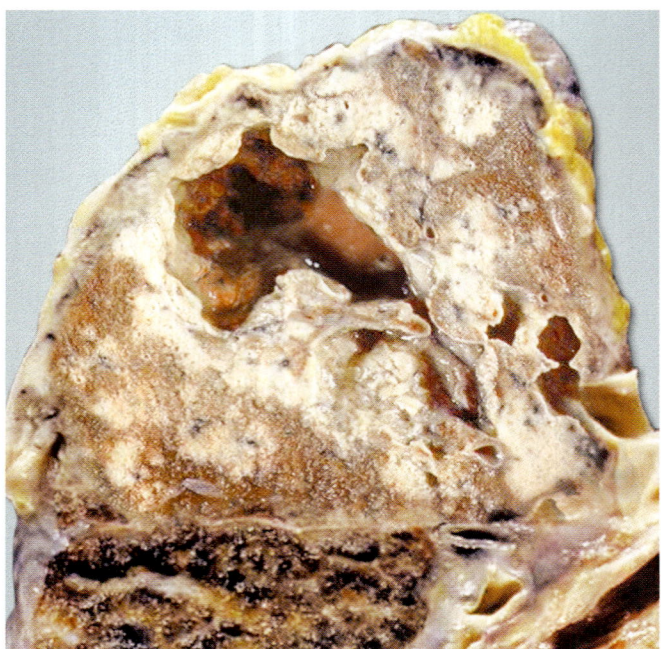

Fig. 18.17: Lung showing cavity in a case of secondary tuberculosis.

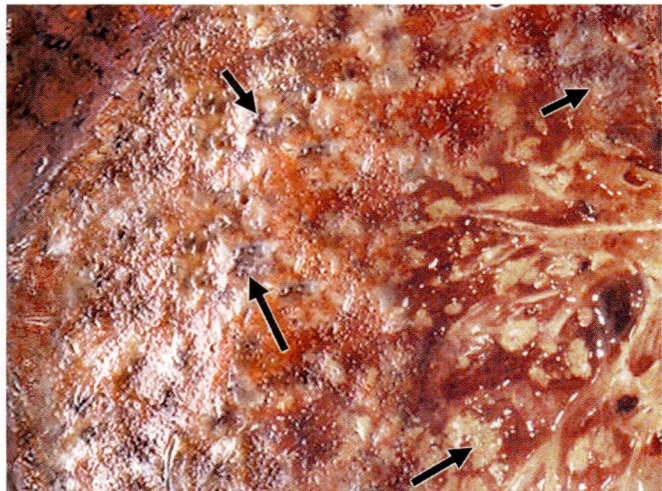

Fig. 18.18: Miliary tuberculosis. Lung showing millet-like seedlings of tuberculosis (arrows).

Chest radiograph reveals very small nodules throughout the lungs that look like millet seeds. It occurs shortly after primary infection in immunocompromised persons (Fig. 18.18).

Other Complications

Patient may also develop tubercular laryngitis, bronchopleural fistula, bronchiectasis, vertebral tuberculosis, i.e. Pott's disease, amyloidosis, scar carcinoma of lung and granulomatous hepatitis.

Clinical Features

Patient presents with cough, expectoration, hemoptysis (blood-tinged sputum), night sweats, evening rise of temperature, anorexia, loss of weight, lassitude, and chest pain.

Fever is probably caused by the absorption of toxic products from the site of infection and synthesis of cytokines (TNF-α and IL-1) by macrophages.

On clinical examination, percussion note is dull over the affected area. On auscultation, one can hear *bronchial breath sounds, crepitant crackles and wheeze*. Sound is heard through stethoscope, when the patient whispers, it is known as *whispered pectoriloquy*.

TUBERCULOSIS IN HIV CASES

Mycobacterium avium intracellulare (MAC) infection is a progressive systemic disorder, often occurring in patients who have AIDS. Approximately 33% of all patients develop overt disease due to depletion of CD4+ T cells.

CD4+ T Cells Count <200/cu mm

- Immunosuppression is more severe. Consolidation occurs in lower and middle lobe of lungs. Lymphadenopathy occurs in 50% cases. This pneumonia is characterized by an extensive infiltrate of macrophages.
- Lesions range from epithelioid granulomas containing a few organisms to loose aggregates of foamy macrophages.
- Clinical presentation associated with *Mycobacterium avium intracellulare* resembles those of tuberculosis.

CD4+ T Cells Count >300/cu mm

Immunosuppression is less severe. Apical regions of lungs are affected. Extrapulmonary organs involvement occurs in 15% cases.

CHRONIC OBSTRUCTIVE PULMONARY DISEASE

OVERVIEW

Chronic Obstructive Pulmonary Diseases

Chronic obstructive pulmonary diseases (COPD, or airway diseases) are characterized by chronic obstruction of airflow (partial or complete obstruction).

Examples of diffuse COPD are chronic bronchitis, bronchiectasis, emphysema, and bronchial asthma. On the other hand, restrictive pulmonary diseases caused by interstitial or infiltrative lesion of lung and skeletal abnormalities like kyphoscoliosis is characterized by decrease in both FEV1 and FVC resulting in a normal FEV1: FVC ratio.

- *Obstruction of air respiratory passages:* There is increased resistance to airflow from the trachea and large bronchi to the terminal and respiratory bronchioles due to increased luminal secretions (cystic fibrosis or smoking), thickening of airway wall (edema or hypertrophy), or loss of the elastic recoil of the airway (parenchymal destruction).
- *Respiratory volumes:* Patients show a marked decrease in the forced expiratory volume (FEV1) and an increased or normal forced vital capacity resulting in a decreased FEV1: FVC ratio.

Differences between obstructive and restrictive lung diseases are shown in Table 18.9.

Categories of COPD

- *Local obstructive pulmonary disease:* Obstruction due to tumor or inhalation of foreign body causes distal lung collapse. It may be complicated by lipid pneumonia or lobar pneumonia. Pulmonary function tests are normal.
- *Diffuse chronic obstructive pulmonary disease:* Obstruction occurs in bronchi and bronchioles. Pulmonary function tests are abnormal revealing obstructive pathology.

Chronic obstructive pulmonary disease is caused by chronic bronchitis, emphysema, bronchiectasis, and bronchial asthma. Spectrum of chronic obstructive pulmonary diseases is shown in Table 18.10.

CHRONIC BRONCHITIS

Chronic bronchitis is an inflammation of bronchi caused by prolonged inhalation of tobacco smoke (most common) and air pollutants.

It is characterized by *persistent cough* with *sputum production* for at least 3 months for 2 consecutive years in the absence of identifiable cause.

Table 18.9: Differences between obstructive and restrictive lung diseases

Characteristics	Obstructive lung diseases	Restrictive lung diseases
Definition	Increased resistance to airway owing to partial or complete obstruction at any level from trachea, large bronchi to terminal bronchioles	Reduced lung capacity (expansion) of lung either due to chest wall or skeletal abnormality or infiltrative parenchymal diseases
FEV1	Decreased	Decreased
FVC	Increased	Decreased
FEV1: FVC ratio	Decreased	Normal
Associated with	Chronic bronchitis, bronchiectasis, emphysema and bronchial asthma	Chest wall disorders (kyphoscoliosis) and acute respiratory distress syndrome

Table 18.10: Spectrum of chronic obstructive pulmonary diseases

Clinical entity	Anatomic site	Age group	Pathological changes	Etiology	Clinical manifestations
Chronic bronchitis	Bronchi	Adults	Mucous gland hyperplasia, hypersecretion and increased Reid index, bronchial wall thickened	Tobacco smoke, air pollutants causing impaired mucociliary apparatus	Cough, sputum production for at least 3 months for 2 consecutive years
Bronchiectasis	Bronchi	Adults	Abnormal permanent dilation of bronchi associated with scarring	Bronchial obstruction, persistent infections, α_1-antitrypsin (antiprotease) deficiency damaging bronchi	Cough, copious foul smelling sputum and fever
Bronchial asthma	Bronchi	Adults and children	Smooth muscle hyperplasia, increased mucus, inflammation, mucus plugs in bronchioles	Immunological mechanism (IgE-sensitized mast cells) and undefined etiology causing bronchospasm	Episodic wheezing, cough and dyspnea
Emphysema	Acinus	Adults	Enlargement of airspaces along with destruction of alveolar walls	Tobacco smoke and α_1-antitrypsin (antiprotease) deficiency	Severe progressive exertional dyspnea, crackles and wheezing
Bronchiolitis (small airways disease)	Bronchiole	Children	Decreased synthesis of surfactant, occluded bronchiole	Viral infections and pollutants	Cough and breathlessness

Productive cough occurs due to hyperplasia and hypersecretion of bronchial submucosal glands.

These patients are called blue bloaters due to decreased O_2 saturation from hypoxemia.

Pathogenesis

Chronic bronchitis is caused by tobacco smoke (90%), pollen grains, cotton, silica dust, air pollution and infectious agents such as bacteria and viruses.

> **Gross Morphology**
> Bronchi are hyperemic and swollen. Lumen shows mucinous or mucopurulent secretions.
>
> **Light Microscopy**
> Pathology includes hyperplasia of bronchial submucosal glands, leading to increased Reid index, ratio of the thickness of the gland layer to that of the bronchial wall.
> - *Bronchi:* Bronchi show chronic inflammation with lymphocytic infiltrate), squamous metaplasia, goblet cell hyperplasia, fibrosis and loss of cilia resulting in narrowing of bronchi.
> - *Bronchial submucosal glands:* These glands undergo hyperplasia and hypertrophy and secrete abundant mucus responsible for sputum overproduction and retention in air passages.
> - *Reid index:* It is increased in chronic bronchitis. Increase in size of the mucosal gland layer is assessed by Reid index.
>   Ratio of thickness of mucous gland layer to the thickness of bronchial wall (epithelium to cartilage) is called Reid index. Normal Reid index is 0.4 (Fig. 18.19).

Consequences

- *Chronic obstructive airway disease:* Patient develops wheezing due to narrowing of the terminal bronchioles by mucus plugs. Resistance to airflow in the small airways leads to severe ventilation-perfusion imbalance and decreased arterial oxygenation.
- *Cor pulmonale and heart failure:* Patient develops exertional dyspnea, cyanosis and cor pulmonale. The combination of cyanosis and edema secondary to cor pulmonale has led to the label *blue bloaters* (cyanosis) for such patients. Hypoxia induced erythropoiesis by erythropoietin increases hemoglobin.
- *Cyanosis:* Though the amount of hemoglobin is high, yet oxygenation is low, therefore, cyanosis is evident. Patient may develop respiratory acidosis.
- *Dysplastic change:* Respiratory epithelium may undergo dysplasia or metaplasia.

Chest Radiograph

It shows prominent vessels with an enlarged horizontally oriented heart and increased bronchial markings.

Clinical Features

Patients present with productive cough, dyspnea in late cases, cyanosis of skin and mucous membranes, hypoxemia due to decreased O_2 saturation, expiratory wheezing, sibilant rhonchi, and cor pulmonale.

Complications

Complications of chronic bronchitis include cor pulmonale, bronchiectasis, bronchopneumonia and bronchogenic carcinoma.

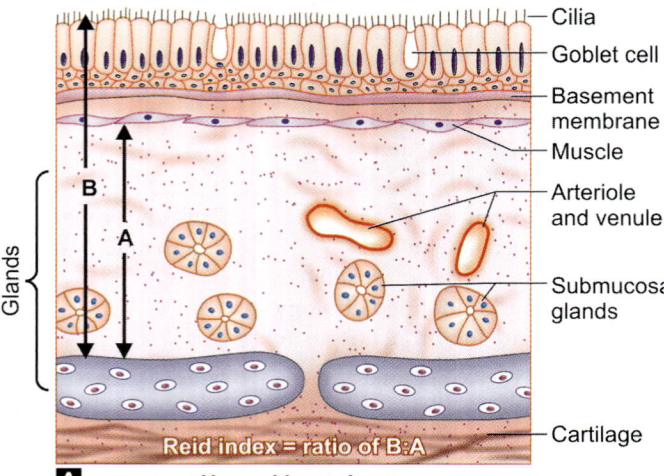 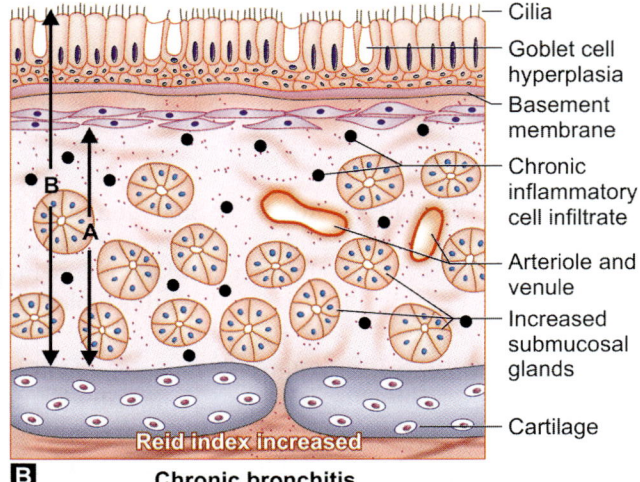

Fig. 18.19: Chronic bronchitis. The lumen of the bronchus shows marked thickening of the mucous glands approximately twice the normal. Squamous metaplasia of epithelium may also occur.

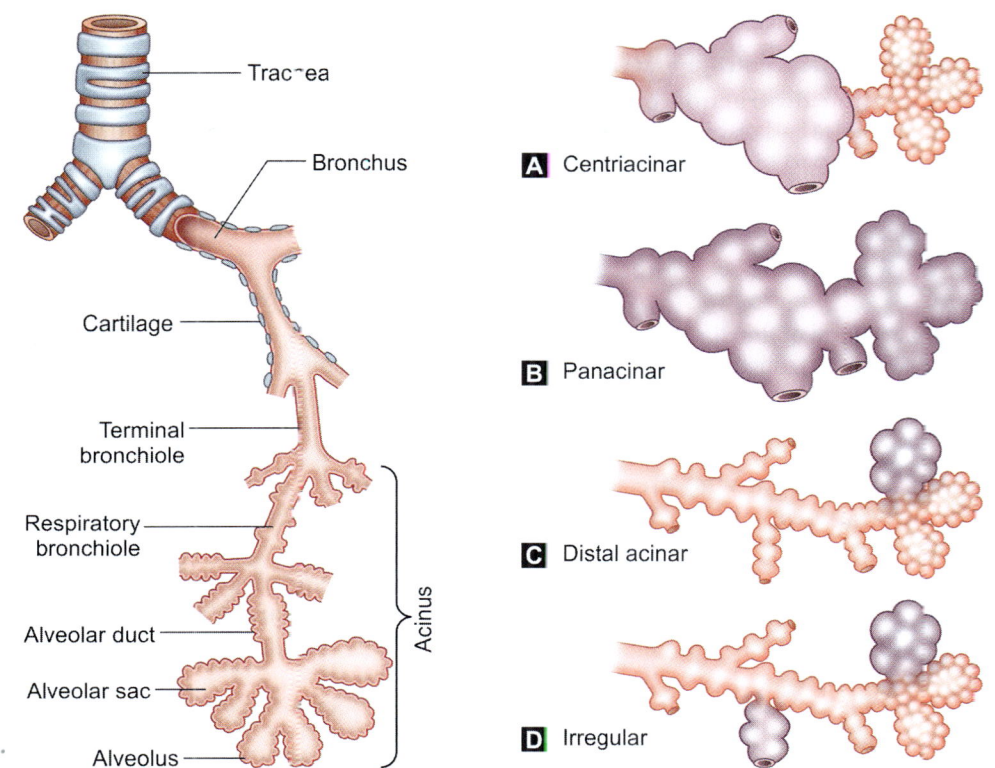

Fig. 18.20: Types of emphysema.

EMPHYSEMA

Emphysema is a chronic lung disease characterized by abnormal permanent enlargement of the airspaces, i.e. respiratory bronchioles, alveolar ducts and alveoli distal to the terminal bronchiole associated with destruction of the alveolar walls without obvious fibrosis and inflammation. Patients develop dyspnea due to impaired oxygen–carbon dioxide exchange.

Types of Emphysema

Centriacinar and panacinar emphysema are most common. Paraseptal emphysema may risk of spontaneous pneumothorax. Irregular emphysema may associated with fibrosis.

Centriacinar and panacinar emphysema cause clinically significant airflow obstruction (Fig. 18.20).

Etiopathogenesis

Emphysema occurs as a consequence of protease–antiprotease; and oxidant–antioxidant imbalances. Tobacco smoking is most common cause of emphysema followed by α_1-antitrypsin deficiency (Fig. 18.21).

α_1-antitrypsin (antiprotease)

- Normally, α_1-antitrypsin (antiprotease) inhibits elastases activity. The α_1-antitrypsin is a protein encoded on the proteinase inhibitor locus (Pi) on chromosome 14.

Normal amounts of α_1-antitrypsin are synthesized by liver in normal genotype persons (PiMM phenotype). It is a major inhibitor of a variety of proteases including elastase, and responsible for 90% of antiproteinase activity in the blood.

- Homozygous PiZZ genotype has decreased synthesis of α_1-antitrypsin. Serum electrophoresis reveals absence of α_1-globulin peak. Most patients with

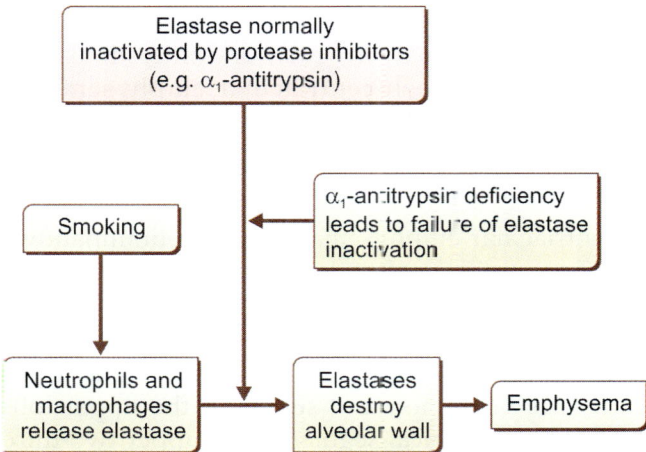

Fig. 18.21: Pathogenesis of emphysema. Under physiological state, proteases synthesized by inflammatory cells are inactivated by extracellular proteases especially α_1-antitrypsin. If proteases are not inactivated, these cause destruction of lung parenchyma. Imbalance of activity of proteases and protease inhibitors is responsible for emphysema.

Table 18.11: Differences between centriacinar emphysema and panacinar emphysema

Characteristics	Centriacinar (centrilobular) emphysema	Panacinar (panlobular) emphysema
Sites	Targeting destruction of the distal terminal bronchioles and respiratory bronchioles (proximal or central part of the acini of respiratory unit)	Targeting destruction of terminal bronchioles and the entire respiratory unit
Frequency	More common	Less common
Lobes affected	Apical segments of upper lobes	Basal parts of lower lobes
Risk factors	Tobacco smoking or coal workers pneumoconiosis	Patients with α_1-antitrypsin deficiency (an autosomal dominant disorder)
Mechanism	Destruction of the distal terminal bronchioles and respiratory bronchioles	Destruction of terminal bronchioles and the entire respiratory unit
Gross morphology	Not significant	Voluminous lungs overlapping heart and hiding it

clinically diagnosed emphysema who are younger than 40 years of age have α_1-antitrypsin (PiZZ phenotype) deficiency.
- Intravenous purified pooled human plasma is recommended to enhance α_1-antitrypsin levels in these patients.

Tobacco smoking: Tobacco smoke inhibits synthesis of α_1-antitrypsin, and increases the activity of the macrophage's elastases resulting in destruction of alveolar walls.

- *Free radicals:* Tobacco smoke comprises free radicals, which antagonize antioxidant mechanisms leading in tissue damage.
- *Reactive oxygen species:* Tobacco smoke contains abundant reactive oxygen species, i.e. free radicals, which deplete these antioxidant mechanisms, thereby inciting tissue damage.

Classification

Classification of emphysema includes centriacinar, panacinar, periacinar, irregular and interstitial types. Differences between centriacinar emphysema and panacinar emphysema are shown in Table 18.11.

CENTRIACINAR EMPHYSEMA

- Centriacinar emphysema occurs predominantly in heavy smokers, often in association with chronic bronchitis.
  It initially affects the respiratory bronchioles and then involve central portion of acinus. The lesions are more common and severe in the upper lobes especially in apical segments (i.e. upper two-thirds of the lungs).
- Tobacco smoke induces an inflammatory reaction as a result of synthesis of serine elastase and free radicals by neutrophils and macrophages.
- Elastases cause destruction of the walls of the respiratory unit, by promoting splitting peptide bond hydrolysis.
- Free radicals inactivate α_1-antitrypsin (antiprotease) and antioxidant glutathione leading to destruction of walls of respiratory unit.

PANACINAR EMPHYSEMA

- Panacinar emphysema initially affects peripheral structures of acinus (i.e. the alveolus and alveolar duct), and then extends to involve the respiratory bronchioles.
- It tends to occur more commonly in the lower zones as well as anterior margins of the lung.
- The acini are uniformly distended from the level of the respiratory bronchiole to the terminal bronchiole. It is usually more severe at the bases of the lung. It affects equally men and women.

DISTAL ACINAR (PARASEPTAL) EMPHYSEMA

- In distal (paraseptal) emphysema, the proximal portion of the acinus is normal, but the dilation predominantly involves distal part of the respiratory unit, i.e. alveoli and alveolar ducts in subpleural region and interlobar septa.
- The characteristic of morphological findings includes multiple, continuous enlarged airspaces measuring <0.5 cm to >2.0 cm in diameter sometimes forming cyst-like structures (bullae) in subpleural region due to focal destruction of alveolar walls with confluence of multiple alveoli.
- There is increased risk of spontaneous pneumothorax as a result of rupture of bullae.

IRREGULAR EMPHYSEMA

- The acinus is irregularly involved. It is almost invariably associated with scars from healed inflammatory process.

- It is most common form of emphysema. Patients are asymptomatic and clinically insignificant.

INTERSTITIAL EMPHYSEMA

Interstitial emphysema occurs as a result of entrance of air into the connective tissue of lung, subcutaneous tissue or mediastinum in settings of penetrating chest injury, chronic bronchitis, and obstruction to airflow. Children with whooping cough are prone to interstitial emphysema.

Differences between emphysema and chronic bronchitis are shown in Table 18.12.

Gross Morphology
- In centriacinar emphysema, upper two-thirds of the lungs are more severely affected than the lower lungs.
- In panacinar emphysema, lungs are pale and voluminous obscuring heart.

- Distal emphysema shows bullae in subpleural region due to focal destruction of alveolar walls with confluence of multiple alveoli leading to spontaneous pneumothorax (Figs 18.22 to 18.24).

Light Microscopy
- Alveolar walls show thinning and destruction. Adjacent alveoli become confluent creating large airspaces.
- There is loss of elastic tissue in the surrounding alveolar septate, number of alveolar capillaries is diminished.
- Ischemia is probably a factor in rupture of alveoli. Special stains show loss of elastic tissue (Fig. 18.25).

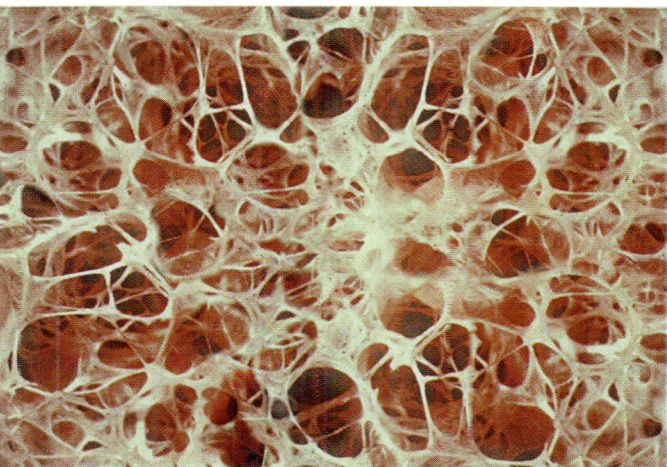

Fig. 18.23: Panacinar (panlobular) emphysematous lung. Cut surface shows dilated airspaces in all lung fields. Panacinar emphysema occurs with loss of all portions of the acinus from the respiratory bronchiole to the alveoli. This pattern is typical for α_1-antitrypsin deficiency. On the other hand, centrilobular (centriacinar) involves primarily the upper lobes and occurs with loss of the respiratory bronchioles in the proximal portion of the acinus, with sparing of distal alveoli especially in smokers.

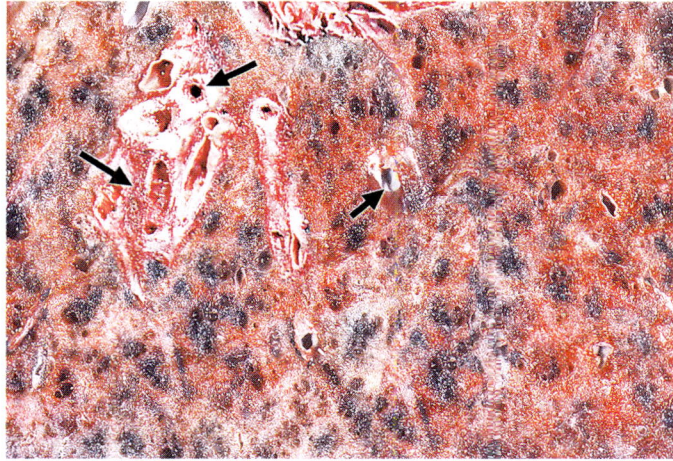

Fig. 18.22: Centriacinar emphysema. Central areas show marked emphysematous damage (arrows), surrounded by relatively spared alveolar spaces.

Table 18.12: Differences between emphysema and chronic bronchitis

Parameters	Emphysema	Bronchitis
Age group	50–75 years	15–40 years
Onset and severity of dyspnea	Early onset and severe	Late onset but mild
Cough	Late but scanty sputum	Early and copious sputum
Infections	Occasional	Common
Respiratory insufficiency	Terminal event	Repeated events
Cor pulmonale	Rare and in terminal stage	Common
Airway resistance	Normal or slightly increased	Increased
Elastic recoil	Low	Normal
Chest radiograph	Hyperinflation of lungs with small heart	Prominent blood vessels and large heart
Clinical appearance	Pink puffer	Blue bloater

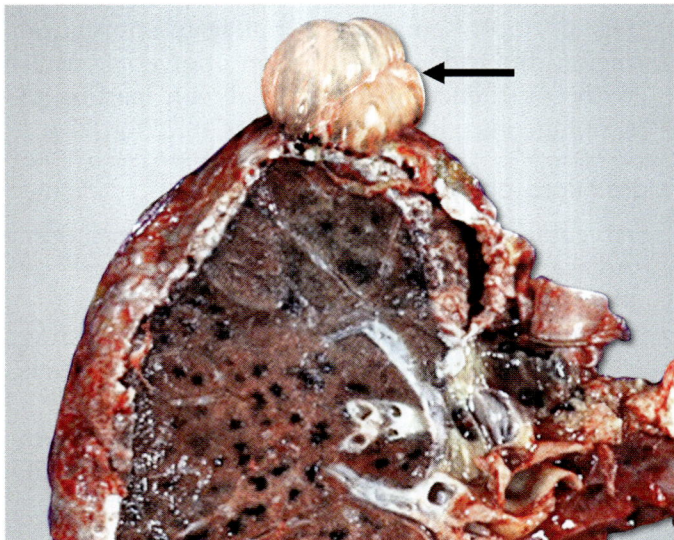

Fig. 18.24: Distal (paraseptal) emphysema. The characteristics of morphological findings include multiple, continuous enlarged airspaces measuring <0.5 cm to more than 2.0 cm in diameter sometimes forming cyst-like structures (bullae) in subpleural region due to focal destruction of alveolar walls with confluence of multiple alveoli. There is increased risk of spontaneous pneumothorax as a result of rupture of bullae. Large bullous is seen on subpleural region (arrow).

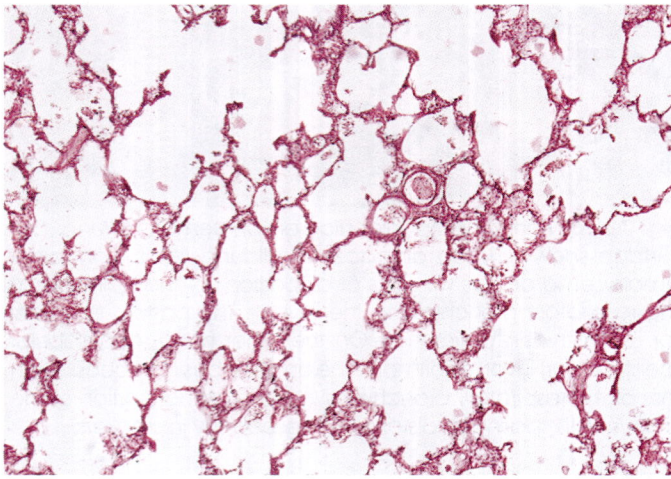

Fig. 18.25: Pulmonary emphysema. There is marked enlargement of airspaces with thinning and destruction of alveolar septa. Tobacco smoking and a_1-antitrypsin antiprotease are important predisposing risk factors (400X).

Clinical Features

The classic presentation of emphysema (centriacinar or panacinar) is *pink puffer* who develops tachypnea, severe progressive exertional dyspnea and prolonged forced expiration, cough, crackles and wheezing on inspiration and barrel-shaped chest. Breath sounds are diminished due to hyperinflation.

Chest expansion is decreased. Tactile fremitus is decreased. Centriacinar emphysema frequently coexists with chronic bronchitis. Cor pulmonale is uncommon. Pulmonary function tests reveal reduction of ratio of FEV1 to FCV.

Chest Radiograph

It shows hyperlucent lung fields, increased antero-posterior diameter producing barrel shaped chest, vertically oriented heart and depressed diaphragms due to hyperinflated lungs.

Complications

The complications of emphysema are interstitial emphysema, pneumothorax, cor pulmonale, respiratory acidosis, and coma. Expansion of emphysema into the interstitial tissues of the chest wall occurs as a results of acute overinflation of the lungs with rupture and perforation in multiple airspaces in interstitial fibrous septa.

Functional Effects of Emphysema

It is categorized into two groups depending on tolerance to hypoxia or not.

- *Blue bloaters tolerate hypoxia.* Patient develops severe hypoxemia, hypercapnea, right ventricular hypertrophy, cor pulmonale with peripheral edema, and secondary polycythemia.
- *Pink puffers do not tolerate hypoxia.* Patient develops severe dyspnea, hyperventilation, and relatively normal blood gases.

BRONCHIECTASIS

Bronchiectasis is abnormal permanent (irreversible) dilation of bronchi and bronchioles caused by chronic necrotizing infections resulting in destruction of cartilage and elastic tissue. The bronchi and bronchioles are filled with mucus and neutrophils. Cough and expectoration of copious amounts of purulent sputum are characteristic findings. Obstruction and infection result in bronchiectasis. It more frequently affects young persons than adults.

SALIENT FEATURES

- Normally, airways cannot be traced beyond 2–3 cm from pleural surface. Bronchiectasis is more common in vertical airways especially distal bronchi or bronchioles of lower lobes extending up to pleural surface. Upper lobes are affected in pulmonary tuberculosis.
- These airways undergo four times dilation than normal size, and lumen is filled with suppurative exudates.

- The dilation is permanent and should not be confused with a transient mild cylindrical dilatation, which occurs in viral or bacterial pneumonia or collapsed lung; in which the changes become reversible within six weeks.
- Aspergillus species may also grow in pre-existing cavities caused by bronchiectasis. They proliferate to form fungus balls, which are also referred to as *aspergillomas* or *mycetomas*.

PATHOGENESIS

Obstruction and chronic persistent infection cause damage to bronchial walls leading to weakening and permanent dilation of bronchial tree. Obstructive secretions and inflammations are present throughout the wall of bronchi. Congenital causes usually affect both lungs. These patients are asymptomatic and superadded infection appear late in life.

Congenital Causes

- *Kartagener's syndrome:* It is autosomal recessive disorder characterized by sinusitis, bronchiectasis and situs inversus, sometimes with male sterility and hearing loss. Structural defect occurs in the dynein arms known as *primary ciliary dyskinesis*. Impaired ciliary activity predisposes to infection in the sinuses and bronchi and results in bronchiectasis. Male infertility is an important manifestation of ciliary dyskinesia.
- *Cystic fibrosis:* Cystic fibrosis is autosomal recessive disorder of exocrine glands characterized by synthesis of thick secretions in their ducts. It is also known as *mucoviscidosis or fibrocystic disease* of the pancreas.

    Normally, transmembrane conductance regulator (CFTr) gene located on long arm of chromosome 7 codes for a membrane protein that participates in the movement of chloride and other ions across membranes. Mutation of CFTr gene causes malfunction of exocrine glands and results in increased viscosity of mucus and increased chloride concentration in sweat and tears.
- *Chronic granulomatous disease of childhood.* It is X-linked disorder with defect in NADPH oxidase activity in neutrophils. It leads to failure of synthesis of superoxide anion and hydrogen peroxide during phagocytosis. Disease is characterized by phagocytic cells that ingest but unable to kill certain microorganisms.
- α_1-*antitrypsin deficiency:* α_1-antitrypsin synthesized by liver in normal genotype persons (PiMM phenotype) is a major inhibitor of a variety of proteases, including elastase. α_1-antitrypsin is a protein encoded on the proteinase inhibitor locus (Pi) on chromosome 14. Its deficiency may be associated with bronchiectasis.
- *Williams-Campbell syndrome:* It is characterized by bronchial cartilage deficiency leading to bronchiectasis.

Acquired Causes

Bronchial obstruction (partial or complete) and post-inflammation play an important role in pathogenesis of bronchiectasis.

- *Bronchial obstruction:* It occurs due to neoplasm, foreign body, aspiration and compression due to lymph node.
- *Post-inflammation (non-obstruction):* Bronchiectasis results from repeated episodes of pneumonia especially during first two decades of life.

    Patient with immunodeficiency states may develope *superadded infection* due to *Haemophilus influenzae* (most common), measles, whooping cough, tuberculosis and allergic bronchopulmonary aspergillosis. Traction bronchiectasis occurs from pulmonary fibrosis.

> **Gross Morphology**
> - Bronchiectasis most commonly affects pulmonary lower lobes.
> - Bronchi and bronchioles reveal destruction of wall with replacement by scar tissue.
> - Dilated airways may take various shapes, i.e. cylindrical, fusiform, varicose (numerous constriction and dilation) and saccular (bead-like bulge on one side).
> - Dilated airways are easily visible up to <3 mm from the pleural surface. Normally, bronchi are traceable up to 2–3 cm from the pleural surface.
> - Bronchi and bronchioles are dilated and filled with pus, which impairs normal inflow of O_2 in lungs and outflow of CO_2 (Fig. 18.26).

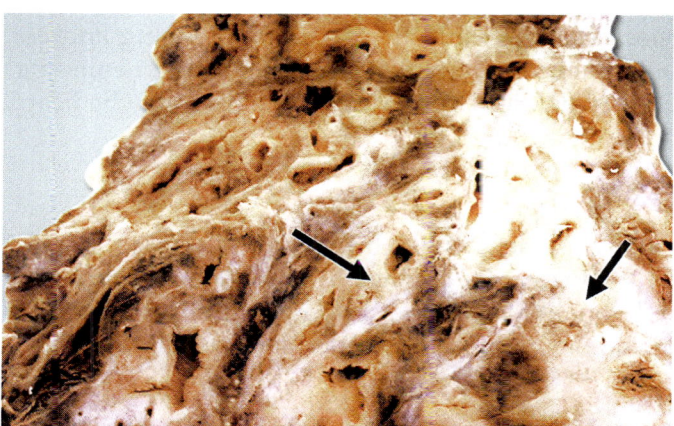

Fig. 18.26: Bronchiectasis shows abnormal permanent dilatation of bronchi of variable sizes filled with pus (arrows).

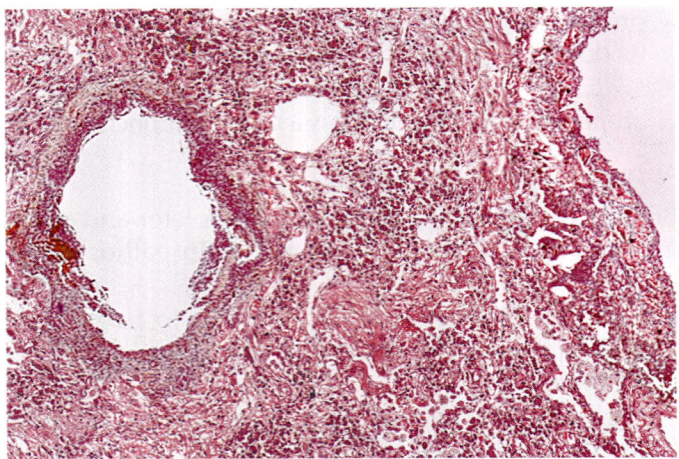

Fig. 18.27: Bronchiectasis. Bronchial wall is infiltrated by acute and chronic inflammatory cells (400X).

Light Microscopy

- *Intense inflammation:* The wall of bronchi and bronchioles are infiltrated by acute and chronic inflammatory cells, composed of neutrophils, lymphocytes, plasma cells and macrophages. Mature lymphoid follicles may also be present.
- *Desquamation of lining epithelium:* Mucosa of airways shows extensive areas of necrotizing ulceration. Remaining lining epithelium may show squamous metaplasia.
- *Granulation tissue:* In more advanced cases, there is presence of granulation tissue and fragmentation of cartilage. Mucous glands persist longer than other structures.
- *Fibrosis:* Fibrosis occurs in bronchi and bronchioles walls. Peribronchial fibrosis is also evident (Fig. 18.27).

CLINICAL FEATURES

Patient presents with constant cough, foul smelling sputum, hemoptysis (in some cases), wheezing, shortness of breath, fever, digital clubbing and cor pulmonale. Some patients may develop pneumonia. On auscultation, moist crackling noises may be heard in the chest.

COMPLICATIONS

Patient presents with bronchiectasis may develop lung abscess, pneumonia, bronchopleural fistula, cor pulmonale, necrotising brain abscess, lung abscess, meningitis, amyloidosis and squamous cell carcinoma.

DIAGNOSIS

A complete medical history and physical examination by a physician is necessary.

- *Imaging techniques:* Chest X-ray, bronchography, and CT may reveal evidence of bronchiectasis.
- *Sputum examination:* Sputum will need to be collected and cultured (grown in a laboratory dish), in order to examine it microscopically for the specific type of organism responsible for infection.
- *Pulmonary function tests:* These are performed to determine the presence and severity of abnormal airflow out of the lungs.
- *Diagnostic techniques:* A careful search for other underlying diseases is important, looking in particular for ciliary abnormalities, cystic fibrosis, or immunoglobulin deficiencies.

BRONCHIAL ASTHMA

Bronchial asthma results from bronchospasm of bronchi and terminal bronchioles. Airways are obstructed due to increased mucus secretion and mucosal edema. It is mediated by type 1 hypersensitivity reaction or undefined causes. Patient presents with episodic reversible wheezing, cough, dyspnea and respiratory alkalosis.

ETIOLOGY

It occurs due to air-pollutants, viral induced respiratory infections (rhinovirus, parainfluenza virus, and respiratory syncytial virus), aspirin sensitivity, stress, cigarette smoke and fungus spores of *Aspergillus flavus*.

MECHANISM

Bronchial asthma occurs by two mechanisms: Extrinsic (immune) or intrinsic (nonimmune) asthma. Extrinsic asthma is typically a childhood disease, whereas intrinsic asthma usually begins in adults.

- *Extrinsic (immune) asthma:* It is mediated by type 1 hypersensitivity reaction involving IgE bound to mast cells. It occurs due to exposure to allergens. Disease starts in childhood. There is family history of allergy.
- *Intrinsic (nonimmune) asthma:* Bronchial asthma is associated with chronic bronchitis, exercise or cold induced asthma. Disease most often begins in adult life. There is no family history of allergy.

AGE GROUP

It is most common chronic respiratory disease in children (<10 years) in 50% cases than adults. Adult males and females are equally affected.

PATHOLOGICAL CHANGES

These include bronchial smooth muscle hypertrophy, hyperplasia of bronchial submucosal glands and goblet cells, airways plugged by viscid mucus containing, *Curschmann spirals*, eosinophils, and *Charcot-Leyden crystals in sputum*.

PATHOGENESIS

There are early and late phase reactions in pathogenesis of bronchial asthma. Late phase reactions occur 4–8 hours after a symptom-free period.

Early Phase Reactions

- *First exposure to allergen:* Allergen may enter through nose by inhalation (most common) and ingestion (mouth). It is absorbed in the tissues and triggers immune response. T helper cells release interleukins (IL-4 and IL-5). IL-4 stimulates B cells to synthesize IgE, which binds to the mast cells on mucosal surfaces.
- *Second exposure to allergen:* Allergen re-enters the nose and mouth. Inhaled antigens cross-link IgE antibodies on mast cells on mucosal surfaces. It triggers mast cells to release histamine and leukotrienes. These chemical mediators cause bronchospasm, mucus secretion, smooth muscle contraction, deposition of plasma proteins in the bronchial submucosa due to increased vascular permeability, and influx of leukocytes (LTB4).

Late Phase Reactions

- *Chemokine (eotaxin) synthesis:* Eotaxin synthesized by leukocytes participates in emigration of eosinophils in the tissues.
- *Leukotrienes synthesis:* Synthesis of leukotrienes (LTC4, LTD4, and LTE4) by mast cells cause prolonged bronchoconstriction. Acetylcholine synthesis further causes bronchospasm (Fig. 18.28).

Light Microscopy

- *Bronchi/bronchiole changes:* These include bronchial smooth muscle hypertrophy, hyperplasia of goblet cells, thickening and hyalinization of basement membranes.
- *Bronchial wall:* It is infiltrated by eosinophils, mast cells, macrophages and lymphocytes.
- *Bronchial lumen:* Bronchial mucosa shows edema, focal ulceration. Bronchial lumen is occluded with mucus plugs containing whorl-like accumulations of epithelial cells.
- *Curschmann spirals* and crystalloids of eosinophils derived *major basic protein and cationic proteins* coalesce to form *Charcot-Leyden crystals* demonstrated in the sputum of bronchial asthma patients.

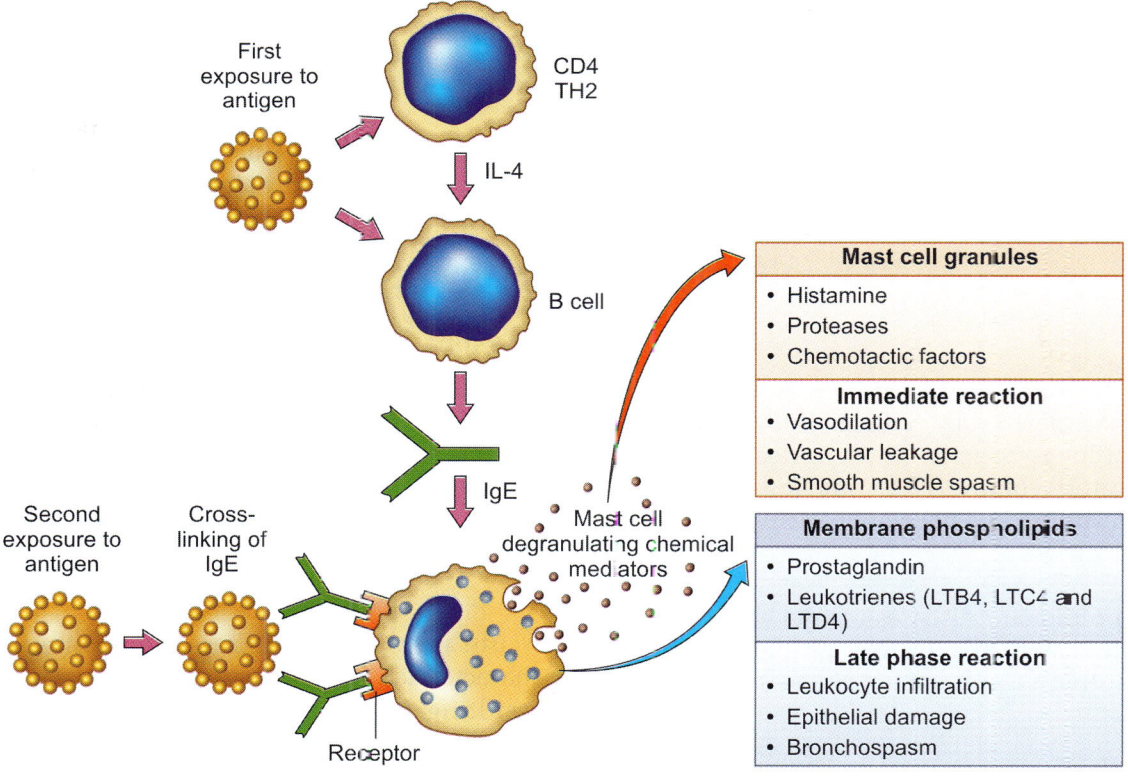

Fig. 18.28: Type 1 hypersensitivity reaction. The antigen stimulates B cells to produce IgE. IgE binds to mast cells or basophils *via* its Fc fragment, causing them to be *sensitized*. Further exposure to antigen causes cross-linking of bound IgE on mast cells, resulting in degranulation.

CLINICAL FEATURES

Breathlessness

Bronchial asthma attack may last for hours or even days. Due to narrowing of airways, patient presents with sudden dyspnea, episodic expiratory wheezing, i.e. inspiratory in severe cases, tightness in the chest, nocturnal coughing, and tachypnea with use of accessory muscles for breathing.

Prolonged Coughing

After the bronchial asthmatic attack is over, there is prolonged coughing up of tenacious secretions. Anteroposterior diameter of chest is increased due to air trapping and increase in residual volume.

Initially, patient develops respiratory alkalosis. If bronchospasm is not relieved, patient may develop respiratory acidosis. Such patients need tracheal intubation and mechanical ventilation.

COMPLICATIONS

Patient may develop pneumothorax, pneumomediastinum, status asthmaticus and fatal outcome. When severe acute asthma is unresponsive to therapy, it is referred to as status asthmaticus.

Light microscopy of lung in status asthmaticus often shows a bronchus containing a luminal mucous plug, submucosal gland hyperplasia, smooth muscle hyperplasia, basement membrane thickening, and increased numbers of eosinophils (Table 18.13).

Table 18.13: Comparison of extrinsic and intrinsic asthma

Characteristics	Extrinsic asthma	Intrinsic asthma
Definition	It is caused by type 1 hypersensitivity reaction induced by exposure to an extrinsic antigen	It is caused by diverse non-immune mechanisms as a result of intrinsic stimuli
Age of clinical presentation	Childhood	Adult
Family history	Present	Absent
Preceding allergic reactions	It is present in the form of rhinitis, urticaria, and eczema	Absent
Drug hypersensitivity	Absent	Present
Serum IgE level	Increased	Normal
Skin test	Positive skin test	Negative skin test
Emphysema	Unusual	Common
Associated chronic bronchitis	Absent	Present
Examples	Atopic/allergic asthma Occupational asthma Allergic bronchopulmonary aspergillosis	Aspirin ingestion, pulmonary infection especially viral, cold, inhaled irritants, stress, exercise

RESTRICTIVE PULMONARY DISEASES

OVERVIEW

Restrictive pulmonary diseases comprise group of disorders characterized by reduced lung expansion as well as total lung capacity. There is decrease in both forced expiratory volume (FEV1) and forced vital capacity (FVC) resulting in a normal FEV1:FVC ratio.

Etiology

Restrictive pulmonary diseases restrict expansion and often interfere with respiratory gaseous exchange. Causes of restrictive pulmonary diseases are shown in Table 18.14.

Pathogenesis

Gas exchange barrier consists of alveolar epithelial cells, capillary endothelial cells, basement membrane and interstitial tissue. Initial injury occurs to endothelial and epithelial cells. It is followed by interstitial fibrosis leading to dyspnea. Damage to epithelium and alveolar capillaries leads to impaired ventilation-perfusion leading to hypoxia, cyanosis and cor pulmonale.

ACUTE RESTRICTIVE PULMONARY DISEASES

ACUTE RESPIRATORY DISTRESS SYNDROME IN ADULTS

Acute respiratory distress syndrome in adults is characterized by pulmonary edema (noncardiogenic) resulting from *acute alveolar-capillary damage*. It is also known as *shock lung*. It can quickly lead to acute respiratory failure with fatal outcome within 48 hours in 50–70% cases. *Highest rates of mortality are aspiration of gastric contents, bacteremia and pneumonia.*

Lung

Table 18.14: Causes of restrictive pulmonary diseases

Etiology	Disorders
Chest wall abnormality	Deformities (kyphoscoliosis)
	Neuromuscular disorder
Acute primary lung disease	Acute respiratory distress syndrome
Chronic primary lung disease	*Occupational lung diseases:* Asbestosis, silicosis, coal worker's pneumoconiosis
	Interstitial lung disease (interstitial pneumonia), idiopathic pulmonary fibrosis
	Immune diseases: Sarcoidosis, systemic lupus erythematosus, rheumatoid arthritis, Wegener's granulomatosis and Goodpasture syndrome
	Physical injury: Radiation induced injury
	Drugs: Chemotherapeutic agents, methotrexate

- Normally, surfactant reduces tension in alveoli and keeps alveoli open. Decrease in synthesis of surfactant by type 2 pneumocytes causes acute respiratory distress syndrome.
- Patient develops a clinical syndrome characterized by refractory hypoxemia not responsive to oxygen therapy, reduction in lung compliance, normal oncotic pressure, normal capillary pulmonary wedge pressure and chest radiograph suggestive of bilateral pulmonary edema.

Etiopathogenesis

It may follow direct or indirect lung injury. Sepsis is most common cause of acute respiratory distress syndrome (ARDS). Other causes include pulmonary contusions, severe trauma and shock. *Etiology of acute respiratory distress syndrome* is shown in Table 18.15.

- *Direct lung injury:* Hantavirus, oxygen toxicity, inhalation of chemical irritants (chlorine), smoke inhalation, pneumonia, aspiration of gastric contents and post-lung transplant cause acute alveolar-capillary damage (>30% of cases). Coronavirus destroys type 2 pneumocytes and causes diffuse alveolar damage.
- *Indirect lung injury:* Various systemic disorders cause indirect alveolar-capillary damage. Examples are septicemia (40%), severe trauma with shock (20%), acute hemorrhagic pancreatitis, therapeutic drug (bleomycin), overdose with street drug (heroin), multiple blood transfusions, cardiopulmonary bypass, disseminated intravascular coagulation, fat embolism, complicated abdominal surgery, and radiation injury.

Table 18.15: Etiology of acute respiratory distress syndrome

Lung damage	Disorders
Primary lung damage	Aspiration of gastric contents (35%)
	Bacterial and viral pneumonias (12%)
	Inhalation of smoke and chlorine
	Oxygen toxicity
	Radiation-induced injury
	Drug-induced lung injury (salicylates, bleomycin)
	Paraquat poison
Secondary lung damage	Disseminated intravascular coagulation (22%)
	Traumatic shock (5%)
	Multiple blood transfusions (5%)
	Extensive burns
	Septicemia (4%)
	Acute pancreatitis
Highest prevalence of acute respiratory distress syndrome in decreasing frequency occurs due to aspiration of gastric contents, disseminated intravascular coagulation, pneumonias, traumatic injury, and multiple blood transfusions.	
Highest rates of mortality are aspiration of gastric contents, bacteremia and pneumonia	

Pathogenesis

Following alveolar-capillary damage, alveolar macrophages synthesize IL-1, IL8, TNF-α and macrophage inhibiting factor (MIF). Chemical mediators IL-1, IL8, and TNF-α cause sequestration of neutrophils into the alveolar spaces, and aggregation of platelets.

Activation of the coagulation cascade is suggested by the presence of microemboli containing aggregate of platelets in alveolar capillaries. Pathogenesis of acute respiratory distress syndrome is shown in Fig. 18.29.

Exudative phase: Lung becomes dark, red and firm within 7 days. Histamine released by platelets increases the pulmonary capillary permeability resulting in pulmonary edema.

Neutrophils synthesize chemical mediators like *leukotrienes, oxidants, proteases and platelet-activating factor,* resulting in damage to type 1 and 2 pneumocytes.

Damage to type 2 pneumocytes leads to inactivation of surfactant (lecithin-rich surface-active lipid) and atelectasis (collapse of alveoli).

- It leads to pulmonary edema and fibrinous exudation. Fibrinous exudates form hyaline membranes lining alveoli, which appear bright, pink in hematoxylin and eosin stained sections.
- *Macrophage inhibitory factor* (MIF) released into the local milieu sustains the ongoing pro-inflammatory response. These pathological changes result in impairment of respiratory gas exchange with consequent severe hypoxia.

Proliferative phase: This phase begins about one week after the initial injury. It is marked by the proliferation of macrophage within alveolar walls. Alveolar macrophages digest the remnant of hyaline membranes and other cellular debris. TGF-β and PDGF synthesized by macrophages cause proliferation of fibroblasts leading to mild fibrosis. This mild fibrosis resolves in mild cases.

Fibrotic phase: In severe cases, it may progress to restructuring of the pulmonary parenchyma and cyst formation. Alveolar walls are thickened. Progressive fibrosis may produce honeycomb appearance in rare cases.

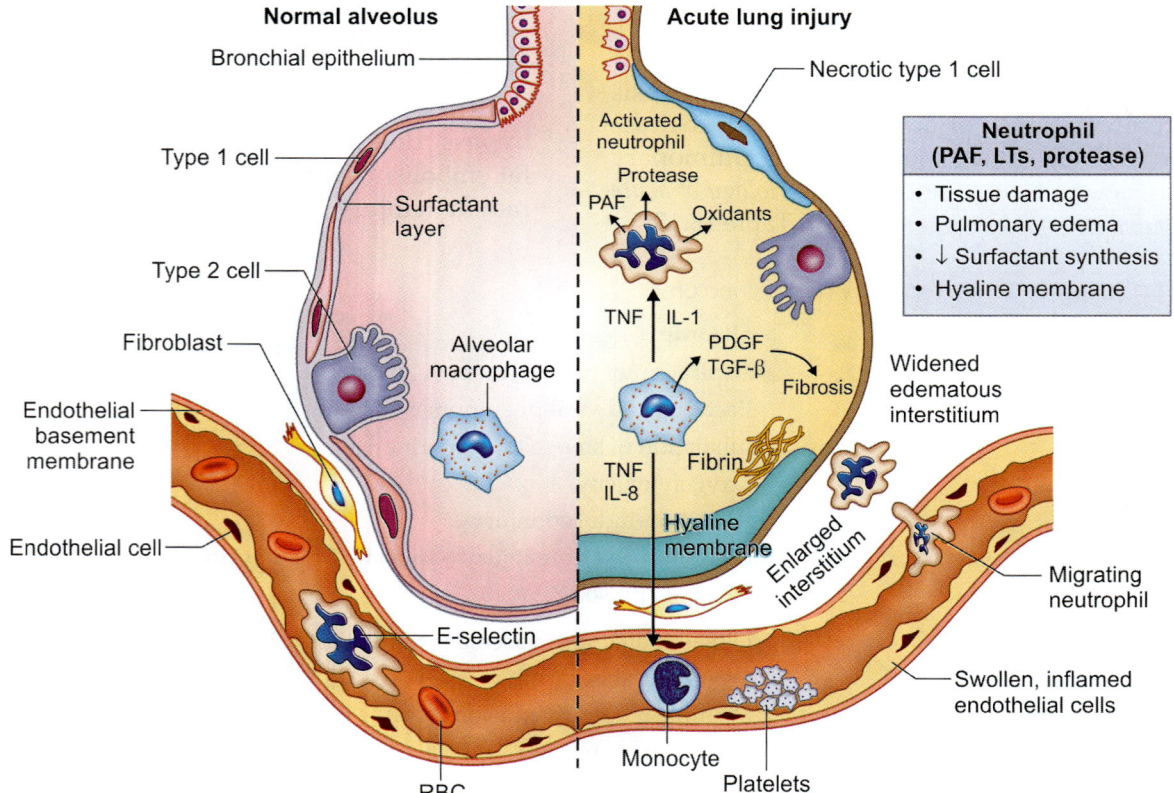

Fig. 18.29: Pathogenesis of acute respiratory distress syndrome. Normal alveolus is seen on left half of figure. Synthesis of IL-8 and TNF by macrophages and neutrophils occurs in the alveoli. Leukotrienes, oxidants, proteases, and platelet-activating factor (PAF) synthesized by neutrophils produce local tissue damage, pulmonary edema, surfactant inactivation, and hyaline membrane formation. Fibrogenic factors (PDGF and TGF-β) synthesized by macrophages stimulate fibroblast growth and collagen deposition associated with the healing phase of injury.

Gross Morphology

Lungs are heavy, diffusely firm, solid, dark red and rubbery due to diffuse alveolar damage.

Light Microscopy

ARDS in adults comprises two stages, i.e. acute exudative stage and proliferative stage.

- *Acute exudative stage:* Lung shows congestion of capillaries, interstitial edema, and fibrinous exudates in alveoli. The alveolar walls are lined with hyaline membranes.
- *Proliferative stage (fibrosis):* Fibrinous exudates undergo organization leading to alveolar fibrosis and thickening of the alveolar septa. There may be superimposed bronchopneumonia in fatal cases. Light microscopy of diffuse alveolar damage is shown in Fig. 18.30.

Chest Radiograph

Initially it shows bilateral interstitial infiltrates followed by extensive consolidation in 80%.

Clinical Features

- *Respiratory system:* Patient has rapid, shallow breathing, dyspnea, intercostal and suprasternal retraction crackles, rhonchi, respiratory and metabolic acidosis, and sometimes respiratory failure. Pulmonary edema in acute respiratory distress syndrome does not resolve, however, it resolves in cases of congestive heart failure.
- *Cardiovascular system:* Patient develops arterial hypoxemia refractory to oxygen therapy, cyanosis, tachycardia, and hypotension.

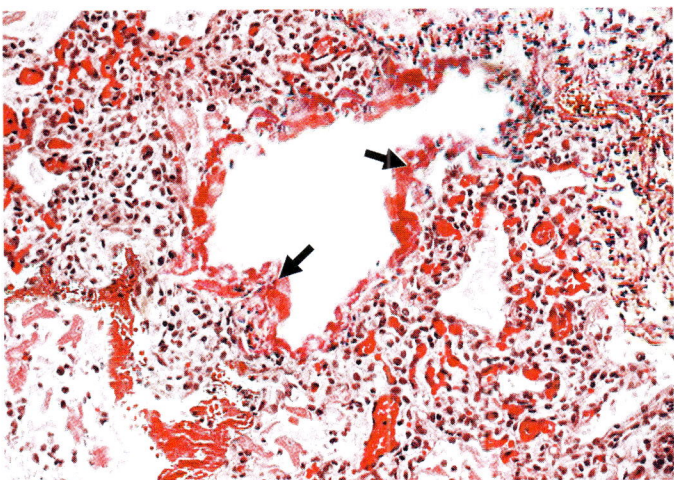

Fig. 18.30: Diffuse alveolar damage. Acute exudative phase showing protein-rich hyaline membranes, interstitial edema and inflammation (arrows).

- *Central nervous system:* Patient develops restlessness, apprehension, mental sluggishness, and motor dysfunction.
- *Urinary system:* Patient has decreased urinary output.

Prognosis

Patient with acute respiratory distress syndrome is frequently fatal (60%). Approximately 30–40% of cases with good intensive care may survive. High concentration of oxygen therapy may further cause damage due to oxygen toxicity. Old age, multisystem failure and high levels of IL-1 indicate poor prognosis.

RESPIRATORY DISTRESS SYNDROME IN THE INFANTS

The pathogenesis of respiratory distress syndrome of the newborn is intimately linked to a *deficiency of surfactant*. It leads to collapse of the alveoli followed by leakage of fibrin-rich fluid into the alveoli from injured vascular bed resulting in respiratory failure in newborn.

Normally surfactant, lecithin-rich lipid synthesized by pneumocytes 2 prevents collapse (atelectasis) of the alveoli during expiration by lowering the surface tension of the alveoli at low lung volumes and keeps alveoli open. Cortisol increases the synthesis of surfactant, while insulin inhibits its synthesis.

Clinical Features

The first symptom of respiratory distress syndrome usually appearing within an hour of birth is cyanosis, increased respiratory effort, with forceful intercostal retraction and the use of accessory neck muscles in newborn.

Despite advances in neonatal intensive care, the overall mortality of RDS is about 15%, and 33% of infants born before 30 weeks of gestational age die of this disorder.

Predisposing Factors

These include prematurity, maternal diabetes mellitus, neonatal amniotic fluid aspiration and birth by cesarean section.

- *Premature newborn:* Premature newborn is unable to synthesize surfactant. To reduce the potential for developing respiratory distress syndrome in newborn, woman is administered glucocorticoids to enhance fetal surfactant synthesis.
- *Maternal diabetes mellitus:* Fetal hyperglycemia increases the insulin release. Good blood sugar control of maternal diabetes by insulin reduces the risk of respiratory distress syndrome in newborn.

- *Neonatal amniotic fluid aspiration:* Amniotic fluid aspiration in newborn leads to severe damage to alveolar-capillary membrane resulting in impaired respiratory gases exchange.

Pathogenesis

There is decreased synthesis of surfactant in the immature lungs of premature newborn infants. Immature lungs and decreased surfactant cause decreased lung compliance, atelectasis and hypoxia.

Hypoxia produces acute respiratory distress syndrome in infants by two mechanisms. It causes vasoconstriction of pulmonary vasculature leading to pulmonary hypertension and decreased pulmonary perfusion.

Hypoxia simultaneously increases pulmonary capillary permeability leading to alveolar exudation and formation of hyaline membrane. *Pathogenesis of acute respiratory distress syndrome* in infant is shown in Fig. 18.31.

Gross Morphology
Lungs are dark red, airless heavier than usual, with areas of atelectasis alternating with occasional dilated alveoli or alveolar ducts.

Light Microscopy
- The alveolar ducts and alveoli are lined by conspicuous, eosinophilic, fibrin-rich, amorphous material, termed hyaline membranes.
- Pulmonary capillaries are congested.

Complications

Intraventricular hemorrhage is a major complication of respiratory distress syndrome in newborn. Thin-walled veins in the periventricular germinal matrix are dilated as a result of anoxia resulting in rupture.

Intraventricular hemorrhage reflects anoxic injury to the periventricular capillaries, dilation of thin-walled veins, thrombosis and impaired autoregulation.

Diagnostic Tools

Examination of amniotic fluid by flow cytometry and immunofluorescence polarizing microscopy is used to assess fetal pulmonary maturity.
- Previously, lecithin to sphingomyelin ratio greater than 2.1 in amniotic fluid was estimated indicating fetal maturity.
- Currently, phosphatidylglycerol concentration is estimated in amniotic fluid as well as blood, because it is reliable in spite of meconium contamination.

SEVERE RESPIRATORY DISTRESS SYNDROME

Severe acute respiratory syndrome (SARS) is a viral (*corona virus*) respiratory tract infection that can progress to pneumonia and, eventually, death. Incubation of SARS virus is 2 to 10 days.

Mode of Transmission

Coronavirus is transmitted by respiratory droplets produced when an infected person coughs or sneezes. These droplets are inhaled by the nearby person and get deposited on the mucous membranes of the mouth, nose, or eyes. It is also transmitted by using viral contaminated objects on mouth, nose, or eyes.

Risk Factors

SARS includes close contact with an infected person, exhaled droplets and body secretions, and traveling to endemic areas.

Pathogenesis

The SARS virion attaches to receptors on the host cell membrane. It then releases enzymes and weakens

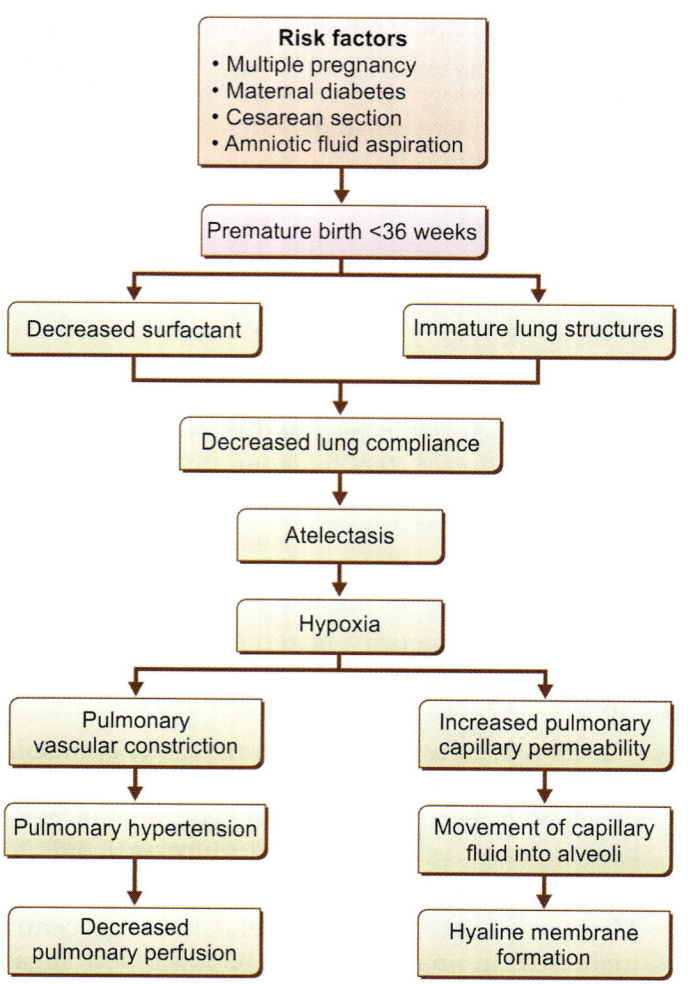

Fig. 18.31: Pathogenesis of neonatal acute respiratory distress syndrome in the infant.

the cell membrane. SARS virion penetrates the cell membrane, and removes the protein coating that protects its genetic material resulting in replication and maturation. It then escapes from the cell by budding from the plasma membrane. The infection then can spread to other host cells.

Clinical Features

Patient initially presents with fever, fatigue, headache, chills, myalgia, malaise, anorexia, and diarrhea. Later, patient develops dry cough, dyspnea, progressive and hypoxemia, and respiratory failure.

DIFFUSE ALVEOLAR DAMAGE (DAD)

Diffuse alveolar damage is nonspecific injury to alveolar epithelial and endothelial cells caused by variety of acute insults. These injurious agents include respiratory infections, sepsis, shock, aspiration of gastric contents, inhalation of toxic gases, near-drowning, radiation pneumonitis, and a large assortment of drugs and other chemicals.

The clinical counterpart of severe DAD is acute respiratory distress syndrome. In this disorder, a patient with apparently normal lungs sustains pulmonary damage and then develops rapid progressive respiratory failure (Table 18.16).

CHRONIC RESTRICTIVE PULMONARY DISEASES

PNEUMOCONIOSIS

Pneumoconiosis is inhalation of mineral dust into the lungs. Dust particles are phagocytozed by alveolar macrophages, which then collect and drain into peribronchial lymphatic channels and hilar lymph nodes.

Mineral dusts include *coal dust, silica, asbestos* and *beryllium*. These account for 25% cases of chronic interstitial lung disease. Some dusts are apparently inert and cause a little or no damage. Certain dusts are antigenic and cause damage through immunological reactions. Exposure to asbestos may predispose to tuberculosis or neoplasia. Occupational causes of the lung disease is shown in Table 18.17.

Predisposing factors: The factors which determine the extent of damage caused by an inhaled dust include its *size, shape, solubility, concentration, and duration of exposure, effectiveness of mucociliary mechanism* and co-existence of other lung diseases.

- *Size:* The size of the inhaled dust particles determines site of deposition in lung alveoli. Dust particles measuring 1–5 micron are most dangerous, which reach alveoli and cause lung damage. Dust particles measuring <1.00 micron are suspended in respiratory tract and exhaled. Dust particles measuring >5 micron

Table 18.16: Etiology of diffuse alveolar damage (DAD)

Category	Selected agents
Infectious agents	Viruses, Mycoplasma, opportunistic infections in immunocompromised persons
Inhaled toxins	Oxygen toxicity, smoke
Therapeutic agents	Chemotherapeutic drugs, amiodarone, nitrofurantoin
Shock	Traumatic, cardiogenic shock
Sepsis	Any organism
Miscellaneous conditions	Radiation, burns, cardiopulmonary bypass, pancreatitis

Table 18.17: Occupational causes of lung disease

Occupation	Agent	Disease
Mining	Coal dust	Pneumoconiosis
Quarrying (Stone crushing)	Silica dust	Silicosis
Foundry work	Silica dust	Silicosis
Asbestos: Mining, heating, building, demolition	Asbestos fibers	Asbestosis—mesothelioma, lung cancer
Farming	Actinomycetes	Alveolitis
Paint spraying	Isocyanates	Bronchial asthma
Plastics manufacture	Isocyanates	Bronchial asthma
Soldering	Colonophony	Bronchial asthma

trapped in the mucus of nasopharynx, trachea, and bronchi are cleared by mucociliary apparatus.
- *Shape:* Long and thin fibers of asbestos may reach the alveoli and cause lung damage.
- *Solubility:* Finely divided dust may induce exudative reactions. Large particles resist dissolution, hence may persist within lung parenchyma for years together and produce fibrosis in lungs.
- *Concentration:* Increased concentration of dust particles produces more lung damage.
- *Duration of exposure:* Exposure to dust particles for longer period in mine workers increases risk of lung damage.
- *Mucociliary mechanism:* Normally, mucus secretion and mucociliary apparatus participate in clearance of dust particles. Damage to mucociliary apparatus by cigarette smoking predisposes to the accumulation of mineral dusts in lungs resulting in lung damage.

Radiological findings: These are related to the degree of associated fibrosis. Highest atomic number (56) of mineral dust gives a denser chest radiograph than least atomic number (carbon 12), given the same amount of particles inhaled.

Coal Worker's Pneumoconiosis

Deposition of coal dust, i.e. anthracotic pigment derived from coal mines and tobacco smoke in the interstitial tissue of lungs and hilar nodes is known as *coal worker pneumoconiosis*. Alveolar macrophages laden with anthracotic pigment are called as *dust cells*. Pathological lesions depend upon duration of exposure and magnitude of coal dust.

- *Forms of coal dusts:* Coal dust exists in various forms—anthracite (most fibrogenic) and least fibrogenic bituminous, sub-bituminous. There is no study on lignite.
- *Pathogenesis:* Inhalation of massive amount of coal dust is engulfed by alveolar macrophages. These macrophages transmit the dust to interstitium of the lung and form aggregates around respiratory bronchioles. *Coal worker's pneumoconiosis in lung* is shown in Fig. 18.32.

Clinical features

- *Asymptomatic anthracosis:* Coal dust is deposited in connective tissue along lymphatic channels and draining hilar lymph nodes without perceptible cellular reaction.
- *Simple coal worker's pneumoconiosis:* Deposition of coal dust produces fibrotic opacities measuring <1.00 cm in upper lobes as well as upper region of lower lobes. Accumulation of coal dust near respiratory bronchioles produce centrilobular emphysema.

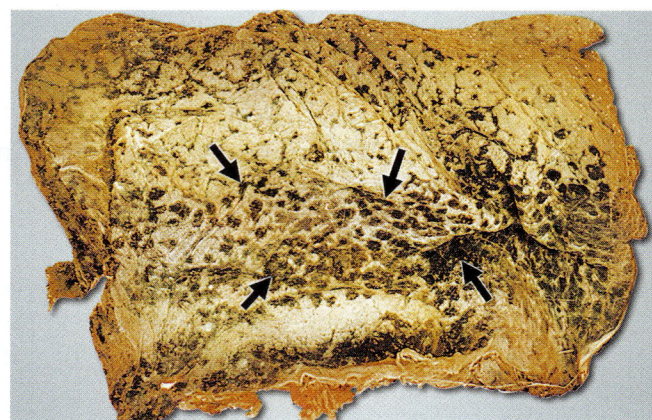

Fig. 18.32: Coal worker's pneumoconiosis shows deposition of coal dusts in lung (arrows).

- *Complicated coal worker's pneumoconiosis:* It is also known as *pulmonary progressive massive fibrosis* (PMF) or black lung disease. Accumulation of coal dust produces fibrotic opacities measuring >1–2 cm with or without necrotic centers in posterior part of upper lobes and upper segment of lower lobe. Patients may develop cor pulmonale.

  There is no increased risk of tuberculosis or lung cancer. Patient may develop *Caplan syndrome* characterized by coal worker pneumoconiosis forming large cavities and rheumatoid arthritis (Table 18.18).

Silicosis

Deposition of silica dust in lung parenchyma producing silicotic nodular opacities is known as *silicosis*. The greater the degree of exposure to silica and increasing length of exposure determine the amount of *silicotic nodule* formation and the degree of restrictive lung disease.

It is most common occupational disease across world. *An occupational history is of importance in establishing the diagnosis. In silicosis, opacities contain collagen and quartz.*

Forms of silica: Silica exists in three forms, i.e. crystalline, cristocrystalline and amorphous silica.

- *Crystalline silica:* Examples are quartz, tridymite and cristobalite. Quartz is derived from foundries, i.e. casting material, sandblasting and mines. At higher temperature (800–1400°C), quartz gets converted into tridymite and cristobalite. Inhalation of these products is more potent than quartz in producing fibrosis in upper lobes.
- *Cristocrystalline silica:* It contains minute crystals of flint, chert, opal, chalcedomy. Higher temperature converts cristocrystalline silica into tridymite, which is potent in producing fibrosis.
- *Amorphous silica:* It comprises glass, kaolin and diatomite.

Table 18.18: Features of simple and complicated coal worker's pneumoconiosis

Lesions	Simple coal worker's pneumoconiosis	Complicated coal worker's pneumoconiosis
Fibrosis	Absent	Present
Size of lesion	<1.0 cm (macules 1–2 mm) and nodules <5 mm	Nodules >2.0 cm (usually 5–10 cm)
Region of lung	Upper region	Upper lobe (posterior region) Lower lobe (upper segment)
Pulmonary functions	Normal	Impaired
Emphysema	Focal	Centriacinar or panacinar emphysema
Pulmonary vessels	Normal	Thickened
Chronic bronchitis	Absent	Present
Cor pulmonale	Absent	Present
Cavitation	Absent	Present (containing inky fluid)

Pathogenesis

- *Pronged exposure to quartz:* It results in formation of *silicotic nodule* in lung composed of concentric layers of collagen with or without central cavitation. There is a minimal inflammatory reaction. Quartz polarizes in the nodules. *Egg shell* dystrophic calcification is present in *hilar nodes*.

- *Prolonged exposure to tridymite and cristobalite:* It causes activation and cytolysis of alveolar macrophages, which release cytokines, which stimulate fibrosis. Radiograph study in early phase reveals fine nodularity imparting *snowstorm appearance*; and later *diffuse pulmonary fibrosis with irregular emphysema* (Fig. 18.33).

Clinical features: These depend on lesions present in simple or complicated silicosis. Patients may develop cor pulmonale and *Caplan syndrome*. There is increased risk for developing lung cancer and tuberculosis.

Asbestosis

Deposition of asbestos fibers in the respiratory unit, i.e. respiratory bronchioles, alveolar ducts, alveoli is known as *asbestosis*. Occupational hazards occur due to asbestos and its products after a long exposure of 10 years. *Lower lobes of lungs are severely affected*.

Source of asbestos: Asbestos occurs as silica compounds throughout earth. It is widely used in flooring, roofing materials, insulating conduits (i.e. sewer, water), brake linings, and clutch castings as well as a fire retardant. It is inconsumable air and water pollutant.

Asbestos fibers: Asbestos fibers measure 5–300 micron in length and 0.25–0.5 micron in width. There are two types of asbestos fibers, i.e. serpentine fibers and most dangerous amphibole fibers. Types of asbestos fibers are shown in Table 18.19 and grading of asbestosis is shown in Table 18.20.

- *Serpentine fiber:* These are composed of *chrysolite fibess*, i.e. white asbestos. These are curly and flexible fibers,

Table 18.19: Types of asbestos fibers

Characteristics	Serpentine fibers	Amphibole fibers
Composition	Chrysolite fibers (white asbestos)	Crosidolite fibers (blue asbestos) Amosite fibers (brown asbestos)
Fibers shape	Curled	Straight fibers
Fibers texture	Flexible	Stiff
Fragmentation	No fragmentation	Fragmentation occurs
Site of deposition	Upper respiratory tract (alveoli spared)	Respiratory unit (terminal bronchioles, acini and alveoli)
Lesions	These do not produce lung lesions	Pleural effusion (recurrent) Pleural plaques Lung extensive fibrosis Mesotheliomas Lung cancer (adenocarcinoma and squamous cell carcinoma) Cancers of gastrointestinal tract and larynx Other lesions such as emphysema, bronchiectasis and pulmonary hypertension

Table 18.20: Grading of asbestosis

Criteria	Grade
Amount of lung parenchyma involved	A: Lung parenchyma not involved B: <25% of lung parenchyma involved C: 25–50% of lung parenchyma involved
Severity of fibrosis and distortion of lung parenchyma	Zero to 4: Zero (no fibrosis) and 4 (severe fibrosis)

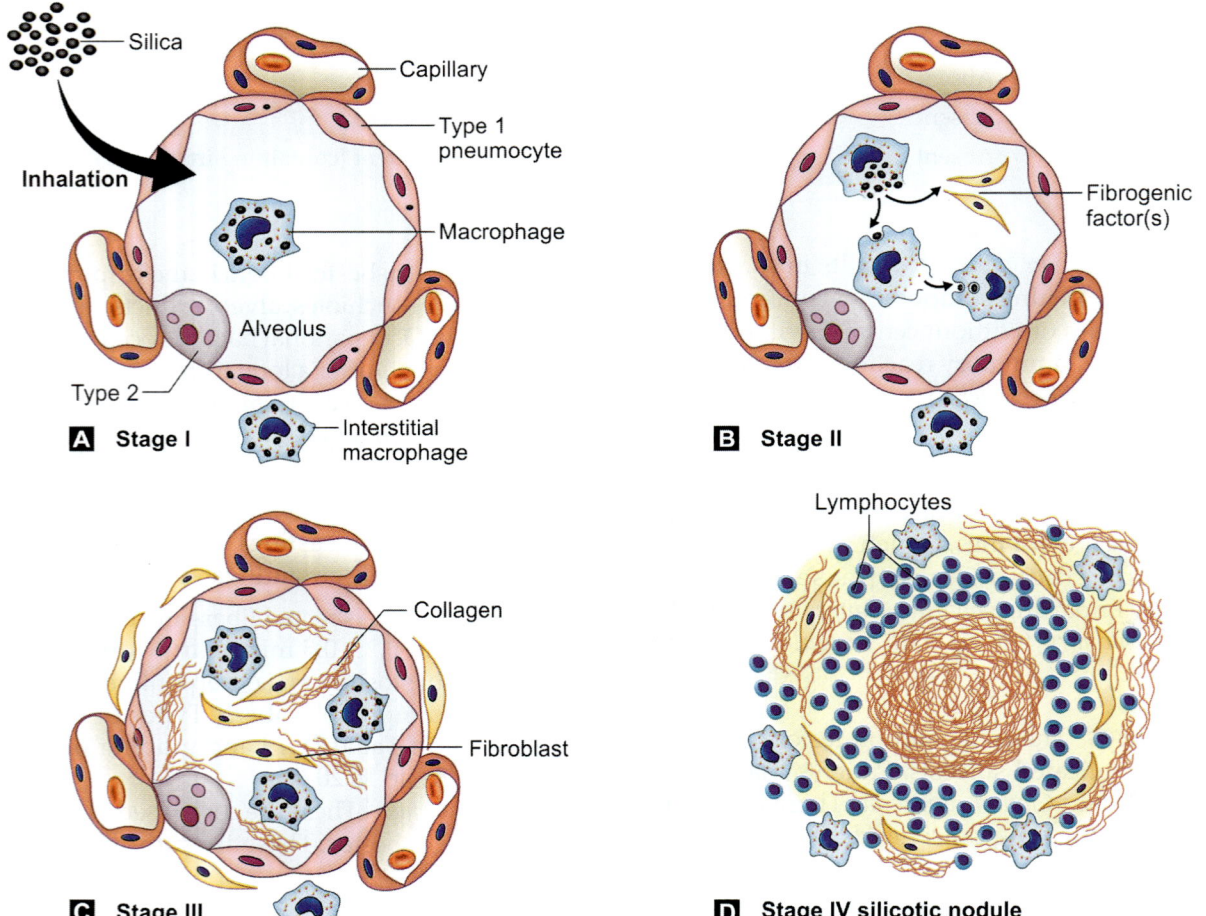

Fig. 18.33: Pathogenesis of pneumoconiosis by silicosis. Inhaled silica particles are toxic to the alveolar macrophages, which die and release a fibrogenic factor. The released silica is again engulfed by alveolar macrophages. The process leads to formation of silicotic nodule.

which reach the upper respiratory tract without fragmentation. These do not produce lung fibrosis.

- *Amphibole fibers:* These are composed of *crosidolite fibers*, i.e. blue asbestos and *amosite fibers*, i.e. brown asbestos. These are straight and rigid fibers, which undergo fragmentation and reach the alveoli. These fibers are most dangerous responsible for pathological lesions.

Pathogenesis: Straight and rigid amphibole fibers undergo fragmentation and reach the alveoli and produce recurrent pleural effusions, pleural plaques, mesothelioma, bronchogenic carcinoma, other cancers (GIT, larynx), emphysema, bronchiectasis and pulmonary hypertension. Pathogenesis of asbestosis lung is shown in Fig. 18.34.

Pathological lesions: Serpentine fibers of asbestos coated with iron, i.e. ferritin and proteins are phagocytozed by macrophages. These form golden brown beaded *ferruginous bodies;* demonstrated in sputum or in distal, small airways. Amphiboles asbestos fibers have been associated with cancerous and non-cancerous lung diseases.

- *Pleural effusion:* Patient exposed to asbestosis develops recurrent and bilateral pleural effusion.

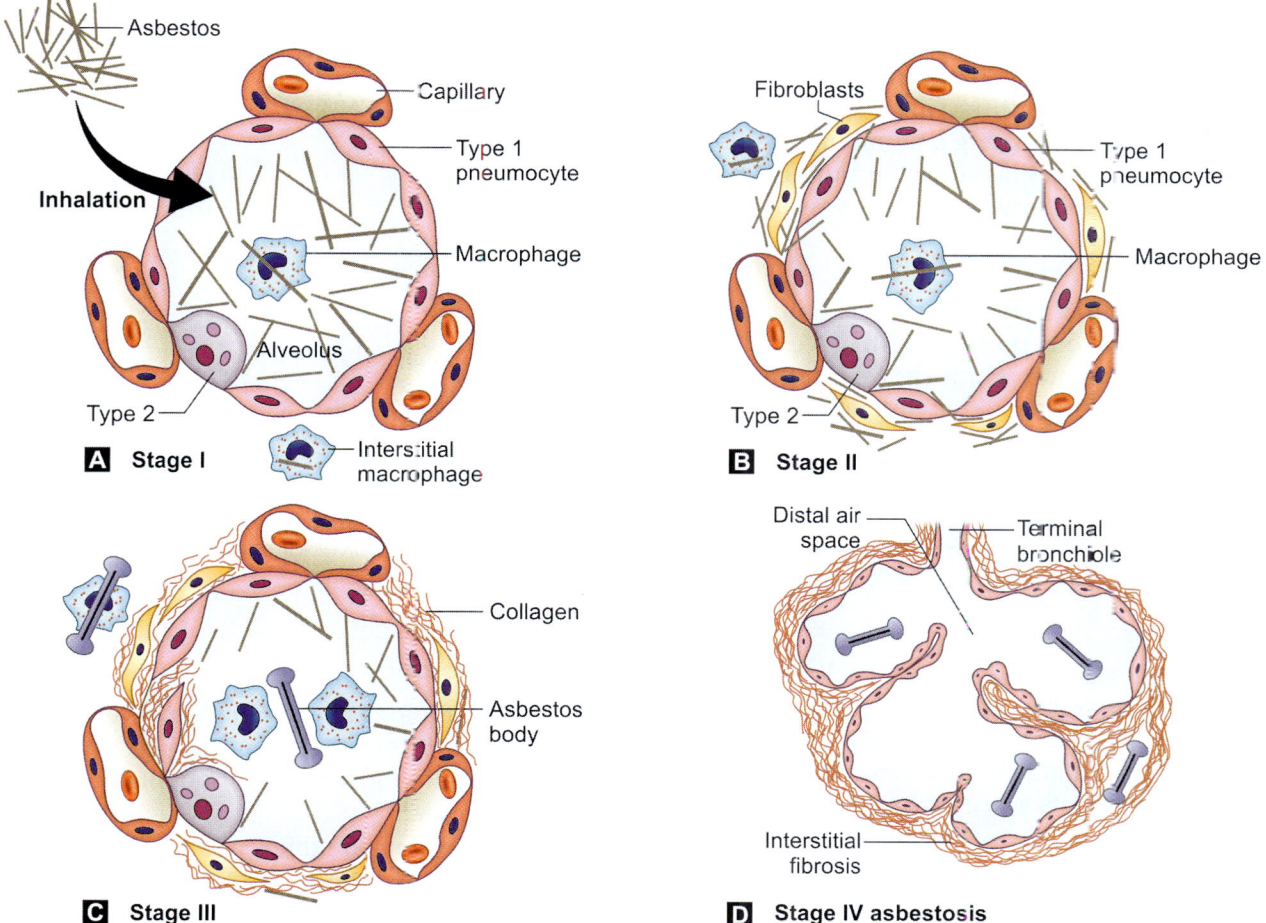

Fig. 18.34: Pathogenesis of pneumoconiosis by asbestos fibers. Asbestosis is characterized by inhalation of small amount of dust producing extensive pulmonary fibrosis.

- *Pleural plaques:* Benign pleural plaques are most common lesions in asbestosis. These are well circumscribed tan-white *benign pleural plaques* containing calcium over the domes of diaphragm and costophrenic angles. They do not contain asbestos bodies.
- *Mesothelioma:* Mesothelioma arises from visceral layer of pleura and peritoneum. It occurs in 5–10% cases, 25 to 40 years after first exposure. Tumor is dense white bulky filling the cavity. Patient presents with dyspnea, pain and effusion. Malignant mesothelioma arises from serosa of pleura encasing the lung.
- *Lung cancer:* Bronchogenic carcinoma is most common asbestos related cancer such as adenocarcinoma (most common) and squamous cell carcinoma. Cigarette smoking increases the risk for lung cancer manifold.
- *Other malignancies:* There is increased risk of cancer of gastrointestinal, tract larynx and lymph nodes.
- *Other lesions:* Patients may develop emphysema, bronchiectasis and pulmonary hypertension.

Berylliosis

Deposition of beryllium (mineral dust, fumes) in the lungs is known as *berylliosis*. There is increased risk of *cor pulmonale* and *lung cancer*.

Source: Grinding, heating, melting of beryllium metal and alloys produce dangerous particles in the form of beryllium oxide. These are inhaled and produce two types of lesions in respiratory tract.

Pathological lesions: Inhalation of *beryllium oxide*, patient develops *acute non-specific chemical tracheobronchopneumonia*. Later on, the patient develops *diffuse interstitial fibrosis* and noncaseating epithelioid cell granuloma entrapping *birefringent crystals*. These may become 50 micrometer in size called *Schumann bodies* similar to sarcoidosis. In biopsy, other causes of noncaseating epithelioid cell granulomatous disorders must be excluded.

DRUGS ASSOCIATED WITH INTERSTITIAL FIBROSIS

Prolonged therapeutic administration of amiodarone, bleomycin, busulfan, cyclophosphamide, methotrexate, methysergide, nitrosourea and nitrofurantoin cause chronic interstitial pulmonary fibrosis. Pulmonary manifestations of drug reactions include diffuse interstitial pneumonia, diffuse alveolar damage, bronchiolitis obliterans organizing pneumonia, eosinophilic pneumonia, pulmonary hemorrhage, pulmonary veno-occlusive disease and large and small vessel vasculitis.

RADIATION INDUCED INTERSTITIAL LUNG DISEASE

Acute pneumonitis may occur 1 to 6 months after radiotherapy. Patient presents with fever, dyspnea, pleural effusions. Radiograph shows infiltrates. Some patients develop chronic radiation pneumonitis.

IDIOPATHIC PULMONARY FIBROSIS

Idiopathic pulmonary fibrosis accounts for 15% cases of chronic interstitial diseases. Men are more affected than women in 40–70 years of age group.

Pathogenesis

Unknown agent triggers repeated cycles of alveolitis resulting in alveolar fibrosis and proximal dilation of the small airways. IL-8, FGF, TGF-β, PDGF synthesized by macrophages stimulate fibroblasts resulting in alveolar fibrosis. Lung exhibits *honeycomb* appearance.

Clinical Features

Patient presents with fever, breathlessness, chronic non-productive cough, late inspiratory crackles, hypoxemia and cyanosis. Patient has poor prognosis with mean survival of 4–6 years.

> **Gross Morphology**
>
> Normal architecture of lungs is impaired showing extensive fibrosis. Gross morphology of lung is shown in Fig. 18.35.

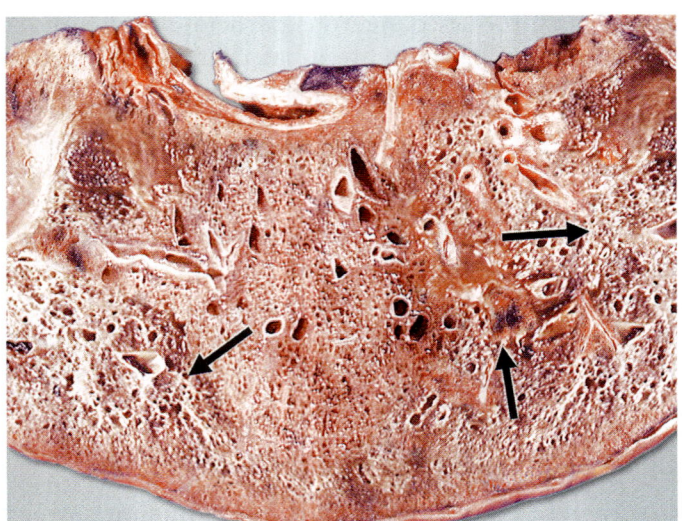

Fig. 18.35: Lung shows extensive fibrosis (arrows).

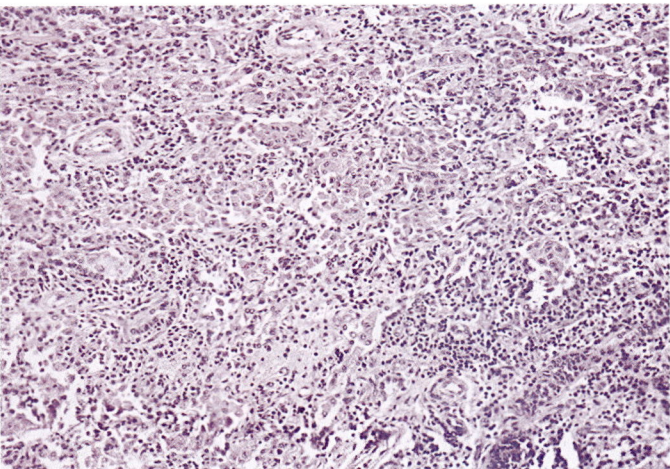

Fig. 18.36: Idiopathic pulmonary fibrosis showing desquamative pneumonia. Alveolar septa are thickened by fibrosis. Capillaries are diminished. Interalveolar septa are infiltrated by chronic inflammatory cells (100X).

> **Light Microscopy**
>
> - Histopathological examination reveals interstitial fibrosis, interstitial pneumonia, desquamative pneumonia and bronchiolitis obliterans organizing pneumonia.
> - Alveolar septa are thickened by fibrosis.
> - Capillaries are diminished. Interalveolar septa are infiltrated by chronic inflammatory cells (Fig. 18.36).

SARCOIDOSIS

Sarcoidosis is a noncaseating granulomatous disease of unknown etiology. It becomes clinically apparent in teenagers and young adults. It is more common in women than men.

Organs Involved

Noncaseating granulomas are seen in lymph nodes, bone marrow, spleen and skin.

- *Lung:* It shows pulmonary interstitial fibrosis and respiratory failure. Symptoms of pulmonary disease include dyspnea, cough, and wheezing.
- *Skin lesions:* Patient develops rashes on the nose and cheeks (lupus pernio), lateral painful nodules on extremities, i.e. erythema nodosum and inflammation of subcutaneous fat.
- *Anterior uveitis:* It results in blurred vision, glaucoma and corneal opacities. Angiotensin-converting enzyme (ACE) synthesized by epithelioid macrophages is elevated in the blood.
- *Liver:* Patient develops granulomatous hepatitis.

Chest radiograph: It reveals bilateral hilar lymphadenopathy and interstitial lung disease manifesting as diffuse reticular densities.

Laboratory diagnosis: Tuberculin test is negative. Blood γ-globulins and calcium levels are raised with hypercalciuria.

Definitive diagnosis requires biopsy demonstrating noncaseating granulomas, laminated calcium concretions, i.e. Schaumann bodies and star-shaped inclusions called asteroid bodies.

COLLAGEN VASCULAR DISEASE

Collagen vascular diseases (i.e. scleroderma and systemic lupus erythromatosus) accounts for 10% of chronic interstitial pulmonary fibrosis. Approximately 50% of patients with systemic lupus erythematosis produce chronic interstitial pulmonary fibrosis, pleuritis with pleural effusions.

RHEUMATOID ARTHRITIS

Rheumatoid arthritis may produce pulmonary interstitial fibrosis, nodules undergoing cavitation, pleuritis and pleural effusion. Caplan syndrome comprises rheumatoid nodules and pneumoconiosis.

EOSINOPHILIC GRANULOMA

Eosinophilic granuloma in lung is characterized by localized proliferation of histiocytes closely related to the Langerhans' cells of the skin. These histiocytes contain *Birbeck granules* resembling tennis rackets.

Histiocytes are admixed with lymphocytes and eosinophils. Patient develops pneumonitis. It most often occurs in the lung or ribs.

EOSINOPHILIC PNEUMONIA

Eosinophilic pneumonia refers to accumulation of eosinophils and macrophages in alveolar spaces due to allergens. The alveolar septa are thickened by the presence of numerous eosinophils and hyaline membranes are present.

It is classified as either idiopathic or secondary to an underlying illness. Patient with acute eosinophilic pneumonia responds dramatically to corticosteroids than chronic eosinophilic pneumonia.

HYPERSENSITIVITY PNEUMONITIS

Extrinsic allergic alveolitis associated with exposure to a known *inhaled thermophilic Actinomyces*, i.e. *Saccharopolyspora rectivirgula* antigen in moldy hay. Patient develops farmer's lung.

Pathogenesis: On first exposure to thermophilic Actinomyces antigen, patient's blood IgG antibodies level is increased. On subsequent exposure to antigen, antigen-antibody complexes are formed resulting in inflammatory reaction in lung tissue due to type III hypersensitivity response.

Later, patient develops granulomatous inflammation on lungs due to type IV hypersensitivity. Persons handling moldy hay should use facial mask. These patients respond well to corticosteroid therapy.

GOODPASTURE SYNDROME

Goodpasture syndrome is an autoimmune disorder, i.e. *in situ* immune complex mediated disorder involving kidneys and lungs. Hemorrhagic pneumonitis and glomerulonephritis are caused by antibodies (IgG) directed against glomerular basement membrane, i.e. noncollagenous domain of type IV collagen.

Local complement activation results in the recruitment of neutrophils, tissue injury, pulmonary hemorrhage, and glomerulonephritis. Patient presents with hematuria due to glomerular involvement and hemoptysis, i.e. pulmonary hemorrhage.

BYSSINOSIS

Exposure to bacterial endotoxin from gram-negative bacteria growing on the cotton, linen or hemp products in textile factories produces *byssinosis*. It occurs in workers in textile factories. Patient presents with breathlessness due to pulmonary involvement.

SILO FILLER'S DISEASE

Inhalation of wheat weevil protein causes Silo filler's disease due to immediate hypersensitivity reaction resulting in dyspnea. Patient responds to corticosteroid therapy.

LYMPHANGIOLEIOMYOMATOSIS

It is a rare interstitial lung disease that occurs in women of childbearing age. Patient develops widespread abnormal proliferation of smooth muscle in the lung, mediastinal and retroperitoneal lymph nodes, and the major lymphatic ducts.

> **Gross Morphology**
> On gross examination, the lungs show bilateral, diffuse enlargement, with extensive cystic changes resembling those of emphysema.

Treatment

Hormonal ablation through oophorectomy and antiestrogen and progesterone therapy has shown some promise.

PULMONARY ALVEOLAR PROTEINOSIS

Pulmonary alveolar proteinosis (PAP) is also termed as lipoproteinosis. It is an uncommon disease of unknown etiology, in which the alveoli are filled with a granular, proteinaceous and eosinophilic amorphous material, which are PAS-positive, diastase resistant, and rich in lipids. This material sometimes appears to be surfactant.

Acquired PAP: Recent studies have revealed that alveolar proteinosis is associated with compromised immunity, leukemia and lymphoma, respiratory infections, and exposure to environmental inorganic dusts. Light microscopy shows homogenous, agranular precipitate within the alveoli producing focal to confluent consolidation with minimal inflammation. The patients are treated by repeated bronchoalveolar lavage that may halt progression of the disease.

Congenital PAP: It is a rare cause of immediate onset neonatal respiratory distress syndrome. It has a fatal outcome shortly after birth. Without lung transplantation, death occurs between 3 and 6 months.

PNEUMOTHORAX AND ATELECTASIS LUNG

PNEUMOTHORAX

Pneumothorax is the presence of air outside the lung, within the pleural space. It leads to partial or complete lung collapse. It may be due to traumatic perforation of the pleura or may be spontaneous.

Spontaneous pneumothorax occurs when the visceral pleura ruptures without an external traumatic injury or iatrogenic etiology. Pneumothorax causes collapse of a previously expanded lung, a condition that is termed atelectasis. The most common types of pneumothorax are open, closed, and tension.

OPEN PNEUMOTHORAX

In open pneumothorax, there is loss of negative intrathoracic pressure. In spontaneous pneumothorax, trachea deviates to side of spontaneous pneumothorax (Fig. 18.37).

Etiology

- Penetrating wounds or rib fracture results in open pneumothorax. Due to penetrating injury, atmospheric air flows directly into the pleural cavity (negative intrapleural pressure).
- As the air pressure in the pleural cavity becomes positive, the lung collapses on the affected side, resulting in decreased total lung capacity, vital capacity, and lung compliance.
- Iatrogenic induced open pneumothorax occurs as a result of aspiration of pleural fluid (thoracocentesis) or pleural or transbronchial lung biopsies.

Clinical Features

Patient presents with tachycardia. On clinical examination, breath sounds are absent on affected side. Chest rigidity is seen on affected side. Crackling is observed beneath skin on palpation.

CLOSED PNEUMOTHORAX

Closed pneumothorax develops in a spontaneous manner especially in smokers in adults 30–40 years of age. It is more common in men than women. It may recur in the opposite lung in 25% cases within 2 years.

Types

- *Primary pneumothorax:* It occurs in young age group. The condition runs in families. *Rupture of paraseptal emphysema is the most common cause of closed*

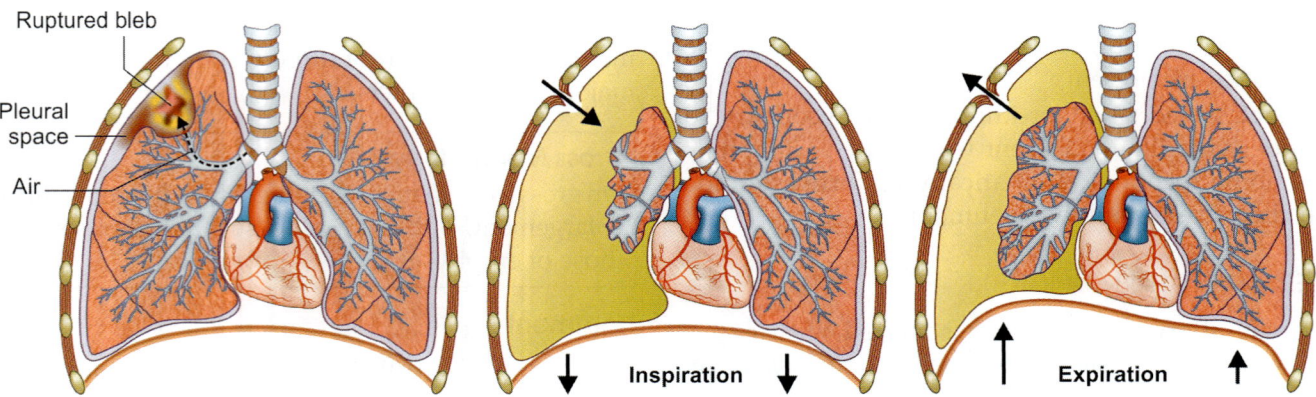

Fig. 18.37: Open pneumothorax. Air enters into the pleural cavity leading to lung collapse.

pneumothorax. It may also occur due to rupture of apical subpleural bleb.

Patient presents with sharp pleuritic pain and breathlessness. Clinical course is self-limited. *Chest drain is not required*, if patient is not in respiratory distress.

- *Secondary pneumothorax:* It occurs as a result of visceral pleural leakage in tuberculosis, necrotizing tumors and lung diseases with cavities.

Clinical Features

Patient presents with shortness of breath, respiratory distress, cyanosis and sudden onset severe pleuritic pain enhanced by coughing, breathing, and chest movement. On clinical examination, there is asymmetrical chest wall movement. Percussion note is hyperresonant. Trachea deviates to same side of spontaneous pneumothorax due to loss of negative intrathoracic pressure.

Upright Chest X-ray

It reveals white visceral pleural line and absence of vessel markings in the peripheral region of visceral pleural line.

TENSION PNEUMOTHORAX

There is increase in pleural cavity pressure in tension pneumothorax. Trachea deviates to contralateral side in tension pneumothorax (Fig. 18.38).

Pathogenesis

- Tension pneumothorax occurs as a result of trauma to pleura in mechanically ventilated patients. Each inspiration results in rushing out of air from alveoli and enters the pleural space through punctured site.
- It acts as a one-way check valve, but cannot escape as the rupture site closes on expiration. Each inspiration keeps on increasing intrapleural pressure resulting in lung collapse, i.e. atelectasis. It forces mediastinal structures, i.e. heart, trachea, esophagus, and great vessels to opposite side.
- Heart and opposite lung are compressed resulting in impairment of venous return. Trachea deviates to opposite side due to increase in pleural cavity pressure. The diaphragm is flattened.

Clinical Features

Patient presents with sudden onset of severe dyspnea, pleuritic chest pain, hypotension, decreased cardiac output and cardiac arrest. On auscultation, breath sounds are absent. Percussion note is resonant due to presence of air in the pleural cavity or the affected side.

Treatment

Pressure in pleural cavity is relieved by inserting a needle into the second intercostal space on the mid-clavicular line or putting a chest tube.

SURGICAL EMPHYSEMA

Presence of air in the tissues during surgical procedure is known as *surgical emphysema*. It requires a breach of an air-containing viscus in communication with soft tissues, and the generation of positive pressure to push the air along tissue planes. It occurs due to rupture of esophagus. Mediastinal surgical emphysema can also occur due to bronchial asthma or barotrauma from positive pressure ventilation.

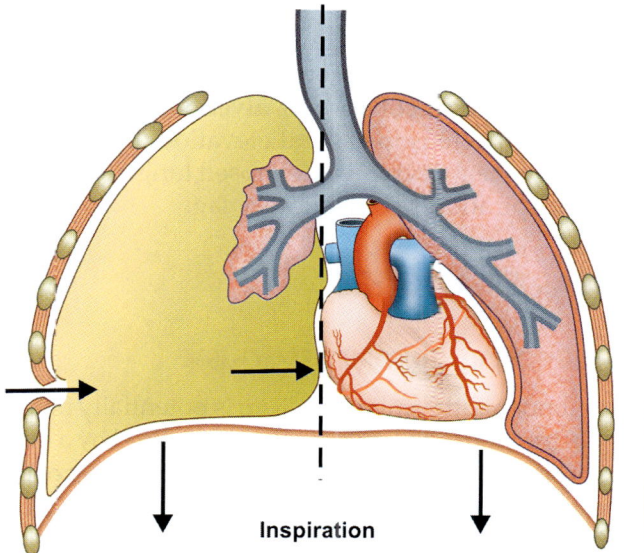 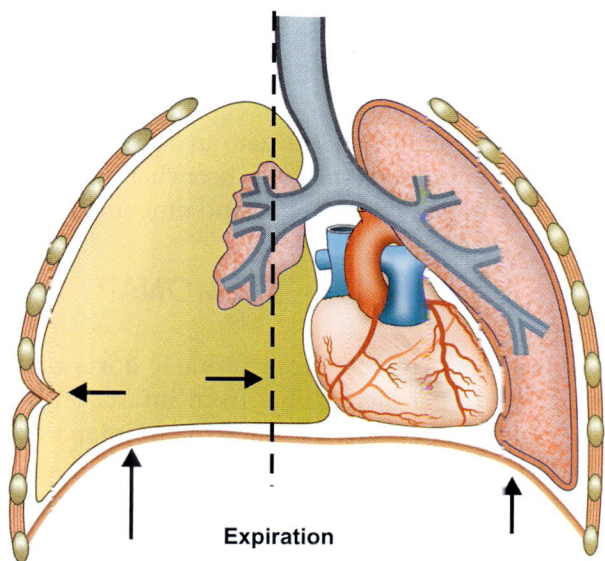

Fig. 18.38: Tension pneumothorax. Each inspiration results in rushing out of air from alveoli and enters the pleural space through punctured site. It acts as a one-way check valve, but cannot escape as the rupture site closes on expiration (arrows).

ATELECTASIS OR LUNG COLLAPSE

Atelectasis refers to incomplete expansion of the lungs or the collapse of previously inflated lung substance. Severe atelectasis significantly reduces oxygenation and predisposes to infection. Obstruction of airways causes resorption atelectasis, while air or fluid in pleural cavity under increased pressure results in compression atelectasis.

Etiopathogenesis

Acquired Atelectasis

It is generally encountered in adults and may be divided into following categories: obstructive or resorption atelectasis, compression atelectasis, patchy atelectasis and contraction atelectasis. Atelectasis is a reversible disorder except that caused by contraction.

Atelectasis Neonatorum

- It is failure of alveolar spaces to expand adequately at birth. Primary atelectasis is failure of initial aeration of the lungs at birth. The alveoli remain collapsed and respiration is never fully established. It is associated with premature birth and intrauterine hypoxia.
- It occurs due to deficient synthesis of surfactant phosphatidylcholine (lecithin) synthesized by type 2 pneumocytes and stored in lamellar bodies. Surfactant reduces surface tension in the small airways. Synthesis of surfactant begins in 28th week of gestation.
- Cortisol and thyroxine increase its synthesis while decreased by insulin.
- Secondary neonatal atelectasis is collapse of previously aerated bronchi.

Types of Atelectasis

Obstructive Atelectasis

- It involves parts of the lung distal to an obstruction in cases of aspiration of foreign bodies, bronchial centrally located bronchogenic carcinoma, and mucopurulent plugs after postoperative states, bronchial asthma, chronic bronchitis, and bronchiectasis.
- Airway obstruction by thick secretions prevents air from reaching the alveoli. It occurs due to obstruction of bronchi, segmental bronchi, or terminal bronchioles.

Compression Atelectasis

- It usually involves the entire lung. The pleural space is filled with fluid compressing the lung, which has retracted towards the hilus.
- Similar findings can be produced by pneumothorax, except in this case the lung collapses because of entry of air into the pleural space.
- Collapse occurs due to lack of air and distal resorption of pre-existing air through the pores of Kohn in the alveolar walls, involving all or part of a lung.
- Air or fluid in the pleural cavity under increased pressure collapses small airways beneath the pleura. In tension pneumothorax, air compresses the lung. Accumulation of fluid in the pleural cavity compresses the lung.

Patchy Atelectasis

Patchy atelectasis is characterized by presence of airless irregular patches in small segments of both lungs. It occurs in neonatal as well as adult respiratory distress syndrome.

Contraction Atelectasis

Contraction atelectasis occurs when local or generalized fibrotic changes in the lungs or pleura prevent full expansion of the lung parenchyma, especially in subpleural regions.

Clinical Features

Patient presents with fever and dyspnea, both usually occur within 24 to 36 hours of collapse. Percussion note is dull due to collapse of alveoli. Breath sounds are absent. There is ipsilateral elevation of the diaphragm and tracheal deviation. Collapsed lung does not expand on inspiration, i.e. inspiratory lag.

PULMONARY VASCULAR DISORDERS

Bronchial arteries originate from thoracic aorta and intercostal arteries; protect lungs from infarction. A pulmonary embolus produces a hemorrhagic infarction in 10% of cases.

Patient with decreased bronchial artery as well as blood flow and obstructive lung disease will likely result in a hemorrhagic infarct, hence increases the risk of morbidity and mortality.

PULMONARY THROMBOEMBOLISM

Pulmonary thromboembolism is potentially fatal. It is an obstruction of the pulmonary arterial bed by a dislodged thrombus. Patient presents with abrupt onset of pleuritic pain, shortness of breath and hypoxia. Bronchial arteries protect lungs from infarction.

Dyspnea and tachypnea are common symptoms in cases of pulmonary infarction.

Lung

Etiology

Most pulmonary emboli arise from the *deep veins of the lower extremities in 50% cases*. It may originate in *femoral* and *pelvic veins* in many cases. Rarely, it can be due to nonthrombotic particulate material such as fat, amniotic fluid, clumps of tumor cells or bone marrow, or foreign matter, such as bullet fragments.

Risk Factors

These include stasis of venous blood flow on prolonged bed rest or immobilization, thrombophlebitis, varicose veins, hypercoagulable states due to use of hormonal contraceptives, and pregnancy.

Consequences

The size of the embolus determines pulmonary vessel that is occluded. Large emboli occluding the major vessels are known as *saddle embolus*. Small emboli occlude medium-sized and small pulmonary arteries. Occlusion of pulmonary artery decreases the perfusion of lung parenchyma and resulting in hemorrhagic pulmonary infarction with fatal outcome (Fig. 18.39).

Morphology of hemorrhagic lung infarct: Hemorrhagic lung infarct is raised, wedge-shaped area with red blue discoloration that extends to the pleural surface. Majority of pulmonary infarct are located in the lower lobes. Perfusion is greater than ventilation in the lower lobes (Fig. 18.40).

Clinical Features

Approximately 50% of patients with mild pulmonary thromboembolism are asymptomatic. But in rest 50%, massive pulmonary thromboembolism results in obstruction of pulmonary arterial circulation.

Patient develops dyspnea or pleuritic chest pain on inspiration, expiratory wheezing, tachycardia, productive cough, blood-tinged sputum, low-grade fever and pleural effusion with fibrinous exudate.

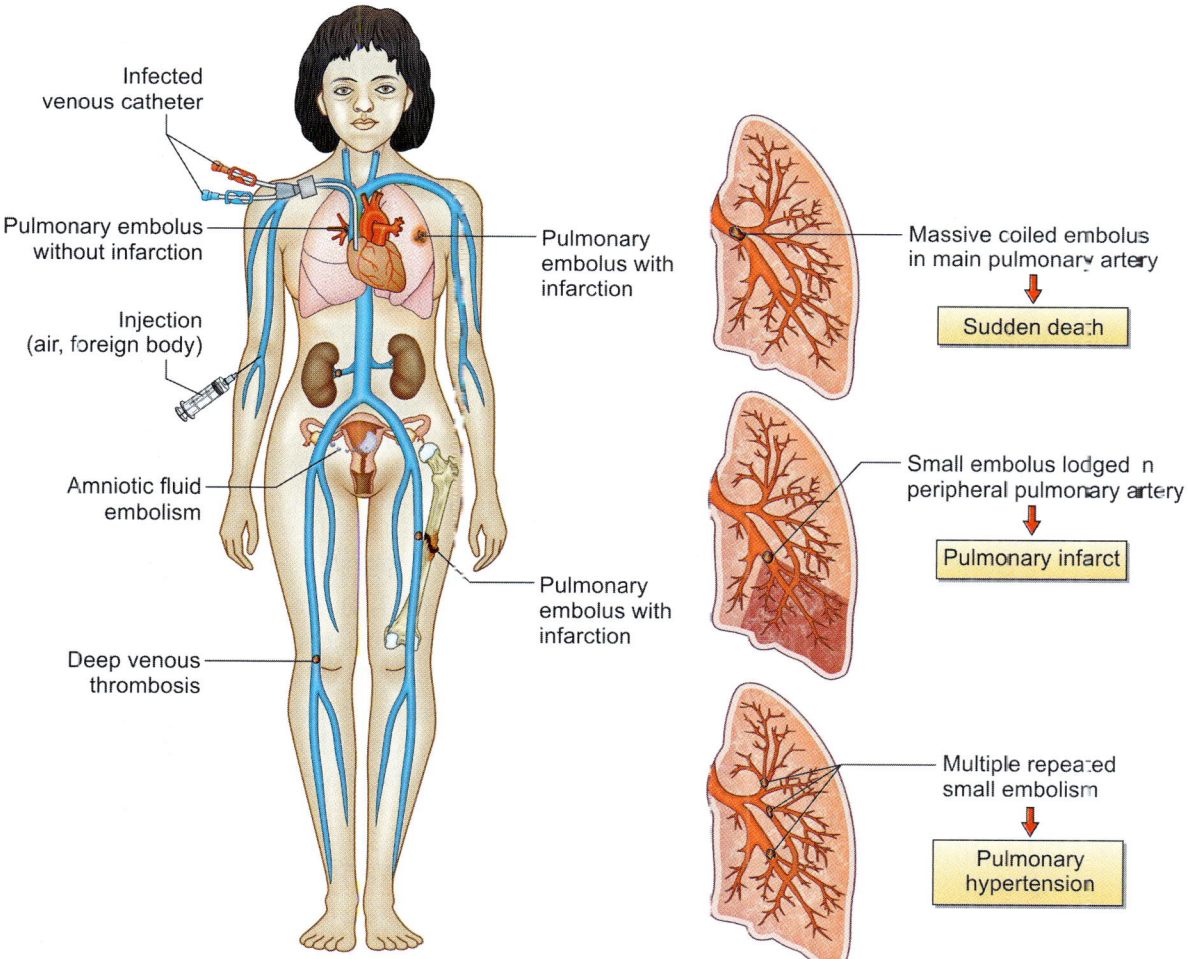

Fig. 18.39: Pathogenesis and consequences of pulmonary thromboembolism. Massive embolus in main pulmonary artery leading to sudden death. Small embolus in peripheral branches of pulmonary artery causes pulmonary hemorrhagic infarct. Multiple repeated small emboli lead to pulmonary hypertension.

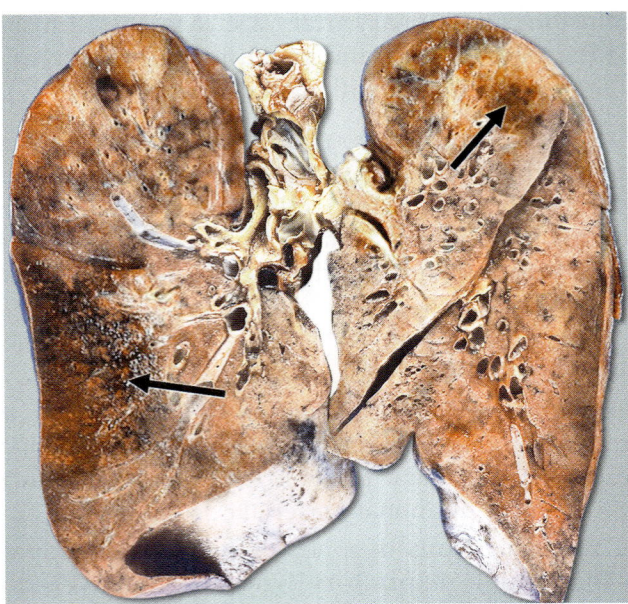

Fig. 18.40: Pulmonary hemorrhagic infarct (arrows).

Imaging Techniques

- *Chest radiograph:* It shows pleural effusion; *cut-off* sign of one or more pulmonary arteries. Hypovascularity is demonstrated beyond the blocked vessel. Wedge-shaped area of consolidation seen is known as *Hampton's hump*.
- *Radionuclide scan:* It shows abnormal perfusion radionuclide scan. Ventilation scan is normal, but the perfusion scan is abnormal.
- *Pulmonary angiogram:* It is gold standard confirmatory test. It is expensive and not readily available in smaller hospitals.
- *Spiral (helical) CT:* It is excellent if pre-existing lung disease is present.
- *Positive O-dimer:* It is usually performed in conjunction with ventilation/perfusion scan or spiral CT.

Prognosis

Overall survival rate is 80%. Hemorrhagic infarct resolves without treatment in 60% cases. In 90% cases, the lesion resolves with treatment.

FAT EMBOLISM SYNDROME

Fat embolism syndrome is a rare but potentially fatal problem. Pulmonary, cerebral, and cutaneous manifestations occur within 24 to 48 hours after a traumatic injury of bone. Fat emboli comprise fat microglobules in the circulation.

Etiopathogenesis

Fat embolism syndrome most often occurs as a consequence of *severe trauma with long bone fractures* such as femur with abundant fatty marrow. It can also be seen with *extensive trauma* to fat laden tissues, burns, and very rarely with orthopedic procedures.

Pathogenesis

On fracture, bone marrow fatty globules enter the circulation, lodge in small blood vessels of the lung, skin, kidneys, brain and other organs producing ischemia and hemorrhage. It results in the clinical manifestations.

Fat microglobules are converted into fatty acids, which damage vascular endothelium resulting in formation of platelet thrombi in areas of injury.

Capillary permeability is increased. Lung surfactant is activated, allowing protein-rich fluid to leak into the alveoli, resulting in pulmonary edema.

Clinical Features

Patient develops fat embolism syndrome within 24 to 72 hours. It is characterized by pulmonary distress, cutaneous petechial hemorrhages, and various neurologic manifestations with fatal outcome.

- *Pulmonary manifestations:* Patient develops dyspnea and tachypnea due to presence of fat microglobules in pulmonary capillaries causing hypoxemia.
- *Petechial hemorrhage:* Patient develops petechial hemorrhage over the *chest* and *upper extremities* due to thrombocytopenia from platelets adhesion to microglobules of fat.
- *Neurologic manifestations:* Numerous petechial hemorrhages are produced by fat emboli to the brain, particularly in white matter known as *brain purpura*.

Patient develops neurologic manifestations such as loss of consciousness, cerebral edema and herniation within a week in less than 10% of cases with fatal outcome (Fig. 18.41).

Laboratory Diagnosis

Fatty acids released from fat emboli are taken by alveolar macrophages. Bronchoalveolar lavage is performed in suspected cases of fat embolism syndrome.

Smears are stained with fat stains (Sudan III, Sudan IV, Sudan black and Oil red O). Positivity of smears with fat stains is suggestive of fat embolism syndrome.

PULMONARY HYPERTENSION

Primary pulmonary hypertension is a rare disorder of unknown etiology that arises in the absence of heart or lung disease with poor prognosis.

It is characterized by thickening of the media of pulmonary muscular arteries. As pulmonary

Lung

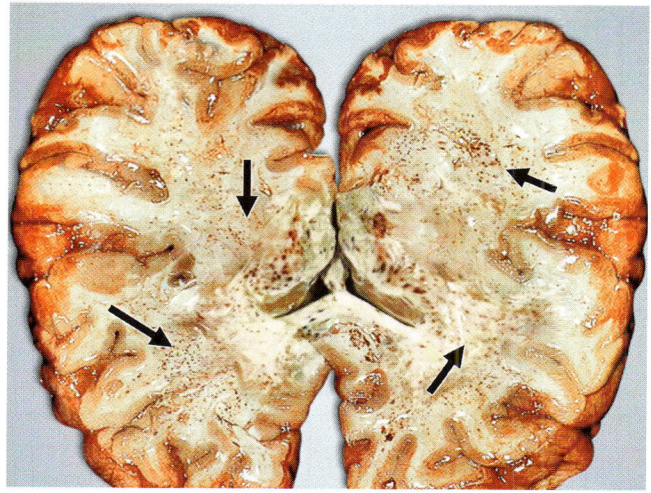

Fig. 18.41: Fat embolus. The patient was in a motorcycle accident and sustained multiple fractures of both legs. The fat emboli caused petechial hemorrhages in the white matter throughout the brain, resulting in coma and death. The macroscopic appearance of cerebral malaria is identical to this (arrows).

hypertension becomes more severe, there is extensive intimal fibrosis and muscle thickening within arteries and arterioles, which may be occlusive.

Etiopathogenesis

- *Primary pulmonary hypertension:* It is characterized by mean pulmonary artery pressure >25 mm Hg at rest and >30 mm Hg with exercise. It is most common in young women. Gene mutation is associated with synthesis of transforming growth factor (TGF) which causes proliferation of smooth muscle cells of pulmonary artery.
- *Secondary pulmonary hypertension:* It is more common than primary pulmonary hypertension. Hypoxemia and respiratory acidosis stimulate vasoconstriction of pulmonary arteries.

Hypoxemia occurs in chronic obstructive pulmonary disease (COPD), congenital left-to right shunt, mitral stenosis, recurrent pulmonary thromboembolism and increased blood viscosity from polycythemia.

Vasoconstriction is caused by increased synthesis of endothelin vasoconstrictor and loss of nitric oxide vasodilator.

Pathology

Pulmonary hypertension imposes an increased afterload on the right ventricle resulting in right ventricular hypertrophy.

Histopathological changes in muscular arteries in pulmonary hypertension may show media hypertrophy, cellular intimal proliferation, plexiform, angiomatous

Table 18.21: Grading of pulmonary vascular lesions

Grade	Pathologic lesions
Grade 1	Medial hypertrophy
Grade 2	Grade 1 + cellular intimal proliferation
Grade 3	Grade 2 + intimal fibrosis
Grade 4	Grade 3 + plexiform lesion
Grade 5	Grade 4 + dilatation (angiomatous lesions)
Grade 6	Grade 5 + necrotizing lesions

and necrotizing lesions. Changes seen in muscular arteries in the lung in pulmonary hypertension are shown in Fig. 18.42. Grading of pulmonary vascular lesions is shown in Table 18.21.

Clinical Features

Patient presents with dyspnea on exertion, chest pain and left parasternal heave, sign of right ventricular hypertrophy. On auscultation, there is accentuation of P2 as a result of pulmonary hypertension. Features of right-sided heart failure occur due to cor pulmonale.

Laboratory Diagnosis

Chest radiograph shows enlargement of main pulmonary arteries and tapering of the distal vessels. Catheterization is done to measure mean pulmonary artery pressures at rest and after exercise.

PULMONARY EDEMA

Pulmonary edema refers to intra-alveolar accumulation of fluid. Pulmonary edema is a common complication of left heart failure. Normally, pulmonary capillary hydrostatic pressure, capillary oncotic pressure, capillary permeability, and lymphatic drainage are in balance. This prevents fluid infiltration to the lungs. When this balance changes, or if the lymphatic drainage system is obstructed, pulmonary edema results.

Etiology

- Left ventricular failure is caused by acute myocardial infarction, cardiomyopathies, hypertensive, or valvular heart disease (mitral stenosis, aortic stenosis), left atrial myxoma.
- Pulmonary edema may occur due to increased alveolar capillary permeability caused by inhalation of irritant gases, pneumonia, shock, sepsis, pancreatitis, uremia, or drug overdose. It may also occur as a result of rapid ascent to high altitude.

Pathophysiology

- Blood pools in the ventricle and atrium and eventually backs up into the pulmonary veins and capillaries.

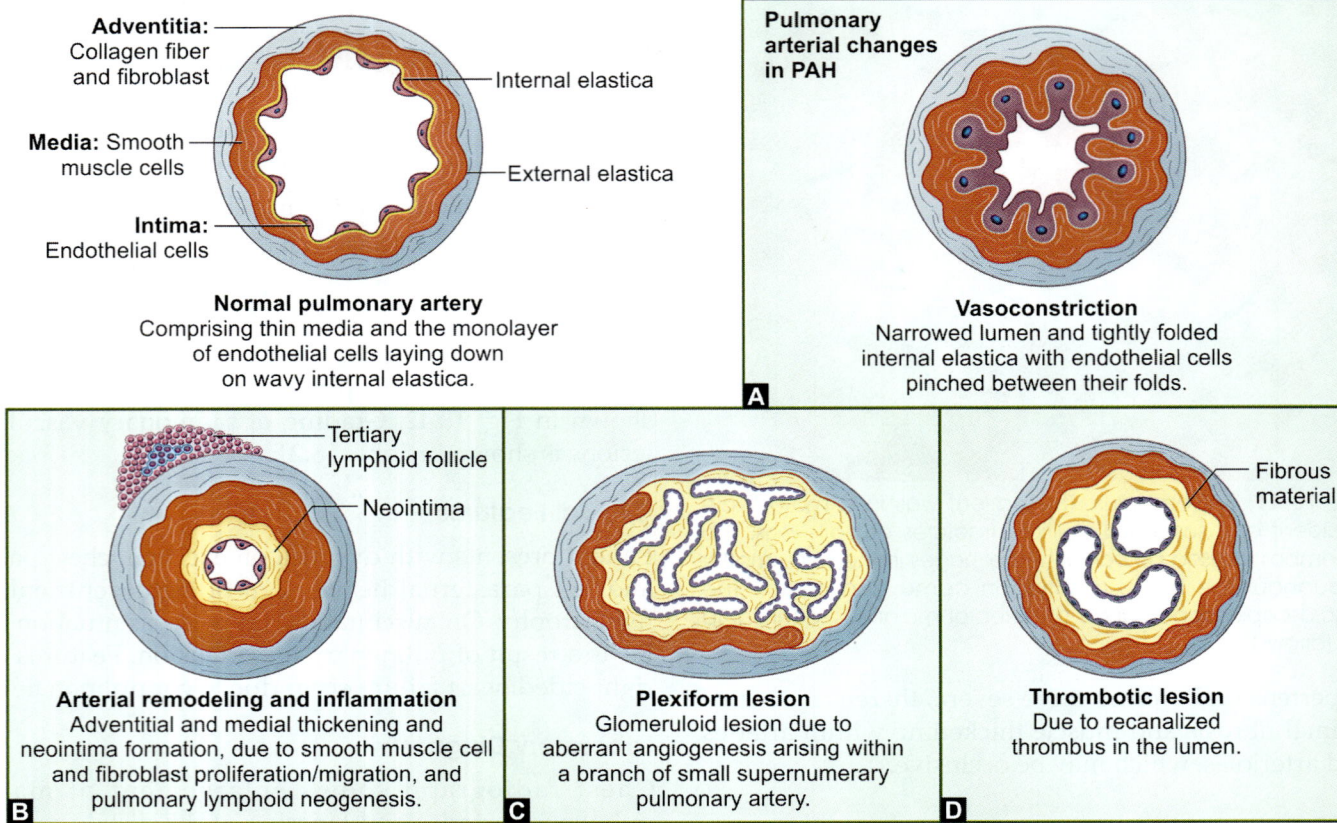

Fig. 18.42: Changes seen in muscular arteries of the lung in pulmonary hypertension.

- Rising capillary pressure pushes sodium and water into the interstitial space, causing pulmonary edema.
- Because the left ventricle cannot handle the increased venous return, fluid pools in the pulmonary circulation, worsening pulmonary edema. Decreased breath sounds, dullness on percussion, crackles, and orthopnea.
- The right ventricle may now become stressed because it is pumping against greater pulmonary vascular resistance and left ventricular pressure (Fig. 18.43).

Light Microscopy

The alveoli in this lung are filled with a smooth to slightly floccular pink material characteristic of pulmonary edema. Capillaries in the alveolar walls are congested with many red blood cells (Fig. 18.44).

Clinical Features

- *Dyspnea:* It is an early symptom from pulmonary congestion. On auscultation, crackles and wheeze breath sounds are heard. Pulmonary vascular congestion and proteinaceous pink staining intra-alveolar fluid can be seen in this manifestation of left-sided heart failure.
- *Orthopnea:* Patient cannot breathe unless sitting up.
- *Cough:* Patient has frothy pink or white sputum.
- *Edema:* Pleural effusion with hydrothorax most often occur. Reduction in renal perfusion activates renin-angiotensin-aldosterone system leading to retention of salt and water. Cerebral anoxia is less frequent.
- *Cool moist skin:* Patient has weak pulse, cool moist skin as the peripheral vasoconstriction shunts blood to vital organs.

Assay of B-type Natriuretic Peptide

Assay of B-type natriuretic peptide is elevated in heart failure. Natriuretic peptide elevation may aid in the distinction of heart failure from other disorders such as acute coronary syndrome, bronchial asthma, chronic obstructive pulmonary disease, or pulmonary thromboembolism phenomenon, which may also present with dyspnea or edema.

PULMONARY VASCULITIS

Patient with vasculitis and related lesions often present with alveolar hemorrhages. These include Good-Pasture syndrome, idiopathic rapidly progressive glomerulonephritis, Wegener's granulomatosis, microscopic polyarteritis, systemic lupus erythematosus and toxins.

Patient may develop pulmonary hemorrhagic syndromes as shown in Table 18.22.

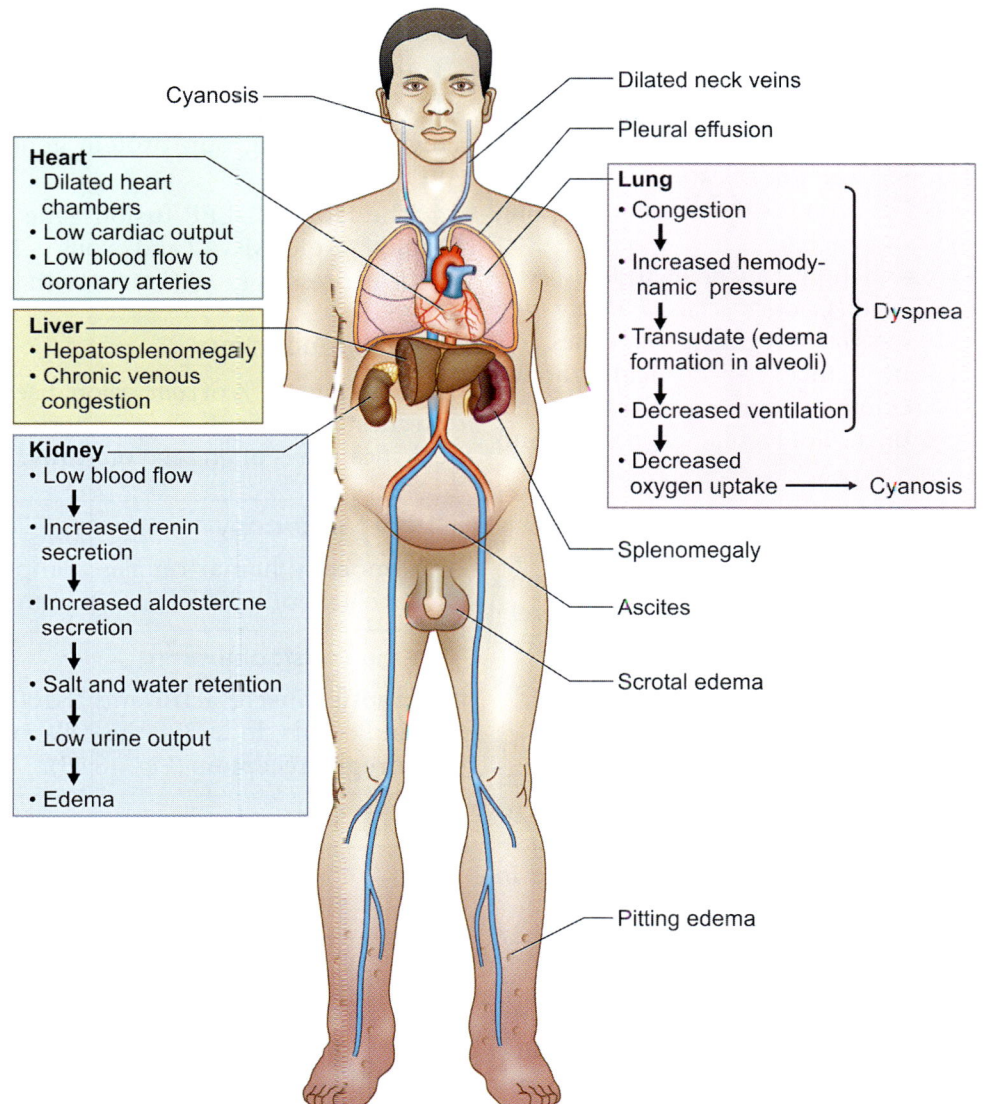

Fig. 18.43: Clinical manifestations in heart failure. Left heart failure is associated with retention of salt and water, pulmonary congestion, dyspnea, cyanosis, generalized edema, ascites, hydrothorax and scrotal edema. Right heart failure is associated with systemic venous congestion, peripheral pitting edema over ankles and hepatosplenomegaly.

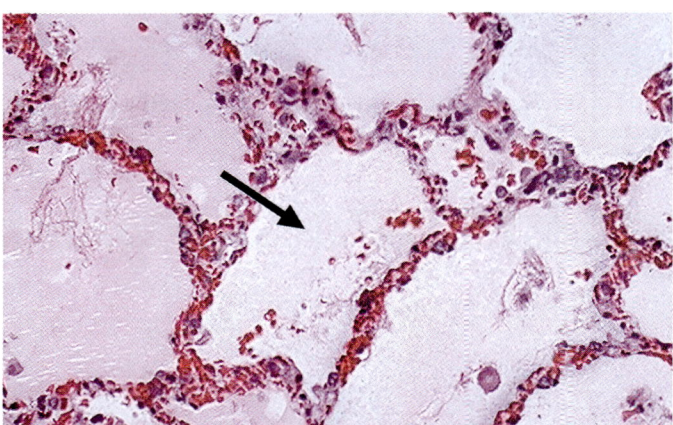

Fig. 18.44: Pulmonary edema. The alveoli in this lung are filled with a smooth to slightly floccular pink material. Alveolar capillaries are congested (arrow) (400X).

Table 18.22: Pulmonary hemorrhagic syndromes

Syndrome	Inflammation of capillaries	Immunofluor-escence study
Goodpasture syndrome	+/−	Linear staining
Idiopathic rapidly progressive glomeru-lonephritis	+	Granular staining
Wegener's granulo-matosis	+	−
Microscopic poly-arteritis	+	−
Collagen vascular disease (SLE)	+	+
Toxins	−	−

LUNG TUMORS

Many benign and malignant tumors originate in the lungs. Approximately 90–95% are malignant tumors, 5% carcinoid tumors and 2–5% mesenchymal and tumor-like disorders. *Cigarette smoking* remains the most important risk factor for the development of lung cancer across world.

Other risk factors for lung cancer include *asbestos exposure, radiation, chemicals, heavy metals, fibrosing lung disorders, immunosuppression* and *genetic syndromes*.

Most common lung cancers in clinical practice include small cell carcinoma, squamous cell carcinoma, adenocarcinoma, bronchioloalveolar carcinoma and large cell carcinoma.

BENIGN TUMORS

Benign tumors of lung include bronchial adenoma and hamartomas (most common). These are relatively uncommon. Size of tumor remains constant for >2 years, but may exhibit dystrophic calcification on chest radiograph.

Patient with tumor in peripheral region is usually asymptomatic, until it is large. But centrally located benign tumor may present with hemoptysis and signs of bronchial obstruction. According to WHO classification, primary benign lung tumors are classified in Table 18.23.

PULMONARY HAMARTOMA

Hamartoma is disorganized benign mature tissue with altered architecture found in their normal anatomic location.

Age and Sex Predilection

It affects adults over 40 years of age, with a peak in the sixth decade of life.

Molecular Genetics

Chromosomal anomalies such as rearrangements of *12q14–15* or *6p21* suggest that pulmonary hamartoma is a neoplastic process.

It has a high frequency of the translocation *t(3; 12)(q27–28; q14–15)*, resulting in gene fusion of the high mobility group protein gene HMGA2 and the LPP gene.

The HMGA2–LPP fusion gene usually consists of exons 1–3 of HMGA2 and exons 9–11 of LPP and seems to be expressed in all tumors with this translocation.

Imaging Technique

It constitutes 10% of *coin* lesion discovered incidentally on chest radiograph. A characteristic *popcorn* pattern of calcification is often seen on X-ray.

> **Light Microscopy**
> Pulmonary hamartoma is composed of cartilage, bronchial epithelium, and smooth muscle cells.
>
> **Immunohistochemistry**
> **Smooth muscle actin** and **S-100** are expressed in spindle cells. In males, the cells express **ER, PR** and **androgen receptors** (Fig. 18.45).

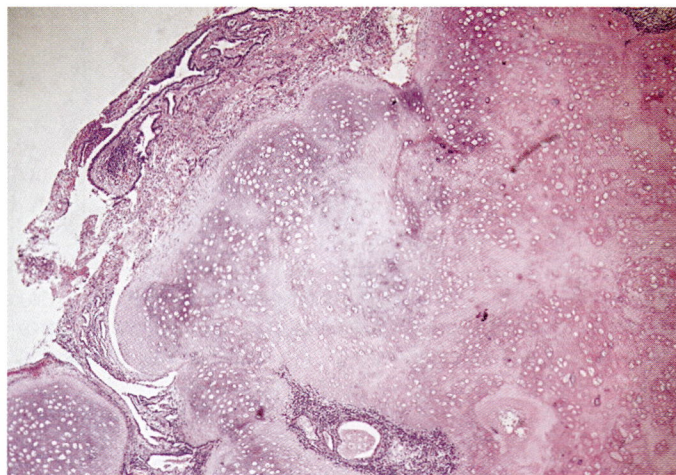

Fig. 18.45: Pulmonary hamartoma is composed of cartilage, bronchial epithelium, and smooth muscle cells (100X).

Table 18.23: WHO classification of benign lung tumors

Origin	Tumors and tumor-like lesions
Epithelial origin	*Bronchial adenoma:* Alveolar, papillary, mucinous or mucous variants* *Bronchial papilloma:* Squamous cell type, glandular type or mixed type
Mesenchymal origin	Pulmonary hamartoma* Chondroma Congenital peribronchial myofibroblastic tumor Inflammatory myofibroblastic tumor Epithelioid hemangioendothelioma

*Bronchial adenoma and pulmonary hamartoma are most common benign tumors

BRONCHOPULMONARY CARCINOIDS

Carcinoid tumors of lung are derived from *pluripotent neuroendocrine cells* of major bronchial epithelium constituting up to 2% of primary lung tumors. These are not associated with cigarette smoking.

Carcinoid tumors also contain neuroendocrine granules, but the tumor cells are arranged in a distinctive pattern. Cushing's syndrome is often encountered in patients with small cell carcinoma, but not carcinoid tumor.

Behavior

These are slow growing highly vascular tumors. About 85% tumors are benign in nature. These do not metastasize but may spread by direct extension. In approximately 15% of cases, metastasis may occur.

Age Group

It is most common solitary primary tumor in children located in central region, but may affect elderly persons.

Location

Bronchopulmonary carcinoid tumor may be located in *central, peripheral* and *midportion of lung*. Centrally located carcinoid tumor appears as fleshy, smooth polypoid growth protruding into bronchial lumen. It obstructs bronchial lumen which results in pneumonia.

Clinical Features

Patient with carcinoid tumor confined to lung presents with hemoptysis (most common), cough, and carcinoid syndrome associated with synthesis of neuropeptide in <1% cases. Regional lymph node metastases occur in 20% of patients.

Light Microscopy

Histological variants of bronchopulmonary carcinoids include classic and atypical.

- *Classic carcinoid tumor:* It is slow growing tumor that does not metastasize and has excellent prognosis with appropriate surgery (5-year survival in 90%). Tumor is composed of monomorphic round to oval cells with salt and pepper nuclei and eosinophilic granular cytoplasm. The tumor cells are arranged in small groups or nests, cords or tubular structures separated by thin fibrous septa (Fig. 18.46).
- *Atypical carcinoid tumor:* Presently this variant is reclassified alongside small cell lung carcinoma as part of the spectrum of neuroendocrine carcinoma. On histological examination, tumor shows **5 to 10 mitotic figures** *per 10 high power fields*, pleomorphism with hyperchromatic nuclei and tumor necrosis.

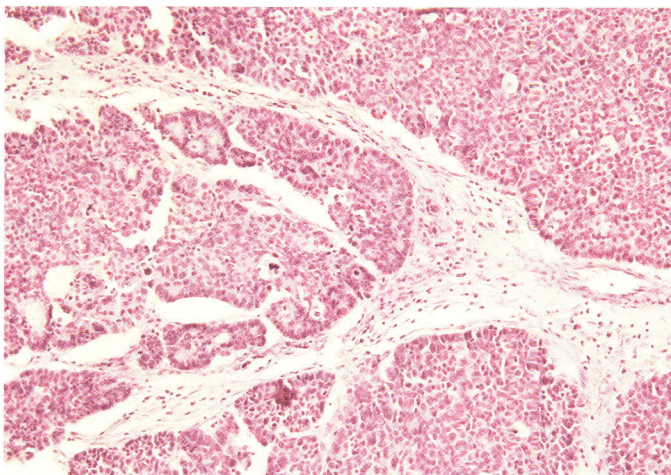

Fig. 18.46: Bronchopulmonary carcinoid is composed of monomorphic round to oval cells with salt and pepper nuclei and abundant eosinophilic granular cytoplasm arranged in small groups or nests, cords or tubular structures and separated by thin fibrous septa (100X).

Histochemistry

Silver stain shows black granules in the cytoplasm, which may be argentaphilic or argyrophilic in nature.

- *Argentaffin cells:* These reduce silver salts to metallic silver (**black color**) without the help of reducing agent.
- *Argyrophil cells:* These reduce silver salts to metallic silver (**black color**) only after addition of a reducing agent.

Immunohistochemistry

Panel of markers is used to analyze expression in bronchopulmonary carcinoid on histopathological sections (Table 18.24).

Table 18.24: Immunohistochemistry used in bronchopulmonary carcinoid

Tumor marker	Expression
Nonspecific enolase (NSE)	Positive
Chromogranin (neural marker)	Positive
Synaptophysin (neural marker)	Positive
Cytokeratin	Positive
CDX2*	Negative

*CDX2 is positive in GIT carcinoids

PRIMARY PULMONARY MALIGNANT TUMORS

Lung cancer is the most common fatal malignancy in both men and women in the age group above 50 years. Lung cancers are rare under age of 30 years. Surgical excision has limited role in management, as majority of

Table 18.25: Chemical and occupational carcinogens associated with lung cancers

Etiological agent	Associated cancers
Polycyclic hydrocarbons	
Tobacco smoke and consumption of smoked meat and fish	*Lung carcinoma* Oral carcinoma Esophagus carcinoma (middle and distal region) Pancreas carcinoma Renal pelvis transitional cell carcinoma Urinary bladder transitional cell carcinoma
Occupational exposure	
Asbestos (used in building material)	*Lung carcinoma* Mesothelioma Gastrointestinal cancers
Uranium mine workers	*Lung carcinoma*
Beryllium and its compounds (used in missile fuel, nuclear reactors, aerospace application and light weight alloys)	*Lung carcinoma*
Nickel (used plating ceramics, ferrous alloys, batteries and stainless steel welding)	*Lung carcinoma* Nasal cavity carcinoma
Arsenic (used in alloys, medication, preparation of fungicides and herbicides (occupational exposure)	*Lung carcinoma* or liver angiosarcoma Squamous cell carcinoma of skin Basal cell carcinoma of skin
Chromium (used in paints, pigments and preservatives)	*Lung carcinoma*

cases report to hospital very late with locally advanced disease or wide dissemination (Table 18.25).

Risk Factors

- *Tobacco smoking:* Tobacco smoking accounts for 80–90% of lung cancers. Lung cancer correlates with duration and cumulative amount of exposure and depth of inhalation of tobacco smoke. Neutral fraction of tobacco smoke contains polycyclic hydrocarbons, which bind to nuclear DNA and exert mutagenic effect. Acidic fraction of tobacco smoke contains tumor promoting benzopyrene compound. Well differentiated **squamous cell carcinoma, small cell carcinoma, large cell carcinoma** and to some extent adenocarcinoma all demonstrate an increased incidence with increasing tobacco smoke consumption. Approximately 25% of lung cancers in nonsmokers have been attributed to passive tobacco smoke. Many genetic alterations are caused by tobacco smoking.
- *Occupational exposure:* Occupational exposure to pollutants during metal refining and smelting processes such as arsenic, nickel, iron oxides, chromium, asbestos, beryllium, cadmium, mustard gas, pesticides, and uranium increases the risk of lung cancer in 10% of cases.
- *Asbestos exposure:* Asbestos exposure is the best recognized occupational risk factor of lung cancer. Tobacco smoking is synergistic risk factor in asbestos-exposed persons to manyfolds in the development of lung cancers such as **adenocarcinoma** (most common) and **squamous cell carcinoma**. Asbestos fibers act as promoter and cigarette smoke as initiator as well as promoter in lung carcinogenesis.
- *Uranium exposure:* Incidence of lung cancer is increased in uranium workers. Uranium exposure emits particulate products and radon gas. Patient develops lung cancer after 17 years of exposure to uranium.
- *Exposure to ionizing radiation:* It can cause DNA mutations and chromosomal abnormalities resulting in lung cancer. Japanese are at increased risk of lung cancers, i.e. squamous cell carcinoma, adenocarcinoma and small cell carcinoma after atom bomb explosion in Hiroshima and Nagasaki.
- *Exposure to chemicals:* Chloromethyl ether is a potent carcinogen causing small cell lung carcinoma. Combustion of coal and other fossils releases polycyclic aromatic hydrocarbon benzopyrene, which increases risk for lung cancer.
- *Diffuse pulmonary fibrosis:* Diffuse pulmonary fibrosis in tuberculosis has been associated with increased risk of lung cancer.
- *Chronic obstructive pulmonary disease:* Risk of lung cancer increases in chronic bronchitis and diffuse pulmonary fibrosis. Proposed mechanisms of

increased risk include decreased clearance of inhaled carcinogens and epithelial metaplasia.

- *Genetic predisposition:* In general, relatives of persons with lung cancer have higher risk of development of lung cancer. Defects in specific oncogenes, specific HLA antigens, and enzyme and tumor suppressor genes increase the risk of development of lung cancer. Mutation of p53 tumor suppressor gene is common in both small cell lung cancer (70%) and non-small lung cancer cells (30%).

Precursor Lesions

The 'term' precursor lesion does not imply that it definitely progress to lung cancer. Four types of epithelial precursor lesions are squamous dysplasia and carcinoma *in situ*, atypical adenomatous hyperplasia, adenocarcinoma *in situ* and diffuse idiopathic pulmonary neuroendocrine cell hyperplasia.

Classification

Lung carcinomas have been classified by World Health Organization based on their histopathological appearances. Majority of lung cancers are classified by WHO criteria into small cell and non-small cell carcinomas in the ratio of 1:4.

These are clinically and genetically distinct. These vary in their primary site, invasion, spread and biological behavior. WHO classification of lung tumors is shown in Table 18.26. Histological variants of primary lung cancers are shown in Fig. 18.47.

- *Small cell lung carcinoma (SCLC):* It constitutes 20–25% of lung cancers. It is most aggressive lung cancer arising in central region of lung and causing paraneoplastic syndrome. It often metastasizes widely before the primary tumor mass in the lung reaches a large size leading to bronchial obstruction and lung collapse. It is usually treated by chemotherapy rather than radiotherapy or surgery. Prognosis is very poor.
- *Non-small cell lung carcinomas (NSCLC):* These include squamous cell carcinoma (25–40%), adenocarcinoma (30–50%), and large cell carcinoma (10–20%). These tumors invade stroma and pre-existing structures. Histological characteristics of non-small cell lung cancers are much less significant, but pathological staging is critical to treatment and prognostic outcome.

These tumors are treated by surgery, if tumor is limited to lung. Bronchioloalveolar carcinoma (10%) is a subtype of adenocarcinoma characterized by spreading along the alveolar septa in *lepidic*

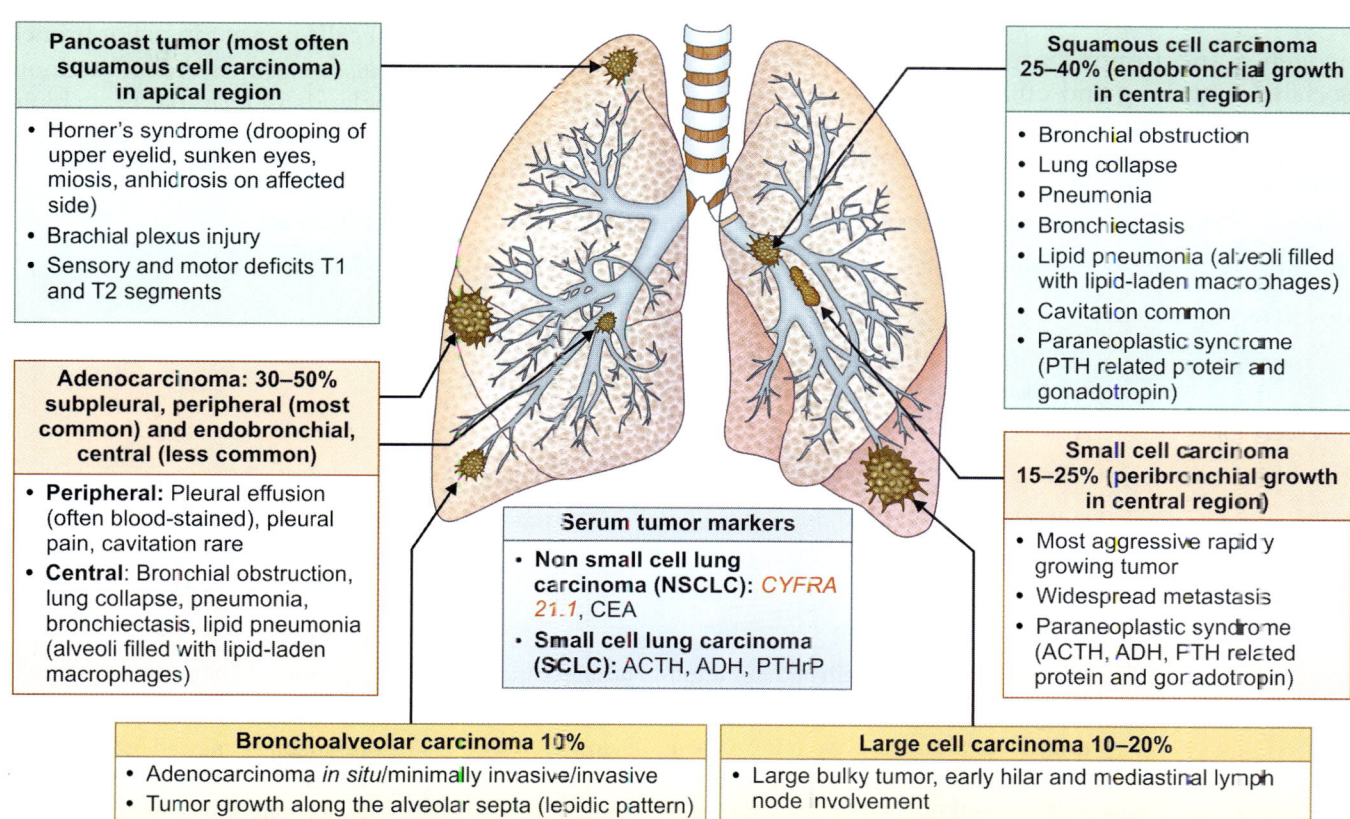

Fig. 18.47: Histological variants of primary lung cancers. Clinical features of lung cancer depend on site of lesion, invasion of neighboring structures and extent of metastases.

Table 18.26: WHO classification of lung tumors

Lesion/Tumor	Light microscopic findings
Preinvasive lesions	Atypical adenomatous hyperplasia, squamous dysplasia, carcinoma *in situ* and diffuse idiopathic pulmonary neuroendocrine cell hyperplasia (lesions <5 mm and multiple)
Squamous cell carcinoma	Keratinizing, nonkeratinizing, papillary, clear cell, small cell and basaloid variants
Adenocarcinoma	Acinar, papillary or mixed, solid variants
Bronchioloalveolar carcinoma	Mucinous or non-mucinous or mixed variants
Large cell carcinoma	Neuroendocrine, basaloid, clear cell, rhabdoid variants
Small cell carcinoma	Neuroendocrine tumor
Adenosquamous carcinoma	Both glandular and squamous elements
Sarcomatoid carcinoma	Pleomorphic, spindle cell, giant cell variants and carcinosarcoma
Carcinoid tumor	Typical and atypical carcinoid tumor
Carcinoma of salivary gland type	Mucoepidermoid carcinoma, adenoid cystic carcinoma

pattern without invading stroma and pre-existing structures.
- *Uncommon malignant tumors:* These include bronchopulmonary carcinoids, mucoepidermoid carcinoma, adenoid cystic carcinoma, angiosarcoma, hemangioendothelioma and malignant lymphoma.

Molecular Genetics

Oncogenes and tumor suppressor gene mutations associated with lung and other cancers are shown in Table 18.27 and gene mutations in various histological variants of lung cancers are shown in Table 18.28.

Origin

Lung cancer arises from cells capable of cell division in lower respiratory tract.
- *Neuroendocrine argentaffin cells or Kulchitsky cells:* Small cell carcinoma arises from Kulchitsky cells in central region of chest.
- *Basal cells in major bronchi:* Squamous cell carcinoma originates from basal cells present in major bronchi.
- *Mucous glands in terminal bronchioles:* Adenocarcinoma arises from mucous glands in terminal bronchioles. Approximately 72% of adenocarcinomas are located in subpleural region.

Table 18.27: Oncogenes and tumor suppressor gene mutations associated with lung and other cancers

Category	Proto-oncogenes	Mode of action	Associated cancers
Growth factor receptors			
EGF receptor	ERBB1 (EGFR) Erb-B2 (avian erythroblastosis)	Amplification	Lung adenocarcinoma
ALK receptor	ALK	Point mutation	Lung adenocarcinoma
Signal-transduction proteins			
GTP-binding proteins	K-RAS	Point mutation	Lung carcinoma Colon carcinoma Pancreatic carcinoma
Cell cycle progression inhibitors (tumor suppressor gene)			
Gene	Functions of pRB protein and mutation	Familial cancers	Associated sporadic cancers
RB gene (locus 13p14)	RB gene codes for pRB protein inhibiting G1 to S of cell cycle and nuclear transcription factor (mutation by deletion and nonsense)	Retinoblastoma and osteosarcoma	Lung carcinoma Retinoblastoma and osteosarcoma Breast carcinoma Colon carcinoma Prostatic carcinoma Urinary bladder carcinoma

Table 18.28: Gene mutations in specific lung cancers

Lung cancer	Gene mutations
Small cell lung carcinoma	Oncogene C-MYC *Tumor suppressor gene:* RB gene (80–100%) and TP53 gene (50–80%) Anti-apoptotic BCL2 gene (90%)
Squamous cell carcinoma	*Oncogenes:* EGFR1 (80%), and ERBB2 (Her2 neu) (30%) *Tumor suppressor genes:* TP53 (60–80%), RB gene (15%) and p16 Cyclin dependent kinase inhibitor gene—$CDKN_2A$ (loci 3p, 9p)
Adenocarcinoma	*Oncogenes:* K-RAS, EGFR, ERBB2 (Her2 neu), ALK, ROS, MET and RET *Tumor suppressor genes:* p53 gene, RB and p16 gene

Table 18.29: Origin of lung cancers

Cell of origin	Location	Lung cancer
Kulchitsky cells (neuroendocrine cells)	Central region of lung	Small cell carcinoma
Basal cells	Major bronchi (lobar or segmental)	Squamous cell carcinoma
Mucous glands	Terminal bronchioles	Adenocarcinoma
Clara cells	Terminal bronchioloalveolar region	Bronchioloalveolar carcinoma

- *Clara cells in terminal bronchioloalveolar region:* Bronchioloalveolar carcinoma originates from clara cells (Table 18.29).

Location

- *Central region:* Squamous cell carcinoma and small cell carcinoma are centrally located. Squamous cell carcinoma shows endobronchial growth. Small cell carcinoma shows peribronchial growth.
- *Peripheral region:* Adenocarcinoma, bronchioloalveolar carcinoma and large cell carcinoma are located in peripheral region.
- *Central or peripheral:* Some patients with adenocarcinoma may develop tumor in the central portion of lung that grows as endobronchial growth invading bronchial cartilage. Local and systemic manifestations of lung carcinoma are shown in Table 18.30.

Table 18.30: Local and systemic manifestations of lung carcinoma

Clinical manifestations	Pathological basis
Hemoptysis	Involvement of central airways
Chest pain	Hemorrhage from lung carcinoma in bronchial airways
Dyspnea	Extension of lung carcinoma into mediastinum, pleura or chest wall
Dysphagia	Obstruction of airways
Lipid pneumonia	Accumulation of cellular lipid in foamy macrophages due to obstruction of airways by tumor
Pneumonia, lung abscess, lobar collapse	Obstruction of airways
Pleural effusion	Tumor invading pleura
Hoarseness of voice	Recurrent nerve paralysis
Rib destruction	Invasion of chest wall by tumor
Superior vena cava syndrome	Compression of superior vena cava by tumor
Diaphragm paralysis	Phrenic nerve paralysis
Horner syndrome (ptosis, sunken eye, miosis, loss of sweating on affected site	Invasion of sympathetic ganglia by lung cancer
Pericardial effusion/cardiac tamponade	Involvement of pericardium by tumor
Paraneoplastic syndrome	Hormones synthesized by lung cancer

Imaging Techniques

- Primary lung cancers are poorly circumscribed, solitary undergoing cavitation and calcification.
- Tumors metastasizing to lung are sharply circumscribed and multiple. These usually lack cavitation and calcification. Presence of calcification in the tumor indicates metastases from osteosarcoma and chondrosarcoma.

Therapeutic Correlation

Small cell lung carcinoma (SCLC) initially responds to chemotherapy. Non-small cell lung carcinoma (NSCLC) confined to lung is curable by surgery. Small cell lung carcinoma is most often metastatic than non-small cell lung carcinoma.

Paraneoplastic Syndrome

Paraneoplastic syndromes occur in small cell carcinoma, squamous cell carcinoma, adenocarcinoma and large cell carcinoma. Paraneoplastic syndromes in lung cancer are shown in Table 18.31.

Neuromuscular Manifestations

Nonmetastatic neuromuscular abnormalities associated with lung cancer are shown in Table 18.32.

Table 18.31: Paraneoplastic syndromes in lung cancer

System	Clinical manifestations
Neuroendocrine manifestations	
General symptoms	Weight loss, fever and anorexia
Skin manifestations	Acanthosis nigricans, dermatomyositis, tylosis (marked hyperkeratosis of palms and soles)
Vascular manifestations	Thrombophlebitis migrans, non-infective thrombotic endocarditis, disseminated intravascular coagulation
Skeletal system	Hypertrophic osteodystrophy, clubbing of fingers
Nervous system	Myasthenia-like syndrome, peripheral neuropathies, cerebellar syndrome, myositis, and encephalopathy
Endocrine and neuroendocrine manifestations	
ACTH-like synthesis in small cell carcinoma	Cushing's syndrome (facial edema, cachexia, low serum potassium and alkalosis)
ADH-like synthesis in small cell carcinoma	Inappropriate secretion of antidiuretic syndrome (high urine osmolality and low serum sodium, confusion, weakness and seizures (if extreme)
Parathormone-like effects in squamous cell carcinoma	Serum calcium high, weakness, polyuria, polydipsia, constipation, abdominal pain and coma (if extreme)
Gonadotropin-like effects due to estrogens in squamous cell carcinoma, carcinoma, adenocarcinoma, small cell carcinoma and large cell carcinoma	Gynecomastia and testicular atrophy

Endocrine and neuroendocrine products of lung cancers: These include ACTH, calcitonin, parathormone-related peptide, melanocyte-stimulating hormone, growth hormone, chorionic gonadotropin, insulin, gastrin, renin, glucagon, estradiol, erythropoietin, histaminase, DOPA-decarboxylase, carcinoembryonic antigen, α-fetoprotein, bombesin and neuron-specific enolase.

Table 18.32: Nonmetastatic neuromuscular abnormalities associated with lung cancer

Neuromuscular abnormalities	Features
Peripheral neuropathy (motor, sensory or mixed)	Muscle weakness, muscle wasting, loss of tendon reflexes, glove and stocking type of loss of sensation
Autonomic neuropathy	Gastrointestinal and urinary bladder disturbances, and or postural hypotension
Cerebellar ataxia	Nystagmus, dysarthria, impaired coordination
Eaton-Lambert syndrome	Differs from myasthenia gravis in muscle function with improvement due to repeated effort monitored by electromyography
Polymyositis–dermatomyositis	Weakness of proximal region with pain and tenderness, purple facial rash, arthralgia, dysphagia and Raynaud's phenomenon
Acute transverse myelopathy	Flaccid paraparesis with sensory loss, sphincter functional loss

Table 18.33: Intrathoracic manifestations of bronchial carcinoma

Location	Clinical manifestations
Apical region	Pancoast syndrome Horner's syndrome Sensory and motor deficits of T1 and T2 segments
Peripheral region	Pleural effusion (often blood stained), pleural pain
Central region	Bronchial obstruction Lung collapse Pneumonia Bronchiectasis Lipid pneumonia (alveoli filled with lipid-laden macrophages)

Intrathoracic Manifestations

Intrathoracic manifestations of bronchial carcinoma are shown in Table 18.33.

SMALL CELL LUNG CARCINOMA

Small cell lung carcinoma (previously referred to as *oat cell* carcinoma) is rapidly growing highly malignant epithelial tumor of the lung that exhibits neuroendocrine features.

It constitutes 15–25% of lung cancers. It is strongly associated with **cigarette smoking**. It is more common in men than women. It is commonly associated with **paraneoplastic syndrome**.

Patient develops tumor in hilar or parahilar region. Extensive peribronchial growth causes bronchial narrowing. Lymph nodes are enlarged. Metastases are demonstrated in >90% of cases at diagnosis.

- Tumor causes extensive peribronchial invasion in the hilar or parahilar region.
- Bronchial narrowing, marked mediastinal lymphadenopathy and early widespread metastases are present in 90% of cases at diagnosis. It is a common cause of superior vena cava syndrome. Prognosis is very poor.
- The tumor is responsive to chemotherapy. The median survival is measured in months. Small cell carcinoma of lung showing risk factors, gene mutations, clinical manifestations, immunohistochemistry and metastases is shown in Fig. 18.48.

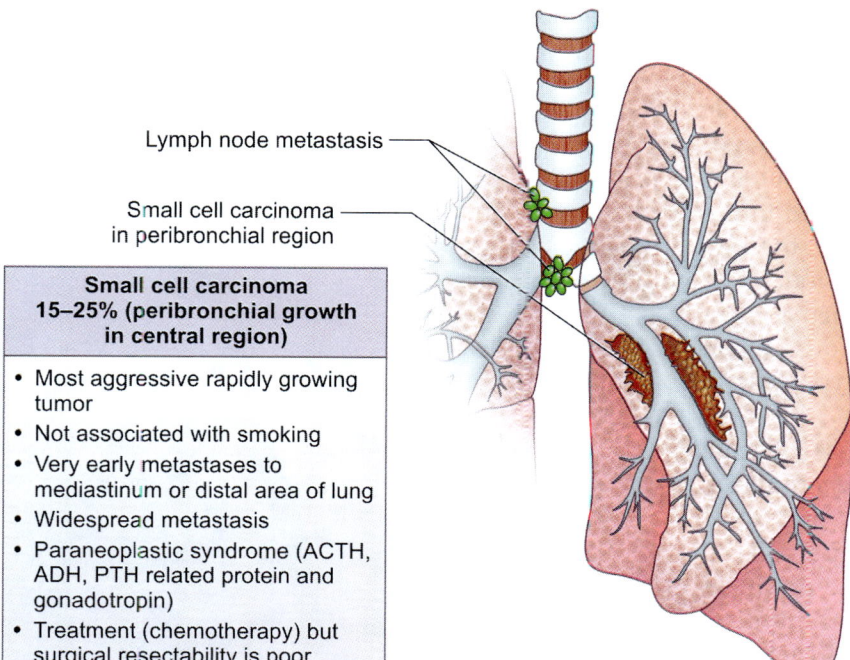

Fig. 18.48: Small cell carcinoma of lung shows risk factors, genes mutations, clinical manifestations, immunohistochemistry and metastases.

Origin

It arises from neuroendocrine argentaffin cells (Kulchitsky cells) near central portion of chest. It accounts for 20% of all lung cancers.

Molecular Genetics

Small cell lung carcinoma exhibits mutations of both C-MYC oncogene and tumor suppressor gene, i.e. RB gene (80–100%), p53 gene (50–80%) and 3p deletion. There is expression of anti-apoptotic BCL2 gene in 90%. There is low expression of pro-apoptotic BAX gene in small cell lung carcinoma. Gene mutations in small cell lung carcinoma are shown in Fig. 18.48.

Paraneoplastic Syndrome

Paraneoplastic syndrome most often occurs in small cell carcinoma. The tumor synthesizes polypeptide hormones such as ACTH, ADH, parathormone-like peptide, gonadotropins, insulin-like growth factor and calcitonin.

- *Eaton-Lambert syndrome:* It is characterized by muscular weakness of pelvic girdles, wasting, and fatigability of the proximal limbs and trunk. It is usually associated with **small cell carcinoma** of the lung (65%).

    Under physiological state, calcium channels are necessary for release of acetylcholine. The pathogenic IgG autoantibodies are formed against voltage-sensitive calcium channels in motor nerve terminals.

    The calcium channels are greatly reduced in the presynaptic membrane in these patients, thereby interfering with neuromuscular transmission.
- *Peripheral neuropathy:* IgG autoantibodies against anterior and lateral horns of central nervous system cause motor and sensory loss resulting in peripheral neuropathy.
- *Cerebellar degeneration:* Autoantibodies cause subacute cerebellar degeneration presenting with severe ataxia, vertigo and dysarthria.
- *Corticotropic effects:* ACTH synthesized by small cell lung cancer stimulates adrenal gland and produces cortical hormones. Patient presents with atypical Cushing's syndrome, facial edema and cachexia. Serum calcium is decreased.
- *ADH effects:* Small cell lung cancer synthesizes ADH, which acts on kidney collecting ducts and produces high urine osmolarity and low serum osmolarity resulting in decreased serum sodium level. Patient becomes irritable and develops convulsions and seizures.
- *PTH-related protein:* Tumor ectopically secretes PTH-related protein resulting in hypercalcemia. Patient presents with constipation, abdominal pain, polyuria and polydipsia.
- *Gonadotropic substances:* Tumor ectopically synthesizes estrogens which cause development of gynecomastia and testicular atrophy.

Gross Morphology

Tumor is lobulated and soft in consistency. Cut surface of this tumor has a white to tan appearance (Fig. 18.49).

Light Microscopy

- *Cell morphology:* Tumor is composed of small anaplastic oval to spindle cells with scanty cytoplasm and ill-defined borders, nuclear molding and inconspicuous nuclei. Nuclear chromatin is finely granular exhibiting *salt and pepper* pattern. *It shows 6 to 7 mitoses per high power fields.*
- *Cells arrangement:* These cells are arranged in sheets, cords, or small aggregates that exhibit neither squamous nor glandular differentiation.
- *Necrosis:* Extensive necrosis is often seen in Fig. 18.50.

Immunohistochemistry

Panel of markers is used to analyze expression in small cell carcinoma on histopathological sections. These comprise **chromogranin, synaptophysin, Leu7** and **neuron-specific enolase** (specific marker) (*see* Fig. 18.48).

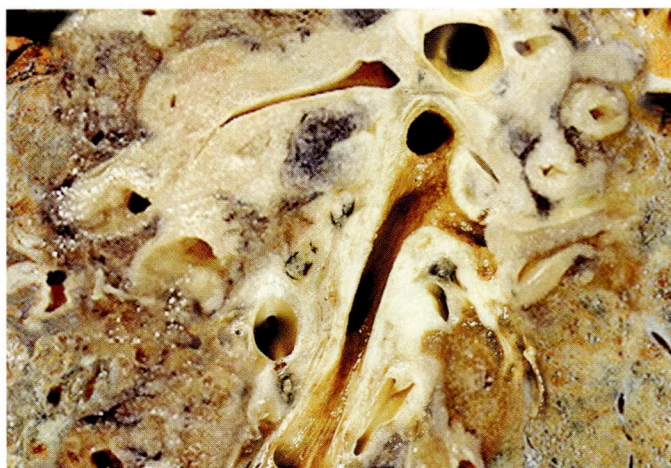

Fig. 18.49: Small cell lung carcinoma. This most aggressive tumor arises centrally, spreads extensively along the bronchi. It often metastasizes widely before the primary tumor mass in the lung reaches a large size leading to bronchial obstruction and lung collapse. The cut surface of this tumor has a soft, lobulated, and white to tan appearance. Black rounded areas represent hilar lymph nodes with metastatic carcinoma. It is usually treated by chemotherapy rather than radiotherapy or surgery. Prognosis is very poor.

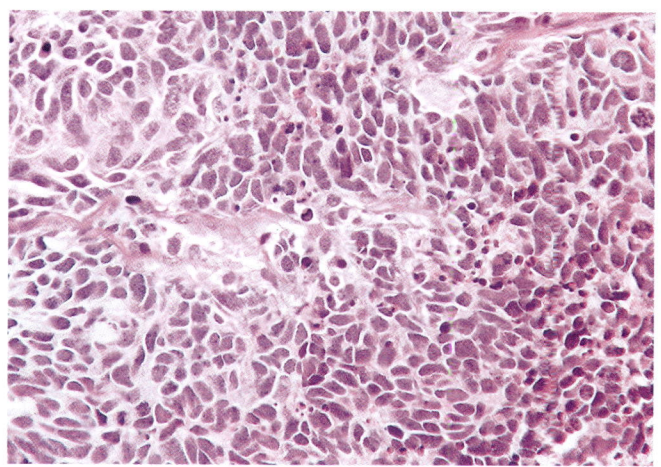

Fig. 18.50: Small cell carcinoma. It is composed of small dark blue cells with minimal cytoplasm (400X).

Electron Microscopy

Dense-core neurosecretory granules 100 nm are present in tumor cells in 66% cases. The granules are similar to those found in the neuroendocrine Kulchitsky cells scattered along the bronchial epithelium particularly in fetus and neonates. These neurosecretory granules synthesize ectopic polypeptide hormones.

Mode of Spread

- *Direct spread:* Tumor appears as a perihilar mass that spreads along the bronchi in the circumferential manner. Hence, it does not obstruct the bronchus lumen. On reaching a large size, it may cause bronchial obstruction and lung collapse.
- *Lymphatic route:* It spreads to hilar tracheobronchial lymph nodes with extension to mediastinal lymph nodes in >50% of cases. It may also involve cervical lymph nodes.
- *Hematogenous spread:* Approximately 66% cases have metastasized to extranodal location at time of diagnosis. It metastasizes to adrenal gland, liver, brain, bone, spinal cord, kidneys, and pancreas. Adrenal gland involvement is usually asymptomatic (Table 18.34).

Therapeutic Correlation

Small cell carcinoma grows rapidly and spreads so quickly that is generally treated with **chemotherapy** (most effective) and radiation alone, surgery has no chance to eradicate the tumor.

Targeted chemotherapies for lung cancer include the use of biologically engineered monoclonal antibodies that kill cancer cells.

Prognosis

It is the most aggressive type of lung cancer and has the worst prognosis, i.e. 12 weeks without treatment.

Table 18.34: Sites of metastases from lung cancers

Location	Frequency
Hilar tracheobronchial lymph nodes	80%
Extrathoracic lymph nodes (mediastinum and cervical region)	66%
Liver	50%
Adrenal glands (asymptomatic)	50%
Bone	30%
Kidney	25%
Brain	20%
Spinal cord	Uncommon
Pancreas	Uncommon

SQUAMOUS CELL CARCINOMA LUNG

Squamous cell carcinoma is the most common variant of lung cancer also known as *epidermoid carcinoma* affecting 55–75 years of age group. It accounts for 25–40% of cases. It is strongly associated with **tobacco smoking**. Squamous dysplasia is precursor lesion for squamous cell carcinoma.

- *Origin:* It arises from **basal cell** of major bronchi in majority of cases in hilar portion of chest; and bronchioles in a few patients.
- *Growth:* Endobronchial growth caused bronchial obstruction. It then invades bronchial wall and then adjacent lung parenchyma or blood vessels. *Atelectasis, bronchiectasis and consolidation are common.* Tumor appears as solitary hilar mass. **Central necrosis** and **cavitation** are more common than with other cell types.
- *Symptoms:* Endobronchial growth of tumor causes early symptoms. It is detected on sputum cytological examination before being radiographically visible. It metastasizes late, hence has relatively good prognosis. Risk factors, gene mutations, clinical manifestations, immunohistochemistry and metastases of squamous cell carcinoma of lung are shown in Fig. 18.51.

Etiology

- *Cigarette smoking:* Cigarette smoking is important cause of lung cancer, i.e. small cell lung carcinoma and squamous cell carcinoma.
- *Asbestosis:* Adenocarcinoma (most common) and squamous cell carcinoma are asbestos related lung cancers in 34% cigarette smokers. Asbestos fibers act as promoter in carcinogenesis.
- *Ionizing radiation:* Japanese are at increased risk of lung cancers (squamous cell carcinoma, adenocarcinoma and small cell carcinoma) after atom bomb explosion in Hiroshima and Nagasaki.
- *Uranium miners:* Uranium exposure emits particulate products and radon gas. Inhalation of particulate

products may cause lung cancer after 17 years of exposure.
- *Metals:* Metal refining and smelting processes of nickel, chromium, arsenic, cadmium exposure result in lung cancer.

Molecular Genetics

Proto-oncogenes participate in normal cellular growth and development. Tumor suppressor genes inhibit this process. When proto-oncogenes undergo mutations, they are referred as *oncogenes*. Tobacco smoking harbors genetic abnormalities, i.e. chromosomal deletions involve tumor suppressor loci of 3p, 9p and 17p. Chromosome 3p and 9p deletions involving site of CDKN2A gene in 65% of cases. Chromosome 17p deletion involves TP53 gene. TP53 gene mutation is demonstrated in squamous dysplasia in 10–50% and squamous cell carcinoma in 60–80% of cases. FGFR1 gene encoding fibroblast growth factor receptor tyrosine kinase is overexpressed in squamous cell carcinoma. Her 2neu is overexpressed in 30% of cases. Gene mutations in squamous cell carcinoma of lung are shown in Fig. 18.51.

Gross Morphology
- Tumor is solid with cut surface pale white to tan, firm in consistency. Large tumors are necrotic, granular giving cheesy appearance as seen in tuberculosis.
- Hilar tumors are solid in central located tumor. Peripheral tumors are small, far away from pleura and showing cavitation.

Light Microscopy
- Well differentiated squamous cell carcinoma is composed of polygonal cells forming nests with hyperchromatic angular nuclei, pink cytoplasm with distinct cell borders.

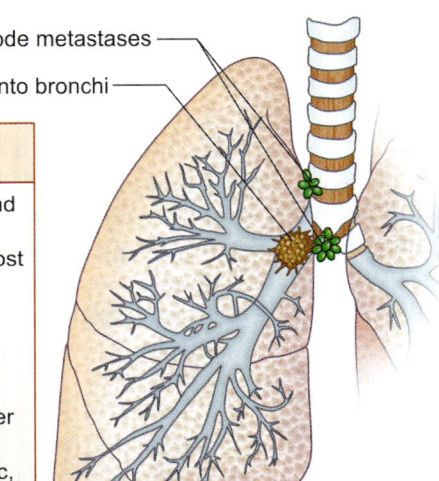

Risk factors of squamous cell carcinoma
- Cigarette smoking (squamous and small cell carcinoma)
- Asbestosis [adenocarcinoma (most common) and squamous cell carcinoma]
- Ionization radiation (squamous, small cell carcinoma, adeno-carcinoma)
- Uranium miners (lung cancer after 17 years)
- Metals (nickel, chromium, arsenic, cadmium exposure results in lung cancer)

Clinical features of squamous cell carcinoma
- Cough (75% cases)
- Hemoptysis (<50% cases)
- Dyspnea (pleural effusion, phrenic nerve invasion)
- Hoarseness of voice (recurrent laryngeal nerve involvement)
- Superior vena cava syndrome
- Cardiac tamponade
- Paraneoplastic syndrome (PTH-related protein causing increased serum calcium; gonadotropin leading to gynecomastia and testicular atrophy)
- Lung manifestations (bronchial obstruction, collapse, pneumonia, bronchiectasis and lipid pneumonia)

Gene mutations in squamous cell carcinoma of lung		
Genes	Examples	Frequency
Oncogenes	FGFR1	80%
	Her2 neu	30%
Tumor suppressor genes	p53 gene	60–80%
	RB gene	15%

Immunohistochemistry of squamous cell carcinoma	
Marker	Expression
p40, p63 and cytokeratins	Positive
Carcinoembryonic antigen (CEA)	Positive
Epithelial membrane antigen (EMA)	Positive
Cytoplasmic and intranuclear surfactant	Positive

Sites of metastases from lung cancers			
Location	Frequency	Location	Frequency
Hilar tracheobronchial lymph nodes	80%	Bone (pathological fracture)	30%
Extrathoracic lymph nodes (mediastinum and cervical region)	66%	Kidney	25%
		Brain (epileptic siezures)	20%
Liver	50%	Spinal cord	Uncommon
Adrenal glands (asymptomatic)	50%	Pancreas	Uncommon

Fig. 18.51: Squamous cell carcinoma of lung shows risk factors, gene mutations, clinical manifestations, immunohistochemistry and metastases.

- It displays intercellular bridging and keratin pearls, which appear as a small round nest of brightly eosinophilic aggregates of keratin surrounded by concentric (*onion skin*) layers of squamous cells (Figs 18.52 and 18.53).
- Basaloid variant of squamous cell carcinoma has poor prognosis.

Immunohistochemistry
Panel of markers is used to analyze expression in squamous cell carcinoma on histopathological sections (*see* Fig. 18.51).

Clinical Features
Patient with squamous cell carcinoma may present with history of cough (75%), hemoptysis (<50%), severe chest pain (40%), dyspnea (20%) wheeze, stridor, hoarseness of voice, weight loss, paraneoplastic syndrome (ectopically secrete PTH-related protein resulting in hypercalcemia).

- *Cough:* It is common presentation (75%) in lung cancer involving central airways.
- *Hemoptysis:* It occurs in <50% of patients at initial presentation (Table 18.35). It occurs due to hemorrhage from a tumor located in central airways.
- *Severe chest pain:* It suggests invasion of chest wall with intercostal nerves. Brachial plexus is involved in pancoast tumor located in apical portion.
- *Dyspnea:* Patient develops dyspnea due to loss of functioning lung parenchyma, invasion of lymphatics and pleura (massive pleural effusion). Hemorrhagic pleural effusion indicates invasion of pleura.
- *Digital clubbing:* It occurs due to reactive periosteal changes in the underlying bones in non-small cell lung cancers (e.g. squamous, adenocarcinoma, and large cell carcinomas). Mechanism is unknown. It may resolve with excision of the primary lesion.
- *Invasion of mediastinum:* Patient may develop hoarseness of voice due to involvement of recurrent laryngeal nerve supplying vocal cords, dysphagia due to invasion or extrinsic pressure on esophagus and superior vena cava syndrome. Obstruction of the superior vena cava leads to venous congestion in head and neck.

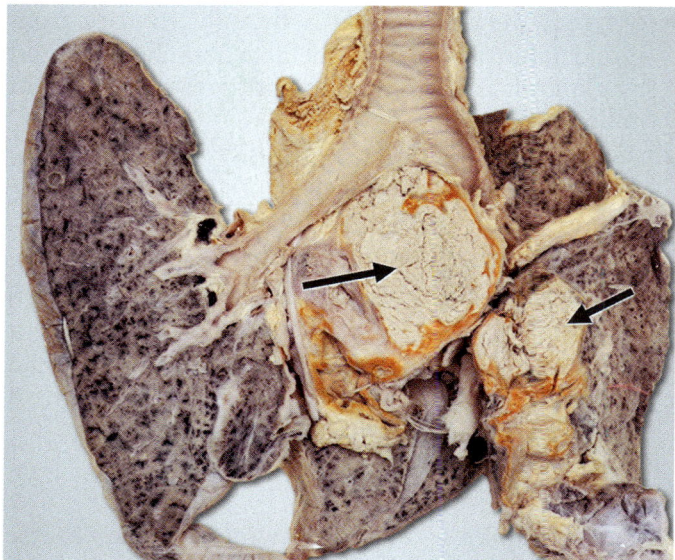

Fig. 18.52: Squamous cell carcinoma of lung. It is arising centrally and obstructing the left main bronchus. The neoplasm is very firm and has a pale white to tan cut surface (arrows).

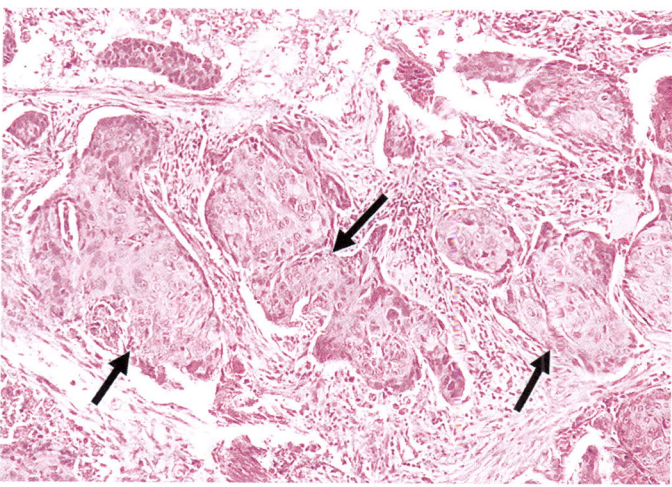

Fig. 18.53: Squamous cell carcinoma of lung showing well differentiated polygonal tumor cells with pink cytoplasm with distinct cell borders and intercellular bridges. The nuclei are hyperchromatic and angular with many mitoses (arrows) (400X).

Table 18.35: Causes of hemoptysis

Etiology	Disorders
Inflammatory lesions	Tuberculosis*
	Bronchiectasis*
	Pneumonias*
Neoplastic lesions	Primary lung cancers*
	Metastatic lung cancers*
	Bronchopulmonary adenoma
Other lesions	Pulmonary embolism and infarction*
	Mitral stenosis
	Left ventricular failure
	Anticoagulant therapy
	Bronchial adenoma
	Idiopathic pulmonary hemosiderosis

*Most common causes of hemoptysis are tuberculosis, bronchiectasis, pneumonias, bronchogenic carcinoma, pulmonary embolism and infarction.

- *Difficulty in respiration:* Phrenic nerve invasion causes paralysis of diaphragm.
- *Cardiac tamponade:* Tumor may cause erosion of major blood vessels and produce massive bleeding in pericardial cavity.
- *Lung lesions:* Patient with squamous cell carcinoma obstructing the bronchial lumen becomes symptomatic earlier. Complete bronchial obstruction may lead to pneumonia, bronchiectasis, lung collapse and lung abscess. Partial bronchial obstruction results in emphysema. Lipoid pneumonia occurs due to accumulation of cellular lipid in foamy macrophages especially obstruction caused by lung cancer.
- *Paraneoplastic syndrome:* It ectopically secretes PTH-related protein resulting to hypercalcemia. Patient presents with constipation, abdominal pain, polyuria and polydipsia.
  Serum calcium levels are increased. Gonadotropin synthesized by tumor leads to development of gynecomastia and testicular atrophy.

Pancoast Tumor

Apical primary lung cancer (usually squamous cell carcinoma) is known as *Pancoast tumor* can involve structures of the neck. It may invade cervical sympathetic chain (Horner's syndrome), brachial plexus and ribs.

- *Horner's syndrome:* Involvement of the cervical sympathetic chain causes Horner's syndrome (e.g. ptosis-drooping of upper eyelid, enophthalmos (sunken eyes), miosis (constriction of pupil), and anhidrosis (loss of sweating) on the affected side.
- *Brachial plexus injury:* Apical tumor in superior sulcus may destroy brachial plexus.
- *Chest wall invasion:* Apical tumor in superior sulcus may destroy neighboring ribs.

Mode of Spread

- *Direct spread:* It appears as a perihilar mass that spreads along the bronchi in the circumferential manner. Hence, it does not obstruct the bronchus lumen. On reaching a large size, may cause bronchial obstruction and lung collapse.
- *Lymphatic route:* It spreads to hilar tracheobronchial lymph nodes with extension to mediastinal lymph nodes in >50%. It may also involve cervical lymph nodes.
- *Hematogenous spread:* Approximately 66% cases have metastasized to extranodal location at time of diagnosis. It metastasizes to adrenal gland, liver, brain, bone, spinal cord, kidneys, and pancreas. Adrenal gland involvement is usually asymptomatic.

Therapeutic Correlation

Most often it is treated surgically. It responds to radiotherapy.

ADENOCARCINOMA LUNG

Adenocarcinoma is the most common lung cancer in elderly women. Its association with tobacco smoking is relatively weak. It accounts for 20 to 40% of all lung cancers. It is most common lung cancer in the United States. Early metastases are common. Tumor is present in peripheral region of lung most often on **upper lobe** in 75% of cases. *Speculated appearance of the tumor is demonstrated on radiograph.*

- *Origin:* Adenocarcinoma is thought to arise from bronchial or alveolar epithelium and characterized by glandular differentiation with presence of mucin in the tumor cells.
- *Cell population:* Cell population may comprise columnar cells, goblet cells, Clara cells or mucous glands. Tumor shows glandular differentiation with presence of mucin in the tumor cells.
- *Invasion:* Invasion of lung parenchyma is most often present.
- *Metastases:* Early metastasis is more common than squamous cell carcinoma especially to central nervous system and adrenal glands.

Location

Adenocarcinoma is a slow growing irregular tumor measuring <4.0 cm in diameter in peripheral or central regions of lung. Large tumor may completely replace the entire lobe of the lung. It is often associated with fibrosis. It may arise in relation to pre-existing pulmonary fibrosis.

- *Peripheral subpleural mass:* Approximately 75% of patients present as a peripheral subpleural solitary nodule in peripheral region. It is often associated with pleural fibrosis and subpleural scars, now recognized as desmoplastic response to tumor.
- *Central endobronchial growth:* In a few cases, adenocarcinoma originates within major bronchi in the central region of upper lobes. Tumor grows as endobronchial growth invading bronchial cartilage.

Etiology

Ionizing radiation may cause lung cancer. Japanese are at increased risk of lung cancers (squamous cell carcinoma, adenocarcinoma and small cell carcinoma) after atom bomb explosion in Hiroshima and Nagasaki.

Molecular Genetics

Gene mutations in adenocarcinoma of lung are shown in Table 18.36.

Table 18.36: Molecular genetics in adenocarcinoma of lung

Gene mutations	Examples
Oncogene mutation	K-RAS oncogene EGFR oncogene (80%) *ERBB2 (Her2 neu)* oncogene (30%) ALK ROS MET RET

Gross Morphology

Tumor measures 2–5 cm in diameter. Cut section is gray white and glistening depending on amount of mucin production.

Light Microscopy

There are four histological variants of adenocarcinoma of lung: acinar, papillary, solid and bronchoalveolar variants.
- Tumor cells are arranged in acinar, papillary, micropapillary, and solid containing mucin.
- Well differentiated adenocarcinoma is composed of tumor cells forming glandular elements

Histochemistry

Mucin production present in tumor cells may be demonstrated by **mucicarmine, alcian blue** and **periodic Schiff stain** (Figs 18.54 and 18.55).

Immunohistochemistry

Panel of markers is used to analyze expression in adenocarcinoma of lung on histopathological sections is shown in Table 18.37.

Mode of Spread

Early metastasis is more common than squamous cell carcinoma especially to central nervous system and adrenal glands. Sites of metastases from lung cancers via hematogenous route are may be demonstrated in hilar tracheobronchial lymph nodes, extrathoracic lymph nodes (mediastinum and cervical region), liver, adrenal glands (asymptomatic), bone, kidney, brain, spinal cord and pancreas.

Therapeutic Correlation

Patient with stage I adenocarcinoma confined to lung, who undergoes complete surgical excision has a 5-year survival (50 to 80%).

Differences between squamous cell carcinoma and adenocarcinoma of lung are shown in Table 18.38.

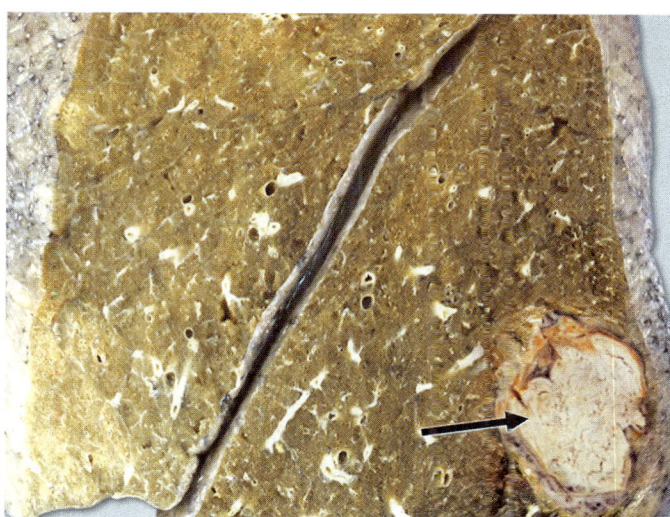

Fig. 18.54: Peripheral adenocarcinoma of lung. It tends to occur more peripherally in lung. It occurs more often in non-smokers and in smokers who have quit. Resection would have a greater chance for cure. The solitary appearance of this neoplasm suggests that the tumor is primary rather than metastatic (arrow).

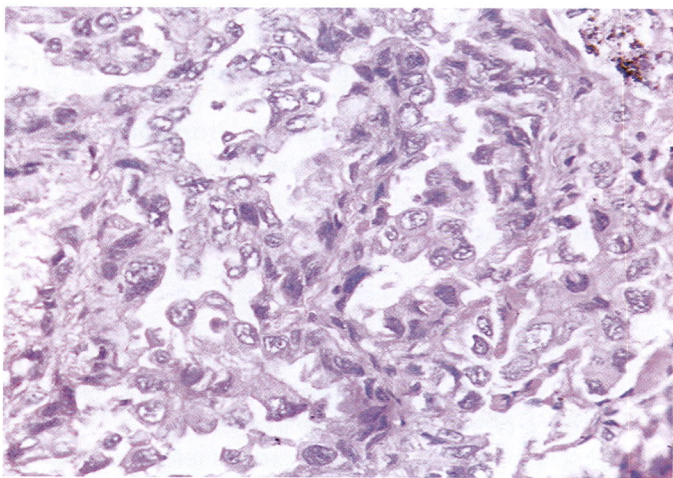

Fig. 18.55: Adenocarcinoma of lung is showing well differentiated adenocarcinoma (400X).

Table 18.37: Immunohistochemistry in adenocarcinoma of lung

Tumor marker	Expression
Cytokeratin (low molecular weight)	Positive
Epithelial membrane antigen (EMA)	Positive
Napsin A	Positive
TTF1 (Thyroid transcription factor)	Positive
Carcinoembryonic antigen (CEA)	Positive
B72.3 monoclonal antibody reacts with tumor-associated glycoprotein-72 (TAG-72)	Positive
Ber-EP4 monoclonal antibody reacts with glycoproteins of tumor cells	Positive
CD15 (LeuM1) monoclonal antibody reacts with tumor cells	Positive

Table 18.38: Differences between squamous cell carcinoma and adenocarcinoma of lung

Characteristics	Squamous cell carcinoma	Adenocarcinoma
Sex	Male	Female
History of smoking	Associated with smoking	Not associated with smoking
Location	Larger, more central	Tend to be more peripherally located
Growth rate	Rapid	Slow
Local spread	Predominant	Uncommon
Molecular genetics	FGFR 1 (80%), ERBB2 (*Her2 neu*) (30%), TP53 (60–80%), RB gene (15%), p16 and CDKN2K gene	K-RAS, FGFR 1, ALK, ROS, MET and RET genes
Distant metastases	Later stage	Early stage
Light microscopy	Well-differentiated carcinoma showing keratin pearls and intercellular bridges. May be poorly differentiated	Bronchial derived and bronchioloalveolar carcinoma
Immunohisto-chemistry	Cytokeratins, carcinoembryonic antigen (CEA), epithelial membrane antigen (EMA) and cytoplasmic and intranuclear surfactant	Cytokeratins, carcinoembryonic antigen (CEA), epithelial membrane antigen (EMA) and cytoplasmic, intranuclear surfactant, TTF 1 and CD15 (Leu M1)
Size	Larger	Smaller
Scarring	Absent	May be present

BRONCHIOLOALVEOLAR CARCINOMA

Bronchioloalveolar carcinoma is a well-differentiated subtype of adenocarcinoma. It arises from Clara cells present in nonciliated epithelium of terminal bronchioles and spread along the alveolar septa.

Recent Advances
Based on recent WHO classification of lung tumors, the previously designated bronchiolar carcinoma is classified as described under:
- Adenocarcinoma *in situ*: It refers to ≤3 cm tumor growth lacking invasion of stroma, lymphatic vascular or pleura. There is no growth pattern other than lepidic.
- Minimally invasive adenocarcinoma: It refers to ≤3 cm tumor growth with ≤5 cm area of stromal invasion or growth pattern other than lepidic.
- Invasive adenocarcinoma lepidic predominance: It refers to ≥3 cm tumor growth or invasion of lymphatic, vascular and pleura; or tumor necrosis area of >5 mm area of stromal invasion or growth patter other than lepidic.

There is no relationship to smoking. It affects patients of both sexes in all ages from the 20s to the advanced years of life. Noninvasive tumor characterized by lepidic growth has good prognosis. Diffuse or patchy ill-defined tumor showing consolidation has poor prognosis.

- *Noninvasive growth:* Tumor tends to occur in peripheral region of lung. Tumor spreads as a thin layer of cells using the alveoli or bronchial walls as a framework or scaffold in *lepidic pattern*. This pattern of growth does not invade lung parenchyma, pleura or blood vessels. It has excellent prognosis when localized with a 5-year survival rate approaching 100%.
- *Invasive growth*: The growth most often invades and destroys lung parenchyma. Prognosis is poor (Table 18.39).

Gross Morphology
Broncholoalveolar carcinoma has been divided into mucinous and nonmucinous types. Mucinous type has

Table 18.39: Differences between noninvasive and invasive bronchioloalveolar carcinoma

Parameters	Noninvasive tumor	Invasive tumor
Frequency	60%	40%
Growth	Poorly defined nodule	Diffuse or patchy consolidation due to mucus filled alveoli
Invasion of lung, pleura and blood vessels	Absent	Present
Imaging techniques	Pseudocavitation demonstrated in bronchogram	CT angiogram sign
Light microscopy	Lepidic pattern along alveolar and bronchial wall	Mucinous cell type
Prognosis	Excellent	Poor

a glistening appearance on gross examination. Patient presents with solitary coin lesion (>50%) or diffuse form mimicking lobar pneumonia consolidation.

Light Microscopy

Nonmucinous and mucinous subtypes of bronchioloalveolar carcinoma occur in equal numbers. These variants correlate with radiographic appearance.

- *Mucinous bronchioloalveolar carcinoma:* Tumor is composed of well differentiated tall columnar to cuboidal epithelial cells that spread along the framework of alveolar septa and project like papillary formations into the alveolar spaces. This pattern resembles butterfly sitting on fence, i.e. *lepidic pattern*.

  Tumor cells do not invade interstitium. Most tumors are well differentiated and tend to preserve the native septal wall architecture. A similar growth pattern may be seen in metastatic adenocarcinomas. Light microscopy of bronchioloalveolar carcinoma is shown in Fig. 18.56.
- *Nonmucinous bronchioloalveolar carcinoma:* It constitutes 66% of cases and comprises Clara cells and pneumocytes II, growing along alveolar walls. Differences between bronchioloalveolar carcinoma and atypical alveolar hyperplasia are shown in Table 18.40.

Clinical Features

Patient presents with copious watery sputum termed as *bronchorrhea* as a result of extensive mucin production, cough, and pain. Atelectasis and emphysema are infrequent.

Mode of Spread

Hematogenous spread: Approximately 66% cases have metastasized to extranodal location at time of diagnosis. It metastasizes to adrenal gland (50%), liver (30%), brain (20%), bone, spinal cord, kidneys and pancreas. Adrenal gland involvement is usually asymptomatic.

Imaging Technique

This tumor is discovered as a single nodule or multiple nodules or pneumonia-like diffuse infiltrate (ground glass opacities) on the radiograph.

Diffuse lesion may involve several lobes of lung or even bilateral with poor prognosis. After resection, tumor can appear in another lobe or opposite side.

Prognosis

Patient with solitary tumor in stage I has excellent prognosis with 5-year survival after surgical excision. Patient with tumor exhibiting diffuse pattern has poor outcome.

LARGE CELL CARCINOMA LUNG

Large cell carcinoma is peripherally located and accounts for about 10–20% of all lung cancers. It is characteristically aggressive and metastasizes early with fatal outcome. *It is strongly associated with cigarette smoking.* Patient presents as a mass >4 cm in diameter in peripheral region of lung in 60% of cases with early metastasis and poor prognosis.

Imaging Techniques

Radiological appearance is similar to adenocarcinoma except for its large size.

Gross Morphology

Tumor is large >4 cm in diameter.

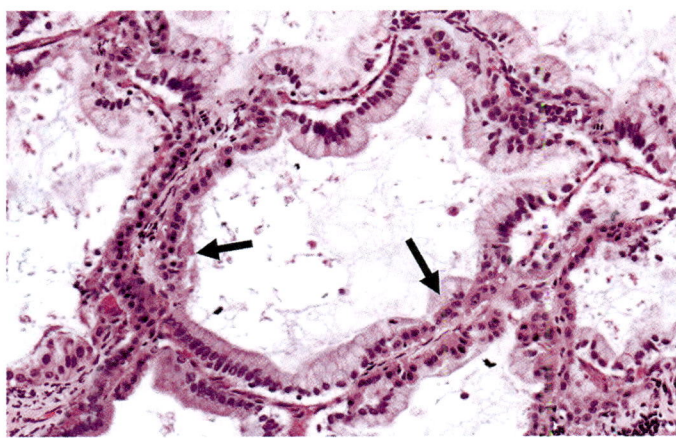

Fig. 18.56: Bronchioloalveolar carcinoma. It is composed of columnar cells that proliferate along the framework of alveolar septa. The cells are well differentiated. It has a better prognosis than most other primary lung cancers (arrows) (400X).

Table 18.40: Bronchioloalveolar carcinoma versus atypical alveolar hyperplasia

Parameters	Bronchioloalveolar carcinoma	Atypical alveolar hyperplasia
Size of lesion	5 mm	Small usually <5 mm
Clinical features	Gross lesion demonstrated on radiographs	Often unsuspected. Atypical hyperplasia may be found in histologic sections of grossly normal lungs
Morphology of cells	Monomorphic cells with mild atypical features	Polymorphic cells with mild atypical features

Light Microscopy

- *Classic variant:* It is composed of large cells with hyperchromatic nuclei and prominent nucleoli. There is minimal squamous or glandular differentiation. It does not express cytokeratin.
- *Tumor with neuroendocrine differentiation:* It is composed of tumor cells arranged in nests, trabecular, forming rosettes and palisading pattern. It suggests neuroendocrine differentiation on histochemical and electron microscopy.
- *Adenosquamous variant:* It has mixed histologic features of both adenocarcinoma and squamous cell carcinoma in 33% of cases. Patient presents with mass in the lung periphery and indistinguishable from adenocarcinoma or large cell carcinoma. *Metastases are common*. It has *aggressive behavior* with *poor prognosis*. Differences between various histological types of lung carcinoma are shown in Table 18.41.

SECONDARY PULMONARY MALIGNANT TUMORS

Pulmonary metastases are more common than primary lung cancers. In one-third of all fatal cancers, pulmonary metastases are evident at autopsy (Figs 18.57 and 18.58).

Morphology

Metastases are seen in lung parenchyma (most common), pleural cavity and lymphatics. Lymphatics may be diffusely involved, leading to the appearance of *lymphangitis carcinomatosa*.

Lung Metastases

Breast carcinoma is most common cause of lung metastases followed by colon cancer, and renal cell carcinoma. Other cancers metastasizing to lungs are salivary glands, thyroid gland, uterus, ovaries, urinary bladder and prostate (Tables 18.42 to 18.44).

Imaging Techniques

Lung metastases demonstrated by imaging techniques may be solitary, cannon balls, poorly differentiated, snow storm and diffuse alveolar patterns are shown in Table 18.45.

Coin Lesion in Lungs

Chest radiograph demonstrates solitary pulmonary nodule <5.0 cm or coin lesion in decreased frequency includes tuberculosis, histoplasmosis, primary lung cancer, bronchial hamartomas, amyloid deposits (pseudotumor), chondroma, lipoma and leiomyoma (*see* Figs 18.57 and 18.58).

DIAGNOSTIC TECHNIQUES

Imaging Techniques

These are chest radiographs, CT scan, MRI, bone scan and positron emission tomography described as under:

- *Chest X-rays:* A chest radiograph will detect most lung cancers.
- *Mediastinoscopy:* It is performed in case of involvement of mediastinum by lung cancer. It helps in evaluating the extent of the tumor.
- *CT scan:* It is most important investigation in suspected lung cancer. It helps surgeon to know, whether the lung cancer is resectable or not.

  Draining lymph nodes measuring >2 cm are likely to be involved due to metastases in 70%. Lymph nodes <1 cm are unlikely to be involved.

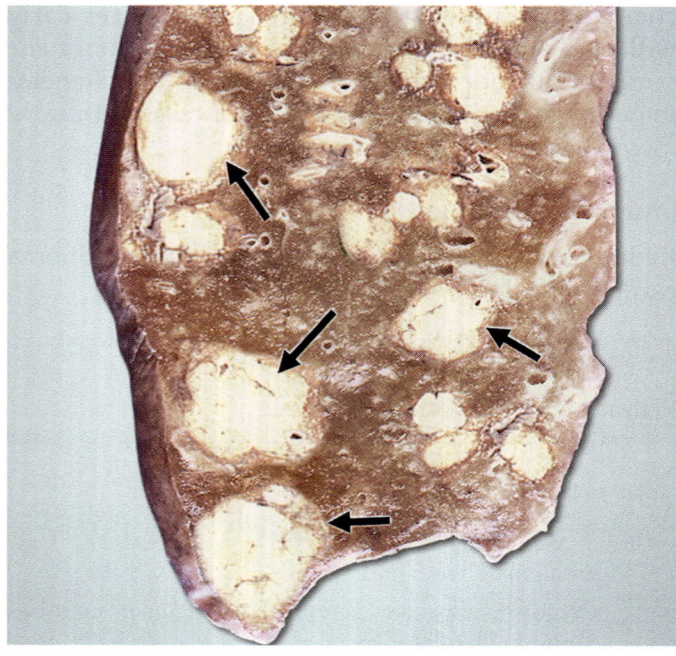

Fig. 18.57: Metastases in lung showing variable sized nodules (arrows).

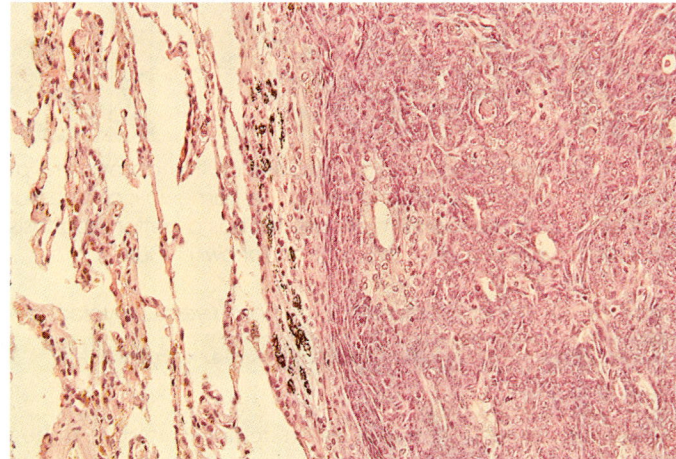

Fig. 18.58: Lung showing metastatic deposit from carcinoma (100X)

Table 18.41: Features of various histopathological variants of lung cancers

Parameters	Small cell carcinoma Lung	Squamous cell carcinoma Lung	Adenocarcinoma Lung	Bronchioloalveolar carcinoma	Large cell carcinoma Lung
Frequency	15–25%	25–40%	30–50%	10%	10–20%
Cell of origin	Neuroendocrine tumor (Kulchitsky cells)	Basal cells of major bronchi	Mucus producing glands near previous scar	Clara cells (nonciliated epithelium) of terminal bronchiole	Showing squamous and glandular differentiation on electron microscopy
Location in lung	Central	Central	Peripheral (75%), central (25%)	Peripheral	Peripheral (65%)
Tobacco smoking	Strong association	Strong association	Weak association	No association	Strong association
Growth rate	Very rapid	Slow	Slow to moderate	Slow	Rapid
Metastasis	Very early to mediastinum or distal area of lung and widespread metastases	Localized metastasis not common or occurs late, usually to hilar lymph nodes, adrenals, liver	Early metastasis throughout lung and brain or to other organs	Late metastasis	Early and widespread metastasis to kidney, liver and adrenals
Molecular genetics	C-MYC, RB gene (80–100%) and p53 gene (50–80%)	EGFR (80%), ERBB2 (Her2 neu) in (30%), TP53 (60–80%) and RB gene (15%)	K-RAS, EGFR, ERBB2 (Her2 neu), p53 gene, RB and p16 gene	K-RAS, EGFR, ERBB2 (Her2 neu), p53 gene, RB and p16 gene	RB and p16 gene
Light microscopy	Small cells, scanty cytoplasm, hyperchromic nuclei (EM showing neurosecretory granules)	Well differentiated SCC with keratin	Tumor cells forming glandular pattern	Lepidic growth pattern or diffuse pattern	Anaplastic or neuroendocrine differentiation or adenosquamous variants
Immunohisto-chemistry	Chromogranin, synaptophysin, Leu7 marker, and neuron-specific enolase	p40, p63, cytokeratins, carcinoembryonic antigen, epithelial membrane antigen	Cytokeratin, epithelial membrane antigen, napsin-A, TTF1, carcinoembryonic antigen, B72.3 monoclonal antibody reacting with TAG-72, Ber-EP4, CD15 (LeuM1)	—	—
Paraneoplastic syndrome	ACTH, ADH parathormone related protein, gonadotropin	Parathormone-related protein, gonadotropin	Gonadotropin	Absent	Gonadotropin
Clinical behavior	Most aggressive wide distant metastasis at diagnosis	Rapidly growing tumor with cavitation with late metastasis, lung collapse, consolidation	Cavitation rare	Solitary coin lesion or diffuse mimicking lobar consolidation	Large bulky tumor <4 cm in diameter
Treatment	Combination chemotherapy, surgical resectability is poor	Surgical resectability is good, if stage I or II	Surgical resectability is good, if stage I or II; chemotherapy, radiation and surgery may be combined for stage III	Chemotherapy and surgical resection or lung	Radiotherapy is palliative but chemotherapy is of limited use

Table 18.42: Immunohistochemistry of primary tumors metastasizing to lung in adults

Primary cancers	Immunoprofiles
Breast carcinoma	ER, PR, *Her2 neu*, CK7, GCDFP-15 (gross cystic disease fluid protein-15), mammoglobulin, Ki-67, p53, CK5, NY-BR and E-cadherin
Renal cell carcinoma	Cytokeratin, vimentin
Colon carcinoma	CK20, CDX2
Thyroid carcinoma	TTF1, thyroglobulin, CA-125 cell surface glycoprotein (monoclonal antibody OC-125
Osteosarcoma	Vimentin
Ewing's sarcoma	CD99 (MIC2 specific marker), vimentin, nonspecific enolase (NSE), neurofilament and cytokeratin (low molecular weight)
Endometrium carcinoma type 1	p53, ER, PR, PTEN
Prostatic carcinoma	PSA (prostatic specific antigen), PSAP (prostatic specific acid phosphatase), PSMA (prostate specific membrane antigen), NXK3.1 and prostein
Non-Hodgkin's lymphoma B cell	LCA, CD10, CD19 and 20
Non-Hodgkin's lymphoma T cell	CD3
Choriocarcinoma	Human chorionic gonadotropin

Table 18.43: Immunohistochemistry of primary tumors metastasizing to lung in children

Primary cancers	Immunoprofiles
Rhabdomyosarcoma	Desmin, vimentin, myoglobin and myoD1

Table 18.44: Differences between primary and secondary tumors

Feature	Primary tumors	Secondary tumors
Lesion	Usually solitary	Usually multiple
Circumscribed	Poorly circumscribed	Sharply circumscribed
Cavitation	Usual	Unusual
Calcification	Usual	Extremely unusual. If calcification present, then it is indicative of chondrosarcoma and osteosarcoma

Table 18.45: Radiological appearances of metastatic deposits in lungs

Type of lesion	Cancers
Solitary lesions	Breast carcinoma,* colon carcinoma, renal cell carcinoma
Cannon ball multiple lesions	Breast carcinoma, colon carcinoma, renal cell carcinoma, testicular germ cell tumors, bone (osteosarcoma) and soft tissue sarcoma
Poorly differentiated multiple lesions	Breast carcinoma, choriocarcinoma
Snow storm pattern (multiple small nodules)	Breast carcinoma, thyroid carcinoma, urinary bladder carcinoma, prostatic carcinoma
Diffuse alveolar consolidation	Breast carcinoma, primary lymphomas (differential diagnosis pneumonias)

*On imaging study, breast carcinoma metastases in lung may show solitary multiple cannon balls, and multiple poorly differentiated nodules or diffuse alveolar consolidation. Multiple nodules are also demonstrated in Wegener's granulomatosis, rheumatoid lung disease, histoplasmosis and coccidioidomycosis.

- *MRI technique:* It is essential to evaluate metastases in brain, spinal cord and other organs.
- *Bone scan:* It is done to evaluate bone metastases.
- *Positron emission tomography:* Presence or absence of metastatic deposits in draining lymph nodes and remote organs (liver, adrenal glands and elsewhere) is critical to management of lung cancer.

Positron emission tomography with radiolabeled *fluorodeoxyglucose* (FDG-PET) and biopsy are essential diagnostic tools. The dye is taken up by all cells, but more avidity with cancer cells. Dye enters Krebs cycle but cannot complete, and accumulates in the malignant cells. A PET scan shows how well the lungs are functioning.

Fiberoptic Bronchoscopy

It is used to take biopsy from representative area from centrally located lung cancers (squamous cell carcinoma and small cell lung carcinoma).

Sputum Examination

Sputum cytology may reveal malignant cells in 85% cases but the false-negative rate is high. Asbestos bodies may be demonstrated in sputum during prolonged exposure to asbestos.

Bronchoalveolar Lavage

Saline is injected in to a lung segment down a bronchoscope. Saline is aspirated and examined for cells and organisms.

Biopsy

- *Bronchial biopsy:* Bronchoscope is introduced to take biopsy to diagnose neoplasia, sarcoidosis and allergic aspergillosis.
- *Transbronchial biopsy:* Forceps is advanced to lung periphery down bronchoscope to take biopsy sample. It is done to diagnose infections, diffuse lung disease and transplant monitoring.
- *Ultrasound or CT-guided percutaneous needle biopsy:* It is performed to take biopsy from localized mass lesions (lung cancer) under ultrasound/CT-guidance.
- *Open biopsy:* It is done in cases of chronic diffuse lung diseases of uncertain origin.

Gross Morphology and Light Microscopy

- Biopsy fixed in 10% formalin is processed in tissue processor. Sections are stained with hematoxylin and eosin.
- Diagnostic features to be reported with resected lung carcinomas include tumor margins, histological type, and grade, lymphatic and blood vessel involvement and staging.

Histochemistry

- Alcian blue, mucicarmine and PAS are used to demonstrate mucin in adenocarcinoma. Epithelial mucins are stained purple or dark blue color.
- Connective tissue mucins are stained as pale blue with alcian blue, but it does not stain with PAS.
- Approximately 75% of lung cancers show positivity with Kreberg's stain.

Immunohistochemistry

Primary lung cancer: Immunohistochemistry plays significant role in differential diagnosis of primary lung cancers described as under.

- *Neuron-specific enolase:* It is specific for neural crest cells of the neuroendocrine series, i.e. *small cell carcinoma*.
- *Cytokeratin:* Squamous cell carcinoma shows positivity for cytokeratin.
- *Carcinoembryonic antigen (CEA):* This is a glycoprotein of heterogeneous composition normally detected in the glycocalyx of fetal epithelial cells, particularly those of mucin-secreting glandular nature. It is mainly used for the differential diagnosis between *adenocarcinoma* (usually positive) and *mesothelioma* (usually negative).
- *B72.3 monoclonal antibody:* It is a monoclonal antibody reacts with a high molecular weight glycoprotein that has been named tumor-associated glycoprotein-72 (TAG-72).

  One of its most common applications is in the differential diagnosis between *mesothelioma* (in which it is usually negative) and *lung adenocarcinoma* (usually positive).
- *Ber-EP4 monoclonal antibody:* It is mainly used for the differential diagnosis between *adenocarcinoma* and *mesothelioma*.
- *Calretinin:* This is a calcium-binding protein. Its main use is in the differential diagnosis between *mesothelioma* (almost always positive except for the desmoplastic variant) and *lung adenocarcinoma* (usually but not always negative).
- *Centromere protein H (CENP-H):* This is one of the fundamental components of the human active kinetochore and is thought to be associated with tumorigenesis. *High CENP-H protein expression has been related to poor outcome in patients with non-small cell carcinoma of lung.*
- *CD15 (LeuM1):* This antibody has been found to react with lung adenocarcinoma. Its main use is in the differential diagnosis between *lung adenocarcinoma* (usually positive) and *mesothelioma* (usually negative).

Serum Tumor Markers in Primary Lung Cancers

Certain tumors liberate products (e.g. cell surface antigens, cytoplasmic proteins, enzymes and hormones) that can be detected in blood samples, thereby acting as tumor markers. Their utility is to confirm the diagnosis.

Blood biochemistry analysis is done to evaluate biochemical alterations in primary and secondary lung cancers. Serum tumor markers analyzed in diagnosing primary lung cancers are shown in Table 18.46.

- *Serum p53:* The p53 alteration is most often demonstrated in human cancer. The p53 protein overexpression is detected by p53 antibodies in 60–70% of lung

Table 18.46: Serum tumor markers analyzed in diagnosing primary lung cancers

Categories	Serum tumor markers	Associated malignancies
Oncofetal proteins	Carcinoembryonic antigen (CEA)	*Lung carcinoma (adenocarcinoma and anaplastic carcinoma)* Nonseminomatous germ cell testicular tumor Colon carcinoma Stomach carcinoma Pancreatic carcinoma Breast carcinoma
Hormones	Adrenocorticotropin hormone (ACTH)	*Small cell carcinoma of lung* Pancreatic carcinoma Neural tumors
	Antidiuretic hormone (ADH) and atrial natriuretic hormone (ANH)	*Small cell carcinoma of lung* Intratracheal neoplasm
	Parathyroid hormone related protein (PTHrP)	*Small cell carcinoma of lung* Squamous cell carcinoma Breast carcinoma Ovarian carcinoma Renal cell carcinoma Adult T cell lymphoma
	Gonadotropin	*Small cell lung carcinoma* *Squamous cell carcinoma of lung* *Adenocarcinoma of lung* *Large cell carcinoma of lung*
	Insulin ectopic hormone	Fibrosarcoma Mesenchymal sarcoma Hepatocellular carcinoma Cerebellar hemangioma Hepatocellular carcinoma Multiple myeloma Malignant lymphoma Liver carcinoma Prostatic carcinoma
Isoenzymes	Neuron-specific enolase (NSE)	Small cell carcinoma of lung Neuroblastoma
Mucins and glycoproteins	Cytokeratin fragment 21.1 (Cyfra 21.1)	Non-small cell lung carcinoma

cancers. The p53 can be used as a precocious marker of p53 alteration before clinical manifestations of lung carcinoma.

- *Serum carcinoembryonic antigen (CEA):* Elevated serum CEA level is demonstrated in patients with extrathoracic lung cancer (adenocarcinoma and anaplastic carcinoma) in 23% of cases.

  Serum CEA is also elevated in *colon, pancreas and breast cancers.*

- *Serum TTF1:* Its concentration is increased in adenocarcinoma of lung and thyroid carcinoma.

- *Serum combined NSE + ProGRP:* In the combined analysis of NSE + ProGRP, sensitivity and specificity in the diagnosis of small cell carcinoma is seen in >80% of cases.

- *Serum combined TSGF + SCCAg + CYFRA21-1:* In the combined examination of serum levels of TSGF + SCCAg + CYFRA21-1 sensitivity and specificity in the diagnosis of squamous cell carcinoma is demonstrated in >80% of cases.

Serum Tumor Markers in Metastatic Lung Cancers

Serum tumor markers analyzed in metastatic lung cancers are shown in Table 18.47.

Table 18.47: Serum tumor markers in metastatic lung cancers

Primary cancers	Immunoprofiles
Breast carcinoma	CA 15.3, CA 27.29, CEA, ER & PR, PS2, *Her2 neu*, p53, DNA ploidy, S phase and EGFR, BRCA gene, CK7, GCDFP-15 (gross cystic disease fluid protein-15), and mammaglobin
Renal cell carcinoma	Erythropoietin
Colorectal carcinoma	CEA and p53
Thyroid carcinoma	TTF1, thyroglobulin
Endometrium carcinoma type 1	ER, PR, PTEN
Prostatic carcinoma	PAP, PSA, DNA ploidy and IGFBP 2
Choriocarcinoma	Human chorionic gonadotropin

PLEURAL DISEASES

Serosal membranes are derived from the mesoderm. These form the visceral and parietal surfaces of pleural, pericardial and peritoneal cavities including tunica vaginalis.

Parietal layer is perforated by lymphatic lacuna that connect with the lymphatic channels, which drain the enclosed cavities. Maximum quantity of fluid is absorbed into the lymphatic channels.

PLEURAL EFFUSION

The pleural cavity contains a small amount of pleural fluid (<10 ml in a 70 kg man). Daily production of pleural fluid is 17 ml. Maximum quantity of fluid is absorbed into the lymphatic channels.

Fluid moves from parietal pleura to pleural space to lungs. Movement depends upon the balance of Starling pressures. Mechanism of formation of pleural fluid is shown in Fig. 18.59.

Causes

Excessive accumulation of fluid in pleural cavity occurs in settings of congestive heart failure, cirrhosis, pneumonia, cancers and coronary bypass surgery. Leading causes of pleural effusions are shown in Table 18.48.

Pathogenesis

Pleuritis (inflammation of the pleura) may result from the extension of any pulmonary infection to the visceral

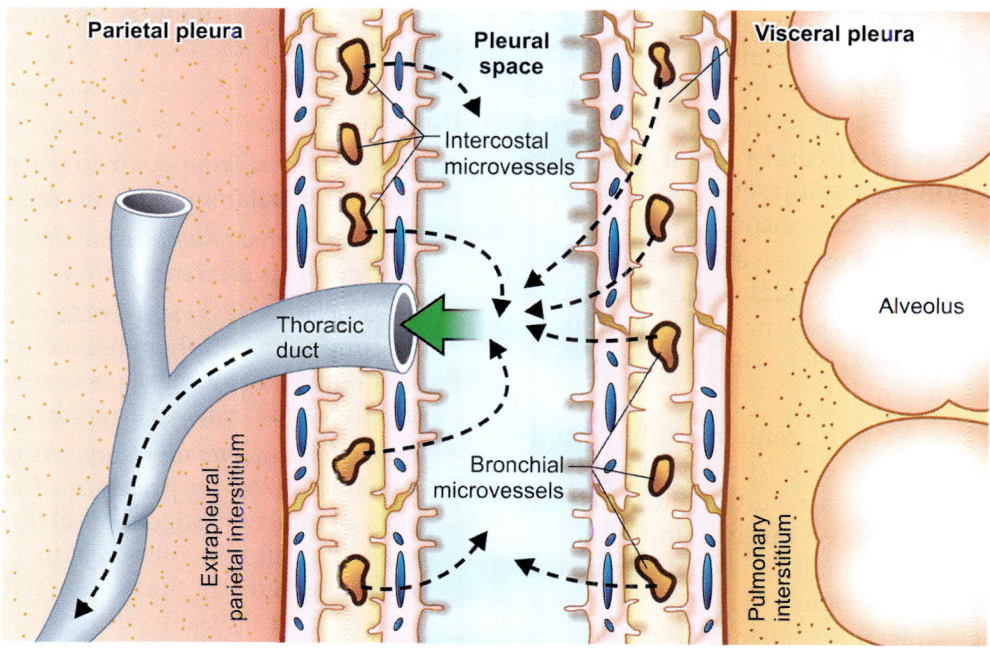

Fig. 18.59: Mechanism of formation of pleural fluid.

Table 18.48: Leading causes of pleural effusions

Etiology	Exudate	Transudate
Congestive heart failure	No	Yes
Cirrhosis	No	Yes
Pneumonia	Yes	No
Cancer	Yes	No
Viral disease	Yes	No
Coronary artery bypass surgery	Yes	No
Pulmonary embolism	Sometimes	Sometimes

pleura. Causes of pleuritis include bacterial infections, viral infections, and pulmonary infarction involving the surface of the lung.

- Pyothorax refers to a turbid effusion containing many neutrophils. Empyema is a variant of pyothorax in which thick pus accumulates within the pleural cavity, often with loculation and fibrosis.
- *Transudative effusions:* Decreased oncotic pressure or increased hydrostatic pressure causes transudative pleural effusions. Transudate is ultrafiltrate of plasma involving disturbances in Starling pressures. Abnormal accumulation of fluid occurs due to imbalance between hydrostatic pressure and or reduction in plasma oncotic pressure. The pleura usually remains normal.

    This is termed as transudative pleural effusion. Increased hydrostatic pressure in visceral pleura occurs in congestive heart failure. Nephrotic syndrome leads to decreased oncotic pressure.
- *Exudative effusions:* It most often results from pathological disorders of pleura resulting in increased vascular permeability and/or impaired fluid reabsorption (e.g. lymphatic obstruction). Increased vessel permeability of visceral pleural capillaries occurs due to pulmonary infarction, pneumonia, tuberculosis and metastatic cancers.

    Tuberculosis and malignancy are most common causes of pleural effusion. Exudate is rich in proteins and inflammatory cells. Obstruction of lymphatic drainage from the visceral pleura by lung cancer also causes pleural effusion.
- *Chylothorax:* Pleural cavity contains milky, lipid-rich turbid lymph fluid due to duct (lymphatic) obstruction. It occurs as a result of thoracic duct (lymphatic) obstruction or rarely lymphomas in the posterior mediastinum. It can be iatrogenic tear during surgery or pathologic.

    Pleural fluid triglyceride >110 mg/dl is diagnostic of chylous effusion. Repeated thoracocentesis leads to malnutrition and compromised immune system. Chylothorax is treated by pleuroperitoneal shunt, surgical ligation of thoracic duct, radiation therapy and chemical pleurodesis.
- *Pseudochylous effusion:* In rheumatoid lung disease, there is excessive accumulation of milky and turbid fluid in pleural cavity due to inflammatory process and necrotic debris.
- *Hydrothorax:* It refers to transudation of edema fluid into the pleural cavity. The elevation of hydrostatic pressure in patients with congestive heart failure causes transudation of edema fluid into the pleural cavity (i.e. hydrothorax).
- *Hemothorax:* It refers to accumulation of blood in the pleural cavity.
- *Urinothorax:* Unilateral pleural effusion is caused by ipsilateral obstructive uropathy.

Diagnostic Approach

Diagnostic approach includes detailed history, physical examination, imaging techniques, pleural fluid analysis and histopathological examination.

- Indications of thoracocentesis include significant pleural effusion of unknown etiology and unilateral pleural effusion persisting for three days.
- Investigative parameters of pleural effusions are physical appearance, smell, total proteins content, LDH, microbiological analysis, cytology, amylase, cholesterol triglyceride ratio, deaminase and PCR.

    Physical parameters of pleural fluid is shown in Table 18.49 and differences between pleural fluid exudates and transudate according to Light's criteria are shown in Table 18.50.

Light Microscopy

Smears prepared from centrifuged pleural fluid are examined for inflammatory and malignant cells.

- *Neutrophil predominant exudates:* Exudate-rich in neutrophils is seen in pyothorax.
- *Lymphocyte predominant exudates:* Exudate-rich in predominant lymphocytes include tuberculosis, lymphomas, chylothorax, sarcoidosis, acute lung rejection and coronary artery bypass surgery.
- *Eosinophil predominant pleural effusion:* Eosinophilia is characterized by presence of eosinophil count >10% of total nucleated pleural fluid cells. Etiology of eosinophil-rich pleural effusions is pneumothorax, benign asbestosis pleural disease, parasitic disease, fungal disease, drug-induced and Churg-Strauss syndrome.

Table 18.49: Physical parameters of pleural fluid

Parameters	Characteristic findings	Probable diagnosis
Color	Pale yellow	Classic paucicellular transudate
	Red (bloody)	Cancers, trauma, benign asbestos effusion, post-cardiac injury syndrome, pulmonary infarction
	Milky white	Chylothorax
	Brown	Amoebic liver abscess rupture, long-standing bloody effusion
	Black	Aspergillosis infection
	Yellow green	Rheumatoid pleurisy
	Green	Bilipleural fistula
Odor	Putrid	Anaerobic empyema

Table 18.50: Differences between pleural fluid exudates and transudate according to Light's criteria

Component	Pleural exudate	Pleural transudate
Pleural fluid/serum protein	>0.5	<0.5
Pleural fluid LDH/serum LDH	>0.6	<0.6
Pleural fluid LDH	>200 Units/L	<200 Units/L

PLEURITIS

Acute Pleuritis

Acute pleuritis is most often associated with bacterial pneumonia. Gram-positive bacteria are most often isolated.

Spontaneous bacterial pleuritis is occasionally seen in a case of cirrhosis. Autoimmune pleuritis may mimic infectious pleuritis.

PLEURAL FIBROSIS

Reactive Pleural Fibrosis

Reactive pleural fibrosis most often occurs as a consequence of prior inflammation or surgery. Pleural fibrosis occurs due to adhesion between parietal and visceral layers of pleura.

Pleural Plaques

Pleural plaques are formed on parietal layer of pleura. Chronic pleural effusions and exposure to asbestos produces raised, discrete, white to gray bilateral pleural plaques. Histopathological examination of pleural plaque shows paucicellular dense collagenous tissue.

Diffuse Fibrosis of Visceral Layer

Diffuse fibrosis of visceral layer occurs due to silicosis, advanced hypersensitivity reactions, connective tissue disorders and empyema.

Gross Morphology

Diffuse fibrosis of visceral layer is difficult to differentiate from desmoplastic mesothelioma.

Light Microscopy

Diffuse fibrosis of visceral layer does not infiltrate the subjacent soft tissue. On the other hand, mesothelioma invades the subjacent soft tissue.

MALIGNANT PLEURAL TUMORS

Diffuse Malignant Mesothelioma

Mesothelioma arises from mesothelial cells of pleura. It occurs in occupational prolonged exposure to asbestos for 30 to 40 years.

Oncogenic SV 40 virus has also been reported as etiological cause in some cases. Rare cases may be related to therapeutic radiation exposure. Widespread metastases can occur.

Pathology

Tumor begins as multiple small nodules on the parietal and visceral pleura encasing lung. It then invades the soft tissues of the chest wall and often extends into the mediastinum and encasing of the pericardial sac. Disease is lethal with 100% mortality.

Clinical Features

Patient with mesothelioma presents with dyspnea, chest pain, and pleural effusion, constitutional symptoms such as weight loss, weakness and fatigue.

Light Microscopy

- *Epitheliod mesothelioma:* Tumor is composed of bland cells with abundant eosinophilic cytoplasm arranged in sheet-like microglandular and tubulo-papillary patterns. In some cases, tumor may show more anaplastic features. Psammoma bodies are occasionally seen.
- *Sarcomatoid mesothelioma:* Tumor is composed of spindle cells arranged in haphazard pattern. Immunohistochemical analysis shows positivity for cytokeratin 5/6. Tumor showing osteosarcoma and chondrosarcoma differentiation express actin, desmin, vimentin and or S-100. Sarcomatoid mesothelioma has aggressive behavior.
- *Desmoplastic mesothelioma:* This variant is most often misdiagnosed as organizing pleuritis in small biopsy specimens. Tumor is composed of scattered atypical cells arranged in storiform pattern in >50% of cases. There is presence of dense collagenous fibers in the background of tumor cells.
- *Biphasic mesothelioma:* This variant comprise mixed epithelioid and sarcomatous patterns.
- By definition, each component should comprise at least 10% of the tumor (Figs 18.60 and 18.61).

Immunohistochemistry

Panel of markers is used to analyze expression in mesothelioma on histopathological sections (Table 18.51).

Immunohistochemistry analysis is done in differential diagnosis of lung adenocarcinoma and mesothelioma (Table 18.52).

Primary Pleural Effusion Lymphoma

Primary pleural effusion lymphoma presents as pleural effusion without an associated tumor mass. It is

Table 18.51: Immunohistochemistry of mesothelioma

Marker	Expression
Calretinin (calcium-binding protein)	Positive
WT1	Positive
Cytokeratin 5/6	Positive
Carcinoembryonic antigen (CEA)	Negative

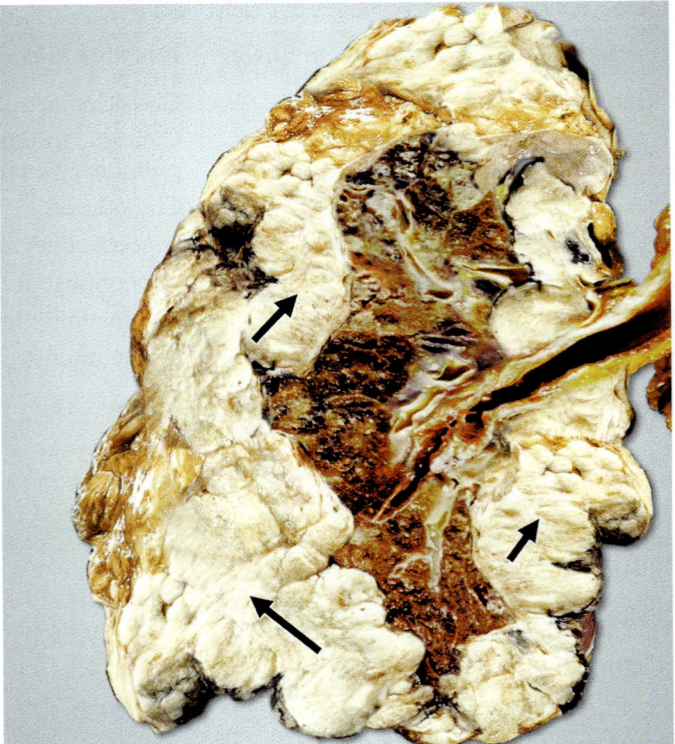

Fig. 18.60: Mesothelioma showing bulky dense white tumor arising from visceral pleura most often associated with prolonged asbestos exposure. Asbestos exposure more commonly predisposes to bronchogenic carcinomas. Smoking increases the 10 times risk for lung cancer (arrows).

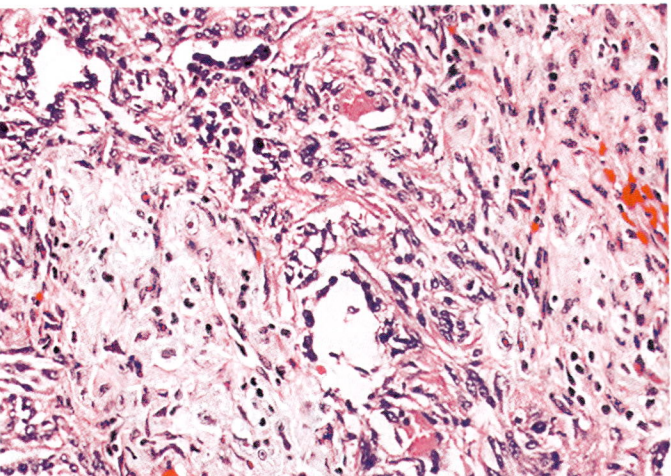

Fig. 18.61: Mesotheliomas showing plump rounded cells with abundant eosinophilic cytoplasm forming gland-like configurations (400X).

associated with human herpes 8 virus and acquired immunodeficiency syndrome. Immunohistochemical analysis reveals that primary pleural effusion lymphoma is of null phenotype, although occasional cases express B cell or T cell markers.

Table 18.52: Immunohistochemistry in differential diagnosis of lung adenocarcinoma and mesothelioma

Monoclonal antibodies	Adenocarcinoma lung	Mesothelioma
Carcinoembryonic antigen (CEA)	Positive	Negative
B72.3 monoclonal antibody	Positive	Negative
Ber-EP4 monoclonal antibody	Positive	Negative
CD15 (LeuM1) monoclonal antibody	Positive	Negative
Calretinin calcium-binding protein	Negative	Positive in mesothelioma except its desmoplastic variant

Pyothorax Effusion Lymphoma

This diffuse large B cell lymphoma arises from pleura in elderly persons, who have long-standing history of pyothorax in the settings of tuberculous pleuritis.

It is strongly associated with Epstein-Barr virus infection.

Immunohistochemical analysis of tumor shows positivity for B cell markers. CD20 is most often negative.

CHAPTER 19

Oral Cavity and Salivary Glands

Learning Objectives

ORAL CAVITY
- Overview
- Congenital Disorders
- Inherited Focal Disorders
- Inflammatory Disorders
- Tumors
- Epithelial Precursor Lesions

SALIVARY GLANDS
- Inflammatory Disorders
- Cystic Disorders
- Tumors of Salivary Glands

JAW
- Dental and Periodontal Disorders
- Cystic Lesions
- Odontogenic and Nonodontogenic Tumors

ORAL CAVITY

OVERVIEW

Oral cavity is lined by stratified squamous epithelium similar to skin. Epithelium of oral cavity varies in respect of keratinization. There are variations in the presence and absence of rete ridges. Rete ridges are absent from the floor of mouth. Rete ridges are well marked in the palate and gums.

CONGENITAL DISORDERS

Facial Clefts

Facial clefts are most common congenital disorders in the oral cavity about 1 per 800 live births. These occur due to failure of fusion of facial processes at 7th week of gestation. This gap is normally bridged by ectomesenchyme. According to recent studies, abnormalities of growth factors may be linked with these malformations.

Harelip

Harelip is the most common congenital defect of upper lip. On the 35th day of gestation, the frontal prominence fuses with the maxillary process to form the upper lip. It results from failure of fusion of the lower part of the median nasal process with the maxillary process. Disturbance in gene expression interferes with proper fusion resulting in cleft lip, with or without cleft palate.

In addition to multifactorial inheritance, developmental anomalies may occur due to teratogenic effects of rubella and anticonvulsants involving chromosomes. Harelip is unilateral in 80% of cases. About two-thirds of patients have left-sided harelip.

Cleft Palate

Cleft palate is less common congenital defect than harelip. It occurs in about 1 per 2500 live births. Unlike harelip, isolated cleft palate is more common in females. It occurs due to failure of fusion of facial processes due to multifactorial inheritance in which multiple genes interact with various environmental factors to produce disease.

It is more common in *Pierre Robin syndrome* characterized by small mandible. Backward displacement of chin and displaced small tongue posteriorly cause upper airway obstruction. Cleft palate may occur as part of trisomies 13 and 18.

Oral Cavity and Salivary Glands

Hemifacial Hypertrophy

Hemifacial hypertrophy is characterized by rapid growth of both hard and soft tissues on one side of the face. The teeth on the affected side and half of tongue with hypertrophied papillae may occur.

INHERITED FOCAL DISORDERS

Fordyce's Granules

Fordyce's granules are small yellowish-white granules located on the lateral aspect of the vermilion of the upper lip or surface of the buccal mucosa in normal adults with no clinical significance. These granules represent ectopic development of sebaceous glands.

Congenital Lip Pits

Congenital lip pits are small fistulae communicating the surface epithelium with underlying mucous glands. These are most often bilateral located on the lower lip. These may be isolated lesions or associated cleft palate, harelip and agenesis of second premolar teeth. Later may be inherited as autosomal disorder.

Endogenous Pigmentation

Endogenous melanin pigment may be deposited on lips, oral mucosa and circumoral skin in various disorders. These include neurofibromatosis, fibrous dysplasia of bone, Peutz-Jeghers syndrome, hemochromomatosis and Addison's disease. Peutz-Jeghers syndrome is characterized by pigmentation of the vermilion of the lips and small intestinal polyps.

Congenital Epulis

Congenital epulis refers non-neoplastic benign lesion of the gingivae especially in females. It is most often a reparative growth rather than a true neoplasm. On histopathological examination, lesion is composed of aggregates of large granular cells covered by well differentiated squamous epithelium. Electron microscopy suggests that lesion either originates from fibroblasts or perivascular pericytes. These cells are negative for S-100 protein.

White Sponge Nevus

White sponge nevus is an autosomal disorder characterized by shaggy, white patches on the oral and buccal mucosae. The thickened squamous epithelium becomes edematous that easily desquamate. Histopathological examination of lesion shows hyperplastic squamous epithelium, in which there is marked intracellular and extracellular edema.

INFLAMMATORY DISORDERS

Inflammatory disorders of oral cavity are caused by bacteria, viruses or fungi. Oral lesions may occur in various systemic disorders (Table 19.1).

Acute Necrotizing Ulcerative Gingivitis (Vincent Angina)

Acute necrotizing ulcerative gingivitis (Vincent angina) represents an infection by two symbiotic organisms; one is a fusiform bacillus, and the other is a spirochete (*Borrelia vincentii*). These organisms are found in oral cavity in normal persons. These organisms multiply under anaerobic conditions and cause tissue breakdown. Malnutrition promotes the risk of development of this order.

Clinical Features

Patient develops acute ulcerative necrotizing gingivitis in persons with decreased resistance to infection as a result of inadequate nutrition, immunodeficiency, or poor oral hygiene. The ulceration tends to spread and involving all gingival margins, which become covered by a necrotic pseudomembrane.

Table 19.1: Oral lesions in systemic disorders

Systemic disorders	Mechanism	Oral lesions
Pemphigus vulgaris	*Autoimmune disorder:* IgG antibodies directed against the intercellular area between keratinocytes	Vesicular lesions
Erythema multiforme	Hypersensitivity to sulphonamide drug	It involves oral mucosa (Stevens-Johnson syndrome)
Addison's disease	Adrenal gland disorder	Oral pigmentation
Amyloidosis	Amyloid deposition in tongue	Macroglossia
Lichen planus	Skin disorder	Fine, lacy white lines on the mucosal surface called *Wickham's striae*
Lead poisoning	Toxic effect	Lead line in oral mucosa

Ludwig Angina

Ludwig angina is potentially life-threatening inflammatory process. It is rapidly spreading cellulitis (phlegmon) in submaxillary or sublingual space. Normal oral bacterial flora is responsible for infection. These microorganisms cause cellulitis following extraction of a tooth, hairline fractures of lingual cortex of the mandible. By following the fascial planes, the infection may dissect into the parapharyngeal space, and from there, into the carotid sheath.

Exudative Pharyngitis

Patient with *Streptococcus pyogenses* develops exudative pharyngitis/tonsillitis in 20–30% cases. Patient presents with painful exudative lesions in the pharynx and tonsils.

Candida Albicans (Oral Thrush)

Candida albicans is a common surface inhabitant of the oral cavity, gastrointestinal tract, and vagina. Patient develops oral thrush including tongue (white pseudomembrane consisting of keratinous debris and yeasts). It most commonly occurs in debilitated infants, children, diabetes mellitus and AIDS in 40 to 90% of cases. About 5–10% of neonates are affected as a result of infection acquired during delivery. In more severe cases, extensive white pseudomembrane formation occurs.

Herpes Simplex Virus 1 Infection

The disease starts with painful inflammation of the affected mucosa, followed shortly by the formation of vesicles due to *ballooning degeneration* of the epithelial cells. Shallow ulcers are formed as a result of rupture of vesicles. The ulcers heal spontaneously without scar formation. It tends to recur with activation by trauma, sunshine, febrile illnesses or menstruation.

Age Group

It affects both children and young adults.

Clinical Features

Patient presents with fever, stomatitis (lips, oral mucosa), blisters on vagina (herpes vaginalis) and cold sores caused by herpesvirus type 1.

> **Light Microscopy**
> - Lesion shows intranuclear inclusion bodies in some epithelial cells.
> - There is presence of multinucleated epithelial cells with *ground glass* homogenized nuclei, often exhibiting nuclear molding at the edge of the ulcer.

Other Viral Infections

Patient with coxsackievirus A infection develops vesicular lesions in oral cavity, hand and feet.

Patient with Epstein-Barr virus infection presents with exudative pharyngitis, leukoplakia located on the lateral side of tongue in HIV positive patients.

Aphthous Stomatitis

Patient presents with recurrent painful erosive, recurrent solitary or multiple ulcerations in the mouth. It may or may not be associated with systemic diseases. Etiology is unknown. Light microscopy shows a shallow ulcer covered by a fibrinopurulent exudate.

TUMORS

SQUAMOUS CELL PAPILLOMA

It is the most common benign tumor of oral mucosa, most often seen on the tongue, lips, gingivae, or buccal mucosa.

SQUAMOUS CELL CARCINOMA

Approximately 95% of the cancers of the head and neck are squamous cell carcinomas. These most often occur in the oral cavity in older age group. Biologically, squamous cell carcinoma in oral cavity is similar to elsewhere in head and neck.

Locations

- Squamous cell carcinoma occurs in *lower lip, floor of mouth, tongue, the palatine* and *lingual tonsils*. Ventrolateral surface of tongue and floor of the mouth are the most frequent sites involved accounting for >50% of cases. Least affected sites are dorsum of the tongue and hard palate.
- Oral mucosa with thin non-keratinized squamous epithelium and poorly developed or absent rete ridges and narrow lamina propria are at greater risk of development of oral cancer. Locations of oral squamous cell carcinoma are shown in Fig. 19.1.

Pathogenesis

Combined abuse of oral tobacco, snuff-dipping or pan chewing and alcohol predispose to oral cancer. Leukoplakia may predispose to oral cancer. In 50% of cases, human papillomavirus (HPV-16) is the etiological agent in oropharyngeal squamous cell carcinoma.

Molecular Genetics

All cell lines derived from squamous cell carcinoma show multiple loss of chromosomes. Short arms of acrocentric chromosomes (13, 14, 15, 21 and 22) are deleted in 70% of cases. Cytogenetic changes in oral cancer are shown in Table 19.2.

Oral Cavity and Salivary Glands

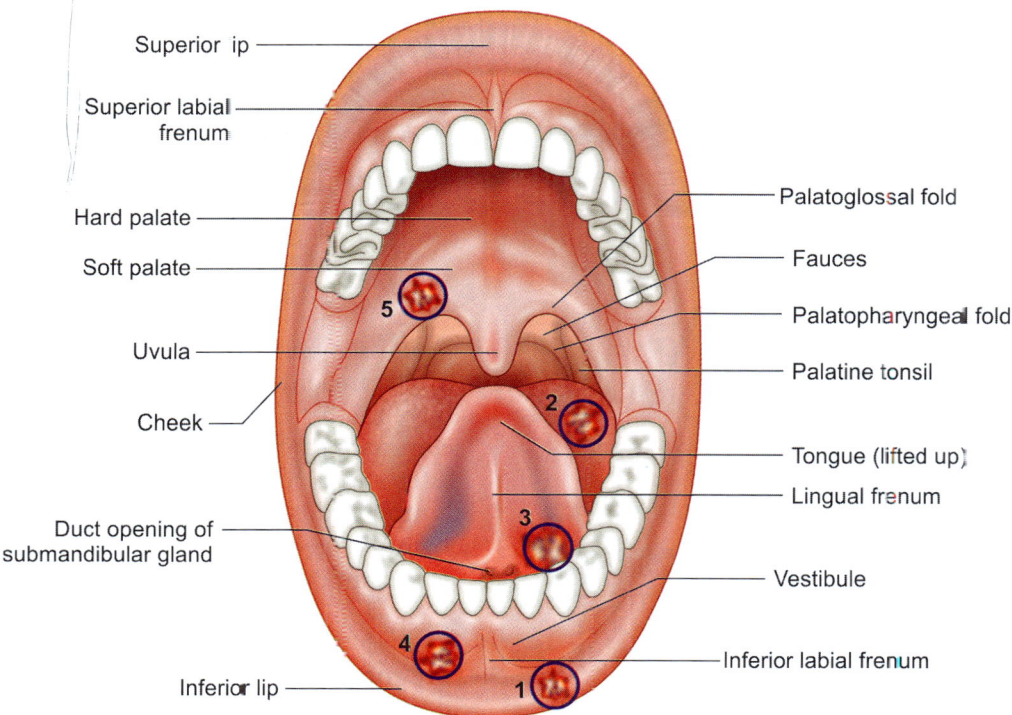

Fig. 19.1: Locations and frequency of oral carcinoma (1–5 most common to least common).

Table 19.2: Cytogenetic changes in oral cancer in descending order

Chromosomal abnormality	Frequency
Chromosome 18q	100%
Chromosome 10p	80%
Chromosome 8p	70%
Chromosome 3p	60%
Chromosome 9p	-
Chromosome 17p	-
Chromosome 4p	-
Chromosome 6p	-
Chromosome 13q	-
Chromosome 14q	-

Molecular Biology

It is a multistep process involving the sequential activation of oncogenes and inactivation of tumor suppressor genes in the clonal population of cells.

At the molecular level, amplification and overexpression have been observed in respect of epidermal growth factor receptor (EGFR), the apoptosis-inhibiting BCL2 gene. The high frequency of these aberrations suggests that these genomic alterations play an important role in the pathogenesis of oral squamous cell carcinoma.

- *Transition from normal to hyperplasia:* First change is loss of chromosomal 9p21 and 3p. Hypermethylation and loss of heterozygosity at this locus leads to inactivation of p16, an inhibitor of cyclin-dependent kinase.
- *Mild/moderate dysplasia to severe dysplasia:* Subsequent loss of heterozygosity at 17p with mutation of p53 tumor suppressor gene progresses to severe dysplasia.
- *Severe dysplasia to SCC:* Finally, amplification and overexpression of the cyclin D1 gene (located on 11q13) and genomic deletions of 4q, 6p, 8p, 13q and 14q progresses to squamous cell carcinoma.

Gross Morphology

It depends on stage of the presentation of oral cancer. Initial lesion is either opaque white or irregular warty areas. Later, the lesion undergoes ulceration. Ulcer has firm rolled edges and indurated bed.

Light Microscopy

- *Squamous cell carcinoma:* It ranges from well differentiated keratinizing to poorly differentiated, sometimes sarcomatoid to basaloid morphology. It may be slow to rapidly growing invading cervical lymph nodes. Low-grade well differentiated squamous carcinoma is associated with smokeless tobacco (Figs 19.2 and 19.3).

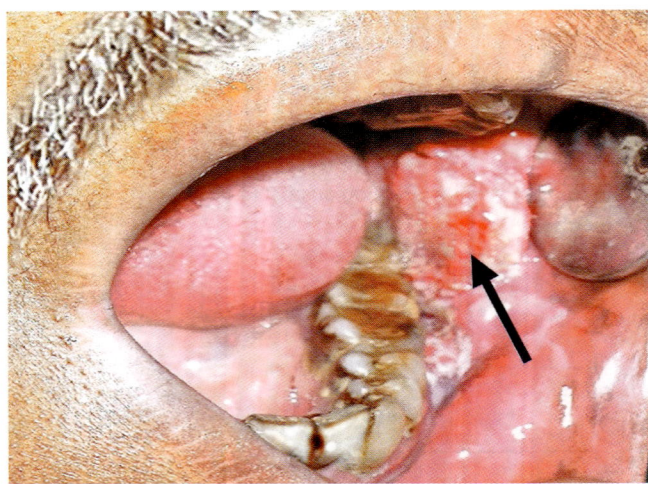

Fig. 19.2: Squamous cell carcinoma of lower lip (arrow).

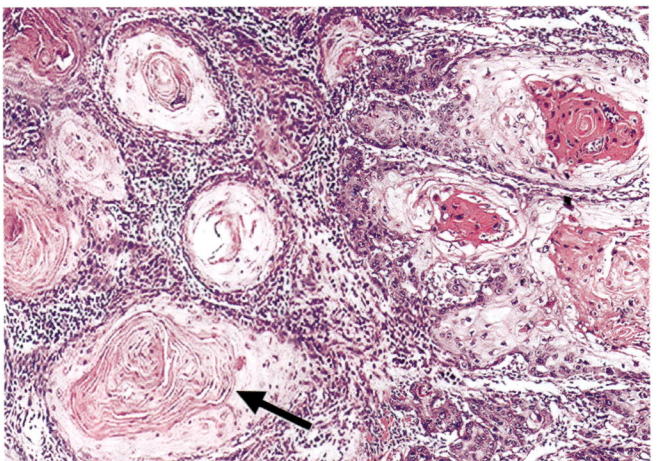

Fig. 19.3: Well differentiated squamous cell carcinoma (arrow) (400X).

- *Verrucous carcinoma:* It occurs in buccal mucosa and gums of lower jaw. Patient presents with bulky, soft, cauliflower-like growth that becomes infected giving foul smell.

  Light microscopy shows well differentiated carcinoma. Rete ridges are markedly thickened and growing down into underlying tissues in a characteristically bullous pattern. At a later stage, tumor invades stroma.

Immunohistochemistry

Panel of markers is used to analyze expression in oral squamous cell carcinoma on histopathological sections (Table 19.3).

Mode of Spread

- *Direct invasion:* Tumor has tendency to invade either deeply or widely within the subepithelial tissue. Invasion of mandible creates obstacle to complete surgical excision.

Table 19.3: Immunohistochemistry of oral squamous cell carcinoma

Markers	Differentiation of tumor	Expression
Cytokeratin 1, 10	Well differentiated keratinized SCC	Positivity
Cytokeratin 4, 13	Well differentiated non-keratinized SCC	Positivity
Cytokeratin 8, 18	Poorly differentiated SCC	Positivity

- *Lymphatic route:* Lymph node metastases are more often present at the time of clinical presentation in relation to oral carcinoma. Lymph nodes most commonly are seen in the submandibular region. At later stage, tumor may metastasize to mediastinal lymph nodes.
- *Hematogenous route:* Oral carcinoma may metastasize to distant organs such as lungs, liver and bones.

Prognosis

- Prognosis of oral carcinoma depends on location, depth of invasion, stage, histological grading, desmoplastic reaction, tissue eosinophilia, lymph node metastases and DNA ploidy.
- Presence of florid desmoplastic reaction in squamous cell carcinoma of lip is associated with increased incidence of metastases and aggressive behavior.
- Tumor infiltrated by eosinophils has favorable prognosis. Lymph node metastases are used in staging system. Extracapsular spread is an indicator of poor prognosis.
- The nondiploid tumors tend to be clinically more advanced than diploid tumors.
- Overexpression of p16 has favorable prognosis.
- Overexpression of p21 gene and TROP2, loss of H antigen and amplification of 3q26.3 is associated with poor prognosis.

KAPOSI'S SARCOMA

Kaposi's sarcoma occurs due to herpesvirus 8 in the oral cavity. It is most frequently associated with AIDS and located on the palate. It is locally aggressive endothelial tumor. Survival rate and staging are shown in Tables 19.4 and 19.5.

Table 19.4: Overall 5-year survival rate of oral carcinoma

Location	Survival rate
Lower lip	90%
Anterior aspect of tongue	60%
Posterior part of tongue, floor, tonsil, gum, hard palate	40%
Soft palate	20–30%

Table 19.5: Stage grouping of oral carcinoma

Stage	Tumor	Lymph node metastases	Distant metastases	5-year survival
Stage 0	Tis (Tumor in situ)	N0	M0	100%
Stage I	T1 (≤2 cm)	N0	M0	90%
Stage II	T2 (>2 to 4 cm)	N0	M0	77%
Stage III	T1, T2	N1 (≤3 cm)	M0	61%
	T3 (>4 cm)	N0, N1	M0	
Stage IVA	T1, T2, T3	N2 (>3–6 cm single or)	M0	32%
	T4a (Advanced invading tissue)	N0, N1, N2	M0	
Stage IVB	T4b	Any N	M0	25%
	Any T	N3 (>6 cm)	M0	
Stage IVC	Any T	Any N	M1	3.5%

Immunohistochemistry

Lining cells of vascular structures are positive for **CD31, CD34, podoplanin** and **nuclear expression** of **HHV8**.

Prognosis

Evolution of disease is modified by treatment that includes surgery radiotherapy and chemotherapy.

EPITHELIAL PRECURSOR LESIONS

Leukoplakia

Leukoplakia is a clinical term describing irregular white mucosal patches of oral mucosa. On clinical examination, lesion be homogenous, nodular, erythroplakia or proliferative verrucous leukoplakia. WHO criteria used in diagnosis of dysplasia are shown in Table 19.6.

Pathogenesis

It results from hyperkeratosis, usually secondary to chronic irritation. It is caused by oral tobacco products and excessive alcohol intake.

Pathology

Leukoplakia is usually benign. However, it may represent dysplasia (mild, moderate or severe) or carcinoma *in situ* progressing to squamous cell carcinoma. Oral intraepithelial neoplasia is categorized into grade I (mild dysplasia), grade II (moderate dysplasia) and grade III (severe dysplasia or carcinoma *in situ*). Biopsy is required to rule out squamous dysplasia or squamous cell carcinoma (Fig. 19.4).

Granuloma Pyogenicum

Granuloma pyogenicum (Fig. 19.5) is a reactive vascular lesion most commonly seen on tongue, lips, or buccal mucosa especially in pregnant women. Minor trauma to these tissues permits invasion of microorganisms.

Table 19.6: WHO criteria used in diagnosis of dysplasia

Histological architecture
Irregular epithelial stratification
Loss of polarity of basal cells
Drop-shaped rete ridges
Increased number of mitoses
Abnormally superficial mitoses
Premature keratinization in single cells (dyskeratosis)
Keratin pearls within rete ridges
Cytological features
Anisocytosis (variation in size)
Cellular and nuclear pleomorphism
Anisonucleosis (abnormal variation in nuclear size) with prominent nucleoli
Increased nucleocytoplasmic ratio
Atypical mitotic figures

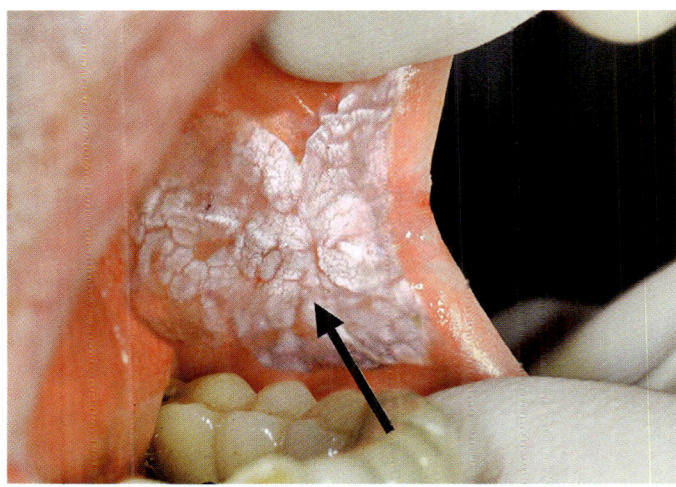

Fig. 19.4: Leukoplakia of the oral cavity (arrow).

Clinical Features

Patient presents with small <1.0 cm elevated, red or purple, soft mass, with a smooth, lobulated, ulcerated surface in the oral cavity most frequent on the gingiva.

Light Microscopy

Histopathological examination shows nodule composed of highly vascular granulation tissue that shows varying degrees of acute and chronic inflammation. This lesion later transforms to less vascular mass resembling fibroma.

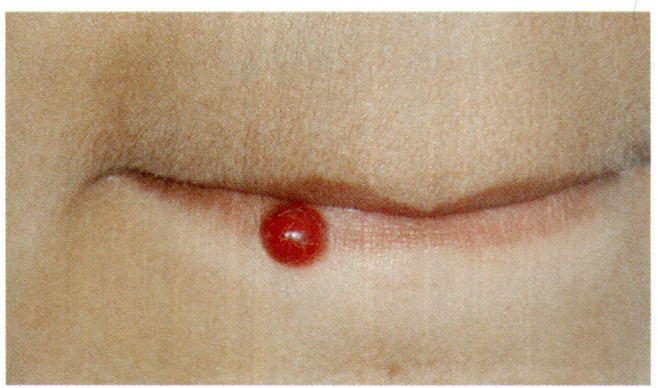

Fig. 19.5: Granuloma pyogenicum on the lip.

SALIVARY GLANDS

The salivary gland system comprises three pairs of major glands—parotid, submandibular and sublingual and many minor glands dispersed in the submucosa of oral cavity, lips, gingiva, floor of the mouth, cheek, hard and soft tongue, tonsillar areas and oropharynx (Figs 19.6 and 19.7).

The functional unit of salivary glands is the secretory acinus and related ducts, and myoepithelial cells. Acini may be serous, mucous or mixed.

The parotid gland is almost purely serous and the parenchyma is divided into lobules by fibrous septa.

The gland is divided into superficial and deep portions by the facial nerve. Each gland drains via a main duct (Stenson's duct) and enters into the mouth.

The submandibular glands are located in the groove between the lower jaw and tongue. These drain via Whartson's duct into the mouth.

The sublingual glands are situated in the sublingual tissue of the mandible. Each gland drains via Bartholin's duct into the mouth. In some cases, sublingual gland's main excretory duct joins the main submandibular duct.

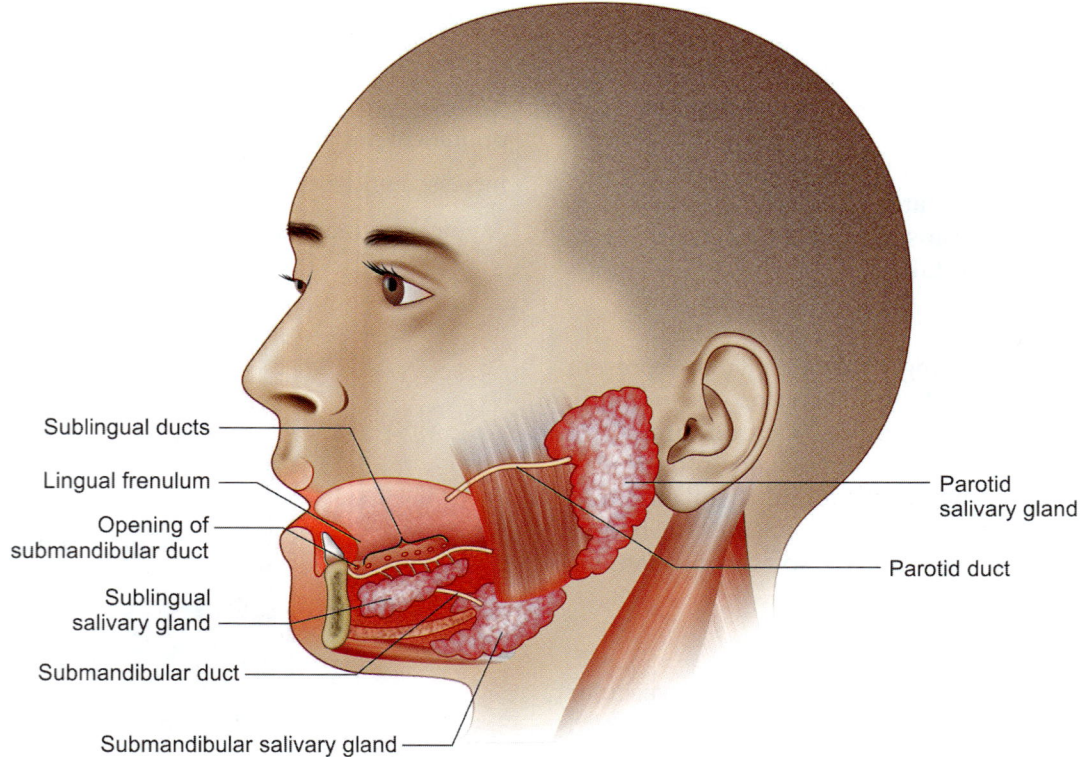

Fig. 19.6: Salivary glands.

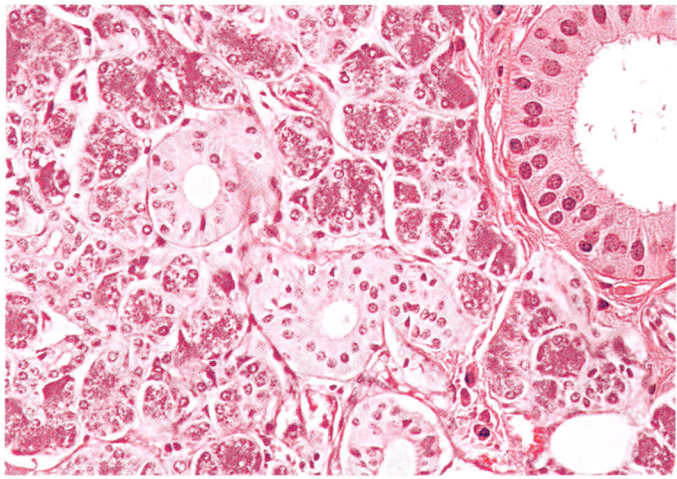

Fig. 19.7: Normal salivary gland (400X).

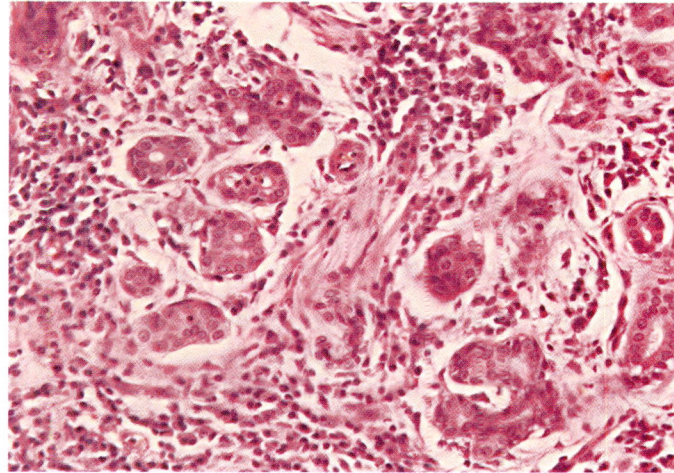

Fig. 19.8: Chronic sialadenitis.

INFLAMMATORY DISORDERS

Sialadenitis may be caused by infection (viral or bacterial), immune-mediated mechanisms, or occlusion of the salivary ducts by stones (sialolithiasis).

ACUTE SIALADENITIS

Acute sialadenitis is most often caused by bacterial or viral infection. Oral cavity is the source of bacterial infection. Bacterial sialadenitis occurs when saliva flow through the affected duct is decreased due to salivary calculi. Nowadays, acute sialadenitis is seen mainly in association with chronic xerostomia. Causative organisms include *Staphylococcus aureus* followed by *Streptococcus viridans*.

Clinical Features

Patient presents with painful enlargement of one or both salivary glands. Examination of the duct orifices may show the presence of pus discharging into the oral cavity. Acute sialadenitis leads to abscess formation.

> **Light Microscopy**
> It shows purulent exudate and bacterial colonies.

VIRAL SIALADENITIS

Mumps is the most common cause of deafness in 80% of cases among the postnatal viral infections. It causes bilateral parotitis with increased serum amylase most commonly in children <14 years of age. The incubation period is 16 to 18 days.

> **Light Microscopy**
> Surgical specimen shows infiltration by chronic inflammatory cells (Fig. 19.8).

Complications

These include orchitis (unilateral; no sterility risk), oophoritis, aseptic meningitis (most common extra-salivary complication) and pancreatitis with increased serum amylase.

AUTOIMMUNE SIALADENITIS

Autoimmune sialadenitis is relatively common. Sjögren's syndrome is a chronic inflammatory disease of the salivary and lacrimal glands. It is characterized by keratoconjunctivitis sicca (dry eyes), and xerostomia (dry mouth), due to lymphocytic infiltration and parenchymal destruction of the parotid and lacrimal glands. It may be associated with a systemic collagen vascular disease. Malignant lymphoma is a frequent complication.

Etiology

It is most likely of autoimmune origin associated with rheumatoid arthritis.

> **Light Microscopy**
> Parotid and lacrimal glands show infiltration by lymphocytes. Late in the course of the disease, the affected glands become atrophic, with fibrosis and fatty infiltration of the parenchyma.

Antibodies

Autoantibodies demonstrated in Sjögren's syndrome are anti-SS (Ro), anti-SS (La), rheumatoid factors, antisalivary gland and rheumatoid arthritis precipitinin.

CHRONIC OBSTRUCTIVE SIALADENITIS

Chronic obstructive sialadenitis most often occurs in the submandibular gland, producing a characteristic histological morphology.

> **Light Microscopy**
>
> Dilated ducts contain eosinophilic glycoproteins. Squamous metaplasia is demonstrated in ducts. There is expansion of interlobular connective tissue resulting in fibrosis. The acini shows marked atrophy. A mild to moderate chronic inflammatory infiltrate is seen.

CHRONIC RECURRENT PAROTITIS

Chronic recurrent parotitis occurs between the ages of 5–15 years. Girls are more commonly affected than boys. Patient presents with swelling, tenderness over parotid glands, fever and malaise lasting for 7–10 days.

> **Light Microscopy**
>
> Affected parotid gland shows acinar atrophy and fibrosis.

CYSTIC DISORDERS

MUCOCELE

This cyst-like pool of mucus, lined by granulation tissue, develops near a minor salivary gland. It results from mucus leakage caused by rupture of obstructed or traumatized ducts. Ranula is a large mucocele of salivary gland origin, characteristically localized to the floor of the mouth.

TUMORS OF SALIVARY GLANDS

Salivary gland tumors have diverse histopathology. These are relatively uncommon constituting 2–6% of all head and neck neoplasms. Their histological and behavioral diversity as well as their proximity to important head and neck structures that pose considerable management challenges.

Fine needle aspiration cytology is the popular method for diagnostic evaluation of salivary gland masses due to their superficial nature and easy accessibility for the procedure.

The majority of tumors of the parotid gland are benign; in contrast, about 50% of the tumors of the submandibular gland are malignant. Pleomorphic adenoma is the most common benign salivary gland tumor. Mucoepidermoid carcinoma is the most common malignant tumor of salivary gland. Recurrence after surgical removal is common, because remnants of tumor may be left behind.

Distribution

- *Parotid glands:* The majority of salivary gland tumors occur in the parotid gland (80%) overall. Approximately 80% tumors are benign and 20% malignant.
- *Submandibular glands:* Approximately 15% of tumors occur in submandibular glands. Tumors may be benign in 50% and malignant in 50% of cases.
- *Sublingual and minor salivary glands:* Approximately 5% of salivary glands tumor occur in these glands. Around 40% are benign and 60% are malignant.

Risk Factors

Irradiation is only etiologic factor of salivary gland tumors. Adults or children receiving therapeutic irradiation in head and neck are at greater risk of development of salivary gland tumors. An increase in the incidence of salivary gland tumors has also been reported amongst survivors of the nuclear bomb attacks on Hiroshima and Nagasaki in Japanese population.

A number of viruses has been implicated in the pathogenesis of salivary gland tumors. There is a strong association between Epstein-Barr virus (EBV) and lymphoepithelial carcinomas, but this appears to be largely restricted to Asian patients (Fig. 19.9).

Classification

WHO classification of salivary gland tumors is shown in Table 19.7. Salient features of malignant tumors of salivary glands are shown in Table 19.8.

Table 19.7: WHO classification of salivary gland tumors

Benign epithelial tumors	Pleomorphic adenoma; *monomorphic adenoma:* basal cell adenoma (most common in parotid gland), canalicular adenoma (minor salivary glands multifocal in origin), sebaceous adenoma, glycogen-rich adenoma and clear cell adenoma Warthin tumor (papillary cystadenoma lymphomatosum or adenolymphoma) Oncocytoma (oxyphilic), myoepithelioma, ductal papilloma
Malignant epithelial tumors	Mucoepidermoid carcinoma, adenoid cystic carcinoma, acinic cell carcinoma, adenocarcinoma, squamous cell carcinoma, carcinoma ex-pleomorphic adenoma, carcinosarcoma
Non-epithelial tumors	Capillary hemangiomas
Hematolymphoid malignancies	Hodgkin's disease, diffuse large B cell lymphoma, extranodal marginal B cell lymphoma
Secondary tumors	Uncommon tumors

Oral Cavity and Salivary Glands

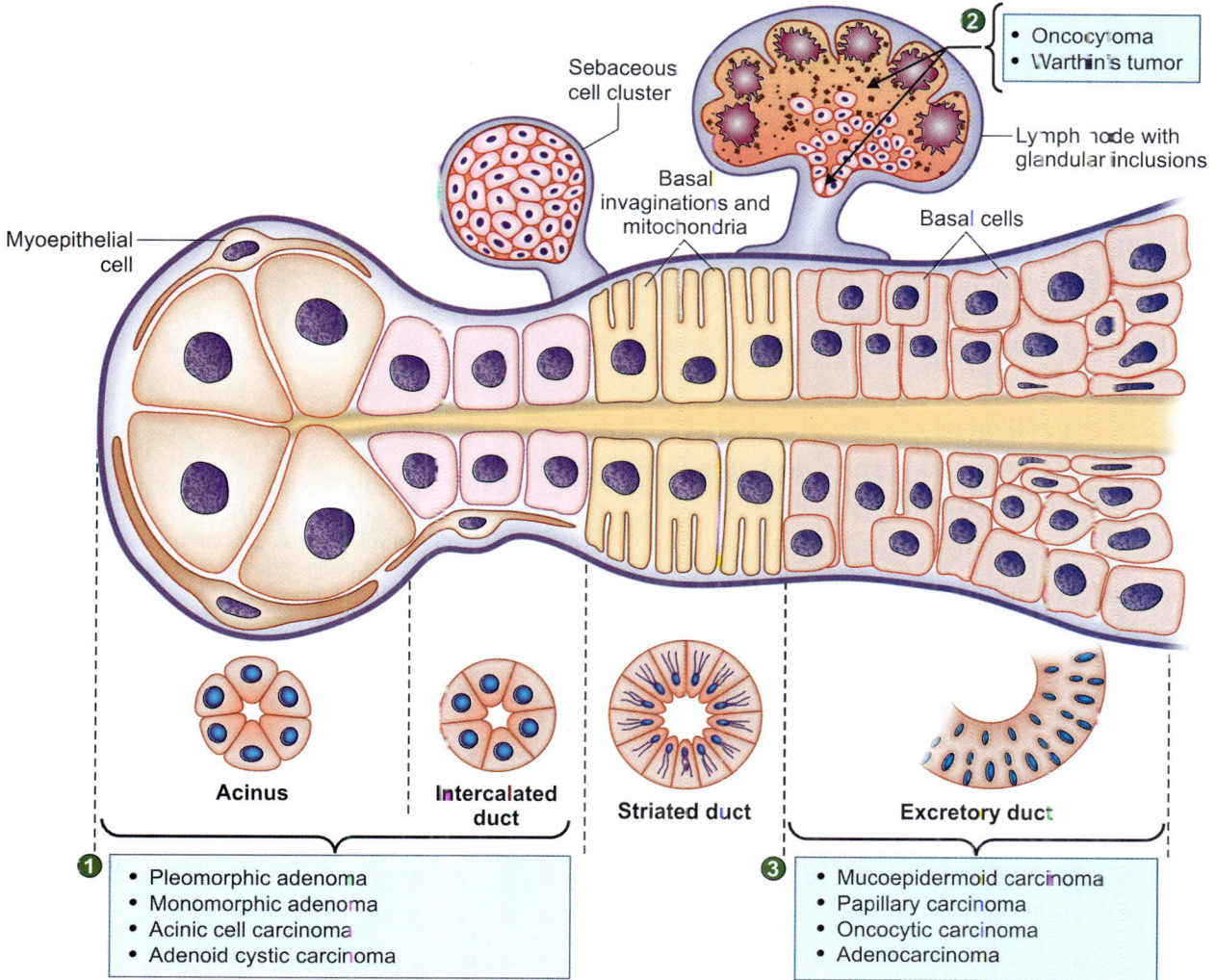

Fig. 19.9: Tumors of salivary glands.

Table 19.8: Salient features of important malignant tumors

Tumor	Sites	Age group	Molecular genetics	Features	Light microscopy	Markers
Muco-epidermoid carcinoma	Parotid and minor salivary glands	Young to elderly	Translocation 11q21, 19p13	Slow growing mass, spreads by direct invasion, lymphatic and hematogenous route	Low to high grade	MUC4 positivity better prognosis
Adenoid cystic carcinoma	Submandibular, minor salivary and parotid glands	5th decade	Losses of 12p, 6p23q, 13q21	Tumor invades perineural space	Cribriform or solid pattern	CEA, keratin, S-100 protein, muscle specific actin and KI-67
Acinic cell carcinoma	Parotid glands	5th decade	–	Clinical course variable, spreads via lymphatic and hematogenous route	Solid or papillary cystic or follicular pattern	The acinic cells show PAS positive diastase resistant granules. These cells are negative for mucin stains
Polymorphous low grade carcinoma	Minor salivary glands	4th decade	–	Mass in palate	Tumor cells forming glandular structures	Keratin, vimentin, S-100 protein, CEA, GFAP, muscle specific actin, EMA. Galectin-3 and BCL2

PLEOMORPHIC ADENOMA

Pleomorphic adenoma is commonest salivary gland tumor. It is slow growing painless mass. **Parotid gland** is the most common site followed by minor salivary glands. It was called mixed salivary gland tumor because the stroma showing areas mimicking cartilaginous differentiation.

It has a biphasic appearance, which represents an admixture of epithelial and chondromyxoid stromal elements. Mesenchymal chondroid areas occur due to metaplastic changes in the adenoma. It is rarely becomes malignant.

Age and Sex Distribution

It affects between 40 and 60 years of age. It is more common in women than men (4:1).

Location

It most frequently occurs in major salivary gland usually in superficial parotid gland above the facial nerve (90%) and deep part of parotid gland below facial nerve in 10% of cases. It also occurs in submandibular gland (45%) and minor salivary glands, e.g. palate, upper lip and mucosa (45%).

Molecular Genetics

Chromosomes 3p21, 8q12 and 12q13-15 rearrangements and the PLAG-1 and HMGI-C genes are demonstrated in pleomorphic adenomas.

Clinical Features

Patient presents with *slow growing, painless* and *firm nontender mass* in parotid gland. *Lateral palate is the most common site in minor salivary gland.* In all locations, small tumors are *nontender* and *mobile on palpation.* These may become fixed with advanced growth. *Facial nerve paralysis in association with pleomorphic adenomas almost never occurs,* even with extremely large tumors.

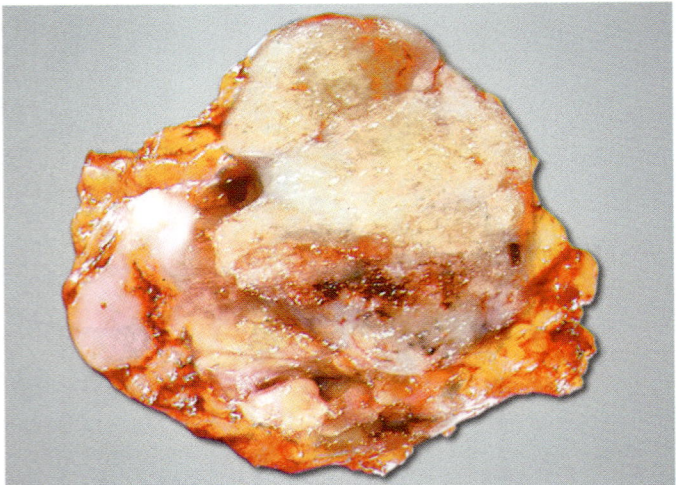

Fig. 19.10: Pleomorphic adenoma of parotid gland. The multilobulated appearance of this tumor is shown. It must be removed together with some surrounding parotid gland, or else some of the irregular projections around its margins will be left behind and the tumor will recur.

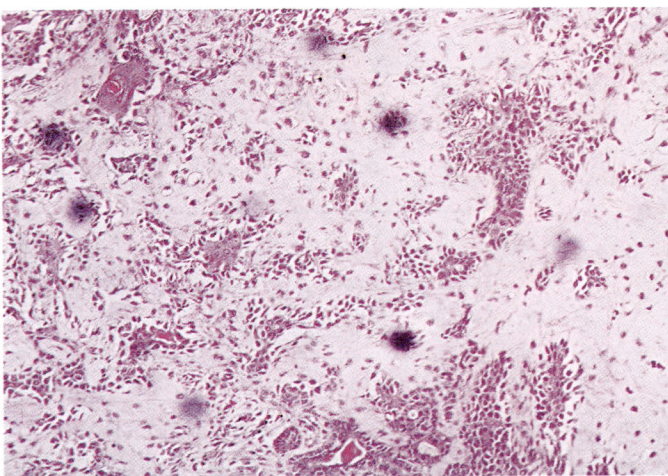

Fig. 19.11: Pleomorphic adenoma. It is composed of gland-like epithelial component surrounded by a myxomatous stroma often containing foci of bone or cartilage (100X).

Gross Morphology

- Pleomorphic adenoma in parotid gland is *encapsulated smooth* or *lobulated tumor,* clearly demarcated from the surrounding normal salivary gland.
- The tumor often shows small projections. If the tumor is enucleated, these projections are left behind resulting in recurrence of tumor after excision.
- Cut surface is *solid, rubbery and containing areas of gelatinous myxoid stroma.*
- Pleomorphic adenoma arising in minor salivary glands is never encapsulated (Figs 19.10 and 19.11).

Light Microscopy

There is considerable variation in the histologic features within single tumor. Therefore, multiple samples are necessary to study the complete morphology of the tumor. Tumor may be composed of epithelial and stromal component in varying proportions.

- *Epithelial component:* Epithelial component is believed to originate from intercalated ducts. Tumor is composed of gland-like epithelial component surrounded by a myxomatous stroma often containing foci of bone or cartilage. Epithelial cells are arranged in nests, solid sheets, some forming duct-like structures.

> - *Stromal component:* These epithelial cells are embedded in chondromyxoid stroma. The stroma shows accumulation of basophilic material with the staining reaction of connective tissue mucins. The myxoid stroma may be bulky invaded by stromal cells.

Malignant Potential

Malignancy in pleomorphic adenoma encompasses these entities: carcinoma ex pleomorphic adenoma and carcinosarcoma. *Staining for Her2 neu can be used to detect early carcinoma in a pleomorphic adenoma.* Carcinosarcoma has poor prognosis.

Metastasizing Pleomorphic Adenoma

Metastasizing pleomorphic adenoma is defined as a histologically benign pleomorphic adenoma that manifests local or distant metastases in multiple organs such as bone, lung, lymph nodes and rarely kidneys.

Therapeutic Correlation

Often, the tumor is difficult to remove completely because of its proximity to the facial nerve, and it is likely to recur after resection due to tumor spillage in the wound. Recurrence of pleomorphic adenoma represents local growth and does not reflect malignancy.

WARTHIN'S TUMOR

Warthin's tumor accounts for 8% of all tumors in the parotid glands. It is a multicentric tumor, also known as papillary cystadenoma lymphomatosum or adenolymphoma. The term adenolymphoma should not be confused with any form of lymphoma. This is monomorphic adenoma with heavy lymphocyte infiltrate in the stroma. Recurrence after excision of tumor is rare. Rarely, squamous cell carcinoma or lymphoma may arise from this tumor.

Origin

It most often occurs in parotid glands. It arises from hydrotropic salivary duct epithelium within the immediately subjacent lymph node or it may be due to cystic changes of the epithelium in the inflammatory infiltrate.

Age and Sex Predilection

It is the only tumor of the salivary glands that is more common in men (especially smokers) than in women. It generally occurs after the age of 30, with most arising after age 50 years. Bilateral tumors occur in 10% of cases.

Molecular Genetics

Translocations of chromosomes 11q21 and 19p13 in Warthin tumor.

Clinical Features

Patient presents with slow growing painless firm or rubbery or nodular mass. A few patients may present with rapidly growing tumor associated with pain or pressure symptoms.

Imaging Technique

Radionuclide scanning (Tc 99m) is helpful in patients with Warthin's tumor and oncocytoma.

> **Gross Morphology**
> - Tumor forms soft well circumscribed encapsulated brown mass usually located superficially within the parotid gland.
> - Cut surface shows irregular multiple cysts of variable diameter containing variably viscous fluid.
> - The lymphoid component makes up the solid areas of the tumor (Figs 19.12 and 19.13).

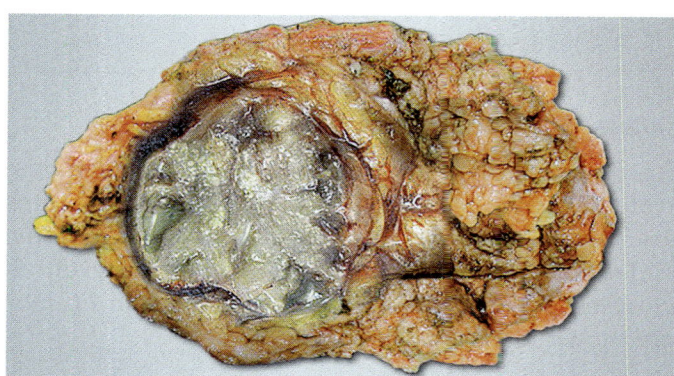

Fig. 19.12: Warthin's tumor (adenolymphoma) of the parotid gland. Cut surface of this benign tumor is multicystic. The cysts are filled with mucus. It is the second most frequent tumor of the parotid gland, after pleomorphic adenoma.

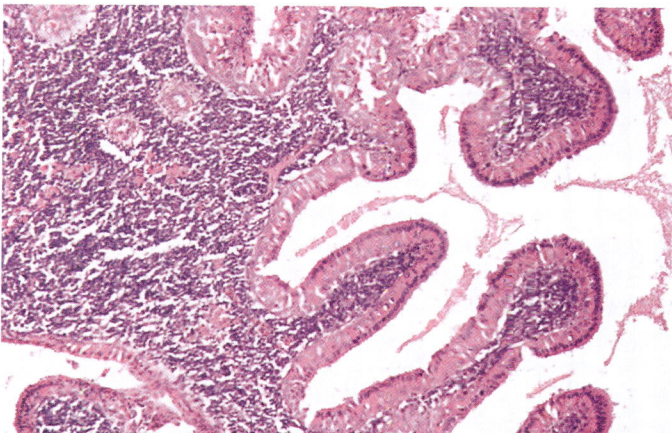

Fig. 19.13: Warthin's tumor is composed of mixture of epithelial and lymphoid elements. Clefts and cysts are lined by pink staining double layer epithelium. These epithelial cells are forming papillary projections into cystic glandular spaces embedded in dense lymphoid tissue (400X).

Light Microscopy

Tumor is composed of mixture of epithelial and lymphoid elements.

- *Epithelial element:* Clefts and cysts are lined by pink staining double layer epithelium. Inner layer consists of tall columnar cells with granular cytoplasm (oncocytes) towards the luminal aspect lining the cystic spaces. Outer layer is composed of cuboidal cells along the basement membrane. Electron microscopy reveals presence of large number of mitochondria accounting for the granular cytoplasm, suggesting common feature for oncocytes in all epithelial tissues.
- *Stromal lymphoid tissue:* These epithelial cells are forming papillary projections into cystic glandular spaces embedded in dense lymphoid tissue. The stroma contains florid lymphoid infiltrate in which some normal lymphoid follicles with germinal centers are present. The cyst fluid has a characteristic 'motor oil' quality.

Differential Diagnosis

It is worth mentioning that oncocytes are also demonstrated in oncocytic tumors. Lymphoid aggregates are demonstrated in lymphoepithelial cyst, chronic sialadenitis and Sjögren's syndrome. Differences between pleomorphic adenoma and Warthin's tumor are shown in Table 19.9.

Therapeutic Correlation

It is treated by surgical resection with preservation of facial nerve.

ONCOCYTOMA

Oncocytoma is rare benign salivary gland tumor affecting elderly men and women. Recurrence rate is low after surgical excision (Fig. 19.14).

Site of Origin

It is mainly located in parotid gland (80%), submandibular gland (10%) and rest in minor salivary glands (palate, buccal mucosa or tongue).

Clinical Features

Patient presents with *slow growing painless, firm, mobile nontender mass* in superficial lobe of parotid gland.

> **Gross Morphology**
> Tumor is homogenous with a smooth surface. It may be divided into lobules by fibrous septae.

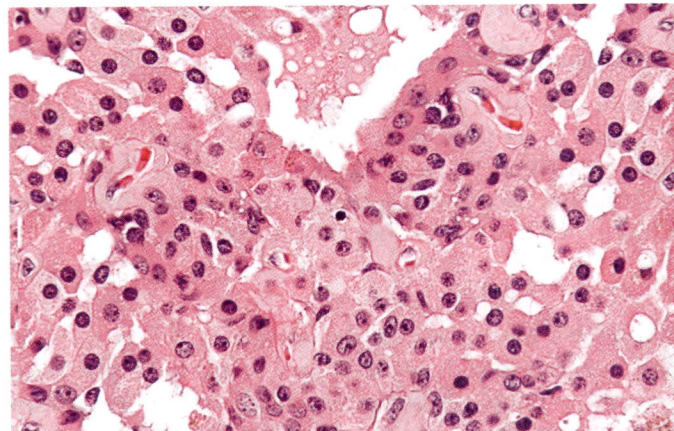

Fig. 19.14: Oncocytoma is composed of cords of uniform polyhedral cells with distinct cell membrane, granular eosinophilic cytoplasm, central round vesicular nuclei, and thin fibrous stroma (400X).

Table 19.9: Differences between pleomorphic adenoma and Warthin's tumor

Parameters	Pleomorphic adenoma	Warthin's tumor
Origin	Intercalated ducts	Striated ducts
Glands involved	Parotid gland and minor salivary glands, e.g. palate, upper lip and mucosa (10%)	Parotid gland
Frequency	70–80%	10%
Sex predilection	Females preponderance	Males > females
Number	Solitary (90%)	Solitary (90%) and multiple (10%)
Laterality	Unilateral (most often)	Unilateral (most often)
Clinical features	Nodular firm inconsistency	Smooth soft and cystic lesion
Histology	Epithelial cells are embedded in chondromyxoid stroma	Double layer pink stationing epithelium and lymphoid aggregates
Recurrence	Common after surgical excision	Uncommon after surgical excision

Light Microscopy
Tumor is composed of uniform epithelial cells arranged in sheets or cords. These cells contain abundant mitochondria constituting 60% of the cell volume, which impart a brightly eosinophilic look.

Electron Microscopy
Tumor cells contain hyperplasia of mitochondria constituting 60% of cell volume.

MYOEPITHELIOMA
Myoepithelioma is a rare benign tumor arising in parotid and minor salivary glands (hard or soft palate). It is occasionally seen in the submandibular glands. Local recurrence is more common than pleomorphic adenoma after surgical excision.

Age and Sex Predilection
It equally affects men and women over 50 years of age.

Clinical Features
Patient presents with slow growing asymptomatic mass.

Gross Morphology
Tumor is well circumscribed similar to a pleomorphic adenoma but without the myxoid stroma.

Light Microscopy
Histologic variants of myoepithelioma include spindle cell type, hyaline type, plasmacytoid type or clear cell type.
- *Spindle cell variant*: It occurs in parotid gland. It is composed of spindle cells arranged in sheets and cords.
- *Plasmacytoid pattern*: It is less common but the most frequently encountered pattern in palate tumors.
- *Combined pattern*: It demonstrates a combination of the spindle and plasmacytoid cells. This variant is uncommon.

Immunohistochemistry
Panel of markers is used to analyze expression in myoepithelioma on histopathological sections (Table 19.10).

Table 19.10: Immunohistochemistry of myoepithelioma

Markers	Expression
S-100 protein	Positivity
Pancytokeratin	Positivity
Smooth muscle actin	Positivity
p63	Positivity

MONOMORPHIC ADENOMA
Monomorphic adenoma is rare salivary gland tumor affecting 60–70 years of age group. Histologic variants of monomorphic adenoma include *basal cell adenoma* (most common in parotid gland), *canalicular adenoma* (minor salivary glands multifocal in origin), *sebaceous adenoma*, *glycogen-rich adenoma* and *clear cell adenoma*. Tumor is easily excised. Recurrence is rare after surgical excision.

Clinical Features
Patient presents with slow growing painless firm to fluctuant 1–2 cm nodule.

Gross Morphology
Tumor is well circumscribed solid to cystic without capsule. Cut surface is tan to pink.

Light Microscopy
Light microscopy shows various histologic patterns. It is composed of cords of cells forming duct-like structures in a background of fibrous stroma. Canalicular adenoma is composed of two rows of cells opposed to each other giving beaded appearance.

Immunohistochemistry
Panel of markers is used to analyze expression in canalicular adenoma on histopathological sections (Table 19.11).

Table 19.11: Immunohistochemistry of canalicular adenoma

Markers	Expression
S-100 protein	Positivity
Cytokeratin	Positivity

MUCOEPIDERMOID CARCINOMA
Mucoepidermoid carcinoma is most common malignant glandular epithelial neoplasm of the salivary glands. It most often occurs in the parotid glands. It may arise in minor salivary glands.

It is characterized by mucous, intermediate, epidermoid cells, columnar, clear cells and oncocytic features. All mucoepidermoid carcinomas are potentially malignant with metastatic potential regardless of their microscopic appearance.

Age Group
It occurs more frequently in women than in men affecting young to elderly persons.

Molecular Level Subdivisions
Translocations of chromosomes *11q21 and 19p13* are demonstrated in mucoepidermoid carcinoma resulting in MECT-MAMAL2 fusion. The median survival of

fusion positive patients is >10 years. On the other hand, median survival of fusion negative patients is 1.6 years.

Elevated Her2 neu gene expression and gene amplification have been demonstrated in mucoepidermoid carcinoma.

Clinical Features

Patient presents with slow growing asymptomatic mass in salivary glands, very similar to that of benign tumor.

Gross Examination

Tumor is well circumscribed partially encapsulated with infiltrative edges. Cut surface is firm, smooth with cystic areas.

Light Microscopy

Mucoepidermoid carcinoma may be low, intermediate or high grade. Histopathologic features and grading mucoepidermoid carcinoma are based on cystic appearance, necrosis, neural invasion, mitotic figures and anaplasia (Tables 19.12 and 19.13).

- *Low grade mucoepidermoid carcinoma* (Fig. 19.15) is composed of mixture of squamoid (epidermoid), mucus-secreting cells (eccentric nuclei), and *intermediate cells* (Fig. 19.16). The proportion of different cell types and their architectural configuration (including cyst formation) varies. These cells are arranged in sheets, nests and duct-like patterns. It is cystic and well differentiated tumor. Keratin pearl formation may be seen in occasional case.
- *High grade mucoepidermoid carcinoma* shows solid growth pattern with predominant epidermoid cells and increased cellularity with cellular atypia and frequent mitotic figures. It may be mistaken for squamous cell carcinoma (Fig. 19.17).

Table 19.12: Histopathologic features and scores of mucoepidermoid carcinoma

Light microscopic findings	Scoring system
Cystic component >20%	2
Neural invasion	2
Necrosis	3
Mitotic figures 4 or greater than/high power field	3
Anaplasia	4

Table 19.13: Tumor grading and scoring of mucoepidermoid carcinoma

Tumor grade	Scoring system
Low grade neoplasm	0–4
Intermediate grade neoplasm	5–6
High grade neoplasm	7 or more

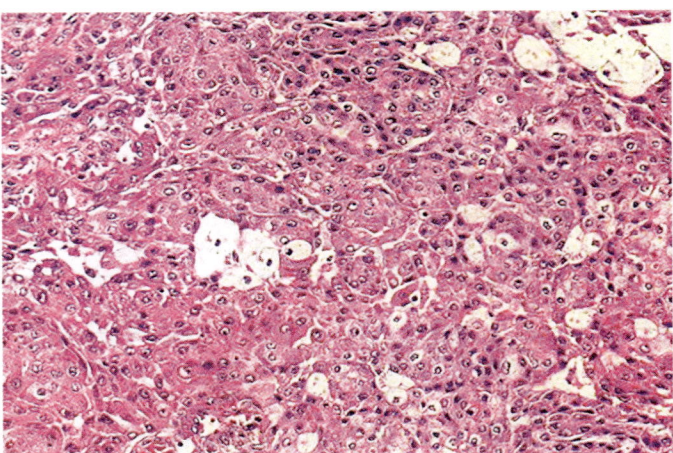

Fig. 19.16: Mucoepidermoid carcinoma (intermediate grade tumor). It is composed of mucus and squamoid cells in equal proportion. Tumor cells are pleomorphic and showing mitotic figures (400X).

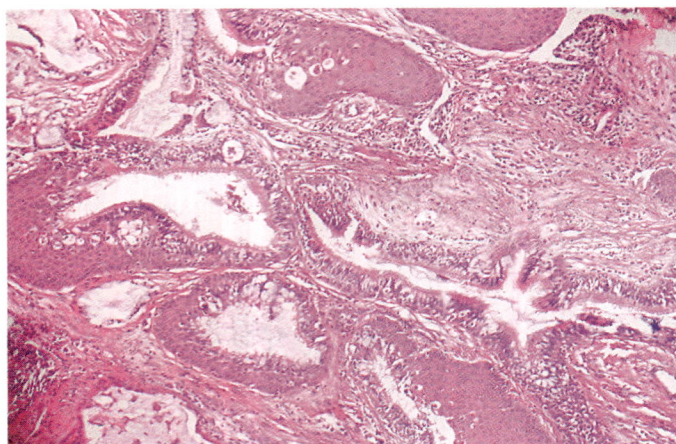

Fig. 19.15: Mucoepidermoid carcinoma (low grade tumor). It is chiefly composed of mucus cells. Epidermal cells are less than mucus cells (400X).

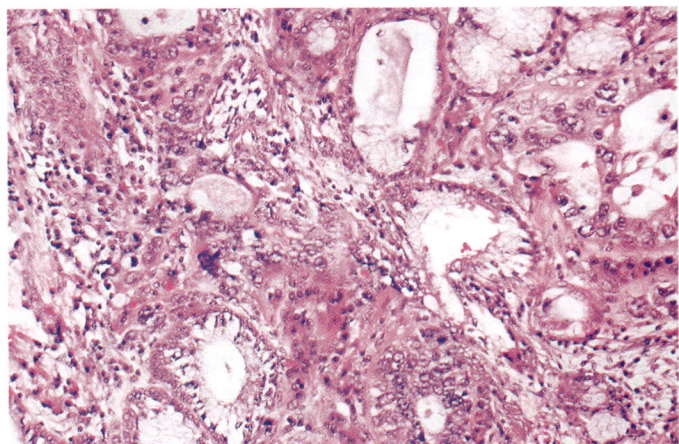

Fig. 19.17: Mucoepidermoid carcinoma (high grade tumor). It is chiefly composed of squamoid cells and smaller population of mucus cells (400X).

Oral Cavity and Salivary Glands

Table 19.14: Mode of spread of mucoepidermoid carcinoma located in various locations

Location of tumor	Mode of spread	Metastases
Parotid gland (most common site)	Lymphatic route	Pre-auricular and submandibular lymph nodes
Submandibular gland	Lymphatic route	Submandibular and upper jugular lymph nodes
Palate	Direct invasion	Upper respiratory tract and base of skull
Lip	Lymphatic route	Submental lymph modes
Oral cavity	Lymphatic route	Submandibular, post-auricular and upper accessory nodes in neck level II then to levels III, IV and V

There may be widespread metastases to lung, liver, bone, and brain.

Histochemistry

Positive histochemical staining for mucin is seen in mucoepidermoid carcinoma rather than squamous cell carcinoma. *Tumor with MUC4 positivity has better prognosis than MUC1.*

Mode of Spread

Mucoepidermoid carcinoma may spread by direct invasion, lymphatic route and hematogenous route (Table 19.14).

Prognosis

Low grade cases have an excellent prognosis (5-year survival: 90%), but high grade tumors do poorly (5-year survival: 20 to 40%).

ADENOID CYSTIC CARCINOMA

Adenoid cystic carcinoma is second most common salivary gland malignant tumor. It most often invades *perineural spaces* (Figs 19.18 to 19.20).

It has a relentless clinical course with *fatal outcome*. Growth pattern is most commonly in part, infiltrative and hence recurrence is common after surgical excision.

Location

Tumor occurs in *submandibular* (15%), *parotid gland* (2%), *sublingual* and *minor salivary glands* (15–20%). It is a *slow growing tumor* with extensive perineural invasion causing pain.

Age and Sex Predilection

It affects equally men and women with peak in the 5th decade. It tends to recur after surgery.

Molecular Genetics

Frequent losses at 12q (33%) 6q23-q, 13q21-q22 and 19q regions (40%) have been reported.

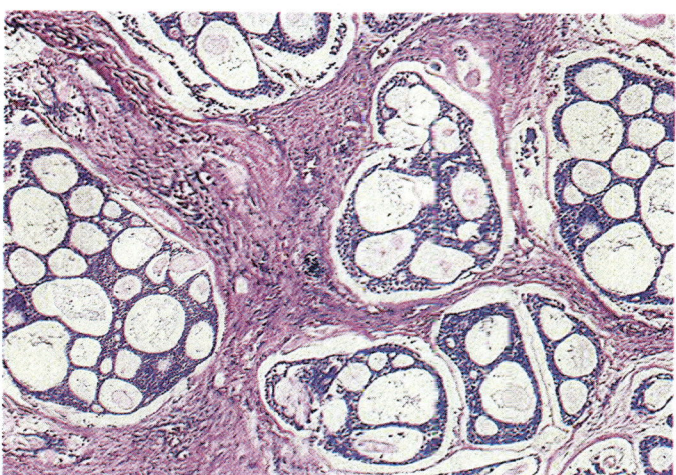

Fig. 19.19: Adenoid cystic carcinoma. It is composed of inner ductal cells and outer myoepithelial cells (400X).

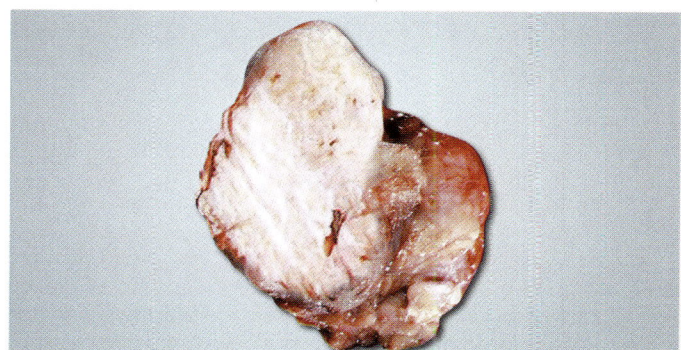

Fig. 19.18: Adenoid cystic carcinoma. It is well circumscribed solid tumor light tan with infiltrative margins.

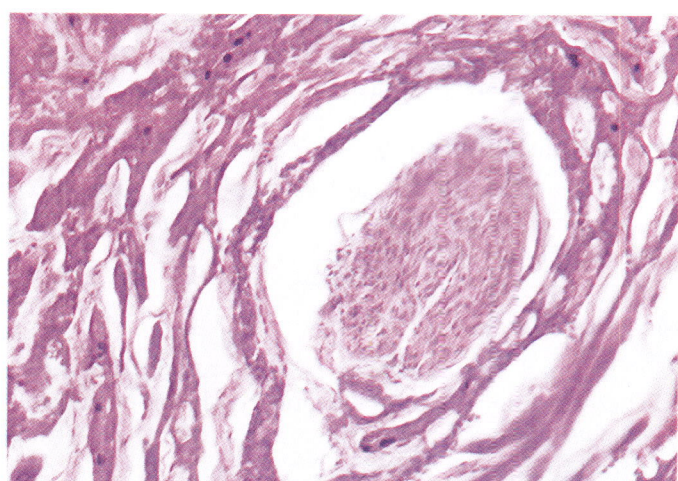

Fig. 19.20: Adenoid cystic carcinoma shows perineural invasion (400X).

Clinical Features

Patient with tumor in major salivary gland especially in submandibular gland presents with asymptomatic slow growing mass but highly malignant neoplasm followed by *pain due to perineural invasion.*

Hypoglossal nerve involvement leads to impairment of tongue movements.

Lingual nerve invasion causes tingling sensation of tongue. Facial nerve paralysis may also occur.

Minor salivary gland involvement is characterized by a submucosal mass with or without pain and ulceration.

Gross Morphology

Tumor is well circumscribed but without capsule. It is invariably infiltrative tumor invading surrounding normal tissue.

Despite its name, it is solid tumor that rarely displays obvious cystic spaces on cut surface.

Light Microscopy

Tumor is a basaloid tumor consisting of epithelial and myoepithelial cells in variable morphological configurations.

It shows three patterns: cribriform (most common), tubular or solid.

- *Cribriform pattern:* If the cystic spaces are large and numerous, it is termed as cribriform pattern. It is often referred to as *swiss cheese* pattern. The tumor cells are small monomorphic with scant cytoplasm arranged in nests around cylindrical spaces that may contain mucinous or hyalinized material.
- *Solid pattern:* It is composed of sheets of tumor cells with no intervening spaces. The tumor is graded as 1, 2 and 3. Grade 1 tumor is composed of tubular and cribriform pattern. Grade 2 tumor contains 30–70% solid areas. Grade 2 comprises >70% solid areas has poor prognosis.

Immunohistochemistry

Panel of markers is used to analyze expression in adenoid cystic carcinoma on histopathological sections (Table 19.15).

Mode of Spread

- *Direct invasion:* Adenoid cystic carcinoma invades surrounding connective tissue involving perineural spaces. Tumor may permeate bones and penetrate through nose or antrum.
- *Hematogenous route:* Tumor may metastasize to distant organs especially lungs.

Table 19.15: Immunohistochemistry of adenoid cystic carcinoma

Markers	Expression
Carcinoembryonic antigen (CEA)	Positivity in ductal cells
Cytokeratin	
S-100 protein	Positivity around pseudoglandular spaces
Muscle specific actin	
Ki-67	

Prognostic Factors

Factors that influence survival include histologic patterns, location of tumor, clinical stage, bone involvement and status of surgical margins.

- Tubular and cribriform patterns have less aggressive course.
- Tumor with solid pattern of cells, tumor suppressor p53 gene mutation and foci of dedifferentiation has poor prognosis.

Therapeutic Correlation

It is treated by complete surgical excision and postoperative radiation therapy. Since it shows perineural invasion, hence *facial nerve is also sacrificed along with tumor.*

ACINIC CELL CARCINOMA

Acinic cell carcinoma (Fig. 19.21) is rare malignant tumor accounting for 2–3% of tumors in parotid glands, in which at least neoplastic cells demonstrate serous acinar cell differentiation with PAS-diastase positive zymogen secretory granules. Salivary ductal cells are also a component of this neoplasm. Approximately 80–90% of these tumors occur within *parotid glands*.

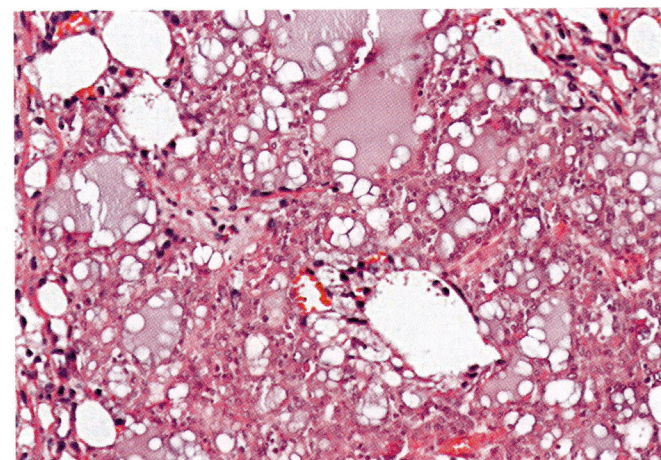

Fig. 19.21: Acinic cell carcinoma shows vacuolated cells similar in size to intercalated duct-type cells but have clear cytoplasmic vacuoles, which sometimes distend the cellular membranes (400X).

Age Group

It is low grade malignancy of salivary glands especially in children and young age group. Peak incidence is in the 5th decade especially women.

Clinical Features

Patient presents with slow growing asymptomatic tumor in parotid glands. Acinic cell carcinoma may transform to high grade adenocarcinoma or poorly differentiated carcinoma presenting with rapid growth, pain and facial nerve palsy. Clinical course is characterized by metastases (8–10%) and local recurrence after surgical excision in 12–20% of patients. Treatment is surgical excision.

Gross Morphology

Tumor is well circumscribed without a capsule measuring 1–3 cm in largest dimension. Cut surface appears lobular with gray white, friable, solid and cystic areas.

Light Microscopy

- *Tumor is composed of acinic cells arranged in:* solid or papillary cystic or follicular pattern. The acinic cells show close resemblance to serous acini of salivary glands.
- Tumor cells show differentiation towards acinar cells and ductal cells; but lack myoepithelial differentiation. But there is loss of normal lobular architecture and lacking normal ducts in the tumor nodule.
- The surrounding stroma often shows presence of lymphoid infiltrate.

Histochemistry

The acinic cells show *PAS positive diastase resistant granules*. These cells are negative for mucin stains.

Mode of Spread

Acinic cell carcinoma initially metastasizes to cervical lymph nodes and subsequently to more distant organs especially in the lungs.

Prognostic Factors

Histological grading has been unsuccessful to predict prognosis. Poor prognostic factors include *necrosis, extraglandular extension, increased pleomorphism, high mitotic rate,* and *prominent infiltration of nerves and blood vessels.*

Prognosis

Circumscribed well differentiated acinic cell carcinoma with abundant lymphoid aggregates has excellent prognosis.

POLYMORPHOUS LOW GRADE ADENOCARCINOMA (PLGA)

Adenocarcinoma (Fig. 19.22) is second common tumor of minor salivary glands. Approximately 60% of the cases have involved the palate. Other locations are buccal mucosa, retromolar region, upper lip, and the base of the tongue. It affects over 40 years of age with equal frequency in men and women. It has infiltrative growth pattern with low metastatic potential.

Clinical Features

Painless mass in the palate is the most common clinical sign. Bleeding or ulceration of the overlying mucosa occurs occasionally.

Gross Morphology

Tumor is solid firm circumscribed with irregular border invading into surrounding tissue. Cut surface is lobulated with yellow tan.

Light Microscopy

Tumor is composed of tumor cells forming glandular structures.

Immunohistochemistry

Panel of markers is used to analyze expression in polymorphous low grade adenocarcinoma on histopathological sections (Table 19.16).

Metastases

Tumor may metastasize to regional lymph nodes and distant organs (*lung and bone*).

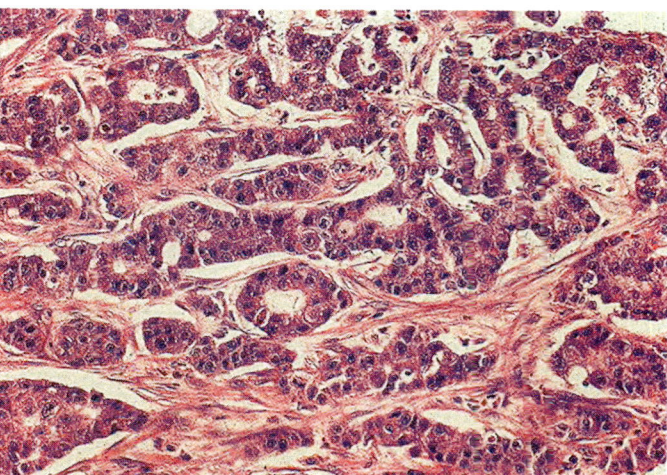

Fig. 19.22: Adenocarcinoma shows presence of glandular structures and absence of squamoid cells (400X).

Table 19.16: Immunohistochemistry of polymorphous low grade adenocarcinoma

Markers	Expression
Cytokeartin	Positivity (100%)
Vimentin	Positivity (100%)
S-100 protein	Positivity (97%)
Carcinoembryonic antigen (CEA)	Positivity (54%)
Glial fibrillary acidic protein (GFAP)	Positivity (15%)
Muscle specific actin	Positivity (13%)
Epithelial membrane antigen	Positivity (12%)
Galectin-3	Positivity in significant number of cases
BCL-2	Overexpression in most cases

CARCINOSARCOMA

Carcinosarcoma is a rare aggressive malignant tumor composed of epithelial and mesenchymal components. It may occur in pleomorphic adenoma and malignant tumors (undifferentiated and adenocarcinoma) *except acinic cell carcinoma*.

Most commonly this will be in the form of an undifferentiated carcinoma (30%) or adenocarcinoma (25%).

Approximately, 25% of patients will have lymph node metastasis on presentation. Currently recommended treatment includes radical surgery, neck dissection for palpable nodes and postoperative radiotherapy.

SQUAMOUS CELL CARCINOMA

Squamous cell carcinoma is rare malignant tumor of salivary gland seen over 60 years of age. Men are more affected than women. High grade mucoepidermoid carcinoma, metastatic squamous cell carcinoma to the gland or intraglandular nodes and direct extension of a squamous cell carcinoma must first be excluded to establish diagnosis.

Gross and histologic appearance is similar to squamous cell carcinoma seen in other sites. It varies from well differentiated with keratinization to poorly-differentiated without keratinization. It is an aggressive tumor, which may metastasize to regional lymph nodes.

Treatment consists of surgical resection, neck dissection and postoperative radiation.

JAW

OVERVIEW

Jaw harbors odontogenic apparatus of deciduous and permanent dentitions. The teeth gums are composed of enamel, dermal papillae and tooth follicle. The enamel organ is composed of ectodermally derived epithelial cells, the ameloblasts. The dental papillae are derived from ectomesenchyme, forming dentine. The tooth follicle is also derived from ectomesenchyme that surrounds developing tooth and provides support to tooth and perichondrium. Odontogenic tissue may be source of cysts and tumors. Normal structure of tooth is shown in Fig. 19.23.

DENTAL AND PERIODONTAL DISORDERS

Dental Caries

Dental caries is the most prevalent chronic disease of the calcified tissues of the teeth. It begins with the disintegration of the enamel prisms, accumulation of debris and superadded *Streptococcus mutans* infections. These changes produce a small pit or fissure in the enamel (Fig. 19.24).

Cavity Formation

Reaching of infection at dentinoenamel junction leads to spread of infection laterally penetrating the dentin along the dentinal tubules. It leads to formation of cavity in the dentin producing a flask-shaped lesion with a narrow orifice. Microorganisms may invade vascular pulp of the tooth.

Clinical Features

Patient may develop pulpitis results to periapical granulation tissue and periodontitis of the marginal gingiva.

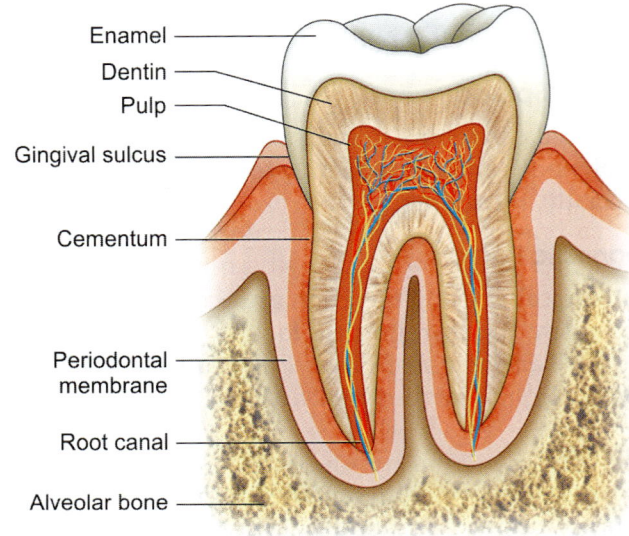

Fig. 19.23: Normal structure of tooth.

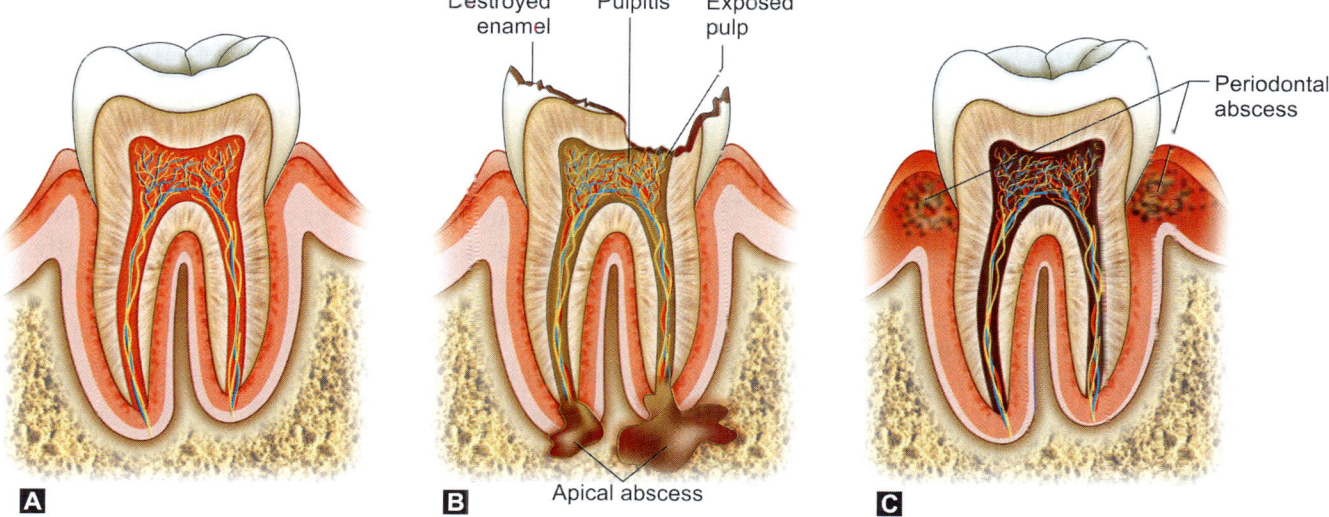

Fig. 19.24: Pathogenesis of dental caries. (A) Normal structure of tooth, (B) apical abscess, (C) periodontal abscess.

Periodontal Disease

Periodontal disease refers to acute and chronic disorders of the soft tissues surrounding the teeth. It leads to the loss of supporting bone. Adults with poor oral hygiene develop chronic periodontal disease. There may be a strong family history of periodontal disease. Chronic periodontitis causes loss of more teeth in comparison to caries.

CYSTIC LESIONS

Odontogenic and nonodontogenic cysts are shown in Tables 19.17 and 19.18.

Dentigerous Cyst (Follicular Cyst)

Dentigerous cyst is a unilocular cyst. It forms in association with the crown of an impacted molar or canine tooth. Enucleation and excision of the associated tooth are the treatment of choice.

Patient presents with asymptomatic, well defined expansile radiolucent lesion. On light microscopy, dentigerous cyst is lined by cuboidal to flattened epithelial cells. There is presence of focal keratinization, mucous cells, inflammatory cells and *dystrophic calcification*.

Keratocystic Odontogenic Tumor (Odontogenic Keratocyst)

Odontogenic keratocyst is symptomatic unilocular cyst in the mandible or maxilla affecting 2nd to 4th decades of life. Cyst contains keratinous debris. On light microscopy, cyst shows palisading basal cells covered by a few layers of squamous cells under parakeratotic surface. Lack of rete ridges is diagnostic feature. Rarely carcinoma may arise from the cyst.

Table 19.17: Odontogenic cysts

Developmental odontogenic cysts
Dentigerous cysts (follicular cyst)
Keratocystic odontogenic tumor (odontogenic keratocyst)
Lateral periodontal cyst
Gingival cyst of adults
Calcifying cystic odontogenic tumor (calcifying odontogenic cyst, Gorlin cyst)
Glandular odontogenic cyst
Inflammatory odontogenic cysts
Periapical (radicular) cyst
Residual periapical (radicular) cyst

Table 19.18: Nonodontogenic cysts

Epithelial-lined nonodontogenic cysts (fissural cyst)
Nasopalatine duct cysts (fissural cysts)
Globulomaxillary cyst
Median palatal cysts
Nonepithelial-lined nonodontogenic cysts
Simple bone cysts
Aneurysmal bone cysts

Lateral Periodontal Cyst

Lateral periodontal cyst occurs in lateral surface of roots of mandibular premolar teeth during 5th to 7th decades. Cyst is well demarcated, radiolucent on radiograph. On light microscopy, cyst shows a thin layer of nonkeratinized epithelium with focal thickening. There is no inflammation surrounding the cyst.

Gingival Cyst

Gingival cyst occurs in the buccal gingiva of the mandible near the premolar and molar teeth during 5th to 6th decades. Cyst may be single measuring <1 cm in diameter or multiple. On light microscopy, cyst is lined by a thin layer of epithelium. There is no inflammation in surrounding soft tissue.

Calcifying Odontogenic Cyst

Calcifying odontogenic cyst occurs as a radiolucent asymptomatic lesion in maxilla or mandible during 2nd and 3rd decades of life. On light microscopy, cyst shows a proliferating layer of columnar palisaded basal cells similar to ameloblasts. Superficial layer has large cells with eosinophilic cytoplasm lacking nuclei (ghost cells). Calcification may be seen. Recurrence is uncommon after enucleation of cyst.

Glandular Odontogenic Cyst

Glandular odontogenic cyst is referred to sialo-odontogenic cyst. It occurs as a radiolucent lesion in anterior region of mandible or maxilla. Patient most often presents with painful swelling.

On light microscopy, cyst contains nonkeratinized epithelium, mucus secreting cells and focal solid areas. There may be presence of ghost cells and hyaline bodies. Surgical excision is the treatment of choice.

Radicular (Periapical Cyst)

Radicular cyst is associated with nonviable carious teeth. It occurs in the apical third of tooth root during 3rd to 7th decades of life.

Patient presents with painful swelling. On light microscopy, cyst shows inflammation surrounding the nonkeratinizing epithelium.

There is presence of cholesterol clefts, foamy macrophages, dystrophic calcification, and intraepithelial hyaline bodies (*Rushton bodies*). Residual cyst is a variant of radicular cyst occurring at the site of extracted tooth.

Nasopalatine Duct Cyst

Nasopalatine duct cyst is the most common lesion affecting 4th to 6th decades of life. It arises from moderate-sized nerves and small muscular arteries within incisive canal.

Patient presents with swelling of the anterior palate, with pain. It is well circumscribed radiolucent lesion demonstrated on radiograph.

On light microscopy, cyst may be lined by stratified squamous, pseudostratified columnar cells within the incisive canal. Surgical enucleation is the treatment of choice.

Globulomaxillary Cyst

Globulomaxillary cyst originates from epithelium entrapped during fusion of the globular portion of the medial nasal process within maxillary process especially between the lateral incisors. Cyst is well circumscribed radiolucent demonstrated on radiograph.

On light microscopy, cyst is lined by stratified squamous epithelium. Occasionally, it is lined by pseudostratified columnar ciliated epithelium. Enucleation is the treatment of choice.

Median Palatal Cyst

Median palatal cyst is believed to originate from epithelium entrapped along the embryonic line of fusion of the lateral palatal shelves of the maxilla affecting young adults.

Patient presents with firm or fluctuant swelling in the midline of the hard palate posterior to the incisive papilla. It is well circumscribed radiolucent lesion in the midline of the hard palate demonstrated on radiograph.

On light microscopy, cyst is lined by stratified squamous epithelium. Surgical enucleation is the treatment of choice.

Simple Bone Cyst

Simple bone cyst is known with multiple names such as unicameral bone cyst or solitary bone cyst, progressive bone cyst, traumatic bone cyst or hemorrhagic bone cyst. It is well circumscribed osteolytic lesion in the posterior mandible in young <20 years of age. Maxilla may be affected in some cases.

On light microscopy, cyst is lined by fibrovascular tissue with hemosiderin laden macrophages. There is presence of reactive bone and osteoclasts.

Aneurysmal Bone Cyst

Aneurysmal bone cyst is rapidly enlarging blood-filled cystic lesion affecting first three decades of life. It occurs in mandible (60%) or maxilla (40%). This cystic lesion may be isolated or associated with chondroblastoma or osteoblastoma.

On light microscopy, aneurysmal bone cyst shows fibrotic stroma with multinucleated giant cells, macrophages and hemosiderin granules. There may be presence of ossification (Fig. 19.25).

ODONTOGENIC TUMORS

Odontogenic tumors are derived from epithelial, ectomesenchymal and or mesenchymal elements of the tooth forming apparatuses. It is worth mentioning that peripheral (extraosseous) equivalents of most central odontogenic tumors located in the mandibular or

Oral Cavity and Salivary Glands

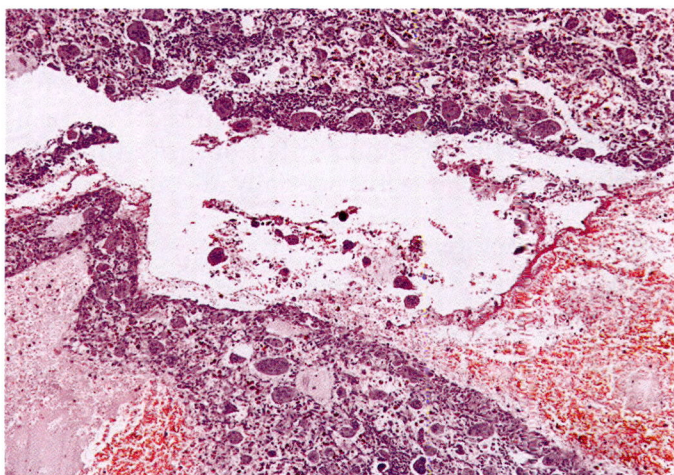

Fig. 19.25: Aneurysmal bone cyst shows fibrotic stroma with multinucleated giant cells, macrophages and hemosiderin granules (100X).

maxillary gingiva arising either from surface mucosa or dental lamina nests in the submucosa or in the sinonasal tract. Classification of the tumors of jaw is shown in Table 19.19.

Table 19.19: Classification of jaw tumors

Benign tumors
Adenomatoid odontogenic tumor (adenoameloblastoma)
Calcifying odontogenic tumor
Ameloblastic fibroma
Odontoma (complex odontoma, compound odontoma and odontoameloblastoma)
Cementoma
Borderline tumors
Ameloblastoma (adamantinoma)
Malignant tumors
Ameloblastic carcinoma
Odontogenic carcinoma
Ameloblastic fibrosarcoma

ADENOMATOID ODONTOGENIC TUMOR

Adenomatoid odontogenic tumor most often occurs in anterior maxilla. It affects especially females during second decade of life. It is slow growing tumor with progressive growth. Tumor is composed of odontogenic epithelium embedded in a mature connective tissue.

Gross Morphology
Tumor is predominantly cystic simulating an odontogenic cyst.

Light Microscopy
Tumor is composed of numerous duct-like structures lined by cuboidal or columnar cells. Hyaline and calcified deposits may be scattered throughout epithelial lining duct-like structures.

CALCIFYING EPITHELIAL ODONTOGENIC TUMOR (PINDBORG TUMOR)

Calcifying epithelial odontogenic tumor most often occurs in mandibular premolar-molar area in association with an embedded tooth. Tumor may occur in gingiva. It occurs during 4th and 5th decades with no sex predilection. Tumor may be invasive. It may recur after surgical excision. It is less aggressive tumor than ameloblastoma.

Gross Morphology
Tumor is solid. Cystic variety has been reported.

Light Microscopy
- Tumor is composed of closely packed polyhedral epithelial cells and scanty stroma.
- Tumor cells show mild pleomorphism.
- There is presence of eosinophilic homogenous amyloid-like material that becomes calcified.

SQUAMOUS ODONTOGENIC TUMOR

Squamous odontogenic tumor is a benign tumor. It occurs in anterior maxilla and posterior mandible. Tumor in the maxillary region tends to be more aggressive. On radiograph, tumor appears as a well-circumscribed semicircular radiolucency surrounded by sclerotic border.

Light Microscopy
Tumor is composed of nests and islands of well differentiated squamous epithelium lacking atypia located within a collagenous stroma of low to moderate cellularity.

AMELOBLASTIC FIBROMA

Ameloblastic fibroma most often affects younger age group. It has benign clinical behavior.

Gross Morphology
Tumor is solid. But cystic variant has been reported.

> **Light Microscopy**
> - Tumor is composed of neoplastic fibrous stroma enclosing thin strip of ameloblastic epithelium. The presence of mesenchymal component is the diagnostic feature of this tumor.
> - Epithelial component has two layers of cells.
> - There may be presence of hard tooth structures such as dentin. Occasionally stellate reticulum is present.

ODONTOMA

Odontoma features production of calcified parts of teeth. It occurs in the alveolar ridge of the mandible or maxilla. There are three variants: complex, compound and ameloblastic odontomas.

Complex Odontoma

Complex odontoma most often occurs in molar areas of the mandible especially of females. It is a benign poorly differentiated tumor forming enamel, dentin or cementum in uncoordinated fashion. It is incidentally detected on routine radiographic examination.

Compound Odontoma

Compound odontoma most often occurs in the anterior region of maxilla. It is a benign well differentiated tumor composed of masses of small denticles.

Ameloblastic Odontoma

Ameloblastic odontoma is aggressive tumor. It is currently regarded as immature complex odontoma. Tumor is solid and cystic. Tumor is composed of prominent epithelial component resembling ameloblastoma. It recurs after surgical excision.

CEMENTOMA

Cementoma is relatively common non-neoplastic disorder. It most often occurs in mandibular incisor region especially affecting females. It is restricted to small region surrounding apices of teeth. Lesion is asymptomatic and does not require treatment.

> **Light Microscopy**
> Lesion is composed of curvilinear trabeculae resembling *ginger root* or irregularly shaped cementum-like masses. It should be differentiated from cemento-ossifying fibroma, which shows thin isolated trabeculae with prominent osteoblastic rimming.

ODONTOGENIC MYXOMA, MYXOFIBROMA AND FIBROMA

Odontogenic myxoma is derived from dental papilla (tooth germ origin), hence qualifies for odontogenic origin. It is related to malformed or missing teeth. It occurs during 2nd and 3rd decades in mandible and maxilla. It is cystic lesion demonstrated on radiograph. Recurrence is common after surgical removal. Odontogenic fibroma most often occurs in maxilla anterior to the molar teeth especially affecting females.

> **Gross Morphology**
> Tumor is cystic in consistency.

> **Light Microscopy**
> Tumor is composed of loose stellate cells with long branching odontogenic epithelium.

> **Immunohistochemistry**
> - Tumor cells of odontogenic myxoma are immunoreactive for **vimentin** but *negative for S-100 protein*.
> - Odontogenic fibroma differs from myxoma by the presence of fibrous tissue and odontogenic epithelial rests.
> - Myxofibroma is composed of myxomatous and fibrous components in equal proportion.

AMELOBLASTOMA (ADMANTINOMA)

Ameloblastoma is the most common of the epithelial odontogenic tumors. It constitutes 1% of tumors and cysts of jaw affecting 3rd to 5th decades.

Origin

It arises from epithelial lining of dentigerous cyst, remnants of the dental lamina and enamel organ or basal layer of oral mucosa. Over 80% occur in the mandible and 70% in the molar ramus area.

> **Gross Morphology**
> Traditionally, ameloblastoma has been divided into solid and multicystic, but this distinction is arbitrary.

> **Light Microscopy**
> Histologic variants of ameloblastoma are follicular, plexiform, acanthomatous, papilliferous-keratotic, granular cell, desmoplastic, vascular and dentino-ameloblastoma. Two or more histologic patterns may coexist within the same tumor. Out of these follicular and plexiform histological variants are more common.
> - *Follicular variant:* Tumor is composed of outermost tall columnar cells with polarization of the nuclei away from basement membrane resembling inner dental epithelium of the developing tooth follicle (ameloblastic layer). The inner (central) portion of the epithelial island is composed of loose network of cells resembling stellate reticulum. Squamous metaplasia within the stellate reticulum gives rise to the acanthomatous variant.

- *Plexiform variant:* Tumor is composed of irregular nests and interdigitating cords of epithelial cells with a minimum of stroma (Figs 19.26 and 19.27).

Immunohistochemistry

Panel of markers is used to analyze expression in ameloblastoma on histopathological sections. Granular cell ameloblastoma is positive for **cytokeratin** and **CD68** but *negative for S-100 protein.* Tumor cells exhibit strong reactivity for cytokeratins (Table 19.20).

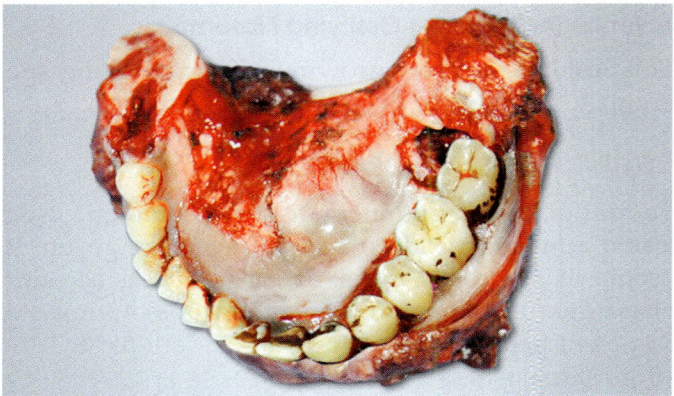

Fig. 19.26: Ameloblastoma of maxilla. Tumor is multilocular and located in maxilla arising from the enamel organ.

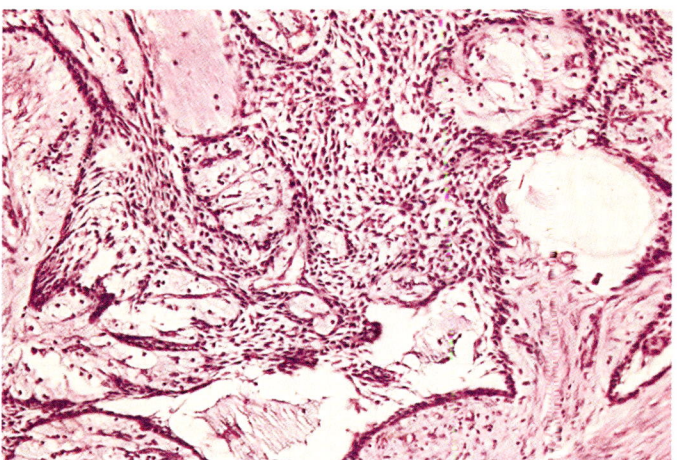

Fig. 19.27: Ameloblastoma. Tumor is composed of outermost tall columnar cells with polarization of the nuclei from basement membrane. The inner (central) portion of the epithelial island is composed of loose network of cells resembling stellate reticulum (100X).

Table 19.20: Immunohistochemistry of ameloblastoma

Markers	Expression
CK5, CK14 CK8, CK18, CK19	Positivity
Calretinin	Positivity (stellate reticulum areas)
S-100 protein	Negative

Electron Microscopy

On electron microscopy study, tumor cells exhibit clear cut evidence of epithelial differentiation in the form of tonofilaments and complex desmosomes.

Mode of Spread

Ameloblastoma has invasive property and tendency to recur after surgical excision. It is due to these properties, this is placed under borderline (low grade malignant) tumor category by oral pathologists and WHO classification. Distant metastases have been documented and are rare instances.

Differential Diagnosis

Ameloblastoma has to be differentiated from focal reactive hyperplasia in a dentigerous cyst, unicystic ameloblastoma. Minimal criteria for diagnosis of ameloblastoma is presence of a palisaded basal layer with stellate reticulum-like epithelium above. Immunoreactivity for calretinin supports the diagnosis.

Management

Enucleation of the tumor is most often curative. Local recurrence may occur after surgical excision if ameloblastic islands remain embedded in the cyst wall.

AMELOBLASTIC CARCINOMA

Ameloblastic carcinoma has microscopic architectural features of ameloblastoma with additional malignant component. Tumor shows lack of differentiation, increased cellularity, marked atypia, numerous mitoses, vascular and neural invasion.

ODONTOGENIC CARCINOMA

Odontogenic carcinoma is restricted to primary intraosseous carcinoma lacking ameloblastic-like pattern. It is considered to be of odontogenic origin either *de novo* or arising in a odontogenic cyst.

Clear Cell Odontogenic Carcinoma

Clear cell odontogenic carcinoma most often occurs in jaw. It simulates metastatic clear cell carcinoma of salivary gland. Tumor is composed of clear cells arranged in nests surrounded by mature collagenous stroma. Tumor cells lack glycogen and mucin.

Sclerosing Odontogenic Carcinoma

Sclerosing odontogenic carcinoma is composed of polygonal monomorphic epithelial cells arranged in small nests and thin cords embedded in abundant sclerosing hyaline stroma. These tumor cells exhibit skeletal muscle and neural infiltration.

AMELOBLASTIC FIBROSARCOMA

Ameloblastic fibrosarcoma morphology is similar to ameloblastic fibroma except it shows increased cellularity, cytological atypia and aggressive clinical course. It has diminished or absent epithelial component. Some tumors containing combined features of ameloblastic carcinoma and fibrosarcoma are termed as ameloblastic carcinosarcoma.

NONODONTOGENIC TUMORS

Nonodontogenic tumors are classified in Table 19.21.

Table 19.21: Nonodontogenic tumors

Benign fibro-osseous lesions
Fibrous dysplasia
Juvenile ossifying fibroma: Trabecular and psammomatoid variants
Cementosseous fibroma: Periapical or florid variants
Giant cell lesions
Central (intraosseous) giant cell granuloma
Brown tumor of hyperparathyroidism
Cherubism
Aneurysmal bone cyst

FIBROUS DYSPLASIA

Fibrous dysplasia may be polyostotic or mono-ostotic associated with somatic mutation of **GNAS1 gene**. Polyostotic form is associated with **Albright syndrome.** Mean age at the time of diagnosis is 25–35 years.

Clinical Features

Patient presents with painless unilateral swelling of maxilla or mandible.

Imaging Technique

On radiograph, lesion varies from cystic or translucent to sclerotic or radiopaque with ill-defined margins.

Light Microscopy

Fibrous dysplasia is composed of C-shaped or Chinese figure-like trabeculae of woven or immature bone within proliferating fibroblastic stroma. These trabeculae lack rimming by osteoblasts. Two morphological variations represented are described as under.

Immunohistochemistry

Fibrous dysplasia shows stronger immunoreactivity for osteocalcin.

FIBROMA GROUP LESIONS

Fibroma group lesions are derived from periodontal ligament. These have predilection for molar-premolar region of mandible. These lesions are more amenable to surgical enucleation or curettage. These lesions are differentiated from fibrous dysplasia.

Ossifying Fibroma

Lesion is composed of lamellar bone with osteoblastic rimming.

Cementifying Fibroma

Lesion is composed of rounded psammoma-like masses resembling cement.

Juvenile (Aggressive) Ossifying Fibroma

This lesion is actively growing affecting young age group. It is composed of cellular fibrous stroma.

CENTRAL GIANT CELL GRANULOMA

Central giant cell granuloma is most common cystic lesion affecting children and younger age group. It occurs in mandible or maxilla. It occurs as a result of trauma resulting to organization of slow minute recurrent hemorrhages. These lesions are treated by surgical removal or curettage.

On the other hand, peripheral giant cell granuloma is characterized by development of cystic mass on the gingiva or the alveolar process as a result of unusual proliferative reaction to local injury. It is seen as a mass covered by mucous membrane, which can be ulcerated.

Light Microscopy

This cellular lesion is composed of numerous multinucleated giant cells embedded in a fibrous stroma that also contains ovoid or spindle-shaped mesenchymal cells. Osteoclast-like giant cells have patchy distribution usually associated with areas of hemorrhage.

CHERUBISM

Cherubism is hereditary autosomal dominant disorder characterized by intraosseous fibrous swellings of the jaw. *The gene responsible for cherubism has been mapped on chromosome 4p16.3.* On light microscopy, it is indistinguishable from central giant cell granuloma. Young patient may present with bilateral involvement of mandible and maxilla.

BROWN TUMOR OF HYPERPARATHYROIDISM

Osteoclastic bone resorption results to *osteitis fibrosa cystica* (also known as *brown tumor*) in jaw and long bones. The lesion is expansile and multilocular with solid and cystic areas. Cystic areas have a brown color due to presence of abundant hemosiderin.

CHAPTER 20

Gastrointestinal Tract

Learning Objectives

ESOPHAGUS
- Inflammatory Lesions
- Non-neoplastic Disorders
- Tumors of Esophagus

STOMACH
- *Helicobacter pylori* Induced GI Disorders
- Inflammatory Diseases
- Peptic Ulcer Disease
- Primary Tumors

SMALL INTESTINE
- Anatomy
- Congenital Anomalies
- Malabsorptive Disorders
- Infectious Diseases
- Obstructive Diseases
- Vascular Diseases
- Polyps and Tumors

LARGE INTESTINE
- Anatomy and Physiology
- Neuromuscular Disorders
- Diverticular Diseases
- Obstructive Diseases
- Inflammatory Bowel Disease
- Vascular Disorders
- Polyps and Tumors of Large Intestine
- Multiple Polyposis Syndromes
- Hereditary Nonpolyposis Colon Cancer (Lynch Syndrome)
- Colorectal Carcinoma

APPENDIX
- Acute Appendicitis

ANUS AND PERIANAL REGION
- Vascular Disorders
- Non-neoplastic Diseases
- Malignant Tumors

PERITONEUM
- Non-neoplastic Lesions
- Primary and Secondary Neoplasms

GENERAL CONSIDERATIONS

EMBRYOLOGY

Gastrointestinal tract (GIT) is derived from endoderm. Endoderm layer is innermost of the three layers forming the developing embryo. During fetal life, GIT is divided into foregut, midgut and hindgut. Foregut is supplied by coeliac trunk, midgut by superior mesenteric artery and hindgut by inferior mesenteric artery. These parts develop into definite parts of GIT.

Developmental Anomalies

- *Atresia (absence of lumen):* The normal gastrointestinal system is a tube that develops from cords of embryonic cells. The cells forming the central part of these cords undergo apoptosis, and a lumen is thus formed.

  If the centrally located cells do not undergo apoptosis, the lumen never forms and the affected part of the GI system will be atretic (i.e. unpassable).

- *Duodenal atresia:* It is most commonly associated with *Down's syndrome*. It is characterized by vomiting of *bile stained material at birth* and an abdominal radiograph with the *double bubble sign*.
- *Stenosis:* It refers to narrowing of GIT lumen.
- *Diverticulosis:* It refers to formation of outpouchings in intestinal tract.
- *Fistula:* It refers to connection between the lumen of the GI tract and another tubular systems, e.g. an esophageal-tracheal fistula.

HISTOLOGY

Entire gastrointestinal tract has a relatively uniform structure. It consists of four layers, i.e. innermost mucosa, submucosa, muscular coat and outermost serosa (adventitia). Adventitia in esophagus is linked with other thoracic organs.

Gut Divisions

Depending on the innervation of GIT, pain is referred in different regions.

- *Foregut:* It extends from esophagus to second part of duodenum, where common bile duct enters in this region. It comprises esophagus, stomach and duodenum. Visceral pain arising from foregut is referred to epigastrium.
- *Midgut:* It starts from the duodenum just distal to entry of common bile duct and extends to middle and distal thirds transverse colon known as *Cannon's point*. It includes terminal ileum, tip of the appendix, and adjacent colon. Visceral pain arising from midgut radiates to periumbilical region.

    Pain in acute appendicitis is felt around periumbilical region (midgut). Pain in acute appendicitis is localized to right iliac fossa due to inflammation of the peritoneum.
- *Hindgut:* It starts from Cannon's point to distal structures of GIT. It includes small portion of transverse colon, descending colon and rectum. Visceral pain arising from hindgut radiates to suprapubic region.

DISEASES OF GIT

Main diseases of the gastrointestinal tract include: development disorders (e.g. atresia, stenosis, diverticulosis and fistula), inflammatory (e.g. esophagitis, inflammatory bowel disease), functional disorders, circulatory disorders and tumors.

Obstructive disorders of gastrointestinal tract are shown in Table 20.1.

Signs and Symptoms

Most important symptoms and signs pertaining to the GI system include dysphagia, vomiting, hematemesis, hematochezia, melena, colics, diarrhea and constipation.

Table 20.1: Obstructive disorders of gastrointestinal tract

Disorder	Features
Duodenal atresia	Duodenal atresia, most commonly associated with Down's syndrome, is characterized by vomiting of bile stained material at birth and an abdominal radiograph with the *double bubble sign*
Hirschsprung's disease (congenital megacolon)	It is characterized by congenital absence of ganglion cells due to gene mutation (endothelin-3) usually in the submucosal and muscular coat of large bowel Aganglionic segment of colon is permanently contracted causing intestinal obstruction. This obstruction leads to dilatation of proximal normal (ganglionic) segment Rectum is always involved, and this is the preferred site for biopsy. Sigmoid colon and proximal are involved, but entire colonic involvement is very rare
Acquired megacolon	It may be associated with Down's syndrome and Chagas' disease
Adhesions	These are commonly acquired from previous abdominal surgery
Direct inguinal hernia	Direct inguinal hernia occurs through the posterior wall of the inguinal canal in the centre of Hesselbach's triangle
Indirect inguinal hernia	Indirect inguinal hernia is most common cause of intestinal obstruction, in which small bowel extends into the scrotal sac, lateral to the triangle of Hesselbach
Umbilical hernia	Umbilical hernias occur in children and adults. Ascites and pregnancy precipitate hernias in adults
Incisional hernia	Ventral hernias occur in previously surgical incision sites

Contd...

Table 20.1: Obstructive disorders of gastrointestinal tract (Contd...)

Disorder	Features
Intussusception	An intussusception is an invagination of one segment of proximal bowel (usually the terminal ileum) into the distal bowel (usually the cecum), causing intestinal obstruction and ischemia of inner loop: ileocecal (most common), jejunojejunal, ileoileal and colocolic It primarily affects children due to active peristalsis and lymphoid hyperplasia. In adults, pedunculated polyps are common cause of intussusception
Volvulus	Volvulus is twisting of a mobile loop of the intestine (usually the sigmoid colon) around its own mesenteric root with subsequent obstruction and infarction. It is also found in the small intestine It occurs in small intestine and sigmoid colon Complications include strangulation, gangrene and obstruction
Malrotation of intestine	During fetal life, defective rotation of intestine occurs. As a result, large bowel does not descend into right iliac fossa. These patients are prone to develop volvulus and internal hernia
Paralytic ileus	Paralytic ileus is a lack of intestinal peristalsis associated with stagnation of intestinal contents The most common causes include abdominal surgery persisting for 2–3 days, peritonitis, shock and vascular collapse
Gallstone ileus	Gallstone ileus occurs when a chronically inflamed gallbladder forms a fistula with the small intestine at ileocecal valve
Meconium ileus	Meconium ileus is a potential complication of a newborn with cystic fibrosis

ESOPHAGUS

GENERAL CONSIDERATIONS

ANATOMY

Esophagus is a long hollow muscular tube. It consists of four layers. With the exception of infradiaphragmatic portion, esophagus is lined by non-keratinized stratified squamous epithelium. The lining epithelium well marked basal layer constitutes 15% of total thickness of epithelium. The lower two-thirds of the esophagus possesses thick muscularis mucosa. Gastroesophageal reflux leads to thickness of this epithelial layer.

PHYSIOLOGY

Esophagus participates in propulsion of food from the mouth to the stomach. It also prevents reflux of gastric contents from the stomach back into esophagus.

DEVELOPMENTAL ANOMALIES

Tracheoesophageal fistula is a congenital disorder characterized by direct communication between trachea and esophagus. Food passing through fistula enters the trachea, causing choking, coughing and cyanosis on attempts at food intake soon after birth.

Newborn may develop pneumonia as a result of milk reflux into the lungs resulting indistention of the stomach by air. This disorder requires immediate surgical correction. It occurs in three distinct variants.

- Upper esophagus ends in a blind pouch (esophageal atresia). *The lower portion of esophagus communicates with the trachea near the tracheal bifurcation.* It is the *most common variant* (90%). *Maternal polyhydramnios* (increased amniotic fluid) is a frequently associated abnormality.
- In second most common variant of esophageal atresia, only the *upper portion of esophagus communicates with the trachea.* The lower esophageal segment is not connected to the upper esophagus.
- In a third variant, there is a *fistulous connection between the trachea and a completely patent esophagus.*

CLINICAL SYMPTOMS

- *Dysphagia:* It refers to difficulty in swallowing of solid food (sign of obstruction) or solids as well as liquids (motor dysfunction). Obstruction of esophagus occurs due to strictures, webs, rings, tumor or functional disorders (achalasia or paralysis).
- *Odynophagia:* It refers to pain on swallowing. Most common causes include gastroesophageal reflux disease (GERD) and infectious esophagitis (e.g. virus and fungi).
- *Heartburn:* It refers to burning sensation in retrosternal region as a result of regurgitation of acid in mouth. It is most often associated with gastroesophageal reflux disease.

Section III: Systemic Pathology

Table 20.2: Gross handling and tissue handling of esophagus

Procedure	Characteristics
Standard endoscopic biopsy	Several small tissue fragments measuring 1 to 5 mm consist of mucosa and muscularis mucosae
Endoscopic biopsy with jumbo forceps	Several tissue fragments measuring 4 to 8 mm consist of mucosa and submucosa
Endoscopic mucosal resection (EMR)	En block resection of superficial malignant and premalignant lesions measuring 1 to 2 mm
Esophagectomy	Tissue specimens consist of esophagus, proximal stomach and attached soft tissue with lymph nodes

GROSS EXAMINATION AND TISSUE HANDLING

Various esophageal diseases are studied by tissue sections obtained by standard endoscopic biopsy, endoscopic mucosal resection (EMR) and esophagectomy (Table 20.2).

INFLAMMATORY LESIONS

ESOPHAGITIS

The esophagus is covered by squamous epithelium, which is relatively resistant to infection. Esophagitis occurs due to gastroesophageal reflux disease, chemicals, cytotoxic drugs, uremia and irradiation.

In immunocompromised host in AIDS, various opportunistic infectious agents cause esophagitis such as herpes simplex type I, and cytomegalovirus. *Candida albicans* causes white mucosal painful patches in esophagus in debilitated persons. Eosinophilic esophagitis involves midesophagus in children.

Differences between reflux and eosinophilic esophagitis are shown in Table 20.3.

GASTROESOPHAGEAL REFLUX DISEASE (GERD)

Under physiological state, lower esophageal sphincter (LES) prevents the entry of the gastric contents in the esophagus. Gastroesophageal reflux disease is popularly known as *heartburn*.

GERD describes chronic backflow of digestive juices (hydrochloric acid and bile) into the esophagus due to transient relaxation of lower esophageal sphincter resulting in damage to epithelial lining of esophagus. Gastroesophageal reflux disease is shown in Fig. 20.1.

Predisposing Factors

These include hiatus hernia (most common), reflex esophagitis, incompetent lower esophageal sphincter, increased intra-abdominal pressure (pregnancy), scleroderma, decreased lower esophageal sphincter tone as a result of alcohol, smoking and caffeine.

Pathogenesis

Gastroesophageal reflux causes breach in mucosal barrier, which may allow infectious agents (e.g. *Candida albicans*, herpes simplex virus or cytomegalovirus and bacteria) resulting in acute inflammation of the lower-third of esophagus as well as metaplastic change in lining epithelium.

Clinical Features

Patient with GERD presents with acute epigastric pain at night (when reflux is worse), nocturnal cough, nocturnal asthma and hematemesis. Symptoms are relieved by antacids.

Table 20.3: Differences between reflux and eosinophilic esophagitis

Parameters	Reflux esophagitis	Eosinophilic esophagitis
Age group	Adults	Children
Sex predilection	Male and female equally affected	Males > females
Symptom	Heartburn	Dysphagia
Endoscopic findings	Variable	Stricture, ring
Histopathological examination	<5 Eosinophils per high power field	>20 Eosinophils per high power field Eosinophilic microabscesses
Treatment	Anti-reflex therapy	Topical steroids
Complications	Barret esophagus, stricture	Stricture

Gastrointestinal Tract

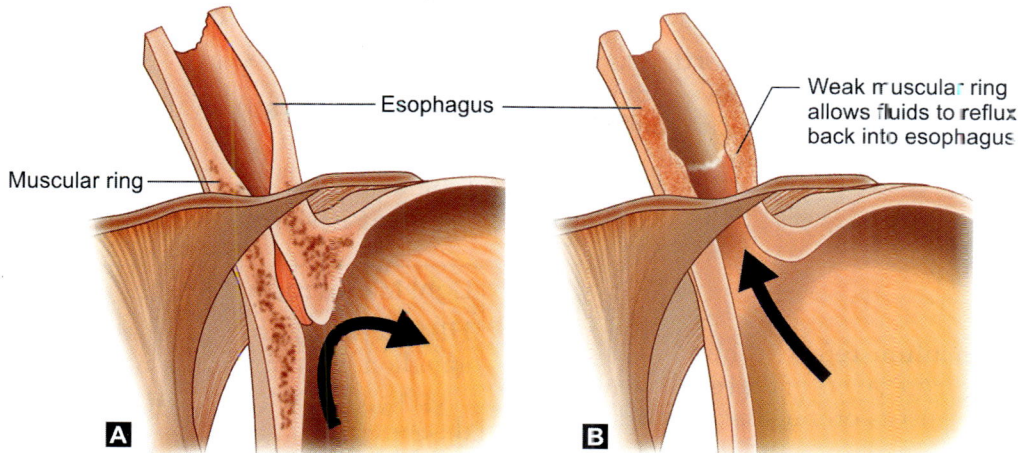

Fig. 20.1: Gastroesophageal reflux disease. (A) Normal esophagus, (B) esophagus is involved as a result of gastroesophageal reflux.

Complications

Chronic irritation of the esophageal epithelium due to gastroesophageal reflux disease (GERD) may cause several complications: Barrett esophagus, esophageal ulcers, stricture formation and respiratory injury described as under.

- *Barrett esophagus:* It refers to replacement of the esophageal squamous epithelium by glandular columnar epithelium resembling gastric or colonic epithelium.
- *Esophageal ulcers:* These lesions may bleed or undergo superadded infection.
- *Stricture formation:* Chronic irritation to esophageal lining results in fibrosis forming esophageal stricture.
- *Respiratory injury:* Aspiration of gastric contents in the airways cause injury to larynx and lungs.

BARRETT ESOPHAGUS

Barrett esophagus is a pathological change characterized by replacement of the esophageal squamous epithelium by glandular columnar epithelium resembling gastric or colonic epithelium. There is increased risk for adenocarcinoma of esophagus in 5–10% of cases.

Pathogenesis

Chronic gastroesophageal reflux disease induces esophagitis and glandular metaplasia in distal third of esophagus due to gastric contents (acid, bile). Healing occurs by ingrowth of immature pluripotent stem cells resulting in replacement of esophageal squamous epithelium by columnar epithelium (similar to gastric or intestine) in distal third. It is known as *Barrett esophagus.* Endoscopy reveals salmon red patches, replacing the normal squamous esophageal epithelium.

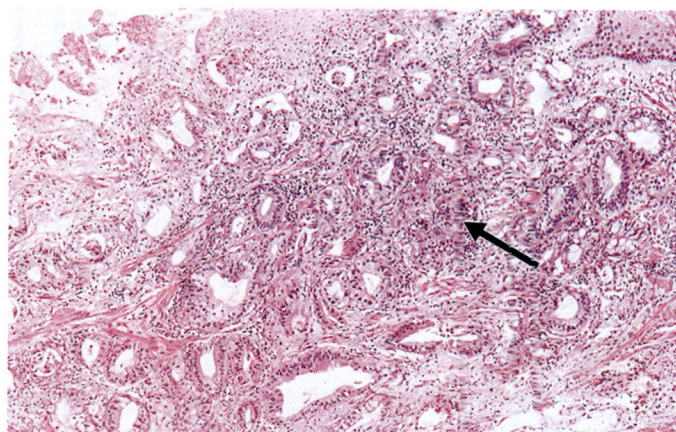

Fig. 20.2: Barrett esophagus showing dysplasia of gastric type of mucosa as a result of metaplasia. Goblet cells in columnar mucosa are seen (arrow).

Light Microscopy

- Histopathological examination reveals replacement of the esophageal squamous epithelium by glandular columnar epithelium (similar to gastric or intestinal columnar epithelium) in a patchy or circumferential manner, known as *Barrett esophagus*.
- Underlying connective tissue usually shows signs of chronic inflammation. Barrett esophagus showing glandular metaplasia is shown in Fig. 20.2.

Clinical Features

Patient presents with painful swallowing (odynophagia), ulceration, hematemesis, and esophageal stricture.

Diagnostic Approach

On endoscopy, Barrett esophagus has *salmon pink* appearance. Patients with Barrett esophagus undergo surveillance endoscopy and biopsy to monitor for the development of dysplasia, as it may undergo malignant transformation.

Complications

Barrett esophagus is a definite risk factor for development of adenocarcinoma in 5–10% cases. Severe dysplasia must be followed up clinically in every case, and partial resection of the esophagus is recommended in some cases.

NON-NEOPLASTIC DISORDERS

ESOPHAGEAL DIVERTICULI

Esophageal diverticulum refers to herniation (outpouching) of one or more layers of the esophageal wall. True diverticulum consists of mucosal, muscular, and serosal layers.

False (pulsion) diverticulum is created by increased intraesophageal pressure results is herniation of mucosa, submucosa and muscularis propria through weak wall. Esophageal diverticula occur in three characteristic locations.

Zenker's Diverticulum

It is most common esophageal diverticulum; present above the upper esophageal sphincter due to defect in the cricopharyngeus muscle. It affects older than 60 years.

Traction Diverticulum

It is present near the midpoint of the esophagus due to motor abnormalities.

Epiphrenic Diverticulum

It is located above the lower esophageal sphincter due to motor abnormalities associated with achalasia (persistent constriction of the lower esophageal sphincter).

ACHALASIA

During swallowing, vasoactive peptides synthesized by ganglion cells in myenteric plexus result in relaxation of lower esophageal sphincter. Achalasia refers to loss of esophageal peristalsis and relaxation of lower esophageal sphincter resulting in dysphagia.

Pathogenesis

- *Congenital:* Absence of ganglion cells in myenteric plexus in lower esophageal sphincter causes loss of esophageal peristalsis and relaxation of lower esophageal sphincter, it is known as *achalasia*. *Proximal esophagus* above LES (lower esophageal sphincter) is dilated.
- *Acquired causes:* Trypanosoma cruzi infection (Chagas' disease) is the most important cause of achalasia in South America. Food is retained within the esophagus, and esophagus undergoes hypertrophy and dilatation.

Clinical Features

Patient presents with dysphagia for solids and liquids. Achalasia may lead to esophageal squamous cell carcinoma in about 5% of cases.

> **Light Microscopy**
>
> Histopathological examination reveals absence of ganglion cells in the myenteric plexus of the lower esophageal sphincter, analogous to Hirschsprung's disease.

HIATUS HERNIA

Hiatus hernia is a protrusion of the stomach through an enlarged esophageal hiatus in the diaphragm. Patient presents with heartburn and regurgitation. Large herniation carries a risk of gastric volvulus or intrathoracic gastric dilation. There are two types of hiatal hernia—*sliding* and *paraesophageal*.

Sliding Hiatal Hernia

It refers to protrusion of the proximal stomach upward above the diaphragm through a widened diaphragmatic hiatus (most common in 90%). Patient presents with nocturnal epigastric distress, hematemesis, and dysphagia (stricture formation). Patient may develop Barrett's esophagus (glandular metaplasia) resulting in risk for adenocarcinoma in 5–10% of cases.

Paraesophageal Hernia

The gastroesophageal junction is in the normal location, but only small portion of the stomach rolls up (less common in 10%) and may be strangulated by the diaphragm (Fig. 20.3).

SCLERODERMA

Scleroderma is an autoimmune disease associated with systemic increased synthesis of collagen in blood vessels, skin and internal organs. **Anti-Scl-70 antibodies** to nuclear topoisomerase are virtually *specific for this autoimmune disease.*

Lower esophageal sphincter is relaxed and dilated. There is absence of peristalsis in the proximal esophagus (dysphagia).

CREST Syndrome

The CREST syndrome, a variant of progressive systemic sclerosis, is also associated with esophageal motility problems.

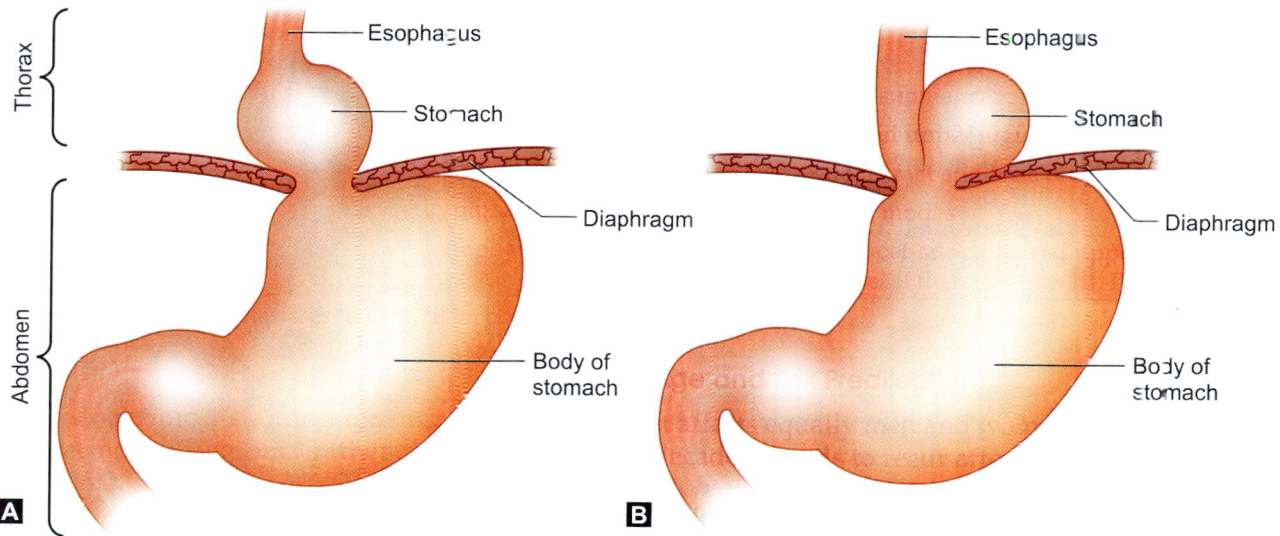

Fig. 20.3: Hiatal hernia. (A) Sliding hiatal hernia, (B) paraesophageal hiatal hernia.

Clinical features: Patient presents with dysphagia, intermittent episodes of ischemia of the fingers, marked by pallor, paresthesia and pain (Raynaud phenomenon).

ESOPHAGEAL STRICTURE

Esophageal stricture most often results from prolonged esophageal gastric acid reflux. It may also be caused by accidental ingestion of corrosive alkali or acid (suicidal or accidental).

Strong acid produces coagulative necrosis, and strong alkali results in liquefactive necrosis. It heals with stricture formation in esophagus, and marked by progressive dysphagia.

POSTCRICOID WEBS (RINGS)

Postcricoid webs are thin mucosal membranes that project into the lumen of the esophagus most common seen in Plummer-Vinson syndrome also known as *Paterson-Kelly syndrome.*

Clinical Features

Patient develops iron deficiency anemia, postcricoid webs in the esophagus resulting in dysphagia, glossitis, leukoplakia, koilonychia (spoon nails) and achlorhydria. There is increased risk of development of carcinoma of oropharynx and upper esophagus in Plummer-Vinson syndrome.

ESOPHAGEAL VARICES

Left gastric vein drains blood from distal esophagus and proximal stomach into the portal vein. Portal hypertension causes esophageal varices due to dilatation of left gastric vein.

Esophageal veins are dilated veins immediately beneath the mucosa in the lower-third of esophagus in cirrhosis. These veins are linked to the portal system through gastroesophageal anastomoses. Left gastric vein is also dilated in these patients.

Varices >5 mm in diameter are prone to rupture and life-threatening hemorrhage. Endoscopy is the primary tool for confirming esophageal varices and treated by sclerotherapy.

SCHATZKI RING

Patient develops subepithelial semicircular fibrous stand in the wall of the esophagus resulting in narrowing of lumen at gastroesophageal junction. Patient presents with dysphagia. The lesion may be demonstrated by endoscopy.

VATER'S SYNDROME

Vater's syndrome is characterized by vertebral abnormalities, atresia, tracheoesophageal fistula, renal disease and absent radius.

BOERHAAVE'S SYNDROME

Boerhaave's syndrome is characterized by rupture of distal esophagus due to vomiting or retching (forceful vomiting).

MALLORY-WEISS SYNDROME

Mallory-Weiss syndrome is characterized by mucosal tear of distal esophagus and upper stomach due to violent retching leading to bleeding. It is typically encountered in chronic alcoholics.

TUMORS OF ESOPHAGUS

Leiomyoma, squamous cell carcinoma and adenocarcinoma are common tumors of esophagus. Histological examination of esophageal carcinoma reveals squamous cell carcinoma (60%) and adenocarcinoma (40%). Squamous cell carcinoma occurs worldwide. Primary melanoma of esophagus is extremely rare, but melanoma from other site may metastasize to esophagus.

BENIGN POLYPS

Fibrovascular Polyps

These are pedunculated intraluminal growth filling esophageal lumen. On histopathological examination, polys are composed of fibrovascular core covered by benign squamous mucosa.

Inflammatory Polyps

These are often related to GERD and present near the squamocolumnar junction. On endoscopy, inflammatory polyp resembles adenocarcinoma. On histopathological examination, polyp is composed of inflamed squamous and/or foveolar mucosa.

Squamous Papilloma

It is often related to GERD. On histopathological examination, it is composed of fibrovascular core covered by benign reactive squamous epithelium with varying degrees of inflammation.

SQUAMOUS CELL CARCINOMA

Squamous cell carcinoma is most common malignant tumor of the esophagus. It frequently affects 50–60 years old age group and is more common in men than women. Esophageal carcinoma most often occurs in lower portion (30%) followed by middle portion (50%) and upper portion (20%). Distribution of esophageal carcinoma is shown in Fig. 20.4.

Risk Factors

- *Cigarette smoking* (most common) and *alcohol* are two important well-known risk factors.

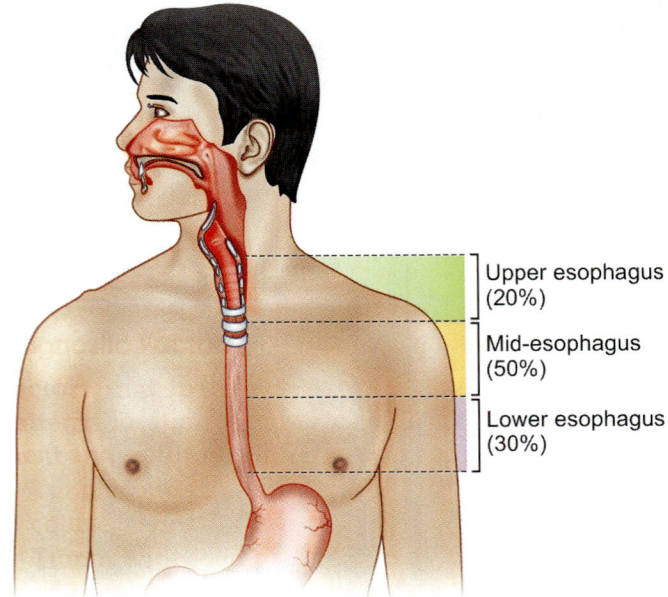

Fig. 20.4: Distribution of esophageal carcinoma.

- Other predisposing factors include *Plummer-Vinson syndrome, achalasia* and *Barrett esophagus*. Human papillomavirus plays an etiologic role in esophageal carcinogenesis.
- *Polycyclic hydrocarbons* are aromatic hydrocarbons derived from animal fat by process of broiling of meats (e.g. *smoked meat* and *fish*). Ingestion of smoked meat containing polycyclic hydrocarbons undergoes hydroxylation in liver forming *epoxides*, results in forming covalent adducts. These bind to cellular DNA, RNA and proteins and alter the genome. Exposure to polycyclic hydrocarbons may produce cancers of oral cavity, *esophagus (upper- and middle-third)* and *pancreas* (Table 20.4).

Molecular Genetics

Mutation of p53 tumor suppressor gene plays role in the pathogenesis of squamous cell carcinoma. Epidermal growth factor is strongly expressed in squamous cell carcinoma. Mutation of cyclins (CCND1/cyclin D1) by translocation or amplification is associated with esophageal carcinoma.

Table 20.4: Chemical carcinogens associated with esophageal carcinoma

Chemical carcinogen	Examples	Associated cancers
Polycyclic hydrocarbons	Tobacco smoke, ingestion of smoked meat and fish	*Esophagus carcinoma* (middle and distal)
		Oral carcinoma
		Pancreas carcinoma
		Lung carcinoma
		Renal pelvis transitional cell carcinoma
		Urinary bladder transitional cell carcinoma

Gastrointestinal Tract

Table 20.5: Oncogenes, their mode of activation and associated with esophageal carcinoma

Category	Proto-oncogene	Mode of activation	Associated malignancies
Cyclins and cyclin-dependent kinases (cell cycle regulators)			
Cyclins	CCND1 (cyclin D1)	Amplification	*Esophageal cancers*
		Amplification	Multiple myeloma, Breast carcinoma
		Translocation	Mantle cell lymphomas

Table 20.6: Tumor suppressor gene mutation associated with esophageal carcinoma

Gene	Protein	Function	Familial tumors	Sporadic cancers
Cell cycle progression inhibitors				
CDKN2A	p16^{INK4a} and p14 ARF	p16 inhibits CDK, p14 indirectly activates p53 tumor suppressor gene	Familial melanoma	*Esophageal carcinoma*, Pancreas carcinoma, Breast carcinoma

Normally, cyclins and cyclin-dependent kinases act as cell cycle regulatory proteins and control the expression of several genes. Oncogene activation and tumor suppressor gene mutation associated with esophageal carcinoma are shown in Tables 20.5 and 20.6.

Locations

- Tumor may occur in any portion of esophagus. But it most commonly develops in the middle region (most common) and lower-thirds in areas of normal anatomic constrictions. Distally located tumor often invades the stomach. It is an aggressive cancer with rapid progression and short survival.
- Growth protrudes into the esophageal lumen, with spread by local extension into adjacent structures, i.e. trachea, bronchi, or aorta, or diffuse infiltration into the esophageal wall.

Clinical Features

Patient presents with dysphagia, weight loss, and anorexia. Occasionally, pain or hematemesis may occur.

Gross Morphology

- The tumor is usually circumferential and often ulcerated (most common) with sharply demarcated margins. It may be a fungating growth obstructing esophageal lumen.
- Cut surface of tumor is gray white, which invades muscular wall, extends out and involves trachea (Fig. 20.5).

Light Microscopy

Histopathological examination shows a range from well-differentiated carcinoma with *epithelial pearls* to poorly differentiated carcinoma that lack evidence of squamous differentiation (Fig. 20.6).

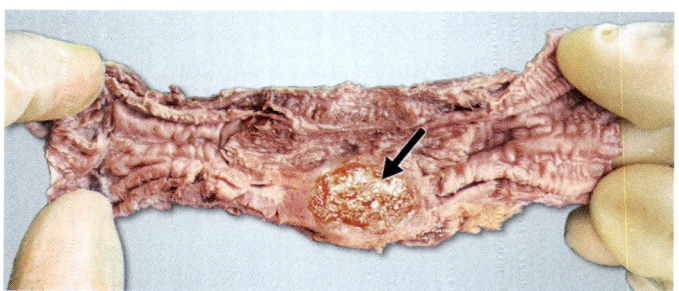

Fig. 20.5: Squamous cell carcinoma of esophagus showing fungating growth invading wall (arrow).

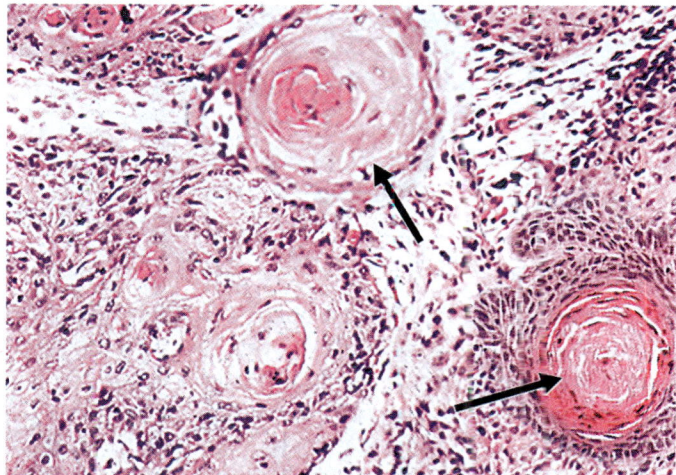

Fig. 20.6: Squamous cell carcinoma of esophagus showing keratin pearls (arrows) (400X).

Immunohistochemistry

Presence of **cytokeratin** in tumor cells is related to the degree of differentiation of the tumor. Some tumors may express **vimentin**. Centromere protein H (**CENP-H**) is one of the fundamental components of the human active kinetochore.

High CENP-H protein expression has been related to poor outcome in patients with esophageal cancer. Panel of markers is used to analyze expression in squamous cell carcinoma of esophagus on histopathological sections (Table 20.7).

Table 20.7: Immunohistochemistry of esophageal squamous cell carcinoma

Tumor marker	Expression
Cytokeratin	Positive
Vimentin	Positive in some tumors
CENP-H protein (high expression has poor prognosis)	Positive

Mode of Spread

- *Local spread:* The tumor invades in longitudinal and transverse directions. Longitudinal spread may involve gastric region. There may be formation of tracheoesophageal fistula.
- *Lymphatic spread:* Esophagus has abundant lymphatic drainage. It first spreads beneath the mucosa, then locally by lymphatic channels that drain into *periesophageal area below the diaphragm and upward into the cervical lymph nodes.*

  The tumor may also metastasize to *submucosa of stomach,* probably through the submucosal lymphatic channels. *These nodal metastases occur early in the course of the disease.* This is the main reason for treatment failure.
- *Hematogenous spread:* It metastasizes via hematogenous route to the *liver, lungs and adrenal glands.*

ADENOCARCINOMA

Adenocarcinoma most often occurs in the lower-third of the esophagus especially in the setting of Barrett esophagus. Gastroesophageal reflux disease plays key role in the pathogenesis of Barrett disease.

Barrett esophagus is a pathological change characterized by replacement of the esophageal squamous epithelium by glandular columnar epithelium resembling gastric or colonic epithelium. There is increased risk for adenocarcinoma of esophagus in 5–10% of cases.

Gross Morphology
Tumor is a small polypoidal, elevated, flat, occult or even depressed lesion. It is located close to gastroesophageal junction.

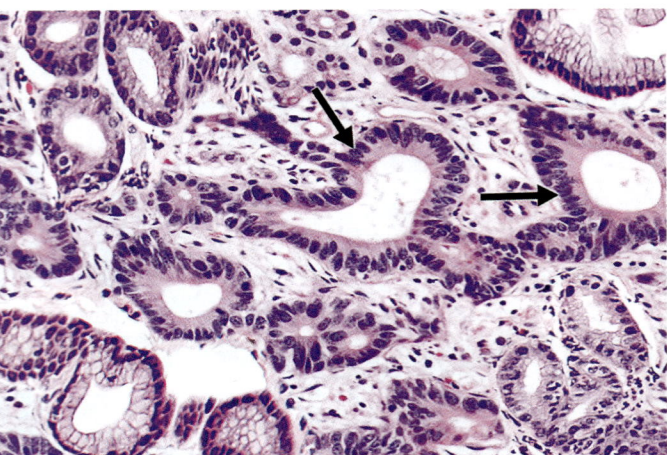

Fig. 20.7: Adenocarcinoma of esophagus (arrows) (400X).

Light Microscopy
- Tumor is composed of infiltrative tubular or papillary structures. Signet ring cells with mucin production may be demonstrated. Presence of signet cell must be differentiated from signet ring cell gastric carcinoma (composed of >50% signet cells).
- Esophageal adenocarcinoma may be well differentiated (>95% of tumor composed of glands), moderately differentiated (50–90%) and poorly differentiated (<50%). Well differentiated carcinoma poses diagnostic challenge (Fig. 20.7).

Immunohistochemistry
More than 90% of esophageal adenocarcinoma express **CK7**. Approximately 40% of these tumors also express **CK20**.

NEUROENDOCRINE TUMORS

Neuroendocrine tumors most often occur in distal esophagus. These tumors may be small or polypoid, or large fungating, ulcerated and deeply invasive.

Light Microscopy
Neuroendocrine tumor is composed of uniform bland cells arranged in solid, acinar or trabecular pattern with areas of necrosis.

MESENCHYMAL TUMORS

Leiomyoma

Leiomyoma is the most common mesenchymal tumor of esophagus. It is demonstrated as an intramural, well circumscribed growth in the middle to distal esophagus. Cut surface is gray white. Histopathological examination reveals benign smooth muscle bundles arranged in whirling pattern.

Gastrointestinal Stromal Tumor

Gastrointestinal stromal tumor occurs as intraluminal mass in distal portion of esophagus. The tumor is **CD117 positive.**

Granular Cell Tumor

Granular cell tumor is demonstrated as incidental submucosal lesion. On histopathological examination, tumor is composed of bland cells arranged in sheets and nests with granular cytoplasm. Cytoplasm shows positivity with **S-100** and **PAS.**

Vascular Tumors

Capillary or cavernous hemangiomas appear as polypoidal intramural masses. Lymphangiomas are small sessile to pedunculated growth in the middle- to lower-third of esophagus.

OTHER TUMORS

Melanoma

Primary melanoma most often occurs as pigmented, polypoidal mass in the middle or distal portion of esophagus.

Lymphoma

Primary lymphoma rarely occurs in esophagus. On histopathological examination, diffuse large B cell lymphoma, mucosa associated lymphoid tissue lymphoma and T cell lymphoma have been described.

Metastases

Esophagus is uncommonly involved due to metastases. Breast carcinoma, lung carcinoma and melanoma may metastasize to the esophagus.

STOMACH

GENERAL CONSIDERATIONS

ANATOMY AND PHYSIOLOGY

Stomach is divided into five regions: cardia, fundus, body (corpus), antrum and pylorus. The pylorus ends in a strong muscular sphincter at the gastroduodenal junction. The pylorus is a muscular zone of stomach controlling passage of food into duodenum. Cardiac region is poorly defined extending up to 5 cm distal to gastroesophageal junction. Stomach also has lesser and greater curvatures.

HISTOLOGY

Stomach has five layers: mucosa, submucosa, smooth muscle, subserosa and serosa. Mucosa of the entire stomach is composed of tubular glands. The cardia region consists of mucus secreting glands. Fundus and body regions of stomach consist of glands that synthesize acid pepsin juices. Pylorus region consists of endocrine cells, which synthesize gastrin hormone.

Gastric Glands in Body of Stomach

Gastric gland consisting of surface mucosal cells form gastric pits of foveola. Gastric gland consists of three portions: isthmus, neck and base. Parietal cells are located in isthmus. Neck of stomach contains parietal cells, mucosal cells and stem cells.

- *Chief cells (zymogenic cells):* These cells synthesize pepsinogen. Hydrochloric acid synthesized by parietal cells converts pepsinogen into pepsin. Pepsin breaks certain peptide bonds in proteins. These cells secrete gastric lipase, which splits short chain triglycerides into fatty acids and monoglycerides.
- *Parietal cells (oxyntic cells):* Parietal cells secrete intrinsic factor, which is needed for absorption of vitamin B_{12}, required for erythropoiesis. Deficiency of vitamin B_{12} causes macrocytic anemia. Parietal cells also secrete hydrochloric acid, which kills microorganisms in food, denatures proteins and converts pepsinogen into pepsin.
- *Mucus surface and neck cells:* These cells secrete mucus, which forms a protective barrier that prevents digestion of stomach wall.
- *Enteroendocrine (G cells):* These cells stimulate chief cells to secrete pepsinogen and parietal cells to secrete HCl. It provides acidic pH (pH 1.8). It converts proenzyme pepsinogen into active pepsin. Pepsin converts proteins into peptides. Rennin is a proteolytic enzyme found in stomach of infants which helps in the digestion of milk proteins.
- *Brunner's glands* present in the duodenum synthesize *alkaline fluid to buffer gastric acid* and mucus for protection and lubrication.

VESSELS AND NERVES

Blood Supply

Most of the blood supply to stomach is derived from the coeliac artery. Left and right gastric arteries are present along the lesser curvature. Left and right gastroepiploic arteries are present along great curvature. Proximal stomach also receives blood supply from inferior phrenic and short gastric arteries.

Venous Drainage

Venous drainage parallels the arterial supply of stomach. Left and right gastric veins drain into the portal vein.

Right gastroepiploic veins drain into superior mesenteric vein, while left gastroepiploic vein into the splenic vein.

Lymphatic Drainage

Lymphatic drainage from superior gastric, suprapyloric, pancreaticoduodenal and inferior gastric/subpyloric regions of stomach drain into coeliac group of lymph nodes and thoracic duct.

Innervation

Stomach is supplied by vagus nerve (parasympathetic) and sympathetic *via* the coeliac plexus.

HELICOBACTER PYLORI INDUCED GI DISORDERS

Helicobacter pylori is transmitted by feco-oral route. The bacterium resides within the mucosal layer lining pits beneath the bicarbonate-rich mucous barrier, where the pH approaches neutrality. *Helicobacter pylori* does not survive in metaplastic glands. Mucus and bicarbonate secretion are defense mechanisms against acid and pepsin (Fig. 20.8). Role of *Helicobacter pylori* in gastrointestinal disorders is shown in Table 20.8.

HELICOBACTER PYLORI INDUCED MUCOSAL INJURY

Helicobacter pylori induces mucosal injury by following mechanisms. Role of *Helicobacter pylori* in gastrointestinal disorders is shown in Fig. 20.9.

Table 20.8: Role of *Helicobacter pylori* in gastrointestinal disorders

Gastrointestinal disorder	Frequency
Gastritis (acute/chronic)	100%
Peptic ulcer disease	10%
Gastric atrophy	5%
Gastric adenocarcinoma	1%
MALT lymphoma (mucosa associated lymphoid tissue lymphoma of stomach)	<1%

Attachment of Helicobacter Pylori to Mucosal Cells

The pathogen attaches to mucosa with the help of its adhesin molecules.

Role of VacA Exotoxin

VacA exotoxin released by the pathogen participates in the formation of vacuoles, induction of apoptosis as a result of leakage of mitochondrial cytochrome c, *disruption of epithelial functions and blockage of T cell response*.

Role of DNA Segment (CagA) Effector Molecules

CagA effector molecules alter signaling pathway and tight junctions. These also induce IL-8 synthesis.

Role of Immunologic T and B Cells

These cells synthesize thrombotic PAF, which acts on bacterial gene products of *Helicobacter pylori* resulting in synthesis of *proteases, phospholipases, and urease* responsible for mucosal injury.

Role of Urease

- Urease of Helicobacter bacteria derives energy from urea. Urease converts urea *into ammonia and CO_2*. Ammonia neutralizes hydrogen ions present in mucus layer of gastric mucosa and provides favorable microenvironment for growth of *Helicobacter pylori*.
- Ammonia *stimulates gastrin*, which enhances hydrochloric acid production resulting in mucosal injury due to impaired duodenal bicarbonate levels.
- Myeloperoxidase converts *ammonia into monochloramine*, which causes mucosal injury.

Role of Protease Enzyme

Protease breaks down mucus glycoproteins and destroys mucosal barrier.

Role of Phospholipase

Phospholipase *damages surface epithelial cells*. It also enhances *release of leukotrienes*, which attract polymorphonuclear cells resulting in release of *myeloperoxidase*.

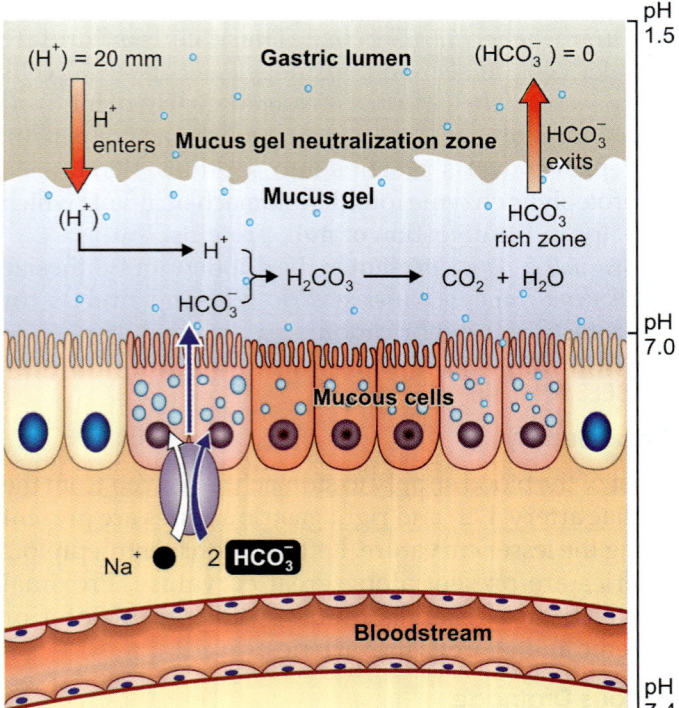

Fig. 20.8: Mucus and bicarbonate secretion as defense mechanisms against acid and pepsin.

Gastrointestinal Tract

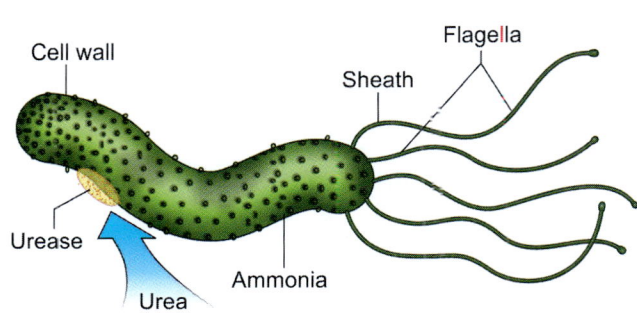
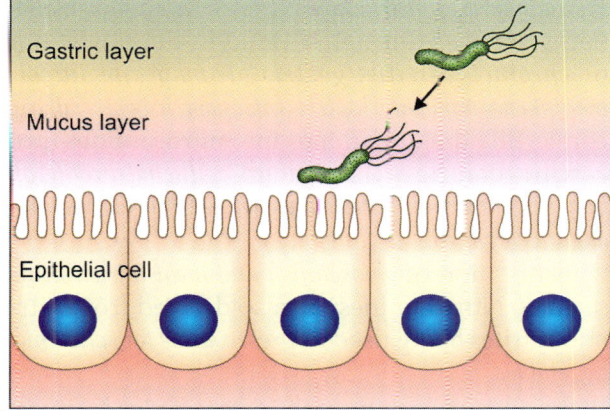
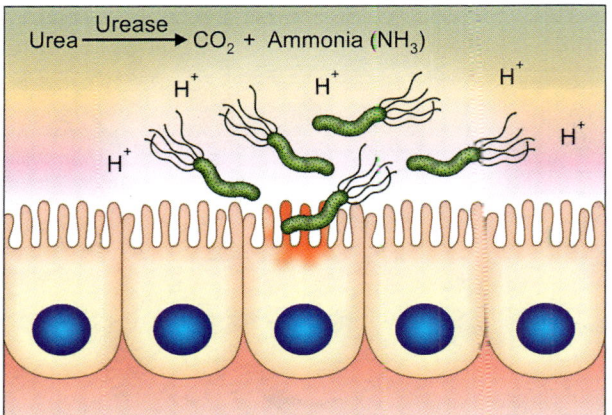
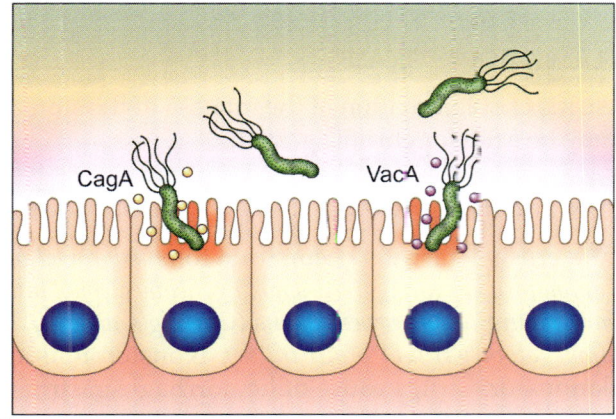
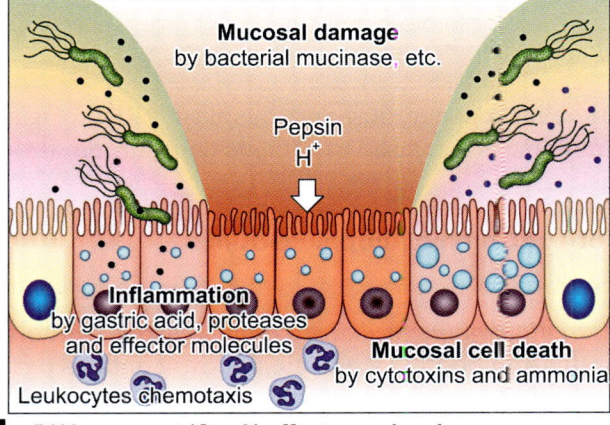
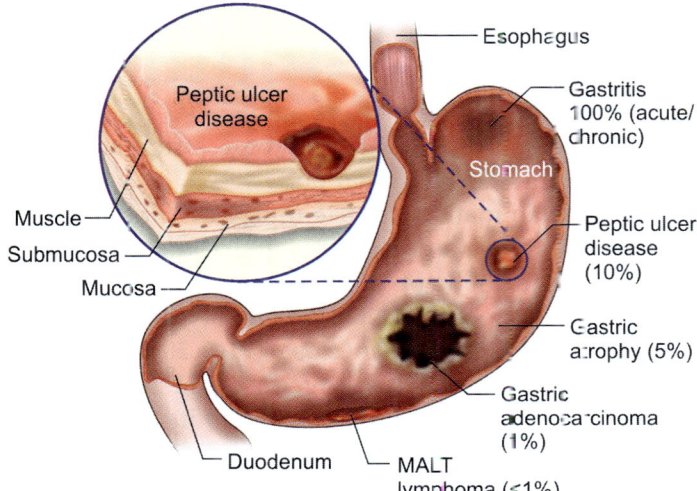

Fig. 20.9: Role of *Helicobacter pylori* in gastrointestinal disorders.

HELICOBACTER PYLORI INDUCED GIT MALIGNANCIES

World Health Organization has designated *Helicobacter pylori*—a potential human carcinogen. It is strongly associated with *gastric adenocarcinoma (lower portion) and gastric B cell lymphoma* of the mucosa associated lymphoid tissue (MALT) type.

- *Helicobacter pylori* causes *gastric adenocarcinoma (lower portion)* through its role in the development of *chronic gastritis, gastric atrophy and intestinal metaplasia, hypochlorhydria, intragastric bacterial growth converting dietary amines into nitrosamines (potent carcinogenic agent), sustained epithelial proliferation, genomic mutation, dysplasia, early gastric carcinoma and advanced gastric carcinoma.*
- Consumption of *smoked fish and meat is rich in nitrosamines*. Nitrosamines are also derived from nitrates and nitrites being used as *preservative for salted pickled vegetables.*
- In the advanced stage of the disease; *urea breath test or antibody test for Helicobacter pylori* must be performed.

INFLAMMATORY DISEASES

Gastritis is inflammation of the mucosa of the stomach. It may be acute or chronic gastritis.

ACUTE EROSIVE GASTRITIS

Acute erosive gastritis occurs due to *nonsteroidal anti-inflammatory drugs, cigarette smoking, heavy alcohol intake, biliary regurgitation, severe burns (Curling's ulcer), AIDS (cytomegalovirus) and brain injury*. Nonsteroidal anti-inflammatory drugs cause of hemorrhagic gastritis by *disrupting bicarbonate-rich mucous barrier*.

Light Microscopy

Gastric mucosa shows multiple erosions not extending beyond the muscularis mucosa. It shows acute inflammation, necrosis, and hemorrhage.

CHRONIC GASTRITIS

Chronic gastritis refers to atrophy of gastric glands secondary to chronic inflammation.

On gross examination, gastric mucosa is inflamed (Fig. 20.10). On histopathological examination, chronic gastritis reveals atrophy of the gastric glands as well as lamina propria, intestinal metaplasia and lymphocytic infiltrate in the atrophic mucosa (Fig. 20.11). As *Helicobacter pylori* does not survive in the metaplastic intestinal glands, hence not demonstrated in biopsies. Histopathological types of chronic gastritis include type A, type B and type AB.

Atrophic Gastritis

This pathological term is reserved for *chronic gastritis with intestinal metaplasia*. The crypts of the gastric corpus are replaced by intestinal glands with goblet cells. There is *elongation of glandular necks* with extended epithelial regeneration and dysplasia. Risk of gastric carcinoma is increased in patients with chronic atrophic gastritis.

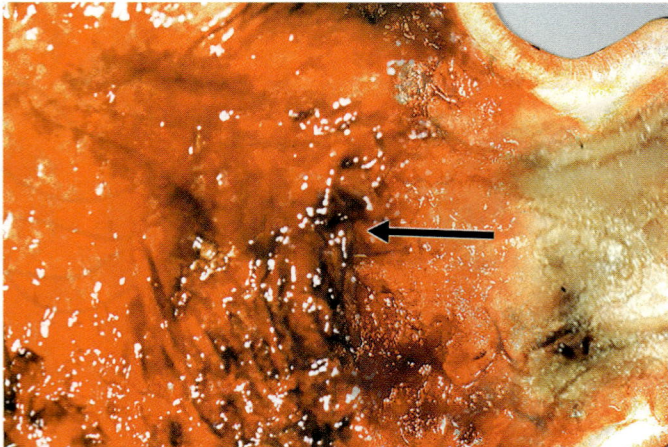

Fig. 20.10: Chronic gastritis showing inflamed gastric mucosa (arrow).

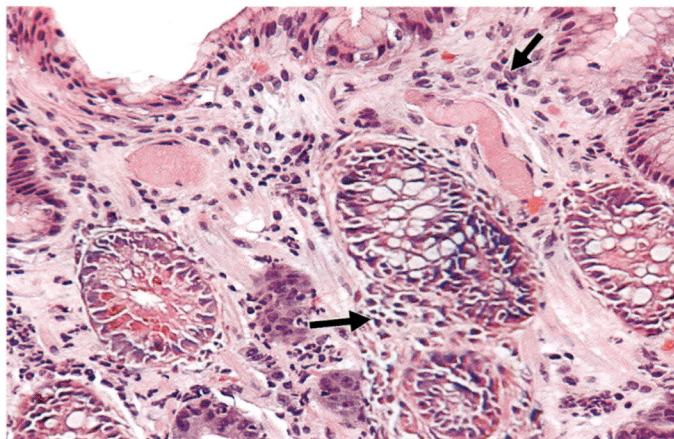

Fig. 20.11: Chronic gastritis light microscopy showing chronic inflammatory infiltrate in gastric region with intestinal metaplasia (arrows) (400X).

Types of Chronic Atrophic Gastritis

Chronic Gastritis Type A

It is *autoimmune mediated chronic gastritis* involving fundus and body of stomach. Fundus contains parietal cells, which synthesize hydrochloric acid and vitamin B_{12} binder intrinsic factor.
- *Pathogenesis:* Immunological destruction of parietal cells by autoantibodies results in achlorhydria and pernicious anemia. Bone marrow and peripheral smear display features of megaloblastic anemia due to destruction of intrinsic factor. Serum gastrin level is increased as a result of gastric G cell hyperplasia.
- *Complications:* Patient with autoimmune mediated chronic gastritis may develop gastric adenocarcinoma (10%), *carcinoid tumors and chronic thyroiditis.*

Table 20.9: Differences between chronic atrophic gastritis type A and type B

Parameters	Chronic atrophic gastritis A (autoimmune)	Chronic atrophic gastritis B (non-autoimmune)
Patient population	Older age group (white women)	Adults (worldwide)
Pathogenesis	Autoimmune mechanism Autoantibodies against parietal cells and intrinsic factor	Nonimmune mechanism *Helicobacter pylori*
Clinical manifestations	Pernicious anemia (megaloblastic erythropoiesis) Decreased gastric acid secretion	Abdominal pain and dyspepsia Upper gastrointestinal bleeding
Light microscopy	Chronic gastritis Progressive destruction of glands in fundus region Intestinal metaplasia (pyloric region) and enterochromaffin cells hyperplasia	Chronic gastritis Destruction of glands absent Intestinal metaplasia (pyloric region, if body involved)
Serum gastrin level	Elevated	Normal or low
Complications	Gastric adenocarcinoma (10%) Carcinoid tumors Chronic thyroiditis	Gastric adenocarcinoma (lower gastric region) MALT lymphoma (mucosa associated lymphoid tissue lymphoma) Gastroduodenal ulcers
Clinical course	Chronic aggressive course	Chronic less aggressive course

Chronic atrophic gastritis type AB caused by *Helicobacter pylori* and dietary factors predisposes to gastric adenocarcinoma. Eosinophilic gastritis is related to allergens and characterized by transmural infiltration by eosinophils and muscular hypertrophy.

Chronic Gastritis Type B

Helicobacter pylori resides in the gastric antrum and pylorus. *It is associated with chronic gastritis type B.*

These patients are also associated with *gastroduodenal ulcers, gastric adenocarcinoma and MALT (mucosa associated lymphoid tissue) lymphoma.* Differences between chronic gastritis type A and type B are shown in Table 20.9.

Chronic Gastritis Type AB

Chronic gastritis type AB is associated with combination of *Helicobacter pylori* and dietary factors. It predisposes to gastric adenocarcinoma.

PEPTIC ULCER DISEASE

Peptic ulcer disease occurs in *duodenum, stomach, lower end of the esophagus or Meckel's diverticulum* Helicobacter pylori is most often associated with duodenal ulcers (90%) and gastric ulcers (65%). *Eradication of Helicobacter pylori contributes to the healing of peptic ulcers.*

Peptic ulcer disease is most often solitary, but may be multiple in 20% of cases. Vagotomy is used only in the treatment of complicated persistent duodenal ulcers resistant to other treatment modalities. Pathogenesis and clinical course of peptic ulcer disease are shown in Fig. 20.12.

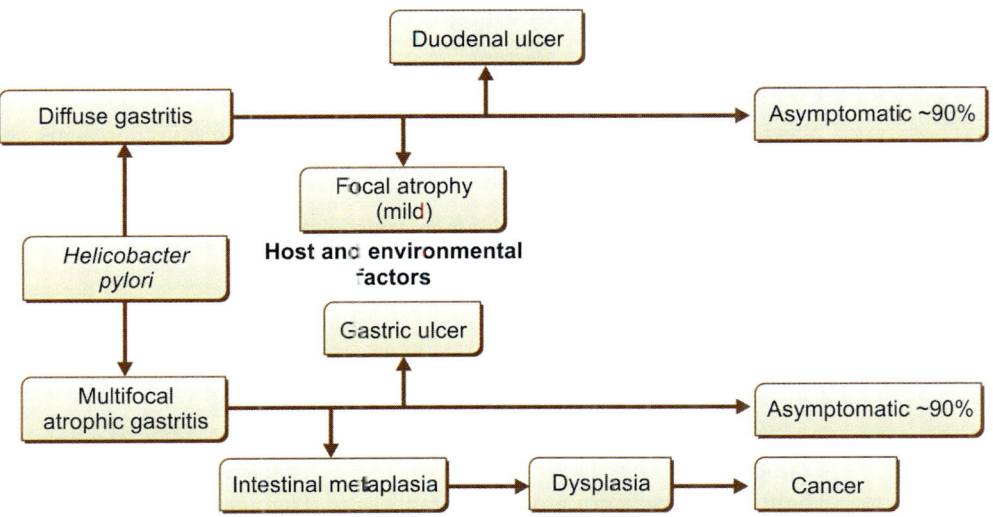

Fig. 20.12: Pathogenesis and clinical course of peptic ulcer disease.

LOCATIONS

Duodenal peptic ulcer most often occurs in first portion of the **duodenum** *just close to the pylorus*. It is associated with hypersecretion of gastric acid and pepsin and *Helicobacter pylori* infection.

Helicobacter pylori increases gastric acid secretion and impair mucosal defenses. Gastric peptic ulcer most often occurs at lesser curvature just at the junction of the body and pyloric antrum. Differences between duodenal and gastric peptic ulcer are shown in Table 20.10.

ETIOPATHOGENESIS

Since the gastric acid of ulcer patients does not contain unusually high quantities of hydrochloric acid or pepsin, it is postulated that glands are damaged by a **back-diffusion of hydrogen ions** (most important). *Helicobacter pylori*, spicy food, alcohol and drug aspirin disrupt mucosal barrier resulting in mucosal injury due to back diffusion of hydrogen ions. *Campylobacter pylori*, a common cause of gastritis has been associated with peptic ulcer disease and gastric carcinoma.

Table 20.10: Differences between duodenal and gastric peptic ulcers

Parameters	Duodenal ulcer	Gastric ulcer
Age group	25–50 years of age	More than 50 years
Sex predilection	Men > women	Men and women equally affected
Risk factors	MEN 1, cirrhosis, chronic obstructive pulmonary disease, chronic renal failure, hyperparathyroidism	Smoking delays healing of ulcer
Frequency	More often (75% cases)	Less often (25%)
Increased incidence	Blood group O	Blood group A
Etiology	*Helicobacter pylori* responsible for defective mucosal barrier in 80–90% of cases	Due to disruption of mucosal barrier due to mucosal ischemia (reduced PGE), bile reflux, delayed gastric emptying
Basal acid out (BAO) and maximal acid output (MAO)	Acid levels high	Normal to low. May be increased due to enhanced gastrin secretion
Number of ulcer	Solitary	Solitary
Location	Anterior portion of first part of duodenum in 90% cases and posterior portion	Lesser curvature of antrum (same location for cancer)
Perforation	Ulcer present in posterior portion of duodenum may perforate into pancreas results in pancreatitis	Perforation is less common
Clinical findings	Burning epigastric pain 1–3 hours after eating. Epigastric pain relieved by eating	Epigastric pain exacerbated by eating
Malignant transformation	Duodenal ulcers never undergo malignant transformation	More common
Complications	Bleeding from gastroduodenal artery, perforation (air under diaphragm, pain radiates to left or right shoulder) Gastric outlet obstruction and pancreatitis	Bleeding from left gastric artery Perforation
Endoscopy accuracy	90–95%	90–95%
Upper GI barium study	Diagnostic in 70–80% cases	Diagnostic in 70–80% cases
Histopathological examination	Not essential as not undergoing malignant transformation	Essential to rule out malignant transformation in 1–4% cases
Treatment	Avoid NSAIDs, alcohol, smoking Eradication of *Helicobacter pylori* Highly selective vagotomy in resistant cases	Avoid NSAIDs, alcohol, smoking Eradication *Helicobacter pylori* Hemigastrectomy without vagotomy in resistant cases

Helicobacter Pylori

- This pathogen increases *gastric acid secretion and apparently impair both gastric and duodenal mucosal defenses* resulting in duodenal ulcer (90%) and gastric ulcer (65%).
- *Helicobacter pylori* synthesizes *urease, phospholipase and protease* that cause breakdown of glycoproteins resulting in defective mucosal barrier.

  Increased permeability of the gastric mucosa to hydrogen ion, leads to back diffusion of hydrogen ions resulting in injury to the gastric mucosa (mucosal ischemia due to reduced PGE). Eradication of *Helicobacter pylori* infection is curative of peptic ulcer disease in most patients.

Bile Reflux and Delayed Gastric Emptying

These may also cause peptic ulcer disease.

Dietary Factors and Acid Secretion

Alcohol, spicy food, and substances that stimulate acid secretion may play a pathogenetic role. *Duodenal ulcer is always associated with hypersecretion of gastric acid and pepsin.*

- Due to increased parietal cell mass, basal acid output (BAO) and maximal acid output (MAO) are increased in duodenal ulcer.
- On the other hand, basal acid output (BAO) and maximal acid output (MAO) are normal to low in gastric ulcer.

NSAIDs

Drug such as aspirin inhibits prostaglandin synthesis resulting in damage to mucosal barrier resulting in ulcer.

Tobacco Smoking

The incidence of peptic ulcer is two-fold greater in smokers.

Zollinger-Ellison Syndrome

Recurrent intractable peptic ulcer disease or peptic ulcer in aberrant sites, i.e. the jejunum is characteristic of the Zollinger-Ellison syndrome with excess gastrin production, most often from a gastrinoma (islet cell tumor of the pancreas).

Genetic Factors

Increased frequency of occurrence of peptic ulcer disease in persons with blood group O suggests that genetic factors may play a role.

Hyperparathyroidism

Peptic ulcer disease is sometimes associated with primary hyperparathyroidism.

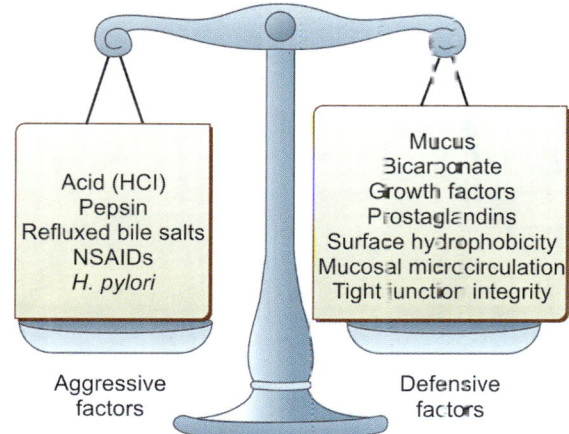

Fig. 20.13: Defensive and aggressive factors in relation to peptic ulcer disease.

Multiple Endocrine Neoplasia I

Peptic ulcer disease may occur in MEN I, an autosomal dominant disorder characterized by adenomas or hyperplasia of pituitary, thyroid, parathyroid, adrenal cortical, and pancreatic islet cell.

Hypercalcemia increases serum gastrin, thereby stimulating gastric acid secretion. Defensive and aggressive factors in relation to peptic ulcer disease are shown in Fig. 20.13.

CLINICAL FEATURES

Patient with gastric ulcer presents with epigastric pain just after food intake. While pain occurs within 1–3 hours after food intake in duodenal ulcer.

Gross Morphology

Morphological features of peptic ulcer disease are described in Fig. 20.14.

- *Size and shape:* Most peptic ulcers are small round or oval defect of the mucosa measuring 1–2 cm in diameter, and rarely exceeding 4 cm size.
- *Base of the ulcer:* It is *smooth and clean* due to action of hydrochloric acid and pepsin, but it may be covered with fibrin.
- *Margin of ulcer:* Gastric ulcer shows radiating folds of gastric mucosa starting at the *ulcer punched out margins* appearing as radiating fold in a *spoke-like fashion, in contrast to gastric carcinoma,* which often has an irregular necrotic base and firm, raised margins.

  The distinction between gastric peptic ulcer and ulcerated gastric carcinoma must be established by biopsy. In contrast to malignant gastric ulcer, peptic ulcer disease usually heals with conservative management.

20 Section III: Systemic Pathology

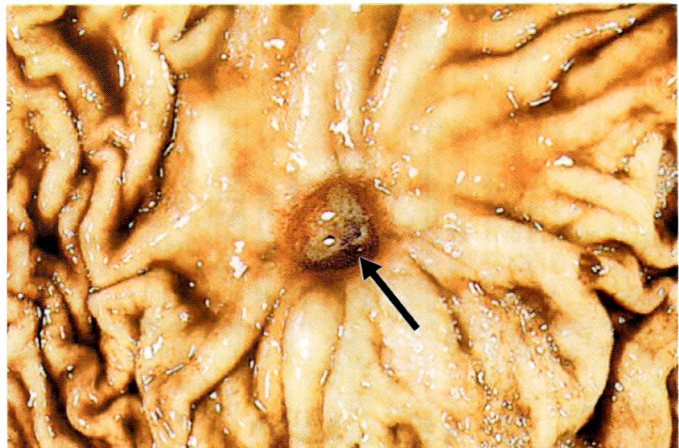

Fig. 20.14: Chronic peptic ulcer. A partial gastrectomy was performed because of hematemesis. There was a bleeding artery in the base of the ulcer (arrow).

Light Microscopy

On histopathological examination, peptic ulcer shows following four zones from superficial layer to deep base. The mucosal defect may extend all the way to the muscle layer (Figs 20.15 and 20.16).

- *Floor/base:* It is superficial zone of peptic ulcer composed of necrotic fibrinous amorphous debris.
- *Zone of acute inflammatory exudates:* This zone is infiltrated by numerous neutrophils. Inflammation is present beneath floor/base of ulcer, and merges with granulation tissue.
- *Granulation tissue:* It is composed of *blood vessels, fibroblasts, macrophages, lymphocytes* and *plasma cells.* It gradually transforms into a zone of fibrous scarring.
- *Zone of fibrous scarring:* Granulation tissue rests on a solid fibrous or collagenous scar. If the ulcer extends into the muscle layer, it may erode blood vessels and cause bleeding.

COMPLICATIONS

Complications of peptic ulcer disease include hemorrhage, perforation, stenosis, pancreatitis and malignant transformation described as under.

Hemorrhage

It is the most common complication of peptic ulcer. Patient presents with *hematemesis* with *melena* (black stools containing blood). Ulcer erodes the wall of arteries supplying to the region. *Gastroduodenal artery bleeds in duodenal ulcer.*

Whereas *bleeding occurs from left gastric artery in gastric ulcer.* Severe bleeding is life-threatening in 10–20% of patients. Melena is commonly seen in patients who suffer from chronic peptic ulcer disease.

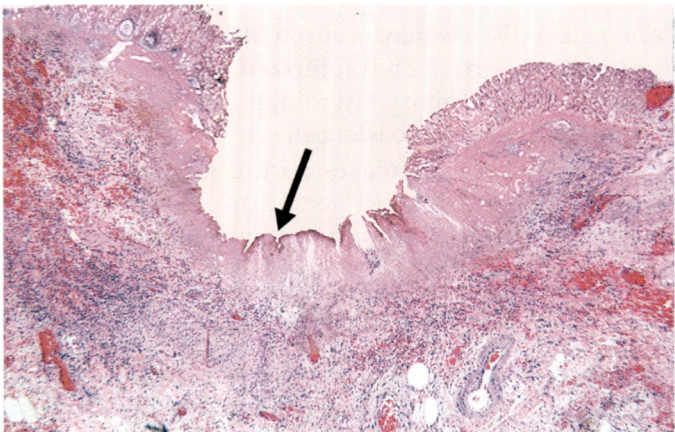

Fig. 20.15: Chronic peptic ulcer microscopy showing base composed of necrotic fibrinous amorphous debris, overlying inflammatory infiltrate, granulation tissue and fibrous tissue (arrow) (100X).

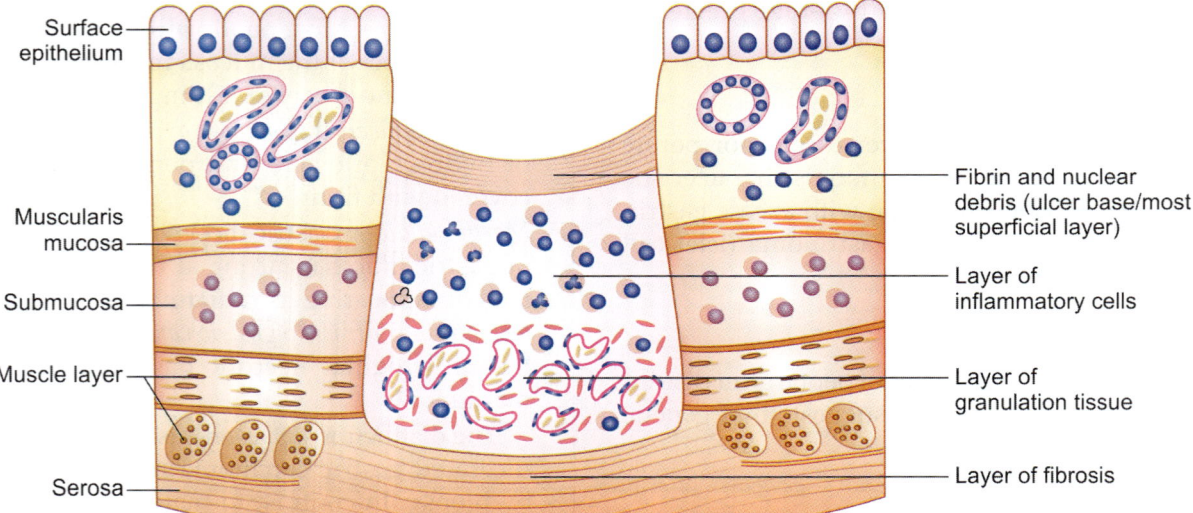

Fig. 20.16: Peptic ulcer disease showing four zones from superficial layer to deep base: superficial floor/base, zone of inflammatory exudate, zone of granulation and zone of fibrous scarring.

Gastrointestinal Tract

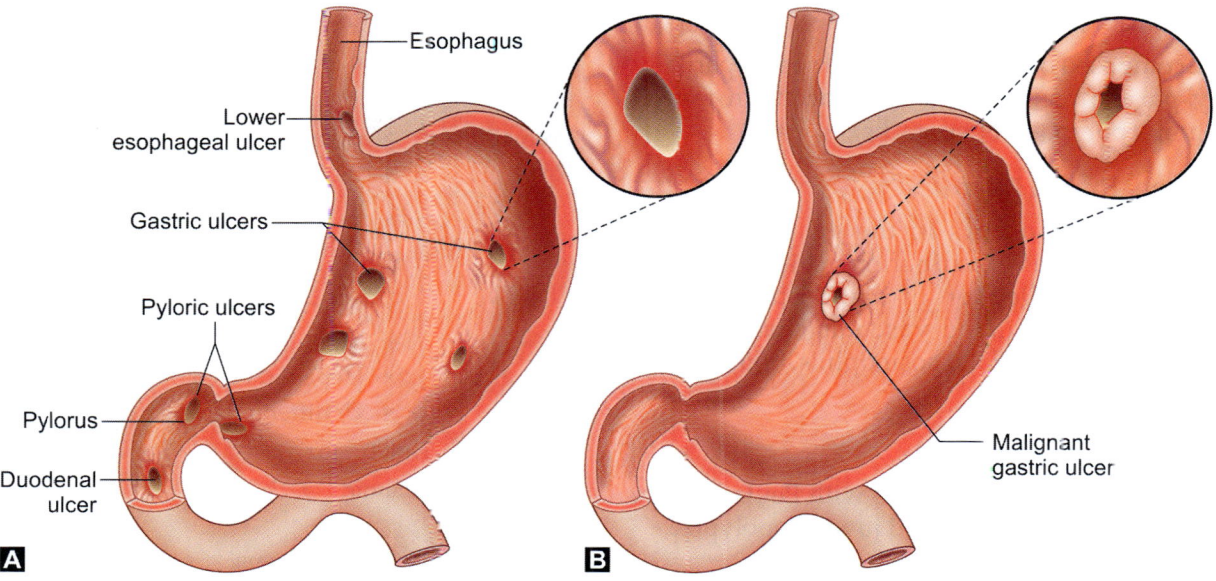

Fig. 20.17: (A) Peptic ulcer disease showing distribution of ulcers in stomach and duodenum, (B) malignant gastric ulcer.

Table 20.11: Differences between benign and malignant gastric ulcers

Parameters	Benign gastric ulcer	Malignant gastric ulcer
Age group	Younger age group	Older age group
Gender	Male predominance	Male and female equally affected or male predominance
Site of ulcer	Along lesser curvature of stomach	Along greater curvature of stomach
Base of ulcer	Clear and hemorrhagic	Necrotic debris
Gastric mucosal folds	Radiating mucosal folds	Interrupted mucosal folds
Margins of ulcer	Sharply punched out	Irregular heaped up
Barium meal study	Sharp punched out lesion	Irregular lesion
Light microscopy	Composed of necrotic floor base, numerous neutrophils, granulation tissue and fibrosis	Showing features of malignancy, that may disseminate to distant organs

Perforation

Duodenal ulcer most often perforates than gastric ulcer in 10% of cases. Patient develops *peritonitis* and *paralytic ileus*.

Air is demonstrated under the diaphragm (*pneumoperitoneum*) by imaging techniques. Perforation with severe hemorrhage is responsible for shock with fatal outcome.

Hourglass Deformity and Pyloric Stenosis

Fibrosis around the healed ulcer leads to stenosis of the area in 5% of patients. Fibrosis around healed gastric ulcer causes narrowing in center of the stomach giving *hourglass deformity*. Patient with healed ulcer in duodenum develops pyloric stenosis.

Pancreatitis

Perforation of posterior wall of duodenal ulcer may cause peritonitis or involvement of liver. Pancreatitis is accompanied by dull pain and elevated *serum amylase and lipase*.

Malignant Transformation

Most gastric ulcers are benign, but small percentage may undergo malignant transformation. *Duodenal ulcers never undergo malignant transformation.*

Peptic ulcer disease showing distribution of benign ulcers in stomach and duodenum and malignant gastric ulcer are shown in Fig. 20.17.

Differences between benign and malignant ulcers are shown in Table 20.11.

GASTRIC POLYPS

Hyperplastic Polyps

These are composed of elongated, dilated, branching foveola and inflamed lamina propria. These may occur in Osler-Weber-Rendu syndrome.

Polyps in Fundal Region

These are composed of cystically dilated spaces partially lined by parietal cells. These may occur in famial adenomatous polyposis or sporadic.

Inflammatory Fibroid Polyp

It most commonly occurs in the gastric antrum. On histopathological examination, it is composed of a submucosal collection of bland spindle cells in a background of dilated vascular channels and inflammatory cells especially eosinophils. Spindle cells are CD34 positive.

Hamartomatous Polyps

These are demonstrated in patients with Peutz-Jeghers syndrome, Cowden's disease and juvenile polyposis.

PRIMARY TUMORS

Primary gastric tumors are classified into benign and malignant. These include adenocarcinoma (95%) and lymphomas (3%), carcinoids and neuroendocrine carcinomas (1%), stromal tumors and leiomyomas (1%). Intestinal metaplasia is precursor lesion of gastric adenocarcinoma. Leiomyoma is most common benign tumor of stomach.

Primary cancers of stomach involve mucosa whereas secondary tumors (e.g. carcinoma breast, malignant melanoma and leukemic infiltration) involve submucosa and muscularis. WHO classification of gastric tumors is shown in Table 20.12.

GASTRIC ADENOCARCINOMA

Gastric adenocarcinoma is the most common. It constitutes 90–95% of all gastric cancers. It is often discovered at advanced stage. Practically all gastric carcinomas arise from generative or basal cells of foveolae. Intestinal metaplasia is precursor lesion of gastric adenocarcinoma. Locations and distribution of gastric carcinoma are shown in Table 20.13. Distribution of gastric carcinoma is shown in Fig. 20.18.

Predisposing Risk Factors

Gender

Gastric carcinoma is more common in men than in women.

Age Group

There is a sharp increase in gastric carcinoma rates in people over the age of 50 years especially in men. Most people are diagnosed with gastric carcinoma in their late 60s and 80s.

Table 20.12: WHO classification of gastric tumors

Origin	Examples
Epethial tumors	
Premalignant lesions	• Adenoma • Intraepithelial neoplasm (low or high grade)
Carcinoma	• Adenocarcinoma (papillary tubular, mucinous, poorly cohesive and mixed) • Adenosquamous • Medullary carcinoma • Hepatoid carcinoma • Undifferentiated carcinoma
Neuroendocrine tumor	
	• NET G1 carcinoid • NET G2 • Neuroendocrine carcinoma • Mixed adenoneuroendocrine carcinoma • EC cell, serotonin producing NET • Gastrin producing NET (gastrinoma)
Mesenchyal tumors	
	• Glomus tumor • Granular cell tumor • Leiomyoma • Plexiform fibromyxoma • Gastrointestinal, stromal tumor • Kaposi sarcoma • Leiomyosarcoma • Synovial sarcoma
Lymphoid tumor	
	• Lymphomas
Secondary tumors	
	• Breast carcinoma • Melanoma • Leukemic infiltration

Table 20.13: Location and frequency of gastric carcinoma

Locations	Frequency
Pyloantrum region (anterior and posterior walls and lesser curvature of stomach)	50–60%
Cardiac region of stomach	25%
Body and fundus region	25%
Greater curvature of stomach	12%

Geography

Incidence of gastric carcinoma is higher in Japan, Finland, and Iceland, Chile, Russia, China and Southern and Eastern Europe, but low in USA. Its incidence is higher in South India than rest of the country.

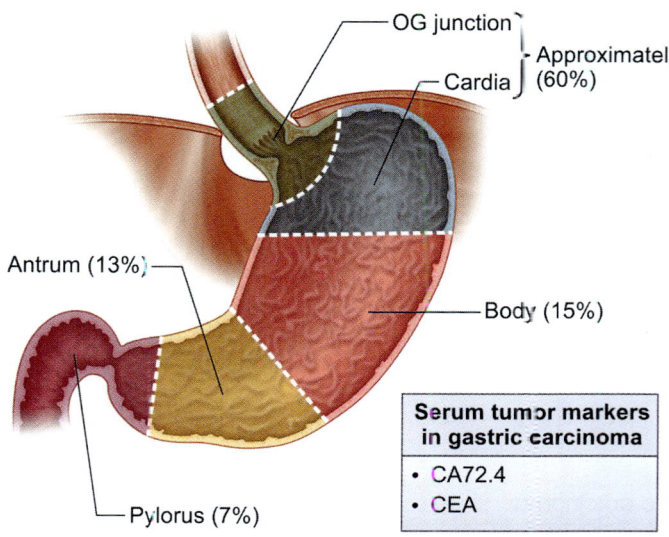

Fig. 20.18: Distribution of gastric carcinoma.

Helicobacter Pylori

Incidence of gastric cancer in the lower (distal) part of the stomach parallels the presence of chronic gastritis secondary to *Helicobacter pylori*. Persistent infection by *Helicobacter pylori* is associated with *chronic atrophic gastritis, sustained epithelial proliferation, genomic mutation, dysplasia, early gastric carcinoma and advanced gastric adenocarcinoma*, MALT (mucosa associated lymphoid tissue) lymphoma and carcinoid tumors. *Helicobacter pylori* induces mucosal injury and converts dietary amines into nitrosamines (carcinogenic agent).

Dietary Factors

Diet rich in nitrosamines increases the risk of gastric cancer. Consumption of *smoked fish and meat* is rich in *nitrosamines*. Nitrosamines are also derived from nitrates and nitrites being used as *preservative for salted pickled vegetables*.

Dietary nitrates and nitrites substances are converted to nitrosamines by *Helicobacter pylori*. On the other hand, eating lots of fresh fruits and vegetables appears to lower the risk of stomach cancer. Green leafy vegetables and citrus fruits act as antioxidants and thus are protective against gastric cancer. A high intake of animal fat has also been considered a protective factor against gastric cancer.

Tobacco Chewing or Smoking

Tobacco smoking or chewing increases cancer risk in the upper portion of the stomach near the esophagus. The rate of stomach cancer is about double in smokers.

Blood Group A

For unknown reasons, people with blood group A have a higher risk of getting stomach cancer in 4% of these cases.

Previous Stomach Surgery

Partial gastrectomy performed in peptic ulcer disease increases risk of gastric carcinoma after many years of surgery. It is due to *decreased secretion of gastric acid*, which allows more *nitrite-producing bacteria* to be present. *Reflux of bile* from the small intestine into the stomach after surgery may also increase the risk of gastric cancer.

Pernicious Anemia

Intrinsic factor synthesized by parietal cell is required for absorption of vitamin B_{12}. Autoantibodies formed against intrinsic factor cause megaloblastic anemia. Risk of gastric carcinoma increases in patients suffering from pernicious anemia.

Ménétrier Disease (Hypertrophic Gastropathy)

This disorder is characterized by excessive growth of gastric lining resulting in large mucosal folds. There is low level of gastric acid in this disorder. Due to unknown reason, there is increased risk of gastric cancer.

Inherited Cancer Syndromes

Some inherited conditions may raise a person's risk of stomach cancer. Gene mutations such as *E-cadherin, β-catenin, APC tumor suppressor gene, fibroblast growth factor, DNA repair genes and FGF3* participate in the pathogenesis of gastric carcinoma. Oncogenes, tumor suppressor gene mutations and chemical carcinogens associated with gastric carcinoma are shown in Tables 20.14 to 20.16.

- *Germline defects of E-cadherin (CDH1):* Under physiological state, E-cadherin (CDH1) participates in adhesion of intercellular junctions of gastric mucosal cells. A minority of gastric carcinoma cases is related to germline defects of E-cadherin (CDH1).

  Mutation of this gene causes impairment of intercellular junctions of gastric mucosal cells. It seems a key step in development of gastric signet ring adenocarcinoma with diffuse infiltration resulting in a *linitis plastica* (leather bottle) gross appearance.

- *Mutation of β-catenin:* Under physiological state, β-catenin, a protein binds to E-cadherin. Mutation of β-catenin is associated with *gastric signet ring adenocarcinoma* (**linitis plastica variant**) There is increased risk of development of *lobular carcinoma breast*.

- *Hereditary non-polyposis colorectal cancer (HNPCC):* This inherited genetic disorder is also known as *Lynch syndrome* which increases risk of gastric carcinoma (linitis plastica). In most cases, this disorder is caused by a defect in either the *MLH1* or *MSH2* gene, but

Table 20.14: Oncogenes, their mode of activation associated with gastric carcinoma

Category	Proto-oncogene	Mode of activation	Associated malignancies
Growth factors			
Fibroblast growth factors (FGFs)	FGF3	Amplification	Osteosarcoma *Gastric carcinoma* Bladder cancer Breast cancer Melanoma
Growth factor receptors			
Receptor for KIT ligand	KIT	Point mutation	*Gastrointestinal tumors* Seminoma Leukemia

Table 20.15: Tumor suppressor gene mutations associated with gastric carcinoma

Gene	Protein	Function	Familial tumors	Sporadic cancers
Mitogenic signaling pathway inhibitors				
APC	Adenomatous polyposis protein (locus 5p21) Mutation by deletion or nonsense	APC inhibits WNT signaling activator pathway, thus prevents nuclear transcription. It degrades catenin	Familial polyposis coli with malignant transformation	*Gastric carcinoma* Colon carcinoma Pancreas carcinoma Thyroid carcinoma Melanoma
Inhibitors of invasiveness and metastases				
CDH1	E-cadherin	Participates in cell adhesion and inhibits cell motility	*Gastric carcinoma*	*Gastric carcinoma* Breast lobular carcinoma

Table 20.16: Chemical carcinogens and associated with gastric carcinoma

Chemical carcinogen	Examples	Associated cancers
Nitrosamines	Nitrates and nitrites widely used as fertilizers and as food additives converted to nitrosamines by gut bacteria in hypochlorhydria	*Gastric carcinoma*
Occupational asbestosis	Asbestos in building material	*Gastric carcinoma* Lung carcinoma Mesotheliomas

other genes can cause HNPCC, including *MLH3, MSH6, TGFBR2, PMS1,* and *PMS2.*

- *Familial adenomatous polyposis (FAP):* It is caused by mutations in the APC gene. People with this disorder are at increased risk of colorectal cancer and gastric carcinoma.
- *BRCA1 and BRCA2 mutations:* Women who carry mutations of the inherited breast cancer genes BRCA1 or BRCA2 may also have a higher rate of gastric carcinoma.
- *Li-Fraumeni syndrome:* Li-Fraumeni syndrome is caused by a mutation in the TP53 gene. There is increased risk of gastric carcinoma at young age in patient suffering from this syndrome.

- *Peutz-Jeghers syndrome:* This syndrome is caused by mutations in the *gene STK1*. This disorder is characterized by hamartomatous polyps in the stomach, intestines, nose, airways and lungs and dark freckle-like spots on the lips and inner cheeks. The patient with Peutz-Jeghers syndrome is at increased risk of development of cancers of the *breast, colon, pancreas, stomach,* and *several other organs.*
- *A family history of stomach cancer:* People with first-degree relatives (parents, siblings, or children) who have had gastric carcinoma are more likely to develop this disease.
- *Common variable immunodeficiency (CVID):* People with CVID have an increased risk of gastric carcinoma. The

immune system in these patients *fails to synthesize antibodies against pathogens*. There is increased risk of atrophic gastritis, pernicious anemia, gastric carcinoma and gastric MALT lymphoma.
- *Occupational exposure:* Workers in the *coal, asbestos, and rubber industries* seem to have a higher risk of gastric carcinoma.

Classification of Gastric Carcinoma

Gastric carcinoma is classified on the basis of depth of invasion (e.g. early and advanced gastric carcinoma), *macroscopic growth pattern* (e.g. flat mucosal lesions, exophytic, ulcerative and diffuse infiltrating types) and *histologic types* (e.g. *intestinal adenocarcinoma and diffuse infiltrative type, e.g. linitis plastica*).

According to Depth of Invasion

According to depth of invasion, gastric carcinoma has been divided into early and advanced gastric carcinoma. Approximately 5-year survival rate after surgical resection in early gastric carcinoma has been found to be 93 to 99%, in comparison with 5 to 15% in advanced gastric carcinoma.
- *Early gastric carcinoma:* Early gastric carcinoma is *confined to the mucosa or submucosa* without penetration of the muscularis coat regardless of the lymph node status of the patient; the superficial type has an excellent prognosis. It takes 8 years to become more invasive. It is diagnosed by barium study or endoscopy and biopsy.
- *Advanced gastric carcinoma:* When gastric carcinoma *infiltrates the muscular coat or beyond*, it is termed as advanced gastric cancer with poor prognosis.

According to Growth Patterns

Based on gross appearance, gastric carcinoma has been classified into following types.
- *Flat mucosal lesions:* Early intramucosal carcinomas may present in the form of mucosal patches or loss of rugae. Flat mucosal lesions are not visible on endoscopy. High risk people are screened yearly with *endoscopy* and cytological examination of gastric brushings for early detection of gastric cancer especially in Japan.
- *Exophytic carcinomas:* Intestinal type of gastric adenocarcinoma is polypoidal or fungating growth (cauliflower) protruding into the lumen of the stomach.
- *Ulcerated carcinoma:* It is most often >2 cm in diameter along the *lesser curvature, pylorus* and *antrum* in majority of cases. Ulcerated carcinoma also known as *malignant ulcer* has rolled elevated edges (Crate-like) and not clearly demarcated from the normal mucosa.

Benign peptic ulcers have sharp regular margins. *Biopsy is essential to differentiate benign gastric ulcer from malignant ulcer.*
- *Diffuse infiltrating carcinoma/linitis plastica:* It is also known as *linitis plastica*. It is diffuse infiltrative type of cancer converting the gastric wall into rigid thick structure known as *leather bottle* appearance.

Histological Variants

According to Lauren's classification, two major categories of gastric carcinoma exists, which have been designated *intestinal type* (53%), *diffuse infiltrative type* (33%) and the remainders are heterogeneous in composition.

Extracellular mucin release in either types of gastric carcinoma can result in formation of large mucin lakes that dissect tissue planes. Intestinal adenocarcinoma and diffuse infiltrative (linitis plastica) carcinoma of stomach are described as under.

Differences between intestinal type and diffuse type gastric carcinoma based on Lauren's classification are shown in Table 20.17.

Intestinal Type Gastric Adenocarcinoma

Intestinal type of gastric carcinoma arises from precursor lesions in stomach. It is associated with autoimmune-mediated chronic gastritis (type A), *Helicobacter pylori* associated chronic gastritis (type B), dietary nitrosamines and smoked food ingestion.

> **Gross Morphology**
>
> Tumor is solid polypoidal (fungating) mass projecting into the lumen of the stomach. It may undergo ulceration (Figs 20.19 and 20.20).
>
> **Light Microscopy**
> - On histopathological examination, gastric adenocarcinoma may exhibit papillary, tubular, mucinous, poorly cohesive or mixed patterns.
> - Tumor is composed of malignant cells with hyperchromatic nuclei and arranged in well defined glandular and papillary structures
> - These glandular structures are lined by tall columnar cells containing mucin resembling colonic adenocarcinoma (Fig. 20.21).
>
> **Immunohistochemistry**
>
> Panel of markers is used to analyze expression in intestinal type of gastric adenocarcinoma on histopathological sections are **cytokeratin, epithelial membrane antigen** (EMA) and **carcinoembryonic antigen** (CEA).

Table 20.17: Differences between intestinal type and diffuse type gastric carcinoma based on Lauren's classification

Characteristics	Intestinal variant of gastric carcinoma	Linitis plastica (diffuse infiltrative type) of gastric carcinoma
Age group	>55 years	Younger age group
Male to female sex	M:F — 2:1	M:F — 1:1
Frequency	53%	33%
Precursor lesion	Present (chronic gastritis type A)	Absent
Helicobacter pylori role	Present	Absent
Role of dietary nitrosamines and smoked fish	Present	Absent
Location of tumor	Lesser curvature of pylorus and antrum (50 to 60% of cases) Cardia (25% of cases) Fundus and body (along less common)	Diffuse involvement of stomach Pyloric obstruction common
Gastric peristalsis	Present	Absent
Gross morphology	Polypoidal or ulcerated growth	Diffuse infiltration of malignant cells in the stomach wall giving leather bottle appearance
Light microscopy	Malignant cells resembling intestinal type arranged in glandular pattern	Shows signet ring cells infiltrating the stomach wall Submucosal fibrosis with or without mucosa ulceration Inflammation +
Immunohistochemistry	Cytokeratin + Epithelial membrane antigen Carcinoembryonic antigen	– – –
Metastases	Regional lymph nodes and distant organs	*Krukenberg tumors of ovaries* due to transcoelomic spread
Molecular genetics	APC gene mutation p16 and p53	E-cadherin

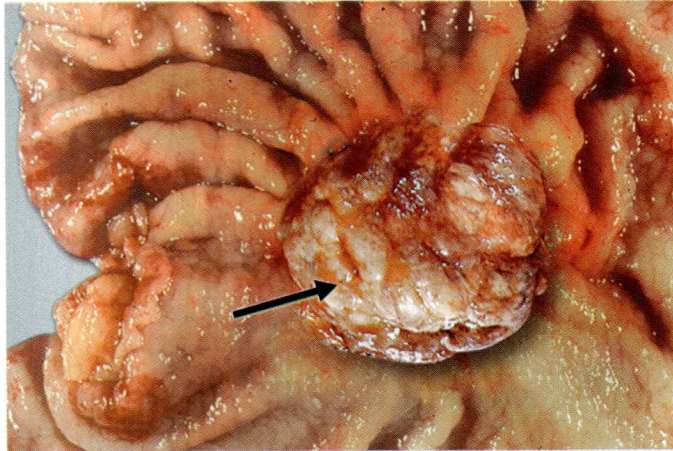

Fig. 20.19: Polypoid adenocarcinoma of the stomach. The patient was treated by partial gastrectomy (arrow).

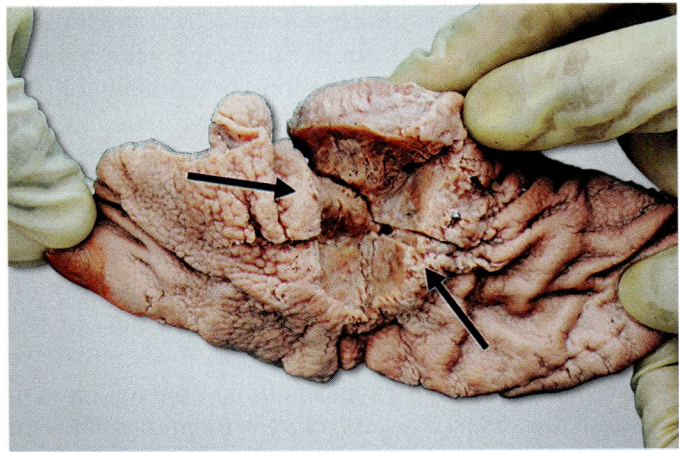

Fig. 20.20: Gastric carcinoma showing ulceroproliferative growth (arrows).

Gastrointestinal Tract

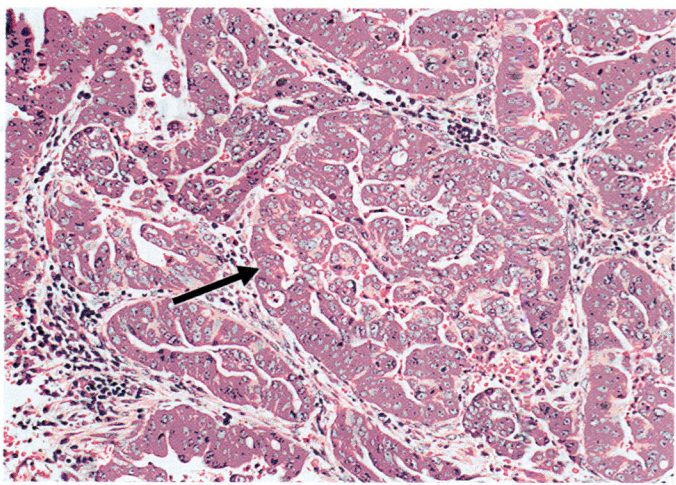

Fig. 20.21: Gastric adenocarcinoma (arrow) (100X).

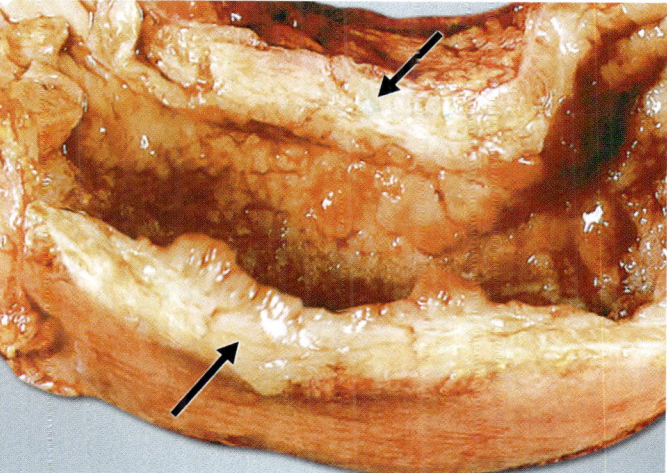

Fig. 20.22: Linitis plastica. In this type of adenocarcinoma of the stomach, the tumor cells infiltrate beneath the mucosa and produce marked fibrosis and thickening of the stomach wall (arrows).

Diffuse Infiltrative Type Gastric Adenocarcinoma

Diffuse infiltrative variant of gastric carcinoma does not develop from precursor lesions in stomach. It is not associated with *Helicobacter pylori*. It constitutes 10% of all gastric carcinomas. No true tumor mass is seen macroscopically.

Gross Morphology
- The stomach becomes stiff rigid walls due to infiltration of tumor cells in all gastric layers and extensive fibrosis (desmoplastic reaction) giving radiologic *leather bottle* appearance of stomach. It has been referred to as a *linitis plastica*.
- Peristalsis is absent in stomach (Fig. 20.22).

Light Microscopy
- Tumor is composed of small cells, containing abundant *mucin* pushing the nuclei to the periphery called *signet ring cells*. Glandular differentiation is not seen.
- These cells permeate mucosa as well as gastric wall individually or in small clusters.
- These are often confused with macrophages. Submucosal fibrosis is present with or without mucosa ulceration (Fig. 20.23).

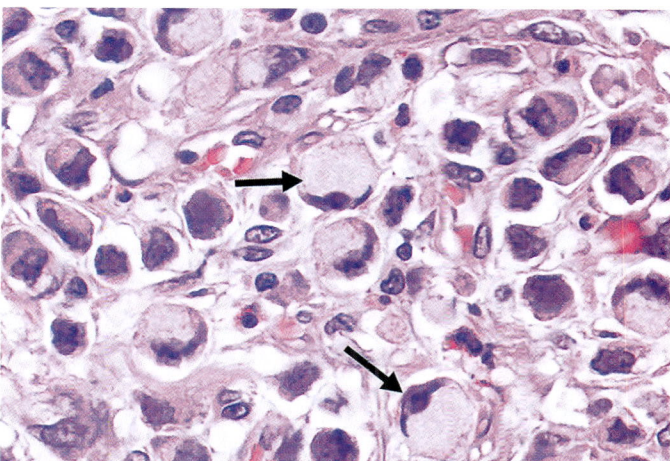

Fig. 20.23: Linitis plastica (diffuse infiltrative type) gastric adenocarcinoma showing tumor cells containing abundant mucin pushing the nuclei to the periphery called *signet ring cells* (arrows) (400X).

Mode of Spread

Gastric carcinomas spread by direct extension, lymphatic, hematogenous and transcoelomic routes described as under.

- *Direct spread:* All gastric carcinomas spread by invasion of full thickness of the wall resulting in *peritoneal dissemination* especially in *diffuse type carcinoma*.
- *Lymphatic spread:* Gastric carcinoma may spread to regional and distant lymph nodes. *Supraclavicular lymph node* metastases are called *Virchow's sign*. Virchow node is *supraclavicular lymph node*, which filters the lymph from the thoracic duct prior to its entry into the systemic veins.
- *Hematogenous spread:* Blood-borne metastases to liver, lung or brain are usual with intestinal type carcinoma.
- *Transcoelomic spread:* Involvement of the both ovaries by metastatic carcinoma (diffuse infiltrating growth pattern) of the *stomach, breast* and *colon* is referred to as **Krukenberg tumors**. The tumor cells often contain abundant mucin, displacing the nucleus to one side and resulting in so-called signet ring cells.

Clinical Features

Symptoms

Weight loss and epigastric pain are the most common symptoms. Other symptoms include vomiting, hematemesis or melena, anorexia, abdominal mass, dysphagia, diarrhea and iron deficiency anemia. Patient develops symptoms depending on involvement of organs due to metastases.

Clinical Signs

Clinical signs include cachexia, anemia, epigastric mass, hepatomegaly, palpable supraclavicular lymph node. Virchow node is supraclavicular lymph node, which filters the lymph from the thoracic duct prior to its entry into the systemic veins.

Laboratory Diagnosis

Gastric carcinomas are diagnosed by following diagnostic tools described as under.

Serum Tumor Markers

CA 72.4 and carcinoembryonic antigen (CEA) are used to detect gastric carcinoma. Serum CA 72.4, is also increased in colon carcinoma. Serum CEA is also increased *nonseminomatous germ cell testicular tumor, colon carcinoma,* gastric carcinoma, pancreatic carcinoma, lung carcinoma and breast carcinoma.

Exfoliative Cytology

Examination of tumor cells obtained by gastric lavage is a diagnostic tool. Gastric lavage with chymotrypsin softens mucous over gastric cancer.

Endoscopy

It is performed to know the extent of lesion and obtain biopsies from representative areas.

Imaging Techniques

Barium meal study is useful in diagnosis of *linitis plastica*. It shows persistent, irregular, filling defect. *USG, CT scan and MRI are done to rule out secondary deposits in coeliac lymph nodes* and distant organs, i.e. liver and ovaries.

Double contrast barium swallow has 90% accuracy, but it is difficult to differentiate between malignant and benign ulcers. *CT scan is useful for evaluation of distant disease.*

Histopathological Examination

Biopsies are processed and sections are examined. Histochemical stain mucicarmine demonstrates mucin.

Immunohistochemistry and FISH

Gastric carcinomas that are Her2 neu positive can be treated with drugs that target the Her2 neu protein, such as trastuzumab (Herceptin®).

The biopsy sample may be tested in 2 different ways.
- *Immunohistochemistry (IHC):* In this test, special antibodies that stick to the Her2 neu protein are applied to the sample, which cause cells to change color if many copies are present. This color change can be seen under a microscope. The test results are reported as 0, 1 +, 2 +, or 3 +.
- *Fluorescent in situ hybridization (FISH):* This test uses fluorescent pieces of DNA that specifically stick to copies of the Her2 neu gene in cells, which can then be counted under a special microscope.

Serum Pepsinogen Level

It is a specific marker for intestinal metaplasia precursor of gastric carcinoma.

Gastric Function Tests

Gastric hydrochloric acid is decreased in gastric adenocarcinoma resulting in achlorhydria or hypochlorhydria.

GASTRIC MALT LYMPHOMA

Gastric lymphoma is the most common form of extranodal lymphoma of B cell origin (mucosa associated lymphoid tissue). It originates from the mucosa associated lymphoid tissue (MALT). It is low grade lymphoma associated with *Helicobacter pylori* infection.

Demonstration of light chain restriction is helpful in differentiating MALT lymphoma from reactive lesions.

Predisposing Factors

These include AIDS, celiac disease and Mediterranean α-heavy chain disease.

Pathogens and Gastrointestinal Cancers

- World Health Organization has designated *Helicobacter pylori*—a potential human carcinogen. *Helicobacter pylori* is strongly associated with gastric adenocarcinoma (lower half of gastric region) and low grade B cell lymphoma of the mucosa associated lymphoid tissue (MALT) type. *Some of these lymphomas regress after eradication of Helicobacter pylori infection with antibiotics.*
- *Borrelia burgdorferi*, a spirochete and *Campylobacter jejuni* have been associated with gastrointestinal tract lymphoma.

Clinical Features

Patient presents with nonspecific symptoms such as weight loss, dyspepsia, and abdominal pain.

Gastrointestinal Tract

Gross Morphology
Gastric lymphoma replaces normal mucosa (Fig. 20.24).

Light Microscopy
- Gastric mucosa and submucosa are infiltrated by small cleaved forming follicles, lymphoepithelial lesion and Dutcher bodies.
- Lymphoepithelial lesion consists of >3 lymphocytes, that displacing adjacent epithelial cells and destroying the gastric gland.
- Gastric mucosa may show erosion, intestinal metaplasia, atrophy and *Helicobacter pylori* (Fig. 20.25).

Immunohistochemistry
Panel of markers is used to analyze expression in gastric MALT lymphoma on histopathological sections (Table 20.18). Differences between MALT lymphoma and chronic gastritis on histological examination are shown in Table 20.19.

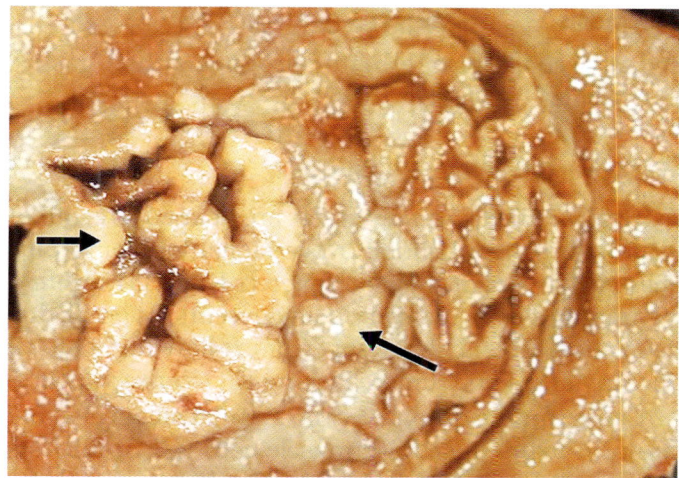

Fig. 20.24: Gastric lymphoma replacing most of normal gastric mucosa (arrows).

Table 20.18: Immunohistochemistry of gastric MALT lymphoma

Marker	Expression
CD20	Positive
CD79a	Positive
CD21	Positive
CD35	Positive

Some gastric MALT lymphomas are also positive for CD43
Gastric MALT lymphoma is negative for CD5, CD10, CD23, BCL2 and cyclin D1

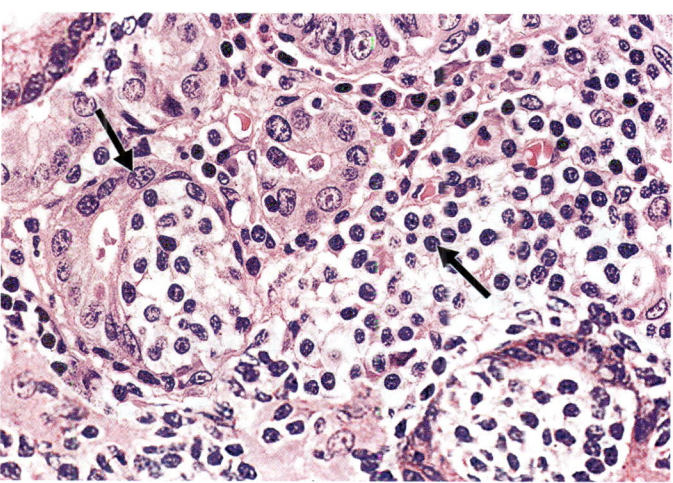

Fig. 20.25: Gastric lymphoma (arrows) (400X).

Table 20.19: Differences between MALT lymphoma and chronic gastritis on histological examination

Parameters	MALT lymphoma	Chronic gastritis
Lymphoid follicle	Frequent	Infrequent
Follicular colonization	May be present	Absent
Interfollicular lymphocytes	Immature lymphocytes with irregular nuclear contour	Mature lymphocytes
B cells (CD20)	Predominant, present in lymphoid follicles and interfollicular region (CD43 positive)	Sparse, present in lymphoid follicles (CD43 negative)
T cells (CD3)	Scattered in variable in number	Diffusely present in lamina propria
Plasma cells	Present in variable number beneath surface lining epithelium showing light chain restriction	Present diffusely in lamina propria and lacking light chain restriction
Lymphoid cells infiltration in muscularis mucosa	May be present	Absent
Helicobacter pylori	May be demonstrated	May be demonstrated

MALT (mucosa associated lymphoid tissue)

Prognosis

It has a considerably better prognosis than gastric carcinoma (45% 5-year survival).

GASTROINTESTINAL STROMAL TUMORS

Gastrointestinal stromal tumors are defined as cellular, spindle cells, epithelioid or occasionally pleomorphic mesenchymal tumors, which express **Kit (C117) protein** by immunohistochemistry a few exceptions occur due to fixation defects, sampling errors, following STI-571B therapy and some tumors lacking Kit expression.

These tumors originate from stromal stem cells that are precursors of smooth muscle cells (**GI fibroblasts or pacemaker cells of Cajal controlling peristalsis**). These may be associated with *neurofibromatosis* and *Carney's triad* (GIST, paraganglioma and pulmonary chondroma).

Locations

These tumors occur in entire gastrointestinal tract such as *stomach (50%), small intestine (25%), large intestine (10%)*, and extragastrointestinal sites. Gastric stromal tumors are usually *submucosal and covered by intact mucosa*.

Molecular Genetics

Approximately 75–80% of GISTs have *Kit mutations*. Mutations in platelet-derived growth factor receptor α (*PDGFRα*) have been demonstrated in 10% of cases.

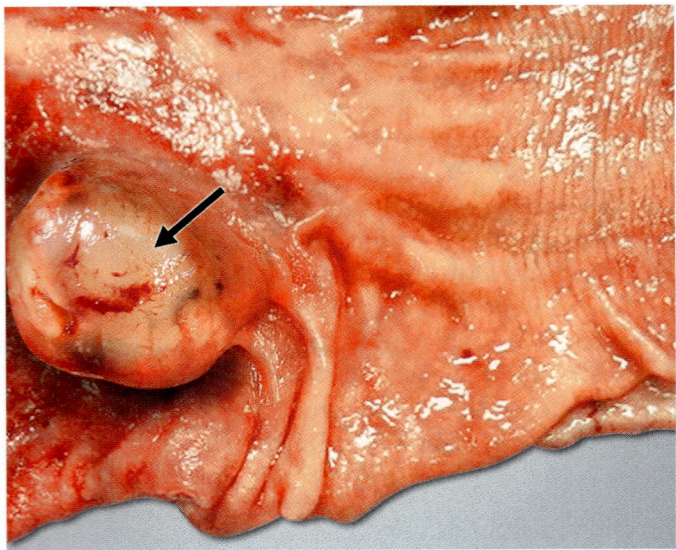

Fig. 20.26: Gastrointestinal stromal tumor showing well circumscribed tumor projecting towards lumen (arrow).

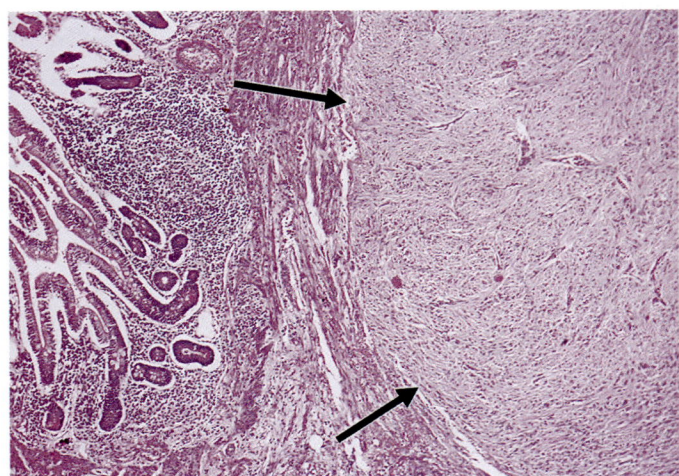

Fig. 20.27: Gastrointestinal stromal tumors (arrows) (100X).

Gross Morphology

GISTs range from a few mm to >40 cm with mean size of 6 cm. Tumor is well circumscribed. Cut surface is smooth, lobulated with whorled-silk appearance. Prominent fibrohyaline areas undergoing calcification may be demonstrated (Fig. 20.26).

Light Microscopy

Gastrointestinal stromal tumors are classified into three categories based on histopathological examination: spindle cell, epithelioid or mixed cell variants (Fig. 20.27).
- Tumor may be composed of fascicles and bundles of spindle cells or epithelioid cells with vacuolated cytoplasm or mixture of spindle and epithelioid cells with focal pleomorphism.
- Benign gastrointestinal stromal tumors are small measuring 2–5 cm and showing a few mitoses.

- Malignant stromal tumors measure >6 cm and show hemorrhage, necrosis, high mitoses and features of anaplasia. Proposed guidelines for assessing malignant potential of gastric GISTs are shown in Table 20.20.

Immunohistochemistry

Panel of markers is used to analyze expression in gastrointestinal stromal tumors on histopathological sections (Table 20.21).

Phenotype Categories

A stromal tumor showing histologic sign of smooth muscle differentiation is called *leiomyoma or leiomyosarcoma*.

Table 20.20: Proposed guidelines for assessing malignant potential of gastric GISTs

Tumor size	Mitoses	Predictable behavior
≤2 cm	≤5 mitoses/50 HPFs	Benign, metastasis rate or tumor-related mortality: 0%
>2 cm ≤10 cm	5 mitoses/50 HPFs	Very low malignant potential, metastasis rate or tumor-related mortality: <3%
>10 cm	≤5 mitoses/50 HPFs, or ≤5 cm, >5 mitoses/50 HPFs	Low to moderate malignant potential, metastasis rate or tumor-related mortality: 12–15%
>5 cm	>5 mitoses/50 HPFs	High malignant potential, metastasis rate or tumor-related mortality: 49–86%

Table 20.21: Immunohistochemistry of gastrointestinal stromal tumors

Tumor marker	Expression
c-kit oncogene (CD117) encoding tyrosine kinase	Positive (95%)
DOG1 (protein of unknown function)	Positive (most specific marker)
CD171 (cell adhesive molecule)	Positive
Protein kinase C theta	Positive
Vimentin	Positive
Smooth muscle actin encoded by ACTA2 gene located on 10q–24q	Positive
CD34	Positive
Desmin	Positive (5%)

GIST showing neural differentiation in autonomic nervous system is known as *GANT*. GISTs may show dual smooth muscle and neural differentiation.

Behavior
Mitotic count, size, and location help in predicting the behavior of these tumors. Stromal tumors in small intestine most often behave like leiomyosarcoma as opposite to the stomach. GISTs are considered to be of low malignant potential and removed surgically.

Management
Surgical resection of tumor and treatment with *imatinib* cure the patients, therapeutic agent *imatinib* inhibits the tyrosine kinase activity of c-kit and PDGFRα.

CARCINOID TUMORS
Carcinoid tumors are present in *stomach* (body and fundus) and *proximal duodenum*. These tumors synthesize *histamine, stomatosin* and *serotonin*. Gastric carcinoids are associated with chronic atrophic gastritis or MEN I.

Duodenal carcinoid tumors are associated with Zollinger-Ellison syndrome or neurofibromatosis 1 or sporadic. Carcinoid tumors are discussed in details under small intestinal tumors.

NON-NEOPLASTIC DISEASES

CONGENITAL PYLORIC STENOSIS
Congenital pyloric stenosis is a male-dominant disorder and more common in identical twins. It is characterized by hypertrophy of the circular smooth muscle in the pyloric region of the stomach resulting in obstruction of the outlet of stomach. The only consistent microscopic abnormality is *hypertrophy of the circular muscle coat*.

Clinical Features
Patient presents with projectile vomiting of non-bile stained fluid 2–4 weeks after birth On clinical examination, palpable mass is observed through the abdominal wall in the epigastric region. Surgical resection within first 6 months of life gives excellent results.

MÉNÉTRIER DISEASE
Ménétrier disease (giant hypertrophic gastritis) is characterized by extreme enlargement of gastric rugae (*greater curvature in the fundus and body of the stomach*) and sometimes by severe loss of plasma proteins from the altered mucosa. The disease occurs in children due to cytomegalovirus and adults. Overexpression of TGF-α is seen in adulthood form. Affected patients have an increased risk of stomach cancer.

PANCREATIC HETEROTROPIC RESTS

Pancreatic heterotropic rests most commonly occur in the wall of the stomach.

HYPERPLASTIC (REGENERATIVE) POLYPS

Hyperplastic (regenerative) polyps are non-neoplastic polyps that may be associated with chronic blood loss.

TRICHOBEZOAR

Trichobezoar is usually seen in long-haired girls or young women who eat their own hair as a nervous habit. Such a trichobezoar may grow by accretion to form a complete cast of the stomach. Strands of hair may extend into the bowel as far as the transverse colon (Rapunzel syndrome) (Fig. 20.28).

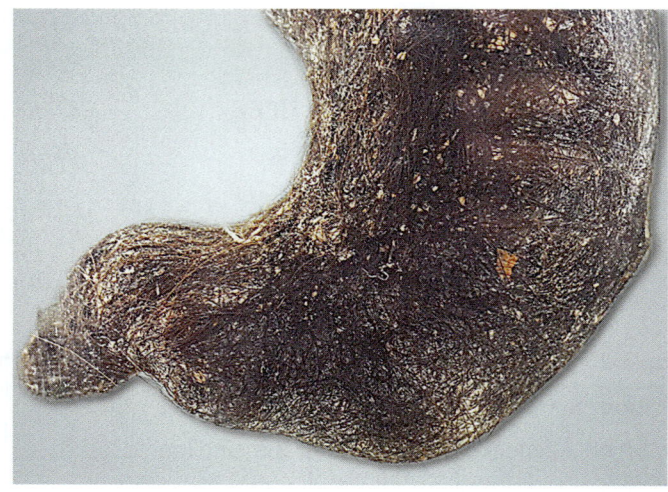

Fig. 20.28: Trichobezoar.

SMALL INTESTINE

ANATOMY

Small intestine is 6 to 7 meters long. It comprises duodenum, jejunum and ileum. It begins at the distal gastric pylorus and ends at ileocecal region. It consists of mucosa, submucosa, muscular coat and serous coat. It is lined by villus mucosa.

The individual villus consists of finger-like projections. It is lined by tall columnar absorptive cells, goblet cells, crypt cells, neuroendocrine cells and Paneth cells. The lamina propria contains plasma cells. Payer's patches composed of aggregates of lymphocytes are distributed throughout the mucosa of small intestine.

Duodenum contains Brunner's glands. The entire mucosa rests on muscularis mucosae. The smooth muscle layer delineates the lamina propria from the submucosa.

CONGENITAL ANOMALIES

MECKEL'S DIVERTICULUM

Vitelline (omphalomesenteric) duct remnant causes outpouching of small intestine known as *Meckel's diverticulum*. Congenital diverticulum is a rare occurrence in the duodenum and jejunum.

Etiopathogenesis

It is the most common congenital anomaly of the *small intestine. It occurs due to failure of closure of embryonic vitelline (omphalomesenteric) duct.*

It occurs due to outpouching of all the four layers of small intestine (true diverticulum) in the antimesenteric aspect of ileum, *within 60–100 cm from ileocecal valve.*

Gross Morphology
Meckel's diverticulum showing outpouching of small intestine is shown in Fig. 20.29.

Light Microscopy
Diverticulum may contain heterotropic rests such as pancreatic tissue, gastric, duodenal, or colonic mucosa (Fig. 20.30).

Clinical Features
Most patients are generally asymptomatic. Patient may develop bleeding in Meckel's diverticulum owing to the presence of *heterotropic rests of gastric or pancreatic mucosa.*

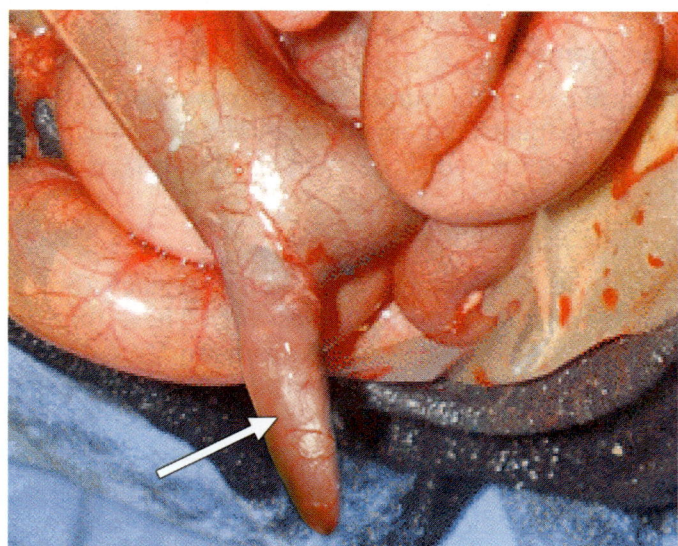

Fig. 20.29: Meckel's diverticulum showing outpouching of small intestine (arrow).

Gastrointestinal Tract

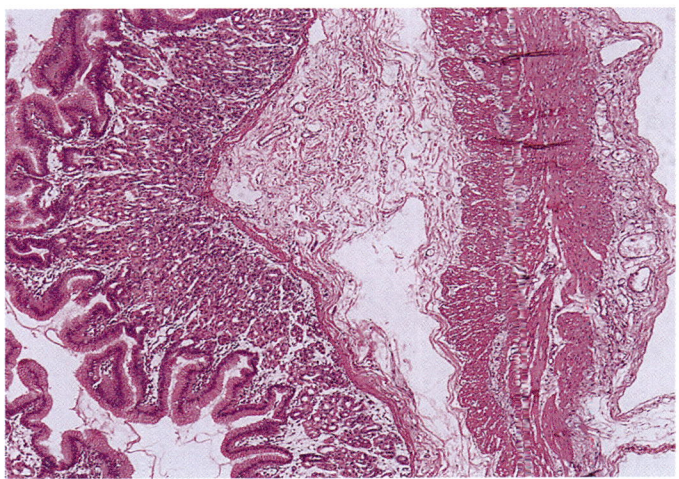

Fig. 20.30: Meckel's diverticulum showing heterotropic rests of gastric mucosa (100X).

Complications

Approximately 2% of patients may develop *ectopic peptic ulcers, ileoumbilical fistula, intussusception, volvulus, intestinal obstruction, perforation, diverticulitis* and *mucocele*.

HETEROTROPIC GASTRIC MUCOSA

Presence of heterotropic gastric full thickness fundic type oxyntic mucosa produces small nodule or sessile polyp in the duodenal bulb. This entity differs from foveolar surface metaplasia of duodenal mucosa seen secondary to inflammation of duodenum by *Helicobacter pylori*.

HETEROTROPIC PANCREAS

Patient with heterotropic pancreas presents with mass in duodenum. On histopathological examination, the lesion is composed of *pancreatic ducts* and *acini* with or without islet's of Langerhans.

MALROTATION OF SMALL INTESTINE

During fetal life, defective rotation of intestine occurs. As a result, large bowel does not descend into right iliac fossa. These patients are prone to develop volvulus and internal hernia.

DUPLICATION OF SMALL INTESTINE

Duplication of the small intestine may be tubular or cystic. Approximately 75% are not contagious with the lumen of the associated segment of small intestine. Duplications comprise all the layers of the segment.

MALABSORPTIVE DISORDERS

Malabsorption is defined as increased fecal excretion of fat with concurrent deficiencies of vitamins, minerals, carbohydrates, and proteins. Bile salts and fatty acids are required to micellarize monoglycerides and fatty acids. Small intestinal villi are required to reabsorb micelles. Deficiency of pancreatic lipase leads to malassimilation of the fats in the small bowel.

Etiology

Malabsorption syndrome is caused by pancreatic insufficiency (e.g. chronic pancreatitis), bile salts/bile acid deficiency (e.g. cirrhosis, cholestasis) and small bowel disease (e.g. celiac disease).

Other causes include Whipple disease, Crohn's disease and diseases obstructing the intestinal lymphatics. Small bowel disorders producing malabsorption syndrome include *celiac disease, refractory sprue, collagenous sprue, autoimmune enteropathy, common variable immunodeficiency, microvillus inclusion disease, lymphangiectasia, disaccharidases deficiency* and *abetalipoproteinemia*.

Causes and clinical manufestations of malabsorption syndrome are shown in Tables 20.22 and 20.23.

Table 20.22: Causes of malabsorption syndrome

Primary causes	Secondary causes
Celiac disease	Mucosal damage (Crohn's disease, tubercular intestine, NHL intestine, radiation)
Whipple disease	Chronic pancreatitis causing pancreatic insufficiency
Refractory sprue	Liver disorders (cirrhosis, cholestasis causing bile salts/bile acid deficiency)
Collagenous sprue	Surgical resection of small intestine
Autoimmune enteropathy	Parasitic infestations (hookworm, roundworm, Giardia)
Common variable immunodeficiency	Drugs administration (methotrexate, neomycin)
Microvillus inclusion disease and disaccharidases deficiency	Impaired transport (lymphangiectasia and abetalipoproteinemia)

Table 20.23: Clinical manifestations of malabsorption syndrome

Dietary constituents	Site of absorption	Essential requirement	Clinical manifestations
Carbohydrates			
Starch	Small intestine	Amylase Maltase Isomaltase-α-dextrin	Diarrhea Flatulence Abdominal discomfort
Sucrose	Small intestine	Sucrase	–
Lactose	Small intestine	Lactase	–
Fats			
Fat	Upper jejunum	Pancreatic lipase Bile salts Functioning lymphatic channels	Weight loss Steatorrhea Fat-soluble vitamins deficiency
Proteins	Small intestine	Pancreatic enzymes (e.g. trypsin, chymotrypsin, elastin)	Edema, loss of muscle mass, weakness
Water and electrolytes	Mainly small intestine	Osmotic gradient	Diarrhea, dehydration, muscle cramps
Vitamins			
Vitamin B_{12}	Ileum	Intrinsic factor	Megaloblastic anemia, glossitis, peripheral neuropathy
Folic acid	Upper jejunum	Absorption may be impaired by anticonvulsant drugs	Glossitis, chelosis
Vitamin A	Upper jejunum	Bile salts	Night blindness, exophthalmia, corneal irritation
Vitamin D	Upper jejunum	Bile salts	Bone pain, fractures, tetany
Vitamin K	Upper jejunum	Bile salts	Easy bruising and bleeding
Vitamin E	Upper jejunum	Bile salts	Uncertain
Minerals			
Calcium	Duodenum	Vitamin D and parathormone	Bone pain, fractures, tetany
Iron	Duodenum and jejunum	Normal pH (hydrochloric acid)	Iron deficiency anemia, glossitis

Clinical Features

Patient presents with steatorrhea, weight loss, diarrhea, and malnutrition. Steatorrhea denotes passage of excessive sticky stools that float as a result of maldigestion of fats by small bowel as a result of pancreatic insufficiency.

Complications

Patient develops manifestations as result of deficiencies of vitamins (e.g. fat soluble and water soluble), pitting edema (e.g. hypoproteinemia), and recurrent infections, and dimorphic anemia (e.g. iron and folate deficiency).

Laboratory Diagnosis

General screening tests for malabsorption include 24 hours faecal fat and serum β-carotene. The gold standard test to document fat malabsorption is the quantitative 72 hours stool test for fat. *Decreased absorption of D-xylose indicates small bowel disease.* It is useful in identifying assimilation of proteins in the small bowel (decreased uptake of the pentose sugar).

CELIAC DISEASE

Celiac disease is an autoimmune disease caused by *sensitivity to gluten in cereal products.* Autoantibodies to gluten result in flattening or destruction of intestinal villi. It is also known as *celiac sprue*, nontropical sprue or gluten induced enteropathy. Genetic and immune-mediated mechanisms may be involved in the pathogenesis of celiac disease. Patient presents with chronic diarrhea, abdominal distention and malabsorption syndrome.

Genetic Predisposition

Incidence increases in association with human leukocyte antigens (HLAs), HLA-B8 and HLA-DW3, type I diabetes mellitus and dermatitis herpetiformis, an autoimmune (IgA-mediated) vesicular disease of skin, with celiac disease. Genetic factors in celiac disease are shown in Table 20.24.

Etiopathogenesis

Gluten is a name for group of proteins present in grains such as wheat, oat, rye, barley and spelt.

Physiological state: Normally, digestive enzymes split gluten into small chains of amino acids resulting in absorption of gluten by intestinal villi.

Pathological state: In celiac disease, digestive enzymes split gluten into long chain amino acid known as *gliadin*. Disease producing gliadin is absorbed into intestinal villi.

Autoantibodies to gliadin result in triggering inflammatory response. Intestinal biopsy (e.g. proximal jejunum and distal ileum exhibiting villus atrophy) is essential for diagnosis. Pathogenesis of celiac disease is shown in Fig. 20.31.

Table 20.24: Genetic factors in celiac disease

Categories	Examples
Human leukocyte antigens (HLAs)	HLA DQ2 (Class II)
	HLA DQ8 (Class II)
	HLA-DW3
Polymorphism of immune regulatory genes determining mucosal epithelial cell polarity	IL-2
	IL-21
	CCR3
	SH2B3
Associated disorders	Diabetes mellitus type 1
	Sjögren's syndrome
	Ataxia-telangiectasia
	Autism
	IgA nephropathy
	Down's syndrome
	Turner's syndrome
	Dermatitis herpetiformis

Light Microscopy

- Normal intestinal villi are slender and much longer than crypts. In celiac disease, intestinal biopsy shows *villus atrophy* (complete loss of villi), elongation of crypts due to hyperplasia.
- Overall thickness of the mucosa may not be reduced significantly as a result of crypt hyperplasia. *Enterocyte damage* may be evidenced by flattening and or cytoplasmic vacuolization.
- Lamina propria shows infiltration by *macrophages, lymphocytes and plasma cells*. These changes can revert to normal in response to a gluten-free diet.
- Light microscopy of celiac disease is shown in Fig. 20.32. Disorders that may mimic gluten-sensitive enteropathy are shown in Table 20.25.

Table 20.25: Disorders that may mimic gluten-sensitive enteropathy

Disorders
Celiac disease/gluten-sensitive enteropathy
Tropical sprue
Helicobacter pylori infection
Bacterial overgrowth
Autoimmune enteropathy
Nonsteroidal anti-inflammatory drug administration
Dermatitis herpetiformis
HIV enteropathy
Food allergies
Giardiasis
Crohn's disease
Zollinger-Ellison disease
Systemic autoimmune diseases
Viral enteritis

Clinical Features

Children present with diarrhea (pale, bulky, frothy, foul-smelling stools), failure to thrive, growth retardation, weight loss, weakness and abdominal distension with *nonspecific* symptoms or anemia.

Complications

Celiac disease is complicated by splenic atrophy and less commonly, large *T cell lymphoma* of the small bowel and small intestinal obstruction.

Laboratory Diagnosis

Diagnostic modalities include 24 hours fecal fat excretion, *D-xylose test, anti-tissue transglutaminase circulating autoantibodies* and *intestinal biopsy*. Demonstration of autoantibodies in serum may also be used for screening prior to definitive diagnosis by biopsy.

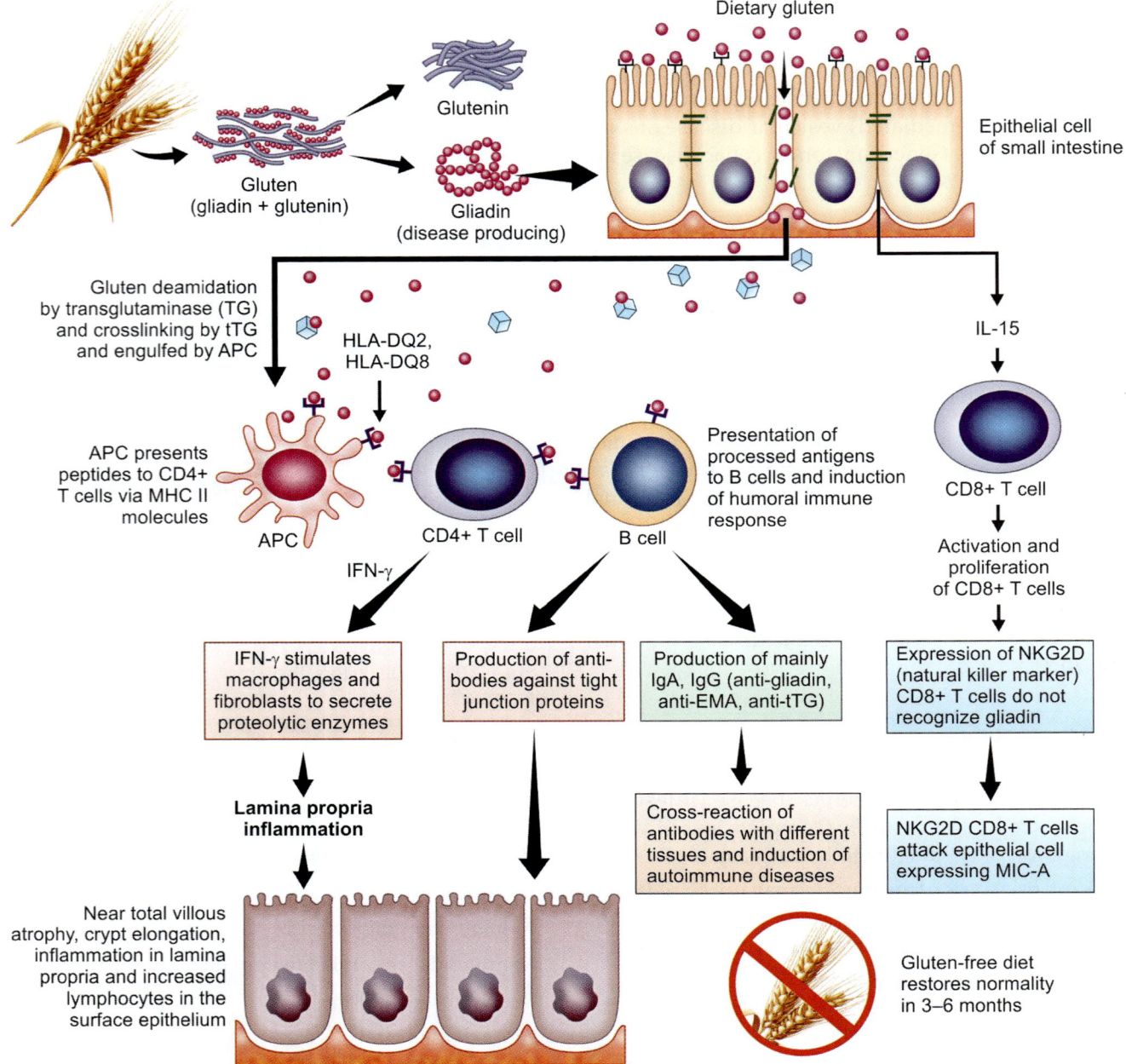

Fig. 20.31: Pathogenesis of celiac disease. Sensitivity to gliadin (disease producing) causes villus atrophy due to epithelial cell destruction, crypt hyperplasia due to expansion of epithelial cells in the proliferative compartment at the bases of the crypts inflammation of lamina propria and increased number of natural killer cells and CD8+ T cells in the epithelium.

Treatment

A gluten-free diet cures celiac disease. *Gluten is not present in corn, quinoa, potatoes, nuts, rice or soy.* Flour made from these foods, vegetables and meat deficient in gluten are advised in celiac disease.

REFRACTORY SPRUE

Refractory sprue refers to unresponsiveness to a gluten free diet. Relapse of symptoms occurs despite gluten restriction. It is not distinguishable from classic celiac disease. Some gastroenterologists regard refractory sprue as type of T cell lymphoma. There may be presence of numerous neutrophils.

COLLAGENOUS SPRUE

Collagenous sprue is characterized by flattening of mucosal villi and deposition of collagen fibers in subepithelial region.

AUTOIMMUNE ENTEROPATHY

Autoimmune enteropathy shares clinical and histopathological features with celiac disease. It involves

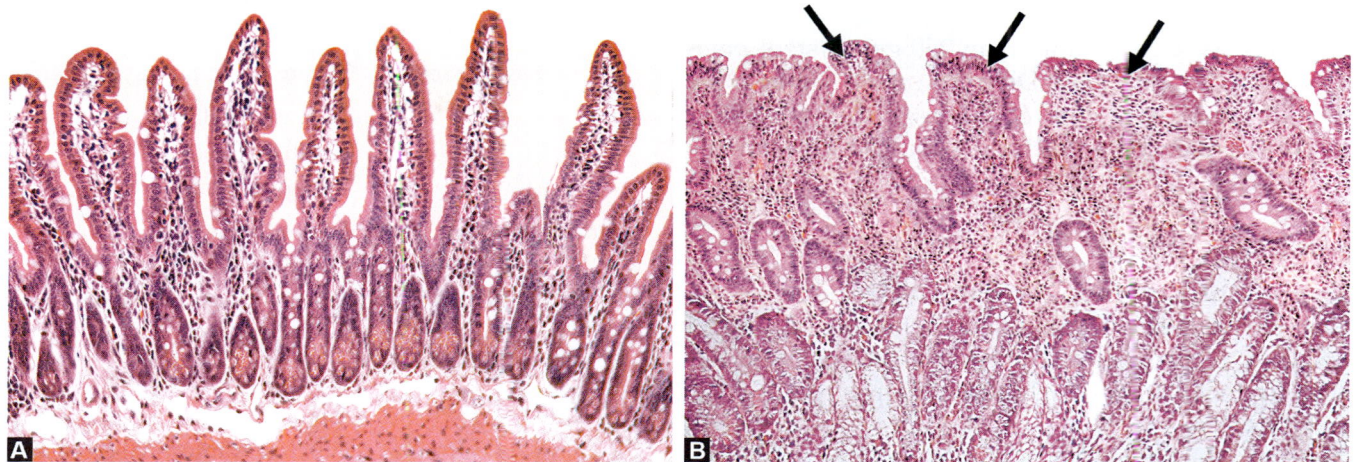

Fig. 20.32: Celiac disease. (A) Showing normal villi of small intestine, (B) Showing villus atrophy and chronic inflammatory cells in lamina propria in celiac disease (arrows) (100X).

both small intestine and large intestine. Clinical response to steroids may help to establish diagnosis.

Light Microscopy

On histopathological examination, villus shows flattening and dense lamina propria infiltration by lymphocytes and plasma cells. Apoptotic bodies are apparent.

EOSINOPHILIC GASTROENTERITIS

Eosinophilic gastroenteritis involves stomach and intestine. Mucosal involvement is common. On histopathological examination, the mucosa shows *infiltration by eosinophils.* There is presence of *cryptitis* and *crypt abscess formation.* Parasitic infestations, food allergy to cow's milk protein, drug reaction, connective tissue disorders and tumors must be excluded.

COMMON VARIABLE IMMUNODEFICIENCY

Common variable immunodeficiency is characterized by loss of plasma cells in lamina propria. Histopathological examination shows *variable degree of blunting of villi, lymphocytic infiltration in epithelium and lymphoid aggregates.* Giardia should be searched in the biopsies.

MICROVILLUS INCLUSION DISEASE

Microvillus inclusion disease is an autosomal recessive disorder causing *diarrhea in infancy.* Basic defect is loss of normal brush border on the luminal surface of the enterocytes as a result of incorporation of brush border into the cytoplasm appearing as apical microvillus inclusions. The histopathological features are demonstrated by *periodic acid–Schiff (PAS) stain, electron microscopy and immunohistochemistry (carcinoembryonic antigen, CD10 or villin).* *Histopathological examination shows diffuse villus atrophy lacking inflammatory response.*

LYMPHANGIECTASIA

Intestinal lymphangiectasis is characterized by abnormal dilated lymphatic channels of small intestine. It may be congenital or secondary. It is additional cause of malabsorption syndrome. It leads to *marked gastrointestinal protein loss* with resultant hypoproteinemia and *generalized edema.*

DISACCHARIDASE DEFICIENCY

Lactose is one of the most common disaccharides in dairy products. The intestinal brush border contains disaccharidases that are important for cleavage of lactose to free glucose and galactose for absorption.

Acquired Disaccharidase Deficiency

Acquired disaccharidase deficiency is a widespread disorder of carbohydrate absorption. It leads to milk intolerance. The symptoms of this disease typically begin in adolescence, when patients complain of *flatulence and diarrhea* after the ingestion of dairy products. Histopathological changes in the intestine are not significant.

Congenital Lactase Deficiency

Congenital lactase deficiency is rare but may be lethal if not recognized.

ABETALIPOPROTEINEMIA

No characteristic features are present in the intestine. Circulating *acanthocytes (red cells with spiny projections)* suggest the diagnosis of β-lipoprotein deficiency caused by hereditary deficiency of *apoprotein-β.*

DIARRHEA

Diarrhea is passage of more than 250 gm of stool per day (normal 100 gm/day). Diarrhea may be acute (<3 weeks duration) and chronic (>4 weeks). Signs and symptoms associated with chronic diarrhea are shown in Table 20.26.

MICROBIAL PATHOGENS ASSOCIATED WITH DIARRHEA

- *Rota virus:* It is the most common childhood cause of watery diarrhea without blood in children <2 years of age. It is transmitted by the *fecal-oral route*. Rotavirus is demonstrated in duodenal biopsy specimens in 50% of cases.
- *Norwalk virus:* It is most common cause of diarrhea in childhood and adults.
- *Food poisoning:* Patient presents with gastroenteritis from ingestion of contaminated food. Microbial pathogens include *Staphylococcus aureus*, *Clostridium botulinum* (in canned foods; toxins block cholinergic nerves in infants), *Bacillus cereus* (contaminated fried rice, *Clostridium perfringens* and *Salmonella*.
- *Clostridium difficile:* Patient develops pseudomembranous colitis caused by *Clostridium difficile* due to antibiotic-induced (most commonly *ampicillin* and *clindamycin*). It is best diagnosed by toxin assay of stool. *It is treated with metronidazole.*
- *Shigella sonnei:* It is transmitted by the fecal-oral route. Patient presents with bloody diarrhea as a result of pseudomembranous inflammation in the ileum and colon.
- *Salmonella typhimurium:* It is transmitted by fecal-oral route from animal reservoirs (poultry turtles). Patient develops enterocolitis.
- *Salmonella typhi:* It is transmitted by fecal-oral route. Pathogen invades Peyer's patches and produces septicemia during the first week. Blood is the best culture medium for isolation. Second week of the infection is marked by diarrhea.

  In addition, patient has classic triad of bradycardia, absolute neutropenia, and hepatosplenomegaly. It may produce a chronic carrier state. The organism persists in gallbladder for one year after infection.
- *Campylobacter jejuni:* It is contracted by eating contaminated poultry or drinking contaminated milk. It is the most common invasive bacterial enterocolitis in the United States. Patient presents with bloody diarrhea with crypt abscesses, and the ulcers resembling ulcerative colitis.
- *Vibrio cholerae:* It produces a powerful enterotoxin that stimulates *adenyl cyclase* in the small bowel, leading to a severe secretory diarrhea (*rice water stool*). It is best treated with a glucose/electrolyte solution.

Table 20.26: Signs and symptoms associated with chronic diarrhea

Signs and symptoms	Chronic diarrheal syndrome
Arthritis	Ulcerative colitis Crohn's disease Whipple's disease
Liver disease	Ulcerative colitis Crohn's disease Colon carcinoma with metastases
Fever	Ulcerative colitis Crohn's disease Amoebic colitis Tubercular intestinal disease Whipple disease
Neuropathy	Amyloidosis Diabetic diarrhea
Severe weight loss	Malabsorption syndrome Inflammatory bowel disease
Lymphadenopathy	GIT lymphoma AIDS Ulcerative colitis Crohn's disease Whipple's disease
Erythema nodosum	Ulcerative colitis Crohn's disease
Dermatitis herpetiformis	Celiac disease
Flushing	Carcinoid tumors
Pyoderma gangrenosum	Ulcerative colitis

- *E. coli:* Pathogen produces toxin induced and invasive diarrheas. Heat labile strain stimulates cyclic AMP producing secretory diarrhea. Enetroinvasive strain is associated with an invasive enterocolitis.

  Enterohemorrhagic strain associated with the O157:H7 serotype contaminating raw ground beef, may produce hemolytic uremic syndrome and hemorrhagic or pseudomembranous colitis. Enteropathogenetic strain produces mild diarrhea in infants and children.

TYPES OF DIARRHEA

Osmotic Diarrhea

Nonabsorbable osmotic substances (e.g. mannitol, sorbitol, sugar-free gum or magnesium sulfate from Epton salt) stimulate osmotic influx of water and electrolytes into the intestinal lumen producing osmotic diarrhea. Intake of milk products by children due to genetic deficiency of lactase enzyme causes withdrawing of water into the lumen, resulting in a hypotonic diarrhea without mucosal inflammation.

Secretory Diarrhea

In secretory diarrhea, the intestinal cells secrete more water than they can absorb. *Vibrio cholerae* without causing intestinal mucosal inflammation secretes toxin that activates the adenyl cyclic AMP dependent water pump in the cell membrane.

The intestinal cells secrete chloride accompanied by water into the lumen producing secretory diarrhea. *E. coli* toxin that is heat stable toxin stimulates water influx through mechanisms that are not cyclic AMP dependent.

Other causes of secretory diarrhea include Rotavirus, Norwalk virus. Neuroendocrine tumors (e.g. carcinoids and pancreatic islet cell tumors) synthesize vasoactive amines (e.g. serotonin and other polypeptides) responsible for secretory diarrhea.

Exudative (Invasive) Diarrhea

Exudative diarrhea is caused by pathogens (e.g. *E. coli*, *Clostridium difficile* and *Shigella*). The organisms cause inflammation of intestinal mucosa with production of inflammatory exudates. Fecal smears show leukocytes. Other causes include ulcerative colitis, Crohn's disease, lymphomas and carcinomas.

INFECTIOUS DISEASES

TROPICAL SPRUE AND BACTERIAL OVERGROWTH

Tropical sprue and bacterial overgrowth simulate celiac disease. These may involve the entire small intestine with more severe disease in distal segment. Clinical history and travel history are important in establishing diagnosis.

WHIPPLE DISEASE (TROPICAL SPRUE)

Tropical sprue is also known as *Whipple disease*. It is of probable infectious origin (*Tropheryma whippelii*) in Far East; often responds well to tetracycline. It may involve the *entire small intestine* with more severe disease in distal segment. It may resemble celiac disease, but megaloblastic anemia dominates the clinical picture. Intestinal biopsy shows only partial villus atrophy.

Etiopathogenesis

Whipple disease is caused by *Tropheryma whippelii* bacteria. It usually affects *30–60 years of age group*, involving multiple organs such as small intestine (*jejunum and ileum*), joints (*arthralgia*) and *cardiac* and *neurologic manifestations*. These organisms block lymphatic channels of small intestine and uptake of fat (malabsorption). Draining mesenteric *lymph nodes, liver, lung, heart, brain, bone* and synovial membrane are also infiltrated with *macrophages carrying organisms*.

Clinical Features

Patient presents with fever, chronic diarrhea, joint pain, gray-brown skin pigmentation, and generalized lymphadenopathy; antibiotics are curative.

Gross Morphology

Small intestinal wall is thickened and edematous with dull-colored serosa. Mesentery is thickened and indurated with mesenteric lymphadenopathy.

Light Microscopy

- Histopathological examination shows blunting and widening of the villi of jejunum and ileum.
- Lamina propria is infiltrated by large number of foamy macrophages widening of the villi. Histopathological changes in Whipple disease are shown in Fig. 20.33.

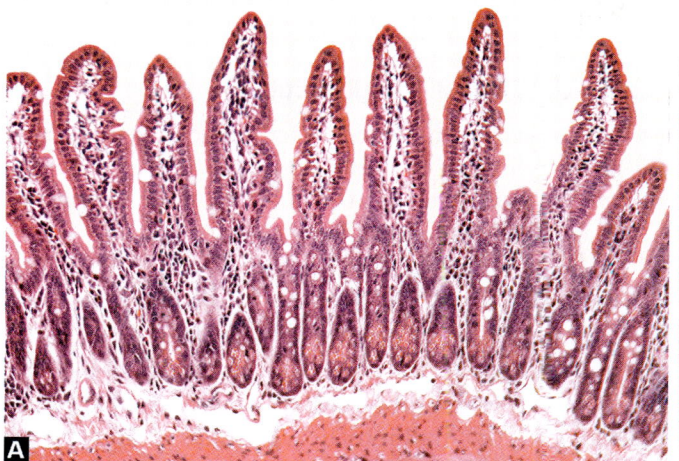
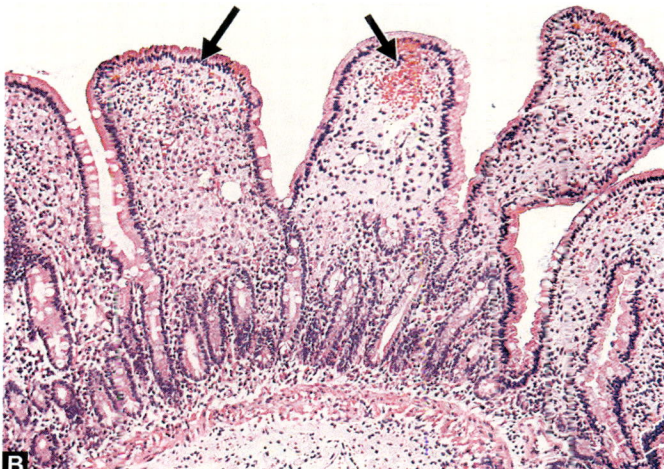

Fig. 20.33: Whipple disease. (A) Showing normal villi of small intestine, (B) showing blunting and widening of the villi of jejunum and lamina propria is infiltrated by large number of foamy macrophages (arrows) (100X).

Histochemistry

These organisms are present in macrophages of intestinal mucosa, which are visualized by *diastase resistant* **PAS stain** and **Gomori's methenamine silver** as *rod-shaped structures*. Draining mesenteric *lymph nodes, liver, lung, heart, brain, bone* and *synovial membrane* are also infiltrated with organisms carrying macrophages. These organisms may demonstrated by *polymerase chain reaction and electron microscopy*.

Treatment

These patients are treated by antibiotics therapy.

GIARDIASIS

Giardiasis is caused by *Giardia lamblia*. It does not induce significant villus architectural changes. The parasite is demonstrated at the luminal surface of normal appearing mucosa on histopathological examination. The parasite is mistaken as cytoplasmic debris. **Giemsa stain** and **trichrome stain** highlight the parasite. Histopathological findings demonstrating *Giardia lamblia* is shown in Fig. 20.34.

ASCARIS STRONGYLOIDIASIS

Strongyloidiasis is a human disease caused by nematode roundworm called *Strongyloides stercoralis*. It most often infects small intestine and rarely colon. The parasite is diagnosed by demonstration of *larvae, eggs and adult worms embedded in the crypts*. Eosinophils, sometimes with Charcat-Leyden crystals may be present. Gastric strongyloidiasis may occur in association with human T-lymphotropic virus causing adult *T cell lymphoma*. Multiple roundworms of *Strongyloides stercoralis* are shown in Fig. 20.35.

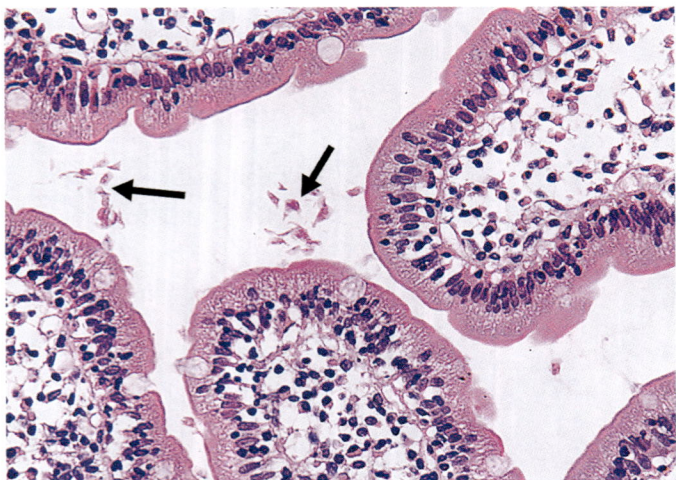

Fig. 20.34: Giardiasis. *Giardia lamblia* parasites are seen on the mucosal side of intestine (arrows).

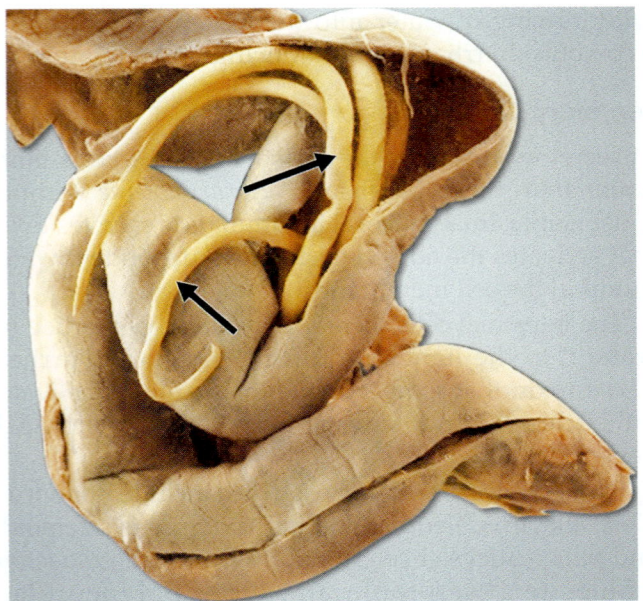

Fig. 20.35: *Ascaris strongyloides stercoralis* (roundworm nematode) causing gangrene of small intestine (arrows).

TUBERCULAR INTESTINAL ULCER

Tuberculosis is worldwide health problem caused by tubercle bacilli (homis strain). It is transmitted by inhalation of droplets (most common), ingestion of infected milk and skin inoculation (handling infected specimens).

Mycobacterium tubercle bacilli reach the intestine by either ingestion of infected sputum or *ingestion of unpasteurized milk*. Tuberculosis affects terminal ileum and most often *ileocecal region*.

Primary Intestinal Tuberculosis

Mycobacterium tubercle bacilli (bovis stain) reach the intestine due to *ingestion of unpasteurized milk*. Draining lymph nodes of small intestine are enlarged and matted with caseous necrosis known as *tabes mesenterica*. It most often heals by *fibrosis* and *dystrophic calcification*.

Secondary Intestinal Tuberculosis

- Mycobacterium tubercle bacilli reach the intestine by swallowing of *infected sputum in a case of pulmonary tuberculosis*. Intestinal lesions are more prominent than draining lymph nodes.
- The tubercular lesions begin in the Peyer's patches (lymphoid follicles) and spread through lymphatic channels resulting in tubercular ulcer in terminal ileum especially in **ileocecal region**.
- It produces circumferential ulcers perpendicular to long axis of small intestine. Fibrosis in this region is responsible for *stricture formation*. Stricture formation in the intestine is shown in Fig. 20.36.

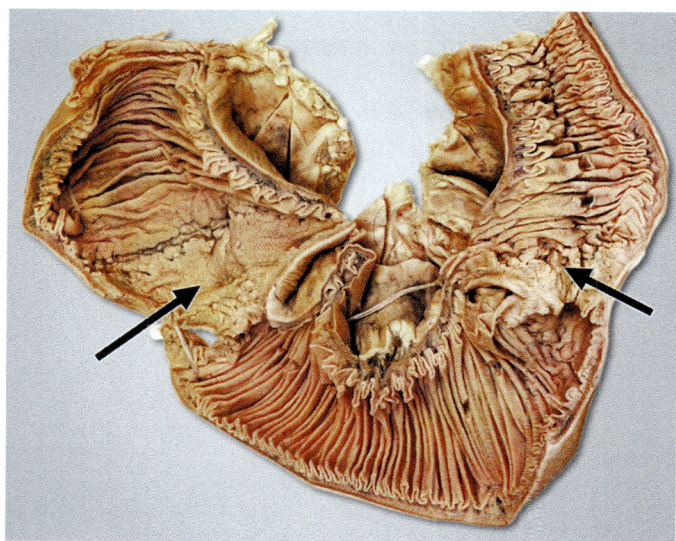

Fig. 20.36: Tubercular stricture of intestine (arrows).

Hyperplastic Ileocecal Tuberculosis

It is a variant of intestinal tuberculosis characterized by thickening of terminal ileum, cecum and ascending colon with mucosal ulceration. On clinical examination, hyperplastic ileocecal tuberculosis is *palpable and mistaken for caecal carcinoma*.

Light Microscopy

- Histopathological examination reveals epithelioid granulomas, caseous necrosis and Langhans' giant cells.
- Crohn's disease also produces stricture formation, in which segmental involvement of intestine occurs with skip areas thickened wall resembles pipe-like and shows irregular linear ulcers in the mucosa.

TYPHOID INTESTINAL ULCERS

Typhoid fever is a systemic disease caused by *Salmonella typhi* bacilli. Patient presents with continued fever with relative bradycardia, abdominal symptoms and psychosis. There is involvement of mononuclear phagocytic system with nodule formation in the Peyer's patches of lower ileum.

Transmission

Salmonella typhi has three antigenic structures: O antigens, H antigens and Vi antigens. The organism is transmitted by fecal-oral route.

Clinical Features

Patient may present with *step-ladder rise of fever* during *first week* and *continued during second and third week*, headache, nausea, vomiting, abdominal tenderness, rose spots (2–4 mm on trunk) and hepatosplenomegaly.

Clinical manifestations and laboratory findings in typhoid fever are shown in Table 20.27. Differences between tubercular and typhoid ulcer are shown in Table 20.28.

Extraintestinal Lesions

Proliferation of reticuloendothelial cells occurs in *spleen* (sinus histiocytes), *liver* (Kupffer's cells), *lymph nodes* and *bone marrow*. Patient develops splenomegaly, hepatomegaly and lymphadenopathy.

Pathogenesis

Ingested pathogen invades the mucosa, engulfed by macrophages and transported to regional lymph nodes. Multiplication of pathogen occurs in the lymphoid tissue resulting in bacteremia. These organisms reinfect lymphoid tissue and liberate endotoxin leading to delayed hypersensitivity reaction. *Erythrophagocytosis is demonstrated in histopathological examination of tissue sections*.

Intestinal Pathology

Terminal ileum and cecum are involved. There are four stages lasting for 4 weeks.

Table 20.27: Clinical manifestations and laboratory findings in typhoid fever

Clinical features	First stage (1st week)	Second stage (2nd week)	Third stage (3rd week)	Fourth stage (4th week)
Rose spots	Present on 5th day	Persists till 10th day	Absent	Absent
Splenomegaly	Slightly palpable on 6th day	Moderate enlarged	Moderate enlarged	Moderate enlarged
Psychosis and confusion	Absent	Present on 10th day	Present	Absent
Leukopenia	Present on 5th day	Present	Present	Absent
Blood culture	+++	+++	+/–	–
Stool culture	–	+	+++	–
Widal reaction	–	++	+++	–

Table 20.28: Differences between tubercular and typhoid ulcer

Characteristics	Tubercular ulcer	Typhoid ulcer
Causative organism	Mycobacterium tubercle bacilli	*Salmonella typhi*
Site of gut involvement	Ileocecal region	Terminal ileum (most common), may occur in jejunum or colon
Lymphoid involvement	Peyer's patches	Peyer's patches and also lymphoid follicles
Arrangement of ulcers	Transverse axis of intestine	Longitudinal axis of intestine
Size of ulcer	Large	Small
Margin	Irregular ulcer may encircle gut	Regular well circumscribed
Base of ulcer	Caseous material (creamy white)	Black due to sloughing of mucosa
Perforation of ulcer	Absent	Common
Bleeding from ulcer	Absent	Common
Stricture formation	Present as a result of fibrosis	Absent
Light microscopy	Caseous necrosis, epithelioid granulomas, Langhans' giant cells and demonstration of acid fast bacilli	Erythrophagocytosis and presence of organisms in macrophages

- *Hyperplasia of Peyer's patches (first week):* In the first week of infection, hyperplasia of Peyer's patches (lymphoid tissue) of terminal ileum occurs in the mucosa and extending to submucosa in the terminal ileum. Mucosa is projecting on the surface. *Blood culture is positive but stool culture is negative.*
- *Necrosis (second week):* Necrosis of Peyer's patches occurs from center to periphery exhibiting yellow or greenish-brown discoloration. *Blood culture and stool culture are positive.*
- *Ulceration (third week):* In the third week of infection, mucosal surface of ileum shows round to oval deep ulcers along the long with axis of intestine on gross examination. *Stool culture and Widal reaction are positive.* These ulcers may **perforate** leading to hemorrhage.
- *Healing (fourth week):* Healing of ulcers occurs in the 4th week of infection. Widal reaction is positive. Typhoid ulcers in small intestine are shown in Figs 20.37 and 20.38.

OBSTRUCTIVE DISEASES

Partial or complete obstruction of lumen of small intestine is a serious clinical disorder.

It is of three types: simple, strangulated (interrupting blood supply) and closed loop type (isolating from rest of small intestine).

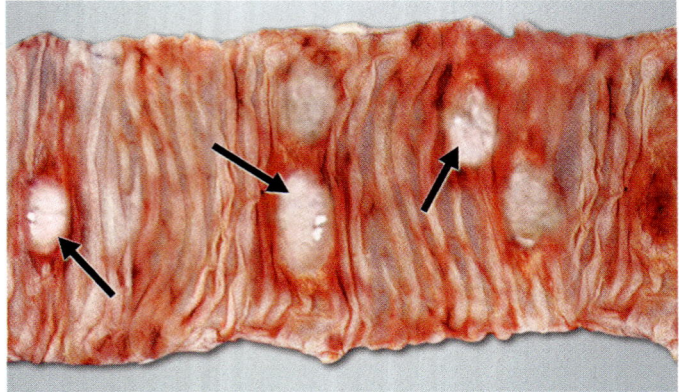

Fig. 20.37: Typhoid ulcers in small intestine. The Peyer's patches are prominent. Round to oval ulcers with hemorrhage are present along the long axis of intestine (arrows).

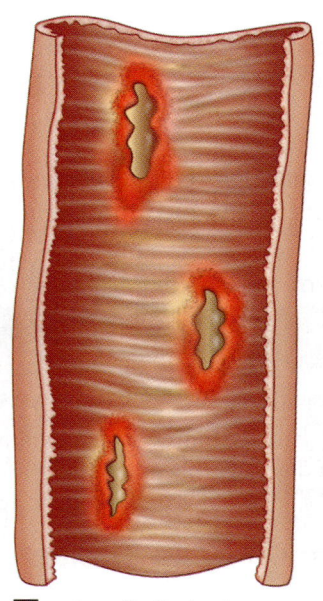
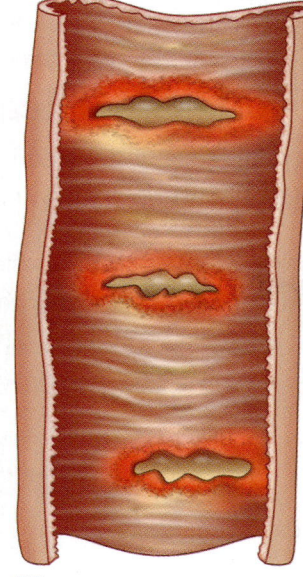

A   Longitudinal axis   B   Horizontal axis

Fig. 20.38: Ulcers in small intestine. (A) Typhoid ulcers, (B) tubercular ulcers.

Etiology

Most common cause of small bowel obstruction is adhesions from previous surgery. It may also occur due to congenital bowel deformities. Intestinal obstructions are of three kinds: *intraluminal* (e.g. tumor, foreign bodies), *intramural* and *extra-intestinal*.

DUODENAL ATRESIA

Duodenal atresia represents either a failure of the gut to canalize or a failure of a segment to develop during fetal growth. The normal GI system is a tube that develops from cords of embryonic cells. The cells forming the central part of these cords undergo apoptosis, and a lumen is thus formed. If the centrally located cells do not undergo apoptosis, the lumen never forms and the affected part of the GI system will be atretic (i.e. unpassable).

Duodenal atresia, most commonly associated with *Down's syndrome*, is characterized by vomiting of *bile stained material at birth* and an abdominal radiograph with the *double bubble sign*.

MECONIUM ILEUS

Meconium ileus in babies with cystic fibrosis may be complicated by volvulus and intestinal atresia.

INTESTINAL INTUSSUSCEPTION

Intussusception is an invagination of one segment of proximal bowel (usually the terminal ileum) into the distal bowel (usually the caecum), causing intestinal obstruction. Intussusception is a common cause of intestinal obstruction in children due to active peristalsis between *3 months and 6 years of age*.

In adults, intussusception occurs due to organic cause such as pedunculated polyps or cancerous growth. Small pedunculated tumors carried by peristalsis may pull forward the loop to which such a tumor is attached.

Based on the location, these may be ileocecal (most common), jejunojejunal, ileoileal and colo-colic. The inner loop of the gut may become necrotic unless the invagination is everted surgically.

Pathology

Intussusception progresses to tissue necrosis of segment of intestine as a result of decreased blood flow, swelling and inflammation. It can lead to intestinal perforation and infection. Shock and dehydration can occur very rapidly. Gross morphology of intussusception is shown in Fig. 20.39.

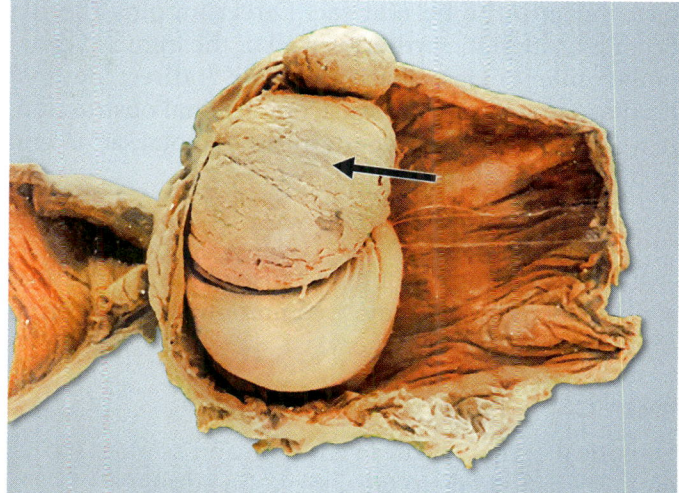

Fig. 20.39: Intussusception showing invagination of one segment of proximal bowel (usually the terminal ileum) into the distal bowel (arrow).

Clinical Features

Child presents with signs of obstruction (paroxysmal abdominal colicky pain) and rectal bleeding (*currant jelly stools*) from bowel infarction. On clinical examination, *abdominal distension and decreased bowel sounds* are observed. Features of dehydration include rapid pulse, pallor and marked sweating.

Diagnostic Evaluation

Abdominal radiograph may show *absence of gas in right upper quadrant*. Ultrasonography may be done to locate area of telescoped bowel.

PARALYTIC ILEUS

Paralytic ileus is a lack of intestinal peristalsis associated with stagnation of intestinal contents. The most common causes include *abdominal surgery persisting for 2–3 days, peritonitis, shock and vascular collapse*.

GALLSTONE ILEUS

In some cases of gallstone disease, gallstone erodes through the gallbladder into the adjacent small bowel forming cholecystoenteric fistula. Gallbladder stone enters ileum through the *fistulous tract and blocks the intestine known as gallstone ileus*. It can be very serious and requires immediate surgery. It primarily occurs in patients over age 65, and can sometimes be fatal.

INGUINAL HERNIA

The hernial contents are intestine, omentum, or other abdominal contents that pass through the hernial opening into the hernial sac. Direct inguinal hernia occurs through the posterior wall of the inguinal canal in the center of Hesselbach's triangle. Indirect inguinal hernia is most common cause of intestinal obstruction, in which small bowel extends into the scrotal sac, lateral to the triangle of Hesselbach.

ADHESIONS

Adhesions are most common cause of gastrointestinal obstruction. These are most commonly acquired from previous abdominal surgery.

UMBILICAL HERNIA

Umbilical hernias occur in children and adults. Ascites and pregnancy precipitate hernias in adults.

VENTRAL HERNIA

Ventral hernias (incisional hernias) occur in previous surgical incision sites.

VASCULAR DISEASES

SMALL BOWEL INFARCTION

Occlusion of superior mesenteric artery is most common cause of small bowel infarction. *Small intestine is supplied by superior mesenteric artery. Colon receives blood from inferior mesenteric artery.* Atheromatous plaques are common in superior mesenteric artery due to its oblique origin from the aorta.

Etiology

Causes of decreased blood supply to small intestine include thrombus over an atheromatous plaque in supply vessel, emboli from left heart, hypovolemia shock, vasospasm (digitalis), venous thrombus (polycythemia) or mechanical obstruction (volvulus). Systemic arterial thrombi may embolize to mesenteric arteries resulting in intestinal infarction.

Clinical Features

Patient presents with diffuse abdominal pain and bloody diarrhea.

Complications

In transmural gut infarction; there is danger *of gut perforation with mucosal ulcerations* and *pseudomembrane formation.*

POLYPS AND TUMORS

Tumors of the small intestine make up a small percentage of gastrointestinal neoplasms. The most common malignant tumors are neuroendocrine (carcinoid) tumors, lymphoma, adenocarcinoma, and GISTs.

Non-neoplastic lesions are more common in small intestine. WHO classification of small intestinal tumors is shown in Table 20.29.

Table 20.29: WHO classification of small intestine tumors

Categories	Polyps and tumors
Adenomas	Tubular adenoma Villus adenoma Tubulovillus adenoma
Dysplasia (intraepithelial neoplasia)	Low grade dysplasia High grade dysplasia
Hamartomas	Peutz-Jeghers polyp Juvenile polyp
Carcinomas	Mucinous adenocarcinoma Signet cell adenocarcinoma Squamous cell carcinoma Adenosquamous carcinoma Medullary carcinoma Undifferentiated carcinoma
Neuroendocrine tumors	Net G1 (carcinoid tumor) Net G2 Neuroendocrine carcinoma (small cell or large cell type)
Mesenchymal tumors	Leiomyoma Lipoma Gastrointestinal stromal tumor Leiomyosarcoma Angiosarcoma Kaposi sarcoma
Lymphoid tumors	Burkitt's lymphoma B cell lymphoma Diffuse large B cell lymphoma Follicular lymphoma T cell lymphoma
Secondary tumors	Metastases from other organs

ADENOCARCINOMA

Adenocarcinoma of small intestine is much less common than in colon. Approximately 40–50% of cases occur in the duodenum in the region of ampulla of Vater. It may occur in jejunum or ileum.

Gross Morphology
- Duodenal adenocarcinoma is relatively circumscribed with polypoidal appearance and central ulceration.
- Adenocarcinoma in jejunum or ileum shows circumferential involvement with extensive ulceration and annular appearance.

> **Light Microscopy**
>
> Tumor is well differentiated adenocarcinoma producing mucin. Scattered neuroendocrine cells may be present.

NEUROENDOCRINE (CARCINOID) TUMORS

Carcinoid tumors are neuroendocrine tumors of low-grade malignancy. These are most commonly located in the *submucosa of the intestinal tract, e.g. appendix (40%), terminal ileum (25%), colon, rectum (10–20%), duodenum (2–5%)* and affecting esophagus and stomach.

The tumors are *multicentric in stomach and ileum*. Peak incidence is in the sixth decade. These tumors are well differentiated tumors composed of cells similar to those of normal counterparts.

Goblet cell carcinoid consisting of mucin secreting and goblet-like cells is known as adenocarcinoid tumor with aggressive behavior than classic carcinoid tumor. Features of carcinoid tumors in gastrointestinal tract are shown in Table 20.30.

Neuroendocrine Cells

Neuroendocrine cells of the gut utilize amino acids, or derivatives of amino acids, as chemical messengers mediating paracrine and neuroendocrine effects. They are known as *APUD* (amine precursor uptake and decarboxylation).

- *Enterochromaffin cells:* These cells are named after for their staining after chromate fixation. These are found in groups at the bases of the intestinal crypts small intestine. These cells synthesize 5-HT (5-hydroxytryptamine) and kallikrein.
- *Non-chromaffin enteroendocrine cells.* These are dispersed as single cells in the crypt and villus epithelium, and in the bowel wall.

Categories

These tumors are categorized into three grades (G1, G2 and G3) according to *mitotic count* and *Ki-67 proliferative index*. The term neuroendocrine carcinoma is reserved for poorly differentiated neuroendocrine tumor with marked nuclear atypia and high mitotic rate (>20/high power field). Classification and grading of neuroendocrine tumors (carcinoids) of the GI tract are shown in Table 20.31.

Table 20.30: Features of carcinoid tumors in gastrointestinal tract

Parameters	Foregut carcinoids (proximal to ligament of Treitz)	Midgut carcinoids	Hindgut carcinoids
Structures	Stomach (body and fundus) Proximal duodenum but rare in esophagus	Terminal ileum Jejunum	Tip of appendix Colorectal region
Size	1–2 cm or more	<3.5 cm	Appendix (up to 1 cm) and colon up to 5 cm
Frequency	2–5%	60–80%	10–20%
Substances synthesized	Histamine, somatostatin and serotonin	Serotonin, substance P and polypeptide YY	Serotonin, substance P
Clinical course	Asymptomatic	Aggressive course due to greater depth of local invasion, necrosis and mitosis with poor outcome	Rectal carcinoids producing polypeptide hormones, colonic carcinoid may metastasize
Tumor cells	Argyrophilic cells	Argentaphilic cells	Argyrophilic cells
Carcinoid syndrome	Rare	Most common	Rare

Table 20.31: Classification and grading of neuroendocrine tumors (carcinoids) of the GI tract

Classification	Grade	Cytological features	Mitotic count
Neuroendocrine tumor	1	Cytological bland	<2 per HPF and or 2% ≤Ki-67 index
	2	Cytological bland	2–20% per HPF and or 3–20% Ki-67 index
			>20 per 10 HPF and or >20% Ki-67 index
Neuroendocrine carcinoma (NEC)	3	Tumor displaying at least 30% component of adenocarcinoma	
Hyperplastic or preneoplastic lesions	–	–	

Grading requires mitotic count in at least 50 HPFs and Ki-67 percentage in at least 500–2000 cells within the area of strongest nuclear labeling.

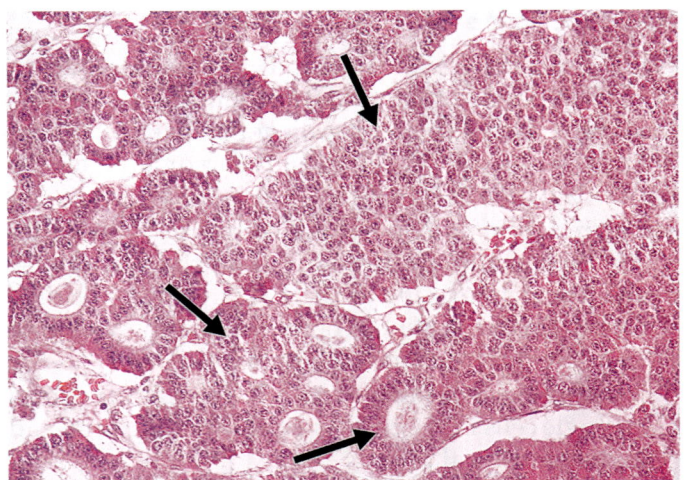

Fig. 20.40: Neuroendocrine tumor of ileum is composed of uniform cells with stippled chromatin (arrows) (400X).

Gross Morphology
Following formalin fixation, tumor acquires yellow color. Infiltration of the submucosa by tumor is the rule.

Light Microscopy
- These are low-grade tumors composed of neuroendocrine cells.
- Tumor cells are round with uniform nuclei, scanty cytoplasm and indistinct cell borders. These are arranged in solid nests, cords separated by thin fibrous septa.
- Tumor cells may form rosettes around blood vessels, which secrete hormones into the systemic circulation (Fig. 20.40).

Histochemical Staining
Silver staining demonstrates black granules in the cytoplasm. Argentaffin cells containing granules have the property of reducing silver salts without the help of reducing agent, while argyrophil cells reduce silver salts to metallic silver (black color) only after addition of a reducing agent.

Electron Microscopy
Tumor cells show cytoplasmic granules, which are stained red with eosin, yellowish brown with chrome salts, black with iron-hematoxylin and metallic black with silver salts.

Immunohistochemistry
Panel of markers is used to analyze expression in small intestinal neuroendocrine tumors on histopathological sections (Table 20.32).

Metastases
Carcinoids of appendix and rectum are seldom malignant. Most carcinoids invade submucosa and muscularis and sometimes penetrate bowel wall. Metastases may be seen in 5% of cases having tumor <1.0 cm size. However, large carcinoid tumor >2 cm size in ileum and appendix has tendency to spread to regional lymph nodes and distant organs such as liver, lungs and bones in 66% of cases.

Carcinoid Syndrome
Neuroendocrine tumors metastasizing to the liver can lead to carcinoid syndrome as a result of synthesis of 5-HT (5-hydroxytryptamine), serotonin, and bradykinin. 5-HT increases gut motility resulting in diarrhea, excessive bowel sounds (borborygmi) and abdominal pain.

Kallikrein produces flushing of skin, bronchospasm and diarrhea. 5-HT is inactivated in the liver by monoamine oxidase to form 5-hydroxyindole acetic acid (5-HIAA), and this is excreted in the urine.

Urinary 5-hydroxyindole acetic acid may be elevated. Patient presents with cutaneous flushing, watery diarrhea, abdominal cramps, bronchospasm and valvular lesions of the right side of the heart. Clinical manifestations of carcinoids of small intestine are shown in Table 20.33.

Carcinoid Heart Disease
The products synthesized by carcinoid tumor such as 5-HT, serotonin, and bradykinin enter into hepatic

Table 20.32: Immunohistochemistry in intestinal carcinoid tumors

Tumor marker	Tumor location	Expression
Chromogranin (neural marker)	Small intestine	Positive
Synaptophysin (neural marker)	Small intestine	Positive
Neuron-specific enolase	Small intestine	Positive
CDX2 (diffuse nuclear staining)	Small intestine and duodenum	Positive
PAX8 (polyclonal antibody)	Duodenum	Positive

Intestinal carcinoid tumors are negative for thyroid transcription factor 1 (TTF 1), PAX8 and ISL 1.

Gastrointestinal Tract

Table 20.33: Clinical manifestations of carcinoids of small intestine

Organs involved	Clinical manifestations
Liver	Metastases
Vascular phenomenon	Flushing, cyanosis and telangiectasia
Respiratory system	Bronchoconstriction
Heart	Pulmonary and tricuspid valve heart disease
Blood and tissue cells	5-Hydroxytryptamine (5-HT) and serotonin
Urine analysis	5-Hydroxyindole acetic acid (5-HIAA) is increased
Skin	Hyperpigmentation
Legs	Edema

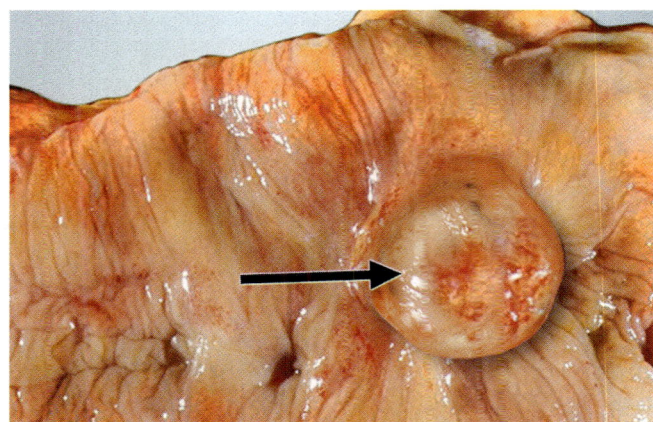

Fig. 20.41: Gastrointestinal stromal tumor showing well circumscribed tumor projecting towards lumen of intestine (arrow).

veins and affect the right side of the heart. The patient develops *tricuspid valve incompetence* and *pulmonary valve stenosis* as a result of formation of fibrous plaques. Smooth muscle cells within endocardium may undergo proliferation as a result of stimulation by kallikrein.

GASTROINTESTINAL STROMAL TUMORS

Gastrointestinal stromal tumors (GISTs) are the most common mesenchymal tumors of the small intestine. These most often affect adults with a peak incidence of seventh decade and equal sex predilection.

Locations

These tumors occur in entire gastrointestinal tract such as *stomach* (50%), *small intestine* (25%), *large intestine* (10%), and extra gastrointestinal sites. *Gastric stromal tumors are usually submucosal* and covered by intact mucosa.

Molecular Genetics

Approximately 75–80% of GISTs have Kit mutations. Mutations in platelet-derived growth factor receptor-α (PDGFR-α) have been demonstrated in 10% of cases.

Gross Morphology
- Small intestinal GISTs vary from small mural nodule to large exophytic pedunculated masses.
- Duodenal tumor measures 5 cm in diameter.
- Tumors in jejunum and ileum measure 7 cm in diameter (Fig. 20.41).

Light Microscopy
- Tumor is composed of fascicles of bland spindle cells with abundant fibrillary cytoplasm.
- Skeinoid fibers are typical of such tumors in small intestine (Fig. 20.42).

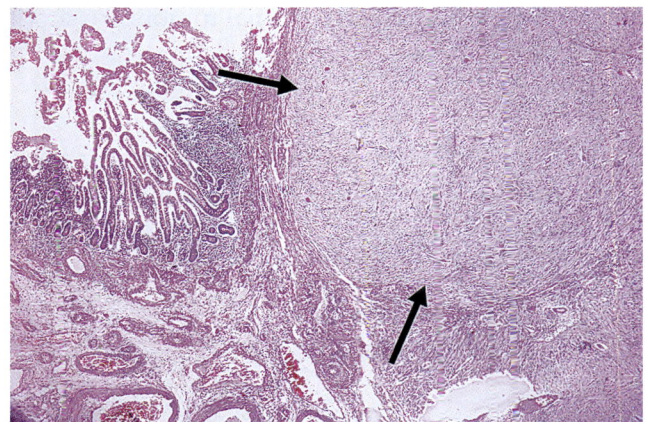

Fig. 20.42: Gastrointestinal stromal tumors (arrows) (100X).

Immunohistochemistry

Panel of markers is used to analyze expression in gastrointestinal stromal tumors on histopathological sections (Table 20.34).

Table 20.34: Immunohistochemistry of gastrointestinal stromal tumors

Tumor marker	Expression
C-Kit oncogene (CD117) encoding tyrosine kinase	Positive (95%)
DOG1 (protein of unknown function)	Positive (most specific marker)
CD171 (cell adhesive molecule)	Positive
Protein kinase C theta	Positive
Vimentin	Positive
Smooth muscle actin encoded by ACTA2 gene located on 10q–q24	Positive
CD34	Positive
Desmin	Positive (5%)

Table 20.35: Proposed guidelines for predicting malignant behavior of gastrointestinal stromal tumors

Tumor size	Light microscopy	Clinical behavior	Metastases and mortality
≤ 2 cm	≤ 5 mitoses/50 HPF	Benign course	Prognosis excellent
≤ 2 cm and ≥ 5 cm	≤ 5 mitoses/50 HPF	Low malignant potential	Metastases and fatal outcome (4%)
≥ 5 cm and ≤ 10 cm	≤ 5 mitoses/50 HPF	Moderately malignant	Metastases and fatal outcome (25%)
> 10 cm	≤ 5 mitoses/50 HPF	Highly malignant	Metastases and fatal outcome (50–90%)

Clinical Behavior

Mitotic count, size, and location help in predicting the behavior of these tumors. Stromal tumors in small intestine most often behave like leiomyosarcoma as opposite to the stomach. GISTs are considered to be of low malignant potential and are removed surgically. Proposed guidelines for predicting malignant behavior of gastrointestinal stromal tumors are shown in Table 20.35.

DIFFUSE LARGE B CELL LYMPHOMA

Diffuse large B cell lymphoma (DLBCL) can arise from the abundant lymphoid tissue of the small intestine. It accounts for 50% of all lymphomas. Patient may present with malabsorption when there is diffuse involvement.

Gross Morphology
Large polypoidal or ulcerated circumferential tumor mass is seen in small intestine (Fig. 20.43).

Light Microscopy
Tumor is composed of sheets of large lymphoid cells with vesicular chromatin, prominent nucleoli, irregular contours and scanty cytoplasm (Fig. 20.44).

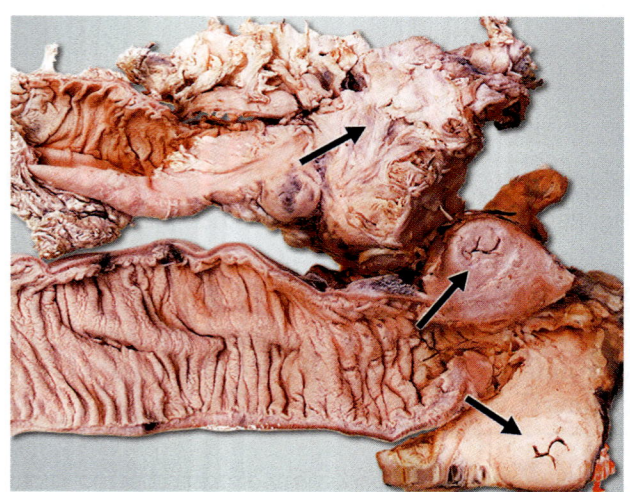

Fig. 20.43: Large polypoidal or ulcerated circumferential lymphoma tumor mass is seen in small intestine (arrows).

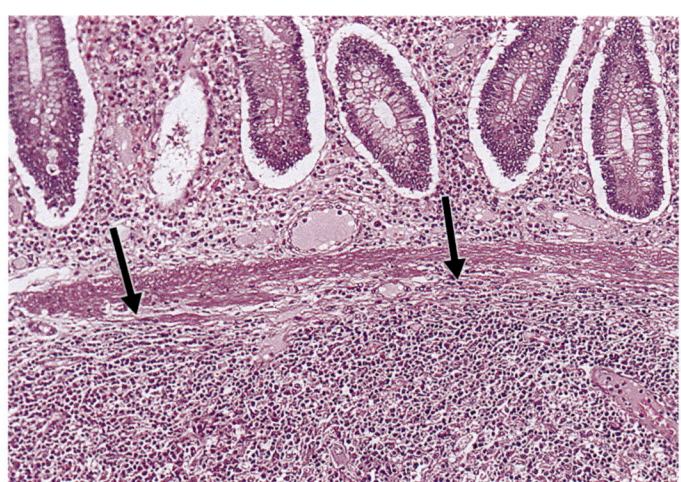

Fig. 20.44: Diffuse large cell lymphoma infiltrating intestinal mucosa (arrows) (400X).

LARGE INTESTINE

ANATOMY AND PHYSIOLOGY

Large intestine measures 1.5 to 1.8 meters in length extending from ileocecal valve to dentate line of the anal canal. It consists of right and left colon. Right colon is subdivided into caecum, ascending colon and proximal transverse colon.

Left colon consists of distal transverse colon, descending colon, sigmoid colon and rectum. Rectum measures 10.5–12 cm in length. Transverse colon always has mesentery. Mesentery is seen in ascending colon in 12% and descending colon in 22%.

BLOOD SUPPLY

Superior mesenteric artery supplies blood to the *right colon as far as distal transverse colon.* Inferior mesenteric artery supplies blood to *left colon and rectum.* Remainder of the rectum and anal canal supplied by middle rectal arteries and branches of the pudendal arteries.

HISTOLOGY

Large intestine consists of mucosa, submucosa, muscular coat and serous coat. Mucosa of colon is lined by simple columnar epithelium with a thin brush border and numerous goblet cells. The crypts of Lieberkühn are straight and branched lined by goblet cells. At the base of the crypts endocrine and undifferentiated cells are present.

Mucosa absorbs some ions, soluble compounds and maintains water balance. It secretes mucus, which lubricates colon and protects mucosa. It breaks down undigested carbohydrates, proteins, and amino acids into products that can be expelled in feces or absorbed and detoxified by liver.

It synthesizes certain vitamins of B complex and vitamin K. Muscular layer moves contents along length of colon into sigmoid colon and rectum by contractions of circular and longitudinal muscles.

NEUROMUSCULAR DISORDERS

HIRSCHSPRUNG'S DISEASE

Hirschsprung's disease is also referred to as congenital megacolon. It is characterized by *congenital absence of ganglion cells usually in the submucosal and muscular coat of large bowel (distal sigmoid colon and rectum)*. It most often affects male infants in 80% of cases (Fig. 20.45).

Predisposing Factors

Hirschsprung's disease is associated with *Down's syndrome* and *Waardenburg syndrome*. Waardenburg syndrome is characterized by *congenital deafness, gut malrotation, gastric diverticulum, intestinal atresia, urogenital abnormalities* and *cardiovascular abnormalities*. Acquired megacolon may be associated with Chagas' disease.

Molecular Genetics

RET gene (located on 10q11.2) is the most common gene mutation demonstrated in Hirschsprung's disease. Other gene mutations seen associated with this disorder include *EDNRB gene (located on 13q22), SOX10 (located on 22q13), SIP1 gene (located on 2q22), PHOX2B gene (located on 4q12) and neuregulin gene (located on 8)*.

EDNRB gene present on surface of cells encodes protein that connects the neural crest cells to digestive tract. *Interaction of endothelin-3 with endothelin receptor type B protein is essential for development of enteric neurons*. Gene mutations in Hirschsprung's disease are shown in Table 20.36.

Table 20.36: Gene mutations in Hirschsprung's disease

Gene	Located on chromosome
RET gene	10q11.2
EDNRB gene	13q22
SIP1 gene	2q22
PHOX2B	4q12
Neuregulin gene	8

Pathogenesis

Marked dilation of the colon (ganglionic segment) occurs proximal to the stenotic rectum (aganglionic segment), with clinical signs of intestinal obstruction.

Physiological state: During intrauterine life, the neural crest cells migrate into upper alimentary tract and then follow caudally via vagus nerve fibers by 12 weeks of gestation. These ganglion cells are present in submucosa (Auerbach's plexus) and between muscular coats (Meissener's plexus). These are responsible for the peristaltic moment of the intestine in postnatal life.

Pathological state: Failure of migration of ganglion cells in the submucosal (Auerbach's plexus) and muscular coat (Meissener's plexus) in the large intestine, especially rectum results in Hirschsprung's disease. Immune-mediated neuronal necrosis has been suggested in the

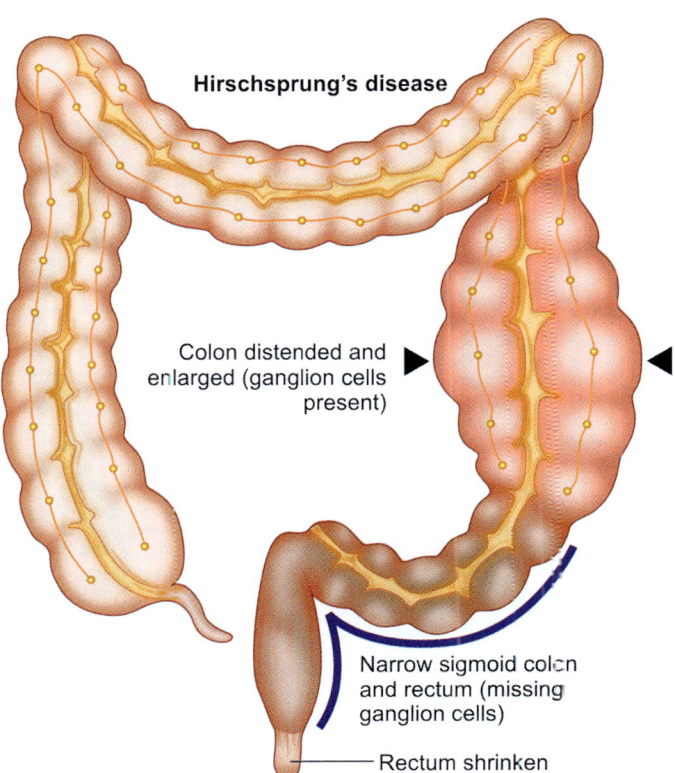

Fig. 20.45: Hirschsprung's disease showing narrow sigmoid colon absence of ganglion cells and dilated normal colon with presence of ganglion cells proximal to constricted segment.

pathogenesis of Hirschsprung's disease, that shows aberrant expression of MHC class II molecules in colon responsible for recurrence of disease after surgery.

Sites Involved

Rectum is always involved, and this is the preferred site for biopsy. *Sigmoid colon and adjacent proximal colon* are involved, but entire colonic involvement is very rare. *Aganglionic segment of colon is permanently contracted* causing intestinal obstruction. This obstruction leads to dilatation of proximal normal (ganglionic) segment.

Classification

Based on length of large intestine involved, infant has *classic segment* (<40 cm colon), *long segment* (colon involvement extending to small intestine), *short segment* (a few cm of colon involved), *ultra-short* (<2 cm colon involved) and *zonal form* (skip areas in colon).

Clinical Features

Newborn develops delayed passage of meconium, severe constipation, vomiting and abdominal distension. There may be electrolyte imbalance, peritonitis, superimposed enterocolitis, toxic megacolon and perforation.

On examination, *anal canal and rectum are small devoid of stool with tight anal sphincter. Abdominal distension,* radiograph and barium enema findings in Hirschsprung's disease are shown in Fig. 20.46.

Gross Morphology

- Sigmoid colon and rectum (aganglionic bowel) are narrowed due to absence of ganglion cells.
- Proximal segment of colon (ganglionic bowel) is dilated (Fig. 20.47).

Light Microscopy

Narrowed distal segment shows complete absence of ganglion cells in submucosa (Auerbach's plexus) and muscular coat (Meissener's plexus). It is accompanied by hypertrophy of nerves (Fig. 20.48).

Immunohistochemistry

- Identification of ganglion cells may be difficult in neonates due to immaturity of the ganglion cells. *Ganglion cells are positive for neuron-specific enolase.* Hypertrophied nerve bundles are positive for **S-100**, and **cathepsin-D**.
- Another promising marker is **calretinin**, a vitamin D-dependent calcium binding protein, absence of which has been seen in Hirschsprung's disease.

Laboratory Diagnosis

The diagnosis is made clinically (chronic constipation in a young child) but must be confirmed by biopsy, which typically shows an absence of ganglion cells.

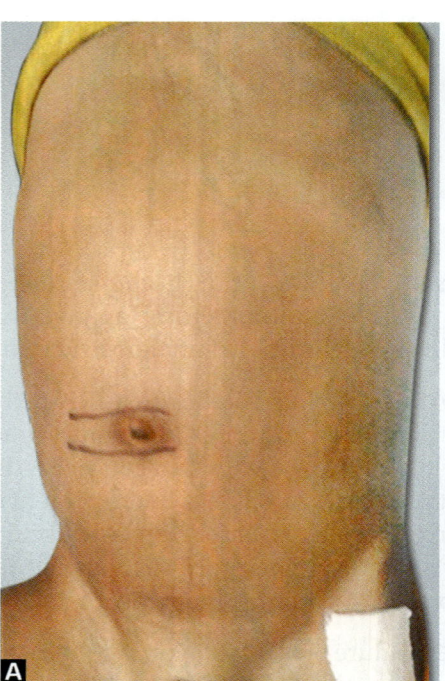
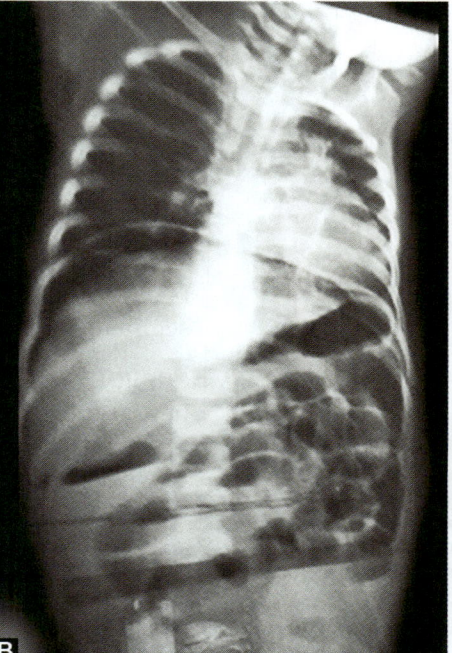
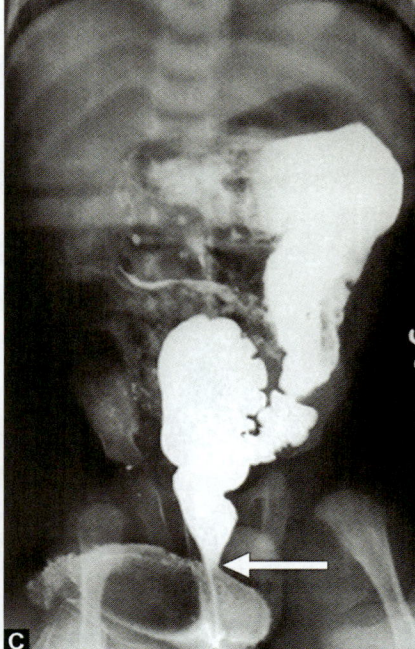

Fig. 20.46: Hirschsprung's disease. (A) Child showing abdominal distension, (B) abdominal radiograph showing dilated loops with multiple air fluid levels suggestive of intestinal obstruction, (C) barium enema showing cone-shaped transition zone at the rectosigmoid junction (arrow).

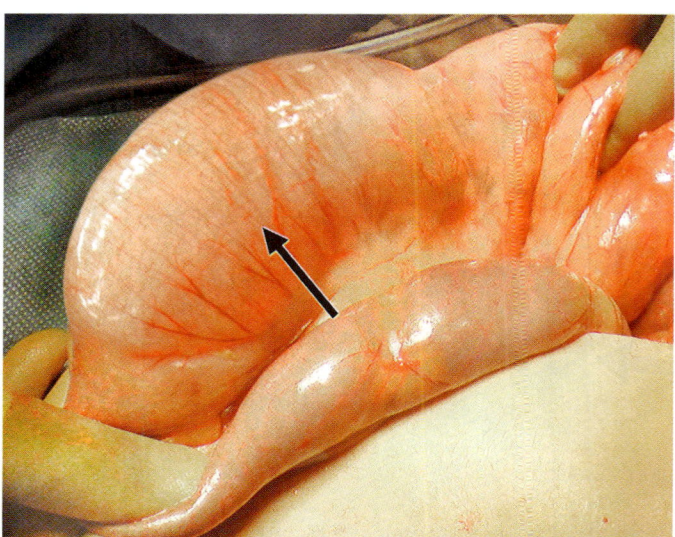

Fig. 20.47: Hirschsprung's disease. The baby of one week had been constipated since birth and exhibited signs of intestinal obstruction. Barium enema showed a narrowed lower rectal segment with dilated rectum above it. There were no ganglion cells in the narrowed segment (arrow).

- *Rectal biopsy:* Rectum is always involved, and this is the preferred site for biopsy *at least 2 cm above anal verge in infants* and *3 cm above anal verge in children.*
- Light microscopy shows absence of ganglion cells in the affected segment of intestine.
- *Imaging techniques:* Barium enema-contrast material flows into an unexpanded distal segment, then passes through a cone-shaped area and finally enters the dilated proximal bowel.
- *Electromanometry:* It is only useful to confirm the diagnosis in cases of *ultra-short segment of Hirschsprung's disease.*
- *Frozen section:* Acetylcholinesterase is used to demonstrate marked increase in thick nerve fibers in the wall of affected intestine. Ratio of acetylcholinesterase to butyryl cholinesterase is increased in Hirschsprung's disease.

Surgical Treatment

The part of the intestine that does not contain ganglion cells must be resected.

PSEUDO-OBSTRUCTION SYNDROME

Pseudo-obstruction syndrome is a heterogeneous group of neuromuscular disorders characterized by colonic inertia and constipation.

Diagnosis is really a challenge. Careful evaluation of nerves or muscle fibers of the muscularis propria on histopathological examination, special stains and clinical correlation help in establishing diagnosis.

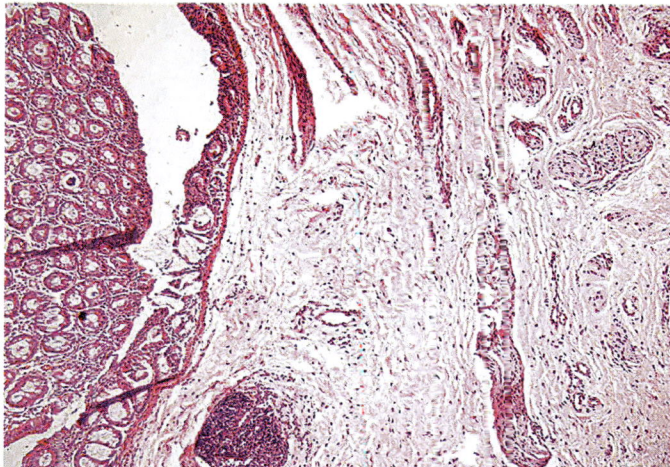

Fig. 20.48: Hirschsprung's disease. Punch biopsy from the rectosigmoid region showing increase in the number and size of nerve bundles in the submucosa with conspicuous absence of ganglion cells (100X).

DIVERTICULAR DISEASES

DIVERTICULOSIS

Diverticulum is pulsion (or false) herniation of pockets of *mucosa and submucosa* through the defects in weakened muscular propria throughout the colon along the antimesenteric taeniae coli, where arteries penetrate the muscular propria.

Locations

Diverticula are almost always multiple. Diverticulosis is most common in the sigmoid colon (85%). Sigmoid diverticular disease is the most common cause hematochezia (bright red blood in stool) from lower intestinal tract and colovesical fistulas. Diverticulum disease is shown in Fig. 20.49.

Pathogenesis

Diverticuli occur due to increased intraluminal pressure (presumably low fiber content in diet) especially in older persons. These are pulsion diverticula that form two rows along the antimesenteric taeniae coli at the site where arteries perforate the muscular propria. These are most common in men older than age 40 and in people who eat a low-fiber diet.

Clinical Features

Patient with diverticulosis is most often asymptomatic and will remain so unless diverticulitis develops. Diverticulitis results from the irritation caused by retained fecal material that obstructs the lumen of a diverticulum.

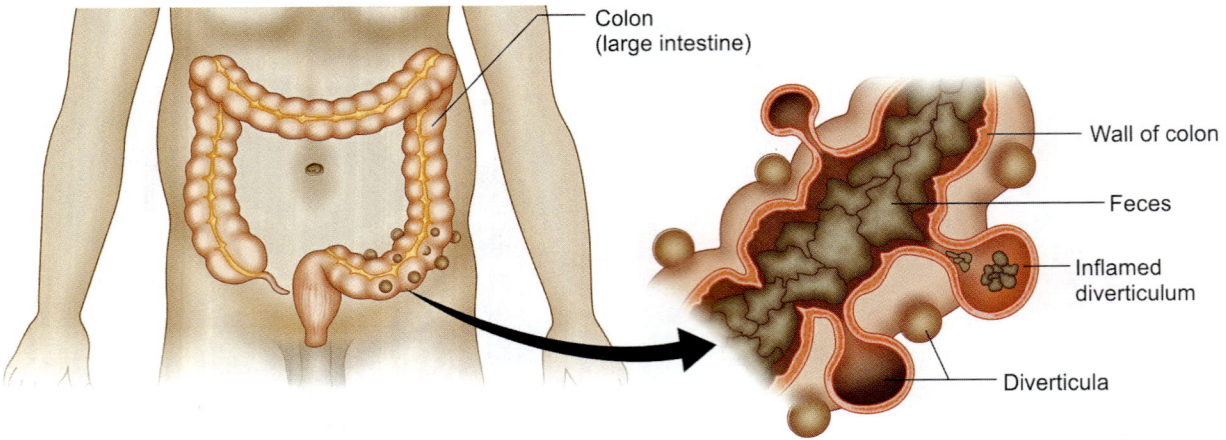

Fig. 20.49: Diverticulum disease.

Long-standing cases present with ribbon-like stools, intermittent diarrhea, abdominal distension, abdominal rigidity and pain, nausea, vomiting with diminishing or absent bowel sounds. Clinical features of diverticular disease are shown in Table 20.37

Complications

Complications of diverticular disease include acute inflammation, perforation, fistula, stricture and bleeding. Complications of diverticular disease are shown in Table 20.38.

Diagnosis

Diverticular disease is diagnosed by double contrast barium enema and colonoscopy. Fistulas are demonstrated by **barium enema** examination. Most diverticular abscesses are confirmed by ultrasonography.

Radionuclide imaging and **arteriography** are performed to localize the source of bleeding as well as angiodysplasia.

DIVERTICULITIS

Diverticulitis refers to inflammation of diverticula. It commonly affects older persons. In diverticulitis, retained undigested food and bacteria accumulate in the diverticular sac.

Pathogenesis

Colonic bacteria attack the thin walls of the diverticulum resulting in perforation, abscess, peritonitis (most serious complication), abscess formation, bowel obstruction, or hemorrhage. Occasionally, the inflamed colon segment may adhere to the bladder or other organs and cause a fistula.

Clinical Features

Patient presents with *lower abdominal pain, tenderness, and bright red rectal bleeding* (most frequent finding). Patient has other signs of acute inflammation such as fever and leukocytosis.

Table 20.37: Clinical features of diverticular disease

Disorder	Clinical features
Diverticulosis	Asymptomatic Colicky abdominal pain Altered bowel habit
Acute diverticulitis	Constant abdominal pain Fever Nausea and vomiting Bleeding Altered bowel habit Localized or generalized abdominal pain

Laparotomy is performed for generalized peritonitis to remove pus and feces.

Table 20.38: Complications of diverticular disease

Complications	Clinical findings
Acute inflammation	Abscess formation Peritonitis (local or generalized)
Perforation	Local fecal peritonitis Generalized fecal peritonitis
Fistula	Colovesical fistula Colovaginal fistula
Stricture	Stricture formation
Bleeding	Bleeding from diverticuli

OBSTRUCTIVE DISEASES

Intestinal obstruction refers to partial or complete obstruction of the bowel lumen. Obstruction of small intestine is more serious.

Gastrointestinal Tract

Pathology

In initial phase of intestinal obstruction peristalsis temporarily increases in attempt to force contents past obstruction. Intestinal distension impedes venous blood supply to bowel, halting normal absorptive processes.

Bowel wall swells and becomes edematous as water, sodium, and potassium are secreted into intestine and not absorbed from it. Gas-forming bacteria collect above obstruction enhancing distension. Untreated patient develops severe hypovolemia and sepsis with fatal outcome.

Etiology

Most common cause of small bowel obstruction is adhesions from previous surgery. It may also occur due to congenital bowel deformities. Intestinal obstructions are of three kinds: intraluminal (e.g. tumor, foreign bodies), intramural and extra intestinal.

Clinical Features

Patients with bowel obstruction present with colicky pain followed by a pain-free interval accompanied by constipation and inability to pass gas (flatus). Untreated complete obstruction of the small or large bowel can cause death within hours due to shock and vascular collapse. Ultimately, intestinal obstruction may lead to ischemia, necrosis, and death.

VOLVULUS

Volvulus is twisting of a mobile segment of the intestine on its mesenteric root. It occurs in sigmoid colon (*most common site*) and small intestine. The twist is *counterclockwise* in most cases. Volvulus is always a consequence of *congenital anomaly*.

Pathology

During intrauterine life, *defective intestine rotation* results in abnormal positions of the small intestine and colon, anomalous attachments, and bands. *Kinking of bowel interrupts the blood supply* resulting in *infarction, intestinal gangrene* and *obstruction*. Volvulus showing twisting of a mobile segment of the intestine on its mesenteric root is shown in Fig. 20.50.

INTUSSUSCEPTION

An intussusception is an invagination of one segment of proximal bowel (usually the terminal ileum) into the distal bowel (usually the cecum), causing intestinal obstruction. *Colocolic intussusception is relatively uncommon.* The inner loop of the gut may become necrotic unless the invagination is everted surgically.

- Intussusception is most common cause of intestinal obstruction in children younger than age 2 years due to active peristalsis.
- In adults, intussusception occurs due to organic cause such as pedunculated polyps or cancerous growth. Small pedunculated tumors carried by peristalsis may pull forward the loop to which such a tumor is attached.

Clinical Features

Child presents with signs of obstruction (colicky pain) and rectal bleeding (*currant jelly stools*) from bowel infarction.

INFLAMMATORY BOWEL DISEASE

GENERAL CONSIDERATIONS

Inflammatory bowel disease (IBD) comprises two diseases: *ulcerative colitis* (most common) and *Crohn's disease* of

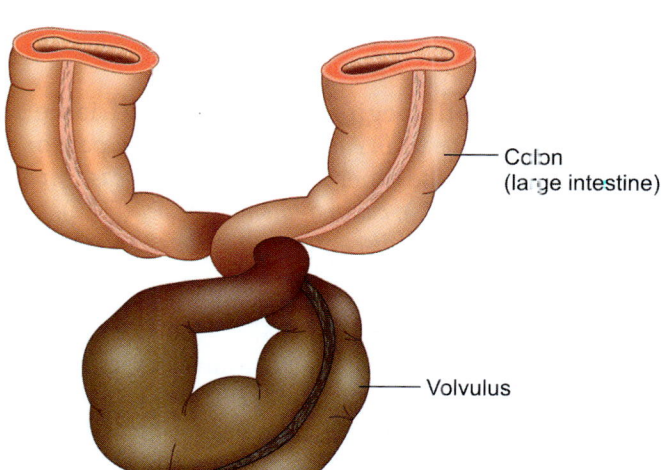
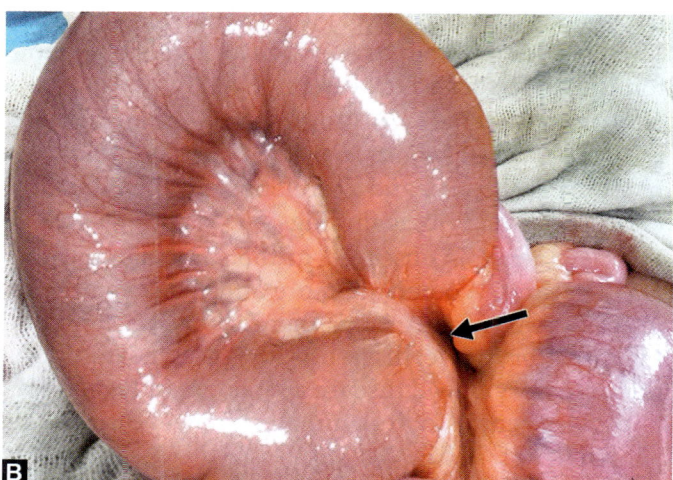

Fig. 20.50: Volvulus showing twisting of a mobile segment of the intestine on its mesenteric root (arrow).

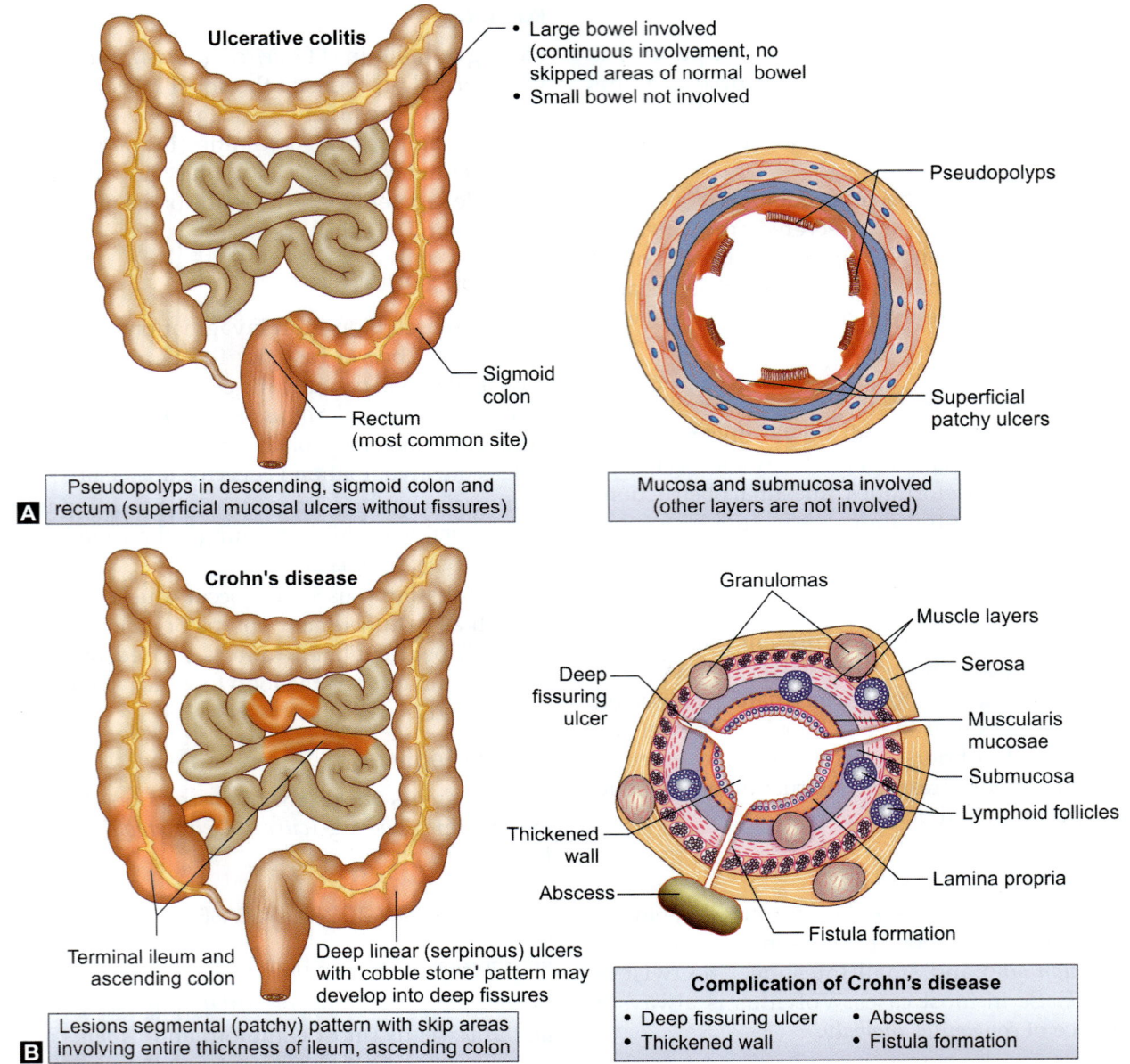

Fig. 20.51: Features of inflammatory bowel disease (IBD). (A) Showing ulcerative colitis, (B) showing Crohn's disease.

unknown etiology. But psychological, infectious and autoimmune factors have been implicated.
- *Ulcerative colitis and Crohn's disease share many features, but may differ from one another.* The diagnosis is made by exclusion and correlating all the clinical, endoscopic, radiologic findings.
- Peak incidence is observed in the same age group (15–25 years). Women are more affected than males in 20–25 years of age group. There is family history of inflammatory bowel disease in 20% cases. Features of inflammatory bowel disease are shown in Fig. 20.51 and pathogenesis of inflammatory bowel disease is shown in Fig. 20.52.
- Inflammatory bowel disease is associated with GIT complications and extraintestinal manifestations.

Locations

Ulcerative colitis begins in the *rectum* (friable red mucosa) and *extends in continuity* to involve part or the entire colon. On the other hand, *Crohn's disease involves terminal ileum (30%), colon and small bowel (50%),* colon alone (20%) having *discontinuous/skipped* involvement of the bowel.

Gross Morphology
- In ulcerative colitis, mucosa and submucosa of the rectum, colon and appendix show ulcerations forming pseudopolyps. There is absence of fistulae formation. Anus is not commonly involved.
- Crohn's disease involves all layers of small or large intestine.

Gastrointestinal Tract

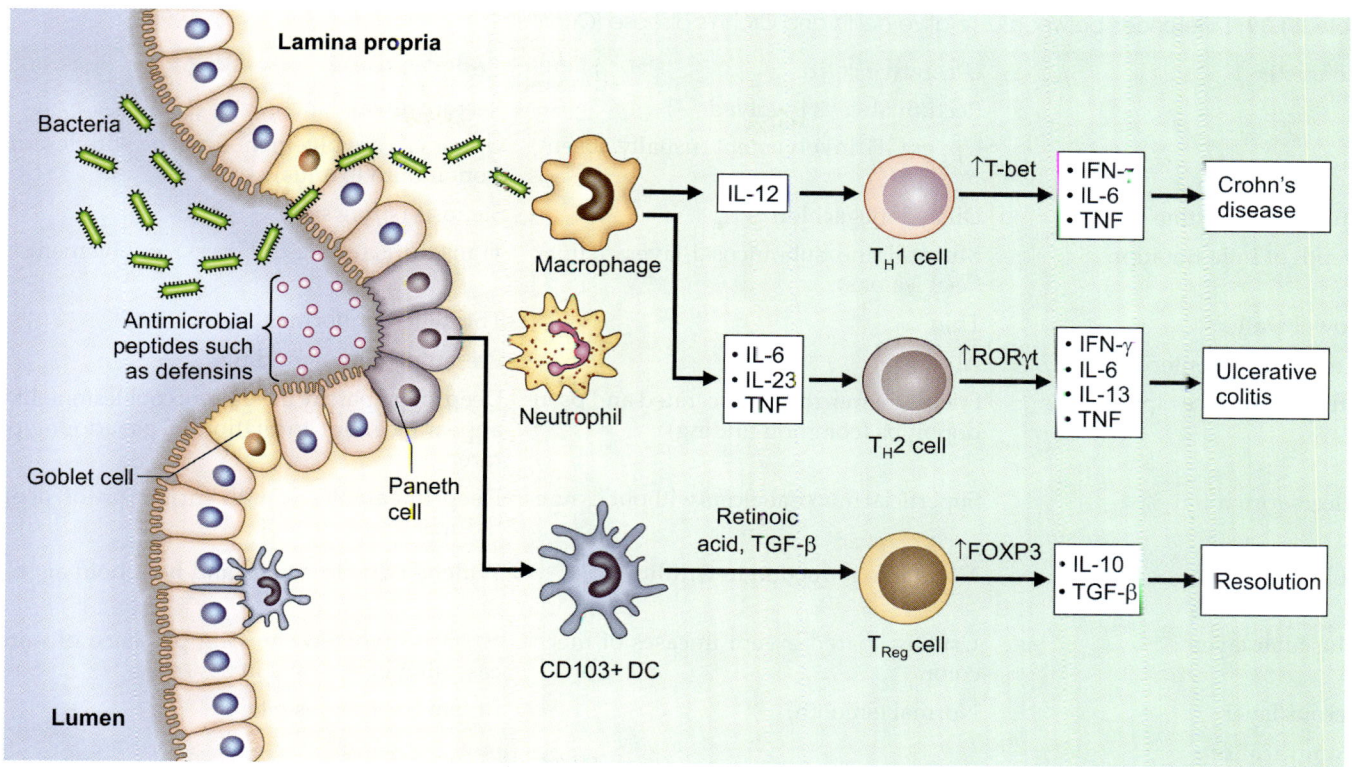

Fig. 20.52: Pathogenesis of inflammatory bowel disease.

Endoscopy

Ulcerative colitis produces *ulceration with pseudopolyp formation* due to bulging of inflamed mucosa surrounded by areas of ulceration.

Crohn's disease produces linear ulcers, cobble stoning, luminal narrowing (string signs on barium studies), and fistula formation.

Light Microscopy

- Ulcerative colitis produces crypt abscesses due to accumulation of neutrophils resulting in rupture and crypt atrophy.
- Crohn's disease is associated with noncaseating granulomas (50% cases), lymphoid aggregates, and aphthoid mucosal ulcers. Involvement of the ileum also favors Crohn's disease.

Complications

Ulcerative colitis is more likely to result in adenocarcinoma (increased risk with duration), HLA-B27 positive ankylosing spondylitis, toxic megacolon, and sclerosing pericholangitis.

Crohn's disease is more likely to involve other areas of gastrointestinal tract from mouth to anus (fissures and fistulas).

Clinical Features

Patient with ulcerative colitis presents with abdominal cramps, diarrhea with blood and mucus, rectal bleeding, and tenesmus (ineffective and painful straining of stool).

On the other hand, patient with Crohn's disease presents with right lower quadrant colicky pain (obstruction) with diarrhea and anal bleeding. Differences between ulcerative colitis and Crohn's disease are shown in Table 20.39.

Table 20.39: Differences between ulcerative colitis and Crohn's disease

Character	Ulcerative colitis	Crohn's disease
Gross morphology		
Distribution	Diffuse pattern (continuous without skip lesions)	Segmental (patchy) pattern with skip lesions
	Sigmoid colon (common)	Terminal ileum and ascending colon (common)
	Ileum involvement (<10%)	Ileum involvement common

Contd...

Table 20.39: Differences between ulcerative colitis and Crohn's disease (Contd...)

Character	Ulcerative colitis	Crohn's disease
	Rectum always involved	Rectum always spared
	Upper GIT involvement (usually absent)	Upper GIT involvement (may be with lesions from mouth to anus)
Lumen of intestine	Dilated megacolon	Stenosis (*string sign*)
Depth of inflammation	Mucosal and submucosal layers (superficial lesions)	Transmural (entire thickness) involvement
Bowel wall	Thin	Thickened or normal
Creeping mesenteric fat	Absent	Present (common finding)
Mucosal surface appearance	Friable, hemorrhagic, ulcerated and pseudopolyps (common finding)	Deep linear patchy ulceration; cobblestone-like appearance, but formation of pseudopolyps rare
Ulcers formation	Superficial mucosal ulcers without fissures	Deep linear ulcers with formation of deep fissures
Submucosa	Normal to reduction in width	Widened due to edema and lymphoid aggregates
Muscular layer	Usually spared except in cases of megacolon	Always involved showing presence of non-caseating granuloma in 60% cases
Serous layer	Normal (smooth)	Inflammation present
Complications		
Ulceration of mouth and stomach	Absent	May be present in 1–5% cases
Fibrous strictures	Never	Common due to fibrosis
Fistula formation and sinus tracts	Extremely rare	Internal and external fistulas in 10% cases
Toxic megacolon	Present (hypotonic and distended bowel)	Absent
Perianal abscess and fistula	Absent	Present in 50%
Malignant change	May occur infrequently in disease of more than 10 years duration	Present in 1% cases
Type of malignancy	Carcinoma is more common than lymphoma	Lymphoma is more common than carcinoma
Light microscopy		
Crypt abscess	Present in mucosa	Absent in mucosa
Inflammatory cells	Nonspecific acute and chronic inflammatory cells (e.g. lymphocytes, plasma cells, neutrophils, eosinophils and mast cells) confined to mucosa and submucosa	Chronic inflammatory cells (e.g. lymphocytes, plasma cells and macrophages) forming lymphoid aggregates are seen involving all layers of intestine (transmural)
Well-formed granulomas	Absent	Most often present in 60% cases in muscular coat
Transmural lymphoid aggregates	Absent	Common
Immunologic features		
Lymphocytes	CD4+, T_H2	CD4+, T_H1
Cytokines	IL-4, IL-5, IL-13 and TGF-β	IL-12, TNF-α and IFN-γ
ANCA-P antibodies	Positive in most cases	Positive in a few cases
Clinical features		
Age group	Young adults	Young adults
Gender predilection	No gender predilection	Women > men
Clinical findings	Recurrent left-sided abdominal cramping with bloody diarrhea and mucus	Recurrent right lower quadrant colicky pain (obstruction with diarrhea)

Gastrointestinal Tract

ULCERATIVE COLITIS

Ulcerative colitis is chronic superficial inflammatory disease that affects the mucosa and submucosa of the colon and rectum resulting in mucosal ulcerations, pseudopolyps (mucosal remnants of previous severe ulceration) formation. Disease is of unknown etiology. It *begins in the rectum and sigmoid colon*, rarely affecting terminal ileum. The disease cycles between exacerbation and remission.

Age Group

Ulcerative colitis occurs primarily in young adults (15–30 years) and then 55–65 years of age.

Clinical Features

Patient presents with *recurrent bloody diarrhea with mucus* (hallmark), abdominal cramping, tenesmus (ineffective and painful straining of stool), weight loss, anorexia, nausea, vomiting, and weakness.

Gross Morphology

- Ulcerative colitis is characterized by superficial ulcerations limited to mucosa and submucosa of large intestine.
- It begins in the rectum (friable red mucosa) and extends in continuity to involve part or the entire colon.
- It does not involve the mucosa of the anal transitional zone or the anal canal.
- It is continuous in its distribution, so skip lesions are not encountered (Fig. 20.53).

Light Microscopy

Colonic changes are confined to mucosa and submucosa in ulcerative colitis. Histopathological changes depend on progression of disease (Fig. 20.54).

- *Abscesses formation:* Rectum and colon show extensive ulceration of mucosa and submucosa. Mucosa shows hyperemia resulting in mucosal friability. Exudative inflammation leads to crypt abscesses formation in colon. Polymorphonuclear cells are particularly evident as aggregates within distended crypts (crypt abscess) of Lieberkühn resulting in rupture and atrophy. Initially, the colon's mucosal surface becomes dark, red, and velvety.

- *Ulcers formation:* Abscesses form and coalesce into ulcers. The ulcers are irregular in outline involving mucosa and submucosa, but in severe cases there is extension into the main muscular coat and perforation is likely. The ulcers expand and coalesce involving large areas. Ulcerations are continuous unlike Crohn's disease. Sloughing of mucosa results into bloody mucus filled stools.

- *Healing stage:* The intestinal wall becomes thickened and fibrosed. As granulation tissue replaces the muscle layer, the colon narrows, shortens, and loses its characteristic pouches (haustral folds). Colon shows formation of pseudopolyps (mucosal remnants of previous severe ulceration).

Complications

HLA-B27 positive persons develop ankylosing spondylitis, toxic megacolon, and sclerosing pericholangitis.

- *Acute complications:* These include *toxic megacolon (medical emergency-marked dilation of colon), perforation, hemorrhage,* and *dehydration* due to electrolytes imbalance.

- *Chronic complications:* Patient may develop *anemia* (bloody diarrhea) and *colon adenocarcinoma* (increased risk with duration 5 to 10% per decade of pancolitis). HLA-B27 positive persons develop *ankylosing spondylitis, and sclerosing pericholangitis*.

Presence of ulcerative colitis-associated dysplasia is usually indication for colectomy. Complications of ulcerative colitis are shown in Table 20.40.

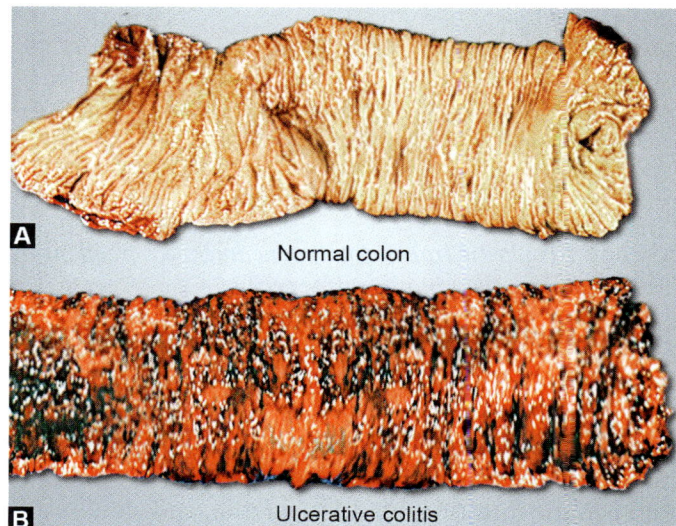

Fig. 20.53: Ulcerative colitis. (A) Showing normal colon, (B) showing ulcerative colitis with pseudopolyps formation as a result of intense inflammation of mucosa and submucosa. Inflammation begins in the rectum involving sigmoid colon and extends upward and around to the ascending colon.

Laboratory Diagnosis

The diagnosis of ulcerative colitis is made by exclusion and correlating all the clinical, endoscopic, radiological, and pathological findings.

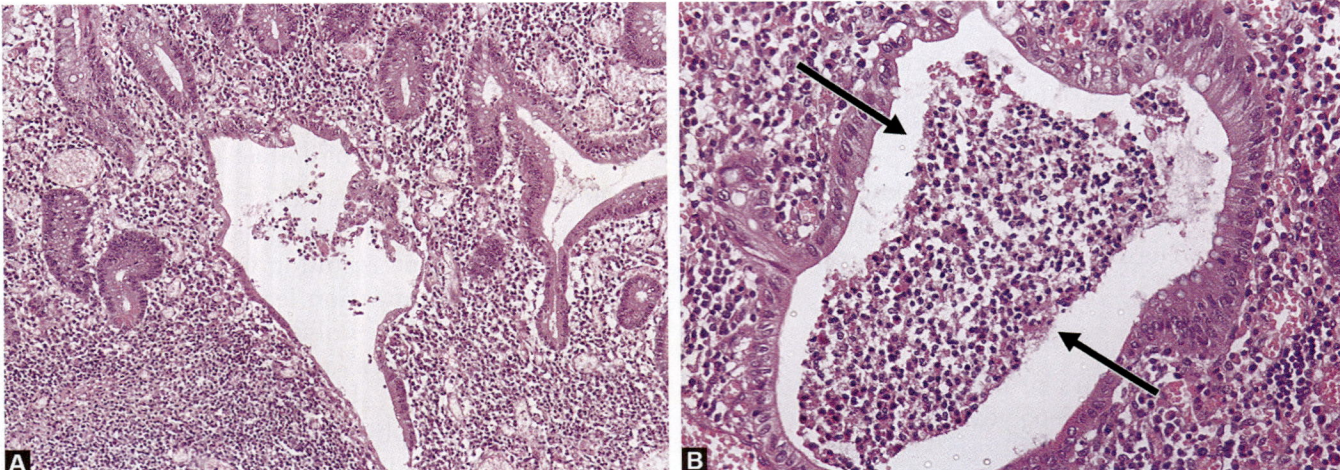

Fig. 20.54: Ulcerative colitis. The intense inflammation of ulcerative colitis is confined primarily to the mucosa and submucosa. The colonic mucosal epithelium demonstrates loss of goblet cells. Crypt abscesses are a histologic finding more typical with ulcerative colitis (arrows) (400X).

Table 20.40: Complications of ulcerative colitis

Complications	Common findings
Blood loss	May be acute hemorrhage
	Chronic hemorrhage leading to anemia
Electrolyte disturbances	Due to severe diarrhea in acute phase
Toxic megacolon	May develop insidiously
Colorectal cancer	Increased risk of colorectal carcinoma, if patient develops disease in childhood, with clinically severe attack, total involvement of the colon and continuous rather than intermittent symptoms
Skin	Erythema nodosum (subcutaneous inflammation)
Liver	Pericholangitis (inflammation around bile ducts)
	Sclerosing cholangitis (fibrous constriction and obliteration of bile ducts)
	Cholangiocarcinoma
	Chronic active hepatitis
Eye	Iritis
	Uveitis
	Episcleritis
Joints	Increased incidence of ankylosing spondylitis

CROHN'S DISEASE

Crohn's disease refers to transmural chronic inflammation of terminal ileum (most common), ascending and sigmoid colon. Disease is of unknown etiology and may involve lymph nodes and supporting membranes. Presence of noncaseating granulomas in ileum favors Crohn's disease.

Age Group

Crohn's disease affects men and women equally in *20–40 years of age group*, although no age group is exempt. It also tends to run in families up to 20% of patients. It occurs most frequently in people of Jewish descent. *Neoplastic transformation is much less frequent in Crohn's disease than in ulcerative colitis.*

Clinical Features

Patient presents with *generalized abdominal pain* especially in *right lower quadrant, diarrhea, fever, malabsorption, weight loss, intestinal obstruction* resulting from fibrous stricture, and *fistulas* between loops of intestine and between the intestine, bladder, vagina, and skin.

Pathogenesis

Chronic inflammation involves all layers of the intestinal wall (transmural involvement) in Crohn's disease described as under:

Gastrointestinal Tract

- *Cobblestone appearance of mucosa:* Lymphatic channels of submucosa blocked by enlarged lymph nodes results in edema linear mucosal ulcers oriented along long axis of intestine. Elevation of surviving mucosa between the ulcers gives nodular **cobblestone appearance**. Submucosal edema, abscesses, later fibrosis and fissures are also seen.
- *String sign:* Fibrosis of intestinal wall causes thickening and narrowing of the lumen. Intestinal lumen showing narrowing is demonstrated as 'string sign' on barium studies.
- *Noncaseating granulomas:* These are seen in 50% cases.
- *Skipping lesions:* Crohn's disease has skipping lesions (ulcerations) on the mucosa while ulcerative colitis has continuous lesions.
- *Oval elevated patches in mucosa:* Peyer's patches of small intestine are also inflamed, exhibiting oval elevated patches.
- *Inflammation of serous coat:* Serous coat of intestine is inflamed, that gets adhered to other intestinal loop.
- *Strictures:* These are formed in the involved bowel due to thickening, shortening and narrowing.
- *Fistulous tract:* Narrow fissures formed may penetrate deep and forms fistulous tract with adjacent loop of gut.

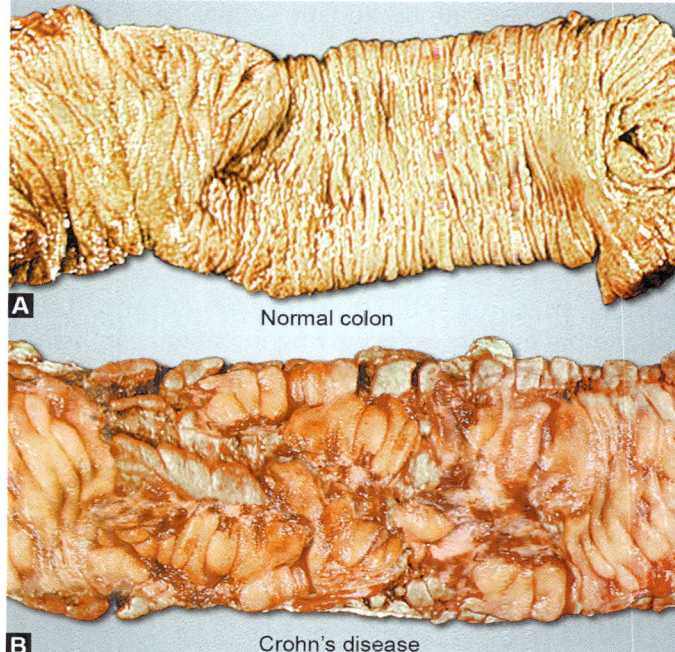

Fig. 20.55: Crohn's disease of the terminal ileum showing thickening of the wall and irregular nodular 'cobblestone' appearance of the mucosal surface. The patient presented with recurrent attacks of lower abdominal pain and vomiting for 6 weeks. A mass was palpable in the right iliac fossa.

Gross Morphology
- Wall of the gut shows thickening due to *inflammation, fibrosis and hypertrophy of the muscular coat* giving *rubbery* appearance and *stricture formation*.
- Crohn's disease produces *skipped lesions*. Linear mucosal ulcers are oriented along long axis. Mucosa between the ulcers gives nodular *cobblestone appearance*. Narrow fissures formed may penetrate deep and form *fistulous tract* with adjacent loop of gut (Fig. 20.55).

Light Microscopy
- Histopathological examination shows transmural inflammation composed of lymphocytes, plasma cells and histiocytes.
- Submucosa and subserosa of the gut show noncaseating granulomas, lymphoid aggregates, which may be seen in regional lymph nodes (Fig. 20.56).

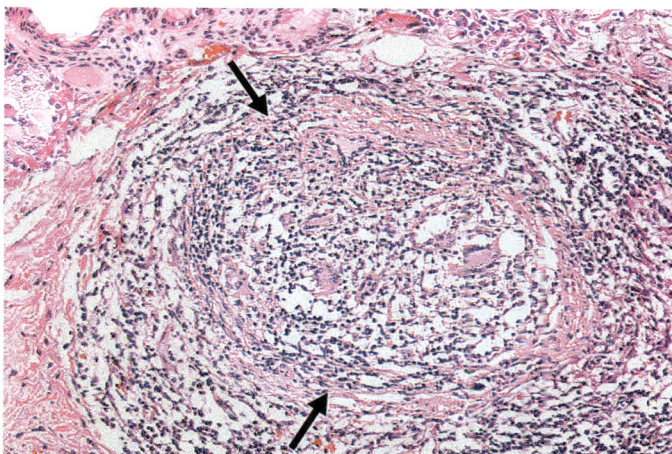

Fig. 20.56: Crohn's disease showing transmural inflammation with lymphocytes, epithelioid granulomas and giant cells (100X). Special stains for organisms were negative (arrows) 100X.

intestinal bacterial flora. There is formation of pseudomembrane composed of superficial plaque-like irregular grayish mucosal fibrinous exudates. *Rectosigmoid colon is the most common site.*

OTHER CAUSES OF COLITIS

PSEUDOMEMBRANOUS COLITIS

Pseudomembranous colitis is potentially fatal acute mucosal reaction of colon to toxins produced by *Clostridium difficile*. Most cases are associated with prior administration of *antibiotics* resulting in loss of normal

Pathogenesis

Administration of broad-spectrum antibiotics suppresses the normal flora of intestine and causes overgrowth of *Clostridium difficile*.

- *Clostridium difficile* exotoxin causes acute inflammation of colonic mucosa. Increased vascular

permeability leads to exudation of proteins especially fibrinogen, which gets polymerized to fibrin.
- Fibrin admixed with mucus from the colonic glands and necrotic tissue forms pseudomembrane attached loosely to the remnants of mucosa beneath it. *Forceful removal of pseudomembrane leaves behind bleeding ulcerations.*

Clinical Features
Patient presents with diarrhea, fever, and lower abdominal tenderness occurring in patients on broad-spectrum antibiotic therapy.

Therapeutic Correlation
Specific administration of antibiotics (vancomycin, metronidazole), hydration and discontinuation of antibiotics are effective measures to eradicate *Clostridium difficile*.

Diagnostic Approach
Lesions can be demonstrated by endoscopy. *Clostridium difficile* toxin is demonstrated in the stool.

AMOEBIC COLITIS
Amoebic colitis is caused by *Entamoeba histolytica* transmitted by *fecal-oral route*. The parasite invades colonic mucosa (intestinal amoebiasis) or by hematogenous route reach the *liver, lung* and *brain* leading to extraintestinal amoebiasis (amoebic abscess).

Pathogenesis
Cysts of *Entamoeba histolytica* ingested become small trophozoites in the alkaline medium of intestine. Small trophozoites develop into adult trophozoites, *move to cecum and become highly invasive pathogen*. These trophozoites lyase the host tissue. These are converted to cysts.
- Direct extension of the liver abscess through the diaphragm into the right lobe of lung.
- Patient may present with amoebic dysentery and low grade fever. Comparison of typhoid fever, bacillary dysentery and intestinal amoebiasis is shown in Table 20.41.

Gross Morphology
- Amoebic ulcers are most often seen in cecum. Less common sites of involvement include ascending colon, sigmoid colon, rectum and appendix.
- Ulcers range from pinpoint sized to flask-shaped in cecum. Ulcers give reddish brown hue resembling *anchovy paste* (Fig. 20.57).

Light Microscopy
- *Entamoeba histolytica* is demonstrated in the base and at the margins of ulcers, chiefly in the submucosa. Some red blood cells are phagocytosed by the trophozoites (erythrophagocytes).
- Intestine biopsy showing large number of trophozoites of *Entamoeba histolytica* is shown in Fig. 20.58.

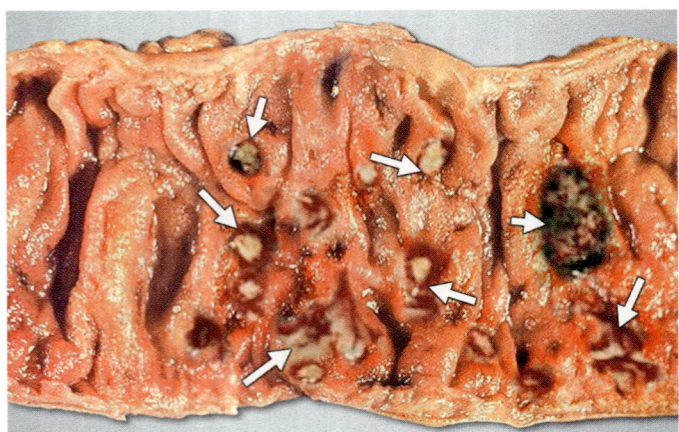

Fig. 20.57: Large bowel showing flask-shaped amoebic ulcers with reddish brown hue resembling anchovy paste (arrows).

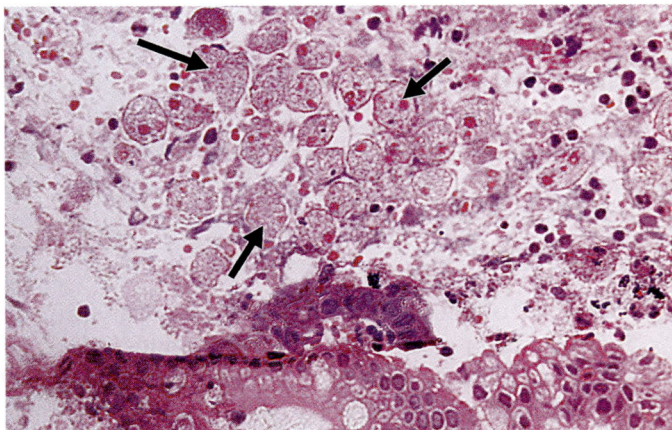

Fig. 20.58: Intestine biopsy showing large number of trophozoites of *Entamoeba histolytica* (arrows) (400X).

Table 20.41: Comparison of typhoid fever, bacillary dysentery and intestinal amoebiasis

Causative organisms	*Salmonella typhi*	*Clostridium difficile* exotoxin	*Entamoeba histolytica*
Intestinal involvement	Lower ileum and cecum	Sigmoid and rectum	Cecum
Inflammation	Typhoid granuloma	Fibrinous pseudomembrane	Necrosis
Location of ulcers	Longitudinal axis of intestine	Map-like ulcer	Flask-like ulcers
Clinical features	Continued fever, diarrhea, confusion and bradycardia	Bloody mucoid diarrhea and tenesmus	Reddish brown hue resembling anchovy paste and diarrhea with bleeding

CHOLERA

Vibrio cholerae without causing mucosal inflammation (small bowel, colon) secretes toxin that activates the **adenyl cyclic AMP dependent water pump** in the cell membrane. The intestinal cells secrete chloride accompanied by water into the lumen producing secretory diarrhea.

RADIATION COLITIS

Radiation colitis occurs as a result of radiation therapy given in prostate and cervical cancers. Radiotherapy produces lesions ranging from reversible injury of the intestinal mucosa to chronic inflammation, ulceration, and fibrosis of the intestine.

DIVERSION COLITIS

Diversion colitis refers to an inflammatory response in the blind segment, most often the rectum (**Hartmann pouch**) following ileostomy or colostomy formation. This process is caused by deficiency of short-chain fatty acids.

Pathological findings include *granular friable mucosa with marked lymphoid hyperplasia and cryptitis mimicking inflammatory bowel disease*. Clinical history is most important to exclude other causes.

COLLAGENOUS COLITIS

Collagenous colitis refers to presence of thick collagen layer at the subepithelial region. Thickness of the collagen layer is variable. There is presence of capillaries and inflammatory cells entrapped in collagenous fibers. Evaluation requires well-oriented sections in difficult case. Masson's trichome stain may be useful to demonstrate collagen fibers.

STERCORAL ULCER

Incomplete evacuation of the feces in debilitating disease or old persons may lead to fecal impaction. Fecal impaction causes pressure necrosis of the mucosa resulting in stercoral ulcer. Complications include *rectal bleeding* and *perforation*.

VASCULAR DISORDERS

LARGE BOWEL INFARCTION

Large bowel has arterial blood supply from more than one artery. *Splenic flexure and rectosigmoid junction* are the most common sites of infarcts in colon. These are less vascularized areas known as **watershed regions.**

Locations

Watershed regions include splenic flexure (junction of the superior and inferior mesenteric arteries) and rectosigmoid junction (junction of left colic and sigmoid-superior rectal branches of the inferior mesenteric artery).

Large bowel infarction with watershed areas is shown in Fig. 20.59. Causes of intestinal ischemia are shown in Table 20.42.

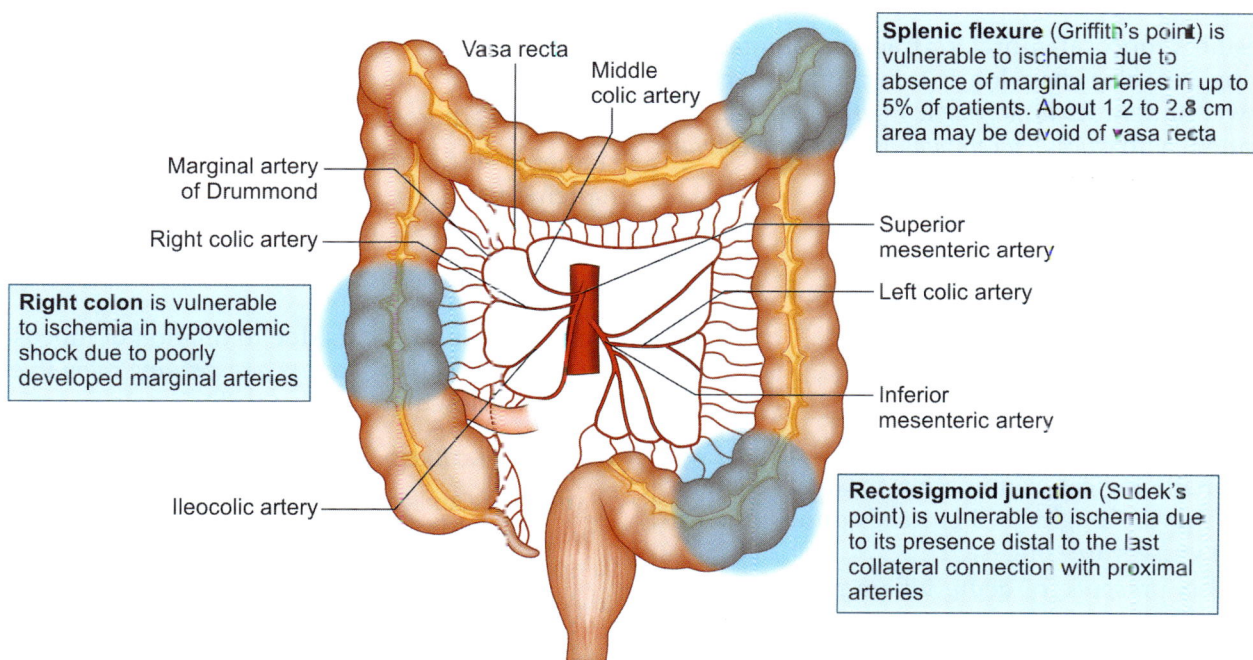

Fig. 20.59: Large bowel infarction showing watershed areas.

Table 20.42: Causes of intestinal ischemia

Categories	Disorders
Acute vascular occlusion	Thrombosis or embolism
Nonocclusive mesenteric ischemia	Necrotizing enterocolitis
Blood vessels diseases	Vasculitides and vasculopathies
Vascular compression	Volvulus Intussusception Celiac axis compression
Hypercoagulable states	Pancreatic carcinoma Myeloproliferative syndromes Antiphospholipid antibodies (APAs) Hyperhomocysteinemia Heparin-induced thrombocytopenia
Drugs	Chemotherapeutic agents
Infections	*Clostridium difficile* *Escherichia coli* Staphylococcal enterocolitis Cytomegalovirus *Aspergillus flavus* Candida species

Mucosal ischemic colitis is caused by *Clostridium difficile*, *Escherichia coli*, nonsteroidal anti-inflammatory drugs, Crohn's disease, radiation and collagen colitis.

Pathology

The result is mucosal, mural, or transmural infarction involving the wall of the colon. In transmural infarctions, the bowel undergoes *hemorrhagic infarction* (danger of perforation) with *mucosal ulcerations* and *pseudomembrane formation*.

Gross Morphology

Morphology of ischemic bowel disease is variable depending on duration and severity of vascular compromise. Ischemic bowel segment shows *dusky appearance* (Fig. 20.60).

Light Microscopy

- Histopathological examination in acute ischemic state shows sloughing of surface epithelium. The blood vessels are congested.
- There is presence of acute inflammatory cells in the wall. Chronic bowel ischemia shows atrophic surface epithelium and fibrotic lamina propria (Fig. 20.61).

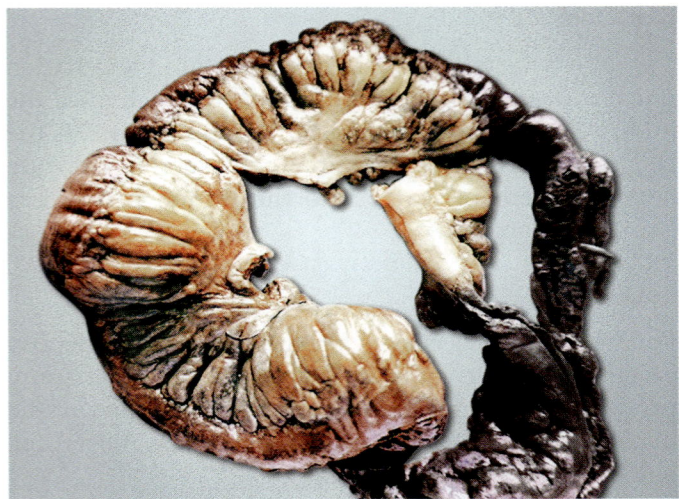

Fig. 20.60: Ischemic bowel disease showing dusky blackish discoloration.

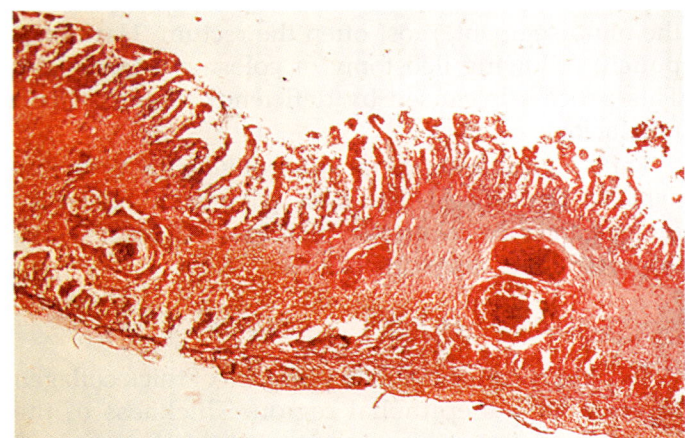

Fig. 20.61: Ischemic bowel disease showing sloughing of epithelium, congested blood vessels and acute inflammatory cells (100X).

Clinical Features

Patients with ischemic colitis present with pain in splenic flexure region and bloody diarrhea. Repair occurs by fibrosis may eventuate is ischemic strictures.

ANGIODYSPLASIA

Angiodysplasia occurs due to dilation of mucosal and *submucosal venules of cecum or ascending colon* in elderly persons. Mesenteric angiography is a diagnostic tool.

Clinical Features

Patient presents with *unexplained lower bowel bleeding* (bright red blood in stool known as *hematochezia*). It is associated with aortic stenosis and von Willebrand's disease due to unknown etiology.

It is the second most common cause of *hematochezia* after diverticulosis. Causes of gastrointestinal hemorrhage are shown in Table 20.43.

Table 20.43: Causes of gastrointestinal hemorrhage	
Age group	Disorders
Children	Meckel's diverticulum Juvenile polyp Ulcerative colitis Crohn's disease
Adults	Ulcerative colitis Crohn's disease Adenomatous polyp Gastric carcinoma Colorectal carcinoma Arteriovenous malformations Hereditary telangiectasia Nonsteroidal anti-inflammatory drugs Infective colitis Hemorrhoids Solitary rectal ulcer Anal fissure
Elderly persons	Diverticular disease Angiodysplasia Adenomatous polyp Gastric carcinoma Colorectal carcinoma Ischemic colitis Ulcerative colitis Crohn's disease Radiation proctitis

POLYPS AND TUMORS OF LARGE INTESTINE

Adenomatous polyps are polypoidal structures distributed throughout the large intestine. Approximately 40% are located in the right colon, 40% in the left colon and 20% in rectum. Sigmoid region is the most common site for gastrointestinal polyps.

These are more common in men than women. These may be pedunculated (attached by stem) or sessile (broad base attachment). Hyperplastic polyp, pedunculated tubular adenoma and sessile villus adenoma are shown in Fig. 20.62.

Large intestine harbors most malignant lesions. Colorectal carcinoma is currently the most common tumor affecting men and women with peak in 7th decade. Rectum is the most common site for adenocarcinomas followed by sigmoid colon.

Moderately differentiated adenocarcinomas are the most common histological variant of adenocarcinoma of colon. Patient with colorectal carcinoma has varied clinical presentation depending on the primary location in the large intestine. WHO classification of tumors of large intestine is shown in Table 20.44.

NON-NEOPLASTIC POLYPS

Hyperplastic Polyps

Hyperplastic polyps are most common intestinal polyps. These are often found in the colon (*rectosigmoid*). Hyperplasia of colonic epithelium leads to formation of elongated glands with *saw tooth appearance* on cross section. These are clinically insignificant. There is *no malignant potential.*

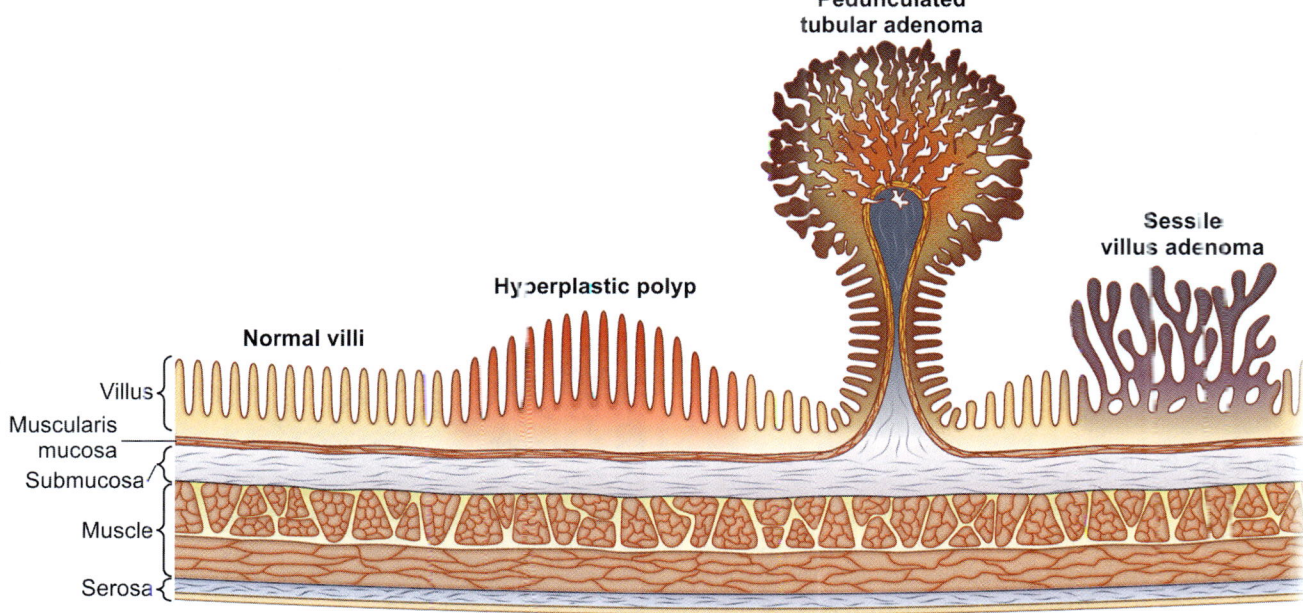

Fig. 20.62: Showing hyperplastic polyp, pedunculated tubular adenoma and sessile villus adenoma.

Table 20.44: WHO classification of tumors of large intestine

Categories	Polyps and tumors
Adenomas	Tubular adenoma Villus adenoma Tubulovillus adenoma
Dysplasia (intra-epithelial neoplasia)	Low grade dysplasia High grade dysplasia
Hamartomas	Peutz-Jeghers polyp Juvenile polyp (children) Cowden disease associated polyps
Serrated lesions	Hyperplastic polyp (adults) Sessile serrated polyp Traditional serrated adenoma
Carcinomas	Adenocarcinoma (cribriform, comedo, mucinous and medullary variants) Signet cell adenocarcinoma Squamous cell carcinoma Adenosquamous carcinoma Spindle cell carcinoma Undifferentiated carcinoma
Neuroendocrine tumors	Net G1 (carcinoid tumor) Net G2 Neuroendocrine carcinoma (small cell or large cell type)
Mesenchymal tumors	Leiomyoma Lipoma Gastrointestinal stromal tumor Leiomyosarcoma Angiosarcoma Kaposi sarcoma
Lymphoid tumors	Burkitt's lymphoma B cell lymphoma Diffuse large B cell lymphoma Follicular lymphoma Mantle cell lymphoma T cell lymphoma
Secondary tumors	Metastases from other organs

Inflammatory Polyps

Inflammatory polyps include benign lymphoid polyps and inflammatory pseudopolyps consisting of granulation tissue and remnants of mucosa, caused by chronic inflammatory bowel disease. Rectal mucosa is most common site. It may be a reaction to local irritation.

Inflammatory Pseudopolyps

Inflammatory pseudopolyps are associated with ulcerative colitis and other inflammatory diseases of the colon. These consist of granulation tissue and residual and regenerating mucosa.

Juvenile (Retention) Polyp

Juvenile polyp is a *solitary hamartomatous pedunculated polyp also known as retention polyp affecting children* <5 years of age.

Locations

Juvenile polyp occurs in rectum (most common), small intestine and colon. It may be associated with the juvenile polyposis syndrome.

Molecular Genetics

Gene mutations of SMADA and BMPR1 have been demonstrated in juvenile polyps. Autosomal dominant variant has 10% risk of malignancy.

Malignant Potential

There is increased risk of cancers of stomach, small intestine and colon.

Gross Morphology

Juvenile polyp has smooth surface and gelatinous on cut section.

Light Microscopy

Histologically, it is composed of *mucus-filled cystic glands* and edematous, usually inflamed stroma (Fig. 20.63).

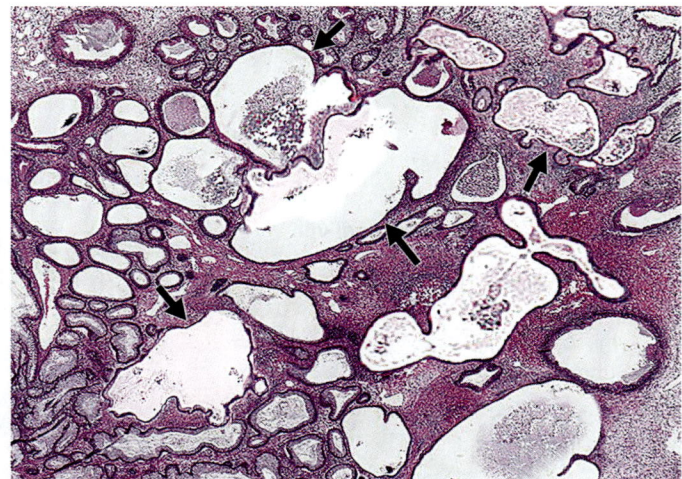

Fig. 20.63: Juvenile polyp showing mucus-filled cystic glands and edematous, usually inflamed stroma (arrows) (100X).

Peutz-Jeghers Syndrome

Peutz-Jeghers syndrome is an autosomal dominant disorder due to **LKB1/STK11 gene mutations** in young children of 10–15 years of age. It is characterized by multiple hamartomatous polyps in *small intestine* (most common), *stomach and colon* in decreasing frequency; *melanotic pigmented macules* (1–5 mm) of *lips, perioral skin, hands and genitalia*.

Malignant Potential

There is increased risk of cancers of gastrointestinal tract, thyroid, breast, lung, pancreas, gonads, and urinary bladder.

Light Microscopy

On histological examination, polyp is composed of *branching network of smooth muscle fibers continuous with the muscularis mucosa* that *support irregularly arranged glands of the polyp*.

Cowden Syndrome

Cowden syndrome is nonhereditary disorder affecting >50 years of age. It is characterized by *hamartomatous polyps in colon*. There is presence of crypt dilatation and edema in nonpolypoidal mucosa. There is increased risk of *benign and malignant tumors of thyroid and breast*.

NEOPLASTIC POLYPS

Adenomatous polyps are true neoplasms arising from the mucosal epithelium. These occur in colon especially *rectosigmoid colon*. These are rarely seen in small intestine. Patients are most often asymptomatic, but rectal bleeding may occur.

These are subdivided into *tubular adenomas* (most common *raspberry on a stalk*), *villus adenomas, tubulovillus* (mixture of tubular and villus); and *sessile serrated adenomas* (serrated epithelium lining the crypts).

All adenomas are precancerous lesions. The risk for malignant transformation parallels the percentage of the villus component (finger-like projections) in the polyp and size >2 cm increases the risk. There is *increased risk for developing colon cancer (e.g. rectosigmoid region) in villus adenoma*.

Tubular Adenomas

Tubular adenomas are most common benign neoplastic polyps in the *colon* (90%) and *rectosigmoid region* (50%). Most *polyps* (99%) are excised through endoscopy.

Gross Morphology

Tubular adenomas are usually multiple and pedunculated attached to the intestine by a stalk. These are generally <2 cm in size (Fig. 20.64)

Light Microscopy

- Tubular adenoma is composed of closely packed tubular glands forming the *head of the polyp* lined by mucus secreting columnar epithelium.
- More than 80% of tumor cells form glandular and tubular arrangement (Fig. 20.65).

Malignant Transformation

Adenocarcinomas arise in 1–3% cases. Risk of cancer is *proportional to the increasing size and number of polyps*.

Villus Adenomas

Villus adenomas account for 10% of neoplastic polyps. These are more than 2 cm in size in diameter with *velvety surface showing finger-like villus structures and high potential for malignant change*. Large villus adenomas may secrete *copious electrolyte-rich mucus*, resulting in decreased serum potassium level and acute renal failure.

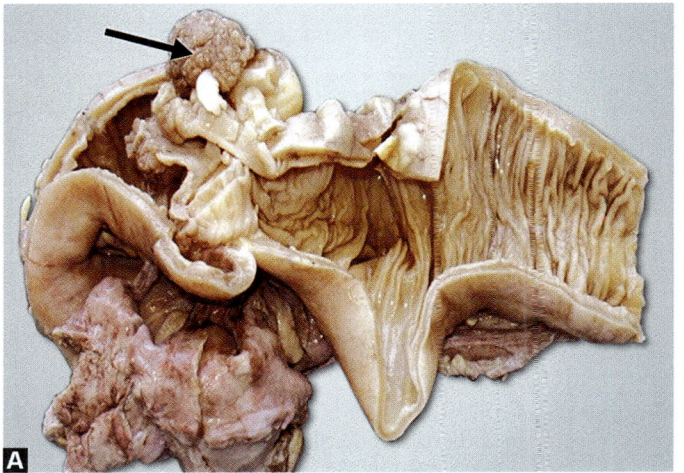
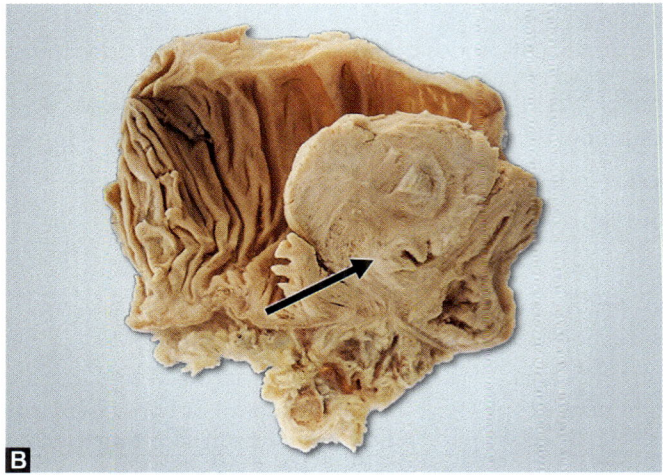

Fig. 20.64: Tubular adenoma in intestine. (A and B) Showing pedunculated polyp (arrows).

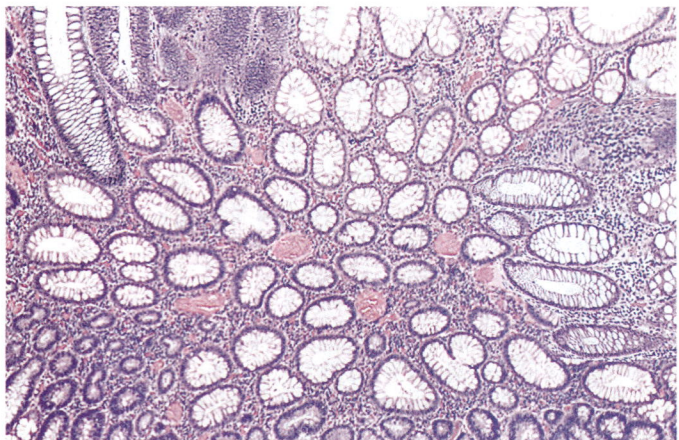

Fig. 20.65: Tubular adenoma showing closely packed tubular glands lined by mucus secreting columnar epithelium (100X).

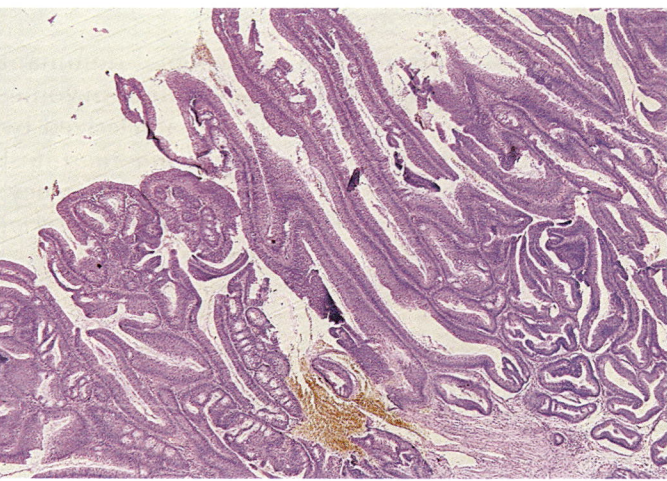

Fig. 20.66: Villus adenomas showing finger-like protrusions lined with columnar epithelium (100X).

Gross Morphology
- Villus adenomas are *solitary, sessile with broad base* measuring ≥1–5 cm in diameter.
- These are most often located in the rectum extending over a wide area as thick, carpet-like growth.
- Finger-like projections (villi) protrude from the base of the polyps into the lumen of the intestine.

Light Microscopy
- These are composed of villi (i.e. finger-like protrusions lined with columnar epithelium).
- More than 80% of tumor cells form villus projections (Fig. 20.66).

Tubulovillus Adenomas

Tubulovillus adenomas constitute 15% of adenomatous polyps. These tumors represent an intermediate step between tubular and villus adenomas in all respects.

If the *tubular adenoma component* constitutes >40% of the total tumor mass or 20–80% villus component, it is known as *tubulovillus adenoma*.

Light Microscopy
Tubulovillus adenoma shows tubular and villus components (Fig. 20.67).

Malignant Potential

Approximately 50% of all villus adenomas undergo malignant transformation to adenocarcinomas. Differences between tubular and villus adenomas are shown in Table 20.45.

Malignant Potential

Risk of colon carcinoma in neoplastic polyps is shown in Table 20.46.

Table 20.45: Differences between tubular and villus adenomas

Parameters	Tubular adenoma	Villus adenoma
Definition	Consisting of >75% tubular appearance	Consisting of >50% villus appearance
Occurrence	90–95% of total adenomas	<1% of total adenomas
Location	Colon (90%)	Rectum Rectosigmoid region
Age group	Earlier age group	Elderly persons
Gross morphology	Small, pedunculated	Large sessile velvet-like appearance projecting above normal mucosa
Light microscopy	Stalk composed of fibrovascular tissue covered by benign mucin secreting mucosal cells	Frond-like villus structures covered by dysplastic and disordered columnar epithelial cells
Risk of malignancy	Uncommon	Relatively common

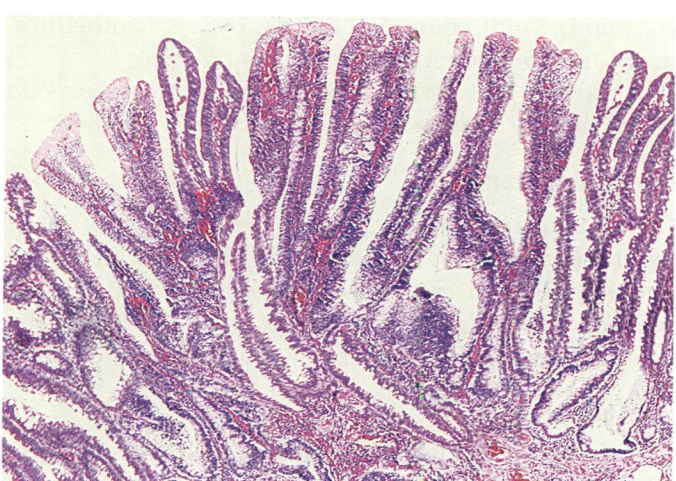

Fig. 20.67: Tubulovillus adenoma showing tubular and villus components (100X).

Table 20.46: Risk of colon carcinoma in neoplastic polyps

Neoplastic polyp	Size (<1 cm)	Size (1–2 cm)	Size (>2 cm)
Tubular adenoma	1%	10.2%	34.7%
Tubulovillus adenoma	3.9%	7.4%	45.8%
Villus adenoma	9.5%	10.3%	52.8%
Risk of development of colon carcinoma is higher in villus adenoma			

Sessile Serrated Adenomas

Sessile serrated adenomas resemble hyperplastic polyps, but unlike hyperplastic polyps, these may undergo malignant transformation.

These most often occur in right colon. These demonstrate microsatellite instability. Sessile serrated adenomas can be very subtle and are easily missed on endoscopy.

MULTIPLE POLYPOSIS SYNDROMES

Multiple polyposis syndromes are associated with a greatly increased *risk of malignant transformation*.

FAMILIAL ADENOMATOUS POLYPOSIS COLI

Familial adenomatous polyposis coli is an autosomal dominant disorder associated with inactivation of the **APC gene** (adenomatous polyposis gene) located on chromosome **5q21**. It is characterized by development of >100 tubular adenoma polyps (ranging **500 to 2500**) in **colon** and **rectum**, particularly in the *rectosigmoid region*.

Polyps are not present at birth. These appear in childhood and become clinically evident in *second decade of life*. Familial adenomatous coli with multiple polyps covering entire mucosa is shown in Fig. 20.68.

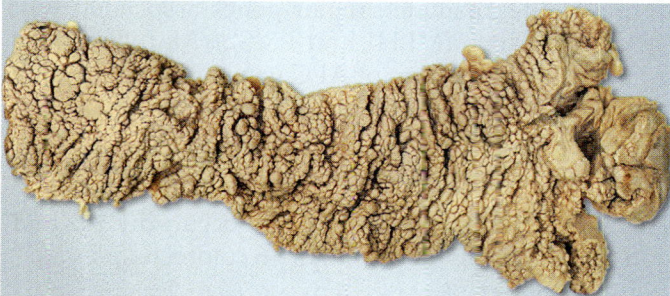

Fig. 20.68: Familial adenomatous coli showing multiple polyps covering virtually the whole of the mucosal surface of the colon >100 tubular adenoma polyps (ranging 500 to 2500).

Molecular Genetics

Progression from adenoma to adenocarcinoma involves a series of steps. Patient with adenomatous polyposis coli has *mutation in the APC tumor suppressor gene located on long arm of chromosome 5*.

Further *new mutations occur in 30–50%* of patients. These include mutation of *p53 tumor suppressor gene on chromosome 17 and point mutation of RAS oncogene*.

Malignant Potential

The risk of malignant transformation approaches 100%. *The risk of malignancy is related to the size of adenoma, amount of villus component, grade of epithelial dysplasia and family history.*

Dysplastic foci show stratification, hyperchromatic nuclei, mitotic figures in upper crypts and surface epithelium.

Management

By the 40 years, all the patients develop adenocarcinoma, hence need *prophylactic total colectomy*.

GARDNER'S SYNDROME

Gardner's syndrome is a variant of familial polyposis syndrome due to APC gene mutation. It is autosomal dominant disorder affecting children 10–15 years of age.

It is associated *with numerous adenomatous polyps along with osteomas in the mandible and abdominal desmoid*.

TURCOT'S SYNDROME

Turcot's syndrome is autosomal dominant disorder due to **APC gene mutation (5q21)**. It is characterized by *multiple adenomatous colon polyps* with increased risk of *colorectal cancer* and brain cancers (*medulloblastoma or glioblastoma multiforme*). It may be associated with familial adenomatous polyposis or Lynch syndrome.

Molecular Basis

Molecular basis is either due to mutation of *APC gene located on long arm of chromosome 5q21 or mutation* in one of the mismatch repair genes associated with Lynch syndrome (MLH1 and PMS2). *Medulloblastoma* occurs due to mutation of APC gene and glioblastoma multiforme due to mutation of mismatch repair genes.

JUVENILE COLI

This autosomal dominant syndrome occurs due to mutation of PTEN. Patient develops >6 colorectal polyps.

CRONOKITE-CANADA SYNDROME

Cronokite-Canada syndrome is *nonhereditary disorder* affecting >50 years of age. It is characterized by *multiple hamartomatous polyps in stomach, small intestine and colorectal region with protein losing enteropathy and cutaneous hypopigmentation.* Patient presents with diarrhea, weight loss, abdominal pain and weakness.

TUBEROUS SCLEROSIS

Tuberous sclerosis is caused by mutation in the TSC1 or TSC gene, which encode *hamartin and tuberin* proteins, respectively. Tuberous sclerosis is associated with multiple hamartomas in rectum, brain (as cortical tubers subependymal hamartomas), face, and kidneys (renal angiomyolipoma in 80% cases). Gastrointestinal polyposis syndromes are shown in Table 20.47.

HEREDITARY NONPOLYPOSIS COLON CANCER

Hereditary nonpolyposis colon cancer (HNPCC) is also known as *Lynch syndrome.* There is increased risk of development of carcinoma of endometrium (most common), right colon carcinoma, ovary, urothelium, brain and stomach in these patients.

A variant that involves a propensity for sebaceous tumors of the skin is known as *Muir Torre syndrome.*

Molecular Genetics

Lynch syndrome occurs due to *inactivation of DNA mismatch repair genes* (principally MLH1, MSH2, MSH6, and PMS2); that cannot correct errors in nucleotide pairing. *Microsatellite instability* is seen in 90% of the tumors that develop in these patients.

Pathology

Colon carcinoma is often preceded by serrated adenomas, rather than tubular adenomas seen in the traditional APC tumor pathway. Extensive history and screening for early development of these cancers is required in the management of these patients.

COLORECTAL CARCINOMA

Colorectal carcinoma is second most common cancer killer in both men and women. It is most common malignancy in developed countries. It may be *sporadic* (99%) and *familial* (1%).

Colorectal carcinoma begins as a small polyp, detectable through regular screening by colonoscopy. Histopathological study is the gold standard for the diagnosis. *Early detection, surgery, radiation and or chemotherapy can be effective treatment.* Colorectal carcinomas showing distribution, risk factors, serum tumor markers and immunohistochemistry are shown in Fig. 20.69.

Table 20.47: Gastrointestinal polyposis syndromes

Syndrome	Age group	Gene mutations	Lesions
Familial adenomatous polyposis	10–15	APC (5q21)	Multiple adenomatous polyps in >100 *tubular adenoma polyp*s (ranging 500 to 2500) in colon and rectum, particularly in the rectosigmoid region leading to malignant change by 40 years.
Gardner syndrome	40–50	APC (5q21)	Multiple adenomatous polyps, *osteomas in the mandible and abdominal desmoid soft tissue*
Turcot syndrome	10–15	APC (5q21)	Multiple adenomatous polyps, medulloblastoma or glioblastoma multiforme
Cronokite-Canada syndrome	>50 years	Nonhereditary disorder	Multiple hamartomatous polyps in stomach, small intestine and colorectal region, cutaneous hypopigmentation
Tuberous sclerosis	Children to adult age group	TSC1 (encoding *hamartin*) or TSC (encoding *tuberin* proteins)	Multiple hamartomas in rectum, brain associated with renal angiomyolipoma
Peutz-Jeghers syndrome	10–15 years	LKB1/STK1	Arborising polyps in small intestine, colon, stomach in decreasing frequency associated with skin macules and increased risk of GIT, thyroid, breast, lung, pancreas, gonads and urinary bladder

Gastrointestinal Tract

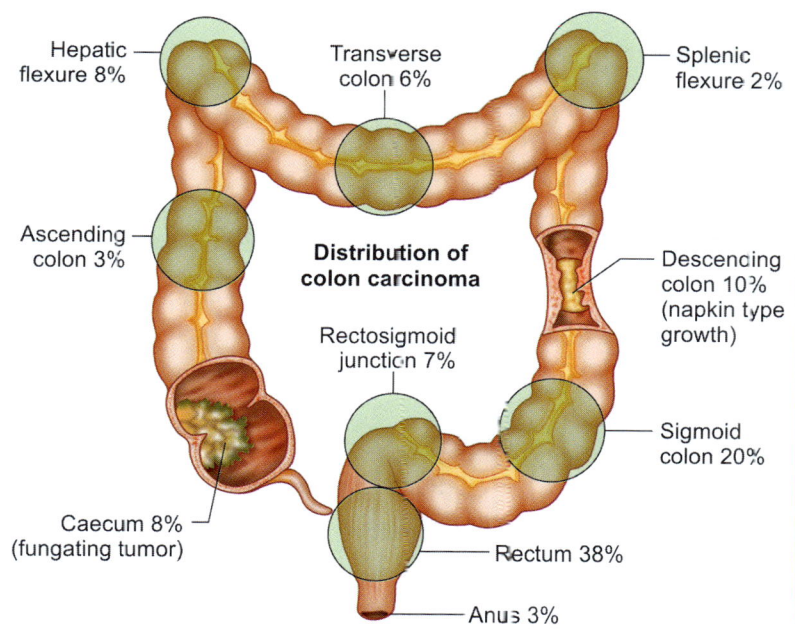

Distribution of colon carcinoma:
- Hepatic flexure 8%
- Transverse colon 6%
- Splenic flexure 2%
- Ascending colon 3%
- Descending colon 10% (napkin type growth)
- Rectosigmoid junction 7%
- Sigmoid colon 20%
- Caecum 8% (fungating tumor)
- Rectum 38%
- Anus 3%

Risk factors (colon carcinoma)
- Age >50 years
- High fat, low fiber diet
- Ulcerative colitis and Crohn's disease
- Familial adenomatous polyposis (FAP)
- Hereditary nonpolyposis colorectal cancer (HNPCC)
- Adenomas (villous, tubular and tubulovillous)
- Peutz-Jeghers syndrome
- Family history of colorectal cancer

Immunohistochemistry (colorectal carcinoma)

Tumor marker	Expression
Carcinoembryonic antigen (CEA)	Positive
CK20	Positive
CDX2 (transcription factor)	Positive
SAT2 (transcription factor)	Positive
p53	Positive
β-catenin	Positive
CK7	Focally positive

Serum tumor markers used to detect colon carcinoma

Category	Tumor marker	Cancers	Category	Tumor marker	Cancers
Oncofetal proteins	Carcinoembryonic antigen (CEA)	• Colon carcinoma • NSGCT of testis • Gastric carcinoma • Pancreatic carcinoma • Lung carcinoma • Breast carcinoma	Mucins and glycoproteins	CA 19.9	• Colon carcinoma • Pancreatic carcinoma
				CA 72.4	• Colon carcinoma • Gastric carcinoma

Fig. 20.69: Colorectal carcinomas showing distribution, risk factors, serum tumor markers and immunohistochemistry.

Risk factors for development of colorectal carcinoma are shown in Table 20.48. Frequency of colorectal carcinoma is shown in Table 20.49. Dietary factors associated with colorectal carcinoma are shown in Table 20.50. Dietary fibers in common food are shown in Table 20.51.

Table 20.48: Risk factors for colorectal carcinoma

Risk factors
Elderly persons
Familial adenomatous polyposis
Inflammatory bowel disease (ulcerative colitis and Crohn's disease)
Hereditary nonpolyposis colorectal cancer (HNPCC also known as Lynch syndrome)
History of colorectal neoplasms
Obesity
Tobacco smoking
Nonsteroidal anti-inflammatory drugs
Dietary factors (consumption of red meat, animal fat, saturated fat, refined carbohydrate)
Chronic alcoholism

Distribution

Rectosigmoid is the most common site for colon cancer (38%), sigmoid colon (20%), descending colon (10%), cecum (8%), hepatic flexure (8%), transverse colon (5%), ascending colon (3%), and anal region (3%).

Left-sided colon cancer most likely to obstruct lumen, while right-sided colon cancer more likely to bleed. Distribution of colon cancer in decreasing frequency is shown in Table 20.52.

Molecular Genetic Alterations

Colorectal cancer is a slow growing adenocarcinoma. It develops through a set of anatomic changes progressing

Table 20.49: Frequency of colorectal carcinoma

Cases	Frequency
Sporadic cases	65–85%
Familial cases	10–30%
Hereditary nonpolyposis colorectal cancer (HNPCC)	5%
Familial adenomatous polyposis	1%
Rare colorectal syndrome	0.1%

Table 20.50: Dietary factors associated with colorectal carcinoma

Dietary constituents	Mechanism
Red meat, animal fat and saturated fat in diet	Enhancing bile acid synthesis, which gets converted to potential carcinogens by bacteria
Low fiber content in diet	Decreasing stool bulk
	Increasing fecal transit time (e.g. constipation), altering bacterial flora with formation of malignant potential toxic oxidative byproducts of carbohydrate
Low intake of vitamins A, C, E	Decreasing radical scavenger activity
High content of refined carbohydrates	Potential carcinogens

Table 20.51: Dietary fibers in common food

Categories		Content (gram/kg)	Categories		Content (gram/kg)
Flour	Bran	440	Cereals	Purified wheat	154
	Whole meal	96		Shredded wheat	123
	Brown flour	75		Cornflakes	110
	White flour	30		Muesli	74
Fruits	Apricots (dried)	240		Porridge	8
	Figs (dried)	185	Boiled vegetables	Peas (frozen)	120
	Prunes (dried)	161		Spinach	63
	Banana	34		Sweetcorn	57
	Oranges	20		Beans-broad	42
	Apple (peeled)	20		Beans-french	32
	Pears	17		Potato chips	32
	Peaches	14		Carrots	31
Nuts	Coconut (desiccated)	325		Brussel sprouts	29
	Almonds	143		Potato-old/baked	25
	Peanuts	81		Cabbage	25
Bread	Wholemeal bread	85		Beetroot	25
	Brown bread	51		Turnips	22
	White bread	27		Celery	22
				Potato-new	20
				Cauliflower	18

Table 20.52: Distribution of colon cancer in decreasing frequency

Location	Frequency
Rectosigmoid region	38%
Sigmoid colon	20%
Descending colon	10%
Cecum	8%
Hepatic flexure colon	8%
Transverse colon	5%
Ascending colon	3%
Anal canal	3%

from normal mucosa to adenomatous polyp carcinoma *in situ*, to invasive carcinoma to metastatic tumor. Combination of genetic and epigenetic abnormalities are observed in the development of colorectal carcinoma.

- Two distinct pathways have been described such as APC/β-catenin pathway and classic adenoma-carcinoma sequence with microsatellite pathway. Both pathways involve stepwise accumulation of multiple mutations.
- Oncogenes, their mode of activation and associated with colon carcinoma are shown in Table 20.53.

Gastrointestinal Tract 20

Table 20.53: Oncogenes, their mode of activation and associated with colon carcinoma (signal transduction proteins)

Category	Proto-oncogene	Mode of activation	Associated malignancies
GTP-binding (G) proteins	K-RAS	Point mutation	Colon carcinoma Lung carcinoma Pancreas carcinoma
RAS signal transduction	BRAF	Point mutation Translocation	Colon carcinoma Melanoma Leukemia

Tumor suppressor gene mutations associated with colon carcinoma are shown in Table 20.54. *Morphologic and molecular changes* in the adenoma-colon carcinoma sequence are shown in Fig. 20.70.

APC/β-catenin Pathway

- APC tumor suppressor gene has been mapped on 5q21. Most commonly APC pathway has been presented as a model of tumor progression.

- APC promotes cell migration and cell adhesion. It binds to the cytoskeleton protein β-catenin. β-catenin also acts as oncogene by binding to the TGF-β receptor.

Classic Adenoma-carcinoma Sequence with Microsatellite Pathway

This pathway is associated with *defects in DNA mismatch repair*. It accounts for 80% of sporadic colorectal cancers.

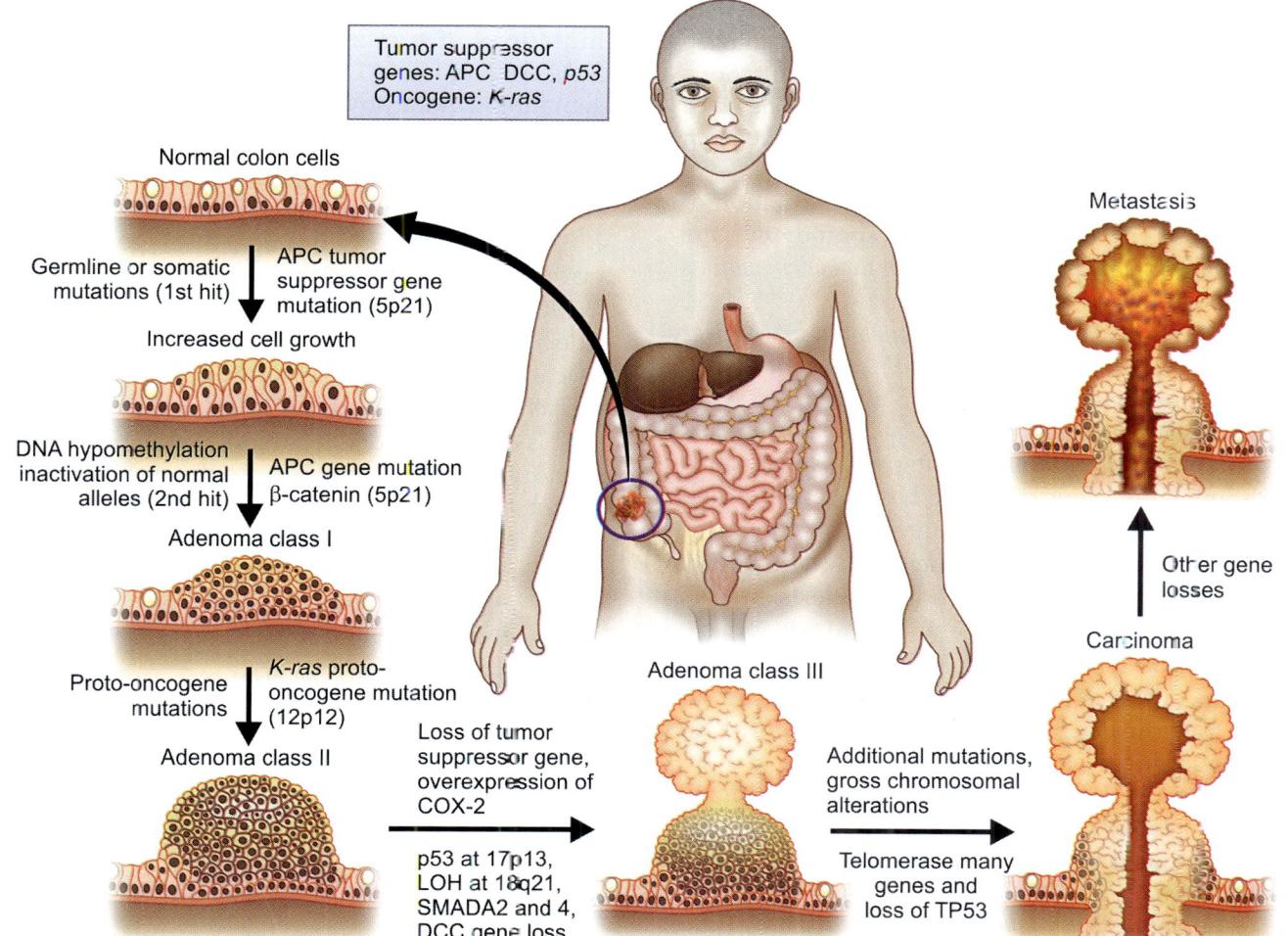

Fig. 20.70: Morphologic and molecular changes in the adenoma-carcinoma sequence. It is postulated by Knudson's hypothesis that loss of normal copy of tumor suppressor APC gene occurs early in life. This is the first hit. Loss of intact copy of APC gene follows (second hit). Other gene mutations include K-RAS, losses at 18q21 involving SMAD2 and SMADA4 and inactivation of tumor suppressor p53 gene. It leads to the emergence of colorectal carcinoma and metastases, in which additional gene mutations occur.

Table 20.54: Tumor suppressor genes associated with colon carcinoma

Gene	Protein	Function	Familial tumors	Sporadic cancers
SMADA-2 SMADA-4	SMADA-2 protein SMADA-4 protein	Both inhibit TGF-β signaling pathway. These repress CDK4 and MYC. These also induce expression of CDK inhibitor	Juvenile polyposis	Colon carcinoma Pancreas carcinoma
RB gene	Retinoblastoma protein (locus 13p14) Mutation by deletion and nonsense	It codes for pRB protein, master brake on cell cycle by inhibiting nuclear transcription and G1 to S transition during cell cycle	Retinoblastoma Osteosarcoma	Retinoblastoma Osteosarcoma Breast carcinoma Colon carcinoma Prostate carcinoma Urinary bladder carcinoma Lung carcinoma
Angiogenesis inhibitors				
STK11	Liver kinase B1 (LKB1) or STK11	It activates AMPK family of kinases. It suppresses cell growth when cell nutrients and energy levels are low	Peutz-Jeghers syndrome: cancers of GIT, pancreas	Diverse carcinomas in 5–20% cases

- *First hit (normal mucosa to mucosa alteration):* Gene mutations in the development of colon cancer may be inherited (germline) or acquired (somatic). Mutations of tumor suppressor *APC gene (5q21)* and mismatch repair genes such as MSH2 at 2p22 participate in alteration of normal mucosa. APC is a key negative regular of β-catenin, a component of WNT pathway. Mutation of APC gene has been demonstrated in sporadic cancers (*colon, stomach and pancreas*) and *familial adenomatous polyposis.*

  Under physiological state, APC gene prevents nuclear transcription by degrading catenin, an activator of nuclear transcription. With loss of function of APC, accumulation of β-catenin activates transcription of genes encoding MYC and cyclin D1 leading to cell proliferation. Additional mutations of K-RAS have been observed in adenomas and invasive colorectal carcinomas.

- *Second hit (altered mucosa to adenoma):* Methylation abnormalities, inactivation of normal alleles of APC, and MSH2 transform altered mucosa to adenoma.

- *Adenoma to colonic malignant transformation:* K-RAS proto-oncogene is located on chromosome 12p—a signal transducing protein. *Point mutation of K-RAS has been identified in colon carcinoma in 50% of cases.* There is as well as homozygous loss of additional cancer suppressor genes (DCC at 18p21, p53 at 17p13) participate in transformation of adenoma to colon carcinoma.

- *Microsatellite instability mechanism:* Additional mutations and gross chromosomal alterations such as *loss of DNA repair genes* mutated TGF-β receptor gene and defective BAX gene produce marked changes in colon cancer growth.

  Neoplastic progression is also associated with mutations of tumor suppressor genes encoding SMADA2 and SMADA4, which are effectors of TGF signaling. Under physiological state, TGF signaling inhibits the cell cycle.

- *Defects in DNA mismatch repair genes:* DNA mismatch repair genes include principally MLH1, MSH2, MSH6, and PMS2. Normally, these genes correct errors in nucleotide pairing.

  Mutations of these cannot correct errors in nucleotide pairing. There is increased risk of development of carcinoma of right colon, known as *hereditary nonpolyposis colon cancer.*

  It is often preceded by serrated adenomas, rather than tubular adenomas seen in the traditional APC tumor pathway. Extensive history of screening of early development of these cancers is required in the management of these patients. Sporadic mismatch repair defects may also occur and are usually related to abnormal methylation.

- *p53 Tumor suppressor gene:* The p53 associated with colon carcinoma. It is a gatekeeper tumor suppressor gene located on chromosome 17. The p53 gene product is a nuclear binding protein that halts cell cycle in G1 by inhibiting nuclear transcription factor, until the mutation is repaired.

Clinical Correlation

Left-sided colon cancer is most likely to obstruct lumen, while right-sided colon cancer is more likely to bleed. Many cancers are within the reach of the finger (during digital rectal examination) or the rectosigmoidoscope.

The patients present with occult bleeding, change in bowel habits, loss of weight, loss of appetite and anemia.

Clinical manifestations according to location of carcinoma in large bowel are shown in Table 20.55. Differences between right- and left-sided colorectal carcinomas are shown in Table 20.56.

Right-sided Colon Cancer
- Adenocarcinoma of ascending and transverse colon tend to be **exophytic, polypoidal growth**, or crater-like **ulcerations** with raised margins, and commonly present with bleeding per rectum. Right-sided colonic carcinomas are more invasive and metastasize early as compared to left-sided lesions.
- Patient presents with black, tarry stools, rectal bleeding, anemia, abdominal aching, pressure, or dull cramps, weakness, fatigue, exertional dyspnea, diarrhea, constipation, anorexia, weight loss and vomiting.

Left-sided Colorectal Cancer
- Adenocarcinoma of the rectum or sigmoid colon often presents as a **circumferential annular/napkin ring configuration** mass narrowing the intestinal lumen. It produces early obstruction of colon lumen.
- Patient presents with black, tarry stools or rectal bleeding, intermittent abdominal fullness or cramping; rectal pressure, constipation, diarrhea or *ribbon-like* stool, and dark or bright red blood in stool; mucus in or on stool.

Gross Morphology
- Colorectal adenocarcinomas show wide range of gross appearances including fungating intraluminal growth, ulcerated growth with heaped up edges and circumferential growth.
- Tumor is firm with grey white appearance.
- Approximately 10% are mucinous adenocarcinomas (Figs 20.71 and 20.72).

Light Microscopy
- Classic colorectal adenocarcinoma is composed of irregularly distributed tubular structures in a desmoplastic stroma. There is presence of complex cribriform architecture and intraluminal necrosis. It shows abundant pool of mucin in 50% of the tumor area.
- Signet ring adenocarcinomas are rare in colon and composed of cells with abundant intracytoplasmic vacuoles arranged in diffuse infiltrative cords, nests and sheets (Fig. 20.73).

Table 20.55: Clinical manifestations according to location of carcinoma in large bowel

Symptoms	Right-sided colon carcinoma (frequency %)	Left-sided colon carcinoma (frequency %)	Carcinoma rectum (frequency %)
Pain abdomen	80	60	5
Mass abdomen	70	40	0
Rectal bleeding	20	20	60
Change in bowel habit	40	60	80
Weight loss	50	15	25
Vomiting	30	10	0
Obstruction	5	20	5

Table 20.56: Differences between right- and left-sided colorectal carcinomas

Characteristics	Right-sided colorectal carcinoma	Left-sided colorectal carcinoma
Location of growth	Cecum and ascending colon	Descending colon and rectosigmoid region
Growth pattern	Usually fungating or polypoid large cauliflower-like, soft friable growth projecting into the lumen (rarely napkin-ring type)	Napkin-ring configuration as a result of fibrosis. It leads to obstruction of lumen
Invasion of growth	More invasive	Less invasive
Clinical correlation	Silent lesion and diagnosed later	Obstructive lesion, so diagnosed early
Histologic features	Similar	Similar
Involvement of other structures	More common such as mesentery, lymph nodes, distant metastases	Less common such as mesentery, lymph nodes, distant metastases
Prognosis	Good	Poor

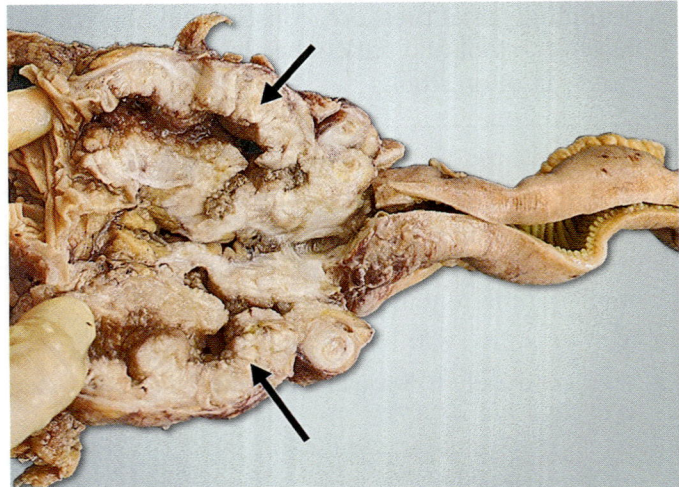

Fig. 20.71: Carcinoma in cecum showing fungating intraluminal growth. Tumor is firm with gray white appearance. Cut surface is gray white (arrows).

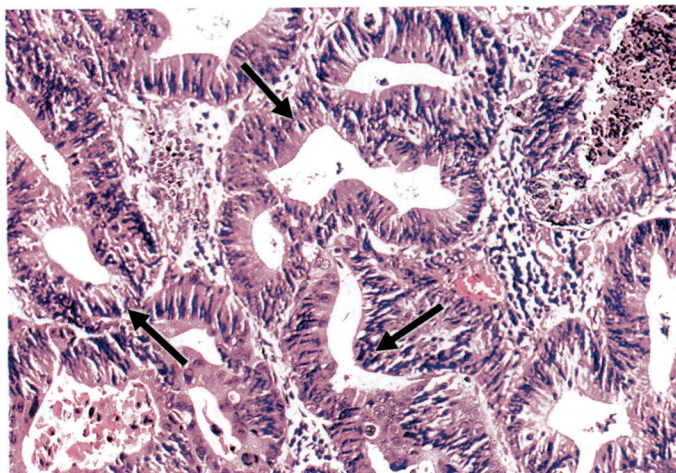

Fig. 20.73: Classic colorectal adenocarcinoma is composed of irregularly distributed tubular structures in a desmoplastic stroma (arrows) (400X).

Table 20.57: Immunohistochemistry of conventional colorectal adenocarcinoma

Tumor marker	Expression
Carcinoembryonic antigen (CEA)	Positive
CK20	Positive
CDX2 (transcription factor)	Positive
SAT2 (transcription factor)	Positive
p53	Positive
β-catenin	Positive (nuclear staining)
CK7	Focally positive in small subsets
Conventional colorectal adenocarcinomas are negative for TTF1, PAX2 and WT1	

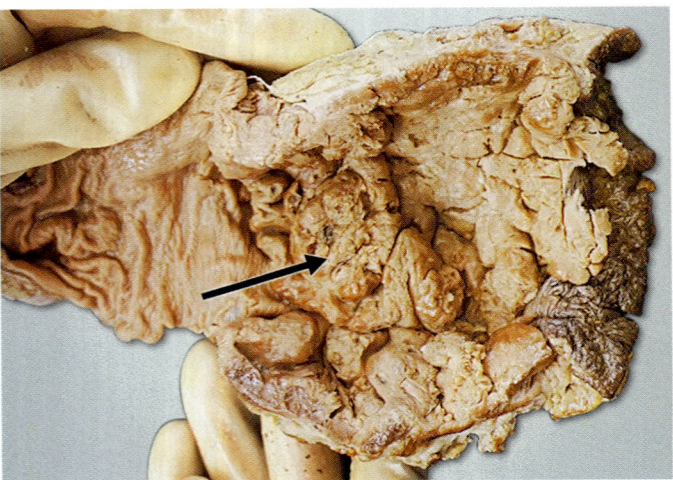

Fig. 20.72: Carcinoma in rectum showing fungating and ulcerated intraluminal growth. Tumor is firm with grey white appearance. Cut surface is gray white with areas of necrosis (arrow).

Immunohistochemistry

Panel of markers is used to analyze expression inconventional (microsatellite stable) colorectal adenocarcinomas on histopathological sections (Table 20.57).

Metastases

Right-sided colonic carcinomas are more invasive and metastasize early as compared to left-sided lesions.

- *Lymphatic route:* Colorectal carcinoma invades lymphatic channels and initially involves the lymph nodes immediately underlying the tumor.
- *Hematogenous route:* Blood-borne metastases from colorectal carcinoma is usually first seen in the *liver and then lungs.* Solitary liver metastasis may be treated by wedge resection giving months to years of symptoms free remission.

Multiple liver metastases are not resectable. These patients may respond to chemotherapy for months/years.

Complications

These include obstruction, hemorrhage, perforation and infection.

Diagnostic Modalities

- *Serum tumor markers:* Serum carcinoembryonic antigen (CEA), CA 19.9 and CA 72.4 levels are increased in colon carcinoma. Serum tumor markers used to detect colon carcinoma are shown in Table 20.58.

Table 20.58: Serum tumor markers used to detect colon carcinoma

Category	Tumor marker	Examples
Oncofetal proteins	Carcinoembryonic antigen (CEA)	Colon carcinoma Nonseminomatous germ cell testicular tumor Stomach carcinoma Pancreatic carcinoma Lung carcinoma Breast carcinoma
Mucins and glycoproteins	CA 19.9	Colon carcinoma Pancreatic carcinoma
	CA 72.4	Colon carcinoma Gastric carcinoma

- *Digital rectal examination:* Digital rectal examination is carried out to feel the growth in the rectum and anal canal.
- *Barium enema:* Barium enema with or without contrast media is used to visualize the local deformities of intestinal topography.
- *Sigmoidoscopy:* Sigmoidoscopy rigid or flexible fiber optic type is performed to visualize rectal tumors or routine screening.
- *Colonoscopy:* Colonoscopy is used to visualize the colon for detection of early polypoidal tumors during preoperative period and recurrences after surgical resection. Multiple biopsies may be obtained for histopathological examination.
- *Computed tomography (CT):* Computed tomography is performed to stage disease and detection of metastases.
- *Magnetic resonance imaging (MRI):* Magnetic resonance imaging is performed to metastatic disease.
- *Transrectal ultrasonography:* Transrectal tomography is an excellent choice for staging rectal carcinoma.
- *Laparotomy:* Laparotomy is performed to detect metastases to abdominal regions especially liver and omentum, that often remains undetected by current imaging techniques.

Therapeutic Correlation

Patient with EGFR positive tumor cells is treated with cetuximab monoclonal antibody targeting EGFR positive tumor cells.

Prognosis

The grade and stage of the tumor (Astler-Coller system) determine the prognosis: location of the tumor, extent of bowel involvement, histological grading and presence or absence of metastasis. The overall 5-year survival regardless of the stage is 35%.

APPENDIX

The appendix is a tubular structure extending from the cecum. It has an average length 7–10 cm. It is lined by colonic-type mucosa, surrounded by submucosa and muscular coats.

In children and young adults the mucosa contains numerous lymphoid follicles. In the elderly, the lumen often shows fibrous obliteration. Appendix fills with food and empties regularly into the cecum. Because appendix empties insufficiently due to its small lumen, therefore, it is prone to obstruction and vulnerable to infection.

ACUTE APPENDICITIS

Acute appendicitis is bacterial infection associated with proximal obstruction of the lumen. It is a common cause of acute abdomen. It is most frequent in adolescents and young adults and has no sex predilection.

Etiopathogenesis

Appendix becomes inflamed and edematous as a result of lumen occlusion by **fecolith** or **carcinoid tumor**. It leads to increase in intraluminal pressure, ischemic mucosal injury, and secondary bacterial infection. Other causes of lumen occlusion include submucosal *lymphoid hyperplasia* in the course of viral infection, *pinworms*, carcinoid tumor of appendix and barium from X-ray studies.

Clinical Features

Patient presents with pain in periumbilical region (central abdomen) radiating to right iliac quadrant. Systemic symptoms include fever, nausea and vomiting. Rebound tenderness may be demonstrated by pushing the abdominal wall at **McBurney's point.**

- Atypical presentation is encountered if the appendix is in retroperitoneal or intrapelvic location.
- Abdominal mass in the right lower quadrant may be palpated following a rupture of appendix and formation of a periappendiceal abscess. Pathological disorders confused with acute appendicitis are shown in Table 20.59.

Gross Morphology

- External surface of appendix is congested appendix and distal half covered by purulent exudate.
- The lumen contains a purulent exudate and often a fecolith (Fig. 20.74).

Light Microscopy

- Diagnostic criteria of acute appendicitis include infiltration of muscular coat of appendix by polymorphonuclear infiltration.
- Acute inflammatory infiltrate extends from the mucosa through the full thickness of the appendiceal wall (Fig. 20.75).

Complications

If untreated by surgical resection, appendicitis most often leads to *perforation or periappendiceal abscess*, or both. Transmural necrotizing inflammation of the appendix results in *peritonitis*. Patient may develop

Table 20.59: Pathological disorders confused with acute appendicitis

Most common disorders	
• Mesenteric lymphadenitis	• Ruptured ovarian follicle
• Acute salpingitis	• Torsion ovarian cyst
• Acute cholecystitis	• Inflammatory bowel disease
• Ectopic pregnancy	• Acute pyelonephritis and urinary tract infection

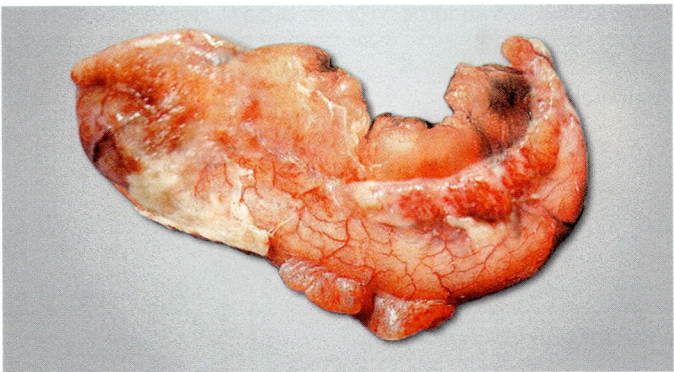

Fig. 20.74: Acute appendicitis showing congestion on the external surface.

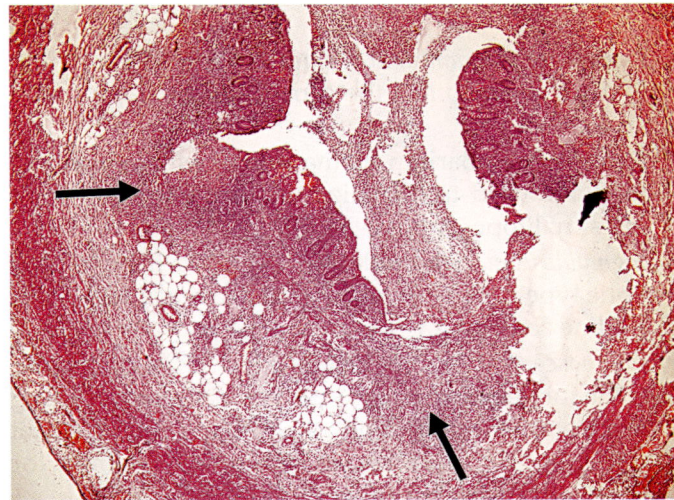

Fig. 20.75: Diagnostic criteria of acute appendicitis showing neutrophilic infiltration in the muscular coat (arrows) (100X).

septicemia resulting in *pylephlebitis* (inflammation of the portal vein), *liver abscess* and *subphrenic abscess*.

Laboratory Diagnosis

Peripheral smear examination shows leukocytosis with increased neutrophil count. Ultrasound and X-ray are performed in atypical cases prior to surgery.

Therapeutic Correlation

The inflamed appendix in acute appendicitis should be surgically removed because of possible devastating complications of perforation or abscess.

Precautions

Yersinia enterocolitica can cause *mesenteric granulomatous lymphadenitis* in children. Patient presents with *pain in the right lower quadrant (pseudoappendicitis), diarrhea, reactive arthritis, erythema nodosum, and septicemia*. Infected children frequently undergo laparotomy due to a mistaken diagnosis of appendicitis.

MUCOCELE OF APPENDIX

Mucocele of appendix refers to a dilated mucous-filled appendix.

Pathogenesis

Mucocele of appendix occurs due to chronic obstruction and mucinous cystadenoma or mucinous cystadenocarcinoma.

Complications

Rupture of a neoplastic mucocele may seed the peritoneal cavity with mucus secreting tumor cells, a condition referred to as *pseudomyxoma peritonei*.

CARCINOID TUMOR

Carcinoids are neuroendocrine tumors of low grade malignancy that are most commonly located in the submucosa of the intestines (e.g. appendix, terminal ileum, and rectum).

The most common appendiceal neoplasm is neuroendocrine (carcinoid) tumor, which is usually detected as an incidental finding. *Tip of the appendix is the most common site.*

Clinical Course

Clinical course of carcinoid tumor of appendix depends on size of the neoplasm.

- *Carcinoid tumor <2 cm:* It is considered benign. It rarely metastasizes. Perineural or lymphovascular is not indicative of malignant potential.
- *Carcinoid tumor >2 cm:* It invades mesoappendix and metastasizes to *regional lymph nodes, liver, lungs and bones in 66% of cases.*

ANUS AND PERIANAL REGION

Anal canal is present at the terminal end of gastrointestinal tract. It measures 3–4 cm in length. The mucosal lining the upper region of the anal canal is extension of rectal mucosa. The mucosa lining the middle region of the anal canal known as *transition zone measuring* 0.5 to 1 cm above the dentate line has features of both metaplastic squamous mucosa and urothelium.

The mucosa of distal portion of anal canal extending from the dentate line to the anal verge, is composed of specialized nonkeratinizing squamous epithelium with melanocytes. Important disorders of anorectal region are shown in Fig. 20.76.

VASCULAR DISORDERS

HEMORRHOIDS

These are painless dilated venous plexuses in the anal canal. All hemorrhoids result from increased portal venous pressure. Precipitating factors include chronic constipation, straining at stool, pregnancy, obesity, chronic liver disease and low fiber diet.

Hemorrhoids should not be diagnosed unless prolapse or bleeding is a dominant symptom. Classification of hemorrhoids is shown in Table 20.60. Investigation of rectal bleeding is shown in Table 20.61.

External Hemorrhoids

These originate from below the anorectal junction. It is covered by anal skin. It occurs as a result of dilation of inferior hemorrhoidal veins.

These are predisposed by a low-fiber diet. When thrombosed, these contain clotted blood.

Table 20.60: Classification of hemorrhoids

Degree	Features
First degree	Bleeding
Second degree	Prolapse and reducing spontaneously
Third degree	Prolapse needing pushing back
Fourth degree	Prolapse permanent

Treatment of hemorrhoids is based on symptoms rather than appearances

Table 20.61: Investigation of rectal bleeding

Symptoms (bright red blood)	Diagnostic tools
Bright red blood seen only on paper	Inspection Rectal examination Proctoscopy Rigid sigmoidoscopy
Bright red blood drippling into pain	Proctoscopy Rigid sigmoidoscopy
Bright red blood mixed with motion	Proctoscopy Rigid sigmoidoscopy Flexible sigmoidoscopy
Dark red blood	Proctoscopy Rigid sigmoidoscopy Flexible sigmoidoscopy Barium meal
Anyone over 40 years of age and family history of colorectal anaplasia	Flexible sigmoidoscopy

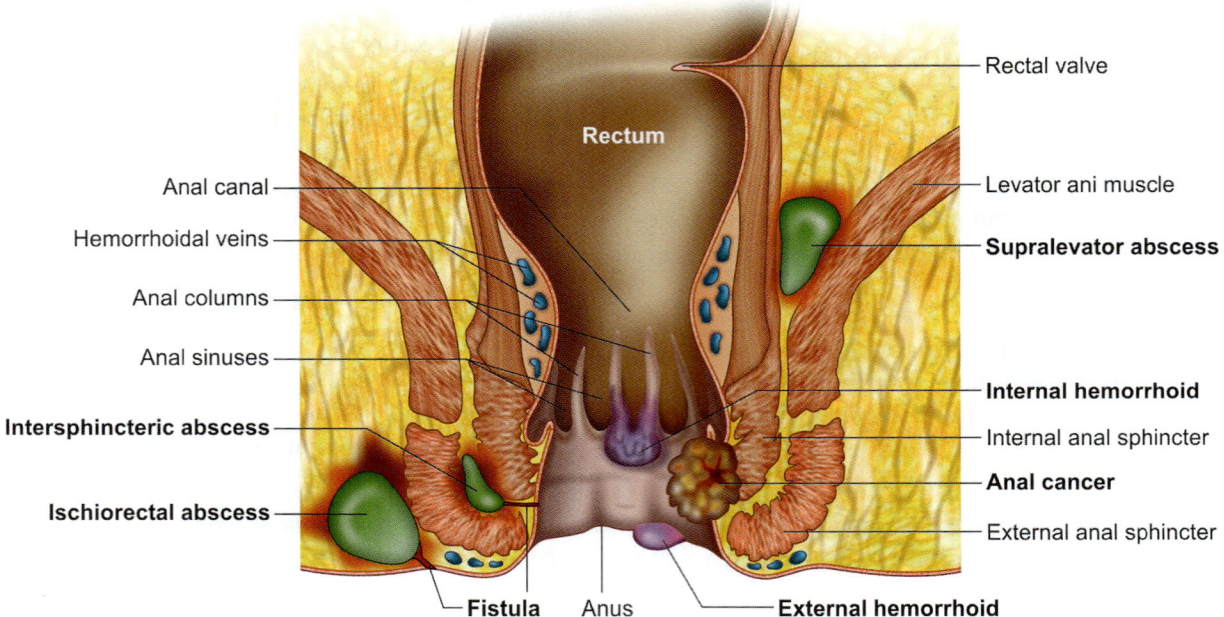

Fig. 20.76: Anorectal region showing important disorders.

These become painful swollen, shiny blue and itchy resulting in bleeding during defecation. Resolution of external hemorrhoids leaves a painless flabby skin sac around the anal orifice.

Internal Hemorrhoids

These originate from dilatation of superior hemorrhoidal veins above the anorectal junction and are covered by mucous membrane.

When the person performs a Valsalva maneuver, these appear as red mucosal mass may protrude from anus. These are not palpable.

NON-NEOPLASTIC DISEASES

PILONIDAL SINUS

Pilonidal sinus is hair containing cyst or sinus located in the midline over the coccyx or lower sacrum. On examination, it opens up as a dimple with visible hair and possibly, an erythematous halo.

It may appear as a palpable cyst. When it is enlarged, it has a palpable sinus tract. Although it is congenital disorder, yet the lesion is diagnosed between the ages of 15 or 30 years.

ANORECTAL FISTULA

Chronic inflammation in anorectal region creates an abnormal passage from inner anus or rectum out to skin surface surrounding anus. It most often occurs due to local abscess. Patient presents with serosanguineous or purulent discharge from red raised tract opening on applying pressure. Bidigital palpation may reveal an indurated cord.

ANAL FISSURE

Anal fissure is a longitudinal tear in the superficial mucosa at the anal margin. More than 90% fissures are located in the posterior midline area. These are accompanied by hyperplastic papule known as *sentinel tag*. Fissures most often results from trauma due to passage of hard stool or irritable diarrheal stool.

Patient presents with pain during and after bowel action, minor bleeding, itching, constipation, and painful spasm of sphincter.

RECTAL PROLAPSE

The rectal mucous protruding through the anus is known as *rectal prolapse*. Rectal prolapse appears as moist red doughnut with radiating lines.

- *Incomplete rectal prolapse:* When prolapse is incomplete, only the mucosa is bulging.
- *Complete rectal prolapse:* When complete rectal prolapse occurs, it includes the anal sphincter following a Valsalva maneuver such as straining at stool or exercise.

Predisposing Factors

Predisposing factors include *constipation, excessive straining at defecation, deep pouch of Douglas, redundant sigmoid colon, decreased sigmoid colon, decreased anal canal sphincter tone and reduced pelvic support.*

Other conditions causing rectal prolapse are large hemorrhoids, prolapsing rectal tumor, anal warts and polyps.

Clinical Features

Patient presents with prolapse related to defecation, mucus discharge, bleeding, and incontinence.

PRURITUS ANI

Pruritus ani is characterized by sensation of itch, burning or pain. It is more common in men than women.

Etiology

It is idiopathic in 50% of cases. Anorectal causes include fissures, fistula, papilloma, skin tags, hemorrhoids and prolapse. Dermatological causes are psoriasis, lichen planus, Paget's disease, candidiasis and threadworms. Dietary factors implicated in pruritus ani include coffee, tea, spices, pork, alcohol, tomatoes and drugs (e.g. antibiotics, laxatives, colchicine, and quinidine).

Clinical Features

Patient presents with slight itch in perianal skin that may progress to severe itch especially during summer.

Management

Secondary causes of pruritus ani should be identified and treated. Patient should be advised about personal hygiene.

MALIGNANT TUMORS

Anal cancer is relatively uncommon. It accounts for about 4% of anorectal malignancies. Various anal neoplasms include squamous cell carcinoma, malignant melanoma, lymphoma and anal gland adenocarcinoma. Overall anal cancers are more common in women. Lesions at the anal margins are more common in men.

PATHOLOGY

Anal cancers arise at or above the dentate line and not visible at the anus. Anal cancers arising below the dentate line are visible at the anus. These behave like basal cell carcinomas and have favorable prognosis than anal canal cancers.

Etiology

There is increased incidence of anal cancer among male homosexuals. Approximately 50% of anal cancers are associated with human papillomavirus infection.

Clinical Features

Patient presents with bleeding, pain, swelling and ulceration around anus. As the anal cancer advances, patient suffers worsening pain, disturbed bowel habit, urinary incontinence and rectovaginal fistula.

Approximately 50% of anal cancers are diagnosed before the malignancy has spread beyond primary site. About 13–25% are diagnosed after the anal cancer has spread to inguinal lymph nodes and 10% to distant organs. Delay in presentation and diagnosis cause direct as well as distant metastases.

Differential Diagnosis

Early anal cancers may be confused with warts, fissures, hemorrhoids leading to delayed diagnosis.

Epidermoid Carcinoma

About 80% of anal cancers are squamous cell carcinoma. These are most frequently encountered in the anus at anorectal junction in the male homosexual population, HPV type 16 and 18 induced squamous cell carcinoma may occur.

Gross Morphology
Anal cancers appear as ulcers or proliferative growth with ulcerated areas.
Light Microscopy
On histopathological examination, tumor varies predominantly well differentiated keratinizing large cell carcinoma at the anal margin to less differentiated nonkeratinizing to small cell carcinoma in the upper anal canal (Fig. 20.77).

Basaloid Carcinoma

It occurs at the squamocolumnar junction or transitional zone, sometimes called cloacogenic carcinoma.

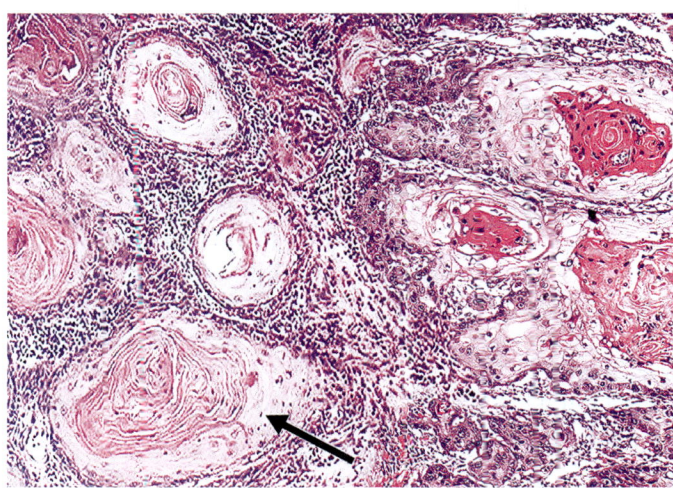

Fig. 20.77: Well differentiated squamous cell carcinoma of anus (arrow) (400X).

PERITONEUM

ANATOMY

Serosal membranes are derived from the mesoderm. These form the visceral and parietal surfaces of pleural, pericardial and peritoneal cavities including tunica vaginalis. On histopathological examination, serous membranes are lined by flat mesothelial cells resting on a basement membrane, below which lies a poorly delimited connective tissue layer.

NON-NEOPLASTIC LESIONS

Acute Peritonitis

Acute peritonitis is caused as a result of perforation of gastric, biliary, intestine or pancreas. Spontaneous bacterial peritonitis most often occurs in children, immunocompromised persons or patients with cirrhosis.

Granulomatous Serositis

Granulomatous serositis presents as small nodules in the setting of disseminated cancers. It may be caused by infections, noninfectious causes, autoimmune and meconium induced. Causes of granulomatous serositis are shown in Table 20.62.

Metaplasia

Metaplasia most often occurs in women in the abdomen and pelvic region. It is due to its close embryologic relationship with müllerian ducts. Pathogenesis of metaplasia of peritoneum is discussed below.

- *Endometriosis:* When endometriosis develops in the wall of intestine, ureter or urinary bladder, the woman presents with signs and symptoms resembling malignancy. On histopathological examination, the lesion is composed of endometrial glands with stroma, dense fibrosis and adhesions.
- *Endocervicosis:* Endocervicosis comprise benign glands resembling endocervical type of epithelium leading to metaplasia of peritoneum.
- *Ectopic decidual metaplasia:* Ectopic decidual metaplasia of peritoneum occurs in pregnant women. There is presence of small gray white nodules on the peritoneal surfaces.
- *Walthard nests:* Walthard nests appear as yellow white nodules on the serosal surface of fallopian tubes. These may undergo cystic change. Histopathological examination reveals transitional metaplasia of peritoneum.
- *Disseminated peritoneal leiomyomatosis:* It is uncommon multifocal proliferation of smooth muscle like cells thought to represent hormone induced metaplasia of peritoneum.

Fibrosis of Peritoneum

Reactive peritoneal fibrosis occurs in the setting of recurrent peritonitis often associated with long-term peritoneal dialysis, cirrhosis, or surgery.

Sclerosing peritonitis occurs as a result of hyperplasia of submesothelial mesenchymal cells covering small intestine, diaphragm, liver, spleen in the setting of peritoneal dialysis, autoimmune disorders and carcinoid tumors.

Eosinophilic Peritonitis

Eosinophilic peritonitis occurs in the settings of childhood atopy, autoimmune collagenous disorders, hypereosinophilic syndrome, lymphomas and metastatic carcinoma.

PRIMARY NEOPLASMS

WHO classification of tumors of peritoneum is shown in Table 20.63.

Well Differentiated Papillary Mesothelioma

Well differentiated papillary mesothelioma is a low grade tumor associated with asbestos exposure. It most often occurs in women during reproductive period in 80% of cases.

Table 20.62: Causes of granulomatous serositis

Categories	Disorders
Infectious causes	Fungal infections (histoplasmosis, Cryptococcus)
	Parasites (Schistosomiasis, Echinococcus or Ascaris)
Noninfectious causes	Sutures or starch
	Implants of keratin derived from mature cystic teratoma, endometrioid adenocarcinoma with squamous differentiation, squamous cell carcinoma of cervix
Autoimmune disorders	Crohn's disease or sarcoidosis
Meconium	Meconium in neonate inducing peritonitis

Gastrointestinal Tract

Table 20.63: WHO classification of tumors of peritoneum

Categories	Tumors
Mesothelial tumors	Well differentiated papillary mesothelioma (low grade tumor associated with asbestos exposure)
	Multicystic mesothelioma (low grade tumor also known as *multilocular peritoneal inclusion cyst*)
	Diffuse malignant mesothelioma
	Adenomatoid tumor
Smooth muscle cell tumors	Leiomyomatosis peritoneal disseminata
Tumors of uncertain origin	Desmoplastic small round cell tumor
Epithelial tumors	Primary peritoneal adenocarcinoma
	Primary peritoneal borderline tumor

Gross Morphology
Tumor is solitary to multifocal <2 cm in diameter. Cut surface is gray white exhibiting nodules and papillary structures.

Light Microscopy
Tumor is composed of papillary fronds with fibrovascular core covered by single layer of bland cuboidal to flattened mesothelial cells.

Clinical Course
Clinical course is indolent.

Multicystic Mesothelioma
Multicystic mesothelioma is a low-grade neoplasm also known as multicystic peritoneal inclusion cyst. On histopathological examination, multilocular cysts are lined by mesothelium with bland cytological features harboring areas of conventional malignant mesothelioma.

Diffuse Malignant Mesothelioma
Diffuse malignant mesothelioma of peritoneum is a rare neoplasm. On histopathological examination, tumor resembles ectopic decidual reaction.

Immunohistochemistry
Panel of markers is used to analyze expression in diffuse malignant mesothelioma on histopathological sections (Table 20.64).

SECONDARY NEOPLASMS
Secondary tumors metastasizing to the peritoneal serosal surface are shown in Table 20.65.

Table 20.64: Immunohistochemistry of diffuse malignant mesothelioma

Tumor marker	Expression
Calretinin	Positive
Thrombomodulin	Positive
WT1	Positive
Cytokeratin 5/6	Positive

MOC-31, Ber-EP4, CA19-9 and CD15 (Leu-M1) markers are negative in diffuse malignant mesothelioma. These are used to distinguish peritoneal epithelioid mesothelioma from peritoneal and ovarian serous carcinomas.

Pseudomyxoma Peritonei
Pseudomyxoma peritonei is clinical term used to designate masses of jelly-like mucus in the abdomen and pelvis.

Most common cause of pseudomyxoma peritonei is low grade mucinous neoplasm of appendix. Less common causes are tumors arising from stomach, ovary, pancreas and hepatobiliary system.

Table 20.65: Metastases to the peritoneal serosal surface

Primary tumors
• Ovarian cancer
• Cervix cancer
• Breast carcinoma
• Biliary tract carcinoma
• Upper gastrointestinal tract cancer
• Sarcomas of female reproductive tract
• Endometrial carcinoma
• Fallopian tube cancer
• Pancreatic carcinoma
• Lung cancer
• Lower gastrointestinal tract cancer

INVESTIGATIONS OF GASTROINTESTINAL DISORDERS

Large bowel disorders include *hyperplastic polyps, neoplastic polyps, neoplasms, inflammatory bowel disease, diverticula, infectious colitis, drug-induced colitis and irritable bowel syndrome*. Investigations of colorectal disorders include detailed history, abdominal examination, anorectal examination, digital examination, proctoscopy, sigmoidoscopy, colonoscopy, barium enema, imaging techniques and feces examination.

Distribution of carcinomas in upper gastrointestinal tract is shown in Fig. 20.78. *Helicobacter pylori* induced gastrointestinal disorders are shown in Fig. 20.79. Appendix disorders include acute appendicitis and carcinoid tumor. Important disorders of large bowel are shown in Fig. 20.80. Symptoms of colorectal disorders are shown in Table 20.66. Differential diagnosis of lower abdominal mass is shown in Table 20.67.

Abdominal Examination

Abdomen should be inspected for *visible peristalsis* and *distension*. *Palpable sigmoid colon* is observed in *constipated patients*. Palpable liver may disclose metastatic deposits from colorectal carcinoma.

Anorectal Examination

Rectum and anus are readily accessible. Findings on anorectal examination include *pruritus ani, perianal warts, perianal abscess, perianal hematoma, prolapsing hemorrhoids, thrombosed hemorrhoids, anal fistula, anal fissures, anal cancer, rectal prolapse, rectocele and fecal soiling of perineum*.

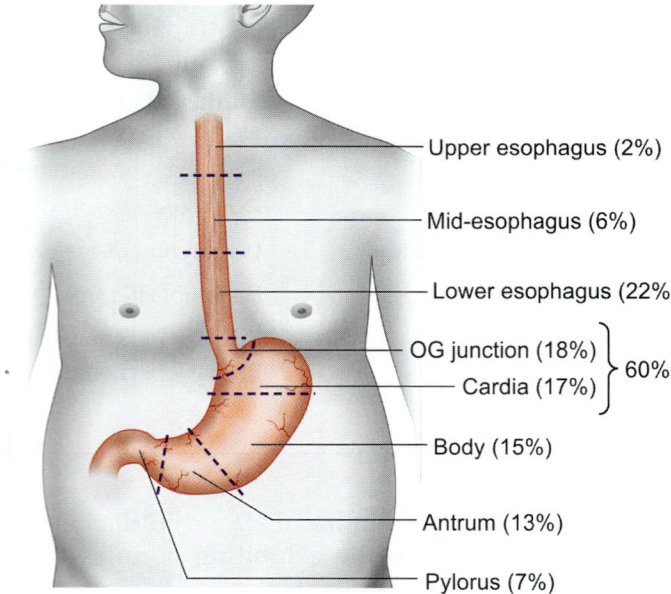

Fig. 20.78: Distribution of carcinomas in upper gastrointestinal tract.

Digital Examination

Digital examination helps in diagnosing skin tags and Crohn's disease. On straining, *prolapsing hemorrhoids, rectal prolapse and tumors* are detected.

Proctoscopy

Fiberoptic proctoscopy helps in visualization of rectal prolapsing mucosa, hemorrhoids, dentate line and anal epithelium.

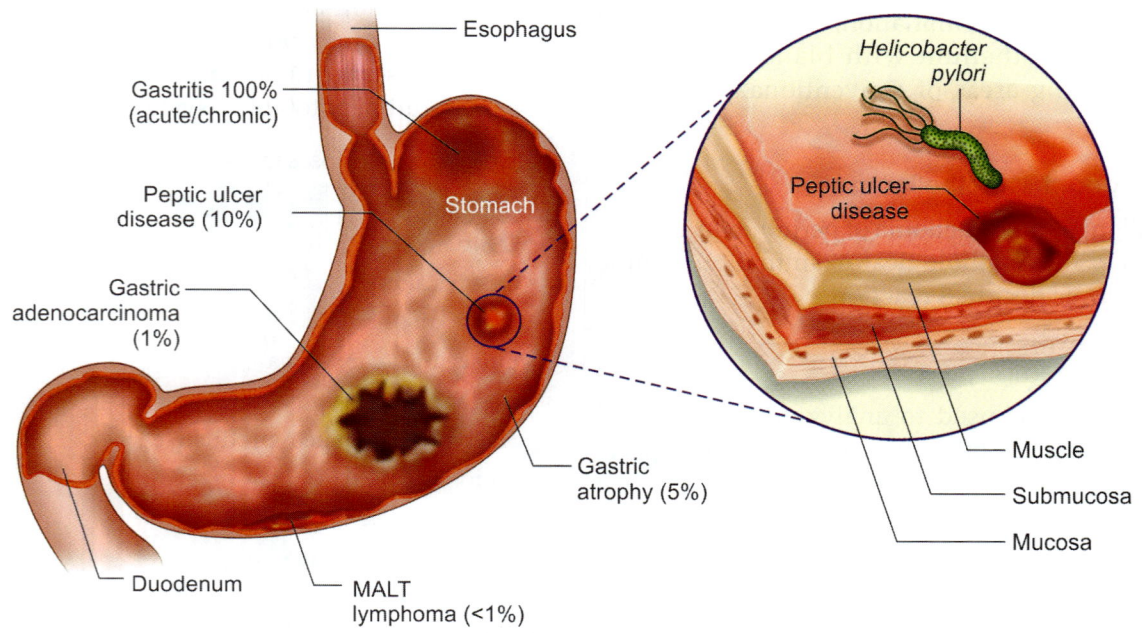

Fig. 20.79: *Helicobacter pylori* induced gastrointestinal disorders.

Gastrointestinal Tract

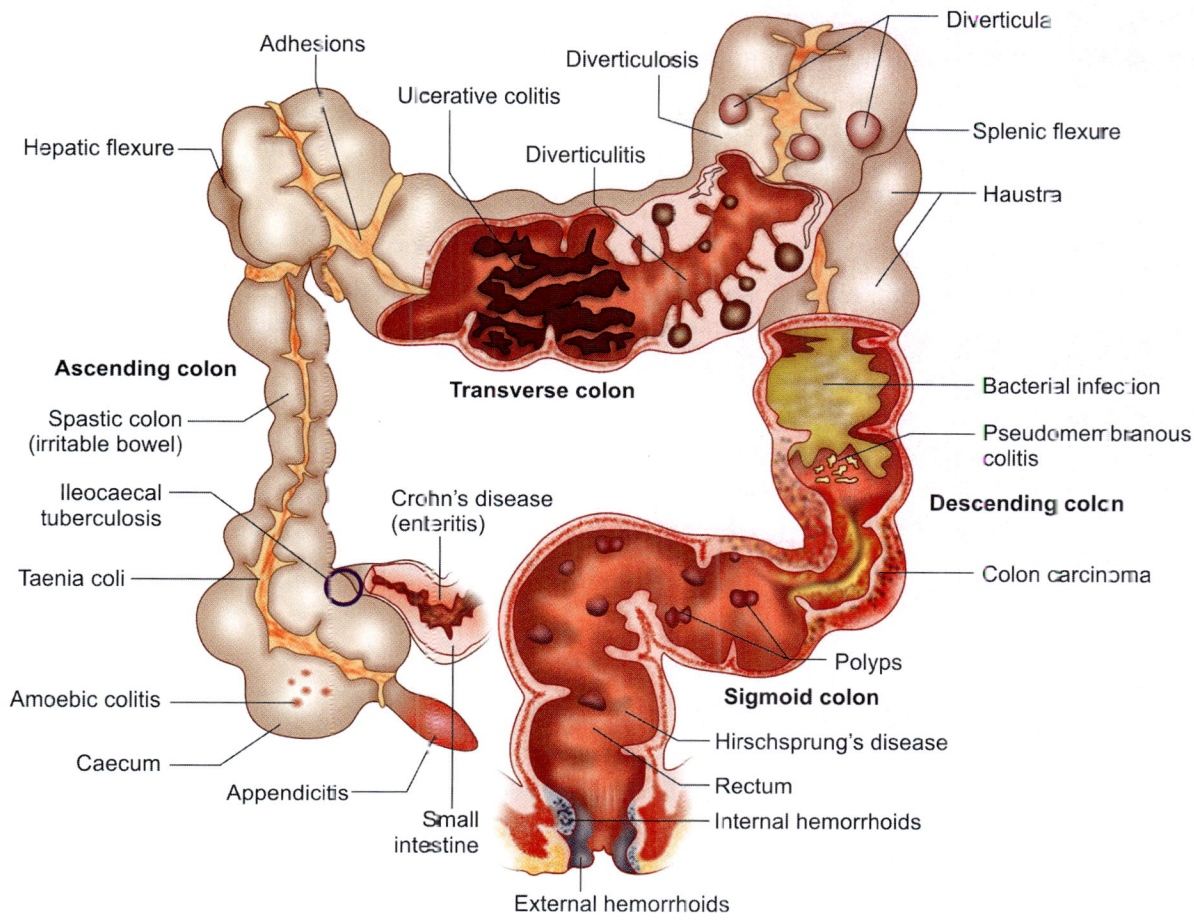

Fig. 20.80: Important disorders of large bowel.

Table 20.66: Symptoms of colorectal disorders

Parameters	Symptoms
Nonspecific symptoms	Malaise
	Vomiting
	Weight loss
Abdominal pain	Constant pain or colic
	Distension
	Borborygmi
Bowel habits	Altered frequency
	Constipation or diarrhea
	Bleeding (bright red or mixed with mucus, dark or altered)
Anal and perianal	Pruritus
	Pain related to defecation
	Prolapse
	Incontinence
	Discharge
	Tenesmus
	Swelling (painful or painless)

Table 20.67: Differential diagnosis of lower abdominal mass

Location	Disorders
Right iliac fossa	Carcinoma of cecum
	Crohn's disease
	Appendicular abscess
	Ileocecal tuberculosis
	Actinomycosis
	Intussusception
Left iliac fossa	Carcinoma of sigmoid colon
	Diverticular disease
Either iliac fossa	Ovarian mass
	Ectopic pregnancy
	Transplanted kidney

Flexible Sigmoidoscopy

Flexible sigmoidoscopy permits examination up to 60 cm from the anal margin. It is performed without sedation in <10 minutes. Approximately 70% of colorectal carcinomas are within reach of flexible sigmoidoscope.

Colonoscopy

Patient should take a low residual diet followed by clear fluids for 48 hours and strong purgative before colonoscopy. Colonoscopy is more sensitive for detecting *fine mucosal abnormalities, biopsy sampling and therapeutic procedures* such as polypectomy.

Double Contrast Barium Enema

In double contrast barium enema, air is pushed after evacuation of barium. It discloses *gross anatomy, extracolonic abnormalities such as fistulas*.

Imaging Modalities

Imaging techniques used to detect colorectal disorders include ultrasonography, CT scan and MRI scan.

- *Ultrasonography:* It may demonstrate clinically *inapparent metastases* in patients with colorectal carcinoma.
- *CT and MRI scans:* Preoperative computed tomography and magnetic resonance scanning give more accurate information in *detection of local extent of rectal carcinoma and hepatic metastases* than ultrasonography. MRI scanning is useful in the assessment of complex anal fistulas.

Feces Examination

Detection of occult blood in the feces is important in the investigation of patients with unexplained iron deficiency anemia.

- *Occult blood:* Feces of patient smeared on a filter paper is impregnated with guaiac acid and then added hydrogen peroxide. Hematin from hemoglobin in the feces catalyzes the oxidation of guaiac acid giving characteristic color change to blue. Immunologic tests for human hemoglobin may prove to be more sensitive.

Table 20.68: Immunohistochemistry analyzed in GIT tumors

GIT tract	Tumor markers
Gastric adenocarcinoma (intestinal type)	Cytokeratin Carcinoembryonic antigen (CEA) Epithelial membrane antigen (EMA)
Gastrointestinal stromal tumors	c-kit oncogene (CD117) encoding tyrosine kinase DOG 1 (most specific marker) CD171 (cell adhesive molecule) Protein kinase C theta Vimentin Smooth muscle actin (encoded by ACTA2 gene located on 10q–q24) CD34 Desmin
Gastrointestinal carcinoids	Chromogranin (neural marker) Synaptophysin (neural marker) Neuron-specific enolase CDX2 (diffuse nuclear staining) PAX8 (polyclonal antibody)
Gastric MALT lymphoma	CD20 CD79a CD21 CD35 CD43
Colorectal adenocarcinoma	Carcinoembryonic antigen (CEA) CK20 CDX2 (transcription factor) SAT2 (transcription factor) p53 β-catenin (nuclear staining) CK7

- *24 hours fecal fat and D-xylose tests:* Diagnostic modalities include 24 hours fecal fat excretion. D-xylose test, anti-tissue transglutaminase circulating autoantibodies and intestinal biopsy.

    These autoantibody tests may also be used for screening prior to definitive diagnosis by biopsy.

- *Culture and sensitivity:* It is done if infection is suspected such as *Entamoeba histolytica* and toxins of *Clostridium difficile* in patients with pseudomembranous colitis.

Helicobacter Pylori Tests

In the advanced stage of *Helicobacter pylori* induced gastrointestinal disorders; *urea breath test or antibody test for Helicobacter pylori* must be performed.

Serum Tumor Markers

Serum carcinoembryonic antigen (CEA), CA 19.9 and CA 72.4 levels are increased in colon carcinoma.

Sampling of Tissue Biopsy

- *Endoscopic biopsy:* Small fragments of mucosal tissue are obtained for histopathological examination.
- *Suction biopsy:* It makes possible to obtain submucosa for study.
- *Polypectomy:* The specimen is bisected or serial sections depending on size of polypoid mass.
- *Endoscopic mucosal resection:* Mucosal resections are obtained by this method.
- *Bowel resection:* Portion of bowel resection is obtained to study various gastrointestinal disorders. Serosal surface is examined to study involvement by tumor. Bowel wall is inspected for tumor involvement, perforation and adhesion.

    Mesentery and soft tissue are dissected to obtain lymph nodes. A minimum of 12 lymph nodes is required for establishing staging criteria.

Immunohistochemistry

Immunohistochemistry has now become the most powerful and widely used ancillary diagnostic tool in surgical pathology, especially in the diagnosis of undifferentiated tumors. Immunohistochemistry analyzed in GIT tumors is shown in Table 20.68.

CHAPTER 21

Liver, Gallbladder and Exocrine Pancreas

Learning Objectives

LIVER
- Patterns of Necrosis

JAUNDICE AND CHOLESTASIS
- Recurrent Jaundice during Pregnancy
- Hereditary Hyperbilirubinemia
- Neonatal Cholestasis

HEPATITIS
- Acute/Chronic Viral Hepatitis
- Hepatotropic Viruses
- Autoimmune Hepatitis (Lupoid Hepatitis)

BACTERIAL AND PARASITIC INFECTIONS OF LIVER
- Bacterial Liver Infections
- Parasitic Infections
- Cholangitis and Liver Abscess
- Drugs and Toxins induced Liver Injury
- Acetaminophen induced Hepatocellular Injury
- Carbon Tetrachloride induced Liver Injury

CIRRHOSIS
- Morphological Classification
- Etiopathogenesis
- Clinical Manifestations
- Portal Hypertension with or without Portal Vein Obstruction
- Massive Splenomegaly
- Hematological Abnormalities

METABOLIC LIVER DISEASES
- Alcoholic Liver Disease
- Nonalcoholic Fatty Liver Disease (NAFLD)
- Hemochromatosis
- Wilson Disease
- α_1-Antitrypsin Deficiency
- Glycogen and Lysosomal Storage Diseases
- Amyloidosis Liver
- Indian Childhood Cirrhosis
- Acute Fatty Liver of Pregnancy
- Reye Syndrome

BILE DUCT DISORDERS
- Primary Biliary Cirrhosis
- Secondary Biliary Cirrhosis
- Primary Sclerosing Cholangitis

VASCULAR DISORDERS
- Impairment of Hepatic Venous Drainage
- Impairment of Arterial Underperfusion
- Miscellaneous Intrahepatic Vascular Conditions

LIVER TUMORS
- Primary Benign Tumors
- Benign or Premalignant Hepatocellular Lesions in Cirrhotic Liver
- Hepatocellular Hyperplasia
- Primary Malignant Tumors
- Metastatic Tumors (Liver Metastases)

GALLBLADDER
- Non-neoplastic Conditions
- Cholelithiasis (Gallstone Disease)

COMMON NEOPLASMS AND PRECURSOR LESIONS OF GALLBLADDER
- Adenoma Gallbladder
- Adenocarcinoma Gallbladder
- Biliary Adenocarcinoma

PANCREAS
- Overview
- Anatomy and Physiology

PANCREATITIS
- Acute Pancreatitis
- Chronic Pancreatitis
- Autoimmune Pancreatitis
- Cystic Fibrosis Pancreas

PANCREATIC TUMORS
- Exocrine Tumors
- Islet Cell Tumors
- Metastatic Tumors

LIVER

NORMAL STRUCTURE

The liver and pancreas are derived as glandular outgrowths of the primitive foregut. The liver is the largest parenchymal organ weighing about 1000 to 1500 gm. It lies just below the diaphragm. The right lobe is larger than the left lobe. The falciform ligament is the rough dividing line between the two lobes. External surface is smooth and brown. Cut surface is brown.

Anatomy of the liver and its relationship to the gallbladder, pancreas and duodenum is shown in Fig. 21.1.

Liver Acinus (Lobule)

Liver is divided histologically into hexagonal or polyhedral lobules. The center of the lobule has central vein. Portal triads are present at the periphery of the lobule (Figs 21.2 and 21.3).

Portal Triad

It consists of branch of bile duct, portal vein and hepatic artery surrounded by fibrocollagenous tissue. The area surrounding central vein is known as *centrilobular area*. The area surrounding portal triad is known as *periportal area*.

Hepatocytes

Liver cells radiate from the portal tracts towards the terminal hepatic venules. Hepatocytes are arranged in columns one-cell thick. Sinusoid is present between each of these columns.

Limiting Plates

Portal tract is bound by a row of hepatocytes known as *limiting plate*. The liver cell plates are *two-cell thick in babies and small children*. By attaining the age of 5 years the normal *one-cell thick* pattern is established. Destruction of limiting plates in hepatitis is known as *piecemeal necrosis*.

Functional Zones of Liver Acinus (Lobule)

Functionally, the liver can be divided into three zones between the portal triad and central vein, based on oxygen and nutrients supply.

Zone 1: It encircles the portal tracts, where the richest content of oxygen and nutrients from hepatic arteries enter.

Zone 2: It is located in between zone 1 and zone 3.

Zone 3: It is located most distant from the portal tract around central veins. It is poor in oxygen and nutrients surrounding the terminal venule.

Hepatic Vasculature

Near the hilum, portal tract contains portal vein, branch of hepatic artery and interlobular bile ducts. Liver

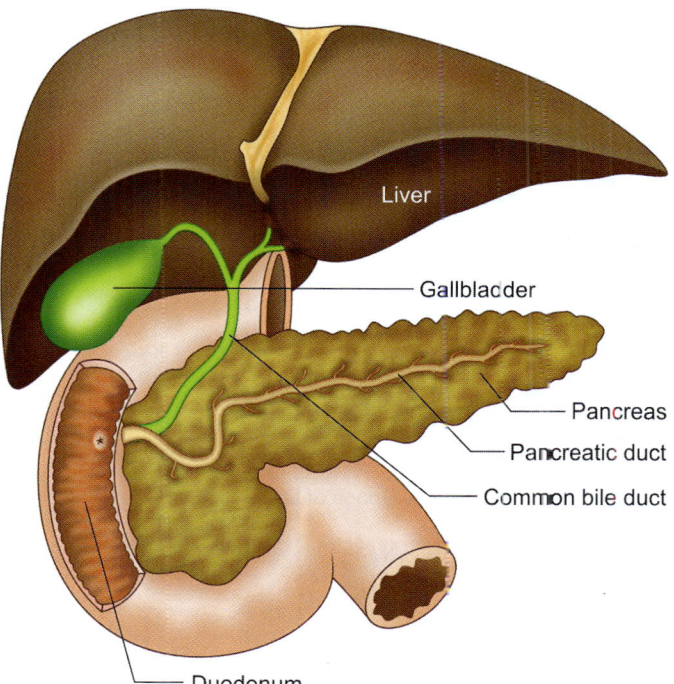

Fig. 21.1: Anatomy of the liver and its relationship to the gallbladder, pancreas and duodenum.

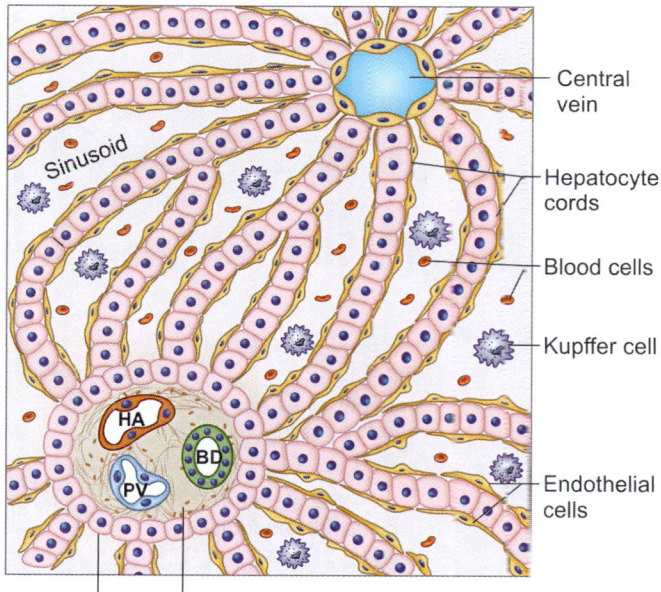

Fig. 21.2: Schematic representation of the normal liver lobule. The portal tract contains branches of the hepatic artery, portal vein, and interlobular bile duct. The liver cell plates converge to the terminal hepatic venule.

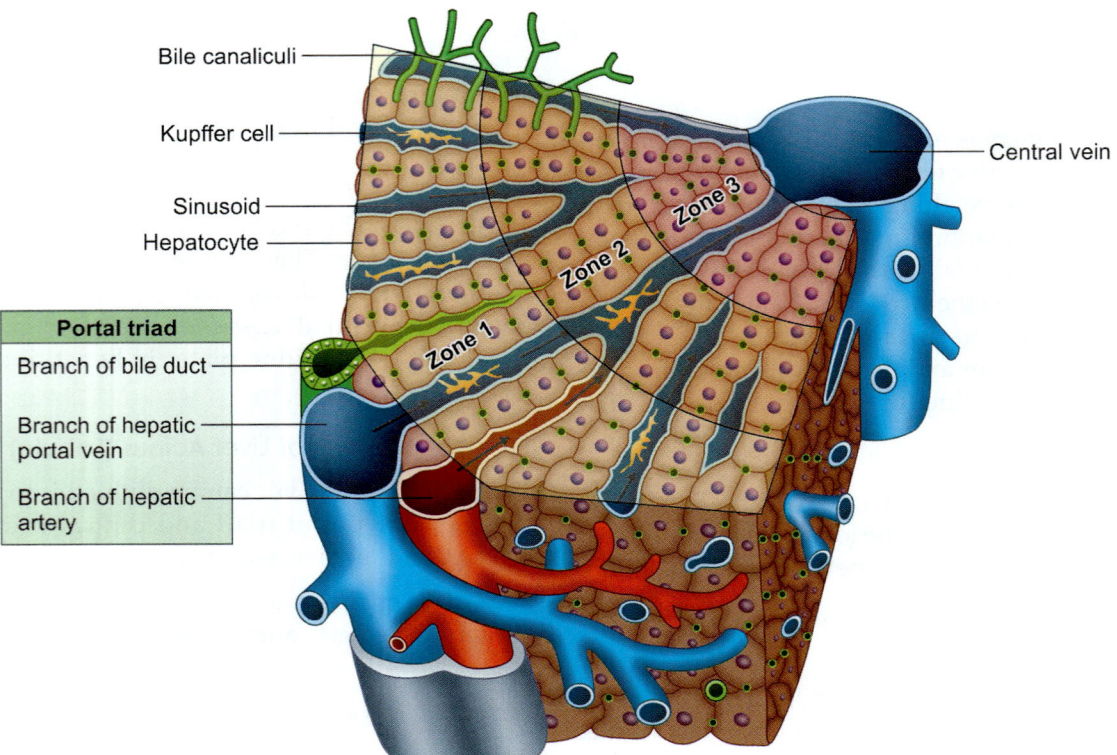

Fig. 21.3: Liver lobule shows cords of hepatocytes, sinusoids and bile ducts in the liver. Blood flows in sinusoids towards the center of the lobule (terminal hepatic vein) and bile in opposite direction draining in the bile ducts.

receives blood supply from portal vein and hepatic artery. The liver cell plates converge to the terminal hepatic venule (Fig. 21.4).

Portal Vein

Liver receives 70–75% blood flow from portal vein. Portal vein is formed by joining of the superior mesenteric and splenic vein. *Normal portal vein pressure is 5–10 mm Hg.*

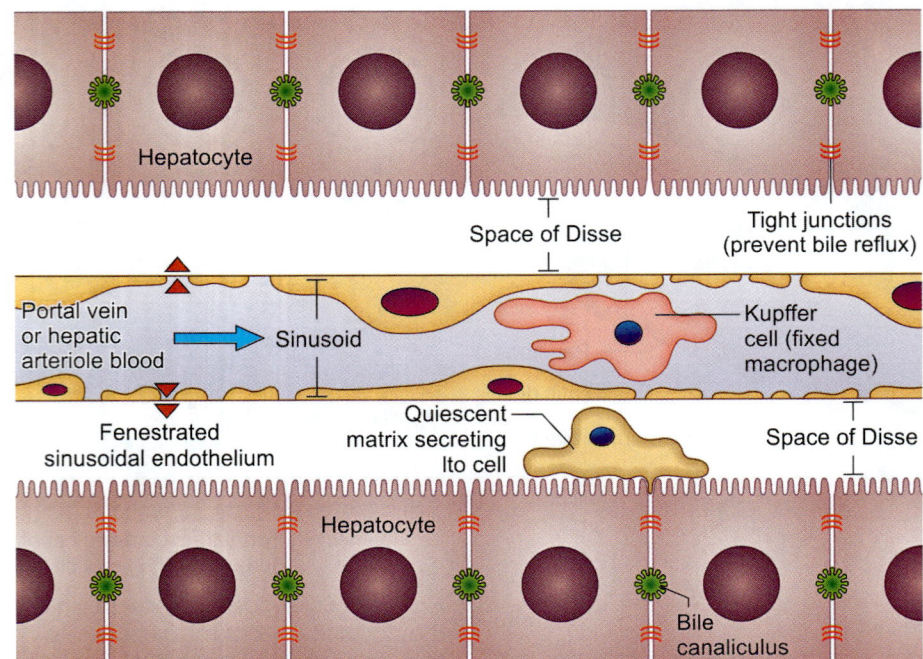

Fig. 21.4: The hepatic sinusoid and perisinusoidal space. Tight junction between hepatocytes prevents escape of bile.

Hepatic Artery

Liver receives 25–30% oxygenated blood flow from hepatic artery. Hepatic artery occlusion does not cause necrosis of hepatocytes except in transplanted liver.

Hepatic Vein

It drains blood from the liver to the inferior vena cava. Hepatic abnormalities include disturbance of blood flow and portal hypertension.

Hepatic Sinusoids

Liver Sinusoids

The liver sinusoids are lined by endothelial cells. Underneath the endothelium, there is a row of hepatocytes. Sinusoidal endothelium lacks tight junctions between endothelial cells and basement membrane under the endothelium.

This anatomical arrangement permits free access of plasma from sinusoidal blood to hepatocytes, thus facilitating two-way exchange of molecules between liver cells and blood.

Space of Disse

The space between the endothelium and hepatocytes is known as *space of Disse*. It contains collagen fibers especially type III, proteoglycans and some fibronectin. Space of Disse consists of Kupffer cells and perisinusoidal stellate cells (Ito cells).

Kupffer Cells

These cells are attached to the endothelium. These function as fixed tissue macrophages and participate in the phagocytosis of gut derived bacteria. *The Kupffer cell population is greatest in zone 1 of the liver cell acinus. Kupffer cells help in metabolism of vitamin A.*

Perisinusoidal Stellate Cells (Ito Cells)

These cells are in close contact with the liver cells. These cells may extend into small recesses between hepatocytes. Most of them contain vitamin A. These cells have myofibroblastic properties and participate in synthesis of collagen fibers during inflammation.

Bile Canaliculi

These are present in between hepatocytes. Bile from bile canaliculi is drained into the bile ducts in portal triad and ultimately into the common bile duct. The canalicular microvilli are surrounded by a meshwork of contractile proteins, which maintain tone within the canalicular system. From the canaliculi, the bile flows into the periductules known as *canals of Hering*.

PHYSIOLOGY

Liver participates in excretion of substances, detoxification of substances, synthesis of vitamin K-dependent clotting factors (II, VII, IX, X), proteins, metabolism of carbohydrates, lipids and proteins; and storage of iron. Functions of the liver are shown in Table 21.1.

Table 21.1: Functions of the liver

Parameters	Liver functions
Lipid metabolism	Oxidation of triglycerides into the fatty acids, further conversion into ketone bodies for fuel, glucose and cholesterol
	Synthesis and excretion of lipoprotein into the blood
	Synthesis of cholesterol and phospholipid
	Synthesis of bile acids
	Synthesis and excretion of cholesterol and bile acids
Carbohydrate metabolism	Conversion of carbohydrates and proteins into triglycerides and fatty acids
	Regulation of blood glucose by glycogenesis, glycogenolysis and gluconeogenesis
Protein metabolism	Synthesis of plasma proteins including albumin and coagulation factors
	Synthesis of non-essential amino acids
	Synthesis of coagulation factors (II, VII, IX, X)
Waste management, detoxification and drug metabolism	Detoxification of metabolic waste products (e.g. deamination of amino acids and production of urea)
Storage	Storage of vitamins, iron, carbohydrate (glycogen) and fat
Intermediate metabolism	Clearance and excretion of drugs, toxins, metabolic byproducts (bilirubin, ammonia and estrogen hormone)
Secretion	Synthesis and secretion of bile
Bile juice contains many of the products of the above processes	

Functions of the liver and clinical manifestations of altered function are shown in Table 21.2.

Carbohydrate Metabolism

Liver participates in conversion of carbohydrates and proteins into triglycerides and fatty acids. It regulates blood glucose concentration by glycogenesis, glycogenolysis and gluconeogenesis. Hepatic pathway of carbohydrate metabolism is shown in Fig. 21.5.

Protein Metabolism

Liver participates in synthesis of plasma proteins (albumin, α and β globulins and fibrinogen), vitamin K-dependent coagulation factors (II, VII, IX, X), and nonessential amino acids. It also synthesizes α_1-antitrypsin and ceruloplasmin (Fig. 21.6).
- Decreased synthesis of albumin leads to edema.
- Decreased synthesis of fibrinogen and vitamin K-dependent coagulation factors leads to coagulation disorders.
- The α_1-antitrypsin deficiency causes panacinar emphysema and cirrhosis.

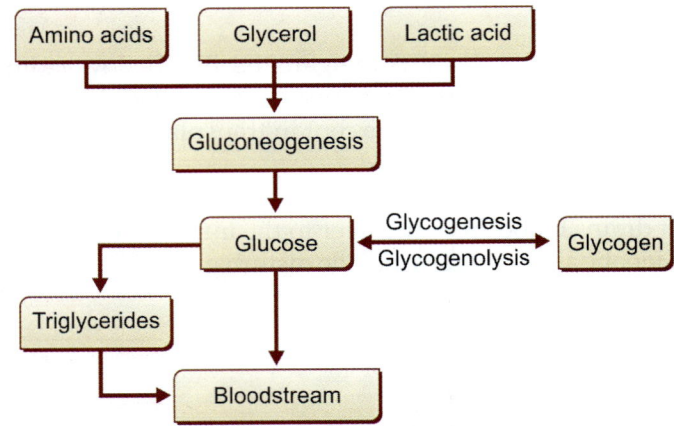

Fig. 21.5: Hepatic pathway for storage and synthesis of glucose and conversion of glucose to fatty acids.

- Deficiency of copper transporting ceruloplasmin protein results in Wilson's disease.

Lipid Metabolism

Liver oxidizes triglycerides into the fatty acids, which can be further metabolized into ketone bodies for

Table 21.2: Functions of the liver and clinical manifestations of altered function

Metabolism	Liver functions	Clinical manifestations of altered function
Carbohydrate metabolism	Glycogen storage and synthesis of glucose derived from amino acids, lactic acid and glycerol	Hypoglycemia due to impaired glycogenolysis and gluconeogenesis. Abnormal glucose tolerance due to impairment of uptake and release of glucose by the liver
Fat metabolism	Lipoprotein synthesis Conversion of proteins and carbohydrates to fat; synthesis, recycling and elimination of cholesterol; formation of ketone bodies from fatty acids	Impaired synthesis of lipoproteins Altered serum cholesterol level
Proteins metabolism	Deamination of proteins and synthesis of urea from ammonia Synthesis of plasma proteins Synthesis of clotting factors (fibrinogen, prothrombin, factors V, VII, IX and X) Synthesis of bile salts Elimination of bilirubin by hepatocytes	Increased blood ammonia level Decreased serum proteins especially albumin resulting in edema Bleeding tendencies due to decreased synthesis of clotting factors Malabsorption of fats and fat soluble vitamins Increased serum bilirubin and jaundice
Metabolism of steroid hormones	Sex hormones Glucocorticoids Aldosterone	Gonadal dysfunction including gynecomastia in male Increased cortisol concentration (Cushing's syndrome) Manifestations of hyperaldosteronism (sodium retention and hypokalemia)
Metabolism of drugs	Drugs metabolism taking place in liver	Decreased metabolism of drug and its binding due to decreased synthesis of albumin
Vitamins and minerals	Storage of vitamins and minerals	Clinical manifestations of fat-soluble vitamins due to deficiency of storage in liver
Filtration and removal of bacteria	Liver Kupffer cells filter and remove bacteria	Increased exposure of coelomic cavities

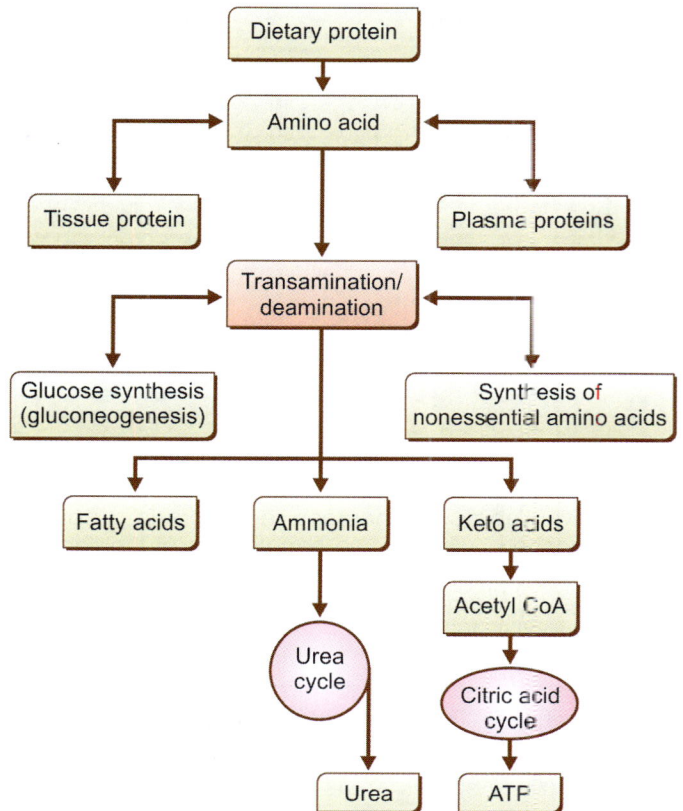

Fig. 21.6: Hepatic pathway of protein metabolism shows conversion of amino acids to proteins, nucleic acids, keto acids and glucose. The urea cycle converts ammonia generated by the deamination of amino acids to urea (acetyl CoA, ATP and adenosine triphosphate).

fuel, glucose and cholesterol. It synthesizes and excretes lipoprotein into the blood. It participates in synthesis and excretion of cholesterol, phospholipid and bile acids. Hepatic lipid metabolism is shown in Fig. 21.7.

Intermediate Metabolism
Liver participates in the clearance and excretion of drugs, toxins metabolic byproducts (bilirubin, ammonia and estrogen hormone).

Waste Management
Liver participates in detoxification of metabolic waste products (e.g. deamination of amino acids and production of urea).

Storage Function
Liver stores vitamins, iron, carbohydrate (glycogen) and fat.

Secretion
Liver participates in synthesis and secretion of bile. Bile juice contains many of the products of the above processes.

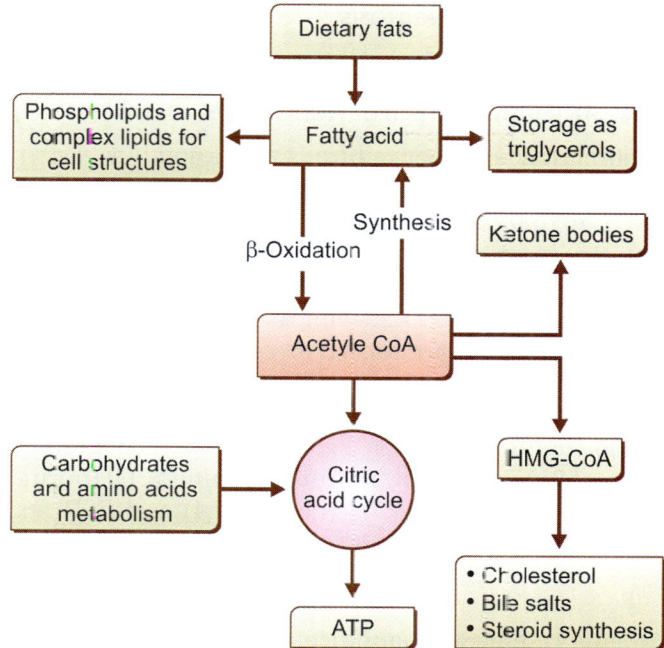

Fig. 21.7: Hepatic lipid metabolism shows β-oxidation breaking fatty acids into two-carbon acetyl CoA units, which are used in the citric acid cycle to generate ATP or synthesis of cholesterol of keto acids leading to their release into blood for utilization by the tissues for energy purpose.

PATTERNS OF NECROSIS

Focal Liver Necrosis
Focal necrosis of liver involves single cell or small group of cells in any area of lobules. But all liver lobules are not affected.

Etiology
Focal necrosis is caused by viral hepatitis, toxic agents and bacteria.

> **Light Microscopy**
> Liver biopsy shows Councilman's bodies (apoptotic bodies) in viral hepatitis. Kupffer cells hyperplasia is seen around necrotic cells.

Zonal Liver Necrosis
Zonal liver necrosis is characterized by involvement of identical region of all hepatic lobules. There are three types of zonal necrosis.

- *Centrilobular necrosis:* It most often occurs due to *cardiac failure, hypotensive shock, viral hepatitis, carbon tetrachloride toxicity* and *chloroform toxicity*.
- *Midzonal necrosis:* It is seen in *yellow fever*.
- *Periportal necrosis:* It occurs due to *phosphorus poison* and *eclampsia of pregnancy*.

Submassive Liver Necrosis

An entire hepatic lobule shows necrosis.

Massive (Fulminant) Liver Necrosis

Fulminant acute liver failure is also known as *massive hepatic necrosis*. It is caused by hepatotropic viruses, drugs, toxins and chemicals. Fulminant acute hepatitis may progress to hepatic encephalopathy within 2–3 weeks of onset of jaundice. Causes of fulminant hepatitis are shown in Table 21.3. Clinical features of fulminant acute liver failure are shown in Table 21.4.

Indications for Immediate Liver Transplantation

These include serum bilirubin level >300 µmol/L (normal 3–17 µmol/L), serum creatinine >300 (normal 70–170 µmol/L), pH <7.3 (normal 7.4) and INR >6.5 (normal 1.0).

Clinical Features

Patient presents with jaundice, bleeding, confusion and disorientation. Marked elevation of ALT and AST are characteristic findings. Serum bilirubin rises rapidly. There is prolonged prothrombin time.

> **Gross Morphology**
> - Liver is soft flabby shrunken in size one-third of its normal weight (500 g) with wrinkled Glisson's capsule.

Table 21.3: Etiology of massive (fulminant) liver necrosis

Categories	Examples
Hepatotropic viruses	HBV, HDV, HEV (20% in pregnant women) and HCV (rare)
Therapeutic drugs	Acetaminophen, methyldopa, isoniazid, halothane, and antidepressants
Toxins	Myotoxin
Chemicals	Carbon tetrachloride and phosphorus

Table 21.4: Clinical features of fulminant acute liver failure

Fulminant liver failure	Clinical manifestations
Hepatic encephalopathy	Grade I: Mild confusion, euphoria or depression
	Grade II: Drowsy and semi-comatose
	Grade III: Stupor (marked confusion but rousable)
	Grade IV: Coma (unrousable)
Jaundice	Yellow discoloration of eyes
Bleeding tendency	Oozing from gastrointestinal tract
Asterixis (flapping tremors)	Demonstrated with the arms outstretched and hands dorsiflexed reflecting uremia

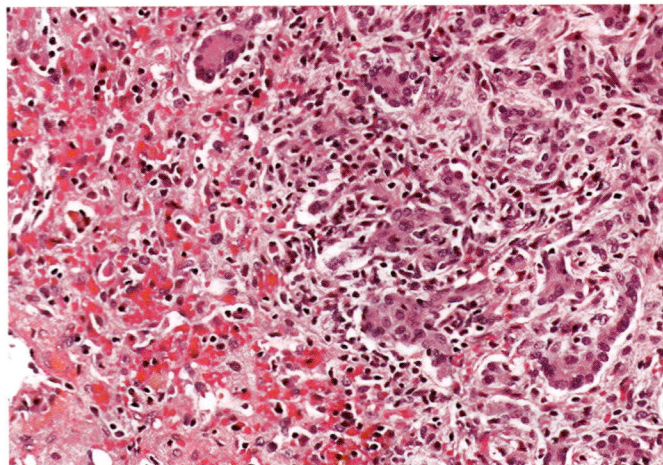

Fig. 21.8: Massive liver necrosis (acute liver failure). There is extensive hepatocyte necrosis seen here in a case of acetaminophen overdose. The hepatocytes at the right are dead, and those at the left are dying. This pattern can be seen with a variety of hepatotoxins. Acute liver failure leads to hepatic encephalopathy (400X).

> - There is presence of patches of greenish bile stained areas.
> - Cut surface shows areas of necrosis and patches of bile stain.

Light Microscopy
- Liver biopsy reveals necrotic liver lobules, leaving a collapsed collagenous and reticulin framework.
- Necrosis and collapse of reticulin framework are responsible for shrinkage of liver.
- The portal tracts appear to be close to each other.
- There may be slight infiltration by chronic inflammatory cells in the portal areas (Fig. 21.8).

Prognosis

Mortality rate is very high in >80% of cases. These patients die unless an emergency liver transplantation is performed. Rest of the patients recover due to regeneration of hepatocytes.

Histological Patterns of Liver Necrosis

Liver cell injuries may occur in isolated or group of cells, periportal piecemeal necrosis and bridging necrosis described as under.

Single cell or group of cells necrosis: This pattern of necrosis of liver cells is seen around terminal hepatic venule. Necrosis of hepatocytes occurs due to viral hepatitis, toxins or obstruction to venous drainage of liver or congestive heart failure (Fig. 21.9).

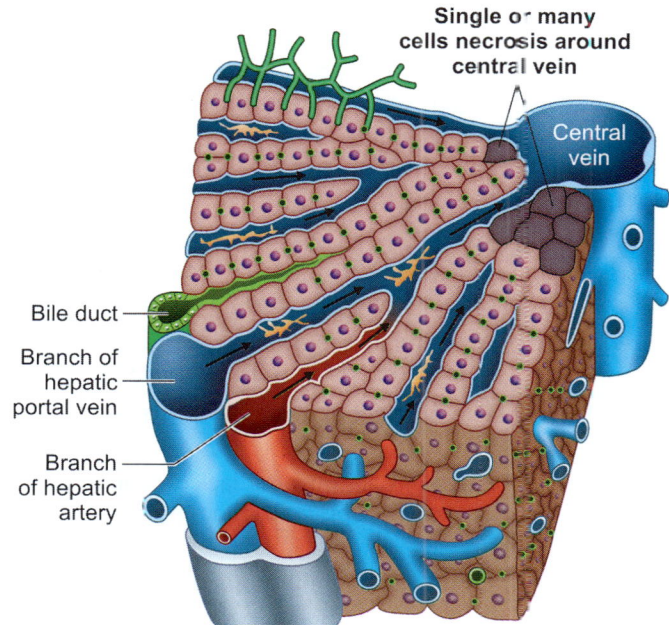

Fig. 21.9: Single cell or group of liver cells necrosis around terminal hepatic venule. This pattern of necrosis of hepatocytes occurs due to viral hepatitis, toxins or obstruction to venous drainage of liver or congestive heart failure.

Periportal piecemeal necrosis: This pattern of necrosis of liver cells is seen around portal tract. It occurs in chronic active hepatitis, autoimmune hepatitis and active cirrhosis (Fig. 21.10).

Bridging necrosis: Bridging necrosis of hepatocytes occurs between portal tract and terminal hepatic venule. It occurs in severe viral infection (Fig. 21.11).

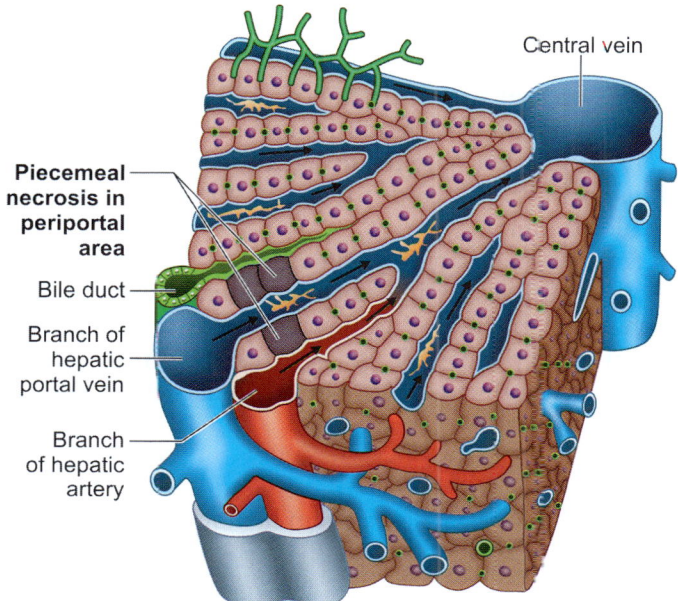

Fig. 21.10: Piecemeal necrosis around periportal area. It occurs in chronic active hepatitis, autoimmune hepatitis and active cirrhosis.

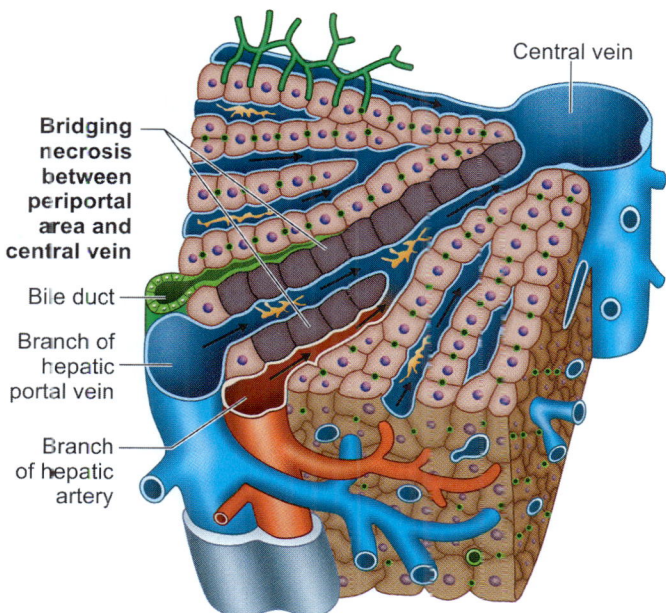

Fig. 21.11: Bridging necrosis of hepatocytes between portal triad and terminal hepatic venule. It occurs in severe viral infection.

Clinical Features

Patient with liver disease shows various clinical manifestations described as under (Table 21.5).

Jaundice

Jaundice refers to yellow discoloration of tissues (sclera) due to deposition of bilirubin pigment as a result of raised serum bilirubin concentration.

Bleeding Tendencies

Patient presents with easy bruising and prolonged clotting time of blood due to failure of synthesis of coagulation factors (II, VII, IX, X).

Edema Legs

Patient presents with edema in dependent parts of lower limb due to decreased synthesis of albumin.

Ascites

Patient presents with ascites due to portal hypertension and decreased albumin synthesis by liver.

Gynecomastia

Patient presents with bilateral gynecomastia due to failure of detoxification of estrogens.

Hepatic Encephalopathy

Patient presents with altered consciousness, lack of coordination, coma and flapping tremors due to failure of detoxification of ammonia and excitatory amino acids derived from protein breakdown.

Table 21.5: Clinical features of liver disease

Clinical signs and symptoms	Mechanism	Clinical features
Jaundice	Failure of uptake, conjugation and excretion of bilirubin	Yellow discoloration of tissues (sclera) due to deposition of bilirubin pigment
Bleeding	Failure of synthesis of vitamin K-dependent coagulation factors (II, VII, IX, X)	Easy bruising and prolonged clotting time of blood
Edema (transudate)	Failure of synthesis of albumin causing decreased oncotic pressure exerted by plasma proteins	Swelling in the dependent part of body due to accumulation of fluid (water) in extracellular compartment
Ascites	Portal hypertension and decreased hepatic synthesis of albumen	Accumulation of fluid in peritoneal cavity, demonstrated by shifting dullness
Gynecomastia	Failure to detoxify endogenous or exogenous estrogens	Enlargement of bilateral breasts
Encephalopathy	Occurs due to failure to detoxify ammonia and excitatory amino acids derived from protein breakdown	Altered consciousness, lack of coordination, coma and flapping tremors
Hematemesis and melena	Portal hypertension	Blood loss in vomitus and stool

Blood Loss in Vomitus and Melena

Patient with portal hypertension presents with bleeding from esophageal varices and melena.

LABORATORY INVESTIGATIONS IN LIVER DISORDERS

Liver function tests frequently give a good idea of the likely cause of liver disease. Serum analysis in liver disorders is carried out to analyze biochemical abnormalities as shown in Tables 21.6 and 21.7. Certain patterns of abnormality suggest a particular type of liver disease, but none is specific.

Alkaline Phosphatase

Alkaline phosphatase enzyme is located on the cell membrane of biliary canaliculi.
- Marked increased level of serum alkaline phosphatase indicates disease of the biliary system (intrahepatic cholestasis, extrahepatic biliary obstruction, or primary biliary cirrhosis).
- Moderate levels are less useful in preceding cause of liver disease.

Transaminases

Transaminases are enzymes located in the hepatocyte cytoplasm.
- Marked increase in level of serum transaminases reflects active necrosis of liver cells from any cause. *ALT is more specific for the liver than AST.*
- Low levels of increase in transaminases may be seen in cholestasis, as well as following induction of enzymes by drugs such as anticonvulsants.
- Elevated *glutamyl transpeptidase* level is a sensitive index of liver cell damage.

Conjugated and Unconjugated Bilirubin

- Conjugated bilirubin is secreted by liver cells. Obstruction of biliary canaliculi causes increased serum bilirubin. But increased conjugated bilirubin is also seen in due to liver cell destruction.
- Unconjugated bilirubin levels increase in disorders causing excessive destruction of red cells.

Albumin

Blood level reflects synthetic properties of the liver. Because of its half-life, low levels of albumin reflect long-standing liver disease, particularly cirrhosis.

Ceruloplasmin

Ceruloplasmin levels are reduced in Wilson's disease. In Wilson's disease mutation of **ATP7B gene** located on chromosome 13 leads to deficiency of a copper transporting ATPase resulting in decrease in copper transport into bile and impairs its incorporation into ceruloplasmin.

Accumulated copper causes toxic injury to organs by free radicals, which displace metals from metalloenzymes. Decreased serum ceruloplasmin, increased hepatic copper (>250 µg/1 g dry weight of liver), and increased urinary copper are consistently seen in Wilson's disease.

Transferrin

Transferrin level is increased in hemochromatosis.

Clotting Abnormalities

Coagulation abnormalities are commonly seen in liver disease due to failure of hepatic synthesis of these proteins. This is a feature of liver failure, as

Table 21.6: Laboratory investigations in liver disorders

Liver disorders	Laboratory investigations	Interpretation
Liver failure	Serum albumin Prothrombin time (normal <15 seconds) measures factors II, V, VII, X	Decreased
Hepatocellular injury	Alanine aminotransferase (ALT) normal <40 IU/L (hepatocellular enzyme) Aspartate aminotransferase (AST) normal <40 IU/L (hepatocellular enzyme) LDH (hepatocellular enzyme) γ-Glutamyltransferase (γ-GT) normal <50 IU/L (plasma membrane enzyme from damage to bile canaliculi) 5′-Nucleotidase (plasma membrane enzyme from damage to bile canaliculi) Serum alkaline phosphatase (plasma membrane enzyme from damage to bile canaliculi)	Increased
Hepatocellular injury, biliary obstruction, liver failure, hemolysis, congenital hyperbilirubinemia	Serum bilirubin (normal 5–12 µmol/L)	Increased
Hepatitis A infection	IgM anti-HAV antibody	Present
Hepatitis B infection or carrier state	HBsAg	Present
Chronic active hepatitis (HBV infection)	HBeAg	Present
HCV exposure	Anti-HCV antibody	Present
HCV induced hepatitis	HCV RNA	Present
Alcoholic cirrhosis	IgA and γ-glutamyltransferase	Increased
Autoimmune hepatitis	IgG, anti-smooth muscle antibody and antinuclear factor	Increased
Primary biliary cirrhosis	IgM, anti-mitochondrial antibody	Increased
Wilson's disease	Ceruloplasmin	Decreased
Hemochromatosis	Ferritin	Increased
Hepatocellular carcinoma	α-fetoproteins (normally undetectable)	Increased
$α_1$-antitrypsin deficiency	$α_1$-antitrypsin	Decreased

Table 21.7: Diagnostic utility of serum autoantibodies in liver disorders

Autoantibodies	Result	Liver disorders
Anti-mitochondrial antibody	Present	Primary biliary cirrhosis (80–90%) Chronic active hepatitis (10–25%)
Anti-smooth muscle antibody	Present	Chronic active hepatitis (20–60%) Primary biliary cirrhosis (10–30%) Alcoholic liver disease (10–15%)
Anti-nuclear antibody	Present	Chronic active hepatitis (20–50%) Primary biliary cirrhosis (15–40%) Drug-induced chronic active hepatitis (10–30%)
Anti-DNA antibody	Present	All types of liver disorders (30–60%)
Hepatocyte membrane antibody	Present	Chronic active hepatitis (40%) Cirrhosis (60%) HBsAg negative acute hepatitis (15%)
Bile canalicular antibody	Present	Chronic active hepatitis (20–40%) Primary biliary cirrhosis (20–40%)

consequence of the end-stage of chronic liver disease such as cirrhosis. *The one-step prothrombin time is a sensitive index of vitamin K-dependent clotting factors (II, VII, IX and X).*

Autoantibodies

Several diseases are associated with abnormal immunological parameters.
- Primary biliary cirrhosis is associated with anti-mitochondrial autoantibodies and raised serum IgM levels.
- Autoimmune chronic hepatitis is associated with anti-smooth muscle antibodies.

Imaging Studies

Imaging studies are valuable as primary investigations of patients with jaundice or tumors and space occupying lesions as part of pre-operative assessment.

Liver Biopsy

Percutaneous Vim Silverman needle biopsy is usually performed to diagnose liver diseases. Blind biopsy of the right side of the liver is used to assess probable diffuse disease processes. CT or ultrasound-guided needle biopsy may be used to sample discrete lesions.

Some liver diseases are diagnosed by considering clinical features, blood tests (LFT), serological tests for viral hepatitis and urine analysis.

Purpose

Liver biopsy is examined to diagnose disease, its severity and progression. Prior to liver biopsy, *prothrombin time estimation is essential*. Prothrombin time is measured to distinguish between hepatocellular jaundice and obstructive jaundice.

Laboratory Investigations

Screening laboratory studies must be carried out 24–48 hours in advance such as complete blood counts, prothrombin time/activated partial thromboplastin time, bleeding time and cross matching for possible transfusion. After liver biopsy, pulse, blood pressure and abdominal girth should be monitored to rule out bleeding. Indications of liver biopsy and complications are shown in Tables 21.8 and 21.9.

Table 21.8: Indications of liver biopsy

Liver cirrhosis
Chronic hepatitis with or without cirrhosis to differentiate chronic persistent and lobular hepatitis
Hepatocellular carcinoma
Metastases in liver
Staging of lymphomas
Persistence of elevated liver enzymes
Cholestasis of unknown etiology
Unexplained splenomegaly
Evaluation of response to treatment

Table 21.9: Complications of liver biopsy

Pain (most common) in <50% of cases. It subsides in 1–2 days
Hemorrhage from puncture site but less frequent
Hemoperitoneum
Subcapsular hematoma in liver
Hemobilia (bleeding in biliary tree)
Bile leakage with peritonitis associated with severe obstruction of the larger bile ducts
Lacerations of kidney, gallbladder, pancreas and other internal organs
Right-sided pneumothorax
Arteriovenous fistula

JAUNDICE AND CHOLESTASIS

Jaundice is also called *icterus*. Clinical jaundice appears when serum bilirubin exceeds 2.5 mg/dl. It causes yellow discoloration of sclerae, skin, and mucous membranes due to accumulation of bilirubin, the catabolic product of the heme moiety of hemoglobin. It is most often associated with *hepatocellular disease, biliary obstruction, or hemolytic anemia*.

BILIRUBIN METABOLISM

After 100–120 days, RBCs are destroyed by reticuloendothelial system and liberate hemoglobin, which dissociates to form heme and globin. Simplified pathway of bilirubin metabolism is shown in Fig. 21.12 and pathogenesis of jaundice is shown in Fig. 21.13.

- Heme consists of porphyrin and iron. Globin goes to amino acid pool. Iron goes to *iron storage sites (bone marrow, spleen and liver) for reutilization.*
- Porphyrin is converted into biliverdin and then unconjugated bilirubin (water insoluble), which goes to liver to form conjugated bilirubin (glucuronyl transferase). Conjugated bilirubin enters bile duct and enters small intestine and excreted in feces.
- Part of bilirubin in intestine is absorbed and goes to liver, which is called *enterohepatic circulation*.
- Rest of conjugated bilirubin is excreted as stercobilinogen in feces. Total normal bilirubin level is 0.3–1.0 mg/dl. Differences between direct and indirect bilirubin are shown in Table 21.10. Deranged

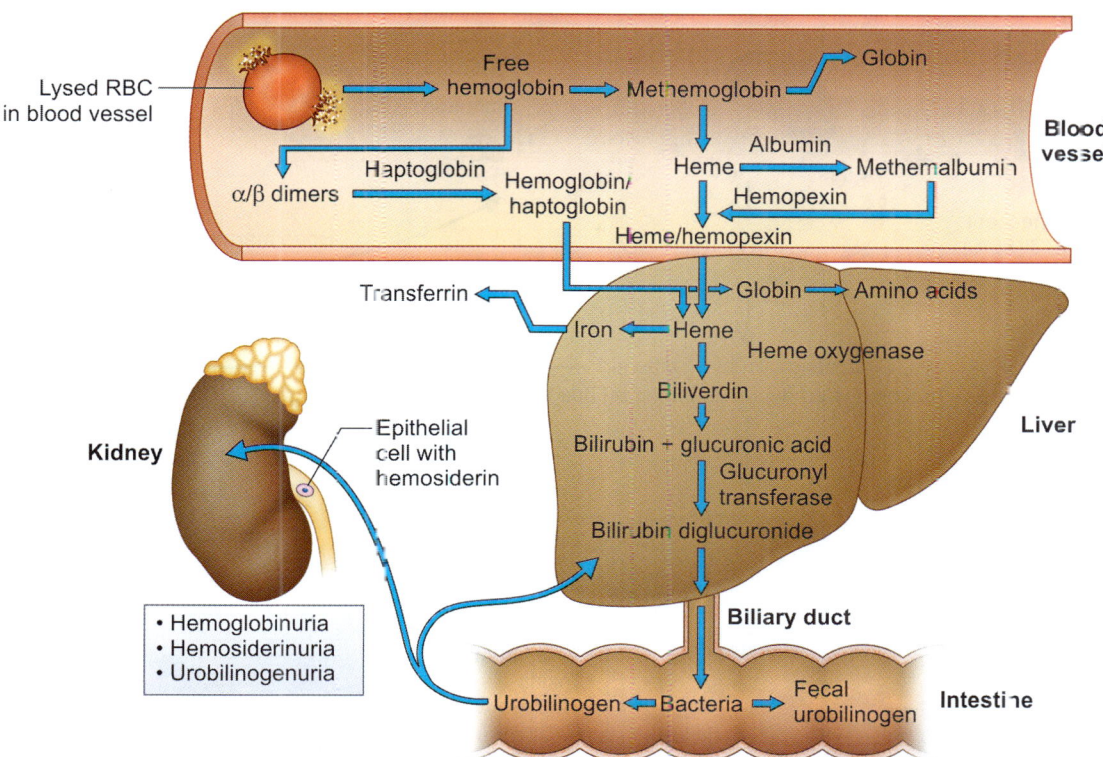

Fig. 21.12: Simplified pathway of bilirubin metabolism. Hemolytic anemia leads to increased biliary excretion of bilirubin. Obstruction of biliary passages will cause regurgitation of conjugated, water-soluble bilirubin into the blood which is then excreted in the urine. Hepatocellular damage in hepatitis will cause impaired biliary excretion of urobilinogen and conjugated bilirubin; these are excreted in the urine, causing it to darken. The enterohepatic circulation returns *cholic acid* and *chenodeoxycholic acid* to the liver; this enhances bile secretion.

Table 21.10: Differences between direct bilirubin and indirect bilirubin

Direct bilirubin	Indirect bilirubin
Normal range (0–0.2 mg/dl)	Normal range (0.3–0.7 mg/dl)
Conjugated bilirubin (direct reacting)	Unconjugated bilirubin (indirect reacting)
Water soluble	Lipophilic and water insoluble
Loosely bound to albumin	Tightly bound to albumin
Easily filtered by glomeruli and excreted in urine	Not filtered by glomeruli, hence not excreted in urine
Unable to cross blood–brain barrier	Able to cross blood–brain barrier and damages brain of the newborn (kernicterus) with erythroblastosis fetalis

bilirubin metabolism in various disorders is shown in Table 21.11.

PHYSIOLOGICAL JAUNDICE

Physiological jaundice is also called *neonatal jaundice*. It is common but clinically insignificant characterized by unconjugated hyperbilirubinemia observed during the first week of life.

Transient jaundice results from both increased bilirubin production and a relative deficiency of glucuronyl transferase in the immature liver especially in premature infants. It is known as *physiological jaundice of newborn*.

It must be distinguished from neonatal cholestasis due to extrahepatic *biliary atresia, α_1-antitrypsin deficiency* and *cytomegalovirus infection*.

CHOLESTASIS

Failure to drain bile leads to the appearance in the plasma of increased concentrations of all constituents of bile such as bilirubin, alkaline phosphatase, IgA and less often cholesterol.

Causes of cholestasis are shown in Table 21.12. Cholestasis due to intrahepatic and extrahepatic causes is shown in Table 21.13.

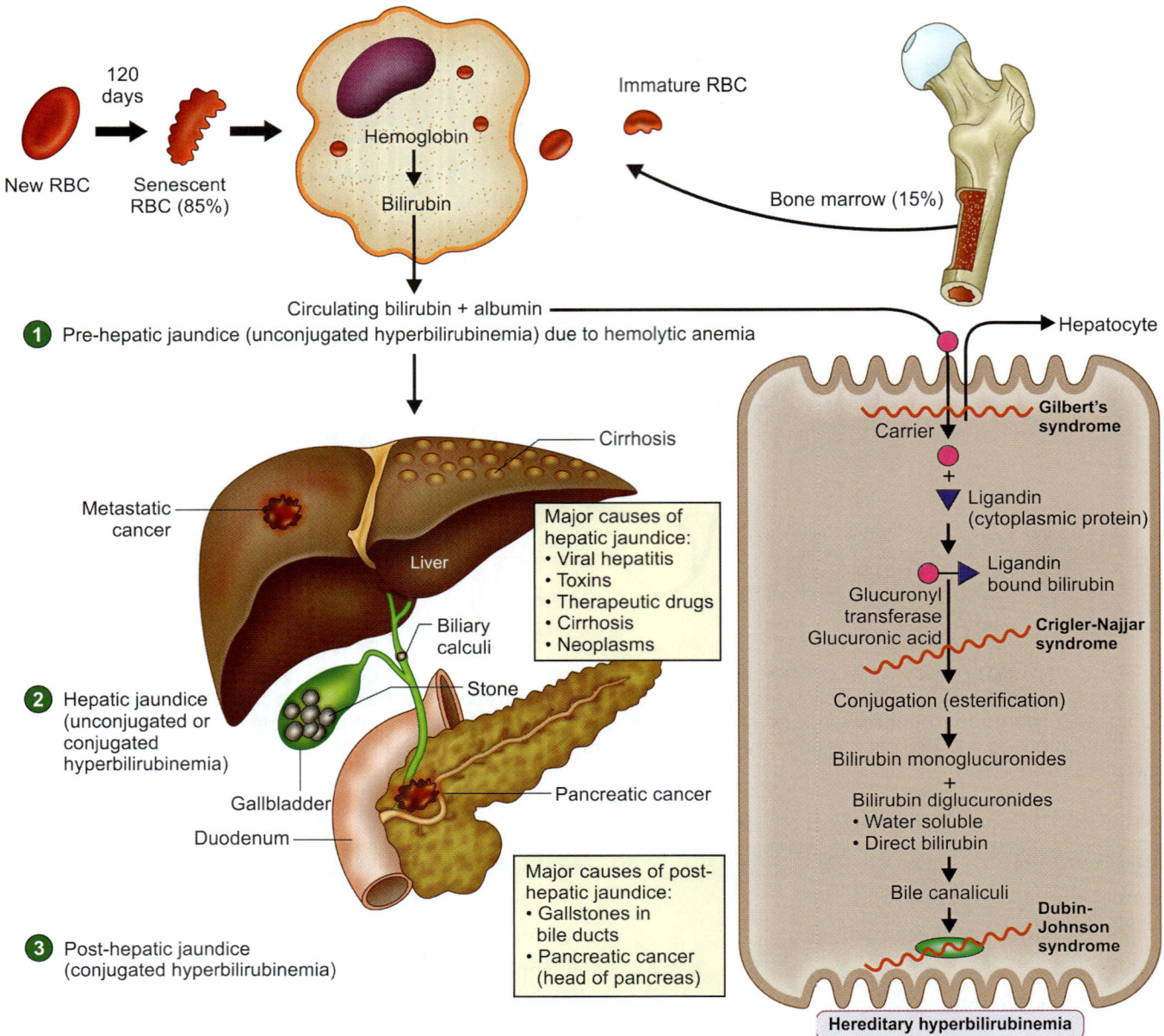

Fig. 21.13: Pathogenesis of jaundice.

Secondary changes resulting from cholestasis

- *Scattered liver cell necrosis:* Increased concentration of bile causes scattered liver cell injury.
- *Cellular debris in macrophages:* Macrophages accumulate bile pigment and cellular debris.
- *Periportal fibrosis and proliferation of bile ductules:* These histological findings are nonspecific.
- *Feathery degeneration of hepatocytes:* Liver cells are swollen due to accumulation of water and bile pigment.
- *Formation of bile lakes:* Long-standing cholestasis may cause liver cell injury. Extravasated bile pigments form brownish-yellow masses admixed with cellular debris.

RECURRENT JAUNDICE DURING PREGNANCY

It most often occurs in the third trimester of pregnancy, after seven months of gestation. Biochemical findings mimic extrahepatic biliary obstruction. Jaundice clears after delivery, which may recur with subsequent pregnancy. Etiology is related to increased levels of estrogens. Complications include stillbirths, prematurity and fetal distress.

HEREDITARY HYPERBILIRUBINEMIA

Under physiological state, after a span of 100–120 days, red blood cells release unconjugated bilirubin. Hepatocytes participate in conjugation of bilirubin and its excretion in biliary ducts.

Table 21.11: Deranged bilirubin metabolism in various disorders

Pathophysiology of hyperbilirubinemia	Causes
Pre-hepatic causes (increased bilirubin production)	Hemolytic anemia
	Aortic aneurysm rupture
	Massive intestinal hemorrhage
	Blood resorption from large hematoma
Hepatic causes (decreased uptake of bilirubin)	Gilbert's syndrome*
	Diffuse hepatocellular injury by HBV and HCV
	Chloramphenicol drug
	Flavaspidic drug used in tapeworm infestations (drug inhibiting uptake of bilirubin by binding to the ligand)
	Contrast media used for cholecystography
Hepatic impaired conjugation of bilirubin (unconjugated hyperbilirubinemia)	Neonatal jaundice
	Crigler-Najjar syndrome (Types I and II)*
	Gilbert's syndrome
	Hepatic impaired excretion of bilirubin (conjugated hyperbilirubinemia)
	Dubin-Johnson syndrome*
	Rotor's syndrome*
	Hepatitis
	Pregnancy associated cholestasis (recurrent jaundice of pregnancy)
	Drugs causing intrahepatic cholestasis such as oral contraceptives and anabolic hormones
	Alcoholic cirrhosis
	Primary biliary cirrhosis
	Hepatic infiltration
	Sepsis
Post-hepatic obstruction of bilirubin outflow in extra-hepatic biliary passages (conjugated hyperbilirubinemia)	Primary sclerosing cholangitis
	Gallstones
	Cholangiocarcinoma
	Portahepatitis lymph nodes
	Biliary atresia
	Surgical induced biliary stenosis
	Carcinoma of head of pancreas
	Carcinoma of ampulla of Vater
	Pancreatitis

*Gilbert's syndrome, Crigler-Najjar syndrome, Dubin-Johnson syndrome, and Rotor's syndrome are examples of hereditary hyperbilirubinemia.

There are three steps: uptake of unconjugated bilirubin by hepatocytes, conjugation of bilirubin by glucuronyl transferase enzyme in hepatocytes and excretion of conjugated bilirubin in biliary ducts. Defects at any level may result in congenital hyperbilirubinemia. Examples are Gilbert's syndrome, Crigler-Najjar syndrome, Dubin-Johnson syndrome and Rotor syndrome. Comparison of various types of hereditary hyperbilirubinemia is shown in Table 21.14.

GILBERT'S SYNDROME

Gilbert's syndrome is familial autosomal dominant as well as recessive disorder. It is characterized by mild, recurrent, unconjugated hyperbilirubinemia (<6 mg/dl) due to impaired clearance of bilirubin in the absence of significant liver disease. This disease is usually detected in later life. Aside from jaundice, patients are asymptomatic.

Table 21.12: Causes of cholestasis

Pathophysiology of cholestasis	Causes
Extrahepatic mechanical obstruction	Primary sclerosing cholangitis
	Gallstones
	Cholangiocarcinoma
	Portahepatitis lymph nodes
	Biliary atresia
	Surgical induced biliary stenosis
	Carcinoma of head of pancreas
	Carcinoma of ampulla of Vater
	Pancreatitis
Intrahepatic mechanical obstruction	Granulomas
	Metastatic neoplasms
	Cystic fibrosis
Mechanical obstruction in infancy	Biliary atresia (extrahepatic or intrahepatic)
Intrahepatic cholestasis without obstruction	Certain infections
	α-Antitrypsin deficiency
	Part of paraneoplastic syndromes in renal cell carcinoma
	Pregnancy
	Viral hepatitis
	Hepatotoxic drugs
	Idiopathic recurrent cholestasis
	Familial progressive cholestasis (Byler's disease)
	Primary biliary cirrhosis
	Other types of cirrhosis

Table 21.13: Cholestasis due to extrahepatic and intrahepatic causes

Liver biopsy (LM)	Extrahepatic cholestasis	Intrahepatic cholestasis
Cholestasis	Severe degree	Mild degree
Bile pigments present	Ducts and ductules	Hepatocytes and Kupffer cells
	Rupture of bile canaliculi leading to bile lake formation	
Acute inflammation (PMNs cells) in bile ducts	Present surrounding bile duct and canaliculi	Absent surrounding bile duct and canaliculi
Feathery degeneration of hepatocytes	Unremarkable	Marked

Etiology

The cause is a combination of decreased bilirubin uptake by liver cells and reduced activity of glucuronyl transferase.

Clinical Features

Patient presents with episodic hyperbilirubinemia precipitated by stress, fatigue, alcohol use, or recurrent infection.

> **Light Microscopy**
> Liver morphology is otherwise unimpaired.

CRIGLER-NAJJAR SYNDROME

Crigler-Najjar syndrome is familial disorder characterized by unconjugated hyperbilirubinemia due to lack of glucuronyl transferase enzyme or its decreased activity in hepatocytes. Differences between Crigler-Najjar syndrome types I and II are shown in Table 21.15. Crigler-Najjar syndrome has two variants described as under:

Crigler-Najjar syndrome type I: It is *most severe disorder*. A total lack of glucuronyl transferase results in early death from kernicterus; damage to the basal ganglia and other parts of the central nervous system caused by unconjugated bilirubin.

Table 21.14: Comparison of various types of hereditary hyperbilirubinemias

Disorder	Inheritance	Bilirubin metabolism defects	Serum bilirubin	Clinical course	Prognosis
Unconjugated hyperbilirubinemia					
Gilbert's syndrome	Autosomal dominant	UDP-glucuronyl transferase activity decreased	<6 mg/dl	Episodic hyperbilirubinemia (marked jaundice)	Excellent
Crigler-Najjar syndrome type I	Autosomal recessive	UDP-glucuronyl transferase activity absent	>20 mg/dl	Fatal outcome during neonatal period (mild jaundice)	Poor
Crigler-Najjar syndrome type II	Autosomal dominant	UDP-glucuronyl transferase activity decreased	<20 mg/dl	Mild course (mild jaundice)	Good
Conjugated hyperbilirubinemia					
Dubin-Johnson syndrome	Autosomal recessive	Impaired bilirubin excretion due to mutation of canalicular multidrug resistance protein 2 (MRP2)	<5 mg/dl	Intermittent mild jaundice, mild hepatomegaly (brown-to-black in hepatocytes)	Excellent
Rotor's syndrome	Autosomal recessive	Decreased hepatic uptake and storage. Decreased biliary excretion	<6 mg/dl	Benign course (mild jaundice)	Good

Table 21.15: Differences between Crigler-Najjar syndrome types I and II

Characteristics	Crigler-Najjar syndrome	
	Type I	Type II
Disorder	Autosomal dominant disorder	Autosomal recessive disorder
Glucuronyl transferase enzyme	Complete deficiency	Deficiency varying from one person to another
Kernicterus	Common	Rarely
Clinical course	Severe type	Mild type
Bilirubin	Unconjugated hyperbilirubinemia	Bile consisting of unconjugated as well as conjugated hyperbilirubinemia
Prognosis	Death during first year	Life is compatible depending on content of glucuronyl transferase enzyme
Response to phenobarbital therapy	No response	Responds well results in synthesis of glucuronyl transferase enzyme

Crigler-Najjar syndrome type II: It is *less severe form* and compatible with life. It *responds to phenobarbital therapy*, which decreases the serum concentration of unconjugated bilirubin.

DUBIN-JOHNSON SYNDROME

Dubin-Johnson syndrome is an autosomal recessive familial disorder. Conjugated hyperbilirubinemia occurs due to defective bilirubin transport. *Liver biopsy shows conspicuous deposition of melanin-like pigment.*

Molecular Genetics

Dubin-Johnson syndrome occurs due to gene mutation of *canalicular membrane protein 2 (MRP2)*. MRP2 participates in ATP dependent excretion of bilirubin mono- and diglucuronides across the canalicular membrane into the bile canaliculi.

Clinical Features

Patient presents with intermittent mild jaundice, hepatomegaly and nonspecific gastrointestinal symptoms.

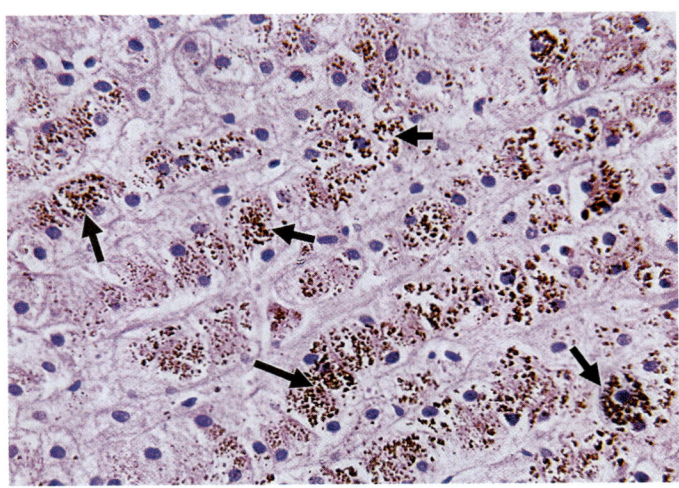

Fig. 21.14: Dubin-Johnson syndrome. Liver shows deposition of brown-to-black melanin-like pigment in hepatocytes and Kupffer cells mainly in centrilobular region (arrows) (400X).

Gross Morphology

It reveals *blackish discoloration* of liver due to accumulation of polymerized epinephrine metabolites.

Light Microscopy

Liver architecture is normal. It shows deposition of brown-to-black *melanin-like pigment in hepatocytes and Kupffer cells mainly in centrilobular region* (Fig. 21.14). This feature differentiates from other congenital conjugated hyperbilirubinemia.

Histochemistry

The chemical nature of this pigment is not clear. The dark pigment is demonstrated by *Masson Fontana stain*.

Laboratory Investigations

Serum bilirubin level is raised between 2 and 5 mg/dl. Serum transaminases and alkaline phosphatase are within normal limits. *Bromsulphthalein excretion* is a diagnostic test for Dubin-Johnson syndrome.

ROTOR SYNDROME

Rotor's syndrome is a relatively benign condition resulting in conjugated hyperbilirubinemia. It is similar to Dubin-Johnson syndrome, but abnormal pigment is not present. Both Dubin-Johnson syndrome and Rotor syndrome cause conjugated hyperbilirubinemia (<6 mg/dl).

NEONATAL CHOLESTASIS

Neonatal cholestasis occurs due to various disorders (Table 21.16).

BILIARY ATRESIA

Extrahepatic biliary atresia is characterized by inflammation with stricture of hepatic or common bile ducts. This leads to marked cholestasis with intrahepatic bile duct proliferation, fibrosis, and cirrhosis. The *liver becomes rock hard*.

Light Microscopy

Histological examination of liver shows numerous brown-green bile plugs, bile duct proliferation, and extensive fibrosis (Fig. 21.15).

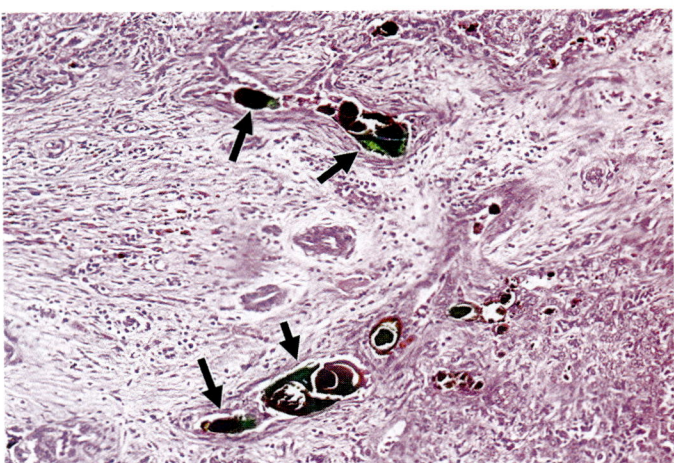

Fig. 21.15: Extrahepatic biliary atresia shows numerous brown-green bile plugs, bile duct proliferation, and extensive fibrosis (arrows) (100X).

Table 21.16: Major causes of neonatal cholestasis

Categories	Etiological agents
Bile duct obstruction	Extrahepatic biliary atresia
Neonatal infection	Cytomegalovirus, bacterial sepsis, syphilis or urinary tract infection
Toxic substances	Drugs like acetaminophen, methyldopa, halothane, antidepressants and isoniazid
Metabolic disorders	Niemann-Pick disease, tyrosinemia, galactosemia, cystic fibrosis, α_1-antitrypsin deficiency or defective bile acid synthetic pathways
Miscellaneous disorders	Indian childhood cirrhosis, Alagille syndrome (paucity of bile ducts) or hypotensive shock
Idiopathic neonatal hepatitis	Unknown

ALAGILLE SYNDROME

Alagille syndrome is a rare genetic autosomal dominant disorder. It can affect the liver, heart and other organs. It is characterized by abnormalities in the bile ducts leading to liver damage. *Mutation in notch signaling pathway is involved in the development of this disorder.*

Patient presents with mild to severe symptoms such as jaundice, pruritus, xanthomas, congenital heart defects, butterfly shape of vertebral column and other bones (radiographs).

DRUGS INDUCED HEPATITIS

Various therapeutic drugs may induce hepatitis. These include acetaminophen, methyldopa, halothane, antidepressants and isoniazid.

> **Light Microscopy**
>
> Liver biopsy shows presence of eosinophils in the portal tracts, evidence of cholestasis, and sometimes granulomas.

CAROLI DISEASE

Caroli disease is autosomal dominant trait disorder. Mutation of PKHD1 gene linked to ARPKD has been demonstrated in patient with Caroli disease. There is history of liver and kidney disease. It is characterized by segmental dilatation of larger intrahepatic ducts associated with bile inspissation.

It is frequently complicated by cholelithiasis and hepatic abscess. There is increased risk of development of cholangiocarcinoma.

NEONATAL HEPATITIS OF UNKNOWN ETIOLOGY

Neonatal hepatitis is of unknown etiology in 50% cases. Approximately 30% of cases are assigned to α_1-antitrypsin deficiency alone. Most of the other known causes can be attributed to chromosomal abnormalities or intrauterine infections or biliary atresia.

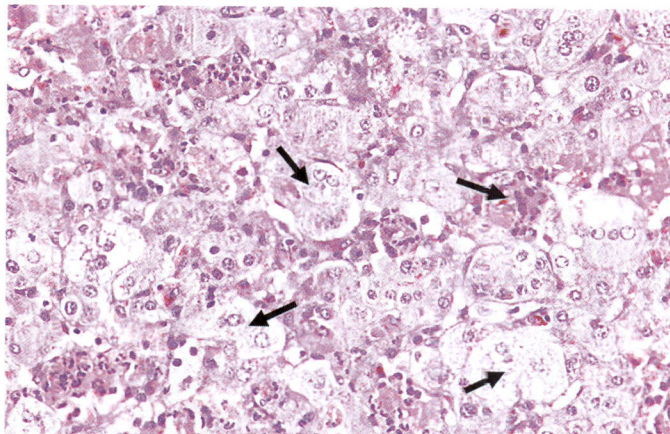

Fig. 21.16: Neonatal hepatitis. Seen here is the major differential diagnosis of biliary atresia: This is neonatal giant cell hepatitis. There is lobular disarray with focal hepatocyte necrosis, giant cell transformation, lymphocytic infiltration, Kupffer cell hyperplasia, and cholestasis (not seen here). Neonatal hepatitis may be idiopathic or of viral origin. Many neonates recover in a couple of months (arrows) (400X).

Clinical Features

Neonatal hepatitis may cause jaundice during the first few weeks of life. Most infants with uncomplicated neonatal hepatitis eventually recover. Untreated biliary obstruction causes progressive fibrosis resulting in secondary biliary cirrhosis.

> **Light Microscopy**
>
> - Liver biopsy shows presence of multinucleated giant cells (characteristic finding).
> - These giant cells contain as many as 40 nuclei and may appear detached from other cells in the liver plate.
> - Hepatocytes may contain bile pigment due to prolonged cholestasis and hemosiderin (Fig. 21.16).

DIFFERENTIAL DIAGNOSIS OF JAUNDICE

Differential diagnosis of jaundice (Table 21.17) and disorders causing type of hyperbilirubinemia (Table 21.18).

Table 21.17: Differential diagnosis of jaundice

Etiology	Serum	Urine	Stool color
Hemolytic anemia	Unconjugated hyperbilirubinemia	Normal	Dark
Hepatocellular jaundice (e.g. acute hepatitis)	Mixed hyperbilirubinemia Increased transaminases	Dark	Pale
Obstructive jaundice (e.g. cholestasis)	Conjugated hyperbilirubinemia Increased alkaline phosphatase Increased transaminases	Dark	Pale
Congenital hyperbilirubinemia (e.g. Gilbert's syndrome)	Unconjugated or conjugated hyperbilirubinemia Other tests normal No evidence of hemolysis	Variable	Variable

Section III: Systemic Pathology

Table 21.18: Disorders causing hyperbilirubinemia

Causes	Alkaline phosphatase and AST/ALT	Hyperbilirubinemia
Gallstone, carcinoma of common bile duct obstruct the bile flow	Alkaline phosphatase level >AST/ALT occurs in obstructive jaundice	Direct (conjugated) bilirubin >15% of total bilirubin
Pancreatic head carcinoma		
Viral hepatitis induced hepatocellular damage	Alkaline phosphatase level <AST/ALT	
Physiological jaundice of newborn	Not applicable	Indirect (unconjugated) bilirubin <15% of total bilirubin
Hemolytic anemia		
Breast milk jaundice due to presence of β-glucuronidase in milk		
Diffuse hepatocellular damage due to cirrhosis, viruses and drugs		
Gilbert's syndrome		
Crigler-Najjar syndrome (types I and II)		

HEMOLYTIC JAUNDICE

Hemolytic jaundice occurs due to rapid destruction of red blood cells resulting in production of excess of bilirubin. Liver is not able to conjugate excess of bilirubin. Hemolytic disease of the newborn most commonly occurs with Rh blood group incompatibility between mother and fetus.

Clinical Features

Patient develops jaundice due to excess of unconjugated bilirubin in blood. This is seen in sickle cell disease, mismatched blood transfusions and some infections.

Urine Analysis

Urine analysis shows increased urobilinogen and absence of bilirubin (acholuria). Degree of urine urobilinogen increase is directly related to increased hemoglobin catabolism.

HEPATOCELLULAR JAUNDICE

This occurs due to hepatitis, congenital hyperbilirubinemia (malfunction of glucuronyl transferase enzyme systems), and hepatocellular carcinoma. Patient develops jaundice due to excess of conjugated and unconjugated bilirubin in blood. Urine analysis may show normal or decreased urobilinogen.

EXTRAHEPATIC JAUNDICE

Extrahepatic jaundice is related to mechanical obstruction outside the liver due to gallstones or pancreatic tumors obstructing pancreatic biliary duct.

Clinical Features

Patient presents with jaundice due to excess of conjugated bilirubin in blood passage of clay-colored stools.

Urine Analysis

Urine analysis shows decreased urobilinogen. Serum enzymes ALT and AST levels are variable.

Blood Biochemistry

Alkaline phosphatase and cholesterol are increased.

HEPATITIS

ACUTE/CHRONIC VIRAL HEPATITIS

Hepatitis refers to inflammation of the liver caused by viruses, autoimmune mechanisms, drugs, toxins or secondary to other systemic disorders.

VIRUSES

The known *hepatotropic viruses* primarily affecting liver cells include hepatitis A virus (HAV), hepatitis B virus (HBV), hepatitis B-associated delta virus (HDV), hepatitis C virus (HCV), and hepatitis E virus (HEV).

Viruses causing systemic disease that can involve the liver include Epstein-Barr virus (infectious mononucleosis), which may cause a mild hepatitis during the acute phase; cytomegalovirus (particularly in newborns and immunosuppressed persons); herpesviruses; and enteroviruses.

CLINICAL COURSE

Infection with hepatotropic viruses may produce clinical manifestations of varying grades of severity ranging from mild jaundice, nausea and anorexia to fulminating illness resulting in acute liver failure with fatal outcome. Some cases may progress to *cirrhosis* with increased risk of development of *hepatocellular carcinoma*. Clinical course of the following viral hepatitis is shown in Table 21.19 and differentiating histological features of acute and chronic viral hepatitis are shown in Table 21.20.

Table 21.19: Clinical course of the following viral hepatitis

Clinical pattern of disease	Viruses
Asymptomatic (most often with HAV infection)	HAV, HBV, HCV, HDV and HEV
Acute hepatitis without jaundice (anicteric hepatitis)	HAV, HBV, HCV, HDV and HEV
Acute hepatitis with jaundice (icteric jaundice)	HAV, HBV, HCV, HDV and HEV
Massive liver necrosis with acute liver failure (rare)	HAV, HBV, HCV, HDV and HEV
Chronic hepatitis	HBV, HCV and HDV
Chronic career state	HBV, HCV and HDV

Table 21.20: Differentiating histological features of acute and chronic viral hepatitis

Parameters	Acute viral hepatitis	Chronic viral hepatitis
Hepatocellular injury		
Hepatotropic virus	HAV (most frequent), HBV, HCV, HDV, HEV	HBV, HCV, HDV
Lobular disarray	Disrupted liver architecture	Disrupted liver architecture
Area involved	Centrilobular zone of liver	Throughout liver lobule
Cell swelling (ballooning degeneration)	Present	Present
Cholestasis (bile plugs)	Present	Present
Fatty change	Present (HCV infection)	Present (HCV infection)
Cytolysis of liver cells	Isolated or cluster of cells	Isolated or cluster of cells
Councilman bodies in sinusoids	Present	-
Portal tract inflammation	Uncommon unless severe inflammation	Common
Spillover inflammation from portal tract into liver acinus causing necrosis of liver cells	Uncommon unless severe inflammation	Common (interface necrosis)
Bridging inflammation and necrosis	Uncommon unless severe inflammation	Common
Piecemeal necrosis	Absent	Present (hallmark of progressive liver damage)
Regeneration of hepatocytes	Present	Present
Sinusoidal cell reactive changes	Kupffer cells accumulating phagocytosed cellular debris	Kupffer cells accumulating phagocytosed cellular debris
	Mononuclear cell infiltration	Mononuclear cell infiltration
Fibrosis	Absent	Portal and periportal fibrosis with formation of bridging fibrous septa
Ground-glass appearance of hepatocytes due to accumulation of HBsAg	Absent	Present due to HBV infection
Bile duct epithelial proliferation and lymphoid aggregates	Absent	Present due to HCV infection
Cirrhosis	Absent	Common with fatal outcome
Hepatocellular carcinoma	Absent	Increased risk

Histological changes shared by acute and chronic viral hepatitis are liver cell injury, necrosis of hepatocytes, apoptosis of liver cells, regeneration of hepatocytes and sinusoidal changes.

- *Acute viral hepatitis:* It is characterized by jaundice and extremely high elevations of *serum enzymes (aspartate and alanine aminotransferases)*. It is diagnosed clinically by serological and biochemical tests. On histopathological study, acute viral hepatitis is characterized by *liver cell injury and regeneration, chronic inflammation but absence of fibrosis*. The presence of viral antigens and their antibodies can be determined through laboratory tests.
- *Chronic viral hepatitis:* Chronicity of the inflammatory process are especially associated with infection with HBV, HCV and HDV. Light microscopy shows *liver cell injury and regeneration, chronic inflammation and presence of fibrosis*.

TERMINOLOGY

- Terminology of chronic hepatitis has evolved. In the past, chronic persistent hepatitis, chronic lobular hepatitis and chronic active hepatitis denoted the severity of chronic hepatitis.
- Current recommendations are to indicate *chronic hepatitis*, the severity of *necroinflammatory activity (grade)*, the *extent of fibrosis (stage)* and etiology.
- Most commonly used systems for grading and staging are the *Ishak Modification of Hepatitis Activity Index and METAVIR system* (Table 21.21).

ETIOPATHOGENESIS

Various viruses may infect the liver. Hepatotropic viruses infecting liver include *HAV, HBV, HCV, HDV and HEV*. Other viruses are *Epstein-Barr virus, cytomegalovirus, rubella, adenovirus and enterovirus*. Acute viral hepatitis shows similar morphology irrespective of their precise etiology.

HAV infection has direct cytopathic effect. Liver cell injury occurs due to attack by cytotoxic T and killer cells followed by antibodies formed against viral neoantigens expressed on virally infected hepatocytes.

The mechanisms of injury have been most closely studied in HBV. It is thought that the extent of inflammation and necrosis depends on the person's immune response.

- *Prompt immune response:* A prompt immune response during the acute phase of the infection may cause liver cell injury but at the same time eliminate the virus.

Table 21.21: Classification of hepatitis based on etiology and histologic activity (grades)

Classification of hepatitis based on etiology	
Hepatotropic viruses	HAV, HBV, HCV, HDV and HEV (most common)
Uncommon viruses	Cytomegalovirus and herpes virus in immunocompromised persons, yellow fever virus (causing mid-zonal necrosis), Epstein-Barr virus, rubella virus, Ebola virus, adenovirus and enterovirus
Parasites	*Entamoeba histolytica, Echinococcus granulosus* infestation and *Schistosoma mansoni* or *japonicum*
Leptospira species	Weil's disease characterized by jaundice, renal failure, and icterohemorrhagic fever
Autoimmune hepatitis	Immune-mediated
Drug-induced hepatitis	Acute hepatitis: sulphonylureas, phenothiazines and tricyclic antidepressants
	Chronic hepatitis: methotrexate, α-methyldopa, nitrofurantoin and oxyphenisatin
Based on histologic activity (grade): necrosis and inflammation	
Portal inflammation	Inflammation confined to portal tract
Periportal inflammation	Inflammation extending from portal tract to surrounding periportal area
Piecemeal necrosis (now known as *interface necrosis*)	Seen in viral hepatitis, autoimmune hepatitis and steatohepatitis characterized by loss of hepatocytes between lobule and limiting plate of portal tracts. New term *toxic necrosis* suggested after the Greek noun meaning *nibbling*
Bridging necrosis	Confluent necrosis bridging adjacent central veins of hepatic lobules and portal triads. Bridging necrosis is characteristic of subacute hepatitis
Classification of hepatitis based on degree of fibrosis (progression of disease)	
Stage 0	Liver does not show fibrosis
Stage 1	Liver showing mild fibrosis confined to portal tract
Stage 2	Liver showing moderate fibrosis in portal and periportal areas
Stage 3	Liver showing severe fibrosis (bridging necrosis)
Stage 4	Liver showing cirrhosis

- *Marginal immune response:* People with marginal immune response and fewer symptoms are less likely to eliminate the virus, and hepatocytes expressing the viral antigens persist, resulting in the chronic or carrier state.
- *Accelerated immune response:* Fulminant hepatitis would be explained in terms of an accelerated immune response with severe liver necrosis.

Hepatocellular Injury

Liver cell injury is marked in centrilobular zone. Ballooning degeneration and Councilman bodies are prominent features.

- *Ballooning degeneration:* Small clusters of hepatocytes show ballooning degeneration with empty look and granules around nucleus. The cytoplasm of liver cells does not bind eosin giving empty appearance.

  This empty appearance of cytoplasm correlates with intracellular edema and consequent dilatation of the endoplasmic reticulum, loss of ribosomes and swelling of the mitochondria. Ballooning degeneration may cause necrosis of some hepatocytes. Effect of this type of injury may be reversible in some cases.
- *Biliary cholestasis:* Bile accumulates in the biliary canaliculi which causes feathery appearance of hepatocytes.
- *Fatty change:* Mild fatty change is seen in hepatocytes especially with HCV infection.

Hepatocellular Necrosis

- *Liver cell necrosis:* Isolated cell or clusters of cells may undergo irreversible cell necrosis. Apoptosis removes viral infected scattered hepatocytes. Apoptotic cells represent membrane-bound cellular chromatin remnants that are extruded into the hepatic sinusoids in cases of viral hepatitis. These are called *Councilman bodies*. These appear as eosinophilic stained structures in hematoxylin and eosin stained sections seen under light microscope.
- *Bridging necrosis:* Severe hepatocellular injury may lead to bridging necrosis (portal-portal, central-central or portal-central).
- *Lobular disarray:* Normal architecture of liver is disrupted.
- *Regenerative changes:* Hepatocytes may show proliferative changes.

Sinusoidal Cell Reactive Changes

Kupffer cells are prominent and increased in number in the sinusoids. These contain phagocytosed cellular debris, bile pigments and lipofuscin pigment. There is influx of lymphocytes, plasma cells and macrophages into sinusoids.

Inflammatory Response with Influx of Mononuclear Cells

- *Portal tract:* Portal tract is also the site of inflammation. Connective tissue of portal tract shows infiltration by lymphocytes, macrophages and plasma cells. Presence of neutrophils and eosinophils are not uncommon. Persistent inflammation and fibrosis is an unfavorable sign of chronic hepatitis progressing to postnecrotic cirrhosis.
- *Liver acinus:* Spillover of chronic inflammatory cells (lymphocytes, macrophages and plasma cells) from portal tract into liver acinus causes liver cell necrosis. Inflammation is most severe in the perivenular region of acinar zone.

Changes in the Connective Tissue Framework

In majority of cases, there is insufficient liver cell necrosis exhibiting normal architecture of liver cell plates. In more severe cases with extensive liver cell necrosis exhibit bridging necrosis extending from portal tract to central vein. There is collapse of reticulin fiber framework in this area. Bridging necrosis is the most serious development, because there is increased risk of subsequent cirrhosis.

Gross Morphology

- Acute viral hepatitis progressing to fulminant acute liver failure leads to reduction in size of the liver.
- Liver capsule shows wrinkling indicating rapid reduction of liver cell mass. Cut surface of such liver exhibits red appearance. It may greenish due to cholestasis.
- In some cases, there is evidence of commencing regeneration of hepatocytes in the form of rounded yellowish areas scattered against the red background of necrotic liver.

Light Microscopy

- Structural changes in acute hepatitis comprise evidence of liver cell necrosis in centrilobular zone, inflammation within the liver acini and portal tract connective tissue.
- Changes in the connective tissue framework most often occurs as a result of extensive severe loss of hepatocytes.
- Acute viral hepatitis has two major features: *lobular disarray and chronic inflammatory infiltrate*.
- Ballooning degeneration and Councilman bodies are prominent features. Morphological features of acute hepatitis are shown in Figs 21.17, 21.18 and Table 21.22.

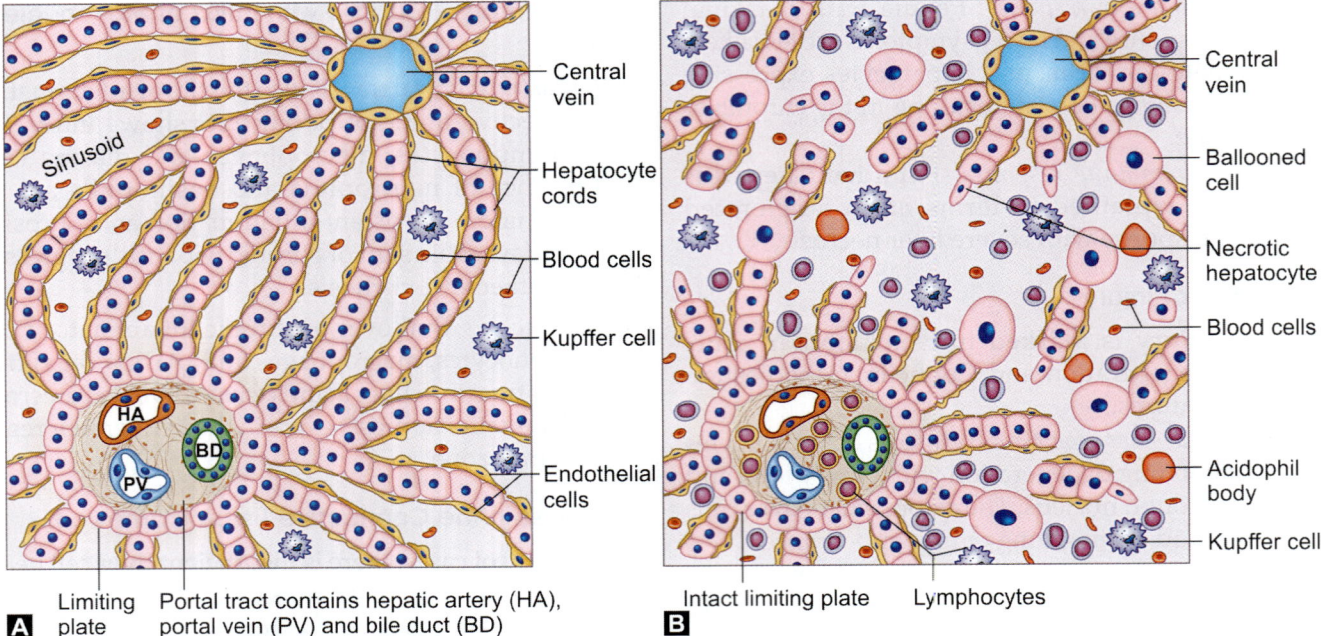

Fig. 21.17: (A) Normal liver acinus, (B) acute viral hepatitis shows scattered necrosis of single hepatocytes and small clusters of hepatocytes, ballooned cells (BC), necrotic cells (NC), and acidophilic bodies free in the sinusoids. The inflammation in the lobules and portal tracts is predominantly lymphocytic, although a few macrophages are also seen. The limiting plate is intact terminal hepatic venule.

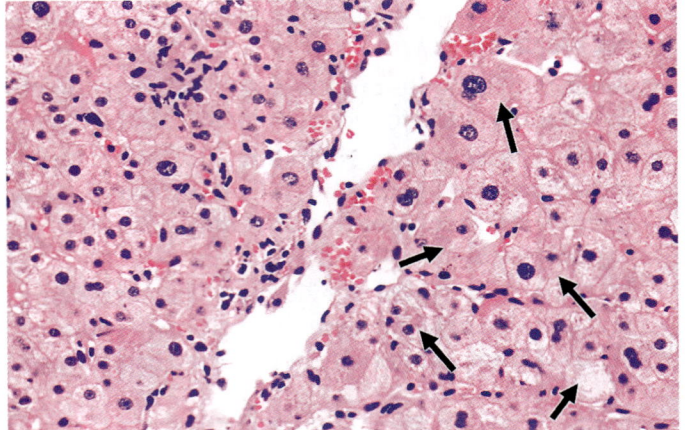

Fig. 21.18: Acute viral hepatitis. Hepatocytes show ballooning degeneration. These contain eosinophilic cytoplasm. There is presence of mononuclear cells infiltration. Hepatitis B can result in a fulminant hepatitis with extensive necrosis. At a later stage, a dying hepatocyte is seen shrinking down to form an eosinophilic *Councilman body* (arrows) (400X).

BIOCHEMICAL ABNORMALITIES

These include serum enzymes, serum bilirubin, urine analysis and serological tests described as under:

- *Serum enzymes:* There are increased levels of transaminases (ALT and AST) three to five times. It may be over 1000 IU/L in severe hepatitis. Transaminases return to normal level over a period of several months. There is modest increase of alkaline phosphatase.
- *Serum bilirubin:* There is variable increase in serum bilirubin concentration.
- *Urine analysis:* Bilirubin is present in urine.
- *Serologic test:* It must be performed to determine which virus has caused the disease.

ACUTE VIRAL HEPATITIS

Incubation period is the period from the time of infection and the first symptoms appear. Acute viral hepatitis has three phases: preicteric phase (prodromal phase), icteric phase (jaundice) and recovery phase (convalescence phase).

- *Preicteric phase:* Patient presents with fever, malaise, lassitude, anorexia, vomiting, right upper quadrant tenderness (hepatomegaly), arthralgia, dark-colored urine and clay-colored stools.

  Approximately 10% of patients with HBV infection show signs of serum sickness, characterized by skin rash, arthralgia, or mild proteinuria.

  Serum transaminases increase steadily and attain peak before clinical jaundice appears. Peripheral blood smear reveals atypical lymphocytosis.
- *Icteric phase (jaundice):* The icteric phase is variable depending on the type of hepatitis. Patient develops itching, jaundice, abdominal pain and tenderness associated with elevation of liver enzymes and bilirubin in blood and acholic stools. Urine analysis

Table 21.22: Morphological features of acute hepatitis

Morphological changes	Light microscopy
Hepatocellular injury	Liver cell swelling (ballooning degeneration)
	Cholestasis (bile plugs)
	Fatty change due to HCV
Hepatocellular necrosis	Liver cell necrosis (isolated or clusters)
	Bridging necrosis in severe inflammation (portal-portal, central-central, portal-central)
	Lobular disarray (loss of normal architecture)
Hepatocytes regeneration	Proliferation of hepatocytes
Sinusoidal cell reactive changes	Accumulation of phagocytosed cellular debris in Kupffer cells
	Influx of mononuclear cells in sinusoids
Portal tracts	Mononuclear inflammatory infiltrate in portal tracts
	Spillover of inflammatory cells into adjoining parenchyma may show liver cell necrosis

shows darkening of urine due to increased bilirubin and urobilinogen. Jaundice is usually accompanied by improvement of constitutional symptoms.

- *Recovery phase:* It is also known as *convalescence phase*. The duration of this recovery phase varies. Symptoms are subsiding like return of appetite and resolution of jaundice.

CHRONIC VIRAL HEPATITIS

Chronic hepatitis refers to chronic inflammatory process that may be associated with continuing necrosis of hepatocytes and which lasts for >6 months. It results from all hepatotropic viruses (HBV, HCV and HDV except HAV or HEV).

Liver may show mild, moderate, or severe injury depending on the extent of injury, inflammation and repair. Depending on course, hepatotropic viruses may cause portal hepatitis (previously known as *chronic persistent hepatitis*), chronic lobular hepatitis and chronic active hepatitis.

PORTAL HEPATITIS

Portal hepatitis was previously known as *chronic persistent hepatitis*. It occurs only in HBV and HCV infections.

Light Microscopy

Liver biopsy shows following features (Figs 21.19 and 21.20).
- *Preservation of normal liver acinar architecture:* Liver acinar architecture is preserved.

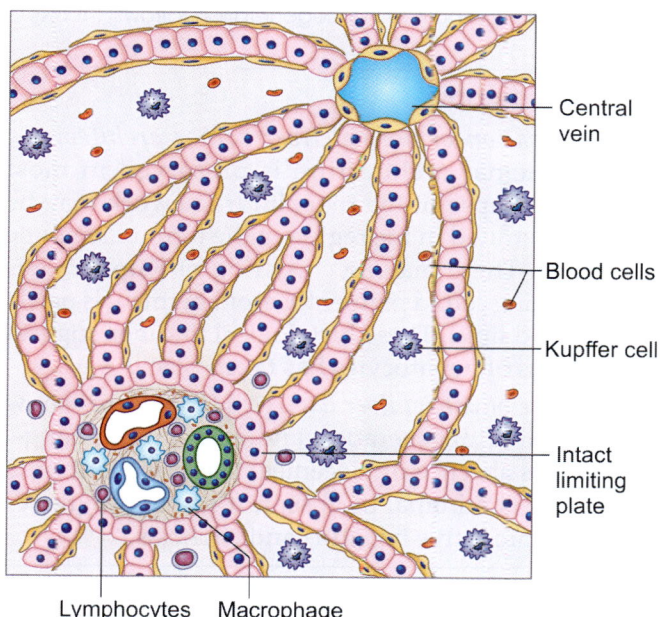

Fig. 21.19: Portal hepatitis (previously known as *chronic persistent*). Chronic inflammation is confined to the portal tracts. Limiting plate is intact. The lobular parenchyma appears normal.

- *Portal tract inflammation:* Chronic inflammation is confined to portal tracts without damaging limiting plates. Connective tissue of portal tracts infiltrated by lymphocytes, plasma cells and macrophages. Limiting plates are intact.
- *Lack of patchy necrosis of hepatocytes:* Hepatocytes do not show evidence of piecemeal necrosis.

CHRONIC LOBULAR HEPATITIS

Chronic lobular hepatitis has been regarded by some authors as a variant of portal hepatitis.

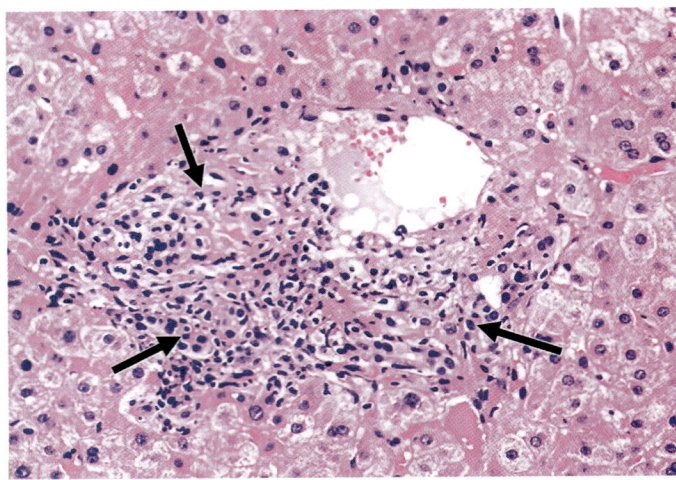

Fig. 21.20: Portal hepatitis (previously known as *chronic persistent*). Chronic inflammation is confined to the portal tracts. Limiting plate is intact. The lobular parenchyma appears normal. Hepatocytes show ballooning degeneration (arrows) (400X).

Light Microscopy

- *Preservation of normal liver acinar architecture:* Liver acinar architecture is preserved in most part. Collapse of the reticulin framework may be demonstrated in the region of the terminal hepatic venule. There may be clustering of Kupffer cells containing ceroid pigment. Ceroid pigment is partly oxidized lipid. These histological findings suggest that loss of hepatocytes has taken place.
- *Evidence of patchy liver damage:* Hepatocytes show ballooning degeneration and acidophilic change. There is absence of piecemeal necrosis. Periportal fibrosis is minimal or absent. It rarely progresses to chronic active hepatitis and cirrhosis.

CHRONIC ACTIVE HEPATITIS

Chronic active hepatitis is the most serious form of chronic hepatitis. *Liver biopsy shows chronic inflammation in portal tracts, damaging the limiting plates and extending into liver lobule.* There is presence of bridging necrosis and periportal fibrosis. Chronic hepatitis most often progresses to cirrhosis.

Effects of Chronic HBV Infection

These depend on whether or not viral replication is occurring. In serological terms, these patients may show following findings (Table 21.23).

- HBsAg and HBV DNA are positive
- HBsAg and HBV DNA are positive, but HBeAg is negative
- HBsAg is positive, but HBV DNA and HBeAg are negative.

Light Microscopy

- *Ballooning degeneration:* The hepatocytes show *ballooning* with scattered apoptotic cells. It depends on whether or not viral replication is occurring. Hepatocytes show ground-glass appearance due to accumulation of HBsAg in the cytoplasm.
- *Biliary cholestasis:* It may be severe as a result of fibrosis or secondary to cirrhosis.
- *Kupffer cell hyperplasia:* Kupffer cells are also prominent and increased in number in the sinusoids. These contain phagocytosed cellular debris, bile pigments and lipofuscin pigment.
- *Piecemeal necrosis:* Hepatocellular necrosis in periportal region is known as *piecemeal necrosis*. It is seen in immunocompetent persons.
- *Bridging necrosis with periportal fibrosis:* In very severe cases, there may be presence of bridging necrosis with periportal fibrosis connecting vascular structures of portal tract to terminal hepatic venules by a thick band of collapsed reticulin.

  Collagen fibers are laid down to replace injured hepatocytes. Fibrous septa may extend into lobules. Coalescence of fibrous strands, associated with regeneration of hepatocytes may lead to cirrhosis.
- *Portal tract chronic inflammation:* It is similar to that seen in portal hepatitis. Portal tracts are infiltrated by large number lymphocytes, macrophages, and plasma cells. These inflammatory cells erode limiting plates and extend into lobular parenchyma.

  It is accompanied by periportal fibrosis. The expanded portal tracts often display proliferated bile ductules.
- *Segmental bile duct lesions:* Both large and interlobular ducts undergo epithelial hyperplasia resulting in narrowing or occlusion (Figs 21.21 and 21.22).

Clinical Features

Patient presents with nonspecific symptoms such as fatigue, anorexia and malaise.

HEPATOTROPIC VIRUSES

HEPATITIS A VIRUS (HAV)

Hepatitis A virus is single-stranded spherical unenveloped RNA icosahedral virus measuring 27 nm in diameter. It is inactivated by boiling for one minute or formaldehyde and chlorine. It is resistant to heat, acid

Liver, Gallbladder and Exocrine Pancreas

Table 21.23: Effects of chronic HBV infection

Chronic HBV	Serology	Pathology
Viral replication of HBV	HBsAg positive and HBV DNA positive HBsAg positive and HBV DNA positive, but HBeAg negative	Light microscopy shows features of chronic viral hepatitis
Chronic carriers of HBV infection	HBsAg positive and HBV DNA negative and HBeAg negative	Serum transaminases normal Light microscopy may show ground-glass hepatocytes but lack inflammation Inflammation absent on light microscopy

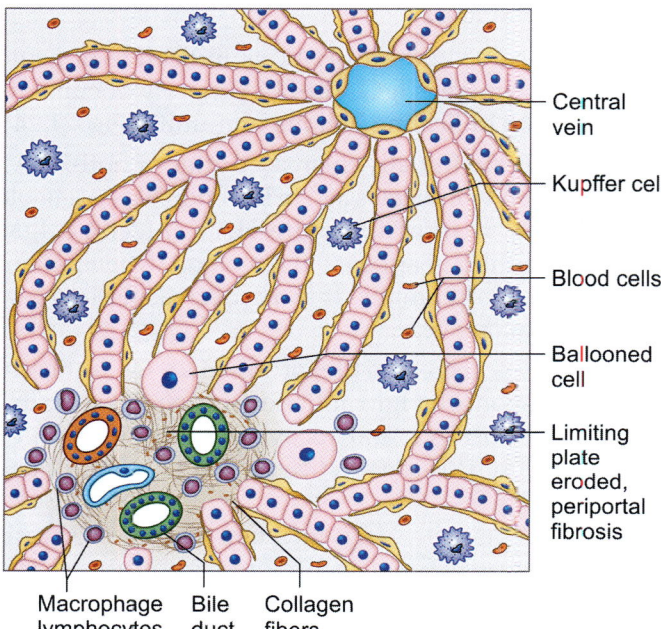

Fig. 21.21: Chronic active hepatitis is marked by severe chronic inflammation in the portal tracts. Periportal necrosis of hepatocytes is conspicuous, ballooned cells are present, and limiting plate is eroded. The inflammation extends into the lobular parenchyma and is accompanied by periportal fibrosis. The expanded portal tracts often display proliferated bile ductules and collagen fibers.

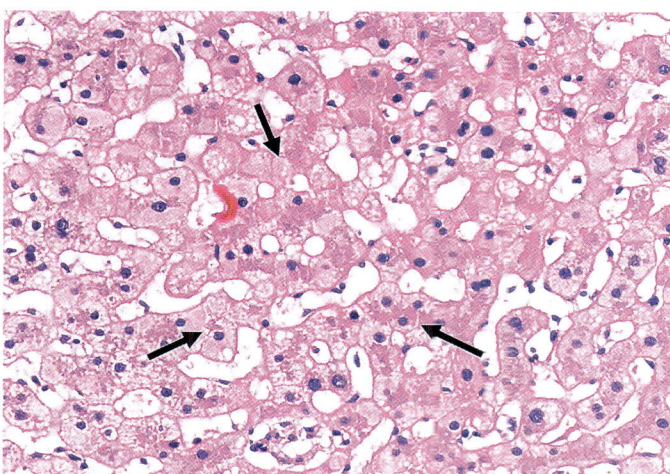

Fig. 21.22: Chronic active hepatitis. Ground-glass hepatocytes in chronic hepatitis. Smooth endoplasmic reticulum of hepatocytes distended with virions (HBsAg) gives *ground-glass appearance of hepatocytes* (arrows) (400X).

of HAV. The fecal shedding of HAV occurs during the first 2 to 3 weeks of the illness before and one week after onset of jaundice. Exposure to HAV gives lifelong immunity. Pathogenesis of HAV induced hepatitis is shown in Fig. 21.23.

and ether. It usually is a benign, self-limited disease, although it can cause acute fulminant hepatitis and death or need for transplantation in 0.15 to 0.2% of cases. There is no carrier state or chronic state.

Etiology

Hepatitis A is contracted primarily by the fecal–oral route. Parenteral infection does not occur. Edible shellfish concentrate the virus in contaminated waters and may also transmit the infection especially in USA. Anal intercourse is a risk factor for homosexual. It has a brief incubation period of 15–45 days.

Pathogenesis

The virus replicates in the liver, is excreted in the bile, and shed in the stool. There is only one antigenic type

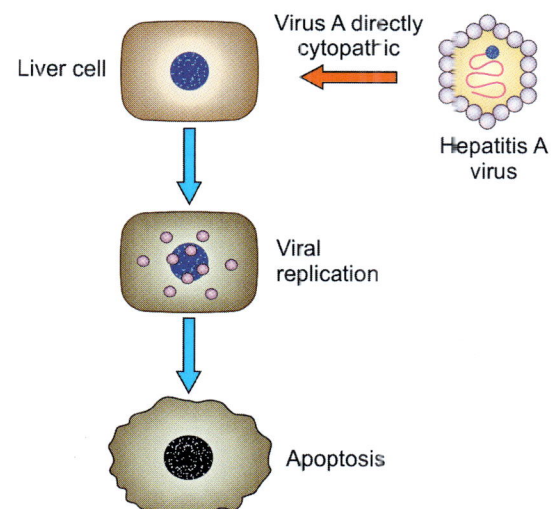

Fig. 21.23: Pathogenesis of HAV induced hepatitis. HAV in contrast to HBV appears to be directly cytopathic.

Age Group

The clinical presentation of symptoms is dependent upon age, with the severity of symptoms increasing in older age groups.

Children below 6 years most often are asymptomatic. Older children and adults are symptomatic with clinical jaundice in 70% of cases. Symptoms usually last approximately 2 months but can last longer.

Clinical Features

There are three phases of hepatitis induced by HAV—*preicteric, icteric and recovery phases* described as under:

- *Preicteric phase:* HAV is present in liver, bile, stool and blood. Patient is asymptomatic in this phase.
- *Icteric phase:* Patient develops *mild jaundice, malaise, nausea, anorexia and fever*. Jaundice appears one week after the onset of symptoms with peak at around 10 days. On clinical examination, liver may become enlarged and tender.

  At this stage, there is clear evidence of damage to hepatocytes in the form of marked *elevation of serum liver enzymes (ALAT) reflecting liver cell necrosis. Serum bilirubin (mostly conjugated) is increased. Serum albumin generally remains normal.*

  Coagulation tests may be abnormal. One stage prothrombin time is sensitive indicator of severity of liver disease. HAV appears in stool 2–3 weeks before jaundice and one week after icteric phase.

- *Recovery phase:* Signs and symptoms generally recover over a period of 3–8 weeks. Complete recovery occurs in most patients with mortality in <1%. Majority of patients recover without progressing to chronic hepatitis. HAV infection is not associated with cirrhosis or hepatocellular carcinoma. It has no carrier state.
- *Fulminant hepatitis:* Only a few patients may develop fulminant hepatitis with mortality in 0.1% of cases.

Serological Studies

The presence of IgM anti-HAV is indicative of acute hepatitis A, whereas IgG anti-HAV merely documents past infection indicating lifelong immunity (Fig. 21.24).

- *IgM antibody:* Initially, increased titer of anti-HAV-IgM antibody indicates active infection. It is a reliable diagnostic marker for acute HAV infection. IgM specific antibody appears in the blood, when patient becomes symptomatic. It starts decreasing in a few months to one year.
- *IgG antibody:* Increased titer of anti-HAV IgG antibody appears soon after IgM antibody in blood. It indicates exposure to HAV and recovery from infection or vaccination. *It is a protective antibody* giving *lifelong immunity.*

  In patients with HAV infection, chronic hepatitis never occurs. There is lifelong immunity. Viral elimination is total without a carrier state.

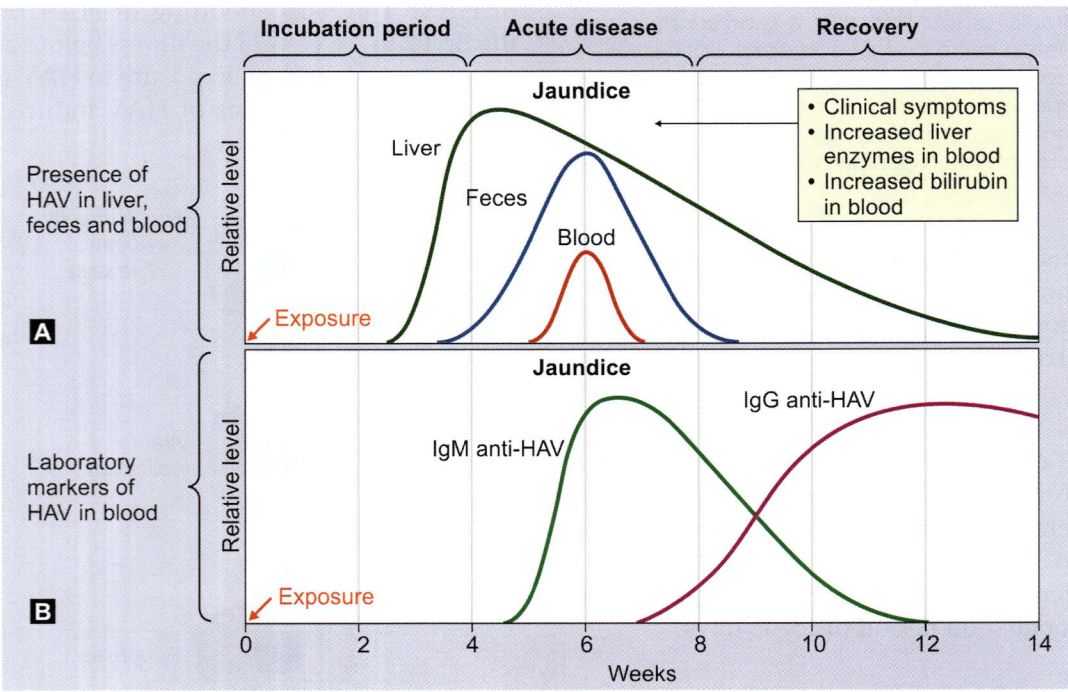

Fig. 21.24: Serological studies in acute viral hepatitis due to HAV. The presence of IgM anti-HAV is indicative of acute hepatitis A, whereas IgG anti-HAV merely documents past infection indicating lifelong immunity. Presence of IgM antibodies coincides with a decline in fecal shedding of the virus.

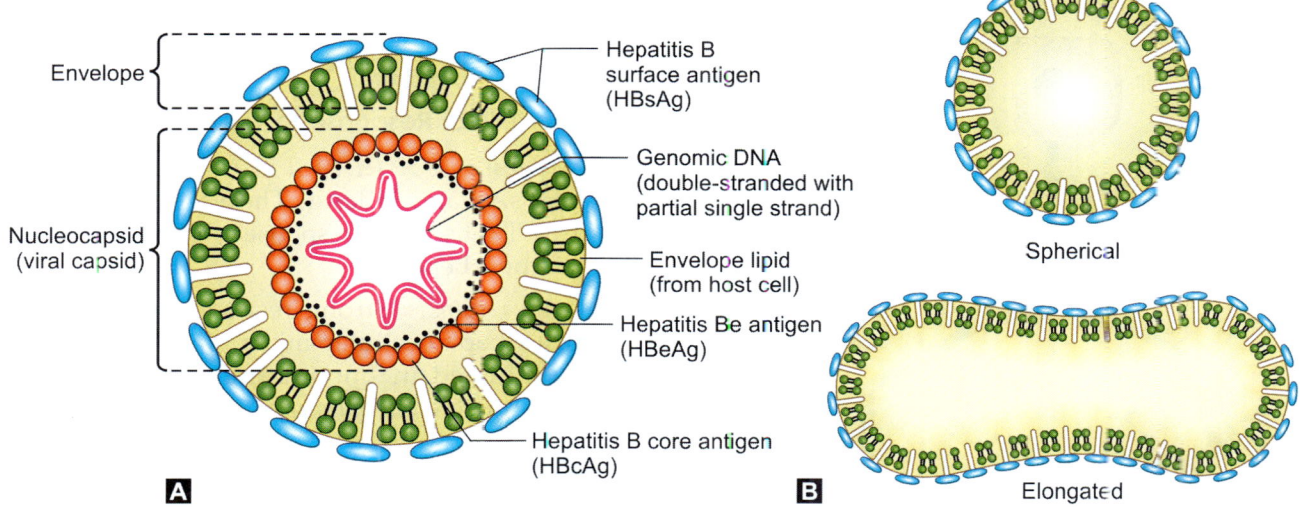

Fig. 21.25: Structure of hepatitis B virus. (A) Hepatitis B virus (Dane particles), and (B) viral envelope particles containing HBsAg.

Light Microscopy

Histological examination of liver biopsy in acute viral hepatitis shows disarray of the liver cell plates accompanied by inflammatory infiltrate and liver cell necrosis.

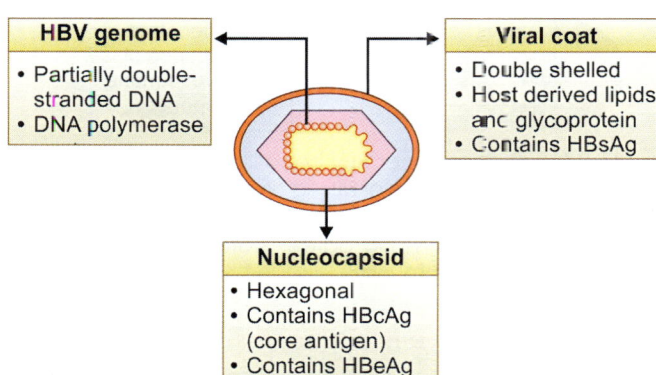

Fig. 21.26: Structure of hepatitis B virus shows HBV genome, viral coat and nucleocapsid.

Vaccination

The vaccine against HAV is available and highly effective. Vaccination is of a little benefit in prevention of hepatitis in people with known *HAV exposure*. It is intended to replace the use of immunoglobulin in people at high-risk for HAV.

HEPATITIS B VIRUS (HBV)

HBV is complete virion measuring 42 nm in diameter. It is known as *Dane particle*. It is hardy virus, which can withstand extremes of temperature and humidity. HBV consists of lipoprotein coat with central core (nucleocapsid).

- *Viral lipoprotein coat:* It consists of central core surrounded by lipoprotein coat containing the hepatitis B surface antigen (HBsAg).
- *Central core (nucleocapsid):* It is hexagonal in shape. It contains double-stranded circular DNA, DNA polymerase, hepatitis B core antigen (HBcAg), and hepatitis Be antigen (HBeAg).

  Presence of HBeAg in the serum *indicates active viral replication, infectivity of serum and progression of liver cell damage* (Figs 21.25 and 21.26).

Mode of Transmission

It is transmitted via transfusion of blood or blood products, hemodialysis, accidental needle-stick (health workers), intravenous drug abuse, homosexual activity, contact with body fluids by shedding of virus in saliva, tears, and breast milk and transplacental transmission from mother to neonate.

Incubation Period

This period is 4 to 26 weeks (average 60 to 90 days or 8 weeks).

Pathogenesis

HBV virions are not directly cytopathic. These integrate into the host DNA and induce hepatic inflammation leading to hepatocellular injury. Smooth endoplasmic reticulum of hepatocytes distended with virions gives *ground-glass appearance of hepatocytes*. It indicates chronic carrier state.

Increased titers of HBeAg, HBV DNA and viral polymerase indicate active viral replication in blood and correlates with infectivity of the blood. Pathogenesis of HBV hepatitis is shown in Fig. 21.27.

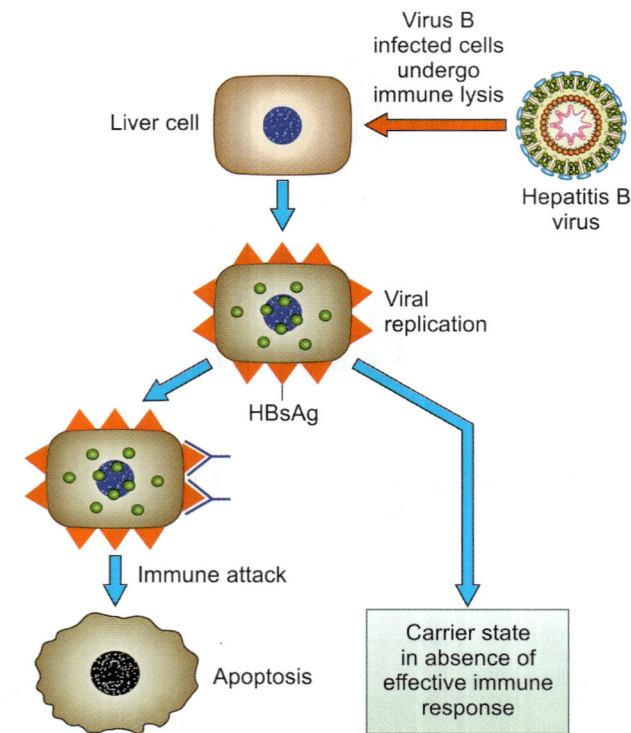

Fig. 21.27: Pathogenesis of HBV hepatitis. The HBV causes liver cell injury due to expression of HBsAg on surface of hepatocytes. The infected liver cells are eliminated by immune-mediated mechanism. Asymptomatic career state can ensure in the absence of specific immunity.

Entry of HBV into the Hepatocytes

HBV entry into the hepatocytes may depend on polymerized human serum albumin (PHSA) serving as a linkage between the putative receptors of virus and hepatocytes. The virus enters the host liver cells. Virion multiplication occurs in hepatocytes as a result of proliferation of HBV DNA.

Processing of Viral DNA

This DNA of virus acts as the template for the formation of RNA, which is termed *pregenomic*. This term is given because this RNA forms the template for the formation of viral DNA through the medium of a virally encoded reverse transcriptase. It leads to formation of complete virions.

Integrative Phase

During integrative phase, virions are not produced; and there is absence of antigens and antibodies.

Hepatocellular Response to Virions

- *Weak response to CD8+ T cells:* There is formation of HBsAg and HBcAg. These sensitize cytotoxic CD8+ T cells. Weak response of CD8+ T cells results in chronic hepatitis.
- *Strong response:* Strong response of CD8+ T cells causes hepatocellular injury. Excess of HBsAg is accumulated in smooth endoplasmic reticulum producing *ground-glass appearance* of hepatocytes.

Extrahepatic Manifestations

HBsAg and anti-HBsAb form immune complex resulting in deposition in blood vessels. It activates complement system resulting in angioedema, arthritis, skin rashes, fever and glomerulonephritis.

Serological Study of Acute HBV Infection

Serological assays may be employed to distinguish between acute and chronic hepatitis due to HBV infection. Most sensitive and specific commercial methods used in diagnosis are **radioimmunoassay (RIA)** and **enzyme-linked immunosorbent assay (ELISA)** by using specific antibodies against various HBV proteins.

Both these methods can detect HBsAg as low as 0.25 ng/ml and anti-HBs antibodies. PCR is used to detect low concentration of HBV DNA present in both blood and tissue samples (Table 21.24 and Fig. 21.28).

- *HBsAg first marker in serum:* Surface antigen (HBsAg) is the first marker appearing in the serum. It is demonstrated in the serum between 1 week to 2 months after exposure and before the appearance of clinical symptoms. It disappears from the blood during convalescence. *Persistence of HBsAg is being used to differentiate acute from chronic hepatitis.* HBsAg persists up to 4 months in acute hepatitis. Persistence of HBsAg longer than 6 months defines chronic hepatitis.

Table 21.24: Serological events in HBV infection

HbsAg	HBeAg	Anti-HBe	Anti-HBc	Anti-HBc IgM	Anti-HBs	Significance
+	+/−	+/−	+	+	−	Acute HBV infection
+	+	−	+	−/Weak positive	−	HBV career (high infectivity)
+	−	+	+	−	−	HBV career (low infective)
−	−	+/−	+	−	+	Past HBV infection
−	−	−	−	−	+	Past HBV immunization

Liver, Gallbladder and Exocrine Pancreas

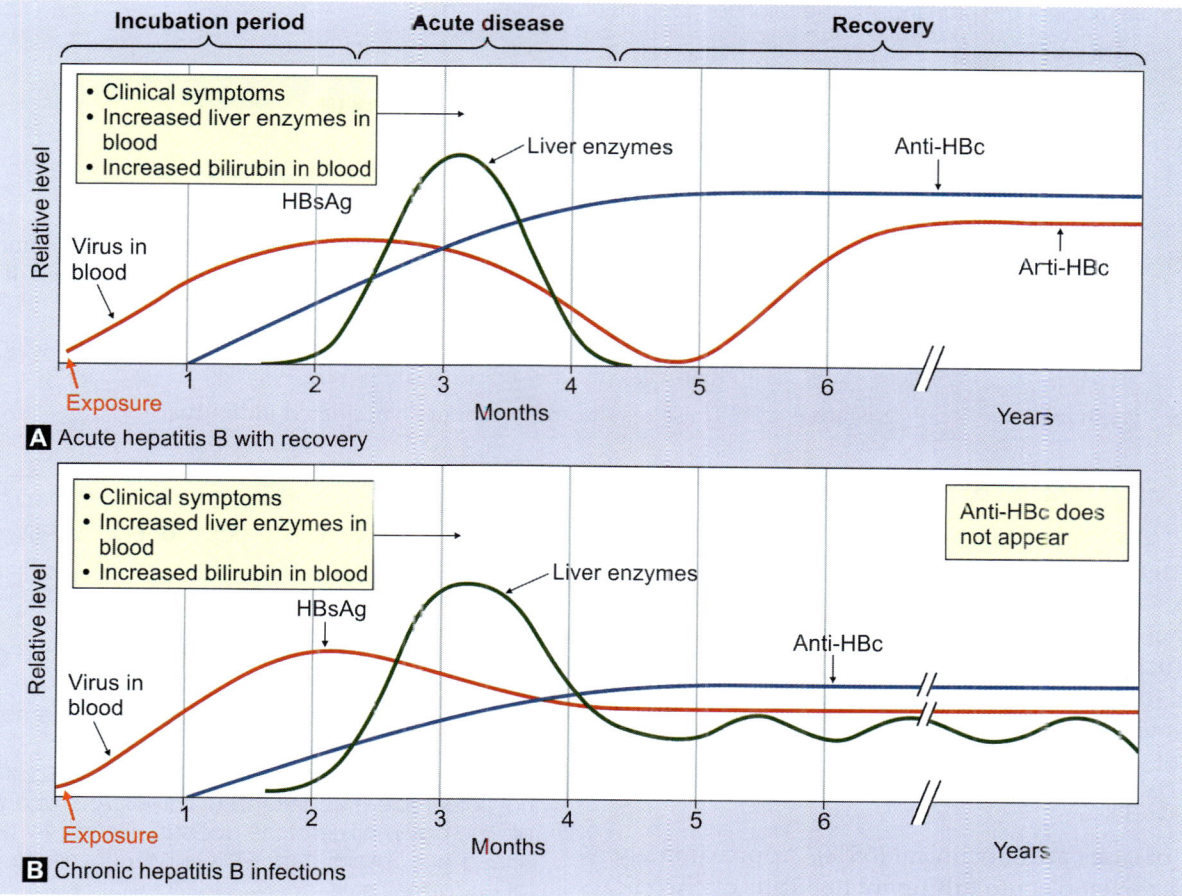

Fig. 21.28: Hepatitis B. (A) Clinical phases and serological markers. Acute infection is characterized by rapid appearance of viremia before clinical symptoms appear. There is disappearance of HBV from the blood and appearance of antibodies against hepatitis B surface antigen (HbsAg). (B) Chronic hepatitis is signaled by continuing onset of jaundice or presence of viremia.

- *HBeAg second marker in serum:* Presence of HBeAg in the serum indicates maximum infectivity and intense viral replication. As with surface antigen (HBsAg), 'e' antigen (HBeAg) appears before the onset of clinical manifestations. It disappears from the serum in two weeks. As the 'e' antigen is cleared from the serum, the antibody to 'e' antigen appears in the serum. But there is a gap between disappearance of the 'e' antigen and demonstration of antibody.

- *Anti-HBc (both IgG and IgM):* With the onset of clinical manifestations, anti-HBc (both IgG and IgM) most often appear in the serum and remain in low concentration for life. It does not play significant role in viral elimination. It rather serves as a marker for infection. It is important to mention that HBcAg is not detectable in serum.

- *Anti-HBs antibody last marker in serum:* Last marker to appear in serum is anti-HBs. It is measured if present in excess concentration. This antibody forms immune complexes with the circulating HBsAg. These antigen antibody complexes may produce extrahepatic complications such as glomerulonephritis, necrotizing vasculitis and serum sickness like syndrome. The antibody to HBsAg participates in elimination of HBsAg.

  There is a *window period* between the appearance of HBsAg and the appearance of the corresponding antibody. IgG anti-HBs is protective antibody to subsequent infection. Its persistence indicates either active or passive immunization against HBV. Recombinant vaccine consists of HBsAg alone.

- *HBV-DNA:* The presence of viral DNA (HBV DNA) in the serum is the most certain indicator of hepatitis B infection. It indicates viral burden and active replication. It evaluates recovery from infection after antiviral therapy. It helps in differentiation of inactive carrier state and chronic hepatitis in HBV infection. Serological markers and interpretation for hepatitis B virus infection are shown in Table 21.25.

Table 21.25: Serological markers and interpretation for hepatitis B virus infection

Presence/absence			Interpretation
HBsAg	Anti-HBsAb	Anti-HBcAb	
Positive	Negative	Negative	Early acute HBV infection
Positive	Positive or negative	Positive	Either acute or chronic HBV infection
Negative	Positive	Positive	Previous HBV infection and current immunity to the virus
Negative	Negative	Positive	Not clear interpretation either due to HBV infection in the remote past, low-level HBV infection, or false-positive/non-specific reactions. If present, anti-HBs help validate anti-HBc reactivity
Negative	Negative	Negative	These results suggest that liver toxicity is due to some other agents other than HBV
Negative	Positive	Negative	These results are typical of a vaccinated individual

Hallmark of Chronicity of HBV Infection

Failure to clear HBsAg from serum after 6 months is the hallmark of chronicity due to HBV infection. It occurs in <5% of cases. Presence of HBeAg, HBV DNA or polymerase in the serum either singly or together indicates active viral replication. In patients where there is no viral replication, the continuing presence of HBsAg correlates with integration of the viral genome into the genome of host hepatocytes.

Clinical Course

Majority of cases are subclinical (65%). Approximately 35% cases develop acute fulminant hepatitis or chronic hepatitis. Approximately 10–30% chronic hepatitis cases develop confluent hepatic necrosis and cirrhosis (<1%) may develop hepatocellular carcinoma.

Clinical course of hepatitis B infection is shown in Fig. 21.29. Differences between hepatitis induced by HAV and HBV are shown in Table 21.26.

Summary of serological studies HBV induced hepatitis
- HBsAg is demonstrated in acute or chronic HBV induced hepatitis.
- Demonstration of IgG anti-HBs and IgG anti-HBc indicates previous exposure to HBV.
- Demonstration of IgG anti-HBs indicates that the person is immunized.
- IgM anti-HBc is the only serological marker demonstrated during window period.
- Window period is a period in which HBsAg and anti-HBsAb is not detectable in the serum, but anti-HBcAb and anti-HBeAb are the only markers of the disease. HbsAg, HBV DNA, and HBeAg are absent. It (anti-HBC-IgM) converts to anti-HBc IgG in 6 months.
- Qualitative marker of HBV replication is HBeAg.
- Quantitative marker (definite) of HBV replication is HBV DNA > HBV DNA polymerase.
- Inactive carrier refers to HBeAg negative with normal ALT levels and undetectable or low level of HBV DNA (<2000 IU/ml).

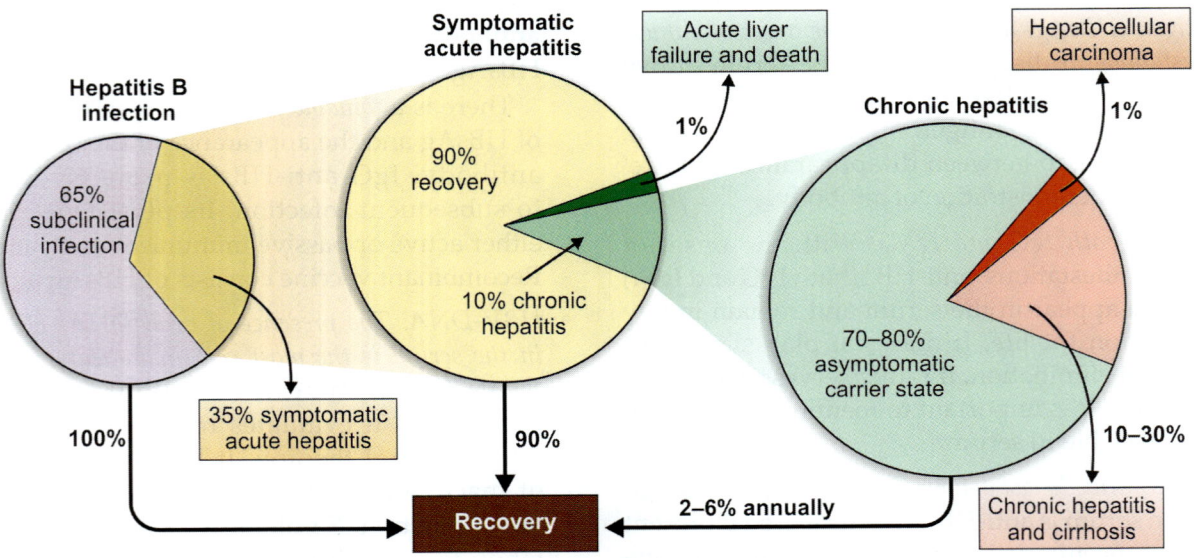

Fig. 21.29: Clinical course of hepatitis B infection. It has subclinical, acute hepatitis, chronic hepatitis or asymptomatic chronic carrier. Fulminant acute hepatitis with massive liver cell necrosis may be seen in 1% of cases. There is increased risk of development of cirrhosis and hepatocellular carcinoma.

Table 21.26: Differences between hepatitis induced by HAV and HBV

Parameters	Hepatitis A infection	Hepatitis B infection
Mode of transmission	Fecal-oral route	Parenteral route and close contact
Carrier state	Absent	Present
Chronic hepatitis	Absent	Present
Age	Children and adolescents	All age group
Viruses in stool and body secretions	Viruses are present in stool 2–3 weeks of after onset of jaundice	Viruses are not excreted in stool. But these are present in body secretions
Viremia	Transient excretion	Viruses remain for prolonged period starting from incubation period, acute hepatitis to chronic hepatitis. Infection transmitted by such blood administration to other persons
Vertical transmission	Absent	Present
Fulminant hepatitis	Rare	More frequent
Risk of hepatocellular carcinoma	Absent	Present
Clinical course	Usually self-limited	Variable, it may be severe with fatal outcome

---

Precore or basic core mutant HBV

- Patient with precore or basic core mutant HBV develops severe and progressive liver disease. There is increased risk of cirrhosis and hepatocellular carcinoma.
- Serological assays reveal HBeAg negative but positive anti-HBe. HBV DNA levels are >10,000 copies/ml.
- Blood biochemistry analysis reveals persistent or intermittent elevations in ALT (alanine aminotransferase) activity.

Clinical Manifestations

Subclinical Acute Hepatitis

It is asymptomatic or clinically unrecognized.

Acute Icteric Hepatitis

HbsAg is the first marker of infection. It appears 2 to 8 weeks after exposure, and persists up to 4 months.

Fulminant Acute Hepatitis with Massive Hepatic Necrosis

It develops in <1% of clinically diagnosed HBV infections. Markedly elevation of ALT and AST are characteristic findings.

- Gross examination reveals soft flabby shrunken liver, and wrinkled Glisson's capsule.
- Light microscopy shows necrotic liver lobules, leaving a collapsed collagenous framework. These patients die unless an emergency liver transplantation is performed.

Chronic Hepatitis

Persistence of abnormal liver function tests and HBsAg in cytoplasm of hepatocytes for longer than 6 months is considered chronic hepatitis.

- *Chronic carriers:* These are otherwise healthy carriers. HBsAg persists longer than 6 months. There is absence of infective particles in 10–15% cases. Anti-HBc IgM converts to anti-HBc IgG.
- *Chronic active hepatitis:* It occurs in 33% cases of chronic carriers. There is presence of infective particles. There is increased risk for post-necrotic cirrhosis (33%) and hepatocellular carcinoma (10%).

Light Microscopy

- Liver biopsy in patient with chronic active hepatitis is performed to assess evidence of fibrosis and inflammatory grade of the disease.
- It shows infiltration of connective tissue of portal tracts by lymphocytes, plasma cells and macrophages.
- There is presence of fibrosis and *piecemeal necrosis of the limiting plate of hepatocytes close to the portal tracts.*
- Hepatocytes with HBsAg show cytoplasmic *ground-glass appearance and sanded nuclei* (Fig. 21.30).

Immunohistochemistry

- Immunohistochemistry reveals HBsAg in cytoplasm. HBsAg is demonstrated by *Shikata's orcein stain, Victoria blue* and *aldehyde fuscin stain.*
- HBcAg is expressed in cytoplasm, membrane or nucleus and its presence indicates active replication and infectivity of the virus.

HEPATITIS C VIRUS (HCV)

HCV is 30–60 nm enveloped single-stranded RNA flavivirus. About 50% of affected persons develop

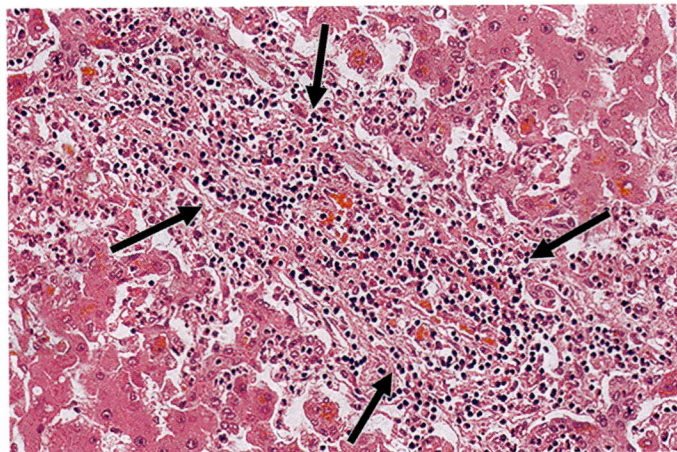

Fig. 21.30: Chronic active hepatitis: viral hepatitis leads to liver cell destruction. A mononuclear inflammatory cell infiltrate extends from portal areas and disrupts the limiting plate of hepatocytes which are undergoing necrosis, the so-called *piecemeal* necrosis of chronic active hepatitis. In this case, the hepatitis B surface antigen (HbsAg) and hepatitis B core antibody (HbcAb) were positive (arrows) (400X).

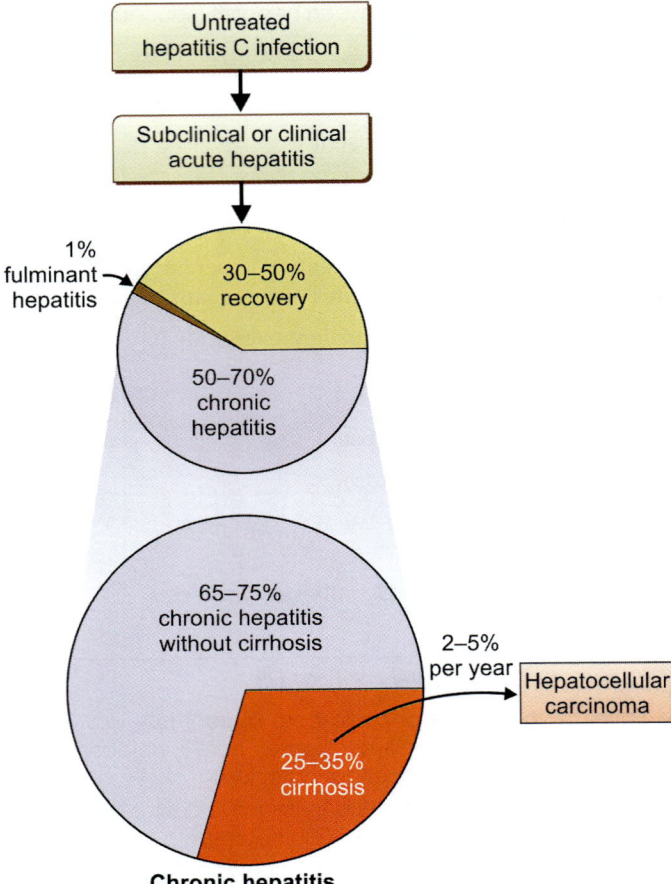

Fig. 21.31: Outcome of untreated hepatitis C infection.

biochemical evidence of chronic liver disease. Approximately 10% of cases develop chronic active hepatitis or cirrhosis.

Coexistent conditions such as hepatitis B infection, alcoholism, hemochromatosis and α_1-antitrypsin deficiency adversely affect the clinical course of HCV infection. Factors associated with spontaneous clearing of HCV infection appear to include younger age, female sex, and certain histocompatibility genes. Outcome of untreated hepatitis C infection is shown in Fig. 21.31.

Incubation Period
It is similar to HBV, i.e. 4 to 26 weeks.

Mode of Transmission
HCV is transmitted by blood-borne parental route, sexual contact, transplacental infection of the fetus and co-infection with HBV described as under:
- *Blood and its products transfusion (parenteral route):* It is transmitted by blood-borne parental route with sharing of needles in drug addicts (blood and its products transfusion). About 60 to 90 percent of intravenous drug users are infected with HCV.
- *Sexual contact:* It can also be transmitted by sexual intercourse with infected person.
- *Transplacental route:* Mother transmits infection to fetus via transplacental route.
- *Co-infection:* Persons with HBV co-infection are also affected.

Clinical Features
Most people infected with HCV have a normal life-span. It is persistent infection due to recurrent relapses is a rule (>85%) and usually mild. The most serious consequences of chronic HCV infection are progressive liver fibrosis leading to *cirrhosis* over 10 to 30, end-stage liver disease, and *hepatocellular cancer*.

Extrahepatic Symptoms
- *Cryoglobulinemia:* Immune response to virus leads to cryoglobulinemia. IgM cryoglobulins precipitate at 4°C and dissolve again at 37°C. These are demonstrated in 35% of patients. Mixed cryoglobulinemia (IgM and IgG) is demonstrated in some patients with hepatitis C infection. These cryoglobulins induce *glomerular and vascular injury*.
- *Membranous glomerulonephritis:* Membranous glomerulonephritis is also mediated by cryoglobulins. Patient may develop *nephrotic syndrome* characterized by massive proteinuria, hypoproteinemia, hyperlipidemia, lipiduria and generalized edema.
- *Purpura or Raynaud phenomenon:* Vasculitis mediated by deposition of cryoglobulins in the vessel wall is associated with purpura or Raynaud phenomenon.

Light Microscopy

In addition to the features common to viral hepatitis, HCV infection may produce the following histological changes:

- *Cytopathic changes in the hepatocytes:* Histopathological examination shows scattered liver cells with intense degree of eosinophilia indicating damage to hepatocytes by HCV. There is no evidence of inflammation.
- *Presence of inflammatory cells within sinusoids:* The sinusoids show infiltration by lymphocytes and macrophages. The intensity of inflammation is out of proportion to the relatively small amount of hepatocytic damage.
- *Presence of inflammatory cells within portal tracts:* Connective tissue of hepatocytes may show lymphoid aggregates.
- *Evidence of intrahepatic bile ducts damage:* Presence of inflammatory infiltrate in bile duct epithelium causes destruction of intrahepatic bile duct in 30% of cases.
- *Focal fatty change:* Sublethal liver cell injury is seen in the form of small droplet fatty change (Fig. 21.32).

Serological Studies

Initially IgM anti-HCV antibody appears. It is followed by appearance of IgG anti-HCV antibodies. Chronic infection shows episodic elevations in serum transaminases with persistent HCV RNA in blood.

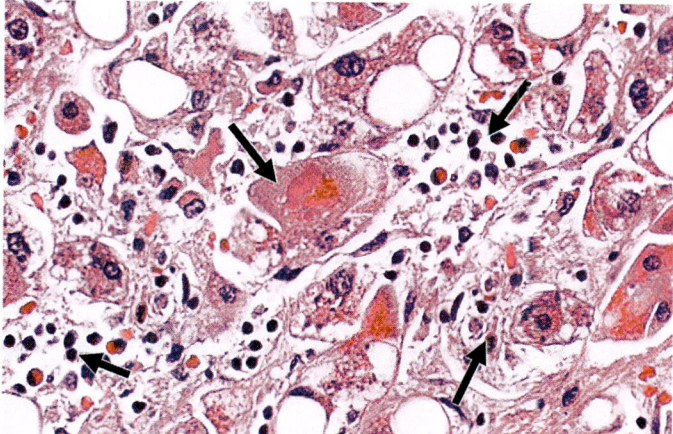

Fig. 21.32: Viral hepatitis C. This is a case of viral hepatitis C, which in half of cases leads to chronic liver disease. The extent of chronic hepatitis can be graded by the degree of activity (necrosis and inflammation) and staged by the degree of fibrosis. In this case, necrosis and inflammation are prominent, and there is some steatosis as well. Regardless of the grade or stage, the etiology of the hepatitis must be sought, for the treatment may depend upon knowing the cause, and chronic liver diseases of different etiologies may appear microscopically and grossly similar (arrows) (400X).

Anti-HCV IgG does not provide immunity due to antigenic variability and genome instability seen in HCV. Direct measurement of HCV in the serum remains the most accurate test for infection.

The viral tests are highly sensitive and specific, but more costly than antibody tests.

- *Screening with enzyme immunoassay:* Presence of anti-HCV IgG indicates infection or recovery. It is not a protective antibody.
- *Confirmatory tests:* These include recombinant immunoblot assay (RIBA) and HCV RNA using polymerase chain reaction (Fig. 21.33).

Treatment

α-Interferon is administered in these patients.

HEPATITIS D VIRUS

Hepatitis D virus is single-stranded spherical RNA virus containing delta protein antigen (HDAg). It is surrounded by a proteinaceous coat of HBsAg. It requires *co-infection* or *superinfection with HBV* for replication. It is infective only when encapsulated by HBV. Incidence with HDV infection is especially high in intravenous drug users.

Pathology

HDV has *direct cytopathic effect* on hepatocytes in contrast to HBV. It produces extensive injury to liver. Liver shows microvesicular *fatty change* and many acidophilic *Councilman bodies*. Chronicity is very rare.

Incubation Period

It is 4–7 weeks in superinfection.

Mode of Transmission

Mode of transmission can be acquired simultaneously with HBV (co-infection) or it may secondarily infect HBV carriers (superinfection). Both co-infection and superinfection may be followed by acute hepatitis (Table 21.27 and Fig. 21.34).

- *Co-infection:* Person receiving infected blood transfusion with HBV and HDV develops acute hepatitis.
- *Superinfection:* Carriers of HBV develop superinfection with HDV.

Serological Studies

Anti-HDV IgM is most reliable marker of acute HDV infection. Anti-HBc IgM is also demonstrated. IgG is not a protective antibody.

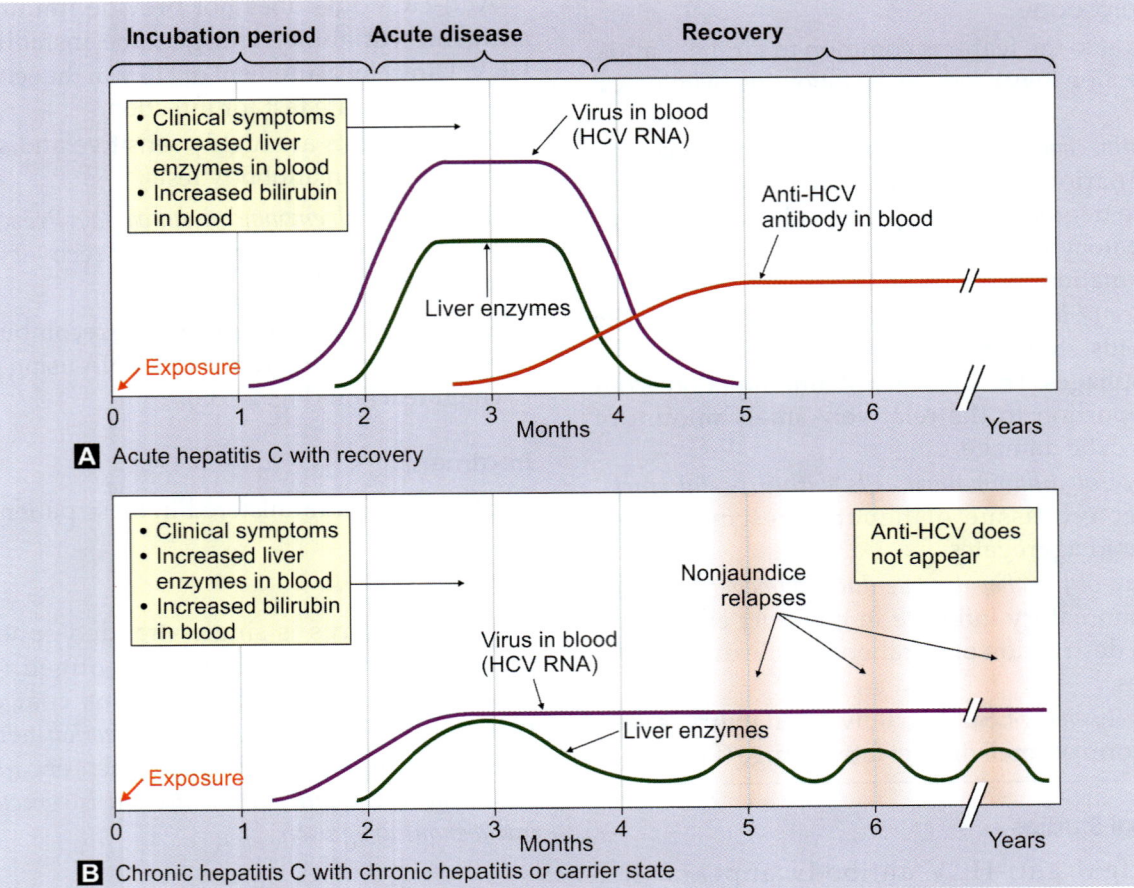

Fig. 21.33: Chronic hepatitis C. (A) Acute hepatitis C with recovery, (B) chronic hepatitis C with chronic hepatitis or carrier state.

Table 21.27: Co-infection and superinfection in relation to hepatitis D infection

Parameters	Co-infection	Superinfection
Status of patient before infection	HDV and HBV in healthy carrier	HDV infection in HBV carrier
Recovery from acute hepatitis with immunity	90%	10–15%
Risk of fulminant hepatitis and death	3–4%	7–10%
Risk of developing chronic hepatitis resulting in cirrhosis	Rare	80%

HEPATITIS E VIRUS (HEV)

Hepatitis E virus has now been cloned and sequenced. It is single-stranded RNA virus measuring 32 to 34 nm. Infection is contracted with recent travel to endemic areas, i.e. Africa, Asia, or Central America.

Infection resembles HAV, but it is *more common in young adults* rather than children. No vaccine has been developed for prophylaxis.

Mode of Transmission

It is transmitted by fecal–oral route. Incubation period is 35 to 40 days.

Clinical Features

Like hepatitis A, hepatitis E usually presents as an acute self-limited illness with low mortality (in 1 to 12% of patient presents with mild hepatitis with jaundice, fever and arthralgia that lasts about 6 weeks.

It does not progress to chronic liver disease. For unknown reasons, infection during pregnancy is associated with high mortality due to fulminant hepatic failure in 20% of cases.

Serological Studies in Hepatitis E Virus

Presence of anti-HBe IgM indicates active infection. Anti-HEV IgG indicates recovery (protective antibody).

HEPATITIS G VIRUS (HGV)

A viral agent similar to HCV has been cloned and was identified as hepatitis G virus (HGV), also referred to as GBV-C. HGV is a flavivirus transmitted parenterally by blood. It is found in 1 to 2% of *blood donors* and at a much

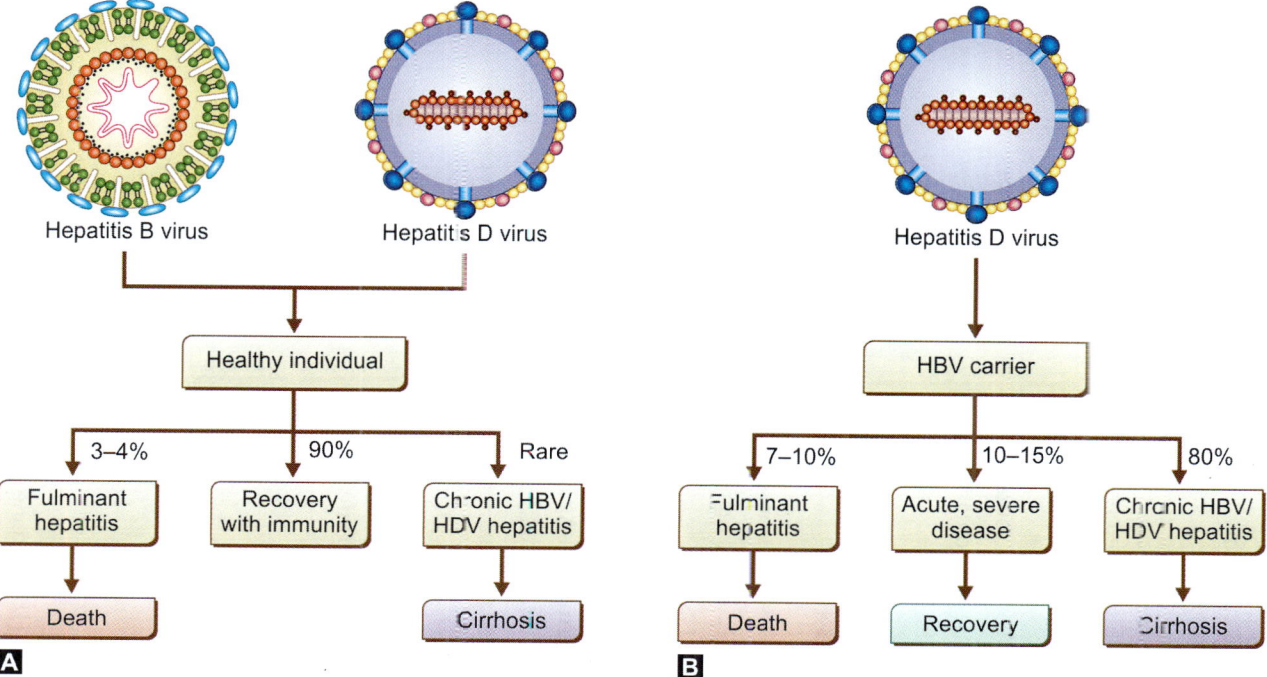

Fig. 21.34: (A) Co-infection, (B) superinfection in relation to hepatitis D infection.

higher rate among *intravenous drug abusers*. It does not lead to chronic hepatitis and has no known *relationship to hepatocellular carcinoma*. Comparison of hepatotropic viruses is shown in Table 21.28.

AUTOIMMUNE HEPATITIS (LUPOID HEPATITIS)

Autoimmune hepatitis is the most common autoimmune chronic progressive disorder of liver especially in young women. This disorder is mediated by CD8+ T cells. Women with autoimmune hepatitis show circulating antinuclear autoantibodies and elevated serum IgG concentration. But there are no serum markers to diagnose this disorder.

Etiology

It is caused by viruses, drugs and in the setting of autoimmune disorders like rheumatoid arthritis, ulcerative colitis and Sjögren's syndrome.

Pathogenesis

A pathogenetic role for immune-mediated mechanisms is suggested by following.

- Positive *LE cell* phenomenon in 10% cases of systemic lupus erythematosus
- *Anti-nuclear antibodies* in >50% of cases
- *Smooth muscle cell autoantibodies* in 40–60% of cases
- Autoantibody against receptor on cell membrane of hepatocytes
- Autoantibodies against microsomes
- Reduction in the number of and functional ability of suppressor T cells
- Heavy plasma cell infiltrate in liver
- Rapid response to treatment with immunosuppressive agents.

Classification

Autoimmune hepatitis is classified into two categories based on the basis of autoantibodies described in Table 21.29.

Clinical Features

Patient presents with jaundice, acne, amenorrhea and hepatosplenomegaly.

> **Light Microscopy**
> Liver shows characteristic infiltration of plasma cells in periportal regions. Entire spectrum of hepatitis is demonstrated.

Prognosis

Untreated patient with autoimmune hepatitis may develop hepatocellular failure and cirrhosis with fatal outcome.

Management

These patients are treated by immunosuppressive therapy. Liver transplantation is recommended for end-stage disease and history of recurrence.

Table 21.28: Comparison of hepatotropic viruses

Characteristics	Hepatitis A	Hepatitis B	Hepatitis C	Hepatitis D	Hepatitis E
Family	Picornavirus	Hepadnavirus	Flavivirus	Unknown	Calciviridae
Year of identification	1973	1965	1989	1977	1995
Genetic material	ssRNA	ssDNA	ssRNA	ssRNA	ssRNA
Morphology	Icosahedral capsid	Double shelled enveloped	Enveloped	Enveloped replication defective	Icosahedral unenveloped
Size	27 nm	42 nm	30–60 nm	35 nm	32–24 nm
Transmission	Fecal-oral route; Male homosexuals	Parental route; Sexual contact; Mother to fetus; Breastfeeding	Parental route; Sexual contact	Parental route; Sexual contact	Fecal–oral route
Incubation period	2–6 weeks	4–26 weeks	2–26 weeks	4–7 weeks	2–8 weeks
Age group	Children and adolescents	Any age	Adults	Any age	Young adults
Onset	Acute onset	Insidious onset	Insidious onset	Insidious onset	Acute onset
Prevalence	Worldwide	Worldwide	Probably worldwide	Endemic region	Only in developing countries
Antigen	HAV (viremia transient)	HbsAg, HbcAg, HbeAg	HCV, C100-3, C-33c, and NS-5	HbsAg, HDV	HEV
Antibodies	Anti-HAV	Anti-Hbs	Anti-HCV	Anti-HbsAg	Anti-HAV
Nature of illness	Mild	Occasionally severe	Moderate	Occasionally severe	Mild except during pregnancy
Fulminant hepatitis	0.1–0.4%	<1%	Rare	3–4%	0.3–3% (20% in pregnant women)
Carrier state	None	0.1–1%	0.2–0.4%	0.1–10%	No carrier state
Chronic hepatitis	Absent	5–10%	>70% cases	<5% (co-infection) and 80 (superinfection)	None
Cirrhosis	None	Yes	Yes	+/−	None
Hepatocellular carcinoma	No	Yes	Yes	Unknown	Unknown
Prognosis	Excellent	Poor	Moderate	Variable	Good
Associated findings	None	Serum sickness (5–10%), polyarteritis nodosa and membranous glomerulonephritis	Post-transfusion hepatitis, MPGN-1, and porphyria cutanea tarda	None	None
Specific prophylaxis	Immunoglobulin administration and vaccination	Immunoglobulin administration and vaccination	Nil	HBV vaccine	Nil

Table 21.29: Autoantibodies formed in autoimmune hepatitis types I and II

Autoimmune hepatitis types	Autoantibodies
Autoimmune hepatitis type I	ANA (antinuclear antigen) most common, SMA (smooth muscle actin antigen) most specific, SLA (soluble liver antigen), LPA (soluble pancreas antigen)
Autoimmune hepatitis type II	LKM1 (liver, kidney microsome), LC-1 (liver cytosol-1 antigen)

BACTERIAL AND PARASITIC INFECTIONS OF LIVER

BACTERIAL LIVER INFECTIONS

Bacterial infections of the liver occur in various ways. These include space-occupying abscess, cholangitis, granulomatous inflammation and peliosis. Liver is the most common site of abscess formation.

Abscess formation is most often seen in right lobe of liver. Abscesses in liver are frequently multiple and seen in older patients or immunocompromised young individuals.

PYOGENIC BACTERIAL LIVER ABSCESS

Etiopathogenesis

Pyogenic liver abscess is caused by staphylococci, streptococci, and gram-negative enterobacteria, i.e. anaerobic inhabitants of the gastrointestinal tract. The bacteria gain access to the liver by direct extension from contiguous organs or through the portal vein or hepatic artery, bile ducts or by direct invasion or inoculation through the Glisson's capsule. The routes of infection are described as under:

- *Arterial route of infection:* Bacteria reach the liver through hepatic artery during sepsis or in septic thromboemboli in bacterial endocarditis. Liver abscess may be caused by a variety of bacteria, such as streptococci, staphylococci, and gram-negative bacteria.
- *Portal vein infection:* Bacteria may originate in infected diverticula or mucosal abscesses. In preantibiotic era, bacterial appendicitis was a common cause of liver abscess; today it is uncommon.
- *Ascending biliary infection:* Bacteria ascending into the liver from the duodenum are most often gram-negative. Such infections usually occur in patients who have bile stones or other diseases of biliary tract.
- *Direct invasion of liver:* Bacterial infection of gallbladder may extend to liver transdiaphragmatic infection or direct entry of bacteria into liver from the infected peritoneum. It is a rare complication of severe infection and usually found in terminally ill patients or those who have had extensive surgery.
- *Direct inoculation of bacteria:* This type of infection is typically found in wounded people.

Gross Morphology
Microabscesses are formed in the liver resulting in hepatomegaly (Fig. 21.35).

Light Microscopy
On histological examination, microabscess of liver contains numerous neutrophils. The beginning of an organizing abscess wall shows some pink fibrin (Fig. 21.36).

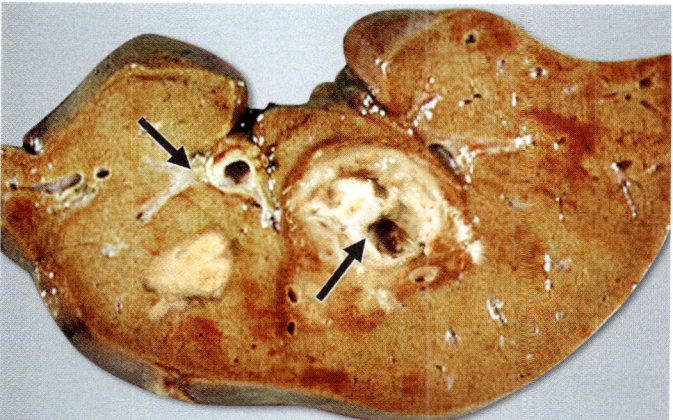

Fig. 21.35: Liver abscesses. This patient died from gram-negative septicemia and the abscesses are a complication of this. The site of the original infection was not found (arrows).

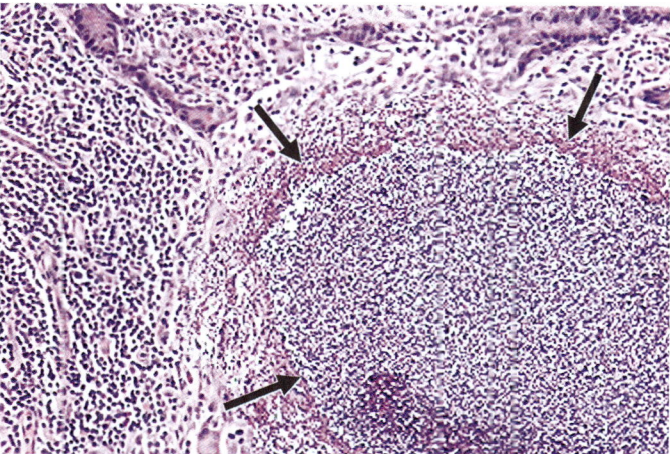

Fig. 21.36: Pyogenic liver abscess. Microscopically, a microabscess of liver contains numerous neutrophils in the center. The beginning of an organizing abscess wall with some pink fibrin is seen here (arrows) (100X).

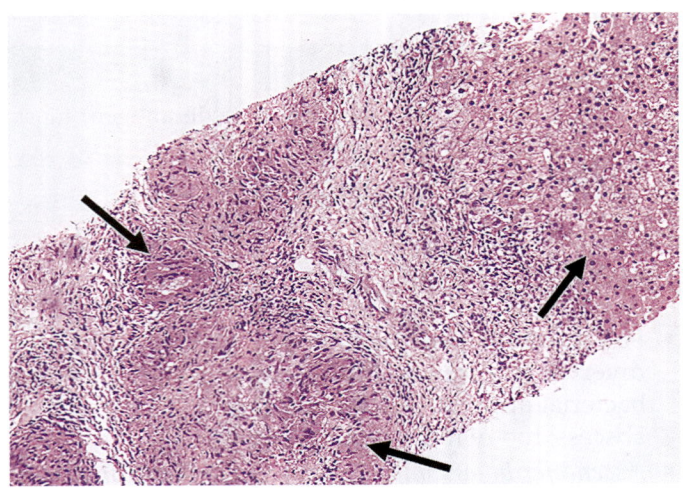

Fig. 21.37: Tuberculosis of liver shows epithelioid cell granuloma. Patient had miliary tuberculosis involving many organs including liver (arrows) (100X).

GRANULOMATOUS LIVER ABSCESS

Granulomatous liver abscess occurs in the settings of tuberculosis, fungal infections and brucellosis. Tuberculous liver abscess most often occurs in developing countries. Tuberculosis is worldwide health problem caused by tubercle bacilli. It is transmitted by inhalation of droplets (most common), ingestion (infected milk) and skin inoculation (handling infected specimens). It may involve multiple systems.

Tubercle bacilli may disseminate via systemic circulation to seed distant organs such as bone marrow, liver, spleen, adrenal glands, retina, meninges, kidneys, fallopian tubes, and epididymis. Light microscopy of tuberculoses of liver is shown in Fig. 21.37.

PARASITIC INFECTIONS

Parasitic and helminthic infections are important in tropical countries. Such infections include malarial parasite, *Entamoeba histolytica*, *Leishmania donovani*, liver fluke (e.g. *Fasciola hepatica* and *Clonorchis sinensis*) and *Echinococcus granulosus*.

AMOEBIC LIVER ABSCESS

Amoebic liver abscess is the most common form of extraintestinal amoebiasis. It most often occurs in *posterosuperior part of right lobe*.

Etiology

Amoebic liver abscess is caused by *Entamoeba histolytica*. Approximately, 30% of patients have a history of antecedent intestinal amoebiasis. It is most often in men than women. The disease is rare in children. Large amoebic abscess presses upon liver capsule resulting in pain.

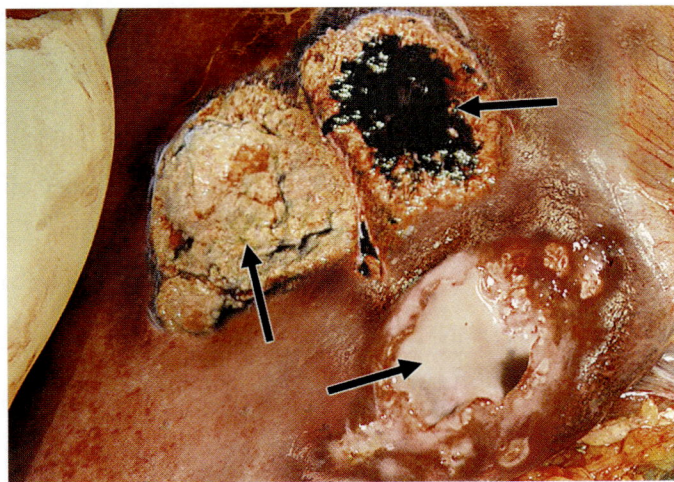

Fig. 21.38: Amoebic liver abscess. This is an amoebic abscess of liver. Abscesses may arise in liver when there is seeding of infection from the bowel, because the infectious agents are carried to the liver from the portal venous circulation (arrows).

Clinical Features

Patient presents with abrupt onset of fever and dull aching abdominal pain in the right upper quadrant or epigastrium, usually lasting <10 days. Jaundice is unusual.

Gross Morphology
Necrosed hepatocytes are admixed with blood resembling *anchovy sauce* (Fig. 21.38).

Light Microscopy
Abscess material on microscopy shows necrotic material with a few neutrophils with clusters of trophozoites of amoeba.

Laboratory Diagnosis

The diagnosis of liver abscess is most often made by radiological or ultrasound in conjunction with serological testing for antibodies to *Entamoeba histolytica*.

Complications

Amoebic liver abscess may be secondarily infected. Abscess can extend and *perforate* into *pleuropulmonary structures*, *subphrenic space*, *peritoneal cavity* and *pericardial sac*. There may be dissemination of amoebic liver abscess to *brain* or *kidney*. Differences between amoebic and pyogenic liver abscesses are shown in Table 21.30.

HYDATID CYST LIVER

Hydatid cyst liver is caused by *Echinococcus granulosus*. It is common in India, right lobe of liver is the commonest site of hydatid cyst followed by lung. Accidental spillage

Liver, Gallbladder and Exocrine Pancreas

Table 21.30: Differences between amoebic and pyogenic liver abscesses

Characteristics	Amoebic liver abscess	Pyogenic liver abscess
Causative organism	*Entamoeba histolytica*	*Escherichia coli*, Pseudomonas and Klebsiella
Liver lobe involved	Posterosuperior part of right lobe	Posterior part of right lobe
Abscess	Single abscess of variable size	Single or multiple abscesses
Gross morphology	The center of abscess has necrotic area containing reddish brown thick pus resembling anchovy or chocolate sauce. Abscess is surrounded by necrotic liver parenchyma	The center of abscess contains pus. Abscess is surrounded by fibrous capsule
Light microscopy	It shows leukocytes, RBCs, necrotic debris and *Entamoeba histolytica*	It shows infiltration by neutrophils
Septicemia	Absent	It may occur due to dissemination of pathogens
Jaundice	Rare	Always present

during fine needle aspiration may cause anaphylactic shock.

Hydatid disease is caused by larval or cystic stage of *Echinococcus granulosus* tapeworm or *Echinococcus multilocularis*. Adult parasites are found in dogs and sheep. Humans are infected after ingestion of eggs. The eggs hatch in the small intestine and their larvae pass to the liver by portal circulation. Most commonly the right lobe is affected although any lobe can be affected.

Echinococcus multilocularis is less common. Cysts are multilocular containing thick pasty material, not surrounded by a fibrous wall. It has a more aggressive clinical disease course in comparison to *Echinococcus granulosus*.

Gross Morphology

Liver contains multiple cysts of various sizes. Color of the cysts is white of an boiled egg (Fig. 21.39).

Light Microscopy

- The cyst is filled with colorless fluid and contains daughter cysts and brood capsules with scolices.
- The cyst wall shows an inner germinal layer (endocyst), outer chitinous (fibrous lamina) ectocyst layer surrounded by either granulation tissue or a fibrous capsule (pericyst).
- The adjacent liver shows portal eosinophilic infiltrate. The scolices having hooklets of 20–40 µm length (Fig. 21.40).

Cytological Examination

Smear shows laminated membranous structures resembling ectocyst of hydatid cyst. Claw-like refractile hooklets are demonstrated in the background (Fig. 21.41).

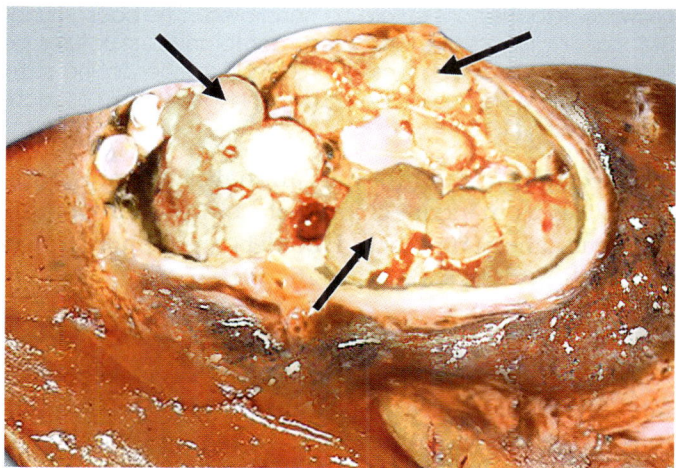

Fig. 21.39: Hydatid cyst of liver. The patient had lived in a sheep-raising area of Australia, but this was an incidental postmortem finding. The outer, thick fibrotic wall of the cyst is clearly seen and the cyst is filled with multiple daughter cysts of varying sizes (arrows).

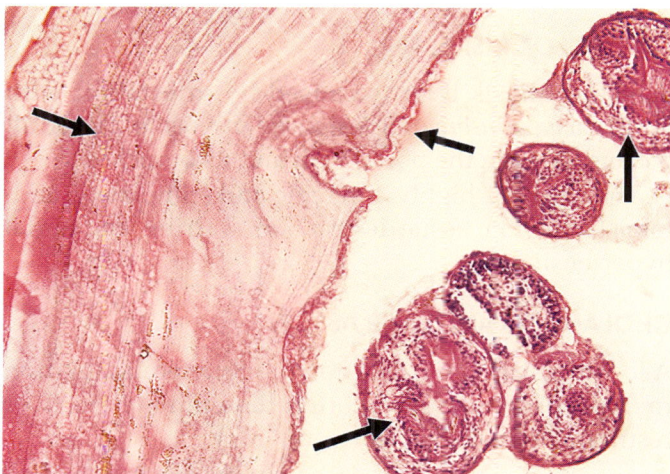

Fig. 21.40: Hydatid cyst of liver. The cyst wall shows an inner germinal layer (endocyst), outer chitinous (fibrous lamina) ectocyst layer surrounded by either granulation tissue or a fibrous capsule (pericyst). Scolices having hooklets are also seen (arrows) (400X).

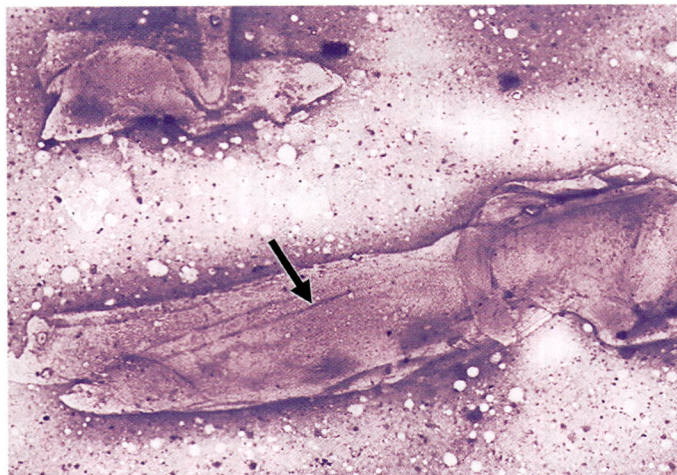

Fig. 21.41: FNAC hydatid cyst of liver. Smear shows laminated membranous structures resembling ectocyst of hydatid cyst. Claw-like refractile hooklets are demonstrated in the background. PAS stain highlights the laminated membranous structures as magenta-colored structures and Gomori methenamine stain black. Hooklets are demonstrated by Ziehl-Neelsen stain as bright purple (arrow) (400X).

PAS stain highlights the laminated membranous structures as magenta-colored structures and Gomori methenamine stain black. Hooklets are demonstrated by Ziehl-Neelsen stain as bright purple.

Complications

Rupture of the cyst into the peritoneal cavity results in fatal anaphylactic reaction. Rupture of cyst can occur into the gallbladder or through the diaphragm into the pleural space and lung.

HEPATOMEGALY DUE TO MALARIA

Hepatic malaria causes hepatomegaly secondary to hypertrophy and hyperplasia of Kupffer cells.

SCHISTOSOMIASIS LIVER

Schistosomiasis liver is caused by infestation with *Schistosoma mansoni* or *Schistosoma japonicum*. The adult worms lodge in the portal vein and its branches.

The eggs are highly antigenic and stimulate granuloma formation, tissue destruction, scarring, and portal hypertension.

CHOLANGITIS AND LIVER ABSCESS

Ascending cholangitis after percutaneous ablation therapy of liver tumors often disseminates to liver resulting in liver abscess.

SUPPURATIVE THROMBOSIS OF PORTAL VEIN

Portal vein thrombosis most often occurs due to intra-abdominal sepsis following perforated appendix, peritonitis or diverticulitis. Infection from portal vein spreads to liver.

Patient presents with fever, rigors and abdominal pain in right upper quadrant. Liver functions are abnormal but clinical jaundice is uncommon. Portal vein thrombosis may cause portal hypertension.

DRUGS AND TOXINS INDUCED LIVER INJURY

Exposure to drugs and industrial chemicals may cause acute liver injury. Chemicals act as systemic poisons and get converted to toxic intermediate leading to centrilobular injury.

Drugs and toxic chemicals may affect one or more of the liver lobular structures such as hepatocytes, bile ductules, bile ducts, blood vessels and mononuclear phagocytes. Lesions affecting hepatocytes are shown in Table 21.31. Lesions affecting bile ductules and bile ducts are shown in Table 21.32.

Pathogensis

Pathogenesis of liver injury by drugs occurs either by direct or idiosyncratic mechanisms.

Direct Injury

It is dose dependent. Drugs may produce intermediate metabolites and free radicals. These cause adverse effects on hepatocytes by peroxidation of cell membrane lipids leading to liver cell injury. Metabolic intermediates may also block the biochemical pathways by impairing mitochondrial oxidation of fatty acids. Therefore, liver shows fatty change.

Idiosyncrasy

Idiosyncrasy mechanism of drugs causing liver injury is not dose dependent.

- *Hypersensitivity:* Metabolites of isoniazid and halothane may cause liver injury by hypersensitivity reaction.
- *Autoantibody synthesis:* Autoantibody synthesized against drug produce adverse effects on cytochrome P450 enzyme.
- *Hapten formation:* Drug or its metabolite binds to cellular proteins and forms a hapten. This hapten acts as antigen leads to hepatocellular injury.

ACETAMINOPHEN INDUCED HEPATOCELLULAR INJURY

Acetaminophen is an important analgesic recommended by clinicians. Excessive consumption is highly toxic to the liver. The toxic dose of acetaminophen after a single acute ingestion is in the range of 150 mg/kg in children and 7 gm in adults. Drug toxicity should be suspected

Table 21.31: Drugs and toxins affecting hepatocytes

Pathological findings	Mode of action	Drugs and toxins
Toxic hepatic coagulative necrosis in zone 3	Reactive metabolites	Paracetamol, carbon tetrachloride poisoning and mushroom *Amanita phalloides* poisonings
Cytosolic spotty necrosis producing intralobular inflammation	Formation of neoantigens as a result of hapten linkage with liver cell proteins	Halothane, erythromycin, isoniazid and α-methyldopa
Acute hepatitis like morphology with cholestasis	Immune-mediated	Sulphonylureas, phenothiazines and tricyclic antidepressants
Chronic hepatitis like morphology	Immune-mediated	Methotrexate, α-methyldopa, nitrofurantoin and oxyphenisatin
Macrovasicular fatty change	Due to decreased proteins synthesis, lack of apoprotein B-100, damage to endoplasmic reticulum, Golgi apparatus or plasma membrane of hepatocytes	Alcohol and methotrexate
Microvesicular fatty change	Reflecting impaired mitochondrial oxidation of fatty acids	Tetracycline, valproic acid (anticonvulsant), Reye's syndrome and poisoning by ingestion of unripe ackee fruit in Jamaica patients
Phospholipid accumulation in lysosomes	Due to inhibition of phospholipase by drugs	Amiodarone
Granulomatous hepatitis	Cell-mediated mechanism	Sulphonamide, allopurinol, carbamazepine, phenylbutazone and quinine
Cirrhosis	Direct toxicity	Ethanol, methotrexate and carbon tetrachloride
Hepatocellular adenoma, hepatocellular carcinoma	–	Estrogens and thormostat contrast dye
Angiosarcoma	–	Vinyl chloride and inorganic arsenic

Table 21.32: Drugs and toxins affecting bile ductules and bile ducts

Pathological findings	Mode of action	Drugs and toxins
Acute cholestasis	Estrogen binding with 17β-glucuronides causing cholestasis	Oral contraceptives, anabolic and androgenic steroids
Prolonged cholestasis with destruction of small bile ducts	Immune-mediated mechanisms	Chlorpromazine, paraquat poisoning and arsenic derivatives
Intrahepatic and extrahepatic stricture resembling sclerosing cholangitis	Mechanism unknown	Infusion of floxuridine into the hepatic artery in the treatment of liver metastases from colorectal carcinoma

in all cases of acute hepatitis. Drug-induced liver injury can be either direct or indirect. Indirect injury is caused by metabolites and free radicals that are produced as byproducts of xenobiotic metabolism.

Physiological State

Normal dose of acetaminophen is rapidly absorbed from the stomach and small intestine and conjugated in the liver to nontoxic metabolite, which then is eliminated in the urine.

Pathological State

In case of acute overdose, normal pathways of acetaminophen metabolism become saturated. Excess acetaminophen is then metabolized in the liver via the mixed function oxidase P450 system located in the smooth endoplasmic reticulum of the liver, yielding oxidative metabolites leading to centrilobular necrosis. Patient may later develop *hepatocellular necrosis*.

CARBON TETRACHLORIDE INDUCED LIVER INJURY

Carbon tetrachloride (CCl_4) is well-studied hepatotoxin. Immune reactions against a chemical or its metabolites are also causes of indirect liver damage. Chemically-induced hepatic injury is classified as *predictable* when toxicity is immediate and dose-dependent and as *unpredictable* or *idiosyncratic* when toxicity occurs without explanation.

Exposure to industrial solvents, such as carbon tetrachloride, causes predictable toxic liver injury, characterized by centrilobular necrosis and elevated serum levels of transaminases.

Mechanism

CCl_4 is metabolized via the mixed function oxygenase system (P450) located in the smooth endoplasmic reticulum of the liver to a chloride ion and a highly reactive trichloromethyl free radical. Like the hydroxyl radical, this radical is a potent initiator of lipid peroxidation, which damages the plasma membrane and leads to cell death.

Light Microscopy

Acute, chemically-induced hepatic injury shows the entire spectrum of liver disease, from transient cholestasis to massive hepatic necrosis.

CIRRHOSIS

Cirrhosis is a manifestation of end stage of chronic liver disease. It is characterized by widespread destruction of hepatocytes, which are replaced by bridging fibrous septae, regeneration of hepatocytes forming nodules resulting into disruption of entire liver architecture with variable degree of portosystemic shunting.

Fibrosis and formation of abnormal parenchymal nodules must be present for establishing diagnosis of cirrhosis. It is especially prevalent among malnourished people older than age 50 with chronic alcoholism; it is also twice as common in men as in women. Etiological classification of cirrhosis is shown in Table 21.33.

CLASSIFICATION

ETIOLOGICAL CLASSIFICATION

Cirrhosis is classified according to etiology described as under.

Alcoholic (Laennec or Nutritional) Cirrhosis

It is most frequently occurring form of cirrhosis associated with alcoholism. Liver shows micronodular pattern evolving in late stages to typical hobnail liver with large and irregular nodules.

Post-necrotic Cirrhosis

Liver shows large, irregular nodules containing intact hepatic lobules; diverse etiologies. This form of macro-nodular cirrhosis is often a sequela of chronic active hepatitis; HBV and HCV. Post-necrotic cirrhosis leads to hepatocellular carcinoma more often than other forms of cirrhosis.

Biliary Cirrhosis

Primary biliary cirrhosis is of probable autoimmune origin caused by *anti-mitochondrial antibodies*; obstructive jaundice. Secondary biliary cirrhosis is the end result of long-standing extrahepatic biliary obstruction (stone, stricture, pancreatitis or pancreatic carcinoma and congenital malformation).

Hemochromatosis Induced Cirrhosis

Primary (hereditary) hemochromatosis is familial defect in control of iron absorption resulting in massive accumulation of hemosiderin in hepatic and pancreatic parenchymal cells, myocardium, and other sites; classic triad of cirrhosis, diabetes mellitus, and increased skin pigmentation; cirrhosis micronodular type. Secondary

Table 21.33: Etiological classification of cirrhosis

Common causes	Rare causes
• Alcohol related liver disease (Laennec's cirrhosis, portal cirrhosis or Hobnail cirrhosis)	• Primary biliary cirrhosis (PBC)
• HBV and HCV (most common in India)	• Wilson's disease
• Non-alcoholic liver disease	• Autoimmune hepatitis
• Secondary biliary cirrhosis (e.g. obstruction of the common bile duct by stone, stricture and pancreatitis or pancreatic carcinoma)	• Primary sclerosing cholangitis
• Hemochromatosis	• Inborn errors of metabolism (α_1-antitrypsin deficiency, galactosemia, glycogen storage disease, fructose intolerance and acid cholesterol ester hydrolase deficiency)
• Methotrexate drug-induced cirrhosis	
• Carbon tetrachloride and ethanol induced cirrhosis	

hemochromatosis is caused by chronic iron overload of diverse etiology.

Wilson's Disease Induced Cirrhosis

It is an autosomal recessive disorder of copper metabolism in which excess copper can be deposited in the liver, kidney tubular cells (aminoaciduria and glycosuria), brain (basal ganglia especially the putamen of the lenticular nucleus impairing extrapyramidal motor functions), and eye cornea (Descemet membrane known as *Kayser-Fleischer ring*).

Ceruloplasmin levels are decreased in Wilson's disease secondary to copper deposition in various organs. Cirrhosis can be micronodular or macronodular.

Inborn Error of Metabolism

Persons with inborn errors of metabolism result in cirrhosis. These include α_1-antitrypsin deficiency, galactose-1-phosphate uridyl transferase deficiency (galactosemia) and glycogen storage disease.

MORPHOLOGICAL CLASSIFICATION

Cirrhosis is classified according to etiology and morphology of nodules. Morphological classification of cirrhosis is purely descriptive. It has no relevance in the clinical presentation and management of these patients.

Micronodular Cirrhosis

It is characterized by nodules measuring <3 mm in size. Liver involvement shows diffuse pattern. Etiology, frequency and light microscopic features in micronodular cirrhosis (Table 21.34).

Macronodular Cirrhosis

It is characterized by nodules measuring >3 mm in size. Liver involvement shows more irregular pattern. Etiology, frequency and light microscopic features in macronodular cirrhosis (Table 21.35).

Micro- and Macronodular Cirrhosis

It is characterized by presence of nodules ranging from <3 to >3 mm in diameter. Some portal tracts and central

Table 21.34: Etiology, frequency and light microscopic features in micronodular cirrhosis

Etiology	Frequency	Light microscopy
Alcoholic cirrhosis	60–70%	Fatty change, neutrophilic infiltration and Mallory's bodies
Primary biliary cirrhosis	5%	Portal tract inflammation (early stage) and granulomas, medium-sized bile duct destruction, cholestasis in zone 1 in periportal region, Mallory's bodies in some cases
Large bile duct obstruction induced cirrhosis	<5%	Marked cholestasis and bile cell proliferation; and irregular outlines of cirrhotic nodules
Hemochromatosis induced cirrhosis	5%	Marked deposition of hemosiderin in hepatocytes, Kuppfer cells and epithelium of ducts
Intestinal bypass	Rare	Marked fatty change, and Mallory's bodies in some cases
Cystic fibrosis induced cirrhosis	Rare	Periodic acid–Schiff material present in proliferated ductules in portal tracts
Indian childhood cirrhosis	Rare	Mallory's bodies

Table 21.35: Etiology, frequency and light microscopic features in macronodular cirrhosis

Etiology	Frequency	Light microscopy
Chronic viral hepatitis (HBV or HCV)	10–20%	Hepatocytes show ground-glass appearance and viral antigens are demonstrated by immunohistochemistry
Cryptogenic cirrhosis	Common	Macronodular cirrhosis of unknown etiology
Wilson's disease	Rare	Excess deposition of copper in hepatocytes demonstrated by rubeanic acid, fatty change and sometimes Mallory's bodies
α_1-Antitrypsin deficiency	Rare	Periodic acid–Schiff stain positive and diastase resistant globules in hepatocytes demonstrated by immunohistochemistry
Drugs and toxins	Rare	Macronodular cirrhosis
Hereditary hemorrhagic telangiectasia	Rare	Large dilated blood vessels in fibrous septa of liver

veins are spared. It is a type of incomplete expression of micronodular cirrhosis.

ETIOPATHOGENESIS

Most important pathways leading to cirrhosis are chronic active hepatitis, steatohepatitis (fatty change with evidence of inflammation), portal fibrosis and fibrosis occurring in acinar zone 3.

Chronic active hepatitis and alcohol liver disease are the most important causes of cirrhosis accounting >60% of cases. The changes that occur in cirrhosis, include irreversible chronic injury of the liver, extensive fibrosis, and nodular tissue growth, resulting from liver cell death; collapse of the liver's supporting structure, distortion of the vascular bed, and nodular regeneration of remaining liver tissue. Toxins stimulate sinusoidal endothelial cells and Kupffer cells (Fig. 21.42).

Activated Kupffer Cells

These release PDGF, TNF-α, TGF-β, ET-1 and MCP-1. PDGF and TNF-α participate in the proliferation of perisinusoidal stellate cells (Ito cells).

PDGF and MCP-1 released by activated Kupffer cells participate in chemotaxis of neutrophils and lymphocytes. Hepatocytes undergo dysfunction and apoptosis.

Perisinusoidal Endothelial Cells

These synthesize endothelin (ET-1) and platelet activating factor. ET-1 stimulates quiescent matrix synthesizing stellate cells (Ito cells).

Stellate (Ito) Cells

These myofibroblast like-stellate cells synthesize collagen fibers. Contraction of stellate cells (Ito cells) causes decreased sinusoidal perfusion resulting in hypoxia.

Morphological Features

Morphological features of cirrhosis are studied on gross examination of liver and histopathological study.

> **Gross Morphology**
>
> - **Early cirrhosis:** Liver is to >2 kg. External surface may show diffuse nodularity. Cut surface shows yellow discoloration (Fig. 21.43).
> - **Late cirrhosis:** Liver is shrunken in size weighing <1 kg. External surface shows nodules (micronodules <3 mm or macronodules >3 mm or mixed pattern). Cut surface shows brown discoloration (Fig. 21.44).

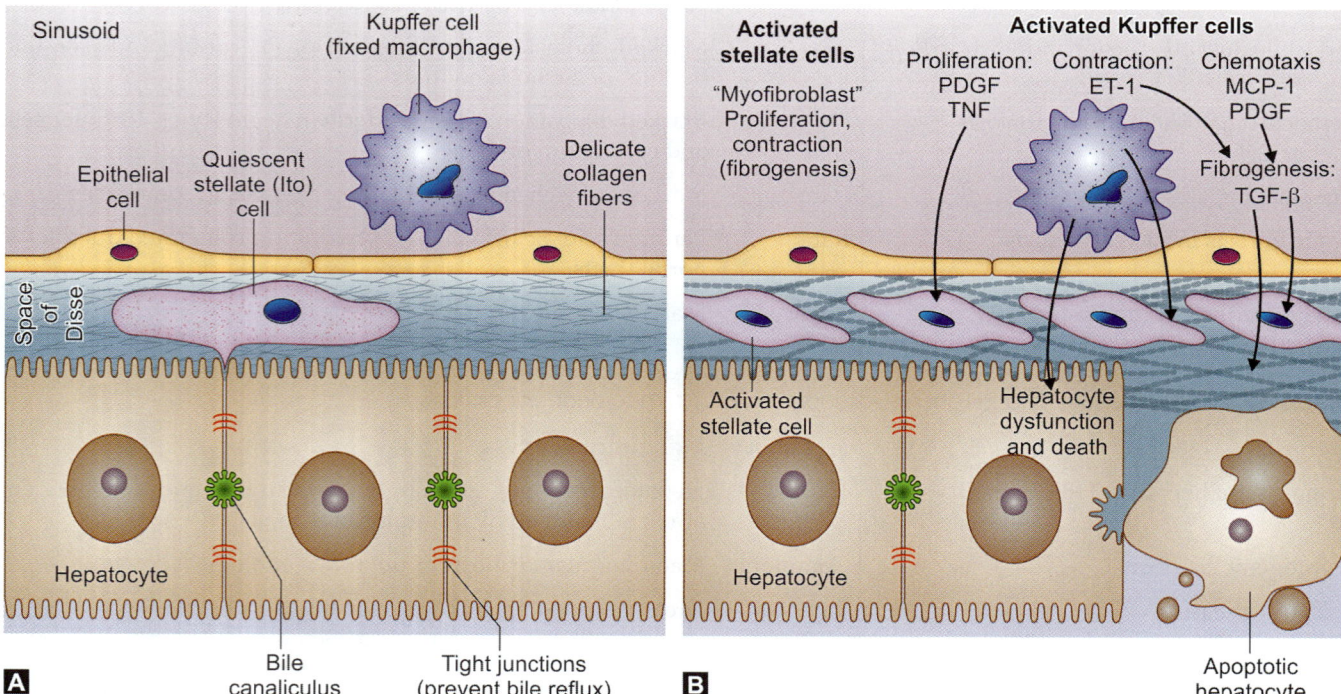

Fig. 21.42: (A) Normal liver morphology, (B) pathogenesis of cirrhosis. Kupffer cell activation and platelet activating factor synthesized by endothelial cells produce cytokines leading to influx of PMNs cells. Endothelial cells synthesize endothelins, which stimulate myofibroblast like Ito cells to synthesize collagen. Contraction of Ito stellate cells results in decreased sinusoidal perfusion and thus cause hypoxia.

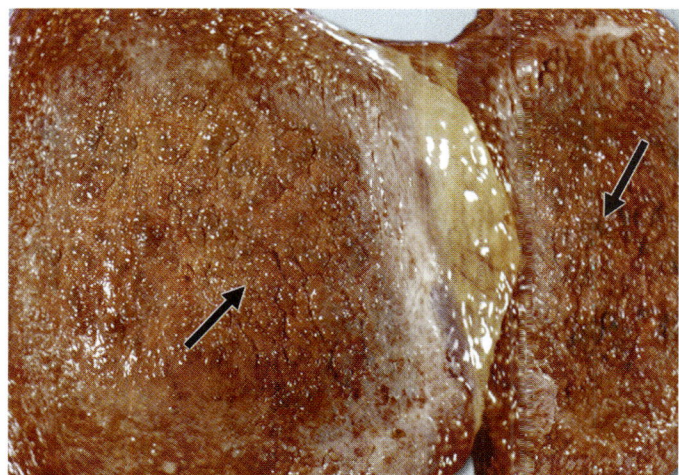

Fig. 21.43: Micronodular cirrhosis. This is an example of a micronodular cirrhosis. The regenerative nodules are quite small, averaging <3 mm in size. The most common cause for this is chronic alcoholism. The process of cirrhosis develops over many years (arrows).

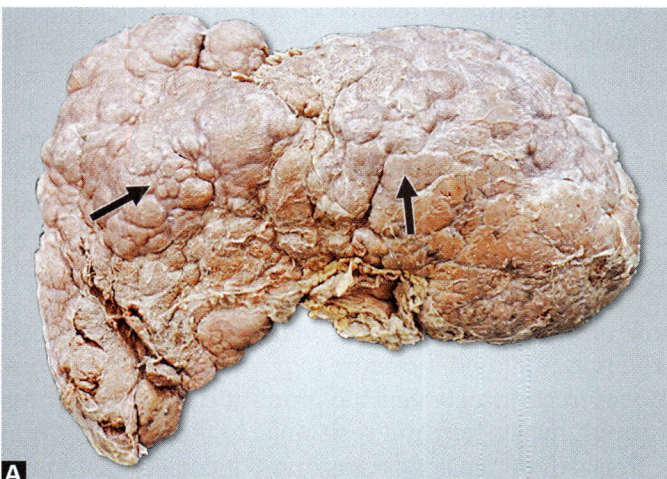

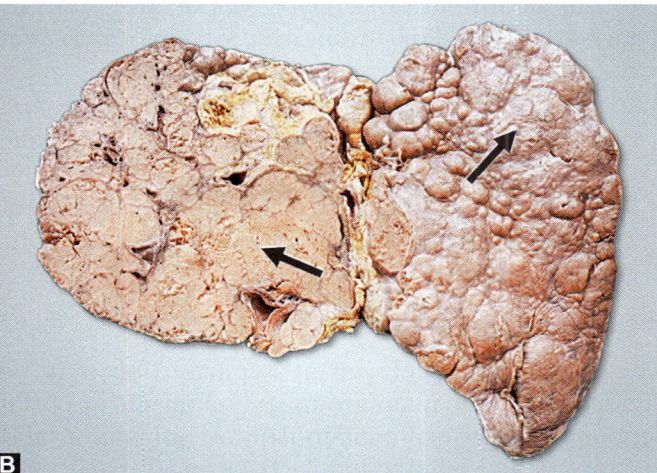

Fig. 21.44: Macronodular cirrhosis. External as well as cut surface of liver shows large nodules >3 mm in diameter. Viral hepatitis (B or C) is the most common cause for macronodular cirrhosis. It may be associated with Wilson's disease and α_1-antitrypsin deficiency (arrows).

Light Microscopy

- Liver architecture is disrupted. It shows regenerating nodules of hepatocytes separated by fibrous bands of variable thickness resulting in disruption of architecture of entire liver.
- Fibrosis occurs as a result of synthesis of collagen by perisinusoidal hepatic stellate cells (Ito cells) (Figs 21.45 and 21.46). Differences between cirrhosis and fibrosis are shown in Table 21.36.

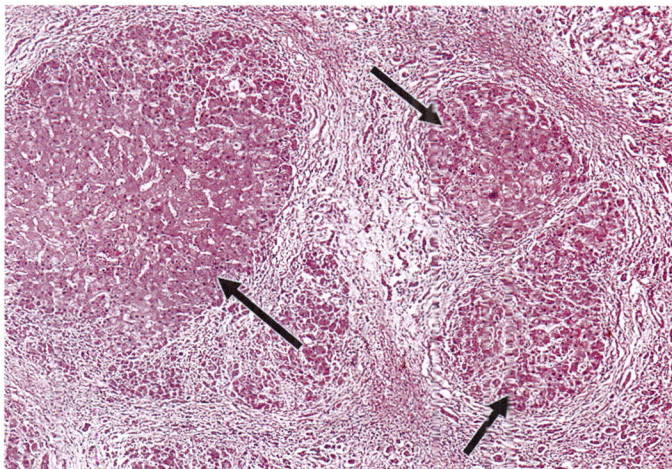

Fig. 21.45: Liver cirrhosis shows regenerative nodules of hepatocytes surrounded by fibrous connective tissue that bridges between portal tracts. Within this collagenous tissue is scattered lymphocytes as well as a proliferation of bile ducts (arrows) (400X).

Table 21.36: Differences between cirrhosis and fibrosis

Parameters	Cirrhosis	Fibrosis
Portal hypertension	Present	Present (marked)
Intrahepatic shunts contributing to portal-systemic shunts	Present	Absent
Impaired hepatocyte functions	Present	Absent
Increased risk of development of hepatocellular carcinoma	Present	Absent

CLINICAL MANIFESTATIONS

These include jaundice, ascites, signs of hyperestrinism (palmar erythema, spider telangiectasia, gynecomastia, and testicular atrophy), and consequences of increased portal venous pressure (esophageal varices, distended abdominal veins (caput medusae), splenomegaly, and consequences of hypoalbuminemia (ascites, peripheral edema). Cirrhosis may lead to *hepatic failure* and *hepatocellular carcinoma* in regenerating nodules. Clinical manifestations of liver cirrhosis are shown in Fig. 21.47 and Table 21.37.

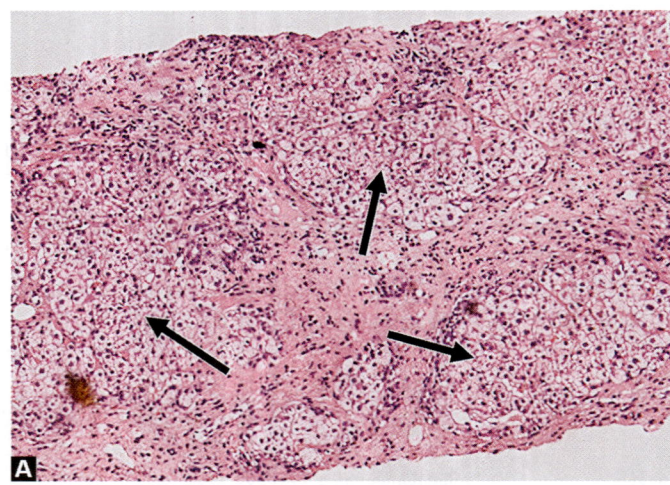
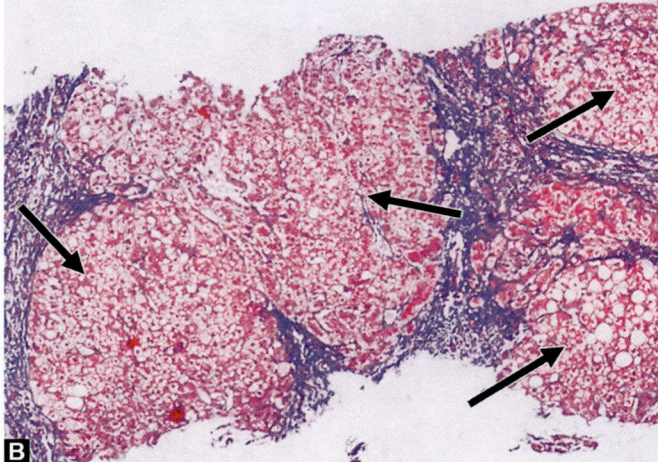

Fig. 21.46: (A) Liver cirrhosis shows regenerative nodules of hepatocytes surrounded by fibrous connective tissue that bridges between portal tracts. Within this collagenous tissue scattered lymphocytes as well as a proliferation of bile ducts (arrows), (B) regenerating nodules surrounded by dense connective tissue stained by Masson trichrome (arrows) (100X).

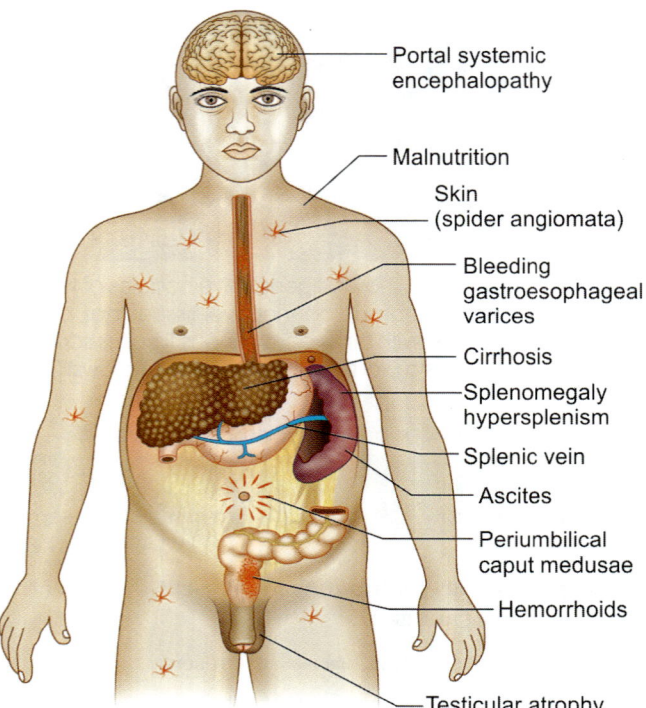

Fig. 21.47: Cirrhosis shows clinical manifestations.

Table 21.37: Clinical manifestations of liver cirrhosis

Clinical sequel	Clinical findings
Portal hypertension	Esophageal varices, splenomegaly, caput medusae, ascites, ankle edema, hypersplenism (anemia, leukopenia and thrombocytopenia) patient develops anemia, hemorrhagic tendencies
Hyperestrinism	Spider nevi, pectoral alopecia, gynecomastia, altered hair distribution, palmar erythema, testicular atrophy

PORTAL HYPERTENSION

Portal hypertension is characterized by the development of venous collaterals with varices in the submucosal veins of the esophagus, hemorrhoidal plexus, and other sites.

Patient with portal hypertension has fatal outcome due to development of hepatic encephalopathy, massive GIT bleeding, recurrent infection, hepatorenal syndrome and hepatocellular carcinoma.

Pathogenesis

Normal pressure in portal vein is 7 mm Hg. As in other vascular bed, pressure in portal vein results from the interaction between the amount of blood flowing through the system and resistance to the blood flow.

- Portal hypertension occurs due to increased resistance to blood flow anywhere in the portal system or increased blood flow through the systemic circulation or combination of both mechanisms.

  In majority of cases, portal hypertension occurs due to resistance to blood flow in prehepatic, hepatic or posthepatic vascular tree.

- Portal hypertension causes significant diversion of blood from the portal circulation into the systemic circulation.

Etiological Classification

At a functional level, portal hypertension may be divided into three main groups based on site of portal venous obstruction (postsinusoidal, sinusoidal and presinusoidal) is shown in Fig. 21.48 and Table 21.38.

- In presinusoidal portal hypertension hepatic venous pressure is normal even though increased pressure in portal vein. Liver functions are normal. Bleeding episode as a rule not followed by liver failure.

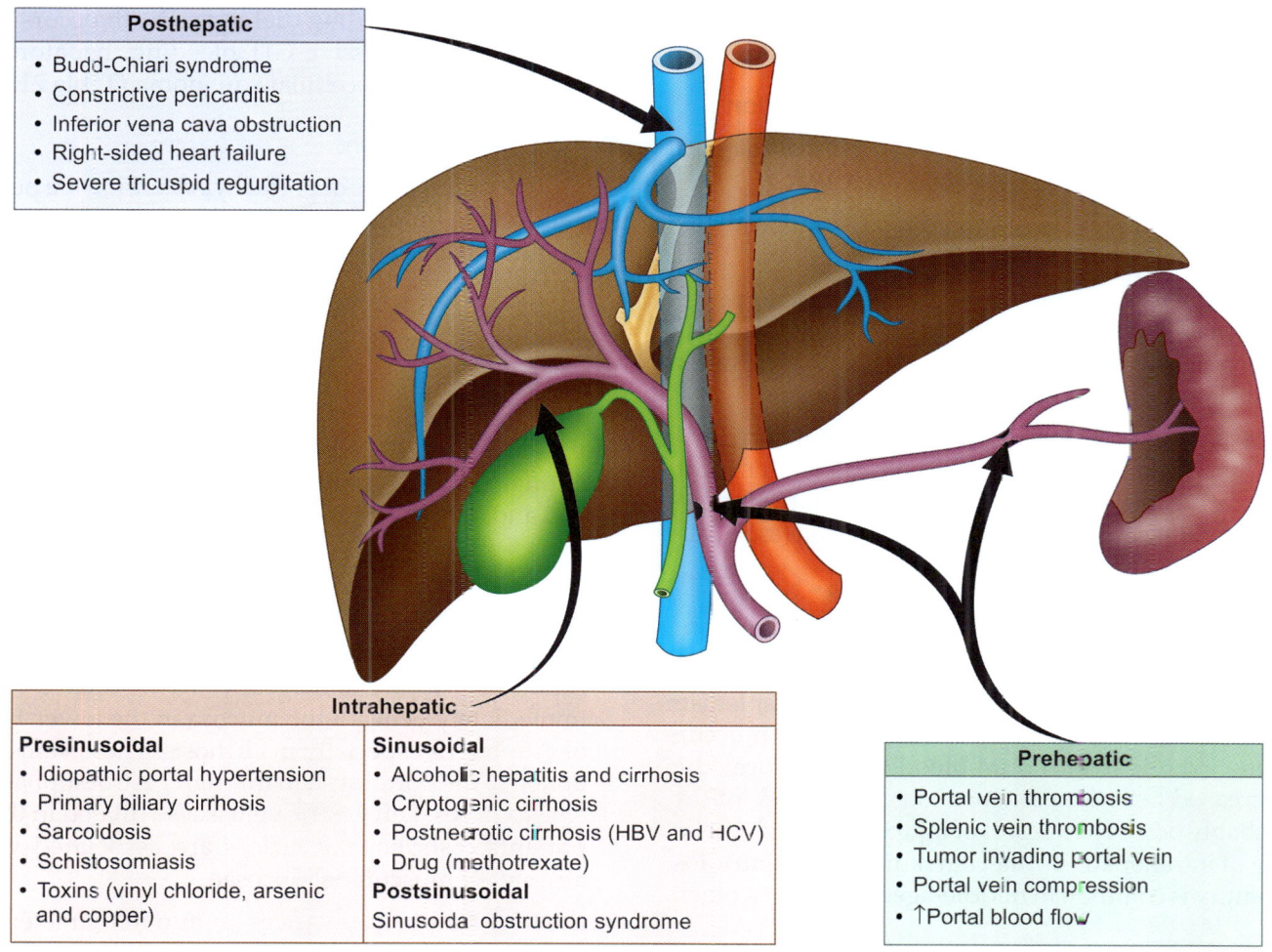

Fig. 21.48: Portal hypertension shows prehepatic, intrahepatic and posthepatic causes.

Table 21.38: Etiological classification of portal hypertension

Site of lesions	Causes
Postsinusoidal etiology	
Heart	Constrictive pericarditis and congestive heart failure
Inferior vena cava	Fibrous tissue webs, thrombosis and tumor invasion
Large extrahepatic veins	Thrombosis (Bud-Chiari syndrome), tumor invasion and fibrous webs
Small intrahepatic veins	Veno-occlusive disorder, alcoholism and central hyaline sclerosis
Sinusoidal etiology	
Intrahepatic lesions	Cirrhosis (most common), acute alcoholic hepatitis, viral hepatitis (HBV and HCV), cytotoxic drug (methotrexate), vitamin A intoxication
Presinusoidal etiology	
Portal tract lesions	Schistosomiasis, early primary biliary cirrhosis, congenital hepatic fibrosis, chronic active hepatitis, toxins (vinyl chloride, arsenic, copper), sarcoidosis, tuberculosis, and idiopathic
Portal and splenic veins	Thrombosis, compression and tumor invasion
Increased portal blood flow	Idiopathic tropical splenomegaly and arteriovenous fistula

- In sinusoidal and postsinusoidal portal hypertension, the resistance to blood flow extends from the central hepatic veins. Hence, pressure in both hepatic and portal veins is increased. Patient with sinusoidal portal hypertension as seen in cirrhosis frequently develop liver failure following a variceal bleed.

PORTAL HYPERTENSION WITH OR WITHOUT PORTAL VEIN OBSTRUCTION

Portal Hypertension with Portal Vein Obstruction

Thrombosis in portal vein is the principal pathological cause of extrahepatic portal vein obstruction.

- *Neonates:* Infection may spread along umbilical vein to reach the left portal vein.
- *Old children:* Intra-abdominal sepsis such as appendicitis may be responsible for portal vein thrombosis. Probable predisposing factors include dehydration associated with gastroenteritis and infection.
- *Adults:* Portal vein thrombosis may occur in ulcerative colitis, Crohn's disease, sclerosing cholangitis, post-operative period, hypercoagulable state (myeloproliferative disorder) and tumor invasion (especially hepatocellular carcinoma).

Portal Hypertension without Portal Vein Obstruction

Presinusoidal portal hypertension is characterized by splenomegaly, functional evidence of hypersplenism without portal vein obstruction. This situation occurs in non-cirrhotic liver. Portal blood pressure rises due to increased hepatic resistance to portal blood inflow. It probably occurs as a result of injury to the endothelial lining of intrahepatic portal vein radicles and sinusoids. This entity is common in middle-aged Japanese women.

Clinical Features

In cirrhosis, liver is unable to receive blood from the gastrointestinal tract and accessory organs. As the pressure in the portal vein rises; blood backs up into the spleen and flows through collateral channels to the venous system, bypassing the liver. Liver fails to synthesize essential vital blood components, filter substances or neutralize toxic substances.

Patient with cirrhosis presents with jaundice, hypoalbuminemia, hyperammonemia (hepatic encephalopathy), fetor hepaticus, palmar erythema, spider angiomas, caput medusae, gynecomastia, respiratory, renal failure and bleeding diathesis. Death occurs due to hepatic coma, massive GIT bleeding, hepatorenal syndrome and hepatocellular carcinoma (Table 21.39).

Clinical Manifestations

Clinical manifestations of portal hypertension are portosystemic shunts, massive splenomegaly and ascites. Later patient develops various complications with fatal outcome.

Portosystemic Shunts

Pressure in the venous system causes distension and varicosity of the veins in esophagus and around umbilicus. Varicose veins can hemorrhage during vomiting, resulting in bloody vomit, internal hemorrhage, and shock with fatal outcome.

Esophageal Varices

In many patients, the first sign of portal hypertension is bleeding esophageal varices.

- *Location of varies:* Esophageal veins are dilated veins immediately beneath the mucosa in the lower-third of esophagus especially in cirrhosis. These veins are linked to the portal system through gastroesophageal anastomoses. Left gastric vein is also dilated in these patients. Esophageal varices are associated with atrophy of muscularis mucosae.
- *Rupture:* Esophageal varices >5 mm in diameter are prone to rupture and life-threatening hematemesis; requiring emergency care to control hemorrhage and prevent hypovolemic shock.
- *Endoscopy:* It is the primary tool for confirming esophageal varices. Varices are graded according to severity. Grade 1 varices can be depressed by pressure exerted by endoscopy. Grade 2 varices cannot be depressed by endoscopy. Grade 3 varices are confluent and extend circumferentially around esophageal lumen.
- *Sclerotherapy:* Esophageal varix is treated by sclerotherapy.

Table 21.39: Clinical manifestations in cirrhosis

Clinical sequelae	Clinical findings
Portal hypertension	Esophageal varices, splenomegaly, caput medusae, ascites, ankle edema, hypersplenism (anemia, leukopenia and thrombocytopenia) patient develops anemia, hemorrhagic tendencies
Hyperestrinism	Spider nevi, pectoral alopecia, gynecomastia, altered hair distribution, palmar erythema, testicular atrophy
Hepatic encephalopathy	Jaundice, hemorrhagic tendencies due to decreased synthesis of coagulation factors, edema due to decreased synthesis of albumin by liver. Asterixis is a flapping tremor associated with hepatic encephalopathy

- *Imaging techniques:* These demonstrate numerous prominent blue venous channels beneath the mucosa of the everted esophagus, particularly above the gastroesophageal junction.

Caput Medusae around Umbilicus

The umbilical vein remnants of fetal circulation present in falciparum ligament. It can become anastomotic link between portal vein and epigastric veins of anterior abdominal wall around umbilicus. Caput medusae results from dilation of the periumbilical venous collaterals as a result of portal hypertension and activation of porto-caval anastomoses.

Hemorrhoids in Rectal Submucosa

Superior and middle hemorrhoidal veins form part of the portal venous drainage, whereas the inferior hemorrhoidal vein drains into the inferior vena cava. Anastomoses formed between these two systems lead to development of rectal varices (hemorrhoids).

- *Internal hemorrhoids:* These are formed due to dilatation of superior hemorrhoidal veins. These may protrude from the anus.
- *External hemorrhoids:* These are formed due to dilatation of inferior hemorrhoidal veins.

Shunting of Blood in Left Renal Vein

Shunting of blood to left renal vein occurs derived directly from splenic vein or pancreatic or gastric veins.

MASSIVE SPLENOMEGALY

Morphological consequences of portal hypertension are esophageal varices and massive splenomegaly.

Gross Morphology
- The spleen is enlarged, as it is unable to drain through portal vein. Due to excess of blood in spleen, the risk of rupture and internal hemorrhage is very high.
- Due to pooling of platelets in enlarged spleen, patient develops thrombocytopenia (Fig. 21.49).

Light Microscopy
- Sinusoids of spleen are dilated and lined by prominent endothelial cells.
- Macrophages are prominent and containing hemosiderin granules.
- Spleen may show small hemorrhages.

ASCITES

Ascites is defined as the accumulation of free fluid in the peritoneal cavity. Clinical examination does not detect ascites if fluid is <500 ml. In clinical practice,

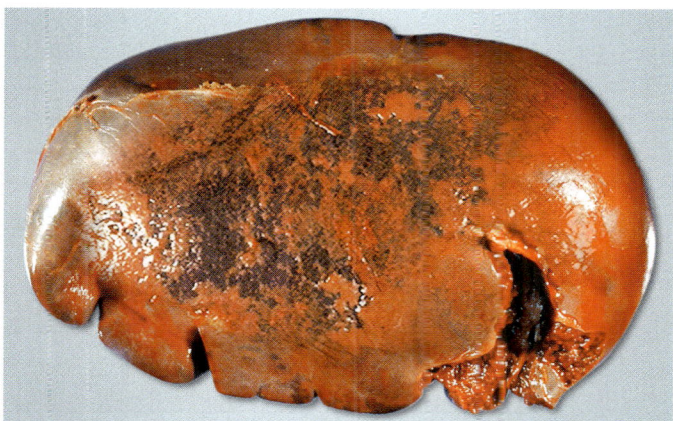

Fig. 21.49: Massive splenomegaly in portal hypertension. The spleen is enlarged from the normal 300 gm or less to between 500 and 1000 gm. Another finding here is the irregular pale tan plaques of collagen over the purple capsule known as *sugar icing* or *hyaline perisplenitis* which follows the splenomegaly and/or multiple episodes of peritonitis that are a common accompaniment to cirrhosis of liver.

patient with decompensated cirrhosis may accumulate excessive fluid in the peritoneal cavity leading to gross distension of the abdominal wall. Protein content of fluid reveals low protein content about 1–2 gm/dl indicating expression of transudate. Higher concentration of protein in the fluid reflects either superadded infection or cirrhosis progressing to hepatocellular carcinoma. Pathogenesis of ascites and generalized edema in liver disease (Fig. 21.50).

Pathogenesis

Patient develops ascites due to sinusoidal hypertension, percolation of hepatic lymph, intestinal capillary fluid leakage and renal retention of Na^+ and water. There is seepage of plasma out of veins and lymphatic channels into the peritoneal space resulting in abdominal distension.

Normal flora of gut may seep out to produce infection in this fluid, resulting in life-threatening spontaneous bacterial peritonitis. Patient with cirrhosis develops peripheral edema, ascites and hydrothorax by the following mechanisms:

- *Increased pressure at the venous end of splanchnic capillaries:* It leads to transudation of fluid from vascular to the extravascular compartment. This mechanism occurs in the presence of sinusoidal portal hypertension as a result of deposition of collagen fibers in the *space of Disse*.
- *Increased formation of hepatic lymph:* Lymphatic channels are dilated at the hilum of the liver. Flow of lymph in thoracic duct is also increased. It is likely that escape of lymph from the liver surface occurs only when the capacity of the thoracic duct is exceeded.

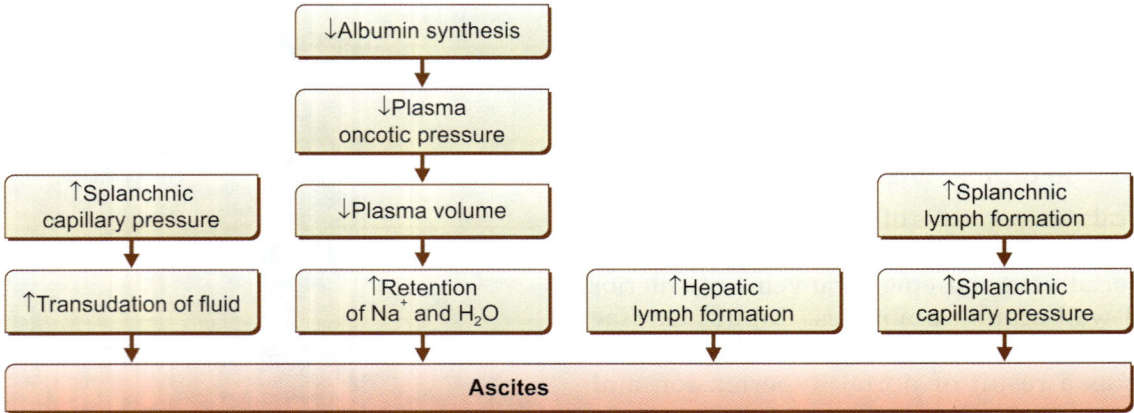

Fig. 21.50: Pathogenesis of ascites and generalized edema in liver disease.

- *Decreased oncotic pressure:* In the setting of cirrhosis, decreased intravascular oncotic pressure due to hypoalbuminemia is also an important factor in the pathogenesis of ascites. Overall, imbalances in Starling forces lead to transudation of fluid into the abdominal cavity.
- *Decreased degradation of aldosterone and angiotensin II:* Concentration of aldosterone and angiotensin II is increased due to decreased degradation in cirrhotic patients. Increased aldosterone level acts on distal convoluted tubules and enhances excessive absorption of sodium and water. It is worth mentioning that angiotensin II stimulates adrenal cortex to synthesize aldosterone.

Complications

Complications of portal hypertension are hepatic encephalopathy, altered metabolic activity, disruption of hormonal inactivation, bleeding and bruising; skin lesions and hematological abnormalities (Figs 21.51 and 21.52).

HEPATIC ENCEPHALOPATHY

Patient with liver disease presenting with neuropsychiatric disturbances is known as *hepatic encephalopathy*. It may occur in a background of chronic liver disease such as cirrhosis in association with massive necrosis of liver leading to acute liver failure. The progressive loss of liver function can lead to liver failure. A person with end-stage liver failure needs liver transplantation for survival.

Clinical Course

- *Acute liver failure:* Patient with acute liver failure due to fulminant hepatitis or drug-induced hepatocellular injury develops rapid hepatic encephalopathy with poor outcome.
- *Chronic liver disease:* Clinical manifestation is different in patient with chronic liver disease. During clinical course, features of gradual hepatic encephalopathy occur.

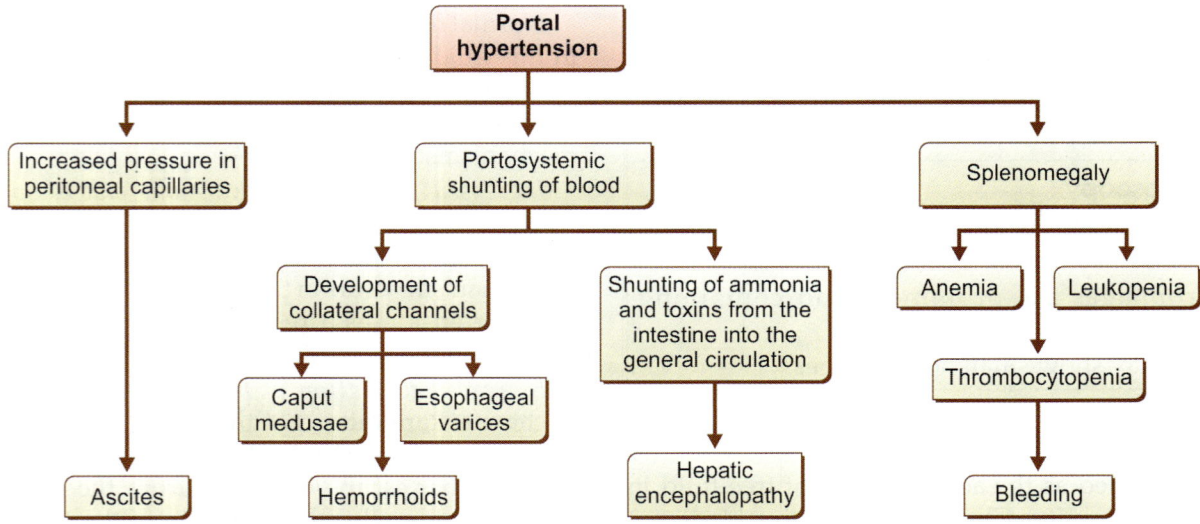

Fig. 21.51: Mechanism of disturbed liver functions related to portal hypertension.

Liver, Gallbladder and Exocrine Pancreas

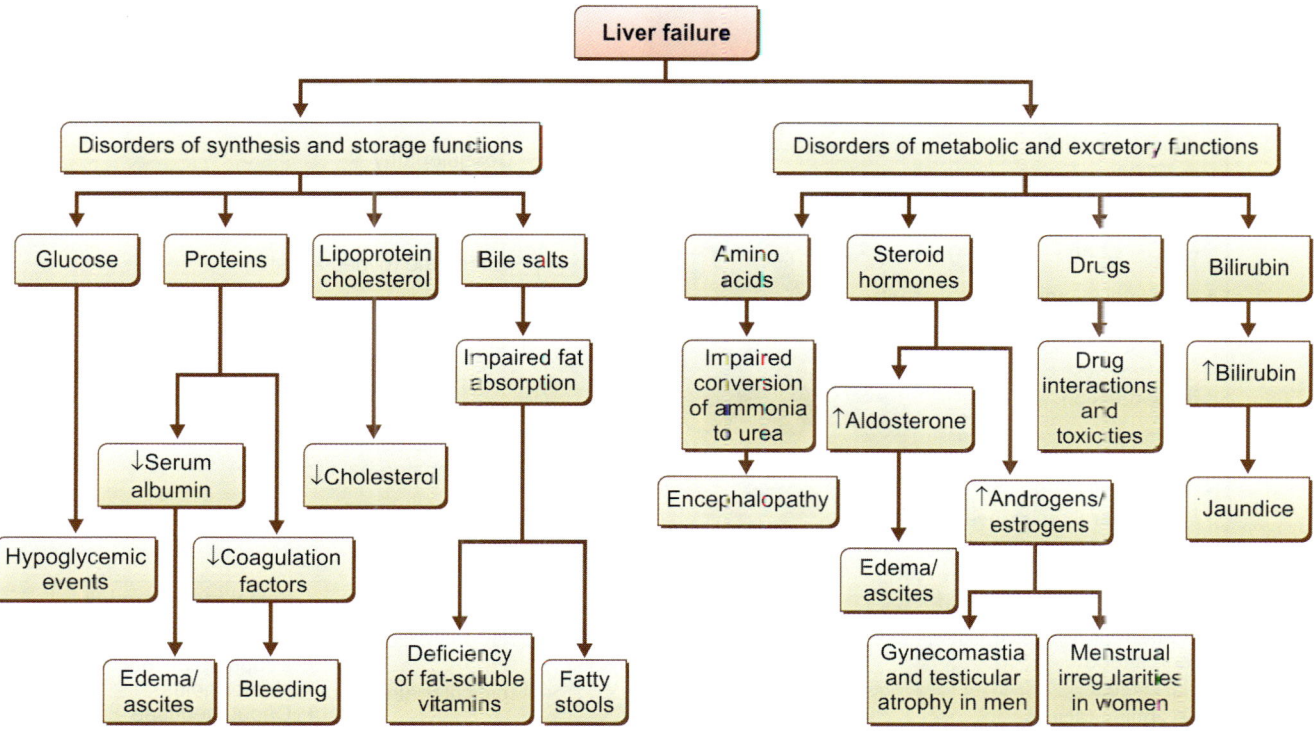

Fig. 21.52: Alterations in liver function and clinical manifestations of liver failure.

Pathogenesis

Central to the development of hepatic encephalopathy is shunting of portal blood to systemic circulation.

- *Functional basis:* Massive liver necrosis resulting from fulminant or toxic damage fails to metabolize the constituents of the portal blood.
- *Anatomically basis:* In patient with cirrhosis, shunting of portal blood to systemic circulation is purely based on disrupted anatomical architecture of liver.

Clinical Features

Patient presents with somnolence, confusion, neck rigidity, flapping tremors of hands (asterixis), hallucinations, and coma with fatal outcome.

Flapping tremors are characteristic of hepatic encephalopathy but not pathognomonic, because these may be seen in patient with uremia, respiratory failure, cardiac failure and hypoglycemia (Fig. 21.53).

Gross Morphology

The brain appears normal. Cerebral edema is seen in patient with fulminant hepatitis in 50% of cases, who have been in coma for some days.

Light Microscopy

- *Early histological changes:* Histopathological examination reveals increase in size and number of protoplasmic astrocytes in the deep cortex, basal ganglion and dentate nucleus in cerebellum. Astrocytes show pale cytoplasm and lobulated nucleus. Such altered astrocytes are also known as *Alzheimer type II cells*.
- *Late histological changes:* In patients with history of recurrent episodes of hepatic encephalopathy over time, the cortex is thinned out due to irreversible loss of neurons and fibers. Demyelination is an occasional finding demonstrated in the spinal tracts producing spastic paraplegia.

Altered Metabolic Activity in Hepatic Encephalopathy

Advanced cases of cirrhosis fail to detoxify toxic substances. Further blood–brain barrier in central nervous system becomes less effective in these patients. Altered metabolic activity in hepatic encephalopathy include increased concentration of ammonia, mercaptans, octapine and γ-aminobutyric acid (GABA).

Toxic substances such as ammonia and other enteric degradation products shunting from liver to

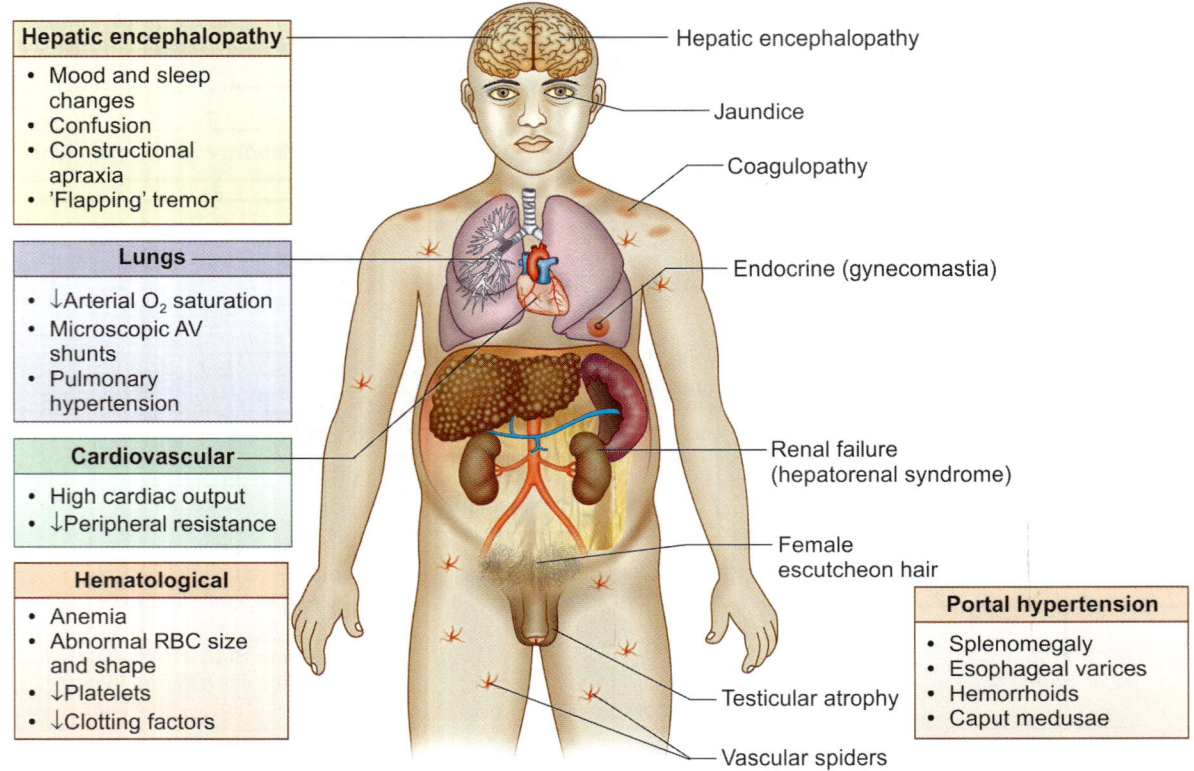

Fig. 21.53: Clinical manifestations and complications of hepatic encephalopathy in a patient of portal hypertension.

the systemic circulation deliver neurotoxic substances and cause brain damage (Fig. 21.54). Factors triggering hepatic encephalopathy are shown in Table 21.40.

Increased Blood Ammonia Concentration

It is not a reliable indicator of hepatic encephalopathy, because some patients with unequivocal coma may show normal blood ammonia concentration.

Mercaptans

Derivatives of aromatic amino acids such methionine, phenylalamine, tyrosine and tryptophan are known as

Table 21.40: Factors triggering hepatic encephalopathy

Factors	Examples
Infections	Bacterial peritonitis, chest infections, urinary tract infections
Hemorrhage	Esophageal varices, peptic ulcer, Mallory-Weiss syndrome (vomiting induced bleeding)
Electrolytes imbalance	Diuretics
Drugs and toxic substances	Morphea, benzodiazepines, barbiturates, and alcohol

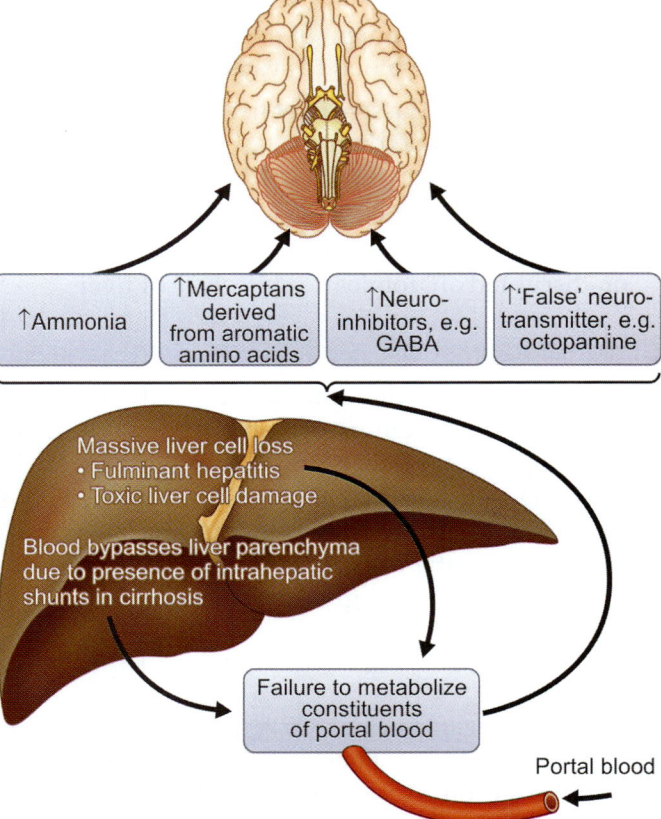

Fig. 21.54: Pathogenesis of hepatic encephalopathy.

mercaptans. These are responsible for the curious odor of breath *fetor hepaticus* in patient with acute liver failure.

Octopamine False Neurotransmitter

Its derived from colon as a result of bacterial infection.

γ-Aminobutyric Acid (GABA) Neurotransmitter

Patient with hepatic encephalopathy exhibits increased binding of benzodiazepines and increased blood concentration of GABA.

Glutamine Concentration in CSF

It is most often increased in hepatic encephalopathy. Its measurement is a *reliable diagnostic tool.* Glutamine in cerebrospinal fluid is derived from aromatic amino acids such as methionine, phenylalamine, tyrosine and tryptophan.

HEPATORENAL SYNDROME

Advanced cirrhosis can impair blood flow to the kidneys resulting in hepatorenal syndrome. Renal leads to oliguria, azotemia, and increased levels of serum creatinine.

Pathogenesis

Renal failure occurs due to vasoconstriction and hypoperfusion of the kidneys mediated by various hormones and vasoactive substances, some of which may not be cleared by the cirrhotic liver. Hepatorenal syndrome is an emergency that requires a liver transplant.

Disruption of Hormones Inactivation

Liver normally inactivates estrogen in men. Male patients with cirrhosis no longer inactivate estrogen.

Hyperestrinism in Men

It manifests with gynecomastia, loss of chest and pubic hair; impotence, testicular atrophy and palmar erythema, spider nevi (capillary telangiectasis) of the face, upper arms, and chest. These findings are attributed to reduced hepatic catabolism of estrogens (i.e. hyperestrogenism).

Hyperestrinism in Women

Women patients present with cessation of menstrual periods, infertility and growth of body hair. Both men and women with cirrhosis can expect a decreased sex drive.

BLEEDING AND BRUISING

Patient with chronic liver disease presents with bleeding and bruise for prolonged periods. Affected person may show several functional bleeding defects. Bleeding and bruise occur by the following mechanisms.

Decreased Synthesis of Proteins

Liver synthesizes inadequate vitamin K-dependent coagulation factors and substrates (II, VII, IX, and X); natural occurring anticoagulants such as protein C, protein S and antithrombin III; and antifibrinolytic protein (plasminogen).

Synthesis of Abnormal Forms of Proteins

Liver synthesizes abnormal forms of vitamin K-dependent clotting factors, fibrinogen, and factor VIII except von Willebrand factor.

Decreased Clearance of Proteins

There is impaired clearance of activated clotting factors, thrombin-antithrombin III complex and plasminogen activators synthesized by endothelium.

SKIN LESIONS

Jaundice

Bilirubin, a product of dead red blood cells is produced in the spleen and then recycled in the liver as a component of bile. Cirrhosis interferes with this process; bilirubin (most often mixed conjugated and unconjugated) is accumulated in the bloodstream. Bilirubin has affinity for sclera giving yellow discoloration.

Spider Nevi

Patient with chronic liver disease may develop spider nevi. These lesions consist of a centrally dilated arteriole from which numerous small vessels radiate. Pressure exerted on the central arteriole causes blanching of the lesions. Number of spider nevi increases in patient with worsening liver disease and the converse is true if liver pathology improves.

Palmar Erythema

Patient with chronic liver disease most often develops warm red palms with eminent thenar and hypothenar regions.

HEMATOLOGICAL ABNORMALITIES

Patient with chronic liver disease may show hematological abnormalities.

Anemia: Patient develops anemia as a result of hypersplenism induced hemolysis, increased plasma volume (sodium and water absorption), recurrent bleeding associated with esophageal varices and bone marrow depression.

RBCs

- *Type of anemia:* Patient may develop macrocytic anemia due to disturbance of vitamin B_{12} and folic acid metabolism. Microcytic anemia occurs as a result of recurrent bleeding.
- *Target cells:* Presence of target cells is associated with increased amounts of cholesterol and phospholipid in the cell membrane.
- *Echinocytes (spiky):* These are associated with binding of an abnormal high density lipoprotein to the red cell surface.
- *Acanthocytes:* These are bizarre cells with many projections on their surfaces. Mechanism of acanthocytes is not known.

WBCs

- *Leukocytosis:* It is associated with fulminant hepatitis, hepatic malignancy, ascending cholangitis and alcoholic liver disease.
- *Leukopenia:* It is associated with alcoholic cirrhosis as a result of hypersplenism and toxic effects on bone marrow.

Platelets

Thrombocytopenia occurs due to increased pooling of platelets in the spleen, shortening of platelet's lifespan and inability of the bone marrow to compensate fully for these defects. There may be abnormality of aggregation defects of platelets.

METABOLIC LIVER DISEASES

ALCOHOLIC LIVER DISEASE

Alcoholic liver disease is the constellation of hepatic changes associated with excessive alcohol consumption. Approximately 60% of chronic alcoholics develop fatty liver. Around 40% develops steatohepatitis, showing inflammation and early fibrosis on histological examination. Approximately 10–15% may develop micronodular cirrhosis over a span of 10–15 years. Only 10% of persons with cirrhosis develop hepatocellular carcinoma. Alcoholic liver disease is shown in Fig. 21.55.

Alcohol intake and increased risk of cirrhosis in men is shown in Table 21.41.

Table 21.41: Alcohol intake and increased risk of cirrhosis in men

Quantity of daily intake of alcohol	Relative risk of cirrhosis
0.2 gm	1
40–60 gm	6
60–80 gm	14

Pathogenesis

Ethanol absorbed by gastrointestinal tract is metabolized in liver by three pathways: alcohol dehydrogenase (most important), microsomal ethanol oxidizing system

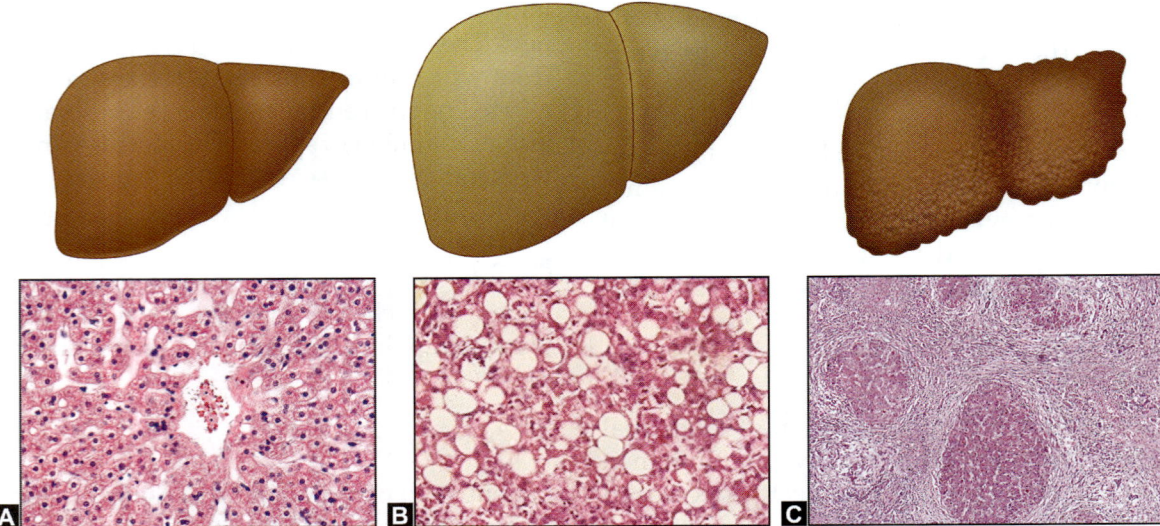

Fig. 21.55: Alcoholic liver disease. Approximately 60% of chronic alcoholics develop fatty liver. Around 40% develop steatohepatitis, showing inflammation and early fibrosis on histological examination. Approximately 10–15% may develop micronodular cirrhosis. Only 10% of persons with cirrhosis develop hepatocellular carcinoma. (A) Normal liver, (B) fatty liver, (C) cirrhosis of liver.

(P450) and catalase. Alcohol mobilizes fatty acids from peripheral adipose tissue.

It alters mitochondrial and smooth endoplasmic reticulum thus inhibits fatty acid oxidation to ketone bodies and CO_2. Alcohol also decreases synthesis of lipoproteins resulting in accumulation of fat in liver cells.

- *Mobilization and biosynthesis of fatty acids:* Ethanol participates in mobilization of fatty acids to liver from peripheral stored fat. Alcohol dehydrogenase generates excessive NADH resulting in biosynthesis of lipid.
- *Mitochondrial dysfunction:* Normally, mitochondria participates in metabolism of ethanol to acetaldehyde. Ethanol disrupts normal functions of mitochondria and microtubules resulting in decreased fatty acid metabolism.
  Fatty acids then accumulate in smooth endoplasmic reticulum of hepatocytes. There is decreased synthesis of lipoproteins, hence liver is unable to release fatty acids to peripheral tissues.
- *Lipid peroxidation by acetaldehyde:* Acetaldehyde, metabolic product of ethanol induces lipid peroxidation with formation of malondiadehyde-acetaldehyde adduct. Autoantibody formed against this adduct results in hepatocellular injury.
- *Role of cytokines in cirrhotic nodules formation:* Ethanol stimulates Kupffer cells to synthesize cytokines such as TNF-α, IL-1, IL-6 and TNF-β, responsible for inflammation in liver. These cytokines stimulate stellate cells to synthesize malondiadehyde-acetaldehyde adduct responsible for *cirrhotic nodules* formation by laying down of collagen fibers.
- *Free radicals induced hepatocellular injury:* Microsomal ethanol oxidizing system (P450) participates in oxidation of ethanol and generation of free radicals leading to hepatocellular injury.

FATTY CHANGE (STEATOSIS) LIVER

Fatty change of the liver is the most frequent morphologic abnormality caused by alcohol. It is characterized by the accumulation of triglycerides within parenchymal cells. It results from an imbalance between the uptake, utilization, and mobilization of fat from liver cells.

The amount of fat deposited varies with the amount of alcohol consumed, as well as the patient's hormonal status, diet, and other factors. Accumulation of triglyceride by itself is not ordinarily damaging, and the condition is fully reversible upon discontinuation of alcohol abuse.

Causes

Alcohol abuse and diabetes mellitus associated with obesity are the most common causes of fatty change in liver. Alcoholic fatty liver may be reversible with complete abstinence from alcohol. Nonalcoholic fatty liver disease (NAFLD) is a related condition unrelated to alcohol consumption. Normal liver metabolism of free fatty acids (FFAs) is shown in Fig. 21.56.

- *Alcohol intake:* It alters mitochondrial and smooth endoplasmic reticulum function and thus inhibit fatty acid oxidation resulting in accumulation of lipids in hepatocytes.
- *Protein malnutrition:* It causes decreased synthesis of lipoproteins. Anoxia inhibits fatty acid oxidation.
- *Starvation:* It leads to mobilization of fatty acids. Diabetes mellitus and obesity may also cause fatty change.

Patterns of Fatty Liver

Pattern and etiology of fatty liver (steatosis) are shown in Table 21.42.

Table 21.42: Pattern and etiology of fatty liver (steatosis)

Microvesicular steatosis	Macrovesicular steatosis
Acute fatty liver of pregnancy in 3rd trimester leads to acute liver failure with fatal outcome	Late alcoholic liver disease
Early alcoholic liver disease	Toxins
Tetracycline drug (hypersensitivity-like reaction in liver)	Diabetes mellitus (insulin resistance)
Reye syndrome	Protein energy malnutrition (kwashiorkor)
Lysosomal acid lipase deficiency	Lipodystrophy
Chronic viral hepatitis	Dysbetalipoproteinemia
Wolman disease	Inflammatory bowel disease
	Syndrome X (diabetes mellitus and obesity with raised lipid level)
	Estrogens and calcium channel blockers

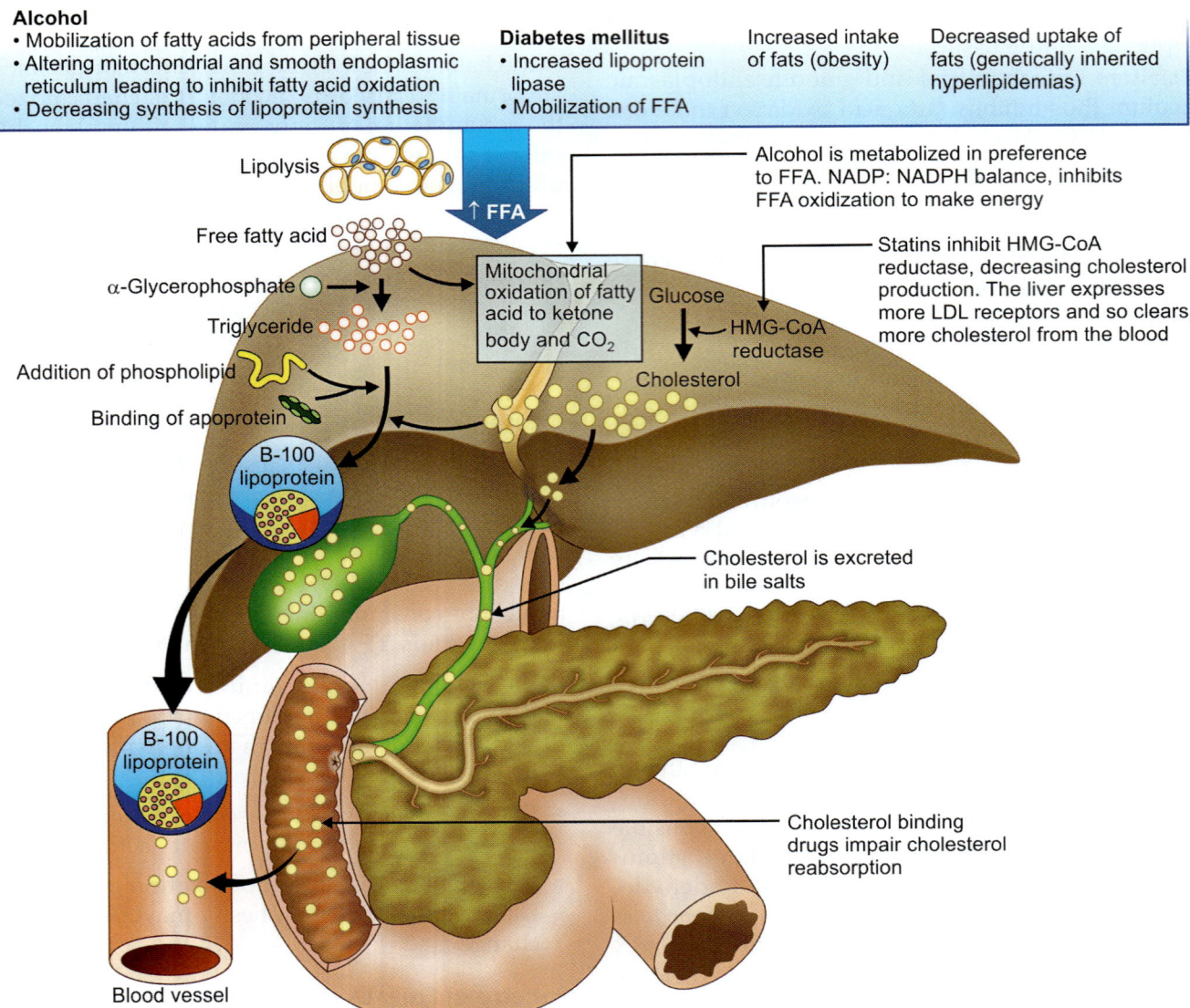

Fig. 21.56: Normal liver metabolism of free fatty acids (FFA). The cholesterol pathway is also shown. Cholesterol is also brought to the liver by high-density lipoproteins (HDL). The point at which alcohol interacts are shown. The effects of drug statin treatment are shown.

- *Microvesicular steatosis:* Minute multiple droplets of fats are present in hepatocytes not displacing nuclei to periphery.
- *Macrovesicular steatosis:* Single large lipid droplet is present in hepatocytes displacing nuclei to periphery.

Pathophysiology

Physiological state: Free fatty acids from adipose tissue or ingested are normally transported into hepatocytes, where these are esterified to triglycerides, converted into cholesterol or phospholipids, or oxidized to ketone bodies. Some of the fatty acids are synthesized from acetate within hepatocytes as well. Egress of the triglyceride requires the formation of complexes with apoproteins to form lipoproteins, which are able to enter the circulation.

Pathological state: Defects in any of the steps of uptake, catabolism, or secretion can lead to accumulation of triglycerides in fatty liver. Hepatotoxins (e.g. *alcohol*) alter mitochondrial and smooth endoplasmic reticulum function and thus inhibit fatty acid oxidation. *Carbon tetrachloride* and *protein malnutrition* decrease the synthesis of apoproteins. *Anoxia* inhibits fatty acid oxidation, and starvation increase fatty acid mobilization from peripheral stores.

Clinical Significance

Mild fatty change has no effect on cellular functions. Severe fatty change may transiently impair cellular functions. But in carbon tetrachloride poisoning, fatty change is irreversible.

Liver, Gallbladder and Exocrine Pancreas

Clinical Features

Patient with fatty liver shows hepatomegaly and mild elevation of serum bilirubin and alkaline phosphatase.

Gross Morphology

Fatty change starts at centrilobular area and progresses to involve whole lobule. Mild fatty change in liver may not affect the gross appearance. Severe fatty change results in enlargement of liver. It becomes progressively yellow on cut surface until it may weigh 3 to 6 kg. This uniform change is consistent with fatty metamorphosis (fatty change). Gross morphology of fatty liver is shown in Fig. 21.57.

Light Microscopy

- *Fatty change:* Initially, hepatocytes show small fat vacuoles around nucleus (mild fatty change or microvesicular) in hematoxylin and eosin stained sections. Progressive accumulation of fat vacuoles in the cytoplasm coalesces to create spaces that displace the nucleus toward periphery (severe fatty change).
- *Fatty cysts:* Occasionally contiguous cells rupture, and the enclosed fat globules unite to produce so-called fatty cysts.
- *Distribution:* Distribution of lipid vacuoles may be diffuse, focal or zonal, midzonal or peripheral depending on severity and etiology (Fig. 21.58).

Fat Demonstration by Frozen Section Technique

In paraffin embedded sections, fat is dissolved during processing of tissue. Fat can be demonstrated by frozen

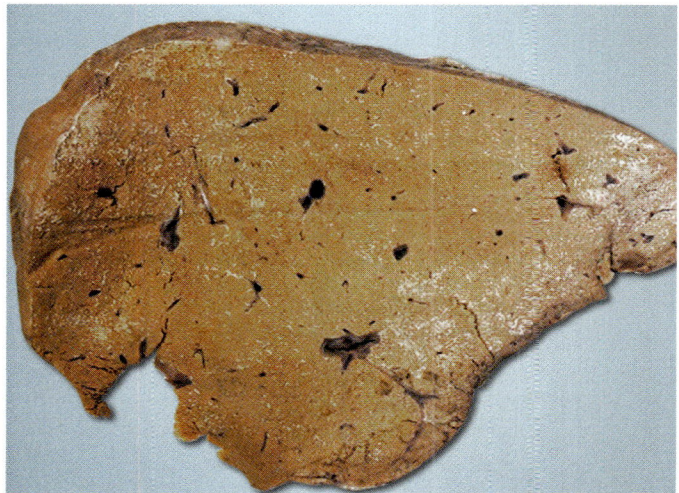

Fig. 21.57: Fatty liver. This is a larger liver with more pronounced fatty change. Such fatty change is most often *nutritional* in etiology when diet is poor in protein and/or when fatty acid metabolism is deranged and/or when liver cell function is impaired.

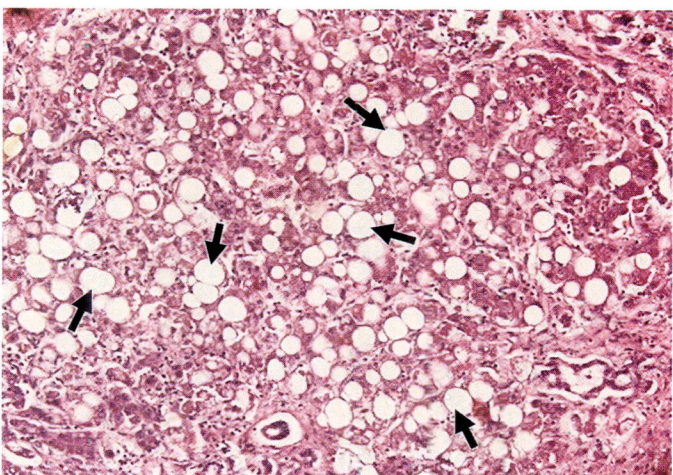

Fig. 21.58: Fatty change in liver. The lipid accumulates in the hepatocytes as vacuoles. These vacuoles have a clear appearance with H&E staining. Alcohol, the most common cause, is a hepatotoxin that interferes with mitochondrial and microsomal function in hepatocytes, leading to an accumulation of lipid. In developing countries, fatty change is seen in kwashiorkor. It is associated with diabetes mellitus, obesity, and severe gastrointestinal malabsorption (arrows) (400X).

section technique with the fat stains such as Sudan III, *Sudan IV, Sudan black, Oil red O* and *osmic acid*.

STEATOHEPATITIS

Acute alcoholic hepatitis is characterized by hepatic steatosis and hydropic swelling of hepatocytes, focal hepatocellular necrosis, infiltration by neutrophils, and cytoplasmic hyaline inclusions within the hepatocytes (*Mallory bodies*), which represent *precipitated intermediate filament proteins* (cytokeratin 8 and 18). Development of irreversible perivenular and peri-sinusoidal fibrosis in acute alcoholic hepatitis may progress to cirrhosis.

Clinical Features

Patient with acute alcoholic hepatitis presents with malaise and anorexia, fever, loss of weight, pain in right upper quadrant due to hepatomegaly, and jaundice. Serum bilirubin and alkaline phosphatase levels are raised with peripheral neutrophilic leukocytosis.

Light Microscopy

Liver biopsy examined under light microscope shows hepatic steatosis and hydropic swelling of hepatocytes, focal hepatocellular necrosis, infiltration by neutrophils, and cytoplasmic Mallory's hyaline inclusions within the hepatocytes (Fig. 21.59).

Section III: Systemic Pathology

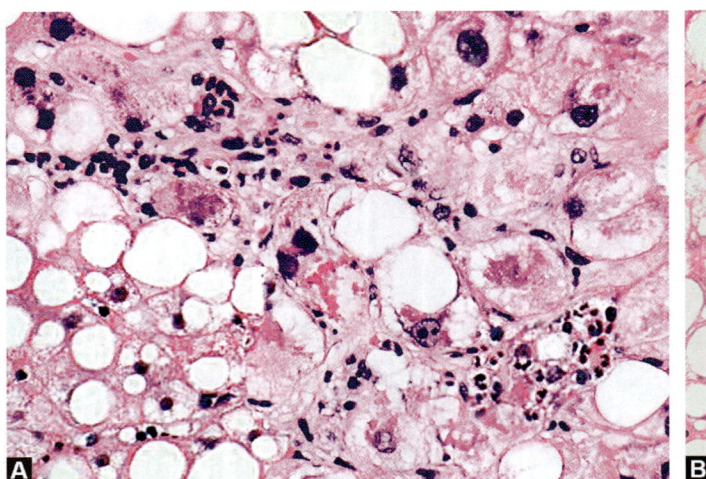
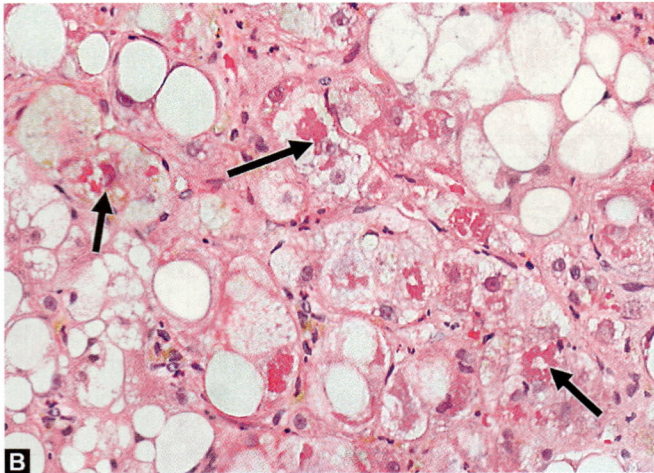

Fig. 21.59: Steatohepatitis. (A) Hepatocytes show an accumulation of fat and Mallory's hyaline. It is infiltrated by neutrophils; (B) Mallory's hyaline. At high magnification can be seen globular red hyaline material. This is Mallory's hyaline, also known as *alcoholic hyaline* because it is most often seen in conjunction with chronic alcoholism. The globules are aggregates of intermediate filaments in the cytoplasm resulting from hepatocyte injury (arrows) (400X).

Electron Microscopy

Giant mitochondria (megamitochondria) is ultrastructural feature of alcoholic liver disease.

Mallory's Denk Hyaline Inclusions

Mallory's hyaline inclusions are also known as *Mallory-Denk hyaline.* These are present in primary biliary cirrhosis but absent in secondary biliary cirrhosis. Mallory's hyaline inclusions are demonstrated in various disorders (Table 21.43).

Table 21.43: Mallory's hyaline inclusions associated disorders

- Alcoholic liver disease
- Primary biliary cirrhosis
- Non-alcoholic fatty liver disease
- Indian childhood cirrhosis
- Chronic cholestatic disease
- Focal nodular hyperplasia of liver
- Hepatocellular carcinoma
- α_1-Antitrypsin deficiency
- Wilson's disease

ALCOHOLIC CIRRHOSIS

Development of irreversible perivenular and perisunusoidal fibrosis in acute alcoholic hepatitis may progress to cirrhosis. Chronic alcoholism is the most frequent cause of cirrhosis.

Initially, patient develops micronodular cirrhosis and later progresses to typical *hobnail liver* with large, irregular nodules (macronodular cirrhosis). Laennec cirrhosis shows replacement of entire liver lobule by tough pale fibrous scar tissue.

Gross Morphology

- The liver may be enlarged or small and shrunken. The pattern is most often micronodular.
- In late stages, the nodules tend to become larger and irregular; this pattern results in a scarred, shrunken liver termed the *hobnail liver* (Fig. 21.60).

Light Microscopy

- Hepatic architecture is obscured by fibrous bands surrounding nodules of distorted liver cell plates.
- These fibrous bands show proliferating bile ducts, lymphocytes and plasma cells (Fig. 21.61).

Consequences

Consequences of intrahepatic scarring with increased portal venous pressure lead to esophageal varices often resulting in upper gastrointestinal hemorrhage, rectal

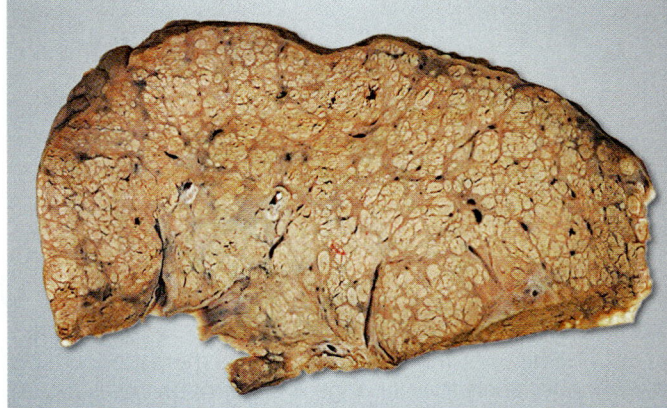

Fig. 21.60: Alcoholic cirrhosis. Cut surface of liver shows nodules of variable size.

Liver, Gallbladder and Exocrine Pancreas

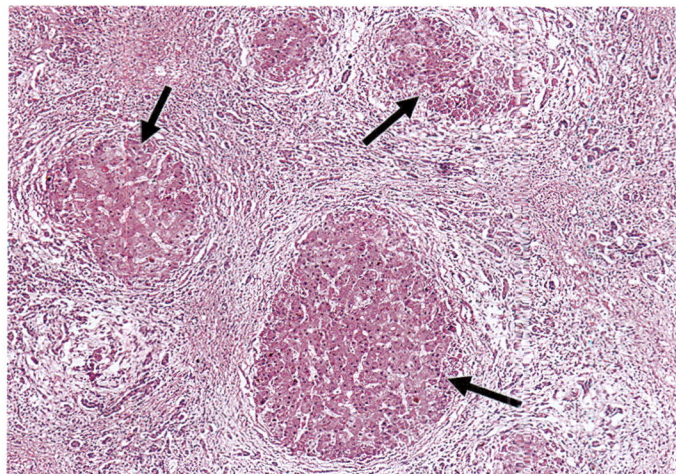

Fig. 21.61: Liver cirrhosis shows regenerative nodules of hepatocytes surrounded by fibrous connective tissue that bridges between portal tracts. Within this collagenous tissue is scattered lymphocytes as well as a proliferation of bile ducts (arrows) (100X).

hemorrhoids, periumbilical venous collaterals (caput medusae) and splenomegaly.

Differences between alcoholic and post-necrotic cirrhosis are shown in Table 21.44.

Clinical Features

Patient presents with jaundice, distended abdomen, esophageal varices, caput medusae, massive splenomegaly with elevated serum transaminases levels and serum alkaline phosphatase. Serum protein levels are decreased. Clinical manifestations associated with hepatocellular damage and liver failure are described as under.

- *Jaundice:* It is most often mixed conjugated and unconjugated.
- *Hypoalbuminemia:* It is caused by decreased albumin synthesis in damaged hepatocytes.
- *Decreased synthesis of coagulation factors:* Liver synthesizes less coagulation factors with the exception of von Willebrand factor.
- *Hyperestrinism:* It manifests as palmar erythema; spider nevi (capillary telangiectasia) of the face, upper arms, and chest; loss of body and pubic hair; testicular atrophy; and gynecomastia.
- *Peripheral edema, ascites or hydrothorax:* These occur by various mechanisms. Liver fails to synthesize albumin leading to decreased plasma oncotic pressure. Increased portal venous pressure leads to increased production of hepatic lymph, retention of sodium and water. It occurs as a result of decreased hepatic degradation of aldosterone, activation of the renin-angiotensin system, or both.
- *Hepatic encephalopathy (portal-systemic encephalopathy):* It is facilitated by shunting from the portal to the systemic circulation, with delivery of neurotoxic substances, such as ammonia and other enteric degradation products, directly into the systemic circulation. *Neurological manifestations varying from slight confusion to deep coma along with asterix (flapping tremor of hands) are characteristic features.*

Table 21.44: Differences between alcoholic and post-necrotic cirrhosis

Parameters	Alcoholic cirrhosis	Post-necrotic cirrhosis
Nodules		
Size of nodules in liver	Initially micronodular cirrhosis later mixed micronodules and macronodules giving *hobnail appearance*	Macronodules
Gross morphology		
External surface	Initially, liver yellow-tan in color, later brown colored	Liver small, shrunken and distorted. It shows irregular coarse scars and nodules
Cut surface	Cut surface showing multiple nodules of variable sizes	Cut surface revealing macronodules of variable sizes
Light microscopy		
Fibrous septa	Initially delicate and later thick	Generally thick
Inflammatory cells	Sparse infiltration of fibrous septa by macrophages, lymphocytes and plasma cells	Heavy infiltration of fibrous septa by macrophages, lymphocytes and plasma cells resulting in formation of lymphoid follicles
Mallory's body	May be present but rare	Absent
Proliferation of bile ducts	Minimal proliferation	Extensive proliferation
Fatty change	May show fatty change	Absent

NONALCOHOLIC FATTY LIVER DISEASE

Nonalcoholic fatty liver disease (NAFLD) is so named because it closely resembles alcoholic fatty liver. This condition represents a spectrum of liver injuries that initially display steatosis, with or without hepatitis. This disorder may progress to bridging fibrosis and cirrhosis of liver.

It is consistently associated with metabolic syndromes characterized by *central obesity, type 2 diabetes mellitus, dyslipidemia, and microalbuminuria*.

Pathogenesis

- *Hepatic steatosis:* It arises due to insulin resistance and from diminished exercise and genetic/epigenetic mechanisms.
- *Liver cell necrosis:* Oxidative and inflammatory injury resulting from *dysfunctional visceral adipose tissue secreted inflammatory mediators (TNF-α, IL-6)* leads to liver cell necrosis.
- *Fibrosis: TNF-α, TGF-β, NK cell mediated stellate cell activation* leads to connective tissue deposition.

> **Light Microscopy**
> - Steatosis is pathologically defined as involving *>5% of hepatocytes*. In comparison to alcoholics steatohepatitis, *Mallory-Denk bodies, neutrophils are less prominent* and mononuclear cells predominate in NAFLD.
> - Hepatic inflammation, hepatocyte death, or scarring vary according to the stage of the disease.
> - *Cirrhosis may develop after many years* (Fig. 21.62).

Grading and Staging of Nonalcoholic Fatty Liver Disease

Grading and staging of nonalcoholic fatty liver disease (NAFLD) is shown in Tables 21.45 and 21.46.

Table 21.45: Component scores for grading nonalcoholic fatty liver disease (NAFLD)

Stage	Steatosis	Lobular inflammation	Hepatocellular ballooning
Stage 0	<5%	None	None
Stage 1	5–33%	<2/20 × field	Mild (few)
Stage 2	34–66%	2-4/20 × field	Moderate to marked
Stage 3	>66%	>4/20 × field	Moderate to marked

NAFLD activity score: NAS 0–8 (steatosis + lobular inflammation + ballooning)

Table 21.46: Fibrosis scoring: Based on Masson trichrome stain for nonalcoholic fatty liver disease (NAFLD)

Stage	Masson trichrome
Stage 0	None
Stage 1a	Delicate zone 3 perisinusoidal fibrosis and requires trichrome stain
Stage 1b	Dense zone 3 perisinusoidal fibrosis, visible on hematoxylin and eosin
Stage 1c	Portal/periportal fibrosis
Stage 2	Zone 3 perisinusoidal and portal fibrosis
Stage 3	Bridging
Stage 4	Cirrhosis

HEMOCHROMATOSIS

Hemochromatosis is characterized by excessive accumulation of iron (hemosiderin) in parenchymal cells of liver, pancreas and myocardium.

Disease manifests when body storage iron exceeds 20 gm. It occurs in the settings of hereditary or acquired hemochromatosis.

Basic Defect

Primary (hereditary) hemochromatosis occurs due to mutations in the HFE gene leading to uncontrolled iron absorption and accumulation in various organs. Secondary hemochromatosis is caused by chronic iron overload of diverse etiology.

Distribution of normal iron in adults is shown in Table 21.47. Causes of primary and secondary hemochromatosis are shown in Table 21.48.

Regulation of Iron

Hepcidin is main regulator of iron absorption.

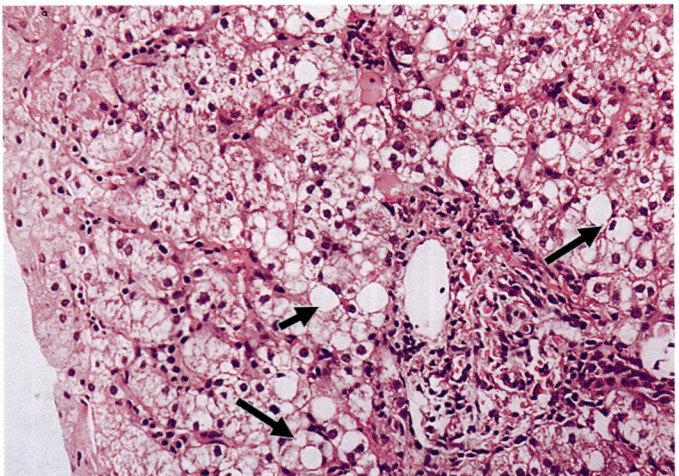

Fig. 21.62: Nonalcoholic fatty change. Steatosis is pathologically defined as involving more than 5% of hepatocytes. It shows infiltration by lymphocytes, plasma cells and macrophages (arrows) (400X).

Table 21.47: Distribution of normal iron in adults

Iron	Sites	Values of total body iron (3.0–5.0 gm)
Functional iron	Hemoglobin	1.5–3.0 gm
	Essential/functional/non-available iron	Myoglobin: 0.3 gm
		Enzymes of cellular respiration: 0.05 gm
Storage/available tissue iron	Ferritin	1.2–2.0 gm
	Hemosiderin	
Plasma iron	Transferrin bound iron for transport	3–4 mg

Genetic hemochromatosis refers to >50 gm of total body iron. Normal liver contains 0.5 gm in 98% of hepatocytes

Table 21.48: Causes of primary and secondary hemochromatosis

Causes	Disorders
Genetic hemochromatosis	Mutation of HFE gene on chromosome 6
Secondary hemochromatosis	
Parenteral iron overload due to frequent blood transfusions and iron dextran injections	Aplastic anemia
	Leukemias
	Sickle cell anemia
	Myelodysplastic syndrome
	Long-term hemodialysis
Ineffective erythropoiesis with increased erythroid activity	β-Thalassemia
	Sideroblastic anemia
	Pyruvate kinase deficiency
Increased oral intake of iron	Bantu siderosis also called *African iron overload*
Chronic liver disease	Chronic alcohol disease
	Porphyria cutanea tarda
Congenital atransferrinemia	Hereditary disorder
Neonatal hemochromatosis	–

It is also known as liver expressed antimicrobial peptide or LEAP1, encoded by the HAMP gene.

PRIMARY (HEREDITARY) HEMOCHROMATOSIS

Hereditary hemochromatosis is autosomal recessive disorder of iron absorption by the intestinal mucosa.

The disease is most often caused by a mutation in the HFE gene located on chromosome 6p23 in close linkage with the HLA locus. It is characteristically familial rather than sporadic. Inheritance of this gene results in excessive absorption of iron.

Four types of primary hemochromatosis are shown in Table 21.49.

Organs Involved

Clinical manifestations occur due to deposition of hemosiderin in the cytoplasm of liver (cirrhosis and hepatic failure), pancreas (diabetes mellitus), myocardium (congestive failure), joint linings (arthritis), endocrine glands and skin in decreasing order of severity resulting in organ dysfunction. Parenchymal hemosiderin is demonstrated by *Prussian blue staining*.

Table 21.49: Types of primary hemochromatosis

Type	Disorder	Gene mutation
Type I	Autosomal recessive	HFE gene located on chromosome 6
Type IIA	Autosomal recessive	Hemojuvelin gene located on chromosome 1
Type IIB	Autosomal recessive	HAMP (hepcidin) gene located on chromosome 19
Type III	Autosomal recessive	Transferrin receptor (TFR2) gene located on chromosome 7
Type IV	Autosomal dominant	SLC40A1 (ferroprotein) gene located on chromosome 2

Bronze Diabetes

Bronze diabetes is triad of *micronodular cirrhosis*, *diabetes*, and *hyperpigmentation* seen in primary hemochromatosis. These patients develop portal hypertension and hepatocellular carcinoma.

Organs Involved

Many organs are involved in primary hemochromatosis (Fig. 21.63).

- *Liver:* It shows features of micronodular cirrhosis. Hepatocytes as well as Kupffer cells show excessive deposition of brown granules of hemosiderin. *Liver iron concentration is >400 µg/100 mg of wet liver. Normal wet liver contains iron concentration <30 µg/100 mg.* Prussian blue iron stain demonstrates the blue granules of hemosiderin in hepatocytes and Kupffer cells (mononuclear phagocyte system). Most common causes of death are **cirrhosis** and **hepatocellular carcinoma.**
- *Pancreas:* Excessive deposition of iron in *islets of Langerhans* causes *diffuse interstitial fibrosis* resulting in diabetes mellitus.
- *Myocardium:* Excessive deposition of iron in myocardium may cause *restrictive myocarditis, arrhythmias and congestive heart failure.*
- *Endocrine glands:* Excessive deposition of iron in thyroid gland, parathyroid, pituitary and adrenal glands may lead to endocrinal gland dysfunction.
- *Joints:* Excessive iron is deposited in synovial linings of joints in 30 to 50% of cases. *Cartilage damage* leads to disabling polyarthritis.
- *Skin pigmentation:* Skin pigmentation on face, neck and extensor surface of forearms occurs due to deposition of melanin and hemosiderin in 70 to 90% of patients. It is component of bronze diabetes mellitus.
- *Testes:* Small atrophic testes (hypogonadism) in hemochromatosis occur due to *impairment of*

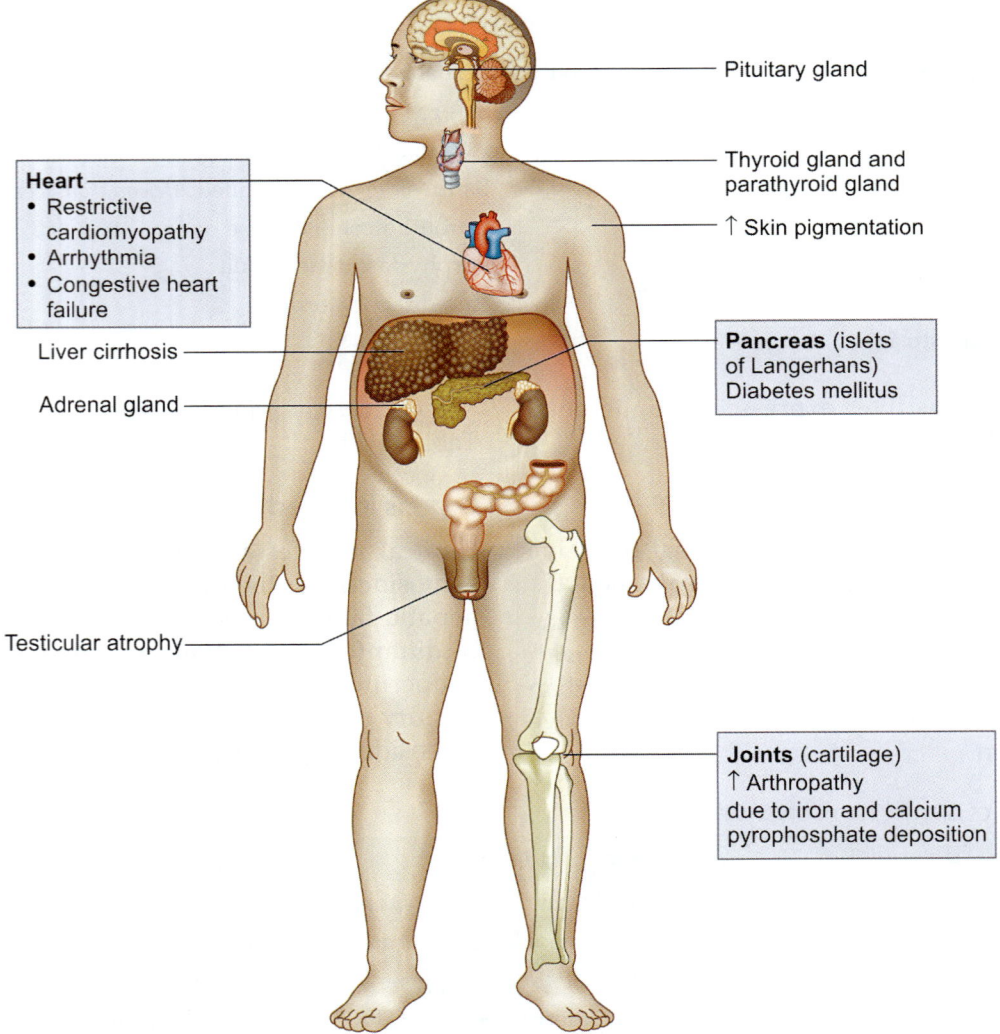

Fig. 21.63: Primary hemochromatosis shows involvement of multiple organs due to deposition of iron.

hypothalamopituitary function by iron deposition and not due to excessive deposition of iron in testes.

Clinical Features

Patient presents with *hepatomegaly, abdominal pain, skin pigmentation, diabetes mellitus or deranged glucose metabolism, cardiac dysfunction, amenorrhea in females, decreased libido and impotence in males.* Cause of death is due to development of hepatocellular carcinoma, cardiac disease and liver failure. Chelating agent desferrioxamine is administered in patients with severe anemia and hypoproteinemia.

> **Light Microscopy**
>
> Hepatocytes as well as *Kupffer cells* show excessive deposition of brown granules of hemosiderin (Fig. 21.64).

Screening Tests

The recommended screening test for hemochromatosis is increased serum transferrin saturation, which is increased. In selected cases, molecular testing is done to demonstrate mutations in the HFE gene in tissues. Early detection and occasional phlebotomy can prevent multiorgan failure attributed to iron accumulation in tissues.

Laboratory Diagnosis

- There is marked increase in serum iron and modest reduction in total iron-binding capacity (TIBC, transferrin). This combination results in increased transferrin iron saturation (100%).
- Serum ferritin levels are increased >500 ng/ml (normal value is <150 ng/ml) in these patients.

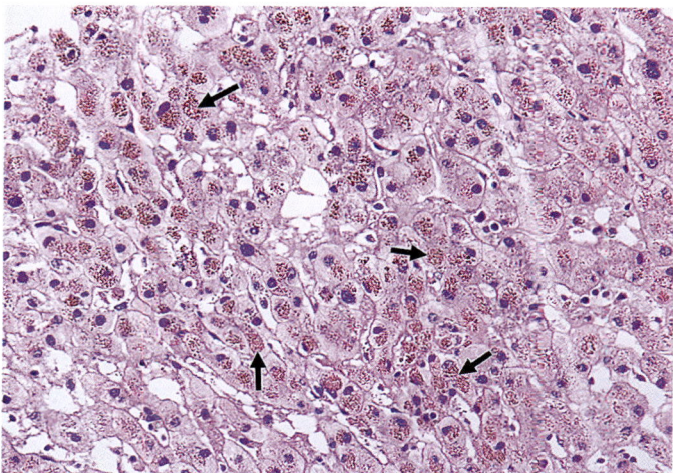

Fig. 21.64: Hemochromatosis in liver. Hepatocytes as well as Kupffer cells show excessive deposition of brown granules of hemosiderin (arrows) (400X).

- Blood biochemistry such as blood sugar and urine analysis should be done in patients with *bronze diabetes*. Iron is demonstrated by Prussian blue reaction in the tissues.

SECONDARY HEMOCHROMATOSIS

Secondary hemochromatosis is most often associated with a combination of ineffective erythropoiesis and multiple transfusions in *thalassemia major*, high intake of iron and *Bantus siderosis* due to consumption of traditional beer home-brewed in steel drums.

Excessive iron is deposited largely in the mononuclear phagocytic system, which is some instances, may spill over into parenchymal cells, producing a hybrid condition.

WILSON DISEASE

Wilson disease is an autosomal recessive disorder of copper metabolism in which excess copper can be deposited in the liver and brain. It occurs due to impaired transport of copper across lysosomal membrane or bile canaliculi. Ceruloplasmin levels are decreased in Wilson disease secondary to copper deposition in *liver, basal ganglion* and *corneal limbus*.

Normal Metabolism

Copper absorbed from proximal small intestine is bound to apoceruloplasmin in liver to form ceruloplasmin, that is secreted into the blood which is taken up by liver and broken down in lysosomes. Released copper is then excreted through the bile.

Pathogenesis

In Wilson disease *mutation of ATP7B gene located on chromosome 13 leads* to deficiency of a *copper transporting ATPase* resulting in decrease in copper transport into bile and impairs its incorporation into ceruloplasmin. Accumulated copper causes toxic injury to organs by free radical mediated injury and displacing of metals from metalloenzymes.

Pathology

Accumulation of copper in various organs results in liver (*chronic hepatitis to micronodular or macronodular cirrhosis*), brain (basal ganglia especially the putamen of the lenticular nucleus impairing extrapyramidal motor functions), kidney tubular cells (aminoaciduria and glycosuria), and eye (Descemet membrane known as *Kayser-Fleischer ring*).

Clinical Features

Patients present with neuropsychiatric symptoms and movement disorders, rigid dystonia as a result of basal ganglia involvement. Patients may also present with symptoms of acute or chronic liver disease and ocular *Kayser-Fleischer ring*.

> **Light Microscopy**
> - Liver biopsy shows chronic hepatitis and fatty change. Liver cell nuclei are vacuolated.
> - Mallory bodies in periportal hepatocytes and piecemeal necrosis are present in the cytoplasm.
> - Stainable copper is present in liver cells.
> - Cirrhosis occurs following chronic hepatitis.

Histochemistry

Excessive copper in tissues can be demonstrated by *rhodamine stain for copper and orcein stain for copper associated protein*.

Laboratory Findings

Decreased serum ceruloplasmin, increased hepatic copper (>250 μg/1 g dry weight of liver) and increased urinary copper are consistently seen (Table 21.50).

α_1-ANTITRYPSIN DEFICIENCY

The α_1-antitrypsin deficiency is the most common genetic cause of liver disease in infants and children. It is the most frequent genetic disease for which liver transplantation is indicated. The liver may be involved with or without lung disease in the form of emphysema. *There is increased risk of development of hepatocellular carcinoma.*

Age Group

This disorder may affect infants, children and adults. Liver diseases associated with α_1-antitrypsin deficiency in these age groups are shown in Table 21.51.

Pathogenesis

Physiological state: The α_1-antitrypsin (AAT) is a protein encoded on the proteinase inhibitor locus (Pi) on chromosome 14. It is synthesized by liver in normal genotype persons (PiMM phenotype). This protein prevents enzymes such as elastin from degrading normal host tissue. *It accounts for 90% of antiproteinase activity in the blood.*

Pathological state: The α_1-antitrypsin (AAT) deficiency is an autosomal dominant disorder equally affecting men and women. Most patients with clinically-diagnosed *emphysema* who are younger than 40 years of age have α1-antitrypsin (PiZZ phenotype) deficiency.

Associated Disorders

- Homozygous PiZZ genotype patients deficient in α_1-antitrypsin (AAT) (<11 μm/L) are prone to *panacinar*

Table 21.50: Laboratory diagnosis of Wilson's disease

Test	Results
Ocular findings	Kayser-Fleischer rings
Hepatic copper content (confirmatory test)	250 g copper per 10 g of dried liver tissue
Serum ceruloplasmin level (most specific screening)	Decreased
Urinary excretion of copper	Increased
Rhodamine stain	Used to stain copper
Orcein stain	Used to stain copper associated protein

Table 21.51: Liver diseases associated with α_1-antitrypsin deficiency in age groups

Liver disorder	Clinical features	Light microscopy
Neonatal hepatitis	Cholestasis jaundice	Cholestasis (marked)
		Liver cell necrosis
		Lymphocytes, plasma cells and macrophages infiltration
		Globules of α_1-antitrypsin demonstrated after attaining 6 months of age
		Recovery is common
Childhood cirrhosis	Persistence of jaundice >6 months	Cirrhosis
Adult macronodular cirrhosis (60–70 years)	Only liver involved and lungs spared	Cirrhosis (globules of α_1-antitrypsin demonstrated)
		Hepatocellular carcinoma

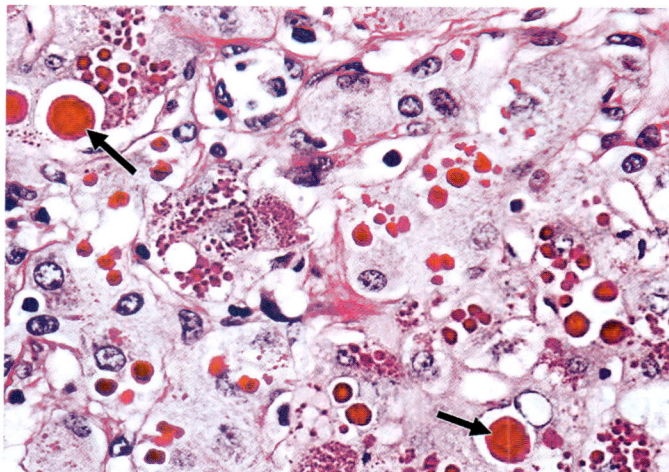

Fig. 21.65: The α_1-antitrypsin (AAT). The periporal red hyaline globules seen here with periodic acid–Schiff (PAS) stain are characteristic for α_1-antitrypsin deficiency (a person with homozygous PiZZ genotype). The globules are intrahepatic collections of α_1-antitrypsin that is not being excreted from the hepatocytes. This may eventually lead to a macronodular cirrhosis. These patients are also prone to develop panlobular emphysema of lungs (arrows) (400X).

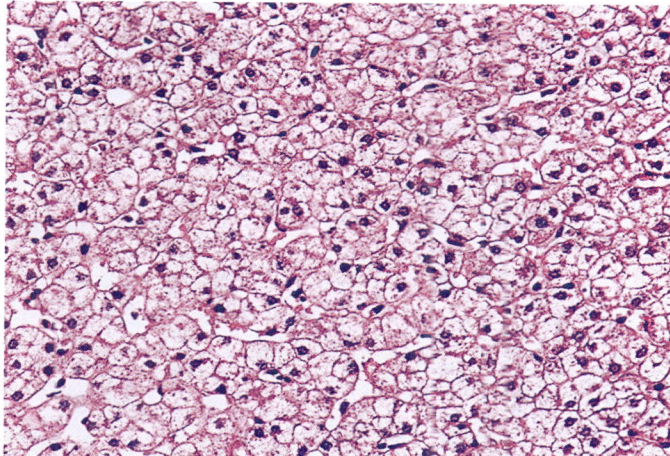

Fig. 21.66: Glycogen storage disease liver shows deposition of glycogen in hepatocytes giving mosaic appearance (400X).

emphysema, cirrhosis, cutaneous panniculitis, neonatal hepatitis, bronchiectasis and *Wegener's granulomatosis*. Serum electrophoresis reveals absence of α_1-globulin peak.

- Smoking appears to be the most important risk factor for the development of panacinar emphysema among AAT deficient persons. Among smokers, even mild to moderate reductions in AAT levels may be associated with panacinar emphysema leading to more rapid decline in lung function.

  Destruction of lung parenchyma and consequent emphysema results from an imbalance between the major natural antiprotease, AAT and inflammatory proteases (especially leukocyte elastase). *Intravenous purified pooled human plasma is recommended to enhance ATT levels in these patients.*

Light Microscopy

- Histological examination shows round-to-oval cytoplasmic globular inclusions of misfolded α_1-antitrypsin PAS positive diastase resistant proteins in hepatocytes.
- These globules stain red with PAS after removing glycogen with diastase (Fig. 21.65).

GLYCOGEN STORAGE DISEASE

Andersen disease, which is also known as *glycogen storage disease type IV*, is an autosomal recessive genetic disease caused by deficiency of a glycogen-branching enzyme. This enzyme deficiency results in the *accumulation of abnormal glycogen (amylopectin)* in the liver, muscle, and other tissues.

Clinical Features

In most affected persons, the condition becomes evident in the first months of life. Patient presents with *failure to thrive and hepatomegaly*. Disease progresses to *hepatic fibrosis leading to cirrhosis and liver failure*.

Light Microscopy

- Histological examination of liver biopsy shows pale distended hepatocytes giving mosaic appearance.
- PAS staining and electron microscopy may help in confirming diagnosis (Fig. 21.66).

LYSOSOMAL STORAGE DISEASE

NIEMANN-PICK DISEASE

Niemann-Pick disease is a hereditary lysosomal storage disease.

Pathogenesis

This disorder caused by deficiency of sphingomyelinase results in *accumulation of sphingomyelin in phagocytes (types A and B Niemann-Pick disease)*. Type C Niemann-Pick disease is caused by defect in a gene involved in *cholesterol transport with cholesterol accumulation* within phagocytes.

Diagnostic hallmark is presence of *foamy histiocytes* containing sphingomyelin in liver, spleen, lymph nodes, and skin.

Clinical Features

Child presents with *hepatosplenomegaly, anemia, fever* and neurologic manifestations.

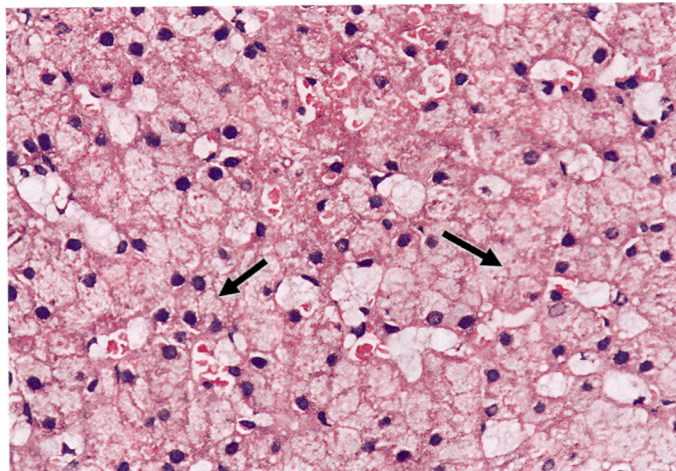

Fig. 21.67: Niemann-Pick disorder. Liver Kupffer cells show *foamy histiocytes* containing sphingomyelin (arrows) (400X).

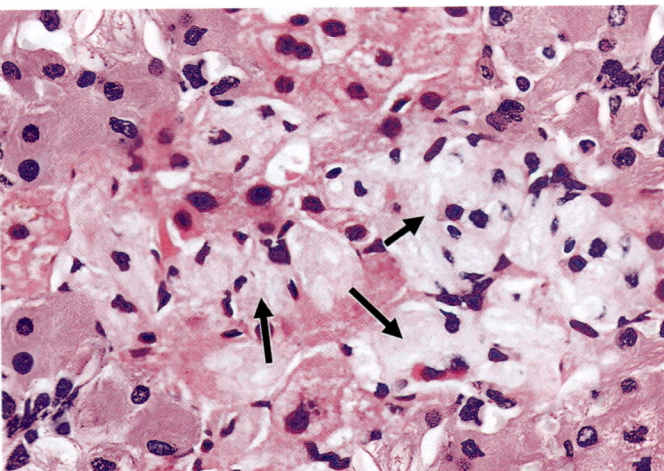

Fig. 21.68: Gaucher's disease shows cell containing cigarette paper-like cytoplasmic appearance and eccentric nuclei, which are lipid-laden macrophages (arrows) (400X).

Approximately 50% of the patients develop cherry red spot in the macula similar to that of Tay-Sachs disease. Death occurs by 3 years of age.

Light Microscopy

Histological examination of liver biopsy shows *foamy histiocytes* containing sphingomyelin in Kupffer cells (Fig. 21.67).

GAUCHER'S DISEASE

Gaucher's disease is autosomal recessive disorder most often seen in persons of European (Ashkenazic) Jewish lineage. It is characterized by accumulation of glucosylceramide (membrane glycosphingolipids) derived from the catabolism of senescent leukocytes, primarily in the lysosomes of macrophages.

The membranes of these cells are rich in the cerebrosides, and when their degradation is blocked by the deficiency of glucocerebrosidase (lysosomal acid β-glucosidase), an intermediate metabolite such as glucosylceramide accumulates.

Clinical Features

- *Adult Gaucher's disease (type 1):* It accounts for 80% of cases. Patient presents with hepatosplenomegaly, bone pain and fracture due to erosion of femoral head and other long bones.
- *Infantile Gaucher's disease (type 2):* Infant develops severe CNS involvement with fatal outcome before 1 year of age.
- *Juvenile Gaucher's disease (type 3):* Its onset usually occurs in early childhood. There is involvement of brain and the viscera. It is less severe than Gaucher's disease (type 2).

Light Microscopy

Histological examination of liver biopsy shows *Gaucher's cells* with a distinctive cigarette paper-like cytoplasmic appearance and eccentric nuclei, which are lipid-laden macrophages present along liver sinusoids (Kupffer cells). Diagnosis is confirmed by presence of Gaucher's cells, and assay of specific enzymes (chitotriosidase and angiotensin-converting enzyme markers of macrophage proliferation) (Fig. 21.68).

AMYLOIDOSIS LIVER

Amyloidosis is a well-known complication of chronic inflammatory disorders such as tuberculosis, bronchiectasis, rheumatoid arthritis, or osteomyelitis. It stimulates the production of amyloid from the serum amyloid A (SAA) protein, an acute phase reactant secreted by the liver. The kidneys (80%), liver, spleen, and adrenals are the most common organs involved.

Gross Morphology

The amyloid liver is usually grossly enlarged (as much as 900 gm), pale, and smooth surface, firm consistency. When sectioned, it shows sharp rigid edges.

Light Microscopy

- Amyloid material is initially deposited in the *space of Disse* between the hepatocytes and vascular sinusoids. As more amyloid accumulates, it compresses the hepatic cords and sinusoids.
- The hepatic cords undergo nutritional and pressure atrophy and become displaced or replaced by bands and nodules of amyloid (Fig. 21.69).

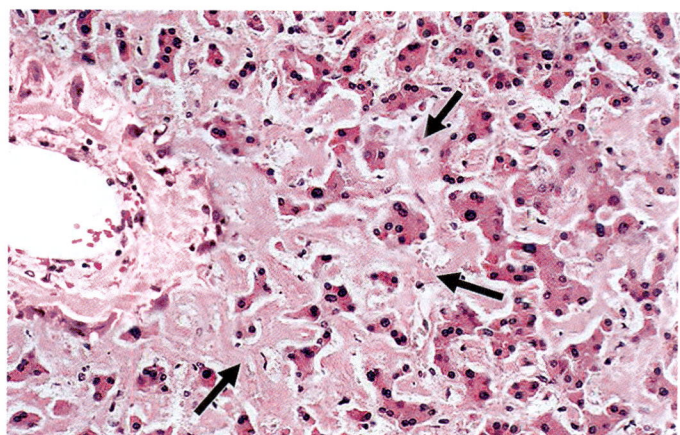

Fig. 21.69: Amyloid liver shows deposition of amyloid material in the *space of Disse* between the hepatocytes and vascular sinusoids leading to compression of hepatic cords (arrows) (400X).

Amyloid Stains

Amyloid material is demonstrated by Congo red staining under light microscopy. Pretreatment of tissue with potassium permanganate stained by Congo red demonstrates AL amyloid only but not AA amyloid. Stains used to demonstrate amyloid material are shown in Table 21.52.

INDIAN CHILDHOOD CIRRHOSIS

Indian childhood cirrhosis most often affects children between 6 months to 5 years in Indian population. Exact etiology is unknown.

It is most often seen in Aggarwal, Brahmin, Kayastha and Sikhs. Serum copper and copper binding protein levels are increased in these patients.

Clinical Features

Child presents with *hepatosplenomegaly and jaundice*. Child develops portal hypertension with fatal outcome.

> **Light Microscopy**
>
> Liver biopsy shows *micronodular cirrhosis, Mallory's hyaline body, and diffuse fibrosis around individual hepatocytes* (known as *creeping fibrosis*), chronic inflammatory cells, bile stasis and ductular proliferation.

ACUTE FATTY LIVER OF PREGNANCY

Acute fatty liver of pregnancy (AFLP) is a rare *life-threatening complication of pregnancy* with fatal outcome. It usually occurs in late third trimester. *Acute hepatic failure is associated with microvesicular fatty liver.*

Clinical Features

Patient develops severe liver dysfunction with hypoalbuminemia, hypofibrinogenemia, prolonged clotting times and hypocholesterolemia.

The most critical component of caring for a woman with AFLP is the delivery of her fetus. While the natural history of the disease is improvement within 24–48 hours of delivery.

REYE SYNDROME

Reye syndrome occurs in children. Patient presents with encephalopathy, coma, and microvesicular fatty liver. Reye syndrome is associated with aspirin administration in children with acute viral infections.

Table 21.52: Stains used to demonstrate amyloid material

Amyloid stain	Color imparted
Congo red with light microscopy	Pink
Congo red with polarizing microscopy	Apple green birefringence (color of a Granny Smith apple)
Methyl violet (metachromatic stain)	Bright pink
Crystal violet (metachromatic stain)	Pink
Fluorescent stains: Thioflavin-T, Thioflavin-S	Greenish (immunofluorescence study)
Von Gieson stain	Khaki color
PAS stain	Magenta color

BILE DUCT DISORDERS

Biliary cirrhosis occurs as primary or secondary disorder. Primary biliary cirrhosis (PBC) is an autoimmune chronic progressive disorder and more frequent than secondary biliary cirrhosis. It is caused by extrahepatic biliary obstruction.

PRIMARY BILIARY CIRRHOSIS

Primary biliary cirrhosis (nonsuppurative destructive cholangitis) occurs due to chronic destruction of intrahepatic bile ducts in the portal tracts. It evolves through ductal lesions, scarring, and eventually cirrhosis. The hallmark of this condition is the presence in serum of antimitochondrial antibodies. These autoantibodies recognize epitopes associated with the mitochondrial pyruvate dehydrogenase complex.

Age Group
It occurs more often in women than in men (10:1 female predominance) between 40 and 50 years of age.

Predisposing Factors
Majority of patients are associated with an autoimmune disorder such as thyroiditis, rheumatoid arthritis, scleroderma, Sjögren syndrome, or systemic lupus erythematosus.

Pathogenesis
Intrahepatic bile duct destruction is caused by circulating *antimitochondrial antibodies* in >95% of patients. These antimitochondrial antibodies play no role in the pathogenesis of the disease. The complement system is chronically activated.

Clinical Features
Patient presents with itching, jaundice, hepatosplenomegaly, passage of clay-colored stool and dark-colored urine. Serum cholesterol level is raised secondary to severe obstructive jaundice. Hypercholesterolemia leads to cutaneous xanthomas formation.

> **Light Microscopy**
> - Liver biopsy shows nonsuppurative inflammation of interlobular ducts (florid duct lesions). The cells surrounding bile duct destruction site include predominant suppressor/cytotoxic CD8+ T cells, macrophages, B cells and plasma cells in some portal tracts.
>   Bile duct destruction is mediated by these suppressor/cytotoxic CD8+ T cells.
> - There may be presence of epithelioid granulomas. Proliferation of bile ductules within portal tracts is common and may be florid.
> - It is worth mentioning that macrophages and B cells cause periductal inflammation but do not mediate epithelial cytotoxicity (Fig. 21.70).

Laboratory Findings
Serum conjugated bilirubin, alkaline phosphatase and cholesterol levels are increased.

Diagnostic Tool
Serum antimitochondrial antibodies (IgM especially M2) are used in the *diagnosis of primary biliary cirrhosis*.

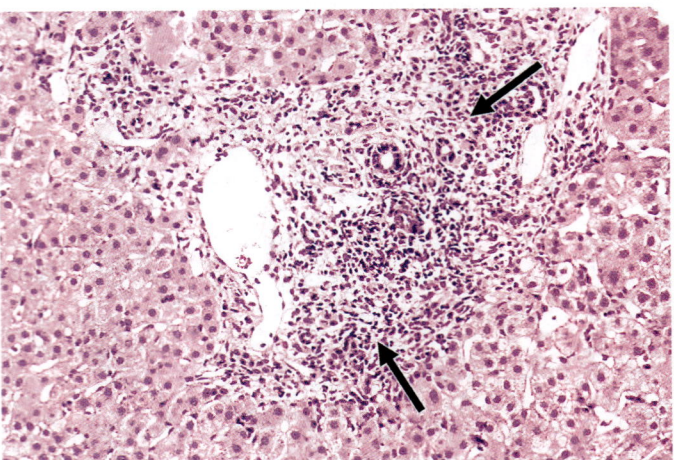

Fig. 21.70: Primary biliary cirrhosis. This is a case of primary biliary cirrhosis, a rare autoimmune disease (mostly of middle-aged women) that is characterized by destruction of bile ductules within the triads of the liver. Antimitochondrial antibody can be detected in serum. Seen here in a portal tract is an intense chronic inflammatory infiltrate with loss of bile ductules. Micronodular cirrhosis ensues (arrows) (400X).

Outcome
Patient with primary biliary cirrhosis may develop micronodular cirrhosis. Hepatocellular carcinoma does not develop.

Most common causes of death are liver failure and variceal bleeding.

Grading and Staging
Grading and staging of primary biliary cirrhosis is shown in Table 21.53.

Table 21.53: Grading and staging of primary biliary cirrhosis

Stages	Scheuer	Ludwig
Stage 1	Florid duct lesion Bile duct damage Portal inflammation	*Portal stage:* Portal inflammation
Stage 2	Ductular proliferation (reaction) Expanded portal tracts Proliferated ductules Piecemeal necrosis	*Periportal stage:* Periportal inflammation ± and piecemeal necrosis
Stage 3	Scarring Fibrosis Loss of ducts	*Septal stage:* Fibrous septa and bridging necrosis
Stage 4	Nodular cirrhosis	Cirrhosis

SECONDARY BILIARY CIRRHOSIS
Secondary biliary cirrhosis is caused by extrahepatic biliary obstruction due to passage of stone in common bile duct or carcinoma head of pancreas.

Persistent obstruction increases the pressure within intrahepatic bile ducts and cholangioles resulting in ductal injury.

Lodgment of stones in the common bile duct leads to obstructive jaundice, cholangitis, and acute pancreatitis. Men and women are equally affected.

Clinical Features

Patient presents with pruritus, jaundice, malaise, diarrhea, steatorrhea, weight loss, dark urine, clay-colored stool and hepatosplenomegaly.

Laboratory Findings

Serum conjugated bilirubin, cholesterol and alkaline phosphatase levels are raised. Urine shows bile salts and bile pigments.

Light Microscopy

- Liver biopsy shows bile stasis and bile lakes, accumulations of bile within hepatic parenchyma.
- Inflammation is seen in ducts and periductal region. Healing occurs by formation of fibrous tissue (Fig. 21.71).

Complications

These include ascending cholangitis and bacterial inflammation of the intrahepatic bile ducts. Differences between intrahepatic and extrahepatic cholestasis are shown in Table 21.54.

PRIMARY SCLEROSING CHOLANGITIS

Primary sclerosing cholangitis is rare pathological progressive fibro-obliterative disorder of unknown etiology. It primarily affects young men between 30 and 50 years of age group.

Men are more affected than women (2:1). Approximately 70% of patients with PSC have long-standing ulcerative colitis indicating autoimmune disorder. It is associated with HLAB-8, DR-3 and DQ-2.

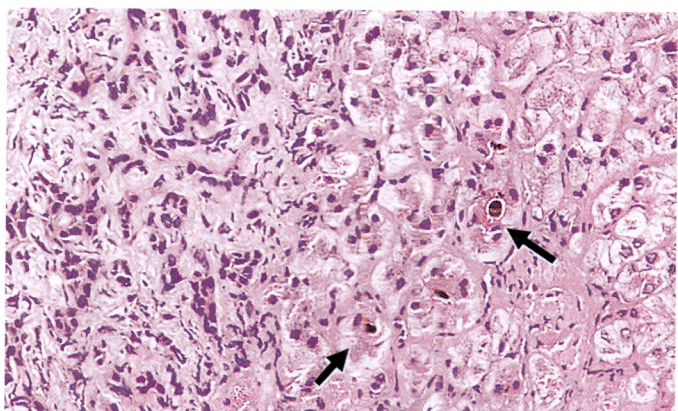

Fig. 21.71: Extrahepatic biliary obstruction shows bile stasis forming bile lakes as a result of accumulation of bile within hepatic parenchyma. Mononuclear inflammatory is seen in ducts and around ducts (arrows) (400X).

Pathology

Primary sclerosing cholangitis is characterized by inflammation, onion skin fibrosis and obliteration of intrahepatic and extrahepatic bile ducts, with dilation of preserved segments. It eventually develops into biliary cirrhosis. Cholangiocarcinoma is a late complication in these patients.

Imaging Techniques

Definite diagnosis of primary sclerosing cholangitis rests on imaging by MRCP and ERCP. Radiograph shows beaded biliary tree, representing sporadic strictures.

Clinical Features

Patient presents with *pruritus, jaundice, malaise, hepatosplenomegaly, passage of clay-colored stool and dark-colored urine*.

Complications are *biliary cirrhosis, chronic pancreatitis, hepatocellular carcinoma and cholangiocarcinoma* (10%).

Table 21.54: Differences between intrahepatic and extrahepatic cholestasis

Characteristics	Intrahepatic cholestasis	Extrahepatic cholestasis
Bile pigment	Bile pigment is present in hepatocytes and Kupffer cells	Bile plugs present in bile ducts and ductules result in rupture of bile canaliculi
Cholestasis severity	Mild degree	Bile lakes present
PMN cells infiltration around bile ducts and canaliculi	Absent	Present
Feathery degeneration of hepatocytes	Marked	Not much marked

Laboratory Findings

Serum conjugated bilirubin, cholesterol, alkaline phosphatase, IgM levels are raised.

Light Microscopy

Liver biopsy shows concentric fibrosis around ducts in *onion skin appearance*, segmental stenosis of extrahepatic and intrahepatic bile ducts. Chronic cholestasis is typical finding (Fig. 21.72).

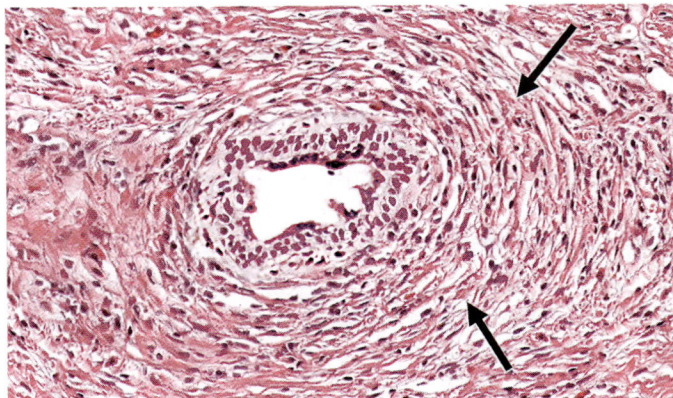

Fig. 21.72: Primary sclerosing cholangitis. Microscopically, this bile duct in a case of sclerosing cholangitis is surrounded by marked collagenous connective tissue deposition (arrows) (100X).

Grading and Staging

Grading and staging of primary sclerosing cholangitis is shown in Table 21.55.

Table 21.55: Grading and staging of primary sclerosing cholangitis

Stages	Scheuer	Ludwig
Stage 1	Portal stage	Portal inflammation or bile duct abnormalities
Stage 2	Periportal stage	Periportal fibrosis or enlargement of portal tract
Stage 3	Septal stage	Fibrous septal or bridging necrosis
Stage 4	Cirrhotic stage	Cirrhosis

VASCULAR DISORDERS

Vascular disorders of liver occur due to impairment of hepatic venous drainage, arterial underperfusion and miscellaneous intrahepatic vascular conditions.

IMPAIRMENT OF HEPATIC VENOUS DRAINAGE
CHRONIC VENOUS CONGESTION LIVER

In long-standing chronic right-sided heart failure, increased venous pressure leads to chronic venous congestion of liver, because hepatic veins drain into inferior vena cava. Pitting edema is seen in lower extremities.

Etiology

Chronic venous congestion of liver occurs due to right-sided cardiac heart failure in patients with chronic obstructive pulmonary disease and thrombosis in hepatic vein or inferior vena cava.

Gross Morphology
- Liver is enlarged, tense, and cyanotic with rounded edges.
- Cut surface of the liver can assume a variegated red and yellow appearance referred to as *nutmeg liver*, with dark red congested centrilobular areas alternating with pale unaffected peripheral portions of the lobules.
- It resembles a cross section of a nutmeg, and so-called as *nutmeg liver*.

Light Microscopy

Macrophages contain iron pigment. Bile stasis within canaliculi may also be seen. Acinar pattern of liver becomes exaggerated due to these changes. Post-congestion fibrosis may produce finely nodular liver known as *cardiac cirrhosis* (Fig. 21.73).

- *Dark areas of the nutmeg:* These are represented by the congested and dilated venous radicles and sinusoids of zone 3 region. These changes cause pressure atrophy of the centrilobular liver cords. In severe cases, the hepatocytes show necrosis.
- *Pale areas of the liver:* These are represented by the hypoxic fatty change in hepatocytes. Hepatocytes in mid-zone show fatty change. Hepatocytes are normal in the peripheral zones. Left heart failure leads to decreased perfusion resulting in centrilobular ischemic necrosis of hepatocytes.
- *Centrilobular hemorrhagic necrosis:* Combination of decreased perfusion and congestion cause centrilobular hemorrhagic necrosis. Liver shows variegated mottled appearance. There is sharp demarcation of viable periportal necrotic centrilobular hepatocytes.
- *Cardiac cirrhosis:* Long standing chronic passive congestion of liver leads to bridging fibrosis in extreme cases resulting in cardiac cirrhosis (Figs 21.74 and 21.75).

Liver, Gallbladder and Exocrine Pancreas

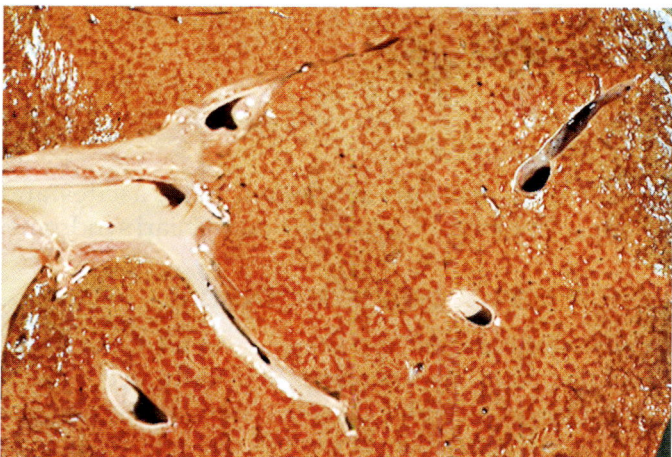

Fig. 21.73: Central venous congestion. Here is an example of a *nutmeg* liver seen with chronic passive congestion of the liver. Note the dark red congested regions that represent accumulation of RBCs in centrilobular regions.

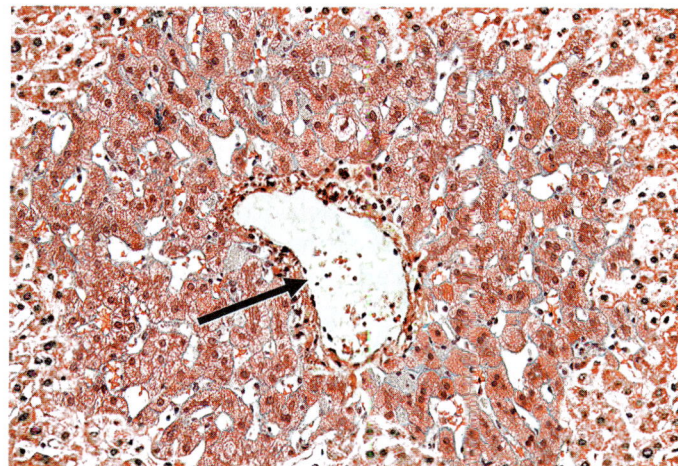

Fig. 21.74: Central venous congestion. Microscopically, the nutmeg pattern results from congestion around the central veins, as seen here. This is usually due to a *right-sided* heart failure (arrow).

BUDD-CHIARI SYNDROME

Budd-Chiari syndrome occurs due to *thrombotic occlusion in major hepatic veins at their origin or inferior vena cava distal to its junction with the hepatic veins*. It is characterized by classic triad: *hepatomegaly, abdominal pain and ascites*. It most often occurs due to *thrombosis or to invasion of the hepatic veins*. Etiology of large hepatic vein thrombosis is shown in Table 21.56.

Clinical Features

Patient presents with abdominal pain, mild jaundice, ascites, and eventual liver failure. Acute hepatic failure and death often occur rapidly. Clinical features and their frequency in Budd-Chiari syndrome are shown in Table 21.57.

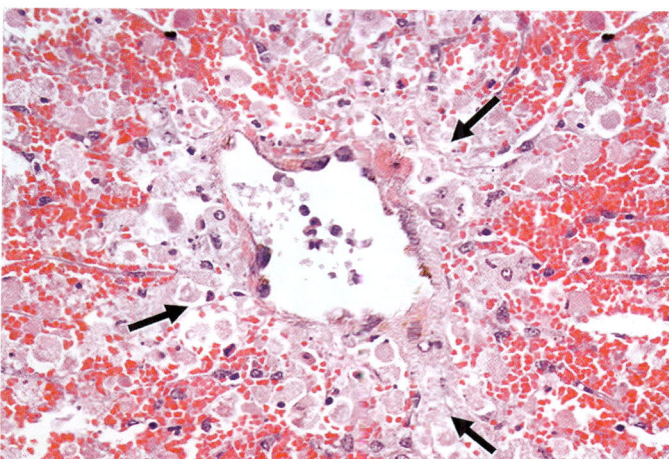

Fig. 21.75: Cardiac cirrhosis. Chronic hepatic passive congestion continues for a long time, a condition called *cardiac cirrhosis* may develop in which there fibrosis is bridging between central zonal regions, as shown below, so that the portal tracts appear to be in the center of the reorganized lobule. This process is best termed *cardiac sclerosis* because, unlike a true cirrhosis, there is minimal nodular regeneration (arrows) (400X).

Table 21.56: Etiology of large hepatic vein thrombosis

- Primary myeloproliferative disorders (polycythemia vera)
- Paroxysmal nocturnal hemoglobinuria
- Promyelocytic leukemia
- Protein C deficiency
- Protein S deficiency
- Antithrombin III deficiency
- Antiphospholipid autoantibodies (lupus anticoagulant)
- Hepatocellular carcinoma
- Behçet's disease
- Allergic vasculitis
- Oral contraceptives
- Pregnancy and postpartum state
- Certain solid tumors
- Idiopathic (10% cases)

Table 21.57: Budd-Chiari syndrome, clinical features and their frequency

Clinical manifestations	Frequency
Ascites	96%
Hepatomegaly	90%
Abdominal pain	80%
Splenomegaly	64%
Edema	46%
Jaundice	44%
Fever	40%
Hepatic encephalopathy	22%
Gastrointestinal bleeding	14%

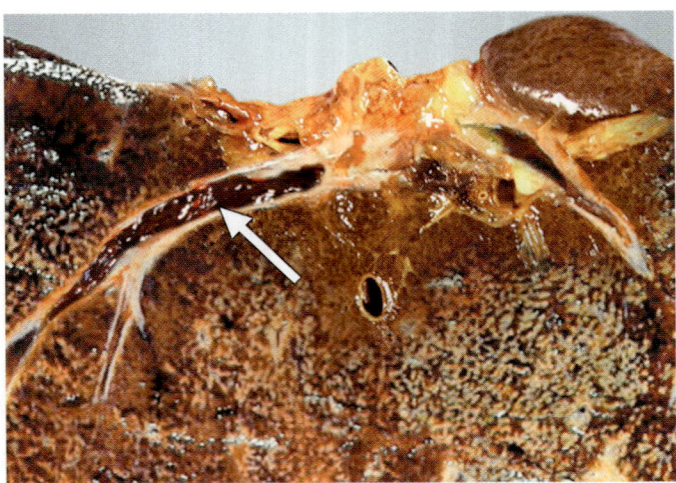

Fig. 21.76: Budd-Chiari syndrome. The liver has been sliced coronally, with the caudate lobe in the middle. Thrombus can be seen in the hepatic veins. This caused obstruction, which resulted in venous congestion of the liver, most marked in the caudate lobe (arrow).

> **Gross Morphology**
> Thrombus in the hepatic veins cause obstruction to blood flow to liver leading to venous congestion of the liver (Fig. 21.76).
>
> **Light Microscopy**
> - Liver biopsy shows severe centrilobular necrosis and hemorrhage.
> - The sinusoids of the central zone are dilated and packed with erythrocytes showing chronic passive congestion as a result of localized obstruction to venous drainage.
> - Rim of hepatocytes in zone 1 shows survival.

SINUSOIDAL OBSTRUCTION SYNDROME (VENO-OCCLUSIVE DISORDER)

Veno-occlusive disorder is also known as *sinusoidal obstruction syndrome*. It is characterized by non-thrombotic luminal narrowing affecting the hepatic vein radicles and sublobular veins.

Narrowing of these blood vessels occurs due to growth of a new layer of subendothelial connective tissue. Predisposing factors of veno-occlusive disorder are described as under:
- Poisoning with pyrrolizidine alkaloids occurs either due to contamination of flour or ingestion of teas derived from alkaloid-containing plants such as Crotalaria and Senecio species.
- Irradiation of liver
- Treatment with anticancer drugs
- Bone marrow transplantation is major cause within 4 weeks in 20% cases due to high doses of chemotherapeutic agents (cyclophosphamide) and total body irradiation
- Graft-versus-host reaction

Clinical Features
Patient presents with abdominal pain, ascites and hepatosplenomegaly similar to Budd-Chiari syndrome.

NONCIRRHOTIC PORTAL HYPERTENSION

Noncirrhotic portal hypertension is also known as *idiopathic portal hypertension*. It usually occurs as a result of presinusoidal causes. It may also occur due to hepatic causes such as sarcoidosis, schistosomiasis or congenital hepatic fibrosis. Clinically liver functions are maintained.

NODULAR REGENERATIVE HYPERPLASIA

It is related to aberrant blood flow. Liver parenchyma is diffusely nodular without fibrosis. Reticulin stain highlights regenerative hepatocytes outlined by atrophic cords.

HEPATOPORTAL SCLEROSIS

It occurs due to intrahepatic portal vein injury and scarring. Portal vein remains initially patent, that later on shows marked thickening with luminal narrowing.

IMPAIRMENT OF ARTERIAL UNDERPERFUSION

FUNCTIONAL UNDERPERFUSION

Infarcts in liver are rare due to its dual blood supply (portal vein and hepatic arteries). Liver receives blood from hepatic arteries and portal vein. Red infarct areas receives constant blood supply from normal spared vessel of liver, allows RBCs to diffuse through necrotic tissue.

STRUCTURAL UNDERPERFUSION

Red or hemorrhagic infarcts in liver occurs due to embolism, sepsis, polyarteritis nodosa, disseminated intravascular coagulation and Budd-Chiari syndrome (portal vein thrombosis).

MISCELLANEOUS INTRAHEPATIC VASCULAR CONDITIONS

PELIOSIS HEPATITIS

Peliosis hepatitis is reversible sinusoidal dilatation of liver of unknown etiology. It is characterized by blood-filled cystic spaces partly lined by endothelial cells.

Etiology

This disorder is associated with tuberculosis, cancers, AIDS, post-transplantation immunodeficiency, therapeutic use of anabolic hormones, oral contraceptives and danazol.

Peliosis has also been observed in patients to control renal transplant rejection with azathioprine.

Clinical Features

Patient presents with hepatomegaly and jaundice.

Light Microscopy

Histological examination of liver shows numerous blood-filled spaces partly lined by endothelial cells.

RENDU-OSLER-WEBER DISEASE

Rendu-Osler-Weber disease is hereditary hemorrhagic telangiectasia. It is autosomal dominant disease characterized by the presence of numerous blood-filled spaces affecting many tissues.

Liver lesions in hereditary hemorrhagic telangiectasia type 2 occurs due to *mutation of alk gene located on chromosome 12*. Patient presents with *noise bleed*.

Gross Morphology

Liver contains subcapsular enlarged blood vessels.

Light Microscopy

Hepatic lesions are composed of *thick-walled veins, scattered dilated sinusoids* and *abnormal-sized portal tracts*.

LIVER TUMORS

Current WHO histological classification of liver and intrahepatic bile ducts are shown in Table 21.58. Most common type is metastases from various organs in noncirrhotic liver. Metastases most often present as multiple nodules in contrast to the single nodules of primary tumors. Metastases to a cirrhotic liver are very uncommon.

PRIMARY BENIGN TUMORS

HEPATOCELLULAR ADENOMA

Hepatocellular adenoma is a rare tumor. One setting for their occurrence is young women taking oral contraceptives. It usually occurs as a *solitary, sharply demarcated encapsulated mass* up to 40 cm in diameter and 3 kg in weight. It is located anywhere in liver *beneath capsule*.

Complication

Subcapsular tumor has a *tendency to rupture* resulting in *severe bleeding in peritoneal cavity especially during pregnancy. It induces* hypovolemic shock that requires emergency treatment.

Pathogenesis

Hepatocellular adenoma has three variants. Each has risk of development of malignant transformation.

- *HNF-α inactivated hepatic adenomas:* It encodes for transcriptional factor. Approximately 80% of these tumors show somatic mutations of HNF-α. Heterozygous germline mutations are responsible for autosomal dominant *MODY-3 (maturity onset diabetes mellitus)*.
- *β-catenin activated hepatic adenomas:* Mutation of β-catenin is associated with adenomas and undergoing *malignant transformation*.
- *Inflammatory hepatic adenomas:* These have small risk of development of malignant transformation. It is associated with gp130 a co-receptor for IL-6, that leads to consecutive *JAK-STAT signaling* and over expression of acute phase reactant.

Gross Morphology

- Hepatocellular adenoma is well circumscribed tumor. The cut surface demonstrates greenish bile staining, indicating that it is of hepatocyte origin.
- Occasionally, tumor has *pseudopods projecting into liver substance mimicking hepatocellular carcinoma* (Fig. 21.77).

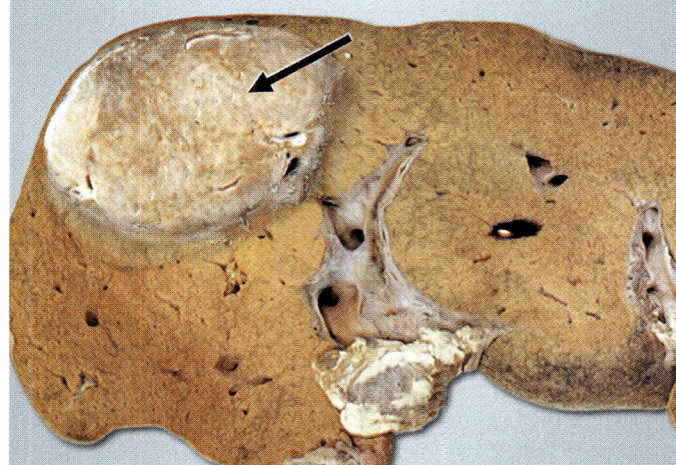

Fig. 21.77: Hepatic adenoma. The cut surface of the hepatic adenoma demonstrates greenish bile staining, indicating that it is of hepatocyte origin (no other neoplasm could accumulate bile pigment). Such neoplasms are rare. One setting for their occurrence is young women taking oral contraceptives (arrow).

Table 21.58: WHO histological classification of liver and intrahepatic bile ducts

Tumors	Origin	Examples
Benign tumors hepatocellular origin	Epithelial origin	Hepatocellular adenoma (HNF1-α mutation, β-catenin activating and gp130 mutation and inflammatory type) Focal nodular hyperplasia Dysplastic nodules
	Mesenchymal tumors	Cavernous hemangioma (*most common benign tumor in liver*) Lymphangioma Hemangioendothelioma
Malignant tumors hepatocellular origin	Epithelial origin	Hepatocellular carcinoma (early hepatocellular, HCC fibrolamellar, HCC scirrhous, and HCC sarcomatoid variants) Hepatoblastoma (most common tumor in children)
Benign and malignant tumors of biliary origin	Epithelial origin	Bile duct adenoma, microcystic adenoma and biliary adenofibroma Biliary intraepithelial neoplasia, grade 3 Intrahepatic cholangiocarcinoma
Malignancies of mixed or uncertain origin	Mixed tumors	Angiosarcoma, carcinosarcoma, combined hepatocellular-cholangiocarcinoma, hepatoblastoma (mixed epithelial-mesenchymal), malignant rhabdoid tumor
Germ cell tumors	Germ cell origin Lymphoid cells	Teratoma and yolk sac tumor (endodermal sinus tumor) Lymphomas Leukemias
Liver metastases (secondaries liver)	Epithelial origin Mesenchymal origin Small round cell tumors	Carcinomas of breast, lung, gastric, colon, rectum, pancreas, prostate, endometrium, thyroid and kidney (RCC) Hemangiosarcomas (multifocal), and rhabdomyosarcoma Wilm's tumor, Ewing's sarcoma, neuroblastoma, and bronchial carcinoid

Light Microscopy

- *Cell morphology:* It is composed of a relatively uniform population of hepatocytes with a normal nucleus to cytoplasm ratio.
- *Arrangements:* Tumor cells are arranged in one- to three-cell-thick plates with intact reticulin framework similar to that in normal liver. The cell plates are usually more irregular and nonlinear than in the normal liver. Portal zones are absent.
- *Naked arterioles:* The presence of arterioles without accompanying bile ducts and surrounded by scant connective tissue is a characteristic feature of hepatocellular adenoma (*naked arterioles*) (Fig. 21.78).

HEMANGIOMA LIVER

Hemangioma liver is the most common benign tumor of the liver. Occasionally spontaneous *bleeding* and rupture and *thrombocytopenia* due to sequestration of platelets.

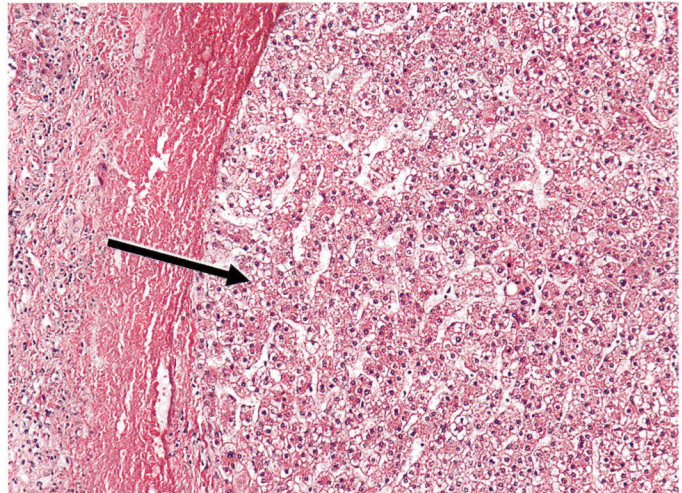

Fig. 21.78: Hepatocellular adenoma. Normal liver tissue with a portal tract is seen on the left. The hepatic adenoma is on the right and is composed of cells that closely resemble normal hepatocytes, but the neoplastic liver tissue is disorganized hepatocyte cords and does not contain a normal lobular architecture (arrow).

Gross Morphology

Tumor is most often <1 cm located just beneath liver capsule. Cut surface is brown (Fig. 21.79).

Light Microscopy

Liver hemangioma is composed of vascular channels lined by endothelial cells (Fig. 21.80)

LYMPHANGIOMA LIVER

Lymphangioma liver occurs in infants and children. Liver involvement occurs as a part of multicentric process affecting other organs.

HEMANGIOENDOTHELIOMA LIVER

Hemangioendothelioma liver is highly cellular tumor in children (87%) especially less than 6 months of age. Tumor is solitary or multiple. *Death occurs due to liver failure.*

MULTIPLE BILIARY HAMARTOMAS (VON MEYENBURG COMPLEX)

Bile duct hamartoma is asymptomatic lesion also known as *von Meyenburg complex*. It shows irregularly dilated bile ducts. It is characterized by multiple bile duct hamartomas and biliary microhamartomas <5 mm.

It is important to distinguish this disorder from multiple hepatic metastases. Women are more affected than men.

Predisposing Factors

It is attributed to ischemia, inflammation or genetic abnormalities. It is known to be associated with *polycystic liver disease and autosomal polycystic disease of kidney*. Several reports suggest that these patients may develop *hepatocellular carcinoma* and *cholangiocarcinoma*.

Gross Morphology

- Liver surface shows creamy nodules mimicking secondary deposits from colon carcinoma.
- Histological examination of the nodules shows proliferations of bile ducts (Fig. 21.81).

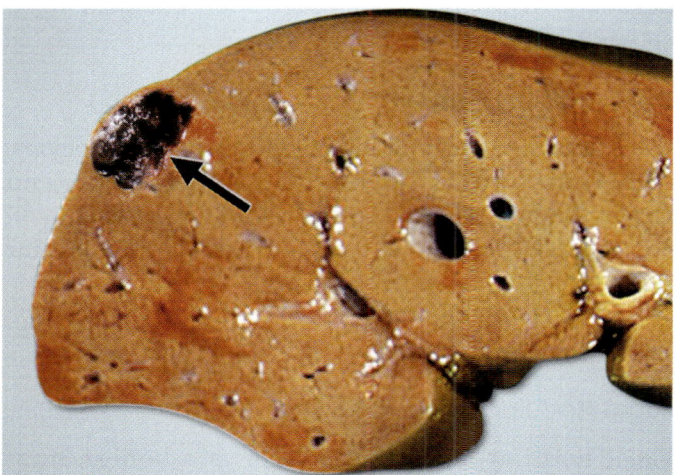

Fig. 21.79: Hemangioma liver. This is a benign hemangioma of the liver just beneath the capsule. Perhaps one person in 50 has such a neoplasm, which is typically just an incidental finding, since most are 1 cm or less. They can sometimes be multiple (arrow).

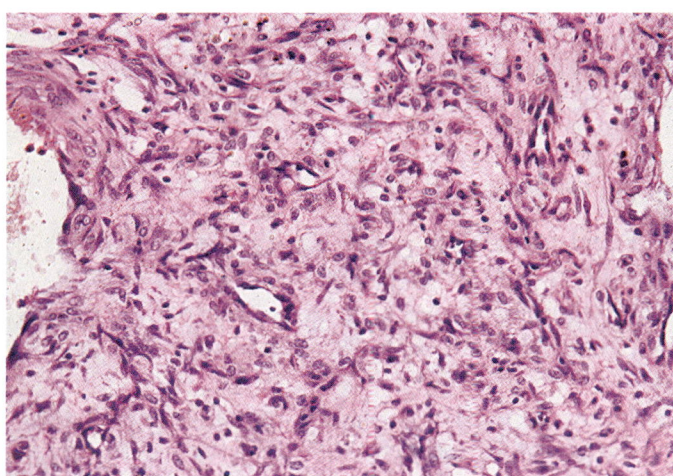

Fig. 21.80: Liver hemangioma shows vascular channels lined by endothelial cells (100X).

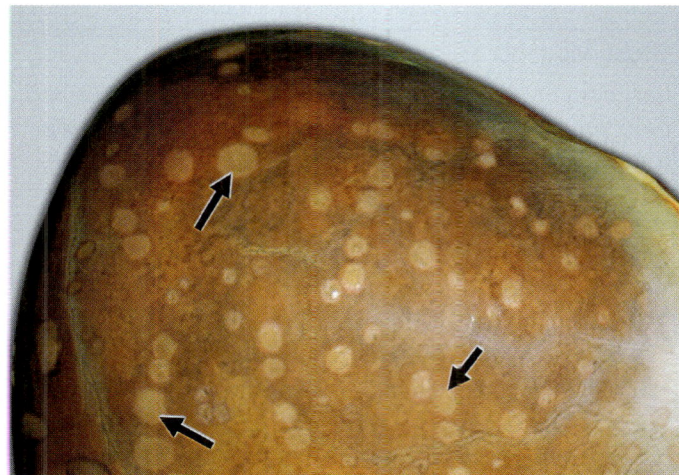

Fig. 21.81: Multiple bile duct hamartomas. Liver surface shows creamy nodules consisting of proliferations of bile ducts. During surgery for bowel cancer, surgeon may consider metastatic deposits in liver. Histopathological examination of one or two nodules confirms diagnosis that these are not secondary deposits (arrows).

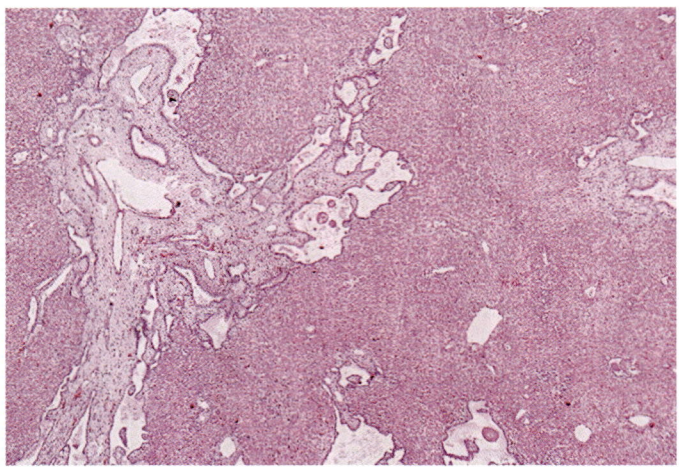

Fig. 21.82: Multiple bile duct hamartomas are also known as *von Meyenburg complex*. Hamartoma is composed of small disorganized clusters of dilated cystic bile ducts lined by columnar cells enclosed within fibrocollagenous stroma (100X).

Light Microscopy

Biliary hamartomas are composed of small disorganized clusters of dilated cystic bile ducts lined by columnar cells enclosed within fibrocollagenous stroma (Fig. 21.82).

BENIGN OR PREMALIGNANT HEPATOCELLULAR LESIONS IN CIRRHOTIC LIVER

LARGE REGENERATIVE NODULES LIVER

Large regenerative nodules formed in liver measure >1 cm. These are almost always <3 cm in greatest diameter. These occur in the *setting of cirrhosis*.

Gross Morphology

Large regenerative nodules are sharply circumscribed pale yellow to tan and may be bile stained. They tend to bulge on cut section.

Light Microscopy

- Large regenerative nodules in liver resemble cirrhotic nodules with an intact reticulin framework similar to that of normal liver, and the cell plates are one to two cells thick.
- Portal tracts are usually present within the nodule, and bile ductular reaction may be prominent. Large regenerative nodules have been associated with an *increased incidence of hepatocellular carcinoma*.

DYSPLASIA LIVER

Two different types of atypical hepatocytes occur in cirrhotic nodules and have been referred to as large cell dysplasia and small cell dysplasia.

Dysplastic Focus

A cluster of dysplastic hepatocytes that is recognized microscopically measuring <1 mm in diameter.

Dysplastic Nodule

It is a large lesion (usually >1 mm) that is grossly or radiologically apparent and is termed dysplastic nodule.

Large Cell Change

This lesion is characterized by nuclear enlargement, hyperchromasia, prominent nucleoli, but with abundant cytoplasm and hence, a normal nucleus to cytoplasm ratio. It may instead represent a regenerative or degenerative phenomenon or a response to prolonged cholestasis.

Small Cell Change

It is characterized by smaller than normal hepatocytes, higher than normal nucleus to cytoplasm ratio, and hyperchromatic nuclei. Small expansive foci of cell change are closely associated with hepatocellular carcinoma than large cell change.

HEPATOCELLULAR HYPERPLASIA

Focal Nodular Hyperplasia Liver

Focal nodular hyperplasia liver is a benign non-neoplastic lesion often diagnosed as an incidental finding during radiological investigations done for other causes. It is commonly seen in young women in 3rd to 4th decades. It is associated with use of anabolic steroid or contraceptives. It shows central stellate fibrous scar with arterial blood vessels. Liver functions are normal.

AFP levels are not raised. It rarely grows or bleeds. It does not undergo malignant transformation. Patient presents with upper abdominal mass.

Gross Morphology

- Focal nodular hyperplasia liver is most often a solitary well circumscribed lesion <5 cm in size.
- It is usually located near the capsule of liver in 80% of cases. Multifocal lesions can also be seen in 20% of cases.
- It may be focal or diffuse. It appears nodular, well demarcated, unencapsulated with lighter color when compared to surrounding liver.
- FNH has a characteristic central scar on gross examination (Fig. 21.83).

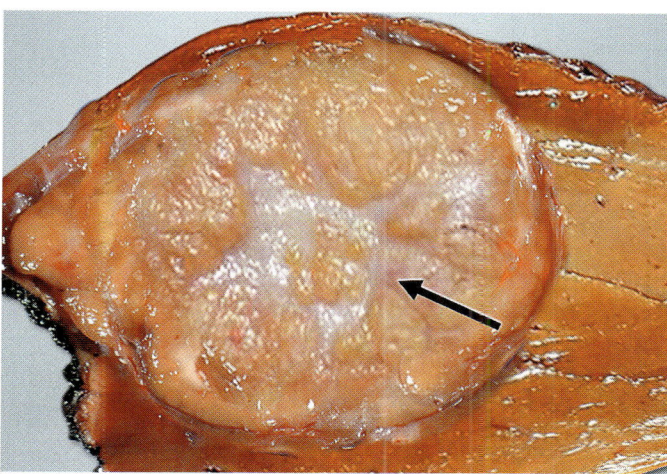

Fig. 21.83: Focal nodular hyperplasia. This well circumscribed mass in the liver is a benign lesion. It is regarded as being a hamartoma and is distinguished from a true adenoma by the presence of the central stellate scar, which contains bile ductules. This is a large example of FNH. The abnormal areas are usually multiple and smaller than this one (arrow).

Light Microscopy

- Focal nodular hyperplasia has normal-appearing hepatocytes arranged in nodules that are separated by fibrous tissue.
- *The cell plates are 2 to 3 cell thick and the reticulin framework is intact similar to normal liver.*
- Rarely foci of mild nuclear atypia and conspicuous nucleoli can be seen.

Immunohistochemistry

Hepatocyte markers such as *Hep Par-1, CAM 5.2,* and *polyclonal CEA* are positive. Glutamine synthetase has a characteristic *map-like pattern* in FNH. AFP is negative.

Prognosis

Focal nodular hyperplasia is a benign lesion with no real evidence for progression to carcinoma. Risk of hemorrhage and rupture is less as compared to hepatocellular adenoma. It is treated by local resection.

Diffuse Hyperplasia Liver

Diffuse hepatocellular hyperplasia occurs *without fibrosis*. It is associated with rheumatoid arthritis (most common), myeloproliferative disorders, hyperviscosity syndromes, transplantation of liver and kidney, HIV infection, vasculitis and drugs (anabolic drugs, cytotoxic drugs).

PRIMARY MALIGNANT TUMORS

HEPATOCELLULAR CARCINOMA

Hepatocellular carcinoma is the most common primary malignancy of the liver. It affects more than 50 years but younger age group may be affected. It is marked by increased serum concentration of α-fetoprotein.

There is a propensity for invasion of vascular channels with hematogenous dissemination. Some tumors may obstruct the biliary ducts results in *increased serum alkaline phosphatase*. It is prone to *hemorrhage and necrosis* resulting in *hemoperitoneum*.

Predisposing Factors

Adenomatous hyperplasia and liver dysplasia are thought to be *precursor* of hepatocellular carcinoma.

Risk Factors

HBV, HCV, chronic alcoholism, tyrosinemia, primary hemochromatosis, nonalcoholic fatty liver disease, cirrhosis, aflatoxin β_1 and azo dyes derivatives of aromatic amines increase risk of hepatocellular carcinoma.

- *Hepatitis B infection:* Genetic material of HBV has been demonstrated in the malignant cells of hepatocellular carcinoma. There is increased risk of hepatocellular carcinoma, if infection has been contracted during infancy or childhood. HBV *activates proto-oncogene and inactivates TP53 suppressor gene* resulting in hepatocellular carcinoma.
- *Hepatitis C infection:* Hepatitis C virus participates in the pathogenesis of hepatocellular carcinoma in 5–10% cases by two mechanisms: it directly induces liver cancers or it first induces post-necrotic cirrhosis resulting in hepatocellular carcinoma.
- *Chronic alcoholism:* Alcoholism along with HBV or HCV increases the risk of liver cancer many folds.
- *Primary hemochromatosis:* It first produces cirrhosis leading to hepatocellular carcinoma.
- *Non-alcoholic fatty liver:* It can lead to cirrhosis and hepatocellular carcinoma.
- *Cirrhosis:* Any etiology responsible for cirrhosis may lead to hepatocellular carcinoma.
- *Aflatoxin β_1:* It is a potent carcinogen synthesized by *Aspergillus flavus* grown on peanuts and grains stored in hot humid conditions. Like the polycyclic aromatic hydrocarbons, aflatoxin β_1 can *bind covalently to DNA and is thought to cause specific point mutations in the p53 tumor suppressor gene* resulting in liver cancer in Asian and African population. It is among the most potent liver carcinogens recognized.
- *Azo dyes derivatives of aromatic amines:* These are derivatives of aromatic amines. Dimethylamino-azobenzene, known as *butter yellow* imparts an appetizing yellow color to margarine causing liver cancer. Pathogens and chemicals participating in pathogenesis of liver carcinoma are shown in Tables 21.59 and 21.60.

Section III: Systemic Pathology

Table 21.59: Pathogens induced liver cell cancers

Organisms	Pathogens	Associated tumors
Viruses	HCV (RNA)	Hepatocellular carcinoma
	HBV (DNA)	
Fungus	*Aspergillus flavus* (aflatoxin β_1 product)	Hepatocellular carcinoma
Parasites	*Clonorchis sinensis* (liver fluke)	Hepatocellular carcinoma Cholangiocarcinoma (bile duct carcinoma) Pancreatic carcinoma
	Opisthorchis viverrini	Cholangiocarcinoma (bile duct carcinoma)
	Fasciola hepatica	

Table 21.60: Indirect acting chemical carcinogens induced liver cancers

Chemical carcinogen	Examples	Associated cancers
Azo dyes derivatives of aromatic amines	Dimethylaminoazobenzene, known as *butter yellow* imparts an appetizing yellow color to margarine	Hepatocellular carcinoma
Natural carcinogens	Aflatoxin β_1 synthesized by fungus *Aspergillus flavus* in growing stored grains, nuts and peanut	Hepatocellular carcinoma
Organohalogen compounds	Polyvinyl chloride, carbon tetrachloride, chloroform, hexachlorobenzene, trichloroethylene	Liver angiosarcoma
Occupational carcinogens	Arsenic used in alloys, medication, preparation of fungicides and herbicides	Liver angiosarcoma, skin squamous cell carcinoma and basal cell carcinoma, lung carcinoma

Molecular Genetics

- *Growth factor baseline activity:* Many cancer cells, acquire the ability to synthesize the same growth factors to which they are responsive, generating an autocrine loop. Increased baseline activity of hepatocyte growth factor (HGF) oncogene product is associated with hepatocellular carcinoma and thyroid carcinoma.
- *Insertional mutagenesis:* It is form of oncogene activation, which occurs due to insertion of a viral gene into the mammalian DNA, resulting in genetic dysregulation and hepatocellular carcinoma. The best example of such an event may be found in hepatitis virus-infected human liver cells.
- *Mutant RAS:* Mutant signal transducing RAS protein has been associated with hepatocellular carcinoma.
- *Translocation and amplification of CCND1/Cyclin D1:* It has been demonstrated in hepatocellular carcinoma.
- *Amplification or point mutation of CDK4 (cyclin-dependent kinase):* It has been demonstrated in hepatocellular carcinoma.

Gross Morphology

- Primary hepatocellular carcinoma is usually a solitary, poorly circumscribed mass, generally in the background of cirrhosis. It may be partially or completely encapsulated tumor.
- Tumor arising in accessory lobe is pedunculated.
- Cut surface has greenish yellow hue with necrosis and hemorrhage.
- Neoplasm <2 cm in diameter is referred to as small HCC lacking gross vascular invasion, necrosis or hemorrhage (Fig. 21.84).

Light Microscopy

Cell morphology: The tumor cells are large polyhedral with hyperchromatic nuclei, prominent nuclei, intracytoplasmic globular hyaline inclusions and atypical mitoses.

Cell arrangement: These cords of tumor cells are much wider than the normal liver plate that is two cells thick arranged in solid, tubular and trabecular patterns.

Well differentiated tumor shows trabecular (sinusoidal—most important diagnostic feature) or glandular pattern (acinar pattern) and also exhibits pseudoglandular pattern.

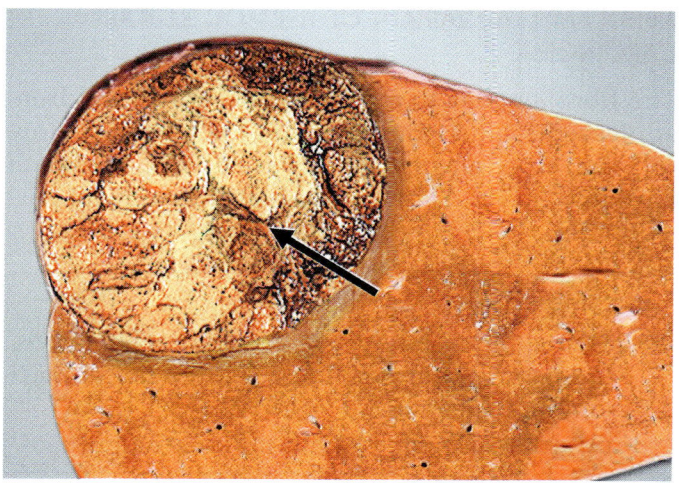

Fig. 21.84: Hepatocellular carcinoma. The satellite nodules of this hepatocellular carcinoma represent either intrahepatic spread of the tumor or multicentric origin of the tumor. Such masses may also focally obstruct the biliary tract and lead to an elevated alkaline phosphatase (arrow).

Undifferentiated hepatocellular carcinoma shows marked pleomorphism, scant cytoplasm, bizarre mitotic figures, tumor giant cells, prominent nuclei with nucleoli.

- *Cell inclusions:* Cytoplasmic inclusions such as *Mallory-Denk bodies,* globular eosinophilic bodies composed of proteins including albumin, fibrinogen, α_1-antitrypsin, or ferritin, may be present. Pale bodies containing fibrinogen are seen in fibrolamellar hepatocellular carcinoma (Fig. 21.85).

Immunohistochemistry

- Panel of markers is used to analyze expression in hepatocellular carcinoma on histopathological sections. Tumor cells are *positive for HBsAg*. Hepatocellular carcinoma should be differentiated from metastatic carcinoma.
- Hepatocellular carcinoma expresses *Arginase-1, Glypican* and *Hep Par-1,* while these are not expressed in metastatic carcinoma.
- Immunohistochemistry of hepatocellular carcinoma is shown in Table 21.61. Immunohistochemistry in hepatocellular and metastatic carcinoma is shown in Table 21.62.

Serum Tumor Marker

Serum α-fetoprotein level is increased in 60–80% cases of hepatocellular carcinoma. Serum α-fetoprotein is also raised in cirrhosis, chronic hepatitis, hepatoblastoma and yolk sac tumor of gonads.

Table 21.61: Immunohistochemistry of hepatocellular carcinoma

Tumor markers	Expression
α_1-Antitrypsin (75% cases)	Positive
α-Fetoprotein (60–80% cases)	Positive
CEA (carcinoembryogenic antigen in 30% cases)	Positive
Arginase-1	Positive
Glypican-3	Positive
Hep Par-1 (hepatocyte paraffin-1)	Positive
Des-gamma carboxyprothrombin (DCP): It is a protein induced by vitamin K abnormality (PIVKA-2)	Positive
Vitamin B_{12} binding protein	Positive
Human hepatocyte growth factor	Positive
Neurotensin is expressed by fibrolamellar variant of hepatocellular carcinoma	Positive
Arginase-1 is a binuclear manganese metalloenzyme that catalyzes the hydrolysis of arginine to ornithine and urea. It has been proposed as a *sensitive and specific marker of hepatocytes and hepatocellular neoplasms.*	

Table 21.62: Immunohistochemistry in hepatocellular and metastatic carcinoma

Tumor marker	Hepatocellular carcinoma	Metastatic carcinoma
Arginase-1 Glypican-3 Hep Par-1 (hepatocyte paraffin-1)	Positive	Negative
Specific markers are used to confirm origin of tumors metastasizing to liver		

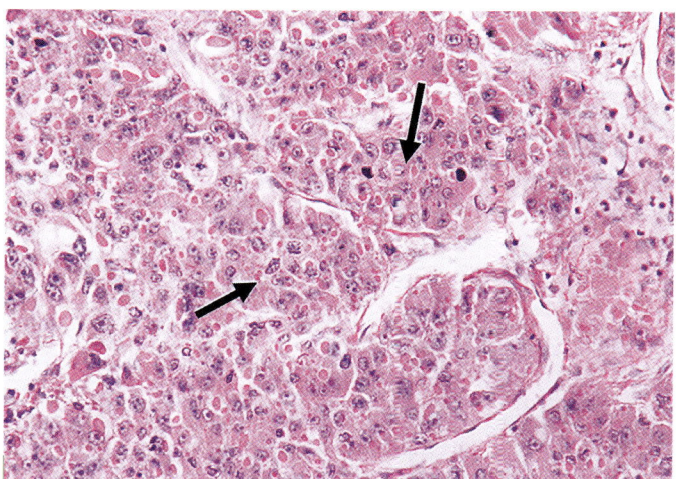

Fig. 21.85: Hepatocellular carcinoma trabecular pattern. Tumor is composed of liver cords that are much wider than the normal liver plate that is two cells thick. Tumor cells are arranged in trabeculae. There is no discernible normal lobular architecture, though vascular structures are present. It is associated with elevated α-fetoprotein (arrows) (400X).

Paraneoplastic Syndrome

Patient with hepatocellular carcinoma may present with hypoglycemia, increased red blood cell count, increased serum calcium level, hypercholesterolemia and porphyria.

Clinical Features

- Clinical symptoms may be masked in the background of chronic hepatitis or cirrhosis. Patient presents with abdominal fullness, upper abdominal pain, weight loss and generalized weakness.

   These patients reach terminal stage characterized by cachexia, gastrointestinal or esophageal variceal bleeding, and liver failure with hepatic coma or rupture of tumor with fatal hemorrhage.
- On clinical examination, liver is enlarged with irregular nodularity surface.

Mode of Spread

- *Lymphatic route:* It spreads by lymphatic route to peripancreatic and para-aortic lymph nodes.
- *Hematogenous route:* Hematogenous spread of hepatocellular carcinoma is relatively less frequent. It may spread by hematogenous route by invading portal vein reaching to right side heart resulting in metastases to lungs, bones, adrenal glands and central nervous system.

Laboratory Investigations

- *Serum des-gamma carboxyprothrombin:* Its positivity is demonstrated in 75 to 90% cases with large tumor. Small tumors do not show positivity.
- *Serum α-fetoprotein:* It is a glycoprotein normally synthesized in the fetus by the yolk sac, liver, and gastrointestinal tract.

   In adults, an elevated serum level of AFP is a useful indicator of *hepatocellular carcinoma* and *germ cell tumors of the testis*.
- *Imaging techniques:* These include ultrasonography, hepatic angiography, CT scan and MRI.
- MRI demonstrates location, invasiveness and presence or absence of multifocality.
- *Fine needle aspiration cytology:* It is cost effective diagnostic tool for early diagnosis.
- *Histopathological examination:* It is performed to confirm diagnosis. Hepatocellular carcinoma should be differentiated from hepatocellular adenoma and focal nodular hyperplasia. Differential diagnosis of hepatocellular carcinoma is shown in Table 21.63.
- *Immunohistochemistry:* Panel of markers is used to study the expression of hepatocellular carcinoma and metastases.

FIBROLAMELLAR VARIANT OF HEPATOCELLULAR CARCINOMA

The fibrolamellar variant HCC occurs in children, adolescents, and young adults (50% cases below 35 years) especially females. It has no association with HBV infection and cirrhosis. It is associated with *good prognosis*.

Gross Morphology

- It is single large, hard scirrhous tumor with fibrous bands running through it. Sometimes tumor may show encapsulation.
- Cut surface of tumor reveals multiple nodules.

Light Microscopy

Collagen fibers are arranged in lamellar fashion around the large polygonal tumor cells arranged in nests and cords (Fig. 21.86). Differences between hepatocellular carcinoma and fibrolamellar variant hepatocellular carcinoma are shown in Table 21.64.

Immunohistochemistry

Neurotensin is tumor marker for fibrolamellar variant of hepatocellular carcinoma.

Clinical Course

Death occurs due to GIT bleeding and liver failure.

Mode of Spread

It spreads by lymphatic route.

Prognosis

Prognosis is better than classic hepatocellular carcinoma.

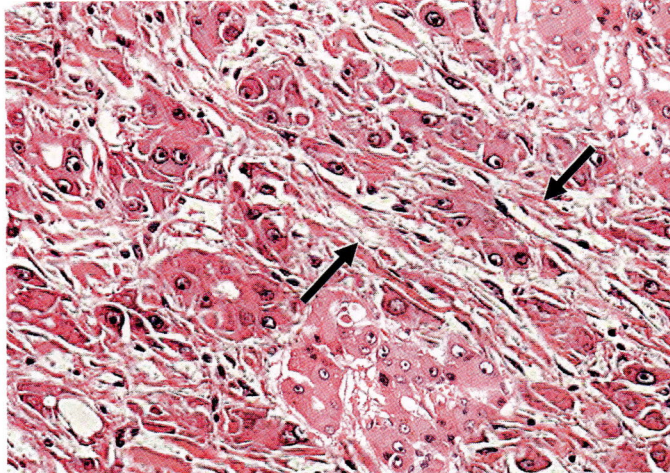

Fig. 21.86: Fibrolamellar variant of hepatocellular carcinoma shows tumor cells surrounded by fibrocollagenous tissue (arrows) (400X).

Table 21.63: Differential diagnosis of hepatocellular carcinoma

Parameters	Hepatocellular adenoma	Focal nodular hyperplasia	Hepatocellular carcinoma
Age and sex	Women, 3rd–4th decades	All ages and young women	Men
AFP	Normal	Normal	Often elevated
Background liver	Normal	Normal	Cirrhotic
OCP use	Common	Occasional	Absent
Other associations	DM, alcohol, obesity, male hormone use	Vascular abnormalities	HBV, HCV, alcohol, drugs and toxins
Capsule	May be present	Absent	May be present
Number	Solitary or multiple	Usually solitary	Solitary or multiple
Bile	Present	Absent	Present
Central scar	Absent	Present	Absent
Interlobar bile ducts	Absent except at periphery	Absent except at periphery	Absent
Bile ductular reaction	Present	Present (prominent)	Absent
Arterioles	Naked arterioles	Aberrant arterioles with myointimal thickening	Naked arterioles
Cell plates	1–3 cells thick	1–3 cells thick	More than 3 cells thick
Hemorrhage or necrosis	Present in larger adenomas	Absent	Present
Kupffer cells	Reduced or absent	Present	Absent
Nuclear pleomorphism	Absent or minimal	Absent	Present
Nucleoli	Absent	Absent	Present
Reticulin framework	Normal	Normal and more prominent	Decreased or absent
Glutamine synthetase IHC	Perivenous pattern	Map-like pattern	Variable
Beta-catenin (IHC)	Positive	Absent	Positive in 10% cases
Molecular genetics	Monoclonal	Polyclonal	Monoclonal

Table 21.64: Differences between hepatocellular carcinoma and fibrolamellar variant HCC

Parameters	Hepatocellular carcinoma	Fibrolamellar variant HCC
Age group	50–60 years	20–30 years
Sex predilection	More common men than women	Men and women equally affected
Etiology	Cirrhosis	Not arising in cirrhotic liver
Involvement of liver lobe	Right lobe	Left lobe
Gross morphology	Solitary or nodular tumor Central necrosis common	Solitary or nodular tumor Central necrosis uncommon
Light microscopy	Basic structure is trabecular pattern with acidophilic cytoplasm and large nucleoli	Collagen fibers arranged in lamellar fashion around the large polygonal tumor cells arranged in nests and cords
Immunohistochemistry	α_1-Antitrypsin (75%), α-fetoprotein (60–80%), carcinoembryogenic antigen (30%), arginase-1, glypican-3, Hep Par-1 (hepatocyte paraffin-1), des-gamma carboxyprothrombin (DCP) and human hepatocyte growth factor	Neurotensin
Resectability rate	Less	More
Prognosis	Poor	Good

CHOLANGIOCARCINOMA

Cholangiocarcinoma is also known as *bile duct carcinoma*. It is less common than hepatocellular carcinoma. It is never associated with HBV infection or cirrhosis.

Origin

It arises from epithelium lining intrahepatic biliary ducts at the porta hepatis to the smallest bile ductules at the periphery of the hepatic lobules.

Locations

- *Extrahepatic cholangiocarcinoma:* It is most common type seen in 90% cases. Perihilar type is most common type seen in 60% and known as *Klatskin tumor located at the junction of left and right hepatic ducts*. It may be located in distal bile ducts in 20–30% cases.
- *Intrahepatic cholangiocarcinoma:* It is less common type seen in 10% cases.

Risk Factors

- *Clonorchis sinensis (liver fluke):* It is transmitted through consumption of raw or undercooked vegetables. It resides in the biliary tree resulting in cholangiocarcinoma in far East population.
- *Opisthorchis viverrini:* It may cause cholangiosarcoma of the bile ducts.
- *Thorostat contrast medium:* Sometimes, it occurs as a late complication of thorium dioxide (thorostat) administration.
- *Primary sclerosing cholangitis:* It is associated with ulcerative colitis. There is increased incidence of cholangiocarcinoma.
- *Caroli's disease:* It is also known as *choledocal cyst*. It is congenital fibropolycystic disease of biliary system.
- *Chronic alcoholic disease:* There may be increased risk of development of cholangiocarcinoma.
- *Hepatitis C virus (HCV):* Patient with hepatitis C infection may develop cholangiocarcinoma.

Molecular Genetics

Upregulation of IL-6 activates AKT results in over expression of MCL-1 (anti-apoptotic protein).

There is *upregulation of K-RAS and downregulation of p53 tumor suppressor gene*.

Clinical Features

Patient presents with *painless lump, jaundice, pruritus, weight loss and acholic stools*.

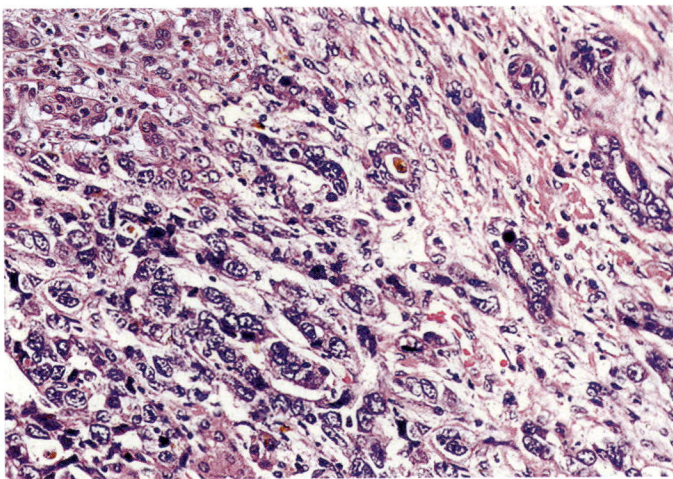

Fig. 21.87: Cholangiocarcinoma shows glandular appearance. It does not make bile, but the cells do make mucin, and they can be almost impossible to distinguish from metastatic adenocarcinoma on biopsy or fine needle aspirate (400X).

Light Microscopy
Tumor is composed of small cuboidal cells with intracytoplasmic mucin arranged in glandular pattern. Desmoplastic stroma is present (Fig. 21.87).
Immunohistochemistry
The tumor cells express **CK7** and **CK19**.

Differential Diagnosis

Tumor cells are not bile stained, as bile is synthesized by hepatocytes. It is worth mentioning that hepatocellular carcinoma tumor cells show bile. It does not make bile, but the cells do make mucin, and they can be almost impossible to distinguish from metastatic adenocarcinoma on biopsy or fine needle aspirate. *Fibrolamellar variant of hepatocellular carcinoma consists of fibrous septa but negative for CK7 and CK19.*

Mode of Spread

Like hepatocellular carcinoma, it has a propensity for early invasion of vascular channels.

HEPATOBLASTOMA

Hepatoblastoma is uncommon malignant liver cancer in infants and children <3 years of age. It is composed of tissue resembling fetal liver cells or bile ducts. It is diagnosed during first year of childhood.

Origin

It originates from immature liver precursor cells. The tumor is usually unifocal affecting right lobe of liver more often than left lobe.

Predisposing Factors

Persons with familial adenomatous polyposis frequently develop hepatoblastoma.

Molecular Genetics

β-Catenin has been demonstrated in 70% cases of hepatoblastoma. *Activation of Wnt signaling pathway may play important role in the pathogenesis of hepatoblastoma.*

Clinical Features

Patient presents with abdominal mass and failure to thrive. It is usually associated with nephroblastoma, cleft palate, hemihypertrophy, renal or cardiac malformations.

Light Microscopy

- *Fetal variant tumor:* It is composed of polygonal cells with central round nuclei and prominent nucleoli. The 2–3 cells thick plates are arranged in sheets, trabeculae and solid groups. There may be foci of hematopoiesis.
- *Embryonal variant:* Tumor cells are arranged in sheets, ribbons, acinar and rosettes.
- *Macrotrabecular variant:* Tumor is composed of >10 cells thick plates arranged in trabecular fashion.
- *Small cell (undifferentiated) variant tumor:* It has more primitive histology with predominance of small to medium-sized cells arranged in loose clusters.
- *Epithelial-mesenchymal variant tumor:* It consists of teratoid features, comprising of spindle or oval cells with osteoid, cartilage or other sarcomatoid characteristics. *It is worth mentioning that there is absence of portal tracts in hepatoblastoma.* The tumor cells show pleomorphism and mitoses in comparison to minimal pleomorphism and low mitotic figures. Light microscopy of hepatoblastoma is shown in Fig. 21.88.

Immunohistochemistry

Panel of markers is used to analyze expression in hepatoblastoma on histopathological sections as shown in Table 21.65.

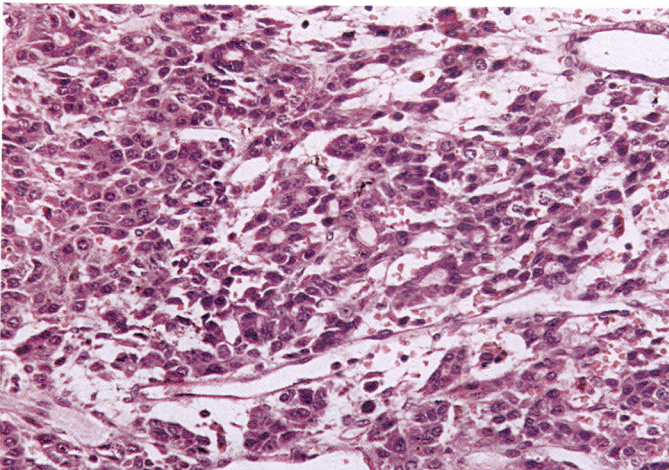

Fig. 21.88: Hepatoblastoma. It is composed of polygonal cells with central round nuclei and prominent nucleoli. The 2–3 cells thick plates are arranged in sheets, trabeculae and solid groups. There may be foci of hematopoiesis (400X)

Table 21.65: Immunohistochemistry in hepatoblastoma

Tumor markers	Expression
α-Fetoprotein (AFP)	Positive
Hep Par-1	Positive
HCG	Positive
Keratin	Positive
Carcinoembryonic antigen (CEA)	Positive
Glycipan-3	Positive
Epithelial membrane antigen (EMA)	Positive
Vimentin	Positive

Children with fetal variant have better prognosis with survival for an average of 9 years. Complete surgical resection remains key treatment for achieving long-term survival.

Prognostic Factors

Prognosis of hepatoblastoma is better than hepatocellular carcinoma. The α-fetoprotein (AFP) levels are commonly elevated. When AFP is not raised at diagnosis, the prognosis is poor.

Patient with <1 year of age, histologic variants (macrotrabecular and small cell types) are associated with poor prognosis.

ANGIOSARCOMA LIVER

Liver angiosarcoma is a rare malignant vascular tumor of liver. It most often occurs in adults. It may also affect children.

Risk Factors

These include macronodular cirrhosis or hemochromatosis due to polyvinyl chloride (PVC) exposure for 16 years, thorium dioxide exposure for 20 years and arsenic exposure for prolonged period.

Immunohistochemistry

Factor VIII related antigen is demonstrated in all cases.

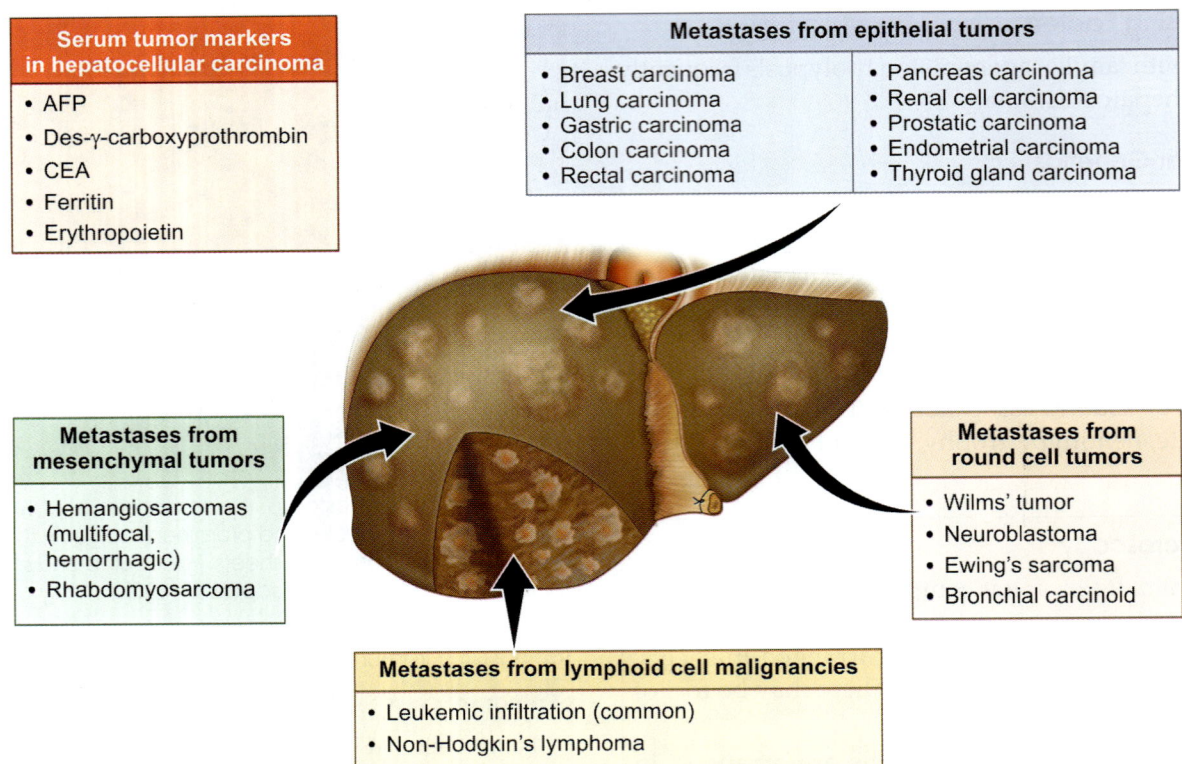

Fig. 21.89: Liver metastases from epithelial, mesenchymal and round cell tumors.

METASTATIC TUMORS (LIVER METASTASES)

Despite all the foregoing material, hepatic malignancies are commonest. Such metastases may be present in 40% of adults with malignant disease elsewhere. Metastatic deposits are visible on the capsular surface of the liver. These deposits show multiple nodules of variable sizes with central depression as a result of tumor necrosis.

Liver metastases arising from epithelial, mesenchymal and round cell tumors are shown in Fig. 21.89 and Table 21.66.

Mode of Metastases

- *Direct spread:* Liver may be involved by direct spread from malignant neoplasms in the vicinity such as *pancreas, extrahepatic bile duct, stomach and gallbladder.*

Table 21.66: Immunohistochemistry of malignant tumors metastasizing to liver

Tumor	Immunohistochemistry
Liver metastases from epithelial tumors	
Breast carcinoma	ER, PR, Her2 neu, CK7, GCDFP-15 (gross cystic disease fluid protein-15) and mammoglobulin, Ki67, eK5, NY-BR1, E-cadherin
Lung carcinoma	EMA, CK7 and TTF1
Gastric carcinoma	Cytokeratin, EMA and CEA
Colorectal carcinoma	CK20, CDX2, CEA and β-catenin
Pancreas carcinoma	Vimentin, α_1-antitrypsin and α_1-antichymotrypsin
Renal cell carcinoma	Coexpression of cytokeratin and vimentin
Prostate carcinoma	Prostate specific antigen (PSA), prostate specific alkaline phosphatase (PSAP), NXK31, prostein and p63
Endometrium carcinoma type 1	ER, PR and PTEN
Thyroid gland carcinoma	TTF1, thyroglobulin, CA 125 and cell surface glycoprotein

Contd...

Table 21.66: Immunohistochemistry of malignant tumors metastasizing to liver (Contd...)

Tumor	Immunohistochemistry
Liver metastases from lymphoid cell malignancies	
NHL B cell (*common*)	CD10, CD19 and CD20
NHL T cell (*common*)	CD3
*Leukemias (*common*)	Cytochemistry, flow cytometry and cytogenetics
Liver metastases from mesenchymal tumors	
Rhabdomyosarcoma	Desmin, myogenin, myoglobin, MyoD1 and vimentin
Metastases from round cell tumors	
Wilm's tumor	WT1 and WT2
Neuroblastoma	Nonspecific enolase (NSE), neurofilament, chromogranin, synaptophysin
Ewing's sarcoma	CD99 (MIC2 specific marker), vimentin and NSE
Bronchial carcinoid tumor	NSE, chromogranin, synaptophysin and cytokearatin

Hemangiosarcomas (multifocal, hemorrhagic) may also metastasize to liver.

- *Hematogenous route:* Most common malignancies metastasizing to liver in adults include large gut, lung, breast, kidney, stomach and malignant melanoma. Metastases confined to liver are more probable in association with tumors drained by portal vein. Blood-borne spread from colorectal carcinoma is most often seen in the liver. *Multiple metastases in liver* are shown in Fig. 21.90. *Solitary liver metastasis* is shown in Fig. 21.91.

Clinical Features

Patient presents with massive hepatomegaly with nodules at the free edges, jaundice at a later stage as a result of massive liver involvement and obstruction of major hepatic ducts. There is unexplained increase in the serum concentration of alkaline phosphatase.

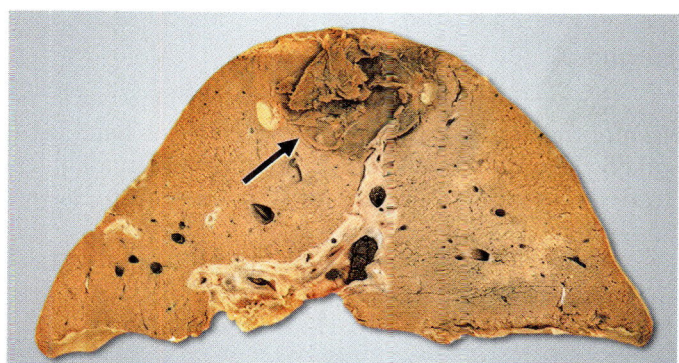

Fig. 21.91: Liver metastasis. Solitary metastasis is seen in liver (arrow).

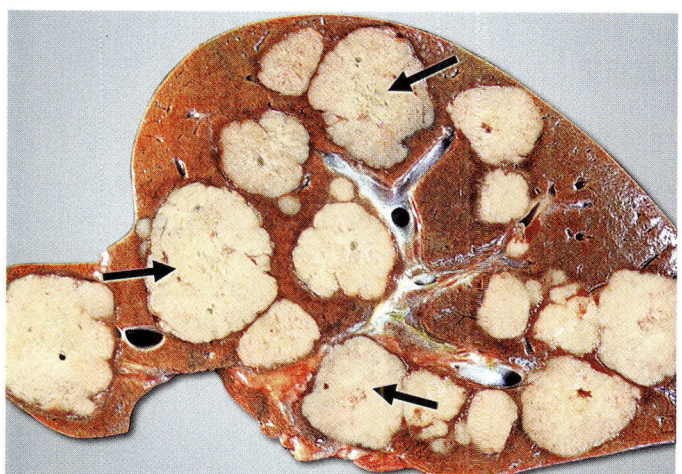

Fig. 21.90: Multiple metastases in liver. Note the numerous mass lesions that are of variable size. Some of the larger ones demonstrate central necrosis. The masses are metastases to the liver. The obstruction from such masses generally elevates alkaline phosphatase, but not all bile ducts are obstructed, so hyperbilirubinemia is typically not present. Also, the transaminases are usually not greatly elevated (arrows).

Imaging Technique

Tumors metastasizing to liver are most often multiple, however solitary deposit may also be demonstrated by imaging technique. Computed tomographic (CT) scan with contrast of the abdomen in transverse view demonstrates metastases in liver (Fig. 21.92).

Light Microscopy

Histological study is done on biopsy obtained from liver metastatic deposits. Liver metastases from breast carcinoma is shown in Fig. 21.93. Liver metastasis from squamous cell carcinoma is shown in Fig. 21.94.

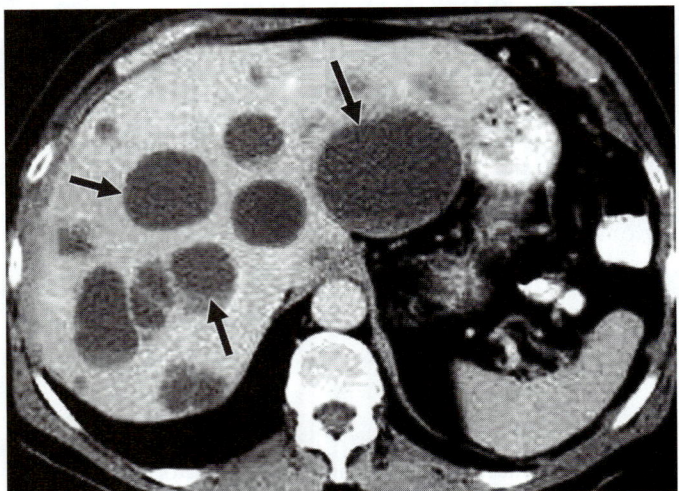

Fig. 21.92: Liver metastases. This computed tomographic (CT) scan with contrast of the abdomen in transverse view demonstrates multiple mass lesions representing metastases from a colonic adenocarcinoma. A normal spleen appears at the lower right in the image (on the patient's left) (arrows).

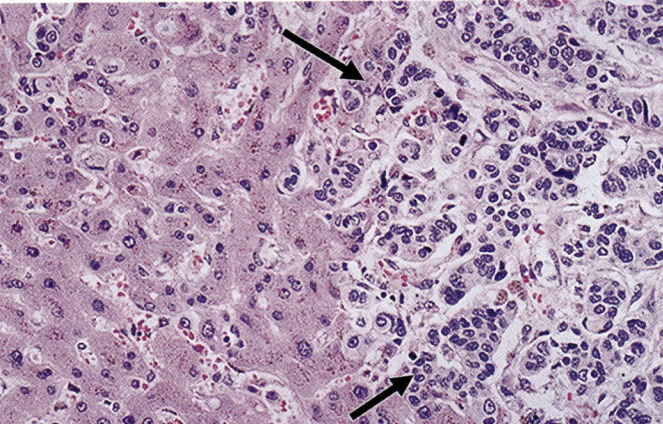

Fig. 21.93: Liver metastases from breast carcinoma. Microscopically, metastatic infiltrating ductal carcinoma from breast is seen on the right, with normal liver parenchyma on the left (arrows) (400X).

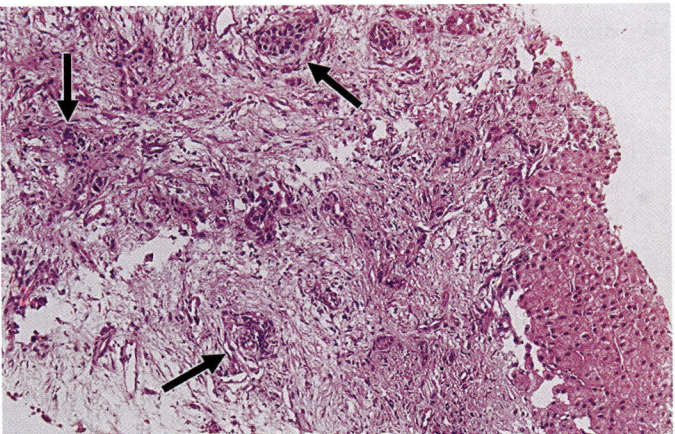

Fig. 21.94: Liver metastasis shows metastatic deposits from squamous cell carcinoma (arrows) (100X).

Prognosis

Median survival in untreated cases varies between 4 and 15 months. Patient with solitary metastasis has longer survival. Solitary metastasis in liver may be treatable by wedge resection, giving months/years symptoms-free remission.

Multiple liver metastases are not resectable. These may respond to chemotherapy.

GALLBLADDER

OVERVIEW

ANATOMY

Gallbladder consists of fundus, body and neck. It is covered by serosa except the portion in the liver fossa which merges with liver parenchyma. It is located in the right upper quadrant, under the costal margin at the level of the 9th costal cartilage. The level of the 9th costal cartilage can be palpated as a distinct notch.

The extrahepatic ducts include the right and left hepatic ducts, which join to form common hepatic duct in the porta hepatis. Common hepatic duct is joined by cystic duct to form common bile duct. The bile duct and the pancreatic duct join and open into the duodenum as the common hepatopancreatic duct which is guarded by a sphincter called the *sphincter of Oddi*.

HISTOLOGY

Gallbladder consists of a layer of folded columnar epithelium and lamina propria of loose connective tissue that directly rests on muscularis propria. The muscularis propria rests on irregularly arranged smooth muscle bundles. External surface of gallbladder is covered by layer of serosa.

PHYSIOLOGY

Bile juice composed of bile salts, sodium taurocholate and sodium glycolate, cholesterol and phospholipids secreted by the hepatic cells passes through the hepatic ducts and is stored and concentrated by gallbladder.

Stimuli are received from vagus nerve, secretin, mucus, water and electrolytes for synthesis of bile juice.

Bile salts are necessary for emulsification and absorption of fats. Bile juice also activates lipase.

SAMPLING

Cholecystectomy is usually performed for cholelithiasis. Porcelain gallbladder is uniformly firm and associated with flattened mucosal surface and submitted to rule out adenocarcinoma.

Endoscopic retrograde cholangiography (*ERCP*) is performed to take biopsy for stricture and overt neoplasm. *Frozen section* is done to evaluate bile duct margins during pancreatoduodenectomy or liver resection for bile duct adenocarcinoma.

NON-NEOPLASTIC CONDITIONS

CHOLECYSTITIS

Cholecystitis is associated with cholelithiasis in >90% of the cases. Classical signs of cholecystitis results from obstruction of the cystic duct by gallstones. It leads to enlarged painful gallbladder distension. Abnormal cholesterol metabolism and bile salts play important role in the pathogenesis of gallstones. The acute form of cholecystitis is most common during middle age; the chronic form occurs most often in elderly people.

ACUTE CHOLECYSTITIS

Acute cholecystitis is characterized by full thickness edema, congestion and serosal fibrinopurulent exudate. It is most often caused by pyogenic bacteria. It may also occur due to poor or absent blood flow to the gallbladder. Stone impacted in neck or cystic duct results in obstruction of bile flow into the duodenum.

Clinical Features

Patient presents with nausea, vomiting, fever, jaundice (if stone in bile duct), and leukocytosis associated with right upper quadrant and epigastric pain and tenderness. *Murphy sign is associated with acute cholecystitis.*

Gross Morphology

- The gallbladder lumen is filled with fibrin, frank pus and hemorrhage. Gallbladder becomes enlarged and tense. Accumulation of pus in lumen is known as *empyema gallbladder*.
- Patient may also develop gangrenous cholecystitis characterized by hemorrhage, transmural necrosis, and or perforation. Serosal surface is covered with inflammatory exudates. Subserosal region exhibits bright red areas of hemorrhages to green-black discoloration.

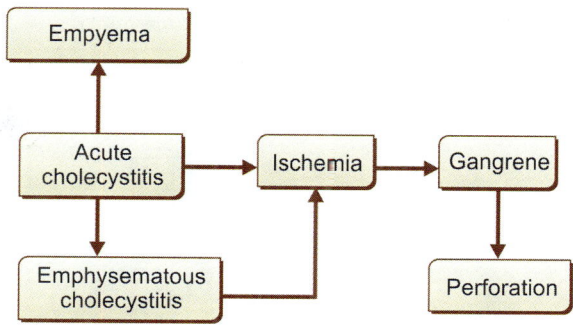

Fig. 21.95: Complications of acute cholecystitis.

Light Microscopy

Histopathological examination of acute cholecystitis shows transmural edema, congestion, serous fibrinopurulent exudate composed of fibrin and polymorphonuclear cells.

Treatment

Acute cholecystitis is initially treated with intravenous fluids and antibiotics which lead to a resolution of the acute inflammation in 70–80% of patients.

Complication

Empyema gallbladder is characterized by accumulation of pus seen in 2–3% of patients with acute cholecystitis. Necrosis of gallbladder results in perforation, abscess formation and peritonitis. *Complications of acute cholecystitis* is shown in Fig. 21.95.

- *Pathogenesis:* Acute inflammation of gallbladder causes edema, vascular compromise and superadded infection resulting in gallbladder empyema (a pus-filled gallbladder).
- *Clinical features:* Patient usually experiences severe abdominal pain for more than 7 days.

CHRONIC CHOLECYSTITIS

Chronic cholecystitis is associated with hypertrophy of *muscle bundles, fibrosis, chronic inflammatory* infiltrate and formation of *Rokitansky-Aschoff sinuses*. Gallbladder is thickened by fibrosis and is relatively rigid.

Etiology

Chronic cholecystitis may develop insidiously or after repeated episodes of acute cholecystitis. It is invariably associated with gallstones.

Clinical Features

Patient may be asymptomatic or symptomatic. Patient may present with constant or an excruciating *colicky* pain. Biliary colic and jaundice occur due to obstruction of the biliary system.

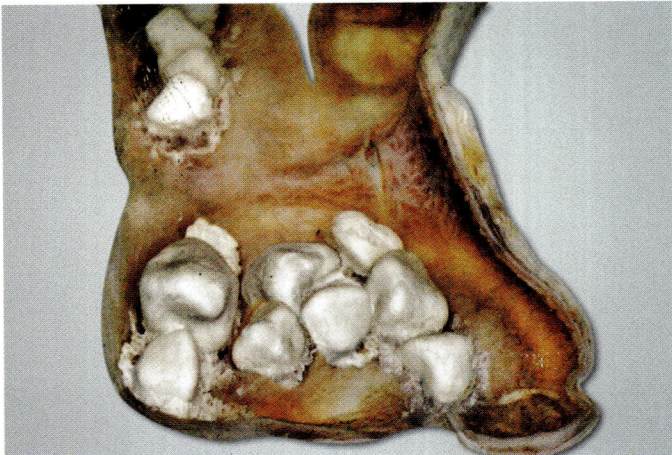

Fig. 21.96: Gallstones. Cut opened specimen of gallbladder shows multiple faceted white-colored stones. Wall of the gallbladder is thickened.

Infection of static bile causes cholangitis and liver abscess. There is increased risk in development of gallbladder carcinoma in cholelithiasis.

Gross Morphology

Gallbladder is thickened by fibrosis exhibiting gray white in color. The wall is thickened from 2 mm to 1 cm depending on fibrosis.

Mucosa may be ulcerated. Gallbladder lumen may contain stones impacted in bile (Fig. 21.96).

Light Microscopy

- *Epithelium:* It shows formation of *Rokitansky-Aschoff sinuses* due to herniation of the lining mucosa into the muscle layers. Rupture of *Rokitansky-Aschoff sinuses may lead to xanthogranulomatous cholecystitis containing lipid-laden macrophages* and giant cells mimicking clear cell carcinoma. It is prone to give rise to fistulae. Muscularis mucosa is absent.
- *Muscular coat:* It is replaced by fibrosis. *Muscle bundles are hypertrophied.* All the coats are infiltrated by chronic inflammatory cells composed of *lymphocytes, macrophages* and *plasma cells. Perimuscular fibrosis* is evident.
- *Serous coat:* It shows fibrosis. The wall may be markedly thickened, porcelain gallbladder occurs due to calcification. Light microscopy of chronic cholecystitis is shown in Fig. 21.97.

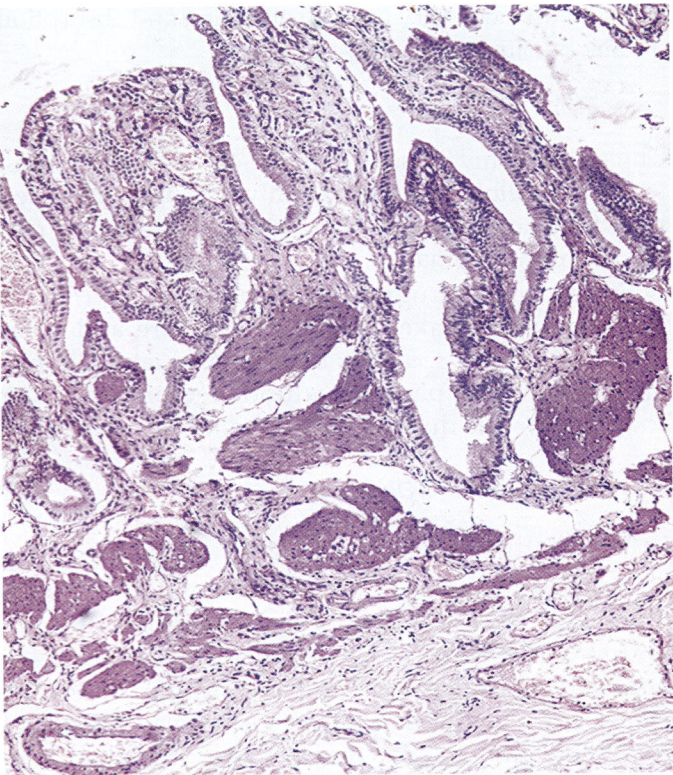

Fig. 21.97: Chronic cholecystitis. It is almost always seen in association with gallstones, though precipitation of bile alone may be sufficient to produce inflammation. There may not be a history of bouts of acute cholecystitis. It shows ulceration of mucosa formation of Rokitansky-Aschoff sinuses due to herniation of the lining mucosa into the muscle layers. There is presence of perimuscular fibrosis (100X).

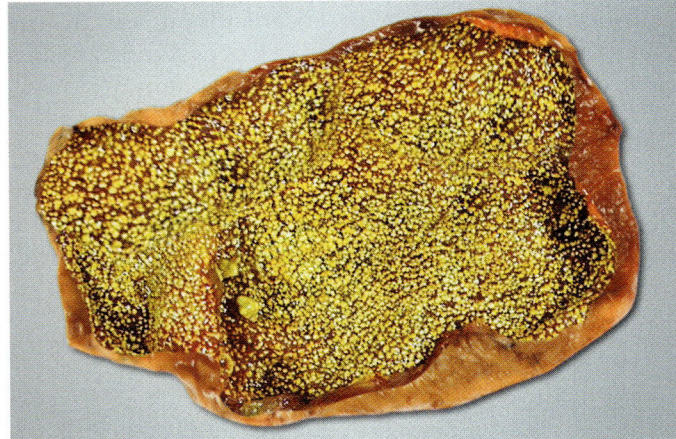

Fig. 21.98: Strawberry (cholesterolosis) gallbladder. Mucosal surface of cut opened gallbladder shows yellow speckled appearance.

CHOLESTEROLOSIS (STRAWBERRY GALLBLADDER)

Cholesterolosis of gallbladder is characterized by yellow mucosal speckled appearance known as *strawberry gallbladder.* Gross morphology of cholesterolosis is shown in Fig. 21.98.

Light Microscopy

- Histological examination shows presence of cholesterol laden macrophages in the lamina proria of the gallbladder mucosa.

Liver, Gallbladder and Exocrine Pancreas

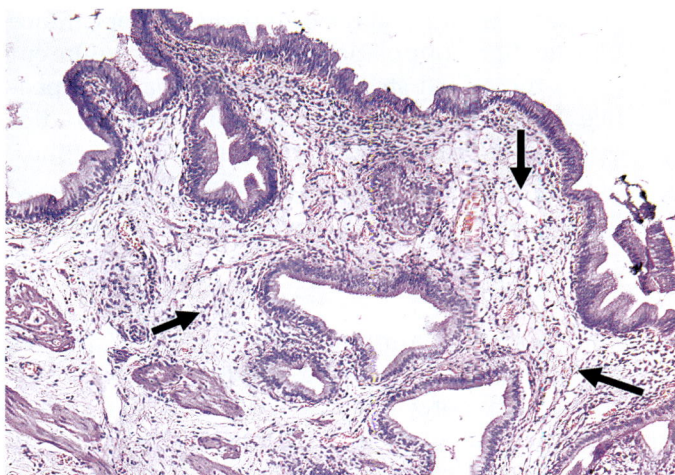

Fig. 21.99: Cholesterolosis (strawberry) gallbladder. Mucosa shows presence of cholesterol laden foamy macrophages in the lamina propria of the gallbladder mucosa (arrows).

- There is no association with inflammatory changes or presence of gallstones.
- This finding is incidental without clinical significance (Fig. 21.99).

MUCOCELE OF GALLBLADDER

Mucocele of gallbladder occurs as a result of sterile long-standing obstruction of the cystic duct by a gallstone. The gallbladder is distended with clear, mucus, watery fluid results to flattening of mucosa and thinning of wall. There is absence of bile in lumen and inflammatory changes in the wall. Mucocele of gallbladder is shown in Fig. 21.100.

During surgical removal, thin wall of gallbladder demands to avoid spillage of mucus into the peritoneal cavity, so that *pseudomyxoma peritonei* is prevented. Pseudomyxoma peritonei becomes seeded with mucus-producing epithelial cells and the cavity fills with mucus.

Complications

Mucocele of gallbladder may cause cholangitis, perforation with local abscess, diffuse peritonitis, cholecyst enteric fistula and multiorgan failure.

CHOLEDOCHAL CYST

Choledochal cyst is a form of fibropolycystic disease leading to dilatation of the common bile duct assuming fusiform or spherical shape. Entire lesion should be excised and submitted for histopathological examination to exclude biliary intrahepatic neoplasm or adenocarcinoma.

CHOLELITHIASIS (GALLSTONE DISEASE)

Gallstone disease is a major cause of morbidity and mortality throughout the world. It has a higher incidence in women and is often associated with obesity and multiple pregnancies. Patients with gallstones are most often asymptomatic. Fatty food intolerance is characteristic. It produces diverse histopathological changes in gallbladder mucosa, namely acute inflammation, chronic inflammation, granulomatous inflammation, hyperplasia, cholesterolosis, dysplasia and carcinoma.

COMPOSITION OF BILE JUICE

The liver synthesizes bile continuously, and enters the gallbladder via hepatic ducts. The gallbladder concentrates and stores it until the duodenum transmits signals to gallbladder to release bile into the duodenum for digestion of fat. Bile juice consists of cholesterol, bile salts, bile acids, phospholipids, proteins, bilirubin, sodium bicarbonate and water. Normal bile solutes are shown in Fig. 21.101 and Table 21.67.

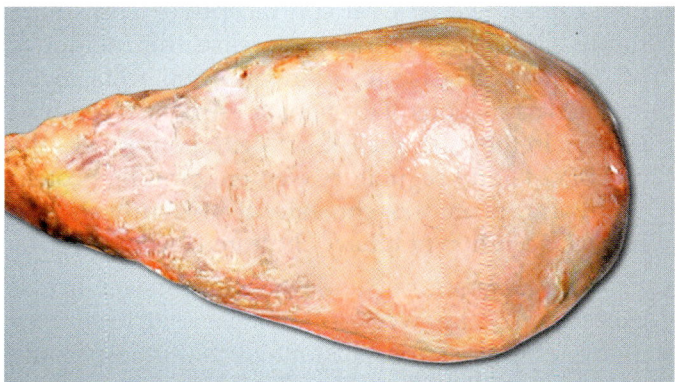

Fig. 21.100: Mucocele of gallbladder. It is filled with mucus watery fluid.

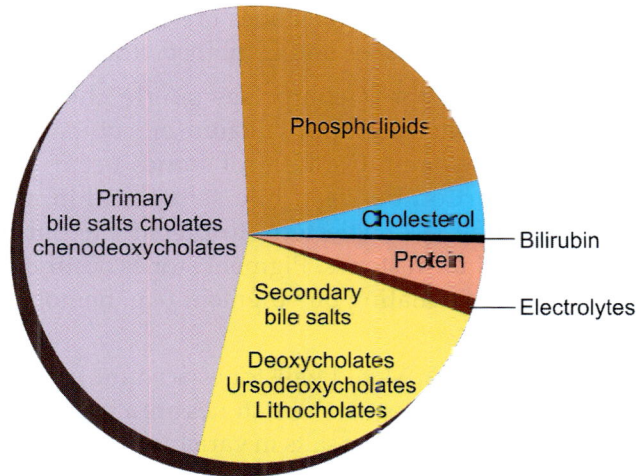

Fig. 21.101: Components of bile.

Table 21.67: Bile solutes

Bile solute	% of solute present in bile solute
Water	97%
Bile salts (cholic acid, chenodeoxycholic acid and deoxycholic acid)	67%
Phospholipids (mainly lecithin)	22%
Protein	4.5%
Cholesterol	4%
Bilirubin	0.3%
Sodium bicarbonate	Present in small fraction

- *Cholesterol:* Bile contains 4% of cholesterol. It is kept soluble by bile salts and lecithin.
- *Bile salts/acids (cholic acid/chenodeoxycholic acid):* Bile salts are derived from the catabolism of cholesterol. These are linked with taurine or glycine to form the bile salts. These constitute 67% of bile. These are mostly reabsorbed in terminal ileum (enterohepatic circulation).
- *Phospholipids (mainly lecithin):* It increases solubility of cholesterol.
- *Proteins:* Bile contains 4.5% of proteins.
- *Bilirubin:* It is a by-product of haem degradation.
- *Inorganic salt (sodium bicarbonate):* It keeps bile alkaline to neutralize gastric acid in duodenum.
- *Water:* Bile contains 97% of water.

CATEGORIES OF GALLSTONES

Vast majority of gallbladder stones are classified into three groups: cholesterol stones (20%), pigment stones (5%) and mixed stones (75%). Depending on chemical constituents in calculus, gallstones are of three types: pure stones, mixed stones and combined stones.

- *Pure gall calculus:* It comprises single chemical constituent (cholesterol or calcium bilirubinate or calcium carbonate). Cholesterol stones occur due to disproportion between bile salts/lecithin and cholesterol allows cholesterol to precipitate out of solution and form stones. Pigment stones occur due to excess of circulating bile pigment (e.g. hemolytic anemia).
- *Mixed gall calculi:* Mixed gallstones account for 85% of all gallstones. Most of these stones are a mixture of cholesterol and calcium salts in variable proportions. These stones have similar pathophysiology as cholesterol stones.

These are multiple and faceted external appearance owing to tight opposition with one other. On cut section, the mixed stones exhibit laminated appearance. Mixed stones can often be visualized on radiograph due to presence of calcium salts in the stones.

- *Combined gallstones:* These are composed of mixture of salts forming a nucleus surrounded by a shell.

RISK FACTORS

Gallstone disease is a multifactorial disease. Changes in composition of bile during synthesis in liver and absorptive ability of gallbladder epithelial lining participate in the pathogenesis of gallbladder. Risk factors of gallstones are described as under:

- *Race:* Native Americans or Mexican Americans have the highest incidence of gallstones of any specific racial groups.
- *Gender:* Women most common develop gallstones than men especially during the fertile years.
- *Obesity:* Obesity, particularly abdominal or centripetal obesity, is a well-established risk factor for gallstone disease. Obesity is associated with an increased activity of the rate-limiting step in cholesterol synthesis, the hepatic enzyme, 3-hydroxyl-3-methyl-glutaryl co-enzyme A (HMG-CoA) reductase, leading to increased cholesterol synthesis in the liver, its secretion into bile and storage in the gallbladder.
- *Female sex hormones:* During pregnancy, female sex hormones are endogenously raised; these adversely influence hepatic bile secretion. Estrogen increases amount of cholesterol in bile and decreases gallbladder activity. These changes allow the cholesterol to crystallize in gallbladder. Estrogen levels may be related to contraceptive pills, or hormone replacement therapy. Progesterone acts by reducing bile salt secretion and impairing gallbladder emptying leading to stasis.
- *Oral contraceptives:* Oral contraceptives with three months estrogen therapy increase the incidence of gallstone disease in younger women. Estrogen augments functions of the hepatic estrogen receptor-α (ER-α). In the liver, the ER-α receptor stimulates the SREBP-2 (sterol regulatory element binding protein pathway), promotes cholesterol biosynthesis and hepatic secretion of biliary cholesterol.
- *Rapid weight loss:* Low caloric diet or rapid weight loss exceeding 1.5 kg/week following bariatric surgery increases the risk for gallstone formation especially during the first 6 weeks. These factors reduce gallbladder emptying, so bile becomes concentrated and cholesterol precipitates out into stones.

- *History of gallstones:* People who have gallstones in the past are more likely to develop gallstones in future.
- *Role of liver:* Obesity and estrogen imbalance especially in women (40 years) causes liver to synthesize bile that is high in cholesterol or lacking proper concentration of bile salts. When the gallbladder concentrates this bile, inflammation may occur. Excessive reabsorption of water and bile salts makes the bile less soluble.
- *Diabetes mellitus:* Diabetics have high levels of triglycerides, which increase the risk of gallstones.
- *Liver disease:* Advanced cirrhosis is a well-established risk factor for gall pigmented stones. It is related to altered pigment secretion, abnormal gallbladder motility and/or increased estrogen levels.
- *Crohn's disease:* There is increased risk of development of gallstones in patients with Crohn's disease. Terminal ileum is not able to transport bile acids, so these enter the colon. Biological detergents solubilize unconjugated bilirubin resulting in absorption and return to the liver. The liver then secretes excessive pigment that subsequently precipitates as gallstones. Fasting in Crohn's disease or altered bacterial colonic flora may enhance the deconjugation of bilirubin, which is passively absorbed resulting in increased enterohepatic cycling of the bile pigment.
- *Cystic fibrosis:* Similar to ileal Crohn's disease, cystic fibrosis is associated with bile acid malabsorption due to its binding to undigested dietary nutrients. Gallstone prevalence in cystic fibrosis is increased by 10 to 30%.
- *Sickle cell disease:* In sickle cell disease, chronic hemolysis leads to excessive bilirubin excretion with the formation of black pigment stones composed of calcium bilirubinate.
- *Cholesterol lowering drugs:* The drugs that are designed to lower blood cholesterol help to concentrate cholesterol in the gallbladder, increasing the risk of forming stones.
- *Octreotide drug:* It is a long-acting analogue of somatostatin that inhibits cholecystokinin release, resulting in decreased motility of gallbladder and small intestine. Bile stasis enhances synthesis of deoxycholic acid (bile acid) and cholesterol resulting in precipitation and crystallization of cholesterol.
- *Thiazide diuretics:* Thiazide treatment may increase biliary cholesterol saturation leading to gallstones formation.

PATHOGENESIS

Bile salts, cholesterol and lecithin are present in the form of mixed micelles and vesicles in gallbladder.

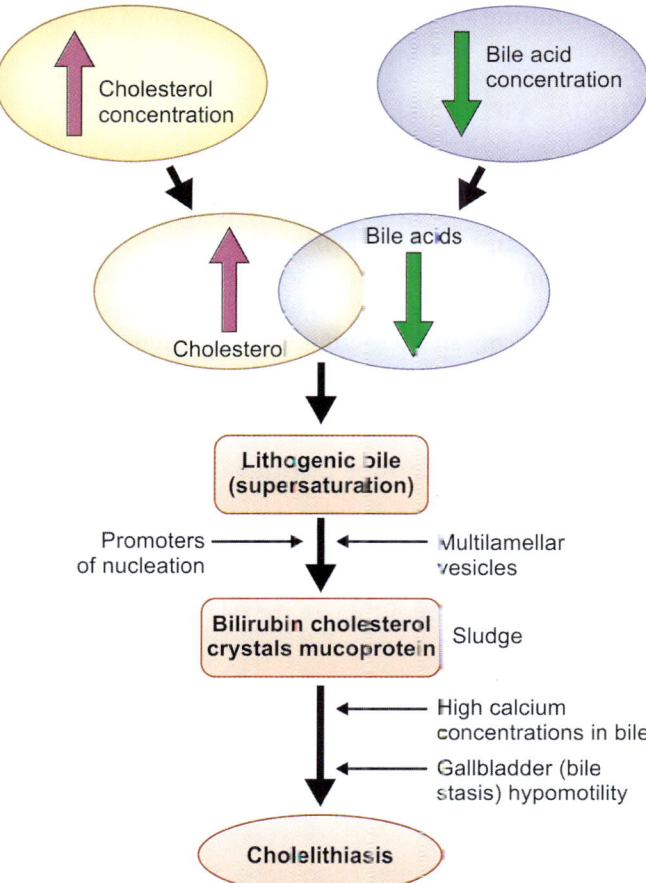

Fig. 21.102: Pathogenesis of gallstone formation.

Pathological changes in gallbladder epithelium may play an important role in the process of gallstone formation. *Pathogenesis of gallstone formation* is shown in Fig. 21.102.

Formation of Multilamellar Vesicles

Supersaturation of these constituents (bile salts, cholesterol and lecithin) form multilamellar vesicles. The amount of cholesterol in the bile is supposed to increase with age. This is caused by dyslipoproteinemia that results in a linear increase in cholesterol excretion into the bile and by the reduced synthesis of bile acids due to the dropped activity of the enzyme cholesterol 7α-hydroxylase.

Nucleation

Gallbladder hypomotility and cholesterol nucleation convert multilamellar vesicles to cholesterol monohydrate filaments, which are arranged in plates.

Promotion

Promoters (mucus hypersecretion, gallbladder hypomotility, calcium salts) act on cholesterol monohydrate plate resulting in accretion (nucleation) and formation of cholesterol stones.

CLINICAL ASPECTS

Asymptomatic/Silent Gallstones

Most patients are unaware of gallstone disease and remain asymptomatic for life. They never experience biliary pain or complications such as acute cholecystitis, cholangitis, or pancreatitis. Hence, most gallstones are clinically *silent*, an incidental finding often discovered during abdominal ultrasound being performed for another reason.

Symptomatic Gallstones Disease

Gallstones can produce a variety of symptoms depending on their anatomical site. These patients require surgical cholecystectomy. Most complications associated with cholelithiasis are related to obstruction of the biliary tree.

Additional rare complications include empyema of the gallbladder, perforation, fistula formation, bile peritonitis, and gallstone ileus. In most cases, gallstones are associated with chronic cholecystitis. Natural history of gallstone disease is shown in Table 21.68.

Table 21.68: Natural history of gallstone disease

Symptom	% of patients
Asymptomatic	40%
Cholangitis	20%
Jaundice	20%
Biliary colic	15%
Pancreatitis	5%

Functional (Acalculus) Gallbladder Disease

Biliary pain in acalculus gallbladder seemingly results from increased intraluminal pressure, as the gallbladder contracts against an obstructed outlet. Biliary colic occurs due to lack of coordination between gallbladder contraction and sphincter of Oddi relaxation, or visceral hypersensitivity.

A clue to its existence is impaired gallbladder emptying, reliably estimated by cholecystokinin-cholescintigraphy. Ultrasonography shows empty gallbladder lacking gallstone disease.

Patient presents with acute abdominal pain in the right upper quadrant that may radiate to the back, between the shoulders, or to the front of the chest, colic, nausea and vomiting, chill, low-grade fever, jaundice, belching, flatulence, indigestion and light-headedness.

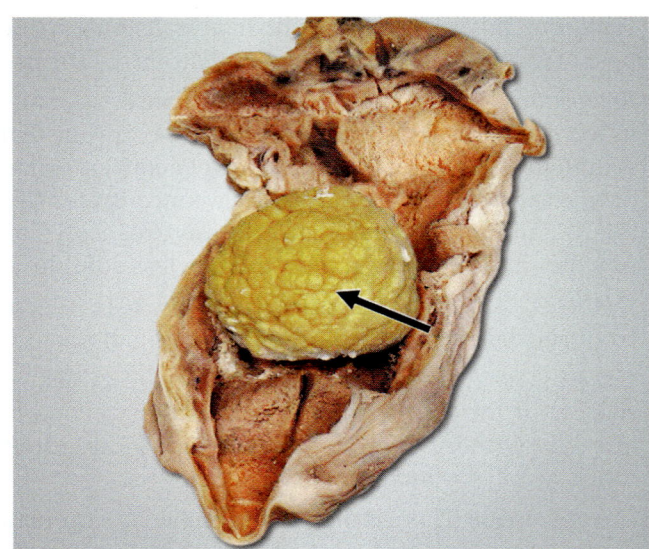

Fig. 21.103: Cholesterol stones. Gallbladder shows solitary cholesterol stone (arrow).

CHOLESTEROL GALLSTONES

More than 75% of gallstones contain significant amount of cholesterol. Cholesterol stones are *round or faceted, yellow to tan*, and may be *single or multiple*. These stones are *too large to enter the cystic duct or the common bile duct*. Cholesterol stones are *radiolucent* and not demonstrated on radiograph. But these are *demonstrated by ultrasonography* (Fig. 21.103).

Composition

- *Cholesterol stone:* Gallstone contains 90% of cholesterol. It is most often single, large stone >2.5 cm, pale or white in color. It has soft consistency and can be cut easily. Cut surface has radiating structure made up of cholesterol crystals.
- *Mixed stones:* Gallstones contain 50% of cholesterol and rest mucoproteins, calcium and bilirubin. These are usually multiple but smaller than pure cholesterol stones measuring 0.5–2.5 in diameter. Mixed gallstones account for 85% of all gallstones. These exhibit characteristic *faceted appearance*.

Predisposing Factors

During their reproductive years, women are up to three times more likely to develop cholesterol gallstones than men. Risk factors for cholesterol stones include female sex, diabetes mellitus, pregnancy, estrogen therapy, hyperlipidemia, bile stasis and inborn disorders of bile acid metabolism.

In obese women, cholesterol secretion by the liver is increased. Impaired gallbladder motor function is another risk factor that leads to gallstone formation. In this case, stasis permits the formation of biliary sludge, which then progresses to macroscopic stones. These stones are more prevalent in Americans.

Pathogenesis

Supersaturation of cholesterol, hypomotility of gallbladder and mucins in gallbladder participate in the pathogenesis of cholesterol stones.

- *Supersaturation of cholesterol:* If the bile juice contains excess cholesterol or is deficient in bile acids, it becomes supersaturated with cholesterol and precipitates to form stones (lithogenic bile). Cholesterol nucleation is accelerated in bile and mucous hypersecretion in the gallbladder.
- *Hypomotility:* Gallbladder motility is decreased in pregnancy, rapid weight loss and long-term starvation. Gene polymorphisms increase the rate of cholelithiasis due to impaired gallbladder motility.
- *Mucins in gallbladder:* Mucin-glycoprotein gel is one of the most important and identified pronucleators. Secretory mucins are gel-forming and may increase bile viscosity.

An increased expression of gel-forming mucins such as MUC5AC and MUC2 has been associated with hepatobiliary gallstones, indicating a gene-gene interaction that might affect the accumulation of mucin gel and cholesterol gallstones formation. Pathophysiology of cholesterol stones is shown in Fig. 21.104.

PIGMENT GALLSTONES

Pigment gallstones occur in 10% of Western population. These are more common in Asian population. Precipitation of excess insoluble unconjugated bilirubin results in the formation of pigment stones.

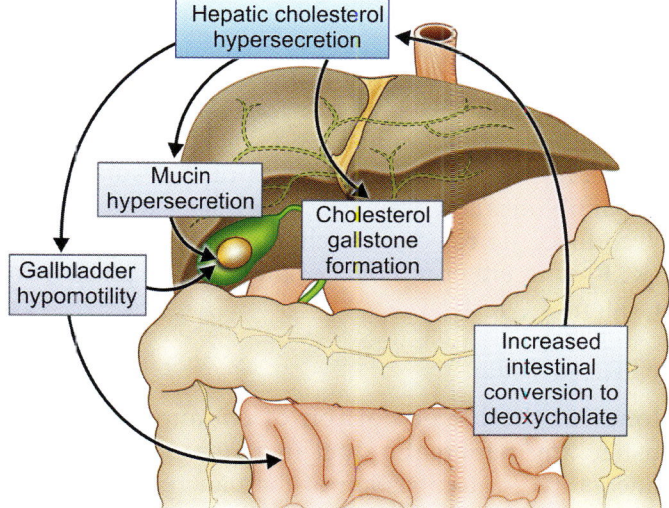

Fig. 21.104: Cholesterol stone formed by hypersecretion leading to formation of cholesterol stone.

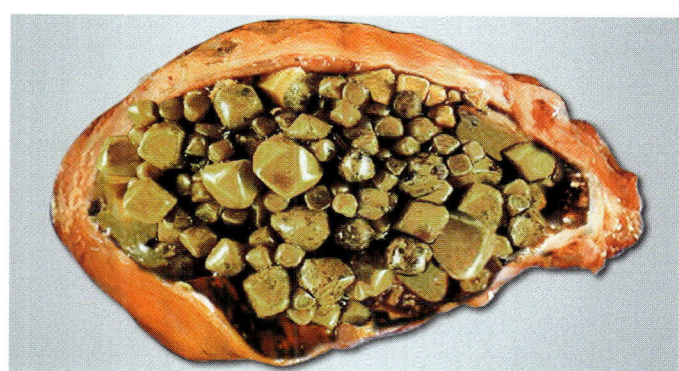

Fig. 21.105: Pigmented stones. Gallbladder shows multiple faceted yellow tan gallstones. Stone may exit via the cystic duct or common bile duct and obstruct bile flow. It may obstruct at the ampulla of Vater and produce a pancreatitis. Biliary tract obstruction leads to jaundice with increased total and direct bilirubin in serum.

These are most often associated with hemolytic anemia and bacterial infection. *Pigmented stones in gallbladder showing multiple faceted yellow tan gallstones are shown in Fig. 21.105.*

Categories

Pigment stones are classified into two main categories.

- *Black pigment gallstones:* These stones are commonest and associated with hemolysis and cirrhosis. These are confined to the gallbladder. Bile is sterile. These stones consist of large amounts of polymerized degradation product of oxidized bilirubin.
- *Brown pigment gallstones:* These stones contain large amount of calcium bilirubinate. These have soft consistency. Cut surface shows laminated appearance. These are formed in either gallbladder or bile ducts. The bile is most often infected.

Predisposing Factors

There is increased frequency in Crohn's disease, ileal resection or bypass, cystic fibrosis with pancreatic insufficiency. Pigment stones are more common in Asian than Western population.

Pathogenesis

Chronic intravascular hemolysis is the cause of pigment stones.

> **Gross Morphology**
> - Bile pigment stones are usually multiple measuring <1.5 cm in diameter found in sterile bile.
> - These are composed of calcium salts of unconjugated bilirubin (calcium bilirubinate), mucin glycoprotein, less cholesterol monohydrate crystals.

Table 21.69: Differences between various types of gallstones

Parameters	Cholesterol gallstones	Black pigment stones	Brown pigment stones	Biliary sludge (microlithiasis)
Composition	Cholesterol (50–100%)	Calcium bilirubinate polymer	Unconjugated bilirubin, calcium soap of fatty acids, cholesterol and mucin	Pigment (calcium bilirubinate) cholesterol microcrystals and mucin
Location	Gallbladder ± common bile duct	Gallbladder ± common bile duct	Bile ducts	Gallbladder
Detection	Ultrasound	Ultrasound	Cholangiography	Abdominal or endoscopic ultrasonography
Clinical association	Family history (genetic), obesity, female sex and aging (excessive cholesterol secretion)	Increased or altered bilirubin excretion in hemolysis, cirrhosis, cystic fibrosis, Crohn's disease and advanced age (excessive bilirubin excretion)	Infection, inflammation and infestation (stasis and strictures)	Fasting total parenteral nutrition (TPN) and pregnancy

- These are radiopaque in 50 to 75% cases (imaging technique). Differences between various types of gallstones are shown in Table 21.69.

COMPLICATIONS

Most common complications of cholelithiasis include severe biliary colic (stone in cystic duct), obstructive jaundice (common bile duct obstruction), ascending cholangitis and acute pancreatitis. Less common complications are acute cholecystitis, empyema, perforation in gallbladder, gallstone ileus, porcelain gallbladder, mucocele gallbladder, risk of squamous cell carcinoma, extension of inflammation in the biliary tree, *Mirizzi's syndrome* and *Bouveret's syndrome*.

SEVERE BILIARY COLIC

If a stone lodges in the cystic duct, the gallbladder contracts but cannot empty. Passage of stones into the cystic duct often causes severe biliary colic. Fat entering the duodenum causes the intestinal mucosa to secrete the hormone cholecystokinin, which stimulates the gallbladder to contract and empty.

Clinical Features

Patient presents with sudden pain in right upper quadrant that may radiate to scapular region, lasts for 2–4 hours following ingestion of fatty meals, alcohol, and caffeine. It is associated with nausea and vomiting.

> **Light Microscopy**
> Mild inflammatory change of the gallbladder wall can occur with biliary colic; with recurrent episodes leading to chronic cholecystitis.

OBSTRUCTIVE JAUNDICE

Lodgement of stones in the common bile duct leads to obstructive jaundice, cholangitis, and acute pancreatitis. Biliary narrowing and swelling of the tissue around the stone can also cause irritation and inflammation of the common bile duct.

Clinical Features

Patient presents with obstructive jaundice with conjugated hyperbilirubinemia, hypercholesterolemia, and increased alkaline phosphatase.

ASCENDING CHOLANGITIS

Infection in the common bile duct from obstruction is common and serious. It results from secondary bacterial infection facilitated by obstructed bile flow as a result of gallstone in common bile duct.

Clinical Features

Patient presents with *Charcot's triad* of fever, jaundice and right upper abdominal pain. This potentially life-threatening complication requires urgent supportive care, antibiotics and drainage of the biliary tree, usually by endoscopic retrograde cholangiopancreatogram (ERCP) with either removal of the stone or placement of a stent.

ACUTE PANCREATITIS

Stones in the lower portion of common bile duct obstructing pancreatic duct increases risk of acute pancreatitis. Autodigestion of the pancreas occurs by the lipase enzyme, which normally secretes into the duodenum. These lipids then form soaps (saponification) with calcium, leading to hypocalcemia.

Clinical Features

Patient presents with rapid onset of upper abdominal pain and vomiting. Gallstone pancreatitis can be a life-threatening disease and requires correction of hypovolemia, antibiotics and the early consideration of endoscopic sphincterotomy via ERCP in severe cases.

ACUTE CHOLECYSTITIS

Acute cholecystitis occurs due to complete obstruction of the cystic duct by a gallstone in 95% of gallstone disease. Acalculus cholecystitis occurs in remainder 5% of cases.

The most serious complication of acute cholecystitis is infection, which develops in about 20% of cases. It is extremely dangerous and life-threatening if it spreads to other parts of the body leading to septicemia and surgery is often required.

Untreated cases of acute cholecystitis may result in formation of abscesses, gangrene and necrosis. These are encountered in elderly diabetic patients.

EMPYEMA GALLBLADDER

Empyema gallbladder is characterized by accumulation of pus seen in 2–3% of patients with acute cholecystitis.

Acute inflammation of gallbladder causes edema, vascular compromise and superadded infection resulting in gallbladder empyema (a pus-filled gallbladder). Necrosis of gallbladder results in perforation, abscess formation and peritonitis.

Clinical Features

Patient usually experiences severe abdominal pain for more than 7 days.

Treatment

Acute cholecystitis is initially treated with intravenous fluids and antibiotics which lead to a resolution of the acute inflammation in 70–80% of patients.

PERFORATED GALLBLADDER

An estimated 10% of acute cholecystitis results in a perforated gallbladder, which is a life-threatening condition. Perforation of the gallbladder is most common in people with diabetes.

The risk also increases with a condition called emphysematous cholecystitis, due to infection with gas forming bacteria (*E. coli* and *Clostridium welchii*).

Once the gallbladder has perforated, pain may temporarily decrease. This is a dangerous and misleading sign, because peritonitis develops afterward.

GALLSTONE ILEUS

In some cases of gallstone disease, gallstone erodes through the gallbladder into the adjacent small bowel forming cholecystenteric fistula. Gallbladder stone enters ileum through the fistulous tract and blocks the intestine known as *gallstone ileus*.

It can be very serious and requires immediate surgery. It primarily occurs in patients over age 65, and can sometimes be fatal.

RISK OF SQUAMOUS CELL CARCINOMA

It most often arises in the setting of chronic inflammation, with most patients (75%) having pre-existing gallstones and cholecystitis. The presence of gallstones increases the risk of gallbladder squamous cell carcinoma by 4 to 5 folds.

Pathology

Chronic irritation of gallbladder induced by gallstones leads to squamous metaplasia of columnar mucosa leading to squamous cell carcinoma (exophytic or infiltrative growth).

Clinical Features

Patient developing squamous cell carcinoma is most often asymptomatic until the disease has reached an advanced stage. Patient presents with weight loss, anemia, recurrent vomiting and abdominal lump.

PORCELAIN GALLBLADDER

Gallbladder is referred to as porcelain when their walls become calcified (due to calcium deposits) appears like porcelain on radiograph. It has been associated with a high risk for cancer. This condition may develop from a chronic inflammatory reaction that may actually be responsible for the cancer risk.

MUCOCELE OF GALLBLADDER

Gallbladder is distended with mucus secondary to sterile long-standing obstruction of the cystic duct by a gallstone. During surgical removal, thin wall of gallbladder demands to avoid spillage of mucus into the peritoneal cavity, so that *pseudomyxoma peritonei* is prevented. Pseudomyxoma peritonei becomes seeded with mucus-producing epithelial cells and the cavity fills with mucus.

> **Gross Morphology**
>
> Gallbladder is distended with clear, mucus and watery fluid.

> **Light Microscopy**
> - Accumulation of clear, mucus and watery fluid in gallbladder leads to flattening of mucosa and thinning of wall.
> - There is absence of bile in lumen and inflammatory changes in the wall.

Complications

Mucocele may cause cholangitis, perforation with local abscess, diffuse peritonitis, cholecyst enteric fistula and multiorgan failure.

EXTENDING INFLAMMATION IN BILIARY TREE

Inflammation can progress up the biliary tree into any of the bile ducts. This causes scar tissue, fluid accumulation, cirrhosis, portal hypertension, and bleeding.

MIRIZZI'S SYNDROME

Impaction of gallstones in the gallbladder neck (*Hartmann's pouch*) can lead to compression of the common hepatic duct producing jaundice, which is termed Mirizzi's syndrome. It is rare presentation of gallstone disease. It may be complicated by fistula formation (cholecystocholedochal fistula), which usually requires surgical repair.

BOUVERET'S SYNDROME

Gallstones can rarely erode through the gallbladder wall and stomach resulting in cholecystogastric fistula formation. Gallstone impaction in the stomach or duodenum leads to gastric outlet obstruction; known as *Bouveret's syndrome*.

Differential diagnosis of pain in right upper quadrant includes gallbladder disease (and its related complications), gastritis/duodenitis, peptic ulcer disease/perforated peptic ulcer, acute pancreatitis, right lower lobe pneumonia and myocardial infarction (Table 21.70).

LABORATORY DIAGNOSIS

Laboratory investigations carried out in diagnosing gallbladder disease include complete hemogram, blood biochemistry and imaging techniques. Approximately 10% gallstones are radiopaque.

Ultrasonography

Ultrasonography is the first line investigation in gallbladder disease for diagnosing cholelithiasis. Dilatation of biliary tree calibre suggests stone in common bile duct (normal CBD <8 mm). Thickening of wall of gallbladder suggests chronic cholecystitis.

Table 21.70: Differential diagnosis of pain in right upper quadrant

Pathological entity	Clinical history	Clinical examination	Laboratory investigations
Biliary colic	Intermittent pain (minutes to hours) in right upper quadrant/radiating to back and right shoulder	Tenderness in right upper quadrant, afebrile and no peritonism	LFT, CRP and WBCs count normal
Acute cholecystitis	Constant pain in right upper quadrant, radiating to back and right shoulder	Tenderness in right upper quadrant, Murphy's sign and febrile	CRP and WBCs raised, LFT normal or mild elevation
Empyema	Constant pain in right upper quadrant, radiating to back or right shoulder	Tenderness in right upper quadrant, peritonism, Murphy's sign +ve, pyrexia, more septic than acute cholecystitis	WBCs and CRP raised, LFT normal or mild elevation
Obstructive jaundice	Yellow discoloration of eyes, passage of pale stool and dark urine, painless or mild pain in right upper quadrant	Jaundice, non-tender right upper quadrant, no peritonism, afebrile, Murphy's sign negative	WBCs and CRP normal, LFT (serum bilirubin and alkaline phosphatase raised)
Ascending cholangitis	Beck's triad (pain in right upper quadrant, jaundice and rigors)	Jaundice, tenderness in right upper quadrant, peritonism, spiking high pyrexia, and may develop septic shock	WBCs and CRP normal, LFT (serum bilirubin and alkaline phosphatase raised)
Acute pancreatitis	Severe constant pain upper abdominal pain, radiating to back and profuse vomiting	Tenderness in right upper abdomen or generalized peritonism and afebrile	WBCs and CRP raised, LFT normal, serum amylase raised and DIC (complication)

Magnetic Resonance Cholangiopancreatography (MRCP)

It is noninvasive diagnostic tool much more accurate than ultrasonography. It visualizes biliary tree accurately. It is used to look for biliary dilatation and any stones in biliary tree.

Endoscopic Retrograde Cholangiography (ERCP)

This invasive technique has diagnostic and therapeutic utility in biliary obstruction. It visualizes biliary tree dilatation and stones in biliary tree.

Stones can be extracted to unobstruct the biliary tree and perform sphincterotomy. There is increased risk of development of pancreatitis and duodenal perforation.

Percutaneous Transhepatic Cholangiography (PTC)

This invasive technique is used to unobstruct biliary tree when ERCP has failed. It has higher complication rate than ERCP.

CT Scan

It is not the first line investigation used if suspicion of gallbladder empyema, gangrene, or perforation and in acute pancreatitis.

COMMON NEOPLASMS AND PRECURSOR LESIONS OF GALLBLADDER

Benign tumors of the gallbladder are rare. The most common primary tumor of the gallbladder is adenocarcinoma, which is often associated with gallstones. Carcinoma of the extrahepatic biliary ducts and the ampulla of Vater is less common than carcinoma of the gallbladder. WHO histological classification of gallbladder and extrahepatic bile duct tumors is shown in Table 21.71.

Clinical Features

Patient suffering from adenocarcinoma gallbladder presents with progressive, relentless obstructive jaundice and palpable gallbladder.

Tumor obstructing the common bile duct leads to an enlarged, distended gallbladder. On the other hand, stone obstructing common bile duct does not cause enlarged gallbladder (*Courvoisier sign*).

Gallbladder carcinoma is almost always adenocarcinoma.

ADENOMA GALLBLADDER

Adenoma of gallbladder is a rare benign solitary polypoidal lesion. Small adenoma is low malignant potential. Large adenoma may harbor foci of high grade BilIN3 and invasive carcinoma. Histological examination of the lesion shows tubular or papillary or tubulopapillary appearance.

BILIARY INTRAEPITHELIAL NEOPLASIA

Biliary intraepithelial neoplasia may be grades 1, 2 or 3. Grade 3 intraepithelial neoplasia may be associated with invasive carcinoma. Therefore, thorough sampling of the cystic duct and margins of the lesion should be carried out to exclude malignancy. Cholecystectomy

Table 21.71: WHO histological classification of gallbladder and extrahepatic bile ducts

Categories	Neoplastic lesions
Premalignant epithelial lesions	*Adenoma:* Tubular, papillary and tubulopapillary
	Biliary intraepithelial neoplasia (BilIN): Grades 1, 2 and 3
	Intracystic (gallbladder) or intraductal (bile ducts) papillary neoplasms: Low, intermediate or high grade
	Mucinous neoplasms: Low, intermediate or high grade
Malignant epithelial neoplasms	Adenocarcinoma (biliary, gastric foveola, intestinal, clear cell and signet ring cell types), adenosquamous carcinoma, squamous cell carcinoma and undifferentiated carcinoma
Neuroendocrine neoplasms	Neuroendocrine tumor (NET G1 and NET G2), neuroendocrine carcinomas (small and large cell), mixed adenoneuroendocrine carcinoma, tubular carcinoid and goblet cell carcinoid
Mesenchymal tumors	Granular cell tumor, leiomyoma, leiomyosarcoma, Kaposi's sarcoma and rhabdomyosarcoma
Lymphoid cells	Lymphomas
Secondary tumors	Metastases from various organs

is curative. Grade 3 intraepithelial neoplasia shows overexpression of p53.

ADENOCARCINOMA GALLBLADDER

Gallbladder carcinoma (GBC) can develop in obese women, cholelithiasis, porcelain gallbladder and primary sclerosing cholangitis. The prognosis with adenocarcinoma of the gallbladder is usually poor, because they have often invaded and metastasized by the time they are discovered.

Pathogenesis

- *Metaplasia:* Metaplasia of gallbladder mucosa occurs as a result of irritation by *solitary gallstone*. It is widely accepted that metaplastic epithelium is more susceptible to *malignant transformation*.
- *Low grade dysplasia:* It occurs in 40% and high grade in 16% of cases with cholelithiasis. Carcinoma *in situ* has been observed in 3.5% of *cholelithiasis specimens*. The great majority of *in situ* carcinoma is grossly indistinguishable from cholecystitis and can easily be overlooked on microscopic examination. Dysplasia, carcinoma *in situ* and invasive carcinoma of gallbladder have been associated with multiple stones.

Molecular Genetics

Changes of the E-cadherin/β-catenin complex during cell to cell interactions result in the loss of cell adhesion and may account for the ability of cancer cells to metastasize.

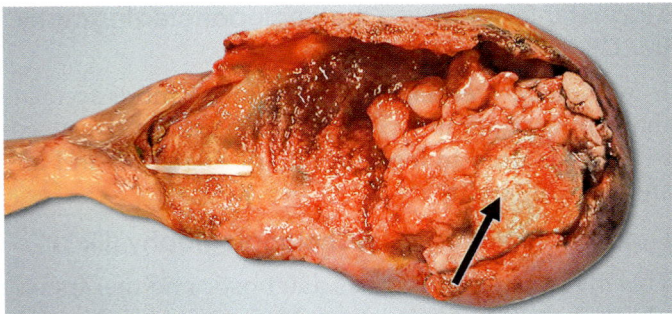

Fig. 21.106: Gallbladder carcinoma shows fungating growth (arrow).

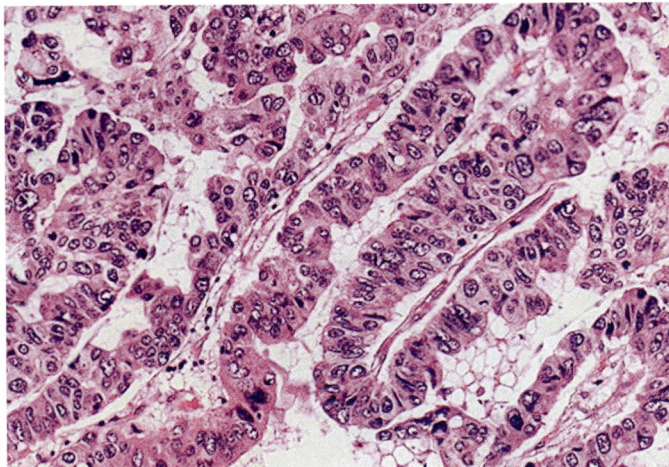

Fig. 21.107: Gallbladder adenocarcinoma. It is composed of columnar cells forming glandular and papillary structures. The prognosis with adenocarcinoma of the gallbladder is usually poor, because they have often invaded and metastasized by the time they are discovered (400X).

Gross Morphology

The thickness of the gallbladder wall may be normal or minimally thickened. Mucosal induration mimics chronic cholecystitis. The mucosa may appear granular, slightly nodular or trabecular pattern in carcinoma *in situ* and invasive carcinoma. It gives support to the idea that carcinoma *in situ* grows slowly and is a precursor lesion of invasive gallbladder cancer. Gross morphology of carcinoma of gallbladder is shown in Fig. 21.106.

Light Microscopy

- *Well differentiated adenocarcinoma:* Tumor is composed of columnar cells forming glandular and papillary structures invading gallbladder wall. The mucosal surface shows massive ulceration and necrosis. Perineural invasion, and vascular emboli may be observed. Sometimes acidophilic secretion is demonstrated within the lumen. Histological features of well differentiated carcinoma of gallbladder are shown in Fig. 21.107.
- *Undifferentiated adenocarcinoma:* It shows presence of clusters of tumor cells with numerous mitoses surrounded by sclerohyaline stroma.
- *Squamous cell carcinoma:* Cholelithiasis causing squamous metaplasia of columnar epithelium leads to squamous cell carcinoma (exophytic or infiltrative growth). It comprises islands of tumor cells with keratinization and keratin pearls. In some islands of tumor cells, partial necrosis lesions and a polymorph inflammatory reaction were observed.
- *Mucin secreting adenocarcinoma:* It is composed of tumor cells arranged in glandular pattern. There is presence of abundant mucus secretion in the cells identified as *signet ring cells* and out side glands compressing clusters of malignant cells. Numerous tumor emboli in lymphatic channels predict unfavorable prognosis.

- *Papillary adenocarcinoma:* It is composed of exuberant surface proliferation forming villous structures. The tumor cells invade the gallbladder wall. There is presence perineural invasion by tumor cells. Lymphatic channels show presence of tumor emboli.

Klatskin Tumor

This slow growing tumor originates from confluence of hepatic ducts near hilum.

BILIARY ADENOCARCINOMA

Biliary adenocarcinomas may be composed of intestinal, goblet and neuroendocrine cells. Tumors are composed of intestinal type cells are most often K20 and CDX2 immunoreactive.

ADENOCARCINOMA OF EXTRAHEPATIC BILE DUCTS

Adenocarcinoma has been classified as perihilar or distal. Each of these entities has its own staging system. These tumors show thickening of the wall. Therefore, thorough sampling is required to evaluate margins and local extension.

Perihilar Adenocarcinomas

The tumors originate proximal to cystic duct. These account for 60% of adenocarcinomas.

Distal Adenocarcinomas

The tumors arise between the junction of the cystic duct and common bile duct and the ampulla of Vater. These account for 30% of adenocarcinomas. Anatomic boundaries for classification of adenocarcinomas of extrahepatic bile ducts are shown in Fig. 21.108.

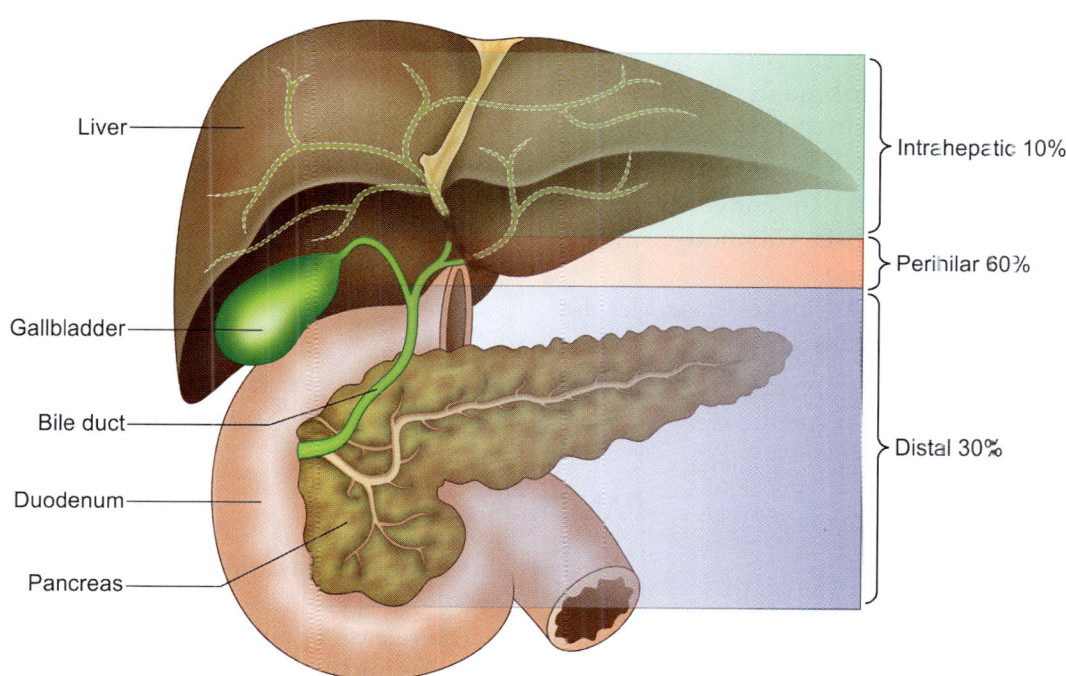

Fig. 21.108: Anatomic boundaries for classification of adenocarcinomas of extrahepatic bile ducts.

PANCREAS

OVERVIEW

ANATOMY AND PHYSIOLOGY

Pancreas is located in retroperitoneal region. It measures 15–20 cm and weighs 85–120 gm. It consists of head, neck, body and tail.

It is compound gland, i.e. exocrine and endocrine glands. Islets of Langerhans comprise three types of cells (α, β and δ cells) constituting 1–2% of pancreatic tissue.

Duct System

Exocrine pancreas has duct system. Acinar cells drain into intercalated ducts, intralobular ducts, interlobular ducts and main pancreatic duct of Wirsung and accessory duct of Santorini.

Blood Supply and Lymphatic Drainage

It receives blood supply from branch from coeliac trunk and superior mesenteric artery. Lymphatic drainage of pancreas occurs to lymph nodes around coeliac trunk.

Annular Pancreas

Annular pancreas is a congenital condition in which the head of the pancreas surrounds the second portion of the duodenum.

It may be associated with duodenal atresia. Infants present with feeding disorders and growth retardation.

Pancreatic Juice

It contains amylase, lipases and nucleases. It also contains inactive enzymes in the form of trypsinogen, chymotrypsinogen and procarboxypeptidases.

- *Pancreatic amylase:* It converts starch into maltose and alpha dextrins.
- *Pancreatic lipase:* It converts triglyceride (fats and oils) into fatty acids and monoglycerides, triglyceride (fats and oils) have already been emulsified by bile salts.
- *Pancreatic trypsin:* Enterokinase converts trypsinogen into trypsin. Trypsin converts proteins into peptides.
- *Pancreatic chymotrypsin:* Trypsin converts chymotrypsinogen into chymotrypsin. Chymotrypsin also converts proteins into peptides.

    Trypsin converts proelastase into elastase. Elastase converts proteins into peptides.
- *Pancreatic carboxypeptidase:* Trypsin converts procarboxypeptidase into carboxypeptidase. Carboxypeptidase converts terminal amino acid at carboxyl acid end of peptides into peptides and amino acids.
- *Pancreatic ribonuclease:* It converts ribonucleic acids into nucleotides.
- *Pancreatic nucleosidase:* It converts nucleotides into nucleosides.

Disorders

Pathological lesions seen in clinical practice include pancreatitis and neoplastic lesions of exocrine and endocrine components of pancreas.

Pathological lesions of pancreas in clinical practice are shown in Fig. 21.109.

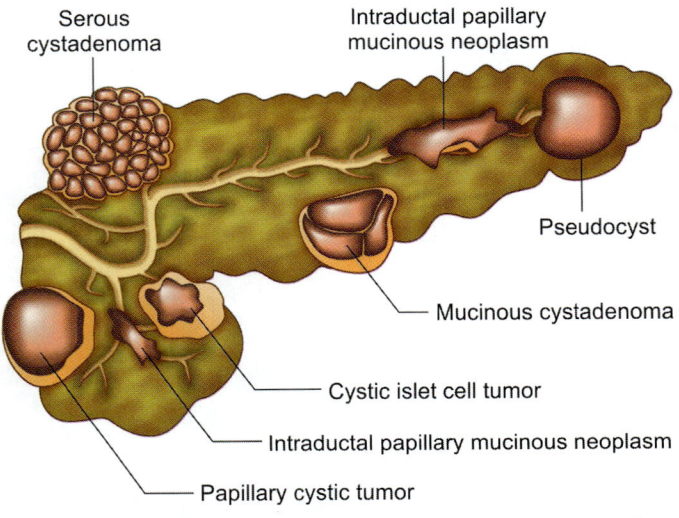

Fig. 21.109: Pathological lesions of pancreas in clinical practice.

PANCREATITIS

ACUTE PANCREATITIS

Acute pancreatitis is an inflammatory condition of the exocrine pancreas that results from injury to acinar cells. Pancreatic enzymes autodigest the gland.

Predisposing Factors

Cholelithiasis and excess alcohol are most common causes of acute pancreatitis. Approximately 45% of all cases with acute pancreatitis are associated with gallstones.

Chronic alcoholism is responsible for 33% cases of acute pancreatitis. Other causes include therapeutic agents such as anticancer drugs, immunosuppressive agents, sulfonamides, and diuretics.

Pathogenesis

Injury to acinar cells activates pancreatic enzymes, resulting in autodigestion of panaceas. Pancreas shows hemorrhagic fat necrosis with deposition of calcium soaps.

The release of amylase and lipase from the injured pancreas into the serum provides a sensitive marker for monitoring injury to acinar cells.

Pseudocysts are formed late in the course of acute pancreatitis.

Gross Morphology

Pancreas is swollen and edematous. Hemorrhages are seen in severe injury. Chalky white fat necrosis is evident.

Light Microscopy

- Histopathological examination shows preservation of parenchyma, interstitial edema, leukocytic infiltration, calcification and extensive necrosis in severe cases.

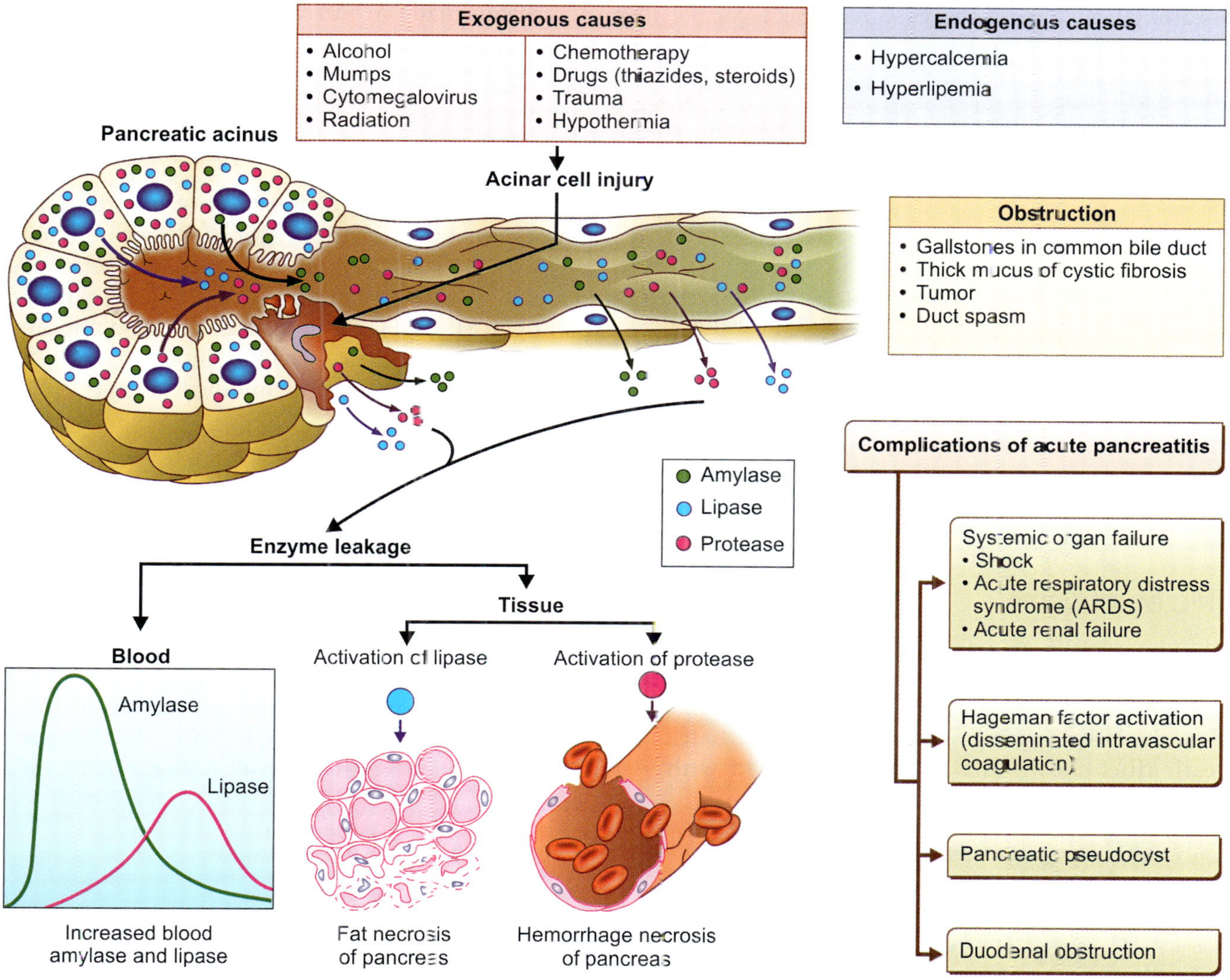

21 Liver, Gallbladder and Exocrine Pancreas

Fig. 21.110: Pathogenesis of acute pancreatitis shows causes of pancreatic injury implicated and complications.

- Microscopic examination of fat necrosis of pancreas reveals irregular islands of necrotic fat cells, which lose their outlines and become indistinct.
- There is presence of inflammatory cells, macrophages filled with fat and calcium deposits. Deposition of calcium around the periphery of necrotic fat cells gives a basophilic tinge (100X).
- Pathogenesis of acute pancreatitis with causes of pancreatic injury implicated and complications is shown in Fig. 21.110. Light microscopy of pancreatic fat necrosis is shown in Fig. 21.111.

Clinical Features

Patient presents with sudden severe constant pain in epigastrium and left hypochondrium radiating to back, severe nausea and vomiting. Retroperitoneal hemorrhage is associated with radiation of pain in flank and periumbilical region.

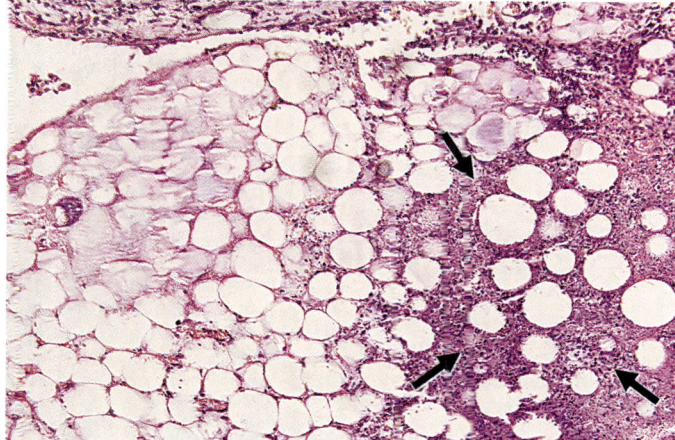

Fig. 21.111: Fat necrosis of pancreas. Microscopic examination reveals irregular islands of necrotic fat cells, which lose their outlines and become indistinct. There is presence of inflammatory cells, macrophages filled with fat and calcium deposits. Deposition of calcium around the periphery of necrotic fat cells gives a basophilic tinge (arrows) (100X).

On examination, patient shows signs of tachycardia, hypotensive shock and tenderness in upper abdomen.

Laboratory Findings

Serum amylase and lipase levels are increased. Calcium fatty acid soaps formed in acute pancreatitis results in hypocalcemia.

Complications

Acute pancreatitis can be superimposed on chronic pancreatitis. Pancreatic pseudocysts, a late complication of acute pancreatitis is lined by connective tissue and contain blood, necrotic debris. It occurs as a result of liquefaction of pancreas by pancreatic enzymes (peptidases, lipases, and amylase). Pseudocysts may enlarge to compress and even obstruct the duodenum. They may become secondarily infected and form an abscess.

CHRONIC PANCREATITIS

Chronic pancreatitis is characterized by irreversible destruction of exocrine parenchyma of pancreas, acinar atrophy, chronic inflammatory infiltrate, irregular fibrosis and relative sparing of the islets of Langerhans. Pancreatic duct shows dilatation, lumen filled with proteinaceous material and calcification. Later on islets of Langerhans show destruction (Fig. 21.112).

Etiology

It has strong association with chronic alcoholism in 70% of cases.

Other causes include obstruction of bile duct and pancreatic duct as a result of stones, hyperlipidemia, hyperparathyroidism, and hereditary chronic pancreatitis due to germline mutations in cationic trypsinogen (PRSS1), cystic fibrosis transmembrane conductance regulator (CFTR), chymotrypsin C, calcium-sensing receptor, and anionic trypsin (PRSS2).

Pathology

Focal calcification in head of pancreas and intraductal calculi may be demonstrated by imaging techniques. Pseudocysts may be evident in pancreas. Pancreatic insufficiency results in malabsorption syndrome.

Clinical Features

These are extremely variable and include abdominal and back pain, progressive disability, and steatorrhea, which is a manifestation of pancreatic insufficiency with lipase deficiency. Fat malabsorption due to chronic

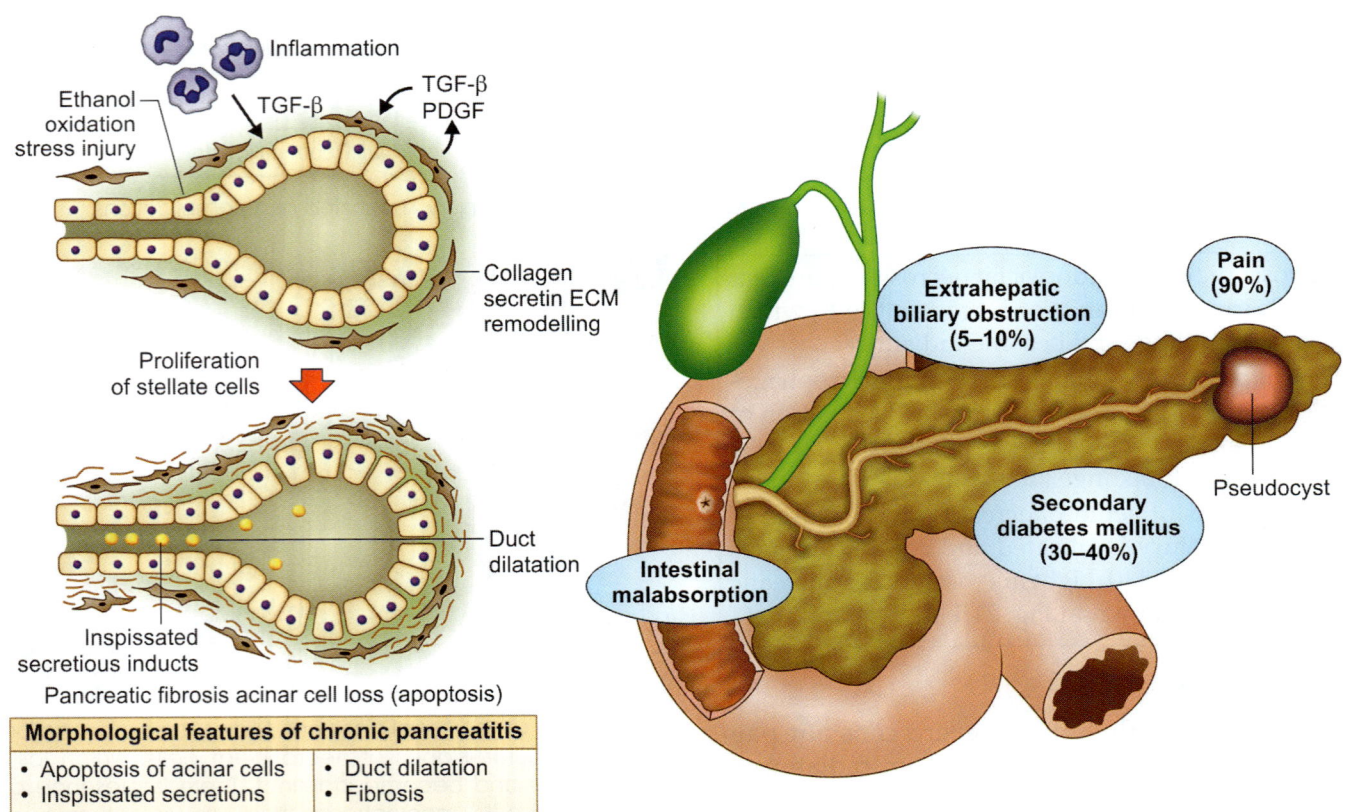

Fig. 21.112: Morphological and clinical manifestations of chronic pancreatitis.

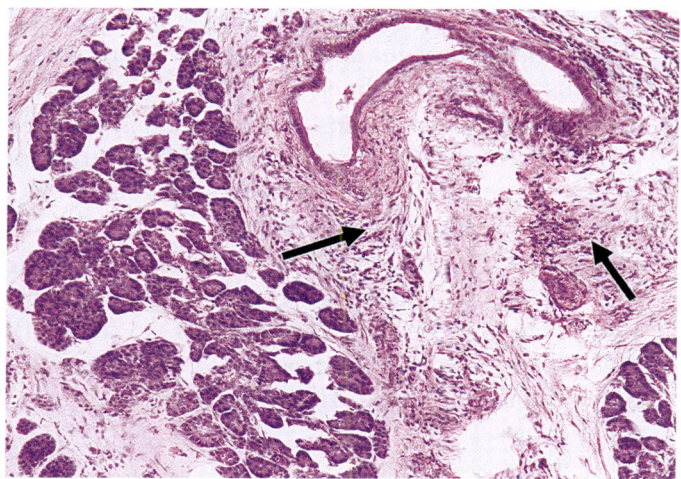

Fig. 21.113: Chronic pancreatitis shows infiltration by chronic inflammatory cells. Fibrosis is evident (arrows) (100X).

pancreatitis is most often associated with steatorrhea, the fecal matter is foul smelling and floats because of a high fat content.

Long-standing malabsorption is accompanied by nutritional deficiency, including weight loss, anemia, osteomalacia (vitamin D deficiency), and a tendency to bleed.

Light Microscopy

Histological examination of pancreas shows infiltration by lymphocytes, plasma cells and macrophages. There is presence of extensive fibrosis (Fig. 21.113).

Diagnostic Approach

Endoscopic retrograde cholangiopancreatography (ERCP) or biopsy may help to differentiate inflammation from malignant processes.

AUTOIMMUNE PANCREATITIS

Pancreas is involved as a result of systemic immunoglobulin G4 (IgG4) related sclerosing diseases such as inflammatory bowel disease and primary sclerosing cholangitis.

This systemic disorder affects other organs (50–85%) such as salivary glands, lungs, lymph nodes, bile duct system, kidney, retroperitoneum, and prostate. Autoimmune pancreatitis mimics pancreatic carcinoma.

Diagnostic Approach

Serum immunoglobulin G (IgG) and IgG4 levels are frequently high in autoimmune pancreatitis. However, IgG4 is more than sensitive than total IgG for diagnosing autoimmune pancreatitis.

Dense IgG4 plasma cells are observed on immunohistostaining of the affected organs.

Clinical Features

When autoimmune pancreatitis appears as a discrete mass (usually at pancreatic head), it can be mistaken for pancreatic cancer.

Light Microscopy

Histopathological examination shares periductal inflammation, however type 1 shows interlobular inflammation and obliterative phlebitis.

Autoimmune pancreatitis is further categorized into two types. Differences between type 1 and type 2 autoimmune pancreatitis are shown in Table 21.72.

- *Autoimmune pancreatitis type 1:* The number of IgG4 positive plasma cells are >50 per high power field in 88% of cases.
- *Autoimmune pancreatitis type 2:* The number of IgG4 positive plasma cells are 7 per high power field in 88% of cases.

CYSTIC FIBROSIS PANCREAS

Cystic fibrosis pancreas is autosomal recessive disorder of exocrine glands that causes their secretions (mainly mucus, digestive enzymes, bile and sweat) to become abnormally thick and viscous. It is also known as mucoviscidosis or fibrocystic disease of the pancreas. It is a lethal disease among White population.

Table 21.72: Differences between type 1 and type 2 autoimmune pancreatitis

Parameters	Autoimmune pancreatitis	
	Type 1	Type 2
Organs involved	Systemic involvement	Confined to pancreas
Periductal inflammation	Less marked	More marked
Ductal/lobular abscesses	Less marked	More marked
Obliterative phlebitis	More marked	Less marked
IgG4 plasma cells	>50 per HPF in 88%	>10 per HPF in 88%

Physiological state: Normally, transmembrane conductance regulator (CFTr) gene located on long arm of chromosome 7 codes for a membrane protein that participates in the movement of chloride and other ions across membranes.

Pathological state: Mutation of CFTr gene causes malfunction of exocrine glands results in increased viscosity of mucus and increased chloride concentration in sweat and tears. Pathological effects in cystic fibrosis are shown in Fig. 21.114.

Pathological Lesions

- *Respiratory system:* Patient develops recurrent pulmonary infections such as chronic bronchitis, lung abscess, and bronchiectasis. *Pseudomonas aeruginosa* infection is a common cause of death in cystic fibrosis.

  Other respiratory system changes include development of nasal polyps and chronic sinusitis. Ultimately congestion of lung may alter the pulmonary circulation and to the possibility of right side heart failure.

- *Digestive system:* Newborn develops intestinal obstruction caused by thick viscous meconium known as *meconium ileus*. In adults, cystic fibrosis interferes with the normal synthesis and drainage of bile resulting in gallstones, portal hypertension, splenomegaly, congestion or cirrhosis.

  Decreased synthesis of pancreatic enzymes and bicarbonate may lead to pancreatitis, diabetes mellitus and duodenal peptic ulcer.

- *Skin:* Cystic fibrosis affects sweat glands in the skin resulting in abnormally thick salty perspiration. There is increased risk of heat stroke and salts depletion especially in infants.

- *Reproductive system:* Almost all men with cystic fibrosis are sterile because epididymis cannot synthesize or incomplete formation of vas deferens.

  Women with cystic fibrosis often have normal reproductive system and can have successful pregnancies.

Diagnosis

Sweat chloride test is an important diagnostic tool. Secretion by sweat glands of chloride and sodium is normal, but their reabsorption by sweat ducts is impaired. Molecular testing of CFTR gene mutation is another tool. Screening done by using immunoreactive trypsinogen (IrT) assay shows elevated levels in infants with cystic fibrosis.

Treatment

Inhaled bronchodilators reduce resistance in respiratory airways. Inhaled mucolytic agents and saline help in dissolving mucus. Antibiotics are administered to cover infection.

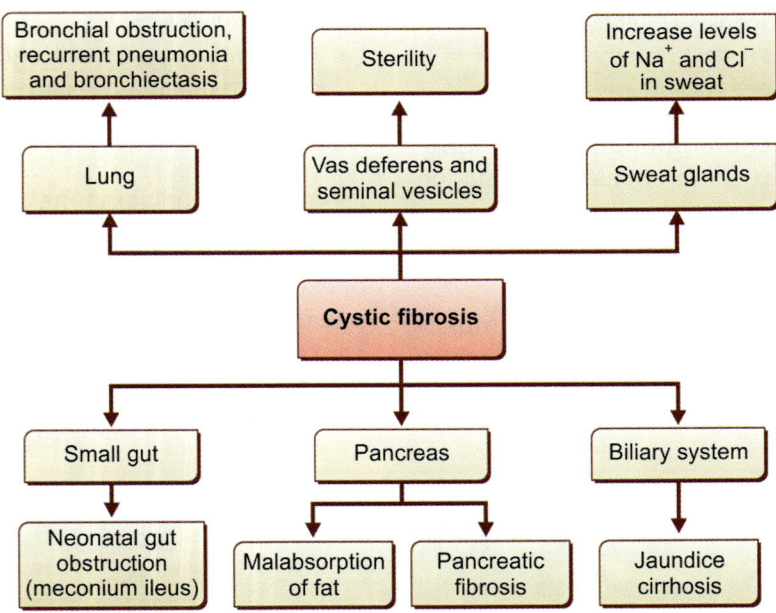

Fig. 21.114: Pathological effects in cystic fibrosis.

PANCREATIC TUMORS

EXOCRINE TUMORS

Exocrine tumors of pancreas include adenocarcinoma. Other pancreatic exocrine tumors include serous cystic neoplasms, mucinous cystic neoplasms, solid pseudopapillary neoplasms, and pancreatoblastomas.

PANCREATIC ADENOCARCINOMA

Pancreatic duct adenocarcinoma is the most common malignancy of gastrointestinal tract with high death rate. The majority of pancreatic carcinomas arise from pancreatic duct epithelium. Acinar cell carcinoma is much less common. It is most often silent before widespread dissemination occurs. Death usually results within 1 year. Ductal carcinomas elicit an intense desmoplastic response.

Predisposing Factors

- *Cigarette smoking:* It is the most important risk factor in the development of pancreatic adenocarcinoma.
- *Chemicals exposure:* Consumption of smoked meat and fish intake containing polycyclic hydrocarbons increases risk of pancreatic carcinoma. *Indirect acting chemical carcinogens associated with pancreatic cancer* are shown in Table 21.73.
- *Parasite:* Schistosoma haematobium also increases risk of pancreatic carcinoma. *Parasite associated with pancreatic carcinoma* is shown in Table 21.74.
- *Other factors:* Chronic pancreatitis, diabetes mellitus and alcoholism have been associated with an increased risk of pancreatic cancer. Consumption of high fat diet has also been implicated but less common.
- *Familial syndromes:* Several familial syndromes increasing the risk of pancreatic adenocarcinoma include Lynch syndrome, Peutz-Jeghers syndrome (STK11/LB1 gene on chromosome 19p13), *hereditary pancreatitis* (PRSS1 gene), *familial atypical mole melanoma syndrome* (p16 gene, chromosome 9p21), BRCA2 *gene mutation* (13q12–q13), *familial pancreatic cancer syndrome* and Fanconi anemia component genes.

Molecular Genetics

Oncogenes, their mode of activation and associated cancers are shown in Table 21.75. *Tumor suppressor gene mutations associated with pancreatic carcinoma* are shown in Table 21.76.

- *K-RAS signal-transducing proteins:* Point mutation of K-RAS (chromosome 12p) has been identified in *pancreas* (90%), *colon* (50%), and *lung* (30%).
- *SMADA4 tumor suppressor gene (chromosome 18q):* SMADA4 tumor suppressor gene is also known as *DPC4*. Mutation of DPC4 (deletion) has been demonstrated in 55% of *pancreatic cancers*.
- *BRCA2 gene (chromosome 13q):* BRCA2 tumor suppressor gene mutation has been associated with pancreatic cancers.

Table 21.73: Indirect acting chemical carcinogens associated with pancreatic cancer

Chemical carcinogen	Examples	Associated cancers
Polycyclic hydrocarbons	Smoked meat and fish intake	Pancreas carcinoma
		Oral carcinoma
	Cigarette smoke	Esophagus carcinoma (middle and distal)
		Lung carcinoma
		Renal pelvis transitional cell carcinoma
		Urinary bladder transitional cell carcinoma

Table 21.74: Parasite associated with pancreatic carcinoma

Parasite	Associated tumors
Schistosoma haematobium	Pancreatic carcinoma
	Squamous cell carcinoma of the urinary bladder

Table 21.75: Oncogenes, their mode of activation and associated cancers (signal-transducing proteins)

Category	Proto-oncogene	Mode of activation	Associated malignancies
GTP-binding (G) proteins	K-RAS	Point mutation	Pancreas carcinoma
			Colon carcinoma
			Lung carcinoma

Table 21.76: Tumor suppressor genes associated with pancreatic carcinoma

Gene	Protein	Function	Familial tumors	Sporadic cancers
Mitogenic signaling pathway inhibitors				
APC	Adenomatous polyposis protein (locus 5p21) Mutation by deletion or nonsense	APC inhibits Wnt signaling activator pathway, thus prevents nuclear transcription. It degrades catenin	Familial polyposis coli with malignant transformation	Pancreas carcinoma Colon carcinoma Gastric carcinoma Thyroid carcinoma Melanoma
SMADA2 SMADA4	SMADA2 protein SMADA4 protein	Both inhibit TGF-β signaling pathway. These repress CDK4 and MYC. These also induce expression of CDK inhibitor	Juvenile polyposis	Pancreas carcinoma (55%) Colon carcinoma
Cell cycle progression inhibitors				
CDKN2A	P16/INK4a and P14ARF	P16 inhibits CDK. P14 indirectly activates p53 tumor suppressor gene	Familial melanoma	Pancreas carcinoma Breast carcinoma Esophagus carcinoma
Angiogenesis inhibitors				
STK11	Liver kinase B1 (LKB1) or STK11	It activates AMPK family of kinases. It suppresses cell growth when cell nutrients and energy levels are low	*Peutz-Jeghers syndrome:* cancers of GIT and pancreas	Diverse carcinomas in 5–20% of cases

- *APC gene (chromosome 5p21):* Mutation of APC tumor suppressor gene (deletion and nonsense) has been demonstrated in sporadic cancers (*colon, stomach and pancreas*) and *familial adenomatous polyposis* developing colon cancer.
- *TGF-β tumor suppressor gene:* TGF-β tumor suppressor gene inhibits G1 to S phase of cell cycle. Mutation of TGF-β has been demonstrated in pancreatic cancer.

Evolution of Pancreatic Adenocarcinoma

Pancreatic carcinoma is a genetic disease of inherited or acquired gene mutations. Accumulation of multiple mutations of various genes is most important than their occurrence in a specific order.

- *Early stage:* It is thought that telomerase shortening and point mutation of K-RAS (12p) oncogene is an early event in most cases of pancreatic intraductal neoplasia in more than 90% of cases.
- *Intermediate stage:* There is inactivation of the p16 tumor suppressor gene (CDKN2A on chromosome 9p) in more than 95% of cases.
- *Late stage:* Inactivation of p53, SMAD4 (DPC4 on chromosome 18q) in 55% and BRCA2 (13q) tumor suppressor gene occurs in 10%. It results in invasive carcinoma. Other less common gene mutations include LKB1/STK11 (19q), MKK4 (17p) and RB1 (13q).

Clinical Features

Patient complains of abdominal dull pain constant in nature in upper abdomen radiating to the back, marked loss of weight and anorexia. Patient also mentions passage of dark-colored urine and clay-colored stool. Locations of adenocarcinoma of pancreas and clinical manifestations are shown in Fig. 21.115.

- *Nonspecific symptoms:* Patient may present with abdominal pain radiating to the back, weight loss and anorexia.
- *Migratory thrombophlebitis:* It occurs probably due to release of thrombogenic substances into the circulation (e.g. serine proteases) that initiate the coagulation cascade in 10% of cases (Trousseau sign).
- *Carcinoma arising in head of pancreas:* It frequently obstructs common bile duct resulting in painless obstructive jaundice in 20% of cases. It is often accompanied by a distended, palpable gallbladder termed as *Courvoisier sign* in this setting.
- *Carcinoma involving the pancreatic tail:* It can cause islet destruction and secondary diabetes mellitus.

Physical Examination

The classic presentations of pancreatic cancer are loss of weight, jaundice, distended palpable gallbladder (*Courvoisier sign*).

- *Migratory thrombophlebitis (Trousseau sign):* It occurs probably due to release of thrombogenic substances

Liver, Gallbladder and Exocrine Pancreas

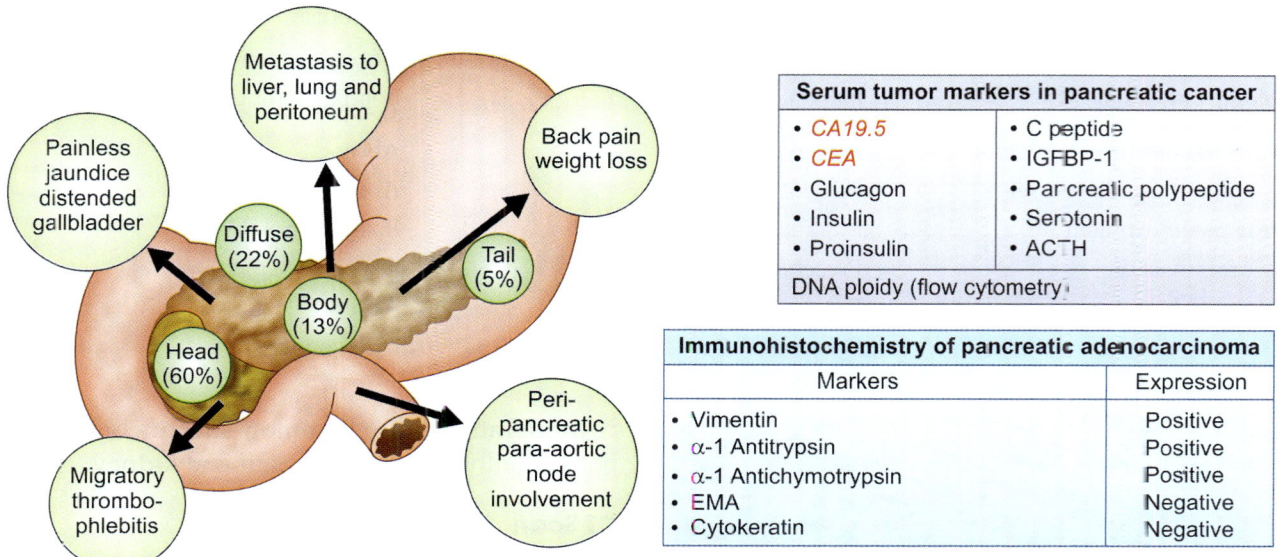

Fig. 21.115: Locations of adenocarcinoma of pancreas and clinical manifestations.

into the circulation (e.g. serine proteases) that initiate the coagulation cascade in 10% of cases.

- *Obstructive jaundice (Courvoisier sign):* Carcinoma arising in head of pancreas frequently obstructs common bile duct resulting in painless obstructive jaundice in 20% of cases.

  It is often accompanied by a distended, palpable gallbladder termed as *Courvoisier sign* in this setting.
- *Secondary diabetes mellitus:* Carcinoma involving the pancreatic tail can cause islet destruction and secondary diabetes mellitus.

Laboratory Findings

Laboratory tests are consistent with obstructive jaundice, i.e. conjugated hyperbilirubinemia with high 5′ nucleosidase (specific marker for bile duct epithelial cell injury) and alkaline phosphatase. CA19-9 tumor marker is most often elevated (normal range <37 IU/ml).

Gross Morphology

- *Pancreatic cancer occurs in various portions of pancreas:* head (60%), body (15%) and tail (5%) of the gland. The tumor diffusely involves the entire gland.
- Tumor is usually hard, satellite, poorly circumscribed and gray-white in color. Gross morphology of carcinoma of pancreas is shown in Fig. 21.116.

Light Microscopy

Most common histologic variant of pancreatic cancer is adenocarcinoma. Less common histologic variants include acinic cell, adenosquamous and poorly differentiated carcinoma.

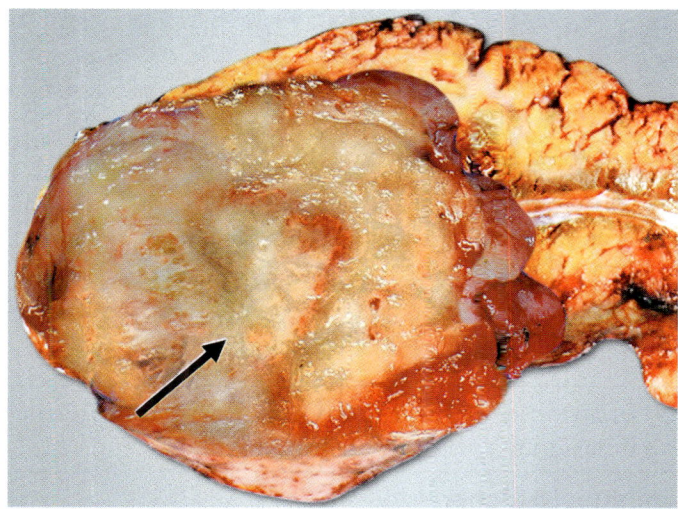

Fig. 21.116: Adenocarcinoma pancreas. Head of pancreas shows gray white tumor with areas of hemorrhage (arrow).

Morphology of pancreatic adenocarcinoma is described as under.

- *Cell morphology:* Tumor is composed of pleomorphic small to bizarre cuboidal to columnar malignant cells forming abortive glandular structures or nests. Light microscopy is shown in Fig. 21.117. Differences between ductal adenocarcinoma of pancreas and chronic pancreatitis are shown in Table 21.77.
- *Differentiation:* Tumor is most often moderately to poorly differentiated adenocarcinoma irrespective of location of tumor in pancreas (well differentiated rare).
- *Fibrosis:* Tumor cells infiltrate the wall resulting in dense stromal fibrosis.

Table 21.77: Differences between ductal adenocarcinoma of pancreas and chronic pancreatitis

Histopathological features	Ductal adenocarcinoma	Chronic pancreatitis
Histologic pattern	Haphazardly arranged	Lobular arrangement
Ruptured or incomplete glands	Present	Absent
Companion muscular vessel	Present	Absent
Nuclear pleomorphism	Marked in the same glands	Insignificant
Perineural invasion	Present	Absent
Invasion of blood vessels	Present	Absent
Mitoses	Frequent	Infrequent

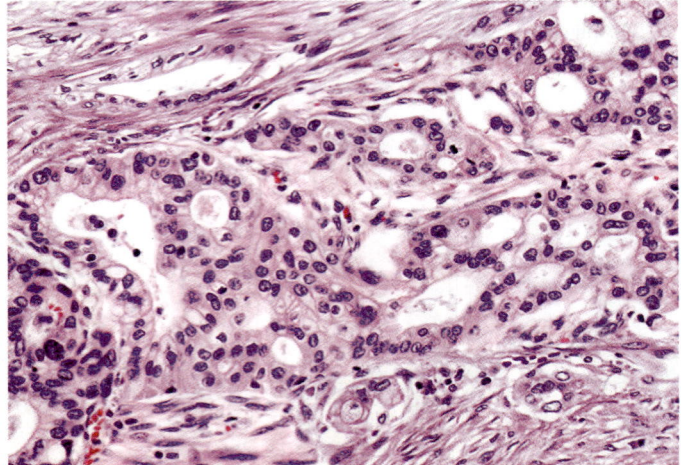

Fig. 21.117: Adenocarcinoma pancreas. Tumor is composed of pleomorphic small to columnar malignant cells forming abortive glandular structures or nests (400X).

- *Invasion:* Perineural invasion and lymphatic invasion may be demonstrated.

Immunohistochemistry

Panel of markers is used to analyze expression in pancreatic adenocarcinoma on histopathological sections as shown in Table 21.78.

Table 21.78: Immunohistochemistry of duct adenocarcinoma of pancreas

Markers	Expression
Vimentin	Positive
α_1-antitrypsin	Positive
α_1-antichymotrypsin	Positive
EMA	Negative
Cytokeratin	Negative

Mode of Spread

Pancreatic adenocarcinoma most often metastasizes to regional lymph nodes, liver, lung, pleura, intestine and peritoneum.

Moderately other common sites include adrenals, bones, gallbladder, diaphragm and kidney.

CT Scan

CT imaging technique highlights early detection of pancreatic cancer, accurate staging and effective treatment of pancreatic cancer.

Surgical Resection

It is the only curative treatment option. Only 10–30% cancers are resectable at the time of presentation with a 5-year survival rate of 18–20%, and a median survival of these patients is 17–21 months.

Patients with locally advanced disease have a median survival of 6–10 months.

PANCREATOBLASTOMA

It is rare malignant pancreatic neoplasm most often affecting children up to 15 years of age.

Light microscopy reveals squamous islands admixed with undifferentiated cells. Prognosis is better in comparison to that of pancreatic ductal adenocarcinoma.

ISLET CELL TUMORS

GLUCAGONOMA

Glucagonoma is rare neuroendocrine tumor of pancreatic α cells of pancreas. It results in secondary diabetes mellitus. Patient with a glucagonoma presents with *necrotizing migratory erythema*, mild hyperglycemia, and anemia.

INSULINOMA

Insulinoma is the most common islet cell tumor derived from β cells of pancreas. It is low-grade malignant neoplasm. It synthesizes excess of insulin resulting in hypoglycemia.

Insulinoma synthesizes insulin by splitting of C-peptide fragment of the proinsulin molecule resulting in increased serum C-peptide level (diagnostic tool).

Purification of commercial insulin preparations is done by splitting of C-peptide fragment of proinsulin. Hence, exogenous administration of insulin does not increase C-peptide.

Clinical Features

Symptoms of hypoglycemia as a result of episodic hyperinsulinemia include hunger, sweating, irritability, epileptic seizures, and coma.

It is known as *Whipple triad*. Glucose administration dramatically causes reversal of central nervous system abnormalities.

GASTRINOMA

This malignant tumor derived from G cells is most often located in the pancreas. It may also occur in duodenum. It synthesizes excess of gastrin resulting in increased serum gastrin levels.

Clinical Features

Gastrinoma of pancreas results in *Zollinger-Ellison syndrome* characterized by gastric hypersecretion of hydrochloric acid, recurrent peptic ulcer disease of the duodenum and sometimes the jejunum, and elevated levels of gastrin in blood.

STOMATOSTATINOMA

Stomatostatinoma is islet cell tumor derived from δ cells of pancreas. Normally, δ cells of pancreas secrete somatostatin hormone that inhibits the release of insulin by pancreas. Somatostatin also inhibits the pituitary release of growth hormone. It decreases secretion, motility and absorption in the digestive tract.

Clinical Features

Excess synthesis of somatostatin hormone by tumor results in mild diabetes mellitus, gallstones, steatorrhea, and hypochlorhydria.

VASOACTIVE INTESTINAL PEPTIDE TUMOR

This rare islet cell endocrine tumor is marked by secretion of vasoactive intestinal peptide (VIP).

Vasoactive intestinal peptide stimulates adenylyl cyclase enzyme that leads to the synthesis of large amounts of cAMP. The cAMP causes increased secretion of potassium and water into the intestinal lumen.

Clinical Features

Patient presents with watery diarrhea (5 liters/day), hypokalemia, low levels of chloride in gastric juice (achlorhydria). These symptoms constitute *pancreatic cholera*.

MULTIPLE ENDOCRINE NEOPLASIA 1 (MEN 1)

Multiple endocrine neoplasia type 1 is also known as *Wermer-Morrison syndrome* caused by mutation of the MEN 1 tumor suppressor gene.

Wermer-Morrison syndrome comprises pituitary adenoma (acromegaly), parathyroid gland hyperplasia (hypercalcemia) or adenoma and pancreas islet cell tumors (insulinoma and gastrinoma). Gastrinoma produces *Zollinger-Ellison syndrome*.

CARCINOID TUMORS

Carcinoid tumors of the pancreas are rare malignant neoplasms that closely resemble intestinal carcinoids.

When confined to the pancreas, serotonin, bradykinin, and histamine synthesized from the tumor into venous blood, induce atypical carcinoid syndrome.

Hepatic metastases cause the full blown carcinoid syndrome.

Patient presents with severe facial flushing, bronchial wheezing, watery diarrhea, abdominal colic, hypotension, periorbital edema, and tearing.

METASTATIC TUMORS

Hematogenous Route

Most common malignant tumors of lung, breast, thyroid gland, kidney and melanoma (skin) via hematogenous route reach the pancreas.

Direct Extension

Malignant tumors of stomach, duodenum, colon, kidney, lymph nodes and adrenal glands may spread to pancreas by direct extension.

CHAPTER 22

Kidney and Ureter

Learning Objectives

ANATOMY
- Overview

PHYSIOLOGY
- Mechanism of Urine Formation

GLOMERULI
- Structure of the Glomerulus • Glomerular Permeability Barriers

GLOMERULONEPHRITIS
- Glomerulonephritis: Terminology, classification, Pathogenesis

NEPHROTIC SYNDROME
- Minimal Change Disease • Focal Segmental Glomerulosclerosis • Membranous Glomerulonephritis • Membranoproliferative Glomerulonephritis • Diabetic Nephropathy and Amyloid Nephropathy

ACUTE NEPHRITIC SYNDROME
- Post-streptococcal Glomerulonephritis • Alport's Syndrome
- IgA Nephropathy (Berger's Disease) • Hemolytic Uremic Syndrome

CHRONIC GLOMERULONEPHRITIS
- Clinical Manifestation • Dialysis Machine

EVALUATION OF RENAL BIOPSY

DISEASES OF THE TUBULES
- Overview of Acute Tubular Necrosis • Acute Tubular Necrosis (Ischemic Type)
- Pathogenesis of Acute Tubular Necrosis • Acute Renal Failure (Azotemia)

TUBULOINTERSTITIAL DISORDERS
- Clinical Manifestation • Dialysis Machine

OBSTRUCTIVE UROPATHY AND HYDRONEPHROSIS

RENAL STONES (NEPHROLITHIASIS AND UROLITHIASIS)

VASCULAR DISORDERS

CYSTIC DISEASES OF KIDNEY

CONGENITAL ANOMALIES OF THE URINARY TRACT

NEOPLASMS OF THE KIDNEY

LABORATORY DIAGNOSIS

ANATOMY

OVERVIEW

- Urinary tract comprises the kidneys, renal pelvises, ureters, urinary bladder and urethra. The kidneys and renal pelvises constitute upper urinary tract; the ureters, urinary bladder and urethra form lower urinary tract.
- Urine produced by nephrons within a renal pyramid empties into the orifices of the terminal collecting ducts (Bellini's ducts) into a minor calyx, major calyx and then funnel shaped renal pelvis.
- The collecting system comprises renal pelvises, urinary bladder and urethra that carry urine from the kidneys to the urethra for urination. Normal urinary tract health depends on smooth unobstructed urine.

FUNCTIONS

- Kidneys participate in excretion of waste metabolic products, adjustment of blood pH by excretion of more or less acid, maintenance of plasma concentration of salts, regulation of blood volume, regulation of blood pressure and hematopoiesis.
- Juxtaglomerular apparatus releases renin into the blood to raise blood pressure through renin-angiotensin-aldosterone system.

Kidney and Ureter 22

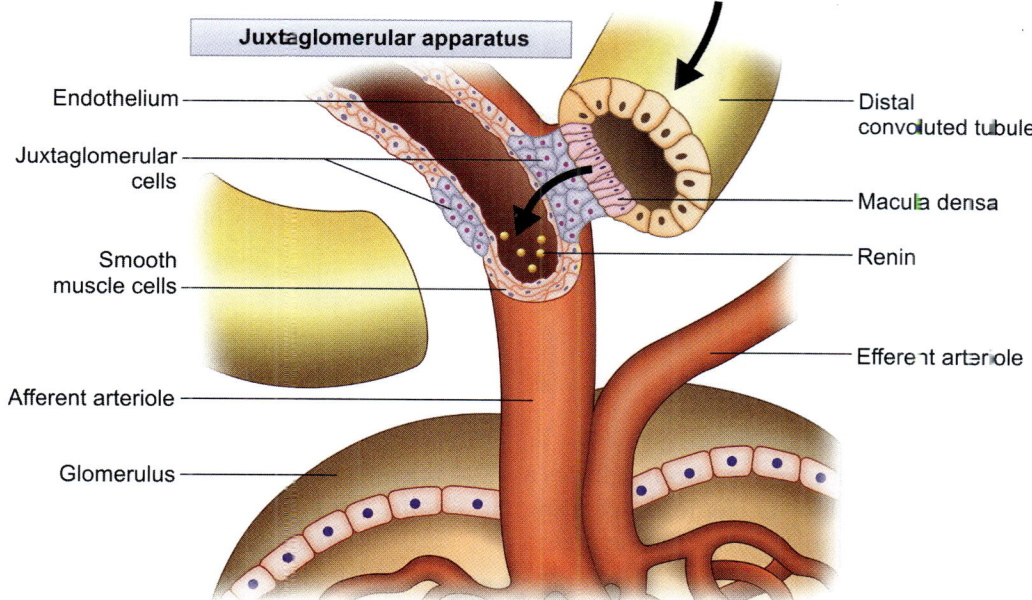

Fig. 22.1: Juxtaglomerular apparatus shows juxtaglomerular cells. Macula densa and nongranular lacis cells (*Courtesy by* Dr Abhijit Das).

JUXTAGLOMERULAR APPARATUS

Juxtaglomerular apparatus is closely related to glomerulus, where afferent arteriole enters. JG apparatus consists of three components (Fig. 22.1).

- *Juxtaglomerular cells:* These are modified smooth muscle cells with granular cytoplasm present in the media of afferent arterioles. These cells contain renin.
- *Macula densa:* It is region of distal tubule, where distal tubule returns to the vascular pole of its parent glomerulus.
- *Nongranular lacis cells:* These are present in area bounded by afferent arterioles, macula densa and glomerulus.

KIDNEYS

Kidneys are bean-shaped encapsulated organs (normal weight 150 gm). Each kidney in the human contains about one million nephrons, each capable of forming urine. These are unable to regenerate new nephrons. Therefore, with renal injury, disorders or normal aging process, there is gradual decrease in number of nephrons.

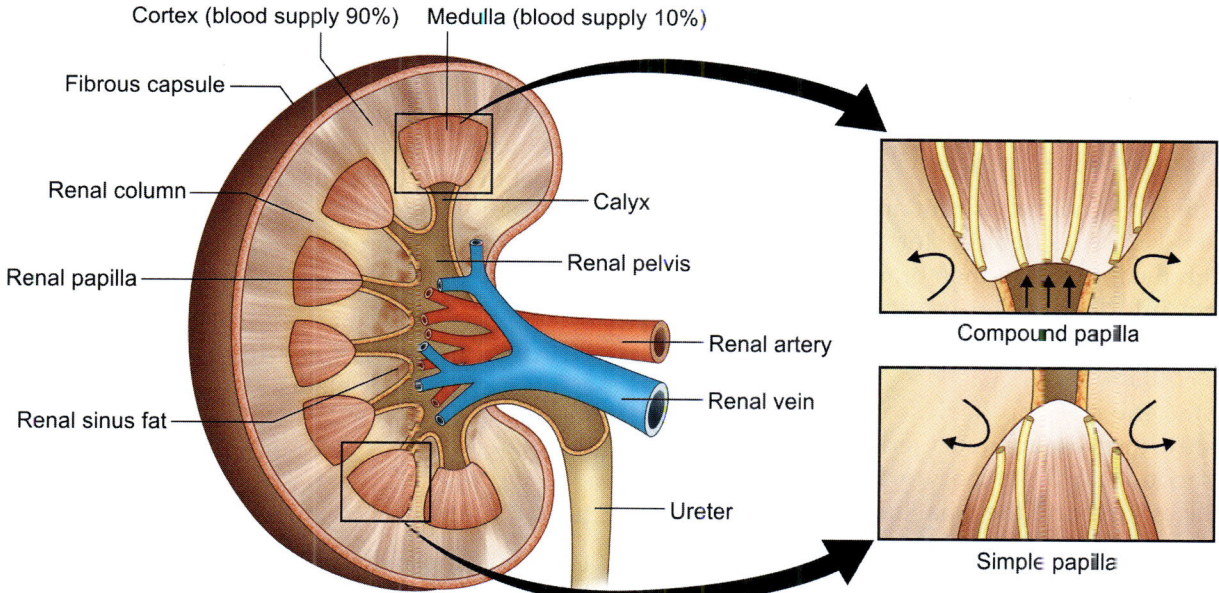

Fig. 22.2: Illustrates the anatomay of kidney. Compound papillae are present in the poles of kidney. Obstruction to urine flow first affect compound papillae. Rest of the papillae are simple (*Courtesy by* Dr Abhijit Das).

Table 22.1: Comparison between renal cortex and medulla

Parameters	Renal cortex (1.2–1.5 cm)	Renal medulla
Blood supply	90%	10%
Number of nephrons	85% They lack vasa recta	15% They possess vasa recta
Nephron's portions	Glomeruli, proximal and distal convoluted tubules	Collecting ducts and loop of Henle
Interstitial tissue	10%	20–30%
Pyramids	Absent	Present
Synthesis of substances	Erythropoietin	Prostaglandins

Renin is synthesized by juxtaglomerular apparatus.

Each nephron derived from the ureteric bud includes a glomerulus, proximal tubule, loop of Henle (descending and ascending limb), distal tubule, connecting segment, and collecting duct (Fig. 22.2).

- *Cut surface:* Each kidney is composed of 8–18 lobes. Each lobe constitutes a conical medullary pyramid capped by cortical tissue. Downward extension of cortical tissue between the pyramids is called columns of Bertini. The cortex is normally about 1.2–1.5 cm thick over the pyramids. Renal columns or columns of Bertini are located where cortical tissue dips into the medulla between the pyramids. Base of pyramid is towards cortex and its papilla pointing towards renal pelvis (Table 22.1).

- *Type of papillae of pyramids:* There are two types of papillae—simple and compound. *Compound papillae* are concave shaped with valveless straight ducts located at the poles. That is the reason that hydronephrotic changes are marked in the polar areas due to presence of compound papillae resulting from obstruction to the urinary flow. Rest of the pyramids contain conical *simple papillae* with obliquely placed ducts having valve like action.

- *Blood supply:* Renal pelvis contains renal artery, renal vein, and nerves. Renal artery enters the kidney through the hilum and then branches progressively to form interlobar arteries, arcuate arteries, and efferent arterioles, resulting in formation of glomerular capillaries.

    Distal ends of capillaries of each glomerulus coalesce to form the afferent arterioles, which progress to a second capillary network. The peritubular capillaries surround the renal tubules. Renal arteries are the end arteries. Obstruction to renal artery results in renal infarction (pale/white infarct).

- *Renal blood flow:* Kidneys receive 25% of cardiac output: 1200 ml of blood (600 ml of plasma) per minute. The glomeruli filter 120 ml of filtrate per minute (GFR=120 ml/minute).

    Approximately, 130–180 liters of filtrate is presented to the tubules each day, which results in production of one liter of urine per day. Renal cortex receives 90% and medulla 10% of arterial blood.

- *Histology:* Kidney is composed of glomeruli, tubules, interstitial tissue (10% in cortex and 20–30% in medulla) and blood vessels. Disease of any one component of kidney affects other components resulting in impairment of renal functions. *Erythropoietin is synthesized by cortical interstitial tissue, while prostaglandins by medullary interstitial tissue.*

RENAL PELVIS

Renal pelvis is a funnel-shaped structure present at the hilum of kidney. It is lined by transitional epithelium. It contains renal artery, renal vein, and nerves. Renal pelvis drains urine into ureter.

URETERS

Ureters are lined by transitional epithelium. Strong muscular contractions within calyces and renal pelvis propel the urine into the ureter. Musculature of ureter and pelvis is continuous. Thus, these allow synchronous peristaltic contractions from kidney to urinary bladder.

URINARY BLADDER

Urinary bladder is lined by transitional epithelium. Capacity of urinary bladder is 300–450 ml. It is supplied by sacral nerves (S2, 3, 4). Urine is forced out of the bladder and through the urethra.

URETHRA

Urethra is approximately 3 cm long in females and 20 cm in males. In males, it consists of prostatic, membranous and penile parts. Women are more prone to urinary tract infection due to short urethra.

PHYSIOLOGY

Homeostasis is defined as a steady state for normal life's metabolic processes. The kidneys regulate the content of blood plasma to maintain the homeostasis of the internal fluid environment, within normal limits. Changes in the water content in the cells beyond range may cause death.

Approximately >12% of the body water loss in humans may even be fatal. All animals possess readily permeable membranes such as respiratory surfaces and oral membranes. Kidneys perform functions by filtration, reabsorption, secretion and excretion.

REABSORPTION OF ESSENTIAL SUBSTANCES

Kidneys absorb essential metabolites by active process such as sodium (50–55%), potassium, amino acids, glucose, phosphates (100%) and bicarbonate (80%).

Water is absorbed in proximal tubules by passive process. Sodium is pumped from tubule cell to interstitial fluid. It drives chloride ions into the interstitial fluid by passive process.

EXCRETION OF HARMFUL PRODUCTS

Kidneys participate in excretion of *waste products*. These include *urea, creatinine, uric acid, guanidino compounds, metabolic end products of nucleic acids, aliphatic amines, middle molecules (polypeptides)*. Normal range of blood urea is 20–40 mg% and serum creatinine 0.6–1.5 mg%. If the renal functions are impaired, accumulation of waste products in the body is termed as '*azotemia*'. If the patient develops clinical manifestations, it is denoted as '*uremia*'.

MAINTENANCE OF ACID–BASE HEMOSTASIS

Distal tubules participate in deamination of amino acids resulting in *ammonia production* that enters the filtrate.

Hydrogen and *potassium ions also enter distal tubular filtrate in exchange of sodium ions* (sodium ions moving out of filtrate). Ammonia combines with hydrogen ions to form ammonium salts.

REGULATION OF WATER AND ELECTROLYTES

Kidneys regulate water by concentrating and diluting urine. These control sodium reabsorption in the proximal and distal collecting tubules. The functioning of the kidneys is efficiently monitored and regulated by hormonal feedback mechanisms involving hypothalamus, juxtaglomerular apparatus and to a certain extent, the heart. Renin-angiotensin-aldosterone system (RAAS), antidiuretic hormone (ADH), and atrial natriuretic factor (ANF) provide an elaborate system of checks and balances that regulate body fluid osmolarity, salt concentrations, blood pressure and blood volume (Fig. 22.3 and Table 22.2).

- *Renin-angiotensin-aldosterone system:* Renin secreted by juxtaglomerular apparatus (JGA) stimulates liver to synthesize angiotensinogen, which gets converted to angiotensin I. This product is converted to angiotensin II (vasoconstrictive action also) in lungs by angiotensin converting enzyme (ACE).

  Angiotensin II stimulates adrenal zona glomerulosa cells to synthesize aldosterone, which acts on distal convoluted tubule resulting in absorption of sodium and water. Thus, blood volume expansion occurs. Aldosterone acts on distal convoluted tubule and helps in absorption of Na^+ and water and completing the feedback circuit by supporting the release of renin. Distal convoluted tubule helps in regulation of blood pH by the reabsorption of HCO_3^-, an important buffer.

- *Role of antidiuretic hormone (ADH):* Osmoreceptors in the hypothalamus are activated by changes in blood volume, body volume and ionic concentration. Excess of loss of fluid from the body leads to synthesis of antidiuretic hormone (ADH) by hypothalamus via posterior pituitary gland. ADH circulates in blood and acts on collecting ducts to absorb water. ADH also acts on the principal cells of collecting ducts and helps absorption of water.

- *Role of atrial natriuretic factor (ANF): Atrial natriuretic factor is a peptide hormone, which opposes the regulation by renin-angiotensin-aldosterone system (RAAS).* The walls of both atria of the heart release atrial natriuretic factor (ANF) in response to an increase in blood volume and pressure. ANF inhibits the release of renin from the JGA, and thereby, inhibits NaCl reabsorption by the collecting duct and reduces aldosterone release from adrenal gland.

MAINTENANCE OF VASCULAR TONE

Kidneys play an important role in *maintaining vascular tone by synthesis of angiotensin II and prostaglandins.* Angiotensin II synthesized in response to renin production by juxtaglomerular cells causes vasoconstriction of peripheral resistance arterioles and efferent arterioles.

Prostaglandins synthesized by renal medulla causes *vasodilation of the afferent arterioles.*

SYNTHESIS OF PRODUCTS

Erythropoietin synthesized in the endothelial cells in the peritubular capillaries (cortex) plays key role in *hematopoiesis.*

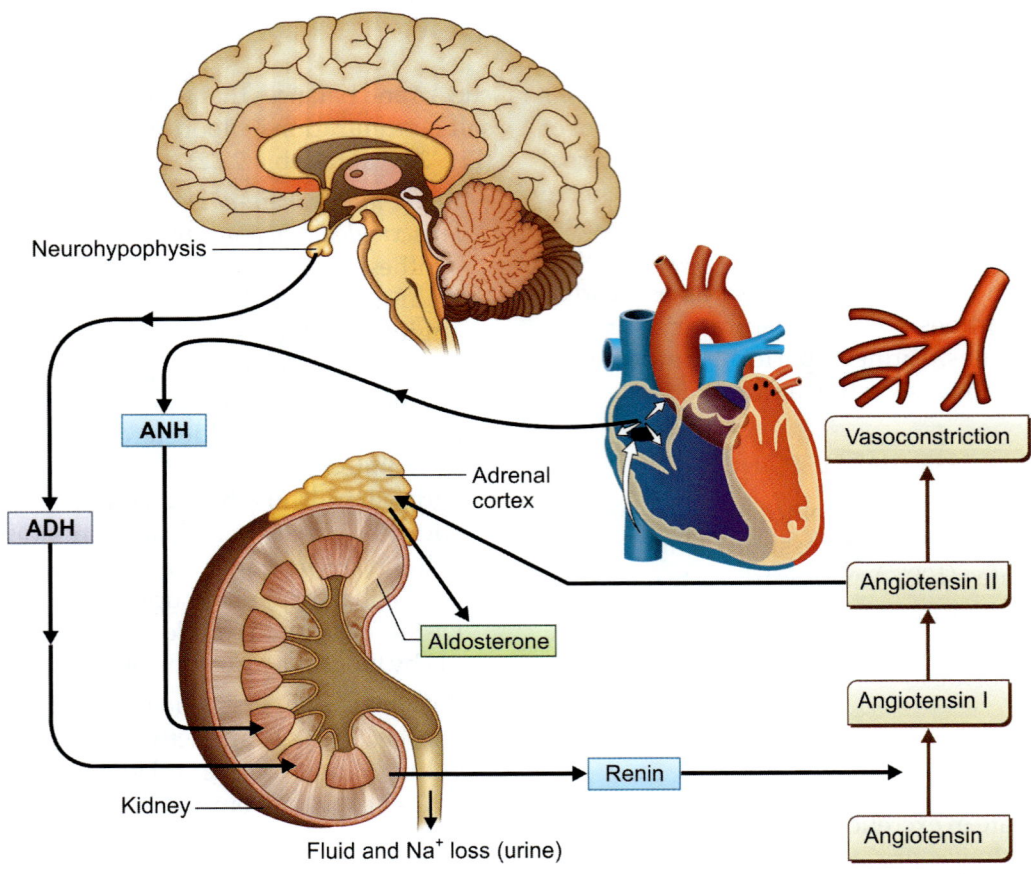

Fig. 22.3: It illustrates regulation of water and electrolytes (*Courtesy by Dr Abhijit Das*).

Table 22.2: Substances that affect renal function

Substance	Source	Actions
Aldosterone	Hypotension stimulates adrenal cortex to release aldosterone	Promotes reabsorption of sodium and water in kidneys to increase plasma volume and blood pressure
Atrial natriuretic factor (ANF)	Atrial myocardial cells release ANF in response to increased blood pressure	Promotes excretion of sodium and water in kidneys to decrease plasma volume and blood pressure
Antidiuretic hormone (ADH)	Hypothalamus releases ADH and concentrated in posterior pituitary gland when blood pressure falls	Promotes water absorption from distal tubules and collecting ducts to conserve water to concentrate the urine
Renin	Renin is synthesized by renal cortex when blood pressure falls	Renin increases angiotensin in blood
Angiotensin	Angiotensinogen protein in the blood is activated by renin	Angiotensin II stimulates synthesis of aldosterone by adrenal cortex. It also causes vasoconstriction and increases peripheral resistance

MAINTENANCE OF CALCIUM HOMEOSTASIS

- *Second hydroxylation of vitamin D:* Proximal renal tubular cells synthesize enzyme 1-α *hydroxylase*, which participates in conversion of vitamin D_2 (25-hydroxycholecalciferol) to vitamin D_3 (1, 25-dihydroxycholecalciferol). *Vitamin D_3 is the active form of vitamin D.*

- *Actions of vitamin D:* Vitamin D increases *gastrointestinal reabsorption of calcium* and *phosphorus*. Vitamin D_3 along with parathormone participate in calcium absorption by distal convoluted tubules, resulting in *bone mineralization*. It increases the production of osteoclasts from macrophage stem cells. Osteoclasts release enzyme alkaline phosphatase, which participates in hydrolysis of pyrophosphate and other inhibitors of calcium-phosphate crystallization, resulting to bone mineralization.

MECHANISM OF URINE FORMATION

Nephrons regulate water and electrolytes, mainly sodium, in the nephrons loop, distal tubule and collecting ducts according to the body's needs (Fig. 22.4).

GLOMERULAR FILTRATION

- Glomerular filtration is the first step in urine formation. Blood pressure inside the glomeruli forces water and dissolved substances into the glomerular Bowman's capsule. Blood cells and proteins remain behind in the blood. Glomeruli comprise size and charge dependent barriers.
- Glomeruli exclude all molecules >3.5 nm in size and negatively charged albumin with 70,000 molecular weight. Blood cells and proteins remain behind in the blood. The smaller diameter of the efferent arteriole as compared with that of afferent arteriole maintains high hydrostatic pressure. Depending on the extent of injury to the glomeruli, excretion of red blood cells and proteins in urine occurs.

TUBULAR REABSORPTION

Tubular reabsorption moves essential substances back into the blood, while keeping waste products in the nephrons to be eliminated in the urine (Table 22.3, Figs 22.5 and 22.6).

TUBULAR SECRETION

Tubular secretion moves additional substances from the blood into the nephrons for elimination Movement of the hydrogen ions is one means by which the pH

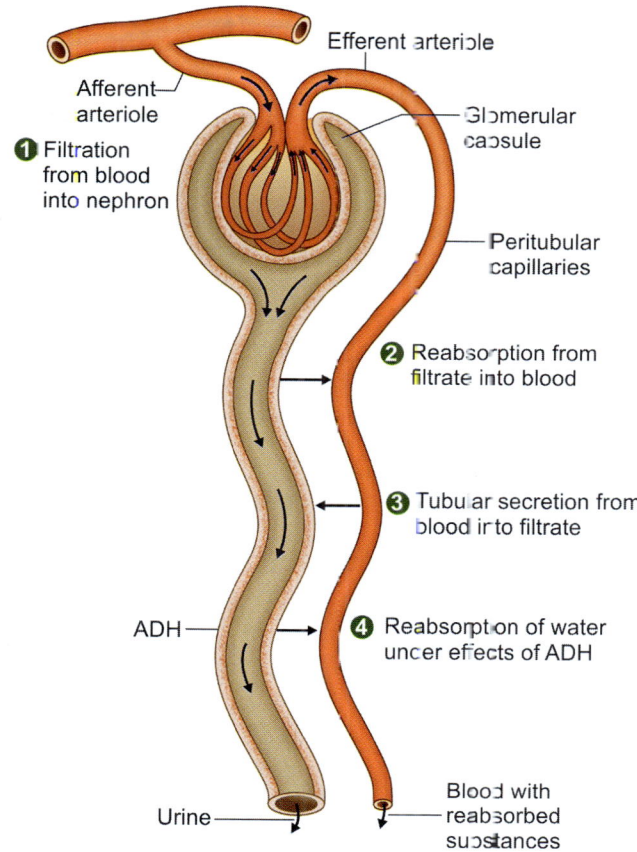

Fig. 22.4: Tubular processing of the glomerular filtrate: under physiological state, the tubule completely reabsorbs from glomerular filtrate all glucose and amino acids. The tubules reabsorb variable quantity of water to adjust plasma osmolarity and secretes variable quantity of hydrogen and electrolytes to adjust plasma pH and electrolyte concentration. Toxins, urea and creatinine are excreted unaltered into urine (*Courtesy by Dr Abhijit Das*).

of body fluids is balanced. Distal tubules participate in deamination of amino acids resulting in ammonia production that enters the filtrate. Hydrogen and potassium ions also enter filtrate in exchange of sodium ions (sodium ions moving out of filtrate). Ammonia combines with hydrogen ions to form ammonium salts.

Table 22.3: Reabsorption of essential metabolites by nephron tubules

Part of nephron	Reabsorption by active process	Reabsorption by passive process
Proximal tubule	Na^+, K^+, Cl^-, HCO_3^-, amino acids, glucose and phosphates	Water (80%)
Loop of Henle	Descending limb is only permeable to water only	Water (10%)
	Ascending limb is only permeable to salts. Reabsorption of Na^+, chloride, K^+, Ca^+, HCO_3^- and Mg^+	Water (Nil)
Distal tubule	Na^+, Cl^-, Ca^+ and Mg^+ (absorption of Na^+, Cl^-, by aldosterone)	Water (5%)
Collecting duct	Water absorption by ADH	Water (5%)

High yield facts: Hydrogen ions and organic acids secreted by proximal tubules enter peritubular network of blood vessels. Hydrogen ions also secreted by distal tubule.

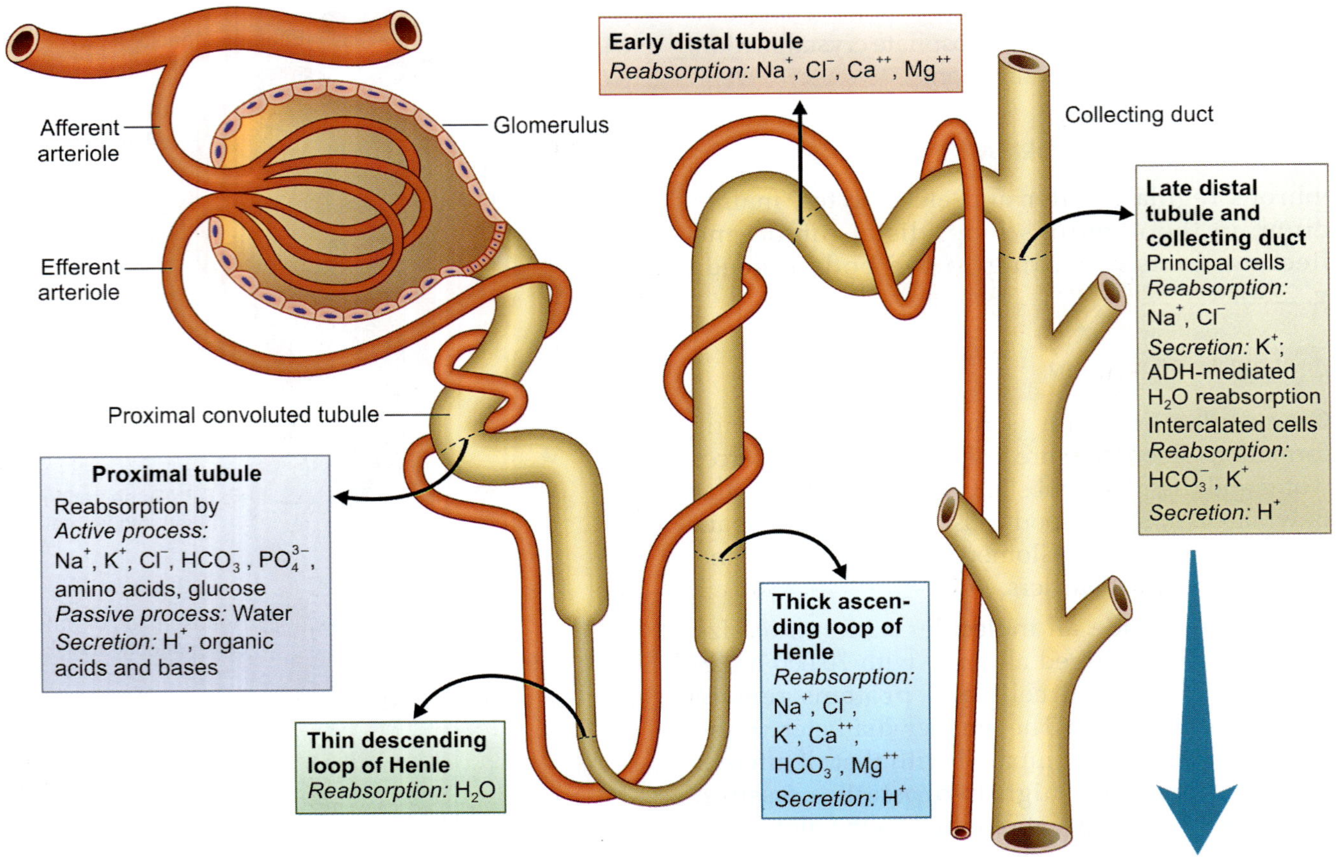

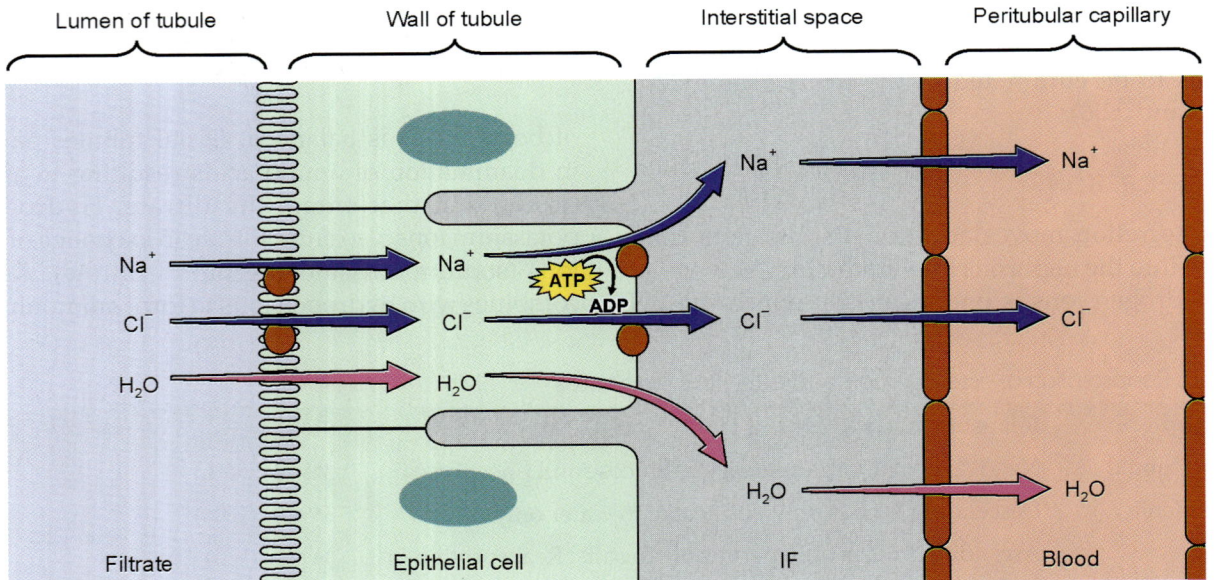

Fig. 22.5: Illustrates site of reabsorption of essential metabolites by nephron tubules. Sites of tubular water (H_2O), glucose, amino acids, Na^+ (sodium), Cl^- (chloride), HCO_3^- (bicarbonate), K^+ (potassium), Ca^{++} (calcium), and Mg^{++} (magnesium) reabsorption, and organic acids and bases, H^+ (hydrogen), and K^+ secretion (*Courtesy by Dr Abhijit Das*).

Fig. 22.6: Mechanism of sodium reabsorption and potassium secretion by principal cells of the late distal and collecting tubules. Aldosterone exerts its action by increasing the activity of the Na^+/K^+-ATPase pump that transports sodium outward through the basolateral membrane of the cell and into the blood at the same time it pumps potassium into the cell. Aldosterone also increases the permeability of the luminal membrane for potassium.

CONCENTRATION OF URINE BY THE COUNTERCURRENT MECHANISM

Human kidneys can produce nearly four times concentrated urine than the initial filtrate formed. Proximity of loop of Henle and vasa recta play an important role in production of concentrated urine by *countercurrent mechanism.*

Fluid is flowing in opposite direction between loop of Henle and vasa recta, and thus forming countercurrent system. Countercurrent mechanism concentrates the urine and reduces the volume excreted. There is increasing concentration of the interstitial fluid moving from the cortex to the medulla (Fig. 22.7).

Urine concentration is regulated by means of exchange of water and electrolytes, mainly sodium, in the loop of Henle, distal tubule and collecting ducts. As urine flows through the collecting ducts, water is drawn and hypertonic interstitial fluid moving from cortex to medulla thus concentrating the urine. ADH increases the permeability of the collecting duct, allowing more water to leave the urine.

COLLECTING DUCTS

These are permeable to urea, but impermeable to salt. Urea diffuses out of collecting ducts and enters into interstitial fluid contributing to high osmolarity of medulla. As the urine flows through the collecting ducts, ADH increases the permeability of the collecting duct, and pushes out water from filtrate into interstitial fluid.

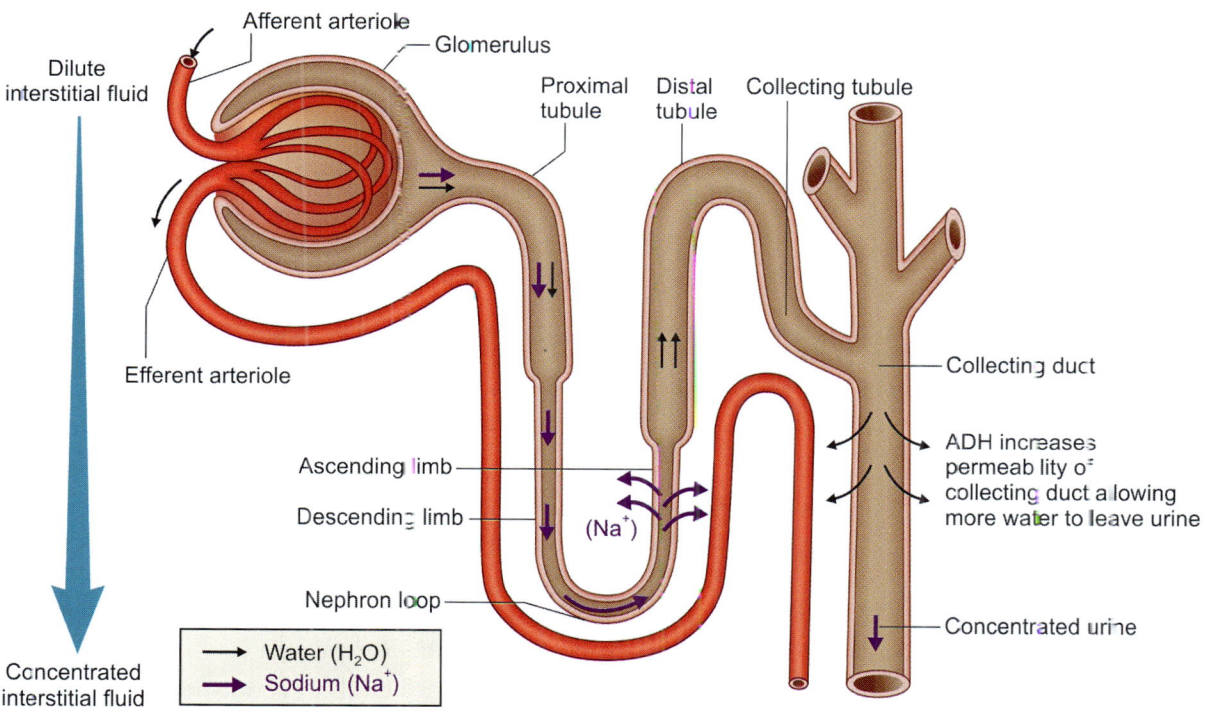

Fig. 22.7: Concentration of urine by the countercurrent mechanism. Urine concentration is regulated by exchange of water and electrolytes mainly sodium in the loop of Henle, distal tubule and collecting duct. As urine flows through the collecting ducts, water is drawn out by the hypertonic interstitial fluid, thus concentrating the urine. ADH increases the permeability of the collecting ducts, allowing more water to leave the urine (*Courtesy by* Dr Abhijit Das).

GLOMERULI

STRUCTURE OF THE GLOMERULUS

Glomerulus comprises *bunch of capillaries, glomerular basement membrane, Bowman's capsule (visceral and parietal epithelial cells) and mesangial cells.* Size and charge on GBM determine protein filtration.

Water, salts, glucose and other small molecules cross glomerular basement membrane from blood into Bowman's space as glomerular filtrate except red blood cells, proteins and other large molecules (Figs 22.8, 22.9 and Table 22.4).

Glomerular Capillaries

Capillaries are lined by thin layer of fenestrated endothelial cells being about 70–100 nm in diameter.

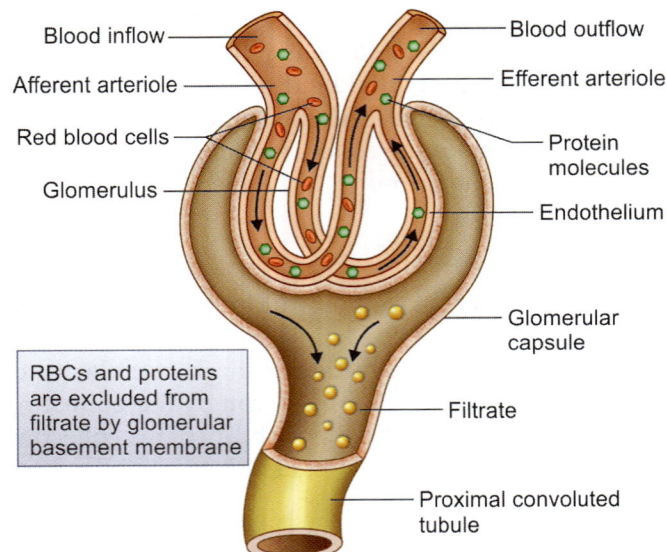

Fig. 22.8: Structure of glomerulus. It shows afferent arteriole and efferent arteriole. Diameter of efferent arteriole is smaller than afferent arteriole. Filtration occurs due to small diameter of efferent arteriole. Hydrostatic pressure in the glomerulus is >60 mm Hg. Blood flow to kidneys is 1200 ml/minute (blood plasma 600 ml/minute). Glomerular filtration is 10% of the total blood flow (*Courtesy by* Dr Abhijit Das).

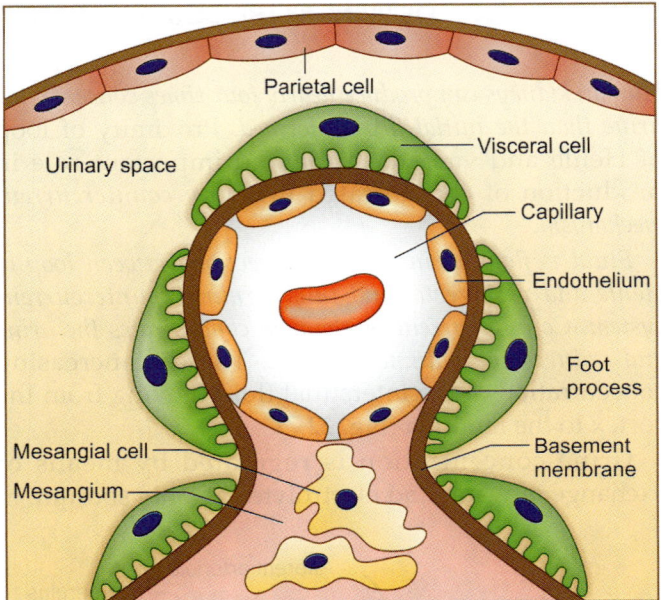

Fig. 22.9: Normal glomerulus: single glomerular loop shows relationship between glomerular cells, glomerular basement membrane and mesangial matrix. Outer portion of fenestrated endothelium is in contact with inner surface of glomerular basement membrane. Central part of fenestrated endothelium is in contact with mesangial cells. Visceral layer of Bowman's capsule covers glomerular basement membrane (*Courtesy by* Dr Abhijit Das).

Table 22.4: Structure of glomerulus

Components	Functions
Glomerular capillary endothelial cells	Exclude molecules >3.5 nm diameter
Glomerular basement membrane	*Composition:* Lamina rara interna, lamina densa and lamina rara externa Negative charge on GBM due to polyanionic proteoglycans and anionic sialoglycoprotein sexcludes negative charged molecules like albumin Collagen IV fibers provide strength to GBM Laminin helps in the attachment of endothelial cells and visceral cells of Bowman's capsule to the matrix
Visceral epithelial cells of Bowman's capsule	Slit pores between podocytes prevent filtration of large size molecules
Parietal epithelial cells of Bowman's capsule	Bowman's capsule is lined by parietal cells
Mesangial cells	Mesangial cells provide mechanical support to the glomerular capillaries and regulate glomerular filtration rate

Glomerular Basement Membrane

Glomerular basement membrane is 250–350 nm in thickness. It consists of central electron dense layer, the lamina densa, thinner electron-lucent lamina rara interna (towards endothelial cells), and lamina rara externa (towards visceral layer of Bowman's capsule).

Composition

Glomerular basement membrane comprises *collagen fiber types IV and V, laminin, fibronectin, proteoglycans and fibroblasts. Proteoglycans consists of glycosaminoglycans linked to protein and calcium.* It regulates connective tissue structure permeability.

There is negative charge on endothelial cells, glomerular basement membrane and visceral epithelial cells (podocytes). As albumin also possesses negative charge, therefore, it is repelled and not filtered in the glomerular filtrate (Fig. 22.10).

- *Collagen IV and V:* These provide *structural strength* to the capillary. These are resistant to collagenase enzymes.
- *Laminin:* Laminin is a cross-shaped molecule. It is distributed along glomerular basement membrane's lamina rara interna and externa. It comprises long arm and short arm. Long arm binds heparan sulfate and short arm with globular ends to collagen.

Kidney and Ureter

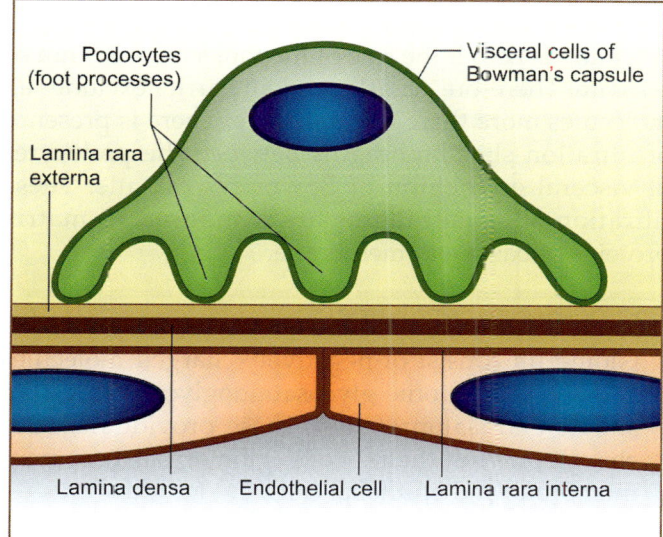

Fig. 22.10: Structure of glomerular basement membrane (GBM) is composed of lamina densa (middle portion), lamina rara interna towards endothelial cells and lamina rara externa towards visceral cells of Bowman's capsule. There is a negative charge on the endothelial cells, GBM and visceral cells. These act as charge dependent barrier for negative charged albumin (*Courtesy by Dr Abhijit Das*).

Laminin has high affinity for collagen and proteoglycans. It is believed to mediate attachment of endothelium and visceral epithelium to connective tissue matrix substrates.

- *Fibronectin:* It is a multifunctional glycoprotein consisting of two dimers held together by disulphide bonds. It is synthesized by fibroblasts, monocytes, endothelial cells and other cells. It binds to collagen, fibrin, heparan, and proteoglycans and on other cells via integrin receptors. *It is involved in interactions of cells with the extracellular matrix.*
- *Polyanionic-proteoglycans:* Proteoglycans comprise heparan sulfate hyaluronic acid, chondroitin, dermatan, and keratin, linked covalently to protein core. Heparan sulfate is present in the form of clusters in lamina densa and along lamina rara interna and externa. These retain fluid and maintain normal shape and structure of GBM. Proteoglycans play diverse role in regulating connective tissue, structure, charge dependent permeability barrier and modulating cell differentiation.
- *Anionic-sialoglycoproteins:* Anionic-sialoglycoproteins coat glomerular endothelial and the visceral epithelial cells. These are responsible for charge dependent glomerular filtration barrier.
- *Fibroblasts:* Fibroblasts synthesize glycosaminoglycans comprising of hyaluronic acid, chondroitin, dermatan, keratin and heparan sulfate. Fibroblasts synthesize elastic fibers. In inflammation, elastase synthesized by bacteria, polymorphonuclear cells degrade elastic fibers resulting in formation of elastic myofibrils and elastin fibers. Elastin fibers are abundant amorphous substance comprising of tropoelastin (polypeptide), desmosine, iododesmosine and tropoelastin.

Visceral Epithelial Cells of Bowman's Capsule

- *Visceral epithelial cells of Bowman's capsule:* These are primarily responsible for production of the glomerular basement membrane. These contain podocytes (foot-like processes). Slit pores between the podocytes 20–30 nm wide are bridged by a thin diaphragm, which serve as a distal major filtration barrier for preventing protein loss in the urine.
- *Proteins associated with podocytes:* Proteins linking podocytes include *nephrin, podocin and CD2 associated proteins*. Integrins span the membrane and anchor the actin cytoskeleton to the collagen type IV in the lamina rara externa of the basement membrane. Effacement of podocytes seen in minimal change disease is responsible for nephrotic syndrome (Fig. 22.11).

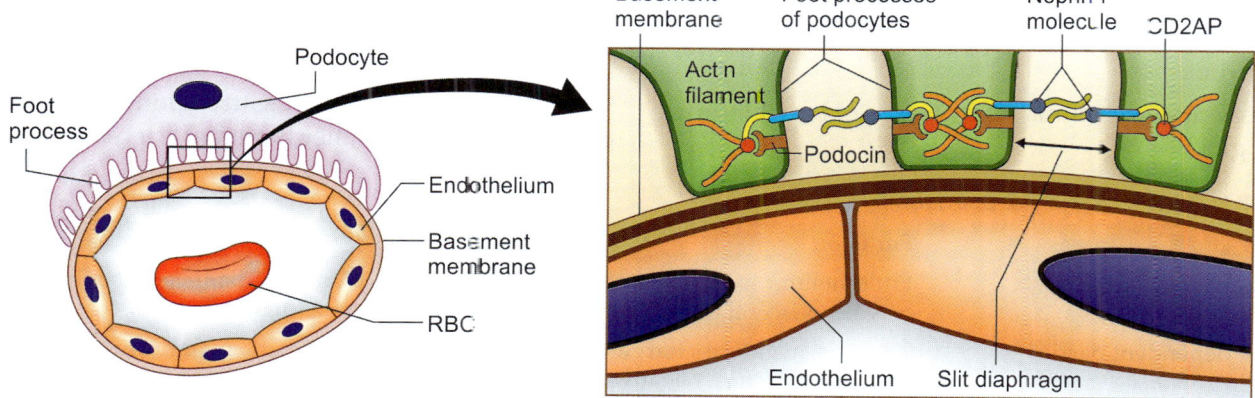

Fig. 22.11: Schematic diagrams of some of the proteins of the glomerular slit diagrams such as CD2AP, CD2 associated proteins (*Courtesy by Dr Abhijit Das*).

Parietal Epithelial Cells of Bowman's Capsule

Parietal epithelial cells line the Bowman's capsule. Due to increased permeability of glomeruli, fibrinogen leaks and stimulates the parietal cells, which undergo proliferation forming *crescents* resulting in destruction of the glomeruli, and impairment of renal functions.

Mesangial Cells

- Normally, mesangial cells are present in small number in mesangial matrix. These provide mechanical support to the glomerular capillaries. These participate in *processing plasma proteins and immune complexes.*
- These *maintain glomerular basement membrane* and matrix elements. These participate in *modulation of glomerular filtration rate.*
- These synthesize *prostaglandins* and *cytokines*, which participate in cell proliferation and chemotaxis of inflammatory cells. These release *inflammatory mediators in IgA nephropathy.*

GLOMERULAR PERMEABILITY BARRIERS

Glomeruli consist of *size and charge dependent barriers. Alteration in size and charge dependent barriers leads to leakage of proteins and blood cells in urine.* The barrier effect of the glomeruli prevents red blood cells, proteins and other large molecules from leaving blood and passing into urine. Glomerulopathy causes impairment of charge dependent barrier resulting in protein loss (Table 22.5).

- *Under physiological state*, albuminuria is <30 mg/24 hours.
- *Microalbuminuria* refers to loss of albumin in the range of 30–300 mg/24 hours. Microalbuminuria is considered as the earliest sign of diabetic glomerulopathy.
- *Overt albuminuria* is defined >300 mg of albumin in urine 24 hours.
- *Selective proteinuria* reveals presence of albumin in the urine.
- *Nonselective proteinuria* refers to loss of both albumin and globulin.

Size-dependent Barrier

Filtration is zero if the size of the molecule is 3.5 nm or >3.5 nm. Therefore, size dependent barrier excludes all molecules more than 3.5 nm in size. There is presence of filtration slit diaphragms between the podocytes of visceral epithelium of Bowman's capsule. These filtration slit diaphragms are composed of matrix proteins of basement membrane.

Charge-dependent Barrier

- Glomeruli consist of negatively charged molecules such as polyanionic glycosaminoglycans (heparan sulfate and sialoproteins). These provide negative charge on endothelial cells, glomerular basement membrane and epithelial cells.
- Glomeruli allow greater penetration of neutral and cationic molecules than anionic molecules of the same size. These exclude negatively charged albumin from glomerular filtrate.

GLOMERULAR FILTRATE RATE (GFR)

- *Kidneys receive 25% of cardiac output:* 1200 ml of blood (600 ml of plasma) per minute. The glomeruli filter 120 ml of filtrate per minute (GFR=120 ml/minute). Almost all of the glomerular filtrate is reabsorbed by renal tubules.
- Glomerular filtration occurs through endothelial cells (85%) and mesangial region (15%). Mesangial cells regulate GFR and have phagocytic action. Glomeruli participate in filtration of substances.
- Glomerular filtration is the first step in urine formation. Blood pressure inside the glomeruli forces water and dissolved substances into the glomerular Bowman's capsule. Blood cells and proteins remain behind in the blood. The smaller diameter of the efferent arteriole as compared with that of afferent arteriole maintains high hydrostatic pressure.

GFR Depends on Various Factors

Glomerular filtration rate depends upon: (a) renal blood flow, (b) hydrostatic pressure glomeruli (normal 60 mm Hg due to smaller lumen of efferent arterioles),

Table 22.5: Type of glomerular permeability barriers

Barrier	Function
Size dependent barrier	Endothelium excludes molecule of 3.5 nm or >3.5 nm in diameter. Diaphragm slits between visceral podocytes exclude are also size dependent barriers
Charge dependent barrier	There is negative charge on endothelial cells, basement membrane and visceral podocytes. Hence, negatively charged albumin is excluded in glomerular filtrate

High yield facts: The barrier effect of the glomerulus prevents RBCs, protein, and other large molecules from leaving blood and passing into urine.

(c) number of functional glomeruli, (d) blood colloidal pressure (normal 25 mm Hg), and (e) back pressure in tubules (normal 15 mm Hg).

Filtration Pressure

- Filtration pressure is necessary to drive fluid across the glomerular basement membrane. It is equal to the difference between the blood pressure in the glomeruli (60 mm Hg) and sum of osmotic pressure exerted by plasma proteins (27 mm Hg) and intratubular pressure (15 mm Hg).
- Filtration pressure = Blood pressure in the glomeruli – (osmotic pressure 27 mm Hg in glomeruli + intratubular pressure 15 mm Hg).
- If the intratubular pressure is high due to obstruction to urine outflow, it adversely affects glomerular filtration rate.

Tubular Processing of the Glomerular Filtrate

- Under physiological state, tubules completely reabsorb from glomerular filtrate all the glucose and amino acid. *Almost all of the glomerular filtrate is reabsorbed by renal tubules and returned to blood.*
- *The tubules reabsorb variable amount of water to adjust plasma osmolality and secrete variable quantity of hydrogen and electrolytes to adjust plasma pH and electrolyte concentration.* Toxins, creatinine and urea pass unaltered into urine.

GLOMERULONEPHRITIS

- Glomerulonephritis is classified according to *involvement of glomeruli* either due to intrinsic cause (primary) or systemic disorders (secondary) and familial glomerulopathy. Almost all primary glomerular diseases occur due to autoimmunity (Table 22.6).
- Immunologic injury to glomerular basement membrane activates complement system that attract inflammatory cells. Hydrolytic enzymes released by inflammatory cells cause glomerular injury without interruption of the filtration barrier.

Primary Glomerular Diseases

These glomerular disorders are intrinsic to the kidney and mediated by immune-complex mechanism. Primary glomerulonephritis is classified based on mechanism of glomerular injury.

- *In situ anti-glomerular membrane disease:* Antibodies circulating in blood attach to native Goodpasture antigen in the glomerular basement membrane (Goodpasture's syndrome).

Table 22.6: Classification of glomerular diseases

Primary glomerulopathy	Secondary glomerulopathy	Familial glomerulopathy
Acute proliferative glomerulonephritis (post-streptococcal GN or non-streptococcal GN)	Diabetes mellitus	Alport's syndrome due to mutations of α-3, α-4 or α-5 chains of collagen type IV
Rapidly progressive glomerulonephritis (crescentic GN)	Multiple myeloma	Fabry's disease
Minimal change disease	Amyloidosis	Thin membrane disease
Membranous glomerulopathy	Goodpasture's syndrome	Nephrosialidosis
Membranoproliferative glomerulonephritis	Microscopic polyarteritis	Congenital nephrotic syndrome due to NPHS1 (nephrin molecules) and NPHS2 (podocin) gene mutations
Focal segmental glomerulosclerosis	Wegener's granulomatosis	Focal segmental glomerulosclerosis due to gene mutation of α-actinin 4 protein (ACTN4) podocyte binding protein or calcium channel regulating TRPC6 (transient receptor potential calcium channel-6)
Mesangial IgA nephropathy	Henoch-Schönlein purpura Bacterial endocarditis Drugs, e.g. penicillamine, gold, street heroin, phenytoin, captopril *Infections:* Malaria, hepatitis B virus, leprosy, syphilis	Congenital membranoproliferative GN due to gene mutations of complement factor-H PPAR-γ

- *Immunecomplex-mediated glomerular diseases:* These immune complexes are formed elsewhere circulate in blood and deposited in the glomerular basement membrane (GBM). Examples are proliferative glomerulonephritis (diffuse or focal), membranous glomerulonephritis, membranoproliferative glomerulonephritis, focal segmental glomerulosclerosis and crescentic glomerulonephritis (rapidly progressive glomerulonephritis).

Secondary Glomerular Diseases

Glomeruli may be damaged in the course of systemic diseases: These may be caused by the following mechanisms:

- *Immune complex mediated GN:* These include *systemic lupus erythematosus, Henoch-Schönlein purpura and infective endocarditis.*
- *Metabolic disorders:* These are *diabetes mellitus, renal amyloidosis and multiple myeloma.*
- *Hematological and vascular disorders:* These include *hypertension, polyarteritis nodosa, Wegener's granulomatosis, hemolytic uremic syndrome, idiopathic thrombocytopenic purpura and disseminated intravascular coagulation.*

Familial Glomerulopathy

- *Congenital nephrotic syndrome:* NPHS1 (nephrin molecules) and NPHS2 (podocin) *regulate slit pores of membrane at birth.* Gene mutations lead to congenital nephrotic syndrome.
- *Alport's syndrome:* It occurs due to mutations of α-3, α-4 or α-5 chains of collagen type IV resulting in *splitting of basement membrane with glomerulosclerosis.*
- *Focal segmental glomerulosclerosis:* TRPC6 cation channel mutation produces focal *segmental glomerulosclerosis* (FSGS) in adulthood.

- *Non-diabetic end stage renal disease:* It occurs due to polymorphism in the gene encoding apolipoprotein-L1 (APOL1) in 70% African Americans.
- *Membranoproliferative GN:* Due to *gene mutation of complement factor-H. PPAR-γ*, patient develops membranoproliferative glomerulonephritis. It is sometimes associated with dense deposit disease.
- *Fabry's disease:* It is lysosomal storage disease due to *deficiency of α-galactosidase deficiency resulting in familial glomerulopathy.*
- *Nephrosialidosis:* It occurs due to deficiency of N-acetyl-neuraminic acid hydrolase causing nephrosialidosis and showing focal segmental glomerulosclerosis (FSGS) (Table 22.7).

GLOMERULONEPHRITIS: TERMINOLOGY

Distribution of disease in kidney is based on glomerular involvement (Fig. 22.12 and Table 22.8).

- *Diffuse proliferative glomerulonephritis:* Almost all the glomeruli (>50–100%) of both kidneys show pathologic change. Glomeruli are hypercellular due to proliferation of glomerular cells and leukocytic infiltration. It is termed as exudative/necrotizing glomerulonephritis.
- *Focal proliferative glomerulonephritis:* It refers to pathological change in some glomeruli (<50% of glomeruli), whereas others are normal. *Examples are Henoch-Schönlein purpura and IgA nephropathy.*
- *Global glomerulonephritis:* All the capillaries of the glomerulus are affected. It is seen in *lupus nephritis (SLE).*
- *Segmental glomerulosclerosis:* It refers to an increase in extracellular matrix (hyalinization) within the mesangial region, involving only a segment of the involved glomerulus. It is seen in *diabetes mellitus.*

Table 22.7: Genetic basis of familial nephrotic syndrome

Genetic	Nephrotic syndrome
NPHS-1 Gene	It is located on chromosome 19q13. It encodes for nephrin protein. It is key component of the slit diaphragm, which regulates glomerular filtration rate. NPHS-1 gene mutation causes congenital nephrotic syndrome (Finnish type)
NPHS-2 Gene	It is located on chromosome 1q. It encodes for podocin protein located in the slit diaphragm. NPHS-2 gene mutation causes steroid resistant nephrotic syndrome in children or autosomal recessive focal segmental glomerulosclerosis
α-Actin 4 protein (ACTN4)	It is a podocyte binding protein. Mutation is responsible for autosomal dominant focal segmental glomerulosclerosis
TRPC6 (transient receptor potential calcium channel-6) gene	It regulates calcium channels. TRPC6 mutation adversely affects function of podocytes by enhancing calcium influx into them. Mutation is also responsible for adult onset focal segmental glomerulosclerosis
Apolipoprotein L-1 gene (APOL1)	It is located on chromosome 22. Gene mutation is associated with increased risk of focal segmental glomerulosclerosis and renal failure

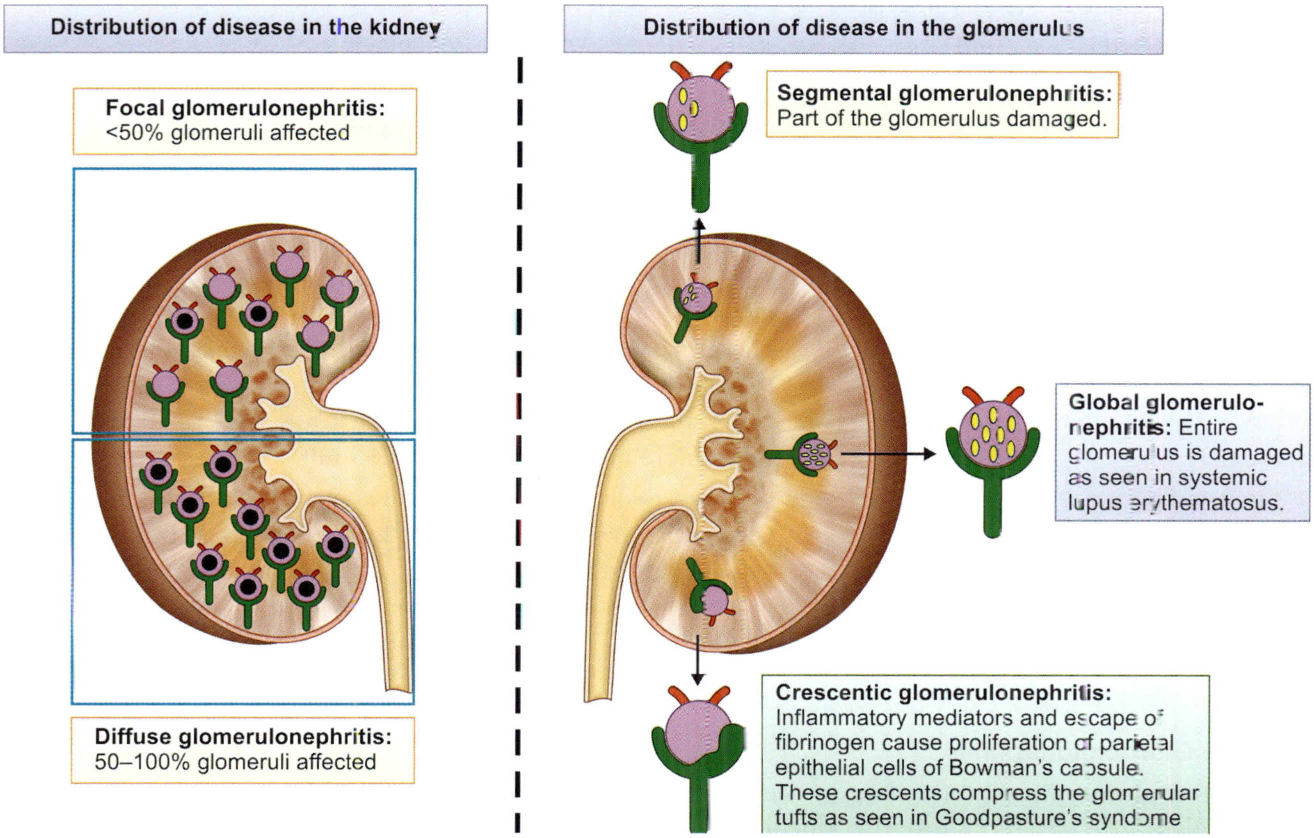

Fig. 22.12: It illustrates distribution of disease in kidney based on glomerular involvement.

Table 22.8: Terminology of glomerulonephritis

Terms	Glomeruli features
Diffuse glomerulonephritis	Glomeruli involvement: >50–100% (bilateral)
Focal glomerulonephritis	Glomeruli involvement: <50% (bilateral)
Global glomerulonephritis	All the capillaries of the glomerulus are affected
Segmental glomerulosclerosis	Segment of glomeruli are affected with hyalinization within the mesangial region
Crescentic glomerulonephritis	Inflamamtory mediators stimulate parietal cells of Bowman's capsule to proliferate and compress glomerular tufts

- *Crescentic glomerulosclerosis:* Inflammatory mediators cause proliferation of parietal epithelial cells in Bowman's syndrome resulting in proliferation of glomerular tuft, e.g. *rapidly proliferative glomerulonephritis* such as Goodpasture's syndrome.

GLOMERULONEPHRITIS: CLASSIFICATION

Glomerulonephritis is classified based on integrity of glomerular basement membrane and cellularity of glomeruli.

These are thin membrane disease, non-proliferative glomerulonephritis and proliferative glomerulonephritis (Table 22.9).

Thin Membrane Disease

It is autosomal dominant benign disorder characterized by thin glomerular basement membrane on electron microscopy.

Patient presents with persistent hematuria and mild proteinuria but overall prognosis is excellent.

Non-proliferative Glomerulonephritis

Injured glomeruli lack increased cellularity. It is seen in *minimal change disease, focal segmental glomerulosclerosis* and *membranous glomerulonephritis*. These glomerular disorders are important causes of nephrotic syndrome.

Table 22.9: Classification of glomerulonephritis

Glomerulonephritis	Features
Thin membrane disease	
Autosomal dominant benign disorder characterized by thin glomerular basement membrane	Persistent hematuria and mild proteinuria but overall prognosis is excellent
Nonproliferative glomerulonephritis	
Minimal change disease	Effacement of visceral epithelial foot processes
Focal segmental glomerulosclerosis	Thickening and wrinkling of glomerular basement membrane, mild increase in mesangial cells and lack of immune complex deposits
Membranous glomerulonephritis	The term membranous is applied to just diffuse thickening of the GBM, without any proliferative change
Proliferative glomerulonephritis	
Endocapillary GN	Cellular proliferation in the capillaries tuft
Extracapillary GN	Cellular proliferation extending into Bowman's capsule
Exudative/necrotizing GN	Glomeruli showing infiltration by leukocytes and necrosis
Membranoproliferative GN	Showing GBM thickening as well as proliferation of endothelial and mesangial cells of glomeruli (hypercellular glomeruli)
Crescentic GN (RPGN)	Involving >80% glomeruli: crescents are proliferations of the parietal cells, which fill Bowman's capsular space around glomeruli

Proliferative Glomerulonephritis

- The injured glomeruli exhibit *increased cellularity (hypercellular glomeruli)*. It occurs either due to proliferation of glomerular cells (*endothelial cells, mesangial cells*) or influx of *inflammatory cells* (neutrophils, macrophages) in glomeruli. *More than 100 nuclei are demonstrated in affected glomeruli (diffuse/focal GN)*.
- Examples of proliferative glomerulonephritis are *endocapillary, GN, extracapillary GN, exudative GN, membranous GN, membranoproliferative GN and crescentic GN.*

GLOMERULONEPHRITIS : PATHOGENESIS

Pathogenesis of glomerulonephritis occurs by three mechanisms: in situ complex mediated, immune complex mediated and ANCA mediated mechanisms. Antigens may be exogenous or endogenous as shown in Fig. 22.13 and Table 22.10.

Table 22.10: Antigens causing glomerulonephritis

Source	Examples of antigens
Exogenous antigens	Bacteria *Viruses:* HBV, HCV *Parasites:* Malarial parasite (falciparum) *Tumors antigens:* Colon cancer, lung cancer and lymphomas *Drugs:* Heroin, gold and penicillamine *Autoimmune:* Systemic lupus erythematosus
Endogenous antigens	Goodpasture's antigen Heymann's antigen

ANTI-GBM-MEDIATED GLOMERULONEPHRITIS

In situ complex-mediated glomerulonephritis, antibodies are directed against GBM antigens (intrinsic/planted). Type II hypersensitivity reaction plays an important role in pathogenesis of *in situ* immune complex-mediated glomerulonephritis (Fig. 22.14).

Antibodies to Endogenous Glomerular Antigen

Goodpasture's syndrome is an autoimmune disorder characterized by rapidly progressive glomerulonephritis (hematuria) and pulmonary hemorrhages (hemoptysis). Antibodies (IgG) are directed against GBM COL4-A3 antigen (Goodpasture antigen) located in non-collagenous domain of type IV collagen fibers. Antibodies are simultaneously directed against pulmonary alveoli (Fig. 22.15).

- *Renal changes:* Over 90% of patients with anti-GBM glomerulonephritis develop crescentic glomerulonephritis. *Glomeruli are hypercellular with crescents and macrophages.* Antibodies directed against the glomerular basement membrane causes rupture of GBM and extravasation of blood and inflammatory cells into the urinary space (i.e. the space between Bowman's capsule and the glomerular capillary tufts). *Fibrinogen stimulates proliferation of Bowman's capsule parietal cells resulting in crescents formation (crescentic glomerulonephritis).* It is worth mentioning that crescentic glomerulonephritis also occurs in Wegener granulomatosis or polyarteritis nodosa (Table 22.11).

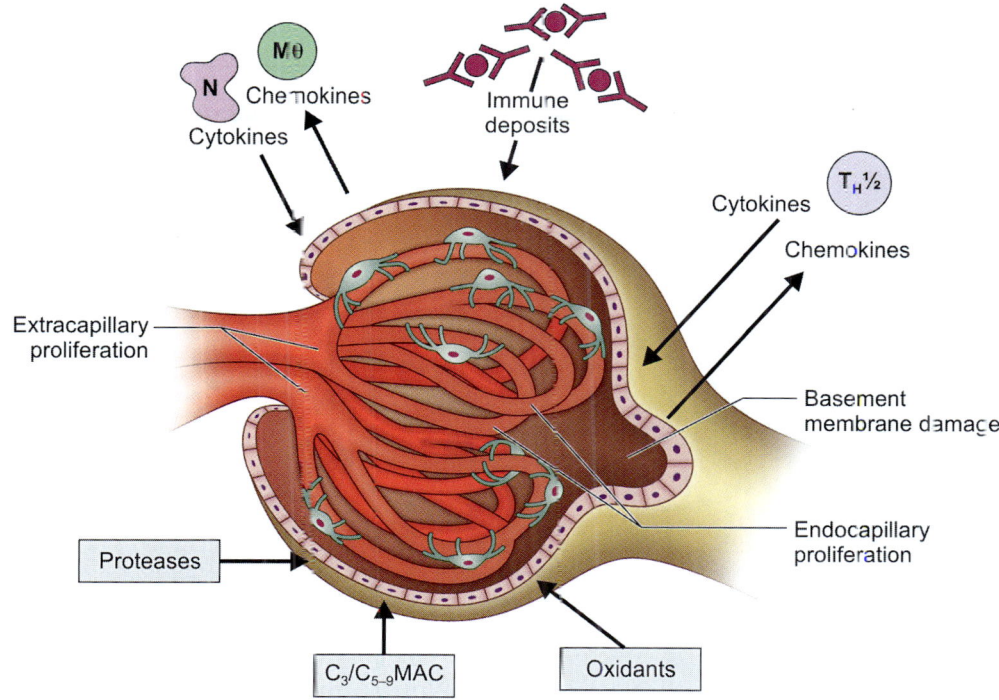

Fig. 22.13: Pathogenesis of glomerulonephritis.

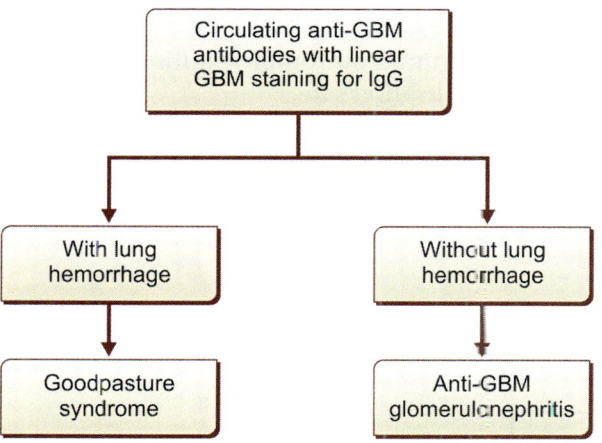

Fig. 22.14: Anti-GBM-mediated glomerulonephritis.

- *Immunofluorescence microscopy:* Diffuse linear immunofluorescence for IgG and C3, fibrin in crescents are seen along the glomerular basement membrane.
- *Clinical course:* Patient presents with *rapidly progressive renal failure, hemoptysis and nephritic syndrome.*

Antibodies to Non-glomerular Planted Antigens

Exogenous antigens derived from *bacterial products, viral products (HBV, HCV), DNA, drugs (penicillamine, gold or heroin), tumors (colon cancer, lung cancer)* and *parasite (malarial parasite)* are planted in glomeruli via *hematogenous route.*

Antibodies are formed against these planted fixed antigens in glomerular basement membrane resulting in immune complex formation that cause glomerular injury.

Immunofluorescence staining: Immunofluorescence staining of renal section reveals *lumpy bumpy granular pattern in subepithelial region of glomeruli.*

IMMUNE COMPLEX-MEDIATED GLOMERULONEPHRITIS

Type III hypersensitivity reaction plays an important role in the immune complex-mediated glomerulonephritis.

Pathogenesis

- Since the preformed immune complexes represent large protein aggregates that cannot pass through the GBM, they are *trapped.*

Table 22.11: Morphological features of anti-GBM-mediated glomerulonephritis (Goodpasture's syndrome)

Parameters	Characteristics
Cell proliferation	Some increase in mesangial cells. Neutrophilic infiltration in affected glomeruli
Glomerular basement membrane alterations	Some thickening and irregularity of glomerular basement membrane.
Immune complex deposition	Deposition of IgG and C3 along basement membrane in a 'linear fashion'. This feature is present in >90% of cases.
Other cases	Approximately 80% of cases show presence of 'crescents' wholly or partially obliterating the urinary space.

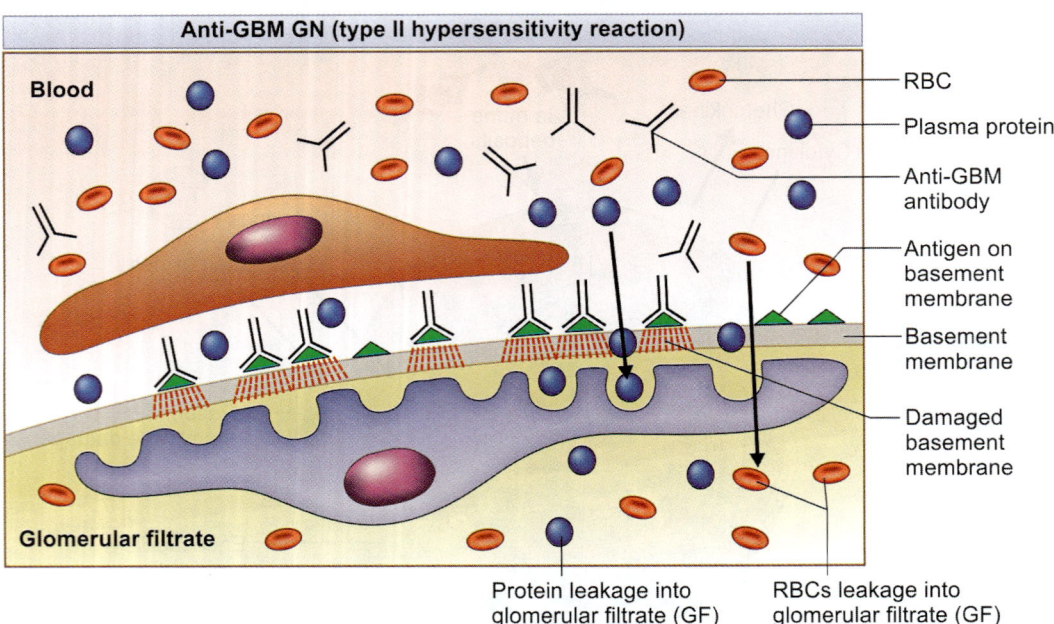

Fig. 22.15: Pathogenesis of anti-GBM-mediated glomerulonephritis.

- Depending on the size, solubility, and electrical charge of the immune complexes, they may get deposited on the subepithelial, or subendothelial, or intramembranous region of GBM or mesangial matrix regions.
- Platelets, basophils, complement and inflammatory cells play an important role in the pathogenesis of immune complex-mediated glomerulonephritis.
- Immune complexes activate complement system. Complement increases glomerular permeability and attracts neutrophils.
- Neutrophils phagocytose immune complexes. Frustrated phagocytosis by neutrophils cause to liberation of hydrolytic enzymes and glomerular damage.
- Platelets form microthrombi resulting in decreased glomerular filtration rate.

Basophils and platelets also release vasoactive amines leading to increased glomerular permeability (Figs 22.16 and 22.17).

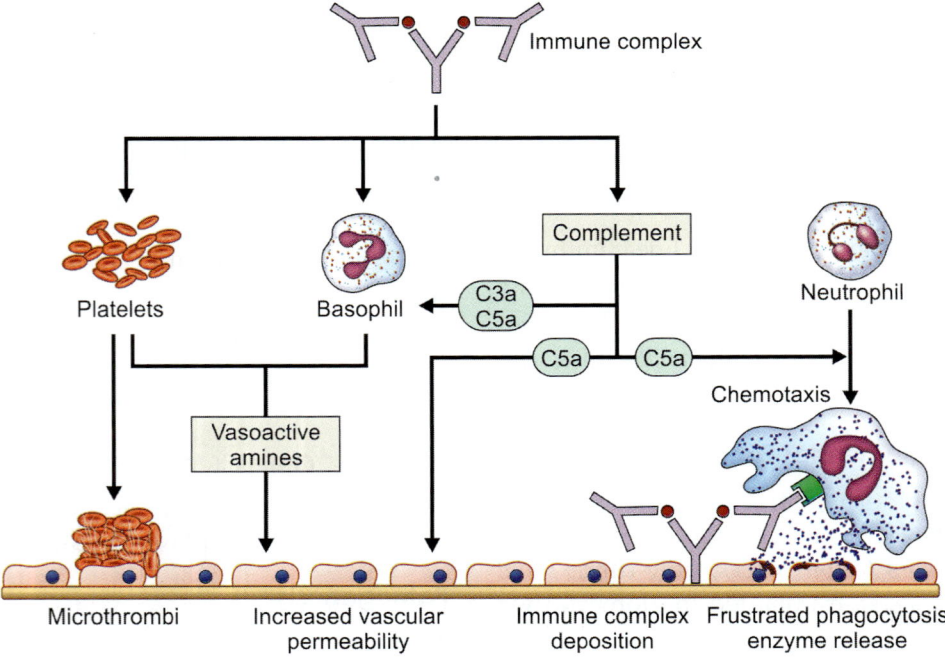

Fig. 22.16: Immune complex-mediated glomerulonephritis. Immune complexes can be trapped in the kidney and elsewhere in the body, can activate complement, and cause other damaging responses.

Kidney and Ureter

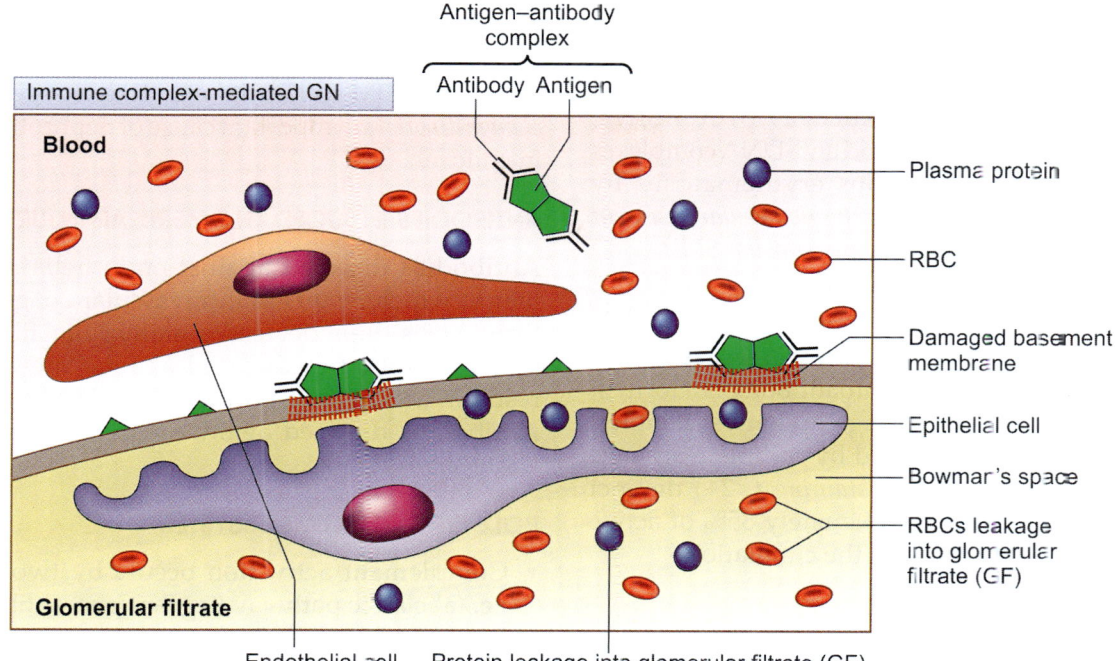

Fig. 22.17: Pathogenesis of immune complex-mediated glomerulonephritis (type III hypersensitivity).

Examples of Immune Complex-mediated GN

These include IgA nephropathy, Henoch-Schönlein purpura, lupus nephritis, acute post-streptococcal glomerulonephritis, membranous glomerulonephritis, and membranoproliferative glomerulonephritis (Fig. 22.18).

Fate of Circulating Immune Complexes

Short-lived antigen antibody complexes are degraded by polymorphonuclear cells, monocytes, macrophages, mesangial cells and endogenous proteases.

Repeated cycle of formation of antigen-antibody complexes formed in circulation, are trapped in glomeruli and causing glomerular injury.

Location of Immune Complexes

- Highly anionic macromolecules are excluded by glomerular basement membrane. These are trapped in *subendothelial region* of kidney.
- Highly cationic immunogens tend to cross *subepithelial region* and bind to anionic sites, DNA nucleosome and other nuclear proteins.
- Neutral charged molecules are trapped in mesangial region. Large circulating complexes are not usually nephritogenic. These are cleared by reticuloendothelial system.

Mechanism of Glomerular Injury

- Immune complexes activate the complement system. C5a is produced which is chemotactic

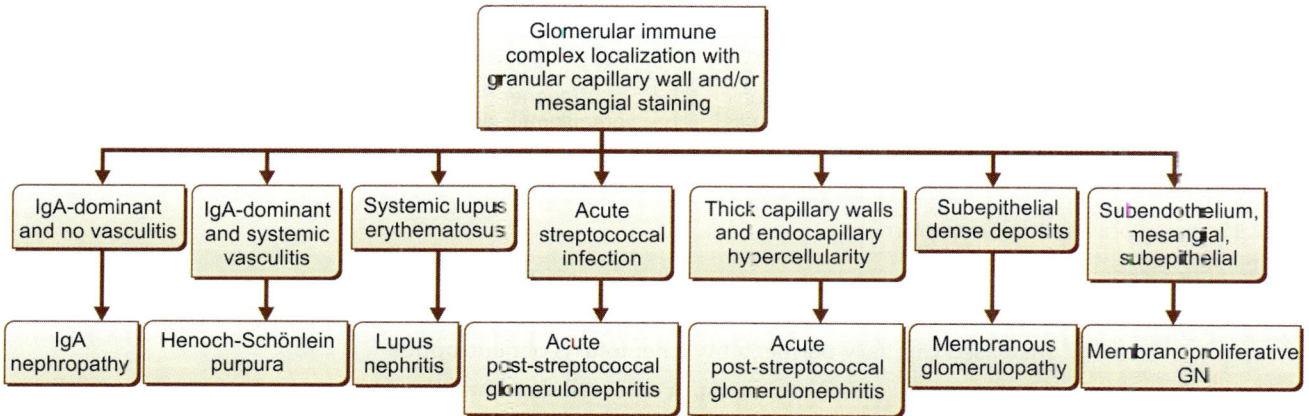

Fig. 22.18: Examples of immune complex-mediated glomerulonephritis.

for neutrophils. Neutrophils damage the glomeruli by *liberating hydrolytic enzymes (frustrated phagocytosis)*.
- Depending on extent of glomeruli injury, patient develops manifestations such as proteinuria, hematuria and uremia. DNA and anti-DNA complexes are formed in systemic lupus erythematosus by forming *granular deposits along the glomerular basement membrane in systemic lupus erythematosus (SLE)*.

ANCA GLOMERULONEPHRITIS

Pauci-immune and ANCA glomerulonephritis and vasculitis: Antineutrophilic cytoplasmic autoantibody is a form of small vessel vasculitis involving capillaries, venules, and arterioles. It is characterized by complete absence or paucity of *ummunoglobulin staining* (<2+) distinct from anti-GBM disease. Approximately 85% of active untreated cases show ANCA in the circulation.

Major Clinicopathologic Expression

The major clinicopathologic expression of pauci-immune and ANCA-associated vasculitis include crescentic glomerulonephritis, microscopic angitis, Wegener's granulomatosis (granuloma with polyangiitis), and eosinophilic granulomtosis with polyangiitis (Churg-Strauss syndrome) (Fig. 22.19).

> **Light Microscopy**
> - Light microscopy shows fibrinoid necrosis and crescent formation.
> - In <10% of cases, glomerulonephritis may be accompanied by necrotizing arteritis (interlobular and vasa recta).

ROLE OF TYPE IV HYPERSENSITIVITY REACTION

Cytokines synthesized by T cells damage podocytes and cause the GBM to lose its negative charge in *minimal change disease,* an important cause of nephrotic syndrome in children.

ANTIBODIES INDUCED GLOMERULAR INJURY

Antibodies directed against endothelial cells cause injury, which results in intravascular coagulation and thrombosis, thus decreases glomerular filtration rate (GFR). Antibodies directed against mesangial cells result in mesangiolysis or mesangial cell proliferation. Antibodies directed against visceral epithelial cells result in proteinuria.

ROLE OF COMPLEMENT SYSTEM

- Complement activation occurs by two pathways, i.e. (a) classic pathway (e.g. antigen-antibody complexes (IgG and IgM), bacterial products, viruses) and (b) alternative pathway (e.g. microorganisms and IgA).
- Chemotactic fragments mediate influx of neutrophils and macrophages.
- Complement (C3–C5) may also increase the permeability of the GBM and cause mechanical lesions through the action of membrane attack complex (C5–C9) (Table 22.12).

ROLE OF NEPHRITIC FACTORS (Ne-AP AND Ne-CP)

Normally C3 convertase enzyme causes break down of complement. While properdin opposes the action of

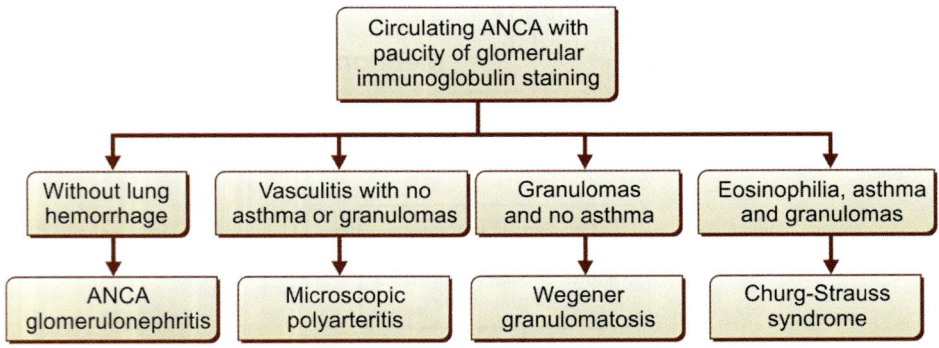

Fig. 22.19: Examples of ANCA glomerulonephritis.

Table 22.12: Biological effects of complement

Complement cascade	Actions
C3a	Increased capillary permeability; opsonization of bacteria and phagocytosis by macrophage
C5a	Increased capillary permeability; chemotaxis of neutrophils
C3a and C5a	Contraction of smooth muscle and mast cell degranulation
C5 to C9	Lysis of pathogens or target cells by the membrane attack complex

C3 convertase. Nephritic factors (Ne-AP and Ne-CP) are the immunoglobulins which inactivate inhibitors of C3 convertase, i.e. properdin. Thus, break down of complement continues; and results in low serum complement levels.

ROLE OF CYTOKINES AND CHEMOKINES

- Cytokines (especially interleukin-1) and chemokines participate in the recruitment of inflammatory cells and their activation. These can directly contribute to the injury to the GBM. Mesangial cells also synthesize various substances, which initiate inflammatory response in the absence of leukocytic infiltration.
- CXC chemokine (α-chemokine) participates in activation and chemotaxis of neutrophils. Neutrophils liberate hydrolytic enzymes resulting in glomerular injury. MCP-1 (monocyte chemotactic protein-1) synthesized by mesangial cells attracts monocytes. RANTES (regulated and named T cell expressed and secreted): synthesized by mesangial cells attracts lymphocytes (Table 22.13).

ROLE OF INFLAMMATORY CELLS

Neutrophils, lymphocytes, monocytes/macrophages and natural killer cells participate in the pathogenesis of glomerulonephritis. Neutrophils and macrophages synthesize proteases oxygen derived free radicals arachiodonic acid metabolite, which decrease GFR. On activation of macrophages, T cells and natural killer cells produce biologically active molecules, which participate in the pathogenesis of glomerulonephritis.

ROLE OF PLATELETS

Platelets possess C3 and Fc receptors. Platelets synthesize eicosanoids and platelet derived growth factor (PDGF). PDGF causes mesangial cell proliferation of glomeruli. Platelet degranulation occurs and release vasoactive peptides (histamine, serotonin), which increase glomerular permeability.

ROLE OF PDGF, FGF-β AND TGF-β

- PDGF synthesized by platelets causes proliferation of mesangial cells. Transforming growth factor-β and fibroblast growth factor produce extracellular matrix deposition and hyalinization of glomeruli.
- Transforming growth factor-β promotes extracellular matrix synthesis and contributes to glomerulosclerosis in later stages of the disease (Table 22.14).

ROLE OF COAGULATION SYSTEM

- Glomerular injury causes activation of clotting factors to produce fibrin. Fibrin traps platelets and form microthrombi, resulting in reduced glomerular filtration rate.
- Macrophages participate in deposition of fibrin. Fibrin acts as a stimulus to form crescents in glomeruli by parietal cells of Bowman's capsule

Table 22.13: Chemokines and their actions

Chemokines	Examples and actions	Net result
C-X-C chemokine (α-chemokine)	α-chemokine	Neutrophils activation and recruitment
C-C chemokine (β-chemokine)	MCP-1 (monocyte chemotactic protein-1) RANTES (regulated and named T cell expressed and secreted) Eotaxin	Monocytes recruitment Lymphocytes recruitment Eosinophils and basophils recruitment
C-chemokine (γ-chemokine), e.g. *lymphotoxin*	Lymphotoxin	Lymphocytes recruitment
CX3C chemokine, e.g. *fractalkine*	Fractalkine participates	Monocytes and T cells recruitment and strong adhesion between monocytes and T cells

Table 22.14: Role of growth factors in the pathogenesis of glomerulopathy

Growth factor	Source/synthesis	Net result
PDGF	Macrophages, smooth muscle cells, endothelial cells, keratinocytes. PDGF is stored in platelets	Proliferation of mesangial cells
FGF-β	Macrophages, T cells, endothelial cells, platelets, many other cells	Deposition of extracellular matrix and hyalinization of glomeruli
TGF-β	Macrophages, T cells, endothelial cells, platelets	Deposition of extracellular matrix and hyalinization of glomeruli

Plasminogen activator inhibitor-1 (PAI-1) inhibits degradation of fibrin and matrix proteins; thereby causing thrombosis and fibrosis.

ROLE OF PROSTAGLANDINS, NITRIC OXIDE AND ENDOTHELIN

- These chemical mediators act on endothelial, mesangial, and epithelial cells and may play key role in regulating the blood flow through the inflamed glomeruli.
- PGD-2 promotes platelets aggregation and causes vasodilation, and increased vascular permeability of glomeruli.
- PGD-2 and PGE-2 modulate leukocytic phagocytic activity. Nitric oxide causes vasodilatation by relaxing vascular smooth muscle cells (Table 22.15).
- Endothelin is potent vasoconstrictor, synthesized by endothelial cells.

SYNDROMES OF GLOMERULAR DISEASES

Glomerular diseases produce various clinical syndromes. These include nephritic syndrome, nephrotic syndrome, rapidly progressively glomerulonephritis, chronic renal failure and end stage renal disease.

Other disorders are asymptomatic hematuria or asymptomatic proteinuria detected on routine urine examination (Tables 22.16 and 22.17).

Table 22.15: Pathogenesis of glomerulonephritis

In situ complex-mediated glomerulonephritis	Antibodies to endogenous (intrinsic) Goodpasture's antigen
	Antibodies to exogenous (planted) antigen
Immune complex-mediated glomerulonephritis (type III hypersensitivity reaction)	Immune complexes formed elsewhere are trapped in glomeruli
ANCA glomerulonephritis	It also participates in pathogenesis of glomerulonephritis
Role of type IV hypersensitivity reaction	It also participates in pathogenesis of glomerulonephritis
Role of antibodies	Injury to glomerular endothelial cells, mesangial cells and visceral endothelial cells
Role of complement system	C3a and C5a increase glomerular permeability. C5a attracts neutrophils. During phagocytosis, neutrophils liberate hydrolytic enzymes leading to glomerular injury
Role of nephritic factors (Ne-AP and Ne-CP)	Nephritic factors inactivate properdin, that normally stabilizes C3 convertase leading to unchecked breakdown of complement
Cytokines: IL-1 and chemokines	Recruitment of inflammatory cells at site of glomerular injury
Role of inflammatory cells	Release of hydrolytic enzymes and synthesis of chemical mediators
Role of platelets	Platelets release histamine and serotonin leading to increased glomerular permeability
Role of growth factors	PDGF causes proliferation of mesangial cells. FGF-β and TGF-β cause deposition of extracellular matrix deposition and hyalinization of glomeruli
Role of coagulation factor	Glomerular endothelial injury activate clotting factors leading to formation of microthrombi and hence reduction in GFR
Role of chemical mediators	PGD2 promotes platelets aggregation and increases glomerular permeability

Table 22.16: Syndromes of glomerular disease

Syndrome	Mechanism	Clinical manifestation
Nephritic syndrome	Glomerular perfusion failure (usually transient)	Hematuria, proteinuria <3.5 gm/24 hours (most often <2 gm/day), azotemia, oliguria, periorbital edema and hypertension
Nephrotic syndrome	Glomerular permeability	Massive proteinuria ≥3.5 gm/24 hours, lipiduria, hypoproteinemia, hyperlipidemia, and generalized edema
Rapidly progressive glomerulonephritis (RPGN)	Crescents formation (Bowman's capsule parietal cells proliferation) as a result of leakage of fibrinogen	Nephritic syndrome progressing to renal failure

Contd...

Table 22.16: Syndromes of glomerular disease (Contd...)

Syndrome	Mechanism	Clinical manifestation
Chronic renal failure (GFR <20% of normal)	Chronic irreversible nephron failure both glomerular and tubular failure. There is progressive parenchymal destruction	Azotemia progressing to uremia over months to years
End stage renal disease (GFR <5% of normal)	Glomeruli are markedly sclerosed, tubular atrophy with thyroidization, interstitial fibrosis and vascular thickening	Terminal stage with uremic manifestations

Other disorders are asymptomatic hematuria or asymptomatic proteinuria detected on routine urine examination: if GFR is 50% of normal, patient is asymptomatic but prone to uremia. If GFR is 20–50% of normal, kidney's concentrating ability is decreased and patient is prone to uremia.

Table 22.17: Comparison between nephritic syndrome and nephrotic syndrome

Parameters	Nephritic syndrome	Nephrotic syndrome
Proteinuria	<2.0 g/day	≥3.5 g/day
Serum proteins	Total serum proteins decreased up to lesser extent *Albumin:* Globulin normal	Total serum proteins markedly decreased *Albumin:* Globulin is reversed (normal albumin/globulin is 2:1)
Hyperlipidemia	Uncommon	Common due to increased synthesis of lipoproteins by liver to compensate protein loss in urine
Edema	Mild around periorbital region	Severe generalized edema (pitting edema legs, pleural effusion, ascites)
Hypertension	Present	Less frequent
Serum complement	Decreased	Most often normal
Urine analysis	*24 hours urine output:* Oliguria *Color:* Smoky-colored due to hematuria *Specific gravity:* Increased due to proteins in urine *Urinary sediment:* Dysmorphic RBCs and RBCs casts	*24 hours urine output:* Normal *Color:* Milky or frothy due to lipiduria *Specific gravity:* Increased due to proteins in urine. Sugar is present in diabetic nephropathy. In diabetic nephropathy, sugar present in urine also raises specific gravity. *Urinary sediment:* Hyaline casts
Etiology	Post-streptococcal GN Post-nonstreptococcal GN (post infectious) IgA nephropathy Goodpasture's syndrome Wegener's granulomatosis Henoch-Schönlein purpura	Minimal change Membranous GN Membranoproliferative GN Focal segmental glomerulosclerosis Diabetic nephropathy Amyloid nephropathy
Prognosis	Recovery occurs in 95% cases of post-streptococcal glomerulonephritis. A few cases develop rapidly progressive glomerulonephritis	Prognosis is excellent in minimal change disease, as it responds to corticosteroid therapy. Prognosis is variable in other disorders

NEPHROTIC SYNDORME

Nephrotic syndrome is characterized by heavy proteinuria (>3.5 g protein/24 hours), hypoproteinemia (resulting from proteinuria), hyperlipidemia (compensatory synthesis of lipoproteins by liver), generalized edema (resulting from decreased plasma colloid oncotic pressure) and lipiduria.

Nephrotic syndrome occurs due to increased basement membrane permeability, permitting the urinary loss of plasma proteins, particularly low molecular weight proteins, such as albumin. Glomerular diseases associated with nephrotic syndrome and its pathogenesis are shown in Table 22.18 and Fig. 22.20.

Table 22.18: Glomerular diseases commonly associated with nephrotic syndrome

Disorder	Light microscopy	Immunofluorescence patterns	Electron microscopy findings	Prognosis
Minimal change disease	Glomeruli appear normal. Positive fat stains in glomeruli and tubules	No pattern	Effacement of the podocytes of visceral layer of Bowman's capsule	Corticosteroid therapy effective. Prognosis is excellent in 90%
Membranous GN	Diffuse thickening of GBM Reticulin stain demonstrates spikes and domes due to immune complex deposition in subepithelial region	*Granular pattern:* IgG and C3	Subepithelial deposits and fusion of podocytes of visceral layer of Bowman's capsule	About 40–50% patients progress to end stage disease
Focal segmental glomerulosclerosis	Focal segmental disease with sclerosis of glomeruli. Detachment of epithelial cells from GBM is the hallmark of disorder	IgM and C3 in some cases	Fusion of podocytes, but no electron dense deposit	Poor prognosis in 50–80% as patient develops end stage disease within 10 years. There is recurrence after renal transplantation
Membranoprilipherative GN	*Type I:* Diffuse thickening of basement membrane. Special stain shows double contour of GBM (tram track appearance) due to ingrowth of mesangial cells between endothelial cells and GBM *Type II:* Tram track appearance is not prominent	*Type I:* Granular pattern : IgG, IgM, C3, C1q, C4 *Type II:* Granular pattern: C3 present but lack IgG, C1q, C4	*Type I:* Electron dense deposits in subendothelial region *Type II:* Electron dense deposits in within basement membrane	Prognosis is poor. About 50% patients develop chronic renal failure within 10 years Prognosis is poor. About 50% patients develop chronic renal failure within 10 years
Diabetic glomerulo-sclerosis (Kimmelstiel-Wilson disease)	Ball-like deposits are present in the mesangial region. Hyaline arteriosclerosis	Trapping of proteins	No electron dense deposits. It shows fusion of podocytes and thickening of basement membrane	Diabetic nephropathy is important cause of end stage disease. Other lesions are papillary necrosis, acute pyelonephritis and chronic pyelonephritis
Amyloid nephropathy	Thickening of GBM. Congo red stain under polarized microscope reveals apple-green birefringence (color of Grammy Smith apple)	Nonspecific trapping of proteins	Amyloid fibrils in mesangial region, GBM and renal tubules	Renal failure is common cause of fatal outcome
Pre-eclampsia/eclampsia (pregnancy-induced hypertension)	*Diffuse disorder:* Glomeruli are bloodless. Endothelial cells are swollen	Nonspecific deposits of IgG, IgM fibrin	Vacuolated endothelial cells and widening of sub-endothelial spaces	Reversible disorder
Systemic lupus erythematosus-induced nephropathy	*Type IV:* Diffuse proliferative GN: endocapillary and/or extracapillary proliferation in 50% or more glomeruli ('wire loop lesion') *Type V:* Membranous GN: thick glomerular loops and increased cellularity of mesangial cells	Mesangial and glomerular loop + Mesangial and glomerular loop +	Mesangial and subendothelial deposits Numerous subepithelial and scattered mesangial deposits	Nephrotic syndrome progresses to chronic renal failure Nephrotic syndrome progresses to chronic renal failure

Kidney and Ureter

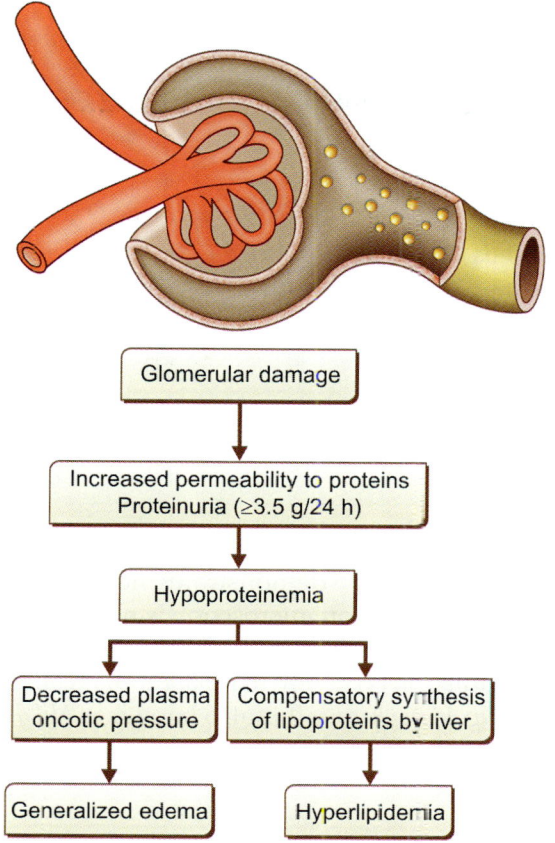

Nephrotic syndrome	
Parameters	Urinary and blood findings
• Proteinuria	≥3.5 g/day
• Generalized edema	It is due to decreased serum albumin levels.
• Hyperlipidemia	The liver synthesizes extra lipoproteins (especially LDL) as a non-specific response to decreased plasma oncotic pressure due to proteinuria.

Note: Urine sediment—analysis, it shows hyaline cast, oval fat body (lipid containing renal tubular cells). Oval fat bodies under polarized microscopy appear as 'maltese-cross' pattern.

Risk factors associated with nephrotic syndrome	
Risk	Mechanism
• Hypercoagulability of the blood with thrombosis of renal and deep veins	Loss of antithrombin III and antiplasmin
• Atheromatous plaques	High LDL and cholesterol levels
• Recurrent infections	Loss of antibodies in the gamma fraction of plasma
• Microcytic hypochromic anemia	Loss of transferrin bound iron

Fig. 22.20: Pathogenesis of nephrotic syndrome.

Proteinuria

Proteinuria occurs in nephrotic syndrome due to damage to glomeruli by the following mechanisms:
- Damage to the integrity of the epithelial cells, as in minimal change disease or *focal segmental glomerulosclerosis*.
- Immune deposition occurs within the capillary wall, as in *membranous glomerulonephritis*.
- Damage to the integrity of the basement membrane by excessive accumulation of abnormal membrane-like material, occurs as in *diabetes mellitus*.
- Deposition of extraneous substances occurs within the wall, as in *amyloid deposition*.

Clinical Correlation

Patient with nephrotic syndrome excrete various essential metabolic products in urine such as proteins, sugar, ketone bodies, immunoglobulins (recurrent infection), transferrin bound iron loss (iron deficiency anemia), antithrombin III, antiplasmin (renal vein thrombosis), thyroxine binding proteins, zinc binding proteins, and copper binding proteins.

Urine Analysis

- *Proteins lost in urine:* These are albumin, globulins, immunoglobulins, thyroxine binding protein, transferrin bound iron, vitamin D binding protein, zinc binding proteins, copper binding protein, antithrombin III, and antiplasmin.
- *Light microscopy:* It reveals hyaline casts, oval fat bodies or pus cells. Oval fat bodies are lipid-containing renal tubular epithelial cells. When examined by polarized light, the lipids in casts are seen as being doubly refractile or birefringent and displaying a symmetric '*Maltese-cross pattern*'.

Biochemistry

Patient should be investigated by estimating total serum proteins, albumin/globulin ratio, lipid profile, blood urea and serum creatinine, serum testing (HbsAg, HIV).

Etiology of Nephrotic Syndrome

Etiology of nephrotic syndrome varies in adults and children (Table 22.19).

Table 22.19: Main causes of nephrotic syndrome in adults and children

Causes of nephrotic syndrome in adults		Causes of nephrotic syndrome in childhood	
Disorder	Frequency (%)	Disorder	Frequency (%)
Diabetes nephropathy	40%	Minimal change disease	60%
Lupus nephritis	-	Focal glomerulosclerosis	10%
Amyloid nephropathy	-	All forms of proliferative glomerulonephritis	10%
Membranous glomerulonephritis	20%	Membranous glomerulonephritis	5%
All forms of proliferative glomerulonephritis	15%	Glomerulopathy secondary to systemic disorders	5%
Minimal change disease	10%		
Focal glomerulosclerosis	10%		
Membranoproliferative glomerulonephritis	5%		

Minimal change disease responds to corticosteroid therapy and prognosis is excellent.

MINIMAL CHANGE DISEASE

Age Group

- Minimal change disease is most common cause of nephrotic syndrome in young children (65%). It can also occur in adults either primary or secondary to Hodgkin's disease (nodular sclerosis), chronic lymphocytic leukemia, or atopic allergies.

- Light microscopy demonstrates normal-appearing glomeruli. Electron microscopy is normal except for the disappearance of epithelial foot processes. Lipid accumulation is present in renal tubular cells referred to as *lipoid nephrosis*. It is also known as *Nil disease*. It responds well to steroid therapy. It does not progress to renal failure (Fig. 22.21).

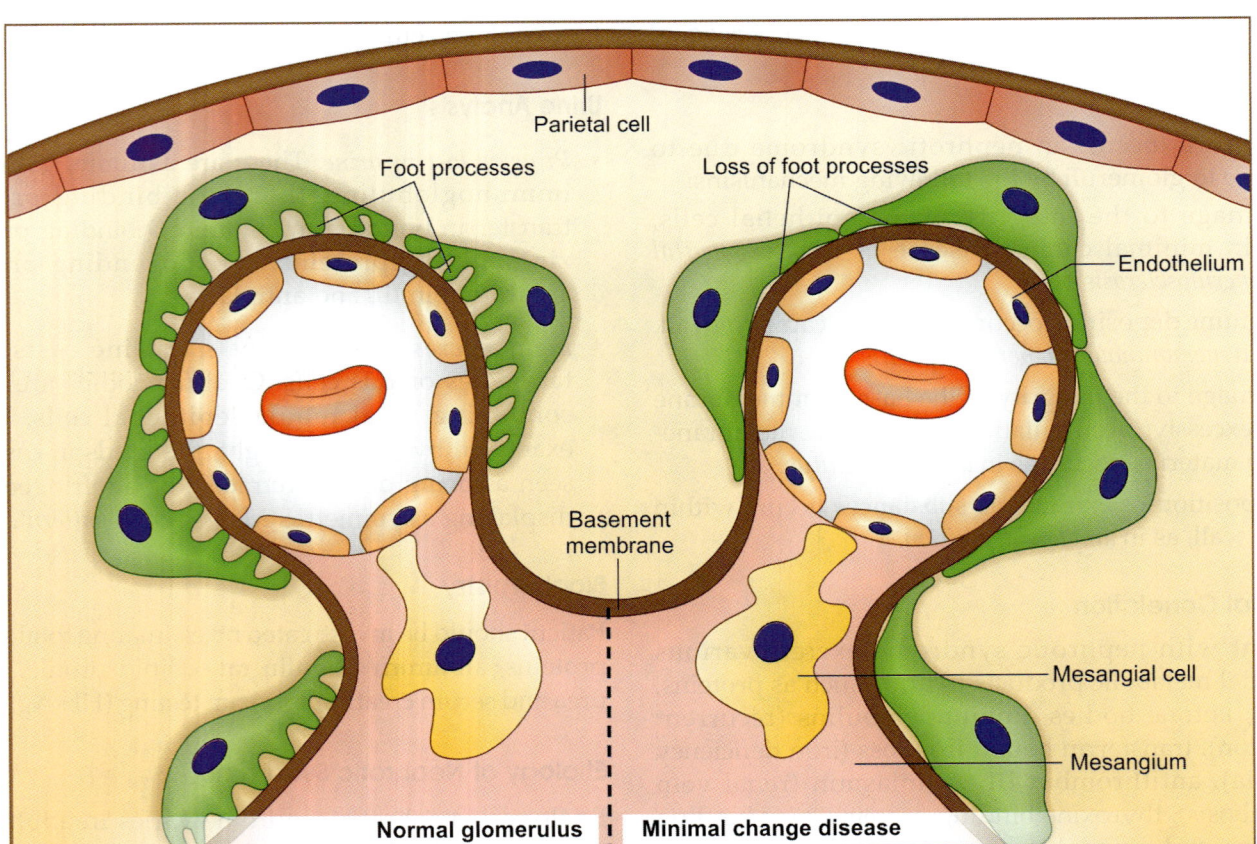

Fig. 22.21: Minimal change disease—this disorder shows effacement of podocytes (foot processes of visceral epithelial cells of Bowman's capsule) on electron microscopy. All other glomerular structures appear intact (*Courtesy by* Dr Abhijit Das).

Etiopathogenesis

- Exact mechanism is unknown. It is thought to be related to upper respiratory infection that alters host response resulting in type IV hypersensitivity reaction or synthesis of cytokines (lymphokines) by abnormal T cells. These lymphokines cause ballooning of visceral epithelial cells resulting in effacement of podocytes and loss of charge dependent barrier of glomerular basement membrane.
  Loss of polyanions proteoglycans leads to massive proteinuria.
- Minimal change disease is associated with atopic history, Hodgkin's disease (nodular) sclerosis, non-Hodgkin's lymphoma and chronic lymphocytic leukemias.

Light Microscopy

Light microscopy reveals normal glomeruli. Fat stains demonstrate presence of lipid in the tubules and glomeruli (Fig. 22.22 and Table 22.20).

Electron Microscopy

It demonstrates total *effacement of visceral epithelial foot processes* with weakening of slit-pore membranes.

This retraction presumably results from extensive cell swelling and occurs in virtually all cases of proteinuria in the nephrotic range.

Immunofluorescent Microscopy

Immunofluorescence study is insignificant in minimal change disease. Occasionally it shows minimal amounts of IgM in the mesangial region.

Clinical Features

The patient with minimal change disease presents with features of nephrotic syndrome; characterized by massive selective proteinuria 3.5 gm or >/24 hours (average 10 gm/24 hours), hypoproteinemia with severe hypoalbuminemia, hypercholesterolemia and generalized edema. It is accompanied by acellular urinary sediment. Less common clinical features include hypertension (30% in children, 50% in adults) and allergic symptoms 40% in children.

Prognosis

Primary responders are patients who have complete remission (<0.2 mg/ 24 hours of proteinuria) after a single course of prednisolone. Approximately 90–95% of children will develop a complete remission after 8 weeks of steroid therapy, and 80–85% of adults will achieve complete remission after a course of 20–24 weeks.

FOCAL SEGMENTAL GLOMERULOSCLEROSIS (FSGS)

- Focal segmental glomerulosclerosis is a pattern of injury seen in many conditions. Glomeruli at the corticomedullary junction are affected without inflammation and immune complex deposits. It refers to glomerular injury, which is focal (involving some glomeruli, but not all), and segmental (involving part of glomerulus).
- It is a major cause of nephrotic syndrome affecting adults as well as children. Renal biopsy from uninvolved glomeruli sometimes leads to a misdiagnosis of minimal change disease (Table 22.21).

Etiology

- It may be due to multiple factors, i.e. mutations, viruses (HIV), intravenous heroin abuse, massive obesity, IgA nephropathy, unilateral renal agenesis and congenital nephrotic syndrome (19q13). Nephropathy associated with HIV infection is a severe and rapidly progressive collapsing form of FSGS (Table 22.22).

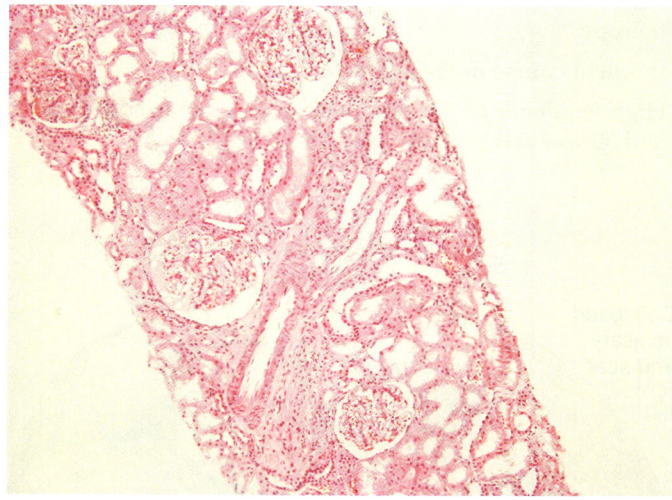

Fig. 22.22: Minimal change disease. Light microscopy reveals normal glomeruli (100X).

Table 22.20: Morphological features in minimal change disease

Parameters	Characteristics
Cell proliferation	Absent
Glomerular basement membrane alteration	Absent
Immune complex deposition	Absent
Other features	Withdrawal of foot processes due to loss of glomerular polyanion demonstrated on electron microscopy

Table 22.21: Working classification of focal segmental glomerulosclerosis (FSGS)

Type	Histologic features	Possible prognostic implication
FSGS NOS (not otherwise specified)	Segmental sclerosis	Typical course
Collapsing FSGS	Collapse of glomerular tuft, visceral epithelial hyperplasia	Poor prognosis
Cellular FSGS	Endocapillary proliferation, often visceral hyperplasia	Early stage lesion Related to tip
Tip lesion FSGS	Sclerosis/adhesion at proximal tubule pole	Better prognosis
Perihilar variant FSGS	Sclerosis and hyalinosis at vascular pole	May reflect a secondary type of FSGS

Table 22.22: Causes of focal segmental glomerulosclerosis

HIV nephropathy
Heroin addiction nephropathy
Sickle cell disease involving kidney
Massive obesity
IgA nephropathy
Reflux nephropathy
Unilateral renal agenesis (congenital)
Congenital nephrotic syndrome linked to chromosome (19q13)
Idiopathic FSGS (10–15%)

Table 22.23: Salient features of idiopathic focal segmental glomerulosclerosis

Incidence: 10–15%
Higher incidence of hematuria, reduced GFR and hypertension
Nephrotic syndrome (30% adults and 10% children)
Persistent proteinuria and progressive decline in renal function
Only patients with tip lesion respond to corticosteroid therapy
Indolent course in FSGS due to obesity
High incidence of developing chronic glomerulonephritis and 50% of cases go into end stage kidney

- Focal segmental glomerulosclerosis may be idiopathic (Table 22.23).
- Patients progress to end stage renal disease in less than a year. In reflux nephropathy, reduction in renal mass causes adaptive stress on the reduced number of nephrons resulting in increased capillary pressure and filtration and enlargement of glomeruli due to functional overwork of glomeruli (Fig. 22.23).

Pathogenesis

Possible mechanisms include T cell-mediated circulating permeability factor, TGF-β mediated cellular proliferation and mesangial matrix synthesis, and vacuolization of visceral epithelial cells (podocytes), associated with genetic mutations.

Light Microscopy
- Glomeruli show sclerotic areas. Visceral epithelial cells show vacuolization.
- Detachment of epithelial cells from GBM is hallmark of disease (Table 22.24 and Fig. 22.24).

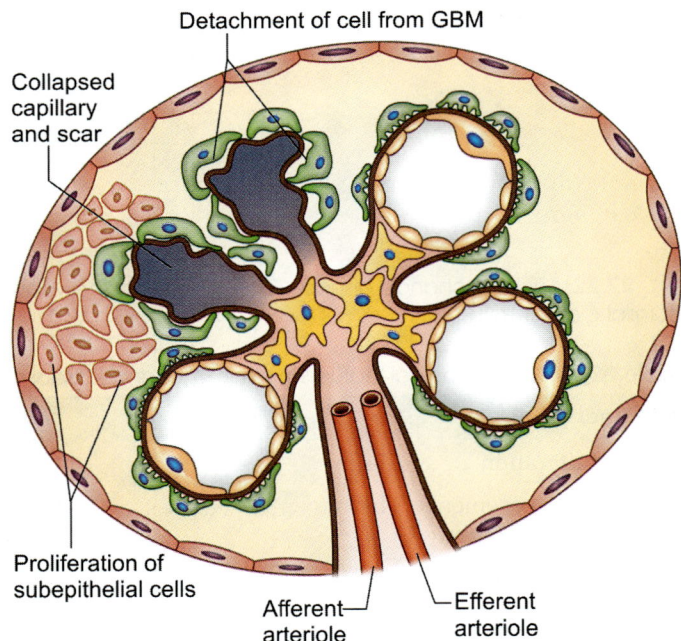

Fig. 22.23: It illustrates focal segmental glomerulosclerosis. Detachment of epithelial cells from GBM is hallmark of disease.

Table 22.24: Morphological features of focal segmental glomerulosclerosis

Parameters	Characteristics
Cell proliferation	Mild increase in number of mesangial cells
Glomerular basement membrane alterations	Thickening and wrinkling of basement membrane
Immune complex deposition	Absent
Other findings	Early stage: Foam cells in glomerular capillaries and focal adhesions to Bowman's capsule
	Acellular, hyaline periodic acid–Schiff (PAS) positive material is distributed segmentally. Affected segment eventually collapse and hyaline masses enlarge
	It shows retraction of foot processes of epithelial cells

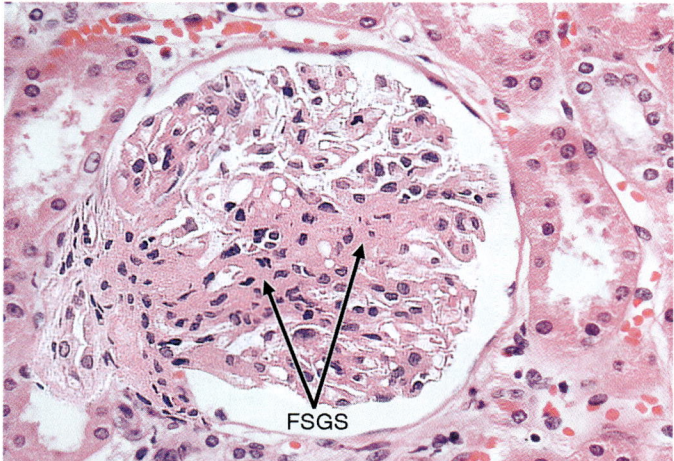

Fig. 22.24: Focal segmental glomerulosclerosis. Light microscopy shows sclerosis of glomerulus. Detachment of epithelial cells from GBM is hallmark of disease (arrows) (400X).

Immunofluorescence Microscopy

It reveals deposition of IgM and C3 in some cases of focal segmental glomeruli.

Electron Microscopy

Glomeruli show fusion of podocytes but lack electron dense deposits.

Clinical Manifestations

Patient presents with nephrotic syndrome in adults (30%) and children (10%). It may be associated with hematuria, and hypertension. It does not respond well to steroid treatment.

Prognosis

Approximately 60–80% of patients develop end stage renal disease (renal failure) within 10 years. Recurrence is common after renal transplant.

MEMBRANOUS GLOMERULONEPHRITIS (MGN)

Membranous glomerulonephritis is a frequent cause of the nephrotic syndrome in adults (30–50 years). It more often affects men than women. It is a slowly progressive disorder. It shows a little response to steroid therapy. Glomerular capillaries are 5–10 times thickened.

Etiology

- *Primary or idiopathic MGN:* Most cases are idiopathic or primary constituting 85% of cases. It is an immune complex-mediated disorder of unknown etiology. Incidence is highest in teenagers and young adults. It is in situ immune complex deposition resembling Heymann's GN in rats with antibody directed against epithelial antigen. Antibodies directed against GP-330 antigen present on brush border of epithelium of proximal convoluted tubules and visceral epithelium.
- *Secondary MGN:* It occurs due to deposition of circulating immune complex in 15% of cases. It is associated with malignancies (breast, lung, colon, malignant melanoma and lymphomas), infectious agents (malaria, leprosy, syphilis, hepatitis B virus, filariasis, schistosomiasis), drugs (captopril, penicillamine, gold, mercury, trimethadione), and autoimmune disorders such as systemic lupus erythematosus, Hashimoto's thyroiditis (thyroglobulin), type I diabetes mellitus, and sarcoidosis or rarely rheumatoid arthritis. Immune complex deposition is found in these conditions.

Pathogenesis

- It is charaterized by deposition of immune complex (immunoglobulin and complement) in diffuse granular fashion (usually referred to as *lumpy bumpy*) in the subepithelial glomerular capillaries and mesangium resulting in GBM thickening.
- The subepithelial location of these complexes indicates that they may be formed locally through the action of antibodies and a local foot process antigen (*megalin or GP-330*) present in coated pits of basal surface of visceral epithelium and brush border of proximal convoluted tubules of kidney, or by the preformed circulating immune complexes (Fig. 22.25 and Table 22.25).

Table 22.25: Membranous glomerulonephritis: Stages

Stage	Features
Stage I	Deposition of immune complexes in subepithelial region initially cause loss of foot processes of visceral epithelial cells
Stage II	Immune complexes start invading glomerular basement membrane exhibiting 'spikes and domes pattern' demonstrated by special stain. There is loss of foot processes of visceral epithelial cells
Stage III	Immune complexes are completely incorporated in the glomerular basement membrane
Stage IV	These immune complexes cause widening and thickening and increased permeability of glomerular basement membrane resulting in massive proteinuria

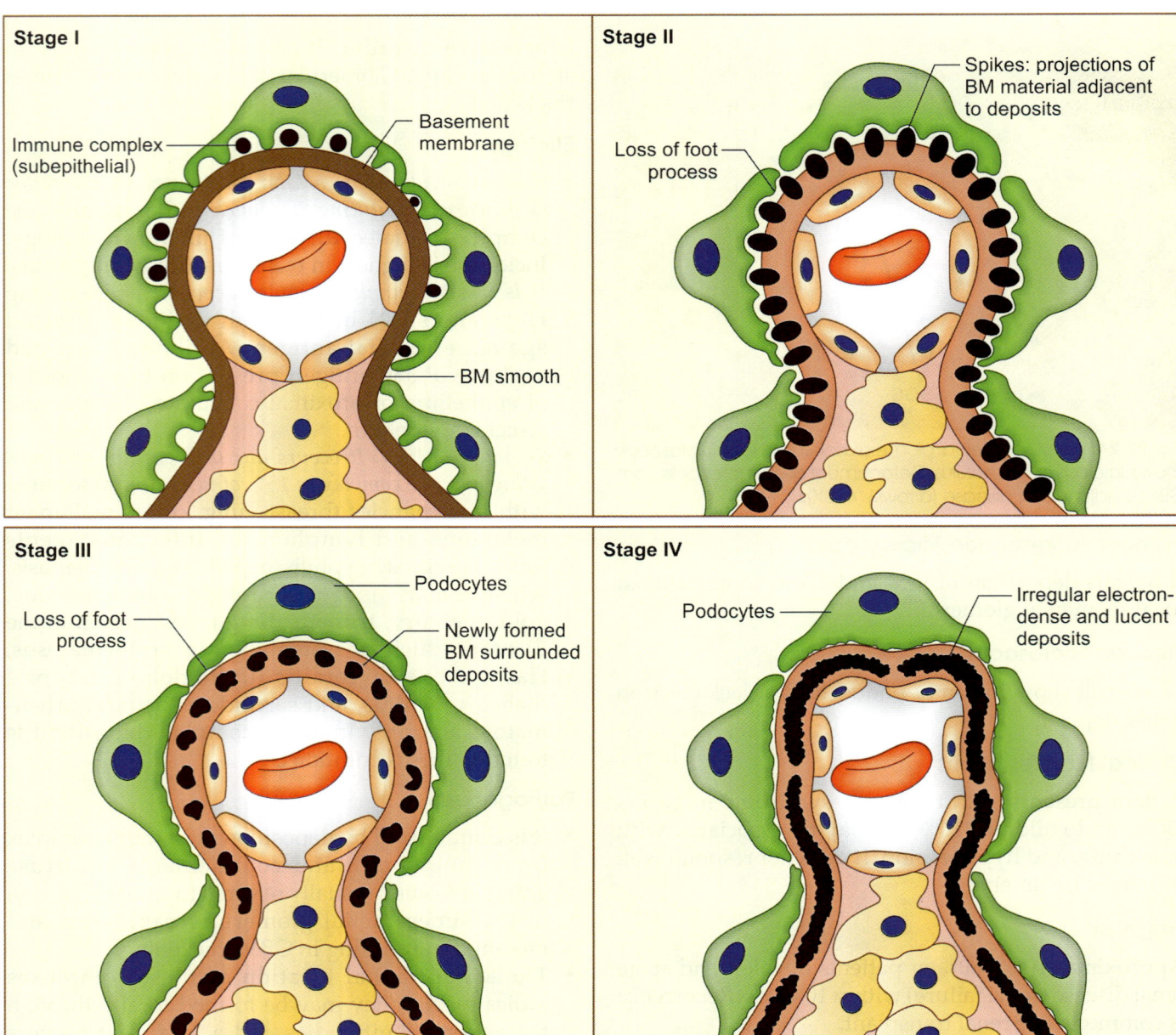

Fig. 22.25: Membranous glomerulopathy—this disorder occurs due to deposition of immune complex in subepithelial regions accompanying changes in the basement membrane. Stage I shows smooth basement membrane with deposition of immune complex in subepithelial region. Stage II shows spikes (projections) due to depositions of immune complex in GBM. In stage III, immune complexes are surrounded by newly formed basement membrane. In stage IV, immune complex has disrupted GBM (*Courtesy by* Dr Abhijit Das).

Light Microscopy

- Examination of hematoxylin and eosin stained section reveals enlargement of glomerular tufts with diffuse thickening of capillary loops without increased cellularity of glomeruli.
- Renal biopsy shows *spikes and domes appearance* of glomerular capillaries that is best visualized with special stains such as silver stain (Fig. 22.26 and Table 22.26).

Silver Methenamine Stain

Silver methenamine stain highlights the proteinaceous basement membranes as black. It shows duplication of glomerular basement membrane with *spikes and domes appearance*. It results from the extension of basement membrane between and around the immune-complex deposits. *The spikes are basement membrane material, and the domes denoting immune complex deposits* (Fig. 22.27).

Immunofluorescence Microscopy

It shows granular deposits of IgG or C3 outlining the glomerular capillary loops. It is a feature of immune complex-mediated glomerulonephritis.

Electron Microscopy

It reveals a *hair-on-end appearance* (correspond with subepithelial deposits of IgG or C3), in which the black basement membrane material appears as projections around the capillary loops. Intramembranous electron-dense immune complex deposits are also appreciated.

Clinical Course

Clinical course of membranous glomerulonephritis is highly variable such as spontaneous remission (25%), persistent proteinuria, hypertension (50%), renal vein thrombosis (due to loss of antithrombin III and antiplasmin in urine) and hematuria, impairment of renal function (50%), and renal failure (25%).

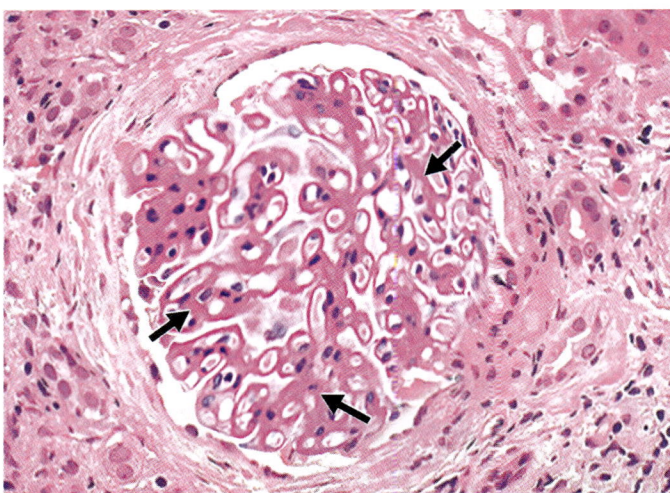

Fig. 22.26: Membranous glomerulopathy—hematoxylin and eosin stained section reveals enlargement of glomerular tufts with diffuse thickening of capillary loops without increased cellularity of glomeruli (arrows) (400X).

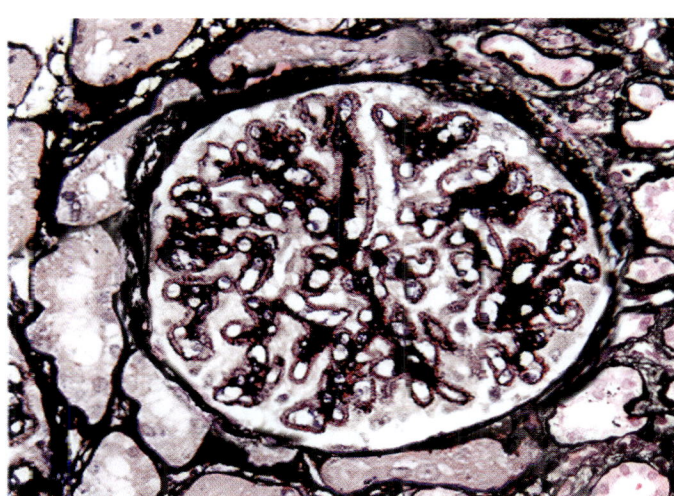

Fig. 22.27: Membranous glomerulonephritis. Silver methenamine stain of glomeruli—characteristic black basement membrane material appears as "spikes" projections around the capillary loops and domes due to immune complex deposits are seen (400X).

Table 22.26: Morphological features of membranous glomerulonephritis

Parameters	Characteristics
Cell proliferation	Absent
Glomerular basement membrane alterations	Uniform thickening of GBM Spikes of new basement membrane material protrude from the epithelial aspect of the GBM between subepithelial immune complexes. These spikes eventually enclose the remains of the immune complexes within glomerular basement membrane
Immune complex deposition	During initial phase of course of the disease, small subepithelial immune complexes are deposited along the glomerular basement membrane. These increase in number and grow larger

MEMBRANOPROLIFERATIVE GLOMERULONEPHRITIS (MPGN)

Membranoproliferative glomerulonephritis is characterized by proliferation of mesangial cells, increase in mesangial matrix and exudation of inflammatory cells. It is slowly progressive disorder. It affects patients between 5 to 30 years of age. It shows a little response to corticosteroid therapy.

The disease occurs in three forms: type I, type II and type III (Fig. 22.28).

Type I MPGN

- *Pathogenesis:* It constitutes 90% of cases. It is an anti-GBM disease. Antibodies are formed against non-collagenous α_3-chain of collagen type IV. It is strongly associated with hepatitis C virus, hepatitis B, or malarial parasite, cytomegalovirus, cryoglobulins, penicillamine drug, neoplasms and systemic lupus erythematosus (10%). Hepatitis C serology should always be performed in type I MPGN.
- *Light microscopy:* Both type I and type II show similar picture. The glomeruli become *hypercellular* and exhibit *lobular appearance*. Mesangial cell proliferation results in *splitting and thickening of glomerular basement membrane,* hence giving Tram track appearance (double contour of GBM due to ingrowth of mesangial region) demonstrated with silver stain. Proliferation of endothelial cells causes decrease in lumina of glomeruli resulting in decreased glomerular filtration rate (Figs 22.29, 22.30 and Table 22.27).
- *Immunofluorescence microscopy:* It reveals granular immune complex deposits comprising of IgG, IgM, C3, C1q and C4. These appear as spherical or ring-shaped deposits in mesangial as well as subendothelial regions of glomeruli.
- *Electron microscopy:* It shows electron dense deposits in subendothelial regions of glomeruli.

Type II MPGN

It is an immune complex mediated glomerulonephritis. It is also known as *dense deposit disease*. It constitutes 10% of cases.

- *Pathogenesis:* It is associated with C3 nephritic factor, an autoantibody that binds to C3 convertase (C3bBb), which prevents degradation of C3 convertase causing sustained activation of C3 resulting in very low serum C3 levels. There is only deposition of complement in the form of irregular ribbon-like or circular aggregates in lamina densa of glomerular basement membrane. Prognosis is very poor.

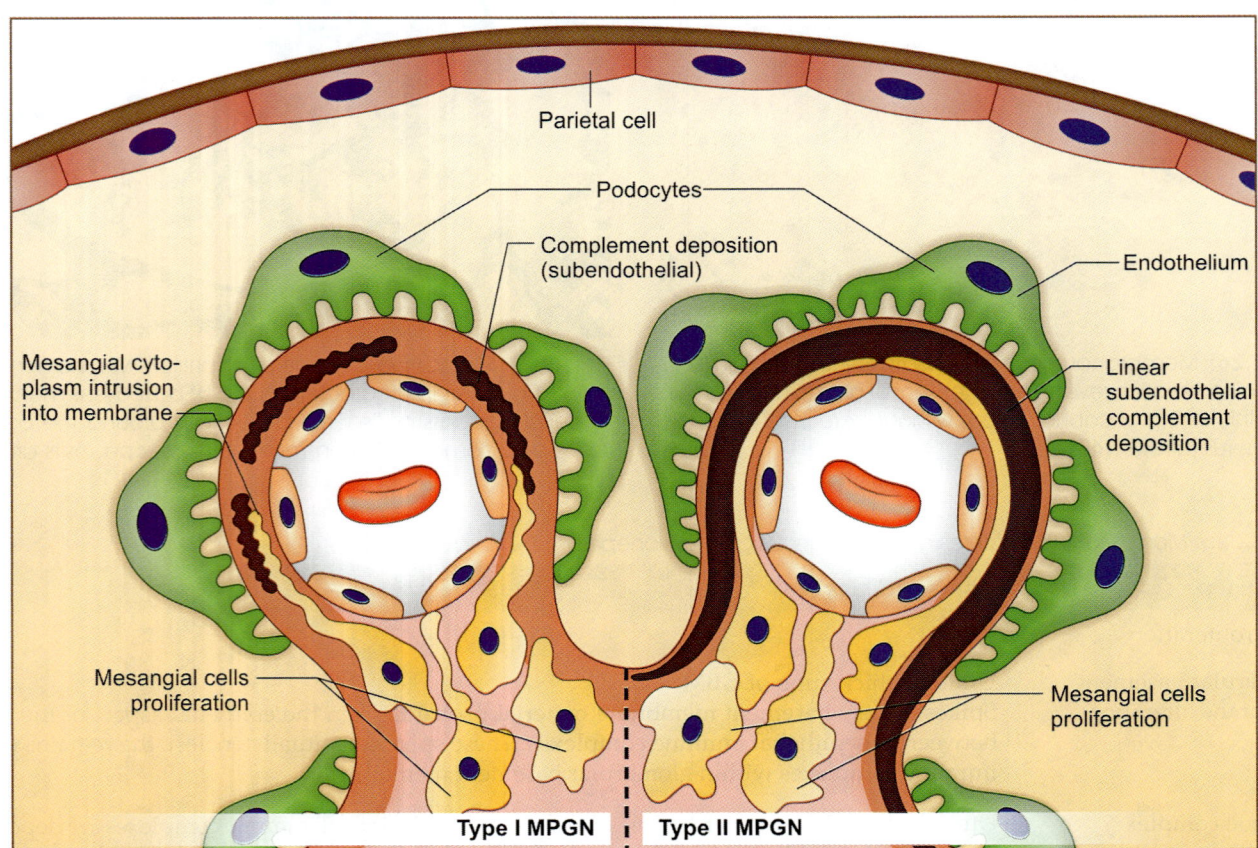

Fig. 22.28: Membranoproliferative glomerulonephritis type I and type II (*Courtesy by* Dr Abhijit Das).

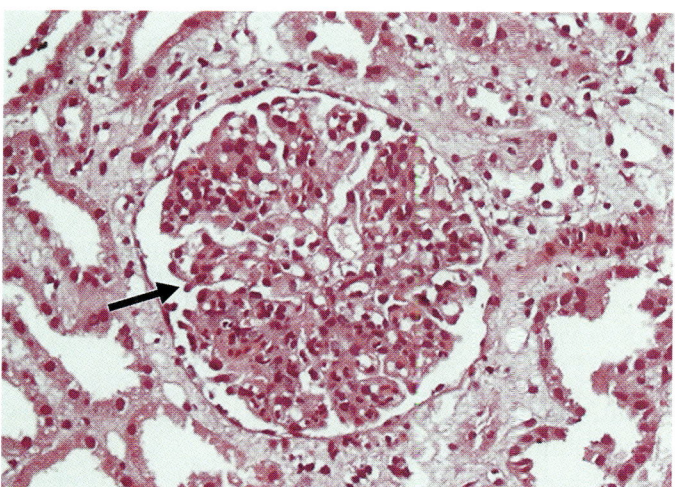

Fig. 22.29: Membranoproliferative glomerulonephritis—the glomeruli become hypercellular and exhibit lobular appearance. Mesangial cells proliferation results in splitting and thickening of glomerular basement membrane, hence giving 'Tram track' appearance (double contour of GBM due to ingrowth of mesangial region) demonstrated with silver stain (arrow) (400X).

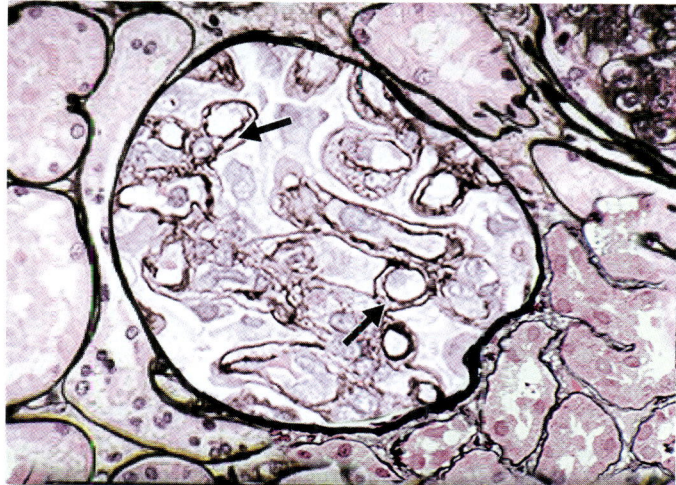

Fig. 22.30: Membranoproliferative GN—type : this silver stain demonstrates a double contour to many basement membranes, or the 'tram-tracking'. It results from basement membrane reduplication (arrows) (400X).

Table 22.27: Morphological features of type I membranoproliferative glomerulonephritis

Parameters	Characteristics
Cellular proliferation	Marked proliferation of mesangial cells in the mesangial region. This feature is responsible for lobular appearance of glomeruli and sometimes nodules in the mesangial region
Glomerular basement membrane alterations	Hematoxylin and eosin stained section shows thickening of glomerular basement membrane in 80% of glomeruli
	Silver stained section shows *tram track* or double contour appearance. This is partly due to the presence of complement deposits and partly to the presence of mesangial cells cytoplasm and matrix, and partly to the formation of new membrane matrix just beneath the endothelial cells
Immune complex deposition	Electron dense deposits are demonstrated in the subendothelial layer of mesangial region in the new basement membrane formed as described above
	Subepithelial immune deposits comprised of C3 are present in 15–20% of cases
Others	If proteinuria is heavy, foot processes (podocytes) of visceral layer may be retracted

- *Immunofluorescence microscopy:* It shows granular C3 and absence of IgG, or C1q or C4 in glomerular basement membrane.
- *Electron microscopy:* It shows electron dense deposits of immune complex deposits within glomerular basement membrane.

Type III MPGN (Pauci-immune Mediated Type)

- It is characterized by deposition of immune complex in subendothelial and subepithelial region.
- There is absence of anti-GBM or immune complex-mediated glomerulonephritis.
- Most patients have circulating anti-neutrophil cytoplasmic antibodies associated with vasculitis, i.e. Wegener granulomatosis, microscopic polyarteritis and polyarteritis nodosa (Table 22.28).

Clinical Features

Patient initially develops nephritic syndrome slowly progressing to nephrotic syndrome and chronic renal failure.

Patient may develop renal vein thrombosis, hypertension and clinical manifestations of uremia.

DIABETIC NEPHROPATHY

Diabetic nephropathy most often occurs in type 1 than type 2 diabetes mellitus. It is the most important cause of end stage renal disease in 55% of cases, diagnostic criteria of diabetes mellitus include: fasting blood sugar >126 mg/dl at least on two different occasions or random blood sugar >200 mg/dl.

Table 22.28: Membranoproliferative glomerulonephritis comparison of types 1, 2 and 3

Parameters	MPGN 1	MPGN 2	MPGN 3
Frequency	90%	10%	Rare
Complement activation pathway	Classic pathway	Alternate pathway	–
Immune complex	IgG, IgM, C3, C1q, C4	C3 but lack IgG and C1q and C4	Nature of immune complex is unknown
Site of deposition of immune complex	Subendothelium (most common), mesangial region and occasionally in subepithelial region of glomeruli	Electron dense deposits: C3 is deposited in the form of ribbon within lamina densa of basement membrane	Immune complex may be deposited in the subendothelial and subepithelial regions of glomeruli

Clinical Features

Microalbuminuria is first sign of diabetic nephropathy; occuring after 10 years. It is defined as urinary albumin excretion of >300 mg/day.

Diabetic nephropathy manifests clinically as the nephrotic syndrome; however, this syndrome is compounded by renal failure and hypertension. Retinopathy parallels nephropathy. Hypertension is treated by captopril antagonist of angiotensin II.

Pathogenesis

Diabetic glomerulosclerosis occurs due to abnormal nonenzymatic glycosylation resulting from attachment of glucose to amino acids of serum proteins, mesangial matrix proteins and glomerular basement membrane. Mechanism of diabetic glomerulopathy is described as under.

- Glucose combines with proteins to form Schiff's base (reversible process), followed by formation of early glycosylated end products (reversible process) or (amadori product); and then advanced glycosylated end products (irreversible process); which resist enzymatic degradation.
- Advanced glycosylated end (AGE) products induce binding of plasma proteins, i.e. immunoglobulins resulting in excessive matrix production.
- These also bind to collagen fibers of glomerular basement membrane as well as tubular basement membrane, resulting in impairment of interaction with laminin, thus resulting in increased capillary proteinuria.
- Overt proteinuria occurs 10 to 15 years after the onset of diabetes and often becomes severe enough to cause nephrotic syndrome. Tubular permeability is also increased.

Light Microscopy

- It shows focal areas of glomerulosclerosis and hyaline arteriosclerosis. It shows initially diffuse glomerulosclerosis progressing to nodular glomerulosclerosis resulting in proteinuria.
- Retinopathy parallels nephropathy. Immunofluorescence microscopy shows trapping of proteins in glomeruli (Table 22.29).

Other renal lesions are pyelonephritis, papillary necrosis, capsular drops and fibrin cap.

- *Diffuse glomerulosclerosis:* It parallels with widening of mesangial areas due to accumulation of basement like stroma in the mesangial region, increased number of mesangial cells in 2–5 years after the onset of diabetes mellitus. Focal effacement of foot processes is common (Fig. 22.31).
- *Nodular glomerulosclerosis:* It is also known as *Kimmelstiel-Wilson disease.* It shows sclerotic nodules in the peripheral region of intercapillary region of glomeruli. *Sclerotic nodules are formed due to*

Table 22.29: Renal lesions in diabetic nephropathy

Diabetic glomerulosclerosis (widening of mesangial areas due to accumulation of basement like stroma in the mesangial region, increased number of mesangial cells in 2–5 years after the onset of diabetes mellitus)
Kimmelstiel-Wilson disease (nodular glomerulosclerosis): sclerotic nodules in the peripheral region of intercapillary region of glomeruli
Hyaline arteriosclerosis
Acute pyelonephritis
Papillary necrosis
Capsular drop (plasma proteins deposition inside Bowman's capsule)
Fibrin cap (plasma proteins deposition in subendothelial region)

accumulation of trapped proteins and synthesis of type IV collagen in mesangial matrix. Glomerulosclerosis leads to renal ischemia, tubular atrophy, interstitial fibrosis and ultimately small contracted kidneys. The remaining glomerular loops show signs of diffuse glomerulosclerosis (Fig. 22.32).

- *Hyaline arteriolosclerosis:* The renal afferent and efferent arterioles may undergo hyalinization resulting in glomerular ischemia and hypertension in diabetic patients (Fig. 22.33).
- *Acute pyelonephritis:* Glucosuria of diabetes in diabetes mellitus predisposes to acute pyelonephritis by

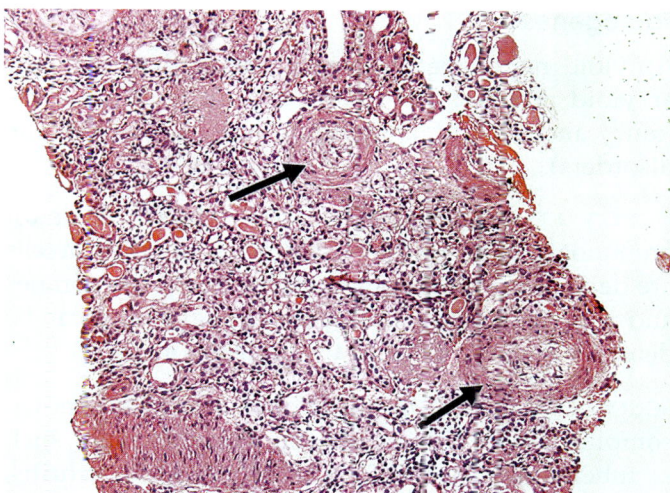

Fig. 22.33: Benign nephrosclerosis shows hyalinization of arterioles in diabetic nephropathy (arrows) (100X)

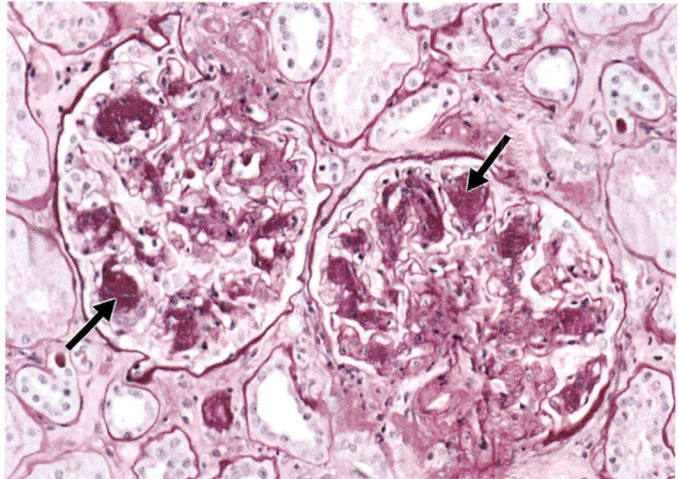

Fig. 22.31: Diffuse glomerulosclerosis in diabetic nephropathy. It shows widening of mesangial areas due to accumulation of basement membrane like stroma in the mesangial region (arrows) (400X).

providing a rich medium for bacterial growth in the renal interstitial tissue. Patient presents with fever, urinary colic, and severe groin and flank pain.

- *Papillary necrosis:* Necrosis of the papillary tips may occur in severe cases. It is serious complication of diabetic nephropathy. It can be seen as a complication of chronic analgesic abuse, infectious pyelonephritis and sickle cell anemia.

  Necrotic papillae in the acute phases could be pale and soft or hemorrhagic. These may become detached from cortical tissues and passed in the urine as tissue fragments. Necrotic papillae that are not detached may resolve as amorphous, fibrotic scarred tissue.

  On light microscopy, it would show necrosis of the cellular elements of the papillae and hemorrhage and inflammatory reactions at the interface with viable areas.

- *Capsular drop:* Accumulation of plasma proteins inside Bowman's capsule is known as *capsular drop*.
- *Fibrin cap:* Accumulation of plasma proteins in the subendothelial region of glomeruli is known as *fibrin cap*.

Electron Microscopy

On electron microscopy, basement membrane of glomeruli and tubules is thickened. It reveals fusion of podocytes and accumulation of glycosylated basement membrane-like material in mesangial region.

AMYLOID NEPHROPATHY

Kidneys are commonly involved in 80% cases of systemic amyloidosis. Patient develops renal failure with fatal outcome.

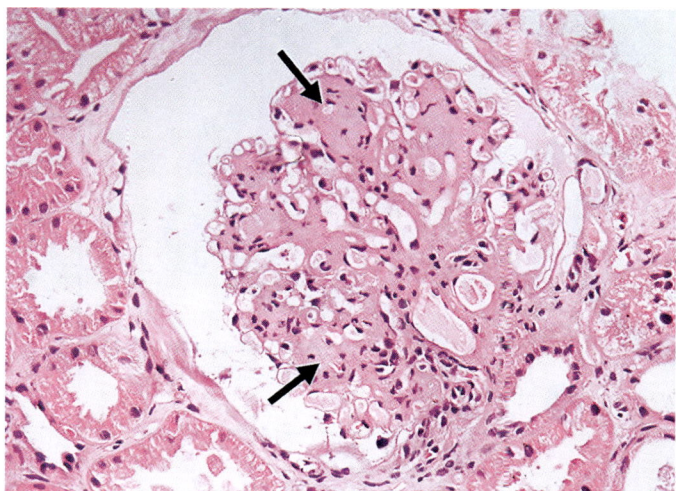

Fig. 22.32: Nodular glomerulosclerosis (Kimmelstiel-Wilson disease) in diabetic nephropathy. It shows sclerotic nodules in the peripheral region of intercapillary region of glomeruli. These nodules are formed due to accumulation of trapped proteins and synthesis of type IV collagen in mesangial matrix (arrows) (400X).

Pathogenesis

Amyloid nephropathy occurs due to deposition of amyloid material in primary (AL in multiple myeloma) and secondary amyloidosis (AA in chronic disorders).

Primary amyloidosis: Kappa (κ) or Lambda (λ) chains of immunoglobulins synthesized by neoplastic plasma cells are deposited in the glomerular basement membranes and mesangial matrix. These immunoglobulins can be detected in serum or urine by electrophoresis.

Secondary amyloidosis: Amyloidosis is a well-known complication of chronic inflammatory disorder such as tuberculosis, bronchiectasis, rheumatoid arthritis, and osteomyelitis. These stimulate the production of amyloid from the serum amyloid A (SAA) protein, an acute-phase reactant secreted by the liver. The kidneys (80%), liver, spleen, and adrenals are the most common organs involved (Fig. 22.34).

Gross Morphology
Cut section of kidneys reveals firm and waxy surface.

Light Microscopy
- Glomeruli show thickening of glomerular basement membrane. Amyloid material appears as amorphous, homogenous and eosinophilic in mesangial region, tubular basement membranes, renal vessels and interstitial tissue.
- Expansion of mesangial region obliterates the glomerular capillary loops rendering the glomerular filter leaky to plasma proteins and impaired renal functions. There is no cellular response to the amyloid deposits (Fig. 22.35).

Amyloid Demonstration
Amyloid material in glomerular mesangial matrix, glomerular and tubular basement membrane is demonstrated by Congo red staining under polarized microscopy, which reveals characteristic **apple-green birefringence** (color of a **Granny Smith apple**). Amyloid material can also be demonstrated by various other stains, i.e. thioflavine-T, thioflavine-S, methyl violet, crystal violet.

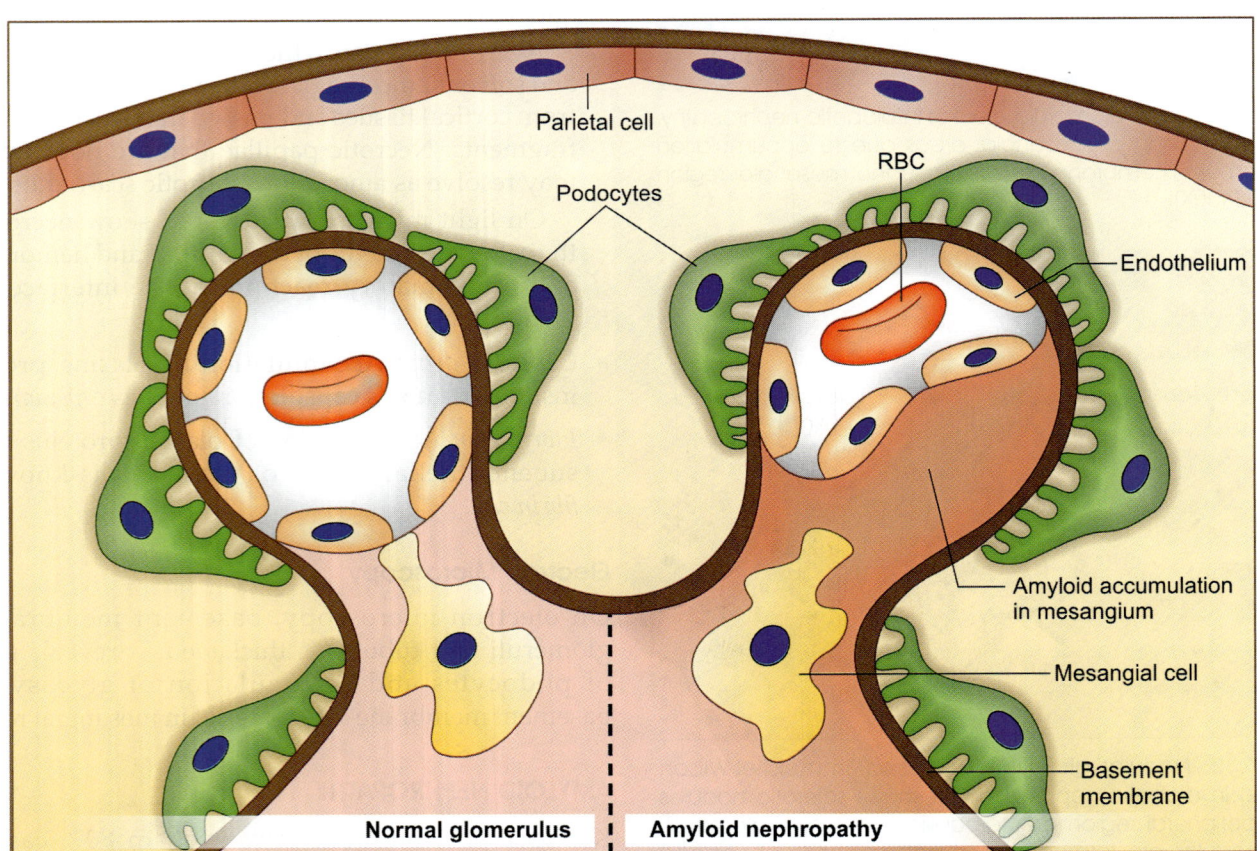

Fig. 22.34: Schematic representation of amyloid nephropathy. On left is normal glomerulus. Right glomerulus shows amyloid deposition in the glomerular mesangial region (*Courtesy by* Dr Abhijit Das).

Kidney and Ureter

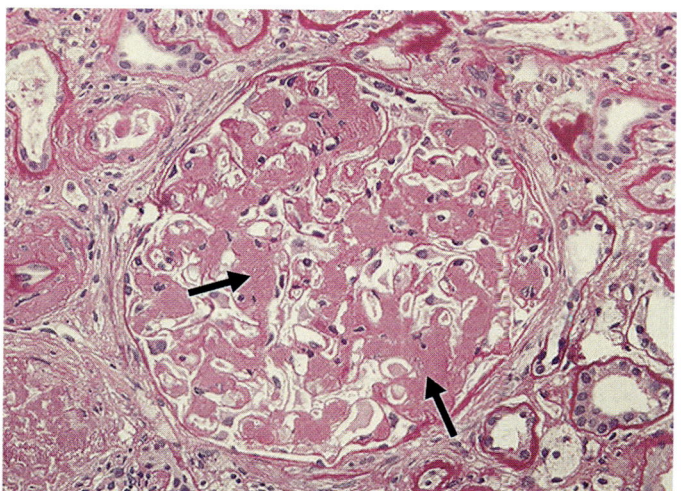

Fig. 22.35: Amyloid nephropathy: initially, amyloid material is deposited in the mesangium and then extending along the inner surface of GBM distorting glomerular lumina. Light microscopy shows amorphous acellular material extending to mesangial matrix and obstructing glomerular lumina (arrows) (400X).

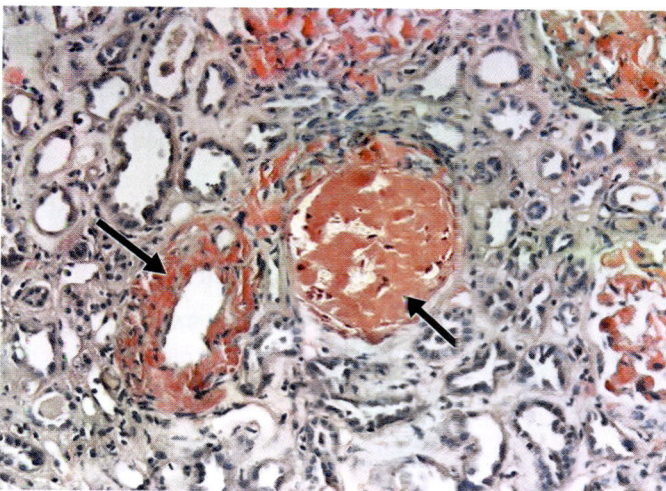

Fig. 22.36: Amyloid nephropathy. Amyloid material is stained by Congo red stain. Nodules in diabetic glomerulosclerosis are PAS positive but negative for Congo red stain (arrows) (400X).

AA Amyloid and AL Differentiation

Pretreatment of tissue with potassium permanganate stained by Congo red demonstrates AL amyloid only but not AA amyloid (Fig. 22.36 and Table 22.30).

Immunofluorescence Pattern

It reveals non-specific trapping of proteins.

Electron Microscopy

It demonstrates 7–10 nm thick amyloid fibrils with periodic beading in mesangial matrix, glomerular basement membrane, tubular basement membrane and arterioles.

Clinical Features

Renal amyloidosis presents with proteinuria (nephrotic or nephritic range) and hypertension in (50%) of cases.

As the disease progresses, there will be renal insufficiency and chronic renal failure (small contracted kidneys) over 2–3 years. Renal manifestations caused by deposition of SAA amyloid are clinically indistinguishable from that related to AL amyloid.

Prognosis

Renal failure is a common cause of death in amyloidosis.

LUPUS NEPHRITIS

Systemic lupus erythematosus (SLE) is an autoimmune disease characterized by a generalized dysregulation and hyperactivity of B cells, with production of auto-antibodies to DNA, RNA, and autologous proteins. Nephritis is one of the most common complications of systemic lupus erythematosus (60–70%) (Table 22.31).

Table 22.30: Stains used to demonstrate amyloid material

Amyloid stain	Color imparted
Methyl violet (metachromatic stain)	Pink
Crystal violet (metachromatic stain)	Pink
Congo red with light microscopy*	Rose-pink
Congo red with polarizing microscopy*	Apple green
Fluorescent stains: Thioflavin-T, Thioflavin-S	Greenish (immunofluorescence study)
von Gieson stain	Khaki color
PAS stain	Magenta color

*Congo red stain is commonly used to demonstrate amyloid deposits in tissue sections.

Table 22.31: Summary of pathological findings of lupus nephritis according to WHO criteria

Class	Frequency	Light microscopy	Immunofluorescence study	Electron microscopy	Clinical syndromes
I	–	Minimal mesangial hypercellularity	Mesangial+	Mesangial deposits	Mild proteinuria and hematuria (asymptomatic)
II	25	Mesangial hypercellularity and increased mesangial matrix	Mesangial+	Mesangial deposits	–
III	20	*Focal proliferative GN:* Endocapillary and/or extracapillary proliferation in <50% or more glomeruli	Mesangial and glomerular loop+	Mesangial and subendothelial deposits	Mild proteinuria with or without hematuria, but normal renal functions
IV	40	*Diffuse proliferative GN:* Endocapillary and/or extracapillary proliferation in 50% or more glomeruli (*wire loop lesion*)	Mesangial and glomerular loop +	Mesangial and subendothelial deposits	Nephritic or nephrotic syndrome
V	15	*Membranous GN:* Thick glomerular loops and increased cellularity of mesangial cells	Mesangial and glomerular loop+	Numerous subepithelial and scattered mesangial deposits	Nephrotic syndrome
VI	–	*Advanced sclerosing glomerulonephritis:* Thickened glomerular loops >90% (segmental glomerulosclerosis), tubular atrophy and interstitial fibrosis	Variable	–	Chronic renal failure

Pathogenesis

- *It occurs by two mechanisms:* (i) immune complexes (DNA-anti-DNA) are formed in circulation, reach the glomeruli or (ii) anti-DNA antibodies are formed against planted DNA (*in situ*) in glomeruli.
- These immune complexes activate classical pathway of complement resulting to injury of to glomeruli, tubules and interstitial tissue.
- Decreased serum C3 level correlates with disease activity. In general, the more immune complex deposition and increased cellular proliferation, indicate poor prognosis. Renal changes are highly variable (Tables 22.32 and 22.33).

Light Microscopy

- Diffuse proliferative GN is the most common lesion seen on light microscopy.
- Endocapillary and/or extracapillary proliferation is seen in 50% or more glomeruli (*wire loop lesion*) (Fig. 22.37).

Immunofluorescence Study

Renal biopsy shows granular deposition of IgG, C3 and fibrin along glomerular basement membrane,

Table 22.32: Active and chronic lesions in lupus nephritis

Lesion	Characteristics
Active lesion	Endocapillary hypercellularity with or without leukocyte infiltration and reduction in lumen size Karyorrhexis Fibrinoid necrosis Crescents, cellular of fibrocellular Subendothelial immune complex deposits identified as *wire loop lesions* Intraluminal immune aggregates (hyaline thrombi)
Chronic lesion	Glomerular sclerosis (segmental or global) Fibrous adhesions Fibrous crescents

in subendothelial and mesangial regions of glomeruli. It is indistinguishable from that of idiopathic membranous nephropathy. It is worth mentioning subendothelial deposits are encountered in lupus nephritis and membranoproliferative glomerulonephritis.

Clinical Features

Severity of renal lesion determines the clinical course. Patient presents with nephrotic syndromes but proteinuria may be in nephritic range. Infection is the most common cause of death.

Table 22.33: Manifestations of systemic lupus erythematosus

Systems involved	Clinical manifestations
Nervous system	Neurologic and mental disorders
Skin and mucous membranes	Skin rashes in malar region and purpuric spots
Cervical lymph nodes	Lymphadenopathy
Respiratory system	Pleuritis
Cardiovascular system	Endothelial cells of blood vessels are swollen without undergoing proliferation Libman-Sack's endocarditis (non-infective cardiac vegetations) and pericarditis
Urinary system	Lupus nephritis
Joints	Arthritis
Blood smear	Normocytic normochromic picture, leukopenia and thrombocytopenia
Blood biochemistry	There is increased γ-globulin Serum albumin is decreased Antinuclear test is positive
LE cell phenomenon in vitro	Lupus cells may be demonstrated in vitro

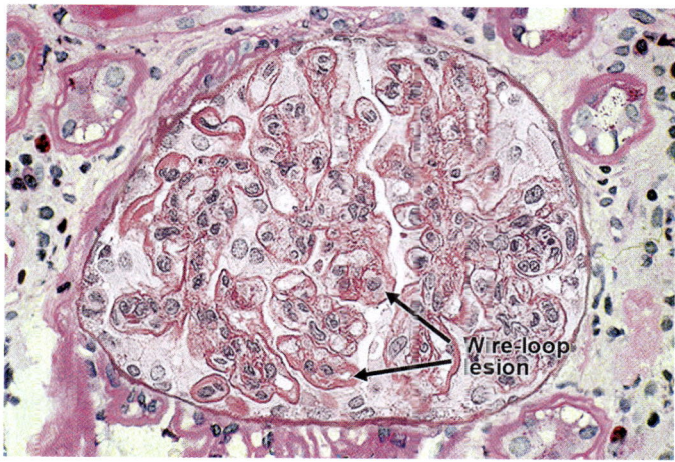

Fig. 22.37: Lupus nephritis shows wireloop lesion (arrows) (400X).

Laboratory Findings

Decreased serum C3 level correlates with disease activity. Demonstration of anti-dsDNA is highly specific for renal disease correlating with disease activity.

Prognosis

Approximately 90% of patients survive for 10 years.

ACUTE NEPHRITIC SYNDROME

Acute nephritic syndrome is characterized by inflammatory rupture of the glomerular capillaries with resultant bleeding into the urinary space, proteinuria and mild periorbital edema.

Patient presents with abrupt onset of hypertension, hematuria (with dysmorphic RBCs), red blood cell casts, mild to moderate proteinuria (<3.5 g/24 hour), oliguria due to reduced glomerular filtration rate, and eventually resulting in uremic symptoms (Table 22.34).

Causes

It occurs in post-streptococcal infection (most important cause in children), non-streptococcal organisms, IgA nephropathy (most common cause in adults), Goodpasture's syndrome, systemic lupus erythematosus (diffuse proliferative type), Wegener's granulomatosis, microscopic polyarteritis, Henoch-Schönlein purpura, and essential cryoglobulinemia.

POST-STREPTOCOCCAL GLOMERULONEPHRITIS

Epidemiology

Acute post-streptococcal glomerulonephritis in underdeveloped countries usually affects children between the ages of 2 and 14 years.

It is more common in boys. Only 10% of the patients are adults >40 years. It may occur at any age, including infancy (Fig. 22.38).

Etiology

It is a common complication of infections typically streptococcal skin infection (impetigo by *Streptococcus β-haemolyticus* group-A Sero M types 47, 49, 55, 2, 60 and 57) rather than streptococcal pharyngitis (*Streptococcus β-hemolyticus* group-A Sero M types 1, 2, 4, 3, 25, 49 and 12).

Post-streptococcal glomerulonephritis develops 1–3 weeks after streptococcal pharyngitis and 2–6 weeks after skin infection (Table 22.35).

Pathogenesis

It occurs by immune-mediated and nonimmune-mediated mechanisms.

Immune-mediated Mechanism

Post-streptococcal glomerulonephritis is an *immune-mediated disease* involving putative streptococcal antigens (zSPEB and NAPLr), circulating immune complexes, and activation of complement in association with cell-mediated injury. Recently these two antigens

Table 22.34: Glomerular diseases commonly associated with nephritic syndrome

Disorder	Light microscopy	Immunofluorescence patterns	Electron microscopy findings	Prognosis
Post-streptococcal glomerulonephritis	*Diffuse proliferative GN:* All cells of glomeruli are increased. Glomeruli are infiltrated by neutrophils	*Granular:* IgG, IgM, C3 (fibrin absent)	Subepithelial deposits or *humps*	Recovery occurs in 95% children and 60% adults. Rarely patients may develop rapidly progressive glomerulonephritis and chronic glomerulonephritis.
Systemic lupus erythematosus	*Diffuse proliferative GN:* Endocapillary and/or extracapillary proliferation in 50% or more glomeruli (*wire loop lesion*)	*Granular:* IgG, C3, fibrin in mesangial and glomerular loop	Subendothelial deposits and also in mesangial region	90% patients survive at 10 years
Alport's syndrome	Foam cells are present in glomeruli and tubules. There is increased mesangial matrix. There is increased thickening of GBM with splitting	No definite pattern. Deposition of IgM, C3	No electron dense deposits. GBM shows lucency	It is end stage renal failure in second or third decade
IgA nephropathy	Focal proliferative glomerulonephritis	*Granular pattern:* IgA and C3 deposition in mesangial region	Electron dense deposits in mesangial region	Patient may develop chronic renal failure and survival rate in 80–90% patients is 10 years
Rapidly progressive glomerulonephritis	About 50% of glomeruli are compressed by crescents filling glomerular spaces	*Goodpasture's syndrome:* Linear IgG, C3, fibrin	*Goodpasture's syndrome:* No electron dense deposits	Majority (90%) progress to chronic renal failure

Table 22.35: Clinical and laboratory findings in post-streptococcal glomerulonephritis

Parameters	Findings
Clinical features	Hypertension, periorbital edema, passage of smoky-colored urine, oliguria, flank pain, fever, malaise, anorexia, nausea, and vomiting and pallor *Physical findings:* Periorbital edema, anemia, blood pressure high
Clinical course	*Children:* Prognosis excellent in 95%, or rapidly progressive glomerulonephritis (RPGN) and chronic glomerulonephritis *Adults:* Prognosis good in 60%. Many develop rapidly progressive glomerulonephritis
Urinary findings	Oliguria <400 ml/day output, smoky-colored urine due to hematuria, colored specific gravity due to proteinuria, proteinuria in nephritic range. Light microscopy shows dysmorphic RBCs and RBCs casts
Blood biochemistry	Serum proteins and complement levels decreased Blood urea and serum creatinine raised Anti-DNAase-B titer, anti-streptolysin titer and anti-hyaluronidase titers raised

have been identified as the potential cause of acute post-streptococcal glomerulonephritis. Exact mechanism of pathogenesis remains to be determined.

- *Nephritogenic streptococcal strains:* Nephritogenic streptococci release two antigens (zSPEB—zymogen precursor streptococcal pyrogenic exotoxin-B) and NAPLr—nephritis associated plasmin receptor into the circulation, streptococcal proteins may alter host immunoglobulin G (IgG) synthesis. Antibodies to streptococcal antigens combine with host immunoglobulin G (IgG). Immune complexes formed are deposited in the *subepithelial regions of glomeruli*. These activate the complement system.

- *Activation of complement system:* These streptococcal antigens (zSPEB, NAPLr) activate complement system by two mechanisms: (a) these antigens

Kidney and Ureter 22

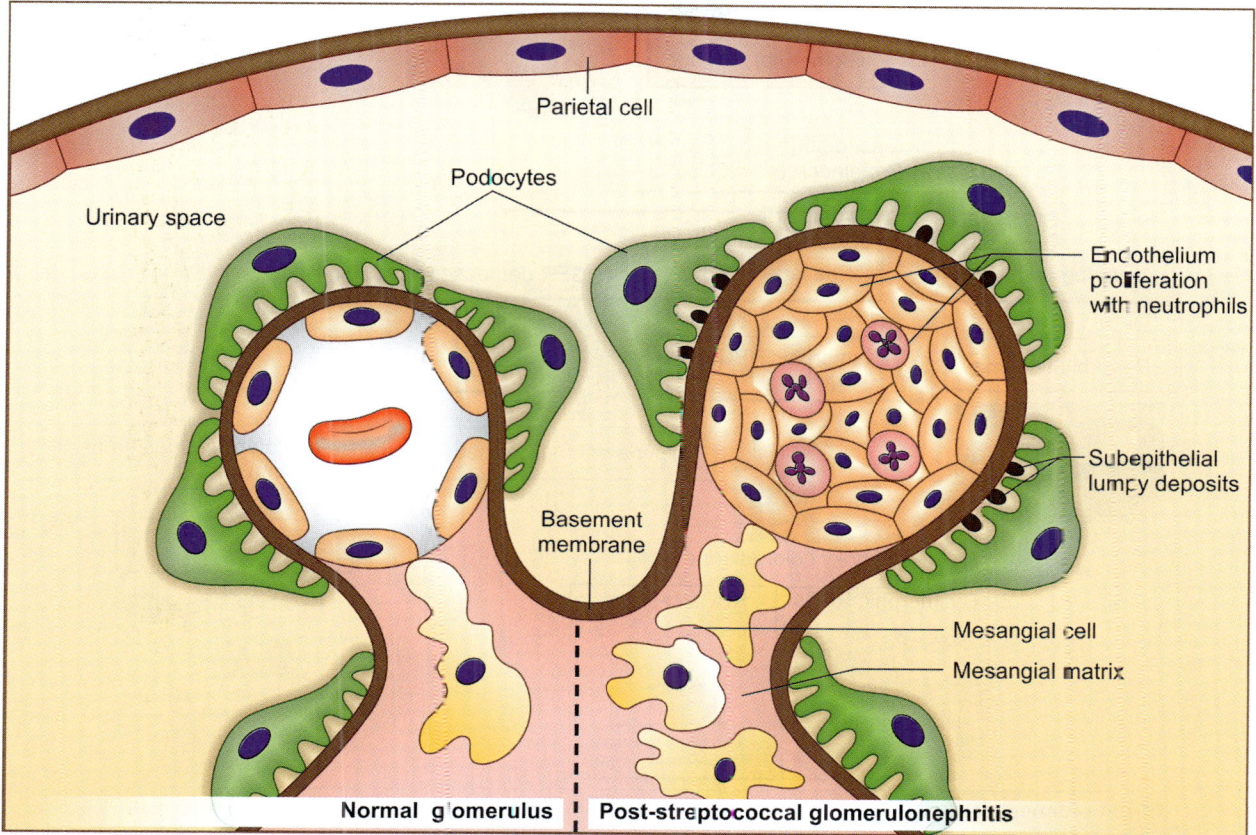

Fig. 22.38: Schematic representation of post-streptococcal glomerulonephritis. Left glomerulus is normal. Right glomerulus is hypercellular due to proliferation of glomerular endothelial cells and infiltration by neutrophils. Glomerular lumen is obliterated reading to reduce glomerular filtration rate. Immune complexes are seen in subepithelial region (*Courtesy by* Dr Abhijit Das .

have biochemical affinity for plasmin, forming complexes resulting in activation of complement system by *alternate pathway*. The nephritogenic antigen, zSPEB, has been demonstrated inside the subepithelial 'humps' on biopsy. (b) these antigens bind to sites within the glomerulus, and activate complement system by *direct pathway* by interacting with properdin.

- *Recruitment of inflammatory cells:* Complement fixation via the classic pathway leads to the generation of additional inflammatory mediators and recruitment of inflammatory cells in the glomeruli. Early in the course of disorder, resident endothelial and mesangial cells undergo excessive proliferation. It is accompanied by infiltration with polymorphonuclear cell and monocytes. Macrophages are effector cells that cause cellular proliferation of glomeruli (Fig. 22.39).

Nonimmune-mediated Mechanism

It has been proposed that delayed-type hypersensitivity, superantigens, and autoimmunity play role in pathogenesis of post-streptococcal glomerulonephritis.

- *Delayed hypersensitivity type IV:* A role of delayed-type hypersensitivity has been implicated in the pathogenesis of this disease. Early in the course of APSGN, resident endothelial and mesangial cells undergo proliferation and accompanied by infiltration with polymorphonuclear leukocytes and monocytes. Macrophages are effector cells that cause resident cellular proliferation. The infiltration of macrophages in the glomeruli is mediated by complement-induced chemotaxis, and most likely, by an antigen-specific event related to delayed type hypersensitivity mediated by helper/inducer T cells.

- *Superantigens:* Streptococcal M proteins and pyrogenic exotoxins can act as superantigens. These cause marked expansion of T cells expressing specific T cell receptor β-chain variable gene segments. Massive T cell activation occurs, with release of T cell-derived lymphokines such as IL-1 and IL-6.

- *Autoimmunity:* Autologous IgG in APSGN becomes antigenic and elicits an anti-IgG rheumatoid factor response, leading to formation of cryoglobulins. Cryoglobulins, rheumatoid factors, and other autoimmune phenomena occur in APSGN and are thought to play a role in the pathogenesis of the disease together with streptococcal superantigens.

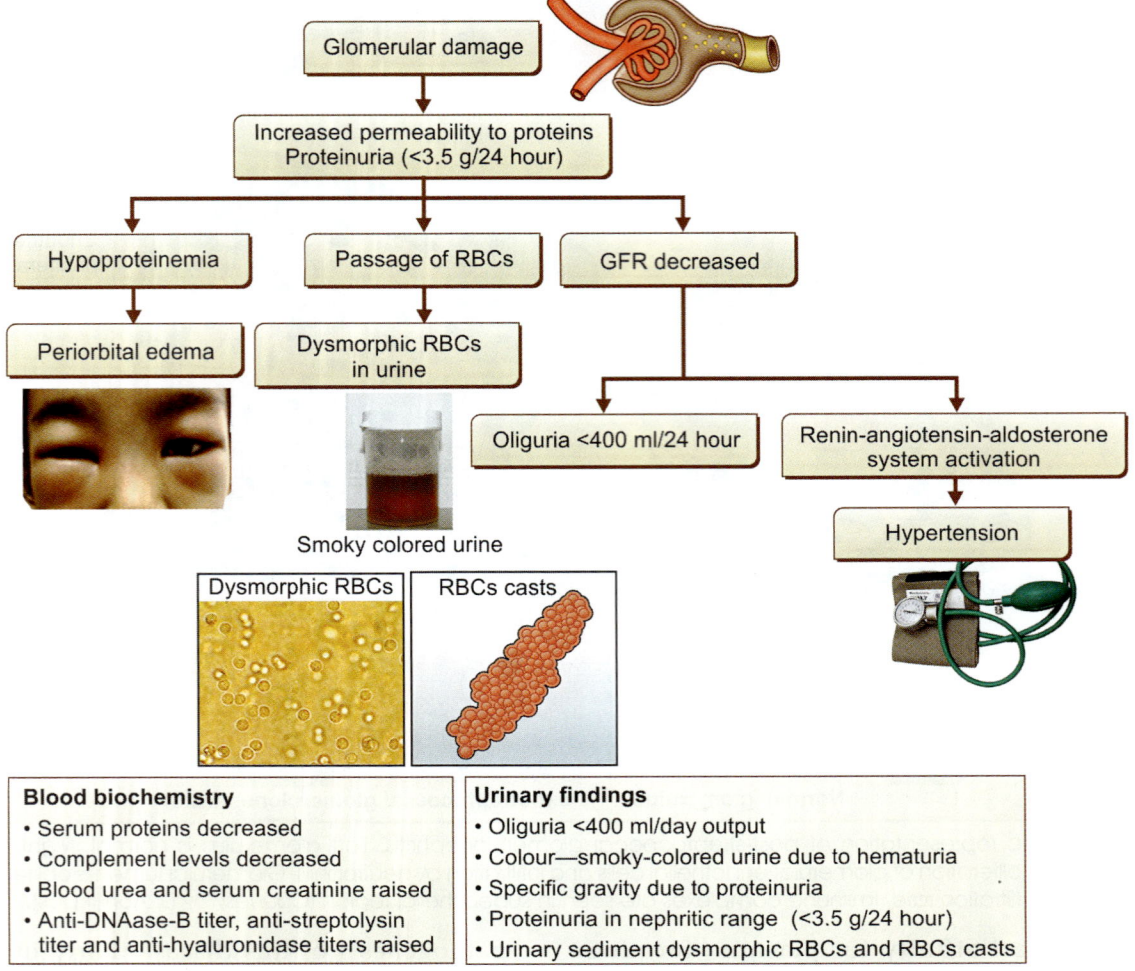

Fig. 22.39: Pathophysiology of post-streptococcal glomerulonephritis.

Gross Morphology

The kidneys may be enlarged up to 50%. The patients may develop acute abdominal pain due to stretching of renal capsule by enlarged kidney.

Light Microscopy

- Glomeruli become hypercellular due to proliferation of mesangial cells; and infiltration by PMN cells and macrophages. Endothelial cells do not proliferate but are swollen. Glomeruli contain red blood cells. These changes reduce glomerular filtration rate.
- Mesangial cell proliferation causes widening of mesangial areas.
- Tubules lumina contain proteinaceous material and red cell casts.
- Interstitial edema and inflammation may be present, indicating that the entire kidney is reacting to the immunologic injury to the glomeruli (Table 22.36 and Fig. 22.40).

Table 22.36: Morphological features of post-streptococcal glomerulonephritis.

Parameters	Characteristics
Cellular proliferation	Glomeruli hypercellular due to proliferation of mesangial cells, neutrophils and macrophages infiltration in glomerular tufts. Endothelial cells do no proliferate but are swollen
Glomerular basement membrane alterations	Basement membrane is not thickened
Immune complex deposition	Large electron-dense immune deposits are most often seen on the epithelial side of basement membrane. These have a characteristic 'dome' shape. There may be small deposits of variable shapes in other locations
Others	Occasional capsular crescents may be demonstrated

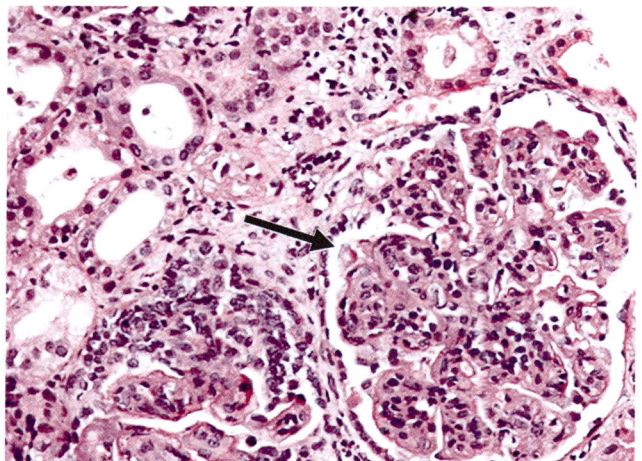

Fig. 22.40: Postinfectious glomerulonephritis shows immune complex deposition as humplike structures in subepithelial region. Immune complex may be deposited in subendothelial region leading to proliferation of endothelial cell and decrease in glomerular filtration rate (arrow) (400X).

Immunofluorescence Study

It shows immune complex deposits of IgG, IgM, C3, C4 and C5–C9 and subepithelial deposits which appear as humps. These subepithelial deposits can also be demonstrated by electron microscopy.

Clinical Features

Usually 2–5 years old child presents with history of sore throat with latent period of up to 3 weeks followed by symptoms: (a) *hypertension* due to salt retention (renin-angiotensin-aldosterone system), (b) passage of *smoky-colored urine* (hematuria due to glomerular injury along with dysmorphic RBCs, (c) abrupt onset of *oliguria* due to reduced glomerular filtration rate (<400 ml/day urine output), (d) *periorbital edema*, (e) systemic symptoms of headache, malaise, anorexia, and *flank pain* due to swelling of the renal capsule in 50% of cases.

- *Hypertension*: Patients develop headache due to mild to moderate hypertension. It occurs due to reduced glomerular filtration rate as a result of decreased glomerular lumina in inflamed glomeruli. It leads to increased synthesis of renin. Activation of renin-angiotensin-aldosterone system cuases hypertension as a result of salt retention and increased peripheral resistance. Severe cases may develop hypertensive encephalopathy and acute pulmonary edema.
- *Hematuria causing anemia*: Patients develop hematuria (smoky-colored urine) due to damaged glomerular basement membrane, which occurs within 1–3 weeks following group-A streptococci infection. Frank hematuria may occur in severe case. Urine contains dysmorphic RBCs with irregular membranes due to inflamed glomeruli from immune complex deposition. *RBCs cast in urinary sediment is a key finding.*
- *Oliguria:* Urine output is <400 ml/day (normal output 600 to 2500 ml/day). It occurs due to decreased GFR from inflamed glomeruli. Tubular function is intact.
- *Periorbital puffiness (edema):* It occurs as a result of proteinuria (nephritic range) and salt retention in the loose skin in periorbital area. Sodium retention increases plasma hydrostatic pressure by activation of renin-angiotensin-aldosterone system. Edema may be migratory, appearing in eyelids in the morning, disappearing in the afternoon, and reappearing around the ankle in ambulatory patients by the end of the day. In some cases, edema starts in the eyelids and face then the lower and upper limbs then generalized.
- *Flank pain:* Patient may present with flank pain due to stretching of renal capsule.
- *Acute renal failure:* Patient develops acute renal failure due to injury of capillary or formation of microthrombi in glomeruli. Patient may develop acute tubular obstruction by formation of hyaline casts in tubules.
- *Other manifestations:* Patient may present with fever, malaise, anorexia, nausea, and vomiting and pallor due to anemia.

Clinical Course

- In children, prognosis is excellent as 95% cases recover in 2–3 months. But <1% may progress to rapidly progressive glomerulonephritis (RPGN) and chronic glomerulonephritis in 1–2%. Approximately 60% of adults recover from disease, but 3–5% may develop rapidly progressive glomerulonephritis.
- With a rapidly progressive GN, the glomerular damage is so severe that fibrinogen leaks into Bowman's space, leading to proliferation of the parietal epithelial cells of glomeruli and formation of a crescent. Crescents are found in >50% of glomeruli. These represent sign of severe glomerular injury.

Urine Analysis

- Total urine output is decreased, i.e. oliguria <400 ml/day.
- Color of urine is smoky-colored due to hematuria (gross or microscopic). It most often occurs after 1–2 weeks of post-streptococcal glomerulonephritis.
- Specific gravity is increased due to presence of proteins in urine. It is estimated by Vogal's urinometer.
- Biochemical analysis reveals mild to moderate proteinuria >150 mg/L but <3.5 gm/24 hours). Five percent of children and 20% of adults have

proteinuria in the nephrotic range. Proteinuria occurs due to increased permeability of the glomerular basement membrane.
- On examination of urinary sediment, RBC casts are key feature along with dysmorphic RBCs. Occasionally WBC casts are also present.

Blood Biochemistry

- *Serum proteins:* Serum proteins are decreased due to loss of albumin in urine. Increased α_2 globulin indicates acute inflammation.
- *Azotemia with a BUN: Creatinine ratio >15:* Tubular function is intact in acute glomerulonephritis. Blood urea and serum creatinine levels are raised.
- *Serum complement:* Decreased serum complement occurs 24 hours before the onset of hematuria. This reflects transient depletion of complement due to immune complex deposits in the kidney.
- *Anti-DNAase-B titer:* This streptococcal antibody is more frequently elevated than is ASO titer following streptococcal skin infections in 70% of cases. DNAase-B provides evidence of a recent streptococcal infection.
- *Antistreptolysin O titer:* Increased antistreptolysin-O (ASO) titer appears 1–3 weeks after infection. It peaks at 3–5 weeks of infection. 50% of patients may show no rise in ASO titer. Height of the titer does not reflect the severity of renal diseases.
- *Anti-hyaluronidase titer:* Anti-hyaluronidase titer is raised in 40%.

ALPORT'S SYNDROME

- It is sex-linked dominant disorder affecting children (M>F). It most often occurs in males than females. It is associated with nephritis, nerve deafness and ocular defects.
- Glomeruli show proliferative and sclerosing changes. Ocular defects include lens dislocation, cataract and corneal dystrophy.
- Males express the full syndrome and present with hematuria and proteinuria. Females are carriers, but manifest with hematuria.
- Rare autosomal recessive and autosomal dominant pedigree also exist, in which males and females are equally susceptible to the full syndrome.

Pathogenesis

Normally, type IV collagen fibers present in glomerular basement membrane gives structural strength. Gene mutation encoding the α_5-chain of collagen type IV results in interference with the assembly and architecture of collagen type IV. It ultimately causes defective synthesis of glomerular basement membrane.

Light Microscopy
- *Glomeruli:* Glomeruli show irregular thickening with splitting of basement membranes. Similar alterations may be seen in the tubular basement membrane with a distinctive basket weave appearance. As the disease progresses, patient develops focal segmental glomerulosclerosis, vascular sclerosis, tubular atrophy and interstitial fibrosis.
- *Tubules:* Renal tubular cells acquire a foamy appearance owing to the accumulation of neutral fats and mucopolysaccharides (foam cells).
- *Mesangial region:* There is increased mesangial matrix.

Immunofluorescence Microscopy

It shows deposition of IgM and C3 with no definite pattern.

Electron Microscopy

Glomerular basement membrane shows lucency.

Clinical Course

Patient presents with hematuria, proteinuria, progressive renal failure, and hypertension later in the course of the disease. End stage renal failure occurs in second or third decade.

IgA NEPHROPATHY (BERGER'S DISEASE)

IgA nephropathy is also known as *Berger disease*. It is the most common form of glomerulonephritis in adults (HLA-DR4). Children may also be affected. It is major cause of chronic renal failure (Fig. 22.41).

Etiopathogenesis

It is caused by deposition of IgA1 immune complex in the mesangial region of glomeruli. It is often initiated by infections (bacteria and viruses) of the respiratory or gastrointestinal tracts.

It most likely activates complement through the alternative pathway. The diagnostic finding is mesangial staining that is more intense for IgA and complement C3. Pathogenesis of IgA nephropathy is shown in Fig. 22.42.

Light Microscopy
It reveals ranging from no discernible light microscopic changes to chronic sclerosing glomerulonephritis (Fig. 22.43).

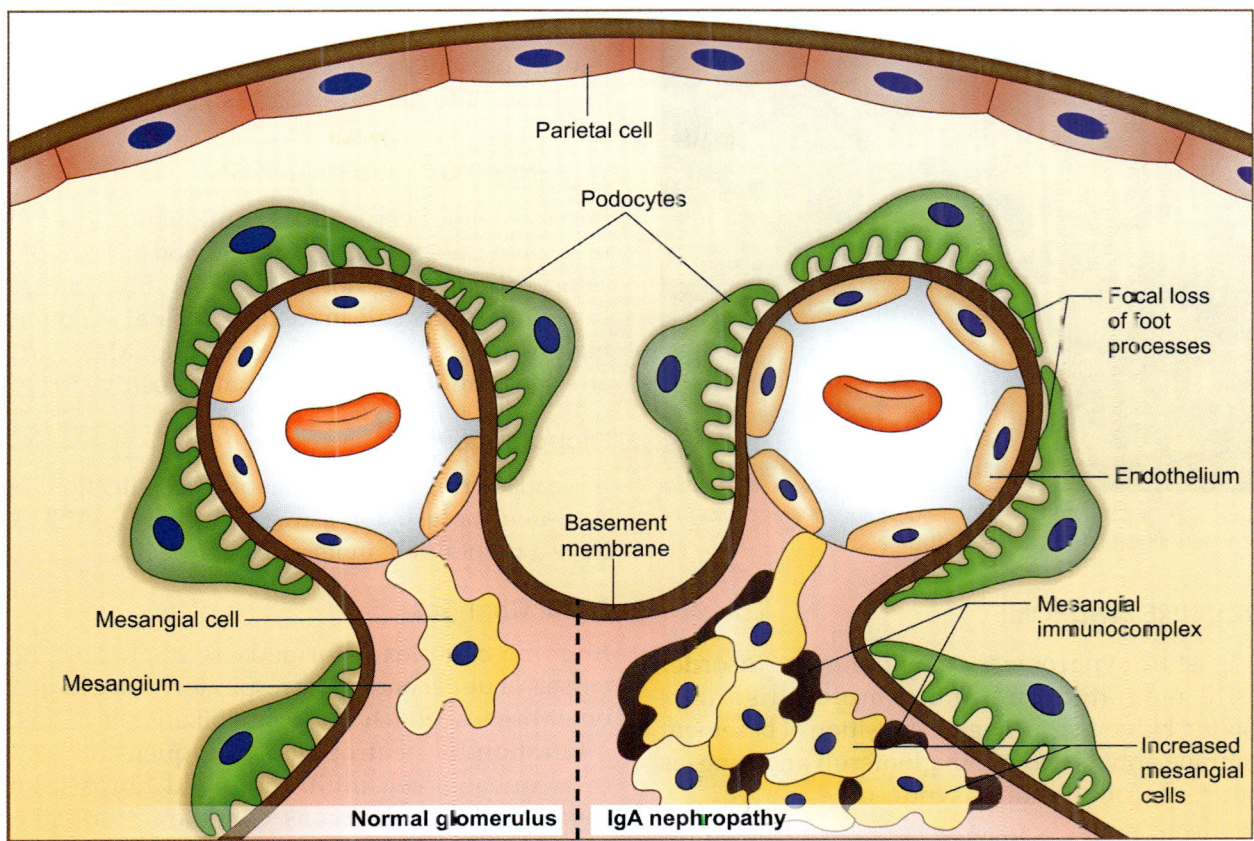

Fig. 22.41: IgA nephropathy. IgA is most commonly deposited in the mesangial region. IgA may also be demonstrated between the mesangial cells and the glomerular basement membrane (*Courtesy by Dr Abhijit Das*).

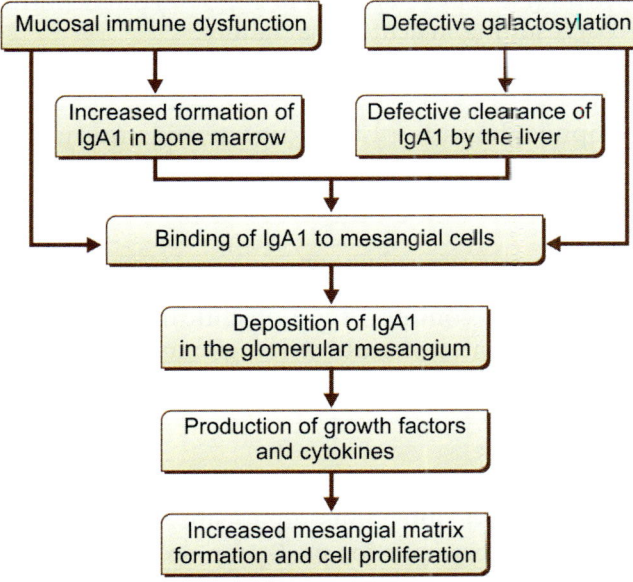

Fig. 22.42: Pathogensis of IgA nephropathy.

Immunofluorescence Microscopy

It shows granular IgA and C3 in the mesangial region of glomeruli (Fig. 22.44).

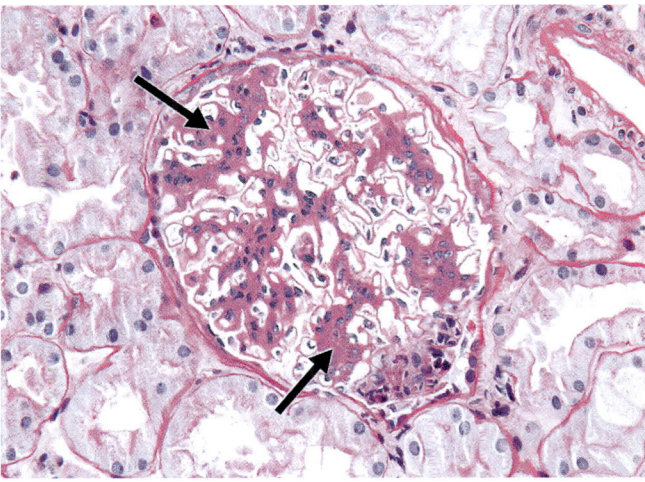

Fig. 22.43: IgA nephropathy—glomerulus shows deposition of IgA (arrows) (400X).

Clinical course

Recurrent hematuria and proteinuria are present early in life. It is followed by progressive renal failure with heavy proteinuria, and hypertension later in the course of the disease in 30–50% of cases. Approximately, 90% of patients develop end stage renal disease after 10 years.

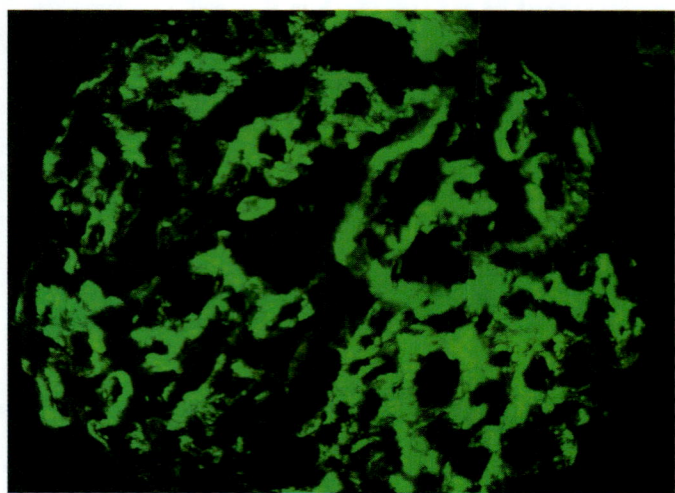

Fig. 22.44: IgA nephropathy—glomerulus shows deposition of IgA on immunofluorescence study (400X).

GOODPASTURE SYNDROME

- Goodpasture syndrome is an autoimmune disorder (*in situ* mediated immune complex disorder) involving kidneys and lungs. Deposition of basement membrane antibody (IgG) in glomeruli and lungs is a feature of Goodpasture's syndrome.
- The antibodies are formed against glomerular basement membranes of the glomeruli (non-collagenous domain of type IV collagen) as well as the pulmonary alveoli.
- Patient presents with hematuria (glomerular involvement) and hemoptysis (pulmonary hemorrhage).

Renal Changes

- Over 90% of patients with anti-GBM glomerulonephritis develop crescentic glomerulonephritis. Glomeruli are hypercellular with crescents and macrophages.
- Antibodies directed against the glomerular basement membrane causes rupture of GBM, extravasation of blood and inflammatory cells into the urinary space, i.e. the space between Bowman's capsule and the glomerular capillary tufts.
- Fibrinogen stimulates proliferation of Bowman's capsule parietal cells resulting in crescents formation (crescentic glomerulonephritis). It is worth mentioning that crescentic glomerulonephritis also occurs in Wegener's granulomatosis or polyarteritis nodosa.

Immunofluorescence Microscopy

Diffuse linear immunofluorescence for IgG is seen along the glomerular basement membrane.

Clinical Course

Patient presents with nephritic signs and symptoms progressing to rapidly progressive renal failure.

WEGENER'S GRANULOMATOSIS

It is a systemic necrotizing granulomatous vasculitis of unknown etiology. It involves blood vessels of respiratory tract such as nose, sinuses and lungs (90–95%). But renal glomeruli involvement is also common. It mainly affects 50–60 years age group. Males are more affected than females. It is usually positive for ANCA.

Etiopathogenesis

It is caused due to inhalation of some infectious agents. Anti-neutrophil cytoplasmic antibodies (c-ANCA type) have a pivotal role in its pathogenesis.

Renal Changes

Immune complexes formed are deposited in small vessels of upper and lower respiratory tract, kidneys and other organs, which cause necrotizing vasculitis, early infiltration by neutrophils, subsequent mononuclear (macrophage) cell infiltration, and fibrosis. Fibrosis occurs with chronic lesions. Granuloma formation with giant cells is prominent.

Clinical Course

Patient may also develop necrotizing glomerulonephritis (–70%) resulting in acute renal failure.

Therapeutic Correlation

Cyclophosphamide plus corticosteroids are useful treatment. In untreated patients, outcome is fatal within one year.

HENOCH-SCHÖNLEIN PURPURA

It is the most common type of childhood immune complex-mediated vasculitis. The glomerular lesion is identical with that of IgA nephropathy.

Etiology

It may be precipitated by exogenous antigens such as drugs, foods, or infectious organisms. It follows an upper respiratory infection post-streptococcal in origin. IgA deposition occurs in vessel of skin often similar to IgA nephropathy.

Clinical Features

Patient presents with nephritic syndrome, skin rashes on extensor surfaces of the arms, legs, and buttocks, painful joints, and gastrointestinal involvement (colicky abdominal pain with melena). Most patients do well, but a few progress to end stage renal disease. In adults, a rapidly progressive (crescentic) glomerulonephritis can occur.

HEMOLYTIC UREMIC SYNDROME

Hemolytic uremic syndrome (HUS) is a disease characterized by hemolytic anemia, acute kidney failure (uremia), and thrombocytopenia. HUS is the most common cause of acute renal failure (Fig. 22.45).

Etiopathogenesis

Ingestion of contaminated food with *Shiga toxin strain of Escherichia coli* is most important cause of hemolytic uremic syndrome. Toxin is injurious to glomerular endothelial cells resulting in thrombotic microangiopathy. Subendothelial electron-lucent material causes narrowing of the lumen of glomerular capillary. Swelling of the endothelial cells also contributes to narrowing of the lumen of glomerular capillary.

Clinical Features

Patient presents with hemorrhagic diarrhea and rapidly progressive renal failure.

RAPIDLY PROGRESSIVE GLOMERULONEPHRITIS

- Rapidly progressive glomerulonephritis (RPG) is also known as crescentic glomerulonephritis. It refers to clinical manifestation characterized by rapid progression to acute renal failure and end stage renal disease in 90% of cases within weeks or months.
- It occurs due to severe glomerular injury resulting in exudation of inflammatory cells through the disrupted, segmentally necrotic basement membrane leads to the formation of crescents between the Bowman's capsule and the glomerular tuft involving >50% of glomeruli (Fig. 22.46).

Pathogenesis

- RPGN is idiopathic in 50% of cases. It is thought to be immune-mediated disorder because most patients have antibodies to neutrophils (ANCA). Though prognosis of post-streptococcal glomerulonephritis is excellent, yet in approximately 5% of cases of RPGN, the disease is of post-streptococcal etiology.
- Other causes include Goodpasture's syndrome, systemic lupus erythematosus, polyarteritis nodosa, Wegener's granulomatosis, IgA nephropathy, Henoch-Schönlein purpura and drug (penicillamine).

Categories of RPGN

RPGN is classified into three categories:

- *Antiglomerular basement membrane (anti-GBM) antibody disease:* Goodpasture's syndrome is characterized by IgG antibodies directed against non-collagenous domain of α_3 type IV collagen in GBM and pulmonary

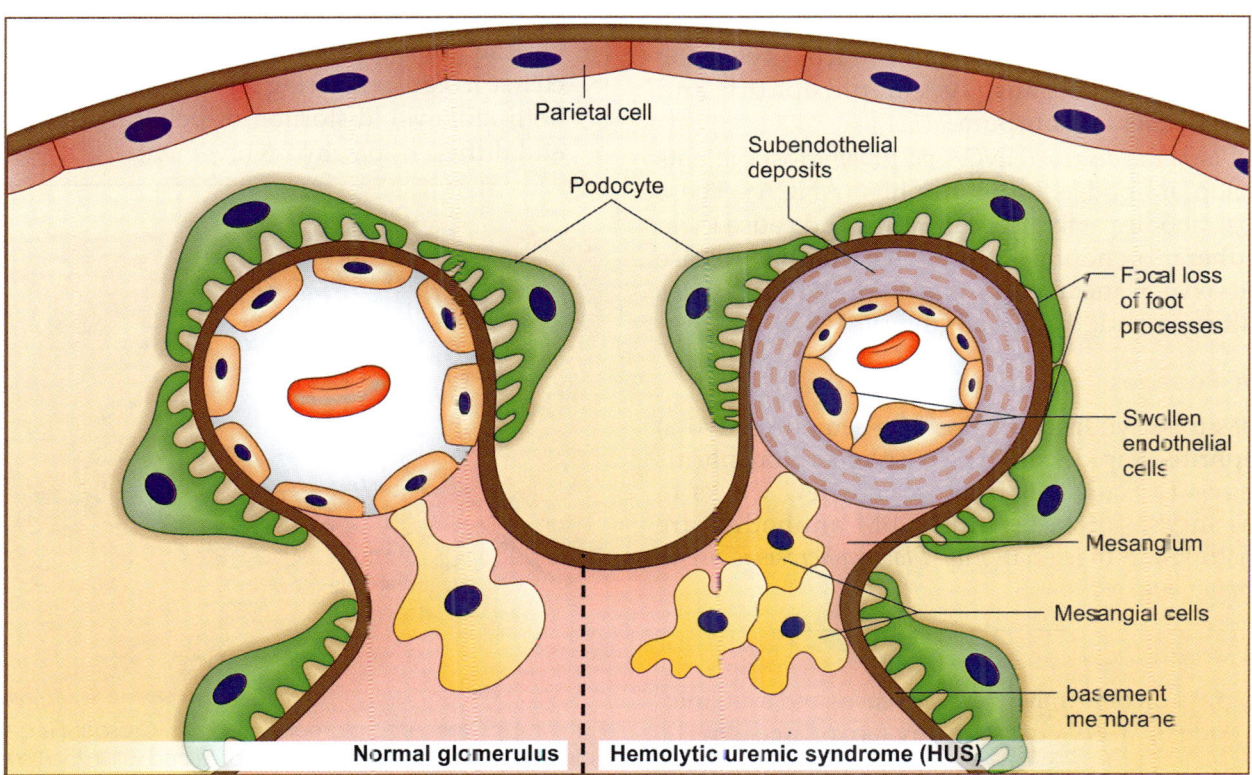

Fig. 22.45: Hemolytic uremic glomerulopathy (*Courtesy by* Dr Abhijit Das).

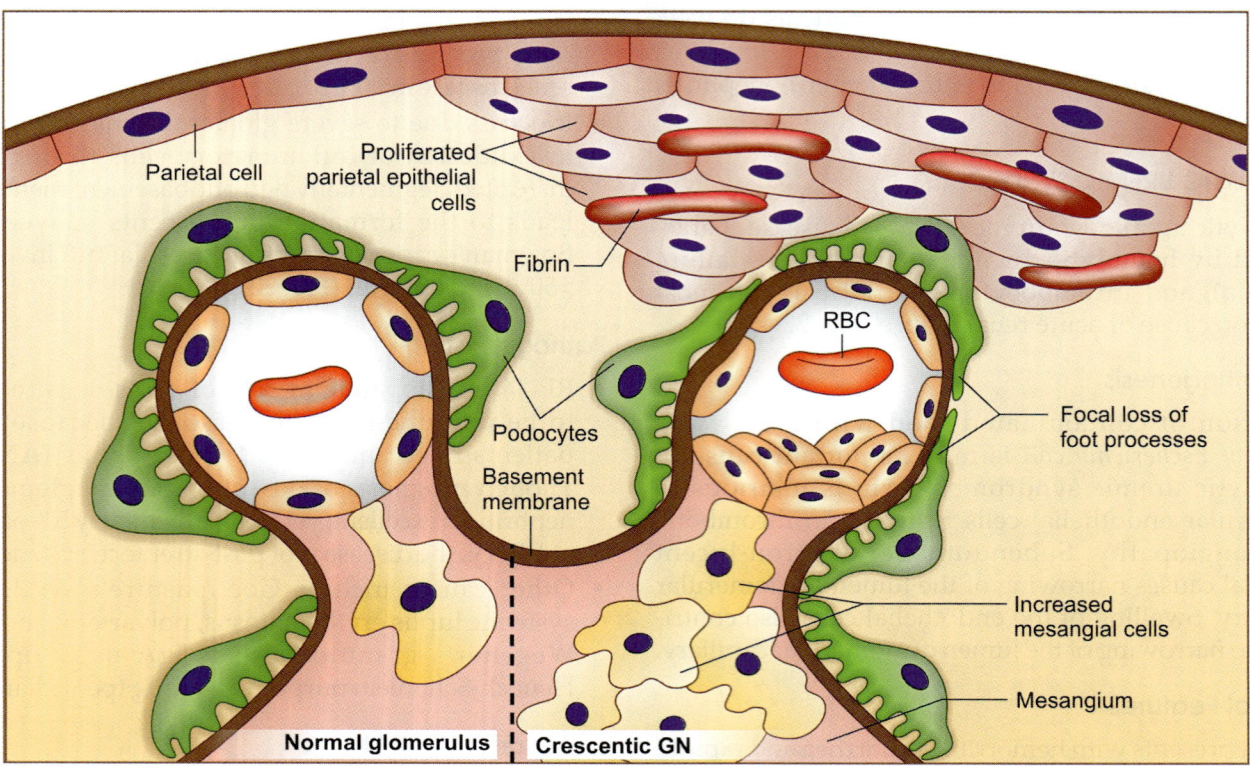

Fig. 22.46: Crescentic glomerulonephritis (RPGN) (*Courtesy by* Dr Abhijit Das).

capillaries. Patient with Goodpasture's syndrome presents with features of acute nephritic syndrome and hemoptysis. *Immunofluorescence microscopy shows liner IgG, C3 and fibrin deposits.*
- *Immune complex-mediated disease:* These include postinfectious glomerulonephritis, systemic lupus erythematosus, IgA nephropathy and Henoch-Schönlein purpura.
- *Pauci-immune disease (ANCA-positive):* Most patients develop antibodies to neutrophils (ANCA). These autoantibodies activate neutrophils and cause them to adhere to endothelial cells. Neutrophils release toxic oxygen metabolites and hydrolytic enzymes resulting in endothelial cells injury.

Clinical Features

Goodpasture's syndrome begins with hemoptysis (70%) and nephritis. Rapidly progressive glomerulonephritis progresses to acute renal failure in a few weeks to months in 90% of cases. Anti-GBM antibodies are demonstrated in these patients. *Plasmapheresis is useful in removing antibodies.*

Gross Morphology
- Progression of primary renal diseases and systemic disorders involving kidneys produce small contracted kidneys. Chronic glomerulonephritis, involving bilateral kidneys shows fine granularity on external surface giving grain leather appearance with lack of demarcation between cortex and medulla on cut surface.
- On the contrary, chronic pyelonephritis shows coarse irregular scarring (U- or V-shaped in one or both kidneys), distortion of pelvicalyceal system and diffuse or patchy involvement.

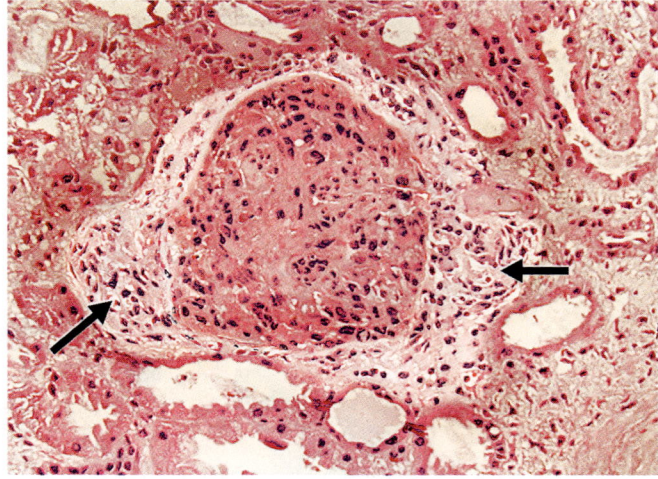

Fig. 22.47: Crescentic glomerulonephritis. Crescent is demonstrated surrounding glomerulur capillaries and within the Bowman's capsule (arrows) (400X).

Systemic diseases such as amyloidosis, diabetic nephropathy and multiple myeloma lead to small contracted kidneys.

Large scars in kidneys occur in healed infarct and polyarteritis nodosa. There is loss of concentrating power of kidneys. *Urine analysis shows fixed specific gravity: 1.010.*

Light Microscopy
- It shows glomeruli, tubules, blood vessels and interstitial tissue.
- Crescent is formed due to proliferation of parietal cells of Bowman's capsule. Crescent is compressing the glomerulus (Fig. 22.47).

CHRONIC GLOMERULONEPHRITIS

Progressive permanent destruction of nephrons in many kinds of kidney diseases eventually leads to chronic renal failure (GFR <20% of normal). Patient with chronic glomerulonephritis progresses to chronic renal failure.

Etiology

These include in descending order of frequency (e.g. rapidly progressive crescentic GN (80–90%), focal segmental glomerulosclerosis (50–80%), and membranoproliferative glomerulonephritis (50%), IgA nephropathy (30–50%), membranous glomerulonephritis (30–40%), diabetic nephropathy and rarely postinfectious glomerulonephritis (1–2%) (Fig. 22.48 and Table 22.37).

Gross Morphology
- Bilaterally symmetrically small contracted *kidneys* due to long-standing injury to the glomeruli.

Table 22.37: Glomerular diseases progressing to chronic glomerulonephritis

Glomerular diseases	Frequency (%)
Post-streptococcal glomerulonephritis	Children 1–2%, adults (majority 40%)
Rapidly progressive glomerulonephritis (RPGN)	90%
Membranous glomerulonephritis	30–50%
Focal glomerulosclerosis	50–80%
Membranoproliferative glomerulonephritis	50%
IgA nephropathy	30–50%

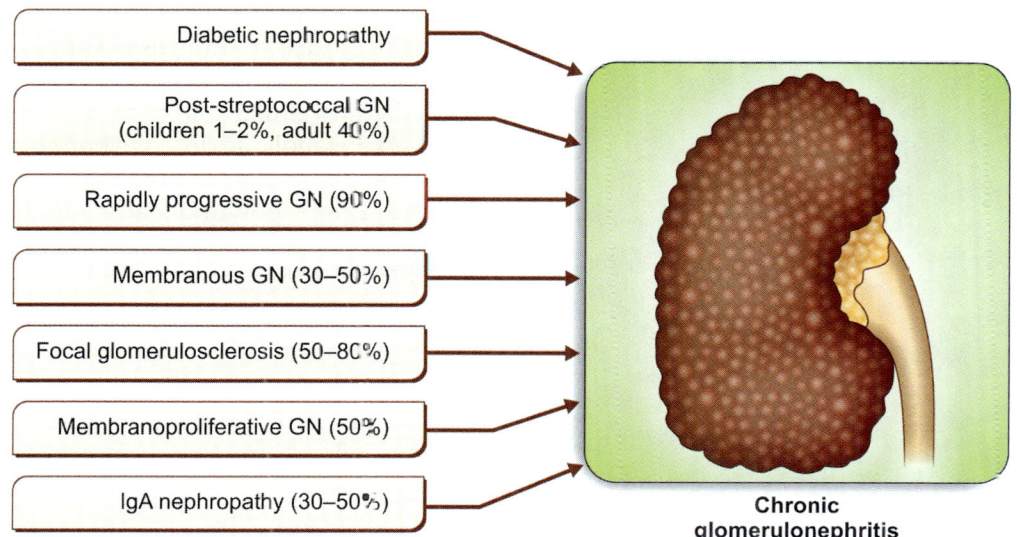

Fig. 22.48: Etiopathogenesis of chronic glomerulonephritis. Kidney is small contracted. External surface shows fine granularity known as 'grain leather' appearance.

- External surface reveals diffuse fine granularity (*grain leather appearance*).
- Cut surface shows thinning of cortex. Peripelvic fat appears to be grossly increased, because of reduced renal parenchyma.

Light Microscopy

It depends upon stage of the disease (Fig. 22.49).

- *Glomeruli:* Hyaline obliteration of glomeruli transforms glomeruli into acellular eosinophilic masses (PAS+). Hyaline represents a combination of trapped plasma proteins, increased mesangial matrix, basement membrane like material and collagen fibers.
- *Blood vessels:* Small- and medium-sized blood vessels: arteriosclerosis and arteriolosclerosis may be conspicuous as a result of accompanying hypertension.
- *Tubules:* These show dilation, atrophy, and loss of renal tubules. When the atrophic tubules contain eosinophilic proteinaceous casts, the resultant similarity in appearance to thyroid follicles is referred to as thyroidization.
- *Interstitial tissue:* It shows marked fibrosis with mononuclear cell infiltration.
- *Mesangial region:* There is increased mesangial matrix.

Clinical Course

- Proteinuria diminishes due to obliteration of glomeruli. Azotemia refers to accumulation of waste products in blood, i.e. BUN, creatinine, urates, guanidino compounds, metabolic end products of nucleic acids, aliphatic amines, middle molecules (polypeptides) and parathormone. Parathormone is toxic to cells by augmenting contraction. Uremia refers to increased concentration of waste products in blood with clinical manifestations.
- Most patients are hypertensive and sometimes the dominant clinical manifestations are cerebral or cardiovascular accidents. Disease is usually progressive.

End Stage Renal Disease

- End stage renal disease has GFR <5% of normal. The microscopic appearance of the *end stage kidney* is similar regardless of cause, which is why a biopsy in a patient with chronic renal failure yields a little useful information.
- The glomeruli are sclerosed. Tubules are often dilated and filled with pink casts and give an appearance of *thyroidization*. Blood vessels are thickened. There are scattered chronic inflammatory cell infiltrates.

CLINICAL MANIFESTATIONS

Chronic renal failure (CRF) is most frequently caused by the following disorders, in descending order of frequency: diabetes mellitus, hypertension, glomerulonephritis, unknown causes, and interstitial nephritis (Fig. 22.50 and Table 22.38).

Uremia is a set of clinical and laboratory findings encountered in patients with end stage kidney disease (Table 22.39). Key laboratory features reflect inadequate excretion of degradation products and minerals described as under.

Water and Electrolytes Imbalance

Electrolyte abnormalities include either sodium loss (early) or sodium retention (late), hyperkalemia producing cardiac arrhythmias (potassium cannot be excreted, transcellular shift related to pH), and increased anion gap metabolic acidosis (retention of organic acids). Due to the diminished concentrating ability of kidney, patient develops polyuria leading to dehydration.

Acid–Base Equilibrium Imbalance

Physiological state: Under physiological state, deamination of amino acids occurs in DCT cells to form ammonia, which enters filtrate.

Potassium and hydrogen ions also enter filtrate in exchange of sodium ions. Ammonia combines with hydrogen ions.

Pathological state: In chronic glomerulonephritis, decreased formation of ammonia in the DCT cells, and decreased serum bicarbonate levels lead to decreased

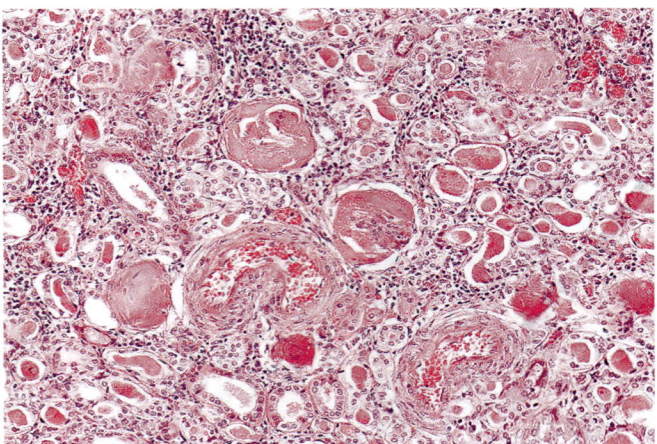

Fig. 22.49: Chronic glomerulonephritis shows sclerosis of glomeruli, thyroidization of tubules, hyalinization of blood vessels and interstitial fibrosis. Mononuclear cells infiltration is seen in interstitial tissue (400X).

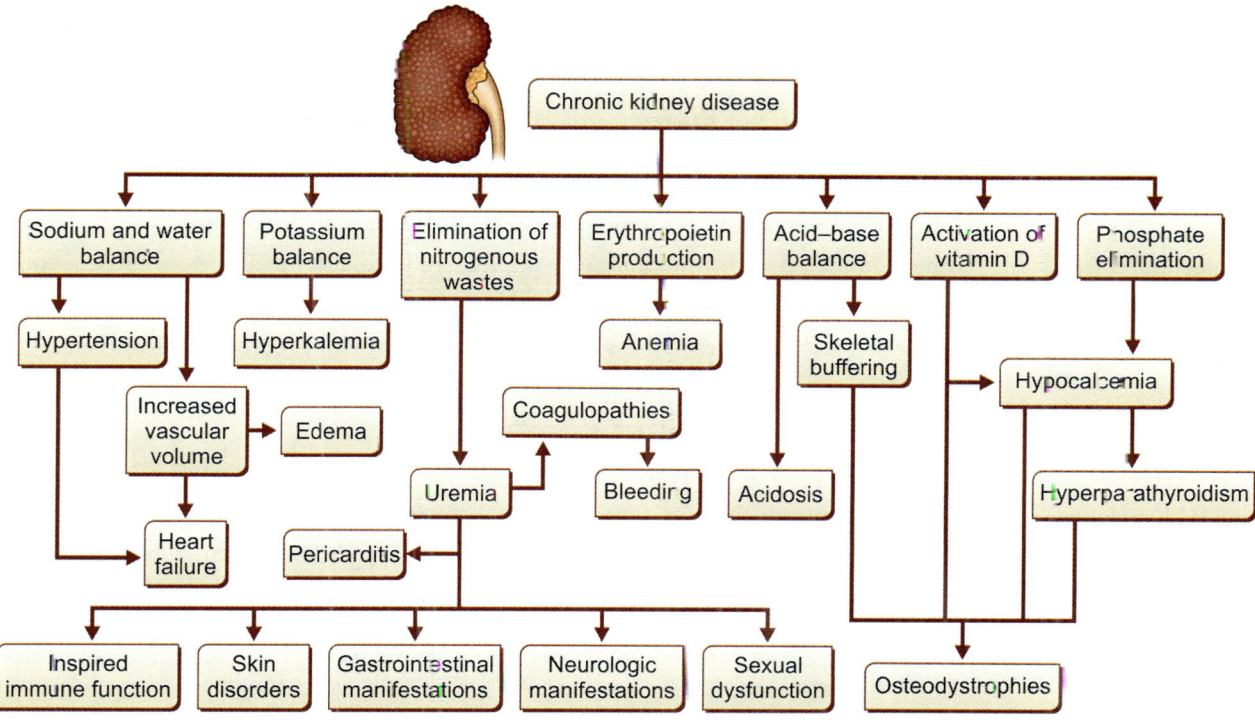

Fig. 22.50: Clinical manifestations of chronic kidney disease.

Table 22.38: Etiology of chronic renal failure

Etiology	Disorders
Primary glomerular diseases	Acute glomerulonephritis, anti-glomerular basement membrane disease, chronic glomerulonephritis, Goodpasture's syndrome, intercapillary glomerulosclerosis, rapidly progressive glomerulonephritis
Primary tubular diseases	Chronic hypercalcemia, chronic potassium depletions, Fanconi's syndrome, heavy metal poisoning (lead and cadmium)
Vascular diseases	Ischemic renal diseases, bilateral renal artery stenosis (congenital or acquired), long-standing nephrosclerosis
Infections	Chronic pyelonephritis, tuberculosis
Obstructive disease	Upper (calculi, neoplasms and retroperitoneal fibrosis), lower (congenital anomalies of bladder or urethra), prostatic enlargement, urethral stricture
Collagen diseases	Diffuse systemic sclerosis (scleroderma), systemic lupus erythromatosus, polyarteritis nodosa
Metabolic renal diseases	Amyloidosis, chronic phenacetin over dosage, gout and hyperuricemic nephropathy, primary hyperparathyroidism, milk-alkali syndromes, sarcoidosis
Congenital anomalies	Hypoplastic kidney, medullary cystic diseases, polycystic kidney

buffering action of hydrogen ions resulting in metabolic acidosis. Patient develops *Kussmaul respiration* (sighing respiration).

Cardiopulmonary Abnormalities

- Patients develop hypertension, congestive heart failure and uremic pericarditis.
- Cardiopulmonary manifestations consist of accelerated atherosclerosis (increased VLDL from decreased catabolism), congestive heart failure with pulmonary edema (volume overload—fine crepitation and dyspnea), hypertension (salt retention, volume overload, renin-angiotensin-aldosterone system) and uremic pericarditis (fibrinous type, often with hemorrhage), and uremic pneumonitis.
- Friction rub is heard on auscultation, which disappears, if the patient gets hemodialysis.

Gastrointestinal Tract Disturbances

- Gastrointestinal disturbances consist of chronic esophagitis, hemorrhagic gastritis, peptic ulcer disease, enteritis, and intractable hiccups. Due to

Table 22.39: Uremic manifestations

Systems	Clinical manifestations
Cardiovascular system	Hypertension
	Serofibrinous pericarditis (occasional)
Respiratory system	Hilar pneumonitis, X-ray shows 'batwing' opacity (uremic lung)
	Respiration: Deep sighing (Kussmaul respiration, urine smell to breath)
Gastrointestinal tract	Tongue is coated with ammoniacal or unpleasant taste, hiccup, anorexia, nausea, vomiting
	Diffuse or patchy ulcerations from mouth to anus results in gastrointestinal bleeding
Nervous system	Headache, lassitude, drowsiness, weakness, muscle wasting, convulsions or coma
Retinal changes	Arteriosclerotic retinopathy or hypertensive retinopathy
Dermal changes	Eyelid swelling, grayish yellow, and pallor face
	Pruritus, purpura and skin infections
Peripheral blood smear	Normocytic normochromic picture with polychromasia. Burr cells may appear
Urinary system	*Urine analysis:* Proteinuria usual. Microscopy reveals pyuria, hematuria, broadcasts
Biochemical abnormalities	Glomerular filtrate rate, urea and creatinine clearance is decreased. There is increased plasma concentration of urea and creatinine. Urine concentrating and diluting ability is decreased. There is disturbance of sodium, potassium, calcium, phosphate, and glucose metabolism. Acidosis present.

diffuse/patchy ulcerations in gastrointestinal tract, i.e. *mouth to anus*, patient presents with bleeding from gastrointestinal tract, nausea and vomiting.

- There is an increased susceptibility to infection (HBV, HCV, CMV, and HIV) owing to functional leukocyte abnormalities and the hazards of hemodialysis.

Hematological Abnormalities

- Normocytic anemias are most frequently due to decreased synthesis of erythropoietin.
- Bleeding time is prolonged, because toxic metabolites cause functional defects of platelets, i.e. platelets aggregation and decreased platelets factor release.
- Patient has gastrointestinal tract bleeding.

Calcium and Phosphate Disturbances

Physiological state: Normally vitamin D_2 to D_3 conversion takes place in kidney. In chronic renal failure, active metabolite D_3 is not formed, hence leads to decreased absorption of calcium at gastrointestinal level. Hence, serum calcium is low.

Pathological state: Hypocalcemia occurs owing to hypovitaminosis-D due to loss of the 1α-hydroxylating enzyme and hyperphosphatemia as a result of decreased excretion, which drives calcium into tissue. Increased phosphates levels in blood reduce blood ionized calcium level, which stimulates parathyroid glands to produce parathormone. Hemodialysis fluid rich in aluminum inhibits calcium deposition in bones resulting in osteomalacia.

Renal Osteodystrophy (Bone Changes in Chronic Renal Failure)

Renal osteodystrophy (skeletal abnormalities) occurs due to deranged calcium and phosphates metabolism. Bone alterations include osteomalacia (decreased bone mineralization), osteoporosis (decreased bone matrix; due to buffering action of metabolic acidosis), and osteitis fibrosa cystica from secondary hyperparathyroidism.

- *Osteomalacia:* It is decreased mineralization of the organic bone matrix (osteoid). Hypovitaminosis causes hypocalcemia leading to decreased bone mineralization. It produces fractures and bone pain.
- *Osteoporosis:* It refers to decreased bone matrix due to metabolic acidosis. Loss of organic bone matrix and minerals causes an overall reduction in bone mass. It produces fractures and bone pain.
- *Osteitis fibrosa cystica:* Hypovitaminosis-D causes hypocalcemia, which stimulates production of parathyroid hormone resulting in secondary hyperparathyroidism. It increases bone resorption and causes cystic lesion in bone (jaw). Hemorrhage into the cysts causes a brown discoloration.

Dermatological Changes

Patients develop *uremic frost*, pruritus, chronic dermatitis, and sallow discoloration of skin due to accumulation of urochrome pigment in skin.

Neuromuscular Disturbances

Patients develop muscle weakness, functional peripheral nerve disease, encephalopathy, seizures and coma.

Urinary Findings

Urinalysis demonstrates isosthenuria fixed specific gravity due to loss of concentration and dilution, proteinuria, presence of waxy and broad casts.

Blood Biochemistry

Blood urea and serum creatinine levels are markedly increased. There is disturbance of sodium, potassium, calcium, and phosphate and glucose metabolism. Acidosis is present.

DIALYSIS MACHINE

Dialysis is the separation of large particles from smaller ones through a selectively permeable membrane. The dialysate draws fluid and waste out of blood as a substitute for nonfunctional kidneys.

- *Hemodialysis:* The patient blood flows through a dialysis machine.
- *Peritoneal dialysis:* The dialysate is introduced into the peritoneal cavity; the peritoneum acts as the dialysis membrane.
- *The principal of dialysis:* Materials flow through a semipermeable membrane based on the concentration on either side of the membrane.

EVALUATION OF RENAL BIOPSY

It has a diagnostic role in renal disorders. Successful renal biopsy is a traumatic procedure; hence the patient's urine consists of RBCs after successful renal biopsy. Renal biopsy must consists of at least five glomeruli for diagnosing renal lesions. Kidney compromises glomeruli, tubules, blood vessels and interstitial tissue.

A renal biopsy specimen is examined by light microscopy (hematoxylin and eosin stain), immunofluorescence studies, and electron microscopy (EM). Routine and specialized stains help classify the glomerular disease as diffuse, focal, membranous, proliferative glomerulonephritis.

In H&E stained section, we should evaluate, overall cellularity, the symmetry and the thickness of the glomeruli. With normal cellularity, cell nuclei are not clustered or overlapping. Clusters of cells in glomeruli, especially away from the hilum, indicate abnormal hypercellularity.

- Normally tubules are arranged back to back. Inflammatory process of kidney widens intertubular space.
- Blood vessels show nephrosclerotic changes in hypertension.
- There is increased extracellular material in glomeruli due to (i) deposition of immune complexes, (ii) thickening or replication of glomerular basement membrane (GBM), (iii) increase in collagen matrix (sclerosis), (iv) insudation of plasma proteins (hyalinosis), (v) fibrinoid necrosis, and (vi) deposition of amyloid.

> ### Light Microscopy
>
> Various stains are used to evaluate renal biopsy (Tables 22.40 and 22.41).
> - *Hematoxylin and eosin stain:* It is used to study the cellularity, symmetry and thickness of glomeruli, tubules, blood vessels and interstitial tissue in renal biopsy section. With normal cellularity of glomeruli, cell nuclei are not clustered or overlapping. Clusters of cells in glomeruli, especially away from the hilum, indicate abnormal hypercellularity.
> - *Periodic acid–Schiff stain (PAS stain):* PAS stains carbohydrate moiety in the glomerular basement membrane, tubular basement membrane and mesangial matrix.
> - *Jones methenamine silver impregnation stain:* It outlines glomerular and tubular basement membrane. The spike and dome appearance is seen in membranous glomerulonephritis. The tram-track appearance is seen in membranoproliferative glomerulonephritis.
> - *Congo red stain:* It is used to demonstrate amyloid in tissue.
> - *Masson's trichrome stain:* It is used to demonstrate collagen deposition, degree of glomerulosclerosis and interstitial fibrosis.
> - *Fat stains:* Sudan III, Sudan IV, Sudan black and oil red O are used to demonstrate fat microemboli in glomeruli.

Glomerular Changes

- *Increased cellularity of glomeruli:* Glomerular cellularity is increased due to proliferation of glomerular capillary cells (endothelial cells and mesangial cells), infiltration of leukocytes in glomeruli, and proliferation of *extracapillary parietal cells* forming crescents (Fig. 22.51).
- *Increased extracellular material:* Extracellular material is deposited in glomeruli due to amyloid deposit, fibrinoid necrosis in malignant hypertension, insudation of plasma proteins in benign hypertension (hyalinosis), and collagen matrix in glomerulosclerosis (Tables 22.42 and 22.43).

Table 22.40: Stains used to evaluate renal biopsy

Stains	Used to demonstrate
Hematoxylin and eosin stain	Cellularity, symmetry and thickness of glomeruli, tubules, blood vessels and interstitial tissue
Periodic acid–Schiff stain (PAS stain)	Glomerular basement membrane, tubular basement membrane and mesangial matrix
Jones methenamine silver impregnation stain	Glomerular basement membrane, tubular basement membrane
Congo red stain	Amyloid material
Masson's trichome stain	Collagen deposition (focal segmental glomerulosclerosis)
Fat stains	Fat microemboli in glomeruli

Table 22.41: Staining characteristics of normal and abnormal renal structures

Renal tissue components	PAS stain	Masson's trichrome stain	Silver methenamine stain
Normal renal structures			
Basement membrane	Red	Deep blue	Black
Mesangial matrix	Red	Deep blue	Black
Interstitial collagen fibers	–	Pale blue	–
Cell cytoplasm	–	Rust/Orange granular	–
Abnormal renal findings			
Immune complex	–/+	Bright red-orange homogenous	–
Fibrin	Weakly +	Bright red-orange fibrillar	–
Amyloid	–	Light blue-orange	–
Tubular casts (Tamm-Horsfall protein)	Red	Light blue	Gray black
Insudative lesions	–/+	Bright red-orange homogenous	–

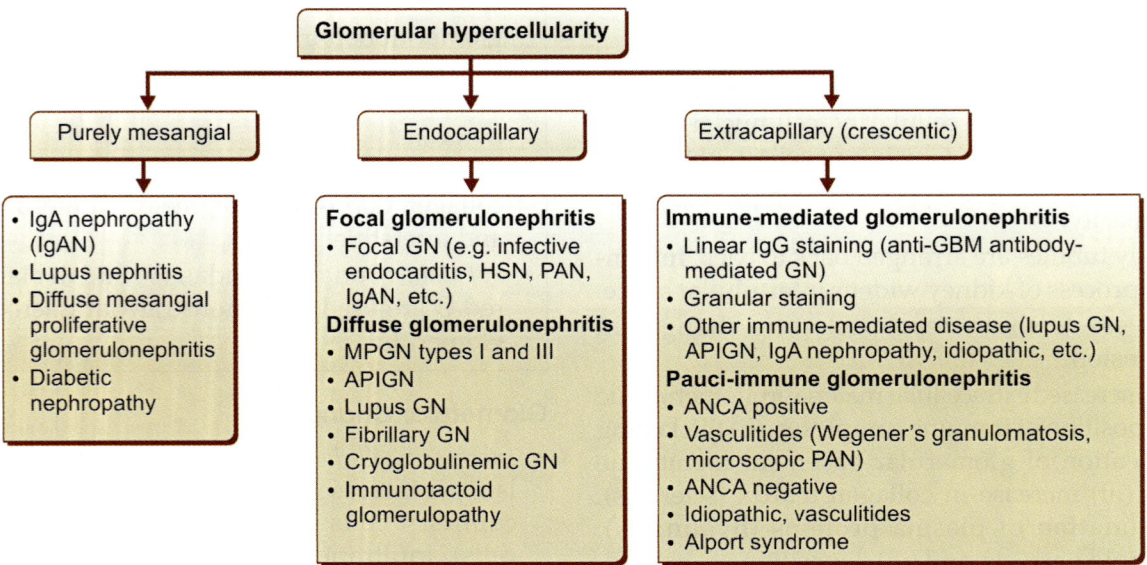

Fig. 22.51: Glomerular hypercellularity shows etiology of proliferation of mesangial cells, endocapillary and exocapillary hypercellularity.

Immunofluorescence Microscopy

Immunofluorescence studies identify immune complex deposits, patterns of deposition of IgG, IgA, IgM, complement (Clq, C3), fibrin, light chains, and albumin (Fig. 22.52).

Location of Immune Complex Deposits

Highly anionic macromolecules are excluded by glomerular basement membrane. These are trapped in subendothelial region of kidney. Cationic molecules bind to anionic sites, DNA nucleosome and other nuclear

Table 22.42: Renal biopsy interpretation

Terminology	Characteristics
Focal involvement	<50% of glomeruli
Diffuse involvement	>50% of glomeruli
Segmental involvement	Part of glomerulus
Global involvement	All of glomerulus
Mesangial hypercellularity	4 or more nuclei in mesangial region
Endocapillary hypercellularity	Increased cellularity internal to the GBM composed of leukocytes, endothelial cells and mesangial cells
Extracapillary hypercellularity	Increased cellularity in Bowman's space (>1 layer of parietal or visceral cells or monocyte/macrophage)
Crescentic glomerulonephritis	Extracapillary hypercellularity other than the epithelial hyperplasia of collapsing variant of FSGS
Fibrinoid necrosis	Lytic destruction of cells and matrix with deposition of acidophilic fibrin-rich material
Sclerosis of glomeruli	Increased collagenous extracellular matrix that is expanding the mesangium, obliterating capillary lumens or forming adhesions to Bowman's capsule
Hyaline change in glomeruli	Glassy acidophilic extracellular material
Membranoproliferative glomerulonephritis	Combined capillary wall thickening and mesangial or endocapillary hypercellularity
Lobular glomerulonephritis	Expansion of segments demarcated by intervening urinary space
Mesangiolysis	Detachment of paramesangial GBM from the meangial matrix or lysis of mesangial matrix

Table 22.43: Major glomerular patterns and differential diagnosis on light microscopy

Parameters on light microscopy	Examples
Minimal changes	Minimal change disease, thin membrane disease, early lupus nephritis, early mild IgA nephropathy, early diabetic nephropathy
Proliferative glomerulonephritis	Postinfectious glomerulonephritis, lupus nephritis, Henoch-Schönlein purpura
Focal segmental glomerulosclerosis	Primary or secondary glomerulonephritis (not otherwise specified)
Mesangial cell proliferation (hypercellular mesangial region)	IgA nephropathy, lupus nephritis (IgM, C1q, C3/IgG)
Thick capillary loops	Membranous glomerulonephritis, diabetic nephropathy, Alport's syndrome and amyloidosis (early stage)
Tram-track appearance	Membranoproliferative glomerulonephritis, Henoch-Schönlein purpura, lupus nephritis
Nodular pattern	Diabetic nephropathy, amyloidosis and monoclonal immunoglobulin deposition disease (MIDD)
Crescents formation	Crescents seen in various types of glomerulonephritis: diffuse pattern of Goodpasture's syndrome, acute diffuse proliferative glomerulonephritis (occasional), diffuse mesangioproliferative glomerulonephritis, Henoch-Schönlein purpura, microscopic polyarteritis, Wegener's granulomatosis, acute scleroderma involving kidney and segmental lupus nephritis with tuft necrosis

proteins. Highly cationic immunogens tend to cross subepithelial region. Neutral charged molecules are trapped in mesangial region (Table 22.44).

- *Subendothelial deposits:* Immune complexes are deposited in subendothelial region in patients with *systemic lupus erythematosus.*
- *Subepithelial deposits:* Lumpy bumpy (large size) immune complex deposits are demonstrated in *post-streptococcal glomerulonephritis and membranous glomerulonephritis.*
- *Intramembranous deposits:* Immune complex deposits are seen within glomerular basement membrane in

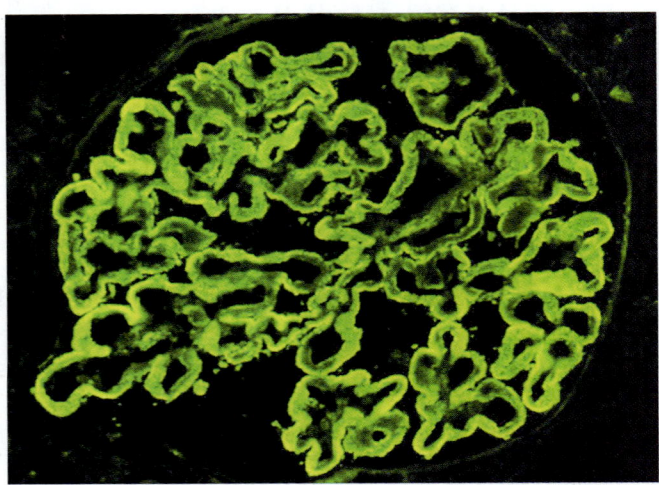 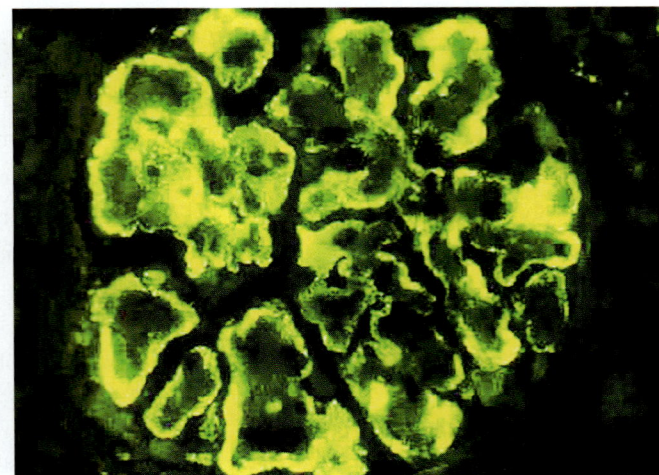

Fig. 22.52: Glomerular immunofluorescence indicating linear (A) and granular (B) capillary wall staining for immunoglobulin G (IgG).

Table 22.44: Immunofluorescence staining used to demonstrate immune deposits in glomerular diseases

Location of immune complex deposition	Disorder
Subendothelial deposits	Systemic lupus erythematosus
Subepithelial *Lumpy bumpy* deposits	Post-streptococcal glomerulonephritis Membranous glomerulonephritis
Intramembranous deposits	Systemic lupus erythematosus Membranoproliferative glomerulonephritis
Mesangial deposits	IgA nephropathy

Immunofluorescence microscopy: Diffuse linear immunofluorescence for IgG and C3, fibrin in crescents are seen along the glomerular basement membrane in Goodpasture's syndrome.

systemic lupus erythematosus and membranoproliferative glomerulonephritis.

- *Mesangial deposits:* Immune complex comprising of IgA1 and complement are deposited in mesangial region of glomeruli in patient with IgA nephropathy.

Patterns of Immune Complex Deposits in Glomerulopathy

Immune complexes deposited in glomeruli may show diffuse linear staining or *lumpy bumpy* or irregular (fluffy) patterns (Tables 22.45 and 22.46).

Table 22.45: Immune complex deposits in renal tissue

Immunofluorescence microscopy	Light microscopy	Electron microscopy
Granular immune complex deposits	Trichrome stain bright red	Electron dense
Linear immune complex deposits	Not visible	Not visible

Table 22.46: Patterns of immune complex deposits in glomerulopathy

Immune complex deposits patterns	Examples
Diffuse linear staining for IgG	Goodpasture's syndrome
Granular *lumpy bumpy* immune complex deposits	Post-streptococcal glomerulonephritis (subepithelial region) Membranous glomerulonephritis (intramembranous and subepithelial regions) IgA nephropathy (mesangial region) Lupus glomerulonephritis (subendothelial region)
Irregular (fluffy) deposits	Monoclonal light chains (AL amyloidosis) AA protein (AA amyloidosis)

- *Diffuse linear staining of GBM:* Diffuse linear staining for IgG is seen along the glomerular basement membrane in *Goodpasture's syndrome*.
- *Granular lumpy bumpy deposits:* Granular *lumpy bumpy* immune complex deposits are demonstrated in *post-streptococcal glomerulonephritis* (subepithelial region), membranous glomerulonephritis (intramembranous and subepithelial regions), IgA nephropathy (mesangial region) and lupus glomerulonephritis (subendothelial region). Their distribution is less uniform owing to differences in their charge, size, and solubility.
- *Irregular (fluffy) deposits:* Irregular (fluffy) staining is associated with monoclonal light chains (AL *amyloidosis*) and AA protein (AA amyloidosis).

Electron Microscopy

Renal biopsy examined under electron microscopy reveals site of immune complex deposits, thickening and replication of glomerular basement membrane, collagen matrix and fibrillary deposits (Table 22.47).

- *Electron dense immune complex deposits:* Electron dense immune complex deposits are demonstrated by electron microscopic study in membranous glomerulonephritis (intramembranous and subepithelial region), IgA nephropathy (mesangial region) and lupus glomerulonephritis (subendothelial region). Electron microscopy identifies structural abnormalities in minimal change disease affecting children responsible for nephrotic syndrome (e.g. *effacement of foot process*).
- *GBM thickening:* Electron microscopy identifies GBM thickening in diabetic glomerulosclerosis.
- *GBM replication:* It is demonstrated in membranoproliferative glomerulonephritis by electron microscopy.
- *Collagen matrix deposition:* Electron microscopy identifies collagen matrix deposition in focal segmental glomerulosclerosis.
- *Fibrillary deposit:* Electron microscopy identifies fibrillary deposit in amyloidosis.

Table 22.47: Electron microscopy in glomerulopathy

Parameters	Examples of glomerulopathy
Electron dense immune complex	Membranous glomerulonephritis (intramembranous and subepithelial region) IgA nephropathy (mesangial region) Lupus glomerulonephritis (subendothelial region) Minimal change disease (effacement of podocytes)
GBM thickening	Diabetic glomerulosclerosis
GBM replication	Membranoproliferative glomerulonephritis
Collagen matrix deposition	Focal segmental glomerulosclerosis
Fibrillary deposit	Amyloid kidney

DISEASES OF THE TUBULES

OVERVIEW OF ACUTE TUBULAR NECROSIS

Acute tubular necrosis (ATN) is caused by ischemia or toxic substances. It is a severe, but potentially reversible, impairment of tubular epithelial function resulting in acute renal failure within 24 hours. Kidneys are not able to excrete waste products (urea and creatinine) and maintain normal fluid and electrolyte homeostasis.

Classification

Tubular epithelial cells are particularly sensitive to anoxia and toxins, which cause cell necrosis. Acute tubular necrosis is divided into ischemic and nephrotoxic. It is accompanied by oliguria in most of cases (<400 ml/24 hours) or anuria. Some cases have polyuria (>800 ml/24 hours) (Table 22.48 and Fig. 22.53).

Table 22.48: Comparison between ischemic and nephrotoxic types of acute tubular necrosis

Parameters	Acute tubular necrosis (ischemic type)	Acute tubular necrosis (nephrotoxic type)
Etiology	Ischemia	Toxic substances
Lesions	Segmental (patchy) in proximal tubules and loop of Henle	Diffuse lesions in proximal tubules and loop of Henle
Regeneration of tubular epithelial cells	Good, if blood supply is restored immediately	Poor

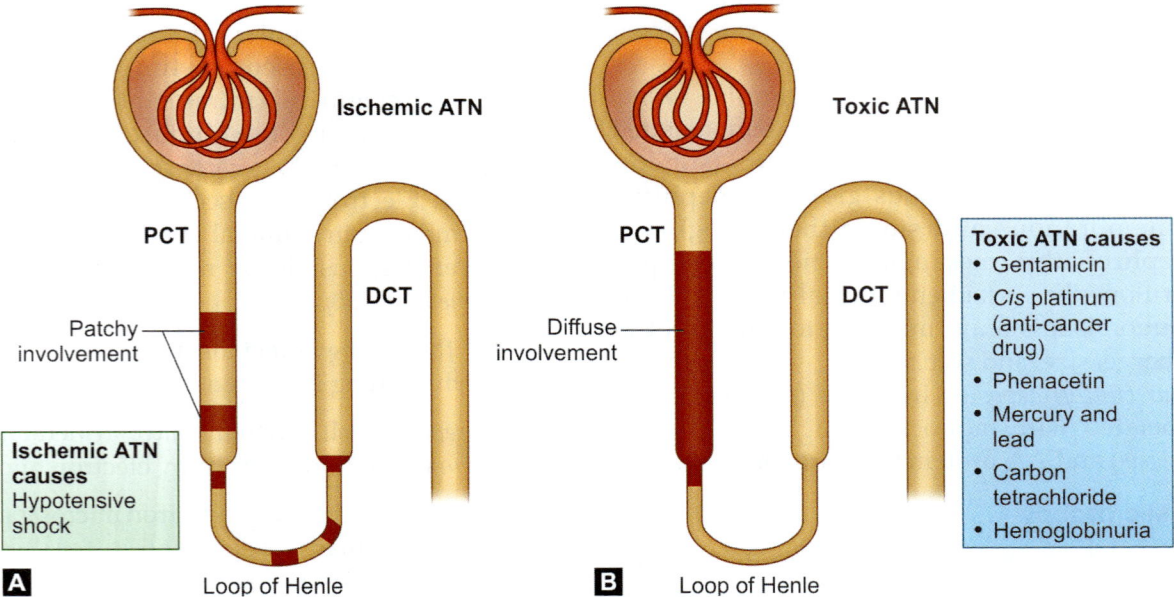

Fig. 22.53: Acute tubular necrosis shows ischemic type and toxic type

ACUTE TUBULAR NECROSIS (ISCHEMIC TYPE)

Etiology

Ischemic ATN results from reduced renal perfusion, usually associated with hypotension following massive hemorrhage, burns and septicemia. Other causes include incompatible blood transfusion, acute pancreatitis and acute intestinal obstruction.

Consequence

Ischemia starts in outer cortex and extends inwards as blood pressure falls. Ischemic changes are marked in the cortical region (proximal tubule straight segment and thick ascending limb of loop of Henle), and medullary region (loop of Henle). Juxtamedullary nephrons usually escape ischemic injury, being closer to main arterial branches.

Pathogenesis

Tubular epithelial cells, with their high rate of energy-consuming metabolic activity and numerous organelles, are particularly sensitive to hypoxia and anoxia.
- *ATP depletion:* Depletion of adenosine triphosphate (ATP) results in accumulation of intracellular calcium.
- *Increased calcium in cells:* Increased intracellular calcium activates cellular enzymes. Phospholipase causes cell membrane injury. Protease causes rearrangement of cytoskeleton.
- *O_2 derived free radicals:* Generation of reactive oxygen species amplify the tubular damage.
- *Role of cytokines:* Release of cytokines leads to recruitment of leucocytes. Influx of neutrophils leads to more tubular injury by liberating hydrolytic enzymes.

Focal denudation of the tubular basement membrane occurs due to necrosis of individual tubular epithelial cells. Necrotic epithelial cells are present in some tubular lumina.

Tubular Lesions

Ischemia causes patchy necrosis of proximal tubules and loop of Henle with intervening skip lesions. Tubular basement membranes are disrupted at these sites, which prevents tubular cell regeneration.

Gross Morphology

The kidneys are swollen. Cut surface reveals pale cortex and a congested medulla. No pathologic changes are seen in the glomeruli or blood vessels.

Electron and Light Microscopy

Initial electron microscopic examination of affected tubules reveals loss of brush border, blebbing of apical cell membrane with hypoxic vacuoles. It is followed by irreversible changes such as detachment of tubular cell membrane. Nucleus undergoes changes such as pyknosis, karyorrhexis and karyolysis demonstrated on light microscopy.

Blood Biochemistry

Patients have increased serum BUN and creatinine (ratio <15).

Urine Analysis

It shows presence of pigmented tubular casts.

Clinical Features

Patient develops anionic gap metabolic acidosis due to increased hyperkalemia. Hypokalemia occurs in diuresis phase.

ACUTE TUBULAR NECROSIS (NEPHROTOXIC TYPE)

Etiology

Chemical induced tubular epithelial injury is the most common cause of acute renal failure. Tubular epithelial cells being metabolically active absorb and concentrate these chemicals. That is the reason that tubular cells are vulnerable to injury due to toxic substances (Table 22.49). These are described below.

Nephrotoxic drugs

- *Antibiotics:* These include gentamicin (most common), penicillin, methicillin, cephalosporins, and polymyxin. Patient with hypersensitivity to penicillin develops tubulointerstitial nephritis by immune-mediated mechanism.
- *Anticancer drug:* Administration of anticancer drug such as cis platinum causes direct toxic injury to tubules.
- *NSAID (phenacetin):* Prolonged intake of analgesic phenacetin causes papillary necrosis by inhibiting prostaglandin synthesis (vasodilator) resulting in ischemia of the renal medulla.
- *Ethylene glycol:* Ingestion of this toxic substance causes acute tubular necrosis. It also causes intratubular deposition of oxalate crystals visualized by polarized microscopy.
- *Radiographic contrast media:* Iodinated contrast media used in radiology is toxic to tubules.
- *Heavy metals:* Exposure to mercury and lead leads to acute tubular necrosis.
- *Organic solvents:* Exposure to nephrotoxic agents, i.e. chloroform, carbon tetrachloride results in acute tubular necrosis.

Table 22.49: Nephrotoxic agents causing acute tubular necrosis

Antibiotics: Gentamicin (most common), penicillin, methicillin, cephalosporins, and polymyxin
Anticancer drug: 'cis platinum'
Nonsteroidal anti-inflammatory drug (NSAID): Phenacetin
Ethylene glycol
Radiographic contrast media
Heavy metals: Mercury and lead
Organic solvents: Chloroform, carbon tetrachloride
Hemoglobinuria
Myoglobinuria

- *Hemoglobinuria and myoglobinuria:* These cause acute tubular necrosis.

Light Microscopy

- Tubules show widespread necrosis of proximal tubular epithelial cells with sparing of distal and collecting tubules.
- Basement membrane of proximal tubules is intact and revealing vacuolation of cytoplasm.

PATHOGENESIS OF ACUTE TUBULAR NECROSIS

Ischemia and toxins cause necrosis of tubular cells as well as endothelial cells (Fig. 22.54). Sequence of events are described as mentioned:

- *Exfoliation of tubular epithelial cells:* Necrosed tubular cells exfoliate and enter into distal tubular lumen. These cells combine with Tam-Horsfall proteins and form *pigmented renal tubular cell casts* in distal tubules.

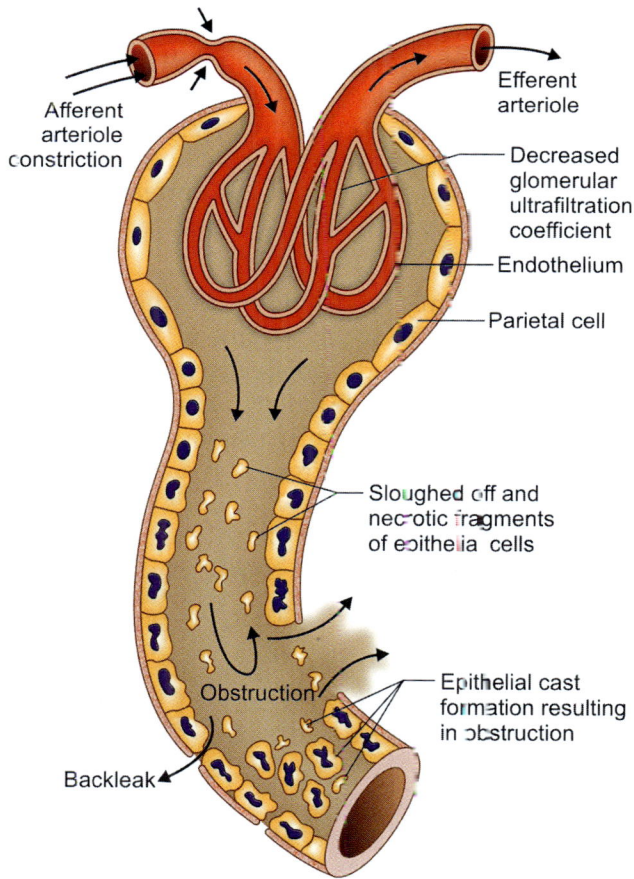

Fig. 22.54: Pathogenesis of acute tubular necrosis. Sloughing and necrosis of tubular epithelial cells lead to formation of cast. Presence of tubular casts cause obstruction and increase intraluminal pressure leading to reduction of glomerular filtration rate. Tubular injury and increased intraluminal pressure are responsible for leakage of fluid from tubular lumen into the interstitium.

- *Obstruction to urine outflow:* Tubular casts obstruct urinary outflow and increase intratubular pressure. Increased intratubular luminal pressure pushes fluid into the interstitium resulting in decreased glomerular filtration rate (oliguria).
- *Vasoconstriction of afferent arterioles:* It plays an important role in oliguria due to decreasing glomerular filtration rate. It occurs as a result of decreased synthesis of vasodilators by injured endothelial cells such as nitric oxide and PGI_2; and increased synthesis of vasoconstrictor angiotensin II.
- *Decreased glomerular filtration rate:* Net result is decreased glomerular filtration rate. All these changes lead to reduced production of urine and cause oliguria. Initially, the changes induced by ischemia or toxins are reversible, but later become irreversible.

ACUTE RENAL FAILURE (AZOTEMIA)

- Acute renal failure is the sudden interruption of renal function. It is critical illness and treated promptly to restore renal functions. It can be caused by poor blood supply to kidney (prerenal etiology), or kidney disease (renal etiology) or obstruction to urine outflow (post-renal etiology). It is potentially reversible, however, if left untreated, permanent damage can lead to chronic renal failure (Table 22.50).
- Hemolytic uremic syndrome occurs due to ingestion of Shiga-toxin-producing strains of *Escherichia coli* results in injury to endothelial cells. It is not associated with angiopathy outside kidney. Patient presents with hemorrhagic diarrhea, microangiopathic hemolytic anemia and rapidly progressive renal failure.

Etiology of Acute Renal Failure

- *Prerenal causes:* Prerenal azotemia implies a reduction in the glomerular filtration rate (GFR) due to hypovolemia in the presence of normal renal function. If uncorrected, it most frequently progresses to ischemic acute tubular necrosis (ATN), which is the most common cause of acute renal failure.

    Decreased renal perfusion occurs due to massive hemorrhage, massive burns, septic shock (gram-negative sepsis), cardiac arrhythmias, cardiogenic shock, heart failure, cardiac tamponade, pulmonary embolism, arterial emboli, thrombi, disseminated intravascular coagulation, eclampsia, vasculitis and malignant hypertension.
- *Intrarenal causes:* Intrinsic renal diseases target the glomeruli (e.g. acute glomerulonephritis, rapidly progressive crescentric glomerulonephritis), tubules (e.g. acute tubular necrosis due to ischemia, toxins), interstitial tissue (e.g. acute pyelonephritis and drug-induced acute interstitial nephritis), or blood vessels (e.g. *malignant hypertension, polyarteritis nodosa), sickle cell disease, systemic lupus erythematosus, transfusion reaction, myeloma nephropathy, crush injuries and papillary necrosis.* The tubular reabsorption is greatly impaired and urinary excretion of sodium is not decreased.
- *Postrenal causes:* Ureteral or urethral mechanical obstruction to urine outflow due to renal calculi, prostatic hyperplasia and invasive cervical cancer may result in acute renal failure (Table 22.51).

Clinical Features

- Patient initially develops oliguria (decreased urine output), azotemia (excess levels of urea in blood), and rarely, anuria (*failure to secrete urine*). It progresses to electrolyte imbalance, metabolic acidosis, uremic

Table 22.50: Parameters in renal failure

Renal reserve	GFR	Characteristics
Diminished renal reserve	GFR: 50% of normal	Blood urea: Normal Serum creatinine: Normal Susceptible to uremia
Renal insufficiency	GFR: 20–50% of normal	Blood urea: Increased Serum creatinine: Increased Sudden susceptible to uremia Azotemia associated with hypertension, decreased concentrating ability of kidneys
Renal failure	GFR: <20% of normal	Blood urea: Increased Serum creatinine: Increased Overt uremic manifestations Kidneys fail to regulate volume, solute composition

Azotemia refers to accumulation of waste products in the body.
Uremia refers to accumulation of waste products in the body with clinical manifestations.

Table 22.51: Renal causes of acute renal failure other than acute tubular necrosis

Renal disorder	Anatomical renal component affected
Various glomerulopathies especially crescentic glomerulonephritis	Glomeruli
Crystal deposition (e.g. oxalates and sulphonamide)	Tubular lumen
Occlusion of renal artery, persistent vasoconstriction of intrarenal vessels, thrombotic thrombocytopenic purpura, malignant nephrosclerosis and bilateral cortical necrosis associated with separation of the placenta	Blood vessels
Acute interstitial nephritis of various type	Interstitial tissue of renal parenchyma

manifestations; renal dysfunction disrupting systemic body systems.
- Patient develops headache, drowsiness, pulmonary edema. Kussmaul's respiration, arrhythmias, heart failure, deranged blood pressure, systemic edema, dry mucous membrane and skin.

Phases of Acute Renal Failure

It has three distinct phases: oliguric, diuretic and recovery (Table 22.52).
- *Oliguric phase:* Patient develops oliguria (decreased urine output <400 ml/24 hours), due to poor renal perfusion (prerenal etiology). It results in impairment of kidney's ability to conserve sodium. There is increased blood urea nitrogen (BUN) and creatinine levels and decreased ratio of BUN to creatinine (from normal levels of 20:1 to abnormal decrease of 10:1).
- *Diuretic phase:* Patient develops slow rise in BUN and creatinine levels. Serum electrolytes (potassium, sodium) are decreased. Body water depletion occurs. Blood pressure falls. If untreated, patient has fatal outcome.
- *Recovery phase:* Well treated patient recovers with restoration of normal BUN and creatinine levels and urine output between 1 and 2 liter/day.

Table 22.52: Urine analysis in acute renal failure

Etiology of acute renal failure	Urinary sediment analysis
Acute tubular necrosis	Dirty brown casts and exfoliated epithelial cells
Acute tubulointerstitial nephritis	White blood cell casts and numerous pus cells
Acute post-streptococcal glomerulonephritis	Red blood cell casts, dysmorphic RBCs and proteinuria in nephritic range <2 gm/day

TUBULOINTERSTITIAL DISORDERS

Tubulointerstitial nephritis is inflammation of tubules and interstitial tissue. It occurs in the settings of infection, toxins, drugs, heavy metals (lead poisoning), irradiation, hypercalcemia, multiple myeloma and autoimmune disorders such as systemic lupus erythematosus, Sjögren's syndrome (Fig. 22.55).

PYELONEPHRITIS

It refers to bacterial infection of the kidney parenchyma and or renal pelvis. Depending on the course of disease, it is categorized as acute pyelonephritis or chronic pyelonephritis. Vesicoureteral reflux (VUR) with ascending bacterial urinary tract infections play an important role in the pathogenesis of pyelonephritis (Tables 22.53 and 22.54).
- *Acute pyelonephritis:* It produces severe symptoms as the kidneys are actively and aggressively attacked by bacteria. In some cases, bacteria may invade glomerular capillaries resulting in potentially life-threatening sepsis. Kidneys show radiating yellowish gray streaks in pyramids and abscess in cortex. There is moderate hydronephrosis and blunting of calyces.
- *Chronic pyelonephritis:* It results from incompletely treated acute pyelonephritis. The organisms continue to multiply and destroy the renal parenchyma. The process is slow and painless. The net result is permanent damage to kidneys with impaired function. Kidneys show wedge-shaped subcapsular scars, thinning of renal parenchyma, blunting of corticomedullary junctions and dilated fibrosed pelvis and calyces in majority of cases.

ACUTE PYELONEPHRITIS (APN)

- It refers to formation of pus (abscess) in the tubules. Vesicoureteral reflux (VUR) with ascending infection is most common cause of acute pyelonephritis.

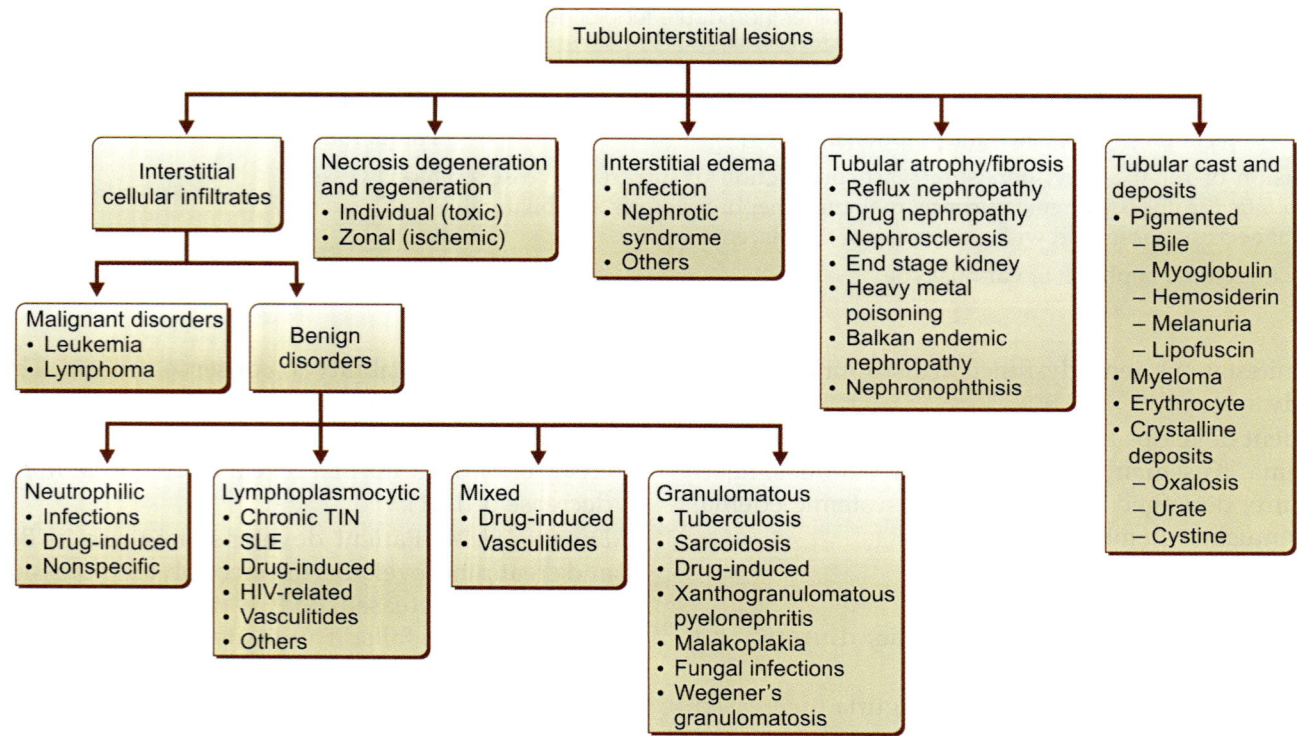

Fig. 22.55: Tubulointerstitial lesions. Etiology and pathological findings.

Table 22.53: Comparison between chronic glomerulonephritis and chronic pyelonephritis

Parameters	Chronic glomerulonephritis	Chronic pyelonephritis
Kidney involvement	Bilateral involvement	Unilateral involvement
Kidney contraction	Moderate contraction	Marked contraction
Glomerular changes	Diffuse involvement of glomeruli Proliferation of glomerular tuft present Thickening of glomerular tuft present Changes in the Bowman's space are not usually present	Patchy involvement of glomeruli Proliferation of glomerular tuft absent Thickening of glomerular tuft rarely Changes in the Bowman's space are relatively greater
Tubular loss	Tubular loss in relation to sclerosed glomeruli present	Tubular loss is not confined to area with glomerular lesion
Interstitial fibrosis	Fine	Coarse
Inflammatory infiltrate	Less	Marked
Pelvis inflammation	Seldom inflamed	Usually inflamed
Vascular changes	Moderate	Marked
Necrotising papillitis	Absent	Present

- Vesicoureteral reflux carries infected urine up to the ureters into the renal pelvis and calyces resulting in entry of the bacteria through the papillae into the renal parenchyma. Bacteriuria is a typical finding in patients with acute pyelonephritis.
- Urinary tract infection is common due to shorter length of the female urethra especially during pregnancy.

Etiology

- *Escherichia coli* from the feces cause distal colonization in the urethra. Ascending urinary tract infection by *Escherichia coli* is the most common cause of acute pyelonephritis in (85%) of cases. Other gram-negative organisms include Proteus, Klebsiella, enterococci.

Table 22.54: Comparison between acute and chronic pyelonephritis

Characteristics	Acute pyelonephritis	Chronic pyelonephritis
Definition	It is characterized by acute suppurative inflammation of kidney caused by bacteria	It is chronic tubulointerstitial disease characterized by chronic inflammation, renal scarring and involvement of calyces and renal pelvis
Etiology	Urinary tract obstruction, instrumentation, catheterization, diabetes mellitus, pregnancy and pre-existing renal diseases	Chronic obstructive pyelonephritis and reflux nephropathy
Pathology	Bacterial infection and renal lesion associated with urinary tract infection	Bacterial infection plays a dominant role but vesicoureteral reflux and obstruction play role in its pathogenesis
Gross morphology	Patch interstitial suppurative inflammation and tubular necrosis	Coarse discrete corticomedullary scarring is present overlying blunted or dilated calyx
Light microscopy	It shows infiltration of neutrophils and bacterial colonies	Tubules show atrophy in some areas and dilation in other areas. Dilated tubules contain eosinophilic material mimicking colloid hence named as *thyroidization* of tubules
Clinical course	Sudden onset of fever, back pain and malaise	Onset is insidious (silent process)

- Gram-positive pyogenic bacteria may cause acute pyelonephritis through hematogenous dissemination (uncommon cause). Infection of the bladder and urethra often precedes acute pyelonephritis.
- Acute pyelonephritis most often occurs in women than men, because women have short urethra injured during sexual intercourse resulting to urethritis and cystitis.

Predisposing Factors

- *Diseases:* These include urinary tract obstruction (e.g. calculi, prostatic hypertrophy), renal cystic diseases, diabetes mellitus, medullary sponge of kidney, vesicoureteral reflux (VUR), previous instrumentation of the urinary tract, pregnancy, sickle cell disease and neurogenic urinary bladder. Diabetic patients with glucosuria are at increased risk for developing acute pyelonephritis.
- *Vesicoureteral reflux:* Intravesical portion of the ureter is normally compressed with micturition, which prevents reflux of urine into the ureters. In vesicoureteral reflux, the intravesical portion of the ureter is not compressed during micturition, as a result urine refluxes into the ureters during micturition. If vesicoureteral reflux persists, infected urine ascends to the renal pelvis and renal parenchyma resulting in acute pyelonephritis and then progressing to chronic pyelonephritis.
- *Residual volume of urine:* There is increased incidence of acute pyelonephritis in patients with atonic bladder or flaccid urinary bladder caused by progesterone therapy; in which residual volume of urine is increased (normal residual volume 2–3 ml). Obstruction to urinary outflow due to nodular hyperplasia prostate is also important cause of acute pyelonephritis.

Gross Morphology

- Acute pyelonephritis is often a focal disease, and much of the kidney often appears normal. The kidneys develop grayish white areas of small microabscesses in tubular lumens and interstitial tissue of cortex as well as medulla on the subcapsular surface (Fig. 22.56).
- Accumulation of pus in the calyces and pelvis causes obstruction to urine outflow resulting in *pyonephros*. Extension of suppuration through the renal capsule leads to formation of perinephric abscess. The urothelium of the renal pelvis and calyces may be hyperemic and covered by a purulent exudate.

Light Microscopy

- Renal biopsy shows an extensive infiltrate of neutrophils in the collecting tubules and interstitial tissue.
- The glomeruli and blood vessels are not involved by purulent infection.
- Molding of neutrophils forms WBCs casts in the tubules, which are passed in the urine along with free neutrophils and bacteria (pyuria).

Clinical Features

- Patient with mild acute pyelonephritis may present with low-grade fever with or without pain in the

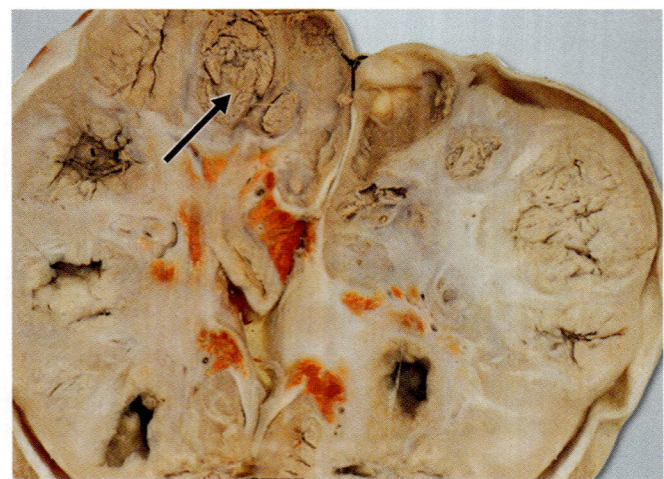

Fig. 22.56: Acute pyelonephritis—acute pyelonephritis is often a focal disease, and much of the kidney often appears normal. The kidney shows multiple grayish white areas of small microabscesses in the renal parenchyma (arrow).

consists of WBCs casts. There is an increased incidence of pyelonephritis during pregnancy.

Complications

Patients with acute pyelonephritis develop various complications, i.e. *chronic pyelonephritis, pyonephrosis* (due to obstruction to urine outflow), *perinephric abscess, renal papillary necrosis and septicemia* (endotoxic shock).

Laboratory Findings

Microscopic examination of urine reveals WBCs casts, pus cells, hematuria and bacteriuria usually *E. coli*. Urine culture in suspected cases is considered as significant, if excess of $(10)^5$ culture forming units/ml is present, which excludes cases of extraneous bacterial contamination.

CHRONIC PYELONEPHRITIS

Chronic pyelonephritis is caused by recurrent and persistent bacterial infection secondary to urinary tract obstruction, vesicoureteral reflux (ascending infected urine from urethritis or cystitis especially in young girls), or both. It usually affects one kidney causing small asymmetric contraction with scarred surface. The patient is usually asymptomatic.

- lower back or costovertebral angle and voiding small quantity of urine at frequent intervals.
- In severe infection, patient presents with sudden onset of spiking fever, flank pain, without gross hematuria, chills, nausea, vomiting, increased frequency of urination and painful urination (dysuria) if associated with lower urinary tract infection. Patient's urine

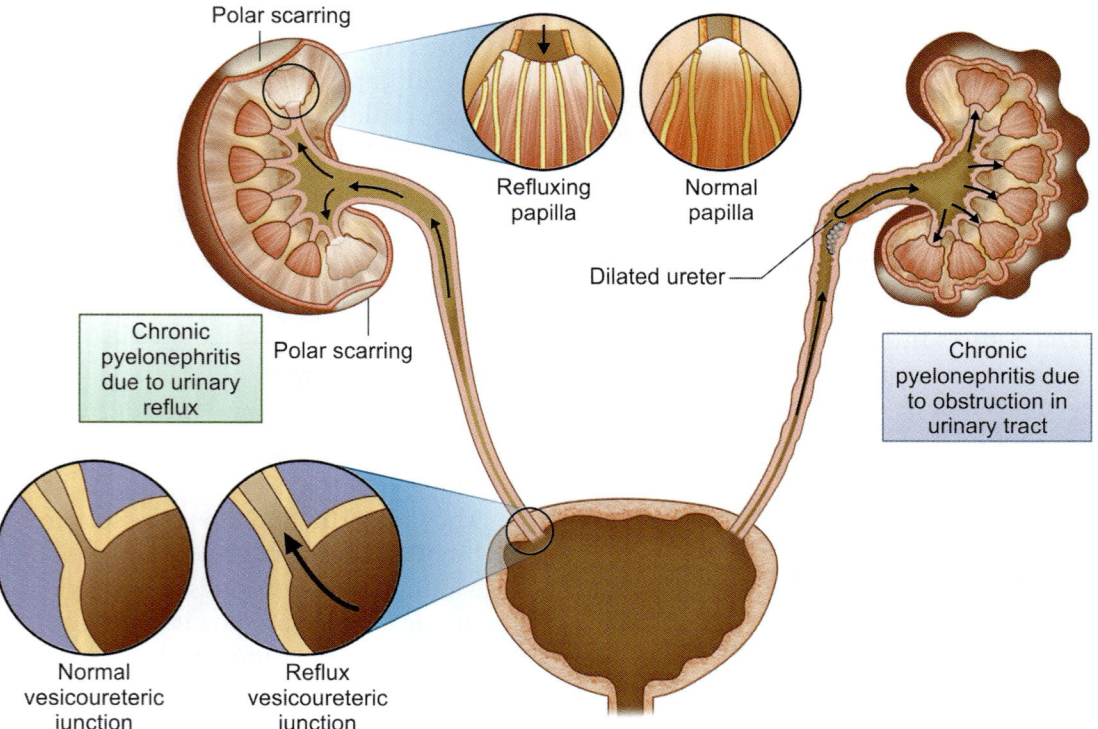

Fig. 22.57: Chronic pyelonephritis due to vesicoureteral reflux with irregular scars at poles. Obstruction of the urinary tract leads to high pressure backflow of urine leading to destruction of all papillae in renal parenchyma. It leads to diffuse scarring of the kidney and thinning of overlying cortex.

Kidney and Ureter

Etiopathogenesis

- *Vesicoureteral reflux:* The intravesical portion of the ureter is not compressed during micturition, as a result urine refluxes into the ureter, renal pelvis and renal parenchyma resulting in acute pyelonephritis and then progressing to chronic pyelonephritis. Vesicoureteral reflux targets children under 5 years old due to an incompetent ureterovesical junction (Fig. 22.57).
- *Urinary tract obstruction:* Obstruction to urinary flow due to renal stones, prostatic hyperplasia or tumors is *associated with inflammation as well as dilatation of the ureter and renal pelvis, calyces especially polar compound papillae containing straight ducts* with absence of valve-like action. It leads to diffuse irregular U-shaped cortical scarring in polar areas. These changes are visible with an intravenous pyelography (IVP) (Fig. 22.58).

Gross Morphology

- Renal parenchyma in chronic pyelonephritis is firm due to extensive fibrosis.
- External surface reveals broad asymmetric U-shaped scars involving cortex and medulla especially in upper pole.
- Cut surface shows deformity of the renal pelvis and calyces (Fig. 22.59).

Light Microscopy

- *Tubules:* Histologic section shows dilation, atrophy, and loss of renal tubules. When the atrophic tubules contain eosinophilic proteinaceous casts, the resultant similarity in appearance to thyroid follicles is referred to as thyroidization (Fig. 22.60).
- *Interstitial stroma:* Interstitial stroma undergoes fibrosis and infiltrated by lymphocytes, plasma cells and macrophages.
- *Glomeruli:* There is presence of secondary glomerulosclerosis.
- *Blood vessels:* Arteries show endarteritis with narrowing of the lumen and fibrosis of media.

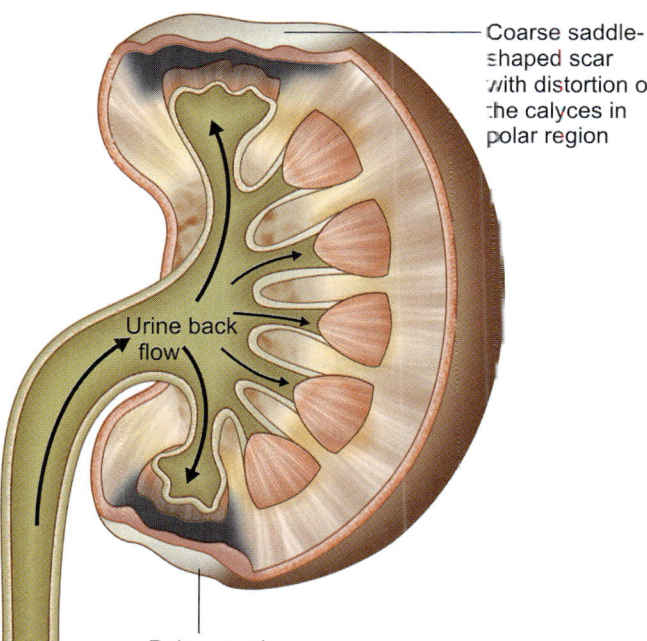

Fig. 22.58: Chronic pyelonephritis caused by vesicoureteral reflux. Vesicoureteral reflux causes infection of the compound papillae located on the poles. Note the relationship of the coarse saddle-shaped scars with distortion of the calyces.

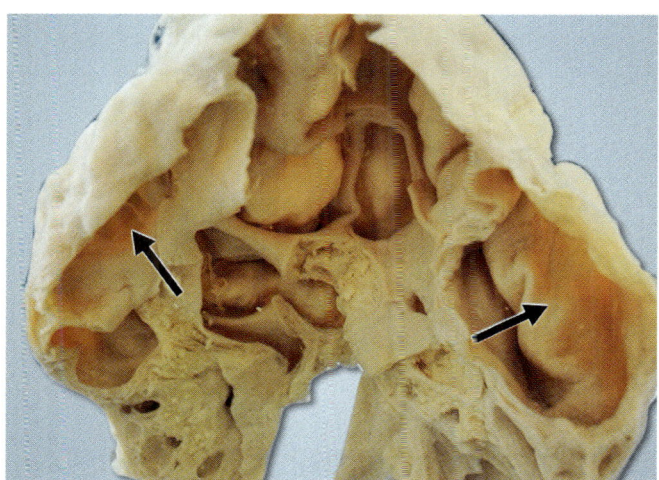

Fig. 22.59: Chronic pyelonephritis with hydronephrosis. Cortical cut surface shows marked dilation of calyces caused by inflammatory destruction of papillae, with atrophy and scarring of the overlying cortex (arrows).

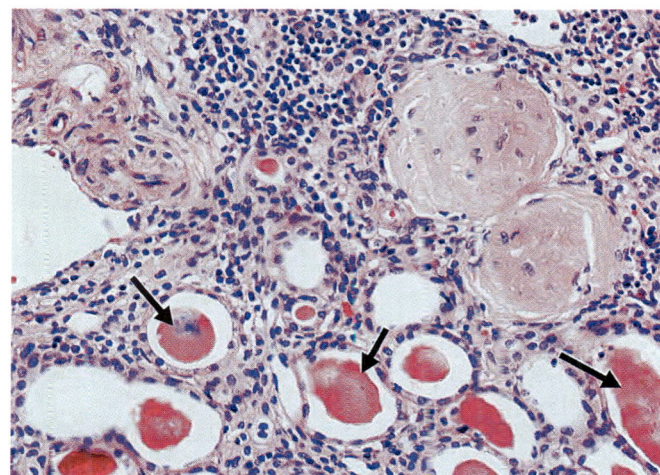

Fig. 22.60: Chronic pyelonephritis with thyroidization of tubules and thickening of blood vessels (arrows) (400X).

Clinical Features

- Patient with chronic pyelonephritis presents with episodic manifestations of urinary tract infection or acute pyelonephritis, such as recurrent fever and flank pain. Patients develop gradual loss of renal function, especially in bilateral involvement.
- Children with reflex nephropathy develop hypertension, flank pain and other vague signs of inflammation resulting in chronic renal failure.

XANTHOGRANULOMATOUS PYELONEPHRITIS

Xanthogranulomatous glomerulonephritis is usually associated with staghorn calculus obstructing urinary outflow together with chronic infection with Proteus infection cause suppurative destruction of renal parenchyma. Sometimes long-standing infection may be localized by forming a mass-like lesion. It can be grossly and microscopically mistaken as clear cell *variant of renal cell carcinoma.*

Light Microscopy

- The histiocytes (clear or foamy) due to breakdown of renal parenchyma are typically admixed with lymphocytes and plasma cells.
- The vascular stroma characteristic of clear cel variant of renal cell carcinoma is missing in xanthogranulomatous pyelonephritis.

TUBERCULAR PYELONEPHRITIS

Kidneys are most common extrapulmonary site in tuberculosis. This can cause asymptomatic pyuria (white blood cells in the urine). It can spread to the reproductive organs and affect reproduction. In men, epididymitis (inflammation of the epididymis) may occur. Urine analysis reveals acidic pH, proteinuria and pus cells.

Gross Morphology

Kidneys are enlarged. Cut surface reveals caseous material filling the renal pelvis (Fig. 22.61).

Light Microscopy

Histopathological examination shows caseous necrosis, epithelioid cell granulomas and Langhans' giant cells.

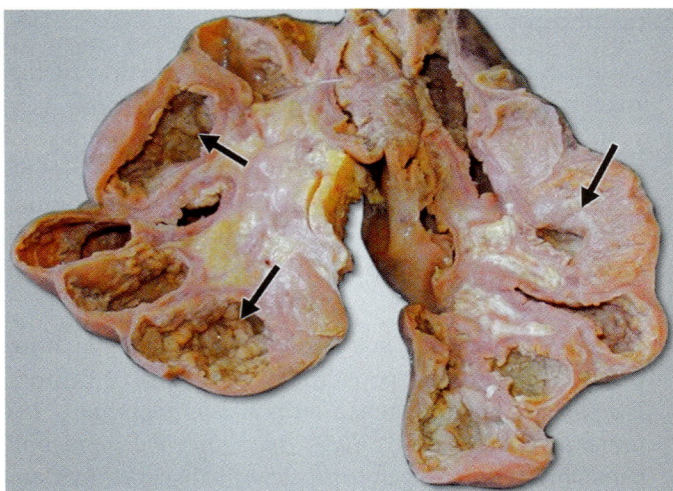

Fig. 22.61: Tubercular pyelonephritis. Fibrous-walled abscess cavity filled with caseous material is shown on cut surface. This patient had a previous well-established history of pulmonary tuberculosis. Section from the patient's nephrectomy specimen shows a tuberculous granuloma, with central caseating necrosis and peripheral scarring (arrows).

URATE NEPHROPATHY

Any condition associated with elevated levels of uric acid in the blood results in deposition of urate crystals in the tubules and interstitium is known as urate nephropathy.

Acute Urate Nephropathy

It occurs due to massive release of nucleic acid purines (uric acid) following aggressive treatment of disseminated cancer with allopurinol (e.g. leukemia and lymphoma) resulting in increased serum uric acid level. Urate crystals are deposited in the tubules and interstitial tissue.

Chronic Urate Nephropathy

It is caused by gout characterized by tubular and interstitial deposition of crystalline monosodium urate. The crystalline monosodium urate, when excreted leads to plug the tubules. It leads to deposition of uric acid crystals in tubules and interstitial tissue in the medulla, forming pale yellowish 'tophi' with surrounding foreign body inflammation, mononuclear cell infiltrates, and fibrosis. Patients with hyperuricemia may also have nephrolithiasis with uric acid stones.

DRUGS INDUCED ACUTE TUBULOINTERSTITIAL DISEASES

Drug-induced acute tubulointerstitial nephritis reflects a cell-mediated immune response. It is characterized histologically by infiltrates of activated lymphocytes (T cells) and eosinophils, a pattern that indicates a type IV cell-mediated immune reaction. Presence of eosinophilia and eosinophiluria indicates a type I hypersensitivity response.

Etiology

The most frequently implicated drugs include penicillin (particularly methicillin), rifampicin, sulfonamides, NSAIDs, allopurinol, and diuretics (thiazides, furosemide). It occurs two weeks after beginning a drug. Withdrawal of the drug usually results in reversal of the disease.

Clinical Features

Patient presents with abrupt onset of fever, skin rash and rapidly progressive renal failure, approximately 2 weeks after drug administration. Eosinophilia and eosinophiluria are highly predictive. Renal functions are impaired with increased blood urea and serum creatinine.

Urine Analysis

It reveals mild to moderate proteinuria, hematuria, and eosinophiluria (eosinophils in the urine). Withdrawal of the drug causes reversal of the disease.

ANALGESIC INDUCED NEPHROPATHY

- Analgesic nephropathy is a common cause of chronic drug-induced interstitial nephritis. It is more common in women than men associated with chronic pain.
- The combination of acetaminophen (a metabolite of phenacetin) and aspirin in the setting of a patient (usually a woman) with chronic headache or pain is responsible for most cases.
- A cumulative analgesics ingestion of 3 kg or daily consumption of 1 gm/day (>2 kg) over a span of 3 years is sufficient to produce analgesic nephropathy.

Mode of Action

- Acetaminophen forms free radicals, which bind with the renal tubular cells and cause oxidative cellular damage of renal tubules in medulla. While aspirin inhibits prostaglandin synthesis, hence eliminating the vasodilator effects of prostaglandins.
- Vasoconstriction of renal vessels causes ischemic injury (coagulation necrosis) in the renal medullary papillae and tubulointerstitial fibrosis.

Pathology

Patient develops papillary necrosis of some or all papillae, which appears pale white infarcts. Papillary necrosis may also occur in sickle cell anemia, diabetes mellitus, acute pyelonephritis, and obstructive uropathy.

Clinical Features

Sloughing of the necrosed renal papillae (renal papillary necrosis) is associated with gross hematuria, proteinuria, and colicky flank pain. An intravenous pyelogram reveals a *ring defect* where one or more papillae used to reside.

Complications

These include renal papillary necrosis, hypertension, renal stones, hematuria, accelerated atherosclerosis, urothelial bladder transitional cell carcinomas (very high risk), tubulointerstitial fibrosis, and end stage renal disease are potential complications.

LIGHT CHAIN CAST NEPHROPATHY IN MULTIPLE MYELOMA

Renal injury is the most common cause of death in multiple myeloma.

Pathogenesis

- *Direct effects of Bence Jones protein:* Bence Jones proteins are the light chain of immunoglobulin filtered through the glomeruli. These are toxic to the tubules. At acidic pH of urine, the light chains of Bence Jones protein bind to Tam-Horsfall glycoproteins, which are synthesized by distal tubular epithelial cells. These casts cause obstruction to urinary flow in the tubules.
- *Amyloidosis:* AL amyloid formed from the light chains of immunoglobulin deposit in glomeruli, blood vessels, and tubular basement membranes of tubules.
- *Light chain nephropathy:* In some instances, the deposits of light chains do not become fibrillar and do not transform into AL amyloid. Nevertheless, these deposits damage the GBM and tubular basement membranes and cause renal failure.
- *Hypercalcemia:* It leads to nephrocalcinosis and urinary stone formation.

Clinical Features

Light chain cast nephropathy may manifest either acute or chronic renal failure. Proteinuria is most often present in variable range (nephritic or nephrotic range). If patient presents with proteinuria in nephrotic range, AL amyloidosis or light chain deposition disease is more likely than light chain cast nephropathy.

Light Microscopy
- The characteristic tubular lesions show numerous dense hyaline casts in the distal tubules and collecting ducts. These casts are brightly eosinophilic with angulated borders.
- These casts induce foreign body reaction, characterized by multinucleated giant cells and macrophages.
- Interstitial tissue is infiltrated by chronic inflammatory cells.
- More chronic lesions show tubular atrophy and interstitial fibrosis. Focal deposition of calcium is demonstrated in interstitial tissue.

Immunohistochemistry
Immunohistochemical staining reveals that the casts containing light chains and Tamm-Horsfall glycoproteins.

RENAL TUBULAR FUNCTIONAL DISORDERS

Fanconi's Syndrome
It refers to generalized dysfunction of the proximal renal tubules. It may be hereditary or acquired. Patient has impaired absorption of glucose, amino acids, bicarbonate and phosphates. Patient presents with glycosuria, increased excretion of phosphates with decreased blood level of phosphates, amino acids and systemic acidosis.

Cystinuria
It occurs in children with hereditary cystinuria, an error of amino acid metabolism resulting in excess of cysteine in the urine due to impaired tubular reabsorption of cysteine. It is associated with cysteine stones.

Hartnup Disease
It refers to genetically impaired tubular reabsorption of tryptophan. Patient develops pellagra like manifestations.

NEPHROCALCINOSIS
- Hypercalcemia may cause nephrocalcinosis or nephrolithiasis or urolithiasis. Nephrocalcinosis may cause tubular defects especially impairment of concentrating ability of kidneys, salt excretion and renal tubular acidosis.
- In hypercalcemia, deposition of calcium in renal parenchyma is an example of metastatic calcification, in contrast to dystrophic calcification demonstrated at the site of renal parenchyma injury due to infarcts or cortical necrosis (Table 22.55).

Pathology
- In patient with nephrosclerosis, extent of calcification varies from microscopic to grossly visible demonstrated on radiograph.
- Hypercalcemia due to primary hyperparathyroidism, results in renal parenchyma shows wedge-shaped scars interspersed with relatively normal renal tissue. These scars are composed of parenchymal atrophy and interstitial fibrosis.

Electron Microscopy
Mitochondria of tubular epithelial cells contains abundant calcium deposits.

Light Microscopy
- Basement membrane of renal tubules especially proximal tubules shows deposition of calcium. Calcium deposition also occurs in the cytoplasm of tubules and interstitial tissue. These tubular epithelial cells laden with calcium slough into the lumina in the form of aggregates as calcified casts.
- Scattered glomeruli show calcification in Bowman's capsule. Intrarenal arteries may also show calcification.
- Calcium deposits appear deeply basophilic in hematoxylin and eosin sections and black with von Kossa stain.

Table 22.55: Etiology of hypercalcemia leading to nephrocalcinosis

Parameters	Causes
Increased resorption of calcium from bone	Primary hyperparathyroidism
	Renal osteodystrophy
	Neoplasms synthesizing parathormone or parathormone-like protein and metastases
Increased intestinal absorption of calcium	Milk-alkali syndrome
	Vitamin D excess
	Idiopathic hypercalcemia
	Sarcoidosis

OBSTRUCTIVE UROPATHY AND HYDRONEPHROSIS

OVERVIEW

Obstruction may occur anywhere in the urinary system (e.g. renal tubules, renal pelvis, ureters, urethra, prostate, and bladder). Patient develops hydronephrosis. In children, the condition is most often congenital (e.g. posterior urethral valves and urethral strictures) and congenital ureteric abnormality (ureterocele). In adults, the condition is most often acquired.

Etiology in Adults

- *Renal causes:* These include staghorn calculus, transitional cell carcinoma of renal pelvis and atrophic scarred cortex.
- *Ureteric causes:* These include ureteral stone, transitional cell carcinoma, retroperitoneal fibrosis, surgical scars, and necrotic debris.
- *Extrinsic compression causes:* These include pregnancy, endometriosis, and carcinoma cervix in women. Obstructive causes in men are carcinoma urinary bladder, benign nodular hyperplasia of prostate, neurogenic bladder (e.g. spinal cord damage) and urethral stricture as a consequence of chronic urethritis (Fig. 22.62 and Table 22.56).

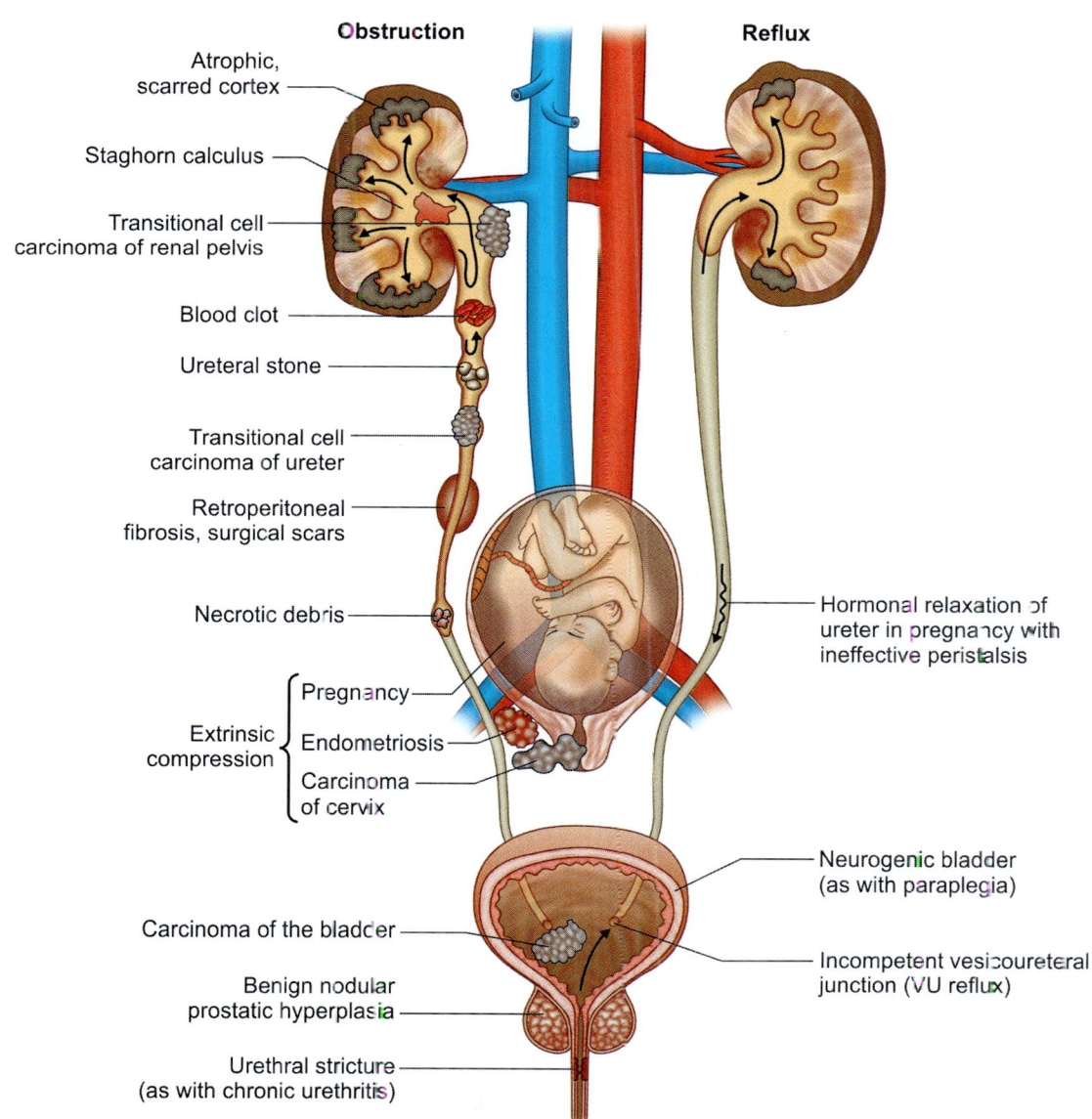

Fig. 22.62: Causes of urinary obstruction.

Clinical Manifestations

- *Hydronephrosis:* It leads to dilatation of the renal pelvis, collecting ducts, proximal and distal convoluted tubules. Calyces undergo atrophic changes and flattening with variable degrees of compression atrophy of the cortex and medulla. Loss of nephrons is accompanied by fibrosis.
- *Renal colic:* Patient with renal stone presents with excruciating pain caused by acute distension of the ureter, usually by the transit of a small stone.
- *Superadded infection:* It is localized proximal to the site of obstruction. It may lead to infection of the renal parenchyma.

Table 22.56: Causes of urinary tract obstruction

Level of obstruction	Cause
Renal pelvis	Renal calculi Papillary necrosis
Ureter	Renal calculi Pregnancy Tumors that compress the ureter Ureteral stricture Congenital disorders of the ureterovesical junction and ureteropelvic junction strictures
Urinary bladder and urethra	Urinary bladder cancer Neurogenic urinary bladder Urinary bladder calculi Prostatic hyperplasia or prostate cancer Urethral strictures Congenital urethral defects

RENAL STONES (NEPHROLITHIASIS AND UROLITHIASIS)

PATHOGENESIS

Nephrolithiasis refers to formation of stones in collecting system of the urinary tract. Renal pelvis and calyces are the most common sites of renal stones. These are more common in men than women. In most cases, the presence of a urinary stone is associated with an increased blood level and urinary excretion of its principal component. More than 90% of stones are radio dense on KUB radiographs (Table 22.57).

Table 22.57: Composition, contributory factors and treatment of kidney stones

Type of stone	Percentage of renal stones	Contributing factors	Treatment
Calcium oxalate or calcium phosphate	75%	Hypercalcemia and hypercalciuria Hyperparathyroidism Vitamin D intoxication Milk alkali syndrome Renal tubular acidosis Intestinal bypass surgery Hyperoxaluria	Treatment of underlying cause, increased fluid intake, thiazide diuretics and dietary restriction of foods rich in oxalates
Magnesium ammonium phosphate (struvite) also called staghorn stone	15%	Urea splitting bacteria	Treatment of urinary tract infection, acidification of urine and increased fluid intake
Uric acid (urate)	3-4%	Formed in acid urine with pH of approximately 5.5, gout, high-purine diet	Increased fluid intake, allopurinol for hyperuricosuria, alkalization of urine
Cystine	Very rare	Cystinuria (inherited disorder of amino acid metabolism)	Increased fluid intake, alkalization of urine

Calcium oxalate stones most often occur in adults and constitute 75–80% of cases.
Calcium phosphate stones are most common type of stones in children (10–20%).

Physiological State

Normally, stone formation is prevented by various mechanisms:

- *Hydration:* Hydration prevents supersaturation of urinary solutes (e.g. calcium, uric acid, oxalates).
- *Citrate:* Citrate chelates calcium constituent in urine.
- *Inhibitors:* Stone formation is prevented by presence of inhibitors in urine such as pyrophosphate, diphosphonate, citrate, glycosaminoglycans and nephrocalcin.

Predisposing Factors

Stones formation is accelerated by following mechanisms:

- Supersaturation of urinary solutes occurs due to low urinary output.
- Deficiency of urinary citrate fails to chelate calcium.
- Hypercalcemia occurs due to increased reabsorption of calcium by intestine; and primary hyperparathyroidism in 10% of cases.
- Hypercalciuria is the most common metabolic abnormality in calcium stone formers.
- Excessive intake of dairy products rich in oxalates and phosphates causes stone formation.
- Recurrent urinary tract infection caused by urea-splitting *Proteus vulgaris*, Proteus, Klebsiella species and Staphylococcus make the urine alkaline resulting in precipitation of ammonium magnesium phosphate stones known as *staghorn stones filling entire renal pelvis and calyceal system*.

TYPE OF RENAL STONES

- Renal stone requires a nidus to form. It comprises mucoprotein matrix (3–5%) and aggregated material derived from precipitation of urinary solutes, which constitutes 95–98% of the stone mass.
- Depending on presence of salt constituents, urinary stones are of four types: (i) calcium containing stones (calcium oxalates or calcium phosphate), (ii) calcium deficient stones such as magnesium ammonium phosphate or (triple stones or struvite stones, which form staghorn calculus), (iii) uric acid stones, (iv) xanthine stones and (v) cystine stones. These are discussed below.

CALCIUM STONES

Most urinary stones contain calcium complexed with oxalate or phosphate, or a mixture of both anions. These constitute 80–85% of urinary stones.

Etiology

These are usually related to idiopathic calciuria, increased absorption of calcium in the intestine, and increased renal excretion of calcium, or hypercalcemia.

Hypercalcemia may be caused by hyperparathyroidism characterized by deposition of calcium in the basement membrane of renal tubules (nephrocalcinosis) and renal parenchyma.

Hypercalcemia often occurs due to osteolytic metastases and ectopic production of parathyroid hormone (often by a squamous cell carcinoma of the lung). Other causes of hypercalcemia include vitamin D intoxication, milk-alkali syndrome and sarcoidosis.

Type of Calcium Stones

Calcium Oxalate Stones

These most often occur in adults and constitute 75–80% of cases. These are *radiopaque*. These occur due to increased absorption of oxalate from the bowel mucosa in Crohn's disease; and intake of certain foods (e.g. spinach, chocolate). *The surface of calcium oxalate stone is rough, brown color probably due to old blood pigment.*

Calcium Phosphate Stones

These are most common type of stones in children (10–20%). These are associated with *consumption of dairy products* with recurrent urinary tract infections or distal renal tubular acidosis. *Consistency of stones is hard/soft*.

Therapeutic Correlation

Hyperchlorothiazide increases renal tubule reabsorption of calcium. Cellulose phosphate binds calcium in intestine.

MAGNESIUM AMMONIUM PHOSPHATE STONES

Magnesium ammonium phosphate stones are the second most common form of renal stones. These are formed in patients with recurrent urinary tract infections by urea-splitting *Proteus vulgaris*, Klebsiella species and Staphylococcus. These constitute 15% of stones (Fig. 22.63).

Mechanism

Urease produced by these organisms convert urea into NH_3, thus causes alkaline pH of urine, resulting in precipitation of magnesium ammonium phosphate (struvite) and calcium phosphate (apatite).

Morphology of Stones

Staghorn calculi fill the entire pelvis and calices. The stone has flaking surface and gray white color.

Section III: Systemic Pathology

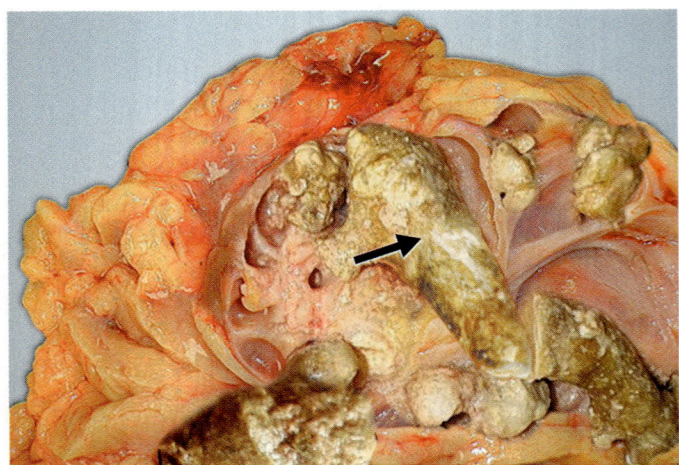

Fig. 22.63: Staghorn stone in kidney (arrow).

Therapeutic Correlation
Because of large size staghorn stone filling entire renal pelvis and calyceal system, surgical removal is done. Antibiotics are given to eliminate urease producing bacteria.

URIC ACID STONES

Etiopathogenesis
Uric acid stones are associated with hyperuricemia in 50% of patients, secondary to gout or increased cell turn over (leukemias or myeloproliferative syndrome). These are associated with intake of diet rich in meat and purines. Long-standing diarrhea leads to small volume of very acidic urine responsible for uric acid stones formation.

Morphology
Uric acid stones are <2 cm size with smooth light yellow-brown color, hard consistency and radiolucent.

Therapeutic Correlation
Allopurinol increases urinary pH and makes uric acid soluble in urine.

CYSTINE STONES
These stones are relatively rare. These occur in children with hereditary cystinuria, an error of amino acid metabolism resulting in excess of cysteine in the urine. These stones are round in shape with smooth surface.

Clinical Course
Most kidney stones are completely silent. Patient with large renal stones presents with an abrupt onset of severe, colicky pain in the flank radiating to the groin; and associated with either microscopic or macroscopic hematuria.

XANTHINE STONES
These are <2 cm, smooth, light yellow color, radiolucent; stones may or may not be visualized with plain X-ray films.

COMPLICATIONS
Patient with urolithiasis may develop hydronephrosis and chronic pyonephrosis (Figs 22.64 and 22.65).
- *Hydronephrosis:* Obstruction to the urinary outflow leads to dilatation of calyceal system. Surface of the calyceal system is smooth.

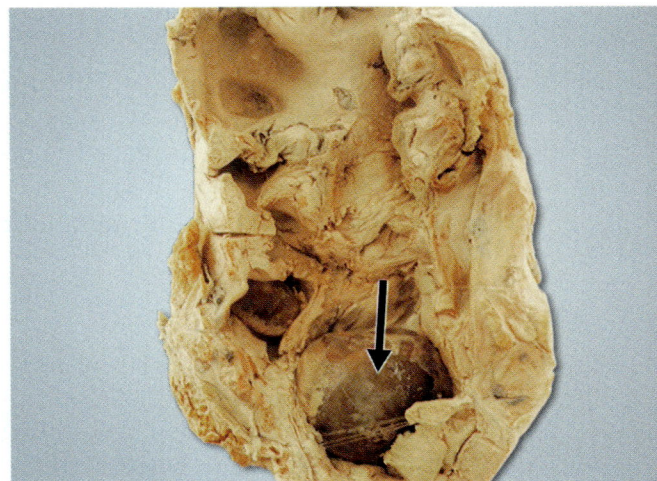

Fig. 22.64: Chronic pyelonephritis with nephrolithiasis (arrow).

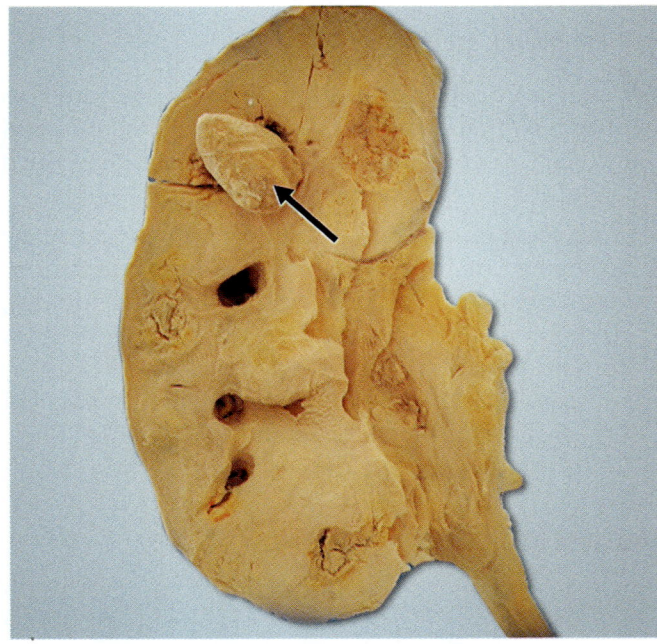

Fig. 22.65: Chronic pyelonephritis with pyonephrosis (arrow).

- *Pyonephrosis:* Obstruction in the renal pelvis or upper part of ureter leads to superadded infection and suppuration of the contents of the calyceal system known as *pyonephrosis*.

  The suppurative exudate fails to drain out due to obstruction. The surface of calyces becomes shaggy due to accumulation of pus.

  Extension of suppurative inflammation through the renal capsule leads to perinephric abscess.

LABORATORY DIAGNOSIS AND MANAGEMENT

Laboratory Diagnosis

- *Urine analysis:* It is performed to demonstrate hematuria and crystals. It is also performed to study the composition of the stone (urine must be strained), since treatment is often tailored to the composition of the stone. Approximately >50% of cases, pass stones in urine within 48 hours. Recurrence of stone formation is seen in 50% of cases.
- *Imaging techniques:* X-rays kidney-ureter-bladder (KUB) **may reveal radiopaque stones** in >80% of patients. Enhanced spiral (helical) CT scan and ultrasonography are done to demonstrate urinary stones. Intravenous urography is helpful to locate urinary stone.
- *Blood biochemistry:* Serum calcium and parathormone levels are increased in hyperparathyroidism.

Surgical Procedures

- *Nephrolithotomy:* It refers to removal of renal stones by making a small tract from the skin to the kidney.
- *ESWL (extracorporeal shock wave lithotripsy):* It is used to remove stones in the kidney or upper ureter. Shock waves are directed by a probe placed on the tummy or back. This shatters the stone into small fragments which then can be passed spontaneously.
- *Surgery:* If ESWL does not work surgery can be used to remove staghorn stone.
- *Cystoscopy:* Bladder stones are removed using a cystoscope, a special instrument which is passed through the urethra into the bladder

VASCULAR DISORDERS

DIFFUSE CORTICAL NECROSIS SECONDARY TO SHOCK

- Diffuse cortical necrosis refers to acute widespread ischemic necrosis limited to the large portions of the renal cortex of both kidneys; the medulla is spared. Bilateral pale infarcts are seen in renal cortex. Massive tubular necrosis leads to fatal outcome. Infarction may be patchy in some cases and compatible with survival.
- Vasa recta arising from juxtamedullary efferent arterioles supply arterial blood to the medulla. Thus, occlusion of the outer cortical vessels leads to cortical necrosis sparing medulla.

Pathogenesis

- Diffuse cortical necrosis occurs in the setting of hypovolemia and endotoxic shock. It most often occurs in pregnant women with pre-eclampsia, eclampsia, or abruptio placentae.
- Pregnant woman develops acute renal failure. It is also associated with septic shock and other causes of vascular collapse. It is thought that the cause is a combination of end-organ vasospasm and disseminated intravascular coagulation. Due to disseminated intravascular coagulation (DIC), necrosis is limited to cortex.

Vascular lesions—histological patterns and their underlying causes are shown in Fig. 22.66.

Gross Morphology

- The extent of cortical necrosis varies from patchy to confluent.
- Complete occlusion of the arterial supply to cortex produce pale/while infarcts.

Light Microscopy

- Kidneys show fibrin/platelets clots in arterioles and glomerular capillaries.
- Glomeruli, proximal and distal tubules are severely affected.
- Cellular outlines are maintained with loss of structural details.
- Patient who survive, dystrophic calcification occurs in areas of cortical necrosis.

Clinical Features

Patient with severe cortical necrosis manifests as acute renal failure. It is initially indistinguishable from that produced by acute tubular necrosis.

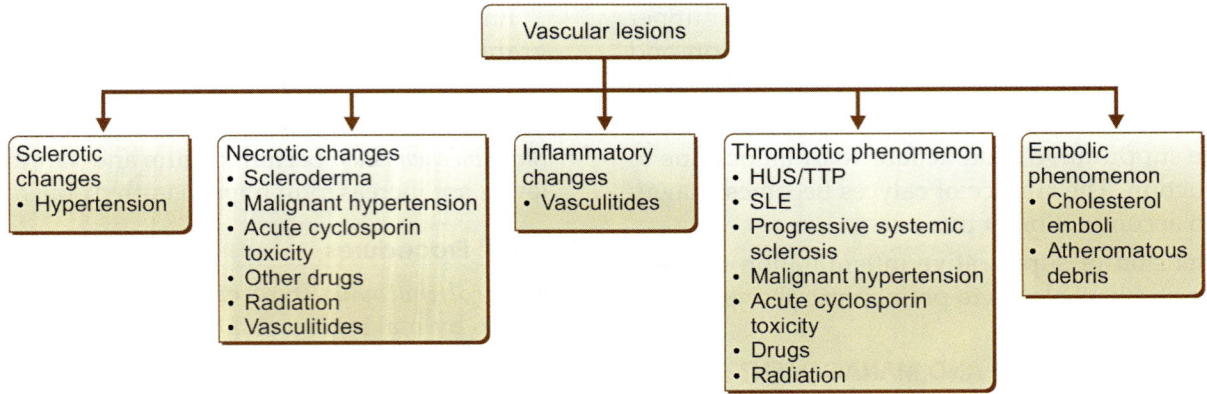

Fig. 22.66: Vascular lesions—histological patterns and their underlying causes.

RENAL INFARCTION

Renal infarction refers to ischemic necrosis due to obstruction interlobar or larger branches of the renal artery.

Pathogenesis

- It most often occurs secondary to thromboembolization from the left heart (90%), embolization of cardiac vegetations or complicated atherosclerotic plaque, nephrosclerosis (benign and malignant), vasculitis (e.g. polyarteritis nodosa), and sickle cell nephropathy.
- Sickle cell nephropathy is the most common organ manifestation of sickle cell disease. Patients with sickle cell disease develop painful, episodic crises. The rigidity of sickled erythrocytes results in obstruction of the microcirculation, with subsequent hypoxia and ischemic injury in many organs.

 The interstitial tissue in which the vasa recta course has a low oxygen tension. As a result, in patients with sickle cell disease, erythrocytes in the vasa recta tend to sickle and occlude the lumina. Infarcts in the medulla and papillae ensue, sometimes severe enough to cause renal papillary necrosis. The glomeruli are conspicuously congested with sickle cells.

Gross Morphology
- Irregular wedge-shaped pale infarcts are present in cortex.
- Old infarcts have a V-shaped appearance due to scar tissue.

Clinical Features

Patient presents with sudden onset of flank pain and hematuria.

SICKLE CELL NEPHROPATHY

Sickle cell nephropathy occurs with sickle cell disease or trait. Sickling of red blood cell may occur in peritubular capillaries in the medulla due to the low O_2 tension in the medulla. Patient develops papillary necrosis and pyelonephritis (Table 22.58).

Clinical Features

Patient presents with asymptomatic hematuria (most common) due to infarction in the medulla. Kidneys lose concentrating ability of urine.

BENIGN AND MALIGNANT NEPHROSCLEROSIS

Hypertension is intermittent or sustained elevation of systolic blood pressure >139 mm Hg or diastolic blood

Table 22.58: Causes of papillary necrosis

Disorder	Papillary necrosis (time course)	Number of papillae affected	Infection	Calcification
Diabetic nephropathy with or without infection	10 years	Several at same stages	80%	Rare
Analgesic abuse most often associated with phenacetin	7 years	All at different stages	25%	Frequent
Sickle cell disease	Variable	Few papillae	+/–	Rare
Lower urinary tract obstruction with or without infection	Variable	90%	90%	Frequent

Kidney and Ureter

Table 22.59: Differences between benign and malignant nephrosclerosis

Parameters	Benign nephrosclerosis	Malignant nephrosclerosis
Pathogenesis	Benign hypertension increases vascular permeability leading to deposition of plasma proteins in subintimal regions	Severe hypertension (>160/110 mm Hg) causes severe endothelial injury leading to intravascular coagulation and rupture of blood vessels
Vascular changes	Hyaline arteriosclerosis Reduplication of elastic lamina	Fibrinoid necrosis with fixed lumina leading to marked reduction of GFR Hyperplastic arteriolosclerosis or onion skin appearance
Morphology of kidneys	Kidney size is decreased due to ischemia	Small contracted kidneys due to marked diffuse glomerular sclerosis
	External surface: grain leather appearance with thinned out cortex	External surface: flea bitten kidney due to rupture of renal small vessels especially capillaries
	Tubular atrophy and increased interstitial fibrosis	Tubular loss in relation to sclerosed glomeruli present
Clinical course	Uremic manifestations are uncommon	Patients develop chronic renal failure with manifestations of uremia

pressure >89 mm Hg. Vascular changes in kidneys due to hypertension are known as benign or malignant nephrosclerosis (Table 22.59).

- *Benign nephrosclerosis:* Mild to moderate hypertension causes hypertensive nephrosclerosis. Approximately 15% hypertensive patients demonstrate benign nephrosclerosis. On gross examination, kidneys involvement shows fine granularity giving '*grain leather appearance*'.
- *Malignant nephrosclerosis:* Malignant hypertension causing necrosis of glomerular endothelial cells results to multiple areas of hemorrhage on the surface of kidney is known as *flea bitten kidney*.

Other causes of flea bitten kidneys are emboli from infective endocarditis, rapidly progressive glomerulonephritis, systemic lupus erythematosus, Goodpasture's syndrome and Henoch-Schönlein purpura (Table 22.60).

BENIGN NEPHROSCLEROSIS LEADS TO OBLITERATION OF GLOMERULI

Pathogenesis

Vascular changes occur in interlobar, arcuate arteries and afferent arterioles located within the cortex of both

Table 22.60: Causes of flea bitten kidneys

Malignant hypertension
Emboli from infective endocarditis
Rapidly progressive glomerulonephritis
Systemic lupus erythematosus
Goodpasture's syndrome
Henoch-Schönlein purpura

kidneys in approximately 15% of patients with benign hypertension. There are two types of vascular changes, i.e. hyaline arteriosclerosis and reduplication of elastic lamina. Similar changes are also seen in elderly persons (normal and hypertensive) and diabetes mellitus.

Due to benign hypertension, persons develop increased permeability of vessels resulting in deposition of plasma proteins in subintimal regions of blood vessels. Lumina of the blood vessels is decreased leading to ischemic changes in organs.

Gross Morphology

- In benign hypertension, kidneys are symmetrically reduced in size due to ischemia.
- External surface of the kidneys is finely granular (grain leather-like appearance), with V-shaped representing infarcts caused by the occlusion of medium-sized renal vessels.
- On cut section, cortex is thinned out.

Light Microscopy

- Renal changes in benign hypertension are known as *benign nephrosclerosis*.
- The interlobar and arcuate arteries exhibit intimal fibrosis, reduplication of the internal elastic lamina, and smooth muscle hypertrophy with narrowing of the lumen, leading to ischemia.
- The afferent arterioles exhibit concentric hyaline arteriolosclerosis (thickening of the wall) with narrowing of lumen resulting in ischemic changes. It results in tubular loss or atrophy, increased interstitial fibrosis replacing nephrons, associated with infiltrates of lymphocytes (no plasma cells).

MALIGNANT NEPHROSCLEROSIS LEADS TO FATAL RENAL DISEASE

- Malignant hypertension refers to a severely elevated blood pressure (diastolic blood pressure >130 mm Hg). It results in rapidly progressive vascular disease.
- It affects the brain (cerebral stroke), heart (left ventricular hypertrophy and failure), kidney (renal failure) and retina (focal retinal hemorrhages and papilledema).
- It can be a complication of either essential (primary) or secondary hypertension. It most often occurs in young African-American males.

Gross Morphology
- Renal changes in malignant hypertension are known as malignant nephrosclerosis.
- Renal arterioles and glomeruli rupture, resulting in *flea-bitten* kidney, multiple pinpoint petechial hemorrhages on the external surface of kidney.

Light Microscopy
Malignant hypertension causes necrotizing arteriolitis and glomerulitis with *fibrinoid necrosis* and hyperplastic arteriolosclerosis (*onion skin* appearance).

Renal tubules show atrophic changes. Tubules contain eosinophilic material (known as *thyroidization of tubules*). There is tubular loss in relation to sclerosed glomeruli present. Patients develop chronic renal failure with manifestations of uremia.

- *Fibrinoid necrosis:* Malignant hypertension injures endothelial cells and causes increased vascular permeability, which leads to insudation of plasma proteins into the vessel wall. Severe endothelial injury causes intravascular coagulation and rupture of blood vessels. Lumen becomes narrow and fixed resulting into ischemia. This morphologic change in renal arterioles is known as *fibrinoid necrosis* (Fig. 22.67).
- *Hyperplastic arteriolosclerosis:* Acute vascular injury is followed by smooth muscle proliferation with an increase in concentric layers of smooth muscle cells that yield the so-called *onion skin* appearance. Smooth muscle hyperplasia occurs as a result of growth factors derived from platelets and inflammatory cells at the site of vascular injury (Fig. 22.68).

Consequence
Poor perfusion of the kidneys stimulates the release of renin, which serves to elevate systemic blood pressure even further by activation of renin-angiotensin-aldosterone system (renovascular hypertension).

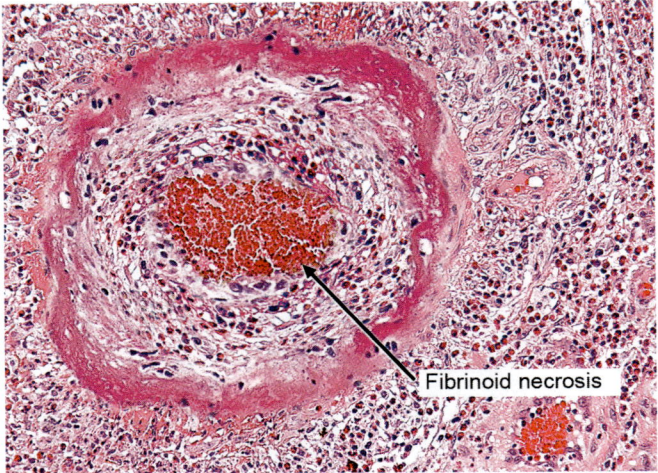

Fig. 22.67: Malignant hypertension leads to fibrinoid necrosis of small arteries as shown here. The damage to the arteries leads to formation of pink fibrin, hence the term '*fibrinoid*' (arrow) (400X).

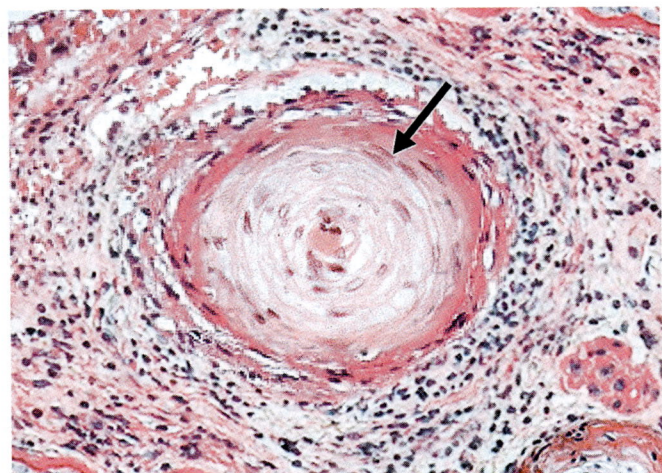

Fig. 22.68: Hyaline arteriosclerosis—smooth muscle proliferation with an increase in concentric layers of smooth muscle cells that yield the so-called *onion skin* appearance (arrow) (400X).

Clinical Features
Patient develops renal failure, vascular stress that may present as myocardial infarct, congestive heart failure, or cerebral strokes and increased intracranial pressure, which often produces symptoms such as seizures, headache, nausea, vomiting, visual impairment, and coma.

Physical Examination
Blood pressure is very high >160/110 mm Hg, pounding heartbeat, and bulging optic disc papilledema.

THROMBOTIC MICROANGIOPATHY

It refers to extensive endothelial damage due to multiple causes such as infections, drugs (e.g. cisplatin chemotherapy), autoimmune diseases, malignant hypertension, and pregnancy.

Table 22.61: Causes of thrombotic microangiopathy

- *Therapeutic agents:* Cisplatin, cyclosporin, mitocin
- *Bacterial infections:* Escherichia coli, Pseudomonas, Shigella
- *Autoimmune disorders:* SLE, scleroderma and antiphospholipid antibody syndrome
- Malignant hypertension
- Pregnancy and post-partum factors

Alterations in blood flow lead to mechanical fragmentation of erythrocytes (schistocytes) and thrombocytopenia. This disorder is known as microangiopathic hemolytic anemia (Table 22.61).

Pathogenesis

Endothelial damage initiates a final common pathway of vascular changes such as thrombus formation resulting in focal ischemic necrosis.

These vascular changes are to those seen in malignant nephrosclerosis.

Light Microscopy

Light microscopy of affected kidneys exhibits arteriolar fibrinoid necrosis, arterial edematous intimal expansion, glomerular congestion, and vascular thrombosis.

Clinical Features

Patients typically present with thrombocytopenia, hypertension, and renal failure.

TOXEMIA OF PREGNANCY INVOLVING KIDNEYS

- Toxemia of pregnancy most often occurs during third trimester of first pregnancy. It most often affects kidneys, liver and brain (hemorrhages) in acute toxemia of pregnancy.
- Clinical triad is hypertension, excessive weight gain and albumen loss in urine. Toxemia of pregnancy exists in two forms—pre-eclampsia and eclampsia.
  - Pre-eclampsia refers to the triad of hypertension, proteinuria, and edema (fluid retention), during the third trimester of pregnancy. It usually begins insidiously after the 20th week of pregnancy.
  - In eclampsia, pregnant women develop convulsion in addition to clinical manifestations observed in pre-eclampsia.

Clinical Features

Proteinuria is >3 gm per day, and renal function declines. It is complicated by convulsions, and disseminated intravascular coagulation in eclampsia with fatal outcome.

Disseminated intravascular coagulation is characterized by formation of fibrin thrombi in the liver, brain, and kidneys. Patient develops puffiness on face, pitting edema and convulsions in true eclampsia.

As the disease progresses the diastolic pressure persistently exceeds 110 mm Hg.

Light Microscopy

- Pre-eclamptic nephropathy or pregnancy induced nephropathy shows marked swelling of glomerular endothelial cells with marked narrowing of lumina.
- Mesangial cells as well as endothelial cells are enlarged and possess multiple vacuoles and vesicular structures (Fig. 22.69).

VASCULITIS INVOLVING KIDNEYS

Renal vessels are involved in various types of vasculitis (Table 22.62).

Small-sized Vessel Vasculitis

- *Immune complex-mediated vasculitis:* Glomeruli are affected in patients suffering from Henoch-Schönlein purpura, cryoglobulinemia and Goodpasture's syndrome.
- *Anti-GBM vasculitis:* Glomeruli are affected in Goodpasture's syndrome.
- *ANCA vasculitis:* Glomeruli, arterioles, interlobular arteries are affected in Wegener's granulomatosis, microscopic polyangiitis and Churg-Strauss syndrome.

Medium-sized Vessel Vasculitis

Interlobular arteries and arcuate arteries are involved in polyarteritis nodosa or Kawasaki disease resulting in renal infarcts and hemorrhage.

Large-sized Vessel Vasculitis

Main renal arteries are affected in giant cell arteritis or Takayasu's syndrome resulting in renovascular hypertension.

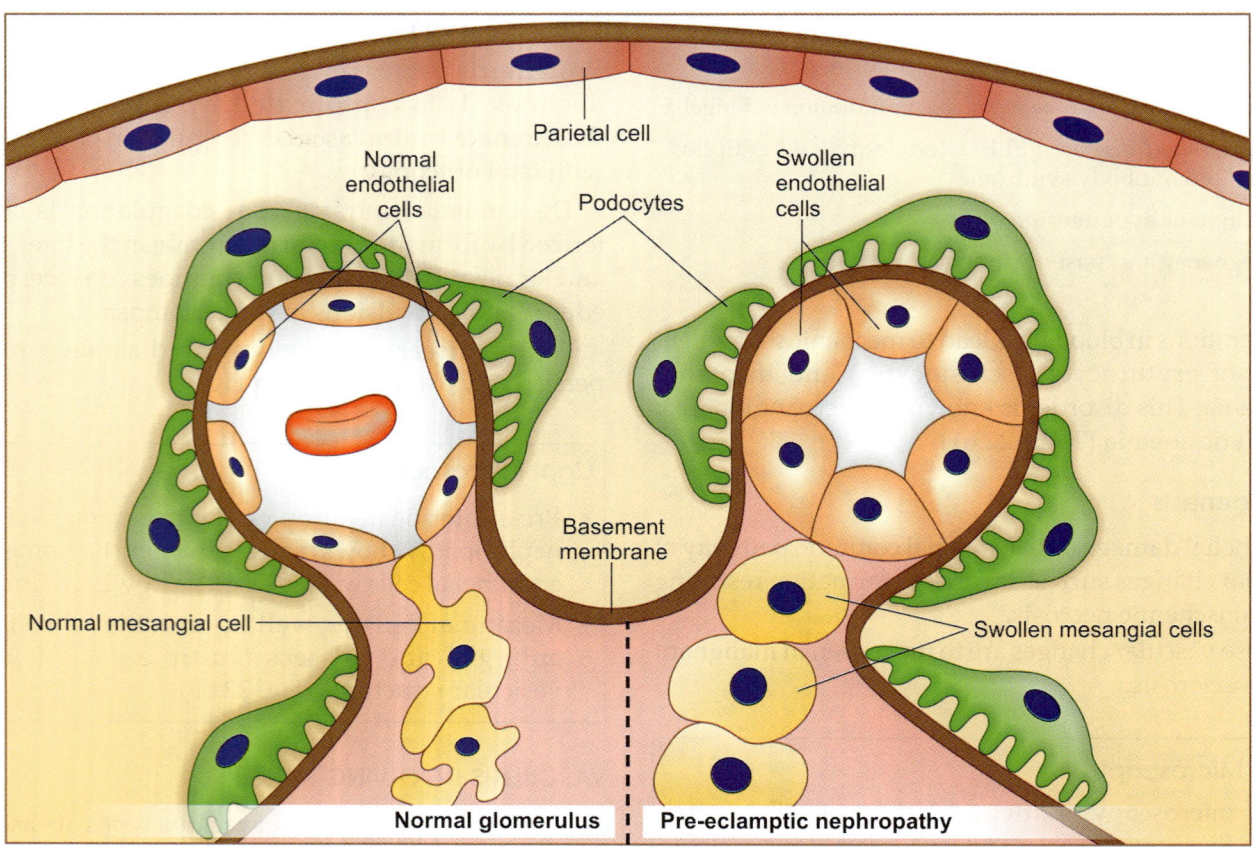

Fig. 22.69: Glomerulopathy in pre-eclampsia of pregnancy (*Courtesy by* Dr Abhijit Das).

Table 22.62: Vasculitis involving kidneys

Size of vessels	Mechanisms	Major types of renal vessels involved	Major renal manifestations
Small-sized vessel vasculitis			
Immune complex mediated vasculitis	Henoch-Schönlein purpura Cryoglobulinemia	Glomeruli	Nephritis
Anti-GBM vasculitis	Goodpasture's syndrome		
ANCA vasculitis	Wegener's granulomatosis Microscopic polyangiitis Churg-Strauss syndrome	Glomeruli, arterioles, interlobular arteries	Nephritis
Medium-sized vessel vasculitis			
	Polyarteritis nodosa Kawasaki disease	Interlobular arteries and arcuate arteries	Renal infarcts and hemorrhage
Large-sized vessel vasculitis			
	Giant cell arteritis Takayasu's syndrome	Main renal artery	Renovascular hypertension

CYSTIC DISEASES OF KIDNEY

ADULT POLYCYSTIC KIDNEYS

It is autosomal dominant polycystic kidney disease. Though the genetic defect is present at birth, yet it manifests between 15 and 30 years of age. That is why this condition has also been called adult polycystic kidney disease.

Patient develops numerous bilateral cysts within the renal parenchyma that replace and ultimately destroy the renal parenchyma resulting in enlargement. It is most often associated with berry aneurysm of the circle of Willis resulting in subarachnoid hemorrhage.

Origin

The cysts originate from the tubules at any level, hence lining of these cysts vary in size. Approximately 33% of patients develop hepatic cysts, whose lining resembles bile duct epithelium.

Molecular Genetics

PKD1, PKD2 and PKD3 gene mutations are associated with adult polycystic kidney disease. PKD1 gene encodes polycystin.

Gross Examination

The kidneys are enlarged up to 3 or 4 kg or more. The affected kidney contains large fluid-filled cysts with areas of organized hemorrhage (Fig. 22.70).

Clinical Features

Patient presents with sense of heaviness in the loins, bilateral flank and palpable renal masses, hypertension, blood clots in the urine (hematuria), progression to end-stage renal failure after the age of 40 years. Secondary polycythemia may occur. In women, it may be diagnosed at an earlier age during antenatal investigations, either as palpable masses or as impaired renal function.

INFANTILE POLYCYSTIC KIDNEY DISEASE

Autosomal recessive polycystic bilateral kidney disease occurs in infants. *In utero*, there is typically oligohydramnios because of poor renal function and failure to form significant amounts of fetal urine.

Origin

Cysts originate from the collecting ducts.

Gross Morphology
- Both kidneys are markedly enlarged and tend to fill the retroperitoneum and displace abdominal contents.
- External surface is smooth. The kidneys tend to be symmetrically enlarged.
- The cysts are quite small and uniform, perhaps 1 to 2 mm on average (Fig. 22.71).

Light Microscopy
The characteristic finding occurs in the later third trimester is cystic change with the cysts elongated and radially arranged. The cysts are lined by cuboidal epithelium. Cysts are smaller and present at right angles to the cortical surface.

Clinical Features

Patient presents with multiple cysts evident at birth. The closed cysts are not in continuity with the

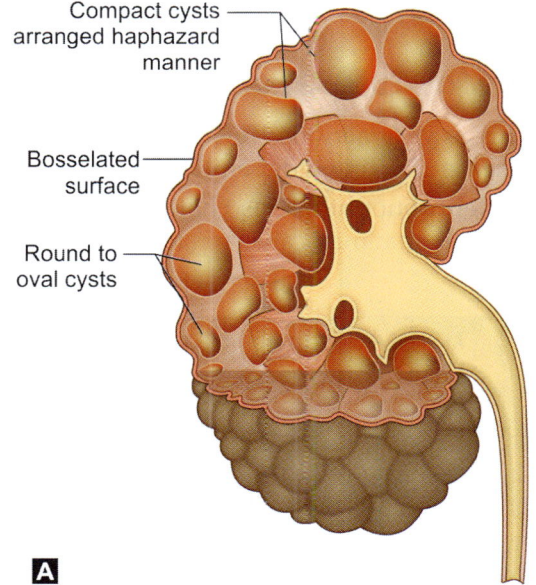

A

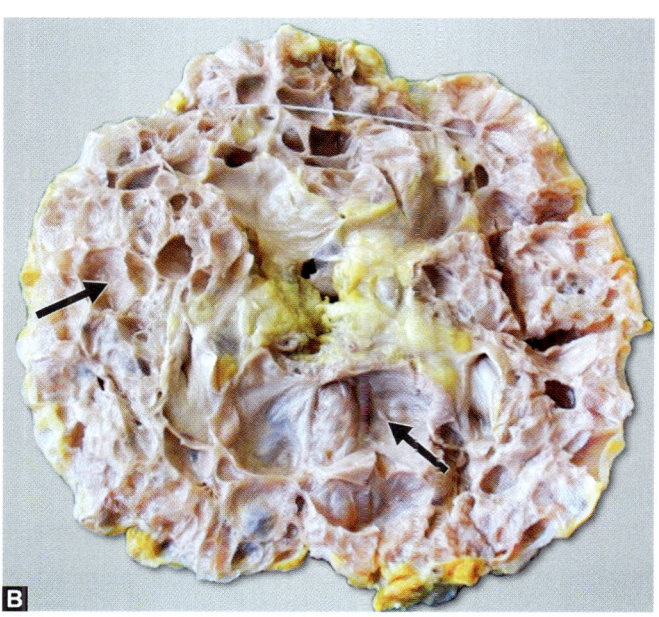

B

Fig. 22.70: Adult polycystic disease of the kidneys. The kidney substance is almost completely replaced by cysts of varying size. The kidneys may be not much bigger than normal, but usually they are quite large. Cut surface shows the cysts with very little normal renal tissue remaining (arrows).

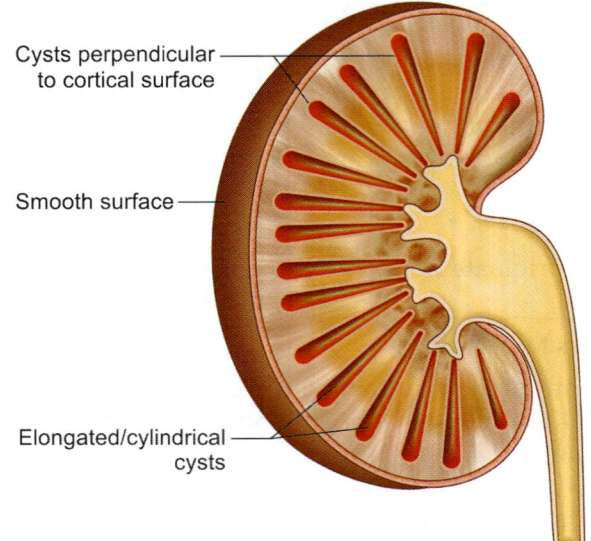

Fig. 22.71: Infantile polycystic kidney disease.

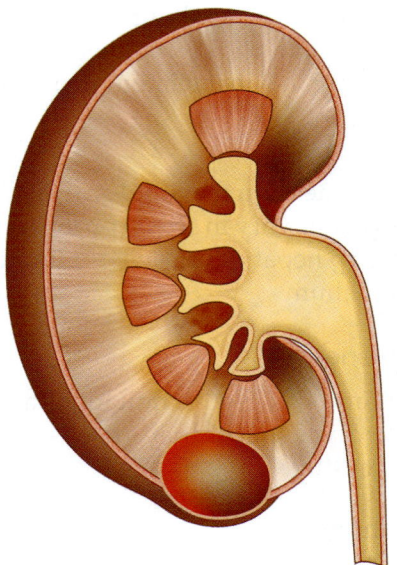

Fig. 22.72: Simple cyst kidney.

collecting system. Death occurs shortly after birth (Table 22.63).

SOLITARY RENAL CYST

Solitary cyst of the kidney is comparatively rare. It is solitary and well defined cyst more common in women than men. It more often involves the lower pole of the kidney.

Abdominal ultrasonography or computed tomography has led to the incidental detection of asymptomatic renal cyst. Complications of simple renal cyst hemorrhage, infection, or rupture result in development of complex cysts with calcification, multiple lobules (Fig. 22.72).

Gross Morphology
- Solitary renal cyst is discrete lesion within kidney located in cortex. It extends outside the renal parenchyma and distorting the renal contour.

- It is oval or circular in shape with well-defined outline.
- External surface is smooth, transparent, avascular, yellowish or bluish white in color.
- It is filled with homogenous clear or straw-colored fluid.

Light Microscopy
Simple renal cyst is lined by a thin layer of fibrous tissue lined by a single layer of flattened or cuboidal epithelium.

UREMIC MEDULLARY CYSTIC RENAL DISEASE

This is very serious (but uncommon) form of cystic disease affecting older children.

Nephronophthisis is characterized by cysts in the medulla that may cause renal failure.

Table 22.63: Comparison of adult and childhood polycystic kidneys

Characteristics	Adult polycystic kidney	Childhood polycystic kidney
Inheritance	Autosomal dominance	Autosomal recessive
Pathologic features	Large, multiple cysts in kidneys are associated with liver cysts and berry aneurysms	Large cystic kidney at the time of birth
Origin of renal cysts	Cortex and medulla	Distal and collecting tubules
Clinical features	Hematuria, flank pain, hypertension	Bilateral abdominal mass
Outcome	Patient develops chronic renal failure at the age of 40–60 years	Child dies during infancy or childhood
Complications	Subarachnoid hemorrhage, colonic diverticulum and mitral valve prolapse	Liver fibrosis, splenomegaly and esophageal varices

MEDULLARY SPONGE KIDNEY

Medullary sponge kidney (also known as Cacchi–Ricci disease) is a congenital disorder of the kidneys. It is characterized by cystic dilatation of the collecting tubules in one or both kidneys. Patients with medullary sponge kidney are at increased risk for development of kidney stones and urinary tract infection. Renal functions are impaired without renal failure (Fig. 22.73).

ACQUIRED CYSTIC RENAL DISEASE

This disease is associated with long-term dialysis therapy. Multiple cysts, glomerular and tubular atrophy, and scarring are characteristic. The incidence of renal cell carcinoma is increased in these patients (Table 22.64).

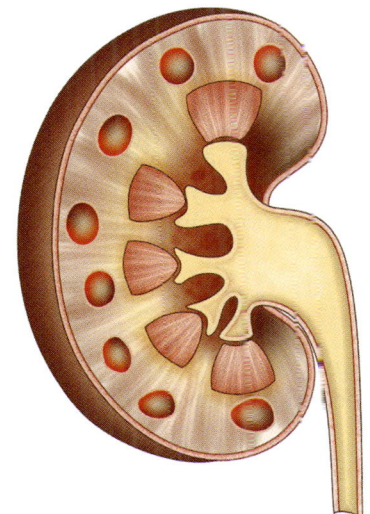

Fig. 22.73: Medullary sponge kidney.

Table 22.64: Cystic diseases of the kidneys

Disorder	Inheritance	Pathology	Clinical manifestations	Clinical course
Adult polycystic kidney disease	Autosomal dominant	Kidneys and liver show large cysts. Berry aneurysm	Renal stones, hematuria, UTI and hypertension	Patient develops chronic renal failure at age of 40–60 years
Childhood polycystic kidney disease	Autosomal recessive	Patient presents with large cystic kidneys at birth	Liver fibrosis	Fatal during infancy and childhood
Adult onset medullary cystic disease	Autosomal dominant	Cysts at the junction of cortex and medulla	Salt wasting polyuria	Patient develops chronic renal failure at age of adulthood
Familial juvenile nephronophthisis	Autosomal recessive	Cysts at the junction of cortex and medulla	Anemia, growth retardation and salt losing polyuria	Patient develops chronic renal failure beginning at childhood
Medullary sponge kidney	None	Medullary cysts	Renal stones, hematuria and UTI	Patient has a benign course
Multicystic renal dysplasia	None	Kidneys are irregular with variable size cysts	It is associated with other renal anomalies	Surgery cures unilateral renal involvement. Patient with bilateral renal involvement develops chronic renal failure

CONGENITAL ANOMALIES OF THE URINARY TRACT

BILATERAL RENAL AGENESIS

- This rare condition is not compatible with life. Both kidneys are absent. Resulting conditions include oligohydramnios, or decreased amniotic fluid, which occurs because the renal system fails to excrete fluid swallowed by the fetus.
- Other resulting conditions include multiple fetal anomalies (e.g. hypoplastic lung, defects in extremities), all caused by oligohydramnios and collectively known as *oligohydramnios*, or *Potter* syndrome characterized by (hyperhydramnios or increased amniotic fluid, is associated with duodenal atresia or with tracheoesophageal fistula of the type in which the upper esophagus ends in a blind pouch and the lower esophagus communicates with the trachea.

UNILATERAL RENAL AGENESIS

One kidney is missing. This condition is much more common than complete renal agenesis.

ECTOPIC KIDNEYS

Kidneys that do not reach the lumbar area but remain in the pelvis or presacral area are considered ectopic. During fetal development, the kidneys initially located in the lower abdomen move upward toward their permanent position in lumbar region.

HORSESHOE KIDNEYS

Fusion of both kidneys at their lower poles results in so-called *horseshoe* kidney. It may cause urinary tract obstruction because of impingement on the ureters.

URETER ANOMALIES

Double ureters may affect the ureters alone or may be part of a duplication of the entire urinary collecting system on one side. Developmental anomalies of the renal pelvis and ureters are found in 2–3% of all persons.

NEOPLASMS OF THE KIDNEY

Renal tumors are classified into the following categories: Primary and secondary tumors (Tables 22.65, 22.66 and Fig. 22.74).

WILMS' TUMOR (NEPHROBLASTOMA)

Wilms' tumor is the most frequent abdominal solid malignant tumor in children. It accounts for 5% of childhood tumor. In most instances of Wilms' tumor, the neoplasm is sporadic (90%) and unilateral. However, in 5% of cases, it arises in the context of several congenital syndromes (10%). WT1 (tumor suppressor gene) is implicated in the development of Wilms' tumor. The tumor is often huge resulting in abdominal distension.

Origin

Wilms' tumor is derived from embryonal mesonephric mesoderm. The tumor is composed of elements that resemble normal fetal tissue: (a) metanephric blastemal (abortive glomeruli, tubules), (b) immature mesenchymal stroma, and (c) immature epithelial elements.

Table 22.65: WHO histologic classification of important primary tumors of the kidney

Primary renal tumors	
Clear cell variant of renal cell carcinoma	Carcinoma of the collecting ducts of Bellini
Papillary renal cell carcinoma	Renal medullary carcinoma
Chromophobe renal cell carcinoma	Xp11 translocation carcinoma
Primary nephroblastic tumors	
Nephroblastoma (Wilms' tumor) common tumor of childhood	
Cystic partially differentiated nephroblastoma	
Metastatic (secondary) tumors to kidney: Breast carcinoma, bronchus carcinoma, malignant melanoma and lymphomas • Metastases to kidneys are multiple involving both kidneys. Metastases exhibit central indentations, or *umbilications*, from necrosis	
High yield facts	
Clinical features in a patient with *renal angiomyolipoma (hamartoma)* initially are similar to renal cell carcinoma	

Table 22.66: Benign renal tumors

Tumor	Gross morphology	Light microscopy
Renal papillary cortical adenoma	Size <2 cm in sub-capsular region. Cut surface is pale yellow to gray	Small uniform cells with clear to eosinophilic cytoplasm forming branching papillary fronds
Renal oncocytoma	Well-circumscribed tumor arising from proximal and distal tubules in poles. Cut surface has a uniform mahogany, brown color due to mitochondrial lipochrome pigments	Tumor comprises large epithelial cells called oncocytes, which have abundant eosinophilic homogeneous or granular cytoplasm (due to mitochondria) and uniform small nuclei
Metanephric adenoma	Small solid lesion in the renal cortex	Tumor is composed of small round cells with bland nuclei and scanty cytoplasm. These are arranged in tubules and papillae with scant stroma. Areas of calcification may be seen

Kidney and Ureter

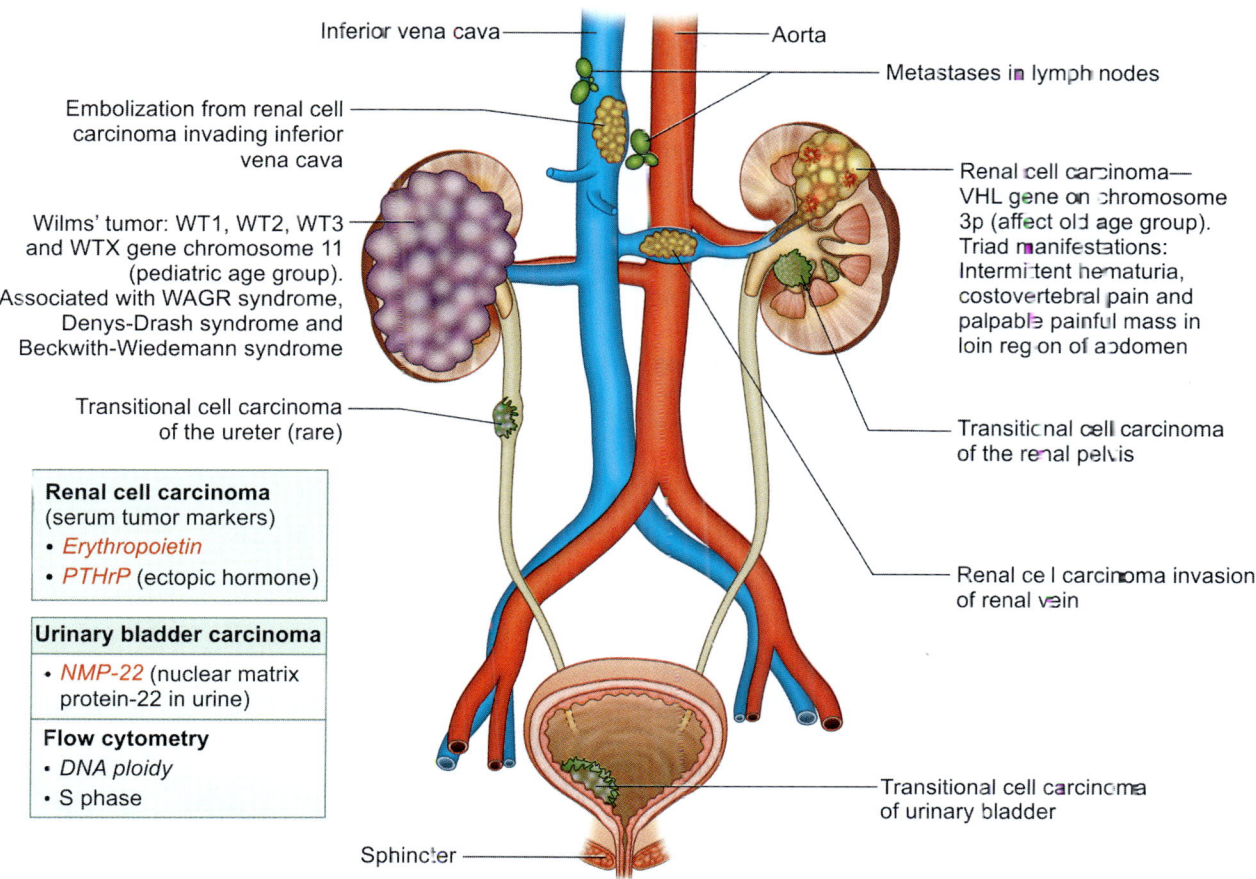

Fig. 22.74: Common malignant tumors of the urinary tract.

Age Group and Sex Predilection

It occurs between 1 to 5 years of age and before 9 years of age in 90% of cases. It rarely occurs after age of 9 years. Males and females are equally affected.

Molecular Genetics

WT1 tumor suppressor gene is located on short arm of chromosome 11 (11p13). Wilms' tumor is caused by deletion or inactivation of WT1 gene. WT1 gene mutation also affects contiguous genes and causes other lesions in familial cases (Table 22.67).

- *Sporadic Wilms' tumor:* WT1 gene mutation has been demonstrated in stromal component of Wilms' tumor in some sporadic cases. It suggests that the stromal component of Wilms' tumor is neoplastic. It raises the possibility that undifferentiated blastema cells are precursors of the stromal and heterologous elements. It has been suggested that in addition to WT1; WT2 gene mutation plays an important role in the genesis of sporadic cases of Wilms' tumors.
- *Association of Wilms' tumor in familial syndromes:* WT1 tumor suppressor gene is located on short arm of chromosome 11 (11p13). Wilms' tumor is caused by deletion or inactivation of WT1 gene. WT1 gene mutation also affects contiguous genes and causes other lesions in familial cases in 10% of cases. Patient with familial syndromes may develop Wilms' tumor.
  - *WAGR syndrome:* The patient presents with Wilms' tumor (WT1 gene mutation), *aniridia* (absence of the iris) due to mutation of contiguous aniridia gene (*PAX6 gene* located on chromosome 11), genitourinary malformations and mental retardation.

Table 22.67: Molecular derangements in Wilms' tumor

Tumor	Cytogenetic abnormality	Implicated genes	Protein role	Related assay(s)
Nephroblastoma	Deletion or mutations involving 11p13, 11p15, or Xp11.1	WT1, WT2, WT3, WTX	Zinc-finger DNA-binding protein; tumor suppressor genes	IPCX for WT1

- *Denys-Drash syndrome (DDS):* The patient presents with Wilms' tumor (WT1 gene mutation), genitourinary malformations, intersexual disorders, tumors of the gonads (ovaries or testes) and glomerulopathy (mesangial sclerosis) resulting in renal failure.
- *Beckwith-Wiedemann syndrome (BWS):* It is associated with Wilms' tumor, unusual 'hemihypertrophy' (ranging from gigantism to asymmetric growth), tumors of the liver and adrenal glands, hepatosplenomegaly, macroglossia, malformations around the ear; and abdominal wall defects near the navel (omphalocele). This is thought to be caused by an overactive copy of an oncogene on chromosome 11, called IGF2. Oncogenes, if becomes overactive; then it results in uncontrolled cell growth.

Clinical Features

Patient presents with unilateral non-tender mass in abdomen, hematuria, hypertension (due to increased renin secretion), and pain abdomen due to pressure exerted by tumor on surrounding structures. Constitutional symptoms are anorexia, loss of appetite, generalized weakness and weight loss.

Gross Morphology

The kidney is extensively replaced by large bulging fleshy, pale white tumor. Cut surface reveals tumor enclosed in a rim of renal cortex and capsule (Fig. 22.75).

Light Microscopy

Wilms' tumor resembles the fetal nephrogenic zone and attempts to form primitive glomerular and tubular structures. Tumor comprises three components (Fig. 22.76).

- *Metanephric blastema:* It shows poorly developed glomeruli and tubules.
- *Immature mesenchymal tissue:* It comprises striated muscle together with myxoid tissue, cartilage, bone and fat and thus creating a rather bizarre mixture.
- *Immature epithelial tissue:* It consists of immature epithelial tissue.

Staging of Wilms' Tumor

Staging is shown in Table 22.68.

Mode of Spread

Wilms' tumor may metastasize to various organs in decreasing frequency: lungs (most common), liver

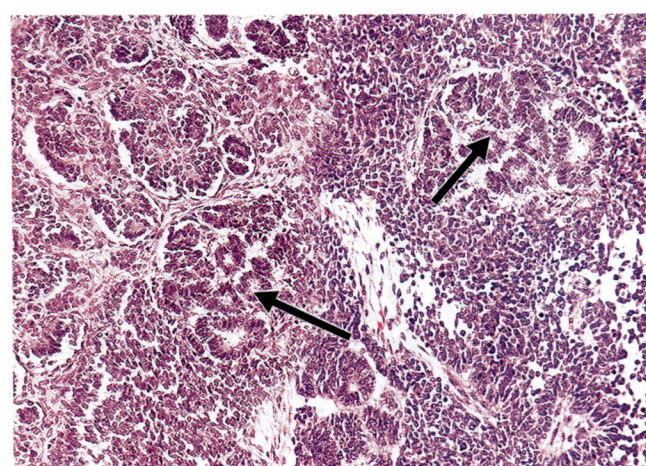

Fig. 22.76. Wilms' tumor—it resembles the fetal nephrogenic zone and attempts to form primitive glomerular and tubular structures (arrows) (100X).

Table 22.68: Staging of Wilms' tumor

Stage I	Tumor limited to the kidney with intact capsule and completely resected. There is no rupture of blood vessels
Stage II	Tumor has invaded renal capsule involving surrounding structures
Stage III	Tumor has spread beyond the kidney area involving abdominal or pelvic lymph nodes. Resection of tumor is not possible
Stage IV	The tumor has spread to distant structures such as the lungs, liver or brain. Metastases of lymph nodes outside abdomen and pelvis
Stage V	Bilateral renal involvement at diagnosis

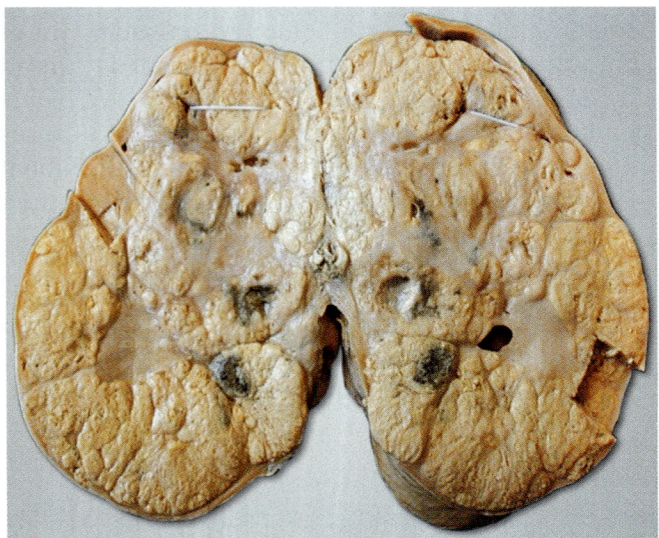

Fig. 22.75: Wilms' tumor. The kidney is extensively replaced by large bulging fleshy, pale white tumor. Cut surface reveals tumor enclosed in a rim of renal cortex and capsule.

and brain. It rarely metastasizes to bones in contrast to neuroblastoma where bone is the principle site. It may metastasize to opposite kidneys (5–10%), adrenal glands, bowel, vertebrae and paraspinal region.

Laboratory Diagnosis

Imaging techniques: These include abdominal ultrasonography, CT scan, and magnetic resonance imaging. Chest X-ray is done to rule out lung metastases. Kidney and liver function tests, FNAC and histopathology are diagnostic tools.

RENAL CELL CARCINOMA (RCC)

Histological Variants

Clear Cell Variant of Renal Cell Carcinoma

It is most common variant and constituting 70–80% of cases. It arises from proximal tubular cells in cortex. von Hippel-Lindau (vHL) gene mutation on chromosome 3 has been demonstrated in sporadic and familial cases. It is bright golden yellow tumor located in pole of kidney. Light microscopy reveals tumor cells with clear cytoplasm containing abundant glycogen and lipids. It expresses both *cytokeratin* and *vimentin*.

Papillary Variant of Renal Cell Carcinoma

It constitutes 10–15% of cases. It arises from distal tubular cells in cortex. It is never associated with vHL gene mutation located on chromosome 3. Trisomy or tetrasomy 7, 16 and 17 are common due to chromosomal gains.

Loss of Y chromosome is seen in familial cases PRCC gene on chromosome 1 fuses with TFE 3 gene on chromosome X. Fusion protein dysregulates mitotic checkpoints allowing abnormal segregation of chromosomes. It has *worst prognosis*.

Chromophobe Variant of Renal Cell Carcinoma

It constitutes 5% of cases. It originates from intercalated cells of collecting ducts in cortex. Multiple chromosomal losses/hypoploidy occur in this variant. It comprises eosinophilic granular cells with prominent cell borders closely mimicking oncocytomas. It has best prognosis.

Collecting Duct Carcinoma in Medulla

It is a rare tumor constituting 2% of cases and arising from collecting ducts in medullary region. Tumor is circumscribed with central areas of necrosis.

Xp11 Translocation Renal Cell Carcinoma

This rare tumor occurs in children. Immunophenotype of renal tumors and comparison of histological variants of renal cell carcinoma are shown in Tables 22.69 and 22.70.

CLEAR CELL VARIANT OF RENAL CELL CARCINOMA

It is the most common histologic variant of renal cell carcinoma. It constitutes 70–80% of cases. It most often occurs in men than women, in the age group of 50–70 years. vHL gene mutation located on chromosome 3 has been demonstrated in sporadic and familial cases. It is *bright golden yellow tumor* located in upper or lower pole of kidney. Light microscopy reveals tumor cells with *clear cytoplasm* containing abundant *glycogen* and *lipids*. It expresses both *cytokeratin* and *vimentin*.

Origin

It arises from proximal tubular cells in cortex. It generally arises in one of the renal poles, frequently the upper pole.

Table 22.69: Immunophenotype of renal tumors

Marker	Clear cell RCC	Papillary RCC	Chromophobe RCC	Oncocytoma	X11p translocation RCC	MTSCC (mucinous tubular and spindle cell carcinoma)	Clear cell papillary RCC
PAX2	+	+	–/+	+	–	+	Not applicable
RCC Ma	+	+	–/+		+	+/–	Not applicable
CD10	+	+	–/+	–	+	–	–
Vimentin	+	+	–	–	+/–	+/–	+
CK7	–	+	+	–	–	+	+
AE1/AE3	+	++	+	+		+	+
KS-cadherin	–/+	–/+	+	+	–/+	–	Not applicable
C-kit (CD117)	–	–/+	+	+	Not applicable	–	Not applicable

Table 22.70: Comparison of histologic variants of renal cell carcinoma

Parameters	RCC clear cell variant	RCC papillary (chromophil) variant	RCC chromophobe variant	Bellini duct carcinoma	Xp11 translocation RCC
Cell of origin	Proximal tubule in cortex	Distal tubule in cortex	Intercalated ducts of collecting tubules in cortex	Collecting duct in medulla	–
Frequency	70–80%	10–15%	5%	Rare	Rare
Cytogenetics	Sporadic: 3p gene mutation. Familial: vHL gene mutation (methylation) t(3:6), t(3:8), t(3:11)	Sporadic: trisomy 7, 16, 17 due to chromosomal gains Pediatric papillary RCC t(X:1) mutated activated MET. Familial: trisomy 7, mutated or activated MET. Loss of Y chromosome is seen in familial cases	Sporadic: loss of multiple chromosome, extreme hypodiploid	Reports on losses of chromosomes 1, 6, 14, 15, and 22 have been reported	Gene fusions involving the TFE3 transcription factor gene. These comprise at least one-third of pediatric RCC
Light microscopy	Large round/polygonal cells with centrally placed round nuclei and abundant clear cytoplasm arranged in solid cords, papillae, tubules or nests or alveolar pattern Tumor cells express cytokeratin and vimentin	Fibrovascular core is lined by tumor cells arranged in papillary pattern Psammoma bodies in fibrovascular core	Polyhedral tumor cells, eccentric nuclei, perinuclear halo, prominent membranes resembling vegetable cells. Electron microscopy study reveals microvesicles 150–300 nm diameter. Hale's colloidal iron reacts with a substance present in the microvesicles	Hobnail pattern and desmoplastic reaction	–
Immunohisto-chemistry	Both keratins (8, 18) and vimentin. Epithelial membrane antigen, α-1 antitrypsin, S-100 and angiotensinogen converting enzyme (ACE). PAX2 or PAX8. PAX2 is the best marker with 50–80% sensitivity	Ki-67	–	Cytokeratin 19, ulex europaeus lectin, and vimentin	–
Prognosis	Relatively in between	Worst prognosis	Best prognosis	Poor prognosis	

High yield facts: Xp11 translocation renal cell carcinomas bear gene fusions involving the TFE3 transcription factor gene. These comprise at least one-third of pediatric RCC. Presence of dense calcifications in tumor resemble renal lithiasis, and obstruction of the renal pelvis promoting extensive obscuring xanthogranulomatous pyelonephritis.

Clinical Features

- Hematuria is the most frequent presenting sign. Malignant cells are rarely detected in the urine in renal cell carcinoma. The tumor spreads most frequently to the lungs and bones. The tumor is often quite large and may result in a palpable mass.
- Oncocytoma and renal angiomyolipoma are often difficult to differentiate from RCC by imaging techniques. The tumor most often invades renal veins and can extend up the vena cava reaching right side of heart with early dissemination.

Predisposing Factors

- *Tobacco smoking:* It is most important risk factor for development of renal cell carcinoma in sporadic cases.
- *Prolonged exposure to polycyclic hydrocarbons:* These are aromatic hydrocarbons originally derived from coal tar, among the most extensively studied carcinogens. These are also derived from cigarette smoke. These bind to cellular DNA, RNA and proteins and alter the genome.
- *Prolonged exposure* to heavy metals (lead), asbestos, petroleum products, coke oven emissions, analgesic abuse (phenacetin) and estrogens therapy increase risk of RCC.
- *Adult polycystic disease* and *hemodialysis* induced *renal cystic disease* are risk factors for RCC.
- *Obese* and *hypertensive persons* are at increased risk of RCC.
- *Association with von Hippel-Lindau (VHL) disease:* Most cases of renal cell carcinoma are sporadic (98%) affecting elderly persons, but about 2% are inherited in younger age group. Loss of one allele of the VHL gene located on chromosome 3 occurs in these cases. This evidence strongly suggests that loss of the tumor suppressor function of the VHL gene product is an important event in the genesis of clear cell RCC (Table 22.71).

VHL Gene

Physiological state: It is a tumor suppressor gene located on chromosome 3p (3p12 to 3p26). It regulates the transcription of *vascular endothelial growth factor* (VEGF) and *platelet-derived growth factor* (PDGF) proteins. It encodes a protein which causes degradation of hypoxia inducible factor-1 (HIF-1).

Pathological state

- *VHL gene mutation in RCC:* VHL causes accumulation of hypoxia inducible factor-1 (HIF-1) resulting in cell growth and angiogenesis through proangiogenic proteins, i.e. *vascular endothelial growth factor* (VEGF), TGF-β and *insulin like-growth factor* (IGF) in renal cell carcinoma. Mutation of one allele of VHL gene is seen in 98% of sporadic renal cell and familial (2%) carcinomas.
- *Mechanism of VHL gene mutation:* It occurs by two mechanisms: (a) *loss of sequences* occur due to loss of sequences on chromosome 3p either by deletion (3p12 to 3p26) or imbalanced translocation, i.e. (3;6, 3;8, 3;11), (b) *hypermethylation of VHL* gene leads to inactivation of VHL gene in about 80% cases.
- *Renal cell carcinoma as a part of VHL disease:* Mutation of one allele of VHL tumor suppressor gene is seen in patients with autosomal dominant VHL syndrome. Approximately 40% of all patients with VHL disease (characterized by retinal hemangiomas and cerebellar hemangioblastomas) develop unilateral clear cell variant of renal cell carcinoma.

Table 22.71: Predisposing factors towards renal cell carcinoma

Risk factors	Description
VHL disease	VHL disease is associated with renal cell carcinoma in 28%. Locus of VHL gene is close to oncogene raf-1 on chromosome 3p25. Mutation of VHL gene causes VHL disease. Normally VHL gene located on 3p25 is a tumor suppressor gene
Acquired cystic disease of kidney	Renal cell carcinoma occurs in acquired cystic disease of kidney associated with dialysis performed in chronic renal failure over a span of 5 years
Cigarette smoking	Cigarette smoking increases risk of development of renal cell carcinoma in 33% of cases
Obesity	Obesity in women increase risk of development of renal cell carcinoma
Inherited	Renal cell carcinoma is associated with 3;8 or 3;11 translocation. Breakpoint is at the proximal end of 3p. Cumulative risk occurs at 60 years in 85%
	Loss of one allele from the short arm of chromosome 3 occurs in 90% of sporadic renal cell carcinoma and is not associated with hereditary cases

Gross Morphology

- Tumor is unilateral solitary tumor in 90% of cases, bilateral involvement is rare. Multicentric tumors occur in 10% of cases. Tumor is well *circumscribed, partially encapsulated* spherical mass. Cut surface shows *variegated* appearance (solid and cystic areas).
- On cut surface, tumor is *golden yellow mass* due to presence of lipids in tumor cells. Areas of *hemorrhage* and *necrosis* are present.
- Tumor may invade the peri-renal fat, adrenal gland, surrounding tissues and renal vein. Invasion of renal vein is a common mode of spread. During processing the nephrectomy specimen, examination of renal vein determines *metastatic potential* of tumor (Figs 22.77 and 22.78).

Light Microscopy

- *Cell morphology:* Tumor is comprised of large round/polygonal cells with centrally placed round nuclei and abundant clear cytoplasm. The cytoplasm of tumor cells appears clear because it is rich in glycogen and fat, which are washed out during histologic processing of the tissue. In some cases, cytoplasm may be granular.
- *Arrangement of cells:* Tumor cells form solid cords, papillae, tubules or nests or alveolar pattern. These cells are demarcated by a network of thin-walled blood vessels in the delicate supporting stroma. The stroma may be reduced, but well vascularized (Fig. 22.79).
- *Nuclear grading:* Fuhrman has described nuclear grading of renal cell carcinoma from grade I to grade IV (Table 22.72).

Histochemistry

Tumor cells are rich in glycogen (PAS positive) and fat. Lipids are dissolved during processing of tissue in paraffin-embedded specimens. Fat can be demonstrated by frozen section technique by applying fat stains (Sudan-III, Sudan-IV, Sudan black or Oil red O). There is absence of mucus in tumor cells.

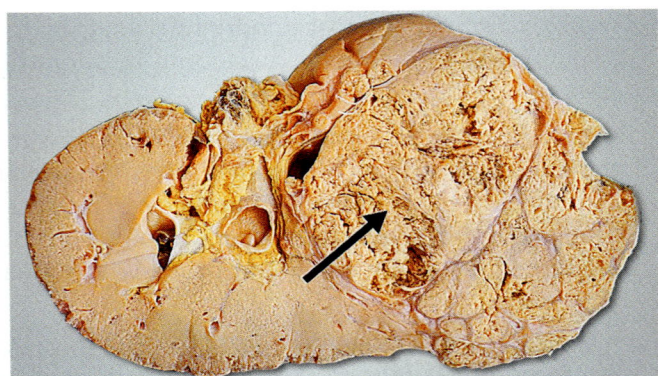

Fig. 22.78: Renal cell carcinoma—tumor is well circumscribed, partially encapsulated spherical mass. Cut surface shows variegated appearance (solid and cystic areas). On cut surface, tumor is golden yellow mass due to presence of lipids in tumor cells. Areas of hemorrhage and necrosis are present (arrow).

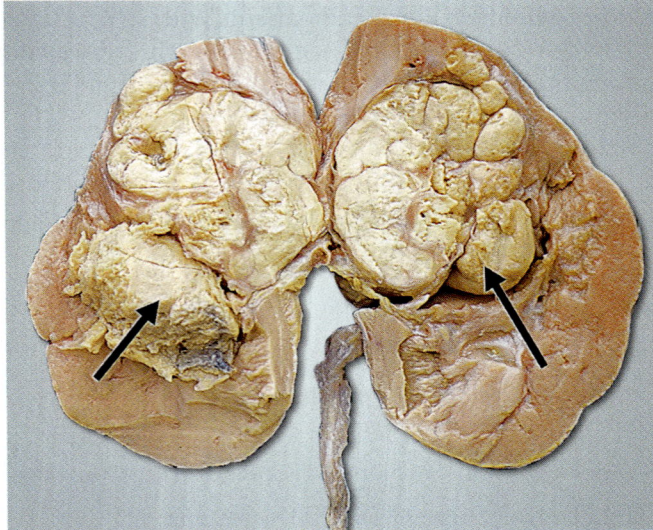

Fig. 22.77: Renal cell carcinoma—tumor is well circumscribed, partially encapsulated spherical mass. Cut surface shows variegated appearance (solid and cystic areas). On cut surface, tumor is golden yellow mass due to presence of lipids in tumor cells. Areas of hemorrhage and necrosis are present (arrows).

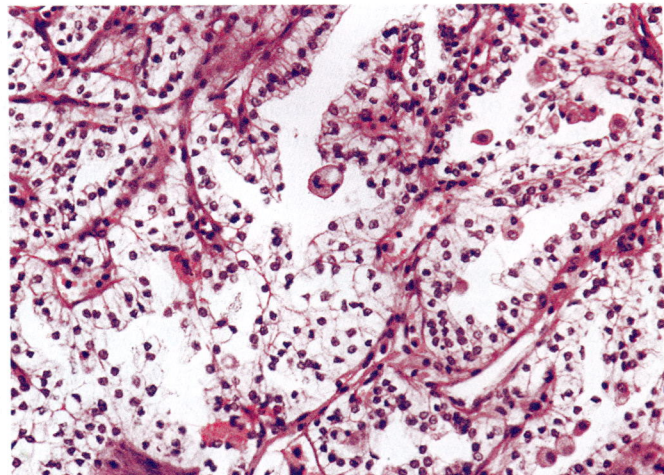

Fig. 22.79: Renal cell carcinoma (clear cell variant). Tumor is comprised of large round/polygonal cells with centrally placed round nuclei and abundant clear cytoplasm. The cytoplasm of tumor cells appears clear because it is rich in glycogen and fat, which are washed out during histologic processing of the tissue. Tumor cells are forming solid cords, papillae, tubules or nests or alveolar pattern. These cells are demarcated by a network of thin-walled blood vessels in the delicate supporting stroma. The stroma may be reduced, but well vascularized (400X).

Table 22.72: Fuhrman's nuclear grading of renal cell carcinoma

Grade	Nuclear features
Grade 1	*Nuclei:* Small round and uniform
	Nucleoli: Not evident
Grade 2	*Nuclei:* Outline irregular
	Nucleoli: Inconspicuous
Grade 3	*Nuclei:* Irregular
	Nucleoli: Identifiable at 100X
Grade 4	*Nuclei:* Large pleomorphic, hyperchromatic
	Nucleoli: Single or multiple

Immunohistochemistry

- Renal cell carcinoma expresses both cytokeratins and vimentins. Conventional renal cell carcinomas express keratins (8, 18) and CD10, while other types express keratins 7 and 19.
- Other markers used include epithelial membrane antigen, α_1-antitrypsin, S-100 and angiotensinogen converting enzyme (ACE). Using immunostains potentially supporting primary or metastatic renal cell carcinoma include PAX2 or PAX8. PAX2 is the best marker with 50–80% sensitivity (Table 22.73).

Clinical Features

- *Triad manifestations:* Patients with 10 cm size tumor present with: (i) intermittent hematuria (50–60%), (ii) costovertebral pain (45%) and (iii) palpable mass with pain in loin region of abdomen (30%).
- *Constitutional symptoms:* These include fever, malaise, weakness, weight loss. Grossly visible painless hematuria should be considered a sign of urinary tract cancer until proven otherwise.

Table 22.73: Immunohistochemistry of renal cell carcinoma (clear cell variant)

Marker	Expression
Cytokeratins (8, 18)	Positive
Vimentin	Positive
CD10	Positive
Epithelial membrane antigen (EMA)	Positive
α_1-antitrypsin	Positive
S-100	Positive
Angiotensin converting enzyme (ACE)	Positive
PAX2	Positive
PAX8	Positive

Physical Examination

- Edema in lower legs occurs due to extension of tumor in the inferior vena cava.
- Sudden onset of left-sided varicocele occurs in old persons due to obstruction of left testicular vein draining directly into left renal vein by the tumor.
- Metastases of renal cell carcinoma to pelvis and femur results to pathological fracture.
- Symptoms related to metastases in lung, opposite kidney, adrenals, gingival, central nervous system, larynx, bronchi, nasal cavity, thyroid gland, skin and soft tissue as first sign of disease (5%).

Paraneoplastic Syndrome

- Tumor synthesizes ectopic hormones in 5% of cases resulting in clinical manifestations—renin (hypertension), erythropoietin (polycythemia), parathormone like peptide (hypercalcemia) and gonadotropins (feminization or musculinization), ACTH (Cushing's syndrome).
- Patient may also develop hepatic dysfunction, acquired dysfibrinogenemia and amyloidosis. Peripheral smear examination may reveal eosinophilia and leukemoid reactions in 5% of cases (Table 22.74).

Mode of Spread

Renal cell carcinoma metastasizes in 30% cases by following routes:

- *Local spread:* Tumor invades renal capsule and peripelvic fat. It has tendency to invade renal vein in 15–20%. The tumor may invade inferior vena cava and extend to right side of heart.
- *Lymphatic route:* Tumor metastasizes to para-aortic and other lymph nodes.
- *Hematogenous route:* In order of decreasing frequency, metastases are seen in lungs (50–75%), osteolytic lesions in bones (33%), liver (18%), skin (8%), and

Table 22.74: Systemic manifestations of renal cell carcinoma

Clinical features	Mechanism
Fever	Prostaglandins
Hypercalcemia	Synthesis of parathyroid hormone related peptide by tumor
Increased RBCs count in 4% of cases	Increased synthesis of erythropoietin by tumor
Amyloidosis in 3% of cases	Stimulation of serum amyloid (SAA) synthesis by liver
Galactorrhea	Ectopic synthesis of prolactin
Hypertension	Increased synthesis of renin
Gynecomastia	Exact mechanism unknown

brain (8%). Renal cell carcinoma may extend into the inferior vena cava known as *carcinomatous thrombus*.

Staging

Stage I : Tumor confined within capsule of kidney has 10 years survival in 70% of cases.
Stage II : Tumor invading perinephric fat.
Stage III: Tumor invading the renal vein or inferior vena cava (A), or regional lymph node involvement (B), or both (C).
Stage IV : Tumor invading adjacent viscera (excluding ipsilateral adrenal) or distant metastases.

Laboratory investigations

- *Hemogram:* Polycythemia due to erythropoietin synthesis by renal cell carcinoma.
- *Urine analysis:* Hematuria (RBCs) is the most common finding. Malignant cells are not frequently demonstrated (uncommon).
- *Biochemistry:* Serum calcium levels may be high, liver and kidney function tests.
- *Imaging techniques:* Ultrasound of the abdomen especially kidneys, intravenous pyelography, renal arteriography, bone scan may show involvement of the bones due to metastases.

CHROMOPHIL (PAPILLARY) VARIANT OF RENAL CELL CARCINOMA

Chromophil (papillary) variant of renal cell carcinoma arises from distal tubular epithelial cells. It may be sporadic or familial and accounts for 10–15% of cases.

It arises from distal tubular cells in cortex. It most often occurs in patients who develop hemodialysis associated cystic disease.

Tumors may be multifocal involving both kidneys. Tumor fungates into calyces, involves renal pelvis, and extends into ureter.

It may also invade the renal vein, inferior vena cava and right atrium. Out of three histologic variants, chromophil renal cell carcinoma has worst prognosis.

Molecular Genetics

- It is never associated with VHL gene mutation located on chromosome 3. Trisomy or tetrasomy 7, 16 and 17 are common due to chromosomal gains. Loss of Y chromosome is seen in familial cases.
- PRCC gene on chromosome 1 fuses with TFE 3 gene on chromosome X. Fusion protein dysregulates mitotic checkpoints allowing abnormal segregation of chromosomes.

Patient develops bilateral hereditary papillary variant of renal cell carcinomas due to overexpression of MET proto-oncogene.

Gross Morphology

It reveals tan-brown colored well-circumscribed tumor. Cut section appears granular due to its papillary architecture. Areas of hemorrhage and necrosis are present in large tumors (Fig. 22.80).

Light Microscopy

- Papillary renal cell carcinoma is composed of varying proportions of papillary and tubular structures. Papillae (fibrovascular core) are lined by a single layer of tumor cells with round uniform nuclei without nucleoli.
- Fibrovascular core usually consists of aggregates of foamy macrophages, and may also show psammoma bodies.
- The stroma is usually scanty but highly vascularized (Fig. 22.81).

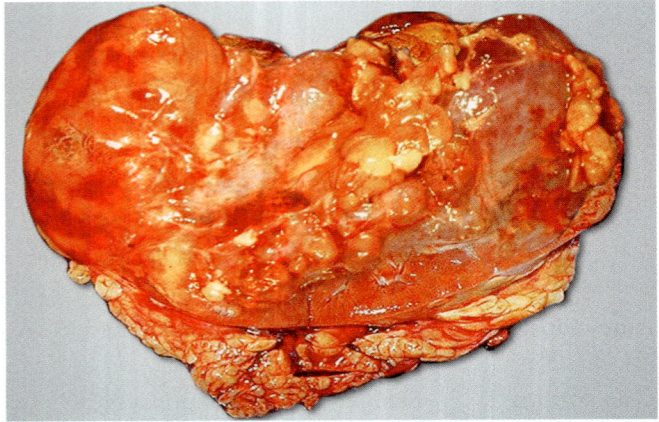

Fig. 22.80: Papillary renal cell carcinoma. Cut surface shows tumor with papillary protrusions. The great majority of papillary renal cell carcinoma has familial predisposition.

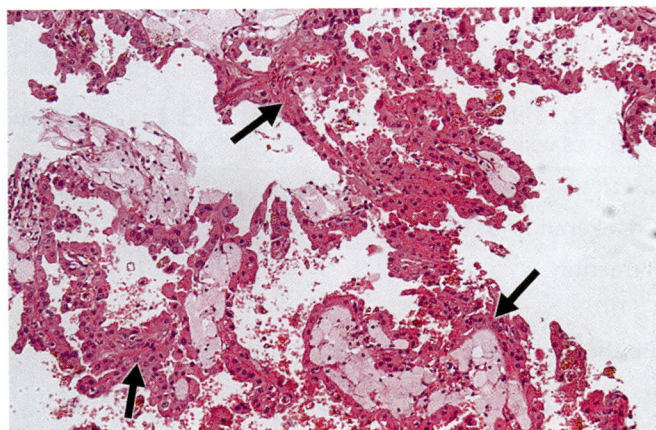

Fig. 22.81: Renal cell carcinoma (chromophil/papillary variant). Tumor shows papillae made of a thin fibrovascular core covered by cuboidal or low columnar cells with round uniform nuclei without nucleoli. The stroma is usually scanty but highly vascularized (arrows).

> **Immunohistochemistry**
> Tumor cells express CK7.

CHROMOPHOBE VARIANT OF RENAL CELL CARCINOMA

Chromophobe variant of renal cell carcinoma arises from intercalated cells of collecting ducts. Out of three histologic variants, prognosis of chromophobe renal cell carcinoma is excellent. Men and women are equally affected.

Chromosomal Abnormalities

Multiple chromosomal losses or extreme hypoploidy is seen on cytogenetic study.

> **Gross Morphology**
> It reveals well-circumscribed, light brown tumor. It is difficult to differentiate it from renal oncocytoma. Hemorrhage and necrosis are rare.
>
> **Light Microscopy**
> - Tumor is composed of polyhedral pleomorphic cells with eccentrically placed nuclei with a perinuclear halo.
> - The nuclei are hyperchromatic with irregular contours.
> - Cytoplasmic membrane of these cells are prominent resembling vegetable cells. Tumor cells are arranged in solid sheets with a concentration of the largest cells around blood vessels (Fig. 22.82).

Histochemistry

Hale's colloidal iron stain reveals strong blue cytoplasmic staining in chromophobe variant of renal cell carcinoma. This staining pattern is absent in clear cell variant and chromophil variant of renal cell carcinoma.

Electron Microscopy

It reveals numerous oval cytoplasmic microvesicles measuring from 150 to 300 nm in diameter. These are not found in any other renal tumor and that are considered diagnostic. It is quite likely that Hale's colloidal iron reacts with a substance present in the microvesicles.

Xp TRANSLOCATION OF RENAL CELL CARCINOMA

It is most often affects young patients. It constitutes at least one-third of pediatric renal cell carcinoma. Presence of dense calcifications in tumor resemble renal lithiasis, and obstruction of the renal pelvis promotes extensive obscuring xanthogranulomatous pyelonephritis.

Molecular Genetics

Xp11 translocation renal cell carcinomas bear gene fusions involving the TFE3 transcription factor gene located at Xp11.2 (Table 22.75).

> **Gross Morphology**
> - Tumor has a fibrous pseudocapsule ranging in size from 3 to 14 cm in diameter.
> - Cut surface is yellow or gray white with varying degree of calcification.
> - Sometimes, tumor imparts egg-shell consistency (Fig. 22.83).
>
> **Light Microscopy**
> - Tumor cells are arranged in nests and papillary formations surrounded by thin-walled capillary vessels.
> - Sometimes central cells in nests are dyscohesive imparting an alveolar or bloody garland appearance.
> - Stromal macrophages and psammoma bodies, if present are limited in number (Fig. 22.84).

Table 22.75: Molecular derangements in translocation carcinomas in children

Translocation carcinomas	Transcriptional activators	Karyotyping
t(x;1) (p11,2;q34)	ASPL-TFE3	IPOX for TFE
t(x;1) (p11,2;q25)	PSF-TFE3	Cathepsin K
t(x;1) (p11,2;q21)	PRCC-TFE3	
t(6;1) (p21;q12)	Alpha-TFEB	

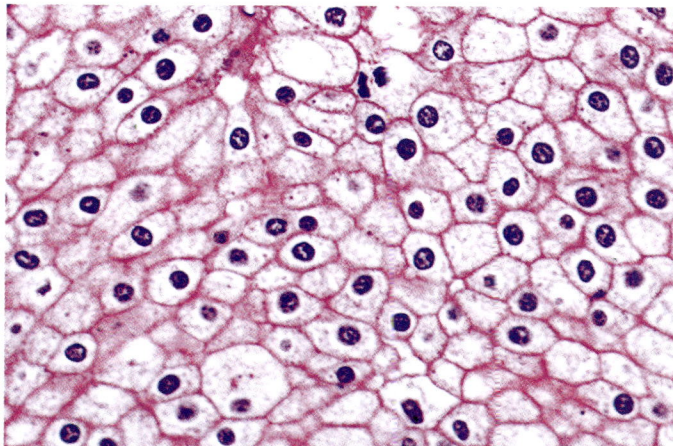

Fig. 22.82: Chromophobe renal cell carcinoma. Tumor is composed of polyhedral pleomorphic cells with eccentrically placed nuclei with a perinuclear halo. The nuclei are hyperchromatic with irregular contours (400X).

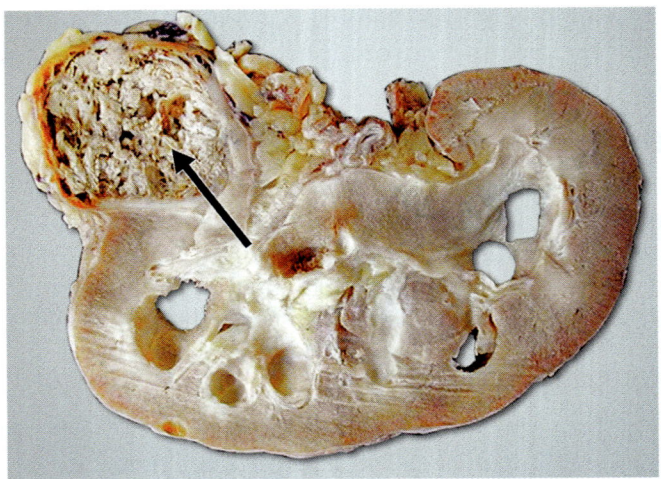

Fig. 22.83: Xp11 translocation renal cell carcinoma. Tumor has a fibrous pseudocapsule. It is located at lower pole. Cut surface is yellow or gray white with varying degrees of calcification. It may sometimes, impart egg-shell consistency (arrow).

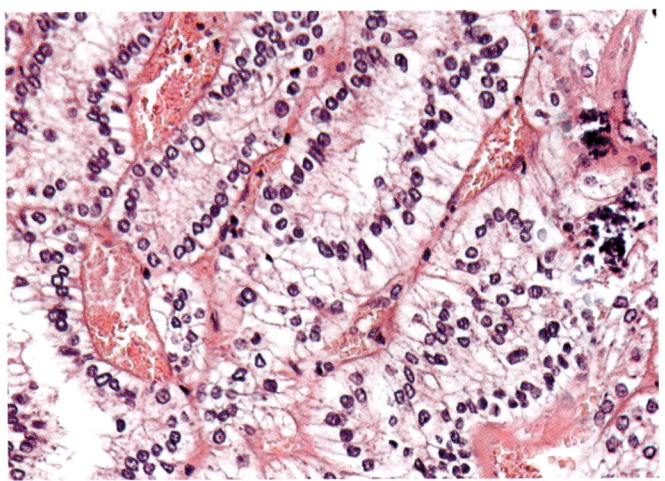

Fig. 22.84: Xp11 translocation renal cell carcinoma. Tumor is composed of nests and papillary structures surrounded by thin-walled vessels.

BELLINI DUCT RENAL CELL CARCINOMA

Bellini duct renal cell carcinoma is a rare tumor (2% of cases) arising from collecting ducts in medullary region. Tumor is circumscribed with central areas of necrosis. However, recent studies show that other renal neoplasms such as oncocytomas and chromophobe RCC most likely originate also in the collecting ducts.

Chromosomal Analysis

Cytogenetic information is still very limited in these tumors, but losses of chromosomes 1, 6, 14, 15, and 22 have been reported.

Immunohistochemistry

It can help to establish the correct diagnosis. It stains positively for cytokeratin 19, ulex europaeus lectin, and vimentin, while urothelial carcinomas stain negatively for vimentin, and RCC stains negatively for ulex europaeus lectin.

RENAL ANGIOMYOLIPOMA (HAMARTOMA)

Renal angiomyolipoma is a hamartoma comprised of fat, smooth muscle and thick-walled blood vessels in varying proportion and haphazardly arranged. It may occur as sporadic or in association of tuberous sclerosis. It is often associated with tuberous sclerosis syndrome. It most often occurs in adults of 50 years of age. It rarely occurs in pediatric age group.

Sporadic Renal Angiomyolipoma

Patients develop multifocal, small and bilateral renal asymptomatic or symptomatic (hematuria) lesions. Occasionally, lymph node involvement occurs but without fatal outcome.

Tuberous Sclerosis Associated Renal Angiomyolipoma

It is caused by mutations in the TSC1 or TSC genes which encode the hamartin and tuberin proteins, respectively. Tuberous sclerosis is associated with multiple hamartomas within brain (as cortical tubers subependymal hamartomas), face, and kidneys (renal angiomyolipoma in 80% of cases).

Molecular Genetics

Renal angiomyolipoma in children exhibits molecular derangements such as 9q34, 16p13.3, 5q, TSC1, TSC2 and tumor suppressor genes.

Clinical Features

Patient may present with flank pain/loin mass and hematuria. Clinical picture mimics like renal cell carcinoma. Light microscopy confirms the diagnosis.

Gross Morphology

Renal angiomyolipoma reveals well circumscribed mass having variegated appearances replaces the upper pole of this kidney. In 25% of cases, the angiomyolipoma may be confused with malignancy because of extension outside the renal capsule (Fig. 22.85).

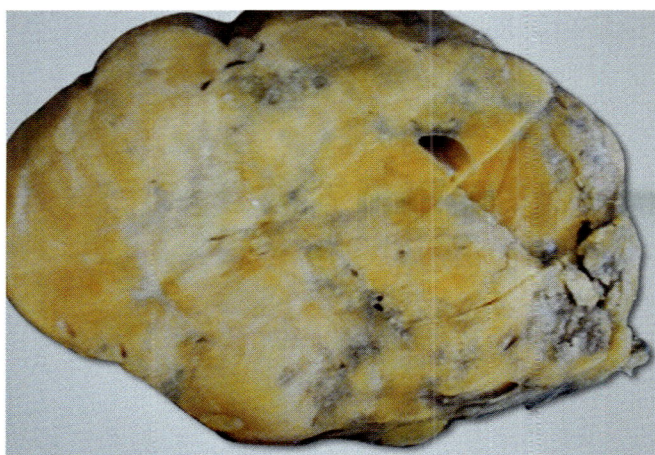

Fig. 22.85: Renal angiomyolipoma. Cut surface shows gray white and yellow tissue.

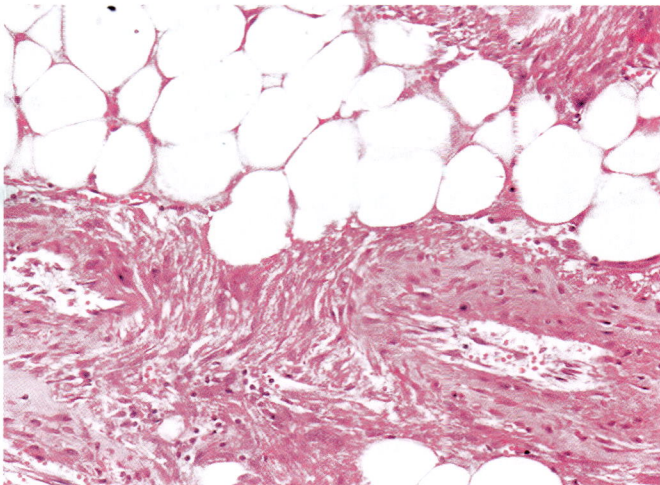

Fig. 22.86: Renal angiomyolipoma. Light microscopy reveals mature adipose tissue, smooth muscle and thick-walled blood vessels in varying proportion and haphazardly arranged.

Light Microscopy

Renal angiomyolipoma comprises mature adipose tissue, smooth muscle and thick-walled blood vessels in varying proportion and haphazardly arranged (Fig. 22.86).

UROTHELIAL CARCINOMA OF RENAL PELVIS

Renal pelvis, ureters and urinary bladder are lined by transitional epithelium. Urothelial tumors of the renal pelvis and ureter are less common. It is most common urothelial tumor affecting adults.

It constitutes 5–10% of primary renal tumors with poor prognosis. It is similar to transitional cell tumors of the urinary bladder.

Approximately 50% have similar tumors elsewhere in the urinary tract.

Risk Factors

- Cigarette smoking is the most common cause of renal pelvis carcinoma. There is increased risk of renal pelvis carcinoma in patients with intake of analgesic drugs (*phenacetin*), *cyclophosphamide* drug for longer period, and prolonged exposure of occupational workers in *aniline dye* and *rubber industries*. Patient presents with hematuria and flank pain.
- Risk factors of tumors of renal pelvis are similar to bladder cancer, suggesting a *field effect*.
- In aniline and rubber industries, prolonged exposure to β-naphthylamine (glucuronide (aromatic amine) urothelial carcinoma. β-naphthylamine absorbed by gastrointestinal tract reaches liver.

In the liver, hydroxylation of β-naphthylamine forms 1-hydroxy-2-naphthylamine (active carcinogenic metabolite), that combines with glucuronic acid and excreted in the urinary tract.

This molecule is deconjugated by bladder mucosal enzyme glucuronidase, thus exposing the urothelium to the active carcinogen results in bladder cancer.

Gross Morphology

- Tumor may be flat and infiltrative. It is most often papillary but may invade renal pelvis wall.
- Tumor may invade renal vein and metastasize to various organs.
- It may result in fragments breaking off from the tips of fronds; and the tumor cells are detected in urine on cytological examination.

Light Microscopy

Transitional cell carcinoma may be well differentiated to anaplastic carcinoma.

Clinical Features

- Patients most frequently present with hematuria and flank pain. Transitional epithelial cells lining papillae may detach and may be found in urine, important for diagnosis.

  Tumor fragmentation may block urinary outflow and cause flank pain and hydronephrotic changes.
- Even a small tumor may cause hematuria, renal colic, or urinary obstruction and can be diagnosed in early stages of development.

  Excision of the entire ureter is necessary because of the high frequency of concurrent and subsequent carcinomas.

LABORATORY DIAGNOSIS

Laboratory investigations in renal deseases are described in Tables 22.76 to 22.79 and Figs 22.87 and 22.88).

Table 22.76: Normal values for routine urinalysis

General characteristics and measurements	Chemical determinants	Microscopic examination of urinary sediment
Color: yellow	Proteins	Casts: negative; occasional
Appearance: clear to slightly hazy	Glucose: negative	Red blood cells: negative
Specific gravity: 1.005–1.025 with normal fluid intake	Ketone bodies: negative	Crystals: negative (none)
pH: 4.5–8.0; average person has pH of about 5 or 6	Blood: negative	White blood cells: negative
Volume: 600–2500 ml/24; average urine volume is 1200 ml/24 hour	Bilirubin: negative Urobilinogen: 0.5-4.0 mg/dl Nitrate for bacteria: negative Leukocyte esterase: negative	Epithelial cells: few (low power field)

Table 22.77: Causes of hematuria

• Glomerulonephritis	• Renal pelvis transitional cell carcinoma	• Calculi in urinary tract
• Interstitial renal disease	• Transitional cell carcinoma of the urter, urinary bladder or urethra	• Tuberculosis of kidney
• Renal papillary necrosis	• Other neoplasms of the urinary bladder, ureter and urethra	• Exacerbation by anticoagulants
• Renal cell carcinoma	• Urinary tract infection	

Table 22.78: Normal blood chemistry levels

Substance	Normal values
Blood urea nitrogen	8.0–20.0 mg/dl (2.9–7.1 mmol/L)
Creatinine	0.6–1.2 mg/dl (50–100 mmol/L)
Sodium	135–145 mEq/L
Chloride	98–106 mEq/L
Potassium	3.5–5 mEq/L
Carbon dioxide (CO_2 content)	24–29 mEq/L
Calcium	8.5–10.5 mg/dl (2.1–2.6 mmol/L)
Uric acid	Male: 2.4–7.4 mg/dl (14–440 μmol/L)
	Female: 1.4–5.8 mg/dl (80–350 μmol/L)
pH	7.35–7.45

Values may vary among laboratories, depending on the method of analysis used.

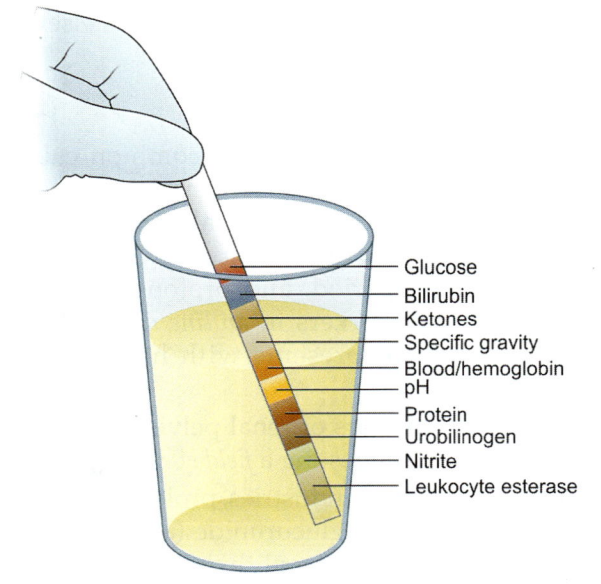

Fig. 22.87: Dipstick is a bedside qualitative estimation of urinary chemical constituents, specific gravity, leukocyte esterase and pH.

Kidney and Ureter 22

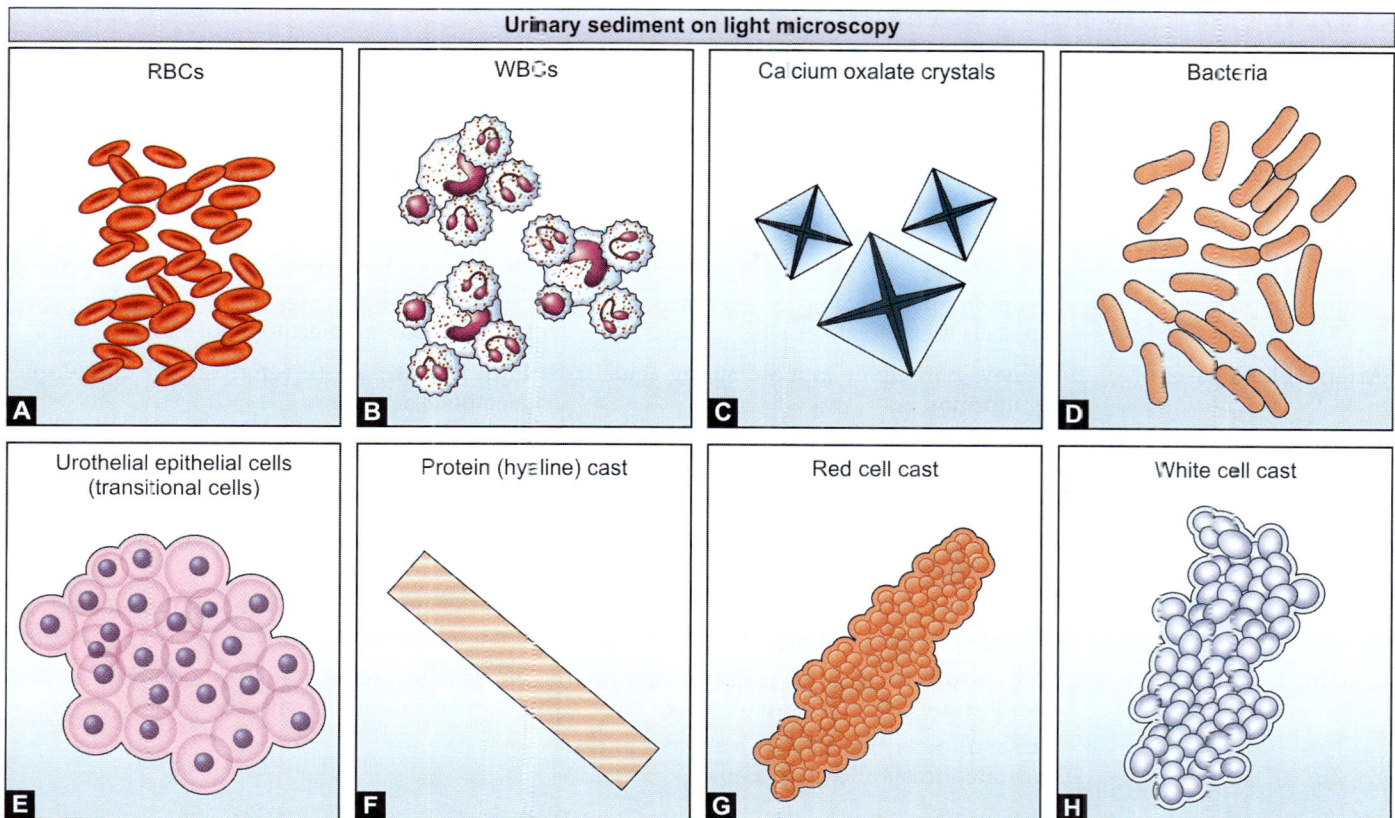

Fig. 22.88: Urinary sediment is examined under light microscopy to demonstrate RBCs, pus cells, calcium oxalate crystals, bacteria, epithelial cast, protein (hyaline) cast and white cell cast in various urinary tract disorders.

Table 22.79: Laboratory investigations used in renal disease

Investigations	Reason	Comments
Serum potassium	The kidneys are the main route of excretion of potassium Hyperkalemia occurs in acute renal failure. Levels may reach life-threatening state	Frequent monitoring of serum potassium levels, is therefore, essential
Serum sodium	Most renal diseases have a little impact on serum sodium levels Serum sodium levels are vital in diabetes insipidus and syndrome of inappropriate ADH secretion (SIADH)	Close monitoring is vital if large volume of fluids are administered in acute renal failure and patient on hemodialysis
Blood urea	Urea is a nitrogenous waste product of proteins synthesized by the liver and excreted by kidneys	Its estimation provides a measure of the severity of the renal insufficiency in acute and chronic renal failure
Serum creatinine	Creatinine is derived from muscle and normal levels exhibit muscle mass and racial variability	Serum creatinine levels are increased in acute and chronic renal failure
Serum proteins	Serum proteins are decreased in nephrotic and nephritic syndrome	Proteins are lost in urine in variable proportion depending on severity of glomerular injury
Serum lipids	Serum lipids are increased in nephrotic syndrome	Liver compensates protein loss by synthesizing lipoproteins leading to increased serum lipid levels

Contd...

Table 22.79: Laboratory investigations used in renal disease (Contd...)

Investigations	Reason	Comments
Blood sugar	Blood sugar levels increased cause diabetic nephropathy	Blood sugar monitoring is essential in diabetes mellitus
Serum calcium and phosphate	Kidneys activate vitamin D. This activation is impaired in chronic renal failure	Hypocalcemia is accompanied by increased parathormone level, as a consequence phosphates levels are raised. Magnesium levels should be monitored
Serum complement	Serum complement may be altered in systemic lupus erythematosus	Serum complement level is decreased in post-streptococcal glomerulonephritis
Arterial blood gases	Kidneys participate in maintaining acid–base equilibrium	Patient with acute renal failure develops metabolic acidosis
Serum autoantibodies	Most relevance to nephrology are ANCA (antineutrophilic cytoplasmic antibody) in vasculitis and ANA (antinuclear antibodies to double-stranded DNA) for systemic lupus erythematosus	Serum ANCA is analyzed in vasculitis leading to glomerulopathy. Serum ANA is analyzed in lupus nephritis
Serum immunoglobulins and electrophoresis	These investigations are carried out in suspected cases of myeloma causing renal impairment	Light chains form casts in tubules leading to renal impairment
Imaging techniques	Plain abdominal radiograph is helpful to demonstrate calculi in urinary tract Ultrasonography evaluates obstruction, hydronephrosis and neoplasms	Nuclear medicine scans provide data of the overall excretory function of kidneys
Hemogram	Erythropoietin level is decreased in chronic renal failure. Patient develops anemia	Transferrin bound iron loss occurs in nephrotic syndrome resulting in iron deficiency anemia
Bleeding and coagulation studies	These are essential prior to renal biopsy	Kidney biopsy is contraindicated in bleeding and coagulation disorders. Hypercoagulable state may occur in nephrotic syndrome
Cystatin C (recent biomarker)	It is encoded by CST3 gene It belongs to type 2 cystine gene family It is found in all tissues It is excreted in urine	Increased concentration in blood indicates impaired glomerular filtrate and renal functions

CHAPTER 23

Urinary Bladder and Male Reproductive System

Learning Objectives

URINARY BLADDER
- Benign Disorders of Urinary Bladder
- Neoplastic Urothelial Lesions
  - Flat Urothelial Lesions with Atypia
  - Invasive Urothelial Neoplasms
  - Botryoides Rhabdomyosarcoma

TESTES
- Anatomy and Physiology
- Testicular Tumors
- Germ Cell Tumors
- Sex Cord-Gonadal Stromal Tumors
- Other Tumors
- Male Hypogonadism and Impotence
- Inflammatory Disorders
- Miscellaneous Disorders
- Male Infertility

PROSTATE GLAND
- Anatomy and Histology
- Inflammatory Disorders of Prostate
- Nodular Hyperplasia of Prostate
- Prostatic Adenocarcinoma

DISEASES OF PENIS
- Inflammatory Disorders
- Carcinoma of Penis
  - Invasive Carcinoma of Penis
- Congenital Anomalies and Miscellaneous Diseases

URINARY BLADDER

BENIGN DISORDERS OF URINARY BLADDER

Benign disorders of urinary bladder include cystitis (acute, chronic, granulomatous, interstitial, hemorrhagic, papillary polypoid, eosinophilic), cystitis glandularis, malakoplakia, extrophy, persistence of the urachal sinus, vesicoumbilical fistula or urachal diverticulum and urinary bladder diverticulum (Table 23.1).

ACUTE CYSTITIS

Ascending infection from the urethra is the most common route of infection causing cystitis. It most often occurs in women because of a short urethra, especially during pregnancy. In acute cystitis, bladder stroma is edematous, hemorrhagic, with neutrophilic infiltrate of variable intensity (Fig. 23.1).

Etiological Agents

Escherichia coli is the most common cause of acute cystitis in 85% of cases. *Proteus vulgaris*, *Klebsiella*, and *Enterococci* are also responsible in some cases. *Staphylococcus saprophyticus*, a coagulase-negative bacterium, is associated with 10–20% of cases in young, sexually active females.

Predisposing Factors

These include bladder calculi, bladder outlet obstruction, diabetes mellitus, immunodeficiency,

Table 23.1: Benign disorders of urinary bladder

Type of inflammation	Etiology
Acute infectious cystitis	Intermittent urinary obstruction in females
	Escherichia coli (85%) of cases. *Proteus vulgaris*, Klebsiella, and Enterococci
Chronic infectious cystitis	Cystoscopy or indwelling catheters for prolonged periods and intermittent urinary obstruction
Granulomatous cystitis	Bacteria, fungi, parasites and intravesical immunotherapy
Chronic interstitial cystitis	Middle-aged and elderly women
Hemorrhagic cystitis	Cyclophosphamide therapy and adenovirus infection in immuno-compromised persons
Papillary and polypoid (bullous) cystitis	Prolonged indwelling catheter
Eosinophilic cystitis	Eosinophils present in lamina propria of urinary bladder due to allergic conditions, parasitic infestations. Eosinophils may be present in the adjoining areas of urothelial carcinomas
Cystitis glandularis	It occurs in a setting of chronic bladder inflammation: bladder exstrophy, chronically infected neurogenic bladder, and bladders chronically irritated by stones or an indwelling catheter
Malakoplakia	Soft yellow mucosal plaque shows abundant epithelioid histiocytes (known as *Hansemann histiocytes*) containing basophilic intracytoplasmic granules known as *Michaellis-Guttmann bodies* containing iron (Perl's stain) and calcium (von Kossa)
Extrophy	Exstrophy of the bladder is absence of the anterior part of the bladder and abdominal wall
Persistence of the urachal sinus	Due to persistence of the urachal sinus, there is drainage of urine from the umbilicus of a newborn
Vesicoumbilical fistula or urachal diverticulum	It occurs due to failure of the urachus to involute
Urinary bladder diverticulum	It occurs due to nodular hyperplasia prostate resulting in obstruction and recurrent infections

prior instrumentation or catheterization, radiation therapy and chemotherapy.

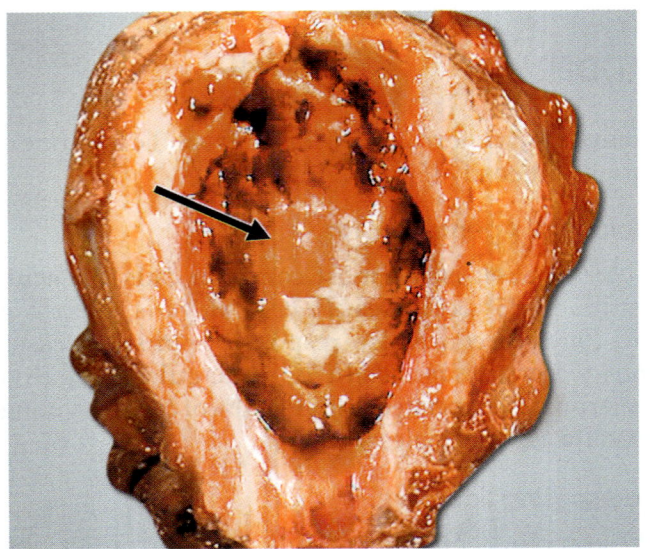

Fig. 23.1: Acute cystitis. The mucosal surface is red and inflamed. The patient had an indwelling catheter for many weeks before death from other pathology (arrow).

Light Microscopy

Urinary bladder is infiltrated by polymorphonuclear infiltrate.

Urine Examination

Examination of the urine usually reveals inflammatory cells. Causative agent can be identified by urine culture. Most cases of cystitis respond well to treatment with antimicrobial agents.

Clinical Features

Patients present with dysuria, increased frequency of urination, a sense of urgency, and discomfort over the bladder.

CHRONIC CYSTITIS

Chronic cystitis is associated with lack of resolution of the inflammatory reaction in patients with acute cystitis. It occurs due to introduction of pathogens into the bladder during *cystoscopy* or *indwelling catheters* remaining for prolonged periods.

Light Microscopy

Bladder stroma shows predominance of lymphocytes and fibrosis of the lamina propria.

GRANULOMATOUS CYSTITIS

Granulomatous cystitis is caused by bacteria, fungi, parasites and intravesical immunotherapy. Light microscopy of urinary bladder shows granulomas and chronic inflammatory cells.

CHRONIC INTERSTITIAL CYSTITIS

Chronic interstitial cystitis is characterized by prolonged transmural chronic interstitial inflammation of the bladder wall. It is occasionally associated with mucosal ulceration known as *Hunner ulcer*. It may be of unknown etiology.

Age Group

It most often affects middle-aged women.

Clinical Features

Patient presents with suprapubic pain, frequency and urgency with or without hematuria.

HEMORRHAGIC CYSTITIS

Hemorrhagic cystitis is caused by *cyclophosphamide* therapy and adenovirus infection in *immunocompromised persons*.

PAPILLARY AND POLYPOID (BULLOUS) CYSTITIS

Papillary polypoid (bullous) cystitis occurs due to prolonged indwelling catheter. Lesion is difficult to differentiate from low grade urothelial neoplasm.

EOSINOPHILIC CYSTITIS

Eosinophilic cystitis is characterized by presence of eosinophils in lamina propria of urinary bladder due to allergic conditions and parasitic infestations. Eosinophils may be present in the adjoining areas of urothelial carcinomas.

CYSTITIS GLANDULARIS

Cystitis glandularis most often occurs in a setting of chronic bladder inflammation: Bladder exstrophy, chronically infected neurogenic bladder and bladder chronically irritated by stones or an indwelling catheter.

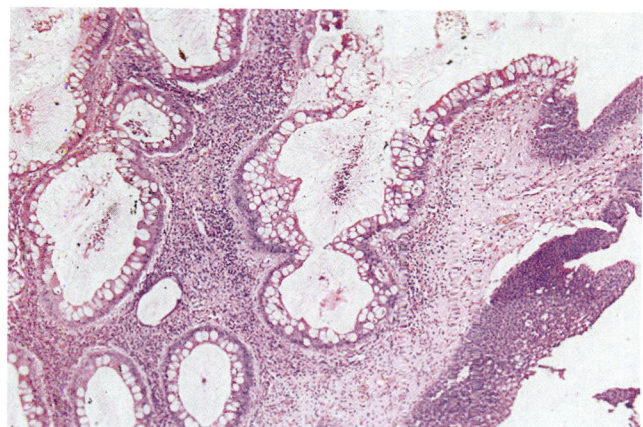

Fig. 23.2: Cystitis glandularis shows intestinal metaplasia (400X).

Gross Morphology

It takes the form of focally or diffusely inflamed edematous or polypoid bladder mucosa, as in this case.

Light Microscopy

Urinary bladder shows chronic inflammation with intestinal metaplasia (Fig. 23.2).

MALACOPLAKIA

Malacoplakia is *granulomatous disorder* of urinary bladder of unknown etiology. Incidence is increased in patients with *immunosuppression, chronic infections,* or *cancer*.

It is associated with accumulation of macrophages resulting in formation of soft yellow-brown plaques on the mucosal surface of the bladder.

The plaques represent mucosa that is expanded by the presence of histiocytes with lysosomal dysfunction.

It may simulate neoplasia, as shown in this endoscopic image from the bladder of a woman with a long history of recurrent urinary infection, and recent hematuria.

Light Microscopy

- Light microscopy reveals large number of macrophages with abundant eosinophilic cytoplasm containing PAS-positive granules.
- Some of these macrophages show laminated, basophilic deposits of calcium termed '**Michaelis-Gutmann bodies**' (Fig. 23.3).

EXSTROPHY OF URINARY BLADDER

Exstrophy of the bladder refers *absence of the anterior part of the bladder and abdominal wall*; that can be recognized at the time of birth. In some male infants, it is associated with *epispadias* (incomplete formation of the penile urethra).

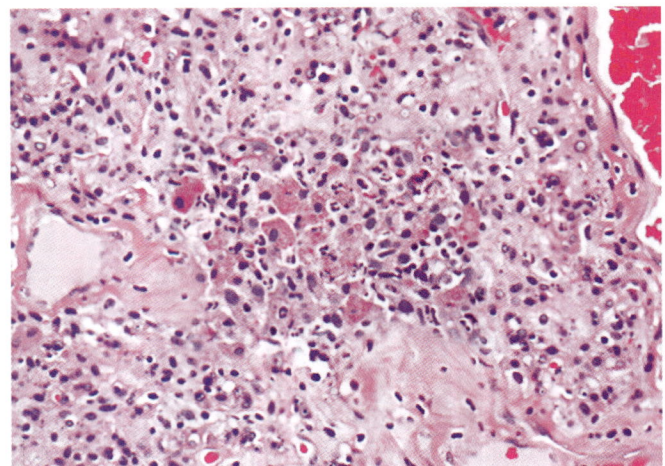

Fig. 23.3: Malacoplakia shows intracellular and extracellular target-like structures termed as Michaelis-Gutmann bodies formed due to deposition of calcium (400X).

Consequence

In patients with exstrophy of the bladder, posterior wall of the bladder undergoes mechanical trauma and undergoes *squamous or glandular metaplasia* and *recurrent infections*.

Despite surgical repair, there is an increased *risk* for *squamous cell carcinoma* or *adenocarcinoma* during 50 to 60 years of age.

PERSISTENCE OF URACHAL SINUS

Due to persistence of the urachal sinus, there is *drainage of urine from the umbilicus of a newborn*. Drainage of fecal matter from the umbilicus occurs due to persistence of the vitelline sinus.

VESICOUMBILICAL FISTULA OR URACHAL DIVERTICULUM

Failure of the urachus to involute may result in vesicoumbilical fistula or urachal diverticulum.

URINARY BLADDER DIVERTICULUM

It most often develops in elderly men in patient with *nodular hyperplasia prostate* resulting in obstruction and recurrent infections. Solitary or multiple sac-like outpouchings are present in bladder wall.

NEOPLASTIC UROTHELIAL LESIONS

Most bladder tumors arise from the urothelium (transitional epithelium) and constitute >98% of all primary tumors of the bladder. These include flat lesions, papillary neoplasms and invasive malignant urothelial cell carcinomas. *Most common malignant tumor* arising from muscle *in children* is *embryonal rhabdomyosarcoma*, also known as *sarcoma botryoides*.

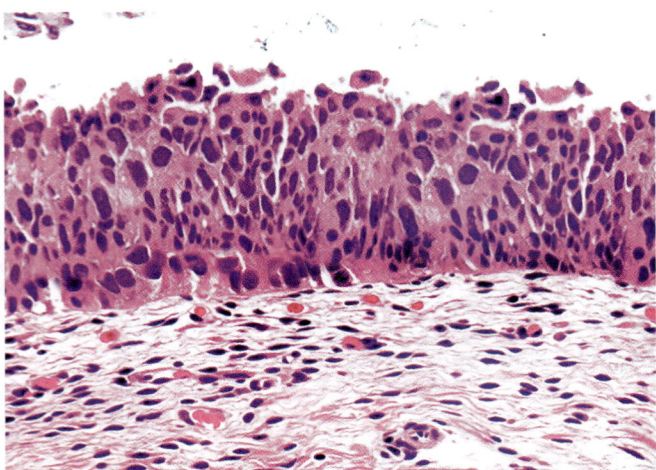

Fig. 23.4: Urothelial dysplasia shows good preservation of cellular polarity with uniform nuclear size and shape. There is presence of mitotic figures in the uroepthelium (400X).

Urothelial lesions may be flat with atypia, papillary and invasive types (Table 23.2).

FLAT UROTHELIAL LESIONS WITH ATYPIA

Urothelial Dysplasia

It is flat lesion in urinary bladder. Urothelial cells show nuclear enlargement, chromatin clumping and loss of polarity (Fig. 23.4).

Urothelial Carcinoma *in situ*

It is flat lesion in urinary bladder. Light microscopy shows cellular atypia of the entire mucosa, from the basal layer to the surface (Fig. 23.5). *Immunohistochemistry study shows positivity for cytokeratin 20, p53, CD44 and Ki-67.*

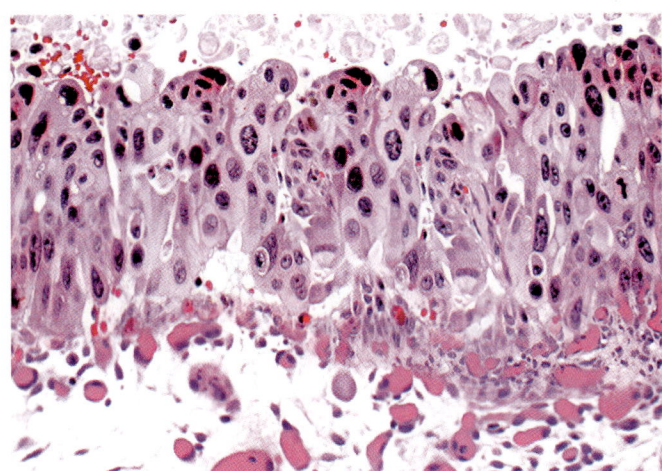

Fig. 23.5: Carcinoma *in situ*. Urothelial cells are pleomorphic with high nucleocytoplasmic ratio, irregular nuclear contours, hyperchromatic nuclei and prominent nucleoli. Cellular polarity is lost. Mitotic figures are atypical. Diagnosis of urothelial carcinoma *in situ* does not require full-thickness involvement. The superficial umbrella cell layer may be intact (400X).

Table 23.2: Urothelial lesions

Urothelial lesion	Morphology on cystoscopy	Light microscopy	Recurrence after surgery (%)	Malignant potential (%)
Flat urothelial lesions with atypia				
• Urothelial dysplasia	Flat lesion	Urothelial cells with nuclear enlargement, chromatin clumping and loss of polarity	–	15%
• Urothelial carcinoma in situ	Flat lesion	Cellular atypia of the entire mucosa, from the basal layer to the surface	–	Malignant entity (immunohistochemistry positive for cytokeratin 20, p53, CD44 and Ki-67)
Papillary urothelial neoplasms				
• Urothelial papilloma	Single papillary frond (2 to 5 cm in diameter), painless hematuria	Tumor is composed of delicate papillary frond with no minimal branching or fusion	<80%	2%
• Inverted papilloma	Polypoidal or sessile growth	Tumor is composed of anastomosing cords of bland urothelial cells with rare mitoses growing towards lamina propria	Rarely recur	No
• Noninvasive papillary urothelial neoplasm of low malignant potential (PUNLMP)	Single papillary frond (2 to 5 cm in diameter)	Tumor is composed of fused papillae with enlarged nuclei. Mitotic figures are rare and basal	25–30%	4%
• Noninvasive papillary urothelial carcinoma (low grade)	Tumor is larger than papilloma. These are more likely multiple tumors	Tumor shows frequent branching and fusion of papillae. There is variation in nuclear size, shape and contour. Mitoses are occasional and seen at any level	64–71%	2–10%
• Noninvasive papillary urothelial carcinoma (high grade)	These frequently invade bladder wall	Tumor is composed of frequent branching and fusion of papillae. Cells are pleomorphic with frequent mitoses	56–18%	18% (high grade)
Invasive urothelial neoplasms				
• Transitional cell carcinoma with squamous or glandular or trophoblastic differentiation	Exophytic (cauliflower-like) or ulcerated lesions	Transitional cell carcinoma may show squamous or glandular or trophoblastic differentiation. These may be well differentiated or moderately differentiated or poorly differentiated carcinomas	Recurrence in all cases	Highly malignant tumor
• Squamous cell carcinoma	Large fungating solitary necrotic tumor	Squamous cell carcinoma	Recurrence in all cases	Highly malignant tumor does not respond to radiotherapy or chemotherapy
• Adenocarcinoma	Most often deeply invasive growth with fatal outcome	Adenocarcinoma (tumor cells show positivity for creatine kinase, uracoplakin and thrombomodulin)	Recurrence in all cases	Highly malignant tumor

INVASIVE UROTHELIAL NEOPLASMS

- Bladder carcinoma most often occurs in 50 to 80 years age group. Men are affected three times more often than women. Most cases of carcinoma *in situ* progress subsequently to invasive carcinoma by invading the lamina propria.
- Invasive urothelial carcinomas may have *papillary, polypoid, nodular* or *ulcerative configurations.*
- Cystoscopy may reveal *multiple, red, velvety, flat patches*. These are high grade tumors.
- Pathological stage depends on *anatomic depth* of *invasion of tumor*. There are several different histological patterns.

Histological Variants

Most urinary bladder carcinomas (90%) are classified as *transitional cell carcinomas*. The remaining histologic variants are squamous cell carcinoma (due to *Schistosoma haematobium* and exstrophy of the bladder) or *adenocarcinoma* (exstrophy of the bladder, foci of cystitis glandularis, and remnants of urachal epithelium) or small cell carcinoma.

- *Squamous differentiation in urothelial carcinoma:* It is seen in 20% of cases. This variant has *poor prognosis*, as it most often *does not respond to radiotherapy or chemotherapy.*
- *Glandular differentiation in urothelial carcinoma:* It is seen in 6% of invasive urothelial carcinomas.
- *Trophoblastic differentiation in urothelial carcinoma:* It shows positivity for hCG with raised serum hCG levels.

Risk Factors

- *Tobacco smoking:* Smoking is a known risk factor for bladder cancer. *Cigarette smoke containing polycyclic hydrocarbons are converted to ultimate carcinogen* (benzo (a) pyrene), which may produce lung carcinoma (local site) and cancers at distant sites (e.g. bladder carcinoma and renal cell carcinoma).
- *Exposure to aromatic amines (azo dyes):* Persons working in aniline dye and rubber industries are heavily exposed to β-naphthylamine. It is absorbed by gastrointestinal tract resulting in bladder carcinoma. In the liver, hydroxylation of β-*naphthylamine* forms 1-hydroxy-2-naphthylamine (water-soluble active carcinogenic metabolite), that combines with glucuronic acid and excreted in the urinary tract.
  This molecule is deconjugated by bladder mucosal enzyme glucuronidase, thus exposing the urothelium to the active carcinogen resulting in bladder carcinoma (Fig. 23.6 and Table 23.3).
- *Schistosoma haematobium:* This *Schistosoma haematobium infection in Egypt* is associated with an increased incidence of squamous cell carcinoma of urinary bladder. Parasite causes foci of squamous metaplasia of the bladder epithelium resulting in squamous cell carcinoma of the bladder.
- *Therapeutic agents:* Administration of drugs, i.e. *cyclophosphamide* and analgesics increases risk of bladder carcinoma.
- *Radiation exposure:* Radiation therapy (for cervical, prostate, or rectal cancer) may increase the risk of urinary bladder carcinoma.
- *Exstrophy of the bladder:* Exstrophy of the bladder is absence of the anterior part of the bladder and

Table 23.3: Indirect acting chemical carcinogens and associated cancers

Chemical carcinogen	Examples	Associated cancers
Polycyclic hydrocarbons	Cigarette smoke, ingestion of smoked meat and fish	*Urinary bladder transitional cell carcinoma* Oral carcinoma Esophagus carcinoma (middle and distal) Pancreas carcinoma Lung carcinoma Renal pelvis transitional cell carcinoma
Aromatic amines	Aniline dye and rubber industries, benzidine-O, anisidine-O and toluidine Unlike polycyclic hydrocarbons, aromatic amines produce no local carcinogenic effect	*Transitional cell carcinoma of urinary bladder* *Mechanism:* Mucosal glucuronidase in the urinary bladder converts β-naphthylamine glucuronide (aromatic amine) to the carcinogenic molecule β-naphthylamine results in urinary bladder cancer
Aromatic hydrocarbons	Benzene present in crude oil (petrochemical), benz (a) anthracene and benz (a) pyrene	*Urinary bladder carcinoma* Acute leukemia Hodgkin's disease

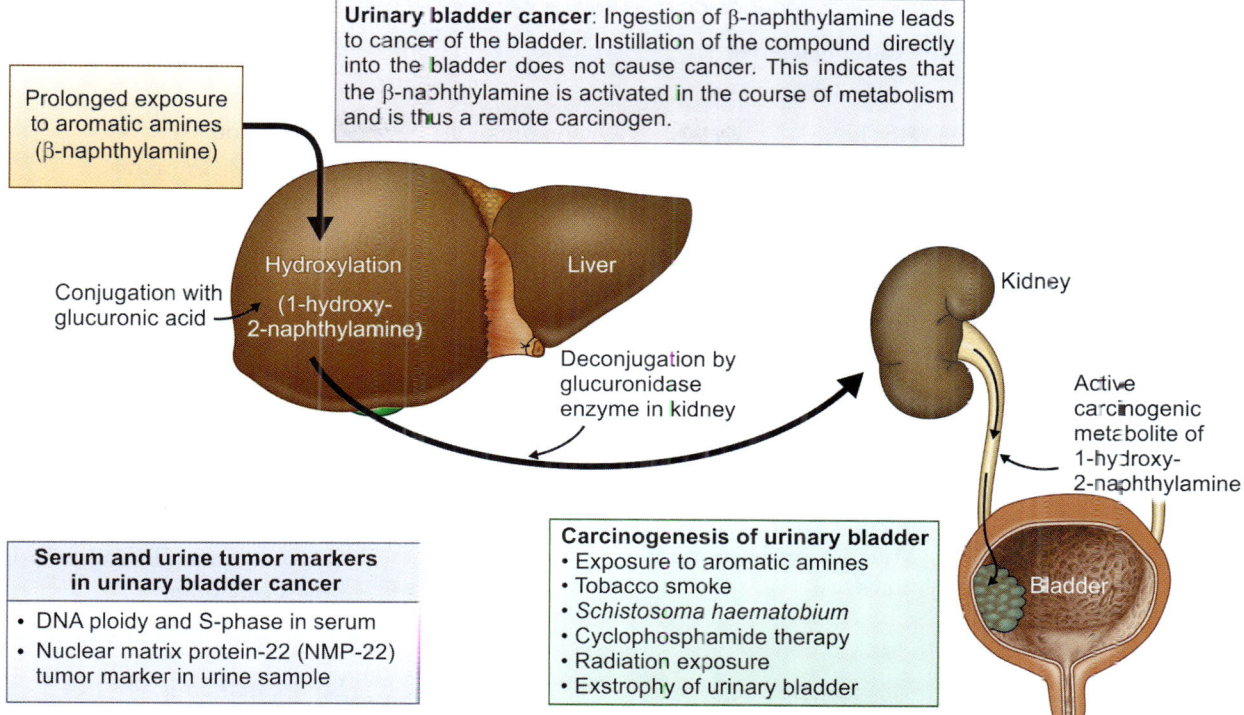

Fig. 23.6: Pathogenesis of urinary bladder carcinoma.

abdominal wall; that can be recognized at the time of birth. In patients with exstrophy of the bladder, posterior wall of the bladder undergoes mechanical trauma resulting in *squamous* or *glandular metaplasia* and *recurrent infections*. Despite surgical repair, there is an *increased risk* for *squamous cell carcinoma* or *adenocarcinoma* in 50 to 60 years of age.

Molecular Genetics

- *FGF3 growth factor:* Amplification of FGF3 has been demonstrated in *urinary bladder carcinoma, breast cancer, stomach cancer and melanoma.* Many cancer cells, acquire the ability to synthesize the same growth factors to which they are responsive, generating an autocrine loop.
- *H-RAS signal-transducing proteins:* It participates in intracellular guanosine triphosphate signaling. Mutant H-RAS has been demonstrated in *urinary bladder carcinoma (6%) and renal cell carcinoma.*
- *Mitogenic signaling pathway inhibitors:* Retinoblastoma protein located on locus 13p14 codes for pRB protein, master brake on cell cycle. It inhibits G1 to S transition during cell cycle. It inhibits nuclear transcription factor. Mutation by deletion of RB gene is associated with *sporadic urinary bladder carcinoma, osteosarcoma, breast carcinoma, colon carcinoma, prostate carcinoma and lung carcinoma.* RB gene mutation is also associated with *familial retinoblastoma and osteosarcoma* (Table 23.4).

Chromosomal Abnormalities

Chromosomal abnormalities have been demonstrated in urinary bladder cancers (Table 23.5).

Clinical Features

The earliest sign of bladder cancer is sudden painless hematuria in urine, which may be red- or rust-colored. In the later stages, the bladder may become irritable with painful urination.

Gross Morphology

- *The lesions in urinary bladder may show various morphological patterns:* flat (carcinoma *in situ*), papillary (small lesion), exophytic (cauliflower-like) or ulcerated lesions.
- Invasive tumor often present as ulceration with indurated margins, that usually invades into the deeper layers of the urinary bladder and extends into the surrounding structures and pelvic organs (Fig. 23.7).

Light Microscopy

Depending on the histologic variants, i.e. transitional cell carcinoma, squamous cell carcinoma, adenocarcinoma or small cell carcinoma, light microscopy reveals cellular atypia of the entire mucosa, from the basal layer to the surface invading the lamina propria.

Table 23.4: Oncogenes and tumor suppressor genes associated with urinary bladder cancers

Category	Proto-oncogene	Mode of activation	Associated malignancies
Growth factors			
Fibroblast growth factors (FGF)	HST1 FGF3	Overexpression Amplification	Osteosarcoma *Urinary bladder cancer* Osteosarcoma Stomach cancer Breast cancer Melanoma
Signal-transduction proteins			
GTP-binding (G) proteins	H-RAS	Point mutation	*Urinary bladder carcinoma* Renal cell carcinoma
Mitogenic signaling pathway inhibitor			
RB tumor suppressor gene	Retinoblastoma protein (locus 13q) Mutation by deletion and nonsense	Deletion and nonsense mutation	*Urinary bladder carcinoma* Retinoblastoma (familial or sporadic) Osteosarcoma (familial or sporadic) Breast carcinoma Colon carcinoma Prostate carcinoma Lung carcinoma

Table 23.5: Chromosome abnormalities in urinary bladder cancer

Chromosome	Abnormality
1	It may represent secondary change
5	Isochromosome formation affects the short arm (p) has been demonstrated in 40% cases of urinary bladder. Isochromosome arises from transverse division of the centromere during meiosis instead of the normal longitudinal division
9	Monosomy of chromosome 9 occurs in 50% of superficial papillary tumors 9q deletion is most common in advanced bladder cancer in 67% of cases. This 9q deletion has not been demonstrated in any other solid tumor
11	Deletion of short arm (p) of chromosome 11 has been demonstrated in 40% of bladder cancer. It represents secondary change related to invasiveness of bladder cancer
17	17p deletion is related to p53 tumor suppressor gene. 17p deletion has been demonstrated in 63% of bladder cancer. It is related to invasiveness of tumor
7	Trisomy of chromosome has been demonstrated in a few cases of bladder cancer The c-erb gene encoding receptor for epidermal growth factor is sited on this chromosome 7. It is expressed in 80% of bladder cancers and in 29% of superficial tumors

Histological Variants

Transitional Cell Carcinoma

The prognosis of transitional carcinoma depends on the grade and stage of the tumor.

- *Well differentiated transitional papillary tumors* are classified as *grade I*, which have good prognosis.
- *Papillary tumors* composed of broad papillae and solid areas are classified as *grade II*, which have an intermediate prognosis.
- *Solid anaplastic tumors* are classified as *grade III*, which have a *poor prognosis*. Tumor cells express **CK7** and **CK20** on immunohistochemical study (Figs 23.8 and 23.9).

> **Immunohistochemistry**
>
> Transitional cell carcinomas show positivity for **p53. Thrombomodulin, uroplakin-III** and **cytokeratin** (high MW) (Table 23.6).

Urinary Bladder and Male Reproductive System 23

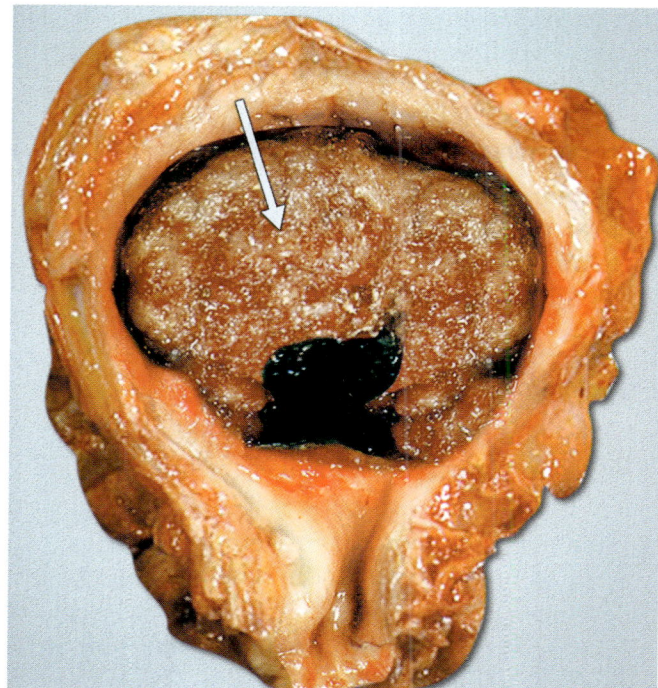

Fig. 23.7: Carcinoma of the bladder. The entire mucosal surface is replaced by a transitional cell carcinoma (arrow).

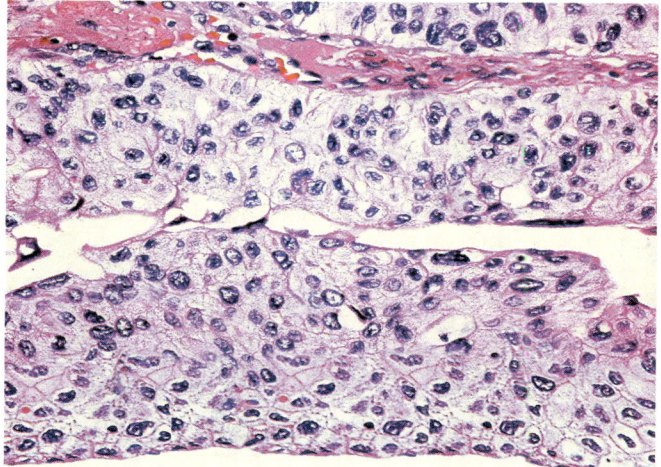

Fig. 23.8: Low grade papillary urothelial carcinoma. At higher power, loss of cellular orientation is evident. Nuclei vary slightly in shape and size. Few mitotic figures may be found (400X).

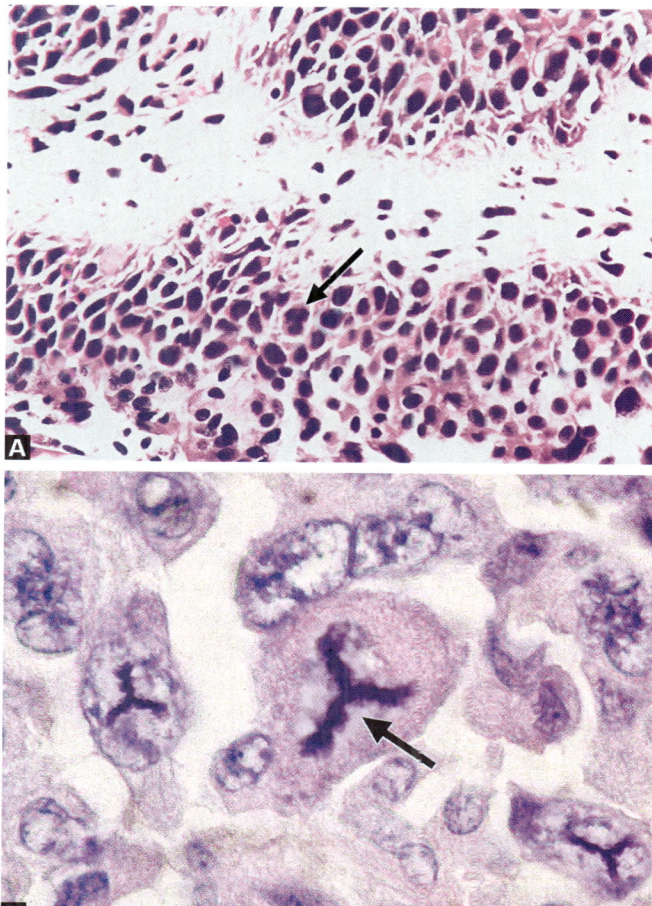

Fig. 23.9: (A) High grade papillary urothelial carcinoma, tumor cells are pleomorphic with hyperchromatic large nuclei and high nuclear to cytoplasmic ratio (arrow). (B) Mitotic figures are frequent. Arrow indicates a tripolar mitosis (400X).

Table 23.6: Immunohistochemistry of transitional cell carcinoma

Marker	Percentage of cases positive
p63	81–96%
Thrombomodulin	69–91%
Uroplakin-III	57%
Cytokeratins (high molecular weight)	65–100%

Squamous Cell Carcinoma

- *Risk factors:* It is associated with *Schistosoma haematobium* parasitic infection especially in Egypt. Predisposing factors include chronic cystitis, long-term indwelling catheters, smoking, diverticula, nonfunctioning urinary bladder, renal transplants cases and exstrophy. *Exstrophy of the bladder may predispose to squamous cell carcinoma or adenocarcinoma.*

- *Gross morphology:* It reveals large fungating solid necrotic tumor that can fill the entire bladder. Verrucous squamous cell carcinoma (exophytic growth) is exclusively associated with *Schistosoma haematobium*.

- *Light microscopy:* Invasive squamous cell carcinoma is well differentiated tumor. It shows well-defined islands of squamous cells with keratinization, keratin pearls, prominent intercellular bridges, and minimal nuclear pleomorphism (Fig. 23.10).

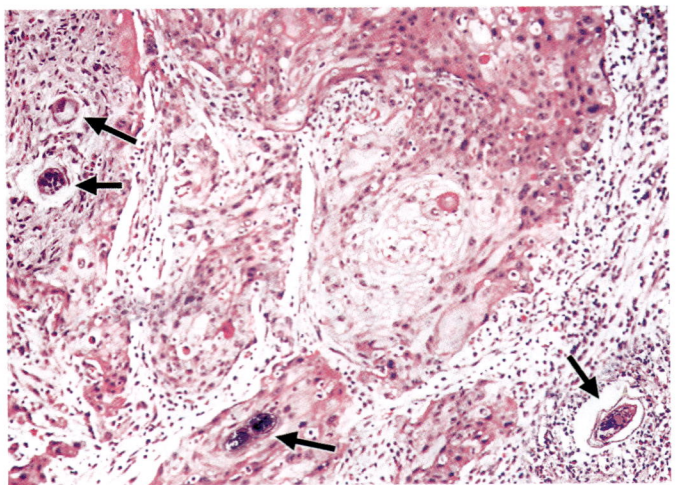

Fig. 23.10: Invasive squamous cell carcinoma is well differentiated tumor. It shows well-defined islands of squamous cells with keratinization, keratin pearls, prominent intercellular bridges, and minimal nuclear pleomorphism. It shows *Schistosoma haematobium* (arrows) (400X).

Adenocarcinoma

- Adenocarcinoma of urinary bladder accounts for 2% of all malignant tumors of the bladder. It arises from foci of *cystitis glandularis or intestinal metaplasia or remnants of urachal epithelium* in the bladder dome.
- It is most often *deeply invasive with fatal outcome*. Exstrophy of the bladder may *predispose to adenocarcinoma or squamous cell carcinoma*.

BOTRYOID RHABDOMYOSARCOMA

It most often manifests in children as *sarcoma botryoides* in urinary bladder. Cystoscopy reveals *grape-like polypoidal lesions on mucosal surface of bladder trigone*. Almost all genitourinary tract cases are of the embryonal rhabdomyosarcoma variant.

Gross Examination

Most embryonal rhabdomyosarcomas of the urinary bladder present as *polypoidal intraluminal masses* resembling cluster of grapes hence named as botryoid type.

Light Microscopy

- Tumor is present in subepithelial region with overlying intact transitional epithelium of urinary bladder wall.
- Tumor is composed of numerous round to oval cells admixed with spindle cells in loose myxoid stroma.
- These tumor cells form cambium layer under the surface urothelium (Fig. 23.11).

Immunohistochemistry

Tumor cells show positivity for **desmin, myogenin, myoglobin** and **myoD1**.

Treatment and Prognosis

Prognosis of this variant has improved with multi-modular treatment. Combined radiation therapy and chemotherapy increase survival rates in these children with this neoplasm.

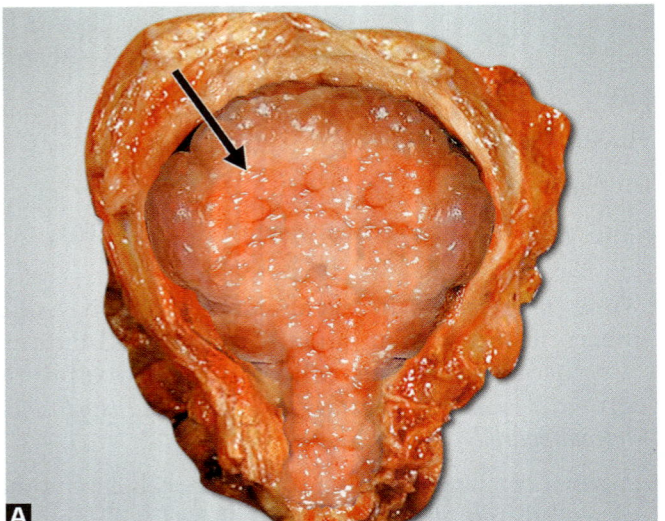
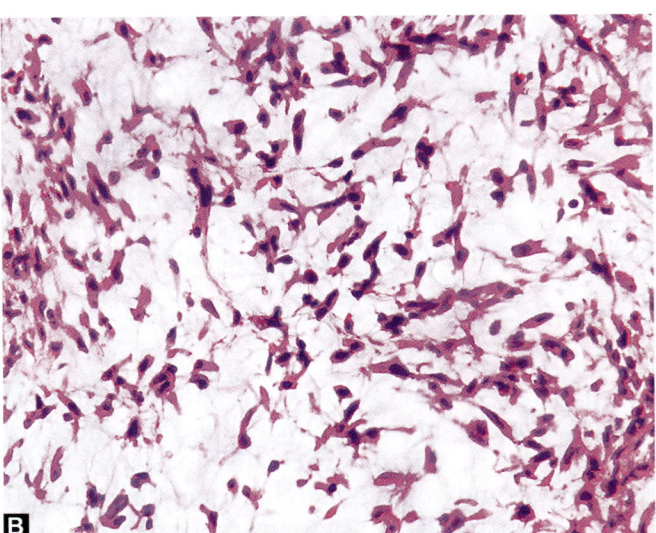

Fig. 23.11: Botryoides rhabdomyosarcoma. Tumor is composed of numerous round to oval cells admixed with spindle cells in loose myxoid stroma (arrow) (400X).

TESTES

ANATOMY AND PHYSIOLOGY

Testes are composed of seminiferous tubules, which are surrounded by a basement membrane (tunica propria) and supported by a delicate fibrovascular stroma, in which Leydig cells are present.

Sertoli cells support germ cells and synthesize estrogens and some androgens. Leydig cells produce testosterone and other androgenic hormones. Normal germ cells to Sertoli cell ratio is 13:1 in seminiferous tubules.

Spermatogenesis

- Under physiological state, various hormones, i.e. growth hormone, testosterone synthesized by Leydig cells play an important role in spermatogenesis.
- Sertoli cells convert some portion of testosterone into estrogens. Estrogens play vital role in spermiogenesis, e.g. maturation of spermatids into spermatozoa.

Sertoli cells synthesize androgen binding protein, which binds and transports both testosterone and estrogens into seminiferous tubules, which promotes maturation of spermatozoa (Fig. 23.12).

Jensen's Score

It refers to score given at each stage of maturation. *Score 10 is given to complete mature spermatogenesis and score 0 to complete absence of germ cells.* Normal spermatogenesis with azospermia indicates obstructive pathology.

TESTICULAR TUMORS

Testicular cancer accounts for 1% of all male cancers. Germ cell tumors (GCT) constitute 95% of testicular tumors. These comprise a heterogeneous group of solid neoplasms that arise in midline locations including the *gonads, retroperitoneum, mediastinum*, and *central nervous system* (called as *germinoma*). These tumors exist in pure form in 40% and mixed forms in 60% of cases.

Classification

- *Origin:* Primary testicular tumors may be derived from *primordial germ cells, Sertoli cells* and *Leydig cells*. Testes may be involved due to metastases from other organs. Germ cell tumors include seminomatous and non-seminomatous tumors. Spermatocytic seminomas arise from primary spermatocytes (Fig. 23.13).

- *Intratubular neoplasia:* Tumor confined to seminiferous tubule is known as *intratubular neoplasia*. Seminoma directly originates from germ cell. Seminoma is not end stage neoplasm, but may also act as precursors of other germ cell tumors such as embryonal carcinoma. Germ cell differentiates into totipotent stem cells. *Tumors arising from totipotent stem cells may show* **embryonic differentiation** (e.g. *embryonal carcinoma* and *teratoma*), and **extra-embryonic differentiation** (e.g. *yolk sac tumor* and *choriocarcinoma*).

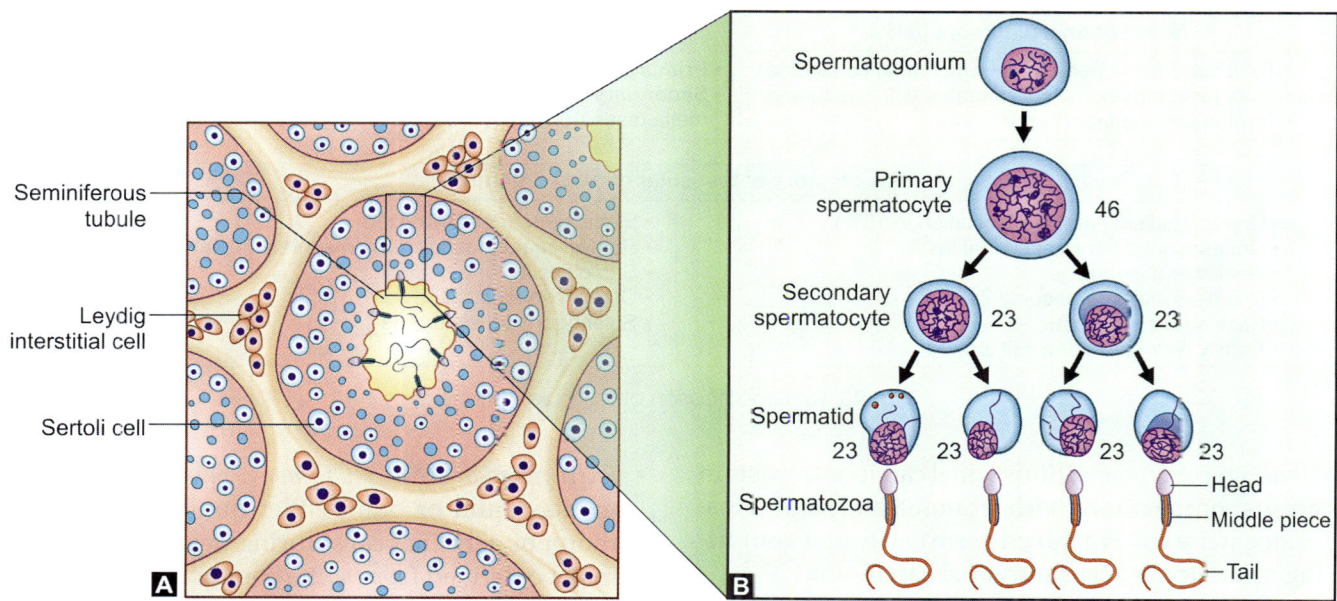

Fig. 23.12: The various stages of spermatogenesis. (A) Cross-section of seminiferous tubule, (B) stages of development of spermatozoa.

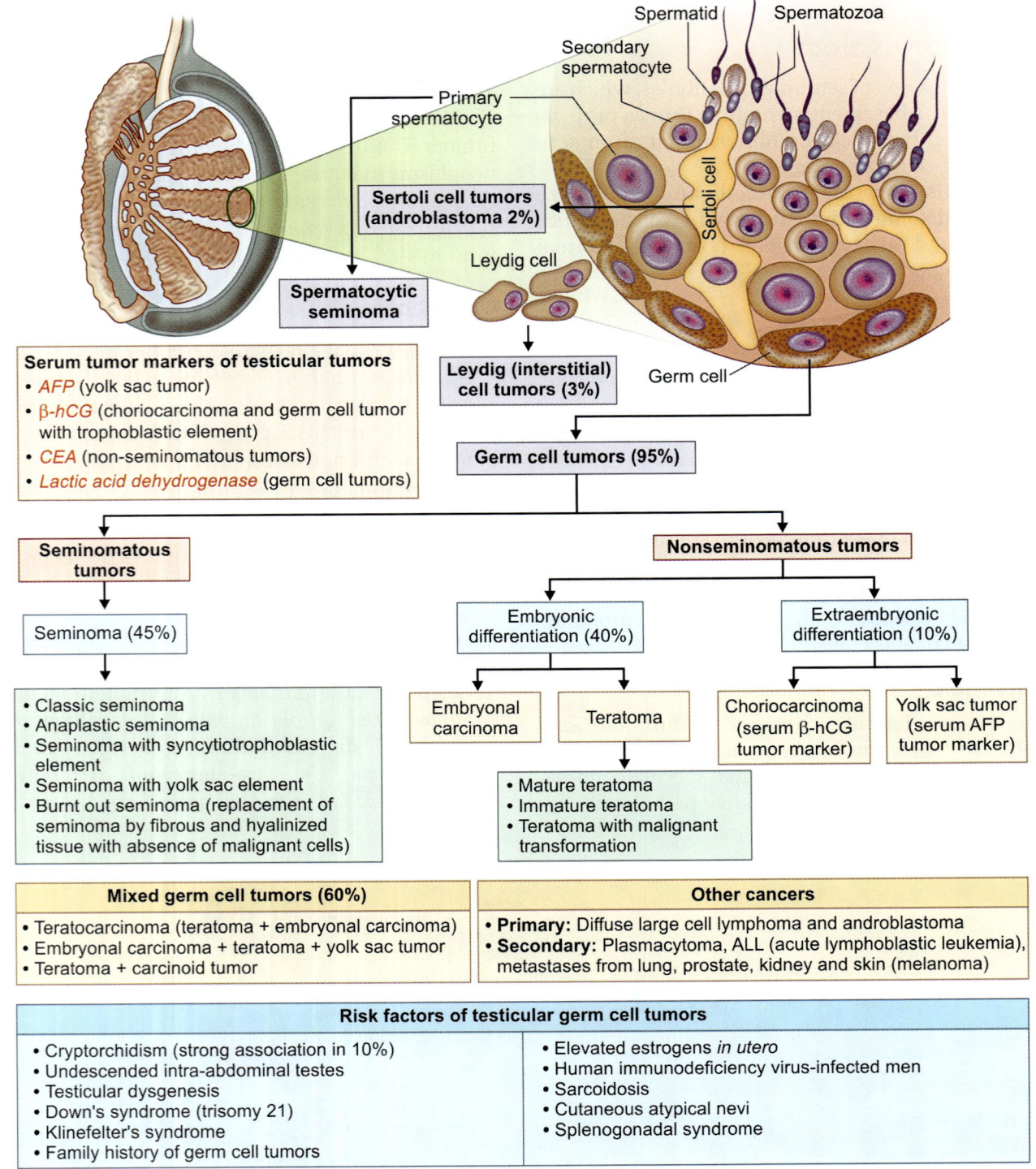

Fig. 23.13: Classification of testicular tumors.

- *Mixed germ cell tumors:* Embryonal carcinoma exists in various combinations with teratoma and seminoma. Teratocarcinoma is a mixed germ cell tumor comprising of teratoma and embryonal carcinoma.

  Teratocarcinoma may also show endodermal sinus tumor.

- *Extragonadal germ cell tumors:* These may occur in mediastinum or brain either due to aberrant migration of germinal cells during development. These may be derived from some common precursor stem cell line that give rise to germinal cells. Treatment can result in long term survival.

GERM CELL TUMORS

Etiology and Pathogenesis

Although the cause of testicular cancer is unknown, there is a possible genetic link and a geographic risk to acquiring this type of cancer. *Approximately 95% of malignant tumors arising in the testis are germ cell tumors.* Various risk factors are shown in Table 23.7.

Molecular Genetics

Molecular genetics in germ cell tumors include isochromosome 12, random gain of chromosomes, novel gene DAD-R gene, aneuploid DNA content and increased telomerase activity (Table 23.8).

Clinical Manifestations

Often the first sign of testicular cancer is a slight enlargement of the testicle that may be accompanied by some degree of discomfort. This may be an ache in the abdomen or groin or a sensation of dragging or heaviness in the scrotum. Pain may be experienced in the later stage as the tumor grows rapidly.

Table 23.7: Risk factors of testicular germ cell tumors

- Cryptorchidism (strong association in 10%)
- Undescended intra-abdominal testes
- Testicular dysgenesis
- Down's syndrome (trisomy 21)
- Klinefelter's syndrome
- Family history of germ cell tumors
- Elevated estrogens *in utero*
- Human immunodeficiency virus-infected men
- Sarcoidosis
- Cutaneous atypical nevi
- Splenogonadal syndrome

Mode of Spread

Testicular germ cell tumors spread by lymphatic and hematogenous routes (Table 23.9). These cancer can spread when the tumor may be barely palpable. Signs of metastatic spread include swelling of the lower extremities, back pain, neck mass, cough, hemoptysis, or dizziness.

Diagnosis

- *Thorough urologic history and physical examination:* A painless testicular mass may be cancer. Conditions that produce an intrascrotal mass similar to testicular cancer include *epididymitis, orchitis, hydrocele,* or *hematocele.* The examination for masses should include palpation of the testes and surrounding structures, transillumination of the scrotum, and abdominal palpation.
- *Ultrasonography:* Testicular ultrasonography can be used to differentiate testicular masses.
- *CT and MRI:* CT scans and MRI are used in assessing *metastatic spread.*
- *Tumor markers:* Tumor markers are used to evaluate testicular mass for diagnosis, staging, monitor response to therapy, detect relapse and assess tumor burden. A potential diagnostic pitfall of new markers is their expression in fetal germ cells.

Tumor markers that measure protein antigens produced by malignant cells provide information about the existence of a tumor and the type of tumor present. These markers may detect tumors that are too small to be found on physical examination or radiographs (Table 23.10).

Molecular Markers

Transcription factor encoded by OCT 3/4 gene is expressed in *primordial germ cells* as well as in *seminoma* and *embryonal carcinoma* estimated by immunoperoxidase technique.

Table 23.8: Molecular genetics in testicular germ cell tumors

Parameters	Characteristics
Isochromosome 12p	It is virtually in all germ cell tumors (90%)
Random gain of chromosomes	Gain of 1, 7, 9, 12, 17, 21, 22, X (70%)
Novel gene DAD-R gene	It prevents apoptosis and plays an important role in pathogenesis of germ cell tumors
Aneuploid DNA content	It is observed in majority of germ cell tumors
	Hyperdiploid and most often triploid or tetraploid
	Mean DNA index in seminoma is higher than NSGCT
	Spermatocytic seminoma is diploid and or near hyperdiploid
Telomerase activity	It is increased in all germ cell tumors except teratoma
	There is inverse relationship between the level of telomerase and differentiation stage of germ cell tumors

Table 23.9: Mode of spread of testicular germ cell tumors

Mode of spread	Metastases in organs	Comments
Lymph nodes involvement	Para-aortic and iliac lymph nodes, later to mediastinal and left supra-clavicular nodes	Germ cell tumors metastasize to lymph nodes
	Retroperitoneal lymph nodes below renal vessels	These lymph nodes are involved on same side in 80–85% cases
		These lymph nodes are involved on both sides in 13–20% cases
	Inguinal lymph nodes	Inguinal lymph nodes are only involved unless tumor invades skin or scrotum
		Inguinal lymph nodes may also be involved in recurrence of tumor in a cutaneous scar, or a history of previous operation in the area
	Para-aortic lymph nodes	These are involved in embryonal carcinoma (adults) and yolk sac tumor (children)
Hematogenous route	Seminoma	Lungs, liver, brain, and bone
	Embryonal carcinoma	It frequently metastasizes early
	Choriocarcinoma	Widespread metastases to lungs, liver, brain, and bones

Mature teratoma in the postpubertal testis is accompanied by metastases. Conversely, mature teratoma of the prepubertal testis has never been shown to metastasize.

Polymerase Chain Reaction

Testicular germ cell tumors show *inactivation of X chromosome* detected by *polymerase chain reaction* (PCR).

Clinical Staging

- The clinical staging (TNM classification) for testicular cancer is as follows: stage I, tumor confined to testes, epididymis, or spermatic cord; stage II, tumor spread

Table 23.10: Tumor markers of germ cell tumors of testes

Tumor markers	Seminoma	Embryonal carcinoma	Yolk sac tumor	Spermatocytic seminoma
LIN28 (RNA binding protein)	++++ (>80%)	++++ (>80%)	++++ (>80%) (excellent marker)	+ (<20%)
SALL4 (+ nuclei)	++++ (>80%)	++++ (>80%)	++++ (>80%) highly sensitive	Variable
PLAP (placental alkaline phosphatase)	++++ (>80%)	++++ (>80%)	++++ (>80%)	+ (<20%)
c-kit (CD117)	++++ (>80%)	+ (<20%)	+ (<20%)	Variable
OCT4	++++ (>80%)	++++ (>80%)	+ (<20%)	+ (<20%)
CD30	++ (<20%)	++++ (>80%)	Variable	+ (<20%)
Vimentin	++++	–	–	–
Lactic dehydrogenase	++++	–	–	–
Podoplanin	++++	–	–	–
α-1 antitrypsin	–	–	++++	–
Cytokeratin (in choriocarcinoma +)	–	++	++++ (consistent)	–
α-fetoprotein (AFP)	–	–	++++	–

α-fetoprotein (AFP) is synthesized by fetal gut, liver and yolk sac. One year after birth, it is less than 16 ng/ml in serum and undetectable except by most sensitive methods. It is increased in cases of yolk sac tumor.
β-hCG is increased in choriocarcinoma and seminoma with syncytiotrophoblastic cells.
Testicular germ cell tumors show inactivation of X chromosome detected by polymerase chain reaction (PCR).

to retroperitoneal lymph nodes below the diaphragm; and stage III, metastases outside the retroperitoneal nodes or above the diaphragm.
- Staging procedures include CT scans of the chest, abdomen, and pelvis; ultrasonography for detection of bulky inferior nodal metastases; and occasionally lymphangiography.

Treatment

- The basic treatment of all testicular cancers includes orchiectomy, which is done at the time of diagnostic exploration. *Surgical therapy* is advantageous because it enables precise diagnosis of the disease.
- Recommendations for further therapy (e.g., *retroperitoneal lymph node dissection, chemotherapy, radiation therapy*) are based on the pathologic findings from the surgical procedure.

   Treatment after orchiectomy depends on the histologic characteristics of the tumor and the clinical stage of the disease. With appropriate treatment, the prognosis for men with testicular cancer is excellent. Comparison between seminomatous and nonseminomatous germ cell tumors is shown in Table 23.11.

Prognosis

Men with stage I and stage II disease do very well. Men who have retroperitoneal lymph node dissection may experience retrograde ejaculation or failure to ejaculate because of severing of the sympathetic plexus. *Infertility may result from retrograde ejaculation or the toxic effects of chemotherapy or radiation therapy. Sperm banking should be considered for men undergoing these treatments.*

SEMINOMA

It is most common malignant germ cell tumor. It is analogous to dysgerminoma, a germ cell ovarian tumor. It accounts for 50% of all testicular tumors. *The tumor replaces the whole testis* and rarely involves tunica vaginalis.

Burnt Out Seminoma

Replacement of seminoma by *fibrous* and *hyalinized* tissue (*sometimes calcification* in scar) and *absence of malignant cells* is termed burnt out seminoma.

Age Group

Peak incidence is in the mid-30s age group (25–45 years of age). It is *highly radiosensitive tumor.*

Predisposing Factor

Undescended (cryptorchid) testis is major predisposing factor.

Molecular Genetics

- The only *consistent* cytogenetic abnormality in testicular germ cell tumors is an *additional fragment of chromosome 12* (isochromosome p12).
- Point mutation is the most common type of mutation, in which a single base substitution in the DNA results in a miscoded protein.

Table 23.11: Comparison of seminomatous and nonseminomatous tumors

Characteristics	Seminomatous tumors	Nonseminomatous tumors
Examples	Seminoma	Embryonic differentiation: these include embryonal carcinoma and teratoma
		Extraembryonic differentiation: these include yolk sac tumor (endodermal sinus tumor) and choriocarcinoma
Diagnosed	70% of patients are diagnosed in stage I	Majority of patients are diagnosed in stage II/III
Mode of spread	Lymphatic spread (retroperitoneal/para-aortic, mediastinal, and supraclavicular lymph nodes) followed by hematogenous route (in lungs, liver, brain and bone)	Lymphatic, hematogenous route (lungs, liver, bones and brain)
Metastasis	Late metastases	Early metastases
Management	Seminoma is radiosensitive tumor	Nonseminomatous germ cell tumors are radio-resistant tumors
	Seminoma stages I and II are treated by irradiation of retroperitoneum up to diaphragm	These tumors are treated by chemotherapy, or retroperitoneal lymph node dissection
	Bulky retroperitoneal or distant metastases of seminoma are treated by chemotherapy	
Prognosis	Good prognosis	Poor prognosis

- For example, mutant KIT ligand growth factor receptors deliver continuous mitogenic signals to the cell, even in the absence of growth factor in seminoma.

Clinical Features

Patient presents with painless unilateral testicular enlargement. *Seminoma with syncytiotrophoblastic element is associated with increased serum human chorionic gonadotropin (hCG)*, the same tumor marker associated with choriocarcinoma and other germ cell tumors.

> **Gross Morphology**
> - Entire testis is replaced by tumor in 50% of cases. The tumor is *well circumscribed, solid, rubbery-firm, bulky mass*, sometimes attains 10 times the size of normal testis.
> - Tunica albuginea is not penetrated by the tumor. Occasionally extension of tumor involves epididymis, spermatic cord or scrotal sac.
> - Cut surface appears *lobulated gray-white homogenous*. Necrosis and hemorrhage is inconspicuous (Fig. 23.14).

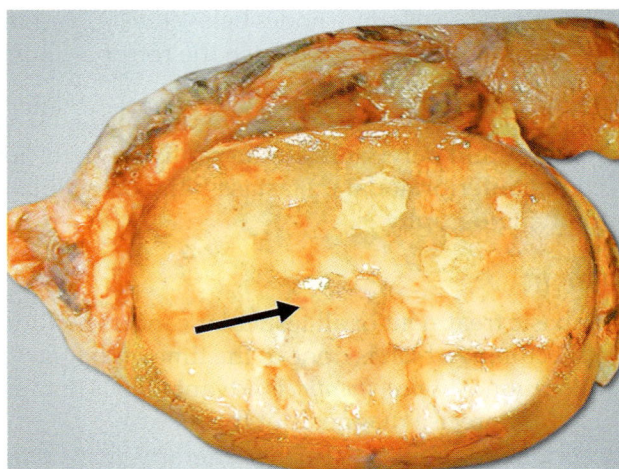

Fig. 23.14: Seminoma of the testis. The testis is enlarged and completely replaced by fleshy, lobulated, homogeneous creamy tissue (arrow).

Histological Variants (Table 23.12)

Classic Seminoma

- *Classic seminoma* accounts for 85–90% of cases.
- *Tumor cells:* Classic seminoma comprises uniform round cells arranged in sheets. The tumor cells contain *clear cytoplasm-rich in glycogen, centrally* located *nuclei* and *prominent nucleoli* with *distinct cell borders*. The nucleolus has characteristics amphophilic staining pattern, apparent multiplicity, elongated shape, and irregular contours. The number of mitoses is highly variable.
- *Fibrous septa:* Fibrous fine to thick septa separate nests (lobules) of tumor cells. These fibrous septa are infiltrated by *T cells (most frequent), plasma cells, macrophages and eosinophils.* A granulomatous reaction containing Langhans' type multinucleated giant cells and epithelioid cells may also be present in 25%. *This immunologic response can obscure the neoplastic nature of the disease.* Host response correlates with a **better prognosis** (Fig. 23.15).
- *Intratubular germ cell neoplasia:* A precursor lesion known as intratubular germ cell neoplasia (ITGCN) is often identified in the background seminiferous tubules (Fig. 23.16A).

Anaplastic Seminoma

It is a histological subtype with *marked cellular pleomorphism* with *6 or more mitotic figures per high power field*. **Prognosis** of this variant is **worse** than classic seminoma (Fig. 23.16B).

Seminoma with Syncytiotrophoblastic Element

- Serum hCG levels, elaborated by syncytiotrophoblastic element present in seminoma, are elevated in about 15% of cases, but these elevations are not as high as those seen in choriocarcinoma.

Table 23.12: Features of histological variants of seminoma

Histologic variants of seminoma	Characteristics
Classic seminoma	Monomorphic tumor cells are arranged in sheets divided by fibrous septa Fibrous septa are infiltrated by chronic inflammatory cells (immunologic response) A granulomatous reaction containing Langhans' type multinucleated giant cells and epithelioid cells may also be present in 25%
Anaplastic seminoma	Marked cellular pleomorphism with 6 or more mitotic figures per high power field. Prognosis of this variant is worse than classic seminoma
Seminoma with syncytiotrophoblastic element	Syncytiotrophoblastic element synthesizes hCG leading to increased serum levels
Seminoma with yolk sac element	Tumor cells show immunoreactivity for α-fetoprotein (AFP)

Urinary Bladder and Male Reproductive System

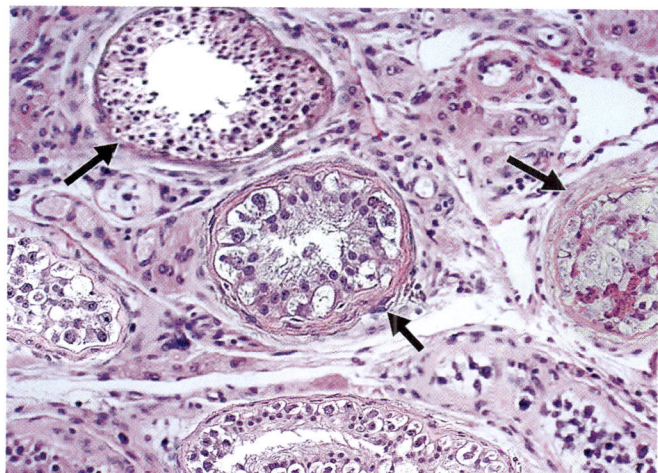

Fig. 23.15: Intratubular seminoma with syncytiotrophoblastic cells. The seminiferous tubules are entirely filled with seminoma cells. In most instances, invasive foci are observed in the specimen (arrows) (400X).

- Presence of syncytiotrophoblastic element around blood vessels reveals foci of hemorrhages around them within the tumor. The **prognosis** of this variant is relatively **poor** (Fig. 23.17).

Seminoma with Yolk Sac Element

- Seminoma exhibits foci consistent with yolk sac differentiation, by virtue of the architectural arrangement, hyaline globules, and *immunoreactivity for α-fetoprotein* (AFP).
- Sometimes yolk sac element is missed during reporting. Seminoma associated with yolk sac elements is usually associated with *increased serum α-fetoprotein* (AFP).

Histochemistry

The tumor cells are rich in glycogen. It can be demonstrated by periodic staining (PAS) with diastase pretreatment.

Immunohistochemistry

Panel of markers is used in surgical specimens of seminoma as shown in Table 23.13.

Metastases

Seminoma spreads by lymphatic channels to *retroperitoneal/para-aortic, mediastinal,* and *supraclavicular lymph nodes.* Blood-borne metastases occur most frequently in *lungs, liver, brain* and *bone.* In combined tumor (seminoma + NSGCT), the latter component is the one more likely to metastasize.

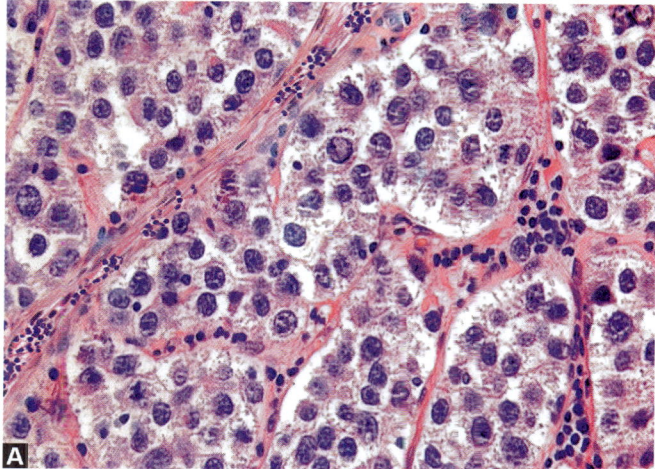

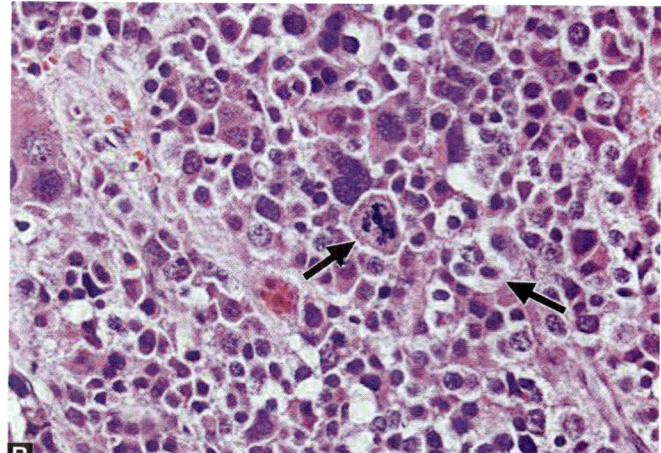

Fig. 23.16: (A) Classic seminoma. Tumor cells grow in sheets separated by fibrous septa containing blood vessels. Lymphoid infiltrates are virtually always present, sometimes imparting a florid reactive appearance with germinal centers, and (B) anaplastic seminoma shows marked cellular pleomorphism with 6 or more mitotic figures per high power field. Prognosis of this variant is worse than classic seminoma (arrows) (400X).

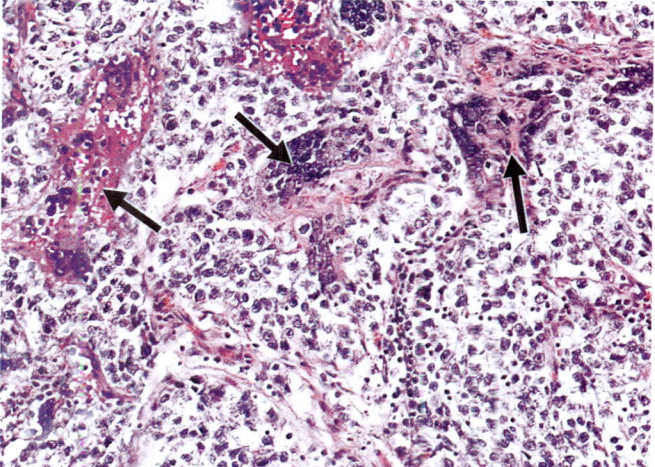

Fig. 23.17: Seminoma with syncytiotrophoblastic element. Syncytiotrophoblasts are found in 4–7% of seminomas, usually randomly scattered (arrows) (100X).

Table 23.13: Immunohistochemistry of seminoma

Immunohistochemistry	Expression in neoplastic cells
Placental alkaline phosphatase (membrane-associated histochemical marker)	Positive
CD117 (c-kit)	Positive
OCT3/4 (transcriptional factor)	Positive
SALL4	Positive
Cytokeratin	Positive
Vimentin	Positive
Angiotensin converting enzyme	Positive
Lactic dehydrogenase	Positive
Ferritin	Positive

Seminoma with syncytiotrophoblastic element shows positivity for *human hCG*. The prognosis of this variant is relatively more aggressive.

Management

The tumor is *highly radiosensitive* and *often curable*, even when presence of metastases to abdominal lymph nodes. Orchidectomy and adjuvant radiotherapy and chemotherapy cures 90% of cases with long-term remission in 50–90% of patients.

SPERMATOCYTIC SEMINOMA

It is a rare *slow growing* tumor seen in older men (>65 years). Despite its name, it is unrelated to conventional seminoma. In contrast to classic seminoma, spermatocytic seminoma is *never seen in combination with NSGCT*. It constitutes 1 to 2% of all germ cell neoplasms. *Prognosis is excellent following simple orchidectomy.*

Origin

It originates from primary spermatocyte and not primordial germ cells.

Molecular Genetics

It expresses **NY-ESO-1** (the product of a *cancer-testis gene*), like normal spermatogonia, primary spermatocytes, and the cells of IGCN, and in contrast to classic seminoma and NSGCT. Numerical chromosomal aberrations are common, and gain of chromosome 9 is characteristic.

> **Gross Morphology**
> - The tumor measures 3–15 cm, which bulges on the cut surface.
> - Cut surface is soft, friable, edematous and gelatinous/mucinous appearance (Fig. 23.18).

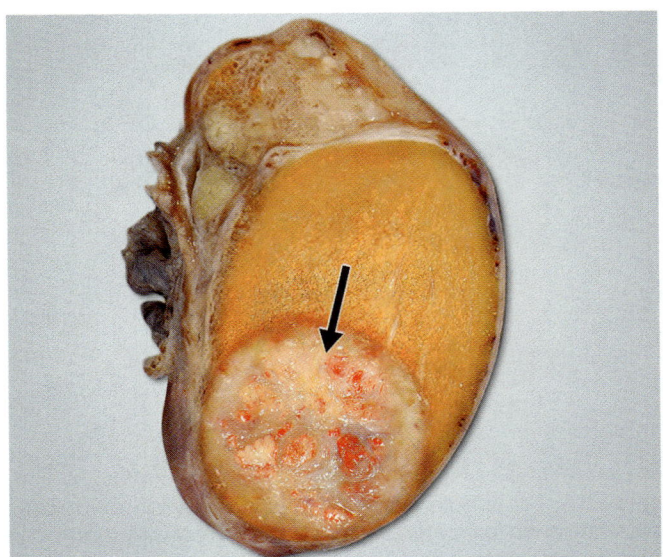

Fig. 23.18: Spermatocytic seminoma ranges from 3 to 15 cm in diameter. It is usually well-circumscribed, soft, and gray-tan. It may be multilobulated or multicentric. The cut surface may be mucoid or friable, and cysts may be present. Hemorrhage and necrosis are limited in extent (arrow).

> **Light Microscopy**
> - The tumor cells resemble primary spermatocytes showing marked degree of pleomorphism, i.e. numerous medium cell 15–18 microns with round nucleus and eosinophilic cytoplasm, small 6–8 microns cell resemble secondary spermatocytes with narrow rim of cytoplasm; and scattered giant cells 50–80 microns.
> - The nuclei exhibit filamentous appearance. The cytoplasm is devoid of glycogen. Its stroma lacks lymphocytes (Fig. 23.19).

> **Immunohistochemistry**
> In contrast to classic seminoma, immunoreactivity for **placental alkaline phosphatase** (PLAP) is most often **absent**.

Metastases

Metastases are practically *non-existing*. Sometimes, the tumor exhibits highly malignant component of sarcomatous appearance and showing *skeletal muscle differentiation* resulting in *widespread metastases*.

Prognosis

It is more commonly bilateral, excellent prognosis. Metastases are practically nonexistent and, therefore, simple orchiectomy may be sufficient therapy. Differences between seminoma and spermatocytic seminoma are given in Table 23.14.

Urinary Bladder and Male Reproductive System

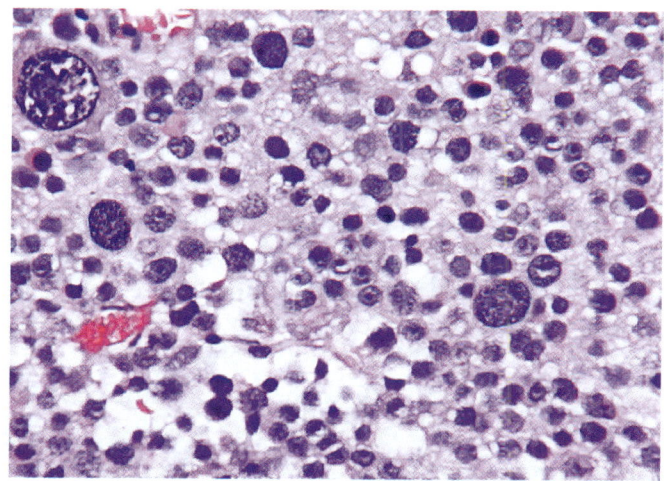

Fig. 23.19: Spermatocytic seminoma. The tumor cells are of three types. Small (6–8 mm), medium (15–20 mm) and large cells (50–100 mm exhibit a filamentous or "spireme" chromatin distribution) (400X).

EMBRYONAL CARCINOMA (NSGCT)

Embryonal carcinoma is a malignant nonseminomatous germ cell tumor. It is analogous to a similar tumor occurring in the ovary. It most often occurs in younger age group between 25 and 35 years of age.

Pure or Mixed Tumor Embryonal Carcinoma

Embryonal carcinoma occurs in pure form in 15–30% of cases. It most often occurs mixed with teratoma in 40% of cases and known as *teratocarcinoma*, that shows an increase in both CEA and α-fetoprotein (AFP) in 90% of cases.

Molecular Genetics

Cytogenetic analysis has confirmed the presence of *isochromosome 12p in many cases.*

Table 23.14: Differences between classic seminoma and spermatocytic seminoma

Parameters	Classic seminoma	Spermatocytic seminoma
Origin	Primordial germ cell	Primary spermatocyte
Frequency	Most common usually unilateral	Uncommon (bilateral)
Age group (peak)	4th decade	>65 years of age
Molecular genetics		NY-ESO-1 (the product of a *cancer-testis gene*)
Growth	Rapid growth	Slow growth
Gross morphology	Complete replacement of testes in 50% of cases	Partial replacement of testis
	Well circumscribed, solid, rubbery-firm, bulky mass, sometimes attains 10 times the size of normal testis	The tumor measures 3–15 cm, which bulges on the cut surface
	Cut surface appears lobulated gray-white homogenous	Cut surface is soft, friable, edematous and gelatinous/mucinous appearance
Histologic variants	Classic seminoma, anaplastic seminoma, seminoma with syncytiotrophoblastic element and seminoma with yolk sac component. Monomorphic tumor cells are divided by fibrous septa	Pleomorphic tumor cells with filamentous nuclear appearance
Histochemistry	PAS positive due to presence of glycogen in tumor cells	PAS negative due to absence of glycogen in tumor cells
Tumor markers		
LIN28 (RNA binding protein)	++++ (>80%)	+ (<20%)
SALL4 (+ nuclei)	++++ (>80%)	Variable
PLAP (placental alkaline phosphatase)	++++ (>80%)	+ (<20%)
c-kit (CD117)	++++ (>80%)	Variable
OCT4	++++ (>80%)	+ (<20%)
CD30	++ (<20%)	+ (<20%)
Prognosis	Good prognosis in classic seminoma. Relatively poor in anaplastic seminoma and seminoma with syncytiotrophoblastic element	Good except tumor showing skeletal muscle differentiation

Clinical Features

Patient most often presents with painless unilateral testicular enlargement. It invades the testis, epididymis, blood vessels and metastasizes to para-aortic abdominal lymph nodes, lungs, liver and other organs. Teratocarcinoma often metastasizes as embryonal carcinoma, and the reverse also occurs.

Gross Morphology
- Embryonal carcinoma is the smallest germ cell tumor (in pure form) averaging 2.5 cm and not replacing entire testis.
- Cut surface reveals *variegated*, gray-white, granular or smooth, bulging surface with areas of hemorrhage and necrosis.
- Approximately, 20% of embryonal carcinomas have invaded the adjacent epididymis or tunica albuginea at the time of excision (Fig. 23.20).

Light Microscopy
- Pure embryonal carcinoma comprises *highly pleomorphic cells* with hyperchromatic nuclei, prominent nucleoli and indistinct cell borders that are similar to cells from early embryos.
- These cells are arranged in glandular, papillary structures or solid pattern and variable areas of undifferentiated sheets of tumor cells exhibiting syncytial growth surrounded by dilated vascular channels filled with red blood cells.
- High mitotic activity with tumor giant cells is frequent.
- Syncytiotrophoblastic element may be present.
- Areas of hemorrhage are also present.
- Peritumoral invasion of blood vessels and lymphatics is important feature to document (Fig. 23.21).

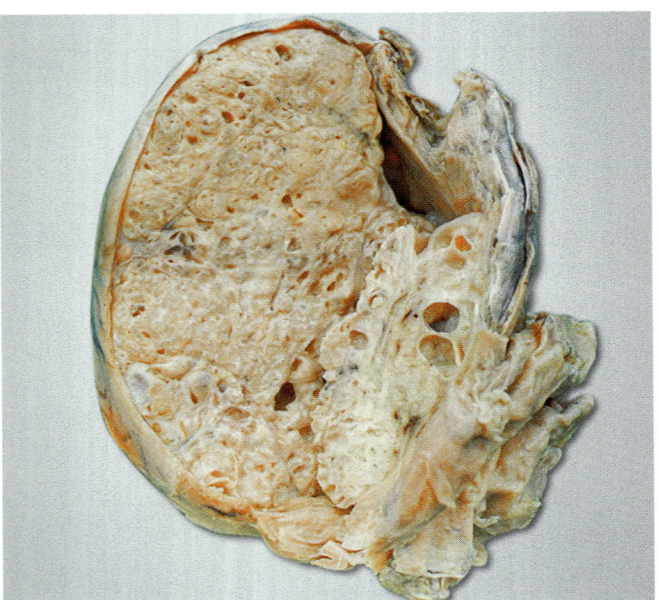

Fig. 23.20: Embryonal carcinoma—in adults, embryonal carcinoma is almost invariably a component of a mixed germ cell tumor. Cut surface reveals variegated, gray-white, granular or smooth, bulging surface with areas of hemorrhage and necrosis.

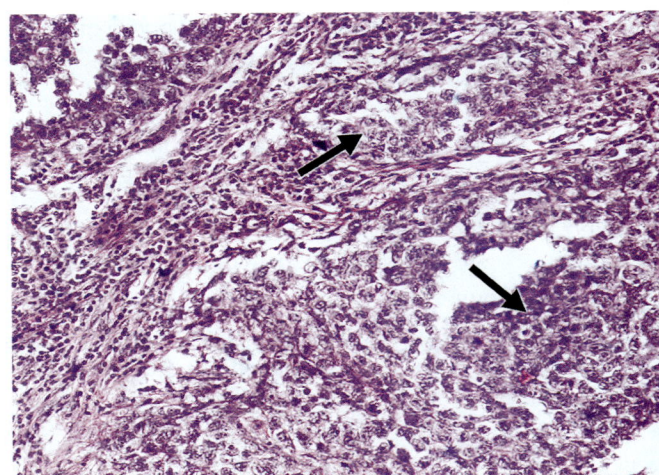

Fig. 23.21: Embryonal carcinoma—tumor architecture is variable. Tumor cells often grow in diffuse sheets and may be arranged to resemble poorly formed glands. Tumor cells are large and tend to overlap one another, and cell membranes are difficult to discern, exhibiting a syncytial appearance to the tumor. Tumor cell nuclei are vesicular with irregular outlines, coarse chromatin, and prominent nucleoli. Mitotic figures and apoptotic cells are abundant (arrows) (200X).

Table 23.15: Immunohistochemistry of embryonal carcinoma

Immunohistochemistry	Expression in neoplastic cells
Placental alkaline phosphatase (membrane-associated histochemical marker)	Positive
Cytokeratin (keratin 19 and high MW)	Positive
CD30	Positive
OCT 3/4	Positive
SALL4	Positive
SOX2	Positive
α-fetoprotein (AFP)	Positive

Serum α-fetoproteins are detectable in 70% of cases of embryonal carcinoma.
Cytogenetic analysis has confirmed the presence of isochromosome 12p in many cases of embryonal carcinoma.

Immunohistochemistry

Panel of markers is used on surgical specimens of embryonal carcinoma (Table 23.15).

Prognosis

It is *less sensitive to radiation* than seminoma and hence more aggressive and *lethal*. The prognosis is much worse than for seminoma.

Treatment

It is *highly sensitive to chemotherapy*, and the cure rates are now over 90%.

TERATOMA

- Teratoma is most frequent malignant nonseminomatous germ cell tumor derived from two or more embryonic layers (ectoderm, endoderm and mesoderm).
- It comprises multiple tissue types, i.e. neural tissue, cartilage islands, ciliated epithelium of bronchi, thyroid tissue, liver cells, embryonic gut, or striated muscle embedded in fibrous or myxoid stroma.
- Prognosis is poor in adults. It is more aggressive than seminoma. Pure teratoma occurs in children, and mixed germ cell tumor in adults.

Pure/Mixed Teratomas

- *Pure teratoma:* Pure teratomas occur in *infants* and *children* (4–12 years). It is second in frequency to yolk sac tumor. *Prognosis is good in infants and children.* But in post-pubertal period, all teratomas are regarded as malignant and capable of metastatic behavior regardless of elements are mature or immature.
- *Mixed teratomas:* Mixed teratomas most often occur in adults (20–30 years). The tumor comprises teratoma and embryonal carcinoma in 45% cases. Teratomas elements may be mature or immature (fetal/embryonal).

  A few teratomas may contain carcinoid tumor component (argyrophil and secretory granules containing neuron-specific enolase, chromogranin, synaptophysin, but not associated with the carcinoid syndrome).

Gross Morphology

- Tumor measures 5–10 cm and shows variegated appearance with solid and cystic areas.
- Presence of hemorrhage necrosis indicates admixture of teratoma with embryonal carcinoma or choriocarcinoma or both (Figs 23.22 and 23.24).

Light Microscopy

It is classified according to the degree and type of differentiation exhibited.

- *Mature teratoma:* It comprises multiple mature tissue types derived from ectoderm, mesoderm, and endoderm, such as neural tissue, cartilage islands, ciliated epithelium of bronchi, thyroid tissue, liver cells, embryonic gut, or striated muscle embedded in fibrous or myxoid stroma. This teratoma is almost always malignant with metastatic potential, whereas the analogous ovarian tumor is almost always benign (Fig. 23.23).
- *Immature teratoma:* Primitive neural elements are often present in this variant, and behavior is malignant (Fig. 23.25).
- *Teratoma with malignant transformation:* This teratoma contains malignant tissue, such as squamous cell carcinoma, mucin secreting adenocarcinoma and sarcoma.

Mode of Spread

- The majority of nonseminomatous germ cell tumors spread by both lymphatic (retroperitoneal, para-aortic, mediastinal and supraclavicular lymph nodes) and hematogenous routes (lungs, liver, brain, bones) and are not radiosensitive,

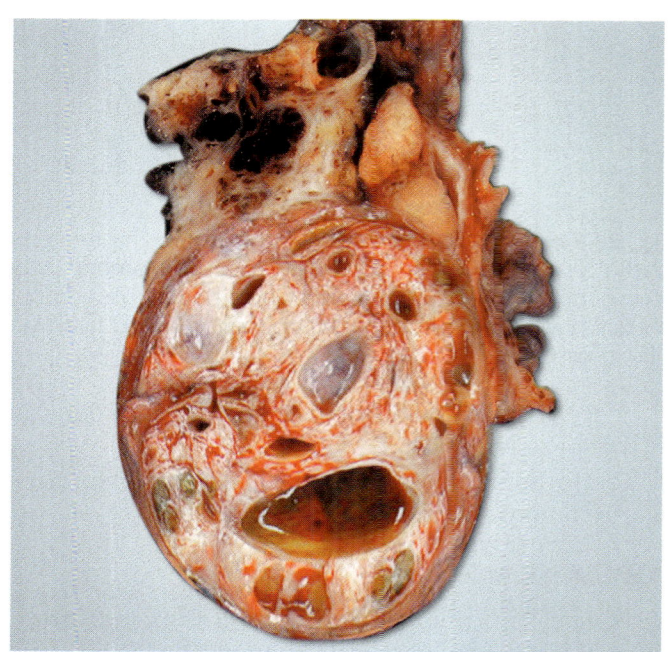

Fig. 23.22: Mature teratoma—teratomas typically have both solid and cystic components. The solid component is sometimes recognizable as cartilage. The material within the cysts may be serous, mucoid, or keratinous. This tumor arose in the testis of a 2-year-old boy, and as such was considered benign. However, teratomas in 20 to 30 years of malignant behavior.

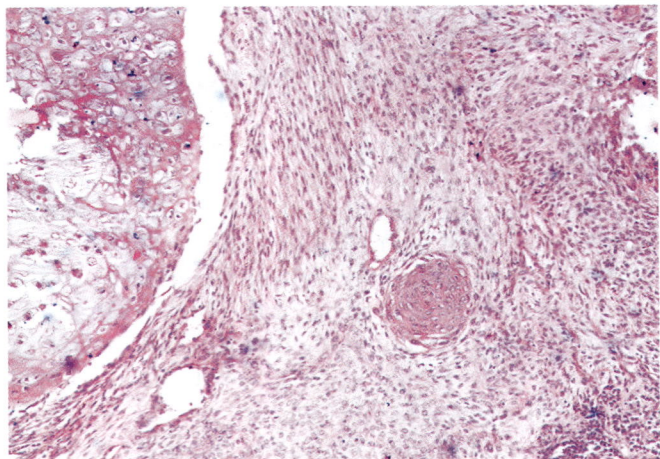

Fig. 23.23: Mature teratoma—cartilage and an island of squamous epithelium set in a fibrous stroma (400X).

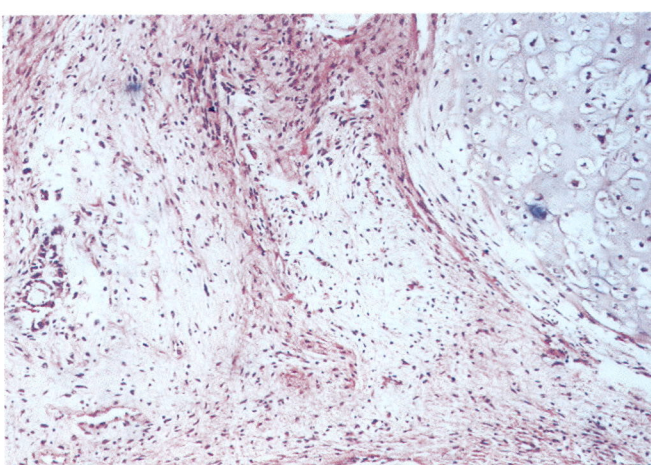

Fig. 23.25: Teratoma with immature elements. This teratoma with mature adipose, cartilage and squamous elements has an area of immature tissue at upper right. Immature elements, if limited, appear to have no influence on prognosis (200X).

Origin

It arises from primordial germ cell showing differentiation towards yolk sac and allantoic membrane.

Pathogenesis

Hypermethylation of the RUNX3 gene promoter is thought to play a pathogenetic role in this neoplasm.

Molecular Genetics

Yolk sac tumor in infants and children commonly shows *loss of 1p and 6q, gain of 1q, 20p, and 12 isochromosome.*

Age Group

The pure form occurs exclusively in infancy and early childhood. Pure yolk sac tumor is very rare in adults. But in adults it most often appears as a component of mixed germ cell tumors.

Serum α-fetoprotein

Its levels are elevated in most preoperative cases.

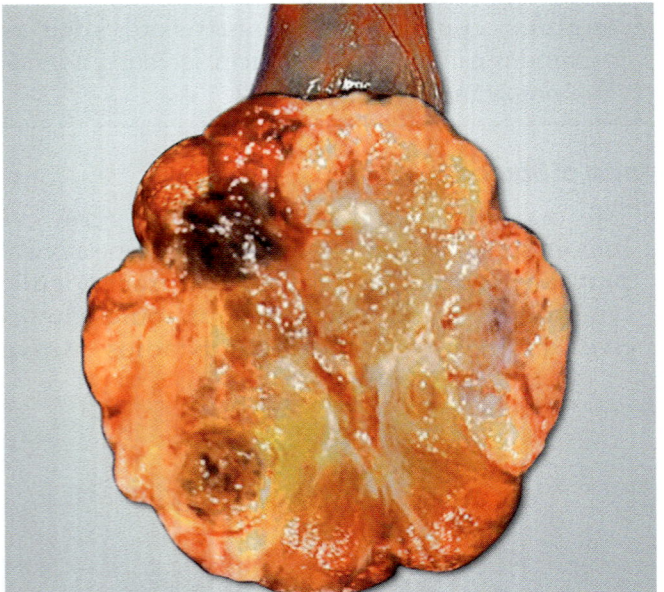

Fig. 23.24: Teratoma with immature elements. This teratoma had a very extensive component of immature elements in the form of primitive neuroectodermal tumor, perhaps accounting for its fleshy bulging encephaloid appearance and the areas of hemorrhage.

hence their natural history is markedly different from that of seminomas.
- Teratocarcinoma often metastasizes as embryonal carcinoma, and the reverse also occurs.

YOLK SAC TUMOR

Yolk sac tumor is the most common malignant nonseminomatous germ cell tumor of the testis during *infancy* and *early childhood* under 4 years of age. It is analogous to endodermal sinus tumor of the ovary. It is usually accompanied by an increase in s*erum α-fetoprotein*. It is also known as *endodermal sinus tumor* or *infantile embryonal carcinoma*.

Gross Morphology
- Tumor is lobulated 2 to 6 cm in diameter and demarcated from surrounding tissues.
- Cut surface reveals yellow solid with mucinous texture and cystic areas.
- Hemorrhage and necrosis may be seen (Fig. 23.26).

Light Microscopy

Yolk sac tumor shows interlacing strands of cuboidal to columnar epithelial cells surrounded by loose myxoid connective stroma.

Urinary Bladder and Male Reproductive System

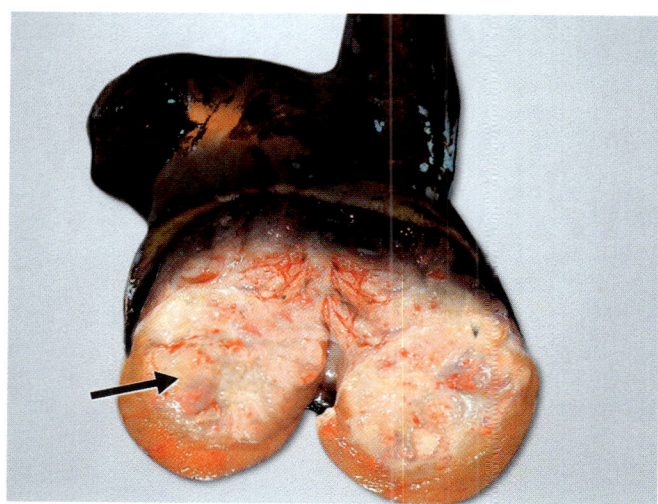

Fig. 23.26: Yolk sac tumor. This is the commonest testicular tumor in children, the majority of whom are <2 years old. In children, yolk sac tumor is typically pure in its makeup. It has completely replaced the normal testicular tissue. It tends to be bulging, shiny, or mucoid (creamy), and may show areas of cystic degeneration. The cut surface of embryonal carcinoma is often somewhat granular in consistency; necrosis and hemorrhage are common and may be extensive. It is typically smaller than seminoma and its interface with adjacent normal parenchyma may be somewhat indistinct (arrow).

- The classic finding is the *Schiller-Duval bodies* attempting to form the yolk sac. The lobular arrangement of cells, surrounded by empty spaces, results in the formation of glomeruloid structures containing a central fibrovascular core referred to as Schiller-Duval bodies.
- Intracellular and extracellular hyaline globules are characteristic of yolk sac differentiation and occur in 85% of cases.
- The presence of α-fetoproteins (AFP) in the tumor cells is highly characteristic of differentiation of tumor into yolk sac cells. It reacts with PAS, and resistant to digestion with diastase (Fig. 23.27).

Immunohistochemistry

Panel of markers is used in surgical specimens of yolk sac tumor (Table 23.16).

Clinical Correlation

Most testicular endodermal sinus tumors of the pure variant occur in infants and children under the age of 3 years. Prognosis is excellent under 3 years of age following timely orchidectomy in a 95% of cases.

Serum Tumor Marker

These tumors produce *α-fetoprotein*, which can be used for *monitoring the recurrence of disease* following surgery by estimating level in serum. This glycoprotein is a

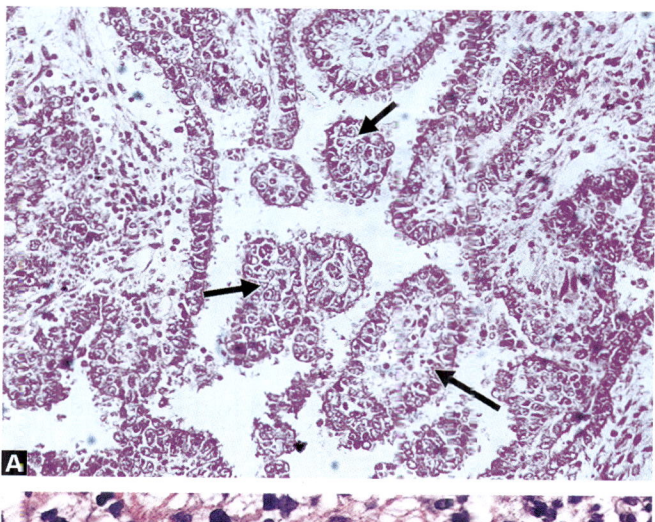

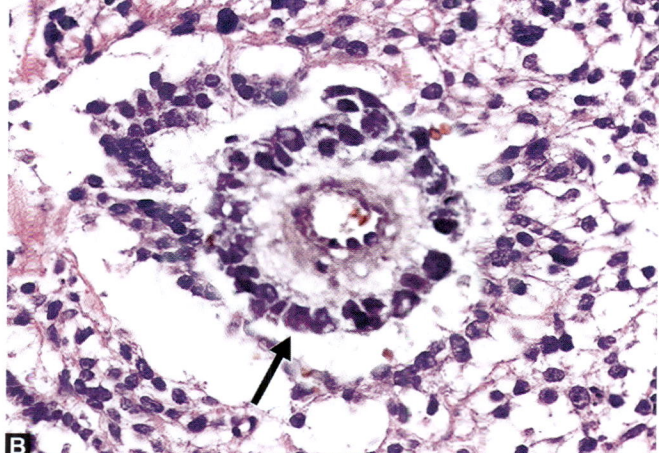

Fig 23.27: Yolk sac tumor. (A) The endodermal sinus pattern of yolk sac tumor is characterized by the presence of irregular interconnecting labyrinthine-like spaces and Schiller-Duval bodies, several of which are nicely illustrated (arrows) and (B) It is showing Schiller-Duval bodies (arrow) (400X).

Table 23.16: Immunohistochemistry of yolk sac tumor

Panel of markers	Expression in neoplastic cells
Cytokeratin (consistent)	Positive
α-fetoprotein	Positive
Placental alkaline phosphatase	Positive
$α_1$-antitrypsin	Positive
A SALL4	Positive (highly reactive)
OCT3/4	Positive (highly reactive)

Yolk sac tumors produce α-fetoprotein, which can be used for monitoring the recurrence of disease following surgery by estimating level in serum.

major plasma component of the fetus, the major sources being the liver and the visceral endoderm of the yolk sac. It is one of the major oncofetal antigens.

CHORIOCARCINOMA

Choriocarcinoma is highly malignant rapidly growing nonseminomatous germ cell tumor. This tumor is analogous to choriocarcinoma of the ovary. *Identical choriocarcinomas are also seen in placenta, ovary, sequestered nests of totipotent cells* in *mediastinum* and *abdomen*. Tumor synthesizes β-hCG representing germ cell differentiation to an extraembryonic structure, namely the placenta. It is *highly chemosensitive tumor.*

Age Group

It most often occurs in the second to third decade.

Clinical Features

Patient presents with widespread metastases via hematogenous routes (lungs, liver, brain, bones) with fatal outcome. Tumor is detected as a small palpable nodule without testicular enlargement.

Gross Morphology

- It is usually small tumor with extensive areas of hemorrhage and necrosis.
- Sometimes, primary tumor is replaced by fibrous scar but widespread metastases.
- The invasive growth of trophoblastic cells in the tumor is associated with hemorrhage (Fig. 23.28).

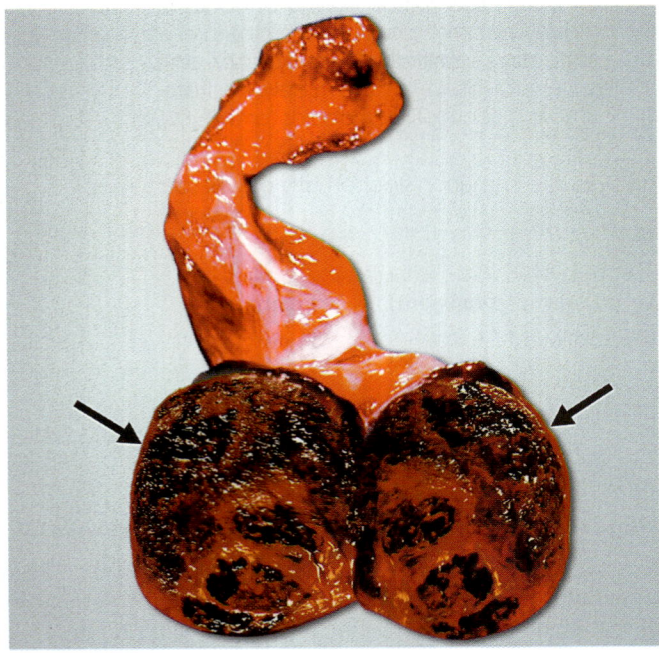

Fig. 23.28: Choriocarcinoma—the testis is replaced by a bloody bulging mass. More typically, choriocarcinoma tends to be somewhat smaller, and may not significantly distort the testis (arrows).

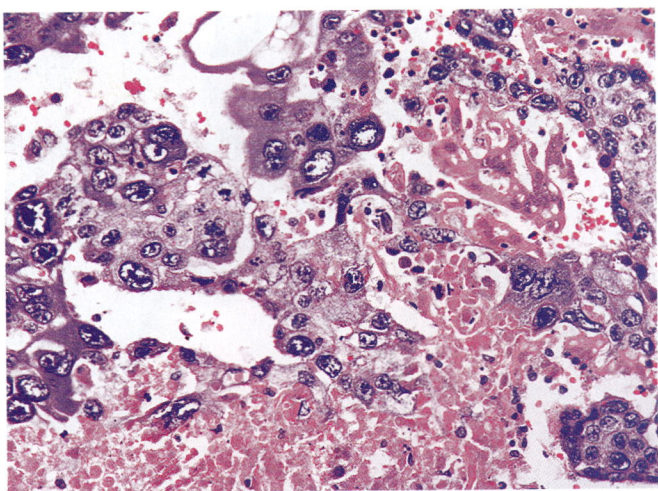

Fig. 23.29: Choriocarcinoma—the tumor is composed of multinucleated syncytiotrophoblastic and cytotrophoblastic cells. The multinucleated syncytiotrophoblasts have voluminous eosinophilic cytoplasm and large darkly staining irregular nuclei with prominent nucleoli. The smaller mononuclear cytotrophoblasts are fairly uniform in size with amphophilic cytoplasm and distinct cellular outlines resembling to the tumor cells of solid yolk sac tumor (400X).

Light Microscopy

- Syncytiotrophoblastic cells cap a cluster of cytotrophoblastic cells. These cells are large multinucleated with many irregular, hyperchromatic nuclei with abundant eosinophilic vacuolated cytoplasm.
- Cytotrophoblastic cells are more regular polygonal cells with single nucleus arranged in cords and masses (Fig. 23.29).

Immunohistochemistry

- Syncytiotrophoblastic element demonstrates the presence of human chorionic gonadotrophin (hCG) within these cells.
- These cells synthesize hCG, hence serum levels are increased.

MIXED GERM CELL TUMORS

Mixed germ cell tumors most often occur in adults (20–30 years). Teratocarcinoma is composed of teratoma and embryonal carcinoma in 45% cases. Teratomas elements may be mature or immature (fetal/embryonal).

A few teratomas may contain carcinoid tumor component (argyrophil and secretory granules containing **neuron-specific enolase, chromogranin, synaptophysin,** but not associated with the carcinoid syndrome).

Mixed germ cell tumor may be composed of teratoma, embryonal carcinoma and yolk sac tumor. In combined tumor (seminoma + NSGCT), the latter component is the one most likely to metastasize (Figs 23.30 and 23.31).

Urinary Bladder and Male Reproductive System

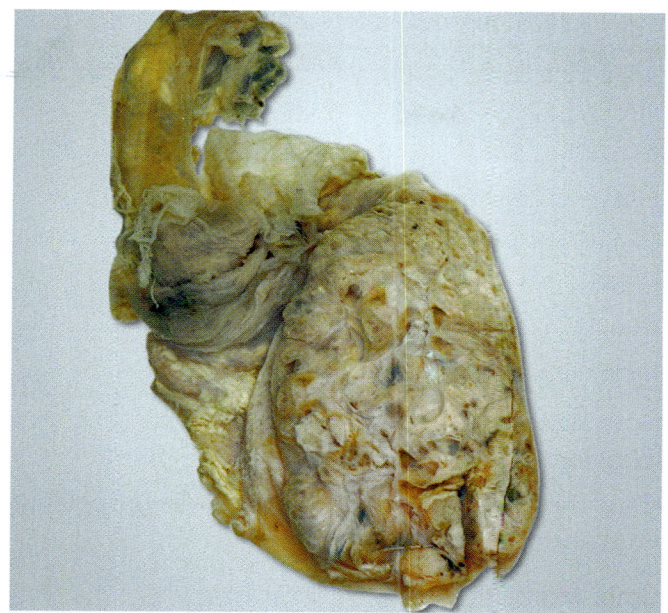

Fig. 23.30: Mixed germ cell tumor of testis. It consists of teratoma, yolk sac and embryonal carcinoma.

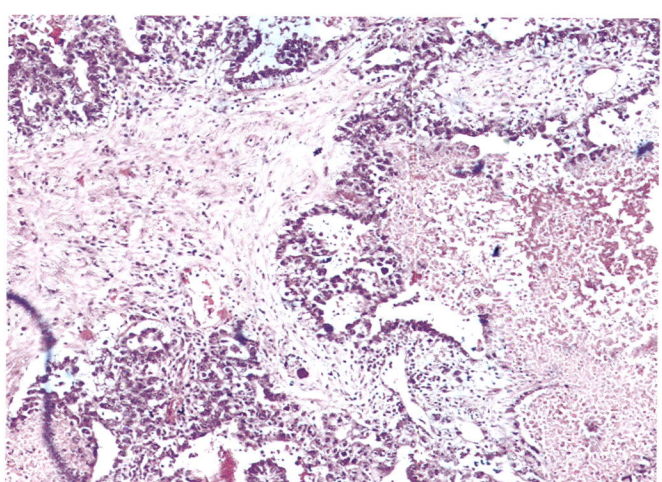

Fig. 23.31: Teratocarcinoma shows components of teratoma and embryonal carcinoma (100X).

SEX CORD-GONADAL STROMAL TUMORS

Sertoli cells support germ cells. These form basement membrane of seminiferous tubules. These synthesize estrogens and up to some extent androgens. Leydig cells produce testosterone and other androgens. Sex cord tumors comprise approximately 5% of testicular tumors.

SERTOLI CELL TUMOR (ANDROBLASTOMA)

It is a non-germ cell tumor derived from the sex cord stroma of testis. It is characterized by a paucity of endocrine manifestations. These tumors are most often benign, but anaplastic in 10% of cases metastasizing to iliac and para-aortic lymph nodes.

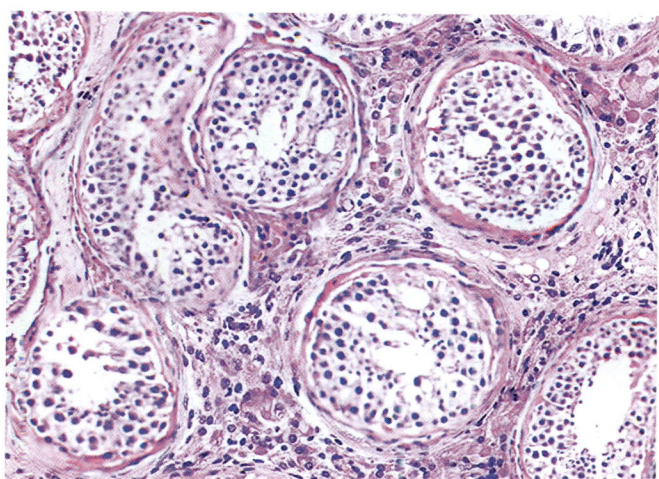

Fig. 23.32: Sertoli cell tumors (100X).

Table 23.17: Immunohistochemistry of Sertoli cell tumor

Marker	Expression
Inhibin	Positive
CD88	Positive
Anti-müllerian hormone	Positive
Vimentin	Positive
Keratin	Positive
α_1-antitrypsin	Positive
Neuron-specific enolase	Positive

Gross Morphology
- Tumor is small and firm well circumscribed nodule.
- Cut surface is gray white to yellow, homogenous cut surface with focal cystic areas.

Light Microscopy
- Tumor is composed of only Sertoli cells or may have a component of granulosa cells.
- These are arranged in distinctive trabeculae with tendency to form tubular structures resembling seminiferous tubules lined by elongated cells having the appearance of Sertoli cells (Fig. 23.32).

Immunohistochemistry
Sertoli cell tumors show reactivity for **inhibin, CD88, anti-müllerian hormone, vimentin, keratin, α-antitrypsin,** and **neuron-specific enolase** (Table 23.17).

LEYDIG (INTERSTITIAL) CELL TUMOR

It is non-germ cell tumor derived from testicular stromal Leydig cells. It is uncommon accounting for 2% of testicular tumors.

Age Group

It most often occurs in adults between 30 and 45 years of age. It may affect any age group. Approximately 25% of all Leydig cell tumors show evidence of malignant behavior in the form of metastatic disease, particularly to lymph nodes, lung and liver.

Clinical Features

The tumor most often synthesizes androgens, but sometimes produces both androgens and estrogens and sometimes corticosteroids. It is most often associated with precocious puberty due to production of androgens in children and with gynecomastia in adults.

Gross Morphology

Tumor is well circumscribed nodule. It forms a golden brown nodule within the body of the testis and homogenous on cut surface.

Light Microscopy

- Tumor comprises large round or polygonal cells with distinct borders, abundant granular deeply eosinophilic cytoplasm and round to oval nuclei.
- These are arranged in sheets or tubules or trabecular pattern.
- These cells contain intracytoplasmic rod-shaped *Reinke crystals* demonstrated with Masson trichrome stain (Fig. 23.33).

Immunohistochemistry

The markers that have proved to be of the greatest utility for the evaluation of these tumors are inhibin, vimentin, calretinin, and Mart-1.

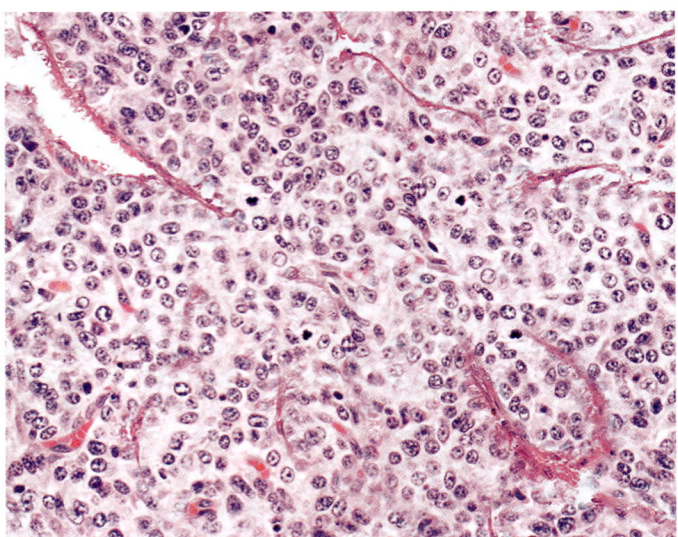

Fig. 23.33: Leydig cell tumor (200X).

Table 23.18: Tumor markers of Leydig cell tumor

Tumor markers	Expression in tumor cells
LIN28	+ (<20%)
SALL4	+ (<20%)
PLAP	+ (<20%) to 80%
c-kit (CD117)	+ (<20%)
OCT4	+ (<20%)
CD30	+ (<20%) to 80%
Inhibin	++++ (>80%)

Behavior

90% of the tumors are benign, while 10% have a potential for invasion and metastases.

Tumor Markers

Leydig cell tumors are inhibin positive. Lipofuscin pigment and Reinke crystals are present in these tumors. Panel of tumor markers is used on surgical specimens of Sertoli-Leydig cell tumors (Table 23.18).

OTHER TUMORS

DIFFUSE LARGE CELL LYMPHOMA

Testicular lymphoma constitutes 5% of testicular neoplasms. Nearly all cases are of non-Hodgkin type. *Bilateral testicular involvement in a patient over 60 years should suggest systemic non-Hodgkin's lymphoma* rather than primary germ cell tumors. A few cases of primary lymphoma of the testis have been reported. It most often occurs in patients over 60 years. Dissemination is common, hence poor prognosis.

Gross Morphology

Large cell lymphoma results in a solid homogeneous replacement of the testicular parenchyma, similar to that of seminoma.

Light Microscopy

- The most common histologic variant is diffuse large B cell lymphoma. But other variants such as small lymphocytic lymphoma, follicular lymphoma, anaplastic large cell lymphoma and NK/T cell lymphoma may also occur.
- The tumor cells surround seminiferous tubules.
- There is a high incidence of vascular invasion (Fig. 23.34).

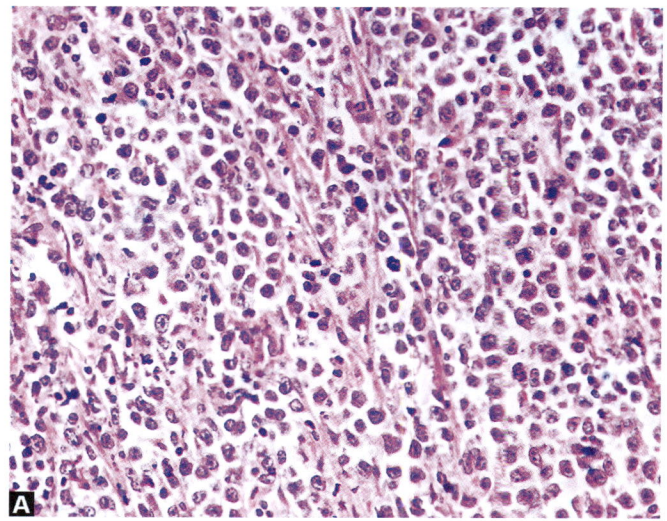

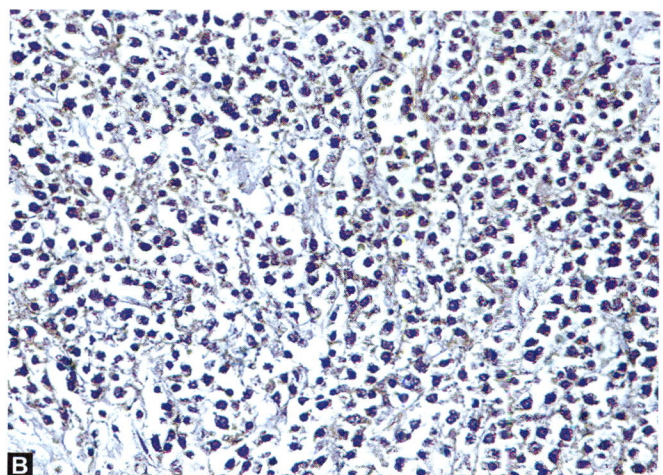

Fig. 23.34: (A) Diffuse large lymphoma of testis (H&E staining 400X) and (B) Neoplastic cells show CD45 positive staining (immunohistochemistry).

Management

Diffuse large cell lymphoma of the testis is treated with orchiectomy and chemotherapy, sometimes combined with radiation therapy.

PLASMACYTOMA TESTES

It may be seen as first clinical manifestation of multiple myeloma or as an isolated lesion.

LEUKEMIC INFILTRATION

Leukemic involvement of the testis is more commonly seen with acute lymphoblastic leukemia in children in 8%, but it also may occur in the myeloblastic types. Often the testis represents the first sign of relapse after bone marrow remission.

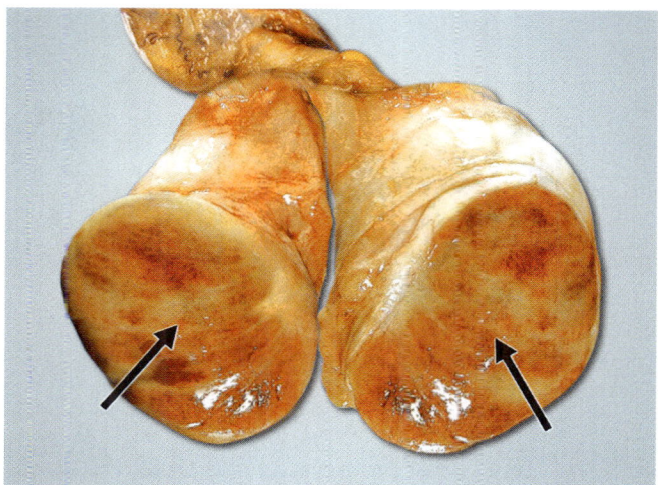

Fig 23.35: Acute lymphoblastic leukemia infiltrating both testes. The normal testicular tissue has been completely replaced by creamy, slightly hemorrhagic tumor tissue. When patients have responded to chemotherapeutic treatment of acute lymphoblastic leukemia, the first manifestation of recurrence is frequently in the testes (arrows).

Immunohistochemistry

It is helpful in identification of residual disease. Radiotherapy is most effective in controlling the testicular involvement, but bone marrow relapse will develop in most cases (Fig. 23.35).

METASTASES IN TESTES

Cancers of lung, prostate, kidney, stomach, or skin (melanoma) may metastasize to testes. Prostatic carcinoma metastasizing to testes has better prognosis than involving penis. In children, the testis can be involved by metastatic neuroblastoma from the adrenal or other sites.

ADENOMATOID TUMOR

Adenomatoid tumor is the most common benign tumor of testicular adnexa. It represents almost 60% of all cases.

Origin

This tumor is of mesothelial origin. It arises in upper or lower pole of the epididymis.

Gross Morphology

Tumor is solitary, round to oval in shape measuring <5 cm in diameter (Fig. 23.36).

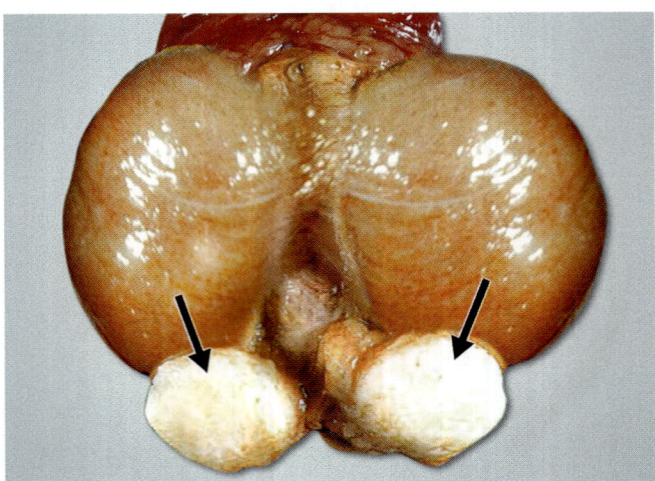

Fig. 23.36: Adenomatoid tumor of the epididymis. There is a creamy, well circumscribed tumor in the epididymis (arrows).

Light Microscopy

- Tumor is composed of round to oval or slit-like tubules in fibrous, hyalinized, and/or muscular stroma.
- The lining cells are columnar or flat having vacuolated cytoplasm (Fig. 23.37).

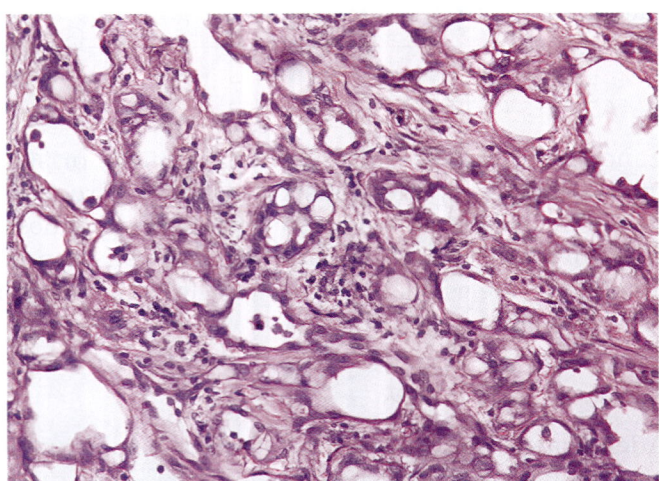

Fig. 23.37: Adenomatoid tumor of the epididymis (100X).

Table 23.19: Immunohistochemistry of adenomatoid tumor

Marker	Expression
Cytokeratin	Positive
Calretinin	Positive
Epithelial membrane antigen (EMA)	Positive
WT1	Positive
Factor VIII related antigen	Negative
CD51	Negative

Immunohistochemistry

Tumor cells are immunoreactive for expression of **cytokeratin, calretinin, EMA** and **WT1**. These cells are negative for *factor VIII-related antigen* and *CD31*, a profile indicating a mesothelial origin rather from vascular endothelium (Table 23.19).

MALE HYPOGONADISM AND IMPOTENCE

MALE HYPOGONADISM

Male hypogonadism refers to failure of the Leydig cells to produce testosterone, failure of seminiferous cells to generate sperm, or an abnormality in androgen receptors. Approximately 90% of male infertility is due to hypogonadism resulting in impaired spermatogenesis in the presence of normal production of testosterone (seminiferous tubule dysfunction).

- *Primary hypogonadism:* It involves testicular problems in synthesizing testosterone in the Leydig cells (increased LH levels, decreased sperm count, normal FSH) or generating spermatozoa in the seminiferous tubules (increased FSH [decreased inhibin], low sperm count, normal LH and testosterone).
- *Secondary hypogonadism:* It refers to disorders in the pituitary or hypothalamic axis or to receptor deficiencies.

MALE IMPOTENCE

Male impotence is defined as persistent inability to obtain an erection during attempted sexual intercourse; it occurs in 10–35% of adult men.

Etiology

- Testosterone deficiency accounts for 15–20% of cases.
- Other causes include psychological problems, autonomic neuropathy, endocrine disease (hypothyroidism, hypopituitarism) or drugs. The most useful finding that excludes an organic cause of impotence is the presence of nocturnal penile tumescence (erections that normally occur during sleep).
- *Drugs:* Drugs associated with impotence include major tranquillizers (phenothiazines), lithium, sedatives (barbiturates or benzodiazepines), antihypertensive drugs (methyl dopa or debrisoquine or cloridine), alcohol, estrogens and drug abuse (heroin or methadone).

INFLAMMATORY DISORDERS

Orchitis is inflammation of the testis. It can result from bacterial or viral infection.

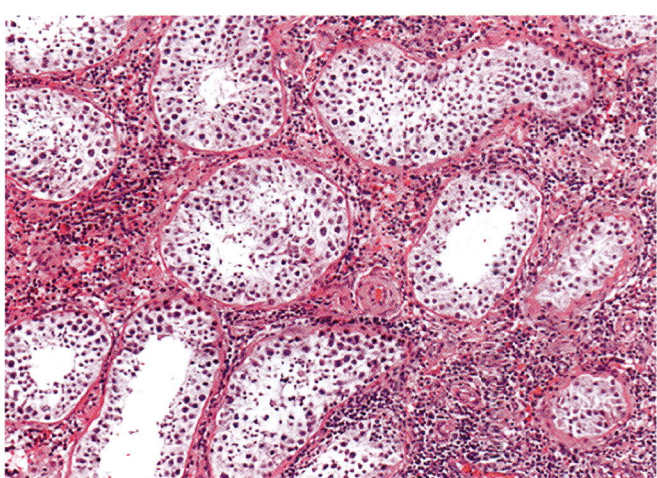

Fig. 23.38: Mumps orchitis. Testes becomes painful and swollen 4–6 days after parotitis. Testes show widespread foci of acute and chronic inflammatory cells destroying seminiferous tubules. Bilateral testes involvement may result in infertility (100X).

MUMPS ORCHITIS

When viral, orchitis is most often due to mumps virus in 20% of adult males. Patient presents with unilateral painful gonadal swelling (Fig. 23.38).

BACTERIAL ORCHITIS

- Epididymitis is more common than orchitis. When bacterial, orchitis is often associated with epididymitis. It is caused by bacterial infection.
- It is sexually acquired infection due to *Neisseria gonorrhoeae* (gonorrhea) or *Chlamydia trachomatis*. *Escherichia coli* associated urinary tract infection is the most common causative agent.
- Patient presents with intrascrotal pain and tenderness, with or without associated fever. When bilateral, orchitis may result in sterility due to atrophy of the seminiferous tubules.
- Serum testosterone is decreased, whereas pituitary follicle-stimulating hormone and luteinizing hormone are increased. Orchitis may be caused by syphilis.

TUBERCULOUS EPIDIDYMITIS

It is usually a complication of pulmonary and renal tuberculosis. The epididymis is enlarged and indurated and usually associated with testicular involvement by the same disease process. Light microscopy reveals caseous necrosis, epithelioid granulomas and occasional Langhans' giant cells (Fig. 23.39).

GRANULOMATOUS ORCHITIS

- It is usually associated with trauma to testis. Some consider it as an autoimmune basis. It affects middle

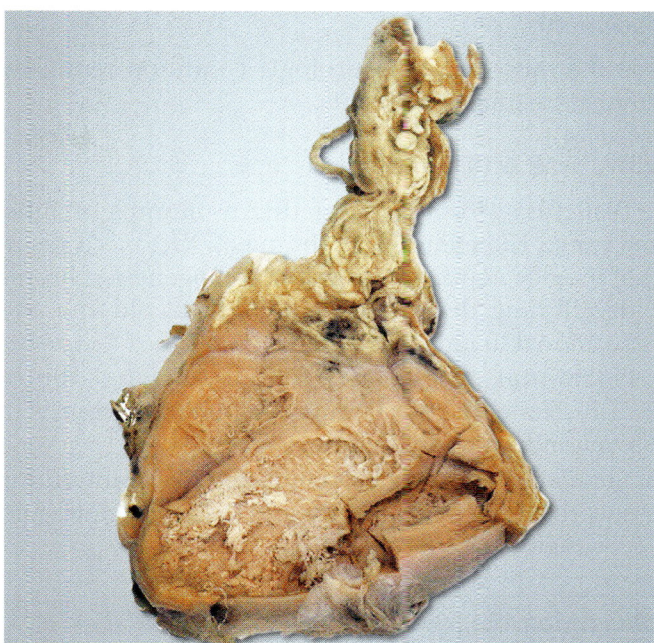

Fig. 23.39: TB epididymo-orchitis. The testis contains multiple rounded granulomatous lesions. The epididymis is almost completely replaced by similar tissue. The patient had disseminated tuberculosis.

aged males. Some cases are associated with urinary tract infections, history of prostatectomy, inguinal hernia repair and trauma.
- Testicular involvement may be total or partial resulting in vaguely nodular, firm painful testicular enlargement associated with fever.
- Light microscopy reveals lymphocytes, plasma cells, macrophages, fibroblasts and scattered multinucleated giant cells.

SYPHILITIC ORCHITIS

Clinically, a syphilitic gumma can resemble a neoplasm.

CRYPTORCHIDISM

- In majority of these infants, the testis will descend into the scrotum during the first year of life.
- Cryptorchidism is developmental failure of a testis to descend into the scrotum especially in premature newborns.
- According to their location, the cryptorchid testes can be classified as abdominal, inguinal, or upper scrotal. Anorchia refers to congenital absence of testes.

Complications

It is associated with testicular atrophy and sterility. There is increased incidence of germ cell tumors such as seminoma and embryonal carcinoma, even if the testis is surgically moved from its ectopic location back to the scrotum.

Treatment

It is the most common urologic condition requiring surgical treatment in infants.

TESTICULAR ATROPHY

- Testicular atrophy occurs due to mumps orchitis, trauma, Klinefelter's syndrome (47XXY) as a result of meiotic nondisjunction during oogenesis, chronic debilitating disease, cryptorchidism, old age and hormonal imbalance.
- Hormonal excess or deficiency occurs due to disorders of hypothalamus or pituitary, cirrhosis of liver and estrogen therapy.
- Klinefelter's syndrome is characterized by infertility, and the testicular atrophy and loss of meiotic and postmeiotic germ cells.

Gross Morphology
Grossly, cryptorchid testes in adults are small and brown.

Light Microscopy
• The testicular seminiferous tubules are atrophic, and their basement membrane is greatly thickened and hyalinized. • Scattered patent seminiferous tubules with markedly thickened walls are present, but may contain only Sertoli cells and absence of germ cell elements. • The Leydig cells are prominent; some of them may be present inside the tubules.

MALE PSEUDOHERMAPHRODITISM

- It is congenital disorder also known as testicular feminization syndrome. It occurs due to a congenital deficiency of the androgen receptor. Males have a normal 46XY karyotype.
- Patient presents with cryptorchid testes, but the external genital organs appear feminine or ambiguously female, with signs of virilization. Patients with congenital adrenal hyperplasia have a normal 46XX karyotype.

MISCELLANEOUS DISORDERS

TESTICULAR TORSION

- Physical trauma results in torsion of the spermatic cord. It occurs in late childhood and early adolescence, rare after 20 years of age. Torsion usually occurs on the left side.

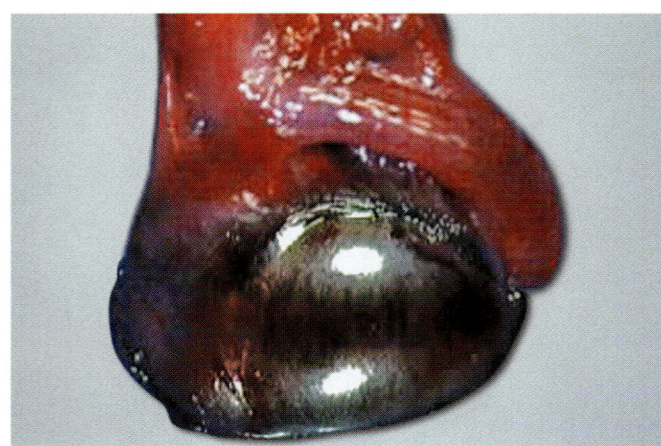

Fig. 23.40: Torsion testis.

- Faulty anchoring of testis on wall of the scrotum allows testis to rotate. Torsion of the spermatic cord cuts off venous outflow while there is continued arterial flow to the testis.
- The resulting increasing vascular congestion leads to vascular rupture, hemorrhage and necrosis.

Clinical Examination

Scrotum is enlarged and swollen. Affected testis (usually left) is higher owing to rotation and shortening. On palpation, spermatic cord feels thick, swollen, and tender. Epididymis may be anterior. Cremasteric reflex is absent on affected side.

Gross Morphology
The testis becomes enlarged, necrotic and hemorrhagic (Fig. 23.40).

Light Microscopy
It reveals hemorrhage and necrosis of seminiferous tubules and interstitial tissue.

Clinical Features

Patient presents with excruciating sudden pain in the testis following trauma.

HYDROCELE

Hydrocele is a serous fluid collection in the scrotal tunica vaginalis. It is most often idiopathic.

- *Congenital hydrocele* occurs due to persistence of continuity of the tunica vaginalis with the peritoneal cavity. It is the most common cause of scrotal swelling in infants often associated with inguinal hernia.
- *Acquired hydrocele* occurs in adults secondary to infection, lymphatic obstruction by tumor or trauma affecting scrotum. Positive transillumination test differentiates hydrocele from testicular tumors.

SPERMATOCELE

Spermatocele is a sperm-containing cyst formed from the protrusions of widened efferent ducts of the rete testis or epididymis. It is located above and posterior to the testis. It is attached to the epididymis, but separate from the testes.

Morphology

Most spermatoceles are small <1 cm; occasionally these may be larger and mistaken for hydrocele. It is most often intratesticular. It contains milky fluid containing spermatozoa. Patient presents with *painless paratesticular nodule* or as a *fluctuating mass*.

HEMATOCELE

Hematocele is an accumulation of blood resulting in distension of tunica vaginalis. It is most often caused by trauma. Testicular tumors and infections may also result in hematocele.

VARICOCELE

- Varicocele results from dilation of the multiple veins of the spermatic cord. Patient presents with nodularity on the lateral side of the scrotum. Most patients are asymptomatic and discovered during routine physical examination. Varicocele is palpated as a bag of worms.
- Varicocele is considered a common cause of *male infertility* and *oligospermia* due to unknown reason. Surgical resection of varicocele by ligation of the internal spermatic vein often improves reproductive function.

MALE INFERTILITY

ANATOMY AND CLINICAL EXAMINATION

Semen Production

Testes (10%), seminal vesicle (60%) and prostate (30%) contribute in the formation of semen. If semen is stored at –100°C, sperms may be preserved for years.

- *Testes:* Both testes produce sperms. Sperms are stored mainly in alkaline medium. In temperate regions, sperms motility is increased but lifespan decreased. Lifespan in female genital system is 1–2 days.
- *Prostate gland:* Prostatic fluid is milky white with alkaline pH, containing citrate ion, calcium, acid phosphatase and profibrinolysin. Alkaline pH neutralizes acidic pH of vas deferens and vaginal acidic pH (3.5–4).

Table 23.20: Normal semen values as suggested by WHO (1999)

Volume	2.0 ml or more
pH	7.2–7.8
Sperm concentration	20 million/ml or more
Total sperm count	>40 million per ejaculate
Motility	50% or more progressive forward motility
Morphology	15% or more normal form
Viability	75% or more living
Leukocytes	Less than 1 million/ml
Sperm agglutination	<2

- *Seminal vesicle:* It synthesizes fructose, prostaglandins and fibrinogen. Fructose provides nutrition to sperms. Prostaglandins play an important role in fertilization by reacting with cervical mucus to make susceptible to sperms and possibly cause reverse peristaltic contraction in the uterus and fallopian tube to move sperms upwards towards ovaries.

Semen Analysis

- Normal sperm count is 60–120 million per ml. In case of infertility, two or more specimens are necessary with two days abstinence. Freshly ejaculated specimen is a coagulum (Table 23.20).
- Prostatic lysozyme and α-amylase liquify the semen in 30 minutes. Coagulum is not formed in patients with underdeveloped seminal vesicle or lacking vas deferens. Fructose levels are below normal in these patients.

Testicular Measurement

Testicular size is measured by commercially available plastic testes models *orchidometer*. Lower limit of normal testis is 20 ml volume and size 4.0 × 2.7 cm. Germinal elements account for over 75% of testicular mass.

CAUSES OF MALE INFERTILITY

Chronic Alcoholism

It causes infertility due to decreased gonadotrophin and testosterone levels.

Drugs

Heroin and *methadone drugs* affect hypothalamic-hypophyseal axis and reduce ejaculate volume as well as sperm count. Exposure to *diethylstilbestrol in utero* can cause epididymal cysts and obstructive changes.

Exposure to DDT (dichlorodiphenyltrichloroethane) and chlordecone results in decreased spermatogenesis. Colchicine, alkylating agents and nitrofurantoin administration result in sperm structure and motility abnormality.

Diabetes Mellitus

It may cause partial or complete retrograde ejaculation or impotence.

Varicocele

Varicocele patients often have semen of poor quality. Approximately one-third of men undergoing varicocele ligation become fertile after numbers in large number in the urine may denote retrograde ejaculation. An elderly patient with ilsolated left-sided varicocele should be investigated for renal cell carcinoma.

Surgical Procedure

Vasectomy, hernia repair, decreased blood supply to testes, vas obstruction and undescended testes are important causes of sterility.

Pathogens

Tuberculosis may cause epididymal obstruction. *Mumps* may result in testicular atrophy. Oligospermia is caused by renal diseases.

Undescended Testes

Fertilization of ovum with sperm from undescended testes results in spontaneous abortion.

PROSTATE GLAND

ANATOMY AND HISTOLOGY

Anatomy

Prostate gland is located below the bladder. The seminal vesicles are located posterior to the prostate. The urethra exits from the bladder and traverses the prostate before exiting to the penile urethra. A thin layer of connective tissue surrounding prostate merges with surrounding soft tissues, including nerves. There is no distinct capsule. Normal weight of prostate gland is 20 gm for ages 20–50 years and 30 gm for ages 60–80 years.

Histology

Prostate is composed of *tubuloalveolar glands* and *supporting fibromuscular* stroma in equal proportions. The glands are radiating from the urethra. The glands are lined by two cell layers, i.e. outer cuboidal cells and inner tall columnar mucin-secreting epithelium, forming inward papillary projections. These glands synthesize laminated concretions of prostatic secretions known as *corpora amylacea* within the glandular lumina.

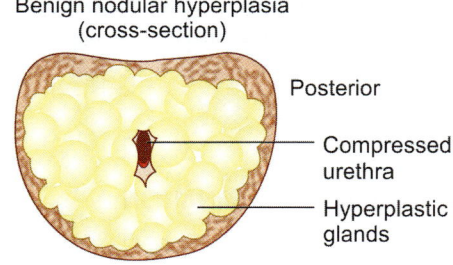

Benign nodular hyperplasia mainly involves center of the prostate gland

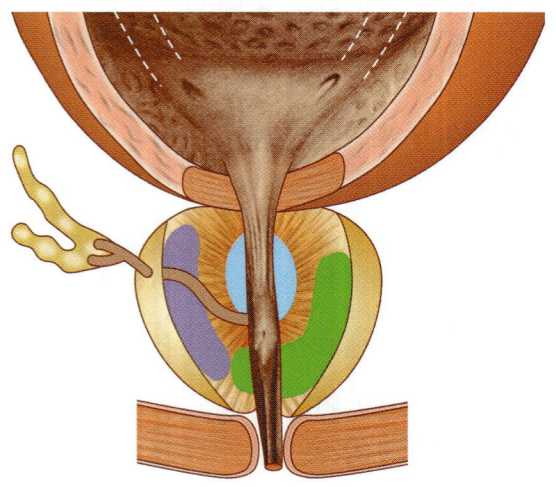

Prostatic carcinoma (serum tumor markers)
- *PSA* (prostate specific antigen)
- *PAP* (prostate acid phosphatase)
- IGFBP2

DNA ploidy (flow cytometry)

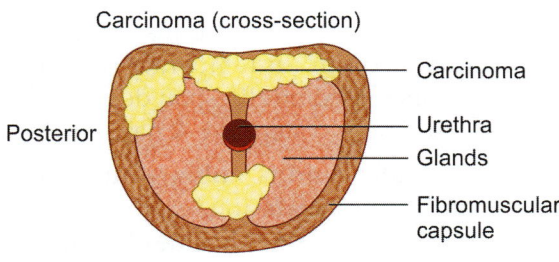

Carcinoma of the prostate usually occurs in the posterior of the gland and may be detectable by DRE

Fig. 23.41: Prostate gland shows site of prostate carcinoma and nodular hyperplasia prostate.

Urinary Bladder and Male Reproductive System

Zones of Prostate

Based on group of glands, the prostate is subdivided into three zones: central zone, transition zone (site for nodular hyperplasia prostate), and peripheral (site for prostate cancer). Dihydrotestosterone (DHT) is the primary androgen responsible for stimulation of glands and stroma in the prostate (Fig. 23.41).

Gross Examination and Sampling

Most common prostatic sampling is done by needle biopsy, transurethral resection of prostate (TURP), fine needle aspirates, open simple and radical prostectomy. Needle biopsy and prostate chips are fixed in 10% neutral buffered formalin.

INFLAMMATORY DISORDERS OF PROSTATE

Asymptomatic Acute Prostatitis

Urinary tract infection by coliform organisms as well as *Neisseria gonorrhoea* results into acute prostatitis. It may be associated with some dysuria. Microscopically, the glands are filled with neutrophils, and the intervening stroma may also contain a few neutrophils (Fig. 23.42).

Chronic Prostatitis

It may follow acute prostatitis. Chlamydial organism may also cause chronic prostatitis. Patient presents with dysuria along with low grade pelvic pain or low back pain. On histopathological examination, lymphocytes, plasma cells, and macrophages appear in the stroma (Fig. 23.43).

Granulomatous Prostatitis

Granulomatous prostatitis can clinically present with increased prostate specific antigen level and or

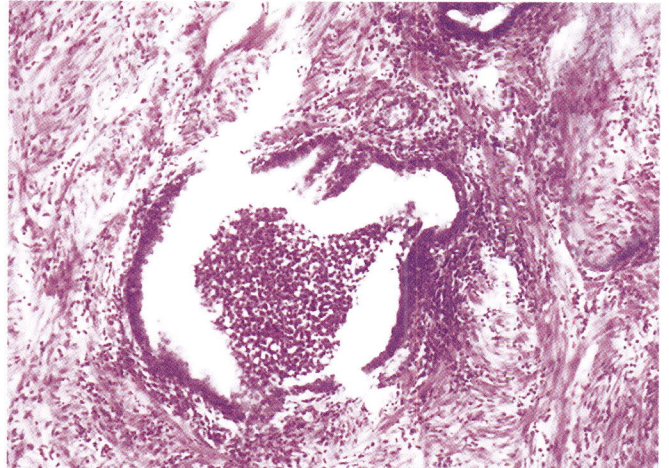

Fig. 23.42: Acute prostatitis—the luminal space is filled with neutrophils.

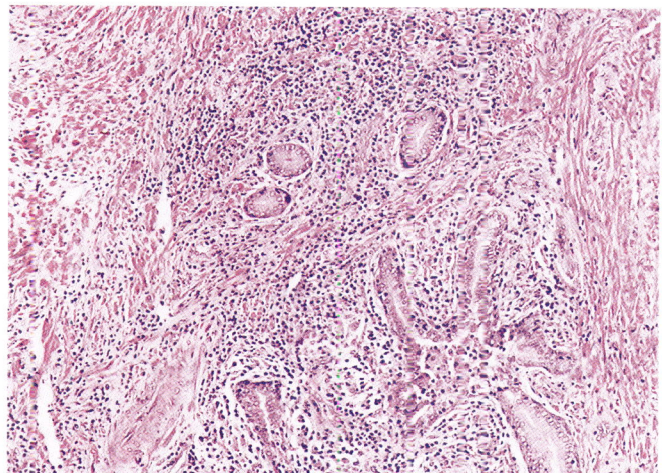

Fig. 23.43: Chronic prostatitis, no specific. There is prominent periductal inflammation. The inflammatory infiltrate is composed of lymphocytes and histiocytes.

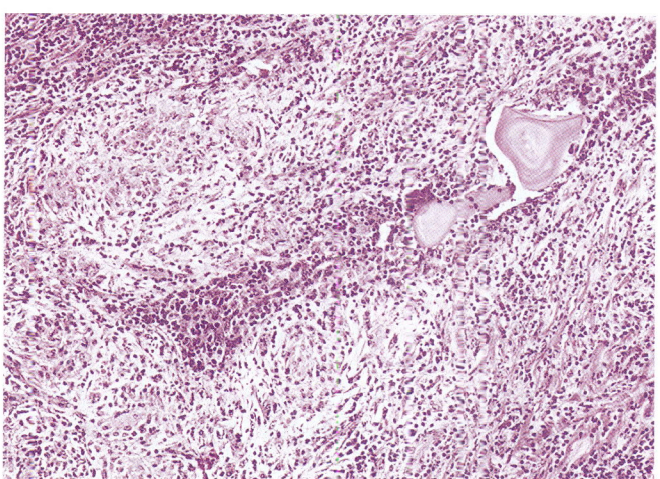

Fig. 23.44: Granulomatous prostatitis nonspecific. There is polymorphous infiltrate of lymphocytes, macrophages, plasma cells, neutrophils, multinucleated giant cells and occasional eosinophils.

palpable abnormality. Nonspecific granulomatous prostatitis probably occurs in response to prostatic secretions released into the prostatic stroma due to rupture of the ducts. Light microscopy reveals noncaseating granulomas, chronic inflammatory cells with giant cells. Rarely fungal infection may cause granulomatous prostatitis (Fig. 23.44). Variants are xanthogranulomatous prostatitis and prostatic xanthoma.

NODULAR HYPERPLASIA OF PROSTATE

It is the most common cause of urinary tract obstruction. It most often affects older men. Rectal examination reveals a firm, enlarged, nodular prostate.

Pathogenesis

- *Dihydrotestosterone (DHT):* It is a major growth factor for prostate gland. It is derived from testosterone by the action of 5α-reductase enzyme. Dihydrotestosterone binds to nuclear DHT receptors and triggers prostatic hyperplasia of both glandular and fibromuscular stromal elements. Therapeutic administration of drug inhibiting 5α-reductase enzyme is useful in the medical management of nodular hyperplasia prostate.
- *Estrogens:* Age-related increase in estrogens level also plays an indirect role by stimulating the production of DHT receptors. These estrogens promote expression of receptors for dihydrotestosterone (DHT) in prostate.
- *α-adrenergic blockers:* The α-adrenergic blockers cause relaxation of smooth muscle in prostate and help in relieving obstruction.

Molecular Genetics

BRCA2 gene (13q) mutation has been associated with **prostate cancer**. BRCA2 regulates DNA repair by binding to RAD51, a molecule that mediates DNA double-strand repair breaks. It encodes protein involved in checkpoint functions related to progression of the cell cycle into S phase.

Clinical Features

Patient's symptoms are related to urethral obstruction of urine outflow. Patient presents with *frequency* of micturition, *difficulty in starting urination, nocturia, dribbling* and *dysuria*. There is increased risk of urinary tract infection, hydroureter, hydronephrosis and renal failure (Fig. 23.45). Urinary obstruction in cases of long duration results in morphological changes in urinary bladder such as distension, bladder diverticula, muscular hypertrophy, and trabeculae formation. Urine retained inside a diverticulum is often infected, a complication that may lead to the formation of bladder stones.

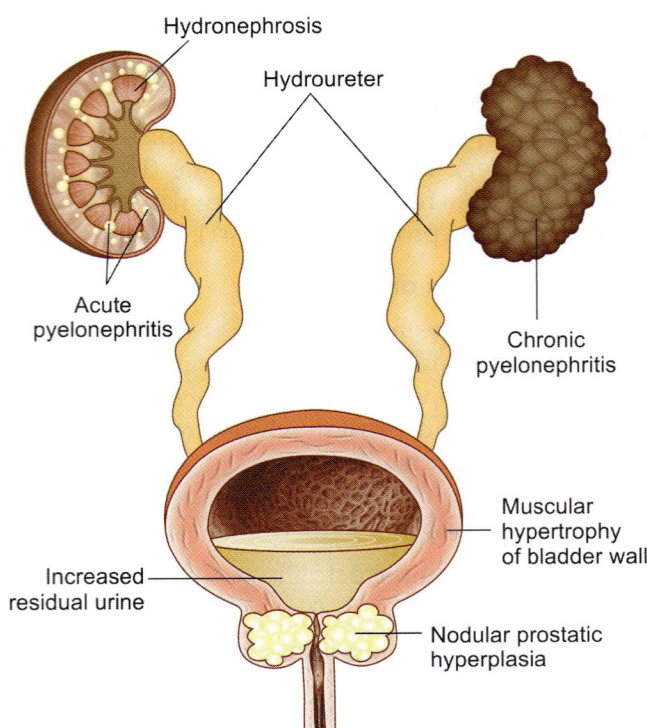

Fig. 23.45: Nodular hyperplasia prostate. It has produced hydroureter, hydronephrosis and pyelonephritis.

Gross Morphology

- Prostate with nodular hyperplasia can weigh 50 to 100 gm (normal 20 to 30 gm).
- Gross examination reveals multiple gray white rubbery nodules of variable sizes in the parenchyma.
- Cut surface shows solid and cystic areas. Benign nodular hyperplasia primarily affects periurethral and transitional zones. Involvement of periurethral portion of the prostate compresses urethra side to side resulting in a vertical slit (Fig. 23.46).

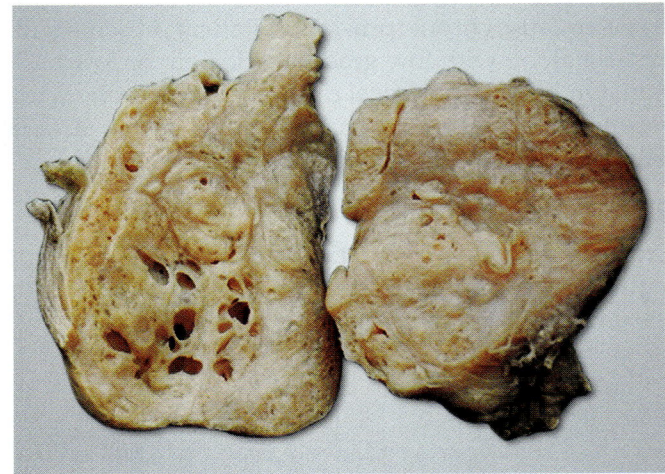

Fig. 23.46: Nodular hyperplasia prostate. The prostate is considerably enlarged. Its cut surface shows a creamy, lobulated solid and cystic areas appearance.

Light Microscopy

Histologically, benign nodular hyperplasia is diagnosed on samples like TURP chips, simple or radical prostatic specimens. It should not be diagnosed in needle biopsy samples. Light microscopy may reveal hyperplasia of glands and stroma in variable proportions (Fig. 23.47).

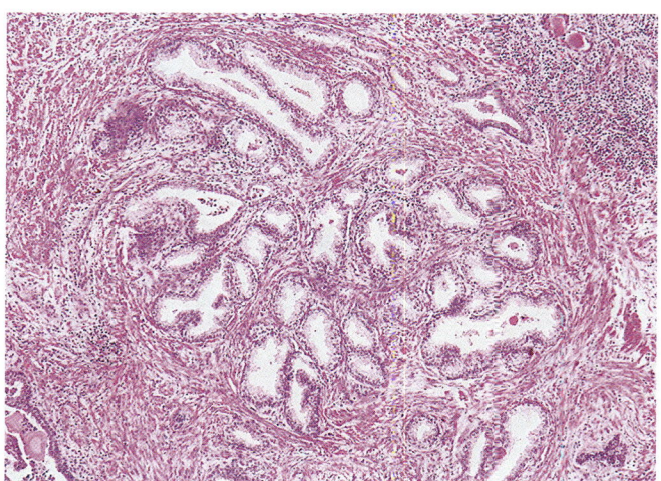

Fig. 23.47: Nodular hyperplasia prostate. The acini are relatively uniform and evenly spaced. The acini are lined by columnar secretory cells. The basal cell layers may be inconspicuous, but may be highlighted by high molecular weight cytokeratin immunostain (400X).

- *Mixed epithelial and stromal hyperplasia:* It is most common with glandular and stromal hyperplasia in various proportions. The glands show irregular sized glandular spaces lined by epithelium, i.e. inner columnar layer and outer flattened myoepithelial cell layer.
- *Pure stromal nodules:* Uncommon is pure nodular stromal hyperplasia composed of hyalinized leiomyomatous nodules with spindled or myxoid (stellate cells).

PROSTATIC ADENOCARCINOMA

Prostate cancer is the most common cancer affecting older men (>50 years). It most often arises from the peripheral group of glands (ducts and acini) of prostate. Established risk factors for adenocarcinoma prostate include age, family history and race. Risk of prostatic carcinoma increases, if father suffered from this disease.

Diagnostic Triad

Adenocarcinoma is the most common malignant tumor of prostate. It is most often diagnosed by rectal examination, ultrasonography and serum prostate specific antigen. *Serum prostate specific antigen is widely used for early detection of prostate cancer.*

Predisposing Factors

There is no evidence that adenocarcinoma originates from nodular hyperplasia prostate.

- *Role of androgens:* Androgens play an important role in pathogenesis of prostate cancer. Prostate cancer cells are dependent on androgen's interaction with androgen receptors resulting in activation of pro-growth and pro-survival genes.

  Androgen receptors with short glutamine repeats are more sensitive to androgens.

  On the other hand, androgen receptors with numerous glutamine repeats are less sensitive to androgens.
- *Precursor lesions:* It is generally accepted that dysplastic lesion progresses to invasive prostatic adenocarcinoma.
- *Increased fat consumption:* Excessive consumption of fat increases risk of prostate cancer. Dietary products, i.e. *vitamin D, selenium, soya products* and *tomato's lycopene* prevent prostate cancer.
- *Cadmium:* It is used in batteries and metal paintings; and associated with prostatic cancer.

Molecular Genetics

Germline Genes

Risk of prostate cancer increases with first degree relative with prostate cancer especially at an early age. BRCA2 mutation is associated with increased risk of prostate cancer.

Acquired Mutations and Epigenetic Changes

- *Chromosomal rearrangements:* Prostate epithelial cells become more sensitive to overexpression of ETS transcription factor.

  ETS transcription factor is formed due to juxtaposition of ETS family, transcriptional factor and adjoining androgen regulated TMPRSS2 promoter gene.
- *Hypermethylation of glutathione S-transferase gene:* It downregulates its expression resulting in increased susceptibility to several carcinogens.
- *Reduced E-cadherin expression:* It is associated with increased expression of the EZH2 transcriptional repressor.

Clinical Features

- Patient is asymptomatic in the initial phase. He becomes symptomatic, when prostatic carcinoma spreads beyond the prostate gland invading surrounding structures, i.e. ejaculatory ducts in the space between the seminal vesicles or perivesicular fascia, bladder and rectum.

  Local invasion into the urethra and bladder neck may cause frequency of micturition and difficulty in passage of urine.

- This is followed by involvement of draining lymph nodes and distant metastases to bones. When disseminated, the cancer may respond to endocrine therapy because tumor growth is partially related to the activity of androgens.
- Gleason system of grading based on differentiation of prostatic carcinoma helps in prediction of course. The prostatic tumor is most often well differentiated adenocarcinoma.

Gross Morphology
Tumor shows gray white to yellowish ill-defined areas when compared to the native parenchyma (Fig. 23.48).

Light Microscopy
Major diagnostic criteria are pattern of growth (infiltrative small glands or cribriform glands), absence of basal cells and nuclear atypia with nucleolar enlargement (Table 23.21). Gleason system of grading based on differentiation of prostatic cancer helps in prediction of course (Table 23.22).

- *Well differentiated carcinoma:* The prostatic carcinoma is most often well differentiated adenocarcinoma. It comprises small glands arranged back-to-back, with a little or no intervening stroma. Tumor cells contain normochromatic nuclei with single prominent nucleolus and mitoses (Fig. 23.49).

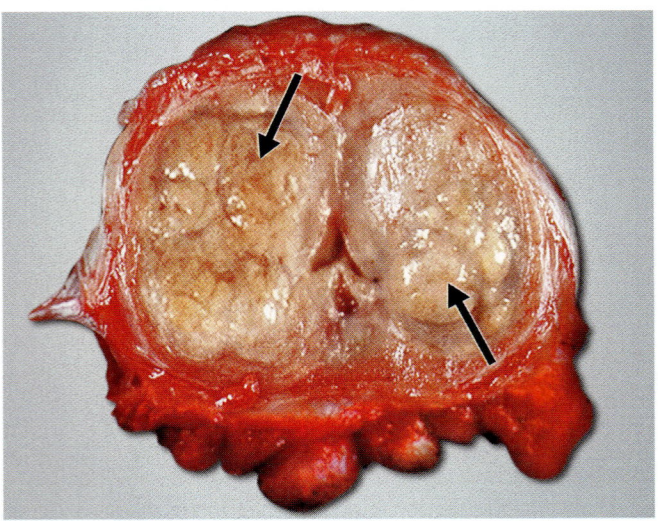

Fig. 23.48: Prostatic adenocarcinoma shows a large yellow tumor present in the posterolateral aspect of the prostate (arrows).

Table 23.22: Gleason system of grading of prostatic carcinoma

Light microscopy	Gleason grade
Well differentiated carcinoma (abnormal glandular arrangements in the form of well-circumscribed nodule with closely packed acini)	1 and 2
Single small infiltrative glands with wide stromal separation	3
Cribriform pattern with fused small acini or poorly formed glands	4
High grade prostatic carcinoma composed of sheets, cords, single cells or comedocarcinoma (glands lined by tumor cells with central necrosis)	5

Table 23.21: Diagnostic criteria for prostatic carcinoma

Major and minor criteria	Light microscopic findings
Major criteria (most important)	*Architectural pattern:* Infiltrative small glands or cribriform glands too large or irregular to represent high grade PIN *Basal cell layer absent:* Basal cells are stained by using antibody 34βE12 against cytokeratins (high molecular weight) *Nuclear atypia:* Nuclear and nucleolar enlargement
Minor criteria	*Intraluminal blue mucin:* blue-tinged or basophilic mucinous secretions Pink amorphous secretions Mitotic figures Intraluminal crystalloids Adjacent high grade PIN Amphophilic cytoplasm

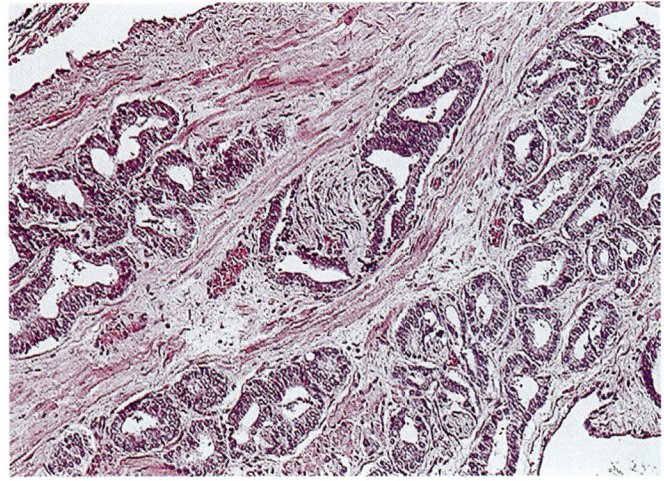

Fig. 23.49: Prostatic adenocarcinoma with perineural invasion. Acid sulfated and nonsulfated mucins are often present in malignant acini, appearing as amorphous or delicate thread-like faintly basophilic intraluminal secretions. Note the haphazard arrangement of acini (400X).

Table 23.23: Immunophenotype of prostatic carcinoma and urothelial carcinoma

Marker	Prostatic carcinoma (% of cases positive)	Urothelial carcinoma (% of cases positive)
PSA (prostate-specific antigen)	94–100%	Negative
PSAP (prostate-specific acid phosphatase)	89–100%	Negative
PSMA (prostate-specific membrane antigen)	92%	Negative
NXK3.1	95%	Negative
Prostein	100%	6%
p63	0–3%	81–96%
Thrombomodulin	0%	69–91%
Uroplakin III	0%	57%
Cytokeratins (high molecular weight) detected by antibody 34βE12	0–10%	65–100%

Note: Mean: 3% prostatic carcinoma cases are positive. Up to 20% of cases of metastatic prostatic carcinoma can be positive.

- *Poorly differentiated carcinoma:* Light microscopy shows fused glands (cribriform glands). These are arranged in solid nests. These glands may contain crystalloids and bluish mucin secretions.

Immunohistochemistry

Markers of prostate carcinoma are PSA (prostate-specific antigen), PSAP (prostate-specific acid phosphatase), PSMA (prostate-specific membrane antigen), NXK3.1 and prostein (Table 23.23).

Prognostic Parameters

Patient with well differentiated adenocarcinoma of prostate with free resected margins, lack of invasion of nerves, blood vessels and Gleason's capsule has good prognosis.

Therapeutic Correlation

Tumor cells exhibit androgen-dependent growth. Chemical castration by the administration of androgenic antagonists (e.g. leuprolide) is used in the treatment of prostate cancer.

Diagnostic Tools

Both prostate-specific antigen (PSA) and serum prostatic acid phosphatase are increased in prostatic carcinoma. Concentration of prostate-specific antigen values in different age groups (Table 23.24).

Table 23.24: Prostate-specific antigen values in different age groups

Age group (years)	Serum prostate-specific antigen in ng/ml
40–49	2.5 ng/ml
50–69	3 ng/ml
70–79	6.5 ng/ml

Note: Older men have higher serum PSA level than younger one.

- *Prostate-specific antigen (PSA):* PSA is a product of prostatic epithelium normally synthesized in the semen. It is serine protease, whose function is to cleave and liquefy the seminal vesicle coagulum formed after ejaculation.

  In most laboratories, normal cut off point of serum level of prostate-specific antigen is 4 ng/ml. Serum PSA levels may be increased in prostatic carcinoma, nodular hyperplasia of prostate, prostatitis, and prostate infarct.

  Prostatic carcinoma is associated with increased total PSA levels in serum and decreased free form. On the other hand, increased total PSA levels in serum with a proportionate increase in the fraction of free PSA suggests nodular hyperplasia prostate (Table 23.25).

- *Serum prostatic acid phosphatase:* Its level increases when prostatic cancer invades capsule and surrounding tissues, but it lacks sensitivity in early disease. Therefore, estimation of serum-prostatic acid phosphatase along with prostate-specific antigen (PSA) is useful in the follow-up cases of widespread metastases.

- *Serum alkaline phosphatase:* Serum alkaline phosphatase is an indicator of bone osteoblastic metastases in advanced disease.

- *α-methylacyl-CoA racemase enzyme:* This mitochondrial and peroxisomal enzymes are overexpressed in prostatic adenocarcinoma and some other carcinomas.

Table 23.25: Percentage of free PSA and total PSA levels in serum

Prostate disorders	Serum free and total PSA levels
Prostate carcinoma	Total serum PSA levels high; Serum free PSA levels less than 10%
Benign nodular hyperplasia	Total serum PSA levels high; Serum free PSA levels >25%

Note: Percentage of free PSA/total PSA levels in serum is lower in men with prostate carcinoma than with benign nodular hyperplasia.

PENIS

INFLAMMATORY DISORDERS

Inflammatory disorders include a number of sexually transmitted infectious processes.

Urethra

Neisseria gonorrhoeae infection manifests with urethral discharge, typically purulent and greenish yellow. *Chlamydia trachomatis* infection leads to urethritis and epididymitis.

Glans Penis and Prepuce

- *Treponema pallidum* causes syphilis, which may present with an elevated, painless, superficially ulcerated, firm papule (chancre) on the glans penis or prepuce that ordinarily heals within 2 to 6 weeks. The organism is demonstrated by dark field examination.
- Bacterial inflammation of the glans penis is known as *balanitis*. Extension of inflammation to the foreskin is called balanoposthitis. Significant complications are stricture of the meatus, phimosis, and paraphimosis. In immunocompromised persons and diabetes mellitus, it can also be caused by fungal infection.

Penis

Herpes simplex virus can cause a vesicular rash on the penis. Human papillomavirus (HPV) is associated with condyloma acuminatum of the penis.

CARCINOMA OF PENIS

Squamous cell carcinoma is the most common cancer of the penis. It occurs in the form of carcinoma *in situ* or invasive squamous cell carcinoma. It is rare in circumcised men.

Etiology

Predisposing factors include poor personal hygiene, accumulation of smegma, uncircumcised men and venereal disease. Disease is often associated with *HPV infection types 16, 18, 31, and 33 in 66% of cases.*

CARCINOMA *IN SITU* OF PENIS

It refers to microscopically full-thickness atypia of the squamous epithelium. It is divided into Bowen disease, erythroplasia of Queyrat, and Bowenoid papulosis.

Bowen Disease

Patient presents with single sharply demarcated erythematous plaque or grayish plaque most often on the shaft of the penis or on the scrotum. It may progress to invasive carcinoma.

Erythroplasia of Queyrat

Patient develops as solitary or multiple, shiny, soft, erythematous plaques on the glans and foreskin.

Bowenoid Papulosis

Patient presents with multiple verrucoid (wart-like) lesions often resembling condyloma acuminatum affecting younger age group.

INVASIVE CARCINOMA OF PENIS

Patient presents with fungating or ulcerative growth most often on shaft of penis. Light microscopy reveals squamous cell carcinoma (Figs 23.50 and 23.51).

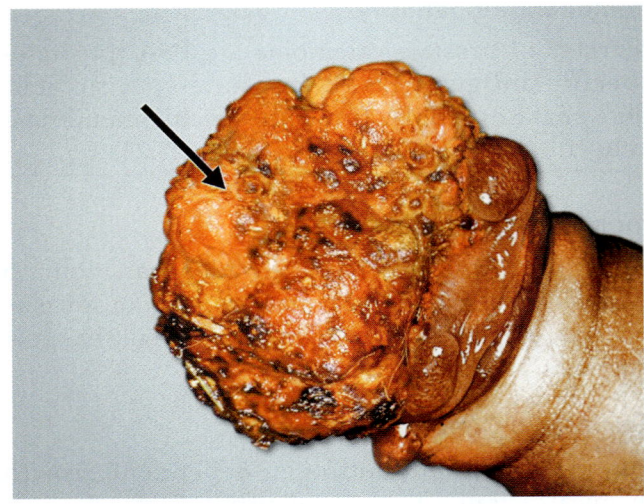

Fig. 23.50: Invasive carcinoma of penis (arrow).

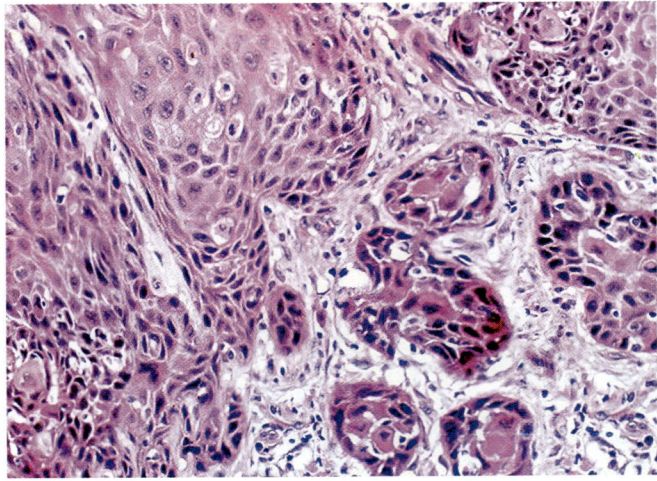

Fig. 23.51: Squamous cell carcinoma of penis (400X).

CONGENITAL ANOMALIES AND MISCELLANEOUS DISEASES

Hypospadias

It refers to location of urethral meatus on the ventral surface of the penis. It results from incomplete closure of the urethral folds of the urogenital sinus. It is repaired by surgical procedure.

Epispadias

It refers to location of urethral meatus on the dorsal surface of the penis. It is less common than hypospadias.

Phimosis

In phimosis, abnormal tight foreskin of penis leads to narrowing of the orifice of prepuce resulting in difficulty to retract over the glans penis. This condition may be congenital or result from inflammation or from trauma.

Paraphimosis

Forceful retraction of narrow prepuce may strangulate the glans and obstruct venous blood flow. This disorder is known as *paraphimosis*.

Peyronie Disease

It results from subcutaneous fibrosis of the dorsum of the penis affecting older persons of unknown etiology.

Priapism

It is an intractable, often painful erection of penis. It is associated with venous thrombosis of the corpora cavernosa, sickle cell anemia, hypercoagulable states, spinal injuries, chronic myeloid leukemia and some drugs.

CHAPTER 24

Female Reproductive System

Learning Objectives

VULVA
- Inflammatory Diseases
- Tumors and Tumor-like Diseases
- Non-neoplastic Disorders

VAGINA
- Inflammatory Diseases
- Malignant Tumors and VIN

CERVIX
- Inflammatory Diseases
- Neoplasms of Cervix and CIN

FALLOPIAN TUBES
- Inflammatory Diseases
- Other Non-neoplastic Diseases
- Neoplastic Diseases

ENDOMETRIUM
- Endometriosis
- Endometrial Adenocarcinoma

OVARY
- General Considerations
- Surface Epithelial Tumors
- Germ Cell Tumors
- Sex Cord Stromal Tumors
- Laboratory Diagnosis of Ovarian Tumors
- Ovarian Cysts

GESTATIONAL TROPHOBLASTIC TUMORS
- Complete and Incomplete Hydatidiform Moles
- Invasive Hydatidiform Mole
- Gestational Choriocarcinoma

PREGNANCY ASSOCIATED DISEASES
- Toxemia of Pregnancy
- Thromboembolism
- Amniotic Fluid Embolism
- Gestational Diabetes Mellitus
- Ectopic Pregnancy
- Sheehan's Syndrome
- Chorioamnionitis
- Abnormalities of Placental Attachment

OVERVIEW

EMBRYOLOGY

- A central principle of genital tract development in both sexes holds that the müllerian tubes will develop along female lines unless specifically impeded by embryonic testicular factors.
- In males, Sertoli cells in the developing testis produce *müllerian-inhibiting substance*, a protein that causes the müllerian ducts to regress.
- Müllerian ducts are the precursors of the fallopian ducts, uterus, and upper-third of the vagina.

Formation of the ovary and vulva is not affected by müllerian inhibitory protein.

ANATOMY

Organs of female genital system include ovaries, fallopian tubes, uterus (corpus cervix), lower genital tract (vagina and vulva) and placenta.

Functions

- Functions of female genital system are conception, delivery of the baby, synthesis of estrogen and progesterone. Ovaries participate in ovulation.

Female Reproductive System

- Fertilization takes place in fallopian tubes. Fertilized ovum is transported from fallopian tubes to uterine cavity.
- Implantation of fertilized ovum and placenta formation occurs in uterine cavity. Ovaries and placenta function as hormonal organs to maintain the pregnancy.
- Induction of labor and delivery of baby occur through vagina.

Female Genital System

- Female genital system consists of a pair of ovaries, along with a pair of oviducts (fallopian tubes), uterus, cervix, vagina and external genitalia (labia majora, labia minora and clitoris) located in pelvic region (Fig. 24.1).
- Mammary glands are integrated structurally and functionally to support the process of ovulation, fertilization, pregnancy, birth and childcare.

Ovaries

- Each ovary measures 3 × 1.5 × 1.0 cm. Ovaries are located in pelvic cavity attached to pelvic wall and uterus by ligaments. It is covered by germinal epithelium.
- On cut section, ovary shows cortex and medulla. Outer surface is lined by epithelium. Cortex contains large number of graafian follicles. Each ovary consists of 2 lacs graafian follicles.

Two Fallopian Tubes

- These are also called uterine tubes or oviducts. Fallopian tube is 10–12 cm in length. Its wall is comprised of mucosa, muscular layer and serous layer.
- Part of fallopian tube closer to ovary is called infundibulum, which possesses finger-like projections called fimbriae. It collects ovum from the ovary after ovulation.
- Part of fallopian tube close to uterus is called isthmus. Wider part of fallopian tube is called ampulla lying between isthmus and infundibulum.
- Fallopian tube is lined by ciliated columnar epithelium as well as secretory cells. Secretory cells produce viscous liquid medium; which provides nutrition and protection to the ovum.

Uterus

- Normal uterus is a pear-shaped hollow organ. It weighs 40–80 gm in adult women. It is divided into upper corpus and lower cervical segments. The uterine cavity is triangular measuring 6 cm in length. It is composed of inner endometrial lining consisting of endometrial glands, middle muscular wall and outer serous coat. Serous coat extends to the peritoneal reflection. The peritoneal reflection is short in anterior region than posterior region. Therefore, it may be used for orienting hysterectomy specimens.
- Cervix has *internal os* and *external os*. Cervix projects slightly into an elastic muscular tube, the vagina. It is a check point of vaginal bacterial flora. It secretes mucin to control bacterial growth in vagina. Cervix prevents preterm labor by acting as stopper for conceptus before term.

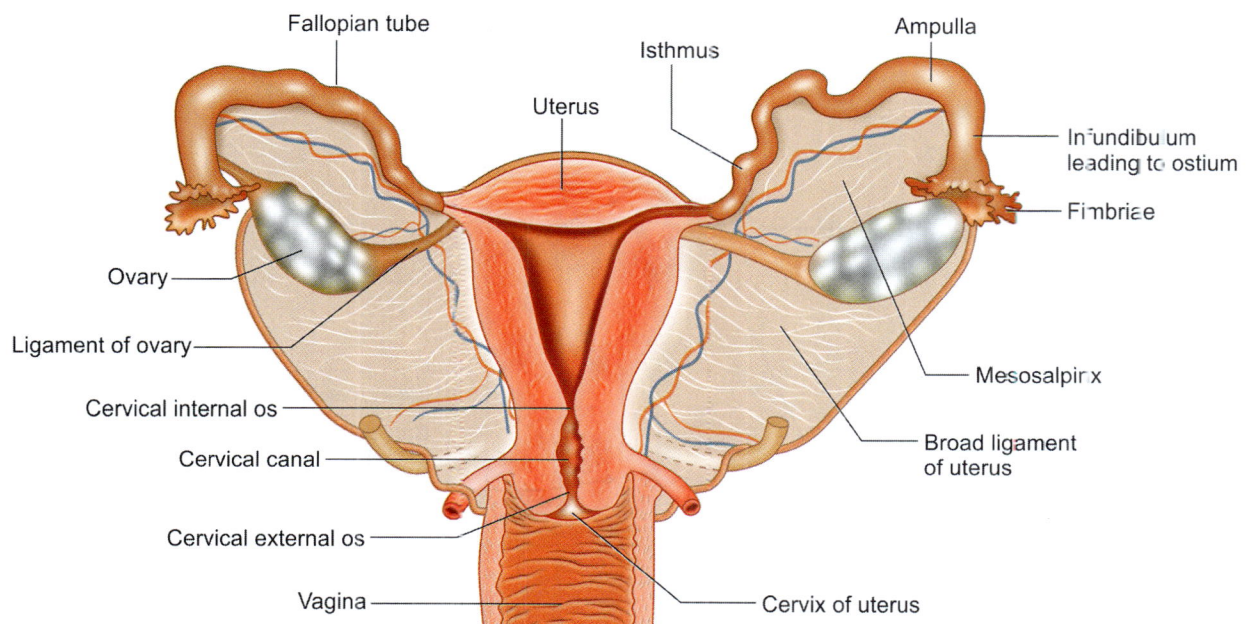

Fig. 24.1: Structure of female genital system.

- Tissue sampling includes endometrial biopsy and curettage specimens, products of conception, and hysterectomy specimens. The samples are processed and examined to establish diagnosis.

Vagina

Vagina consists of mucosa, muscular layer and serous layer without glands. It is covered by hymen, a thin ring of tissue. Vagina is comprised of labia majora, labia minora and accessory genital glands.

External Genital Organs

Mons pubis is fatty tissue covered by skin and pubic hair. Clitoris is tiny finger-like structure lined by stratified squamous epithelium. It is analogous to the male's glans penis.

FERTILIZATION AND DEVELOPMENT OF EMBRYO

Functions of Placenta

- Placenta plays an important role in supporting gestation. It acts as a barrier of maternal immune response and fetus. Cell surface MHC class II protein is involved in immune response.
- It is maternal-fetal interface for molecular exchanges such as gases, inorganic and organic substances, nutrients, hormones and antibodies. It is physical protector of fetus. It participates in elimination of nitrogenous waste products.
- Placenta acts as endocrine gland by secreting human chorionic gonadotropin hormone (hCG), estrogens progesterone, and chorionic corticotrophin.
- hCG stimulates corpus luteum of pregnancy that continues to secrete progesterone until the end of the pregnancy.
- In the later phase of pregnancy, relaxin is synthesized by placenta and ovary. Relaxin facilitates parturition by softening the connective tissue of pubic symphysis.

PATHOLOGICAL DISEASES

Pathological disorders of female genital tract are shown in Fig. 24.2 and Table 24.1.

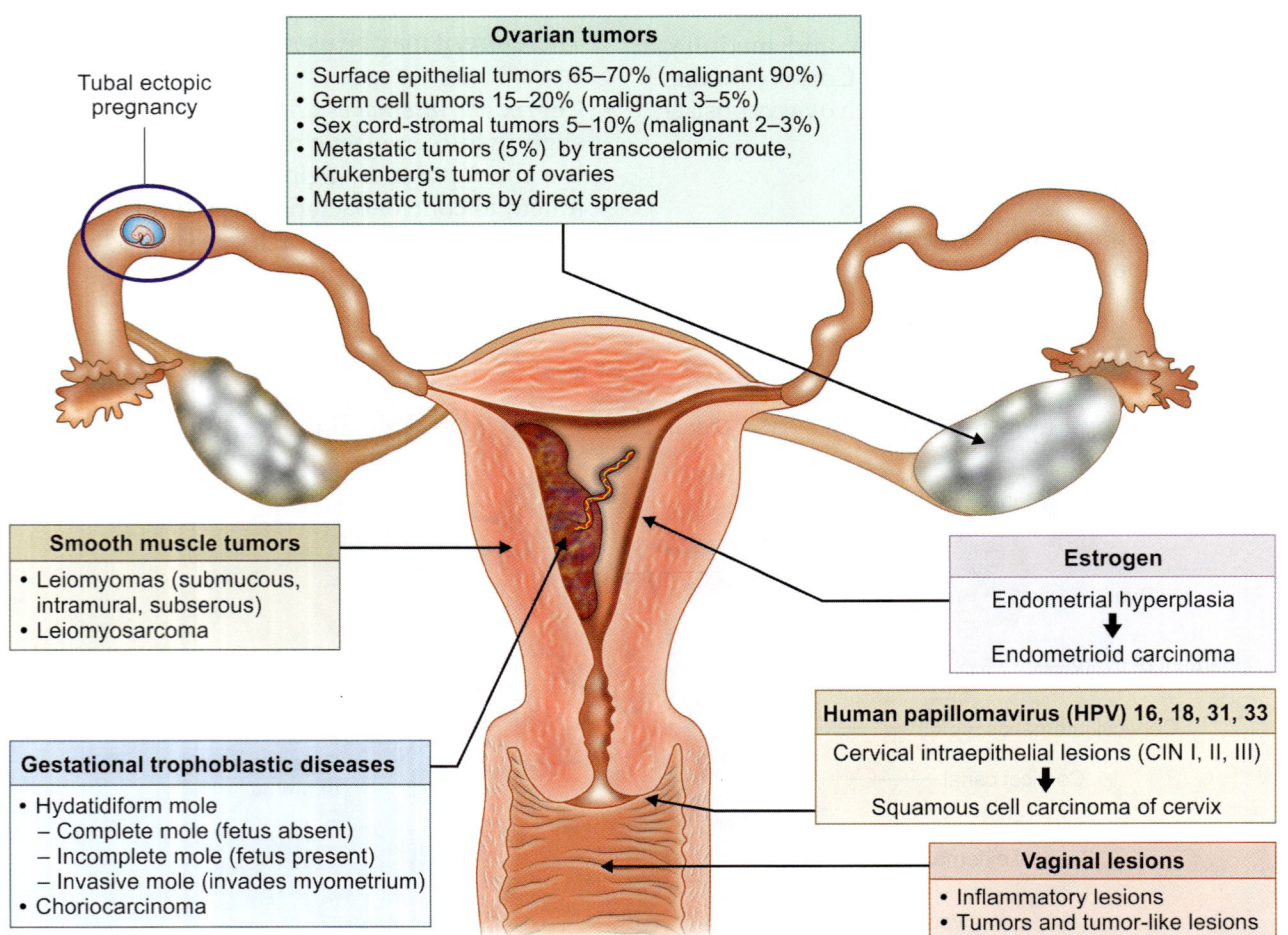

Fig. 24.2: Pathology of female genital system.

Table 24.1: Pathology of female reproductive system

FGS organ	Disorders
Ovaries	Neoplastic diseases, cysts (torsion), endometriosis, hemorrhagic corpus luteum, hormonal imbalance
Fallopian tubes	Infection, tubal pregnancy, neoplastic disease
Uterus corpus	Neoplastic disease, hyperplasia, functional bleeding, infection
Cervix	CIN and cervical carcinoma
Lower genital tract (vagina and vulva)	Squamous intraepithelial neoplasia and carcinoma
Placenta	Abnormality (molar pregnancy), infection, placental dysfunction, neoplastic disease (rare)

VULVA

INFLAMMTORY DISEASES

- Vulval inflammation is common in post-menopausal women. It is related to thin atrophy of the skin, which has very thin epithelial covering at this phase of life and is easily abraded. Inflammation at other periods of life frequently involves Bartholin's gland.
- The duct of Bartholin's glands may become blocked with cyst formation. This may become infected leading to Bartholin's abscess.
- The vulva is most often involved by infections, especially those that flourish in moist areas (e.g. *Candida albicans*), or involve hair follicles (e.g. *Staphylococcus boils*). Skin of the vulva may be involved with any other skin disease, such as psoriasis or eczema.

HUMAN PAPILLOMA VIRAL INFECTION

Human papillomavirus (6, 11) causes vulvar wart known as *condyloma acuminatum* on vagina and cervix.

> **Light Microscopy**
> - Koilocytes (intracytoplasmic vacuolation) are indicative of HPV-infected epithelial cells.
> - These are apparent in cytopathologic (Papanicolaou smear) and histopathologic preparations (Fig. 24.3).

Consequence

It may contribute to the pathogenesis of squamous cell carcinoma of vulva and vagina.

LYMPHOGRANULOMA VENEREUM

Lymphogranuloma venereum is caused by gram-negative *Chlamydia trachomatis* (L1, L2, or L3 serotypes) transmitted by sexual contact.

Clinical Course

a. After a few days to a month, patient develops small papule or ulcer at the site of inoculation such as vulva

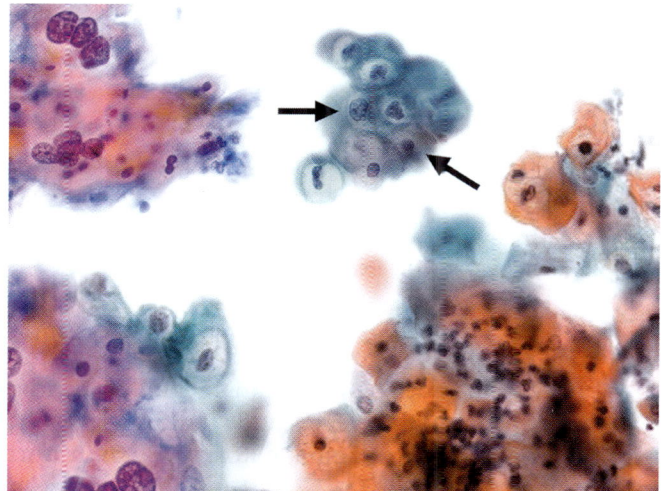

Fig. 24.3: Photomicrograph from a smear showing koilocytosis, the typical appearance of cervical squamous cell infected by human papillomavirus (HPV). There is a *halo* of cleared cytoplasm surrounding an enlarged nucleus (arrows) (400×)

or vagina. It is followed by lymphadenopathy in both inguinal regions and sometimes pelvic region resulting in chronic suppurative fistulas in the pelvic viscera.

- In some untreated patients, lymphatic obstruction leads to genital elephantiasis and rectal strictures.

GRANULOMA INGUINALE

Granuloma inguinale begins as a papule on the vagina, perineum or vagina. It can spread widely, resulting in extensive ulceration and destruction of tissue.

> **Light Microscopy**
> - Histological examination reveals granulomatous lesion.
> - *Donovan bodies* represent macrophages stuffed with numerous *Calymmatobacterium granulomatis* organisms.

CONDYLOMA ACUMINATUM

Etiology

- Condyloma acuminatum is a nonmalignant tumor-like exophytic, papillomatous lesion on the skin or mucous membranes of the lower female genital tract (perineal, vulval and vaginal regions).
- It is caused by HPV types 6 and 11. The median time from infection to first detection of HPV is 3 months. HPV types 6 and 11 are detected in over 80% of macroscopically visible condylomata.

> **Light Microscopy**
> - The vacuolated cells in the cervical biopsy due to HPV types 6, 11 infections are termed koilocytes. These squamous cells show irregular crenated or *raisin-like nuclei* surrounded laterally by clear cytoplasm (*spoon-like cell*).
> - The virus particles can be demonstrated in nucleus by electron microscopy. These are also demonstrable by immunohistochemistry.

HERPES SIMPLEX VIRUS INFECTIONS

Etiology

HSV type 2 infection is transmitted by sexual contact. HSV type 1 is also capable of causing genital infections. HSV 2 produces small vesicles and shallow ulcers that can involve the cervix, vagina, clitoris, vulva, urethra, and perianal skin.

Clinical Features

- These vesicles appear 3–7 days after the intercourse in 30% of women. Ulcers may persist for 1–3 weeks but heal spontaneously without scarring.
- The virus migrates along the nerves to the lumbar ganglia, and remains dormant. The virus can be activated, that may descend to the vulva to produce recurrent vesicles.

> **Light Microscopy**
> Multinucleated giant cells with viral inclusions, nuclear molding, and margination of the chromatin are demonstrated in cytological smears from lesions.

TUMORS AND TUMOR-LIKE DISEASES

PAPILLARY HIDRADENOMA

It is the most common well circumscribed benign tumor of the vulva. It occurs in labia majora and labia minora. It arises from anogenital ectopic breast tissue or apocrine sweat glands.

Clinical Features

Patient presents with labial nodule that may ulcerate and bleed.

> **Light Microscopy**
> - On light microscopy, tumor is composed of cells arranged in complex glandular and papillary pattern with scant stroma.
> - Luminal layer is lined by cuboidal epithelium with apocrine differentiation, and basal layer of myoepithelial cells. Surgical excision cures the patient.

ANGIOMYOFIBROBLASTOMA

It is well circumscribed tumor seen in vulva, vagina or perineal soft tissue.

> **Light Microscopy**
> - On light microscopy, tumor is composed of spindle cells or oval cells with minimal myxoid stroma.
> - The cells are arranged in whirling pattern around blood vessels.
>
> **Immunohistochemistry**
> Immunohistochemistry of tumor cells shows positivity *with desmin and hormone receptors. CD34 expression is demonstrated in 50% cases.*
>
> | Marker | Expression |
> |---|---|
> | Desmin | Positive |
> | ER | Positive |
> | PR | Positive |
> | CD34 | Positive |

LEUKOPLAKIA OF VULVA

Leukoplakia, as implied by its name, is a whitish plaque-like thickening of the mucosa noticed on naked eye examination. Histologic examination shows intraepithelial neoplasia.

BOWEN'S DISEASE OF THE VULVA

Bowen's disease is a multicentric lesion in vulva. It is also known as *vulvar carcinoma in situ*.

SQUAMOUS CELL CARCINOMA OF VULVA

It is the most common malignant tumor of the vulva, that commonly express cytokeratins. It constitutes 85% cancers of vulva.

Etiopathogenesis

- It is the end result of a multistep process that has its origin in vulvar intraepithelial neoplasia.
- Human papillomavirus 16, 18, 31, or 33 (HPV 16 most common) commonly infects vulva in 85% of elderly women.
- Patient develops HPV induced premalignant vaginal intraepithelial neoplasia (grades 1, 2 and 3 lesions) resulting in vaginal invasive squamous cell carcinoma. It may also develop in association with dysplastic precursor known as 'lichen sclerosus'.

Gross Morphology

Growth is exophytic (66%) and others are ulcerative and endophytic (Fig. 24.4).

Light Microscopy

- Tumor shows well-differentiated squamous cell carcinoma with keratin pearls in majority of cases.
- Some may show poorly differentiated (basaloid) carcinoma (Fig. 24.5).

Mode of Spread

- *Local spread:* It spreads slowly and invades contiguous skin, vagina, and rectum.
- *Lymphatic route:* It metastasizes by lymphatic route to the superficial inguinal and then involving the deep inguinal, femoral, and pelvic lymph nodes.
- *Hematogenous spread:* It leads to distant metastases in lung, and liver. The frequency of metastases is related to the size and local extension of tumor.

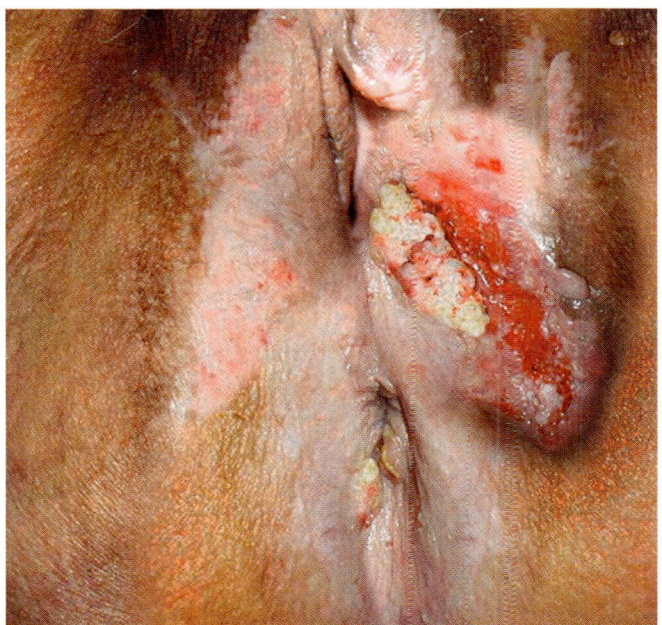

Fig. 24.4: Squamous cell carcinoma of vulva. Fungating growth with ulceration is visible.

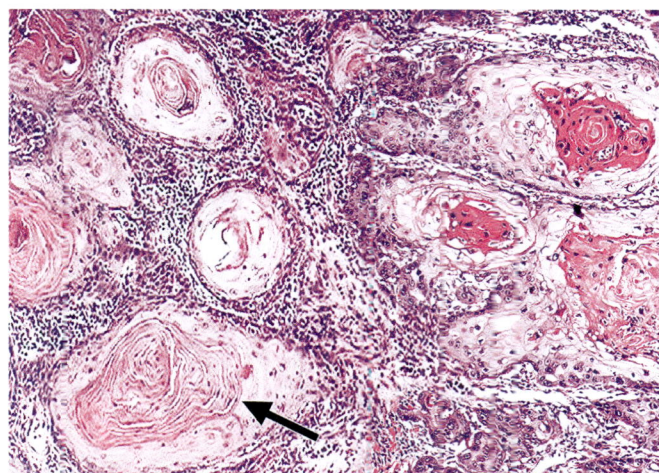

Fig. 24.5: Squamous cell carcinoma of vulva. At high magnification, nests of neoplastic squamous cells are invaded through a chronically inflamed stroma. This cancer is well-differentiated, as evidenced by keratin pearls (400X).

EXTRAMAMMARY PAGET'S DISEASE OF VULVA

Paget disease of the vulva is similar to Paget disease of the breast. It is primarily an intradermal adenocarcinoma derived from multipotent cells in the epidermis, adnexa or anogenital glands. The disorder usually occurs on the labia majora in elderly women.

Associated Lesions

Paget's disease may be associated with underlying adenocarcinoma of Bartholin glands or adenocarcinoma of cervix or transitional carcinoma of urethra and urinary bladder.

Clinical Features

Patient presents with pruritic, eczematous raised rash in the vulvar perianal, or perineal areas. It may persist for decades and often recurs following local excision (Fig. 24.6).

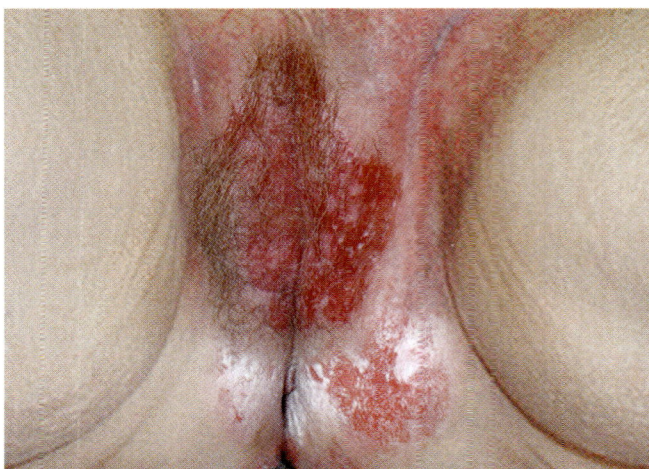

Fig. 24.6: Paget's disease of vulva. Eczematous raised rash is seen in the vulvar region.

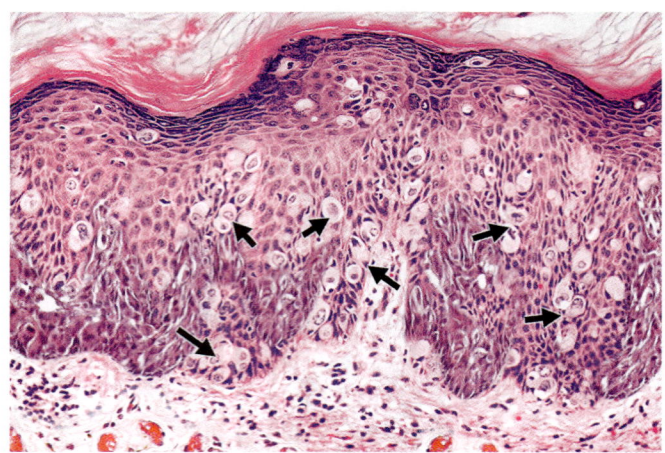

Fig. 24.7: Paget's disease of vulva. The tumor cells in the overlying epidermis are called Paget's cells. These are large cells with abundant clear cytoplasm and large nuclei with prominent nucleoli, arranged singly or in clusters; represent intraepithelial extension of an underlying carcinoma in situ or invasive ductal carcinoma (arrows) (400X).

Light Microscopy
- Paget's disease of the vulva has similar histological features as the Paget's disease of nipple. Tumor cells are large pale containing glycosaminoglycans (mucin) surrounded by a clear, halo-like area of vacuolation (*Paget cells*) (Fig. 24.7).
- These cells are arranged in nests at the epidermal-dermal interface and within the epidermis (pagetoid spread).

Immunohistochemistry
The tumor expresses carcinoembryonic antigen (CEA), epithelial membrane antigen and CK7. But CK20 is negative in tumor cells.

Marker	Expression
Carcinoembryonic antigen (CEA)	Positive
Epithelial membrane antigen (EMA)	Positive
CK7	Positive
CK20	Negative

Histochemistry
Mucopolysaccharides present in the tumor cells are stained with **PAS, mucicarmine** and **Alcian blue**.

MELANOMA

Melanoma of vulva is a rare lesion affecting elderly women (60–70 years). It accounts for approximately 10% of malignant tumors of the vulva.

Clinical Features
Patient presents with spreading pigmented patch or pigmented mass. Spreading pigmented patch resembles extramammary Paget's disease.

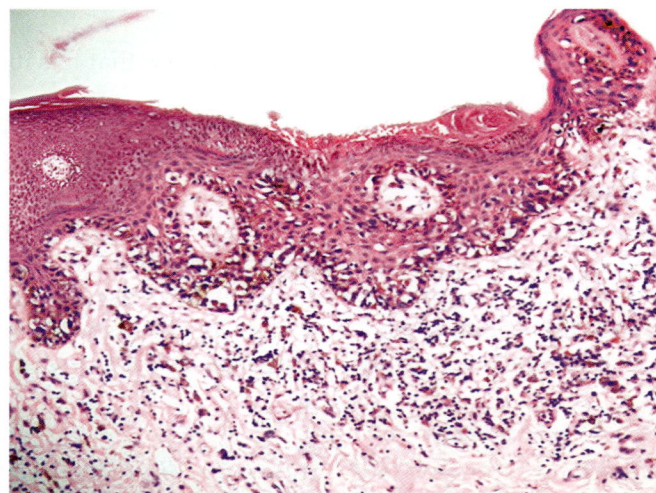

Fig. 24.8: Malignant melanoma. Tumor is composed of melanoma cells (100X).

Light Microscopy
- Tumor is composed of melanoma cells larger than nevus cells. These cells contain large nuclei with irregular contours with eosinophilic nuclei.
- Chromatin is clumped at the periphery of the nuclear membrane (Fig. 24.8).

Immunohistochemistry
It shows positivity for S-100 protein, MART-1 (melan-A), Ki-67, CAM-5.2 and HMB-45. Extra-mammary Paget's disease shows positivity for mucin, but melanoma not.

Marker	Expression
HMB-45	Positive
MART-1 (melan-A)	Positive
Tyrosinase	Positive
Ki-67 (excellent marker)	Positive
S-100	Positive
CAM-5.2	Positive

NON-NEOPLASTIC DISORDERS

BARTHOLIN CYST

- The Bartholin glands produce a clear mucoid secretion that continuously lubricates the vestibular surface.
- Obstruction of Bartholin ducts results in Bartholin cyst. It may be secondarily infected by *Neisseria gonorrhoeae* or staphylococci, Chlamydia resulting in Bartholin gland abscess. It is treated with incision and drainage (Fig. 24.9).

CARBUNCLE

Carbuncle is an exophytic or often ulcerated, polypoid mass of 1 to 2 cm in diameter present near the female

Female Reproductive System

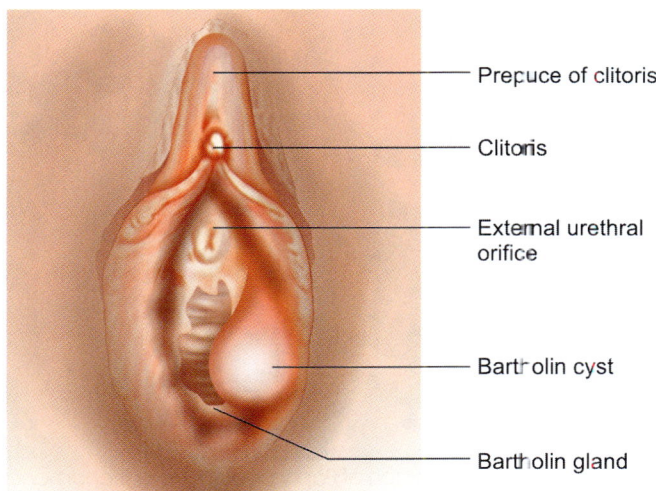

Fig. 24.9: Bartholin cyst.

urethral meatus resulting in pain and bleeding. It most often affects perimenopausal women.

Light Microscopy

Light microscopy reveals acute as well as chronic inflammatory granulation tissue and hyperplasia of lining epithelium.

TOXIC SHOCK SYNDROME

Certain strains of *Staphylococcus aureus* release an exotoxin called *toxic shock syndrome toxin-1*. It causes toxic shock syndrome, an acute sometimes fatal disorder.

Clinical Features

Patient presents with fever, shock, desquamative erythematous rash, vomiting, diarrhea, myalgias, neurologic signs and decreased platelets count. Patient may develop disseminated intravascular coagulation.

LICHEN SCLEROSIS

It is an inflammatory disease of the vulva. It is most often associated with autoimmune disorders such as vitiligo, pernicious anemia, and Hashimoto's thyroiditis.

Clinical Features

Patient presents with pruritus due to development of white plaques and atrophic skin with a *parchment paper* like or crinkled appearance resulting in marked contracture of the vulvar tissues (dyspareunia).

Light Microscopy

- Skin lesion shows hyperkeratosis, epithelial thinning with flattening of the rete pegs and homogeneous, a cellular zone in the upper dermis.
- A band of chronic inflammatory cells typically lies beneath this layer.
- Minority of patients may develop squamous cell carcinoma (15%).

VAGINA

INFLAMMATORY DISEASES

Vaginal discharge is a common complaint in multiparous women. Physiological discharge is scanty, mucoid and colorless. Pathological discharge occurs due to *Trichomonas vaginalis* or *Candida albicans* or bacterial vaginosis.

Transmission

Primary mode of transmission of sexually transmitted infections is through vaginal or anal sex or vertical transmission from mother to fetus. There are however a number of inflammatory conditions which arise primarily in vagina.

BACTERIAL VAGINOSIS

Bacterial vaginosis involves an imbalance in the hormonal and bacterial environment of the vagina. It results in vaginal discharge, irritation and increased risk of transmission of sexually transmitted diseases and pelvic inflammatory diseases and complicated pregnancy (Figs 24.10 and 24.11).

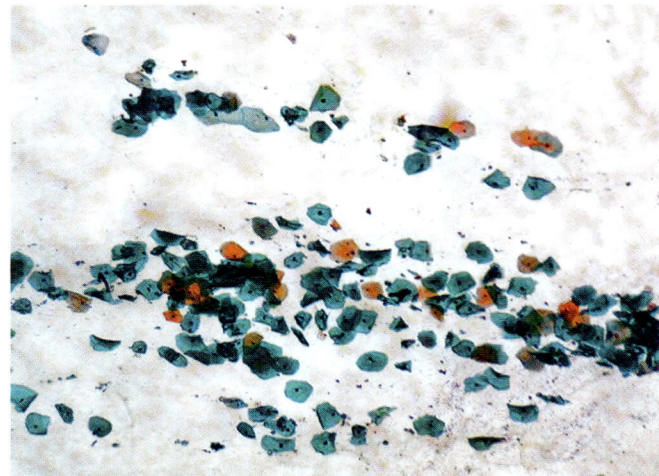

Fig. 24.10: Microphotograph of normal Pap smear showing superficial and intermediate squamous epithelial cells (Pap stain 100X).

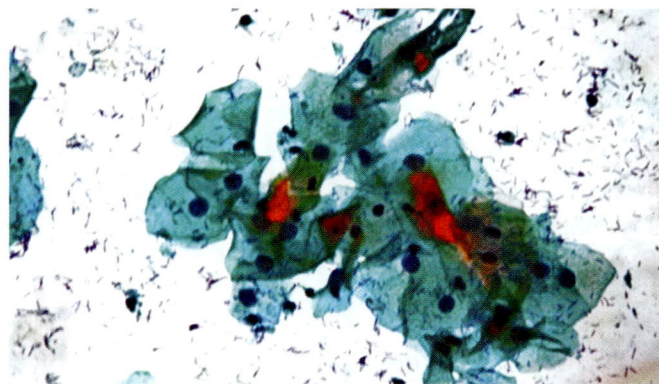

Fig. 24.11: Photomicrograph showing bacterial vaginosis on Pap smear with clue cells (Pap stain 400X).

CANDIDA ALBICANS

Candida albicans causes vulvovaginitis affecting 10% of women. *Candida albicans* is a normal vaginal flora. Infection is commonly associated with pregnancy, diabetes mellitus, broad-spectrum antibiotic therapy, oral contraceptive use, and immunosuppression resulting in fungal growth.

Clinical Features

Patient presents with white curd-like vaginal discharge that may cause intense itching.

Per Vaginal Examination

Per vaginal examination shows white patches on the mucosal surface of vagina covered with vaginal discharge.

Diagnosis

Diagnosis is best made microscopically on wet mounts or Pap smear showing fungal pseudohyphae (Fig. 24.12).

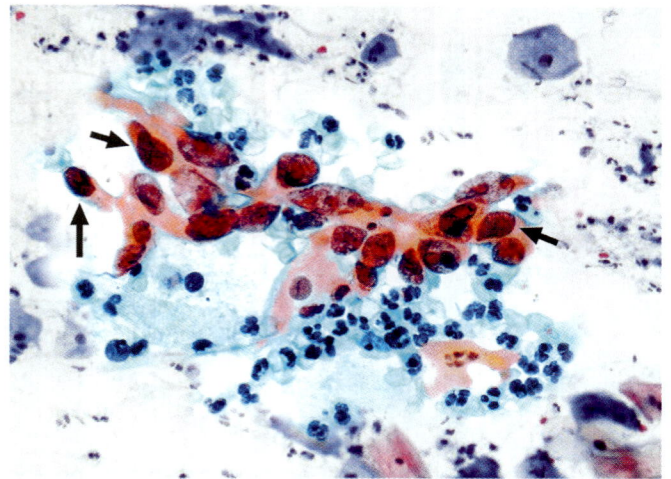

Fig. 24.12: Microphotograph of Pap smear showing *Candida albicans* (arrows) (400X).

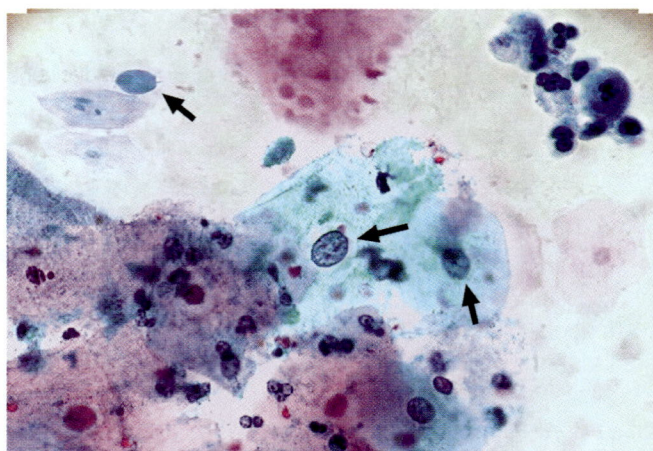

Fig. 24.13: Microphotograph of Pap smear showing *Trichomonas vaginalis* (arrows) (400X)

TRICHOMONAS VAGINALIS

Trichomonas vaginalis is the second most common cause of vaginitis. It is commonly transmitted by sexual contact.

Clinical Features

Patient presents with a profuse opaque or creamy-colored frothy discharge with fishy smell. Discharge may cause vulvar irritation and burning micturition due to urethral inflammation.

Diagnostic Test

These flagellated protozoa are best diagnosed in freshly prepared wet mounts (i.e. smears of unfixed vaginal discharge, in which the protozoa keep moving) (Fig. 24.13).

GARDNERELLA VAGINALIS

Gardnerella vaginalis is a common cause of vaginal discharge. This microbe grows on vagina due to loss of the normal vaginal lactobacilli.

Clinical Features

Patient presents with thin homogeneous vaginal discharge with a malodorous, fishy amine odor, especially on addition of 10% potassium hydroxide.

Diagnosis

The infection is best recognized on Pap smear by appearance of *clue cells* (i.e. squamous cells covered with clumped nuclei, folded cytoplasm, and numerous bacteria attached to their surface).

CHLAMYDIA TRACHOMATIS

Chlamydia trachomatis (serotype D-K) transmitted by sexual contact produces cervicitis and pelvic inflammatory disease.

Clinical Features

The disease is most often asymptomatic. Patient may present with vaginal discharge, vesicles and ulcers on vulva, pelvic pain or pelvic mass, and discomfort during intercourse.

SYPHILIS

Treponema pallidum is a spirochete and the etiologic agent of syphilis. It is transmitted by sexual contact.

Clinical Features

Patient presents with firm, painless ulcer known as a chancre, which is usually not apparent clinically. During secondary syphilis, patient sometimes develops gray, flattened, wart-like lesions known as *condylomata lata*. Syphilis is a hazard during pregnancy because spirochetes can cross the placenta and resulting in fetal malformation.

CHANCROID

After 3 to 5 days of sexual contact with infected partner by *Haemophilus ducreyi*, a gram-negative bacillus causes soft and painful ulcerated lesion known as chancroid on the cervix, vagina, vulva, or perianal region.

Chancroid is a similar lesion to the primary lesion in syphilis, but instead is painful. This disease is most common in tropical areas, but rare in the United States.

Clinical Features

It may be associated inguinal lymphadenopathy, fever, chills, and malaise. It sometimes causes urethral stenosis.

> **Light Microscopy**
> Light microscopy reveals a granulomatous inflammatory reaction.

MALIGNANT TUMORS AND VIN

Malignant tumors of vagina include vaginal intraepithelial neoplasia, squamous cell carcinoma, verrucous carcinoma, sarcoma botryoides, leiomyomas and malignant melanoma.

VAGINAL INTRAEPITHELIAL NEOPLASIA (VIN)

Vaginal intraepithelial neoplasia is a premalignant, HPV associated lesion. It affects women 20–40 years of age (Table 24.2).

Etiopathogenesis

- Risk factors include early age at first intercourse especially with multiple sexual partners. Low grade intraepithelial neoplasia is caused HPV (6, 11) and high grade intraepithelial neoplasia by HPV (16, 31, 33, 35, and 39).
- Approximately 5% cases with low grade intraepithelial neoplasia progresses to high grade dysplasia or invasive carcinoma over span of several years.

> **Gross Morphology**
> Vaginal intraepithelial neoplasia appears as an exophytic growth to verrucopapillary lesion.
>
> **Light Microscopy**
> Squamous epithelium of vaginal intraepithelial neoplasia shows hyperchromatic nuclei and irregular nuclear membrane.

Grading

Grading is based on the extent of thickness of squamous epithelium (VIN-1, VIN-2 and VIN-3) sharing dysplastic changes.

Management

Clinical management of VIN-1 is simple follow-up of the patient. VIN-2 and VIN-3 are treated by simple excision or laser ablation.

Table 24.2: Comparison of VIN types

Parameters	VIN of usual type	Differentiated VIN
Age	Younger age group	Postmenopausal age group
Etiology	HPV related cytopathic effect	Not related to HPV, but associated with lichen sclerosis. No cytopathic effect
Light microscopy	Hyperchromatic nuclei, prominent nuclear membrane and mitoses. Lesion shows warty, basaloid or mixed subtypes	Cells with hyperchromatic nuclei, prominent nuclear membrane, mitoses and eosinophilic cytoplasm
Grading	VIN-1, VIN-2 and VIN-3	VIN-3
Progression	Lower	High keratinizing squamous cell carcinoma

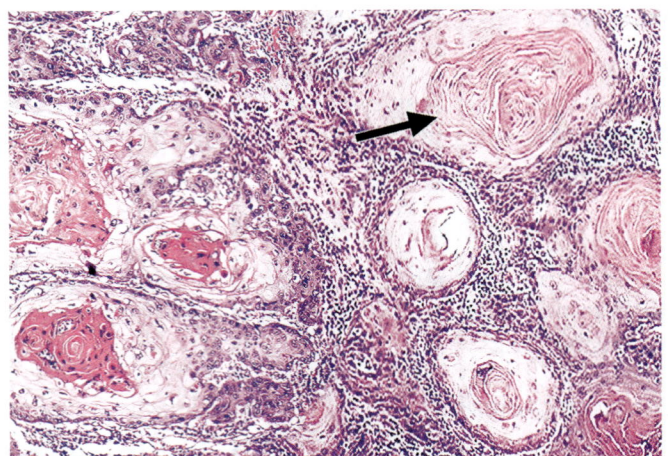

Fig. 24.14: Squamous cell carcinoma of vagina. At high magnification, nests of neoplastic squamous cells are invaded through a chronically inflamed stroma. This cancer is well-differentiated, as evidenced by keratin pearls. However, most cervical squamous carcinomas are non-keratinizing (arrow) (400X).

SQUAMOUS CELL CARCINOMA OF VAGINA

Squamous cell carcinoma of the vagina most often occurs in 60–80 years of age. In younger women, the tumor is usually associated with HPV infections.

Light Microscopy
• Tumor is composed of atypical cells with hyperchromatic nuclei arranged in nests. • Tumor cells form keratin pearls (Fig. 24.14).

Mode of Spread

Squamous cell carcinoma of the vagina spreads to regional lymph nodes, lungs, liver and bones.

VERRUCOUS CARCINOMA

Verrucous carcinoma of the vagina is a slow growing variant of squamous cell carcinoma. Local or distant metastases are very rare.

Gross Morphology
Tumor exhibits warty gross appearance.
Light Microscopy
• It is well differentiated squamous cell carcinoma. • Tumor is composed of nests of tumor cells invading stroma.

CLEAR CELL ADENOCARCINOMA

Clear cell adenocarcinoma is a rare vaginal tumor, most of which found in young daughters of <20 years of age, whose mothers have taken *diethylstilbestrol* (DES) during pregnancy.

Clinical Features

Patient initially develops vaginal adenosis characterized by mucosal columnar epithelium lined crypts in areas normally lined by stratified squamous epithelium. *Vaginal adenosis is thought to be a precursor of clear cell adenocarcinoma.*

Light Microscopy
• Tumor is composed of *pleomorphic cells* with *hyperchromatic nuclei* with *abundant clear cytoplasm*. • Tumor cells are arranged in papillary or tubular or cystic manner. • Hobnailing is a prominent feature. • Metastases to distant organs are demonstrated by imaging techniques.

Mode of Spread

Tumor may spread to *regional lymph nodes* and *lungs*.

BOTRYOIDES RHABDOMYOSARCOMA

Botryoid rhabdomyosarcoma is a subtype of embryonal rhabdomyosarcoma. It is most common vaginal malignant tumor in children <5 years of age. It is most often located in submucosa of vagina.

Gross Examination
Tumor resembles cluster of grapes hence named as botryoid type (Fig. 24.15).
Light Microscopy
• Tumor is composed of numerous round to oval cells with eosinophilic cytoplasm admixed with *spindle cells in loose myxoid stroma*. • At least one microscopic field must exhibit the malignant cells forming a *condensed layer beneath epithelium known as cambium layer* (Fig. 24.16).

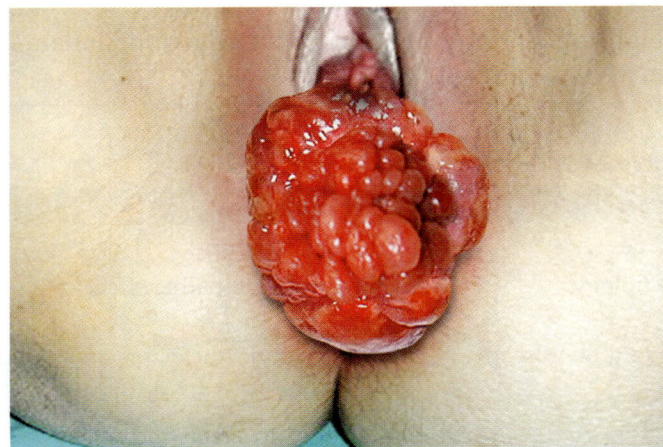

Fig. 24.15: Botryoides rhabdomyosarcoma. Tumor resembles cluster of grapes.

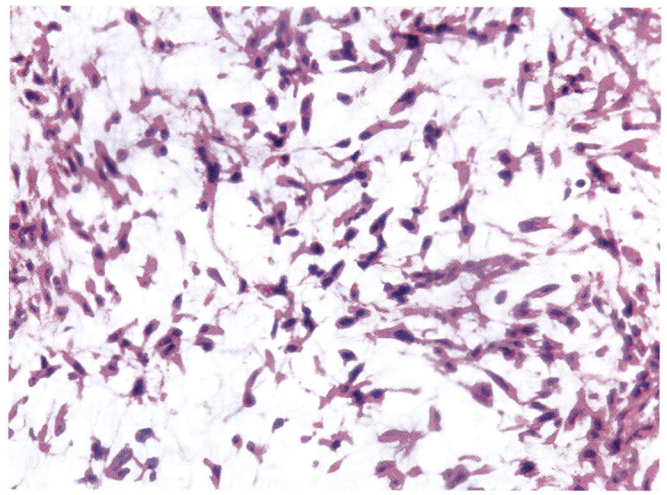

Fig. 24.16: Tumor is composed of numerous round to oval cells admixed with spindle cells in loose myxoid stroma (400X).

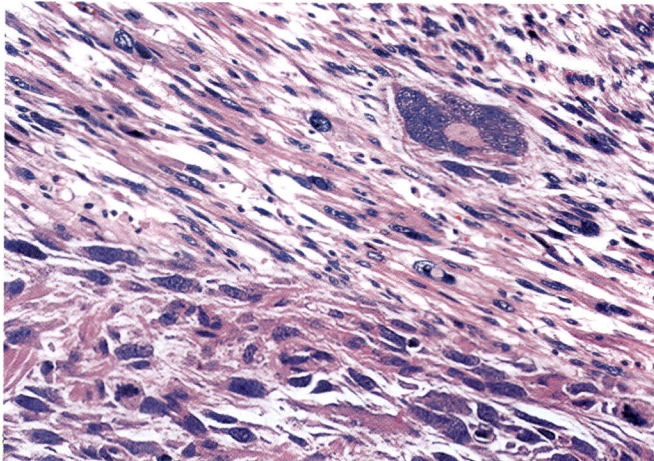

Fig. 24.17: Leiomyosarcoma. As with sarcomas in general, leiomyosarcomas have spindle cells. Several mitoses are seen here, just in this one high power field (400X).

Immunohistochemistry
Tumor cells are immunopositive for skeletal muscle markers such as *actin, desmin, myoD1, vimentin, myoglobin,* and *myogenin*.

Marker	Expression
Desmin	Positive
Myogenin	Positive
Vimentin	Positive
Myoglobin	Positive
MyoD1	Positive
Actin	Positive

Treatment and Prognosis
Combined surgical excision, radiation therapy and chemotherapy increase survival rates in these children with this neoplasm. Prognosis is most often excellent.

LEIOMYOSARCOMA
Leiomyosarcoma is the most common malignant vaginal mesenchymal tumor.

Gross Morphology
- Tumor measures 3–5 cm in diameter.
- Tumor is soft with irregular borders and areas of necrosis on gross examination or not bulging above the surface when cut.
- Single best criterion for predicting the behavior of smooth muscle tumors is mitotic activity.

Light Microscopy
Pleomorphic spindle-shaped tumor cells show moderate to marked nuclear atypia and ≥5 mitoses per high power fields (Fig. 24.17) and foci of necrosis.

Immunohistochemistry
Tumor cells are immunopositive for SMA and S-100.

Marker	Expression
SMA	Positive
S-100	Positive

MELANOMA
Malignant melanoma of the vagina is a rare malignant neoplasm. It most often affects postmenopausal women in the lower-third of the vagina.

Gross Morphology
Tumor is bulky mass with or without pigmentation.

Light Microscopy
- Tumor is composed of melanoma cells larger than nevus cells. These cells contain large nuclei with irregular contours with prominent eosinophilic nucleoli (Fig. 24.18).
- Chromatin is clumped at the periphery of the nuclear membrane.

Immunohistochemistry
It shows positivity for S-100 protein, MART-1 (melan-A), Ki-67, CAM-5.2, and HMB-45. Extra-mammary Paget's disease shows positivity for mucin, but melanoma not.

Marker	Expression
HMB-45	Positive
MART-1 (melan-A)	Positive
Tyrosinase	Positive
Ki-67 (excellent marker)	Positive
S-100	Positive
CAM-5.2	Positive

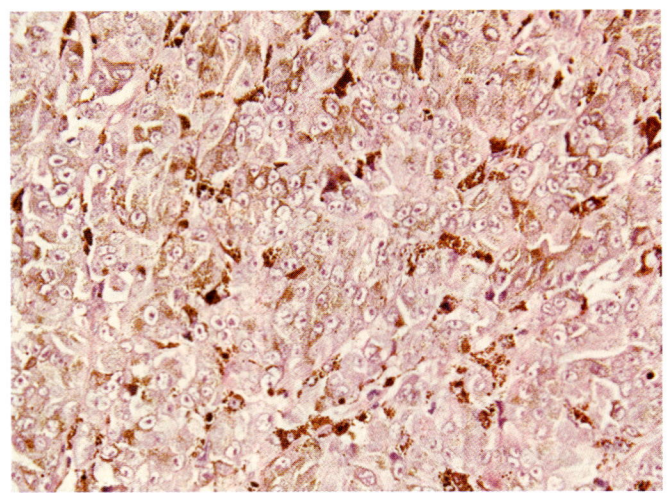

Fig. 24.18: Malignant melanoma. Tumor is composed of melanoma cells (400X).

Clinical Course

Vaginal melanomas are treated by surgical excision, radiotherapy and chemotherapy. Prognosis is very poor with high recurrence rate.

PELVIC INFLAMMATORY DISEASE

Extension of infection from vagina, fallopian tubes or ovaries into pelvis is known as pelvic inflammatory disease. It most often affects women in reproductive age group between 20 and 40 years.

Etiology

- It is most often a complication of sexually transmitted infections (40–45%). It is caused by *Neisseria gonorrhoeae* and *Chlamydia trachomatis*.
- Polymicrobial infections (staphylococci, streptococci, or enteric bacteria) during delivery or abortion are responsible for pelvic inflammatory disease in 45–50% of cases.
- Other causes include tuberculosis (5%), vaginal amoebiasis, and Actinomyces (intrauterine contraceptive device) (Fig. 24.19).

Clinical Features

- Patient presents with abdominal tenderness (direct/rebound), tenderness on movement of cervix and uterus, adnexal tenderness, positive endocervical smear for gonococcal infection, fever, leucocytosis, and purulent material on lapsroscopy or culdocentesis. Infection spreads via periluminal route, hence chances of fertility are bright.

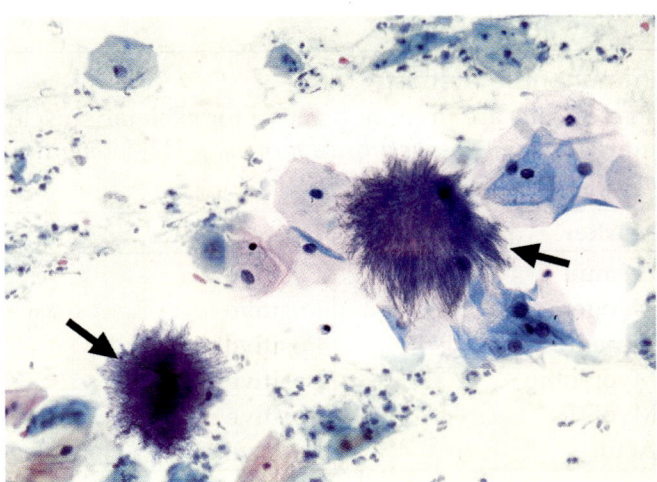

Fig. 24.19: *Actinomyces israelii*. Pap smear shows cotton ball-like pseudofilamentous appearance in woman with intrauterine device (arrows) (400X).

Table 24.3: Characteristics of pelvic pain

Parameters	Uterine pain	Ovarian pain	Pelvic adhesions or infection	Endometriosis
Location	Midline	Left or right iliac fossa	Generalized lower abdominal pain more on one side	Variable
Onset of pain	Before menstrual period	Sudden, intermittent	Pain, acute or chronic	Sudden
Character	Cramping	Gripping pain	Shooting gripping pain	Shooting cramping
Radiation	Lower back and upper thighs	Groin region, if free fluid it radiates to shoulders	–	–
Associated features	Bleeding per vagina	Ovarian cysts, pregnancy or irregular menstrual cycle	Discharge, fever, post-surgery	Infertility
Timing	Pain during menstruation	May be cyclic pain	Acute pain, may be cyclic	Builds up during menstrual period
Exacerbating	–	Positional pain	Movement, clinical examination	Intercourse, cyclical
Severity	Variable spasms	Intense spasm	Intense in waves	Varies

- Tuberculosis as well as Chlamydia spread via intraluminal route hence cause infertility. Patient develops acute or chronic pelvic inflammatory disease depending on the causative organisms.

Complications

- Infertility occurs due to occlusion of fallopian tubes. Patients with chronic nonspecific infection present with fever, malaise, and fatigue.

- Pelvic mass, which is tender and often associated with pain during urinary bladder distension or defecation or intercourse (dyspareunia).
- Patients with spreading infection develop peritoneal adhesions or generalized bacteremia.

Differential Diagnosis

Pelvic pain may occur due to disorders of uterus, ovaries, pelvic adhesions and endometriosis (Table 24.3).

CERVIX

INFLAMMATORY DISEASES

Acute cervicitis is a pattern of inflammation marked by neutrophilic infiltrate in stroma and epithelium. It shows edema and reactive epithelial atypia. Acute cervicitis is caused by bacteria, viruses, fungi and protozoa.

Chronic cervicitis comprises lymphocytes and plasma cells infiltrate. Papillary endocervicitis refers to inflammation of endocervical mucosa forming papillary structures.

NONINFECTIOUS CERVICITIS

Noninfectious cervicitis can occur due to chemical exposure, pessary, tampons and surgical trauma.

> **Light Microscopy**
> Cervix may show infiltration by neutrophils or lymphocytes and plasma cells or granulomatous lesions.

BACTERIAL CERVICITIS

- Bacterial cervicitis is caused by *Neisseria gonorrhoeae* (sexual transmission) and *Chlamydia trachomatis*. Patient presents with mucopurulent discharge. *Chlamydia trachomatis* may produce follicular cervicitis in chronic cases.
- *Actinomyces israelii* infection is associated with intrauterine device use. It is demonstrated in *pseudofilamentous structures* in Pap smears.
- Ophthalmia neonatorum, a neonatal conjunctival infection is acquired at delivery caused by *Neisseria gonorrhoeae*.

CHRONIC CERVICITIS

Chronic cervicitis occurs due to *Candida albicans*, *Trichomonas vaginalis* and *Chlamydia trachomatis*. The latter is associated with reactive lymphoid follicles. Erosion is characterized by columnar epithelium replacing squamous epithelium, grossly resulting in an erythematous area. Sometimes it is a manifestation of chronic cervicitis. The condition is often asymptomatic. It may be manifested by cervical discharge (Figs 24.20 and 24.21).

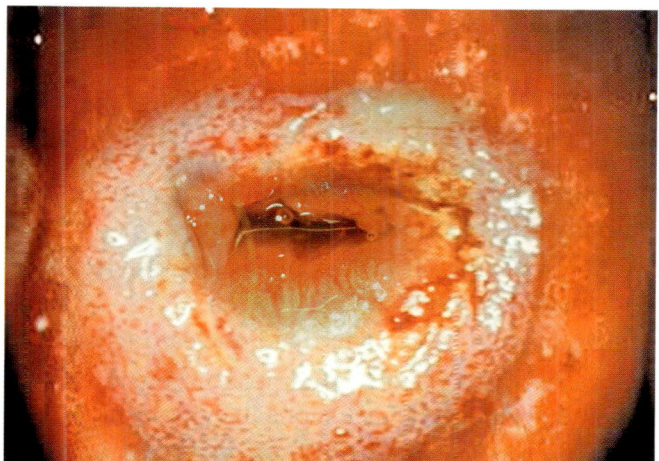

Fig. 24.20: Chronic cervicitis—chronic cervicitis with ectropion of the cervix (columnar epithelium has replaced squamous epithelium). The latter is shown as an extensive reddened zone. The cervix is also scarred and deformed from previous deliveries.

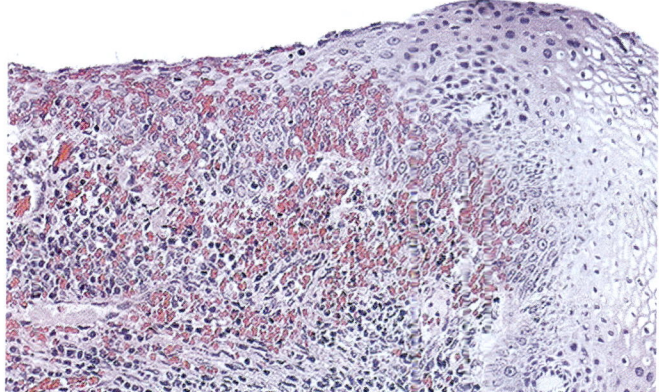

Fig. 24.21: Chronic cervicitis—this is chronic cervicitis at the squamocolumnar junction of the cervix. Small round dark lymphocytes are seen in the submucosa, and there is also hemorrhage. Chronic cervicitis is quite common.

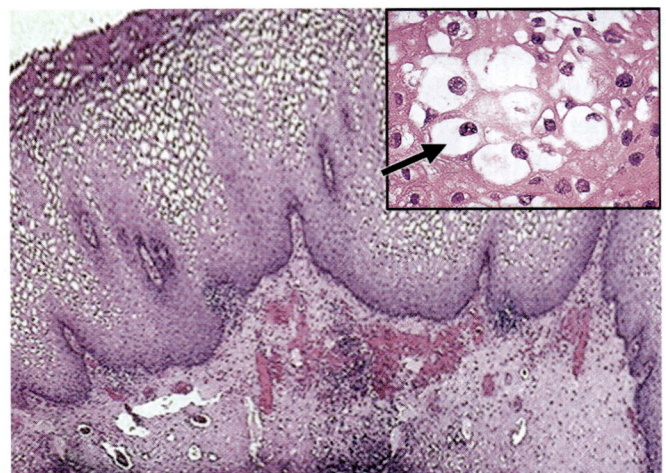

Fig. 24.22: Chronic cervicitis—this cervical biopsy demonstrates a thickened squamous epithelium and the squamous cells have a vacuolated appearance. This is koilocytotic change. A condyloma accuminatum would have a similar appearance (arrow) (100X).

Viral Cervicitis

- *Herpes simplex virus type 2:* It causes ulceration resulting in cervicitis. Light microscopy shows enlarged epithelial nuclei, molding of nuclei, multinucleation, and margination of chromatin in virally infected at the edge of ulcer.
- *Cytomegalovirus:* It causes nuclear and cytoplasmic inclusions in infected cervix.
- *Adenovirus:* It causes smudged nuclear inclusions.
- *Poxvirus:* Molluscum contagiosum generates large round eosinophilic inclusions in cytoplasm.
- *Human papillomavirus (HPV 16, 18, 31, 33 or 45):* It is responsible for cervical intraepithelial neoplasia (CIN I, CIN II, CIN III) and cervical carcinoma (Fig. 24.22).

Granulomatous Cervicitis

Granulomatous cervicitis is caused by *Mycobacterium tuberculosis* and *Treponema pallidum*.

Gross Morphology
Cervix shows extensive reddened areas.

Light Microscopy
- Chronic cervicitis occurs at the squamocolumnar junction of the cervix.
- Submucosa of cervix is infiltrated by chronic inflammatory cells.

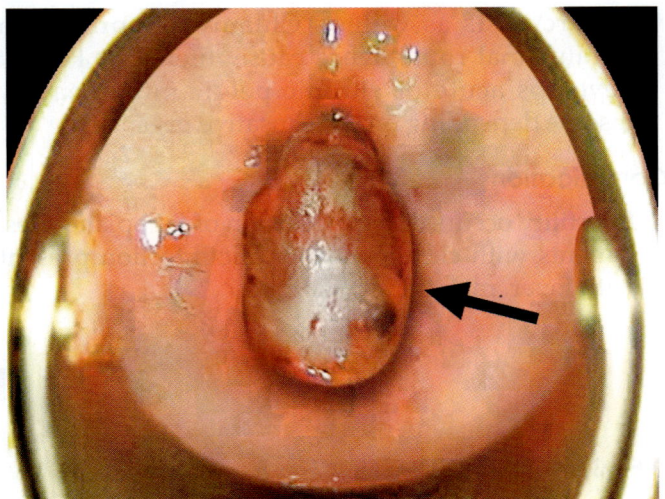

Fig. 24.23: Endocervical polyp (arrow).

NEOPLASMS OF CERVIX AND CIN

ENDOCERVICAL POLYP

It is most common benign cervical growth. Per vaginal examination reveals single smooth or lobulated mass measuring less than 3 cm in greatest dimension (Fig. 24.23).

Clinical Features

Patient presents with vaginal bleeding or discharge as a result of erosions and granulation tissue.

Light Microscopy
- It reveals that polyp is lined by mucinous epithelium with varying degrees of squamous metaplasia.
- It rarely undergoes malignant change in 0.2% of cases.
- Simple excision or curettage is curative (Fig. 24.24).

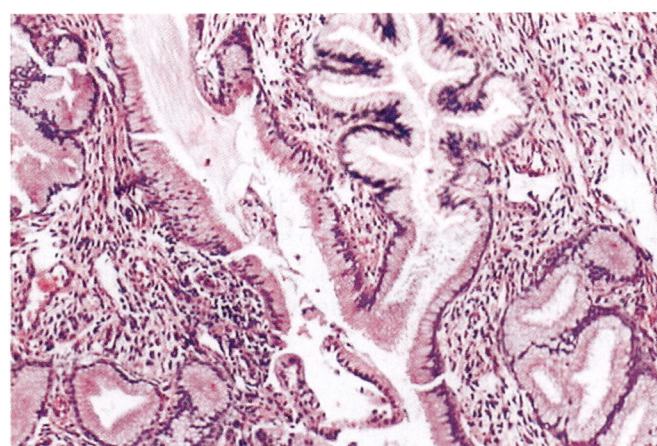

Fig. 24.24: Endocervical polyp (100X).

Female Reproductive System

CERVICAL INTRAEPITHELIAL NEOPLASIA (CIN)

- Cervical intraepithelial neoplasia is disordered epithelial dysplastic lesion manifested by loss of polarity and nuclear hyperchromasia beginning at the basal layer and extending upwards.
- Based on extent of involvement of cervical epithelium, the lesions are sub-classified into three types seen on histopathological examination: CIN I, CIN II, and CIN III.

The principal significance of CIN is its precursor role in the genesis of invasive cervical carcinoma. Genomic integration of HPV DNA sequences, most often types 16, 18, 31, 33 or 45 is associated with CIN, as well as with frank malignant change (Figs 24.25 to 24.28 and Table 24.4).

CIN I (Mild Dysplasia)

- Cervical intraepithelial neoplasia I (CIN I) is a low grade lesion. It affects 20–30 years old women.
- It involves the innermost one-third of the cervical epithelium affecting 20–30 years old women.
- More than 85% of all CIN I regress spontaneously, 10% progress to CIN III, and 2–3% progress to invasive carcinoma.

CIN II (Moderate Dysplasia)

- It involves innermost two-thirds of thickness of epithelium affecting 30–40 years old women.
- It may progress to CIN III in many patients.

CIN III (Severe Dysplasia)

- It involves the full thickness of the cervical epithelium affecting 30–40 years old women. It does not invade the basement membrane.
- Approximately 25% of all untreated cases may progress to invasive carcinoma within 10 years of diagnosis. Such involved cervix must be excised by

Table 24.4: Classification of HPV-associated cervical intraepithelial neoplasia (CIN)

Classification of CIN		Synonym	
CIN I	Low grade CIN	Mild dysplasia	Low grade squamous intraepithelial lesion
CIN II	Moderate CIN	Moderate dysplasia	High grade squamous intraepithelial lesion
CIN III	Severe dysplasia or carcinoma *in situ*	Severe dysplasia	High grade squamous intraepithelial lesion

CIN is a flat lesion. Pap smear examination is done to evaluate cells morphology

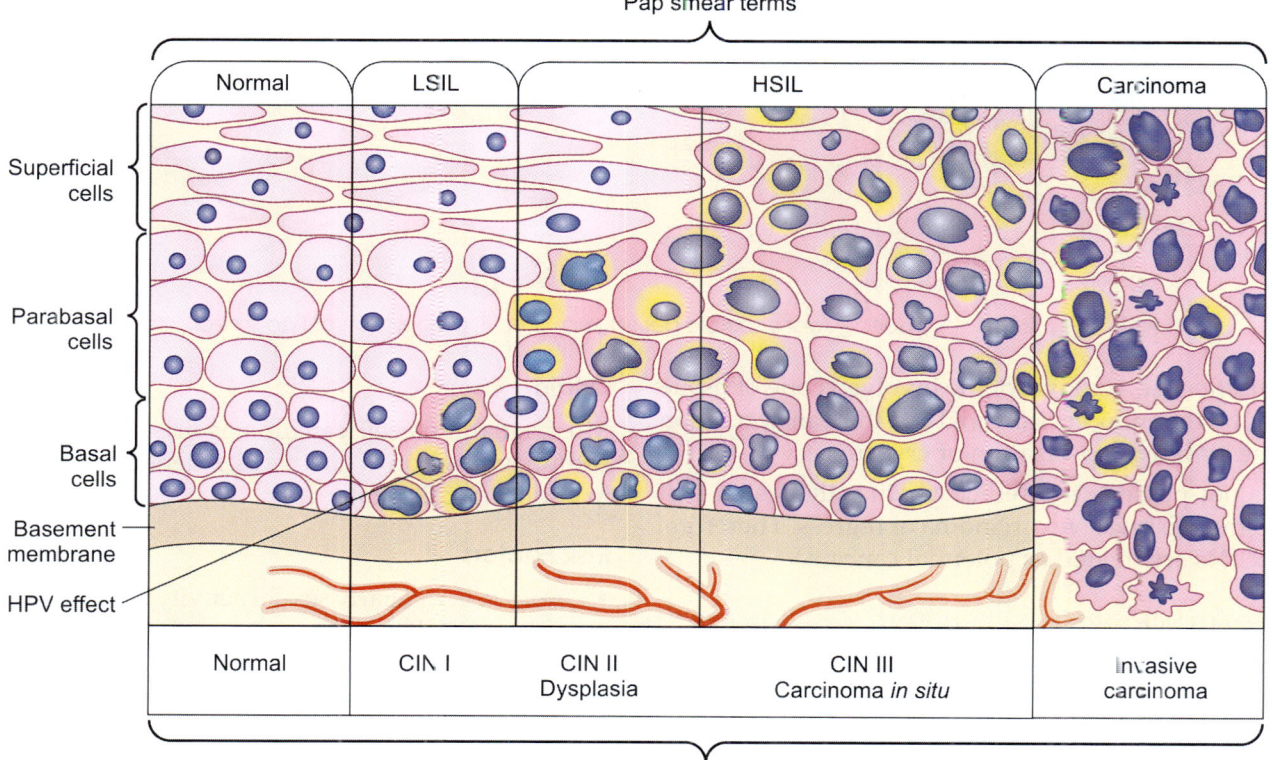

Fig. 24.25: Development of cervical intraepithelial neoplasia (CIN I, CIN II, CIN III) and cervical carcinoma.

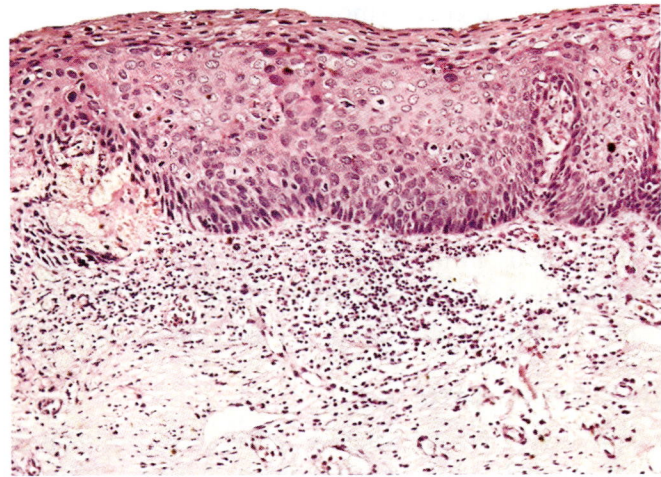

Fig. 24.26: CIN II cervix—moderate dysplastic epithelium, lower two-thirds epithelial layer is undifferentiated. The upper dermis shows dense inflammation (100X).

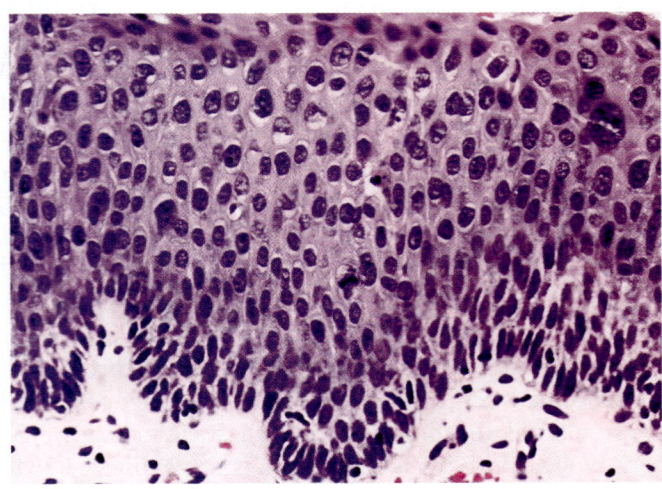

Fig. 24.27: CIN III (cervical intraepithelial neoplasia). This is cervical squamous dysplasia at high magnification extending from the center to the right. The epithelium is normal at the left. Note how the dysplastic cell nuclei are larger and darker, and the dysplastic cells have a disorderly arrangement (400X).

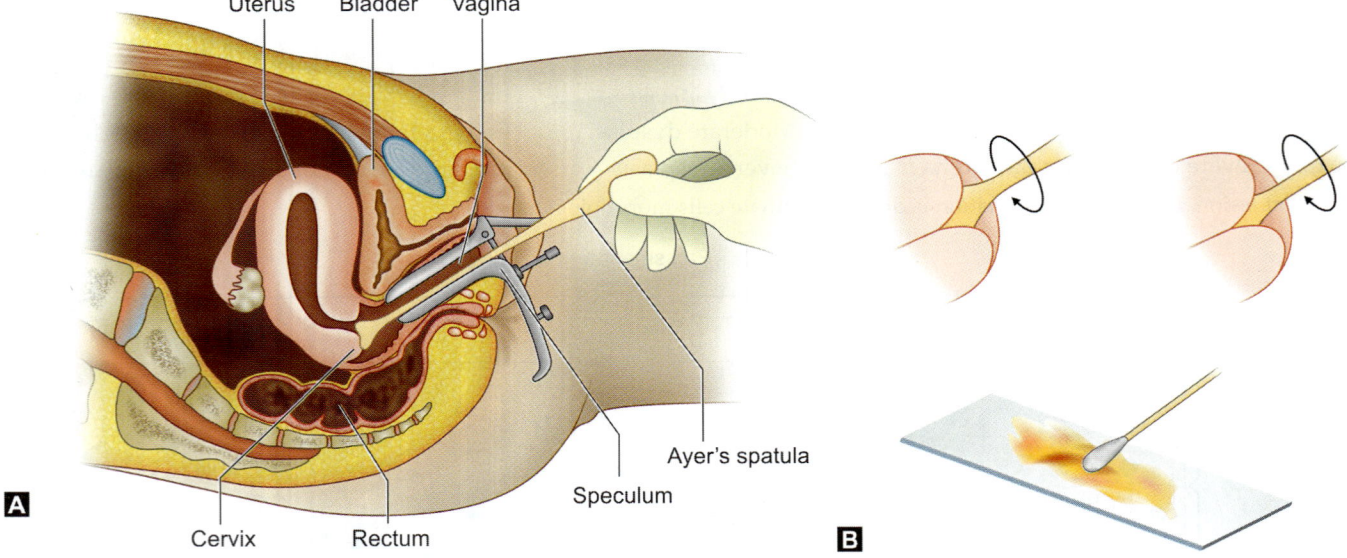

Fig. 24.28: (A) Inserting Ayer's spatule per vagina, and (B) preparation of Pap smear.

conization (i.e. removal of the involved cone of tissue around the endocervical canal and the transformation zone by laser vaporization or cryosurgery).
- It is not possible to predict whether the lesion will progress to invasive carcinoma or regress. Therefore, all CINs are treated as potential cancers.

CERVICAL CARCINOMA

Cervical carcinoma is most common malignant tumor of the female genital tract. It has biphasic age incidence 20–39 years and >50 years. It rarely occurs in those younger than age 20 years. Clinical features depend on stage of the disease.

Origin
Most squamous cell carcinomas arise at the squamocolumnar junction of *external os*. Adenocarcinoma arises in endocervical canal.

Risk Factors
- *Sexual activity:* Early sexual activity (<16 years of age) with multiple partners is associated with cervical cancer.

  There is increased risk of cervical carcinoma in women, who have sexual contact with high risk sexual partners, who had either former wife with cervical carcinoma or penile condylomas.

Female Reproductive System

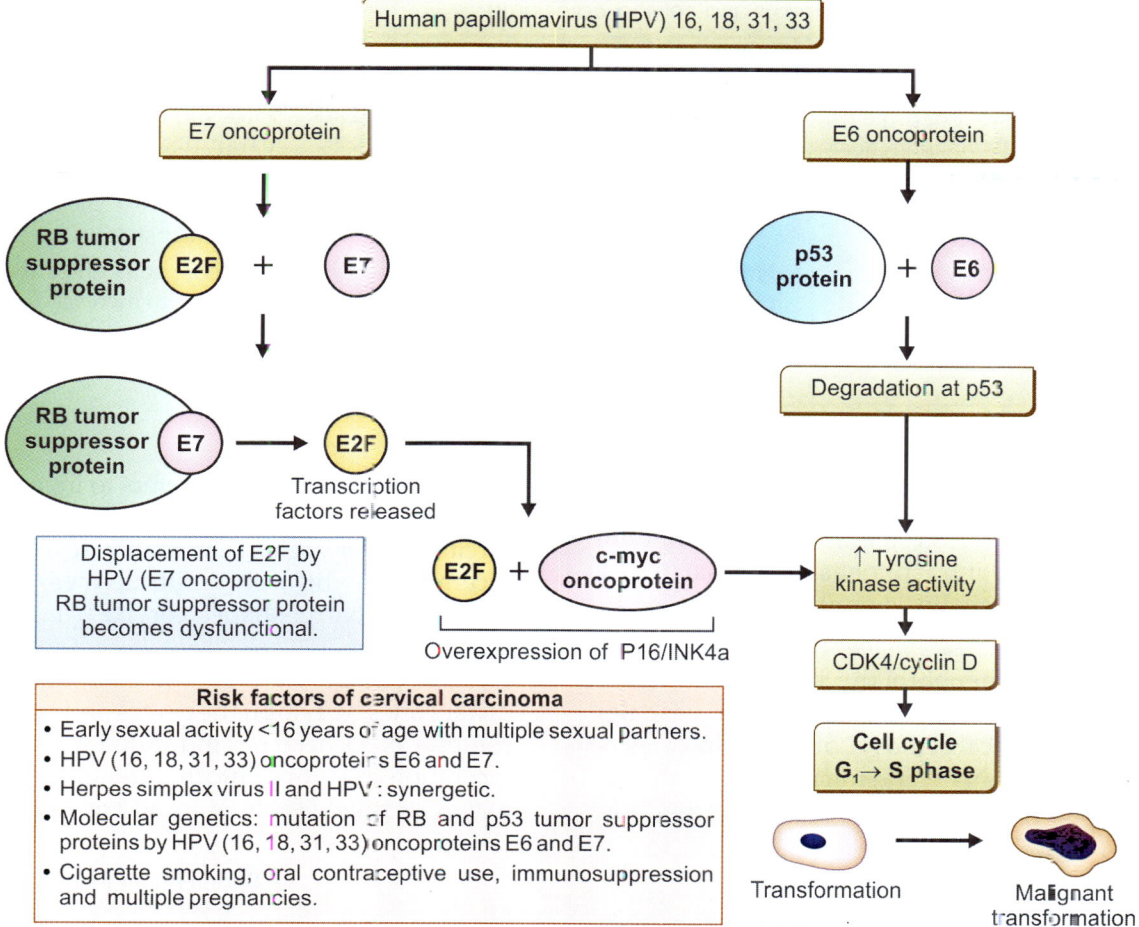

Fig. 24.29: Principles of HPV E6 and E7 oncogene activity in cervical carcinoma.

- *Human papillomavirus:* Genomic integration of HPV DNA sequences, most often types 16, 18, 31, 33 or 45 transmitted by sexual contact is associated with CIN, as well as with cervical carcinoma.

- *Herpes simplex II:* It acts as a promoter. HPV viral proteins E6 and E7 bind and inactivate the gene products of p53 and Rb, respectively. HPV and herpes simplex may be synergetic.

- *Molecular genetics:* Activation of the RAS oncogene and p53 tumor suppressor gene mutation plays an important role in cervical oncogenesis.

- *Cigarette smoking:* It has an important co-carcinogenic role.

- *Oral contraceptive use, immunosuppression and multiple pregnancies:* These increase risk of cervical carcinoma manyfolds.

Human Papillomavirus and Cervical Carcinoma

- HPV 16, 18 are associated with cervical cancer. Vaccines against some of human papillomavirus are available. HPV 16, 18 infect immature epithelial basal cells at the squamocolumnar junction.

- It produces *koilocytic atypia*, consisting of nuclear atypia and a cytoplasmic perinuclear halo.

These viruses cannot infect the mature superficial squamous cells that cover the ectocervix, vagina, or vulva. Human papillomavirus plays an important role in the pathogenesis of cervical carcinoma (Table 24.5, Figs 24.29 and 24.30).

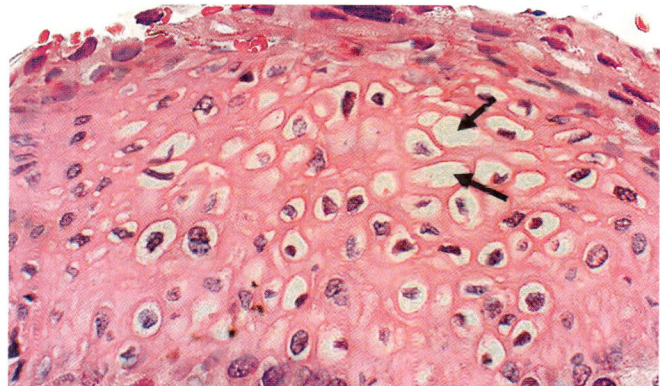

Fig. 24.30: Human papillomavirus in cervix—high power view of HPV infection characterized by cells with pyknotic, irregular nuclei and clear cytoplasm. Moderate squamous dysplasia is also present (arrows).

Section III: Systemic Pathology

Table 24.5: E7 and E6 of human papillomavirus and cervical carcinoma

Mechanism of action	E7 oncoprotein	E6 oncoprotein
• Gene products of HPV 16, 18 viruses inactivate tumor suppressor proteins. Once inside the cells of their host, human papillomavirus (16, 18) synthesizes a protein designated E7 and another designated E6	• It increases activity of CDK4/cyclin D by inactivating CDK inhibitors (p21 and p27). It binds to the RB protein and displaces transcription factor E2F	• It degrades p53 protein. It stimulates the expression of TERT, the catalytic subunit of telomerase resulting in increased tyrosine kinase activity. These changes cause genome instability
• Oncoproteins encoded by the E6 and E7 genes of HPV16 bind p53 and Rb	• Now E2F is free to bind to the promoters of genes (like c-myc) that cause the cell to enter the cell cycle. Therefore, inhibition of p21 and RB-E2F causes increased activity of CDK4/cyclin D results in genome instability	• The host cells enter the cell cycle resulting in increased proliferation

Evolution of Cervical Carcinoma

- *Cervical intraepithelial neoplasia:* Initially, patient developing cervical intraepithelial neoplasia (CIN I, CIN II, CIN III) is usually asymptomatic.
- *Microinvasive cervical carcinoma:* It refers to stromal invasion <5 mm beneath the basement membrane without evidence of lymphatic or vascular involvement. Surgical removal of cervix in cases of severe dysplasia (CIN III) and microinvasive cervical carcinoma is associated with an excellent prognosis.
- *Early invasive carcinoma:* It refers to invasion of basement membrane and underlying stroma by cervical carcinoma. Per vagina examination reveals fungating, ulcerative or diffusely infiltrative cervical growth resulting in barrel-shaped cervix.
- *Advanced invasive carcinoma:* It can spread directly to adjacent pelvic structures or disseminate to distant sites by lymphatic routes and hematogenous routes. Cervix becomes indurated with necrosis and ulceration, resulting information of large fungating mass is formed (Table 24.6 and Fig. 24.31).

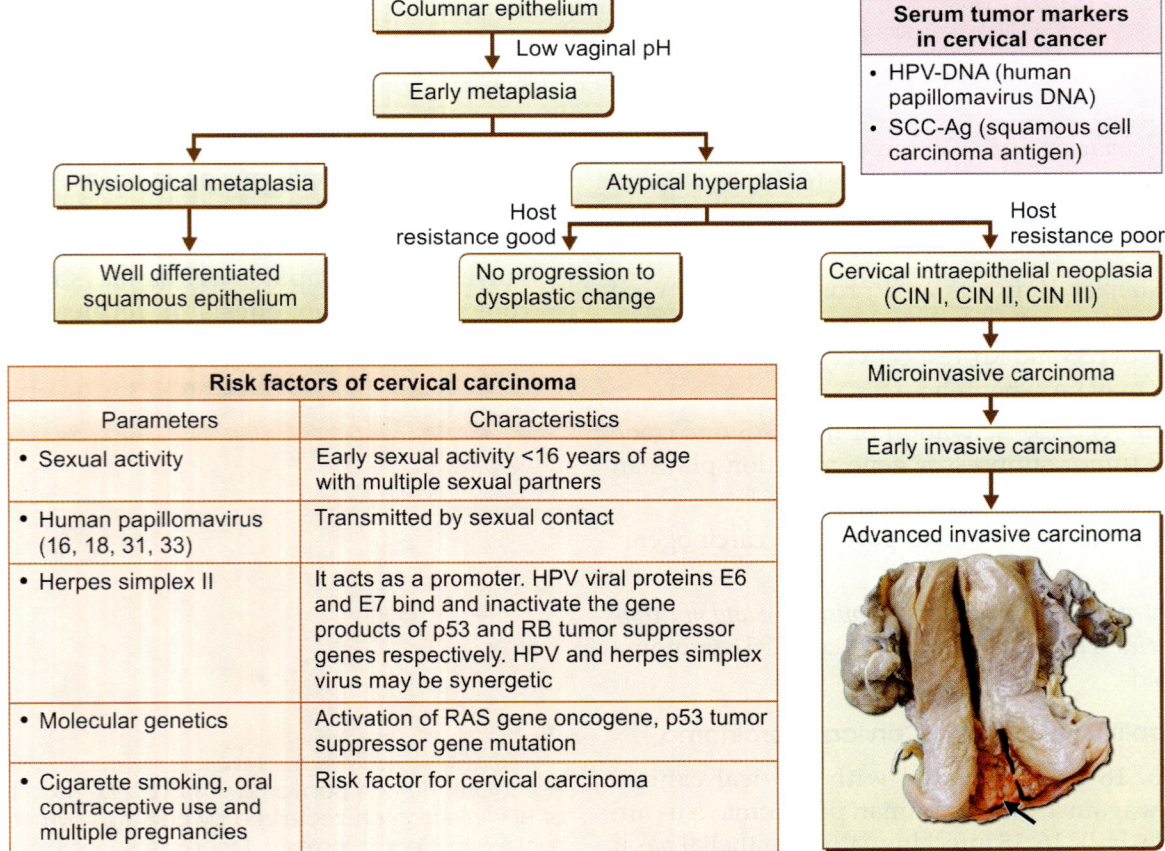

Fig. 24.31. Development of cervical intraepithelial neoplasia (CIN I, CIN II, CIN III) and cervical carcinoma (arrow).

Table 24.6: Evolution of cervical carcinoma

Sequence of evolution	Characteristics
Cervical intraepithelial neoplasia	CIN I, CIN II, CIN III
Microinvasive cervical carcinoma	Stromal invasion <5 mm beneath the basement membrane without evidence of lymphatic or vascular involvement
Early invasive carcinoma	Invasion of basement membrane and underlying stroma by cervical carcinoma
Advanced invasive carcinoma (fungating tumor)	Metastases to adjacent pelvic structures and distant metastases (lungs, liver) by lymphatic routes and hematogenous routes

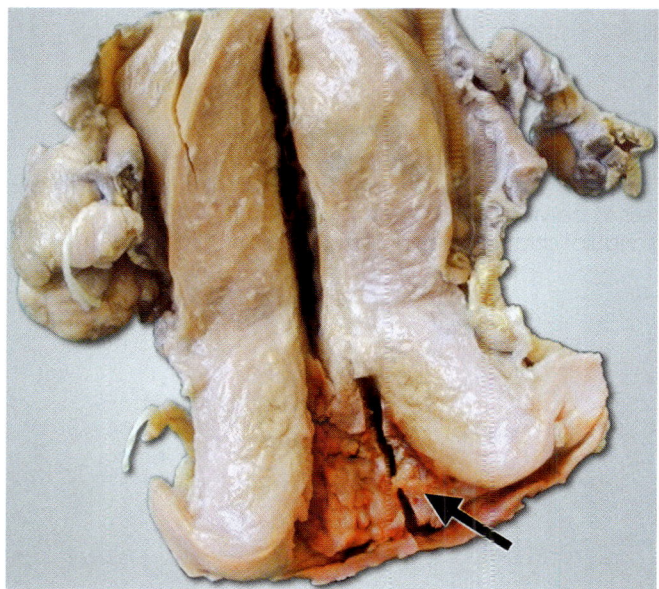

Fig. 24.32: Cervical carcinoma. Growth is seen in cervical region (arrow).

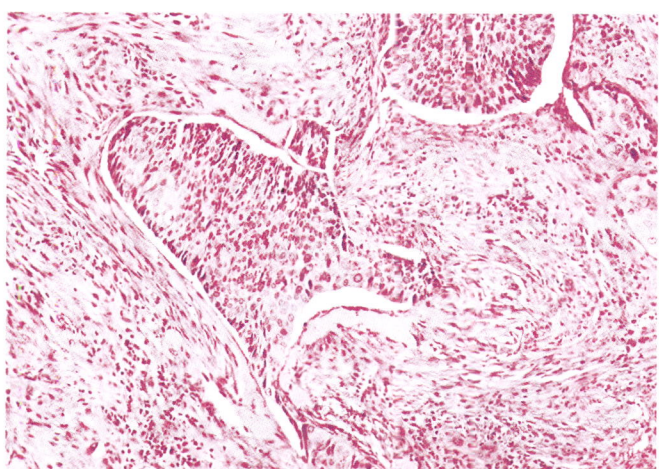

Fig. 24.33: Cervical large cell non-keratinizing squamous cell carcinoma (400X).

Gross Morphology
Early stages of cervical cancer often manifest as poorly defined, granular, eroded lesions or nodular and exophytic mass (Fig. 24.32).

Light Microscopy
Histological variants of cervical carcinoma (Table 24.7) include squamous cell carcinoma (non-keratinizing or keratinizing), adenocarcinoma, adenosquamous or small cell carcinoma (Figs 24.33 to 24.37). Cytomorphological features of cervical squamous cell carcinoma is described in Fig. 24.38.

- *Squamous cell carcinoma:* It accounts for 80–90% of cases. It is further sub-classified as large cell non-keratinizing (most common 65%). Large cell variant producing keratinizing pearls and prickle cells (25%); and small cell type (poor prognosis). In almost all cases, squamous cell carcinoma varies from well differentiated to highly anaplastic carcinoma.

- *Adenocarcinoma:* It accounts for 10–20% of malignant cervical tumors. It arises from mucus producing endocervical glands. It affects elderly women (mean 55 years). It shares etiological factors with squamous cell carcinoma of the cervix and spreads similarly. Malignant cells are frequently infected with HPV types 16 and 18.

Table 24.7: Histological variants of cervical carcinoma

Histological variants	%	Characteristics
Squamous cell carcinoma	80–90%	Large cell non-keratinizing (65%) Large cell keratinizing producing keratinizing pearls and prickle cells (25%) Small cell carcinoma (poor prognosis)
Adenocarcinoma	10–20%	It arises from endocervical glands Malignant cells are frequently infected with HPV types 16 and 18
Adenosquamous carcinoma	<%	It arises from reserve cells in cervix. It has favorable prognosis
Small cell carcinoma	Rare	More aggressive course than the conventional squamous cell carcinoma

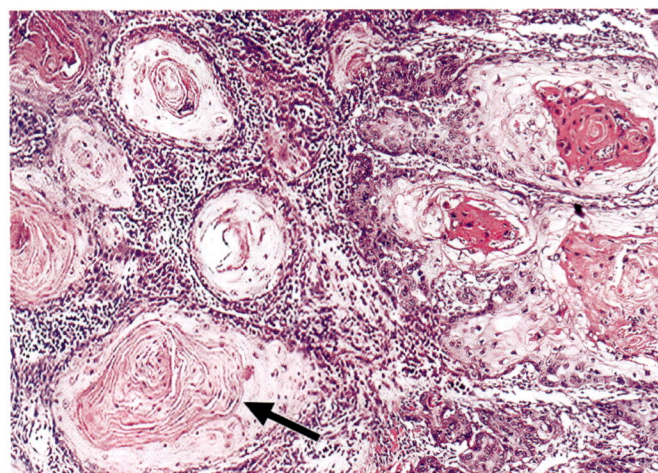

Fig. 24.34: Cervical squamous cell carcinoma. At high magnification, nests of neoplastic squamous cells are invaded through a chronically inflamed stroma. This cancer is well-differentiated, as evidenced by keratin pearls (arrow). However, most cervical squamous carcinomas are non-keratinizing (400X).

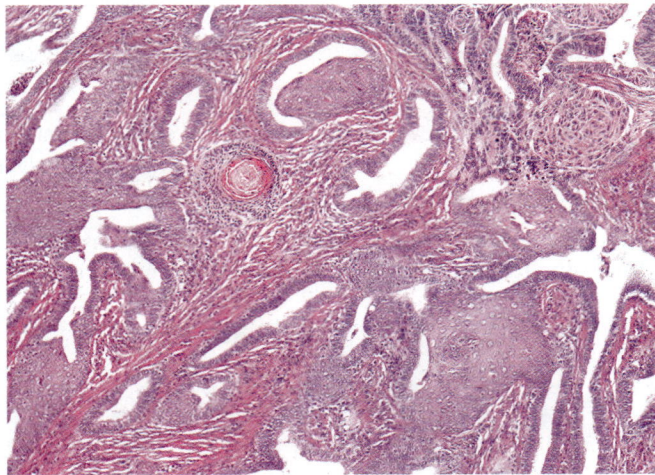

Fig. 24.36: Adenosquamous carcinoma. It arises from reserve cells in cervix with favorable prognosis. Tumor is composed of glandular and squamous components (400X).

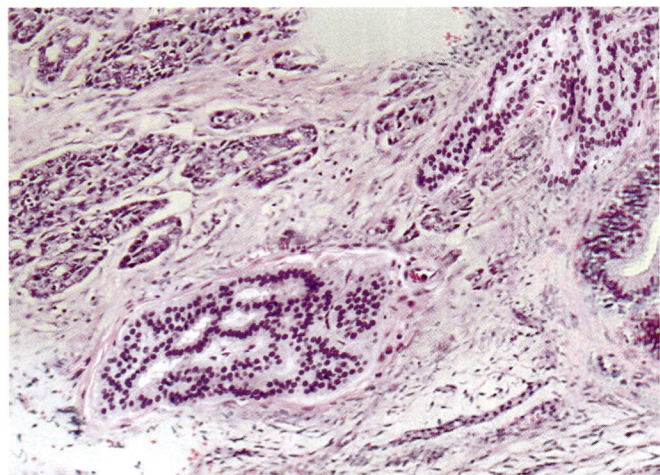

Fig. 24.35: Adenocarcinoma. It arises from mucus producing endocervical glands. Tumor cells are arranged in glandular pattern (400X).

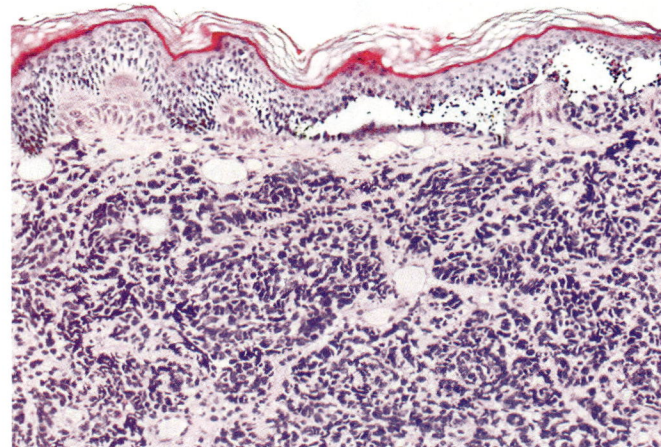

Fig. 24.37: Small cell carcinoma (400X). Tumor is composed of small atypical cells. It has poor prognosis (100X).

- *Adenosquamous carcinoma:* It accounts for 4% of malignant cervical tumors. It arises from reserve cells in cervix with favorable prognosis.
- *Small cell carcinoma:* It is rare having more aggressive course than the conventional squamous cell carcinoma.

Mode of Spread (Table 24.8)

- *Direct invasion:* In early stage, local extension into surrounding tissues (parametrium) leads to ureteral compression. It causes hydroureter, hydronephrosis and ultimately renal failure with fatal outcome in 50% of patients.

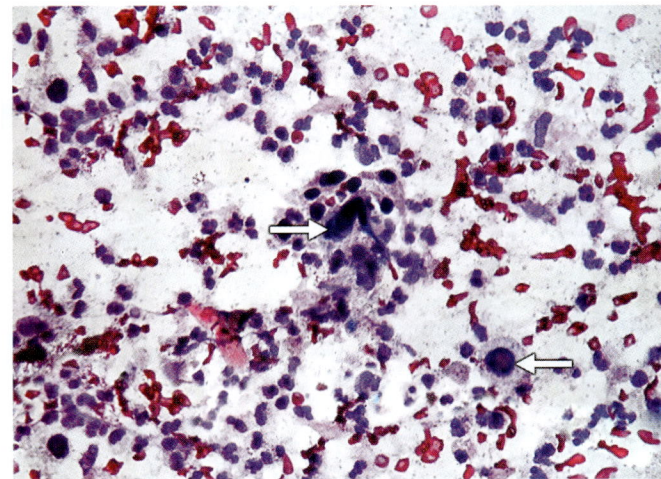

Fig. 24.38: Microphotograph of squamous cell carcinoma with tadpole cell on Pap smear (arrows) (400X).

Table 24.8: Mode of spread of cervical carcinoma

Mode of spread	Characteristics
Direct invasion	Parametrium Compression of ureter causes hydroureter, hydronephrosis and ultimately acute renal failure (50%)
Lymphatic route	Pelvic nodes (e.g. paracervical, obturator, external iliac, internal iliac, common iliac and aortic lymph nodes)
Hematogenous route	Distant metastases to lungs, liver, bones and brain

In later stage, bladder and rectal involvement may lead to fistula formation. Spread along the uterosacral ligaments involves the sacral nerves, causing severe pain. In some cases, the growth encircles the 'external os', and obstructs the cervical canal leading to development of pyometra.

- *Lymphatic spread:* It involves the chains of pelvic nodes (e.g. paracervical, obturator, external iliac, internal iliac, common iliac and aortic lymph nodes). The tumor most commonly extends into contiguous parametrial structures.
- *Hematogenous spread:* In later stages of disease, distant metastases may occur in lungs, liver, bones or brain.

Clinical Features

- Patient is asymptomatic in early stage of cervical carcinoma. Later, patient presents with abnormal persistent bleeding or spotting between menstrual periods or postcoital bleeding and pain.
- In advanced stage, patient presents with pelvic pain, foul smelling vaginal discharge (saprophytic infection), vaginal leakage of stool or urine from a fistula, anorexia, weight loss and anemia.

Laboratory Diagnosis

- *Exfoliative cytology:* Cervical carcinoma and its precursors (cervical intraepithelial neoplasia) can be detected by vaginal exfoliative cytology. Pap smears can be obtained directly or under colposcopic guidance. Positive exfoliative cytology findings need to be confirmed by biopsy. For occult lesions (contact bleeding and vaginal discharge), Pap smear, colposcopic examination and cervical biopsy are performed.
- *Colposcopy:* 3% acetic acid is applied to transformation zone for visualization of vascular alterations of growth.
- *Schiller's test:* Normal cells are rich in glycogen, while absent in malignant cells. Schiller's test is performed by applying Lugol's iodine (a solution of iodine and potassium iodide). Normal cervical cells give mahogony brown discoloration, while cancerous cells fail to take up the stain.
- *Cervical biopsy:* Punch or wedge biopsy is done at 12, 3, 6 and 9 o'clock position.
- *Endocervical curetting:* It is done with cold knife, which is useful in endocervical cancer when portio vaginalis appears healthy and cervix feels barrel shaped.
- *Conization:* It is done with cold knife. It is indicated in following situations: (i) if no visible lesion is seen on colposcopy, (ii) if cytological follow-up is not possible and (iii) if there is discrepancy between vaginal cytology and directed biopsy.
- *Fractional curettage:* It helps to differentiate endocervical cancer from endometrial adenocarcinoma.

Staging

The clinical stage of cervical carcinoma is the most important prognostic factor for survival. Staging has been developed by FIGO as described in Table 24.9.

Management

Radical hysterectomy (Wertheim's hysterectomy) is favored for localized tumor, especially in younger women. Radiation therapy or combinations of the radiation and hysterectomy are used for more advanced tumors.

Table 24.9: Staging of cervical carcinoma developed by FIGO

Stage	Cervical carcinoma involving structures	5-year survival after treatment
Stage 0	Superficial layers of the cervix	100%
Stage I	Cervix (microscopic to 4 cm in diameter)	80–90%
Stage II	Extension from cervix into the surrounding area, vagina or tissues surrounding uterus	75%
Stage III	Lower vagina and/or the pelvic wall. Large growth blocking the outflow of urine through the urethra. Pelvis lymph nodes may be involved	36%
Stage IV	Urinary bladder, rectum or distant organs such as liver, lungs and other organs	10%

FALLOPIAN TUBES

ANATOMY

Fallopian tube consists of interstitial portion (uterine end), isthmus, ampulla (wider portion) and infundibulum and opens as finger-like projections (towards ovary). Salpingitis can predispose to ectopic pregnancy.

INFLAMMATORY DISEASES

ACUTE SALPINGITIS

It is most often associated with inflammation of endometrium, ovaries and pelvic inflammatory disease in young to middle-aged women. In some cases, acute salpingitis occurs due to abortion, puerperal sepsis, trauma and surgical manipulation.

Etiopathogenesis

It is caused by *Escherichia coli, Neisseria gonorrhoeae* (gram-negative diplococci), *Chlamydia trachomatis*, and Mycoplasma, Staphylococcus and streptococci organisms resulting in suppuration. Damage to the fallopian tube results from acute salpingitis may lead to infertility.

> **Gross Morphology**
> Bilateral fallopian tubes are congested, edematous and lumen filled with purulent exudates (pyosalpinx).
>
> **Light Microscopy**
> Fallopian tube epithelium shows marked infiltration by numerous neutrophils with congestion and edema (Fig. 24.39).

Treatment

Antibiotic therapy resolves the inflammation. If resolution of the acute inflammation does not occur, chronic salpingitis follows with formation of tubo-ovarian mass.

CHRONIC SALPINGITIS

Repeated attacks by organisms cause chronic salpingitis with formation of *violin string* adhesion. Hydrosalpinx may be end stage of chronic salpingitis characterized by thin wall with a few plicae and lumen filled with clear fluid. Numerous adhesions occur on the serosal surface.

> **Gross Morphology**
> Fallopian tube is most often enlarged, fibrotic, disordered and adhered to the ovary and surrounding structures.
>
> **Light Microscopy**
> Plicae of fallopian tube show infiltration by lymphocytes and plasma cells. Fusion of plicae may lead to formation of follicle-like spaces known as *salpingitis follicularis*.

GRANULOMATOUS SALPINGITIS

Granulomatous salpingitis may be caused by tuberculosis, sarcoidosis, Crohn's disease and fungal infections.

Tubercular salpingitis occurs as a result of extension of tubercular infection from endometrium. Spread of tubercular infection through intraluminal route causes adhesions of lining epithelium, resulting in infertility.

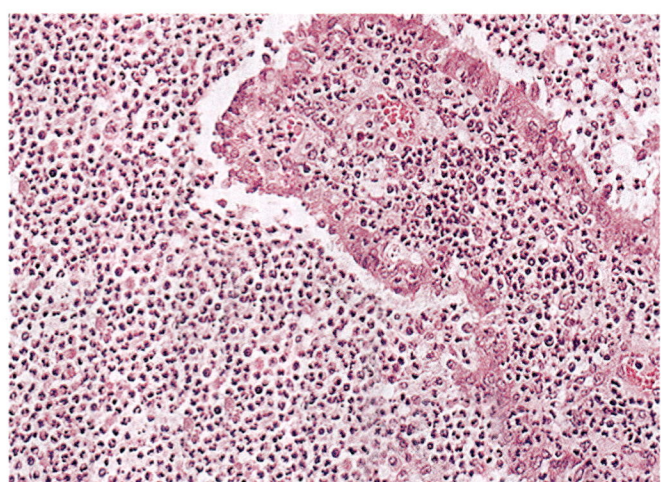

Fig. 24.39: Acute salpingitis. A remnant of tubal epithelium is seen here surrounded and infiltrated by numerous neutrophils. This is acute salpingitis. *Neisseria gonorrhoeae* was cultured.

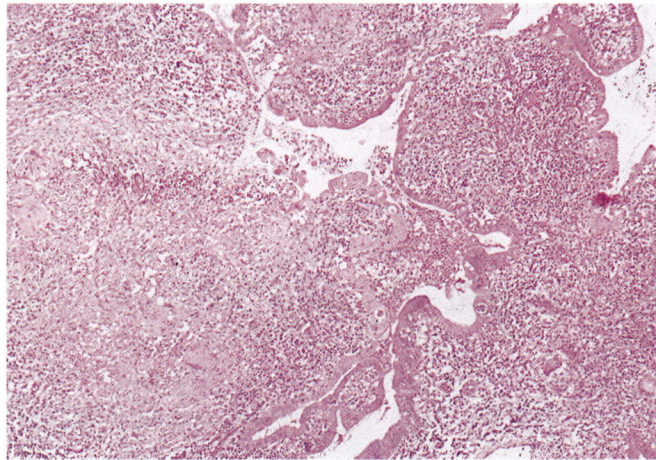

Fig. 24.40: Tubercular salpingitis shows large number of epithelioid cell granulomas, Langhans' giant cells and caseous material. In the background, tubal wall is infiltrated by lymphocytes, macrophages and plasma cells (100X).

Light Microscopy

Fallopian tube shows epithelioid cell granulomas, Langhans' giant cells and caseous necrosis (Fig. 24.40).

SALPINGITIS ISTHMICA NODOSA

Salpingitis isthmica nodosa is most often associated with ectopic pregnancy and infertility in young women. Its pathogenesis is not clear.

Gross Morphology

- Fallopian tubal wall shows a nodule in the isthmus region measuring 1 to 2 cm in diameter.
- Bilateral fallopian tubes are involved in 85% of cases.

Light Microscopy

Fallopian tubal lesion consists if outpouchings of tubal epithelium surrounded by a thickened wall of smooth muscle.

OTHER NON-NEOPLASTIC DISEASES

TUBAL ENDOMETRIOSIS

Presence of normal endometrial glands and stroma in fallopian tubes outside uterine cavity is known as *endometriosis*. Fallopian tubes are most frequently involved due to endometriosis in 1–2% women during reproductive period.

It is an important cause of infertility. Endometriosis regresses after menopause. It is described in details in placental and pregnancy associated disorders.

Gross Morphology

Fallopian tube endometriosis consists of dark brown chocolate-colored serosal nodules.

Light Microscopy

Fallopian tube shows presence of endometrial glands surrounded by endometrial stroma associated with hemosiderin-laden macrophages and chronic inflammatory cells.

ECTOPIC PREGNANCY

Ampulla of the fallopian tube is the most common site of ectopic pregnancy. It is described in details in placental and pregnancy associated disorders.

Risk Factors

These include salpingitis, prior ectopic pregnancy, salpingitis isthmica nodosa, congenital tubal anomalies and endometriosis.

Clinical Features

Patient presents with tubal rupture and shock.

Gross Morphology

Fallopian tube shows dilatation, hemorrhagic, chorionic villi with or without embryo.

Light Microscopy

Fallopian tubal mucosa or wall shows chorionic villi or trophoblast.

NEOPLASTIC DISEASES

ADENOMATOID TUMOR

It is the most common benign tumor of the fallopian tubes. It is derived from mesothelium.

Gross Morphology

Tumor is well circumscribed and white tan-colored seen in tubal wall.

Light Microscopy

Tumor shows slit-like spaces lined by single layer of flattened cuboidal cells (Fig. 24.41).

Immunohistochemistry

Tumor cells are immunopositive for expression of cytokeratin, calretinin, EMA and vimentin. These cells are negative for factor VIII-related antigen and CD31, a profile indicating a mesothelial origin rather from vascular endothelium.

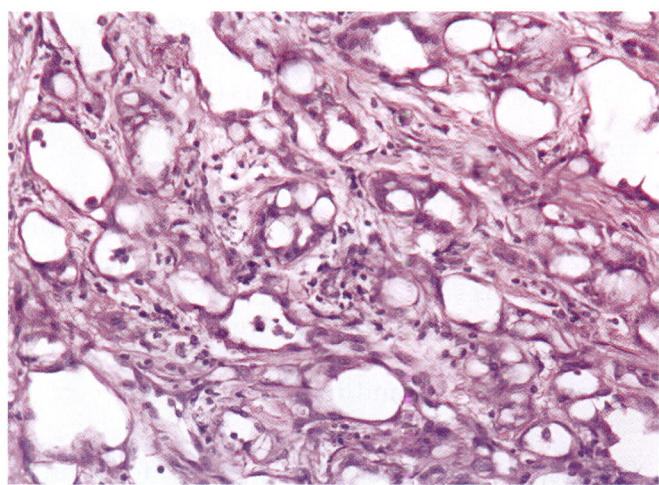

Fig. 24.41: Adenomatoid tumor of the fallopian tube (400X).

Marker	Expression
Cytokeratin	Positive
Calretinin	Positive
Epithelial membrane antigen (EMA)	Positive
Vimentin	Positive
Factor VIII-related antigen	Negative
CD31	Negative

ADENOCARCINOMA

Primary adenocarcinoma of fallopian tube is extremely rare. There is an association with BRCA mutations. In the vast majority of cases, it is associated with bulky tumors extending from the ovary or endometrium. There may be a watery secretion resulting in vaginal discharge.

ENDOMETRIUM

MENSTRUAL (ENDOMETRIAL CYCLE)

Menstrual cycle is stimulated continually by hormones. It denudes its mucosa every month. History of menstrual cycle must be emphasized on age of menarche, length of menstrual cycle, use of contraceptive pills, days of blood loss, number of pads used per day and presence of blood clots. The menstrual cycle (normally 28 days) is sub-divided into the proliferative phase, secretory phase and menstrual phase.

Proliferative Phase

The proliferative phase is associated with gland proliferation and mitoses secondary to estrogen stimulation. During proliferative phase, endometrium becomes 3–4 mm in thickness.

- *Estrogen synthesis:* Estrogen is derived from aromatization of testosterone in the granulosa cells of ovaries. Testosterone and 17-ketosteroids (DHEA and androstenedione) are synthesized in the theca interna of ovary under LH stimulation. Estrogen has a negative feedback on FSH, the later resulting at mid-cycle in the LH surge and the induction of ovulation.
- *Light microscopy:* The epithelium is cuboidal, growing taller as ovulation is approached. The glands are simple. The stromal cells are narrow spindles to begin with, become plump. Glands especially those of cervical region secrete a thin mucus which helps in guiding sperm towards uterus (Fig. 24.42).

Secretory Phase

It starts on the 14th day of menstrual cycle till 21st day under the influence of progesterone hormone. Luteinizing hormone (LH) stimulates ovarian theca interna cells resulting in progesterone synthesis. Progesterone increases the body temperature, which is useful in documenting ovulation. It also increases salt and water retention and inhibits LH. Endometrium becomes 5–6 mm in thickness.

- *Fertilization:* During secretory phase, fertilization occurs in the ampullary portions of the fallopian tube.

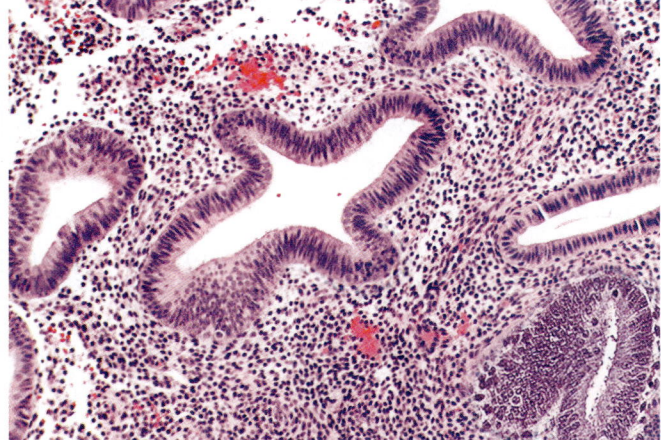

Fig. 24.42: Normal proliferative endometrium. This is the microscopic appearance of normal proliferative endometrium in the menstrual cycle. The proliferative phase is the variable part of the cycle. In this phase, tubular glands with columnar cells and surrounding dense stroma are proliferating to build up the endometrium following shedding with previous menstruation (400X).

It requires 3 days for the embryo to move through the tube and another 2–3 days to implant in the endometrium (day 21).

Syncytiotrophoblastic tissue from the developing placenta synthesizes β-hCG and LH analogue that maintains the production of progesterone by the corpus luteum for 8–10 weeks, after which the placenta takes over hormone production. If fertilization does not take place, secretory phase is followed by menstrual phase.

- *Light microscopy:* Endometrial glands are dilated, tortuous, lined by tall epithelial cells associated with basal nuclei, clear cytoplasm and subnuclear vacuoles (Figs 24.43 and 24.44).

Menstrual Phase

Estrogen eventually declines, the corpus luteum involutes, and progesterone drops, resulting in menstruation. Normal menstrual fluid is non-clotted due to the presence of fibrinolysin. A patient with passage of clots indicates uterine pathology.

Female Reproductive System

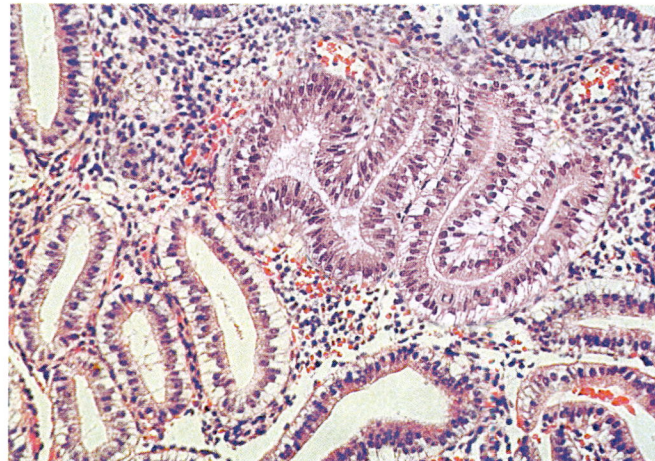

Fig. 24.43: Early secretory endometrium. The appearance with prominent subnuclear vacuoles in cells forming the glands is consistent with post-ovulatory day 2. The histologic changes following ovulation are quite constant over the 14 days to menstruation and can be utilized to date the endometrium (400X).

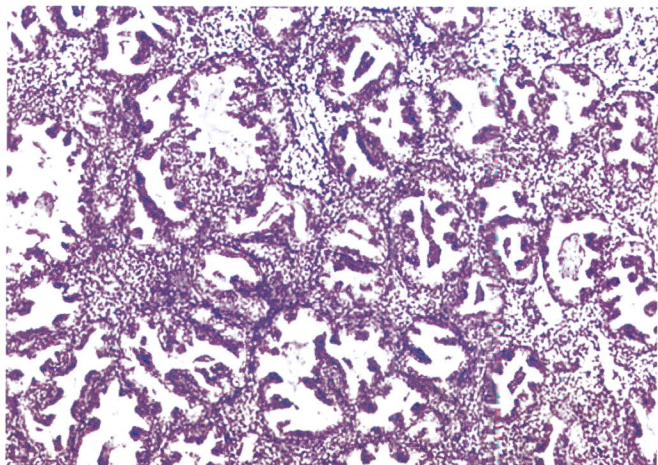

Fig. 24.44: Normal secretory endometrium. This is normal secretory phase endometrium. Note the larger tortuous glands with secretions. The secretory phase starts at 14th day course leading to either implantation of a fertilized ovum or menstruation.

FUNCTIONAL DISORDERS OF MENSTRUAL CYCLE

Functional disorders of menstrual cycle are amenorrhea and dysmenorrhea describes as under.

Amenorrhea

- Amenorrhea is the abnormal absence of menstruation. Absence of menstruation is normal during pregnancy, lactation, before puberty and after menopause. Amenorrhea may be subdivided into primary or secondary.
- Primary amenorrhea is the absence of menarche in an adolescent girls after 16 years of age. Secondary amenorrhea is the absence of menstruation for at least 3 months after the normal onset of menarche.

Etiology

- *Primary amenorrhea:* Imperforate hymen is the most important cause of primary amenorrhea. Dysfunctional hypothalamic-pituitary-ovarian axis causes primary amenorrhea. Turner's syndrome is the most common genetic cause of prepubertal ovarian failure. Anovulation occurs due to deficient synthesis of gonadotropins, estrogens, FSH and LH. Decreased estrogen levels may be secondary to a ypothalamic-pituitary disturbance (low FSH and LH). FSH and LH levels are increased in primary ovarian disorder.
- *Secondary amenorrhea:* Pregnancy and menopause are most common causes of secondary amenorrhea. Hypogonadotropic hypoestrogenic anovulation, endometrial adhesions (Asherman syndrome) and premature ovarian failure cause secondary amenorrhea.

Clinical Features

Patient presents with absence of menstruation, hirsutism, vasomotor flushes and vaginal atrophy. Acne is observed in secondary amenorrhea.

Diagnosis

Radiograph establishes age of the patient. Blood pituitary gonadotropin level, thyroid profile, progesterone, androgen and FSH levels are analyzed. Microscopic examination of cervical mucus is performed to detect *fern test* (estrogenic effect).

Dysmenorrhea

Primary dysmenorrhea (painful menstruation) occurs due to increased production of prostaglandins-F, which increases uterine contractions. Endometriosis is most important cause of secondary dysmenorrhea.

DYSFUNCTIONAL UTERINE BLEEDING (DUB)

Dysfunctional uterine bleeding is defined as bleeding not associated with any structural abnormality in pelvis. The uterus and its appendages are structurally normal. It is presumably related to hormonal changes. The main causes of dysfunctional uterine bleeding include failure of ovulation (anovulatory cycle) and inadequate luteal phase (Table 24.10).

Etiology

- *Anovulatory cycle (failure of ovulation):* It is presumably related to hormonal changes. Dysfunctional uterine bleeding may also be caused by neuroendocrine disturbances (e.g. anxiety and anorexia nervosa), severe malnutrition, and debilitating diseases.

Table 24.10: Causes of vaginal bleeding

Age group	Causes
Pre-puberty	Precocious puberty
Adolescence	Anovulatory cycles
Reproductive age	Complication of pregnancy Organic lesion Anovulatory cycle Dysfunctional uterine bleeding
Peri-menopause	Anovulatory cycle Irregular shedding Organic lesion
Post-menopause	Atrophic endometrium Organic lesion

- *Inadequate luteal phase:* If the corpus luteum does not secrete progesterone in adequate amounts, the level of progesterone may not be sufficient for ful transition of proliferative endometrium to secretory endometrium. Such irregular maturation of the endometrium is usually associated with *spotting*, premature onset of menstrual bleeding or prolonged bleeding.

Pathology

If ovulation does not occur during secretory phase, the endometrium will continue to proliferate until it outgrows its own blood supply. At that point, the surface portion of the endometrium becomes ischemic and starts dying off. This leads to bleeding per vagina, which typically occurs 2 or 3 weeks after the date of the *missed menstruation*.

Clinical Features

Patient may present with menorrhagia (episodes of vaginal bleeding between menstruations) or heavy or prolonged menstruation persisting for longer than 8 days, fatigue due to anemia and infertility as a result of anovulation.

Diagnostic Tests

Ovulatory body temperature monitoring, serum progesterone level and endometrial biopsy are performed. Patient should be investigated to rule out infections, polyps and cancer of the genital tract.

ENDOMETRITIS

Endometritis results from infection of the endometrium. It may be acute or chronic depending on underlying cause.

Acute Endometritis

Acute endometritis is common often caused by *Staphylococcus aureus* or *Streptococcus* species. It is

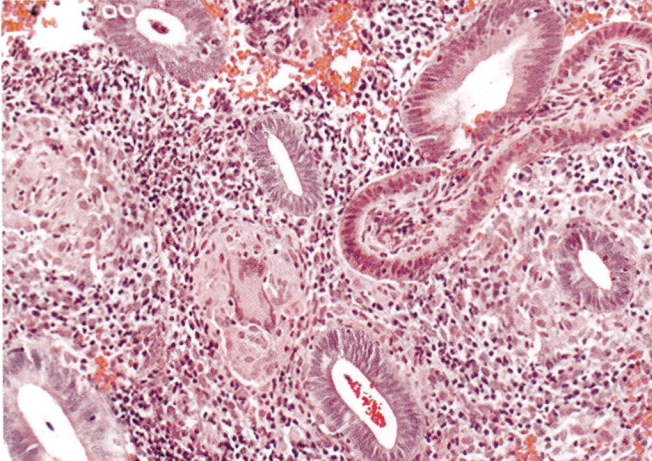

Fig. 24.45: Chronic endometritis. Chronic endometritis can occur in patients with chronic pelvic inflammatory disease, as a postpartum or post-abortion complication, in association with intrauterine devices (IUDs), or with tuberculosis. In a sixth of patients there is no definable cause for chronic endometritis.

most often associated with intrauterine contraceptive devices, intrauterine trauma from instrumentation, and postpartum retention of placental fragments. Cervical stenosis may also result in accumulation of pus in uterine cavity known as *pyometra*.

Light Microscopy

Light microscopy reveals polymorphonuclear cell infiltration.

Chronic Endometritis

Tuberculosis is most important cause of chronic endometritis in endemic regions. *Actinomyces israelii* infection is also responsible for chronic endometritis due to intrauterine contraceptive device.

Patient presents with abnormal bleeding, pain, discharge, fever, and infertility.

Light Microscopy

- Normal endometrium mucosa contains lymphocytes and lymphoid follicles but lack plasma cells.
- Presence of plasma cells in the endometrial stroma is diagnostic of chronic endometritis (Fig. 24.45).

ENDOMETRIAL HYPERPLASIA

Endometrial hyperplasia refers to abnormal proliferation of endometrial glands. It ranges from simple glandular crowding to complex hyperplasia with or without atypia. Complex hyperplasia with atypia is difficult to distinguish from early endometrial carcinoma.

Etiology

Endometrial hyperplasia is usually caused by estrogenic stimulation. It occurs in anovulatory cycles as a result of estrogenic effect not opposed by progesterone. Excess of estrogens also occurs in women with polycystic ovary disease, estrogen-secreting ovarian tumors, i.e. granulosa cell tumor, estrogen replacement therapy and ovarian cortical stromal hyperplasia.

Clinical Features

It may progress to atypical hyperplasia and ultimately endometrial carcinoma and manifest with postmenopausal bleeding. Young women manifest with menorrhagia and anovulation.

Gross Morphology

Uterine endometrium is diffusely thickened due to prolonged action of estrogens (Fig. 24.46).

Light Microscopy

- Endometrial hyperplasia refers to a spectrum that ranges from simple glandular crowding to conspicuous proliferation of atypical glands.
- These changes are often difficult to distinguish from carcinoma.
- Estrogen exposure is thought to be a risk factor for both endometrial hyperplasia and endometrial carcinoma.
- Endometrial hyperplasia is of three types (e.g. simple, complex without atypia and complex with atypia) on histopathologic examination of endometrial biopsy described as under (Figs 24.47 to 24.49).

Histological Patterns

- *Simple (cystic) endometrial hyperplasia*: It contains an increased number of *dilated glands* separated from each other by normal stroma (*swiss cheese pattern*).
- *Complex (adenomatous) endometrial hyperplasia without atypia*: The irregularly shaped glands appear overcrowded and are surrounded by relatively scant stroma. The glandular epithelium is lined by uniform cells showing no atypia. Only 5% of patients with complex hyperplasia without atypia ultimately progress to endometrial carcinoma in a span of 10 years.
- *Complex (adenomatous) endometrial hyperplasia with atypia*: It is characterized by cytologic atypia and marked glandular crowding with stratification of cells that often protrude into the lumen. These glands frequently show back-to-back arrangement.

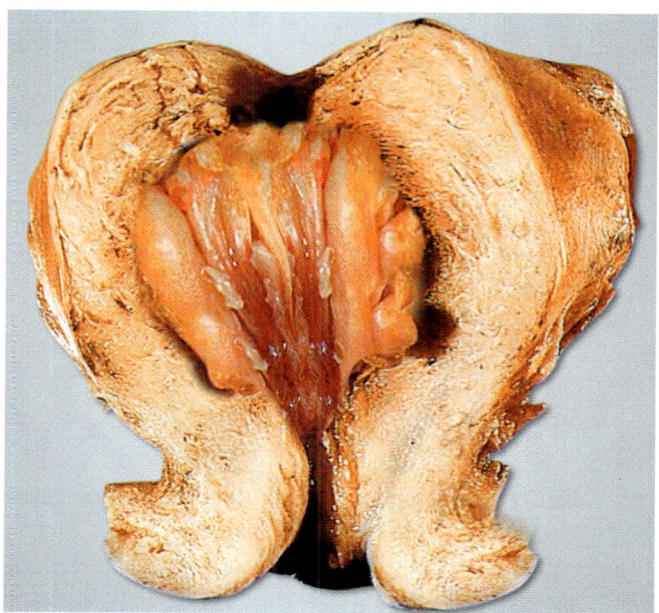

Fig. 24.46: Endometrial hyperplasia. The whole endometrium is involved, rather than there being a discrete polyp. It results with conditions of prolonged estrogen excess. The patient presented with metrorrhagia (uterine bleeding at irregular intervals), menorrhagia (excessive bleeding with menstrual periods), or menometrorrhagia.

Most reliable diagnostic criteria are presence of round rather than oval cells with hyperchromatic nuclei, prominent nucleoli and high nuclear-to-cytoplasmic ratio. Approximately 25% of complex atypical hyperplasia may progress to endometrial carcinoma in a span of 4 years.

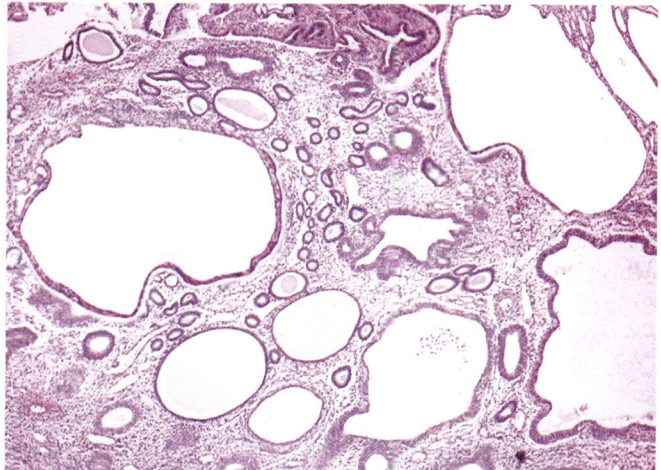

Fig. 24.47: Simple endometrial hyperplasia. This is endometrial cystic hyperplasia in which the amount of endometrium is abnormally increased and not cycling as it should. The glands are enlarged and irregular with columnar cells that lack atypia (100X).

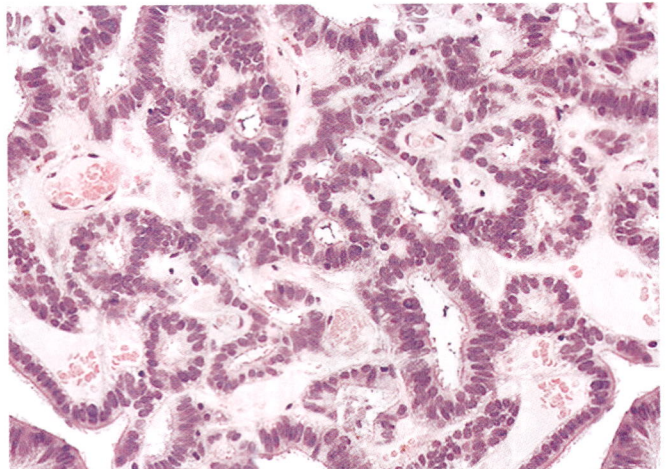

Fig. 24.48: Complex (adenomatous) hyperplasia without atypia (400X).

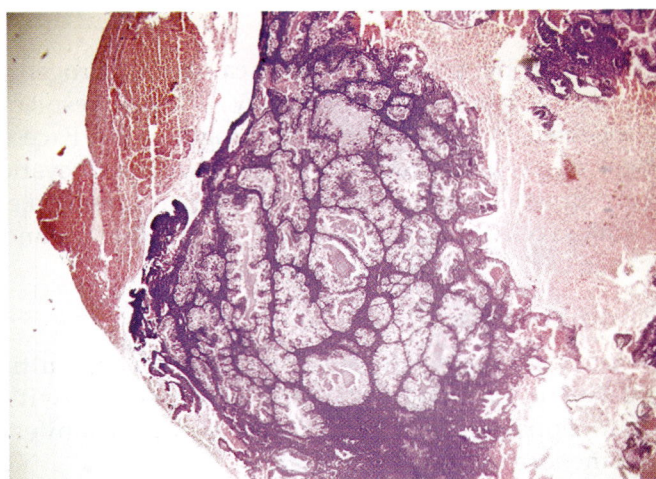

Fig. 24.50: Arias-Stella reaction. Endometrial glands are hypersecretory with back-to-back arrangement. The cells are large with abundant clear or eosinophilic cytoplasm, large hyperchromatic pleomorphic and smudged nuclei. There is presence of decidualized stroma. It may provide initial information of ectopic pregnancy (100X).

- There is presence of decidualized stroma. It may provide initial information of ectopic pregnancy (Fig. 24.50).

ADENOMYOSIS UTERI

Adenomyosis uteri is a term denoting the presence of islands of endometrium in the myometrium. It does not represent a neoplastic process. Approximately, 15–20% of all resected uteri show some evidence of adenomyosis.

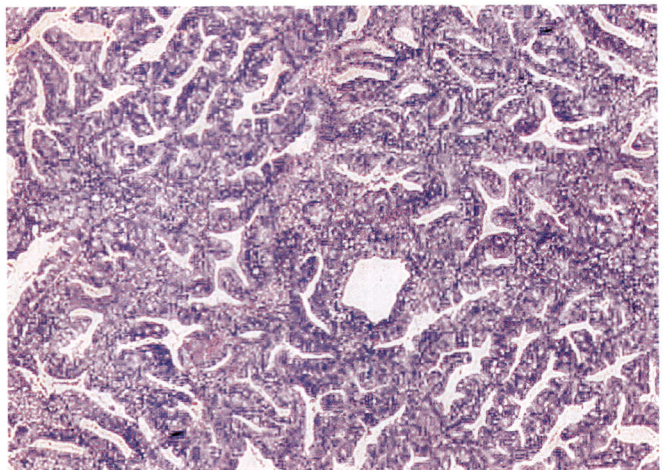

Fig. 24.49: Complex (adenomatous) hyperplasia with atypia (400X).

Gross Morphology

It reveals asymmetrical hyperplasia of uterus. Multiple small hemorrhagic cysts are seen in myometrium (Fig. 24.51).

Light Microscopy

It shows presence of nests of endometrial glands lined by mild proliferative to inactive endometrium, surrounded by endometrial stroma with varying degrees of fibrosis in the myometrium (Fig. 24.52).

ARIAS-STELLA REACTION

Arias-Stella reaction is hormone induced gestational endometrial hyperplasia due to intrauterine pregnancy, ectopic pregnancy, exogenous hormonal therapy, hydatidiform mole, choriocarcinoma and endometriosis. It may provide initial information of ectopic pregnancy.

Light Microscopy

- Endometrial glands are hypersecretory with back-to-back arrangement. The cells are large with abundant clear or eosinophilic cytoplasm, large hyperchromatic pleomorphic and smudged nuclei.

Clinical Features

Many patients with adenomyosis are asymptomatic. Patient may present with dysmenorrhea and dyspareunia, which increases with subsequent cycles.

Female Reproductive System

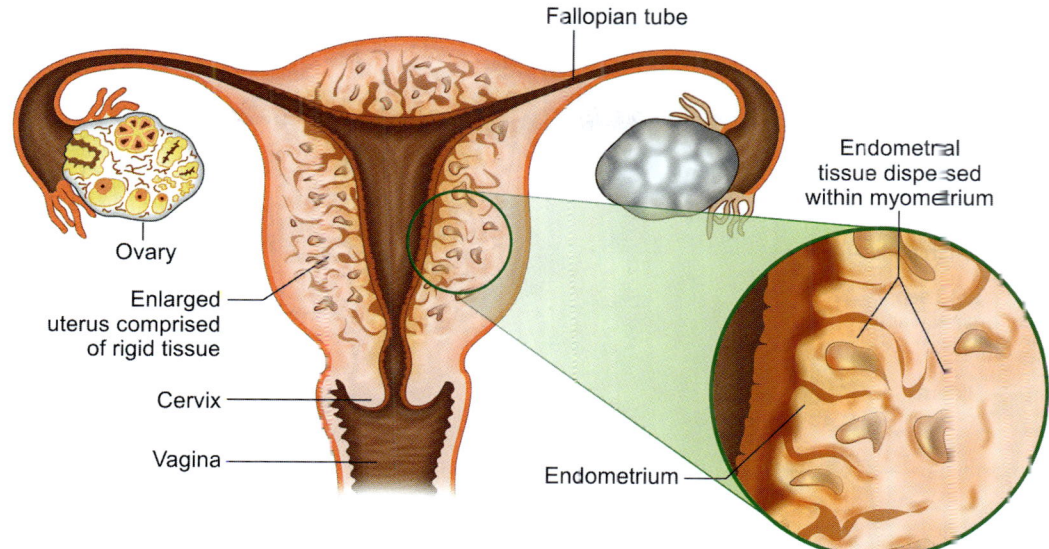

Fig. 24.51: Adenomyosis uterus. The thickened and spongy appearing myometrial wall of this sectioned uterus is typical of adenomyosis. This condition leads to uterine enlargement and irregular bleeding.

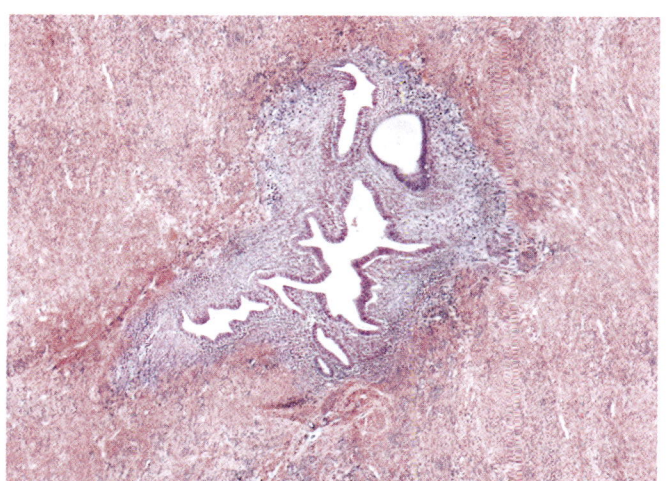

Fig. 24.52: Adenomyosis uterus. Adenomyosis occurs when endometrial glands and stroma are found in the myometrium, not just in the endometrium where they belong. This condition leads to uterine enlargement and irregular bleeding (100X).

ENDOMETRIOSIS

Endometriosis is presence of benign endometrial glands and stroma outside the uterus. It is an important cause of infertility. It affects 5 to 10% of women of reproductive age and regresses after menopause.

Pathogenesis

- Endometriosis occurs either by retrograde dissemination of endometrial fragments through fallopian tubes during menstruation, resulting in implantation on the ovary, or lymphatic-hematogenous dissemination of endometrial fragments.
- Uterine as well as ectopic endometrial glands respond to estrogen and progesterone during each menstrual cycle resulting in sloughing and bleeding in ectopic endometrial glands forming large cysts. It leads to inflammation and fibrosis.

Locations

- The ovaries are the most common sites (80%), followed by the uterine ligaments, fallopian tubes, rectovaginal septum, rectosigmoid colon, and pelvic peritoneum (Table 24.11).
- Since the fimbrial openings of fallopian tubes are in the posterior area of pelvis, most ectopic endometrial glands are generally confined to the pelvic region.

Table 24.11: Location of endometriosis

• Ovaries (80%) most common site
• Cul de sac (most common site)
• Broad ligament (most common site)
• Fallopian tubes (fimbrial openings)
• Umbilical region
• Urinary bladder
• Ileum
• Abdominal wall operated scar
• Vulva
• Perineum
• Lymph nodes
• Kidneys
• Liver
• Diaphragm

Section III: Systemic Pathology

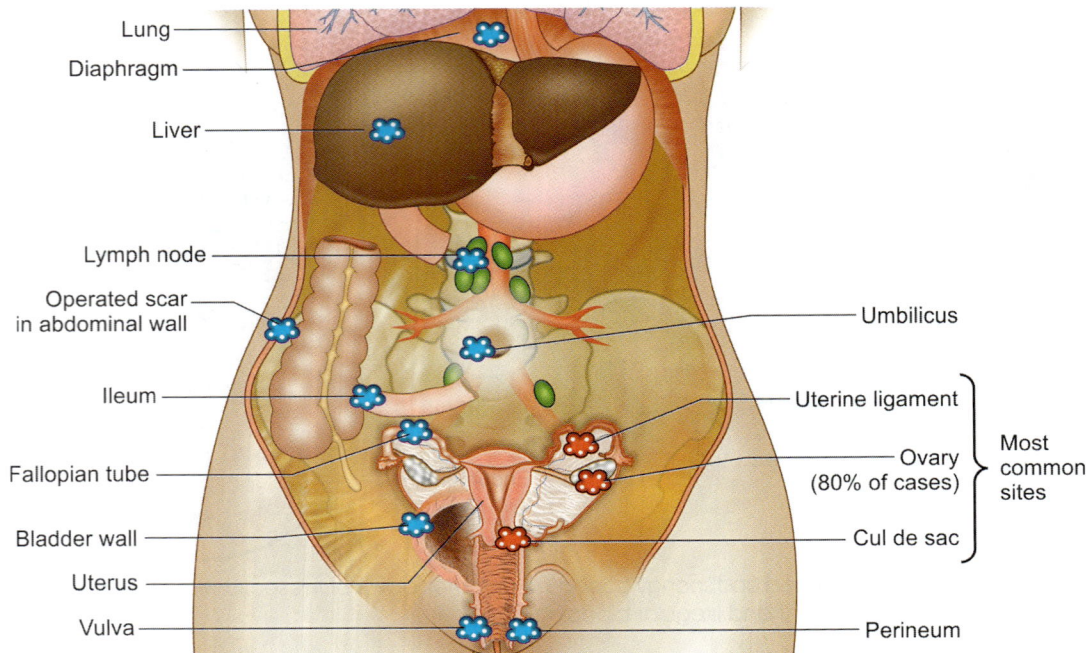

Fig. 24.53: Endometriosis—the drawing shows some of the sites where endometrial deposits can occur. Red highlights the three most common sites; ovary, uterine ligaments and cul de sac.

- Other sites include urinary bladder, lung, pleura, kidneys, extremities and operated scars of abdomen (Fig. 24.53).

Gross Morphology
Menstrual-type bleeding occurs into the ectopic endometrial glands resulting in formation of blood filled cysts up to 15 cm in diameter containing chocolate-colored material (*chocolate cysts*) (Fig. 24.54).

Light Microscopy
- The diagnosis of endometriosis is based on finding endometrial glands, stroma, and hemosiderin in the stroma on microscopy of biopsy tissue.
- Foci of healed endometrium in the form of hemosiderin on the peritoneal surface are referred to as *powder burns* (Fig. 24.55).

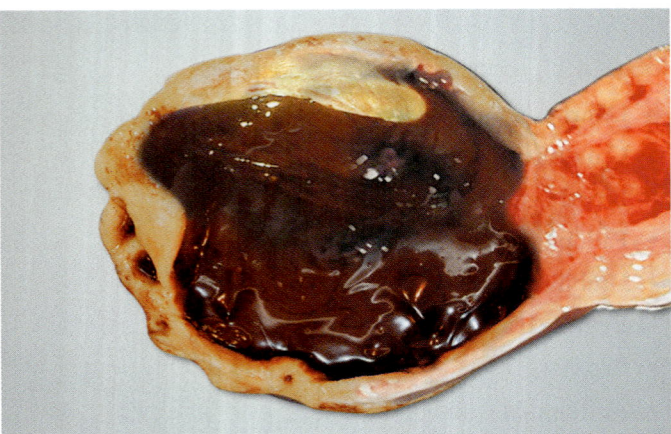

Fig. 24.54: Chocolate cyst in endometriosis. This is a section through an enlarged 12 cm ovary to demonstrate a cystic cavity filled with old blood typical for endometriosis with formation of an endometriotic, or *chocolate* cyst. The hemorrhage from endometriosis into the ovary may give rise to a large *chocolate cyst* so named because the old blood in the cystic space formed by the hemorrhage is broken down to produce much hemosiderin and a brown to black color.

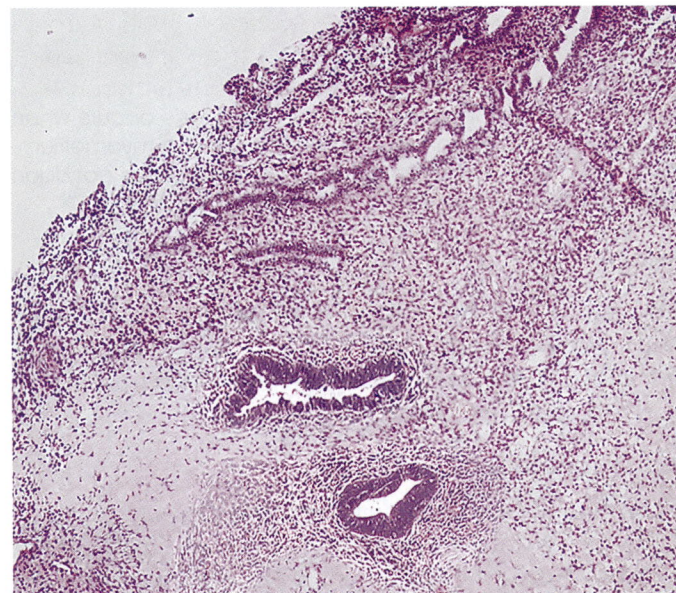

Fig. 24.55. Endometriosis—endometrial glands and stroma are seen at high magnification in the wall of the colon. Endometriosis is symptomatic during reproductive years when patients may present with dysmenorrhea, pelvic pain, and infertility (100X).

Female Reproductive System

Clinical Features

- Patient presents with severe menstrual-related pelvic pain due to inflammation and fibrosis in areas around ectopic endometrial glands. Pain begins 5 to 7 days before menstruation peaks and lasts for 2 to 3 days. Patient may develop painful sexual intercourse.
- The inflammation causes fibrosis and adhesions often resulting in infertility. Endometriosis in colon causes abdominal cramps, pelvic pain, painful defecation, constipation and bloody stools. Urinary bladder endometriosis causes suprapubic pain, dysuria and hematuria.

Diagnostic Technique

Laparoscopy is the gold standard for screening. It shows red-blue to yellow-brown nodules measuring 1–5 mm. In occasional case, the ovarian chocolate cysts are formed measuring 20 cm in diameter.

ENDOMETRIAL POLYP

Endometrial polyps most often occur in the perimenopausal period. These are solitary finger-like benign lesions found in the uterine cavity. Most polyps are diagnosed in perimenopausal women complaining of spotting or irregular bleeding. Polyps are easily removed by curettage (Fig. 24.56).

Pathogenesis

It is thought that endometrial foci are hypersensitive to estrogenic stimulation or unresponsive to progesterone. Hence, these foci do not slough during menstruation and continue to progress. Patient presents with spotting or irregular bleeding.

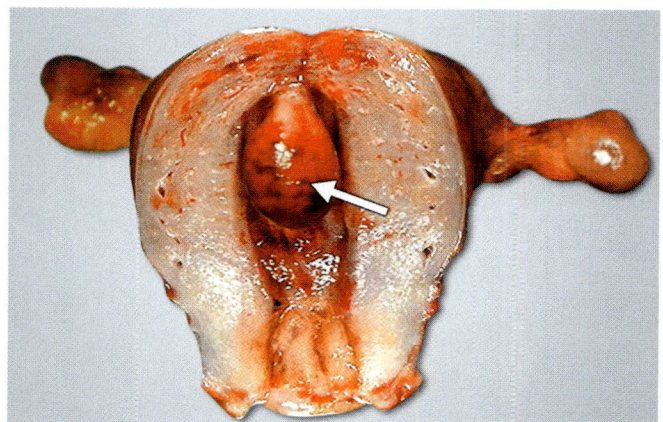

Fig. 24.56: Endometrial polyp protrudes into the uterine cavity. The lesions are believed to arise from endometrial foci that are hypersensitive to estrogen stimulation and that fail to slough with menstruation. Such benign polyps may cause uterine bleeding (arrow).

Light Microscopy

- *Endometrial polyp consists of core* covered by surface endometrium.
- Core of polyp comprises dilated and hyperplastic endometrial glands embedded in fibrous endometrial stroma containing thick-walled, coiled, dilated blood vessels.

ENDOMETRIAL ADENOCARCINOMA

Endometrial adenocarcinoma is most common invasive gynecological cancer. It originates in the endometrium or lining of the uterus.

Morphological subtypes include serous papillary and clear cell carcinoma. Annual manual pelvic examination is performed to search for uterus enlargement, pelvic masses or induration. Endometrial biopsy is a reliable diagnostic tool.

- Type I endometrioid adenocarcinoma is associated with estrogen stimulation. Incidence is 35%. It affects obese, diabetic and hypertensive women. Light microscopy shows well differentiated endometrial adenocarcinoma. It has good prognosis.
- Type II non-endometrioid adenocarcinoma is not associated with estrogen stimulation.

Age Group

It most common affects postmenopausal women (50 to 60 years).

Molecular Genetics

Loss of function of PTEN tumor suppressor gene occurs in 65% of cases of endometrial carcinoma. It is an informative biomarker for endometrial carcinogenesis.

Clinical Features

Patient presents with enlargement of uterus, persistent and unusual bleeding per vagina, pain and weight loss.

TYPE I ENDOMETRIOID ADENOCARCINOMA

Morphologically, these tumors resemble normal endometrium. It occurs due to prolonged estrogenic stimulation and carries a good prognosis. It most often occurs in premenopausal and perimenopausal women, and carries a good prognosis.

Etiology

- *Hormonal imbalance:* Most postmenopausal women who develop uterine cancer have a history of anovulatory menstrual cycles or other hormonal imbalance such as estrogen-producing tumors (granulosa cell tumors of ovary), estrogen hormonal replacement therapy, prolonged reproductive period (early menarche and late menopause) and obesity.

- **Obesity:** In obese women, adipose tissue converts androgens into estrogens, fueling the proliferation of endometrial tissue.

Predisposing Factors

- It is associated with a higher frequency in diabetic, hypertensive, infertile women and familial endometrial carcinoma and hereditary non-polyposis colorectal cancer (HNPCC), or Lynch syndrome. Lynch syndrome is characterized by development of adenocarcinoma of the endometrium, colon, and breast).
- Endometrial carcinoma may develop in these patients before gastrointestinal malignancies. Strong family history in women >50 years of age should prompt investigation for mismatch repair defects.

TYPE II ENDOMETRIOID ADENOCARCINOMA

Type II endometrioid adenocarcinoma accounts for 15% of cases. It is not associated with estrogen stimulation. It occurs in the settings of thin, slim, normotensive women with precursor atrophic endometrium. Light microscopy shows poorly differentiated endometrioid adenocarcinoma with poor prognosis.

Gross Morphology

Patient with endometrial carcinoma develops three types of growth (e.g. exophytic polypoid, diffuse thickening and invasive)
- Exophytic polypoid growth protrudes within the uterine cavity (Fig. 24.57).
- Diffuse thickening of the endometrium is a superficial carcinoma without invading the myometrium.
- Invasive adenocarcinoma extends through the myometrium into the serosa.

Light Microscopy

The tumor has many histological variants: endometrioid carcinoma (85%), squamous differentiation (adenoacanthoma, adenosquamous), papillary, serous, and clear cell types.

- *Adenocarcinoma or endometrioid adenocarcinoma:* It accounts of 85% cases—tumor is composed of well-formed, closely packed glands with cytologic atypia that bear resemblance to endometrial glands, hence known as endometrioid adenocarcinoma.

  Approximately >50% tumors are well to moderately differentiated adenocarcinoma (type I endometrioid adenocarcinoma). Rest 50% of tumors show poor differentiation (type II endometrioid adenocarcinoma) (Fig. 24.58 and Table 24.12).
- *Squamous differentiation in adenocarcinomas:* These include adenoacanthoma and adenosquamous carcinoma in some cases.
- *Less common varients:* These include papillary serous carcinoma, or clear cell adenocarcinoma, which account for minority of cases. These have poorer prognosis. There is possible genetic influence. Both variants are associated with atrophy in adjacent endometrium without hyperplasia.

Immunohistochemistry

CA 125 is a cell surface glycoprotein originally identified in mucinous epithelial ovarian tumors. It is also expressed in adenocarcinoma of endometrium; cancers of *gastrointestinal tract*, *thyroid* and *breast*.

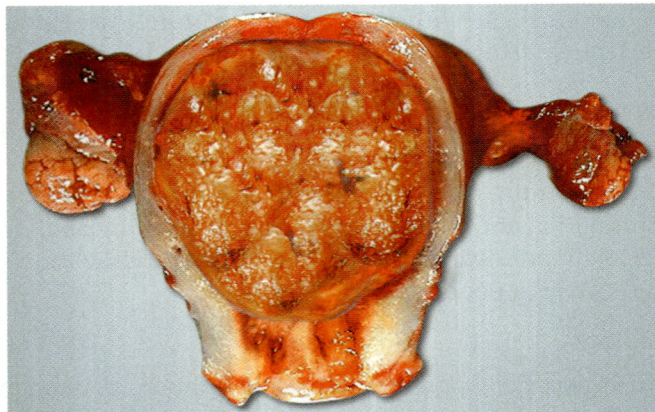

Fig. 24.57: Endometrial carcinoma. This uterus is not enlarged, but there is an irregular mass in the upper fundus that proved to be endometrial adenocarcinoma on biopsy. Such carcinomas are more likely to occur in postmenopausal women. Thus, any postmenopausal bleeding should make you suspect that this lesion may be present.

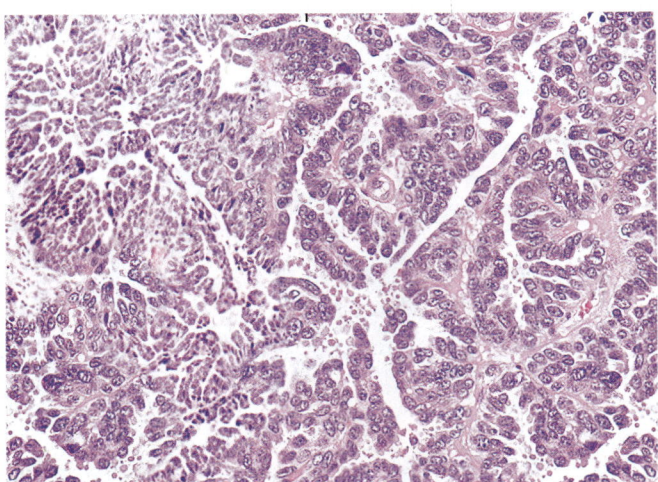

Fig. 24.58: Endometrial adenocarcinoma. This is endometrial adenocarcinoma which can be seen invading into the smooth muscle bundles of the myometrial wall of the uterus. This neoplasm has a higher stage than a neoplasm that is just confined to the endometrium or is superficially invasive (100X).

Table 24.12: Endometrial carcinomas and comparison of its variants

Parameters	Type I: Endometrioid carcinoma (adenocarcinoma)	Type II: Endometrioid carcinoma (papillary serous carcinoma)
Incidence	85%	15%
Clinical settings	Obese women Diabetic women Hypertensive women Unopposed action of increased estrogen levels Endometrial hyperplasia	Thin slim women Not diabetic women Normotensive women Relative low level of estrogen levels Endometrial atrophy
Precursor lesion	Endometrial hyperplasia	Atrophic endometrium with development of carcinoma *in situ*
Light microscopy	Well differentiated carcinoma resemble normal endometrium	Poorly differentiated carcinoma with papillary epithelial pattern
Molecular profile	ER/PR: positive p53 mutation: absent Microsatellite instability: ++ (20–30%) PTEN mutation: + (34–53%) K-RAS mutation: present TP53 P13K mutation: present FGF-2 (growth factor) mutation: present β-catenin mutation: present PTEN ARID1A (regulator of chromatin)	ER/PR: negative p53 mutation: present Microsatellite instability: + (11%) PTEN mutation: absent K-RAS mutation: absent TP53 Aneuploidy P13K mutation: absent FGF-2 (growth factor) mutation: absent β-catenin mutation: absent FBX W7 (regulator of MYC, cyclin E) CHD4 (regulator of chromatin)
Mode of spread	Lymphatic route	Lymphatic route and intraperitoneal spread
Behavior	Indolent behavior	Aggressive behavior
Prognosis	Good	Poor

Mode of Spread

Endometrial carcinoma spreads by local invasion, tubal, lymphatic and hematogenous routes described as under.

- *Local invasion:* It may take place in several directions i.e. tube, myometrium and periuterine structures, cervix, vagina and urinary bladder.
- *Tubal spread:* It may spread to fallopian tube, ovaries and peritoneum.
- *Lymphatic route:* It metastasizes to pelvic lymph nodes (e.g. internal iliac and para-aortic lymph nodes), but some tumor cells may skip the pelvic lymph nodes; and involve peri-aortic lymph nodes.
- *Hematogenous route:* Metastatic deposits may occur in the vagina and ovaries via hematogenous route. Distant metastases are found in lungs, liver, bone and brain in advanced disease in 40% of cases.

Staging

Staging is a clinical exercise that classifies tumors according to their size, invasiveness and spread. Tumors are staged according to the TNM system (T: tumor size, N: lymph node involvement, M: metastases to distant organs). Schemes for TNM classification vary according to tumor type and organ involved (Table 24.13 and Fig. 24.59).

Table 24.13: Staging of endometrial carcinoma

Stage	Tumor
Stage I	Tumor confined to uterine endometrium or showing only superficial invasion of myometrium
Stage II	Tumor confined to corpus and cervix. Tumor invading deeply into the myometrium
Stage III	Extends outside uterus but confined to pelvis
Stage IV	Invasion of urinary bladder or rectum or metastases to lymph nodes and distant metastases to lungs, liver, bone and brain

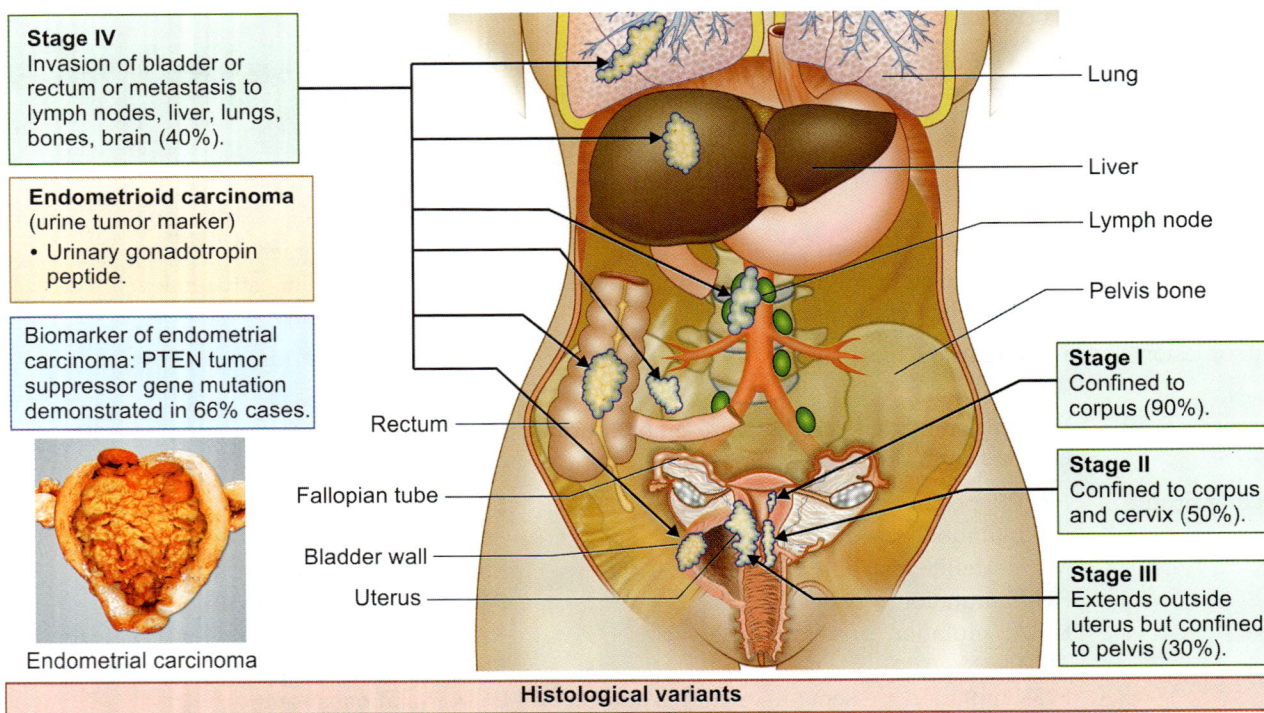

Stage IV
Invasion of bladder or rectum or metastasis to lymph nodes, liver, lungs, bones, brain (40%).

Endometrioid carcinoma (urine tumor marker)
- Urinary gonadotropin peptide.

Biomarker of endometrial carcinoma: PTEN tumor suppressor gene mutation demonstrated in 66% cases.

Endometrial carcinoma

Stage I Confined to corpus (90%).

Stage II Confined to corpus and cervix (50%).

Stage III Extends outside uterus but confined to pelvis (30%).

Histological variants
• Type I Endometrioid carcinoma: It is associated with estrogen stimulation. It has good prognosis.
• Type II Endometrioid carcinoma: It most often occurs in older age group. It is not associated with estrogen stimulation. It has poor prognosis. Morphologic subtypes include serous papillary and clear cell carcinoma.

Mode of spread of endometrial carcinoma	
Mode of spread	**Organs involved**
1. Local invasion	Fallopian tube, myometrium, cervix, vagina and urinary bladder
2. Tubal spread	Fallopian tube, ovaries and peritoneum
3. Lymphatic route	Pelvic lymph nodes (e.g. internal iliac and para-aortic lymph nodes), but some tumor cells may skip the pelvic lymph nodes; and involve peri-aortic lymph nodes.
4. Hematogenous route	Lungs, liver, bone and brain

Fig. 24.59: Endometrial adenocarcinoma. It illustrates types of endometrial adenocarcinoma, mode of spread and staging (approximate five-year survival percentage is shown for various stages).

ENDOMETRIAL STROMAL TUMOR

- These are rare low grade or high grade tumors. Low grade tumors infiltrate extensively through the lymphatics of the myometrium. The tumor cells are bland and showing few mitoses.
- High grade endometrial stromal sarcomas show a vascular supporting framework with spindle-shaped neoplastic cells concentrically arranged around blood vessels. These are much rarer than leiomyosarcomas. It difficult to separate these tumors from uterine leiomyosarcoma.

CARCINOSARCOMA (MIXED MÜLLERIAN TUMOR)

Carcinosarcoma is a mixed tumor with malignant epithelial and stromal components. It is highly malignant tumor also known as *malignant mixed müllerian tumor*. It affects postmenopausal women.

Origin

It is derived from multipotential stromal cells.

Clinical Features

Patient presents with bleeding per vagina. On per vaginal examination, tumor is soft, bulky and fleshy protruding through the cervix into the vagina.

Light Microscopy

On histological examination, tumor comprises malignant glandular and stromal components. It usually *metastasizes as adenocarcinoma*.

Female Reproductive System

MYOMETRIUM

SMOOTH MUSCLE CELL TUMORS

Smooth muscle cell tumors of the uterus are leiomyomas (most common) and leiomyosarcomas.

LEIOMYOMA (FIBROID/FIBROMYOMA/MYOMA)

Leiomyomas are most common benign tumors of smooth muscle origin, also known as *fibroids*. These usually occur in the uterine corpus (intramural, submucous and subserous regions). These may arise in cervix or uterine ligaments.

It most often occurs during reproductive period and most regresses after the menopause. Leiomyomas can cause painful menstruation and contribute to infertility.

Estrogen Sensitivity

- The tumors are estrogen-sensitive. Estrogen promotes the growth of leiomyomas, although it does not initiate them. Both estrogen and progestin receptors are present in leiomyomas.
- Elevated estrogen levels may cause leiomyoma's enlargement during first trimester of pregnancy.

Molecular Genetics

Leiomyomas show clonal abnormalities of 12q/7q and 6p resulting in rearrangement of genes.

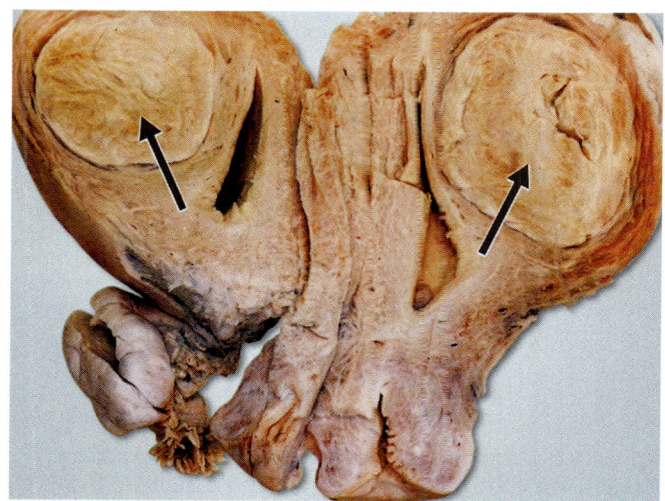

Fig. 24.60: Leiomyoma—cut surface of intramural leiomyoma reveals whorled pattern reflecting the fact that these are composed of smooth muscle bundles (arrows).

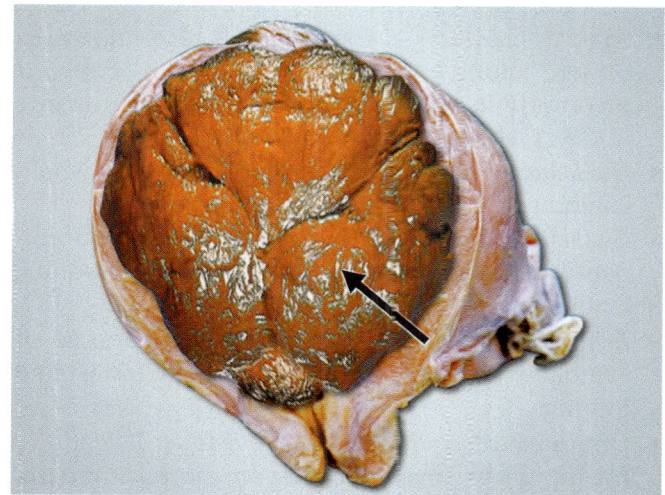

Fig. 24.61: Leiomyoma shows red degeneration (red meat appearance) (arrow).

Gross Morphology

Leiomyomas are discrete, firm, pale gray, sharply circumscribed and varying in size without encapsulation.

- *Cut surface:* Cut section reveals whorled pattern reflecting the fact that these are composed of smooth muscle bundles. Most leiomyomas are present within wall (intramural), but some are pedunculated and present in submucosal and subserosal region (Fig. 24.60).
- *Secondary changes in large leiomyomas:* These are yellow-brown to red softening (cystic degeneration), atrophy, hyaline degeneration, cystic degeneration, fatty change, dystrophic calcification, red degeneration, and chondroid/osteoid metaplasia (Fig. 24.61).

Light Microscopy

- Leiomyoma comprised of whorled bundles of smooth muscle cells that resemble the uninvolved myometrium.
- Individual smooth muscle cells are uniform in size and shape containing oval nucleus and long, slender bipolar cytoplasmic processes. Mitotic figures are sparse.
- These cells are arranged in whorled fashion (Fig. 24.62).

Histological Variants

- *Cellular leiomyoma:* It is also known as *apoleptic leiomyoma* shows areas of hemorrhage. It may rupture resulting in hemoperitoneum. Cellular leiomyoma occurs in pregnant women or young females on oral contraceptives.

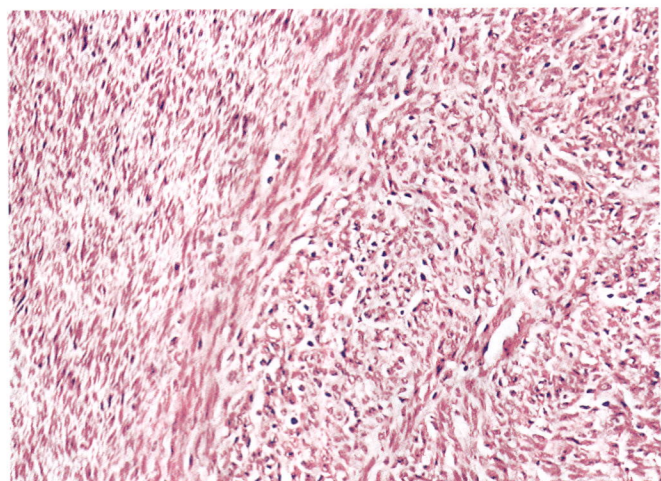

Fig. 24.62: Leiomyoma. The microscopic appearance of a benign leiomyoma. Normal myometrium is at the left, and the neoplasm is well-differentiated so that the leiomyoma at the right hardly appears different. Bundles of smooth muscle are interlacing in the tumor mass (400X).

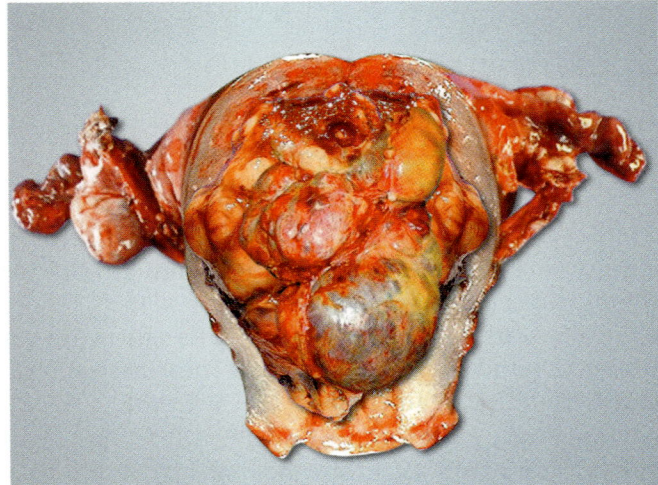

Fig. 24.63: Leiomyosarcoma of the uterus. The uterus is expanded by a massive, fleshy, partly necrotic and hemorrhagic-looking malignant tumor.

- *Symplasmic (bizarre) leiomyoma:* It also known as bizarre leiomyoma. It is composed of scattered pleomorphic cells with irregular hyperchromatic nuclei, giant cells with a low mitotic index.
- *Lipoleiomyoma:* It refers to classic leiomyoma which contains islands of mature adipocytes.
- *Epithelioid leiomyoma:* It is composed of predominantly epithelioid cells with clear to eosinophilic cytoplasm and nuclei with fine chromatin.
- *Benign metastasizing leiomyoma:* It is composed of tumor invading blood vessels and metastasizing to lungs.
- *Disseminated peritoneal leiomyomatosis:* It leads to formation of small nodules on the peritoneum. These tumors are considered benign despite their unusual behavior.

Clinical Features

In most instances, leiomyomas are asymptomatic and discovered by gynecologists during routine pelvic examination.

- *Intramural large leiomyoma:* It may compress the bladder and rectum; resulting in feeling of heaviness, pain, incontinence of urine and urgency of defecation.
- *Subserosal leiomyomas:* It undergoes torsion due to twisting of pedicle, and detachment resulting in pain and signs of peritonitis.
- *Submucosal leiomyoma:* It is pedunculated tumor, which increases the endometrial surface area. Patient presents with excessive uterine bleeding.

LEIOMYOSARCOMA

Leiomyosarcoma is a highly malignant tumor of smooth muscle cell origin *de novo*, and unrelated to pre-existing leiomyoma. Single best criterion for predicting the behavior of smooth muscle tumors is mitotic activity.

Gross Morphology

One should suspect leiomyosarcoma, if an apparent smooth muscle tumor is soft with irregular borders and areas of necrosis on gross examination. On cut section, tumor is not bulging above the surface (Fig. 24.63).

Light Microscopy

- *Diagnostic criteria:* It includes following features on light microscopy: (1) 10 or more mitoses per 10 high-powered field (HPF); (2) 5 or more mitoses per 10 HPF, with nuclear atypia and necrosis; and (3) myxoid and epithelioid smooth muscle tumors with 5 or more mitoses per 10 HPF (Fig. 24.64).
- *STUMP:* Some tumors that meet some, but not all, of the diagnostic criteria for leiomyosarcoma are considered 'STUMP' (smooth muscle tumors of uncertain malignant potential).

Mode of Spread

It spreads by local invasion and hematogenous route resulting in distant metastases.

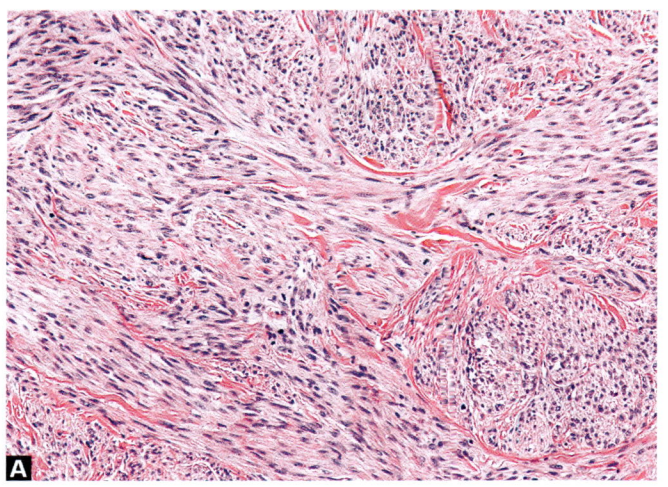 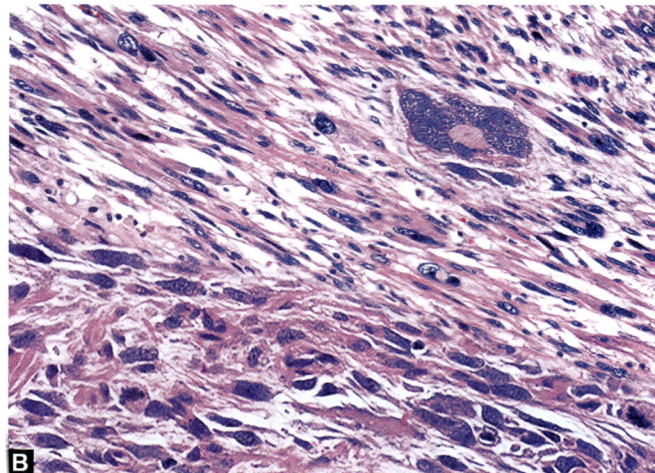

Fig. 24.64: Leiomyosarcoma. As with sarcomas in general, leiomyosarcomas have spindle cells. Several mitoses are seen here, just in this one high power field (400X).

OVARY

GENERAL CONSIDERATIONS

- Ovarian cancer is the second most common malignancy of the genital tract. It is the second most common cause of death due to late diagnosis.
- Most of the ovarian tumors are of epithelial origin. These occur after the age of 35 years with increasing incidence as age advances.
- Approximately 3% of ovarian tumors occur before 35 years of age. These are mostly non-epithelial in origin as germ cell tumors.
- Primary ovarian tumors are classified according to the World Health Organization (WHO) classification, which divides primary tumors into three main groups based on line of differentiation—surface epithelium (müllerian epithelium), germ cell (ovum), and sex cord stroma (ovarian stroma) (Fig. 24.65 and Table 24.14). Differences between benign and malignant ovarian tumors are shown in Table 24.15.

Table 24.14: Histological classification of ovarian tumors

Surface epithelial tumors: 65–70% (malignant 90%)	*Serous tumors:* Serous cystadenoma, borderline tumors (low malignant potential, or with microinvasion) and serous cystadenocarcinoma	
	Mucinous tumors: Mucinous cystadenoma, borderline tumors and mucinous cystadenocarcinoma	
	Endometroid carcinomas	
	Clear cell carcinoma	
	Brenner tumors: Benign, borderline, malignant tumors and transitional cell carcinoma	
Germ cell tumors: 15–20% (malignant tumors 3–5%)	• Dysgerminoma • Teratomas • Embryonal carcinoma	• Endodermal sinus tumor (yolk sac tumor) • Choriocarcinoma • Mixed germ cell tumors
Sex cord stromal tumors: 5–10% (malignant 2–3%)	• Granulosa cell tumor • Thecoma • Fibroma • Sertoli-Leydig cell tumor	• Pure Leydig cell tumor • Androblastoma • Pregnancy luteoma
Metastatic tumors (5%)	*Transcoelomic route of extra-müllerian origin:* Krukenberg's tumor is ovarian cancer due to metastases from gastric mucin secreting carcinoma (75%), colon mucin secreting carcinoma and lobular carcinoma of breast, biliary tract and pancreas	
	Müllerian origin (endometrial and fallopian tube carcinoma)	

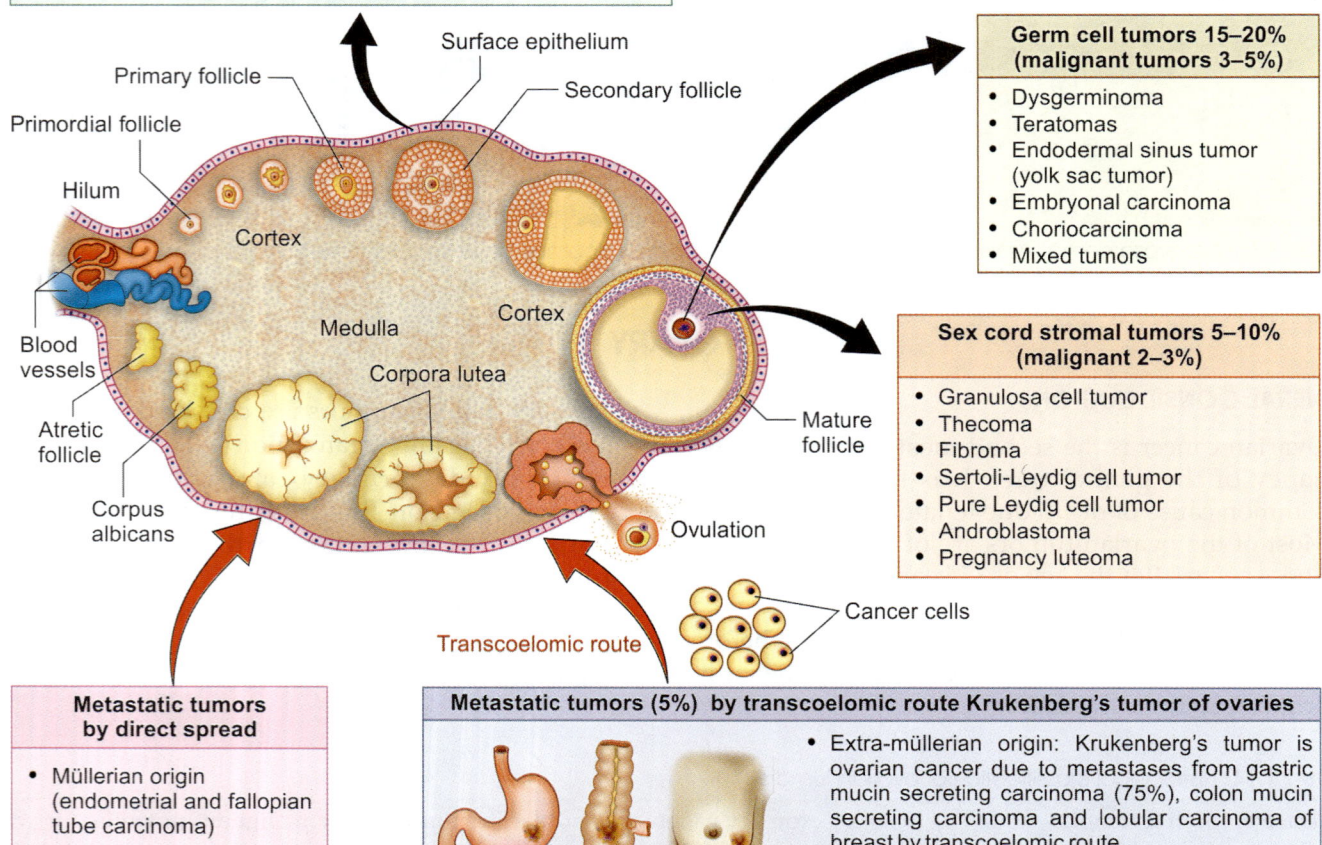

Fig. 24.65: Classification of ovarian tumors.

Table 24.15: Differences between benign and malignant ovarian tumors

Parameters	Benign ovarian tumors	Malignant ovarian tumors
Clinical examination		
Mobility	Mobile	Fixed large lump
Consistency	Cystic	Solid and cystic
Laterality	Unilateral	Bilateral
Cul de sac	Smooth on per vagina examination	Nodular on per vagina examination
Intraoperative findings	Unilateral cyst with intact capsule	Ovarian capsule breached
Imaging technique findings		
Size	Most often, 10 cm size	Size varies
Septate	<2 mm thickness	Multiple septate >3 mm
Calcification	Calcification (teratoma)	Calcification absent
Omental involvement	Absent	Present
Ascites	Absent (present in fibroma presenting as Meig's syndrome)	Present

Female Reproductive System

KRUKENBERG'S TUMOR (METASTATIC TUMOR)

Krukenberg's tumor is the metastatic carcinoma of ovaries. The stomach (mucin secreting adenocarcinoma) is the primary site in 75% of cases, followed by colon (mucin secreting adenocarcinoma) and lobular carcinoma breast.

Metastases occur by transcoelomic spread. One should suspect metastatic carcinoma in bilateral involvement of ovaries with multiple nodules.

Gross Morphology
- Tumor shows multiple solid nodules.
- Cut surface shows gray white, gelatinous, areas of extensive necrosis and cystic spaces (Fig. 24.66).

Light Microscopy
It is characterized by ovarian metastases, in which the tumor shows *nests of mucin-filled signet ring epithelial cells with eccentric nuclei within a cellular stroma* derived from the ovary (Fig. 24.67).

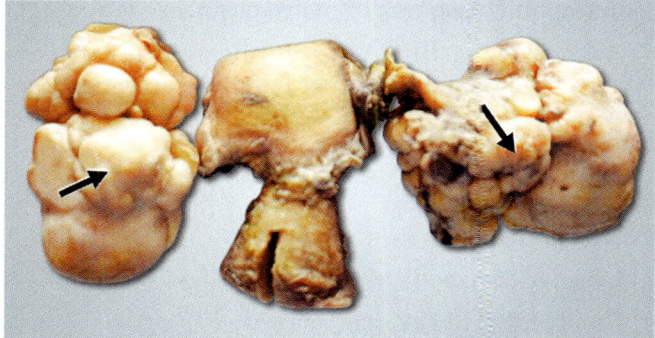

Fig. 24.66: Krukenberg's tumor: Both ovaries show involvement as a result of metastases from primary cancers of stomach or colon or breast (arrows).

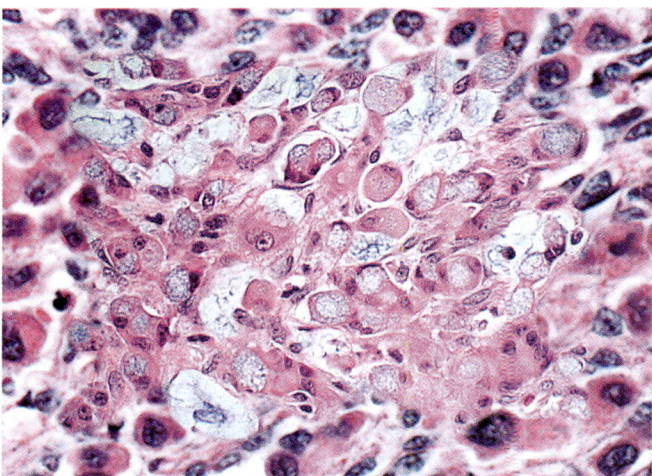

Fig. 24.67: Krukenberg's tumor showing nests of mucin-filled *signet ring* epithelial cells with eccentric nuclei within a cellular stroma (200X).

Immunohistochemistry
- Metastatic gastric carcinoma is immunoreactive with **cytokeratin, CEA** and **EMA**.
- Metastatic colon carcinoma shows *positivity with* **CK20** but negative for **CK7**.
- Metastatic labular carcinoma of breast shows positivity with **ER, PR** and **Her2 neu**.

SURFACE EPITHELIAL TUMORS

This group, which accounts for 65–70% of all ovarian tumors, comprises serous, mucinous, endometrioid, clear cell, and transitional (Brenner) tumors.

Histogenesis

During embryonic life, the coelomic cavity is lined by a mesothelium. This mesothelium gives rise to müllerian ducts, from which uterus, fallopian tubes, and vagina originate. Pluripotency of the ovarian surface epithelium accounts for the spectrum of histological tumor variants seen in this location.

Differentiation of Surface Epithelium

Surface epithelium has potential to differentiate to ciliated columnar epithelium resembling tubal epithelium, tall mucus-secreting non-ciliated epithelium resembling endocervix, uterine endometrial glands and transitional epithelium resembling urinary bladder (Table 24.16).

Histological Variants

Benign Surface Epithelial Tumors

Surface epithelial benign tumors include serous cystadenoma, mucinous cystadenoma and Brenner tumors. Serous tumors account for approximately 20% of all ovarian tumors. Serous epithelial tumors are most often bilateral. These are more common than mucinous tumors.

Borderline Surface Epithelial Tumors

Approximately 10% of ovarian surface epithelial tumors are borderline malignant. These tumors show varying degree of nuclear atypia and increased mitotic activity. These remain confined to the ovary. Rarely, these may metastasize to peritoneum.

- *Serous borderline tumors:* These most often occur in 20–50 years of age group. Cells may shed from the surface and implant on peritoneum, possibly reflecting multifocal origin. S-100 protein is positive in particularly borderline tumors.
- *Mucinous borderline tumors:* These most often occur in younger women. Hart Norris criteria of borderline mucinous tumor include atypical epithelial cells

Table 24.16: Surface epithelium of ovary has potential to differentiate into various tumors

Lining epithelium	Similar to epithelial lining	Examples of ovarian tumors
Ciliated columnar epithelium	Fallopian tube	Serous tumors
Tall mucus-secreting non-ciliated epithelium	Endocervix	Mucinous tumors
Epithelium similar to uterine endometrial glands	Uterine endometrial glands	Endometrioid tumors
	Uterine endometrial glands during pregnancy	Clear cell tumors (glycogen rich)
Transitional epithelium	Urinary bladder	Brenner tumors

>4 layers thick, showing pleomorphism and arranged in cribriform pattern. There is lack of fibrovascular cores.

- *Borderline endometrioid tumors:* These exhibit well differentiated adenocarcinoma with lack of stromal invasion. Borderline Brenner tumor is composed of cysts and papillae. These papillae are projecting in cystic spaces and lined by stratified lining. Stromal invasion is absent.

Malignant Surface Epithelial Tumors

Well differentiated surface epithelial tumors tend to be associated with early stage disease. Mucinous and endometrial tumors have better prognosis than serous cystadenocarcinomas. Serous epithelial tumors are most often bilateral with malignant potential in 30% of patients.

Clinical Course

Clinical course of benign and malignant ovarian tumors are described as under (Table 24.17).

Risk Factors

Definite risk factors can be identified only in minority of cases and include ovarian dysgenesis, family cancer syndrome, and BRCA1 and BRCA2 gene mutations linked with an increased incidence of breast cancer (Table 24.18).

- *Age group:* As a group, younger patients have a better outcome due to occurrence of higher percentage of borderline, well-differentiated, and stage I tumors in this age group.
- *Nulliparity:* It is dangerous because repeated disruption and repair of the epithelial surface. It occurs during normal cyclic ovulation in nulliparous. Conversely, suppression of ovulation in multiparous women is protective due to repeated pregnancy, lactation and oral contraceptive pills.
- *Long fertile period:* Early menarche (>12 years age), late menopause and long-term estrogen replacement therapy increase risk of ovarian cancer.
- *Family history:* BRCA1 is implicated in cancer of breast and ovary. If mother had ovarian cancer then

Table 24.18: Risk factors of ovarian cancer

- Elderly age group
- Nulliparity
- Long fertile period
- Family history of ovarian cancer
- Gonadal dysgenesis
- Superovulation therapy for infertility treatment
- BRCA1 tumor suppressor gene mutation
- ERBB2 (Her2 neu)
- SMADA4 tumor suppressor gene mutation
- DNA mismatch repair genes inactivation

Table 24.17: Clinical course of surface epithelial ovarian tumors

Benign surface epithelial ovarian tumors	Malignant surface epithelial ovarian tumors
These constitute 80% of ovarian tumors	These affect elderly women (40–65 years)
Most ovarian tumors are benign and non-functional and so do not produce clinical effects until they have grown to a large size and present with increasing mass or girth	Malignant tumors rapidly spread outside the ovary by local extension or surface seeding and occasionally through lymphatic route and bloodstream involving extra-abdominal organs such as lung at the time of diagnosis
	Patient presents with abdominal mass, ascites, cachexia, and pleural effusion, signs of increased pressure on neighboring organs such as urinary frequency, constipation, torsion, feminizing or masculinizing effects
	These often have poor prognosis

daughter is at increased risk of developing cancer of breast and ovary.

- *Gonadal dysgenesis:* Patient develops ovarian childhood malignancies and rarely gonadoblastoma.
- *Superovulation therapy for infertility treatment:* It may also be a predisposing factor (controversial).
- *BRCA1 tumor suppressor gene:* Mutation of BRCA1 has been implicated in familial cancers of ovary (50%) and breast. These patients tend to develop ovarian cancer considerably earlier than women who have sporadic ovarian cancer.
- *ERBB2 (Her2 neu):* Gene amplification of ERBB2 (Her2 neu) is demonstrated by immunohistochemistry (monoclonal antibody) on the cell membrane or using fluorescent *in situ* hybridization. Mutation of ERBB2 (Her2 neu) is observed in 30% of ovarian cancers. Herceptin is administered to treat ovarian cancers.
- *SMADA4 tumor suppressor gene:* Mutation of DPC4 (deletion) has been demonstrated in 55% of pancreatic cancers and rarely seen in breast and ovaries.
- *DNA mismatch repair genes inactivation:* There is increased risk of development of carcinoma of endometrium (first most common cancer), right colon and ovary in patients with hereditary non-polyposis colon cancer (Lynch syndrome).

Immunohistochemistry

Panel of markers is used on histological sections of surgical specimens of surface epithelial ovarian tumors.

Markers	Expression
CA 125 (cell surface glycoprotein most important marker recognized by the monoclonal antibody OC 125)	Positive (mucinous epithelial ovarian tumors) Positive (cancer of) cervix, endometrium, gastrointestinal tract, thyroid, and breast
Vimentin	Positive
Ber-EP4	Positive
Desmoplakin	Positive
Estrogen and progesterone receptors (ER, PR)	Positive
Epidermal growth factor	Positive
Follicle-stimulating hormone	Positive

Mode of Spread of Surface Epithelial Carcinomas

- *Serous and mucinous cystadenocarcinoma and endometrioid carcinoma:* These metastasize to pleura, diaphragm, lymph nodes, liver, stomach, omentum, serosa of bowel, pelvic peritoneal implant and opposite ovary.

Table 24.19: Mode of spread of surface epithelial carcinomas of ovary

Route	Ovarian carcinomas	Organs involved
Direct extension	Serous or mucinous cystadenocarcinoma	Omentum or pelvic peritoneum, the serosa of the uterine corpus, fallopian tube and ovary (auto implants) and opposite ovary Stomach, sigmoid colon, caecum, liver, spleen due to spread from peritoneum Entire peritoneal cavity covered by tumor implants <1 cm simulating miliary tuberculosis
	Borderline serous tumors	Peritoneal implants (16–47%) Psammoma bodies more numerous in noninvasive carcinoma than invasive peritoneal implants
Peritoneal dissemination	Serous cystadenocarcinoma Mucinous cystadenocarcinoma Endometrioid carcinoma	Peritoneal involvement resulting in ascites (most common) } Peritoneal involvement less common
Distant metastases	Papillary serous cystadenocarcinoma	Lungs, pleural cavity (pleural effusion)
Lymphatic route	Papillary serous cystadenocarcinoma	It most often usually spreads by lymphatic route Contralateral ovary, omentum peritoneal cavity, lymph nodes (*para-aortic* and *pelvic*), and liver An umbilical metastasis ('*Sister Joseph's nodule*') may be the first manifestation of the disease Intestinal obstruction (intestine involvement) and hydronephrosis (ureter involvement)
	Mucinous cystadenocarcinoma	It rarely spreads by lymphatic route

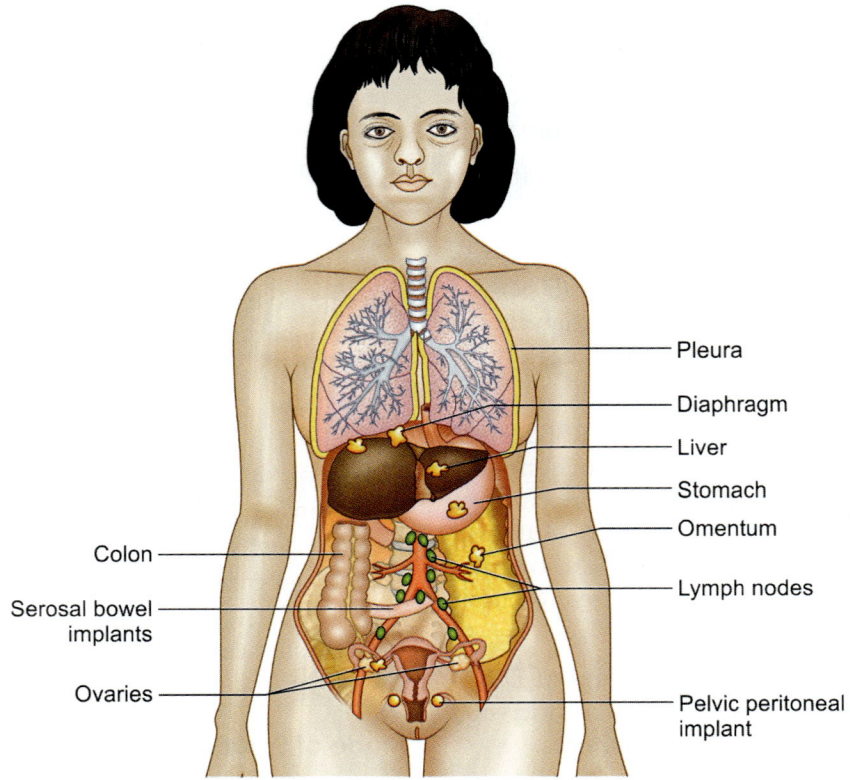

Fig. 24.68: Metastases of surface epithelial ovarian carcinoma.

- *Mucinous and endometrioid ovarian carcinomas:* These have less tendency to early and widespread peritoneal involvement in comparison to serous cystadenocarcinoma.
- *Serous cystadenocarcinoma:* It most often spreads by lymphatic route.
- *Mucinous cystadenocarcinoma:* It rarely spreads by lymphatic route.

Mode of spread of surface epithelial ovarian carcinomas is described in Table 24.19 and Fig. 24.68).

SEROUS SURFACE EPITHELIAL TUMORS

Serous tumors account for approximately 20% of all ovarian tumors. These are more common than mucinous tumors. These are most often bilateral with malignant potential in 30% of patients.

These occur in women during reproductive age group (20–50 years). Therefore, mucinous tumors have better prognosis.

Histological Types

These include serous cystadenoma, borderline tumor and serous cystadenocarcinoma.

The tumor cells from serous borderline tumor may shed from the surface and implant on peritoneum, possibly reflecting multifocal origins. The tumor cells show positivity for S-100.

Electron Microscopy

Ultrastructurally, cilia are often found in ovarian benign and borderline tumors, but usually absent in carcinomas.

> **Immunohistochemistry**
> - The neoplastic cells are always reactive to keratins (**CK7+/CK20**). These also express **EMA** and **CK18**. **S-100** protein is positive in particularly borderline tumors.
> - WT1 stains diffusely most ovarian serous carcinomas, ascertaining the site of origin of serous carcinomas within the female genital tract.
> - PAX8 is commonly positive in serous tumors of the ovary.
> - Various monoclonal antibodies have been produced against epithelial (mainly serous) ovarian tumors, such as CA 125 and SMO47.

Serous Cystadenoma

Serous cystadenoma is most common tumor affecting 20–40 years of women.

Gross Morphology

- Bilateral ovarian involvement is very common. This benign tumor is unilocular cyst measuring 10–15 cm and filled with clear serous fluid.
- Cyst is either covered by smooth glistening capsule or partly by papillary excrescences (Figs 24.69A and B).

Light Microscopy

- The tumor is composed of fibrovascular core lined by single layer ciliated tall columnar epithelium similar to fallopian tube epithelium, without atypia.
- There is presence of *psammoma bodies* with concentric layers of calcification (calcification of necrotic cells) in the fibrovascular core in 30% cases.
- Surgical excision of cystadenoma cures the patient (Fig. 24.69C).

Borderline Serous Tumors of Low Malignant Potential

Approximately 10% of ovarian surface epithelial tumors are borderline malignant. These tumors are predominantly cystic and seen in perimenopausal women. Light microscopy shows varying degree of nuclear atypia and increased mitotic activity. These remain confined to the ovary. Rarely, cells may shed from the surface and implant on peritoneum, possibly reflecting multifocal origin. **S-100 protein** is positive in particularly borderline tumors (Fig. 24.70).

Borderline Serous Tumors with Microinvasion

Occasional borderline serous tumor may exhibit microinvasion involving <3 mm stroma. It is considered progression of the disease.

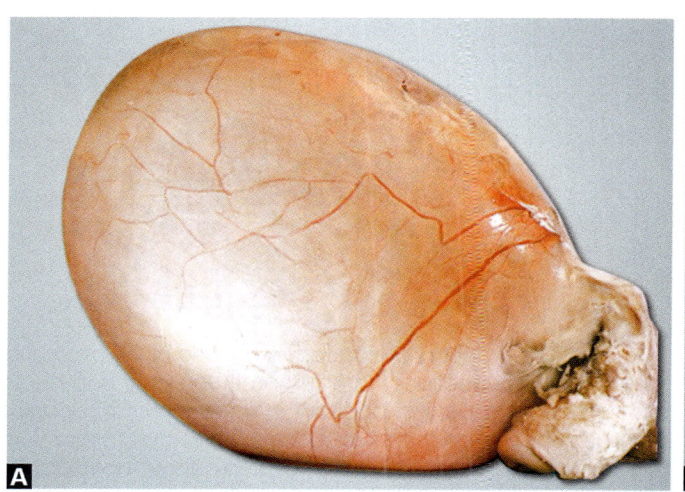
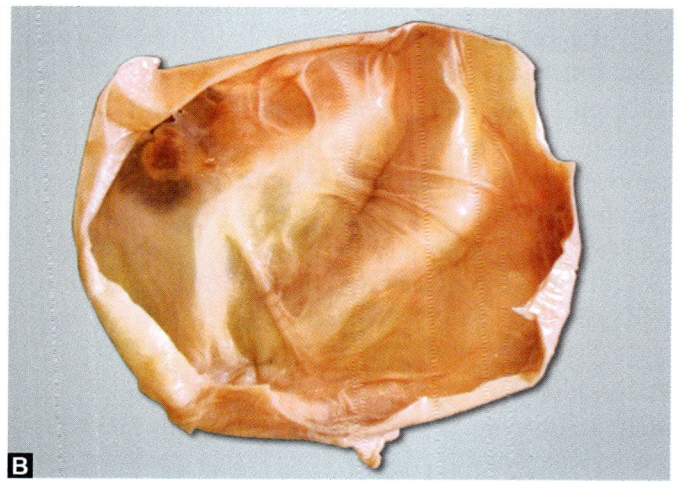

Fig. 24.69: (A) Serous cystadenoma, and (B) unilocular, thin-walled cyst containing clear fluid.

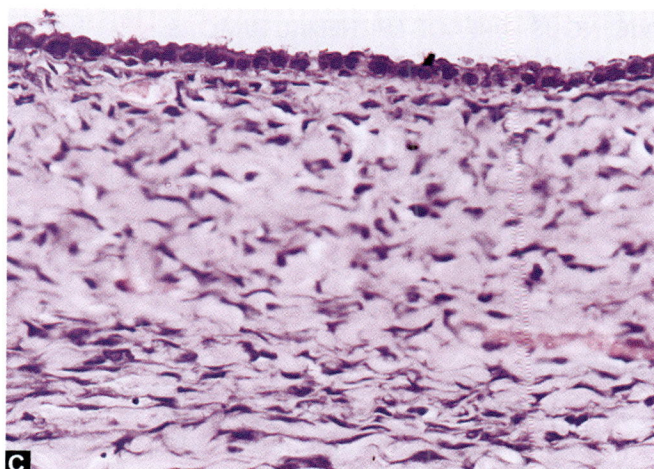

Fig. 24.69C: Tumor comprises fibrovascular core lined by single layer ciliated tall columnar epithelium similar to fallopian tube epithelium, without atypia (100X).

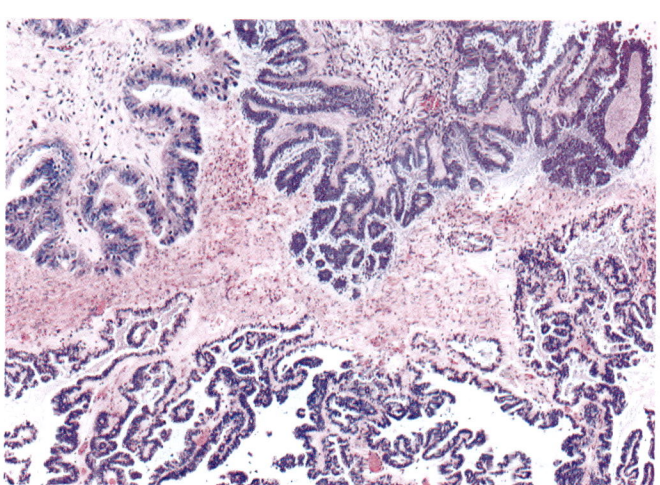

Fig. 24.70: Serous borderline tumor. Tumor shows nuclear atypia and increased mitotic activity. It is confined to be ovary (100X).

Serous Cystadenocarcinoma

This malignant tumor accounts for approximately 50% of ovarian carcinomas and is frequently bilateral. The criteria of malignancy are stromal invasion. Presence of psammoma bodies in a patient with ascites is most compatible with the diagnosis of papillary serous cystadenocarcinoma of the ovary (Table 24.20).

Gross Morphology
- Serous cystadenocarcinoma has both solid and cystic element. It has papillary pattern with stromal invasion.
- Tumor is solid with papillary projections and foci of necrosis.
- The outgrowth of tumor cells through the capsule of the tumor is an ominous sign (Fig. 24.71A).

Light Microscopy
- The tumor is composed of multilayered cells with solid papillae formation, cytologic atypia and psammoma bodies.
- Stromal invasion by tumor cells is evident.
- The presence of tumor nodules on the peritoneum and ascites fluid that contains tumor cells is other sign of malignancy.
- Glandular tissue may be present. Tumor could be demonstrated at any stage of differentiation (Fig. 24.71B).

Clinical course
Patient undergoes rapid deterioration with fatal outcome.

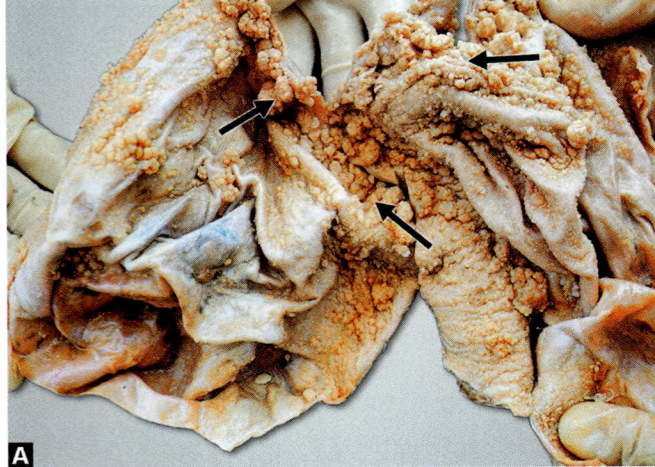
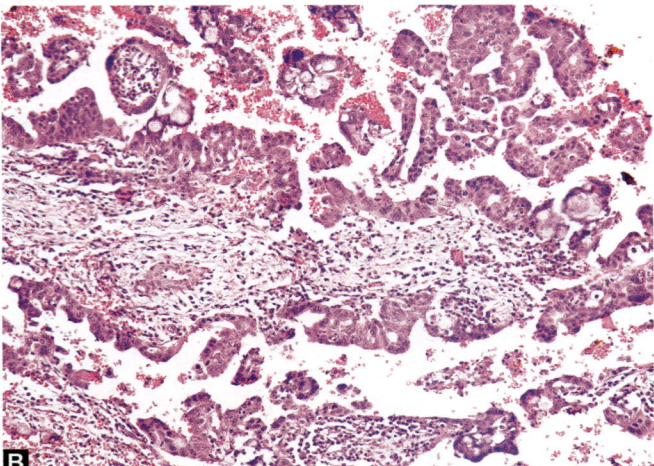

Fig. 24.71: (A) Papillary cystadenocarcinoma of the ovary. Note the papillary projections in the lumen of the cyst, and also on its surface. In a benign papillary cystadenoma, the papillae are present only on the inner surface of the cyst (arrows), and (B) the tumor is composed of multilayered cells with solid papillae formation, cytologic atypia and psammoma bodies. Stromal invasion by tumor cells is evident (100X).

Table 24.20: Immunohistochemistry in serous cystadenocarcinoma of ovary

Panel of markers	Expression in tumor cells
CA 125	Positive
CK7	Positive
CK20	Positive
SMO47	Positive
B72.3	Positive
CEA	Positive
Ber-EP4	Positive
PAX8	Positive
Placental alkaline phosphatase (PLAP)	Positive
Hormone receptors	Positive
WT1	Positive

MUCINOUS SURFACE EPITHELIAL TUMORS

Mucinous tumors are less common than serous tumors. These constitute 25% of all ovarian tumors. These are more often unilateral in 80% and bilateral in 20% of cases. Mucinous tumors are larger and usually multilocular filled with viscous mucus.

Age Group
These occur in middle-aged women.

Categories
Like serous tumors, mucinous tumors can be classified as benign mucinous cystadenoma (80%), borderline tumor (10–15%) and mucinous cystadenocarcinoma (5–10%). Mucinous tumors may be lined by endocervical or intestinal type of epithelium.

Mucinous Cystadenoma

Mucinous cystadenoma can reach a very large size. It is multilocular cystic lesion filled with viscous mucus. It is most often unilateral, but bilateral in 25% of cases. It may undergo torsion, rupture, borderline tumor or mucinous cystadenocarcinoma. Surgical excision of mucinous cystadenoma cures the patient.

Gross Morphology
- Mucinous cystadenoma reveals large multilocular cyst.
- Cut surface shows multiple cystic spaces filled with viscous mucus. In a few cases, it may reach truly massive proportion, exceeding 50 cm in diameter (Fig. 24.72).

Light Microscopy
Tumor is lined by tall mucus-secreting non-ciliated endocervical like epithelium with apical vacuolation (Fig. 24.73).

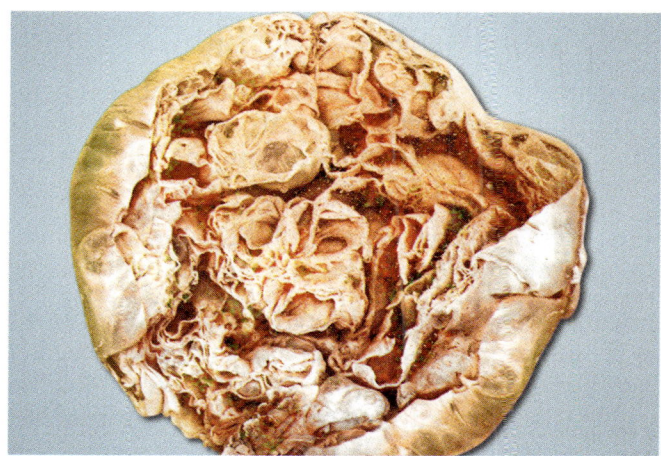

Fig. 24.72: Mucinous cystadenoma showing multiple cystic spaces filled with viscous mucus.

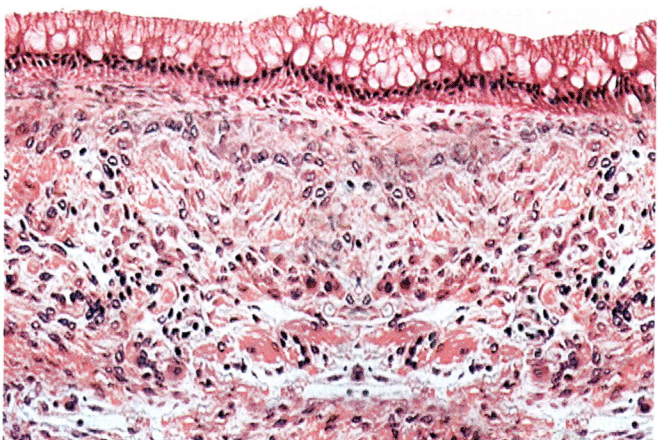

Fig. 24.73: Mucinous cystadenoma (100x).

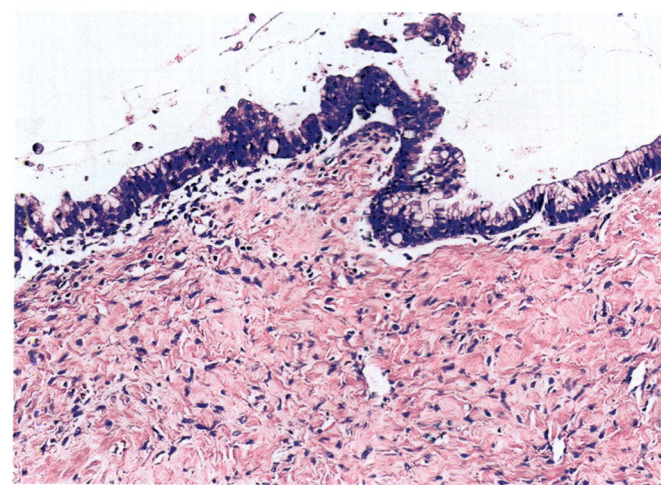

Fig. 24.74: Mucinous borderline tumor showing varying degree of nuclear atypia and increased mitotic activity confined to epthelium. There is no invasion of stroma by tumor cells (100X).

Mucinous Borderline Tumor

Light microsocpy shows varying degree of nuclear atypia and increased mitotic activity confined to epthelium. There is no invasion of stroma by tumor cells (Fig. 24.74).

Mucinous Cystadenocarcinoma

Mucinous cystadenocarcinoma account for 10% of malignant ovarian tumors. These are most often unilateral, multilocular cysts and largest tumors of the ovary. A cyst diameter of 25 cm is common. Thin-walled cysts are containing mucinous fluid.

Age group
Mucinous cystadenocarcinoma most often occurs in perimenopausal women.

Clinical feature
- Approximately 5% of women with mucinous tumor presents with *pseudomyxoma peritonei* known as *jelly belly*, a condition characterized by filling of peritoneal cavity with pool of mucin due to peritoneal tumor implants.
- Most mucinous tumors in the ovary associated with *pseudomyxoma peritonei* are metastatic in origin. It is worth mentioning that pseudomyxoma peritonei may also occur in mucocele of appendix.
- Accumulated mucinous contents may cause intestinal adhesions resulting in fatal outcome.

Gross Morphology
Mucinous cystadenocarcinoma is large multilocular tumor. Cut surface shows multiple cystic spaces filled with mucinous fluid (Fig. 24.75).

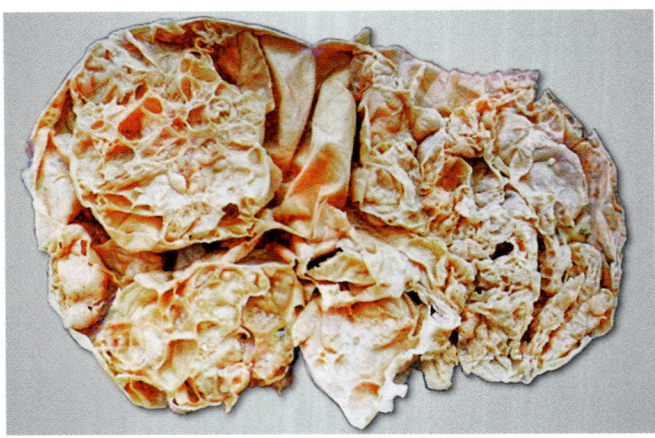

Fig. 24.75: Mucinous cystadenocarcinoma shows multilocular cysts containing mucinous material. Solid areas are malignant.

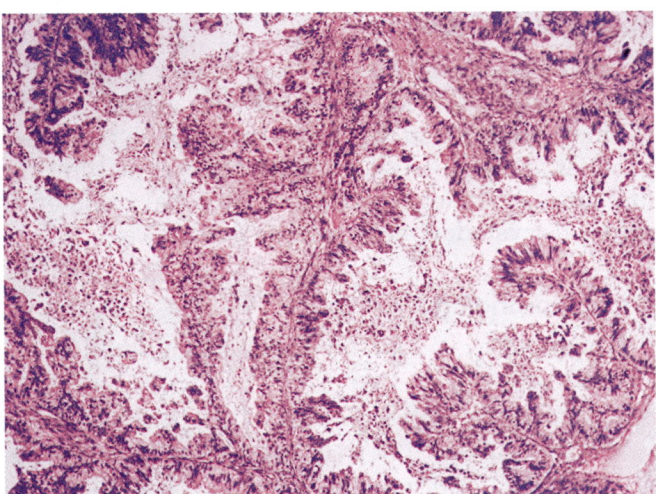

Fig. 24.76: Mucinous cystadenocarcinoma.

Light Microscopy

Frank stromal invasion by tumor cells is demonstrated in histological sections. Two patterns of invasion are recognized—expansile and destructive.

- *Expansile pattern:* It shows multilayered atypical epithelial cells arranged in crowded glandular fashion, a little stroma and sometimes a cribriform architecture.
- *Destructive pattern:* It shows single glands or individual atypical cells invading >3 mm in two linear dimensions or >10 mm in 2 areas (Fig. 24.76).

Mucinous cystadenocarcinoma of ovary should be differentiated from metastatic colorectal adenocarcinoma metastasizing to ovaries (Table 24.21).

Immunohistochemistry

Ovarian mucinous cystadenocarcinomas show positivity with **CA 125** and **CK7**. Metastatic colorectal adenocarcinomas show positivity with CK20 and CEA.

Clinical Course

Mucinous adenocarcinomas rarely spread by lymphatics. These are clinically silent; hence the majority of patients have advanced metastatic disease at diagnosis.

ENDOMETRIOID ADENOCARCINOMA

- *Endometrioid adenocarcinoma* histologically resembles well differentiated carcinoma of endometrium. Majority of endometrioid tumors of the ovary are carcinomas. Squamous differentiation may be seen in all types of endometrioid tumors.
- *Origin:* It is a surface epithelial ovarian tumor arising from the coelomic epithelium. It constitutes 10% of the malignant ovarian tumors affecting perimenopausal age group.
- *Association:* Approximately 10–20% are associated with endometriosis and endometrial carcinoma.
- *Benign endometrioid tumors* (adenofibromas/cystadenofibromas) are rare. These are composed of endometrial glands arranged in fibrous stroma. These are distinguished from endometriosis by lack of associated endometrial stroma and hemosiderin-laden macrophages.

Origin

This surface epithelial ovarian tumor arises from the coelomic epithelium.

Table 24.21: Comparison between mucinous cystadenocarcinoma and metastatic colorectal mucinous carcinomas

Parameters	Mucinous cystadenocarcinoma	Metastatic colorectal adenocarcinomas to ovaries
Ovary involvement	Unilateral involvement	Bilateral involvement
Light microscopy	Multilayered atypical epithelial cells arranged in crowded glandular fashion, a little stroma	Garland pattern of glands lining cystic spaces
	Destructive pattern shows single glands or individual atypical cells	These contain dirty necrosis (abundant karyorrhectic debris)
Immunoreactivity	CK7 and CA 125	CK20 and CEA

Gross Morphology
- Endometrioid adenocarcinoma is more often *solid cystic* tumor in contrast to serous and mucinous tumors.
- The content tends to be *hemorrhagic turbid brown fluid* rather than serous or mucinous. Visible papillary formations are usually absent or inconspicuous.
- It is mostly unilocular cystic tumor containing turbid brown fluid.

Light Microscopy
- *Endometrioid* adenocarcinoma of ovary resembles endometrial adenocarcinoma.
- Most are well differentiated, with or without papillary formations. Some cases (50%) may show squamous cell differentiation to form adenoacanthoma (Fig. 24.77 and Table 24.22).
- Similarly, some tumors have foci resembling serous or mucinous carcinomas.

Histochemistry
Mucin present within lumen or surface of epithelium is demonstrated by **mucicarcmine**.

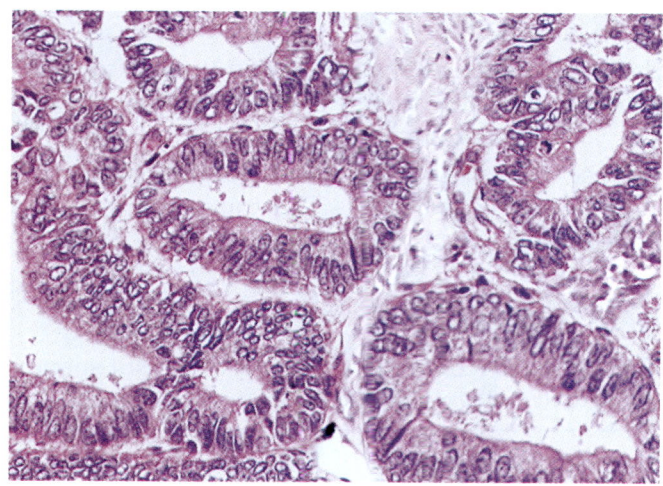

Fig. 24.77: Endometrioid carcinoma (100X).

Prognosis
Endometrioid carcinoma has better prognosis when compared with serous cystadenocarcinomas or mucinous cystadenocarcinomas comparison of serous and mucinous and endometricid carcinomas is given in Table 24.23.

Table 22.22: FIGO grading system for endometrioid adenocarcinoma

Grade	Differentiation	Growth	Histological features
Grade 1	Well differentiated	<5% solid growth	Well-formed glands
Grade 2	Moderately differentiated	6–50% solid growth	More complex glandular architecture with increased stratification
Grade 3	Poorly differentiated	>50% sold growth	Poorly formed glands with large sheets of cells

Table 24.23: Comparison of serous and mucinous and endometrioid carcinomas

Characteristics	Serous cystadenocarcinoma	Mucinous cystadenocarcinoma	Endometrioid carcinoma
Age group	Reproductive age	Middle adult age	Perimenopausal women
Relative frequency	60–80% (more common)	5–15% (less common)	10–25%
Ovary involvement	30–50% (often bilateral)	10–20% (mostly unilateral)	15–30%
Tumor	Unilocular cyst	Multilocular cysts	Solid or cystic
Size	Moderate	Often large size	Moderate
Fluid content	Serous fluid	Mucinous fluid	Hemorrhagic fluid
Coexistent endometrial hyperplasia or carcinoma	Exceptional	Exceptional	15–30%
Torsion	Common	Absent	Absent
Pseudomyxoma peritonei	Absent	Most often	Absent
Lining epithelium	Cuboidal	Columnar, with basally located nucleus	Columnar, with centrally located nucleus
Mucin	Present only in luminal border	Abundant mucin present in cytoplasm	Mucin is present in luminal border
Squamous metaplasia	Exceptional case	Exceptional case	50% cases
Cilia	Frequent	Absent	Rare
Psammoma bodies	30%	Exceptional case	Exceptional case

CLEAR CELL CARCINOMA

Clear cell carcinoma (mesonephroid tumor) is the *least common* tumor. Majority of clear cell tumors are frank *high grade adenocarcinomas*.

These have *strong association to ovarian endometriosis* and *endometrioid carcinomas*. This tumor is always high grade and carry a *poor prognosis*.

Gross Morphology

Tumor reveals combination of solid and cystic spongy areas. Cut surface is white tan to yellow (Fig. 24.78).

Light Microscopy

- *Tumor cells morphology:* In the solid area of tumor, it comprises large tumor cells with clear cytoplasm containing glycogen, mucin, and fat. Some of the nuclei protrude into the lumina, resulting in hobnail configuration.
- *Arrangement of tumor cells:* These cells are arranged in solid sheets, tubular and papillary fashion. The cores of the papillae often exhibit prominent hyalinization and lack epithelial stratification. In cystic areas, it shows neoplastic cells lining the spaces (Fig. 24.79).

Histochemistry

Cells may exhibit positivity with periodic acid–Schiff (PAS), diastase-resistant hyaline globules.

Immunohistochemistry

Panel of markers is used in surgical specimens of clear cell carcinoma (Table 24.24).

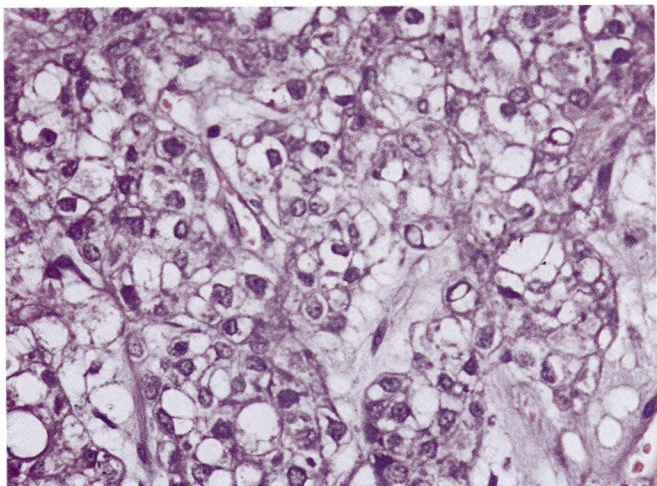

Fig. 24.79: Clear cell carcinoma showing large tumor cells with clear cytoplasm arranged in solid sheets, tubular and papillary fashion (400X).

Table 24.24: Immunohistochemistry of clear cell carcinoma of ovary

Panel of markers	Expression in tumor cells
CA 125	Positive
CEA	Positive
PAX8	Positive
CK7	Positive
CAM	Positive
EMA	Positive
CD15 (Leu-M1)	Positive
Vimentin	Positive
BCL-2	Positive
p53	Positive
ER and PR receptors	Variable reactivity

Clinical Course

These tumors are always *high grade* and carry a *poor prognosis*. Approximately 50% cases have 5 years survival rate, when the tumor is confined to the ovaries.

BRENNER TUMOR

Brenner tumors constitute between 1% and 2% of all ovarian neoplasms.

Origin

Brenner tumor is derived from surface epithelium of ovary. *Most often Brenner tumors are benign in nature.* Rarely, these tumors may be borderline and malignant.

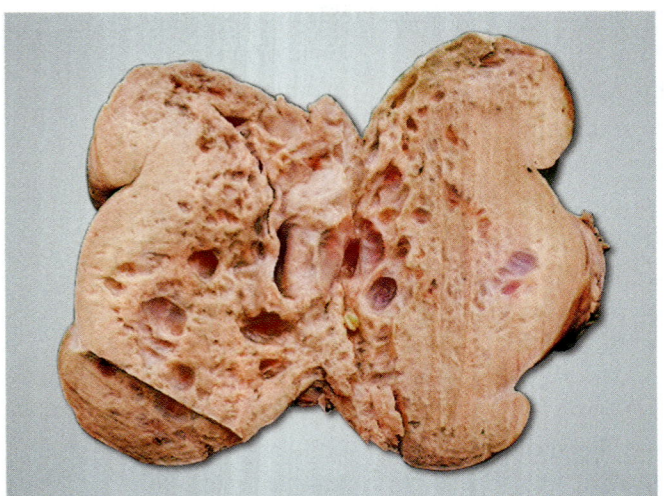

Fig. 24.78: Clear cell carcinoma showing solid and cystic areas.

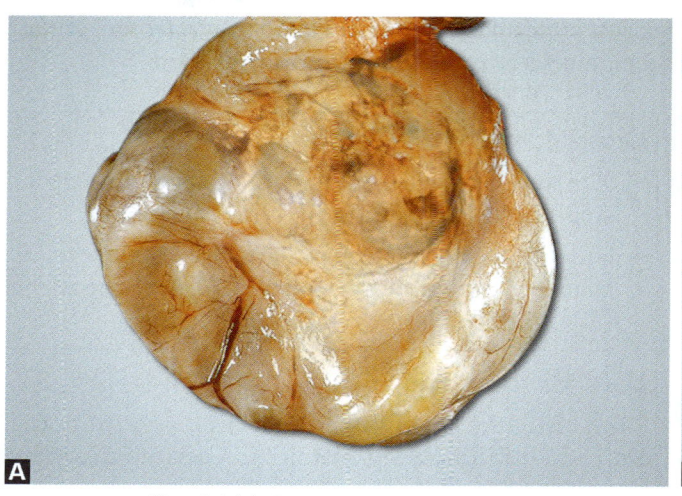
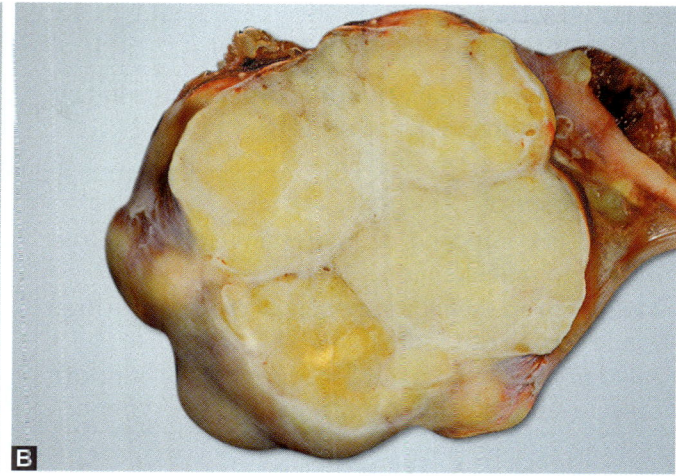

Fig. 24.80: Brenner tumor is encapsulated solid cut surface is white or yellow with form consistency.

Age Group

It occurs in premenopausal (70%) and postmenopausal women.

Clinical Features

Some cases are accompanied by signs of *hyperestrinism*, such as *uterine bleeding* from endometrial hyperplasia in the postmenopausal women.

Gross Morphology

Brenner tumor is encapsulated solid tumor variable in size usually *unilateral, firm, white or yellowish* resembling fibroma but contain small cystic areas filled with opaque, viscous, yellowish-brown fluid (Fig. 24.80).

Light Microscopy

- *Benign Brenner tumor:* It comprises well-formed nests (solid pattern) of transitional epithelium resembling transitional epithelium of urinary bladder. The tumor cells are small, oval with pale cytoplasm and oval nuclei with longitudinal groove (coffee bean appearance). Most often, mucinous glands are present in their center scattered throughout the dense fibrous stroma, resembling that of an ovary. Such neoplasm may have hormonal activity.
- *Borderline Brenner tumor:* This variant is low malignant potential. Tumor is composed of cysts and papillae. These papillae are projecting in cystic spaces and lined by stratified lining. Stromal invasion is absent.
- *Malignant Brenner tumor:* It consists of atypical large pleomorphic cells arranged in large nests with irregular borders. Stromal invasion is present.

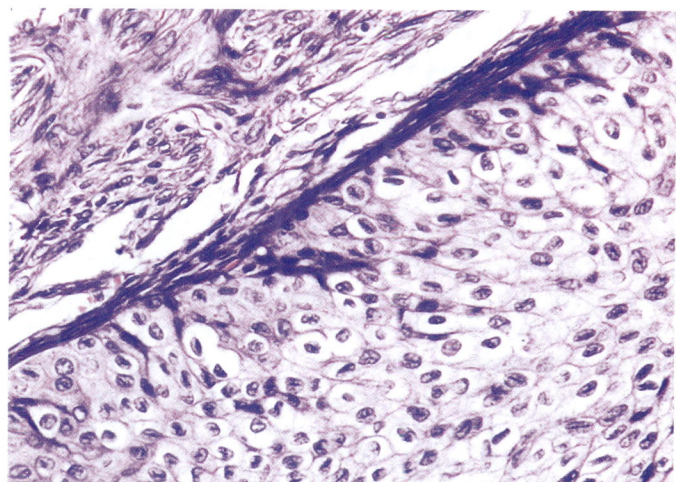

Fig. 24.81: Benign Brenner tumor showing solid and cystic nests of epithelial cells with oval nuclei, small nucleoli in a fibrous stroma. Many of these cells exhibit longitudinal grooves (400X).

- *Transitional cell carcinoma:* It closely resembles transitional cell carcinoma of urinary bladder with same grading (Fig. 24.81).

Histochemistry

The tumor cells may contain *glycogen, mucin, and lipid*. Lipid is present in larger amounts in the stromal cells in the cases accompanied by hyperestrinism.

Immunohistochemistry

The tumor cells are reactive to **cytokeratin, EMA,** and **CEA** (the latter also present in the lumen of the cysts).

Marker	Expression
Cytokeratin	Positive
EMA	Positive
CEA	Positive

CARCINOSARCOMA (MALIGNANT MIXED MÜLLERIAN TUMOR)

Occasionally this primary tumor of ovary occurs in postmenopausal women. Prognosis is very poor.

Light Microscopy
- Tumor is composed of malignant epithelial and mesenchymal elements.
- Malignant epithelial component is most often a high grade serous carcinoma.
- Mesenchymal component consists of smooth muscle, endometrial stroma, cartilage and bone.

GERM CELL TUMORS

Germ cell tumors constitute approximately 25% of all ovarian tumors. These are the most common tumors in children, accounting for 60–70% of all ovarian tumors in these age group especially mature cystic teratomas.

Classification

These include dysgerminoma, germ cell tumors with embryonic differentiation (embryonal carcinoma, teratoma) and extraembryonic differentiation (yolk sac tumor, choriocarcinoma). There may be mixed germ cell tumors (dysgerminoma + benign cystic teratoma). Except mature cystic teratomas, the proportion of malignant germ cell tumors (especially immature teratomas, yolk sac tumors, and dysgerminomas) is much greater than in adults (Table 24.25).

Table 24.25: Germ cell tumors of ovary

Tumor	Examples
Dysgerminoma	Classic dysgerminoma
	Dysgerminoma with syncytio-trophoblastic element
	Dysgerminoma with yolk sac element
	Anaplastic dysgerminoma
Germ cell tumor with embryonic differentiation	Embryonal carcinoma
	Teratomas: Mature, immature
Germ cell tumor with extra-embryonic differentiation	Yolk sac tumor
	Choriocarcinoma

DYSGERMINOMA

This malignant tumor is analogous to testicular seminoma constituting *50% of germ cell tumors* and 2% of all ovarian tumors. It affects *10–30 years* of age group especially second and third decades. It is extremely *radiosensitive*, and most often unilateral in 80–90% cases. Incidence is more in Turner's syndrome, gonadal dysgenesis and pseudohermophroditism.

Gross Morphology
- The tumor is well encapsulated varying in size, i.e. small nodules to filling up entire abdomen.
- Cut surface is *gray white to yellowish, homogenous or lobulated* appearance with solid *rubbery consistency* (Fig. 24.82).

Light Microscopy

Like testicular seminoma, ovarian dysgerminomas may exhibit following histologic variants described as under.

- *Classic dysgerminoma:* Tumor is composed of large nests of monotonously uniform round or oval cells with deeply staining nuclei and abundant clear glycogen-filled cytoplasm. These tumor cells are separated by fibrous septa containing mostly T-lymphocytes (Fig. 24.83).
- *Dysgerminoma with syncytiotrophoblastic element:* It shows scattered hCG-positive syncytiotrophoblastic cells around proximity to blood vessels or to hemorrhagic foci. It may be accompanied by serum elevation of hCG and tissue immunoreactivity for this marker.
- *Dysgerminoma with yolk sac element:* It shows abortive yolk sac elements. Serum α-fetoprotein is raised and tissue cells are reactive for this marker.
- *Anaplastic dysgerminoma:* It shows increased mitotic activity over *30 mitoses per 10 high power fields*. This variant is reactive for keratin.

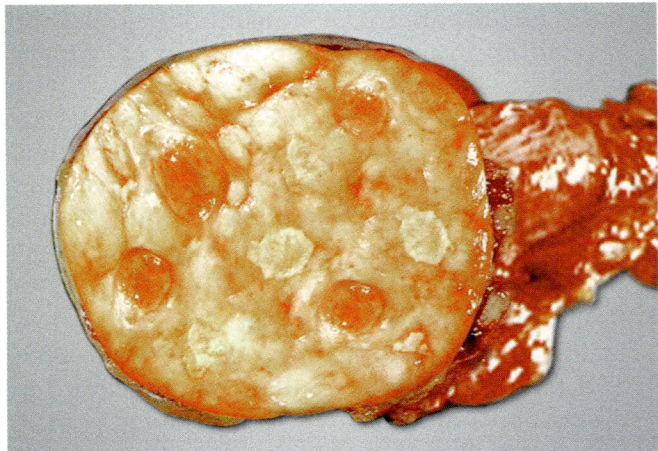

Fig. 24.82: Dysgerminoma of the ovary. The tumor has a cream-colored, fleshy appearance on its cut surface, with some areas of hemorrhage. This tumor has the same microscopic appearances as a seminoma of the testis.

Female Reproductive System

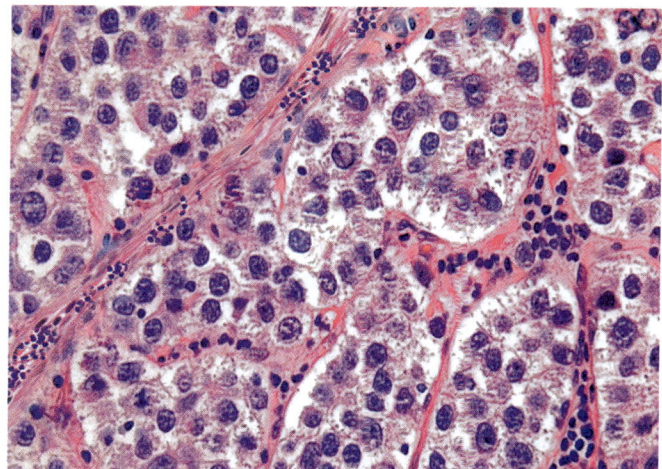

Fig. 24.83: Dysgerminoma—tumor cells grow in sheets separated by fibrous septa containing blood vessels. Lymphoid infiltrates are virtually always present, sometimes imparting a florid reactive appearance with germinal centers (400X).

Immunohistochemistry

Panel of markers is used in surgical specimens of dysgerminoma (Table 24.26).

Table 24.26: Immunohistochemistry in dysgerminoma

Panel of markers	Expression in tumor cells
Placental alkaline phosphatase (PLAP)	Positive
CD117	Positive

Serum Markers

LDH isoenzymes 1 and 2 are increased in 95% of cases.

Metastases

Dysgerminoma usually metastasizes more commonly in the contralateral ovary, retroperitoneal nodes, and peritoneal cavity. Involvement of peritoneum decreases survival rate.

Prognosis

Tumor is extremely responsive to radiotherapy and chemotherapy. Prognosis is excellent in 95% of stage I cases, if tumor is unilateral and salpingo-ophrectomy is done.

EMBRYONAL CARCINOMA

Embryonal carcinoma is highly malignant germ cell tumor affecting young women (mean age 15 years). At surgery, there is extension of the tumor beyond the ovary in 40% of cases. Tumor is generally large with a median diameter of 17 cm.

Serum Markers

Serum α-fetoprotein level is often elevated as a result of its association with yolk sac tumor. Serum human chorionic gonadotropin (hCG) level is invariably high.

Gross Morphology
- Median diameter of this tumor is 17 cm. External surface is smooth and glistening.
- Cut surface is predominantly solid and variegated, with extensive areas of *necrosis* and *hemorrhage*.
- The tumor is variably demarcated from surrounding ovary and structures (Fig. 24.84).

Light Microscopy
- *Tumor cells morphology:* Tumor has a similar morphology to the embryonal carcinoma of the adult testis. It is composed of solid sheets and nests of large primitive cells, occasionally forming glandular and papillary structures. The tumor cells show hyperchromatic pleomorphic nuclei with prominent sometimes multiple nucleoli.
- Areas of hemorrhage and necrosis are seen. *Syncytiotrophoblast-like tumor cells* are frequently seen scattered among the smaller cells. These are immunoreactive for hCG. Embryonal carcinomas largely composed of embryoid bodies are referred to as 'polyembryomas' (Fig. 24.85).

Immunohistochemistry

Panel of markers is used in surgical specimens of embryonal carcinoma (Table 24.27).

Clinical Features

Patient presents with ovarian mass (average 17 cm), precocious puberty (47%), vaginal bleeding (33%), amenorrhea (7%) and hirsutism.

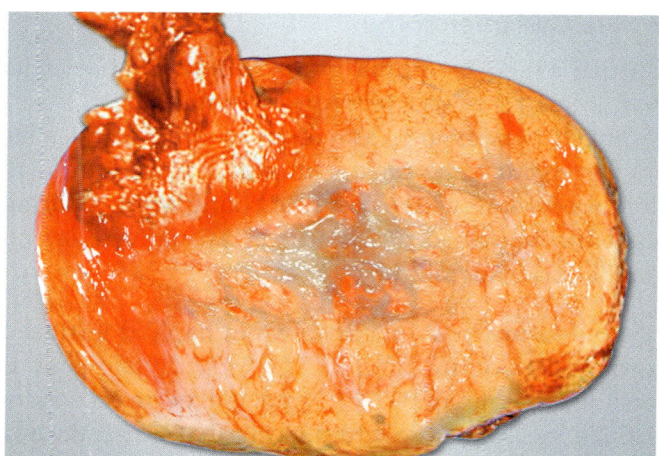

Fig. 24.84: Embryonal carcinoma. Cut surface shows variegated apperance.

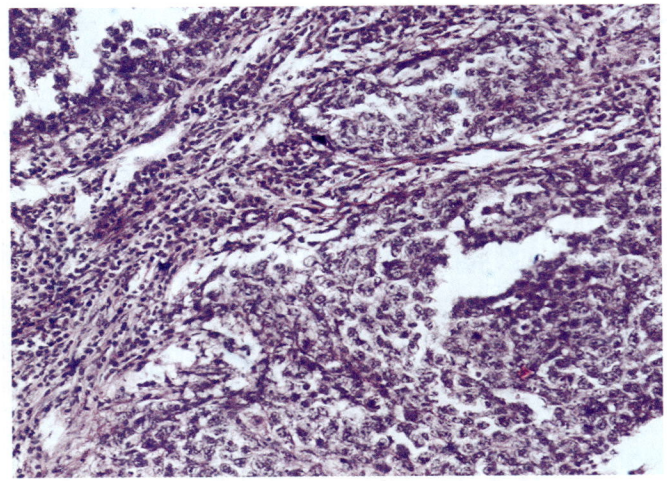

Fig. 24.85: Embryonal carcinoma shows solid sheets of large anaplastic cells with hyperchromatic nuclei (400X).

Table 24.27: Embryonal carcinoma: immunohistochemistry

Panel of markers	Expression in tumor cells
Pankeratin	Positive
CD30	Positive
OCT 3/4	Positive
SALL4	Positive
α-fetoprotein (AFP)	Variable focal staining

TERATOMAS

Teratomas demonstrate tissue elements derived from two or three embryonic layers.

These are observed in distinct forms: mature cystic teratoma, mature solid teratoma, immature teratoma and monodermal specialized teratomas (struma ovarii, carcinoid tumor, struma carcinoid tumor, and tumors with malignant transformation).

Mature Cystic Teratoma

Mature cystic teratoma is also known as *dermoid cyst*. Mature cystic teratomas constitute 90% of germ cell tumors and 20% of all ovarian neoplasms. They constitute the most common ovarian tumor in childhood. It most often occurs in young women during reproductive period. Dermoid cyst is usually unilateral in 75% and bilateral in 25% of cases.

Origin: Mature teratoma arises from haploid fertilized germ cell (? ovum after 1st meiotic division). It is considered that haploid (post-meiotic) germ cells auto-fertilize, yielding diploid tumor cells that are genetically female (46XX). The *radiographic calcifications* are highly suggestive of dermoid cyst.

Gross Morphology
- *External surface:* Mature cystic teratomas are well encapsulated multiloculated containing sebaceous, greasy pultaceous/cheesy material and measure 10–15 cm in diameter. Dermoid cysts are unilocular with an eminence on one aspect from which hairs grow.
- *Cut surface:* It shows thin grey white wrinkled epidermis/cyst wall containing tufts of hair shafts, teeth and areas of calcification. Teeth are often present in a well-defined nipple-like structure covered with hair, known as Rokitansky's protuberance.
- *Fetiform teratomas:* Some tumor may exhibit an imperfectly formed mandible or partial human body-like structure known as fetiform teratomas.
- *Associated tumors:* Mature cystic teratomas may coexist with mucinous cystadenoma, Brenner tumor, and fibrothecoma (Fig. 24.86).

Light Microscopy
- The cysts are lined by stratified squamous epithelium, sebaceous glands, hair shafts and other adnexal structures. Well-formed teeth are common. Many tumors exhibit *cartilage, bone, teeth, smooth muscle, and respiratory tract epithelium.*
- Tissues such as gut, thyroid, and brain are encountered less frequently (Fig. 24.87).

Malignant transformation
- An element of mature cystic teratoma may undergo malignant transformation in about 1% of cases usually *squamous cell carcinoma (most common)*, followed by carcinoid tumor, adenocarcinoma, thyroid carcinoma, melanoma and osteosarcoma, carcinosarcoma, glioblastoma multiforme. This

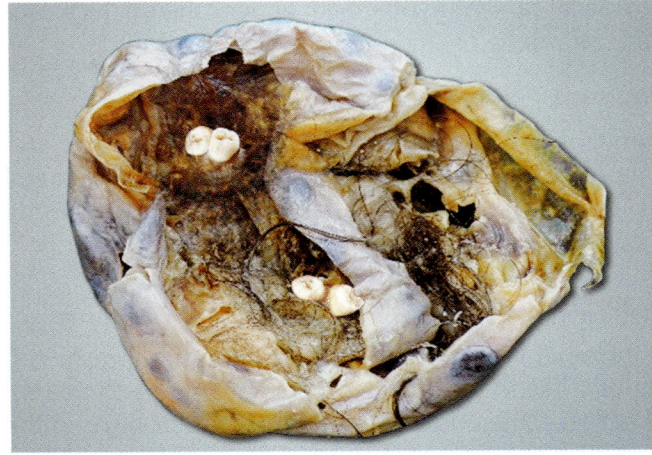

Fig. 24.86: Mature cystic teratoma shows hair and teeth.

Female Reproductive System

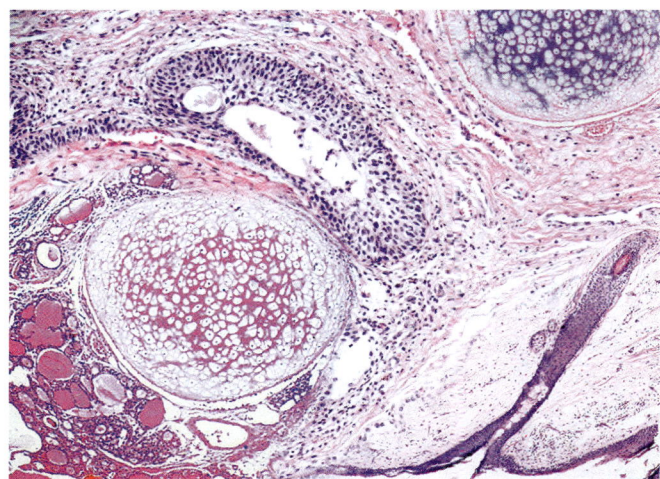

Fig. 24.87: Solid teratoma.

malignant transformation is accompanied by complex chromosomal aberrations.
- Teratomas are graded I, II and III based on the presence of immature neuroepithelium in the tumor.

Karyotyping by banding technique: The tumors show 46XX chromosomal patterns. Some believe that these tumors arise from an ovum after first meiotic division.

Clinical features: These tumors are freely mobile, most often undergoing torsion and subsequent hemorrhagic infarction, leading to abdominal pain.

Mature Solid Teratoma

This rare neoplasm occurs in young women, predominantly in the second decade. Structures of this uncommon variant are derived from all germ layers unlike *dermoid cyst* that mainly comprised structures derived from ectoderm. This tumor is difficult to differentiate from malignant immature teratoma. The prognosis is excellent, even if peritoneal implants (also mature and for the most part glial in composition) are present.

Gross Morphology
The tumor has a predominantly solid gross appearance, but multiple small cystic areas also are present.

Light Microscopy
Mature solid teratoma is composed entirely of adult tissues derived from all three germ layers such as skin, hair, sebaceous gland, teeth, neural and retinal tissues, cartilage, bone, muscle, hemopoietic tissue, bronchial glands, gastrointestinal mucosa, salivary tissue, thyroid tissue and pancreatic tissue.

Karyotyping by banding technique: The tumors show 46XX chromosomal patterns. Some believe that these tumors arise from an ovum after first meiotic division.

Immature Teratoma

Immature teratoma most often occurs in children and adolescents age group (average 18 years). It is rare but *aggressive malignant* tumor. Prognosis is poor except for stage I disease.

Gross Morphology
Tumor is solid bulky with smooth external surface. Capsular penetration by the tumor is usual. Cut surface is solid with multiple minute cysts, or predominantly cystic. Hair, bone, cartilage and calcification may be seen (Fig. 24.88).

Light Microscopy
- Tumor is composed of a mixture of embryonal and adult tissues derived from all three germ layers, regardless of its gross appearance, which are most often primitive neural elements, but mesodermal elements are also common.
- Some tumors are predominantly composed of endodermal derivatives, including esophagus, liver, and intestinal structures.
- Embryonal component of the tumor resembles tissues from an embryo or fetus than an adult. *Immature cartilage, glands, bone, muscle, neural rosettes are present* (Fig. 24.89).

Immunohistochemistry
- Staining for *GFAP* is helpful in the identification of mature and immature glial tissue. Drawback is GFAP is also detectable in chondrocytes.
- Immature and mature neural tissue is reactive for long-chain polysialic acid moiety of the *neural cell adhesion molecule (NCAM)*.

Marker	Expression
GFAP (identification of mature and immature glial tissue)	Positive
NCAM (neural cell adhesion molecule)	Positive

Clinical features
- Patient presents with rapidly growing tumor with local and distant metastases. Recurrence occurs within two years of excision, prognosis depends on grade of tumor. Chemotherapy in low grade tumor may induce maturation of the immature elements.
- *Metastases:* The risk of extraovarian spread depends on the amount of immature tissue present. It is rapidly growing tumor, which penetrates capsule and local and widespread metastases are present.

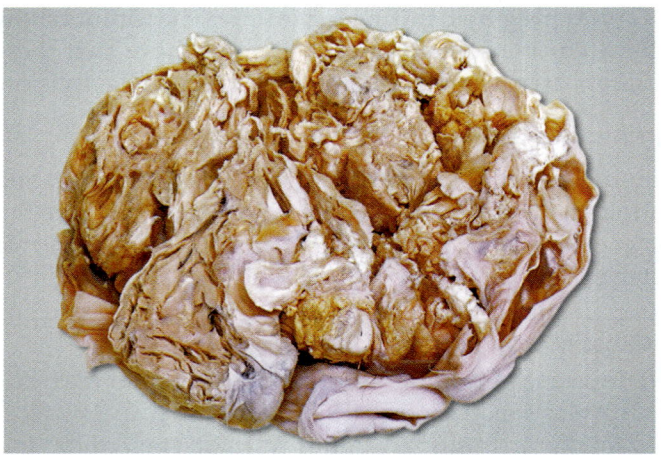

Fig. 24.88: Mature teratoma. Cut surface shows variegated appearance.

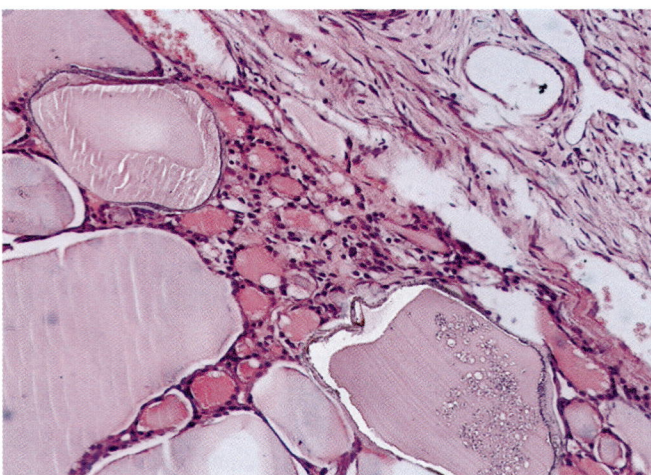

Fig. 24.90: Struma ovarii shows thyroid follicles of variable size filled with colloid material (100X).

Behavior: Benign course (95%), but may develop thyroid carcinoma (5%).

Carcinoid Tumor

Origin: Carcinoid tumor is monodermal specialized functional teratoma. It arises from intestinal epithelium. It synthesizes 5-HT (5-hydroxytryptamine and causes carcinoid syndrome.

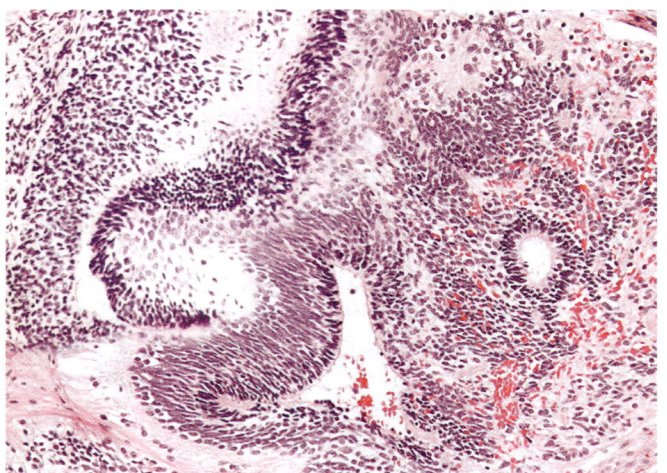

Fig. 24.89: Immature teratoma.

Struma Ovarii

Struma ovarii is a monodermal (specialized) teratoma composed of functional ectopic thyroid tissue. These are most often unilateral tumors and bilateral in a few cases.

Light Microscopy
The tumor is composed of mature thyroid follicles (Fig. 24.90).

Immunohistochemistry
Immunohistochemical studies for **TTF-1** and **thyroid hormones** have established thyroid in nature of this lesion.

Clinical features: Patient presents with features of hyperthyroidism due to thyroxine production by the tumor.

Gross Morphology
Tumor is solid with yellowish discoloration measuring mean diameter of 10 cm. External surface is smooth. Cut surface is predominantly solid, firm, tan to yellow, homogeneous with a few cystic spaces. Primary tumors are unilateral. But metastatic intestinal tumors involve both ovaries.

Light Microscopy
Tumor shows argentaffin cells which reduce silver salts. Rarely there may be mixed tumor comprising of struma ovarii and carcinoid tumor.

Immunohistochemistry
Panel of markers is used in surgical specimens of carcinoid tumor (Table 24.28).

Table 24.28: Immunohistochemistry of carcinoid tumor

Panel of markers	Expression in tumor cells
Neuron-specific enolase (NSE)	Positive
Chromogranin	Positive
5-HT	Positive

YOLK SAC TUMOR

Yolk sac tumor is highly malignant germ cell tumor with extraembryonic differentiation. It is also known as *endodermal sinus tumor* analogous to endodermal sinus tumor of the testis. It histologically resembles mesenchyme of the primitive yolk sac.

Serum Marker

Tumor produces α-fetoprotein. Its detection in the blood is useful both for diagnosis and for monitoring the effectiveness of therapy.

Age Group

It most often affects children and young women (10–30 years). It has also been reported in the elderly women.

Clinical Features

Patient presents with abdominal pain due to rapidly growing pelvic mass. Untreated cases have poor prognosis with two years survival.

Gross Morphology

Tumor reveals variable sized, partly solid tumor measuring 15 cm in diameter. External surface is smooth and glistening. Cut surface shows variegated appearance, partially cystic and often containing large foci of hemorrhage and necrosis (grayish brown).

Light Microscopy

Tumor shows a network of embryonal cells and connective tissue structures arranged around blood vessels as the endodermal sinus of rat placenta *Schiller-Duval bodies* (glomeruloid). Intracellular and extracellular hyaline globules/droplets (PAS positive) are present in all tumors (Fig. 24.91).

Immunohistochemistry

Panel of markers is used in surgical specimens of yolk sac tumor (Table 24.29).

Table 24.29: Immunohistochemistry of yolk sac tumor

Panel of markers	Expression in tumor cells
α-fetoproteins	Positive
α₁-antitrypsin	Positive
Pankeratin	Positive

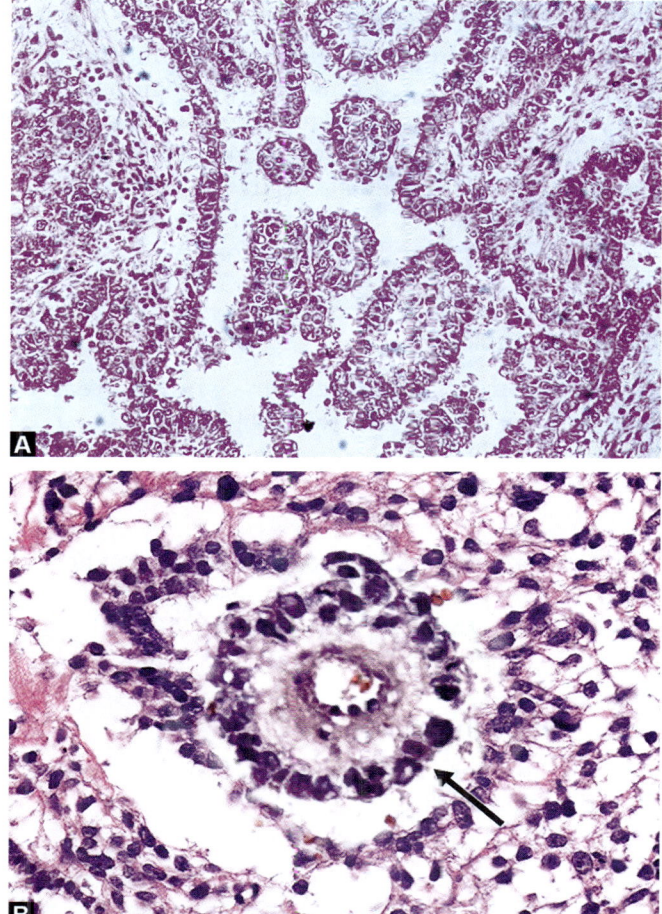

Fig. 24.91: Yolk sac tumor. (A) The endodermal sinus pattern of yolk sac tumor is characterized by the presence of irregular interconnecting labyrinthine-like spaces and Schiller-Duval bodies, several of which are nicely illustrated (200X), and (B) it is showing Schiller-Duval bodies (arrow) (400X).

CHORIOCARCINOMA

Choriocarcinoma of the ovary is a rare malignant germ cell tumor with extraembryonic differentiation. It mimics the epithelial covering of placental villi (cytotrophoblast and syncytiotrophoblast).

Association

Most choriocarcinomas occur in combination with other germ cell tumors. Pure ovarian choriocarcinomas are rare.

Origin

It most often develops *de novo* (98%) and patients after evacuation of complete hydatidiform mole in 2%.

Serum and Urine Marker

Chroriocarcinoma synthesizes human chorionic gonadotropin (hCG). There is increased hCG in serum and urine in these women.

Clinical Features

This tumor most often occurs in prepubertal girls. These young girls present with precocious sexual development, menstrual irregularities, and rapid breast enlargement. On the other hand, women of reproductive age may represent metastasis in lung, liver, brain. In some cases, choriocarcinoma only becomes evident 10 or more years after the last pregnancy.

Gross Morphology

Ovarian pure choriocarcinoma shows areas of hemorrhage and necrosis (Fig. 24.92).

Light Microscopy

Tumor shows an admixture of malignant cytotrophoblast and syncytiotrophoblast. The syncytial cells of choriocarcinoma synthesize hCG, which accounts for the frequent finding of a positive pregnancy test result (Fig. 24.93).

Immunohistochemistry

Panel of markers is used in surgical specimens of choriocarcinoma (Table 24.30).

Table 24.30: Immunohistochemistry of choriocarcinoma

Panel of markers (immunohistochemistry)	Expression in tumor cells
hCG (most specific)	Positive
Keratin 7 (expressed in trophoblastic cells)	Positive
LK26 (a folate-binding protein) also expressed in other ovarian malignancies	Positive

Serum and urine marker: Concentration of human chorionic gonadotropin (hCG) synthesized by choriocarcinoma is increased in serum and urine.

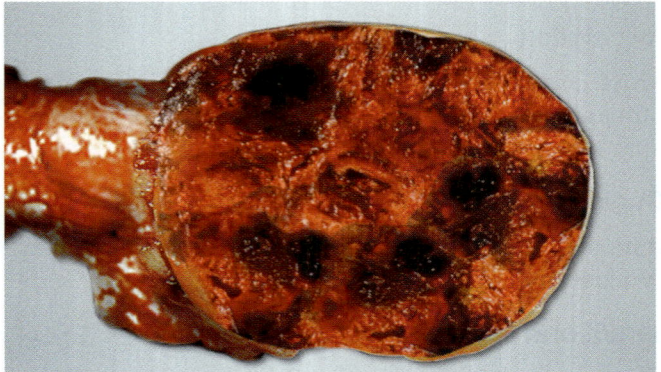

Fig. 24.92: Choriocarcinoma. The testis is replaced by a bloody bulging mass. More typically, choriocarcinoma tends to be somewhat smaller, and may not significantly distort the ovary.

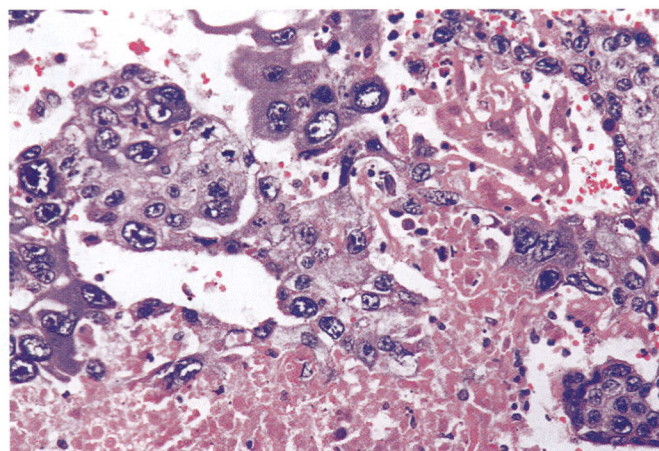

Fig. 24.93: Choriocarcinoma—the tumor is composed of multinucleated syncytiotrophoblastic and cytotrophoblastic cells. The multinucleated syncytiotrophoblasts have voluminous eosinophilic cytoplasm and large darkly staining irregular nuclei with prominent nucleoli. The smaller mononuclear cytotrophoblasts are fairly uniform in size with amphophilic cytoplasm and distinct cellular outlines resembling to the tumor cells of solid yolk sac tumor (400X).

Management

These patients do not respond to chemotherapy and prognosis is therefore poor. Placental choriocarcinoma is responsive to chemotherapy.

POLYEMBRYOMA

It is rare but highly malignant ovarian neoplasm. It is most often a component of mixed germ cell tumor.

Gross Examination

Tumor is solid with areas of hemorrhage and necrosis.

Light Microscopy

Tumor is composed of embryoid bodies (embryonic discs lined by endoderm on one side, ectoderm on opposite side and associated with yolk sac and amniotic cavities).

MIXED GERM CELL TUMORS

Mixed germ cell tumors constitute 10% of germ cell tumors. Most common combination is dysgerminoma and yolk sac tumor, although any combination may occur.

SEX CORD STROMAL TUMORS

Sex cord stromal tumors constitute 10–25% of cases.

Origin

These are derived from ovarian sex cords of embryonic gonads.

Classification

These tumors may be divided into two broad groups, i.e. (a) estrogen producing granulosa cell tumor and the coma; and (b) androgen producing Sertoli-Leydig cell tumors, hilus cell tumors and lipid cell tumors. Except fibromas, all these tumors are endocrinologically functional.

Clinical Course

Most sex cord stromal tumors are benign. Approximately 25% of all granulosa cell tumors are prone to recur or metastasize during the 10-year period after diagnosis and are considered low-grade malignant. Highly malignant tumors are extremely rare.

GRANULOSA CELL TUMORS

- Granulosa cell tumor is potentially malignant ovarian tumor associated with estrogen production. The tumor is derived from sex cord stromal cells.
- Approximately 75% of granulosa cell tumors secrete estrogens. These tumors synthesize weak androgens. Excess of estrogen causes endometrial hyperplasia (most common finding) that may progress to endometrial adenocarcinoma if the functioning granulosa cell tumor remains undetected.

Chromosomal Aberrations

Tumor shows consistent trisomy of chromosome 12. Trisomy of chromosome 14 and 22 has also been demonstrated. All adult granulosa cell tumors show somatic mutation in the FOXL2 gene, flow cytometry reveals DNA polyploidy.

Clinical Features

- Most granulosa cell tumors occur in postmenopausal women and associated with endometrial hyperplasia or endometrial carcinoma or fibrocystic disease of breast.
- *Juvenile granulosa cell tumor* affecting children and young women results in excess estrogens and isosexual precocious puberty.
- *Flow cytometry* reveals greater percentage of aneuploidy in juvenile than adult granulosa cell tumor variety, but without prognostic significance.

Gross Morphology

Granulosa cell tumor is unilateral solid tumor, microscopic size to large solid, cystic encapsulated masses, usually not firm as fibromas and thecomas (Fig. 24.94).

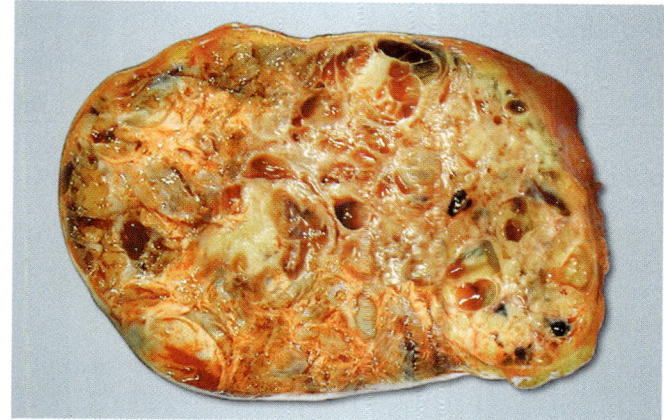

Fig. 24.94: Granulosa cell tumor of the ovary. These tumors, too, are usually yellow. Positive diagnosis depends on the microscopic appearances. They sometimes secrete estrogen.

Light Microscopy

- *Tumor cells morphology:* The tumor is composed of small cuboidal to polygonal, deeply staining granulosa cells arranged in sheets and strands.

  Call-Exner bodies are formed by tumor cells forming rossette-like structures (small follicles) filled with eosinophilic secretion arranged in a circular pattern resembling an ovarian immature follicle.

  Another variant is luteinized granulosa cell tumor comprised of plump granulosa theca cells with ample cytoplasm.
- Granulosa cell tumor chiefly composed of theca cell is almost never malignant (Fig. 24.95).

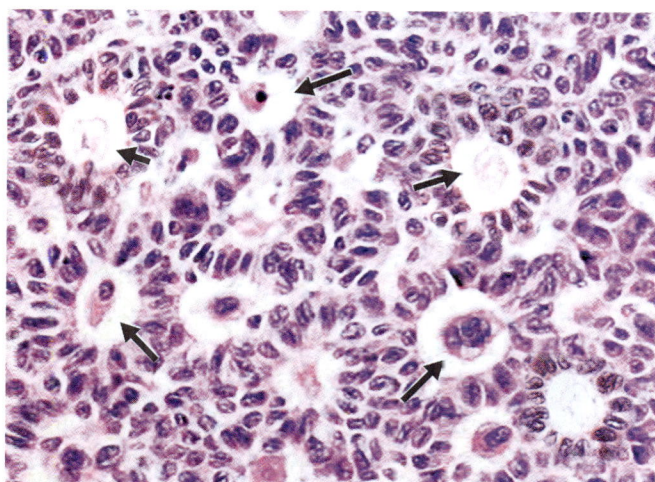

Fig. 24.95: Granulosa cell tumor ovary. Tumor consists of small cuboidal to polygonal, deeply staining granulosa cells arranged in sheets and strands. Call-Exner bodies are formed by tumor cells forming rossette-like structures (small follicles) filled with eosinophilic secretion arranged in a circular pattern resembling an ovarian immature follicle (arrows) (400X).

Immunohistochemistry

Panel of markers is used in surgical specimens of sex cord stromal tumor (Table 24.31).

Table 24.31: Sex cord stromal tumors of ovary: immunohistochemistry

Panel of markers	Expression in tumor cells
Calretinin (most sensitive than inihibin)	Positive
Inhibin	Positive (except fibroma)
A103	Positive
Melanocytic marker Melan-A (Mart-1)	Positive
Estrogen and progesterone receptors	Positive
Other markers include vimentin, desmoplakin, follicle regulatory proteins and S-100 protein (50%)	Positive

Clinical Course

It is difficult to predict biologic behavior on histological evaluation of tumor. *All granulosa cell tumors are potentially malignant.* These may recur or metastasize in 25% cases during the 10-year period after diagnosis and are considered low-grade malignant. 10-year survival is in 85% of cases.

THECOMA

- This benign functional ovarian tumor occasionally synthesizes estrogens. It most often affects 30–50 years of women. In most cases, it produces signs of estrogen synthesis. The tumor is unilateral in 90% of cases and bilateral in 10%.
- Thecomas are *almost always benign*. Some tumors in young women are heavily calcified.

Molecular Genetics

Cytogenetically, it shows *trisomy of chromosome 12.*

Gross Morphology

- Thecomas are solid tumors of 5 to 10 cm in diameter. These are spherical, gray white encapsulated tumors, covered by glistening intact ovarian serosa. Cut surface appears yellow due to presence many lipid-laden theca cells.
- Pure thecomas are rare. Many tumors contain a mixture of fibroma and thecoma components, hence called as fibroma-thecoma (Fig. 24.96).

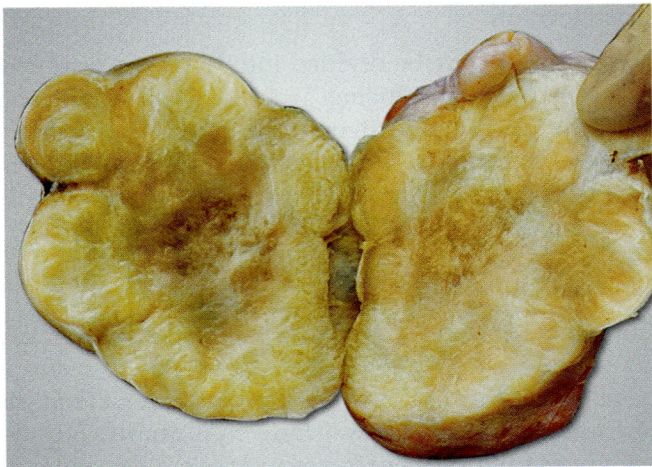

Fig. 24.96: Thecoma of the ovary. This is distinguished from fibroma by the presence of lipid, which gives it a yellow color.

Light Microscopy

- This tumor is composed of round lipid-containing theca cells in addition to fibroblasts. Theca cells contain fat and synthesize estrogens.
- Bands of hyalinized collagen separate nests of theca cells. Lipids in theca cells may be demonstrated by frozen section technique and sections are stained with fat stains such as *Sudan-III, Sudan-IV, Sudan black and oil red-O.*
- Silver stains demonstrate reticulin fibers surrounding individual cells (as opposed to granulosa cell tumor, in which the reticulin surrounds clusters of cells).

Clinical Features

Excess of estrogen synthesis by tumor commonly menstrual irregularities and breast enlargement in premenopausal women. Endometrial hyperplasia and cancer are well-recognized complications.

FIBROMA

It most common benign ovarian stromal tumors. It occurs at all ages, with a peak in the perimenopausal period, and is virtually always benign.

Molecular Genetics

Cytogenetically, it shows trisomy of chromosome 12.

Clinical Features

It may be associated with **Meigs' syndrome**, a triad of ovarian fibroma >8.0 cm in size, ascites, and hydrothorax in 40% of cases. Rarely, it may undergo malignant change and present as fibrosarcoma.

Clinical Features

It is androgen (dehydroepiandrosterone) secreting tumor associated with virilism (masculinization). Due to excess of androgens, approximately 50% of patients initially present with breast atrophy, amenorrhea, and loss of hip fat followed by hirsutism, male escutcheon, enlarged clitoris, and deepened voice.

PURE LEYDIG CELL TUMOR

It is a benign tumor present in the hilus or the ovary. It may synthesize androgens.

Clinical Features

Due to excess androgens, patient presents with musculinization, hirsutism, voice changes, and clitoris enlargement.

Gross Examination
Tumor is small yellow-colored, unilateral less than 3 cm in diameter.
Light Microscopy
The tumor is composed large lipid-laden cells with distinct borders. A typical cytoplasmic structure characteristic of Leydig cells (Reinke crystalloid) is usually present.

Urine Analysis

There is increased excretion of 17-ketosteroid unresponsive to cortisone suppression.

Treatment

Surgical excision cures the patient.

ANDROBLASTOMA

This tumor is unilateral affecting all ages but peak in second and third decades. It has musculinization effect or defeminization effect. This biphasic tumor contains cells resembling testicular Sertoli and Leydig cells interspersed with stroma. It constitutes <5% of cases.

Clinical Features

This tumor synthesizes androgens. It causes atrophy of breasts and external genitalia, amenorrhea, infertility, deepening of the voice, male distribution of hair on face and chest; and hypertrophy of clitoris.

Gross Morphology
Tumor is unilateral small tumor and resembles granulosa theca cell tumor. Cut surface is gray to golden brown.

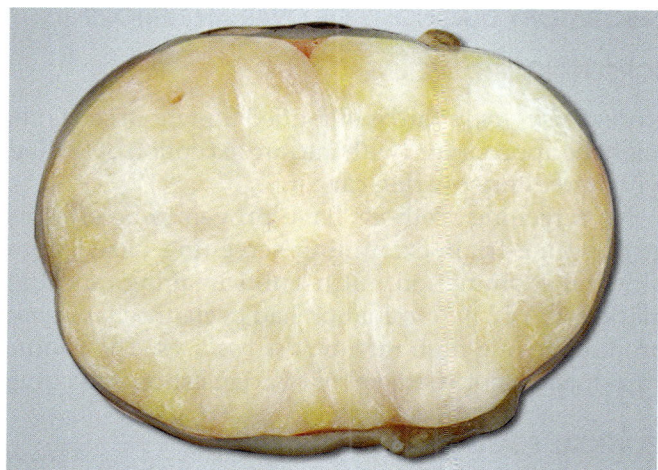

Fig. 24.97: Fibroma of the ovary. The cut surface of the tumor shows a homogeneous white appearance

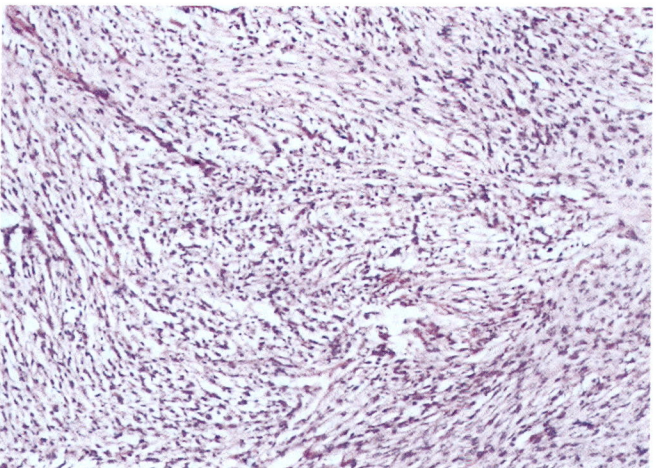

Fig. 24.98: Fibroma of the ovary (100X).

Gross Morphology
The tumors are solid, firm, and gray white. There is absence of hemorrhage and necrosis (Fig. 24.97).
Light Microscopy
Tumor cells resemble the stroma of the normal ovarian cortex. It is composed of well-differentiated bundles of spindle-shaped fibroblasts and variable amounts of collagen (Fig. 24.98).

SERTOLI-LEYDIG CELL TUMOR

It is a rare mesenchymal neoplasm of the ovary of *low malignant potential*. It resembles the embryonic testis.

Age Group

It occurs at all ages but is most common in young women of childbearing age.

> **Light Microscopy**
> - Tumor is a well differentiated tumor composed of Sertoli cells or Leydig cells interspersed with stroma. Intermediate differentiated tumor is composed of immature tubules and large eosinophilic Leydig cells.
> - Poorly differentiated tumor shows sarcomatous pattern, disorderly disposition of epithelial cell cords and absence of Leydig cells.
> - Heterologous elements like mucinous glands, bone and cartilage are present.

GONADOBLASTOMA

It is uncommon tumor. It occurs in individuals with abnormal sexual development and in gonads of indeterminate nature. 80% of patients are phenotypic females and 20% are phenotypic males with undescended testicles and female internal secondary organs.

> **Light Microscopy**
> Tumor is composed of mixture of germs cells and sex cord derivatives resemble immature Sertoli and granulosa cells. A co-existent dysgerminoma occurs in 50% of cases.

PREGNANCY LUTEOMA

Ovary in pregnancy may exhibit nodular proliferation of theca cells, in response to gonadotrophins. Rarely a frank tumor may develop termed as *pregnancy luteoma* that resembles corpus luteum of pregnancy.

Clinical Features

These tumors have been associated with virilization in pregnancy patients and in their respective female infants.

DIFFERENTIAL DIAGNOSIS

- *Functional luteal cysts (regress in 4–6 weeks):* Follicular cysts, corpus luteal cysts and theca lutein cysts.
- Subserous leiomyoma
- Pregnancy and extrauterine pregnancy
- Hydrosalpinx
- Appendicular mass
- Tubercular abdomen
- Hydatid cyst
- Ascites

LABORATORY DIAGNOSIS OF OVARIAN TUMORS

SCREENING PROCEDURES

No *high risk groups* can be identified for whom screening might be appropriate (with the rare exception of families with hereditary ovarian cancer.

No screening methods have proven to be effective at this time-trials examining screening based upon physical examination, ultrasound imaging, and biomarker (CA 125) examination had been unreliable, and productive of a high rate of *false positives*. The routine Pap smear is not effective for ovarian cancer screening.

CLINICAL FEATURES

Ovarian tumors are mainly asymptomatic. 25% of ovarian neoplasms are malignant. Adnexal tumor over 6.0 cm; if persisting/increasing in size in a postmenopausal woman, ovarian tumor be suspected. Benign tumor is usually slow-growing, unilateral, cystic-free mobile.

A solid/cystic, bilateral, rapidly growing tumor associated with pressure symptoms especially in postmenopausal woman is very likely to be malignant. In *hormones producing tumors;* clinical history, vaginal cytology, endometrial histology, estimation of hormone levels in blood and urine are significant.

PER VAGINA AND PER RECTAL EXAMINATION

Physical examination, including examination of the vagina and rectum can detect most important ovarian masses.

IMAGING TECHNIQUES

Radiograph has diagnostic utility in cases of dermoid cyst and serous cystadenoma. Pelvic ultrasound can be very valuable in determining the characteristics of ovarian and other pelvic masses.

FLUID CYTOLOGY

Ascitic fluid cytology is done to demonstrate malignant cells.

> **Light Microscopy**
> - A tissue sample is necessary to make an unequivocal diagnosis, this may be obtained by exploratory laparotomy (surgical incision of the abdominal wall to examine the contents of the peritoneal cavity) or laparoscopy.
> - Surgeons take care to avoid rupturing ovarian masses when a diagnosis of cancer is suspected, so as not to spread the disease.

SEROLOGICAL MARKERS

- *CA 125:* It is a glycoprotein often produced by surface epithelial ovarian tumors. It may help characterize ovarian masses and monitor the extent of disease.
- *Estrogen levels:* These are increased in thecomas and granulosa cell tumors.
- *Androgen levels:* These are increased in Sertoli-Leydig and hilar tumors.
- *α-fetoproteins:* These are demonstrated in yolk sac tumors.
- *Human chorionic gonadotropin (hCG-β) levels:* These are increased in choriocarcinomas.

STAGING

Staging is a clinical exercise that classifies tumors according to their size, invasiveness and spread. Tumors are staged according to the TNM system (T: tumor size, N: lymph node involvement, M: metastases to distant organs).

Schemes for TNM classification vary according to tumor type and organ involved. Grading classifies tumor according to their light microscopic characteristics (Fig. 24.99 and Table 24.32).

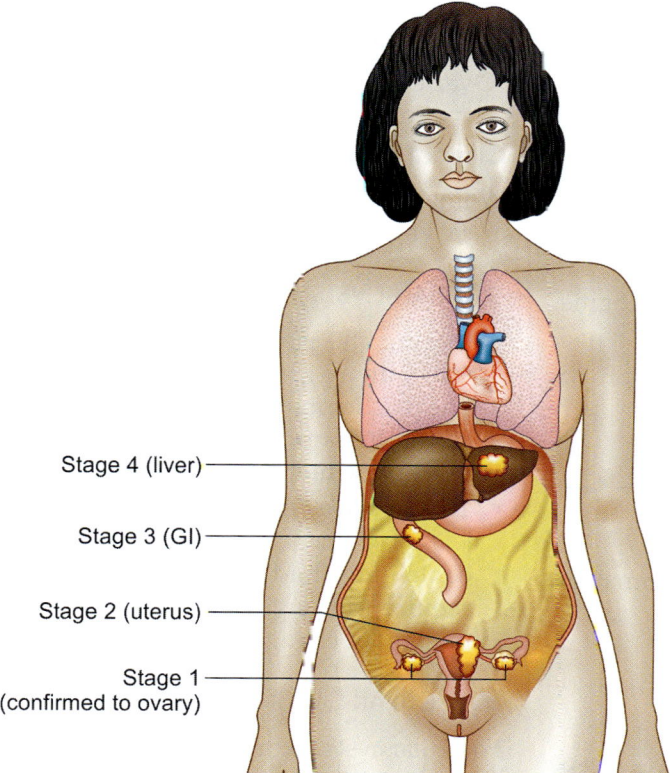

Fig. 24.99: Staging of ovarian cancers.

Table 24.32: Stage of ovarian cancers

Stage	Extent of growth
Stage I	Growth limited to ovaries
Stage II	Growth in one or both ovaries with pelvic extension
Stage III	Tumor involving one or both ovaries with peritoneal implants outside the pelvis and/or positive retroperitoneal or inguinal nodes or superficial liver metastases
Stage IV	Growth involving one or both ovaries with distant metastases, if a pleural effusion is present there must be positive cytology; parenchymal (internal) liver metastases—stage IV

Table 24.33: Inflammatory diseases of ovaries

Parameters	Underlying causes	Light microscopy	Clinical course
Acute oophoritis	Salpingitis Systemic infections Tubo-ovarian abscess Ascending pelvic inflammatory disease	Polymorphonuclear infiltration in ovaries	Subsequent fibrosis, scarring from pelvic inflammatory disease leading to infertility
Autoimmune oophoritis	Autoimmune disorders associated with oligomenorrhea and infertility	Lymphocytes and plasma cells infiltration in developing follicles (ovaries normal size)	Premature ovarian failure and premature menopause
Noninfectious granulomatous oophoritis	Sarcoidosis or foreign body granulomas following pelvic or abdominal surgery	Granulomas	Incidental findings

BENIGN DISORDERS OF OVARY

INFLAMMATORY DISEASES

Inflammatory diseases of ovaries include acute, autoimmune and noninfectious granulomatous oophoritis (Table 24.33).

ACUTE OOPHORITIS

Infection of ovary is almost accompanied by salpingitis, tubo-ovarian abscess and systemic infections.

> **Light Microscopy**
> Ovary is infiltrated by polymorphonuclear cells.

Clinical Course

Subsequent fibrosis, scarring from pelvic inflammatory disease leads to infertility.

AUTOIMMUNE OOPHORITIS

Ovary

Autoimmune disorders of ovaries are associated with oligomenorrhea and infertility.

> **Light Microscopy**
> Ovaries are of normal size and show lymphocytes and plasma cells infiltration in developing follicles.

Clinical Course

Women develop premature ovarian failure and premature menopause.

NONINFECTIOUS GRANULOMATOUS OOPHORITIS

Noninfectious granulomatous oophoritis is seen as incidental finding secondary to sarcoidosis.

> **Light Microscopy**
> Ovaries show granulomas.

Clinical Course

Women with noninfectious granulomatous oophoritis are asymptomatic.

OVARIAN CYSTS

- During the proliferative phase of the menstrual cycle, many graafian follicles are released but only one reaches maturity progressing to development of corpus luteum. It eventually undergoes degeneration during the menstrual cycle.
- *There are two types of functional ovarian cysts (follicular and luteal cysts):* These are small non-neoplastic sacs containing fluid or semisolid material. These cysts require thorough investigation as possible sites of malignant change (Table 24.34).

FOLLICULAR CYSTS

Follicular cysts occur in the first 2 weeks of the menstrual cycle during prepubescent or reproductive age group. When the graafian follicle fails to rupture, it continues to grow and resulting in follicular cyst. It is sometimes associated with hyperestrinism and endometrial hyperplasia.

> **Gross Morphology**
> Follicular cysts are unilateral measuring 2.5–10 cm in diameter. Normal follicle measures up to 1 cm. Follicular cysts contain serosanguineous fluid.

> **Light Microscopy**
> Follicular cysts are lined by inner granulosa cells and outer theca cells.

Table 24.34: Ovarian cysts

Parameters	Age group	Morphology	Light microscopy	Clinical course
Follicular cysts	Prepubescent or reproductive age group	2.5–10 cm in diameter unilateral cysts containing serosanguineous fluid (normal follicle measures up to 1 cm)	Follicular cysts are lined by inner granulosa cells and outer theca cells	Abdominal mass, rupture. Follicular cysts may be associated with polycystic ovarian syndrome or McCune-Albright syndrome
Corpus luteal cysts	Reproductive age group	>3 cm in diameter containing hemorrhagic fluid	Corpus luteal cysts show granulosa cells interspersed with peripheral theca cells similar to normal corpus luteum	Menstrual irregularity, occasionally with intraperitoneal hemorrhage
Polycystic ovarian syndrome	20–30 years	Ovaries are enlarged with thickened, collagenized cortical surface	Multiple uniform follicles and absence of corpus lutea (indicating infrequent ovulation)	Anovulation, infertility hirsutism and increased incidence of endometrial hyperplasia and adenocarcinoma
Surface epithelial inclusion cysts	Reproductive age group	These are formed as a result of repeated invaginations of ovarian epithelium secondary to rupture with ovulation. Size of cysts are <1 cm	These are lined by single layer of cuboidal or columnar cells. Psammoma bodies may be present	These surface inclusion cysts may be precursor of benign, borderline and low grade serous epithelial neoplasms
Paraovarian or paratubal cysts	Reproductive age group	Cysts are derived from mesonephric (Wolffian) or paramesonephric (Müllerian) ducts and found in the hilar region of the ovary	Mesonephric cysts are lined by simple or stratified epithelium with prominent muscular walls Paramesonephric cysts are lined by columnar epithelium with mixture of ciliated and nonciliated cells similar to epithelial inclusion cysts	Asymptomatic
Endometriosis (endometrial glands and stroma outside uterus most often in ovary)	Reproductive age group	Ovaries show thickened cortex, surface adhesion. Cysts are filled with thick brown fluid resembling chocolate syrup, the so-called chocolate cysts	Endometrial glands and stroma associated with hemosiderin-laden macrophages and fibroblasts. These cysts may contain atypical cytologic features and acute inflammation raising suspicious of malignancy	Menstrual cycle associated pain and infertility
Theca luteal cysts	These cysts are formed due to gonadotropin stimulation in patients associated with choriocarcinoma and hydatidiform mole	Ovarian cysts are small	These are lined by luteinized theca cells	Women with choriocarcinoma and hydatidiform mole develop these cysts

Clinical Course

Patient presents with abdominal mass, rupture. Follicular cysts may be associated with polycystic ovarian syndrome or McCune-Albright syndrome.

CORPUS LUTEAL CYSTS

Corpus luteal cysts occur in the second half of the cycle during reproductive age group. Hemorrhage into a persistent mature corpus luteum results in formation of corpus luteal cyst.

Gross Morphology
Corpus luteal cysts measure >3 cm in diameter and contain hemorrhagic fluid.

Light Microscopy
Corpus luteal cysts show granulosa cells interspersed with peripheral theca cells similar to normal corpus luteum.

Clinical Course

Women with corpus luteal cysts are usually associated with *menstrual irregularity*, occasionally with intraperitoneal hemorrhage.

POLYCYSTIC OVARIES (STEIN-LEVENTHAL SYNDROME)

Clinical manifestations of Stein-Leventhal syndrome are related to *excess synthesis of androgenic hormones (amenorrhea or oligomenorrhoea)*, persistent an ovulation (important cause of infertility), and small subcapsular cysts in ovaries, *obesity*, and *hirsutism* in *young women of 20–30 years* of age group.

Etiology

Patient synthesizes excess of luteinizing hormone (LH) and androgens. Increased synthesis of androgens occurs by two mechanisms:
- LH may stimulate follicular theca-lutein cells, with consequent increased synthesis of androgens.
- Hyperinsulinemia in insulin resistance diabetes mellitus may lead to increased ovarian androgen production, which then may cause increased LH synthesis.

Gross Morphology
- Both ovaries are enlarged. Cut section reveals thickened collagenized cortex surface.
- Numerous cysts measuring 2 to 8 mm in diameter are arranged peripherally around a dense core of stroma.

Light Microscopy
- Ovaries show multiple uniform follicles lined by granulosa cells and absence of corpus lutea (indicating infrequent ovulation).
- Ovaries show marked thickened ovarian capsule and cortical stromal fibrosis with islands of focal luteinization.

Complications

Women develop *anovulation, infertility and hirsutism*. Unopposed acyclic estrogen synthesis in women with Stein-Leventhal syndrome leads to increased incidence of endometrial hyperplasia and adenocarcinoma.

SURFACE EPITHELIAL INCLUSION CYSTS

Surface epithelial inclusion cysts are seen during reproductive period. These are formed as a result of repeated invaginations of ovarian epithelium secondary to rupture with ovulation.

Gross Morphology
Surface epithelial inclusion cysts are <1 cm in diameter.

Light Microscopy
- These cysts are lined by single layer of cuboidal or columnar cells.
- Psammoma bodies may be present. Paramesonephric cysts are lined by columnar epithelium with mixture of ciliated and nonciliated cells similar to epithelial inclusion cysts.

Clinical Course

These surface inclusion cysts may be *precursor of benign, borderline and low grade serous epithelial neoplasms*.

PARAOVARIAN OR PARATUBAL CYSTS

Paraovarian or paratubal cysts are formed during reproductive age group. Cysts are derived from mesonephric (Wolffian) or paramesonephric (müllerian) ducts and found in the hilar region of the ovary.

Gross Morphology
Paraovarian or paratubal cysts are of small size.

Light Microscopy
- Mesonephric cysts are lined by simple or stratified epithelium with prominent muscular walls.
- Paramesonephric cysts are lined by columnar epithelium with mixture of ciliated and nonciliated cells similar to epithelial inclusion cysts.

Female Reproductive System

Clinical Course

Women are asymptomatic.

ENDOMETRIOSIS (CHOCOLATE CYSTS)

Endometriosis represents endometrial glands and stroma outside uterus during reproductive period. *The ovary is the most frequent site of endometriosis. Hemorrhage into endometriosis* focus results in formation of blood-filled cysts on the ovary termed *chocolate cysts*.

Gross Morphology
- Ovaries show thickened cortex, surface adhesion.
- Cysts are filled with thick brown fluid resembling chocolate syrup, the so-called chocolate cysts (Fig. 24.100).

Light Microscopy
- Endometrial glands and stroma associated with hemosiderin-laden macrophages and fibroblasts.
- These cysts may contain atypical cytologic features and acute inflammation raising suspicious of malignancy (Fig. 24.101).

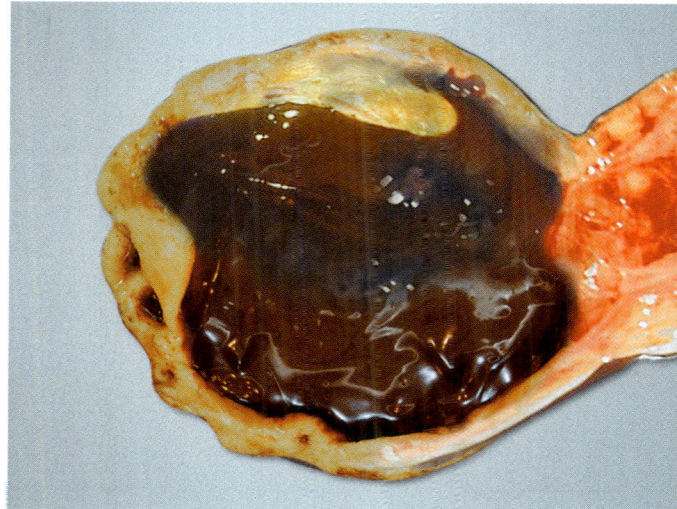

Fig. 24.100: Chocolate cyst in endometriosis. This is a section through an enlarged 12 cm ovary to demonstrate a cystic cavity-filled with old blood typical for endometriosis with formation of an endometriotic, or *chocolate* cyst. The hemorrhage from endometriosis into the ovary may give rise to a large *chocolate cyst* so named because the old blood in the cystic space formed by the hemorrhage is broken down to produce much hemosiderin and a brown to black color.

Clinical Course

Endometriosis is associated *pain during menstrual cycle.* It is *frequent cause of infertility.*

THECA LUTEAL CYSTS

Theca luteal cysts are most often multiple and bilateral. These are lined by luteinized theca cells. These cysts are formed due to gonadotropin stimulation in patients associated with choriocarcinoma and hydatidiform mole.

Gross Morphology
Ovaries contain multiple small cysts of variable diameter.

Light Microscopy
Theca luteal cysts are lined by luteinized theca cells.

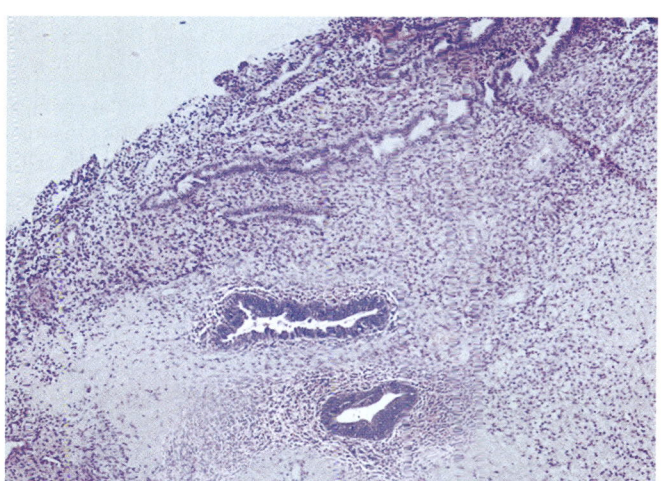

Fig. 24.101: Endometriosis—endometrial glands and stroma are seen at high magnification in the wall of the colon. Endometriosis is symptomatic during reproductive years when patients may present with dysmenorrhea, pelvic pain, and infertility (100X).

GESTATIONAL TROPHOBLASTIC TUMORS

Gestational trophoblastic disease includes abnormal placenta, hydatidiform mole (complete, incomplete and invasive), benign tumor-like diseases of the trophoblast (placental site nodule) and choriocarcinoma, latter being the only malignant tumor, but responsive to chemotherapy.

HYDATIDIFORM MOLE

Hydatidiform mole represents abnormal placenta during pregnancies. It results from faulty fertilization. It is characterized by cystic swelling of the chorionic villi with accompanied by variable trophoblastic proliferation. It occurs in two variants—*complete and partial*

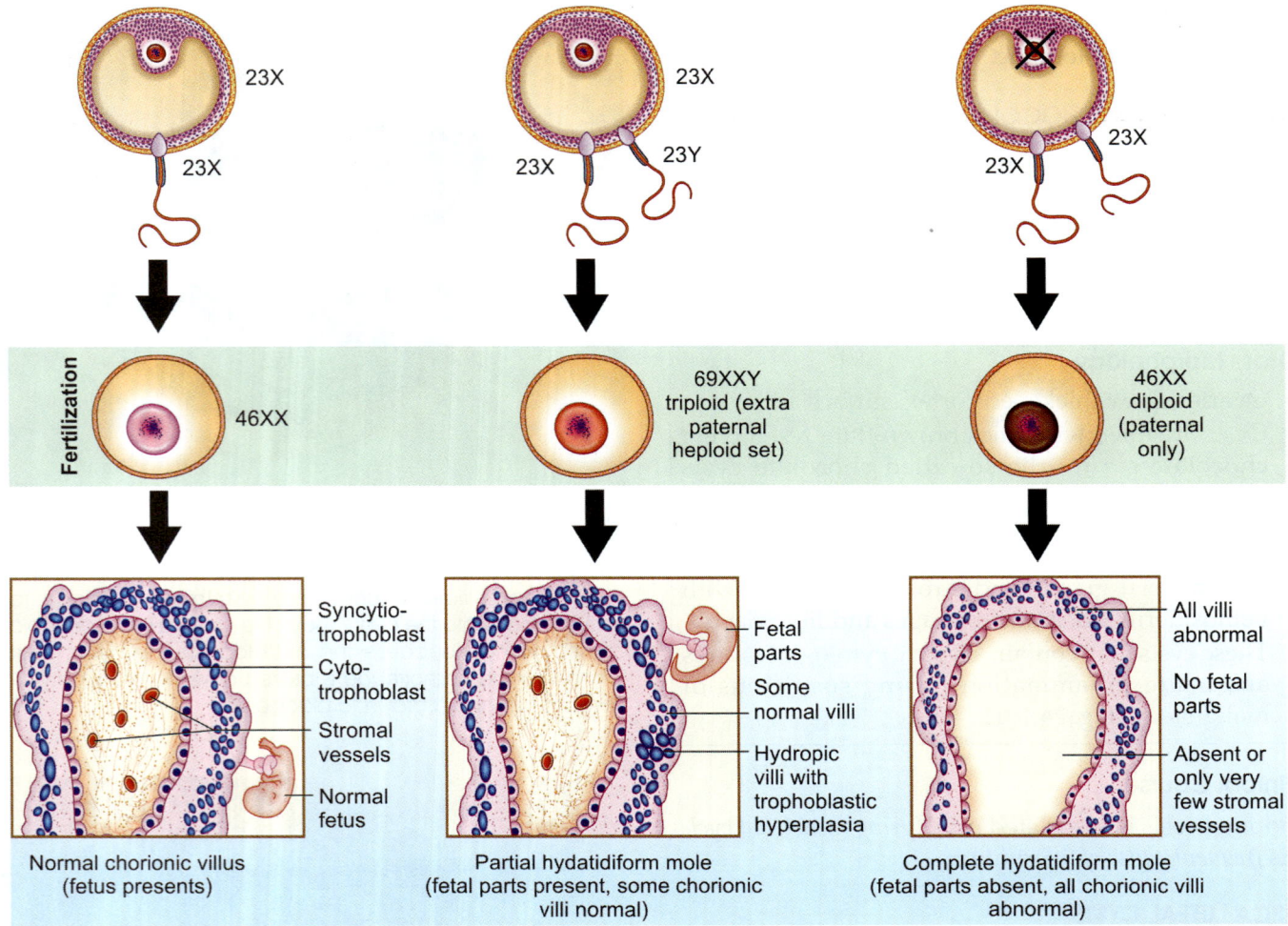

Fig. 24.102: Hydatidiform mole. Genetic analysis, partial moles are triploid and result from fertilization of one ovum by two spermatozoa. Complete moles are diploid, but comprise only paternal chromosomes.

hydatidiform mole. Invasion of hydatidiform mole into myometrium is termed as invasive mole (Fig. 24.102). Differences between complete and partial mole are given in Table 24.35.

Table 24.35: Differences between complete and incomplete hydatidiform mole

Features	Complete hydatidiform mole	Incomplete hydatidiform mole
Normal villi	Absent	May be present
Villous edema	All villi are edematous	Some villi are edematous
Capillaries	Few: no fetal RBCs	Many: fetal RBCs
Trophoblastic hyperplasia	Diffuse and marked	Focal: minimal to moderate
Embryo (fetal parts)	No cord, amnion or fetus	Abnormal fetus (may be present) is viable for a few weeks
Gestational age	8–16 weeks	10–26 weeks
Karyotype	46XX/46XY (diploid)	Triploid 69XXX, tetraploid 92XXXY
Chromosomal pattern	Paternal chromosome only	Maternal and paternal chromosome
Serum hCG	Increased ++++	Increased +
hCG in tissue	++++	+
Pathogenesis	Fertilization of empty egg by ½ sperms	Fertilization of egg by 2 sperms
Malignant transformation	Choriocarcinoma in 2% of cases	Choriocarcinoma rare

Female Reproductive System

COMPLETE HYDATIDIFORM MOLE

Molar changes occur as early as in 4th week but most cases present in 4–5th months of pregnancy. Since the embryo dies at a very early stage, *fetal parts are absent*. Chorionic villi show florid trophoblastic proliferation and hydropic change. *It resembles bunches of grapes*. It exhibits *diploidy (46XX Karyotype)*. It shows only *paternal chromosomes*. Ratio of paternal to maternal chromosomes is 2:0.

Age Group

It most often affects young females <20 years or multiparous >40 years of low socioeconomic group.

Pathogenesis

- Complete hydatidiform mole results from the *fertilization of an empty ovum that lacks functional DNA*, by haploid (23X) set of paternal chromosomes duplicates to 46XX. All the chromosomes are of paternal origin (paternal androgenesis).
- Most molar pregnancies are diagnosed by ultrasound in the early stages of pregnancy and can be completely evacuated by curettage. *Still, approximately 10% of complete moles become locally invasive*.
- Malignant transformation (choriocarcinoma) develops in about 2% of cases.

Gross Morphology

Grossly swollen chorionic villi resemble bunch of grapes pearly white, translucent vesicles measuring a few mm to 2–3 cm (Fig. 24.103).

Light Microscopy

- Chorionic villi are enlarged with irregular scalloped borders, lined with variable degrees of trophoblastic proliferation. The blood vessels are absent or in adequate in loose edematous myxomatous stroma.
- Hydropic change occurs due to abnormal angiogenesis and decreased blood vessels in the chorionic villi resulting in lack of vascular drainage and accumulation of fluid (Fig. 24.104).

Clinical Features

- Patient presents with *history of amenorrhea of less than 24 weeks of gestation, passage of grape-like* structures (vesicles) per vagina, *abdominal pain*, and *hyperemesis*.
- A hydatidiform mole can be mistaken for a normal pregnancy, but the uterus is often too large for the supposed state of gestation.
- Hyperstimulation of ovaries by human chorionic gonadotropin synthesis is responsible for *bilateral ovarian luteal cysts associated with trophoblastic tumors*.
- Normal trophoblastic tissue synthesizes hCG-β, estrogen, progesterone and TSH-like hormones. Excess of TSH production causing hyperthyroidism is seen in 2% cases.

Complications

These include hemorrhage, anemia, uterine sepsis, uterine perforation, choriocarcinoma, and DIC (disseminated intravascular coagulation).

Laboratory Diagnosis

- *Ultrasonography:* It snow-storm/speckled appearance. Doppler study reveals absent fetal heart sounds. X-ray chest is done to rule out metastatic choriocarcinoma.

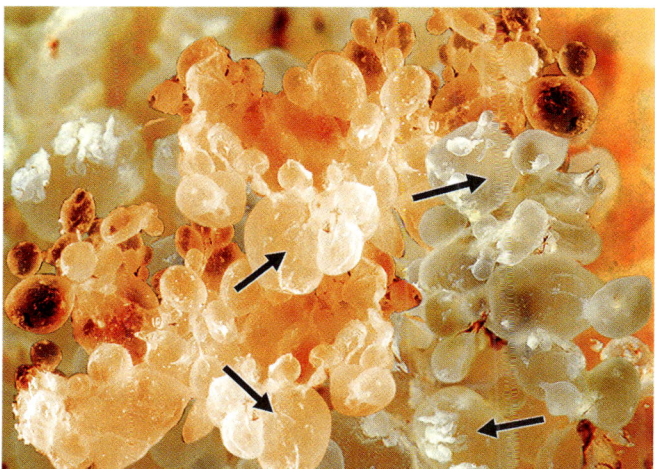

Fig. 24.103: Complete hydatidiform mole. Uterine cavity is occupied by a mass of abnormal chorionic villi resembling a bunch of grapes. Each villus is distended by fluid to reach a diameter of about 1 to 3 mm. No fetus is present (arrows).

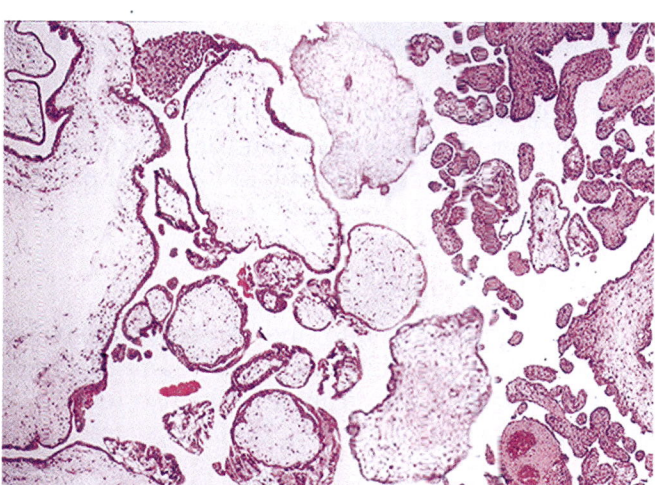

Fig. 24.104: Hydatidiform mole. Histology shows fluid-filled, avascular villi with overlying hyperplastic trophoblast that shows cellular atypia (100X).

Human chorionic gonadotropin level is more than 100,000 IU/24 hours urine.

- *Serum human chorionic gonadotropin level:* It is raised, and monitored at intervals. The patient should be followed up by estimation of serum human chorionic gonadotropin up to 2 years to rule out choriocarcinoma.

Management

Suction and evacuation is done.

Therapeutic Correlation

Chemotherapy should be given to the patients, who have persistent uterine bleeding despite curettage, elevated serum hCG levels remain even after 12 weeks of post-evacuation; and choriocarcinoma on endometrial biopsy.

INCOMPLETE HYDATIDIFORM MOLE

- Partial mole exhibits *partially formed fetal parts*, normal and abnormal hydropic chorionic villi with irregular scalloped borders and variable degree of proliferation.
- Fetus associated with partial mole usually dies after 10 weeks of gestation followed by *abortion of the mole shortly thereafter*.
- Partial moles generally *do not predispose to choriocarcinoma*.

Pathogenesis

- Partial moles result from fertilization of a normal ovum (23X) by two normal spermatozoa each carrying 23 chromosomes—a process called *dispermy*.
- By alternate mechanism, it results from fertilization of a normal ovum (23X) by single spermatozoon that has not undergone meiotic reduction and bears 46 chromosomes.
- The zygote is triploid (69XXY or 69XYY) with two sets of paternal chromosomes and one set of maternal chromosome or rarely tetraploidy. Ratio of paternal to maternal chromosomes is 2:1.

INVASIVE HYDATIDIFORM MOLE

Invasion of molar villi into underlying myometrium, or parametrium, broad ligament and vagina is termed as invasive hydatidiform mole. It is also termed as chorioadenoma destruens (Fig. 24.105).

Clinical Features

- Invasive hydatidiform mole may cause uterine perforation. It may embolize to lung, brain, but

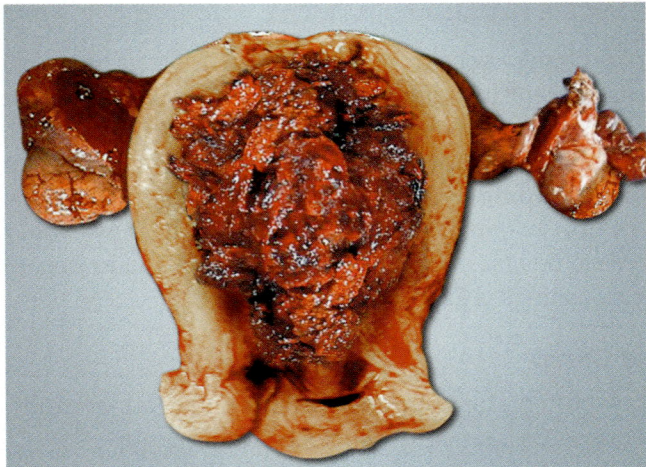

Fig. 24.105: Invasive hydatidiform mole invading myometrium.

does not grow there. hCG-β levels are persistently increased in invasive hydatidiform mole and chroriocarcinoma. It *responds well to chemotherapy*.

- hCG-β subunit levels in blood 70–90 days after normal pregnancy is 120–160 IU/ml. But hCG-β subunit after 70–90 days after hydatidiform mole is 1000 IU/ml.

GESTATIONAL CHORIOCARCINOMA

Gestational choriocarcinoma lack chorionic villi. It is highly invasive epithelial malignant tumor of trophoblast. It *shows widespread metastases*. It is derived from *hydatidiform mole (50% of cases), previous abortion (25%), normal pregnancy (22%)*, and ectopic pregnancy. It develops in 1 of 30,000 pregnancies.

Age Group

It occurs more often in Asian women especially younger than 20 and older than 40 years. Very young and older women (younger than 20 and older than 40 years) are most commonly affected.

Gross Morphology

- Tumor is soft, fleshy, yellow white, large pale areas, ischemia, necrosis, foci of cystic softening with extensive hemorrhage.
- It does not classically produce a large bulky mass (Fig. 24.106).

Light Microscopy

- Tumor is composed of abnormal proliferation of syncytiotrophoblast and cytotrophoblast.
- It does not form chorionic villi. Areas of hemorrhage and necrosis are present (Fig. 24.107).

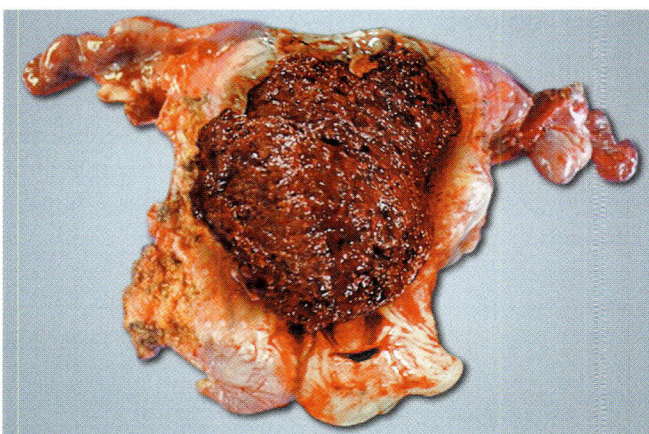

Fig. 24.106: Gestational choriocarcinoma showing extensive hemorrhage and necrosis.

Metastases

- The tumor invades the underlying myometrium, extends uterine serosa, lymphatic channels and blood vessels. It is associated with extensive hemorrhage and necrosis.
- *Distant metastases*: In fatal cases, metastases are seen in *lung (50%), vagina (30%) brain, bone marrow, liver, kidney and other organs*. In occasional case, primary tumor has undergone total necrosis, while the patient has clinical features due to metastases.

Clinical Features

Patient presents with *irregular bloody, foul smelling discharge per vagina, fever, cachexia with raised serum hCG level*. Rapidly growing tumor causes ischemic necrosis, hemorrhage and secondary infection. If infection presence of infection reveals foul smell discharge per vagina.

Management

- Evacuation of uterine contents, surgery and chemotherapy (*methotrexate, actinomycin-D and etoposide*). It responds well to chemotherapy. *Choriocarcinoma arising from the placenta carries paternal gene that are foreign to the host. In contrast, choriocarcinoma arising from the host's own germ cells has the same genes as the host.*

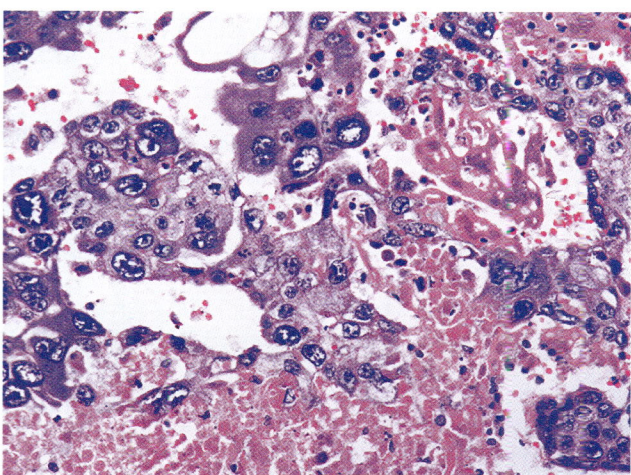

Fig. 24.107: Gestational choriocarcinoma—the tumor is composed of multinucleated syncytiotrophoblastic and cytotrophoblastic cells. The multinucleated syncytiotrophoblasts have voluminous eosinophilic cytoplasm and large darkly staining irregular nuclei with prominent nucleoli. The smaller mononuclear cytotrophoblasts are fairly uniform in size with amphophilic cytoplasm and distinct cellular outlines resembling to the tumor cells of solid yolk sac tumor (400X).

- This accounts for the fact that the gestational choriocarcinomas are readily curable with chemotherapy. It probably stimulates the host immune system in the defense against the choriocarcinoma cells. On the other hand, germ cell choriocarcinomas are incurable.

Prognosis

It is very good with 100% cure rate/remission

PLACENTAL SITE TROPHOBLASTIC TUMOR

It constitutes <2% of gestational trophoblastic tumors. It consists of polygonal cells infiltrating endomyometrium. It is preceded by normal pregnancy in 50% in <2-year period, spontaneous abortion. hCG level is increased. Urine biomarker (mel-cam-9D Ki-67) is used for diagnosis.

Prognosis

Prognosis is poor, if the tumor develops after 4 years interval from prior pregnancy. In 10% of cases, widespread metastases are seen.

PREGNANCY ASSOCIATED DISEASES

TOXEMIA OF PREGNANCY

- Toxemia of pregnancy most often occurs during third trimester in women with first pregnancy. It most often affects *kidneys, liver* and *brain* (hemorrhages) in acute toxemia of pregnancy.

- Patient develops *puffiness on face, pitting edema* and *convulsions in true eclampsia*. Toxemia of pregnancy exists in two forms: preeclampsia or eclampsia. It refers to the *triad of hypertension, proteinuria, and edema (fluid retention)*, complicates the third trimester of pregnancy. It usually begins insidiously after the 20th week of pregnancy (Table 24.36 and Fig. 24.108).

Eclampsia adversely affects *kidneys*, *liver* (subcapsular hemorrhages and periportal necrosis), and *brain* (hemorrhages). Patient may also develop *placental infarcts*.

Clinical Features

- As the disease progresses the *diastolic pressure persistently exceeds 110 mm Hg. Proteinuria is >3 gm* per day, and renal function declines. It is complicated by *convulsions*, and *disseminated intravascular coagulation* the term eclampsia is applied, that can be fatal.

Table 24.36: Differences between preeclampsia (mild) and eclampsia (severe)

Parameters	Preeclampsia	Eclampsia
Diastolic blood pressure	<100 mm Hg	>110 mm Hg and systolic >160 mm Hg
Proteinuria	Traces to mild	Moderate to marked proteinuria
Urine output	Normal	Oliguria
Headache	Absent	Present
Cerebral and visual disturbances	Absent	Present
Upper abdominal pain	Absent	Present
Convulsions	Absent	Present
Serum creatinine	Normal range	Elevated
Thrombocytopenia	Absent	Present
Pulmonary edema	Absent	Present
Fetal growth retardation	Absent	Present

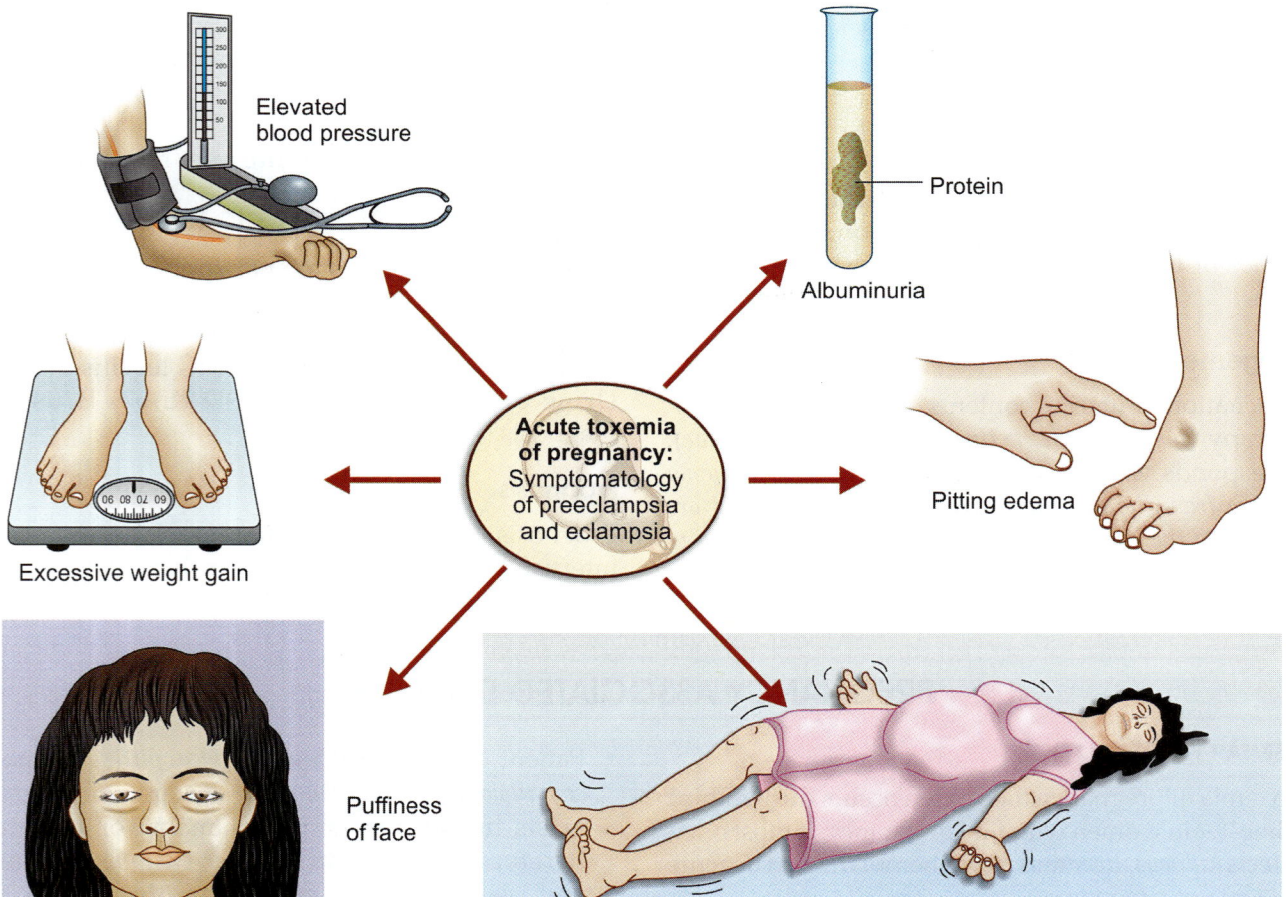

Fig. 24.108: Toxemia of pregnancy: Clinical manifestations in preeclampsia and eclampsia.

- *Disseminated intravascular coagulation* is characterized by formation of *fibrin thrombi in the liver, brain, and kidneys*. Patient may develop subcapsular hemorrhage in liver.

Treatment

The definitive therapy is the removal of the placenta, hopefully by normal delivery.

THROMBOEMBOLISM

There is increased risk of deep vein thrombosis resulting in pulmonary embolism during pregnancy and postpartum period. *The weight of the fetus on femoral vessels slows blood venous return*. Hormonal changes and stress precipitates thrombi formation. Thromboplastin released from amniotic fluid results in activation of coagulation system.

Location

Venous thrombi are present in *deep veins in the lower extremities below knee joint* (most common in 90%), superior saphenous, ovarian or uterine veins.

Clinical Features

- Patient with deep vein thrombus results in pain and distal edema (*Homar's sign*). Patient may develop *migratory thrombophlebitis* and *pulmonary embolization. Ileofemoral venous thrombus is formed during puerperium*.
- Venous thrombi formed in the lower extremities propagate (extend) toward the heart may cause *pulmonary artery embolization*.
- Deep vein thrombosis is entirely asymptomatic in 50% of affected patients. It is recognized only after thrombus is embolized.

AMNIOTIC FLUID EMBOLISM

- The cause of amniotic fluid embolism is a tear in the placental membranes and rupture of maternal veins. This condition is characterized by *sudden peripartal respiratory difficulty, progressing to shock* and often to *death*.
- Amniotic fluid embolism and abruptio placentae are well-known causes of DIC. It is marked by *masses of debris* and *epithelial squamous cells in the maternal pulmonary microcirculation*.
- Amniotic fluid embolism should not be confused with the amniotic fluid aspiration syndrome seen in neonates.

Neonatal Amniotic Fluid Aspiration Syndrome

- It is a disease of the neonate, not of the mother. Inability to expel amniotic fluid at birth is frequently associated with prematurity.
- It is characterized by squamous epithelial cells of amniotic origin in fetal terminal air spaces and larger bronchi.

GESTATIONAL DIABETES MELLITUS

Pregnancy associated transient diabetes mellitus known as gestational diabetes mellitus. Gestational diabetes mellitus is usually identified in the 24–28 weeks of gestation. A woman, who develops gestational diabetes mellitus, has high risk to develop type II diabetes mellitus later in life.

Pathogenesis

- During pregnancy, **anti-insulin hormones** are synthesized by placenta such as *estrogen, prolactin, human chorionic somatomammotropin, cortisol*, and *progesterone*.
- Human chorionic somatomammotropin regulates carbohydrate and protein metabolism of the mother to ensure delivery to the fetus of glucose for energy and protein for fetal growth.

Diagnostic Approach

- Gestational diabetes mellitus is diagnosed with a glucose tolerance test, in which the woman drinks 50 gm glucose. Blood glucose level after an hour >140 mg/dl is considered positive.
- The confirmatory test is a 3-hour, 100 gm glucose tolerance test in which the blood glucose values are set at highest sensitivity. Urine analysis is done for sugar.

Complications

- Due to increased fetal birth weight, there is increased indication of cesarean section. There is *increased fetal birth weight, brachial plexus injuries*, and *neonatal respiratory distress syndrome (hyaline membrane disease)*.
- During intrauterine life in diabetic mothers, fetus develops is let β-*cell hyperplasia* in response to hyperglycemia and increased demand of insulin during early gestation. Pancreatic β-cells, which may secrete insulin autonomously and cause *hypoglycemia at birth*.

ECTOPIC PREGNANCY

Implantation (gestation) of the fertilized ovum outside the normal uterine cavity. Ectopic pregnancy is usually discovered early in a suspected pregnancy when ultrasound examination reveals the uterus to be empty.

Predisposing Factors

Pelvic inflammatory disease (15–50%) with chronic salpingitis often gonorrheal infection leading to partial blockage, peritubal adhesions. There has been increased incidence of ectopic pregnancy in women fitted with IUCD (50%) with normal tubes.

Location

Over 95% of ectopic pregnancies occur in the fallopian tube. *Ampullary implantation of the fallopian tube is commonest* followed by distil/middle-third of tube and isthmus. Other uncommon sites of implantation are ovary, cervix and abdominal cavity.

Clinical Features

Patient presents with severe abdominal pain about 6 weeks after previous normal menstrual period. Tubal rupture causes bleeding in tube (hematosalpinx) and pelvis resulting in hypotensive shock. Tubal pregnancy is suspected when a tubal hematoma is present.

Tubal Changes

The fertilized ovum implants in tubal wall with minimal decidual reaction. *By 12th week of gestation*, the *trophoblast easily penetrates the mucosa* and thin tubal wall *resulting in rupture and intratubal* as well as *intraperitoneal hemorrhage*. Less commonly tubal pregnancy may regress spontaneously with resorption of the entire gestation (Fig. 24.109).

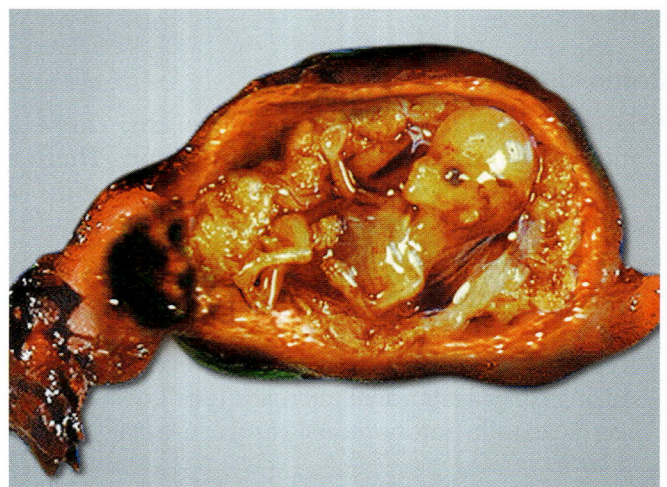

Fig. 24.109: Tubal ectopic pregnancy.

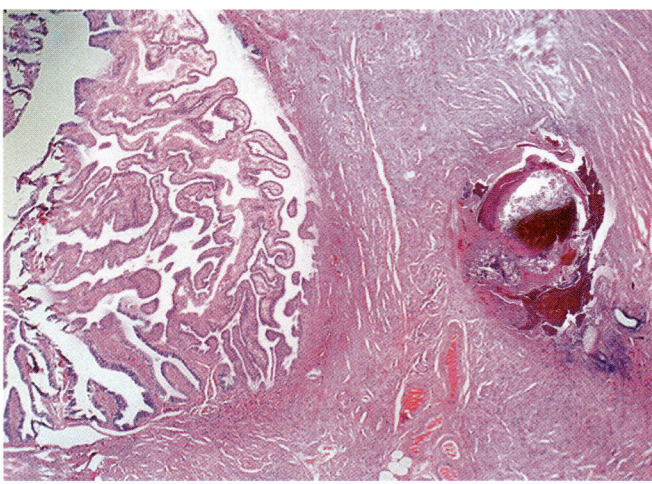

Fig. 24.110: Ectopic tubal pregnancy. A positive pregnancy test (presence of human chorionic gonadotropin), ultrasound, and culdocentesis with presence of blood are helpful in making the diagnosis of ectopic pregnancy. Seen here is tubal epithelium at the right, with rupture site and chorionic villi at the lower left (100X).

> **Light Microscopy**
> Excised tissue shows products of gestation (Fig. 24.110).

Diagnostic Tools

USG, estimation of blood hCG levels and laparoscopy aid in diagnosis.

SHEEHAN'S SYNDROME

During postpartum period, woman develops necrosis of anterior pituitary gland (Fig. 24.111). It is associated with obstetric blood loss, with resultant ischemia of anterior pituitary resulting in hypopituitarism over weeks and months following delivery.

CHORIOAMNIONITIS

Chorioamnionitis often follows premature rupture of membranes. It is most often caused by *ascending infection from the vagina or cervix*. Inflammation of umbilical cord is known as *funisitis*. It can have devastating consequences for both the mother and the child (Fig. 24.112).

ABNORMALITIES OF PLACENTAL ATTACHMENT

Abnormal adherence of the placenta to the uterine wall is categorized according to the depth of villous invasion into the myometrium.

- *Abruptio placentae:* It is premature separation of the placenta. This is an important cause of antepartum bleeding and fetal death. It is often associated with *disseminated intravascular coagulation* (DIC).

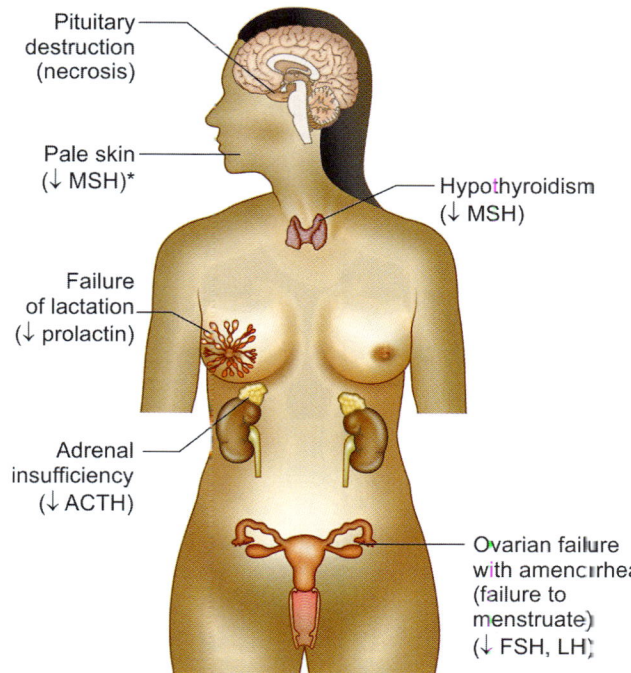

* MSH: melanocyte-stimulating hormone.
MSH is a breakdown product of ACTH.
Excess of MSH produces dark skin.

Fig. 24.111: Clinical manifestations of Sheehan's syndrome. Sheehan's syndrome is caused by hemorrhagic destruction of the pituitary in pregnancy.

- *Placenta accreta:* Placenta accreta is an abnormal adherence of the placenta to the underlying uterine wall without further invasion; the decidual layer is defective. It most often occurs in inflamed endometrium and old scars from prior cesarean sections or other surgery. Most patients have a normal pregnancy and delivery. Impaired placental separation leads to severe bleeding in the third trimester before delivery.

- *Placenta increta:* It defines villi invading the underlying myometrium.

- *Placenta percreta:* It refers to penetration of placental villi into full thickness of the uterine wall.

- *Placenta previa:* It is an attachment of the placenta to the lower uterine segment, partially or completely covering the cervical os. This may coexist with placenta accreta. It is often manifested by bleeding.

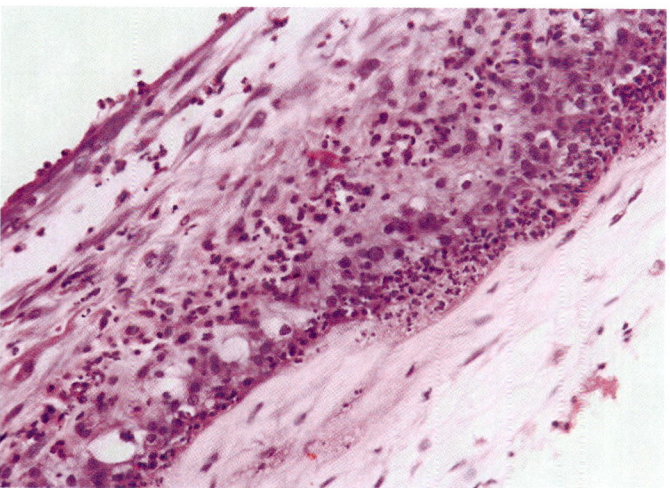

Fig. 24.112: Chorioamnionitis (400X).

CHAPTER 25

Breast

Learning Objectives

FEMALE BREASTS
- Anatomy and Physiology
- Breast Lumps and their Anatomical Correlation
- Clinical Presentation
- Clinical Examination

INFLAMMATORY DISORDERS
- Acute Mastitis
- Periductal Mastitis
- Granulomatous Mastitis

FIBROCYSTIC DISEASE

WHO CLASSIFICATION: BREAST TUMORS
- Stromal Tumors
- Phyllodes Tumor
- Benign Epithelial Tumors

BREAST CARCINOMA
- General Considerations
- Risk Factors
- Major Molecular Pathways in Evolution of Breast Carcinoma
- Histological Variants of Breast Carcinoma
- Mode of Spread of Tumors
- Prognostic and Predictive Factors
- Miscellaneous Diseases of the Female Breast
- Laboratory Diagnosis of Breast Lumps

MALE BREASTS
- Gynecomastia
- Invasive Ductal Carcinoma

FEMALE BREASTS

ANATOMY AND PHYSIOLOGY

The female breasts are modified sweat glands. The breast tissue develops from the milk line. At birth there is no difference between male and female breasts. Pubertal growth is due to glandular and fibrofatty proliferation. The amount of fibroglandular tissue decreases with age. Multiple hormonal stimulation significantly increases the volume of the breast tissue during pregnancy (Fig. 25.1).

Structure

Each breast is comprised of 15–20 lobes interspersed with adipose tissue and connective tissue arranged in radial fashion extending from the *nipple*. The nipple is situated in the center of a darker area of skin called the *areola*. The *areola* contains *small glands*, called *Montgomery glands*, which *lubricate the nipple* during *breastfeeding*.

There are no muscles in the breasts, but the *pectoral muscles* lie under each breast and cover the ribs.

Terminal Duct Lobular Unit (TDLU)

- The lobules of each breast consist of acini or glands lined by an outer myoepithelial cells and an inner secretory cells, also known as *luminal cells*. Each lobe of the breast has one unique terminal duct lobular unit (functional unit), which drains via a *branching duct system*, i.e. *intralobular ducts, interlobular ducts* and *lactiferous sinuses outside through the nipple*. Duct system *carries milk* to the nipples. Each duct has a lining epithelium surrounded by a thin myoepithelial cell layer responsive to *oxytocin*, the hormone that stimulates lactation.

- During pregnancy (30 weeks), each breast shows controlled proliferation of lobular acini lined by cells

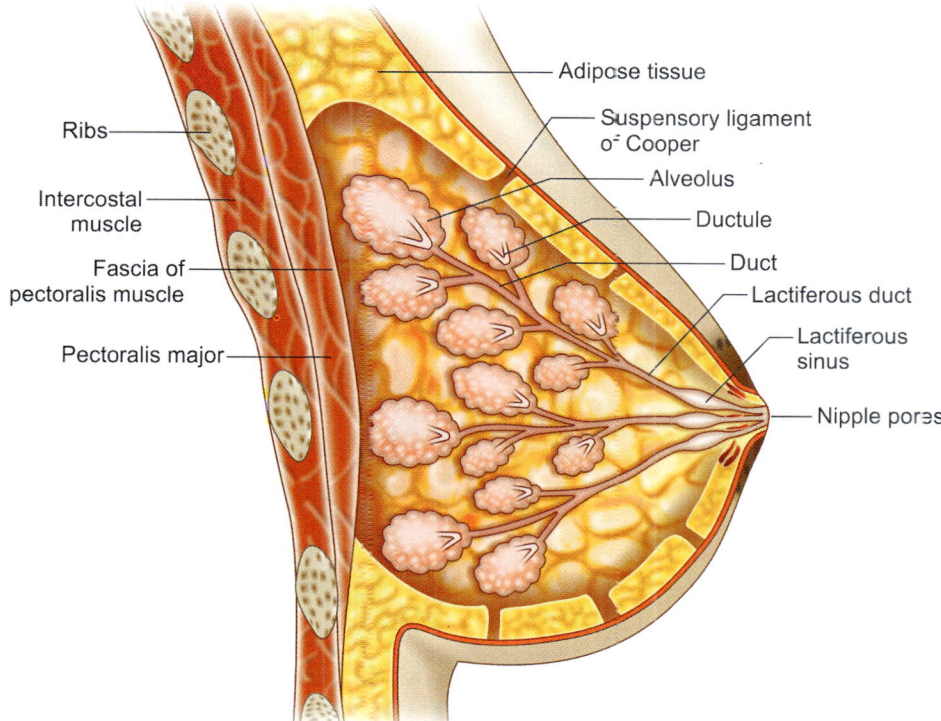

Fig. 25.1: Structure of the adult female breast, showing major components and their functions (*Courtesy by* Dr Abhijit Das).

containing *secretory vacuoles* and secretions in their lumina. Breast milk comprises *casein*, *α-lactalbumin* and *milk fat globule* derived from the luminal surface of ductal cells.
- The acinus is lined by epithelial cells surrounded by myoepithelial cells and the basement membrane. On immunohistochemistry, myoepithelial cells show positivity for **S-100**, *α-smooth muscle actin (α-SMA)*, **p63**, *glial fibrillary acidic protein* and **GFAP**. Myoepithelial cells are most often demonstrated in benign breast tumors. But myoepithelial differentiation is demonstrated in high-grade invasive ductal carcinomas with large central acellular zones (Fig. 25.2).
- Benign breast diseases and carcinomas arise in the terminal duct–lobular unit.

Blood Supply

The vascular supply of the breast is from internal mammary and lateral thoracic artery. There is communication between lymphatic and venous drainage in subclavicular region (Fig. 25.3).

Lymphatic Drainage

The breast has extensive lymphatic drainage. Breast has lymphatic node groups: axillary nodes and internal thoracic lymph nodes. Approximately 75% of the lymphatic drainage occurs to the axillary lymph nodes. So there is greater frequency of tumor metastases to these lymph nodes. Approximately 25% of lymphatic drainage from inner quadrants of breast is drained to *internal mammary* (parasternal) lymph nodes and skin lymphatic channels. To a lesser extent lymph is also drained to nodes adjacent to the vertebra.

There are five groups of axillary lymph nodes:
- *Central axillary nodes:* These are located high up in the middle of the axilla, over the ribs and serratus anterior muscle. These receive lymph from the other three groups of lymph nodes.
- *Pectoral (anterior) nodes:* These are located along the lateral edge of the pectoralis major muscle, just inside the anterior axillary fold.
- *Subscapular (posterior) nodes:* These are situated along the lateral edge of the scapula, deep in the posterior axillary fold.
- *Lateral lymph nodes:* These are situated along the humerus inside upper arm.
- *Apical lymph nodes:* These are situated in the apical region of axilla (Fig. 25.4).

Role of Hormones in Breasts Development

The female breast depends on a variety of hormones for its normal activity. It exhibits structural and functional variation throughout life, especially during puberty, pregnancy, lactation, the normal menstrual cycle, and at the menopause.

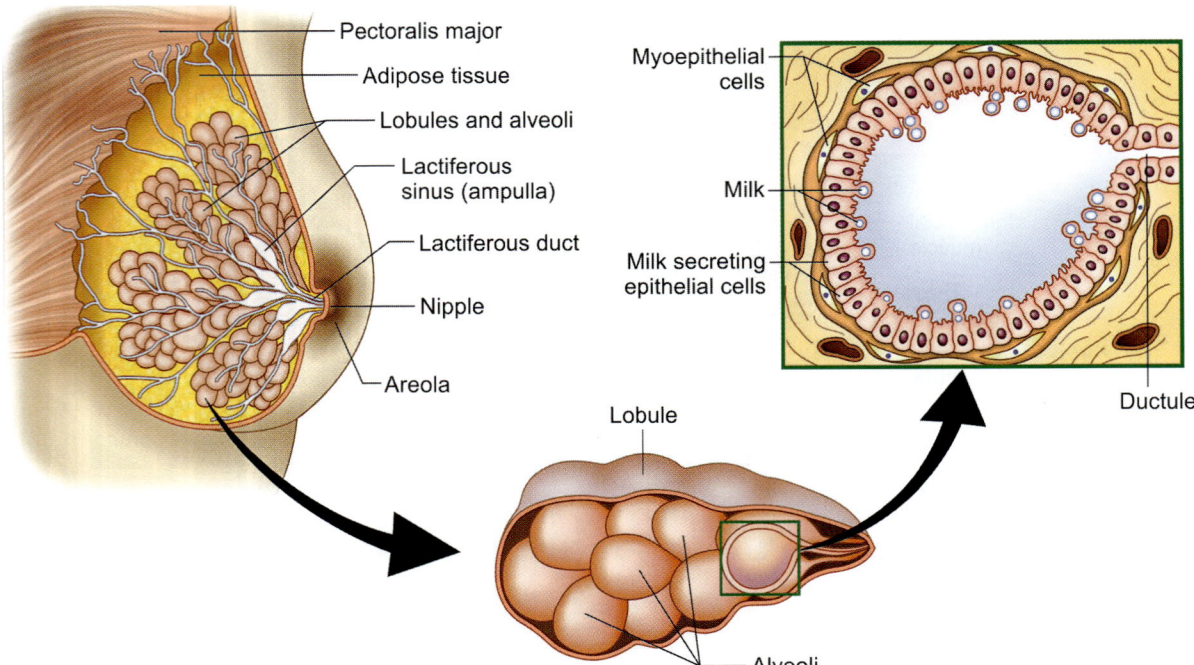

Fig. 25.2: Female breast. Each lobe of the breast has one unique terminal duct lobular unit (functional unit), which drains via a branching duct system, i.e. intralobular ducts, interlobular ducts and lactiferous sinuses outside through the nipple. Duct system carries milk to the nipples. Each duct has a lining epithelium surrounded by a thin myoepithelial cell layer responsive to oxytocin, the hormone that stimulates lactation.

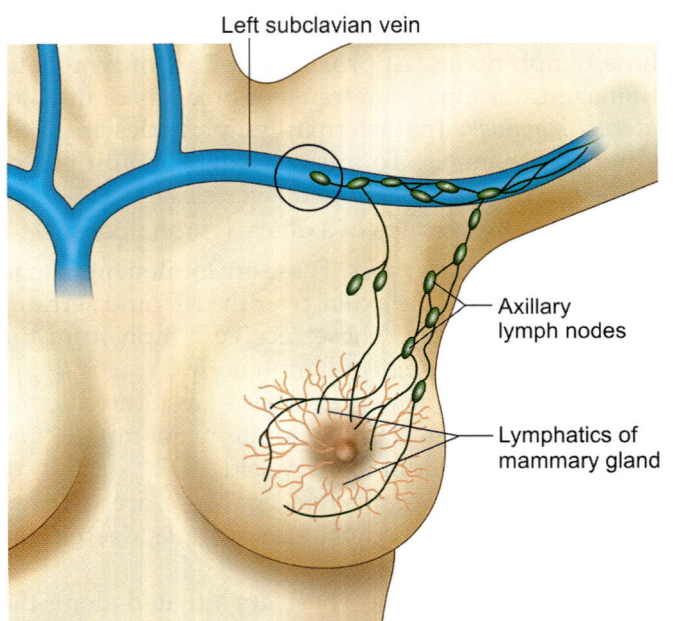

Fig. 25.3: Indicate a chain of the lymph nodes near the axilla and breast. Another point of contact between the two circulations (lymphatic and venous circulation).

- *Hormones and breast development:* Breast development and function depend on the ovarian hormones *estrogen* and *progesterone*. Hormones reaching breast via blood stream either interact with *membrane receptors (prolactin)* or *nuclear receptors (estrogen)*. The hormone receptor interaction activates DNA synthesis of factors responsible for proliferation and differentiation of terminal duct lobular unit. *Estrogen elongates the ducts* and causes them to create side branches. *Progesterone increases the number and size of the lobules* in order to prepare the breast for nourishing a baby. *Growth hormone, insulin and glucocorticoids also participate in proliferation of lobules.*

- *Breast changes during pregnancy:* After ovulation, progesterone makes the breast cells grow and enlargement of blood vessels filled with blood. At this time, the breasts often become engorged with fluid. These may become tender and swollen. The female breast during pregnancy undergoes lobular hypertrophy; so that lactation can occur by the action of prolactin. Breast histology from a woman 30 weeks pregnant, shows the lobular acini lined by cells containing secretory vacuoles and with pink secretions in their lumens.

BREAST LUMPS AND THEIR ANATOMICAL CORRELATION

Frequency of Breast Lumps

A breast mass in a woman is likely to be in decreasing frequency *due to fibrocystic change (40%), miscellaneous benign lesions (13%), carcinomas (10%) or fibroadenomas (7%) and no disease (30%).* The presence of myoepithelial cells in breast epithelial structures typically indicates a benign disease and useful in diagnosis. The **p63** *is a*

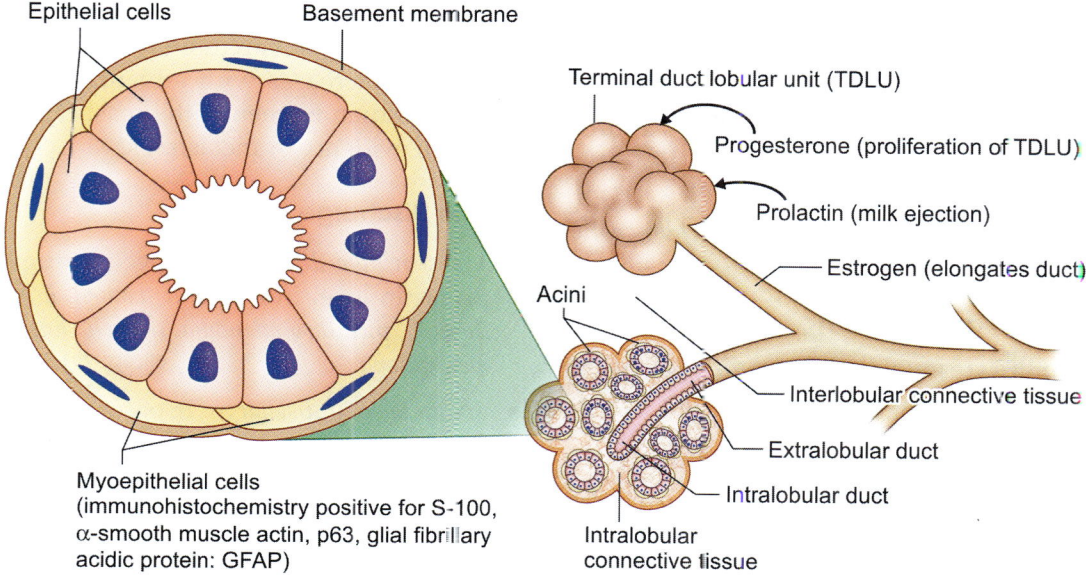

Fig. 25.4: A breast lobule showing the different components. The acinus is lined by epithelial cells surrounded by myoepithelial cells and the basement membrane.

reliable marker for myoepithelial cells. Other myoepithelial cell markers include **S-100, GFAP (glial fibrillary acidic protein)** and **α-smooth muscle actin**. Structure of the adult female breast showing major components and location of various lesions (Fig. 25.5).

Nipple

The nipple may be site of Paget's disease (ductal carcinoma involving nipple skin), nipple adenoma and breast abscess.

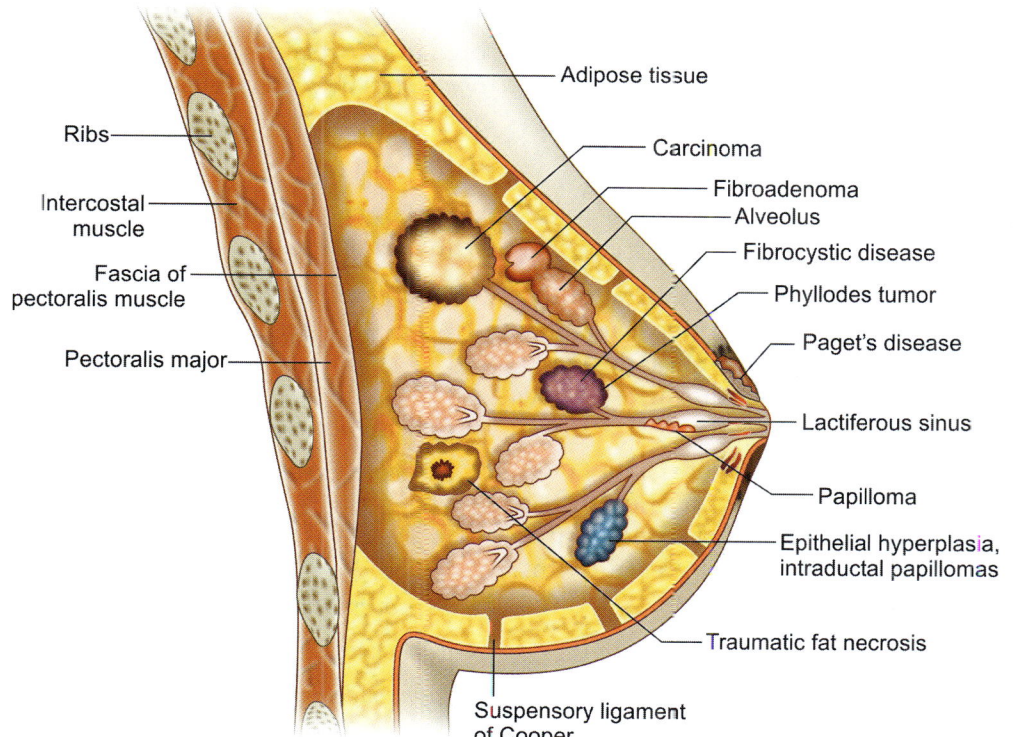

Fig. 25.5: Structure of the adult female breast showing major components and location of various lesions (Courtesy by Dr Achit Das).

Lactiferous Ducts and Sinuses

The lactiferous ducts are the most common site of *intraductal papilloma, galactocele (blocked lactiferous duct in a lactating woman), breast abscess, or plasma cell mastitis*.

Large Ducts

Large ducts are the most common site for *fibrocystic change and most ductal carcinomas*.

Terminal Duct Lobular Unit (TDLU)

The terminal lobules are involved in *sclerosing adenosis (a variant of fibrocystic change), lobular and tubular carcinomas*.

Interlobular or Intralobular Stroma of the Breasts

The breast *interlobular stroma* is the source of *phyllodes tumor*. On the other hand, *fibroadenoma* is derived from *intralobular stroma*.

CLINICAL PRESENTATION

- *Woman* with breast disease most often complains of pain, a palpable lump without a discrete lump and nipple discharge. It is most important to evaluate these women because of the possibility of breast carcinoma.
- Patient with breast carcinoma may present with breast lump, change in the symmetry of the breast, change in the nipple (itching, burning, erosion or retraction), pathological fractures and increased serum calcium levels.
- A spontaneous nipple discharge of any kind in a non-breastfeeding and non-lactating woman warrants investigation (Table. 25.1).

Painful Breasts

- *Premenopausal women:* These present with cyclic pain in bilateral breasts, increasing severity from mid-cycle onwards, and pain improving at menstruation. Women often report fullness, heaviness, areas of tenderness and increased breast size during 3–7 days before each menstruation.
- *Postmenopausal women:* These present with continuous localized breast pain not related to cyclic changes. Approximately 90% of painful breast diseases are benign and 10% of breast carcinoma present with pain.

Breast Lumps

The most common palpable lumps are *fibrocystic disease, fibroadenoma and invasive breast carcinoma*. Premenopausal women most often develop benign palpable masses in 90% and breast carcinoma in 10%. Risk of breast carcinoma increases with advancing age. In clinical practice, Indian women with breast carcinomas report late with evidence of metastases.

Nipple Discharge

- *Milky nipple discharge:* It occurs due to increased prolactin level in *pregnant women, oral contraceptive therapy, pituitary adenoma, tricyclic antidepressant and methyldopa*.
- *Serous/bloody discharge:* It occurs due to *intraductal papilloma or breast carcinoma*.
- *Eczema-like lesion with blood stained discharge:* A rash, often eczema-like lesion, on the nipple or surrounding area and blood stained discharge from nipple is seen in *Paget's disease of nipple* (ductal carcinoma involving overlying skin).

Nipple Retraction

Indrawing (retraction) of the nipple due to *desmoplasia* in an underlying advanced scirrhous breast carcinoma is a late feature. Nipple retraction also occurs due to fibrosis in *chronic inflammation* of the breast.

Overlying Skin Edema

The *"peau d'orange"* (skin edema) appearance of the breast skin occurs due to *obstruction of the dermal lymphatics* by tumor cells.

CLINICAL EXAMINATION

Clinician should note these characteristics in women with breast diseases:

- *Location:* Quadrants
- *Size:* Dimensions
- *Shape:* Lump oval, lobulated or indistinct
- *Consistency:* Soft, firm or hard
- *Movable:* Freely movable or fixed
- *Distinction:* Solitary or multiple
- *Nipple:* Displaced or retracted or nipple discharge
- *Skin over the lump:* Erythematous, dimpled or retracted
- *Tenderness:* Tender on palpation or not
- *Lymphadenopathy:* Lymph nodes palpable or not
- *Distant metastases:* Organs involved

Table 25.1: Pathological basis of breast signs and symptoms in women

Clinical presentation	Pathological correlation
Breast lump frequency	Fibrocystic change (40%) No disease (30%) Miscellaneous benign lesions (13%) Breast carcinomas (10%) Fibroadenomas (7%)
Onset of lump	Fat necrosis-associated with trauma Fibrocystic disease-associated with menstrual cycle Duration and rate of growth of lump (fibroadenoma showing slow growth no apparent change in size in 6+ months and rapid growth in breast carcinoma)
Pain and tenderness in breasts	Mastitis (acute or chronic) Mammary duct ectasia Breast abscess Galactocele Fibrocystic disease (cyclic pain)
Nipple discharge	*Milky nipple discharge (galactorrhea)* occurs due to increased prolactin level during pregnancy, pituitary adenoma, oral contraceptive therapy, tricyclic antidepressant, methyldopa) Serous/Bloody (intraductal papilloma/cancer) Nipple shows rash, eczema-like or blood stained discharge in Paget's disease of nipple (ductal carcinoma involving overlying skin)
Manual examination of breasts	*Diffuse:* Fibrocystic disease *Discrete:* Neoplasm or cyst *Mobile lump:* Fibroadenoma *Bulky tumor:* Phyllodes tumor and giant fibroadenoma *Immobile lump:* Invasive breast carcinoma
Nipple retraction	Breast carcinomas Inflammatory breast lesions undergoing fibrosis Fat necrosis of breast
Skin features	*Peau d' orange:* Lymphatic blockage by cancer cells and puckering *Tethering:* Due to invasion of Cooper's ligament in breast cancer *Erythema:* Acute mastitis and Paget's disease of nipple
Microcalcifications on mammography	Dystrophic calcification associated with fibrocystic changes such as cysts and adenosis Carcinoma *in situ* or invasive carcinoma
Metastases	Lymph nodes involvement in axillary and supraclavicular regions Visceral metastases Bone pain and pathological fractures occur due to metastases

INFLAMMATORY DISORDERS

> **Key Facts**
> - Inflammatory diseases of the breast are rare. Acute infection occurs only in the lactating breast.
> - Periductal mastitis is also known as Zuska's disease or squamous metaplasia of lactiferous ducts.
> - Fat necrosis occurs due to trauma to breast especially in obese women.
> - Duct ectasia shows many thick-walled dilated ducts filled with yellow-brown cheesy secretions.
> - Granulomatous mastitis occurs in systemic granulomatous disease, e.g. tuberculosis, sarcoidosis, Wegener's granulomatosis, fungal infection, breast implants or unknown etiology. There is involvement of lobular epithelium.
> - Lipogranulomas are caused by rupture of a paraffin-filled polythene sac implanted silicone prosthesis previously as a device for breast augmentation.

ACUTE MASTITIS

Milk stasis is the main predisposing factor of lactation mastitis. If not treated appropriately, lactation breast abscesses can recur, which may be complicated by a fistulous tract. It is caused by *Staphylococcus aureus* that can enter the breast tissue through *cracks and fissures in the nipple*. This disorder is usually secondary to obstruction of the duct system by inspissated secretions. Complications of duct ectasia include abscess formation, fistulous tract and nipple retraction. Associated fibrosis and calcification in duct ectasia can simulate breast carcinoma.

Age Group

Breast infection of overlying skin commonly affects women aged between 18 and 45 years, which may be primary or secondary due to infected sebaceous cyst in overlying skin. Females with *pituitary prolactinomas* occasionally are associated with galactorrhea.

Clinical Features

The breast becomes tense, hot, and very painful. Axillary lymph nodes may become enlarged and tender.

Therapeutic Correlation

It may be treated by mechanical suction, frequent emptying of the breasts, and administration of antibiotics.

PERIDUCTAL MASTITIS

Periductal mastitis is also known as *Zuska's disease* or squamous metaplasia of lactiferous ducts.

Age Group

Periductal mastitis occurs especially in smokers.

Pathogenesis

Tobacco use alters the epithelium of lactiferous sinuses. Keratin is trapped into ducts. Nipple inversion occurs due to fibrosis. Recurrences are common.

> **Light Microscopy**
> Histological examination reveals chronic and granulomatous inflammation.

MAMMARY DUCT ECTASIA

Duct ectasia of major subareolar ducts is characterized by inflammation and dilation of the major ducts. The ducts are filled with debris, resulting in dilatation, rupture and inflammation. Possible etiological factors of duct ectasia are infections and cigarette smoking.

Clinical Features

Some women present with greenish brown cheesy nipple discharge, slit-like nipple retraction, or palpable lump simulating cancer that may be hard or doughy. There is no increased risk for breast carcinoma.

> **Gross Morphology**
> - When cut across it shows many thick-walled dilated ducts filled with yellow brown cheesy secretions.
> - In women above 50 years of age, frequent incidental pathological finding is fibrocystic change in 30–40% of cases in surgically excised breast tissue and in autopsy specimens.
>
> **Light Microscopy**
> It shows dilated ducts with fibrosis of wall, inflammatory cell infiltrate with plasma cells, and inspissation of lipid-rich material within duct lumen.

Management

Antibiotics and surgical removal of dilated duct cures these patients.

FAT NECROSIS

Fat necrosis of breast most often occurs in women >55 years. It is most common chronic inflammatory lesion which follows foreign body giant cell reaction and fibrosis due to lipid released from traumatized adipocytes.

Pathogenesis

Trauma to the breast is most common cause of fat necrosis, followed by prior surgical intervention and radiation therapy. It occurs when *lipase enzyme breaks down intracellular triglycerides into free fatty acids.* These free fatty acids combine with *sodium, magnesium* or *calcium* ions to form **soaps**. *The tissue becomes opaque and chalky white.*

Clinical Features

Patient develops unilateral localized breast mass, which may be painful in acute stage. Clinical examination of affected breast reveals a firm, superficial irregular mass, erythema of the overlying skin, dimpling and nipple retraction mimics carcinoma.

Radiological Findings

Breast shows calcified lesion.

Gross Morphology

- It shows chalky white areas of fat saponification. Variegated color and areas of hemorrhage are demonstrated on the cut surface of this lump.
- It is gritty to cut because of the presence of spotty calcification.

Light Microscopy

- In the response to fat necrosis there is an initial acute inflammatory reaction consisting of necrosis of adipocytes and hemorrhage. It is followed by chronic inflammatory response in which numerous plasma cells are seen.
- Macrophages phagocytose lipid released from adipocytes, forming multinucleate giant cells, as well as foam cells, also termed '*lipophages*'.
- There is presence of foreign body giant cells and dystrophic calcification demonstrated by imaging techniques.
- Fibroblastic proliferation leads to fibrosis resulting in extension to the surrounding tissue. As a result, an irregular, fixed, hard mass may ensue and clinically resemble breast carcinoma. Thus, the lesions often require biopsy to establish their benign character.

GRANULOMATOUS MASTITIS

It is a group of immunologic mediated disorder of breast lobules. It leads to alteration in the lobular epithelium during lactation resulting in hypersensitivity reaction in multiparous women.

Etiology

It occurs in systemic granulomatous disease, e.g. tuberculosis, sarcoidosis, Wegener's granulomatosis, fungal infection, breast implants and unknown etiology. There is involvement of lobular epithelium.

Light Microscopy

Breast lobules show granulomas, histiocytes, lymphocytes, plasma cells and giant cells by sparing interlobular stromal region.

- *Breast tuberculosis:* Breast tuberculosis usually occurs due to extension from rib in females. Patient presents with breast abscess and fever. On cut section, breast abscess contains caseous material.

  Light microscopy reveals epithelioid granulomas, caseous necrosis and Langhans's type of giant cells.

- *Sarcoidosis:* Breast sarcoidosis is an idiopathic disorder in which abnormal immune system leads to formation of *noncaseating granulomas* and collection of macrophages.

  These trigger an inflammatory response that causes extensive tissue damage and scarring. It shows noncaseating granuloma and collection of macrophages.

  Kveim test is performed by intracutaneous injection of saline suspension of human sarcoidal spleen or lymph nodes which cause appearance of erythematous nodules.

- *Wegener's granulomatosis:* It is a systemic necrotizing granulomatous vasculitis of unknown etiology or due to inhalation of some infectious agents.

  Antineutrophil cytoplasmic antibodies (c-ANCA type) play a pivotal role in its pathogenesis. Immune complexes formed are deposited in small vessels resulting in necrotizing vasculitis.

SILICONE BREAST IMPLANTS

- Silicone implants in breast are used for *cosmetic augmentation*. Silicone is a polymer of silica, O_2 and hydrogen. Due to leakage of silicone implants, chronic inflammation takes place.
- Lipogranulomas are caused by rupture of a paraffin-filled polythene sac implanted prosthesis previously as a device for breast augmentation. This is a very old-fashioned type of breast implantation.

SCLEROSING LYMPHOCYTIC LOBULITIS

- Sclerosing lymphocytic lobulitis is also known as *lymphocytic mastopathy*. It most often occurs in women with type I diabetes mellitus or autoimmune thyroid diseases. It is considered to be an autoimmune disorder.
- Patient presents with hard palpable lumps. It is difficult to obtain tissue with needle biopsy due to presence of dense collagenous stroma. It should be differentiated from breast carcinoma.

FIBROCYSTIC DISEASE

Fibrocystic breast disease is the most common benign disorder of the female breasts. It is caused by abnormal response of breast to ovarian hormones. Patient develops painful multifocal lumps in both breasts. The frequency of fibrocystic change decreases progressively after menopause.

Although it is a benign condition, the gross and mammographic appearance may mimic carcinoma, and is often difficult to distinguish from carcinoma on frozen section (Fig. 25.6).

Key Facts of Fibrocystic Disease
- It is caused by abnormal response of breast to ovarian hormones.
- Fibrocystic changes occur in glands and stroma. These include fibrosis, duct ectasia, apocrine metaplasia, duct hyperplasia and sclerosing adenosis.
- There is increased risk of development of breast carcinoma related to the presence of atypical hyperplasia of the glands.
- Sclerosing adenosis can be clinically and radiologically confused with breast carcinoma.

Age Group

It affects women in 20 to 50 years of age. About 10% of women have clinically evident disease. It is uncommon before adolescence or after menopause. Approximately 60–90% of breasts show fibrocystic change at autopsy.

Etiology

It is postulated that it results due to hormonal imbalance, i.e. *increased uncontrolled response of estrogens on terminal duct lobular unit* or to decreased progesterone activity. This hormonal imbalance occurs in *functional ovarian granulosa cell tumors and anovulatory cycles*. Environmental toxins inhibiting cyclic guanosine monophosphate enzymes by methylxanthines (e.g. caffeine, tea, chocolate), tyramine (e.g. cheese, wine, nuts) and tobacco may also cause fibrocystic change.

Clinical Features

Patient presents with bilateral breast palpable lumps (irregular nodularity) with mid-cyclic tenderness

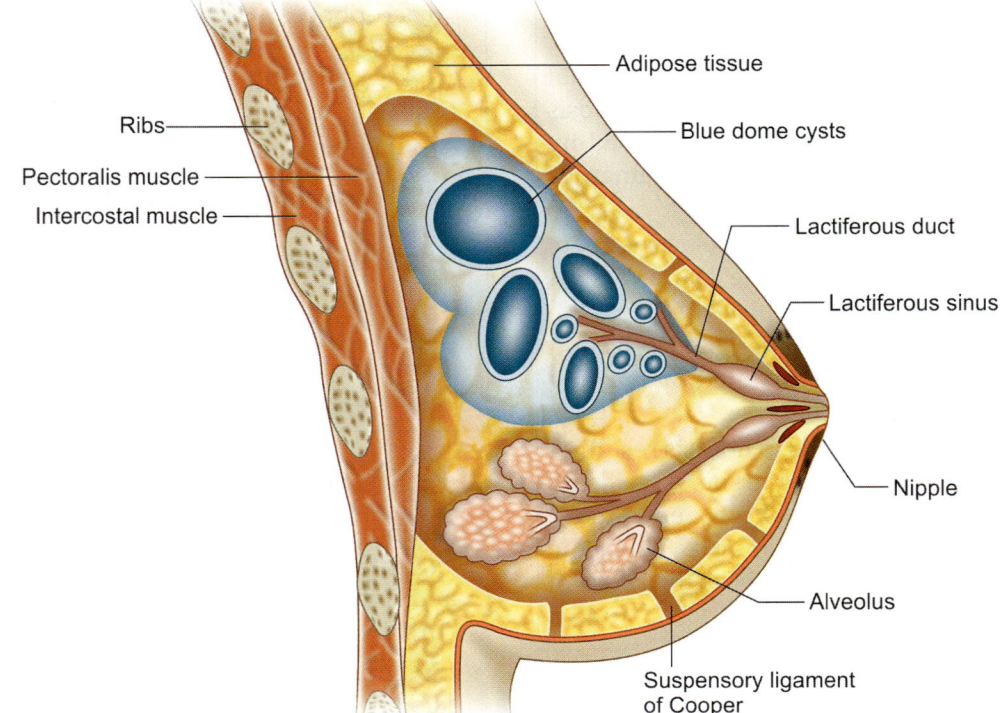

Fig. 25.6: Fibrocystic disease of breast. Structure of the adult female breast showing fibrocystic disease in 45-year-old woman showing one large cyst and multiple smaller ones, with areas of fibrosis (*Courtesy by* Dr Abhijit Das).

varying during the menstrual cycle. *Pain* is present in the *upper outer quadrant* of bilateral breasts. Occasionally, there is history of greenish brown to black nipple discharge containing fat, proteins, ductal cells and erythrocytes.

Gross Morphology
- Cut surface is firm grey white fibrous tissue.
- Some cysts may be quite large, which undergo hemorrhage into the cyst fluid called *blue domed cysts*.
- These cysts vary in size with the menstrual cycle.
- These are most often enlarged and tender one week before menstruation.

Light Microscopy
- Fibrocystic changes occur in glands and stroma, which include fibrosis, duct ectasia, apocrine metaplasia, duct hyperplasia and sclerosing adenosis.
- Histology of fibrocystic disease shows cystic dilatation of the terminal ducts with increased surrounding collagen fibers.
- Fibrocystic changes may be nonproliferative or proliferative.

Histopathological Changes

Nonproliferative Fibrocystic Changes

Nonproliferative fibrocystic changes include dense fibrous stroma encompassing a number of *variable size cystic dilatation of the terminal ducts (duct ectasia) and mild hyperplasia*. Alteration of epithelial lining is termed as '*apocrine metaplasia*'. Apocrine cells are large and more eosinophilic than that usually line the ducts and resemble apocrine sweat gland epithelium. On clinical examination, the breasts are lumpy. There is *no risk of development of breast carcinoma* (Figs 25.7 to 25.11).

Proliferative Fibrocystic Changes

These are associated with epithelial hyperplasia of ducts and lobules, with or without features of atypia, and sclerosing adenosis. *Atypical hyperplasia of ducts and lobules is associated with a five-fold increase* in the risk of developing *ductal carcinoma*. When associated with a family history of breast carcinoma; the risk of development of breast carcinoma is ten-fold.

- *Fibrosis:* Rupture of cysts with extravasation of fluid in the stroma results in inflammation and fibrosis. Dense fibrous interlobular stroma expands into the lobules, and replaces the loose intralobular connective tissue. Strands of fibrous tissue constrict the ducts, so that the normal secretions cannot pass out. Terminal ducts become dilated resulting in formation of cysts containing secretions.
- *Duct ectasia:* Paste-like material in subareolar ducts produces *sticky purulent discharge* that may be *white, gray, brown, green or bloody*. It is caused by stagnation of cellular debris and secretions in the ducts. Cysts filled with bluish fluid are known as *blue dome cysts* when examined through cyst wall. Light microscopy shows cysts lined by uniform benign cuboidal to columnar epithelial cells of variable height with

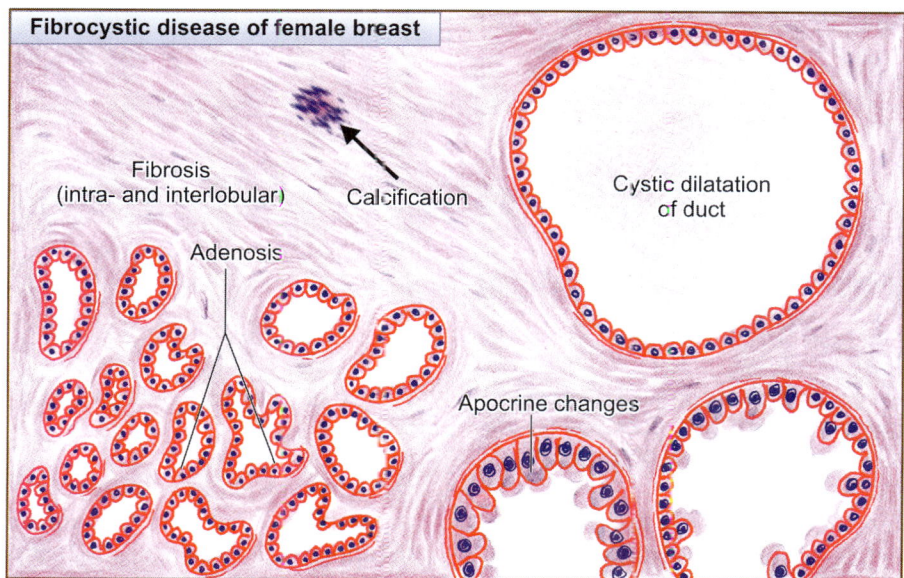

Fig. 25.7: Structure of the adult female breast showing fibrocystic disease (e.g. cystic dilatation of ducts, apocrine change, fibrosis and sclerosing adenosis). In sclerosing adenosis, there are glandular structures with intervening cords of cells in a fibrous stroma. Areas of calcification (arrow) are also present; these would render the lesion visible on mammography (*Courtesy* by Dr Abhijit Das).

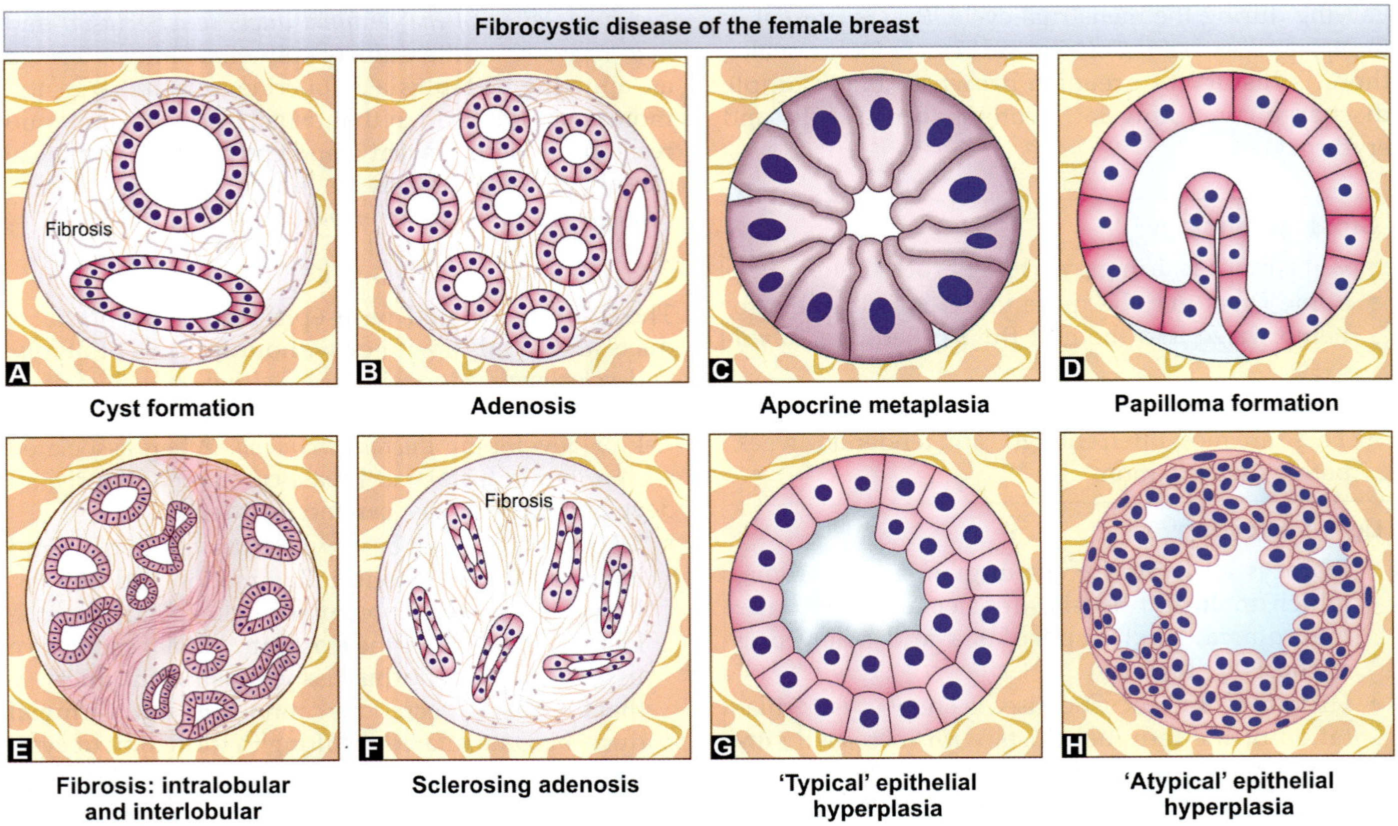

Fibrocystic disease of the female breast

A Cyst formation
B Adenosis
C Apocrine metaplasia
D Papilloma formation
E Fibrosis: intralobular and interlobular
F Sclerosing adenosis
G 'Typical' epithelial hyperplasia
H 'Atypical' epithelial hyperplasia

Fig. 25.8: Fibrocystic disease of breast. It shows (A) cyst formation, (B) adenosis, (C) apocrine metaplasia, (D) papilloma formation, (E) fibrosis (intralobular and interlobular), (F) sclerosing adenosis, (G) typical epithelial hyperplasia, and (H) atypical epithelial hyperplasia. In epithelial hyperplasia, the duct lumen is filled by hyperplastic epithelium. In atypical hyperplasia, there is increased risk of development of breast cancer.

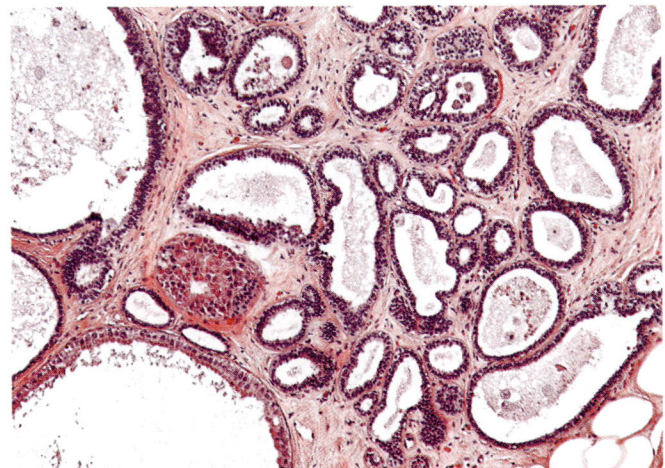

Fig. 25.9: Spectrum of morphological changes in fibrocystic disease of the breast showing duct dilatation, adenosis, fibrosis (intralobular and interlobular), and apocrine change (400X).

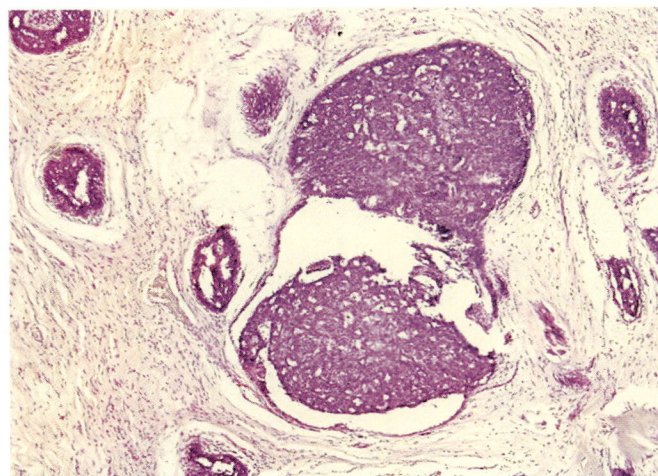

Fig. 25.10: Fibrocystic disease shows typical ductal hyperplasia.

microcalcifications in their lumen. *These cysts do not have malignant potential.* On clinical examination of breast, these lesions reveal *cystic feel.*

- *Apocrine metaplasia:* The cells lining large cysts undergo change consisting of *tall, pink, columnar benign epithelial cells* with small nuclei and brightly *eosinophilic cytoplasm.* **Chromosomal abnormalities** in apocrine epithelium suggest possible precursor of **apocrine carcinoma.**
- *Sclerosing adenosis:* Sclerosing adenosis with fibrosis of the intralobular stroma resulting in compression

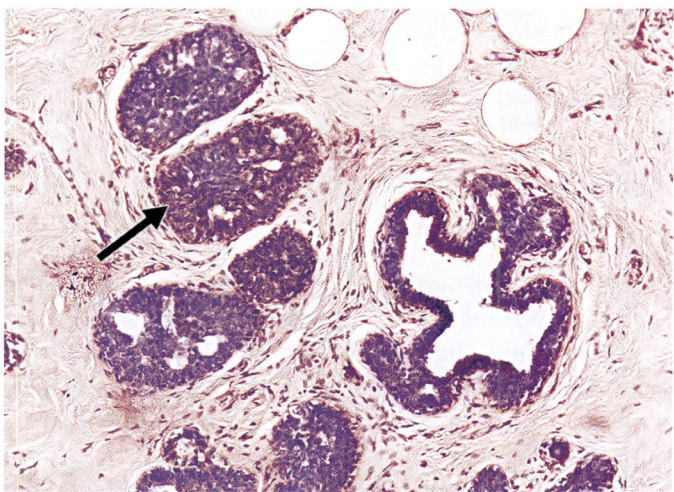

Fig. 25.11: Fibrocystic disease shows atypical ductal hyperplasia (arrow) (100X).

of the epithelial structures to give a pseudoinfiltrative growth pattern. The number of acini per terminal duct is more than double the normal found in normal lobules. *Tubules are lined by two layers of epithelial cells giving lobular configuration.* There is more often presence of numerous microcalcifications. Sclerosing adenosis lesions have become significant in modern clinical practice, as these lesions can be confused with breast carcinoma on **mammographic screening**.

- *Ductal epithelial hyperplasia:* As the ducts are estrogen sensitive, florid ductal epithelial hyperplasia occurs within areas of fibrocystic changes. *The epithelial cells are multilayered, filling and expanding the ducts or acini.* There is a slightly increased risk (1.5 to 2 times) of development of breast carcinoma.
- *Atypical ductal hyperplasia:* It occurs in ducts and lobules lined by **multilayered pleomorphic atypical cells** with hyperchromatic nuclei resembling carcinoma *in situ* of ducts (DCIS) or lobules (LCIS). These atypical cells do not fill the entire lumen of ducts or lobules. These atypical changes are indicative of an increased risk for subsequent breast malignancy (Table 25.2).

Diagnostic Tools

Since the introduction of mammographic and ultrasound imaging of the breast, this condition can be diagnosed without having to perform surgical excision. Ultrasonography is done to distinguish cystic fluid filled lesions in fibrocystic disease from solid masses. Fine needle aspiration cytology of bloody aspirate is done to rule out malignant change. Histopathological examination distinguishes benign from malignant changes.

Table 25.2: Comparison of histological features of ductal hyperplasia and ductal carcinoma *in situ* (DCIS)

Histological features	Ductal hyperplasia (usual type)	Atypical hyperplasia/DCIS (low nuclear grade)
Size	Variable size, rarely extensive when associated with papilloma or radical scar	May be extensive, rarely <3 mm
Cellular composition	Epithelial cells along with spindle cells, lymphocytes, macrophages. Myoepithelial cell hyperplasia around periphery	Single cell population. Absence of spindle cells. Myoepithelial cells around periphery
Architecture	Variable	Well-developed micropapillary, cribriform or solid patterns
Lumina	Lumina irregular often ill-defined slit-like spaces common	Lumina well-delineated, regular, punched out in cribriform pattern
Cell orientation	Streaming pattern with long axis of nuclei arranged parallel to direction of cellular bridges, which often have a 'tapering appearance	Micropapillary structures with indiscernible fibrovascular cores or smooth, well-delineated geometric spaces. Cell bridges 'rigid' in cribriform type with nuclei oriented towards the luminal type
Nuclear spacing	Uneven	Even
Epithelial cell character	Small ovoid with variation in shape	Small uniform monotonous appearance
Nucleoli	Indistinct	Single small
Mitoses	Infrequent	Infrequent, abnormal form
Necrosis	Rare	If present, confined to small particulate debris in cribriform and/or luminal spaces

WHO CLASSIFICATION: BREAST TUMORS

World Health Organization has classified breast tumors as shown in Table 25.3.

STROMAL TUMORS

FIBROADENOMA

Fibroadenoma is the most common benign neoplasm of the breast derived from *intralobular stroma* (Fig. 25.12). It affects females <25 years of age. In some teenagers, it may reach enormous size (10–15 cm), so-called juvenile fibroadenoma. It is cured by local surgical excision. Complex fibroadenomas are associated with an increased risk of subsequent breast carcinoma.

Pathogenesis

Proliferation of intralobular stroma leads to compression of the ducts. It also synthesizes growth factors, which may cause proliferation of ducts. The basis of ductal proliferation is not clear; perhaps the neoplastic stromal cells secrete growth factors that induce proliferation of epithelial cells. It develops in 50% of women who receive *cyclosporine after renal transplantation* due to synthesis of growth factor by intralobular stroma.

Molecular Genetics

It reveals that the stromal cells are monoclonal and representing the neoplastic element of these tumors.

Clinical Features

Patient presents with *solitary, well-circumscribed, firm rubbery* and *painless* lump most often in the *upper outer quadrant*. It may be present in any quadrant. Multiple or bilateral fibroadenomas may be seen in 10–15% of patients. There is no dimpling or retraction of overlying skin.

During menstrual cycle, *pregnancy* and *lactation*, fibroadenoma may undergo *transient enlargement* with some pain in response to increasing *estrogen/progesterone* levels. It may regress and calcify after menopause.

> **Gross Morphology**
> - Fibroadenoma is delineated from adjacent breast tissue.
> - Cut surface is *gray white, smooth, firm with rubbery consistency*.

Table 25.3: WHO classification of breast tumors

Epithelial Tumors	
Adenomas: Tubular adenoma, lactating adenoma, apocrine adenoma, ductal adenoma and pleomorphic adenoma	
Carcinomas	Invasive ductal carcinoma (not otherwise specified), invasive lobular carcinoma (*in situ*/invasive), inflammatory carcinoma, medullary carcinoma, colloid (mucinous) carcinoma, tubular carcinoma, cribriform carcinoma (*in situ*/invasive), invasive papillary carcinoma, invasive micropapillary carcinoma, microinvasive carcinoma, secretory carcinoma, metaplastic carcinoma (chondroid or bone formation or squamous differentiation), apocrine carcinoma, lobular neoplasia (lobular carcinoma *in situ*), lipid rich carcinoma, adenoid cystic carcinoma, and sebaceous carcinoma
	Intraductal proliferative neoplasms: usual ductal hyperplasia, flat epithelial atypia, atypical ductal hyperplasia and ductal carcinoma *in situ*
Fibroepithelial tumors: Fibroadenoma, phyllodes tumor, periductal stromal sarcoma (low-grade) and mammary hamartoma	
Tumors of nipple: Nipple adenoma, Paget's disease of nipple (ductal carcinoma involving skin overlying nipple, syringomatous adenoma	
Myoepithelial lesions: Myoepitheliosis, adenomyoepithelial adenosis, adenomyoepithelioma, malignant myoepithelioma	
Mesenchymal tumors: Hemangioma, angiosarcoma, angiomatosis, hemangiopericytoma, leiomyoma, leiomyosarcoma, lipoma, liposarcoma, angiolipoma, neurofibroma, schwannoma, osteosarcoma, inflammatory myoblastoma, granular cell tumor, fibromatosis (aggressive)	
Malignant lymphomas	
Metastatic tumors	

Fibroadenoma, phyllodes tumor, invasive ductal carcinoma (65–80% and infiltrating lobular carcinoma (5–14%) are significant in clinical practice. Uncommon breast cancers are medullary carcinoma, mucinous (colloid) carcinoma, Paget's disease, papillary carcinoma and tubular carcinoma.

Breast 25

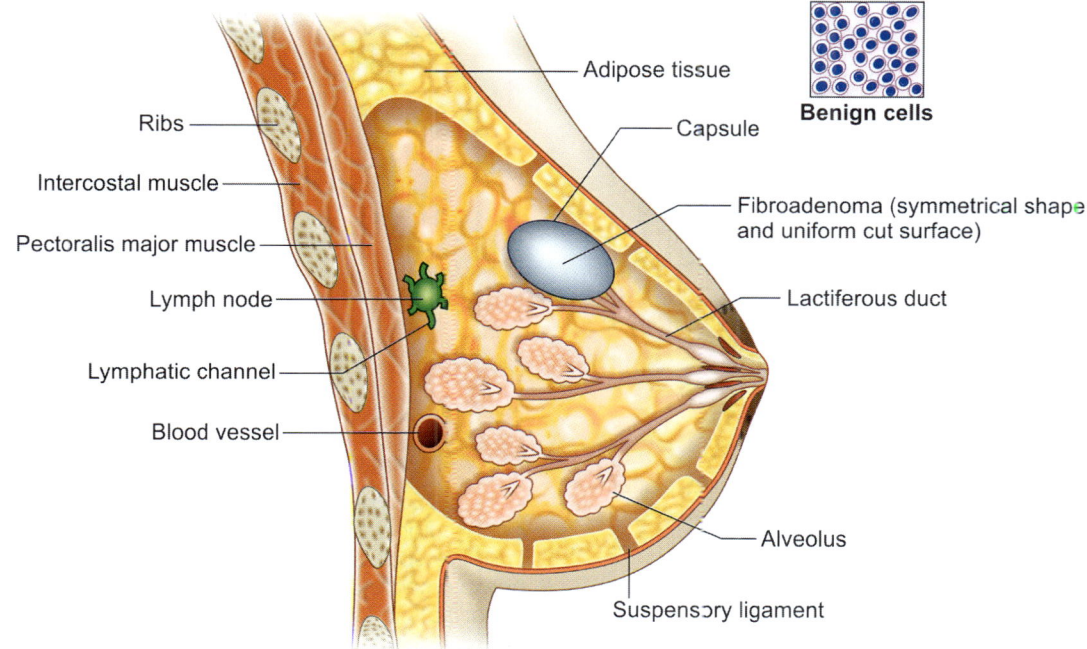

Fig. 25.12: Structure of the adult female breast showing fibroadenoma (well circumscribed tumor) in young female (*Courtesy by* Dr Abhijit Das).

- It most often varies in size 1–3 cm in diameter, but may grow larger. Rarely tumors growing >10 cm in diameter are called giant fibroadenoma (Fig. 25.13).

Light Microscopy

Fibroadenoma showing proliferation and expansion of the stroma is of usually low cellularity. The ductal element sometimes forms an *intracanalicular pattern* with a *leaf like pattern* (Figs 25.14 to 25.16).

Delicate loose fibrous stroma encloses the epithelial component consisting of gland-like or duct-like spaces lined by cuboidal or columnar cells. The stromal cells of loose fibrous stroma are neoplastic, and the epithelial cells lining ducts to be reactive.

Tumor shows biphasic patterns: intracanalicular and pericanalicular patterns.
- *Intracanalicular pattern:* Excessive proliferation of intralobular stroma compressing and distorting glands (ducts) and forming slit-like spaces is known *intracanalicular pattern* with a *leaf-like pattern*.
- *Pericanalicular pattern:* The glands (ducts) retain round shape. Because ducts are not compressed by fibrosis resulting in *pericanalicular pattern*.

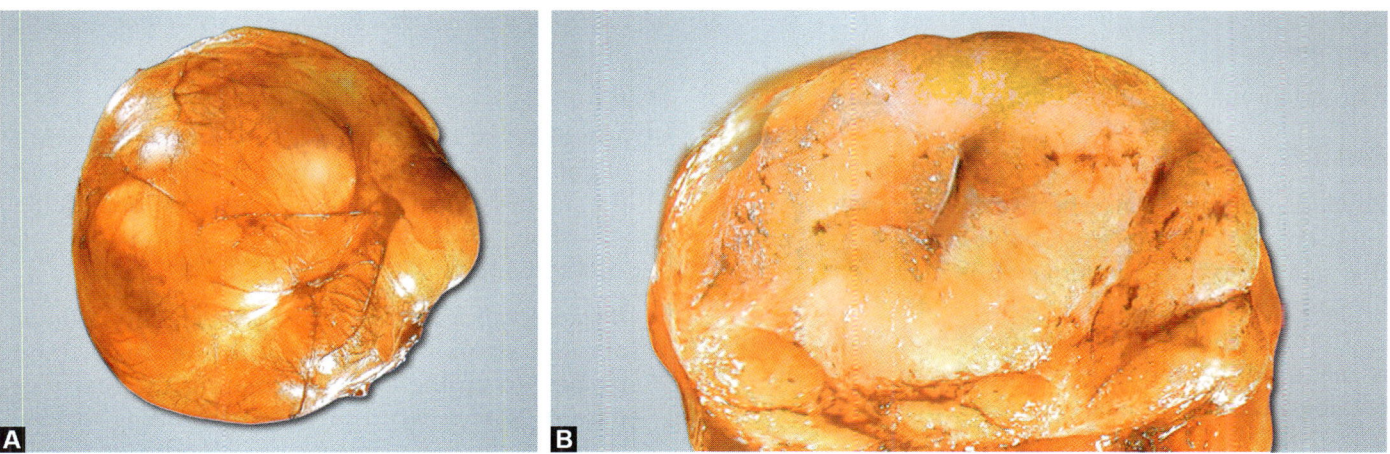

Fig. 25.13: Fibroadenoma—this well circumscribed mobile lump was removed surgically. Cut surface shows lobulated appearance of tumor bulging outwards. Cut surface is gray white, smooth, firm with rubbery consistency. It most often varies in size from 1 to 3 cm in diameter.

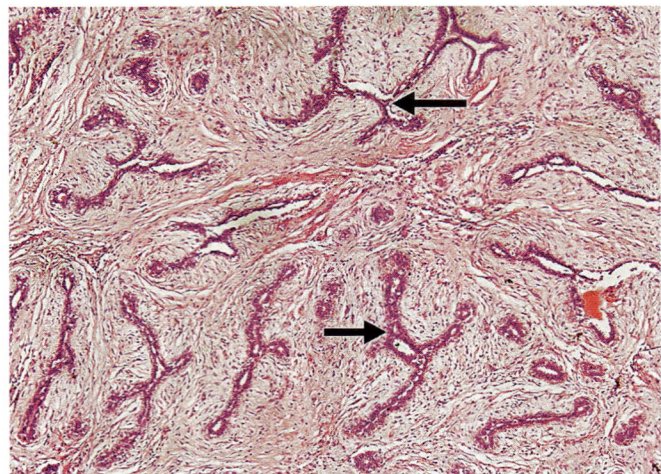

Fig. 25.14: Fibroadenoma breast with intracanalicular pattern—light microscopy shows intracanalicular pattern with glands compressed as cords to form slit-like spaces in fibrotic stroma (arrows) (100X).

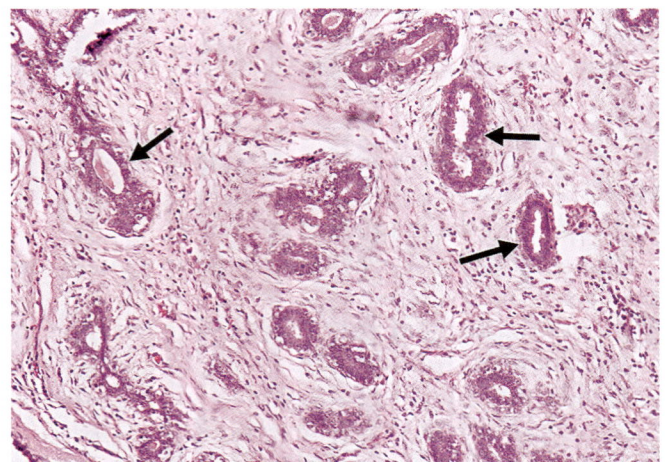

Fig. 25.15: Fibroadenoma breast with pericanalicular pattern—the glands (ducts) retain round shape. Because ducts are not compressed by fibrosis results in 'pericanalicular pattern' (arrows) (100X).

Treatment

Fibroadenoma is treated by surgical excision.

PHYLLODES TUMOR

Phyllodes tumor is a large fleshy bulky tumor measuring 10–15 cm *distorting the breast, and overlying skin ulceration.* It is related to fibroadenomas. It is more cellular than fibroadenoma.

The distinction of phyllodes tumor from fibroadenoma is made not on the size, but on the histological and cytological characteristics of the stromal component.

Origin

It demonstrates proliferation of stromal cells. It is most often low-grade neoplasm arising from interlobular

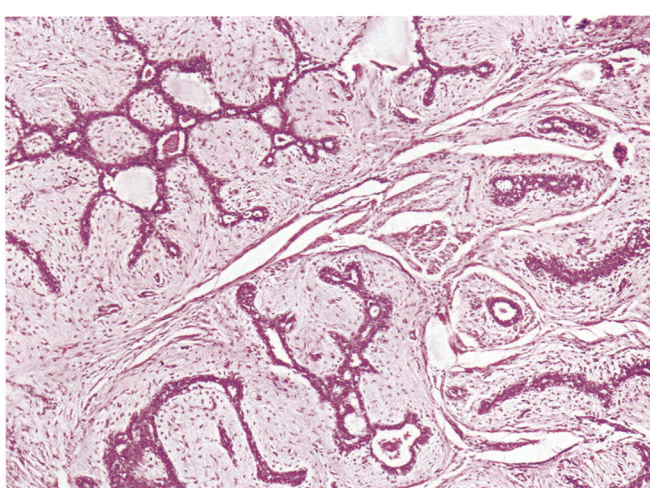

Fig. 25.16: Fibroadenoma shows intracanalicular and pericanalicular patterns. Glands compressed by stroma results in slit-like spaces known as intracanalicular patten. Ducts not compressed by stroma have round shape known as pericanalicular pattern (100X).

stroma accompanied by a benign growth of ductal structures.

Age Group

It most often occurs in older age group. It may affect 30 to 70 years aged women.

Clinical Features

Patient presents with bulky lump distorting the breast with overlying skin ulceration.

Gross Morphology

- Like fibroadenoma, benign phyllodes tumor is sharply circumscribed, lobulated large size tumor measuring 10–15 cm. *Cut surface is firm, glistening, and grayish white with cystic spaces containing leaf-like extensions.*
- *Benign phyllodes tumor has pushing margin.*
- *Malignant phyllodes tumor has infiltrating margin.* It is poorly circumscribed tumor with invasion into the surrounding breast tissue (Figs 25.17 and 25.18).

Light Microscopy

- *Benign phyllodes tumor:* It comprises highly cellular myxoid stroma projecting into the ducts lined by benign epithelial cells, creating the **leaf-like pattern** (Greek word phyllodes meaning *leaf-like clefts and slits*) and presence of **<5 mitoses per 10 HPF in the stroma.** *The stroma is more cellular than a fibroadenoma.*

Breast

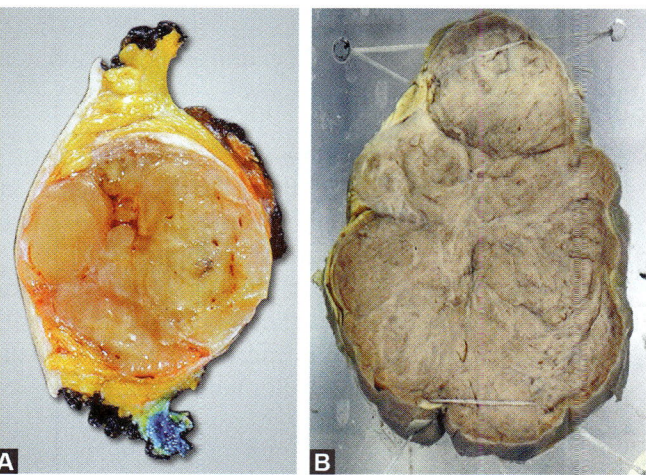

Fig. 25.17: Phyllodes benign tumor—tumor is large bulky with pushing margin. Cut surface is firm, glistening, and grayish white with cystic spaces containing leaf-like extensions.

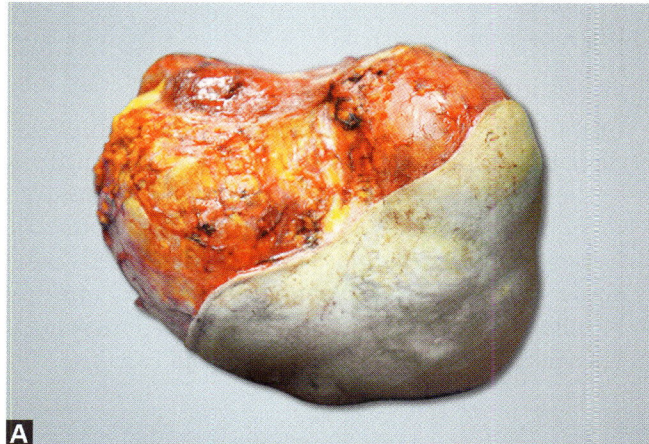

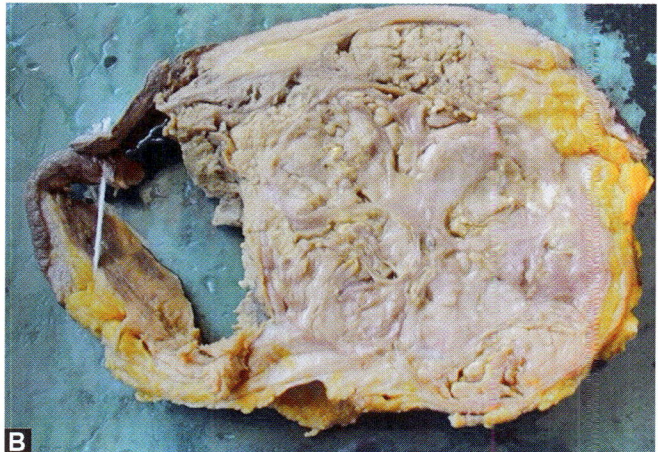

Fig. 25.18: Phyllodes malignant tumor—tumor is large bulky distorting breast with areas of hemorrhage and necrosis. On right side, surgical excised tumor shows firm, glistening, and grayish white with cystic spaces containing leaf-like extensions.

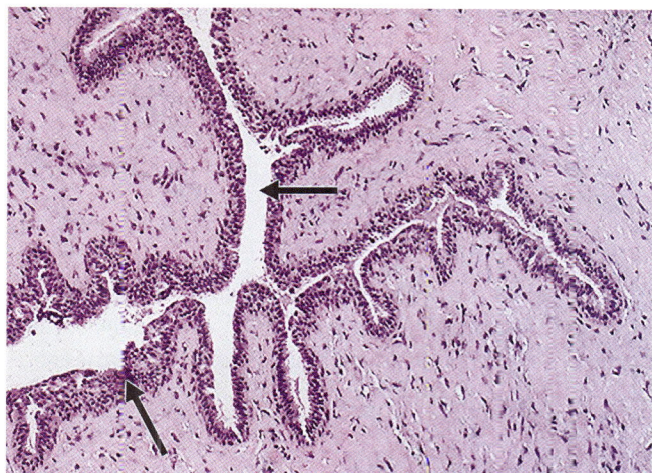

Fig. 25.19: Phyllodes tumor—it comprises highly cellular myxoid stroma projecting into the ducts creating the leaf-like pattern (Greek word *phyllodes* meaning leaf-like clefts and slits) and presence of <5 mitoses per 10 HPF in the stroma. The stroma is more cellular than a fibroadenoma (arrows) (400X).

- *Borderline phyllodes tumor:* Light microscopy shows **5–10 mitoses per 10 HPF.**
- *Malignant phyllodes tumor:* A malignant phyllodes tumor has a sarcomatous stroma that predominates over the ductal elements and invades the breast. It has **abundant mitotic activity.** *Stromal component is abundant in comparison to benign duct elements.*

  Light microscopy shows malignant change in the stromal component of tumor, numerous mitoses **>10 per 10 HPF** in the stroma, hemorrhage and necrosis (Fig. 25.19).

Biologic Behavior

It is difficult to predict biologic behavior. It may *recur locally after incomplete excision.* These rarely high-grade lesions resulting in *metastasize* to *lymph nodes* or *lung* in 33% of cases.

Management

Treatment is wide excision of tumor with wide margin of normal surrounding tissue. In adequate excision of tumor results in recurrences.

Juvenile Papillomatosis

Juvenile papillomatosis is also known as ('Swiss cheese disease') affecting young girls. Patient presents with solitary, unilateral breast lump. The lesion is often mistaken for a phyllodes tumor clinically. It is a marker for families at risk for breast carcinoma coincidentally or later.

Gross Morphology
- The lesion is circumscribed, but not encapsulated containing large multiple cysts. It strongly resembles fibrocystic disease of the breast.
- Differential diagnosis also pubertal macromastia, and juvenile fibroadenoma.

Light Microscopy
Juvenile papillomatosis shows dilated breast ducts lined by a proliferation of highly atypical-looking epithelium that would be regarded as precancerous in an older woman.

BENIGN EPITHELIAL TUMORS

INTRADUCTAL PAPILLOMA

Intraductal papilloma occurs in the *subareolar lactiferous ducts* of female breast. The lesion is rounded and present within a large ductal space. Patient presents with *bleeding from the nipple associated with a breast lump*. A large breast duct contains a fleshy tumor arising from its wall (Fig. 25.20).

Key Facts: Intraductal Papilloma
- It is less common tumor occurring in middle-aged women.
- Patient presents with blood-stained discharge.
- It is usually a solitary lesion occurring in large ducts.
- Tumor is composed of fibrovascular core covered by benign ductal epithelial cells.

Age Group
It occurs in middle-aged (30–50 years) and older women.

Locations
- *Central intraductal papilloma:* It is benign solitary tumor. It usually causes *nipple discharge* (*serous* or *hemorrhagic* due to tearing of tumor) in 80% of cases. It does not undergo malignant change.
- Peripheral intraductal papillomas are most often multiple but smaller in size. These do not present with nipple discharge. There is increased risk of breast carcinoma in multiple papillomas.

Clinical Features
Patient may also present with blood stained nipple discharge, breast lump beneath nipple and nipple retraction. It is cured by local surgical excision.

Gross Morphology
The tumor is tan-pink, friable, usually <1.0 cm in size.

Light Microscopy
- Intraduct papilloma is attached to the wall of the duct by a fibrovascular stalk. It shows multiple branching papillae composed of *thin fibrovascular core lined by cuboidal to columnar ductal cells toward lumen and outer myoepithelial cells*. Ductal cells may show squamous metaplasia or apocrine change.
- Papilloma with <3 mm focus of atypical hyperplasia is termed as ductal carcinoma *in situ*.

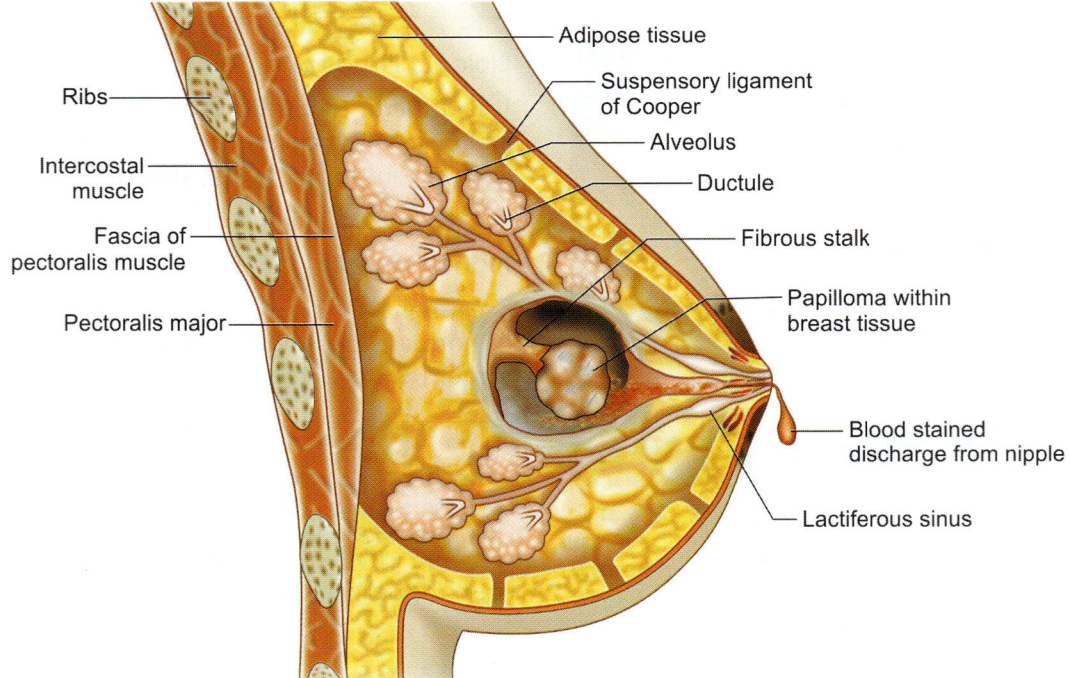

Fig. 25.20: Breast intraductal papilloma has a stalk. Tumor is present within breast substance (*Courtesy* by Dr Abhijit Das).

Table 25.4: Comparison of intraductal papilloma and noninvasive papillary carcinoma

Parameters	Intraductal papilloma	Noninvasive papillary carcinoma
Cell morphology	Benign cells with normochromatic nuclei	Atypical cells with hyperchromatic nuclei
Myoepithelial cells	Present	Absent
Apocrine change	Present	Absent
Adjacent stroma	Thick prominent stroma	Delicate stroma
Sclerosing adenosis	Unusual	Usual

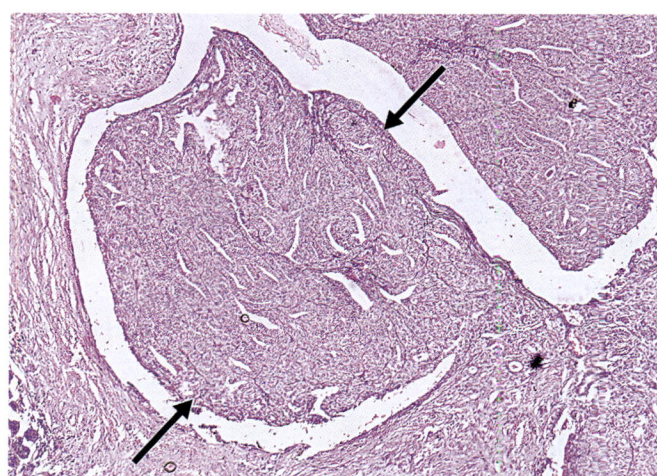

Fig. 25.21: Breast intraductal papilloma shows multiple branching papillae composed of thin fibrovascular core lined by cuboidal to columnar ductal cells toward lumen and outer myoepithelial cells (arrows) (200X).

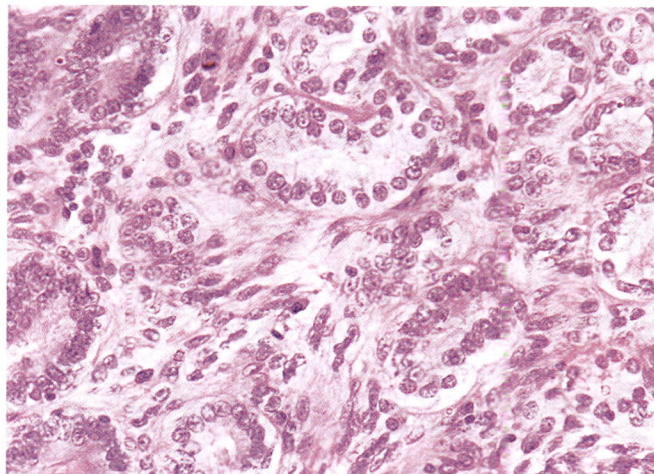

Fig. 25.22: Tubular adenoma shows densely packed uniform round tubules lined by luminal cuboidal epithelial and outer myoepithelial cells without cytological atypia. There is scant intervening stroma without compression of ducts (400X).

- Myoepithelial cells are absent in ductal carcinoma *in situ* occurring in papillomas.
- This lesion must be distinguished from papillomatosis, occurring in the peripheral ducts as a component of proliferative fibrocystic change (Fig. 25.21).
- It should be differentiated from noninvasive papillary carcinoma of breast (Table 25.4).

Immunohistochemistry

Myoepithelial cells in papilloma are positive for **S-100, p63, glial fibrillary acidic protein (GFAP), α-smooth muscle actin (α-SMA)** and **smooth muscle myosin**.

TUBULAR ADENOMA

Tubular adenoma is a benign circumscribed mass in breast. It most often occurs in young women.

Gross Morphology

It is well circumscribed mass, sharply demarcated but without capsule.

Light Microscopy

- Tumor is composed of densely packed uniform round tubules lined by luminal cuboidal epithelial and outer myoepithelial cells without cytological atypia.
- There is scant intervening stroma without compression of ducts (Fig. 25.22).

LACTATING ADENOMA

Lactating adenoma may represent the same lesion under different physiologic conditions. Lactating adenoma has been identified in post-partum biopsies of masses that first presented during pregnancy.

Light Microscopy

On light microscopy, lactating adenoma is composed of large glands lined by large nuclei with clear to vacuolated cytoplasm and intraluminal structures (Fig. 25.23).

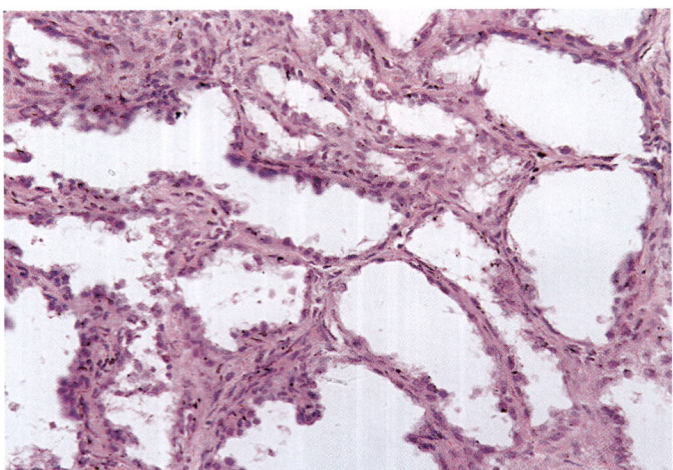

Fig. 25.23: Lactating adenoma is composed of large glands lined by large nuclei with clear to vacuolated cytoplasm and intraluminal structures (200X).

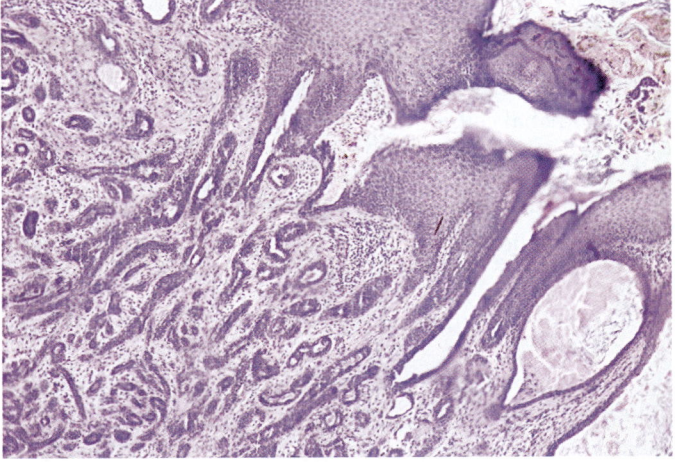

Fig. 25.24: Adenoma of the nipple is on light microscopy, it is composed of duct-like structures associated with collagenous stroma (400X).

COMPLEX ADENOMA

Complex adenoma shows features of fibroadenoma with cysts measuring >3 mm in size, sclerosing adenosis, apocrine change and calcification.

JUVENILE FIBROADENOMA

Juvenile adenoma occurs in young females. It is uncommon to find palpable lump. Tumor is composed of ducts lined by epithelial cells in cellular stroma.

ADENOMA OF THE NIPPLE

This benign tumor most often presents with serous or bloody discharge, ulceration and reddening of nipple, clinically confused with Paget's disease of the nipple.

Light Microscopy

On light microscopy, tumor is composed of duct-like structures associated with collagenous stroma (Fig. 25.24).

Immunohistochemistry

Myoepithelial cells around duct-like structures are demonstrated by *S-100, α-smooth muscle actin (α-SMA), p63 and glial fibrillary acidic protein (GFAP).*

BREAST CARCINOMA

GENERAL CONSIDERATIONS

The most important disease is breast carcinoma especially in postmenopausal women. It is second most frequent cause of death in women. Most breast diseases present as palpable lump. It is important to distinguish cases of breast carcinoma from benign breast disease.

True nature of a breast lump is ascertained by histopathological examination of many areas of the excised lump. Good idea of nature of breast lump before surgery may be obtained by clinical features (size, texture, relation to adjoining tissues), mammographic examination of the affected breast, and cytological examination of smears obtained by fine needle aspiration cytology.

Early detection is the most important factor in breast carcinoma survival. Most important risk factors for breast carcinoma are estrogen stimulation of breasts by ovarian hormones and advancing age. Breast carcinoma arises by accumulation of DNA mutations.

Clinical Features

Breast lump is the presenting symptom in 85–90% of patients with breast carcinoma. Approximately 60% of breast masses are discovered by patient on self-examination. *Clinical breast examination is a necessary complement to screening mammography.*

Distribution

Most glandular tissue is located in the upper outer quadrant and beneath the nipple. Thus, breast carcinoma is most commonly located in upper outer quadrant. It occurs most commonly in the left breast than right.

Location

Breast carcinoma in decreasing frequency is located in upper outer quadrant (50%), central region beneath nipple (20%), lower outer quadrant (10%), upper inner quadrant (10%) and lower inner quadrant (10%), respectively.

Origin

Breast carcinomas are derived from the epithelial cells that line the terminal duct lobular unit. These are classified according to their site of origin into *ductal* and *lobular*. Ductal carcinoma is the most common subtype followed by lobular carcinoma second most common (most often bilateral) with distant metastases. Histological type and frequency are shown in Table 25.5.

- *In situ (noninvasive) breast carcinoma:* Ductal carcinoma *in situ* and lobular carcinoma *in situ* feature neoplastic cells confined within the basement membrane of ducts and lobules, respectively. *Myoepithelial cells can be demonstrated in carcinoma in situ unlike invasive carcinoma.*

  Noninvasive breast carcinomas include ductal carcinoma *in situ*, lobular carcinoma *in situ*, mixed intraductal carcinoma and lobular carcinoma *in situ* and papillary carcinoma and comedocarcinoma

Table 25.5: Histological type and frequency of breast carcinoma

Histological type	Frequency
Carcinoma *in situ*	
• Ductal carcinoma *in situ*	3.6%
• Lobular carcinoma *in situ* (LCIS)	1.6%
• Intraductal and lobular carcinoma *in situ*	0.2%
• Comedocarcinoma with central necrosis	0.3%
Invasive carcinoma	
• Ductal carcinoma (not otherwise specified)	70–75%
• Lobular carcinoma	5–15%
• Ductal and lobular carcinoma	1.6%
• Tubular carcinoma	5%
• Mucinous (colloid) carcinoma	2–3%
• Medullary carcinoma	1–2%
• Micropapillary carcinoma	1–2%
• Metaplastic carcinoma	1%
• Papillary carcinoma	0.8%

Paget's disease constitutes 1.0% of breast cancer. It is may be ductal carcinoma *in situ* or invasive ductal carcinoma involving nipple epidermis.

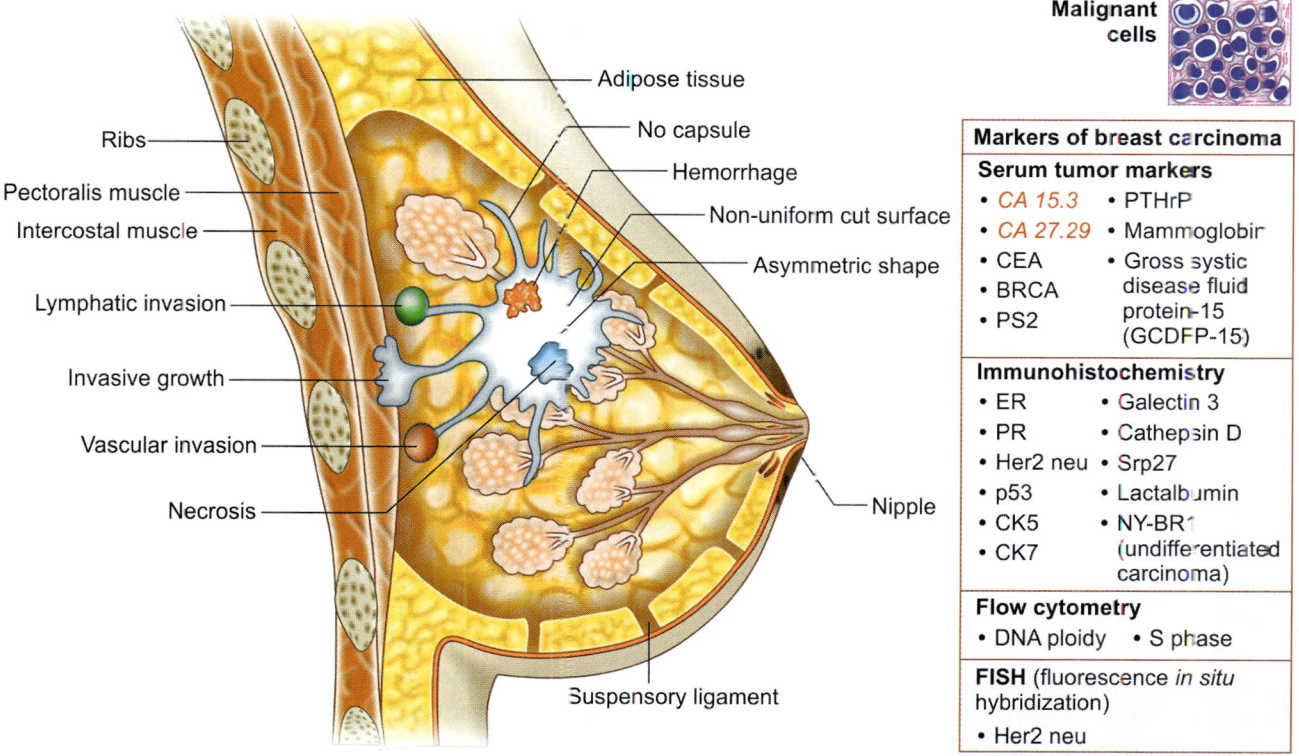

Fig. 25.25: Breast cancer shows invasive duct carcinoma with infiltrating margins and areas of hemorrhage and necrosis (Courtesy by Dr Abhijit Das).

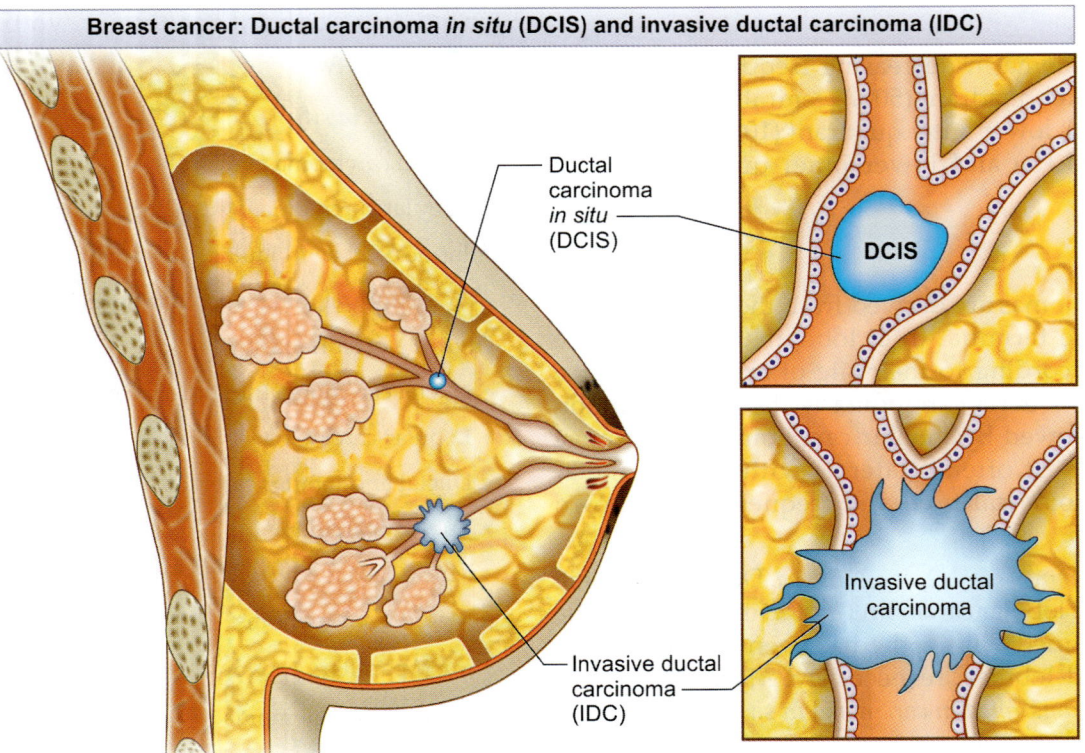

Fig. 25.26: Breast cancer—it shows ductal carcinoma *in situ* in lower inset and invasive duct carcinoma with infiltrating margins in upper inset (*Courtesy by* Dr Abhijit Das).

(ductal carcinoma *in situ* with central necrosis). Ductal carcinoma *in situ* is detected by screening mammography.

- *Invasive breast carcinoma:* When ductal/lobular carcinoma breaches basement membrane and invades the normal breast parenchyma, it is termed as invasive breast carcinoma. Lobular carcinomas are usually multifocal in origin.

CA 125 is a cell surface glycoprotein originally identified in mucinous epithelial *ovarian* tumors. It is also expressed in carcinomas of *endometrium, gastrointestinal tract, thyroid,* and *breast* (Figs 25.25 and 25.26).

Key Facts: Myoepithelial Cells

- The acinus is lined by epithelial cells surrounded by myoepithelial cells and the basement membrane.
- On immunohistochemistry, myoepithelial cells show positivity for **S-100, α-smooth muscle actin (α-SMA), p63, glial fibrillary acidic protein (GFAP)** and **keratin 14.**
- Myoepithelial cells are most often demonstrated in benign breast tumors and carcinoma *in situ*.

RISK FACTORS

POSITIVE FAMILY HISTORY

Incidence of breast carcinoma is greatly increased in *first-degree female relatives* of patients (mother, sister, or daughter) with carcinoma of the breast at a younger age.

Family members may also transmit the abnormal susceptible gene (autosomal dominant with limited penetrance) without developing breast carcinoma themselves. Approximately 5% of cases are associated with a penetrant dominant genetic predisposition. Prophylactic mastectomies are performed in familial positive history of breast carcinomas.

BRCA1 Tumor Suppressor Gene Mutation

All families with strong family history of breast carcinoma may have mutation of *BRCA1*. *It is a tumor suppressor gene located on chromosome 17p2*. It regulates DNA repair by binding to RAD51, a molecule that mediates DNA double-strand repair breaks.

BRCA1 gene mutation is responsible of *52% familial* and rare cases of sporadic breast carcinomas (medullary carcinoma and metaplastic carcinoma). This is also associated with development of carcinoma of the ovary and prostate.

BRCA2 Tumor Suppressor Gene Mutation

BRCA2 gene is a tumor suppressor gene located on chromosome 13q12–13. It regulates DNA repair by binding to RAD51, a molecule that mediates DNA double-strand repair breaks. BRCA2 gene mutation is responsible for 32% familial breast carcinoma. BRCA2 gene mutation is rarely demonstrated in sporadic breast carcinoma.

p53 Tumor Suppressor Gene Mutation

Approximately 5% *of families* with breast carcinoma have mutation of p53 tumor suppressor gene.

GENETIC DISORDERS

Women with genetic disorders are at increased risk of development of breast carcinoma. These are described as under.

Li-Fraumeni Syndrome

Germline mutations of TP53 tumor suppressor gene cause Li-Fraumeni syndrome. Patients may develop multiple cancers such as breast carcinoma, leukemia, sarcoma, brain tumors, adrenal tumors, laryngeal and lung cancer.

Cowden Disease

PTEN gene is located on chromosome 10q. Phosphatase and tensin homologue are proteins of PTEN gene. Normally, PTEN gene products inhibit AKT/PI3K signaling pathway. PTEN gene mutation leads to Cowden disease characterized by fibroadenomas, fibrocystic lesions, ductal epithelial hyperplasia, and nipple malformations. There is increased risk of breast carcinoma in Cowden disease.

Inherited Ataxia-telangiectasia

Under physiological state, ATM gene is a caretaker tumor suppressor gene located on chromosome 11p22. It downregulates tyrosine kinase activity. Patients with ATM gene mutation have reduced capacity to repair DNA breaks resulting in accumulation of numerous genetic mutations overtime. Patient develops inherited ataxia-telangiectasia characterized by cerebral ataxia, immunodeficiency and dilations of small blood vessels. There is increased risk of breast carcinoma, gastric carcinoma, leukemia and lymphomas.

AGE GROUP

Advancing age is the second most important factor for breast carcinoma. Incidence of breast carcinoma increases with advancing age more than 30 years until menopause.

LONGER REPRODUCTIVE SPAN

Early menarche and late menopause increase duration of reproductive life and associated hormonal activity. Prolonged exposure to endogenous estrogen increases risk of breast carcinoma.

NULLIPAROUS WOMEN

Nulliparous women are at greater risk for breast carcinoma. Women who had their first child over age 30 are at greater risk. Pregnant women are at lower risk.

AGE OF WOMEN AT FIRST PREGNANCY

Women who had their first child over age 30 are at greater risk for breast carcinoma. An early age at birth of a second child further reduces the risk of breast carcinoma.

OBESITY

Postmenopausal obesity and increased dietary fat increases the risk of breast carcinoma due to aromatization of androstenedione to estrogens in adipose tissue.

EXCESSIVE EXPOSURE TO ESTROGENS

- Postmenopausal estrogen therapy and oral contraceptive use increase the risk of breast carcinoma. Use of oral contraceptives for >4 years by younger women before their first term pregnancy almost increases risk of postmenopausal breast caracinoma.
- Risk of breast carcinoma increases in women, who receive hormonal replacement therapy for a period of 10–15 years. Hormonal replacement therapy increases breast density, which make detection of breast carcinomas more difficult.
- Hormones via blood circulation interact either with nuclear estrogen receptors of breast terminal duct lobular unit. The hormone-receptor interactions cause activation of DNA response elements leading to proliferation and differentiation factors.

ATYPICAL DUCTAL HYPERPLASIA

Presence of atypical changes in ductal epithelium in fibrocystic disease does increase the risk of breast carcinoma.

HISTORY OF BREAST CARCINOMA IN OPPOSITE BREAST

It is associated with increased incidence of involving opposite breast.

HISTORY OF ENDOMETRIAL CARCINOMA

Women with history of endometrial or ovarian carcinoma are at increased risk for breast carcinoma.

RADIATION EXPOSURE

During Second World War, risk of breast carcinoma among teenage girls has been observed due to low level ionizing radiation later in life.

DIETARY FACTORS

Diet high in animal fat increases five times risk of breast carcinoma in the United States than in Japan.

BREASTFEEDING

Longer period of breastfeeding reduces the risk of breast carcinoma. Lactation suppresses ovulation and may trigger terminal differentiation of luminal cells.

MOLECULAR GENETICS

Approximately 12% of breast carcinomas occur due to inherited gene mutations. Most of the genes play interrelated roles in maintaining genome integrity (Tables 25.6 and 25.7).

Table 25.6: Oncogenes associated breast carcinomas

Category	Proto-oncogene	Mode of activation	Associated cancers
Growth factors			
Fibroblast growth factors	FGF3	Amplification	*Breast carcinoma*, osteosarcoma, gastric carcinoma, urinary bladder carcinoma and melanoma
	INT2	Increased baseline activity	*Breast carcinoma* and melanoma
Growth factor receptors			
EGF-Receptor	ERBB2 (Her2 neu) ERBB2	Amplification	*Breast carcinoma* (marker of aggressiveness)
Signal transduction proteins			
Notch signal transduction	Notch1	Point mutation, translocation	*Breast carcinoma:* Leukemia and lymphoma
Cyclin and cyclin-dependent kinase (cell cycle regulators)			
Cyclin-dependent kinase	CCND1 (cyclin D1)	Amplification	*Breast carcinoma*, multiple myeloma and esophageal cancer

Table 25.7: Tumor suppressor gene associated with breast carcinomas

Gene	Proteins	Function	Familial tumors	Sporadic cancers
Mitotic signaling pathway inhibitors				
PTEN	Phosphatase and tensin homologue	It inhibits AKT/PI3K signaling pathway	*Cowden syndrome* (cancers of breast, endometrium and thyroid gland)	Lymphoid neoplasms, carcinomas
Cell cycle progression inhibitors				
CDKN2A	P16/INK4a and P14ARF	P16 inhibits CDK. P14 indirectly activates p53 tumor suppressor gene	Familial melanoma	Breast carcinoma, pancreas carcinoma, and esophagus carcinoma
RB gene	Retinoblastoma protein (locus 13p14) mutation by deletion and nonsense	It codes for pRB protein, master brake on cell cycle. It inhibits G1 to S transition during cell cycle. It inhibits nuclear transcription factor	Retinoblastoma, osteosarcoma	Breast carcinoma, osteosarcoma, colon carcinoma, prostate carcinoma, urinary bladder carcinoma and lung carcinoma
Inhibitors of invasiveness and metastases				
CDK1	E-Cadherin	It participates in cell adhesion. It inhibits cell motility	Gastric carcinoma	Breast lobular carcinoma and gastric carcinoma

There is increased risk of breast and endometrial cancers in women on oral contraceptive therapy.

Breast

Sporadic breast carcinomas are associated with hormone exposure, age of menarche, age of menopause, reproductive history, hormone replacement therapy and breastfeeding. Estrogen has been identified as promoter of breast caracinomas. Estrogen stimulates breast growth during puberty, menstrual cycles and pregnancy, thereby increasing breast cells potential to malignant change.

BRCA1 Tumor Suppressor Gene

- *Location:* BRCA1 is a tumor suppressor gene located on chromosome 17p21.
- *Function:* BRCA1 regulates DNA repair by binding to RAD51, a molecule that mediates DNA double-strand repair breaks.
- *Gene mutation:* It is responsible for 52% familial and 1–2% of all breast caracinomas. Risk is increased in age group by 70 years. Mutation of BRCA1 occurs by methylation. BRCA1 gene mutation is rare in sporadic medullary carcinoma and metaplastic carcinoma.
- *Associated carcinomas:* BRCA1 gene mutation may occur in cancers of ovary, *male breast, prostate, pancreas and fallopian tube;* but less than BRCA2.

BRCA2 Tumor Suppressor Gene

- *Location:* BRCA2 is a tumor suppressor gene located on chromosome 13q12–13.
- *Function:* BRCA2 regulates DNA repair by binding to RAD51, a molecule that mediates DNA double-strand repair breaks.
- *Gene mutation:* BRAC2 gene mutation is rare in sporadic cases.
- *Associated cancers:* BRCA2 gene mutation also occurs in cancers of ovary, *male breast, prostate, pancreas, stomach, gallbladder, bile duct, pharynx and melanoma.*

TP53 Tumor Suppressor Gene

- *Location:* It is tumor suppressor gene located on chromosome 17p13.1.
- *Function:* TP53 gene product halts cell cycle in G1 phase by inhibiting nuclear transcription factor, until the DNA is repaired. It activates BAX gene induced cell suicide (apoptosis). It interacts with at least 17 cellular and viral proteins.
- *Gene mutation:* TP53 is responsible for 3% of familial and 20% in sporadic breast carcinomas. There is increased risk of breast carcinoma in 90% cases by the age of 70 years.
- *Associated cancers:* TP53 gene mutations are also demonstrated in *pancreas (50–70%), lung, colon, and breast.* TP53 gene mutation also occurs in *Li-Fraumeni syndrome (breast carcinoma, sarcoma, leukemia, brain tumors and adrenal gland cancer).*

CHEK2 Tumor Suppressor Gene

- *Location:* CHEK2 is a tumor suppressor gene located on chromosome 22q12.1.
- *Function:* CHEK2 induces cell cycle arrest. It repairs damaged DNA. It activates BRCA1 and p53 tumor suppressor genes by phosphorylation.
- *Gene mutation:* Gene mutation is responsible for 5% of familial as well as sporadic breast caracinomas. Due to gene mutation, there is increased risk of breast caracinoma in 10–20% cases by 70 years of age especially after radiation exposure. It is worth mentioning that gene mutation is also demonstrated in cancers of *prostate, thyroid* and *kidney.*

RB Tumor Suppressor Gene

- *Location:* It is a gatekeeper tumor suppressor gene. It is located on long arm of chromosome 13p14. Normal people have two alleles of the RB gene.
- *Mechanism:* RB gene codes for pRB protein, master brake on cell cycle. Dephosphorylated RB gene inhibits cell division. *When the Rb gene is phosphorylated, cell division takes place.*
- *Associated cancers:* Rb gene mutation is demonstrated in *breast carcinoma, familial/acquired retinoblastoma, and familial/acquired osteosarcoma.* Rb gene mutation is also associated with cancers of colon, prostate and urinary bladder.

FGF3 (Fibroblast Growth Factor 3)

- *Physiological state:* FGF3 belongs to growth factor category. Many cancer cells, acquire the ability to synthesize the same growth factors to which they are responsive, generating an autocrine loop.
- *Associated cancers:* Amplification of FGF3 is associated with *breast carcinoma, osteosarcoma, stomach carcinoma, bladder carcinoma and melanoma.*

INT2 Oncogene

- *Physiological state:* INT2 belongs to growth factor category. Many cancer cells acquire the ability to synthesize the same growth factors to which they are responsive, generating an autocrine loop.
- *Associated cancers:* Increased baseline activity of INT2 has been demonstrated in breast carcinoma and melanoma.

ERBB2 (Her2 neu) Oncogene

- *Physiological state:* ERBB2 (Her2 neu) belongs to growth factor receptor family. It encodes for an epithelial growth factor receptor on the cell membrane that delivers continuous mitogenic signals to the cells.

- *Gene mutation:* Amplification of ERBB2 (Her2 neu) delivers continuous mitogenic signals to the breast carcinoma cells even in the absence of growth factor in the environment. *It is most often observed in ductal carcinoma and rarely in lobular carcinoma.*
- *Immunohistochemistry:* ERBB2 (Her2 neu) is demonstrated by immunohistochemistry on the cell membrane or using *fluorescent in situ hybridization (FISH).* It is marker of aggressive breast carcinoma.

Notch1 Oncogene

- *Physiological state:* Notch1 gene belongs to Notch signal transduction protein category.
- *Gene mutation:* Point mutation or translocation of Notch1 gene is associated with *breast carcinoma, leukemia* and *lymphomas.*

RAS (RAT Sarcoma) Oncogene

- *Physiological state:* It activates several intracellular signal transduction pathways and activation of the transcription factors 'fos' and 'jun'.
- *Associated cancer: RAS* gene mutation is associated with breast carcinoma.

C-MYC Oncogene (Nuclear Transcription Factor)

- *Physiological state:* C-MYC is nuclear regulatory protein that controls the expression of several genes.
- *Associated cancer:* Mutation of C-MYC is demonstrated in breast carcinoma

BCL-1 Cell Cycle Regulatory Gene

BCL-1 codes for cyclin D1, acts as stimulatory protein of the cell cycle. Mutation of BCL-1 causes loss of regulation of cell cycle resulting in breast carcinoma.

Cyclins and Cyclin-dependent Kinase

- *Physiological state:* CCND1 and cyclin D1 are cell cycle regulators.
- *Gene mutation:* CCND1 and cyclin D1 are activated by translocation and amplification. Deregulation of cyclins due to mutation is associated with breast carcinoma.

E-Cadherins

- *Physiological state:* E-Cadherins belong to CDH1 category. E-Cadherins are inhibitors of invasiveness and metastases.
- *Gene mutation:* E-Cadherins are *irreversibly lost in invasive lobular breast carcinoma,* but expressed in *invasive ductal breast carcinoma.* Germline and somatic mutations of cadherin play an important role in the pathogenesis of *gastric carcinoma (diffuse type).*

PTEN Tumor Suppressor Gene

- *Physiological state:* PTEN gene is located on chromosome 10q. It is inhibitor of mitogenic signaling pathway.
- *Gene mutation and thyroid gland:* PTEN gene mutation is associated with **Cowden disease** characterized by fibroadenoma, fibrocystic disease, ductal epithelial hyperplasia, nipple malformations, breast carcinoma and endometrial carcinoma.

Galectin 3

- *Physiological state:* Galectin 3 is a member of lectin family. It is encoded by LGALS3 gene located on chromosome 14, locus q21–q22. It is expressed in the nucleus, cytoplasm and extracellular space.
- *Overexpression:* Its overexpression promotes neoplastic transformation and the maintenance of transformed phenotypes as well as enhances adhesion of tumor cells to the extracellular matrix in breast carcinoma.

MAJOR MOLECULAR PATHWAYS IN EVOLUTION OF BREAST CARCINOMA

There are three major pathways of development of breast carcinomas (Table 25.8).

ER POSITIVE MOLECULAR PATHWAY (LUMINAL A AND LUMINAL B)

Salient Features

ER positive breast carcinomas are termed as *luminal* as these cancers resemble normal breast luminal cells in terms of their mRNA expression regulated by estrogen. Breast carcinoma is caused by inheritance of germ line BRCA2 gene mutation associated with gain of 1q chromosome, loss of 16q. *ER positive pathway is the most common expressing estrogen receptors* (Figs 25.27 and 25.28).

- *Luminal type A:* It is low-grade tumor with low proliferative rate seen in <50% cases. Recurrence rate is low. *Immunohistochemistry shows positivity for ER/PR and cytokeratin (8, 18).* These patients respond to endocrine therapy (estrogen blocking drug *tamoxifen* and *aromatase inhibitors*). Prognosis is good.
- *Luminal type B:* This type of breast carcinoma is seen in <15% cases. It has **higher proliferative rate** than luminal A type. *Recurrence is high.* Tumor cells may show *low expression of ER/PR.* Immunohistochemistry shows cytokeratin positivity (8, 18). Prognosis may not be as good as in luminal type A.

Sequence of Events

- *Development of flat lesion:* Patient develops flat lesion in breast as a result of gain of 1q chromosome and loss of 16q.

Table 25.8: Molecular subtypes of breast cancer

Molecular subgroup and frequency	Luminal A (50%)	Luminal B (20%)	Her2 neu enrich (15%)	Basal type (up to 15% in African women)
ER	+++	+	–	–
PR	+	+	–	–
Her2 neu	–	–/+	++	–
Proliferation index	Low	Moderate	High	Very high
Distant metastases	Bones, viscera and brain	Bones, viscera and brain	Bones, viscera and brain	Bones, viscera and brain
Gene mutations	GATA-3, LIV-1, CCND-1, FOX-1	–	Amplification of gene located on 17q12	Basal epithelial genes, TP53, BRCA1
Others	CK8/18 (cytokeratin)	CK8/18 (cytokeratin)	Androgen receptors	CK5/6, CK14, vimentin, EGFR, c-kit
Ki-67	+ (<14%)	+ (<14%)	+ (<14%)	+ (<14%)
CD20	+	+	+	+
Prognosis	Excellent (recurrence low)	Intermediate (recurrence high)	Poor (recurrence high)	Poor (recurrence high)
Treatment	Hormonal therapy	Hormonal + chemotherapy	Trastuzumab (herceptin) and anthracyclines	Platinum- and anthracycline-based chemotherapy, PARP inhibitors

PARP, poly (adenosine diphosphate-ribose) polymerase, ER (estrogen), PR (progesterone)
Histological variants of luminal A: low-grade invasive ductal carcinoma (NOS), classic lobular, tubular and cribriform carcinomas
Histological variants of luminal B: invasive ductal carcinoma and micropapillary carcinoma
Histological variants of Her2 neu enrich: invasive ductal carcinoma NOS (not otherwise specified)
Histological variants of basal type: invasive ductal carcinoma NOS (not otherwise specified), medullary and metaplastic carcinomas

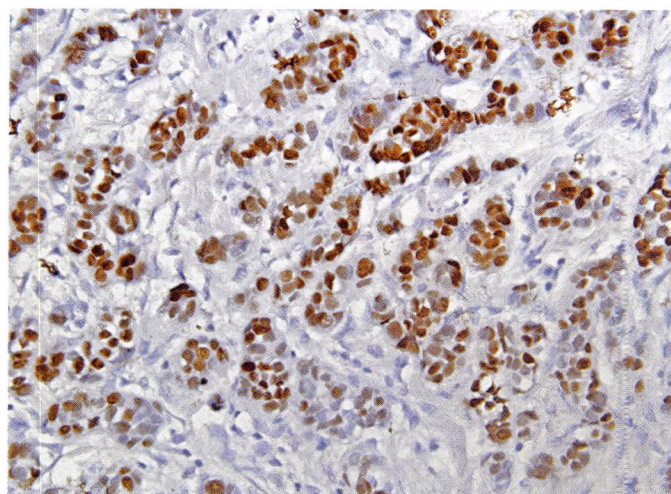

Fig. 25.27: Breast cancer—infiltrative duct carcinoma shows estrogen receptor positivity. Hormone therapy with tamoxifen is used to block the effects of estrogen that may otherwise help breast cancer cells to survive and grow. Most women with breast cancers expressing estrogen or progesterone on their surface benefit from treatment with tamoxifen (400X).

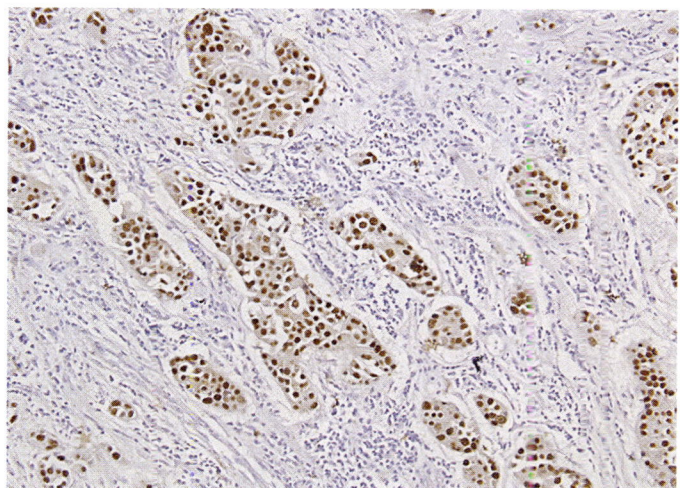

Fig. 25.28: Breast cancer—infiltrative duct carcinoma shows progesterone receptor positivity (100X).

- *Progression to breast carcinoma:* Due to mutation of PIK3CA gene, flat lesion progresses to atypical hyperplasia of breast, ductal carcinoma *in situ* and invasive breast carcinoma. PIK3CA gene product encodes phosphoinositide-3 kinase (PI3K), major component of signal pathway, down regulating growth factor receptor.

Immunohistochemistry

Immunohistochemistry of luminal type A and B breast carcinoma.

- Immunohistochemistry of luminal type A breast carcinoma shows positivity for ER/PR and cytokeratin (8; 18).
- Immunohistochemistry of luminal type B breast carcinoma shows low expression of ER/PR. Tumor cells are immunoreactive to cytokeratin (8; 18).

Marker	Luminal type A	Luminal type B
Estrogen receptor (ER)	+++	+
Progesterone receptor (PR)	++	+
Her2 neu	–	–/+
Cytokeratins (8; 18)	+	+

HER2 NEU ENRICHED MOLECULAR PATHWAY

Salient Features

Her2 neu is located on chromosome 17q. Amplification of Her2 neu is responsible for 20% cases of breast carcinomas. It is the most common type of breast carcinoma in patient with germline mutations in TP53 (Li-Fraumeni syndrome). Patient develops atypical ductal hyperplasia progressing to ductal carcinoma *in situ* resulting in invasive breast carcinoma (Fig. 25.29).

Clinical Course

Her2 neu enriched invasive duct carcinoma is high-grade tumor with higher proliferative rate and poor prognosis. It most often shows involvement of axillary lymph nodes.

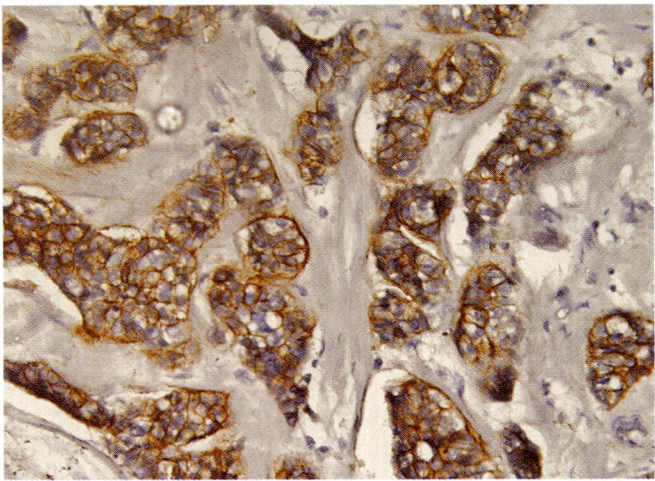

Fig. 25.29: Breast cancer—infiltrative duct carcinoma shows Her2 neu positivity. These patients are treated with herceptin (400X).

Immunohistochemistry

Immunohistochemistry of Her2 neu enriched molecular pathway of breast carcinoma shows Her2 neu positivity. Tumor cells may be ER positive/negative.

Marker	Expression
Her2 neu	Positive
Estrogen receptor (ER)	Positive or negative

Treatment

These patients respond to herceptin and anthracycline based chemotherapeutic agents.

ER AND HER2 NEU NEGATIVE MOLECULAR PATHWAY

Salient Features

It is least understood pathway due to inheritance of BRCA1 gene mutation responsible for 15% of breast carcinomas. These tumors have a *basal-like* pattern of mRNA expression in normal myoepithelial cells.

Basal cell type of breast carcinoma has **high proliferative rate** with positive lymph nodes and high recurrence rate. **TP53 gene mutation** is very common. These breast carcinomas show high expression of basal epithelial genes and TP53 gene mutations, dysfunction of **BRCA1 gene. Ki-67** is expressed in <14% cases.

Progression of DCIS to Invasive Breast Carcinoma

TP53 gene mutation and inactivation of BRCA1 directly cause ductal carcinoma *in situ* progressing to invasive breast carcinoma.

Immunohistochemistry

These tumors are triple negative, i.e. ER/PR and Her2 neu negative.

Marker	Expression
Estrogen receptor (ER)	Negative
Progesterone receptor (PR)	Negative
Her2 neu	Negative

Treatment

These patients do not respond to endocrine therapy (tamoxifen), aromatase inhibitors or herceptin. Prognosis is poor. Trials are going onto treat these patients with platinum-based chemotherapy or PARP inhibitors.

HISTOLOGICAL VARIANTS OF BREAST CARCINOMA

Salient Features

More than 90% of breast carcinomas are adenocarcinomas. These arise in ducts or lobules as carcinoma *in situ*

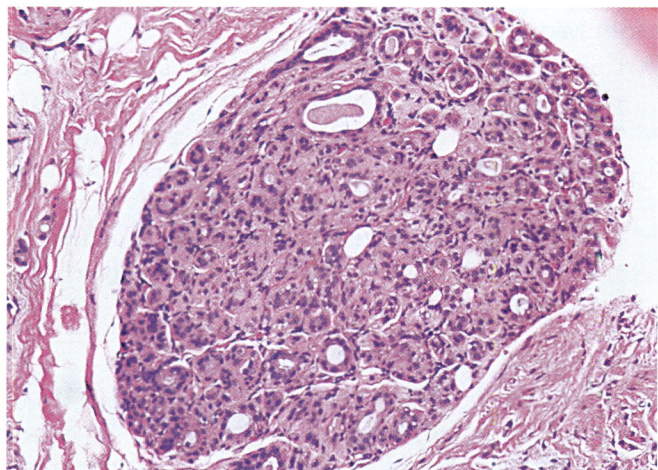

Fig. 25.30: Comedocarcinoma breast. It is high-grade ductal carcinoma *in situ* with highly pleomorphic tumor cells present within and distending the duct space, associated with central comedonecrosis (cheesy material) (400X).

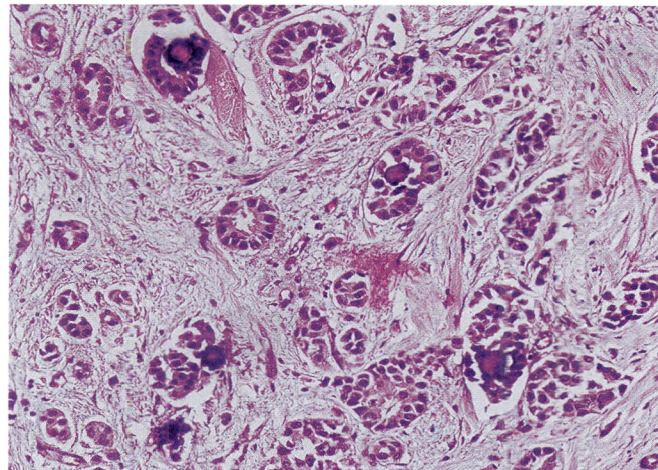

Fig. 25.32: Breast carcinoma shows invasive ductal carcinoma with microcalcifications. Tumor is composed of pleomorphic atypical cells with hyperchromatic nuclei. The cells are arranged in clusters and sheets invading surrounding stroma (400X).

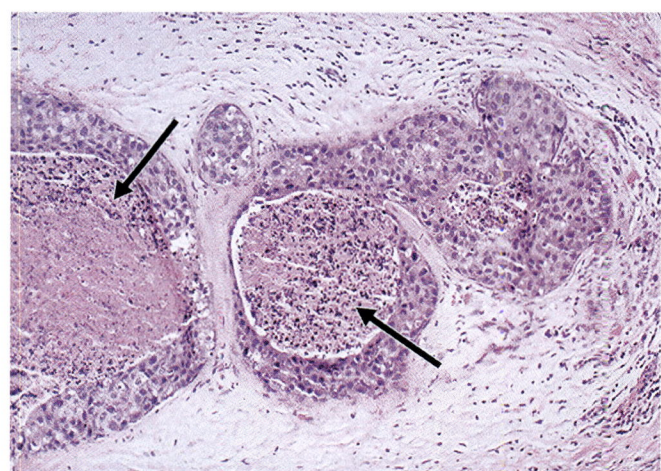

Fig. 25.31: Breast comedocarcinoma. It shows ductal carcinoma *in situ* with central necrosis (arrows) (400X).

(DCIS) (Figs 25.30 and 25.31). When malignant epithelial cells invade the basement membrane and extends in surrounding tissue, it is known as invasive ductal carcinoma. Ductal carcinoma *in situ* is associated with the development of small calcified deposits in the breast demonstrated by mammography.

DUCTAL CARCINOMA

Ductal Carcinoma *in situ*

Ductal carcinoma in situ has two histological variants: comedocarcinoma and non-comedocarcinoma. Tumors may be low, intermediate and high-grades. Low-grade DCIS shows monomorphic cells with nuclei polarized towards luminal spaces, occasional mitosis. Nuclei are not polarized towards luminal spaces.

High-grade DCIS is composed of pleomorphic cells with vesicular hyperchromatic nuclei prominent nucleoli. Intermediate-grade DCIS has intermediate features.

- *Comedocarcinoma:* It is high-grade ductal carcinoma *in situ* with *highly pleomorphic tumor cells* present within and distending the duct space, associated with central comedonecrosis (cheesy material). It may show *lymph node metastases*. The ducts are lined by pleomorphic cells with hyperchromatic irregular nuclei, prominent nucleoli and abundant eosinophilic cytoplasm. These cells are arranged in solid pattern with *central necrosis in the ducts*. The necrotic debris may undergo *dystrophic calcification*. The tumor cells incite chronic inflammatory cells infiltration and fibroblastic response in the surrounding stroma.
- *Non-comedocarcinoma:* This variant shows carcinoma *in situ without central necrosis*. Malignant cells have regular outlines and small nuclei in contrast to comedocarcinoma. These may be arranged in solid pattern or cribriform (multiple lumens within duct) or micropapillary pattern with delicate fibrovascular cores lined by tumor cells.

Invasive Ductal Carcinoma

It is most common breast carcinoma constituting 65–80% of all breast carcinomas. It breaches basement membrane and invades the normal breast at random. Its precursor lesion is ductal carcinoma *in situ*. Its architecture ranges from tubule formation to solid sheets (Fig. 25.32).

LOBULAR CARCINOMA

Lobular carcinoma is most common cancer in the terminal duct lobular unit. These lesions are often *bilateral* and *multifocal* in 20–50% of cases. On light microscopy, lobular carcinoma may be classified as *in situ* or invasive types.

Lobular Carcinoma *in situ* (LCIS)

It is considerably less common (1%) than ductal carcinoma *in situ* (DCIS). It is characterized by distension of the terminal lobules by small to intermediate-sized cells with a few mitoses. Approximately untreated 20 to 30% of cases, patients with lobular carcinoma *in situ* develop invasive lobular carcinoma (Fig. 25.33).

Invasive Lobular Carcinoma

It is less common breast carcinoma constituting 5–10% of cases. Its precursor lesion is lobular carcinoma *in situ*. Although microcalcifications are uncommon, yet *mammography detects the lesion. It is luminal A type of breast carcinoma*. It shows *low proliferative rate*. Recurrence rate is low. Immunohistochemistry shows positivity for ER/PR and cytokeratin (8; 18). These patients respond to tamoxifen, aromatase inhibitors and herceptin. Prognosis is good.

Molecular Genetics

Amplification of ERBB2 (Her2 neu) is rarely detected in noninvasive or invasive lobular carcinoma. It is demonstrated by immunohistochemistry on the cell membrane or using fluorescent *in situ* hybridization (FISH).

Gross Morphology
Lobular carcinoma *in situ* is rubbery poorly circumscribed, firm to hard tumor or not readily palpable.

Light Microscopy
• Classic variant tumor comprises small- to moderately-sized atypical cells that lack cohesion. • These cells are individually dispersed singly in linear fashion *single Indian file pattern* through fibrous tissue around preexisting benign ducts. • Presence of mucin in malignant cells pushes the nucleus against the membrane creating *signet ring* appearance (Fig. 25.34).
Histological Variants
Lobular invasive carcinoma shows five histological types: classic, alveolar (aggregates of more than 20 cells), tubuloalveolar (cells in cords and microtubules), pleomorphic, solid (cells arranged in diffuse sheets) and mixed (70% cells in Indian file pattern) variants.
Immunohistochemistry
It shows ER, PR and cytokeratin (8; 18) positivity in all cases of invasive lobular carcinomas of breast. In addition, a substantial number of these tumors is reactive for carcinoembryonic antigen (CEA).

Marker	Expression
Estrogen receptor (ER)	Positive
Progesterone receptor (PR)	Positive
Cytokeratin (8; 18)	Positive
Carcinoembryonic antigen (CEA)	Positive

Clinical Correlation

Patient presents with bilateral multiple breast lumps in 20–50% of cases. Tumor may spread to axillary lymph nodes and distant organs such as lungs, liver, and

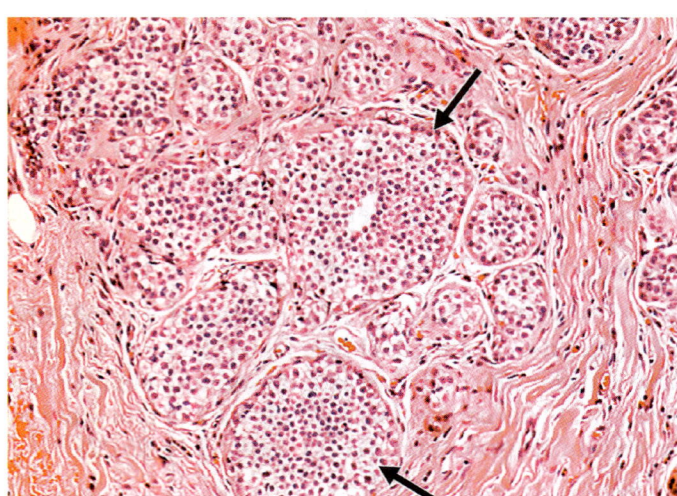

Fig. 25.33: Lobular carcinoma *in situ* of breast. It shows distension of the acini by a uniform population of small round cells with bland nuclear features. The growth pattern is solid (arrows) (400X).

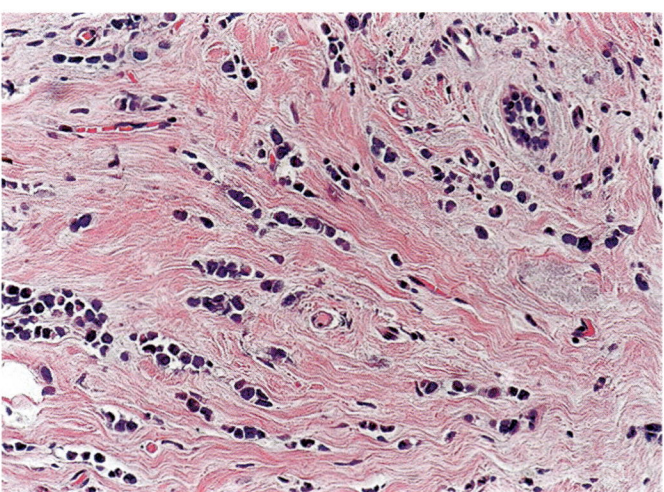

Fig. 25.34: Lobular carcinoma breast shows tumor cells is arranged in Indian file pattern. Left image (100X) and right image (400X).

bone, cerebrospinal fluid, ovaries (*Krukenberg tumor*) and uterus.

Management

It depends on stage with treatment similar to that with invasive duct carcinoma. These patients respond well to tamoxifen, aromatase inhibitors and herceptin.

INVASIVE DUCTAL CARCINOMA (NOS)

Invasive ductal carcinoma (not otherwise specified) is commonest type of breast carcinoma. Most invasive ductal carcinomas may evoke a *dense fibroblastic response* (proliferation of fibroblasts producing collagen fibers) in the host tissue that adds to the lesion's bulk.

It replaces normal breast fat. Prognosis is stage dependent. *Tumor has firm to hard consistency (schirrhous), and chalky white discoloration due to desmoplasia.* **Nipple retraction** due to desmoplasia in an underlying advanced breast carcinoma is a late feature of breast carcinoma.

Clinical Features

Patient presents with poorly defined solitary, non-tender breast lump of variable consistency and mobility with nipple retraction. *It is solid hard, dense and fixed to the underlying tissues or skin* due to invasion of breast carcinoma.

Nipple Retraction

A recent retraction suggests breast carcinoma, which causes fibrosis of the whole duct system and pulls in the nipple, known as *retraction of the nipple.* Fibrosis also contracts the suspensory ligament, that pulls the nipple inward is known as dimpling (also called a skin tether) (Fig. 25.35).

Overlying Skin

The *peau d'orange* (skin edema) appearance of the breast skin occurs due to obstruction of the dermal lymphatics by cancer cells (Fig. 25.36).

Gross Morphology

- Tumor is firm to hard, irregular, and fibrous extension into the adjacent breast stroma that create stellate (crab-like) outline measuring 1–4 cm (rarely 4–5 cm).
- Cut section reveals gray chalky white tissue yellow crab-like satellites extending into the yellow fat tissue.
- Skin surface may show retraction of nipple (Fig. 25.37).

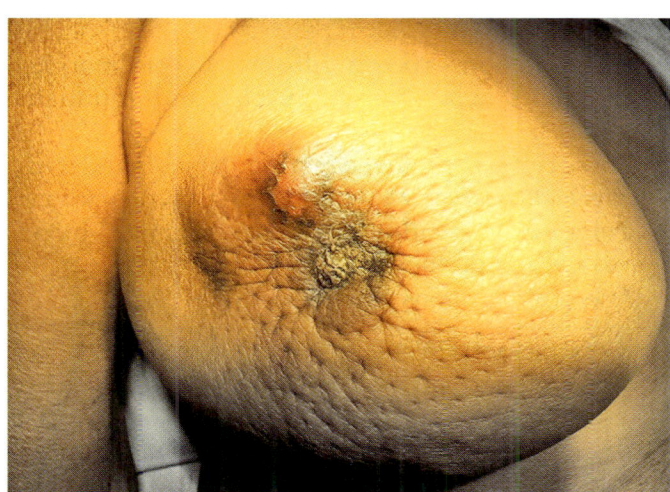

Fig. 25.36: Breast carcinoma—Peau d' orange appearance and nipple retraction. Peau d' orange appearance occurs due to obstruction of dermal lymphatics by tumor cells.

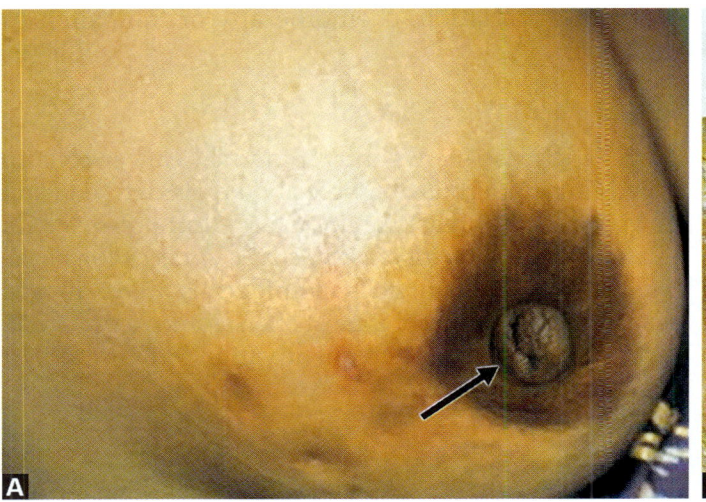
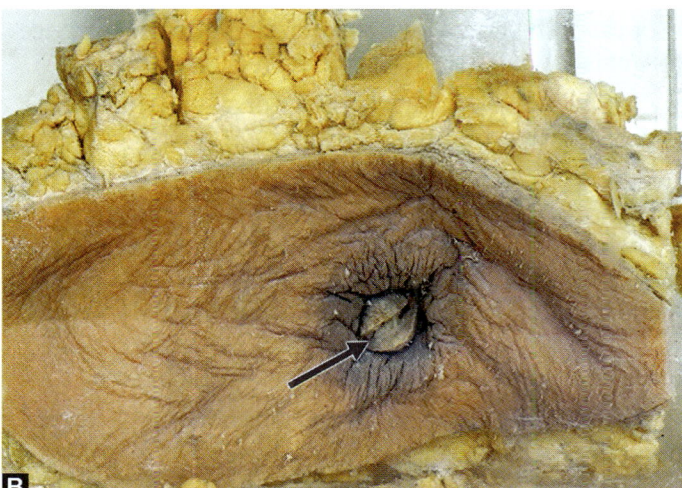

Fig. 25.35: Breast carcinoma. (A) Photograph shows a tumor that has caused nipple retraction (arrow), (B) mastectomy specimen shows nipple retraction (arrow).

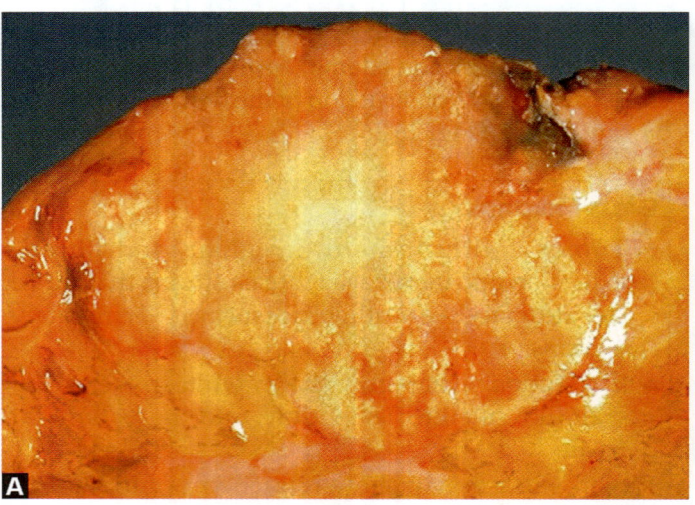 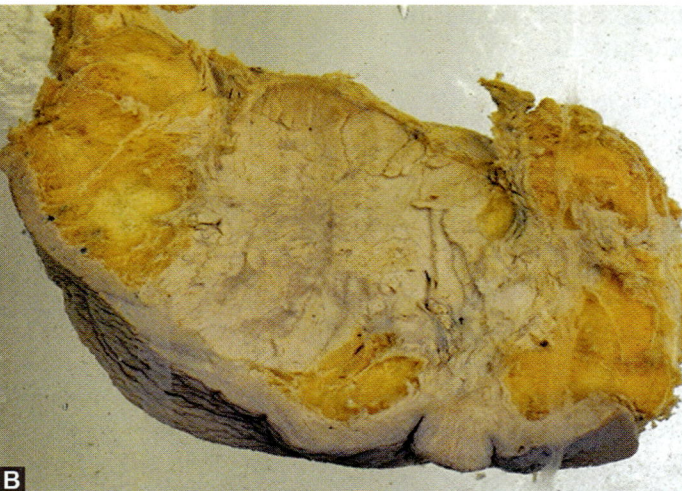

Fig. 25.37: Breast carcinoma (A) and (B) Cut surface shows gray white tumor with infiltrating margins.

Light Microscopy
- Tumor comprises poorly differentiated pleomorphic cells with *hyperchromatic nuclei*, and abundant mitoses.
- These cells are arranged in irregular *nests* and *cords* or *glandular structures* within a dense fibrous stroma.
- Tumor cells invading lymphatic channels, blood vessels and perineural spaces may be seen.
- Microcalcifications may be seen.

Immunohistochemistry
- The cadherin family of cell adhesion molecules is a group of transmembrane glycoproteins located in desmosomes.
- **E-Cadherins** are present in ductal carcinoma and absent in lobular carcinoma of the breast.

Molecular Pathways
- *Luminal type A:* It is low-grade tumor seen in <50% of cases. It shows low proliferative rate. Recurrence rate is low. Prognosis is good.
- *Luminal type B:* It is seen in <15% of cases. It has higher proliferative rate than luminal A type. Recurrence is high. Prognosis may not be as good as in luminal type A.
- *Herceptin enriched:* It is seen in <20% of cases. It is high-grade tumor with higher proliferative rate. It most often shows involvement of axillary lymph nodes. These patients respond to herceptin- and anthracycline-based chemotherapeutic agents.
- *Basal type:* It is high-grade variant of invasive ductal carcinoma. It has high proliferative rate with positive lymph nodes. Recurrence rate is high. TP53 gene mutation is very common. It shows dysfunction of BRCA1 gene. Ki-67 is expressed in <14% of cases.

On immunohistochemistry, it is triple negative, i.e. ER, PR and Her2 neu negative. These patients do not respond to endocrine therapy (tamoxifen, aromatase inhibitors and herceptin). Prognosis is poor. Trials are going onto treat these patients with platinum-based chemotherapy or PARP inhibitors.

Prognostic Implications
Tumor grade, DNA content and proliferative index, and presence of ERBB2 (Her2 neu) amplification also have prognostic implications.

Metastases
Tumor spreads to *axillary lymph nodes* and then to lungs, liver and bones.

Management
It depends on tumor size, grade, metastases status to lymph nodes or distant organs, estrogen and progesterone receptor status. The patients are managed by surgery, irradiation, chemotherapy or tamoxifen or herceptin.

PAGET'S DISEASE OF BREAST
Paget's disease shows intraepidermal cancer cells in overlying epidermis of nipple and areola derived from an intraductal breast carcinoma. *Patient presents with eczematous lesion with crusted, eroded surface over nipple and areola.* Malignant cells in epidermis are known as Paget's cells. The tumor is most often *poorly circumscribed.* This condition is more frequently found in *older women* (Figs 25.38 and 25.39).

Etiopathogenesis
The production by keratinocytes of heregulin-α, which acts via the Her2 neu receptor, may play a role in its pathogenesis.

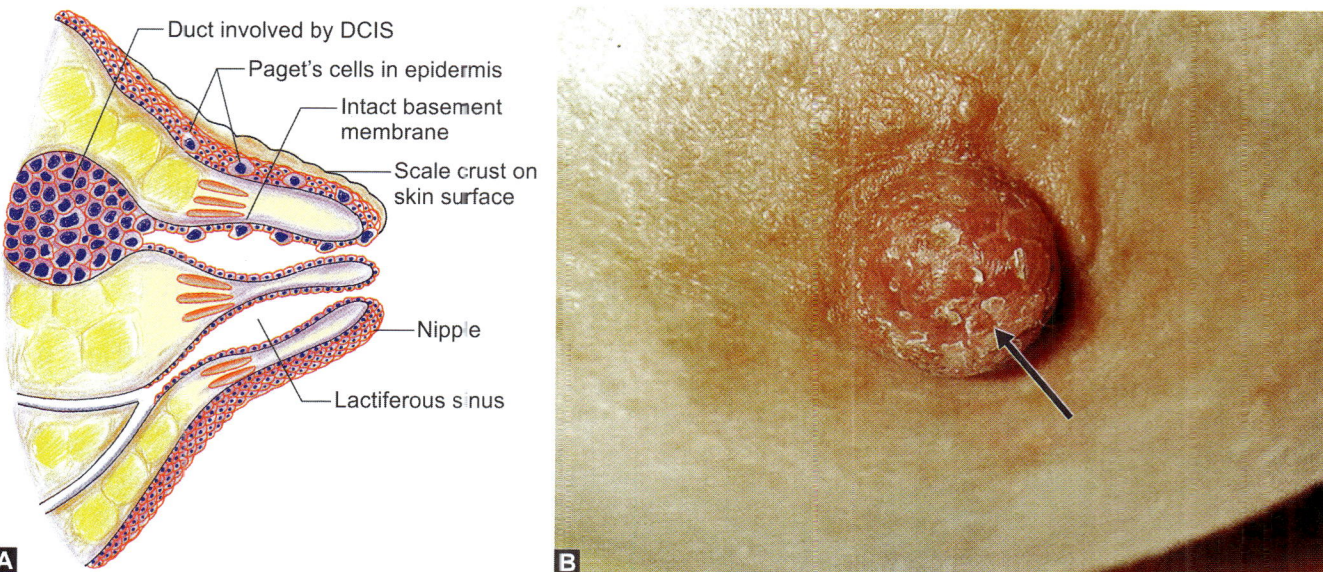

Fig. 25.38: Paget's disease of breast. (A) Structure of the adult female breast showing Paget's disease of the breast. Malignant cells infiltrating overlying epidermis are known as Paget's cells. (B) eczematous lesion with crusted, eroded surface over nipple and areola (arrow) (*Courtesy by* Dr Abhijit Das).

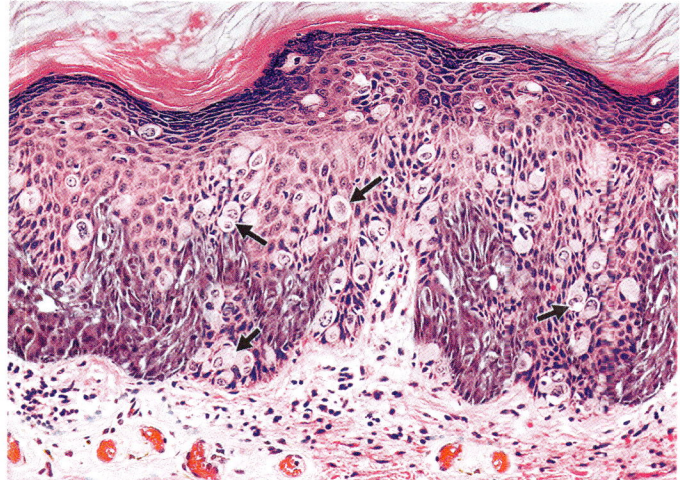

Fig. 25.39: Paget's disease of breast. The tumor cells in the overlying epidermis are called as Paget's cells. These are large cells with abundant clear cytoplasm and large nuclei with prominent nucleoli, arranged singly or in clusters; represent intraepithelial extension of an underlying ductal carcinoma *in situ* or invasive ductal carcinoma (arrows) (400X).

Molecular Genetics

Amplification of ERBB2 (Her2 neu) is observed in Paget's disease of breast. It encodes for an epithelial growth factor receptor (EGFR) on the cell membrane that delivers continuous mitogenic signals to the cell resulting in breast carcinoma, even in the absence of growth factor in the environment. It is demonstrated by monoclonal antibody on the cell membrane or using fluorescent *in situ* hybridization (FISH).

Clinical Features

Paget's disease of the breast affects the nipple from the start, whereas eczema affects the **areolar region first** and only rarely affects the nipple skin, which eventually leads to *erosion and ulceration of the nipple* in elderly women. On examination, a painless mass is palpable in the underlying breast in 50% of cases, and often associated with *delay in diagnosis*.

Light Microscopy

- Histopathological examination reveals either *in situ* or invasive ductal carcinoma, which involves overlying epidermis of nipple and areola.
- The tumor cells in the overlying epidermis are called as Paget's cells.
- Paget's cells within the surface epithelium of the nipple and areola are large cells with abundant clear cytoplasm and large nuclei with prominent nucleoli, arranged singly or in clusters; represent intraepithelial extension of an underlying ductal carcinoma *in situ* or invasive ductal carcinoma (Fig. 25.39).

Histochemistry

PAS stain demonstrates mucin within the Paget's cells of Paget's disease of the breast in right section. This is evidence for their origin from an underlying ductal carcinoma.

Immunohistochemistry

By immunoperoxidase staining, they will also be **cytokeratin positive** (low molecular weight) and *epithelial membrane antigen* (EMA) positive.

Marker	Expression
Cytokeratin (low M.W.)	Positive
Epithelial membrane antigen (EMA)	Positive

Mammography

If Paget's disease is suspected on clinical examination, mammography should be performed to determine if there is an underlying lesion.

Diagnosis

Diagnosis is established by cytology (e.g. smears from imprint and scrapping) or wedge biopsy of nipple.

INFLAMMATORY CARCINOMA

Rapidly growing breast carcinoma metastasizing in dermal lymphatic channels results in thickened, erythematous (red), rough, swollen, hot skin as a consequence of inflammatory process. Edema usually begins in the skin *around and beneath the areola*, the most dependent area of breast (Fig. 25.40).

Prognosis

Prognosis is **poor** in inflammatory breast carcinoma. Patient is treated by chemotherapy followed by surgery and irradiation.

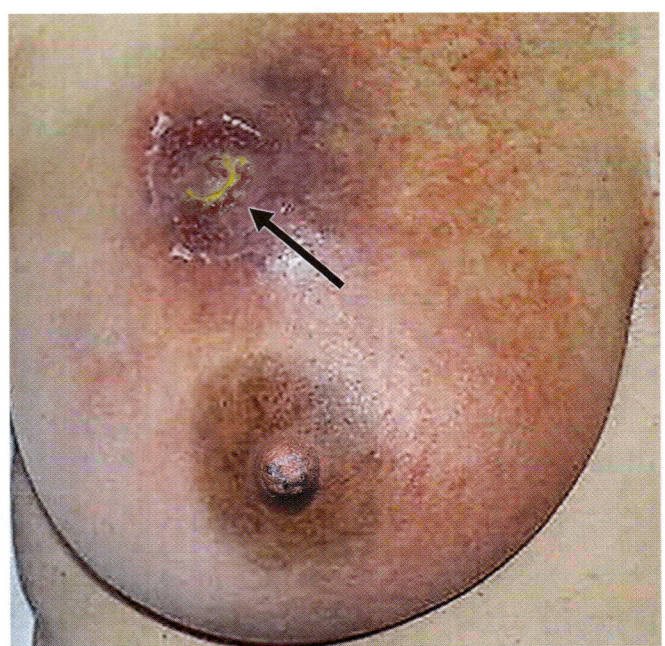

Fig. 25.40: Breast cancer shows inflammatory carcinoma (arrow).

MEDULLARY BREAST CARCINOMA

It is uncommon breast carcinoma affecting young females. Patient presents with fleshy, *bulky tumor measuring 5 to 10 cm in diameter*. It is *basal like subtype of breast* carcinoma. It has high proliferative rate with positive lymph nodes. **Recurrence** rate is **high**.

Molecular Genetics

BRCA1 gene mutations are observed in some cases. TP53 gene mutation is very common. Ki-67 is expressed in <14% cases. Amplification of ERBB2 (Her2 neu) is not seen.

Gross Morphology

- The tumor is *well circumscribed*, with a *soft, fleshy* and *uniform consistency* with rounded *pushing margins*.
- There is no evidence of a fibrous reaction. It most often measures between 1 and 4 cm in diameter.

Light Microscopy

It has three diagnostic features based on histology and gross morphology (Fig. 25.41):
- *Cells morphology:* It comprises pleomorphic atypical cells arranged in interconnecting sheets, forming a syncytial network. Cells contain hyperchromatic nuclei with scant to moderate cytoplasm arranged in sheets forming **syncytial network**. *It shows large bizarre nuclei with high mitotic count.*
- *Intervening stroma with immune cells:* The intervening stroma is scant. There is presence of lymphocytes and plasma cells (immune response) around tumor cell groups (and not between individual tumor cells). Foci of necrosis and hemorrhage may be found.

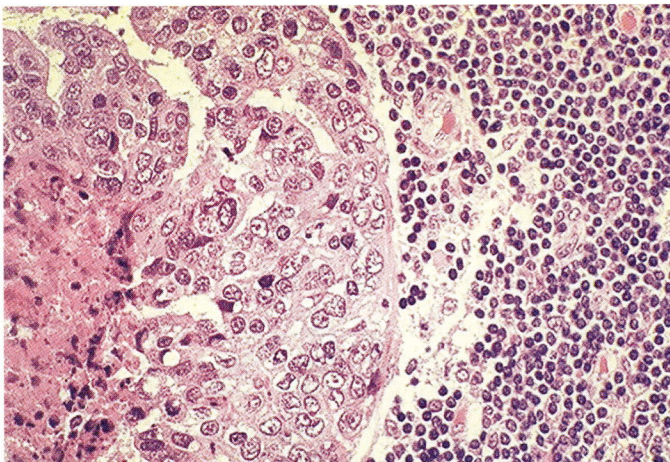

Fig. 25.41: Medullary carcinoma of breast. Carcinoma with medullary features showing a rounded margin and an intense lymphocytic infiltrate at the periphery. The tumor cells form a sheet-like pattern with high degree of nuclear pleomorphism and brisk mitotic activity (400X).

Immunohistochemistry

Approximately 50–65% cases of breast carcinoma are *positive* for **ER** and *negative* for **Her2 neu**.

Marker	Expression
Estrogen receptor (ER)	Positive (50–60%)
Her2 neu	Negative

Treatment

Patients do not respond to tamoxifen, aromatase inhibitors and herceptin. Trials are going onto treat these patients with platinum based chemotherapy or PARP inhibitors.

Prognosis

It has much better prognosis than usual duct carcinoma even with lymph node metastases. Approximately 70% of patients have overall 10-year survival.

COLLOID (MUCINOUS) CARCINOMA

Colloid breast carcinoma accounts for 1–4% of breast carcinomas. It features abundant mucin production.

Molecular Genetics

BRCA1 gene mutation is demonstrated in some cases. Amplification of ERBB2 (Her2 neu) is seen in some cases.

Clinical Features

It is uncommon slow-growing neoplasm primarily seen in elderly women as a small well circumscribed mass.

Gross Morphology

- Tumor is well circumscribed tumor with soft consistency measuring 1–5 cm in diameter with an average of 2.8 cm.
- Cut surface of tumor is completely replaced by glistening gelatinous blue to gray-colored mucoid material (Fig. 25.42).

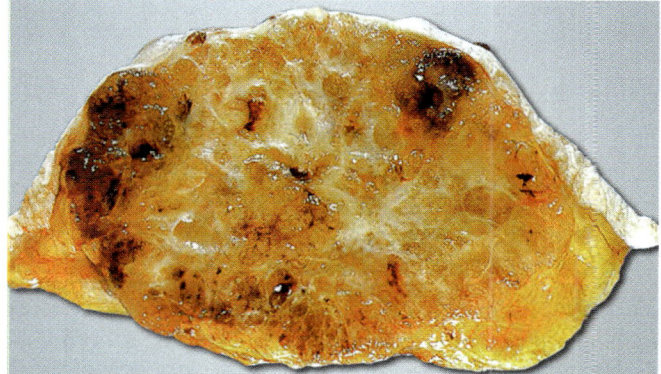

Fig. 25.42: Colloid carcinoma of the breast. This sagitta slice of the breast shows that it is completely replaced by mucoic tumor.

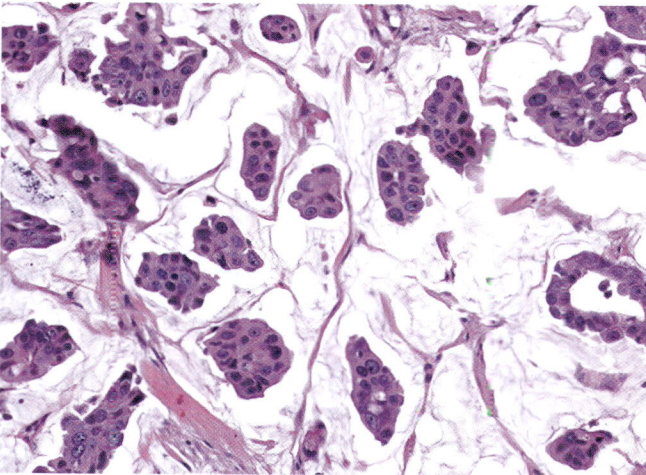

Fig. 25.43: Mucinous/colloid carcinoma of breast Mucinous carcinoma shows large sheets of low-grade malignant cells present within pools of accumulated extracellular mucinous material (400X).

Light Microscopy

- Tumor is composed of small islands or clusters of generally uniform, round epithelial cells (10–20 cells) arranged in trabeculae, nests, sheets or acini with glandular lumen, floating within extensive *lakes of extracellular mucin pool* synthesized by tumor cells.
- Mucin dissects into the surrounding stroma. Tumor contains >90% of mucinous component (Fig. 25.43).

Immunohistochemistry

Most tumors express hormone ER (estrogen receptors) in 80%.

Prognosis

It is *low-grade malignant* tumor with *low incidence of metastases* It has better prognosis than conventional ductal carcinoma.

TUBULAR BREAST CARCINOMA

It accounts for 1 to 4% of invasive breast carcinomas. A higher frequency (up to 19%) has been reported in small and screen-detected breast carcinomas in whites compared with blacks. It affects younger age at onset (40s). *It is luminal A type low-grade invasive ductal cell carcinoma.* It shows *low proliferative rate. Recurrence rate is low.*

Molecular Genetics

Amplification of ERBB2 (Her2 neu) is unusual.

Clinical Features

Patient presents with breast lump measuring 2 mm to 1.5 cm in diameter. Most are 1 cm or less, but rarely examples of 2 cm or above is encountered.

Gross Morphology
- The tumor is usually small (<2 cm), firm to hard in consistency, and often detected on mammography.
- There is increased incidence of cancer in opposite breast in 10–40% of cases.

Light Microscopy
- Diagnosis is made when 75% of neoplasm shows well-formed small duct structures embedded in cellular stroma.
- Tumor shows bland-looking tumor cells arranged in tubules that possess widely patent lumens lined by low-grade single cell layer.
- Myoepithelial cells are absent, and the malignant tubules are arranged in an irregular stellate pattern.
- The intervening stroma is densely fibrotic. Mitoses are rare.
- It may be difficult to separate from sclerosing adenosis or radial scar but generally spread outside the confines of enlarged lobules (Fig. 25.44).

Immunohistochemistry
Virtually all tubular carcinomas express **ER** and **PR** hormone receptors and **cytokeratin (8; 18)**.

Marker	Expression
Estrogen (ER)	Positive
Progesterone (PR)	Positive
Cytokeratin (8; 18)	Positive

Treatment
These patients respond to tamoxifen, aromatase inhibitors and herceptin.

Prognosis
Prognosis is **better** despite multifocal nature and bilateral involvement. Lymph node metastases are rare.

PAPILLARY BREAST CARCINOMA
It constitutes approximately 1–2% of breast carcinoma.

Clinical Features
Approximately 50% tumors are located beneath the nipple (associated with bloody nipple discharge).

Gross Morphology
- The tumor is usually 2–3 cm in size, and well-circumscribed.
- Cystic lesions contain brown mixture of blood clot and neoplastic tissue.

Light Microscopy
- The tumor is composed of delicate fibrovascular tissue lined by atypical epithelial cells with hyperchromatic nuclei and mitoses forming papillary structures with the absence of an outer myoepithelial cell layer.
- It must be differentiated from papilloma that is characterized by thick fibrovascular tissue and presence of myoepithelial cells.
- Periphery of cystic tumor is fibrotic and distinguishing invasion may be difficult unless neoplasm reaches fat (Fig. 25.45).

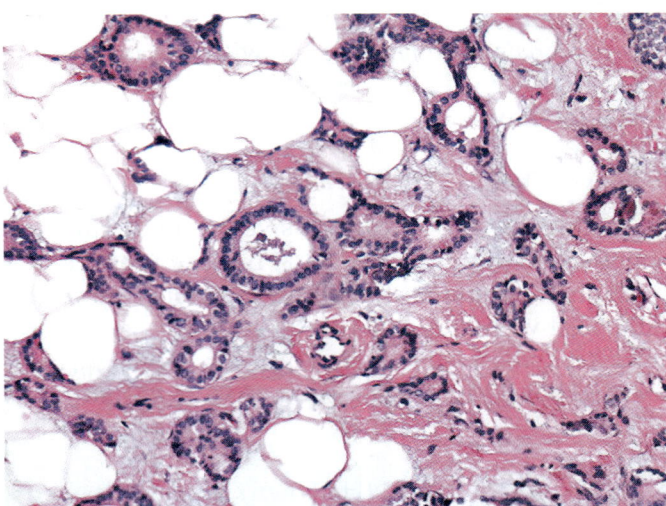

Fig. 25.44: Tubular carcinoma of breast. Tubular carcinoma shows bland-looking tumor cells arranged in tubules that possess widely patent lumens. Myoepithelial cells are absent, and the malignant tubules are arranged in an irregular stellate pattern. The intervening stroma is densely fibrotic (400X).

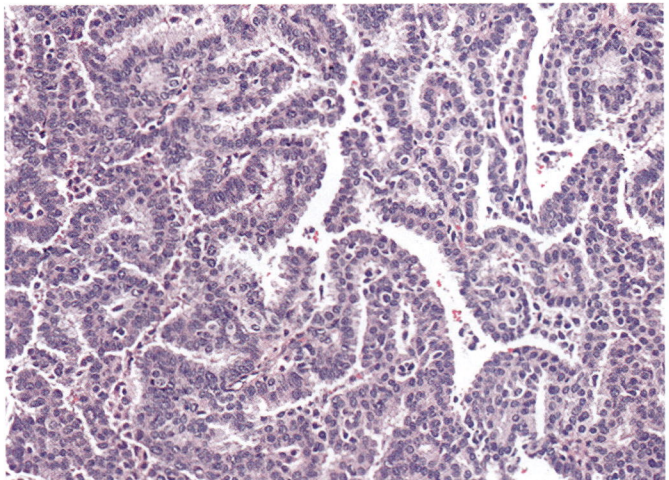

Fig. 25.45: Invasive papillary carcinoma breast is comprised of delicate fibrovascular tissue lined by atypical epithelial cells with hyperchromatic nuclei and mitoses forming papillary structures with the absence of an outer myoepithelial cell layer (400X).

Table 25.9: Comparison of breast intraductal papilloma and noninvasive ductal papillary carcinoma

Parameters	Ductal papilloma	Noninvasive ductal papillary carcinoma
Cell morphology	Benign cells with normal nuclear chromatin	Atypical cells with hyperchromatic nuclei
Myoepithelial cells	Present	Absent
Apocrine changes	Present	Absent
Surrounding stroma	Thick prominent stroma	Delicate stroma
Sclerosing adenosis	Unusual	Usual

INVASIVE MICROPAPILLARY BREAST CARCINOMA

It is luminal type B invasive breast carcinoma: It is seen in <20% of cases. It has **higher proliferative rate** than luminal A-type. **Recurrence is high**. It should be differentiated from duct papilloma (Table 25.9).

Light Microscopy
Invasive micropapillary carcinoma shows rounded groups of tumor cells with a peripheral clear rim and lacks true fibrovascular core (Fig. 25.46).

Immunohistochemistry
Tumor cells may show *low expression of ER and PR*. Immunohistochemistry shows *cytokeratin positivity (8; 18)*.

Marker	Expression
Estrogen receptor (ER)	Low expression
Progesterone receptor (PR)	Low expression
Cytokeratins (8; 18)	Positive

Prognosis
Prognosis may not be as good as in luminal type A.

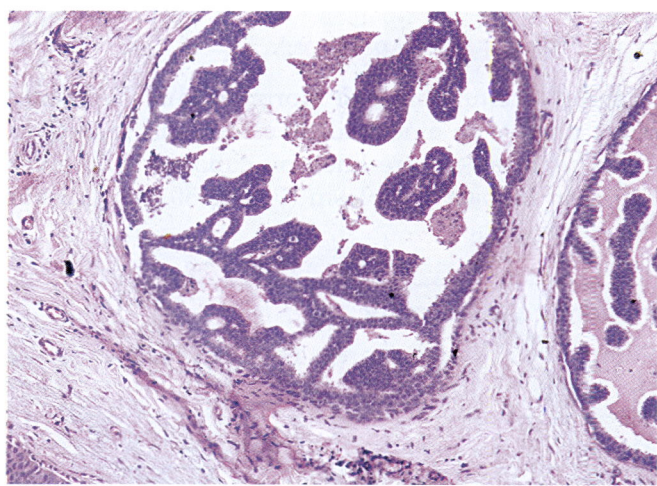

Fig. 25.46: Micropapillary carcinoma of breast. It shows large duct with micropapillary tufts of epithelial cells lacking true fibrovascular core (400X).

METAPLASTIC BREAST CARCINOMA

- Metaplastic carcinoma of the breast is a form of breast carcinoma that shows *differentiation towards malignant squamous epithelium, cartilaginous, or bony tissue.* This term is used to describe a heterogeneous group of neoplasms. It is also known as carcinosarcoma.
- It is *basal like subtype* of breast carcinoma. It has *high proliferative rate* with positive lymph nodes. Recurrence rate is high.

Molecular Genetics
- **TP53 gene** mutation is very common. It shows dysfunction of BRCA1 gene.
- **Ki-67** is expressed in <14% cases.

Treatment
Patients do not respond to tamoxifen, aromatase inhibitors and herceptin. Trials are going onto treat these patients with platinum-based chemotherapy or PARP inhibitors.

Light Microscopy
- Metaplastic carcinoma includes monophasic or biphasic sarcomatoid carcinoma.
- Tumor is admixture of malignant epithelial component (adenocarcinoma grade 2 or 3) with malignant *mesenchymal* elements including cartilage, bone, and myxoid stroma, and/or squamous or spindle cell elements (Figs 25.47 and 25.48).

Immunohistochemistry
- It shows co-expression of *cytokeratin (5; 6)* and *vimentin* in spindle cell elements of metaplastic carcinomas.
- Tumor cells are *triple negative* for *estrogen* and *progesterone receptors* as well as Her2 neu.

Marker	Expression
Cytokeratins (5; 6)	Positive
Vimentin	Positive
Estrogen receptor (ER)	Negative
Progesterone receptor (PR)	Negative
Her2 neu	Negative

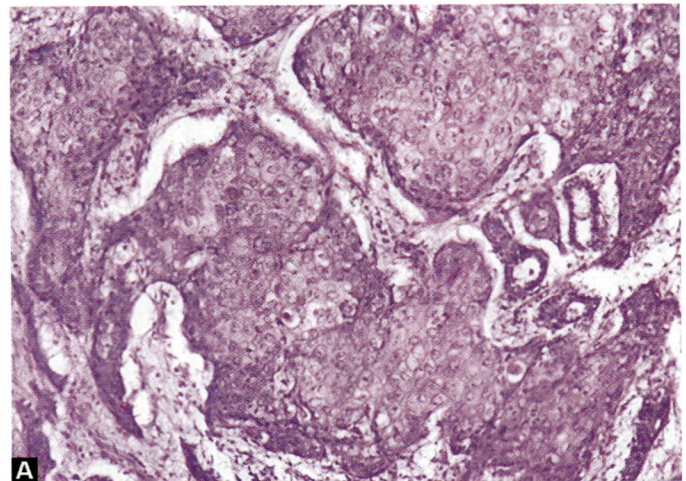
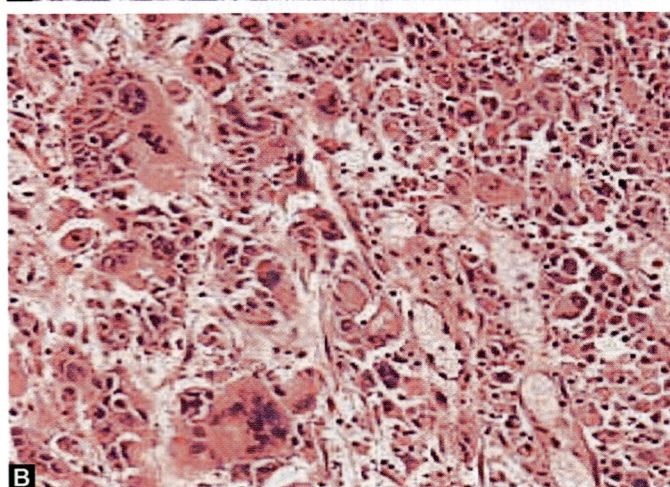

Fig. 25.47: Metaplastic carcinoma of breast with squamous differentiation. (A) Tumor shows mixed squamous cell carcinoma and ductal carcinoma components, (B) the intervening areas show malignant spindle cell proliferation. It is high-grade breast cancer with poor prognosis (400X).

APOCRINE BREAST CARCINOMA

This variant of breast carcinoma consists of tumor cells with apocrine morphology in >90% cells.

Light Microscopy
Tumor is composed of large cells with well-defined cellular outlines, vesicular nuclei, prominent nucleoli, abundant granular cytoplasm and foci of necrosis (Fig. 25.49)
Electron Microscopy
Tumor contains *prominent mitochondria* with *abnormal cisternae, large membrane bound vesicles* and *dense cores*.

Prognosis

It has similar prognosis that of infiltrating duct carcinoma (NOS) of similar grade.

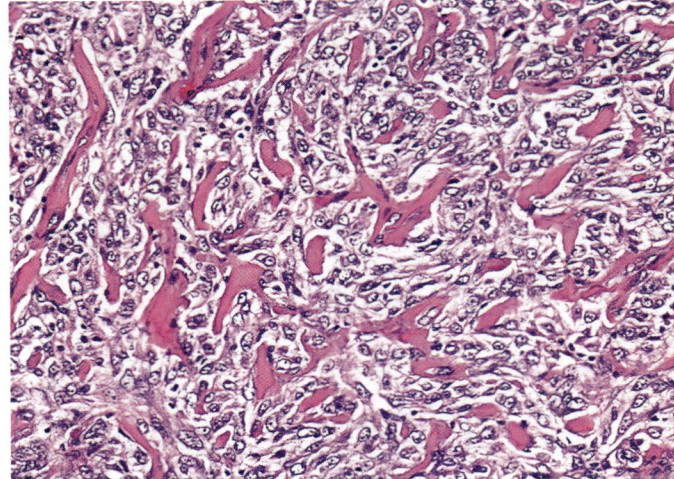

Fig. 25.48: Metaplastic carcinoma of breast (400X).

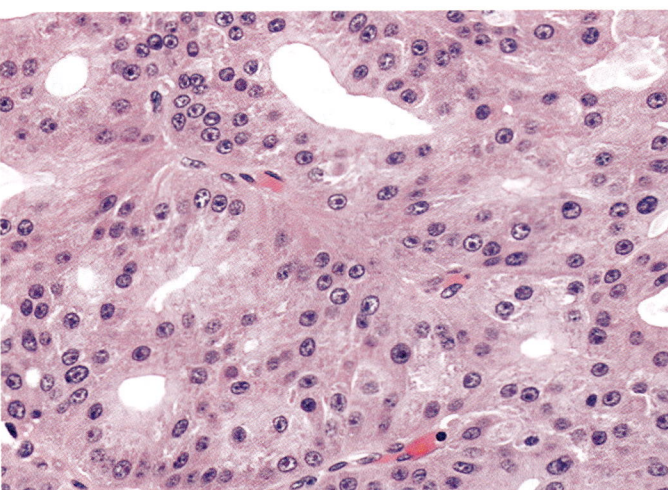

Fig. 25.49: Apocrine breast carcinoma is composed of large cells with well-defined cellular outlines, vesicular nuclei, prominent nucleoli, abundant granular cytoplasm and foci of necrosis (400X).

SECRETORY BREAST CARCINOMA

It mimics lactating breast by forming multiple dilated spaces filled with amorphous eosinophilic secretions. These cystic spaces are lined by cuboidal epithelium with clear or pale cytoplasm (Fig. 25.50). It occurs in young age group.

Immunohistochemistry	
Tumor cells do not express estrogen receptors and Her2 neu.	
Marker	Expression
Estrogen receptors	Negative
Her2 neu	Negative

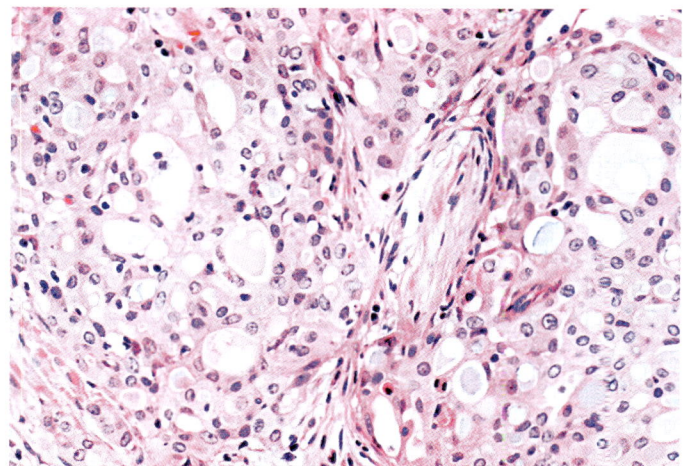

Fig. 25.50: Secretory carcinoma of breast mimics lactating breast by forming multiple dilated spaces filled with amorphous eosinophilic secretions. These cystic spaces are lined by cuboidal epithelium with clear or pale cytoplasm (400X).

CRIBRIFORM BREAST CARCINOMA

It is luminal A type low-grade invasive ductal cell carcinoma. It shows low proliferative rate. Recurrence rate is low. These patients respond to endocrine therapy (tamoxifen, aromatase inhibitors and herceptin. Prognosis is good.

Immunohistochemistry	
Immunohistochemistry shows positivity for ER, PR and cytokeratin (8, 18).	
Marker	**Expression**
Estrogen receptor (ER)	Positive
Progesterone receptor (PR)	Positive
Cytokeratin (8, 18)	Positive

ANGIOSARCOMA BREAST

Radical mastectomy is performed for treatment of a breast carcinoma. Women develops gross lymphedema of the arm, which is a usual consequence of this radical surgery. Occasionally, angiosarcomas arise in the skin and subcutaneous tissue of these grossly edematous arms some years after the surgery. Angiosarcoma of the breast is seen as a *reddish, cavitated hemorrhagic tumor within the subcutaneous mammary tissue.*

Light Microscopy
• Malignant phyllodes tumor showing highly pleomorphic malignant stromal cells, with bizarre cells adjacent to benign ductal epithelium.
• Atypical mitotic figures are seen within the malignant stromal cells.

Summary of major histological types of invasive breast carcinoma is shown in Table 25.10.

MODE OF SPREAD OF TUMORS

- Most breast carcinomas arise from lining epithelium of ducts, which becomes invasive and metastasizes early to axillary *lymph nodes, lungs, liver, bones, brain, adrenal glands* and *ovaries* (**Krukenberg** tumor).
- Women presenting with an isolated enlarged axillary node must be taken seriously because 33 to 50% will have occult breast carcinoma. Mode of spread of breast carcinoma by various routes is described as under.

LOCAL EXTENSION

Invasive breast carcinoma can infiltrate and cause fixation to adjacent structures. If the tumor is deep, fixation may occur to the pectoralis muscles; if superficial, the skin may be involved. Skin involvement can also result in nipple retraction and inversion when the tumor arises near the central zone.

Invasion and obstruction of small cutaneous lymphatic channels results in edema of the skin giving it the appearance of the surface of an orange peel (*peau d'orange*). Once skin fixation occurs, cutaneous ulceration may follow. Breast carcinoma may spread to opposite breast.

LYMPHATIC ROUTE

Breast lymphatic drainage occurs via axillary and internal mammary nodes. Approximately 75% of breast lymphatic drainage takes place in axillary lymph nodes, while rest 25% via internal mammary lymph nodes adjacent to vertebrae and skin lymphatic channels. That is the reason that occult breast carcinoma presents with isolated axillary lymph node enlargement (Fig. 25.51).

Axillary Lymphatic Drainage

- Axillary group consists of approximately 21 lymph nodes, which lie below the axillary vein. These

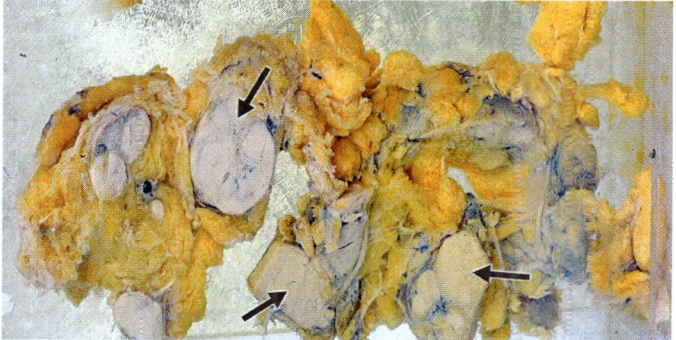

Fig. 25.51: Breast carcinoma—axillary lymph nodes show metastases (arrows).

Table 25.10: Diagnostic features of major histologic types of invasive breast carcinoma

Histologic type	Incidence (%)	Clinical/gross findings	Light microscopy	Prognosis	Typical biomarkers
Invasive ductal carcinoma NOS (not otherwise specified)	70–75	Speculated mass, variable	Variable, devoid of special type histologic features	Variable	Variable
Invasive lobular carcinoma	5–15	Architectural distortion, density (no distinct mass), multifocal/bilateral	Uniform cells, eccentric nuclei, intracytoplasmic lumina, Indian filing, targetoid pattern	Unfavorable	ER (+), PR (+), Her2 neu (−)
Tubular carcinoma	5	Speculated mass, small size	Angulated tubules with tapered ends, open lumina, dense stroma	Favorable	ER (+), PR (+), Her2 neu (−)
Mucinous or colloid carcinoma	2–3	Well-circumscribed lobulated mass, gelatinous cut surface	Tumor cells floating in pools of extracellular mucin	Favorable	ER (+), PR (+), Her2 neu (−)
Medullary carcinoma	1–2	Young women, well-circumscribed mass, no calcifications	Syncytial growth, pushing borders, infiltrated by lymphocytes and plasma cells, high nuclear grade	Favorable (if pure)	Triple negative: ER (−), PR (−), Her2 neu (−); (triple negative)
Micropapillary carcinoma	1–2	Similar to IDC, not otherwise specified (NOS)	Tumor clusters within empty spaces, reverse polarity, no fibrovascular cores	Higher rate of LN metastasis	Variable
Metaplastic carcinoma	<1	Large tumor	Tumor transformation to squamous or mesenchymal (bone, cartilage) elements	Lower LN metastasis; prognosis is very poor	Triple negative: ER (−), PR (−), Her2 neu (−) ER and PR can be positive in glandular elements, coexpression of cytokeratin (5, 6) and vimentin

include anterior, apical, internal (Rotter's nodes), central and lateral lymph nodes.
- *Divisions:* Axillary group lymph nodes are divided into three groups in relation to pectoralis minor muscle proceeding from **Level I (13 nodes)** lateral to muscle, **Level II (5 nodes)** behind muscle and **Level III (3 nodes)** medial to pectoralis minor muscle. Level I and level II lymph nodes are removed in the standard axillary dissection of breast carcinoma.

Sentinel Lymph Node

The sentinel node is usually in level I. It is unusual for the breast carcinoma to skip to higher levels of lymph nodes without involving the lower levels.

Skip Metastases

Skip metastases are seen <5% of patients with axillary lymph node involvement. It is due to lymphatic drainage from level II to level III under surface of pectoralis minor muscle.

HEMATOGENOUS ROUTE

It occurs as a result of vascular permeation in the region of the breast carcinoma, in areas of lymph node metastases with the neoplastic tissue breaking into adjacent tissue and involving blood vessels, or tumor overwhelming the lymph node barrier and reaching the systemic circulation.

Organs involved: Vascular metastases usually occur to *lungs, pleura, liver* and *bone*. Not infrequently, vascular metastases may also be seen in *adrenal glands* and *brain*.

Bone lesions due to metastases: Breast carcinoma metastasizing to bones may show either *osteolytic* or *osteoblastic* lesions.

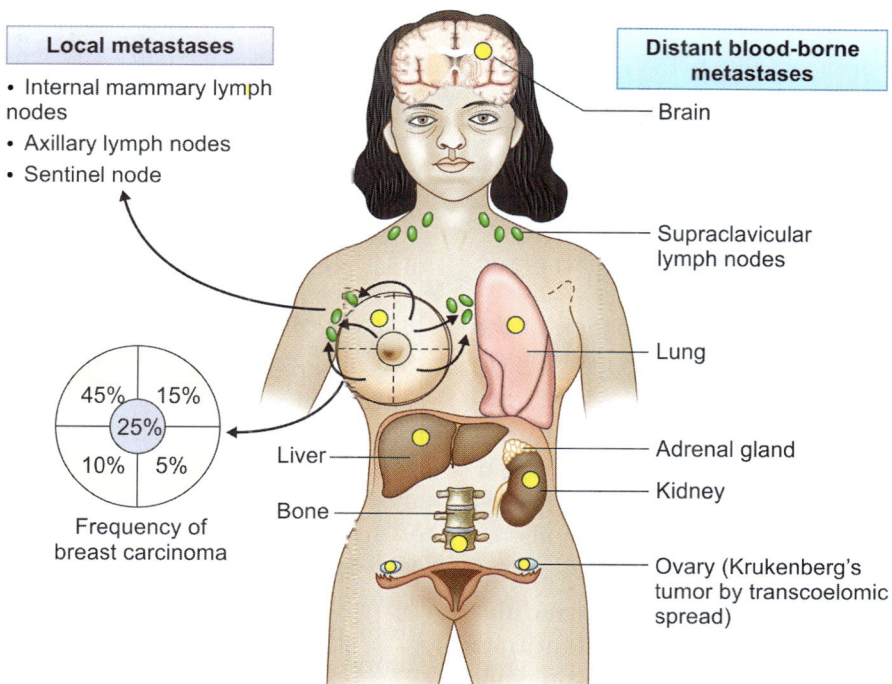

Fig. 25.52: Breast carcinoma—mode of spread of breast cancer. It also shows frequency of breast cancer in various quadrants of breast. Breast carcinoma spreads by local invasion, lymphatic, hematogenous and transcoelomic routes (*Courtesy by Dr Abhijit Das*).

Transcoelomic Route

Breast carcinoma spreading to ovaries by transcoelomic route (retrograde lymphatic channels) in elderly women. It is known as *Krukenberg tumor*. It is rapidly developing bilateral ovarian metastases from cancers of breast, stomach and intestine (Fig. 25.52).

Gross Morphology
- Tumor is large, solid, lobulated, with smooth surface and freely mobile.
- Cut surface is gray white, gelatinous, areas of hemorrhage and cystic spaces.

Light Microscopy

Tumor shows sheets of malignant epithelial cells in a dense fibromyxomatous stroma.

PROGNOSTIC AND PREDICTIVE FACTORS

There are a number of pathologic parameters capable of predicting prognosis and guiding new strategies or treatment in cases of breast carcinoma. Prognosis depends on molecular features or histological type, extent of spread of breast carcinoma (stage) at the time of diagnosis.

Invasiveness of Tumor

Breast carcinoma *in situ* (ductal or lobular) has better prognosis after surgery than invasive carcinoma. Exception is comedocarcinoma, a ductal carcinoma *in situ* (DCIS) with central necrosis and lymph node metastases.

Histological Variant of Tumor

Breast carcinomas, i.e. tubular, papillary, mucinous, microinvasive, medullary and adenoid cystic are associated with better prognosis. Patients with scirrhous type, Paget's disease of breast, secretory carcinoma and apocrine carcinoma have poor prognosis.

Distant Metastases

Breast carcinoma metastases via hematogenous route to *lungs, pleura, liver, bones, brain, adrenal glands* and *ovaries* (Krukenberg tumor) with **fatal outcome**.

Status of Axillary Lymph Nodes

The single best prognostic factor is the presence or absence of axillary nodal metastases in breast carcinoma. There is a direct correlation between survival and the number of axillary lymph nodes involved. Breast carcinoma involving beyond the axillary or internal mammary lymph nodes has a poor prognosis. Breast carcinoma limited to only supraclavicular nodes has a good prognosis.

Tumor Size

Tumor size correlates directly with survival. Patients with smaller tumors <2 cm have better survival rate than those with large tumors. Large size breast carcinoma invades locally into skeletal muscles adjoining breast.

Grading and Staging

Grading classifies tumors according to their light microscopic characteristics. Staging is a clinical exercise that classifies tumors according to their size, invasiveness and spread. Tumors are staged according to the TNM system (T:tumor size, N:lymph node involvement, M:metastases to distant organs). Schemes for TNM classification vary according to tumor type and organ involved (Fig. 25.53).

A grading system (Nottingham modification of the Bloom Richardson Grading System) utilizes histological characteristics of the breast carcinoma.

- *Basis:* It is based on assessment of entire tumor differentiation (e.g. glandular formation), nuclear pleomorphism and frequency of mitotic figures studied in formalin fixed H & E stained sections.
- *Scoring:* For example, a tumor with >75% glandular differentiation would score 1, 10–75% glandular differentiation as score 2, and <10% glandular differentiation would score grade 3. These values are combined and converted into three groups: grade I (scores 3–5), grade II (scores 6–7), and grade III (scores 8 and 9). This histological grade is often known as **Nottingham modification of the Bloom and Richardson Grading System** (Tables 25.11 to 25.13).

Invasion of Lymphatics and Blood Vessels

Invasion of lymphatic channels and blood vessels is demonstrated in 25% breast carcinoma on light microscopy. These patients have poor prognosis.

Age of the Patient

Younger women <35 age have a poorer prognosis than older patients with cancer of equivalent stage.

Markers of Proliferation

Breast carcinoma with high rate of proliferation of cancer cells in S-phase of cell cycle is associated with local recurrence and fatal outcome in comparison to slow proliferative rate of tumor. *S-phase fraction above 5% has poor prognosis*. It is estimated by the use of monoclonal antibodies such as **Ki-67, KiS1**, and **MIB-1**; and identification of proliferating cells by the use of tracers such as **bromodeoxyuridine**. Measurement of proliferation of cancer cells alone does not give complete information, but *prognosis also depends on the metastatic potential of a breast carcinoma*.

DNA Content of the Tumor

Amount of DNA content in breast carcinoma cells measured by **flow cytometry** provides indication of

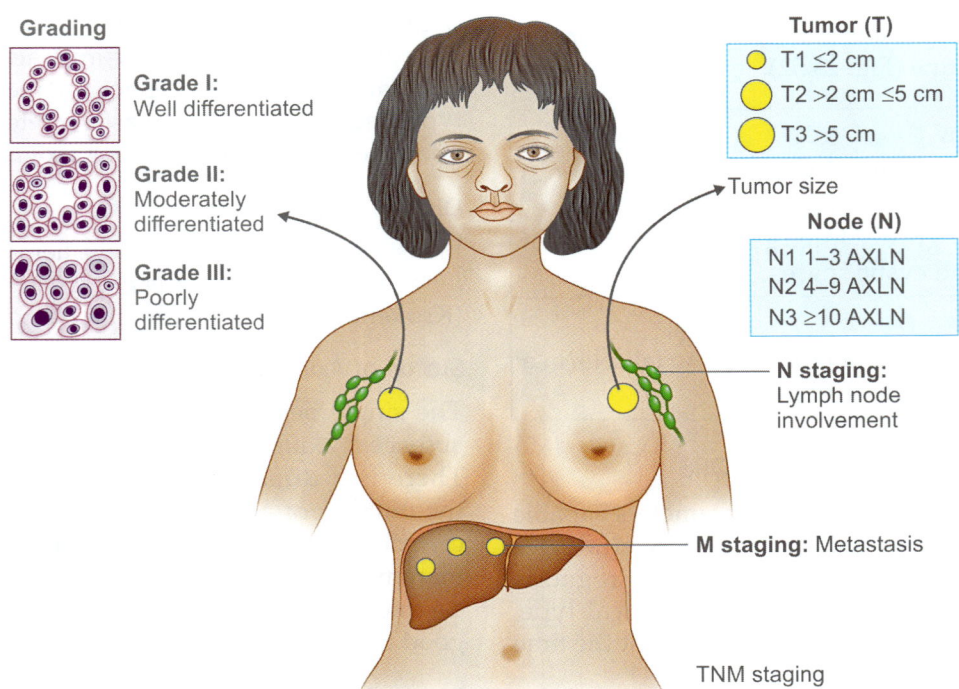

Fig. 25.53. Breast cancer shows grading and staging. TNM stands for tumor, lymph node metastases and distant metastases. Grading and staging of breast carcinoma [grading classifies tumor according to their light microscopic characteristics. Staging is a clinical exercise that classifies tumors according to their size, invasiveness and spread. Tumors are staged according to the TNM system (T: tumor size, N: lymph node involvement, M: metastases to distant organs). Schemes for TNM classification vary according to tumor type and organ involved].

Table 25.11: Nottingham modification of the Bloom and Richardson Grading System

Histology	Characteristics	Scores	Comments
% of tubules formation by tumor cells	>75%	1	Based on assessment of entire tumor
	10–75%	2	
	<10%	3	
Nuclear pleomorphism	Small uniform cells	1	Based on the worst area of tumor
	Moderate increase in size of cells	2	
	Marked variation in size of cells	3	
Mitotic count per 10 HPF	Up to 6	1	Mitotic count at the leading edge of tumor growth
	7–13	2	
	14 or above	3	

The grading is calculated by adding the above scores.

Table 25.12: Correlation of grade and survival rate

Grade	Score	Differentiation of tumor	5-Year survival (%)	7-Year survival (%)
1	3 to 5	Well differentiated tumor	95	90
2	6 or 7	Moderately differentiated tumor	75	65
3	8 or 9	Poorly differentiated	50	45

Table 25.13: Staging of breast carcinoma

Stage	Primary tumor (T)	Positive axillary lymph nodes (N)	Distant metastases	5-Year survival
0	DCIS (Ductal carcinoma *in situ*) LCIS (Lobular carcinoma *in situ*)	None	None	93%
I	Invasive carcinoma, ≤2 cm	None	None	88%
II	Invasive carcinoma, >2 cm Invasive carcinoma, <5 cm	1–3 nodes 1–3 nodes	None	74–81%
III	Invasive carcinoma, >5 cm Invasive carcinoma, any size Invasive carcinoma, attached to skin or chest wall or inflammatory carcinoma	≥4 nodes ≥4 nodes 0–>10 nodes	None None None	41–67%
IV	Any invasive carcinoma • IVa: Pectoralis major muscle involvement • IVb: Skin involvement: skin shows ulceration, satellite nodule and peu d' orange • IVc: Combination of IVa + IVb • IVd: Inflammatory breast carcinoma	Any lymph node status	Present	15%

their malignant potential. Homogenous population of cells with a *euploid* DNA content is seen in normal or benign cells. Poorly differentiated breast carcinoma shows increased DNA content. Breast carcinoma cells with *aneuploid* have a poor outcome. *Diploid tumor has better prognosis than aneuploid tumor.*

Internalized Factors

Chromosomal aneuploidy and proliferative index parameters determined by **flow cytometry** or **FISH** technique provide data on the aggressiveness of the tumor. Flow cytometry performed on the cells obtained by fine needle aspiration, excisional biopsy, or resection from a breast carcinoma can be analyzed to determine the characteristics of the DNA content. The presence of an increased proliferative rate (high S-phase) and aneuploidy in the flow cytometric pattern of breast carcinoma, suggest a worse prognosis.

Hormone Receptors

The hormone receptor status (*estrogen and progesterone*) of the breast carcinoma cells can be useful information for treatment and prognosis. *Breast carcinoma with positive estrogen receptor (ER) treated by estrogen receptor blocker such as tamoxifen has better prognosis.* In general ER positive breast carcinoma has progesterone positive status. Significance of progesterone status is less well understood.

Amplification of Proto-oncogenes

There is increased expression of oncogenes in breast carcinoma; which include Her2 neu, INT2, and C-MYC.

Her2 neu Gene

Physiological state: It encodes for an epithelial growth factor receptor on the cell membrane that stimulates cellular proliferation. Amplification of Her2 neu oncogene is associated with poorly differentiated tumors (high nuclear grade), metastasizing to lymph nodes, with high rate of recurrence, a small chance of survival and aneuploidy (abnormal number of chromosome).

Associated carcinomas: Amplification of Her2 neu is identified in 10 to 35% of primary breast carcinoma (high-grade tumors). It has also been demonstrated in carcinomas of the lung, ovary, and stomach.

Immunohistochemistry: It is demonstrated as c-erbB2 protein by immunohistochemistry on the cell membrane or by analysis of the Her2 neu gene using fluorescent *in situ* hybridization. These patients exhibiting Her2 neu gene amplification are treated with a monoclonal antibody (herceptin that selectively binds to the extracellular domain of the protein.

Galectin 3

Physiological state: Galectin 3 is a member of lectin family. It is encoded by LGALS3 gene located on chromosome 14, locus q21–q22. It is expressed in the nucleus, cytoplasm and extracellular space.

Pathological state: Galectin overexpression promotes neoplastic transformation and the maintenance of transformed phenotypes as well as enhances adhesion of tumor cells to the extracellular matrix in breast carcinoma.

Tumor Suppressor Gene Mutations

Physiological state: NM23, p53 and RB are tumor suppressor genes.

Pathological state: Mutations of these genes lead to overexpression of oncogenes resulting in breast carcinoma. These gene mutations are significantly related to poor differentiation, disease recurrence, diminished survival and absence of steroid hormone receptors.

Associated cancer: RB tumor suppressor gene mutation is also seen in retinoblastoma, breast carcinoma, osteosarcoma glioblastoma, bladder carcinoma and small cell carcinoma lung.

Epidermal Growth Factor Receptors (EGFR)

Physiological state: It is a polypeptide expressed within membrane of breast carcinoma cells. It participates in cell growth.

Pathological state: Breast carcinoma with over-expression of EGFR is associated with poor survival. There is no role of estrogen receptor blocker (tamoxifen) in these patients.

Alterations in Cell Structure

There is increased expression of vimentin, and decreased expression of 'fodrin' in some cases of breast carcinoma.

Loss of Cell Adhesion Molecules

There is loss of integrin in poorly differentiated breast carcinoma; and E-cadherin in lobular variant of breast carcinoma in some cases.

Protease (Cathepsin D)

Physiological state: It is an estrogen induced acidic lysosomal protease 16 demonstrated in the cytoplasm of nonductal carcinomas of breast. It is also found in the stroma between the cells. It has growth promoting activity and extracellular proteolytic activity.

Pathological state: Overexpression of cathepsin D is associated with lymph node metastases and poor prognosis.

Stress Response Proteins (Heat Shock Protein 27)

Physiological state: It is estrogen related heat shock protein or stress response protein (Srp 27).

Pathological state: Overexpression of Srp 27 is associated with nodal and widespread hematogenous metastases to distant organs.

Secondary Messenger Systems

Physiological state: Cyclic AMP binding proteins are the regulatory subunits of a major second messenger system—protein kinase A.

Pathological state: These are overexpressed in 10–15% of cases. Breast carcinoma expressing high concentration of cyclic AMP is associated with poor outcome.

Prognostic and predictive factors are shown in Table 25.14.

Table 25.14: Prognostic and predictive factors of breast carcinoma

Features	Good prognosis	Poor prognosis
Age group	30–50	<30 and >50
Diagnosis	Early	Late
Treatment	Early	Late
Metastases	Absent	Present
Histologic types of breast carcinoma	Ductal carcinoma *in situ* except comedo-carcinoma	Invasive ductal carcinoma
	Low-grade invasive ductal carcinoma (NOS): luminal type A	High-grade invasive ductal carcinoma (NOS): it is Her2 neu enrich breast carcinoma. Her2 neu is sensitive to herceptin. It may be of *basal type* of breast carcinoma
	Lobular carcinoma *in situ*/invasive: luminal type A	Paget's disease of breast with IDC
	Tubular carcinoma: luminal type A	Micropapillary carcinoma: luminal type B
	Cribriform carcinoma: luminal type A	Metaplastic carcinoma: basal type and luminal type B
	Colloid carcinoma	Medullary carcinoma: basal type
	Papillary carcinoma	Secretory carcinoma
Tumor morphology	<2 cm size	>2 cm size
	Pushing margin	Infiltrative margin
	Absence of necrosis	Presence of necrosis
Hormonal status	Estrogen positive	Estrogen negative
	Progesterone positive	Progesterone negative
C-erbB2	Negative	Positive
p53	Negative	Positive
Srp 27	Negative	Positive
Cathepsin D	Negative	Positive
EGFR	Negative	Positive

MISCELLANEOUS DISEASES OF THE FEMALE BREAST

Congenital Hypoplasia of the Breast

Absence of the underlying pectoralis muscles is often associated with this condition.

Juvenile Hypertrophy of the Left Breast

The redness of breast occurs due to cellulitis from ulceration caused by wearing a bra that is too tight. This benign lesion is removed followed by reconstruction of breast (Fig. 25.54).

Accessory Nipple

Accessory nipples occur in both sexes and may be found anywhere on the 'milk line' from the axilla to the groin.

LABORATORY DIAGNOSIS OF BREAST LUMPS

Clinical History

History of lump, mode of onset, duration of symptoms, rate of growth, pain in breast, nipple discharge and bone pain.

Clinical Examination

Nipple, areola, overlying skin, swelling and draining lymph nodes should be examined.

- *Nipple retraction:* It occurs in association with both breast carcinoma and inflammatory conditions.
- *Skin dimpling or a change in contour.* It is present in a high percentage of patients with breast carcinoma.

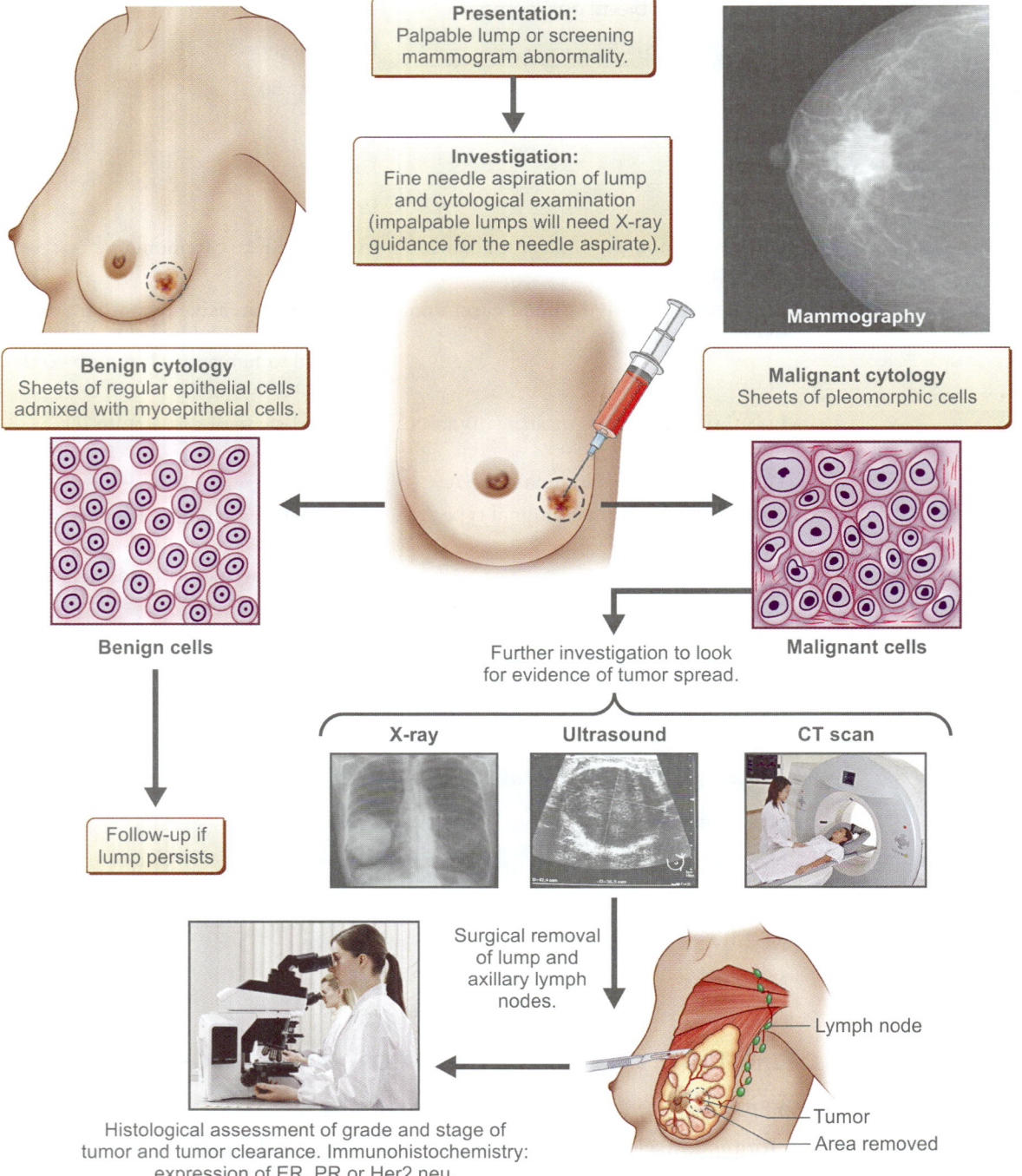

Fig. 25.54: Investigation of a breast lump.

- *Nipple and areola eczema:* Paget's disease affects the nipple from the start, whereas eczema affects the areolar region first and only rarely affects the nipple skin, which eventually leads to erosion and ulceration of the nipple in elderly women. Eczema also occurs due to inflammation in the region.
- *Peau d'orange skin: Inflammatory carcinoma* is a descriptive term referring to a clinical appearance resembling diffuse acute mastitis. It implies dermal lymphatic channels invasion by underlying usually infiltrating ductal carcinoma.
- *Axillary lymph nodes:* These are palpable in 40% of patients with breast carcinoma.

Imaging Diagnostic Tools

Digital Mammography

Digital mammography is screening procedure to detect non-palpable 2–3 mm breast masses. Most mammographic calcification in benign lesions is indeterminate. A few benign lesions such as oil cysts, calcified fibroadenomas and vascular calcification have diagnostic mammographic features. Directional vacuum-assisted core biopsies can remove small benign calcified lesions. BIRADS system (breast imaging and radiological analysis data system) is used for reporting mammograms (Table 25.15, Figs 25.55 and 25.56).

- Microcalcifications most often occur in ductal cancer *in situ* and sclerosing adenosis. The risk of carcinoma increases with increase in the number of calcium specks in a cluster.
- Presence of 5 or more tightly clustered microcalcifications with in 1 cm area of breast lump is considered a threshold for suspicion of cancer. Fibroadenoma shows popcorn calcification.

Table 25.15: BIRADS system used for reporting mammograms

Seven categories	BIRADS system is used for reporting mammograms: It has seven categories	Management	Likelihood of breast carcinoma
0	Incomplete assessment: it needs to additional imaging or prior examinations	Recall for additional imaging and/or await prior examinations	Not applicable
1	Negative assessment	Routine screening	Essentially 0%
2	Benign lesion	Routine screening	Essentially 0%
3	Probably benign lesion	Short interval follow-up for 6 months and then continued	>0% and <2%
4	Suspicious lesion	Tissue diagnosis	4a. Low suspicion for malignancy (>2% to <10%)
			4b. Moderate suspicion of malignancy (>10% to <50%)
			4c. High suspicion of malignancy (>50% to <95%)
5	Highly suspicious of malignancy	Tissue diagnosis	>95%
6	Biopsy proved breast carcinoma	Surgical excision when clinical appropriate	Not applicable

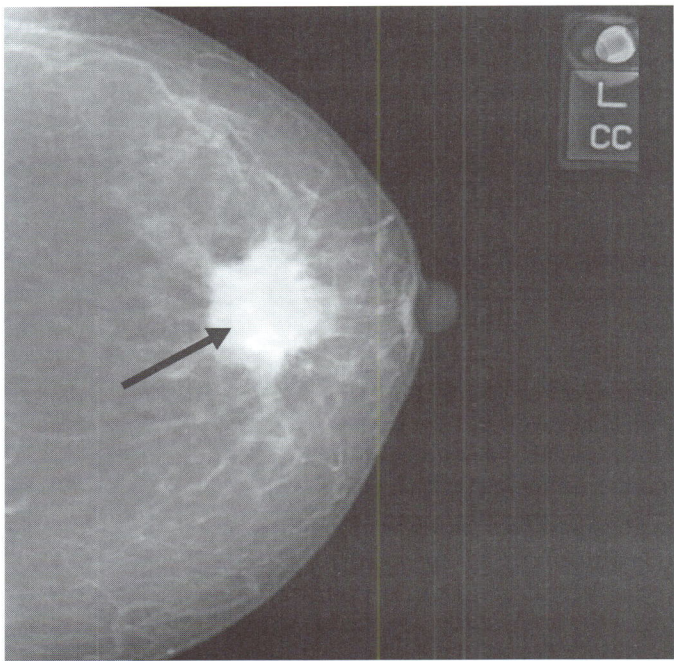

Fig. 25.55: Mammogram shows breast carcinoma: BIRADS 5 (highly suspicious) (arrow).

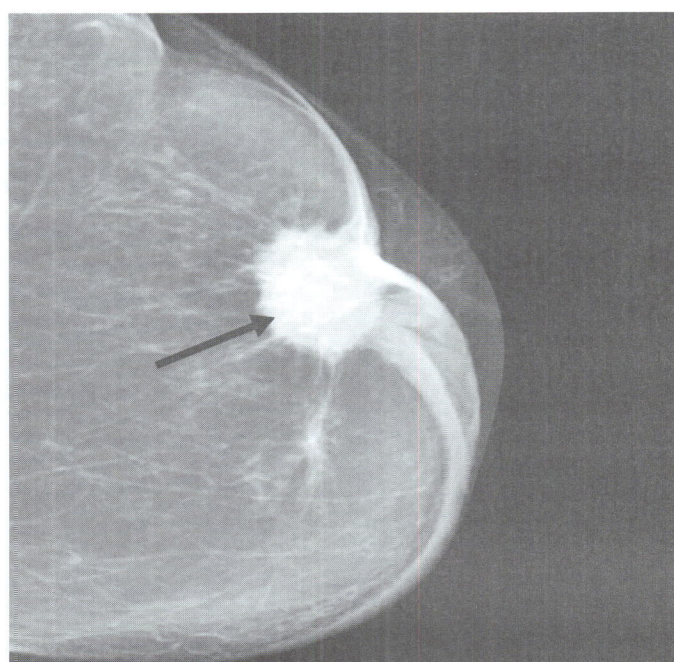

Fig. 25.56: Mammogram shows breast infiltrating carcinoma (biopsy proved breast carcinoma: BIRADS 6) (arrow).

- Mammographic densities are formed due to replacement of adipose tissue with radio-dense tissue. Fibrocystic disease shows rounded densities. Breast carcinoma form irregular masses.
- Approximately 10% breast carcinoma are not detected by mammography.

Ultrasonography

Ultrasound is the best investigation to differentiate cysts (transparent lesion) from solid lesions such as benign lesions (well demarcated) and breast carcinomas (indistinct outlines).

Bone Scan

It is also known as **bone scintigraphy**. It is done to evaluate breast metastases in bone by injecting radioactive substance by intravenous route. After 2–4 hours of absorption of radioactive substance, body scans (films) are taken. This radioactive substance is collected in areas of new bone formation formed by metastases. These areas appear as dark patches on the film. Any part of the bone may be affected by the cancer.

CT Scan

It can detect breast carcinomas and permit visualization of both axillary and internal mammary lymph nodes. High cost and irradiation exposure are drawbacks.

Magnetic Resonance Imaging

MRI is better for assessing lesions in dense breasts than other methods. It is used for evaluation of breast carcinoma, staging of disease (metastases in lungs, bones, liver, brain and ovaries) and detection of silicon prosthesis.

Color Doppler

It gives a picture showing the blood supply to the lump. Imaging techniques are given in Table 25.16.

Triple Assessment

It is the combination of clinical examination, imaging (e.g. mammography for women aged 35 or over and ultrasonography for women under 35), and fine needle aspiration cytology.

Fine Needle Aspiration Cytology

Fine needle aspiration cytology is commonly done to aspirate breast lesions. The smears are stained by May-Grünwald Giemsa (MGG) stain (Figs 25.57 to 25.60) and Papanicolaou stain.

Breast Biopsies

- *Core biopsy:* A small core is removed from the mass by means of a cutting needle technique. It is to interpret results on small biopsy measuring 2 cm in length and 1.0 mm wide.

Table 25.16: Imaging techniques used to detect breast lesions

Imaging techniques	Interpretation
Digital mammography: It detects 2–3 mm lesion. BIRADS system is used for reporting mammograms. Seven categories are described	• Assessment incomplete: 0 • Negative assessment: 1 • Benign lesion assessment: 2 • Probably benign lesion: 3 • Suspicious lesion assessment: 4 • Highly suspicious of malignancy: 5 • Biopsy proved breast carcinoma: 6
	Note: Popcorn calcification is seen in fibroadenoma. Breast tumor showing 5 or more dense calcified deposits in 1 × 1 cm area is highly suspicious of cancer.
Ultrasonography	• It detects cysts (transparent lesion), benign lesions (well demarcated) and breast carcinomas (indistinct outlines)
Bone scan	• It is used for staging of breast carcinoma
CT scan	• Detection of breast carcinoma and involvement of draining axillary and internal mammary lymph nodes
MRI	• Evaluation of breast carcinoma and staging disease (metastases in lungs, bones, liver, brain and ovaries)
Color Doppler	• Visualization of blood supply to the lump

Breast

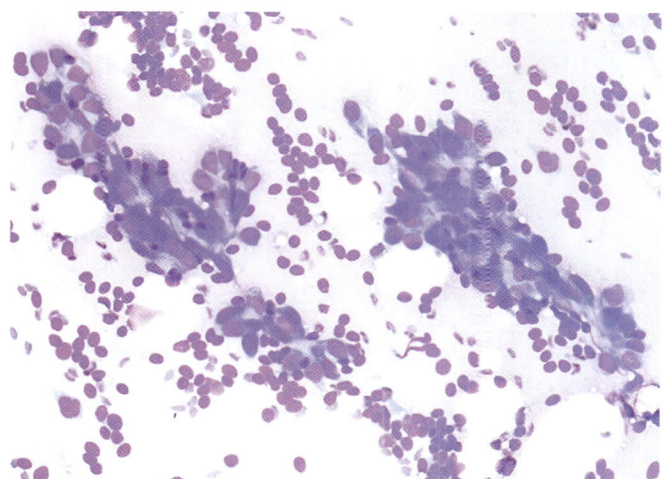

Fig. 25.57: Fibroadenoma breast—fine needle aspirate smear shows benign ductal cells arranged in clusters. Stromal cells are also seen (400X).

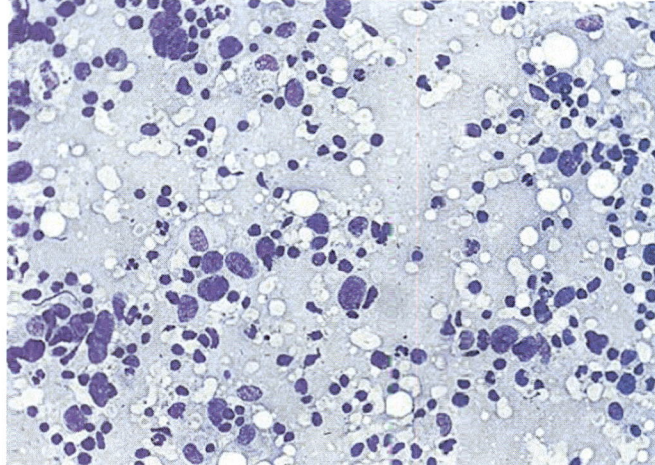

Fig. 25.59: Breast medullary carcinoma—fine needle aspirate smear shows pleomorphic atypical cells with hyperchromatic nuclei and prominent nucleoli arranged in clusters and dissociated forms. In the background, there is presence of lymphocytes (400X).

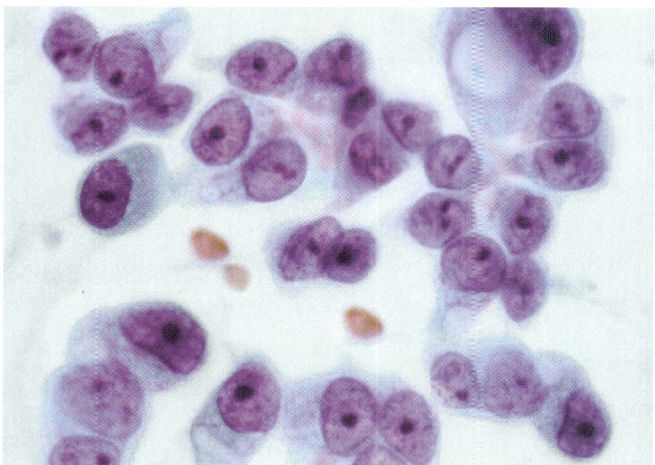

Fig. 25.58: Breast cancer—fine needle aspirate smear shows pleomorphic atypical cells with hyperchromatic nuclei and prominent nucleoli arranged in clusters and dissociated forms (400X).

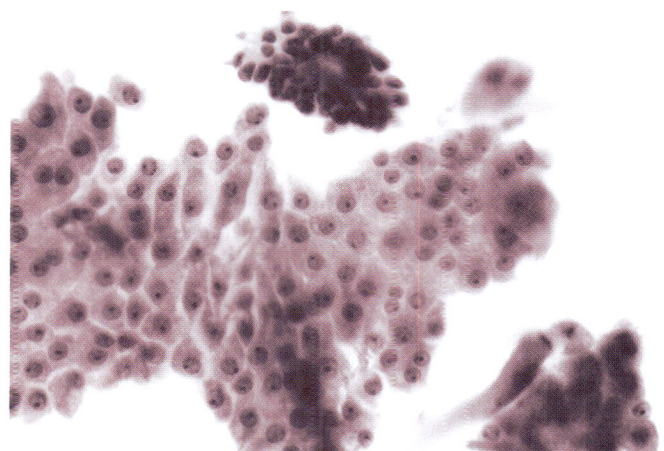

Fig. 25.60: Fibrocystic disease of breast—fine needle aspirate smear shows benign ductal cells arranged in clusters. Apocrine change is seen in the ductal cells (400X).

- *Open biopsy:* Open biopsy should be performed only in patients who have been appropriately investigated by imaging, fine needle aspiration cytology, and, if appropriate, core biopsy. The specimen is fixed in 10% buffered formalin to obtain paraffin sections. Hematoxylin and eosin stained sections are studied by light microscopy. Freshly prepared 2% buffered glutaraldehyde is recommended for fixation of tissues for electron microscopy.
- *Skin biopsy:* Skin biopsy from areola or nipple is important in diagnosing Paget's disease of breast (ductal carcinoma involving epidermis) and inflammatory carcinoma in which dermal lymphatic channels are involved.
- *Sentinel lymph node biopsy:* Sampling of initial node that drains the tumor is done. If negative for metastases, the other nodes in that group are usually negative. If positive for metastases, there is a one-third chance that other nodes in the group have metastases.

Frozen Section Technique

It is a rapid diagnostic technique before proceeding to definite surgery to confirm breast carcinoma, assessment of margins around tumor, and lymph node involvement. Tissues are quickly frozen, sectioned, mounted on slides, stained and interpreted within a few minutes, which enable surgeon to take appropriate decisions about the extent of surgery.

Diagnostic difficulties occur in the presence of papillary lesions, sclerosing adenosis, florid adenosis, atypical ductular hyperplasia, fat necrosis, and lobular carcinoma *in situ* cause diagnostic problems on frozen section evaluation. These lesions are best diagnosed with paraffin embedded sections.

Histological Examination

- *Processing of specimen:* Tru cut biopsy, biopsy; lumpectomy and mastectomy specimens including lymph nodes are fixed in *10% buffered formalin*. Sections obtained from *paraffin embedded blocks* are stained with hematoxylin and eosin.
- *Hormonal study:* The presence of *estrogen* and *progesterone receptors* in nodal metastases is highly suggestive of the presence of primary occult disease in breast.
- *Immunohistochemistry:* It plays an important role in differentiating poorly differentiating carcinoma from lymphoma and benign from malignant lesions. It has diagnostic role in staging breast carcinoma to evaluate tumor markers in fluids and other tissues.

  Various tumor markers used in breast carcinoma include ER, PR, c-erbB2/Her2 neu, cytokeratin CK-7 (high molecular weight), epithelial membrane antigen, milk fat globule membrane antigen, α-lactalbumin (human milk), and *lactoferritin* (Table 25.17).
- *Serum tumor markers:* CA 15.3 is a cell surface glycoprotein originally identified in mucinous epithelial ovarian tumors and recognized by the monoclonal antibody OC 125. Other serum markers for diagnosis of breast carcinoma are GCDFA-15 (gross cystic disease fluid protein-15). CA 27–29, carcinoembryonic antigen (CEA), BRCA, PS2, PTHrP, gross cystic disease fluid protein-15 (FCDFA-15) and mammaglobin.

Recent Advances

Until recently, prognosis and treatment of breast carcinoma were based on clinicopathological analysis of the mastectomy specimen and lymph node status. Breast carcinoma was classified according to tumor type (ductal *vs* lobular infiltrating carcinoma), histological grade (I to III), hormone receptor and Her2 neu status (positive *vs* negative), involvement of the lymph nodes and distant metastasis. But these factors alone were insufficient to reflect the biological heterogeneity fo breast malignancies. Molecular testing of breast carcinoma has focussed on identifying patients at high risk of relapse or who can be benefited from adjuvant therapy even in node negative hormone positive tumors. Some of the well established gene signature tests widely in use are *Mammaprint score, Oncotype Dx and Prosigna kit.* All these tests are aimed at subclassifying early breast carcinoma.

- Mamma print is the first FDA approved gene microarray based prognostic score the utilizes fresh frozen tissue. Top 70 genes that regulate cell cycle, invasion, metastasis, and angiogenesis are evaluated. Tumor has been classified either as high-risk or a low-risk.
- Oncotype Dx assay is a RT-PCR-based assay can be performed on formalin fixed specimens. It analyses 21 genes that include oncogenes and housekeeping genes. The assy computes a recurrence score from 0 to 100, which can be categorized into low risk (<18), intermediate risk (18–30) and high risk (score ≥31). It also predicts and risk of recurrence after 10 years of surgery.
- Prosigna kit utilises formalin fixed paraffin embedded tissue to check for mRNA expression of 50 genes used

Table 25.17: Tumor markers of breast carcinoma

Evaluation method	Marker
Serum tumor marker	• CA 15.3 • CA 27.29 • Carcinoembryonic antigen (CEA) • BRCA • PS2 • PTHrP • Mammaglobin • Gross cystic disease fluid protein-15 (GCDFA-15)
Immunohistochemistry (ductal cell)	• Estrogen receptor (ER) • Progesterone receptor (PR) • Her2 neu • p53 • Galectin 3 • Cathepsin D • Stress respone protein 27 (Srp 27) • Milk fat globule membrane antigen • Lactalbumin • CK5 • CK7 • NY-BR1 (highly undifferentiated breast carcinoma)
Immunohistochemistry (myoepithelial markers)	• p63 • S-100 • α-smooth muscle actin (α-SMA) • Glial fibrillary acidic protein (GFAP)
Flow cytometry	• DNA ploidy • S-phase
FISH (fluorescence *in situ* hybridization)	• Her2 neu

in the PAM50 molecular classification algorithm and five other housekeeping genes. Qualitative *in vitro* diagnostic tool that utilized gene expression data with clinical variables like tumor size and nodal status. This test can be performed in decentralised laboratories too unlike the first two tests. It calculates increase risk of recurrence and probability of distant recurrence.

Next generation sequencing has revolutionised breast carcinoma genomics and is expected to provide insights on personalised treatment of breast carcinoma patients. With its increasing use, novel therapeutic tragets are expected to be identified.

MANAGEMENT OF BREAST CARCINOMA

Treatment of breast carcinoma depends on the stage of the disease. Several options for treatment are most often used in combination for best results. These are described as under.

Surgical Procedures

Surgical procedures include lumpectomy, mastectomy (partial, total, or radical).

Lumpectomy

It is a segmental mastectomy with microscopically free margins, plus sentinel node and low level I and II axillary node resection (breast conservative therapy) that is followed by radiation therapy.

Modified Radical Mastectomy

It is removal of all ipsilateral breast tissue, the pectoralis minor muscle, the nipple-areola complex, and level I, II and III axillary lymph nodes below axillary vein.

Lymph nodes are examined for signs of further metastases. A winged scapula may occur due to damage of the long thoracic nerve. There is also a danger for developing lymphedema.

Radiation Therapy

Radiation therapy can be directed at the tumor, the breast, the chest wall, or other tissues known or suspected to have remaining cancer cells. Radiation therapy is aimed to slow or shrink tumor to make surgery easier.

Chemotherapy

Chemotherapy is used to reduce the size of growth for making surgery easier. It is used to help eliminate cancer cells that may still remain in the breast or that may have already spread to other parts of the body.

Hormonal Therapy

Hormone therapy with tamoxifen is used to block the effects of estrogen that may otherwise help breast carcinoma cells to survive and grow.

Most women with breast carcinoma expressing estrogen or progesterone on their surface benefit from treatment with tamoxifen.

Aromatase Inhibitors

A new class of medicines called *aromatase inhibitors*, such as aromasin has been shown to be as good as or possibly even better than tamoxifen in women with stage IV breast carcinoma.

Biological Therapy

Monoclonal antibodies may be administered to attack potential cancer cells and reduce the risk of recurrence. Herceptin monoclonal antibody binds *Her2 neu* on tumor cell surface and induces receptor internalization.

MALE BREASTS

GYNECOMASTIA

Gynecomastia is enlargement of the male breast analogous to juvenile hypertrophy of the female breast. This condition occurs most commonly at about puberty, presumably resulting from mild hormonal imbalance. It may occur also during adult life. It is morphologically similar to juvenile hypertrophy of the female breast.

Etiopathogenesis

- Unilateral gynecomastia is most often idiopathic. Only very occasional cases of gynecomastia are caused by an endocrine tumor. It is most often bilateral due to secondary causes. It occurs due to excess of circulating estrogens or a relative increase in the estrogen and androgen ratio. Estrogen excess relative to androgens results in proliferation of both ducts and stroma.
- *Gynecomastia is associated with:* (i) hormone-secreting adrenal or testicular neoplasms (estrogenic), (ii) paraneoplastic production of gonadotropins by cancers, (iii) Klinefelter's syndrome, and (iv) liver cirrhosis is characterized by increased conversion of androstenedione into estrogens.
- Liver normally inactivates estrogen in men. Male patients with cirrhosis no longer inactivate estrogen.

Hyperestrinism, in men manifests gynecomastia, loss of chest and pubic hair, impotence, testicular atrophy and palmar erythema (liver palms); spider nevi (capillary telangiectasis) of the face, upper arms, and chest.

Light Microscopy
- Histological examination shows active epithelium within a proliferation of mammary ducts with piling of nuclei in the ducts, periductal fibrosis with numerous fibroblast nuclei.
- No lobules are found in the male breast.

Clinical Features
The patient presents with unilateral or bilateral breast enlargement initially in the subareolar region.

INVASIVE DUCTAL CARCINOMA
Invasive ductal carcinoma is uncommon breast carcinoma in males. Prognosis is poor to that of female breast carcinoma.

Risk Factors
Klinefelter's syndrome and BRCA1 mutation increase risk of breast carcinoma in men.

Clinical Features
Patient usually presents as a painless, firm subareolar mass or a mass in the outer quadrant of the breast. Male breast carcinoma tends to present at advanced clinical stages and with more lymph node metastasis due to paucity of breast tissue in males. *The tumor invades the chest wall muscles.* The clinical presentation of breast carcinoma in males is similar to that in females, except for higher median age at presentation in males.

Light Microscopy
- Approximately 85% of male mammary carcinomas are of the infiltrating duct type.
- Tumor is composed of pleomorphic atypical cells with hyperchromatic nuclei and prominent nucleoli. Cells are arranged in sheets and clusters with presence of mitotic figures.

Immunohistochemistry
These tumors are ER positive in 81% of cases. ER positive invasive ductal carcinoma has better prognosis than ER negative.

Management
Modified radical mastectomy followed by external radiation therapy is the standard treatment for male breast carcinoma. Hormonal therapy, as an adjuvant treatment, is the first-line approach in a majority of patients, and chemotherapy is reserved for patients with poor prognostic factors.

CHAPTER 26

Endocrine System: Pancreas, Thyroid, Parathyroid, Adrenal and Pituitary Glands

Learning Objectives

ENDOCRINE PANCREAS
- Anatomy and Physiology

DIABETES MELLITUS
- Pathophysiology of Diabetes Mellitus
- Mechanism of Organs Damage
- Laboratory Diagnosis

THYROID GLAND
- Anatomy
- Physiology
- Thyroiditis
- Hypothyroidism
- Hyperthyroidism
- Goiter
- Neoplasms of Thyroid Gland
- Thyroid Gland Anomalies
- Thyroid Function Tests

DISEASES OF PARATHYROID GLANDS
- Anatomy and Physiology
- Regulation of Calcium Metabolism
- Calcium Metabolism
- Vitamin D Metabolism
- Hyperparathyroidism
- Hypoparathyroidism
- Pseudohypoparathyroidism
- Neoplasms

DISEASES OF ADRENAL GLANDS
- Adrenal Hyperfunction
- Adrenal Cortical Insufficiency
- Adrenal Virilism (Adrenogenital Syndrome)
- Neoplasms of Adrenal Medulla
- Neoplasms of Adrenal Cortex

PITUITARY GLAND
- Anatomy and Physiology
- Hypofunctioning of Anterior Pituitary Gland
- Hypofunctioning of Posterior Pituitary Gland

ENDOCRINE PANCREAS

ANATOMY AND PHYSIOLOGY

Pancreas is a compound gland, i.e. exocrine and endocrine glands. Islets of Langerhans comprise three types of cells (α, β and δ cells) constituting 1–2% of pancreatic tissue.

Annular pancreas is a congenital condition in which the head of the pancreas surrounds the second portion of the duodenum. It may be associated with duodenal atresia. Infants present with feeding disorders and growth retardation (Fig. 26.1).

Functions of Islets of Langerhans

α Cells of Pancreas

Low blood glucose stimulates release of glucagon by α cells of pancreas. Glucagon acts on liver and adipose tissue, increases blood sugar levels by glycogenolysis and gluconeogenesis. Hyperglycemia inhibits release of glucagon.

- *Glycogenolysis:* Glucagon acts on hepatocytes resulting in breaking down glycogen into glucose (Fig. 26.2).

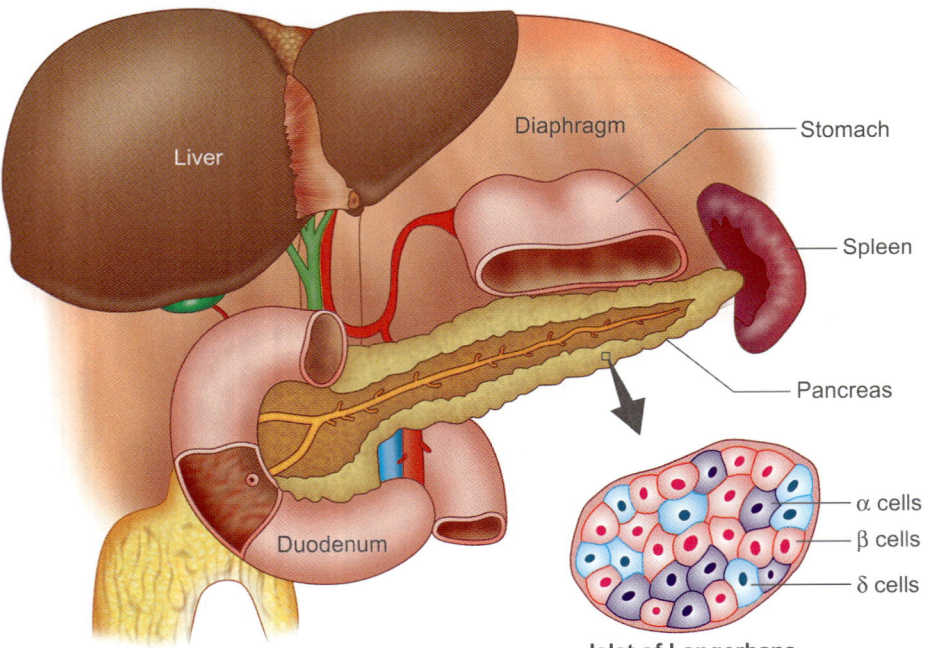

Fig. 26.1: Pancreas (islets) arrangement of the various cell types in a typical islet of Langerhans.

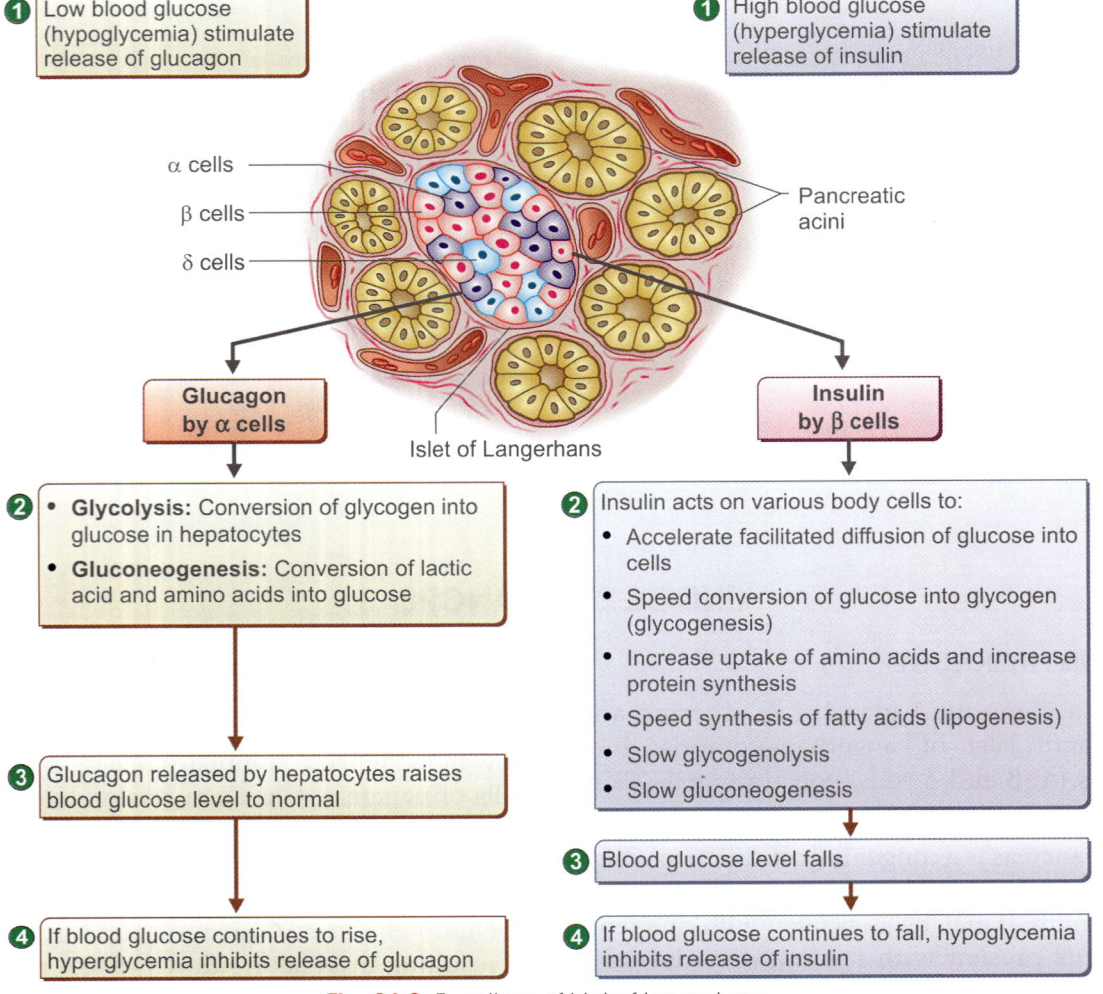

Fig. 26.2: Functions of islet of Langerhans.

- *Neoglucogenesis:* Lactic acid and certain amino acids are converted into glucose in liver by glucagon.

β Cells of Pancreas

β cells situated around capillaries within pancreatic lobules synthesize insulin.

High blood glucose level (hyperglycemia) stimulates release of insulin. *Insulin acts on principal target tissues, i.e. liver, adipose tissue and skeletal muscles.*

It accelerates facilitated diffusion of glucose into the cells resulting in decreased blood sugar levels. Actions of insulin and glucagon on glucose, fat and proteins metabolism are given in Table 26.1.

- *Carbohydrate metabolism:* Insulin speeds conversion of glucose into glycogen (glycogenesis) in liver and muscles. It inhibits glycolysis and gluconeogenesis.
- *Fat metabolism:* Insulin speeds synthesis of fatty acids (lipogenesis) from glucose derived from adipose tissue. It inhibits metabolic breakdown of fat.
- *Protein metabolism:* Insulin increases uptake of amino acids and protein synthesis by liver. It inhibits protein breakdown.

δ Cells of Pancreas

- These cells secrete somatostatin hormone, and inhibit the release of insulin by pancreas. It decreases secretion, motility and absorption in the digestive tract.
- Somatostatin also inhibits the pituitary release of growth hormone.

Synthesis of Insulin

- Rough endoplasmic reticulum of pancreatic β cells synthesize inactive form pre-proinsulin. It is transferred to Golgi apparatus. Pre-proinsulin gets cleaved into insulin and C-peptide.
- **C peptide levels** are marker of endogenous synthesis of insulin. Its estimation is used to *distinguish type 1 diabetes mellitus from type 2 diabetes mellitus* (Table 26.2). Pathogensis of type 1 diabetes mellitus is shown in Fig. 26.3.

Function of Insulin

Normally, insulin molecules bind to the receptors on the body's cells. It allows glucose entry into the cells, where it is converted to glycogen to be utilized for

Table 26.1: Actions of insulin and glucagon on carbohydrate, fat and protein metabolism

Parameters	Insulin	Glucagon
Carbohydrate metabolism (glucose)		
Glucose transport	Insulin enhances glucose transport to skeletal muscle and adipose tissue	–
Glycogen synthesis	Increased glycogen synthesis	Enhances glycogen breakdown
Gluconeogenesis	Decreases gluconeogenesis	Increases gluconeogenesis
Fat metabolism		
Fatty acids and triglycerides synthesis	Promotes fatty acid and triglycerides by the liver	–
Fat storage in adipose tissue	Increases fatty acid into adipose tissue	–
	Increases the conversion of fatty acids into triglycerides by increasing availability of α-glycerol phosphate through increased transport of glucose in adipose tissue	–
	Maintains fat storage by inhibiting breakdown of stored triglycerides by adipose cell lipase	Activates adipose cell lipase, making increased amounts of fatty acids available to the body for use as energy
Proteins metabolism		
Amino acids transport	Increases active transport of amino acids into the cells	Increases amino acids uptake by liver cells and their conversion to glucose by gluconeogenesis
Protein synthesis	Increases protein synthesis by increasing transcription of messenger RNA and accelerating protein synthesis by ribosomal RNA	–
	Decreases protein breakdown by increasing the use of glucose and fatty acids as fuel	–

Table 26.2: C-peptide levels in type 1 and type 2 diabetes mellitus

Parameters	Type 1 diabetes mellitus	Type 2 diabetes mellitus
β cell mass	β cell mass is reduced	β cell mass is normal
Endogenous insulin synthesis	It is absent or reduced	There is normal synthesis of insulin. But peripheral tissue shows resistance to insulin
Blood C-peptide level	Absent or low level	Increased level

energy. It also stimulates protein synthesis and free fatty acid storage in adipose tissue. *Insulin deficiency blocks tissues access to essential nutrients for fuel and storage.*

Insulin Receptor Substrate Molecules

Insulin receptor substrate molecules (IRS-1, IRS-2, IRS-3 and IRS-4) play central role in insulin signaling and maintenance of basic cellular functions, i.e. growth, survival and metabolism.

IRS-1 and IRS-2 participate in glucose production in liver, glucose uptake in skeletal muscle and adipose tissue; and insulin synthesis by pancreatic β cells.

IRS-1 plays central role in glucose production in skeletal muscle. IRS-2 participates in regulation of insulin uptake by liver. It also takes part in development and survival of pancreatic β cells.

IRS-3 and IRS-4 play central role in insulin signaling. IRS-1 defect has been demonstrated in type 2 diabetes mellitus.

DIABETES MELLITUS

Diabetes mellitus is a metabolic disease of carbohydrate, fat and protein brought about by impaired β cell synthesis or release of insulin, or the inability of tissues to utilize insulin leading to hyperglycemia.

Uncontrolled diabetes mellitus is associated with increased risk of **life-threatening complications,** i.e. macrovascular diseases (*atherosclerosis*) like coronary artery disease, cerebral vascular disease, peripheral vascular disease (gangrene) and microvascular diseases like *retinopathy, nephropathy* and *neuropathy.*

Diagnostic Criteria of Diabetes Mellitus

Euglycemic individual (normal person): Fasting blood glucose <100 mg/dl is considered as normal and <140 mg/dl is considered as normal after oral glucose tolerance test (OGTT) (Table 26.3). Diagnostic criteria of diabetes mellitus is any one of the following:

- *Fasting blood glucose level ≥ 126 mg/dl (7 mmol/L):* Fasting is defined as no caloric intake for at least 8 hours.
- *Random blood glucose level ≥ 200 mg/dl (11.1 mmol/L):* Patient has classical signs and symptoms of diabetes mellitus.
- *Abnormal blood sugar level after oral glucose tolerance test (OGTT):* Two-hour plasma glucose level is estimated after a glucose challenge of 1.75 g/kg (maximum dose of 75 g) is ≥ 200 mg/dl (11.1 mmol/L).
- *Impaired oral glucose tolerance test (OGTT):* Individuals with fasting blood glucose between 100 and 126 and OGTT between 140 and 200 mg/dl are considered pre-diabetics. *There is increased risk of development of diabetes mellitus in 5–10% of cases.*
- *HbA1c (Glycated hemoglobin):* Hemoglobin A1c is ≥ 6.5% is accepted additional criteria for diagnosing diabetes mellitus. *Glycosylated HbA1c is formed by non-enzymatic combination of glucose with globin of hemoglobin. Its estimation is used for diagnosis and monitoring diabetes mellitus (Table 26.4).*

Table 26.3: Diagnostic criteria of diabetes mellitus (any one of these criteria) adapted from the American Diabetes Association

Test	Normoglycemic state	Diabetes mellitus
Fasting blood sugar*	<100 mg/dl (5.6 mmol/L)	≥126 mg/dl (7 mmol/L)
Two-hour OGTTs	<140 mg/dl (7.8 mmol/L)	≥200 mg/dl (11.1 mmol/L)
HbA1c (glycated hemoglobin)	–	≥ 6.5%
Classic symptoms of hyperglycemia or hyperglycemic crisis and blood sugar level	–	≥200 mg/dl (11.1 mmol/L)

*Fasting is defined as no caloric intake for at least 8 hours.
One of the preceding first three criteria must be present on a subsequent day to confirm the diagnosis of diabetes mellitus.
In the absence of unequivocal hyperglycemia, fasting blood sugar and HbA1c (glycated hemoglobin) should be confirmed by repeat testing.

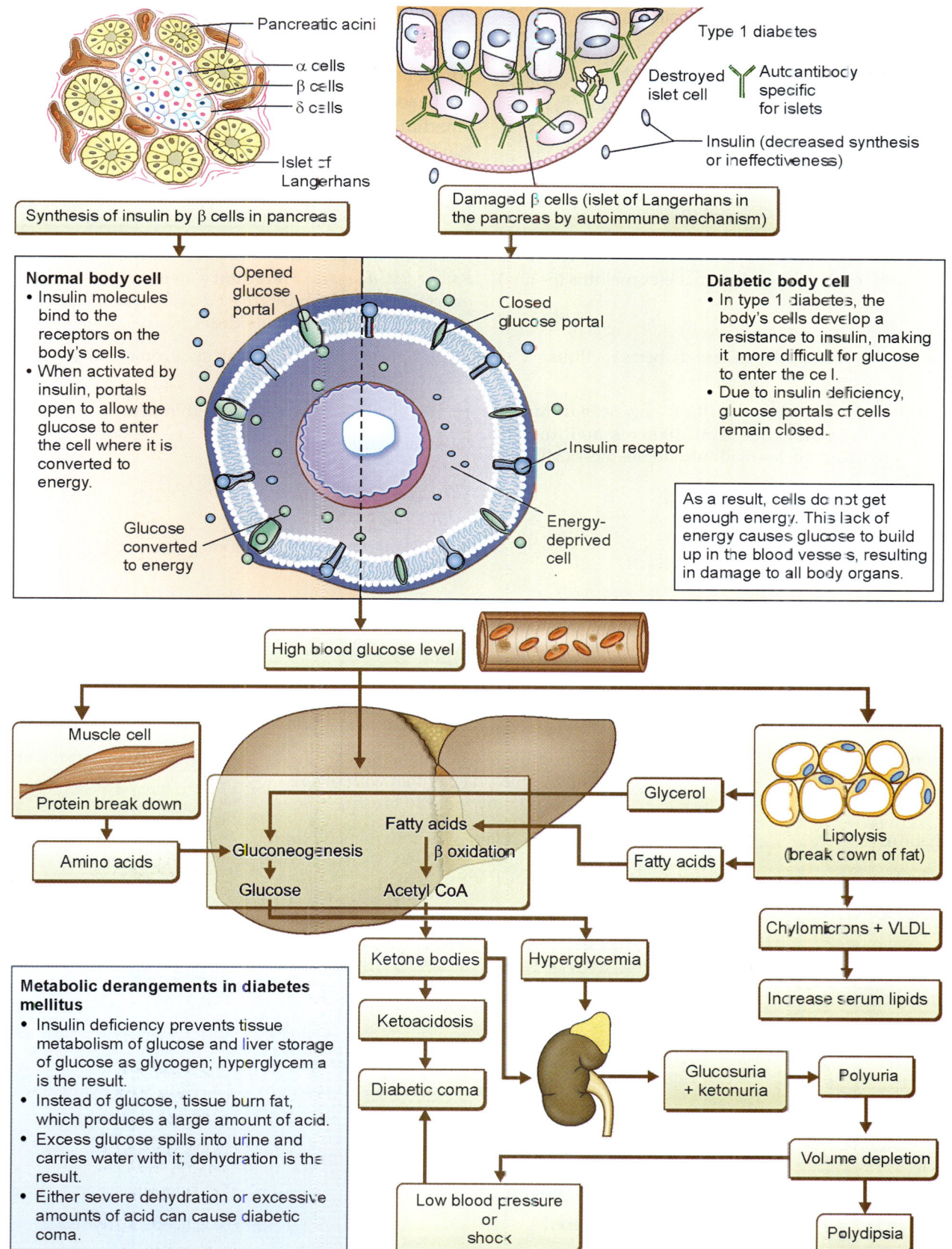

Fig. 26.3: Pathogensis of type 1 diabetes mellitus.

Table 26.4: Glycosylated HbA1c levels: interpretation

Parameters	Level	Percentage
Normal glucose tolerance test	HbA1c	<5.6%
Pre-diabetes mellitus	HbA1c	5.7–6.4%
Diabetes mellitus	HbA1c	≥6.5%

Classification of Diabetes Mellitus

Diabetes mellitus is classified as primary or secondary diabetes mellitus.

Based on pathogeneses, it may be type 1 (immune mediated) or type-2 (non-immune mediated) (Tables 26.5 to 26.7).

Table 26.5: Classification of diabetes mellitus

Primary diabetes mellitus	Secondary diabetes mellitus
Juvenile onset insulin-dependent diabetes mellitus (5–10%)	*Pancreatic diseases:* Hereditary hemochromatosis, acute pancreatitis, cystic fibrosis related diabetes mellitus, pancreatic carcinoma of α cells, amyloidosis pancreas
Adult onset non-insulin-dependent diabetes mellitus	*Adrenal gland diseases:* Cushing syndrome and pheochromocytoma
Maturity onset diabetes mellitus of the young: MOD1, MOD2, MOD3, MOD4, MOD5, neonatal diabetes mellitus and maternal inherited diabetes mellitus and deafness (MIDD)	*Thyroid gland disorders:* Hyperthyroidism
	Gestational diabetes mellitus
Gestational diabetes mellitus	*Therapeutic agents administration:* Glucocorticoids, thiazide drugs, cyclosporine
	Infectious agents: Mumps, cytomegalovirus, HIV infections

Table 26.6: Differences between type 1 and type 2 diabetes mellitus

Parameters	Type 1 diabetes mellitus	Type 2 diabetes mellitus
Prevalence	5 to 10%	90 to 95%
Age on onset	Children and adolescents <20 years	Adults >30 years
Type of onset	Rapid (abrupt), symptomatic polyuria, polydipsia, polyphagia often with severe ketoacidosis (fruity odor to breath)	Gradual often symptomatic
Body habitus	Normal, recent loss of weight (usually thin)	Usually obese (80%)
Family history	Uncommon (<20%)	Common (>60%)
Monozygotic twins	50% concordant	90% concordant
HLA association	Present	Absent
Insulin gene VNTR (variable number of tandem repeats)	Present	Absent
Diabetogenic and obesity related candidate genes	Present	Absent
Islet lesions	Early inflammation, late fibrosis and atrophy	Late fibrosis and atrophy
Islet cell autoantibodies	Present	Absent
β cells mass	Markedly reduced	Normal to slightly reduced
Circulating insulin status	Lack of insulin	Peripheral resistance to insulin
Insulin in blood	Decreased	Normal or increased
C-peptide in blood	Decreased	Increased
Hyperglycemia	Common	Uncommon

Table 26.7: Differences between diabetic ketoacidosis and hyperosmolar hyperglycemic state

Parameters	Diabetic ketoacidosis	Hyperosmolar hyperglycemic state
Prevalence	Type 1 diabetes mellitus	Type 2 diabetes mellitus
Age	Younger age group	Older age group
Prodromal symptoms appear	<24 hours	Several days
Abdominal pain of Kussmaul's respiration	Yes	No
Acidosis	Moderate/severe	Absent
Blood glucose	>250 mg/dl	High (>600 mg/dl)
Serum bicarbonate	<15 mEq/L	>15 mEq/L
Blood/urine ketones	++++	+/−
β-hydroxybutyrate	High	Normal or raised
Arterial blood pH	Low (<7.3)	Normal (>7.3)
Effective serum osmolarity	Variable	Increased (>320)
Anionic gap	>12	Variable

JUVENILE ONSET INSULIN-DEPENDENT TYPE 1 DIABETES MELLITUS

Juvenile onset insulin-dependent type 1 diabetes mellitus is less common than type 2 disease. It is the most common form of diabetes in *children*. It often begins before 30 years of age (juvenile or ketosis-prone diabetes mellitus).

Etiology

Pancreatic β cells of the islets of Langerhans synthesize very little or no insulin at all (absolute deficiency).

Pathogenesis

In genetically susceptible persons, a triggering event possibly a viral infection causes production of autoantibodies against β cells of pancreas.

Incidence is increased with a specific point mutation in the HLA-DQ gene with HLA-DR3- and HLA-DR4 positive persons.

Destruction of β cells (>90%) leads to absolute deficiency of insulin. These patients require insulin for their survival.

Light Microscopy

- The islets of Langerhans are small with decrease in number or absence of β cells.
- There is heavy lymphocytic infiltrates in and around islets.

Consequence

Unless insulin is replaced in type 1 diabetes mellitus, patient develops marked carbohydrate intolerance with hyperglycemia, resulting in polyuria, polydipsia, and weight loss despite increased appetite, ketoacidosis, coma, and death.

Ketoacidosis results from increased catabolism of fat, with production of *ketone bodies* (principally β-hydroxybutyric acid, acetoacetic acid along with small quantities of acetone) by liver. It is worth mentioning that ketoacidosis is not limited to type 1 diabetes mellitus. Ketoacidosis may also seen in starvation.

NON-INSULIN-DEPENDENT TYPE 2 DIABETES MELLITUS

Non-insulin-dependent diabetes mellitus (NIDDM), is also known adult-onset, or ketosis-resistant diabetes mellitus. It is much more common than type 1 disease. It begins later in life, most often in middle age. Obesity and sedentary lifestyle accelerate the onset. It is characterized by decreased response of peripheral tissues to insulin and β cells dysfunctional.

Pathogenesis

NIDDM2 occurs due to increased insulin resistance mediated by *decreased peripheral cell membrane insulin receptors* or *post-receptor dysfunction* (insulin-resistant).

It may be associated with *impaired processing of proinsulin to insulin by β cells, decreased sensing of glucose by β cells, or impaired function of intracellular carrier proteins.*

The plasma insulin concentration is normal and often increased. Central obesity (abdominal fat deposition) is strongly related with insulin resistance.

Peripheral tissue resistance to insulin by NEFAs

- *Accumulation of non-esterified fatty acids (NEFAs):* These are increased in liver and muscle in obese persons.

These are correlated with peripheral tissue resistance to insulin. Toxic intermediates of NEFAs such as *ceramide* and *diacylglycerol* decrease signaling response and adversely affect insulin receptors. These toxic intermediates compete with glucose for substrate oxidation and cause feedback inhibition of glycolysis.

- *Role of adipokines synthesized by adipose tissue:* These include retinol binding protein 4 and resistin. *Antiglycemic adipokines* are leptin and adiponectin. These increase tissue sensitivity by activating AMP and AMPK (protein kinase) and enhance fatty acid oxidation.
- *Role of pro-inflammatory cytokines:* IL-6 and tumor necrosis factor-α may also reduce insulin sensitivity.

Role of β cells dysfunction: **TCF7L2** gene and other genes cause β cells of pancreas dysfunctional. These β cells synthesize more insulin to maintain blood sugar in type 2 DM with increased peripheral resistance to insulin. Amyloid deposition may be directly toxic to β cells of pancreas.

> **Light Microscopy**
> The islets of Langerhans show focal fibrosis and hyalinization due to deposition of amylin also known as *islet amyloid polypeptide* (IAPP).

Consequence

Ketoacidosis is unusual, but does occur due to unusual stress such as infection and surgical procedure.

Therapeutic Correlation

These patients are managed by diet and oral antidiabetic agents. *Insulin therapy is not usually required*. Patients may do reasonably well on diet, exercise and oral hypoglycemic agents for years before they need insulin.

MATURITY ONSET DIABETES MELLITUS OF THE YOUNG (MODY)

This autosomal dominant syndrome is characterized by mild hyperglycemia and *hyposecretion of insulin* but *without loss of β cells*. It has an earlier onset than type 2 diabetes mellitus. It is caused by a diverse group of single gene defects described in Table 26.8.

MONOGENIC FORM OF DIABETES MELLITUS

These are uncommon causes of diabetes mellitus due to genetic defects in function and action of β cells. It is autosomal dominant disorder. Early onset of diabetes mellitus may occur in non-obese young age group <25 years of age and even neonates. Autoantibodies are not demonstrated in these patients (Table 26.9).

Table 26.8: Genetic defects of maturity onset diabetes mellitus

Maturity onset diabetes mellitus	Genetic defects
MODY-1	Hepatocyte nuclear factor-4α (HNF-4α)
MODY-2	Glucokinase (GCK)
MODY-3	Hepatocyte nuclear factor-1α (HNF-1α): it is most common type of MODY in 60% cases
MODY-4	Pancreas and duodenal homeobox-1 (PDX-1)
MODY-5	Hepatocyte necrotic factor-1β (HNF-1β)
Neonatal diabetes mellitus	KCNJ11 and ABCC8 gene mutations
Maternally inherited diabetes mellitus and deafness (MIDD)	Mitochondrial DNA mutations in 3243A-G

MODY denotes maturity onset diabetes mellitus of the young.

Table 26.9: Monogenic forms of diabetes mellitus: mechanisms

Genetic defects of β cells of pancreas
• *Maturity onset diabetes mellitus of the young:* It is the largest subgroup in this category
• *Maternally inherited diabetes mellitus with deafness:* It occurs due to mutations of mitochondrial DNA. It leads to decreased ATP production resulting in diminished insulin release. These develop diabetes mellitus with sensorineural deafness
Genetic defects of action of insulin
• Mutations of several genes adversely affect synthesis of receptors on tissues, insulin binding and intracellular signaling These persons are associated with acanthosis nigricans, polycystic ovaries and increased androgens levels
• Lipoatrophic diabetes mellitus is accompanied by loss of subcutaneous adipose due to mutation of OPAR-γ

GESTATIONAL DIABETES MELLITUS

Pregnancy associated transient diabetes mellitus is known as *gestational diabetes mellitus*. Gestational diabetes mellitus is usually identified in the 24–28 weeks of gestation. Woman, who develops gestational diabetes mellitus, has high risk for development of type 2 diabetes mellitus later in life.

Etiopathogenesis

During pregnancy, **anti-insulin hormones** are synthesized by placenta such as *estrogen, prolactin, human chorionic somatomammotropin, cortisol,* and *progesterone.*

Human chorionic somatomammotropin regulates carbohydrate and protein metabolism of the mother to ensure delivery of glucose and protein for fetal growth. It is also known as *chorionic growth hormone-prolactin,* or *placental lactogen.*

Complications

- *Maternal complication:* Due to increased fetal birth weight, there is increased indication of cesarean section.
- *Neonatal complications:* There is increased fetal birth weight, brachial plexus injuries, and neonatal respiratory distress syndrome (hyaline membrane disease).

  During intrauterine life in diabetic mothers, fetus develops islet β cells hyperplasia in response to hyperglycemia and increased demand of insulin during early gestation. Pancreatic β cells, which may secrete insulin autonomously and cause hypoglycemia at birth of newborn.

Diagnostic Approach

Gestational diabetes mellitus is diagnosed by oral glucose tolerance test, in which the woman drinks 75 gm glucose. Blood glucose level after an hour >140 mg/dl is considered significant.

The confirmatory test is a 3-hour, 100 gm glucose tolerance test in which the blood glucose values are set at highest sensitivity. Urine analysis is done for sugar.

PATHOPHYSIOLOGY OF DIABETES MELLITUS

HYPERGLYCEMIA

Hyperglycemic symptoms commonly include polyuria, polydipsia, and nocturia. Recent weight loss is less frequently reported in children who present with type 2 diabetes compared to those with type 1 disease.

Hyperglycemia is the key factor that produces organ damage caused by decreased insulin, increased glucagon and epinephrine.

Increased gluconeogenesis and glycogenolysis in liver as well decreased glucose uptake by muscle and adipose tissue result in hyperglycemia.

DIABETIC KETOACIDOSIS (DKA)

Diabetic ketoacidosis is mainly a complication of type 1 diabetes mellitus. Children with type 2 diabetes can also present with DKA; characterized by hyperglycemia, ketonuria, and acidosis.

DKA is precipitated by medical illness or omission of insulin resulting in hyperglycemia. It produces severe volume depletion due to loss of sodium and water with osmotic diuresis. Patient becomes unconscious. Diabetic ketoacidosis occurs by the following mechanisms.

Mechanism

- *Lipolysis:* Unchecked hormone-sensitive lipase increases lipolysis with release of fatty acids (Fig. 26.4).
- *β-oxidation of fatty acids:* It results in increased production of acetyl CoA.
- *Conversion of acetyl CoA into ketone bodies:* It results in increased production of ketone bodies, i.e. *acetoacetic acid, β-hydroxybutyric acid* and *acetone* in liver, giving a fruity odor to the breath.

HYPEROSMOLAR HYPERGLYCEMIA STATE

Hyperosmolar hyperglycemia state (HHS) was earlier known as *hyperosmolar nonketotic coma*. It is a condition similar to DKA, characterized by *marked hyperglycemia* (plasma glucose >600 mg/dl) and *severe dehydration* but *little or no ketonuria.*

It is usually seen in adult patients with poorly controlled type 2 diabetes mellitus, but has been reported in adolescents.

Recognition of HHS is important because it is characterized by more severe dehydration than DKA, with high morbidity and mortality (20 to 50%) if not adequately treated.

HYPERLIPIDEMIA

Lack of insulin decreases capillary lipoprotein lipase activity in peripheral blood resulting in accumulation of chylomicrons and VLDL in blood. It may precipitate acute pancreatitis and eruptive xanthoma in the skin (called the *hyperchylomicronemia syndrome*).

Hyperlipidemia in diabetes mellitus (insulin-dependent or non-insulin-dependent) accelerates *atherosclerosis* at an early age. The risk of cerebrovascular disease is high and frequency to develop *gangrene of foot* is about 100 times increased.

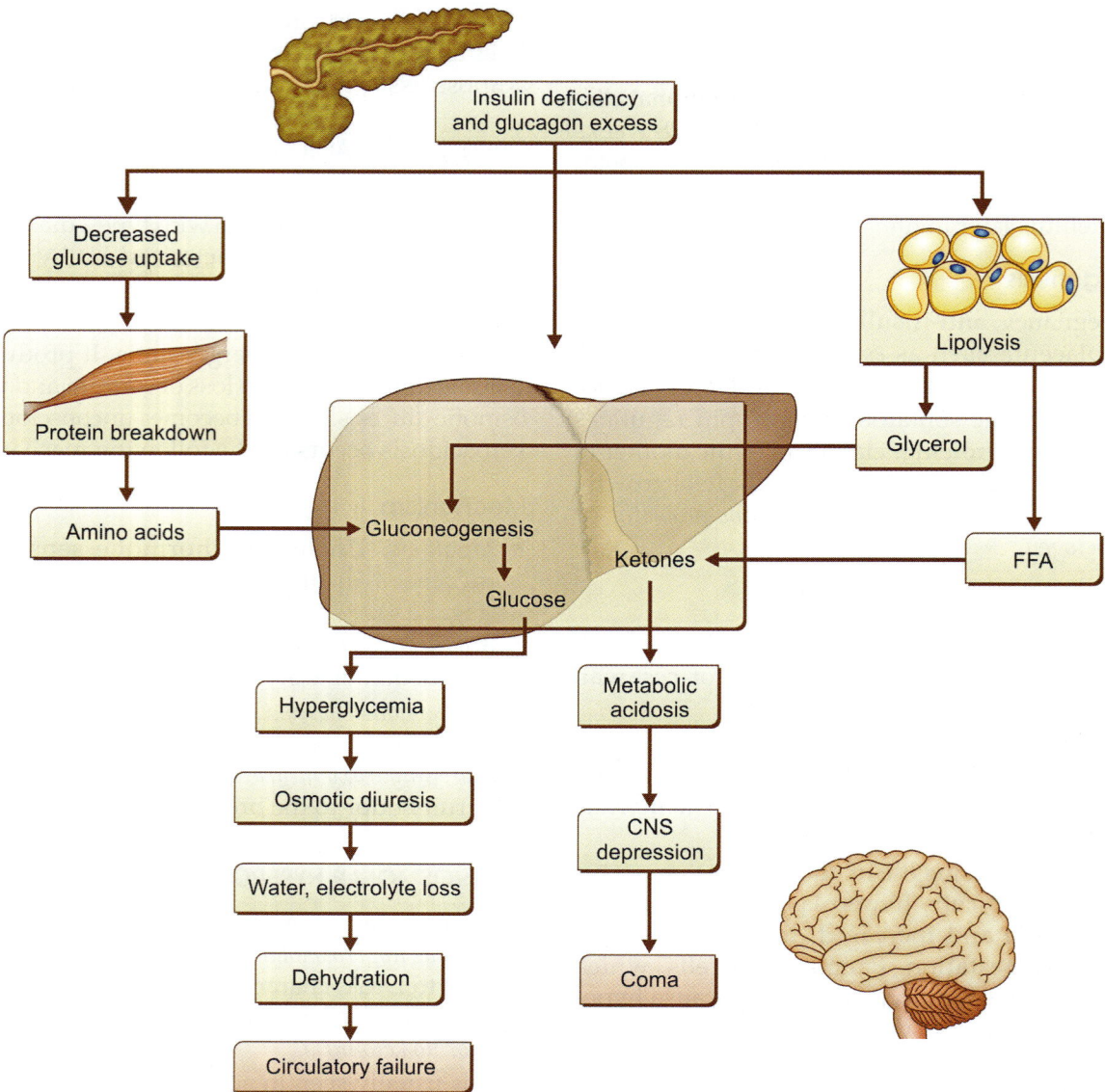

Fig. 26.4: Mechanisms of diabetic ketoacidosis (DKA). DKA is associated with very low insulin levels and extremely high levels of glucagon, catecholamines, and other counter-regulatory hormones. Increased levels of glucagon and catecholamines lead to mobilization of substrates for gluconeogenesis and ketogenesis by the liver. Gluconeogenesis in excess of that needed to supply glucose for the brain and other glucose dependent tissues produces a rise in blood glucose levels. Mobilization of free fatty acids (FFA) from triglyceride stores in adipose tissue leads to accelerated ketone production and ketosis (CNS: central nervous system).

MUSCLE WASTING

Muscle wasting occurs due to increased protein degradation in muscles.

SEVERE VOLUME DEPLETION

Diabetes mellitus produces severe volume depletion and coma due to loss of sodium and water with osmotic diuresis.

DILUTIONAL HYPONATREMIA

Serum sodium is decreased in diabetes mellitus. Glucose overrides sodium in controlling the osmotic gradient. Hence, water shifts out of the intracellular fluid compartment into the extracellular compartment resulting in dilutional hyponatremia.

HYPERKALEMIA

Hyperkalemia occurs due to transcellular shift as excess H^+ ions enter cells in exchange of potassium.

METABOLIC ACIDOSIS

Metabolic acidosis in uncontrolled type 1 diabetes mellitus occurs due to ketoacidosis and lactic acidosis. Blood pH is <7.35.

PRERENAL AZOTEMIA

Prerenal azotemia in diabetes mellitus occurs due to volume depletion resulting in accumulation of waste products in the body.

MECHANISM OF ORGANS DAMAGE

The pathological abnormalities associated with diabetes mellitus are the result of: (i) non-enzymatic glycosylation and (ii) osmotic damage (enzymatic mechanism).

The duration and severity of disease are key factors underlying the clinical presentation of diabetes mellitus. Controlling blood sugar reduces the onset of severity of complications related to retinopathy, nephropathy and neuropathy.

NON-ENZYMATIC GLYCOSYLATION MECHANISM

Glycosylation refers to glucose attaching to amino acids of the basement membrane of vessels rendering them permeable to proteins.

- *Glycosylated end products:* Glucose combines with proteins and forms Schiff's base. It leads to formation of early glycosylated end products (amadori product) and then advanced glycosylated end products (irreversible change), which resist enzymatic degradation.
- *Mechanism of damage by glycosylated end products:* Advanced glycosylated end products cause increased permeability of glomerular basement membrane, hyaline arteriosclerosis of small vessels in kidney; and atherosclerosis of large elastic and medium-sized arteries.
- *Blood vessels involved:* Arteries affected include abdominal aorta, coronary, cerebral, anterior tibial, posterior tibial and popliteal vessels. Atheromatous plaques are formed in these blood vessels resulting in decreased blood supply to the organs.

ENZYMATIC GLYCOSYLATION MECHANISM

Osmotic damage occurs due to conversion of glucose to sorbitol and fructose by aldose reductase and sorbitol dehydrogenase respectively. Both sorbitol and fructose are osmotically active, and draw water into tissue leading to permanent damage.

Complications associated with osmotic damage include peripheral neuropathy (damage to Schwann cells leading to demyelization), cataracts, and microaneurysms in retina (damage to pericytes weakens the vessel wall).

Table 26.10: Complications of uncontrolled diabetes mellitus

Complication	Organ affected
Macrovascular disorders	
Coronary artery disease	Heart
Cerebral vessel disease	Brain
Peripheral vascular disease	Blood vessels of legs and feet Small blood vessels
Microvascular disorders	
Nephropathy	Kidney
Neuropathy	Nerves
Retinopathy	Eye
Skin disorder	
Dermatopathy	Skin

COMPLICATIONS

Chronic complications of diabetes mellitus result from elevated blood glucose levels, impairment of metabolic pathways of glucose, fat and proteins (Fig. 26.5).

Chronic complications of diabetes mellitus are best prevented by measures aimed at tight control of blood glucose levels, control of hypertension and maintenance of normal lipid levels. Effective control of diabetes reduces the incidence of renal, and perhaps retinal disease (Table 26.10).

Macrovascular Disorders

Advanced glycosylated end (AGE) products bind to collagen of blood vessels in uncontrolled diabetes mellitus. These also trap LDL resulting in atherosclerosis of *aorta, coronary, cerebral and popliteal arteries.*

Macrovascular disorders such as coronary artery disease, cerebral stroke and peripheral vascular disease reflect the combined effects of unregulated blood glucose levels, elevated blood pressure and hyperlipidemia. The most common cause of death with diabetes mellitus is myocardial infarction.

Microvascular Disorders

Microvascular disorders include nephropathy, neuropathy and retinopathy.

ANGINA PECTORIS AND ACUTE MYOCARDIAL INFARCTION

Atheromatous plaque in coronary arteries may cause angina, acute myocardial infarction and cardiac failure. Patients become symptomatic if vessels consisting of atherosclerotic plaque involve >75% of lumen. Treatment of acute myocardial infarction includes angioplasty, stents and coronary bypass surgery.

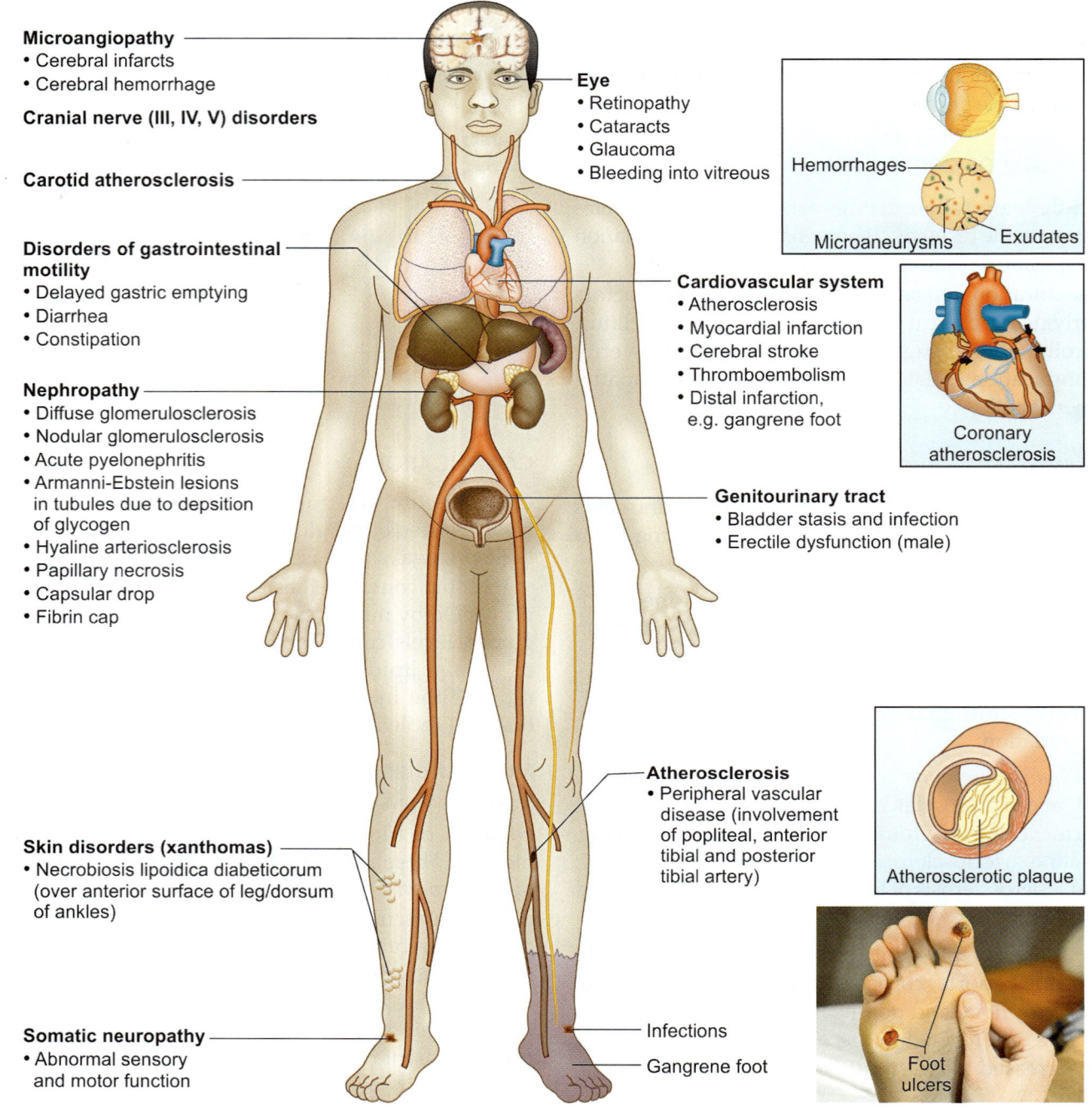

Fig. 26.5: Complications of diabetes mellitus.

CEREBRAL VASCULAR DISEASE

Cerebral vascular disease refers to diseased arteries in the brain. Partial blockage may result in temporary reduction of blood supply to a part of the brain (**transient ischemic attacks**).

A complete loss of blood supply to an area of the brain due to clogging or breaking of a blood vessel results in cerebral vascular stroke.

PERIPHERAL VASCULAR DISEASE

Diabetic patients develop atheromatous plaque in popliteal arteries, anterior and posterior tibial arteries resulting in peripheral vascular disease. In arteriosclerosis, atheromatous plaques buildup in a vessel and limit the blood flow to the organs and limbs.

Partial or complete blockage adversely affects the circulation to lower extremities.

Clinical Features

Patient with partial blockage of vessels presents with *intermittent claudication* (cramps, pain in legs when walking). Complete vessel blockage causes gangrene foot. It is made worse through the development of diabetic neuropathy, resulting in propensity for injury.

DIABETIC NEPHROPATHY

Uncontrolled diabetes mellitus adversely affects glomeruli, tubules, blood vessels and interstitial tissue of kidneys. Renal lesions include diabetic glomerulosclerosis, Kimmelsteil-Wilson disease (nodular glomerulosclerosis), hyaline arteriosclerosis, acute or chronic pyelonephritis, papillary necrosis, capsular drops and fibrin cap (Table 26.11).

Table 26.11: Renal lesions in diabetic nephropathy

- *Diabetic glomerulosclerosis* (widening of mesangial areas due to accumulation of basement like stroma in the mesangial region, increased number of mesangial cells in 2–5 years after the onset of diabetes mellitus)
- *Kimmelsteil-Wilson disease (nodular glomerulosclerosis):* Sclerotic nodules in the peripheral region of intercapillary region of glomeruli demonstrated by PAS staining
- Hyaline arteriolosclerosis
- Acute pyelonephritis
- Papillary necrosis
- Capsular drop (plasma proteins deposition inside Bowman's capsule)
- Fibrin cap (plasma proteins deposition in subendothelial region)
- Armanni-Ebstein lesions in tubules due to deposition of glycogen

Advanced glycosylated end (AGE) products bind to collagen fibers of glomerular basement membrane. It leads to impairment of interaction of laminin, thus resulting to increased capillary permeability. Increased width of glomerular basement membrane is the earliest and most common renal manifestation.

Glomeruli

Diffuse and nodular glomerulosclerosis occur due to increased synthesis of type IV collagen in glomerular basement membrane and mesangium resulting in massive proteinuria and ultimately chronic renal failure. Exudative lesion, i.e. capsular drop due to deposition of plasma proteins especially fibrin is also seen. Glomeruli show increased synthesis of type IV collagen in glomerular basement membrane and mesangial region.

- *Diffuse glomerulosclerosis:* PAS stain demonstrates diffuse glomerulosclerosis associated with long-standing diabetes mellitus. Accumulation of basement like stroma in the mesangium parallels the diffuse thickening of the basement membrane. These changes gradually advance until the entire glomerulus becomes sclerotic. Focal effacement of foot processes is common. Changes of glomerulosclerosis with diabetes mellitus take a decade or longer to develop (Fig. 26.6).

- *Nodular glomerulosclerosis:* It is also known as *Kimmelstiel-Wilson disease*. It comprises nodules in long-standing diabetes, regardless of type. As a result of non-enzymatic glycosylation of proteins, nodular pink hyaline material (PAS positive) is formed in the mesangial matrix due to increased type IV collagen synthesis and trapped proteins, between capillary loops. Intercapillary glomerulosclerosis leads to renal ischemia, tubular atrophy, marked interstitial fibrosis, increased mesangial region, arteriolosclerosis and ultimately small contracted kidney (Fig. 26.7).

Tubules

Armanni-Ebstein lesions due to deposition of glycogen in renal tubules are seen in uncontrolled hyperglycemia. These can occur in either type of diabetes mellitus due to increased permeability of tubules.

Blood Vessels

Hyaline arteriosclerosis of renal arterioles is the main cause of renal microangiopathy in diabetic patients (Fig. 26.8).

Capsular Drop

Accumulation of plasma proteins inside Bowman's capsule is known as *capsular drop* (Fig. 26.9).

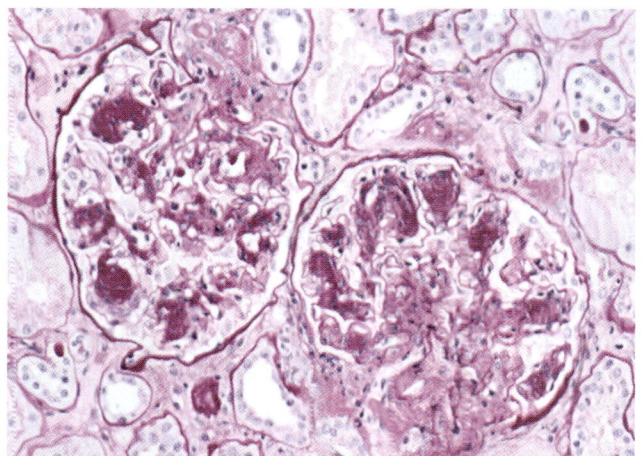

Fig. 26.6: Diffuse glomerulosclerosis in diabetic nephropathy. It shows widening of mesangial areas due to accumulation of basement-like stroma in the mesangial region (400X).

Section III: Systemic Pathology

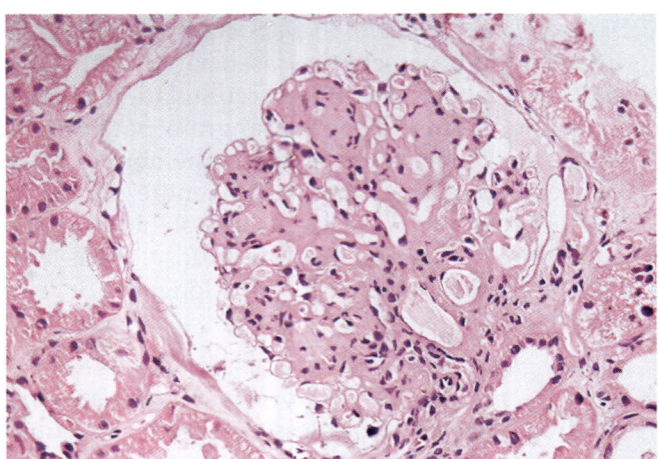

Fig. 26.7: Nodular glomerulosclerosis (Kimmelsteil-Wilson disease) in diabetic nephropathy. It shows sclerotic nodules in the peripheral region of intercapillary region of glomeruli. These nodules are formed due to accumulation of trapped proteins and synthesis of type IV collagen in mesangial matrix (400X).

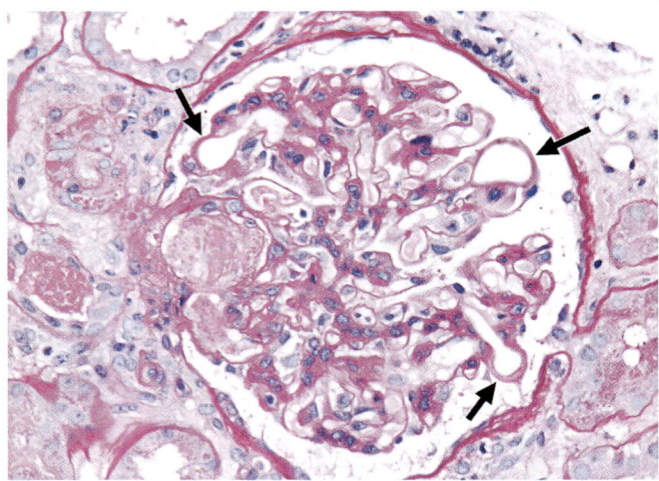

Fig. 26.8: Microaneurysm (arrows).

Fibrin Cap

Accumulation of plasma proteins in the subendothelial region of glomeruli is known as *fibrin cap*.

Papillary Necrosis

Diabetic glomerulosclerosis leads to ischemia of papillae (papillary necrosis). Necrotic papillae may detach and pass in the urine as tissue fragments. Undetached papillae may resolve by fibrosis. It may be noted that **papillary necrosis** can be seen as a complication of **chronic analgesic abuse, diabetic nephropathy, infectious pyelonephritis** and **sickle cell anemia** (Fig. 26.10).

Tubulointerstitial Tissue

Acute pyelonephritis is most frequently secondary to infection by bacteria or fungi. It is characterized by formation of pus in the tubule resulting in abscess

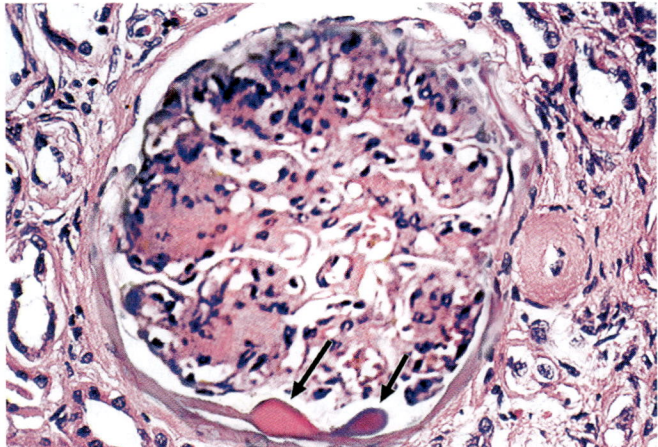

Fig. 26.9: Capsular drop in glomerulus (arrows).

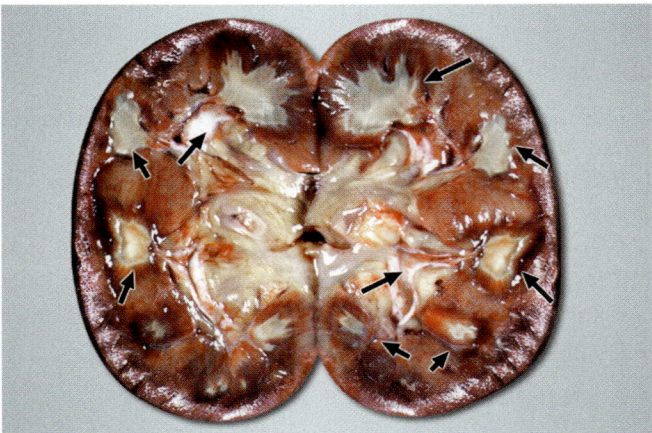

Fig. 26.10: Renal papillary necrosis (arrows).

formation. Microscopic urine analysis shows the presence of numerous pus cells and white blood cell (WBC) casts (Figs 26.11 and 26.12).

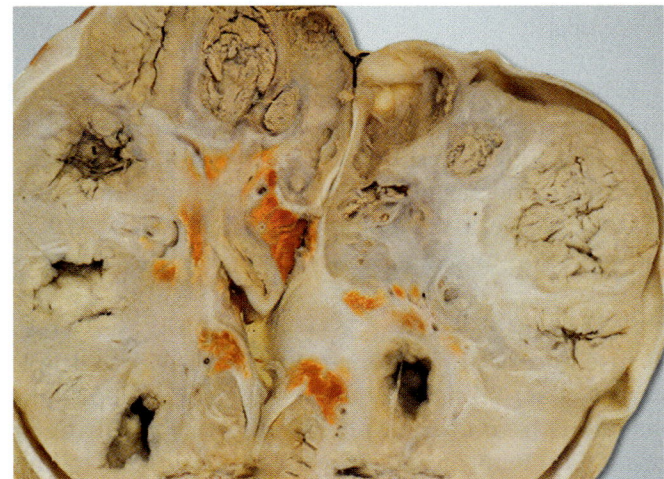

Fig. 26.11: Acute pyelonephritis. Acute pyelonephritis is often a focal disease, and much of the kidney often appears normal. The kidney shows multiple grayish white areas of small microabscesses in the renal parenchyma.

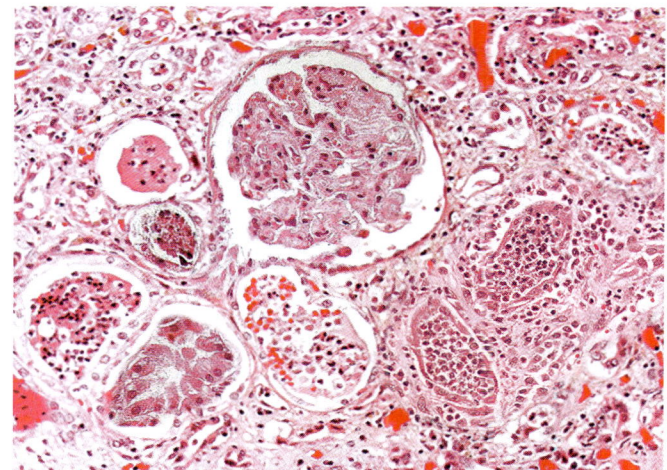

Fig. 26.12: Renal parenchyma is infiltrated by polymorphonuclear cells (100X).

OCULAR DISORDERS

Cataract formation is common. Proliferative retinopathy characterized by retinal exudates, edema, hemorrhages, and microaneurysms of small vessels can lead to blindness (Table 26.12).

Diabetic Retinopathy

There is increased risk of retinopathy (irreversible cause of blindness due to retinal detachment), cataract and glaucoma in type 1 or type 2 diabetes mellitus, usually a decade or so after the onset of diabetes mellitus.

Annual ophthalmic examination is mandatory. Diabetic retinal microangiopathy may be non-proliferative or proliferative.

- *Non-proliferative retinopathy:* It is an early stage without any apparent symptoms in most patients. Retinal vessels develop microaneurysms, which may rupture and form soft cotton wool exudates (microinfarcts). Later on exudate is formed as a result of deposits of protein that have leaked from damaged capillaries. These findings can be viewed with the *ophthalmoscope*. **Macula**, part of the retina where central vision occurs, becomes swollen, resulting in **distorted vision**. The retinopathy also includes increased capillary permeability, edema, and diffuse thickening of basement membranes (microangiopathy). Retinopathy is related to the duration of the disease, occurring in most patients with diabetes mellitus after 10 years.
- *Proliferative retinopathy:* It occurs in uncontrolled both forms of diabetes mellitus. Retinal newly formed vessels are formed (**neovascularization**). These vessels become fragile, and rupture into vitreous and retina. Scar formation in vitreous pulls on the retina leading to its detachment. *Proliferative retinopathy is treated with laser surgery (photocoagulation).*

Glaucoma

In severe retinopathy, neovascularization may lead to *adhesions* (**synechiae**) *between iris and cornea* or iris and lens. *Neovascularization of the iris* leads to *secondary glaucoma* resulting in blindness.

Cataracts

Cataracts are more common in diabetics. Hyperglycemia leads to accumulation of sorbitol that results in osmotic damage to the crystalline lens.

Bleeding into Vitreous

When massive bleeding into the vitreous has occurred, a vitrectomy may be performed. In this surgical procedure, the bloody vitreous is removed and replaced with clear, sterile fluids to restore vision.

PERIPHERAL NEUROPATHY

Osmotic damage to Schwann cells affect both motor (muscle weakness) and sensory (paresthesia) nerves of peripheral nerves in type 1 and type 2 diabetes mellitus (70%). Patient develops ulcerations at pressure points (neuropathic pressure ulcers) on the plantar surfaces of both feet (Table 26.13).

AUTONOMIC NERVOUS SYSTEM NEUROPATHY

Patient may develop gastroparesis (delayed gastric emptying), cardiac arrhythmias and impotence. Diabetic bladder dysfunction occurs when damage to the nerves of the bladder results in incomplete emptying of the bladder. Urine that remains in the bladder is stagnant, and bacteria grow in it. The bacteria travel up to the kidney and cause acute pyelonephritis.

CRANIAL NERVE DISORDERS

Cranial nerves (III, IV, and V) are most commonly affected in long standing cases of diabetes mellitus.

Table 26.12: Ocular disorders in diabetes mellitus

Ocular pathology	Consequence
Diabetic retinopathy	Non-proliferative retinopathy with formation of microaneurysms
	Proliferative retinopathy: scar formation
Glaucoma	Blindness
Cataract	Osmotic damage to the crystalline lens
Bleeding into vitreous	It hampers vision

Table 26.13: Classification of diabetic neuropathies

	Nerves involved	Clinical manifestations
Somatic nerves	Polyneuropathies (bilateral sensory)	Paresthesias, including numbness and tingling
		Impaired pain, temperature, light touch, two-point discrimination and vibratory sensation
		Decreased ankle and knee-jerk reflexes
	Mononeuropathies	Involvement of a mixed nerve trunk that includes loss of sensation, pain, and motor weakness
	Amyotrophy	Associated with muscle weakness, wasting, and severe pain of muscles in the pelvic girdle and thigh
Autonomic nerves	Impaired vasomotor function	Postural hypotension
	Impaired gastrointestinal function	Gastroparesis
		Diarrhea, often postprandial and nocturnal
	Impaired gastrourinary function	Paralytic bladder
		Incomplete voiding
		Erectile dysfunction
		Retrograde ejaculation
	Cranial nerve involvement	Extraocular nerve paralysis
		Impaired pupillary responses
		Impaired special senses

INFECTIOUS DISORDERS

Increased glucose in tissues and body fluids provides favorable growth of conditions for bacteria and fungi. *Diabetes mellitus impairs the function of neutrophils.* Angiopathy caused by diabetes leads to tissue ischemia. Such ischemic tissues are more prone to infections.

Patients develop vulvovaginitis (Candida), external otitis (*Pseudomonas aeruginosa*), cutaneous infections (*Staphylococcus aureus*), and rhinocerebral mucormycosis spreading to face, orbit, skull, and frontal lobe of brain.

SKIN DISORDERS

Patient develops well demarcated yellow plaques over **anterior surface of the leg/dorsum of ankles** known as *necrobiosis lipoidica diabeticorum*. It occurs due to increased synthesis of fat at insulin injection site. Patient may develop xanthomas due to collections of lipid-laden macrophages in the dermis.

MUCORMYCOSIS

Diabetic ketoacidosis helps to potentiate the growth of mucormyosis. Most common site is typically nasopharyngeal region, but the infection can spread to involve *soft tissues and bone of the face, orbit, skull and brain.*

FATTY LIVER

Fatty change refers to abnormal accumulation of triglycerides within parenchymal cells. It is commonly seen in liver, the major organ involved in fat metabolism. The lipid accumulates when lipoprotein transport is disrupted.

Gross Morphology

- Mild fatty change in liver may not affect the gross appearance.
- Severe fatty change results in enlargement of liver. It becomes progressively yellow on cut surface until it may weigh 3 to 6 kg.
- This uniform change is consistent with fatty metamorphosis (fatty change).

Light Microscopy

- *Mild fatty change:* Initially, hepatocytes show small fat vacuoles around nucleus (mild fatty change or microvesicular) in hematoxylin and eosin stained sections.
- *Severe fatty change:* Progressive accumulation of fat vacuoles in the cytoplasm coalesces to create spaces that displace the nucleus toward periphery (severe fatty change).

- *Fatty cysts:* Occasionally contiguous cells rupture, and the enclosed fat globules unite to produce so-called fatty cysts. Distribution of lipid vacuoles may be diffuse, focal or zonal, midzonal or peripheral depending on severity and etiology.
- *Frozen section technique:* In paraffin embedded sections, fat is dissolved during processing of tissue in tissue processor. Fat can be demonstrated by frozen section technique with the fat stains such as Sudan III, Sudan IV, Sudan black, oil red O and osmic acid.

LABORATORY DIAGNOSIS

BLOOD SUGAR

Fasting ≥ 126 mg/dl and random ≥ 200 mg/dl. Values are diagnostic estimated at different occasions.

GLUCOSE TOLERANCE TEST

Glucose tolerance is impaired in a patient, who does not fit in the established criteria of diabetes mellitus, but has increased risk of developing complications involving medium and large elastic arteries (e.g. atherosclerosis of aorta, coronary, cerebral and popliteal arteries) and neuropathy (Table 26.14).

GLYCOSYLATED HEMOGLOBIN (HbA1c)

Serum hemoglobin A1c is an indicator of long-term blood glucose control in diabetes mellitus. In the normal individual, about 3–6% of adult hemoglobin is glycosylated, which accumulates in the RBCs. The percentage of glycosylated hemoglobin is increased depending upon the degree of hyperglycemia. A value >6.5 is diagnostic of diabetes. It is directly related to the average concentration of glucose in the blood. Its estimation evaluates long-term glycemic control.

LIPID PROFILE

Accumulation of chylomicrons and VLDL in blood leads to deranged lipid profile.

SERUM PROTEINS

Total serum proteins are decreased with reversal of albumin/globulin ratio (normal 2:1).

BLOOD UREA (20–40 mg/dl)

It is increased in diabetic nephropathy. Never use anticoagulant containing ammonium salt as it increases urea concentration.

SERUM CREATININE (NORMAL 0.6–1.5 mg %)

It is increased in diabetic nephropathy.

SERUM Na^+

The levels are decreased due to dilutional hyponatremia.

SERUM K^+

The level of serum potassium is increased.

URINE ANALYSIS

Diabetes nephropathy may show *proteins, glucose, ketone bodies, pus cells, hyaline casts, fatty casts* and *oval fat bodies* (lipid-containing renal tubular epithelial cells).

Free fat droplets, fatty casts, and oval fat bodies; when examined by polarized light, the lipids in casts are seen as being doubly refractile or birefringent and they display a symmetric '**maltese-cross pattern**'.

Renal Biopsy

Renal biopsy should consist of at least five glomeruli to comment.

Table 26.14: Glucose tolerance test

Parameter	Normal blood sugar level	Impaired fasting glucose	Diabetes mellitus
Fasting (8 hours)	<100 mg/dl	100–125 mg/dl	≥126 mg/dl
Oral glucose tolerance test (2.2. hours)	<140 mg/dl	<140 mg/dl	≥200 mg/dl

THYROID GLAND

ANATOMY

Location

Thyroid gland consists of two lateral lobes connected in the midline by a broad isthmus just below the larynx. It weighs 20–25 gm in adults.

Structure

Thyroid gland is composed of thyroid follicles lined by cuboidal epithelium and containing colloid. Fibrovascular stroma is present in between the thyroid follicles.

- *Thyroid follicular cells:* These synthesize thyroxine (T_4) and triiodothyronine (T_3), which are needed to keep the body functioning at its normal rate. The thyroid gland needs a regular supply of iodine (which is added to table salt and found in fish and milk) in order to produce thyroid hormones.
- *Parafollicular cells or C cells of thyroid gland:* These synthesize thyrocalcitonin (TC), which lowers the blood level of calcium ions by transporting calcium in the bones. Calcitonin secretion is controlled by calcium ion level in the blood.

PHYSIOLOGY

Response of Thyroid Gland to Stimuli

Thyroid gland responds to many stimuli as in a constant state of adaptation. *Follicular epithelium proliferates and becomes more active during puberty, pregnancy and physiological stress.* When the stress abates, involution occurs and the follicular cells resume their normal size and architecture.

Regulation of Thyroid Hormones

- Low blood levels of T_3 and T_4 or low basal metabolic rate stimulate release of TRH by hypothalamus.
- TRH, carried by hypophyseal portal veins to anterior pituitary gland, stimulates release of TSH by thyrotrophs.
- TSH released into blood stimulates thyroid follicular cells.
- Thyroid hormones (T_4 and T_3) are synthesized from iodine and tyrosine within thyroglobulin (TBG) and transported in the blood bound to plasma proteins, mostly thyroid binding protein (TBG).
- Elevated T_3 and T_4 inhibit release of TRH and TSH by negative feedback mechanism, i.e. inhibiting synthesis of TRH by hypothalamus and TSH synthesis by anterior pituitary gland.

Synthesis of Thyroid Hormones

Synthesis of thyroid hormones thyroxine (T_4) and triiodothyronine (T_3) depend on sufficient quantities of iodine from dietary sources. Thyroid stimulating hormone (TSH) regulates the rate of extraction of iodine from the bloodstream, synthesis of T_4 and T_3, release from storage (as thyroglobulin) and secreted into the bloodstream.

Feedback mechanisms regulate TSH synthesis by pituitary gland. Serum T_4 and T_3 are bound to thyroid-binding globulin (TBG) as shown in Fig. 26.13.

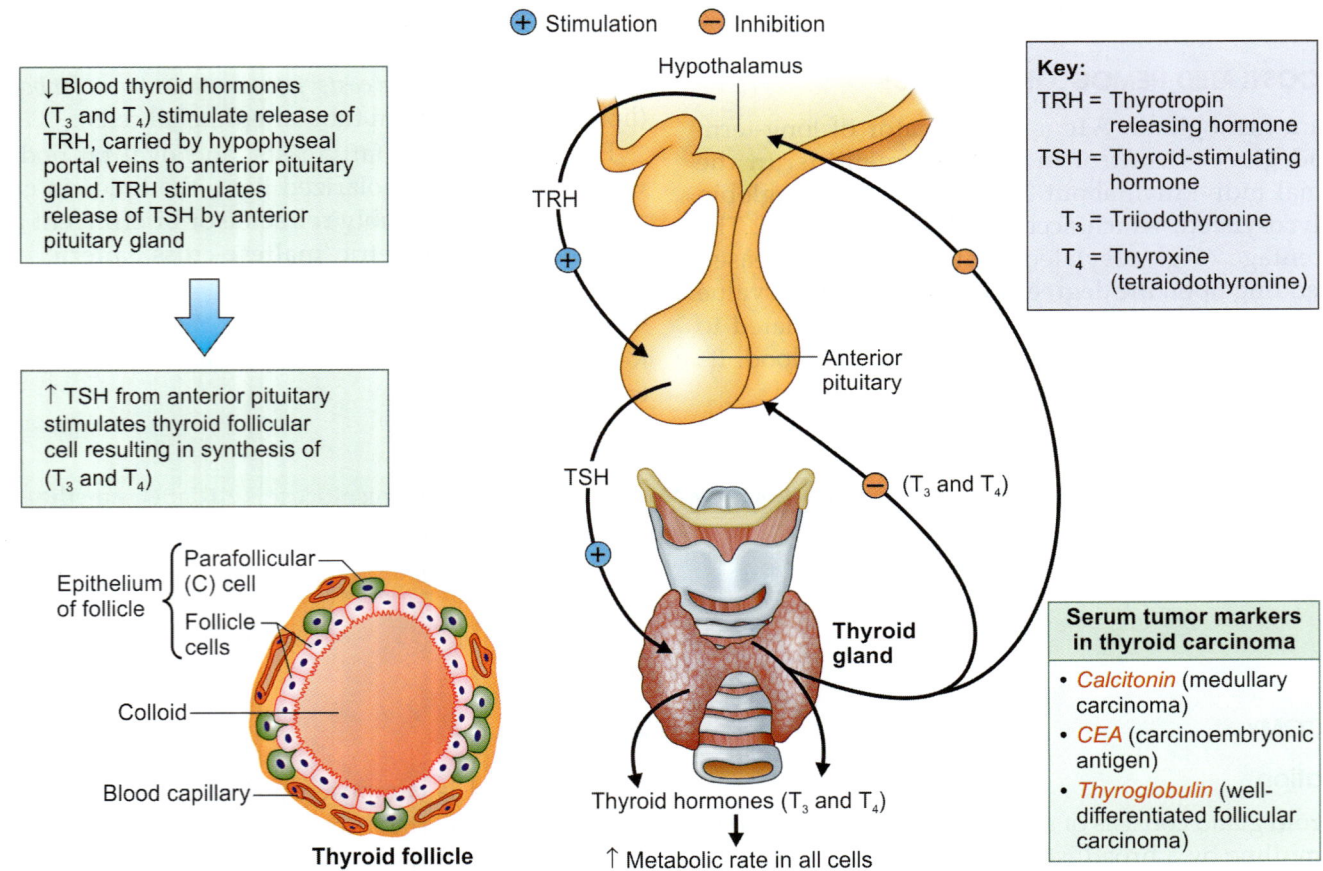

Fig. 26.13: Regulation of thyroid hormones.

Endocrine System: Pancreas, Thyroid, Parathyroid, Adrenal and Pituitary Glands

Steps of Synthesis of Thyroid Hormones

- *Trapping of iodide:* TSH participates in trapping of iodide in thyroid follicular cells.
- *Oxidation of iodides to iodine:* Peroxidase enzyme converts iodide to organically bound iodine in thyroid follicular cells.
- *Organification:* TSH participates in incorporation of iodine into tyrosine resulting in formation of MIT (monoiodotyrosine) and DIT (diiodotyrosine).
- *Coupling of MIT (monoiodotyrosine) and DIT (diiodotyrosine):* **Halogenase** enzyme participates in coupling of MIT and DIT. Coupling of two molecules of DIT forms T_4. Coupling of one molecule of MIT and DIT synthesizes T_3.
- *Storage in thyroid hormones in follicles:* Thyroid hormones (T_4 and T_3) are stored as colloid.
- *Proteolysis of colloid:* It occurs by lysosomal enzyme. It is TSH-mediated process.
- *Binding of thyroid hormones to TBG:* T_4 and T_3 bind to thyroid binding globulins (TBG), prealbumin and albumin. One-third of TBG binding sites are normally occupied (Fig. 26.14).

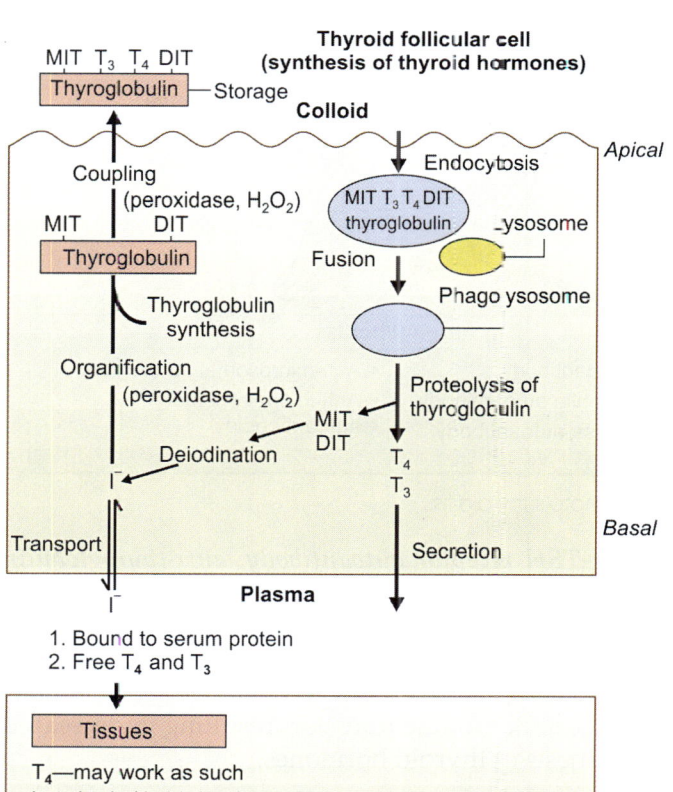

Fig. 26.14: Mechanism of synthesis of thyroid hormones.

Thyroid Hormones in Circulation and Tissues

- *Synthesis of thyroid hormones in circulation:* Thyroid gland synthesizes T_4 (80 microgram) and triiodothyronine T_3 (6 microgram) daily.
- *Conversion of T_4 to T_3 in various tissues:* Only a small fraction of thyroid hormones circulate in free form. Outer ring of 5-deiodinase enzyme converts T_4 to T_3 mainly in *liver, kidneys* (80%) and *dendritic cells* of nervous system (some conversion).
- *Mechanism of actions of T_4 to T_3 on various tissues:* T_3 is metabolically active hormone. It acts on nuclear receptors thus increases messenger RNA and protein synthesis.

Actions of Thyroid Hormones

- *Central nervous system:* Thyroid hormones are essential for *axonal, dendritic development* and *myelinization of CNS* especially in early first year of postnatal life.
  Deficiency of thyroid hormones during intrauterine life results in *mental retardation* due to *non-myelinization of central nervous system* and causes *cretinism* in children.
- *Maturation of growing epiphyseal region and skull:* Thyroid hormones enhance synthesis of *growth hormones* and *insulin-like growth factor;* which is necessary for *maturation of growing epiphyseal region* (linear growth), *skull; tooth eruption and dentition.*
- *Peripheral vasodilatation:* Thyroid hormones enhance synthesis of β-*adrenergic receptors* and cause vasodilatation.
- *Basal metabolic rate:* Thyroid hormones increase basal metabolic rate resulting in increased oxygen consumption.
- *Regulation of metabolism:* Thyroid hormones regulate *carbohydrate, fat* and *protein metabolism.*
- *Maintenance of water and electrolyte balance:* Thyroid hormones maintain water and electrolyte balance.
- *Hematopoiesis:* Thyroid hormones play an important role in hematopoiesis.

THYROIDITIS

HASHIMOTO'S THYROIDITIS

Hashimoto's thyroiditis is an autoimmune disease. Autoantibodies such as *antithyroid peroxidase antibody, antithyroglobulin antibody* and *anti-TSH antibody* are implicated in its pathogenesis. Infiltrates of lymphocytes with germinal center formation are seen in Hashimoto's thyroiditis (Figs 26.15 to 26.17).

Age Group

It occurs more often in **women** (30–50 years) than men.

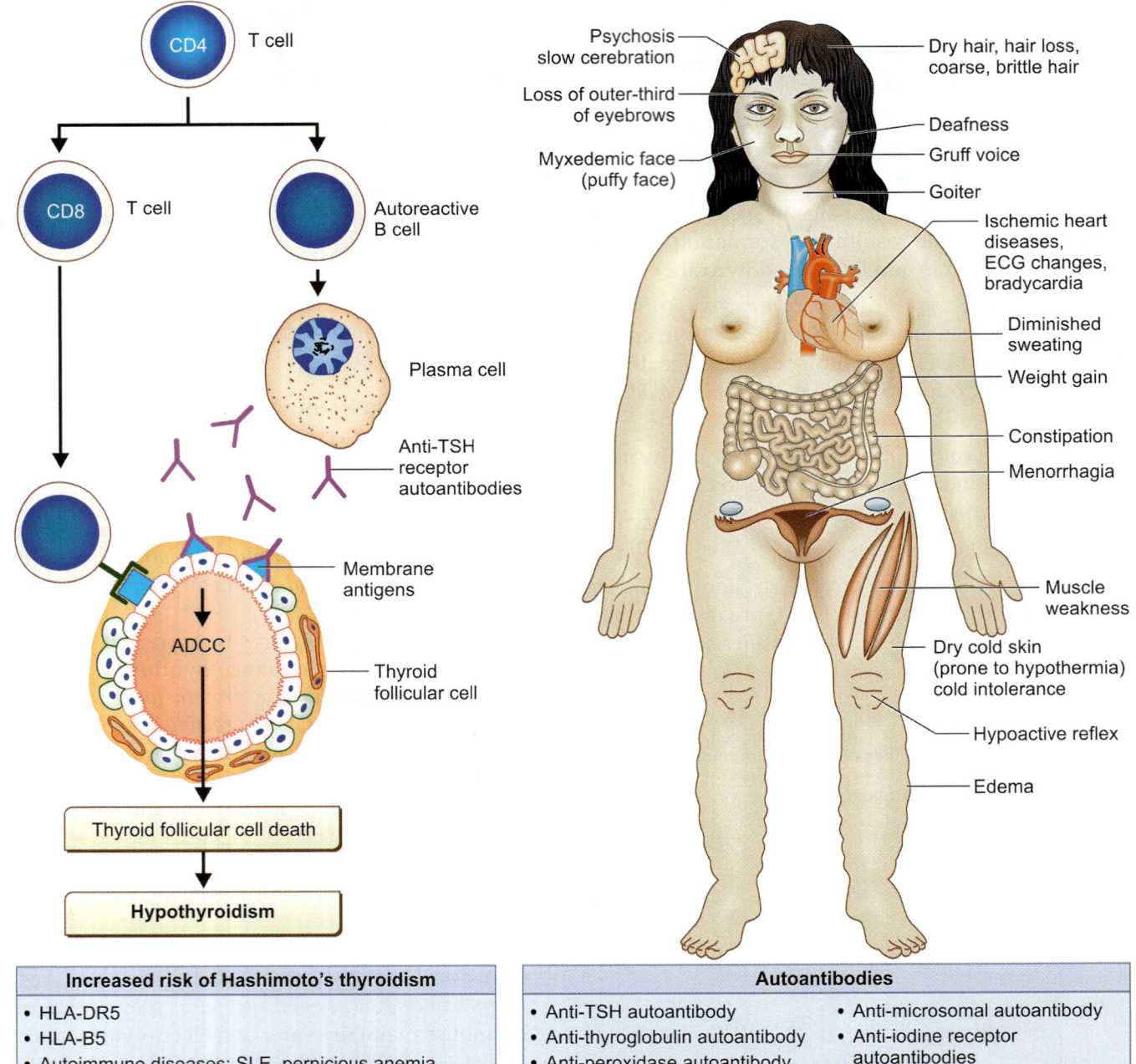

Fig. 26.15: Pathogenesis of Hashimoto's thyroiditis.

Incidence

Its incidence is increased in *HLA-DR5*, *HLA-B5* and autoimmune disorders, i.e. *systemic lupus erythematosus, rheumatoid arthritis, pernicious anemia, Sjögren's syndrome,* adult onset *diabetes mellitus* (type 1), *chronic active hepatitis* and *adrenalitis*.

Pathogenesis

- *Type 2 hypersensitivity reaction:* Loss of activity of T-suppressor cells in Hashimoto's thyroiditis results in formation of *autoantibodies (IgG or IgM)* such as *anti-TSH receptor autoantibody, anti-thyroglobulin autoantibody, anti-peroxidase autoantibody* (peroxidase enzyme located in the apical region of follicular cells), *anti-microsomal autoantibody* and *anti-iodine receptor autoantibody*. Anti-TSH receptor autoantibody inhibits intracellular iodine transport resulting in decreased synthesis of thyroid hormones.

Mechanism: Fc portion of IgG or IgM binds to Fc receptors of cytotoxic leukocytes, i.e. natural killer cells (most important), macrophages, neutrophils and eosinophils which destroy sensitized cells. These

- *Type IV hypersensitivity reaction:* It plays key role in pathogenesis of Hashimoto's thyroiditis. (i) *Cytotoxic T cells destroy thyroid follicular cells and induce apoptosis through the Fa = FasL system.* (ii) *Helper T cells synthesize cytokines that cause chemotaxis of macrophages.* These macrophages cause destruction of thyroid gland. Initially, patient develops hyperthyroidism due to release of thyroid hormones, and eventually hypothyroidism as a result of depleted thyroid hormones.

Gross Morphology

Thyroid gland is diffusely enlarged and firm, weighing 60 to 200 gm. Cut surface is fleshy, pale tan, exhibiting a vaguely nodular pattern.

Light Microscopy

Thyroid gland displays following histological features:

- *Inflammatory infiltrate:* It comprises lymphocytes, plasma cells and macrophages. The inflammatory infiltrates are focally arranged in the form of lymphoid follicles, often with germinal centers.
- *Destruction of follicles:* Extensive destruction and atrophy of the thyroid follicles occurs due to heavy inflammatory infiltrate of CD8+ cytotoxic T cells, CD4+ T cells, recruited macrophages and cell-mediated cytotoxicity by antithyroid antibodies. The remaining thyroid follicles vary in size and shape.
- *Oxyphil metaplasia:* The persistent follicular epithelium is transformed into so-called *Hürthle cells* or *oncocytes* or *Askanazy cells* (oxyphilic metaplasia).
  These have an abundant brightly eosinophilic granular cytoplasm packed with mitochondria and lysosomes. Hürthle cells produce a little or absence of T_3, T_4 and thyroglobulin.
- *Interlobular fibrosis:* Variable interlobular fibrosis is seen in long-standing cases. Fibrosing variant of Hashimoto's thyroiditis shows extensive dense fibrosis within the capsule of thyroid gland with atrophy of thyroid follicles. It should be differentiated from Riedel's thyroiditis.
  It is worth mentioning that Riedel's thyroiditis invades the surrounding structures with extensive fibrosis and scant thyroid tissue.

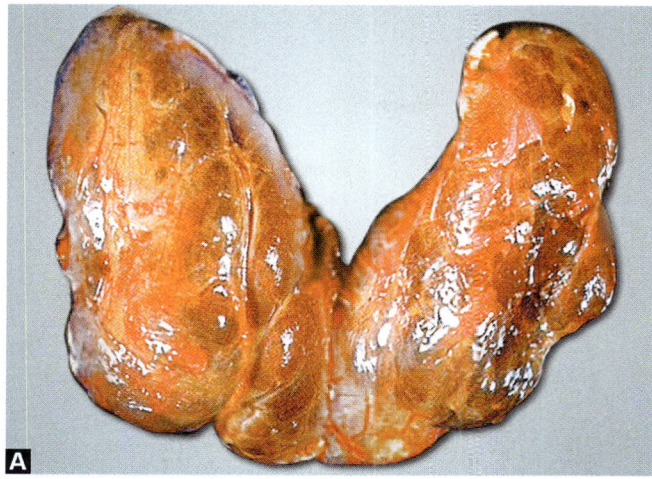
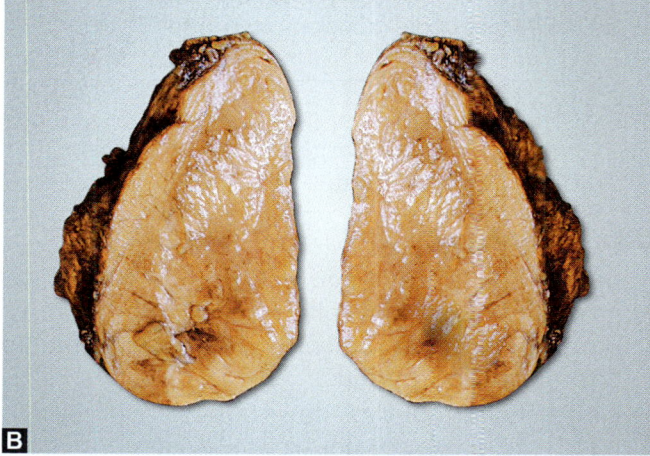

Fig. 26.16: Hashimoto's thyroiditis. Cut surface is fleshy, pale tan, exhibiting a vaguely nodular pattern.

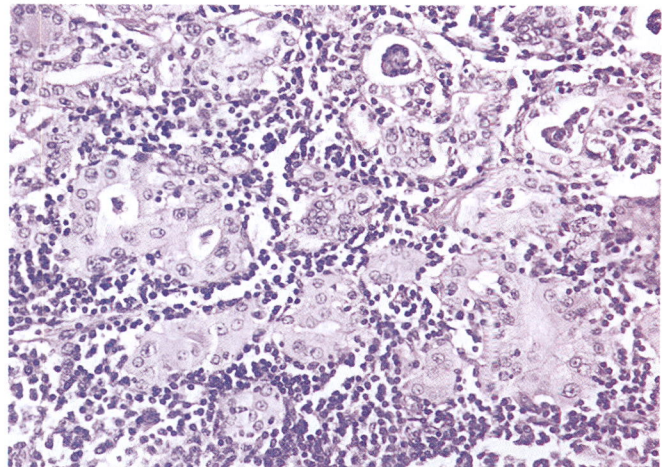

Fig. 26.17: Hashimoto's thyroiditis. Thyroid follicles show destruction due to infiltration by chronic inflammatory cells. Hürthle cell change in follicular cells is seen (400X).

cytotoxic leukocytes release hydrolytic enzymes and oxygen-derived free radicals resulting in tissue damage.

Clinical Features

Early in the course of disease, there may be transient hyperthyroidism from excessive release of thyroid hormones from damaged thyroid follicles, but later hypothyroidism due to depletion of thyroid hormones in 40–50% of cases.

Patient presents with painless diffuse enlargement of thyroid gland, sometimes appear lobulated mass mimicking a tumor. Due to destruction of the thyroid follicles over the years, thyroid gland undergoes marked atrophy, which is often not palpable.

Risk of Malignancy

There is increased risk for subsequent development of primary *B cell non-Hodgkin's lymphoma, papillary carcinoma of thyroid and Hürthle cell neoplasms*.

Laboratory Diagnosis

Diagnostic tests include detection of circulating autoantibodies against the tissues involved anti-microsomal (90%), anti-thyroglobulin (50%), and antiperoxidase are analyzed in Hashimoto's thyroiditis.

Presence of antibody in the lesion (biopsy) is demonstrated by immunofluorescence. TSH is markedly increased in these patients.

SUBACUTE PAINLESS LYMPHOCYTIC THYROIDITIS

Etiology

It is an autoimmune disorder developing during postpartum period. Thyroid gland lacks germinal follicles.

Clinical Features

Patient presents with *abrupt onset of thyrotoxicosis* due to gland destruction, *painless enlarged thyroid gland*. It progresses to primary hypothyroidism in 40 to 50% of cases. It lacks immunological markers as seen in Hashimoto's thyroiditis.

SUBACUTE GRANULOMATOUS THYROIDITIS

It most often affects women of 40–50 years old. It is also known as *de Quervain granulomatous, or giant cell thyroiditis*. It is associated with HLA-B35. It is a self-limited course of several weeks' duration. It is characterized by *granulomatous inflammation with multinucleated giant cells resulting in focal destruction of thyroid gland* (Fig. 26.18).

Etiology

The disease typically occurs after upper respiratory tract infections caused by *influenza virus, adenovirus, echovirus, and coxsackievirus*. Thyroid gland destruction initially results in hyperthyroidism, i.e. increased serum T_4 and decreased TSH. Permanent hypothyroidism is uncommon.

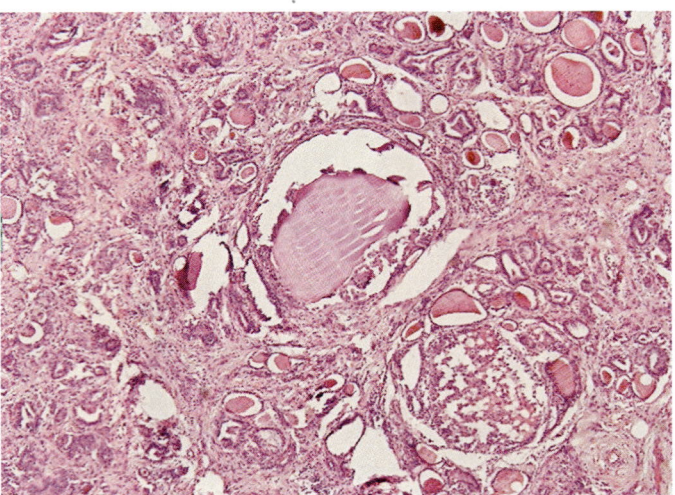

Fig. 26.18: Subacute granulomatous thyroiditis (400X).

Gross Morphology

The thyroid gland is enlarged to 40 to 60 g, and the cut surface is firm and pale.

Light Microscopy

- Initially, it shows acute inflammation with microabscesses. It is followed by infiltration by lymphocytes, plasma cells, and macrophages throughout the thyroid.
- Destruction of follicles allows the release of colloid, which elicits a conspicuous granulomatous reaction.

Clinical Features

Initially the patient may develop transient hyperthyroidism with decreased uptake of ^{123}I followed by hypothyroidism in late stage. Patient presents with *painful tender enlarged thyroid gland* often preceded by an upper respiratory tract infection.

RIEDEL'S THYROIDITIS

Etiology

In Riedel thyroiditis, the thyroid gland is replaced by fibrous tissue and can clinically mimic carcinoma. It may cause *tracheal obstruction*. Extension of fibrous tissue occurs in soft tissues of the neck, progressing in retroperitoneum, mediastinum and orbit. Surgical treatment is required to relieve tracheal or esophageal obstruction.

Gross Morphology

Part or the entire thyroid is hard and is described as *woody*.

Clinical Features

It most often affects only one lobe of thyroid gland. Patient presents with inspiratory stridor (tracheal obstruction), dysphagia (esophagus compression) and hoarseness due to involvement of recurrent laryngeal nerves. Patient may develop hypothyroidism.

ACUTE THYROIDITIS

Etiology

It is caused by *Staphylococcus aureus*. It is treated by course of antibiotics. Thyroid gland destruction initially results in hyperthyroidism (e.g. increased serum T_4 and decreased TSH). Permanent hypothyroidism is uncommon. ^{123}I uptake is decreased.

Clinical Features

Patient presents with fever, tender gland with cervical lymphadenopathy.

HYPOTHYROIDISM

Hypothyroidism manifests as cretinism in children or myxedema in adults.

CRETINISM (THYROID DWARF)

Cretinism results from deficiency of thyroid hormone during fetal development and during postnatal life. Cretinism denotes physical and mental insufficiency secondary to congenital hypothyroidism in children. Cretinism may be endemic, sporadic, or familial and is twice as frequent in girls as in boys.

Physiological state: Thyroid hormones are *essential for brain development*, i.e. axonal and dendrite development especially myelination of central nervous system (formation of myelin sheath around a nerve) in post-natal period in the first two years of life. Thyroid hormones are also necessary for linear growth (maturation of growing epiphyseal region of bones), closure of fontanellae skull and tooth eruption elicitation (Fig. 26.19).

Pathological state: Deficiency of thyroid hormones cause defective development due to non-myelination of nervous system and maturation of the growing fetus leading to stunted growth called cretinism.

Etiology

Most important cause of cretinism is maternal hypothyroidism before development of fetal thyroid gland. Transplacental transfer of antithyroid antibodies from a mother suffering from autoimmune thyroid disease may produce cretinism.

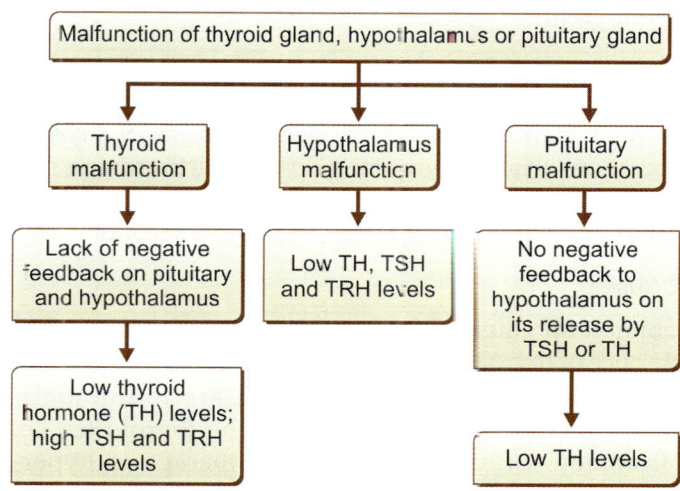

Fig. 26.19: Pathogenesis of hypothyroidism.

It may also be caused due to deficiency of iodine and enzymes required for the synthesis of thyroid hormones. Other causes include maldevelopment of the thyroid gland and failure of the fetal thyroid to descend from its origin at the base of the tongue.

Clinical Features

- Initial manifestations of congenital hypothyroidism appear in the early weeks of life such as sluggishness, slow reflexes (*severe mental retardation*), large *protuberant abdomen* often with *umbilical herniation* flattened broad nose, thick protuberant tongue, *hoarse husky voice*, coarse dry skin, *periorbital edema*, eyes seem widely spaced and low body temperature.
- Later on impairment of physical growth with retarded bone development results in *dwarfism*. There is delay in closure of *fontanelle*, delay in *eruption of* deciduous *teeth* and refractory anemia.
- Mental retardation, stunted growth, and characteristic facies become evident. If thyroid hormone replacement therapy is not promptly provided, congenital hypothyroidism results in mentally retarded dwarf.

Laboratory Diagnosis

The diagnosis of congenital hypothyroidism is confirmed in infants, by decreased serum free T_4 and increased TSH. If maternal antibody transfer is suspected, then tests for antithyroid antibody testing can be performed in both the mother and child.

Therapeutic Correlation

Hypothyroid newborns attain normal development, if early hormonal therapy is started. If it is delayed by 6–12 months, then mental retardation becomes permanent due to brain damage.

MYXEDEMA

Hypothyroidism manifests as myxedema in adults primarily after age of 40 years. It is more common in women than in men. Decreased synthesis of thyroid hormones triiodothyronine (T_3) or and thyroxine (T_4) slows down metabolic processes resulting in hypothyroidism. It is classified as primary or secondary.

Causes

Congenital causes of myxedema include congenital absence of thyroid gland or inborn errors of metabolism.

Acquired causes of myxedema are iodine deficiency (endemic goiter), autoimmune thyroiditis, i.e. Hashimoto's thyroiditis, post-radiotherapy to hyperthyroidism, post-surgical thyroidectomy, antithyroid drugs (carbimazole), and primary tumors of thyroid.

Classification

- *Primary hypothyroidism:* Primary (idiopathic) hypothyroidism most often occurs due to autoimmune mechanism. Approximately 75% of patients with primary hypothyroidism have circulating antibodies to thyroid antigens, suggesting that these cases represent the end stage of autoimmune thyroiditis. Nongoitrous hypothyroidism may also result from antibodies that block TSH itself or the TSH receptor, without activating the thyroid. Some cases are associated with Hashimoto's disease, amyloidosis, sarcoidosis and irradiation.
- *Secondary hypothyroidism:* It is a disorder of the thyroid gland, in which there is failure to stimulate normal thyroid function. It occurs due to: (i) hypothalamus fails to release thyrotropin-releasing hormone (TRH). (ii) Anterior pituitary gland fails to secrete thyroid stimulating hormone (TSH). (iii) Thyroid gland is not able to synthesize thyroid hormones due to iodine deficiency (usually dietary). (iv) Patient receiving antithyroid drugs for the treatment of hyperthyroidism (Table 26.15).

Clinical Features

Early manifestations: Patient presents with insidious onset symptoms due to decreased metabolic rate such as fatigue, cold intolerance, unexplained weight gain, low pitch voice, progressive constipation (decreased GIT motility), anorexia, and muscle cramps.

Late manifestations: With progression of disease, the patient develops systemic manifestations:

- *Periorbital puffiness and non-pitting edema:* Patient develops periorbital puffiness and non-pitting edema legs due to subcutaneous accumulation of mucopolysaccharides and hyaluronic acid.
- *Tongue:* Tongue becomes dry and thick causing hoarseness, slow and slurred speech.
- *Hair loss:* There is hair loss in axillary region, pubic region and lateral aspect (outer-third) of the eyebrows.
- *Skin manifestations:* Skin becomes dry, inelastic, coarse and yellow due to less conversion of carotene into retinoic acid.
- *Congestive heart failure:* Patient develops flabby congestive heart, bradycardia, and poor peripheral circulation, pleural and pericardial effusions.
- *Serum lipid level:* Serum cholesterol level is increased due to decreased synthesis of low-density lipoprotein (LDL) receptors.
- *CNS manifestations:* Patient develops nervous system manifestations such as ataxia (loss of coordination), delayed recovery of 'Achilles reflex' (increase in relaxation phase of deep tendon reflexes), behavioral changes ranging from slight mental slowness to severe impairment (dementia).
- *Infertility:* There is impaired fertility in these patients. Women with hypothyroidism suffer ovulatory failure, progesterone deficiency, decreased libido and irregular and excessive menstrual bleeding (menorrhagia). Erectile dysfunction and oligospermia are common symptoms of hypothyroidism in men.

Table 26.15: Differences between primary and secondary hypothyroidism

Parameters	Primary hypothyroidism	Secondary hypothyroidism
Etiology	Hashimoto's thyroiditis	Pituitary gland disorder
Serum TSH	Increased	Increased
Free T_4	Decreased	Decreased
Thyrotropin-releasing hormone stimulation test	Increased response	No response
Autoantibodies	Anti-TSH receptor autoantibody Anti-thyroglobulin autoantibody Anti-peroxidase autoantibody Anti-microsomal autoantibody Anti-iodine receptor autoantibody	Absent

Laboratory Findings

Increased TSH level and low level of T4 establish hypothyroidism elevated in hypothyroidism. Hypercholesterolemia occurs due to decreased synthesis of low-density lipoprotein (LDL) receptors in hypothyroidism.

Treatment

Patient is put on levothyroxine in small increments every 6–8 weeks to bring serum TSH to the normal range (euthyroid state).

HYPERTHYROIDISM

TOXIC NODULAR GOITER

Increased synthesis of thyroid hormone creates a metabolic imbalance, i.e. increased metabolic rate called hyperthyroidism or thyrotoxicosis. Thyrotoxicosis describes excess of thyroid hormones regardless of etiology. Excess thyroid hormone can be due to various thyroid disorders, i.e. *Graves' disease* (most common) and *toxic nodular goiter* (Fig. 26.20 and Table 26.16).

Clinical Features

Patient presents with weight loss, increased appetite, recent onset of heat intolerance, warm, moist, flushed skin especially hot sweaty palms, nervousness, fine tremors, bounding peripheral pulses, cardiac arrhythmias (atrial fibrillation), dyspnea on exertion, and menstrual abnormalities (amenorrhea or oligomenorrhea).

Males develop impaired fertility, decreased libido and gynecomastia.

GRAVES' DISEASE

Graves' disease is an autoimmune disease. It is associated with decreased TSH activity. TSH receptors are stimulated by TSI, an IgG autoantibody, not by TSH. These autoantibodies such as TSI mimic, the action of TSH, but are not regulated by natural negative feedback controls.

TGI autoantibodies stimulate glandular hyperplasia resulting in thyroid enlargement. Patient develops diffuse toxic goiter, hyperthyroidism, and exophthalmos. Onset is initiated by infection, iodide excess and postpartum.

Epidemiology

It occurs more often in women than in men (young age group). The incidence is increased in HLA-DR3 and HLA-B8 positive individuals. CTL4 and PTPN22 gene mutations increase the risk of Graves' disease. Thyroid acropatchy is associated with digits with clubbing and swelling in patient with Graves' disease.

Pathogenesis

Hypersensitivity reaction type 2 plays an important role in its pathogenesis. T cells induce B cells resulting in synthesis of thyroid-stimulating immunoglobulin

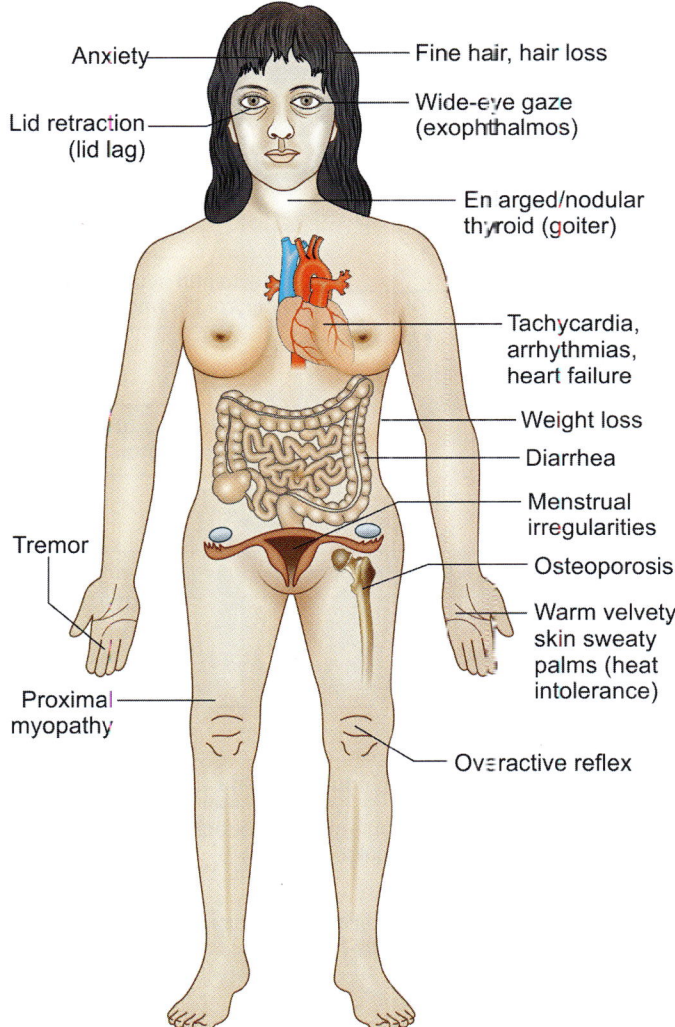

Fig. 26.20: Clinical features of thyrotoxicosis.

Table 26.16: Comparison of Graves' disease and thyroid toxic goiter

Parameters	Graves' disease	Toxic nodular goiter
Sex predilection	Women > Men	Women = Men
Eye signs	Exophthalmos most severe common finding	Exophthalmos less severe
Heart	Tachycardia and fibrillation	Angina
Weight	May lose weight	Often profound

(TSI), an IgG antibody that reacts with TSH receptors and activates adenyl cyclase resulting in increased production of thyroid hormones.

Synthesis of thyroid growth immunoglobulin (TGI) stimulates glandular hyperplasia and thyroid enlargement. In addition to TSI and TGI, anti-microsomal and anti-thyroglobulin autoantibodies are also present (Figs 26.21 and 26.22).

Clinical Features

Patient presents with *non-tender diffuse symmetric thyroid enlargement with features of thyrotoxicosis*. It is associated with exophthalmos in 60–90%, dermatopathy and constitutional symptoms. Thyroid gland and retrobulbar ocular muscles are infiltrated with B cells.

- *Exophthalmos:* Extraocular muscles and retro-orbital tissues are infiltrated by chronic inflammatory cells. There is deposition of *hydrophilic mucopolysaccharides, fibrosis and contractures of extraocular muscles* resulting in incoordination of eye movements.
  Patient presents with *proptosis, lid lag, upper lid retraction, weakness of eye muscles, diplopia, and periorbital edema.*
- *Dermatopathy:* Skin over dorsum of legs or feet becomes edematous and thick orange peeling. It may also show discrete plaque-like lesions in 10–15% of cases. Pretibial dermal swelling occurs due to excessive deposition of glycosaminoglycans in 1–2% of cases.
- *Constitutional symptoms:* These include *weight loss, warm skin, fine tremors* particularly when hands are

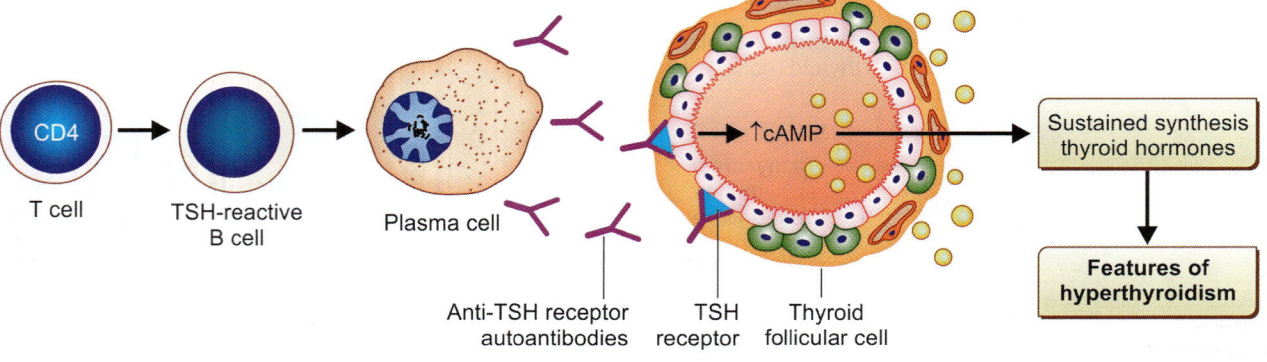

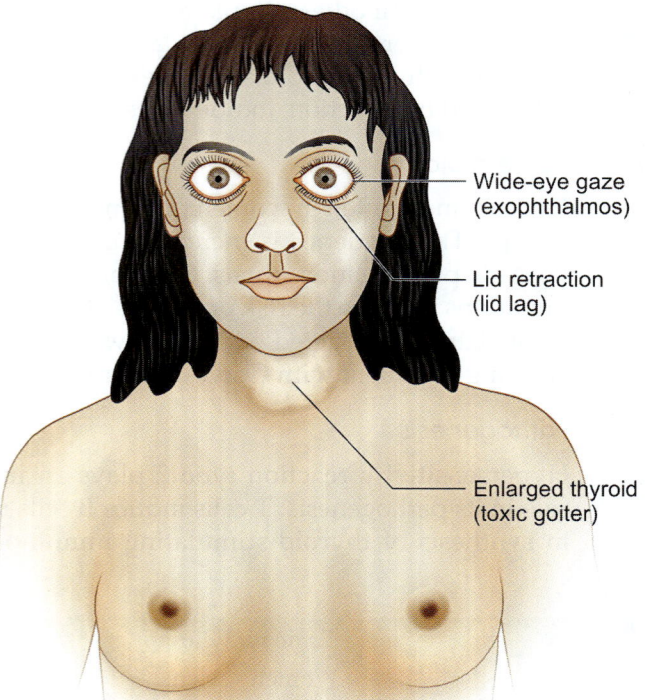

Increased risk factor in Graves' disease
• Young women
• HLA-DR3 and HLA-B8
• CTL4 or PTPN22 gene mutation

Clinical manifestations
• Exophthalmos (lid lag, upper lid retraction, weakness of extraocular muscles).
• Dermatopathy
• Constitutional symptoms (weight loss, warm skin, fine tremors, increased heart rate).

Demonstration of autoantibodies in blood
• TGI: Thyroid growth immunoglobulin stimulates glandular hyperplasia and enlargement.
• TSI: Thyroid-stimulating immunoglobulin mimics TSH and reacts with TSH receptors resulting in sustained synthesis of thyroid hormones.
• Anti-microsomal autoantibodies.
• Anti-thyroglobulin autoantibodies.

Fig. 26.21: Pathogenesis of Graves' disease.

Endocrine System: Pancreas, Thyroid, Parathyroid, Adrenal and Pituitary Glands

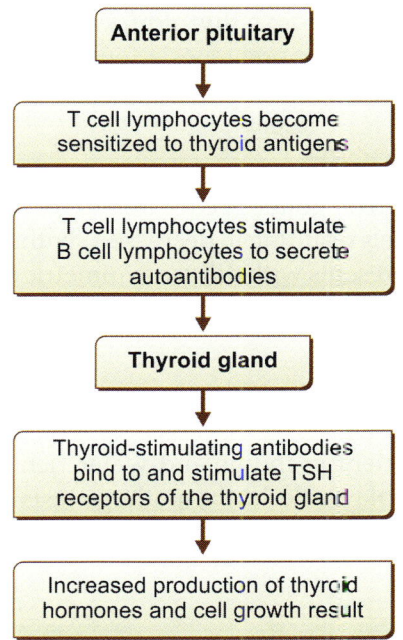

Fig. 26.22: Pathogenesis of Graves' disease.

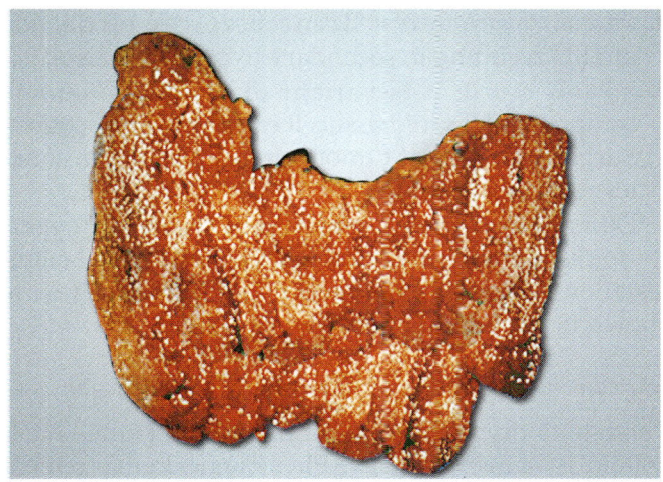

Fig. 26.23: Graves' disease. Cut surface shows a hyperemic, meaty, shiny appearance.

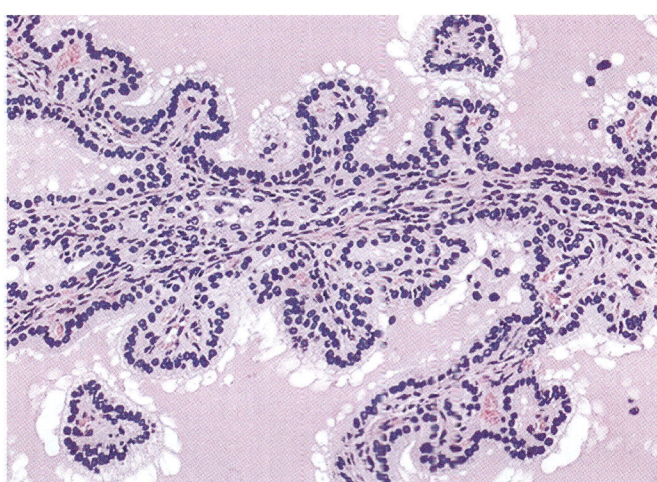

Fig. 26.24: Graves' disease. Light microscopy shows resorption induced scalloping of the margins of the colloid. Antibody mediated hyperplastic papillary epithelial infoldings results from the lining cells becoming columnar in shape and increased in number (400X).

stretched, heat intolerance, diarrhea, anxiety, lid stare due to increased sympathetic stimulation of eyelid muscles; cardiac symptoms (e.g. sinus tachycardia, increased risk for atrial fibrillation, systolic hypertension, high-output heart failure due to increased synthesis of α-adrenergic receptors in the heart).

Gross Morphology
- The thyroid is diffusely enlarged weighing 80 to 90 gm.
- Cut surface reveals soft, red brown, meaty appearance closely resembling cross-section of normal muscle.
- Preoperative iodine administration causes accumulation of colloid and alters the gross appearance.

Light Microscopy
- Marked glandular hyperplasia with micropapillary infoldings, thin colloid with peripheral scalloping of the colloid and lymphocytic infiltration in stroma between thyroid follicles are prominent features.
- Peripheral scalloping occurs as a result of increased proteolysis of colloid and rapid uptake of thyroglobulin by the hyperfunctioning thyroid cells (Figs 26.23 and 26.24).

Laboratory Findings
The best screening tests for Graves' disease are *free T_4 (elevated in Graves' disease) and TSH (greatly decreased in Graves' disease)*. Blood sugar is raised due to glycogenolysis. Peripheral blood shows absolute lymphocytosis.

Treatment
Administration of β-blockers decreases adrenergic effects. Thionamides decrease thyroid hormone synthesis.

OTHER CAUSES OF HYPERTHYROIDISM
- *Plummer disease:* It is a combination of hyperthyroidism, nodular goiter, and absence of exophthalmos. The 'hot' nodules can be adenomas or non-neoplastic areas of nodular hyperplasia.

- *Pituitary hyperfunction:* It can cause excess production of TSH resulting in secondary hyperthyroidism.
- *Struma ovarii:* It is variant of ovarian teratoma composed of thyroid tissue. It can be hyperfunctional. Surgical excision of tumor brings thyroid hormones level to normal range.

Differences between primary and secondary hyperthyroidism are shown in Table 26.17 and clinical manifestations of hypothyroid and hyperthyroid states are shown in Table 26.18.

GOITER

Persistent thyroid gland enlargement from excess colloid is known as *goiter.* Physiological enlargement is not uncommon in puberty and pregnancy. Other causes of goiter include iodine deficiency (endemic or sporadic), Hashimoto's thyroiditis, goitrogens (drugs, food) and dyshormonogenesis (enzyme deficiencies) are shown in Table 26.19.

NONTOXIC GOITER

Simple nontoxic goiter occurs due to increased thyroglobulin levels resulting in decreased synthesis of T_3 and T_4. Patient presents with diffuse symmetric enlargement of thyroid. Females are more affected than males.

Etiology

Dietary factors

- Diet deficient in iodine and water rich in Ca^{++} and fluoride play role in the pathogenesis of nontoxic goiter.

Table 26.17: Differences between primary and secondary hyperthyroidism

Parameters	Primary hyperthyroidism	Secondary hyperthyroidism
Etiology	Graves' disease, toxic adenoma, toxic multinodular goiter	Pituitary gland
Serum TSH	Low	Normal
Free T_4	Increased	Increased
Autoantibodies	TGI (thyroid growth immunoglobulin) TSI (thyroid-stimulating immunoglobulin) Anti-microsomal autoantibody Anti-thyroglobulin autoantibody	Absent

Table 26.18: Clinical manifestations of hypothyroid and hyperthyroid states

Level of organization	Hypothyroidism	Hyperthyroidism
Basal metabolic rate	Decreased	Increased
Sensitivity to catecholamines	Decreased	Increased
Clinical features	Myxedema features Deep voice Impaired growth in children	Exophthalmos in Graves' disease Lid lag Accelerated growth in children
General behavior	Mental retardation (infant) Physical and mental sluggishness Somnolence	Restlessness Hyperkinesis Wakefulness
Cardiovascular system	Decreased cardiac output Bradycardia	Increased cardiac output Tachycardia and palpitation
Gastrointestinal tract	Constipation Loss of appetite	Diarrhea Increased appetite
Respiratory system	Hypoventilation	Breathlessness
Muscle tone and reflexes	Decreased	Increased with tremor and twitching
Temperature tolerance	Cold intolerance	Heat intolerance
Skin and hair	Decreased sweating Coarse and dry skin and hair	Increased sweating Thin silky skin and hair
Weight	Gain	Loss
Blood cholesterol	Increased	Decreased

Endocrine System: Pancreas, Thyroid, Parathyroid, Adrenal and Pituitary Glands

Table 26.19: Classification of goiters morphology, functional activity and iodine deficiency

Parameters	Goiters
Based on morphology	*Diffuse goiter:* It is also known as simple or colloid goiter without thyroid hormone dysfunction
	Nodular goiter: It occurs in the late stage of simple goiter and results to irregular thyroid enlargement either consisting of single nodule or multiple nodules. Most nodular goiters become hyperplastic and do not take up radioactive iodine (*'cold nodules'*)
Based on functional activity	*Nontoxic goiter:* It is also termed simple, colloid, or multinodular goiter. It refers to an enlargement of the thyroid that is not associated with functional, inflammatory, or neoplastic alterations. It occurs due to increased thyroglobulin levels resulting in decreased synthesis of T_3 and T_4. Patient presents with diffuse symmetric enlargement of thyroid. Females are more affected than males
	Toxic goiter: It is associated with hyperthyroidism as seen in Graves' disease
Based on iodine deficiency	*Endemic goiter:* It occurs in iodine deficient geographical areas. Without sufficient iodine, thyroid hormones are not produced and the pituitary continuously secretes thyroid stimulating hormone (TSH)
	Sporadic goiter: It occurs in non-iodine-deficient geographical areas. It is caused by enzyme deficiency, goitrogens, puberty, and pregnancy. Females are more affected than males

- Goitrogens present in vegetables include cabbage, turnips, cassava (e.g. containing thiocyanate inhibits iodine transport), brussels, sprouts (young shoot of a plant), turnips, brassica plants, cruciferae plants and soya beans.

Goitrogenic drugs: The most commonly used goitrogenic drug is lithium, which is used in the management of manic-depressive states. Therapeutic administration of drugs (e.g. salicylates, cyanates, thiocyanates, resorcinol, lithium chloride and cobalt chloride) may result into nontoxic goiter.

Enzyme deficiency
- Deficiency of *peroxidase enzyme* inhibits conversion of iodide to organically bound iodine process and patient develops goiter.
- *Dehalogenase deficiency* inhibits conversion of MIT and DIT to form T_3 and T_4, and results in goiter.

Pathogenesis

Goiter is caused by absolute or relative deficiency of thyroid hormones. There are two stages, i.e. (a) hyperplasia/hypertrophy of thyroid follicles and (b) involution stage. Enlarged thyroid gland weighs 100–150 gm. Initial diffuse thyroid enlargement is followed by multinodular goiter.

- *Hyperplastic stage:* Absolute or relative deficiency of thyroid hormones increase synthesis of TSH by anterior pituitary gland. TSH acts on thyroid follicles, which may undergo hyperplasia/hypertrophy with formation of new thyroid follicles, which attempt to increase thyroid hormones synthesis. This stage is followed by involution stage.
- *Involution stage:* Accumulation of abundant colloid leads to flattening of the epithelium of thyroid follicles. Thyroid gland fails to sustain synthesis of thyroid hormones.

Clinical Features

Patient presents with thyroid enlargement, respiratory distress and dysphagia (Fig. 26.25).

> **Gross Morphology**
> - During involution stage, cut surface of goiter shows numerous cystic nodules filled with gelatinous glistening excess colloid.
> - Areas of hemorrhages are seen into many of these cysts (Fig. 26.26).

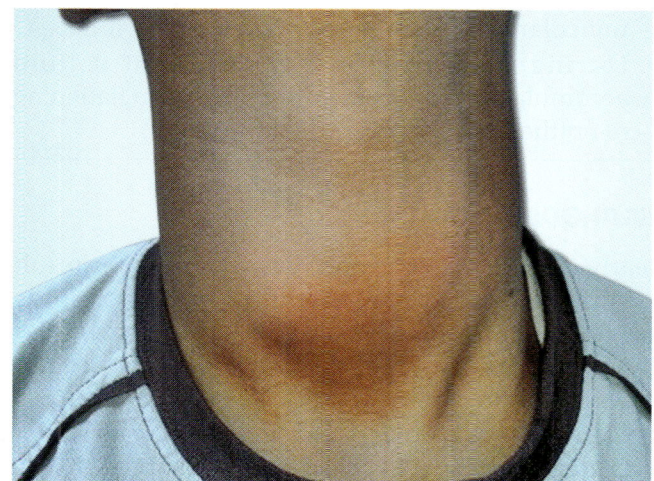

Fig. 26.25: Diffuse goiter. Diffuse enlargement of thyroid gland in male.

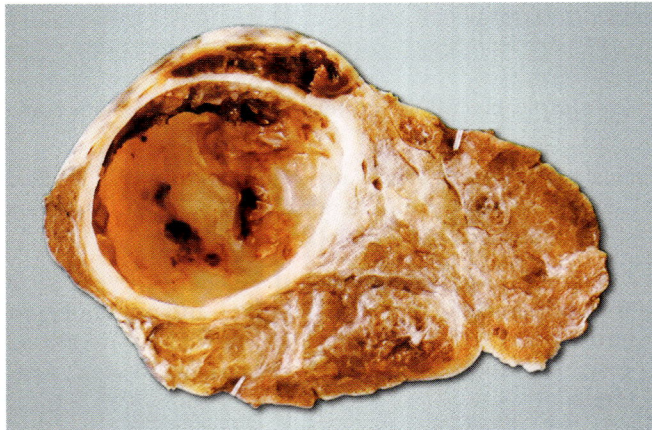

Fig. 26.26: Thyroid nodular goiter with cystic degeneration.

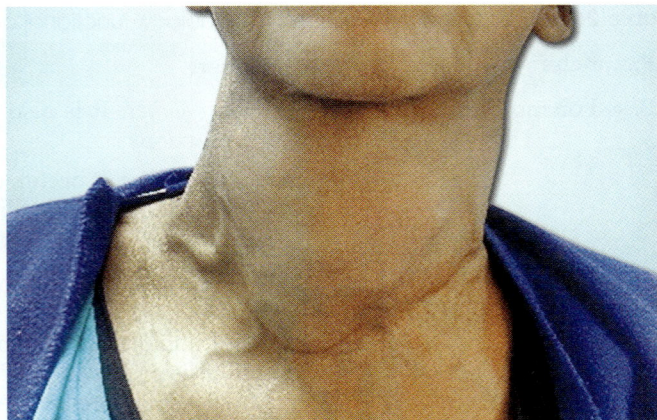

Fig. 26.28: Multinodular goiter obstructing superior vena cava. Dilated veins are seen due to superior vena cava (SVC) syndrome.

compression of trachea (dyspnea), and compression of great vessels of neck (Fig. 26.28).

Pathogenesis

- Absolute or relative deficiency of thyroid hormones stimulates increased synthesis of TSH. It results in hyperplasia and hypertrophy of thyroid follicles, with formation of new follicles and colloid accumulation.
- Uneven accumulation of colloid throughout thyroid follicles leads to tension and stress within thyroid gland resulting in rupture of thyroid follicles and blood vessels.
- Fibrosis further adds to tension within thyroid gland. Sometimes areas of dystrophic calcification are seen.

Clinical Features

- Patient presents with inspiratory stridor (compression of trachea), dysphagia (compression of esophagus). Hoarseness may result from recurrent laryngeal nerve compression. Compression of jugular vein leads to dizziness or syncope known as *Pemberton's sign*, when the patient raises arms above head.
- Hemorrhage into colloid nodule causes sudden painful enlargement of thyroid. Features of hypothyroidism or toxic nodular goiter (TSH-independent *'hot'* nodule) may be present. Dominant nodule in multinodular goiter has 2–5% risk of malignancy.

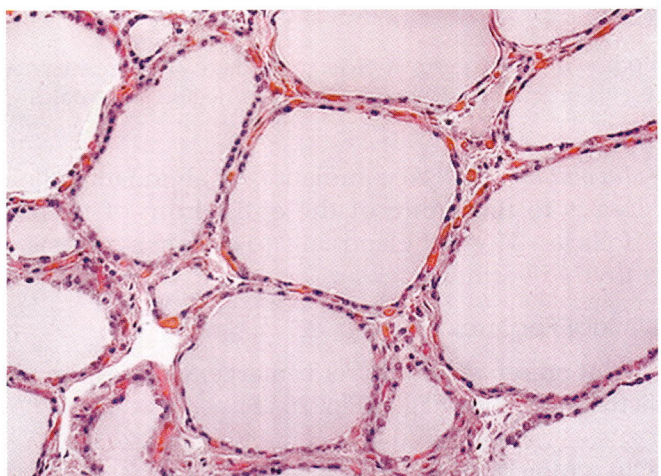

Fig. 26.27: Simple colloid goiter. Thyroid follicles are filled with colloid material. Lining epithelium is flattened (400X).

Light Microscopy

- During hyperplastic stage, thyroid follicular cells show hyperplasia and hypertrophy of thyroid follicular cells, with regeneration of new follicles.
- During involution stage, abundant colloid accumulation in thyroid follicles results in flattening of epithelium (Fig. 26.27).

MULTINODULAR GOITER

Nearly all cases of long-standing simple goiter results in multinodular goiter. It commonly affects older age group. Women are more affected than men (8:1). Dominant nodule in multinodular goiter has 2 to 5% risk of malignancy.

There is uneven proliferation, nodules, scar formation, cysts, degeneration and calcification. Enlarged thyroid gland weighs up to 500–1000 gm. Patient presents with neck mass, compression of esophagus (dysphagia),

Gross Morphology

- Most goiters weigh >40 gm (some <25 gm).
- Cut surface is heterogenous with areas of scaring and calcification.
- Condensation about themselves creates appearance of complete encapsulation so-called adenomatous goiter and multiple colloid adenomatous goiters (Fig. 26.29).

Endocrine System: Pancreas, Thyroid, Parathyroid, Adrenal and Pituitary Glands

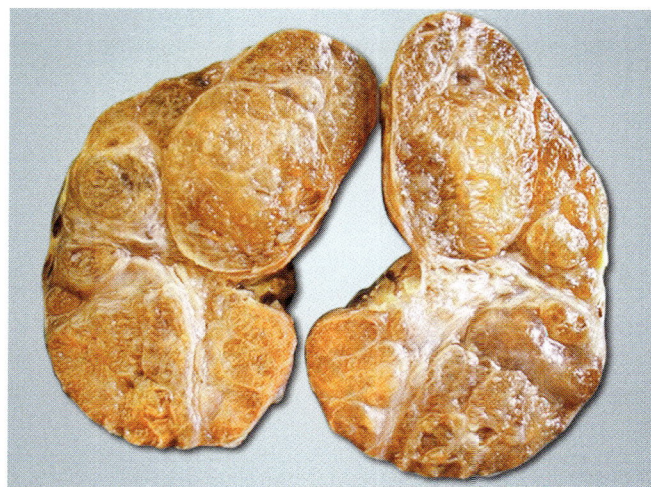

Fig. 26.29: Multinodular goiter in thyroid gland. Cut surface shows multiple nodules filled with colloid material.

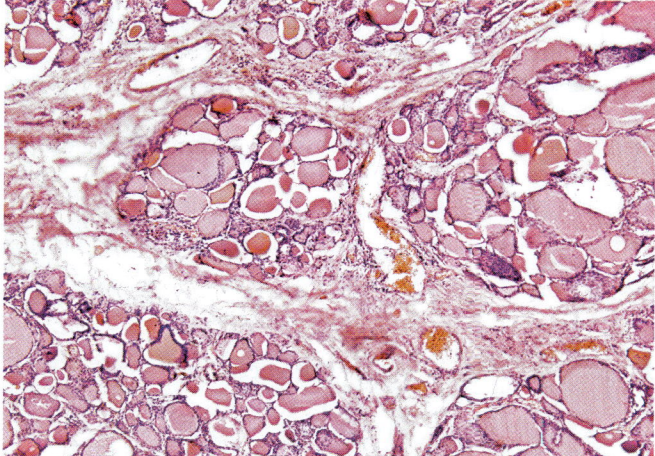

Fig. 26.30: Multinodular goiter showing variable sized thyroid follicles, random irregular scarring with focal areas of hemorrhage and calcification (400X).

> **Light Microscopy**
>
> Histopathological examination reveals variable sized thyroid follicles, random irregular scarring with focal areas of hemorrhage, calcification, microcysts formation; macrophages and foreign body giant cells (Fig. 26.30).

NEOPLASMS OF THYROID GLAND

Classification of Thyroid Tumors

- Thyroid tumors are classified into primary (benign or malignant) and secondary. Thyroid adenoma is a benign tumor. Primary malignant tumors are papillary carcinoma, follicular carcinoma, medullary carcinoma and undifferentiated carcinoma. Papillary carcinoma accounts for 50% of all thyroid cancers.
- Malignant tumors of thyroid gland are more common in women than men over 40 years of age. Thyroid nodule is well circumscribed gray white solitary nodule delineated from surrounding normal thyroid tissue.
- Majority of thyroid nodules are neoplastic in nature. Toxic (hyperfunctioning) nodule concentrates iodine. Such nodules may be benign or malignant tumors.
- WHO histological classification of thyroid tumors is shown in Table 26.20.

Risk Factors

Risk factors of thyroid cancers are iodine deficiency, radiation exposure, high doses of X-rays and hereditary. Gene mutations associated with thyroid cancer are shown in Table 26.21.

Clinical Course

Papillary carcinoma is least aggressive neoplasm with slow metastases. Follicular carcinoma is less common but spreading early to lymph nodes and distant organs. Medullary carcinoma synthesizes thyrocalcitonin, histaminase, prostaglandins and ACTH.

Prognosis

Prognosis is good in children (>70%) with 10 years survival. Rapid growth suggests malignancy.

Patient presents with fixation of growth or cervical lymphadenopathy (70%) or pulmonary metastases (15%) suggest malignancy. thyroid cancers metastasizing to various organs show positivity for thyroglobulin and thyroid transcriptional factor-1 (TTF-1).

THYROID ADENOMA

Thyroid adenoma is most common benign tumor derived from follicular epithelium. Adenomas are cold nodules in comparison with adjacent thyroid tissue. *Somatic mutations in the TSH receptor complex and Gsa genes are demonstrated in up to 40% of adenomas.*

Origin

It originates from thyroid follicular cells. It exhibits follicular differentiation.

Clinical Features

Patient presents with nonfunctional solitary *cold nodule*. Secondary changes may occur in large adenoma, i.e. hemorrhage, edema, fibrosis, calcification and bone formation.

Malignant Potential

Approximately 10% of follicular adenoma may progress to follicular carcinoma.

Table 26.20: WHO histological classification of thyroid tumors

Benign thyroid tumors	
Follicular adenoma	Simple adenoma Colloid adenoma Fetal adenoma Embryonal adenoma Hürthle cell variant of adenoma
Hyalinizing trabecular neoplasm	
Hyalinizing trabecular neoplasm	It shows hyalinization and invasion of capsule
Malignant thyroid tumors	
Primary malignant tumors	Papillary carcinoma Follicular carcinoma *Medullary carcinoma:* Familial or sporadic Poorly differentiated carcinoma *Undifferentiated anaplastic carcinoma:* Small cell variant, carcinosarcoma variant and giant cell carcinoma *Rare tumors:* Mixed follicular and medullary carcinoma, squamous cell carcinoma, mucoepidermoid carcinoma, sclerosing mucoepidermoid carcinoma, mucinous carcinoma, spindle cell tumor with thymus-like differentiation and carcinoma shows thymus-like differentiation *Uncommon tumors:* Teratoma, primary lymphomas, plasmacytoma, ectopic thymoma, angiosarcoma, smooth muscle tumors, paraganglioma, solitary fibrous tumor, follicular dendritic cell tumor, Langerhans cell histiocytosis and secondary tumors

Follicular adenoma, papillary carcinoma, follicular carcinoma and undifferentiated anaplastic carcinoma are important in clinical practice.

Table 26.21: Gene mutations associated with thyroid carcinoma

Category	Proto-oncogene	Mechanism	Associated cancers
Growth factors			
HGF (hepatocyte growth factor)	HGF	Overexpression	Thyroid carcinoma Hepatocellular carcinoma
Growth factor receptors			
Receptors for neurotrophic factors	RET	Point mutation	*Multiple endocrine neoplasia:* MEN IIa, MEN IIb familial thyroid medullary carcinoma
Mitogenic signaling pathway inhibitors (tumor suppressor genes)			
APC	Adenomatous polyposis protein (locus 5p21). Mutation by deletion or nonsense	APC inhibits WNT signaling activator pathway, thus prevents nuclear transcription. It degrades catenin	*Sporadic cancers:* Thyroid carcinoma, colon carcinoma, gastric carcinoma, pancreas carcinoma and melanoma

Low doses of ionization radiation (radiotherapy) in head and neck region can cause or enhance DNA mutations and chromosomal abnormalities.

Diagnostic Criteria

- Thyroid adenoma is surrounded by a complete capsule without evidence of capsular or vessel invasion.
- There is uniform histopathological pattern inside capsule.
- It exhibits distinct architecture of thyroid follicles inside and outside capsule.
- It causes compression of surrounding parenchyma.
- There is lack of multinodularity in remaining thyroid gland.

Histological Variants

- *Simple (normofollicular) adenoma:* It is an encapsulated neoplasm in which the cells are arranged in follicles resembling normal thyroid tissue.
- *Colloid (macrofollicular) adenoma:* It shows large thyroid follicles containing colloid.
- *Fetal (microfollicular) adenoma:* It is commonest variant of thyroid adenoma. It is composed of closely packed small thyroid follicles with scant colloid arranged in edematous fibrovascular stroma.
- *Embryonal (trabecular or solid) adenoma:* It shows thyroid epithelium arranged in solid trabecular pattern or branching cords.
- *Hürthle cell variant of adenoma:* It is composed of large granular cells forming cords containing a little colloid), which have no clinical significance.

Gross morphology and *light microscopy* of thyroid follicular adenoma are shown in Figs 26.31 and 26.32.

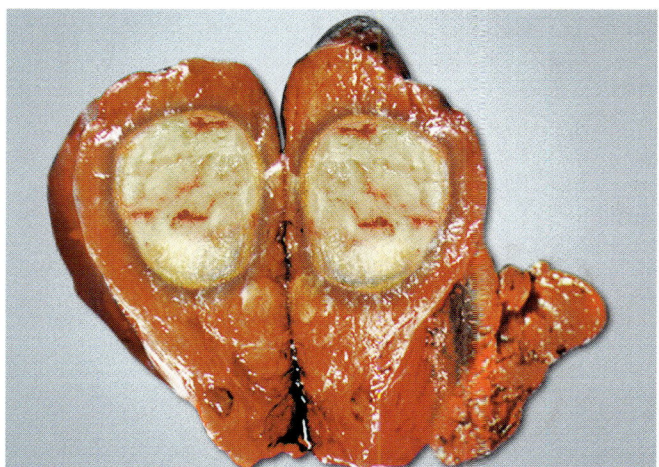

Fig. 26.31: Gross morphology of thyroid follicular adenoma.

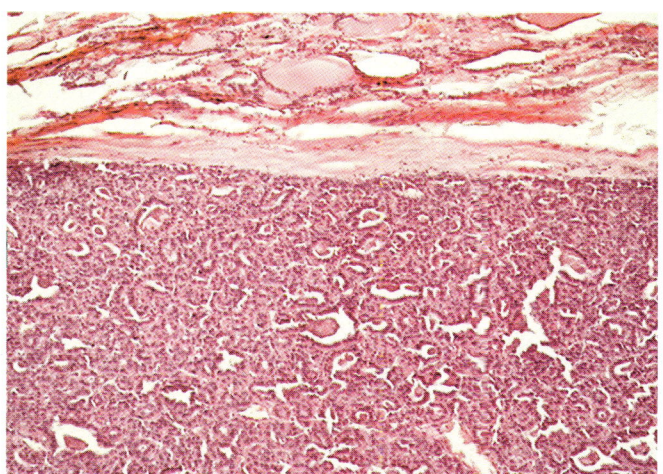

Fig. 26.32: Thyroid follicular adenoma. Tumor is completely surrounded by capsule. Uniform histopathological pattern of thyroid adenoma cells is seen. Tumor has compressed surrounding parenchyma.

HYALINIZING TRABECULAR NEOPLASM

Origin

It originates from thyroid follicular cells.

Light Microscopy

- Tumor is composed of follicular cells without atypia arranged in trabecular pattern with marked hyalinized vascular stroma.
- These features along with invasion of capsule and blood vessels are termed as hyalinizing trabecular carcinoma.

Immunohistochemistry

- Tumor cells show positivity for MIB1.
- It stains membrane and cytoplasm of tumor cells.

PAPILLARY CARCINOMA

Papillary carcinoma thyroid is the commonest thyroid cancer. It accounts for 70–80% of all thyroid cancers. It most often affects young women (20–30 years of age group). It is usually multifocal in origin within the gland and least aggressive thyroid cancer.

Tumor most often remains localized to the thyroid and adjacent tissues for many years. It has a slow tendency to metastasize to regional lymph nodes, but distant metastases are rare. Prognosis is excellent even when adjacent lymph nodes are involved.

Diagnostic Features

Histological features of papillary carcinoma thyroid are presence of true papillae, psammoma bodies, dark red colloid, crowded nuclei, optically clear chromatin (Orphan Annie appearance), irregular nuclear contours, nuclear groove and intranuclear cytoplasmic inclusions.

Radionuclide Scan

Tumor is almost always nonfunctional. It invariably produces a cold nodule by radionuclide scanning.

Risk Factors

Hashimoto's thyroiditis and radiation exposure to the neck increases risk of papillary carcinoma in 5–10% of cases. Ionizing radiations pose a potential worldwide threat in this nuclear age. Low doses of ionizing radiation can cause DNA mutations and chromosomal abnormalities results in cancer. Large doses of radiation can inhibit cell division. Ionizing radiation also can enhance the effects of genetic abnormalities.

Molecular Genetics

- *RET-PTC oncogene:* In some instances, papillary carcinoma may be associated with changes in chromosome 10. Either there is paracentric inversion of chromosome 10, or a reciprocal translocation between chromosomes 10 and 17.

  These chromosomal changes activate the tyrosine kinase domain of RET. These novel fusion genes are referred to as RET-PTC oncogene. Mutations in B-type RAS kinase (BRAF) are also common and predictive of tumor behavior and progression.

- *Hepatocyte growth factor (HGF):* Many cancer cells, acquire the ability to synthesize the same growth factors to which they are responsive, generating an autocrine loop. Increased baseline activity of HGF oncogene product is associated with hepatocellular carcinoma and thyroid cancer.

Clinical Features

The patient presents with slow growing painless occult (<1.5 cm in diameter) to palpable solitary or multifocal thyroid nodule. In some cases, thyroid papillary carcinoma is not palpable (occult), patients present with lymphadenopathy nearby thyroid gland called *Delphian node* containing metastases in 50–70%. Distant metastases are uncommon, i.e. lungs and bone in 10% cases.

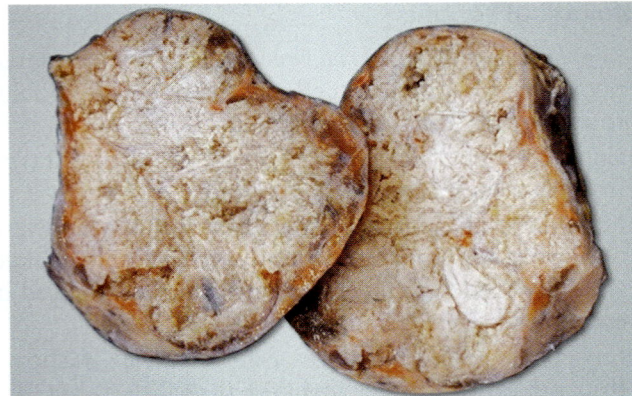

Fig. 26.33: Papillary carcinoma thyroid. On cut surface, tumor is solid grey white with small cystic spaces.

Gross Morphology

- Tumor may be small microscopic occult lesion <1 cm to large 10 cm nodule. Multifocal areas are observed in 20–75%.
- On cut surface, tumor is usually solid gray white and sometimes cystic mass.
- Tumor is clearly invading the capsule.
- Approximately, <10% of cases, tumor is surrounded by a complete capsule (Fig. 26.33).

Light Microscopy

Tumor is composed of fibrovascular stroma lined by tumor cells exhibiting branching tree-like pattern.

- Tumor cells contain optically clear *ground glass nuclei* giving (*Orphan Annie*) appearance. The nuclei show longitudinal nuclear groove and intranuclear pseudoinclusions due to cytoplasmic invagination into the nuclei. Fibrovascular stroma is edematous and infiltrated by lymphocytes, foamy histiocytes and hemosiderin.
- Fibrovascular stroma shows laminated calcific spherules called *Psamomma bodies* formed due to necrosis of cells with dystrophic calcification in 50% of cases. Their presence is strong indicator of papillary carcinoma of thyroid (Figs 26.34 to 26.36).

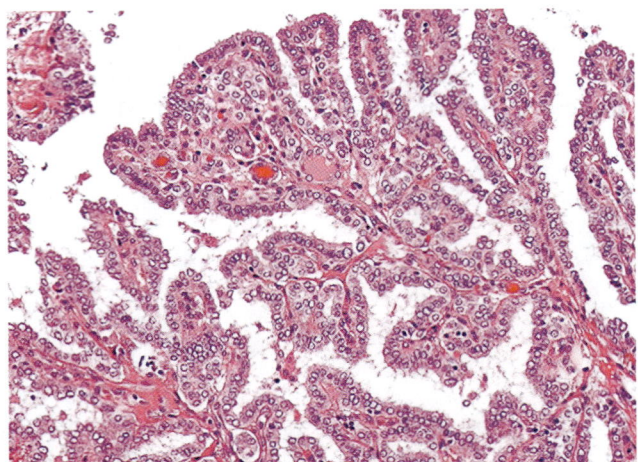

Fig. 26.34: Papillary carcinoma of thyroid.

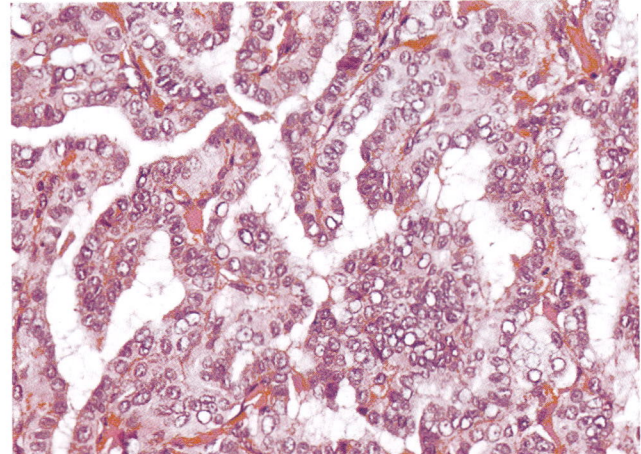

Fig. 26.35: Papillary carcinoma of thyroid. Tumor is composed of fibrovascular core lined by neoplastic cells with optically clear nuclei exhibiting overcrowding (200X).

Histological Variants

- *Follicular variant:* It consists of neoplastic follicular component and psammoma bodies. Prognosis is similar to conventional papillary carcinoma thyroid.

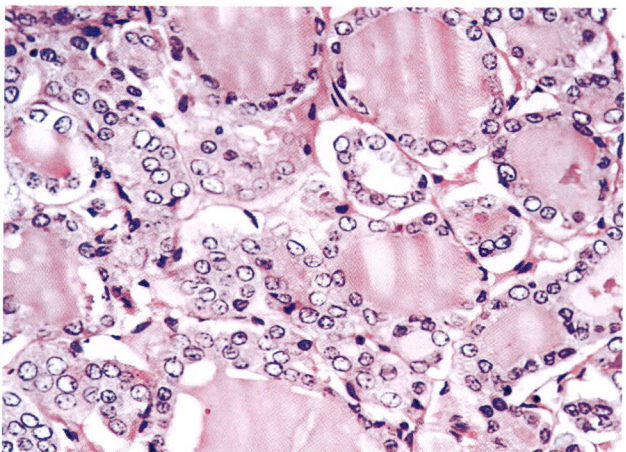

Fig. 26.36: Papillary carcinoma thyroid (follicular variant). Tumor is composed of neoplastic cells with optically clear nuclei exhibiting nuclear grooves (400X).

Diagnostic Criteria

Diagnosis relies on the identification of capsular and/or lymphovascular invasion by neoplastic cells.

Risk Factors

These include iodine deficiency, female gender, elderly persons and radiation exposure.

Molecular Genetics

RAS gene mutations are common. Somatic rearrangements of the tyrosine kinase portion of the RET proto-oncogene with fusion of other genes such as PAX8 and PPARg1 can result in the RET/PTC oncogene that is present in many follicular neoplasms.

Clinical Features

The patient presents with slow growing painless unifocal mass in thyroid region.

- *Encapsulated variant:* It is well encapsulated tumor associated with lymph node metastases but no distant metastases. Prognosis of this variant is excellent.
- *Diffuse sclerosing variant:* It is characterized by diffuse sclerosis, numerous psammoma bodies, squamous metaplasia and inflammation. It is associated with lymph node and distant lung metastases. Prognosis is poor than conventional papillary carcinoma thyroid.
- *Tall cell variant:* Tumor cells consist of abundant eosinophilic cytoplasm and lymphocytic infiltrate. It has worse prognosis than conventional papillary carcinoma thyroid.
- *Columnar variant:* Tumor cells contain tall columnar cells with nuclear stratification.

Clinical Correlation

Patient with papillary carcinoma without evidence of metastasis has an excellent prognosis especially in persons younger than 45 years of age. Prognosis is good with 10-year survival rate in 80–90% of cases. Cure rate is nearly 100% in young patient with small focus of cancer. Relapses occur 20–35 years after treatment.

FOLLICULAR CARCINOMA

Follicular carcinoma thyroid accounts for 15–20% of all thyroid cancers. It most common affects older women over 50–60 years. It is purely follicular without papillary or other elements. It is characterized histologically by relatively uniform follicles. Tumor is capsulated with vascular invasion. This tumor may transform to aggressive anaplastic carcinoma. It may metastasize to the lungs, liver, brain and bones.

Gross Examination

- It is difficult to differentiate between well circumscribed follicular carcinoma and follicular adenoma. Some follicular carcinomas bulge from the confines of its capsule. These show invasion of capsule and surrounding tissues, thus distinguished from follicular adenoma.
- Minimally invasive follicular carcinoma is seen grossly as a well-defined, unifocal encapsulated soft tumor.
- Cut surface is gray white soft with areas of hemorrhage (tan), necrosis and cyst formation (Fig. 26.37).

Light Microscopy

- Tumor is composed of variable sized thyroid follicles lined by tumor cells with normochromatic/hyperchromatic nuclei with oxyphil/clear cytoplasm. These are arranged in cords and invading capsule.
- Minimally invasive follicular carcinoma, which shows only capsular invasion without vascular invasion has better prognosis (Fig. 26.38).

Histological Variants

- *Encapsulated follicular carcinoma variant:* It is well encapsulated with minimal capsular invasion or invasion of blood vessels and distant metastases in 15% of cases.

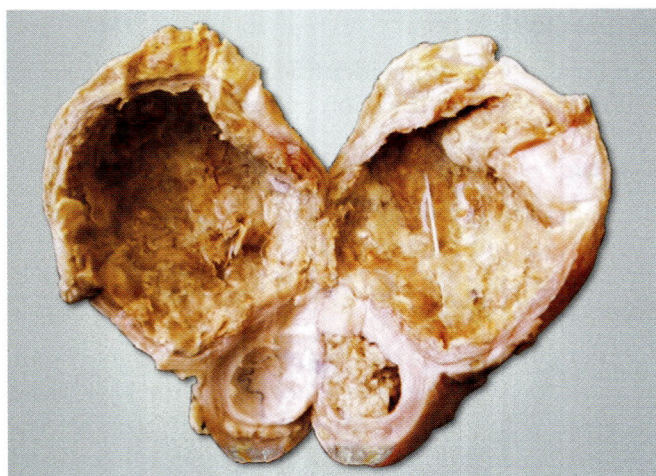

Fig. 26.37: Follicular carcinoma thyroid gross morphology. Cut surface is grey white with areas of hemorrhage and necrosis and cyst formation.

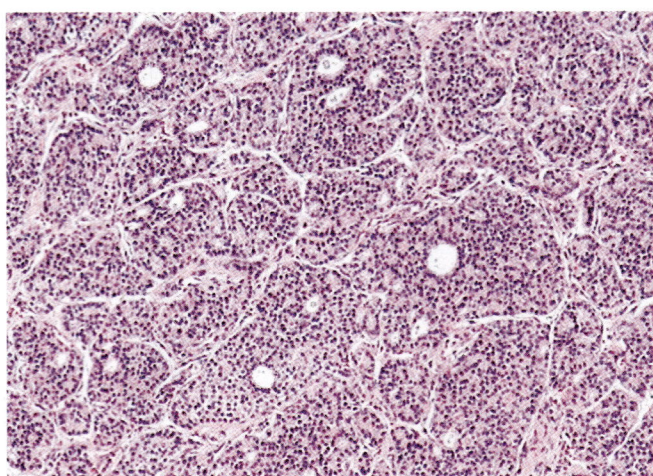

Fig. 26.39: Follicular carcinoma thyroid (insular variant). Tumor shows broad trabeculae of small cells with evenly distributed chromatin with inconspicuous nucleoli and scanty cytoplasm. Tumor cells are arranged around blood vessels with numerous mitosis (200X).

Immunohistochemistry

- Thyroglobulin (Tg) can be used as a tumor marker for well differentiated follicular carcinoma.
- Follicular carcinoma with or without metastases show significant overexpression of **Ki-67** proliferative marker.

Metastasis

It mainly spreads by hematogenous route to *liver, lungs* and *bones*. Lymphatic spread to regional lymph nodes may also occur.

Prognosis

It depends upon stage and histological variant of the tumor. It has a poorer prognosis than papillary carcinoma. It is more likely to recur after surgical removal. Prognostic factors of papillary carcinoma thyroid are shown in Table 26.22.

Treatment

Surgical removal is done in stage I and II. TSH administration is followed by radioactive iodine in stage III and IV. Comparison of papillary and follicular carcinoma of thyroid gland is shown in Table 26.23 and histological features differentiating solitary benign follicular and malignant follicular lesions are shown in 26.24.

MEDULLARY CARCINOMA

Medullary carcinoma thyroid accounts for 5–8%, i.e. third most common of all thyroid cancers. It is most common in females except for inherited cancers. It is

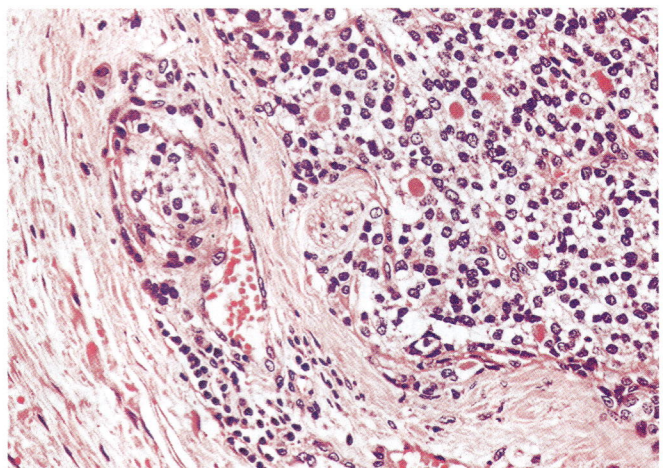

Fig. 26.38: Follicular carcinoma thyroid: Tumor is composed of variable sized thyroid follicles lined by tumor cells with normochromatic/hyperchromatic nuclei with oxyphil/clear cytoplasm. These are arranged in cords and invading capsule (400X).

- *Langhans' struma variant:* It is sluggish tumor compressing respiratory airways.
- *Insular type of follicular carcinoma:* It is rare poorly differentiated variant of follicular carcinoma. Its phenotype is similar to the *pancreatic insulinoma*. It is more aggressive tumor, which shows positivity for thyroglobulin, but negativity for calcitonin.

    Light microscopy shows broad trabeculae of small primitive cells with evenly distributed chromatin with inconspicuous nucleoli and scant cytoplasm. Tumor cells are arranged around blood vessels with numerous mitosis and extrathyroid involvement of lymph nodes (Fig. 26.39).

Table 26.22: Prognostic factors of papillary carcinoma thyroid

Parameters	Good prognosis	Poor prognosis
Sex predilection	Female patients	Male patients
Age group	<40 years of age especially children	>40 years of age
Location	Unicentric (unifocal) tumor	Multicentric (multifocal) tumor
Tumor differentiation	Well differentiated carcinoma	Poorly differentiated carcinoma
Extension of tumor	Tumor is confined within thyroid gland	Tumor is extending outside thyroid gland
Aneuploidy	Absent	Present

Table 26.23: Comparison of papillary and follicular carcinoma of thyroid gland

Parameters	Papillary carcinoma	Follicular carcinoma
Role of radiation	Present	Absent
Encapsulation	Rare	Common
Invasion	Strongly invasive, invades in small islands	Variably invasive in large islands with pushing borders
Multiple tumor foci	Common	Rare
Blood vessel invasion	Rare	Common
Cellular pattern	Papillae, follicles, solid cell group	Follicles, trabeculae no papillae, pseudo-papillary infoldings may occur
Psammoma bodies	Present in 50% in fibrovascular stroma	Absent, but calcified colloid may occur
Nuclear features	Ground glass (*Orphan Annie*) appearance, grooves, pseudoinclusions, often overlapping	Normochromatic or hyperchromatic, no grooves, no overlap

Table 26.24: Histological features differentiating solitary benign from malignant follicular lesions

Benign follicular neoplasm	Follicular carcinoma
Complete but delicate capsule	Dense circumferential fibrosis
Entrapped or sequestered thyroid in/near capsule	Transcapsular *'mushrooming'* invasion
Juxtaposed or prolapsed thyroid tissue near vessels, but with intact endothelium	Adherence of thyroid tissue to endothelium with associated fibrosis

not associated with radiation exposure. These tumors resist radiation and metastasize quickly.

Origin

- Medullary carcinoma of the thyroid is a calcitonin-producing tumor of parafollicular C cells of the thyroid. Parafollicular 'C' cells are abundant in upper lateral lobe of the thyroid gland.
- Altered calcitonin contributes to amyloid deposition within the tumor in majority of cases, demonstrated by Congo red. Serum calcitonin is sometimes used to screen for medullary carcinoma of the thyroid.

Neuroendocrine Features

Medullary carcinoma thyroid possesses neuroendocrine features. Parafollicular C cells synthesize thyrocalcitonin, which is a tumor marker for medullary carcinoma thyroid in 90% of cases. Tumor can synthesize also prostaglandins, histamine, serotonin, ACTH (producing Cushing's syndrome), somatostatin, and gastrin releasing peptides (bombesin).

Age Group

It may be sporadic (80%) or familial (20%). Sporadic cases affect 40–60 years of age. Untreated cases progress rapidly.

Molecular Genetics

- Both familial (90%) and sporadic (50%) medullary carcinomas are associated with **RET proto-oncogene** mutations (chromosome 10) involving exons 10, 11, and 13.
- RET proto-oncogene codes for a transmembrane receptor tyrosine kinase. It is mutated in the MEN IIa

and MEN IIb syndromes, as well as in sporadic cases of medullary carcinoma of the thyroid.
- Mutant neurotropic growth factor receptors deliver continuous mitogenic signals from mutant proto-oncogene RET to the cells, even in the absence of growth factor in the environment.

Prophylactic Thyroidectomy

Patients who carry the RET proto-oncogene should be offered prophylactic total thyroidectomy, which is curative in most cases.

Sporadic Medullary Carcinoma

These patients present with solitary tumor located in mid-portion or upper half of thyroid gland corresponding to a greater concentration of parafollicular 'C' cells in this region. Hormones (e.g. calcitonin, prostaglandins, serotonin, or VIP) synthesized by the tumor increase gastrointestinal secretion and motility responsible for diarrhea in 33% of cases.

Familial Medullary Carcinoma

Familial medullary carcinoma has a better prognosis than sporadic type. It is associated with pheochromocytoma, and completely curable when detected before it causes symptoms. It is associated with autosomal dominant MEN IIa (Sipple syndrome), MEN IIb and inherited medullary carcinoma without associated endocrinopathies. Patients with multiple endocrine neoplasia syndromes have gene mutations that make them susceptible to neoplasia or hyperplasia in multiple organs.

- *MEN IIa syndrome:* It is also known as *Sipple syndrome*. It comprises medullary carcinoma thyroid, parathyroid adenoma or hyperplasia (hyperparathyroidism (33%) and bilateral pheochromocytomas. Hirschsprung's disease (congenital megacolon) and a variety of neural crest tumors (e.g. glioma) are also seen in patients with MEN IIb, the RET oncogene, a transmembrane receptor of the tyrosine kinase family. When a diagnosis of pheochromocytoma is made, demonstration of RET oncogene would justify prophylactic thyroidectomy keeping in view of fatal outcome of medullary carcinoma thyroid.
- *MEN IIb syndrome:* It is associated with medullary carcinoma, bilateral pheochromocytomas, and multiple mucosal ganglioneuromas in lips/tongue. In contrast to MEN IIa, it does not induce hyperparathyroidism. It is linked to different mutations in the RET oncogene compared with MEN IIa. Poor prognostic factors in these patients include age >50, male, distant spread (metastases).
- Inherited medullary carcinoma without associated endocrinopathies is the least aggressive with peak incidence in the ages of 40 and 50.

Clinical Features

Patient presents with symptoms related to endocrine secretion, including carcinoid syndrome (serotonin) and Cushing's syndrome (ACTH). Watery diarrhea occurs in 33% of cases due to secretion of vasoactive intestinal peptide.

Gross Morphology
- Tumor is well circumscribed, solid, firm with gray white to yellow brown. Foci of hemorrhage necrosis are seen in large tumors.
- Tumor diameter 1 cm or less is referred to as medullary microcarcinoma (Fig. 26.40).

Light Microscopy
- The tumor is composed of round to polyhedral granular cells arranged in trabecular, glandular, carcinoid-like patterns.
    The tumor cells are separated by a distinctly fibrovascular stroma containing amyloid material representing deposition of procalcitonin.
- Amyloid material may elicit a florid foreign body type of giant cell reaction.
    This material is eosinophilic with the hematoxylin and eosin stain and takes up the Congo red stain.
    The stroma may be scanty, hemorrhagic or ossified or edematous (Fig. 26.41).

Immunohistochemistry

Tumor cells show positivity for calcitonin, creatine kinase, neuron-specific enolase, chromogranin, synaptophysin, TTF-1 and carcinoembryonic antigen.
    Carcinoembryonic antigen is an oncofetal glycoprotein. It is present in large quantities in medullary carcinoma of thyroid.
    Monoclonal antibodies offer a greater degree of tumor specificity.

Marker	Expression
Calcitonin	Positive
Neuron-specific enolase (NSE)	Positive
Chromogranin	Positive
Synaptophysin	Positive
Thyroid transcription factor-1 (TTF-1)	Positive
Creatine kinase	Positive
Carcinoembryonic antigen (CEA)	Positive

Endocrine System: Pancreas, Thyroid, Parathyroid, Adrenal and Pituitary Glands

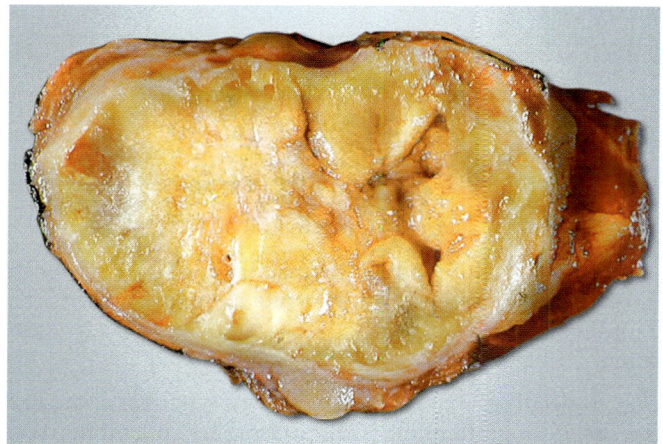

Fig. 26.40: Medullary carcinoma thyroid gross morphology. Tumor is well circumscribed, fleshy, solid, grey white to yellow brown, firm inconsistency, foci of hemorrhage necrosis are seen.

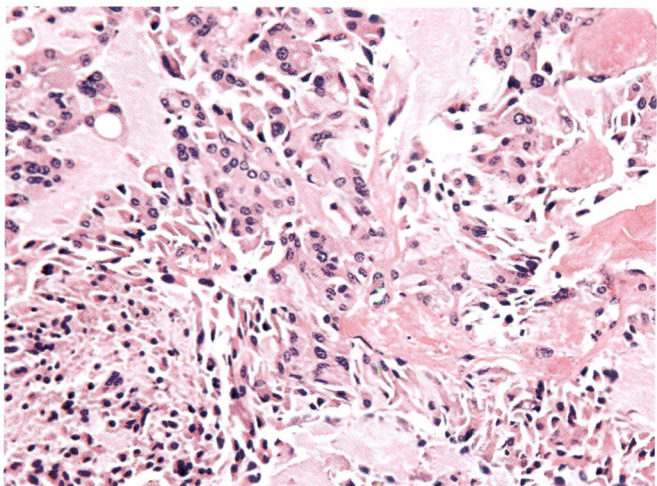

Fig. 26.41: Medullary carcinoma thyroid. The tumor is composed of round to polyhedral granular cells arranged in trabecular, glandular, carcinoid-like patterns. The tumor cells are separated by a distinct fibrovascular stroma containing amyloid material representing deposition of procalcitonin (400X).

Mode of Spread

Medullary carcinoma thyroid extends by direct invasion into soft tissues and metastasizes to the *regional lymph nodes* (cervical and mediastinal) and distant organs such as *lungs, liver, bone, brain,* and *adrenal medulla* by hematogenous route.

Surgical Correlation

Prior to thyroid surgery in MEN IIa and MEN IIb, 24-hour urinary catecholamine estimations are done to confirm pheochromocytomas. Prior to thyroidectomy, pheochromocytoma must be surgically excised first to prevent the risk of severe hypertensive episodes.

Residual disease (following surgery) or recurrence: It can be detected by measuring calcitonin. Comparison of papillary and follicular carcinoma of thyroid gland is shown in Table 26.25.

ANAPLASTIC CARCINOMA

It is the least common thyroid malignancy. It mostly occurs in older patients. It has a very poor prognosis. Invasion beyond capsule, blood vessel involvement and foci of infarct necrosis highlight the aggressive rapid growth of these neoplasms.

Etiology

It occurs as a result of anaplastic transformation of a pre-existing well differentiated tumor usually papillary carcinoma, but also follicular carcinoma (insular variant) and Hürthle cell carcinoma. Approximately 50% of cases arise in the setting of a multinodular goiter.

Clinical Features

Rapidly growing tumor in neck region invades esophagus (dysphagia symptom) or trachea (dysphonia symptom) and vocal cord paralysis. Extrathyroid extension is encountered at the time of initial presentation in most cases. Presence of cervical lymph node metastases is responsible for high recurrence.

Molecular Genetics

A mutated p53 tumor suppressor gene is often demonstrated.

Gross Morphology
The tumor is solid with areas of hemorrhage and necrosis.
Light Microscopy
• The tumor does not make follicles, papillae, or even trabeculae, but it still retains epithelial (squamoid) appearance on morphological and immunohistochemical grounds.
• Presence of admixture of follicular and papillary element may represent residua of previously existing low grade thyroid carcinoma (Fig. 26.42).
Histological Variants
• *Small cell carcinoma:* The tumor is composed of compact, closely packed cuboidal to polygonal cells growing in cords or clusters and numerous mitoses; separated by a fibrous stroma.   It should be differentiated from malignant lymphoma.
• *Carcinosarcoma:* It is composed of malignant epithelial and mesenchymal component.

Table 26.25: Comparison of papillary and follicular carcinoma of thyroid gland

Parameters	Papillary carcinoma	Follicular carcinoma	Medullary carcinoma
Incidence	70–80%	17%	6%
Age group	20–30 years	50–60 years	Middle age
Etiology	Irradiation	Endemic goiter	Sporadic or familial
Encapsulation	Rare	Common	Circumscribed
Gross morphology	On cut surface, tumor is usually solid gray white and sometimes cystic mass	Cut surface is gray white soft with areas of hemorrhage (tan), necrosis and cyst formation	Circumscribed, solid, firm with gray white to yellow brown
Cellular pattern	Papillae, follicles, solid cell group	Follicles, trabeculae, no papillae, pseudopapillary in foldings may occur	Round to polyhedral granular cells arranged in trabecular, glandular with carcinoid-like patterns and separated by fibrovascular stroma containing amyloid material representing deposition of procalcitonin
Psammoma bodies	Psammoma bodies are present in fibrovascular stroma (50%)	Psammoma bodies are absent, but calcified colloid may occur	Psammoma bodies are absent
Nuclear features	Ground glass (*Orphan Annie*) appearance, grooves, pseudoinclusions, often overlapping	Normochromatic or hyperchromatic, no grooves, no overlap	Normochromatic or hyperchromatic, no grooves, no overlap
Amyloid material in tumor	Absent	Absent	Present
Invasion	Strongly invasive, invades in small islands	Variably invasive in large islands with pushing borders	Invades locally
Multiple tumor foci	Common	Rare	Rare
Blood vessel invasion	Rare	Common	Common
Metastases	Lymph nodes	Lungs, liver, bones	Lungs, liver, bones, brain, and adrenal medulla
Prognosis	Excellent	Good	Poor

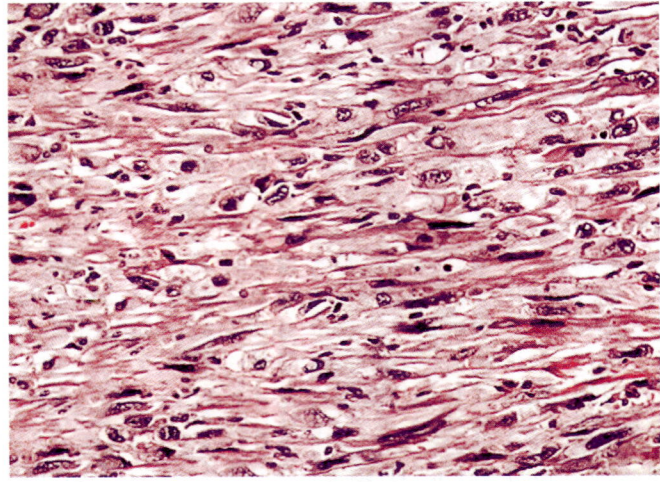

Fig. 26.42: Thyroid anaplastic carcinoma (400X).

- *Giant cell carcinoma:* The tumor is composed of highly anaplastic cells having multiple or multilobate nuclei.
  Other cells may assume spindle shape or elongated with numerous mitoses. Bizarre mitoses and giant cells are characteristic.

THYROID GLAND ANOMALIES

THYROGLOSSAL DUCT CYST

During its normal development, the thyroid gland descends from the base of the tongue to its final position in the neck. Thyroglossal cyst, a remnant of the thyroglossal duct is the most common thyroid anomaly. It may occur anywhere along the path of descent. It is midline cystic swelling that is close to or within the hyoid bone. Patient presents with dysphonia, sore throat and midline swelling evident during adolescence and pregnancy. Patient does not develop endocrine complications. Surgery with removal of the proximal duct along with hyoid bone cures it.

ECTOPIC THYROID TISSUE

It may be found anywhere along the course of the thyroglossal duct.

LINGUAL THYROID

It occurs due to failure of descent of thyroid gland from the base of the tongue. Patient presents with dysphagia for solids and swelling in the base of tongue. ^{123}I is a diagnostic tool to locate the lesion. Lingual thyroid is usually hypofunctional. The lesion is ablated with thyroxine. Surgery is indicated, if lesion is obstructive.

THYROID FUNCTION TESTS

In many patients with thyroid disease, the gland produces excessive amounts of thyroid hormone (hyperthyroidism) or insufficient amounts of thyroid hormone (hypothyroidism). The pituitary hormone TSH stimulates the thyroid gland to synthesize and release the thyroid hormone. When thyroid hormone levels decrease, the TSH rises and *vice versa*. Basically, a normal TSH excludes primary thyroid disease. The TSH assay is able to separate hypothyroid and hyperthyroid patients from normal individuals. Thyroid carcinoma rarely occurs in a hyperfunctioning nodule.

SERUM TSH, T$_4$ AND T$_3$ LEVELS

The pituitary hormone TSH stimulates the thyroid gland to make and release the thyroid hormone. When thyroid hormone levels (T$_4$ and T$_3$) decrease, the TSH rises and *vice versa*.

Table 26.26: Thyroid function tests in various disorders

Parameters	Total T$_4$ (µg/dl)	Total T$_3$ (µg/dl)	TSH (total T$_4$ (µl/ml))	% Radioactive iodine uptake by thyroid gland in 24 hours (µg/dl)	Comments
Normal range	5–12	95–190	0.3–5	10–30	
Thyrotoxicosis					
Primary hyperthyroidism (untreated cases)	Increased	Increased	Decreased	Increased	Thyroid stimulating immunoglobulin increased in Graves' disease
Secondary hyperthyroidism	Increased	Increased	Increased	Increased	
Thyrotoxicosis due to treated cases with overdose of T$_4$	Increased	Decreased	Decreased	Decreased	
Thyrotoxicosis due to treated cases with overdose of T$_3$	Decreased	Increased	Decreased	Normal or increased	
Hypothyroidism					
Primary hypothyroidism untreated cases	Decreased	Decreased	Increased	Decreased	
Secondary hypothyroidism untreated cases due to pituitary failure	Decreased	Decreased	Decreased	Decreased	
Euthyroid					
Euthyroid patient treated with T$_4$	Normal	Varies	Normal to decreased	Decreased	
Patient on iodine therapy	Normal	Normal	Normal	Decreased	Correct dosage determined by clinical effects
Euthyroid sick syndrome	Normal to decreased	Normal	Varies	Decreased	No clinical evidence of hypothyroidism

Table 26.27: Thyroid profile

Parameters	Reference range
Total serum T_4	5.0–12 μg/dl
Free serum T_4	0.7–1.9 ng/dl
Total serum T_3	80–180 ng/dl
Free serum T_3	2.3–4.2 pg/ml
Radioactive iodine uptake	10–30%

Increased serum TSH level is suggestive of hypothyroidism. Decreased serum TSH level suggests hyperthyroidism. Thyroid function tests are described in Tables 26.26 and 26.27.

THYROID HORMONE BINDING PROTEINS (TBP)

Antithyroglobulin and antimicrosomal proteins are thyroid binding proteins. Free portion of TBP is active at tissue level. *Increased serum level of TBP occurs due to pregnancy, contraceptive pills and increased estrogen level. Increased serum TBP results in increased synthesis of T_4 and T_3 by body.*

IMAGING TECHNIQUES

Ultrasonography

Ultrasonography detects 2–3 mm thyroid lesion. Cystic nodules are seldom malignant. Approximately 80% of thyroid carcinoma do not show cystic change.

Solitary nodules in adult women occur as cysts in goiter (60%) or a follicular adenoma (25%). Approximately 85–90% are euthyroid. Presence of irregular poorly defined margins and microcalcifications are suggestive of thyroid cancers.

CT Scan

CT scan defines extent of thyroid lesion, metastases, tracheal and retrosternal involvement.

Radioactive Iodine Uptake and Thyroid Imaging

^{131}I, ^{123}I or ^{99}Tc scanning play major role in evaluation of metastatic disease and in treatment of well-differentiated thyroid cancer. Patient is advised to stop levothyroxine drug prior to radionuclide scan.

Although its sensitivity is variable, its specificity in follow-up of thyroid cancer is very high (96–100%). Most solitary thyroid nodules are cold (95%). Most thyroid carcinomas arise in cold nodules. Risk of cancer in a cold nodule is 10–15%; while negligible in a hot nodule.

Scintigraphy

It is of minimal use in evaluation of solitary thyroid nodules; but useful in recurrent thyroid swellings and retrosternal goiters.

FINE NEEDLE ASPIRATION CYTOLOGY (FNAC)

Fine needle aspiration cytology plays an important role in diagnosing colloid goiter, Hashimoto's thyroiditis (Fig. 26.43), papillary carcinoma (Fig. 26.44) and medullary carcinoma (Fig. 26.45).

HISTOPATHOLOGICAL EXAMINATION

Thyroid biopsy is confirmatory. The specimens are processed, stained by hematoxylin and eosin and examined under microscope.

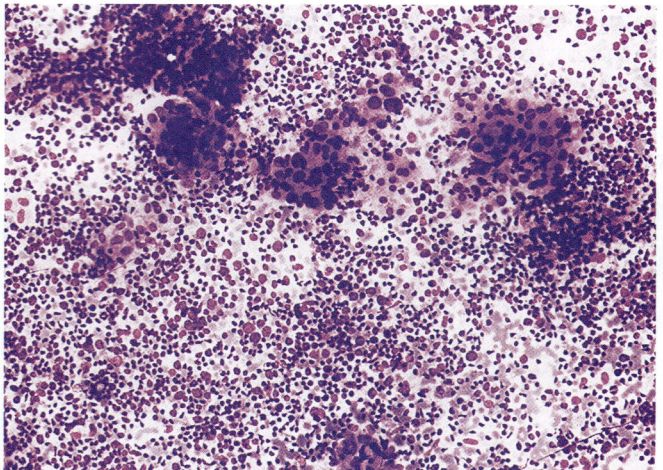

Fig. 26.43: Hashimoto's thyroiditis. Plump epithelioid-like oxyphil or histiocytic cells forming a granuloma-like cluster (MGG, 400X).

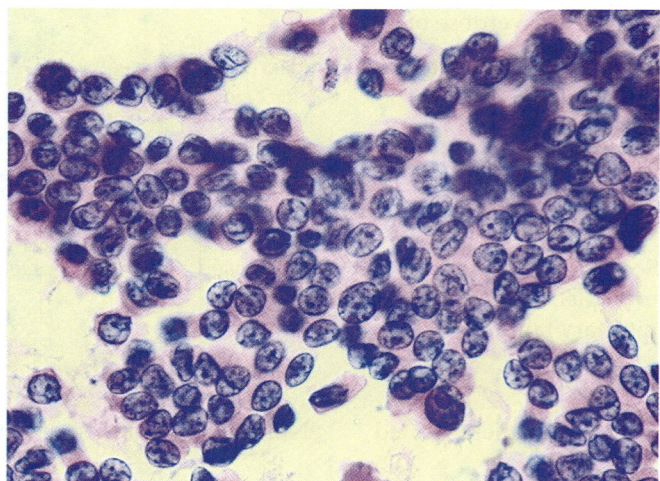

Fig. 26.44: Papillary carcinoma of thyroid—cells forming syncytial aggregates and sheets focally with a distinct 'anatomical border', nuclear crowding and overlapping, intranuclear cytoplasmic inclusions and nuclear grooves, dense cytoplasm, distinct cell borders (400X).

Endocrine System: Pancreas, Thyroid, Parathyroid, Adrenal and Pituitary Glands

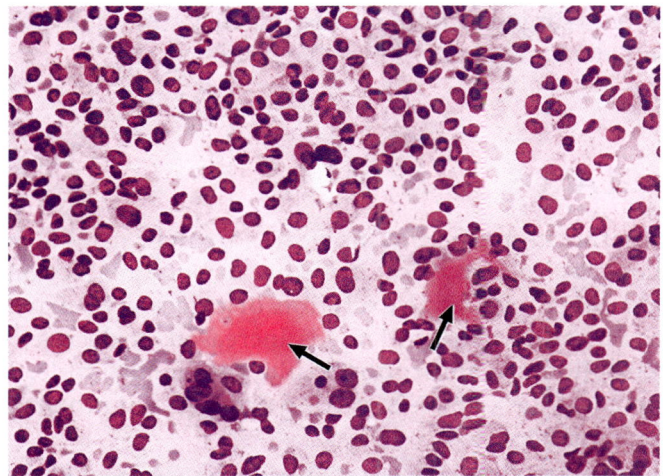

Fig. 26.45: Medullary carcinoma of thyroid. Arrows show amyloid deposits (400X).

GENETIC TESTING

Mutations of the RET proto-oncogene are also responsible for familial medullary thyroid cancer and MEN IIb. Prophylactic thyroidectomy is performed in these cases.

TUMOR MARKERS

Calcitonin

Plasma calcitonin, the product of the parafollicular cells, is the most sensitive marker for diagnosis and monitoring of medullary thyroid carcinoma. It should be measured when medullary carcinoma is suspected in a patient with a positive family history.

Thyroglobulin

It is a reliable marker of diagnosing papillary carcinoma cases. It shows positivity for tumor cells in primary site including recurrent disease or secondary sites as lymph nodes, distant metastases.

Carcinoembryonic Antigen (CEA)

There is increased expression of CEA and calcitonin in medullary carcinoma. CEA is excellent marker for residual disease.

Table 26.28: Antibodies used in diagnosis of thyroid cancers

Antibody	Specificity	Immunoreactivity	Interpretation
Thyroglobulin	Thyroid follicular differentiation	Follicular adenoma/follicular carcinoma, papillary carcinoma, poorly differentiated carcinoma	Anaplastic carcinoma is negative for thyroglobulin. This marker is invaluable for confirming thyroid origin of metastatic tumor
Calcitonin	Parafollicular C cells	Medullary carcinoma	Calcitonin immunoreactivity in metastatic medullary carcinoma
Chromogranin	Pan-neuroendocrine tumor marker	Medullary carcinoma, paraganglioma. Intrathyroid–parathyroid tumor, metastatic neuroendocrine tumor	Chromogranin supports a diagnosis of medullary carcinoma thyroid
Synaptophysin	Pan-neuroendocrine most sensitive and specific marker	Similar to chromogranin (medullary carcinoma, paraganglioma. Intrathyroid-parathyroid tumor, metastatic neuroendocrine tumor)	Similar to chromogranin supports a diagnosis of medullary carcinoma thyroid
Thyroid transcription factor (TTF-1)	TTF-1 is a transcriptional factor	Follicular carcinoma (100%), papillary carcinoma (100%), medullary carcinoma (100%), anaplastic carcinoma (0–50%)	TTF-1 is also positive in lung cancers (adenocarcinoma, small cell carcinoma and carcinoid tumor)
Cytokeratin	Epithelial marker	Follicular epithelial tumors, intrathyroid–parathyroid tumors	Neuroendocrine tumors positive
Leukocyte common antigen (LCA)	Leukocyte-specific marker	Lymphoma, leukemia	Useful in work up of undifferentiated thyroid tumors
S-100 protein	Expressed in normal thyroid follicular cells and especially Hürthle cells	Many thyroid tumors are positive for S-100 protein	Not used in diagnosis of thyroid cancers
Parathormone	Specific for parathyroid cells	Intrathyroid–parathyroid tumors	Most useful in diagnosis of tumors of parathyroid origin tumors

PARATHYROID GLANDS

ANATOMY AND PHYSIOLOGY

ANATOMY

There are two each superior and inferior parathyroid glands embedded on the posterior surfaces of the lateral lobes of the thyroid gland. There are derived from fourth pharyngeal and the third pharyngeal pouch, respectively.

These consist of principal/chief and oxyphil cells arranged in cords; supported by a network of reticulin fibers. Numerous sinusoids lie in close relationship to the cells.

PHYSIOLOGY

Principal/chief cells synthesize parathormone, which regulates the homeostasis of calcium and phosphate ions by increasing blood calcium level and decreasing phosphate level. Secretion is controlled by calcium level in the blood. Secretion of parathormone is not under control of pituitary gland.

REGULATION OF CALCIUM METABOLISM

Parathormone (PTH)

Decreased plasma concentration of ionized calcium stimulates principal cells to synthesize parathormone. Parathormone maintains ionized calcium level in blood by release of calcium due to bone resorption, and retarding renal excretion of calcium in urine. Thus, serum calcium level is increased. It decreases phosphorus reabsorption in the proximal tubule. It increases the synthesis of 1α-hydroxylase in proximal renal tubules.

This enzyme converts 25-hydroxycholecalciferol (vitamin D_2) to 1, 25-dihydroxycholecalciferol (vitamin D_3). Decreased serum calcium and increased phosphate levels stimulate the synthesis of parathormone (Fig. 26.46).

Calcitonin

Increased plasma calcium concentration stimulates thyroid parafollicular cells (C cells) to synthesize calcitonin. Calcitonin promotes deposition of calcium into bone matrix. With respect to regulation of blood Ca^{++} level, calcitonin and parathormone are antagonists.

CALCIUM METABOLISM

Total body calcium in adults is approximately 1.0 kg. It is present in cellular compartment such as bones (995 gm) and skeletal muscles (4–5 gm). Calcium is circulating in blood in three forms.

24 HOURS URINARY CATECHOLAMINES ASSAY

Suspicion of MEN II syndrome will need 24-hour urinary catecholamine estimation to exclude pheochromocytoma prior to surgery. Antibodies used in diagnosis of thyroid carcinomas are shown in Table 26.28.

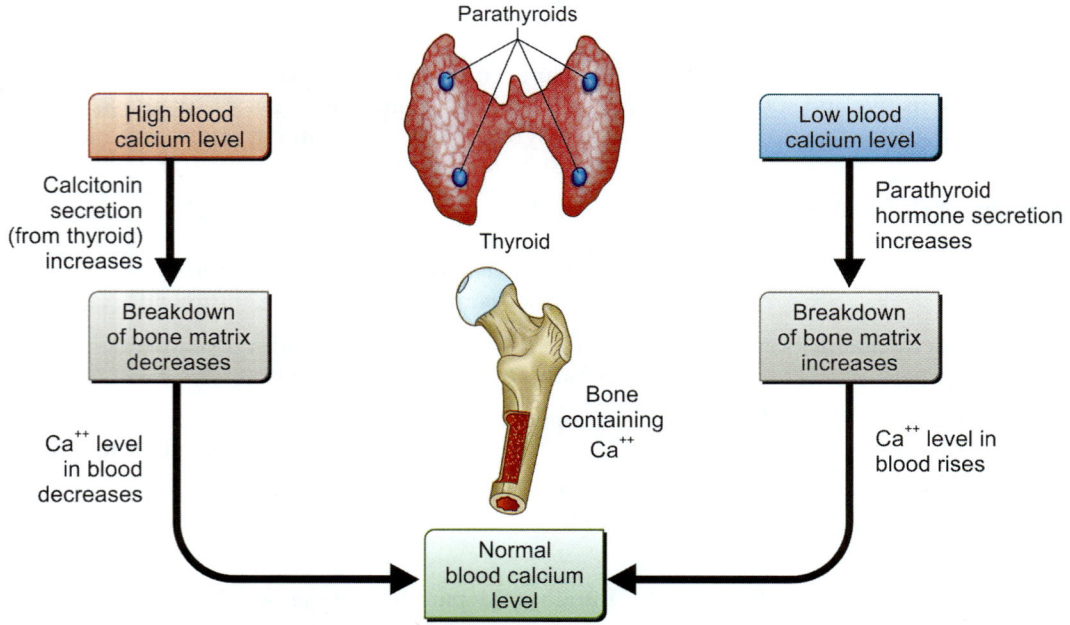

Fig. 26.46: Regulation of calcium by parathormone and calcitonin.

Calcium in Blood

- *Albumen bound calcium (45%):* It is physiologically inactive form.
- *Calcium complexed with citrates and phosphates (5%):* It is diffusible, non-ionized, but physiologically inactive.
- *Free ionized calcium (50%):* It is diffusible metabolically active form. Normal free ionized calcium maintains normal parathormone levels.

Absorption

- Gastric hydrochloric acid makes it in ionic form and hence gets easily absorbed by whole length of small intestine.
- Calcium absorption is increased in younger and normal secretion of bile.
- While absorption is decreased due to aging process, phosphates in diet and decreased bile secretion, which results in increased fatty acids in the gut which form calcium salts.

Calcium Functions

Calcium participates in bone calcification, excitation/contraction of muscles, stabilization of cell membranes, release of neurotransmitters, secretion of material from glands, synthesis of nucleic acids and proteins, promotion of mitosis in thymus and bone marrow, activation and regulation of enzymes and blood coagulation.

VITAMIN D METABOLISM

Physiology

Vitamin D is normal requisite for normal mineralization of bone and cartilage. It maintains normal blood levels of calcium and phosphates.

Vitamin D collaborates with parathormone in mobilizing calcium from bone and stimulates parathormone-dependent reabsorption of calcium in distal renal tubules. It stimulates intestinal absorption of calcium independent of phosphorus.

Sources

Preformed vitamin D in the diet (20%) consists of cholecalciferol (sea fish) and ergocalciferol (vitamin D_2) in plants, and grains. Endogenous synthesis of vitamin D in the skin occurs by photoconversion of 7-dehydrocholesterol via sunlight to vitamin D_3 (cholecalciferol). Dietary source is reabsorbed by small intestine.

Transport

Plasma vitamin D: Vitamin D binds with vitamin D binding proteins and complex carried to liver.

Metabolism

- *Liver:* In liver, first hydroxylation of vitamin D conversion to 25-hydroxyvitamin D occurs in cytochrome. This conversion is augmented by calcium. 25-hydroxyvitamin D is 5–10 times more active than parent vitamin D.
- *Kidney:* In kidneys, second hydroxylation of vitamin D occurs by 1α-hydroxylase enzyme synthesized in the proximal renal tubule cells. The enzyme converts 25-hydroxycholecalciferol (D_2) to calcitriol (D_3).

Storage

Vitamin D is stored in adipose tissue.

Functions of vitamin D_3 (calcitriol)

- Vitamin D attaches to nuclear receptors in target tissues. It increases reabsorption of calcium in the duodenum, and phosphorus in jejunum and ileum.
- It increases bone mineralization by alkaline phosphatase derived from osteoclasts. Alkaline phosphatase participates in bone mineralization by hydrolysis of inhibitors (pyrophosphate), which prevent calcium phosphate mineralization.
- Vitamin D increases the production of osteoclasts from macrophage stem cells. Parathormone and vitamin D_3 act on distal convoluted tubules, hence Ca^{++} absorption occurs.

Causes of vitamin D deficiency

- These include low dietary intake, decreased synthesis of vitamin D, malabsorption of fats, and deranged metabolism of vitamin D in chronic renal failure.
- Depending on severity, duration, stresses on bones and age of the patients, vitamin D deficiency causes failure of bone mineralization resulting in excessive formation of mineralized matrix and abnormally wide osteoid seams.

HYPERPARATHYROIDISM

Hyperparathyroidism can be primary as a result of autonomous proliferation of chief cells or may be secondary, in which case it is a compensatory mechanism.

PRIMARY HYPERPARATHYROIDISM

Primary hyperparathyroidism is most common cause of hypercalcemia. It occurs in postmenopausal women. More than 50% of patients are asymptomatic. Primary hyperparathyroidism is diagnosed when an asymptomatic patient has increased serum calcium levels in routine laboratory tests. Women are more affected than men over 40 years of age. Pathophysiology of hyperparathyroidism is shown in Fig. 26.47.

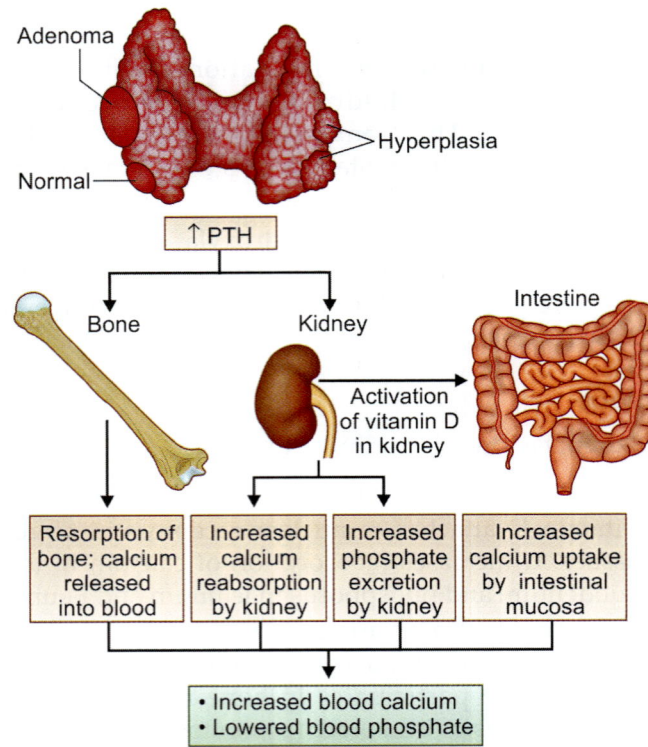

Fig. 26.47: Pathophysiology of hyperparathyroidism.

Etiology

Primary hyperparathyroidism occurs due to parathyroid adenoma (80% most common), hyperplasia (20%), or carcinoma (rarely). Primary hyperparathyroidism can occur as part of MEN I and MEN IIa. Parathormone like hormone may be synthesized by bronchogenic squamous cell carcinoma or renal cell carcinoma.

Clinical Features

Clinical manifestation of hyperparathyroidism is shown in Fig. 26.48.

Patient develops symptoms due to increased bone resorption (osteitis fibrosa cystica) by osteoclasts resulting in increased serum calcium levels. Skeletal manifestations are less common. Patient presents with bone pains and pathological fractures due to generalized demineralization of skeleton.

- *Bone lesions:* Osteoclastic bone resorption results in *osteitis fibrosa cystica* (also known as *brown tumor*) in jaw and long bones. When this lesion is generalized, it is called *von Recklinghausen disease* of bone. The lesion is expansile and multilocular with solid and cystic areas. Cystic areas have a brown color due to presence of abundant hemosiderin.
- *Radiologic examination:* It reveals decrease in bone densities (osteoporosis), bone deformities, chondrocalcinosis (pseudogout), and fractures. Subperiosteal bone resorption occurs along margins of middle phalanges (radial aspect) of fingers and tooth sockets. X-ray skull shows *salt and pepper* appearance.
- *Light microscopy:* Tissue section reveals loss of osseous tissue, poorly calcified immature bone formation, numerous osteoclasts associated with cystic areas and hemosiderin-laden macrophages.

Metastatic Calcification

It occurs in various tissues such as kidney, lungs, cornea, blood vessels, fundal glands of stomach and heart. Blood vessels show metastatic calcification in media and internal elastic lamina.

- *Renal changes:* Calcium stones are most common presentation. Metastatic calcification occurs in tubular epithelial cells and basement membranes in acute cases, while in chronic cases, calcification occurs in whole nephron including collecting ducts (*nephrocalcinosis*) with formation of calcific casts, foci of fibrosis, nephron atrophy and chronic inflammatory cells infiltration, thereby *calcium oxalate calculi* are formed which may cause *hydronephrosis* and *chronic pyelonephritis*.
- *Gastrointestinal tract:* Hypercalcemia predisposes to duodenal peptic ulcer. Calcium stimulates gastrin, which increases gastric acid secretion.
- *Acute pancreatitis:* Calcium activates phospholipase that causes acute pancreatitis. Patient may develop constipation. Serum amylase is analyzed in these patients.
- *Diastolic hypertension:* It occurs due to hypercalcemia. Electrocardium shows shortening of QT interval.
- *Ocular changes:* Patient develops band keratopathy in the limbus of the eye due to metastatic calcification.
- *Central nervous system:* Patient may develop psychosis, confusion, anxiety and coma.

Diagnostic Approach

- Serum PTH analysis is the best initial screening test. Patient with bone metastases has increased serum calcium level with normal PTH.
- Technetium 99m sestamibi radionuclide scan is done to localize parathyroid adenoma. Serum calcium, phosphorus and alkaline phosphatase are increased.
- Urine analysis shows increased excretion of calcium. Decreased tubular reabsorption of phosphorus and increased excretion of phosphorus results in decreased serum phosphorus levels.

Endocrine System: Pancreas, Thyroid, Parathyroid, Adrenal and Pituitary Glands

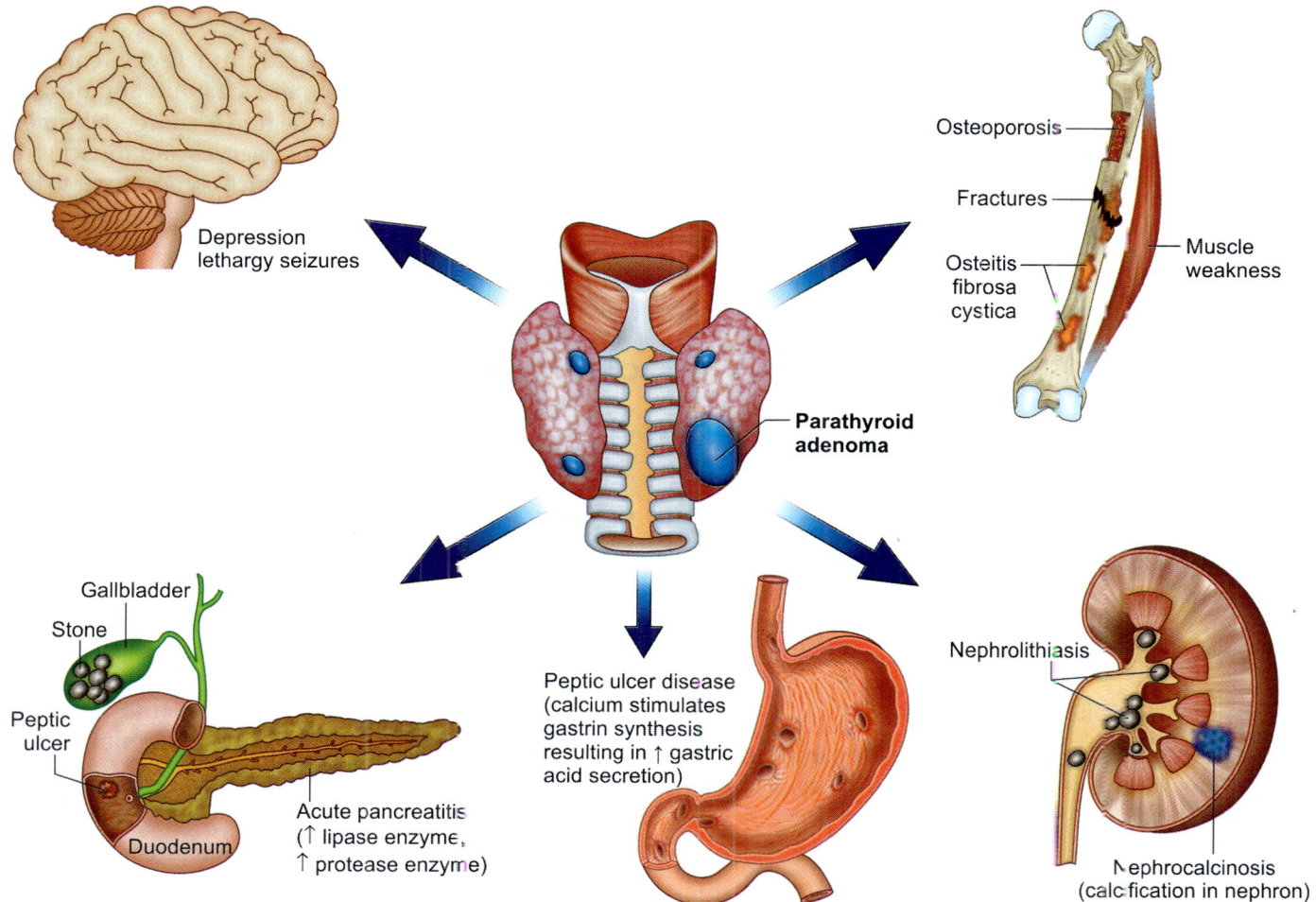

Fig. 26.4B: Clinical manifestations of hyperparathyroidism.

SECONDARY HYPERPARATHYROIDISM

Decreased concentration of serum ionized calcium due to renal retention of phosphate causes compensatory hyperplasia of all four parathyroid glands resulting in secondary hyperparathyroidism.

Etiopathogenesis

Chronic renal failure and intestinal malabsorption are important causes of secondary hyperparathyroidism. Diabetic glomerulosclerosis is a major cause of renal insufficiency. Uncommon causes of secondary hyperparathyroidism are Fanconi syndrome, and renal tubular acidosis. Advanced renal disease contributes to reduction in serum calcium. Other causes are rickets and vitamin D deficiency.

Physiological state: Normally, 1α-hydroxylase enzyme synthesized in the proximal renal tubule cells converts 25-hydroxycholecalciferol (D_2) to 1, 25-dihydroxycholecalciferol (D_3) also called *calcitriol*.

Pathological state: In chronic renal failure, kidneys fail to convert 25-hydroxycholecalciferol (D_2) to 1, 25-dihydroxycholecalciferol (D_3). Deficiency of vitamin D_3 impairs reabsorption of calcium in the duodenum, and phosphorus in jejunum and ileum. It also impairs reabsorption of calcium by distal tubules. Decreased serum calcium level stimulates parathormone.

Bone changes in chronic renal failure are known as *renal osteodystrophy*. Bone changes such as diffuse osteoclastic bone disease and metastatic calcification are similar to those seen in primary hyperparathyroidism. It may develop tertiary hyperparathyroidism. Parathyroid glands become autonomous regardless of calcium level. It may bring serum calcium into normal or increased range.

Blood vessels show metastatic calcification in media and internal elastic lamina. It is more severe in secondary hyperparathyroidism. Some patients develop ischemic muscle pains in extremities and even gangrene. Stomach, heart, lungs and eyes also show ischemic changes.

Diagnostic Approach

Radioimmunoassay determination of circulating parathormone is roughly proportionate to the severity of renal failure. Serum calcium is decreased. There is increased serum levels of phosphorus, alkaline phosphatase and parathormone.

TERTIARY HYPERPARATHYROIDISM

This persistent parathyroid hyperfunction occurs in spite of correction of hypocalcemia and pre-existing secondary hyperparathyroidism. Most often, the cause is development of an adenoma in a previously hyperplastic gland.

α-HYDROXYLASE DEFICIENCY (VITAMIN D RESISTANT RICKETS)

Patient has increased secretion of parathormone. But congenital deficiency of 1α-hydroxylase in renal tubular cells impairs hydroxylation of 25-hydroxycholecalciferol. Kidneys are not able to reabsorb calcium, in spite of increased plasma parathormone levels.

HYPOPARATHYROIDISM

Hypoparathyroidism causes deficiency of parathormone resulting in decreased plasma calcium level (hypocalcemia).

Etiology

Most common cause of hypoparathyroidism is accidental surgical excision of parathyroid glands during thyroidectomy. Autoimmune hypothyroidism is common cause.

DiGeorge syndrome is characterized by congenital thymic hypoplasia (pure T cell deficiency) as a result of failure of descent of third and fourth pharyngeal pouches.

Hypomagnesemia occurs due to diarrhea, aminoglycosides, diuretics and alcoholism. Magnesium is a cofactor for adenyl cyclase. Cyclic adenosine monophosphate (cAMP) is required for parathormone activation.

Clinical Features

Patient may develop tetany, cataracts, loss of hair, abnormal nail growth, increased bone density, convulsions, papilloedema, gastrointestinal disturbances, and calcification of blood vessels of basal ganglia of nervous system. Increased phosphorus level drives calcium into the brain tissue.

TETANY

Patient's total serum calcium remains normal. But serum free ionized calcium level is decreased.

Etiopathogenesis

Decreased serum ionized calcium level leads to increased neuromuscular hyperexcitability. Binding of free ionized calcium to the negative charge albumen causes partial depolarization of nerves and muscles. It lowers the threshold potential, which comes closer to the resting membrane potential. Hence, a smaller stimulus is required to initiate an action potential.

Patient presents with muscle twitches, spasms and convulsions. This condition is called *hypocalcaemic tetany*.

Clinical Features

- *Trousseau's sign:* Patient develops *carpopedal spasm*, i.e. flexion of wrist and thumb. Thumb flexes into the palm along with extension of the fingers.
- *Chvostek's sign:* Taping over facial nerve at the angle of jaw results in quick contraction of the ipsilateral facial muscles known as *Chvostek's sign*.

Laboratory Diagnosis

There are increased serum levels of calcium and phosphates. There are decreased plasma levels of parathormone level and 1, 25-hydroxyvitamin D_3.

PSEUDOHYPOPARATHYROIDISM

Pseudohypoparathyroidism is characterized by end-organ unresponsiveness to parathormone.

Molecular Genetics

It is related to gene mutation, whose product couples hormone receptors to the stimulation of adenylyl cyclase. Gene mutation impairs the synthesis of cAMP by renal tubular epithelium resulting in inadequate resorption of calcium from the glomerular filtrate.

Clinical Features

These patients develop *Albright hereditary osteodystrophy*, characterized by short stature, obesity, mental retardation, subcutaneous calcification, and a number of congenital anomalies of bone.

NEOPLASMS

Tumors of parathyroid glands are parathyroid adenoma, parathyroid carcinoma and secondary tumors. WHO histological classification of parathyroid tumors is shown in Table 26.29.

PARATHYROID ADENOMA

Parathyroid adenoma usually involves right inferior parathyroid gland. It is the cause of 85% of all cases of

Endocrine System: Pancreas, Thyroid, Parathyroid, Adrenal and Pituitary Glands

Table 26.29: WHO histological classification of parathyroid tumors

Primary tumors	Secondary tumors
Parathyroid adenoma (accounts for 80% cases of hyperparathyroidism)	Breast carcinoma, renal cell carcinoma, lung carcinoma or melanoma
Parathyroid carcinoma	

primary hyperparathyroidism. It arises sporadically or as a part of multiple endocrine neoplasia (MEN I and MEN IIa, 20% of cases).

In a small number of cases of sporadic adenoma, genetic analysis has identified rearrangement and overexpression of the cyclin D proto-oncogene.

Gross Morphology
Tumor appears as a circumscribed, encapsulated, reddish brown, solitary mass, measuring 1 to 3 cm in diameter.

Light Microscopy
- Tumor comprises sheets of neoplastic chief cells in a rich capillary network with no intervening adipose tissue.
- A rim of normal parathyroid tissue is usually evident outside the tumor capsule and distinguishes adenoma from parathyroid hyperplasia.

PARATHYROID CARCINOMA

Parathyroid carcinoma is a rare neoplasm. Most patients present with hyperparathyroidism and hypercalcemia of more than 16 mg% with secondary nephrolithiasis, renal insufficiency, osteopenia and/or brown tumor of bone, weakness, fatigue and depression.

Gross Morphology
Tumor is usually large, poorly circumscribed and adherent to surrounding structures especially thyroid gland. It ranges from 1.5 to 6 cm or larger with average weight 6.7 kg.

Light Microscopy
Parathyroid carcinoma has thick capsule, fibrous bands, invasion of capsule, extension in soft tissue, necrosis, vascular invasion, perineural invasion, marked atypia, mitotic figures and tumor cell spindling.

ADRENAL GLANDS

ANATOMY
Each adrenal gland consists of cortex and medulla.

Adrenal Cortex
- *Zona glomerulosa:* It secretes mineralocorticoids mainly aldosterone and deoxycorticosterone. Aldosterone acts on distal convoluted tubules, which results in absorption of Na^+, Cl^- and water; and hence controls electrolyte and water metabolism. In exchange K^+ enters the tubules.
- *Zona fasciculata:* It synthesizes cortisol (mainly) corticosterone and cortisone. These hormones participate in gluconeogenesis in the liver resulting in increased blood glucose level. These hormones cause breakdown of fat (lipolysis) and proteins (proteolysis). These inhibit cellular uptake and utilization of amino acids. These are anti-inflammatory and immunosuppressant.
- *Zona reticularis:* It synthesizes sex hormones (androgens and estrogens) and glucocorticoids. Their main actions on gonads result in development of secondary sexual characteristics, particularly those of the male (growth of axillary hairs, pubic hairs and facial hairs) during puberty. Concentrations of these hormones in adults are so low that their effects are usually insignificant (Figs 26.49 to 26.51).

Adrenal Medulla
Adrenal medulla synthesizes catecholamines (adrenaline and noradrenaline), also called *emergency hormones* or *hormones of fight* and flight in response to stress.

- *Adrenaline (epinephrine):* It mainly acts on skeletal muscles, cardiac muscles, smooth muscles, blood vessels and fat cells. It coverts liver glycogen into glucose, thus blood glucose is increased. It raises blood pressure; accelerates heart rate and force of heartbeat. It causes constriction of capillaries of skin and visceral smooth muscle; dilation of arterioles of heart and skeletal muscles; increase in oxygen consumption; erection of hairs (piloerection); dilation of pupils and initiation of stress responses.
- *Noradrenaline (epinephrine):* It also mainly acts on skeletal muscles, cardiac muscles, smooth muscles, blood vessels and fat cells. It converts liver glycogen into glucose, resulting in increased blood glucose. The functions of noradrenaline are similar to adrenaline.

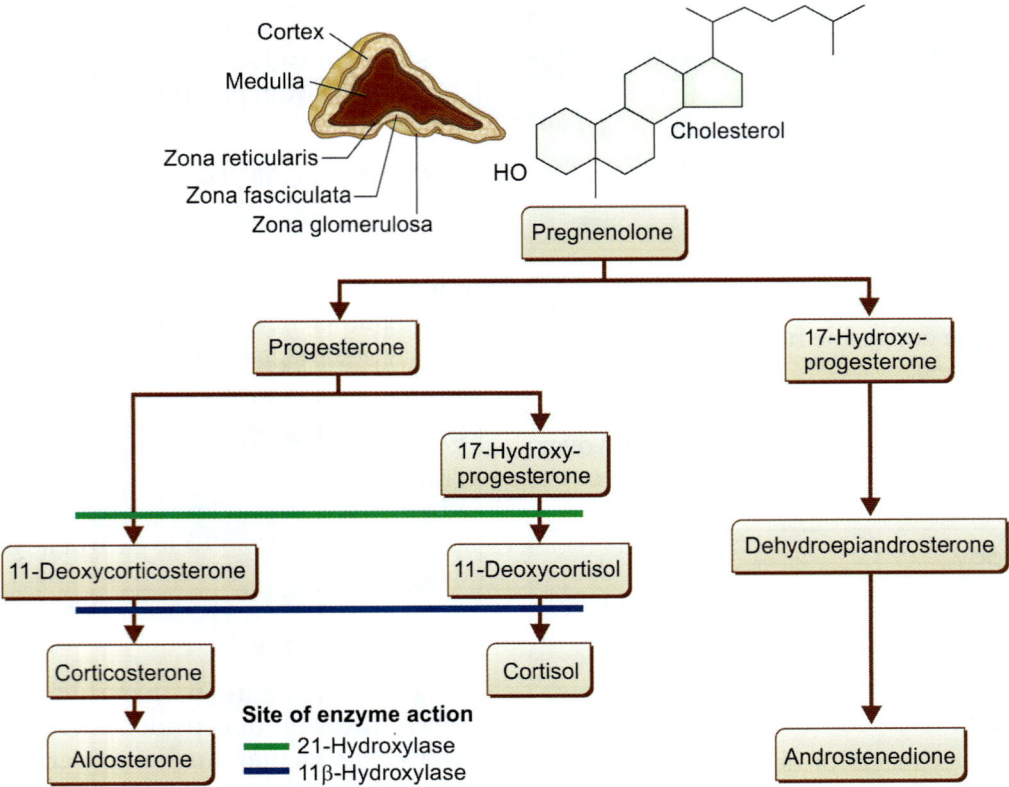

Fig. 26.49: The adrenal gland showing the medulla and the three layers of the cortex. Outer layer of the cortex (zona glomerulosa) is primarily responsible for mineralocorticoid production, and the middle layer (zona fasciculata) and the inner layer (zona reticularis) produce the glucocorticoids and the adrenal androgens.

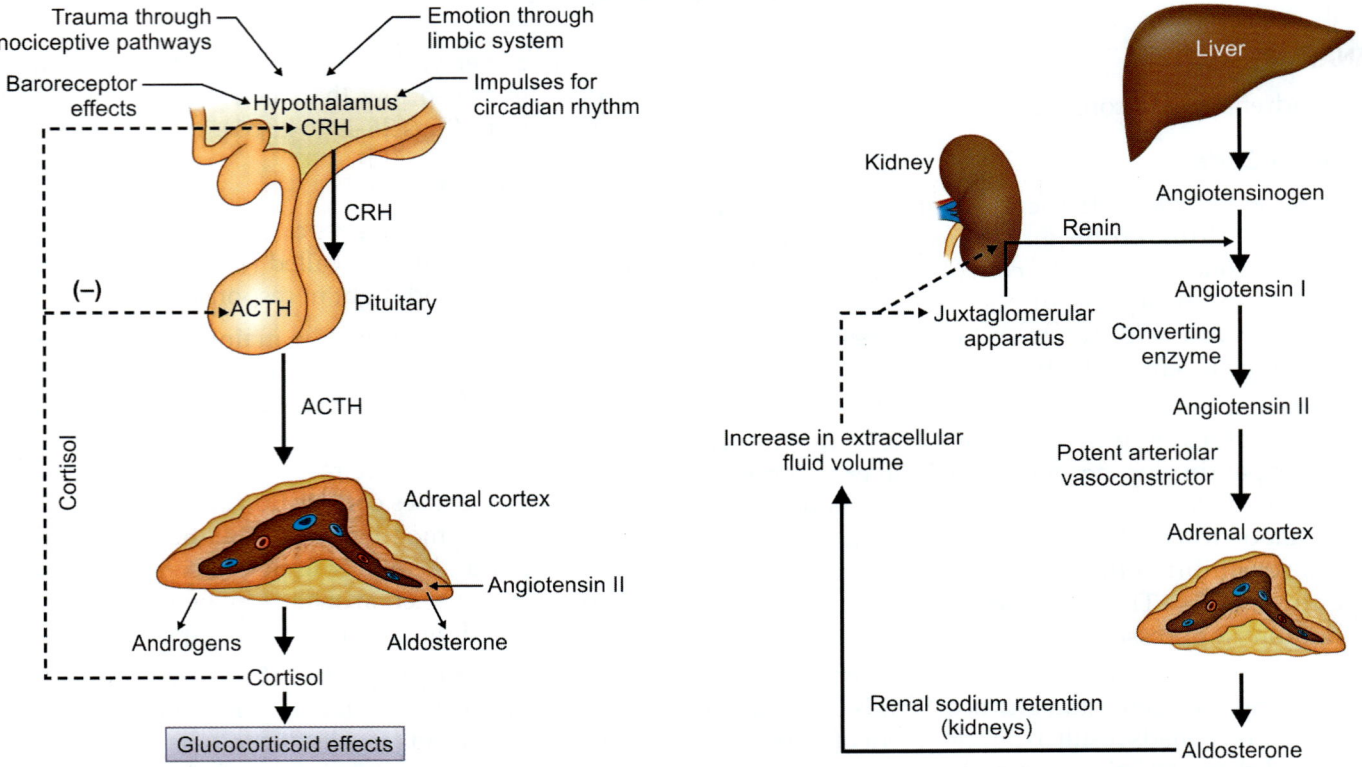

Fig. 26.50: Regulation of glucocorticoids.

Fig. 26.51: Renin-angiotensin-aldosterone system.

Predominant biosynthetic pathways of the adrenal cortex. Critical enzymes in the biosynthetic process include 11β-hydroxylase and 21-hydroxylase.

A deficiency in one of these enzyme blocks the synthesis of hormones.

ADRENAL HYPERFUNCTION

Excessive synthesis of corticosteroids occurs due to adrenal cortical adenoma and carcinoma. Cushing's syndrome and Conn's syndrome are disorders of adrenal cortex due to excess of corticosteroids and aldosterone respectively.

Cushing's disease is reserved for excess synthesis of ACTH by pituitary corticotroph tumors.

CUSHING'S SYNDROME

Cushing's syndrome results from excess of circulating glucocorticoids (primary cortisol).

Cushing's disease due to pituitary disorders is five times more common than Cushing's syndrome. Cushing's syndrome most often occurs in females between 20 and 45 years of age than men.

Etiology

- *Therapeutic administration of corticosteroids:* Most common cause of Cushing's syndrome in USA is the prolonged administration of corticosteroids in the treatment of immunological and inflammatory diseases. Long-term administration of corticosteroids causes increased bone resorption and decreased bone formation, thereby resulting in osteoporosis. Approximately 20% of patients with Cushing's syndrome suffer compression fractures of the vertebrae.
- *Adrenal glands:* Adrenal cortical adenoma, carcinoma and hyperplasia synthesize corticosteroids resulting to Cushing's syndrome.
- *Pituitary disorders:* Pituitary corticotroph microadenoma, adenoma and hyperplasia synthesize excess of corticosteroids resulting in Cushing's disease. Cushing's disease is reserved for excess synthesis of ACTH by pituitary corticotrope tumors.
- *Respiratory system:* Small cell carcinoma and bronchial carcinoid tumor synthesize ectopic corticosteroids leading to Cushing's syndrome (Table 26.30).

Clinical Features

These clinical manifestations depend on the degree and duration of excessive corticosteroid levels, as well as on the levels of adrenal androgens and mineralocorticoids.

Patient presents with redistribution of subcutaneous fat with round moon face, dorsal *buffalo hump* and diabetes mellitus (Fig. 26.52).

Physical Examination

Physical examination reveals relatively thin extremities caused by muscle wasting (muscle weakness); skin atrophy with easy bruising and purplish striae, especially over the abdomen, and hirsutism.

Other manifestations include osteoporosis, amenorrhea, hypertension and psychiatric dysfunction.

Diagnostic Approach

In addition to dexamethasone suppression test, ACTH determinations are useful diagnostic measures in determining the cause of hypercorticism.

ACTH is increased in pituitary hypercorticism and ectopic ACTH production. ACTH is low in hypercorticism of adrenal origin. Half of patients exhibit absolute lymphopenia. Dexamethasone suppression test in Cushing's syndrome is shown in Fig. 26.53.

HYPERALDOSTERONISM

Urine aldosterone is elevated in both primary and secondary aldosteronism. There is decreased plasma renin level in primary aldosteronism. Secondary aldosteronism has increased blood renin level. These are described as under.

Table 26.30: Causes of Cushing's syndrome

Etiology	Disorders	ACTH dependent or independent
Therapeutic administration of corticosteroids	Corticosteroid administration in immunological and inflammatory disorders	-
Adrenal causes	Adrenal hyperplasia, adrenal cortical adenoma, adrenal cortical carcinoma	ACTH independent
Pituitary gland causes	Corticotrope microadenoma, corticotrope adenoma, corticotrope hyperplasia	ACTH dependent
Respiratory system	Small cell carcinoma of lung, bronchial carcinoid tumor	ACTH dependent

Cushing's disease is reserved for excess synthesis of ACTH by pituitary corticotrope tumors.

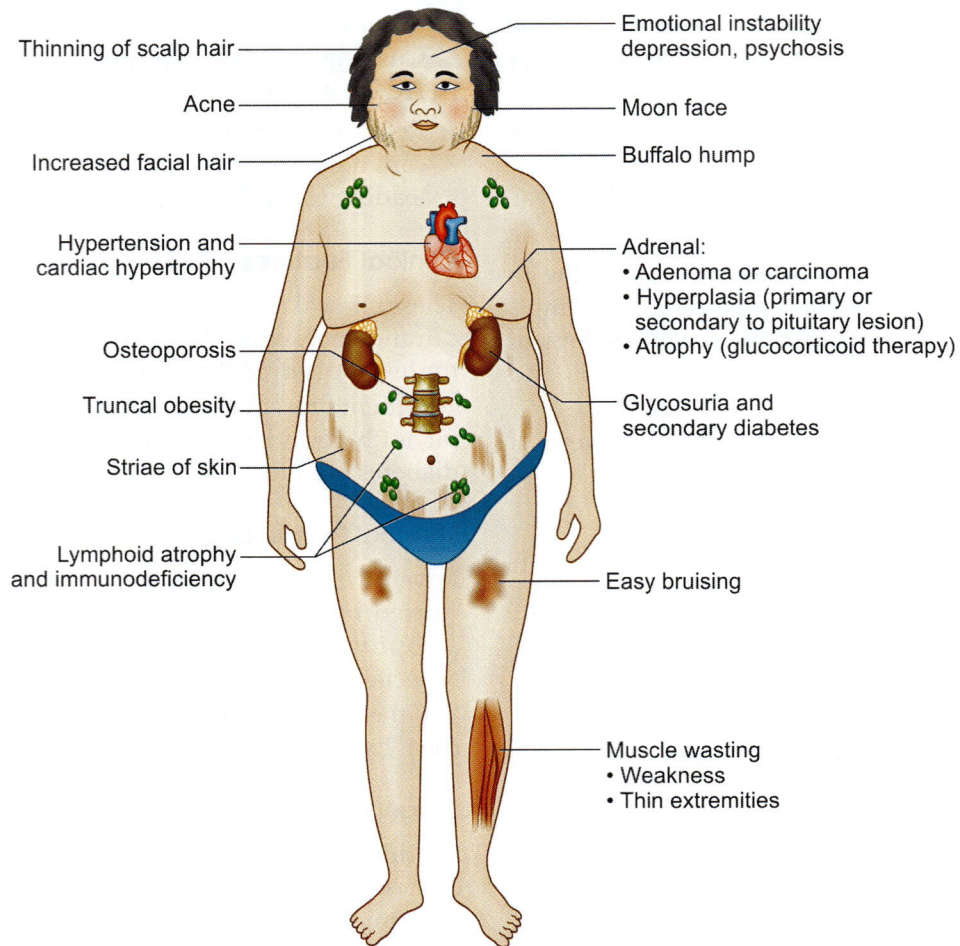

Fig. 26.52: Clinical manifestations of Cushing's syndrome.

Primary Aldosteronism

Etiology

It is also known as *Conn's syndrome*. It reflects in appropriate secretion of aldosterone by an adrenal adenoma (75%) or hyperplastic adrenal glands. Rarely, it may be caused by adrenocortical carcinoma.

Clinical Features

Patient presents with asymptomatic diastolic hypertension, persistent hypokalemia with alkalosis and slightly elevated serum sodium.

Muscle weakness and fatigue are produced by the effects of potassium depletion on skeletal muscle.

Decreased serum renin occurs due to negative feedback of increased blood pressure on renin secretion.

The diagnosis can be confirmed by demonstration of increased aldosterone, lack of response of aldosterone to sodium loading, and decreased serum renin.

Secondary Aldosteronism

This condition is secondary to renal ischemia, renal tumors, and edema (e.g. cirrhosis, nephrotic syndrome, cardiac failure).

The cause is stimulation of the renin-angiotensin system. Serum renin is increased, in contrast to primary aldosteronism.

Renin synthesized in the juxtaglomerular apparatus of the kidney promotes the conversion of angiotensinogen to angiotensin I, which is converted catalytically by angiotensin-converting enzyme (mainly in the lung) to angiotensin II. The release of aldosterone is facilitated by angiotensin II.

Glucocorticoid-remediable Aldosteronism (GRA)

It is autosomal dominant disorder characterized by ectopic production of aldosterone by zona fasciculata of adrenal cortex.

Endocrine System: Pancreas, Thyroid, Parathyroid, Adrenal and Pituitary Glands

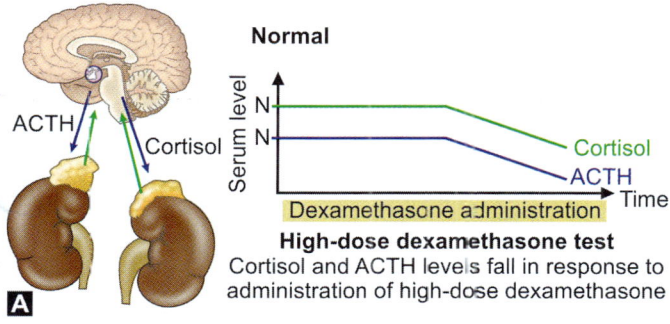

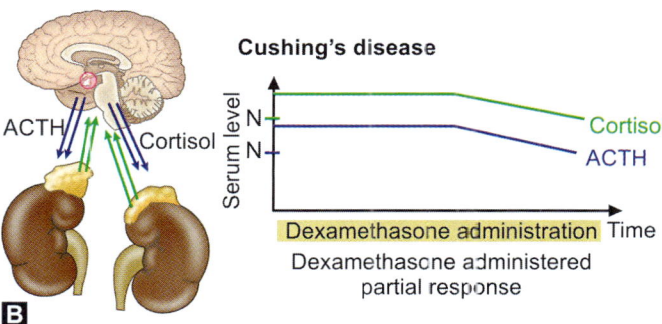

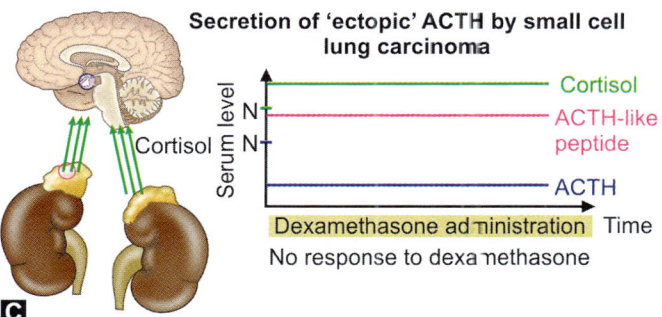

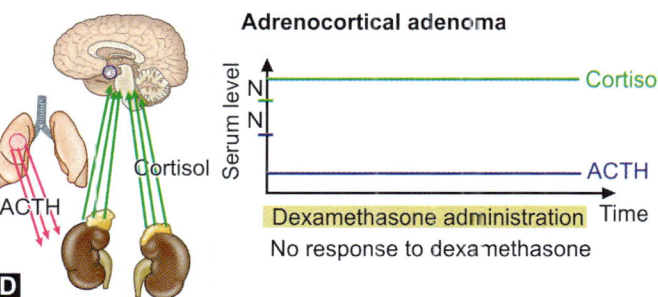

Fig. 26.53: Dexamethasone suppression test in Cushing's syndrome has many causes. Cushing's disease is caused by a pituitary adenoma. The dexamethasone suppression test can help to identify the underlying problem. The principles of the test are shown here.

Physiological state: Aldosterone-synthetase gene and 11β-hydroxylase gene are present on chromosome 8. Aldosterone-synthetase acts on zona glomerulosa to synthesize aldosterone hormones. 11β-Hydroxylase gene controls the synthesis of cortisol by zona fasciculata of adrenal glands.

Pathological state: Mutations of aldosterone-synthetase gene and 11β-hydroxylase gene present on chromosome 8 form hybrid genes resulting in ectopic production of aldosterone by zona fasciculata of adrenal cortex. It leads to expansion of blood volume resulting in hypertension.

ADRENAL CORTICAL INSUFFICIENCY

Hypocorticism can be of primary adrenal cause or secondary to hypothalamic or pituitary dysfunction. Deficiency of glucocorticoids (primarily cortisol), is often associated mineralocorticoid deficiency.

Examples of hypocorticism are Addison's disease and Waterhouse-Friderichsen syndrome described as under.

ADDISON'S DISEASE
(PRIMARY ADRENOCORTICAL DEFICIENCY)

Etiology

Primary chronic adrenal insufficiency (Addison's disease) most often reflects autoimmune destruction of the adrenal gland in 70% of cases. Until recently the most frequent cause was *tuberculosis*.

Addison's disease may be caused due to metastatic tumor, and various infections. Atrophic adrenal gland fails to produce glucocorticoids, mineralocorticoids, and androgens.

Clinical Features

More than 90% of the adrenal gland must be destroyed before the symptoms of chronic adrenal insufficiency appear.

Patient presents with weakness, weight loss, gastrointestinal symptoms, hypotension, electrolyte disturbances (decreased serum sodium, bicarbonate, chloride and increased serum potassium), and hyperpigmentation resulting from compensatory hypothalamic production of proopiomelanocortin, the precursor peptide of both corticotropin and melanocyte-stimulating factor. Clinical manifestations of Addison's disease are shown in Fig. 26.54.

WATERHOUSE-FRIDERICHSEN SYNDROME

Etiology

It occurs due to dissemination of *meningococcal infection*, most often in association with meningococcal meningitis.

Clinical Features

Patient presents with vascular collapse due to hemorrhagic necrosis of the adrenal cortex. It is often associated with *disseminated intravascular coagulation*.

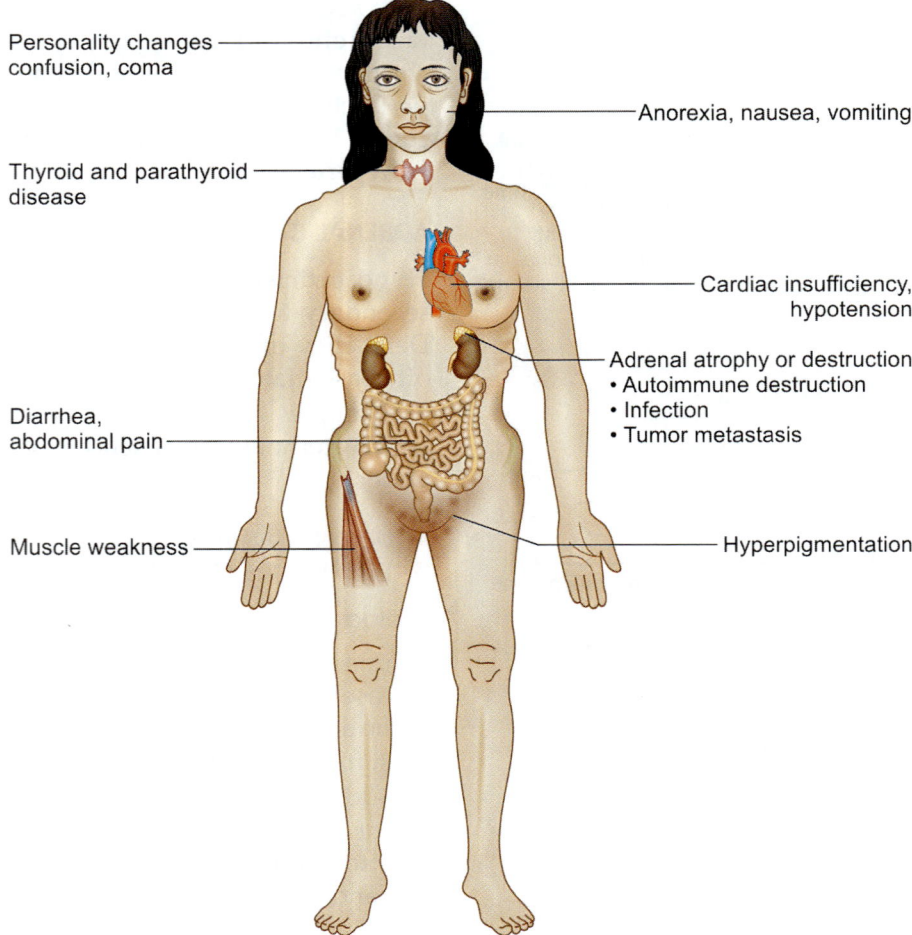

Fig. 26.54: Clinical manifestations of Addison's disease.

ADRENAL VIRILISM (ADRENOGENITAL SYNDROME)

Congenital deficiency of 21-hydroxylase is most common cause of adrenogenital syndrome. It is characterized by decreased cortisol, decreased mineralocorticoids, and an increase in androgenic steroid sex hormones, with resultant salt-losing hypotension and virilization (masculinization). Compensatory increased ACTH leads to resultant adrenal hyperplasia.

Etiology

Adrenogenital syndrome may also be caused by functional adrenocortical adenomas (hormone-producing), common component of MEN I, Carney complex, and McCune-Albright syndrome.

Sporadic adrenocortical carcinoma may result in adrenogenital syndrome, seen in Li-Fraumeni and Beckwith-Wiedemann syndromes.

Clinical Features

Adrenogenital syndrome is associated with virilization, ambiguous genitalia such as hypertrophic clitoris and partial fusion of labioscrotal folds in female infants (pseudohermaphroditism).

Male infants show normal external genitalia, but develop precocious puberty. Eventually, high levels of adrenal androgens lead to premature closure of the epiphyses and stunted growth.

NEOPLASMS OF ADRENAL MEDULLA

PHEOCHROMOCYTOMA

Origin

Pheochromocytoma is a rare tumor derived from chromaffin cells of the adrenal medulla. The tumor releases excess of epinephrine and norepinephrine. There is increased levels of their metabolites like VMA and metanephrin. Tumor arising from extra-adrenal chromaffin cells is called *paraganglioma*.

Clinical Course

It has most often benign course in 90% of cases. The 10% rule of pheochromocytoma includes 10% malignant,

10% familial, 10% bilateral, 10% children involvement and 10% extra-adrenal.

Association

Pheochromocytoma can be part of MEN IIa (Sipple syndrome) or MEN IIb. It can also be associated with neurofibromatosis or with von Hippel-Lindau disease.

Pheochromocytoma associated with MEN IIa and MEN IIb

- *MEN IIa syndrome (Sipple syndrome):* Patient with familial form of medullary carcinoma thyroid is associated with bilateral pheochromocytomas and primary hyperparathyroidism (parathyroid adenoma or hyperplasia).
- *MEN IIb syndrome:* It is associated with medullary carcinoma, bilateral pheochromocytomas, and multiple mucosal ganglioneuromas in lips/tongue. In contrast to MEN IIa, it does not induce hyperparathyroidism. It is linked to different mutations in the RET oncogene compared with MEN IIa. Poor prognostic factors in these patients include age >50, male, and distant spread (metastases).

Gross Morphology

Pheochromocytoma fixed in dichromate solution gives brown discoloration (Fig. 26.55).

Light Microscopy

- Tumor is composed of large polygonal cells with abundant granular cytoplasm with eccentric nuclei arranged in alveolar, nests, trabecular or solid patterns.
- These nests of tumor cells are separated by thin vascular septa.
- The tumor cells contain inclusions.
- Cytoplasm may show pink hyaline diastase resistant PAS positive globules (Fig. 26.56).

Immunohistochemistry

Tumor cells show positivity for synaptophysin, chromogranin-A, neuron-specific enolase (NSE), S-100 and N-CAM (CD56).

Marker	Expression
Synaptophysin	Positive
Chromogranin-A	Positive
Neuron-specific enolase (NSE)	Positive
N-CAM (CD56)	Positive
S-100	Positive

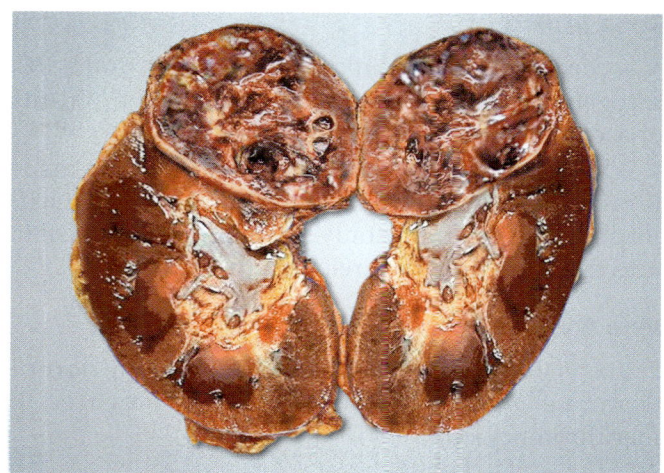

Fig. 26.55: Pheochromocytoma in adrenal glands.

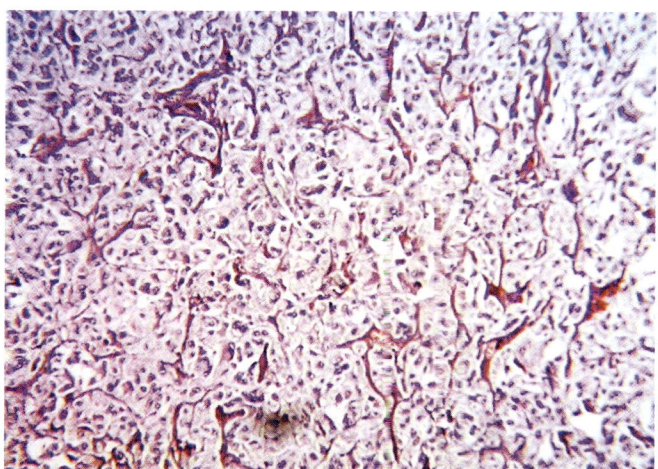

Fig. 26.56: Pheochromocytoma—tumor is composed of large polygonal cells with abundant granular cytoplasm with eccentric nuclei arranged in alveolar, nests, trabecular or solid patterns. These nests of tumor cells are separated by thin vascular septa (400X).

Composite Pheochromocytoma

Pheochromocytoma admixed ganglioneuroma or neuroblastoma or ganglioneuroblastoma or malignant nerve sheath tumor is known as *composite pheochromocytoma*.

Clinical Features

Approximately 66% of patients are asymptomatic. One-third cases show *fluctuating (paroxysmal or episodic) hypertension and tachycardia* due to excessive secretion of catecholamines (epinephrine and norepinephrine) by the tumor. Patient is resistant to antihypertensive therapy.

Patient may also develop hyperglycemia, malignant hypertension (e.g. encephalopathy, papilledema, and proteinuria), myocardial infarction, aortic dissection, and convulsions.

Gene Testing

Pheochromocytoma is linked to mutations in the RET oncogene, a transmembrane receptor of the tyrosine kinase family in sporadic cases (25–70%).

When a diagnosis of pheochromocytoma is made, demonstration of RET oncogene would justify prophylactic thyroidectomy keeping in view of fatal outcome of medullary carcinoma thyroid.

Urine Analysis

Urinary vanillylmandelic acid (**VMA**), a norepinephrine metabolite, is markedly elevated in pheochromocytoma.

NEUROBLASTOMA

Neuroblastoma is a *highly malignant* catecholamine-producing tumor of *neural crest origin* (adrenal medulla or sympathetic ganglia). It is composed of neoplastic neuroblasts. *In situ* neuroblastoma reported in infancy, has higher frequency of apparent spontaneous regression.

Occasionally it converts into a more differentiated form termed ganglioneuroma.

Origin

Tumor originates from the precursor cells of the autonomic nervous system. It is closely related to neuroblastoma of the adrenal medulla or sympathetic ganglia. It is much less common than peripheral neuroblastoma.

Associations

Neuroblastoma may be seen in patients with Beckwith-Wiedemann syndrome, neurofibromatosis, Hirschsprung's disease and fetal hydantoin syndrome.

Sites

Adrenal medulla is the most common site of tumor in 50–80% of cases. Posterior mediastinum in paravertebral regions is next common site. Rare sites include pelvis, lower cervical sympathetic chain, and posterior cranial fossa. In some cases, having heredofamilial basis, both adrenal glands and multiple extra-adrenal sites are involved.

Age Group

It most often affects children under 5 years with peak incidence is in the first 3 years of life. Adults are rarely affected.

Molecular Genetics

Tumor reveals amplification of the N-myc oncogene. Multiple copies of the N-myc oncogene are demonstrated as homogeneously staining regions or as extra chromosomal double minute chromatin bodies. A greater degree of amplification correlates with worse prognosis.

N-myc Nuclear Regulatory Proteins

Physiological state: The 'myc' protein acts as a transcription factor and it controls the expression of several genes. It is activated by gene rearrangement (breaking and sealing of chromosomes) or amplification.

Pathological state: Neuroblastoma reveals amplification of the N-myc oncogene forming thousands of N-myc oncogene copies per cell in neuroblastoma (30% cases).

Multiple copies of the N-myc oncogene are demonstrated as homogeneously staining regions (HSRs) or as extrachromosomal double minute chromatin bodies.

A greater degree of amplification correlates with worse prognosis. The malignant cells of neuroblastoma sometimes differentiate into benign cells, and this change is reflected by a marked reduction in gene amplification.

Mutant ALK Receptor

Physiological state: ALK (anaplastic lymphoma kinase) gene is located on chromosome 2. As a result of the (t2; 5) chromosomal translocation it is fused with the NPM (nucleophosphin) gene, leading to the production of a hybrid NPM–ALK protein.

Pathological state: Mutant receptors deliver continuous mitogenic signals to the cell, even in the absence of growth factor in the environment. It is associated with anaplastic large cell lymphoma (most important), rare cases of lung adenocarcinoma, and neuroblastoma. These cancers synthesize excessive ALK receptors.

Gross Morphology

- Neuroblastoma grows rapidly to become lobular, soft, retroperitoneal masses, undergoing hemorrhage and necrosis.
- Calcification is common finding demonstrated on radiograph (Fig. 26.57).

Light Microscopy

This tumor comprises small round blue tumor cells (neuroblasts) forming characteristic rosette-like structures (*Homer Wright* pseudorosettes) around small vessels (Fig. 26.58).

Immunohistochemistry

Tumor cells show positivity for neuron-specific enolase (NSE), neurofilament, chromogranin-A, and synaptophysin.

Endocrine System: Pancreas, Thyroid, Parathyroid, Adrenal and Pituitary Glands

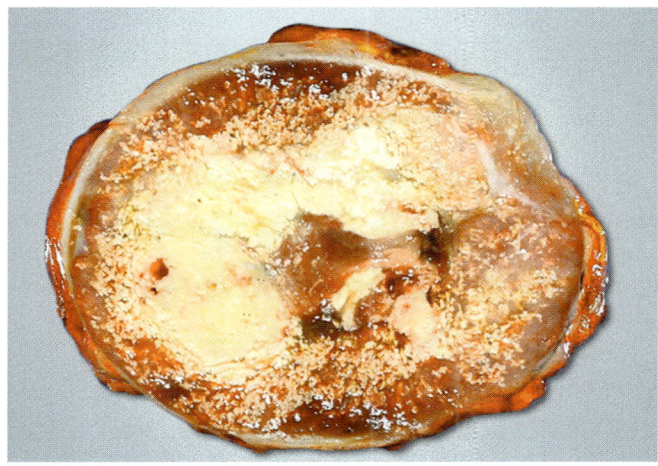

Fig. 26.57: Gross morphology of neuroblastoma of adrenal cortex.

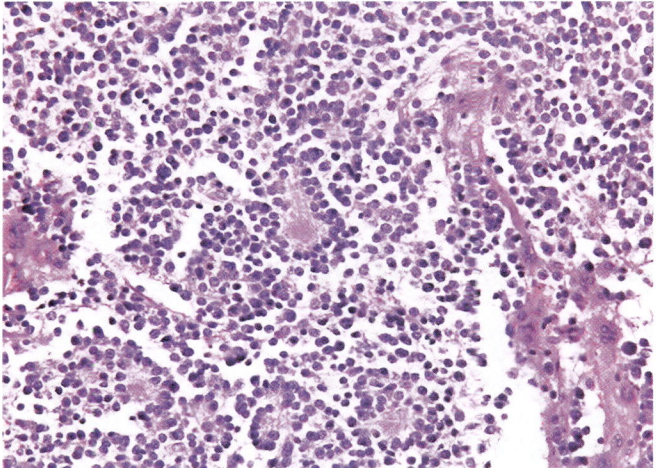

Fig. 26.58: Histology of neuroblastoma (400X).

Marker	Expression
Neuron-specific enolase (NSE)	Positive
Neurofilament	Positive
Chromogranin-A	Positive
Synaptophysin	Positive

Clinical Features

Patient often presents as a large abdominal mass, malaise, fever, pallor and loss of weight. Tumor synthesizes catecholamines (norepinephrine) in 90% of cases, but it rarely causes hypertension.

On local examination, tumor has knobby contour in contrast to smooth contour of Wilm's tumor. As the tumor enlarges, it crosses midline.

Metastasis

Neuroblastoma spreads to the liver, bones (skull, orbit, scalp), lymph nodes, subcutaneous tissue, intraspinal extension or kidney. Bone metastases are multiple and sometimes symmetric.

- *Pepper type of neuroblastoma:* It is characterized by primary tumor as well as secondaries including liver metastases on right side of body
- *Hutchinson's type of neuroblastoma:* It is characterized by left side primary tumor and spreading upward by lymphatic spread and metastases in the orbit and skull.

Urine Analysis

More mature descendants of tumor cells in the adrenal medulla may secrete catecholamines. These compounds are metabolized and excreted as urinary vanillylmandelic acid in the urine. Urinary catecholamines and catecholamine metabolites are the same as in pheochromocytoma.

Prognostic Factors

Amplification of N-myc, gain of 17q, deletion of 1p, and high expression of neuron-specific enolase are associated with poor prognosis. Prognostic factors of neuroblastoma are shown in Table 26.31.

NEOPLASMS OF ADRENAL CORTEX

ADRENOCORTICAL ADENOMA

The patient shows signs and symptoms of Cushing's syndrome (upper truncal obesity and hypercortisolism).

Gross Morphology
The surgical specimen reveals a circumscribed tumor of the adrenal cortex.
Light Microscopy
Tumor is composed of nests of clear, lipid-laden epithelial cells.

ADRENOCORTICAL CARCINOMA

Adrenocortical carcinoma is a rare neoplasm affecting any age group. It is most often *functional tumor* associated with clinical manifestations in contrast to nonfunctional adrenocortical adenoma. *Tumor has strong tendency to invade adrenal vein, inferior vena cava and lymphatic channels.*

Lung adenocarcinoma *frequently metastasizes to adrenal glands.* It is difficult to differentiate from primary adrenocortical carcinoma.

Table 26.31: Prognostic factors of neuroblastoma

Features	Good prognosis	Bad prognosis
Age	Less than 2 years	More than 2 years
Site of tumor	Extra-adrenal tumor	Adrenal gland
Stage	Tumor confined to organ	Tumor extending outside organ
DNA ploidy	Hyperdiploid or near triploid	Diploid near diploid or near tetraploid
N-myc amplification	Absent	Present
Gain of chromosome 17q	Absent	Present
Loss of chromosome 11q	Absent	Present
Telomerase overexpression	Absent	Present
MRP expression	Absent	Present
Trk-B expression-B	Absent	Present
Trk-B expression-A	Present	Absent
CD44 expression	Present	Absent
Lymphocytes around tumor	Present	Absent
S-100 protein expression in tumor cells	Present	Absent
Ratio of vanillylmandelic acid to homovanillic acid	Ratio >1	Ratio <1
Serum ferritin level	Low	High
Serum LDH	<1500 U/ml	>1500 U/ml
Neuron-specific enolase levels (cut of value is 15 ng/ml)	Low	High
Creatine kinase BB (normal cut of less than 1 ng/dl)*	Increased	Highest in stage IV

*Creatine kinase level is highest in stage IV of neuroblastoma.

Clinical Course

- *Lymphatic route:* Tumor spread to para-aortic lymph nodes.
- *Hematogenous route:* Tumor invades blood vessels and spread to *lungs* and *liver*. Bone metastases are unusual.

Gross Morphology
- Tumor is large and poorly circumscribed replacing adrenal gland.
- Cut surface is partially fleshy with cystic areas. There is presence of hemorrhage and necrosis (Fig. 26.59).

Light Microscopy
It shows well differentiated tumor with bizarre nuclei (Fig. 26.60).

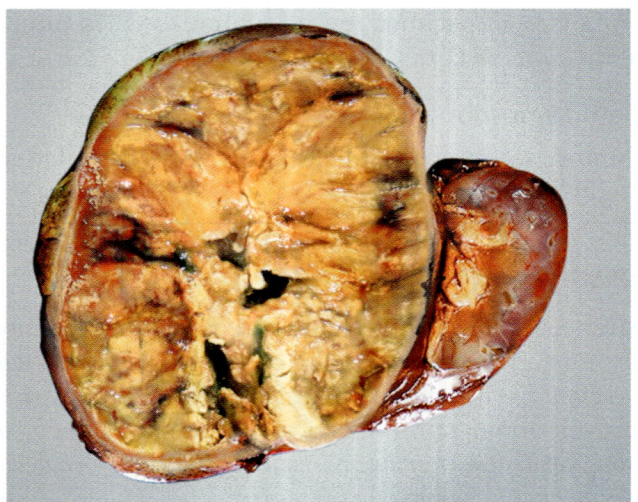

Fig. 26.59: Gross of carcinoma of the adrenal cortex presenting as a large, fleshy partially necrotic tumor that has completely replaced adrenal gland.

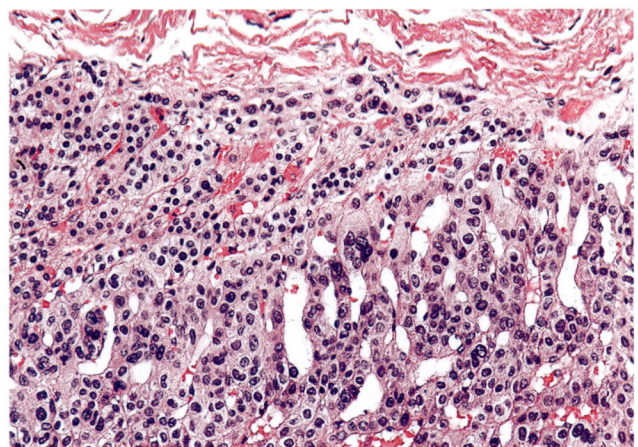

Fig. 26.60: Histology of carcinoma of the adrenal cortex (400X).

Endocrine System: Pancreas, Thyroid, Parathyroid, Adrenal and Pituitary Glands

PITUITARY GLAND

ANATOMY AND PHYSIOLOGY

Divisions

Pituitary gland consists of adenohypophysis (anterior pituitary or pars distalis), pars intermedia and neurohypophysis (posterior pituitary or pars nervosa).

Anterior Pituitary Gland

Hormones synthesized by anterior pituitary are growth hormone, prolactin, thyroid-stimulating hormone (TSH), adrenocorticotrophic hormone (ACTH), follicle-stimulating hormone (FSH) and luteinizing hormone (LH).

Pars Intermedia

It is merged with anterior pituitary gland. It synthesizes melanocyte-stimulating hormone (MSH).

Posterior Pituitary Gland

Hypothalamic neurons synthesize oxytocin and antidiuretic hormone (ADH) or vasopressin, which pass through axons and released at nerve endings. These hormones reach the posterior pituitary gland through portal circulatory system and regulate the functions of the posterior pituitary gland. Posterior pituitary is under the direct neural regulation of the hypothalamus.

Hormones synthesized by anterior pituitary gland and their actions are shown in Table 26.32. Pituitary gland consists of anterior and posterior divisions (Fig. 26.61).

HYPOFUNCTIONING OF ANTERIOR PITUITARY GLAND

Partial or complete forms of hypopituitarism most often affects children and adults. This disorder may cause dwarfism and delayed puberty. Initially, there is decreased FSH and LH levels leading to hypogonadism, impotence in men and menstrual disturbances in women.

Growth hormone deficiency leads to short stature, delayed growth and delayed puberty in children. There is subsequent decrease in TSH and ACTH.

PRIMARY HYPOPITUITARISM

Primary hypopituitarism of anterior pituitary is caused by non-secretory adenoma, Sheehan's syndrome

Table 26.32: Hormones synthesized by anterior pituitary gland and their actions

Cells in pituitary	Hormone synthesis by anterior pituitary	Target organs	Actions on target cells	Net result
Somatotropes (basophilic cells)	Growth hormone (acidophilic cells)	Skeletal system	Growth promoting and anti-insulin actions	Linear bone growth in children
Corticotropes (basophilic cells)	ACTH	Adrenal glands	Synthesis of aldosterone and corticosteroids	Regulate carbohydrate, fat and proteins
Thyrotropes (basophilic cells)	TSH (basophilic cells)	Thyroid gland	T_4, T_3	Regulation of metabolism of carbohydrate, fat and proteins
Lactotropes (acidophilic cells)	Prolactin (PRL)	Female breasts	Synthesis and ejection of milk	Controls reproduction, osmoregulation, growth and metabolism
Gonadotropes (basophilic cells)	FSH, LH	Testes	FSH: spermatogenesis	Increased sperms count
			LH: acts on Leydig cells to synthesize testosterone	Growth, development, maturation of spermatozoa and development of secondary characters
		Ovaries	FSH	Stimulates formation of graafian follicles
			LH	Triggers ovulation, and formation of corpus luteum
Melanophores	Melanocyte-stimulating hormone (MSH)	Skin	Synthesis of cutaneous pigmentation	Subcutaneous dispersion of melanin granules

Somatostatin inhibits synthesis of growth hormone by anterior pituitary gland.

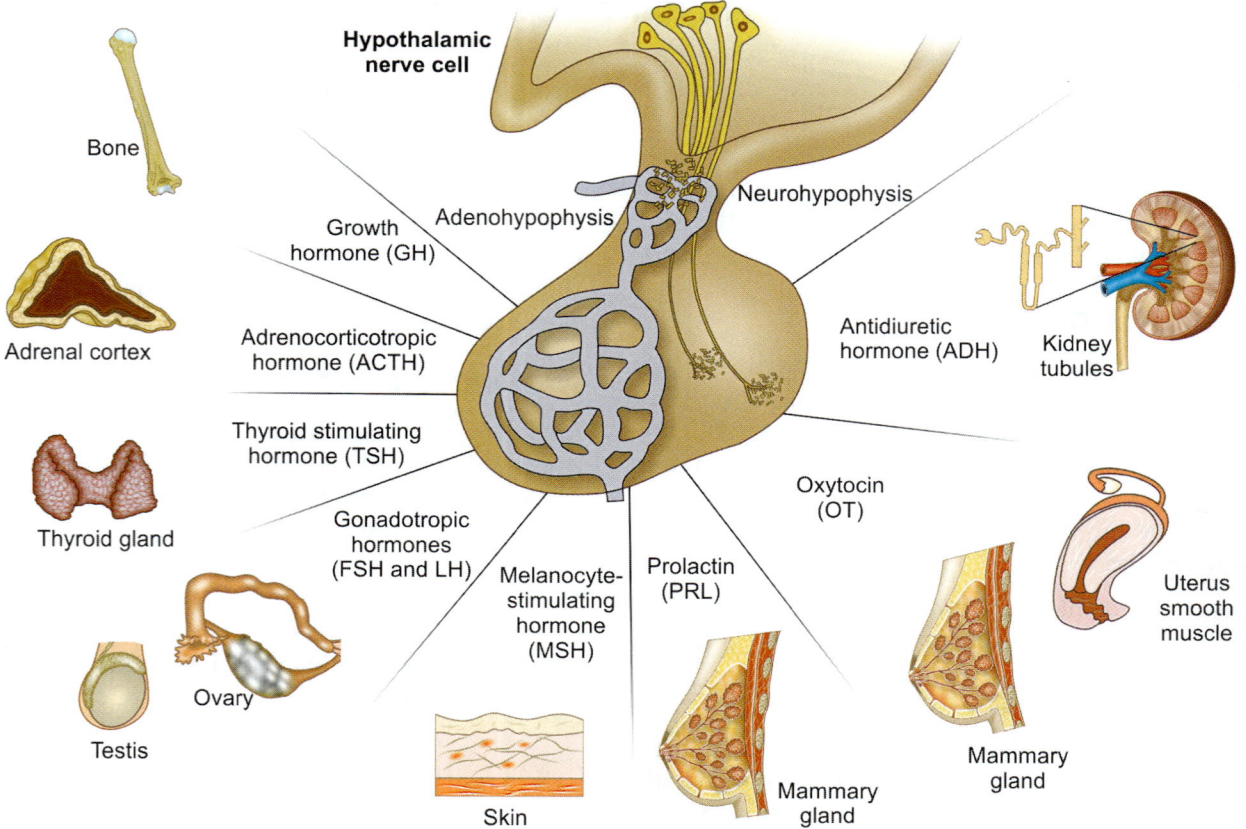

Fig. 26.61: Pituitary gland consists of anterior and posterior divisions.

(post-partum pituitary necrosis), empty-sella syndrome, partial or total hypophysectomy and TB meningitis, irradiation, hemochromatosis and Hand-Schüller-Christian disease.

Etiopathogenesis

Simond's Disease

Patient presents with cachexia (marked wasting) due to destruction of pituitary gland by *pituitary tumors* usually adenomas in more than 50% of cases.

Sheehan's Syndrome

Sheehan's syndrome refers to *infarction of anterior pituitary gland* due to postpartum hemorrhage and shock during childbirth. During pregnancy, pituitary gland becomes enlarged, that renders it vulnerable to a reduction in blood flow.

Clinical features: Patient presents with *adrenal cortical insufficiency, and ovarian failure* (gonadotropin deficiency) with decreased FSH and LH, pallor (decreased MSH), secondary hypothyroidism (thyrotropin deficiency) with decreased TSH, and failure of lactation (decreased prolactin). Clinical manifestations of Sheehan's syndrome are shown in Fig. 26.62.

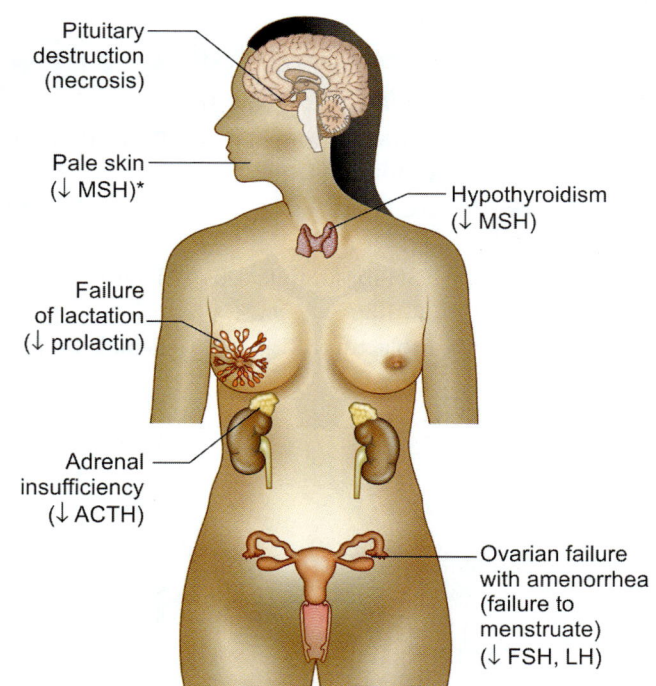

* MSH: Melanocyte-stimulating hormone. MSH is a breakdown product of ACTH. Excess of MSH produces dark skin.

Fig. 26.62: Sheehan's syndrome. Clinical manifestations of Sheehan's syndrome is caused by hemorrhagic destruction of the pituitary gland during pregnancy or postpartum period.

Iatrogenic Hypopituitarism

Pituitary gland may be damaged due to *radiation therapy in the head or neck region* and intracranial neurosurgical procedures.

Traumatic Injury to Skull

Basal skull fractures and trauma to the sella turcica may cause damage to the pituitary gland.

Infiltrative Diseases

Pituitary gland may be damaged by bacterial or viral infections. Hemochromatosis of pituitary may cause panhypopituitarism. Hand-Schüller-Christian disease most often causes diabetes insipidus, but may also cause hypopituitarism.

Molecular Genetic Defects

Mutation of Pit1 gene (3p11), PROP1 gene (5q) or HSEX1 gene (3p21) cause hypopituitarism (Table 26.33).

Clinical Manifestations

- *Growth hormone deficiency:* Deficiency of growth hormone in children results in growth retardation (pituitary dwarfism). In adults, patient develops increased insulin sensitivity with hypoglycemia, decreased muscle strength, and anemia.
- *Gonadotropin deficiency:* In preadolescent children, gonadotropia deficiency results in retarded sexual maturation. Adult men present with loss of libido, impotence, inhibition of spermatogenesis, loss of muscular mass, and decreased facial hair. Women develop amenorrhea and vaginal atrophy.
- *TSH deficiency:* Deficiency of TSH results in secondary hypothyroidism. Patient presents with weight gain, constipation, cold intolerance, fatigue and coarse hair.
- *Prolactin deficiency:* Patient presents with lactation dysfunction in women or gynaecomastia in men. Serum ACTH, FSH, LH, and TSH levels are analyzed. CT scan and MRI of pituitary gland and target glands are essential diagnostic tools.
- *ACTH deficiency:* Deficiency of ACTH results in secondary adrenal failure. It does not result in hyperpigmentation of the skin, probably because of the lack of both ACTH and β-melanocyte-stimulating hormone; this is in contrast to primary adrenal failure (Addison's disease), in which ACTH is increased and hyperpigmentation is the rule.

Patient presents with weakness, fatigue, hypoglycemia, loss of hair in axillae and pubic regions, hypotension, and decreased sodium level.

OTHER CAUSES OF HYPOPITUITARISM

- *Empty-sella syndrome:* It is caused by conditions that destroy all or part of the pituitary gland.
- *Nelson syndrome:* Nelson syndrome involves the development of large pituitary adenomas following bilateral adrenalectomy. This is thought to be due to loss of feedback inhibition on growth of pre-existing pituitary microadenoma.
- *Growth hormone insensitivity (Laron syndrome):* This autosomal recessive disorder is characterized by extreme resistance to growth hormone resulting in short stature and obesity. Biochemical analysis shows high levels of serum growth hormone and low level of insulin like growth factor-1 (IGF-1).
- *Isolated gonadotropin deficiency (Kallmann syndrome):* It occurs due to mutation of KAL1 gene resulting to failure of migration of gonadotropin releasing hormone (GnRH) from its origin in olfactory anlage to their normal location in hypothalamus.

HYPOFUNCTIONING OF POSTERIOR PITUITARY GLAND

Hormones are synthesized in the hypothalamus and transported via axons to the posterior pituitary.

Oxytocin induces uterine contraction during labor and ejection of milk from mammary alveoli. Antidiuretic hormone (ADH, vasopressin) promotes water retention through action on the renal collecting ducts.

ADH DEFICIENCY

Antidiuretic hormone (ADH) participates in determining the concentration of urine by affecting water reabsorption in the distal renal tubules.

- Low ADH activity results in dilute urine and free water excretion. Decreased synthesis of ADH by posterior pituitary results central diabetes insipidus.

Table 26.33: Molecular genetic defects in hypopituitarism

Gene mutations	Deficiency of hormones
Pit1 gene (3p11)	Growth hormone, prolactin and thyroid stimulating hormone
PROP1 gene (5q) transcription factor	Inactivation of FSH, LH, prolactin and thyroid stimulating hormone
HSEX1 gene (3p21) participates in development of optic nerves and pituitary gland	Growth hormone and ADH

- Kidneys unresponsive to ADH results in nephrogenic diabetes insipidus.

Central Diabetes Insipidus

Etiology

- Central diabetes insipidus may be caused by trauma that damages the posterior lobe of the pituitary (neurohypophysis) and interrupts the secretion of ADH.
- Approximately 25% of cases occur due to brain tumors such as *craniopharyngioma* and *germ cell* tumor. Other causes include inflammatory processes, lipid storage disorders resulting in damage to the neurohypophysis or hypothalamus.

Clinical Features

Patient presents with polyuria, with consequent dehydration and insatiable thirst. Patient drinks water constantly to avoid feeling dehydrated. On clinical examination, patient appears dehydrated.

Treatment

Central diabetes insipidus is with ADH.

Nephrogenic Diabetes Insipidus

Kidneys unresponsive to ADH results in nephrogenic diabetes insipidus. *Demeclocycline* and *lithium* are potential causes of nephrogenic diabetes insipidus.

SYNDROME OF INAPPROPRIATE ADH (SIADH) SECRETION

SIADH most often occurs due to ectopic production of ADH by small cell carcinoma of lung (most common). It is also reported with carcinomas of the prostate, gastrointestinal tract, and pancreas, thymomas, NHL, Hodgkin's disease, trauma, and infections.

Clinical Features

SIADH results in retention of water with consequent dilutional hyponatremia, reduced serum osmolality, and inability to dilute the urine. Water intoxication with hyponatremia, result in altered mental status, seizures, coma, and sometimes death.

TUMORS

PITUITARY ADENOMAS

Adenomas be functional (secretory) or non-functional. Secretory adenomas may secrete hormones. Clinical manifestations depend on synthesis of hormones by pituitary adenomas.

Molecular Genetics

Guanine nucleotide binding protein, alpha stimulating (GNAS) is a cytoplasmic signal-transducing protein. Alteration of GNAS is associated with pituitary adenoma and other endocrinal tumors.

Frequency

Frequency of pituitary adenomas is described in Table 26.34.

Pathogenesis

Pituitary adenomas may be part of multiple endocrine neoplasia type I (MEN I). Acquired adenomas may occur due to mutation of cyclin D1, CREB, RAS, and pituitary tumor transforming gene (PTTG).

Histological Classification

Pituitary adenomas of anterior lobe have been classified according to the functional properties of cells.

- *Chromophil adenomas:* Acidophil adenoma synthesizes excess of growth hormone and prolactin. Basophil adenomas synthesize excess of ACTH, TSH, FSH and LH.
- *Chromophobe adenomas:* These are nonfunctional tumors without synthesis of hormones.

Consequences

Microadenoma is small <1 cm in diameter. It does not produce symptoms unless they secrete hormones.

Table 26.34: Frequency of adenomas of anterior pituitary gland

Cell type	Hormone	Frequency (%)
Lactotrope	Prolactin	32
Somatotrope	Growth hormone	21
Corticotrope	ACTH (adrenocorticotropic hormone)	13
Lactotrope/somatotrope	Mixed PRL/GH	6%
Gonadotropes	FSH (follicle-stimulating hormone)	<4
	LH (luteinizing hormone)	
Thyrotrope	TSH (thyroid-stimulating hormone)	
Nonfunctional tumors	–	25

Macroadenoma has space occupying clinical effects such as visual disturbances and increased intracranial pressure. Tumor synthesizing hormones leading to gigantism, acromegaly, Cushing's syndrome, Nelson's syndrome and increased prolactin.

- *Visual disturbances:* Tumor erodes the sella turcica and impinges on adjacent cranial structures such as the optic chiasm resulting in bitemporal hemianopia and loss of central vision.
- *Cranial nerve palsy:* Tumor invading the cavernous sinuses leads to oculomotor palsies and headache.
- *Hyperphagia and loss of temperature regulation:* Tumor invading hypothalamus results in loss of temperature regulation, hyperphagia, and hormonal syndromes because they interfere with the normal hypothalamic input to the pituitary.

Light Microscopy

- Pituitary adenomas of anterior pituitary gland lack the normal reticulin-rich acinar structure.
- Tumor cells are large with round to oval nuclei and delicate stippled (salt and pepper) chromatin and inconspicuous nuclei.
- Tumor cells may appear without definite pattern, i.e. pseudorossette-rich, papillary or organized fashion.

LACTOTROPE ADENOMA (PROLACTINOMA)

This is *most common prolactin-secreting* benign tumor of the pituitary gland. It constitutes 30% of pituitary tumors. Staining is usually chromophobic. Tumor is generally small in 90% of cases. Large tumor impinges on adjacent structures, and bitemporal hemianopia from pressure on the optic chiasm is common (Fig. 26.63).

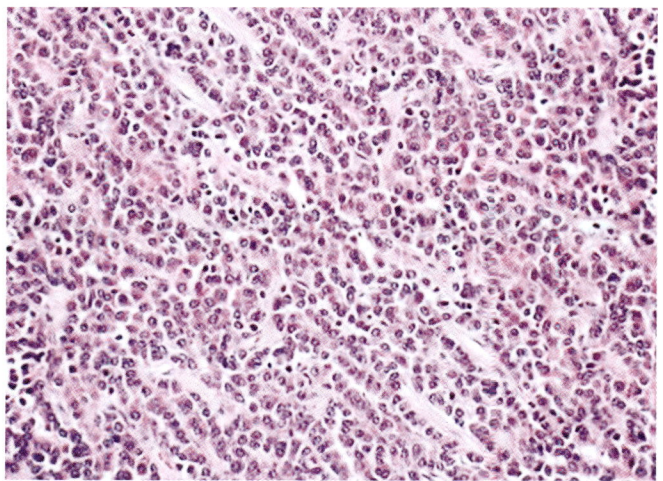

Fig. 26.63: Lactotrope adenoma (prolactinoma) (100X).

Age and Sex Predilection

It occurs more common in men than women (20 to 50 years). Increased synthesis of prolactin can be caused by hypothalamic lesions or by medications (methyldopa, reserpine) that interfere with dopamine (prolactin-inhibitory factor) secretion. It can also be associated with estrogen therapy.

Clinical Features

Young women present with amenorrhea, galactorrhea and infertility. There is increased concentration of serum prolactin level. Increased prolactin level inhibits LH essential for ovulation.

Men present with decreased libido and erectile dysfunction.

Management

Functional lactotrope adenoma is treated with dopamine agonists to inhibit prolactin synthesis. Macroadenoma may require surgery or irradiation.

Tumor resected post-therapy usually shows interstitial fibrosis and reduction in size. Tumor cells show low proliferative index and focally positive for prolactin.

SOMATOTROPIC ADENOMA

This is the second most common pituitary tumor. It secretes growth hormone, causing acromegaly or gigantism.

Most cases of acromegaly are diagnosed in the fourth and fifth decades. Gigantism most often affects infants and children.

Adenoma arising before epiphyseal closure in children or adolescents cause *gigantism*. However, adenoma originating after the fusion of epiphyses of the long bones leads to acromegaly in adults. Expansion of the tumor within the sella turcica may cause local compression effects.

Patient develops clinical manifestations of acromegaly due to combined effects of growth hormone, somatomedin-C and insulin-like growth factor-1, such as headache, and symptoms due to compression of optic chiasma. Patient develops generalized enlargement of viscera.

Growth Hormone

- Growth hormone is synthesized by somatotropes in the anterior pituitary gland. This hormone has growth promoting and anti-insulin actions. This hormone is essential for linear bone growth in children.
- This hormone also participates in increasing rate at which cells transport amino acids across cell membranes. It increases rate of utilization of fatty

acids. It decreases the utilization of carbohydrates (Fig. 26.64 and Table 26.35).

Clinical Features

Clinical manifestations of acromegaly (Fig. 26.65).

- *Head and neck:* Patient has prominent frontal and orbital ridges, coarsened features, recurrent serous otitis media, macroglossia, prominent jaw and thyroid enlargement.
- *Axilla:* There is increased perspiration in axillae.
- *Cardiovascular system:* Patient presents with hypertension, heart failure, cardiomegaly, edema and breathlessness.
- *Skeletal system:* Patient presents with barrel chest, enlarged hands, paresthesia in hands, broad feet, joint pain, degenerative arthritis, peripheral neuropathy, and myopathy.

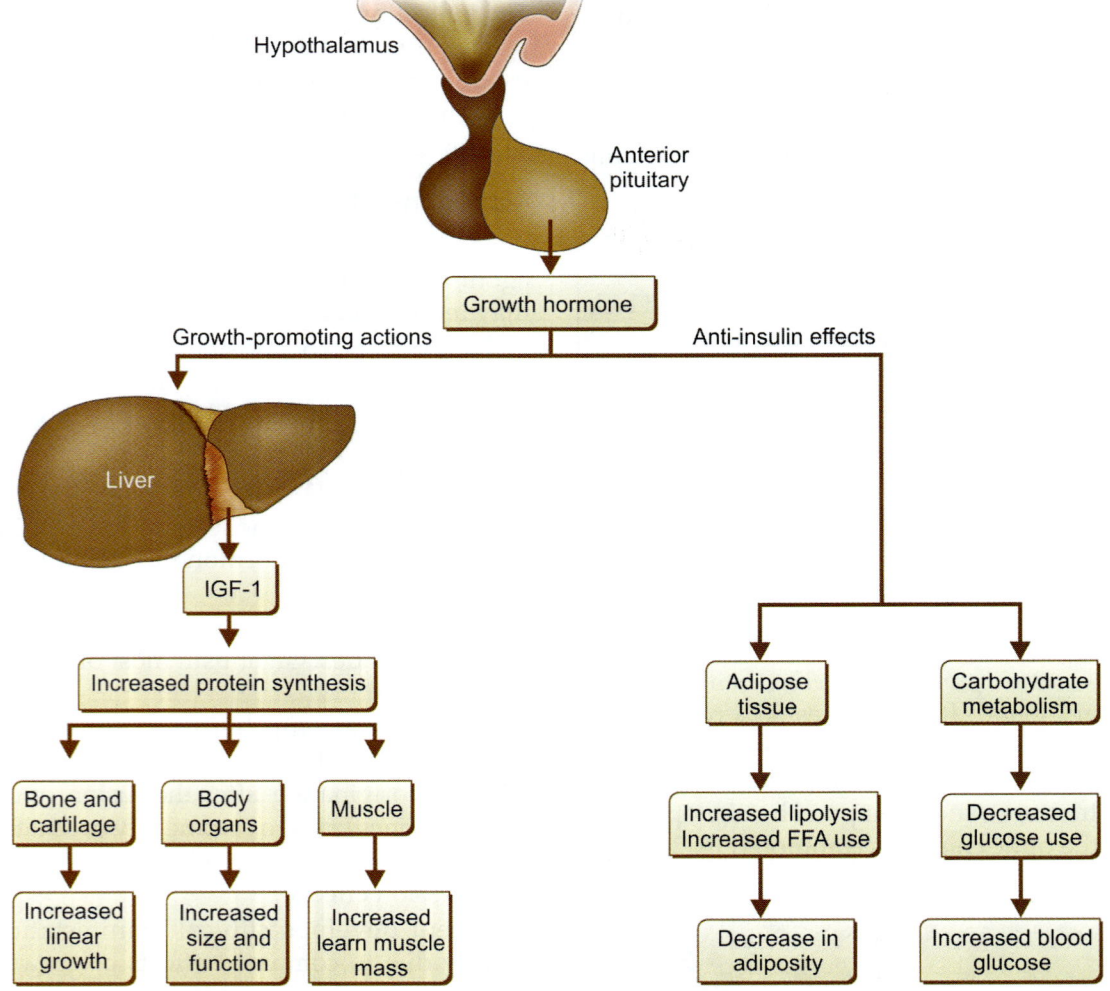

Fig. 26.64: Growth promoting and anti-insulin effects of growth hormone (FFA, free fatty acids; IGF-1, insulin-like growth factor-1).

Table 26.35: Mechanism of action of growth hormone

Actions	Effects
Growth promoting actions Growth hormone stimulates liver to synthesize IGF-1 (insulin-like growth factor-1). IGF-1 participates in protein synthesis	*Bone and cartilage:* IGF-1 increases linear growth *Body organs:* IGF-1 participates in increase in size of organs and their functions *Muscles:* IGF-1 increases lean muscle mass
Anti-insulin actions Growth hormone has anti-insulin actions	*Adipose tissue:* Growth hormone promotes lipolysis, utilization of fatty acids leading to decrease in adiposity *Carbohydrate metabolism:* Growth hormone decreases utilization of glucose leading to increased blood sugar level

Endocrine System: Pancreas, Thyroid, Parathyroid, Adrenal and Pituitary Glands

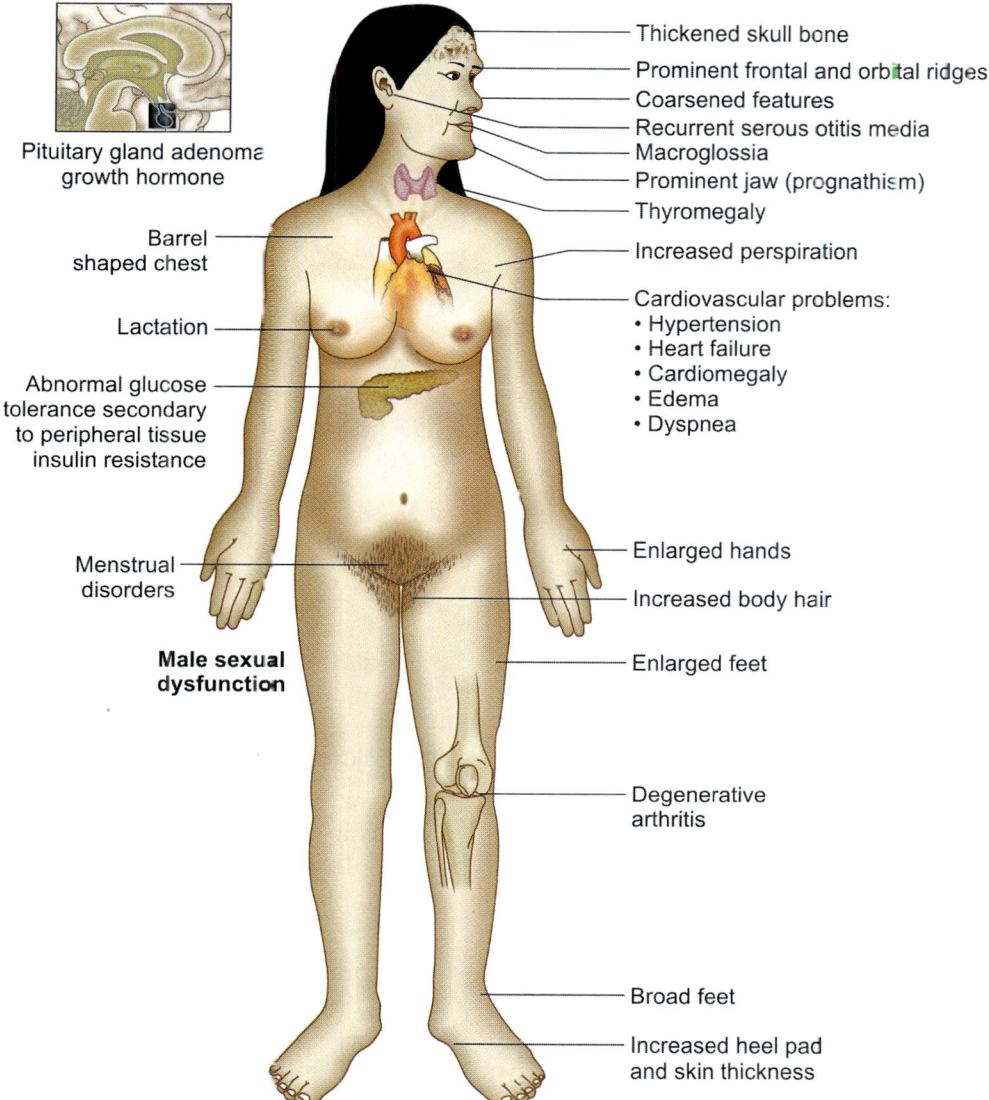

Fig. 26.65: Clinical manifestations of acromegaly.

- *Skin:* Patient develops pigmentation and thickened skin.
- *Sexual problems:* Male develops sexual dysfunction. Female presents with menstrual disturbances.

Diagnostic Marker

Growth hormone excess causes elevation in concentration of insulin-like growth factor-1 (somatomedin-C) by the liver, measurement of which is a reliable indicator of disease activity.

CORTICOTROPIC ADENOMA

Corticotropic adenoma secretes excess of ACTH, resulting in Cushing's syndrome of pituitary origin (Cushing's disease). It is five times more frequent than adrenal tumor associated Cushing's syndrome.

Clinical Features

Patient develops hypercorticism most often of pituitary and less often of adrenal origin. It is worth mentioning that ectopic ACTH production occurs in small cell carcinoma of lung.

Dexamethasone Suppression Test

It distinguishes between ACTH-dependent and ACTH-independent forms of Cushing's syndrome.

Dexamethasone suppresses pituitary secretion of corticotrophin, whereas it has no effect in cases of adrenal hyperplasia or functional adrenal tumors.

MIXED SOMATOTROPH–LACTOTROPH ADENOMA

It consists of two types of cells: *somatotropic cells synthesize growth hormone* and *lactotropic cells secrete prolactin*.

Clinical Features

Approximately 50% of tumors with acromegaly, excess synthesis of prolactin causes loss of libido and erectile dysfunction in men.

Management

These patients are treated with dopamine agonists, which inhibit prolactin secretion.

CRANIOPHARYNGIOMA

Craniopharyngioma is an infiltrative epithelial tumor located in the region of the pituitary fossa above the sella turcica. It does not secrete hormones.

Origin

It is derived from remnants of Rathke's pouch located above the sella turcica, the embryological source of the anterior pituitary gland. It is similar to ameloblastoma of the jaw.

Pathology

Clinical manifestations vary depending on destruction or pressure caused by tumor. Destruction of either or both lobes of pituitary gland result in hypopituitarism. It causes local destruction replacing the midline structures in the region of the hypothalamus.

Clinical Features

- Tumor compresses the pituitary gland and damages the overlying hypothalamus and optic chiasma, presenting with either hypopituitarism or visual disturbances bilateral hemianopia (loss of peripheral visual fields) or hydrocephalus and headaches in children between 10 and 20 years. Cranial nerve damage by tumor causes palsies.
- Patient often presents with *diabetes insipidus* (ADH deficiency), which characterized by an inability to concentrate the urine, with consequent chronic water diuresis, thirst, and polydipsia.
- Approximately 25% of cases of central diabetes insipidus are associated with brain tumors, particularly craniopharyngioma.

Gross Morphology

- Tumor shows solid and cystic areas. It also shows areas of calcification.

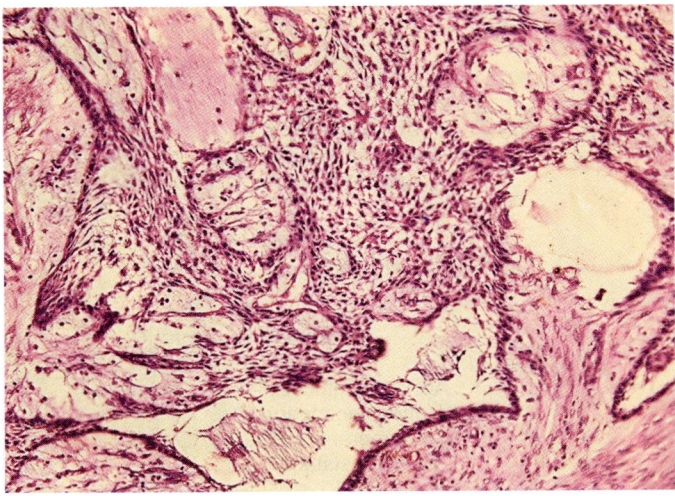

Fig. 26.66: Craniopharyngioma—tumor is composed of solid and cystic areas (400X).

- The cyst is filled with thick fluid containing lipid derived from breakdown of the lining epithelium.

Light Microscopy

- Tumor is composed of solid and cystic areas. Cystic areas are lined by nests and cords of squamous or columnar cells in a loose stroma, closely resembling the appearance of the embryonic tooth bud enamel organ.
- It is most often lined by flat or columnar cells resulting in papillary projections (Fig. 26.66).

Immunohistochemistry

β-Catenin is also useful in the diagnosis of *colorectal adenocarcinoma* (versus adenocarcinomas of other sites), craniopharyngioma, solid and pseudopapillary tumor of the pancreas, and other neoplasms.

Radiological Analysis

Calcification apparent on radiograph is often prominent; facilitating diagnosis.

Recurrence

Although craniopharyngiomas are benign, local recurrence is often a problem because of inability to completely excise infiltrative tumors.

CHAPTER 27

Bones and Joints

Learning Objectives

BONES
- Structure of Bone

OSTEOMYELITIS
- Pyogenic Osteomyelitis
- Tubercular Osteomyelitis

METABOLIC BONE DISEASES
- Renal Osteodystrophy
- Osteitis Fibrosa Cystica
- Peget's Disease of Bone (Osteitis Deformans)

BONE TUMORS
- Bone Forming Tumors
- Cartilaginous Tumors

- Tumors Arising from Undifferentiated Cells
- Osteoclastic Giant Cell-rich Tumor
- Histiocytic Tumors
- Notochord Derived Tumors
- Fibrous/Fibrohistiocytic Malignant Tumors
- Diagnosis of Bone Disorders

JOINTS
- General Considerations
- Arthritis of Probable Autoimmune Origin
- Degenerative Joint Disease
- Arthritis of Metabolic Origin
- Infective Arthritis
- Miscellaneous Disorders of Joints

BONES

STRUCTURE OF BONE

Bone comprises osteocytes, osteoblasts and osteoclasts, which are related to formation, maintenance, and resorption of the bone matrix.

Bone also contains fibroblasts, and blood vessels. The joint space of the mature bone and the growth plate of the growing long bones contain cartilage cells. The bone marrow contains hematopoietic and fat cells. Osteoblast derived proteins of bone matrix are shown in Table 27.1.

Table 27.1: Osteoblast derived proteins of bone matrix

Categories	Examples
Collagen fibers	Collagen fibers type I
Cell adhesion proteins	Osteopontin, thrombopontin and fibronectin
Proteins participating in mineralization	Osteocalcin
Calcium binding proteins	Osteonectin, bone sialoprotein
Enzymes	Alkaline phosphatase, collagenase
Growth factors	Insulin-like growth factor (IGF), TGF-β, platelet derived growth factor (PDGF)
Cytokines	IL-1, IL-6

Normal Bone Cells

- *Osteocytes:* These are mature resting cells involved in the maintenance of the basic functional and anatomic units of bone, called *osteons*. Osteocytes participate in the maintenance of the blood concentration of calcium and phosphate.
- *Osteoblasts:* These are bone forming cells, which synthesize osteoid and participate in its calcification. These can be stimulated by parathyroid hormone, vitamin D, and estrogens.
- *Osteoclasts:* These participate in resorption of bone. These are closely related to macrophages. Thus, they are derived from the same bone marrow precursors responding to granulocyte macrophage-colony stimulating factor (GM-CSF). In contrast to mononuclear macrophages, these cells are multinucleated.

Histology

- *Woven bone:* It is newly formed bone in growing children, composed of haphazardly arranged strands of collagen, appears like woven cloth when examined microscopically under polarized light.
- *Lamellar bone:* Woven bone gradually transforms into lamellar bone, composed of parallel arrays of mineralized osteoid, which is stronger and more resistant to stress, is a typical component of adult bones.

Diseases of Bone

- Bones are affected by numerous developmental, metabolic, infectious and neoplastic diseases and are also prone to mechanical trauma. *Most common site of infection and tumors is the fastest growing site of the long bones.* Genetic disorders may result in the formation of short, deformed, or structurally abnormal bones.
- Patient presents with focal pain in fracture/trauma, osteomyelitis, or osteoid osteoma. Diffuse pain occurs due to bone metastases, osteoporosis, and osteomalacia. Focal or diffuse pain is observed in bone metastases and Paget's disease of bone. Salient features of non-neoplastic bone disorders are shown in Table 27.2.

Table 27.2: Salient features of non-neoplastic bone disorders

Tumor/Lesion	Location	Age	Radiological findings	Pathological findings	Differential diagnosis
Congenital/developmental disorders	Diffuse, sometimes localized; usually symmetrical	<10	Modeling abnormality	Disease-dependent	Very broad
Traumatic disorders	Any part of bone	Any	Fracture lines; dislocation	Hemorrhage; organization; women bone and chondroid matrix	Osteosarcoma and chondrosarcoma
Circulatory disorders					
Avascular necrosis	Convex ends of long bones	5–40	Wedge-shaped radio-density: crescent sign; collapse of articular cartilage	Necrotic marrow and bone; subarticular plate fracture	None
Idiopathic infarction	Medulla of long bones	>20	Serpiginous radio-opacities	Necrotic marrow and bone; calcification and ossification of marrow fat	Enchondroma
Paget's disease of bone	Any portion of any bone; almost always extending to articular end	>50	Early: Bone resorption in wedge shaped edge. Later: Coarse trabeculation: loss of cortico-medullary differentiation	Osteoclastic resorption + increased vascularity and marrow fibrosis: Mosaic cement lines in middle to late stages	Hyperparathyroidism; myelodysplasia and myelofibrosis; metastatic carcinoma
Infectious disorders					
Hematogenous	Cortex of long bones	2–15	Early: ↑Uptake on bone scan; change of marrow signal on MRI Later: Mixed sclerosis and radiolucency	Marrow fibrosis with osteonecrosis and exudate/mixed inflammatory cell infiltrate	Round cell tumors and Langerhans' cell histiocytosis
Direct	Any; open trauma or deep ulcer	Varies	Mixed sclerosis and radiolucency		

OSTEOMYELITIS

Osteomyelitis is inflammation of bone marrow by bacteria. Infectious organisms may reach the bone through the bloodstream. It primarily affects the *metaphyseal area of the long bones of extremities around knee, ankle, and hip joints* because of the unique vascular supply in this region.

Normally, arterioles entering the calcified portion of the growth plate form a loop, and then drain into the medullary cavity without establishing a capillary bed. Slow blood flow into vascular loop allows more time for the bacteria to invade the walls of the blood vessels and establish an infective focus within the bone marrow.

PYOGENIC OSTEOMYELITIS

Pyogenic osteomyelitis may affect neonates, children, adolescents and adults described as under.

Age Group

Children and adolescents

- *Staphylococcus aureus* is the most common cause of hematogenous osteomyelitis due to penetrating injuries and post-surgical wounds.
- In growing bones of children, most bone infection begins predominantly in the highly vascularized growth plate (metaphyseal region) of long bones, with greatest blood flow by nutrient artery, where they exit in intercellular spaces.
- It most often involves femur (distal end), tibia (proximal end) and humerus (proximal end). Salmonella is frequent in association with sickle cell anemia.

Adults

- Osteomyelitis occurs usually as a complication of a compound fracture or sequelae of surgery. Osteomyelitis is an uncommon complication of a closed fracture. Osteomyelitis in adults most often begins in epiphyseal and subchondral locations due to hematogenous dissemination of Staphylococcus pathogen.
- Hematogenous dissemination of *Escherichia coli*, Pseudomonas and Klebsiella species occurs in urinary tract infection and intravenous drug addicts.
- *Pseudomonas aeruginosa* infection also occurs through nail puncture in persons wearing rubber footwear.
- Patient may develop osteomyelitis due to extension from contiguous sites (e.g. periodontal abscess).

Neonates

Haemophilus influenzae, Escherichia coli and Streptococci group B (β-hemolyticus) are responsible for osteomyelitis in neonates.

Anatomical Aspect

Metaphyseal arteries give terminal branches and forming loops irregular afferent venous sinusoids at growth plate. Blood flow is slow and turbulent at growth plate in metaphyseal region of bone predisposing to bacterial seeding.

In addition, lining cells have a little or no phagocytic activity. This area becomes a catch basin for bacteria and forms an abscess.

Pathogenesis

Focus of infection in the metaphysis of long bones attracts polymorphonuclear cells. Entire bone cavity space becomes edematous due to exudates. In the acute stage, pyogenic osteomyelitis may resolve with antibiotic therapy.

Chronic osteomyelitis results from persistent suppurative acute infection of bone. Sequence of events in the pathogenesis of osteomyelitis are shown in Fig. 27.1.

Sequestrum Formation

- Due to rigid structure and limited bone space, inflammatory exudates in bone cavity compress the endosteal blood vessels and impair the inflow of blood.
- Abscess, limited by growth plate, spreads transversely along Volkmann haversian canals elevates the periosteum.
- It will further compress the perforating blood vessels of periosteum in subperiosteal region. Then it extends subperiosteally and may invade shaft in infants less than one year of age.
- Some metaphyseal arterial branches pass through growth plate, and infection may invade epiphysis and joints.

Lytic enzymes detach dead bone from main bone that floats inside the abscess cavity. The necrotic bone is called a *sequestrum* (Fig. 27.2).

Involucrum

Involucrum is the periosteal reactive viable bone that surrounds necrotic bone (sequestrum) in osteomyelitis (Fig. 27.3).

Section III: Systemic Pathology

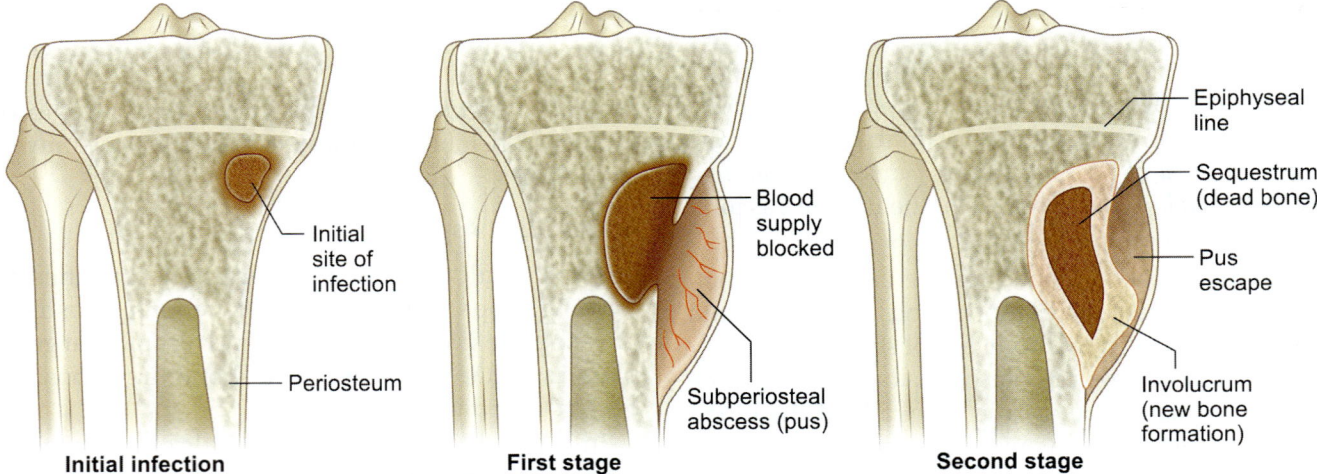

Fig. 27.1: Osteomyelitis shows stages of abscess formation, sequestrum and involucrum.

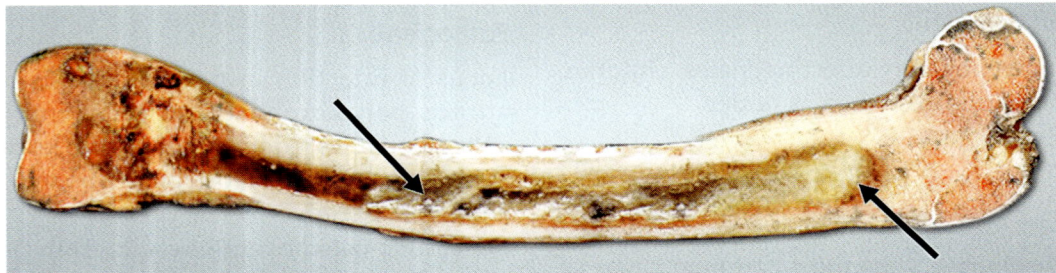

Fig. 27.2: Acute osteomyelitis. There is a large collection of pus in the medullary cavity of the shaft of the femur (arrows).

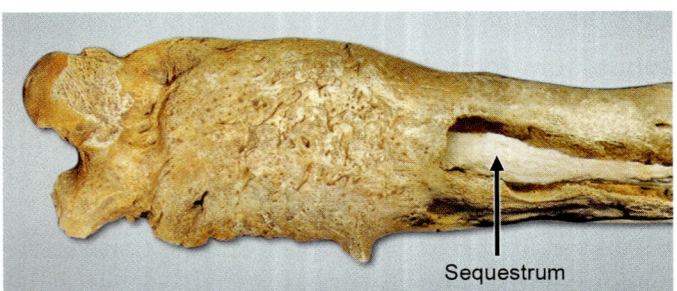

Fig. 27.3: Chronic osteomyelitis. This specimen shows death of shaft of the tibia. This has separated completely as a sequestrum. New bone—an involucrum has formed around the dead bone. Lacunae open through the involucrum and result in discharging sinuses on the skin surface (arrow).

Brodie Abscess

It is a chronic bone abscess. Brodie abscess consists of dense reactive bone from the periosteum and the endosteum that surrounds and contains the infection.

Cloacae

Cloaca is the hole found in the bone during formation of a draining sinus. Infection process may erode periosteum and form sinus to the skin surface of the body through holes in bones. Process is influenced by virulence of organism, resistance or host administration of antibiotics and fibrotic and sclerotic responses.

Radiographic Signs

Initially, bony lesion is osteolytic. Sclerosis appears only after disease has progressed >2 months. Early diagnosis of osteomyelitis is made by Indium-labeled leukocytic scintigram showing focal signal increase in the site of infection.

Clinical Features

Patient with osteomyelitis of long bone presents with fever, pain and tenderness (most common), swelling in acute cases; later followed by discharging sinuses to the skin surface, effusions in adjacent joints and limitation of joint movement. In acute osteomyelitis, peripheral blood shows leukocytosis and blood culture may be positive.

Systemic manifestations in vertebral involvement are usually milder. Pain may be principal manifestation especially in adults.

Complications

- About 5–25% of acute cases fail to resolve and go on to chronic osteomyelitis. The weakened bone is prone to fracture. A fracture complicated by osteomyelitis fails to heal, with development of pseudoarthrosis.
- The disorder may be complicated by secondary (reactive systemic) amyloidosis. An uncommon complication is development of draining sinus tract.

Development of squamous cell carcinoma may occur within sinus tract.

TUBERCULAR OSTEOMYELITIS

Tubercular osteomyelitis is most commonly secondary to hematogenous extension from a primary focus in the lung. It principally targets the vertebral column, called *Pott's disease* in 1 to 3% of people. Vertebral body destruction may result in impingement on the spinal cord (Fig. 27.4). It also targets hip bone, long bones (femur, tibia) and small bones (hands, feet).

Clinical Features

Patient presents with fever, fatigue, bone pain, soft tissue swelling and discharging sinuses (Fig. 27.5).

> **Light Microscopy**
> Bone marrow shows fibrosis infiltrated by chronic inflammatory infiltrate composed of lymphocytes, macrophages and plasma cells. Caseous necrosis and epithelioid cell granulomas are present.

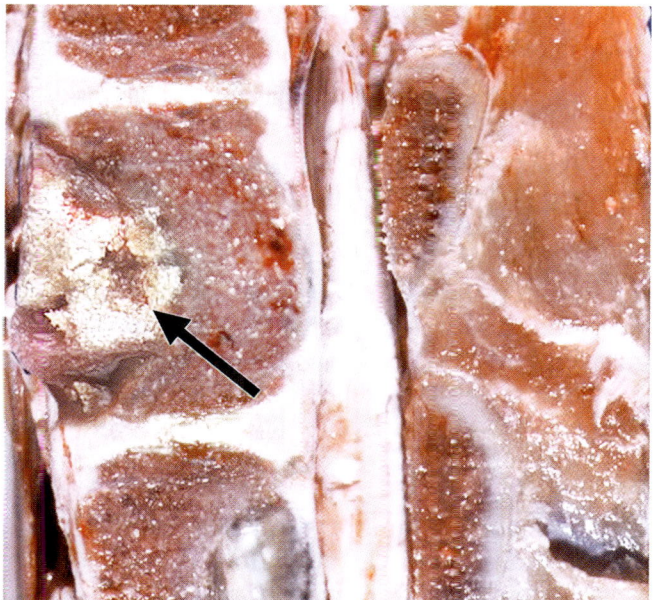

Fig. 27.5: Tuberculous psoas abscess. Two lumbar vertebrae involved by tuberculosis with extension of the caseation into the psoas muscle. When such infection spreads along the psoas, the abscess may *point* in the groin (arrow).

Complications

Patient may develop many complications such as deformities of bones, pathological fractures, secondary amyloidosis or squamous cell carcinoma. The skin at the edges of sinus tracts draining the pus from the infected bone may undergo malignant transformation.

Laboratory Diagnosis

- Pus culture and sensitivity performed in patients with tubercular osteomyelitis may demonstrate pyogenic bacteria due to superadded infection.
- These patients do not respond to antibiotics therapy. Biopsy may not demonstrate epithelioid cell granulomas.
- Therefore, in every case of osteomyelitis with discharging sinuses, blood culture on LJ medium should be done. Imaging techniques are employed as diagnostic tools.

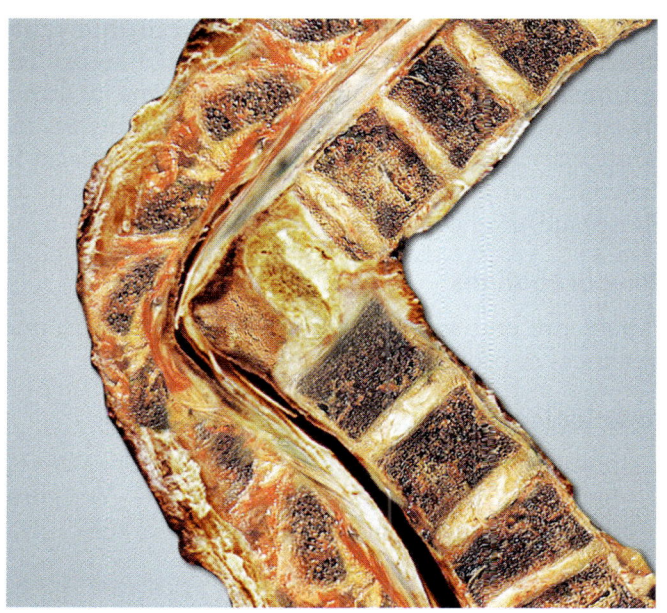

Fig. 27.4: Tuberculosis in the spine of a young boy (Pott's fracture of the vertebrae).

METABOLIC BONE DISEASES

Metabolic bone disease refers to osteopenia (diffuse radiolucency of bone). It occurs due to abnormalities in vitamin D metabolism, phosphate deficiency and defects in the mineralization process. Vitamin D deficiency causes rickets in children and osteomalacia in adults.

Bone Ossification

- *Intramembranous ossification:* Mesenchymal cells form osteoblasts, and results in formation of collagenous osteoid matrix.
- *Endochondral ossification:* It occurs in the development of long tubular bones. Growing cartilage at epiphyseal

plate is mineralized, and then resorbed. It is replaced by osteoid matrix and then mineralized to form bone.

VITAMIN D

Vitamin D occurs in two forms, i.e. vitamin D_2 (ergocalciferol) and vitamin D_3 (cholecalciferol).

Sources

It may be endogenous (80%) or exogenous (20%). Endogenous source exists in the form of dehydrocholesterol in the skin. When skin is under exposure to ultraviolet rays, dehydrocholesterol is converted into vitamin D_3 (cholecalciferol).

Metabolism

After absorption, vitamin D combines with α-globulin and 2-hydroxyvitamin D (vitamin D_2) is formed in the liver. Vitamin D_2 to vitamin D_3 (active form of vitamin D) conversion takes place in kidneys. Low level of serum calcium augments the conversion of vitamin D_2 to vitamin D_3. Vitamin D is stored in adipose tissue.

Functions

- Vitamin D maintains normal plasma levels of calcium and phosphorus.
- It enhances calcium absorption by small intestine.
- It collaborates with parathormone in mobilization of calcium from bone.
- It stimulates parathormone dependent absorption of calcium in distal tubular cells parathormone.
- It is requisite for normal mineralization of epiphyseal cartilage and osteoid.

RICKETS

Etiology

This disorder is caused by failure of action of calcitriol (1,25-dihydroxycholecalciferol), the active form of vitamin D in children. It occurs due to diet deficient in vitamin D, lack of exposure to sunlight, intestinal malabsorption, renal and liver disease.

Pathogenesis

The bony abnormalities in rickets are caused by decreased bone mineralization (calcification). It results in excess accumulation of unmineralized matrix (osteoid), wide osteoid seams, increased thickness of the epiphyseal growth plates and other skeletal deformities. During infancy, head and neck are under greatest stress; hence changes are marked in these areas. Clinical features are shown in Table 27.3.

OSTEOMALACIA

Osteomalacia (soft bones) is a disorder of adults. It is characterized by inadequate mineralization (calcification) of newly formed bone matrix. These bones are susceptible to fracture, but a few deformities.

Etiology

Vitamin D deficiency in adults occurs due to malabsorption syndrome (commonest cause), chronic renal disease (renal osteodystrophy) and PTH like protein synthesized by squamous cell carcinoma of lung, breast carcinoma, ovarian carcinoma (paraneoplastic syndrome) and Fanconi's syndrome. Osteomalacia in Fanconi's syndrome occurs due to renal wastage of phosphate, amino acids and glucose in urine.

Clinical Features

Patient presents with bone pain and tenderness, and weakness of proximal limb muscles.

Radiological Findings

- Spontaneous incomplete fractures (*Looser's zones*) often occur in the long bones or pelvis. Vertebral bodies are typically biconcave because of the central

Table 27.3: Clinical features of rickets

Terms	Clinical findings
Craniotabes	There is thinning and softening of occipital and parietal bones. There is late closure of fontanelles
Frontal bossing	Frontal bone is squared due to increased formation of osteoid
Rachitic rosary	Thickening of costochondral junction occurs due to overgrowth of cartilage and osteoid tissue results in a string of beads-like appearance
Harrison's groove	A depression occurs along the line of insertion of the diaphragm into the rib cage due to inward pull of diaphragm
Pigeon-shaped chest	Anterior protrusion of sternum occurs due to inward pull of metaphyseal areas of ribs by respiratory muscles
Pelvis bones	These are deformed
Spine deformity	Lumbar lordosis occurs, when child is ambulatory

compression of softened vertebrae by intervertebral discs.
- These changes can be reversed by supplementing the diet with adequate amounts of vitamin D and by normalizing the metabolism of calcium.

> **Light Microscopy**
> - In osteomalacia, the bony trabeculae are normal in thickness and rimmed by broad bony spicules of osteoid (incompletely calcified) lined by osteoclasts.
> - Central portion of bony spicules are normally calcified, but their peripheral portion uncalcified.
> - On the other hand, the bone spicules in osteoporosis are thin but normally mineralized.

Blood Biochemistry

Blood calcium is decreased. Serum alkaline phosphatase is increased due to increased activity of osteoblasts (e.g. remember these biochemical changes are absent in osteoporosis).

RENAL OSTEODYSTROPHY

Bone changes in chronic renal failure are known as renal osteodystrophy.

Patient develops clinical, radiological or pathological evidence of bone diseases, i.e. osteoporosis, osteomalacia, bone necrosis, and soft tissue calcification.

Mechanism

- In chronic renal failure, kidneys fail to convert vitamin D_2 to vitamin D_3 (active form) essential for calcium absorption. Prolonged hemodialysis inhibits calcification of osteoid leading to osteomalacia.
- High level of serum phosphates inhibits renal enzymes catalyzing formation of $1,25(OH)2D_3$.
- Therapeutic administration of steroid in patients with chronic glomerulonephritis causes osteoporosis and avascular necrosis of bone.

Pathogenesis

Physiological state: In chronic renal failure, kidneys fail to convert vitamin D_2 to vitamin D_3 (active form). Normally, vitamin D_3 participates in absorption of calcium by intestine.

Pathological state: Nonavailability of vitamin D_3 results in decreased ionized calcium in serum. Decreased serum calcium stimulates parathyroid glands to synthesize parathormone. Parathormone causes resorption of bone resulting in osteomalacia. Disordered remodeling of such bones leads to alternating areas of thickened bone (osteosclerosis) and osteoporosis. In renal osteodystrophy, spine shows *Rugger Jersey* appearance.

Calcification

Deposition of calcium in tissues is demonstrated by imaging technique and light microscopy.
- Nephrocalcinosis can cause interstitial nephritis further aggravating renal failure.
- Calcium deposition occurs in joint cartilage (chondrocalcinosis) and periarticular region at the junction of metacarpals and proximal phalanges. It occurs in intra-articular and periarticular region of shoulders.
- Calcium deposits in cornea are demonstrated by slit-lamp examination revealing band keratitis.
- Medial calcification occurs in tunica media of medium, small size arteries, aorta and major branches.

OSTEITIS FIBROSA CYSTICA

Osteitis fibrosa cystica occurs in primary hyperparathyroidism as a result of bone resorption by parathormone.

Pathogenesis

- Osteoclasts lining subperiosteum and endosteum invade the cortex. As the disease progresses, trabecular bone resorption occurs resulting in replacement of marrow by loose fibrosis and cystic degeneration.
- These areas contain reactive woven bone, and hemosiderin-laden macrophages and often display many giant cells, which are actually osteoclasts.
- The lesion has been termed a *brown tumor*.
- This is not a true tumor, but rather a repair reaction.

Clinical Features

Patient may present with nephrolithiasis, nephrocalcinosis, calcification in blood vessels, epulis (mouth), codfishing of vertebrae, limbus keratopathy, peptic ulcer, pancreatitis and multiple adenomas in pituitary, thyroid gland, pancreas and adrenal glands. Clinical manifestations of osteitis fibrosa cystica are shown in Table 27.4.

Laboratory Findings

Laboratory findings in metabolic bone disorders are shown in Table 27.5.

OSTEOPOROSIS

Osteoporosis is characterized by decreased bone mass but otherwise normally mineralized bone.

Table 27.4: Clinical manifestations

• Kidneys	Nephrolithiasis, nephrocalcinosis	• Blood vessels	Calcium deposition
• Skull (X-ray)	Salt and pepper appearance	• Eye	Limbus keratopathy
• Bone	Cyst formation and fractures	• GIT	Peptic ulcer
• Mouth	Epulis	• Pancreas	Pancreatitis
• Vertebrae	Codfishing of vertebrae	• Miscellaneous	Multiple adenomas in endocrines

Table 27.5: Laboratory findings in metabolic bone disorders

Disorders	Serum calcium	Serum phosphate	Alkaline phosphatase	Parathormone (PTH)	Vitamin D
Osteoporosis	Normal	Normal	Normal	Normal	Normal
Osteomalacia	Low	High/Low	High	Normal	Low/Normal
Hyperparathyroidism	High	Low	Normal/High	High	Normal
Renal osteodystrophy	Normal/High	High	High	High	Normal

It occurs either due to impaired synthesis of bone matrix or increased resorption of bone matrix protein. Bone loss and eventually fractures (hip, wrist, and vertebrae) are the hallmarks of osteoporosis. Serum calcium and phosphate levels are typically normal.

Osteoporosis can be classified as primary (type 1 and type 2) or secondary described as under.

Primary Osteoporosis

Type 1: It is more common in women with postmenopausal state (estrogen deficiency). It is due to an absolute increase in osteoclast activity.

Type 2: It occurs in elderly persons of both sexes. It reflects decreased osteoblast activity.

Secondary Osteoporosis

It results from a variety of identifiable conditions that may include: hyperparathyroidism, cancers (multiple myeloma or metastatic carcinoma), malnutrition, drug therapy (corticosteroids), prolonged immobilization and weightlessness with space travel.

Clinical Features

The affected bones are unable to bear weight. Patient commonly develops compression fractures of the vertebrae resulting in spinal deformity (kyphosis most common) and shortened stature.

- *Axial osteoporosis:* Patient develops vertebral compression fractures in mid-thoracic or mid-lumbar region progression to thoracic kyphosis.

  Patient presents with continuous pain in acute phase and intermittent pain in chronic phase.

- *Appendicular osteoporosis:* Patient develops fractures caused by minimal trauma in proximal femur (intertrochanteric or intracapsular region), proximal humerus and distal radius.

Laboratory Diagnosis

Radiographic measurement of bone density is the best diagnostic tool. It shows diffuse radiolucency of bone. Increased risk for fracture correlates with decreasing bone density.

Various imaging diagnostic techniques include single-photon absorptiometry, dual-photon absorptiometry, quantitative computed tomography, and dual X-ray absorptiometry.

PAGET'S DISEASE OF BONE (OSTEITIS DEFORMANS)

Paget's disease is an increased thickness of abnormal bone architecture caused by increased osteoclastic and osteoblastic activity.

It results from disordered remodeling, in which excessive bone resorption initially results in lytic lesions, followed by disorganized and excessive bone formation.

There is marked increase in serum alkaline phosphatase (a manifestation of osteoblastic activity) and normal serum calcium and phosphorus.

Diagnostic Hallmark in Late Disease

It is characterized by abnormal arrangement of lamellar bone containing islands of irregular bone formation. It resembles pieces of a jig-saw puzzle, are separated by prominent cement lines known as *mosaic pattern*.

Morphologic Phases

There are three phases of disease process: osteolytic, mixed and late phases described as under:

- *Osteolytic phase:* It causes resorption of bone.
- *Mixed phase:* Osteoblastic and osteoclastic lead to new bone formation resulting in *mosaic pattern*.
- *Late phase:* It is characterized by increased bone density, thickened trabeculae with prominent 'mosaic pattern'.

Age Group

It begins after the age of 40 years and mainly affects elderly males.

Etiology

It is of unknown etiology. Viral etiology has been suggested by presence of intranuclear inclusions in osteoclasts demonstrated by electron microscopy. The studies suggest the possible role of a slow virus infection by a paramyxovirus.

Pathogenesis

The majority of patients are first recognized by the presence of an unexpectedly high serum alkaline phosphatase level on biochemical analysis. There are three stages in the development of Paget's disease of bone described as under:
- *Osteoclastic stage:* In this phase, there is excessive resorption of bones.
- *Osteoblastic stage:* Resorption of bones is followed by bone formation with raised alkaline phosphatase activity.
- *Osteosclerotic stage:* Osteoblastic phase is followed by production of thick bone without a normal lamellar bone. The bones are weak in osteosclerotic stage.

Bones Involvement

Patients with Paget's disease of bone usually involve multiple bones (polyostotic) in 85% of cases and single bone (monostotic) in 15% of cases.
- *Polyostotic lesions:* These occur in spine (70%), pelvis (65%), skull (frontal and occipital regions), sacrum, femur, tibia or humerus.
- *Monostotic lesion:* In decreasing order of frequency, bones involved include tibia, pelvis, skull (frontal and occipital regions), femur, vertebrae and humerus. Bone changes begin in subchondral ends of tibia, femur and humerus.

Complications

- *Microfractures:* Although the affected bone is thick but it lacks strength. Affected bone becomes painful due to microfractures.
- *Anterior bowing of leg bones:* Anterior bowing of tibia and femur is common deformity.
- *Hearing loss:* It occurs due to narrowing of the auditory foramen and compression of the eighth cranial nerve or direct involvement of middle ear bones (malleus, incus, and stapes).
- *Frontal bossing:* It occurs due to head enlargement.
- *Narrowing of foramen magnum:* It occurs due to flattening of base of skull (platybasia) resulting in compression of spinal cord.
- *Osteosarcoma:* Approximately 1% of cases may develop osteosarcoma in a focus of Paget's disease, usually in the femur, humerus, or pelvis.
- *CVS manifestations:* High output cardiac failure may result from multiple functional arteriovenous shunts within highly vascular early lesions.

SCURVY

Scurvy occurs due to deficiency of vitamin C. It is characterized by defective formation of mesenchymal tissue and osteoid matrix; defective wound healing; hemorrhagic phenomena.

Vitamin C is required for hydroxylation of proline and lysine, which are essential for collagen synthesis. It participates in the synthesis of reticulin and collagen fibrils from mucopolysaccharide ground substance in wound healing.

Source

Vitamin C is derived from fruits, vegetables, milk, liver and fish. It is not synthesized endogenously. It is stored in the body (normal range 1.5–4.0 gm).

Causes

Deficiency may be observed in elderly individuals and alcoholics. Peritoneal and hemodialysis patients and infants on processed milk may develop scurvy.

Clinical Features

Hemorrhages and healing defects in both children and adults.

Bleeding (hemorrhages)

- Defective connective tissue also leads to fragile capillaries, resulting in abnormal bleeding.
- Infants and children present with hemorrhages in mucocutaneous and muscles along fascial planes at mechanical stress points due to loosened endothelial cells from capillaries especially in nail beds, subperiosteal hematomas, bleeding into spaces: joints, retrobulbar, subarachnoid, and intracerebral hemorrhages. In adults, ulceration and hemorrhage in gums occur due to loosening of teeth.

Skeletal changes
- Bone changes in scurvy are secondary to defective osteoid matrix formation. Insufficient production of osteoid matrix results in cartilaginous overgrowth, widening of epiphysis, bowing of the long bones and chest deformity.
- Osteoporosis is seen especially at the metaphyseal ends of bone.

Other changes

Patient presents with gingival swelling and periodontal infection, impaired wound healing, and anemia.

BONE TUMORS

Bone matrix producing and fibrous tumors are most common. Bone tumors are classified as primary solitary (benign or malignant) or multifocal (secondary).

Classification

Bone tumors are classified as *primary* (benign or malignant) or *secondary* tumors (metastatic tumors). Primary bone tumors and their locations according to age group predilection are depicted in Fig. 27.6, WHO classification of primary bone tumors is shown in Table 27.6. Tumors metastasizing to bones in adults and children are shown in Table 27.7.

Frequency

Primary benign tumors are seven times more common than malignant tumors. Benign tumors such as osteochondroma and osteoid osteomas are most frequent. Most frequent malignant tumors in decreasing frequency include multiple myeloma, osteosarcoma, chondrosarcoma, Ewing's sarcoma, and giant cell tumor of bone.

Age Predilection

Most tumors show an age-dependent occurrence. Benign bone tumors occur within the first three

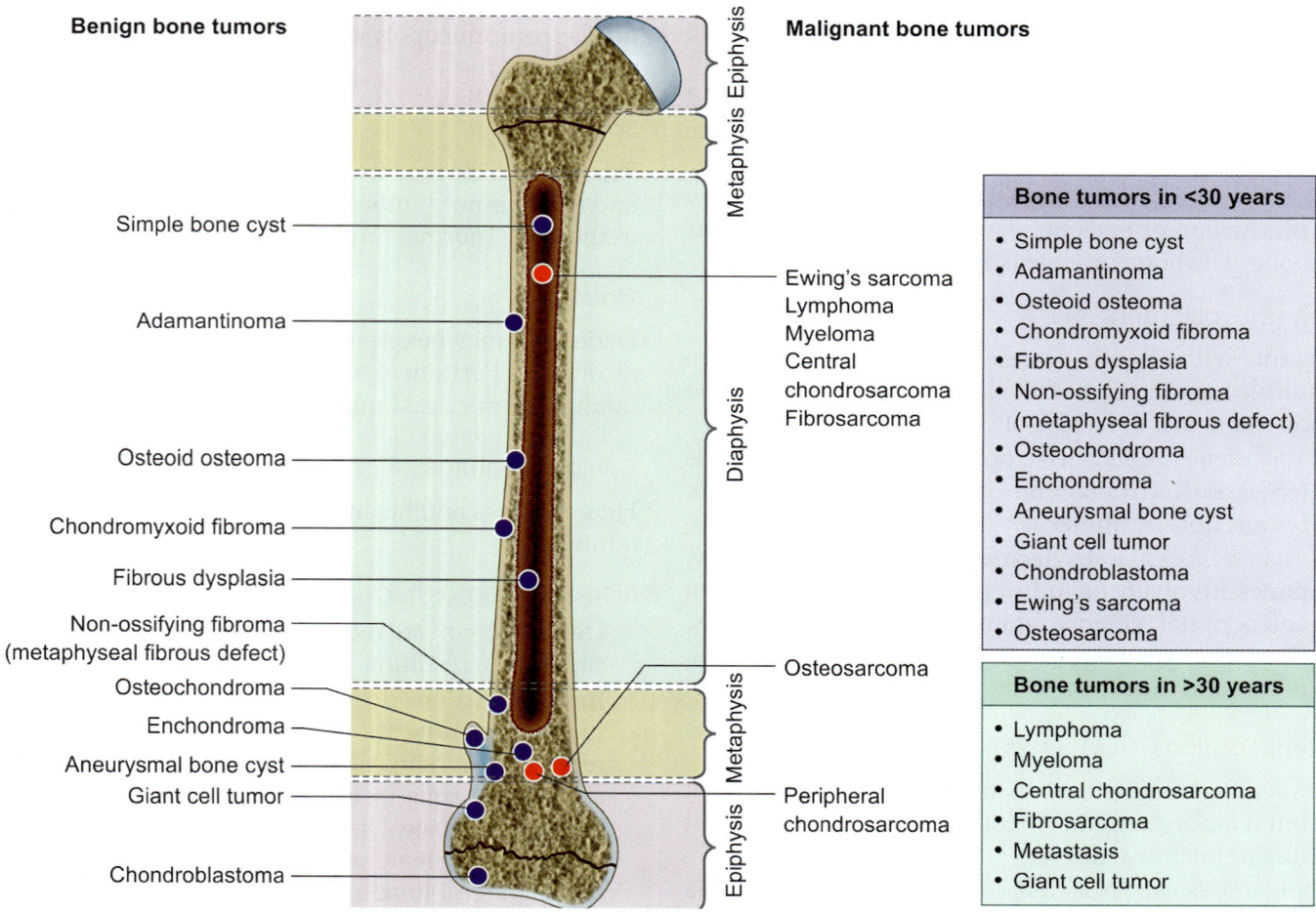

Fig. 27.6: Primary bone tumors and their locations according to age group predilection.

Table 27.6: WHO classification of primary bone tumors

Categories	Examples
Osteogenic tumors	Osteoid osteoma, osteoblastoma
	Osteosarcoma: Conventional, chondroblastic, fibroblastic, telangiectatic, low grade central, parosteal, periosteal, high grade surface osteosarcomas
Cartilaginous tumors	Osteochondroma, chondroma, enchondroma, periosteal chondroma, multiple chondromatosis, chondroblastoma, chondromyxoid fibroma
	Chondrosarcoma: Central (primary or secondary), peripheral, dedifferentiated, mesenchymal and clear cell chondrosarcomas
Ewing's sarcoma/primitive neuroectodermal tumor	Ewing's sarcoma
Giant cell tumor	Giant cell tumor (derived from osteoclasts)
	Malignant change in giant cell tumor
Hematopoietic tumors	Plasma cell myeloma, malignant lymphoma
Notochord tumors	Chordoma
Fibrogenic tumors	Desmoplastic fibroma
	Fibrosarcoma
Fibrohistiocytic tumors	Benign fibrous histiocytoma, malignant fibrous histiocytoma
Miscellaneous tumors	Adamantinoma
	Secondary tumors (metastases in bone)
Vascular tumors	Hemangioma, angiosarcoma
Smooth muscle tumors	Leiomyoma, leiomyosarcoma
Lipogenic tumors	Lipoma, liposarcoma
Neural tumors	Neurilemmoma
Langerhans' cell histiocytosis	Letterer-Siwe disease, Hand-Schüller-Christian disease and eosinophilic granuloma
Miscellaneous lesions	Aneurysmal bone cysts, simple bone cyst, fibrous dysplasia, metaphyseal defect (non-ossifying fibroma), osteofibrous dysplasia, Erdheim-Chester disease, chest wall hamartoma

Table 27.7: Cancers metastasizing to bones (bone metastases) in adults and children

Age group	Examples
Adult age group	Prostatic carcinoma
	Urinary bladder carcinoma
	Breast carcinoma
	Small cell carcinoma of lung
	Renal cell carcinoma
	Gastric carcinoma
	Colon carcinoma
	Thyroid gland carcinoma (follicular type)
Children age group	Neuroblastoma
	Rhabdomyosarcoma
	Retinoblastoma

decades. The most common primary bone tumors in order of increasing age are Ewing's sarcoma (5–20 years), osteosarcoma (10–20 years) and chondrosarcoma (40–60 years).

Anatomic Sites

- *Osteomas:* Osteomas are solitary benign tumors of skull bones.
- *Enchondromas:* These are most common tumors in the short bones of hands and feet.
- *Osteosarcomas:* Osteosarcomas occur predominantly in the long bones of extremities around knee joints in 60% of all cases, e.g. lower end of femur and upper end of tibia.
- *Chondrosarcomas:* Chondrosarcomas tend to involve the axial skeleton of the body (i.e. bones of the pelvic girdle, shoulder girdle, trunk and vertebrae). Pelvic bones are affected in 25–30%.
- *Hematopoietic marrow tumors:* These include Ewing's sarcoma (10–20 years), multiple myeloma, leukemia/lymphoma and metastatic cancers (older age) (Fig. 27.7 and Table 27.8).

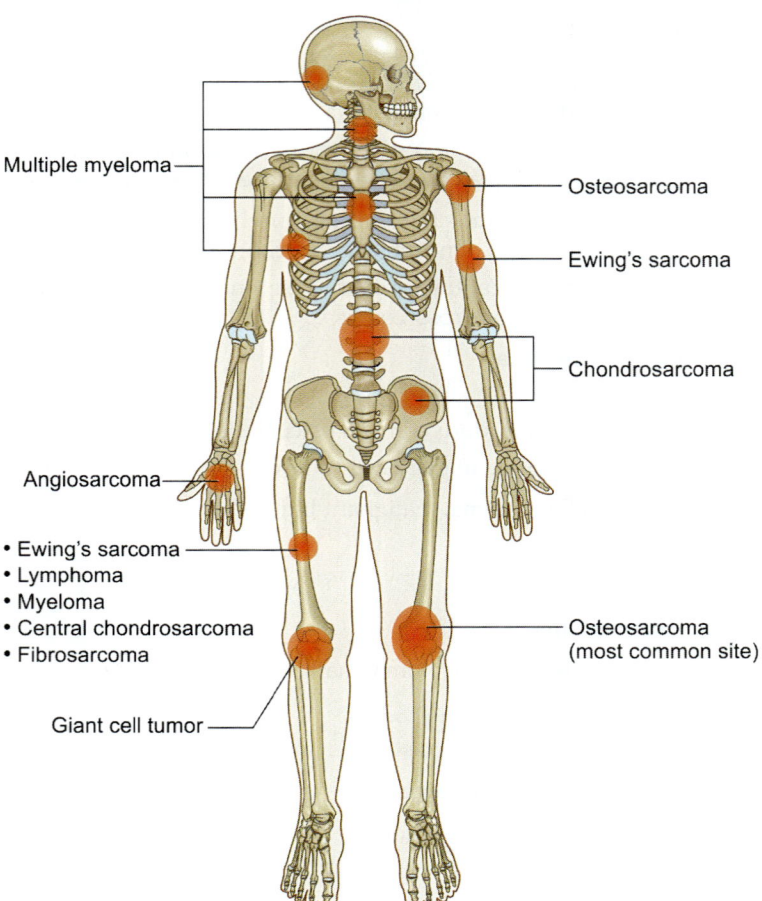

Fig. 27.7: Primary malignant bone tumors and their sites of occurrence.

Table 27.8: Salient features of common primary malignant tumors of bone

Bone tumor and % of all bone tumors	Origin	Age and sex (male to female ratio) predilection	Bones most often involved	Clinical behavior	Treatment and cure rate
Osteosarcoma (30%)	Active bone growth	10–20 years (adolescents) 3:2	Knee joint (60%) (distal femur, proximal tibia) and jaw	Rapid growth, pain, swelling and distant metastases	Surgery, chemotherapy (40%)
Chondrosarcoma (15%)	Cartilage	35–60 years 2:1	Pelvis, vertebrae, proximal long bones	Slow growth, vascular invasion	Surgery (75%)
Ewing's sarcoma (7%)	Bone marrow of growing bone	10–20 years (80% in <20 years) 1:1	Long bones in diaphysis	Widespread metastases	Surgery, chemotherapy (50%)
Fibrosarcoma and malignant fibrous histiocytoma (20%)	Fibrous tissue of bone	30–40 years 3:2	Long bones in diaphysis (femur, tibia, humerus and pelvis)	Local growth, vascular invasion	Surgery (40%)

Origin of Tumor

- *Epiphysis:* Tumors arising from epiphysis include giant cell tumor of bone, benign chondroblastoma, aneurysmal bone cyst and chondrosarcoma. Epiphysis is the most common site for giant cell tumors of bone in 20–40 years of age group. It is practically never seen in children or patients older than 60 years.
- *Metaphysis:* Osteosarcoma and nonossifying fibroma (tumor-like lesion) tend to occur in the metaphysis of long bones.

Table 27.9: Origin of bone tumors in long bones

Bone tumors	Age group	Location
Epiphyseal origin		
Giant cell tumor of bone	20–40 years	Knee area, distal radius (65%). It is practically never seen in children or patients older than 60 years
Chondroblastoma	10–20 years	Knee joint (most common site), skull, ribs, vertebrae and small bones of feet
Chondrosarcoma	35–60 years	Axial skeleton of the body (i.e. bones of the pelvic girdle, shoulder girdle, trunk and vertebrae. Pelvic bones are affected in 25–30%
Metaphyseal origin		
Osteosarcoma	10–20 years	Long bones of extremities around knee joints in 60% Lower end of femur is the most common site Upper end of tibia
Osteosarcoma arising in Paget's disease of bone	>40 years	Upper end of tibia (most common site), humerus and upper end of femur (occasional sites)
Metaphyseal fibrous defect (nonossifying fibroma)		
Diaphyseal origin		
Ewing's sarcoma	Children	Hematopoietic marrow sites in the axial skeleton
Malignant lymphoma	Older age group	Hematopoietic marrow sites in the axial skeleton
Multiple myeloma	Older age group	Hematopoietic marrow sites in the axial skeleton
Ameloblastoma/adamantinoma	Young adults	Long bone, jaw

- *Diaphysis:* Ewing's sarcoma, lymphoma, myeloma and adamantinoma involve diaphysis.

Ewing's develops in the diaphysis of long bones of children and young individuals. It is extremely unusual in middle-aged patients (Table 27.9).

Clinical Features

- *Incidental findings:* Generally, small-sized benign bone tumors tend to be asymptomatic and represent incidental findings.
- *Pain:* Patient may present with pain, a nonspecific symptom that may help in differential diagnosis. Pain occurs in locally aggressive growing lesions, e.g. aggressive osteoblastoma and giant cell tumor, and malignant tumors.
- *Pathological fractures:* Patient may develop pathological fractures complicating benign lesions as well as malignant tumors.
- *Local reaction of tumors:* There may be significant local tissue reaction to the tumor.

BONE FORMING TUMORS

Benign bone forming tumors are characterized by production of bone by neoplastic cells. Tumor bone is usually deposited as woven trabeculae (except osteoma) and is invariably mineralized.

Bone forming benign and malignant tumors are shown in Table 27.10. Salient features of commonest benign bone tumors are shown in Table 27.11.

Table 27.10: Bone forming benign and malignant tumors

Tumors		Frequency (%)
Benign tumors	Osteoid osteoma	13%
	Osteoblastoma	
Malignant tumor	Osteosarcoma	87%

Table 27.11: Salient features of commonest benign bone tumors (bone forming tumors)

Tumor	Locations	Age group	Pathological features
Osteoma	Facial bones	Adults	Mineralized compact bone
Osteoid osteoma	Cortex of long bones	10–30	*Nidus* of immature bone surrounded by sclerotic bone
Osteoblastoma	Vertebrae; cortex of long bones	10–30	Identical to osteoid osteoma but larger, often no sclerosis

OSTEOMA

Osteoma is a benign tumor. It is more common in males than females. Patient develops sessile periosteal or endosteal mass in the skull and facial bones, which may grow into the paranasal sinuses in adults.

Molecular Genetics

Patient with Gardner's syndrome caused by APC gene mutation develops multiple osteomas, colonic polyps and soft tissue tumors.

> **Light Microscopy**
> - Osteoma is composed of mature, irregularly laid down broad bony trabeculae, i.e. a dense mixture of woven and lamellar bone.
> - Intertrabecular spaces are filled with fibrous tissue, which is sometimes highly vascularized and even contain foci of hemopoiesis (Fig. 27.8).

OSTEOID OSTEOMA

Osteoid osteoma is a small, painful, benign tumor of bone. It is composed of osseous tissue (the nidus) and surrounded by a halo of reactive bone formation. It most often occurs during 5–25 years of age.

Origin

Tumor frequently arises in the cortex of the diaphysis of the tubular bones of the lower extremity (femur, tibia, humerus, radius, fibula, phalanges, talus, and calcaneus).

The most common site for an osteoid osteoma is the upper end of the tibia.

Despite their size (usually smaller than 2.0 cm), these can produce considerable pain owing to their prostaglandin synthesis, which can be blocked by non-steroidal anti-inflammatory drug such as aspirin.

Age Group

It most often occurs in young persons in the second or third decade. Males are more affected than females.

> **Gross Morphology**
> - Osteoid osteoma is a 1 cm spherical, hyperemic soft nidus surrounded by reactive, sclerotic bone. It is located in intracortical region of small bones.
> - It may arise close to endosteum or within cancellous bone. It is considerably softer in consistency than the surrounding bone (Fig. 27.9).

> **Light Microscopy**
> - Tumor shows a small focus (nidus), initially composed of irregular and delicate reactive woven bone, rimmed by numerous osteoblasts, and enclosed by a highly vascularized spindle cell stroma.
> - In later stages, tangled islands and trabeculae of partially mineralized osteoid within the fibrous stroma, and densely packed irregular bone trabeculae are seen (Fig. 27.10).

Radiological Findings

X-ray shows <1.5 cm radiolucent focus (nidus) surrounded by densely sclerotic calcified bone in the cortex region. Reaction in surrounding bone, sclerosis of adjacent cortex and periosteal bone thickening are seen.

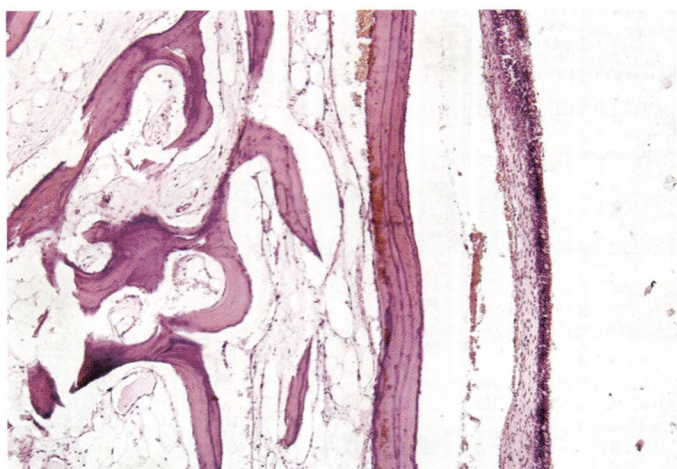

Fig. 27.8: Osteoma of frontal sinus shows mature, irregularly laid down broad bony trabeculae (woven and lamellar bone). Spaces between bony trabeculae are filled with fibrous tissue (400X).

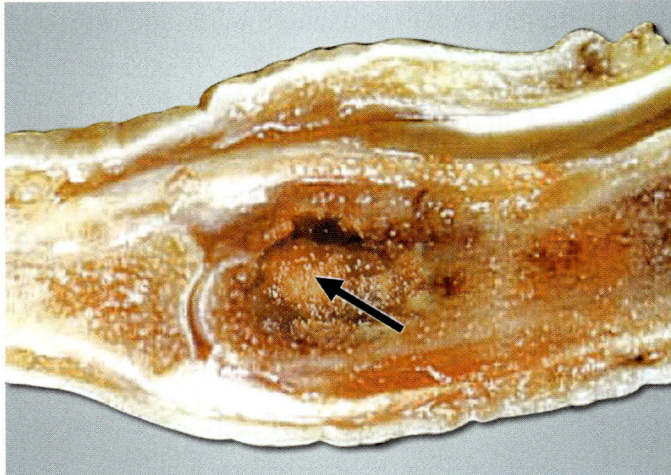

Fig. 27.9: Osteoid osteoma in the proximal phalanx of a finger. There is a benign, well circumscribed tumor within the cortex. The treatment of choice is local curettage. The commonest site for an osteoid osteoma is the upper end of the tibia (arrow).

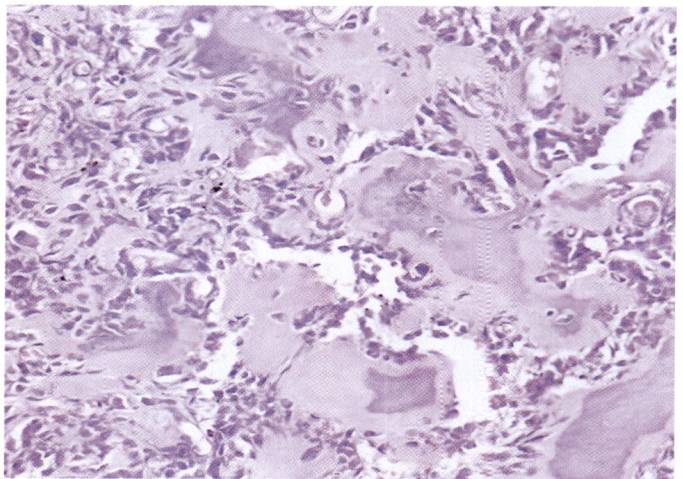

Fig. 27.10: Osteoblastoma is composed of irregular reactive trabeculae of woven bone lined by osteoblasts and osteoclasts separated by fibrovascular tissue (400X).

OSTEOBLASTOMA

Osteoblastoma is a benign neoplasm that is histologically similar to osteoid osteoma. It affects 5–25 years of age. Differences between osteoid osteoma and osteoblastoma are shown in Table 27.12.

Locations

Tumor is a well-circumscribed, painless mass >2.0 cm in size located invertebrae and medulla of long bones (metaphysis and diaphysis) or iliac bones, accompanied by a little or no reactive bone formation.

Clinical Features

Children and young adults are affected. Patient presents with dull pain in affected bone during night with minimal response to aspirin.

The lesions are benign and cured by local resection. Incomplete resection may lead to recurrence without malignant transformation.

Radiological Findings

Osteoblastoma is predominantly lytic lesion with rim of sclerosis demonstrated on radiographs.

> **Light Microscopy**
> - Osteoblastoma is identical to giant osteoid osteoma. The nidus is composed of irregular reactive trabeculae of woven bone lined by osteoblasts and osteoclasts separated by fibrovascular tissue.
> - There is absence of mitoses and atypical cells.

OSTEOSARCOMA

Osteosarcoma is the most common primary malignant tumor of bone. It constitutes 20% of primary bone cancers. In osteosarcoma, malignant osteoblasts produce variable amount of osteoid collagen and mineralized bone matrix. Serum alkaline phosphatase is increased two- to three-fold.

Origin

Histological variants are shown in Table 27.13. Osteosarcoma locations, age and salient pathological features are shown in Table 27.14.

Prognostic Factors

Prognostic factors in patients with osteosarcoma are shown in Table 27.15.

Table 27.12: Differences between osteoid osteoma and osteoblastoma

Parameters	Osteoid osteoma	Osteoblastoma
Age group	<25 years in 75%	5–25 years
Sex (M:F)	2:1	1:1
Size of tumor	<2.0 cm	>2.0 cm
Site of tumor	Femur and tibia (50%) in cortex	Spine
Nocturnal pain (PGE synthesis)	Pain relieved by aspirin	Dull pain with minimal response to aspirin
Radiological findings	Marked bony reaction encircling tumor (nidus small lucent invariably mineralized)	Predominantly lytic lesion with rim of sclerosis
Gross morphology	Well circumscribed round to oval tumor, with hemorrhagic gritty tan tissue	Well circumscribed round to oval tumor, with hemorrhagic gritty tan tissue
Light microscopy (identical in osteoid osteoma and osteoblastoma)	Randomly interconnecting trabecular of woven bone rimmed by osteoblasts with surrounding vascular stroma	Randomly interconnecting trabecular of woven bone rimmed by osteoblasts with surrounding vascular stroma
Surgical excision	Recurrence	Recurrence

Table 27.13: Histological variants of central and peripheral osteosarcoma

Central osteosarcoma	Peripheral osteosarcoma
Conventional intramedullary osteosarcoma (predominant matrix production)	Parosteal osteosarcoma
Low grade osteosarcoma	Periosteal osteosarcoma
Telangiectatic osteosarcoma	High grade surface osteosarcoma
Small cell carcinoma	

Table 27.14: Osteosarcoma locations, age and salient pathological features

Histological variant	Location	Age group	Pathological features
Conventional osteosarcoma	Medullary cavity of long bones (metaphysis)	10–20 years	Osteoid bone formed directly by malignant cells
Low grade central osteosarcoma	Medullary cavity (metaphysis)	10–20 years	Mild fibroblastic proliferation with thick bone trabeculae
Telangiectatic osteosarcoma	Medullary cavity	10–20 years	Blood-filled spaces with fibrous septa and highly malignant osteoid tissue
Parosteal osteosarcoma	Cortex outside periosteum	10–20 years	Mild atypical fibroblastic proliferation with thick bone trabeculae
Periosteal osteosarcoma	Cortex inside periosteum	10–20 years	Abundant cartilage matrix with variable osteoid element
Osteosarcoma	Jaw bone	>40 years	Osteoid bone formed directly by malignant cells

Table 27.15: Factors affecting prognosis in patients with osteosarcoma

Parameters	Clinical significance
Osteosarcoma arising in Paget's disease of bone	Highly malignant clinical course with fatal outcome
Multifocal osteosarcomas	Poor prognosis
Location of osteosarcoma	Osteosarcoma of jaw (5-year survival in 80%)
	Osteosarcoma below knee joint has better than located in proximal sites
	Vertebral and skull osteosarcomas except in jaw having poor prognosis
Parosteal and periosteal osteosarcoma	Better prognosis than conventional intramedullary osteosarcoma
Telangiectatic osteosarcoma	Poor prognosis

Conventional Intramedullary Osteosarcoma

Age and sex predilection: It most often occurs in 10 to 20 years of age. Males are affected more than females.

Predisposing factors: Precursors of bone malignancy are shown in Table 27.16.

Locations: Conventional intramedullary osteosarcoma most often occurs *around knee joint* (distal end of femur or proximal end of tibia) in 60% cases. In patients over 25 years of age may develop osteosarcoma in *hip bone* (15%), *proximal humerus* (10%) and *mandible* (8%). Occasionally, it may occur in *upper end of femur*.

The tumor extends into epiphysis, joint space and soft tissues. Osteosarcoma arising in bones distal to the wrists and ankles is extremely unusual. Sites of occurrence of osteosarcoma are shown in Table 27.17 and Fig. 27.11.

Molecular genetics: Molecular genetics in osteosarcomas (Table 27.18); oncogenes and tumor suppressor genes involved in osteosarcomas and associated cancers (Table 27.19) and radiation associated cancers are shown in Table 27.20.

Clinical features: The first clinical manifestation is often short-term mild, intermittent pain as the progressive enlarging tumor breaks the bone cortex and lifts off the periosteum, which may sometimes cause pathologic fracture in the proximal tibia or distal femur (about the knee). Patient may also develop symptoms due to metastases in lungs. Some cases may show elevated level of serum alkaline phosphatase.

Radiological findings: Codman triangle is a triangular shadow between cortex and raised ends of perisoteum) is an X-ray finding of a bone involved in osteosarcoma.

Bones and Joints

Table 27.16: Precursors of bone malignancy

High risk precursor lesions	Moderate risk precursor lesions	Low risk precursor lesions
Familial retinoblastoma syndrome	Multiple osteochondromas	Fibrous dysplasia
Ollier disease (enchondromatosis)	Paget's disease of bone (polyostotic) causing parosteal osteosarcoma	Bone infarct
Maffucci syndrome (enchondromatosis associated hemangiomas)	Previous exposure to irradiation radio-isotopes (phosphorus)	Chronic osteomyelitis
Rothmund-Thomson syndrome (RTS)	Previous exposure to irradiation radio-isotopes (phosphorus)	Metallic and polyethylene implants
		Osteogenesis imperfecta
		Giant cell tumor
		Osteoblastoma
		Chondroblastoma
		Chondroma
		Werner's syndrome
		Li-Fraumeni syndrome (germline mutations of TP53 tumor suppressor gene)

Table 27.17: Locations of conventional intramedullary osteosarcoma and frequency

Location	Frequency (%)
Around keen joint (distal end of femur or proximal end of tibia)	60%
Hip bones	15%
Proximal humerus	10%
Mandible	8%
Upper end of femur	Occasional

It occurs due to reactive bone formation adjacent to tumor, which lifts the periosteum. Bony spicules formed by tumor cells give *sunburst pattern* of growth on X-ray.

Gross Morphology
- Conventional intramedullary tumor is firm, gray white with gritty areas.
- Cut surface of the tumor is not homogenous because the cellular areas composed of malignant osteoblasts are admixed with osteoid, blood vessels, and areas of necrosis (Fig. 27.12).

Light Microscopy
- *Cells morphology:* Conventional intramedullary osteosarcoma is composed of *polyhedral or spindle-shaped neoplastic cells*. Tumor cells are *pleomorphic with hyperchromatic nuclei and numerous mitoses*. In 50–60% patients, there may be considerable histological variation with in a single tumor, and metastases may not exactly resemble the primary site microscopic appearance.

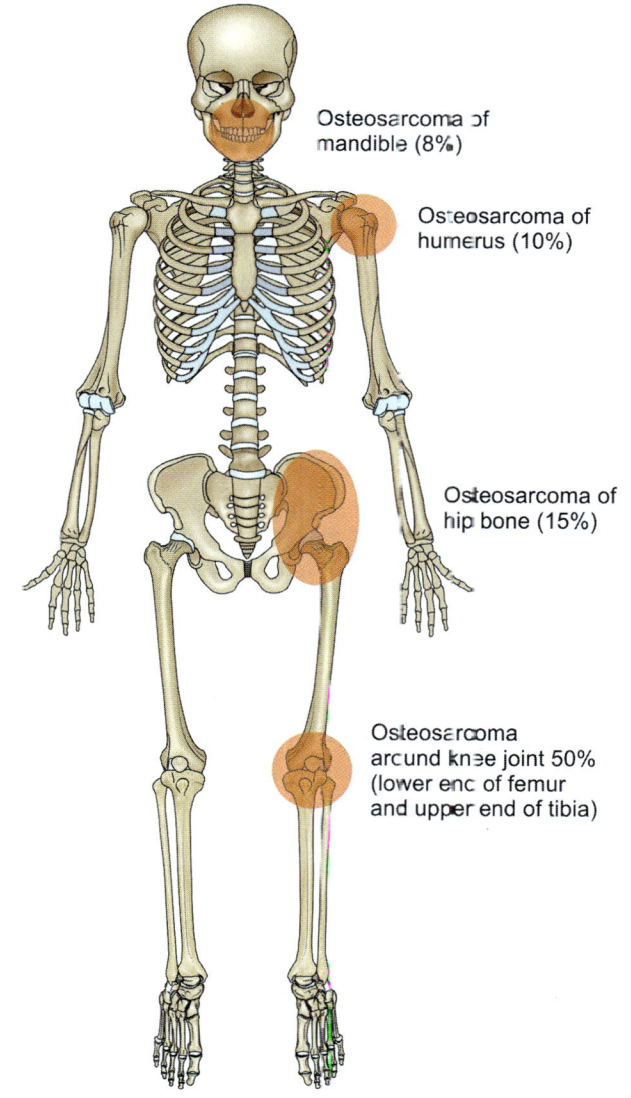

Fig. 27.11: Osteosarcoma and common sites of occurrence.

Table 27.18: Molecular genetics in osteosarcomas

- Mutation of RB tumor suppressor gene encoding 13p14 (familial and sporadic osteosarcoma)
- Mutations of p53, CDK4, p16 and cyclin-D1 genes in most sporadic cases
- Increased baseline activity of FGF3, PDGFB and HST1 genes encoding protein synthesizing growth factors
- Inactivation of *INK4a* gene encoding p16 and p14

Table 27.19: Oncogenes and tumor suppressor genes associated cancers

Growth factors (oncogenes)			
Category	Proto-oncogene	Mode of activation	Associated malignancies
PDGF-β chain	PDGFB (sis-Simion sarcoma)	Over expression	Osteosarcoma Astrocytoma
Fibroblast growth factors (FGFs)	HST1 FGF3	Over expression Amplification	Osteosarcoma Osteosarcoma Gastric carcinoma Bladder carcinoma Breast carcinoma Melanoma

Cell cycle progression inhibitors (tumor suppressor genes)			
Category	Retinoblastoma protein	Familial cases	Sporadic cases
RB gene	Retinoblastoma protein (locus 13p14) Mutation by deletion and nonsense	Retinoblastoma Osteosarcoma	Retinoblastoma Osteosarcoma Breast carcinoma Colon carcinoma Prostate carcinoma Urinary bladder carcinoma Lung carcinoma

Table 27.20: Radiation associated cancers

Exposure to radiation	Associated cancers
Occupational exposure to radium in watch-dial workers	Osteosarcoma
Survivors of bomb blast	AML, CML (but not lymphoid leukemia)
Head and neck radiotherapy	Thyroid cancer
Ultraviolet radiation (UV B: 290–320 nm)	Skin cancers in xeroderma pigmentosum
	Sporadic skin cancers such as basal cell carcinoma, squamous cell carcinoma and melanoma

- *Bone formation:* Formation of fine lace-like pattern of neoplastic bone by tumor cells is diagnostic. These neoplastic cells form islands of reactive new woven bone (pinkish *lace-like osteoid* and *calcified bone spicules*) in response to the infiltration and destruction of the normal bone by the tumor (Fig. 27.13).

Histological Variants

Histologically, osteosarcomas are subclassified on the basis of predominant matrix production such as conventional osteoblastic forming bone, chondroblastic forming cartilage (Fig. 27.14), fibroblastic forming fibrous tissue (mistaken for reactive process) or telangiectatic forming blood filled spaces.

Bones and Joints

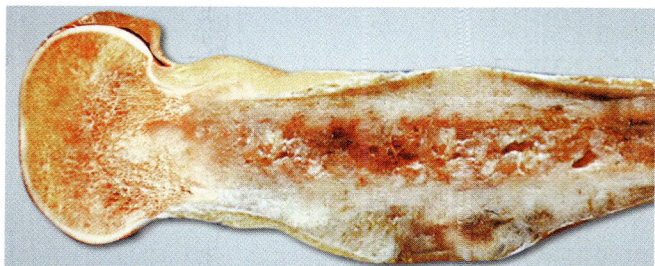

Fig. 27.12: Osteosarcoma—the creamy tumor has involved the lower end of the femur and has broken through the cortical bone and caused elevation of the periosteum.

Mode of metastases: Osteosarcoma invades locally and metastasizes via hematogenous route to the lungs.

Local spread

- *Soft tissue invasion:* Tumor spreads extensively within medullary cavity replacing bone marrow, eventually eroding through cortical plate and extending into soft tissue.
- *Joint involvement:* Tumor usually does not cross the epiphyseal plate, and thus sparing joint cavity involvement. Joint involvement may occur due to extension of tumor cells along tendino-ligamentous structures or through the attachment site in the joint capsule.

Hematogenous route

- *Early hematogenous spread:* Tumor metastasizes to the lungs (20% cases at diagnosis).
- *Late hematogenous spread:* Metastases may later spread to liver, bone and brain or elsewhere.

Management: Preoperative chemotherapy has improved 5-year survival rate in 20–80% cases. Combined chemotherapy with surgery is curative in 80% of childhood and adolescent tumors; old age osteosarcomas have a less favorable response to therapy. Long-term survival is seen in 60–70% cases treated with chemotherapy and limb amputation.

Low Grade Osteosarcoma

Low grade osteosarcoma is a rare variant of central osteosarcoma constituting 1–2% of cases. It most often occurs during 3rd and 4th decades of life with equal sex predilection. Most common sites are femur and tibia (med and distal parts).

Clinical features: Patients give history of pain without swelling for many years.

Imaging technique: Imaging shows a large intramedullary poorly demarcated mass that either is sclerotic or shows trabeculations. Generally no periosteal reaction is seen.

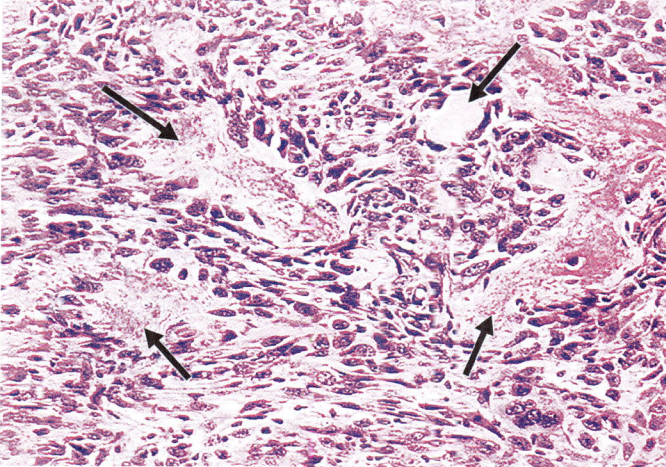

Fig. 27.13: Osteoblastic osteosarcoma. Tumor is composed of pleomorphic polyhedral or spindle-shaped neoplastic cells with hyperchromatic nuclei and mitoses. Formation of fine lace-like pattern of neoplastic bone by tumor cells is diagnostic (arrows) (400X).

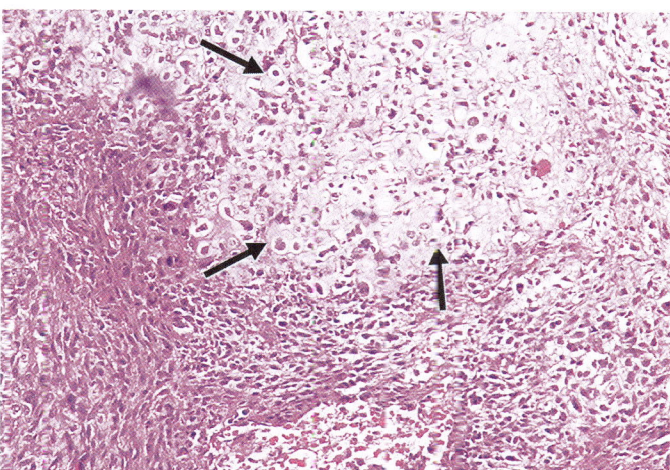

Fig. 27.14: Chondroblastic osteosarcoma. Tumor is composed of pleomorphic polyhedral or spindle-shaped neoplastic cells with hyperchromatic nuclei and mitoses. Formation of chondroid islands by tumor cells is diagnostic (arrows) 400X.

Gross Morphology
- Tumor shows a gritty grey medullary mass that may contain fibrous and fleshy areas. Some tumors show cortical destruction.
- Tumor may extend along the length of bone with poor demarcation between tumor and uninvolved medullary bone.

Light Microscopy
- Tumor is composed of spindle cells in variable proportion lacking cellular atypia.
- There is presence of bone formation showing irregular thick branching bone trabeculae.

Clinical course: It has an indolent course compared with conventional osteosarcoma. If adequately excised, tumor shows high recurrence rate.

Telangiectatic Osteosarcoma

Telangiectatic osteosarcoma is a variant of central osteosarcoma. It occurs during 2nd decade of life with male preponderance. Most common sites are distal femur, proximal tibia and proximal humerus. This variant is more prone to pathological fractures. This tumor is sensitive to chemotherapy.

Imaging technique: Radiograph demonstrates radiolucent expansile mass in metaphysis resembling aneurysmal bone cyst. It has infiltrative destructive margin.

> **Light Microscopy**
> Tumor shows large blood-filled spaces separated by highly cellular fibrous septae that contain pleomorphic tumor cells with variable amount of osteoid production.

Treatment: This aggressive variant is very sensitive to radiotherapy.

Small Cell Osteosarcoma

Small cell osteosarcoma is a variant of central osteosarcoma.

Imaging technique: Tumor is radiolucent on radiographs.

> **Light Microscopy**
> Tumor comprises small round blue cells resembling Ewing's sarcoma except that small cell osteosarcoma shows evidence for bone formation on light microscopy.
>
> **Immunohistochemistry**
> - Small cell osteosarcoma shows membrane positivity for **CD99**. Therefore, some authors consider it a variant of Ewing's sarcoma with diverge differentiation.
> - Ewing's sarcoma shows positivity with CD99, but lacks osteoid element.
> - Lymphoma shows LCA (leukocyte common antigen) positivity, but lacks osteoid element.

Parosteal Osteosarcoma

Parosteal osteosarcoma is a variant of surface osteosarcoma. It involves posterior distal femur associated with periosteum wrapping around bone.

> **Light Microscopy**
> Cartilaginous differentiation is also common.

Clinical course: Prognosis is similar to conventional low grade osteosarcoma. This tumor may undergo dedifferentiation with prognosis similar to conventional intramedullary osteosarcoma.

Periosteal Osteosarcoma

Periosteal osteosarcoma arises between cortex and overlying periosteum. It most often occurs in the diaphysis of tibia or femur during 2nd and 3rd decades with male predominance.

Clinical features: Patient presents with pain and swelling for less than one year duration.

Imaging technique: Imaging shows a surface radiolucent tumor with spiculated calcification, perpendicular to long axis of bone.

> **Gross Morphology**
> - Periosteal osteosarcoma shows lobulated mass. It exhibits cartilaginous appearance over bony surface.
> - Bone may show cortical erosion, but not extending into medullary cavity.
>
> **Light Microscopy**
> Tumor contains abundant cartilaginous matrix. Tumor cells show cytologic atypia.

High Grade Surface Osteosarcoma

High grade surface osteosarcoma arises on bone surface during 3rd and 4th decades with male predominance.

Locations: Most common sites are distal and mid-femur, proximal humerus and fibula.

Clinical features: Patient presents with pain and swelling.

Imaging technique: Imaging finding is like periosteal osteosarcoma except mineralization. Radiograph shows a surface radiolucent tumor with spiculated calcification, perpendicular to long axis of bone.

> **Gross Morphology**
> - High grade surface osteosarcoma shows large lobulated soft to firm mass.
> - There may be hemorrhagic areas.
> - Rarely, tumor may extend into medullary cavity.

Light Microscopy

On light microscopy, this tumor is identical to conventional intramedullary osteosarcoma.

Prognosis: Prognosis is similar to that of conventional intramedullary osteosarcoma.

Differential diagnosis: These include myositis ossificans, osteoblastoma, callus, chondrosarcoma and metastases. In young patients, bone malignancies showing prominent cartilaginous differentiation are almost assuredly chondroblastic osteosarcomas, rather than chondrosarcomas. Conventional chondrosarcomas occur almost exclusively in older patients. Prostatic and breast carcinoma may show osteoblastic reaction. Immunohistochemistry helps in establishing metastases.

CARTILAGINOUS TUMORS

Benign cartilaginous tumors include osteochondroma, chondroma, chondroblastoma and chondromyxoid fibroma (Table 27.21). Chondrosarcoma is malignant tumor derived from cartilage.

CHONDROMA

Solitary chondroma is a benign, intraosseous tumor composed of well differentiated hyaline cartilage. Enchondroma arises within medullary cavity. Juxtacortical chondroma arises from cortical surface of bone.

Locations

Solitary chondroma occurs in metaphysis of tubular bones of hands and feet between 20 and 40 years.

Molecular Genetics

Enchondromas are most common intraosseous cartilaginous tumors. These occur due to mutations of IDH1 and IDH2 genes (isocitrate dehydrogenase).

Imaging Techniques

Chondroma shows radiolucent nodule of cartilage with thin central calcification and intact cortex.

Gross Morphology

Chondroma is <3 cm in diameter. Cut surface shows translucent gray blue appearance (Fig. 27.15).

Light Microscopy

Tumor is composed of well differentiated benign hyaline cartilage (Fig. 27.16).

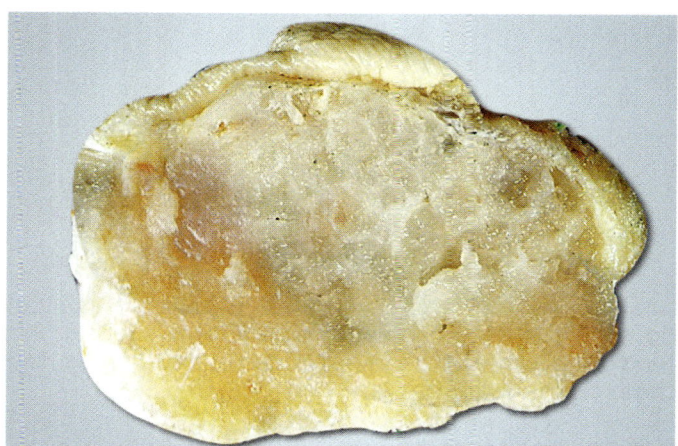

Fig. 27.15: Benign chondroma. This small cartilage tumor was resected from the tibia.

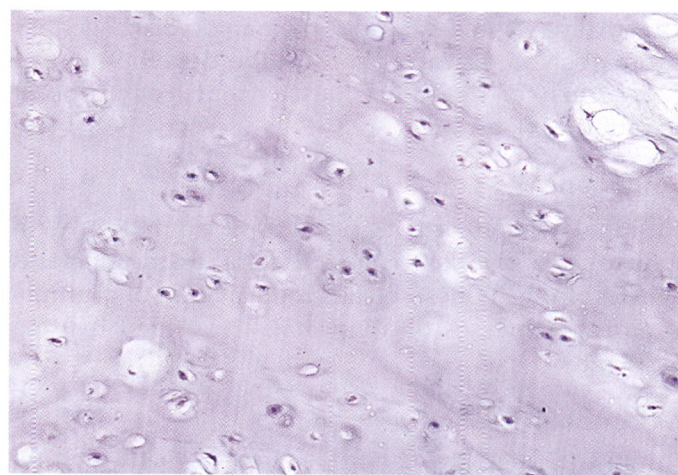

Fig. 27.16: Chondroma—tumor is composed of hyaline cartilage (100X).

Table 27.21: Salient features of commonest benign cartilage forming tumors or tumor-like lesions

Tumor/lesion	Locations	Age predilection	Salient pathological features
Osteochondroma	Metaphysis of long bones	10–30 years	Cartilage-capped bony protrusion
Chondroma	Hands/feet; medulla of long bones	Any group	Variably cellular hyaline cartilage
Chondroblastoma	Epiphysis/apophysis of long bones	10–20 years	Chondroid-like matrix; S-100 positive cells with grooved nuclei
Chondromyxoid fibroma	Metaphysis of long bones	10–30 years	Hypocellular chondromyxoid lobules surrounded by more cellular spindle cell areas

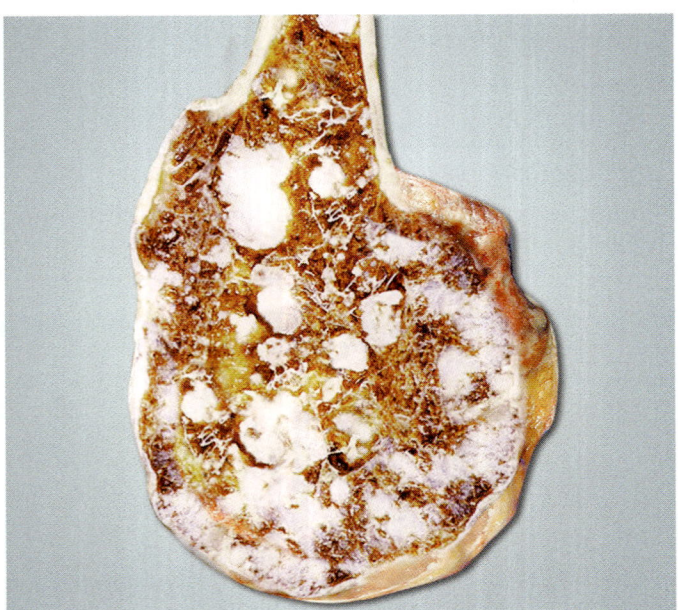

Fig. 27.17: Multiple enchondromata (Ollier's disease). The head of the humerus is greatly expanded by the intramedullary chondromas.

ENCHONDROMATOSIS

Ollier disease is a syndrome characterized by multiple enchondromas. Maffuci syndrome refers to multiple chondromas associated with hemangiomas. Enchondromatosis is characterized by the development of numerous cartilaginous masses that lead to bony deformities (Fig. 27.17).

Pathogenesis

Residual hyaline cartilage or cartilage from the growth plate does not undergo endochondral ossification and remains in the bones. It leads to formation of multiple tumor-like masses of abnormally arranged hyaline cartilage.

Malignant Potential

Enchondroma has strong tendency to undergo malignant change into chondrosarcomas in adult life. Solitary chondroma is a benign, intraosseous tumor composed of well-differentiated hyaline cartilage.

OSTEOCHONDROMA (EXOSTOSIS)

It is the most common benign tumor of bone in young adults (<25 years). It is also known as exostosis. It is mushroom-shaped small outgrowth of bone capped with cartilage.

Cartilaginous cap <2 cm in thickness in osteochondroma is considered as benign tumor.

Cartilaginous irregular cap >2 cm in thickness may indicate malignant potential.

Locations

It most often arises from metaphysis of long bones around knee joints. Lateral aspect of lower end of femur and upper end of tibia are most common sites.

Molecular Genetics

- Recent studies reveal osteochondroma is a true neoplasm. Presence of loss of heterozygosity (LOH) and aneuploidy in osteochondroma indicate a clonal origin for the cartilaginous tissue of osteochondroma.
- Inactivation of both alleles of EXT1 located on 8q22–24.1 in chondrocytes of the cap participates in pathogenesis of solitary osteochondroma or multiple osteochondromas.
- The EXT1 proteins are involved in the biosynthesis of heparan sulphate.

Clinical Features

Lesion starts growing in childhood and becomes clinically apparent in late adolescence. The lesion may become painful because of nerve compression or fracture.

> **Gross Morphology**
> - Osteochondromas may be pedunculated with stalk or sessile (flat). Many osteochondromas are cauliflower shaped.
> - The cartilage cap merges into the underlying spongiosa. The spongiosa of the stalk is continuous with the underlying cancellous bone (Fig. 27.18).

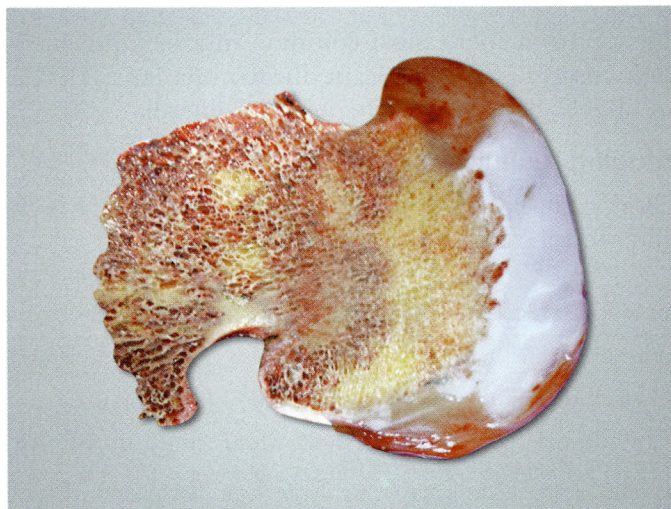

Fig. 27.18: Osteochondroma on a rib. This is a common benign tumor which usually occurs in the region of the epiphyses of long bones. It is characterized by having a distinct cartilage cap. Such tumors are easily excised.

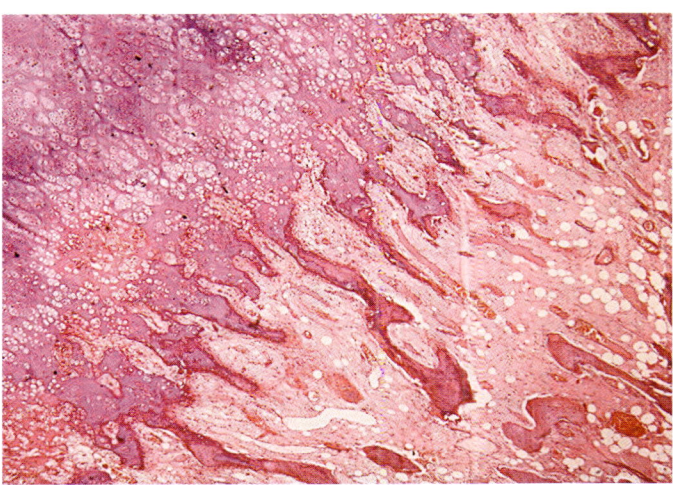

Fig. 27.19: Osteochondroma (100X).

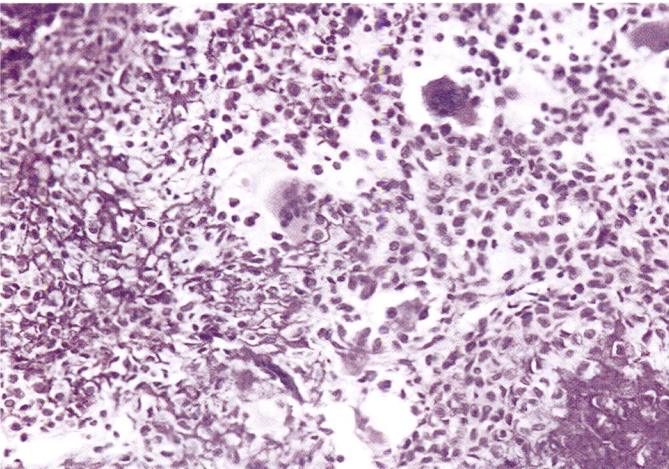

Fig. 27.20: Chondroblastoma—tumor is composed of round or polyhedral chondroblasts with well-defined outlines, grooved round nuclei and pale cytoplasm. It shows chicken wire mesh-like calcification and scattered multinucleated giant cells. Mitoses and atypia are absent (400X).

Light Microscopy
- Chondrocytes are arranged according to an epiphyseal growth plate.
- Benign chondrocytes contain single small nucleus.
- Chondrocytes may contain two nuclei during active bone growth (Fig. 27.19).

Complications
It rarely undergoes malignant transformation. Malignant transformation is frequent in familial osteochondromatosis involving multiple bones.

CHONDROBLASTOMA
Chondroblastoma, a rare tumor is derived from the epiphyseal cartilage before the closure of the epiphysis. It features primitive chondroblasts and cartilage matrix.

Location
It occurs at the epiphyseal ends of long bones adjacent to epiphyseal cartilaginous plate. Occasionally it extends into adjacent metaphysis. Most common site is knee joint. Other sites include skull, ribs, vertebrae and small bones of feet. It may erode through cortex.

Age Group
It commonly occurs in the first two decades. Males are more affected than females.

X-ray Findings
It is well circumscribed osteolytic lesion with multiple areas of calcification.

Gross Morphology
Chondroblastoma has granular texture and gray white appearance with focal areas of calcification. Focal blue gray areas resemble chondroid matrix (Fig. 27.20).

Light Microscopy
- *Cells morphology:* This cellular tumor is composed of round or polyhedral chondroblasts with well-defined outlines, grooved round nuclei and pale cytoplasm. Mitoses and atypia are absent. These chondroblasts merge with areas of hyaline cartilage.
- *Calcification:* There is presence of chicken wire mesh like calcification.
- *Multinucleated giant cells:* Few scattered multinucleated giant cells are present.
- *Vascular spaces:* In some instances, typical areas of chondroblastoma alternate with large amount of blood filled vascular spaces reminiscent of aneurysmal bone cysts. These are referred as *cystic chondroblastomas*.

CHONDROMYXOID FIBROMA
Chondromyxoid fibroma is a benign cartilaginous aggressive tumor affecting adolescents and young adults between 2nd and 3rd decades. Recurrence occurs in 25% of cases after surgical excision.

Sites
Upper end of tibia is the most common site. It may also occur in lower end of femur, bones of feet and jaw. It may extend into soft tissue. Size rarely exceeds 5 cm.

Imaging Technique

X-ray shows eccentric lesion, sharply outlined radiolucent area causing expansion of bone. Calcification is not common.

> **Gross Morphology**
>
> Chondromyxoid fibroma shows solid, lobulated and yellow white tan color. Translucency suggests cartilaginous origin.
>
> **Light Microscopy**
>
> - Tumor consists of lobules, which are separated by bands of fibrous tissue.
> - Lobules are composed of a variable number of multinucleated giant cells with the appearance of osteoclasts; and immature cartilage with a prominent myxoid pattern chondroblasts alternate with stellate myxoid cells and scattered large pleomorphic cells.
> - Mitoses are exceptional. Rarely, tumors representing hybrids between chondromyxoid fibroma and chondrobastoma are encountered (Fig. 27.21).

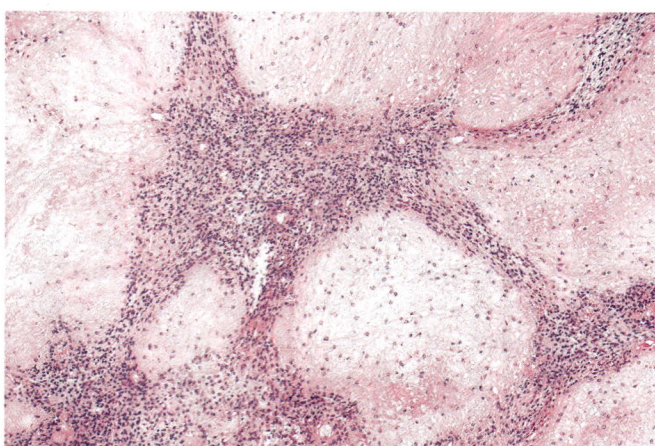

Fig. 27.21: Chondromyxoid fibroma shows lobules containing multinucleated giant cells, immature cartilage, myxoid cells separated by bands of fibrous tissue (100X).

CHONDROSARCOMA

Chondrosarcoma is second most common primary malignant bone tumor. It constitutes 15% of all primary malignant bone tumors.

Salient features of chondrosarcoma are shown in Table 27.22.

- *Central chondrosarcoma:* It arises centrally in bone.
- *Peripheral chondrosarcoma:* It originates within cartilaginous cap of osteochondroma.
- *Periosteal chondrosarcoma:* It occurs in shaft of long bone, showing foci of calcification and endochondral calcification.
- *Chondrosarcoma in skull base:* Sometimes, chondrosarcoma may arise in base of skull.

Origin

Most tumors develop in *de novo*, but some occur in pre-existing enchondroma and may be familial osteochondromatosis.

Age Group

Peak incidence is in the 30–60-year-old age group with male predominance. Conventional chondrosarcomas occur almost exclusively in older patients. Bone malignancy in young patients showing prominent cartilaginous differentiation is almost chondroblastic osteosarcoms, rather than chondrosarcoma.

Locations

- Chondrosarcomas most often originate in the medulla of flat bones such as pelvic girdle (25%), shoulder girdle (scapula), ribs, and vertebral column.
- These may arise from epiphyseal cartilage along the superior metaphyseal and diaphyseal regions of long bones (e.g. proximal parts of the femur, humerus and radius) and around knee joints (lower end of femur or upper end of tibia).

Table 27.22: Salient features of chondrosarcoma

Tumor/lesion	Locations	Age predilection	Salient pathological features
Chondrosarcoma	Flat bones; metaphysis, and epiphysis of long bones	20–80 years	Variably cellular hyaline cartilage permeating bone
Conventional (not otherwise specified)	Metaphysis	20–80 years	Variably cellular hyaline cartilage permeating bone
Dedifferentiated chondrosarcoma	Metaphysis	>30 years	Conventional chondrosarcoma + high grade spindle cell sarcoma
Mesenchymal chondrosarcoma	Metaphysis	20–50 years	Undifferentiated small cell tumor + hyaline cartilage
Clear cell chondrosarcoma	Epiphysis	20–70 years	Conventional tumor with abundant large clear tumor cells

Bones and Joints

Clinical Course

- Most of chondrosarcomas are low grade and *slow growing tumors* with symptoms present for a decade or more.
- Larger tumors are more aggressive than smaller ones. These often reach a large size, expanding the bone and eventually breaking through the periosteum into surrounding soft tissue, but usually maintaining a clearly defined border. These metastasize very late in most cases.

Gross Examination

The tumor appears nodular, irregular, expansile with white to bluish glistening translucent and myxoid appearance (Fig. 27.22).

Light Microscopy

- Tumor is composed of atypical cells within cartilaginous lacunae. There is increased cellularity showing >2 cells with hyperchromatic nuclei per lacunae.
- Features of malignancy especially mitoses are best demonstrated at the edge of the tumor.
- Permeation of bone marrow is the most important criteria of this tumor (Fig. 27.23).

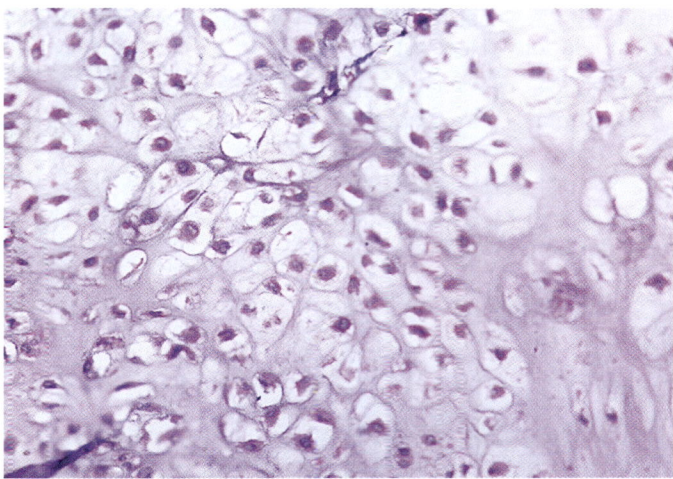

Fig. 27.23: Chondrosarcoma—tumor is composed of atypical cells within cartilaginous lacunae. Each cartilaginous lacunae contains >2 cells with hyperchromatic nuclei (400X).

Histological Variants

These include clear cell chondrosarcoma, myxoid chondrosarcoma, mesenchymal chondrosarcoma and dedifferentiated chondrosarcoma.

Grading

- High grade tumors show tumor cells with marked pleomorphism and high mitotic activity. The tumors are histologically graded (I–IV), depending on degree of differentiation.
- Grade I tumors are well differentiated and histologically resemble normal cartilage. On the other hand, grade IV tumors are poorly differentiated, which grow rapidly with early blood-borne metastases.

Prognosis

Untreated chondrosarcomas generally have a better prognosis than osteosarcoma. *Chondrosarcomas do not respond well to chemotherapy.* Prognosis depends on the *resectability of the tumor*, its *histological grade*, and the presence or absence of *hematogenous metastases*.

TUMORS ARISING FROM UNDIFFERENTIATED CELLS

EWING'S SARCOMA/PRIMITIVE NEUROECTODERMAL TUMORS (PNET)

Ewing's sarcoma is second most common tumor of bone in children and adolescents (5–20 years) after osteosarcoma. It is an osteolytic tumor. Ewing's sarcoma and PNET are defined as round cell sarcomas that show varying degrees of neuroectodermal differentiation. Males are more affected than females. White persons are slightly more affected, while blacks rarely affected.

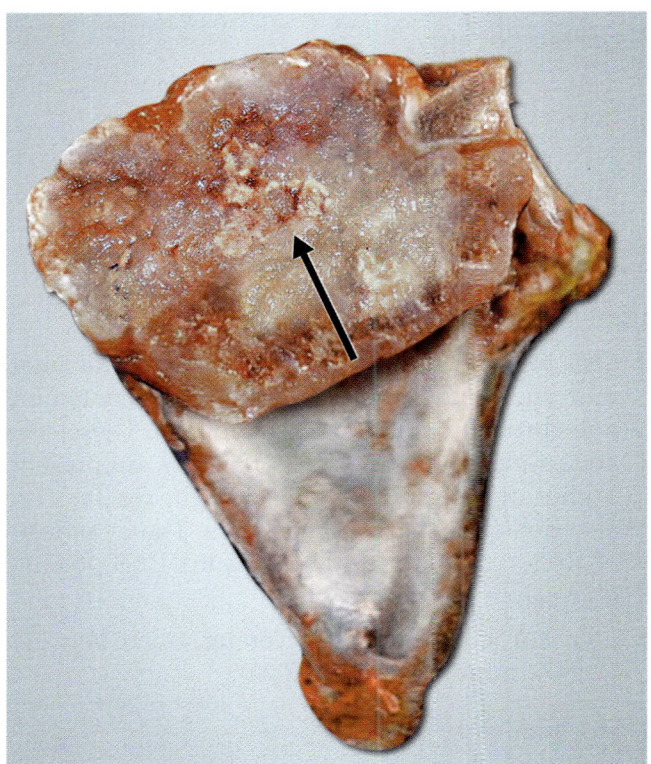

Fig. 27.22: Chondrosarcoma arising in the scapula. This tumor had grown rapidly. Its cut surface shows a lobulated pattern with the white, glistening appearance of cartilage (arrow).

Table 27.23: Salient features of Ewing's sarcoma (primitive neuroectodermal tumors)

Ewing's sarcoma	Diaphysis or metaphysis of long bones, pelvis and ribs	5–20	Small round blue cells ± rosettes; characteristic IHC; translocation
Rare sites of Ewing's sarcoma are skull, scapula and short tubular bones of hands and feet			

Salient features of Ewing's sarcoma are shown in Table 27.23.

Origin

- It arises from primitive bone marrow elements or immature mesenchymal cells of long bones (diaphysis) such as femur and flat bones of pelvis. However, it can also occur in extraskeletal sites.
- Ewing's sarcoma and primitive neuroectodermal tumor (PNET) have similar molecular origin, but the PNET has more neuronal differentiation. *Neural type rosettes* are seen in both lesions.

Molecular Genetics

- *t(q11;22):* Virtually 90% of these tumors have a reciprocal *translocation between chromosomes 11 and 22 (11:22)*, which results in the fusion of the amino terminus of the EWS1 gene to the FLI-1 gene, which encodes a nuclear transcription factor to drive cellular proliferation.
- *t(q24;12):* Approximately 5–15% of these tumors have *q22; q12 translocation*.
- *t(21; 22):* Occasionally *translocation (21; 22)* may also be seen.

  This translocation differentiates this tumor from neuroblastoma.

Locations

It develops most often in the *medullary portion of diaphysis of long bones of extremities* (e.g. proximal femur), but it may involve the ribs and pelvic bones as well.

Imaging Techniques

The tumor cells penetrate into the cortical bone, and then raising the periosteum forming multilayered reactive bone (periosteal reaction) in a typical concentric manner, giving the bone an *onion skin appearance on radiograph*.

Cortex overlying the tumor is irregularly thinned out or thickened. Expansile bone destruction exhibiting *soap bubble* appearance may be seen.

Clinical Features

Patient presents with fever and anemia. Initially, Ewing's sarcoma may clinically mimic acute osteomyelitis.

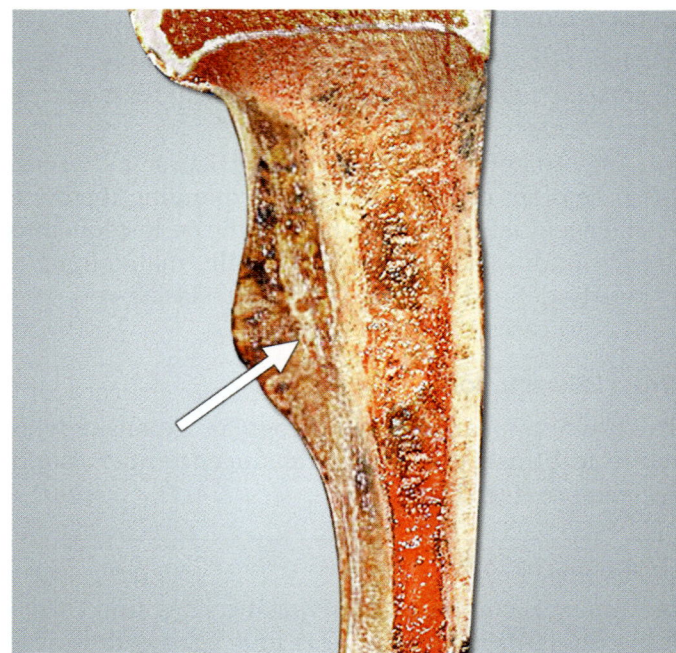

Fig. 27.24: Ewing's sarcoma. A large tumor in the upper diaphysis of the tibia has eroded the cortical bone and extended beneath the periosteum. There is a pathological fracture through the tumor (arrow).

Laboratory investigations show leukocytosis and anemia (Fig. 27.24).

Gross Morphology

- Tumor is tan gray with areas of hemorrhage and necrosis.
- Necrotic yellowish and semi-fluid material obtained from intramedullary or subperiosteal lesion on open biopsy erroneously interpreted as pus by surgeons.

Light Microscopy

- *Cells morphology:* The tumor is composed of small uniform round cells with round nuclei containing fine chromatin and scanty cytoplasm. These cells are arranged in solid sheets. Mitoses are present. Tumor cells forming Homer Wright rosette's are also demonstrated in some cases. The cytoplasm of tumor cells most often contains PAS positive glycogen.
- *Stroma:* There is a little intervening stroma between nests of tumor cells (Fig. 27.25).

Histochemistry

Tumor cells contain glycogen in their cytoplasm; which may be demonstrated by **PAS stain (diastase sensitive)**.

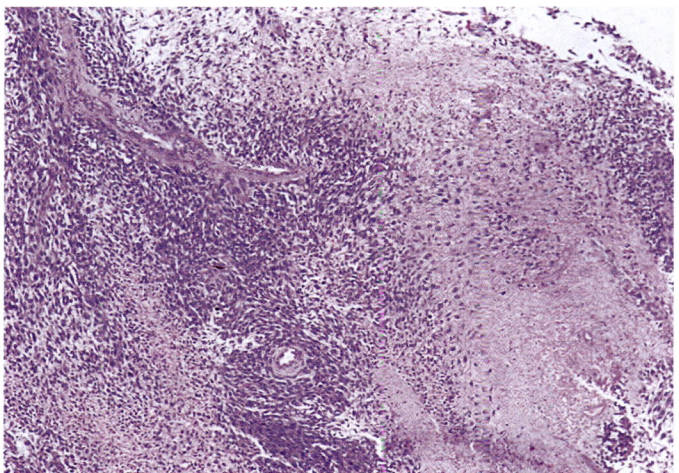

Fig. 27.25: Ewing's sarcoma shows tumor small uniform round cells with round nuclei with fine chromatin and scanty cytoplasm arranged in solid sheets. Mitosis is present. Tumor cells forming Homer Wright rosette's are also demonstrated in some cases. The cytoplasm of tumor cells most often contains PAS positive glycogen (100X).

Immunohistochemistry

Panel of markers is used to analyze expression in Ewing's sarcoma on histopathological sections (Table 27.24).

Metastases

Ewing's sarcoma follows an extremely malignant course with early metastases. It may metastasize early to other bones and thus appear multifocal. Metastases to the lungs, liver, brain, and other organs are common.

Table 27.24: Immunohistochemistry of Ewing's sarcoma

Tumor markers	Expression
MIC2 (most specific marker)*	Positive
Vimentin	Positive
Nonspecific enolase (NSE)	Positive
CD99	Positive
Neurofilament	Positive
Cytokeratins (low molecular weight)	Positive (sometimes)

*MIC2 is the most specific marker of Ewing's sarcoma.

Prognostic Factors

Prognostic factors of Ewing's sarcoma include the stage, anatomic location and size of tumor. Prognosis is poor in tumors originating from pelvis with metastases. In addition to diagnostic utility, EWS/FLI-1 fusion status also provides prognostic information. Tumor responds well to chemotherapy in 75% of cases with 5-year survival.

Differential Diagnosis

Ewing's sarcoma has morphologic resemblance to malignant lymphoma. It should also be differentiated from neuroblastoma. These may also involve the bones of children and adolescents. Histochemistry and chromosomal abnormalities are diagnostic tools in this situation.

OSTEOCLASTIC GIANT CELL-RICH TUMOR

GIANT CELL TUMOR (OSTEOCLASTOMA)

Giant cell tumor of bone is potentially low grade locally aggressive malignant tumor. It accounts for 20% of all bone tumors and has a monocyte-macrophage lineage.

Tumor is composed of multinucleated, osteoclastic giant cells embedded in a supporting spindle-celled stroma. Evidence of malignant component occurs in the form of numerous mitoses in stromal component. It often recurs after local curettage and rarely metastasizes. Salient features of giant cell tumors are shown in Table 27.25.

Age Group

It most often affects 20 and 45 years of age. It is more common in women than in men.

Origin and Locations

It most often arises in epiphysis mostly around knee joint (distal femur or proximal tibia). The tumor expands into the metaphysis results in erosion of the cortical bone. It is confined proximally by the growth plate and is limited to the metaphysis. As the tumor expands, it produces a bright rim of overlying reactive new bone.

Table 27.25: Salient features of giant cell tumor

Tumor	Locations	Age group	Pathological features
Giant cell tumor	Epiphysis/metaphysis of long bones	20–45 years	Evenly placed giant cells among mononuclear cells with identical nuclei; normal serum calcium/phosphate/blood urea nitrogen/creatinine

Radiological Findings

Tumor gives *soap bubble appearance* on radiograph. It shows a large osteolytic eccentric lesion, which erodes into the subendosteal bone plate.

Overlying cortex is destroyed producing a bulging soft tissue mass delineated by a thin shell of reactive bone. The margins of the lesion are well circumscribed, which seldom show sclerosis.

Clinical Features

The expansion of this tumor near a joint can produce arthritic pain. The weakened bone may undergo pathological fracture or deformity occasionally.

Gross Morphology
- The tumor is large, red brown in color frequently undergo cystic degeneration.
- Areas of hemorrhage and necrosis are common expanding and destroying the normal bone.
- Hemosiderin deposition is present. Reactive bone formation also occurs (Fig. 27.26).

Light Microscopy
- *Tumor cells:* Tumor is composed of mononuclear uniform tumor cells with indistinct cell membrane growing in a syncytium as stromal cells.
- *Giant cells:* Numerous multinucleated osteoclast like giant cells containing more than 100 nuclei are scattered among mononuclear stromal cells. The nuclei of stromal cells have identical features to that of the multinucleated cells. Mitoses are frequent. Transforming growth factor-β (TGF-β) osteoprogerin participate in formation of multinucleated osteoclast like giant cells in osteoclastoma (Fig. 27.27).

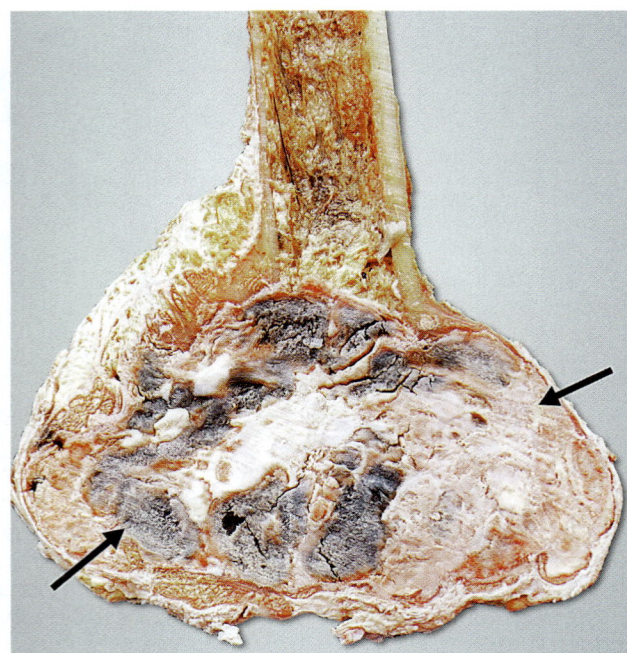

Fig. 27.26: Giant cell tumor in the lower end of the femur. It is a hemorrhagic tumor expanding the lateral condyle and destroying the normal bone (arrows).

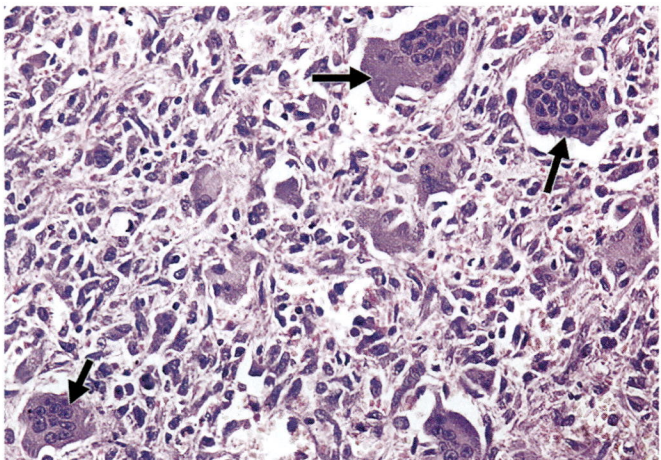

Fig. 27.27: Giant cell tumor of bone is composed of mononuclear uniform tumor cells with indistinct cell membrane growing in a syncytium and stromal cells. Multinucleated giant cells containing >100 nuclei are scattered among mononuclear stromal cells. The nuclei of stromal cells have identical features to that of the mononuclear cells (arrows) (400X).

Prognostic Factors

Giant cell tumor is capable of locally aggressive behavior. It may show metastases in lungs in 4% of cases. Light microscopy does not predict the extent of aggressive behavior of the tumor.

Differential Diagnosis

Giant cell tumor of bone should be differentiated from brown tumor of hyperparathyroidism, giant cell reparative granuloma, metaphyseal fibrous defect, nonossifying fibroma, aneurysmal bone cyst, chondroblastoma, chondromyxoid fibroma and pigmented villonodular synovitis.

Giant cells in these disorders are irregularly distributed in the lesions. Giant cells seen in bone tumors and tumor-like conditions are shown in Table 27.26.

Behavior

Unpredictability of giant cell tumor of bone complicates their management.

Management

Conservative surgery—curettage is associated with 40–60% recurrence rate. Lung metastases are seen up to 4% cases. Morphology of primary and secondary giant cell tumor is similar.

Bones and Joints

Table 27.26: Giant cells seen in bone tumors and tumor-like conditions

Categories	Examples
Benign tumors or tumor-like conditions	Chondroblastoma Osteoclastoma Benign fibrous histiocytoma Chondromyxoid fibroma Fibrous dysplasia Metaphyseal fibrous defects (nonossifying fibroma) Aneurysmal bone cyst
Malignant tumors	Malignant fibrous histiocytoma Fibrosarcoma Giant cell variant of osteosarcoma

HISTIOCYTIC TUMORS

Langerhans' cell histiocytosis (formerly termed histiocytosis X) can occur in various sites, including bone. This group of disorders shows proliferation of histiocytic cells that closely resemble the Langerhans' cells of the epidermis. These cells are tennis racket-shaped containing Birbeck granules.

Salient features of histiocytic tumors are shown in Table 27.27.

Distinctive surface antigens also characterize these Langerhans-like cells. It includes Letterer-Siwe disease, and eosinophilic granuloma.

Light Microscopy

Langerhans' cell histiocytosis is composed of large number of histiocytes resembling Langerhans' cells of skin (Fig. 27.28).

LETTERER-SIWE DISEASE (XANTHOMA SEMINATUM)

Letterer-Siwe disease is acute disseminated Langerhans' cell histiocytosis affecting infants and small children. Disease has rapid aggressive course with fatal outcome.

Clinical Feature

Patient presents with *painless, yellow brown maculopapular skin lesions scattered over face*, especially around eyes, mouth, trunk, perineum, axillae, and recurrent infection as a result of widespread histiocytic proliferation.

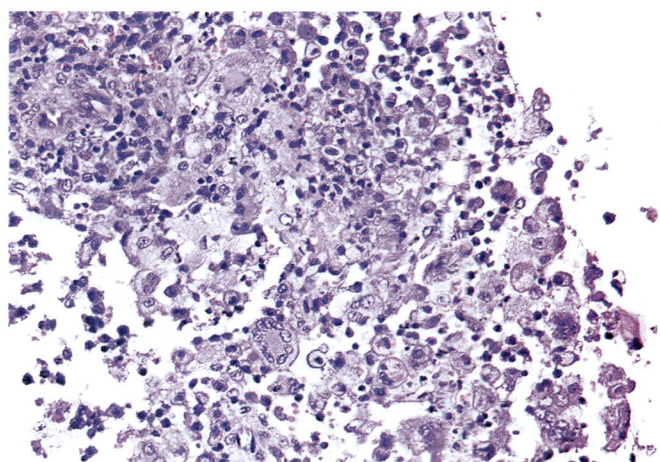

Fig. 27.28: Langerhans' cell histiocytosis shows large number of histiocytes (100X).

Physical Examination

Physical examination reveals *hepatosplenomegaly, lymphadenopathy, pulmonary involvement (honeycomb appearance, spontaneous pneumothorax and pleural effusion)*.

Light Microscopy

Lesion is composed of histiocytes lacking lipids. Foci of necrosis are present.

HAND-SCHÜLLER-CHRISTIAN DISEASE

Hand-Schüller-Christian disease is acute onset followed by chronic progressive histiocytosis affecting infants to

Table 27.27: Salient features of histiocytic tumors

Tumor	Locations	Age group	Pathological features
Langerhans' cell histiocytosis	Skull, jaw, metaphysis and diaphysis of long bones	5–15 years	Mixed inflammatory cells and eosinophils and S-100/CD1a-positive cells with grooved/multilobated nuclei
Benign fibrous histiocytoma	Long bones, pelvis	>20 years	Identical to nonossifying fibroma but variable
Erdheim-Chester disease	Long bones	>40 years	Foamy histiocytes and fibrosis

elderly persons. It most often presents before 5 years of age. It has a better prognosis than Letterer-Siwe disease.

Clinical Features

Disorder has classic triad of skull lesions (orbit, toothbearing area of mandible, mastoid bone), diabetes insipidus due to destruction of sella turcica, and exophthalmos caused by involvement of the orbit.

Various sites are skull orbit, toothbearing area of mandible, mastoid bone, femur, pelvis, ribs, humerus towards end of shaft, spine, lung, skin and mucosa. Hepatosplenomegaly and lymphadenopathy may occur in 25–50% of cases.

Light Microscopy

Lesion shows histiocytic proliferation mixed with inflammatory cells in bone, especially the skull, liver, spleen, and other tissues.

EOSINOPHILIC GRANULOMA

Eosinophilic granuloma may be unifocal or multifocal lesion affecting all ages, i.e. 16 months to 61 years. It has the best prognosis within the group. The lesion sometimes heals without treatment.

Organs Involved

Patient most often presents with solitary lesion in bone. Locations of solitary eosinophilic granuloma are shown in Table 27.28. In some patients, multiple lesions may be present.

Clinical Features

- Patient with bone lesion most often presents with pathological fracture or vertebral collapse. Extraskeletal involvement is most often limited to the lung and sometimes gastrointestinal tract.
- Patient with lung lesion presents with sudden onset, and has cough, weight loss, dyspnea and pneumothorax.
- Lesion in gastrointestinal tract is solitary, which may simulate polyps, gastric carcinoma or duodenal ulcer.

X-ray Findings

There is presence of rarefaction in medullary areas of membranous or long bones. As the lesion enlarges, it

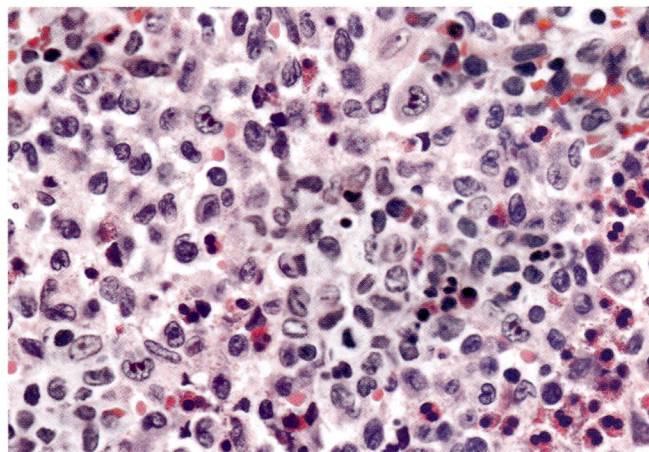

Fig. 27.29: Eosinophilic granuloma shows large number of histiocytes admixed with numerous eosinophils, and lymphocytes (400X).

erodes the inner table of the cortex and resembles a cyst. In some patients, reactive sclerosis may develop.

Light Microscopy

The lesion is composed of proliferation of histiocytes admixed with numerous eosinophils, macrophages, and lymphocytes (Fig. 27.29).

Electron Microscopy

Birebeck granules are demonstrated in histiocytes.

Immunohistochemistry

The tumor cells show positivity for **S-100, CD1a** and **CD207 (langerin)**.

HEMATOGENOUS MALIGNANCIES

MULTIPLE MYELOMA

Myeloma is the most common malignant neoplasm of bone. The majority of patients with myeloma are diagnosed on examination of bone marrow aspirate or bone biopsy specimen.

Majority of patients present with multiple myeloma. Solitary myeloma most often occurs in younger age group progressing to multiple myeloma.

Clinical Features

Patient most often presents with bone pain (65% of cases) and pathological fracture. Spine involvement

Table 27.28: Solitary eosinophilic granuloma locations

Organs involved	Adults	Children
Bones	Ribs, ramus of mandible, vertebral bodies, orbit	Head region and femur
Other organs	Lung and gastrointestinal tract	+/–

causes spinal cord compression. Polyneuropathy most often resolves with treatment of underlying myeloma.

Other symptoms are weight loss and fatigue. Many patients with myeloma develop hypercalcemia. Myeloma kidney is caused by waxy casts of precipitated, nephrotoxic, monoclonal light chains blocking the tubules. Lambda light chains are more than kappa ones.

Prognosis

Patient with solitary plasmacytoma and osteosclerotic myeloma may have prolonged clinical course.

Imaging Technique

Radiograph shows multiple punched out, purely osteolytic lesions in the bone. The lesions are most prominent in the skull bone, ribs, sternum, vertebrae (i.e. bones that contain hematopoietic tissue), and pelvic girdle.

Myeloma rarely associated with bony sclerosis has been termed *osteosclerotic myeloma* (Fig. 27.30).

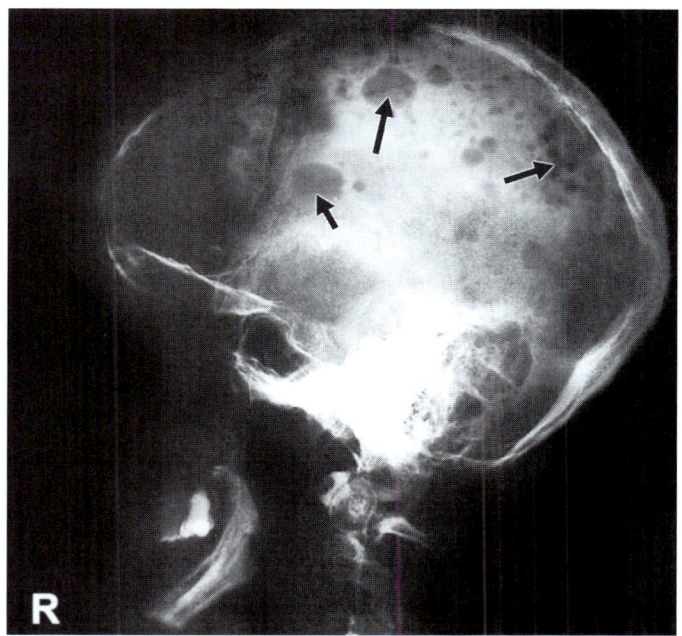

Fig. 27.30: Multiple myeloma. A lateral X-ray of the skull showing the punched-out lytic lesions of multiple myeloma (arrows).

Laboratory Diagnosis

Peripheral blood smear examination shows microcytic hypochromic anemia and rouleaux formation of RBCs.

Erythrocyte sedimentation rate is increased. Monoclonal protein may be demonstrated in serum or urine or both in almost all patients of myeloma.

Gross Morphology

- Tumor resembles *currant jelly*. The lesion is soft and red.
- However, many myeloma tumors may show *fish-flesh* appearance, typical of malignant lymphoma (Fig. 27.31).

Light Microscopy

- Tumor is composed of sheets of plasma cells. These cells have abundant blue to pink cytoplasm and an eccentrically placed round nucleus with clumped chromatin. Binucleated plasma cells are most often present.
- Plasma cells frequently show cytologic atypia. Occasionally, tumor showing pleomorphic cells should be differentiated from malignant lymphoma.
- Approximately 10–15% of myelomas contain amyloid deposits in the wall of blood vessels or among tumor cells eliciting giant cell reaction (Fig. 27.32).

Differential Diagnosis

Myeloma should be differentiated from chronic osteomyelitis (Table 27.29). Occasionally, myeloma shows clustering growth pattern simulating metastatic carcinoma. Metastatic carcinoma shows positivity with cytokeratins.

NOTOCHORD DERIVED TUMORS

CHORDOMA

Chordoma originates from remnants of primitive notochord. Once the notochord develops, it behaves as a mesodermal derivative. Notochord remnants in

Table 27.29: Differences between chronic osteomyelitis and myeloma

Histological parameters	Chronic osteomyelitis	Myeloma
Population of cells	Plasma cells, lymphocytes and neutrophils	Plasma cells
Proliferation of capillaries in the background	Present forming granulation tissue	Absent
Immunohistochemistry	Plasma cells (polyclonal)	Plasma cells (monoclonal), hence diagnostic role

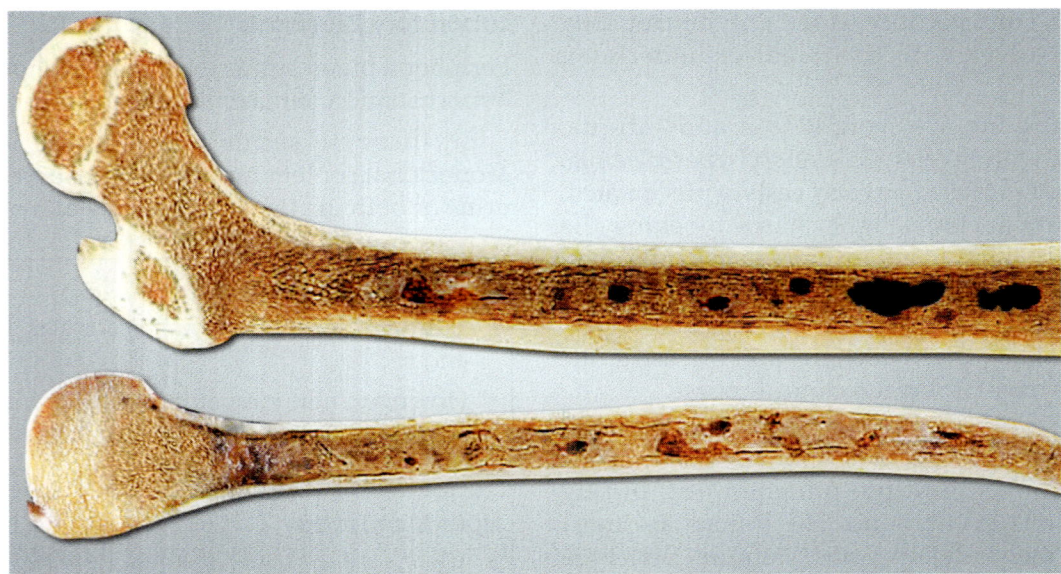

Fig. 27.31: Multiple myeloma. Humerus and femur showing localized areas of deposition of myeloma in the long bones.

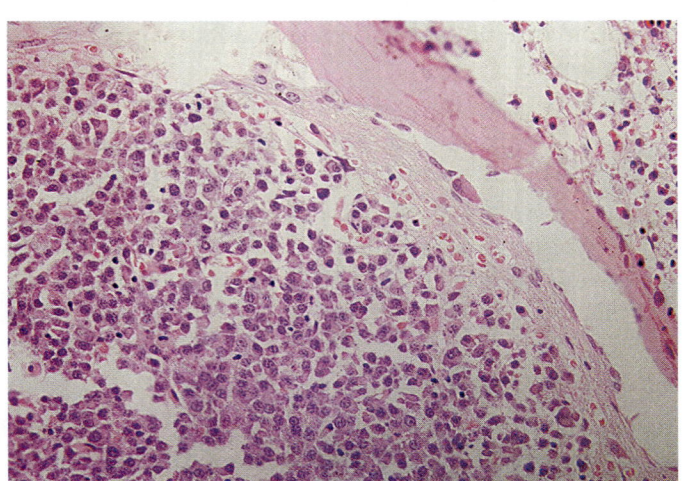

Fig. 27.32: Multiple myeloma shows sheets of myeloma cells containing pinkish cytoplasm and eccentrically placed nucleoli (400X).

adults are represented by parts of *nucleus pulposus of the intervertebral discs.*

Age Group

It affects *infancy to older age group*, but incidence is more in 5th–6th decade. *Females are more affected than males. Chondroid variant of chordoma* closely resembles chondrosarcoma and equally affecting both sexes.

Locations

Chordoma arises in or near the *vertebral bodies* and the *bones of the base of skull.* Nasopharyngeal chordoma arise from ectopic residues of chorda dorsalis.

Extraosteal growths develop in soft tissues around sacrum completely independent of bony origin. But it is difficult to be sure that a tumor in either situation does not have a long filament osseous attachment.

Locations of chordoma affecting various age groups are shown in Table 27.30.

Table 27.30: Locations of chordoma in various age groups

Locations	Frequency (%)	Age group
Spheno-occipital region	35	20–40 years
Upper end of notochord	40–60	
Sacrococcygeal region	30–50	40–60 years
Spinal region	10	

Behavior

Chordoma may be benign or malignant depending on the clinical course.

Clinical Features

Patient presents with multiple cranial palsies due to lesion in posterior cranial fossa, i.e. bilateral hemianopia due to compression of optic chiasma.

Other symptoms due to mass in intranasal, sinuses and nasopharyngeal regions.

Gross Morphology

The tumor is hemorrhagic and has a rather mucoid cut surface (Fig. 27.33).

Light Microscopy

Tumor is composed of large round to polygonal physalipherous cells, as well as many transitional cells with central round nuclei and abundant vacuolated cytoplasm in myxoid stroma (Fig. 27.34).

Bones and Joints

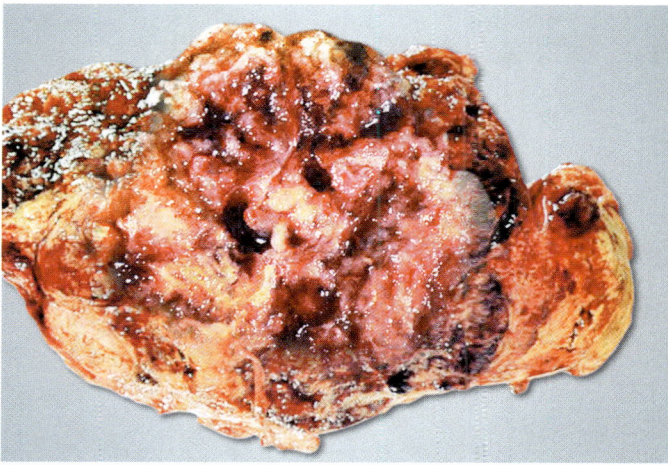

Fig. 27.33: Chordoma removed from the pelvis anterior to the sacrum. The tumor is hemorrhagic and has a rather mucoid cut surface.

Metastases

In 10% cases, metastases are seen in regional lymph nodes, other parts of skeletal system, liver, adrenals, soft tissues of thoracic cage and extremities.

Radiological Findings

Lesions are usually osteolytic but rarely osteoblastic.

Histochemistry

Tumor cells contain *glycogen* demonstrated by *PAS* and *mucicarmine*. Staining for fat is negative.

Immunohistochemistry

Panel of markers is used to analyze expression in chordoma on histopathological section (Table 27.31).

FIBROUS/FIBROHISTIOCYTIC MALIGNANT TUMORS

Fibrous/fibrohistiocytic malignant tumors of bone include fibrosarcoma and malignant fibrous histiocytoma (Table 27.32).

FIBROSARCOMA

Fibrosarcomas of bone originate from metaphysis of long bones and constitute up to 5% of all primary bone tumors. Other frequent sites are proximal femur, distal humerus and proximal tibia. It most often occurs in 20–60 years of age with equal sex predilection.

Clinical Features

Patient presents with painful swelling. Approximately 30% of patients develop pathological fracture.

Imaging Technique

Fibrosarcoma usually appears as a destructive geographic lesion. It may have an ill-defined permeative *moth-eaten* appearance with cortical destruction with soft tissue extension.

Gross Morphology

Well differentiated tumors produce large amount of collagen fibers resulting in firm consistency. Cut surface is gray white with circumscribed margins.

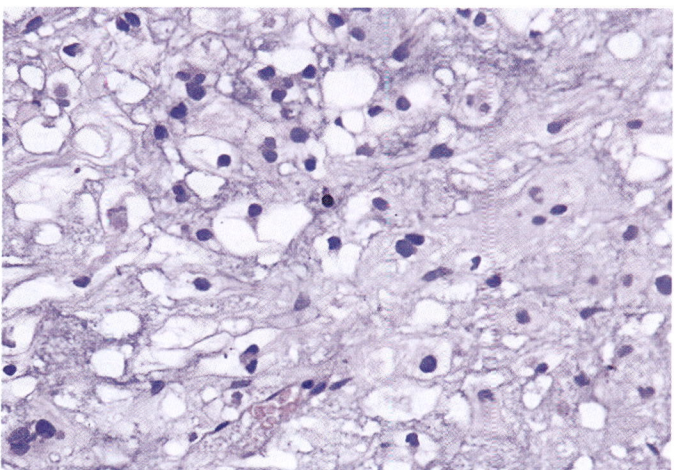

Fig. 27.34: Chordoma. Tumor is composed of large round to polygonal physalipherous cells, with central round nuclei and abundant vacuolated cytoplasm in myxoid stroma (400X).

Table 27.31: Histochemistry of chordoma

Marker	Expression
Neuron-specific enolase (NSE)	Positive
S-100 protein	Positive
Epithelial membrane antigen (EMA)	Positive
Nucleotidase	Positive (strong positivity in membrane of tumor cells)
Carcinoembryonic antigen (CEA)	Positive (rarely)

Table 27.32: Fibrous/fibrohistiocytic malignant tumors of bone

Tumors	Locations	Age group	Histological features
Fibrosarcoma	Metaphysis of long bones; may extend to end of bone	20–60 years	Malignant spindle cells in a fascicular pattern
Malignant fibrous histiocytoma	Metaphysis of long bones; may extend to end of bone	20–80 years	Malignant spindle cells in storiform pattern + histiocytic cells (other patterns may be seen)

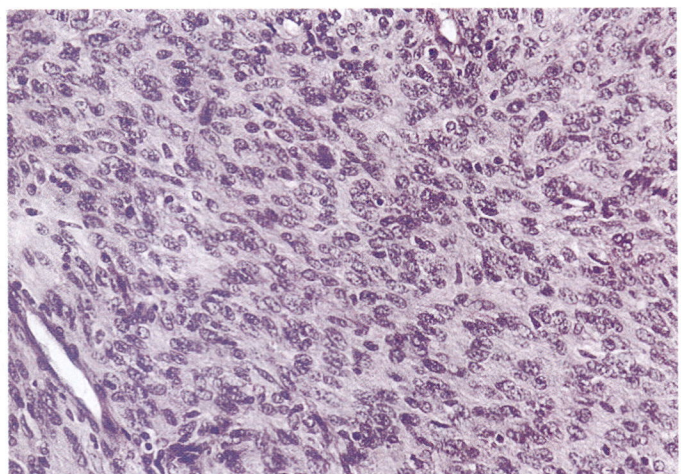

Fig. 27.35: Fibrosarcoma. Tumor is composed of monomorphic spindle cells arranged in long sweeping fascicles in a *herring-bone pattern* (400X).

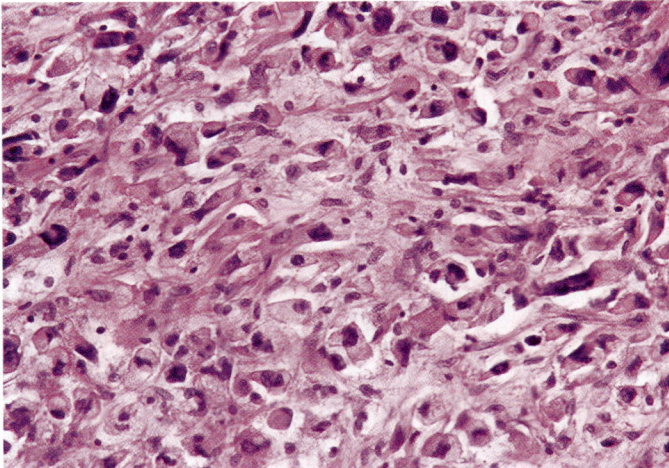

Fig. 27.36: Malignant fibrous histiocytoma shows atypical spindle cells arranged in storiform pattern (400X).

Light Microscopy
- Tumor is composed of uniform population of spindle cells arranged in fascicular or *herring-bone pattern* with varying amount of collagen fibers production.
- High grade tumors tend to be more cellular with greater nuclear atypia and increased mitoses, but less production of collagen fibers. Areas of necrosis may be seen in Fig. 27.35.

Prognostic Factors
Most important prognostic factor is histological tumor grade. Overall, 5-year survival is seen in 34% of cases.

MALIGNANT FIBROUS HISTIOCYTOMA
Malignant fibrous histiocytoma (MFH) arises in metaphysis of long bones. It is composed of fibroblasts and pleomorphic cells with prominent *storiform pattern*. It contains foci of histiocytic (macrophage) differentiation. It most often occurs in 20–80 years of age.

Locations
Primary malignant fibrous histiocytoma most often occurs in the metaphysis of long bones of lower extremities especially femur followed by tibia. Tumor may occur in humerus.

Clinical Features
Patient presents with painful swelling.

Imaging Technique
Tumor is most often osteolytic in nature. However, sclerotic areas may be demonstrated.

Gross Morphology
- Tumor varies from tan to gray white and soft to firm in consistency.
- Margins are irregular with cortical destruction and soft tissue infiltration.

Light Microscopy
- Tumor is composed of malignant spindle cells. The spindle cells tend to be well differentiated and resemble fibroblasts.
- These spindle cells are arranged in an irregularly whorled *storiform pattern*.
- Different histological variants of tumor described include storiform—pleomorphic, histiocytic, myxoid, giant cell and inflammatory types (Fig. 27.36).

Prognostic Factors
Favorable prognostic factors are younger age, low grade and presence of prominent chronic inflammatory cells. Prominent desmoplasia and metastases are poor prognostic factors.

EPITHELIAL TUMORS

ADAMANTINOMA
Adamantinoma most often occurs in cortex of tibia and/or fibula during 20–35 years of age with no sex predilection (Table 27.33).

Table 27.33: Features of adamantinoma

Adamantinoma	Cortex of tibia and/or fibula	20–35 years	Epithelial cells + fibroblasts + woven or lamellar bone

Gross Morphology
Decortication reveals a firm, multilocular mass.

Imaging Techniques
Tumor shows unilocular or multilocular cysts (honeycomb appearance) on radiograph. CT scan usually shows an expansile, radiolucent, multiloculated cystic lesion with characteristic soap bubble appearance.

Light Microscopy
- Tumor is composed of epithelial cells, fibroblasts and woven or lamellar bone. The epithelium consisted of peripheral tall columnar basal cells showing cytoplasmic vacuolization and reverse polarization of the nuclei.
- These epithelial cells surround loose epithelium, resembling the stellate reticulum of the developing teeth. Squamous metaplasia may be seen.

Treatment
Adequate surgical excision is often curative.

SECONDARY TUMORS (BONE METASTASES)
Metastatic carcinoma is the most common tumor of bone after 40 years of age. Skeletal metastases are found in at least 85% of cancer cases in clinical course. Tumor cells usually arrive in the bone by way of the bloodstream.

Bone Metastases
Vertebral column is the most common site of metastases in hematopoietic bone marrow; followed by pelvis, ribs, skull and proximal long bones.

Skeletal metastases are *uncommon below knee or elbow joints*. It is worth mentioning that basal cell carcinoma, gliomas and soft tissue sarcomas except embryonal rhabdomyosarcoma rarely metastasize to bone (Tables 27.34 and 27.35).

Table 27.34: Frequency of metastases in bone hematopoietic marrow in descending order

- Vertebral column (most common site)
- Pelvis
- Ribs
- Skull
- Humerus (proximal end)
- Femur (proximal end)
- Skeletal metastases are uncommon below knee or elbow joints

Table 28.35: Tumors rarely metastasizing to bones

- Basal cell carcinoma
- Gliomas
- Soft tissue sarcomas except embryonal rhabdomyosarcoma

Clinical Anatomy
- Batsons' paravertebral venous plexus has connection with the vena cava and vertebral venous system. Vertebral venous system is extensive and valveless, and has constant connection to breast, thyroid, lung, and prostate.
- In addition, the plexuses are connected to dural sinuses and vasa vascrum of humerus and femur. There are numerous interconnections between vascular and lymphatic system.

Age Group
Bone metastases in adults and children are shown in Table 27.36.
- *Adults:* Cancers of prostate, urinary bladder, breast, lung (small cell type), kidney, gastrointestinal tract, thyroid gland and malignant melanoma most often metastasize to bone in adults.
- *Children:* Neuroblastoma, rhabdomyosarcoma, and retinoblastoma most often metastasize to bones in children.

Table 27.36: Bone metastases in adults and children

• Bone metastases in adults	Prostate carcinoma
	Urinary bladder carcinoma
	Breast carcinoma
	Lung carcinoma (small cell type)
	Kidney carcinoma
	Gastrointestinal tract carcinoma
	Thyroid carcinoma
	Malignant melanoma
• Bone metastases in children	Neuroblastoma
	Rhabdomyosarcoma
	Retinoblastoma

Solitary or multiple bone metastases: Solitary and multifocal bone metastases are shown in Table 27.37.
- *Solitary metastases:* Cancers of lung, kidney and thyroid gland produce solitary metastatic deposit in bones.
- *Multifocal metastases:* Metastatic deposits in bones are usually multiple except renal cell carcinoma, which may be confused with primary bone tumor. Multiple lesions of bones in children may be a feature of neuroblastoma.

Table 27.37: Solitary or multifocal bone metastases

• *Solitary bone metastases*	Lung carcinoma
	Renal cell carcinoma
	Thyroid carcinoma
• *Multifocal bone metastases*	Breast carcinoma
	Gastrointestinal tract cancers
	Lung carcinoma
	Neuroblastoma

Type of Metastases

Metastases in bones may produce osteoblastic or osteoclastic lesions. Breast carcinoma may produce either osteoblastic or osteoclastic lesions (Table 27.38).

- *Osteolytic lesions:* Some tumors (thyroid, gastrointestinal tract, kidney, neuroblastoma, breast, lung and malignant melanoma) produce mostly lytic lesions. These stimulate the synthesis of prostaglandins and cytokines leading to osteoclastic bone resorption.

  It leads to increased serum calcium level, hypercalciuria, and increased hydroxyproline containing peptides excretion reflecting matrix destruction. Serum alkaline phosphatase may be normal or slightly increased.

- *Osteoblastic lesions:* A few neoplasms (prostate, breast, lung, stomach, Hodgkin's disease) stimulate osteoblastic components to make bone. These are associated with increased levels of serum alkaline phosphatase and sometimes decreased calcium levels.

- *Osteolytic/osteoblastic lesions:* Breast carcinoma metastasizing to bones may also show osteoblastic or osteoclastic lesions.

Clinical Features

Patient with metastatic deposits to bone presents with pain, swelling, deformity, encroachment of hemopoietic tissue in the bone marrow, compression of spinal cord or nerve roots and pathological fractures.

NON-NEOPLASTIC LESIONS

ANEURYSMAL BONE CYST

Origin

It is non-neoplastic lesion arising in epiphysis of long bones, vertebral column and flat bones. The lesion is of expansile nature resulting in a ballooned-out distension of the bone.

Age Group

It affects less than 30 years of age.

Clinical Features

Patient presents with bone pain and swelling.

Secondary aneurysmal bone cyst may be seen in association with fibrous dysplasia, osteoblastoma, chondroblastoma, chondrosarcoma and giant cell tumor.

Radiological Features

Aneurysmal bone cyst shows epiphyseal–metaphyseal region with erosion of bone cortex.

Table 27.38: Osteolytic and osteoblastic lesions due to metastases

	Mechanism	Serum
Osteolytic lesions		
Thyroid carcinoma Breast carcinoma* Gastrointestinal tract cancers Kidney carcinoma Neuroblastoma Lung carcinoma Malignant melanoma	Bone resorption due to synthesis of prostaglandins and cytokines leading to hypercalcemia	Serum alkaline phosphatase normal or slightly raised
Osteoblastic lesions		
Prostate carcinoma Breast carcinoma* Lung carcinoma Gastric carcinoma Hodgkin's disease	Osteoblastic activity increased	Serum alkaline phosphatase raised

*Breast carcinoma may produce either osteolytic or osteoblastic lesion.

Gross Examination

It forms a spongy, hemorrhagic mass that may extend into the soft tissues and covered by a thin shell of reactive bone (Fig. 27.37).

> ### Light Microscopy
> The lesion is composed of cystic spaces lined by fibrous septa containing osteoid and numerous osteoclast like multinucleated giant cells. These cystic spaces lined by fibrous septa lack endothelial cells (Fig. 27.38).

Differential Diagnosis

Telangiectatic osteosarcoma shows large blood-filled spaces, atypical cells with high nucleocytoplasmic ratio, numerous mitoses in close vicinity of the osteoid tissue and foci of necrosis.

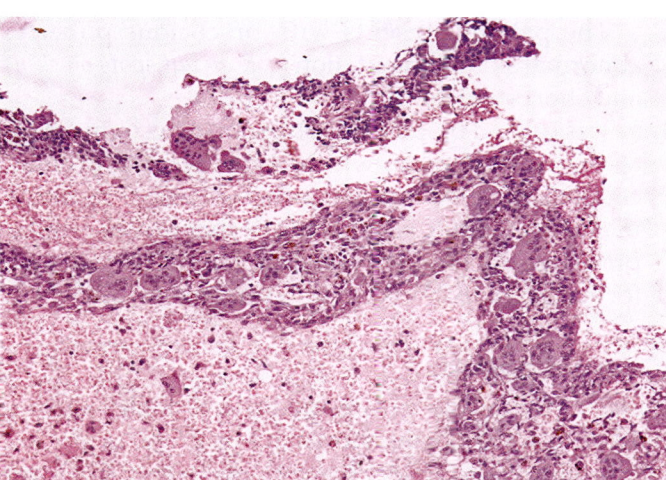

Fig. 27.38: Aneurysmal bone cyst shows cystic spaces lined by fibrous septa containing osteoid and numerous osteoclast like multinucleated giant cells (400X).

FIBROUS DYSPLASIA

Fibrous dysplasia is a developmental abnormality of the skeleton characterized by replacement of portions of bone with fibrous tissue. Lesion is composed of disorganized mixture of fibrous and osseous elements in the interior of the affected bones. It primarily affects children and young adults.

Variants

Depending on the bone involved, it is of three types: *Monostotic, polyostotic* and *McCune-Albright syndrome* (Table 27.39).

- *Monostotic fibrous dysplasia:* It is a solitary lesion in *ribs, femur or cranial bones*.
  Patient is usually asymptomatic. But it may result in spontaneous fractures with pain, swelling, and deformity.
- *Polyostotic fibrous dysplasia:* Patient develops lesions in multiple bones (femur, skull, tibia and humerus).
  It can be associated with severe deformity especially facial involvement in 50% of cases.
- *McCune-Albright syndrome:* This syndrome is *polyostotic fibrous dysplasia*. It most often occurs in very young girls.

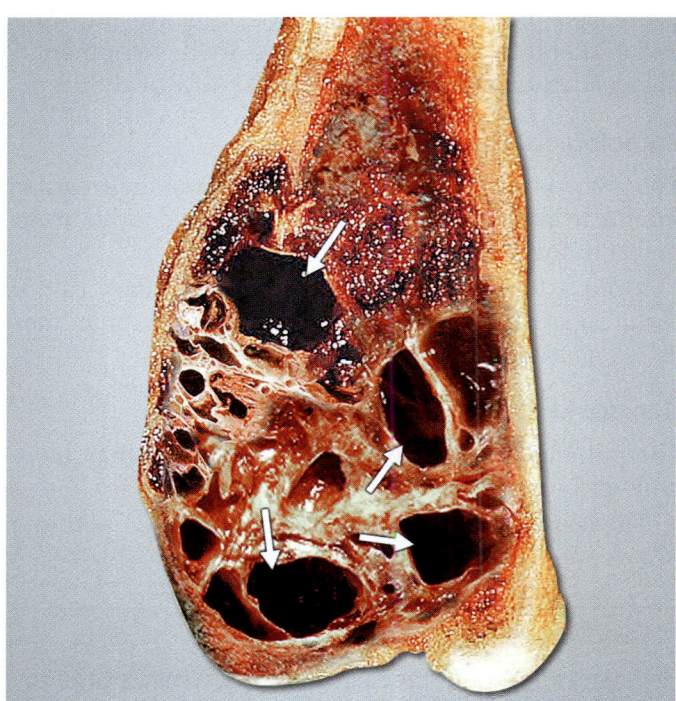

Fig. 27.37: Aneurysmal bone cyst in the lower end of the right ulna. The large angiomatous spaces are expanding the cortex of the bone, hence the name *aneurysmal* (arrows).

Table 27.39: Types of fibrous dysplasia

Type and frequency	Age group	Locations
Monostotic fibrous dysplasia (70%)	Older children and adolescents	Ribs, femur, maxilla, mandible and humerus
Polyostotic fibrous dysplasia (25%)	Young children	Femur, skull (facial involvement in 50% causing deformity), tibia and humerus
Polyostotic fibrous dysplasia associated with McCune-Albright syndrome (3–5%)	Young children	

The patient presents with precocious puberty, abnormal skin pigmentation (*café au lait spots on skin*) and short stature.

It is caused by post-zygotic somatic cell mutation of the GNAS1 gene, which codes for a G-protein-coupled receptor activating *adenyl cyclase*, resulting in *excess adenosine monophosphate* that drives cellular proliferation. It is genetic but not hereditary. Transformation of this process into sarcoma is rare.

Gross Morphology
Fibrous dysplasia in the medullary cavity of the midshaft of the tibia is shown in Fig. 27.39.

Light Microscopy
- The lesion is composed of irregular spicules of woven bone in a cellular stroma that lacks the normal lamellar pattern.
- Lesion produces weak area that can produce deformity and fracture (Fig. 27.40).

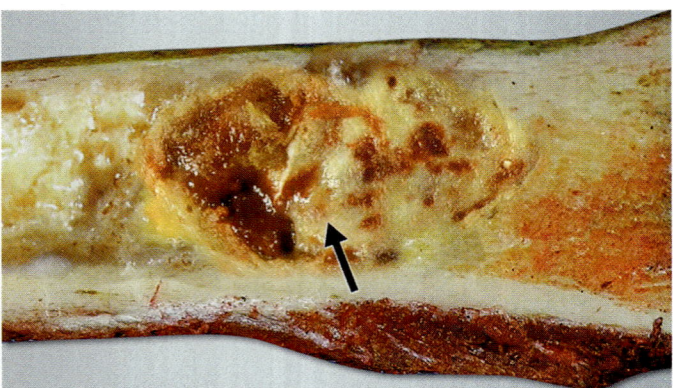

Fig. 27.39: Fibrous dysplasia in the medullary cavity of the midshaft of the tibia (arrow).

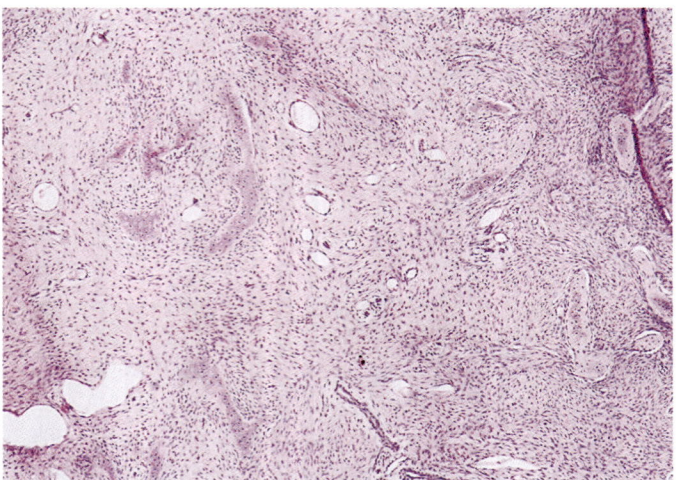

Fig. 27.40: Fibrous dysplasia shows irregular spicules of woven bone in a cellular stroma that lacks the normal lamellar pattern (100X).

METAPHYSEAL FIBROUS DEFECT (NONOSSIFYING FIBROMA)

Metaphyseal fibrous defect and nonossifying fibroma are essentially the same disease except for a difference in size.

Metaphyseal fibrous defect measures 1–4 cm and nonossifying fibroma 5–10 cm. These lesions never undergo malignant transformation.

Age Group
Both lesions are non-neoplastic and affects children.

Pathogenesis
Metaphyseal fibrous defect is unclear and it may be either some developmental aberration at the epiphyseal plate or probably histiocytic origin. It originates in the subperiosteal cortex of metaphysis of long bones such as femur (lower end), both ends of tibia, and fibula in decreased order of frequency. Lesions are multiple and bilateral in 50% of cases. These are developmental defects demonstrated on X-ray in 30–40% of children.

Radiological Findings
The lesion is recognized radiographically as an irregular minute to large defects, sharply demarcated radiolucent defect in the metaphysis.

More extensive lesions involving medullary cavity resulting in a fusiform expansion of bone are sometimes called *nonossifying/nonosteogenic fibroma*.

Clinical Features
The patients are usually asymptomatic but may have pain and fracture.

The lesions often disappear spontaneously within a few years.

Gross Morphology
Gross examination reveals soft, gray white, granular and brown or black lesion within the cortex with an intact shell of overlying bone.

Light Microscopy
- Microscopic examination shows cellular masses of fibrous tissue with a *storiform growth pattern* with *scattered osteoclast like giant cells, hemosiderin laden macrophages* and foamy cells.
- Cellular whorled fibroblasts sometimes form palisading arrangement (Fig. 27.41).

Treatment
These can be cured by curettage.

Bones and Joints

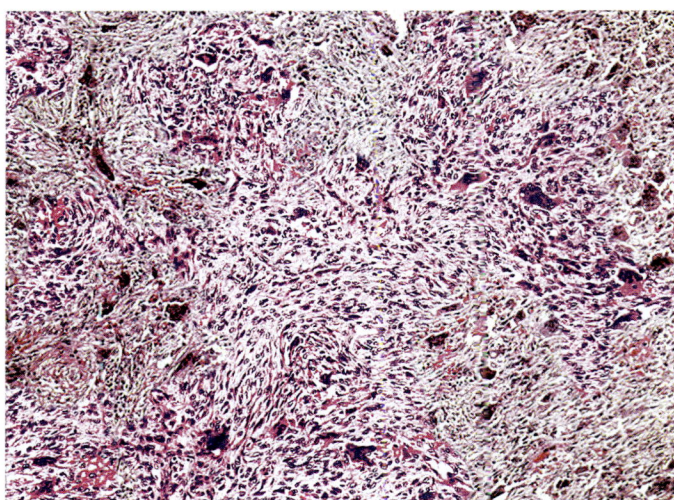

Fig. 27.41: Metaphyseal fibrous defect shows fibrous tissue with a storiform growth pattern with scattered osteoclast like giant cells, hemosiderin laden macrophages and foamy cells (100X).

ACHONDROPLASIA

It is autosomal disorder characterized by short-limbed dwarfism and macrocephaly. These limb bones become short and thick. It represents a failure of normal epiphyseal cartilage formation.

Pathogenesis

Achondroplasia occurs due to mutation of fibroblast growth factor receptor 3 (FGFR 3) located at 4p16.3. This gene mutation arrests chondrocyte proliferation, differentiation and development of epiphyseal plates.

Narrowing of epiphyseal plates, and bony sealing off of the area between the epiphyseal plate and the metaphysis lead to failure of elongation of limb bones. A defective growth hormone receptor is responsible for rare cases of dwarfism (Laron dwarfism).

OSTEOGENESIS IMPERFECTA

Osteogenesis imperfecta is autosomal dominant disorder known as brittle bone disease.

Physiological state: Normally collagen genes (COL1A1 and COL1A2 genes) encode the α_1 and α_2 chains of type I procollagen fibers result in synthesis of collagen fibers, the major structural protein of bone.

Pathological state: Collagen gene mutation leads to defective collagen synthesis in various organs such as skeleton (brittle bones), joints, ears, ligaments, teeth, sclerae, and skin.

The genetic defects in the four types of osteogenesis imperfecta are heterogeneous, but all affect the synthesis of type I collagen fibers.

Clinical Features

- Fractures with minimal trauma of many bones occur during infancy and at the time the child learns to walk. Such children are described as being as *fragile as a China doll* (brittle bone disease). Deficiency of collagen fibers in sclerae imparts translucence to the sclera overlying the choroids (blue sclerae).
- Patients develop hearing loss because fractures and fusion of bones of the middle ear restrict their mobility.

OSTEOPETROSIS

Osteopetrosis is inherited disorder also known as *marble disease* or *Albers-Schönberg disease*. It occurs in two major clinical forms: an autosomal recessive variant that is usually fatal in infancy and a less severe autosomal dominant variant.

Age Group

It affects infants and children. The disorder occurs due to mutations in genes that govern osteoclast formation or function.

Pathology

- Osteopetrosis results in increased bone density (thickened cortex), lack of funnelization of the metaphysis and retention of the primary spongiosum with its cartilage cores. Decreased bone marrow space results in anemia. Due to narrowing of foramina results in blindness, deafness, due to pressure on cranial nerves.
- Patient develops multiple fractures in spite of increased bone density (Figs 27.42 and 27.43).

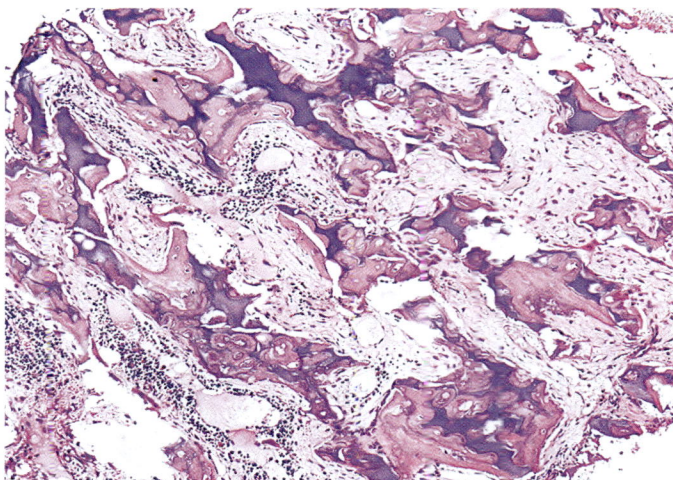

Fig. 27.42: Osteopetrosis shows increased bone density (thickened cortex) and decreased bone marrow space (100X).

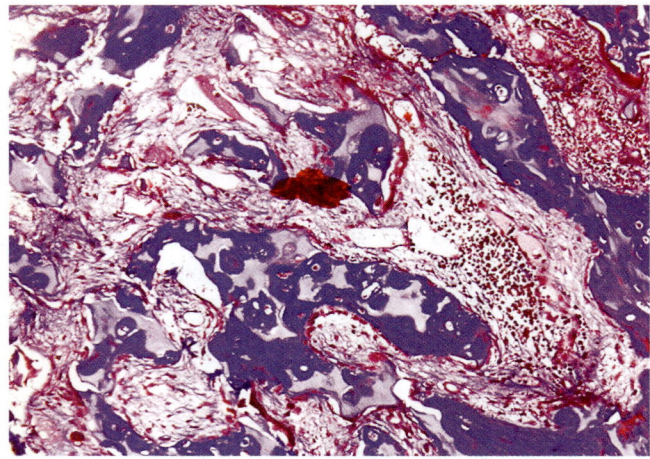

Fig. 27.43: Osteopetrosis—Masson's trichome stain.

OSTEONECROSIS (AVASCULAR NECROSIS)

Osteonecrosis refers to the death of bone marrow in the absence of infection. Growing bones of children and adolescents are often affected.

Etiology

It is caused by trauma, thromboemboli, sickle cell anemia, decompression syndrome or *the bends,* in adults. These lead to interruption of blood supply to bone marrow (Table 27.40).

Pathological Entities

- *Legg-Calvé-Perthes disease:* It refers to osteonecrosis in the femoral head in children. Collapse of the femoral head may lead to joint incongruity and severe osteoarthritis.
- *Osgood-Schlatter disease:* It refers to osteonecrosis of tibial tubercle.
- *Köhler bone disease:* It is avascular necrosis of navicular bone.

Table 27.40: Causes of osteonecrosis

• Mechanical disruption of blood vessels
• Vessel injury
• Vasculitis
• Bone fractures
• Thromboembolism
• Sickle cell disease
• Nitrogen bubbles in decompression
• Gaucher disease
• Corticosteroid therapy
• Radiation therapy
• Legg-Calvé-Perthes disease
• Blount disease
• Systemic lupus erythematosus
• Rheumatoid arthritis
• Chronic pancreatitis
• Tumors
• Epiphyseal disorders

DIAGNOSIS OF BONE DISORDERS

IMAGING TECHNIQUES

Imaging techniques help in determination of location and extent of tumor, i.e. aggressiveness.

- *Plain radiograph:* It is usually the first imaging technique for a suspected bone lesion since it is inexpensive and easily obtainable.

  It is also the best for assessment of general radiological features of the tumor. It is difficult to assess the permeative pattern of destruction or anatomic site, e.g. sacrum. Radiological findings in bone lesions are shown in Table 27.41.

- *Computed tomography:* It is easy to assess the permeative pattern of destruction or anatomic site, e.g. sacrum. In addition, CT is the best technique in assessment of matrix mineralization, cortical detail, and detection of the cystic and fatty lesions.

- *MRI:* It is a method of choice for local staging. It is superior to CT in the definition of medullary and extracortical spread and of the relationship of the tumor to critical neurovascular structures.

- *Bone scintigraphy:* It is a highly sensitive but relatively nonspecific technique. Its main role is in detection of suspected metastases in the whole skeleton. It may detect osteoid osteoma by demonstration of *double density sign* in 50% of cases of osteoid osteoma.

BIOCHEMICAL PARAMETERS

Increased serum alkaline phosphatase level is associated with osteomalacia, bone tumors, bone metastases, Paget's disease of bone and hyperparathyroidism.

Its level is also raised in liver or biliary disorders, late in pregnancy (derived from placenta) and normal bone growth.

HISTOPATHOLOGICAL DIAGNOSIS

Light microscopy has diagnostic value in most primary malignancies of bone.

Histological grade is the most important prognostic feature of bone sarcomas and is a key component of the major staging systems of bone neoplasm. Salient features of most common benign and malignant tumors are shown in Tables 27.42 and 27.43.

Table 27.41: Radiological findings in bone lesions

Bone lesions	Radiological findings
Osteoid osteoma	Radiolucent nidus surrounded by bone sclerosis
Osteosarcoma	Sun-ray appearance (sunburst speculation) and Codman's triangle
Ewing's sarcoma	Onion peel appearance
Giant cell tumor (osteoclastoma)	Soap-bubble appearance
Chondrosarcoma	Mottled calcification within tumor
Aneurysmal bone cyst	Expansile osteolytic lesion with fluid-fluid levels
Fibrous dysplasia	Ground glass appearance
Round cell tumors	Permeative pattern/moth-eaten
Cartilage tumors	Popcorn balls
Osteogenesis imperfecta	Gracile bones
Neurofibromatosis	Scallops from without
Rickets/osteomalacia	Looser's lines
Fibrosarcoma	Bear bite
Eosinophilic granuloma	Punched-out lesion
Congenital syphilis	Rat-bite lesions
Round cell tumors	Permeative pattern or moth-eaten
Medullary infarct	Smoke goes up a chimney

Table 27.42: Salient features of most common benign bone tumors and tumor-like lesions

Tumor/lesion	Locations	Age predilection	Salient pathological features
Cartilage forming tumors or tumor-like lesions			
Osteochondroma	Metaphysis of long bones	10–30 years	Cartilage-capped bony protrusion
Chondroma	Hands/feet; medulla of long bones	Any group	Variably cellular hyaline cartilage
Chondroblastoma	Epiphysis/apophysis of long bones	10–20 years	Chondroid-like matrix; S-100 positive cells with grooved nuclei
Chondromyxoid fibroma	Metaphysis of long bones	10–30 years	Hypocellular chondromyxoid lobules surrounded by more cellular spindle cell areas
Bone forming tumors			
Osteoma	Facial bones	Adults	Mineralized compact bone
Osteoid osteoma	Cortex of long bones	10–30 years	*Nidus* of immature bone surrounded by sclerotic bone
Osteoblastoma	Vertebrae; cortex of long bones	10–30 years	Identical to osteoid osteoma but larger; often no sclerosis
Fibrous tissue derived lesions			
Fibrous dysplasia	Ribs, jaw, long bones—medullary	10–30 years	Irregular woven bone within fibroblastic stroma
Osteofibrous dysplasia	Tibial cortex	<20 years	Similar to fibrous dysplasia but with appositional osteoblasts
Desmoplastic fibroma	Long bones, jaw, pelvis	20–30 years	Fibromatosis-like proliferation
Nonossifying fibroma	Long bones	5–15 years	Bland spindle cells in storiform pattern + histiocytes + giant cells

Contd....

Table 27.42: Salient features of most common benign bone tumors and tumor-like lesions *(Contd...)*

Tumor/lesion	Locations	Age predilection	Salient pathological features
Histiocytic tumors			
Benign fibrous histiocytoma	Long bones, pelvis	>20 years	Identical to nonossifying fibroma but variable
Langerhans' cell histiocytosis	Skull, jaw, metaphysis and diaphysis of long bones	5–15 years	Mixed inflammatory cells and eosinophils and S-100/CD1a-positive cells with grooved/multilobated nuclei
Erdheim-Chester disease	Long bones	>40 years	Foamy histiocytes and fibrosis
Giant cell tumor	Epiphysis/metaphysis of long bones	20–45 years	Evenly placed giant cells among mononuclear cells with identical nuclei and normal serum calcium/phosphate/blood urea nitrogen/creatinine
Miscellaneous lesions			
Aneurysmal bone cyst	Vertebrae, flat and long bones	10–20 years	Blood-filled spaces separated by fibrous septae and giant cells
Simple cyst	Metaphysis of long bones	10–20 years	Fluid-filled *cysts* lined by connective tissue
Hemangioma	Vertebrae, flat and long bones	20–50 years	Capillary and/or cavernous-sized vessels

Table 27.43: Salient features of most common primary malignant bone tumors

Tumor/lesion	Locations	Age predilection	Salient pathological features
Cartilaginous derived malignant tumors			
Chondrosarcoma	Flat bones, metaphysis and epiphysis of long bones	20–80 years	Variably cellular hyaline cartilage permeating bone
Conventional (not otherwise specified)	Metaphysis	20–80 years	Variably cellular hyaline cartilage permeating bone
Dedifferentiated chondrosarcoma	Metaphysis	>30 years	Conventional chondrosarcoma + high grade spindle cell sarcoma
Mesenchymal chondrosarcoma	Metaphysis	20–50 years	Undifferentiated small cell tumor + hyaline cartilage
Clear cell chondrosarcoma	Epiphysis	20–70 years	Conventional tumor with abundant large clear tumor cells
Bone forming malignant tumors			
Osteosarcoma	Metaphysis of long bones, jaw	10–20 years, >40 bimodal	Osteoid formed directly by malignant cells
Conventional osteosarcoma	Medullary		Osteoid formed directly by malignant cells
Low grade central osteosarcoma	Medullary		Mildly atypical fibroblastic + thick bone trabeculae
Telangiectatic osteosarcoma	Medullary		Blood-filled spaces + fibrous septae + highly malignant osteoid

Contd...

Table 27.43: Salient features of most common primary malignant bone tumors *(Contd...)*

Tumor/lesion	Locations	Age predilection	Salient pathological features
Parosteal osteosarcoma	Cortex outside periosteum	10–20 years, >40 bimodal	Mildly atypical fibroblastic proliferation + thick bone trabeculae
Periosteal osteosarcoma	Cortex inside periosteum		Abundant cartilage matrix with variable malignant osteoid
Ewing's sarcoma (primitive neuroectodermal tumors)			
Ewing's sarcoma	Diaphysis of long bones	5–20 years	Small round blue cells ± rosettes, characteristic IHC translocation
Fibrous/fibrohistiocytic malignant tumors			
Fibrosarcoma	Metaphysis of long bones, may extend to end of bone	20–60 years	Malignant spindle cells in a fascicular pattern
Malignant fibrous histiocytoma	Metaphysis of long bones, may extend to end of bone	20–80 years	Malignant spindle cells in storiform pattern + histiocytic cells (other patterns may be seen)
Hematolymphoid malignant tumors			
Myeloma	Skull, vertebrae, pelvis, long bones	>40 years	Variably atypical (monoclonal) plasma cells
Lymphoma	Any bone	Any age group	Lymphoid proliferations similar to non-bony lesions
Notochord derived tumors			
Chordoma	Base of skull, sacrum	>30 years	Lobules of vacuolated cells embedded in myxoid matrix
Blood vessels derived malignant tumors			
Angiosarcoma and hemangioendothelioma		20–60 years	Anastomosing vascular channels lined by highly atypical cells or vacuolated cells in myxoid background; characteristic immunochemistry staining
Miscellaneous tumors			
Adamantinoma	Cortex of tibia and/or fibula	20–35 years	Epithelial cells + fibroblasts + woven or lamellar bone
Metastatic cancers	Any bone	>40 years	IHC confirmatory

JOINTS

GENERAL CONSIDERATIONS

Joints are classified into three categories described as under:

- *Synarthroses joints:* These fibrous immovable joints do not allow any movement. Examples are *coronal suture of skull and root of teeth in socket.*
- *Amphiarthroses joints:* These are cartilaginous or lightly movable joints. The bones involved are joined together with the help of cartilages. These permit limited movements. Examples are *intervertebral joints and pubic symphysis.*
- *Diarthroses joints:* These synovial joints contain synovial fluid in synovial cavity between the articulating surfaces of the two bones.

Such an arrangement allows considerable free movements. Examples of synovial joints are shown in Table 27.44.

Table 27.44: Salient features of diarthroses (synovial joints)

Diarthroses (synovial joints)	Examples
Ball and socket joints	Shoulder joint (between humerus and pectoral girdle)
Hinge joint	Knee and elbow joints
Pivot joint	Atlas rotation around axis vertebrae
Gliding joint	Joint between carpal bones of upper limb
	Joint between navicular and tarsus bone of foot
Saddle joint	Joint between trapezium and metacarpal of thumb
Condyloid joint	Joint between carpals and radius

Synovial Joints

Synovium is a glistening white membrane with villous projections. Synovium lines the inner surface of the joint capsule.

Factors affecting movement of diarthroses include structure or shape of the articulating bones, strength and tension of the joint ligaments and arrangement, and tension of the skeletal muscles around the joints (Fig. 27.44).

Arthroscopy

Arthroscopy is a procedure that involves examination of the interior of joint especially knee to determine the nature and extent of injury.

ARTHRITIS OF PROBABLE AUTOIMMUNE ORIGIN

RHEUMATOID ARTHRITIS

Rheumatoid arthritis is a chronic multisystem disorder of unknown cause. Its hallmark is persistent inflammatory synovitis involving bilateral peripheral joints (*proximal interphalangeal and metacarpophalangeal joints of the hands*) in a symmetric distribution. Surrounding muscles, tendons, ligaments, blood vessels and knee joints may be involved.

Age Group

It is potentially crippling disease affecting more often in women between 20 and 50 years of age. It occurs most often in HLA-DR4-positive individuals.

Hallmark of Disorder

Subcutaneous nodules and *rheumatoid factor (autoantibodies principally IgM or IgG or IgA)* are hallmarks of disease. These autoantibodies are directed against the Fc fragment of IgG.

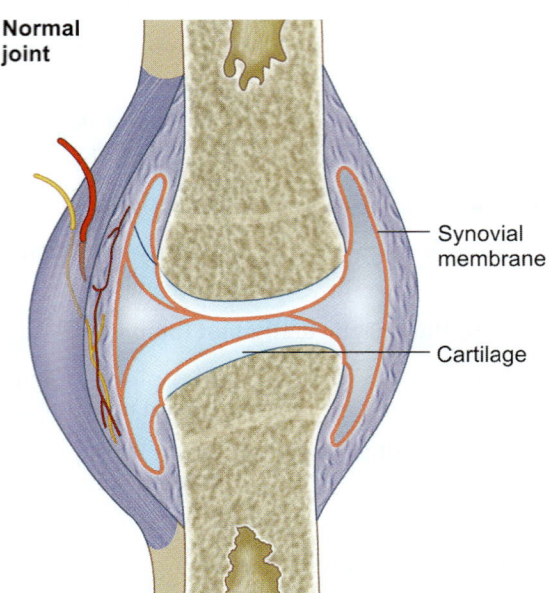

Fig. 27.44: Synovial joint is most common type of diarthrodial joints, which is covered by hyaline articular cartilage composed of collagen proteoglycans and water. This joint is enclosed in capsule. Joints are affected mostly by inflammatory and degenerative diseases.

Rheumatoid factor is demonstrated in the serum in 80% of classic rheumatoid arthritis patients. Rheumatoid factor is useful in diagnosis. Significant titers of RF may also be demonstrated in related collagen vascular diseases, such as *systemic lupus erythematosus, scleroderma, and dermatomyositis*.

Pathological Changes

Pathological changes in rheumatoid arthritis are shown in Fig. 27.45.

- *Inflammatory stage:* Synovitis develops from *congestion and edema of the synovial membrane and joint capsule*. Initially, it shows *acute inflammation* followed by infiltration by lymphocytes and plasma cells. *Synovial cells undergo hyperplasia and hypertrophy with formation of numerous villi and frond-like folds.*

- *Formation of pannus (thickened layers of granulation tissue):* It covers and invades articular cartilage and subchondral bone. It eventually erodes and destroys the joint capsule and bone.

- *Fibrous ankyloses:* It occurs as a result of fibrous invasion of the pannus and scar formation that occludes the joint space. Bone atrophy and misalignment cause visible deformities and restrict movement, causing muscle atrophy, imbalance, and possibly partial dislocations.

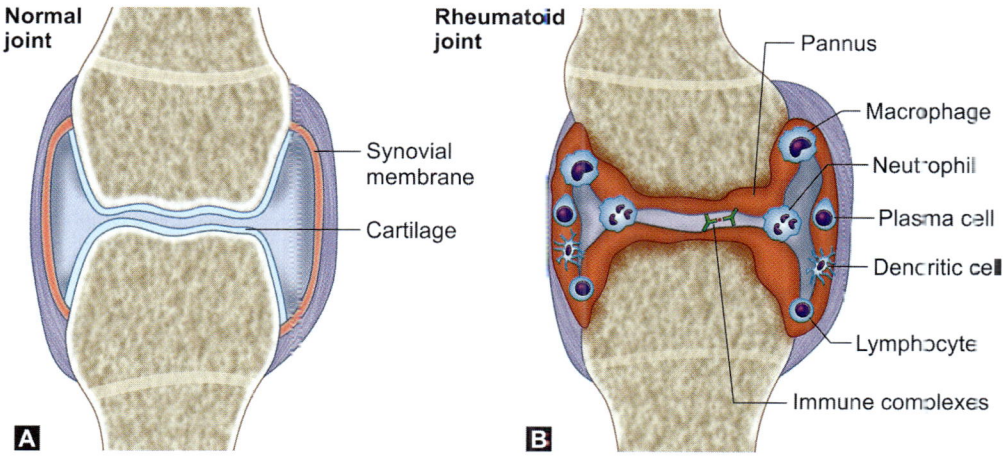

Fig. 27.45: Rheumatoid arthritis—(A) normal synovial joint, (B) pathological changes.

- *Bony ankyloses:* Fibrous tissue calcifies, resulting in bony ankylosis (fixation of a joint) and total immobility. Pain associated with movement may restrict active joint use and cause fibrous or bony ankylosis, soft tissue contractures, and joint deformities. Subcutaneous nodules develop in approximately one-third of patients.

Clinical Features

- *Acute phase:* Patient presents with fatigue, malaise, anorexia, weight loss, fever, and myalgia, bilateral symmetrical swelling and stiffness of joints especially in the morning or after inactivity.
- *Chronic phase:* Patient develops flexion contracture resembling curve of a *swan-neck* as a result of flexion of metacarpophalangeal joints and distal interphalangeal joints.

  Boutonnière deformity occurs as a result of flexion of proximal interphalangeal with compensatory hyperextension of distal interphalangeal joints.

  Patient develops *ulnar deviation (drift) of fingers* resulting from stretching of the articular capsule and muscle imbalance.

  Minimal radial deviation of the wrist may occur. Rheumatoid nodules are formed in metacarpophalangeal joints and distal interphalangeal joints (Figs 27.46 and 27.47).

Extra-articular Manifestations

These include effusions (pleura, pericardium), vasculitis, and anemia of chronic disease, neurologic manifestations, lymphadenopathy and secondary reactive amyloidosis.

Association of Rheumatoid Arthritis

- *Sjögren syndrome:* Patient with Sjögren syndrome is associated with rheumatoid arthritis. It is a chronic inflammatory disease of the salivary (xerostomia) and lacrimal glands (keratoconjunctivitis sicca). It may be associated with a systemic collagen vascular disease. Malignant lymphoma is a frequent complication.
- *Felty syndrome:* It is characterized by splenomegaly, neutropenia, and rheumatoid arthritis.
- *Still disease (juvenile rheumatoid arthritis):* Approximately 20% of children with juvenile arthritis (polyarticular) present with fever, rash, hepatosplenomegaly, lymphadenopathy, pleuritis, and anemia.

  Many children with juvenile arthritis develop ankylosing spondylitis, rheumatoid arthritis, psoriatic arthritis, and other connective tissue diseases.

Light Microscopy

- Histopathological changes occur due to destruction of the joint.
- Synovium undergoes hypertrophy and hyperplasia along with lymphocytes and plasma cells infiltration.
- Lymphoid follicles, acute fibrinous surface exudate, synovial giant cells may be seen.
- Destruction of cartilage and joint fusion (ankylosis) may occur due to the formation of pannus.
- Pannus is composed of inflamed synovium and granulation tissue over the surface of overlying cartilage (Fig. 27.48).

Section III: Systemic Pathology

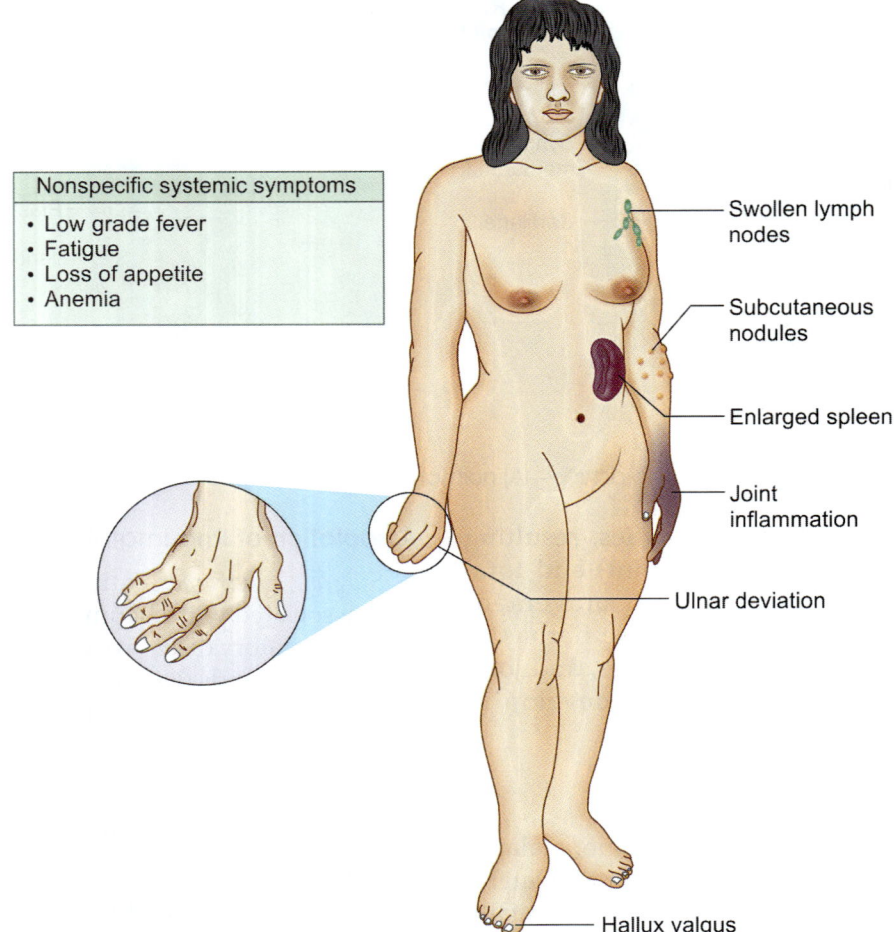

Fig. 27.46: Rheumatoid nodules over an interphalangeal joint of a patient with rheumatoid arthritis.

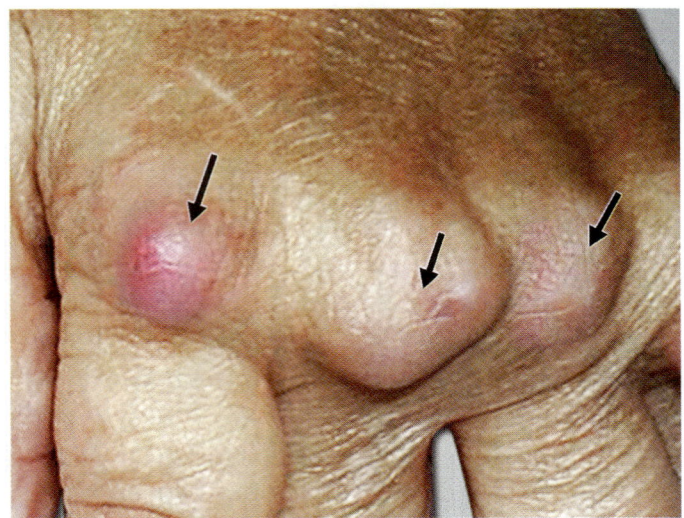

Fig. 27.47: Rheumatoid nodule (arrows).

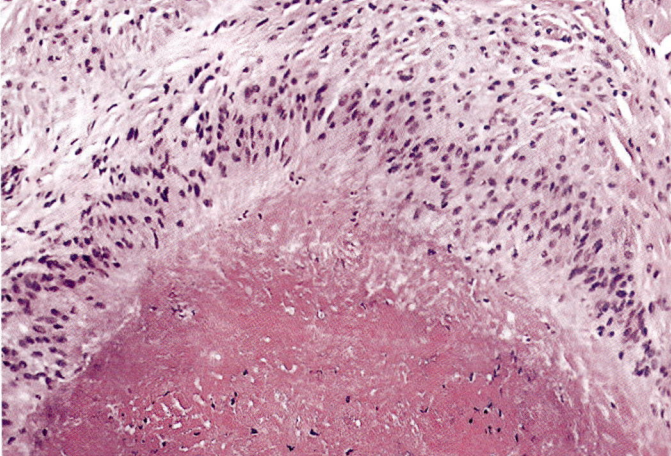

Fig. 27.48: Rheumatoid nodule. It is composed of lymphocytes, plasma cells, lymphoid follicles, acute fibrinous surface exudate, synovial giant cells may be seen (100X).

ANKYLOSING SPONDYLITIS

Ankylosing spondylitis is probably autoimmune disorder with genetic component. It most often affects vertebral column and sacroiliac joints especially in young men. Bony fusion (ankylosis) causes rigidity and fixation of the spine (Fig. 27.49).

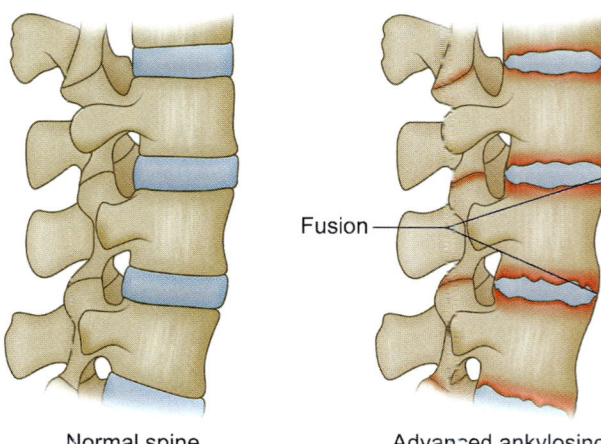

Fig. 27.49: Ankylosing spondylitis shows fusion of vertebrae.

Etiology

Ankylosing spondylitis occurs in various settings.
- *Genetic predisposition:* Almost all patients are positive for HLA-B27 antigen in 90% of cases
- *Reiter syndrome:* It is triad that includes seronegative polyarthritis, conjunctivitis, and urethritis. It is often associated with venereal or bacillary dysentery in men. It is also associated with HLA-B27 antigen in up to 90% of patients.
- *Psoriatic arthritis:* It occurs in approximately 10% of patients with psoriasis. Patient develops peripheral arthritis or ankylosing spondylitis complicating psoriasis.
- *Arthritis associated with inflammatory bowel disease:* Patient develops peripheral arthritis or ankylosing spondylitis complicating ulcerative colitis or Crohn's disease.

DEGENERATIVE JOINT DISEASE

OSTEOARTHRITIS

Osteoarthritis is a slowly progressive destruction of the articular cartilage. Primary osteoarthritis is of unknown etiology and related to mechanical injury (*wear-and-tear*) and genetic predisposition. Secondary osteoarthritis occurs due to mechanical factors, ochronosis and inflammatory disorders.

Age Group

It involves weight-bearing joints and interphalangeal joints especially in women more than 50 years of age.

Pathogenesis

Articular cartilage loses its elasticity results to fragmentation, which floats into synovial fluid. Floating cartilage erodes bone, which exhibits polished, ivory-like appearance (eburnation). It is accompanied by new bone formation (osteocytes) subchondrally and at the margins of the affected joint.

Clinical Examination

Osteophytes (bony spurs) are formed at points of ligamental attachment to bone.

Osteophytes formed at distal interphalangeal joints are known as *Heberden nodes and Bouchard nodes* at proximal interphalangeal joints. Osteophytes undergo fracturing and floating into synovial fluid known as *joint mice*.

> **Gross Morphology**
> - Gross examination reveals cartilaginous thinning, disruption and fibrillation.
> - There is complete loss of cartilage which causes exposure of underlying bone exhibiting dense polished marble-like appearance
>
> **Light Microscopy**
> - Histopathological examination shows characteristic vertical clefts in the cartilage.
> - There may be associated chronic inflammation of synovium and villus hyperplasia.
> - Later findings should not be confused with rheumatoid arthritis.

ARTHRITIS OF METABOLIC ORIGIN

GOUTY ARTHRITIS

Gout is a metabolic disorder of disturbed purine metabolism, associated with elevated serum uric acid. It occurs primarily in men over 40 years of age.

The deposition of monosodium urate crystals leads to formation of gouty tophi in metatarsophalangeal joint of the great toe (podagra), cartilage of helix and antihelix of the ear, and the Achilles tendon.

Joint involvement is extremely painful acute arthritis and bursitis.

Pathogenesis

- When sodium urate crystals precipitate from supersaturated body fluids, these absorb fibronectin, complement, and other proteins on their surfaces. It initiates intense inflammatory reaction with opsonization of crystals by IgG.
- Neutrophils phagocytose urate crystals resulting in release of proteolytic lysosomal enzymes and oxygen derived free radicals. It mediates tissue injury and promotes an inflammatory response. It eventually leads to the formation of nodular tophi.

- *Gouty tophus* is an extracellular soft tissue deposit of urate crystals surrounded by fibrous connective tissue, foreign body giant cells and mononuclear cells.

Variants of Gout

- *Primary gout:* Primary gout, the most common type of gout (85%). It is characterized by hyperuricemia without evident cause affecting middle-aged men.
- *Secondary gout:* It is much less common and characterized by hyperuricemia with evident cause, such as multiple myeloma, leukemia, myeloproliferative syndromes. Patient with chronic renal disease has decreased urate excretion.

  Lesch-Nyhan syndrome is an X-linked disorder due to deficiency of hypoxanthine-guanine phosphoribosyl transferase (HGPRT) which produces hyperuricemia with severe neurological manifestations.

Clinical Features

Patient presents with features due to acute gout arthritis and urate nephropathy described as under:

- *Acute gouty arthritis:* Acute gout usually involves first the metatarsophalangeal joint. Clinical examination reveals redness, swelling, heat and extreme tenderness. In this characteristic location is known as *podagra*. A large meal or alcohol intake, both of which may increase hyperuricemia, often precipitates an exacerbation of the disorder.
- *Urate nephropathy:* Gout often leads to urate nephropathy characterized by interstitial deposition of urate crystals and obstruction of collecting tubules by urate crystals and by formation of urate and calcium stones.

> ### Light Microscopy
> - Chronic accumulation of uric acid crystals leads to the formation of nodules (tophi) that contain granuloma-like aggregates of macrophages.
> - Gouty tophus is composed of multiple irregular foci of amorphous pink stained material by surrounded foreign body giant cells reaction (Fig. 27.50).
> - These tophi may show secondary calcification and ossification. Gouty tophi may be demonstrated by *De Galantha (silver impregnation) stain*.

Diagnosis

The diagnosis is based on the finding of hyperuricemia along with urate crystals and neutrophils in synovial fluid or with biopsy evidence of tophaceous deposits; urate crystals are needle-shaped and negatively birefringent under polarized light.

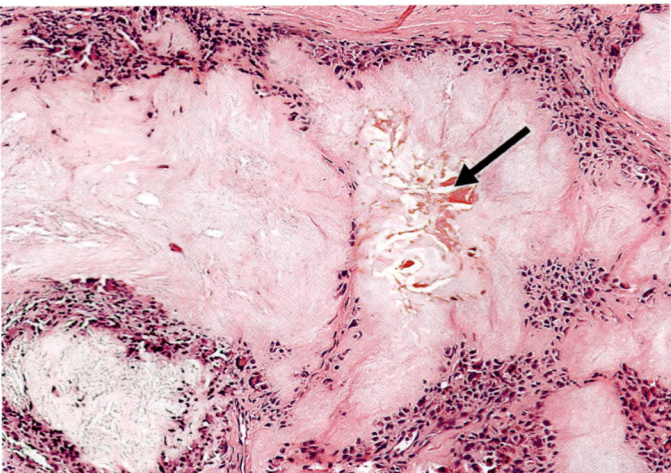

Fig. 27.50: Gouty tophus shows multiple irregular foci of amorphous pink stained material of surrounded foregin body giant cells reaction (arrow) (100X).

CHONDROCALCINOSIS (PSEUDOGOUT)

Chondrocalcinosis (pseudogout) occurs due to deposition of calcium pyrophosphate dihydrate crystals in the synovial membranes (pseudogout), joint cartilage, ligaments, and tendon; which elicits an inflammatory reaction in cartilage. *Under polarized light, these rhomboidin shaped crystals are positively birefringent.*

Pseudogout clinically resembles gout. It refers to self-limited attacks of acute arthritis lasting from 1 day to 4 weeks and involving one or two joints. It most often affects older than 85 years.

Clinical Features

Patient presents with acute onset of gout-like symptoms, manifesting as inflammation and swelling of the knees, ankles, wrists, elbows, hips, or shoulders.

OCHRONOSIS OF JOINTS

Ochronosis is deposition of polymerized homogentisic acid, a black pigment, which is the product of incomplete degradation of tyrosine and phenylalanine occurring due to inborn metabolism of enzyme homogentisic acid oxidase.

Joints Involved

Homogentisic acid is deposited in articular cartilage of vertebral column and later hips, knees and shoulder joints.

Cartilage of nose and ears is also affected. Larger joints may be distended by effusions, which is usually non-inflammatory and synovium is hypertrophied.

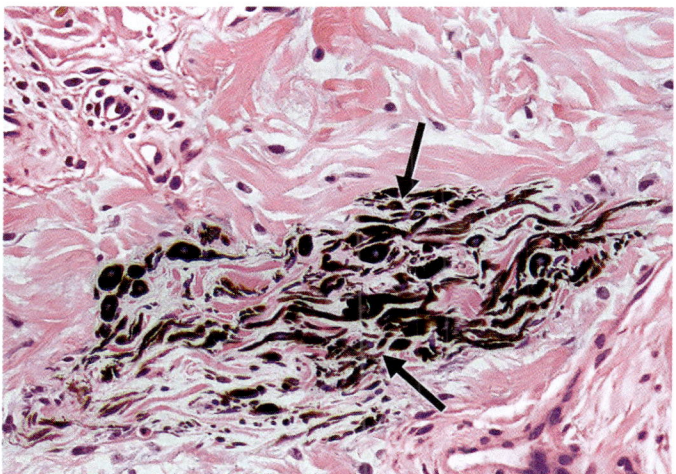

Fig. 27.51: Ochronosis showing deposition of homogentisic acid in cartilage (400X).

> **Light Microscopy**
>
> It shows granular pigment in chondrocytes and matrix is diffusely stained. Synovium shows evidence of acute or chronic inflammation (Fig. 27.51).

INFECTIVE ARTHRITIS

Infective arthritis is characterized by purulent synovial fluid.

GONOCOCCAL ARTHRITIS

Gonococcal arthritis is caused by *Neisseria gonorrhoeae*. It is the most common form of bacterial arthritis (monoarticular). It most often involves knee joint. Other joints such as wrist and small joints of the hand may also be affected.

LYME DISEASE

Spirochete *Borrelia burgdorferi* transmitted by a tick causes Lyme disease.

Clinical Features

Patient presents with erythema chronicum migrans with central fading (bull's eye lesion), polyarticular arthritis involving larger joints (especially knee joints). It can also lead to myocardial, pericardial, or neurologic changes as late sequelae.

Diagnosis

It is diagnosed by demonstration of IgM serum antibodies to *Borrelia burgdorferi*.

Treatment

Response to early treatment with antibiotics is good.

TUBERCULAR ARTHRITIS

Hip joint is most often involved in tuberculosis. There is fullness of groin and lower buttocks with loss of gluteal fold on affected side, flexion of hip or thigh and pain on pressure.

MISCELLANEOUS DISORDERS OF JOINTS

HYPERTROPHIC OSTEOARTHROPATHY

Hypertrophic osteoarthropathy is associated with systemic diseases such as chronic lung disease, congenital cyanotic heart disease, cirrhosis of liver, and inflammatory bowel disease.

Patient develops clubbing of the fingers (most frequent), inflammation of distal end of the radius and ulna. Patient presents with painful swelling and tenderness of the peripheral joints.

GANGLION CYST

This small cystic nodule arising in the tendon sheath or the joint capsule of the wrist is thought to be caused by myxoid degeneration of connective tissue.

PSEUDOARTHROSIS

If a fracture site does not heal, the condition is termed nonunion. It occurs due to interposition of soft tissues at the fracture site, excessive motion, infection, and poor blood supply.

Continued movement at the unhealed fracture may produce pseudoarthrosis. This joint-like material must be surgically excised for the fracture to heal properly.

CHAPTER 28

Soft Tissue Tumors and Skeletal Myopathies

Learning Objectives

SOFT TISSUE TUMORS

- Adipocytic Tumors
- Fibroblastic/Myofibroblastic Reactive Lesions and Tumors
- Fibrohistiocytic Tumors
- Skeletal Muscle Tumors
- Smooth Muscle Tumors
- Perivascular Tumors
- Tumors of Uncertain Origin
- Neural Tumors
- Vascular Tumors

SKELETAL MUSCLES

- Skeletal Muscle Atrophies
- Skeletal Muscle Dystrophies
- Congenital Myopathies
- Inflammatory Myopathies

SOFT TISSUE TUMORS

Soft tissue tumors originate in fibrous connective tissue, adipose tissue, skeletal muscle, joint tissue, blood vessels, lymphatic channels and the peripheral nervous system (neuroectoderm). Benign soft tissue tumors are more common than malignant counterpart. Classification of soft tissue tumors (Table 28.1).

General Principles of Diagnosis

- *Location:* Deep seated soft tissue tumors tend to be malignant than located in superficial region.
- *Size:* Large-sized soft tissue tumors most often tend to be malignant.
- *Growth pattern:* Rapidly growing soft tissue tumors with infiltrative margins are malignant in nature.
- *Metastases:* Soft tissue tumors metastasizing to distant organs are malignant.

Approach to Diagnosis

Soft tissue tumors are diagnosed by histopathological examination, special stains, immunohistochemistry, cytogenetic study, molecular analysis and electron microscopy. Immunohistochemistry study includes *cytokeratin, vimentin, smooth muscle cell actin, desmin, S-100 protein, CD31 and CD34.*

Molecular Genetics

Cytogenetic aberrations in soft tissue sarcomas are shown in Table 28.2.

Etiopathogenesis

Etiology of most of the soft tissue tumors is known. Some of these are associated with radiation therapy, chemical burns, heat burns or trauma; and exposure to phenoxyherbicides and chlorophenols.

Kaposi sarcoma has been documented in patients with AIDS. Most soft tissue sarcomas occur sporadically. However, minority of these tumors are associated with neurofibromatosis type I (neurofibroma, malignant schwannoma), Li-Fraumeni syndrome (soft tissue sarcoma), Gardner's syndrome (fibromatosis) and Osler-Weber-Rendu syndrome (telangiectasis).

Soft Tissue Tumors and Skeletal Myopathies

Table 28.1: Classification of soft tissue tumors

Histological type	Benign tumors	Malignant tumors
Adipose tissue	Lipoma	Liposarcoma
Fibrous tissue	Fibroma Desmoid type fibromatosis Myositis ossificans Nodular fasciitis	Adult and infantile fibrosarcoma
Fibrohistiocytic tumors	Tenosynovial giant cell tumor Benign fibrous histiocytoma	Malignant fibrous histiocytoma
Skeletal muscle	Rhabdomyoma	Rhabdomyosarcoma
Smooth muscle	Leiomyoma	Leiomyosarcoma
Vascular tissue	Hemangioma Lymphangioma	Angiosarcoma Kaposi sarcoma
Peripheral nerves	Schwannoma Neurofibroma Granular cell tumor	Malignant peripheral nerve sheath tumor
Perivascular tumors	Glomus tumors	–
Uncertain histiogenesis	–	Synovial sarcoma Clear cell sarcoma of soft tissue Alveolar soft part sarcoma Epithelioid sarcoma

Table 28.2: Cytogenetic aberrations in soft tissue sarcomas

Tumor type	Cytogenetic changes	Gene rearrangement	Reason for testing
Ewing's sarcoma/peripheral primitive neuroectodermal tumour	t(11;22) (q24;q12) t(21;22) (q22;q12) t(7;22) (q22;q12) t(17;22) (q12;q12) t(2;22) (q33;q12) t(16;22) (p11;q22)	FLI-1-EWSR-1 ERG-EWSR-1 ETV-1-EWSR-1 EIAF-EWSR-1 FEV-EWSR-1 FUS-ERG	Differentiate from other small round cell tumors
Alveolar rhabdomyosarcoma	t(2;13) (q35;q14) t(1;13) (p36;q14)	PAX-3-FOXO1A PAX-7-FOXO1A	Better prognosis Poor prognosis
Myxoid/round cell liposarcoma	t(12;16) (q13;q11) t(12;22) (q13;q11-12)	DDIT-3-FUS DDIT-3-EWSR-1	Diagnostic
Desmoplastic small round cell tumor	t(11;22) (p13;q12)	WT-1-EWSR-1	Poor prognosis
Synovial sarcoma	t(X;18) (p12.2;q11.2)	SSX-1-SS-18 SSX-2-SS-18	Diagnostic
Clear cell sarcoma	t(12;22) (q13;q12) t(2;22) (q33;q12)	ATF-1-EWSR-1 CREB-1-EWSR-1	Distinguishing from cutaneous melanoma
Extraskeletal myxoid chondrosarcoma	t(9;22) (q22;q12) t(9;17) (q22;q11)	NR4A3-EWSR-1 NR4A3-TAF-15	Diagnostic
Dermatofibrosarcoma protuberans	t(17;22) (q22;q13)	PDGFB-COL1A1	Diagnostic and excellent prognosis
Infantile fibrosarcoma	t(12;15) (p13;q25)	ETV-6-NTRK-3	Differentiate from more aggressive adult fibrosarcoma
Alveolar soft part sarcoma	t(X;17) (p11;q25)	ASPL-TFE-3	Diagnostic
Low grade fibromyxoid sarcoma	t(7;16) (q33;p11) t(11;16) (q13;p11)	FUS-CREB3L2 FUS-CREB3L1	Prognosis variable

Contd...

Table 28.2: Cytogenetic aberrations in soft tissue sarcomas (Contd...)

Tumor type	Cytogenetic changes	Gene rearrangement	Reason for testing
Inflammatory myofibroblastic tumor	t(2;1) (p23;p23) t(2;19) (p23;p13) t(2;17) (p23;q23) t(2;11) (p23;p15) t(2;2) (p23;q13)	ALK-TPM-3 ALK-TPM-4 ALK-CLTC ALK-CARS ALK-RANBP-2	-
Myxoinflammatory fibroblastic sarcoma	t(1;10) (p22;q24q)	TGFBR-3-MGEA-5	-
Myoepithelial carcinoma	t(6;22) (p22;q12) t(1;22) (q23;q12) t(19;22) (q13;q12)	EWSR-1-POU5F-1 EWSR-1-PBX-1 EWSR-1-ZNF-444	-
Epithelioid hemangioendothelioma	t(1;13) (p36.3;q25)	WWTR-1CAMTA-1	-
Mesenchymal chondrosarcoma	t(8;8) (q21.1;q13.3)	HEY-1-NCOA-2	-
Undifferentiated (Ewing-like) sarcoma	t(4;19) (q35;q13.1) t(4;10) (q35;q26)	CIC-DUX-4 CIC-DUX-4	-
Atypical lipomatous tumor/well-differentiated liposarcoma	12q rings and giant markers	HMGA(2), CDK4, and MDM-2 amplification	-

Grading

Malignant soft tissue tumors are graded into three types: low, intermediate and high grades. Well differentiated liposarcoma and myxoid liposarcoma are considered as low grade neoplasms.

High grade malignant soft tissue tumors are rhabdomyosarcoma, synovial sarcoma, mesenchymal chondrosarcoma and extraskeletal Ewing's sarcoma.

ADIPOCYTIC TUMORS

LIPOMA

It is the most common soft tissue tumor of mature adipose tissue. It is well encapsulated mass of mature adipocytes. It varies considerably in size. It is soft, mobile and painless lump. It is cured by surgical excision

Locations

It most often appears in the subcutaneous tissues of the upper half of the body, especially on the trunk and neck in adults. Infrequently, lipomas are large and circumscribed located in intramuscular tissue.

Molecular Genetics

Conventional lipomas often show rearrangements of HMGA2 gene localized to 12q14–15, 6p and 13q. Spindle cell and pleomorphic variants of lipomas have rearrangements of 16q and 13q.

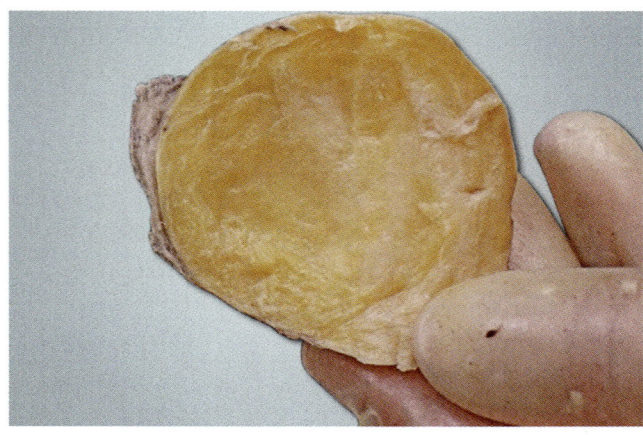

Fig. 28.1: Lipoma. Tumor is encapsulated. Cut surface is yellowish.

Gross Morphology
Tumor is encapsulated. Cut surface is yellowish (Fig. 28.1).

Light Microscopy
- Histologically, a lipoma is often indistinguishable from normal adipose tissue.
- It is composed of lobules of well differentiated adipocytes. There is no pleomorphism (Fig. 28.2).
- Lipomas can occasionally have areas of bone formation (osteolipoma), abundant fibrous tissue (fibrolipoma) or cartilage (chondrolipoma).

Soft Tissue Tumors and Skeletal Myopathies

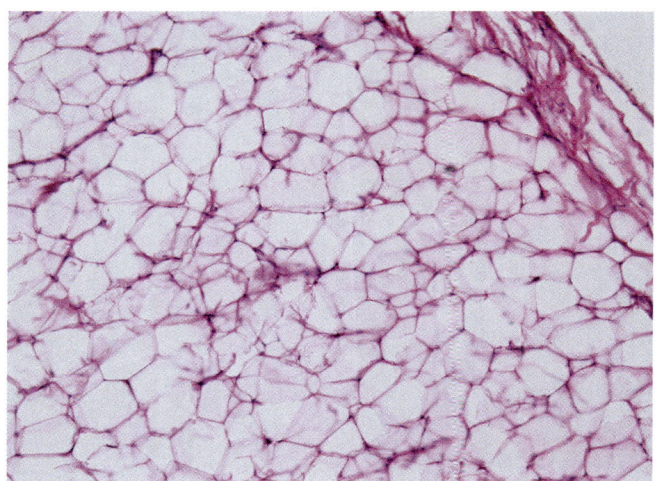

Fig. 28.2: Lipoma. It is composed of lobules of well differentiated adipocytes (400X).

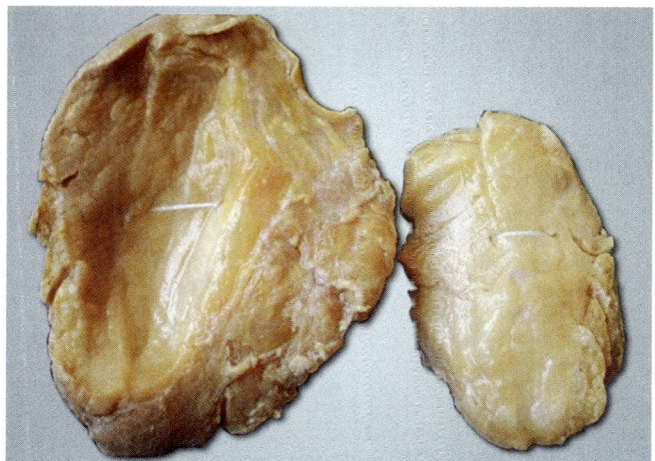

Fig. 28.3: Hibernoma. Cut surface of this lobulated tumor is tan-yellow.

HIBERNOMA

Hibernomas are rare benign encapsulated and richly vascularized adipose tumor seen in young adults in 3rd to 4th decades of life.

Locations

Thigh followed by trunk/chest, upper extremity and head and neck.

Gross Morphology
Hibernoma is lobulated well demarcated tan-yellow to red-brown having a spongy cut surface (Figs 28.3 and 28.4).

Light Microscopy
Hibernoma contains a large number of brown fat cells with multi-vacuolization, granular cytoplasm and small central nucleus. Tumor cells are positive for **S-100 protein**.

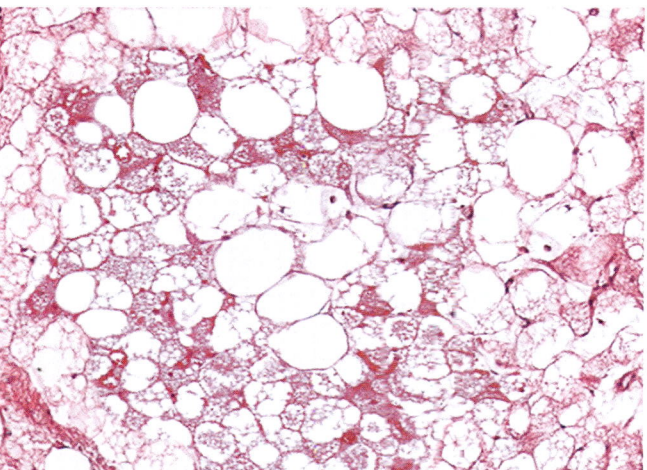

Fig. 28.4: Hibernoma. The cells have numerous small fatty vacuoles, and the small round nuclei often are centrally located. Some cells have a more granular cytoplasm. Genetically, hibernomas have rearrangements at 11q13 (100X).

Molecular Genetics

All hibernomas have breakpoints in 11q13 with many translocation partners.

Prognosis

It is benign tumor with no significant potential for recurrence after surgical excision.

LIPOSARCOMA

Liposarcomas are one of the malignant tumors of adipose tissue of adults during 4th to 6th decades of life. These most often arise in the deep soft tissues of the proximal extremities and retroperitoneal region. *Histological variants include well differentiated, myxoid, round cell and pleomorphic types.*

Light Microscopy
Histologically liposarcomas can be divided into four subtypes: • *Well differentiated liposarcoma:* It is composed of adipocytes with atypical hyperchromatic stromal cells (Fig. 28.5). • *Myxoid liposarcoma:* It shows abundant extracellular basophilic mucin creating a pulmonary edema like growth pattern with arborizing *chicken wire capillaries* and primitive cells at various stages of differentiation resembling fetal fat. Myxoid and round cell variants have the same translocations. Most have t(12;16) (q13;p11) resulting in FUS-DDIT3 fusion, and a minority harbor t(12;22) (q13;q12) rearrangement with EWSR-DDIT3 fusion (Fig. 28.6).

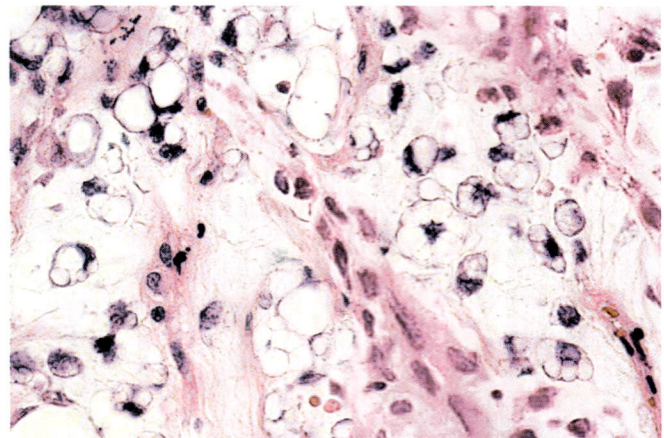

Fig. 28.5: Well differentiated liposarcoma. It is composed of adipocytes with atypical hyperchromatic stromal cells (400X).

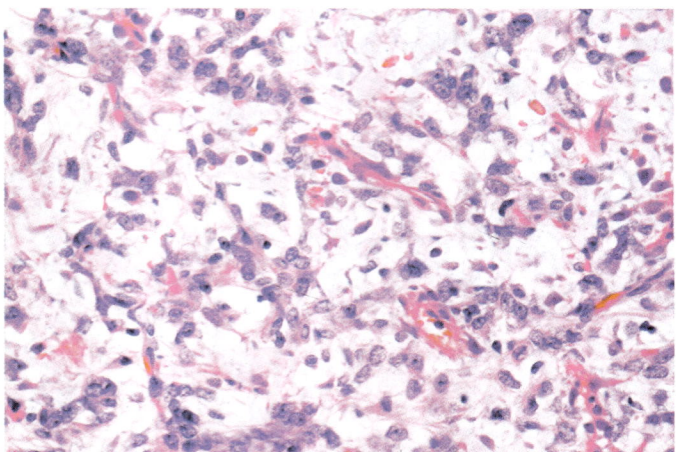

Fig. 28.6: *Myxoid*/round cell liposarcoma. This tumor has small. Uniform spindle cells that are closely related to the capillary blood vessels that are arranged in a characteristic plexiform or *chicken-wire* pattern. Myxoid/round cell liposarcoma occurs in adults mainly in the proximal limbs, especially the thigh and groin and very rarely in the abdomen. Myxoid and round cell variants both have the same translocations. Most have t(12;16)(q13;p11) leading to FUS-DDTIT3 fusion, and a minority harbor t(12;22)(q13;q12) rearrangement with EWSRI-DDIT3 fusion (400X).

- *Pleomorphic liposarcoma:* It shows variable proportion of pleomorphic lipoblasts in a background of a high grade pleomorphic sarcoma (Fig. 28.7).
- *Dedifferentiated pleomorphic liposarcoma:* It constitutes 10% of well differentiated liposarcomas undergoing dedifferentiation to usually an undifferentiated pleomorphic sarcoma or intermediate to high grade myxofibrosarcoma (Figs 28.8 and 28.9).

Prognosis
- All liposarcomas recur locally. Well differentiated liposarcomas are indolent in nature except when located in the retroperitoneum where recurrence is more common.

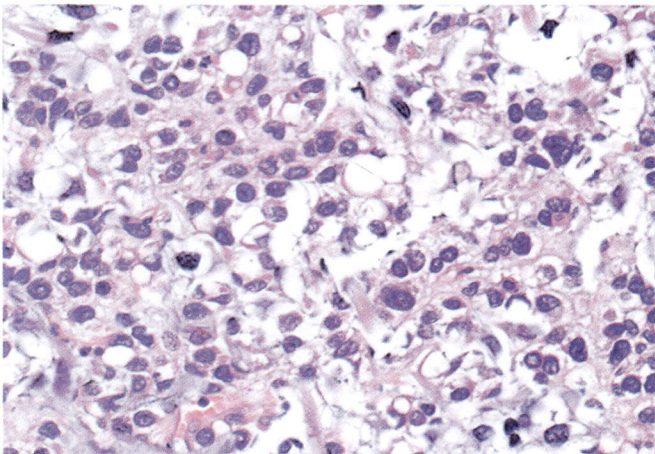

Fig. 28.7: Pleomorphic cell liposarcoma. It shows lipoblasts with minimal pleomorphism. Immunohistochemistry study reveals expression of S-100 protein. Presence of lipoblasts, at least focally, usually is necessary to make the diagnosis of round cell liposarcoma, especially if molecular diagnostic facilities are not available (400X).

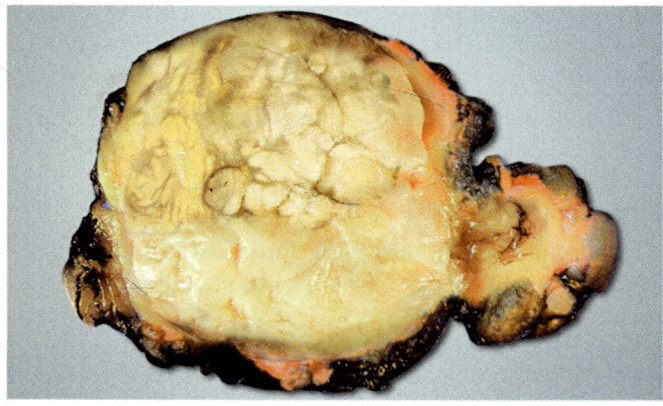

Fig. 28.8: Dedifferentiated liposarcoma. It is most common intra-abdominal neoplasm. Tumor is solid. Clinical course has more aggressive behavior, including metastatic potential.

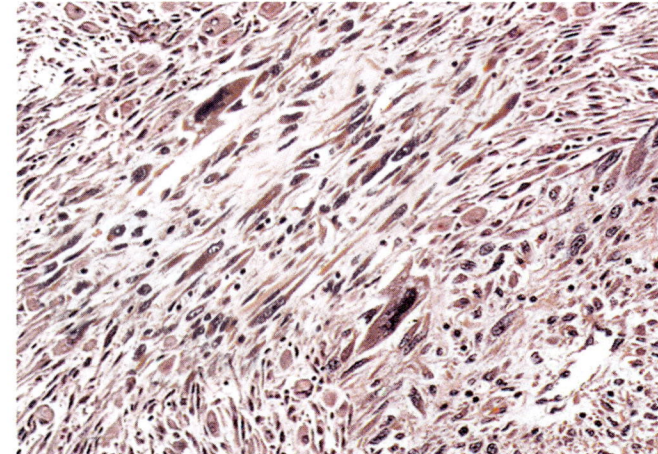

Fig. 28.9: Dedifferentiated pleomorphic liposarcoma. Tumor shows pleomorphic cells, mitoses admixed with inflammatory cells (400X).

- Pleomorphic liposarcomas undergo frequent metastases and behave aggressively whereas myxoid liposarcomas are intermediate in its malignant behavior.

FIBROBLASTIC/MYOFIBROBLASTIC REACTIVE LESIONS AND TUMORS

Reactive lesions include keloid, fibromatosis colli, nodular fasciitis, superficial fibromatosis and deep-seated fibromatosis. Fibroblastic/myofibroblastic tumors include adult/infantile fibrosarcoma and myxoid fibrosarcoma.

KELOID

It is an exaggerated response to injury that produces abundant collagenous soft tissue, forming a large nodular scar.

Etiology

It often follows trauma to the skin, i.e. *ear-piercing* or *surgical wounds*. It most often occurs in dark-skinned persons especially of African lineage. *It tends to recur after resection.*

> ### Light Microscopy
> - On histopathological examination, keloid is composed of dense bundles of collagen fibers in the dermis.
> - These collagen fibers undergo hyalinization and appear as highly eosinophilic acellular material.
> - Keloid should be differentiated from hypertrophic scar (Fig. 28.10 and Table 28.3).

FIBROMATOSIS COLLI

Fibromatosis colli is an uncommon condition characterized by *diffuse fibrous replacement of one sternocleidomastoid muscle*, most often the right. It is also known as *sternomastoid tumor* or *torticollis*. *Antenatal position in utero* appears to be of prime pathogenetic importance.

> ### Light Microscopy
> Histopathological examination reveals diffuse infiltration and replacement of skeletal muscle by hypocellular, often hyalinized, fibrous scar tissue (Fig. 28.11).

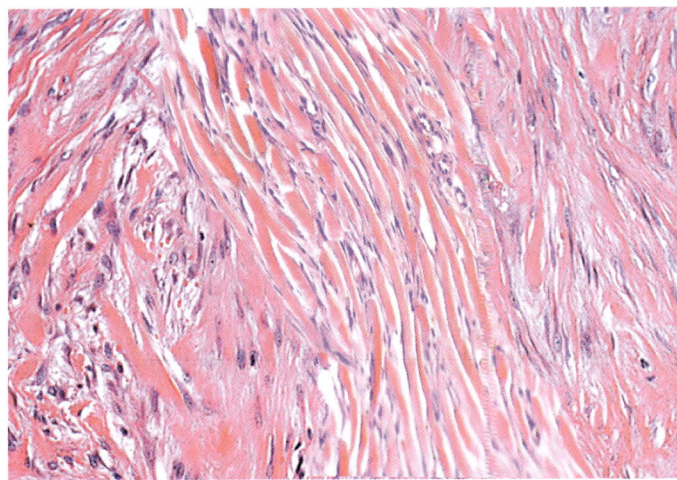

Fig. 28.10: Keloid scar. Thick eosinophilic collagen fibers are a characteristic feature (100X).

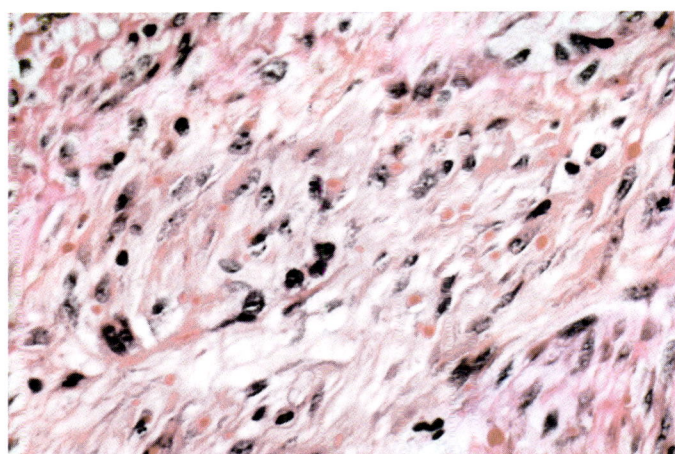

Fig. 28.11: Fibromatosis colli. Cellular fibrous tissue infiltrates fibers of the sternomastoid muscle. It shows late stage of the disease with hypocellular fibrosis (400X).

Table 28.3: Differences between keloid and hypertrophic scar

Parameters	Keloid	Hypertrophic scar
Locations	Face, neck, sternum, forearms and lobes of ear	No predilection
Sex predilection	Females > Males	No sex predilection
Itching and tenderness	Present in smooth lesions	Asymptomatic
Extension beyond the margins of antecedent trauma	Present	Absent
Light microscopy	Cellular fibrous stroma in early stage, later collagen fibers undergo hyalinization and appear as brightly eosinophilic acellular	Persist as relatively cellular fibrous tissue and collagen fibers not undergoing hyalinization
Recurrence	Tend to recur after excision	Occasional recurrence

Prognosis

Many cases resolve spontaneously or with the help of physiotherapy.

NODULAR FASCIITIS

Nodular fasciitis is a self-limiting fibrous pseudo neoplasm that occurs in subcutaneous tissue in young adults.

Location

Upper extremity and trunk are commonly involved.

Gross Morphology

It is poorly circumscribed or infiltrative unencapsulated mass with myxoid or fibrous cut surface.

Light Microscopy

- Nodular fasciitis is composed of plump regular spindle shaped fibroblasts lacking nuclear atypia separated by myxoid stroma giving a torn, feathery or tissue culture like character. Mitotic figures may be present.
- Focally keloidal collagen bundles can be seen.
- Small vessels are numerous giving a resemblance to granulation tissue (Fig. 28.12).

Immunohistochemistry

Smooth muscle actin (SMA) is positive in the fibroblasts.

Prognosis

Recurrence is occasionally observed after incomplete excision.

SUPERFICIAL FIBROMATOSIS

Palmar, plantar or penile fibromatosis constitute small group of superficial fibromatosis. These are characterized by nodular or poorly defined fascicles of mature appearing fibroblasts surrounded by abundant dense collagen fibers. Immunohistochemical and electron microscopy studies indicate that these cells are myofibroblasts. Examples of superficial fibromatosis are *palmar fibromatosis* and *Dupuytren's contracture*.

DESMOID/DEEP-SEATED FIBROMATOSIS

Biologically, deep-seated fibromatosis occurs in the interface between exuberant fibrous proliferations and low grade fibrosarcoma. Three main biologic groups identified: sporadic, i.e. associated with FAP (familial adenomatous polyposis), and multicentric or familial. Patient presents with large infiltrative mass, which does not metastasize.

Gross Morphology

Anatomically, three main subsets are seen: extra-abdominal, abdominal wall and intra-abdominal.

Light Microscopy

Lesion is composed of banal well differentiated fibroblasts (Fig. 28.13).

DERMATOFIBROSARCOMA PROTUBERANS

Dermatofibrosarcoma protuberans is slow growing, solitary or multiple polypoid nodules on the trunk and extremities affecting 20–50 years of adults. It is locally aggressive tumor, which rarely metastasizes.

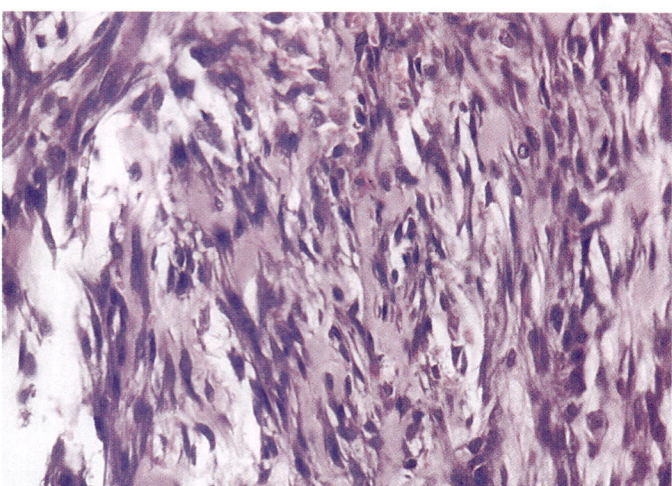

Fig. 28.12: Nodular fasciitis. It shows spindle-shaped fibroblasts separated by myxoid stroma giving a torn, feathery or tissue culture like character. Small vessels are numerous giving a resemblance to granulation tissue (400X).

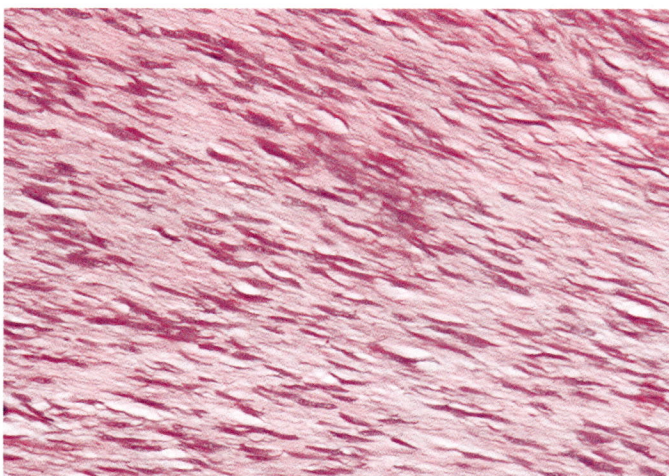

Fig. 28.13: Desmoid tumor. Lesion is composed of banal well differentiated fibroblasts (400X).

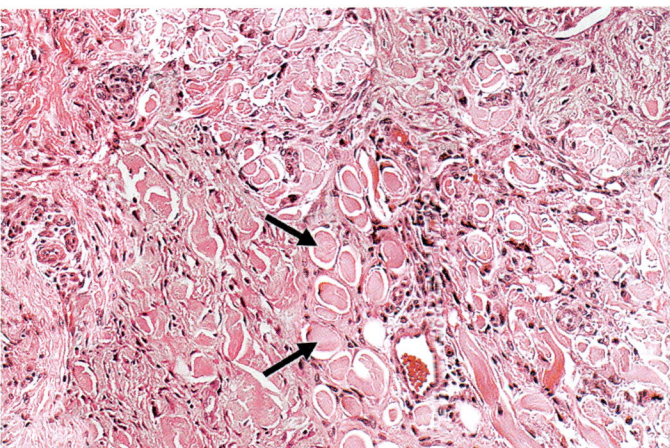

Fig. 28.14: Dermatofibrosarcoma protuberans shows spindle cells forming small storiform pattern or cartwheel appearance extending into the periphery entrapping fat, numerous mitoses and thinned out epidermis (arrows) (400X).

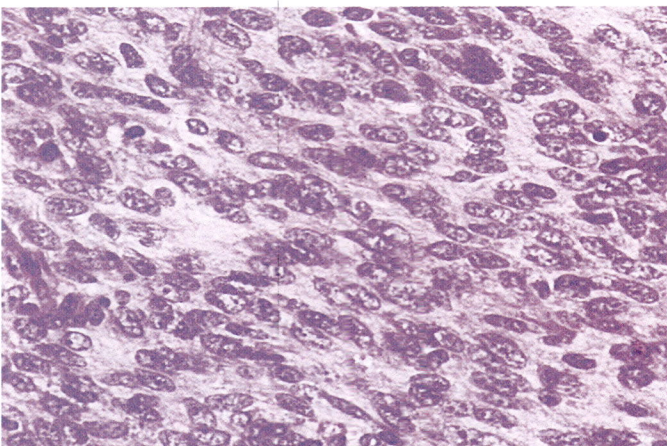

Fig. 28.15: Fibrosarcoma. Tumor is composed of monomorphic spindle cells arranged in long sweeping fascicles in a 'herring-bone pattern' (400X).

Molecular Genetics

Tumor exhibits translocation of t(17;22) (q22;q13) which results in production of a COLLIA1-PDGFB fusion protein.

Light Microscopy

- This cellular tumor is composed of spindle cells forming small *storiform pattern* or *cartwheel appearance* extending into the periphery entrapping fat, numerous mitoses and thinned out epidermis.
- There may be presence of occasional mitotic figures with mild atypia. Overlying epidermis is normal, atrophic, or ulcerated (Fig. 28.14).

Immunohistochemistry

The tumor cells show positivity for **CD34** at periphery of tumor but negative for factor XIIIa.

Differential Diagnosis

Storiform pattern is also demonstrated in dermatofibrosarcoma protuberans, malignant fibrous histiocytoma, liposarcoma, leiomyosarcoma, nerve sheath tumors and occasionally nodular fasciitis.

Prognosis

Prognosis is most often excellent after surgical excision. Metastasis is demonstrated in 5% of cases. Lymph node metastasis may occur in 1% of cases. Recurrence is seen in 11–33% of cases.

ADULT AND INFANTILE FIBROSARCOMA

Fibrosarcoma is a malignant tumor of fibroblasts characterized by spindle-shaped cells demonstrating a *herring-bone pattern*.

Locations

Fibrosarcomas may occur anywhere in the body. Most common sites are *retroperitoneal region, thigh, knee and distal extremities*.

Molecular Genetics

The infantile fibrosarcomas have a specific t(12;15) (p13;q25) translocation, resulting in ETV-6–NTRK-3 fusion (Fig. 28.15).

Gross Morphology

Tumor is unencapsulated infiltrative, and soft fleshy. A little difference is seen between the two groups: adult and infantile fibrosarcoma.

Light Microscopy

Tumor is composed of monomorphic spindle cells arranged in long sweeping fascicles in a *herring-bone pattern*.

MYXOFIBROSARCOMA

Myxofibrosarcoma is a malignant fibroblastic neoplasm with variably prominent myxoid stroma, cellular pleomorphism. It is the most common soft tissue sarcoma of adults in the 6th to 8th decades. The high grade, poorly differentiated end of this spectrum resembles unclassified pleomorphic sarcoma ('MFH') and hence it was also called *myxoid MFH*.

Locations

Limb girdles are affected. *Lower extremities* are more affected than upper extremities.

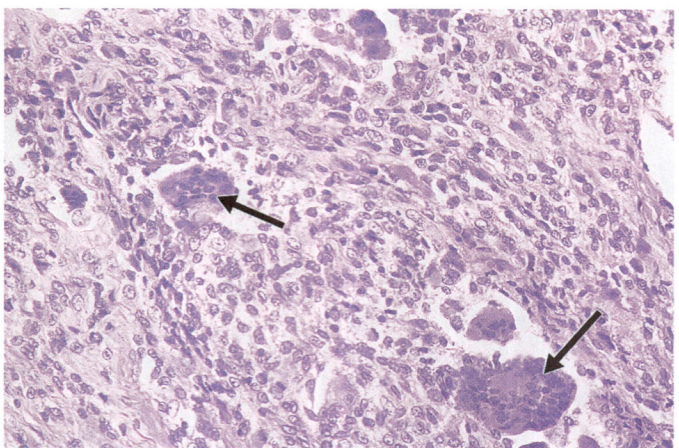

Fig. 28.16: Giant cell tumor of the tendon sheath. Multinucleated cell vary in number from frequent to scanty (arrows) (400X).

Light Microscopy
- Tumor is composed of multinodular pattern with hypocellular areas containing thin-walled curvilinear vessels, atypical, hyperchromatic small spindle and stellate cells with poorly defined, sometimes vacuolated cytoplasm (pseudolipoblasts).
- Tumor can be low grade, intermediate or high grade (Fig. 28.16).

Prognosis
Metastases and mortality are related to the grade of the tumor.

FIBROHISTIOCYTIC TUMORS

LOCALIZED TENOSYNOVIAL GIANT CELL TUMOR

The localized type of tenosynovial giant cell tumor often known in the past as localized nodular tenosynovitis, or giant cell tumor of tendon sheath, is very common. The age at presentation is between 20 and 40 years.

Locations
Digits are affected more commonly.

Gross Morphology
Localized giant cell tumor most often is a well circumscribed, lobulated mass with a variably yellow, tan, or whitish cut surface.

Light Microscopy
Histologically it is composed of rounded eosinophilic mononuclear cells with vesicular nuclei, *osteoclast type multinucleate giant cells*, foamy macrophages, siderophages, and chronic inflammatory cells, sometimes cholesterol clefts and a few osteoclasts.

Prognosis
After local excision, a few cases recur locally.

GIANT CELL TUMOR OF SOFT TISSUE

Giant cell tumor of soft tissue occurs over a wide age range but most frequently in adult.

Location
GCT of soft tissue arises most often in the dermis or subcutis of the limbs.

Gross Morphology
Tumor is well circumscribed and measuring <5 cm.

Light Microscopy
- Histologically, the majority of these tumors are characterized by multiple small nodules that are indistinguishable from giant cell tumor of bone.
- These nodules are distributed in a cellular fibroblastic stroma showing variably prominent hemorrhage and hemosiderin deposition.
- Tumor cells often show frequent mitoses.

Prognosis
Tumors of this type are generally benign but may recur locally. Very rare cases may metastasize.

SKELETAL MUSCLE TUMORS

Rhabdomyosarcomas are the most common malignant tumor exhibiting striated muscle differentiation. These may affect *children* and *adults*. There are several histological variants: *embryonal, alveolar, botryoid* and *pleomorphic rhabdomyosarcomas*.

Overall embryonal rhabdomyosarcoma is the most common variant. Differences between various histological variants of rhabdomyosarcomas are shown in Table 28.4.

EMBRYONAL RHABDOMYOSARCOMA

Embryonal rhabdomyosarcoma is the most common histological variant. It most often occurs in *young children and adolescents especially in head and neck* (orbit).

Light Microscopy
- The tumor is composed of rhabdomyoblasts.
- These appear round strap-shaped, tennis-raquet and spider forms.
- Rhabdomyoblasts exhibit striations (Fig. 28.17).

Table 28.4: Differences between various histological variants of rhabdomyosarcomas

Histological variant	Age group	Features	Immunohistochemistry
Embryonal rhabdomyosarcoma	Children	Some resemblance to developing muscle	Desmin, vimentin, MyoD1, myoglobin
Botryoid rhabdomyosarcoma	Children	Term botryoid (grape-like) polypoid mass with myxoid consistency in mucosa lined organs	Desmin, MyoD1, myoglobin
Alveolar rhabdomyosarcoma	Children and teenagers (10–20 years)	Located in extremities. Small cells arranged in sheets or nests separated by fibrous septa	Myogenin positivity
Pleomorphic rhabdomyosarcoma	6th–7th decades	Lower extremities (usually intra-muscular)	Desmin, MyoD1, myogenin

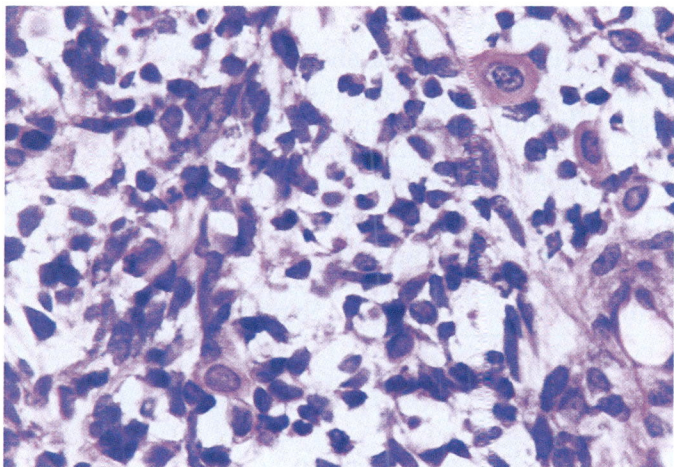

Fig. 28.17: Embryonal rhabdomyosarcoma shows round strap and tennis-raquet shaped rhabdomyoblasts exhibiting striations (400X).

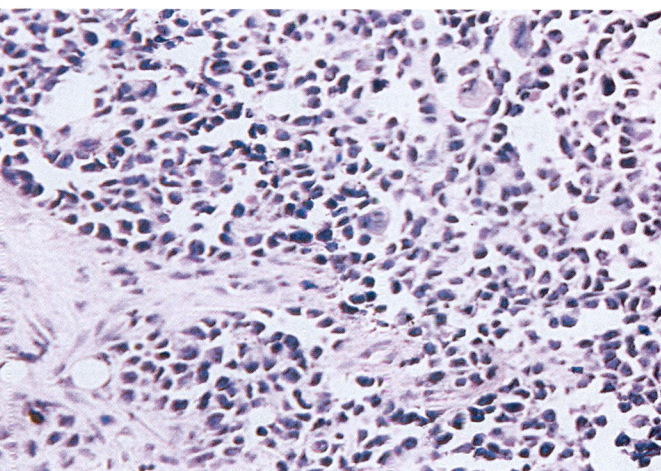

Fig. 28.18: Alveolar rhabdomyosarcoma. Tumor is composed of large round undifferentiated cells arranged in an alveolar pattern (400X).

Immunohistochemistry

Tumor cells show positivity for intermediate filaments like *desmin, vimentin, MyoD1, myoglobin and myogenin.*

Marker	Expression
Desmin	Positive
Vimentin	Positive
MyoD1	Positive
Myoglobin	Positive
Myogenin	Positive

ALVEOLAR RHABDOMYOSARCOMA

It most often affects older children and teenagers. It most often occurs in extremities. It is associated with t(12;13) or t(1;13).

Locations

Extremities are affected more commonly followed by paraspinal and perineal regions.

Gross Morphology

ARMS presents as rapidly growing expansile soft tissue tumor with fleshy appearance and grey-tan color.

Light Microscopy

- Alveolar rhabdomyosarcoma is composed of large, more rounded undifferentiated cells with larger nuclei admixed with variable numbers of eosinophilic rhabdomyoblasts and multinucleate giant cells with peripheral (wreath-like) nuclei.
- These cells are most often arranged in an *alveolar pattern*, such that they line or cover collagenous septa and tend to be *shed* in a discohesive manner into the centre of these alveolar spaces (Fig. 28.18).

Immunohistochemistry

Alveolar rhabdomyosarcomas typically show distinctive strong and diffuse *myogenin* positivity.

Prognosis

Tumor is more aggressive than embryonal rhabdomyosarcoma.

BOTRYOID RHABDOMYOSARCOMA

Botryoid variant of this tumor arises in the mucosal cavities such as urinary bladder, vagina, nasopharynx and middle ear. Cystoscopy of urinary bladder reveals *grape-like polypoidal lesions* on mucosal surface of bladder trigone.

Gross Morphology
Most embryonal rhabdomyosarcomas of the urinary bladder present as *polypoidal intraluminal masses* resembling cluster of grapes hence named as botryoid type.

Light Microscopy
Tumor is composed of linear aggregates of round to oval tumor cells admixed with spindle cells in loose myxoid stroma. These tumor cells form cambium layer under the surface urothelium (Fig. 28.19).

Immunohistochemistry
Tumor cells show positivity for *desmin, vimentin, myogenin, myoglobin* and *MyoD1*.

Marker	Expression
Desmin	Positive
Vimentin	Positive
MyoD1	Positive
Myogenin	Positive
Myoglobin	Positive

Treatment and Prognosis
Prognosis of this variant has improved with multi-modular treatment. Combined radiation therapy and chemotherapy increase survival rates in these children with this neoplasm.

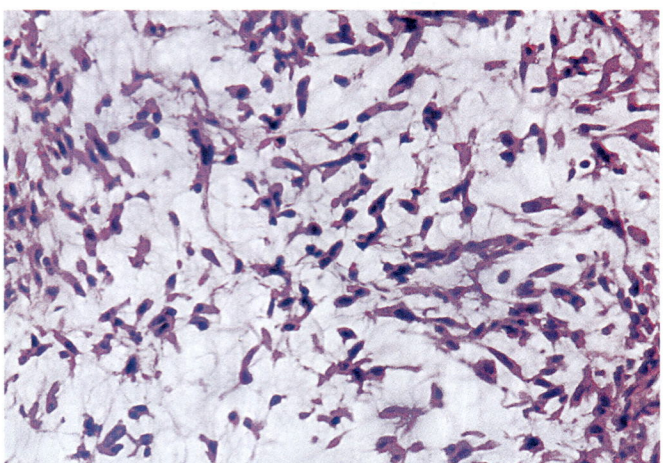

Fig. 28.19: Tumor is composed of numerous round to oval cells admixed with spindle cells in loose myxoid stroma (400X).

PLEOMORPHIC RHABDOMYOSARCOMA

Pleomorphic RMS is a high grade sarcoma with bizarre polygonal, round and spindle cells with skeletal muscle differentiation affecting adults in 6th to 7th decades.

Locations
It arises more commonly in deep soft tissue and most commonly in *lower extremity*.

Gross Morphology
Tumor is well circumscribed with a pseudocapsule and fleshy cut surface (Fig. 28.20).

Light Microscopy
Tumor is composed of sheets of large atypical and multinucleated polygonal eosinophilic cells. Cross striations are rarely seen in Fig. 28.21.

Immunohistochemistry
Tumor cells express desmin, vimentin, MyoD1, myogenin and myoglobin.

Marker	Expression
Desmin	Positive
Vimentin	Positive
MyoD1	Positive
Myogenin	Positive
Myoglobin	Positive

Prognosis
This aggressive tumor shows frequent metastases.

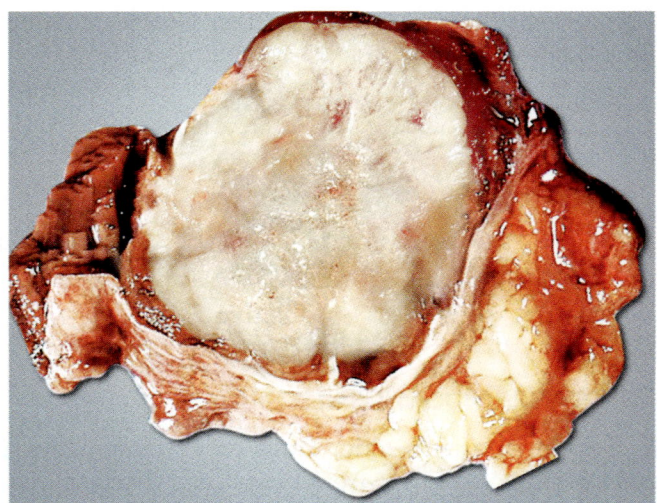

Fig. 28.20: Rhabdomyosarcoma. This tumor was removed from the forearm with a good margin of muscle around it. The tumor is brown, with a central area of hemorrhage. Wide local resection, wherever possible, is currently accepted as the treatment of choice for malignant soft tissue tumors.

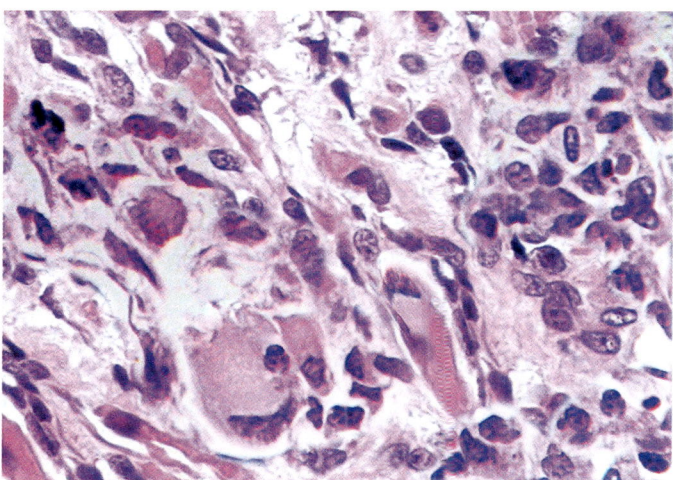

Fig. 28.21: Pleomorphic rhabdomyosarcoma shows atypical multinucleated polygonal cells (400X).

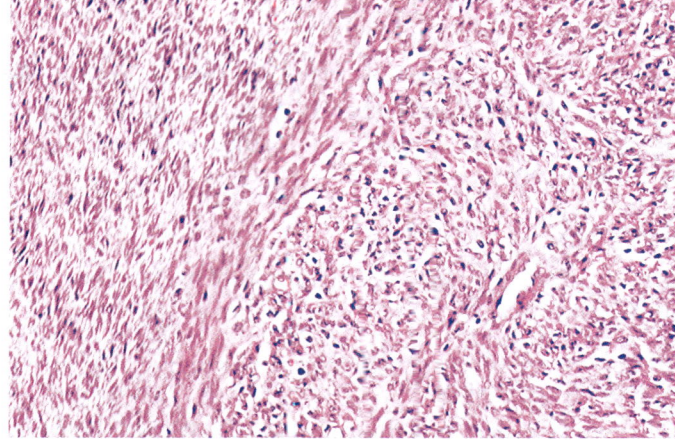

Fig. 28.22: Leiomyoma. Bundles of smooth muscle are interlacing in the tumor mass (100X).

SMOOTH MUSCLE TUMORS

LEIOMYOMA

Cutaneous pilar leiomyoma arises from arrector pili muscle. It occurs mainly in young adults of either sex. Leiomyoma of deep soft tissue is very uncommon.

Locations

Leiomyoma is often multiple than solitary. Patient presents as small, painful pink papules in the limbs and trunk.

> **Light Microscopy**
> - Leiomyoma is composed of bundles and fascicles of smooth muscle cells with eosinophilic cytoplasm and blunt-ended, cigar-shaped nuclei arranged in an irregular manner in the reticular dermis.
> - *Mitotic activity of up to one per 10 per high power field can be seen in pilar leiomyomas whereas mitotic activity of up to one per 50 per high power field in deep leiomyoma. Mitotic activity above this would suggest a malignant behavior of neoplasm* (Fig. 28.22).

LEIOMYOSARCOMA

Leiomyosarcoma is a malignant neoplasm showing smooth muscle differentiation. It occurs in middle-aged *adults* and *older persons*.

Locations

Leiomyosarcomas of soft tissue can arise intra-abdominally, in the vascular wall, subcutaneous or deep soft tissue and cutaneous.

> **Gross Morphology**
> Tumor is fleshy gray white to tan mass with whorled appearance with areas of hemorrhage, necrosis and cystic change.

> **Light Microscopy**
> Histopathological examination is similar to leiomyoma. But the nuclear pleomorphism and mitosis (>4 mitoses/50 HPF) are readily notable. Epithelioid cytomorphology and osteoclast like giant cells can also be seen in Fig. 28.23.

Prognosis

Leiomyosarcomas of soft tissue are capable of local recurrence and metastases.

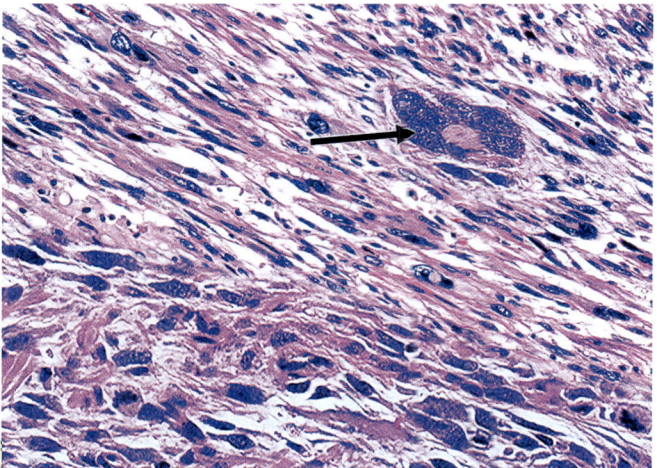

Fig. 28.23: Leiomyosarcoma. As with sarcomas in general, leiomyosarcomas have spindle cells. Several mitoses are seen here, just in this one high power field (arrow) (400X).

PERIVASCULAR TUMORS

GLOMUS TUMORS

Glomus tumors are mesenchymal tumors with cells resembling modified smooth muscle cells of normal glomus body. Glomus tumor commonly occurs in young adults.

Locations

Most common locations are subungual region, the hand, wrist and foot.

> **Gross Morphology**
>
> Typically cutaneous glomus is small <1 cm red blue nodules with history of pain.
>
> **Light Microscopy**
>
> - Glomus cells are small rounded with centrally placed round nucleus and amphophilic cytoplasm and distinct cell borders.
> - Malignant glomus tumor shows marked nuclear atypia, atypical mitotic figures.
> - Glomus tumors of uncertain malignant potential are tumors not fulfilling the above criteria and having a size >2 cm or deep location (Fig. 28.24).
>
> **Immunohistochemistry**
>
> Tumor cells are positive for SMA (smooth muscle actin) and have abundant pericellular type IV collagen.

Prognosis

Malignant glomus tumors are aggressive with metastases and death occurs from disease in up to 40% of patients.

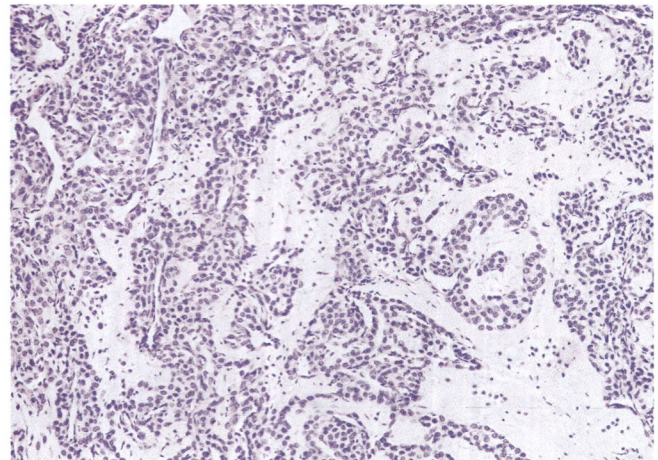

Fig. 28.24: Glomus tumor. It is composed of small rounded with centrally placed round nucleus and amphophilic cytoplasm and distinct cell borders (100X).

TUMORS OF UNCERTAIN ORIGIN

SYNOVIAL SARCOMA

Synovial sarcoma is highly malignant soft tissue tumor. It often occurs in the *lower extremities*. It most often originates in the region of a *joint*, rather than with in a joint cavity. It has no etiologic or direct anatomic relationship to the synovium.

Age Group

It occurs principally in adolescents and young adults of 20–50 years.

Molecular Genetics

This chromosomal *translocation t(X;18)* is seen in synovial sarcoma. Its demonstration is required to confirm the diagnosis. *Chromosomal translocation t(X;18) produces SS-18-SSX1-SSX2 or SSX4 fusion gene. However, this translocation is not entirely specific* for synovial sarcoma.

Clinical Features

Patient presents with painful or tender mass in the vicinity of a large joint, particularly the knee in parapatellar area. Other sites include parapharynx, abdominal wall and pleura (Fig. 28.25).

> **Light Microscopy**
>
> Synovial sarcoma shows two histological patterns: *biphasic* and *monophasic*.
>
> - *Biphasic pattern of synovial sarcoma:* It is more common comprising of both cuboidal-like epithelial forming glandular spaces lined by cuboidal cells in a spindled cell background demonstrable on both light microscopy and immunohistochemistry.
>
>   Glandular spaces are lined by epithelial cells show positivity with monoclonal antibodies to *keratin* and *epithelial membrane antigen* are presumably epithelial (Fig. 28.26).
>
> - *Monophasic pattern of synovial sarcoma:* It is comprised exclusively of the spindled component without obvious epithelial differentiation on hematoxylin and eosin staining.
>
>   Scattered *cytokeratin* positive cells may be seen on immunohistochemistry, suggesting that there is divergent epithelial differentiation in these cases too.
>
> **Histochemistry**
>
> The epithelial component of tumor cells in clefts or glandular spaces are outlined by *PAS, alcian blue, reticulin stain* and *colloidal iron*.

Soft Tissue Tumors and Skeletal Myopathies 28

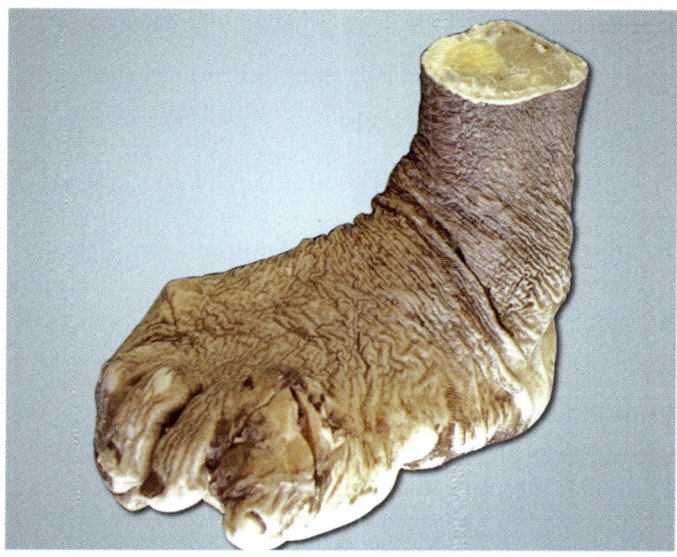

Fig. 28.25: Synovial sarcoma. Amputation of limb was done.

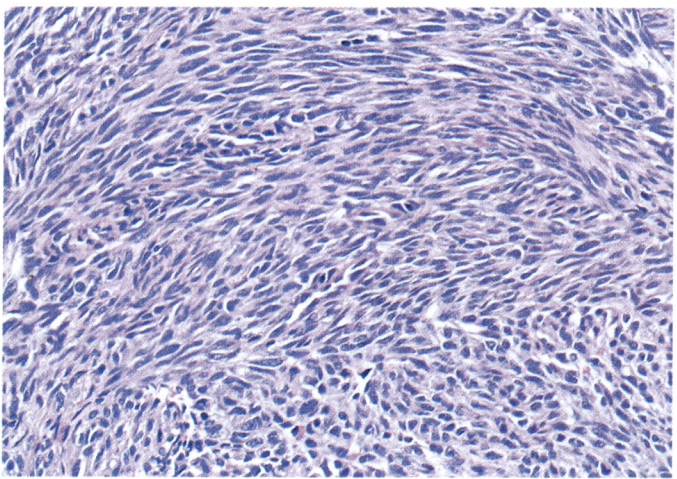

Fig. 28.26: Synovial sarcoma tumor shows both cuboidal-like epithelial forming glandular spaces lined by cuboidal cells in a spindled cell background (400X).

Immunohistochemistry
- Tumor cells show positivity for **CD99** and **BCL2** but negative for CD34.
- Epithelial component of tumor cells show positivity with *cytokeratin* and *epithelial membrane antigen*. *Spindle cells component express vimentin*.

Metastases
Tumor >5 cm in diameter with mitoses 10/HPF in patients >40 years most often metastasizes to distant organs. Prognostic factors of synovial sarcoma are shown in Table 28.5.

ALVEOLAR SOFT PART SARCOMA
Alveolar soft part sarcoma (ASPS) is a rare sarcoma characterized by ASPS CR1-TFE3 fusion gene. It occurs at any age but more commonly seen in 15 to 35 years of age.

Molecular Genetics
Cytogenetically ASPS shows der(17)t(X:17)(p11;q25).

Locations
These tumors are usually situated deep within soft tissues. Frequency in descending orders, these tumors are located in *buttocks and thighs (40%), popliteal region, chest* and *trunk and forearm*.

Gross Morphology
Tumor tends to be poorly circumscribed, pale gray in color with soft consistency and areas of necrosis and hemorrhage.
Light Microscopy
• Tumor shows an organoid or nesting pattern separated by delicate fibrovascular septa. Loss of cellular cohesion and necrosis of centrally located cells gives a pseudoalveolar pattern. • The cells contain rhomboid or rod-shaped intracytoplasmic inclusions better seen on **PAS stain** (Fig. 28.27).

Immunohistochemistry
Tumor shows strong nuclear staining for **TFE3** antibody.

Electron Microscopy
The most distinctive feature of ASPS is membrane bound rhomboid or rectangular crystals that are

Table 28.5: Prognostic factors of synovial sarcoma

Parameters	Good prognosis	Unfavorable prognosis
Tumor size along longest axis	<4 cm	>4 cm
Calcification in tumor	Present	Absent
Vascular invasion	Absent	Present
Mitotic rate	<2 mitoses/per high power field	>2 mitoses/per high power field
Age group	Children	Adults

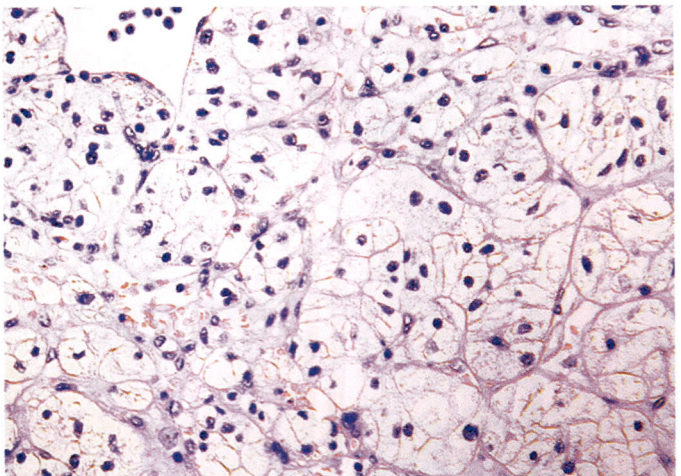

Fig. 28.27: Alveolar soft part sarcoma. Tumor is composed of cells arranged in nests separated by delicate fibrovascular septa giving pseudoalveolar pattern (400X).

composed of periodic lattice work of rigid fibrils with 5–7 nm diameter and 10 nm periodicity. Granules associated with crystal formation are shown to contain *monocarboxylate transporter protein 1* and its *cellular chaperone CD147*.

Prognosis

ASPS seldom recurs locally after complete resection but metastases are common.

UNDIFFERENTIATED PLEOMORPHIC SARCOMA

It is most common in older adults. It does not show specific evidence of lineage differentiation. It was previously known as *malignant fibrous histiocytoma*. It contains foci of histiocytic (macrophage) differentiation. It is the most frequent sarcoma encountered after radiation therapy.

Light Microscopy
It displays a highly variable morphological pattern, with areas of well differentiated spindle-shaped tumor cells resembling fibroblasts arrayed in an irregularly whorled (storiform) pattern adjacent to pleomorphic fields.

EPITHELIOID SARCOMA

It is a malignant tumor exhibiting epithelioid cytomorphology. Two clinicopathological subtypes are recognized: classic or distal and proximal or large cell variant. *The tumor arises in the deep dermis* and *subcutis*. Distal type in young adults whereas the proximal type in older population.

Light Microscopy
• Tumor is composed of pale staining epithelioid cell, spindle cells with pink cytoplasm arranged in aggregates. • Hyaline cytoplasmic (rhabdoid) inclusions are seen in these cells. • Multiple foci of necrosis (granuloma-like pattern of necrosis) are present within tumor. • There is presence of lymphocytes around periphery of tumor cells.

Immunohistochemistry	
Tumor cells show positivity for *cytokeratin, vimentin, epithelial membrane antigen (EMA)* and *CD34*.	
Marker	**Expression**
Cytokeratin	Positive
Vimentin	Positive
Epithelial membrane antigen (EMA)	Positive
CD34	Positive

Prognosis

Epithelioid sarcoma tends to recur repeatedly and metastasize frequently to *lung and lymph nodes*.

CLEAR CELL SARCOMA OF SOFT TISSUE

Clear cell sarcoma of soft tissue is a malignant neoplasm involving deep soft tissue of the extremities. It is also known as *malignant melanoma of soft parts*. It affects young adults.

Location

Majority occur in the extremity with *foot/ankle being* the commonest location.

Gross Morphology
Clear cell sarcoma is usually relatively small (<5 cm). Cut surface is lobulated gray white well circumscribed with pushing margin.

Light Microscopy
• Tumor shows a characteristic nested growth pattern with collagenous bands. • Cells have a pale eosinophilic cytoplasm with vesicular nuclei and macronucleoli, nuclear pleomorphism.

Histochemistry
Melanin is often detected in *Masson fontana stain*.

Immunohistochemistry

Tumor cells are positive for *S-100, HMB-45, MITF* and other melanoma antigens.

Marker	Expression
S-100	Positive
HMB-45	Positive
MITF	Positive

Molecular Genetics

The genetic hallmark is the presence of a *reciprocal translocation t(12;22)(q13;q12)* resulting in fusion of EWSR1 with ATF1.

Prognosis

It is associated with poor prognosis due to metastases in *lymph nodes, lung* and *bones*.

NEURAL TUMORS

NEUROFIBROMA

These firm nodules may be solitary and sporadic or multiple and part of *von Recklinghausen's* disease (neurofibromatosis). There may be overlying hyperpigmentation. With neurofibromatosis, an autosomal dominant disorder, there can be multiple *café au lait* spots (six or more pale brown pigmented macules each >1.5 cm in size). Tumor is well defined but nonencapsulated mass (Fig. 28.28).

> **Light Microscopy**
> Microscopically, tumor is composed of wavy spindle cells with a lot of intervening collagen fibers (Fig. 28.29).

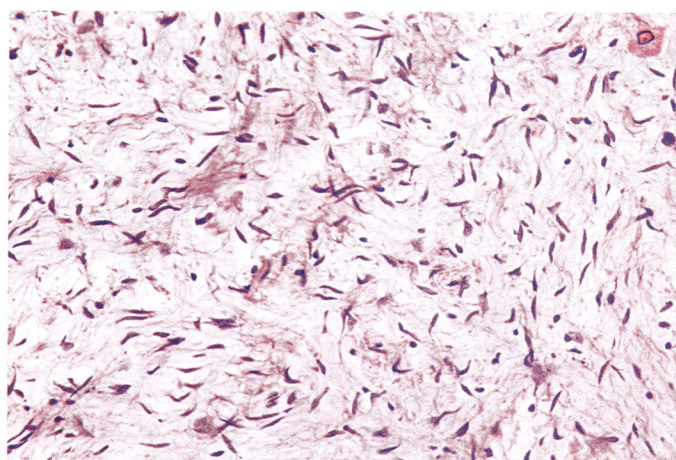

Fig. 28.29: Neurofibroma. Tumor is composed of wavy spindle cells with a lot of intervening collagen fibers (100X).

SCHWANNOMA

Schwannoma or neurilemmoma is a benign tumor of nerve sheath occurring in 4th to 6th decades of life.

Bilateral schwannomas of the acoustic nerve are the cardinal (or pathognomonic) feature of neurofibromatosis type-2 (NF-2).

Locations

The anatomic distribution is very wide, including *cranial nerves, bone, gastrointestinal tract*, particularly the *stomach*. Majority of cases develop in subcutaneous tissue.

Pathogenesis

Mutation of NF-1 and NF-2 is associated with schwannoma (Table 28.6).

> **Light Microscopy**
> Classical schwannoma is an encapsulated neoplasm having two components, known as *Antoni A* and *B tissue*.
> • Antoni A tissue is cellular and consists of monomorphic spindle-shaped Schwann cells, with poorly defined eosinophilic cytoplasm and pointed basophilic nuclei, set in a variably collagenous stroma show nuclear palisading surrounding pink areas known as *verocay bodies*.
> • Antoni B areas are also composed of Schwann cells, but their cytoplasm is inconspicuous, and the nuclei appear suspended in a copious myxoid, often microcystic, matrix (Fig. 28.30).

Immunohistochemistry

Schwannomas show diffuse and strong S-100 protein positivity.

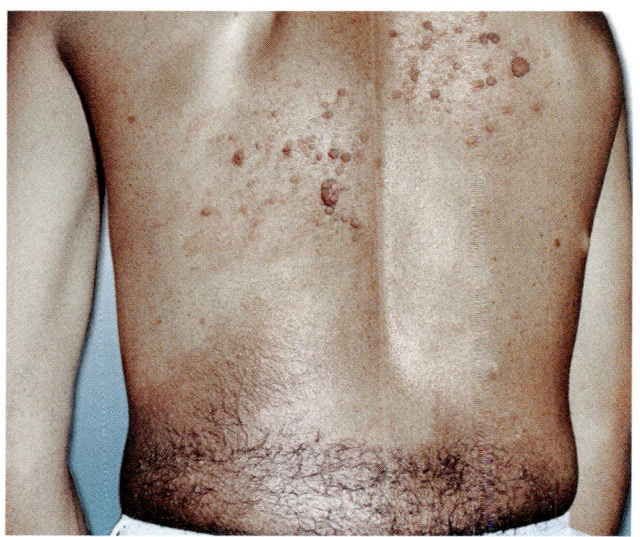

Fig. 28.28: Neurofibroma. Multiple neurofibromas are seen in neurofibromatosis.

Table 28.6: Tumor suppressor genes associated with *schwannoma* (mitogenic signaling pathway inhibitors)

Gene	Protein	Function	Familial tumors	Sporadic cancers
NF-1	Neurofibronin-1 (locus 13p11) Mutation occurs by deletion	NF-1 inhibits RAS/MAP-kinase signaling activator pathway	Neurofibromatosis type 1 (neurofibroma and malignant peripheral nerve tumors)	Schwannoma Juvenile myeloid leukemia Neuroblastoma
NF-2	Merlin (locus 22q) Mutation by deletion or nonsense mutation	NF-2 stabilizes cytoskeleton membrane linkage	Neurofibromatosis type 2 (acoustic schwannoma and meningioma)	Schwannomas

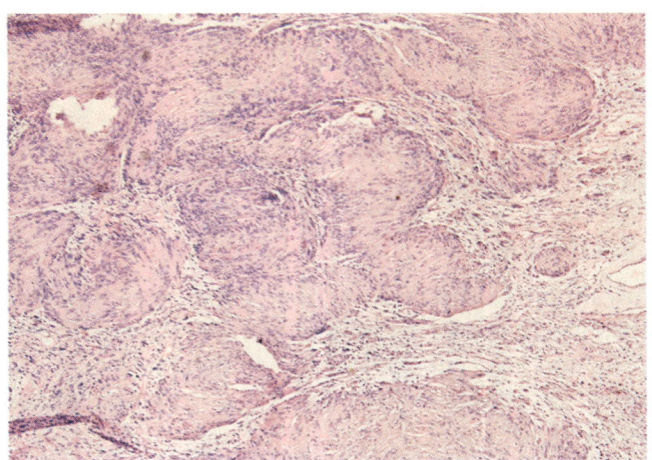

Fig. 28.30: Neurilemmoma. Tumor is composed of cells with palisading nuclei arranged in compact whorls and fascicles (Antoni type A), interspersed with less cellular loosely structured myxomatous appearing areas designated Antoni type B areas (100X).

MALIGNANT PERIPHERAL NERVE SHEATH TUMOR (MPNST)

MPNST is the term given for sarcomas of nerve sheath type. It can arise from a previous nerve sheath tumor or in a patient with NF type 1 (neurofibromatosis type 1). It occurs in patients aged 20 to 50 years.

Locations

Tumor arises in extremities, trunk, head and neck region.

Gross Morphology

Large fusiform mass involving a major nerve with tan yellow cut surface and areas of necrosis.

Light Microscopy

- MPNST can have diverse patterns. Typical tumor is composed of spindle cells in a fascicular pattern often with branching hemangiopericytomatous pattern with hypercellular and hypocellular areas.
- Heterologous elements like cartilage, bone, blood vessels can also be seen.

Immunohistochemistry

S-100 protein positivity is seen in 50% of cases.

Prognosis

MPNSTs are *aggressive tumors* with poor prognosis.

VASCULAR TUMORS

HEMANGIOMA

Hemangiomas are sometimes considered being a hamartoma rather than a neoplasm. These can be variable in size from a few millimeters up to several centimeters in diameter. A hemangioma can be a congenital benign neoplasm. It may cause serious problems if it is large and poorly resectable.

Major Forms

Vascular malformations include capillary (portwine stains).

Clinical Features

Patient presents with bright red to blue, usually level with the surface of the skin, or slightly elevated. *Port-wine stain* variant of capillary hemangioma is purple-red area on the face or neck.

Strawberry capillary hemangioma appears as bright-red raised lesion. *Cherry hemangioma* is small, dome-shaped red papule. Hemangiomas may be part of other syndromes described as under (Fig. 28.31).

Hemangiomas associated with syndromes

- *Sturge-Weber syndrome:* This disorder involves port-wine stain of the face, ipsilateral glaucoma, vascular lesions of ocular choroidal tissue, and extensive hemangiomatous involvement of meninges. Patient presents with convulsions, mental retardation, and retinal detachment.
- *von Hippel-Lindau syndrome:* This disorder involves multiple vascular tumors and other tumors and cysts that are widely scattered throughout many organ systems.

28 Soft Tissue Tumors and Skeletal Myopathies

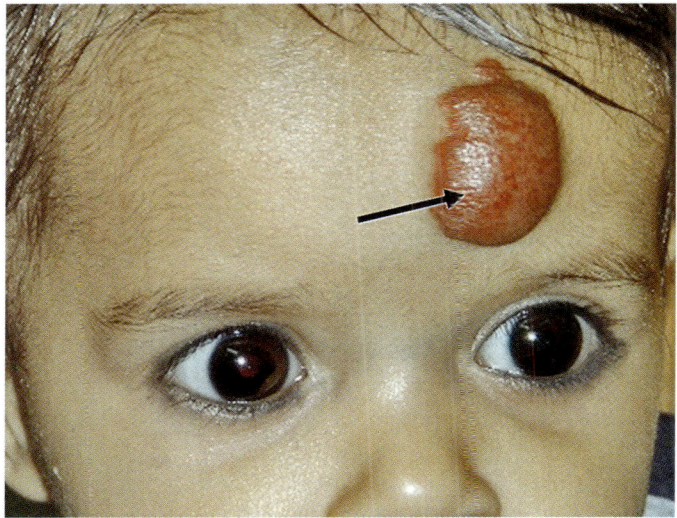

Fig. 28.31: Compressible lesion of hemangioma (arrow).

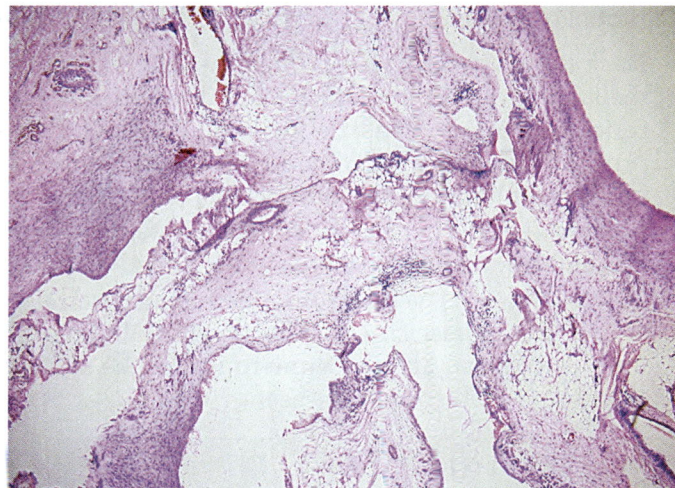

Fig. 28.33: Lymphangioma. Tumor is composed of large lymphatic channels (100X).

Locations

Cystic lesions are most common in *neck*, *axilla* and *groin*. *Cavernous type* is common in *oral cavity, upper trunk*.

Gross Morphology
Multicystic spongy mass with cavities containing watery/milky fluid.

Light Microscopy
Lymphangiomas are characterized by thin-walled dilated lymphatic vessels of varying sizes lined by flattened endothelium and surrounded by lymphoid aggregates (Fig. 28.33).

Immunohistochemistry
Endothelial cells express podoplanin, CD31, PROX1.

Marker	Expression
Podoplanin	Positive
CD31	Positive
PROX1	Positive

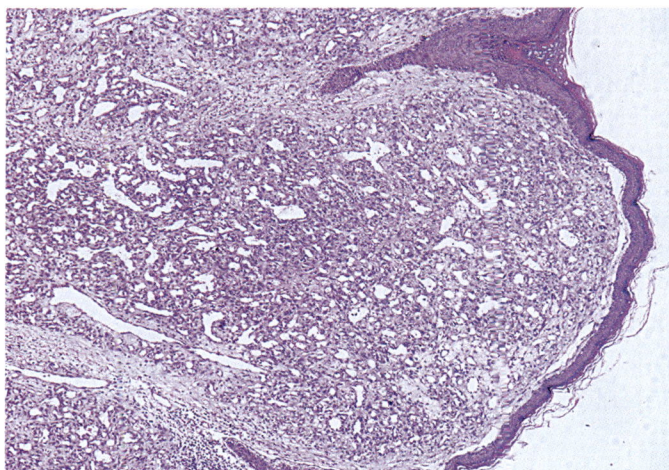

Fig. 28.32: Capillary hemangioma. It is made up of closely packed aggregations of thin-walled capillaries lined with a single layer of endothelium, usually blood-filled, separated by scant connective tissue stroma (100X).

Light Microscopy

- Capillary hemangioma is usually well defined but lacking capsule. It is made up of closely packed aggregations of thin-walled capillaries lined with a single layer of endothelium, usually blood-filled, separated by scant connective tissue stroma. The vascular lumina may be partially or completely thrombosed and organized.
- Cavernous hemangioma is large, endothelium-lined spaces in the dermis and subdermis (Fig. 28.32).

LYMPHANGIOMA

Benign cavernous or cystic vascular lesion composed of dilated lymphatic channels are commonly seen in pediatric age group (first years of life).

Prognosis

Rare recurrences occur due to incomplete surgical removal.

KAPOSI SARCOMA

Kaposi sarcoma is a locally aggressive endothelial tumor-like lesion that usually presents with cutaneous lesions. The disease is associated with HHV8 infection.

Locations

Skin is most typically involved. Sometimes mucous membranes, visceral organs and lymph nodes can be involved.

Clinical Features

- *Patch stage:* Vascular spaces lined by flattened endothelial cells dissect the collagen bundles in the upper reticular dermis. Pre-existing blood vessels may protrude into the lumen of new vessels. An admixed infiltrate of lymphocytes and plasma cells is seen.
- *Plaque stage:* All characteristics of patch stage is exaggerated with vascular spaces showing jagged outlines.
- *Nodular stage:* It is well circumscribed cellular nodules of intersecting fascicles of spindle cells with no or a little cytological atypia. Numerous slit-like spaces containing erythrocytes are seen.

Gross Morphology
Skin lesions (patches, plaques, nodules) vary in size.

Light Microscopy
Four different epidemiological-clinical types of KS identified: These include classic indolent KS, endemic African KS, iatrogenic KS and AIDS associated KS. All show similar morphological features.

Immunohistochemistry
Lining cells of vascular structures are positive for **CD31, CD34, podoplanin,** and show nuclear expression of **HHV8**.

Prognosis
Evolution of disease is modified by treatment that includes surgery, radiotherapy or chemotherapy.

SKELETAL MUSCLES

SKELETAL MUSCLE ATROPHIES

Denervation atrophy is associated with muscle denervation. This type of change involves both type 1 (red) and type 2 (white) fibers, which may appear small and angular on cross section, target fibers, which have a central darker area reminiscent of the bull's eye of a target, may also be seen.

After reinnervation occurs, fiber-type grouping, a cluster of type 1 fibers adjacent to a cluster of type 2 fibers, may be seen.

This contrasts with the mixture of individual type 1 and type 2 fibers characteristic of normal muscle. Disuse atrophy is associated with prolonged immobilization.

It is characterized histologically by angular atrophy, primarily of type 2 fibers. Differences between type 1 and type 2 muscle fibers are shown in Table 28.7.

SKELETAL MUSCLE DYSTROPHIES

This group of genetically determined progressive disorders is characterized by degeneration of skeletal

Table 28.7: Differences between type 1 and type 2 muscle fibers

Features		Type 1 (muscle fiber)	Type 2 (muscle fiber)
Prototype muscle		Soleus muscle	Pectoral muscle
Action and duration		Sustained force, prolonged duration	Sudden movement, short duration
Contraction rate		Slow	Fast
Glycogen content		Scant amount	Abundant amount
Lipid content		Abundant amount	Scant amount
Staining properties	ATPase at pH 4.2	Dark staining	Light staining
	ATPase at pH 9.4	Light staining	Dark staining
	NADH-TR	Dark staining	Light staining
Myoglobin		Yes	No
Ultrastructure findings		Many mitochondria, Wide Z-band	Lesser mitochondria, narrow Z-band
Physiology		Slow-twitch	Fast-twitch
Aerobic energy production		High	Low
Anaerobic energy production		Low	High
Fatigue		Slow	Fast
Energy utilization		Low	High
Color		Red	White
Function		Weight bearing	Purposeful motion

Soft Tissue Tumors and Skeletal Myopathies

muscle and profound wasting and weakness. These are differentiated by age of onset, muscle groups involved, and mode of inheritance.

Increased serum activities of creatine kinase (CK) and other muscle enzymes derived from degenerating muscle fibers are characteristic findings.

Nonspecific degenerative changes on muscle biopsy are also characteristic. Although nonspecific, the muscle biopsy findings are helpful in distinguishing dystrophies from abnormalities secondary to denervation. Examples of muscle dystrophies are shown in Fig. 28.34 and Table 28.8.

DUCHENNE MUSCULAR DYSTROPHY

This X-linked genetic disorder is the most common and severe variety of the disease due to deletion of one or many exons in the *dystrophin gene (DMD gene)* located on the short arm of the X-chromosome (Xp21).

Dystrophin links the subsarcolemmal cytoskeleton to the exterior of the cell through a transmembrane complex of proteins. Boys with disorder cannot produce dystrophin at all. Dystrophin deficient muscles of pelvic and *shoulder girdles* predispose to death of myocytes during contraction. Serum levels of creatine kinase are markedly increased (Fig. 28.35).

Clinical Features

Children fail to walk by 18 months of age due to weakness in the proximal muscles of the extremities, progressing to muscle necrosis, wasting, muscle contracture with fatal outcome in their teens.

Patient develops pneumonia due to weakness of respiratory muscles. More than 90% of afflicted boys are wheelchair bound by the age of 10 years and bedridden by age 15 years.

The most common causes of death are complications of *respiratory insufficiency* caused by muscular weakness or cardiac arrhythmia due to myocardial involvement.

BECKER MUSCULAR DYSTROPHY

It is less common and less severe disorder affecting boys. It is clinically similar to Duchenne muscular dystrophy. In this disease, some dystrophin is produced as a result of segmental deletion of dystrophin gene. It does not cause a coding frameshift.

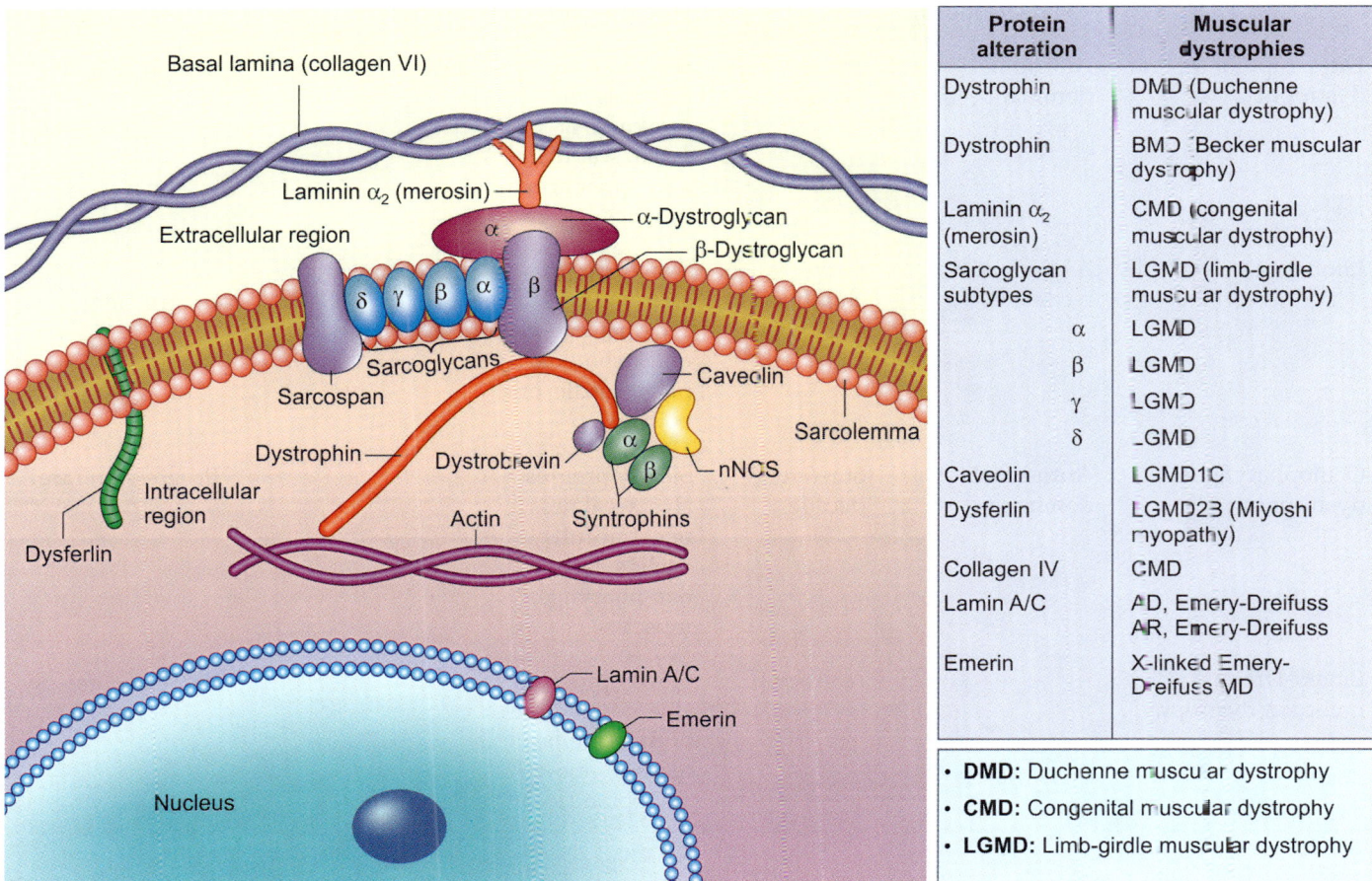

Protein alteration	Muscular dystrophies
Dystrophin	DMD (Duchenne muscular dystrophy)
Dystrophin	BMD (Becker muscular dystrophy)
Laminin α$_2$ (merosin)	CMD (congenital muscular dystrophy)
Sarcoglycan subtypes	LGMD (limb-girdle muscular dystrophy)
α	LGMD
β	LGMD
γ	LGMD
δ	LGMD
Caveolin	LGMD1C
Dysferlin	LGMD2B (Miyoshi myopathy)
Collagen IV	CMD
Lamin A/C	AD, Emery-Dreifuss AR, Emery-Dreifuss
Emerin	X-linked Emery-Dreifuss MD

- **DMD:** Duchenne muscular dystrophy
- **CMD:** Congenital muscular dystrophy
- **LGMD:** Limb-girdle muscular dystrophy

Fig. 28.34: Dystrophin associated protein complex and other proteins involved in muscular dystrophies.

Table 28.8: Salient features of skeletal muscular dystrophies

Type	Inheritance	Age onset	Clinical features	Other systems involved	Clinical course
Duchenne's muscular dystrophy	X-linked recessive due to mutation of dystrophin gene (DMD gene) located on (Xp21)	By age of 5 years	Pelvic and shoulder girdles, pneumonia due to failure of respiratory muscles	Low intelligence and cardiac arrhythmias	Fatal outcome due to respiratory failure by 20 years of age
Becker's muscular dystrophy	X-linked recessive due to segmental deletion of dystrophin gene (DMD gene) located on (Xp21)	By 2nd decade	Slowly progressive weakness of girdle muscle (minor variant of Duchenne's type)	Cardiomegaly	Benign course
Myotonic dystrophy	Autosomal dominant disorder due to increased number of trinucleotide repeats (50–1000) in the myotonin protein kinase gene (normal is <30 nucleotides)	Any decade	Slowly progressive myotonic stiffness or spasm following muscle contraction of eyelids	Cardiac conduction defects, GIT muscles, mental impairment, endocrine glands, cataracts, frontal baldness and gonadal atrophy	Benign course
Facioscapulohumeral dystrophy	Autosomal dominant	2nd–4th decade	Slowly progressive weakness of facial, scapular and upper arm muscles	Hypertension	Benign course
Limb girdle dystrophy	Autosomal recessive	Early childhood to adulthood	Slowly progressive weakness of proximal muscles of the shoulder, pelvic girdle, or both	Cardiomyopathy	Variable progression
Oculopharyngeal dystrophy	Autosomal dominant	5th–6th decade	Slowly progressive weakness of extraocular eyelids, face and pharyngeal muscles	–	Progression rare
Emery-Dreifuss muscular dystrophy	–	Any age	Slowly progressive contractures of the Archilles tendon, elbow and spine	–	Benign course

Soft Tissue Tumors and Skeletal Myopathies

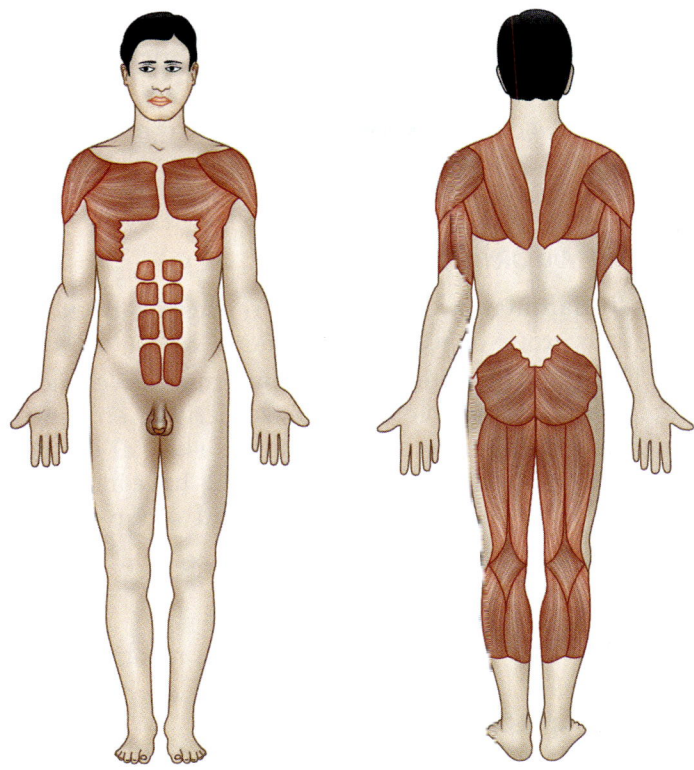

Fig. 28.35: Muscular dystrophy. Initial muscle involvement of Duchenne muscular dystrophies.

MYOTONIC MUSCULAR DYSTROPHY

This disorder demonstrates an autosomal dominant mode of inheritance. It is the most common variety of adult onset muscular dystrophy.

Basic Defect

This disorder is caused by an increased *number of trinucleotide repeats (50–1000) in the myotonin protein kinase gene* (normal is less than 30 nucleotides).

Clinical Features

Its primary symptom is myotonic stiffness or spasm following muscle contraction. Patient is unable to relax muscles once contracted. It is a progressive disorder that affects heart, smooth muscles (gastrointestinal tract), central nervous system, endocrine glands, testes (atrophy) and eyes (cataract).

FACIOSCAPULOHUMERAL MUSCULAR DYSTROPHY

It is autosomal disorder primarily affects the muscles of the face, scapular area, and upper arm. It has slow progressive course with normal life expectancy (Fig. 28.36).

LIMB-GIRDLE DYSTROPHY

This disorder demonstrates autosomal recessive inheritance. It involves the proximal muscles of the shoulder, pelvic girdle, or both (Fig. 23.37).

EMERY-DREIFUSS MUSCULAR DYSTROPHY

It is characterized by contractures of the Achilles' tendon, elbow and spine.

OCULOPHARYNGEAL MUSCULAR DYSTROPHY

It affects muscles of the eyes and pharyngeal muscles.

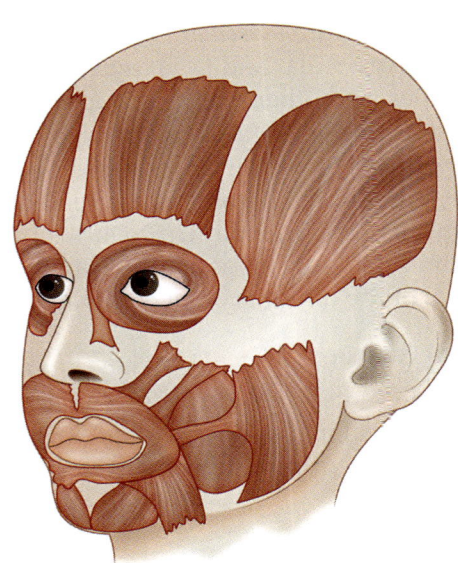
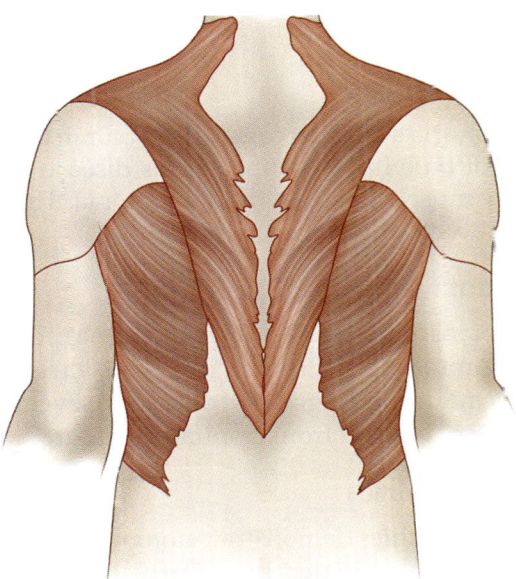

Fig. 28.36: Muscular dystrophy. Initial muscle involvement of facioscapulohumeral muscular dystrophies

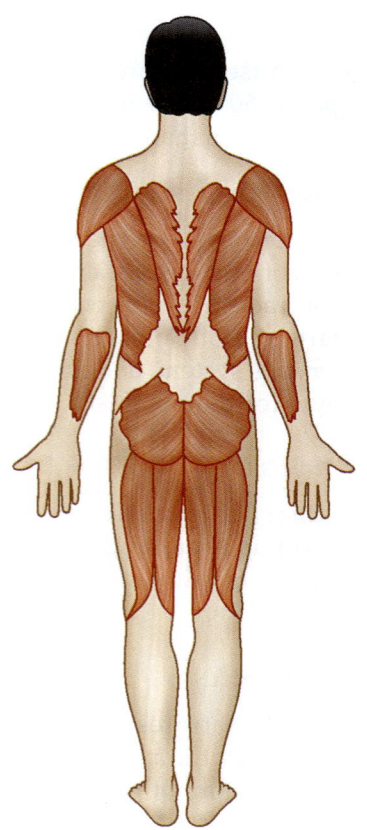

Fig. 28.37: Muscular dystrophy. Initial muscle involvement of limb girdle muscular dystrophies.

CONGENITAL MYOPATHIES

Congenital myopathies with specific histological changes. These disorders are often characterized by floppy infant syndrome, marked hypotonia at birth. They can be distinguished from dystrophies by the combination of specific histological changes, often with normal serum creatine kinase.

Central Core Disease

A loss of mitochondria and other organelles occur in the central portion of type I muscle fibers. This disease is characterized by muscle weakness and hypotonia. The affected infants eventually become ambulatory.

Nemaline Myopathy

This disease demonstrates tangles of small rod-shaped granules, predominantly in type I fibers. It varies clinically from a mild, nonprogressive disease to severe weakness resulting in death from respiratory failure.

Mitochondrial Myopathies

Mitochondrial myopathies demonstrate nonmendelian inheritance. These are mediated by maternally transmitted *mitochondrial DNA abnormalities* (most often deletions).

They may be characterized by a ragged red appearance of muscle fibers and by various mitochondrial enzyme or coenzyme defects.

Kearns-Sayre syndrome is characterized by ophthalmoplegia, pigmentary retinopathy, heart block, cerebellar ataxia, and an exclusively maternal mode of transmission.

INFLAMMATORY MYOPATHIES

The inflammatory myopathies represent a heterogeneous group of acquired disorders.

This group has symmetric proximal muscle weakness, increased serum levels of muscle-derived enzymes, and nonsuppurative inflammation of skeletal muscle. Patients with inflammatory myopathies have increased serum levels of creatine kinase and other muscle enzymes.

Etiology

These are thought to have an autoimmune origin.

> **Light Microscopy**
>
> The inflammatory myopathies show inflammatory cells, necrosis and phagocytosis of muscle fibers, a mixture of regenerating and atrophic fibers, and fibrosis.

MISCELLANEOUS DISORDERS

MYASTHENIA GRAVIS

Myasthenia gravis is an autoimmune disorder more frequent in women than in men. It occurs due to formation of *autoantibodies to postsynaptic acetylcholine receptors of the neuromuscular junction (motor endplate)*. It involves extraocular and facial muscles, muscles of the extremities, and other muscle groups.

The thymoma clearly plays an important role in the pathogenesis of myasthenia gravis. For unexplained reasons, myasthenia gravis is associated with thymic hyperplasia or thymoma. Up to 40% of patients with thymoma develop myasthenia gravis, and surgical removal of the tumor is often curative.

Clinical Features

Patient presents with ptosis, diplopia, and difficulty chewing, speaking, or swallowing. This disease can be complicated by respiratory failure due to diaphragmatic weakness.

Therapeutic Correlation

Patient improves dramatically with administration of drugs with anticholinesterase activity.

LAMBERT-EATON SYNDROME

Lambert-Eaton syndrome is a paraneoplastic disorder. It is also termed as myasthenic-myopathic syndrome. It manifests as muscular weakness of pelvic girdles, wasting, and fatigability of the proximal limbs and trunk.

Association with Cancers

Although it is most commonly associated with *small cell carcinoma of lung*, yet it may also occur in patients with other malignant diseases.

Like myasthenia gravis, the disease seems to have an autoimmune basis because it can be transferred to mice by IgG from patients and it responds to treatment with corticosteroids.

Pathogenesis

The pathogenic IgG autoantibodies recognize voltage-sensitive calcium channels that are expressed both in motor nerve terminals and in the cells of the lung cancer. The calcium channels, which are necessary for release of acetylcholine, are greatly reduced in the presynaptic membrane in these patients, thereby interfering with neuromuscular transmission.

MYOSITIS OSSIFICANS

It most often affects young persons. It is a benign condition but mimics a malignant neoplasm.

The lesion typically results from *blunt trauma to the muscle and soft tissues, usually of the lower limb*.

Over a short time, peripheral revascularization occurs in the hematoma results in formation of bone spicules in the soft tissue.

It often occurs near a bone, on radiography, *it may be misdiagnosed as a malignant bone-forming tumor* (Fig. 28.38).

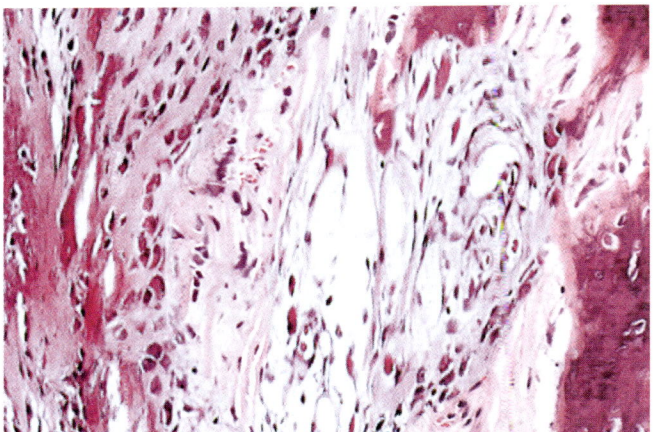

Fig. 28.38: Myositis ossificans. As the lesion matures, the stroma becomes less cellular. Cartilage formation may be seen.

RHABDOMYOLYSIS

Rhabdomyolysis refers to the dissolution of skeletal muscle fibers and the release of myoglobin into the circulation, an event that may result in myoglobinuria and acute renal failure.

Etiology

Rhabdomyolysis may occur due to heat stroke or malignant hyperthermia after administration of an anesthetic such as halothane.

> **Light Microscopy**
>
> It shows active, non-inflammatory myopathy, with scattered necrosis of muscle fibers and varying degrees of degeneration and regeneration.

Clinical Course

The disorder rhabdomyolysis may be acute, subacute, or chronic. During acute phase, the muscles are swollen, tender, and profoundly weak.

CARNITINE PALMITYL TRANSFERASE DEFICIENCY

Patients with carnitine palmityl transferase deficiency cannot metabolize long-chain fatty acids because of an inability to transport these lipids into the mitochondria, where they undergo β-oxidation.

Clinical Features

Patient presents with muscular pain after prolonged exercise, which may progress to myoglobinuria. After such an episode, fibers regenerate and restore muscle structure.

> **Light Microscopy**
>
> It shows no microscopic abnormalities.

Diagnosis

Diagnosis depends on the *biochemical assay* for *carnitine palmityl transferase activity*.

SKELETAL MUSCLE HYPERTROPHY

Skeletal muscle hypertrophy of type II fibers occurs due to androgenic steroids. Stimulation of skeletal muscle type II fibers elicits a faster, shorter, and more powerful contraction than occurs in type I fibers. Skeletal muscle type II fibers rapidly contract for brief duration and react to strength training with hypertrophy. Skeletal muscle does not respond to an increased workload by increasing the number of fibers (hyperplasia).

POMPE'S DISEASE

Pompe disease is autosomal recessive glycogen storage disorder characterized by an inability to degrade glycogen due to *acid maltase deficiency*. It is the most severe form and occurs in the neonatal or early infantile stage.

Many tissues are affected, but the most significant involvement is in *skeletal and cardiac muscle,* the central nervous system, and the liver.

Clinical Features

Patient presents with severe hypotonia and areflexia. Sometimes, the patient has an enlarged tongue and cardiomegaly and die of cardiac failure. Child usually dies within the first 2 years of life.

CHAPTER 29

Skin

Learning Objectives

NORMAL SKIN
- Epidermis
- Dermis
- Subcutaneous Tissue
- Nails
- Skin Disorders: Overview

INFLAMMATORY DISORDERS
- Eczematous Dermatitis
- Impetigo
- Neurodermatitis
- Scabies

CUTANEOUS INFECTIONS
- Molluscum Contagiosum
- Verruca Vulgaris (Common Wart)
- Herpetic Dermatitis (Herpes Simplex Virus)
- Varicella (Chickenpox)
- Superficial Fungal Infections

AUTOIMMUNE DISORDERS
- Psoriasis
- Pemphigus Vulgaris
- Bullous Pemphigoid
- Dermatitis Herpetiformis
- Erythema Multiforme
- Lichen Planus

NONMELANOCYTIC LESIONS AND TUMORS
- Seborrheic Keratosis
- Actinic Keratosis
- Keratoacanthoma
- Squamous Cell Carcinoma *in situ* (Bowen's Disease)
- Invasive Squamous Cell Carcinoma
- Basal Cell Carcinoma

PIGMENTATION DISORDERS AND MELANOCYTIC TUMORS
- Pigmentation Disorders
- Melanocytic Tumors

FIBROUS AND FIBROHISTIOCYTIC TUMORS
- Dermatofibroma
- Dermatofibrosarcoma Protuberans

NEURAL AND NEUROENDOCRINE TUMORS
- Neurofibroma
- Traumatic Neuroma
- Merkel Cell Carcinoma

VASCULAR TUMORS
- Hemangioma

TUMORS OF CUTANEOUS APPENDAGES
- Chondroid Syringoma
- Nodular Hidradenoma
- Pilomatrixoma

CUTANEOUS METASTASES

MISCELLANEOUS DISORDERS
- Fibroepithelial Polyp
- Epidermal Inclusion Cyst
- Acanthosis Nigricans
- Xanthomas
- Granuloma Pyogenicum
- Keloid
- Acne

NORMAL SKIN

HISTOLOGY

Normal skin is composed of two layers—epidermis and dermis and rests on a bed of subcutaneous fat. The epidermis is the surface layer. It is composed of keratinocytes, which produce keratin, a stiff protein.

The deepest layer is composed of basal cells (epidermal stem cells), from which arise new squamous cells. The basal layers undergo mitosis producing keratinocytes that change their size as they move upward.

This journey from the basal layer to the surface (epidermal turnover or transit time) takes about 30 days. Keratocytes make up about 85% of cells in the epidermis.

EPIDERMIS

The epidermis rests on a basement membrane, a thin, acellular film of protein, which separates the epidermis from the dermis below.

Epidermis is composed of stratum germinativum (basal cells), stratum spinosum (prickle layer), stratum granulosum and stratum corneum. Stratum lucidum is present between stratum corneum and stratum granulosum.

As the epidermal cells mature, these undergo flattening with accumulation of keratin to form stratum corneum. This layer is barrier to infectious agents.

Epidermis is very thin in most of regions. It may be 10 to 20 cells thick in some. It is considerably thicker on the palms and soles because of the extra thickness of the surface layer of dead cells of the stratum corneum (Figs 29.1 and 29.2).

Stratum Germinativum

The basal layer, the deepest layer, rests on a basement membrane, which attaches it to the dermis.

Stratum Spinosum (Prickle Layer)

Stratum spinosum is composed of keratinocytes. These are firmly attached to each other by small interlocking cytoplasmic processes, abundant *desmosomes*, and cadherins.

Desmosomes bind adjacent keratinocytes to one another. These are composed of transmembranous desmoglein–desmocollin pairs, which bind to the tonofilaments via desmoplakins, plakoglobin and plakophilin-1.

Desmoglein-1 (Dsg-1) is expressed in the upper epidermis while Dsg-3 is mostly expressed in the basal epidermis (Fig. 29.3).

Stratum Granulosum

This layer contains lamellar granules. It synthesizes phospholipids, cholesterol and glucosylceramides.

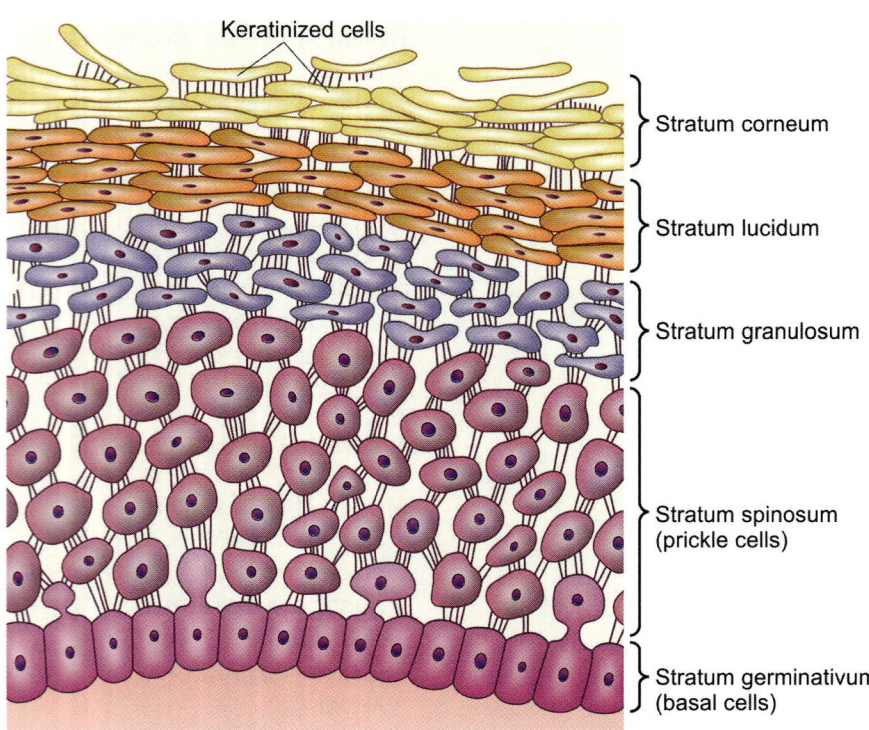

Fig. 29.1: Epidermis. The basal layers undergo mitosis producing keratinocytes that change their size as they move upward, replacing cells that are lost during normal cell shedding.

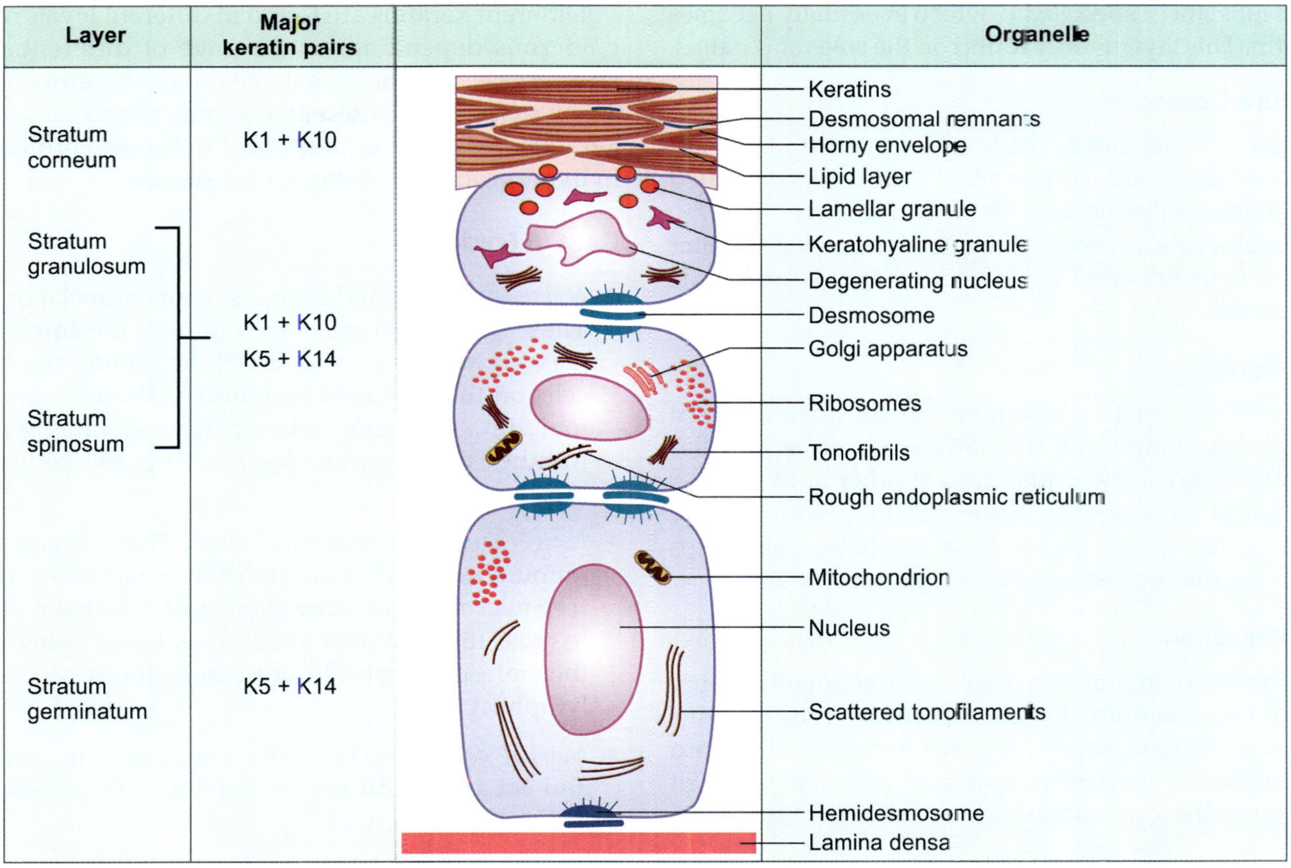

Layer
Major keratin pairs
Organelle
Stratum corneum
K1 + K10
Stratum granulosum
K1 + K10
K5 + K14
Stratum spinosum
Stratum germinatum
K5 + K14
Keratins
Desmosomal remnants
Horny envelope
Lipid layer
Lamellar granule
Keratohyaline granule
Degenerating nucleus
Desmosome
Golgi apparatus
Ribosomes
Tonofibrils
Rough endoplasmic reticulum
Mitochondrion
Nucleus
Scattered tonofilaments
Hemidesmosome
Lamina densa

Fig. 29.2: A representation of the components of various layers of the skin with a depiction of major keratin pairs.

Thus, it helps in the barrier function. It also participates in process of keratinization.

Stratum Lucidum

It is a thin, clear layer of dead skin cells in the epidermis, and is named for its translucent appearance. It contains a

Epidermis
Desmosome
(desmoglein-1 and -3,
desmoplakin)
Basal keratinocyte
(keratins 5 + 14)
Tonofilaments
(keratin)
Hemidesmosome
(BPAg, collagen XVII,
α6, β4 integrin)
Basal cell
membrane
Lamina lucida
(laminin-1)
Anchoring filament
(laminin-5)
Lamina densa
(type IV collagen)
Anchoring fibril
(collagen VII)
Sublamina densa
Dermis

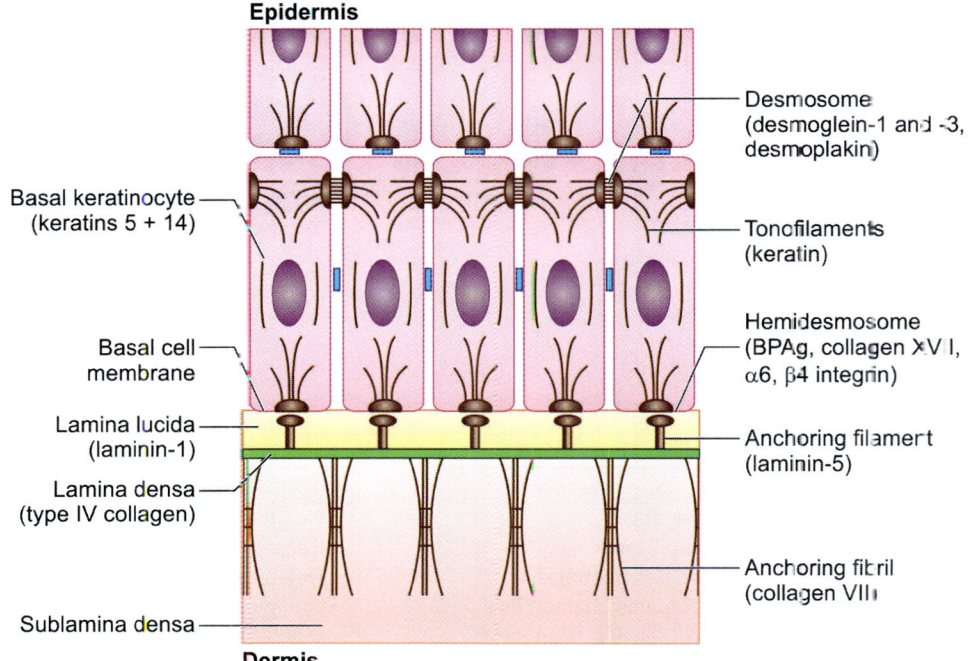

Fig. 29.3: Diagram detailing components of stratum spinosum and basement membrane zone.

clear substance called *eludin*, which eventually becomes keratin. This layer is only found on the soles and palms.

Stratum Corneum

It has no nuclei and is made up of piled-up layers of flattened dead cells (corneocytes)—the bricks separated by lipids and the mortar—in the intercellular space.

Together these provide an effective barrier to water loss and to invasion by infectious agents and toxic chemicals.

Skin Barrier

The *skin barrier* is consequent to the formation of ceramides, cholesterol, free fatty acids (from lamellar granules) and smaller quantities of other lipids.

Natural moisturizing factor (NMF), predominantly made up of amino acids and their metabolites, also helps maintain the properties of the stratum corneum.

Keratinization

The process of maturation of cells with change in quality and type of keratins is called kertinization. Keratins (from the Greek keras meaning *horn*) are the main intermediate filaments in epithelial cells. These are of two types basic and acidic and are always in pairs.

Different keratins are found at different levels of the epidermis depending on the stage of differentiation and disease. Normal basal cells make keratins 5 and 14, but terminally differentiated suprabasal cells make keratins 1 and 10. Keratins 6 and 16 become prominent in hyperproliferative states, i.e. psoriasis.

Cells in Epidermis

- *Melanocytes:* The epidermis also contains melanocytes. These specialized cells, derived from the embryonic nervous system (neural crest), lie among the basal cells on the basement membrane. These synthesize melanin. A single melanocyte associates with a number of keratinocytes forming an epidermal melanin unit.

- *Langerhans' cells (dendritic cells):* These specialized immune system cells are voracious phagocytes. These trap microbes and other alien materials that manage to cross the basement membrane. Langerhans' cells then present captured antigen to immune system lymphocytes.

- *Merkel cells:* Merkel cells are found in normal and act as transducers for fine touch (Figs 29.4 and 29.5).

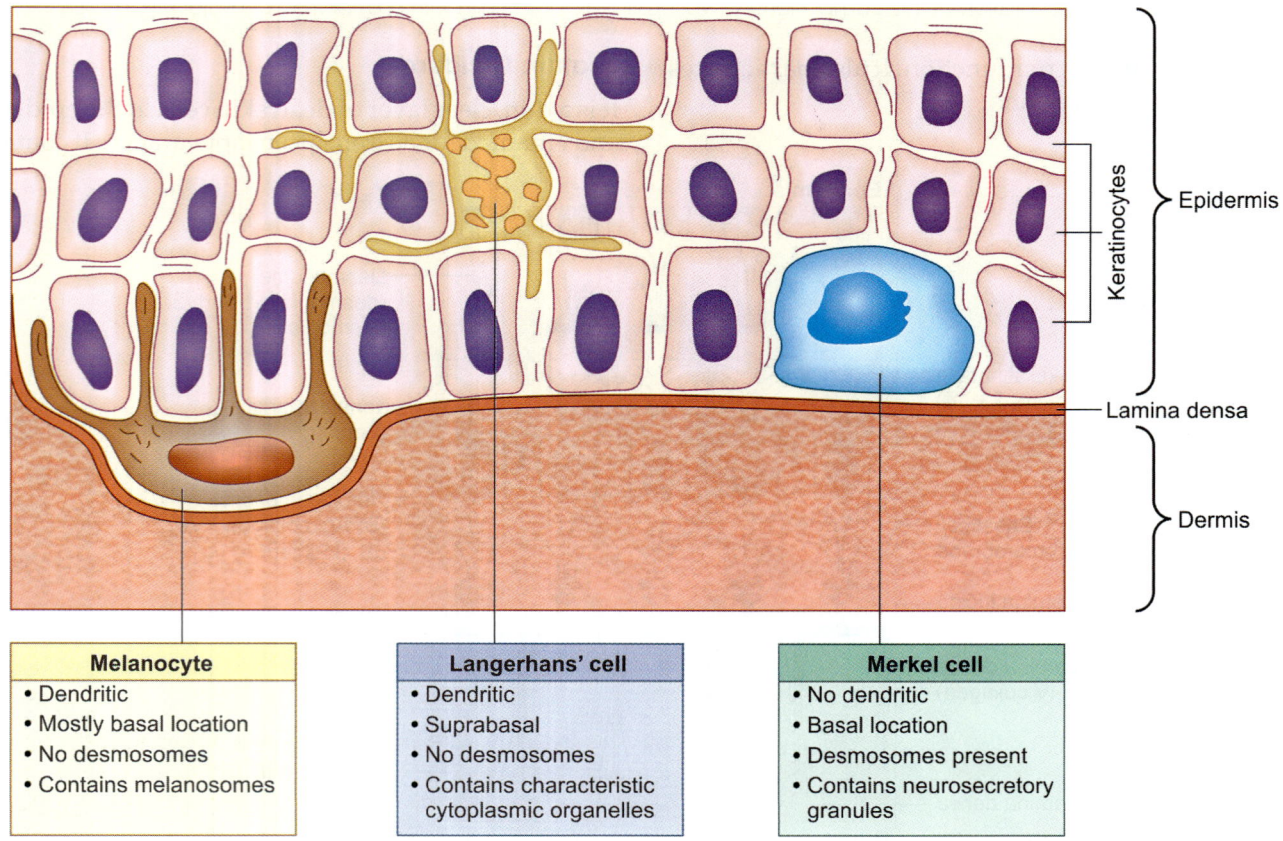

Fig. 29.4: A representation of epidermis and dermis. Epidermis shows melanocyte, Langerhans' cell and Merkel cell.

Skin

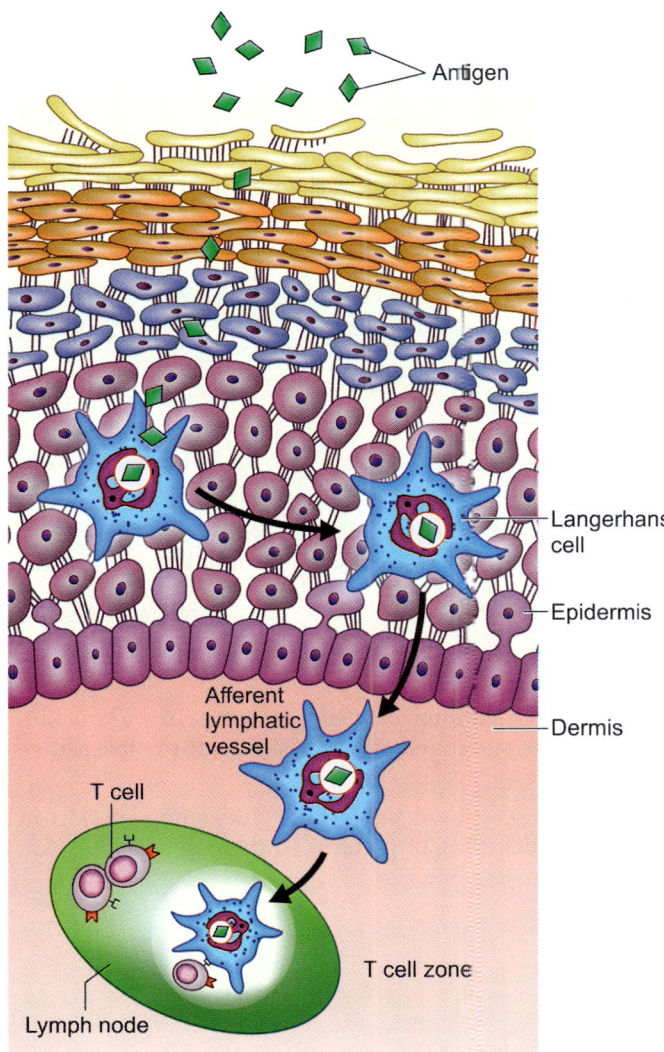

Fig. 29.5: A representation of Langerhans' cells and their function.

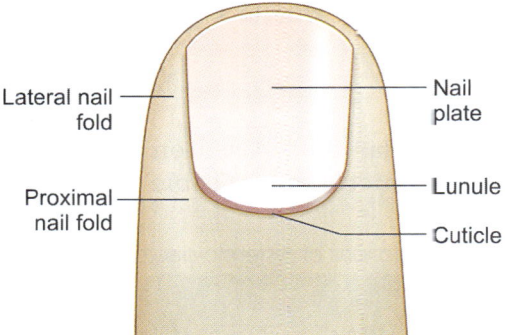

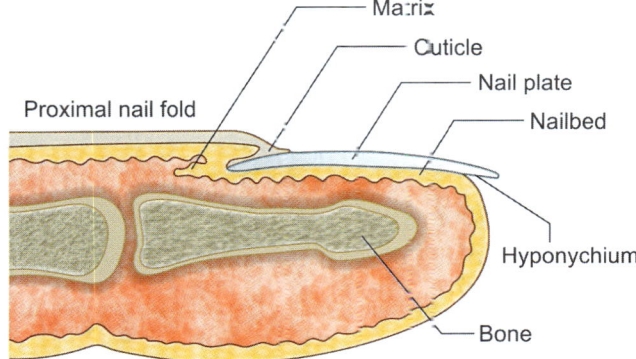

Fig. 29.6: Structure of the nail.

DERMIS

The dermis is a framework of fibrous and elastic tissue. It lies beneath the basement membrane. It contains nerves, specialized sensory nerve endings, blood vessels, and skin appendages (adnexa), such as sweat glands, sebaceous glands and hair follicles. The dermis is usually about 1–2 mm thick, much thicker than the epidermis.

Cells

- *Fibroblasts:* The main cell in the dermis is the fibroblast, which produces the collagen and elastin fibers that account for skin toughness and resiliency.
- *Dermal dendritic cells:* These are similar to epidermal Langerhans' cells.

SUBCUTANEOUS TISSUE

Below the dermis is a pelt of fatty subcutaneous tissue. It serves as insulation and cushioning of some hair follicles. Below subcutaneous fat is a layer of dense fascia that sheaths the entire body and covers bone, muscle, and other deep structures.

NAILS

Structure

The hard keratin of the nail plate is formed in the nail matrix, which lies in an invagination of the epidermis (the nail fold) on the back of the terminal phalanx of each digit. The matrix runs from the proximal end of the floor of the nail fold to the distal margin of the lunula. From this area, the nail plate grows forward over the nailbed, ending in a free margin at the tip of the digit.

Functions

The cuticle acts as a seal to protect the potential space of the nail fold from chemicals and from infection. The nails provide strength and protection for the terminal phalanx. Their presence helps with fine touch and with the handling of small subjects. The structure of the nail and nailbed is shown in Fig. 29.6.

SKIN DISORDERS: OVERVIEW

Skin disorders may be primary or secondary. Primary disorders of the skin include inflammatory, pigment disorders, autoimmune disorders, dermatoses, thermal injuries, and skin cancers (squamous cell carcinoma, basal cell carcinoma and malignant melanoma). Skin manifestations may occur due to systemic disorders (Table 29.1).

Classification

Skin disorders are classified based on histological findings on light microscopy (Table 29.2). Skin tumors may be primary (benign or malignant) and secondary. These are classified according to cell of origin (Table 29.3).

Terminology

Terminology is used in skin disorders (Table 29.4).

Table 29.1: Skin manifestations of systemic disorders

Disease	Skin manifestations
Sarcoidosis	Erythema nodosum, lupus pernio, nodules in scar
Scleroderma	Thickened tight skin (especially fingers), skin telangiectasis, and calcified nodules
Hyperlipidemia	Xanthelasmata of eyelids, xanthomas of elbows, knuckles, buttock, soles, palms and Achilles tendon
Diabetes mellitus	Necrobiosis lipoidica—symmetric plaques on shins with atrophic yellow appearance and waxy feel, cutaneous Candida, ulcers on feet
Cushing's syndrome	Purple striae, thin skin, easy bruising
Inflammatory bowel disease (ulcerative colitis and Crohn's disease)	Pyoderma gangrenosum—large ulcer
Dermatomyositis	Edema and mauve discoloration of eyelid, erythema of the knuckles and other bony points, such as elbow and shoulder to photosensitive butterfly rash on face
Cancers	Acanthosis nigricans—brown velvet-like thickening of skin in axilla, and groin—thickening or painless ichthyosis—fish-like skin appearance

Table 29.2: Classification of skin disorders based on light microscopy

Involving skin component	Disorders
Epidermis	Psoriasis, pemphigus vulgaris
Dermal-epidermal interface	Bullous pemphigoid, erythema multiforme, lupus erythematosus
Superficial and deep vascular bed	Cutaneous vasculitis, contact dermatitis
Dermal connective tissue	Systemic sclerosis
Panniculus adiposus	Erythema nodosum, erythema induratum
Skin neoplasms	Squamous cell carcinoma, basal cell carcinoma, intradermal nevus, malignant melanoma

Table 29.3: Classification of skin tumors

Origin in skin	Tumors
Keratinocytes	Squamous cell carcinoma, basal cell carcinoma
Melanocytes	Intradermal nevus, malignant melanoma
Merkel cells	Merkel cell carcinoma
Langerhans' cells	Langerhans' cell histiocytosis
Skin appendages	Pilomatrixoma, chondroid syringoma
Connective tissue	Hemangioma
Hematopoietic and lymphoid cells	Lymphoma of skin

Table 29.4: Terminology of skin lesions

Lesion	Morphology
Macule	Flat lesion <1 cm (discoloration of skin)
Patch	Flat lesion >1 cm (discoloration of skin)
Papule	Solid elevation of skin <5 mm in diameter
Nodule	Solid elevation >5 mm
Plaque	Palpable elevation >1 cm
Vesicle	Small, fluid-containing blister <5 mm
Bulla	A fluid filled blister >5 mm
Pustule	Visible collection of pus in blister
Crust	Dried exudate, e.g. serum, blood or pus, on the skin surface
Hyperkeratosis	Increased thickness of the stratum corneum
Parakeratosis	Hyperkeratosis with retention of nuclei of keratinocytes
Acanthosis	Thickening of the epidermis
Spongiosis	It refers to epidermal intercellular edema with widening of intercellular spaces
Acantholysis	There is separation of epidermal cells, one from the other; cells appear to float within extracellular fluid
Lichenification	It refers to accentuation of skin markings caused by scratching

Note: Terms are arranged in loosely related groups, generally in order of increasing severity.

INFLAMMATORY DISORDERS

Inflammatory disorders of skin include lichenoid/interface, psoriasiform, spongiotic, vesicobullous, granulomatous, vasculopathic and panniculitis dermatoses (Table 29.5).

Table 29.5: Inflammatory dermatoses terminology and examples

Light microscopy	Examples	Skin lesions
Lichenoid/interface dermatoses		
Damage to basal keratinocytes	Lichen planus	Multiple papules and plaques on skin, hair, nails and mucous membrane
Lymphocytic infiltration in the upper dermis	Lichen planus like keratosis	Single red scaly plaque on sun-exposed regions
	Erythema multiforme (Stevens-Johnson syndrome)	Symmetrical cutaneous sloughing lesions on palms and soles
	Lupus erythematosus	Butterfly shaped skin lesions and organs involvement
	Graft-versus-host disease (acute and chronic)	Acute GVHD: eruptions on palms, soles, head and neck Chronic GVHD: it may resemble lichen planus or lichen morphea
Psoriasisform dermatoses		
Elongation of the rete ridges	Psoriasis	Erythematous plaques with thick skin on extensor surfaces of elbows and knees
	Lichen simplex chronicus	Thick hyperkeratotic plaques on back of neck, extensors of forearms, legs and genital regions
Spongiotic dermatoses		
Expanded space between adjacent keratinocytes of the spinous layer of epidermis	Eczema/atopic dermatitis	Erythematous scaly plaques with variable distribution
	Pityriasis rosea	Erythematous scaly plaques (Christmas tree-like pattern) on back
	Eosinophilic spongiosis	Lesions vary based on etiology

Contd...

Table 29.5: Inflammatory dermatoses terminology and examples (Contd...)

Light microscopy	Examples	Skin lesions
Vesicobullous dermatoses		
Vesicles or bullae formation	Bullous pemphigoid	Generalized tense blisters on erythematous base in elderly
	Pemphigus vulgaris	Painful oral erosions and flaccid cutaneous blisters that extend with lateral pressure (Nikolsky's sign)
	Porphyria cutenea tarda	Blistering of skin-exposed on hand and face
	Epidermolysis bullosa acquisita	Blisters on site of trauma
	Dermatitis herpetiformis	Pruritic small vesicles
Granulomatous dermatoses		
Epitheliod cell granuloma	Necrobiotic granuloma (e.g. granuloma annulare)	Erythematous plaques or subcutaneous nodules on localized or generalized sites
	Necrobiosis lipoidica	Plaques with depressed yellow center in diabetes mellitus
	Sarcoidosis	Variable lesions (annular, hypopigmented spots, ichthyosis-like, alopecia, subcutaneous nodules)
Vasculopathic dermatoses		
Damage to endothelial cells (dysfunctional endothelial cells)	Acute vasculitis (leucocytoplastic vascultis)	Palpable purpura on extremities
	Granuloma faciale	Reddish brown plaques on face
	Lymphocytic vasculitis	Variable morphology
	Vaso-occlusive vasculopathies	Purpura, ulcer or infarct
	Neutrophilic dermatosis (Sweet's syndrome)	Erythematous plaques, abrupt onset on head, neck and upper extremities
	Urticaria	Pruritic wheals
	Pigmented purpuric dermatosis	Multiple clinical variants
	Non-inflammatory purpura	Purplish erythematous discoloration
Panniculitis dermatoses		
Inflammatory changes to the septa or lobules of the subcutaneous adipose tissue	Erythema nodosum (septal)	Single or multiple painful erythematous nodules on anterior leg (shin)
	Erythema induratum/nodular fasciitis	Multiple erythematous plaques on posterior leg (calf)
	Subcutaneous fat necrosis of the newborn	Firm, nodular areas of body
	Membranous lipodystrophy	Variable lesions on lower extremities

ECZEMATOUS DERMATITIS

It is a heterogeneous group of pruritic inflammatory disorders. These include infection, chemicals and allergy (atopy).

Pathogenesis

Eczematous dermatitis frequently occurs in persons with type I anaphylactic-type hypersensitivities, such as hay fever or bronchial asthma (Fig. 29.7).

Chemical can directly injure skin or may act as antigens. Type IV cell-mediated hypersensitivity reaction plays key role in eczema due to chemical contact resulting from cooperation of skin macrophages (Langerhans' cells) and helper T lymphocytes.

The skin manifestations in atopic patients are most often caused by type IV rather than type I hypersensitivity.

Light Microscopy

Morphology of the eczematous lesion depends on the activity of disease.
- *Acute stage:* Lesion shows spongiosis with vesicle formation.

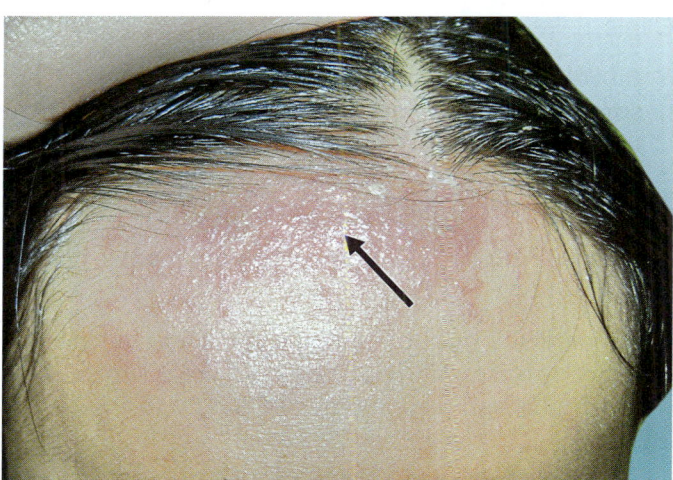

Fig. 29.7: Eczematous allergic contact dermatitis. A patient with itching, erythema and oozing following use of hair dye (arrow).

- *Chronic stage:* Lesion shows acanthosis, hyperkeratosis, lichenification, and focal lymphocytic dermal infiltrates.
- *Subacute stage:* Lesion shows intermediate changes between acute and chronic; less spongiosis and vesiculation than in acute; less acanthosis and hyperkeratosis than in chronic eczematous dermatitis.

IMPETIGO

Impetigo occurs due to bacterial infections (usually *Staphylococcus aureus* or Group A Streptococcus) of the superficial layers of epidermis of exposed skin (face and hands) (Fig. 29.8).

Clinical Features

Patient presents with an erythematous macule. Multiple small pustules rapidly supervene. As pustules break, shallow erosions form, covered with drying serum, giving the characteristic clinical appearance of honey-colored crust. If the crust is not removed, new lesions form about the periphery and extensive epidermal damage may ensue.

Light Microscopy
- Impetigo lesion shows accumulation of neutrophils beneath the stratum corneum, often with the formation of a subcorneal pustule.
- Gram stain reveals the presence of bacteria in these foci.
- Nonspecific, reactive epidermal alterations and superficial dermal inflammation accompany these findings.

NEURODERMATITIS

Neurodermatitis is also known as lichen simplex chronicus. This lesion is clinically indistinguishable from chronic eczematous dermatitis. It produces anatomic changes entirely secondary to scratching. The cause of the pruritus is unknown but may be psychogenic. It is secondary to chronic, habitual rubbing and scratching.

Clinical Features

Patient presents with well-defined hyperpigmented to erythematous leathery plaques with exaggerated skin lines (lichenification) on *posterior neck, genitalia, extensor aspect of arms and legs* (Fig. 29.9).

SCABIES

Scabies caused by the mite *Sarcoptes scabiei*), manifests as burrows under the stratum corneum of the hands, periareolar and genital skin.

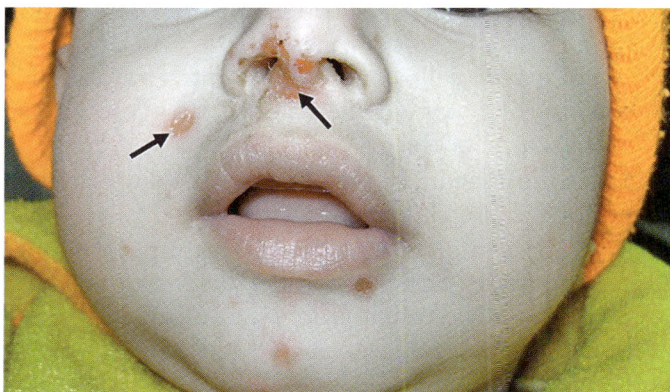

Fig. 29.8: Impetigo. A child with lesions of impetigo on the face with the serum giving rise to the classic golden-yellow, "honey-crusted" lesion (arrows).

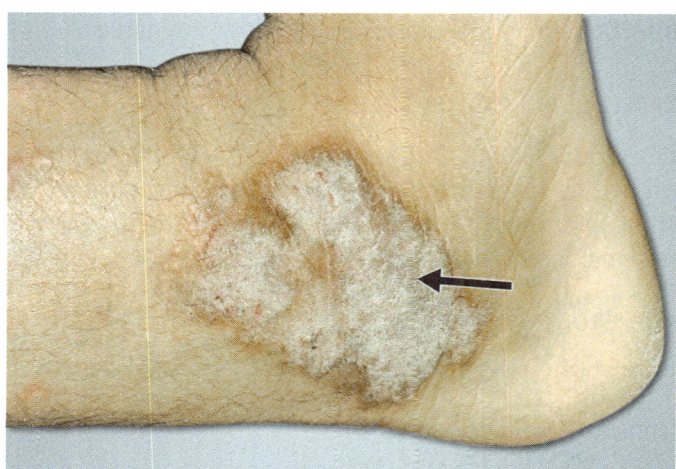

Fig. 29.9: Neurodermatitis. Chronic scratching leads to a thick raised plaque with increase in surface markings (lichen simplex chronicus) (arrow).

Pathogenesis

Sarcoptes scabiei is a mite that lives only on humans. Transmission occurs by close personal contact, i.e. mother–child, siblings, or sexual partners.

Female mites burrow in the epidermis just below the stratum corneum, depositing eggs and feces as they move along.

The first infestation remains asymptomatic for a period of weeks, until an immune response develops and pruritus results.

Upon re-infestation, the symptoms appear in a matter of days.

Clinical Features

- *Burrows:* Female mites are found in slightly raised, sometimes erythematous, irregular lines with a terminal swelling. Typical sites include *interdigital spaces, sides of the hands and feet, flexural surface of the wrist, anterior axillary line, penis, and nipples.*
- *Intense pruritus:* Patient presents with intense itching at night.
- *Dermatitis:* Immune reaction (type IV) to mites leads to both pruritus and diffuse exanthema. Typical sites are thighs, buttocks, and trunk (Figs 29.10 and 29.11).

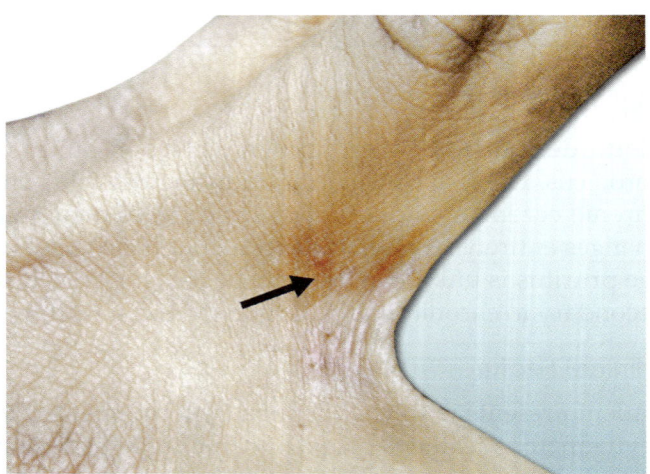

Fig. 29.10: Scabies. Pathognomonic involvement of the web spaces in a case of scabies (arrow).

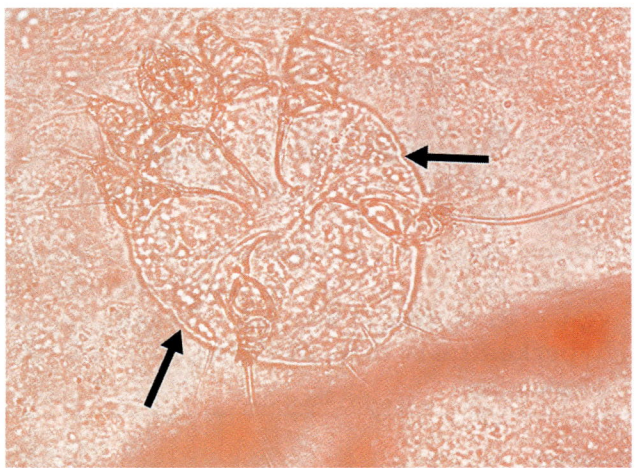

Fig. 29.11: Scabies mite is demonstrated on wet mount preparation (arrows).

CUTANEOUS INFECTIONS

Common cutaneous infections are caused by viruses and fungi (Table 29.6). Molluscum contagiosum and condyloma acuminatum have viral etiology. Fungal infections may be cutaneous and angioinvasive.

MOLLUSCUM CONTAGIOSUM

It is viral infection of the skin caused by DNA poxvirus. MCV-1 is transmitted by direct skin-skin contact or sharing infected clothes. MCV-2 is transmitted via sexual contact in adults.

Age Group

It most often occurs in children and adolescents.

Clinical Features

Patient presents with umbilicated, dome-shaped papules over body, arms and legs. Average incubation period is 6 weeks.

Umbilication of lesion occurs as a result of intra-cytoplasmic viral inclusions extruding infected cell on the surface with central pore (Fig. 29.12).

> **Light Microscopy**
> - Epidermis grows deeper down into the dermis and form closely packed lobules.
>   Epidermal cells contain large intracytoplasmic eosinophilic stained inclusion bodies known as molluscum bodies.
> - These **molluscum bodies** displace the nuclei at the periphery of epidermal cells.
>   In the center of the lesion, stratum corneum disintegrates and release the *molluscum bodies* together with keratinous debris resulting in formation of central crater.
> - Dermis shows prominent acute and chronic inflammatory infiltrate and foreign body giant cells (Fig. 29.13).

Table 29.6: Cutaneous infections caused by viruses and fungi

Examples	Skin lesions
Viral infections	
Molluscum contagiosum	Single or multiple 1–2 mm umbilicated papules in children
Verruca vulgaris	Single or multiple hyperkeratotic lesions
Verruca plana	Multiple small flesh-colored to pinkish papules on face and hands at any age
Condyloma acuminatum	HPV 16, 18 induced single or multiple flesh-colored papules on external genitalia, perineum and anus
Deep palmoplantar wart	Single or multiple hyperkeratotic papules
Herpes simplex	Clinical variable lesions form painful vesicular lesions
Fungal infections	
Dermatophytosis (variable pustules)	*Tinea corporis:* Annular erythematous plaques
	Tinea capitis/Tinea barbae: Folliculitis of scalp or face
	Tinea faciei: Itchy scaly rash over face
	Onychomycosis: Thickened or discolored nails
Angioinvasive fungus	Necrotic papules/plaques in immunocompromised persons
Traumatic implanted fungus/ dematiaceous fungus	Scaly and erythematous nodules at the site of traumas

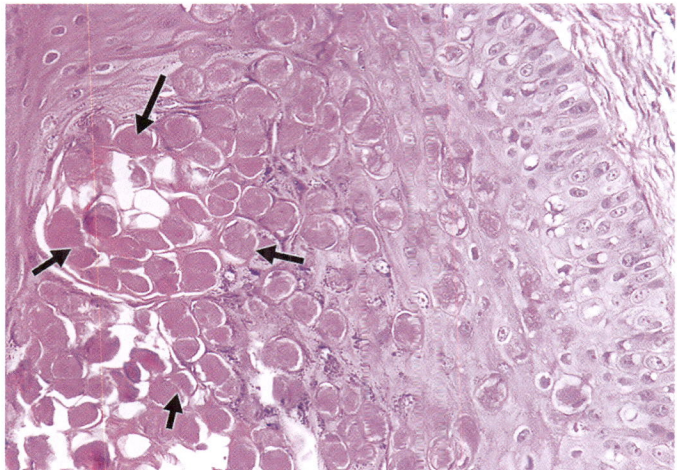

Fig. 29.13: Molluscum contagiosum—epidermal cells contain large intracytoplasmic eosinophilic stained inclusion bodies known as *molluscum bodies* (arrows) (400X).

VERRUCA VULGARIS (COMMON WART)

Etiology
Warts are caused by DNA containing papillomavirus.

Transmission
Transmission involves direct contact between individuals, or autoinoculation.

Clinical Course
Generally, these warts are self-limited lesions, often regressing spontaneously within six months to two years. These strains are distinct from HPV strains associated with gynecologic neoplasms (Fig. 29.14). Classification of warts morphology and distribution is shown in Table 29.7.

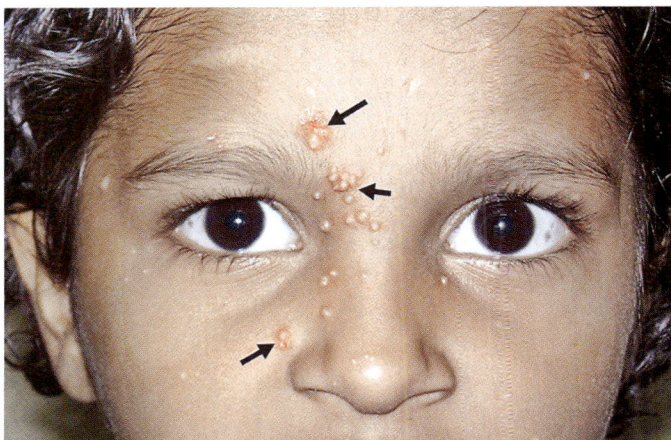

Fig. 29.12: Molluscum contagiosum. This is a typical distribution of lesions on a child's face. Note the eyelid lesions (arrows).

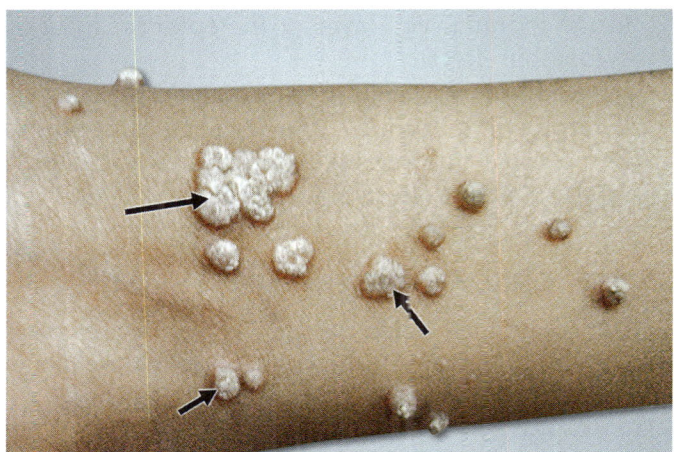

Fig. 29.14: Verruca vulgaris—common warts (verruca vulgaris). This patient has multiple common warts (arrows).

Table 29.7: Classification of warts, distribution and morphology

Lesion	Regions	Morphology
Verruca vulgaris	Hands	These are white to tan, flat to convex 0.1 to 1.0 cm papules with a rough, pebble-like surface
Verruca plana	Face, dorsal surfaces of hands	These are slightly elevated, flat, smooth, tan papules that are generally smaller than V. vulgaris
Verruca plantaris	Sole of foot	These are rough, scaly lesions may reach 1 to 2 cm in diameter, coalesce, and be confused with ordinary calluses
Verruca palmaris	Palm of hand	These are rough, scaly lesions may reach 1 to 2 cm in diameter, coalesce, and be confused with ordinary calluses
Condyloma acuminatum (venereal)	Penis, female genitalia, urethra, perianal area, and rectum	These may reach several cm in diameter and are soft, tan and cauliflower-like

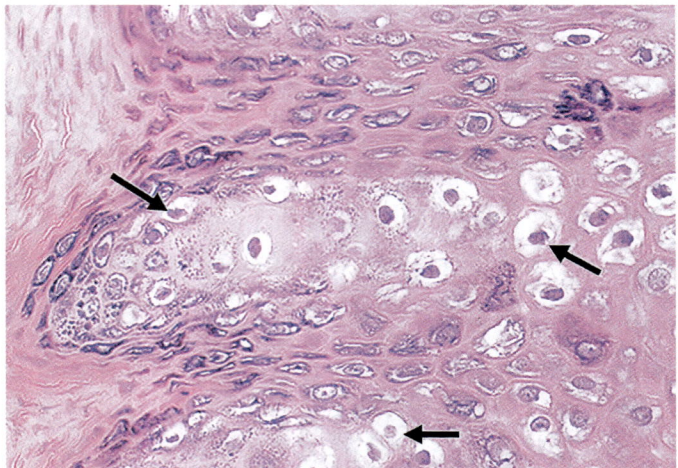

Fig. 29.15: A common wart, or verruca vulgaris. At higher magnification, the vacuolization of the epidermal cells (koilocytotic change) in this verruca vulgaris is seen. It indicates the viral origin of this lesion. One type of human papillomavirus (HPV) is associated with appearance of warts (arrows).

Light Microscopy
- Skin lesion shows vacuolated cells (koilocytes) in the granular cell layer of the epidermis (viral cytopathic effect).
- Infected cells can demonstrate prominent condensed keratohyaline granules and jagged eosinophilic intracytoplasmic keratin aggregates as a result of viral cytopathic effects (Fig. 29.15).

HERPETIC DERMATITIS (HERPES SIMPLEX VIRUS)

This is sometimes called *Shingles* and it occurs most often in immunocompromised patients or in the elderly.

Clinical Features
Crops of painful clear vesicles can appear in perineal-genital area (HSV-II) or produce tender lip, tongue, or buccal sores (*cold sores* from HSV-I). Another pattern produced by herpes zoster (also called varicella zoster virus) is the appearance of painful, clear vesicles on large areas of skin, usually on a dermatomal distribution (Figs 29.16 and 29.17).

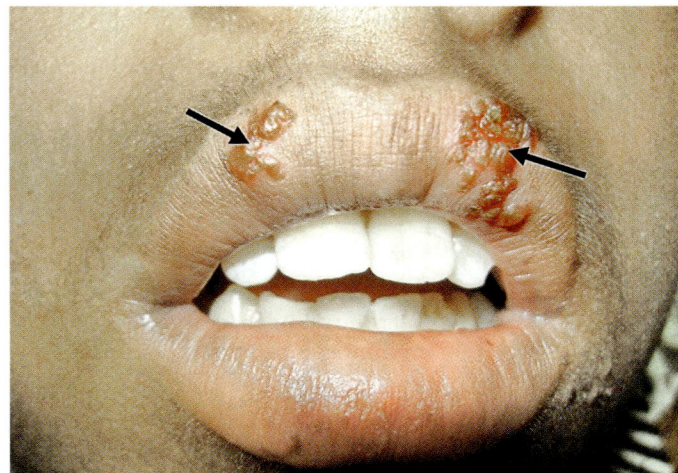

Fig. 29.16: Herpetic dermatitis—a case of recurrent HSV infection on the face in a female with grouped vesicles (arrows).

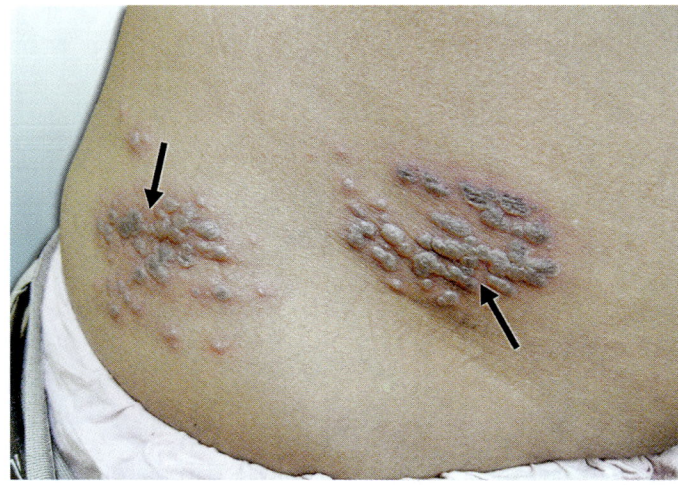

Fig. 29.17: Herpetic dermatitis. Grouped, erythematous, vesicles are seen here in a *zosteriform* distribution (arrows).

Skin

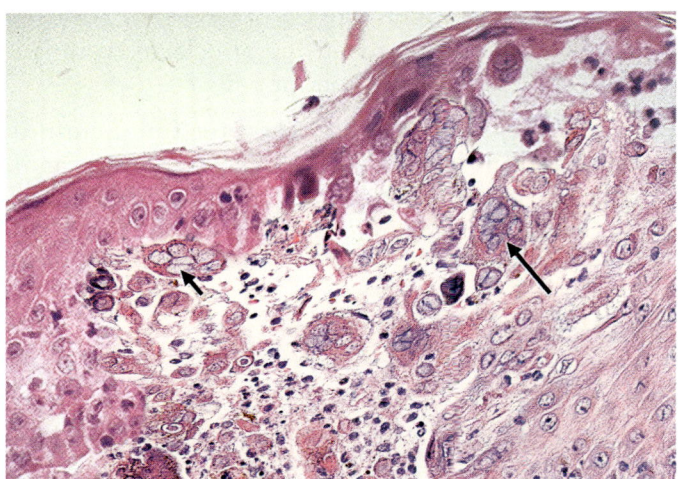

Fig. 29.18: Herpes simplex viral infection. Seen here are cells with multinucleation (long arrow) and steel gray to mauve inclusions (short arrow) typical for herpes simplex infection.

Light Microscopy

Within the lesions on biopsy or cytologic smear are intraepidermal vesicles with dead keratinocytes and multinucleated cells with large nuclei having *inclusions* or at least a change in color of the nucleus on H&E stain (i.e. viral particles inside) (Fig. 29.18).

VARICELLA (CHICKENPOX)

Chickenpox is a viral infection of childhood. It is caused by the varicella-zoster virus.

Clinical Features

Patient presents with fever and generalized vesicular eruptions (rashes). Following overt varicella, the virus can remain latent for years in dorsal root ganglia (Fig. 29.19).

SUPERFICIAL FUNGAL INFECTIONS

These are often confined to the stratum corneum, where they are caused primarily by dermatophytes. These organisms grow in the soil and on animals.

The genera most often causing dermatophytosis include *epidermophyton, microsporum*, and *trichophyton*. They can produce a number of diverse and characteristic clinical lesions according to the area involved.

Tinea Corporis

Tinea corporis is commonly referred to as *ringworm*, annular or ring-like eruption on the body.

It may spread from other infected humans. It may be autoinoculated from other areas of the body infected by tinea pedis or tinea capitis.

Another common method of transmission of tinea corporis is noted in wrestlers. *M. canis, T. rubrum,* and *T. mentagrophytes* are the usual pathogens. Lesions are generally annular with peripheral enlargement and central clearing (Fig. 29.20).

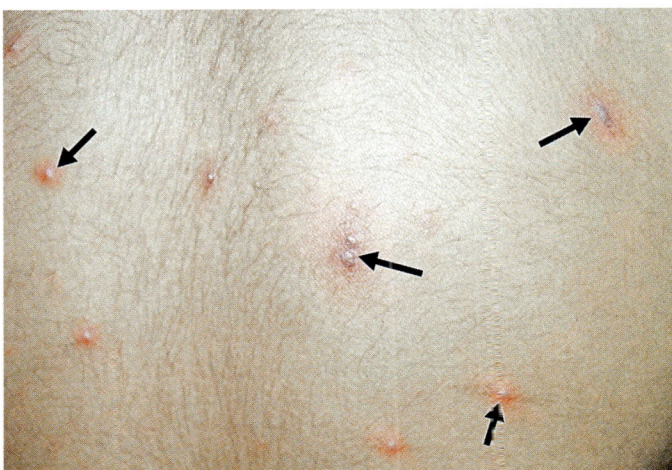

Fig. 29.19: Generalized vesicular eruptions (rashes) in varicella-zoster virus infection (arrows).

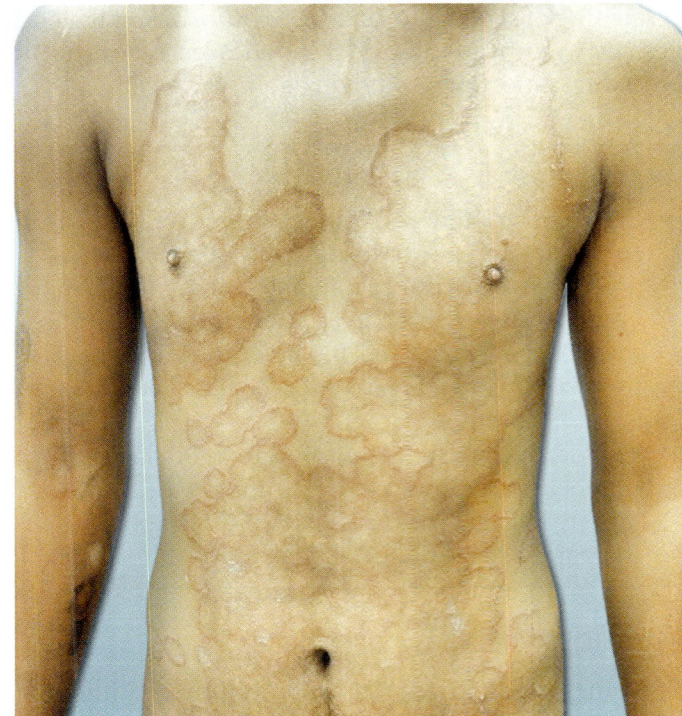

Fig. 29.20: A classic case of tinea corporis showing erythematous raised scaly advancing margins with central clearing showing increased activity of the fungus at the margins and presence of host immune response which clears the fungus from the center.

Light Microscopy
- A scraping with KOH mount can be utilized to identify these fungi. Fungal cell walls are rich in mucopolysaccharides and stained with PAS resulting in bright pink to red appearance. Involved areas of skin and nails may fluoresce under ultraviolet light.
- The fungi are present in the anucleate cornified layer of lesional skin, hair, or nails.
- Therefore, scrapings are taken for fungi culture and definite classification. Reactive epidermal changes may produce a pattern that mimics a mild eczematous dermatitis.

AUTOIMMUNE DISORDERS

PSORIASIS

Psoriasis is a chronic nonpruritic disease of the dermis and epidermis. It is characterized by persistent epidermal hyperplasia resulting in sharply demarcated erythematous plaques covered with a silvery scale commonly on the dorsal extensor cutaneous surfaces. It may be of autoimmune etiology. **Cw6 gene** has the strongest association with psoriasis.

Location

It most often involves *extensor surfaces of the elbows* and *knees, as well as the scalp and sacral area* (Fig. 29.21).

Auspitz Sign

Scratching of scaly lesion causes rupture of small blood vessels in suprapapillary thinned area resulting in pinpoint hemorrhages known as *Auspitz sign*.

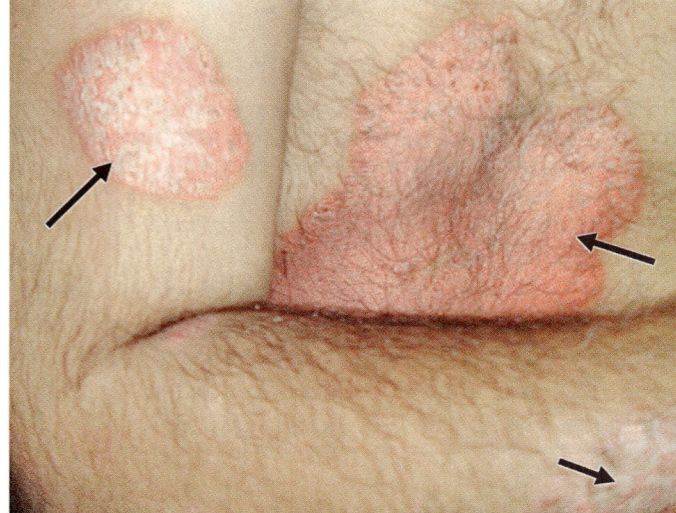

Fig. 29.21: Psoriasis. Multiple erythematous plaques of psoriasis (arrows).

Light Microscopy
- Skin biopsy shows thickening of epidermis several folds, hyperkeratosis, parakeratosis, regular acanthosis and suprapapillary thinning (portion of epidermis over papillae thinned out). Neutrophils may become localized in the epidermal spinous layer or in small '*Munro microabscesses*' in the stratum corneum.
- The dermis below the papillae exhibits a varying number of mononuclear inflammatory cells around the superficial vascular plexuses. The capillaries of the papillae are dilated and tortuous (Fig. 29.22).

PEMPHIGUS VULGARIS

Pemphigus vulgaris is an autoimmune acantholytic disease caused by autoantibody (desmoglein-3) to a keratinocyte antigen. The formation of severe intra-epidermal bullae is due to loss of cell-to-cell adhesion of epidermal cells.

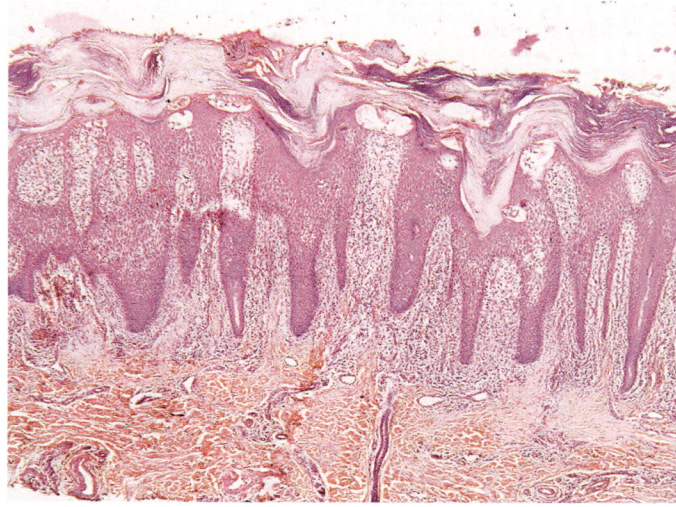

Fig. 29.22: Psoriasis is characterized by downward elongation of the rete ridges with thinning of overlying stratum granulosum, with parakeratosis above this. Small aggregates of neutrophils with surrounding spongiform change are seen in the superficial epidermis. Capillaries within dermal papillae are brought close to the surface (100X).

Age Group

It most often occurs in persons 30 to 60 years of age.

Pathogenesis

Circulating IgG antibodies in patients with pemphigus vulgaris react with an epidermal surface antigen called desmoglein-3, a *desmosomal protein.*

Antigen-antibody complex results in dyshesion. It is augmented by the release of plasminogen activator, hence plasmin. This proteolytic enzyme acts on the intercellular substance and may be the dominant factor in dyshesion.

Clinical Features

Patient initially develops lesions in the oral mucosa followed by extensive involvement of skin. Lesions often rupture, leaving large denuded surfaces subject to secondary infection (Fig. 29.23).

Light Microscopy

- In pemphigus vulgaris, distinctive rounded keratinocytes (termed acantholytic cells) are shed into the vesicle during the process of dyshesion.
- Lesion shows prominent intraepidermal acantholysis with intact basal layer as a floor and the remaining epidermis as a roof. The blister contains lymphocytes, macrophages, eosinophils, and neutrophils (Fig. 29.24).

Immunofluorescence Study

It shows deposition of IgG and C3 around cell membranes highlighting intercellular pattern of staining exhibiting *honeycomb appearance.*

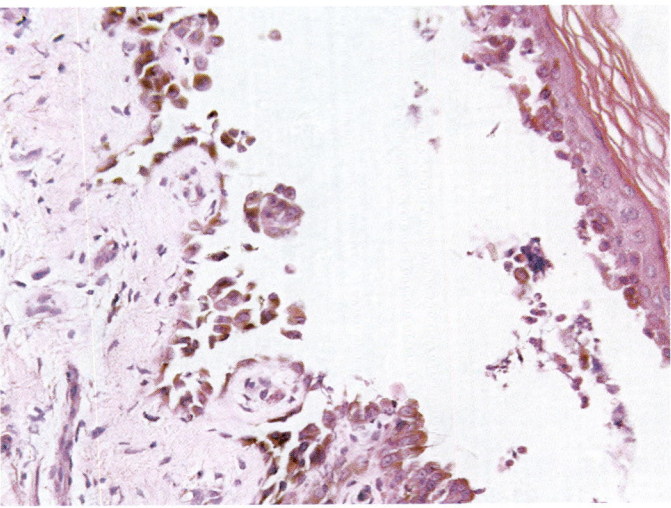

Fig. 29.24: Pemphigus vulgaris (400X).

BULLOUS PEMPHIGOID

This autoimmune blistering disorder resembles pemphigus vulgaris, but of less severity. Acantholysis is absent in bullous pemphigoid but present in pemphigus vulgaris.

Before blisters develop, pruritus, and urticarial lesions may be present. The blisters tend to develop in these areas. Since the entire epidermis forms the blister roof, hence the blisters become very stable.

They are tense, often have a fluid level, and can reach 10 cm in diameter. Oral mucosal involvement occurs in 20%; rarely presenting sign (Fig. 29.25).

Pathogenesis

Complement-fixing IgG antibodies are directed against two basement membrane proteins, BPAG1 and BPAG2.

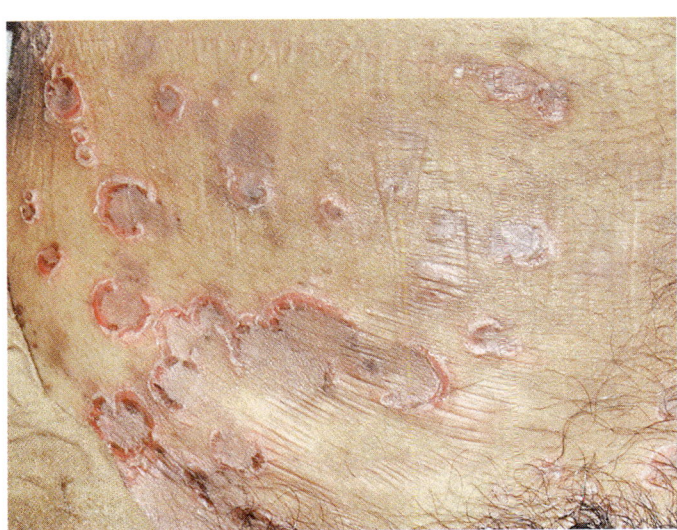

Fig. 29.23: Pemphigus vulgaris. Raw, erythematous and crusted lesions of pemphigus vulgaris.

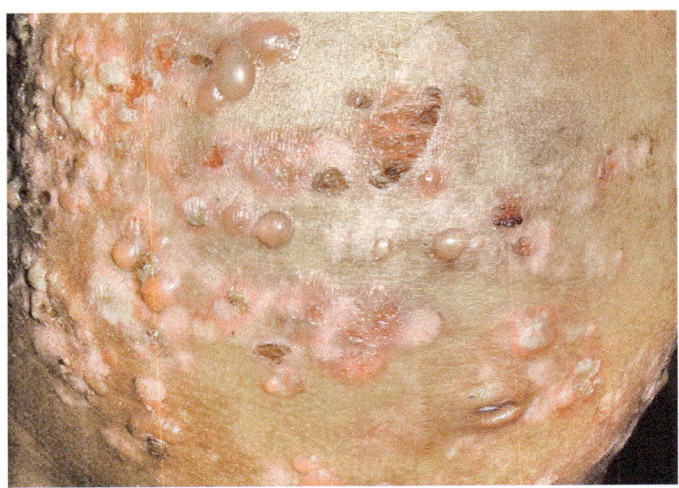

Fig. 29.25: Bullous pemphigoid. Tense blisters on an erythematous base in a case of BP.

Section III: Systemic Pathology

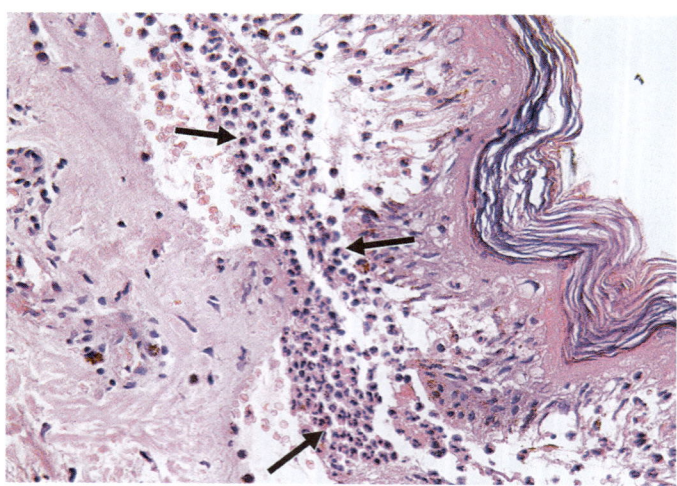

Fig. 29.26: Bullous pemphigoid (arrows) (400X).

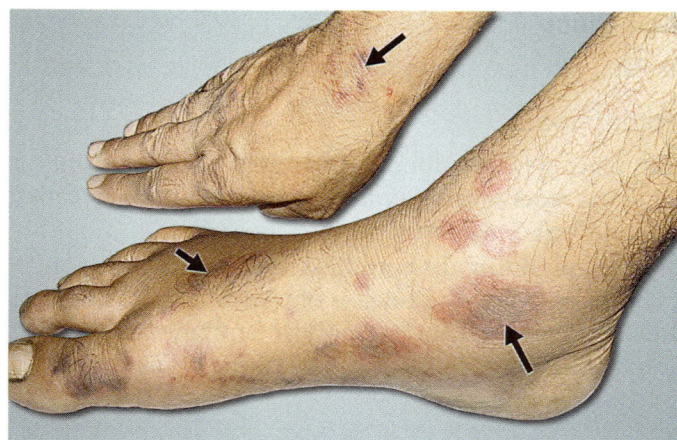

Fig. 29.27: Erythema multiforme. Center cyanosis surrounded by red ring in this case (arrows).

Light Microscopy

Skin biopsy shows subepidermal bullae, with a characteristic inflammatory infiltrate of eosinophils in the surrounding dermis (Fig. 29.26).

Immunofluorescence Study

In contrast to pemphigus vulgaris, immunofluorescent studies demonstrate deposition of C3 and IgG along the epidermal basement membrane.

DERMATITIS HERPETIFORMIS

Dermatitis herpetiformis is an intensely pruritic cutaneous eruption related to *gluten sensitivity* affecting 20–40 years of age.

Pathogenesis

IgA antibodies formed against gluten in the intestine gain access to the circulation and get deposited in the skin. Release of lysosomal enzymes by inflammatory cells cleave the epidermis from the dermis.

Clinical Features

Patient presents with urticaria-like plaques and vesicles over the extensor surfaces of knees and elbows, scalp, upper back, and sacral area. Patient improves when patients are placed on gluten-free diets.

Light Microscopy

Skin biopsy shows dermal microabscesses with neutrophils and eosinophils at the tips of dermal papillae, which become subepidermal blisters, blisters tend to occur in groups.

Immunofluorescence Study

Deposits of IgA are demonstrated at the tips of dermal papillae.

ERYTHEMA MULTIFORME

Erythema multiforme is characterized by development of variegated skin lesions, i.e. macules, papules, and vesicles. It is most often associated with a *target* lesion resembling an archer's bull's eye (Fig. 29.27).

Pathogenesis

There is usually hypersensitivity to coexistent infectious agents, various drugs, a concomitant connective tissue disorder, associated malignancy.

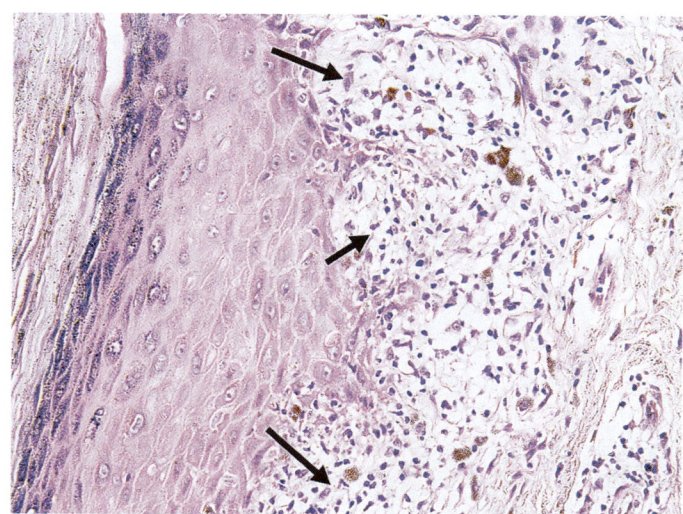

Fig. 29.28: Lichen planus shows lymphoid aggregates along epidermis–dermis junction destroying basal layer of epidermis (arrows) (400X).

LICHEN PLANUS

Lichen planus is considered to be mediated by T cells (Fig. 29.28).

Clinical Features

Patient presents with papules on the inner side of the wrist or blisters on palms and soles.

Light Microscopy

Histopathological examination of skin or oral and genital mucosa consists of band-like lymphoid infiltrates along the epidermal–dermal junction, destroying the basal layer of the epithelium (Fig. 29.28).

NONMELANOCYTIC LESIONS AND TUMORS

SEBORRHEIC KERATOSIS

Seborrheic keratosis is characterized by scaly, frequently pigmented, raised papules or plaques, tan to dark brown in color with velvety to granular surface on the head, neck, trunk, and extremities.

These scales are easily rubbed off. The lesions slowly enlarge and/or increase in number over the years (Fig. 29.29).

Age Group

It most often occurs on middle-aged to older individuals. The sudden appearance of numerous seborrheic keratosis has been associated with internal malignancies (sign of Leser-Trálet), especially gastric adenocarcinoma.

Light Microscopy

Skin biopsy shows broad anastomosing cords of mature stratified squamous epithelium with abrupt area of hyperkeratosis, acanthosis, focal hypergranulosis, and papillomatosis formation of adjacent to normal epidermis. It is associated with formation of small pseudohorn keratin cysts (Fig. 29.30).

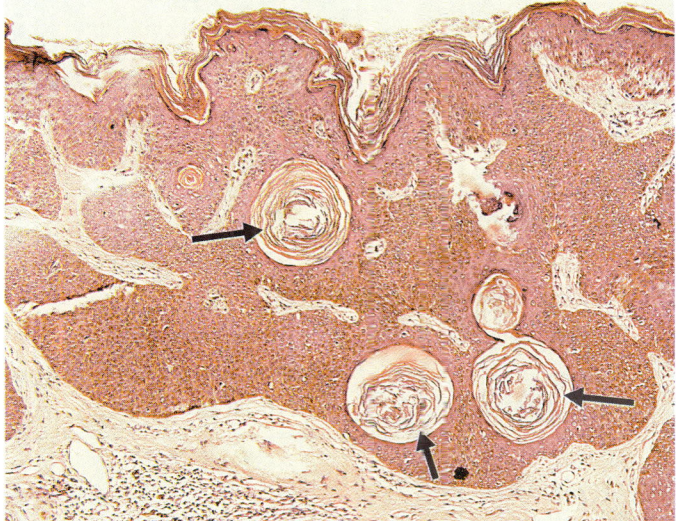

Fig. 29.30: Seborrheic keratosis shows pseudohorn cysts (arrows) (100X).

ACTINIC KERATOSIS

Actinic keratosis is caused by chronic excessive exposure to sunlight. With time, it may evolve into squamous cell carcinoma *in situ*, and finally, resulting in invasive squamous cell carcinoma. However, lesion may remain stable or regress.

Molecular Genetics

TP53 mutation and overexpression of cyclin D1 are demonstrated in 50% of cases. Activation of RAS is seen in 16% of cases. There is presence of loss of heterozygosity on chromosome 9p, 9q, 13q, 17p and 17q. Human papillomavirus has been detected in 41% of cases.

Clinical Features

Patient presents with scaly erythematous papules or nodules <1 cm in diameter on *sun-exposed skin of the face, neck, dorsum of hands and lower extremities* especially in fair-skinned persons. Consistency of lesions is *sandpaper-like*. Some lesions may produce so much keratin that a *cutaneous horn develops* (Fig. 29.31).

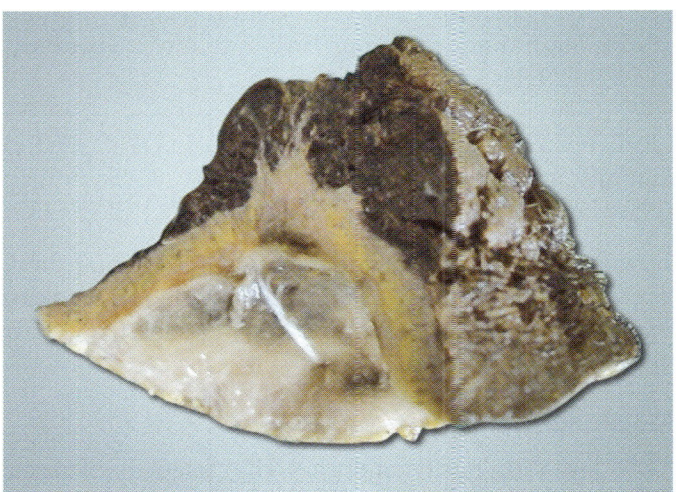

Fig. 29.29: Gross morphology of seborrheic keratosis.

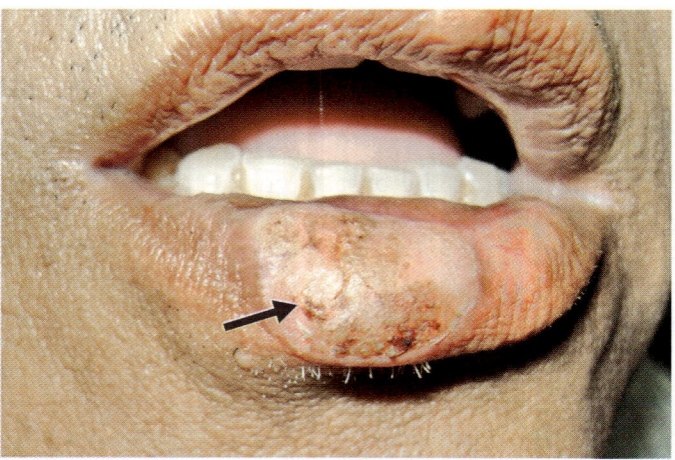

Fig. 29.31: Actinic keratosis. Lesion of actinic keratosis is present on the lip (arrow).

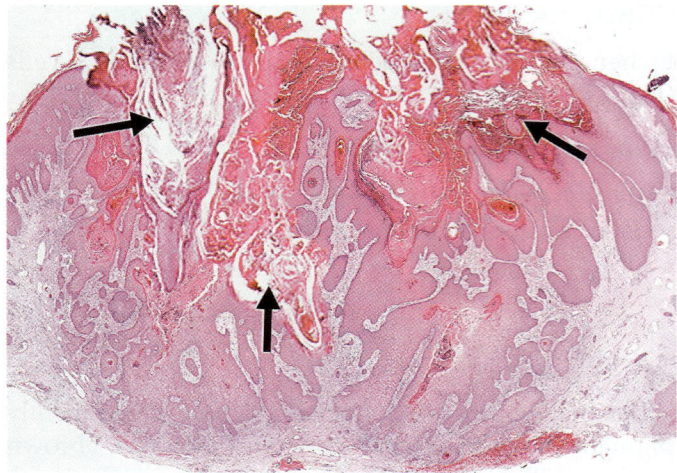

Fig. 29.32: Keratoacanthoma (arrows) (100X).

Light Microscopy

- Histological examination of skin shows patchy parakeratosis and agranulosis.
- Dyskeratotic cells are sometimes present.
- Dysplasia does not involve full thickness of the epidermis. Solar elastosis is most often seen.

KERATOACANTHOMA

This cutaneous low grade tumor is considered as variant of squamous cell carcinoma. It is rapidly growing lesion with central keratin plug. Cytological pleomorphism is less common with glassy pale eosinophilic cytoplasm. There is an abrupt transition between the lesion and adjacent epidermis.

Predisposing Factors

These include trauma, radiotherapy, laser resurfacing, and at the donor site after skin grafting.

Locations

It has predilection for cheeks, nose, ears, and dorsa of hands on sun-exposed areas.

Age Group

Men are more often affected than women in elderly age group.

Clinical Features

This flesh-colored, dome-shaped nodule grows rapidly and attains 1–2 cm with a central crater filled with keratinaceous material, over one to two months. It heals spontaneously after several weeks leaving atrophic scar without treatment.

Gross Morphology

The lesion is solitary nodule with central keratin plug.

Light Microscopy

- This exoendophytic lesion is composed of central, keratin-filled crater, surrounded by keratinizing well differentiated squamous epithelium. There is marked acanthosis and hyperkeratosis.
- Cells in the center of lesion have glassy eosinophilic appearance of cytoplasm. These cells extend upward over the sides of the crater and downward into the dermis as irregular tongues or nests of squamous cells.
- Prominent inflammatory cells are present around the lesion.
- *Microabscesses* are present at the edge of lesion.
- Tumor does not extend beyond sweat glands. Perineural and vascular invasion may be present (Fig. 29.32).

SQUAMOUS CELL CARCINOMA *IN SITU* (BOWEN'S DISEASE)

Bowen's disease is characterized by sharply demarcated, scaly, often hyperkeratotic macule or plaque on skin-exposed regions on face and legs especially in fair skinned person.

Molecular Genetics

TP53 mutation has been observed in majority of cases. Allelic deletion of one or more chromosome has been detected in occasional cases.

Light Microscopy

- Histopathological examination of skin shows enlarged keratinocytes, hyperchromatic nuclei confined to full thickness of epidermis.
- Above the basal layer, there is presence of hyperkeratosis, dyskeratosis, mitoses and loss of maturation.

INVASIVE SQUAMOUS CELL CARCINOMA

Squamous cell carcinoma is a common malignant skin tumor associated with excessive sun exposure. It is most often locally invasive.

Locations

Most common sites include the *lower part of face* and *back of the hands*.

Clinical Features

Patient initially presents with firm or erythematous nodules. Later lesions become shallow ulcers with firm elevated or indurated surroundings, sometimes with crust or scale especially in fair-skin persons as well as immunocompromised adults (Figs 29.33 and 29.34).

Risk Factors

Squamous cell carcinoma frequently originates in a pre-existing actinic keratosis. It most often occurs in sun-exposed areas. It is also associated with chemical carcinogens, such as arsenic, and radiation or radiologic exposure.

Exposure to ultraviolet radiation causes genetic mutation in p53 suppressor gene resulting in squamous cell carcinoma, basal cell carcinoma and skin melanoma. It also releases TNF-α (tumor necrosis factor-α) in exposed skin, possibly diminishing immune response. It induces dimer formation between neighboring thymine pairs in DNA.

Squamous cell carcinoma may be induced by such dimer formation in xeroderma pigmentosum, an autosomal recessive disorder due to failure of DNA excision repair mechanisms.

Repair genes correct errors in nucleotide pairing, excise pyrimidine dimmers in ultraviolet-damaged skin. Mutations of repair genes allow cells with lethal damage to proliferate, which increases the risk of cancer. Carcinogens associated with squamous cell carcinoma is shown in Table 29.8.

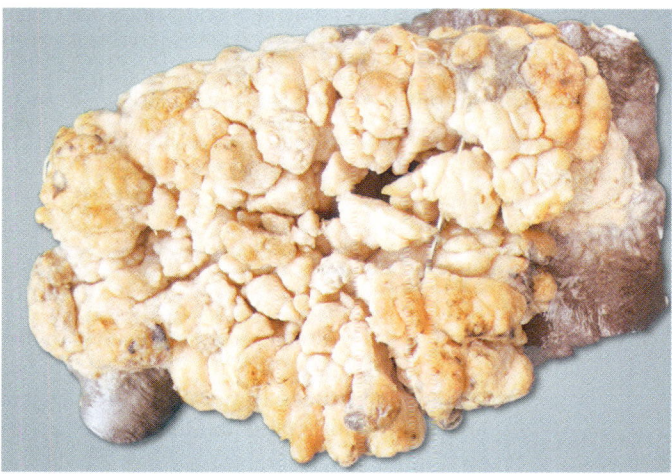

Fig. 29.34: Gross morphology of squamous cell carcinoma.

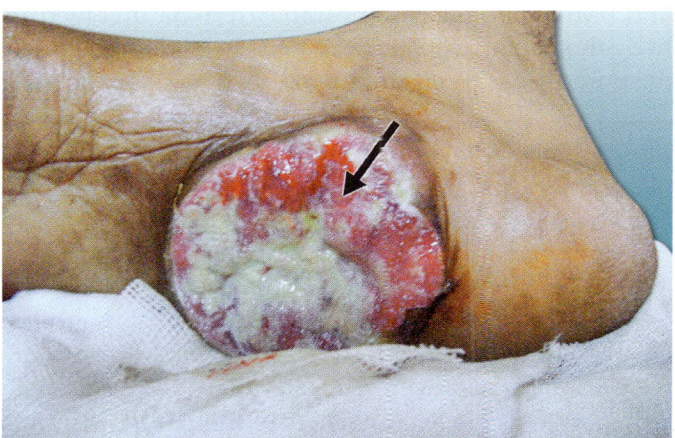

Fig. 29.33: Squamous cell carcinoma. Chronic ulcer on the sole in a case of SCC (arrow).

Light Microscopy

- Highly atypical cells are found at all levels of the epidermis beneath basement membrane. Invasive squamous cell carcinoma shows variable degree of differentiation.
- Tumor is composed of polygonal cells arranged in orderly lobules and exhibiting numerous large zones of keratinization forming squamous or keratin pearls to highly anaplastic, rounded cells with foci of necrosis and only abortive, single-cell keratinization (dyskeratosis) (Fig. 29.35).

Metastasis

Metastasis occurs in fewer than 5% of cases, because most of these lesions are discovered early and cured by ablative therapy.

Table 29.8: Carcinogens associated with squamous cell carcinoma

Chemical carcinogen	Examples	Associated cancers
Indirect acting chemical carcinogens and associated with cancers		
Occupational carcinogens	Arsenic used in alloys, medication, preparation of fungicides and herbicides	*Squamous cell carcinoma (skin)* *Basal cell carcinoma (skin)* Lung carcinoma Liver angiosarcoma
Radiation exposure associated cancers		
Ultraviolet radiation (UV B: 290–320 nm)	It causes p53 gene mutation TNF-α released by exposed skin diminishes immune response It induces dimer formation between neighboring thymine pairs in DNA	*Sporadic skin cancers:* Squamous cell carcinoma, basal cell carcinoma, and melanoma Skin cancers in xeroderma pigmentosum
Injury induced carcinogenesis		
Patient with third-degree burn scars may develop squamous cell carcinoma. Squamous cell carcinoma may develop at the orifices of chronically draining sinuses in patients with chronic osteomyelitis		

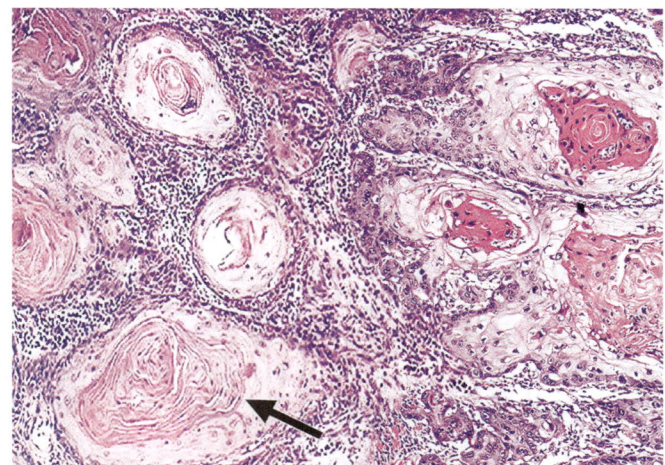

Fig. 29.35: Squamous cell carcinoma shows anaplastic cells forming keratin pearls (arrow) (100X).

BASAL CELL CARCINOMA

Basal cell carcinoma is the most common slow growing malignant tumor in persons with fair skin that rarely metastasizes.

There is a direct correlation between total exposure to sunlight on *head and neck region* resulting in basal cell carcinoma, squamous cell carcinoma and melanoma. In contrast to squamous cell carcinoma, it tends to involve the upper part of the face (Fig. 29.36).

Pathogenesis

Exposure to ultraviolet radiation causes genetic mutation in p53 suppressor gene resulting in basal cell carcinoma, squamous cell carcinoma and skin melanoma. Exposure to sunlight also releases tumor necrosis factor-α (TNF-α) in exposed skin, possibly diminishing immune response (*see* Table 29.8).

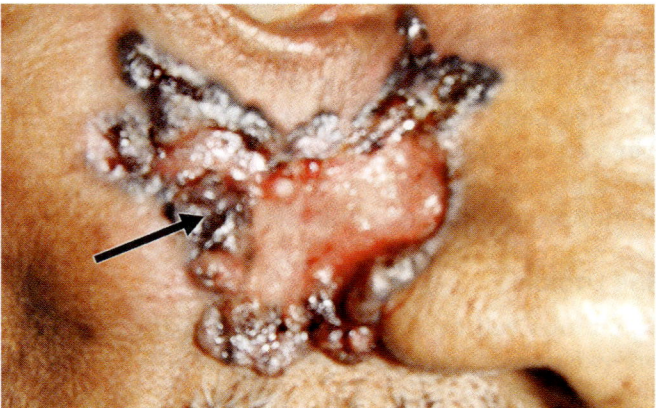

Fig. 29.36: Basal cell carcinoma. A case of pigmented BCC on the face in a farmer (arrow).

Molecular Genetics

Mutations of PTCH1 gene on chromosome 9q22.3 and SMD gene on chromosome 7q31–32 involved in hedgehog signaling pathway have been demonstrated in sporadic basal cell carcinoma.

Gross Morphology
Tumor is pearly papule, often with central ulceration. and overlying telangiectatic vessels.

Light Microscopy
- Tumor is composed of infiltrative deeply basophilic epithelial (basaloid) cells with narrow rims of cytoplasm arranged in clusters.
- These clusters are attached to the epidermis and protruding into the subjacent papillary dermis. Nuclei in the periphery of the clustered cells are arranged in palisading manner (Fig. 29.37).

Skin

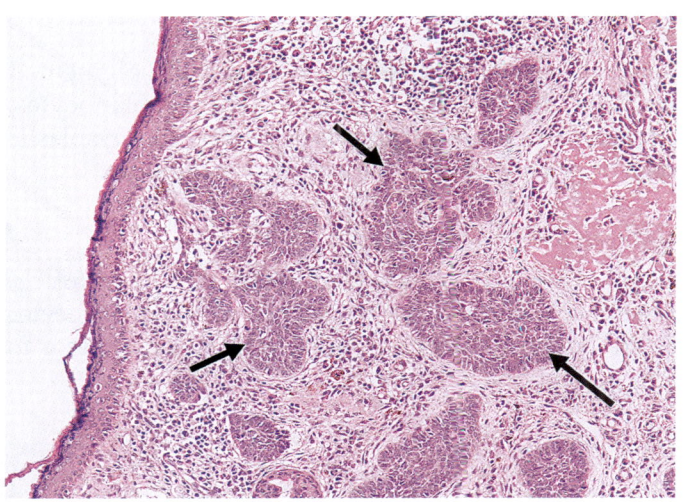

Fig. 29.37: Basal cell carcinoma (arrows) (400X).

Clinical Features

Patient presents with pearly papules containing dilated subepidermal blood vessels. Some contain melanin pigment and appear similar to nevi or melanomas. It is locally aggressive tumor extending in facial tissues, including bone. It almost never metastasizes. It is usually curable by surgical resection.

Treatment

Basal cell carcinoma is treated by surgical excision, radiotherapy, cryotherapy, curettage, electrodesiccation and Mohs micrographic surgery. Recurrence rate for non-Mohs modalities is nearly four times higher than Mohs micrographic surgery. The 5-year recurrensce rate for Mohs micrographic surgery is approximately 6%.

PIGMENTATION DISORDERS AND MELANOCYTIC TUMORS

PIGMENTATION DISORDERS

ALBINISM

Albinism is a failure of pigment production by otherwise intact melanocytes. It occurs in two variants.
- *Ocular albinism* is a melanin dysfunction that is limited to the eyes. This condition is an X-linked disorder.
- *Oculocutaneous albinism* is an autosomal recessive disorder characterized by melanin synthetic defect that involves the eyes, skin, and hair.

Risk Factors

There is increased risk of development of actinic keratosis, basal and squamous cell carcinoma, and malignant melanoma. It is due to sensitivity of skin to sunlight. It occurs due to failure of conversion of tyrosine to dihydroxyphenylalanine (DOPA), an intermediary in melanin synthesis.

VITILIGO

Vitiligo is an acquired loss of melanocytes in discrete areas of skin. These appear as depigmented white patches. It may be of autoimmune etiology.

It is sometimes associated with autoimmune disorders, such as Graves' disease and Addison disease.

Antimelanocyte antibodies are sometimes demonstrable. Toxic substances may cause destruction of melanocytes resulting in vitiligo (Fig. 29.38).

FRECKLE (EPHELIS)

It is produced by an increase of melanin pigment within basal keratinocytes.

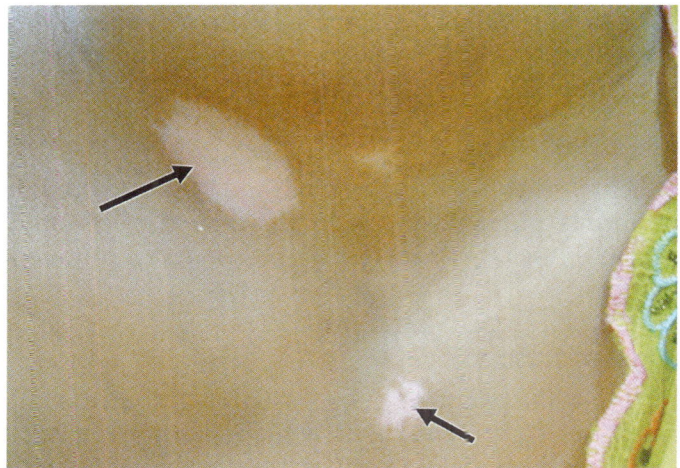

Fig. 29.38: Vitiligo—two macules of vitiligo on the neck (arrows).

LENTIGO SIMPLEX

It is a pigmented macule caused by melanocytic hyperplasia in the epidermis.

MELANOCYTIC TUMORS

MELANOCYTIC NEVUS

It is also known as common mole. It is considered benign tumor or hamartoma. Nevus cells derived from melanocytes and ordinarily occur in clusters or nests. Congenital melanocytic nevus in newborn is shown in Fig. 29.39.

Variants

- *Junctional nevus:* In *junctional nevus,* nevus cells confined to the epidermal–dermal junction.

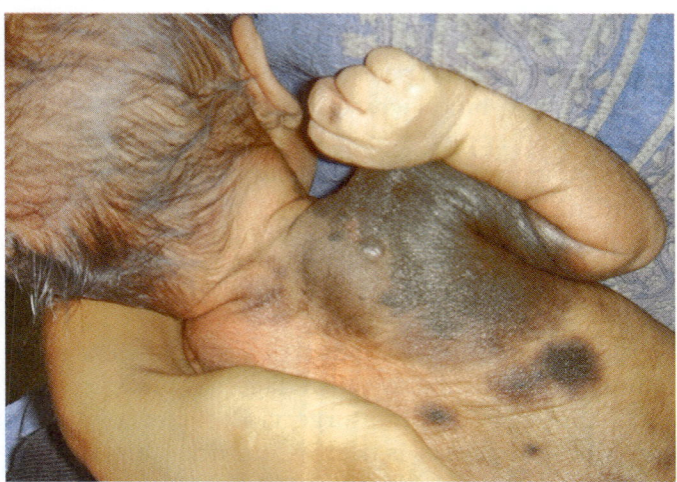

Fig. 29.39: Congenital melanocytic nevus.

- *Compound nevus:* In *compound nevus*, nevus cells are present both at the epidermal–dermal junction and in the dermis.
- *Intradermal nevus:* Intradermal nevus, nevus cells are confined to clusters within the dermis. These nevus cells are often nonpigmented.

Clinical Features

Patient presents with pigmented, and are tan to brown, uniformly pigmented, small <1 cm, areas of elevated skin (papules, or *moles*) with well defined, rounded borders.

Light Microscopy

Nevi are histologically composed of round to oval melanocytes forming either round aggregates arranged in nests or sheets of cells in the epidermis in junctional nevus, dermis in dermal nevus or both in compound nevus (Fig. 29.40).

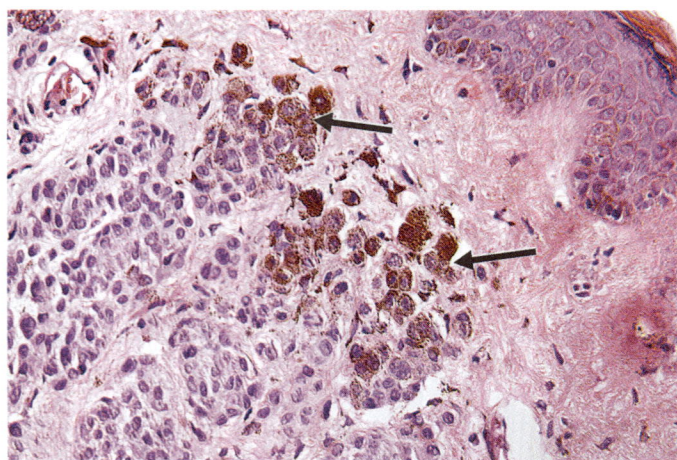

Fig. 29.40: Intradermal nevus showing aggregates of melanocytes (arrows) (400X).

DYSPLASTIC NEVUS

Dysplastic nevus is an atypical, irregularly pigmented lesion with disorderly proliferation of melanocytes, dermal fibrosis, and lymphocytic infiltration. Dysplastic nevi may transform into malignant melanoma.

LENTIGO MALIGNA

Lentigo maligna is also known as *Hutchinson freckle*. Lentigo maligna is characterized by atypical melanocytes at the epidermal–dermal junction. It is a precursor to lentigo maligna melanoma.

BLUE NEVUS

This condition is present since birth. It is characterized by nodular foci of dendritic, highly pigmented melanocytes in the dermis; the blue external appearance results from the dermal location.

SPITZ NEVUS

Spitz nevus is also known as *juvenile melanoma*. It most often affects children. It is most often benign disorder. Atypical variant with borderline behavior exists. Spitz nevus is most often characterized by spindle-shaped cells. It can be confused with malignant melanoma.

MALIGNANT MELANOMA

Malignant melanoma is most common in fair-skinned persons. It is most often associated with *excessive exposure to sunlight.* Metastastes in lymph nodes are shown in Fig. 29.41.

Origin

This disorder arises from melanocytes or nevus cells.

Predisposing Factors

Exposure to ultraviolet radiation causes genetic mutation in p53 suppressor gene resulting in *squamous cell carcinoma, basal cell carcinoma* and *skin melanoma*. It also releases tumor necrosis factor-α (TNF-α) in exposed skin, possibly diminishing immune response. It induces dimer formation between neighboring thymine pairs in DNA.

Molecular Genetics

Molecular genetics of malignant melanoma are described in Tables 29.9 to 29.11.

Clinical Variants

- *Lentigo maligna melanoma:* It is also known as Hutchinson melanotic freckle. Patient presents with large pigmented macule on *sun-exposed skin.*

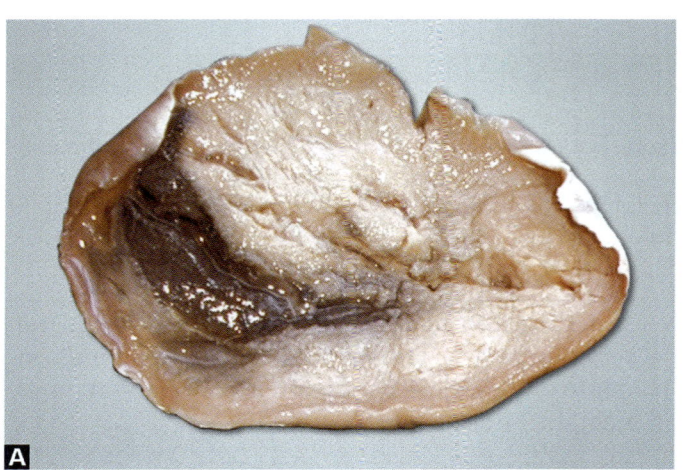
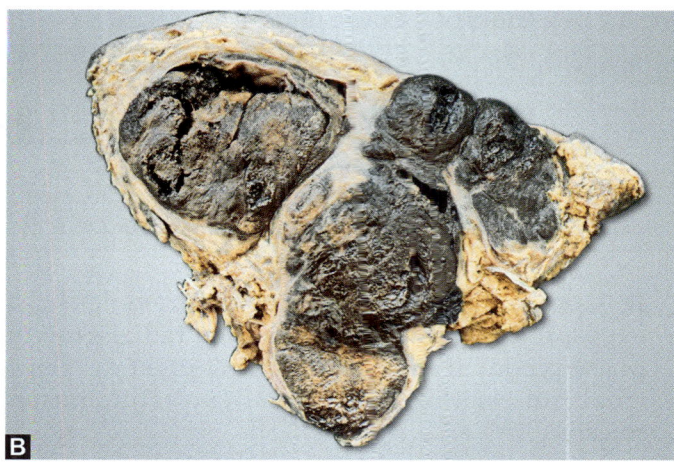

Fig. 29.41: Malignant melanoma. (A) Tumor arises from skin, (B) lymph node metastases.

Table 29.9: Molecular genetics (oncogenes, their mode of activation and associated cancers)

Category	Proto-oncogene	Mode of activation	Associated malignancies
Growth factors			
Fibroblast growth factors (FGFs)	FGF3	Amplification	*Melanoma* Osteosarcoma Gastric carcinoma Bladder carcinoma Breast carcinoma
	INT2	Increased baseline activity	*Melanoma* Breast carcinoma
Signal-transduction proteins			
GTP-binding (G) proteins	N-RAS	Point mutation	*Melanoma* Hematologic malignancies
N-RAS signal transduction	BRAF	Point mutation translocation	*Melanoma* Leukemia Colon carcinoma
Cyclins and cyclin-dependent kinases (cell cycle regulators)			
Cyclin-dependent kinase	CDK4	Amplification or point mutation	*Melanoma* Glioblastoma multiforme Sarcoma
Brain-2 (BRN2): This transcription factor commonly cooperates with transcription factors of the Sry-box (SOX) family by binding to a nearby DNA site necessary for their action. BRN2 is an early marker of melanoblasts and has been implicated in the development of the melanocytic lineage and melanoma. Its clinical relevance is not yet clear.			

Table 29.10: Tumor suppressor genes

Gene	Protein	Function	Familial tumors	Sporadic cancers
Mitogenic signaling pathway inhibitors				
p16 tumor suppressor gene	It is located on chromosome 9p21	It inhibits cyclin-D dependent kinase activity	Familial melanoma	Melanoma, Mesotheliomas Astrocytoma
APC	Adenomatous polyposis protein (locus 5p21) Mutation by deletion or nonsense	APC inhibits WNT signaling activator pathway, thus prevents nuclear transcription. It degrades catenin	Familial polyposis coli with malignant transformation	Melanoma Colon carcinoma, gastric carcinoma, pancreatic carcinoma, thyroid carcinoma

Table 29.11: Radiation exposure associated cancers

Etiology	Mechanism	Associated cancers
Ultraviolet radiation (UV B: 290–320 nm)	It cause p53 gene mutation TNF-α released by exposed skin diminishes immune response It induces dimer formation between neighboring thymine pairs in DNA	Sporadic skin cancers Melanoma, basal cell carcinoma or squamous cell carcinoma Skin cancers in xeroderma pigmentosum

It is probably related to chronic ultraviolet light exposure especially in whites. The radial growth phase predominates initially; most often develops from pre-existing lentigo maligna (Hutchinson freckle).

- *Superficial spreading melanoma:* This variant is common on *trunk and extremities*. It is the most common of the variants. Patient presents with a flat growth in a radial fashion with irregular border and variegated dark brown pigmentation.
- *Nodular melanoma:* It begins with the vertical growth phase. It has the *poorest prognosis* of the clinical variants.
- *Acral lentiginous melanoma:* It most often appears on the hands and feet of dark-skinned persons. It is generally limited to the palms, soles, and subungual regions. A similar tumor occurs on the mucous membranes known as *mucosal lentiginous melanoma*.

Light Microscopy
- *Dermo-epidermal lesion:* Melanoma cells are usually considerably larger than nevus cells. These cells contain large nuclei with irregular contours with eosinophilic nuclei.
  Chromatin is clumped at the periphery of the nuclear membrane. All melanomas start as *in situ* lesion involving only the epidermis.
  Nests of melanoma cells are present at the dermoepidermal junction.
- *Pagetoid spread:* The lesion progresses to involve all layers of the epidermis known as *epidermal tropism* or *Pagetoid spread*.
- *Radial growth:* As melanoma cells expand laterally (so-called radial growth phase), the area of involved skin enlarges. It grows in all directions predominantly lateral within epidermis and papillary zone of the dermis. There is presence of numerous lymphocytes. It does not metastasize, hence prognosis is good.
- *Vertical growth:* Eventually, melanoma cells invade the dermis and the so-called *vertical growth phase* begins (which indicates the progression from *in situ* to *invasive* melanoma). It extends into the reticular dermis or beyond. Prognosis depends on depth of the lesion. It may spread by lymphatic and hematogenous routes.

Electron Microscopy
Sometimes a melanoma will not be well-differentiated enough to show the typical melanin pigmentation. Electron microscopy shows *oval premelanosomes* structures.

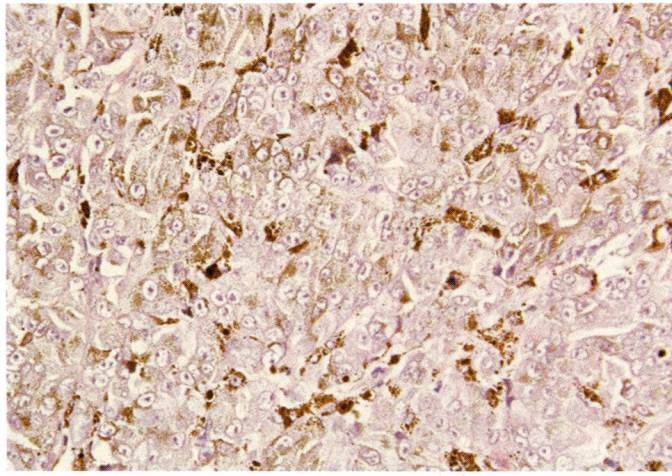

Fig. 29.42: Malignant melanoma (400X).

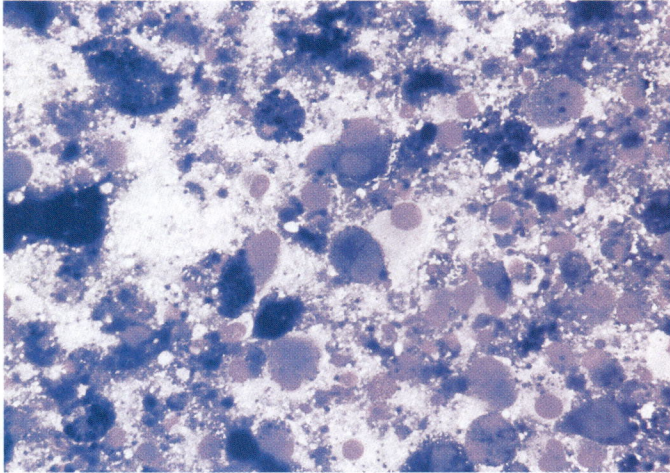

Fig. 29.43: Malignant melanoma. Lymph node metastases are demonstrated by FNAC.

Immunohistochemistry

HMB-45, MART-1 (Melan-A), Ki-67, CAM 5.2, turasinase, and S-100 are markers for malignant melanoma (Figs 29.42 and 29.43).

Marker	Expression
HMB-45	Positive
MART-1 (Melan-A)	Positive
Ki-67	Positive
S-100	Positive
CAM 5.2	Positive
Tyrosinase	Positive

Prognostic Factors

The most important prognostic variable is tumor thickness. Superficial variant of melanoma has better prognosis than vertical variant. Ulceration, high mitotic rate, absence of significant lymphocytic response are poor prognostic indicators.

FIBROUS AND FIBROHISTIOCYTIC TUMORS

DERMATOFIBROMA

Skin lesions are tan to brown, firm dermal papules <1 cm in diameter located most often on the legs of young adults. These lesions dimple inward upon lateral compression (Fig. 29.44).

Gross Morphology

Tumor is well circumscribed. Cut surface is gray white (Fig. 29.45).

Light Microscopy

- Histologically, tumor is composed of homogenous spindle-shaped fibroblasts, histiocytes and blood vessels.
- At the periphery, collagen bundles are surrounded by fibroblasts.
- The overlying epidermis shows acanthosis, basal keratinocyte hyperpigmentation and broad flattened rete ridges or basaloid proliferation, which may be mistaken for basal cell carcinoma (Fig. 29.46).

Electron Microscopy

Tumor cells show positivity for factor XIIIa, but negative with CD34.

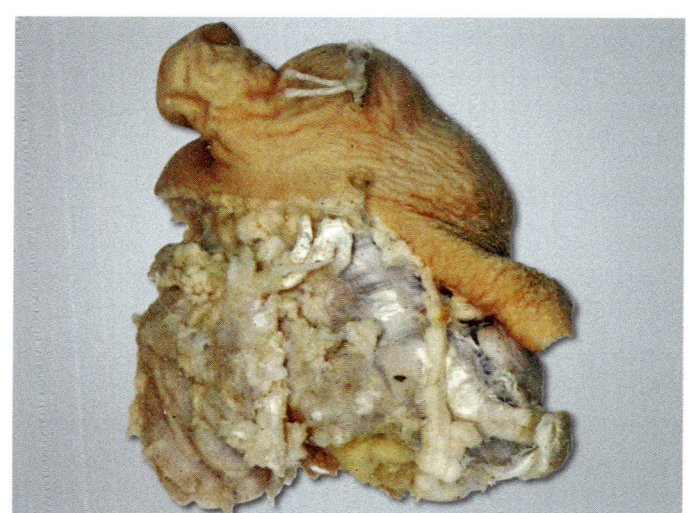

Fig. 29.45: Dermatofibroma (gross morphology).

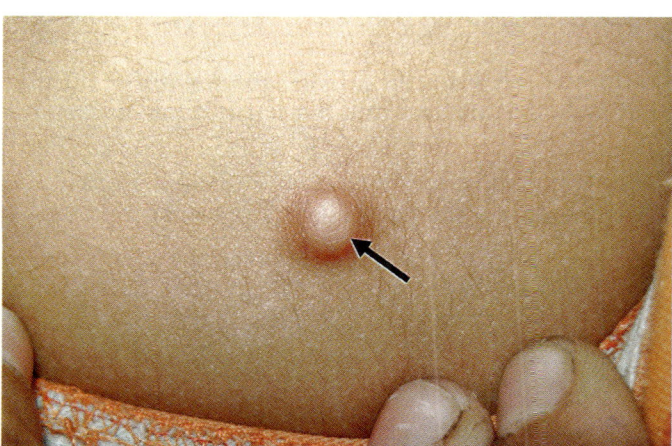

Fig. 29.44: Dermatofibroma (a lesion of dermatofibroma in a child) (arrow).

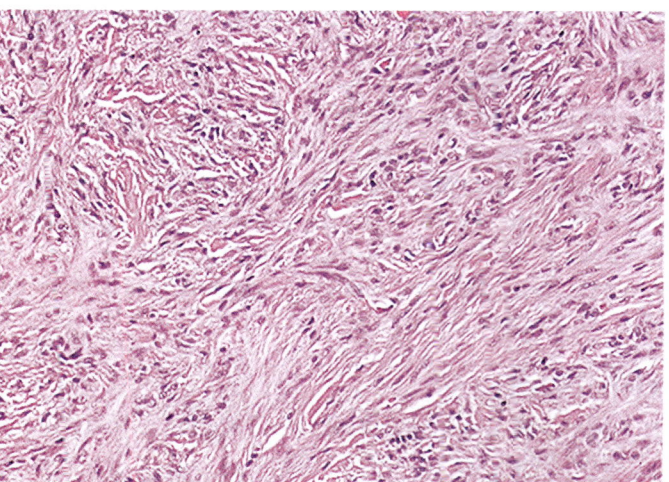

Fig. 29.46: Dermatofibroma—shows the whorling fibroblasts with collagen bundles (100X).

Section III: Systemic Pathology

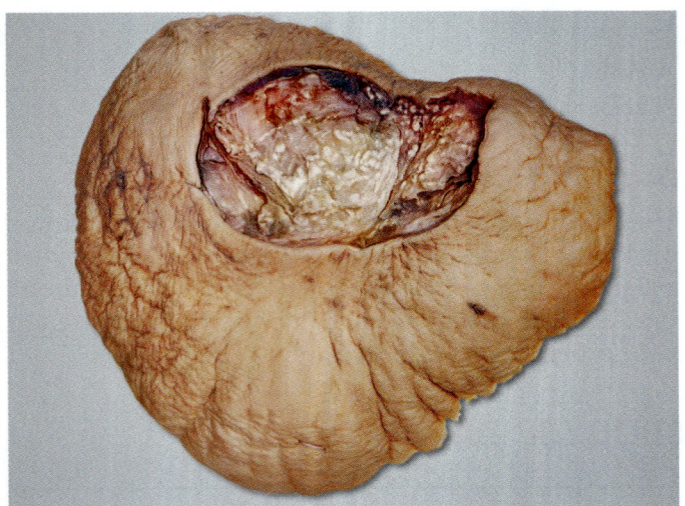

Fig. 29.47: Dermatofibrosarcoma protuberans.

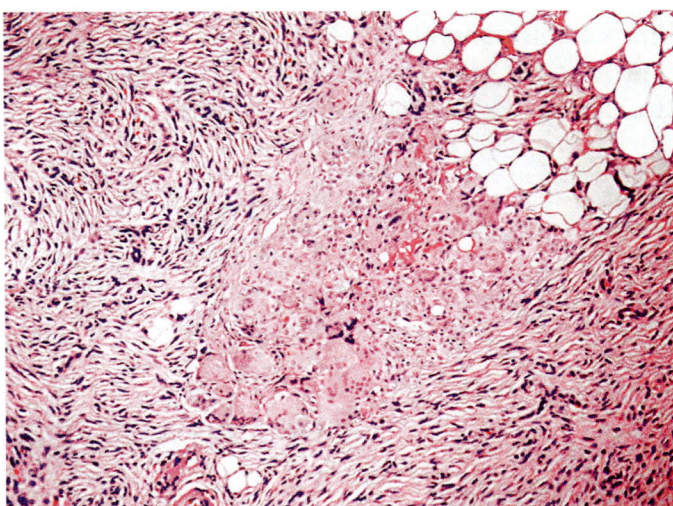

Fig. 29.48: Dermatofibrosarcoma protuberans. Tumor is composed of spindle cells arranged in a storiform or cartwheel appearance (400X).

DERMATOFIBROSARCOMA PROTUBERANS

Dermatofibrosarcoma protuberans is slowly growing, solitary or multiple polypoid nodules on the trunk and extremities of adults. It is slow growing locally aggressive tumor, which rarely metastasizes (Fig. 29.47).

Molecular Genetics

Tumor exhibits translocation of t(17; 22) (q22; q13) which results in production of a COLLIA1-PDGFB fusion protein.

Light Microscopy
- This cellular tumor is composed of homogenous spindle cells arranged in a *storiform or cartwheel pattern.*

- These tumor cells infiltrate between adnexa, extending into the subcutis with fat trapping.
- There may be presence of occasional mitotic figures with mild atypia.
- Overlying epidermis is normal, atrophic, or ulcerated (Fig. 29.48).

Immunohistochemistry
Tumor cells show positivity with **CD34** but negative for factor XIIIa.

Diffential Diagnosis
Storiform pattern is demonstrated in dermatofibrosarcoma protuberans, malignant fibrous histiocytoma, liposarcoma, leiomyosarcoma, nerve sheath tumors and occasionally nodular fasciitis.

NEURAL AND NEUROENDOCRINE TUMORS

NEUROFIBROMA

These firm nodules may be solitary and sporadic or multiple and part of von Recklinghausen's disease (neurofibromatosis). There may be overlying hyperpigmentation. With neurofibromatosis, an autosomal dominant disorder, there can be multiple *café au lait* spots (six or more pale brown pigmented macules each >1.5 cm in size) (Figs 29.49 and 29.50).

Light Microscopy
- Histopathological examination shows well defined but non-encapsulated masses.
- Tumor is composed of wavy spindle cells with a lot of intervening collagen (Fig. 29.51).

TRAUMATIC NEUROMA

Traumatic neuroma is a firm small painful nodule present in the subcutis and deep soft tissue as a result of injury.

The lesion develops most commonly in the soft tissue of the mental foramen area, lower lip and tongue.

Light Microscopy
- Traumatic neuroma is composed of irregularly arranged nerve fascicles embedded in fibrous scar tissue.
- Each fascicle is surrounded by fibrous tissue and perineural cells. There is presence of scattered mast cells.

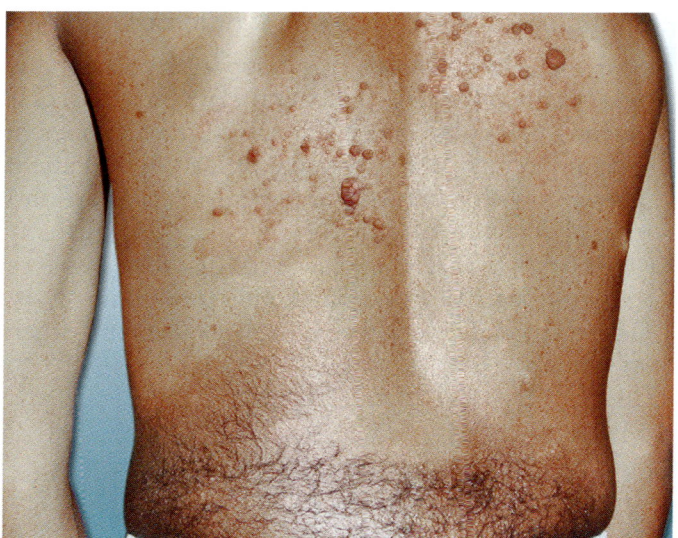

Fig. 29.49: Multiple neurofibromas in neurofibromatosis.

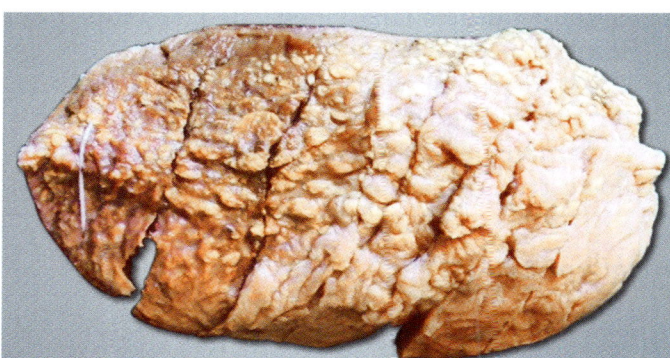

Fig. 29.50: Plexiform neurofibroma. Plexiform neurofibroma (WHO grade I) is pathognomonic of neurofibromatosis type 1 (NF-1) involving single or multiple nerve fascicles of major nerve branches.

MERKEL CELL CARCINOMA

Merkel cell carcinoma is an aggressive neuroendocrine malignancy that typically arises on the head and neck skin of the elderly and grossly appears as a red or violaceous nodule or plaque.

Molecular Genetics

Deletion of chromosome 1p36 and trisomy 6 are most often demonstrated.

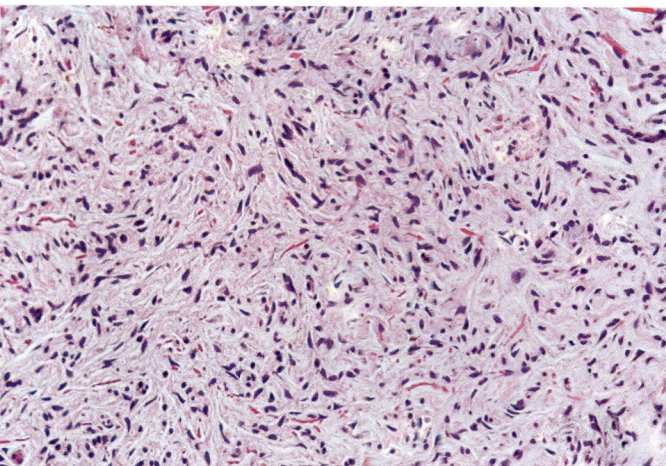

Fig. 29.51: Neurofibroma. Tumor is composed of elongated wavy cells with small dark oblong nuclei. This lesion is benign. However, persons with neurofibromatosis have a long-term risk for development of malignant neoplasms: neurofibrosarcomas, malignant schwannomas, gliomas.

Light Microscopy
- Tumor is composed of small cells with vesicular nuclei, scant cytoplasm, and indistinct borders.
- These are arranged in trabeculae, nests and sheets.
- These invade the dermis and subcutis.

Immunohistochemistry
- In addition to immunostaining for neuroendocrine markers (*synaptophysin, chromogranin*), perinuclear *dot-like* staining with *cytokeratin 20* is characteristic.
- These are negative for S-100 and TTF-1, permitting distinction from melanocytic tumors and small cell lung carcinoma.

Marker	Expression
Non-specific enolase	Positive
Chromogranin	Positive
Synaptophysin	Positive
Cytokeratin-20	Positive

VASCULAR TUMORS

HEMANGIOMA

Hemangiomas are sometimes considered being a hamartoma rather than a neoplasm. These can be variable in size from a few millimeters up to several centimeters in diameter. It may cause serious problems if it is large and poorly resectable (Fig. 29.52). Hemangiomas are most often found in the skin or liver.

Major Forms

Vascular malformations include capillary (portwine stains).

Clinical Features

Patient presents with bright red to blue, usually level with the surface of the skin, or slightly elevated.

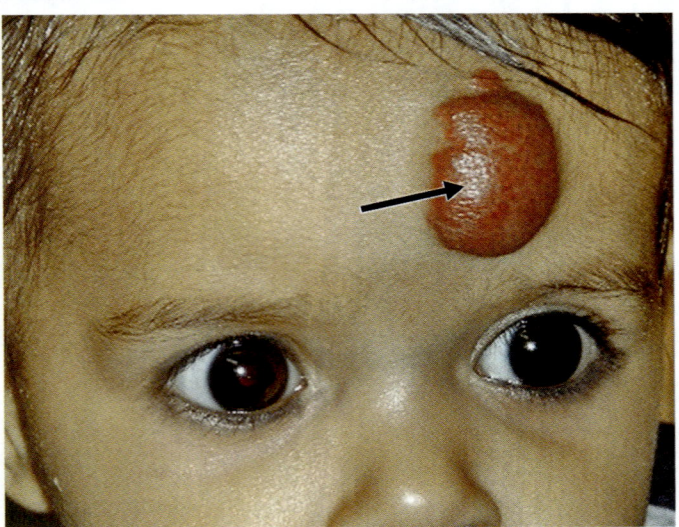

Fig. 29.52: Compressible lesion of hemangioma.

Hemangiomas Associated with Syndromes

- *Sturge-Weber syndrome:* This disorder involves port-wine stain of the face, ipsilateral glaucoma, vascular lesions of ocular choroidal tissue, and extensive hemangiomatous involvement of meninges. Patient presents with convulsions, mental retardation, and retinal detachment.
- *von Hippel-Lindau syndrome:* This disorder involves multiple vascular tumors and other tumors and cysts. These are widely scattered throughout many organ systems.

> **Light Microscopy**
> - Capillary hemangioma is usually well defined but lacking capsule.
> - It is made up of closely packed aggregations of thin-walled capillaries lined with a single layer of endothelium, usually blood-filled, separated by scant connective tissue stroma.
> - The vascular lumina may be partially or completely thrombosed and organized.
> - Cavernous hemangioma is large, endothelium-lined spaces in the dermis and subdermis.

Portwine stain variant of capillary hemangioma is purple-red area on the face or neck.

Strawberry capillary hemangioma appears as bright-red raised lesion. Cherry hemangioma is small, dome-shaped red papule. Hemangiomas may be part of other syndromes described as under.

TUMORS OF CUTANEOUS APPENDAGES

Tumors of the cutaneous appendages are arising from hair follicle, eccrine glands, sebaceous glands.

CHONDROID SYRINGOMA

Chondroid syringoma is a solitary firm tumor located in dermis or subcutaneous tissue on head and neck.

> **Light Microscopy**
> - Tumor is well circumscribed and composed of small epithelial cells arranged in solid nests, small clusters and ducts in the myxoid, chondroid or fibrous stroma.

NODULAR HIDRADENOMA

Nodular hidradenoma is a solitary tumor measuring 0.5–2.0 cm or more. It has no predilection.

> **Light Microscopy**
> - Tumor is circumscribed and nonencapsulated. It is composed of solid and cystic areas.
> - Tumor cells are round, fusiform or polygonal with clear to eosinophilic cytoplasm.

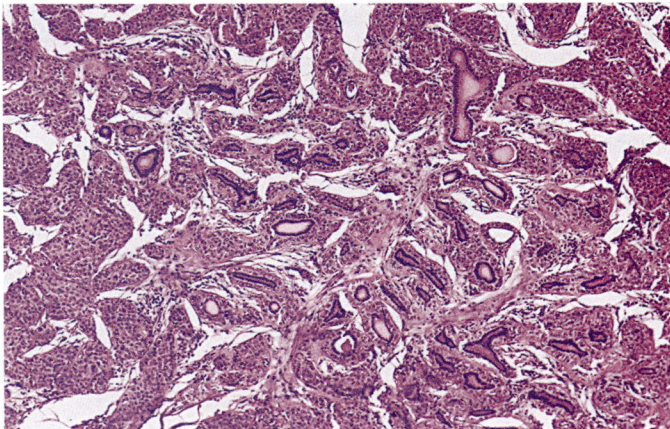

Fig. 29.53: Nodular hidradenoma. Tumor cells are round, fusiform or polygonal exhibiting squamous appearance (100X).

> - Duct-like structures are prominent exhibiting squamous appearance.
> - The stroma varies from fine to dense fibrous tissue to dense hyalinized collagen fibers (Fig. 29.53).

PILOMATRIXOMA

Pilomatrixoma is also known as *calcifying epithelioma* of Malherbe. It arises from hair follicle (Fig. 29.54).

Skin

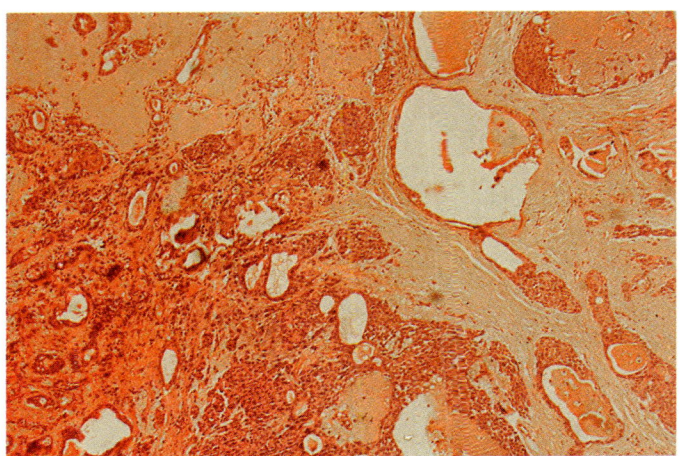

Fig. 29.54: Pilomatrixoma. Tumor is composed of small epithelial cells arranged in solid nests, small clusters and ducts in the mesenchymal components (100X).

Clinical Features

Patient presents with firm nodule deeply located on the face and upper extremities especially during childhood.

Light Microscopy

- Tumor is sharply demarcated in the lower dermis most often the subcutis. It is composed of two types of cells: basaloid and shadow (ghost) cells.
- Basaloid cells resemble the cells of basal cell carcinoma.
- Shadow cells have eosinophilic cytoplasm, distinct cell borders and no nuclear staining. These cells occupy the center of tumor.

CUTANEOUS METASTASES

In adults, cutaneous metastases are seen in cancers of bronchus, large bowel, malignant melanoma, oral squamous cell carcinoma, breast, large bowel, malignant melanoma and rhabdomyosarcoma. Cutaneous metastases occur in children with neuroblastoma.

Immunohistochemistry

Panel of markers is employed on histological sections to find out primary cancers metastasizing to skin (Table 29.12).

Table 29.12: Immunohistochemistry of cutaneous metastases

Panel of markers	Positivity in cancers
CK7	Carcinoma of lung, breast, ovary, and endometrium and pancreaticobiliary tract
CK20, CDX-2, CEA, β-catenin, SAT2, p53, CK7	Colon carcinoma
CK7, GCDFP-15, mammoglobulin, ER, PR and Her2 neu	Breast carcinoma
HMB-45 and S-100, melan (MART-1), CAM 5.2	Malignant melanoma

MISCELLANEOUS DISORDERS

FIBROEPITHELIAL POLYP

Fibroepithelial polyp is also known as *skin tag* or *acrochordon*. It most often occurs on the face near eyelids, neck, axilla, trunk and intertriginous regions. Patient presents with soft, fleshy-colored and bag-like lesion attached to the skin by a small slender stalk.

Light Microscopy

On histological examination, lesion consists of fibrovascular core covered by benign squamous epithelium (Fig. 29.55).

EPIDERMAL INCLUSION CYST

It is a subcutaneous, well circumscribed, firm and often movable, fluctuant nodule.

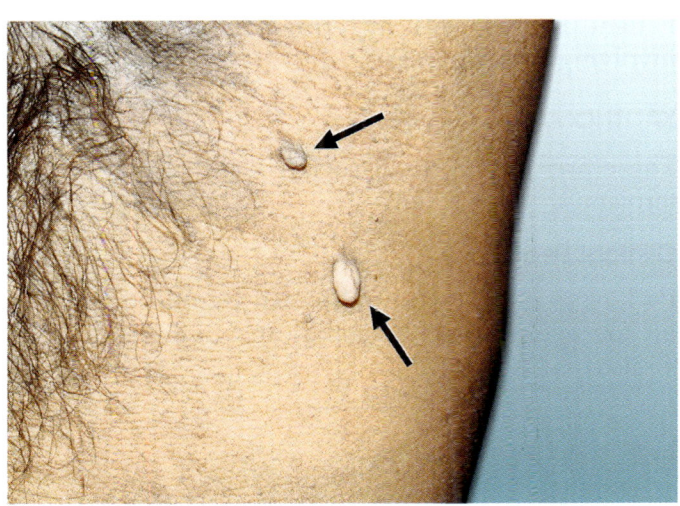

Fig. 29.55: Fibroepithelial polyp (arrows).

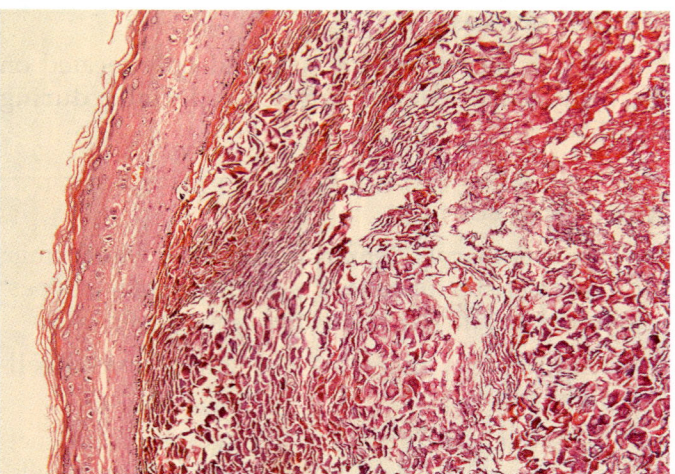

Fig. 29.56: Epidermal inclusion cyst.

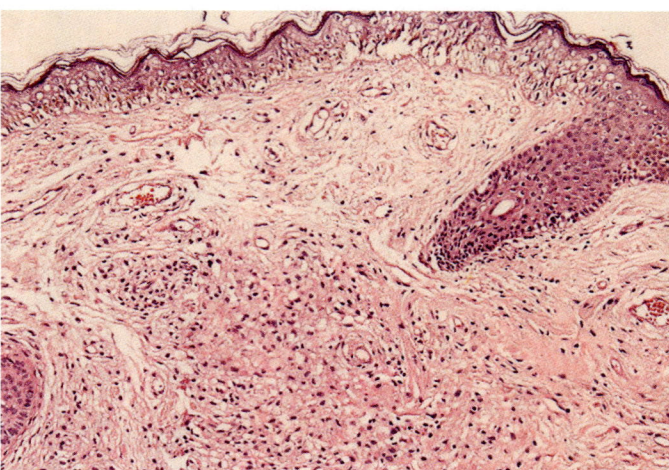

Fig. 29.57: Xanthoma. It is composed of focal dermal collections of lipid-laden histiocytes (100X).

When large, it often becomes painful upon traumatic rupture resulting in release of soft gray-white material.

Light Microscopy

- Histopathological examination reveals a cyst lined by stratified squamous epithelium and is filled with laminated strands of keratinous material.
- A clinically similar lesion seen on the scalp is called a pilar cyst. The pilar cyst lacks a granular layer and is filled with more amorphous material. If ruptured, these surrounding intense acute and chronic inflammatory reaction is seen in Fig. 29.56.

ACANTHOSIS NIGRICANS

This disorder is sometimes a marker of visceral malignancy (stomach, lung, breast, and uterus). It is most often seen in the setting of diabetes mellitus and other endocrinopathies.

Clinical Features

Patient presents with hyperpigmentation most often involving flexural areas.

XANTHOMAS

These are most often associated with hypercholesterolemia.

Clinical Features

Patient presents with yellowish papule or nodule on the eyelids (xanthelasma) and over tendons or joints.

Light Microscopy

Light microscopy of lesion reveals focal dermal collections of lipid-laden histiocytes (Fig. 29.57).

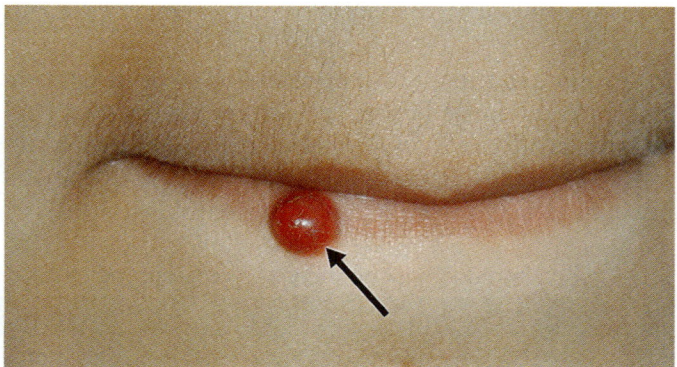

Fig. 29.58: Granuloma pyogenicum (arrow).

GRANULOMA PYOGENICUM

Granuloma pyogenicum is vascular pedunculated lesion characterized by numerous capillaries and edematous stroma. It is common in skin or mucous membranes. It most often develops following trauma (Fig. 29.58).

KELOID

Keloid is an exaggerated response to injury that produces abundant collagenous soft tissue, forming a large nodular scar (Fig. 29.59).

Etiology

It often follows trauma to the skin, such as ear-piercing or surgical wounds. It most often occurs in dark-skinned persons especially of African lineage. It tends to recur after resection.

Light Microscopy

On histopathological examination, keloid is composed of dense bundles of collagen in the dermis (Fig. 29.60).

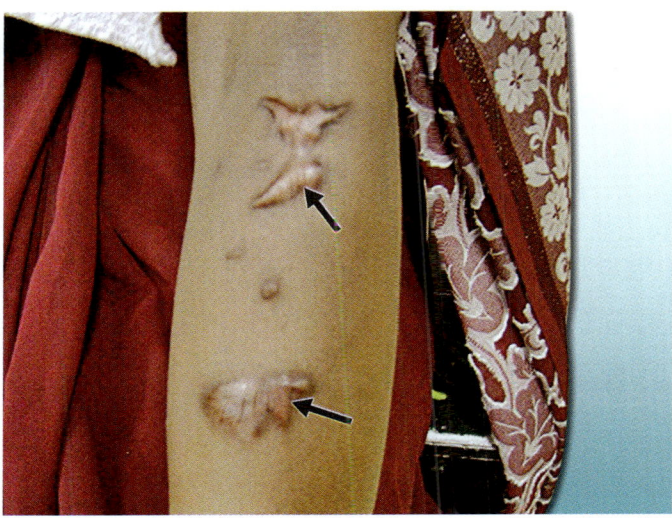

Fig. 29.59: Keloid. Multiple keloids are visible (arrows).

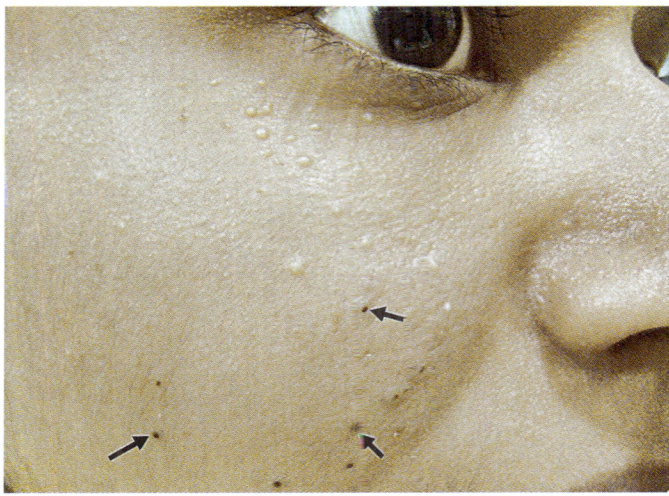

Fig. 29.61: Acne. Multiple black heads or open comedones on the face (lower side), the lesions around the eyes are milias (arrows).

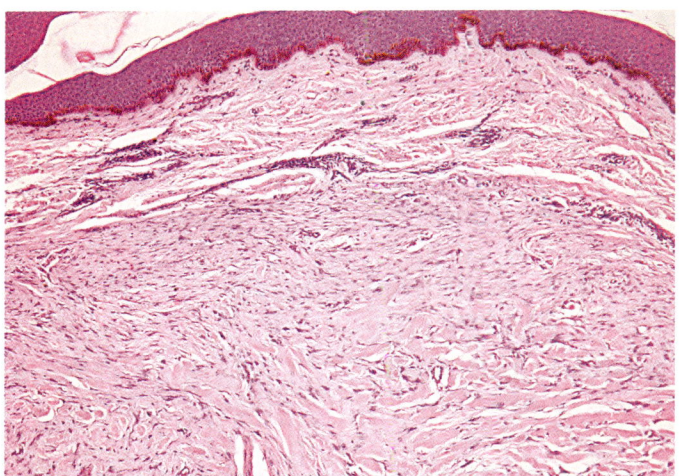

Fig. 29.60: Keloid. It is composed of dense bundles of collagen in the dermis.

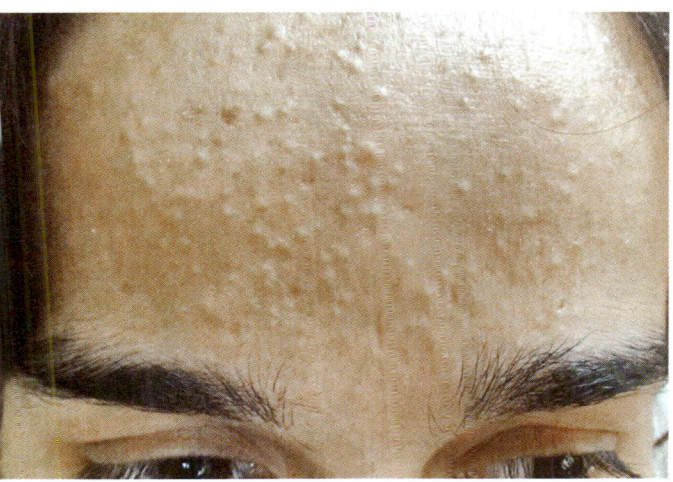

Fig. 29.62: Acne. Closed comedone multiple whiteheads on the forehead.

ACNE

Age Group
It is most often seen in adolescents and young adults.

Locations
It involves hair follicles in areas of face, upper chest, and upper back. Lesions may be open or closed comedones.

The most common lesion is the *comedo* that involves hair follicles (Figs 29.61 and 29.62).

Type of Acne
- *Open comedone:* It consists of a distended hair follicle. It contains a central black keratin plug.
   This color is due to oxidation of melanin pigment (not dirt).
- *Closed comedone:* The lesion is plugged follicles without a visible central opening. It most often ruptures into the dermis resulting in inflammation. Inflammatory acne is characterized by erythematous papules, nodules, and pustules.

CHAPTER 30

Nervous System

Learning Objectives

CNS INFECTIONS
- Meningitis
- Encephalitis

CNS TUMORS
- General Considerations
- Secondary Tumors
- Neuroepithelial Tumors
- Meningeal Tumors
- Tumors of the Cranial and Paraspinal Nerves
- CNS Germ Cell Tumors
- Primary CNS Lymphoma
- Neuronal Tumors
- Multiple Neuromas

REACTION OF CNS TO INJURY

CEREBROVASCULAR DISEASES
- Cerebral Infarction
- Cerebral Hemorrhage
- Subarachnoid Hemorrhage
- Transient Ischemic Attacks
- Fat Embolism

HEAD INJURIES
- Epidural Hematoma
- Subdural Hematoma

DEMYELINATING DISORDERS
- Multiple Sclerosis
- Acute Disseminated Encephalomyelitis
- Guillain-Barré Syndrome

CONGENITAL DISORDERS
- Neural Defects
- TORCH Complex
- Hydrocephalus
- Arnold-Chiari Malformation
- Agenesis of the Corpus Callosum
- Fetal Alcohol Syndrome
- Tuberous Sclerosis Syndrome

ANATOMY

CENTRAL NERVOUS SYSTEM

Central nervous system consists of cerebrum, cerebellum, brainstem, spinal cord, 12 cranial nerves and blood vessels supplying these structures. Brain and spinal cord are covered by meninges. Meninges are composed of outer dense fibrous dura mater and delicate leptomeninges (pia and arachnoid mater). Falx cerebri divides cerebrum into left and right hemispheres. Supratentorial compartment consists of cerebral cortex (frontal, temporal, parietal and occipital lobes), white mater and deep nuclei, i.e. basal ganglion, thalamus, and hypothalamus.

NEUROAXIS

Neuroaxis term denotes brain and spinal cord. Lesions that involve brain parenchyma are said to *intra-axial* (e.g. astrocytoma, central neurocytoma or ependymoma). Lesions located outside the parenchyma are referred to as *extra-axial*, i.e. meningiomas, hemangiopericytoma, schwannoma. Similarly, terms used for spinal lesions are intramedullary or extramedullary.

HISTOLOGY

Central nervous system is composed of gray and white mater that differ quantitatively on gross and histopathological examination. It is composed of *neurons, glial supporting cells* (e.g. astrocytes, oligodendrocytes, ependymal cells), *microglial cells, connective tissue* in meninges and blood vessels.

NEURONS

Central nervous system consists of 100 billion polarized neurons. These cannot divide and hence have limited regeneration. These respond to physical and chemical stimuli; conduct electrical impulses and release chemical regulators.

Structure

- A neuron is a microscopic structure composed of three major parts, namely cell body (perikaryon), dendrites and axon.
- Neuronal cell bodies and dendrites reside in the gray mater (cortex and deep gray mater). Axons create the framework of the white mater.
- Neuroglial cells (astrocytes, oligodendrocytes and microglia) are present in different proportions in these tissues.
- Oligodendrocytes are present in abundance in the white mater, and their processes form myelin sheath that insulin CNS axons.
- Neuropil is a fibrillary material between cell bodies. It is formed by the processes of neurons (axons and dendrites) and glial cells.

NEUROGLIAL CELLS

Neuroglial Cells in CNS

- *Astrocytes:* These are present in white mater of cerebral cortex. These participate in *metabolism of neurotransmitters*. These form *blood–brain barrier* by providing a link between neuron and blood vessels.
- *Microglia cells:* These participate in phagocytosis of microbes and cellular debris.
- *Ependymal cells:* These form links between the ventricles of the brain and the central canal of spinal cord. These participate in *synthesis of cerebrospinal fluid* in choroid plexus and its circulation.
- *Oligodendrocytes:* These form a supporting network by forming myelin sheath around neurons in CNS.

Neuroglial Cells in Peripheral Nervous System

- *Neurilemmocytes or Schwann cells:* Each cell produces part of myelin sheath around a single axon of peripheral nervous system neuron forming insulating myelin sheath forming node of Ranvier.
- *Satellite cells:* These cells support neurons in ganglia of peripheral nervous system.

Blood–Brain Barrier

Processes wrapped astrocytes around blood capillaries isolate neurons various potentially waste products in blood by synthesizing chemical substances tht maintain selective permeability of the endothelial cells of the capillaries.

The endothelial cells create a blood–brain barrier, which prevents the movement of the substances between the blood and the interstitial fluid of the central nervous system (Fig. 30.1).

CONNECTIVE TISSUE

Connective tissue is present in meninges.

BLOOD VESSELS

The brain receives the blood through two *internal carotid arteries* and *vertebral arteries*, which fuse to form the basilar artery. The basilar artery bifurcates into two posterior cerebral arteries which interconnect with branches of the carotid arteries to form the 'circle of Willis' at the base of the brain. The blood vessels are

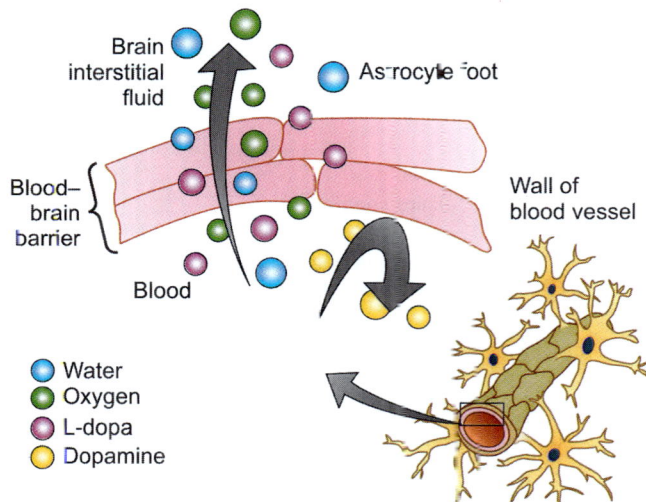

Fig. 30.1: Blood–brain barrier.

non-fenestrated and showing tight junctions with adjacent cells.

INTRACRANIAL COMPARTMENTS

Intracranial compartments are epidural space, subdural space, cerebral parenchymal compartment and intraventricular space described as under.

EPIDURAL SPACE

This is a virtual space between the inner aspect of the cranial bones and the dura mater. The epidural space contains the *middle meningeal arteries* and three main branches, which are *grooved* into the inner surface of the temporal parietal bones.

SUBDURAL SPACE

Subdural space is located between the arachnoid and pia mater and is *filled with CSF*. It is contiguous with the perivascular *Virchow-Robin spaces* surrounding the blood vessels penetrating from the meninges into the brain.

CEREBRAL PARENCHYMAL COMPARTMENT

Cerebral parenchymal compartment is occupied by the neural, glial, and vascular cells.

INTRAVENTRICULAR SPACE

Intraventricular space includes the lateral ventricles, the third and fourth ventricles, and the aqueduct of Sylvius. This compartment is filled with CSF.

Most of CSF is produced by choroid plexuses in the lateral cerebral ventricles at a rate of approximately 500 ml per day. The choroid plexus stretches along the roof of the third ventricle and then angles posteriorly to span the lateral ventricles.

Circulation

CSF flows from its intraventricular origin to sites of reabsorption, principally through the arachnoid villi, into the dural sinuses. From the ventricles, the CSF flows via the cerebral aqueduct and enters the subarachnoid space through the foramen of *Luschka and Magendie*. CSF is absorbed by the arachnoid villi, which provide the *outlet* for CSF to flow into the major dural spaces (Figs 30.2 and 30.3). Normal values of CSF are given in Table 30.1.

Functions

Cerebrospinal fluid supports and protects the brain and spinal cord. It acts as a cushion and *shock absorber*. It acts as a reservoir to regulate the contents of the cranium.

It keeps the brain and spinal cord moist. It may act as a medium for the interchange of metabolic substances between nerve cells and CSF.

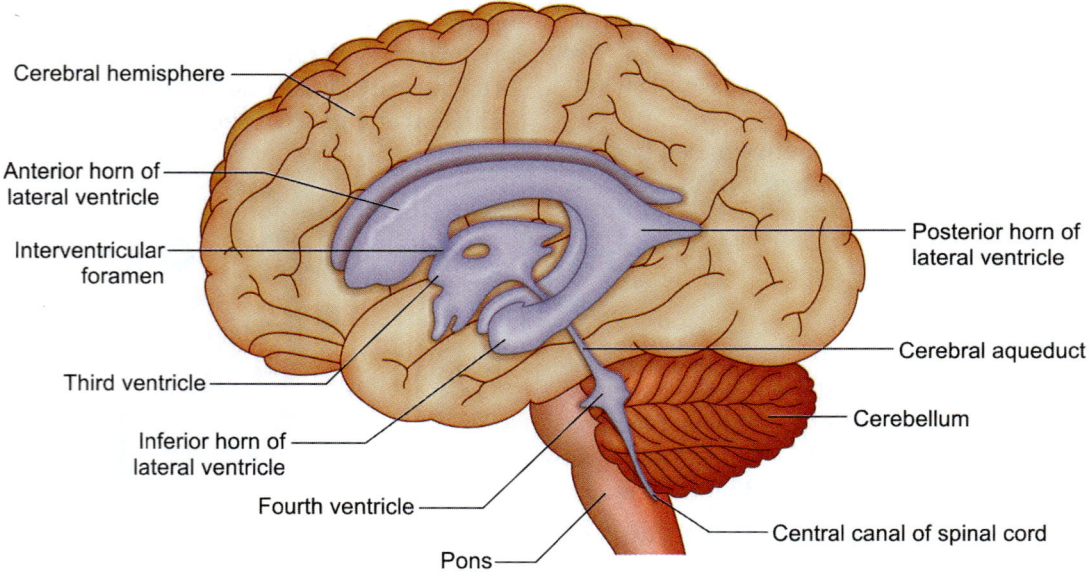

Fig. 30.2: CSF flow in CNS ventricles.

Nervous System

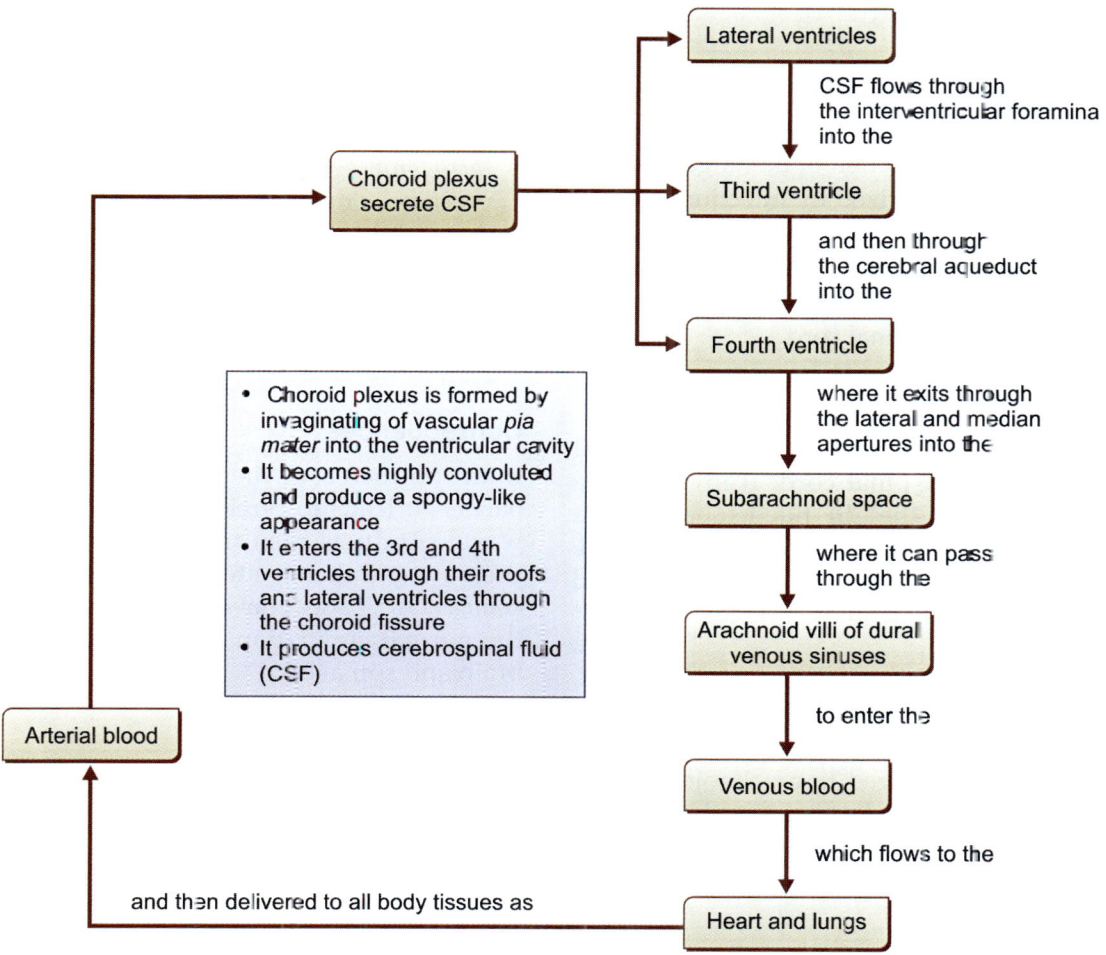

Fig. 30.3: CSF circulation in central nervous system.

Table 30.1: Normal values of CSF

CSF	Normal values
Volume	90 to 150 ml
Pressure	80 to 180 cm of water (20 drops/minute)
Specific gravity	1.006 to 1.008
pH	7.30 to 7.40
Colloids	Poor
Total solids	0.85 to 1.70 gm/dl
Bilirubin	Absent
Proteins	Total 20 to 40 mg%
	Albumin: 50 to 70%
	α_1 globulin: 3 to 9%
	α_2 globulin: 4 to 10%
	β-globulin: 4 to 10%
	γ-globulins: 3 to 9%
	Fibrinogen: nil

CSF	Normal values
Sugar	40 to 80 mg%
Chloride	118–132 mEq/L
Sodium	144–154 mEq/L
Potassium	2.0–3.5 mEq/L
Thyroxine	0.1–0.2 mg/dl
Iron	1.0–2.0 mg/dl
Glutamine	6–16 mg/dl
Urea	6–16 mg/dl
Uric acid	0.5–4.5 mg/dl
Creatinine	0.5–1.2 mg/dl
Cholesterol	0.2–0.5 mg/dl
Light microscopy	0–4 lymphocytes/cu mm
Culture and sensitivity	Sterile

CNS INFECTIONS

CNS infection may be classified into meningitis, encephalitis and brain abscess.
- *Meningitis:* It refers to infection of meninges.
- *Encephalitis:* It is characterized by infection of brain parenchyma.
- *Myelitis:* It refers to infection of spinal cord.
- *Encephalomyelitis:* It is characterized by infection of brain parenchyma and spinal cord.

MENINGITIS

Meningitis is inflammation of the meninges that surround the brain and spinal cord. It involves pia mater, the arachnoid and the CSF-filled subarachnoid space. Inflammation spreads rapidly because of CSF circulation around the brain and spinal cord. It is caused by an infection, but chemical meningitis can occur.

Meninges Involved

Patchy meningitis denotes an inflammatory process restricted to dura mater. Leptomeningitis denotes an inflammatory process localized to arachnoid and pia mater. The infection may be limited to subarachnoid space. It may spread into the brain resulting in meningoencephalitis.

Age Group

Most infections occur in children <5 years of age, young adults and elderly persons. *Otitis media is most important risk factor for meningitis in children.* Such infection can be acute or chronic. The pia mater is the layer most commonly affected.

Etiology

Meningitis is most often caused by bacteria and viruses. Rarely fungi or *Entamoeba histolytica* may also cause meningitis.
- *Bacteria: Escherichia coli*, Salmonella, *Haemophilus influenzae*, Neisseria, streptococci, pneumococci and *Mycobacterium bacilli* cause bacterial meningitis.
- *Viruses:* Viruses causing meningitis include enteroviruses (ECHO virus 3, 7, 9, 11, 21, 30), EB virus, cocxsackievirus (B1–5 and A–9), herpes II virus and mumps virus. Viruses are most often transmitted by fecooral route. *Viral meningitis is less severe than bacterial meningitis.*
- *Fungi: Cryptococcus neoformans* causes meningitis in immunocompromised persons. It is demonstrated by India ink preparation of CSF in a black background. Capsule of *Cryptococcus neoformans* is demonstrated by mucicarmine stain (magenta colored) and silver stain (black color).
- *Iatrogenic agents:* Therapeutic administration of procaine or methotrexate in neurosurgical procedures may produce sterile chemical meningitis.
- *Cancers:* Carcinomatous meningitis occurs due to tumor deposits on the covering of the brain. It occurs in 5% patients with leukemia, lymphoma, melanoma, skin cancer, lung cancer and breast cancer.

Consequences

Infection increases the permeability of blood–brain barrier. It leads to cerebral edema and influx of toxic waste products resulting in increased intracranial pressure and damage to cranial nerves especially *VIII cranial nerve*. Patient develops hydrocephalus that limits the normal circulation of cerebrospinal fluid within brain and spinal cord.

CSF Findings

The presence of neutrophils in the CSF is the most definitive index of bacterial meningitis. By contrast, lymphocytes are the hallmark of tuberculosis and the viral meningitis, as well as some other chronic infections. In untreated cases, delirium gives way to coma and death.

BACTERIAL MENINGITIS

Etiology

Most cases of bacterial meningitis are caused by *Streptococcus pneumoniae* (the pneumococcus-3) or *Neisseria meningitidis* (the meningococcus) in adults. *Escherichia coli*, Salmonella, *Haemophilus influenzae* may also cause meningitis. *Neonates are infected by Escherichia coli, Salmonella and group B streptococci.*

Risk Factors

Risk factors associated with contracting meningitis include head trauma with basilar skull fractures, otitis media, sinusitis or mastoiditis, neurosurgery, dermal sinus tracts, systemic sepsis, or immunocompromised persons.

Portal of Entry

- *Hematogenous spread:* Hematogenous spread is most common. Most infectious agents reach the brain and meninges through the arterial bloodstream. Venous blood may serve as a carrier of infectious agents from the infected periocular and perinasal tissues (e.g. bacterial endocarditis and bronchiectasis). It is worth mentioning that *CNS has no lymphatic channels.*

- *Trauma:* Bacteria may be inoculated directly into the brain by bullets and sharp objects, such as a knife, or by direct entry through an open or surgical wound or skull fracture.
- *Local spread:* It occurs from spread of infection from paranasal sinuses, middle ear (drum perforation), and dental infections.
- *Spread via nerves:* Herpes residing in the trigeminal ganglion of latently infected people can also spread into the brain. Some viruses, such as rabies, ascend into the brain along the axons of peripheral nerves.
- *Ascent of infection:* Infection may ascend by various procedures like cystoscopy.
- *Iatrogenic infection: Staphylococcus epidermidis* is most common organism.

Age Group Predilection

In bacterial meningitis, majority of the organisms originate in nasopharynx. Causative organisms and age group predilection for meningitis (Table 30.2).

- *Neonates: Escherichia coli* is the prime cause of meningitis in the newborn, whose resistance to gram-negative bacteria has not fully developed. The transplacental transfer of maternal IgG imparts protection to the newborn against many bacteria. *Salmonella* also cause meningitis in neonates.
- *Infants and young children: Streptococcus pneumoniae* or *Neisseria meningitidis* cause pyogenic meningitis in this age group. Pyogenic meningitis caused by Neisseria meningitidis may develop *Waterhouse-Friderichsen syndrome*, characterized by hemorrhagic destruction of the adrenal cortex, acute hypocorticism with circulatory collapse, and disseminated intravascular coagulation.
- *Adults <30 years: Heamophilus influenzae* and *Neisseria meningitidis* cause meningitis at a later age.
- *Adults >30 years:* Adults >30 years develop meningitis caused by *Streptococcus pneumoniae*. Mycobacterium tubercular bacilli may affect any age group.

Pathology

- *Organism's entry:* In the pathophysiological process of bacterial meningitis, the bacteria replicate and undergo lysis in the cerebrospinal fluid, releasing endotoxins or cell wall fragments.
- *Release of chemical mediators.* These organisms' products lead to release of inflammatory chemical mediators resulting in movement of glucose and neutrophils across the capillary wall into CSF.
- *Purulent exudate in the subarachnoid space:* Entry of pathogens into the subarachnoid space leads to formation of cloudy purulent exudate. Purulent exudate in the subarachnoid space is characteristic. *CSF findings of diagnostic significance include numerous neutrophils, decreased glucose (<2/3rds of the serum glucose concentration) and increased protein.*
- *Leptomeningeal venulitis:* Thrombophlebitis occur in dural sinuses and bridging veins. Obliteration of arterioles by inflammation leads to vascular congestion, hemorrhagic infarction and cerebral abscess in the surrounding tissues. *Net result is thickening of the meninges and formation of adhesions.*
- *Reactive fibroblastic arachnoiditis with scarring:* Formation of adhesions may impunge on the cranial nerves resulting in cranial nerve palsy. Adhesions may impair the outflow of cerebrospinal fluid causing to hydrocephalus.

Gross Morphology
- The brain is edematous and congested. The subarachnoid space is filled with purulent exudates.
- The pus is most obvious in the sulci and subarachnoid cisterns at the base of the brain (Fig. 30.4).

Light Microscopy
The exudate in meninges consists predominantly of live and dead neutrophils (pus).

Clinical Features
- The most common symptoms of acute bacterial meningitis are fever (>40°C) and chills; severe headache localized to the forehead; stiff neck;

Table 30.2: Causative organisms and age group predilection for meningitis

Age group	Organisms
Neonates	*Escherichia coli, Salmonella*
Infants and young children	*Streptococcus pneumoniae, Neisseria meningitidis*
Adults <30 years	*Haemophilus influenzae, Neisseria meningitidis*
Adults >30 years	*Streptococcus pneumoniae,* Mycobacterium tubercular bacilli

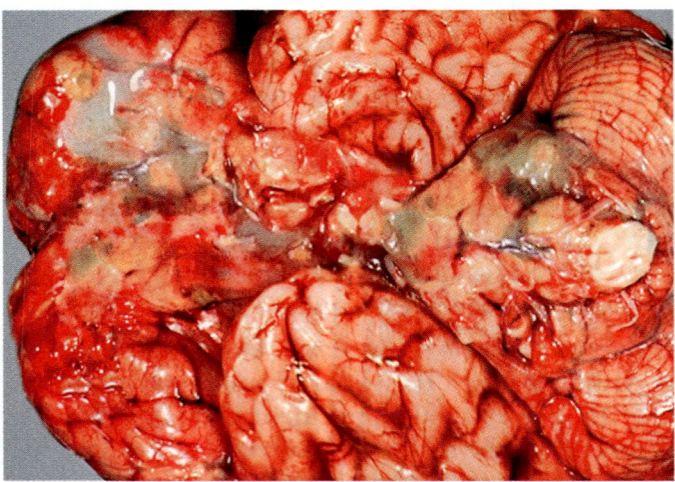

Fig. 30.4: Acute meningitis. One cause for acute swelling is infection. The yellow-tan exudate of acute bacterial meningitis seen here obscures the sulci.

back, abdominal, mental confusion, somnolence, photophobia, seizures, neurologic symptoms, extremity pains; nausea and vomiting.
- Patient experiences knee pain on flexion of hip joint is called *Kernig's sign*. Upon flexion of the neck, there is spontaneous similar movement of the hips and knees are known as *Brudzinski's sign*. Complications of bacterial meningitis are shown in Table 30.3.

Table 30.3: Complications of bacterial meningitis

- Cerebral infarction
- Obstructive hydrocephalus
- Cerebral abscess
- Subdural empyema
- Epilepsy (seizures) and focal neurological deficits
- Cranial nerve palsies
- Sensorineural hearing loss
- Communicating and non-communicating hydrocephalus

Laboratory Diagnosis

- Diagnosis of bacterial meningitis is based on the history and physical examination, along with laboratory data. CSF findings in pyogenic meningitis are shown in Table 30.4.
- Lumbar puncture findings are necessary for accurate diagnosis. These include a cloudy and purulent CSF under increased pressure.
- The CSF typically contains large numbers of polymorphonuclear neutrophils (up to 90,000/mm^3), increased protein content, and reduced sugar content.
- Bacteria can be seen on smears and can easily be cultured with appropriate media. Occasionally, previous antibiotic use limits culture sensitivities, in which case *latex agglutination* can be used, or *polymerase chain reaction* (PCR) testing for *Neisseria meningitidis*, *Haemophilus influenzae*, and *Listeria* species.

Vaccination

Effective *polysaccharide vaccines* are available to protect against meningococcal groups A, C, Y, and W-135. These vaccines are now recommended for *military recruits* and *college students*, who are at increased risk for invasive meningococcal disease.

TUBERCULOUS MENINGITIS

Tuberculous meningitis has insidious onset and may last for weeks or months. It is secondary to tuberculous infection occurring elsewhere in the body.

Locations

Tuberculosis has a predilection for the base of the brain. Basal cisterns and the lateral sulci that contain gelatinous whitish gray material. Inadequately treated tuberculous meningitis results in meningeal fibrosis, communicating

Table 30.4: CSF findings in pyogenic meningitis

Features	Pyogenic meningitis	Normal CSF
Causative organisms	*E. coli*, Salmonella, *Haemophilus influenzae*, *Neisseria meningitidis*, streptococci or pneumococci	No organisms
CSF pressure	Increased	80 to 180 cm of H_2O (20 drops/minute)
Color	Opaque and turbid to frank pus	Clear, colorless
CSF proteins	Increased due to vascular permeability	Normal 15–40 mg%
CSF sugar	Decreased or absent due to consumption by pyogenic bacteria. *CSF sugar:* Blood sugar ratio is <0.4	50–80 mg% *CSF sugar:* Blood sugar ratio is 0.6
CSF white blood cells	Polymorphonuclear cells 90,000/mm^3	0–4 lymphocytes/mm^3
CSF culture	Positive in 70–80%	Sterile
Gram staining	Sensitivity in 75–80%	Organisms absent, hence insignificant

Table 30.5: CSF findings in tubercular meningitis

Features	Tubercular meningitis	Normal CSF
Causative organism	Mycobacterium tubercle bacillus	No organisms
CSF pressure	Increased	80 to 180 cm of H_2O (20 drops/minute)
Color	Straw colored	Clear, colorless
CSF proteins	Increased due to vascular permeability	Normal 15–40 mg%
CSF sugar	Normal range	50–80 mg%
CSF white blood cells	Lymphocyte count increased	0–4 lymphocytes/mm^3
CSF culture	Bacterial growth on LJ medium	Sterile
ZN staining	Acid-fast bacteria demonstration	Organisms absent, hence insignificant

hydrocephalus and vasculitis. Inflammation of striate arteries results in cerebral infarcts.

Light Microscopy
The lesion consists of epithelioid cell granulomas, caseous necrosis and Langhans' giant cells.

CSF Findings
Lumbar puncture reveals increased pressure yielding *straw-colored* CSF. *Protein's content is markedly increased*. Light microscopy of CSF shows numerous *lymphocytes*. Acid-fast bacteria may be grown on culture media. CSF findings in tubercular meningitis are shown in Table 30.5.

VIRAL MENINGITIS
Viral meningitis is less severe than bacterial meningitis. Viral infections are limited to the meninges. It seldom involves the brain or spinal cord. Viruses are most often transmitted by *fecal-oral route*. The acute viral meningitides are self-limited and usually require only symptomatic treatment, except for herpes simplex virus (HSV) type 2, which responds to intravenous acyclovir.

Etiology
Viral meningitis may be caused by many different viruses, most often enteroviruses (ECHO virus 3, 7, 9, 11, 21, 30), including coxsackievirus (B1-5 and A-9), poliovirus, and echovirus. Others include Epstein-Barr virus, mumps virus, HSV, and West Nile virus. The manifestations of viral infections of CNS parenchyma are heterogeneous, owing to viral tropism to specific regions of the brain.

Light Microscopy
The classic hallmark of most CNS viral infections is the presence of perivascular lymphocytes around arteries and arterioles.

Laboratory Diagnosis
There are lymphocytes in the cerebrospinal fluid rather than polymorphonuclear cells. Protein content is only moderately elevated, and the sugar content usually is normal. Although often the virus cannot be identified, newer assays are emerging that allow in some circumstances for rapid identification of *viral ribonucleic acid* (RNA) in CSF. CSF findings in viral meningitis are shown in Table 30.6.

FUNGAL MENINGITIS
Meningitis caused by fungi has insidious onset and may last for weeks or months.

Table 30.6: CSF findings in viral meningitis

Features	Viral meningitis	Normal CSF
Causative organism	Enteroviruses (ECHO virus 3, 7, 9, 11, 21, 30), including coxsackievirus (B1–5 and A–9), poliovirus, and echovirus. Others include Epstein-Barr virus, mumps virus, HSV, and West Nile virus	No organisms
CSF pressure	Increased	80 to 180 cm of H_2O (20 drops/minute)
Color	Clear colorless	Clear, colorless
CSF proteins	Increased due to vascular permeability	Normal 15–40 mg%
CSF sugar	Normal range	50–80 mg%
CSF white blood cells	Lymphocyte count increased	0–4 lymphocytes/mm^3

Etiology

- *Fungi: Cryptococcus neoformans, Coccidioides immitis,* Aspergillus, or *Histoplasma capsulatum* involve the brain substance or the meninges in immunocompromised persons.

- *Cryptococcus neoformans:* It is the most common virulent fungi causing meningitis in immunocompromised persons especially AIDS. It produces sparse tissue response in meninges. It is demonstrated by mixing a drop of infected CSF with India ink.

Light Microscopy

Histopathological examination shows a clear halo about the encapsulated organism.

Differences between pyogenic, tubercular and viral meningitis are given in Table 30.7.

ENCEPHALITIS

VIRAL ENCEPHALITIS

Inflammation of the brain parenchyma is most often caused by viruses. It may be diffuse/localized inflammation of brain.

The nervous system is subject to invasion by many viruses, such as arbovirus, poliovirus, and rabies virus. Person contracts arbovirus infection from reservoirs such as horses, birds and mosquitoes.

Herpes simplex encephalitis is most common in teenagers and young adults. Herpes simplex targets the temporal lobes by binding on the plasma membranes of CNS cells. The virus has ability to remain latent or selective replication in distinct intracellular microenvironments.

Mode of Transmission

The mode of transmission may be the bite of a mosquito (arbovirus), a rabid animal such as dogs, foxes and bats

Table 30.7: Differences between various types of meningitis

Features	Pyogenic meningitis	Tubercular meningitis	Viral meningitis	No organisms
Causative organisms	E. coli, Salmonella, Haemophilus influenzae, Neisseria meningitis, streptococci or pneumococci	Mycobacterium tubercle bacillus	Enteroviruses (ECHO virus 3, 7, 9, 11, 21, 30), including coxsackievirus (B1–5 and A–9), poliovirus, and echovirus. Epstein-Barr virus, mumps virus, HSV, and West Nile virus	60–150 cm H_2O
CSF pressure	Increased	Increased	Increased	80–160 cm H_2O (20 drops/minute)
Color	Opaque and turbid to frank pus	Straw colored	Clear or colorless	Clear, colorless
CSF proteins	Increased	Increased rich in fibrinogen. When allowed to stand forms *cobweb turbidity* (fibrinogen → fibrin)	Increased	Normal 15–40 mg%
CSF sugar	Decreased or absent due to consumption by pyogenic bacteria CSF glucose: serum glucose = <0.4	Decreased It starts rising on ATT therapy	Normal except in mumps and herpes	50–80 mg%
CSF culture	Positive in 70–80%	Detection of AFB antigens by CSF chromatography, ELISA and PCR	Amplification of viral DNA or RNA from CSF by PCR amplification CSF IgG/serum IgG antibody titer >1.5	0–4 lymphocytes/mm^3
Staining technique	Gram staining	ZN staining	Not stained by Gram stain or ZN stain	Insignificant

(rabies virus present in saliva), or ingestion (poliovirus). Common causes of encephalitis in the United States are HSV and West Nile virus. Patient develops severe encephalitis with increased excitability of the CNS.

Clinical Features

Patient presents with hydrophobia (fear from water) characterized by violent muscle contractions and convulsions. It is usually fatal once clinical signs develop.

> **Light Microscopy**
> - Light microscopy of affected brain shows eosinophilic intracytoplasmic inclusions (*Negri bodies*) in the hippocampus and Purkinje cells of the cerebellum.
> - Brainstem and spinal cord show neuronal degeneration, perivascular accumulations of mononuclear cells.

PARASITIC ENCEPHALITIS

Parasitic encephalitis include neurocysticercosis, cerebral malaria, amoebic encephalitis and toxoplasmosis.

Neurocysticercosis

Neurocysticercosis is a common CNS parasitic infection and seizures worldwide caused by *Taenia solium*. Death of the parasite triggers granulomatous inflammatory response. Inflammation subsides over months to years and cyst becomes small fibrotic calcified nodule.

Cerebral Malaria

Cerebral malaria is caused by lodging of parasitized RBCs within the microvasculature of the brain. It is accompanied by petechial hemorrhages in the white mater around necrotic blood vessels. Prompt treatment with corticosteroids and antimalarial drugs reduces mortality.

Amoebic Encephalitis

Amoebic encephalitis is caused by *Naegleria fowleri*, *Balamuthia mandrillaris* and *Acanthamoeba* species. *Naegleria fowleri* enters CNS through cribriform plates during swimming. Patient develops acute meningitis progressing to coma and death. Organisms are demonstrated in subarachnoid space. *Entamoeba histolytica* causes brain abscess.

Cerebral Toxoplasmosis

Toxoplasma gondii is a parasite causing brain infection. It is one of the *TORCH* infections. It is transmitted via transplacental route in neonates, and ingestion of contaminated food due to urine or feces of household cats and pets. *Newborn manifests with hydrocephalus, mental retardation, neurologic abnormalities such as cerebral cortex, basal ganglia, and retinae, involvement of heart, lungs, and liver. Calcification in periventricular area is demonstrated on radiograph.* Immunocompromised adults present with lymphadenitis and CNS involvement.

CEREBRAL ABSCESS

Cerebral abscess is localized purulent infection caused by bacteria, protozoa and fungi. Abscess may be solitary or multiple.

Etiology

Cerebral abscess can result from penetrating skull injuries or from the spread of infection originating elsewhere; sources of infection include the paranasal sinuses or middle ear (most common source), bronchopulmonary infections, infective endocarditis, and other sites.

Pathology

Damaged brain tissue and immunosuppression contribute is some cases. Cerebral abscess matures over two weeks' period. Initially endothelial swelling occurs within 1–2 days followed by neutrophilic infiltration over 3–4 days.

Chronic inflammatory cells composed of macrophages, lymphocytes and plasma cells are present over days 5 to 7. Granulation tissue is formed over days 8 to 14. It is followed by fibrosis (gliosis).

TABES DORSALIS

Tabes dorsalis is a manifestation of tertiary syphilis involving the lumbar spinal cord. Patient develops chronic fibrosing syphilitic meningitis, compression of the posterior nerve roots (carrying sensory nerves) resulting in lancinating pain in extremities.

It also damages the transmission of proprioceptive impulses, causing gait disturbances (ataxia). Joint deformities are common and known as *Charcot joints*.

> **Gross Morphology**
> Focal irregular thickening is seen around spinal cord but may be seen over the convexity of the brain or over the cerebellum.
>
> **Light Microscopy**
> - Tertiary syphilis may also present in the form of granulomatous inflammation (*gumma syphilis*).
> - Meninges contain infiltrates of lymphocytes and plasma cells, typically arranged around the meningeal blood vessels.

CNS TUMORS

GENERAL CONSIDERATIONS

Primary brain tumors account for 2% of all cancer deaths. Metastases to the brain develop in 10 to 15% of cancer people. Most primary tumors of central nervous system occur in intracranial region. *Tumors of the spinal cord are much less frequent. Primary malignant CNS tumors rarely metastasize.* Collectively, neoplasms of astrocytic origin are the most common type of primary brain tumor in adults, followed by primary CNS lymphoma (Figs 30.5 to 30.7).

Basic Types

Intracranial tumors can be divided into three basic types.

- *Primary CNS tumors:* These are derived from neurons and neuroglia.
- *Primary other CNS tumors:* Primary intracranial tumors that originate in the skull cavity but are not derived from the brain tissue itself (e.g. meninges, pituitary gland, pineal gland, primary CNS lymphoma).
- *Metastatic tumors:* In adults, metastases in brain occur from thyroid gland, breast, lung, kidney, colon, NHL and skin melanoma. Acute lymphoblastic leukemia may metastasize to brain in children. In young adults, metastases from osteosarcoma, Ewing's sarcoma and rhabdomyosarcoma may metastasize to brain.

Age Group Distribution

- *Primary CNS tumors in adults:* In adults, the majority of intracranial tumors (70%) are supratentorial. In order of frequency, these include glioblastoma multiforme, meningioma, ependymoma and acoustic neuroma.
- *Primary CNS tumors in children:* In children, the majority of intracranial tumors are infratentorial. In order of frequency, these include cerebellar astrocytoma, medulloblastoma, glioma in brainstem, and ependymoma (in the fourth ventricle).

Risk Factors

Risk factors associated with an increased incidence of brain tumors include Turcot's syndrome, neurofibromatosis, neuromas and cigarette smoking.

Pathogenesis

Mutation of oncogenes and tumor suppressor genes participate in the pathogenesis of brain tumors. Mutator genes (MLH1, MSH2, MSH6, and PMS2), when combined with oncogenes or defective tumor suppressor gene lead to accumulation of genetic mutations resulting in malignant transformation.

Normally, MLH1, MSH2, MSH6, and PMS2 are caretaker genes. Their gene products participate in DNA replication and repairs.

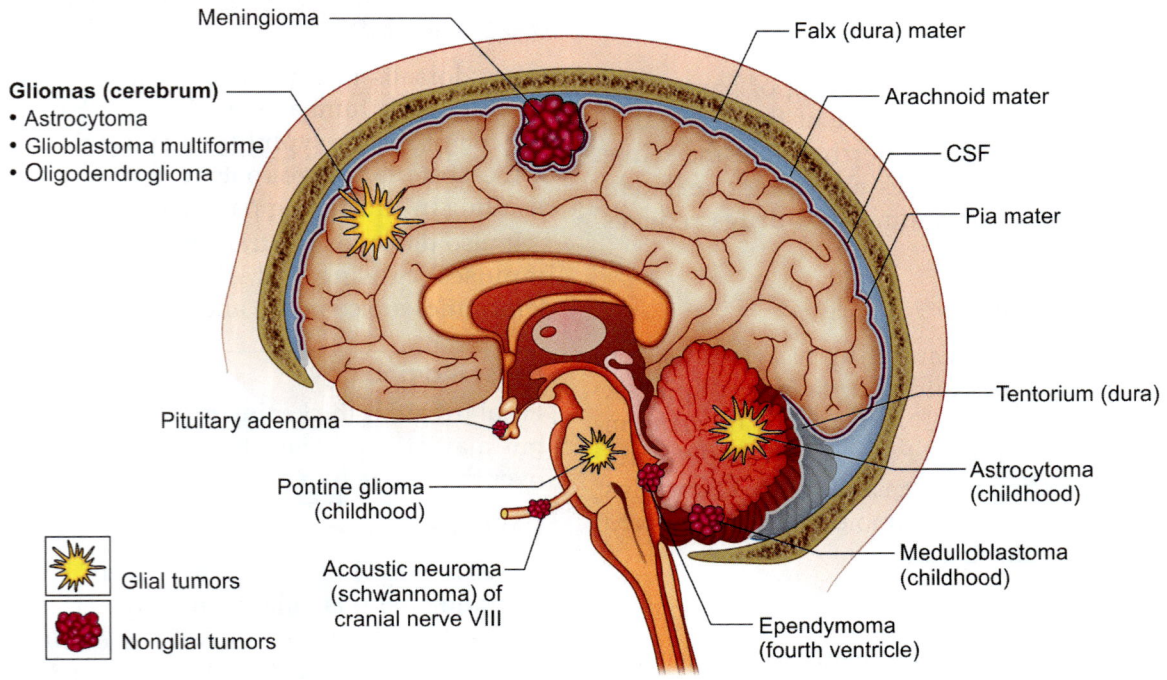

Fig. 30.5: Most common intracranial tumors.

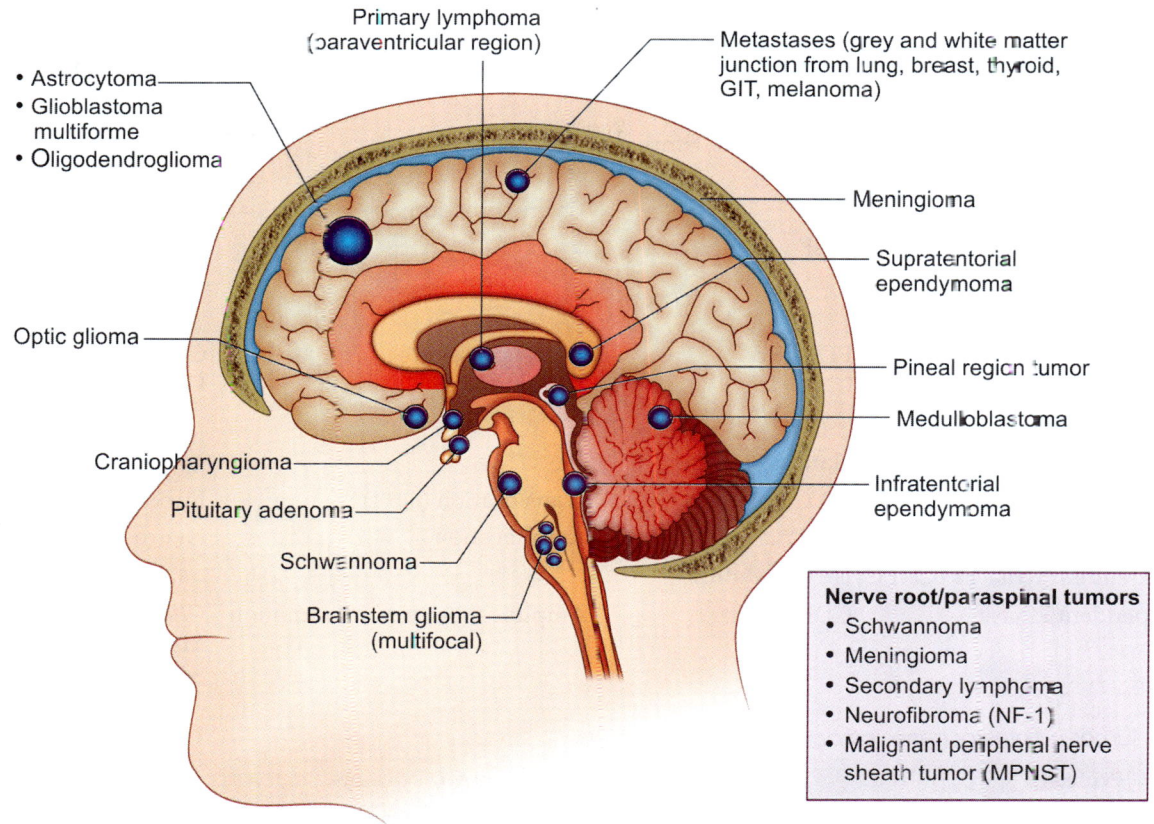

Fig. 30.6: Common primary CNS tumors in adults (*Courtesy:* Dr Abhijit Das).

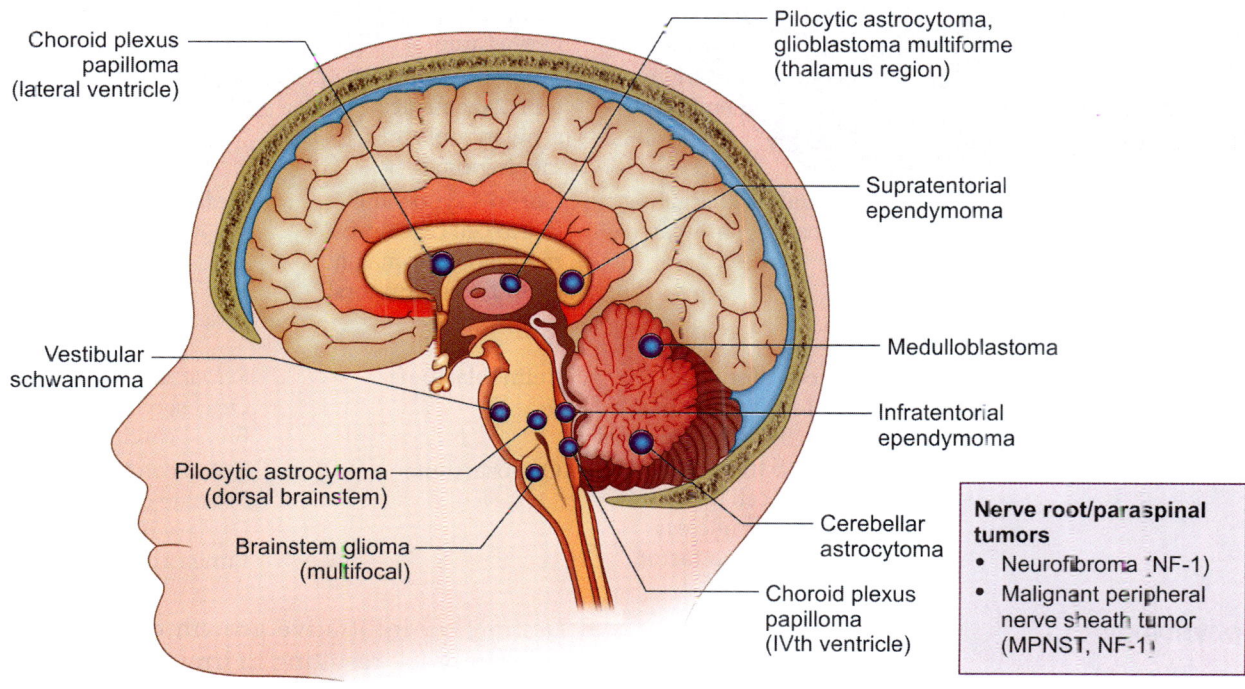

Fig. 30.7: Common primary CNS tumors in children (*Courtesy:* Dr Abhijit Das).

Mutations of these mutator genes (MLH 1, MSH 2, 6 and PMS 2 are associated with increased risk of development of hereditary non-polyposis colon cancer, stomach cancer, urothelial cancer, brain cancer in these patients.

Mutation of oncogenes and tumor suppressor genes associated with CNS tumors and associated tumors are shown in Tables 30.8 and 30.9.

Table 30.8: Oncogenes associated with CNS tumors

Category	Proto-oncogene	Mode of activation	Associated malignancies
Growth Factors			
PDGF-β chain	PDGFB (sis-Simion sarcoma)	Overexpression	*Astrocytoma* Osteosarcoma
TGF-α	TGFA		*Astrocytoma*
HGF (hepatocyte growth factor)	HGF		Hepatocellular carcinoma Thyroid carcinoma
Growth Factor Receptors			
PDGF receptor	PDGFRB	Overexpression Translocation	*Gliomas* Leukemias
Signal-Transduction Proteins			
Transcription Factors (Nuclear Regulatory Proteins)			
MYC (myelocytomatosis) Transcriptional factor	MYC N-MYC	Translocation (8; 14) Amplification	Burkitt's lymphoma Neuroblastoma
Cyclin-dependent Kinases (Cell Cycle Regulators)			
Cyclin-dependent kinase	CDK4	Amplification or point mutation	*Glioblastoma multiforme* Melanoma Sarcoma

Table 30.9: Tumor suppressor genes associated with CNS tumors

Gene	Protein	Function	Familial tumors	Sporadic cancers
Mitogenic Signaling Pathway Inhibitors				
NF-1	Neurofibronin-1 (locus 13p11) Mutation occurs by deletion	NF-1 inhibits RAS/MAP: kinase signaling activator pathway	Neurofibromatosis type 1 (neurofibroma and malignant peripheral nerve tumors)	*Schwannoma* Neuroblastoma Juvenile myeloid leukemia
NF-2	Merlin (locus 22q) Mutation by deletion or nonsense mutation	NF-2 stabilizes cytoskeleton membrane linkage	Neurofibromatosis type 2 (acoustic schwannoma and meningioma)	*Schwannomas* *Meningiomas*
PTCH	Patched	It inhibits Hedgehog signaling pathway	Gorlin's syndrome (basal cell carcinoma, medulloblastoma and other benign tumors)	*Medulloblastoma* Basal cell carcinoma
Cell Cycle Progression Inhibitors				
RB gene	Retinoblastoma protein (locus 13p14) Mutation by deletion and nonsense	It codes for pRB protein, master brake on cell cycle. It inhibits G1 to S transition during cell cycle It inhibits nuclear transcription factor	Retinoblastoma Osteosarcoma	*Retinoblastoma* Osteosarcoma Breast carcinoma Colon carcinoma Prostate carcinoma Urinary bladder carcinoma Lung carcinoma

Pathophysiology

Intracranial neoplasms exert their effects via a combination of the following mechanisms:

- *Compression:* Expansile growth of intracranial tumors compresses the adjacent brain tissue resulting to neurological deficits. Surgical excision of tumor reverses neurological deficits.

- *Destruction:* Infiltrative growth causes destruction of brain tissue resulting in irreversible neurological deficits even after surgical excision.

- *Obstruction to CSF flow:* Tumor present in posterior cranial fossa obstructs foramen of Monro resulting in hydrocephalus. Tumors causing obstruction to CSF flow include choroid plexus, papilloma, ependymoma and pineal region tumor.

- *Cerebral edema:* Patient with malignant intracerebral tumor develops cerebral edema due to neoangiogenesis and defective blood–brain barrier.
- *Focal epileptic seizures:* Expansile or infiltrative growth may cause focal epileptic seizures.

WHO Classification of Brain Tumors

The WHO system is the most widely used classification system for brain tumors. It is based on histopathological characteristics (Table 30.10), immunohistochemistry categories of CNS tumors (Table 30.11) and selected nervous system tumors are shown in Table 30.12.

Table 30.10: Classification and grading of CNS tumors

Tumors	Grade I	Grade II	Grade III	Grade IV
Neuroepithelial Tumors Arising from Neuroglial Cells				
Astrocytic tumors				
Subependymal giant cell astrocytoma and pilocytic astrocytoma	*			
Diffuse infiltrating astrocytoma		*		
Anaplastic astrocytoma			*	
Glioblastoma multiforme				*
Oligodendroglial tumors				
Oligodendroglioma		*		
Anaplastic oligodendroglioma			*	
Ependymal tumors				
Subependymoma and myxopapillary ependymoma	*			
Anaplastic ependymoma			*	
Oligoastrocytic tumors				
Oligoastrocytoma		*		
Anaplastic oligoastrocytoma			*	
Choroid plexus tumors				
Choroid plexus papilloma	*			
Atypical choroid plexus papilloma		*		
Choroid plexus carcinoma			*	
Other neuroepithelial tumors				
Angiocentric glioma	*			
Choroid glioma of the third ventricle		*		
Primitive neuroectodermal tumors (PNET)				
Medulloblastoma (derived from ganglion cells in abdomen), esthesio-neuroblastoma of the nasal mucosa, cerebral neuroblastoma, retinoblastoma, pineoloblastoma, atypical rhabdoid tumor				*
Non-neuroepithelial Tumors				
Meningeal tumors				
Meningoepithelial, fibroblastic, transitional, and psammomatous meningiomas	*			
Metaplastic, chondroid, clear cell and atypical meningiomas		*		
Papillary, rhabdoid and anaplastic meningiomas			*	
Tumors of the cranial and paraspinal nerves				
Schwannoma, neurofibroma and perineuroma	*			
Malignant peripheral nerve sheath tumor (MPNAST)		*	*	*
Tumors of the seller region				
Craniopharyngioma, granular cell tumor of the neurohypophysis and spindle cell oncocytoma of the adenophysis	*			
Primary CNS lymphoma				
Primary CNS lymphoma: B cell/T cell, large cell, NK/T cell				*
Germ cell tumors				
Germinoma, embryonal carcinoma, endodermal sinus tumor (yolk sac tumor), choriocarcinoma, teratoma				

* Neuroepithelial tumors of nervous system show grade of the tumor

Table 30.11: Immunohistochemistry categories of CNS tumor markers

Category	Tumor markers	Tumors	Characteristics
Glial markers	Glial fibrillary acid protein (GFAP)	Glial tumors: choroid plexus tumors, medulloblastoma, neuroectodermal tumors (PNETs) and gangliogliomas Nonglial tumors: nerve sheath and cartilaginous tumors	GFAP is intermediate filament specific for glial differentiation
Neuronal markers	Synaptophysin (more specific) and chromogranin	More primitive neuronal tumors: medulloblastoma and PNETs Others: ganglion cells, pituitary adenomas and carcinomas, carcinoid tumors, neurocytomas and paragangliomas	Synaptophysin is more specific marker for more primitive neuronal tumors
	Neurofilament (NF)	Neurons and axons: gangliogliomas	NF highlights entrapped axons in infiltrative growth pattern. NF is negative in medulloblastoma
	Neu-N	NF highlights neuronal nuclei and cell bodies in identifying cortical dysplasia, neuronal loss, and neurons entrapped in infiltrative growth	NF marker of neuronal differentiation
Epithelial markers	Cytokeratin (CK; AE1/AE3)	Metastatic carcinoma, craniopharyngiomas, chordomas, and choroid plexus tumors	Cross reactivity in glioblastoma multiforme
	CAM 5.2	Metastatic carcinoma	No cross reactivity in glioblastoma multiforme
	Epithelial membrane antigen (EMA)	Meningiomas and ependymomas	EMA is useful along with CD99 and D_2-40 in diagnosing ependymomas
Neuroectodermal marker	S-100 protein	Neuroectodermal cells, melanocytes, glia, Schwann cells, chondrocytes present in paraganglioma, pheochromocytoma and olfactory neuroblastoma, peripheral nerve sheath tumors	Marker of Schwann cell differentiation
Proliferative marker	Ki-67	Marker for tumor grade and prognosis	Ki-67 is proliferative marker
Molecular test markers	INI1/BAF-47 deletions	Mutations observed in atypical teratoid/rhabdoid tumors	Used as surrogate for genetic testing to demonstrate biallelic inactivation of the gene
	Isocitrate dehydrogenase (IDH1/IDH2) mutations	Immunohistochemistry helpful in differentiating low grade gliomas from gliosis	IDH1 monoclonal antibodies used

Table 30.12: Selected central nervous system tumors

Histological variants	Age predilection	Most frequent site	Characteristics
Glioblastoma multiforme	Older persons (40–70 years)	Cerebral hemispheres frontal lobe, crossing corpus callosum involving opposite cerebral hemisphere	• Most common primary highly malignant intracranial tumor • Butterfly-shaped tumor on MRI • Increased intracranial pressure and seizures • Dual loss of 1p 19q associated with good prognosis • Surgical resection impossible, but treated by radiotherapy and chemotherapy
Pilocytic astrocytoma	Children	Cerebellum, optic nerve, brainstem	• Low grade tumor with good prognosis • Immunohistochemistry (GFAP)
Oligodendroglioma	Middle age group	Cerebral hemisphere frontal lobe white matter	• Prone to spontaneous hemorrhage owing to delicate vasculature • Calcification seen on radiograph • Translocation (1p,19q) • Chemosensitive tumor
Medulloblastoma	Most often 15–35 years, may occur in children (<15 years)	Cerebellum (close to 4th ventricle)	• Highly malignant intracranial tumor • Chromosome 17 alteration • Seeding CSF • Resection difficult, highly radiosensitive with poor prognosis • Immunohistochemistry (synaptophysin or nestin, neuron-specific enolase and GFAP)
Ependymoma	Most common in first two decades	4th ventricle of brain	• Histological variants (well differentiated, myxopapillary and anaplastic) • Immunohistochemistry (GFAP, S-100, vimentin) • Increased intracranial pressure, hydrocephalus
Choroid plexus	Children	Lateral ventricle, 4th ventricle of brain	• Uncommon neuroectodermal tumor but seeding CSF • Hydrocephalus
Metastatic tumors	Variable age	Metastases from lung, breast, kidney, colon, thyroid, skin melanoma	• Metastatic tumors are more common than primary intracranial tumors
Meningioma	20–40 years (more common in women)	Convexity of cerebral hemispheres, falx cerebri, olfactory groove beneath frontal lobe, lesser wing of sphenoid wing, sella turcica, foramen magnum, thoracic region of spinal cord	• Second most common primary intracranial neoplasm (grade I) • Aggressive menigiomas (clear cell and chondroid variant grade II, papillary and rhabdoid variant grade III) • Benign tumor is present external to the brain hence easy resection
Schwannoma (neurilemmoma)	Middle to later life	8th cranial nerve (when schwannoma is intracranial)	• Acoustic schwannoma, common intracranial tumor, ranking third after glioblastoma multiforme and meningioma, most often benign tumor is usually resectable
Retinoblastoma	Young children (<3 years)	Retina, bilateral and multifocal in familial form; unilateral and unifocal in sporadic forms	• Most common eye tumor of young children; linked to Rb gene deletion or inactivation

SECONDARY TUMORS

Metastatic tumors are more common than primary intracranial tumors of the CNS. These occur in adults (30% of cases) and children (6–10% of cases). Common sources of metastases in adults include lung carcinoma, breast carcinoma, skin melanoma, renal cell carcinoma, colon carcinoma, thyroid carcinoma and NHL.

In children, sources of metastases include acute lymphoblastic lymphoma, osteosarcoma, Ewing's sarcoma and rhabdomyosarcoma (Figs 30.8 and 30.9).

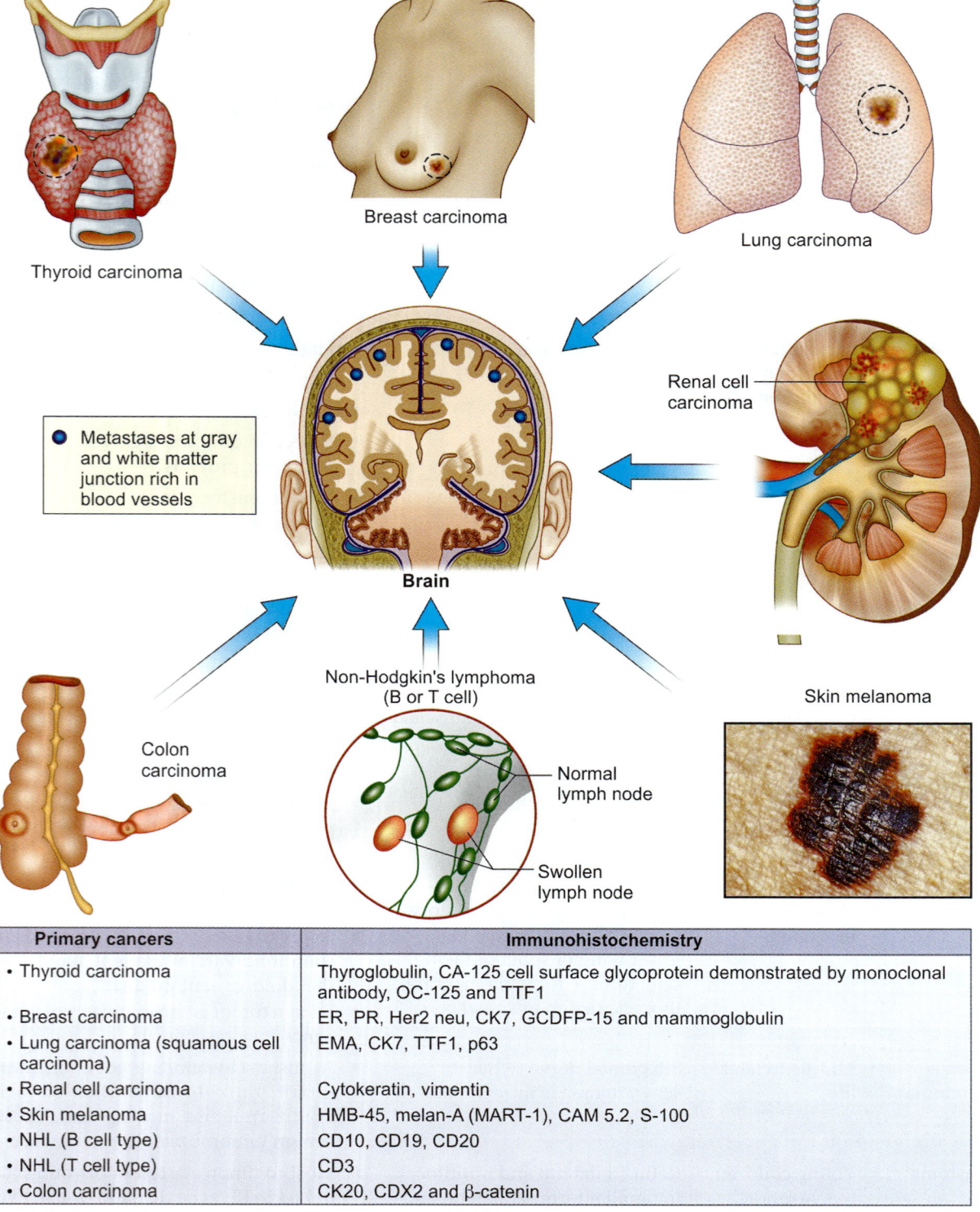

Primary cancers	Immunohistochemistry
• Thyroid carcinoma	Thyroglobulin, CA-125 cell surface glycoprotein demonstrated by monoclonal antibody, OC-125 and TTF1
• Breast carcinoma	ER, PR, Her2 neu, CK7, GCDFP-15 and mammoglobulin
• Lung carcinoma (squamous cell carcinoma)	EMA, CK7, TTF1, p63
• Renal cell carcinoma	Cytokeratin, vimentin
• Skin melanoma	HMB-45, melan-A (MART-1), CAM 5.2, S-100
• NHL (B cell type)	CD10, CD19, CD20
• NHL (T cell type)	CD3
• Colon carcinoma	CK20, CDX2 and β-catenin

Fig. 30.8: Common brain metastases in adults from thyroid, breast, lung, kidney, colon, skin melanoma and NHL.

Nervous System 30

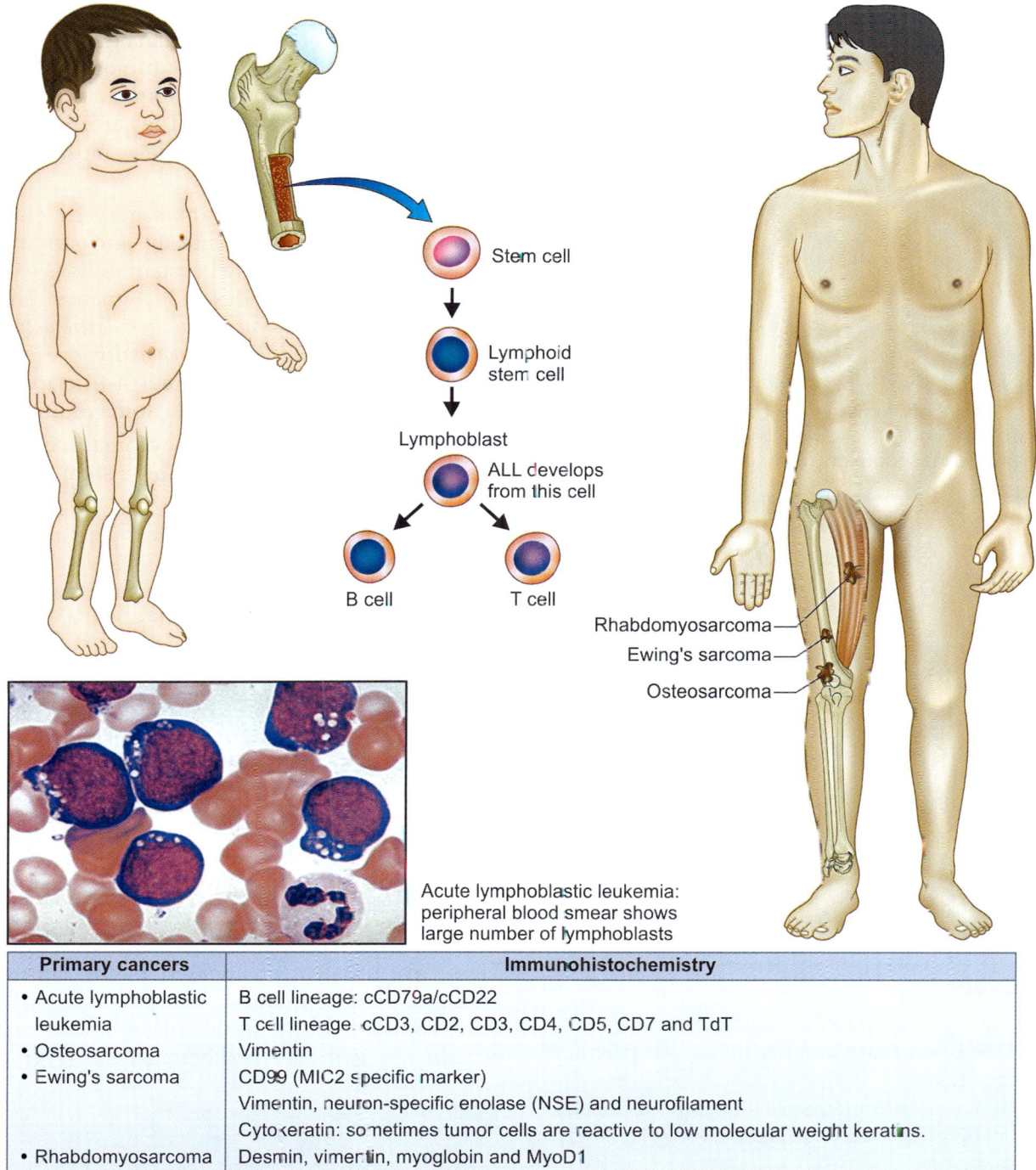

Fig. 30.9: Common brain metastases in children and young adults from acute lymphoblastic leukemia, Ewing's sarcoma, osteosarcoma and rhabdomyosarcoma.

Location of Metastases

Most metastatic lesions seed to the *gray-white junction, reflecting the rich capillary bed in this area*. The borders of a metastasis tend to be more discrete than those of a primary glioma.

These tumors involve subarachnoid space and cause meningitis (Fig. 30.10).

Imaging Technique

Metastasis in brain appears as *discrete, globoid shape lesion*, and prominent halo of edema in contrast to primary glioma or medulloblastoma.

Spinal cord involvement is uncommon. If present, then *metastatic deposits are seen in extradural space of spinal cord*.

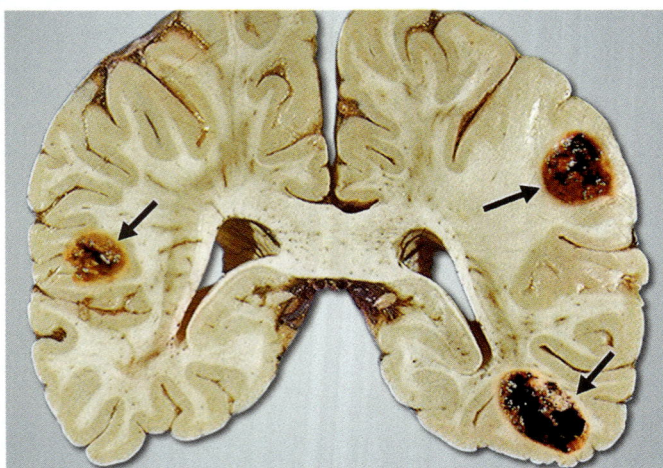

Fig. 30.10: Secondary tumor in the brain. Secondary tumor deposits are usually multiple and well circumscribed. Pigmented secondaries indicate secondary melanoma (arrows).

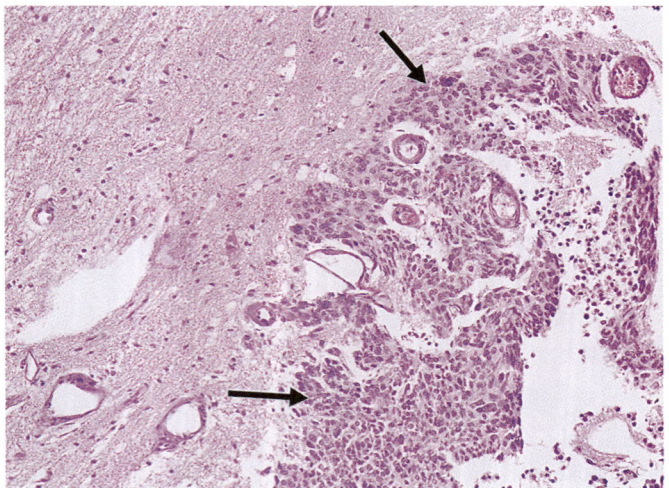

Fig. 30.11: Metastases in brain from carcinoma (arrows) (100X).

Light Microscopy
- A biopsy is required to differentiate these lesions. A solitary brain mass in an adult can be primary or metastatic.
- In some cases, the metastases become clinically apparent before primary site is observed (Fig. 30.11).

Immunohistochemistry
It is useful to confirm source of primary cancers metastasizing to central nervous system.

NEUROEPITHELIAL TUMORS

ASTROCYTIC TUMORS

Astrocytomas are the most common primary brain tumors constituting 70% of all CNS tumors. Peak occurrence is in the late middle-age group. These tumors originate from astrocytes in the cerebral hemisphere, cerebellum, optic nerve and brainstem. For purposes of classification, astrocytic tumors can be subdivided into fibrillary (infiltrating) astrocytic tumors and pilocytic astrocytomas. Fibrillary astrocytomas account for 80% of adult primary brain tumors. They are most common in middle age. Pilocytic astrocytomas most often occur in cerebellum in children.

- *Classification:* Astrocytomas may be classified based on their invasion into the surrounding brain tissue. A commonly used system divides astrocytic tumors into three grades of malignancy. These are *well differentiated astrocytoma, anaplastic astrocytoma (invasive tumor) and glioblastoma multiforme (high grade invasive tumor)*. Many low grade astrocytomas may progress to high grade glioblastoma multiforme.
- *Behavior:* Low grade astrocytoma arising from cerebellum, optic nerve and brainstem in children has good prognosis.
- *Histological grading:* Histological grading is based on *nuclear atypia*, *mitotic activity*, *endothelial cells or microvascular proliferation* and *necrosis* in tumor. Astrocytoma lacks true rosettes, cell-cell junctions and microvilli lined lumina.

Pilocytic Astrocytoma

Pilocytic astrocytomas are distinguished from other astrocytomas by their cellular appearance and their benign behavior. It is grade I tumor.

Age Group

Typically, they occur in children and young adults.

Locations

These are most often located in the cerebellum. These also can be found in the floor and walls of the third ventricle, in the optic chiasm and nerves, and occasionally in the cerebral hemispheres (Fig. 30.12).

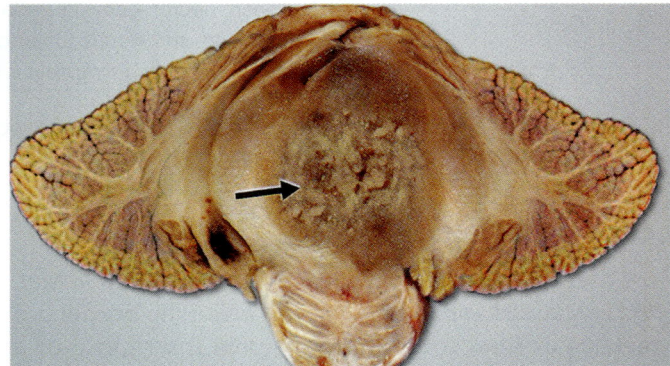

Fig. 30.12: Cerebellum containing a large astrocytoma. The majority of the brain tumors in children occur below the tentorium cerebelli (arrow).

Light Microscopy

Pilocytic astrocytoma is composed of long hair like cells cytoplasmic processes.

Immunohistochemistry

Glial fibrillary acidic protein (GFAP) is an intermediate filament protein. It is variable expressed in variable proportions in astrocytic tumors. Tumor cells also show positivity with *PTAH*.

Prognosis

The prognosis of people with pilocytic astrocytomas is influenced primarily by their location. The prognosis is usually better for people with surgically resectable tumors, such as those located in the cerebellar cortex, than for people with less accessible tumors, such as those involving the hypothalamus or brainstem.

Anaplastic Astrocytomas

Anaplastic astrocytomas have a peak incidence in the sixth decade. Although they usually are found in the cerebral hemispheres. These also can occur in the cerebellum, brainstem, or spinal cord. These are considered to arise from previously well differentiated astrocytomas.

Location

These most often occur in the cerebral hemispheres of adults.

Clinical Features

Clinically, infiltrating astrocytic tumors present with symptoms of increased ICP (e.g. headache) or focal abnormalities related to their position (e.g. seizures).

Prognosis

Anaplastic astrocytomas are associated with poor prognosis than well differentiated astrocytomas, but better prognosis when compared to glioblastoma multiforme.

Gross Morphology

- The tumor has arisen in the right hemisphere and extends through the genu of the corpus callosum into the left hemisphere.
- There is hemorrhage and necrosis in the tumor, indicating that it is a high-grade malignancy (Fig. 30.13).

Light Microscopy

- Tumor is composed of large number of pleomorphic cells and increased mitotic figures.
- Blood vessels are more prominent than usual due to proliferation of endothelial cells (Fig. 30.14).

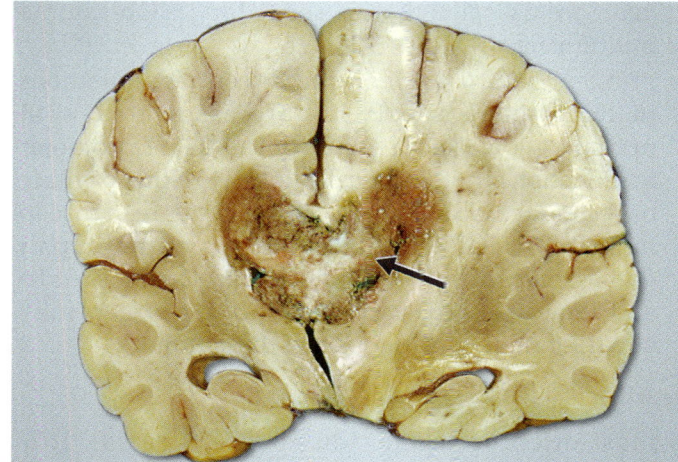

Fig. 30.13: Astrocytoma. Brain slice examined from its posterior aspect. The tumor has arisen in the right hemisphere and extends through the genu of the corpus callosum into the left hemisphere. There is hemorrhage and necrosis in the tumor, indicating that it is a high-grade malignancy. It has extended into the third ventricle, obstructing the interventricular foramina and resulting in hydrocephalus, as shown by the dilatation of the anterior horns of both lateral ventricles (arrow).

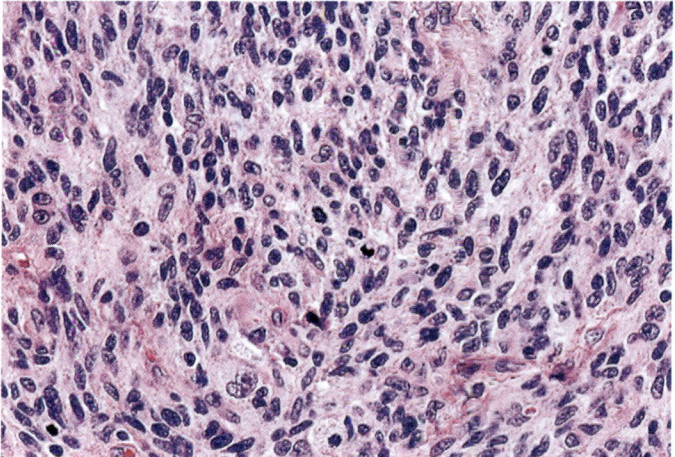

Fig. 30.14: Astrocytoma anaplastic type (400X).

Glioblastoma Multiforme

Glioblastoma multiforme arising in cerebrum is the most common and highly malignant primary intracranial neoplasm (grade IV). *Most patients die within one year of diagnosis.* These tumors have ill-defined margins and grow irregularly into the surrounding brain tissue and, therefore, it is difficult to eradicate the tumor. These increase intracranial pressure.

Origin

It may either arise *de novo* or from dedifferentiation of a low-grade astrocytoma in young patients, as primary tumor of CNS.

- *Secondary glioblastoma multiforme:* Amplification of PDGF-A and inactivation of p53 tumor suppressor

gene are associated with secondary glioblastoma multiforme.
- *Primary glioblastoma multiforme:* In contrast, mutations in EGFR-gene and PTEN are associated with primary glioblastoma multiforme. MGMT promoter methylation is not specifically linked to either primary or secondary GBM, but it predicts better response to treatment in GBMs because tumors cannot repair damage caused by alkylating agents. Dual loss of 1p and 19q can also be seen in astrocytomas, generally a marker of good prognosis in these tumors.

Age Group

It most often occurs in adults (40–70 years). It is extremely rare in children.

Location

It occurs in frontal lobes, crosses corpus callosum and extends into opposite cerebral hemisphere. MRI shows butterfly shaped tumor.

Oncogenesis

Oncogenesis of astrocytomas is shown in Table 30.13.

Clinical Features

Clinically, infiltrating astrocytic tumors present with symptoms of increased ICP (e.g. headache) or focal abnormalities related to their position (e.g. seizures).

Gross Morphology

It is poorly circumscribed tumor. As the tumor invades and causes obliteration of vessels, the tumor features patchy (multifocal areas) yellow areas of necrosis and red zones of hemorrhage (Fig. 30.15).

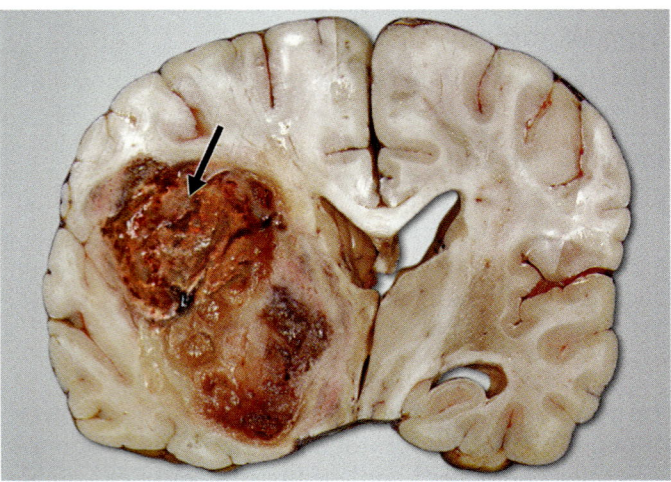

Fig. 30.15: Glioblastoma multiforme (GBM). This is the worst possible form of glioma, a glioblastoma multiforme (GBM). These neoplasms are quite vascular with prominent areas of necrosis and hemorrhage. Note how this one has crossed the midline to the opposite hemisphere (arrow).

Light Microscopy

- *Cellular morphology:* Tumor comprises highly pleomorphic astroglial cells with hyperchromatic nuclei, multinucleated giant cells, mitosis and marked proliferation of endothelial cells.
- *Capillary endothelial proliferation:* It is striking histological features. The abnormal blood vessels have thick-walled branches terminating in a triangle of capillaries. These vessels have similar appearance to renal glomeruli called *glomeruloid areas*.
- *Pseudopalisading pattern:* Rod-shaped nuclei of tumor cells are arranged in palisading pattern around prominent vessels perpendicular to the necrotic areas.

Table 30.13: Oncogenes associated with glioblastoma multiforme

Category	Proto-oncogene	Mode of activation	Associated malignancies
Growth factors			
PDGF-β chain	PDGFB (*sis*-Simion sarcoma)	Overexpression	*Astrocytoma* Osteosarcoma
TGF-α	TGFA	Overexpression	*Astrocytoma*
Hepatocyte growth factor (HGF)	HGF	Overexpression	Hepatocellular carcinoma Thyroid carcinoma
Growth factor receptors			
PDGF receptor	PDGFRB	Overexpression Translocation	*Gliomas* Leukemias
Transcription factors (nuclear regulatory proteins)			
Cyclin-dependent kinase (cell cycle regulatory proteins)	CDK4	Amplification or point mutation	*Glioblastoma multiforme* Melanoma Sarcoma

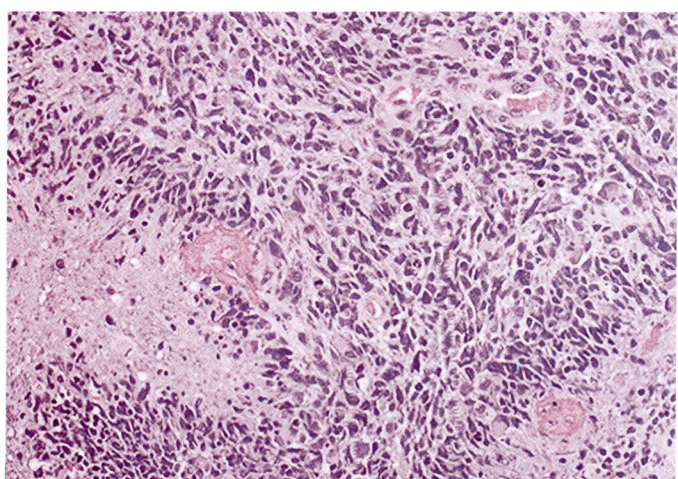

Fig. 30.16: This glioblastoma multiforme (GBM) demonstrates marked cellularity with marked hyperchromatism and pleomorphism. Note the prominent vascularity as well as the area of necrosis at the left with neoplastic cells palisading around it (400X).

- *Small rod-shaped anaplastic cells:* These tumor cells are frequently demonstrated in glioblastoma multiforme. These are actively dividing cells (12–19%) demonstrated by *radioactive thymidine uptake studies.*
- *Hemorrhage and necrosis:* Areas of hemorrhage and necrosis are common (Fig. 30.16).

Metastases

The neoplastic cells can infiltrate widely, particularly along white mater tracts, seeding CSF, and rarely metastasizes outside the CNS.

Treatment

Surgical resection of tumor is impossible, but radiation and chemotherapy may add months to patient's survival.

OLIGODENDROGLIOMA

Oligodendroglioma is *benign slow growing ill-defined* tumor arising from oligodendrocytes in the white mater of *frontal lobe of cerebral hemispheres* of middle age group. It represents 5 to 20% of glial tumors affecting middle age group. It may feature presenting both oligodendrocytes and astrocytes.

Radiograph

It most often shows *calcification*, visible on X-rays in 40% of patients. The patients may present clinically with *epilepsy*.

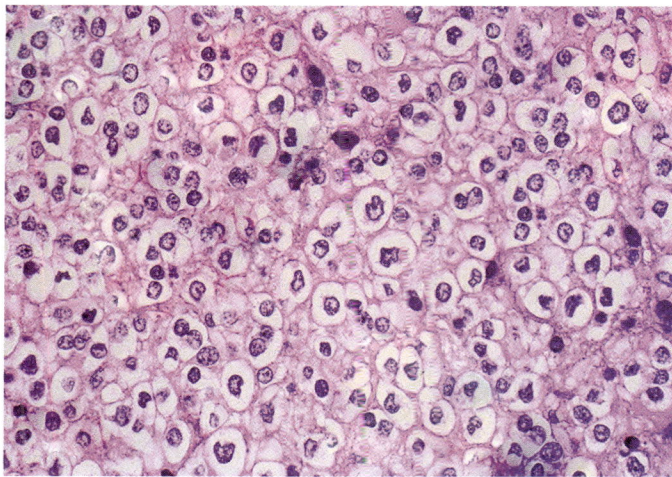

Fig. 30.17: Oligodendroglioma. The tumor cells show acute swelling of the perinuclear zones giving them a characteristic *poached egg-like* appearance (400X).

Molecular Genetics

A translocation between chromosomes 1p and 19q is the characteristic molecular finding.

- Well differentiated tumor is composed of closely packed small, round and uniform nuclei similar to normal oligodendrocytes surrounded by a clear cytoplasm and prominent cell membrane (*fried egg appearance*).
- Tumor is divided into groups of cells by delicate capillary strands. Small foci of calcification are common and visualized on radiograph.
- These *calcospherites* are occasionally scattered randomly throughout the lesion (Fig. 30.17).

Prognosis

Prognosis of patient with oligodendroglioma depends on the histological grade of the tumor, its location, and recognition of molecular features that can be linked to chemosensitivity. *Oligodendroglial tumors are prone to spontaneous hemorrhage owing to their delicate vasculature.*

EPENDYMOMA

Ependymomas are derived from the single layer of epithelium that lines the ventricles and spinal canal. *It most often occurs in the 4th ventricle,* where papillary growth produces obstruction and results in hydrocephalus (Fig. 30.18). Distribution of ependymomas is shown in Table 30.14.

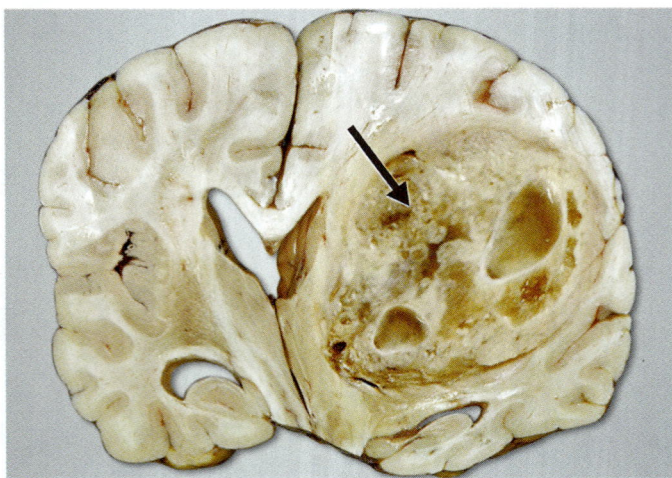

Fig. 30.18: Ependymoma in the right lateral ventricle. The tumor is well circumscribed and apparently confined to the ventricle. It has compressed the CSF pathways, causing dilatation of the third ventricle and the left lateral ventricle. The macroscopic appearance of this tumor suggests an ependymoma, but microscopic confirmation would be required (arrow).

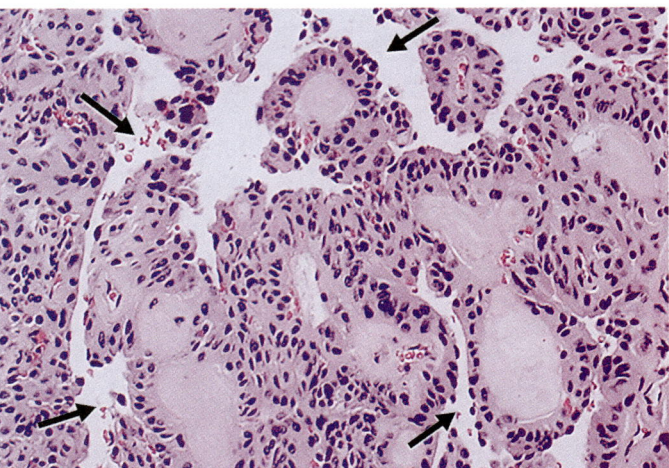

Fig. 30.19: This is a myxopapillary ependymoma, which is typically found arising in the filum terminale of the spinal cord. Note the cells around papillations that have a myxoid connective tissue core. Surgical removal is made easier if this tumor has not grown around nerve roots of the cauda equina (arrows) (400X).

Table 30.14: Distribution of ependymomas

Location	Frequency
Floor of fourth ventricle	38%
Cerebral ventricles	20%
Cervicothoracic spinal cord	14%
Cauda equina	28%

Age Group

Although they can occur at any age. These are most likely to occur in the first two decades of life. Spinal cord is the most common site for ependymomas occurring in middle age.

Clinical Features

The clinical features depend on the location of the neoplasm. Intracranial tumors are often associated with hydrocephalus and evidence of increased intracranial pressure (ICP).

Light Microscopy

- *Well differentiated ependymoma:* Most ependymomas are well differentiated giving epithelial appearance similar to that of normal ependymal cells and glial differentiation. Tumor is composed of *round to oval cells forming tubules* with *carrot-shaped nuclei* with abundant granular cytoplasm. A characteristic finding is the orientation of ependymal cells around vascular channels forming pseudorosettes.
- *Myxopapillary ependymoma:* A special variant, myxopapillary ependymoma may also originate from the lining of the central canal of the spinal cord and the filum terminale in lumbosacral portion region. Extensive invasion of adjacent CNS structures is uncommon. Light microscopy shows myxoid background.
- *Anaplastic variant:* Tumor is highly cellular and composed of numerous mitoses, blood vessel proliferation and necrosis with infiltrative vascularized cores lined by elongated cells forming papillary structures (Fig. 30.19).

Immunohistochemistry

Panel of markers is used to analyze expression in ependymoma on histopathological sections (Table 30.15).

Table 30.15: Immunohistochemistry of ependymoma

Panel of markers	Positivity
GFAP	+++
S-100	+++
Vimentin	++++
Luminal surface of rosettes shows positivity with epithelial membrane antigen (EMA).	

CHOROID PLEXUS PAPILLOMA

Choroid plexus papilloma is an uncommon tumor. It originates from neuroectodermal cells adjacent to embryonic lateral and fourth ventricle. It leads to increased intracranial pressure due to obstruction to CSF flow resulting in *obstructive hydrocephalus*. There is little tendency of local infiltration. *It spreads via CSF. It commonly affects children.*

Light Microscopy

- Tumor is composed of benign cuboidal to columnar cells arranged in tubules and acini.
- Tumor cells exhibiting pleomorphism, numerous mitoses, invasion and lack of papillary pattern indicate malignant behavior.

PRIMITIVE NEUROECTODERMAL TUMORS (PNETs)

These are small blue tumors of the nervous system. These include medulloblastoma, neuroblastoma arising from autonomic ganglia in the abdomen, cerebral neuroblastoma, retinoblastoma, pineoblastoma and esthesioblastoma arising from nasal mucosa.

Light Microscopy

- These primitive neuroectodermal tumors show similar morphology.
- Tumor cells possess high nucleocytoplasmic ratio. These have fibrillary processes demonstrated by silver staining technique. Nuclei are small, oval and darkly stained.
- Mitoses are common.
- Many tumors show evidence of neuronal, glial or ependymal differentiation.

Retinoblastoma

Retinoblastoma is a malignant retinal tumor of childhood. The tumor is sporadic (60%) and familial (40%). Sporadic tumors are unilateral and monocentric in origin. Familial tumors are more often bilateral and multicentric in origin. Some inherited cases also develop pinealoblastoma (so-called trilateral retinoblastoma).

Origin

It arises from the retina in children under 3 years. Around 40% of cases are inherited and the tumor may be bilateral. Remaining cases arise sporadically and are usually unilateral.

Molecular Genetics

Retinoblastoma gene (RB gene), a tumor suppressor gene situated on the short arm of chromosome 13(13q14). The normal Rb protein prevents cell mitosis. The tumor is the prototype of the *two-hit* hypothesis of Knudson. In first hit, germline deletion inherited mutation occurs in allele 1. In second hit, somatic deletion occurs in remaining normal allele. Both deletions are required for tumor development of familial or sporadic retinoblastoma. Onset of familial retinoblastoma is earlier than sporadic form. Retinoblastoma was mapped to the long arm of chromosome 13 (13p14.1–q14.2) (Figs 30.20, 30.21 and Table 30.16).

Gross Morphology

- Endophytic growth protrudes into the vitreous cavity. Exophytic tumor grows between retina and pigment epithelium.
- Tumor may exhibit endophytic as well as exophytic growth patterns (Fig. 30.22).

Light Microscopy

- Tumor is composed of small round cells with hyperchromatic nuclei and scant cytoplasm, numerous mitoses and formation of *Flexner-Wintersteiner rosettes*.
- These rosettes show central lumen lined by pink material with nuclei away from lumen (Fig. 30.23).

Immunohistochemistry

Panel of markers is used to analyze expression in retinoblastoma on histopathological sections (Table 30.17).

Mode of Spread

The tumor may fill the eye and spread locally into the brain via the optic nerve or systemically after invasion of the choroid. Distant metastases are demonstrated in cranial vault and skeletal system.

Table 30.16: Tumor suppressor genes associated with retinoblastoma (cell cycle progression inhibitors)

Gene	Protein	Function	Familial tumors	Sporadic cancers
RB gene	Retinoblastoma protein (locus 13p14) Mutation by deletion and nonsense	It codes for pRB protein, master brake on cell cycle (G1 to S) by inhibiting nuclear transcription factor	*Retinoblastoma* *Osteosarcoma*	*Retinoblastoma* Osteosarcoma Breast Colon carcinoma Prostate carcinoma Urinary bladder carcinoma Lung carcinoma

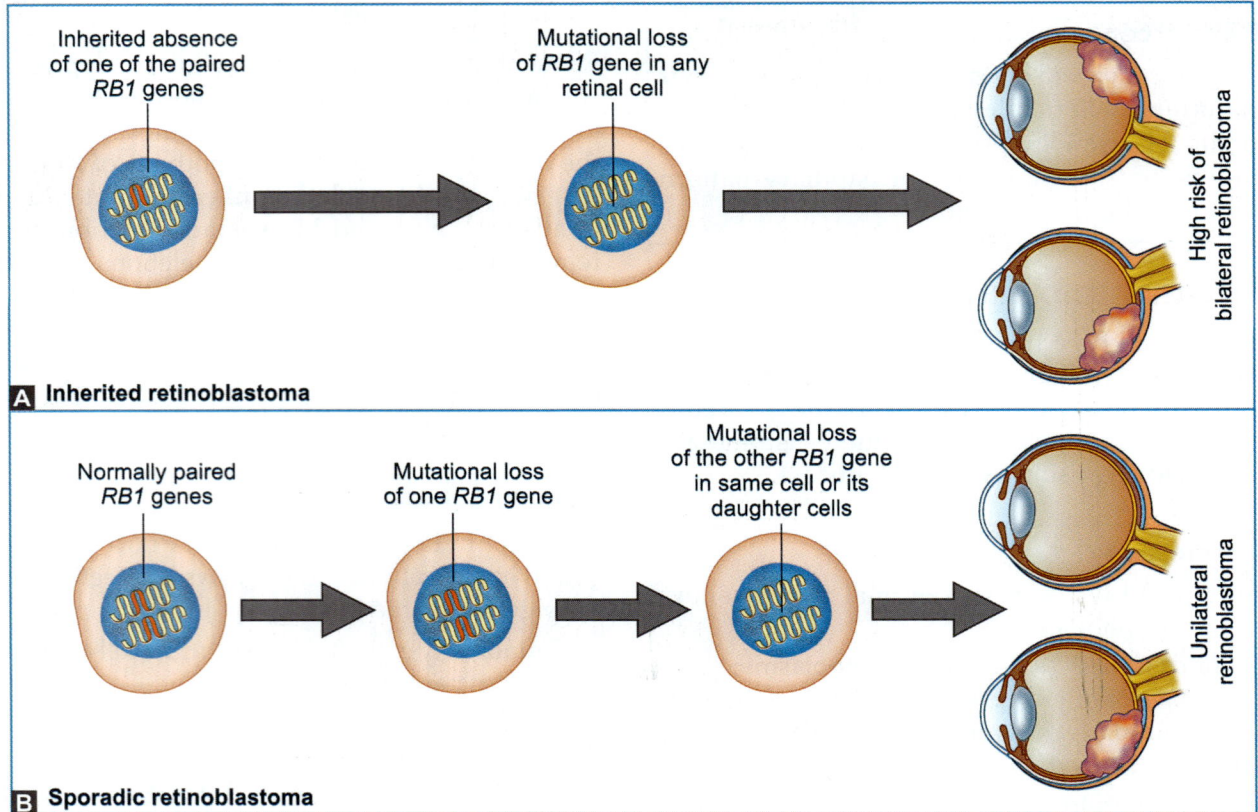

Fig. 30.20: Retinoblastoma is a tumor suppressor gene located on long arm of chromosome 13. Mutation of *RB1* gene predisposes to increased risk of development of retinoblastoma. (A) Germline mutation in one of the paired alleles of the *RB1* gene is required to develop inherited bilateral retinoblastoma, (B) normal individuals without an inherited germline mutation of the *RB1* gene have a low incidence of sporadic unilateral retinoblastoma.

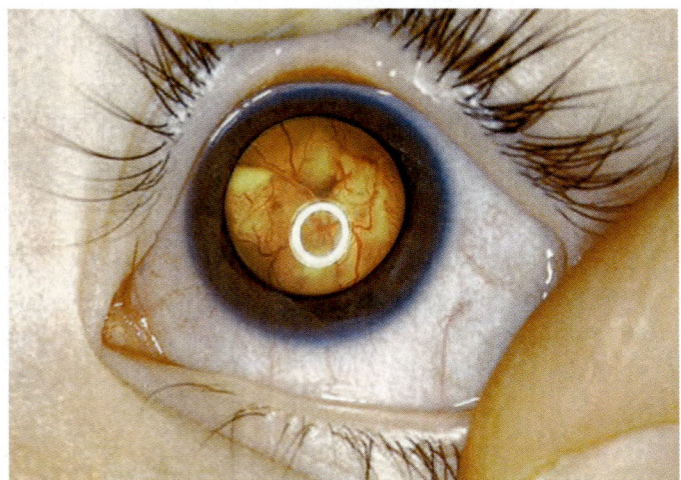

Fig. 30.21: Retinoblastoma. The mother was alerted to the condition by the white color of the pupil. There was also some loss of vision.

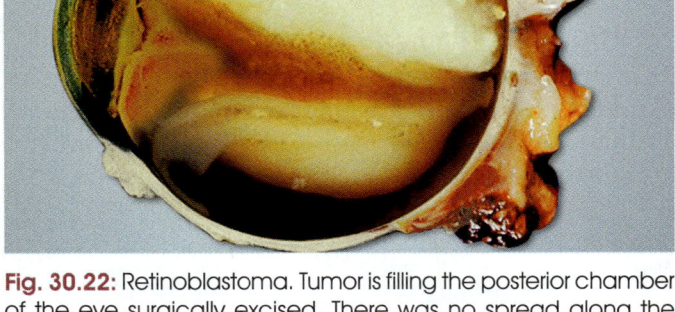

Fig. 30.22: Retinoblastoma. Tumor is filling the posterior chamber of the eye surgically excised. There was no spread along the subdural space around the optic nerve, no tumor in the other eye. There was no family history.

Treatment

Modern therapy is curative in and around 90% of cases. Some inherited cases also develop pinealoblastoma, so-called *trilateral retinoblastoma*.

Medulloblastoma

Medulloblastoma, WHO grade IV is second most common and highly malignant brain tumor of cerebellum. It most often occurs in patients between

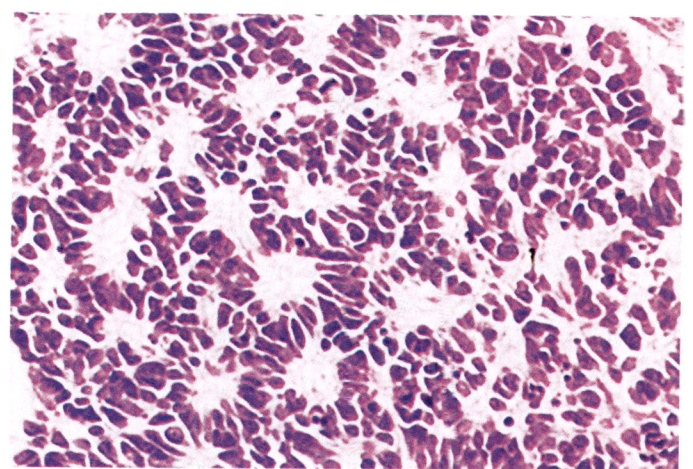

Fig. 30.23: Retinoblastoma shows small round cells with hyperchromatic nuclei and scant cytoplasm, numerous mitoses and formation of *Flexner-Wintersteiner* rosettes. These rosettes show central lumen lined by pink material with nuclei away from lumen (400X).

Table 30.17: Immunohistochemistry of retinoblastoma

Panel of markers	Positivity
GFPA	
S-100	
Neuron-specific enolase (NSE)	+++
Synaptophysin	
Myelin basic protein	

15–35 years, and majority in children <15 years old (Fig. 30.24). Mutation of tumor suppressor gene associated with medulloblastoma is shown in Table 30.18.

Origin
It originates from primitive neuroectodermal cells (fetal external granular layer) within cerebellar vermis (midline) in children; and within cerebral hemispheres in adults.

Clinical Features
Tumor originating within cerebellar vermis most often spreads down the neuraxis and *occludes the fourth ventricle resulting in hydrocephalus.*

Mode of Spread
Distant metastases, most often involving bone and lymph nodes are rare.

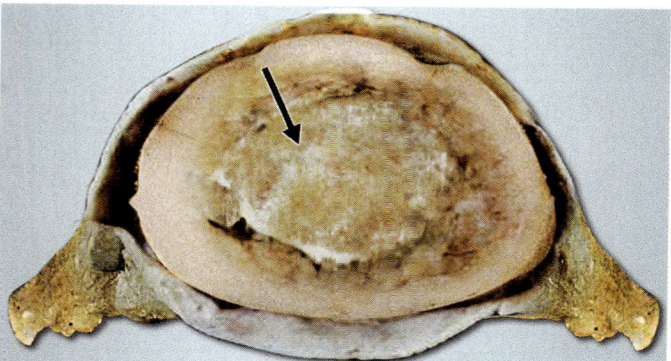

Fig. 30.24: Medulloblastoma—transverse section of spinal cord shows tumor in the subarachnoid space around the cord. This mode of spread is characteristically seen in medulloblastoma (arrow).

Molecular Genetics
Cytogenetic alterations involving **chromosome 17** are common in this tumor.

Histological Variants
These include classic and desmoplastic/nodular medulloblastomas.

Light Microscopy
- Tumor is composed of poorly differentiated small cells with round-to-oval hyperchromatic nuclei and scant cytoplasm.
- Mitotic figures are often present in abundance.
- These cells form *Homer Wright* rosettes, histological feature of neuroblasts (Fig. 30.25).

Immunohistochemistry
Panel of markers is used to differentiate from metastatic epithelial tumors, lymphomas, or other neuroectodermal malignancies (Table 30.19).

Table 30.19: Immunohistochemistry of medulloblastoma

Panel of markers	Positivity
Synaptophysin or nestin	+++
Neuron-specific enolase (NSE)	+++

Metastasis
Since medulloblastoma occurs close to the fourth ventricle, it commonly disseminates into the subarachnoid space and via CSF seeds into the spinal cord.

Table 30.18: Tumor suppressor genes associated with medulloblastoma (mitogenic signaling pathway inhibitors)

Tumor suppressor gene	Protein	Function	Familial tumors	Sporadic cancers
PTCH	Patch	Inhibits Hedgehog signaling pathway	Gorlin's syndrome (basal cell carcinoma, medulloblastoma and other benign tumors)	*Medulloblastoma* Basal cell carcinoma

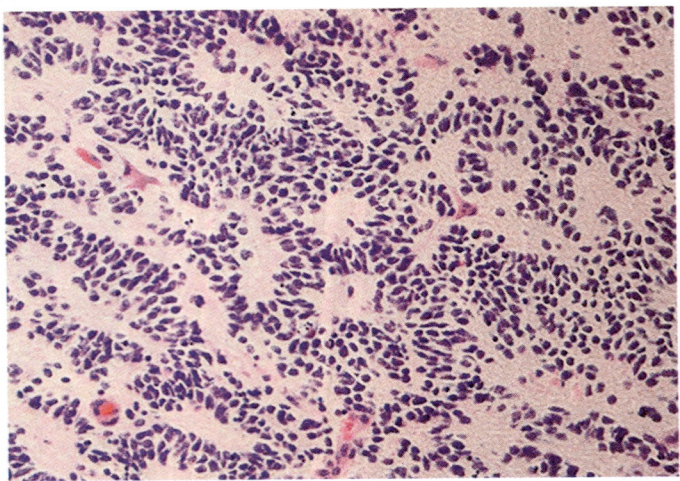

Fig. 30.25: Medulloblastoma consists of small round blue cells (400X).

Treatment

The location of the tumor often makes it difficult to excise completely. Although highly radiosensitive, yet patients have poor prognosis.

MENINGEAL TUMORS

MENINGIOMA

Meningioma is the second most common primary intracranial benign neoplasm of adults.

It most often occurs in women than men between 20 and 60 years of age with a peak incidence around 45. Spinal meningiomas are more common in females than males. It is uncommon in children. It accounts for almost 20% of all primary intracranial neoplasms.

Origin

Meningiomas bear resemblance to the arachnoidal cells that normally inhabit the inner surface of dura mater.

Location

Common locations of meningiomas include convexities of the brain near venous sinuses, parasagittal region along the falx cerebri (most common site), along skull base, or tentorium, olfactory nerve sheath in the groove beneath the frontal lobe, lesser wing of sphenoid wing, sella turcica, foramen magnum and within the spinal cord in thoracic segment. Occasionally, these tumors may arise in the ventricular system.

Histological Variants and Grades

Meningiomas are classified based on grade according to WHO classification. Grade I has benign course. Grades II and III grow rapidly with great propensity to recur following resection. FISH for common genetic changes may also be helpful for grading diagnosis. Histological variants and grading are shown in Table 30.20.

- *Meningiomas grade I:* Examples are meningoepithelial, fibroblastic, transitional and psammomatous meningiomas. These are slow growing benign tumors. Enlargement of tumor growth leads to clinical manifestations like headache, seizures, or focal neurological deficits by compressing adjacent structures. Median survival varies between 5 and 20 years.
- *Meningiomas grade II:* Examples are metaplastic, chondroid, clear cell and atypical meningioma. These rapidly growing tumors recur following excision. Median survival is 5 years.
- *Meningiomas grade III:* Examples are papillary, rhabdoid and anaplastic. These rapidly growing tumors recur following excision. Median survival is <2 years (Table 30.21).

Molecular Genetics

Meningioma is associated with neurofibromatosis type 2 due to mutation of NF2 gene located on long arm of chromosome 22 in person with previous history of irradiation. It is considered to be important for tumor development. Loss of the CDKN2A/p16 region on 9p/21 in anaplastic meningiomas is associated

Table 30.20: Histological variants and grades of meningeal tumors

Histological variants	Grade I	Grade II	Grade III	Grade IV
Meningoepithelial meningioma	*			
Fibroblastic meningioma	*			
Transitional meningioma	*			
Psammomatous meningioma	*			
Metaplastic meningioma		*		
Atypical meningioma (chondroid meningioma and clear cell meningioma)		*		
Anaplastic meningioma (papillary meningioma and rhabdoid meningioma)			*	

Table 30.21: Features of meningiomas

Parameters	Grade I	Grade II	Grade III
Survival rate	5–20 years	5 years	<2 years
Molecular genetics	NF2 (locus 22q) gene mutation		Loss of the CDKN2A/p16 region on 9p/21
Mitotic figures	Nil	4 or more mitoses per 10 high power fields	20 or more mitotic figures per 10 or 40 high power fields

Table 30.22: Tumor suppressor genes associated with meningiomas (mitogenic signaling pathway inhibitors)

Gene	Protein	Function	Familial tumors	Sporadic cancers
NF-2	Merlin (locus 22q) Mutation by deletion or nonsense mutation	NF-2 stabilizes cytoskeleton membrane linkage	Neurofibromatosis type 2 (acoustic schwannoma and meningioma)	Meningiomas Schwannomas

decreased survival. Lack of genetic 9p/21 alteration in meningiomas is associated with long survival (Table 30.22).

Clinical Features

Meningioma is *slow growing*, well circumscribed, and often *highly vascular tumors*. It usually is benign. Complete removal is possible if the tumor does not involve vital structures especially present external to the brain.

Imaging Technique

These often infiltrate overlying bone and cause increased bone density (hyperostosis) seen on X-ray.

Gross Morphology
- The tumors are popcorn shaped, firm, well circumscribed lobulated masses adherent to dura. These invade dura or dural sinuses.
- These may indent the surface of the brain without invading; which is common cause of new onset focal seizures (Fig. 30.26).

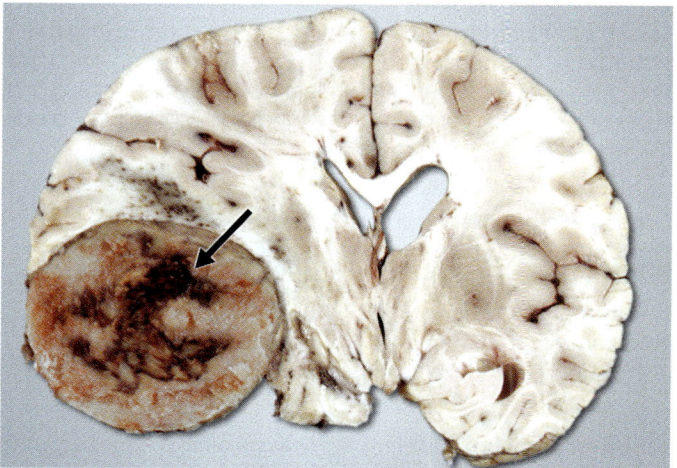

Fig. 30.26: Meningioma. Tumor arises from the dura is well encapsulated. It is cured by surgical excision (arrow).

Light Microscopy

Histological patterns: There are three grades of meningiomas. Grade I includes meningothelial, fibrous and transitional meningiomas.

- *Meningoepithelial (syncytial) meningioma:* Tumor consists of swirling solid masses of polygonal cells with poorly defined cell borders giving syncytial whorled appearance. These cells have round to oval centrally located nuclei with finely granular cytoplasm. Some amount of collagen stroma divides the tumor into irregular lobules.
- *Fibrous (fibroblastic) meningioma:* It is less frequent variant spindle shape cell fibroblastic meningioma. Tumor cells are arranged in parallel or interlacing bundles. Whorled pattern and psammoma bodies are less frequent.
- *Transitional (mixed) meningioma:* It shows features of both meningoepithelial and fibroblastic elements arranged in whorled pattern. Some of whorls contain psammoma bodies due to dystrophic calcification. There may be presence of xanthomatous and myxomatous degeneration. These express estrogen receptors. Meningoepithelial or transitional meningiomas should be differentiated from metastatic carcinoma and fibroblastic meningioma from schwannoma.
- *Meningiomas grade II (atypical meningiomas):* These tumors have a higher mitotic index (4 or more mitoses per 10 high power fields), increased cellularity, increased nucleocytoplasmic ratio, prominent nucleoli. Immunohistochemistry reveals increased Ki-67. These are associated with local invasion and increased risk of recurrence after resection.
- *Meningiomas grade III (anaplastic meningioma):* These tumors must exhibit increased mitoses (20 or more mitotic figures per 10 or 40 high power fields) (Fig. 30.27).

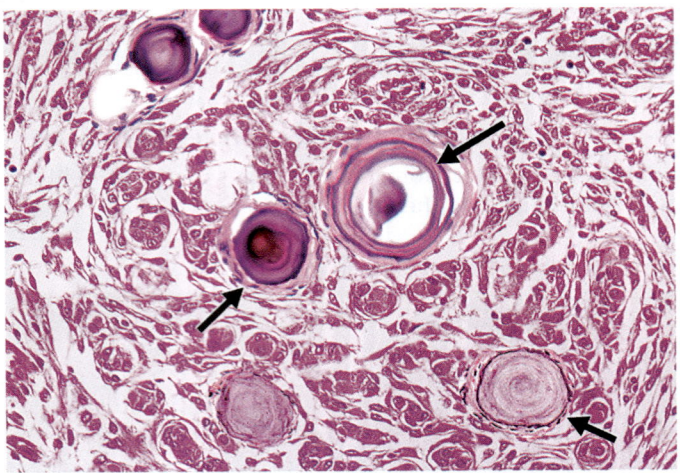

Fig. 30.27: Meningioma. Tumor consists of swirling masses of fusiform meningoepithelial cells with oval nuclei containing dispersed chromatin in a composite solid and whorled pattern. Small foci of calcification (psammoma bodies–calcified bodies) are common (arrows).

Locations

Schwannomas are most often intracranial in cerebellopontine angle with involvement of the vestibulocochlear cranial nerve (acoustic neuroma). Expansion of the tumor results in tinnitus (most common) and sensorineural deafness. These also originate frequently in posterior nerve roots and peripheral nerves.

Light Microscopy

Tumor is composed of compact whorls and fascicles of collagen, and nuclei are arranged in palisading fashion surrounding pink areas known as *Verocay bodies* (Antoni type A), interspersed with less cellular loosely structured myxomatous appearing areas designated Antoni type B areas (the pattern resembles the stripes of a zebra) (Fig. 30.28).

Immunohistochemistry

Schwannomas show diffuse and strong **S-100** *positivity*.

Immunohistochemistry

- Most meningiomas show weak positivity for epithelial membrane antigen and progesterone receptors.
- Immunoreactivity for progesterone receptor is less in grades II and III meningiomas.
- **S-100** immunoreactivity is patchy rather than diffuse in meningiomas.
- Atypical meningiomas exhibit increased **Ki-67** (MIB-1 antibody).

TUMORS OF THE CRANIAL AND PARASPINAL NERVES

SCHWANNOMA (NEURILEMMOMA)

Schwannoma (neurilemmoma) is a slowly growing benign encapsulated tumor. It originates from Schwann cell intimately surrounding axons located on cranial nerves, spinal nerve roots or peripheral nerves.

Pathogenesis

Mutations of NF-1 and NF-2 are associated with schwannoma (Table 30.23).

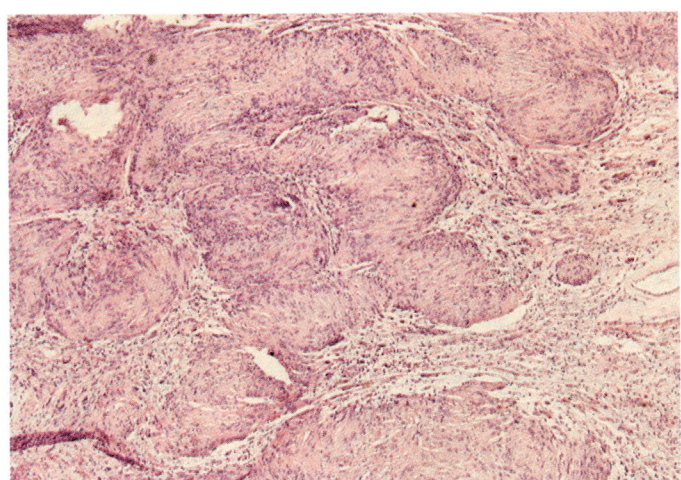

Fig. 30.28: Neurilemmoma. Tumor is composed of cells with palisading nuclei arranged in compact whorls and fascicles (Antoni type A), interspersed with less cellular loosely structured myxomatous appearing areas designated Antoni type B areas (100X).

Table 30.23: Tumor suppressor genes associated with schwannoma (mitogenic signaling pathway inhibitors)

Gene	Protein	Function	Familial tumors	Sporadic cancers
NF-1	Neurofibronin-1 (locus 13p11) Mutation occurs by deletion	NF-1 inhibits RAS/MAP-kinase signaling activator pathway	Neurofibromatosis type 1 (neurofibroma and malignant peripheral nerve tumors)	*Schwannoma* Juvenile myeloid leukemia Neuroblastoma
NF-2	Merlin (locus 22q) Mutation by deletion or nonsense mutation	NF-2 stabilizes cytoskeleton membrane linkage	Neurofibromatosis type 2 (acoustic schwannoma and meningioma)	*Schwannomas* Meningiomas

HEMANGIOBLASTOMA

Hemangioblastoma, WHO grade I tumor occurs most frequently in the *cerebellum, brainstem* and *spinal cord*. It has cellular and reticular variant. It sometimes produces erythropoietin, resulting in secondary polycythemia.

It is a slow growing highly vascular tumor favoring cerebellum in adults.

Molecular Genetics

Tumor shows mutations of von Hippel-Lindau disease (vHL) gene at 3p25–26. Mutation of vHL gene is associated with similar lesions in the retina, pheochromocytoma and renal cell carcinoma (clear cell variant) as part of von Hippel-Lindau disease.

Gross Morphology
- Classic hemangioblastoma is well circumscribed cystic mass with a mural nodule.
- Cyst contains hemorrhagic fluid.

Light Microscopy
- Tumor is composed of thin-walled vascular channels surrounded by large polygonal tumor cells with pale cytoplasm.
- There may be foci of hematopoietic tissue and mast cell infiltration (Fig. 30.29).

Immunohistochemistry

Panel of markers is employed on sections to highlight endothelial cells (Table 30.24).

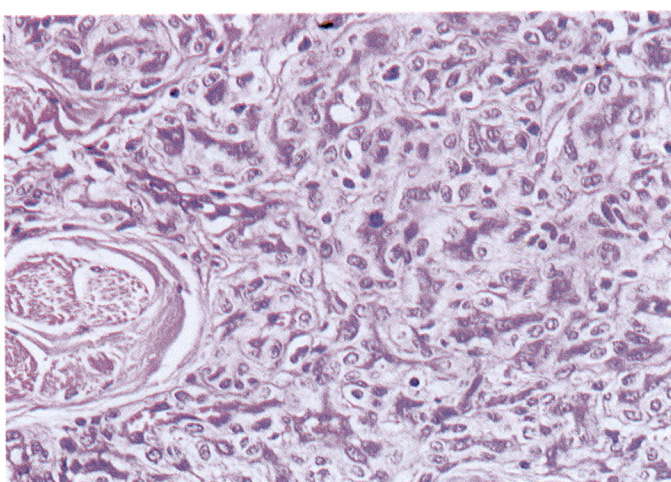

Fig. 30.29: Hemangioblastoma. Tumor is composed of thin walled vascular channels surrounded by large polygonal tumor cells with pale cytoplasm (400X).

Table 30.24: Immunohistochemistry of hemangioblastoma

Panel of markers	Positivity
CD31	+ in endothelial cells
CD34	
CD56	
S-100	+++ in tumor cells
Vimentin	
Nonspecific enolase (NSE)	
Inhibin-α	

CNS GERM CELL TUMORS

Germ cell tumors include germinoma, teratoma, yolk sac tumor, embryonal tumor and choriocarcinoma. These occur in children or young adults.

Clinical Features

Patient with germ cell tumor located in pineal region presents with increased intracranial pressure. Tumor located in suprasellar region is associated with diabetes insipidus and hypopituitarism. Less common sites are basal ganglia and thalamus.

MRI Imaging Technique

Germ cell tumors exhibit heterogenous enhancement. Calcification is seen in teratomas. Hemorrhage is strongly suggestive of choriocarcinoma.

Light Microscopy
Histologically, these tumors are homologous to their gonadal and mediastinal counterparts.

Immunohistochemistry
- *C-Kit immunostaining:* It shows membranous pattern.
- *OCT4 immunostaining:* It shows nuclear pattern.
- *PLAP immunostaining:* Placental alkaline phosphatase immunostaining is seen in cytoplasm and membrane.

Prognosis

Pure germinomas are radiosensitive tumors with excellent prognosis. *Germinoma with syncyriotrophoblastic element has tendency to recur with less favorable prognosis.* Mature teratomas are treated by surgical resection. Yolk sac tumor, embryonal carcinoma and choriocarcinoma have less favorable prognosis

PRIMARY CNS LYMPHOMA

Lymphomas may arise as a primary B cell neoplasm in the brain parenchyma in a manner analogous to its occurrence in the stomach, small bowel, or testis. Non-Hodgkin's lymphomas in CNS are more often primary than metastatic. Metastatic NHL most often spreads to the meninges (epidural, dural or leptomeninges) by sparing brain parenchyma. Death occurs within 2–3 years.

Origin

Primary CNS lymphomas arise in white mater of cerebral hemispheres, commonly in bilateral periventricular positions. It is most often multifocal in distribution involving brain parenchyma especially common in immunocompromised people and associated with the Epstein-Barr virus.

Pathogenesis

EB virus (DNA) plays role in the pathogenesis of primary CNS lymphomas especially in acquired immune deficiency syndrome (Table 30.25).

Table 30.25: Oncogenic DNA virus associated with CNS tumors (viruses)

Pathogens	Associated tumors
EB virus (DNA)	CNS lymphoma in AIDS
	Nasopharyngeal carcinoma
	Hodgkin's disease (mixed cellularity)
	Burkitt's lymphoma
	Extranodal marginal zone B cell NHL

Clinical Features

Most are malignant, and recurrence is common despite treatment. Patient most often presents with behavioral and cognitive changes. Hemiparesis, aphasia, and visual field deficits occur in about 4% of people and seizures occur in 14% of people.

Gross Morphology

Tumor is frequently located in periventricular in location. It appears as nodule or diffuse lesion.

Light Microscopy

- Most primary CNS lymphomas are considered diffuse large B cell lymphomas.
- The neoplastic cells most often have centroblasts like or immunoblasts like morphology.
- Tumor cells are arranged around blood vessels giving angiocentric growth pattern.

Immunohistochemistry

Tumor cells are immunoreactive to **CD20** and **CD79a**.

NEURONAL TUMORS

GANGLIONEUROMA

In some cases, neuronal differentiation proceeds, and mature ganglion cells appear and nerve fibers are formed. In some instances, differentiation is complete; such tumors are found in adult life particularly in the mediastinum where they may grow slowly, eventually causing signs due to their size, but never metastasizing. With intermediate degrees of differentiation the name ganglioneuroblastoma is used.

MULTIPLE NEUROMAS

NEUROFIBROMATOSIS TYPE 1

Neurofibromatosis type 1 is an autosomal dominant disorder caused by mutation in NF-1 gene on chromosome 17. *Plexiform neurofibroma involves multiple nerves.* In few patients, neurofibroma may undergo malignant transformation.

Molecular Genetics

NF-1 tumor suppressor gene is located on chromosome 13p11 on chromosome 17. It codes for protein that inhibits a stimulatory GTPase (RAS) protein. Mutation of NF-1 (deletion) has been demonstrated in sporadic schwannomas (*Ref.* Table 30.25).

Clinical Features

Patient may develop von Recklinghausen neurofibromatosis type 1 characterized by multiple benign neurofibromas, café au lait spots, and iris hamartomas. There is an increased risk of developing fibrosarcomas. Café au lait spots are flat, pigmented melanocytes of the skin. These spots are typically permanent, and may grow or increase in number over time.

NEUROFIBROMATOSIS TYPE 2

NF-2 tumor suppressor gene is located on chromosome 22q. It codes for cytoskeleton membrane linkage. Mutation of NF-2 (deletion and nonsense) has been associated with schwannomas and meningiomas. It is inactivated in persons who have bilateral acoustic neuroma.

Clinical Features

Patient presents with bilateral tumors of the eighth cranial nerve (acoustic neuromas), meningiomas and gliomas. Some schwannomas exhibit deletions or mutations of the NF-2 gene. It is worth mentioning that neurofibromatosis type 1 exhibits neurofibromas but not acoustic neuromas.

REACTION OF CNS TO INJURY

Neurons are most vulnerable cells of the central nervous system. Reactive gliosis is a normal response of the brain to injury and infection but is not visible on the cut surface of the brain at autopsy.

CNS Cells Vulnerable to Hypoxia

The various cells of CNS are not equally sensitive to hypoxia and deficiency of nutrients. Hypoxia affects hippocampus neurons, cerebellar Purkinje cells, pyramidal neurons, and neurons within layers of III and V of neocortex (laminar necrosis).

> **Light Microscopy**
> Affected neurons have pyknotic nuclei and an acidophilic cytoplasm, which stains intensely red with eosin (red is dead) in standard hematoxylin and eosin slides. CO intoxication affects bilateral necrosis of certain neuronal clusters within globus pallidus.

CEREBROVASCULAR DISEASES

Cerebrovascular diseases are the most common group of CNS disorders. It ranks after heart disease and cancer as the third major cause of death in the United States.

CEREBRAL INFARCTION

Cerebral infarction is more frequent than cerebral hemorrhage. Morphological changes in brain depends on duration of deprivation of blood supply. Clinical features depend on the site of vascular obstruction and extent of collateral circulation. Arterial obstruction in this site causes contralateral paralysis, as well as motor and sensory defects and aphasias.

Etiology

Arterial occlusion occurs either due to complicated atheromatous plaques in blood vessels supplying brain (bifurcation of carotid arteries), or emboli arising from cardiac mural thrombi, vegetations of infected endocarditic valves, clumps of tumor cells, bubbles of air, or droplets of fat into middle cerebral artery. Embolism is much less common than thrombosis. Risk factors for cerebral infarction are shown in Table 30.26.

Internal Carotid Artery Occlusion

Thromboembolism is the most important cause of occlusion of internal carotid artery in 80% of patients. Cerebral ischemia occurs when lumen is reduced by 80–90%. Five patterns of ischemic brain damage may be seen as a result of severe stenosis or occlusion of internal carotid artery.

Common sites of aneurysms formation in intracranial arteries are shown in Fig. 30.30 and Table 30.27.

- *Massive cerebral infarction:* It occurs due to involvement of whole territory of middle cerebral artery.
- *Cortex infarction:* It occurs round the sylvian fissure, with or without involvement of internal capsule and basal ganglia.
- *Internal capsule infarction:* Infarction may be restricted to internal capsule.
- *Small infarction within white mater:* It occurs due to involvement of middle cerebral artery supplying white mater.
- *Infarcts in watershed areas:* Infarction occurs in the boundary zone between the territories supplied by middle cerebral and anterior cerebral arteries. Watershed areas of the arterial territory are most remote from the patent arterial stems and thus most vulnerable to the effects of cerebral under perfusion.

Basilar Artery Occlusion

It leads to flaccid quadriplegia, coma and bulbar palsy.

Middle Cerebral Artery Occlusion

This blood vessel is the commonest site of intracranial occlusion. It occurs due to thromboembolic phenomenon in 66% of patients. Occlusion of middle cerebral artery causes contralateral hemiparesis, contralateral cortical type of sensory loss and ipsilateral facial weakness. Patient may develop aphasia and visual defect (hemianopia).

Anterior Cerebral Artery Occlusion

Occlusion in anterior cerebral artery causes contralateral lower extremity weakness and altered mental status.

Posterior Cerebral Artery Occlusion

Occlusion in posterior cerebral artery causes contralateral visual loss.

Table 30.26: Risk factors for cerebral stroke

Risk factors	Comments
Modifiable risk factors	
Hyperlipidemia	*Acquired hyperlipidemia:* High lipid diet and nephrotic syndrome increases risk of atherosclerosis
Hypertension	Persistent high blood pressure causing endothelial dysfunction
Diabetes mellitus	*Diagnostic criteria:* Fating blood sugar >126 mg/dl or random blood sugar >200 mg/dl. Advanced glycosylated end products formed participate in pathogenesis of atheromatous plaque
Tobacco smoking	Tobacco smoking causes endothelial dysfunction, deranged lipids (increased LDL and decreased HDL), platelets activation synthesizing ADP and TxA2, platelets adhesion and arterial wall hypoxia due to accumulation of carbon monoxide in the blood
Sedentary lifestyle	Regular moderate exercise reduces the risk of atherosclerosis by increasing HDL
Minor risk factors	Type 'A' personality with stress factors in lifestyle Increased homocysteine level (>100 μm/L) Hyperuricemia Increased serum ferritin level Methylene tetrahydrofolate reductase mutation Lipoprotein 'a' mutation Hormonal replacement therapy in postmenopausal women Infectious agents demonstrated in atheromatous plaque (*Chlamydia pneumoniae*, herpesvirus and cytomegalovirus)
Non-modifiable risk factors	
Genetic factors	Familial hyperlipidemia: Defective LDL receptor inhibits cholesterol uptake by the liver
Familial predisposition	A family history of premature coronary artery disease is a major risk factor
Racial factors	Blacks have less severe atherosclerosis than Whites
Gender	Women >45 and men >55 years

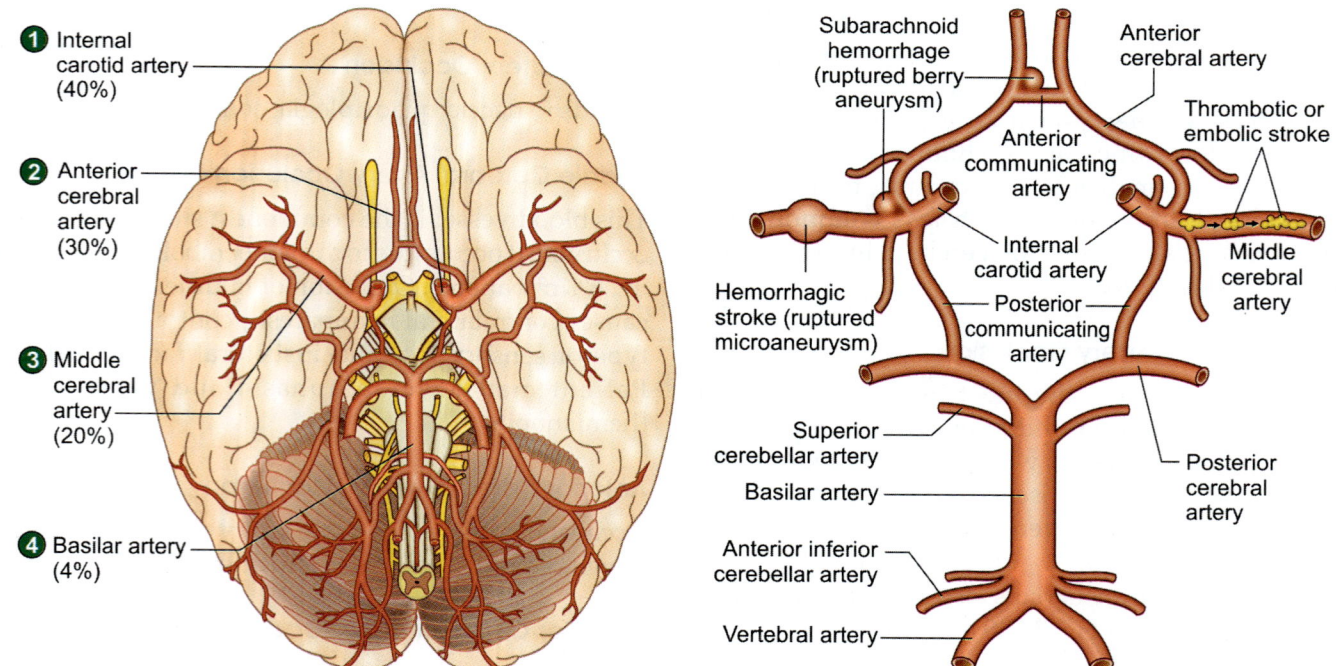

Fig. 30.30: Cerebrovascular diseases. Common sites of aneurysms formation in intracranial arteries.

Nervous System

Table 30.27: Cerebrovascular diseases

Type	Predisposing factors	Common sites
Cerebral infarction		
Thrombus formation	Atherosclerosis	Arterial obstruction of internal and external carotid arteries at the origin in the neck, vertebral arteries, basilar arteries, middle cerebral arteries of circle of Willis
Embolism	Cardiac mural thrombi, valvular vegetation and fat emboli	Middle cerebral is the most frequent site of embolic occlusion
Cerebral hemorrhage		
Intracerebral hemorrhage	Hypertension, coagulation disorders, hemorrhage within a malignant tumor	It may result from rupture of Charcot-Bouchard aneurysms in a long-standing case of hypertension
Subarachnoid hemorrhage	Rupture of congenital berry aneurysm especially in hypertension	Circle of Willis and bifurcation of the middle cerebral artery

Small Cerebral Arteries Occlusion

Obstruction of small cerebral arteries produces lacunar strokes involving motor or sensory areas. Pure motor lacunar stroke most often results from lesions affecting the internal capsule. Pure sensory lacunar stroke most often results from lesions affecting the thalamus.

Light Microscopy

- Brain does not contain proteins; hence ischemia produces liquefactive necrosis and formation of cystic spaces containing creamy liquid necrotic cell debris by hydrolytic enzymes by phagocytes.
- The cyst wall is formed by proliferating capillaries, neutrophils, macrophages and gliosis (proliferating neuroglial cells) (Fig. 30.31).

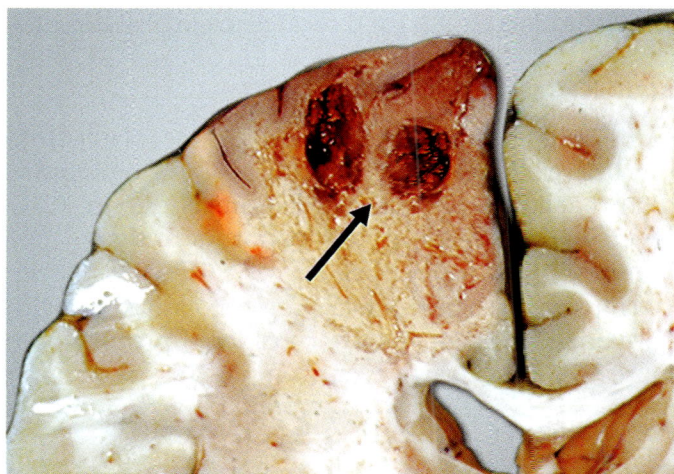

Fig. 30.31: Cerebral infarct. This intermediate infarct of the frontal lobe shows liquefactive necrosis with formation of cystic spaces as resolution begins (arrow).

CEREBRAL HEMORRHAGE

Cerebral hemorrhage consists of hemorrhage into the tissue of cerebral hemispheres. It is most often complicated by long-standing hypertension, coagulation disorders, hemorrhage within brain tumors and Charcot-Bouchard aneurysms. Hemorrhage most often occurs in the basal ganglia/thalamus; other favored sites include the pons, cerebellum, and frontal lobe white mater. Primary cerebral hemorrhage occurs in the region of lentiform nucleus, pons or white mater of the cerebellum.

SUBARACHNOID HEMORRHAGE

Spontaneous subarachnoid hemorrhage accounts for 6% of cerebrovascular disease, with a peak age of 5–60 years. It is commonly associated with rupture of a *congenital berry aneurysm in the circle of Willis* compounded by hypertension. Other causes are mycotic aneurysms, arteriovenous malformations and cavernous hemangiomas. Features and causes of subarachnoid hemorrhage are shown in Tables 30.28 and 30.29.

Table 30.28: Causes of subarachnoid hemorrhage

Etiology	Frequency
Saccular aneurysm rupture in one of the major cerebral arteries	65%
Arteriovenous malformation bleed	5%
Blood dyscrasia	2.5%
Extension of intracerebral bleed into sub-arachnoid space	2.5%
Mycotic aneurysm rupture	Rare
Unknown etiology	25%

Table 30.29: Manifestations of subarachnoid hemorrhage

Features	Frequency
Mortality in first week	30%
Risk of recurrent bleeding in first week	10%
Risk of recurrent bleeding each year	5%
Peak age	55–60 years

Berry Aneurysm

Berry aneurysm is rounded sac like structure involving only part of the circumference of a blood vessel. It throbs and pushes against surrounding structures. Mural thrombus is most often found within aneurysmal sac.

- *Sites:* The most common site of berry aneurysm formation is between the anterior communicating and the anterior cerebral arteries in the circle of Willis. Sites of rupture of berry aneurysm are shown in Table 30.30.
- *Shape:* These develop as saccular lesions (1.0–1.5) at site of congenital defects in smooth muscle distribution at a branch point of the arterial wall.
- *Risk factors:* These include hemodynamic stress, hypertension and coarctation of aorta, autosomal dominant adult polycystic kidney disease, Marfan's syndrome and type 1 neurofibromatosis.
- *Clinical features:* Rupture of berry aneurysm is the most common cause of subarachnoid hemorrhage. Patient presents with history of severe headache, nuchal rigidity from irritation of the meninges. Aneurysms present on the anterior communicating artery may rupture into the third ventricle leading to massive intraventricular hemorrhage. Cerebral infarction is the most common complication. Patient may develop hydrocephalus as result of blockage by blood clot of the channels through which cerebrospinal fluid flows.

Table 30.30: Sites for rupture of berry aneurysm

Site	Frequency
Junction of the internal carotid and the posterior communicating artery	40%
Junction of the anterior cerebral and anterior communicating artery	30%
Main bifurcation of the middle cerebral artery in the sylvian fissure	20%
Point where the basilar artery divides into the posterior cerebral artery	4%

Mycotic Aneurysm

It is caused by infection of the artery wall. Most cases develop mycotic aneurysm due to impaction of infected emboli derived from vegetation occurring within first 5 weeks of development of infective endocarditis in 3–10% of patients.

- *Etiology:* Causative organisms of infective endocarditis include pyogenic bacteria, such as *Streptococcus pyogenes* and *Staphylococcus aureus*. True fungal aneurysms result from fungal meningitis or fungal emboli from cardiac valves. Aspergillus is the species most commonly involved.
- *Clinical features:* Emboli from infective endocarditis may involve cerebral blood vessels which results in hemorrhage in the basal ganglia, extending into the subarachnoid space.

Arteriovenous Fistulas

Arteriovenous (AV) fistulas are abnormal communications (direct shunt) between arteries and veins. Arteriography with thorostat dye establishes the diagnosis.

- *Etiology:* These are often secondary to trauma. Penetrating knife injury is the most common cause of arteriovenous fistula. Most common sites are scalp, arm and leg vessels. Veins are arterialized.
- *Clinical features:* Patient develops increased circumference of the limbs. There is presence of bruits and thrills.

Large AV fistulas reduce systemic resistance and bypass the microcirculation, hence increasing venous return to the heart and producing high output cardiac failure.

Cavernous Hemangiomas

These are located in the white mater of the brain. Patient presents in the 3rd to 5th decades with neurological symptoms such as epilepsy (38%), intracranial bleeding (23%), headache (28%) and focal neurological deficits.

TRANSIENT ISCHEMIC ATTACKS (TIA)

Transient ischemic attacks are brief episodes of impaired focal neurological function caused by a temporary disturbance of cerebral circulation. These are fully reversible and most often last not more than a few minutes.

Transient ischemic attacks are not associated with permanent damage, but are considered precursors to more serious occlusive events.

Pathogenesis

Transient ischemic attacks occur due to breaking of small proportion of mural thrombus from underlying atheromatous plaque. Other causes are sudden decline in cardiac output and hypercoagulable states.

FAT EMBOLISM

Fat embolism is presence of emboli comprising of fat microglobules in the circulation (Fig 30.32).

Etiology

Fat embolism syndrome is most often a consequence of severe trauma with long bone fractures such as femur with abundant fatty marrow. It can also be seen with extensive trauma to fat laden tissues, burns, and very rarely with orthopedic procedures.

Pathogenesis

On fracture, bone marrow fatty fragments enter the circulation, lodge in small blood vessels of the lung, skin, kidneys, brain and other organs producing ischemia and hemorrhage. It results in the clinical manifestations. Fat microglobules are converted into fatty acids, which damage vascular endothelium resulting in formation of platelet thrombi in areas of injury.

Clinical Features

Patient develops potentially fatal fat embolism syndrome within 24 to 72 hours. It is characterized by pulmonary distress, cutaneous petechial hemorrhages, and various neurologic manifestations.

- *Pulmonary manifestations:* Patient develops dyspnea and tachypnea due to presence of fat microglobules in pulmonary capillaries causing hypoxemia.
- *Petechial hemorrhage:* Patient develops petechial hemorrhage over the chest and upper extremities due to thrombocytopenia from platelet adhesion to microglobules of fat.
- *Neurological manifestations:* Numerous petechial hemorrhages are produced by fat emboli to the brain, particularly in white mater known as *brain purpura*.

  Patient develops neurological manifestations such as loss of consciousness, cerebral edema and herniation within a week in less than 10% of cases with fatal outcome (*ref* to Fig. 30.32).

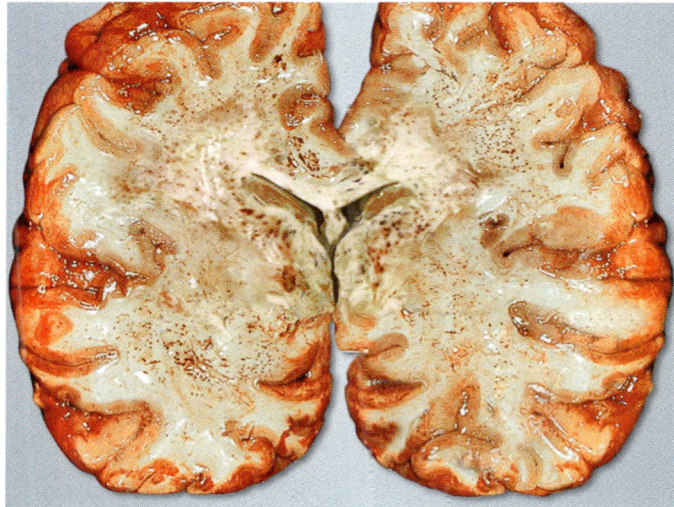

Fig. 30.32: Fat embolus. The patient was in a motorcycle accident and sustained multiple fractures of both legs. The fat emboli caused petechial hemorrhages in the white mater throughout the brain, resulting in coma and death. The macroscopic appearance of cerebral malaria is identical to this.

HEAD INJURIES

Head injuries are caused by penetrating wounds and nonpenetrating injuries. Penetrating wounds cause brain damage predisposing to infection of brain (meningitis, cerebral abscess). Brain injury caused by penetrating injuries producing impact at the site of injury is known as coup injury.

Injury on the opposite side of the brain from the impact is known as *countercoup injury*. Contusions comprise both coup and countercoup injuries. Depending on the anatomic position of the ruptured vessel, bleeding can occur in any of several compartments, including the epidural, subdural, intracerebral, and subarachnoid spaces (Fig. 30.33).

EPIDURAL HEMATOMA

An epidural hematoma is an arterial hemorrhage between the dura and the skull. It results from skull fracture and laceration of the middle meningeal artery. Because bleeding is arterial in origin, rapid expansion of the hematoma compresses the brain.

Clinical Features

Patient presents with short period of consciousness (lucid interval), followed by loss of consciousness and signs of cerebral compression.

SUBDURAL HEMATOMA

A subdural hematoma is venous hemorrhage underneath the dura. Bleeding most often results from laceration of the bridging veins joining the cerebrum to venous sinuses within the dura. Patient presents with gradual signs of cerebral compression occurring hours, days, or weeks after injury.

After cessation of bleeding, the resultant clot can slowly imbibe water, resulting in signs of increasing intracranial pressure (Figs 30.34 and 30.35).

Section III: Systemic Pathology

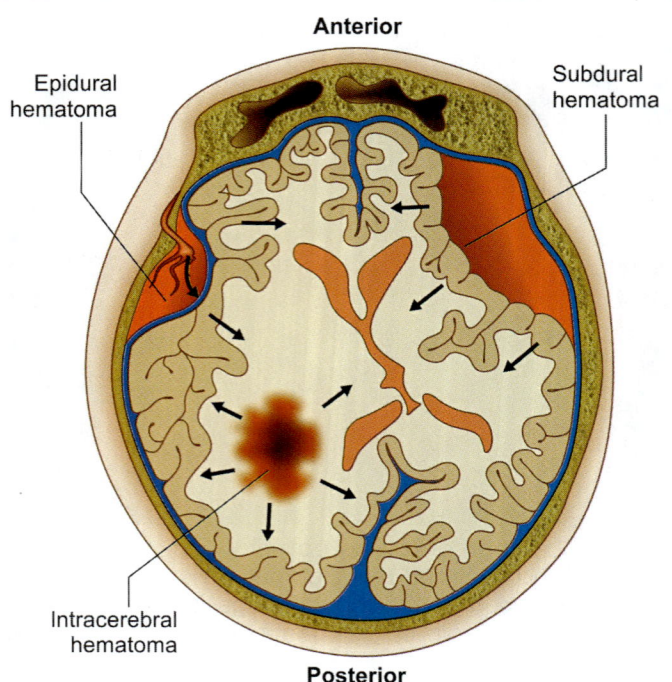

Fig. 30.33: Location of epidural, subdural and intracerebral hematomas.

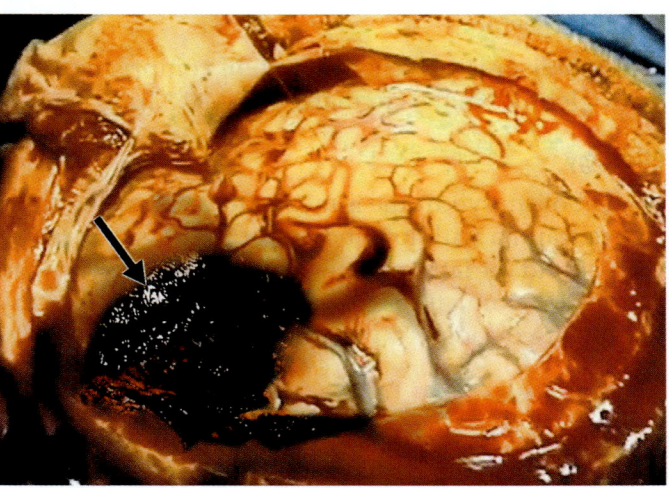

Fig. 30.34: Epidural hematoma. A blood clot is seen over the external surface of the dura. It occurs as a result of trauma to middle meningeal artery (arrow).

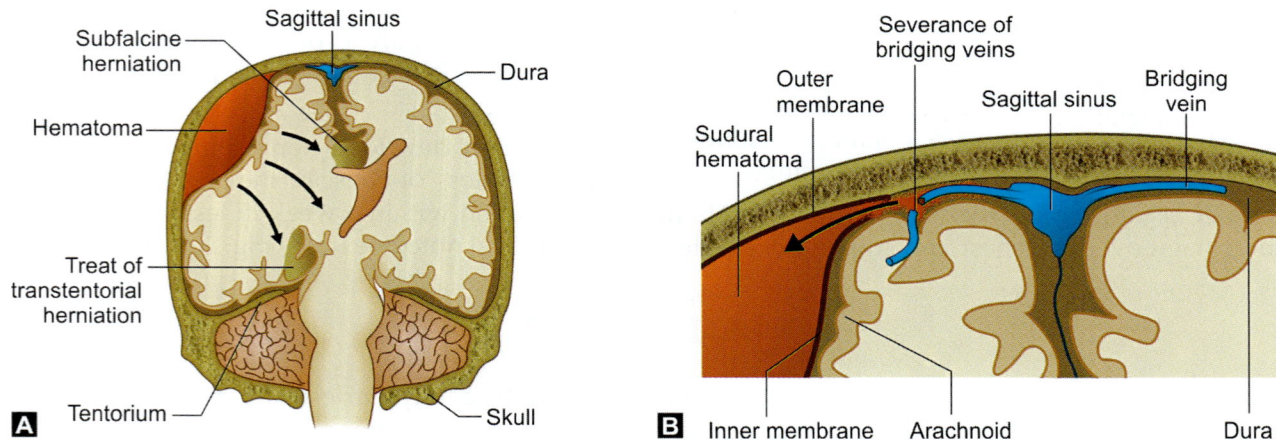

Fig. 30.35: Mechanism of bleeding in subdural hematoma.

DEMYELINATING DISORDERS

MULTIPLE SCLEROSIS

Multiple sclerosis is the most common demyelinating disease of unknown etiology. It is characterized by destruction of myelin sheaths in the spinal cord and brain with relative preservation of axons.

Etiology

It is considered to be autoimmune disorder (probable viral etiology) due to increased incidence in HLA haplotypes (A3, B7, DR2, and DW2).

Pathology

The disease is associated with plaques scattered irregularly throughout the central nervous system. Common sites are the optic nerve, brainstem, and paraventricular areas. Helper CD4+ and cytotoxic CD8+ T cells and macrophages infiltrate plaques; reactive gliosis occurs later. Peripheral nerves are not affected.

Age and Sex Predilection

It begins between 20 and 30 years of age. It most often affects men than women.

Clinical Features

Clinical course is highly variable depending on the site of involvement. Patient may present with numbness, weakness of the lower extremities, visual disturbances and retrobulbar pain, sensory disturbances, and possible loss of bladder control.

The classic Charcot triad (nystagmus, intention tremor, and scanning speech), which is significant for diagnosis, may occur.

CSF Findings

The classic CSF electrophoretic finding is that of multiple oligoclonal bands of immunoglobulin.

Clinical Course

It is characterized by exacerbations and remissions. Clinical course is progressive, leading to increasing disability.

ACUTE DISSEMINATED ENCEPHALOMYELITIS

Acute disseminated encephalomyelitis refers to widespread demyelination. It is preceded by viral illnesses such as measles, mumps, rubella, and chickenpox, and is often known as post-infectious encephalitis. It may be due to delayed hypersensitivity reaction. The course varies from a complete recovery to a fatal outcome.

GUILLAIN-BARRÉ SYNDROME

Guillain-Barré syndrome is autoimmune disorder involving acute inflammation and destruction of myelin sheath of peripheral nerves by macrophages and lymphocytes. It is often preceded by viral infection, immunization, or allergic reactions.

Age Group

It most often occurs in young adults. It has four variants.
- Acute inflammatory demyelinating polyradiculoneuropathy is the most common variant (90%).
- Acute motor axonal neuropathy occurs in children and has good prognosis.
- Acute motor sensory axonal neuropathy affects adults and has poor recovery rate.
- Miller Fisher syndrome is rare variant involving only cranial nerves.

Clinical Features

It usually starts in the extremities and moves toward the trunk, may result in respiratory failure. If cranial nerves are involved, patient has facial weakness, pain, and difficulty in speech.

CSF Examination

It shows increased proteins concentration with only modest increase in cell count, which is an important diagnostic finding.

Treatment

Patients are administered immunomodulators to inhibit antibodies formation, anticoagulants are given to reduce risk of deep vein thrombosis and pulmonary embolism. Nonsteroidal anti-inflammatory drugs are given to relieve pain.

CONGENITAL DISORDERS

NEURAL DEFECTS

Neural tube defects occur due to failure of closure of the neural tube linked with maternal folic acid deficiency.

These can involve vertebrae or skull with or without involvement of the underlying meninges, spinal cord, or brain. In neural tube defects, an increase in α-fetoprotein in both the maternal serum and the amniotic fluid is noted.

Maternal folic acid deficiency has been associated with an increased incidence of neural tube defects, and folic acid has, therefore, been approved for inclusion as a food supplement in commercial flour (Fig. 30.36).

Spina Bifida

Spina bifida is most often asymptomatic entity. It occurs due to failure of posterior vertebral arches to close. It is restricted to the vertebral arches.

Spina Bifida Cystica

It is spina bifida complicated by herniation of meninges through a defect.

Spina Bifida Occulta

It shows spina bifida with no clinically apparent abnormalities. Vertebral arch defect is most often limited to one or two vertebrae.

Meningocele

It is defect in which herniated membranes consist only of meninges, and spina bifida occulta does not manifest any apparent abnormalities.

Meningomyelocele

It is a neural tube defect in which portion of spinal cord along with meninges are protruded in the fluid filled

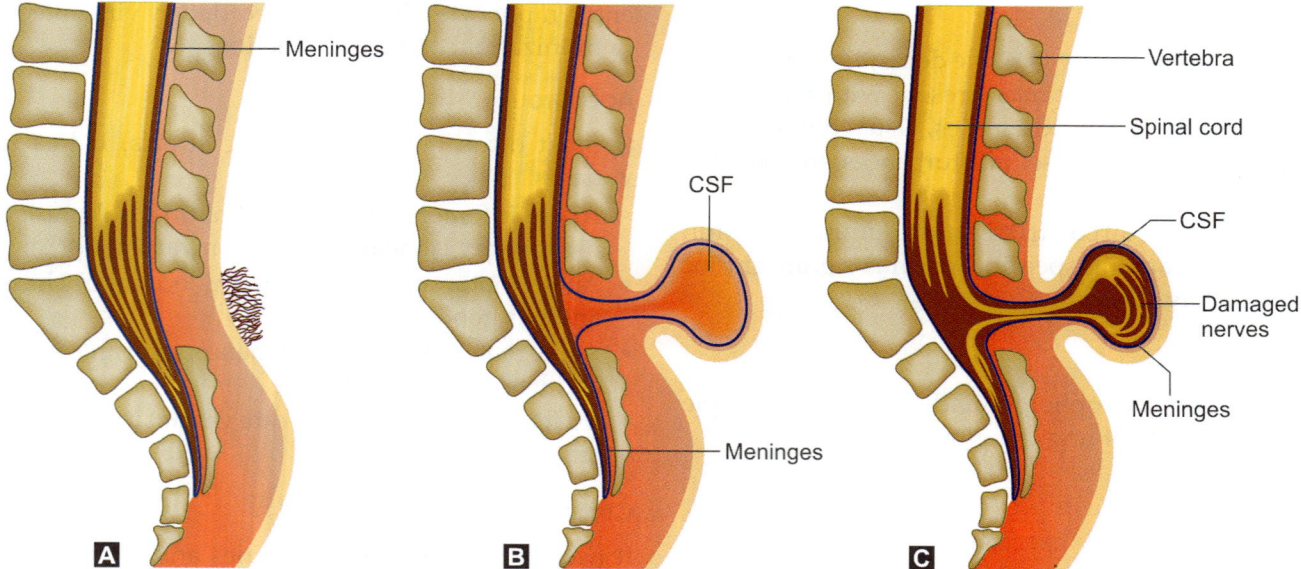

Fig. 30.36: Neural defects. (A) Spina bifida occulta, (B) meningocele, (C) myelomeningocele (*Courtesy:* Dr Akshun Kalia).

herniated tissue. This neural defect exposes the spinal canal and causes the nerve roots to be entrapped.

Anencephaly

It shows marked diminution or absence of fetal brain tissue usually associated with the absence of overlying skull.

- *Holoprosencephaly:* It is a microcephalic brain in which the interhemispheric fissure is absent. The horseshoe-shaped cerebral hemispheres have fused frontal poles, across which the gyri show an irregular horizontal orientation.
- *Hydromyelia:* It is the term for dilation of the central canal of the spinal cord.
- *Syringomyelia:* It is a congenital malformation, in which a tubular cavitation (syrinx) extends for variable distances along the entire length of the spinal cord.
- *Rachischisis:* It is an extreme defect, often without a recognizable spinal cord.
- *Polymicrogyria:* It is a congenital disorder in which the surface of the brain exhibits an excessive number of small, irregularly sized, randomly distributed gyral folds.
- *Arrhinencephaly:* It refers to absence of the olfactory tracts.
- *Lissencephaly:* It refers to congenital disorder in which the cortical surface of the cerebral hemispheres is smooth or has imperfectly formed gyri.
- *Pachygyria:* It is a disorder in which the gyri are reduced in number and usually broad.

TORCH COMPLEX

TORCH complex is a group of infections transmitted from the mother to the fetus. TORCH stands for Toxoplasma, Rubella, Cytomegalovirus, and Herpes simplex virus (and others, such as congenital syphilis). These infections can lead to a syndrome characterized by microcephaly, chorioretinitis, central nervous system (CNS) calcifications, petechial rash, hepatosplenomegaly, and thrombocytopenia.

Pathogenesis

Intrauterine CMV infection is one of the agents of TORCH syndrome. It crosses placenta to induce encephalitis during intrauterine life. These lesions are in proximity to the third ventricle and the aqueduct, the patient is prone to develop hydrocepahalus. Severe CMV infection can cause mental retardation, microcephaly, chorioretinitis, hepatosplenomegaly and periventricular calcifications (Fig. 30.37).

HYDROCEPHALUS

Hydrocephalus denotes increased volume of cerebrospinal fluid (CSF) within the cranial cavity. In infants, it is associated with (sometimes marked) enlargement of the skull.

Etiology

Hydrocephalus is most often caused by obstruction to the CSF circulation by mechanisms such as congenital malformations, inflammation, and tumors. It can also result from overproduction of CSF by choroid plexus papilloma (rare). Intrauterine CMV infection is one of

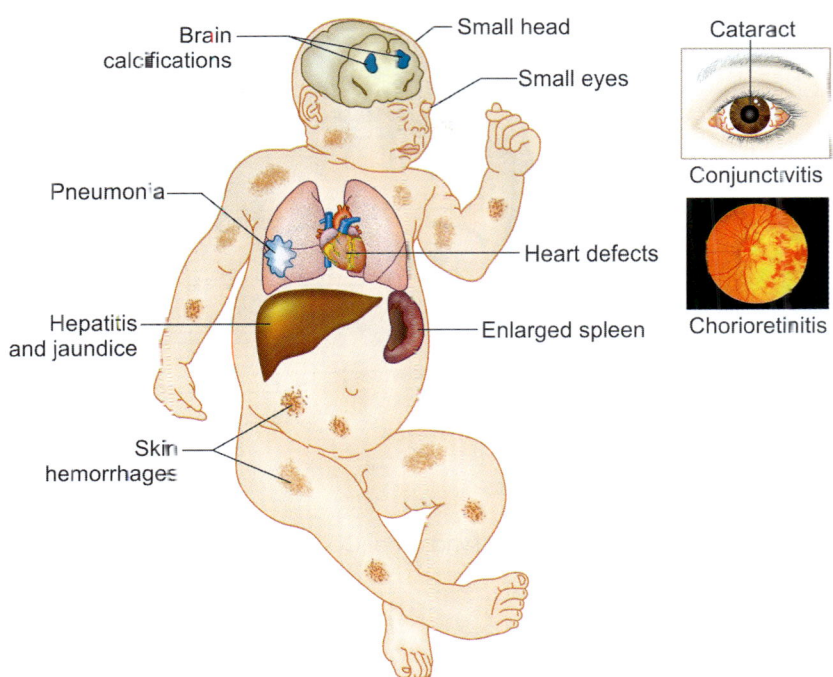

Fig. 30.37: TORCH infections. Fetuses infected in the first trimester by Toxoplasma, rubella, cytomegalovirus, herpesvirus or many other microbes have similar clinical findings as those illustrated in this figure.

the agents of TORCH syndrome. It crosses placenta to induce encephalitis during intrauterine life. These lesions are in proximity to the third ventricle and the aqueduct, the patient is prone to develop hydrocepahalus.

It can also occur as hydrocephalus ex vacuo without obstruction or increased CSF production in disorders characterized by decreased cerebral mass, such as ischemic brain atrophy or advanced Alzheimer disease.

Congenital hydrocephalus refers to an excessive amount of CSF and ventricular enlargement. It is caused by congenital atresia of the *aqueduct of Sylvius*.

Light microscopy of the midbrain may disclose multiple atretic channels or an aqueduct narrowed by gliosis.

Congenital Hydrocephalus

- *Internal hydrocephalus:* The increased volume of CSF is entirely within the ventricles.
- *External hydrocephalus:* The increased volume of CSF is confined to the subarachnoid space.
- *Communicating hydrocephalus:* Free flow of CSF occurs between the ventricles and the subarachnoid space.
- *Noncommunicating hydrocephalus:* Obstructed flow of CSF occurs from the ventricles to the subarachnoid space.

ARNOLD-CHIARI MALFORMATION

Arnold-Chiari malformation is characterized by downward displacement of the cerebellar tonsils and medulla through the foramen magnum. The cerebellar vermis is herniated below the level of the foramen magnum. This malformation results in pressure atrophy of displaced brain tissue.

In addition, it causes hydrocephalus as a result of obstruction of the CSF outflow tract. Presence of a thoracolumbar meningomyelocele is almost always characteristic in this disorder.

AGENESIS OF THE CORPUS CALLOSUM

Agenesis of the corpus callosum can be asymptomatic and is often found in association with other abnormalities.

FETAL ALCOHOL SYNDROME

Fetal alcohol syndrome is the most common acquired cause of mental retardation in the United States. It is associated with excessive maternal alcohol intake during pregnancy (Fig. 30.38).

The common features of fetal alcohol syndrome include intrauterine growth retardation, mental retardation, neurologic impairment, microcephaly, and atrial septal defect.

Children later suffer from mental retardation and minor facial dysmorphic features.

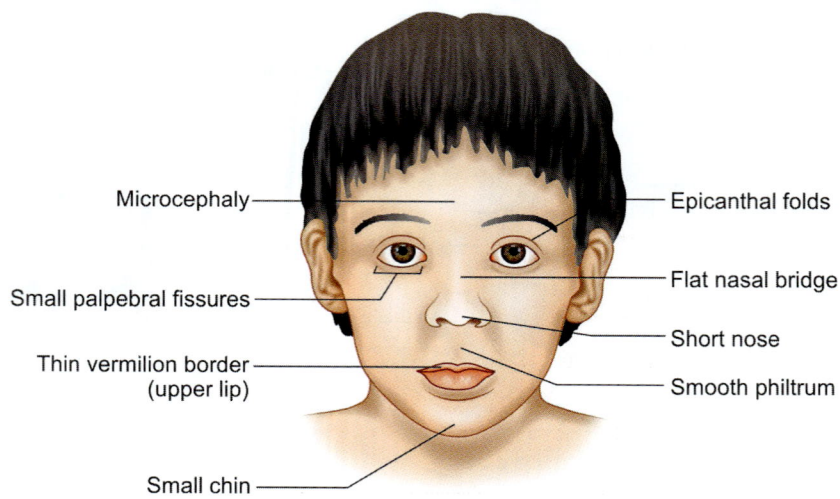

Fig. 30.38: Fetal alcohol syndrome (*Courtesy:* Dr Akshun Kalia).

TUBEROUS SCLEROSIS SYNDROME

This autosomal dominant disorder includes nodular proliferations of multinucleated atypical astrocytes forming tubers (small white nodules scattered in the cerebral cortex and periventricular areas), adenoma sebaceum of the skin, and angiomyolipoma of the kidney. Seizures and mental retardation beginning in infancy are characteristic.

Index

A

α₁-antitrypsin deficiency 38, 46, 302, 883, 879, 1104
α-actin 4 protein (ACTN4) 1162
α-fetoprotein (AFP) 405
α-hydroxylase deficiency (vitamin D resistant rickets) 1456
α-methylacyl-CoA racemase enzyme 1281
α-smooth muscle actin 1361, 1375
α-tocopherol 426
Abetalipoproteinemia 991
Abnormal folding of proteins by reactive oxygen species 22
Abnormal pooling of platelets 604
ABO blood group antigens 302
ABO blood group system 626
ABO blood grouping 632
Acanthosis nigricans 405, 1578
Accelerated phase of chronic myeloid leukemia 567
Accelerated phase of CML (BCR-ABL positive) 567
Accessory nipple 1401
Acetaminophen induced hepatocellular injury 1080
Achalasia 962
Achondroplasia 302, 1513
Acid–base equilibrium imbalance 1198
Acid elution test 527
Acid hydrolase 99, 196
Acid phosphatase 543
Acid serum lysis test 531
Acne 1579
Acquired atelectasis of lung 900
Acquired cystic renal disease 1229
Acquired hypercoagulable state 149, 620
Acquired hyperlipidemia 750
Acquired immunodeficiency syndrome 220
Acquired sideroblastic anemia 531
Acral lentiginous melanoma 1572

Actin filaments 37
Actinic keratosis 13, 1565, 1567
Actinomyces israelii 445, 868
Activated partial thromboplastin time (APTT) 556, 613, 623
Activated prothrombin complex concentrates 635
Activation of leukocytes 64
Active hyperemia 134
Active immunity 179
Acute appendicitis 1029
Acute bacterial endocarditis 812
Acute chest syndrome in sickle cell disease 511
Acute cholecystitis 1127, 1135
Acute cystitis 1245
Acute disseminated encephalomyelitis 1617
Acute endocarditis 812
Acute endometritis 1310
Acute erosive gastritis 970
Acute erythroblastic leukemia 558
Acute fatty liver of pregnancy 1107
Acute fibrinous pericarditis 791
Acute gouty arthritis 1522
Acute graft-versus-host disease (GVHD) 270, 595
Acute Gullain-Barré syndrome 637
Acute heart failure 827
Acute icteric hepatitis 1071
Acute idiopathic thrombocytopenic purpura 602
Acute inflammation 53
Acute iron poisoning 487
Acute lymphangitis 769
Acute lymphoblastic leukemia (ALL) 544, 552
Acute mastitis 1364
Acute megakaryoblastic leukemia 558
Acute myasthenia gravis 637

Acute myeloid leukemia (AML) 547, 550, 552
Acute myocardial infarction 784, 785, 787, 789, 791, 794–797
Acute necrotizing ulcerative gingivitis 933
Acute nephritic syndrome 1187
Acute oophoritis 1346
Acute otitis media 847
Acute pancreatitis 1134, 1140
Acute pericarditis 823
Acute peritonitis 1034
Acute phase reactants 94, 247, 806
Acute promyelocytic leukemia 556
Acute pyelonephritis 1183, 1209, 1421
Acute renal failure 1208, 1209
Acute renal transplant rejection 268
Acute respiratory distress syndrome 160, 886, 887
Acute rheumatic heart disease 802
Acute rhinosinusitis 836
Acute salpingitis 1306
Acute sialadenitis 939
Acute thyroiditis 1431
Acute tubular necrosis 1206, 1207
Acute urate nephropathy 1214
Acute viral hepatitis 1062
Acylating agents 354
Adamantinoma bone 1508
Addison's disease 255, 933, 1461
Adenocarcinoma esophagus 998
Adenocarcinoma gallbladder 1138
Adenocarcinoma lung 918, 966
Adenocarcinoma of extrahepatic bile ducts 1139
Adenocarcinoma—various sites 327
Adenoid cystic carcinoma of salivary gland 947
Adenoma gallbladder 1137
Adenoma of the nipple 1376
Adenoma various sites 324
Adenomatoid odontogenic tumor 953

Adenomatoid tumor of fallopian tube 1307
Adenomatoid tumor of testicular adnexa 1271
Adenomatous polyps of colon 1019
Adenomyosis uteri 1312
Adenosine 235
Adenosine deaminase 218
ADH deficiency 1469
Adhesive pericarditis 825, 826
Adipocytes 419
Adipocytic tumors 1526
ADP 142
Adrenal cortex 1457
Adrenal cortical insufficiency 1461
Adrenal hyperfunction 1459
Adrenal virilism 1462
Adrenocortical adenoma 1465
Adrenocortical carcinoma 1465
Adrenogenital syndrome 1462
Adult and infantile fibrosarcoma 1531
Adult Gaucher's disease (type 1) 1106
Adult polycystic kidney 302, 1226
Adult stem cells 112
Adult T cell leukemia/lymphoma 579, 673
Advanced gastric carcinoma 979
Adverse reactions of blood transfusion 638
Aflatoxin β_1 385, 1117
Agar gel electrophoresis 735
Agenesis of corpus callosum 1619
Agenesis of kidney 13
Air embolism 157, 159, 640
AKT/PI3K signaling pathway 363
Alagille syndrome 1057
Albinism 220, 302, 1569
Alcian blue stain 697 925
Alcohol fixative 692
Alcoholic (Laënnec) cirrhosis 1082, 1098
Alcoholic liver disease 1094
Alder-Reilly anomaly 468, 537
Aleukemic leukemia 540
Alexander Wiener nomenclature blood group system 629
ALK receptors 352
Alkaline phosphatase 698, 1048
Alkaptonuria 310
Alkylating chemotherapeutic agents 384
Allergic polyps 837
Allergic reactions 231, 639
Allergic rhinitis 232
Allogenic grafts 592
Alloimmune hemolytic anemia 519
Alport's syndrome 1162
Alternate pathway of complement activation 210
Alveolar rhabdomyosarcoma 844, 1533
Alveolar soft part sarcoma 377, 1537
Ameloblastic carcinoma 955
Ameloblastic fibroma 953
Ameloblastic fibrosarcoma 956
Ameloblastic odontoma 954
Ameloblastoma 954
Amenorrhea 1309

Amniotic fluid embolism 157, 160, 1355
Amoebic colitis 1014
Amoebic encephalitis 1589
Amoebic liver abscess 1078
Amorphous ground substance 124
Amyloid adrenal gland 279
Amyloid associated 275
Amyloid gastrointestinal tract 279
Amyloid heart 279
Amyloid laboratory diagnosis 280
Amyloid light-chain 273
Amyloid liver 278, 1106
Amyloid nephropathy 277, 1183
Amyloid nervous system 280
Amyloid of aging 277
Amyloid P component 273
Amyloid respiratory system 279
Amyloid skin 279
Amyloid spleen (lardaceous and sago) 279, 680
Amyloid stains 281, 1107, 1185
   Congo red stain examined under light microscope 281
   Congo red stain examined under polarizing microscope 281
   crystal violet (metachromatic stain) 281
   fluorescent stains (thioflavin-T, thioflavin-S) 281
   methyl violet (metachromatic stain) 281
Amyloid β-protein 276
Amyloidosis 47, 273, 933
Amylopectin 1105
Anaerobic glycolysis 20, 21
Anal fissure 1032
Analgesic induced nephropathy 1215
Analogous antigens 190
Anaphylactic shock 176, 211
Anaphylatoxins (C3a, C5a) 81
Anaphylaxis 232, 639
Anaplastic astrocytoma 1599
Anaplastic dysgerminoma 1334
Anaplastic large T cell lymphoma 674
Anaplastic seminoma 1260
Anatomical barriers to pathogens 185
Anatomical dead space refers 860
ANCA glomerulonephritis 1168
Ancylostoma duodenale 455
Anderson disease 309
Androblastoma (Sertoli cell tumor) of testis 1269
Androblastoma—ovary 1343
Androgen induced prostatic carcinoma 391
Anemia of chronic disease 531
Anencephaly 1618
Aneuploidy 295
Aneurysm of sinus of Valsalva 759
Aneurysmal bone cyst 952, 1510
Aneurysms 755, 756, 759, 760
Angelman (happy puppet) syndrome 292
Angina pectoris (>12 hours) in AMI 795
Angina pectoris 783
   stable (typical) angina 784

   unstable (crescendo/pre-infarction) angina 784
   variant (Prinzmetal) angina 784
Angiodysplasia 1016
Angiogenesis 127, 372
Angiogenic factors 334, 372
Angiomyolipoma 771
Angiosarcoma 682, 771
Angiosarcoma breast 1395
Angiosarcoma liver 1123
Angiostatin 335
Angiotensin 334
Angiotensin aldosterone system 422
Angular stomatitis 428
Anionic-sialoglycoproteins 1159
Anitschkow cells 800
Ankylosing spondylitis 255, 1520, 1521
Ankyrin proteins in RBC membrane 500
Annular pancreas 1140, 1409
Anorectal fistula 1032
Anterior cerebral artery occlusion 1611
Anterior pituitary gland 1467
Anti-angiogenic factors 335, 372
Antiapoptotic genes 319
Antibodies induced glomerular injury 1168
Antibodies of ABO system 634
Antibody-dependent mediated cytotoxicity 238
Anticardiolipin antibodies 620
Anticoagulants 476, 477
Anti-D antibody (RhoGAM) administration 630
Antidiuretic hormone (ADH) 1153
Anti-DNA antibody 1049
Anti-DNAase 799
Anti-DNAase-B titer 1192
Anti-DNase-B/anti-hyaluronidase titer 805
Anti-GBM-mediated glomerulonephritis 1164
Antigen presenting cells (APCs) 198
Antigen-responsive T cells 193
   CD4+ T cells 193
   CD8+ T cells (natural killer cells) 193, 402, 534
   CD8+ T cells (suppressor cells) 193
Antigens 187
Antigens ABO blood group system 627
Antigens of Rh system 629
Anti-HBc (both IgG and IgM) in serum 1069
Anti-HBs antibody marker in serum 1069
Anti-HDV IgM in serum 1073
Anti-hyaluronidase titer 1192
Anti-inflammatory agents 85, 94
Anti-mitochondrial antibody 1049
Anti-nuclear antibody 1049
Antinuclear autoantibodies against SS-B 262
Antiphospholipid antibodies 150, 261
Antiphospholipid antibody syndrome 150, 620
Anti-receptor antibody-mediated type II hypersensitivity reaction 241

Index

Anti-smooth muscle antibody 1049
Antistreptolysin-O (ASO) titer 799, 805, 1192
Antistreptozyme test 805
Antithrombin III 147, 148, 150, 600, 619
Antithrombotic properties of endothelium 139, 140
Aortic coarctation 834
Aortic stenosis 820
Aortic valve insufficiency/regurgitation 820
APC tumor suppressor gene 362
APC/β-catenin pathway 1025
Aphthous stomatitis 934
Aplasia of bone marrow 14
Aplastic anemia 528, 512, 541
Apocrine breast carcinoma 1394
Apocrine metaplasia in fibrocystic disease 1368
Apolipoprotein L-1 gene (APOL1) 1162
Apoptosis 16, 32, 33
Apoptotic gene 319
Appendicular osteoporosis 1482
Applications 691
Aqueduct of Sylvius 1582
Arachidonic acid metabolite pathways 82, 84
Arias-Stella reaction 1312
Armanni-Ebstein lesions in tubules 1421
Arnold-Chiari malformation 1619
Aromatase inhibitors 1407
Aromatic amines 384, 385
Array CGH technique 712
Arrhinencephaly 1618
Arrhythmogenic right ventricular cardiomyopathy 811
Arterial thrombi 152
Arteriovenous fistula 760, 1614
Arthritis of metabolic origin 1521
Arthroscopy 1518
Arthus reaction 243
Asbestosis 887, 893, 908
Ascaris strongyloidiasis 994
Ascending cholangitis 1134
Aschoff's nodule 800, 803
Ascites 169, 829, 1047, 1089
Aspergilloma 434
Aspergillus flavus 385, 451
Aspergillus fumigatus 868
Aspirin (NSAIDs) 85
Assay of B-type natriuretic peptide 827, 904
Asterixis (flapping tremors) 1046
Astrocytes 1581
Astrocytic tumors 1598
Astrocytomas 1598
Asymptomatic acute prostatitis 1277
Asymptomatic/silent gallstones 1132
Ataxia hemorrhagic telangiectasia 608
Ataxia-telangiectasia 219, 343, 374, 541, 1379
Atelectasis neonatorum 900
Atelectasis or lung collapse 900

Atheroembolism due to atherosclerosis 157
Atherosclerosis 45, 138, 743, 744, 747, 748, 751, 752, 754, 778, 1419
Atherosclerotic aneurysms 756
ATM tumor suppressor gene 369
Atopic dermatitis 232
ATP 142
ATP7B gene 1048, 1103
ATPase 20
Atrial myxoma 830
Atrial natriuretic factor 1153
Atrial septal defects 833
Atrial thrombi 793
Atrophy—various organs 4, 6
Atypical alveolar hyperplasia 921
Atypical chronic myeloid leukemia (aCML) 562
Atypical ductal hyperplasia 1369, 1379
Auer rods in myeloblasts 553
Auspitz sign in psoriasis 1562
Austin Flint murmur in syphilitic aortitis 756
Autoantibodies in liver disorders 1049
Autocrine signaling 118, 119
Autoimmune disorders 255, 297
Autoimmune enteropathy 990
Autoimmune hemolytic anemia 256, 405, 516
Autoimmune hepatitis (lupoid hepatitis) 1075
Autoimmune oophoritis 1346
Autoimmune pancreatitis 1143
Autoimmune pericarditis in AMI 794
Autoimmune sialadenitis 939
Autoimmune thrombocytopenic purpura 256
Autologous blood transfusion 637
Autonomic nervous system neuropathy 1423
Autosomal codominant inheritance 302
Autosomal dominant inheritance 290, 302, 303
Autosomal recessive inheritance 290, 302, 303, 306
Autosplenectomy 512, 679
AV node conduction system heart 782
Avascular necrosis of femoral head in sickle cell disease 511
Axial osteoporosis 1482
Axillary lymph nodes 1359, 1395, 1396, 1402
Azathioprine immunosuppressive drug 272
Azo dyes derivatives of aromatic amines 385

B

β-hCG 1268
β-microglobulin 577
B cell lymphoma (DLBCL) 663
B cell prolymphocytic leukemia 672

B cells 534
B cells dysfunction role in diabetes mellitus 1416
Bacillary angiomatosis 771
Bacteria induced carcinogenesis 390
Bacterial cervicitis 1297
Bacterial liver infections 1077
Bacterial meningitis 1584, 1586
Bacterial orchitis 1273
Bacterial pneumonias 862
Bacterial products 195
Bacterial vaginosis 1291
Bactericidal permeability increasing protein 69
Balanced polymorphism 291
Ballooning angioplasty 787
Ballooning degeneration 1061
Band 3 (anionic channel) in RBC membrane 500
Band 4.1 in RBC membrane 501
Band 4.2 proteins (pallidin) in RBC membrane 500
Barium enema 1029
Barr bodies 296, 313
Barrett esophagus 961
Barriers to pathogens 185
Bartholin glands 1290
Basal cell carcinoma of skin 326, 1568
Basaloid carcinoma 1033
Basilar artery occlusion 1611
Basophilia 536
Basophilic stippling 465, 479, 480, 561
Basophils 534
BCL family 371
BCL-1 cell cycle regulatory gene 1382
BCR-ABL hybrid (fusion) protein product 376, 564
Becker muscular dystrophy 303, 312, 1543
Beckwith-Wiedemann syndrome (BWS) 1232
Bellini duct renal cell carcinoma 1240
Benign Brenner tumor—ovary 1333
Benign epithelial tumors 322
Benign mesenchymal tumors 324
Benign monoclonal gammopathy 588
Benign nephrosclerosis 1223
Benign phyllodes tumor—breast 1372
Benign surface epithelial tumors—ovary 323
Benign tumors 906
BER-EP4 monoclonal antibody 925
Bernard-Soulier syndrome 142, 606, 622
Berry aneurysm 138, 755, 758, 1614
Berylliosis 895
Bilateral renal agenesis 1229
Bile canalicular antibody 1049
Bile canaliculi 1043
Bile duct disorders 1107
Bile duct hamartoma 1115
Bile juice composition 1129
Biliary adenocarcinoma 1139
Biliary atresia 1056

Biliary cholestasis 1061
Biliary cirrhosis 1107, 1082
Biliary intraepithelial neoplasia 1137
Bilirubin pigment 39
Biological immunosuppression 272
Biological therapy in breast carcinoma 1407
Biotin 428
BIRADS system used for reporting mammograms 1403
Bite cells 480, 515,524
Bitot's spots in eyes 425
Bland infarct (non-infective) infarct 162
Blast crisis in CML 566, 567, 568
Bleeding diathesis 427, 620, 621, 622, 623
Bleeding into vitreous 1423
Bleeding time 623
Blood components therapy 631, 634, 635
Blood cross-matching 634
Blood culture 806
Blood group A 626
Blood group AB 627
Blood group B 627
Blood group O 626
Blood group systems 626
Blood group systems other than ABO and Rh 631
Blood sampling 526, 735
Blood transfusion reactions 240, 638
Blood–brain barrier 1581
Bloom syndrome 541
Blue bloaters tolerate hypoxia 882
Blue nevus 1570
Boerhaave's syndrome 963
Bombay blood group (Oh) 628
Bone and joint crises in sickle cell disease 511
Bone forming tumors 1487
Bone fracture healing 121
Bone marrow 575, 579
Bone marrow aspirate 472, 565, 578, 588
   abnormal cells 472
   cellularity 472
   erythropoiesis 472
   leukopoiesis 472
   megakaryopoiesis 472
   myeloid to erythroid ratio 472
   other bone marrow cells 472
Bone marrow aspiration needles 470
   Klima needle 470
   Salah needle 470
Bone marrow failure syndromes 528
Bone marrow harvesting 593
Bone marrow hyperplasia 10
Bone marrow stem cells 112
Bone marrow stromal cells (MSCs) 113
Bone marrow trephine biopsy 578, 587
Bone metastases 1509
Bone scan in malignancy 1404
Bone tumors 1484
Borderline Brenner tumor 1333
Borderline endometrioid tumors 1324
Borderline phyllodes tumor 1373

Borderline serous tumors of low malignant potential of ovary 1327
Borderline serous tumors with micro-invasion 1327
Borderline surface epithelial tumors of ovary 1323
Borrelia burgdorferi 390, 982
Botryoid rhabdomyosarcoma 1254, 1294, 1534
Bouin's fluid fixative 692
Bouveret's syndrome 1136
Bowen disease of penis 1282
Bowen disease of the vulva 1288
Bowenoid papulosis 1282
Bowman's capsule 1159, 1160
B-prolymphocytic leukemia (PLL) 578
Brachial plexus injury induced by Pancoast tumor 918
Bradykinin 81
BRAF increasing RAS signal transduction protein pathway 354
Brain purpura 902, 1615
Branchial cyst 853
BRCA1 tumor suppressor gene 342, 368, 1325, 1378, 1381
BRCA2 tumor suppressor gene 342, 368, 1145, 1379, 1381
Breast carcinoma 1376
Breast carcinoma—prognostic and predictive factors 1397
Breast lumps 1362
Breast lumps frequency 1360
Breast sarcoidosis 1365
Breast tuberculosis 439, 1365
Breasts during pregnancy 10
Brenner tumor of ovary 1332
Bridging necrosis liver 1047, 1061
Brilliant cresyl blue stain 474, 515
Broad group of cells 111
Brodie abscess 1478
Bromsulphthalein excretion 1056
Bronchial adenoma 906
Bronchial asthma 232, 233, 877, 884
Bronchial biopsy 925
Bronchial hamartoma 331
Bronchial papilloma 906
Bronchiectasis 876, 877, 882
Bronchiolitis 877
Bronchioloalveolar carcinoma 920, 921
Bronchoalveolar lavage 439, 925
Bronchopneumonia 862, 866, 867
Bronchopulmonary carcinoids 907
Bronze diabetes 41, 1102
Brown atrophy of organs 6
Brown tumor of hyperparathyroidism 956
Brucellosis 535
Brudzinski's sign 1586
Bruton's agammaglobulinemia 67
Budd-Chiari syndrome 135, 1111
Bullous pemphigoid 255, 1563
Bundle of His and its branches of heart 782
Burkitt's lymphoma 376,389, 546, 661, 664

Burr cells 480
Byssinosis 897

C

C peptide levels 1411
C5a 195
C5a 63
Cabot's ring 479, 480
Cachexia 6, 400
Cadherins 126
CagA effector molecules 968
Calcific aortic stenosis 821
Calcification 42
Calcifying epithelial odontogenic tumor 953
Calcifying odontogenic cyst 952
Calcinosis 42, 262
Calcitonin 1451, 1452
Calcium 142, 609
Calcium and phosphate disturbances 1200
Calcium metabolism 1452
Calcium oxalate stones—kidney 1219
Calcium phosphate stones—kidney 1219
Calcium pump 20
Calcium stones—kidney 1219
Calcospherites 1601
Call-Exner bodies in granulosa cell tumor of ovary 1341
Calretinin 843, 925
CAM 5.2 843
Cambium layer 1294
Campylobacter jejuni 390, 982, 992
Cancer testis antigens 373
Cancers in AIDS 225
Candida albicans 451, 868, 934
Capillary hemangioma 770,154
Capillary microaneurysms 760
Capsular drop in diabetic nephropathy 1183, 1421
Caput medusae in portal hypertension 1089
Carbon tetrachloride induced liver injury 1081
Carbuncle 1290
Carcinoembryonic antigen (CEA) 405, 925, 1406, 1451
Carcinogenesis 347
Carcinoid heart disease 1000
Carcinoid syndrome 404, 1000
Carcinoid tumor 985, 1031, 1149, 1338
Carcinoma *in situ* 320
Carcinoma of penis 1282
Carcinosarcoma (malignant mixed müllerian tumor) of ovary 1334
Carcinosarcoma of salivary gland 950
Cardiac arrhythmias in AMI 422, 791
Cardiac cirrhosis 135, 1110
Cardiac enzymes in AMI 796
Cardiac hemolytic anemia 522
Cardiac hypertrophy 7, 777, 829
Cardiac imaging techniques in AMI 797

Cardiac muscle stem cells 114
Cardiac rhabdomyoma 831
Cardiac tamponade 822
Cardiac transplantation 809
Cardiac troponins (Tn I and Tn T) in AMI 796
Cardiac tumors 830
Cardiac valves 818
Cardiac vegetations 812, 813
Cardiac vegetations—comparison 817
Cardiogenic shock 171, 173, 791
Cardiomyopathies 807, 808
Carnitine palmityl transferase deficiency 1547
Carnoy's fluid fixative 692
Carotid angiography 855
Carotid body tumor 855
Carprofen drug 85
Cartilaginous tumors 1495
Caseating granulomas 106
Caseous necrosis 26, 28, 432
Caspases and apoptosis 35
Castleman disease 643
Catalase 25
Cataracts 1423
Catarrhal inflammation 73
Categories of birefringence 690
Categories of delayed hypersensitivity reactions 248
Caterpillar cells 800
Cathepsin D 20, 968, 1004, 1400, 1400
Cauliflower ear 846
Causes of valvular diseases 818
Cavernous hemangioma 324, 770, 1614
CD15 (LeuM1) 925
CD2 associated proteins 1159
CD31 62
CD55 522
CD59 522
CDE (Fisher-Race) nomenclature system 629
CDKN2A tumor suppressor gene 363
Celiac disease 988
Cell (forward) blood grouping 632
Cell adhesion proteins 125
Cell cycle 114
Cell cycle inhibitors 341
Cell injury 15
Cell-mediated immunity (CMI) 191
Cell surface receptors 119
Cells in epidermis 1552
Cellular aging 48
Cellular changes in acute inflammation 61
Cellular proteins in blood 19
Cellulose acetate electrophoresis 735
Cementifying fibroma 956
Cementoma 954
Central core (nucleocapsid) 1067
Central core disease 1546
Central diabetes insipidus 1470
Central giant cell granuloma 956
Central nervous system 1580

Central tolerance 250, 252
Centriacinar emphysema 880
Centrilobular emphysema 1041
Centrilobular necrosis liver 045
Centromere enumerating probes (CEPs) 718
Centromere protein H (CENP-H) 925
Cerebral abscess 1589
Cerebral edema 169
Cerebral hemangioblastoma 464
Cerebral infarction 1611
Cerebral malaria 1589
Cerebral parenchymal compartment 1582
Cerebral strokes 748
Cerebral toxoplasmosis 1589
Cerebral vascular disease 1420
Cerebrospinal fluid 1582
Ceruloplasmin 25, 1048
Cerumic gland adenoma 846
Cervical biopsy 1305
Cervical carcinoma 1300
Cervical intraepithelial dysplasia 12
Cervical intraepithelial neoplasia (CIN) 1299
Cervical intraepithelial neoplasia 320, 1299
Cervical lymphadenopathy 643
CFTr gene 7, 883
Chancroid 1293
Charcot joints 1589
Charcot-Leyden crystals in sputum 455, 534, 884
Chédiak-Higashi syndrome 38, 67, 93, 220, 537
Cheilosis 428
CHEK2 tumor suppressor gene 370, 1381
Chemical carcinogens 381
Chemical defenses against pathogens 186
Chemical mediators 73, 235
Chemifluorescence 705
Chemilumiescence 705
Chemokines 195, 431
Chemotactic factors 63
Chemotaxis 61, 63
Chemotherapeutic agents 408
Chemotherapy 567, 1407
Chemotherapy-induced leukemias 541
Cherry hemangioma 1576
Cherubism 956
Chest radiographs 652
Chest wall invasion by Pancoast tumor 918
Chlamydia trachomatis 1292
Cholangiocarcinoma 1122
Cholangitis and liver abscess 1080
Cholecystitis 1127
Choledochal cyst 1129
Cholelithiasis (gallstone disease) 1129
Cholestasis 1050, 1051
Cholesteatoma 847
Cholesterol gallstones 1132
Cholesterol granuloma 847
Cholesterolosis (strawberry gallbladder) 45, 1128

Chondroblastoma 1497
Chondrocalcinosis (pseudogout) 1522
Chondroid syringoma 1576
Chondroma 1495
Chondromyxoid fibroma 1497
Chondronectin 129
Chondrosarcoma 329, 1498
Chordoma 1505
Choreoathetoid movements 608
Chorioamnionitis 1356
Choriocarcinoma 1268, 1339
Choroid plexus 1582
Choroid plexus papilloma 1602
Chromogranin-A 843
Chromophobe variant of renal cell carcinoma 1233
Chromosomal banding techniques 314
    C-banding 314
    G-banding 314
    Giemsa stain 314
    Q-banding 314
    R-banding 314
Chromosomal disorders 292
Chromosomal rearrangements 375
Chromosome instability syndrome 343
Chromothripsis 377
Chronic active hepatitis 1064, 1071
Chronic active myocarditis 807
Chronic bronchitis 876, 877
Chronic carriers in hepatitis 1071
Chronic cervicitis 1297
Chronic cholecystitis 1127
Chronic cystitis 1246
Chronic endometritis 1310
Chronic eosinophilic leukemia 569
Chronic gastritis type A, B and AB 970, 971
Chronic glomerulonephritis 1197
Chronic graft-versus-host disease (GVHD) 270, 595
Chronic granulomatous disease of childhood 68, 537, 883
Chronic granulomatous inflammation 103
Chronic heart failure 827
Chronic hepatitis 1071
Chronic idiopathic thrombocytopenic purpura 603
Chronic interstitial cystitis 1247
Chronic ischemic heart disease 798
Chronic lobular hepatitis 1063
Chronic lymphocytic leukemia (CLL) 574, 662
Chronic lymphocytic leukemia 517, 667
Chronic lymphoproliferative disorders 574
Chronic myeloid leukemia 376, 563
Chronic myeloid leukemia *vs* leukemoid reactions 569
Chronic myelomonocytic leukemia 562
Chronic myeloproliferative disorders 541
Chronic neutrophilic leukemia 569, 570
Chronic obstructive pulmonary disease 876, 908
Chronic obstructive sialadenitis 939

Chronic otitis media 847
Chronic pancreatitis 824, 1142
Chronic prostatitis 1277
Chronic pyelonephritis (CPN) 1212
Chronic recurrent parotitis 940
Chronic renal transplant rejection 269
Chronic rheumatic heart disease 803
Chronic salinities 1306
Chronic sinusitis 837
Chronic urate nephropathy 1214
Chronic venous congestion of liver 135, 1110
Chronic venous congestion of lung 136
Chronic viral hepatitis 1063
Churg-Strauss syndrome 766
Chylothorax 928
Chylous effusion 769
Cip/Kip (Cip/WAF family) 341
    INK4a/ARF family 341
Circulatory overload 639
Circumferential myocardial infarct 784
Cirrhosis 1082
Citrate agar electrophoresis 736
Classes of RNAs 286
Classic dysgerminoma 1334
Classic galactosemia 309
Classic hemophilia 311
Classic seminoma 1260
Classical Reed-Sternberg cells 650
Classification of antibodies 698
Classification of common neoplasms 321
Classification of diabetes mellitus 1414
Classification of hemolytic anemias 495
Classification of soft tissue tumors 1525
Classification of the vasculitides 761
Clear cell adenocarcinoma 1294
Clear cell carcinoma 1332
Clear cell odontogenic carcinoma 955
Clear cell sarcoma of soft tissue 1538
Clear cell variant of renal cell carcinoma 1233
Cleft palate 932
Clinical features in primary HIV infection 227
Cloaca 1478
Clonal deletion 252
Clonal energy 252
Clonal selection 191
Clone deletion of T cells by apoptosis 254
Clonorchis sinensis (liver-fluke) 391
Closed comedon 1579
Closed pneumothorax 898
Clostridium difficile 992
Clot dissolution 146
Clot retraction 146, 600
Clot retraction test 624
Clotting time 613
CML vs atypical CML (aCML) 568
C-MYC oncogene 1382
CNS cells vulnerable to hypoxia 1611
CNS lymphoma in AIDS 390
CNS tumors 1590

Coagulation cascade 143
Coagulation disorders in hepatic disease 618
Coagulation factors 610
Coagulation profile 623
Coagulation system 75, 599
Coagulative necrosis 26
Coal dust 42
Coal worker's pneumoconiosis 892, 887
Coarctation of aorta 834
Cobblestone appearance of mucosa 1013
Cobweb turbidity in CSF 1588
Coccidioides immitis 452, 868
Coding regulatory RNA 287
Codman triangle in osteosarcoma 1490
Codominant inheritance 303
Co-infection in hepatitis 1073
COL1A1 gene 1513
COL1A2 gene 1513
Cold agglutinin disease 518
Cold agglutinin hemolytic anemia 637
Collagen fibers 123
Collagen fibers breakdown products 195
Collagen IV and V 1158
Collagen matrix deposition 1205
Collagen vascular diseases 897
Collagenous colitis 1015
Collagenous sprue 990
Collecting duct carcinoma in renal medulla 1233
COLLIA1-PDGFB fusion protein 1531
Colloid breast carcinoma 1391
Colloidal iron 697
Colonoscopy 1029, 1038
Colorectal carcinoma 1022
Colposcopy 1305
Columnar metaplasia in Barrett's esophagus 11
Combined gallstones 1130
Comedocarcinoma—breast 1385
Common variable immunodeficiency 215, 991
Commonly used stains in histopathology 695, 696
Communicating hydrocephalus 1619
Comparative genomic hybridization (CGH) 712
Compensatory mechanisms 496
Competitive ELISA 723
Complement actions 211
Complement classical pathway 210
Complement-mediated phagocytosis of target cells 240
Complement system 76, 77, 209, 210
Complement system defects 93
Complete carcinogens 382
Complete hydatidiform mole 1351
Complete resolution 32, 69
Complex adenoma 1376
Complex (adenomatous) endometrial hyperplasia with atypia 1311
Complex (adenomatous) endometrial hyperplasia without atypia 1311

Complex odontoma 954
Complications of acute myocardial infarction 795
Component 273
Composite pheochromocytoma 1463
Compound odontoma 954
Compound papillae 1152
Compression atelectasis 900
Condyloma acuminatum 1288
Confined placental mosaicism 296
Congenital dyserythroblastopoietic anemia (CDA) 531
Congenital epulis 933
Congenital heart diseases 831
Congenital hydrocephalus 1619
Congenital hypoplasia of the breast 1401
Congenital lactase deficiency 991
Congenital lip pits 933
Congenital myopathies 1546
Congenital nephrotic syndrome 1162
Congenital pyloric stenosis 985
Congestion 134
Congestive cardiomyopathy 808
Congestive heart failure 791, 826
Congestive heart failure in AMI 791
Congestive splenomegaly 137, 678
Congo red stain 281
Congo red stain for amyloid 280, 1201
Conization of cervix 1305
Connective tissue mucins 925
Constrictive pericarditis 439, 825
Constrictive pericarditis—clinical features 825
Contact dermatitis 248, 250
Contraction atelectasis 900
Conventional osteosarcoma 1490
Coombs' test 501, 517, 525, 576
Corbovinum 756
Cord factor 431
Core biopsy 1404
Coronary artery bypass graft (CABG) 787
Coronary artery disease 422
Coronary care units 787
Cor pulmonale 830
Corpus luteal cysts 1348
Corticotropic adenoma 1473
Councilman bodies 34, 1045, 1061
Covert myeloma 583
Cowden disease 1379
Cowden syndrome 1019
Cranial nerve disorders 1423
Craniopharyngioma 1474
Craniotabes in rickets 425
C-reactive proteins 94, 797
Creatine kinase-MB (CK-MB) 796
Creeping fibrosis 1107
Crescentic glomerulonephritis 1163
CREST syndrome 262, 962
Cretinism (thyroid dwarf) 1431
Cri du chat syndrome 293, 298
Cribriform breast carcinoma 1395
Crigler-Najjar syndrome 1054, 1055

Crohn's disease 104, 249, 1012
Cronokite-Canada syndrome 1022
Cryoglobulinemia 637, 1072
Cryoglobulinemia vasculitis 765
Cryoprecipitate 635, 636
Cryostat 687, 688
Cryptococcus neoformans 452, 472, 868
Cryptorchidism 1273
Crystal violet (metachromatic stain) 281
CST3 gene 1244
Current genetic analysis nomenclature system 630
Curschmann spirals 884
Cushing's syndrome 404, 1459
Cutaneous infections 1558, 1559
Cutaneous metastases 1577
Cw6 gene 1562
Cyanocobalamin 428
Cyclic nucleotides 235
Cyclin D and Cdk-4 synthesis 115
Cyclins and cyclin-dependent kinase 357, 1382
Cyclooxygenase pathway 82, 93
Cyclosporine A immunosuppressive drug 272
Cylindrical aneurysm 755
Cystatin aasay in renal diseases C 1244
Cystic diseases of kidney 1226
Cystic fibrosis of pancreas 291, 302, 310, 837, 883, 1143
Cystic hygroma 770
Cystic infarct in brain 165
Cysticercosis 452
Cystine kidney stones 1220
Cystinuria 1216
Cystitis glandularis 1247
Cystoscopy 1221
Cytochemistry in ALL and AML 543
Cytogenetic aberrations in soft tissue sarcomas 1525
Cytogenetic analysis 709–715
Cytokeratin 925
Cytokines 86, 190
Cytokine receptors 65
Cytomegalovirus 449, 472, 868
Cytoskeleton abnormalities 37
Cytoskeleton filaments 23

D

2,6-dichlorophenolindophenol test (DCIP) 527
DAF (decay accelerating factor) 521
Dane particle 1067
DDAVP (desmopressin 1-sesamino-8 arginine vasopressin) 614
Decalcification 693
Decalcifying solutions 693
Decay accelerating factor (DAF) 521
Decompression sickness 157, 159
Decreased erythropoiesis 806
Decreased platelet production 601

Dedifferentiated pleomorphic liposarcoma 1528
Deep vein thrombosis 422, 768, 1355
Defensins 69
Degenerative joint disease 1521
Delayed wound healing 613
Deletion of chromosome 288
Delphin lymph nodes 643
Dementia 428
Demyelinating disorders 1616
Dendrites 1581
Dendritic cells 198
Dengue hemorrhagic fever 604
Dental caries 950
Dental procedures 613
Dentigerous cyst 951
Denys-Drash syndrome (DDS) 1232
Deoxyadenosylcobalamin 489
Dermal dendritic cells 1553
Dermatitis 428
Dermatitis herpetiformis 1564
Dermatofibroma 1573
Dermatofibrosarcoma protuberans 1530, 1574
Dermatomyositis 257, 262, 405
Dermatopathy 1434
Dermis 1553
Desmoglein-1 (Dsg-1) 1550
Desmoglein–desmocollin 1550
Desmoid/deep-seated fibromatosis 1530
Desquamative interstitial pneumonia (DIP) 868
Destructive bone disease 43
Detection of carrier of hemophilia A 614
Detection systems of immuno-chemistry 699
Dexamethasone suppression test 1473
Diabetes insipidus 1469
Diabetes mellitus 751, 1412
Diabetes mellitus pathophysiology 1417
Diabetic glomerulosclerosis 1421
Diabetic ketoacidosis 1415, 1417
Diabetic nephropathy 1181
Diabetic retinopathy 1423
Diabetic vascular disease 766
Diagnosis of allergy 237
Diagnostic criteria—hairy cell leukemia 578
Diagnostic features—Langerhans' cell histiocytosis 591
Diagnostic utility of serum autoantibodies in liver disorders 1049
Dialysis principle 1201
Diamond-Blackfan syndrome 541
Diethylstilbestrol (DES) 391
Diffuse alveolar damage (DAD) 891
Diffuse and nodular glomerulo-sclerosis 1421
Diffuse cortical necrosis 1221
Diffuse glomerulonephritis 1163
Diffuse glomerulosclerosis 1182, 1421

Diffuse hyperplasia liver 1117
Diffuse infiltrative type gastric adeno-carcinoma 981
Diffuse large B cell lymphoma (DLBCL) 665, 1002
Diffuse linear staining of GBM 1205
Diffuse malignant mesothelioma 929, 1035
Diffuse proliferative glomerulo-nephritis 1162
Diffuse pulmonary fibrosis 908
DiGeorge/velocardiofacial syndrome 218, 298, 683, 1456
Digital mammography 1402
Dihydrotestosterone (DHT) 1278
Dilutional hyponatremia 1418
Dilutional thrombocytopenia 640
Dipalmitoyl-phosphatidyl-choline 858
Direct acting carcinogens 382
Direct Coombs' test 525
Direct immunofluorescence micro-scopy 704
Disaccharidase deficiency 991
Discoid lupus erythematosus 257
Disorders of complement system 79, 219
   hereditary angioneurotic edema 79
   recurrent infections 79
   systemic lupus erythematosus 80
Disorders of complement system cascade 93
Disorders of intermediate filaments 38
Disorders of microtubules 38
Disrupted atheromatous plaque in AMI 787
Dissecting hematoma 138, 755, 757, 777
Disseminated intravascular coagulation (DIC) 95, 151, 160, 404, 549, 616
Distal adenocarcinomas 1139
Distal (paraseptal) emphysema 880
Divalent metal transporter-1 (DMT-1) 482
Diversion colitis 1015
Diverticulitis 1006
Diverticulum 1005
DMT-1 (divalent metal transporter-1) 482
DNA content of the tumor 1398
DNA defects 48
DNA double helix molecule 282
DNA gyrase 287
DNA helicases 287
DNA ligase 287
DNA oncogenic viruses 389
DNA polymerase 287, 1067
DNA probe analysis 415
DNA repair genes 319, 368
DNA replication 287
DNA sequences methods 724–730
DNA single-stranded binding proteins 287
DNA strands 287
DNA-adduct formation 383
Double contrast barium enema 1038
Down's syndrome 295, 297, 541
DPC4 (MADH4/SMAD4) tumor sup-pressor gene 369

Dressler's syndrome 794
Driver mutations 347
Drug-induced acute tubulointerstitial diseases 1214
Drug-induced autoimmune hemolytic anemia 240
Drug-induced hemolytic anemia 519
Drug-induced hepatitis 1057
Drug-induced platelet dysfunction 606
Drug-induced thrombocytopenia 240, 604
Drug-induced vasculitides 766
Drugs and toxins induced liver injury 1080
Drugs associated with interstitial fibrosis 895
Dry beriberi 427
Dry gangrene 31
Dubin-Johnson syndrome 1055
Duchenne muscular dystrophy 303, 312, 1542
Duct ectasia 1367
Ductal carcinoma of breast 1385
Ductal epithelial hyperplasia of fibrocytic disease 1369
Ductus arteriosus 834
Duodenal atresia 997
Duodenal peptic ulcer 972
Duplication of small intestine 987
Durck's granuloma 108
D-Xylose test in malabsorption 1039
Dyserythropoiesis 561
Dysfunctional leukocytes 38
Dysfunctional uterine bleeding 1309
Dysgerminoma 1334
Dysmegakaryopoiesis 561
Dysmenorrhea 1309
Dysmyelopoiesis 561
Dysparaproteinemias and uremia 607
Dysphagia 959
Dysplasia 12, 320
Dysplasia in bronchial epithelium 13
Dysplasia liver 1116
Dysplastic nevus 1570
Dysplastic proliferations 343
Dystrophic calcification 32, 42, 433
Dystrophin gene 312, 1543

E

E selectins 126
Early gastric carcinoma 979
Eaton-Lambert syndrome 241, 243
E-Cadherins 1382
Ecchymosis 137
Echinococcus granulosus 454, 1079
Echocardiography two-dimensional 797
Ectopic kidneys 1229
Ectopic pregnancy 1307
Ectopic thyroid tissue 1449
Eczematous dermatitis 1556
Edible shellfish 1065
EDNRB gene 1003
EDTA (ethylene diamine tetra acetic acid) 476

Edward's syndrome (trisomy 18) 299
Effacement of visceral epithelial foot processes 1175
Efferocytosis 36
Ehlers-Danlos syndrome 302, 305, 608, 757
Electrocardiogram 805
Electrocardiogram (12 leads) in AMI 795
Electron dense immune complex deposits 1205
Electron microscopy (EM) 414, 688–690
    comparison of light and electron microscope 689
    scanning electron microscopy 688
    transmission electron microscopy 688
Electrophoresis 734–737
    cellular acetate electrophoresis 725
    citrate agar electrophoresis 726
    gel electrophoresis 737
Elephantiasis 455
ELISA (enzyme-linked immunosorbent assay) 237, 721–724
Emboli from tumors 160
Embolism 156
Embryonal carcinoma 1263, 1335
Embryonal rhabdomyosarcoma 1532
Embryonic stem cells 112
Emery-Dreifuss muscular dystrophy 1545
Emigration 60
Emphysema 876, 877, 879
Empty-sella syndrome 1469
Empyema 928
Empyema gallbladder 1127, 1135
Encephalitis 1588
Enchondromatosis 1496
End stage renal disease 1198
Endocarditis 802, 811
Endocarditis in intravenous drug abuse 815
Endocarditis in prosthetic valves 815
Endocarditis in rheumatic heart disease 816
Endocarditis of carcinoid syndrome 817
Endocervical curetting 1305
Endocervical polyp 1298
Endocrine associated amyloidosis 277
Endocrine pancreas 1409
Endocrine signaling 119
Endodermal sinus tumor 1266
Endogenous antigens 189
Endogenous melanin 933
Endogenous pigmentation 933
Endometrial hyperplasia 10, 1310, 1311
Endometrial stromal tumor 1318
Endometrioid adenocarcinoma 1330
Endometriosis 1313
Endometriosis (chocolate cysts) 1349
Endometritis 1310
Endoparasites induced carcinogenesis 390
Endophytic papilloma 839
Endoscopic retrograde cholangiography (ERCP) 1137
Endostatin 335
Endothelial adhesion molecule 62
    CD4 62
    E selectin 62

    GlyCam-1 62
    PECAM (CD31) 62
    P selectin 62
    VCAM-1 (Ig family) 62
Endotoxic shock 171
Entamoeba histolytica 454
Enterobius vermicularis 455
Enterochromaffin cells 999
Enzymatic glycosylation mechanism 1419
Enzyme-linked immunosorbent assay (ELISA) 237, 721–724
Eosinophilia 535
Eosinophilic chemotactic factor-A (ECF-A) 235
Eosinophilic cystitis 1247
Eosinophilic gastroenteritis 991
Eosinophilic granuloma 592, 897, 1504
Eosinophilic myocarditis 807
Eosinophilic peritonitis 1034
Eosinophilic pneumonia 897
Eosinophils 534
Ependymal cells 1581
Ependymomas 1601
Epidermal growth factor (EGF) 116, 753
Epidermal growth factor (EGF) receptors 351
Epidermal inclusion cyst 1577
Epidermis 1550
Epidermis stem cells 113
Epidermoid carcinoma 1033
Epidermophyton 1561
Epidural hematoma 1615
Epidural space 1582
Epigenetic changes 377
Epiphrenic diverticulum 962
Epispadias 1283
Epistasis 289
Epithelial mucins 925
Epithelial-mesenchymal transition (EMT) 393
Epithelioid granulomas 431
Epithelioid sarcoma 1538
Epsilon aminocaproic acid (EACA) 614
Epstein-Barr virus 538
Epstein-Barr virus associated cancers 389
Equine gait in hemophilia 612
ER and Her2 neu negative molecular pathway in breast carcinoma 1384
ERBB2 (Her2 neu) oncogene 1325, 1381
ERCP (endoscopic retrograde cholangiography) 1137
Erythema 137
Erythema marginatum 805
Erythema multiforme 933, 1564
Erythematous macule 1557
Erythroblastosis fetalis 240
Erythroplasia of Queyrat 1282
Erythropoiesis 464
Erythropoietin 462, 1153
Erythropoietin secreting tumors 464
    cerebral hemangioblastoma 464
    hepatocellular carcinoma 464

Index

leiomyoma 464
renal cell carcinoma 464
Esophageal diverticulum 962
Esophageal dysmotility 262
Esophageal stricture 963
Esophageal varices 767, 963, 1088
Essential hypertension 773
Essential thrombocythemia 571
Essential thrombocytosis 562
ESWL (extracorporeal shock wave lithotripsy) 1221
Etiology of large hepatic vein thrombosis 1111
Etiopathogenesis 616
Euglin lysis time 616
Euglobulin lysis test 625
Evasion of apoptosis of cancer 370
Evasion of immune surveillance in cancer 395
Evolution of cervical carcinoma 1302, 1303
Ewing's sarcoma/primitive neuroectodermal tumors (PNET) 376, 1495
Exchange of gases 858
Executioner caspases 36
Exfoliative cytology 413, 1305
Exocrine glands atrophy 7
Exocrine tumors 1145
Exophthalmos 1434
Exophytic carcinomas of gastric carcinoma 979
Exophytic papillomas of nasal cavity 838
Expansion of myocardial infarct area in AMI 795
Expansion of trinucleotide repeat 289
Expiratory reserve volume 860
Exposure to chemicals 908
Exposure to ionizing radiation 908
Exstrophy of urinary bladder 1247
External hemorrhoids 1031, 1089
External hydrocephalus 1619
Extracellular accumulations 47
Extracorporeal shock wave lithotripsy (ESWL) 1221
Extrahepatic jaundice 1058
Extramammary Paget's disease of vulva 1289
Extranodal marginal zone B cell lymphoma 390, 663, 671
Extranodal NK cell/T cell lymphoma 675
Extrapulmonary tuberculosis 437
Extravascular RBCs destruction 497
Extrinsic (death receptor) pathway 35
Extrinsic pathway of coagulation 143
Exudate 57, 166
Exudative diarrhea 993
Exudative effusions 928
Exudative pharyngitis 934

F

11β-hydroxylase gene 774
24 hours fecal fat test in malabsorption syndrome 1039
FAB classification of leukemias 540
Fabry disease 303, 312, 1162
Facial clefts 932
Facioscapulohumeral muscular dystrophy 1545
Factor IX (high purity) 635
Factor IX concentrate 637
Factor V 142
Factor V Leiden 148, 150, 619
Factor VII 635
Factor VIII (antihemophilic globulin) 610
Factor VIII and VWF synthesis 610
Factor VIII assay 613
Factor VIII concentrate 636
Factor XI 635
Factors influencing infarction 160
Failure of engraftment 595
Familial adenomatous polyposis (FAP) 302, 342, 978, 1021
Familial amyloidosis 277
Familial glomerulopathy 1162
Familial hypercholesterolemia 302, 304
Familial hyperlipidemia 750
Familial medullary carcinoma of thyroid 1445
Fanconi anemia 374, 528, 541
Fanconi's syndrome 1216
Farmer's lung 244
Fasciola hepatica 391
Fasting blood glucose level 1412
Fat embolism 157, 158, 1615
Fat embolism syndrome 902
Fat necrosis 26, 29, 1364
Fat necrosis of breast 1364
Fat stains 1097, 1201
Fate of thrombus 155
Fat-soluble vitamins 423, 424
Fatty change liver (steatosis) 17, 1095, 1424, 1844
Fatty cysts liver 1097
Fatty streaks 743
FDP D-dimer 623
Febrile non-hemolytic transfusion reactions 639
Feces examination 1038
Felty syndrome 1519
Female genital system 1285
Female pseudohermaphrodite 312
Fenton reaction 22
Fernandez reaction 442
Ferritin 25, 483
Fetal alcohol syndrome 1619
Fetal hemoglobin 507
FGF3 (fibroblast growth factor 3) 1251, 1381
Fiberoptic bronchoscopy 925
Fibrillary deposit 1205
Fibrillin 608
Fibrin cap in glomeruli 1183, 1421
Fibrin generation 599
Fibrin stabilizing factor 599
Fibrinogen 63, 142, 556
Fibrinogen degradation product (FDP D-dimer) 195, 556, 623
Fibrinoid necrosis 26, 31, 743, 776, 1224
Henoch-Schönlein purpura 31
lupus erythematosus 31
polyarteritis nodosa 31
malignant hypertension 31
Fibrinolysin gene 148
Fibrinolytic system 74, 600
Fibrinous inflammation 71
Fibrinous or serofibrinous pericarditis 779, 791, 323
Fibroadenoma—breast 1370
Fibroblast growth factor (FGF) 99, 196, 334, 350, 753
Fibroblast growth factor 3 (FGF3) 1251, 1381
Fibroblastic growth factor-β 117
Fibroblasts 1159, 1553
Fibrocongestive splenomegaly 678
Fibroepithelial polyp 1577
Fibrohistiocytic tumors 1532
Fibrolamellar variant of hepatocellular carcinoma 1120
Fibroma 1342
Fibroma group lesions 956
Fibromatosis colli 1529
Fibronectin 63, 123, 129, 195, 1159
Fibrosarcoma 1507, 1531
Fibrosis of peritoneum 1034
Fibrous (fibroblastic) meningioma 1607
Fibrous dysplasia 956, 1511
Fibrous dysplasia of bone 933
Fibrovascular polyps 964
FIGLU test 493
Firm adhesion 61
First line of host defense 182
FISH and Mc FISH techniques 314
FISH probes and probe development 718
FISH procedure 716
Fistulous tract 1013
Fite stain 445
Fixatives 691
FLAER (fluorescent aerolysin) test 522
Flapping tremors in liver failure 1091
Flat mucosal lesions 979
Flexible sigmoidoscopy 1037
Flow cytometry 315, 415, 501, 522, 527, 579, 705
Fluorescein 698
Fluorescence in situ hybridization (FISH) 314, 716, 719
Fluorescent like stains 440
Fluorescent spot test 516
Fluorescent stains (thioflavin-T, thioflavin-S) 281
Focal glomerulonephritis 1163
Focal liver necrosis 1045
Focal nodular hyperplasia liver 1116
Focal proliferative glomerulonephritis 1162
Focal segmental glomerulosclerosis 1162, 1175
Folic acid 429, 487
Folic acid in DNA synthesis 490

Follicular carcinoma of thyroid 1443
Follicular center cell lymphoma 376
Follicular cysts 1346
Follicular lymphoma 663, 668, 670
Food poisoning 992
Foramen of Luschka and Magendie 1582
Forbers-Cori disease 309
Fordyce's granules 933
Foreign body granuloma 106
Formaldehyde 691, 692
Formation of ABH antigen 627
Formulated peptides 63
Fractional curettage 1305
Fragile X syndrome 289, 303
Frameshift mutations 288
Freckle (ephelis) 1569
Free radical injury 48
Fresh frozen plasma 635, 636
Friedler's myocarditis 807
Friedreich ataxia 809
Frontal bossing in rickets 425
Frozen section technique 414, 687, 688, 1405
Frustrated (regurgitated) phagocytosis 69
Fulminant acute hepatitis with massive hepatic necrosis 1071
Fulminant hepatitis 1066
Fulminant liver necrosis 1046
Fulminant myocarditis 807
Function of insulin 1411
Functional (acalculus) gallbladder disease 1132
Functional residual capacity 860
Functional zones of liver acinus (lobule) 1041
Functions of placenta 1286
Fungal infections 838
Fungal meningitis 1587
Fungal pneumonias 862
Fungal sinusitis 838
Fusiform aneurysm 755

G

G6PD deficiency 291, 303, 514
Galactokinase deficiency 309
Galectin 3 1382, 1400, 1406
Gallbladder 1126
Gallstone ileus 997
Gallstones 1130
Gallstones in sickle cell disease 512
Gamma irradiated red blood cells 635
Gamna-gandy bodies 137, 678, 829
Ganglioneuroma 1610
Gangrene 31
Gangrenous inflammation 73
Gangrenous necrosis 26, 30
Gardner's syndrome 1021
Gardnerella vaginalis 1292
Gas gangrene 31
Gastric adenocarcinoma 976, 981
Gastric adenocarcinoma—intestinal types 979

Gastric carcinoma (linitis plastica variant) 332
Gastric lavage 439
Gastric MALT lymphoma 982
Gastric peptic ulcer 71, 972
Gastrinoma 1149
Gastroesophageal reflux disease (GERD) 960
Gastrointestinal stromal tumors (GIST) 984, 1001
Gastrointestinal tract bleeding 612
Gaucher's cells 680, 1106
Gaucher's disease 307, 480, 589, 680, 1106
GBM replication 1205
GBM thickening 1205
Gel electrophoresis 737
Gene amplification 375
Gene mutation 288, 515
Generalized lymphadenopathy 644
Genetic code 285
Genetic predisposition 798
Genetic variations 291
Genetics terminology 283
Genitourinary system bleeding 612
Genomic stability 374
Germ cell tumors 1334
Germinoma 1609
Gestational choriocarcinoma 1352
Gestational diabetes 422
Gestational diabetes mellitus 422, 1355, 1417
Gestational trophoblastic tumors 1349
GFAP (glial fibrillary acidic protein) 1361
Ghon's focus 432, 873
Giant Aschoff's bodies in rheumatic fever 801
Giant cell tumor (osteoclastoma) of bone 326, 1501, 1502
Giant cell tumor of soft tissue 1532
Giant cells seen in bone tumors and tumor-like conditions 1503
Giardiasis 454, 994
Giemsa stain 477
Gilbert's syndrome 1053
Gingival cyst 952
Glandular metaplasia 343
Glandular odontogenic cyst 952
Glanzmann disease (thrombasthenia) 142, 622
Glaucoma 1423
Gleason system of grading of prostatic carcinoma 1280
Glial fibrillary acidic protein (GFAP) 1361, 1375, 1406
Glioblastoma multiforme 1599
Glisson's capsule 1046
Global glomerulonephritis 1162, 1163
Globin chain electrophoresis 527
Globulomaxillary cyst 952
Glomangioma 770
Glomerular basement membrane (GBM) 1158, 1205

Glomerular capillaries 1157
Glomerular filtrate rate (GFR) 1160
Glomerular filtration pressure 1161
Glomerular permeability barriers 1160
Glomerulonephritis 1164
Glomerulus 1157
Glomus tumors 1536
Glucagonoma 1148
Glucocerebrosidase 680
Glucocorticoid-remediable aldosteronism 774, 1460
Glucocorticoids 85, 94
Glucose tolerance test 1425
Glucuronyl transferase 1051
Glutamyltranspeptidase 1048
Glutaraldehyde 692
Glutathione peroxidase (GPX) 25
Glycocalyx 598
Glycogen storage disease 37, 46, 302, 309, 1105
Glycoprotein IIb/IIIa 598
Glycosaminoglycans 124, 127, 167
Glycosylated hemoglobin (HbA1c) 751, 1425
GNAS1 gene 1512
Goblet cell carcinoid 999
Goiter 1436
Gomori methenamine stain 454, 1080
Gonadal dysgenesis 1325
Gonadoblastoma 1344
Gonococcal arthritis 1523
Good immunogens 189
Goodpasture's syndrome 240, 256, 264, 637, 897, 1194
Gouty arthritis 1521
Gouty tophus 1522
Grades of NHL 659
Grading and staging 402, 1398
Graft rejection 247
Graft-versus-host disease (GVHD) 269, 593
Grain leather-like appearance— kidney 1223
Granular cell tumor 967
Granular lumpy bumpy deposits in glomeruli 1205
Granulation tissue 102
Granuloma formation 105
 breakdown of granuloma 105
 maintenance of granuloma 105
Granuloma inguinale 1287
Granuloma pyogenicum 937, 1578
Granulomatous cervicitis 1298
Granulomatous cystitis 1247
Granulomatous inflammation 103, 248, 249, 680
Granulomatous liver abscess 1078
Granulomatous lymphadenitis 642
Granulomatous mastitis 1365
Granulomatous orchitis 1273
Granulomatous prostatitis 1277
Granulomatous salpingitis 1306
Granulomatous serositis 1034

Index

Granulomatous T cell-mediated hypersensitivity reactions 250
Granulosa cell tumor of ovary 1341
Granzyme B protease 36
Graves' disease 241, 242, 255, 264, 1433
Grenza zone 444
Grocott's methenamine silver stain 838
Growth factors 116
Growth hormone insensitivity (Laron syndrome) 1469
Guillain-Barré syndrome 249, 250, 637, 1617
Gumma syphilis 1589
Gummatous necrosis 31
Gut associated lymphoid tissue (GALT) 181
Gynecomastia 1047, 1407

H

Haber-Weiss reaction 22
Hairy cell leukemia 577, 662, 672
Hairy cells 578
Hallmarks of cancer 345
Halogenase 1427
Ham's test 522
Hamartoma 331
Hamartomatous polyps 976
Hamazaki-Weissenberg bodies 42
HAMP gene 482
Hand and foot syndrome in sickle cell 511
Hand-Schüller-Christian disease 591, 1503
Happy puppet (Angelman) syndrome 292
Hapten 189
Haptoglobin 498, 524
Harelip 932
Harrison's groove in rickets 425
Hartnup disease 428, 1216
Hashimoto's thyroiditis 104, 255, 1427
Hassall corpuscles in thymus 682
HbA1c (glycated hemoglobin) 1412
HbE thalassemia 484
HBeAg 1069
HbH disease 484
HBV-DNA 1069
Head injuries 1615
Healing by primary intention 131
Healing of bone fractures 121
Heart anatomy and physiology 782
Heart failure 136, 827
Heart failure cells 136
Heat shock protein 27, 1400, 1406
Heinz bodies in RBCs 479, 480, 515
Helicobacter pylori 390, 968
Helicobacter pylori tests 1039
Helly's fluid fixative 692
Helmet cells 480
Hemangioblastoma 844, 1609
Hemangioendothelioma 771, 1115
Hemangioma 1114, 1540, 1575
Hemangiopericytoma 771
Hemarthrosis 138, 612, 615
Hematemesis 138
Hematin pigment 41

Hematobilia 138
Hematocele 1275
Hematocephalus 138
Hematochezia 138
Hematocrit values 474
Hematogenous spread of cancer 396
Hematological findings in AML (M3) 556
Hematological findings of CLL 575
Hematological findings of CML 565
Hematoma 138
Hematopoiesis 459, 496
Hematopoietic CD34+ stem cells infusion 594
Hematopoietic growth factors 462
Hematopoietic microenvironment 461, 462
Hematopoietic stem cell transplantation 592
Hematopoietic stem cells (HSCs) 112, 461, 533, 539, 592
Hematoxylin and eosin stain 694, 1201
Hemifacial hypertrophy 933
Hemochromatosis 41, 933, 1100
Hemochromatosis induced cirrhosis 1082
Hemodialysis 1201
Hemodialysis associated amyloidosis 277
Hemoglobin C inclusions 479
Hemoglobin E disorders 514
Hemoglobin electrophoresis 507, 513, 525, 526, 734
Hemoglobin H inclusions 479, 508
Hemoglobin S 291
Hemoglobin synthesis 475, 476, 524
Hemoglobinemia 498
Hemoglobinuria 498
Hemolytic anemia 240, 495
Hemolytic disease of newborn 240, 519
Hemolytic jaundice 40, 495, 1058
Hemolytic transfusion reaction 521, 638
Hemolytic uremic syndrome 523, 604, 1195
Hemopericardium 138, 822
Hemopexin 498, 524
Hemophilia A 303, 609
Hemophilia B 303, 615
Hemophilia with inhibitors 637
Hemoptysis 138
Hemorrhage 137, 138
Hemorrhagic (red) infarct 27, 164
Hemorrhagic cystitis 1247
Hemorrhagic disease of newborn 427, 616
Hemorrhagic inflammation 73
Hemorrhagic lung infarct 901
Hemorrhagic pericarditis 823
Hemorrhoids 1031, 1089
Hemosiderin pigment 40
Hemosiderinuria 498, 524
Hemosiderosis 41, 680
Hemostasis 139
Hemothorax 928
Henoch-Schönlein purpura 607, 766, 1194
Heparin 477
Heparin anticoagulant 477
Heparin induced thrombocytopenia (HIT) syndrome 151, 604

Heparin-like molecules 596
Hepatic encephalopathy 1047, 1090
Hepatic sinusoids 1043
Hepatic vasculature 1041
Hepatitis 1058
Hepatitis A virus (HAV) 1064
Hepatitis B core antigen (HBcAg) 1067
Hepatitis B surface antigen (HBsAg) 1067
Hepatitis B virus (HBV) 1067
Hepatitis B virus associated carcinoma 390
Hepatitis Be antigen (HBeAg) 1067
Hepatitis C virus (HCV) 1071
Hepatitis C virus 389
Hepatitis D virus 1073
Hepatitis E virus 1074
Hepatitis G virus (HGV) 1074
Hepatoblastoma 1122
Hepatocellular adenoma 1113
Hepatocellular carcinoma 464, 1117
Hepatocellular hyperplasia 1116
Hepatocellular jaundice 1058
Hepatocellular necrosis 1061
Hepatocyte growth factor (HGF) 117, 351
Hepatocyte membrane antibody 1049
Hepatocytic embryonic stem cells 112
Hepatomegaly 829
Hepatomegaly due to malaria 1080
Hepatoportal sclerosis 1112
Hepatorenal or von Gierke disease type I 46
Hepatorenal syndrome 1093
Hepatotropic viruses 449, 1058, 1064
Hepatotropic viruses comparison 1076
Hepcidin 482
Her2 neu enriched molecular pathway 1384
Hereditary amyloidosis 277
Hereditary angioneurotic edema 79, 219
Hereditary hemorrhagic telangiectasia 302, 304, 608, 770
Hereditary hyperbilirubinemia 1052
Hereditary hypercoagulable state 148, 619
Hereditary nonpolyposis colorectal cancer (HNPCC) 342, 977, 1022
Hereditary ovalocytosis 501
    band 3 (anion channel) 501
    band 4.1 501
Hereditary sideroblastic anemia 530
Hereditary spherocytosis 302, 304, 499
    ankyrin proteins 500
    band 3 (anionic channel) 500
    band 4.2 proteins (pallidin) 500
    gallstones 500
    jaundice 500
    leg ulcers 500
    spectrin proteins 500
    splenomegaly 500
Hereditary stomatocytosis 502
Hereditary thrombophilia 148, 618
Hermaphroditism 312
Herpes simplex encephalitis 448
Herpes simplex virus 934, 1288, 1560
Herpetic dermatitis 1560

Herring-bone pattern in fibrosarcoma 1508, 1531
Heterologous antigens 190
Heterophilic IgM antibodies 538
Heterotropic gastric mucosa 987
HFE gene 1100, 1103
Hiatus hernia 962
Hibernoma 1527
High grade surface osteosarcoma 1494
High performance liquid chromatography (HPLC) 52, 507, 513, 733, 734
High resolution MRI 797
Highly reactive hydroxyl molecule 68
Hippel-Lindau disease 306
Hirschsprung's disease 1003
Histamine 80, 234, 235
Histiocytic tumors 1503
Histochemical stains 691–697
Histological classification of ovarian tumors 1321
Histological patterns of liver necrosis 1046
Histoplasma capsulatum 452, 472, 868
HIV evasion methods 223
HIV testing for high risk persons 227
HIV vaccines 229
HLA antigens 302
HLA classes (class I and class II) 200
HLA system 264
    Class I HLAs 264
    Class II HLAs 265
    HLA associated diseases 266
    organ transplants 266
HMGA2 1526
Hodgkin's disease 389, 517, 579, 648
Hodgkin's disease—morphologic subtypes 654
Holoprosencephaly 1618
Homar's sign 1355
Homogentisic acid 41
Homologous antigens (ISO-antigens) 190
Hormone induced carcinogenesis 391
Hormone therapy 1407
Hormones and breast development 1360
Horner's syndrome 918
Horseradish peroxidase 698
Horseshoe kidneys 1230
Host defenses 182
Hourglass deformity and pyloric stenosis 975
Howell-Jolly bodies 465, 479, 480, 561
HPV E6/E7 oncogene activity in cancer 365
H-RAS signal-transducing proteins 1251
HTLV 1 (human T-lymphotropic virus type 1) 389
Human chorionic gonadotropin (hCG) 1339
Human factor VIII 635
Human factor VIII (high purity) 635
Human genome 282
Human leukocyte antigen 265
Human papillomavirus 390, 449, 1287, 1301
Humoral immunity 191

Hunter syndrome 303, 311
Huntington disease 289
Huntington's chorea 302
Hurler's syndrome 37, 308
Hutchinson melanotic 1570
Hutchinson-Gilford progeria 49
Hyaline arteriolosclerosis 742, 1183, 1421
Hyaline change 17, 18
Hyaluronidase 799
Hydatid cyst 454, 1078
Hydrocele 1274
Hydrocephalus 1618
Hydrogen peroxide 22
Hydromyelia 1618
Hydronephrosis 1217
Hydropericardium 822
Hydropic change 18
Hydrops fetalis 509
Hydrothorax 169, 928
Hydroxyl radicals 22
Hyperacute graft rejection 267
Hyperaldosteronism 1459
Hypercalcemia 404
Hyperemia 134
Hyperestrinism in women 1093
Hyperhomocystinemia 619, 797
Hyper-IgM syndrome 217
Hyperlipidemia 749
Hyperosmolar hyperglycemia state in DM 1417
Hyperparathyroidism 1453
Hyperplasia 4, 9
Hyperplastic arteriolitis 743
Hyperplastic arteriolosclerosis 776, 1224
Hyperplastic ileocecal tuberculosis 438, 995
Hyperplastic polyps 975, 1017
Hyperplastic (regenerative) polyps 986
Hypersensitivity pneumonitis 868, 897
Hypersensitivity reactions 230–249
    type I hypersensitivity reactions 231
    type II hypersensitivity reactions 237
    type III hypersensitivity reactions 243
    type IV hypersensitivity reactions 245
Hypersensitivity reactions—comparison 230
Hypersplenism 679
Hypertension 772
    benign hypertension 772
    cardiovascular disorders 774
    cardiovascular manifestations 777
    cerebral hemorrhage 777
    CNS disorders 775
    determinants of hypertension 772
    endocrine disorders 774
    essential hypertension 772
    liver manifestations 780
    malignant hypertension 772
    peripheral edema 780
    renal manifestations 780
    renovascular hypertension 774
    retinopathy 777
    role of hormones 774

    secondary hypertension 772
    toxemia of pregnancy 775
Hyperthyroidism 404, 1433
Hypertrophic cardiomyopathy 809
Hypertrophic osteoarthropathy 405, 1523
Hypertrophy 4, 7
Hypertrophy of endoplasmic reticulum 37
Hyperviscosity syndrome 585
Hypervitaminosis D 43
Hypochlorous acid 22
Hypochlorous acid (bleach) 99
Hypoglycemia 404
Hypoplasia 14
Hypoplasia of megakaryocytes 604
Hypoplastic left heart syndrome 835
Hypospadias 1283
Hyposplenism 679
Hypothyroidism 1431
Hypovolemic shock 171, 172
Hypoxia inducible factor (HIF) 92

I

Iatrogenic hypopituitarism 1469
ICAM (intercellular adhesion molecule-1) 752
Idiopathic giant cell myocarditis 807
Idiopathic pulmonary fibrosis 896
Idiopathic thrombocytopenic purpura 602
Idiosyncrasy 1080
IL-1 and TNF-α 117
Ileofemoral venous thrombus 1355
Imaging techniques 805
Immature platelet fraction (IPF) 605
Immature teratoma 1337
Immotile cilia syndrome 38
Immune complex mediated glomerulonephritis 256, 1162
Immune dysfunction in HIV 223
Immunity 178
Immunoassay 527
Immunofluorescence microscopy 261, 703, 704
Immunoglobulin classes 207
    IgA 207
    IgD 207
    IgE 207
    IgG 207
    IgM 207
Immunohistochemistry 415, 698–703
    immunohistochemistry protocol 700, 701
    panel of monoclonal antibodies in common malignancies 701
Immunologic tolerance 250–254
    central tolerance 252
    peripheral tolerance 253
Immunological mediated granulomas 106
Immunophenotyping of chronic lymphoproliferative disorders 576
Immunosuppressive drugs 272
    azathioprine 272
    biological immunosuppression 272

Index

cyclosporine A 272
rapamycin 272
tacrolimus (FK506) 272
Impetigo 1557
In situ anti-glomerular membrane disease 1161
In situ (noninvasive) breast carcinoma 1377
Inactivation of free radicals 25
Inappropriate secretion of antidiuretic hormone 404
Inclusions in red blood cells 479
    basophilic stippling 479
    Cabot's ring 479
    Heinz bodies 479
    hemoglobin C inclusions 479
    hemoglobin H inclusions 479
    Howell-Jolly bodies 479
    siderotic nodules/Pappenheimer bodies 479
Incomplete carcinogens 382
Incomplete hydatidiform mole 1352
Increased cellularity of glomeruli 1201
Increased extracellular material 1201
Increased platelet destruction 601
Increased vascular permeability 56, 211
Indeterminate leprosy 443
Indian childhood cirrhosis 1107
Indications for stem cell transplantation 592
Indirect acting carcinogens 382
Indirect Coombs' test 525
Indirect ELISA 722
Indirect immunofluorescence microscopy 704
Infantile embryonal carcinoma 1266
Infantile Gaucher's disease (type 2) 1106
Infantile polycystic kidney disease 1227
Infarction 160
Infections 595
Infectious mononucleosis 538, 642
Infective endocarditis 811, 813
Infertility 422
Inflammation and infection 836
Inflammatory bowel disease 1007
Inflammatory bowel disease (Crohn's disease) 250
Inflammatory carcinoma 1390
Inflammatory dermatoses terminology and examples 1555
Inflammatory fibroid polyp 976
Inflammatory myopathies 1546
Inflammatory polyps 964, 1018
Infusion of hematopoietic stem cells 594
Ingestion of smoked meat and fish 384
Inguinal hernia 997
Inheritance of monogenic disorders 289
Inherited ataxia-telangiectasia 343, 1379
Inherited cancer syndromes 977
Inhibitors of coagulation 600
Initiator caspases in apoptosis 36
Insertion 288
Insertional mutagenesis 377

Inspiratory reserve volume 860
Insulin receptor substrate molecules 1412
Insulin resistant diabetes mellitus 241, 243
Insulin-like growth factor 117, 422
Insulinoma 1148
INT2 oncogene 1381
Integrin family 59, 62, 126
    $\beta 1$ integrin 126
    $\beta 2$ integrin (LeuCAMs) 126
    $\beta 3$ integrin (cytoadhesions) 126
Integrin receptors 120
Intercellular adhesion molecule-1 (ICAM-1) 752
Interferon-α (IFN-α) 88
Interferon-β (IFN-β) 88
Interferon-γ (IFN-γ) 88
Interleukins 99
Intermediate filaments 38
Internal carotid artery occlusion 1611
Internal hemorrhoids 1032, 1089
Internal hydrocephalus 1619
Interpretation 526
Interstitial emphysema 881
Interstitial pneumonia 862, 866
    gross morphology 867
    hypersensitivity pneumonitis 867
    light microscopy 867
    lymphocytic interstitial pneumonia 867
    mycoplasma pneumoniae 867
    viral pneumonias 867
Intestinal epithelium stem cells 114
Intestinal hemorrhagic infarct 164
Intestinal intussusception 997
Intestinal tuberculosis 438
Intestinal type gastric adenocarcinoma 979
Intracanalicular pattern in fibroadenoma 1371
Intracellular accumulations 44
Intracellular microbial killing 6, 68
Intracoronary stenting 787
Intracranial compartments 1582
Intraductal papilloma 1374
Intramembranous deposits in glomeruli 1203, 1204
Intrathoracic manifestations of bronchial carcinoma 913
Intrauterine toxoplasma infection 42
Intravascular RBCs destruction 498
    plasma haptoglobin level 498
    plasma hemoglobinemia 498
    hemoglobinuria 498
    hemosiderinuria 498
    plasma hemopexin 498
    plasma methemalbumin 498
Intraventricular space 1582
Intrinsic factor 490
Intrinsic mitochondrial pathway 35
Intrinsic pathway of coagulation 143
Invasion and metastases 326, 392
Invasive breast carcinoma 1378
Invasive carcinoma of penis 1282

Invasive ductal carcinoma breast 1385, 1387, 1408
Invasive hydatidiform mole 1352
Invasive lobular carcinoma 1386
Invasive micropapillary breast carcinoma 1393
Invasive squamous cell carcinoma 1567
Invasive urothelial neoplasms 1250
Involucrum formation in osteomyelitis 1477
Iron deficiency anemia 483, 484, 486
Iron metabolism 481, 482
Irregular (fluffy) deposits in glomeruli 1205
Irregular emphysema lung 879, 880
Irreversible cell injury 15, 18
Ischemic infarct 27
Ischemic/reperfusion injury 15
Islet β cells hyperplasia of the pancreas 10
Islet cell tumors 1148
Isochromosome formation 296
Isoelectric focusing (IEF) 527
Isolated gonadotropin deficiency 1469
Isolated IgA deficiency 217
Ito cells in liver 1043

J

JAK/STAT RAS signal transduction protein pathway 356
JAK2 mutation 571
Janeway's lesions in acute bacterial endocarditis 814
Jaundice 1050
Jaundice—differential diagnosis 1057
Jaw lesions 950
Jenner's stain 477
Jensen's score 1255
Jones diagnostic criteria in rheumatic fever 801, 805
Jones methenamine silver impregnation stain 1201
Jugular venous pressure 829
Junctional nevus 1569
Juvenile (aggressive) ossifying fibroma 956
Juvenile adenoma 1376
Juvenile coli 1022
Juvenile Gaucher's disease (type 3) 1106
Juvenile hypertrophy of the left breast 1401
Juvenile myelomonocytic leukemia 561
Juvenile onset insulin-dependent type 1 diabetes mellitus 1415
Juvenile papillomatosis breast (Swiss cheese disease) 1373
Juxtacrine signaling 119
Juxtaglomerular apparatus 1151
Juxtaglomerular cells 1151

K

Kallikrein (kinin) 63, 74
Kallmann syndrome 1469
Kaposi sarcoma 771, 936, 1541

Kartagener's syndrome 38, 837
Karyolysis 26
Karyorrhexis 26
Karyotyping 314, 315
Karyotyping techniques 314
Kawasaki disease 764
Kayser-Fleischer ring eye 1083, 1103
Keloid 1529, 1578
Keratinization 1552
Keratoacanthoma 1566
Keratomalacia 425
Ketoacidosis 1415
Kidney infarct 163
Kikuchi disease 643
Killed vaccine 211
Killing of cancer cells 247
Kimmelsteil-Wilson disease in diabetes nephropathy 1421
Kimura's disease 643
Kininogenase 235
KIT ligand receptors 352
KIT mutations 1001
Kleihauer-Betke test (acid elution test) 527
Klinefelter's syndrome 299, 541
Köhler bone disease 1514
K-RAS signal-transducing proteins 1145
Kreberg's stain 925
Krukenberg's tumor of ovaries 400, 981, 1323
Kupffer cells 1043, 1061, 1106
Kwashiorkor 418

L

L selectin (CD62L) 62, 126
Labile cells 111
Laboratory diagnosis of AML 553
Laboratory testing in HIV 227
Lack of costimulatory signal to T cells 254
Lactalbumin 1406
Lactate dehydrogenase (LDH) 796
Lactating adenoma 1375
Lactiferous ducts and sinuses 1362
Lactoferritin 25, 69
Lactotrope adenoma (prolactinoma) 1471
Lacunar type Reed-Sternberg cells 651
Lambert-Eaton syndrome 405, 1547
Laminar blood flow 597
Laminin 124, 129, 1158
Langerhans' cell histiocytosis 591
Langerhans' cells (dendritic cells) 198, 1552
Langerhans' cells of the skin 198
Langhans' giant cells 438
Lardaceous spleen in amyloidosis 47, 279
Large bowel infarction 1015
Large cell carcinoma lung 921
Large regenerative nodules liver 1116
Large-sized vessel vasculitis 1225
Laron syndrome 1469
Laryngeal edema 79
Laryngeal swab 439
Laryngeal tuberculosis 439

Larynx lesions 856
Lateral periodontal cyst 951
LE cell phenomenon 261
Lectins 126
Left heart failure 139, 827, 830
Left ventricular hypertrophy 829
Left-sided colorectal cancer 1027
Leg ulcers in sickle cell disease 512
Leg vein thrombosis 793
Legg-Calvé-Perthes disease 1514
Leiomyoma 324, 464, 966, 1319, 1535
Leiomyosarcoma 329, 1295, 1320, 1535
Leishman stain 477
Leishmania donovani bodies 472
Leishmaniasis 455, 472
Lentigo maligna melanoma 1570
Lentigo simplex 1569
Lepromatous leprosy 443, 444
Lepromin test 442
Leprosy 440
Leptin 420
Leptocytes 480
Leptomeningeal venulitis 1585
Lesch-Nyhan syndrome 312
Letterer-Siwe disease 1503
Leukemia 539
Leukemoid reaction 95
Leukemoid reactions 569
Leukocyte adhesion 211
Leukocyte adhesion receptors 62
Leukocyte chemotaxis 211
Leukocyte reduced red blood cells 635
Leukocyte transmigration 211
Leukocytes induced injury 69
Leukocytes reduced blood component 636
Leukocytosis 95
Leukoplakia 937
Leukoplakia of vulva 1288
Leukopoiesis 466, 533
Leukotrienes (LTC4, LTD4 and LTE4) 83, 84, 99, 196, 235
Leydig (interstitial) cell tumor 1269
Libman-Sacks endocarditis in SLE 815
Lichen planus 933, 1565
Lichen sclerosis 1291
Licorice 774
Liddle syndrome 774
Li-Fraumeni syndrome 978, 1379
Light chain cast nephropathy in multiple myeloma 1215
Limb-girdle dystrophy 1545
Limitations of microarray analysis 715
Limiting plates of liver 1041
Lineage markers of AML analyzing on flow cytometry 553
Lingual thyroid 1449
Linitis plastica variant 332
Lipid deposition 20
Lipid peroxidation 23
Lipoarabinomannan 431
Lipofuscin pigment 41
Lipogranulomas 1365

Lipoidoses 302
Lipoma 1526
Lipooxygenase pathway 83
Liposarcoma 1527
Lipoxins (LXA4, LXB4) 84
Liquefactive necrosis 26, 27, 28
Liquefactive necrosis in brain 28
Liquefactive necrosis in lungs 28
Lissencephaly 1618
Lithopodion 42
Live vaccines 211
Liver abscess 1077
Liver acinus (lobule) 1041, 1061
Liver amyloidosis 47
Liver cell necrosis 1061
Liver metastases 1124
Liver necrosis—histological patterns 1046
Liver regeneration 121
Liver stem cells 113
Lobar pneumonia 512, 862, 863, 867
    congestion 863
    grey hepatization 865
    organization (carnification) 865
    pathogenesis 863
    red hepatization 863
    resolution 865
    risk factors 863
Lobular carcinoma breast 1385
Lobular carcinoma *in situ* (LCIS) 1386
Lobular disarray 1061
Local scleroderma 261
Localized amyloidosis 277
Localized lymphadenopathy 644
Localized reaction 243
Localized tenosynovial giant cell tumor 1532
Locally malignant tumors 326
Location of stem cells 113
    canals of Hering 113
    hair follicle bulge 113
    hematopoietic stem cells 113
    marrow stem cells 113
    satellite cells 113
    subventricular zone (SVZ) dentate nuclei 113
Locus specific identifier (LSI) probes 719
Long noncoding RNA 288
Looser's zones 1480
Low grade central osteosarcoma 1490, 1493
Lowenstein-Jensen culture medium 440
Ludwig angina 934
Lumpectomy 1407
Lumpy bumpy deposits in glomeruli 1204
Lung abscess 869
Lung capacities 859
Lung consolidation 435
Lung consolidation in tuberculosis 874
Lung tumors 906
Lung volumes and capacities 860
Lungs 857
Lupoid hepatitis 1075
Lupus anticoagulant 620

Lupus anticoagulant syndrome 150
Lupus nephritis 1185
Lyme disease 1523
Lymph nodes 182, 641
Lymphangiectasia 991
Lymphangioma 1541
Lymphangioma liver 1115
Lymphatic spread 396
Lymphatic system 769
Lymphedema 167, 769
Lymphoblast 552
Lymphoblastic leukemia 568
Lymphocyte-depletion variant of Hodgkin's disease 655
Lymphocyte-rich variant of Hodgkin's disease 654
Lymphocytes 534
Lymphocytic-histiocytic Reed-Sternberg cells 651
Lymphocytopenia 536
Lymphocytosis 534, 535
   brucellosis 535
   syphilis 535
   tuberculosis 535
Lymphogranuloma venereum 1287
Lymphoid hyperplasia 642
Lymphoid organs 181
   bone marrow 181
   gut associated lymphoid tissue (GALT) in Peyer's patches 181
   lymph nodes 181
   mucosa associated lymphoid tissue (MALT) 181
   skin associated lymphoid tissue (SALT) 181
   spleen 181
   thymus gland 181
Lymphomatoid granulomatosis 767
Lysosomal dysfunction 37
Lysosomal enzyme 69, 81
Lysosomal hydrolytic enzymes 66
Lysosomal storage disease 307, 1105
LYST gene 93, 220

M

B72.3 monoclonal antibody 925
M spike in multiple myeloma 581
Macronodular cirrhosis 1083
Macrophage chemotactic protein-I (MCP-I) 99, 195
Macrophage inhibitory factor (MIF) 888
Macrophage products 99, 196
Macrovesicular steatosis liver 1096
Macula densa kidney 1151
Magnesium ammonium phosphate stones 1219
Magnetic resonance cholangiopancreatography (MRCP) 1137
Major basic proteins 69
Major diagnostic criteria 801
Major histocompatibility complex 200, 265
Major molecular pathways in evolution of breast carcinoma 1382
Malabsorption syndrome 987
Malacoplakia 1247
Malarial parasite 454, 472
Male hypogonadism 1272
Male impotence 1272
Male infertility 255, 1275
Male pseudohermaphrodite 312, 1274
Male sterility 38
Malignant Brenner tumor 1333
Malignant fibrous histiocytoma 1508
Malignant lymphoid neoplasms 645
Malignant melanoma 1570
Malignant mixed müllerian tumor 1334
Malignant nephrosclerosis 1223, 1224
Malignant peripheral nerve sheath tumor (MPNST) 1540
Malignant phyllodes tumor 1373
Malignant surface epithelial tumors 1324
Malignant tumors 325
Mallory hyaline 38
Mallory's Denk hyaline inclusions 1098
Mallory-Weiss syndrome 963, 1092
Malrotation of small intestine 987
Maltese-cross pattern 1173
Mammaglobin 1406
Mammalian sirtuin system 49
Mannose-binding lectin (MBL-2) 798
Mantle cell lymphoma 663, 670
Mantoux test 870
Marasmus 418
March hemolytic anemia 523
Marfan's syndrome 302, 304, 608, 757
Marginal zone lymphoma 671
Margination of leukocytes 57, 60, 61
Marker chromosome 296
Massive (fulminant) liver necrosis 1046
Massive splenomegaly 1089
Masson's trichrome stain 1201
Mast cells 233, 235
Mature callous formation in bone fracture 121
Mature cystic teratoma of testis 1336
Mature solid teratoma of testis 1337
Mature T cell and NK cell NHL 673
Maturity onset diabetes mellitus of the young (MODY) 1416
May-Grunwald stain 477
May-Grunwald-Giemsa stain 440
May-Hegglin anomaly 468, 537
ME-lectin pathway of complement 210
McArdle syndrome 37, 46, 309
McBurney's point abdomen 1030
McCallum plaque in RHD 803
McCune-Albright syndrome 1511
MDS/myeloproliferative disorders 561
Mean corpuscular hemoglobin (MCH) 474
Mean corpuscular hemoglobin concentration (MCHC) 474
Mean corpuscular volume (MCV) 474
Mechanism of apoptosis 33
Meckel's diverticulum 986
Meconium ileus 997
Median palatal cyst 952
Mediastinal (thymic) large B cell lymphoma 664
Mediterranean fever 277
Medium-sized vessel vasculitis 1225
Medullary breast carcinoma 1390
Medullary carcinoma thyroid 1444–1447
Medullary sponge kidney 1229
Medulloblastoma 1604
Megakaryoblastic crisis in CML 568
Megaloblastic anemia 423, 428, 487, 489
Megaloblastic macrocytic anemia 487
Meigs' syndrome 1342
Melanin pigment 39
Melanocytes 1552
Melanocytic nevus 331, 1569
Melanocytic tumors 1569
Melanoma 843, 1295
Melanoma of sinonasal region 843
Melena 138
Meloxicam drug 85
Membranoproliferative glomerulonephritis 1180
Membranous glomerulonephritis 1177
MEN 1 tumor suppressor gene 343, 369
MEN IIa syndrome (Sipple syndrome) 1463
MEN IIb syndrome 1463
Mendelian traits 303
Ménétrier disease 977, 985
Meningeal tumors 1606
Meningioma 1606, 1607
Meningiomas grade II (atypical meningiomas) 1607
Meningiomas grade III (anaplastic meningioma) 1607
Meningitis 512, 1584–1588
   bacterial meningitis 1584
   tubercular meningitis 1586
   viral meningitis 1587
Meningocele 1617
Meningoepithelial (syncytial) meningioma 1607
Meningomyelocele 1617
Menstrual cycle 1308
Mercaptans 1092
Mercurials 692
Merkel cell carcinoma of skin 1575
Merkel cells in epidermis 1552
Mesangial cells 1150
Mesangial deposits in glomeruli 1204
Mesenteric granulomatous lymphadenitis 1030
Mesothelioma 930
Messenger RNA (mRNA) 286, 288
Metabolic acidosis 1418
Metabolic bone disease 1479
Metachromatic stain 281, 697
Metalloproteinases (MMPs) 99, 129, 196
Metaphase CGH technique 712
Metaphase FISH technique 711

Metaphase fluorescence *in situ* hybridization 711
Metaphyseal fibrous defect (nonossifying fibroma) 1512
Metaplasia 5, 11, 1034
Metaplasia in neoplasm 12
Metaplastic breast carcinoma 1393
Metastases in bones 397
Metastases in brain 399
Metastases in liver 397
Metastases in lungs 397
Metastases in spleen 682
Metastases in testes 1271
Metastasis signature genes 393
Metastasis suppressor genes 393
Metastatic calcification 43, 1454
Methemalbumin 498
Methods for DNA sequences 724
Methyl green pyronine stain 587
Methyl violet (metachromatic stain) 281
Methylene blue stain 515
Methylenetetrahydrofolate gene 148
Microalbuminuria 1160
Microangiopathic hemolytic anemia 523
Microarray analysis 713, 715
Microcolumn chromatography 527
Microglia 1581
Microglia cells 1581
Microinvasion 320
Micronodular cirrhosis 1083
Microorganisms invading bone marrow 472
Microplate method 632
Micro-RNA (miRNA) 287
Micro-RNA in cancer 378
Microscopic polyarteritis 766
Microspherocytes 480
Microsporum 1561
Microtomy 694
Microtubules 38
Microvesicular steatosis 1096
Microvillus inclusion disease 991
Mid-diastolic murmur 819
Middle cerebral artery occlusion 1611
Midzonal necrosis–liver 1045
Migratory polyarthritis in rheumatic fever 801
Migratory thrombophlebitis 404, 1355
Mikulicz syndrome 576
Miliary tuberculosis 436, 875
Milk alkali syndrome 43
Milk fat globule membrane antigen 1406
Milroy disease 769
Minimal change disease of glomeruli 1174
Mirizzi's syndrome 1136
MIRL (membrane inhibitor reactive lysis) 521
Missense gene mutations 288
Mitochondrial dysfunction 21, 37, 1095
Mitochondrial inheritance 290
Mitochondrial myopathies 1546
Mitogenic signaling pathway inhibitors 1251

Mitral valve insufficiency 819
Mitral valve prolapse 820
Mitral valve stenosis 819
Mitsuda reaction in leprosy 442
Mixed cellularity variant of Hodgkin's disease 657
Mixed connective tissue disease 257, 263
Mixed gall calculi 1130
Mixed germ cell tumors 1268, 1340
Mixed germ cell tumors of ovary 1340
Mixed germ cell tumors of testis 1268
Mixed somatotroph–lactotroph adenoma 1473
Mixed teratoma of testis 1265
Mixed tumors of various organs 330
MLH1, MSH2, MSH6, and PMS2 tumor suppressor genes 368
Mode of spread of cancer 579, 652
Modes of cell signaling 119
Modifications of multiplex FISH and SKY 712
Modified radical mastectomy 1407
Molecular carcinogenesis 346
Molecular cytogenetic testing 725
Molecular genetics 574, 580, 581, 591, 910
Molecular genetics in osteosarcomas 1492
Molluscum bodies 448
Molluscum contagiosum 448, 1558
Monckeberg's medial calcific sclerosis 742
Monoclonal antibodies therapy in malignancies 701
Monoclonal antibody-based drugs 208
Monoclonal hypothesis of atherosclerosis 751
Monoclonal property of neoplasia 334
Monocyte chemotactic protein-1 (MCP-1) 196
Monocytes 534
Monocytosis 536
Monomorphic adenoma of salivary gland 945
Mononuclear Reed-Sternberg cells 650
Monosomy 295
Monostotic fibrous dysplasia of bone 1511
Monostotic lesion in Paget's disease of bone 1483
Montelukast 94
Morphological changes in AMI 790
Mosaic antigens 189
Mosaicism 296
MRCP (magnetic resonance cholangio-pancreatography) 1137
Mucicarmine stain 925, 697
Mucin types and their origin 697
Mucinous borderline tumors of ovary 1323, 1329
Mucinous bronchioloalveolar carcinoma 921
Mucinous cystadenocarcinoma of ovary 1329
Mucinous cystadenoma of ovary 1329
Mucinous surface epithelial tumors of ovary 1328

Mucocele 940
Mucocele of appendix 1031
Mucocele of gallbladder 1129, 1135
Mucoepidermoid carcinoma 945
Mucopolysaccharides 302
Mucormycosis 452, 1424
Mucosa associated lymphoid tissue (MALT) 181
Müllerian ducts 1284
Multibacillary (MB) leprosy 441
Multicystic mesothelioma 1035
Multinodular goiter 1438
Multiple endocrine neoplasia 1 (MEN 1) 973, 1149
Multiple myeloma 580, 672, 1504
Multiple myeloma terminology 583
Multiple neuromas 1610
Multiple sclerosis 249, 255, 1616
Multiplex metaphase FISH 712
Multistep carcinogenesis 380
Multisystem autoimmune disorders 257
    dermatomyositis 257
        discoid lupus erythematosus 257
        mixed connective tissue disease 257
        rheumatoid arthritis 257
        scleroderma 257
        Sjögren's syndrome 257
        systemic lupus erythematosus 257
Mumps orchitis 1273
Munro microabscesses 1562
Mural thrombi 793, 794
Mutant ALK receptor 1464
Mutator genes 318
Myasthenia gravis 242, 255, 264, 683, 1546
Mycoplasma pneumonias 862
Myocardial rupture in AMI 792
Myocardial embryonic stem cells 112
Mycobacterium avium intracellulare 437
Mycobacterium lepra bacilli 472
Mycobacterium tubercle bacilli 472, 870
Mycobacterium tuberculosis 28
Mycosis fungoides 676
Mycotic aneurysm 138
Mycotic aneurysms 759
Myelin figures 17
Myeloblast 552
Myeloblastic crisis in chronic myeloid leukemia 568
Myelodysplastic syndrome (MDS) 541, 559
Myelofibrosis 563
Myeloid metaplasia 12
Myeloid sarcoma 558
Myeloma kidney 585, 1505
Myeloperoxidase 543
Myeloperoxidase stain 555
Myeloproliferative diseases 563
    atypical chronic myelogenous leukemia 563
    chronic myelomonocytic leukemia 563
    juvenile myelomonocytic leukemia 563
    MDS/MPN unclassified 563

Index

Myeloproliferative neoplasms 562, 563
    chronic eosinophilic leukemia 563
    chronic myelogenous leukemia 563
    chronic neutrophilic leukemia 563
    essential thrombocythemia 563
    mast cell disease 563
    polycythemia vera (PV) 563
Myocardial infarct 163
Myocardial infarction 149
Myocarditis 806
Myocardium disorders 802
Myometrium 1319
Myotonic dystrophy 289, 302
Myotonic muscular dystrophy 1545
Myotonin protein kinase gene 289
Myxedema 1432
Myxofibrosarcoma 1531
Myxoid liposarcoma 1527
Myxopapillary ependymoma 1602

N

Na^+/K^+ pump 20
Nail disorders 1553
NAP scoring system 566
Nasal adenocarcinoma 844
Nasal plasmacytoma 844
Nasopalatine duct cyst 952
Nasopharyngeal angiofibroma 844
Nasopharyngeal carcinoma 390, 841
Natriuretic peptide B type assay 827, 904
Natural carcinogen 385
Natural killer cells 193, 402, 534
Naxos syndrome 811
Necroptosis 16
Necrosis 26
Negative selection 252
Negri bodies in brain of rabies 1589
Neisseria infections 79
Nelson syndrome 1469
Nemaline myopathy 1546
Neonatal amniotic fluid aspiration syndrome 1355
Neonatal cholestasis 1056
Neonatal hepatitis of unknown etiology 1057
Neonatal hyperbilirubinemia (HDN) 637
Neoplasms of thyroid gland 1439
Neoplastic urothelial lesions 1248
Nephrin molecules 1159
Nephrocalcinosis 1216
Nephrogenic diabetes insipidus 1470
Nephrolithiasis 1218
Nephrolithotomy 1221
Nephrosialidosis 1162
Nephrotic syndrome 1171
NESTROFT test 507
Neural defects 1617
Neural stem cells in brain 113
Neural tumors 1539
Neuregulin gene 1003
Neurilemmocytes 1581

Neurilemmoma 1539, 1608
Neuroaxis 1580
Neuroblastoma 330, 1464
Neurocysticercosis 1589
Neurodermatitis 1557
Neuroectodermal malignancies 330
Neuroendocrine (carcinoid) tumors 999
Neuroendocrine cells 999
Neuroepithelial tumors 1598
Neurofibroma 1539, 1574
Neurofibromatosis 302, 305, 306, 933, 1610
Neurogenic shock 176
Neuroglial cells in CNS 1581
Neuroglial cells in peripheral nervous system 1581
Neurological manifestations in sickle cell disease 512
Neuromuscular abnormalities in lung carcinoma 912
Neuromuscular disturbances 1201
Neuronal cell bodies 1581
Neuronal tumors 1610
Neurons 1581
Neuron-specific enolase (NSE) 843, 925
Neuropeptide Y 420
Neuropeptides (substance P) 91
Neuropil 1581
Neurotensin 1120
Neutral hydrolases 99, 196
Neutropenia (agranulocytosis) 536
Neutrophilia 534
Neutrophils 534
New methylene blue stain 474
Nezelof's syndrome 218
NF1 tumor suppressor gene 362
NF2 tumor suppressor gene 362
NHL-spillover in blood 579
Niacin 428
Niemann-Pick disease 45, 308, 480, 589, 1105
Nil disease 1174
Nipple and areola eczema 1402
Nipple discharge 1362
Nipple retraction 1362, 1387
Nitric oxide 89
Nitroblue tetrazolium (NBT) slide test 68
Nitrosamines 385
N-MYC nuclear regulatory proteins 1464
Nocardiosis 868
Nodal marginal zone lymphoma 671
Nodular fasciitis 1530
Nodular glomerulosclerosis in diabetic nephropathy 1182, 1421
Nodular hidradenoma 1576
Nodular hyperplasia of prostate 1277
Nodular lymphocytic-histiocytic predominant variant HD 657
Nodular melanoma 1572
Nodular regenerative hyperplasia 1112
Nodular sclerosis variant of Hodgkin's disease 656

O

Obesity 419
Obliterative endarteritis 756
Obstructive atelectasis 900
Obstructive hypoventilation syndrome 421
Obstructive jaundice 1134
Obstructive sleep apnea 420
Obstructive uropathy 1217
Occult (hidden) metastases 335
Occult blood 1038
Occupational carcinogens 385
Occupational exposure 908
Ochronosis 1522
Oculopharyngeal muscular dystrophy 1545
Odontogenic carcinoma 955
Odontogenic keratocyst 951
Odontogenic myxoma 954
Odontogenic tumors 952
Odontoma 954
Odynophagia 959
Olfactory neuroblastoma 843
Oligodendrocytes 1581
Oligodendroglial tumors 1601
Oligodendroglioma 1601
Oliguria 1191
Omega-3 fatty acid 85, 94
Oncocytic papillomas 840
Oncocytoma 944
Oncofetal antigens 405
Oncogenes 317
Oncogenesis 317
Onco-micro-RNA (miRNA155, 200, 221) 379
Onco-micro-RNA 379
Open biopsy 925, 1405
Open comedone 1579
Open pneumothorax 898
Opisthorchis viverrini 391
Opportunistic infections in AIDS 223
Opportunistic pulmonary infections 868
Opsoclonus–myoclonus syndrome 405
Opsonin receptors on leukocytes 65
Opsonin receptors on macrophage 195
Opsonization 66, 211
Oral anticoagulants 609
Oral cavity disorders 932, 933
    cleft palate 932
    facial clefts 932
    Fordyce's granules 933
    harelip 932
    hemifacial hypertrophy 933
Oral contraceptives 391
Oral glucose tolerance test (OGTT) 1412
Oral lesions in systemic disorders 933
Orchidometer 1275
Organ transplantation 266
Organohalogen compounds 385
Organs involved 580
Origin 910
Osgood-Schlatter disease 1514
Osler's nodes 814

Osler-Weber-Rendu syndrome 302, 304
Osmoreceptors 1153
Osmotic fragility 501
Osseous metaplasia 11
Osseous metaplasia in myositis ossificans 12
Ossifying fibroma 956
Osteitis deformans 1482
Osteitis fibrosa cystica 1481
Osteoarthritis 423, 1521
Osteoblastic lesions 1510
Osteoblastoma 1489
Osteoblasts 1476
Osteochondroma (exostosis) 1496
Osteoclastic activating factor 582, 583
Osteoclasts 1476
Osteogenesis imperfecta 302, 1513
Osteoid osteoma 1488
Osteolytic lesions 1505, 1510
Osteoma 1488
Osteomalacia 426, 1480
Osteomyelitis in sickle cell disease 512
Osteonecrosis (avascular necrosis) 1514
Osteonectin 129
Osteophytes (bony spurs) 1521
Osteoporosis 1481
Osteosarcoma 329, 1489, 1490
Osteosclerotic myeloma 583
Other blood group systems 630
Other viral infections 934
Otosclerosis 848
Outcome of acute inflammation 69
Outcome of necrosis 32
Ovalocytes 480
Ovarian cysts 1346
Ovarian tumors—histological classification 1321
Overt albuminuria 1160
Oxidant stress 515
Oxidized LDL molecule 754
Oxygen derived free radicals 21, 89
Oxygen-dependent intracellular microbial killing 68
Oxygen-independent microbial killing 69

P

β-pleated sheets of amyloid 273
P selectins 126
p53 tumor suppressor gene mutation 1379
Pacemaker cells of Cajal in GIST 984
Pachygyria 1618
Packed cell volume (PCV) 474
Packed cells transfusion 634
Paget's disease of bone (osteitis deformans) 1482
Paget's disease of breast 1388
Pale (ischemic) infarct 27
Pale infarct undergoing hemorrhagic infarct 164
Palmar erythema 1093
Panacinar emphysema 880
Pancarditis 802

Pancoast tumor of lung 918
Pancreas 1139
Pancreatic amylase 1140
Pancreatic chymotrypsin 1140
Pancreatic duct adenocarcinoma 1145
Pancreatic enzymatic fat necrosis 29
Pancreatic heterotropic rests 986
Pancreatic juice 1140
Pancreatic lipase 1140
Pancreatic trypsin 1140
Pancreatic tumors 1145
Pancreatitis 975, 1140
Pancreatoblastoma 1148
Panel of monoclonal antibodies in common malignancies 701
Papillary breast carcinoma 1392
Papillary carcinoma 1441
Papillary hidradenoma 1288
Papillary necrosis—kidney 1183, 1421
Papillary polypoid (bullous) cystitis 1247
Papillary variant of renal cell carcinoma 1233
Papilloma of various organs 324
Pappenheimer's bodies 479, 480
Para-Bombay blood group 628
Paracrine signaling 118, 119
Paradoxical emboli 158
Paraesophageal hernia 962
Paraffin embedding 694
Parafollicular cells or C cells of thyroid gland 1426
Paraganglioma 855
Paraneoplastic syndrome 402, 684
Paraneoplastic syndromes in lung cancer 912
Paraovarian or paratubal cysts 1348
Paraphimosis 1283
Parasitic encephalitis 1589
Parathormone (PTH) 1452
Parathyroid adenoma 1456
Parathyroid carcinoma 1457
Parietal epithelial cells of Bowman's capsule 1160
Parkinson disease 38
Parosteal osteosarcoma 1490
Paroxysmal cold hemoglobinuria 519
Paroxysmal nocturnal hemoglobinuria 79, 80, 219, 521, 541
Paroxysmal nocturnal hemoglobinuria (PNH)—pathogenesis 521
Partial pressure of gas 859
PAS stain (metachromatic stain) 281, 543, 697, 925, 1201
Passenger mutations 347
Passive immunity 179
Passive venous congestion 134
Patau syndrome (trisomy 13) 299
Patchy atelectasis 900
Patent ductus arteriosus (PDA) 833
Pathogen-associated molecular proteins (PAMPs) 65, 184
Pathological atrophy 6

Pathological calcification 42
Pathological hyperplasia 10
Pathological hypertrophy 7
Pathophysiology of diabetes mellitus 1417
Pavementing of leukocytes 57, 60, 61
PCR (polymerase chain reaction) 3, 15, 440, 724, 1258
Peau d' orange skin 1362, 1402
Pediatric renal cell carcinoma 376
Pedigree construction 313
Peggler-Huet anomaly 468, 537
Peliosis hepatitis 1112
Pelvic bones deformities in rickets 425
Pelvic inflammatory disease (PID) 1296
Pemphigus vulgaris 241, 243, 255, 264, 933, 1562
Peptic ulcer disease 971
Percutaneous transhepatic cholangiography (PTC) 1137
Perforated gallbladder 1135
Perforin 36
Perfusion scintigraphy 797
Pericanalicular pattern of fibroadenoma 1371
Pericardial edema 169
Pericardial effusion 821
Pericarditis 822
Pericarditis complications 804
Pericardium 821
Periductal mastitis 1364
Perihilar adenocarcinomas of extrabiliary duct 1139
Periodic acid–Schiff stain (PAS stain) 543, 697, 925, 1201
Periodontal disease 951
Periorbital puffiness (edema) 1191
Periosteal osteosarcoma 1490, 1494
Peripheral neuropathy (Guillain-Barré syndrome) 250
Peripheral neuropathy 491, 1423
Peripheral tolerance 251, 253
Peripheral vascular disease 748
Periportal area 1041
Periportal necrosis 1045
Periportal piecemeal necrosis 1047
Perisinusoidal endothelial cells 1084
Perisinusoidal stellate cells (Ito cells) 1043
Peritoneal dialysis 1201
Perivascular tumors 1536
Perl's stain 40, 480
Permanent cells in brain, cardiac and skeletal muscle 111
Pernicious anemia 241, 243, 255, 494, 977
Peroxidase enzyme 1427
Peroxidase-antiperoxidase (PAP) method 699
Peroxynitrite 22
Persistence of urachal sinus 1248
Petechial hemorrhages 137
Peutz-Jeghers syndrome 331, 933, 978, 1019
Peyronie disease 1283
Phagocytes 66

Index

Phagocytic receptors 65
Phagocytosis 61, 211
Phagolysosome 66
Pharynx disorders 856
Phases of acute renal failure 1209
Phenylketonuria (PKU) 291, 302, 309
Pheochromocytoma 1462
Philadelphia chromosomal t(9/22) 294, 561, 564, 565
Phimosis 1283
Phlebotomus sandflies 455
Phosphatidyl inositol-3 kinase (PI3k) proteins pathway 355
Phospholipase 20, 968
Photomultiplier tubes 708
PHOX2B gene 1003
Phyllodes tumor of breast 1372
Physiologic atrophy 6
Physiological calcification 42
Physiological hyperplasia 9
Physiological hypertrophy 7
Physiological jaundice 1051
Piecemeal necrosis 1063
PIG-A gene mutation 521
Pigeon-shaped chest in rickets 425
Pigment gallstones 1133
Pigmentation disorders 1569
Pigments 38
Pilocytic astrocytomas 1598
Pilomatrixoma 1576
Pilonidal sinus 1032
Pinealoblastoma 1603
Pink puffers do not tolerate hypoxia 882
Pitocin 1159
Pitting edema 828
Pituitary adenomas 1470
Pituitary gland 1467
PKHD1 gene 1057
Placenta accreta 1357
Placenta increta 1357
Placental abnormal attachments 1356
Placental alkaline phosphatase 1262
Placental site trophoblastic tumor 1353
Plasma 635
Plasma cell leukemia 585
Plasma exchange 637
Plasma products/recombinant concentrates 635
Plasma transfusion 636
Plasmablastic lymphoma 672
Plasmacytoma 844
Plasmacytoma testes 1271
Plasmacytosis 586
Plasmapheresis/plasma exchange 637
Plasminogen 142, 146, 598
Plasminogen activator 394, 600
Plasminogen-plasmin system 147
Platelet activating factor (PAF) 63, 91, 235, 334
Platelet concentrates 635
Platelet count 622

Platelet derived growth factor (PDGF) 63, 99, 116, 142, 195, 196, 350, 597, 753
Platelet derived growth factor (PDGF) receptors 352
Platelet disorders 142, 600, 605
Platelet factor IV 142
Platelet function tests 622
Platelet neutralizing test 620
Platelet products 142
Platelets 141, 597
Platelets adhesion 142, 148, 599, 787
Platelets aggregation 142, 148, 599, 787
Platelets pooling 601
Platelets release reaction 142, 787
Platelets removal 637
Platelets transfusion 636
Platelets' granules 141
Pleomorphic adenoma 942
Pleomorphic liposarcoma 1528
Pleomorphic Reed-Sternberg cells 650
Pleomorphic rhabdomyosarcoma 1534
Pleural effusion 828, 927
Pleural fibrosis 929
Pleuritis 927
Plummer-Vinson syndrome 484
Pneumocystis jiroveci 868
Pneumonias 860, 861, 862
Pneumonias in immunocompromised persons 862
Pneumothorax 898
Point mutation 288, 375
    missense gene mutation 288
    non-missense gene mutation 288
Polarizing light microscope 281, 690, 691
Polarizing microscopy 691
Poliomyelitis 448
Polyanionic-proteoglycans in glomeruli 1159
Polyarteritis nodosa 263, 764
Polychromasia 479
Polycyclic hydrocarbons 384
Polycystic ovaries (Stein-Leventhal syndrome) 1348
Polycythemia 404
Polycythemia vera 570, 571
Polygenic and multifactorial disorders 291
Polymerase chain reaction (PCR) 315, 440, 724, 1258
Polymerized human serum albumin (PHSA) 1068
Polymicrogyria 1618
Polymyositis 262
Polyostotic fibrous dysplasia 1511
Polyostotic lesions 1483
Polyp 324
Polyploidy 295
Polyps in fundal region 976
Pompe disease type II 37, 46, 309
Poor immunogens 189
Porcelain gallbladder 1135
Porcine factor VIII 635
Portal hepatitis 1063

Portal hypertension 1086
Portal tract 1041, 1061
Portosystemic shunts 1088
Positive D-dimer 902
Positive selection 252
Positron emission tomography 924
Post-cricoid webs in iron deficiency anemia 963
Posterior cerebral artery occlusion 1611
Posterior pituitary gland 1467
Postmortem autolysis 31
Postnatal diagnosis 315
Post-necrotic cirrhosis 1082
Post-streptococcal glomerulonephritis 1187
Post-transfusion thrombocytopenia 640
Prader-Willi syndrome 292
PRCC gene 1233
Preauricular sinus 846
Precursor lesions 909
Pregnancy luteoma 1344
Prenatal diagnosis 315, 509
Presbycusis 848
Preservative used in transfusion bags 632
Prevention of transplant rejection 271
Priapism in hematological disorders 512, 1283
Primary aldosteronism 1460
Primary biliary cirrhosis 255, 1107
Primary CNS lymphoma 1609
Primary CNS tumors 1590
Primary complex 432, 872
Primary diabetes mellitus 1414
Primary glomerular diseases 1161
Primary gout 1522
Primary hemochromatosis 41, 1100, 1101
Primary hyperparathyroidism 43, 1453
Primary hypopituitarism 1467
Primary hypothyroidism 1432
Primary immunodeficiency disorders 215
Primary intestinal tuberculosis 994
Primary myelofibrosis 572
Primary neoplasms 830
Primary osteoporosis 1482
Primary other CNS tumors 1590
Primary platelet plug 145
Primary pleural effusion lymphoma 930
Primary pneumothorax 898
Primary pulmonary malignant tumors 907
Primary sclerosing cholangitis 1109
Primary tuberculosis (primary complex) 432, 872, 873
Primary viral myocarditis 807
Primitive neuroectodermal tumors (PNETs) 1603
Prinzmetal angina 784
Proctoscopy 1036
Professional APCs 198
Prognosis of solid tumors 411
Prognostic and predictive factors of breast carcinoma 1397
Prognostic factors of AML (FAB classification) 554

Prognostic factors of synovial sarcoma 1537
Progressive staining 695
Prolactinoma 1471
Proliferative fibrocystic changes 1367
Proliferative glomerulonephritis 1164
Proliferative retinopathy 1423
Prolonged immobilization 43
Prolymphocytic leukemia 662
Proptosis 17
Prostacyclin (PGI$_2$) 83, 84, 596
Prostaglandins 83. 84, 99, 196, 235
Prostate-specific antigen (PSA) 1281
Prostatic adenocarcinoma 1279
Prostatic hyperplasia 10
Prosthetic valve endocarditis 815
Protease (cathepsin D) 20, 968, 1400
Protein C 147, 148, 150, 600, 619
Protein S 147, 148, 150, 600, 619
Protein synthesis 285
Protein–energy malnutrition 417
Proteins associated with podocytes 1159
Proteins in epithelial cells 405
Proteinuria 1173
Proteoglycans 124, 127
Prothrombin 20210 transition 150
Prothrombin complex concentrates 635, 637
Prothrombin G20210A mutation 619
Prothrombin gene 148
Prothrombin time 556, 623, 1050
Prothrombotic factors 140
Prothrombotic properties of endo-
    thelium 139
Proto-oncogenes 317
Prussian blue staining 1101
Pseudoarthrosis 1523
Pseudochylous effusion 928
Pseudogout 1522
Pseudohermaphrodite 312
Pseudohypoparathyroidism 1456
Pseudomembranous colitis 1013
Pseudomembranous inflammation 73
Pseudomyxoma peritonei 1035
Pseudo-obstruction syndrome 1005
Psoriasis 10, 1562
Psoriatic arthritis 1521
PTCH tumor suppressor gene 362
PTEN tumor suppressor gene 363, 1382
Pulmonary alveolar proteinosis (PAP) 898
Pulmonary angiogram 902
Pulmonary artery embolization 1355
Pulmonary edema 169, 903
Pulmonary embolism 157
Pulmonary hamartoma 906
Pulmonary hemorrhagic infarct 164
Pulmonary hypertension 902
Pulmonary manifestations 779
Pulmonary stenosis 821
Pulmonary thromboembolism 157, 900
Pulmonary tuberculosis 432
Pulmonary valve stenosis 821
Pulmonary vascular disorders 900
Pulmonary vasculitis 904

Pulmonary volumes 859
Pure gall calculus 1130
Pure Leydig cell tumor 1343
Pure red cell anemia 529
Pure red cell aplasia (erythroblasto-
    penia) 529
Pure teratoma 1265
Purkinje fibers 782
Purpura 137
Purpura fulminans neonatalis 150
Purulent exudate 823
Purulent or suppurative inflammation 72
Purulent or suppurative pericarditis 823
Pyelonephritis 1209
Pyknosis nucleus 25
Pyogenic bacterial liver abscess 1077
Pyogenic granuloma 770
Pyogenic meningitis—CSF findings 1586
Pyogenic osteomyelitis 1477
Pyothorax 928
Pyothorax effusion lymphoma 931
Pyridoxine 428
Pyruvate kinase deficiency 516

Q

Quinacrine banding technique 314

R

Rabies virus 448
Racemose/cirsoid aneurysm 755
Rachischisis 1618
Radiation carcinogenesis 385
Radiation colitis 1015
Radiation induced interstitial lung
    disease 896
Radiation therapy 1407
Radical hysterectomy (Wertheim's
    hysterectomy) 1305
Radicular cyst 952
Radioactive iodine uptake and thyroid
    imaging 1450
Radioallergosorbent test (RAST) 237
Radiological findings in bone lesions 1515
Radionuclide scan 902, 1441
Radionuclide scanning (99mTc) stannous
    pyrophosphate 797
Ramsay Hunt syndrome 846
Rapamycin immunosuppressive drug 272
Rapidly progressive glomerulonephritis
    (RPGN) 1195
RAS proto-oncogene 353, 1382
Raynaud's phenomenon 262,766
RB tumor suppressor gene 339, 363, 1381
RBCs cast in urine 1191
RBCs fragmentation syndromes 522
Reaction to injury hypothesis 751
Reactive hyperplasia 670
Reactive oxygen species 22
Reciprocal translocation 294
Recombinant factor IX 635

Recombinant factor VIIa 635
Recombinant factor VIII 635
Rectal prolapse 1032
Recurrent infections 79, 219
Recurrent jaundice during pregnancy 1052
Recurrent myocardial infarction 794
Red blood cells 635
Red blood cells removal 637
Red cell indices 474
   hematocrit or packed cell volume
      (PCV) 474
   mean corpuscular hemoglobin
      (MCH) 474
   mean corpuscular hemoglobin
      concentration (MCHC) 474
   mean corpuscular volume (MCV) 474
   red blood cell distribution width
      (RDW) 474
Red infarct 27, 164
Red pulp spleen 677
Reed-Sternberg cells 647, 648
Reed-Sternberg-like cells 651
Refractive index 691
Refractory sprue 990
Regenerative changes 1061
Regressive stain 695
Regulation by suppressive cytokines 254
Regulation of apoptosis 36
Regulation of cell cycle 114
Regurgitation during feeding 69
Reinke crystalloid 1343
Relapsing polychondritis 846
Remodeling of callus formation in bone
    fracture 121
Renal amyloidosis 47
Renal angiomyolipoma 1240
Renal atrophy 7
Renal blood flow 1152
Renal cell carcinoma (RCC) 464, 1233
Renal cell carcinoma—systemic manifesta-
    tions 1237
Renal infarction 1222
Renal lesions in diabetic nephropathy 1421
Renal osteodystrophy 1200, 1481
Renal stones (nephrolithiasis and uro-
    lithiasis) 1218
Renal tubular functional disorders 1216
Renin-angiotensin-aldosterone system
    1153
Repair by fibrosis 32
Repair phase of bone fracture 121
Reperfusion injury in AMI 789
Residual volume 860
Residual volume of urine 1211
Resorption of necrotic tissue 32
Respiratory disorders 859
Respiratory distress syndrome in the
    infants 889
Respiratory system—anatomy 856, 857
Restricrtive cardiomyopathy 811
Restrictive pulmonary diseases 886, 889

Reticulocyte 466
Reticulocyte count 474
Reticuloendothelial cells distribution 97, 98, 194
Reticuloendothelial system 187
Retinoblastoma 330, 1603
Retinoic acid receptor-α (RAR-α) gene 556
Retinoids 25
RET-PTC oncogene 1442
Retroperitoneal hemorrhage 612
Revascularization procedures in AMI 787
Reversible cell injury 15, 17
Reye syndrome 1107
Rh blood group system 628
Rh blood grouping 632
Rh factor incompatibility during pregnancy 630
Rhabdomyolysis 1547
Rheumatic fever and RHD 798
Rheumatoid arthritis 241, 243, 249, 250, 255, 257, 263, 517, 897, 1518
Rheumatoid factor 255, 263
Rhinorrhea 837
Rhinoscleroma 845
Rhinosporidiosis 845
Rhinosporidium seeberi 845
Rhodamine 698
Rhodopsin 424
Riboflavin 428
Ribosomal RNA or rRNA 286
Richardson Grading System 1398
Richter syndrome 576, 665
Rickets 425, 1480
    craniotabes in rickets 425
    deformities of pelvic bones in rickets 425
    frontal bossing in rickets 425
    Harrison's groove in rickets 425
    pigeon-shaped chest in rickets 425
    rachitic rosary in rickets 425
    spine deformity in rickets 425
Riedel's thyroiditis 1430
Right heart failure 827
Right ventricular hypertrophy 830
Right-sided colorectal carcinoma 1027
Ring chromosome 294
Ring sideroblasts 561
Risk factors of AMI 785
RNA oncogenic viruses 387
RNA primase 287
Robertsonian translocation 294
Role of platelets in AMI 787
Rolling of leukocytes 61
Romanowsky stains 477
Rota virus 992
Roth's retinal hemorrhages 814
Rotor's syndrome 1056
Rouleaux formation of RBCs 479
Rugger Jersey appearance 1481
RUNX3 gene promoter 1266
Russell bodies in plasma cells 586
Russell viper venom time test 620

S

S-100 protein 1004, 1361, 1375
SA node in heart 782
Saccharopolyspora rectivirgula 897
Saccular aneurysm 755
Saddle embolus 901
Sago spleen in amyloidosis 47
Salivary gland disorders 938
Salmonella typhi 992
Salmonella typhimurium 992
Salpingitis isthmica nodosa 1307
Sandwich ELISA 723
Saponification 29
Sarcoidosis 896
Sarcoma of various organs 328
Sarcoptes scabiei 1557
Satellite cells in liver 1581
Satellite granuloma 107
Scabies 1557
Scanning electron microscopy (SEM) 688
Schatzki ring 963
Schaumann's bodies 436
Schiller's test 494, 1305
Schiller-Duval bodies in endodermal sinus tumor 1339
Schistosoma haematobium 390
Schistosomiasis liver 1080
Schneiderian sinonasal papillomas 838
Schwann cells 1581
Schwannoma (neurilemmoma) 1539, 1608
Sclerodactyly 262
Scleroderma 255, 257, 261, 897, 962
Sclerosing adenosis 1368
Sclerosing lymphocytic lobulitis 1366
Sclerosing odontogenic carcinoma 955
Sclerotherapy 1088
Scoring system of NAP 566
Scurvy 430, 607, 1483
SDHB and SDHD tumor suppressor genes 365
Sea blue histiocytosis 590
Seborrheic dermatitis 428
Seborrheic keratosis 1565
Second line of host defense 182
Secondary aldosteronism 1460
Secondary biliary cirrhosis 1108
Secondary diabetes mellitus 1414
Secondary glomerular diseases 1162
Secondary gout 1522
Secondary hemochromatosis 41, 1103
Secondary hemostatic plug 145
Secondary hyperparathyroidism 43, 1455
Secondary hypertension 774
Secondary hypothyroidism 1432
Secondary intestinal tuberculosis 994
Secondary messenger systems 1400
Secondary myelofibrosis 573
Secondary neoplasms 830
Secondary osteoporosis 1482
Secondary pneumothorax 899

Secondary polycythemia 571
Secondary pulmonary malignant tumors 922
Secondary thrombocytopenia 603
Secondary tuberculosis 434, 873
Secretory breast carcinoma 1394
Secretory diarrhea 993
Secretory myeloma 583
Seeding/transcoelomic route of carcinomas 400
Segmental glomerulosclerosis 1162, 1163
Selected autoimmune diseases 255
Selectin family 61, 126
    E selectins 61
    L selectins 61
    P selectins 61
Selectins 61, 59, 126, 752
Selection of donor 594
Selective proteinuria 1160
Semen analysis 1275
Seminoma with syncytiotrophoblastic element 1260
Seminoma with yolk sac element 1259
Senile purpura 607
Sentinel lymph node 395, 1396, 1405
Septic (infective) infarcts 162
Septic shock 95, 173
Sequestration crisis 512
Sequestration of antigens 254
Sequestrum formation in osteomyelitis 1477
Serine protease 99, 196
Serofibrinous pericarditis 779, 802, 823
Serotonin 81, 142
Serous borderline tumors of ovary 1323
Serous cystadenocarcinoma of ovary 1328
Serous cystadenoma of ovary 1326
Serous inflammation 71
Serous pericarditis 823
Serous surface epithelial tumors of ovary 1326
Serpentine aneurysm 755
Sertoli cell tumor (androblastoma) of testis 1269
Sertoli-Leydig cell tumor of testis 1343
Serum (reverse) blood grouping 632
Serum alkaline phosphatase 1281
Serum amyloid associated (SAA) level 94
Serum ceruloplasmin 1048
Serum des-gamma carboxyprothrombin 1120
Serum ferritin 486, 1103
Serum fibrinogen 94
Serum iron 486
Serum prostatic acid phosphatase 1281
Serum sickness 243
Serum total iron binding capacity (TIBC) 486
Serum TSH, T4 and T3 levels 1449
Serum α-fetoprotein 1266, 1335
Serum β-microglobulin 586
Sessile serrated adenomas 1021

Seven α-helical transmembrane G-protein coupled receptors 64
Seven transmembrane G-protein coupled receptors 119
Severe acute respiratory syndrome (SARS) 890
Severe biliary colic 1134
Severe combined immune deficiency (SCID) syndrome 218
Sex chromosomal disorders 299
Sex cord stromal tumors of ovary 1340
Sex cord-gonadal stromal tumors of testis 1269
Sézary syndrome 576, 676
Sheehan's syndrome 1356, 1468
Shigella sonnei 992
Shock 170
Sialyl-Lewis X PSGL-1 62
Sickle cell disease 302, 306, 480, 509, 512, 513
Sickle cell nephropathy 1222
Sickle cell thalassemia syndrome 513
   heterozygous (HBS/HBC) disorder 514
   homozygous hemoglobin C disorder 513
Sickling test 480, 513, 524
Sideroblastic anemias 530
Siderotic nodules 479
Sigmoidoscopy 1029
Silicone breast implants 1365
Silicosis 887, 892
Silo filler's disease 897
Silver methenamine stain 1179
Simond's disease 1468
Simon's focus 434
Simple bone cyst 952
Simple bruising 608
Simple cystic endometrial hyperplasia 1311
Simple papillae of kidney 1152
Single cell or group of cells necrosis 1046
Single nucleotide polymorphism (SNP) 291
Sinonasal undifferentiated carcinoma 840
Sinonasal papillomas 838
Sinus histiocytosis 396, 642
Sinusoidal obstruction syndrome 1112
SIP1 gene 1003
Sipple syndrome 1463
Size-dependent barrier of glomeruli 1160
Sjögren's syndrome 255, 257, 262, 939, 1519
Skeletal muscle atrophies 1542
Skeletal muscle atrophy 7
Skeletal muscle dystrophies 1542
Skeletal muscle hypertrophy 1547
Skeletal muscle stem cells 114
Skeletal muscle tumors 1532
Skin associated lymphoid tissue (SALT) 181
Skin barrier to pathogens 1552
Skin biopsy 1405
Skin dysplasia 13
Skin histology 1550–1552
Skin scratch testing 237
Skip metastases 396, 1396
Skipping lesions of Crohn's disease 1013
Slide test for blood grouping 632
Sliding hiatal hernia 962
SMADA4 tumor suppressor gene 1145, 1325
Small bowel infarction 998
Small cell lung carcinoma (SCLC) 909, 913
Small cell osteosarcoma 1494
Small lymphocytic lymphoma 667
Small lymphocytic lymphoma/CLL 667
Small-sized vessel vasculitis 1225
Smoldering (asymptomatic) myeloma 583
Smooth muscle tumors 1535
SNAIL and TWIST genes 393
Sodium dodecyl sulfate polyacrylamide gel electrophoresis 531
Soft tissue bleeding 612
Soft tissue tumors 1524
Solitary plasmacytoma 583
Solitary renal cyst 1228
Somatotropic adenoma 1471
Sources of stem cells 593
Southern blot technique 729
Space of Disse in liver 1043
Special form of granuloma 107
Special stains 695
Specific tolerance 191
Spectrin proteins in RBC membrane 500
Spermatocele 1275
Spermatocytic seminoma 1262
Spermatogenesis 1255
Spider nevi 1093
Spider telangiectasis 769
Spikes and domes appearance in MGN 1179
Spina bifida cystica 1617
Spina bifida occulta 1617
Spine deformity in rickets 425
Spinocerebellar syndrome 427
Spitz nevus 1570
Spleen 677
   angiosarcoma of spleen 682
   autosplenectomy 679
   fibrocongestive splenomegaly 678
   Gaucher's spleen 680
   granulomatous inflammation 680
   hemosiderosis 680
   hypersplenism 679
   hyposplenism 679
   metastases in spleen 682
   red pulp 677
   spleen in amyloidosis 680
   splenectomy 678
   splenic infarct 680
   splenomegal 678
   white pulp 677
Spleen amyloidosis 47
Splenectomy 678
Splenic infarct 163, 680
Splenic lymphoma with villous lymphocytes 580
Splenic marginal zone B cell lymphoma 663
Splenic marginal zone lymphoma 672
Splenomegaly 678, 829
Spontaneous regression of tumors 410
Sporadic medullary carcinoma of thyroid 1446
Sporadic renal angiomyolipoma 1240
Sporadic Wilms' tumor 1231
Squamous cell carcinoma 327, 843, 934, 950, 964
Squamous cell carcinoma *in situ* (Bowen's disease) 1566
Squamous cell carcinoma lung 915
Squamous cell carcinoma of vagina 1294
Squamous cell carcinoma of vulva 1288
Squamous cell papilloma 934
Squamous metaplasia 11
Squamous odontogenic tumor 953
Squamous papilloma 849, 964
Stable (typical) angina 784
Stable cells 111
Staging of CML 566
Staging of Wilms' tumor 1232
Steatohepatitis 1097
Stein-Leventhal syndrome 1348
Stellate (Ito) cells of liver 1084
Stem cell therapy 112
   β cells embryonic stem cells 112
   hepatocytic embryonic stem cells 112
   myocardial embryonic stem cells 112
Stem cell transplantation 592
Stem cells 111, 114, 594
Stem cells in canals of Hering 113
Stem cells in dentate nuclei 113
Stem cells in hair follicle bulge 113
Stem cells in subventricular zone (SVZ) 113
Stercoral ulcer 1015
Steroid receptors 120
Stiff-Person syndrome (SPS) 405
Still disease (juvenile rheumatoid arthritis) 1519
STK11 tumor suppressor gene 365
Stomatocytes 480
Stomatostatinoma 1149
Storage histiocytosis 589
Storiform pattern 1508
Strawberry capillary hemangioma 1576
Strawberry gallbladder 45, 1128
Stress response proteins 27 (Srp27) 27, 1400, 1406
Stricture in Crohn's disease 1013
Stricture in intestinal tuberculosis 438
String sign in Crohn's disease 1013
Strongyloides stercoralis 455
Structural fibrous glycoproteins 123
Structure and functions of platelets 598
Structure of HIV 220
Struma ovarii 1338
Sturge-Weber syndrome 1540, 1576
Subacute bacterial endocarditis 812
Subacute combined degeneration of spinal cord 428, 491

Index

Subacute endocarditis 813
Subacute granulomatous thyroiditis 1430
Subacute painless lymphocytic thyroiditis 1430
Subcellular and cellular alterations 15
Subcellular hypertrophy of liver organelles 8
Subcellular response to injury 37
Subcutaneous edema 169
Subcutaneous necrosis of newborn 32
Subcutaneous nodules 805
Subdural hematoma 1615
Subdural space 1582
Subendocardial infarct 789, 795
Subendocardial myocardial infarct 784, 789
Subendothelial deposits 1203, 1204
Subleukemic leukemia 540
Submassive liver necrosis 1046
Sucrose hemolysis test 522
Sudan black B stain 543
Sudden cardiac death in AMI 791
Sulfated glycosaminoglycans 273
Superantigens 1189
Superficial fibromatosis 1530
Superficial fungal infections 450, 1561
    epidermophyton 450
    microsporum 450
    trichophyton 450
Superficial spreading melanoma 1572
Superinfection 1073
Superoxide anion 22
Superoxide molecule 99, 196
Suppurative fistula 71
Suppurative lymphadenitis 642
Suppurative thrombosis of portal vein 1080
Supravital staining 527
Surface epithelial inclusion cysts 1348
Surface markers of human B and T cells 195
Surfactant phosphatidylcholine (lecithin) 900
Surgical emphysema 899
Surgical implantation 400
Surgical specimens 694
Swan-neck fingers in rheumatoid arthritis 1519
Swiss cheese disease (juvenile papillomatosis breast) 1373
Sydenham's chorea (St. Vitus dance) 805
Symptomatic gallstones disease 1132
Synaptophysin 843
Syndrome of inappropriate ADH (SIADH) secretion 1470
Synovial joints 1518
Synovial sarcoma 377, 1536
Synthesis of insulin 1411
Synthesis of VWF and factor VIII 610, 615
Syphilis 535, 1293
Syphilitic (luetic) aneurysm 756
Syphilitic orchitis 1273
Syringomyelia 1618
Systemic effects of hypertension 777
Systemic effects of inflammation 94
Systemic lupus erythematosus 79, 219, 255, 257, 258, 517, 897
Systemic sclerosis 261
Systemic thromboembolism 157, 158
Systemic venous thrombosis in AMI 795

T

T cells 534
Tabes dorsalis 1589
Tacrolimus (FK506) immunosuppressive drug 272
Takayasu arteritis 763
Tam-Horsfall proteins 1207
Target cells 480
Tattooing 42
Tay-Sachs disease 291, 307
TCF7L2 gene 1416
Telangiectasia 262
Telangiectatic osteosarcoma 1490, 1494
Telomerase activity 334
Temporal (cranial/giant cell) arteritis 763
Tension pneumothorax 899
Teratocarcinoma 1266
Teratoma 330, 1265, 1336
Terminal deoxyribonucleotidyl transferase (TdT) 544
Terminal duct lobular unit (TDLU) 1358
Tertiary hyperparathyroidism 1456
Tertiary syphilis 31
Testicular atrophy 1274
Testicular lymphoma 1270
Testicular torsion 1274
Tetany 1456
Tetrahydrofolate 488
Tetralogy of Fallot 834
TFE 3 gene 1233
TGF-β tumor suppressor gene 370
Thalassemia 302, 502, 504, 505, 507, 508
    α-thalassemia 508
    α-thalassemia trait 494, 508
    β-thalassemia intermedia 484, 508
    β-thalassemia major 484, 504, 505
    β-thalassemia minor 507
Theca luteal cysts 1349
Thecoma ovary 1342
Theories of aging 48
Therapeutic advances in AMI 787
Thermophilic actinomyces 897
Thiamine 427
Thin membrane disease of kidney 1163
Thioflavin-S 281
Thioflavin-T 281
Third line of host defense 185
Thoracic vena cava syndrome 768
Thrombasthenia (Glanzmann's disease) 606
Thrombi in blood vessels 153
Thrombi in heart 152
Thrombin time 623
Thromboangiitis obliterans 764
Thromboasthenia 142, 622
Thrombocytopenia 601, 602

Thrombocytosis 565
Thromboembolism 157, 1355
Thrombomodulin 147
Thrombomodulin molecules 596
Thrombophilia 618
Thrombophlebitis 640, 815
Thrombopoiesis 141, 468
Thrombopoietin 462
Thrombosis 404
Thrombospondin 142, 335, 598
Thrombotic microangiopathy 1224
Thrombotic thrombocytopenic purpura 523, 604, 637
Thromboxane A2 (TxA2) 84
Thymic carcinoma 684
Thymoma 683
Thymus hyperplasia 682
Thyroglobulin 1451
Thyroglossal duct cyst 854, 1448
Thyroid adenoma 1439
Thyroid anaplastic carcinoma 1448
Thyroid binding globulins 1427
Thyroid follicular cells 1426
Thyroid function tests 1449
Thyroid gland 1425
Thyroid gland anomalies 1448
Thyroid gland hyperplasia 10
Thyroid hormone binding proteins (TBP) 1450
Thyroid hormones in circulation and tissues 1427
Tidal volume 860
Tinea corporis 1561
Tissue factor pathway inhibitor 600
Tissue fibrosis 103
Tissue microarray (TMA) 731, 732, 733
Tissue microarray—FISH 718
Tissue processor 694
Tissue typing 267
Tobacco smoking 908
Toll-like receptors (TLRs) on leukocytes 64, 183, 184
Toluidine blue 587
TORCH complex 1618
Total anomalous pulmonary venous return 835
Total lung capacity 860
Toxemia of pregnancy 1225, 1353
Toxic nodular goiter 1433
Toxic shock syndrome 1291
TP53 tumor suppressor gene 340, 366, 1381
Trachea disorders 857
Tracheoesophageal fistula 959
Traction diverticulum 962
Traditional cytogenetic analysis 709
Transaminases 1048
Transbronchial biopsy 925
Transcription factors 356
Transcription of RNA to DNA 287
    coding regulation of RNA 287
    non-coding RNA 287
Transfer RNA or tRNA 286
Transferrin 483

Transforming growth factor-α
    (TGF-α) 63, 116, 196
Transforming growth factor-β
    (TGF-β) 99, 195, 334, 351
Transforming growth factor-β 117, 753
Transfusion associated graft-versus-host
    disease 640
Transfusion hemosiderosis 640
Transfusion related acute lung injury 640
Transient ischemic attacks (TIA) 1614
Transient jaundice 1051
Transitional (mixed) meningioma 1607
Transitional cell carcinoma 328, 1252
Translocation of chromosome 294
Transmigration (diapedesis) 61, 63
Transmission electron microscopy
    (TEM) 688
Transmission of infections 638
Transmission of negative signal to
    T cells 254
Transmural infarct 795, 789
Transmural myocardial infarct 784, 789
Transplant rejection prevention 271
Transplantation immunology 266
    acute renal graft rejection 268
    chronic renal transplant rejection 269
    graft-versus-host disease (GVHD) 269
    hyperacute organ transplant
        rejection 267
    immunosuppressive drugs 272
    organ transplant rejection 267
    organ transplantation 266
Transplanted cells 247
Transport proteins 25
    ceruloplasmin 25
    ferritin 25
    lactoferritin 25
    transferrin 25
Transposition of the great vessels 835
Transthyretin 276
Transudate 57, 165
Transudative effusions 928
Traumatic neuroma 1574
Tree bark appearance in syphilis 756
Trephine bone biopsy 473
Trichobezoar 986
Trichomonas vaginalis 454, 1292
Trichophyton 1561
Tricuspid insufficiency 821
Trilateral retinoblastoma 1603
Triple assessment 1404
Trisodium citrate 476
Trisomy 295
Tropical sprue 993
Troponins (Tn I and Tn T) in AMI 796
TRPC6 (transient receptor potential
    calcium channel-6) gene 1162
True hermaphrodite 312
Truncus arteriosus communism 835
Tubal endometriosis 1307
Tube test 632

Tubercular arthritis 1523
Tubercular effusion 874
Tubercular granulomas 875
Tubercular infection 431
Tubercular intestinal ulcer 994
Tubercular lymphadenitis 439
Tubercular osteomyelitis 438, 1479
Tubercular pericardial effusion 439
Tubercular peritonitis 439
Tubercular pleuritis 435
Tubercular pyelonephritis 438, 1214
Tubercular salpingitis 439
Tuberculin test 248, 870
Tuberculoid leprosy 443
Tuberculosis 430, 535, 870, 871
Tuberculosis in HIV cases 876
Tuberculous cavities 874
Tuberculous disease 431
Tuberculous epididymitis 1273
Tuberculous meningitis 437, 1586
Tuberous sclerosis 302, 306, 1022
Tuberous sclerosis syndrome 1620
Tubular adenoma 1019, 1375
Tubular breast carcinoma 1391
Tubulointerstitial nephritis 1209
Tubulovillus adenomas 1020
Tumor angiogenesis 334
Tumor antigen masking 374
Tumor cell embolization 395
Tumor emboli extravasation 395
Tumor fragment emboli 157
Tumor impingement on nearby
    structures 401
Tumor markers 405
Tumor markers of breast carcinoma 1406
Tumor necrosis factor 88, 431
Tumor necrosis factor-α (TNF-α) 99
Tumor p16 suppressor gene 370
Tumor suppressive micro-RNA 378
Tumor suppressor genes 318
Tumors of blood vessels 769, 770, 771
    angiomyolipoma 771
    angiosarcoma 771
    bacillaryangiomatosis 771
    capillary hemangioma 770
    cavernous hemangioma 770
    cystic hygroma 770
    glomangioma 770
    hemangioendothelioma 771
    hemangiopericytoma 771
    hereditary hemorrhagic telangiec-
        tasia 770
    Kaposi sarcoma 771
    pyogenic granuloma 770
    spider telangiectasis 769
Turcot's syndrome 1021
Turner's mosaicism 296
Turner's syndrome 295, 300
Two-hit hypothesis of Knudson 1603
Tympanosclerosis 847
Type I diabetes mellitus 249, 250

Type I hypersensitivity reactions 231
Type II hypersensitivity reaction 237, 798
Type III hypersensitivity reaction 243
Type IV hypersensitivity reaction 245, 799
Type of electrophoresis 735
Type of immunofluorescence 703
Type of metastases 1510
Typhoid fever 445, 995
Typhoid intestinal ulcers 995
Tyrosinase 373
Tyrosine kinase pathway 352

U

Ulcerated carcinoma 979
Ulcerative colitis 104, 1011
Ultrasound or CT-guided percutaneous
    needle biopsy 925
Umbilical cord blood 594
Umbilical cord blood harvesting 594
Umbilical hernia 998
Undifferentiated pleomorphic
    sarcoma 1538
Unilateral renal agenesis 1229
Unstable (crescendo/pre-infarction)
    angina 784
Urachal diverticulum 1248
Uranium exposure 908
Urate nephropathy 1214, 1522
Urease 968
Uremic medullary cystic renal disease 1228
Ureter anomalies 1230
Uric acid stones 1220
Urinary tract obstruction 1213
Urine electrophoresis 586
Urinothorax 928
Urolithiasis 1218
Urothelial carcinoma *in situ* 1248
Urothelial carcinoma of renal pelvis 1241
Urothelial dysplasia 1248
Uses of flow cytometer 708
Uterine endometrial hyperplasia 10
Uterus muscle hyperplasia during preg-
    nancy 10

V

VacA exotoxin 968
Vaccines 211
Vaginal intraepithelial neoplasia 1293
Variant (Prinzmetal) angina 784
Varicella (chickenpox) 1561
Varicocele 768, 1275
Varicose veins in legs 767
Various types of electrophoresis 737
Vascular cell adhesive molecule I
    (VCAM I) 752
Vascular changes in hypertension 775, 776
Vascular endothelial growth factor
    (VEGF) 117, 334
Vascular endothelium 139
Vascular events in inflammation 55

Vascular purpura 607
Vascular-occlusive episodes in sickle cell disease 511
   acute chest syndrome 511
   autosplenectomy 512
   avascular necrosis of femoral head 511
   bone and joint crises 511
   hand and foot syndrome 511
   priapism 512
   renal papillary necrosis 512
Vasculitis 760, 763
   Churg-Strauss syndrome 766
   cryoglobulinemia vasculitis 766
   diabetic vascular disease 766
   drug-induced vasculitides 766
   Henoch-Schönlein purpura 766
   Kawasaki disease 764
   lymphomatoid granulomatosis 767
   microscopic polyarteritis 766
   polyarteritis nodosa 764
   Raynaud's phenomenon 766
   temporal (cranial/giant cell) arteritis 763
   thromboangiitis obliterans 764
   Wegener's granulomatosis 765
Vasculitis involving kidneys 1225
Vasculostatin 335
Vasoactive amines 80
Vasoactive intestinal peptide tumor 1149
Vasoconstriction 55
Vasodilation 55
Vater's syndrome 963
Veins 767
Vena cava syndrome 768, 769
Veno-occlusive disorder 1112
Venous thrombi 154
Ventral hernia 998
Ventricular aneurysm in AMI 794
Ventricular mural thrombi 793
Ventricular septal defects 833
Verocay bodies 1539
Verruca vulgaris (common wart) 1559
Vesicoumbilical fistula 1248
Vesicoureteral reflux 1210, 1211, 1213
vHL (von Hippel-Lindau) tumor suppressor gene 365, 1235
Vibrio cholerae 992
Villus adenomas 1019
Vim Silverman needle biopsy 1050
Vincent angina 933
Viral carcinogenesis 386
Viral cervicitis 1298
Viral encephalitis 1588
Viral infected cells 247
Viral meningitis 1587
Viral sialadenitis 939
Visceral epithelial cells of Bowman's capsule 1159
Vital capacity 860
Vitamin A 424
Vitamin B_{12} deficiency 489, 491
Vitamin B_{12} in DNA synthesis 490

Vitamin C (ascorbate) 25, 429
Vitamin D 425, 1453, 1480
Vitamin D resistant rickets 1456
Vitamin E (α-tocopherol) 25, 426
Vitamin K 427
Vitiligo 255, 1569
VLA-4 integrin 62
Vocal cord nodule 849
Volvulus 1007
von Gierke disease 37, 146, 309
von Gieson stain 281
von Hippel-Lindau disease 302
von Hippel-Lindau syndrome 306, 1235, 1540, 1576
von Willebrand disease 142, 606, 615
von Willebrand factor 142, 635
Vulnerability of tissues to hypoxia 161

W

WAGR syndrome 1231
Wald's visual cycle 424
Waldenstörm's macroglobulinemia 576, 587, 637
Warburg effect 395
Warm antibody-mediated hemolytic anemia 240, 517
Warthin's tumor salivary gland 943
Warts 1560
Washed red blood cells 635
Water and electrolytes imbalance 1198
Waterhouse-Friderichsen syndrome 1461
Watershed regions 1015
Water-soluble vitamins 427
WBCs qualitative anomalies 468
   Alder-Reilly anomaly 468
   May-Hegglin anomaly 468
   Peggler-Huet anomaly 468
Wegener's granulomatosis 765, 837, 1194
Well differentiated liposarcoma 1527
Well differentiated papillary mesothelioma 1034
Werner syndrome 49
Wernicke-Korsakoff syndrome 427, 428
Wertheim's hysterectomy 1305
Wet beriberi 428
Wet gangrene 31
Whipple disease (tropical sprue) 993
White (pale) infarct 162
White blood cells removal 637
White sponge nevus 933
WHO classification 645
WHO classification of AML (2016) 549
WHO classification of lung tumors 910
WHO classification of lymphoid neoplasms 658
WHO definition of AIDS patient 227
Whole blood 635
Whole blood transfusion 634
Whole chromosome paint (WCP) 718
Willebrand disease 622
Williams-Campbell syndrome 883
Wilms' tumor 1230

Wilms' tumor in familial syndromes 1231
Wilson disease 302, 1103
Wilson's disease induced cirrhosis 1083
Window period 1069
Wire loop lesion in glomeruli in SLE 1186
Wiscott-Aldrich syndrome 219, 541, 606, 683
WNT signal transduction pathway 354
Wound contraction 129
Wound healing by primary intention 10
Wright's stain 477
WT1 tumor suppressor gene 369
Wuchereria bancrofti 455

X

Xanthine stones kidney 1220
Xanthogranulomatous pyelonephritis 1214
Xanthomas 45, 1578
Xeroderma pigmentosum 343, 386
Xerophthalmia 425
X-inactivation 296
X-linked (Bruton) agammaglobulinemia 303
X-linked agammaglobulinemia of Bruton 215, 303
X-linked disorders 303
X-linked dominant inheritance 290
X-linked ichthyosis 303
X-linked recessive disorders 311
X-linked recessive inheritance 290, 303
   Becker muscular dystrophy 303
   Duchenne muscular dystrophy 303
   Fabry disease 303
   Fragile X syndrome 303
   G6PD deficiency 303
   hemophilia A 303
   hemophilia B 303
   Hunter syndrome 303
Xp11 translocation renal cell carcinoma 1233
XXX syndrome (47, XXX) and other multi-X chromosome anomalies 301

Y

Y chromatin 314
Yersinia enterocolitica 1030
Yolk sac tumor of ovary 1339
Yolk sac tumor of testis 1266

Z

Zenker's diverticulum 962
Zenker's fixative 692
Zenker's necrosis 32
Ziehl-Neelsen stain 440
Zileutin drug 94
Zollinger-Ellison syndrome 973
Zona fasciculata of adrenal cortex 1457
Zona glomerulosa of adrenal cortex 1457
Zona reticularis of adrenal cortex 1457
Zonal liver necrosis 1045
Zones of prostate 1277